WITHDRAWN

KT-428-269

WS
KEN
Reference

Staff Library
Singleton Hospital
Tel: 01792 205666 Ext. 5281

Singleton Staff Library
S008543

Rennie and Roberton's Textbook of Neonatology

Content Strategist: *Michael Houston*
Content Development Specialist: *Nani Clansey*
Content Co-ordinator: *Poppy Garraway, Kirsten Lowson, Emma Cole, Alex Jones*
Project Manager: *Annie Victor*
Design: *Kirsteen Wright*
Illustration Manager: *Gillian Richards*
Marketing Manager(s) (UK/USA): *Gaynor Jones*

SINGLETON HOSPITAL
STAFF LIBRARY

Rennie and Roberton's Textbook of Neonatology

Fifth Edition

Editor

JANET M RENNIE MA MD DCH FRCP FRCPCH FRCOG

Consultant and Senior Lecturer in Neonatal Medicine
Elizabeth Garrett Anderson Obstetric Wing
University College Hospital
London
UK

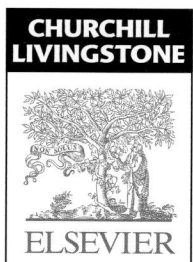

CHURCHILL
LIVINGSTONE

ELSEVIER

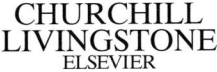

CHURCHILL
LIVINGSTONE
ELSEVIER

An imprint of Elsevier Limited
© 2012, Elsevier Limited. All rights reserved.
Gemma Price: Chapter 28 – Retains copyright to her original figures 11, 12, 20, 21 and 22.
William Reardon: Chapter 31 – Retains copyright to his original figures.

First edition 1986
Second edition 1992
Third edition 1999
Fourth edition 2005

The right of Janet M. Rennie to be identified as author of this work has been asserted by her in accordance with the Copyright, Designs and Patents Act 1988.

No part of this publication may be reproduced or transmitted in any form or by any means, electronic or mechanical, including photocopying, recording, or any information storage and retrieval system, without permission in writing from the publisher. Details on how to seek permission, further information about the Publisher's permissions policies and our arrangements with organizations such as the Copyright Clearance Center and the Copyright Licensing Agency, can be found at our website: www.elsevier.com/permissions.

This book and the individual contributions contained in it are protected under copyright by the Publisher (other than as may be noted herein).

Notices
Knowledge and best practice in this field are constantly changing. As new research and experience broaden our understanding, changes in research methods, professional practices, or medical treatment may become necessary.

Practitioners and researchers must always rely on their own experience and knowledge in evaluating and using any information, methods, compounds, or experiments described herein. In using such information or methods they should be mindful of their own safety and the safety of others, including parties for whom they have a professional responsibility.

With respect to any drug or pharmaceutical products identified, readers are advised to check the most current information provided (i) on procedures featured or (ii) by the manufacturer of each product to be administered, to verify the recommended dose or formula, the method and duration of administration, and contraindications. It is the responsibility of practitioners, relying on their own experience and knowledge of their patients, to make diagnoses, to determine dosages and the best treatment for each individual patient, and to take all appropriate safety precautions.

To the fullest extent of the law, neither the Publisher nor the authors, contributors, or editors, assume any liability for any injury and/or damage to persons or property as a matter of products liability, negligence or otherwise, or from any use or operation of any methods, products, instructions, or ideas contained in the material herein.

ISBN: 978-0-7020-3479-4
E-ISBN: 978-0-7020-5242-2

British Library Cataloging in Publication Data
A Catalogue record for this book is available from the British Library

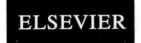

your source for books,
journals and multimedia
in the health sciences
www.elsevierhealth.com

Working together to grow
libraries in developing countries

www.elsevier.com | www.bookaid.org | www.sabre.org

ELSEVIER   BOOK AID International   Sabre Foundation

The publisher's policy is to use **paper manufactured from sustainable forests**

Printed in China
Last digit is the print number: 9   8   7   6   5   4   3   2   1

Table of Contents

Table of Contents

Table of Contents

SINGLETON HOSPITAL
STAFF LIBRARY

Contributors

NEIL AITON MBBS MD MRCPI FRCPCH

Consultant Neonatologist
Trevor Mann Baby Unit
Brighton & Sussex University Hospitals NHS Trust
Royal Sussex County Hospital
Brighton, UK

NICK ARCHER MA FRCP FRCPCH DCH

Consultant Paediatric Cardiologist, Honorary Clinical
Senior Lecturer
Department of Paediatric Cardiology
John Radcliffe Hospital
Oxford, UK

RUTH M AYLING PHD MRCPCH FRCP FRCPATH

Consultant Chemical Pathologist
Clinical Biochemistry
Derriford Hospital
Plymouth, UK

IMELDA BALCHIN BSC MBCHB MSC MRCOG MFSRH MD

Academic Clinical Lecturer and Specialist Registrar
Department of Epidemiology & Public Health
Health Care Evaluation Group
Institute for Women's Health
University College London Hospital NHS Trust
London, UK

PETER G BARTH MD PHD

Emeritus Professor in Paediatric Neurology
University of Amsterdam
Emma's Children Hospital
Amsterdam, Netherlands

ALISON BEDFORD RUSSELL BSC FRCPCH MD

Clinical Lead South West Midlands Newborn Network
  (SWMNN)
Hon Associate Clinical Professor
Warwick Medical School
Neonatal Consultant Birmingham Women's Foundation Trust
Neonatal Unit
Birmingham, UK

NICK BISHOP MB CHB MRCP MD FRCPCH

Professor of Paediatric Bone Disease
Director, Children's Clinical Research Facility
Head, Academic Unit of Child Health
University of Sheffield, Sheffield Children's Hospital
Sheffield, UK

MAGGIE BLOTT FRCOG

Consultant Obstetrician and Labour Ward Lead
Elizabeth Garratt Anderson Wing
Obstretric Service
University College London Hospital NHS Trust
London, UK

ANN BOWRON BSC MSC FRCPATH

Clinical Biochemistry
Bristol Royal Infirmary
Bristol, UK

GERALDINE BOYLAN MA MSC PHD

Professor of Neonatal Physiology
Department of Paediatrics & Child Health
University College Cork and Cork University Maternity
  Hospital
Cork, Ireland

PAMELA CAIRNS MB BCH MRCP MRCPCH DCH MD

Consultant Neonatologist
Department of Child Health
St Michael's Hospital
Bristol, UK

OANA CALUSERIU MD

Medical Genetics Resident, University of Calgary
Alberta Children's Hospital
Department of Medical Genetics
Calgary, Canada

ANDREW J CANT BSC MD FRCP FRCPCH

Professor of Paediatric Immunology
Paediatric Immunology and Infectious Diseases Unit
Great North Children's Hospital
Newcastle-Upon-Tyne, UK

PATRICK H T CARTLIDGE MB CHB DM FRCPCH FRCP

Department of Child Health
Cardiff University
Cardiff, UK

TIM CHEETHAM BSC MBCHB MD MRCP MRCPCH

Institute of Human Genetics, Newcastle University
Children's Out Patient Department
Royal Victoria Infirmary
Newcastle-upon-Tyne, UK

MALCOLM CHISWICK MD FRCP(Lond) FRCPCH FRCOG DCH

Honorary Professor of Neonatal Medicine
University of Manchester, UK
Honorary Consultant in Neonatal Medicine
St Mary's Hospital
Manchester, UK

SIRINUCH CHOMTHO MD PHD

Lecturer, Nutrition Unit
Department of Pediatrics
Faculty of Medicine
Chulalongkorn University
Bangkok, Thailand

IMTI CHOONARA MB CHB MD FRCP

Professor in Child Health
Academic Division of Child Health
  (University of Nottingham)
The Medical School
Derbyshire Children's Hospital
Derby, UK

N M P CLARKE CHM FRCS

Professor and Consultant Orthopaedic Surgeon
University of Southampton and University Hospital
  Southampton NHS Foundation Trust
Southampton General Hospital
Southampton, UK

TIM COLE PHD SCD HONFRCPCH FMEDSCI

Professor of Medical Statistics
MRC Centre of Epidemiology for Child Health
UCL Institute of Child Health
London, UK

SHARON CONROY BPHARM MRPHARMS PHD

Lecturer in Paediatric Clinical Pharmacy
Academic Division of Child Health, University of Nottingham
The Medical School
Derbyshire Children's at the Royal Derby Hospital
Derby, UK

CHRISTOPHER J DARE BSC BM FRCS

Consultant in Paediatric and Spinal Surgery
University Hospital Southampton NHS Foundation Trust
Wessex Neurological Centre
Southampton General Hospital
Southampton, UK

MARK DAVENPORT FRCS

Consultant Pediatric Surgeon
King's College Hospital
London, UK

MARK DENBOW PHD MRCOG

Consultant in Fetal Medicine and Obstetrics
St Michael's Hospital
University Hospitals Bristol NHS Foundation Trust
Bristol, UK

LEIGH DYET MBBS BMEDSCI MRCPCH PHD

Consultant in Neonatal Medicine
University College London Hospital NHS Trust
London, UK

D KEITH EDMONDS MBCH FRCOG FRANZCOG

Consultant Obstetrician and Gynaecologist
Department of Obstretrics and Gynaecology
Queen Charlotte's & Chelsea Hospital
London, UK

KATE FARRER FRCPCH

Consultant Neonatologist
Addenbrooke's Hospital
Cambridge, UK

MARY FEWTRELL MD FRCPCH

Reader in Childhood Nutrition & Honorary Consultant
  Paeditrician
Childhood Nutrition Research Centre
UCL Institute of Child Health
London, UK

BRIAN FLECK BSC (HONS) MBCHB MD FRCSED FRCOPH

Consultant Ophthalmologist
Eye Pavilion
Edinburgh, UK

GRENVILLE F FOX MB CHB FRCPCH

Consultant Neonatologist
Evelina Children's Hospital Neonatal Unit
St Thomas' Hospital
London, UK

ANDREW R GENNERY MD MRCP FRCPCH DCH DIP.MED.SCI

Clinical Reader/Honorary Consultant in Paediatric
  Immunology & HSCT
Children's Bone Marrow Transplant Unit
Great North Children's Hospital
Newcastle upon Tyne, UK

ANDREW GREEN MB PHD FRPI FFPATH(RCPI)

Professor of Medical Genetics
Our Lady's Children's Hospital
Dublin, Ireland

ANNE GREENOUGH MD FRCP FRCPCH DCH

Professor of Neonatology and Clinical Respiratory Physiology
Division of Asthma Allergy and Lung Biology
MRC-Asthma UK Centre in Allergic Mechanisms of Asthma
King's College London
London, UK

FLORIS GROENENDAAL MD PHD

Consultant Neonatologist
Department of Neonatology
Wilhelmina Children's Hospital
University Medical Centre Utrecht
Utrecht, The Netherlands

NEDIM HADŽIĆ MD MSC FRCPCH

Consultant and Honorary Reader in Paediatric Hepatology
Paediatric Liver Service
Department of Child Health
King's College Hospital
London, UK

CORNELIA HAGMANN MD PHD

Consultant in Neonatal Medicine
Clinic of Neonatology
University Hospital of Zurich
Zurich, Switzerland

SIMON HANNAM BSC MD MRCP FRCPCH

Consultant and Honorary Senior Lecturer in Neonatology
Children Nationwide Neonatal Unit
Newborn Unit
King's College Hospital
London, UK

SIAN HARDING MBBS FRCP

Consultant Neonatologist
Neonatal Service
University College London Hospitals NHS Trust
London, UK

JANE HAWDON MA MBBS MRCP FRCPCH PHD

Consultant Neonatologist
Elizabeth Garrett Anderson Wing
University College London Hospitals NHS Foundation Trust
London, UK

ANGELA HUERTAS-CEBALLOS MD MSC FRCPCH

Consultant Neonatologist with Special interest in
  Neurodevelopment
Elizabeth Garrett Anderson Wing
University College London Hospital NHS Foundation Trust
London, UK

PAUL HUMPHRIES MRCP FRCR

Consultant Paediatric Radiologist
University College London Hospital and Great Ormond Street
  Hospital for Children Foundation Trusts
Honorary Senior Lecturer
Institute of Child Health
University College London
London, UK

DAVID ISAACS MBBCHIR MD FRACP FRCPCH

Clinical Professor of Paediatric Infectious Diseases
Department of Infectious Diseases and Microbiology
Children's Hospital at Westmead
Westmead, NSW, Australia

N KEVIN IVES MA MB BCHIR DCH MRCP FRCPCH MD

Honorary Senior Clinical Lecturer
Department of Paediatrics
University of Oxford
Consultant Neonatologist
John Radcliffe Hospital
Oxford, UK

ANOO JAIN FRCPCH MRCP(Ire) DM

Consultant in Neonatal Medicine
University Hospital Bristol NHS Foundation Trust
Regional Intensive Care Nursery
St Michaels Hospital
Bristol, UK

SAMANTHA JOHNSON PHD CPSYCHOL

Department of Health Sciences
University of Leicester
Leicester, UK

SIMON A JONES MB CHB BSC MRCPCH

Consultant in Paediatric Inherited Metabolic Disease
Genetic Medicine
Manchester Academic Health Science Centre
University of Manchester
Central Manchester University Hospitals NHS Foundation
    Trust
St Mary's Hospital
Manchester, UK

STEVE KEMPLEY MA FRCP FRCPCH

Clinical Senior Lecturer in Paediatrics and Honorary
    Consultant Neonatologist
Neonatal Transfer Service for London
Barts and the London School of Medicine and Dentistry
London, UK

GILLIAN KENNEDY MSC MRCSLT

Consultant Speech and Language Therapist
NIDCAP Trainer
Neonatal Unit
Elizabeth Garrett Anderson Wing
University College London Hospital NHS Trust
London, UK

PIPPA KYLE MD FRCOG FRANZCOG CMFM

Consultant Obstetrician, Subspecialist Maternal and
    Fetal Medicine
Women's Services Directorate
Guy's and St Thomas NHS Foundation Trust
London, UK

IAN A LAING MD D UNIV FRCPE FRCPCH

Consultant Neonatologist
Neonatal Unit
Simpson Centre for Reproductive Health
Royal Infirmary of Edinburgh
Edinburgh, UK

CASSIE LAWN MBBS DRCOG MRCGP MRCPCH

Consultant Neonatologist
Trevor Mann Baby Unit
Royal Sussex County Hospital
Brighton, UK

BERTIE LEIGH HON FRCPCH FRCOG AD EUNDEM

Solicitor and Senior Partner
Hempsons
London, UK

ALAN LUCAS MD FRCPCH

Professor
Childhood Nutrition Research Centre
UCL Institute of Child Health
London, UK

ANDREW LYON MA MB FRCP FRCPCH

Consultant Neonatologist
Neonatal Unit
The Simpson Centre for Reproductive Health
Royal Infirmary of Edinburgh
Edinburgh, UK

ALISON MACFARLANE BA DIP STAT CSTAT FFPH

Professor of Perinatal Health
School of Health Sciences
City University London
London, UK

ADNAN MANZUR MBBS FRCPCH

Consultant Paediatric Neurologist
Dubowitz Neuromuscular Centre
Neurosciences
Great Ormond Street Hospital
London, UK

NEIL MARLOW DM FMEDSCI

Professor of Neonatal Medicine
UCL Elizabeth Garrett Anderson Institute of Women's Health
University College London NHS Trust
London, UK

LILA MAYAHI PHD MRCP

Consultant in Acute Medicine, Clinical Pharmacology and
    Therapeutics
St George's NHS Trust
London, UK

HAZEL E MCHAFFIE PHD

Formerly Deputy Director of Research, Institute of Medical
    Ethics and Research Fellow
Department of Medicine
University of Edinburgh
Edinburgh, UK

JOHN MCINTYRE MBCHB DM FRCPCH

Consultant Neonatologist
Derbyshire Childrens Hospital
Derby, UK

JUDITH HELEN MEEK MA (CANTAB) MSC PHD MBBS MRCPCHH

Consultant Neonatologist
University College London Hospital NHS Trust
London, UK

GIORGINA MIELI-VERGANI MD PHD FRCP FRCPCH

Alex Mowat Professor of Paediatric Hepatology
Paediatric Liver Centre
Variety Club Children's Hospital
King's College Hospital
London, UK

ANTHONY D MILNER MD FRCP FRCPCH DCH

Emeritus Professor of Neonatology
Division of Asthma Allergy and Lung Biology
MRC-Asthma UK Centre in Allergic Mechanisms of Asthma
King's College London
London, UK

NEENA MODI MB CHB MD FRCP FRCPCH

Professor of Neonatal Medicine
Imperial College London
Section of Neonatal Medicine
Chelsea & Westminster Hospital
London, UK

COLIN J MORLEY MD FRCPCH

Professor of Neonatal Medicine
The Royal Women's Hospital
Melbourne, Australia and UK
Cambridge, UK

GAVIN MORRISON MA FRCS

Consultant Otolaryngologist
Guy's, St Thomas' and Evelina Children's Hospitals
London, UK

MIRANDA MUGFORD BA(HONS) DPHIL

Professor of Health Economics
Institute of Health
University of East Anglia
Norwich, UK

FRANCESCO MUNTONI MD FRCPCH FMEDSCI

Head, Dubowitz Neuromuscular Centre
UCL Institute of Child Health and Great Ormond Street
   Hospital for Children
Division of Neuroscience
London, UK

EDILE MURDOCH BM MRCP

Consultant Neonatologist
Neonatal Unit
Royal Infirmary of Edinburgh
Edinburgh, UK

NEIL A MURRAY MBCHB MD MRCP MRCPCH

Neonatal Consultant
Homerton Hospital
London, UK

SIMON NEWELL MD FRCP FRCPCH

Consultant and Senior Clinical Lecturer in Neonatal Medicine
Leeds Teaching Hospitals
Vice President, Training and Assessment
Royal College of Paediatrics and Child Health
Leeds, UK

COLM O'DONNELL MB FRCPI MRCPCH FRACP FJFICMI PHD

Consultant Neonatologist
The National Maternity Hospital & Our Lady's Children's
   Hospital
Director of Clinical Research
National Children's Research Centre
Senior Clinical Lecturer
School of Medicine & Medical Science
University College Dublin
Dublin, Ireland

ROGER D PALMER BSC(HONS) PHD MB BCHIR
MRCP(UK) MRCPCH

Medicolegal Advisor
Medical Directorate
Medical Protection Society
London, UK

DHARMINTRA PASUPATHY MSC PHD MRCOG

NIHR Clinical Lecturer in Maternal & Fetal Medicine
Division of Women's Health
Women's Health Academic Centre
KHP King's College London
Guy's & St. Thomas' NHS Foundation Trust
London, UK

DONALD PEEBLES MA MBBS MRCOG MD

Professor of Obstetrics, Honorary Consultant in Maternal/
   Fetal Medicine
Institute for Women's Health
Department of Obstetrics and Gynaecology
Medical School, University College London
University College London Hospital NHS Trust
London, UK

CHINTHIKA PIYASENA MBBCH MRCPCH

Specialist Trainee in Paediatrics
Simpson Centre for Reproductive Medicine
Royal Infirmary of Edinburgh
Edinburgh, UK

NANDIRAN RATNAVEL MRCPCH

Consultant Neonatologist
London Neonatal Transfer Service
Royal London Hospital
London, UK

WILLIAM REARDON MD MRCPI DCH FRCPCH FRCP(LOND)

Consultant Clinical Geneticist
Our Lady's Hospital for Sick Children
Dublin, Ireland

JANET M RENNIE MA MD DCH FRCP FRCPCH FRCOG

Consultant and Senior Lecturer in Neonatal Medicine
University College Hospital
London, UK

STEPHANIE ROBB BMED SCI MD FRCP FRCPCH

Consultant Paediatric Neurologist
Dubowitz Neuromuscular Centre
Institute of Child Health and Great Ormond Street Hospital
Great Ormond Street Hospital
London, UK

IRENE ROBERTS MD FRCP FRCPATH FRCPCH DRCOG

Professor of Paediatric Haematology
Imperial College London, and Consultant Paediatric
  Haematologist
Imperial College Healthcare NHS Trust
London, UK

NICOLA J ROBERTSON PhD FRCPCH

Reader in Translational Neonatal Medicine and Honorary
  Consultant Neonatologist
Institute for Women's Health
University College London
London, UK

MAUREEN ROGERS MBBS FACD

Emeritus Consultant Dermatologist
The Children's Hospital at Westmead
Sydney, Australia

STEVEN M SALE MB CHB FRCA

Consultant in Paediatric Anaesthesia
Bristol Royal Hospital for Children
Bristol, UK

DANIEL J SCHENK BMSC MBCHB MRCPCH

Specialty Registrar of Pediatrics
Neonatal Unit
Royal Victoria Infirmary
Newcastle-upon-Tyne, UK

NEIL SEBIRE MB BS BCLINSCI MD DRCOG FRCPATH

Professor of Pathology
Great Ormond Street Hospital for Children, London
Department of Histopathology
Camelia Botnar Laboratories
Great Ormond Street Hospital
London, UK

DIVYEN K SHAH MBCHB MRCPCH PHD

Consultant Neonatologist and Honorary Senior Lecturer
Royal London Hospital
London, UK

NAIMA SMEULDERS BA MB BCHIR MA MD FRCS(PAED)

Consultant Paediatric Urologist
Department of Paediatric Urology
Great Ormond Street Hospital and
University College London Hospital NHS Trusts
London, UK

GORDON C S SMITH MD PHD FMEDSCI

Professor of Obstetrics and Gynaecology
Department of Obstetrics and Gynaecology
Cambridge University
Cambridge, UK

ALISTAIR G SMYTH BDS MBBS FRCS FDSRCS

Consultant Cleft, Oral and Maxillofacial Surgeon
Northern and Yorkshire Regional Cleft Lip and Palate Service
Department of Cleft Lip and Palate Service
Leeds General Infirmary
Leeds, UK

MARK D STRINGER MS FRCP FRCS FRCS(PAED)

Professor of Anatomy
Department of Anatomy and Structural Biology
Otago School of Medical Sciences
University of Otago
Dunedin, New Zealand

IAN SUGARMAN MBCHB FRCS FRCS(PAED)

Consultant Paediatric Surgeon
Department of Paediatric Surgery
Leeds General Infirmary
Leeds, UK

SUDHIN THAYYIL MD DCH MRCP PHD

Honorary Consultant Neonatologist, Academic Neonatology
Institute for Women's Health, University College London
DoH Fellow
Centre for Cardiovascular Imaging
Great Ormond Street Hospital
London, UK

CARMEN TUROWSKI MD

Trainee Paediatric Surgery
Hannover Medical School
Department of Paediatric Surgery
Hannover, Germany

SUKRUTHA VEERAREDDY MBBS MRCOG PHD

Consultant in Obstetrics
Whittington Hospital NHS Trust
London, UK

MARTIN A WEBER MBCHB MD(Res) DCH (SA) FRCPATH

Consultant Paediatric Pathologist
Department of Histopathology
Great Ormond Street Hospital
London, UK

DUNCAN T WILCOX MBBS MD FRCS

Chair of Pediatric Urology
The Ponzio Family Chair in Pediatric Urology
University of Colorado School of Medicine
Aurora, CO, USA

DAVID WILLIAMS MBBS PHD FRCP

Consultant Obstretric Physician
Institute for Women's Health
University College London Hospital
London, UK

DENISE M WILLIAMS MB FRCP FRCPCH

Consultant Paediatric Oncologist
Department of Paediatrics
Cambridge University Hospital Foundation Trust
Cambridge, UK

JAMES E WRAITH MB CHB FRCPCH

Professor of Paediatric Inherited Metabolic Medicine
Manchester Academic Health Sciences Centre
Genetic Medicine
St. Mary's Hospital
Manchester, UK

JOHN WYATT MB FRCP FRCPCH

Emeritus Professor of Neonatal Paediatrics
Institute for Women's Health
University College London Hospitals NHS Trust
London, UK

ROBERT W M YATES MB BCH BSC(MED) FRCP

Consultant Fetal and Paediatric Cardiologist
Cardiothoracic Unit
Great Ormond Street Hospital
London, UK

Preface

This Fifth Edition of the *Textbook of Neonatology* will be a Silver Jubilee Edition, because it is now 25 years since the First Edition was published in 1986. I have renamed the book *Rennie and Roberton's Textbook of Neonatology* to reflect both the contribution made by Cliff Roberton in establishing the work as a standard text, and my own efforts in keeping it going over the last few editions. My consultant career has spanned those years, and the book has been a constant friend and companion to me during that time. I rely on the content for dependable advice or to start a literature search from a key reference, and I hope that the next generation of neonatologists and neonatal nurses will develop the same loyalty because they too find it indispensable. To that end, I am delighted that this edition will be available on the Web via the Expert Consult site. This will make it possible to keep the bulky copy of the book at home, yet access all the content from anywhere in the world via the internet.

As ever, the preparation of this edition has taken longer than anticipated, and so far it has proved impossible to achieve a gestation period of less than six years between updates. I am glad to report that the UCLH copy of the book is worn out and dog-eared, and whilst that tells me that a new edition is long overdue it also cheers me that the book has been so well used. In the years since the fourth Edition was prepared knowledge has continued to advance at a rapid and sometimes giddying pace, and I am grateful to all the contributors for teaching me much about topics which are outside my particular field of expertise. Reading, checking and re-reading the submissions has been an enjoyable and educational experience. I hope others will find the content equally rewarding, as they continue on their paths to individual learning and in striving to deliver excellent care to the newborn baby.

Janet M Rennie
University College London Hospitals 2012

Acknowledgements

Almost six years have passed since I contemplated the acknowledgements for the Fourth edition, but the number of people to thank remains formidable; far too many to name individually. At Elsevier, Nani Clansey has been wonderful, working tirelessly at reminding those authors who were slipping behind with their chapters, maintaining a grip of vast numbers of illustrations, and sorting muddled reference lists. Without her, the book would probably never have been completed at all. Thanks are also due to Michael Houston, Poppy Garraway, Kirsten Lowson, Emma Cole, Alex Jones and Annie Victor at Elsevier for their support.

As ever, it is the authors of the individual chapters who deserve the most praise. All those who write chapters for textbooks know only too well that the first blush of enthusiasm at being asked to contribute rapidly fades into irritation as the deadline looms, and ends in a phase of frenetic writing and sleepless nights once the actual task of organising the advances in knowledge into a readable piece begins. My requests to squeeze in new information whilst paring down the already minimal word counts, update all the illustrations, use colour, and keep the coverage comprehensive were met with calm, capable professionalism and amused tolerance. I can only imagine the expletives from families and friends, knowing that my suggestions must have incurred significant erosions into the already limited disposable time of busy clinicians.

Some of the original content is now historical, and to reflect that this is the first edition to have a whole chapter devoted to the history of neonatal care. Particular thanks are due to Professor Malcolm Chiswick for taking this on, and for producing such a wonderful and readable account. In short, I cannot thank the contributors enough, and I take this opportunity to thank their partners, families, friends and secretaries on their behalf. I hope they will be pleased with the end product. My colleagues at University College Hospital London have not only put up with my commitment to the book, but they have also contributed chapters, told me of interesting cases, and continued to stimulate my interest in the fascinating world of neonatal medicine. To them, and to Gemma Birchenough our PA, special thanks are due.

Thanks are also due to all the parents who have given permission for images of their baby (or babies) to appear in the book; in particular Bernadette Brent and Alyssa Dale who allowed me to use images of their children on the cover.

Once more, I owe an enormous debt of gratitude to my husband Ian Watts. He has remained supportive and wholly encouraging throughout the many anti-social hours of work involved in editing this Fifth edition, in spite of knowing from bitter experience (based on several previous editions) that it would take far longer than I estimated at the start. I dedicate the book to him, with all my love.

Janet M Rennie
University College London Hospitals, 2012

section 1

Organisation, delivery and outcome of neonatal care

Epidemiology

Alison Macfarlane   Miranda Mugford

Introduction

To set the scene, this chapter defines the epidemiological measures and rates relevant to neonatology and how they can vary within and between populations. This includes outlining the sources of routine collected national data for the UK and Ireland and how they can be compared with those for other European countries. This paves the way for subsequent chapters which describe data collections and research specific to neonatal care.

Births and birth rates

How birth statistics are compiled

There are three main routes through which data about births are collected. These have been described in considerable detail elsewhere (Macfarlane and Mugford 2000) but a brief description and update are given here.

The most frequently used source of data on a national scale is civil registration. In the UK parents are required by law to register a birth with the local Registrar of Births, Marriages and Deaths. As well as issuing a certificate, the registrar passes the information to a central office, which maintains records and, in the past, compiled both national and local statistics. Scotland, Northern Ireland and the Republic of Ireland each have separate General Register Offices. In 1970, the General Register Office for England and Wales was merged with the Government Social Survey to form the Office of Population Censuses and Surveys (OPCS). Then, in April 1996, OPCS merged with the Central Statistical Office and the Labour Market Statistics Group of the former Department of Employment to form the Office for National Statistics, which compiles and publishes a wide range of health, social and economic statistics. In 1999, the Office for National Statistics undertook a major review of

© 2012 Elsevier Ltd

civil registration and proposed wide-ranging changes, including 'through-life records', but these did not get through Parliament (Office for National Statistics 2002; General Register Office 2003). On 1 April 2008, the General Register Office for England and Wales was transferred into the Home Office's Identity and Passport Service, but the Office for National Statistics continues to analyse and publish data derived from civil registration. The General Register Office for Scotland merged with the National Archives of Scotland on 1 April 2011 to become the National Records of Scotland. In Northern Ireland, the General Register Office is part of the Northern Ireland Statistics and Research Agency, which analyses and publishes the data and is itself part of the Northern Ireland Department of Finance and Personnel.

In England, Wales and Scotland, the law originally required all fetal deaths after 28 completed weeks of gestation to be registered as stillbirths. This limit was lowered to 24 weeks on 1 October 1992. All live births at any gestation have to be registered. In Northern Ireland, there is no legal requirement to register a stillbirth, but a system was set up in 1961 to enable next of kin to register them. In the Republic of Ireland there was no system for registration of stillbirths before 1995, although they have been notified to Directors of Community Care since 1957.

The second method of information collection is through birth notification. In the UK all births have to be notified to the local Director of Public Health under a system introduced in 1907 and made compulsory in 1915. This is usually done by midwives immediately after the birth, and must be done within 36 hours. The system was originally devised at an era when most births were at home, so that a health visitor could be informed and then call to see the mother and baby. From the 1960s onwards, local and health authorities developed child health computer systems on which babies' records were initiated by the birth notification and used to administer vaccination and immunisation programmes and to monitor developmental testing.

Since the introduction in England and Wales of the allocation of National Health Service (NHS) numbers for babies at birth in October 2002, the data flows have changed. As the minimum dataset associated with NHS Numbers for Babies is very limited, many maternity units continue to send the fuller dataset used previously in parallel. At the time of writing the NHS Numbers for Babies service is being moved to the NHS Spine, where it will form part of the Personal Demographics Service. In Wales, child health systems have been redeveloped so that data from birth notifications can be aggregated nationally in the National Community Child Health Database and used to produce national birth and perinatal statistics, amongst other purposes.

Despite its limitations, the NHS Numbers for Babies dataset contains key data items, notably gestational age, baby's ethnicity, time of day of birth and birth order of stillbirths as well as live births within multiple births, which are not recorded at birth registration. Following a successful pilot project, linking NHS Numbers for Babies and birth registration data for 2005, these two datasets are now linked routinely by the Office for National Statistics, enhancing the scope and range of data available at a national level (Hilder et al. 2007).

In Northern Ireland, each of the four Health and Social Services Boards had its own child health system. Perinatal data from these were pooled to produce data for the province as a whole, held on the Northern Ireland NHS intranet. These data are now held by the Health and Social Care Board, which superseded the four boards on 1 April 2009. In the Republic of Ireland, a subset of vital statistics data derived from the four-part birth notifications, along with data from birth and death registrations, is analysed and published centrally by the Central Statistics Office. More detailed perinatal statistics, including clinical and sociodemographic data from the third part of the form, are analysed through the National Perinatal Reporting System and published separately by the Economic and Social Research Institute.

The third route for collecting data about births is through hospital-based systems. Traditionally these have collected data at discharge about hospital inpatient stays. More recently, systems have been developed that gather data about a person's episodes of care within a given NHS trust. NHS commissioners should hold information about care given to their residents wherever this is provided. The ways in which this is done are changing rapidly with the development of information technology systems within the NHS.

In England, information about inpatient stays in NHS hospitals is aggregated nationally through the Hospital Episode Statistics (HES) system. There is a separate Maternity HES system to collect information about women delivering in, and babies born in, the maternity departments of NHS hospitals. It should also include babies born at home or in private hospitals, but many of these records are missing. Maternity HES records include the standard admitted patient record plus a 'maternity tail', with a minimum dataset and clinical options. The items in the minimum datasets were specified by the Steering Group on Health Services Information (1985), chaired by Edith Körner. This was known as the Körner Committee and the datasets it recommended are usually referred to as Körner minimum datasets. The clinical options were set out in publications but were never implemented at a national level.

The HES system started in April 1987 and Maternity HES finally got under way in September 1988, but in the mid-1990s it was still very incomplete. By the financial year 1994–95 the system contained maternity tail records for only 67% of deliveries in England (House of Commons Health Committee 1996) and 72% in 2002–3 (Department of Health 2004). By 2009–10, after several years of improvement, data were submitted for between 80% and 90% of the items in the maternity tail. Data from the system are published annually on the Information Centre for Health and Social Care's website (Information Centre for Health and Social Care 2011a). Data are still missing for some units, either because they do not have a computer system in their maternity unit or because maternity systems are not linked to other systems in the hospital so the data in them do not reach Maternity HES (Kenney and Macfarlane 1999). Major changes in data collection have taken place in recent years, with the implementation of the National Care Records Service for individual patient records and of its Secondary Uses Service (Information Centre for Health and Social Care 2011b).

The NHS Information Centre has developed an ambitious new maternity secondary uses dataset for England, with over 1000 data items. It was planned to implement it in stages, with the first starting on 1 April 2011, but the start was delayed by funding decisions (Information Standards Board 2011, Child and Maternal Health Observatory, 2011).

In Wales and Northern Ireland, systems similar to Maternity HES were introduced but very few delivery records have data in the maternity tail. Analyses of data about method of delivery and length of stay have been derived from the Patient Episode Database Wales and published in bulletins on paper and on the Statistics Wales website (Health Statistics Wales 2011). As described above, the dearth of data from maternity tails has led to decisions to use child health systems for collecting more detailed maternity data in Wales.

In England data about episodes of care in neonatal intensive care units are collected, along with data about other episodes in paediatric departments, in the main part of HES. Unfortunately, these data are not routinely linked, at national level at least, to the record of the baby's delivery, but the allocation of NHS numbers to

SINGLETON HOSPITAL
STAFF LIBRARY

babies at birth may make this possible in the future. There is also a lack of consistency in recording levels of special and intensive care in HES and these data are not published routinely. To address this problem a Neonatal Critical Care Minimum Dataset was defined (Information Standards Board 2006). This is described in Chapter 2.

Scotland has had a maternity information system working nationally since the mid-1970s and data about mothers have been collected through the SMR2 Maternity Discharge Sheet. In the past, data about babies were collected through the SMR11 record, which from 1996 covered only sick babies, but this has been superseded by the Scottish Birth Record, described below. Data from SMR2 are published annually in *Scottish Health Statistics*, now published electronically on the Information and Statistics Division Scotland website (Information and Statistics Division 2011a). Data from SMR2 are also combined with those from the Scottish Perinatal and Infant Mortality Survey and published annually on the Information and Statistics Division website in the *Scottish Perinatal and Infant Mortality and Morbidity Report* (Information and Statistics Division 2011b). The report has been administered by a number of different bodies over time. Since 2008, this has been the Reproductive Health Programme of NHS Quality Improvement Scotland, with oversight by the Scottish Perinatal Mortality and Morbidity Review Advisory Group. The report also contains data about the incidence of selected congenital anomalies. The website also has reports on trends over time on topics such as multiple birth and operative vaginal deliveries (Information and Statistics Division 1997, 1998, 2003).

In 2003 Scotland started to implement a completely new system, the Scottish Child Health Information Development project. The first step in this was to implement a web-based Scottish Birth Record and an electronic woman-held record with the later aim of developing links with other systems. The Scottish Birth Record system is a live database, with data entered directly by NHS staff, interfacing with hospital systems where feasible, and available to appropriate NHS staff and to parents.

The other three countries of the UK include data about neonatal care in statistics collected about activity in paediatric departments, but have not so far been able to identify them separately in published data. This gap has led to the implementation of dedicated neonatal systems, linked to the establishment of neonatal networks. The information from them is used in the neonatal audits described in Chapter 2. The Neonatal Data Analysis Unit was set up to oversee these systems and analyse the data.

Trends and variations in birth rates

Definitions

- General fertility rate: the number of live births per 1000 women aged 15–44 years living in the same area.
- Age-specific fertility rate: the number of live births to mothers of each age group per 1000 women in the age group in the same population.
- Total fertility rate: the average number of live children that a group of women would have if they experienced the age-specific fertility rates of the calendar year in question throughout their childbearing lives.

The numbers of live births registered in recent years in each of the four countries of the UK and in the Republic of Ireland are shown in Table 1.1. This shows that, in the late 1980s, the numbers of births rose everywhere except in the Republic of Ireland, before falling again in the early 1990s. After a slight increase in the mid-1990s followed by a further decline, numbers started to rise in 2002 and

2003. This rise continued until 2008, with a slight falling off in 2009, except in the Republic of Ireland. These figures are useful as a measure of the workload of the maternity and paediatric services but shed very little light on the reasons for the increases and decreases. Fluctuations can arise either as a result of changes in the size and age structure of the childbearing population or as a consequence of changes in the birth rate within each age group.

One of the most long-standing measures of birth rate is the general fertility rate. In this the number of live births is expressed as a rate per 1000 women aged 15–44 or, in some cases, 15–49 years. Figure 1.1 shows the general fertility rate for England and Wales since 1838, the first full year after civil registration began in July 1837. The rates for the mid-19th century are probably an underestimate, as birth registration did not become compulsory in England and Wales until 1874. Shortly after this the fertility rate began to decline, a trend that continued steadily until the 1930s. This was interrupted only by a trough during the First World War and a short-lived peak after the war ended. A similar peak followed the Second World War. After this there was a longer term rise in the 1950s and 1960s, followed by a decline through most of the 1970s. After the rate reached a minimum in 1977 it fluctuated, gradually increasing in the late 1980s and decreasing through the 1990s. After rising from 2003 to 2008, it fell slightly in 2009 but rose again in 2010, except for women aged under 20.

This overall rate masks changes since 1977 within age groups. Rates for England and Wales are set out in Table 1.2, which shows birth rates among women in their late teens and 20s rising slightly in the late 1980s as the 'bulge' of women born in the mid-1960s entered the childbearing age range (Craig 1997) and then falling through the 1990s and the early years of the 21st century. In contrast, rates among women in their early 30s rose before levelling off in the mid-1990s, while rates for women in their late 30s and 40s have risen consistently. Since 2003, rates have risen in all age groups except for women aged under 20. They declined in 2009 for all groups aged under 30 while in 2010, they rose for all age groups except women aged under 20.

These age-specific rates can be summed up in a statistic called the 'total fertility rate'. This is a standardised measure that gives the total number of children who would be born to each woman if she experienced the age-specific fertility rates for the year in question throughout her childbearing life. As Table 1.2 shows, the rate for England and Wales rose gradually in the latter half of the 1980s, before falling gradually again, followed by a rise from 2003 to 2008 which tailed off in 2009. Age-specific fertility rates for women aged 30 and over continued to rise in 2009, while those for women aged under 30 fell slightly. Figure 1.2 shows trends over time in total fertility rates in England and Wales, Scotland and the two parts of Ireland, with Scotland having the lowest rates. Rates for local areas, published in national statistical publications for Scotland and Northern Ireland and in the Office for National Statistics Vital Statistics (VS) tables for England, vary considerably between regions and areas. Trends for each local authority area in England can also be seen in interactive maps on the Office for National Statistics website (Office for National Statistics 2011a).

For planning services it would be useful to have some idea of future trends in births, but these are notoriously difficult to predict. Nevertheless, government statisticians attempt to make such projections, combining analyses of past trends with replies to surveys about people's intentions to have children. Population projections for the countries of the UK, formerly produced by the Government Actuary's Department, are now produced by the Office for National Statistics. The 2008-based projections, published in 2010, assumed a peak in fertility in 2008, followed by a fall in 2009 and succeeding years and then a levelling off (Wright 2010).

Table 1.1 Live births in England, Wales, Scotland and Ireland 1975–2010

YEAR	ENGLAND	WALES	ENGLAND AND WALES*	SCOTLAND	NORTHERN IRELAND[†]	REPUBLIC OF IRELAND
1975	568 900	38 030	603 445	67 943	26 130	67 178
1980	618 371	37 357	656 234	68 892	28 582	74 064
1985	619 301	36 771	656 417	66 676	27 427	62 388
1990	666 920	38 866	706 140	65 973	26 251	53 044
1995	613 257	34 477	648 138	60 051	23 693	48 787
1996	614 188	34 894	649 489	59 296	24 382	50 655
1997	608 202	34 520	643 095	59 440	24 087	52 775
1998	602 111	33 438	635 901	57 319	23 668	53 969
1999	589 468	32 111	621 872	55 147	22 957	53 924
2000	572 826	31 304	604 441	53 076	21 512	54 789
2001	563 744	30 616	594 634	52 527	21 962	57 854
2002	565 709	30 205	596 122	51 270	21 385	60 503
2003	589 851	31 400	621 469	52 432	21 648	61 529
2004	607 184	32 325	639 721	53 957	22 318	61 972
2005	613 028	32 593	645 835	54 386	22 328	61 372
2006	635 748	33 628	669 601	55 690	23 272	65 425
2007	655 357	34 414	690 013	57 781	24 451	71 389
2008	672 809	35 650	708 711	60 041	25 631	73 996
2009	671 058	34 937	706 248	59 046	24 910	74 728[§]
2010	687 007	35 952	723 165	58 791	25 315	73 724[§]

*Including births in England and Wales to women normally resident outside England and Wales.
[†]Live birth figures from 1981 are resident births only
[§]Births for Ireland for 2009 and 2010 are year of registration figures and are provisional.
(Data from Office for National Statistics, General Register Office, Scotland, Northern Ireland Statistics and Research Agency, Northern Ireland and Central Statistics Office, Ireland.)

The incidence of preterm birth and low birthweight

Definitions

- Birthweight: the first weight of the newborn or fetus obtained after birth. The actual weight should be recorded to the degree of accuracy to which it is measured.
- Low birthweight: less than 2500 g (up to and including 2499 g).
- Very low birthweight: less than 1500 g (up to and including 1499 g).
- Extremely low birthweight: less than 1000 g (up to and including 999 g).
- Gestational age: the duration of gestation is measured from the first day of the last normal menstrual period. Gestational age is expressed in completed days or completed weeks.
- Preterm: less than 37 completed weeks or 259 completed days of gestation.

In England and Wales, birthweight data have been collected since the mid-1950s through the birth notification system. From 1953 to 1973, each local authority, and from 1974 to 1986 each health authority, submitted a form to central government giving the numbers of low-weight births to women living in their area. Data from this source have been used for these years in Figure 1.3, which shows that the percentage of liveborn babies weighing 2500 g and less, the original definition of 'low birthweight', remained at a similar level of between 6% and 7% from the mid-1950s to the mid-1980s.

The system changed in the early 1980s, when arrangements were made for health authorities to extract birthweights from babies' birth notifications and send them to local registrars of births and deaths to be added to the birth registration. Data flows started to change from 2006 onwards when local register offices moved to registration online. This was an intermittent process, with many teething problems, which could have affected data quality. By July 2009, it was implemented in all register offices in England and Wales. A byproduct of this is that birthweight is now passed

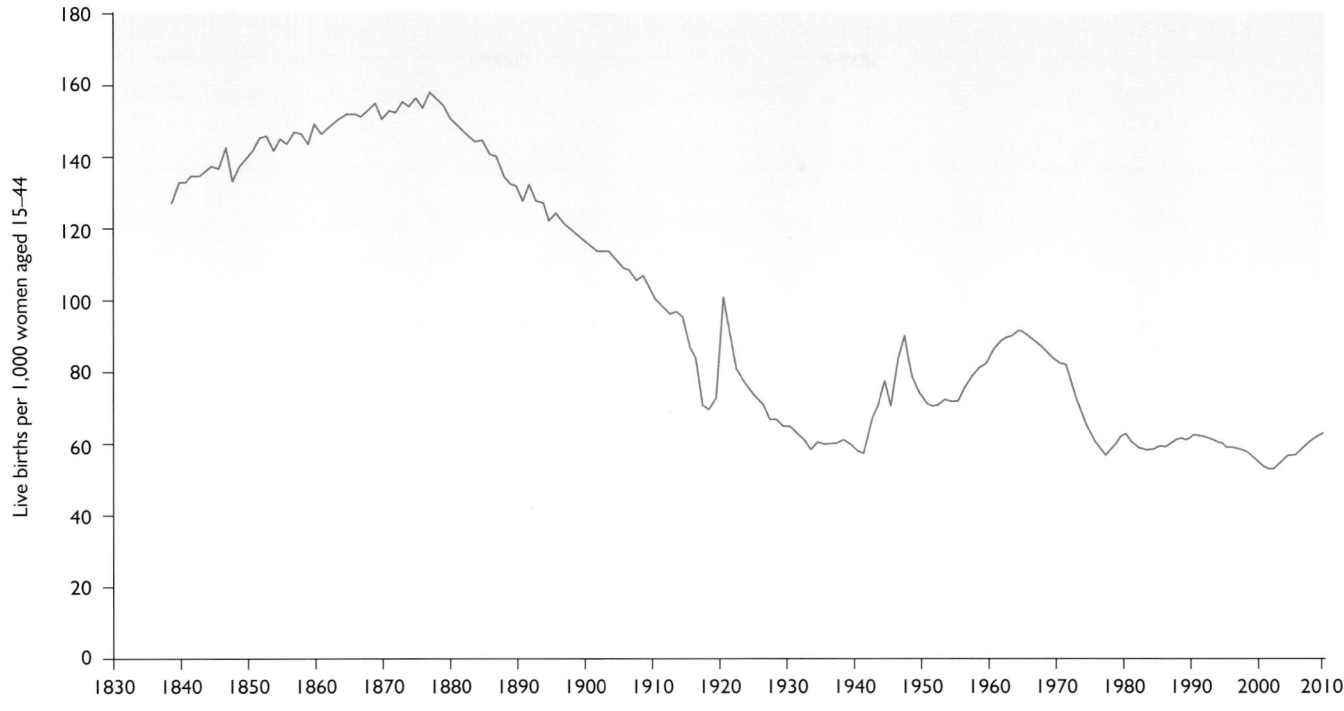

Fig. 1.1 General fertility rate, England and Wales, 1838–2010. *(Data from Office for National Statistics, Birth Statistics.)*

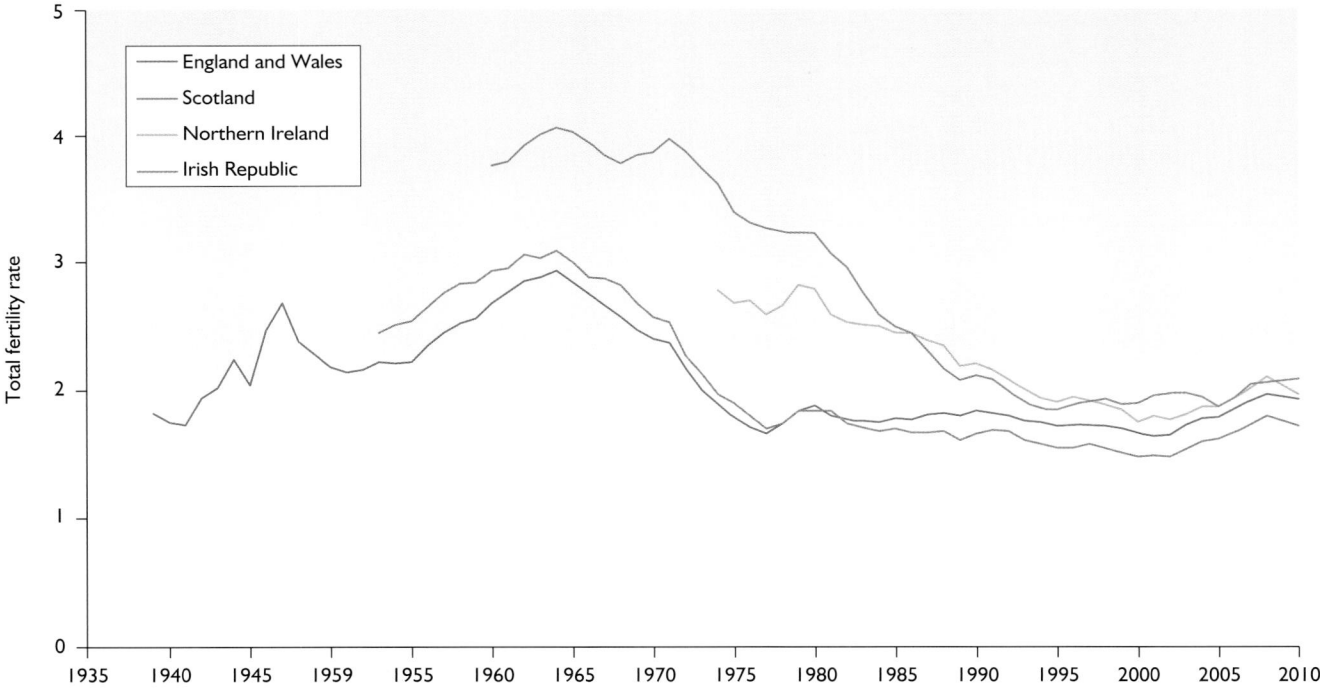

Fig. 1.2 Total fertility rates, UK and Ireland, 1938–2010. *(Data from Office for National Statistics, General Register Office Scotland, Northern Ireland Statistics and Research Agency and Central Statistics Office, Ireland.)*

electronically to the Office for National Statistics from the notification by the midwife or doctor in attendance at the birth.

These data are analysed using the current definition of low birthweight, which was changed in the ninth revision of the *International Classification of Diseases* (World Health Organization 1977) to 'under 2500 g'. Babies weighing under 1500 g at birth are now categorised as 'very low birthweight', and those weighing under 1000 g are described as 'extremely low birthweight' (World Health Organization 1992). These birthweight groups are used in Table 1.3 and in the data for the mid-1990s onwards in Figure 1.3.

Table 1.2 Age-specific fertility rates, England and Wales, 1964–2010

YEAR	LIVE BIRTHS	LIVE BIRTHS PER 1000 WOMEN IN AGE GROUP								TOTAL FERTILITY RATE
		15–44	Under 20	20–24	25–29	30–34	35–39	40–44	45 and over	
1964 (max.)	875 972	92.9	42.5	181.6	187.3	107.7	49.8	13.0	0.9	2.9
1977 (min.)	569 259	58.1	29.4	103.7	117.5	58.6	18.2	4.1	0.3	1.7
1979	638 028	63.3	30.3	111.3	131.2	69.0	21.3	4.3	0.4	1.8
1985	656 417	61.0	29.5	94.5	127.6	76.4	24.1	4.6	0.4	1.8
1990	706 140	64.3	33.3	91.7	122.4	87.3	31.2	5.0	0.3	1.84
1995	648 138	60.5	28.5	76.4	108.7	88.2	36.4	6.5	0.3	1.72
2000	604 441	55.9	29.3	70.0	94.3	87.9	41.4	8.0	0.4	1.72
2001	594 634	54.7	28.0	69.0	91.7	88.0	41.5	8.4	0.5	1.70
2002	596 122	54.7	27.1	69.1	91.5	89.9	43.0	8.6	0.5	1.65
2003	621 469	56.8	26.9	71.3	96.0	95.0	46.4	9.3	0.5	1.73
2004	639 721	58.2	26.8	72.7	97.7	99.7	48.8	9.9	0.5	1.78
2005	645 835	58.3	26.3	71.5	97.9	100.8	50.3	10.3	0.6	1.79
2006	669 601	60.2	26.6	73.0	100.7	104.9	53.9	10.8	0.6	1.86
2007	690 013	62.0	26.0	73.3	103.8	110.2	56.9	11.4	0.7	1.91
2008	708 711	63.8	26.0	74.4	108.1	113.1	58.4	11.9	0.7	1.97
2009	706 248	63.7	25.3	73.9	107.2	113.1	59.0	12.1	0.8	1.96
2010	723 165	65.4	24.2	74	108.0	117.8	61.5	12.5	0.9	2.00

The rates for women of all ages, under 20, and 40 and over are based upon the female population aged 15–44, 15–19 and 40–44 years, respectively. (Data from Office for National Statistics Birth Statistics).

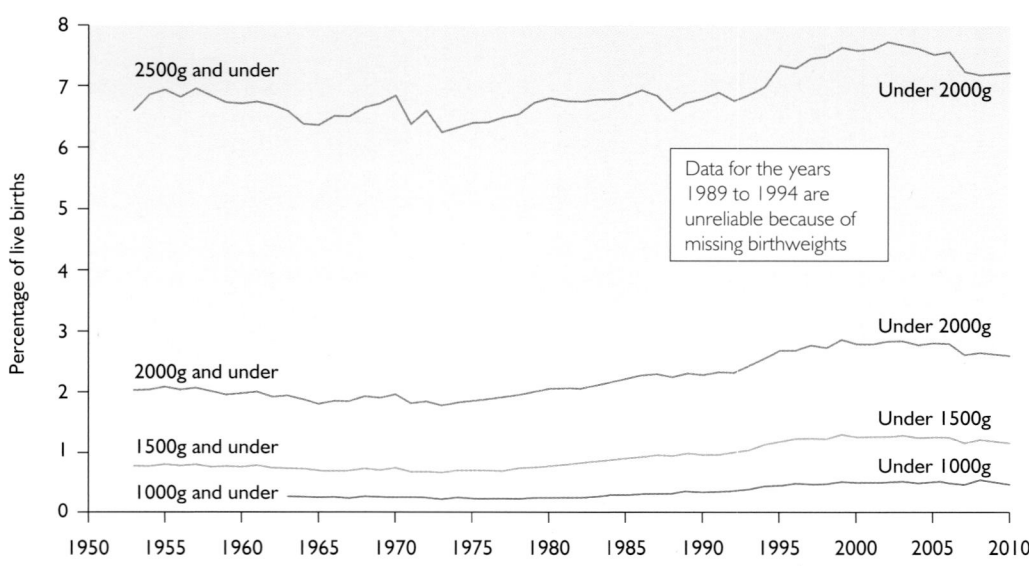

Fig. 1.3 Incidence of low birthweight, England and Wales, 1953–2010. *(Data from LHS 27/1 low birthweight returns and Office for National Statistics mortality statistics. Updated from Birth counts, Tables A3.4.1 and A3.4.2. Macfarlane, Mugford, Henderson et al. 2000)*

Table 1.3 Low-birthweight live births, England and Wales, 1983–2010

YEAR	TOTAL LIVE BIRTHS	LIVE BIRTHS WITH STATED BIRTHWEIGHT	PERCENTAGE OF LIVE BIRTHS WITH STATED BIRTHWEIGHT				
			Less than 1000 g	Less than 1500 g	1500–1999 g	2000–2499 g	Under 2500 g
1983	629 134	628 269	0.27	0.84	1.26	4.60	6.70
1984	636 818	636 006	0.29	0.87	1.28	4.55	6.70
1985	656 417	655 549	0.29	0.90	1.30	4.61	6.81
1986	661 018	660 394	0.31	0.92	1.35	4.66	6.92
1987	681 511	681 009	0.31	0.96	1.33	4.55	6.83
1988	693 577	692 746	0.32	0.94	1.30	4.36	6.59
1989	687 725	666 612	0.37	0.98	1.32	4.45	6.74
1990	706 140	678 374	0.34	0.96	1.32	4.51	6.79
1991	699 217	673 299	0.34	0.96	1.36	4.57	6.89
1992	689 656	663 689	0.36	1.00	1.30	4.51	6.82
1993	674 467	651 166	0.40	1.03	1.40	4.42	6.85
1994	664 726	646 914	0.44	1.12	1.41	4.44	6.98
1995	648 138	645 641	0.44	1.17	1.50	4.65	7.33
1996	649 485	647 948	0.49	1.22	1.45	4.61	7.28
1997	643 095	641 979	0.47	1.23	1.53	4.69	7.45
1998	635 901	635 116	0 48	1.22	1.50	4.76	7.48
1999	621 872	619 963	0.51	1.29	1.56	4.76	7.61
2000	603 421	602 401	0.50	1.25	1.53	4.81	7.59
2001	594 634	593 753	0.51	1.26	1.52	4.82	7.60
2002	596 122	595 213	0.50	1.25	1.57	4.90	7.72
2003	621 469	620 550	0.52	1.28	1.45	4.52	7.67
2004	639 721	638 464	0.49	1.24	1.52	4.75	7.61
2005	645 835	643 591	0.50	1.25	1.55	4.71	7.51
2006	669 601	663 391	0.49	1.24	1.54	4.77	7.56
2007	690 013	682 436	0.47	1.15	1.45	4.62	7.22
2008	708 711	703 214	0.55	1.21	1.43	4.53	7.17
2009	706 248	701 011	0.52	1.19	1.44	4.55	7.18
2010	723 079	715 973	-	1.21	1.39	4.42	7.02

(Data from Office for National Statistics, Mortality statistics, Series DH3 and Childhood mortality.)

Interpreting trends

Both show recent trends in the incidence of low birthweight in England and Wales. Although the percentage of liveborn babies weighing under 2500 g has fluctuated since 1983, the general trend was upwards, followed by a levelling off from 2000 onwards, followed by an apparent drop in 2007. This could be a discontinuity resulting from the change of method of data collection. There were similar patterns in all groups of babies weighing under 2000 g, except that, in the under-1000-g group, the discontinuity in 2007 took the form of an increase.

Between 1983 and 1988 there was no clear trend in the very small proportion of liveborn babies for whom birthweight was missing, and who are known to include a high proportion of small and

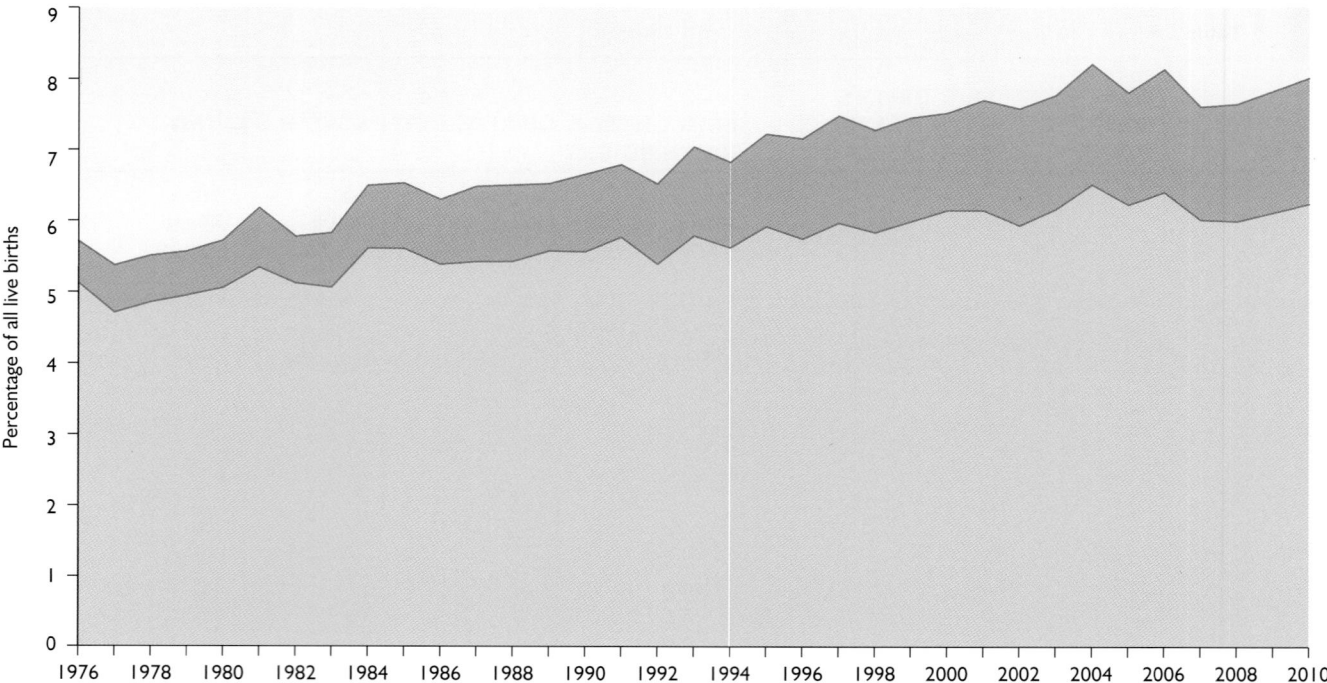

Fig. 1.4 Percentage of live births born before 37 weeks of gestation, by multiplicity, Scotland, 1976–2010. *(Data from Information and Statistics Division Births in Scottish Hospitals.)*

immature babies (Alberman and Botting 1991). In the middle of 1989, financial constraints in the OPCS led to a decline in the completeness of recording of birthweight on birth registration records. Birthweight was missing on up to 4% of records from 1989 to 1994, making the data for these years difficult to interpret. As shown later in Table 1.18, the mortality rate among babies with missing birthweights was well above the overall rate, suggesting that the group included a relatively high proportion of low-birthweight babies. By 1995, the numbers of missing birthweights had declined markedly and the data for 1995 onwards used in Tables 1.3, 1.9, 1.11, 1.13 and 1.18 (see below) and Figure 1.3 became much more reliable than those for the early 1990s. Unfortunately, however, the move to registration online was accompanied by a slight increase in the percentage of missing birthweights, from under 0.2% between 2000 and 2004 to 1.1% in 2007 and 0.74% in 2009.

The reported incidence of low-weight births in 1995 was well above that for 1988 and rose markedly after 1995, as Figure 1.3 shows. Analyses of birthweight data for both England and Wales and Scotland identified two separate trends, however. Although the percentages of low-weight births had increased during the 1980s, there had also been an increase in the proportion of heavier babies (Power 1994; Bonelli and Raab 1997; Maher and Macfarlane 2004). From the 1996s onwards in England and Wales, the proportion of heavier babies levelled off, fluctuating between 11.3% and 11.6% for singleton births.

Although the World Health Organization has published a definition of preterm birth, it has no definition of very preterm or extremely preterm, as a result of the lack of consensus mentioned in Chapter 2. It does, however, recommend groups to be used when publishing data about gestational age. These are under 28, 28–31, 32–36, 37–41 and 42 or more completed weeks and the corresponding numbers of days (World Health Organization 1992). The under-28-week category is often subdivided into less than 24 and 24–27 completed weeks, as has been done in this chapter.

When OPCS made the arrangements in the 1970s to acquire the information about babies' birthweights from birth notification, it also requested gestational age. For reasons that are long forgotten, access to this was refused by clinical organisations. Data about gestational age of babies born in England and Wales only became available at a national level in England and Wales for 2005 onwards via the linkage with NHS Numbers for Babies data (Moser et al. 2007; Hilder and Moser 2008). The data available so far are summarised in Table 1.4 and are published in fuller detail in *Health Statistics Quarterly* and elsewhere on the Office for National Statistics website (Moser et al. 2007, 2008; Moser 2009) As a result, the only data about long-term trends in preterm birth are for Scotland (Macfarlane et al. 1988; Information and Statistics Division Scotland 1997, 2011a; Macfarlane and Mugford 2000). A reported increase in the proportion of preterm births in Scotland can be seen in Figure 1.4 and Table 1.5, which are derived from information in the SMR2 system. Although multiple births have contributed to the rise, preterm singleton births have also increased since the mid-1970s as a proportion of all live births. Table 1.5 also shows a decrease in the rate of postterm births in Scotland and comparison with Table 1.4 suggests that this rate is lower than in England and Wales.

The data for both England and Wales and Scotland suggest that there has been an increase in the reported incidence of very small and very preterm babies. Although the rising incidence of multiple birth, discussed later, has made a major contribution to this rise, it is certainly not the only factor. It has been suggested that an increasing tendency to admit smaller and iller babies to neonatal nurseries has also contributed to the rise. By law all live births should be registered but there is a subjective element in distinguishing between a live birth and a miscarriage, particularly if the baby dies very shortly after birth. In the past some of these very tiny babies would have been regarded as miscarriages and would not therefore have been registered as live births. The lowering of the gestational age

Table 1.4 Live births by gestational age, England and Wales, births in 2005–09

YEAR OF BIRTH	ALL WITH KNOWN GESTATIONAL AGE	PERCENTAGE OF BIRTHS WITH KNOWN GESTATIONAL AGE (WEEKS)						
		Less than 24	24–27	28–31	32–36	All less than 37	37–41	42 and over
All								
2005	640 599	0.1	0.4	0.9	6.2	7.6	88.1	4.3
2006	664 465	0.1	0.4	0.9	6.2	7.6	88.1	4.3
2007	682 021	0.1	0.4	0.8	6.0	7.3	88.6	4.1
2008	701 041	0.1	0.4	0.8	5.9	7.3	88.8	4.0
2009	698 793	0.1	Not available			7.3	88.6	4.1
Singleton								
2005	621 793	0.1	0.3	0.7	5.1	6.2		
2006	644 441	0.1	0.3	0.7	5.1	6.2		
2007	661 442	0.1	0.3	0.7	4.9	5.9		
2008	679 694	0.1	0.3	0.6	4.8	5.8		
2009	676 291	0.08	Not available			5.8	90.0	4.2
Multiple								
2005	18 806	0.7	2.8	7.6	42.2	53.3		
2006	20 024	0.8	2.9	7.3	41.9	53.0		
2007	20 579	0.6	3.1	6.9	41.7	52.3		
2008	21 347	0.6	2.8	7.2	42.7	53.3		
2009	22 502	Not available				52.8	47.1	0.1

(Data from Office for National Statistics. Gestation-specific infant mortality and unpublished data)

limit for registering fetal deaths as stillbirths in all countries of the UK in October 1992 may well have reinforced changes in people's perceptions of which births should be registered as live births.

Another factor that may have contributed to the increase in registration is the growing recognition of parents' need to mourn an unsuccessful outcome of pregnancy. The formalities of registration can sometimes form part of this, together with the process of holding a funeral.

Interpreting differences between areas and countries

The incidence of low birthweight varies both between geographical areas and between sectors of the population, including internationally. Considerable differences were seen in the late 1980s between the countries and parts of countries that took part in the International Collaborative Effort on birthweight, plurality and perinatal and infant mortality (Hartford 1990). Similar differences were seen in the incidences of low birthweight in 1990 (Masuy-Stroobant

1996), in the Peristat perinatal indicator project which used data for the years around 2000 (Buitendijk et al. 2003), and again in the Europeristat project using data for 2004, shown in Table 1.6 and Figure 1.5 (Europeristat 2008). These studies used data collected routinely through the participating countries' vital statistics systems or medical birth registers (Zeitlin et al. 2003; Macfarlane et al. 2003; Gissler et al. 2010).

Although the overall incidence of low birthweight in a population tends to be a reflection of the health of that population in general, and of women of childbearing age in particular, at the bottom end of the birthweight range it is affected by the country's criteria for birth registration. In theory this should not affect live births, as in most countries a live birth is registrable regardless of gestational age or birthweight. There are, however, considerable variations in the criteria for the registration of late fetal deaths as stillbirths. The differences within Europe can be found in Table 3.1 of the Europeristat report (Europeristat 2008). Many countries, including those in the UK, do not follow the World Health Organization's recommendation to use a 22-week cut-off.

Table 1.5 Gestational age of live births in Scotland, years ending 31 March, 1990, 1995, 2000, 2005, 2010

YEAR	TOTAL	PERCENTAGE OF LIVE BIRTHS AT GESTATIONAL AGE (WEEKS)					
		Less than 24	24–27	28–31	32–36	37–41	42+
	All						
1990	63 351	0.0	0.3	0.7	5.3	87.5	5.5
1995	60 261	0.0	0.3	0.8	5.7	88.2	4.7
2000	53 870	0.0	0.3	0.8	6.1	89.4	3.3
2005	53 136	0.0	0.4	0.8	6.3	89.7	2.7
2010[P]	58 051	0.1	0.3	0.8	6.0	89.9	2.9
	Singleton						
1990	61 937	0.0	0.2	0.6	4.6	88.3	5.6
1995	58 712	0.0	0.2	0.7	4.8	89.2	4.9
2000	52 380	0.0	0.3	0.6	5.1	90.5	3.4
2005	51 655	0.0	0.3	0.7	5.2	91.0	2.8
2010[P]	56 185	0.0	0.2	0.6	4.8	91.3	3.0
	Multiple						
1990	1414	0.7	4.1	5.4	39.3	50.6	–
1995	1549	0.6	4.1	5.4	39.3	50.6	–
2000	1490	0.5	2.5	6.0	40.3	50.7	–
2005	1468	0.1	3.8	5.3	47.3	43.6	–
2010[P]	1866	0.7	2.0	6.5	41.9	48.8	–

P, provisional.
(Data from Information and Statistics Division Births in Scottish Hospitals.)
Notes:

1. Excludes home births and births at non-National Health Service hospitals.
2. Where four or more babies are involved in a pregnancy, birth details are recorded only for the first three babies delivered.
3. 2010 data are provisional.
4. Includes births where the birthweight is unknown.

Inevitably, these wide differences in the gestational age at which fetal deaths are registrable as stillbirths can affect decisions about whether a very preterm birth should be regarded as a registrable live birth or as a miscarriage, although the extent to which they do so appears to vary from country to country. As a result, in the Europeristat study, the percentage of live births weighing under 500 g ranged from 0.00% in many countries to 0.05% in Germany and 0.06% in England and Wales. Although these differences have a very limited impact on the comparability of statistics about low birthweight, they have a much larger impact on the comparability of mortality statistics (Buitendijk et al. 2003; Mohangoo et al. 2011). To deal with this problem, the World Health Organization recommends that babies weighing under 500 g or born before 22 completed weeks of gestation are excluded from comparative statistics (World Health Organization 1992). In the Euronatal study, with data for the mid-1990s and common cut-offs, the differences between countries changed when common cut-offs were applied (Graafmans et al. 2001, 2002).

A further factor that has to be taken into account is the extent to which data about gestational age and birthweight are missing, either because the information was not recorded initially or because it was not passed on to population-based data collection systems. This is likely to have affected the trends shown in Figures 1.3 and 1.4, as well as comparisons between countries. Furthermore, where data are almost complete, birthweight is most likely to go unrecorded for babies who die very soon after birth.

Real differences in the low-birthweight rates within countries with the same or similar data collection systems are shown in Table 1.7. In 2009, the incidence of low-weight births in the Government Office regions of England ranged from 6.4% in the South-west region to 8.5% in the West Midlands region. Each of these regions includes a variety of different populations. Differences between local authorities are great. Even though these small babies make up a tiny proportion of all births, they make a considerable contribution to mortality rates. Comparing the countries of the UK, the incidences of low-weight and very-low-weight births in Wales were lower than those for England in 2009, while those for Scotland and Northern Ireland were lower still and the lowest rate of low birthweight shown in Table 1.7 was in the Republic of Ireland.

Differences between smaller areas, such as electoral wards, are even more marked. In each of the countries of the UK, area

Table 1.6 Birthweight distribution of live births in countries participating in the Europeristat European Perinatal indicators project

MEMBER STATE	LIVE BIRTHS		PERCENTAGE OF LIVE BIRTHS WITH STATED BIRTHWEIGHT (G)							
	All	With stated birthweight	Under 500	500–1499	Under 1500	1500–2499	Under 2500	2500–4499	4500 and over	All
Belgium										
Flanders	60 672	60 672	0.00	0.82	**0.82**	5.67	**6.49**	92.49	**1.02**	100.00
Brussels	16 200	15 774	0.02	1.00	**1.01**	5.46	**6.47**	92.75	**0.77**	100.00
Czech Republic	97 671	97 671	0.01	1.05	**1.06**	5.68	**6.74**	92.14	**1.12**	100.00
Denmark	64 521	64 355	0.02	0.91	**0.93**	4.38	**5.30**	91.00	**3.70**	100.00
Germany	646 626	646 380	0.05	1.16	**1.21**	5.87	**7.08**	91.49	**1.43**	100.00
Estonia	13 990	13 954	0.02	0.94	**0.96**	3.31	**4.27**	92.45	**3.28**	100.00
Ireland	62 066	62 042	0.00	0.87	**0.87**	4.10	**4.98**	92.18	**2.84**	100.00
Greece	104 355	104 355	0.01	1.00	**1.01**	7.53	**8.54**	91.05	**0.41**	100.00
Spain	454 591	434 510	0.00	0.78	**0.78**	6.67	**7.45**	91.91	**0.65**	100.00
Valencia	51 047	49 490	0.00	0.84	**0.84**	7.57	**8.42**	90.99	**0.60**	100.00
France	14 572	14 534	0.00	0.85	**0.85**	6.36	**7.22**	91.94	**0.85**	100.00
Italy	539 066	539 066	0.01	0.80	**0.81**	5.85	**6.66**	92.78	**0.56**	100.00
Cyprus*										
Latvia	20 355	20 355	0.00	0.90	**0.90**	4.10	**5.00**	92.98	**2.02**	100.00
Lithuania	29 480	29 480	0.01	0.71	**0.72**	4.02	**4.75**	93.41	**1.84**	100.00
Luxembourg	5 469	5 284	0.00	0.13	**0.13**	4.41	**4.54**	94.72	**0.74**	100.00
Hungary	95 137	95 063	0.06	1.33	**1.39**	6.93	**8.32**	90.51	**1.17**	100.00
Malta	3 887	3 884	0.00	0.90	**0.90**	6.85	**7.75**	91.79	**0.46**	100.00
Netherlands	181 006	180 998	0.03	0.95	**0.98**	5.43	**6.41**	90.68	**2.90**	100.00
Austria	78 934	78 934	0.03	1.01	**1.04**	5.74	**6.77**	92.16	**1.07**	100.00
Poland	356 651	356 647	0.00	0.94	**0.94**	5.17	**6.11**	92.43	**1.46**	100.00
Portugal	109 356	109 049	0.01	0.93	**0.94**	6.67	**7.61**	91.94	**0.45**	100.00
Slovenia	17 846	17 846	0.03	0.88	**0.91**	4.91	**5.83**	93.07	**1.10**	100.00
Slovak Republic	52 388	52 388	0.01	0.89	**0.90**	6.48	**7.38**	91.77	**0.86**	100.00
Finland	57 569	57 544	0.04	0.73	**0.77**	3.39	**4.16**	92.85	**2.99**	100.00
Sweden	100 158	99 915	0.02	0.73	**0.75**	3.46	**4.21**	91.77	**4.02**	100.00
UK										
England and Wales	639 721	638 464	0.06	1.18	**1.24**	6.32	**7.56**	90.76	**1.69**	100.00
Scotland	52 911	52 901	0.04	1.08	**1.12**	6.11	**7.23**	90.69	**2.08**	100.00
Northern Ireland	22 362	22 361	0.02	0.98	**1.00**	4.79	**5.80**	91.74	**2.47**	100.00
Norway	57 111	57 102	0.02	0.89	**0.91**	3.94	**4.85**	90.93	**4.22**	100.00

*Cyprus provided no data on birthweight.
(Data from Europeristat (2008), Table C4_B.)

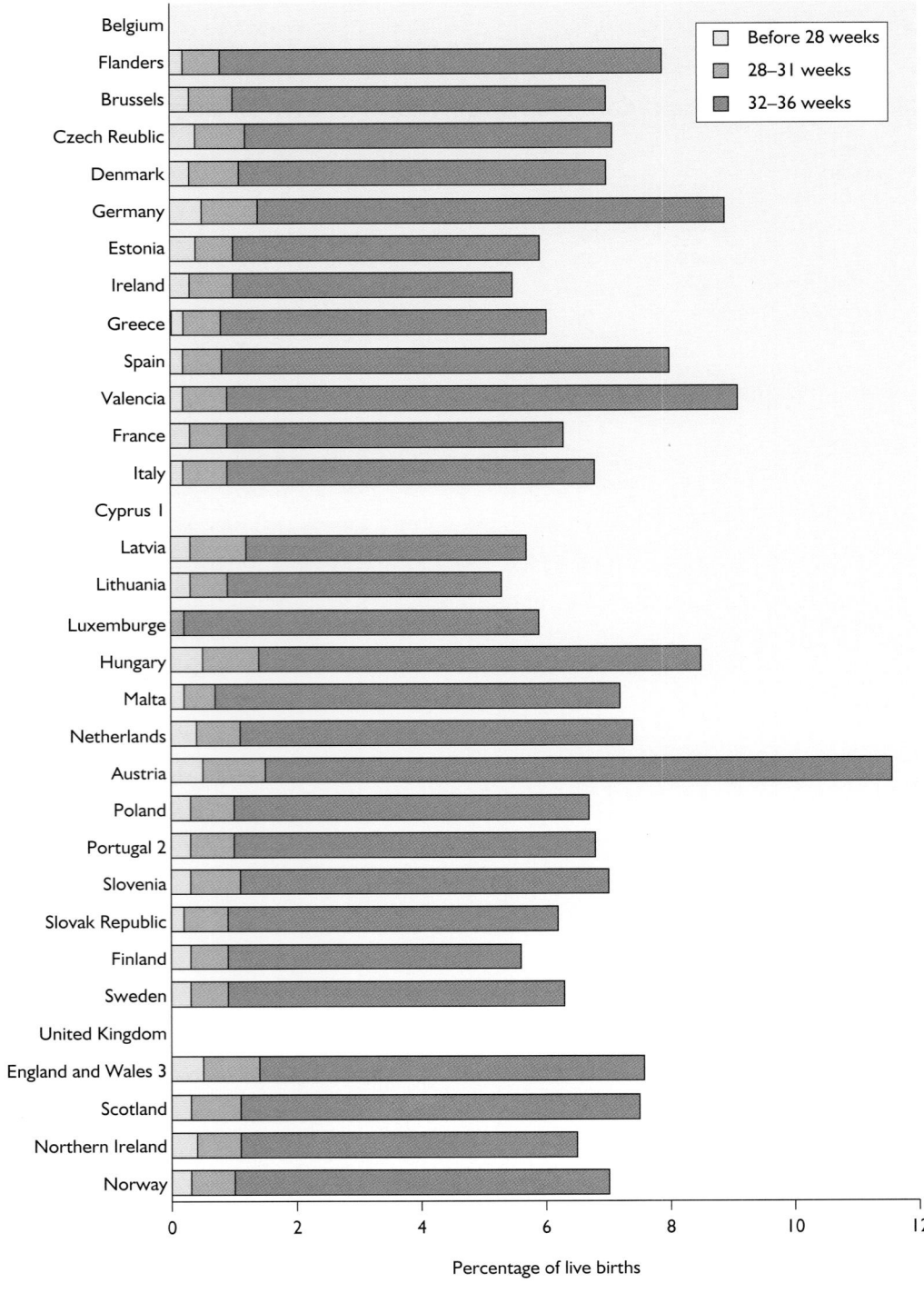

Fig. 1.5 Percentage of live births which were preterm in European Union member states participating in the Europeristat project. *(Data from Europeristat, 2008.)*

deprivation scores have been constructed to classify small areas. These use data from the census and other data, such as unemployment and crime rates, that can be disaggregated to a local level. They can be used to group together areas with similar characteristics within each country, but not for the whole of the UK, given that the composition of the scores is different in England, Wales, Scotland and Northern Ireland (Department of Communities and Local Government 2011).

Social class differences

Definition

- National Statistics Socio-economic class (Table 1.8).

Differences between geographical areas in the incidence of low birthweight reflect, in their turn, differences in the characteristics of the populations and differences between groups within the

Table 1.7 Incidence of low-weight live births in the Government Office regions of England, Wales, Scotland and the Irish Republic, 2009

COUNTRY OR GOVERNMENT OFFICE REGION	NUMBER	NUMBER WITH STATED BIRTHWEIGHT	PERCENTAGE WEIGHING		
			Under 1500 g	1500–2499 g	Under 2500 g
England and Wales	706 248	704 389	1.4	6.1	7.5
North-east	26 261	29 879	1.3	6.1	7.4
North-west	74 588	87 194	1.4	6.1	7.5
Yorkshire and the Humber	55 508	66 159	1.4	6.6	8.0
East Midlands	45 002	53 923	1.4	6.3	7.7
West Midlands	60 985	71 088	1.7	6.9	8.5
East	60 120	71 264	1.4	5.7	7.1
London	105 042	128 817	1.6	6.3	7.9
South-east	88 007	103 536	1.2	5.4	6.7
South-west	49 310	57 700	1.2	5.3	6.4
England	564 823	669 560	1.4	6.1	7.5
Wales	34 937	34 652	1.2	6.1	7.3
Scotland*	57 945	57 883	1.1	5.9	7.0
Northern Ireland	25 034	25 022	1.0	5.1	6.1
Republic of Ireland†	73 996	72 938			5.3

*Year ending 31 March 2009.
†2008.
(Data from Office of National Statistics, published by NCHOD. Information and Statistics Division, SMR2; Perinatal statistics, Northern Ireland; National Perinatal Reporting System, Ireland.)

Table 1.8 Eight-, five- and three-class version of the National Statistics Socio-economic classes

EIGHT-CLASS VERSION	FIVE-CLASS VERSION	THREE-CLASS VERSION

1. Higher managerial, administrative and professional occupations
  1.1 Large employers and higher managerial and administrative occupations
  1.2 Higher professional occupations
2. Lower managerial, administrative and professional occupations
3. Intermediate occupations
4. Small employers and own-account workers
5. Lower supervisory and technical occupations
6. Semiroutine occupations
7. Routine occupations
8. Never worked and long-term unemployed
	1. Higher managerial, administrative and professional occupations
	
	2. Intermediate occupations
	3. Small employers and own-account workers
	4. Lower supervisory and technical occupations
	5. Semiroutine and routine occupations
	*Never worked and long-term unemployed
		1. Higher managerial, administrative and professional occupations
		
		2. Intermediate occupations
		3. Routine and manual occupations
		
		*Never worked and long-term unemployed

(Modified from Office for National Statistics 2010.)

Table 1.9 Low birthweight by National Statistics Socio-economic classification of father and registration status for live births, England and Wales, 2010

SOCIAL CLASS OF FATHER/ REGISTRATION STATUS		PERCENTAGE WEIGHING			NUMBER OF LIVE BIRTHS	
		Under 1500 g	1500–2499 g	Under 2500 g	All*	With stated birthweight
All		**1.19**	**5.99**	**7.18**	**706 248**	**701 011**
Inside marriage or jointly registered, by National Statistics Socio-economic classification of father						
All		**1.16**	**5.83**	**6.99**	**662 509**	**657 610**
1.1	Large employers and higher managerial occupations	0.83	4.98	5.80	45 080	44 820
1.2	Higher professional occupations	1.04	5.59	6.63	64 840	64 360
2	Lower managerial and professional occupations	1.20	5.31	6.50	131 990	131 130
3	Intermediate occupations	1.25	5.17	6.42	38 010	37 710
4	Small employers and own-account workers	0.97	5.76	6.73	95 460	94 750
5	Lower supervisory and technical occupations	1.15	5.42	6.57	82 410	81 730
6	Semiroutine occupations	1.38	6.17	7.55	76 750	76 140
7	Routine occupations	1.30	6.41	7.70	85 520	84 900
Other+		1.62	7.28	8.89	42 870	42 610
Sole registration						
All		**1.63**	**8.44**	**10.07**	**43 739**	**43 401**

*The breakdowns of socio-economic classification do not add to the 'All' figures as they are based on a 10% sample: see Office for National Statistics publication for details.
Students; occupations inadequately described; occupations not classifiable for other reasons; never worked and long-term unemployed.
(Data from Office for National Statistics Infant mortality by social and biological factors, England and Wales, 2010, Table 7.)

population. Table 1.9 shows differences in the incidence of low birthweight in England and Wales when live births are tabulated by the baby's father's social class. The classes used are the eight-class version of the National Statistics Socio-economic classes. The three-, five- and eight-class versions shown in Table 1.8 have been used since 2001, and were modified in 2010 using the Standard Occupational Classification, as revised for use in the 2011 Census (Office for National Statistics 2010). They supersede the Registrar General's social classes, which were used during the 20th century (Macfarlane and Mugford 2000; Rowan 2003).

For babies in each group, and for all birthweights under 2500 g combined, the table shows clear differences between the higher rates of low birthweight among babies with fathers in routine and semiroutine occupation and the lower rates among babies with fathers in professional and managerial occupations. Rates were highest among sole registrations, babies registered by their mother alone. Ideally, these data and those in Table 1.7 should be restricted to singleton births because the birthweight distribution for multiple births is different.

Since 1986, mothers have had the option of recording their occupation on their baby's birth certificate but many mothers still do not do so, either because they are not in paid employment or, in the case of the youngest women, because they do not yet have an occupation. For this reason, tabulations by mother's social class are not routinely published (Macfarlane and Mugford 2000; Rowan 2003).

In Scotland, an analysis of births in the years 1980–4 showed a clear social class gradient in the incidence of preterm births at 20–27, 28–31 and 32–36 weeks (Information and Statistics Division 1987; Macfarlane et al. 1988). In this case, the gestational ages of babies born within marriage were tabulated according to their father's social class, and births outside marriage were grouped into a single category. An analysis of data for the early 1990s, which extended this to include analyses of low birthweight and preterm birth among births outside marriage by mother's social class, found social class differences in low birthweight but not in preterm birth (Macfarlane and Mugford 2000). A subsequent analysis of social class differences in adverse perinatal outcomes, including low

Table 1.10 Preterm birth by National Statistics Socio-economic classification of father and registration status, babies born in England and Wales, 2008

	PERCENTAGE OF LIVE BIRTHS WITH KNOWN GESTATIONAL AGE (WEEKS)					NUMBER OF LIVE BIRTHS	
						All*	With stated gestational age[†‡]
	Under 24	24–27	28–31	32–36	Under 37		
All	0.11	0.36	0.84	5.94	7.25	708 253	701 041
All born within marriage or jointly registered outside marriage[§]	0.10	0.35	0.82	5.85	7.13	662 850	656 304
National Statistics Socio-economic classification of father's occupation[¶]							
Managerial and professional	0.10	0.27	0.74	5.36	6.47	24 397	24 186
Intermediate	0.12	0.47	0.84	5.98	7.41	12 851	12 745
Routine and manual	0.09	0.40	0.84	6.23	7.55	25 017	24 767
Other[¶]	0.25	0.51	0.99	6.37	8.11	4043	3956
Marital/registration status							
Inside marriage	0.10	0.33	0.76	5.75	6.93	387 729	384 276
Joint registration/same address	0.10	0.34	0.84	5.78	7.07	209 941	207 733
Joint registration/different address	0.16	0.52	1.10	6.73	8.51	65 180	64 295
Sole registration	0.16	0.54	1.14	7.27	9.12	45 403	44 737

*Figures for live births in National Statistics Socio-economic classification groups are a 10% sample coded for father's occupation.
[†]Excludes those with low gestational age inconsistent with birthweight, or gestational age not stated, or not linked to an NN4B record.
[‡]Live births of known gestational age only.
[§]Inside marriage and outside marriage/joint registration only, including cases where father's occupation was not stated.
[¶]For births, father's occupation recorded at birth is used; for deaths, father's occupation recorded at infant death is used.
[¶]Students, occupations inadequately described, occupations not classifiable for other reasons, never worked and long-term unemployed.
(Data from Office for National Statistics Gestation-specific infant mortality.)
6 See data quality issues in published articles (Hilder et al. 2007, Hilder, Moser, Dattani et al. 2008, Moser, Macfarlane, Chow et al, 2007)

birthweight, preterm birth and small for gestational age, in Scotland found that, although differences narrowed during the 1980s, they widened during the 1990s (Fairley and Leyland 2006).

Published analyses of data on preterm birth in England and Wales have used the less detailed three-class version of the National Statistics Socio-economic classes. These data, shown in Table 1.10, also show that preterm birth rates are higher in the less advantaged socio-economic groups, except among births before 24 weeks. They are also tabulated by type of registration and show similarities between the rates for births to married parents and births to parents who are not married but give the same address when registering their baby. In contrast, rates for unmarried parents who give different addresses are similar to those for sole registrations. This highlights the differences within the growing category of births outside marriage.

Ethnic origin and country of birth

Birthweight and gestational age distributions are known to differ between ethnic and racial groups (Parsons et al. 1993;

Macfarlane and Mugford 2000; Gagnon et al. 2009; Urquia et al. 2010).

At the time of writing, ethnic origin is not recorded at birth registration, but service users' self-reported ethnicity should be recorded in national NHS data collection systems. Although mothers' ethnic origins had been recorded on most hospital notes and on some districts' birth notification forms for some years, the way it was recorded and classified varied widely. In the mid-1990s, it was decided that the definitions used in the 1991 census should be used universally (National Health Service, Department of Health 1990a, b). These were superseded by the revised classifications used in the 2001 census and will subsequently be replaced by the categories used in 2011. In some cases, the data are incomplete and of questionable quality. Although data on birthweight and method of delivery, collected through the Maternity HES, have been published, black and Asian groups were aggregated in an attempt to overcome problems with data quality, but this obscures known differences within them (Department of Health 2004).

The 1991 population census was the first in which people were asked to indicate how they described their ethnic origin. The categories used in the question were: white, black–Caribbean, black–African, black–other, Indian, Pakistani, Bangladeshi, Chinese, and any other ethnic group. People descended from more than one ethnic or racial group were asked to tick the one to which they considered they belonged, or to tick the 'any other ethnic group' box and describe their ancestry (Office of Population Censuses and Surveys and General Register Office, Scotland 1989). This classification has been criticised on the grounds that it is more an indicator of skin colour than of cultural and social identity (Ahmad and Sheldon 1992).

These questions were revised for use in the 2001 census, when slightly different questions were asked in each of the countries of the UK. In England and Wales, specific categories for people of mixed ethnic background were added, along with the terms black British and Asian British, while Scotland added black Scottish and Asian Scottish categories. The Office for National Statistics has subsequently revised its categories further for use in the 2011 census, in the light of further criticisms, and added a question about national identity within the UK (Office for National Statistics 2003, 2009). In addition, in 2001 and 2011, questions on religion, previously asked only in Northern Ireland, were added in England, Wales and Scotland, where they focused particularly on religions practised by minority ethnic groups.

The ethnic origins of parents are not recorded at birth and infant death registration in England and Wales but their countries of birth are recorded. Although not a measure of ethnic origin, as many women in some minority ethnic groups having babies in the UK today were themselves born in the UK and some were born in other countries to which their parents migrated, it is an approximate measure of migration status. Table 1.11 gives some insight into the differences in the incidence of low birthweight in 2009. As in other years and in particular in an analysis of data for the years 1983–2000, it was highest among babies with mothers born in Pakistan, India and Bangladesh, and nearly as high among babies whose mothers were born in the Caribbean Commonwealth, East Africa and the 'rest of Africa', which is predominantly West Africa. In contrast, the incidence of very low birthweight was markedly higher among babies whose mothers were born in the Caribbean Commonwealth and the 'rest of Africa' (Collingwood Bakeo 2004). For data about births from 2010 onwards, the Office for National Statistics has adopted a new country of birth classification, which is not tied to membership of the British Commonwealth.

The data items recorded on NHS Numbers for Babies notifications include 'baby's ethnicity'. This is somewhat problematic, given that it should be self-reported, but the linkage of this dataset to birth registration has given the opportunity to compare this with the parents' countries of birth. Further linkage with Maternity HES has now enabled comparison with the mother's ethnic origin (Dattani, Datta-Nemdharry and Macfarlane, 2011 and 2012). Analyses of birthweights of babies reported as being of South Asian ethnicities has found little difference in the mean birthweights of those whose mothers were born in the UK and those born in their countries of origin (Leon and Moser 2010). A further analysis has found similarities between rates of preterm birth of babies of Caribbean ethnicity according to whether their mothers were born in the Caribbean or the UK and that, for babies of African ethnicity, rates were similarly high for those whose mothers were born in Western or Middle Africa compared with those whose mothers were born in other parts of Africa (Datta-Nemdharry et al. 2011). This is consistent with the results of studies in the West Midlands, East London, St Denis in northern Paris and with the high rates seen in black women in the USA (Aveyard et al. 2002; Zeitlin et al. 2004; Macfarlane et al. 2005, Goldenberg et al, 2008).

Mother's age

Rates of low birthweight are highest among babies born to women aged under 20 and to women in their 40s and lowest for mothers aged 25–34, as Table 1.12 shows, and rates of preterm birth show a similar but less marked pattern (Moser 2009). The favourable outcome for women in their early 30s is to some extent a consequence of social class differences in childbearing. Although there is a tendency in the population as a whole, both in the UK and in other developed countries, to defer childbearing, women in less skilled occupations are more likely to have their children in their 20s while women in professional occupations are more likely to delay childbearing until their 30s. Women in their late 30s and 40s are more likely to have multiple births and also more likely to experience fertility problems.

These data illustrate the considerable differences that exist between groups within the population in the incidence of low-birthweight and preterm birth and differences within the low-birthweight and preterm birth ranges. The association between these and differences in mortality and morbidity will be discussed later and in Chapter 3, but it is important to remember when interpreting these data that being classified as low birthweight does not necessarily imply that the baby will have clinical problems, particularly at the upper end of the low-birthweight range. On the other hand, the smaller the baby and the shorter its gestational age, the higher the risk of mortality and morbidity. Reviews of the research on the incidence of preterm birth generally conclude that the mechanisms are still poorly understood but that both adverse social conditions and infection are likely to play a part (Kramer et al. 2001; Wadhwa et al. 2001, Kramer and Hogue 2009). The clinical aspects of preterm birth are discussed in Chapter 3.

Multiple births

In England and Wales, multiple births accounted for just over a quarter of babies born alive in 2007 weighing under 1500 g, as Table 1.13 shows. After declining for many years, the incidence of multiple births, shown in Figure 1.6, started to increase from the mid-1970s onwards. The increase continued through the 1980s, from 10.1 multiple births per 1000 maternities in 1982 to 11.4 in 1989, 14.1 in 1995 and 16.2 in 2009 then fell to 15.4 in 2010. There are no data about multiple birth rates for England and Wales for 1981, as multiplicity was not recorded during this year because of industrial action by local registrars of births and deaths.

Multiple birth rates for England and Wales are compared with those for Scotland and Ireland in Table 1.14. Trends in Scotland were similar to those for England and Wales, although rates were slightly lower in Scotland up to the early 1990s. In Northern Ireland the twinning rate was already higher and did not increase in the latter half of the 1980s, but rose considerably in the early 1990s. The rates reached a similar level by the beginning of the 21st century. Since then, they have remained stable in Northern Ireland, but have continued to rise in England and Wales, Scotland and the Irish Republic.

The triplet and higher order birth rates for England and Wales, shown in Figure 1.7, present a rather more dramatic picture than that for multiple births as a whole. After rising slightly during the 1970s, the proportion of triplet and higher order births more than doubled during the 1980s, rising from 12.2 per 100 000 maternities in 1982 to 28.6 in 1989. After a slight pause it rose again sharply to 45.0 in 1995 and 48.3 in 1998, before starting to fall, reaching 21.3 in 2003 and remaining around that level. Rates for Scotland and Northern Ireland, shown in Table 1.14, followed the same

Table 1.11 Low birthweight by mother's country of birth, England and Wales, 2009

MOTHER'S COUNTRY OF BIRTH	ALL	ALL STATED	UNDER 1500 G	1500–2499 G	UNDER 2500 G	UNDER 1500 G	1500–2499 G	UNDER 2500 G
	Numbers of live births					Percentage of live births with stated birthweight		
All	706 248	701 011	8365	41 983	50 348	1.19	5.99	7.18
UK	532 046	528 274	6155	31 614	37 769	1.17	5.98	7.15
England and Wales*	522 808	519 106	6058	31 092	37 150	1.17	5.99	7.16
Scotland	7024	6967	71	416	487	1.02	5.97	6.99
Northern Ireland	2214	2201	26	106	132	1.18	4.82	6.00
Outside the UK	174 202	172 737	2210	10 369	12 579	1.28	6.00	7.28
Irish Republic	2971	2940	32	141	173	1.09	4.80	5.88
Other European Union	44 128	43 752	429	1982	2411	0.98	4.53	5.51
Rest of Europe	7861	7801	96	310	406	1.23	3.97	5.20
Commonwealth								
Australia, Canada								
and New Zealand	4567	4529	41	200	241	0.91	4.42	5.32
New Commonwealth	69 633	69 047	1070	5482	6552	1.55	7.94	9.49
Asia								
Bangladesh	8452	8373	109	773	882	1.30	9.23	10.53
India	12 499	12 400	182	1208	1390	1.47	9.74	11.21
Pakistan	18 394	18 261	226	1567	1793	1.24	8.58	9.82
East Africa	4040	4004	67	292	359	1.67	7.29	8.97
Southern Africa	4654	4625	45	215	260	0.97	4.65	5.62
Rest of Africa	13 026	12 910	292	831	1123	2.26	6.44	8.70
Far East	1361	1349	9	86	95	0.67	6.38	7.04
Caribbean	3457	3414	96	235	331	2.81	6.88	9.70
Rest of the New Commonwealth	3750	3711	44	275	319	1.19	7.41	8.60
USA	3102	3057	32	138	170	1.05	4.51	5.56
Rest of the world and not stated	41 940	41 611	510	2116	2626	1.23	5.09	6.31

*Because of the small number of stillbirths in 'elsewhere' in the UK, all figures for this group have been combined with England and Wales to protect confidentiality.
(Data from Office for National Statistics, Birth Statistics.)

pattern although the timing differed, while rates in the Irish Republic have remained high.

The rising triplet rate was a common feature in most European countries. By 1990, the rates in Belgium and the Netherlands were the highest in Europe, followed by those in West Germany, Italy and France (Masuy-Stroobant 1996). Despite its reputation for high rates of triplet and higher order births, Australia's rate for 1994, 35.0 per 100 000 maternities, was no higher than some of these (Australian Institute of Health and Welfare National Perinatal Statistics Unit 2003). As Table 1.15 shows, triplet rates were still higher than 0.40 per 100 000 maternities in 2004 in the Netherlands, the Brussels region of Belgium, Denmark, Germany, Spain, Italy and Hungary and very much higher among the small numbers of maternities in Cyprus and Malta (Europeristat 2008).

The rise in the incidence of multiple births in general, and triplet and higher order births in particular, is usually attributed to the

Table 1.12 Low birthweight by mother's age, England and Wales, 2009

MOTHER'S AGE (YEARS)	ALL LIVE BIRTHS	ALL WITH STATED BIRTHWEIGHT	PERCENTAGE OF LIVE BIRTHS WITHBIRTHWEIGHT				
			Under 1000 g	1000–1499 g	1500–1999 g	2000–2499 g	Under 2500 g
All	706 248	701 011	0.5	0.7	1.4	4.6	7.2
<20	43 243	42 919	0.6	0.8	1.6	5.0	7.8
20–24	136 012	135 020	0.5	0.6	1.3	4.8	7.3
25–29	194 129	192 728	0.5	0.6	1.3	4.4	6.8
30–34	191 600	190 179	0.5	0.6	1.4	4.3	6.9
35–39	114 288	113 406	0.6	0.8	1.6	4.6	7.5
40 and over	26 976	26 759	0.6	1.0	2.0	5.6	9.2

(Data from Office for National Statistics 2011, childhood mortality statistics 2009 Table 10.)

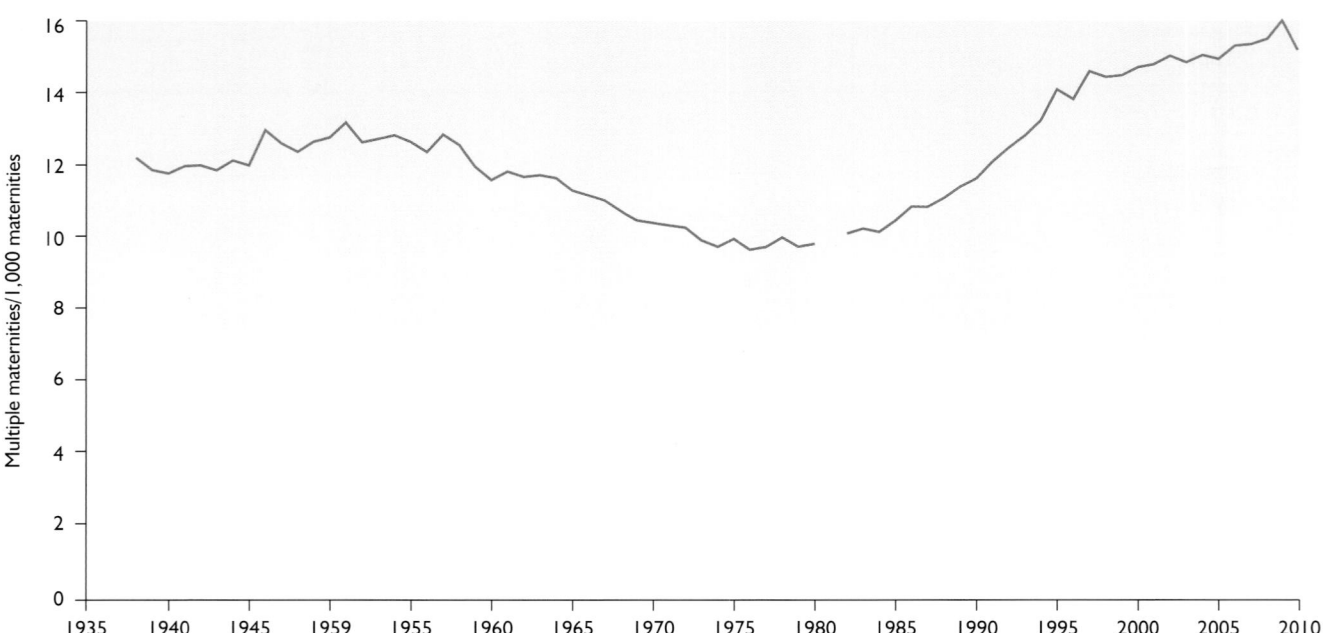

Fig. 1.6 Multiple birth rates, England and Wales, 1938–2010. *(Data from Office for National Statistics, Birth Statistics No data are available for 1981 following industrial action by Registers of Births, Marriages and Deaths.)*

increasing use of drugs for the medical management of subfertility and, since the mid-1980s, to techniques for assisted conception. Unfortunately, there are few data available to quantify their contribution over and above the increase that will have occurred spontaneously as a result of the rising age at childbirth (Blondel and Macfarlane 2003). The National Study of Triplet and Higher-Order Births estimated that 36% of mothers of triplets and 70% of mothers of quadruplet and higher order births born in the years 1980 and 1982–5 had used drugs for the medical management of subfertility (Botting et al. 1990).

The impact of in vitro fertilisation (IVF) was negligible before 1985 (MRC Working Party 1990) but since the 1990s it has become considerable (Human Fertilisation and Embryology Authority 2011). Statistics produced by the Human Fertilisation and Embryology Authority (1994) and its predecessor, the Interim Licensing Authority for Human In Vitro Fertilisation and Embryology (1990), show a clear association between the rise in triplet and higher order births from 1985 onwards and the increasing use of IVF, gamete intrafallopian transfers and associated procedures. Rising rates of multiple births up to the early 1990s in England and Wales coincided with the increasing use of assisted conception and prescriptions for drugs for the medical management of subfertility but the association could not be quantified as it was based solely on routinely collected data (Dunn and Macfarlane 1996). Since then,

Table 1.13 Multiple births as a percentage of all births occurring in 2007, England and Wales

BIRTHWEIGHT (G)	MULTIPLE BIRTHS AS A PERCENTAGE OF		
	Stillbirths	Live births	Infant deaths
Under 1500	10.0	25.4	22.9
1500–1999	9.1	29.7	11.5
2000–2499	6.6	19.5	8.9
Under 2500	9.2	22.5	19.5
2500 and over	1.5	1.4	2.2
All weights	6.7	3.0	13.1

(Data from Office for National Statistics. Birth cohort tables for infant deaths)

prescribing data have been even more difficult to interpret; for example, a decline in the late 1990s may have been a shift to the private sector, about which no statistics are collected routinely, rather than a real decline in use.

The decrease in the triplet rate in the UK followed guidance from the Royal College of Obstetricians and Gynaecologists in 2000 that no more than two embryos should be replaced in IVF procedures involving women under 40. The Human Fertilisation and Embryology Authority included this in its Code of Practice, launched in January 2004. The overall rate of multiple births continued to rise, however, with just under a quarter of births following assisted conception in the UK being multiple (Human Fertilisation and Embryology Authority 2011).

The high rates of multiple births shown in Table 1.14 and in countries where IVF is practised widely led to trials of implantation of just one embryo. A meta-analysis of research on single-embryo transfer concluded that, compared with double-embryo transfer, elective single-embryo transfer resulted in a higher chance of a term singleton live birth, provided that the strategy included an additional cycle with a frozen embryo if the first cycle was unsuccessful (McLernon et al. 2010). It also found that the multiple pregnancy rate after single-embryo transfer was comparable to that in spontaneous pregnancies (McLernon et al. 2010). In the light of this, in

Table 1.14 Multiple birth rates, England and Wales, Scotland and Ireland, 1971–5 to 2006–10

	ENGLAND AND WALES	SCOTLAND	NORTHERN IRELAND	REPUBLIC OF IRELAND
Twins per 1000 maternities				
1971–5	9.9	10	10.7	12.3
1976–80	9.6	9.4	10.1	11.2
1981–5	10.1*	9.9	10.6	10.7
1986–90	10.9	11	10.7	11.5[†]
1991–5	12.6	12.3	12.2	12.4[†]
1996–2000	13.9	13.8	13.8	13.7[†]
2001–5	14.6	15.0	14.5	15.1[†]
2006–10	15.4	15.7	14.6	16.1[‡]
Triplet and higher order births per 1000 maternities				
1971–5	0.11	0.08	0.08	0.12
1976–80	0.13	0.09	0.14	0.13
1981–5	0.14*	0.10	0.12	0.11
1986–90	0.25	0.19	0.14	0.15[†]
1991–5	0.37	0.31	0.31	0.25[†]
1996–2000	0.45	0.36	0.33	0.44[†]
2001–5	0.27	0.19	0.38	0.35[†]
2006–10	0.23	0.19	0.18	0.36[†]

*Excluding 1981.
[†]Based on a revised methodology to take better account of multiple births, including stillbirths.
[‡]2001 only.
(Data from Office for National Statistics; General Register Offices for Scotland and Northern Ireland; and Central Statistics Office, Republic of Ireland, Vital statistics.)

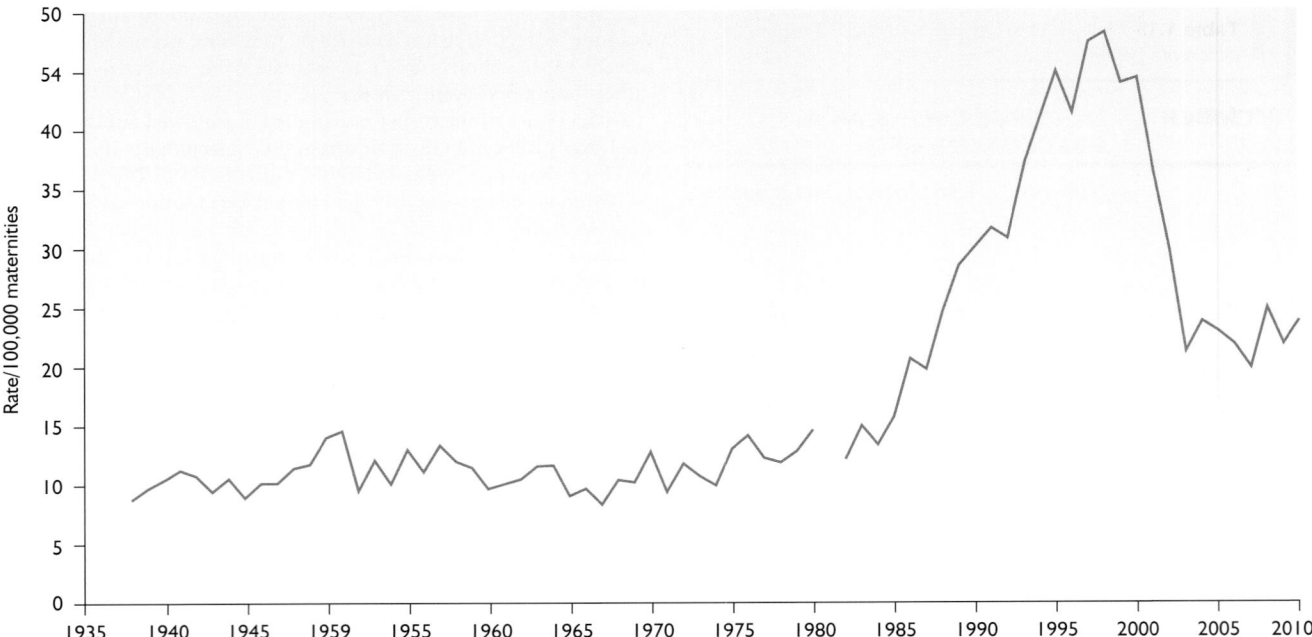

Fig. 1.7 Triplet and higher order births, England and Wales, 1938–2010. *(Data from Office for National Statistics, Birth Statistics. No data are available for 1981 following industrial action by Registers of Births, Marriages and Deaths.)*

January 2009 the Human Fertilisation and Embryology Authority introduced a policy to promote single-embryo transfer and minimise the risk of multiple births from IVF treatment. It started to set a maximum multiple birth rate that clinics should not exceed, with the aim of lowering it each year to attain a multiple target of 10% multiple births. It set up a dedicated system to monitor progress towards this target, with reports published on its website (Human Fertilisation and Embryology Authority 2011). It could be that these policies contributed to the fall in the multiple birth rate in England and Wales in 2010, but no definitive conclusions can be drawn from data for a single year.

Although the HFEA collects data from clinics about all relevant procedures undertaken in the UK, irrespective of whether the women concerned are resident or give birth in the UK, it points out that it does not collect data about the growing numbers of women who go abroad for IVF and then return to the UK to give birth (Human Fertilisation and Embryology Authority 2010).

Mortality in the first year of life

Definitions

- Stillbirth rate: number of stillbirths per 1000 live births and stillbirths.
- Infant mortality rate: number of deaths at age under 1 year per 1000 live births.
- Perinatal mortality rate: number of stillbirths plus number of deaths at age under 7 days per 1000 live births and stillbirths.
- Early neonatal mortality rate: number of deaths at age under 7 days per 1000 live births.
- Neonatal mortality rate: number of deaths at age under 28 days per 1000 live births.
- Postneonatal mortality rate: number of deaths at age 28 days and over, but under 1 year, per 1000 live births.

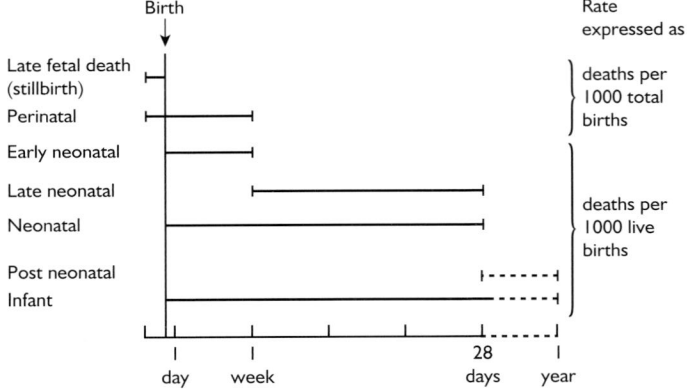

Fig. 1.8 Definition of stillbirth and infant mortality rates.

Trends in mortality rates

The classic indicators of the outcome of pregnancy are stillbirth rates and death rates during the first year of life, defined above and illustrated in Figure 1.8. Trends since 1905 in neonatal and postneonatal mortality rates for England and Wales are illustrated in Figure 1.9. Although the series of infant mortality rates reaches back to the mid-19th century, the current subdivision of the first year of life into the first month and deaths at age of at least 1 month but under 1 year started in 1905. The publication of more detailed analyses started at a time when public concern about infant mortality, stemming from the unfitness of many potential recruits for the Boer War, led to a request to the General Register Office for more detailed statistics (Tatham 1907).

Whereas neonatal mortality rates have decreased relatively steadily during the 20th century, postneonatal mortality, which was initially higher, shows a different pattern. It decreased very rapidly in

Table 1.15 Multiple birth rates in European Union member states and Norway participating in the Europeristat European Perinatal indicators project

EU MEMBER STATE	NUMBER OF WOMEN WITH STATED PLURALITY	RATE PER 1000 MATERNITIES		
		Twins	Triplet and higher order births	All
Belgium				
Flanders	59 956	15.76	0.23	16.00
Brussels	16 009	16.37	0.56	16.93
Czech Republic	96 098	18.64	0.20	18.83
Denmark	63 383	22.48	0.57	23.05
Germany	636 844	17.66	0.51	18.17
Estonia	13 879	12.03	0.07	12.10
Ireland	61 438	15.06	0.33	15.38
Greece*				
Spain	447 784	17.22	0.59	17.82
France	762 378	15.82	0.28	16.10
Italy	534 568	11.50	0.49	11.99
Cyprus	8050	23.48	1.49	24.97
Latvia	20 256	11.45	0.10	11.55
Lithuania	29 306	10.82	0.17	10.99
Luxembourg	5405	13.51	0.37	13.88
Hungary	93 913	16.72	0.69	17.41
Malta	3838	13.03	1.56	14.59
Netherlands	178 774	20.03	0.43	20.46
Austria	77 979	15.39	0.32	15.71
Poland	354 385	10.99	0.19	11.18
Portugal	108 258	13.34	0.38	13.72
Slovenia	17 629	17.64	0.17	17.81
Slovak Republic	51 968	12.10	0.10	12.20
Finland	56 878	14.93	0.28	15.21
Sweden	99 073	13.74	0.15	13.89
UK	709 317	14.74	0.24	14.98
England and Wales	633 728	14.78	0.24	15.02
Scotland	53 502	14.15	0.15	14.30
Northern Ireland	22 087	14.94	0.32	15.26
Norway	56 243	18.67	0.27	18.94

*Greece provided no data on multiple births.
(Data from Europeristat (2008), Table C7.)

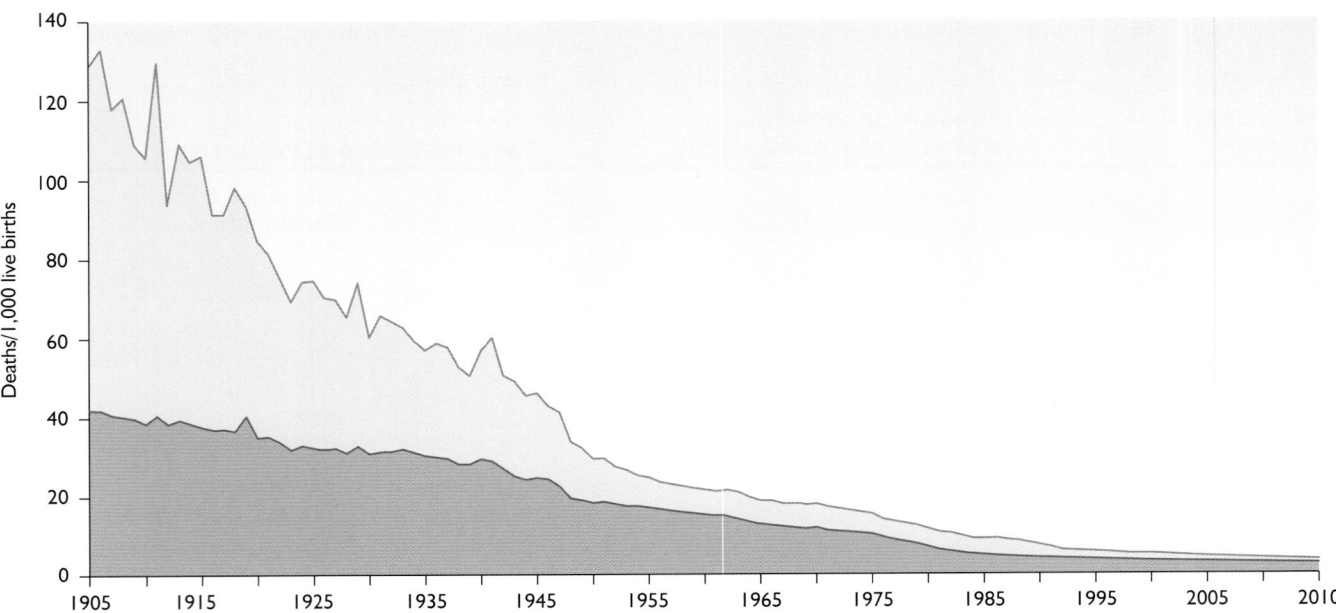

Fig. 1.9 Infant mortality, England and Wales, 1905–2010. *(Data from Office for National Statistics, Mortality Statistics)*

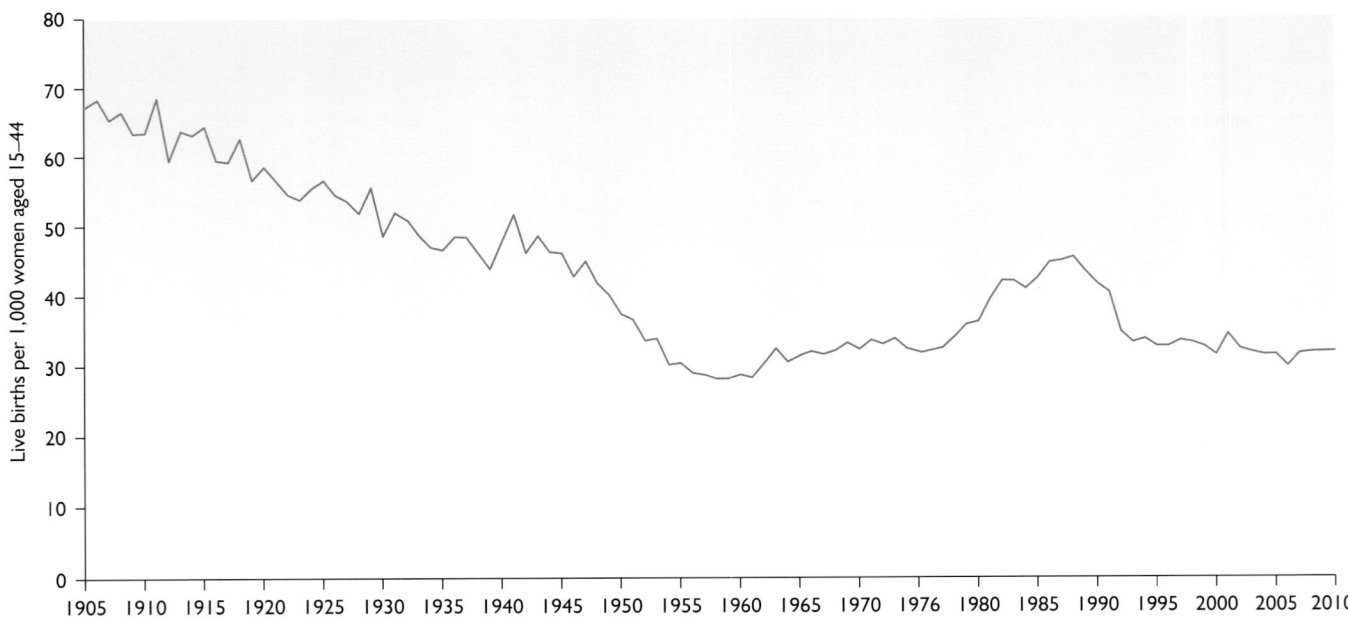

Fig. 1.10 Postneonatal deaths as a percentage of infant deaths, England and Wales, 1905–2010. *(Data from Office for National Statistics, Mortality Statistics.)*

the first half of the century with the decline in fatality from communicable diseases. It showed signs of levelling off between the mid-1970s and mid-1980s. After virtually halving in the late 1980s and early 1990s, the rate levelled off again, before starting to fall more slowly, accounting for about a third of infant deaths, as Figure 1.10 shows.

More recent trends in infant mortality are shown in Figure 1.11, which shows early and late neonatal mortality rates separately. The impact of the change in legislation about stillbirth registration on published stillbirth and perinatal mortality rates is illustrated in

Figure 1.12. The published rates, shown with a dashed line from 1992 onwards, increased. Rates from which stillbirths at 24–27 weeks of gestation have been excluded are plotted as a continuation of the solid line. These showed an apparent halt in the downward trend, with a rise from 2001 to 2004, but subsequently started falling again.

Neonatal, postneonatal and infant mortality rates for England, Wales, Scotland and Ireland in the years since 1970 are shown in Table 1.16. These show continuing small declines in neonatal mortality through the 1990s. As in England and Wales, there was a

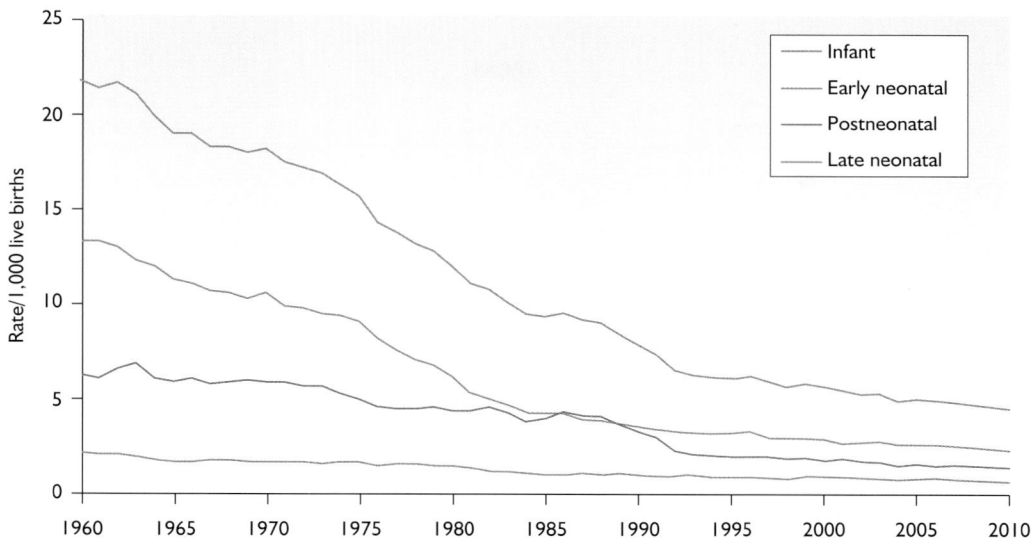

Fig. 1.11 Infant mortality, England and Wales, 1960–2010. *(Data from Office for National Statistics, Mortality Statistics.)*

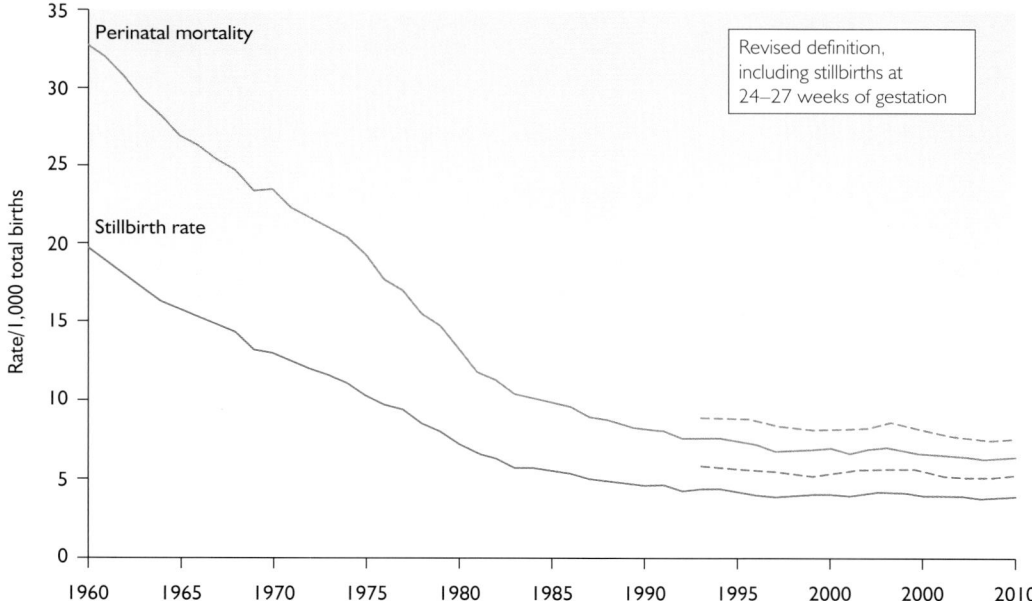

Fig. 1.12 Stillbirth and prenatal mortality rates, England and Wales 1960–2009. *(Data from Office for National Statistics, Mortality Statistics.)*

tendency for the postneonatal mortality rate to level off in the 1980s in each of the other countries, followed by a fall in the late 1980s and from the 1990s onwards. The trends in Scotland, Wales and both parts of Ireland are less clear than those in England and Wales, as they are based on smaller numbers of deaths. As a whole, however, infant mortality continues to decline in most westernised countries, although many European countries have small numbers of deaths, because their populations are small, making trends less apparent.

To what extent do trends in infant mortality in the UK reflect changes in the relative size of high-risk groups, and to what extent has mortality fallen within these groups? Figure 1.3 shows no increase in the incidence of low birthweight in England and Wales between the mid-1950s and mid-1980s, but a rise up to the turn of the century, followed by a fall. Table 1.3 shows a similar picture,

but with an increase in the reported incidence of babies in the lowest birthweight groups, who have the highest mortality. As suggested earlier, the change in definition of stillbirth may have increased the tendency to register very preterm live births, rather than regarding them as miscarriages.

Within birthweight groups, however, trends in mortality look different. A very marked fall between 1963 and 1986 in mortality in the first week after live birth among babies weighing 2500 g and under, followed by a much less dramatic fall since the late 1980s, can be seen in Figure 1.13. A different pattern can be seen in Figure 1.14, which shows a more recent and very marked decline from the late 1970s onwards in mortality rates among babies weighing 1000 g and under, and, after definitions changed in the mid-1980s, among babies weighing under 1000 g. No data about gestational age were available at a national level through most of

Table 1.16 Neonatal, postneonatal and infant mortality rates since 1970, England and Wales, Scotland and Ireland

	ENGLAND	WALES	ENGLAND AND WALES	SCOTLAND	NORTHERN IRELAND	IRISH REPUBLIC
Neonatal mortality						
1970	12.3	12.8	12.3	12.8	15.8	12.8
1975	10.7	10.3	10.7	11.8	13.2	12.0
1980	7.6	7.9	7.7	7.8	8.0	6.7
1985	5.3	5.8	5.4	5.5	5.6	5.3
1990	4.6	3.9	4.6	4.4	4.0	4.8
1995	4.2	3.9	4.2	4.0	5.5	4.8
2000	3.9	3.5	3.9	4.0	3.8	4.3
2001	3.6	3.5	3.6	3.8	4.4	4.0
2002	3.6	3.1	3.6	3.2	3.4	3.6
2003	3.6	3.1	3.6	3.4	4.6	3.8
2004	3.5	3.1	3.5	3.1	3.7	3.4
2005	3.4	2.9	3.4	3.5	5.5	2.7
2006	3.5	2.8	3.5	3.1	4.6	2.7
2007	3.3	3.4	3.3	3.3	3.4	2.2
2008	3.2	3.0	3.2	2.8	3.7	2.7
2009	3.2	3.1	3.1	2.8	4.0	
2010	3.0	2.8	3.0	2.6	4.8	
Postneonatal mortality						
1970	5.9	6.4	5.9	6.9	7.1	6.7
1975	5.3	4.2	5.0	5.4	7.2	5.6
1980	4.4	3.5	4.4	4.3	7.6	3.8
1985	3.9	4.0	4.0	3.9	4.0	3.6
1990	3.3	3.0	3.3	3.3	3.5	3.4
1995	2.0	2.0	2.0	2.2	1.6	1.6
2000	1.7	1.8	1.7	1.8	1.2	1.9
2001	1.8	1.9	1.9	1.7	1.6	1.7
2002	1.7	1.6	1.7	2.1	1.2	1.5
2003	1.7	1.2	1.7	1.7	1.8	1.5
2004	1.6	1.8	1.6	1.9	1.7	1.3
2005	1.6	1.2	1.6	1.7	1.5	1.1
2006	1.5	1.3	1.5	1.4	1.1	1.2
2007	1.4	1.9	1.5	1.5	2.0	1.0
2008	1.4	1.0	1.4	1.4	1.0	1.1
2009	1.4	1.6	1.4	1.2	1.2	
2010	1.4	1.2	1.4	1.2	1.2	

Table 1.16 Continued

	ENGLAND	WALES	ENGLAND AND WALES	SCOTLAND	NORTHERN IRELAND	IRISH REPUBLIC
Infant mortality						
1970	18.2	18.7	18.2	19.6	22.9	19.5
1975	15.7	14.5	15.7	17.2	20.4	17.5
1980	12.0	11.4	12.0	12.1	15.6	10.3
1985	9.2	9.8	9.4	9.4	9.6	8.8
1990	7.9	6.6	7.9	7.7	7.4	8.2
1995	6.1	5.8	6.1	6.2	7.1	6.4
2000	5.6	5.3	5.6	5.7	5.0	6.2
2001	5.4	5.4	5.4	5.5	6.0	5.7
2002	5.3	5.3	4.7	5.3	4.6	5.0
2003	5.3	4.3	5.3	5.1	6.5	5.3
2004	5.1	4.9	5.0	4.9	5.4	4.6
2005	5.0	4.1	5.0	5.2	7.0	3.8
2006	5.0	4.1	5.0	4.5	5.7	3.9
2007	4.8	5.3	4.7	4.7	5.5	3.2
2008	4.7	4.1	4.6	4.2	4.7	3.8
2009	4.6	4.8	4.5	4.0	5.3	
2010	4.3	4.0	4.3	3.7	5.8	

(Data from Office for National Statistics, General Register Offices for Scotland and Northern Ireland and Central Statistics Office, Ireland.)

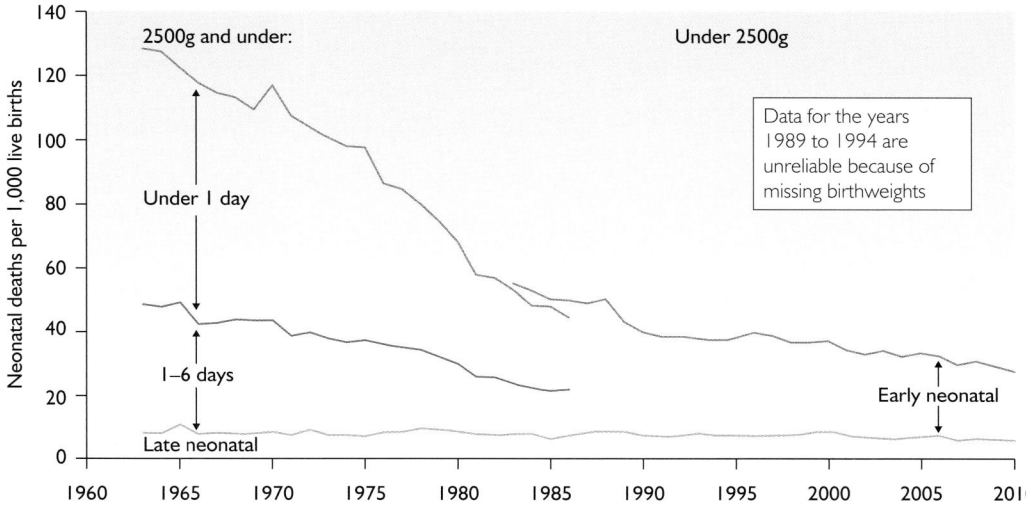

Fig. 1.13 Neonatal mortality among low-birthweight babies, England and Wales, 1963–2010. *(Data from DHSS, LHS 27/1 low birthweight returns and Office for National Statistics; Mortality Statistics. Birth counts, Data updated from Tables A3.5.1 and A3.5.2 Macfarlane, Mugfird, Henderson et al. 2000.)*

this era, but the data for 2005–8, shown in Table 1.17, indicate that mortality is persistently high among babies born before 24 weeks of gestation. Figure 1.17 uses data for 2008 plotted on logarithmic scale to show how neonatal and infant mortality vary by week of gestational age.

The fuller data in Table 1.18 show that neonatal mortality continued to fall in England and Wales from the mid-1980s until the early 1990s, but from the mid-1990s onwards the decline appeared to be confined to babies weighing between 1000 and 2499 g. Trends for the larger babies are far from clear. Table 1.18 also illustrates the

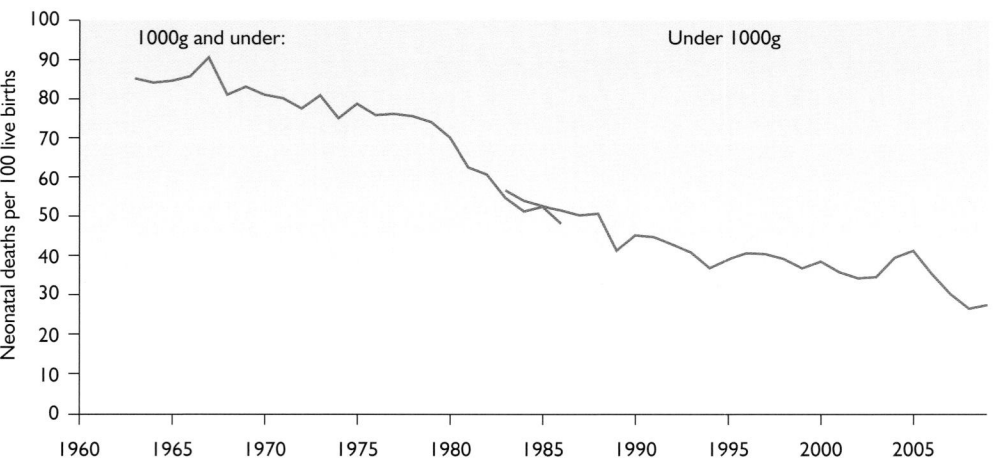

Fig. 1.14 Neonatal mortality among extremely low-birthweight babies, England and Wales, 1963–2009. *(Data from DHSS LHS 27/1 low birthweight returns and Office for National Statistics Mortality Statistic.)*

Table 1.17 Neonatal and infant mortality rates by gestational age, England and Wales, births in 2005–8

YEAR OF BIRTH	ALL BIRTHS	ALL WITH STATED GESTATIONAL AGE	GESTATIONAL AGE (WEEKS)				
			Under 24	24–27	28–31	32–36	37 and over
Neonatal mortality rates per 1000 live births							
2005	3.5	3.4	902.6	236.9	36.6	6.1	0.9
2006	3.4	3.3	848.9	232.4	37.5	5.9	0.9
2007	3.2	3.1	846.9	215.9	36.8	6.3	0.9
2008	3.1	3.0	823.1	199.4	37.8	6.0	0.8
Infant mortality rates per 1000 live births							
2005	5.0	4.9	915.0	298.2	52.2	10.6	1.8
2006	4.9	4.8	883.2	288.5	51.3	9.4	1.9
2007	4.7	4.6	884.4	279.1	50.1	10.1	1.9
2008	4.5	4.4	871.0	270.4	49.2	9.7	1.7
(Data from Office for National Statistics gestation specific infant childhood mortality statistics.)							

impact of the increase in 1989 of the numbers of birth records with missing birthweights. Between 1983 and 1988, when very few birthweights were missing, mortality in this group was very high, suggesting that the babies might not have been weighed because they were very ill or immature.

Between 1989 and 1994 mortality in this group was lower than before, but still markedly higher than average. Thus, mortality in the groups under 2500 g is likely to have been artificially depleted over this period. In 1995, when the proportion of babies with missing birthweights was very much smaller, mortality among them rose, but not to its former level. This means that caution is needed when interpreting the trends in mortality among low-birthweight babies in the late 1980s and early 1990s, shown in Figures 1.13 and 1.14 and Table 1.18. Similar caution is needed in interpreting rates for 2007 onwards, in the light of the recent changes in data flows and increases in the extent of missing birthweights.

Table 1.19 shows neonatal mortality rates by birthweight for singleton babies without lethal anomalies born in Scotland over the years 1985–2002. These are tabulated by gestational age in Table 1.20. Neonatal mortality rates tended to decline, although there was considerable fluctuation because of the smaller numbers of babies involved.

Postneonatal mortality rates for England and Wales, given in Table 1.18, showed no sign of a decline over the years 1983–8, particularly for babies with birthweights under 2500 g. Apart from a possible increase in the 2000–2499-g group, the picture was again one of fluctuation, the extent of which is not surprising, given the relatively small numbers of deaths in each group. This was followed by a sharp decline between 1989 and 1992 in all groups, except for babies weighing under 1000 g. This pattern persisted at a lower level from the mid-1990s onwards.

Putting the neonatal and postneonatal mortality rates together to look at infant mortality as a whole, it can be seen that rates tended

Table 1.18 Neonatal, postneonatal and infant mortality by year of birth and birthweight, England and Wales, births in 1985–2008

YEAR OF BIRTH	ALL WEIGHTS	TOTAL STATED	UNDER 1000 G	1000–1499 G	UNDER 1500 G	1500–1999 G	2000–2499 G	UNDER 2500 G	2500 G AND OVER	NOT STATED
Neonatal mortality rates per 1000 live births										
1985	5.3	5.1	525.5	135	262.0	37.9	12.5	50.3	1.8	156.7
1990	4.4	3.9	444.3	88.4	215	25.1	6.4	39.5	1.3	17.3
1995	4.1	4.0	390.1	63.8	188	17.5	6.5	37.7	1.4	28.4
1996	4.0	3.9	407.3	59.7	198.0	14.9	5.8	39.9	1.1	50.1
1997	3.9	3.8	404.8	60.2	192.6	17.6	5.6	38.8	1.0	60.9
1998	3.8	3.7	389.1	52.6	185.1	15.4	5.3	36.6	1.0	79.3
1999	3.9	3.8	368.8	55.8	180.6	15.8	4.7	36.8	1.1	36.1
2000	3.8	3.7	383.9	46.5	181.9	16.7	5.3	36.7	1.0	51.0
2001	3.6	3.5	360.6	47.4	173.2	14.2	4.8	34.6	1.0	56.8
2002	3.5	3.4	340.6	47.5	165.0	14.0	5.0	32.8	1.0	64.9
2003	3.6	3.5	347.4	46.4	168.9	16.3	4.5	34.3	1.0	53.3
2004	3.4	3.3	333.2	44.3	159.7	13.2	5.2	32.1	1.0	56.5
2005	3.5	3.4	358.1	41.4	168.1	12.7	5.1	33.8	0.9	35.2
2006	3.4	3.3	352.3	40.7	164.1	13.1	4.4	32.4	0.9	20.5
2007	3.3	3.1	300.1	40.0	145.3	14.0	5.9	29.8	1.0	20.2
Postneonatal mortality rates per 1000 live births										
1985	4.1	4.1	53.1	33.2	39.7	19.8	9.9	15.7	3.2	10.4
1990	3.1	3.1	59.6	31.8	41.7	17.1	7.0	13.9	2.3	3.8
1995	2.0	2.0	62.2	20.4	36.3	9.2	5.1	10.9	1.3	6.3
1996	1.9	1.9	48.9	19.3	31.1	9.1	5.9	10.7	1.2	3.3
1997	1.8	1.8	51.9	18.6	31.4	8.7	4.8	10.0	1.2	4.5
1998	1.9	1.9	58.1	18.3	34.0	7.8	5.1	10.3	1.2	2.4
1999	1.8	1.8	55.9	18.7	33.6	8.7	3.9	9.9	1.1	1.6
2000	1.8	1.8	50.6	16.0	29.9	10.5	4.5	9.9	1.1	2.9

Table 1.18 Continued

YEAR OF BIRTH	ALL WEIGHTS	TOTAL STATED	UNDER 1000 G	1000–1499 G	UNDER 1500 G	1500–1999 G	2000–2499 G	UNDER 2500 G	2500 G AND OVER	NOT STATED
2001	1.7	1.7	57.3	12.7	30.6	8.5	4.5	9.6	1.0	1.1
2002	1.8	1.8	59.9	20.1	36.1	8.7	3.9	10.1	1.1	3.3
2003	1.6	1.6	59.8	11.9	31.4	9.5	4.2	9.8	1.0	3.3
2004	1.6	1.6	60.8	16.0	33.9	8.4	3.8	9.7	0.9	3.2
2005	1.5	1.5	54.7	16.4	31.7	8.2	3.9	9.4	0.9	1.3
2006	1.5	1.5	54.8	15.5	31.0	7.0	3.8	8.9	0.9	1.9
2007	1.5	1.5	56.6	14.3	31.4	7.0	3.4	8.6	0.9	3.0
Infant mortality rates per 1000 live births										
1985	9.4	9.2	578.6	168	302	57.6	22.4	66.0	5.0	167.1
1990	7.6	7.0	503.9	120	257	42.2	13.4	53.3	3.6	21.1
1995	6.1	6.0	452.2	84.2	224	26.7	11.5	48.6	2.6	34.7
1996	5.9	5.8	456.2	79.0	229.0	24.0	11.7	50.6	2.3	53.3
1997	5.7	5.6	456.7	78.8	224.0	26.3	10.3	48.8	2.1	65.4
1998	5.7	5.6	447.2	71.0	219.1	23.1	10.4	47.0	2.2	81.7
1999	5.6	5.5	424.8	74.6	214.2	24.5	8.6	46.7	2.2	37.7
2000	5.6	5.5	434.5	62.5	211.8	27.2	9.8	46.6	2.2	53.9
2001	5.3	5.2	417.9	60.2	203.9	22.7	9.3	44.2	2.0	57.9
2002	5.3	5.2	400.5	67.6	201.0	22.6	9.0	42.9	2.0	68.2
2003	5.2	5.2	407.1	58.3	200.3	25.8	8.6	44.1	1.9	56.6
2004	5.0	4.9	394.0	60.3	193.6	21.6	9.0	41.8	1.9	59.7
2005	5.0	4.9	412.8	57.8	199.8	21.0	9.0	43.2	1.8	36.5
2006	4.9	4.8	407.2	56.2	195.1	20.1	8.2	41.4	1.8	22.4
2007	4.7	4.5	356.7	54.3	176.7	21.0	9.3	38.3	1.9	23.2

(Data from Birth counts, Table A 3.5.2, Office for National Statistics mortality statistics, Series DH3 Table 26 and birth cohort infant mortality.)

Table 1.19 Birthweight-specific neonatal mortality rates for singleton babies without lethal anomalies per 1000 live births, Scotland 1994–2010

	BIRTHWEIGHT					
	Under 1500 g	**1500–2499 g**	**2500–3499 g**	**3500–4499 g**	**4500 g and over**	**Total**
1994	176.4	3.6	0.6	0.4	–	2.2
1995	175.5	1.8	0.9	0.3	1.9	2.0
1996	200.0	4.1	0.5	0.6	–	2.2
1997	155.3	2.6	0.7	0.5	–	1.9
1998	159.3	4.1	0.9	0.4	0.0	2.0
1999	171.4	2.3	0.6	0.2	0.9	2.0
2000	182.3	5.6	0.9	0.3	1.0	2.7
2001	178.6	2.6	0.8	0.7	1.0	2.3
2002	145.2	6.1	0.3	0.5	1.0	2.1
2003	139.6	2.5	0.6	0.2	1.0	1.8
2004	129.5	3.5	0.7	0.5	1.8	2.0
2005	147.4	4.6	1.0	0.1	0.0	2.1
2006	125.3	3.3	0.8	0.4	0.0	1.8
2007	175.1	4.2	0.7	0.3	0.0	2.1
2008	109.0	2.9	0.9	0.2	1.5	1.7
2009	115.7	2.4	0.6	0.6	0.0	1.6
2010[p]	113.5	2.5	0.4	0.3	0.8	1.6
	134.4	2.1	0.5	0.4		

[p]Provisional SMR02.
(Data from Information and Statistics Division Scotland, SMR02 and Scottish Perinatal and Infant Mortality and Morbidity Survey.)

to decline up until 1985 and then started to level off. After a decline over the period 1989–93, rates appeared to level off again before declining very slowly from the late 1990s onwards.

It is usual to present birthweight-specific mortality rates in 500-g groups, and mortality rates for babies born in 2007 in singleton and multiple births are compared in Figure 1.15, but there is considerable variation within these groups, particularly at the bottom end of the scale. A fuller picture could be seen of the 'crossover' of rates in an earlier special analysis in which infant mortality rates for the years 1983–7 combined were analysed in 100-g groups (Alberman and Botting 1991). It was necessary to combine 5 years' data to have sufficient numbers of deaths in each group to eliminate the effects of random variation.

Social class differences

Innumerable studies over the years have shown social class gradients in stillbirth and infant mortality rates for the Registrar General's social classes (Macfarlane 1996b; Drever and Whitehead 1997; Macfarlane and Mugford 2000; Macfarlane et al. 2004; Macintosh et al. 2006), as did routine data published annually (Oakley et al. 2009). Neonatal and postneonatal mortality rates for England and Wales, analysed by the National Statistics Socio-economic class of the baby's father, are shown in Figure 1.17. The analysis includes

both births within marriage and those outside marriage registered jointly by both parents, who account for the majority of the rising proportion of births outside marriage. The very high mortality rates among babies registered by the mother on her own are also shown. The data are from the infant mortality-linked file of the Office for National Statistics (Office for National Statistics 2011b).

The most striking feature is that, although there are marked differences between groups, using the current classification does not produce a straightforward gradient. Unlike the Registrar General's classification, which was based on crude assessments of the status of individual occupations, the new classification is based more firmly in sociological theory. In particular, group 4 consists of people working on their own account, who enjoy comparatively low mortality and good health, despite their lack of social status. The explanation advanced is that this results from the amount of autonomy they experience (Rose and O'Reilly 1998). When the groups are amalgamated to form the three-class version of the classification, as has been done in the revised version of the Department of Health's infant mortality target set under the previous UK government, this distinction disappears (Rowan 2003). Another notable feature in Figure 1.17 is the difference between neonatal and postneonatal mortality rates, with the latter showing much wider differences between classes. Deaths attributed to the sudden infant death syndrome show particularly marked social class differences, which

Table 1.20 Gestation-specific neonatal mortality rates for singleton babies without lethal anomalies per 1000 live births, Scotland 1985–2010

	GESTATIONAL AGE (WEEKS)					
	Under 24	24–27	28–31	32–36	37 and over	Total
1985	*	620.4	114.3	6.7	0.6	3.1
1986	*	491.2	94.9	7.8	0.7	2.6
1987	*	477.3	117.6	7.1	0.7	2.8
1988	*	466.1	49.6	7.6	0.5	2.3
1989	*	448.0	94.3	4.2	0.6	2.5
1990	*	392.2	83.9	6.4	0.6	2.7
1991	*	455.1	73.6	5.8	0.6	2.5
1992	*	425.0	44.6	5.4	0.8	2.6
1993	*	349.4	70.4	4.4	0.6	2.1
1994	*	410.1	40.1	3.6	0.5	2.2
1995	*	420.6	56.0	2.9	0.6	2.0
1996	*	433.3	47.9	4.3	0.5	2.2
1997	*	336.1	30.6	2.1	0.5	1.9
1998	*	313.6	28.0	3.6	0.6	2.0
1999	*	345.9	38.6	2.2	0.4	2.0
2000	*	311.6	57.6	6.0	0.6	2.7
2001	*	308.3	36.8	3.4	0.7	2.3
2002	*	359.2	33.5	3.1	0.5	2.1
2003	*	245.8	42.3	2.9	0.3	1.8
2004	*	248.0	36.4	2.6	0.5	2.0
2005	*	279.4	34.5	3.0	0.6	2.1
2006	*	237.4	20.3	3.1	0.6	1.8
2007	*	263.2	57.4	2.4	0.5	2.1
2008	*	162.8	18.2	3.3	0.6	1.7
2009	*	213.9	25.5	2.1	0.6	1.6
2010ᵖ	*	205.6 251.0	25.4 36.6	1.1	0.4	1.6

*Rates not calculated as SMR2 data are incomplete.
ᵖProvisional SMR02.
(Data from Information and Statistics Division Scotland, Scottish Perinatal and Infant Mortality and Morbidity Survey. Data for 1985–93 derived from Birth counts, Table A3.5.5. Macfarlane, Mugford, Henderson et al. 2000)

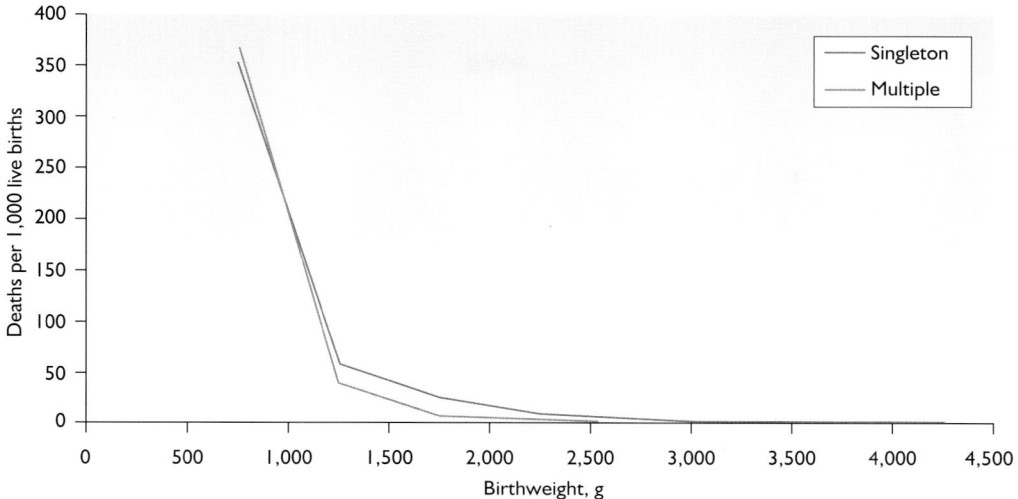

Fig. 1.15 Infant mortality rates for babies from singleton and multiple births born in 2007 in England and Wales. *(Data from Office for National statistics, birth cohort infant mortality.)*

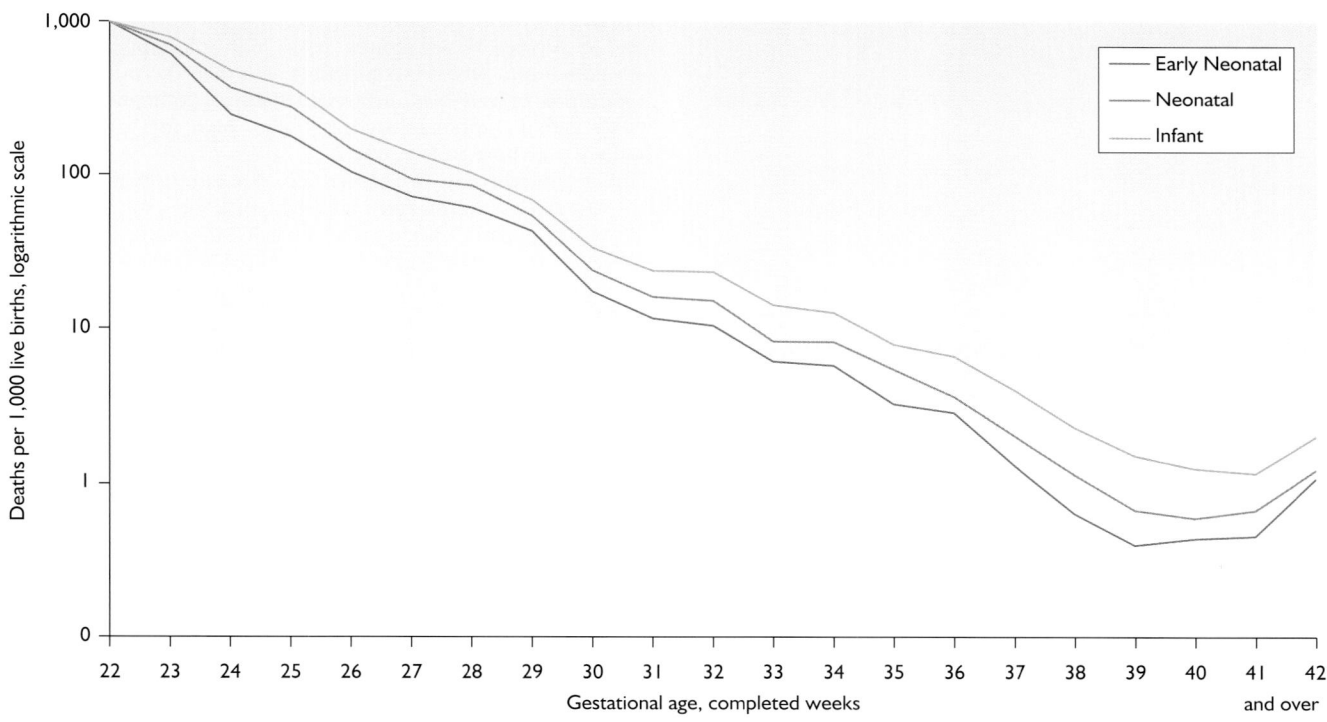

Fig. 1.16 Infant mortality by gestational age, babies born in 2008, England and Wales. *(Data from Office for National Statistics gestation specific infant mortality, unpublished data.)*

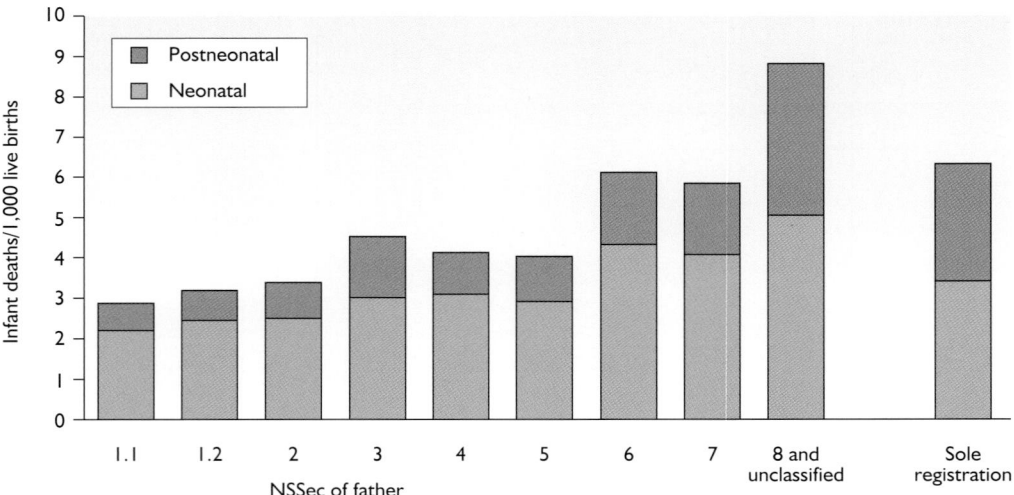

Fig. 1.17 Infant mortality by National Statistics Socio-economic (NSSec) classification of father and sole registrations, England and Wales, 2010. *(Data from Office for National Statistics, Infant and perinatal mortality in England and Wales by social and biological factors, 2010.)*

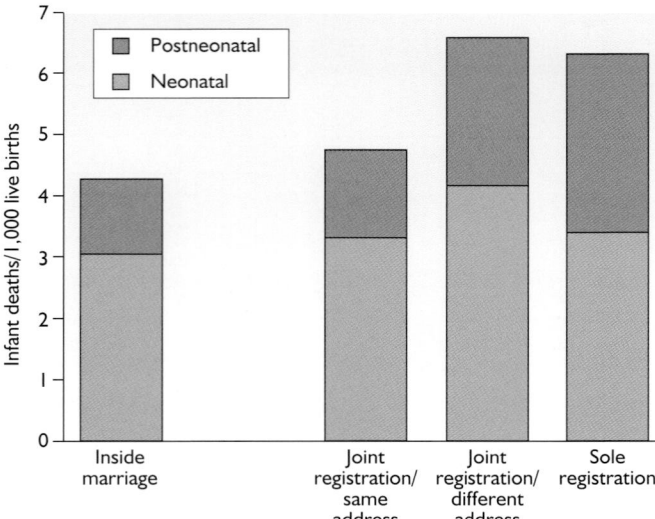

Fig. 1.18 Infant mortality by marital and registration status, England and Wales, 2101. *(Data from Office for National Statistics, Infant and perinatal mortality in England and Wales by social and biological factors, 2010.)*

contribute substantially to the social class differences in postneonatal mortality (Macfarlane and Mugford 2000).

Like low-birthweight and preterm birth, infant mortality varies between babies whose parents gave the same address on their baby's birth registration and those who did not and were therefore unlikely to be living together, as Figure 1.18 shows.

Ethnic origin and country of birth

Neonatal and postneonatal mortality rates for selected mothers' countries of birth for the years 2007–9 combined are shown in Figure 1.19 and tabulated more fully in Table 1.21. As in other years, mortality rates for babies whose mothers were born in Pakistan are markedly higher than those with mothers born elsewhere in the Indian subcontinent, which are much closer to the overall level. This pattern is similar to that apparent in the 1990s, with raised

mortality rates among babies whose mothers were born in Pakistan being associated with congenital anomalies and mortality being relatively high compared with other groups right across the birthweight range (Balarajan and Raleigh 1990). As in earlier years, mortality rates were also relatively high for babies born to women born in the Caribbean Commonwealth and the largely west African 'rest of Africa'. These groups have high mortality associated with immaturity, which is compatible with their exceptionally high proportions of very-low-birthweight babies (Collingwood Bakeo 2004). Perhaps anomalously, rates were high for babies whose mothers were born in East Africa.

Infant mortality rates by babies' recorded ethnicity are shown in Table 1.22. Here again, rates are high for babies stated to be of Pakistani origin and among those of black Caribbean origin. Babies of black African origin had infant mortality rates which were lower, but above those for other groups, reflecting the heterogeneity of this group.

Mother's age and parity

Both neonatal and postneonatal mortality rates are highest for babies born to women aged under 20 or in their 40s, as Table 1.23 shows. In the past, rates were lowest for women in their 20s, but they are now lowest for women in their early 30s. This reflects the extent to which women in the more advantaged socio-economic groups are delaying childbearing until their 30s. Although, at any age, the incidence of clinical problems and consequently mortality rates is highest among women having their first birth, there is a dearth of data on this subject for the UK as, under the Population (Statistics) Acts, in England and Wales, parity has been recorded at birth registration only for births within marriage (Office for National Statistics 2002) successive attempts to change this eventually succeeded and from April 2012, parity, defined as the total number of previous live and still births was recorded for all births registered in England and Wales.

Multiple births

Multiple births accounted for nearly a quarter of infant deaths of babies born in 2007 weighing under 1500 g at birth and well over a tenth of all infant deaths among babies born in that year, as Table

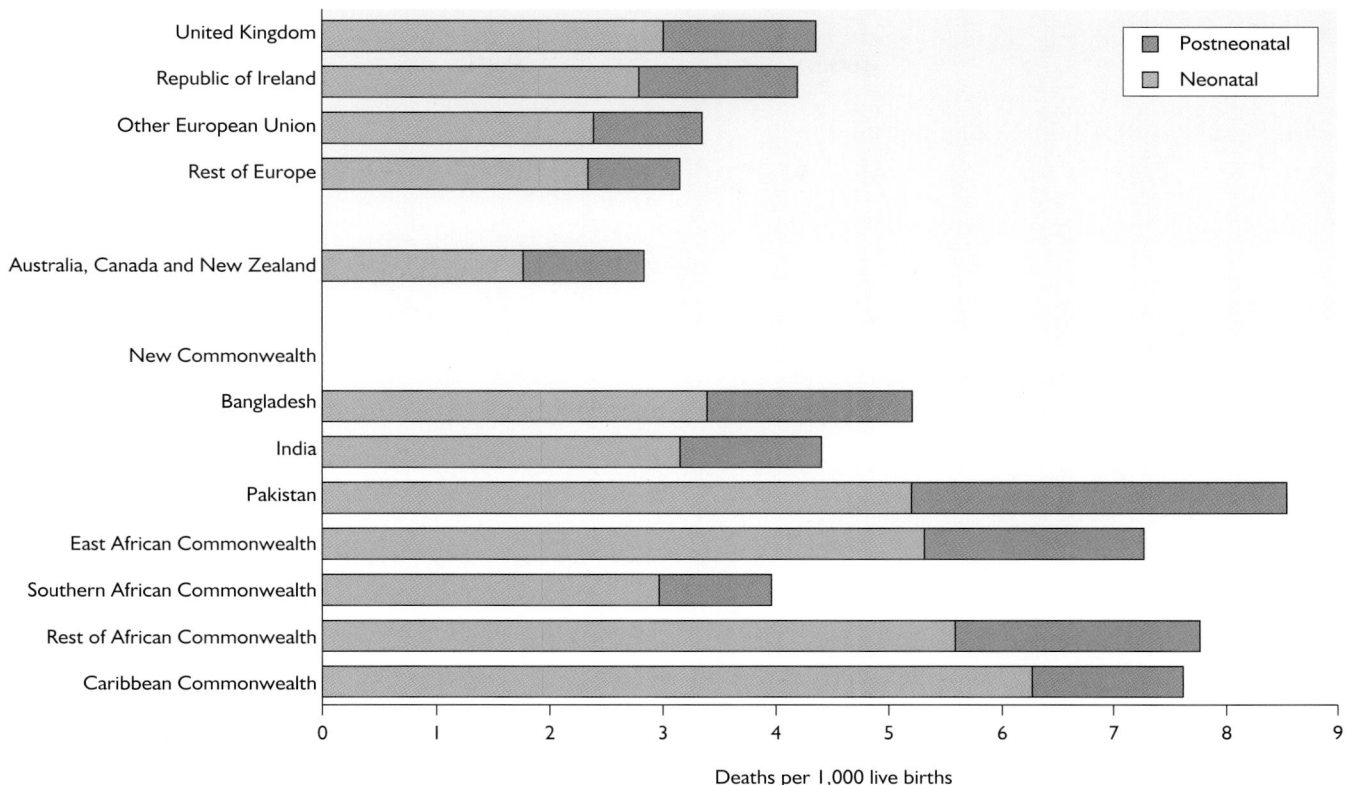

Fig. 1.19 Infant mortality by mother's country of birth, England and Wales, 2007–9. *(Data from Office for National Statistics, Childhood Mortality Statistics.)*

1.13 shows. Figure 1.15 gives an indication of how the relationship between mortality rates for singleton and multiple births changes with birthweight within the category below 1500 g. Overall infant mortality rates are higher for multiple than for singleton births. Not surprisingly, mortality is highest among babies born in triplet and higher order births. This can be seen in Table 1.24, in which infant mortality rates for babies born in multiple births in the years 1975–2007 are compared with those for singletons. Mortality among twins and among triplet and higher order births fell markedly in the 1970s, then fluctuated around a similar level in the 1980s.

Despite year-to-year fluctuations because of the small numbers involved, there was a marked decrease from the early 1990s onwards. No data are available about the extent to which the increasing survival of triplet and higher order births is associated with morbidity in the survivors. These births create problems not only for the staff of neonatal units but for parents faced with the problems of caring for three or more babies of the same age. These have considerable implications for families and for the health and social services so the downturn in the triplet rate has welcome consequences (Botting et al. 1990).

Geographical variations and international comparisons in mortality

Variations from district to district in perinatal and infant mortality rates have always received considerable attention from the press and Parliament (House of Commons Social Services Committee 1988; National Audit Office Maternity Services 1990). Politicians have sometimes assumed that these variations simply reflect differences

in the quality of maternity care. As a result, they have tended to imply that districts and countries with the highest rates simply have to copy the practices of those with the lowest rates and the problem will be solved almost instantly. As a consequence of this, crude perinatal and infant mortality rates and their components have frequently featured over the years in government performance indicators and targets, both as proxy measures of the health of the population and as proxy measures of the quality of healthcare in an area. In recent years, they have been chosen to be two of the key outcome indicators for the NHS in England (Department of Health 2011). Closer inspection of these data shows that these interpretations are oversimplified and that the differences arise from a number of factors.

First, there is the question of which babies to register as births and deaths and which to categorise as miscarriages, which go unrecorded. Decisions about this are likely to reflect cultural, religious and social factors, which may vary from place to place.

Next, it is necessary to consider random variation. Neonatal and infant mortality rates for administrative districts within the UK, such as local authorities in England, are now based on such small numbers of events that what appear to be quite large differences from area to area, or from year to year within an area, are actually no larger than would be expected by chance, as Figure 1.20 shows. In the 1980s, OPCS published perinatal and infant mortality rates for NHS districts in England and Wales based on 3 years' aggregated data in addition to rates for the most recent year. The plethora of boundary changes in the 1990s made it difficult to go on aggregating data. Finally, the Office for National Statistics stopped putting data for NHS areas in the public domain and only NHS staff have access to them, although data for local authority areas are still published.

Table 1.21 Infant mortality by mother's country of birth, England and Wales, 2007–9 combined

MOTHER'S COUNTRY OF BIRTH	LIVE BIRTHS	NEONATAL DEATHS	POSTNEONATAL DEATHS	NEONATAL	POSTNEONATAL	INFANT
	Numbers			Deaths per 1000 live births		
All	2 104 972	6599	2935	3.1	1.4	4.5
UK	1 599 555	4834	2154	3.0	1.3	4.4
Outside the UK	505 417	1765	781	3.5	1.5	5.0
Irish Republic	9267	26	13	2.8	1.4	4.2
Other European Union	118 626	285	114	2.4	1.0	3.4
Rest of Europe	23 376	55	19	2.4	0.8	3.2
Commonwealth						
Australia, Canada and New Zealand	14 039	25	15	1.8	1.1	2.8
New Commonwealth	208 912	924	424	4.4	2.0	6.5
Asia						
Bangladesh	25 856	88	47	3.4	1.8	5.2
India	36 964	117	45	3.2	1.2	4.4
Pakistan	54 868	286	182	5.2	3.3	8.5
East Africa	12 389	66	24	5.3	1.9	7.3
Southern Africa	14 088	42	14	3.0	1.0	4.0
Rest of Africa	38 779	217	84	5.6	2.2	7.8
Far East	4147	*	*	*	*	*
Caribbean	10 512	66	14	6.3	1.3	7.6
Rest of the New Commonwealth	11 309	*	*	*	*	*
USA	9442	27	12	2.9	1.3	4.1
Rest of the world and not stated	121 755	423	184	3.5	1.5	5.0

(Data from Office for National Statistics mortality statistics, Series DH3 and childhood mortality statistics.)

Table 1.22 Infant mortality by baby's ethnicity, England and Wales, births in 2006–8 combined

BABY'S ETHNICITY		LIVE BIRTHS	NEONATAL DEATHS	POSTNEONATAL DEATHS	NEONATAL	POSTNEONATAL	INFANT
		Numbers			Deaths per 1000 live births		
All*		2 066 838	6742	2998	3.3	1.5	4.7
Asian, Asian British	Bangladeshi	27 462	101	56	3.7	2.0	5.7
	Indian	53 494	183	73	3.4	1.4	4.8
	Pakistani	78 955	470	291	6.0	3.7	9.6
Black, black British	African	67 379	366	141	5.4	2.1	7.5
	Caribbean	22 213	136	63	6.1	2.8	9.0
White	White British	1 320 292	3796	1682	2.9	1.3	4.1
	White other	130 792	307	134	2.3	1.0	3.4
All others†		175 142	628	281	3.6	1.6	5.2
Not stated		190 595	736	276	3.9	1.4	5.3

*Information on ethnic group is not available for the 514 births that could not be linked to an NN4B record.
†Chinese, other Asian, other black, other, and all mixed groups.
(Data from Office for National Statistics Gestation specific Mortality Statistics.)

Table 1.23 Infant mortality by mother's age, England and Wales, 2009

MOTHER'S AGE (YEARS)	LIVE BIRTHS	NEONATAL DEATHS	POSTNEONATAL DEATHS	NEONATAL	POSTNEONATAL	INFANT
	Numbers			Deaths per 1000 live births		
All	706 248	2177	961	3.1	1.4	4.4
Under 20	43 243	157	100	3.6	2.3	5.9
20–24	136 012	452	244	3.3	1.8	5.1
25–29	194 129	591	235	3.0	1.2	4.3
30–34	191 600	528	223	2.8	1.2	3.9
35–39	114 288	345	107	3.0	0.9	4.0
40 and over	26 976	104	52	3.9	1.9	5.8

(Data from Office for National Statistics childhood mortality statistics, 2009, Table 10. Office for National Statistics, 2011)

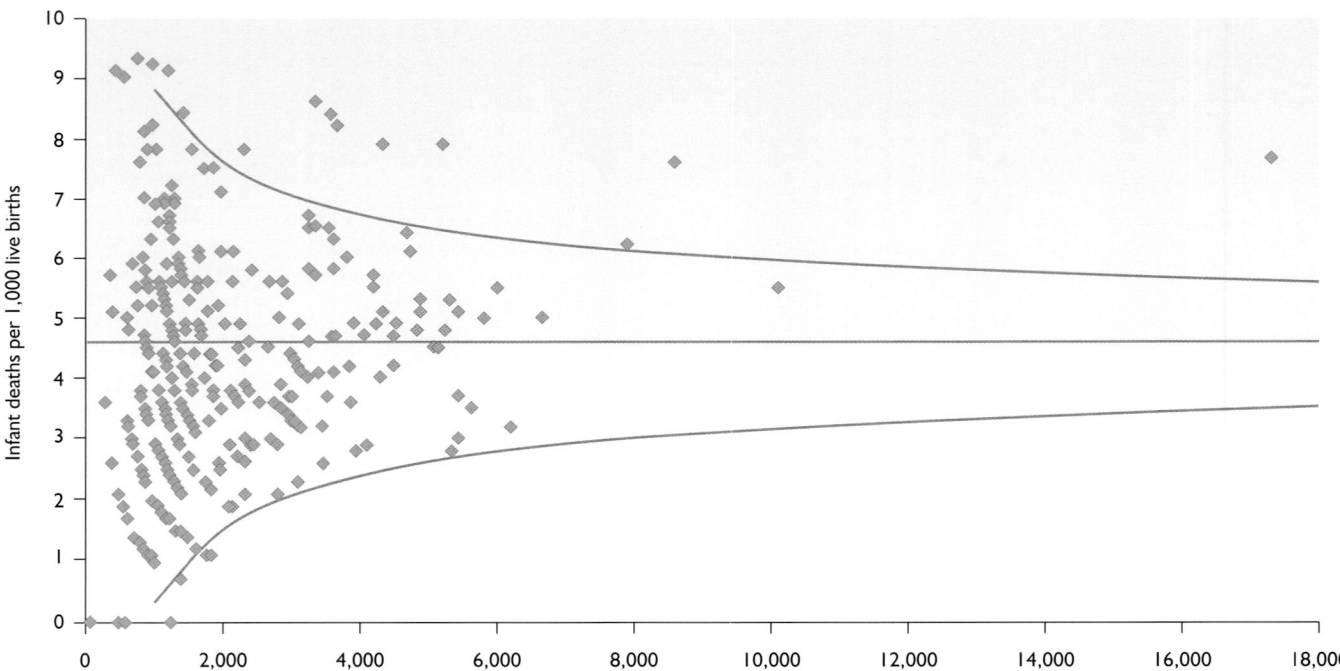

Fig. 1.20 Infant mortality rate by local authority, with 95% control limits for the overall rate based on numbers of live births, England, 2009. Data from the Office for National Statistics published by the National Centre for Health Outcomes Development.

The data shown in Figure 1.20 are therefore based on data for local authorities for a single year (Information Centre for Health and Social Care 2011c). This shows the infant mortality rate for each local authority in England in 2009 plotted against the number of live births to residents in this year. The horizontal line is the rate for England. The curved lines are its 95% control limits for the relevant numbers of live births. It can be seen that in some of the smaller authorities the rates differed considerably from that for England, without going outside the 95% limits. In these instances, the difference between the authority's rate and that for England is no greater than would be expected by chance.

Random variation should also be taken into account when making comparisons between countries, especially when some of them have small populations. Table 1.25 shows neonatal mortality rates for countries participating in the Europeristat project, together with 95% confidence intervals (Buitendijk et al. 2003). These show that even the differences between crude mortality rates are by no means as clear-cut as is commonly assumed and underline the extent to which some countries' rates are based on small numbers of events.

Returning to England and Wales, a special analysis for the years 1983–5 found that the districts whose mortality rates fell below the

Table 1.24 Infant mortality rates for singleton and multiple births by year of birth, England and Wales, 1975–2008

YEAR OF BIRTH	SINGLETON		TWINS		TRIPLETS AND ABOVE	
	Number	Rate	Number	Rate	Number	Rate
1975	8438	14.3	824	71.8	56	249.3
1976	7459	13.0	665	61.8	42	169.4
1977	7697	12.7	586	55.3	26	133.3
1978	7172	12.2	648	56.9	52	248.8
1979	7395	11.8	621	52.3	41	167.3
1980	7057	11.0	583	47.4	43	154.7
1981	NA		NA		NA	
1982	6089	9.9	496	40.8	19	82.6
1983	5786	9.4	492	39.9	21	75.8
1984	5318	8.5	492	39.6	35	138.9
1985	5642	8.8	504	38.3	25	79.4
1986	5508	8.5	611	44.7	38	92.5
1987	5573	8.4	574	40.6	46	113.0
1988	5384	7.9	593	40.4	52	101.2
1989	5065	7.5	562	37.6	58	98.6
1990	4740	6.9	565	36.1	45	71.9
1991	4168	6.1	531	33.0	67	101.4
1992	3858	5.7	473	28.8	49	77.3
1993	3604	5.5	481	29.6	55	75.1
1994	3444	5.3	494	29.8	51	64.4
1995	3399	5.4	493	28.7	66	77.0
1996	3324	5.3	485	28.6	44	55.1
1997	3213	5.1	409	23.3	55	61.8
1998	3134	5.1	426	24.7	50	56.1
1999	3010	5.0	500	27.2	38	47.7
2000	2951	5.0	392	23.4	44	55.8
2001	2686	4.7	417	24.9	30	47.2
2002	2731	4.7	395	23.1	22	43.4
2003	2822	4.7	439	24.3	23	62.2
2004	2786	4.5	398	21.6	26	59.2
2005	2785	4.4	435	23.5	24	55.9
2006	2828	4.4	429	21.7	34	78.9
2007	2843	4.2	407	19.9	20	49.1
2008	2832	4.1	422	20.0	28	54.8

(Data from Office for National Statistics Mortality Statistics, Series DH3, Table 25 and Birth cohort tables for infant deaths (2007 and 2008 cohorts), Table 2.)

Table 1.25 Neonatal mortality rates in countries participating in the Europeristat project, 2004

COUNTRY/ REGION	LIVE BIRTHS	NEONATAL DEATH	NEONATAL MORTALITY RATE PER 1000 LIVE BIRTHS	95% CONFIDENCE INTERVAL	
		Numbers		Lower	Upper
Austria	78 934	215	2.7	2.4	3.1
Belgium					
Brussels	16 200	51	3.4	2.3	4.0
Flanders	60 672	146	2.4	2.0	2.8
Cyprus	8 309	13	1.6	0.7	2.4
Czech Republic	97 671	224	2.3	2.0	2.6
Denmark	64 521	230	3.6	3.1	4.0
Estonia	13 990	59	4.2	3.1	5.3
Finland	57 569	141	2.4	2.0	2.9
France	767 816	1968	2.6	2.5	2.7
Germany	705 622	1892	2.7	2.6	2.8
Greece	104 355	282	2.7	2.4	3.0
Hungary	95 137	423	4.4	4.0	4.9
Ireland	62 066	NA	NA	NA	NA
Italy	539 066	1526	2.8	2.7	3.0
Latvia	20 355	116	5.7	4.7	6.7
Lithuania	29 480	136	4.6	3.8	5.4
Luxembourg	5 469	11	2.0	0.8	3.2
Malta	3 887	17	4.4	2.3	6.4
Netherlands	181 006	631	3.5	3.2	3.8
Norway	57 111	118	2.1	1.7	2.4
Poland	356 697	1731	4.9	4.6	5.1
Portugal	109 356	280	2.6	2.3	2.9
Slovak Republic	52 388	134	2.6	2.1	3.0
Slovenia	17 846	47	2.6	1.9	3.4
Spain	454 591	1199	2.6	2.5	2.8
Sweden	100 158	210	2.1	1.8	2.4
UK					
England and Wales	639 721	2185	3.4	3.3	3.6
Northern Ireland	22 362	66	3.0	2.2	3.7
Scotland	52 911	161	3.0	2.6	3.5

Ireland provided data on early neonatal death.
(Data from Mohangoo et al. (2009).)

lower 95% confidence limit tended to be those with a high proportion of fathers in professional occupations and a low proportion of mothers born in the 'new Commonwealth' or Pakistan (Botting and Macfarlane 1990). Most analyses showed a high correlation between perinatal mortality rates and the proportion of low-weight births.

This study showed that, when mortality was analysed within birth-weight groups, different districts had high and low rates.

These analyses lent support to earlier proposals that birthweight-specific mortality rates were a better proxy measure of the quality of services than crude mortality rates. These had also proposed that multiple births and deaths attributed to congenital anomalies should be excluded. Now that, as a result of both decline in natural incidence and the introduction of screening programmes, mortality attributed to central nervous system anomalies has declined to a much lower level, its inclusion is no longer such a critical factor. In any case, it would be more helpful to use birthweight-specific mortality rates as health service indicators or outcome indicators than to continue the present practice of using crude rates, as successive governments persist in doing. It is also a principle to consider when looking at trends over time and differences between countries.

The extent to which differences in the incidence and reporting of low birthweight can affect international comparisons of infant mortality rates is illustrated in Figure 1.21, which is based on data from the Europeristat project referred to earlier. It shows the contribution of preterm and very preterm births to neonatal deaths in 2004 in the participating countries which had data about gestational age (Europeristat 2008). Because of these differences, the World Health Organization has recommended that babies with gestational age below 22 weeks and birthweight below 500 g should be excluded from comparisons between countries (World Health Organization 1992). Even when a common cut-off is applied, however, birthweight and gestational age-specific mortality vary markedly between countries (Europeristat 2008).

Classification of clinical causes of death

In publications based on death registration, information about causes of death is usually classified to a single underlying cause using the *International Classification of Diseases*, which is revised approximately every 10 years by the World Health Organization. Since the mid-1990s, the 10th revision (ICD-10) has been widely used for most purposes (World Health Organization 1992). The exception is stillbirth and death registration data. Use of ICD-10 for this purpose started in 2000 in Scotland and in 2001 in England, Wales and Northern Ireland. The ICD is designed primarily for use in circumstances in which only limited amounts of clinical information, such as that given on death certificates, is available.

In the perinatal field, other classifications have been developed for use by people with access to the more detailed clinical information found in case notes and pathologists' reports. Perhaps the best known is the classification first developed in Aberdeen in the 1940s by Sir Dugald Baird (Baird and Wyper 1941). This was revised in the early 1980s for use in stillbirth and neonatal mortality surveys in Scotland and the northern region of England, and has separate classifications for conditions in mothers (Cole et al. 1986) and babies (Hey et al. 1986).

A further classification, designed by a pathologist, Jonathan Wigglesworth, is based on externally observable features, supplemented by information from the clinical history (Wigglesworth 1980). A modified version, produced for the International Collaborative Effort on Birthweight, Plurality, Perinatal and Infant Mortality, was designed for use by people who are further removed from the clinical details, and is therefore based on the underlying cause of death coded using the ICD (Cole et al. 1989). It also extended the classification to cover conditions associated with death in the postneonatal period. OPCS used this as a basis for a classification it developed for use on the new form of stillbirth and neonatal death certificate introduced in 1986 (Alberman et al. 1994). These certificates have separate spaces to list conditions in the mother and the baby and other factors relating to the death. The system was further developed for classifying stillbirths (Alberman et al. 1997).

Since then, the classification has been used routinely by the Office for National Statistics in its published tabulations of cause of death. It was revised for use with ICD-10 and extended to postneonatal mortality rates (Dattani and Rowan 2002). It is illustrated in Table 1.26, which shows stillbirth and infant mortality rates for 2009. As described in Chapter 2, there have subsequently been developments in the way the Wigglesworth classification is used to classify information from clinical case notes.

Confidential enquiries

As a result of public concern about levels of perinatal and infant mortality in the late 1970s, many special regional and local surveys and enquiries were set up. These varied in their format. Some were largely restricted to reviews of case notes, whereas others involved interviews with bereaved parents. Some took the form of confidential enquiries, based on the model of the Confidential Enquiries into Maternal Deaths. Some of these initiatives were for a single year or a limited period (Enkin and Chalmers 1980). Others, notably those in Scotland and in the former Northern and South East Thames regions of England, had been in existence for some years.

The rise in infant mortality in England and Wales in 1986 prompted a further enquiry into perinatal, neonatal and infant mortality by the backbench House of Commons Social Services Committee (1988), as it was then called. This recommended 'a targeted programme to reduce perinatal and infant mortality rates, particularly in poorer families where rates are still unnecessarily high'. In addition, it said: 'We recommend that all regions introduce a regular system of confidential inquiries into all unexplained infant deaths and report to the Department of Health on a regular basis. We also recommend that regions and the Department of Health set up a system for monitoring the results of such inquiries and making the lessons learned available to all health districts.'

In its reply, published in 1989, the government announced that it would be setting up a Confidential Enquiry into Stillbirths and Infant Deaths, and the Chief Medical Officer was setting up a working group to consider what form it might take (Department of Health 1989). Secondly, it acknowledged that many regions already conducted epidemiological surveys of stillbirths and neonatal deaths and it had asked the NHS Management Executive to ensure that all regions were doing them by April 1991. Instead of a targeted programme to reduce infant mortality, it stated that: 'Targets need to be set to improve performance' (Department of Health 1989). The Chief Medical Officer's working group reported in 1990 (Department of Health 1990). It recommended a national enquiry, with a regional and district reporting structure, into subsets of individual late fetal losses, stillbirths and infant deaths.

The Confidential Enquiry into Stillbirths and Deaths in Infancy (CESDI) was set up in 1992, with a budget of over £2 million per year for England (Horam 1997), Wales and Northern Ireland to conduct its own enquiries on the same lines, and the data for all three countries are combined. Scotland has been conducting its own enquiries over a much longer period. As the name suggests, the enquiry's brief was to collect information on all late fetal losses at 20–23 weeks of gestation and all stillbirths and deaths in the first year of life, and to try to establish ways in which these deaths might be prevented. It was also to establish panels in each former NHS region to perform enquiries into a designated subset of the deaths.

One of its first priorities was 'sudden unexpected deaths in infancy', a category which went wider than the 'sudden infant death syndrome'. These were the focus of its 1994 report (Confidential Enquiry into Stillbirths and Deaths in Infancy, 1996) and of two papers in the *British Medical Journal* on smoking and sleeping position (Blair et al. 1996a, 1996b). These distracted attention from the

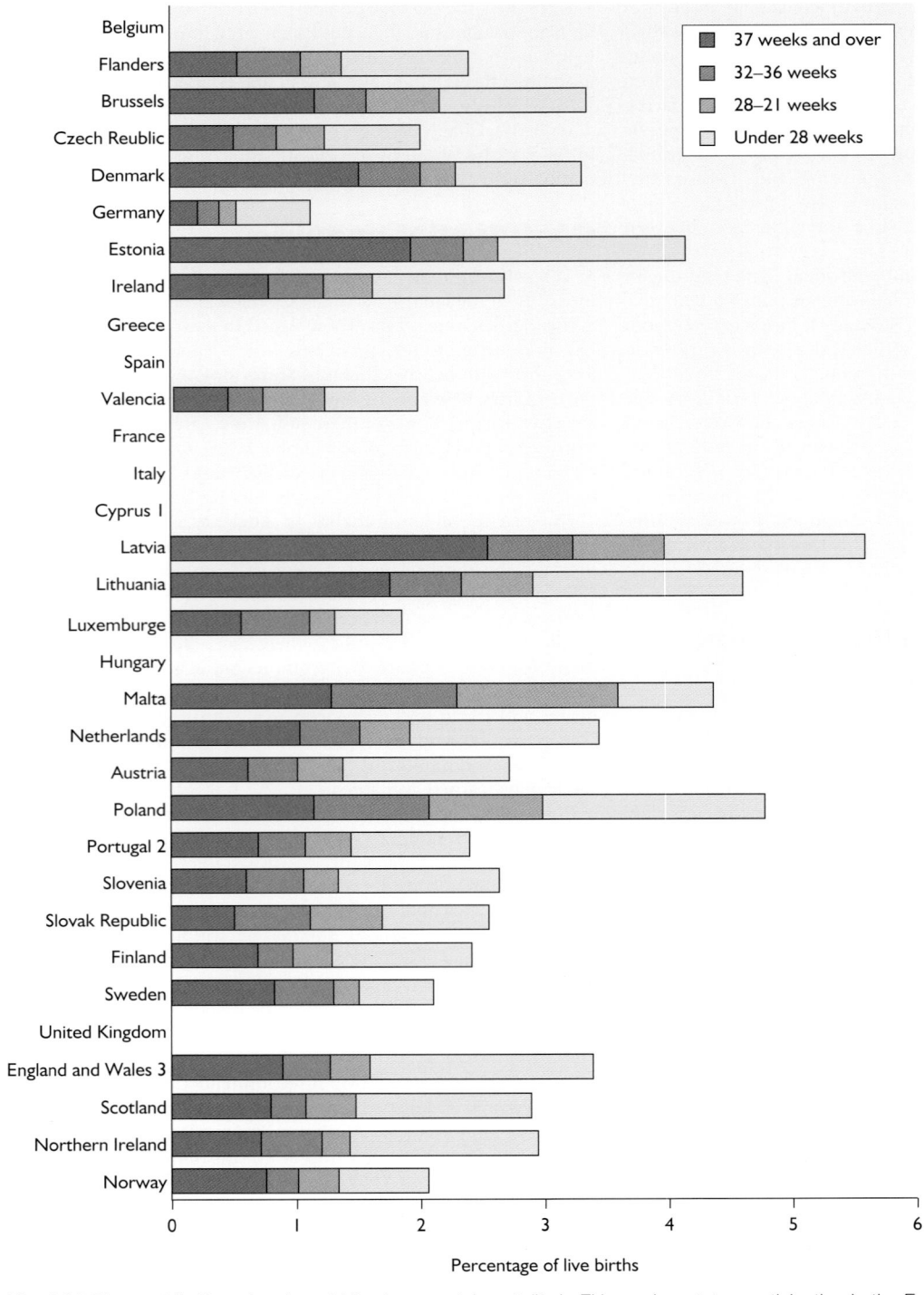

Fig. 1.21 The contribution of preterm births to neonatal mortality in EU member states participating in the Europeristat project. *(Data from Europeristat 2008.)*

fuller data published in the CESDI report, which showed that a high proportion of the babies who died were in very deprived circumstances (Confidential Enquiry into Stillbirths and Deaths in Infancy 1996; Logan et al. 1996; Macfarlane 1996a).

CESDI's other early priority was intrapartum-related deaths of normally formed mature babies. These were the subject of confidential enquiries from 1993 to 1995, the initial results of which

were published in CESDI's report for 1995 (Confidential Enquiry into Stillbirths and Deaths in Infancy 1996, 1997). In 1996 and 1997 the deaths of a random sample of immature babies were the subject of confidential enquiries (Confidential Enquiry into Stillbirths and Deaths in Infancy 1996, 1997). After that, enquiries have focused on large babies, babies born at 27 or 28 weeks of pregnancy, the outcome of diabetic pregnancies (Macintosh et al.

Table 1.26 Stillbirths and infant deaths by Office for National Statistics cause group, England and Wales, 2009

	LIVE BIRTHS	STILLBIRTHS	NEONATAL	POSTNEONATAL	INFANT	STILLBIRTHS	NEONATAL	POSTNEONATAL	INFANT
	Numbers					Rates*			
All causes	706 248	3688	2177	961	3138	5.19	3.08	1.36	4.44
Congenital anomalies		543	606	370	976	0.76	0.86	0.52	1.38
Antepartum infections		31	59	16	75	0.04	0.08	0.02	0.11
Immaturity-related conditions		–	1193	216	1409	–	1.69	0.31	2.00
Asphyxia, anoxia or trauma (Antepartum)		101	201	6	207	0.14	0.28	0.01	0.29
External conditions		10	3	31	34	0.01	0.00	0.04	0.05
Infections		–	36	85	121	–	0.05	0.12	0.17
Other specific conditions		218	17	17	34	0.31	0.02	0.02	0.05
Asphyxia, anoxia or trauma (Intrapartum)		844	–	–	–	1.19	–	–	–
Remaining antepartum deaths		1813	–	–	–	2.55	–	–	–
Sudden infant deaths		–	29	120	149	–	0.04	0.17	0.21
Other conditions		128	33	100	133	0.18	0.05	0.14	0.19

*Stillbirths per 1000 total births and neonatal, postneonatal and infant deaths per 1000 live births.
(Data from Office for National Statistics Child Mortality statistics (2009), England and Wales, Table 7 Office for National Statistics 2011.)

2006) and obesity in pregnancy (Fitzsimons and Modder 2010) and annual reports on perinatal mortality in England, Wales, Northern Ireland, the Channel Isles and the Isle of Man.

After being taken over by the National Institute for Health and Clinical Excellence, which reviewed all the four confidential enquiries, CESDI was merged with the Confidential Enquiry into Maternal Deaths and given a much wider remit as the Confidential Enquiry into Maternal and Child Health. The Enquiry transferred to the National Patient Safety Agency in April 2004 and the organisation subsequently changed its name to the Centre for Maternal and Child Enquiries (CMACE).

In 2010, the National Patient Safety Agency ran a competitive tendering exercise for confidential enquiries, redesignated as the Clinical Outcome Review Programme. The work previously undertaken by CMACE was split into two programmes of work: (1) maternal and newborn; and (2) child health. The contract for the maternal and newborn programme was awarded to a consortium led by the National Perinatal Epidemiology Unit and that for the child health programme was awarded to the Royal College of Paediatrics and Child Health.

In late March 2011 the National Patient Safety Agency decided to discontinue the procurement process for the maternal and newborn confidential enquiry pending a review to be completed by July 2011. The National Patient Safety Agency took steps to try to ensure that data collection continued while this was under. Responsibility passed to the Healthcare Quality Improvement Partnership (HQIP). The review report, published in July 2011, recommended that the programme be re-tendered and that a contractor should be appointed by April 1 2012. This gap is likely to have had some impact on the quality and completeness of the data collected. The award of the contract for the child health programme was unaffected by this.

Morbidity in childhood in relation to circumstances at birth

Although trends in mortality since the mid-1980s are somewhat uncertain, it is clear that over the preceding 20 years there was a dramatic decline in neonatal mortality, particularly among very small and immature babies. This raised the question of whether this fall in mortality was associated with an increase, a decrease or no change in the rate of morbidity among the survivors. Although there are a large number of follow-up studies, it has been difficult to answer this question. This is because information about long-term morbidity has not been collected in a standardised and comparable way, either in the countries of the UK or in most other countries.

There are few routine sources of information on morbidity available and most of these do not routinely link health in childhood to circumstances at birth, although the move towards greater use of record linkage may change this in the future. Because of this gap, data about morbidity in children who were born with low birthweight or preterm or who needed neonatal intensive care for other reasons are available mostly from studies of cohorts of babies cared for in individual hospitals or born to residents in geographically defined populations. Comparisons between these studies and over time is difficult, for a number of reasons, which are described in detail in Chapter 3.

The increasing demand for neonatal care

The increase since the 1960s in the proportion of babies who are born alive and who survive the first few days of life has led to a corresponding increase in the numbers requiring care over and above the normal level of postnatal care given by mothers, with the support of midwives, health visitors, general practitioners and paediatric staff. The likelihood that a baby will need specialist neonatal care is highest among those with the lowest birthweight, and the proportion of babies of low or very low birthweight who survive birth has increased more quickly than the total numbers of live births. The current and planned future organisation of neonatal care and recommendations for data collection in the UK are described in Chapter 2, along with the history of neonatal care. The chapter ends with a description of the data collected routinely in the UK and what they do and do not tell us about trends in the care provided.

Trends in resources for neonatal care

Nationally available data about the NHS include numbers of cots in neonatal units and their use, numbers of paediatric medical staff and numbers of midwifery and nursing staff working in maternity and neonatal units. So far there is little information about the resources needed from health and social services and families once babies leave neonatal units, although these cannot be assumed to be negligible (Mugford 1990; Petrou and Mugford 2000).

Cots for neonatal care

Cots for neonatal care are funded differently depending on the type of care that is expected to be provided: the more intensive the nursing and the more equipment required, the greater the cost of providing the care. As techniques for care change continually, the definitions of levels of care, set out in Chapter 2, need to change in response, so the relevant professional bodies update these definitions from time to time. Until the late 1990s data collected routinely at hospital level counted staffed available cots for care of babies and included relatively little additional evidence about the type of cot or level of care provided.

Data about neonatal cots in England up to 1986 were derived from the SH3 Hospital Return. Numbers of available cots were based on a daily count of staffed available cots in each neonatal unit or special care baby unit (SCBU). Confusion can arise because the numbers of cots counted on the SH3 return were commonly referred to as 'special care cots' and levels of care within the neonatal units were not differentiated. As a result, the total number of cots included those designated for intensive care. The Steering Group on Health Services Information (1985) drew on the reports of the professional bodies mentioned above when compiling the definitions of special and intensive care used in the definition of cots for hospital statistics to be collected from 1987 onwards. Such designation is at best artificial, as it is likely that care considered to be intensive often takes place other than in the intensive care area within a special care nursery.

Data from the SH3 return and its counterparts showed that there was a fall in the absolute numbers of cots in SCBUs in each of the four countries of the UK in the early 1980s. These data, reproduced in *Birth Counts: Statistics of Pregnancy and Childbirth* (Macfarlane et al. 2000), also show decreasing rates of admission and longer lengths of stay for the babies who were admitted. With increasing concern in the 1970s and 1980s about the separation of babies from their mothers, policies of routine admission to special care for many babies changed. The admission rate fell from a high point of about 20% of births in England in the mid-1970s to just over 10% in 1987.

The basis for data collection changed in 1988, and in England the number and use of cots were from that time measured in two different routine systems. Numbers of hospital cots were recorded in the KP70 hospital data system, and the use of cots was derived from the Hospital Episode System, both of which derived data from local health information systems and were administered centrally by the Department of Health. The numbers of cots for neonatal care appear to have continued to decline until 1990, with a levelling of the numbers and rates per 1000 births after that. Since 1996–7, the numbers of cots for intensive neonatal care have been shown separately.

Since 1988 it is no longer the number of admissions but rather the number of 'finished consultant episodes' (FCEs) that is counted. Any baby who is admitted for neonatal care but receives care from different consultants during one admission will be described as receiving more than one FCE during that admission. This can happen if surgery or specialist diagnostic skills are required. Not surprisingly, therefore, numbers of FCEs for babies admitted aged under 28 days and excluding healthy newborns, for 1989–90 until 1995–6, were much higher than the previous numbers of admissions to neonatal units.

Although this analysis of FCEs is not available for subsequent years, the Department of Health published analyses of occupancy,

the percentage of days an available cot is occupied, which show that, although there was a slight increase in the available cots per 1000 live births in the subsequent period, the occupancy was constant at about 70%, suggesting that an increasing number of intensive care cot days was being provided.

Since 1996–7, the KH03 form has listed numbers of intensive care cots in England. Data from that source for the financial years 2000–1 onwards, listed in Table 1.27, show that, although the numbers of cots provided have risen, they have scarcely kept pace with the rising birth rate and that occupancy rates have increased. In contrast, in Wales, where a broader definition of special care beds is used, their numbers have not risen and there are no clear trends in occupancy or length of stay.

Staff for neonatal care

The medical specialty of paediatrics has grown considerably, both in absolute numbers of 'whole-time equivalent' staff and in relation to the numbers of births, as Table 1.28 shows. All staff have been combined, because of changes in categorisation of staff in training.

Table 1.27 Special and intensive care cots, England and Wales, 2000–1 to 2009–10

	AVERAGE DAILY AVAILABLE BEDS	AVERAGE DAILY OCCUPIED BEDS	INPATIENT CASES	PERCENTAGE OCCUPANCY	AVERAGE DURATION OF STAY
Intensive care cots, England					
2000–1	1517	1092		72.0	
2001–2	1543	1088		70.5	
2002–3	1551	1081		69.7	
2003–4	1491	1084		72.7	
2004–5	1523	1120		73.6	
2005–6	1707	1207		70.7	
2006–7	1658	1233		74.3	
2007–8	1734	1257		72.5	
2008–9	1805	1321		73.2	
2009–10	1776	1335		75.1	
Special care beds, Wales					
2000–1	206	114	3012	55.7	13.9
2001–2	202	106	2803	52.5	13.8
2002–3	195	116	3015	59.7	14.1
2003–4	175	115	2862	65.5	14.6
2004–5	184	120	3100	65.6	14.2
2005–6	175	115	2862	65.5	14.6
2006–7	199	121	2826	60.5	15.6
2007–8	204	112	2982	54.9	13.7
2008–9	199	115	3112	57.6	13.5
2009–10	191	114	3138	59.6	13.2

(Data from Department of Health, Health Statistics Wales.)

Table 1.28 Paediatric medical staff in England, Wales, Scotland and Northern Ireland, 1985–2010

YEAR	ENGLAND		WALES		SCOTLAND		NORTHERN IRELAND[‡]	
	wte*	Rate[†]	wte*	Rate[†]	wte*	Rate[†]	wte*	Rate[†]
Paediatrics and paediatric neurology[§]								
1985	1837	2.97	122	3.32	223	3.34	65	2.35
1990	2339	3.51	145	3.73	260	3.94	78	2.94
1995	3892	6.35	228	6.61	321	5.34	126	5.33
2000	4590	8.01	293	9.35	–	–	174	8.10
2001	4600	8.16	293	9.57	536	10.21	187	8.53
2002	5048	8.92	311	10.28	553	10.78	183	8.54
2003	5414	9.18	325	10.33	557	10.62	186	8.57
2004	5893	9.71	367	11.36	576	10.67		
2005	6239	10.18	395	12.11	602	11.06		
2006	6484	10.20	–	–	608	10.92		
2007	6509	9.93	427	12.40	639	11.06		
2008	6912	10.27	425	11.93	601	10.01		
2009	7262	10.82	422	12.07	761	12.89		
2010	7279		441		764			
Paediatric surgery[¶]								
1985	100	0.16	4	0.11	43	0.64	14	0.51
1990	128	0.19	6	0.15	48	0.73	9	0.34
1995	196	0.32	4	0.12	56	0.93	9	0.38
2000	269	0.47	7	0.22	–	–	4	0.18
2001	261	0.46	8	0.26	52	0.99	5	0.22
2002	287	0.51	10	0.33	48	0.94	5	0.22
2003	247	0.42	8	0.26	64	1.23	7	0.31
2004	314	0.52	10	0.30	76	1.41		
2005	328	0.53	9	0.28	57	1.06		
2006	297	0.47	–	–	61	1.10		
2007	274	0.42	14	0.39	54	0.94		
2008	303	0.45	17	0.48	47	0.78		
2009	339	0.50	14	0.40	50	0.85		
2010	341		15		36			

*Whole-time equivalent.
[†]Rate per 1000 live births.
[‡]Figures for Northern Ireland for 1997 onwards are taken from the trust and board human resource management systems. They exclude all agency and bank staff. Bank staff maintain service delivery by covering staff shortfalls and fluctuating workloads. As a consequence their input to the service is difficult to measure. Owing to coding difficulties within the system, it is impossible to identify paediatric neurology staff working within paediatrics. Despite the fact that the attached figures are shown by paediatric departments, it is most probable that all medical staff working within paediatrics are not captured in these figures.
[§]England 2002 onwards does not include paediatric neurology.
[¶]Change in collection in 2001 in Scotland.
(Data from NHS Executive and Department of Health, National Assembly for Wales, ISD Scotland, Department of Health, Personal Social Services and Public Safety, Northern Ireland.)

Table 1.29 Whole-time equivalent nursing and midwifery staff working in maternity care, including neonatal care, England, 1998–2010

YEAR	NURSE CONSULTANT	MODERN MATRON	MANAGER	REGISTERED NURSE – CHILDREN	REGISTERED MIDWIFE	OTHER FIRST LEVEL*	OTHER SECOND LEVEL*	ALL	RATE PER 1000 LIVE BIRTHS
1998			311	328	18 479	3848	442	23 408	38.9
1999			264	330	17 856	4064	405	22 919	38.9
2000			237	375	17 640	4185	339	22 776	39.8
2001	9		232	480	18 011	3604	348	22 684	40.2
2002	18		274	558	18 097	3728	367	23 043	40.7
2003	31		311	611	18 428	4060	317	23 758	40.3
2004	44		376	810	18 835	4169	229	24 463	40.3
2005	49	139	321	772	18 928	4336	204	24 750	40.4
2006	50	141	355	878	18 833	4492	211	24 961	39.3
2007	49	162	380	861	19 278	4732	194	25 654	39.1
2008	55	425	320	857	19 586	4412	137	25,790	38.3
2009	55	412	323	835	20 201	4667	91	26 583	39.6
2010	64	410	409	783	20 760	5018	117	27 561	

(Data from NHS Information Centre, Workforce Statistics.)

Table 1.30 Whole-time equivalent support staff working in the area of maternity care, including neonatal care, England, 1998–2010

YEAR	NURSERY NURSE	NURSING ASSISTANT/ AUXILLARY	HEALTHCARE ASSISTANTS	SUPPORT WORKER	TOTAL	STAFF PER 1000 LIVE BIRTHS
1998	244	3007	928	540	4719	7.8
1999	253	2998	996	545	4792	8.1
2000	263	2914	1074	530	4781	8.3
2001	275	2814	1248	543	4880	8.7
2002	289	2903	1294	500	4986	8.8
2003	300	3065	1410	575	5351	9.1
2004	296	3192	1748	557	5794	9.5
2005	290	2927	1821	627	5665	9.2
2006	284	2787	1864	649	5583	8.8
2007	323	2562	2062	650	5597	8.5
2008	371	2411	2312	779	5874	8.7
2009	435	2582	2458	876	6351	9.5
2010	478	2447	2746	961	6633	

(Data from NHS Information centre, Workforce statistics.)

Data about the division of work between neonatology and other paediatric work are not routinely collected and so it is only possible to comment on the numbers in the specialty of paediatrics as a whole. Data are collected differently from each country's health administration and are not always available on the same basis. Northern Ireland data included community paediatricians and paediatric surgeons in the total figures for paediatrics and paediatric neurology and therefore the totals are not strictly comparable with those from the other countries. Publication of data by specialty appears to have stopped. In England, data about staff in paediatric neurology were not shown separately from 2002 onwards and in Scotland the introduction of a new data collection system in 2001 led to a discontinuity in counting.

The staff numbers are expressed as whole-time equivalents, with each member of staff being counted as the proportion of the full contract hours worked. This avoids the problem of how to count parttime staff, but trends over time can be misleading when nationally agreed hours of work change. It is important to note that changes in the contractual hours of doctors since the 1990s will have reduced the total medical time represented by the whole-time equivalent number of staff.

National data about midwives and nurses can be analysed to indicate how many of them work in maternity areas. These do not show neonatal care separately, although a new system for collecting workforce statistics in England, introduced in 2010, will make this distinction (Information Centre for Health and Social Care 2010). In many maternity units a certain amount of neonatal special care, such as phototherapy, is given in postnatal wards. Because of this blurring of the boundary between different levels of care, it is important to continue to look at the total numbers of maternity unit staff available per birth, as well as the numbers of neonatal unit staff.

The total numbers of qualified hospital nurses and midwives working in the maternity area who were in post on 30 September in each of the years 1998–2010 in England are presented in Table 1.29. Data are shown only for England, as the other countries of the UK do not provide data in this form. In 1980, changes were made in the nationally agreed hours of work for nursing and midwifery staff in the UK. The change in weekly working hours from 40 to 37.5 had the effect of increasing the whole-time equivalents of part-time staff artificially by 6.7% with no actual increase in available staff. Data for the 1980s and 1990s, showed that the numbers of whole-time equivalent midwives and nurses did not increase, and the rate per 1000 live births fell over the period (Macfarlane et al. 2000). This trend is associated with a change in training for nurses under Project 2000. Before 1989 student nurses and midwives were counted as part of the NHS workforce, but students then became supernumerary and were not recorded in staff numbers, but more recently they have been counted as support staff.

From 2003 onwards, there were substantial increases in whole-time equivalent numbers of nurses and midwives in England, but, as Table 1.29 shows, they did not keep pace with the increases in numbers of births. Over this period, there were other changes, with the introduction of consultant nurses and midwives and of modern matrons. Table 1.30 shows that there were also changes in the numbers and designation of support staff in the maternity areas. Most notable was the increase in numbers of healthcare assistants, defined as staff who are trained or under training in the various competencies related to their jobs and who work in specific clinical areas or are part of specific clinical teams. In practice, the work they do varies widely, so it is difficult to quantify their contribution (Sandall et al. 2007).

The need for better data

Although the existing data give a broad picture of the epidemiological context of neonatal care, there are many gaps and inconsistencies. There has been considerable activity in data definition and, more recently, in the development of neonatal systems, but no corresponding expansion in published data. In addition, to interpret these, better data are needed about all births. Here again there are positive developments in plans for data collection and record linkage, but at the time of writing the major concern in the UK is the lack of resources, including for data collection and monitoring services, which means that even the existing data systems are being cut and staff expertise is being lost.

References

Ahmad, W.I.U., Sheldon, T., 1992. 'Race' and statistics. In: Ahmad, W.I.U. (Ed.), The Politics of 'Race' and Health. University of Bradford and Ilkley Community College, Bradford.

Alberman, E., Botting, B., 1991. Trends in prevalence and survival of very low birthweight infants, England and Wales: 1983–7. Arch Dis Child 66, 1304–1308.

Alberman, E., Botting, B., Blatchley, N., et al., 1994. A new hierarchical classification of causes of infant deaths in England and Wales. Arch Dis Child 70, 403–409.

Alberman, E., Blatchley, N., Botting, B., et al., 1997. Medical causes on stillbirth certificates in England and Wales: distribution and results of hierarchical classification tested by the Office for National Statistics. Br J Obstet Gynaecol 104, 1043–1049.

Australian Institute of Health and Welfare National Perinatal Statistics Unit, 2003. Australia's mothers and babies, 2000. Perinatal Statistics Series No 12. AIHW National Perinatal Statistics Unit, Sydney, Australia.

Aveyard, P., Cheng, K.K., Manaseki, S., et al., 2002. The risk of preterm delivery in women from different ethnic groups. Br J Obstet Gynaecol 109, 894–899.

Baird, D., Wyper, J.F.B., 1941. High stillbirth and neonatal mortalities. Lancet 2, 657–659.

Balarajan, R., Raleigh, V.S., 1990. Variations in perinatal, neonatal, postneonatal and infant mortality in England and Wales by mother's country of birth, 1982–85. In: Britton, M. (Ed.), Mortality and Geography: a Review in the mid-1980s in England and Wales. Series DS no 9. HMSO, London.

Blair, P.S., Fleming, P.J., Bensley, D., 1996a. Smoking and the sudden infant death syndrome: results from 1993–95 case-control study for confidential inquiry into stillbirths and deaths in infancy. Br Med J 313, 195–198.

Blondel, B., Macfarlane, A., 2003. Rising multiple maternity rates and medical management of subfertility: better information is needed. Eur J Public Health 13, 83–86.

Bonelli, S.R., Raab, G.M., 1997. Why are babies getting heavier? Comparison of Scottish births from 1980 to 1992. Br Med J 315, 1205.

Botting, B.J., Macfarlane, A.J., 1990. Geographic variations in infant mortality in relation to birthweight 1983–1985. In:

Britton, M. (Ed.), Mortality and Geography: a Review in the mid-1980s in England and Wales. Series DS no 9. HMSO, London.

Botting, B.J., Macfarlane, A.J., Price, F.V. (Eds.) 1990. Three, Four and More: a Study of Triplet and Higher Order Births. HMSO, London.

Buitendijk, S., Zeitlin, J., Cuttini, M., et al., 2003. Indicators of fetal and infant health outcomes. Eur J Obstet Gynecol Reprod Biol 111, S66–S77.

Child and Maternal Health Observatory. 2011. Approval of Maternity and Children's Dataset http://www.chimat.org. uk/resource/item.aspx?RID=119309. Accessed February 8 2012.

Clinical Outcome Review Programme. 2011. Maternal and Newborn Health: Review Panel Report. Chair, Dr Sheila Shribman. http://www.hqip.org.uk/assets/National-Team-Uploads/Maternal-and-Newborn-ReviPanel-FINAL-27-07-11.pdf.

Cole, S.K., Hey, E.N., Thomson, A.M., 1986. Classifying perinatal death: an obstetric approach. Br J Obstet Gynaecol 93, 1204–1212.

Cole, S.K., Hartford, R.B., Bergsjo, P., et al., 1989. International Collaborative Effort (ICE) on birthweight, plurality, perinatal and infant mortality. III. A method of grouping underlying causes of infant death to aid international comparisons. Acta Obstet Scand 68, 113–117.

Collingwood Bakeo, A., 2004. Trends in live births by mother in country of birth in England and Wales 1983–2001. Health Stat Q 23, 25–33.

Confidential Enquiry into Stillbirths and Deaths in Infancy, 1995. Report, 1 January–31 December, 1993. Department of Health, London.

Confidential Enquiry into Stillbirths and Deaths in Infancy, 1996. Third Annual Report, 1 January–31 December, 1994. Department of Health, London.

Confidential Enquiry into Stillbirths and Deaths in Infancy, 1997. Fourth Annual Report, 1 January–31 December, 1995. Maternal and Child Health Research Consortium, London.

Craig, J., 1997. Population review: (9) Summary of issues. Population Trends 88, 5–12.

Dattani, N., Datta-Nemdharry, P., Macfarlane, A., 2011. Linking maternity data for England, 2005–06: methods and data quality. Health Statistics Quarterly 49, 53–76.

Dattani, N., Datta-Nemdharry, P., Macfarlane, A., 2012. Linking maternity data for England, 2007: methods and data quality. Health Statistics Quarterly 53, 4–21.

Datta-Nemdharry P, Dattani N, Macfarlane A, 2011. Birth outcomes for African and Caribbean babies in England and Wales: retrospective analysis of routinely collected data. Submitted for publication.

Dattani, N., Rowan, S., 2002. Causes of neonatal deaths and stillbirths: a new hierarchical classification in ICD 10. Health Stat Q 15, 16–22.

Department of Communities and Local Government, 2011. Indices of Deprivation. Available online at: http://www.imd.communities.gov.uk/.

Department of Health, 1989. Perinatal and Neonatal Mortality. Government Reply to the First Report from the Social Services Committee, Session 1988–1989. Cmd 741. HMSO, London.

Department of Health, 1990. Confidential Enquiry into Stillbirths and Deaths in Infancy. Report of a Working Group set up by the Chief Medical Officer. Department of Health, London.

Department of Health, 2004. NHS Maternity Statistics, England: 2002–2003. Bulletin 2004/10. Department of Health, London.

Department of Health, 2011. Department of Health. The NHS Outcomes Framework 2012/13. Department of Health, London. http://www.dh.gov.uk/prod_consum_dh/groups/dh_digitalassets/documents/digitalasset/dh_131723.pdf.

Drever, F., Whitehead, M., 1997. Inequalities in Health. Series DS No 15. The Stationery Office, London.

Dunn, A., Macfarlane, A.J., 1996. Recent trends in the incidence of multiple births and associated mortality in England and Wales. Arch Dis Child 75, F10–F19.

Enkin, M., Chalmers, I., 1980. Inquiries into perinatal deaths at area health authority level: a status report winter 1979/80. Commun Med 2, 219–224.

Europeristat, 2008. European Perinatal Health Report. Available online at: http://www.europeristat.com/.

Fairley, L., Leyland, A., 2006. Social class inequalities in perinatal outcomes: Scotland 1980–2000. J Epidemiol Community Health 60, 31–36.

Fitzsimons, K., Modder, J., 2010. Setting standards for maternity care for women with obesity in pregnancy. Semin Fetal Neonat Med 15, 100–107.

Fleming, P.J., Blair, P.S., Bacon, C., et al, 1996b. Environment of infants during sleep and risk of the sudden infant death syndrome: results of 1993–95 case-control study for confidential enquiry into stillbirths and deaths in infancy. Br Med J 313, 191–195.

Gagnon, A.J., Zimbeck, M., Zeitlin, J., et al., 2009. Migration to western industrialised countries and perinatal health: a systematic review. Soc Sci Med 69, 934–946.

General Register Office, 2003. Civil Registration: Delivering Vital Change. Office for National Statistics, London.

Gissler, M., Mohangoo, A.D., Blondel, B., et al, 2010. Perinatal health monitoring in Europe: results from the EURO-PERISTAT project. Inform Health Social Care 35, 64–79.

Goldenberg, R.L., Culhane, J.F., Iams, J.D., Romero, R., 2008. Epidemiology and causes of preterm birth. Lancet 371, 75–84.

Graafmans, W.C., Richardus, J.-H., Macfarlane, A., et al, 2001. Comparability of published perinatal mortality rates in Western Europe: the quantitative impact of differences in gestational age and birthweight criteria. Br J Obstet Gynaecol 108, 1237–1245.

Graafmans, W.C., Richardus, J.H., Borsboom, G.J.J.M., et al, 2002. Birthweight and perinatal mortality and seven western European countries. Epidemiology 13, 569–574.

Hartford RB, 1990. Definitions, standards, data quality and comparability. Paper given at the International Symposium on perinatal and infant mortality, Bethesda, Maryland, USA, 30 April–2 May.

Health Statistics Wales, 2011. Maternity Statistics, Wales: Method of Delivery, 2000–2010. Welsh Assembly Government, Cardiff. Available online at: http://wales.gov.uk/docs/statistics/2011/110223sdr272011en.pdf.

Hey, E.N., Lloyd, D.J., Wigglesworth, J.S., 1986. Classifying perinatal death: fetal and neonatal factors. Br J Obstet Gynaecol 93, 1213–1223.

Hilder, L., Moser, K., 2008. Assessing quality of NHS Numbers for Babies data and providing gestational age statistics. Health Stat Q 37, 15–23.

Hilder, L., Moser, K., Dattani, N., et al., 2007. Pilot linkage of NHS Numbers for Babies data with birth registrations. Health Stat Q 33, 25–33.

Horam, J., 1997. Reply to written question from Audrey Wise. Hansard, 20 March col 811. The Stationery Office, London.

House of Commons Health Committee, 1996. Public Expenditure on Health and Personal Social Services. HC 698. The Stationery Office, London.

House of Commons Social Services Committee, 1988. Perinatal, Neonatal and Infant Mortality. HC 54. HMSO, London.

Human Fertilisation and Embryology Authority, 1994. Third Annual Report. HFEA, London.

Human Fertilisation and Embryology Authority, 2004. Code of Practice, sixth ed. HFEA, London.

Human Fertilisation and Embryology Authority, 2010, Treatment Outside UK. Available online at: http://www.hfea.gov.uk/6018.html.

Human Fertilisation and Embryology Authority, 2011. Improving Outcomes for Fertility Patients: Multiple Births. Available online at: http://www.hfea.gov.uk/docs/2011-12-01_-_Multiple_Births_Publication_2011_-_Rationalising_Register_Data_-_FINAL_1.2.DOC.pdf.

Information and Statistics Division, 1987. Birthweight Statistics 1980–1984. Information and Statistics Division, Edinburgh.

Information and Statistics Division, 1997. Births in Scotland 1976–1995. Information and Statistics Division, Edinburgh.

Information and Statistics Division, 1998. Small Babies in Scotland. Information and Statistics Division, Edinburgh.

Information and Statistics Division, 2003. Operative Vaginal Delivery in Scotland: a 20 year Overview with a Chapter on Multiple Pregnancy in Scotland. Information and Statistics Division, Edinburgh.

Information and Statistics Division, 2011a. Births in Scottish Hospitals. Available online at: http://www.isdscotland.org/isd/1018.html.

Information and Statistics Division, 2011b. Scottish Perinatal and Infant Mortality and Morbidity Report (SPIMMR). Available online at: http://www.isdscotland.org/isd/3109.html.

Information Centre for Health and Social Care, 2010. Workforce Census Changes: 2010 and Beyond. Available online at: http://www.ic.nhs.uk/webfiles/publications/workforce/Workforce_Census_Changes_Flyer.pdf.

Information Centre for Health and Social Care, 2011a. Maternity. Available online at: http://www.ic.nhs.uk/statistics-and-data-collections/hospital-care/maternity.

Information Centre for Health and Social Care, 2011b. Maternity Data in HES. Available online at: http://www.hesonline.nhs.uk/Ease/servlet/ContentServer?siteID=1937&categoryID=925.

Information Centre for Health and Social Care, 2011c. Clinical and Health Outcomes Knowledge Base. Available online at: http://www.nchod.nhs.uk/Information.

Information Standards Board, 2006. ISB, 0075. Neonatal Critical Care Minimum Data Set. Available online at: http://www.isb.nhs.uk/documents/isb-0075.

Information Standards Board, 2011. Available online at: http://www.isb.nhs.uk/documents/isb-1513/amd-34-2010/1513342010sub.pdfInterim.

Licensing Authority for Human In Vitro Fertilisation and Embryology, 1990. Fifth Report. Interim Licensing Authority, London.

Kenney, N., Macfarlane, A., 1999. Identifying problems with data collection at a local level: survey of NHS maternity units in England. Br Med J 319, 619–622.

Kramer, M.R., Hogue, C.R., 2009. What causes racial disparities in very preterm birth? A biosocial perspective. Epidemiol Rev 31, 84–98.

Kramer, M., Goulet, L., Lydon, J., et al., 2001. Socio-economic disparities in preterm birth: causal pathways and mechanisms. Paediatr Perinatal Epidemiol 15, 104–123.

Leon, D., Moser, K., 2010. Low birthweight persists in South Asians born in England and Wales regardless of maternal country of birth. Slow pace of acculturation, physiological constraint or both? Analysis of routine data. J Epidemiol Commun Health doi:10.1136/jech.2010.112516.

Logan, S., Spencer, N., Blackburn, C., 1996. Smoking is part of a causal chain (letter). Br Med J 313, 1332–1333.

Macfarlane, A.J., 1996a. Sudden infant death syndrome: more attention should have been paid to socioeconomic factors (letter). Br Med J 313, 1332.

Macfarlane, A.J., 1996b. Inégalités en santé des enfants en Europe: une perspective épidémiologique. In: Santé et mortalité des enfants en Europe. Proceedings of the Chaire Quêtelet, 13–15 September, 1994. Academia-Bruylant, Louvain-la-Neuve.

Macfarlane, A.J., Cole, S., Johnson, A., et al., 1988. Epidemiology of birth before 28 weeks of gestation. Br Med Bull 44, 861–893.

Macfarlane, A.J., Mugford, M., 2000. Birth Counts: Statistics of Pregnancy and Childbirth. Vol 1, second ed. The Stationery Office, London.

Macfarlane, A.J., Mugford, M., Henderson, J., et al., 2000. Birth Counts: Statistics of Pregnancy and Childbirth. Vol 2, second ed. The Stationery Office, London.

Macfarlane, A., Gissler, M., Bolumar, F., Rasmussen, S., 2003. The availability of perinatal health indicators in Europe. Eur J Obstet Gynecol Reprod Biol 111, S15–S32.

Macfarlane, A., Grant, J., Hancock, J., et al., 2005. Early Life Mortality in East London: a Feasibility Study. Summary report. Fetal and Infant Death in East London. City University, London.

Macfarlane, A., Stafford, M., Moser, K., 2004. Social inequalities. In: The Health of Children and Young People. Office for National Statistics, London.

Macintosh, M.C.M., Fleming, K.M., Bailey, J.A., et al., 2006. Perinatal mortality and congenital anomalies in babies of women with type 1 or type 2 diabetes in England, Wales, and Northern Ireland: population based study. Br Med J 333, 177.

Maher, J., Macfarlane, A., 2004. Trends in live births and birthweight by social class and mother's age, 1976–2000. Health Stat Q 23, 34–43.

Masuy-Stroobant, G., 1996. Santé et mortalité infantile en Europe. Victoires d'hier et enjeux de demain. In: Masuy-Stroobant, G., Gourbin, C., Buekens, P. (Eds.), Santé et mortalité des enfants en Europe. Inégalités sociales d'hier et d'aujourd'hui, Chaire Quêtelet, 1994. Academia-Bruylant, Louvain-la-Neuve.

McLernon, D.J., Harrild, K., Bergh, C., et al, 2010. Clinical effectiveness of elective single versus double embryo transfer: meta-analysis of individual patient data from randomised trials. Br Med J 341, c6945.

Mohangoo, A.D., Buitendijk, S.E., Szamotulska, K., et al., 2009. Gestational age patterns of fetal and neonatal mortality in Europe: results from the Euro-Peristat project. Paediatr Perinat Epidemiol 23, 292–300.

Moser, K., 2009. Gestation-specific infant mortality by social and biological factors among babies born in England and Wales in, 2006. Report. Health Stat Q 42, 78–86.

Moser, K., Macfarlane, A., Chow, Y.H., et al., 2007. Introducing new data on gestation-specific infant mortality among babies born in, 2005. in England and Wales. Health Stat Q 35, 13–27.

Moser, K., Leon, D., Stanfield, K., 2008. Birthweight and gestational age by ethnic group, England and Wales, 2005. Health Stat Q 39, 22–31.

MRC Working Party on children conceived by in-vitro fertilisation, 1990. Births in Great Britain resulting from assisted conception. Br Med J 300, 1229–1233.

Mugford, M., 1990. The costs of a multiple birth. In: Botting, B.J., Macfarlane, A.J., Price, F.V. (Eds.), Three, Four and More: a Study of Triplet and Higher Order Births. HMSO, London, pp. 205–217.

National Audit Office Maternity Services, 1990. Report by the Controller and Auditor General. HMSO, London.

National Health Service, Department of Health, 1990a. Working Paper 11. Framework for Information Systems: Overview. HMSO, London.

National Health Service, Department of Health, 1990b. Framework for Information Systems: the Next Steps. HMSO, London.

Oakley, L., Maconochie, N., Doyle, P., et al., 2009. Multivariate analysis of infant death in England and Wales in 2005–06, with focus on socio-economic status and deprivation. Health Stat Q 42, 22–39.

Office for National Statistics, 1999. Registration: Modernising a Vital Service: Births, Marriages and Deaths in the 21st Century. Office for National Statistics, London.

Office for National Statistics, 2002. Civil Registration: Vital Change: Births, Marriages and Deaths in the 21st Century. Cmd 5355. The Stationery Office, London.

Office for National Statistics, 2003. Ethnic Group Statistics: a Guide to the Collection of Ethnicity Data. The Stationery Office, London.

Office for National Statistics, 2009. Final Recommended Questions for the 2011 Census in England and Wales. National Identity. The Stationery Office, London.

Office for National Statistics, 2010. SOC2010 Volume 3 NS-SEC (Rebased On SOC2010) User Manual) Available online at: http://www.ons.gov.uk/about-statistics/classifications/current/soc2010/soc2010-volume-3-ns-sec–rebased-on-soc2010–user-manual/index.html#7.

Office for National Statistics, 2011. Childhood Mortality Statistics, 2009, England and Wales. Available online at: http://www.statistics.gov.uk/downloads/theme_health/child-mortality/child_mort_stats_2009.pdf).

Office of Population Censuses and Surveys and General Register Office, Scotland, 1989. Publication of Draft Census Order. Census newsletter No 11. OPCS, London.

Parsons, L., Macfarlane, A.J., Golding, J., 1993. Pregnancy, birth and maternity care In: Ahmad, W.I.U. (Ed.), Race and Health in Contemporary Britain. Open University Press, Buckingham, pp 51–75.

Petrou, S., Mugford, M., 2000. Predicting the cost of neonatal care. In: Hansen, T., McIntosh, N. (Eds.), Current Topics in Neonatology IV. Harcourt Health Sciences, London, pp. 149–174.

Power, C., 1994. National trends in birth weight: implications for future adult disease. Br Med J 308, 1270–1271.

Rose, D., O'Reilly, K., 1998. The ESRC Review of Government Social Classifications. Office for National Statistics and the Economic and Social Research Council, London.

Rowan, S., 2003. Implications of changes in the United Kingdom social and occupational classifications in 2001 on infant mortality statistics. Health Stat Q 17, 33–40.

Royal College of Obstetricians and Gynaecologists, 2000. National Evidence-Based Guidelines. The Management of Infertility in Tertiary Care. RCOG, London.

Sandall, J., Jill, M., Mansfield, A., 2007. Support workers in maternity services. J Family Healthcare 17, 191–192.

Steering Group on Health Services Information, 1985. Supplement to First and Fourth Reports to the Secretary of State. HMSO, London.

Tatham, J., 1907. Letter to the Registrar General. In: 68th Report of the Registrar General of Births Marriages and Deaths in England and Wales, 1905. Cmd 3279. HMSO, London.

Urquia, M.L., Glazier, R.H., Blondel, B., et al., 2010. International migration and adverse birth outcomes: role of ethnicity, region of origin and destination. J Epidemiol Commun Health 64, 243–251.

Wadhwa, P.D., Culhane, J.F., Rauh, V., et al., 2001. Stress, infection and preterm birth: a biobehavioural perspective. Paediatr Perinat Epidemiol 15 (Suppl 2), 17–29.

Wigglesworth, J.S., 1980. Monitoring perinatal mortality – a pathophysiological approach. Lancet 2, 684–686.

World Health Organization, 1977. Manual of the International Statistical Classification of Diseases, Injuries and Causes of Death, 9th revision. WHO, Geneva.

World Health Organization, 1992. International Statistical Classification of Diseases and Related Health Problems, 10th revision. WHO, Geneva.

Wright, E., 2010. 2008-based national population projections for the United Kingdom and constituent countries. Population Trends 139, 91–114.

Zeitlin, J., Wildman, K., Bréart, G., et al, 2003. Selecting an indicator set for monitoring and evaluating perinatal health in Europe: criteria, methods and results from the PERISTAT project. Eur J Obstet Gynecol Reprod Biol 111, S5–S14.

Zeitlin, J., Bucourt, M., Rivera, L., et al., 2004. Preterm birth and maternal country of birth in a French district with a multiethnic population. Br J Obstet Gynaecol 3, 849–855.

Organisation and evaluation of perinatal care

Neil Marlow

2

CHAPTER CONTENTS

© 2012 Elsevier Ltd

Asphyxia, prematurity, sepsis and malformations remain the major causes of mortality and morbidity identifiable at birth and result in around 4 million deaths each year worldwide. Neonatal intensive care (NIC) has made huge inroads into reducing the mortality and to some extent the morbidity associated with the first three causes, which has resulted in improving survival at increasingly low gestations. Such care, however, is increasingly under pressure as the result of budgetary and skill base constraints.

Within many health systems it is not feasible to provide such expertise and facilities in every setting in which babies are born. Most health services in the developed world have developed increasingly specialised models of neonatal services, concentrating skills and facilities for providing intensive care, ensuring high levels of basic skills close to every birth and dedicated transport facilities to ensure babies receive optimal care in the correct setting to maintain improving outcomes. Such a system is high cost and low throughput compared with many health services, including maternity care.

Concentration is not without problems and increasingly centralised care means much larger delivery units with inherent problems for the obstetric and midwifery teams and pregnant women, and is in conflict with the desire of many groups to provide birth in more 'natural' settings for women at low risk of neonatal complications. These tensions lead to much controversy, which is fuelled by the lack of reliable data with which to evaluate safety in various settings.

In this chapter, therefore, organisation of care will be discussed alongside systems for ensuring that care is safe and effective in different settings and monitored at service, unit and patient level.

Organisation of care

NIC services have developed differently in different health systems, to some extent dependent upon the proximity of the children's and maternity services. In some health systems NIC is located within a children's hospital, which has advantage for paediatric specialist care but places the postpartum mother at a disadvantage and all children have to be transferred in for specialist care. In other systems NIC has developed alongside maternity services, often in isolation from supporting paediatric services. The degree of centralisation of services has also been driven by external factors, either by market forces in privately funded systems or by population distribution. Many health systems mix these structures according to local geography. The relationship between organisational structures and outcome is highly contentious and not easily amenable to study (see below).

Pressures of health economics have driven most services to concentrate intensive care services in fewer expert centres and to review the structure and function of other neonatal services (which care for the majority of babies) in terms of their effectiveness at providing a highly expert resuscitation service or limited intensive care. One example of this is the development of highly centralised NIC in Western Australia, with a land mass 20 times the size of England and a population of 2.2 million compared with 60 million, respectively. There are relatively few large population centres; the whole state is served by two intensive care centres (one in a children's hospital) and a highly developed antenatal and neonatal retrieval service. This contrasts with the 178 neonatal units currently providing intensive care for extremely preterm babies in the UK (Watkinson and Davis 2009). Many European countries have developed NIC within children's hospitals, and thus all babies needing care are transferred in, often from very much smaller and less expert clinics. Slowly this model is being replaced by a centralised system where expertise can be concentrated in fewer and better-resourced maternity/neonatal centres.

Several classifications or categorisations of neonatal units have been used. Most use the concept that a three-tier service is most efficient: the least intensive category of unit provides only short-term stabilisation prior to transfer, the most intensive carries out a full range of intensive care activity, and the intermediate tier provides varying degrees of postnatal support depending on local resources. Evidence is evolving that care in the highest tier centres produces higher survival and less morbidity; the difficulty is how to ensure babies are delivered in an appropriate setting. Current UK definitions are shown in Table 2.1.

Such organisation can only function if units work together as a de facto clinical network and if the health commissioners work to ensure that each network has the capacity and resources to provide for the predicted demand. Parents of babies also need to understand the concept, and the fact that their baby will be moved, should intensive care become necessary, which is against current trends for

care to be delivered in the hospital or setting of choice. Such a working pattern has major potential advantages in terms of high-throughput neonatal intensive care units (NICUs) for the maintenance of clinical skills, high occupancy for intensive care cots permitting efficient use of resources and ability to staff the high-intensity areas.

Within the UK, intensive care resources for adults and for children have been incorporated into managed clinical networks. Services are planned based on a geographic population with different ranges of facilities at each centre. The key issue in the success of these services is the central management of resources across several otherwise independent health service units (trusts). The argument for centralisation of paediatric intensive care has been well made (Ratcliffe 1998) and improved early care, triage and outcome can be anticipated through the underpinning of the network with a strong educational and training base. Despite these structures it remains important in any health system that children access the appropriate level of care (Maybloom et al. 2002).

Overall the demand for NIC has risen (Ch. 1). In parallel, the UK has seen increasing public demand for transparency in the delivery of healthcare, in the wake of several high-profile government reports, and there is a drive to ensure that care is provided by professionals whose expertise is appropriate to the clinical situation. Recent changes in law are leading a reduction in the traditionally overlong working hours for doctors and there is currently a paucity of nursing and specialist doctors to provide specialist neonatal care, fuelling calls for further centralisation.

Current provision of neonatal care in the UK

Women and their families expect that pregnancy, delivery and post-natal care will be delivered in one local centre as close as possible to the family home, and this perception is encouraged by healthcare managers within the National Health Service (NHS) hierarchy. Problems arise when difficulties with either the woman or the fetus develop that cannot be managed by local services. At present further management is dictated by the availability of obstetric and neonatal resources at the referral centre. Central to the planning of care is the

Table 2.1 Types of neonatal services within a network

LEVEL	DESCRIPTION
Level 1	Special care units (SCUs) provide special care for their own local population. Depending on arrangements within their neonatal network, they may also provide some high-dependency services. In addition, SCUs provide a stabilisation facility for babies who need to be transferred to a neonatal intensive care unit (NICU) for intensive or high-dependency care, and they also receive transfers from other network units for continuing special care
Level 2	Local neonatal units (LNUs) provide neonatal care for their own catchment population, except for the sickest babies. They provide all categories of neonatal care, but they transfer babies who require complex or longer term intensive care to a NICU, as they are not staffed to provide longer term intensive care. The majority of babies over 27 weeks of gestation will usually receive their full care, including short periods of intensive care, within their LNU. Some networks have agreed variations on this policy, owing to local requirements. Some LNUs provide high-dependency care and short periods of intensive care for their network population. LNUs may receive transfers from other neonatal services in the network, if these fall within their agreed work pattern
Level 3	Neonatal intensive care units (NICUs) are sited alongside specialist obstetric and fetomaternal medicine services, and provide the whole range of medical neonatal care for their local population, along with additional care for babies and their families referred from the neonatal network. Many NICUs in England are co-located with neonatal surgery services and other specialised services. Medical staff in a NICU should have no clinical responsibilities outside the neonatal and maternity service

Reproduced from Report of the Neonatal Intensive Care Services Review (2009). A Toolkit for Quality Neonatal Services. London, Department of Health.

need to forewarn parents of the likely arrangements if problems develop, so that families are not suddenly faced with the prospect of their care being transferred to another centre, often at some distance, without warning.

In the late 1990s, 246 units provided neonatal care across the UK, 76% of which provided intensive care. This dispersed model had developed as a result of market forces, there being few attempts to centralise care at the time. Since then several national initiatives have effectively centralised care for the extremely preterm baby, using the establishment of managed clinical networks for neonatal care to bring a measure of coordination of care and resources (Marlow and Gill 2007). Currently, neonatal care in England is organised as 22 networks, each centred on one or more lead perinatal centres (usually a university hospital) based on 15 000–25 000 births per annum. The structure of a model neonatal network is shown in Figure 2.1. Management of the network is organised independently of any of the contributing hospitals, in order that resources can be managed effectively and independently of local ambitions. In all networks, care for babies at 26 weeks of gestation or less is centralised, regardless of delivery site, and all have developed a measure of common guidelines and practice.

More recently the NHS has published its framework for NIC (www.dh.gov.uk/en/Publicationsandstatistics/Publications/PublicationsPolicyAndGuidance/DH_107845). This comprehensive document identifies important regional organisation to support NIC and includes a set of quality standards against which neonatal practice can be audited.

With the introduction of the managed clinical network it should be possible to map out a plan for most eventualities, so that a pregnant woman understands the management plan for the anticipated normal pregnancy, what is to happen if a fetal anomaly is discovered, what will happen if very preterm delivery seems likely and what care arrangements are to be made if there is an unanticipated need for NIC. Despite the often-quoted maxim that pregnant women do not wish to travel for their care, all the evidence points to the woman willingly allowing transfer of care if it is clearly in her baby's best interests.

Classification of neonatal care in the UK

One difficulty in determining the size of the workforce needed to staff a neonatal service is the range of activity and case mix of different services. It is thus helpful to define a range of categories of care which may allow the planning of resources.

Within any type of neonatal unit, care for an individual baby can be classified by the level of clinical dependency, which should provide a measure of the resources needed to look after that baby. The definitions of these categories of care will differ between health systems. Within the UK there are several contenders, some of which have been developed using formal studies (Williams et al. 1993), whereas the nationally recommended categories (British Association of Perinatal Medicine 2001, 2010; Report of the Neonatal Intensive Care Services Review 2009) have been developed by professional consensus; we presently recommend that inpatient neonatal care is divided into three categories (Box 2.1).

These categories of care are of value in establishing what level of nurse staffing is necessary to provide cot-side care. Generally, minimum levels specify one nurse to one cot for intensive care, one nurse to two cots for high-dependency cots and one nurse to four cots for special-care cots, although achieving one-to-one nursing is a challenge in the current economic climate with the available workforce skills, and remains aspirational. These minimal requirements do not include managerial and other specialist roles (advanced practice, family care, practice development), which have evolved within the nursing sphere, but require extra resources.

These levels of neonatal care are more tightly defined nationally via the national Neonatal Critical Care Minimum Dataset (http://www.isb.nhs.uk/documents/dscn/dscn2006/142006.pdf) to ensure that there is consistency in definition across the country. The number of intensive care days needed for a particular population will vary depending primarily on the number of low-gestational-age babies cared for, as they utilise the majority of resources. This in

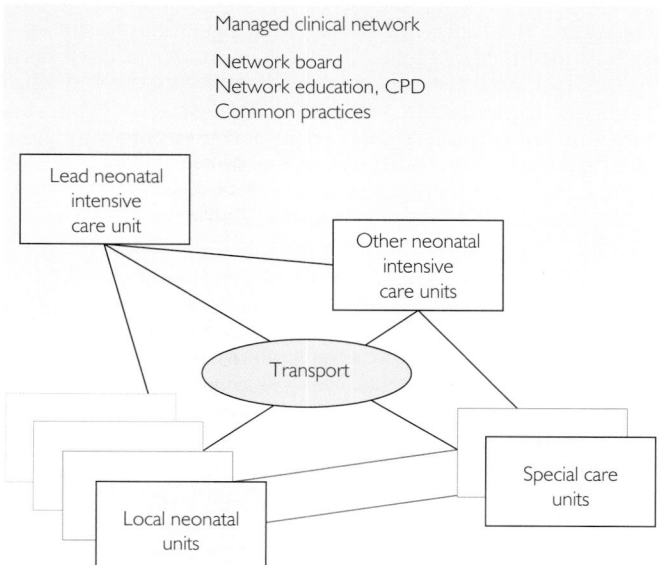

Fig. 2.1 Structure of a neonatal network in England. CPD, continuing professional development. *(Redrawn from Report of the Neonatal Intensive Care Services Review (2009).)*

Box 2.1 Categories of neonatal care

- Special care (SC) is that provided for all other babies who could not reasonably be looked after at home by their mother. Babies receiving special care may need to have their breathing and heart rate monitored, be fed through a tube, supplied with extra oxygen or treated for jaundice; this category also includes babies who are recovering from more specialist treatment before they can be discharged. Special care which occurs alongside the mother is often called 'transitional care' but takes place outside a neonatal unit, in a ward setting

- High-dependency care (HDC) takes place in a neonatal unit and involves care for babies who need continuous monitoring, for example those who weigh less than 1000 g (2 lb 3 oz), or are receiving help with their breathing via continuous positive airway pressure or intravenous feeding, but who do not fulfil any of the requirements for intensive care

- Intensive care (IC) is care provided for babies with the most complex problems who require constant supervision and monitoring and, usually, mechanical ventilation. Because of the possibility of acute deterioration, a doctor must always be available. Extremely immature infants all require intensive care and monitoring over the first weeks, but the range of intensive care work extends throughout the whole gestation period

(Reproduced from Report of the Neonatal Intensive Care Services Review (2009). A Toolkit for Quality Neonatal Services. Department of Health, London.)

turn is dependent upon the social and environmental mix of the population: within the regions of the south-east of the UK, which includes inner city and rural districts, the cot requirement in each region varied between 1.0 and 1.9 intensive care cots per 1000 births, estimated at the recommended 70% occupancy, using older definitions.

To these categories of care, which are dependency based, many hospitals have an intermediate category between the neonatal unit and routine postnatal ward, so-called transitional care. This is primarily aimed at nursing babies who still need 'special care' (for example, gavage feeding) but can be managed in an area alongside their mother and supporting the mother while she provides the majority of care (Ch. 21). In different hospitals this is developed and organised differently and there are no formal definitions to facilitate comparisons. Transitional care has an important effect on neonatal unit activity in that some special care activity is transferred out to a ward staffed primarily by midwives and thus is not always counted in terms of service activity. This may free up staff to assist with the more intensive activity in the neonatal unit, changing the skill mix requirements. In addition, it becomes a local responsibility to determine staffing levels for transitional care and to ensure that adequate support for mothers is available. Despite these difficulties it is a cost-effective and desirable care strategy, encouraging maternal–infant interaction more effectively than remote management on a NICU.

Staffing

Having defined the types of neonatal services and categories of care, the staffing requirements for a neonatal service can be established.

Medical staffing is dependent upon the degree of cross-covering required to run the service and this is in turn dependent on the intensity of care that can effectively be offered:

- For special care units, it is envisaged that no intensive care will take place. Staff will be available in the hospital to attend infrequent emergencies and this cover will be provided as part of an acute paediatric service.
- For local neonatal units, continuous bedside medical support is required, either by a trainee (senior house office (SHO) or resident) or by an advanced neonatal nurse practitioner (ANNP), while middle and consultant tier cover is provided as part of the adjacent acute paediatric service.
- For NIC services, dedicated specialist staff are required with two resident tiers (SHO/ANNP and registrar/consultant), with a supervising consultant available to provide continuity.

In 1996, 25% of units providing intensive care did not have a consultant with more than 50% time dedicated to neonatal care (Tucker et al. 1999). This appears to have somewhat improved by networking. This is clearly unsatisfactory given the huge strides in neonatal care over the past 30 years. As workforce directives reduce the working hours available for all staff, the grade and competency of staff providing first-call care must be examined carefully if we are to continue to provide high-quality care. In some units this is now contributed to by advanced nurse practitioners, who form an intermediate tier of carers outside the clinical practice nursing teams, because of their expertise and wider responsibilities.

Nurse staffing relates to dependency levels and generally is calculated from an estimated establishment for a particular cot number and configuration. Daily monitoring will confirm the adequacy of this. Nurse staffing is the largest part of the unit budget and thus most vulnerable: in 1996, 79% of units had a ratio of nursing

provision to that recommended of less than 1.0 (median 0.84; interquartile range 0.73–0.98), indicating significant underestablishment for the activity that was being carried out, despite taking conservative staffing levels as the norm (1 : 2 intensive care and 1 : 4 for all others) (Tucker et al. 1999). This wide variation in the adequacy of local resources to carry out neonatal care is reflected in the findings of other studies (Parmanum et al. 2000) and has provided the impetus for the current changes in service structure (see below). In a repeat census taken as part of the EPICure 2 study, 73% of units now met this conservative criterion, indicating improved nurse staffing over the 22% found in 1996.

In addition to medical and nursing staff, a range of other supporting skills is required, including allied health professionals (physiotherapy, occupational therapy, speech and language therapy) and other support staff (British Association of Perinatal Medicine 2010). As care for the newborn infant demands different skills from those required for nursing sick older children or adults, specific competencies have been defined for these groups (Report of the Neonatal Intensive Care Services Review 2009; British Association of Perinatal Medicine 2010).

Transfers

Any configuration of neonatal services within a region is dependent upon the availability of both cots and effective patient transport. Transfer of the pregnant woman or her infant is commonplace but within the current service the destination of any transfer cannot be determined with any certainty, as beds are often unavailable at the natural referral centre. Part of the drive to reconfigure services is to remove this lottery.

The relative merits of in utero and postnatal transfer for care require careful consideration. Studies comparing the results of each all have an inherent bias, as the need for intensive care or ventilation cannot be predicted before birth and postnatal transfer will generally be for ongoing ventilator care, although some babies may die before transfer can be effected. Thus a true study on unselected populations is almost impossible to achieve. Nonetheless, within well-centralised systems, with often independent transport services such as in the USA (Bowen 2002) and Australia (Rashid et al. 1999), a more consistent service can be achieved. Even within the UK there is evidence that babies are not placed at significant risk during a well-planned transfer (Leslie and Stephenson 1997, 2003). There are however data that suggest that mortality is increased when transfer is requested but unavailable (Bennett et al. 2002) and babies moved between tertiary centres unable to cope with peaks of demand have poorer outcomes (Parmanum et al. 2000). The key to effective transfer is the establishment of adequate capacity within a clinical network, to allow planned flows of referrals that can be discussed in early pregnancy with all pregnant women.

One study has evaluated the pattern of 'inappropriate transfers' as a measure of the adequacy of capacity in tertiary units (Parmanum et al. 2000). Inappropriate transfers were defined as those out of a perinatal centre. Over 3 months in 1999, 264 in utero transfers and 45 postnatal transfers were recorded in 37 such units. Rates of transfer in each region varied from 0.20 to 5.44 per 1000 live births. The risks and outcomes of these transfers were studied in 242 cases (Bennett et al. 2002). Of in utero transfers, only 61% delivered at the accepting hospital, 12% were moved to a third hospital following delayed delivery and 29% were returned to deliver at their referring hospital. One mother delivered during the journey and nine delivered within 1 hour of arrival. Transfer of mothers and their babies should be a planned process with defined levels of referral and, as far as possible, guaranteed capacity at the natural referral centres.

In utero transfers

It is important to distinguish the urgency with which mothers are referred for specialist care, usually because of impending prematurity, from more elective transfers for expert assessment of fetal malformation or growth restriction. There must be close liaison between both obstetric and the receiving neonatal team before any decision to move a woman is undertaken. The presence of vaginal bleeding, pre-eclampsia or labour and the obstetric history of the woman must be carefully weighed against the need for transfer. Where urgent transfer can be effected safely this must be the best mode of transfer, as both mother and baby will be cared for in the same centre, separation avoided and the baby will be exposed to minimised postnatal risk. However there is a chance of delivery during the journey and a risk of other unforeseen problems, and not infrequently women are moved before birth because of a risk of early delivery and do not deliver. Many services attempt to stratify risk by the use of fetal fibronectin (Bolt et al. 2009) or Actim Partus (Balic et al. 2008) screening, as adjuncts to the diagnosis of preterm labour, in an attempt to avoid unnecessary transfer.

Postnatal transfers

In most areas of the UK, postnatal transfer services initially developed on an ad hoc basis. There are now formalised transport teams in most networks and competencies for staff have been identified (Ch. 13.2). Quality standards for neonatal transfers have been published (Report of the Neonatal Intensive Care Services Review 2009). In the past, such transfers were deemed 'flying squads', where a rapid emergency response team travelled rapidly to support the local team in early-care scenarios. With improvements in care and expertise at local hospitals it should be possible to effect elective transfers at a time that is clinically appropriate for the baby, although robust arrangements need to be put in place for dealing with emergencies arising in units without on-site specialist neonatal staff. No network transport service in the UK currently provides support to standalone midwifery-led units or to home births, where midwives are reliant on calling for help via the standard emergency ambulance service using 999. A centralised service has been shown to be effective in reducing waiting times and quality markers (Kempley et al. 2007).

Relationship of organisational factors to outcome

Given the stress placed above on the structure to support neonatal care, one would anticipate that care organised according to such principles clearly leads to better outcomes. Within the UK system this is far from clear. Several attempts to investigate this relationship have been undertaken. The relationship between organisational issues and mortality is the easiest to undertake but, given the decrease in mortality over the past 10 years, death is a relatively rare event and thus small differences in mortality are more difficult to demonstrate. Furthermore large tertiary units treat a different range of babies from those managed in local services and tend to be overcrowded, with high occupancy rates, and are more likely to be understaffed. Smaller units may also transfer out sick babies soon after birth and the mortality will be attributed to the receiving unit. The complexity of these issues makes it extremely difficult to draw conclusions from comparisons.

Studies of regional outcomes for mixed hospital groups have shown inconsistent effects. In the late 1980s mortality was higher for babies cared for in smaller units in the Trent region of the UK than for babies cared for in larger units. This longitudinal study was reanalysed in the early 1990s following an NHS reorganisation and then demonstrated no difference in mortality by size of unit (Field and Draper 1999). This was ascribed to enhancements in neonatal provision at local hospitals, but clearly the relationship is more complex than that.

Scoring systems for neonatal illness provide one way of correcting for case mix, making adjustment for the illness severity measure when comparing outcomes. The use of such measures is established in paediatric and adult critical care services. In neonatal care the two most frequently used scoring systems are SNAP (Richardson et al. 1993) (plus SNAP-II and SNAPPE-II; Richardson et al. 2001) and CRIB (The International Neonatal Network 1993; Parry et al. 2003), although there are others. Care should be taken when using these measures, as they do not attempt to predict outcome for an individual but are scoring systems describing the clinical condition so that some adjustment between outcomes in a population can be made (Hope 1995; Marlow 2002). These scores require regular review and updating as techniques and interventions change. For example, a tertiary unit that uses delivery-room surfactant or early high-frequency oscillatory ventilation may appear to have low severity of illness scores (based on oxygenation) but similar mortality to other units because the gestational age of the babies cared for is lower. Hence the score itself may partly reflect the care given as much as the underlying characteristics of the baby, i.e. the score may itself be an outcome variable for perinatal care (Marlow 2002).

CRIB originally included data from worst base deficit and highest and lowest inspired oxygen concentrations over the first 12 hours, making it particularly sensitive to changes in early interventions. In contrast, CRIB-II uses temperature on admission and maximal base deficit over the first hour as the clinical variables, which, together with sex, gestational age and birthweight, provide the basis for the score (Fig. 2.2). Using this recently validated model with a high degree of predictive value for mortality (area under the receiver operating characteristic curve: 0.92) in an analysis of the data collected as part of the UK Neonatal Staffing Study, CRIB-II-adjusted mortality did not differ between large and small units in the UK (odds ratio (OR) 1.06; 95% confidence interval (CI) 0.70–1.60) (Tucker 2002).

Nonetheless, corrections for disease severity can provide useful information concerning the relative performance of neonatal services to facilitate the identification of areas for investigation and throw up intriguing questions when applied to cross-national (International Neonatal Network et al. 2000; Field et al. 2002) or national comparisons (Parry et al. 1998). For example, risk-adjusted mortality appears to be significantly higher in Scotland than in England or Australia (International Neonatal Network et al. 2000). The question is raised as to whether this relates to organisation of care, being highly centralised in Australia and devolved in the UK. Caution is required when interpreting these studies as the ethnic, social and demographic profiles of any population may account for more of the variance in outcomes than the perinatal services and the obvious difference, i.e. organisation, may be confounded by population differences. This is emphasised by a further comparison of outcome for babies born at <28 weeks of gestation or <1000 g birthweight between the Trent region of the UK and Denmark (Field et al. 2002). Births in this group were more prevalent in Trent and, despite a higher use of antenatal steroid, babies had higher CRIB scores, received more mechanical ventilation and were more likely to die than those in the Danish population.

The UK Neonatal Staffing Study randomly selected 54 of 186 units in the UK to study the relationship between throughput, consultant and nurse staffing and outcome as mortality, cerebral damage as detected by ultrasound and nosocomial infection (Tucker

The maximum (worst) score for birthweight and gestation is 15, which is obtained for a 22 week male infant of less than 501g birthweight

Male infants

Birthweight (g)	22	23	24	25	26	27	28	29	30	31	32
2751 to 3000											0
2501 to 2750										1	0
2251 to 2500								3	0	0	
2001 to 2250								2	0	0	
1751 to 2000						6	5	3	2	1	0
1501 to 1750			8	6	5	3	3	2	1		
1251 to 1500		12	10	9	8	7	6	5	4	3	3
1001 to 1250		12	11	10	8	7	7	6	6	6	6
751 to 1000	14	13	12	11	10	9	8	8	8		
501 to 750	15	14	13	12	11	10	10				
251 to 500											

Gestational male infants (weeks)

Female infants

Birthweight (g)	22	23	24	25	26	27	28	29	30	31	32
2751 to 3000											0
2501 to 2750										1	0
2251 to 2500								2	0	0	
2001 to 2250								1	0	0	
1751 to 2000						6	4	3	1	0	0
1501 to 1750				7	5	4	3	2	1	1	
1251 to 1500		11	10	8	7	6	5	4	3	3	3
1001 to 1250		11	10	9	8	7	6	5	5	5	5
751 to 1000	13	12	11	10	9	8	8	7	7	7	
501 to 750	14	13	12	11	10	10	10				
251 to 500											

Gestational female infants (weeks)

Temperature at admission (°C)		Base excess (mmol/l):	
≤29.6	5	<−26	7
29.7 to 31.2	4	−26 to −23	6
31.3 to 32.8	3	−22 to −18	5
32.9 to 34.4	2	−17 to −13	4
34.5 to 36	1	−12 to −8	3
36.1 to 37.5	0	−7 to −3	2
37.6 to 39.1	1	−2 to 2	1
39.2 to 40.7	2	≥3	0
≥40.8	3		

Sex, birthweight (g) and gestation (weeks): _____
Temperature at admission (°C): _____
Base excess (mmol/l): _____

Total CRIB-II score [   ]

The logistic regression equation relating CRIB-II mortality (CRIB-II algorithm) is:
Log odds of mortality = $G = -6.476 + 0.450 \times CRIB\text{-}II$
Probability of mortality = $\exp(G)/[1 + \exp(G)]$
The range of possible CRIB-II scores is 0 to 27

Fig. 2.2 Calculation matrix for clinical risk index for babies (CRIB-II). *(Reproduced with permission from Parry et al. (2003).)*

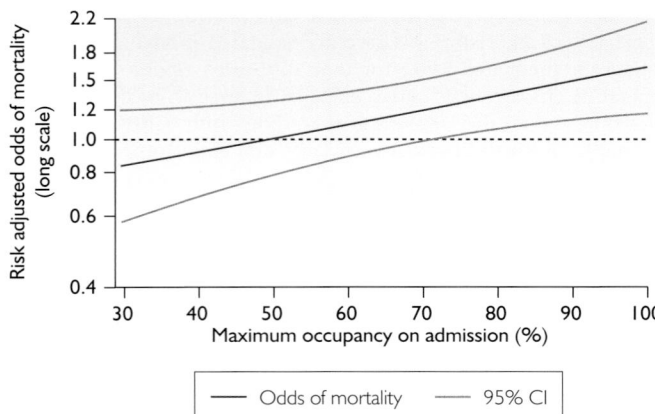

Fig. 2.3 Relationship of risk-adjusted odds of mortality and unit occupancy on day of admission. *(Reproduced with permission from Parry et al. (2003).)*

2002). Data from 13 334 babies were used. High-volume NICUs, treating the sickest babies, had the highest crude mortality but this difference disappeared when risk adjustment was made. However there were important findings relating the risk of dying to the staffing levels on the shift during which a baby was admitted. Babies admitted to a unit working at full capacity were 50% more likely to die than babies admitted to a unit working at 50% capacity (Fig. 2.3). The British Association of Perinatal Medicine (BAPM) has commented that this may be attributable to a number of factors, including inadequate staffing and change of case mix as workload increases. It is crucial that staffing levels and expertise are appropriate to the dependency of the babies.

In a further epidemiological study from the USA, there appeared to be an optimal relationship between neonatologist staffing and mortality (Goodman et al. 2002). The numbers of neonatologists and numbers of cots (expressed in quintiles from the distribution) were related to national statistics of neonatal deaths (in the first 28 days). On average there were 6.2 neonatologists, 33.7 intensive care cots and 17.7 high-dependency cots per 10 000 births. There was lower neonatal mortality where there were 4.8 neonatologists per 10 000 births than with 2.7/10 000 births (OR for death 0.93; 95% CI: 0.88–0.99) but increasing the number above this level did not result in further improvements. Furthermore the availability of neonatal cots was not related to mortality risk and the need for cots (as expressed by the number of babies with birthweight <1501 g) did not relate to cot availability. This must be placed in contrast to the calculated requirement of 10–19 intensive care cots per 10 000 UK births (see above).

In the current EPICure 2 study of births at 26 completed weeks of gestation or less in England during 2006, a time when the network model had become reasonably well established, it was apparent that survival for livebirths in this gestational group was higher overall in NICU services (59%) than in local neonatal units (51%) before (OR 1.51; 95% CI 1.16–1.98) and after adjustment for gestational age and birthweight (OR 1.60; 95% CI (1.17–2.19)). This advantage held when only those babies admitted were included, and this trend was also obvious among smaller and larger NICU services (OR survival livebirths 1.43; 95% CI 1.01–2.01), mainly because of higher survival at 23 and 24 weeks, respectively (EPICure 2 study group unpublished data).

The relationship between organisational factors and simple outcome measures is therefore far from clear but sides on larger services with higher staffing ratios have better outcomes in terms of survival. In the UK it is incumbent on each managed clinical network to ascertain and monitor the availability of cots and staff, and access for its residents to the service when required, and to benchmark these services against other national data.

Philosophy of care and survival

Mortality at low gestations has improved over the past 20 years such that the great majority of babies born at 26 weeks of gestation or more now survive. Attitudes to the resuscitation and continuing care of babies born at lower gestational ages will thus have a profound effect on the rates of survival and thus confound comparisons of different services. These attitudes vary widely across the world. For example, at a time when care was unusual at 24 weeks in the Netherlands, in the UK we were demonstrating about 35% survival at 23–24 weeks and both national studies from Sweden (EXPRESS) (Fellman et al. 2009; EXPRESS Group 2010) and Australia and New Zealand (Donoghue and the ANZNN Executive 2009) report 50% survival for babies admitted for neonatal care (Fig. 2.4). However, the rates of serious neonatal and later morbidity remain very high in these survivors and cannot be ignored (Fellman et al. 2009) and wide variation in the approach to discontinuing care may distort survival further given that so many babies have elective discontinuation of care (Costeloe et al. 2000).

The extent of the differences brought about by extremes of practice was explored by Lorenz and colleagues (2001), who demonstrated marked differences in survival and prevalence of cerebral palsy in two studies with widely differing approaches to outcome (Ch. 3). Indeed, in the UK, regional centres with a proactive approach to the care of extremely low-gestational-age babies report survival at similar levels for babies born at 23 and 24 weeks to the highly centralised Swedish national data (Riley et al. 2008). Without a detailed study of the approach to care at these extremely low gestations the reasons for these differences cannot be explored and it would be incorrect to attribute them to quality of care.

Service evaluation

Clinical governance is the framework in which we as professionals ensure that our care is accountable to our patients and to our host institutions. There is a range of schemes for this and this section

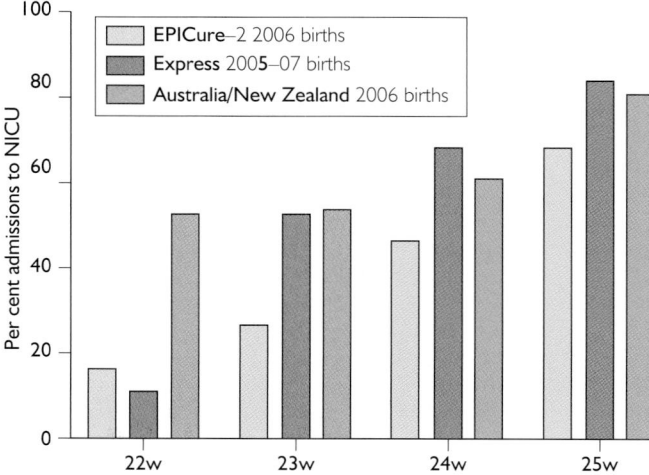

Fig. 2.4 Comparison of survival for babies born at 22–25 weeks admitted for neonatal intensive care in three contemporary studies (note that the small number of 22-week survivors (*n*) accounts for variation in survival rate, and that current UK guidance does not support universal intervention at 23 weeks).

will focus on those applicable to perinatal care under the following headings:

- the clinical governance philosophy
- clinical audit
- standards, guidelines and perinatal audit tools
- benchmarking and evidence-based care.

The clinical governance philosophy

Medical audit was promoted in 1989 by the UK government as a means of protecting the interests of patients in the then new health market, but audit and quality assurance were not new developments. It rapidly became clear that the performance of many services was based upon access and availability, or the personal style directed by consultants, rather than evidence-based practice. The concept was widened to clinical audit, involving multidisciplinary teams, and achieved some limited success. Neonatal and perinatal care provides a prime example of areas of truly multidisciplinary practice where collaboration must occur between doctors, nurses, midwives and other professional groups for a successful service to evolve.

Clinical audit gradually evolved into the wider concept of clinical governance in the late 1990s. The most widely used definition of clinical governance is 'a framework through which NHS organisations are accountable for continually improving the quality of their services and safeguarding high standards of care by creating an environment in which excellence in clinical care will flourish' (Scally and Donaldson 1998). Thus this is designed to introduce a systematic approach to the delivery of NHS care, in which there is corporate accountability for clinical quality and performance. The essential features of the process are not deniable:

- patient-centred care
- widely available information about the quality of care
- reduction in the variations of process, outcomes and access to care
- reduction in risks and hazards to patients
- widespread dissemination and adoption of good and research-based practice.

The key to the delivery of this process is reliable and comprehensive information about the service, something which has been sadly lacking in the NHS. Indeed, the reforms of the mid-1990s may be likened to an experiment without defined outcome measures (Maynard and Bloor 1996). The more recent reforms have increased reporting centrally and hence central control over services which have exacerbated the difficulties of running acute services with unpredictable workloads. The formation of managed clinical networks (see above) should help to resolve some of these issues.

The clinical audit process

Audit is defined as 'an evaluation (esp. by formal, systematic review) of the effectiveness of the management, working practices, and procedures of a company or other professional body' (Oxford English Dictionary 1989).

The key to the audit process is the setting of standards and the appraisal of the clinical service against those standards. This is often assembled into what is commonly called the audit cycle (Fig. 2.5). Standards may be set nationally, regionally or locally and may evaluate three major aspects of care:

1. the structure of the service
2. the process of care
3. the outcome of care or the result of clinical intervention.

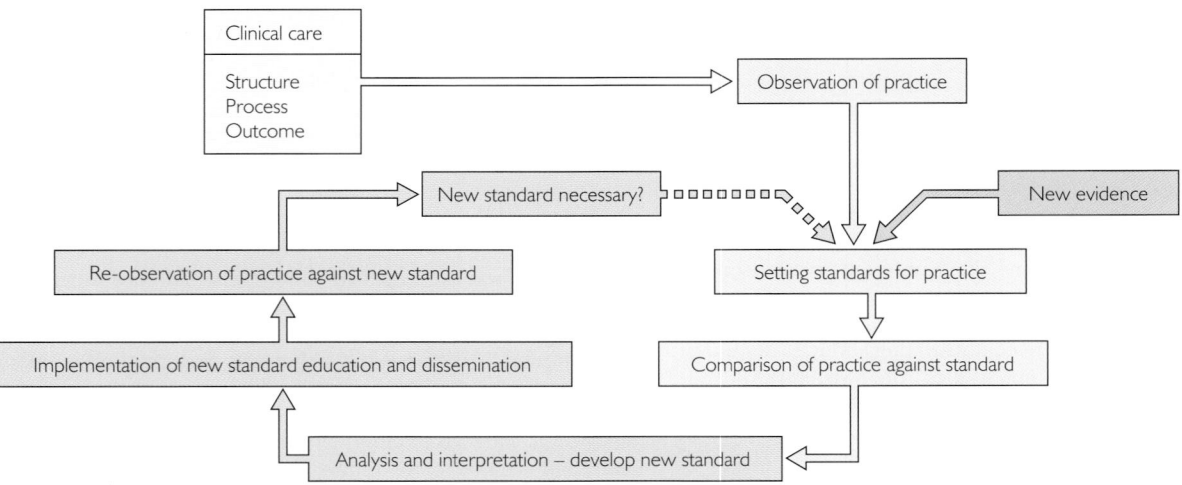

Fig. 2.5 The audit cycle. The cycle commences with the observation of practice and the integration of new evidence into the setting of standards and is completed when a new standard is re-evaluated to confirm the effectiveness of changes in clinical care.

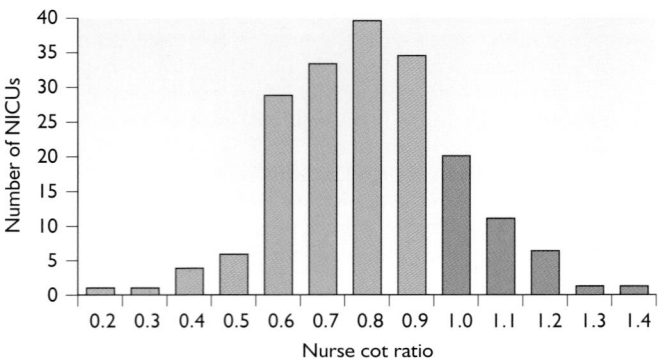

Fig. 2.6 Appropriateness of nursing establishments in all UK neonatal units (actual/recommended numbers of nurses from published standards – lighter bars denote units with lower establishments than required). *(Reproduced with permission from Tucker et al. (1999).)*

The structure of care

This is concerned with the quantity and type of resources and how they are used, for example the number and experience of medical nursing or paramedical staff or the availability of cots. These data are relatively simple to collect and are usually accurate. Standards are produced nationally (see below) and these data can be powerful in the process of bidding for resources. For example, the shortage of neonatal nursing staff was emphasised in the UK Neonatal Staffing Study (Fig. 2.6), which is an example of a national audit of the structure of care.

Audit of structure by itself can only demonstrate potential areas where services may be inadequate and does not form a measure of quality of care until it is matched with patient-based information when it merges with the two other areas of audit. Structural deficiencies may provide one explanation for poor results found during process or outcome audit.

The process of care

The process of care may be considered in three ways:

1. the way patients progress through the system – examples would be admission and discharge procedures, the recording of clinical data in the patient notes and the recording of communication with parents
2. the way particular resources are used – examples would be attendance at delivery by appropriate levels of staff, occupancy and case mix studies and the use of transitional care facilities
3. the way particular conditions are managed – examples here relate to particular admission criteria, diagnostic groups or to interventions. In this area evidence-based practice may be introduced into care via the development of guidelines.

An example of a nationally based audit of the care process is provided by the joint venture between the Royal College of Paediatrics and Child Health (RCPCH), BAPM and Royal College of Ophthalmologists. Standards for screening and treatment of retinopathy of prematurity were issued in 1995. Subsequently a nationwide education programme was undertaken followed by an audit of cases registered as requiring treatment and new guidelines were issued (Haines et al. 2005; Wilkinson et al. 2008).

The outcome of care

The outcome of care (or the result of interventions) provides the final arbiter of success for a service and includes important mortality and morbidity measures. Outcomes may relate to the child (occurrence of death, complications of treatment or longer term neurological development), the parent (satisfaction, breastfeeding rates) or the staff (recruitment, retention, levels of competency or ability to perform procedures).

Mortality rates are clearly defined (Table 2.2), widely available and many are collated nationally (Table 2.3 and Fig. 2.7) or regionally. Although these data offer the opportunity to set local targets and review local performance, extreme care should be exercised in their interpretation as they may be subject to random variation owing to small numbers and systematic variation in methodology of collection. Correction for illness severity has been recommended as a way of avoiding some of these problems (see above).

Choosing outcome measures for specific audit is fraught with difficulty. Outcomes need to be specific, measurable and relevant. For example, babies who receive pulmonary vasodilators to reverse pulmonary hypertension may be audited on their response to treatment, in terms of oxygenation over the period of use and immediately afterwards, but to use duration of ventilation or longer term outcomes (e.g. neurodevelopment) would be inappropriate as

Table 2.2 Perinatal definitions

Livebirth	Baby with signs of life observed after complete expulsion from the mother irrespective of the duration of the pregnancy (signs of life include breathing, heart beat, cord pulsation or voluntary movement)
Stillbirth (or late fetal death)	Fetal death prior to complete delivery of a baby born after the 24th week of pregnancy (168 days after the first day of the last menstrual period (LMP))
Abortion	A conceptus born without signs of life before the end of the 24th week of pregnancy (<168 days after LMP)
Birthweight	The first weight of a fetus or newborn baby obtained after birth (preferably within the first hour after birth)
Gestational age	The duration of gestation measured from the first day of the LMP expressed in completed weeks and days (note that gestational age is never rounded up and thus a baby born at 24 weeks and 6 days is usually considered to be of '24 weeks gestational age')
Preterm	Birth at less than 37 weeks of gestation (<259 days after LMP)
Term	From 37 to 42 completed weeks of gestation (259–293 days after LMP)
Postterm	More than 42 weeks (>293 days after LMP)
The neonatal period	The first 28 days after delivery
Lethal congenital malformation	Death primarily due to congenital malformation

Table 2.3 Total births and deaths for England and Wales 2006 by causes of stillbirth, neonatal and infant death

CAUSE GROUP	BIRTHS		DEATHS			ALL INFANT DEATHS
	Livebirths	Stillbirths	Early neonatal	Neonatal	Postneonatal	
All causes	690013	3598	1716	2207	982	3189
Congenital anomalies		557	413	595	362	957
Antepartum infections		31	33	64	6	70
Immaturity			1026	1241	187	1428
Asphyxia, anoxia, trauma		91	204	224	8	232
External conditions		7	2	6	43	49
Infections			10	26	97	123
Other specific conditions		2	13	19	24	43
Antepartum asphyxia		912				–
Remaining antepartum deaths		1732				–
Sudden infant deaths			3	11	144	155
Other conditions		66	12	21	111	132
(Adapted from Office of National Statistics data: www.statistics.gov.uk.)						

many other things determine these outcomes. The only way to determine the effect of vasodilators on these outcomes is within a randomised controlled trial where comparison groups are tightly matched.

Services should regularly monitor quality aspects of care and it is recommended that these are published as an annual report. Ideally these data would be collated on a regional or national basis and there are excellent examples of this (Fig. 2.8). The minimal content of an annual report has been defined (British Association of Perinatal Medicine 1996) and should also include the monitoring of the rates of disability in defined groups of survivors (see Ch. 3 and Fig. 3.4).

The audit cycle

The audit cycle (Fig. 2.5) comprises a series of processes needed to integrate the results of audit into clinical practice. The identification of topics for audit may be defined within the neonatal team in

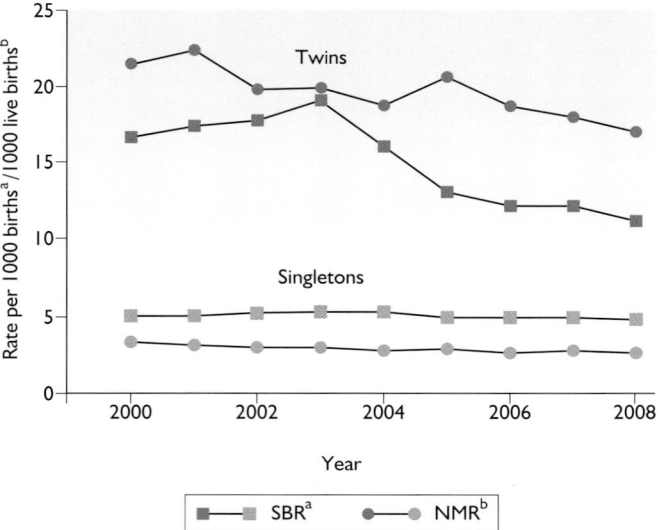

Fig. 2.7 Stillbirths and neonatal death rates 2000–2008 for singletons and twin births in England, Wales, Northern Ireland and crown dependencies. *(Data from Centre for Maternal and Child Enquiries (2010).)*

response to an observation that prompts the initiation of the investigation or the topic may be identified by health commissioners (mortality and disability rates) or regionally/nationally. The American Academy of Pediatrics issues regular statements of policy or guidance that may form the basis for audit. In the UK the medical Royal Colleges have established audit groups and formulate guidance in the specialty. Within neonatology both the RCPCH (www.rcpch.ac.uk – Clinical Effectiveness) and Royal College of Obstetricians and Gynaecologists (www.rcog.org.uk – Good Practice) produce guidance of relevance to neonatal practice, but globally within the UK there are few national neonatal guidelines.

Despite huge investment by the NHS, audit has not won the hearts and minds of many doctors. Part of this is the failure to understand the importance of a scientific base to the collection, analysis and interpretation of audit data, which is as important in the audit process as it is in research. Appropriate support for audit is often not available locally, in terms of either staffing levels or expertise, but investment in the clinical governance process has improved the situation widely over the past 5 years. Correctly supported and executed, audit may make an important contribution to the success of a neonatal service.

Much audit is achieved by examining medical case records. Ideally prospective data collection should be established as variations in recording information may render the audit dataset incomplete. Retrospective audit from case notes should recognise its limitations but it remains an important part of the process. Problems that occur in retrospective and (to a lesser extent) in prospective audit data collection are:

- bias due to poor diagnostic coding
- bias in record retrieval (difficulty in identifying cases, particularly if they have died)
- bias relating to sample size
- reliability of audit data (e.g. variation in recording or definition between patients and errors in filing of investigation results in notes)
- bias due to missing information
- inadequate capture of 'non-routine' data to be used in audit
- case mix and comorbidity

- inability to assess qualitative aspects of care: timeliness, coordination, empathic components and appropriateness.

A good audit design will address these deficiencies in the planning stage and thereby avoid major errors. It will also include and involve staff from outside the immediate neonatal team, who are critical to its success. Once the results are available the critical decision is which of the (any) changes in management that flow from the audit are to be effected. The line of action and responsibility for implementation should be carefully addressed. Financial consequences of audit/changes in practice must be identified and early managerial involvement in implementation is clearly crucial to the success of a project. Medical and nursing education and training for staff in support services must include the development of skills in the audit process.

Finally the audit cycle is a continuous loop: once an audit is complete and the recommendations implemented further audit should be planned to ensure the success of these changes.

Benchmarking

A 'benchmark' was originally a surveying mark placed to allow repeated measurements using a levelling staff; it is thus a point of reference, criterion or touchstone (Oxford English Dictionary 1989). The process of assessing the structure, process or outcome of a service against an externally derived standard is often termed 'benchmarking', in contrast to audit, which is carried out in response to locally derived standards. In effect they are similar processes carried out to different reference points.

Within the professional neonatal community a range of initiatives are designed to benchmark performance against that of other services, regional/network-based groups (e.g. the Trent Neonatal Survey; the Thames Perinatal Group Accreditation Scheme), national initiatives (e.g. the National Neonatal Audit: http://www.rcpch.ac.uk/Research/ce/Clinical-Audit/NNAP) or internationally, using schemes such as the Vermont Oxford Network (www.vtoxford.org) or EuroNeoNet (www.euroneostat.org). One advantage of such schemes is that ongoing benchmarking can identify areas for service improvement strategies, in initiatives such as the Vermont Oxford Network NICQ and the UK National Patient Safety Agency Safer Neonatal Practice programmes (www.nrls.npsa.nhs.uk/resources/clinical-specialty/paediatrics-and-child-health).

Other aspects of clinical governance

Like medical audit, there is a danger that clinical governance will be applied 'top-down' and therefore become irrelevant to many of the staff. Over recent years several hospitals across the UK have encouraged the development of shared governance – a system of encouraging ownership, widening involvement and engagement. With its origins in the US health community, there are several models which have evolved (Burnhope and Edmonstone 2003). Although this is often seen as a nursing development 'which seeks to grant nursing staff control over their professional practice and develop and make a genuine contribution to the wider corporate agenda' (Gavin et al. 1999), the principles can and probably should be extended to multidisciplinary teams such as those that work in neonatal care. Retention and recruitment of nursing staff can be materially enhanced by the inclusion of all grades of staff, enhancing acceptance of responsibility for the service, improving communication and respecting time spent in developing the shared governance process. This process demands a fundamental reappraisal of neonatal teams and is not a 'quick fix' or panacea to aid a failing system.

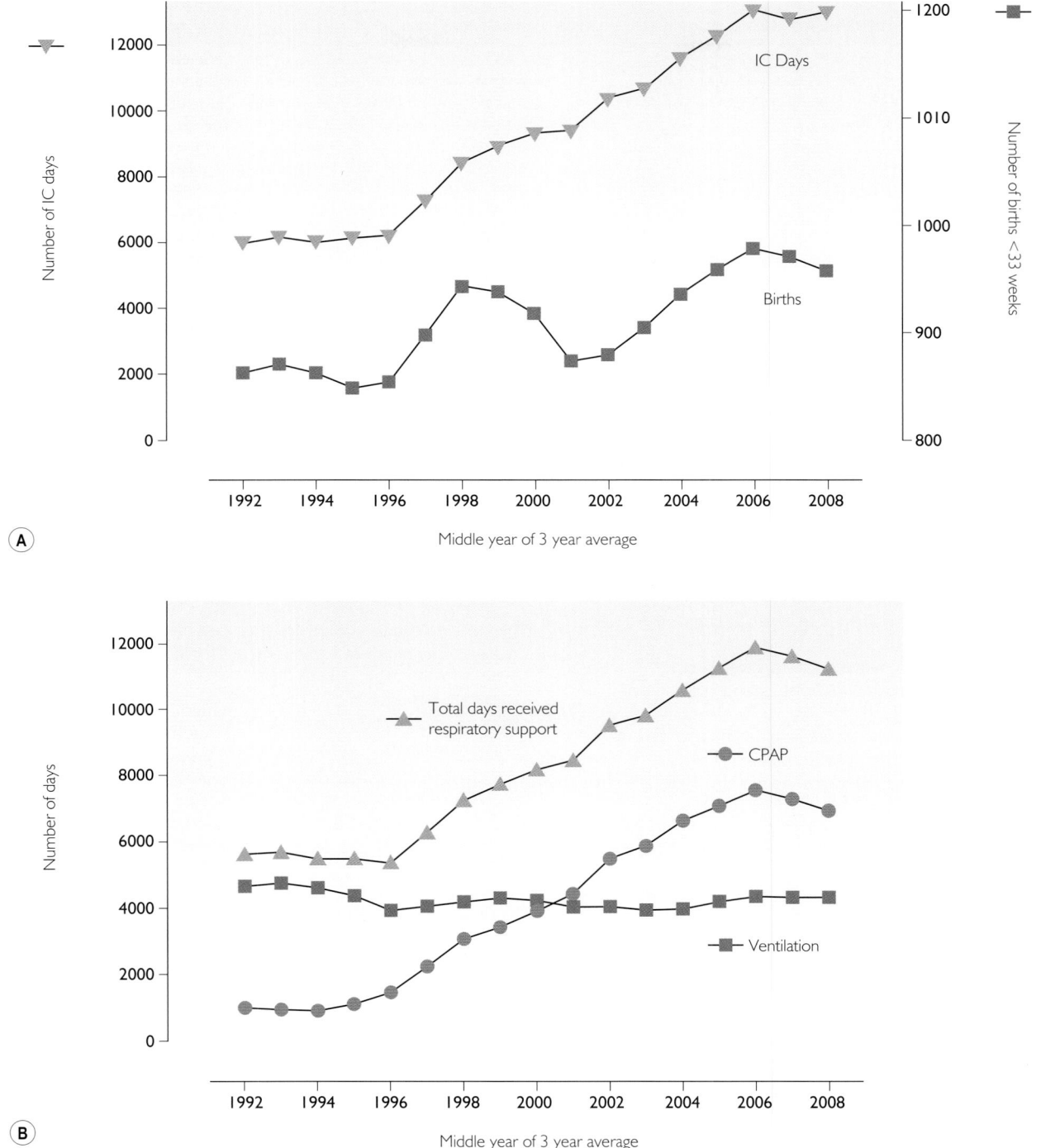

Fig. 2.8 Trent neonatal data.

In a UK health service increasingly driven by elective targets, clinical governance provides a method by which acute services can ensure that their configuration and resources are not passed by. NHS trusts have widely accepted a risk management approach and this needs to be stated and addressed or accepted by the corporate structure. Increasingly, neonatal care is being addressed by a range of corporate agenda such as corporate benchmarking, meeting of standards to minimise the risk of litigation and standard pricing. External reviews of service by NHS-sponsored bodies, such as the Audit Commission, the Clinical Standards Advisory Group, the Department of Health External Review Group and Neonatal Taskforce (Report of the Neonatal Intensive Care Services Review 2009), have been regularly published over the past 10 years. The effect that these initiatives have on the delivery of neonatal care remains to be seen.

Box 2.2 Examples of family-friendly standards for the neonatal intensive care unit

Where admission to a neonatal unit is predicted, a prenatal opportunity to visit the neonatal unit and meet key personnel should be offered to the family

All parents should be introduced to facilities, routines, staff and equipment on admission to a neonatal unit

Every parent should have unrestricted access to his or her baby, unless individual restrictions can be justified in the baby's best interest

Parents should be encouraged and supported to participate in decision-making about the care and treatment of their baby. Written and regularly updated care plans should be shared with parents. Clinical care decisions, including end-of-life decisions, should be made by experienced staff in partnership with the parents and discussions held in an appropriate setting

Parents are encouraged and supported to participate in their baby's care at the earliest opportunity, including:

Regular skin-to-skin care

Providing comforting touch, comfort holding, particularly during painful procedures

Feeding

Day-to-day care, such as nappy changing

Every baby should be treated with dignity and respect:

Appropriate positioning is promoted and encouraged

Clinical interventions are managed to minimise stress, avoid pain and conserve energy

Noise and light levels are managed to minimise stress

Appropriate clothing is used at all times, taking into account parents' choice

Privacy is respected and promoted as appropriate to the baby's condition

All parents will have the opportunity to discuss their baby's diagnosis and care with a senior clinician within 24 hours following admission or a significant change in condition

Written information should be available (in languages and formats appropriate to the local community) to all users of the service on medical and surgical treatments, to permit early and effective communication with parents covering at least:

Condition/diagnosis

Treatment options available

Likely outcomes/benefits of treatment

Possible complications/risks

Possible tests and investigations

Whom to contact with queries or for advice

Where to go for further information, including useful websites

Circumstances requiring consent (written and verbal)

Maternity and neonatal services should encourage breastfeeding and the expression of milk through the provision of information and dedicated support, including:

Whenever possible, initiation of breastfeeding as soon as possible after birth

When necessary, support to start expression as soon after delivery as the mother's condition allows to maximise the benefit of colostrum

The availability of a comfortable, dedicated and discreet area

The facility to express discreetly at the cotside

The availability of breast pumps and associated equipment for every mother who requires them

Supporting breastfeeding as part of the discharge process

Promotion of safe and hygienic handling and storage of breast milk

Possible availability of donor breast milk

(Adapted from Report of the Neonatal Intensive Care Services Review (2009). A Toolkit for Quality Neonatal Services. Department of Health and the Bliss Baby Charter Standards, London. (2009))

Standards and perinatal audit tools

Standards

How do we know that our neonatal services are performing well? This may be done through two main processes – firstly, information is collected about the service and, secondly, a set of quality indicators is used to check that we are performing to a standard. Actually, this is done in reverse, as, once an indicator is defined, the data are then collected to demonstrate performance, or the data collected may not be appropriate. Neonatal services are also expected to be evaluated against a range of local professional health organisation standards, such as record-keeping, as are all other hospital-based areas, but here we consider specific neonatal standards.

The first quality standards for NIC in the UK were published in 1996 and updated in 2001. Where possible statements were based on published evidence but it was recognised that for many none existed. Detailed recommendations covered service size, medical and nurse staffing, support staff, equipment, audit and continuing education within neonatal care. As part of a new Department of Health and NHS initiative, the Neonatal Taskforce, these were redeveloped using a much broader stakeholder base, including parent groups, and are published as an appendix to the *Toolkit for High Quality Neonatal Services* (Report of the Neonatal Intensive Care

Services Review 2009). In this are defined principles or characteristics of a quality service, including organisation, staffing, care of the baby and family experience, transfers, professional competence, education and training, neonatal surgery, clinical governance and data requirements. These are further supported by a revision of the professional standards (British Association of Perinatal Medicine 2010) and have been distilled as National Institute for Health and Clinical Excellence (NICE) *Quality Standards* (NICE 2010). As these reports have only recently been produced it is too early to tell how they will drive service development but for the first time in the UK we have a set of standards that are agreed between service users, providers and managers. An example of standards for family-friendly care is shown in Box 2.2.

Definitions – mortality and morbidity

Conventionally, birthweight is subdivided into low birthweight (LBW: <2501 g), very low birthweight (VLBW: <1501 g) and extremely low birthweight (ELBW: <1001 g). Similar groupings are often used for preterm gestations but there is little agreement as to the definition of very preterm (birth at either ≤30 weeks or ≤32

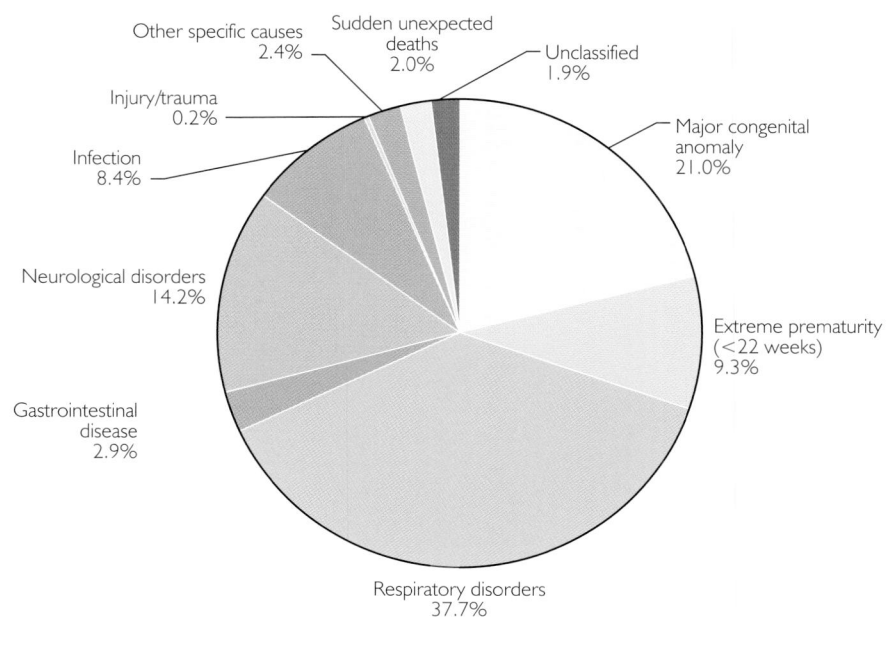

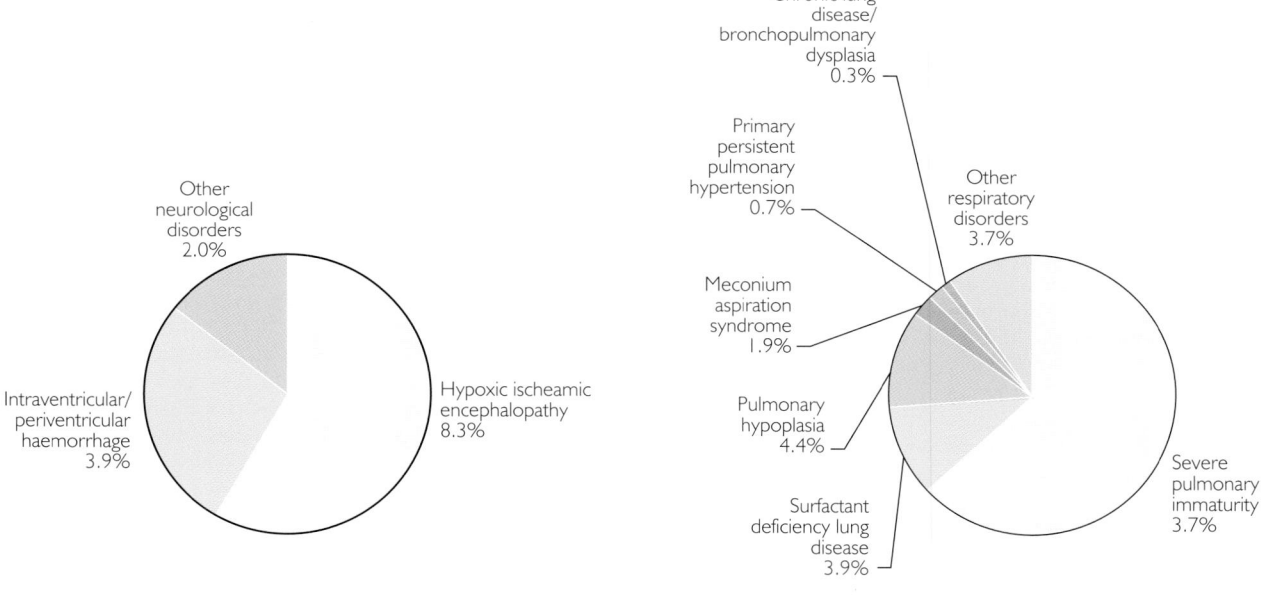

Neurological disorders   **Respiratory disorders**

Fig. 2.9 Primary cause for neonatal deaths 2006 using the Centre for Maternal and Child Enquiries neonatal classification, England and Wales, Northern Ireland and crown dependencies 2008. *(Redrawn from Centre for Maternal and Child Enquiries Perinatal Mortality to 2008. Centre for Maternal and Child Enquiries 2010, London)*

weeks) or extremely preterm (usually birth at 25 or less weeks of gestation). These broad categories are based on risk of death and perinatal complications.

Definition of the causes of perinatal and infant death may help to understand the relationship between specific causes and developments in healthcare. One such classification is that proposed by Wigglesworth, which has been used to classify deaths over several years as part of the Confidential Enquiry into Stillbirths and Deaths in Infancy (CESDI), that has been recently modified (Fig. 2.9) (Centre for Maternal and Child Enquiries 2010). Much of the fall in postneonatal infant mortality has been due to a reduction in the proportion of children ascribed to the sudden infant death syndrome (SIDS) category, initially over the 1980s because of improvements in pathological practice and better diagnosis and then during

Box 2.3 International Federation of Gynecology and Obstetrics (FIGO) recommendations for the international collection of perinatal mortality statistics

Data collection

Collect numbers of births ≥500 g birthweight, early and late neonatal deaths (≤28 days) and identify stillbirths and neonatal deaths with lethal malformations or with birthweight <1000 g

Perinatal statistics

Lethal malformation rate per 1000 births

Stillbirth rate (SBR) per 1000 births

Neonatal mortality rate (NMR) per 1000 livebirths (livebirths dying up to and including 28 days after birth)

Perinatal mortality rate (PNMR) per 1000 births (stillbirths plus livebirths dying up to and including 7 days after birth)

Excluding lethal malformations (include all birthweights)

SBR, NMR, PNMR

Excluding lethal malformations and births <1000 g birthweight

SBR, NMR, PNMR

Excluding births <1000 g birthweight (including lethal malformations)

SBR, NMR, PNMR

Table 2.4 World Health Organization international classification of impairments, disabilities and handicaps

Impairment	Any loss or abnormality of psychological, physiological or anatomical structure or function
Disability	Any restriction or lack (resulting from an impairment) of ability to perform an activity in the manner or within the range considered normal for a human being
Handicap	A disadvantage for a given individual, resulting from an impairment or a disability, that limits or prevents the fulfilment of a role that is normal (depending on age, sex and social and cultural factors) for that individual

the 1990s following the observation that prone lying was associated with SIDS (Fleming et al. 1990), alongside intercurrent illness and parental smoking.

The International Federation of Gynecology and Obstetrics (FIGO) and World Health Organization have defined datasets to facilitate international comparison of neonatal and perinatal morbidity (Box 2.3). In particular the definitions and methods of reporting data recommended by FIGO allow correction for major differences in neonatal service provision, presenting the information as totals and then excluding babies with lethal malformations and those of greater than 1000 g birthweight.

Although these classifications are very helpful on an international stage, providing benchmarking for developing health communities, within a highly developed health service mortality and morbidity at lower gestations and weights have become of equal importance.

Mortality and morbidity rates are critically dependent on the definition of the baseline population and reports of poor outcomes must be clear in their definition for their interpretation and comparison with other reports. For example, a report of outcome for very preterm children will have differing mortality rates if only babies who are admitted for intensive care are considered from a report where all liveborn babies are included, as the latter also includes delivery-room deaths and the former may include postnatal transfers. It is important to attribute deaths appropriately to the unit or population from which the infant derived and not to the unit to which they were transferred. In the EPICure study, livebirth at 20–25 completed weeks of gestation was used and the effect of simply using babies who were admitted for neonatal care results in significantly improved survival rates (Wood et al. 2000). However even this is potentially biased due to differences in the classification of a livebirth and probably the most useful starting point is the population of fetuses who have an audible heart beat at the onset of labour or elective delivery. Babies born at or after 26 weeks of gestation rarely die in the delivery room and differences between outcomes based on babies alive at onset of labour, livebirths or admissions for care become less important.

The definition, use and interpretation of longer term morbidity data are discussed in Chapter 3. The use of standardised definitions of disability (Table 3.2) enhances the ability to benchmark outcomes in one population against another and is to be encouraged. Current international definitions (Table 2.4) have undergone re-evaluation to include broader issues of participation and inclusion but for outcome studies these original definitions suffice (Ch. 3). Historically these data have been collected in high-risk populations by neonatal teams but ideally this information should be available from routine systems to provide a global picture of impairment using the Child Health Computer system or local disability registers. In such situations it is clear that the vast majority of impairment and disability in the community occurs in children who were born at or near full term but birthweight or gestational age-specific rates of disability increase as birthweight and gestation fall. Attempts to harness parental or non-clinical assessment to improve data collection have not been entirely successful.

Neonatal data recording

Population data

Statutory registration of birth and death provides an opportunity for universal data collection that may be targeted at information gathering or to provide ongoing data for subsequent healthcare, e.g. child health systems. This provides basic data in terms of gestation at birth, birthweight, sex and survival. In the UK these have been brought together to provide a comprehensive picture of population variation and trends. Standardisation of more detailed data collection is still not achieved across the UK despite initiatives to enhance it. In the smaller population of Scotland, the SMR-11 birth data collection form has provided an excellent source of population-based information. The development of the rapid reporting form for perinatal death by the CESDI has facilitated a range of investigations into perinatal death and presently continues as an important source of information (www.cemach.org.uk) (see below).

Box 2.4 Summary of current recommended British Association for Perinatal Medicine neonatal dataset (2004)

Patient-based data items

Static data items

Name/code of hospital
Mother's NHS number
Postcode of mother's residence at birth
Planned place of delivery at booking
Place of birth
Baby's NHS number
Date and time of birth
Source of admission to the unit
Date and time of admission
Birthweight
Best estimate of gestation at delivery
Sex
Number of fetuses and birth order
Mother received antenatal steroids
Date of discharge, transfer or death
Time of death
Discharge or transfer destination
Whether postmortem performed
Weight at discharge home
Head circumference at discharge home
Tube feeding at discharge home
Oxygen at discharge home
Surfactant therapy
Chest drain for pulmonary air leak
Date of first retinopathy of prematurity (ROP) screen
Treatment for ROP
Cerebral ultrasound (as per local policy)
Hearing screening (as per local policy)
Shunt surgery for hydrocephalus
Surgery for patent ductus arteriosus
Surgery for necrotising enterocolitis

Daily data items (yes/no except daily weight)

Current weight
Endotracheal tube in situ
Treated with nasal continuous positive airway pressure
Recurrent apnoea requiring frequent (more than 5 in 24 hours) interventions
Intra-arterial or central venous (including umbilical) line in situ
Received:
  Supplemental oxygen

Surfactant
Full or partial exchange transfusion
Peritoneal dialysis
Inotrope, pulmonary vasodilator or prostaglandin
One-to-one nursing care
Any parenteral nutrition
Treatment for convulsions

Unit-based data items

Static data items (annual summary)

Number of:
  Consultants with ≥6 neonatal sessions
  ANNP/nurse consultants in the unit
  Support staff (includes senior nurse manager, ward manager, outreach nurses, family care team, quality and research nurses)
Presence of:
  Senior nurse with managerial responsibility
  Nurse responsible for further education
  Family care team available
  Transport service available
  Physiotherapist, speech therapist, dietician, pharmacist available
Other pressures:
  Average (% whole-time equivalent) annual sickness rate
  Percentage own staff on maternity leave

Daily data items

Number of:
  Nurses involved in direct clinical care with a specialty qualification in neonatal care
  Nurses (excluding students) involved in clinical care without speciality
  Nursing students
  Own staff doing extra shifts
  Number extra nurses supplied from agency
Presence of:
  Resident senior house officer or ANNP with sole responsibility to the neonatal unit
  Resident middle-grade cover from a doctor or ANNP
  Middle grade with sole responsibility for the neonatal unit
  Consultant available during the day with sole responsibility to the neonatal unit
  Consultant on call out of hours with sole responsibility to the neonatal unit

ANNP, advanced neonatal nurse practitioner.

High-risk groups

Statutory recording of data concerning the receipt of NIC is the route by which hospitals are reimbursed for their neonatal unit activity in the National Minimum Data Set (NMDS). These data are collected on a daily basis and provide each hospital with a common process audit. Beyond this there is no system for more structured data collection. Most neonatal services now use a common data platform based on the BAPM Neonatal Dataset (www.bapm.org/publications) using one of three systems (Box 2.4). These are

collated in hospital and network reports. As part of the national drive to acquire reliable and useful neonatal data the National Neonatal Audit Project collects a restricted dataset to determine performance to target in several areas of care provision (Watkinson and Davis 2009).

As an example of good practice, the Australian and New Zealand Neonatal Network has collated information from 22 NICUs from 1994 for babies <32 weeks of gestation or <1500 g birthweight (www.usyd.edu.au/cphsr/anznn). All units are part of a highly developed, regionalised system with centralised care and

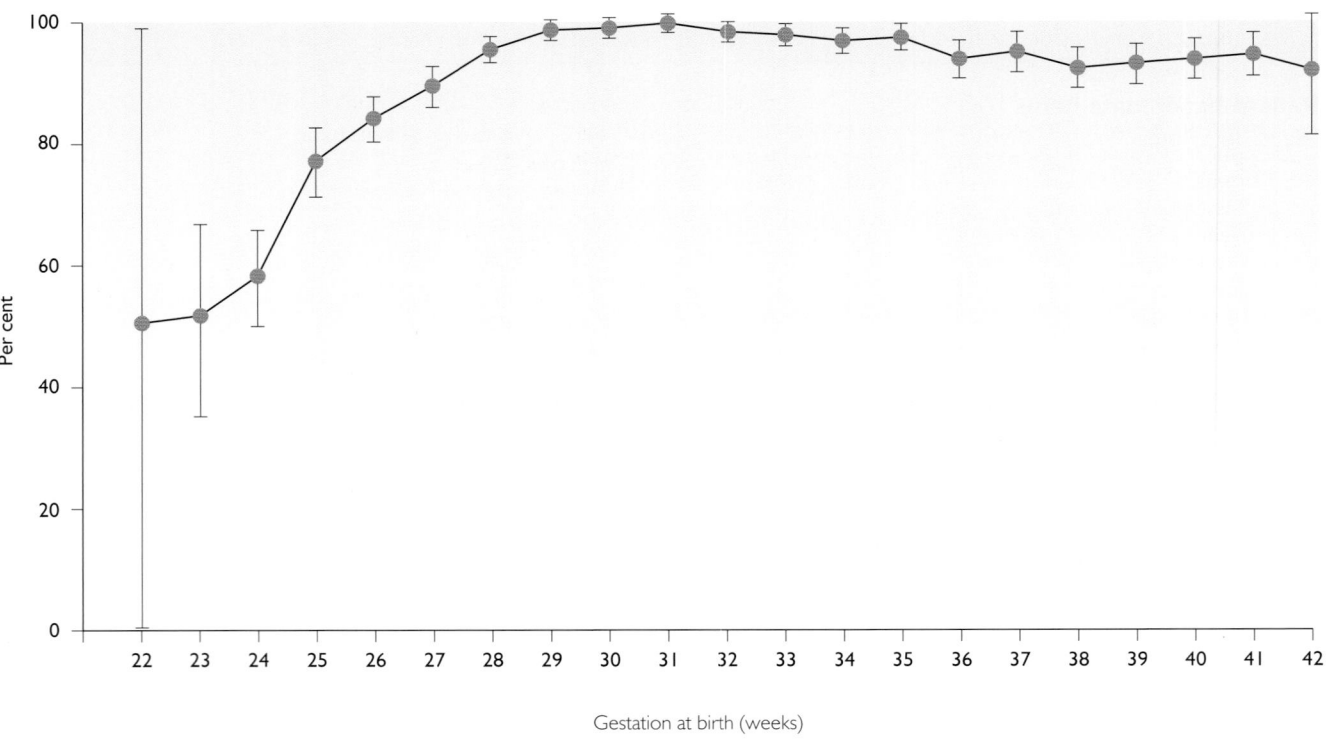

Fig. 2.10 Australia and New Zealand Neonatal Network: survival to discharge by gestational age (with 95% confidence interval). *(Data from Donoghue and the ANZNN Executive (2009).)*

well-organised neonatal retrieval services. In the first report of this collaboration they identified four main objectives:

1. To provide a core dataset that will:
   a. identify trends and variations in mortality and morbidity which warrant further study
   b. enhance the ability to carry out multicentre studies and randomised trials
   c. provide information on neonatal outcomes adjusted for case mix and disease severity to assist with quality improvement.
2. To monitor the use of new technologies.
3. To develop and evaluate a risk score for babies in the network.
4. To develop and assess clinical indicators for perinatal care through neonatal outcomes.

The most recent report (Donoghue and the ANZNN Executive 2009) indicates that most of these aims have been met and that the information provides an excellent set of data against which other neonatal services can be benchmarked. The network also acts as a facilitator for a range of academic activities to ensure that care and outcome continue to improve. The critical mass provided by such collaboration produces narrow confidence intervals for important outcomes (Fig. 2.10).

A further example of international collaboration in this field is the Vermont Oxford Network (www.vtoxford.org). Initially designed to collect and collate patient-based information to facilitate inter-unit comparisons, it now receives data from over 850 neonatal units worldwide and records information on over 50 000 infants, including datasets from over 50% of NICUs in the USA and units in 26 other countries. A smaller international collaboration, EuroPeriStat, is currently evaluating care and implementing quality programmes

in the European Union (www.europeristat.com) as part of an initiative to reduce inequality in outcomes across the European Union.

Guidelines and evidence-based care

Perinatal care is one area of modern medicine which has embraced the concept of the randomised controlled trial and thus in many areas it is possible to base care on secure scientific evidence. The collation of these results has allowed a number of statements to be made about good practice in a wide range of areas, brought together in the Cochrane Collaboration. Neonatal reviews are freely available (www.nichd.nih.gov/cochraneneonatal). Not all areas of practice are however covered by such reviews and clinical practice must take account of a much broader range of evidence and personal experience. Although national and professional bodies may produce guidance for good practice from time to time, clear information is required in the context of the working environment and the local development of guidelines is necessary. The establishment of managed clinical networks poses an opportunity for these to be developed on a network basis, reducing the workload for an individual unit and ensuring a more even delivery of quality care.

Guidelines are not mandatory protocols. Care must be individually tailored to the individual's clinical needs and it may thus be necessary to deviate from unit guidelines if it is deemed necessary in a particular situation. However, default management plans are possible for many areas of care and it is primarily in these areas of care that guidelines make a valuable contribution to good practice.

When guidelines are drawn up it is helpful to identify audit points and methods of audit so that prospective data collection against the standards set may be made.

The process of integrating scientific evidence into practice has been adopted widely as the practice of evidence-based medicine. A full description of this process is outside the remit of this chapter (www.cebm.net). However, the processes of asking answerable questions, assembling and critically appraising the evidence, acting on the evidence and establishing performance against the evidence are central to the audit/guideline philosophy.

Within a single service it is often difficult to demonstrate benefit from the introduction of evidence-based changes in management. Working together as a local network will clearly bring advantages in terms of population size but using the powerful resources of a large organisation such as the Vermont Oxford Network allows a more rapid introduction of change from a broader range of services.

As part of the NICQ 2000 scheme the Vermont Oxford Network facilitated a range of service quality improvements in the areas of nosocomial infection, chronic lung disease, postnatal dexamethasone use, prevention of brain haemorrhage and ischaemic brain injury and family-centred care. This is the first time that such an undertaking has been attempted in the field of clinical care. Each service improvement occurred across a group of neonatal units with variable success. The success of this scheme provides powerful evidence that a facilitated approach, using common methodology across a network of units and evidence-based changes in practice, can be implemented and audited.

In the UK the most effective audit process has been the CESDI. Registered deaths from 20 weeks of gestation until the end of the first postnatal year are reported centrally. Within this system a series of confidential structured enquiries have been organised, each focused around a different theme to identify both avoidable factors and good practice in the management of reported cases. For example, this process was supplemented by the collection of a comparison group of surviving children born at 27 and 28 completed weeks of gestation to provide a national case–control study of factors associated with death (Acolet et al. 2005). The report from this powerful evaluation of practice has important implications for neonatal practice in the UK.

Conclusions

Within a modern health service, neonatal care makes an important contribution to the health of the population, providing critical care support to babies who are seriously ill and taking evidence-based measures to avoid illness and unnecessary intervention. NIC has developed greatly over the past 30 years with demonstrable improvements in survival and morbidity. Organisation of what are now complex services must be demonstrated to be clinically and financially efficient and clinical care must be transparent and evidence-based. These are challenges that are met though clinical governance and service improvement, as described above. These are now key areas of neonatal practice and central to the delivery of improved outcomes in the future.

References

Acolet, D., Elbourne, D., Mcintosh, N., et al., 2005. Project 27/28: inquiry into quality of neonatal care and its effect on the survival of infants who were born at 27 and 28 weeks in England, Wales, and Northern Ireland. Pediatrics 116, 1457–1465.

Balic, D., Latifagic, A., Hudic, I., 2008. Insulin-like growth factor-binding protein-1 (IGFBP-1) in cervical secretions as a predictor of preterm delivery. J Matern Fetal Neonatal Med 21, 297–300.

British Association of Perinatal Medicine, 1996. The BAPM Neonatal Dataset. British Association of Perinatal Medicine, London.

British Association of Perinatal Medicine, 2001. Standards for Hospitals Providing Intensive and High Dependency Care. British Association of Perinatal Medicine, London.

British Association of Perinatal Medicine, 2010. Service Standards for Hospitals Providing Neonatal Care. British Association of Perinatal Medicine, London.

Bennett, C.C., Lal, M.K., Field, D.J., et al., 2002. Maternal morbidity and pregnancy outcome in a cohort of mothers transferred out of perinatal centres during a national census. Br J Obstet Gynaecol 109, 663–666.

Bolt, L.A., Chandiramani, M., De Greeff, A., et al., 2009. Does fetal fibronectin testing change patient management in women at risk of preterm labour? Eur J Obstet Gynecol Reprod Biol 146, 180–183.

Bowen, S.L., 2002. Transport of the mechanically ventilated neonate. Respir Care Clin North Am 8, 67–82.

Burnhope, C., Edmonstone, J., 2003. 'Feel the fear and do it anyway': the hard business of developing Shared Governance. J Nurs Manage 11, 147–157.

Centre for Maternal and Child Enquiries, 2010. Perinatal Mortality 2008. CMACE, London.

Costeloe, K., Hennessy, E., Gibson, A.T., et al., 2000. The EPICure study: outcomes to discharge from hospital for infants born at the threshold of viability. Pediatrics 106, 659–671.

Donoghue, D., the ANZNN Executive, 2009. Report of the Australia and New Zealand Neonatal Network 2006. University of New South Wales, Sydney.

Express Group, 2010. Incidence of and risk factors for neonatal morbidity after active perinatal care: extremely preterm infants study in Sweden (EXPRESS). Acta Paediatr 99, 978–992.

Fellman, V., Hellstrom-Westas, L., Norman, M., et al., 2009. One-year survival of extremely preterm infants after active perinatal care in Sweden. JAMA 301, 2225–2233.

Field, D., Draper, E.S., 1999. Survival and place of delivery following preterm birth: 1994–96. Arch Dis Child Fetal Neonatal Ed 80, F111–F114.

Field, D., Petersen, S., Clarke, M., et al., 2002. Extreme prematurity in the UK and Denmark: population differences in viability. Arch Dis Child Fetal Neonatal Ed 87, F172–F175.

Fleming, P., Berry, J., Gilbert, R., et al., 1990. Bedding and sleeping position in the sudden infant death syndrome. Br Med J 301, 871–872.

Gavin, M., Ash, D., Wakefield, S., et al., 1999. Shared governance: time to consider the cons as well as the pros. J Nurs Manag 7, 193–200.

Goodman, D.C., Fisher, E.S., Little, G.A., et al., 2002. The relation between the availability of neonatal intensive care and neonatal mortality. N Engl J Med 346, 1538–1544.

Haines, L., Fielder, A.R., Baker, H., et al., 2005. UK population based study of severe retinopathy of prematurity: screening, treatment, and outcome. Arch Dis Child Fetal Neonatal Ed 90, F240–F244.

Hope, P., 1995. CRIB, son of Apgar, brother to APACHE. Arch Dis Child Fetal Neonatal Ed 72, F81–F83.

International Neonatal Network, Scottish Neonatal Consultants & Nurses Collaborative Study Group, 2000. Risk adjusted and population based studies of the outcome for high risk infants in Scotland and Australia. Arch Dis Child Fetal Neonatal Ed 82, F118–F123.

Kempley, S.T., Baki, Y., Hayter, G., et al., 2007. Effect of a centralised transfer service on characteristics of inter-hospital neonatal transfers. Arch Dis Child Fetal Neonatal Ed 92, F185–F188.

Leslie, A.J., Stephenson, T.J., 1997. Audit of neonatal intensive care transport – closing the loop. Acta Paediatr 86, 1253–1256.

Leslie, A., Stephenson, T., 2003. Neonatal transfers by advanced neonatal nurse practitioners and paediatric registrars. Arch Dis Child Fetal Neonatal Ed 88, F509–F512.

Lorenz, J.M., Paneth, N., Jetton, J.R., et al., 2001. Comparison of management strategies for extreme prematurity in New Jersey and the Netherlands: outcomes and resource expenditure. Pediatrics 108, 1269–1274.

Marlow, N., 2002. Illness severity measures in neonatal intensive care. Acta Paediatr 91, 367–368.

Marlow, N., Bryan Gill, A., 2007. Establishing neonatal networks: the reality. Arch Dis Child Fetal Neonatal Ed 92, F137–F142.

Maybloom, B., Chapple, J., Davidson, L.L., 2002. Admissions for critically ill children: where and why? Intensive Crit Care Nurs 18, 151–161.

Maynard, A., Bloor, K., 1996. Introducing a market to the United Kingdom's National Health Service. N Engl J Med 334, 604–608.

NICE, 2010. Quality Standards: Specialist Neonatal Care. National Institute for Health and Clinical Excellence, London.

Northern Neonatal Network, 1993. Measuring neonatal nursing workload. Arch Dis Child 68, 539–543.

Oxford English Dictionary, 1989. Oxford University Press, Oxford.

Parmanum, J., Field, D., Rennie, J., et al., 2000. National census of availability of neonatal intensive care. British Association for Perinatal Medicine [see comment]. Br Med J 321, 727–729.

Parry, G.J., Gould, C.R., Mccabe, C.J., et al., 1998. Annual league tables of mortality in neonatal intensive care units: longitudinal study. International Neonatal Network and the Scottish Neonatal Consultants and Nurses Collaborative Study Group. [see comment]. Br Med J. 316, 1931–1935.

Parry, G., Tucker, J., Tarnow-Mordi, W., 2003. CRIB II: an update of the clinical risk index for babies score. Lancet 361, 1789–1791.

Rashid, A., Bhuta, T., Berry, A., 1999. A regionalised transport service, the way ahead? Arch Dis Child 80, 488–492.

Ratcliffe, J., 1998. Provision of intensive care for children. A geographically integrated service may now be achieved. BMJ 316, 1547–1548.

Report of the Neonatal Intensive Care Services Review, 2009. A Toolkit for High Quality Neonatal Services. Department of Health, London.

Richardson, D.K., Gray, J.E., Mccormick, M.C., et al., 1993. Score for Neonatal Acute Physiology: a physiologic severity index for neonatal intensive care. Pediatrics. 91, 617–623.

Richardson, D.K., Corcoran, J.D., Escobar, G.J., et al., 2001. SNAP-II and SNAPPE-II: Simplified newborn illness severity and mortality risk scores. J Pediatr 138, 92–100.

Riley, K., Roth, S., Sellwood, M., et al., 2008. Survival and neurodevelopmental morbidity at 1 year of age following extremely preterm delivery over a 20-year period: a single centre cohort study. Acta Paediatr 97, 159–165.

Scally, G., Donaldson, L.J., 1998. The NHS's 50 anniversary. Clinical governance and the drive for quality improvement in the new NHS in England. BMJ 317, 61–65.

The International Neonatal Network, 1993. The CRIB (clinical risk index for babies) score: a tool for assessing initial neonatal risk and comparing performance of neonatal intensive care units. Lancet. 342, 193–198.

Tucker, J., 2002. Patient volume, staffing, and workload in relation to risk-adjusted outcomes in a random stratified sample of UK neonatal intensive care units: a prospective evaluation. Lancet 359, 99–107.

Tucker, J., Tarnow-Mordi, W., Gould, C., et al., 1999. UK neonatal intensive care services in 1996. On behalf of the UK Neonatal Staffing Study Collaborative Group. Arch Dis Child Fetal Neonatal Ed 80, F233–F234.

Watkinson, M., Davis, K., 2009. Annual Report National Neonatal Audit Programme 2009. RCPCH Science and Research Department, London.

Wilkinson, A.R., Haines, L., Head, K., et al., 2008. UK retinopathy of prematurity guideline. Early Hum Dev 84, 71–74.

Williams, S., Whelan, A., Weindling, A., et al., 1993. Nursing staff requirements for neonatal intensive care. Arch Dis Child 68, 534–538.

Wood, N.S., Marlow, N., Costeloe, K., et al., 2000. Neurologic and developmental disability after extremely preterm birth. EPICure Study Group. N Engl J Med 343, 378–384.

Outcome following preterm birth

3

Neil Marlow   Samantha Johnson

Pregnancies deliver prematurely because of problems with the fetus, the mother or the intrauterine environment; in each of these situations fetal health is compromised before birth and it is perhaps unsurprising that many such children develop later problems, particularly following very preterm birth before 32 weeks of gestation. This period from the middle of the second trimester into the first month of the third trimester is associated with rapid organ growth and development. In the brain, although neuronal migration is mainly complete, cortical structure evolves rapidly and there are important structural elements that develop in this critical period. The processes surrounding preterm birth may interrupt neuronal or oligodendroglial migration and cortical structural development. Furthermore, we understand little of how our clinical care and the effects of the neonatal intensive care unit (NICU) environment interact positively or negatively with these processes. It is, therefore, encouraging that the great majority of survivors develop appropriately and enjoy a good quality of life though to adulthood (Hack et al. 2002; McCormick and Richardson 2002; Cooke 2004; Saigal et al. 2006), but others do develop a range of impairments that interfere with health or education and lead to problems that persist throughout the lifespan. It is these who are the focus of this chapter.

History: early neonatal care

Interest in the care of the newborn has waxed and waned through history. The invention that marked the dawn of 'modern' neonatal care was the incubator, first credited to a French obstetrician, Stéphane Tarnier, derived from an agricultural device to hatch hens' eggs. The introduction into the Paris Maternité hospital in 1878 facilitated the development of the ideas published by Pierre Budin in his classic monograph entitled *Le Nourissant* (*The Nursling*) (Budin 1907). Although mainly concerned with inpatient care, there is one surviving photograph of his 'graduates'.

Martin Couney, a pupil of Budin, requested a chance to exhibit the new incubators in the World Exposition in Berlin in 1896. Permission granted, he conceived the idea of a live exhibit with babies, otherwise destined to die, from a local charitable hospital. These *Kinderbrutanstäldter* (child hatcheries) proved a great success and were soon imitated across the world. Couney himself settled in Cooney Island, where his exhibitions became famous; his own daughter was born prematurely and incubated for 3 months (Silverman 1979).

Couney's influence led Julius Hess to establish the eight-cot premature baby station at the Sarah Morris Hospital, Chicago. This rapidly expanded and led to the first reliable reports of survival and outcome (Hess 1934). No significant deviation from normal term controls was noted in this highly selected population and no effects of birthweight, gestation, sex or maternal illness were found on outcome. Indeed, Gesell and Armatruda (1947), using graduates of Couney's summer exhibitions, concluded: 'prematurity does not

© 2012 Elsevier Ltd

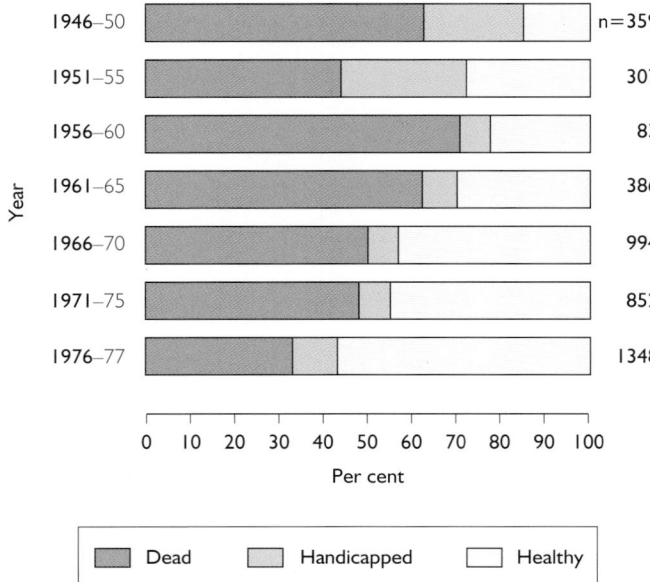

Fig. 3.1 Outcome studies for babies of <1501 g birthweight pooled by quinquennium to show the percentage of babies who died and survived, with and without handicap. *(Redrawn from Stewart et al. (1981).)*

markedly alter the normal course of mental growth. It neither retards nor accelerates'. However, thinking was soon to change.

Over the next decade the importance of the length of gestation was appreciated and increased morbidity in the smaller survivors was noted, leading to questions about care for these vulnerable babies which persist right through to today. For example, Sheridan (1962) observed that improvements in mortality had 'been accompanied by a rising survival of immature, malformed, birth injured and weakly babies' and Drillien (1958) warned that improvements in care might lead to increasing numbers of handicapped children in the community.

Care had up to this point been crude, as exemplified by the uncertainty surrounding the use of oxygen (Cross 1973), but the 1960s heralded the start of more careful and considered interventions such as early feeding with breast milk and more appropriate respiratory interventions. There were conflicting reports as to trends in outcomes during this time. The first important systematic attempt to review trends in outcome for very-low-birthweight (VLBW) births was published by Stewart and colleagues (1981). They indicated some of the difficulties in comparing reports, often from specialist centres reporting selected groups of infants. They summarised outcome from published reports as death, handicapped or healthy survivor and averaged over adjacent 5-year periods over 32 years. From 1960 mortality was found to have fallen progressively, but in each epoch 6–8% of total livebirths had handicaps (Fig. 3.1). There was no evidence, therefore, of an excess of handicapped children in the community as a result of these improvements in care. The same trends applied equally to the subgroup <1000 g birthweight.

The contribution of prematurity to disability in the community

The notion that increased survival brought an additional burden of disability into the population remains even today. The concept of a 'gain' in a healthy survivor is set against a 'loss' as a child with

disability. Overall, the gain in terms of healthy survivors far outweighs the increasing burden of disability in the population. Since the early 1980s there has been an explosion of interest in this area and a huge literature base has evolved. Over short periods of time it is clear that trends in disability rates are hard to demonstrate but mortality has continued to decrease as the gestational age at which birth is considered of borderline viability has fallen, generally without increasing the proportion of survivors with handicap or disability.

The increasing anxiety surrounding the provision of care for the baby of borderline viability persists even today (Nuffield Council on Bioethics 2006) and is now directed to babies born before 25 weeks of gestation, such is survival at later gestational ages. Survival at these low gestations is in part determined by the attitudes of caregivers, some centres preferring not to offer care at these low gestations in the belief that outcome is likely to be so poor that to attempt intensive care is considered wrong. Very few studies have attempted to define the results of different models of care. One important study compares the outcome in a health service with near-universal initiation of intensive care in the USA against selective initiation in the Netherlands; this resulted in 24.1 additional survivors and 7.2 additional cases of cerebral palsy (CP) for each 100 livebirths (Lorenz et al. 2001). Thus the gain and loss account is still in favour of intensive care if CP is used as an outcome; many would argue that cognitive and behavioural impairment is an even more important adverse outcome measure, but one for which the appropriate study has not been done.

Improving survival has been recognised in the UK by the reduction in gestational age for the definition of stillbirth in 1992 from 28 to 24 weeks. Furthermore, as we will see, although most survivors are free of major handicapping conditions, many more subtle (and less easy to predict) conditions in the fields of learning, motor skills and behaviour are now apparent in survivors, closely related to the degree of immaturity at birth. For these more subtle conditions, as for serious disability such as CP, there is a close relationship to gestational age (Fig. 3.2). However it must be emphasised that preterm birth only occurs in a small proportion of the population (6–13% in different countries) and that the groups most often studied with the highest prevalence of disability (very preterm or extremely preterm births) constitute less than 1% of all births. Therefore, the population-attributable risk for all of these conditions is highest in term-born children, followed by late and moderate preterm children and lowest for the very/extremely preterm groups. For example, in terms of special educational needs (SEN), the population-attributable percentage for births 24–27 weeks was 5%, for 28–32 weeks 11%, for 33–36 weeks 20% and 65% from births at full term (MacKay et al. 2010).

Reporting outcomes and study design

Data concerning the progress of neonatal intensive care graduates can be used as part of an ongoing audit of outcome or as part of a hypothesis-based research study. Such a study may explore factors that influence development or developmental trajectories (e.g. social or nutritional factors) or the predictive value of particular observations (e.g. cranial ultrasound appearances). Increasingly, randomised trials of neonatal interventions are including longer term outcomes (usually at 18–24 months) as secondary or even primary outcomes for a range of neonatal treatments and in economic appraisals of such. In an ideal world these would be collected in an agreed fashion for all children using routine systems, but this is as yet not possible.

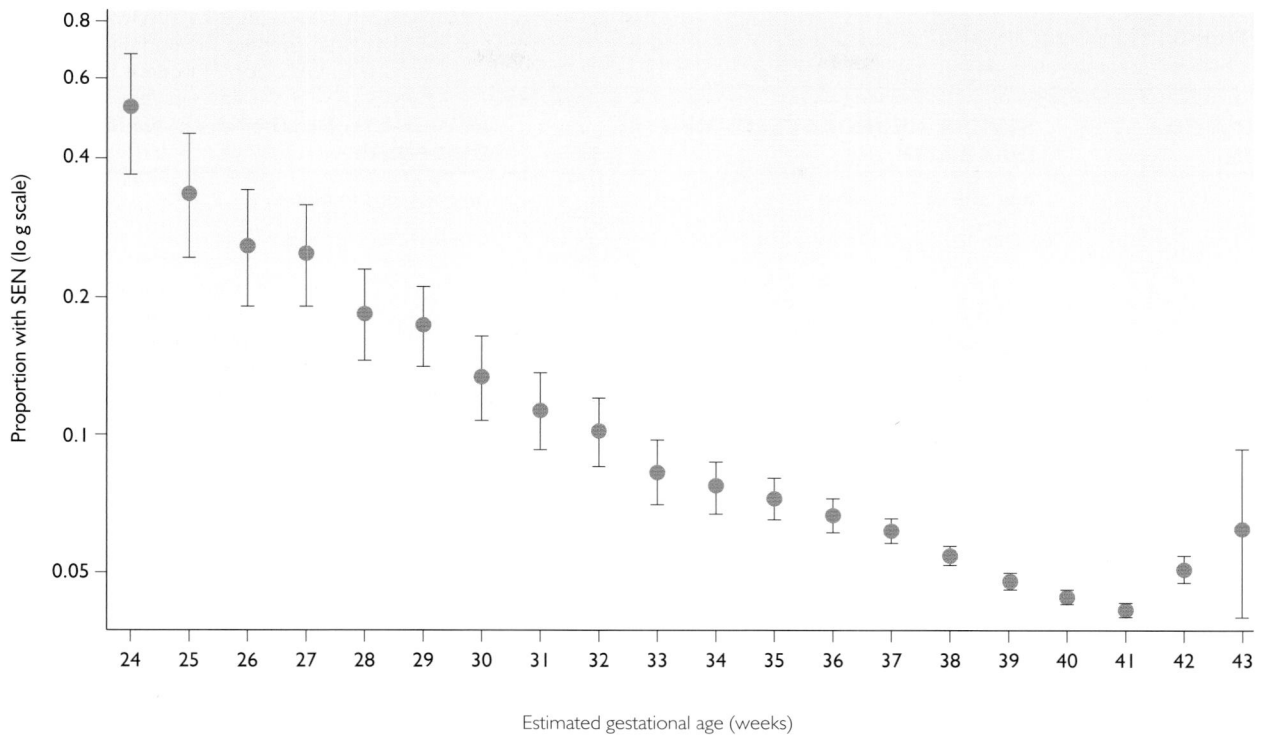

Fig. 3.2 Percentage of children with special educational needs by gestational age at delivery (note the logarithmic scale). *(Redrawn from MacKay et al. (2010).)*

Comparing studies in this area is fraught with methodological problems that often preclude comparison of outcome statistics between studies, despite attempts to do so (see below). It is important, therefore, that the data are presented as fully as possible to facilitate comparison year on year and between studies. Reports of population outcomes should contain as a minimum:

- information on the birth population
  - all births or livebirths in a given geographic population
  - numbers of babies admitted for neonatal intensive care
  - details of transfers for care (in and ex utero)
  - survivors to discharge home
- information on the selection and composition of a comparator population, if applicable
- age at assessment (with range) and correction for prematurity if applied
- proportion of the population assessed and reasons for non-assessment – a diagram similar to that recommended for randomised trials in the CONSORT statement (Schulz et al. 2010) is often the clearest way of displaying this
- measures used to define the performance of a population (e.g. intelligence test), definitions of categories and methods used to classify outcome and the numbers with disability in each domain of outcome (e.g. CP, cognitive function, hearing or visual impairment).

This requirement applies less to targeted studies of interventions but nonetheless the discipline of identifying the sample used by reporting the population as suggested above allows much better understanding of the applicability of the results of studies to routine practice. More detailed descriptions of the requirements for such studies have been published (Kiely and Paneth 1981; Mutch et al. 1989; for a series of reviews see Marlow 2006) and general reporting requirements for cohort studies should be adhered to (von Elm et al. 2007).

In 1994, because of a lack of consistency between studies in definitions for long-term outcomes, guidelines for the categorisation of severely impaired outcome following prematurity were developed in the UK (Anonymous 1995). This was the outcome that was felt to be best predictive of later ongoing disability and ascertainment at 2 years was chosen as the age at which serious CP could be identified with some confidence, bearing in mind the difficulty in interpreting very early assessments. More recently this has been revised to include categories of severe and moderate impairment in both neurodevelopmental and somatic domains (Table 3.1) (Report of a BAPM/RCPCH Working Group 2008). This simple functional classification should serve as a minimum basis for reporting outcomes for preterm populations and may be easily incorporated in routine clinical follow-up. Alongside this the prevalence of CP (see below) should be reported.

There is less consensus regarding the definition of disability at later ages. Formal definitions of impairment, disability and handicap are still very useful and should underpin any scheme (Ch. 2, Table 2.7). However, these definitions have recently been revised to include broader categories of impairment, activity limitations and participation restrictions within society in the International Classification of Function, Disability and Health (ICF), which, although more relevant to society and individuals, makes simple categorisation for outcome studies much less clear.

In pragmatic terms it is usual to continue to categorise impairment across the domains shown in Table 3.1, but with the addition of behaviour (using a relevant behavioural scale) and the inclusion of the Manual Abilities Classification System (Eliasson et al. 2006) alongside the Gross Motor Function Classification System (Palisano et al. 1997). Categorisation on continuous outcomes using

Table 3.1 Summary of definitions for reporting severe and moderate neurodevelopmental disability at 2 years; these may be combined as a single category of neurodevelopmental impairment (NDI), plus additional criteria for other disabilities

CRITERIA FOR DOMAIN	SEVERE NEURODEVELOPMENTAL DISABILITY	MODERATE NEURODEVELOPMENTAL DISABILITY
	Any one of the below	**Any one of the below**
Motor	Cerebral palsy with GMFCS level 3, 4 or 5	Cerebral palsy with GMFCS level 2
Cognitive function	Score < −3 SD below norm (DQ <55)	Score −2 SD to −3 SD below norm (DQ 55–70)
Hearing	No useful hearing even with aids (profound >90 dB HL)	Hearing loss corrected with aids (usually moderate 40–70 dB HL) or Some hearing loss not corrected by aids (usually severe 70–90 dB HL)
Speech and language	No meaningful words/signs or Unable to comprehend cued command (i.e. commands only understood in a familiar situation or with visual cues, e.g. gestures)	Some, but fewer than five, words or signs or Unable to comprehend uncued command but able to comprehend a cued command
Vision	Blind or Can only perceive light or light-reflecting objects	Seems to have moderately reduced vision but better than severe visual impairment or Blind in one eye with good vision in the contralateral eye
Other disabilities (included as additional impairments to SND or NDI)		
Respiratory	Requires continued respiratory support or oxygen	Limited exercise tolerance
Gastrointestinal	Requires TPN, NG or PEG feeding	On special diet or has stoma
Renal	Requires dialysis or awaiting organ transplant	Renal impairment requiring treatment or special diet

(Modified from Report of a BAPM/RCPCH Working Group (2008).)
DQ, Developmental Quotient; GMFCS, Gross Motor Function Classification System; HL, hearing loss; NG, nasogastric; PEG, percutaneous endoscopic gastrostomy; TPN, total parenteral nutrition.

standard deviation bands (−1 to −2 SD; −2 to −3 SD; < −3 SD) to denote, respectively, mild, moderate and severely impaired outcomes is conventional. The use of standardised outcome measures (e.g. cognitive, neurological, motor or behavioural domains) differs widely and, to a large extent, depends upon the hypothesis under investigation. Where there are clear internationally accepted definitions (e.g. Diagnostic and Statistical Manual of Mental Disorders, 4th ed. (DSM-IV)), these should be reported alongside results on measures specific to the individual study. However the research hypothesis will determine the choice and selection of investigation required and the selection of such tests has been discussed in reviews (Salt and Redshaw 2006; Johnson 2007).

Research evaluations in childhood should still, where possible, be focused on a population base, as described above, and data reported in a standardised fashion. The importance of recruiting contemporary comparison groups is stressed as secular upward drifts in IQ scores are well described (Flynn 1999) and the results of categorisation of children's performance will depend on which reference norms are selected with older measures (Wolke et al. 1994). More recently, changes in test structure and standardisation, for example in the new third edition of the Bayley Scales (Bayley-III: Anderson et al. 2010), have made this more important.

The importance of attempting to examine or at least obtain classifying information on all children in a population as far as possible has been stressed. There is some evidence that the non-responders may comprise an excess of severely disabled children (Wolke et al. 1995; Tin et al. 1998; Johnson et al. 2009a), although there is a paucity of data from other studies to support this. Increasingly the issue of research governance and the necessity to respect parents' privacy means that fewer attempts to contact parents for follow-up investigations are justifiable and research ethics committees are mindful to limit these. Difficulties with contacting parents after some time means that the taking of consent for later research evaluations should be done at the point of original entry into the study and contact maintained with newsletters, birthday cards or similar, as this should help to minimise loss to follow-up.

Outcome in early infancy

Motor development

Schemes for neurological examination of the newborn, such as those of Amiel-Tison, Dubowitz and Prechtl, are described in Chapter 40 part 1. Neonatologists must be aware of the different patterns of development over the first year and, where supported by evidence, be prepared to embrace a range of interventions in the nursery and after discharge to optimise a child's development.

Despite the reliance on ultrasound-detected brain lesions for prognosis, clinical assessment of the infant at discharge is of at least equal importance to evaluating the results of cranial imaging. Amiel-Tison and Grenier (1986) have described a simple functional examination to be performed at around 40 weeks' postmenstrual age. At this age, the very preterm baby is quite different from a newborn term infant, particularly if born at a very low gestational age at birth. Ex-preterm babies are more visually active and demonstrate less flexion and more extensor activity. When the examination is optimal and the results of cranial ultrasound show no abnormality, the risk of abnormality at 12 months of age is negligible (Roth et al. 1993). The positive predictive value is less useful as many babies will eventually lose their non-optimal signs early in the first year.

The very preterm baby is hypotonic and weak, with a poorly calcified skeleton. These impart particular vulnerability to external influences on the development of neurological tone and to skeletal deformations. Nursing postures may lead to changes in head and chest shape if they are not varied and prone positioning will encourage extensor posturing and external hip rotation with shortening of the hip adductors (Amiel-Tison and Grenier 1986). This may encourage hip dislocation if the child develops spasticity but may easily be avoided using simple postural management (Downs et al. 1991). The recent interest in nursing positioning will facilitate normal postural development for very preterm infants. Long-term ventilation and chronic lung disease are associated with similar positional issues; neck retraction and truncal extension are features of airway-shortening manoeuvres. Irritability associated with these deformities produces a picture that may be attributed to neurological injury and handling or feeding children with fixed postural deformity is difficult and may lead to problems in maternal attachment.

These influences may all modify the trajectory of development. de Groot and colleagues (1995) have described a group of ex-preterm infants with discrepancies between active and passive muscle tone that are most obvious in the extensor muscles of the trunk and may also be asymmetric (de Groot et al. 1997b). This usually transient dystonia may be a feature of the developing ex-preterm infant independent of positional changes. de Groot and colleagues argue that these tonal abnormalities lead to delay in unsupported sitting and rotation towards the end of the first year. These have implications for transition between postures and also lead to delay in fine motor development (de Groot et al. 1997a, b) and behavioural changes, through impairment of ability to optimise gross motor and hand function in an otherwise normal child because of truncal fixation.

Transient dystonia was described in preterm children by Drillien (1972) as infants with an excess of extensor hypertonicity in the trunk and legs, increased hip adductor tone and delayed supporting reactions. Such changes tend to resolve at around the child's first birthday or over the second year and be initially diagnosed as CP. Other more recent studies have evaluated motor development over the first 18 months. Pederson and colleagues (2000) studied a geographically based cohort of babies <2000 g birthweight. They categorised 29% as dystonic, 10% as hypotonic and 8% as suspected CP. The prevalence of dystonia was 35% in babies <1000 g, 35% for those of 1000–1499 g and 21% in babies 1500–1999 g. The peak prevalence of dystonia was at 7 months of age corrected for prematurity. Of children at 18 months of age with suspected CP, when examined at 7 months, five had been labelled as suspect CP, eight dystonia and one hypotonia. In another study the prevalence of dystonia was 36% of 260 VLBW infants (Pallas Alonso et al. 2000). In a further study, although truncal hyperextension had disappeared by 24–26 months of age, associated abnormalities of arm and hand function appeared to persist, perhaps as precursors of later motor abnormalities (de Vries and de Groot 2002).

Four studies have indicated long-term outcomes for dystonic infants. In Drillien's (1980) original study they were found to have an excess of educational difficulties; in a study of 50 children there was a trend towards more neuromotor difficulties (Sommerfelt et al. 1996); and in a further study dystonic infants had lower cognitive scores and higher disability grades at early school age (Khadilkar et al. 1993).

Cerebral palsy

The definition of CP has been updated to include wider aspects of function (Rosenbaum et al. 2007):

> *Cerebral palsy describes a group of permanent disorders of the development of movement and posture, causing activity limitation, that are attributed to non-progressive disturbances that occurred in the developing fetal or infant brain. The motor disorders of cerebral palsy are often accompanied by disturbances of sensation, perception, cognition, communication, and behaviour, by epilepsy, and by secondary musculoskeletal problems.*

William Little is credited with the observation that cerebral spasticity and paralysis were caused by 'difficulties arising around the time of birth', including preterm birth (and asphyxia), hence the epithet 'Little's disease' applied to diplegia. The specific association between a broad category of bilateral spasticity, which he termed spastic diplegia, and prematurity was first formally described in a paper entitled 'Zum Cerablen Diplegien' published in 1896 by Sigmund Freud, during his work as a paediatric neurologist with Charcot in Paris (Accardo 1982). Thus the increased risk of CP following preterm birth has been known for some time and, indeed, CP is often considered to be the most common and important disability following preterm birth. In fact this is not the case as developmental delay and cognitive impairments are by far the commonest disabilities. Nonetheless CP remains one of the most important outcomes and in the early 1980s spastic diplegia was used as a marker of the success of perinatal services (Hagberg et al. 1996).

The risk of CP is inversely related to gestational age at birth and increased in the presence of fetal growth restriction, at least among moderately preterm children (Blair and Stanley 1990), although the use of fetal growth standards instead of birthweight standards indicates a consistent relationship between prevalence of CP and size at birth across the gestational range (Fig. 3.3) (Jarvis et al. 2003). As many older studies are birthweight-based, the results must be treated with some caution because of the varying proportion of babies born after fetal growth restriction (Ch. 10). Thus the evaluation of secular trends in CP must be related to either birthweight or gestation because of the close links. The evolution of birthweight-specific trends in the prevalence of CP over the time period of introduction of neonatal intensive care in Merseyside, UK, has been described (Pharoah et al. 1996). As birthweight-specific survival increased there was an initial rise in the prevalence of CP within that birthweight band followed by a levelling out. This may relate to the increasing survival of children with CP who would otherwise have died, up to an equilibrium point.

Population trends in the prevalence of CP as a group or in birthweight-specific groupings are difficult to interpret, although towards the late 1990s the rate of CP appeared to be decreasing in Sweden (Himmelmann et al. 2005) and in the Surveillance for Cerebral Palsy in Europe (SCPE) collaboration of CP registers there was a fall in CP prevalence for babies 28–32 weeks from 1981 to 1995 but little change for babies <28 weeks (Fig. 3.4) (Platt et al. 2007). Furthermore, data from the 4Child Register of CP in four UK counties seem to indicate a falling off in CP prevalence for births of less than 28 weeks of gestation through to 2001–2003, demonstrating the value of longitudinal data (Fig. 3.5). These findings are consistent with low prevalence in three recent reports of extremely preterm children from Victoria, Australia (2005: 9.8% 22–27 weeks' gestation: Doyle et al. 2010), from Edmonton, Canada (2000–2003: 1.9% <27 weeks: Robertson et al. 2007) and Cleveland, OH, USA (2000–02: 5% <1000 g birthweight: Wilson-Costello et al. 2005).

The distribution of impairment in CP is determined by the pattern of brain injury. Diplegia, in which the impairment is more

severe caudally, is considered to be the result of damage to the internal capsule as part of periventricular leukomalacia. This usually symmetrical lesion is commonly observed on magnetic resonance imaging (MRI) scans at follow-up even if no neonatal ultrasound evidence of injury was observed (Childs et al. 2001). Diplegia is often associated with relatively mild disability and there is often less severe impairment in other domains compared with other patterns of CP. In the EPICure cohort of babies of 25 weeks' gestational age or less, only 44% (12/27) of children with diplegia had severe disability and thus were likely to have persisting disability at later ages (Wood et al. 2000).

Spastic hemiplegia, where the distribution of impairment is the reverse of diplegia and where there is usually significant asymmetry, results from lesions involving the cortex, such as cerebral venous infarction accompanying germinal matrix and intraventricular haemorrhage. Spastic quadriplegia, where there is four-limb involvement equally distributed in upper and lower limbs, occurs in variable proportions in reports. The distribution of disability in children with diplegia and hemiplegia is not always confined to the legs or to one side of the body and it is a subjective decision as to how to categorise the impairments. This accounts for many of the differences found between different observers. However, the impairment in quadriplegia is more extensive than in the other two and the disability is frequently severe (11/12 in the EPICure cohort). Other types of CP are found less frequently in very preterm populations.

In the discussions of classification of CP the above categories provide a sensible aetiologically relevant categorisation. However, over the years the classification has changed to reflect the prevailing fashion (Morris 2007). Most recently the SCPE group has published a classification and an algorithm, which should be used in future classifications based on three groupings (Table 3.2).

The timing of diagnosis in follow-up reports is important in determining the prevalence of CP; the predictive value of a label of CP increases as the child grows up. There is some consensus that the diagnosis of CP producing significant disability is usually accurate by the age of 2 years (Johnson 1995), but that, before that, abnormal patterns of motor development and dystonia or developmental delay may confuse the unwary. In the National Collaborative Perinatal Project CP was overdiagnosed at 12 months compared with assessment at 7 years, such that half of the children with the

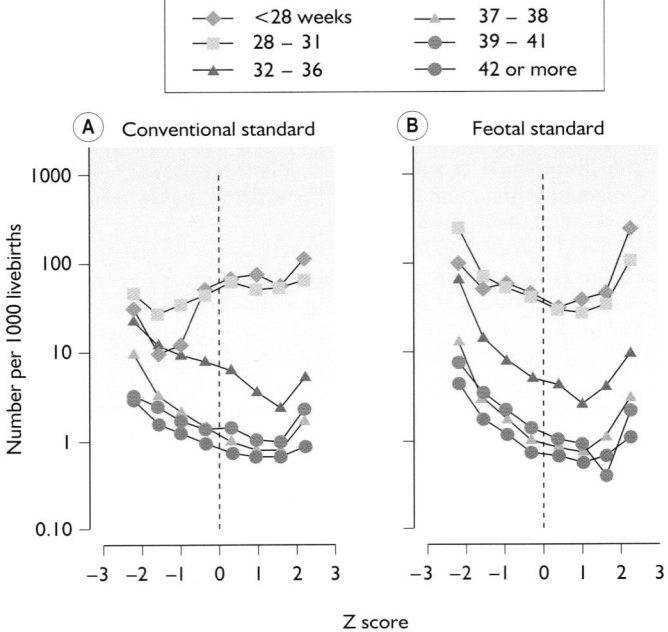

Fig. 3.3 The relationship between birthweight for gestational age based on (A) conventional birthweight standards or (B) fetal growth standards, showing in the latter a consistent relationship over the gestational range. *(Redrawn from Jarvis et al. (2003).)*

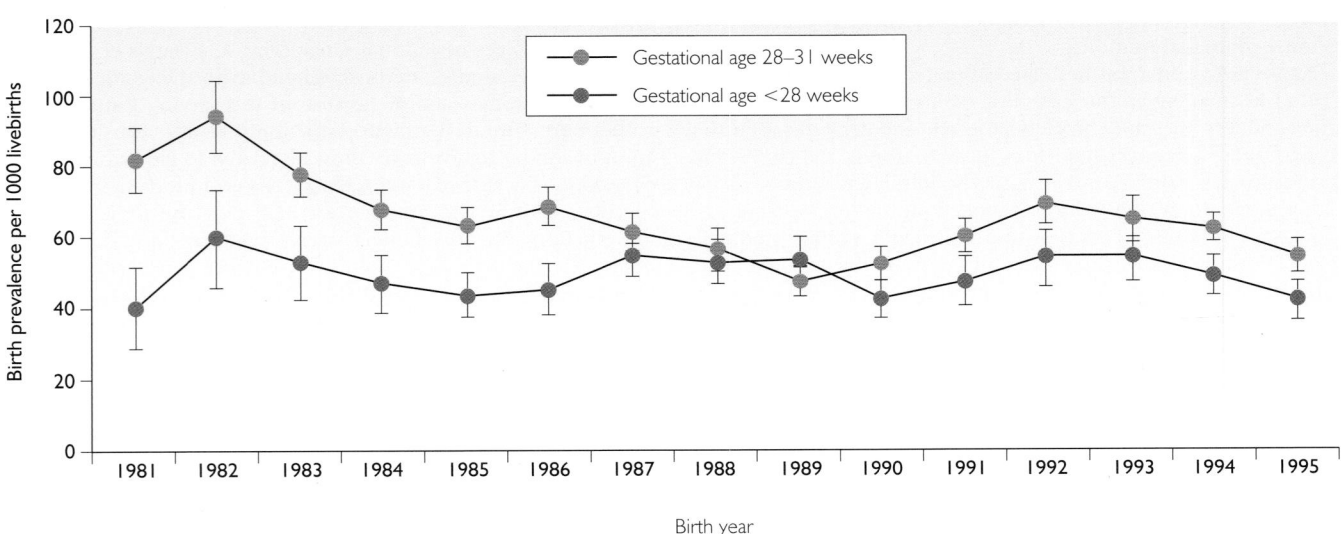

Fig. 3.4 Trends in the prevalence of cerebral palsy from 1981 to 1995 from nine European countries by gestational ages 28–32 weeks and <28 weeks. *(Redrawn from Platt et al. (2007).)*

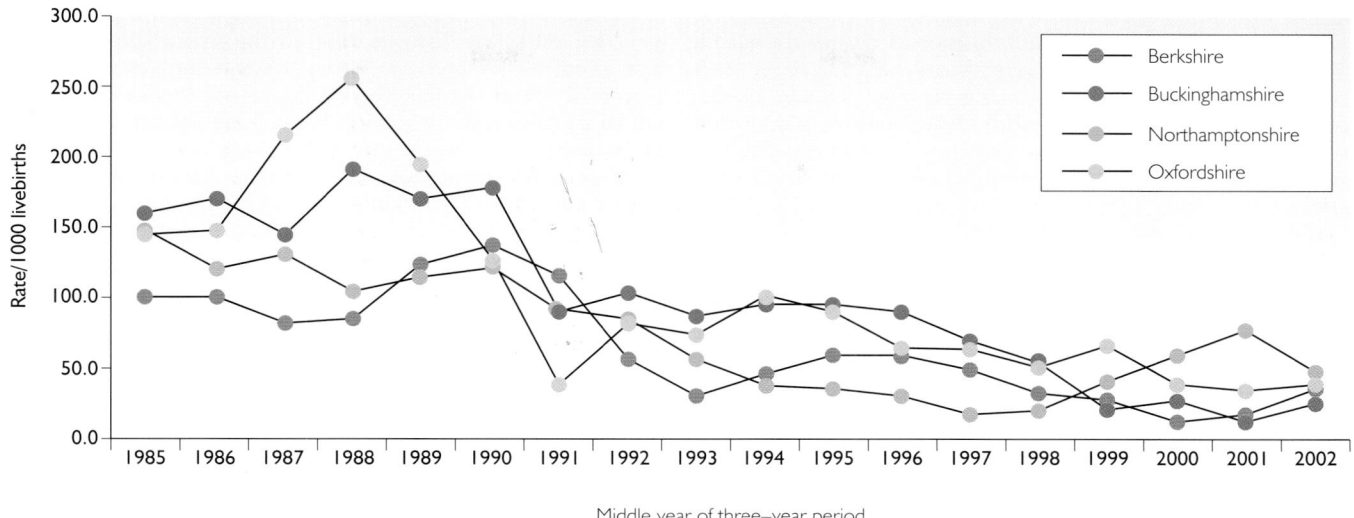

Fig. 3.5 Trends in the prevalence of cerebral palsy for babies born before 29 weeks of gestation in the *4*Child register. *(Data from https://www.npeu.ox.ac.uk/4child.)*

Table 3.2 Categorisation of cerebral palsy based on clinical features

Spastic cerebral palsy

Characterised by at least two of:
- Abnormal pattern of posture and/or movement
- Increased tone (not necessarily constantly)
- Pathological reflexes (hyperreflexia or pyramidal signs, e.g. Babinski response)
  - It may be unilateral (hemiplegia) or bilateral

Ataxic cerebral palsy

Characterised by both of:
- Abnormal pattern of posture and/or movement
- Loss of orderly muscular coordination, so that movements are performed with abnormal force, rhythm and accuracy

Dyskinesic cerebral palsy

Characterised by both of:
- Abnormal pattern of posture and/or movement
- Involuntary, uncontrolled, recurring, occasionally stereotyped movements of affected body parts

Dyskinesic cerebral palsy may be either:
- Dystonic cerebral palsy, dominated by both hypokinesia and hypertonia
- Choreoathetotic cerebral palsy, dominated by both hyperkinesia and hypotonia

(Reproduced from http://www-rheop.ujf-grenoble.fr/scpe2/site_scpe: see website for further details.)

diagnosis at 1 year were free of neurological signs 6 years later (Nelson and Ellenberg 1982). The most common types of CP to resolve were categorised as mild and were of the monoparetic, dyskinetic or diplegic types; resolution was more frequent in black infants. However a significant proportion of the children in whom signs had resolved (13% white and 25% blacks) had an IQ ≤70 at 7 years, emphasising the importance of careful early examination.

Despite the recommendation to wait until 2 years, even at this age there is overdiagnosis (Doyle 2001) and some less severe impairment may not be detectable until early school age (Astbury et al. 1990).

Careful sequential neonatal cerebral ultrasound scanning may identify the majority of children who go on to develop severe CP (de Vries et al. 2004) (Ch. 40.5) and early sequential neuroassessment in infancy is mandatory if CP is to be identified and managed appropriately. The role of other specific investigations is less clear; for example, somatosensory evoked potentials (Pike and Marlow 2000) and Prechtl's assessment of general movements (Einspieler and Prechtl 2005) are good predictors of outcome but have not found a place in routine practice as they are time-consuming and require great skill to do.

Screening vision and hearing

Screening for retinopathy of prematurity (ROP) is addressed in Chapter 33, but this cannot form the basis for screening for visual or ocular impairments. Squints and refractive errors are frequently found at follow-up in infancy and later childhood, thus each assessment must include adequate examination of visual activity and ocular movements. Refractive errors and subtle disorders of vision such as poor stereognosis and contrast sensitivity are found frequently at longer term follow-up (Pennefather et al. 1995; Powls et al. 1997; O'Connor et al. 2002; Johnson et al. 2009a), and should be sought in assessments at school age. In a teenage follow-up of the East Midlands cohort of children who had been screened but not treated for ROP, ophthalmic morbidity was found in 67.8% of children born ≤1000 g, 51.6% of those 1001–1250 g, 44.3% of those 1251–1500 g and 49.5% of those 1501–1750 g compared with 19.5% of their comparison group (O'Connor et al. 2002).

Sensorineural hearing loss is more prevalent in preterm populations, although the aetiology is still obscure and may well be multifactorial (Marlow et al. 2000). Found in 1–4% of VLBW children, this represents a 10-fold increase over unselected populations (Marlow et al. 2000; Hille et al. 2007; Robertson et al. 2009; Coenraad et al. 2010). Because of this, most services have developed targeted neonatal screening policies in which prematurity (either as VLBW or birth ≤32 weeks) is included in the screened population alongside children with a family history of deafness, orofacial anomalies and perinatal central nervous system infection. More recently there has been a move towards universal neonatal hearing screening, predicated on the thesis that early intervention for children with severe or profound hearing loss may improve later language and speech development (Yoshinaga-Itano et al. 1998). Most targeted screening involves automated or manual evoked responses (auditory or brainstem response (ABR)) that will identify children with significant hearing loss. Universal screening in the USA and most European countries involves testing with automated ABR technology, whereas currently in the UK a 'two-step' approach has been adopted using initial screening with otoacoustic emissions and automated ABR for failures. Universal screening has a sensitivity of between 80% and 90% and a specificity of above 90% (Davies 1997) and the median age of detection of severe hearing loss may be as low as 2 months, facilitating early intervention.

Developmental progress

Central to the definition of disability in preterm populations is an estimate of the child's developmental level. Correction of age for prematurity is usually applied up to 2 years, but may be extended to 3 years for extremely preterm children where the correction still makes around 10% difference depending on gestational age (Fig. 3.6). This correction is controversial, as some prefer to assess against chronological age-related norms, claiming that this more correctly identifies those with developmental problems, but as increasingly immature children survive this has fallen out of practice. Correcting for prematurity once the child is in the education system, where he or she is compared with peers, is generally deemed unnecessary.

Clinic assessment using one of the widely available developmental screening tools (e.g. Denver Developmental Screening Test or Schedule of Growing Skills) may indicate normal or very abnormal progress but the diagnostic utility and predictive value are not known; in particular, screening tests are used to identify children for more detailed assessment and are likely to overidentify children with developmental problems.

Most services now evaluate development with a formal assessment using one of the available test instruments. Any scale with

which the assessor is familiar may be used in clinical practice but the commonest ones in current use are the Bayley Scales of Infant and Toddler Development (Bayley-III) and the Griffiths Scales (second edition). Both have had recent standardisations which enhance the value of the results but the Bayley-III was restructured and rescaled in a new manner and this has resulted in relatively high scores (+7 points compared with the second edition – the BSID-II), which makes scores difficult to interpret. Most observers have found that fewer children are identified as low scorers using these scales and recommend that all new preterm cohort studies recruit contemporary term-born comparison children (Anderson et al. 2010), which will add greatly to the logistics and cost of doing such studies. The predictive value of individual developmental score results into childhood is relatively weak, although preterm children appear to track better than normal term-born children. However, in population studies the predictive value of proportions in different outcome categories is much better, hence these scores are useful in categorising outcomes for research purposes. The Bayley-III scales have no values for very poorly performing children (scores < −3 SD) and nominal scores must then be allocated to children who perform below the lower level of the test range; this must be acknowledged in reports as even allocating a score of 50 may produce very different results from allocating a score of −4 SD (40), as is often done.

Using the BSID-II, 30% of the EPICure cohort had scores <70 and 11% <55, representing −2 and −3 SD respectively. Scores were lower in boys but did not vary with gestational age or plurality (Wood et al. 2000). Mean scores were MDI (Mental Development Index) 82 (SD 15) and PDI (Psychomotor Development Index) 83 (SD 16) for those tested but 9.5% of the children assessed failed to complete the BSID-II. Evaluating mean scores of various studies is fraught with difficulty, mainly because exclusions can seriously modify results. It is important to include the whole population in any assessment where possible or to describe why children fail to complete the test.

A formal developmental assessment is expensive and time-consuming for service or research purposes, particularly where a categorisation around one figure is required. Increasingly, 18–24-month assessments are being used as outcome measures for randomised trials and their inclusion adds very significantly to the cost of the project. We have recently validated an adapted parent report questionnaire (Saudino et al. 1998) against the BSID-II at 2 years in very preterm children (Johnson et al. 2003, 2004, 2008; Johnson and Marlow 2011a). This has high correlation ($r = 0.68$) and good diagnostic utility (sensitivity 81%; specificity 81%) for a BSID-II cognitive score <70 and is likely to be as accurate as repeating the developmental assessment with another observer. This has proved a useful tool in the routine follow-up of preterm populations and has been used in multicentre trials, where follow-up is important to the evaluation of the safety and efficacy of an intervention but there are cost constraints. Although the potential cost of overreferrals may be a cause for concern for clinical use of such parental questionnaires, we have shown that very preterm infants with false-positive screens are at greater risk for neurodevelopmental and behavioural problems than those with true negative results and further assessment may be warranted (Johnson et al. 2008).

There are no particular patterns of developmental impairments associated with prematurity, rather as a group scores are globally depressed; this reflects the perhaps surprising lack of specific learning impairments at later ages. Behavioural difficulties are particularly difficult to evaluate in infancy but the knowledge that attention-deficit hyperactivity disorder (ADHD) is a persistent and constant finding in later studies encourages assessment in infancy. Sadly there are no well-respected measures which help to identify

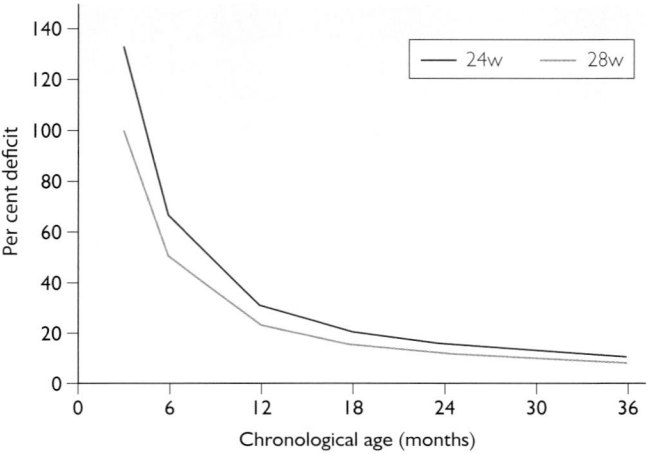

Fig. 3.6 Percentage deficit in developmental terms produced by using chronological age rather than corrected age for 24- and 28-week babies.

children at risk, although direct observation in the clinic does seem to identify a significant proportion of children with inattention and distractibility (Astbury et al. 1990).

Current follow-up practice

Our present practice in University College Hospital is to review children in the multidisciplinary neonatal follow-up clinic until 2 years corrected for prematurity, if they fall into one of three distinct high-risk groups, namely babies of 28 weeks' gestation or less, babies with bronchopulmonary dysplasia and babies who have demonstrated neonatal encephalopathy. Review is by a neonatologist, respiratory nurse, dietician and speech and language therapist, neurologist and a developmental specialist. Children are seen approximately 3-monthly over the first year and then at 2 years. Annual review visits for those with bronchopulmonary dysplasia then are offered until 5 years. A formal neurological assessment (Amiel-Tison and Grenier 1986; Haataja et al. 2001) is done at each visit together with a Bayley-III assessment. Video analysis of general movements (Prechtl et al. 1997) is carried out at 12 weeks postterm. Babies with identified developmental or neurological issues are referred to their local neurodisability team for assessment and intervention.

It should be stressed that this is an environment where we have good community-based family support from health visitors, primary care physicians and community paediatric staff. There is also good support from and easy access to advice from dietetics and locality-based physiotherapy and other family support teams for children with special needs. In other health systems alternative arrangements may be necessary.

Predicting disability in preterm infants

The major determinants of later disability are in essence similar to those predicting perinatal death, often described as part of the continuum of reproductive casualty (Sameroff and Chandler 1975). Perinatal factors increasing risk of disability include male sex (Kraemer 2000; Wood et al. 2000), gestational age and birthweight.

Using simple data such as these one can make broad statements about disability-free survival, which can help inform decisions around the time of birth (Fig. 3.7) (Tyson et al. 2008). A more specific prognosis for serious disability may be derived from brain imaging using ultrasound, MRI or neurosensory assessments (Ch. 40.5) and used to counsel parents on an individual risk basis.

Interventions to improve outcomes for very preterm babies

Children with or at risk of evolving disabilities should be referred for specialist neuroassessment and treatment. However, the knowledge that developmental and cognitive disadvantage is associated with preterm birth has prompted several important efforts to provide developmental or educational therapy for children without overt disabilities. Many of the strategies stem from early attempts

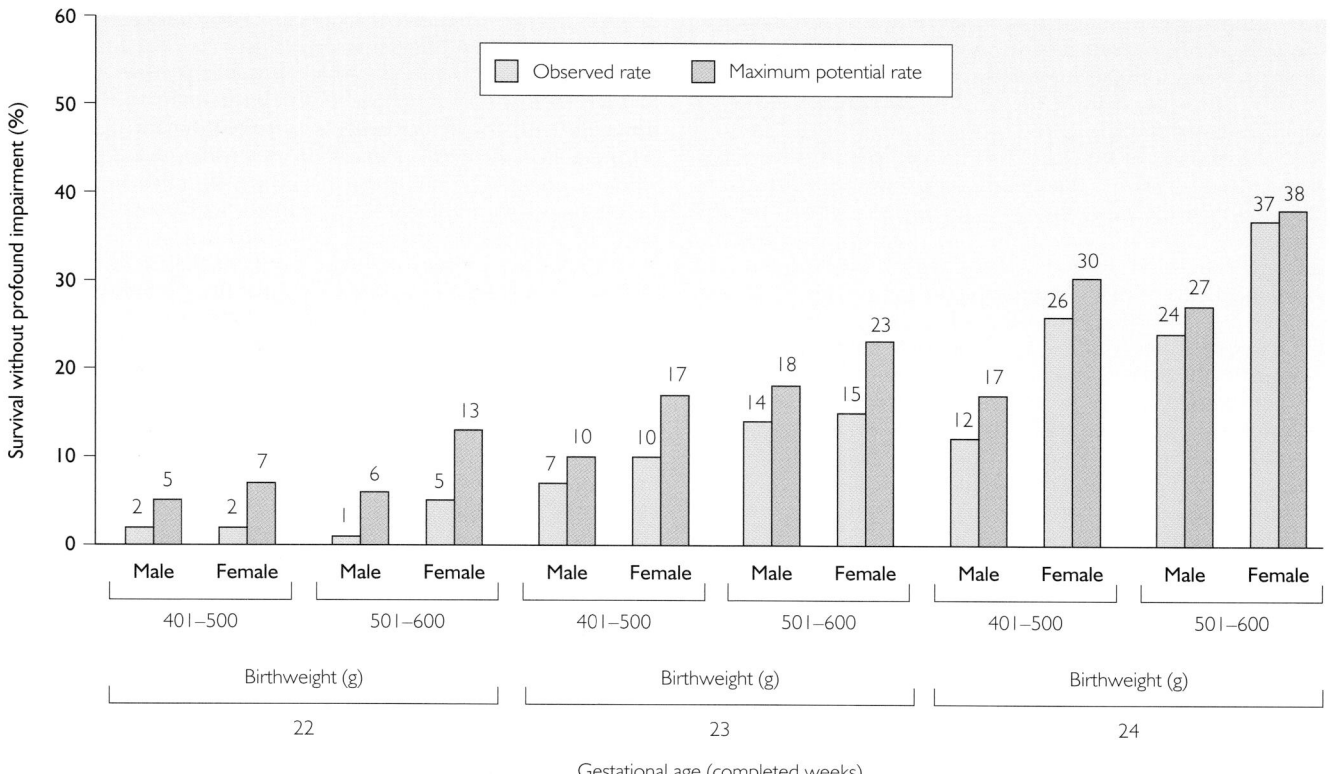

Fig. 3.7 Observed and maximum potential rates of survival without profound impairment at 18–22 months by sex, birthweight and gestational week. *(Redrawn from Tyson et al. (2008).)*

to enhance developmental outcome for children with Down syndrome. Although referral to early education schemes is commonplace, the evidence that these or similar schemes provide benefit in the long term is wanting (Anonymous 1990, 1998; Spittle et al. 2007, 2009; Koldewijn et al. 2010). Nonetheless these schemes may be essential methods of supporting families who are particularly disadvantaged, in whom there are without doubt impressive short-term gains, particularly in the families of heavier and more mature preterm children (Anonymous 1990), but the evidence for long-term benefit in terms of cognitive and learning ability is still lacking (McCarton et al. 1997).

School-age outcomes

There is some degree of continuity across childhood for those with the most severe impairment (Fig. 3.7) and for the most immature children there remains a significant risk of disability even as they enter adolescence. However much of the adverse outcome for such children is dependent upon cognitive and behavioural function, which influences schooling and is discussed next.

Cognitive function and school performance

Preterm birth results in significant cognitive disadvantages for surviving populations. Reports over the last 30 years have consistently identified cognitive impairment as the most common disability at school age. As with other outcomes, interpreting results requires close examination of individual studies and an understanding of the methods and measures used. In particular, the selection of IQ test, criteria for classifying impairment and exclusion of children who are unable to complete assessments affect the reported prevalence of impairment. Although the substitution of a nominal IQ score to quantify performance in those with severe impairment ultimately yields a higher prevalence of impairment, it provides a more accurate estimate of the totality of cognitive deficit for population-based investigations.

The vast majority of studies of very preterm survivors report significantly lower IQ scores than term peers (Johnson 2007). Group mean scores may be within the normal range (–1 SD) and thus the inclusion of a term reference group is crucial for identifying and interpreting the clinical significance of results. In a meta-analysis using pooled data from 1556 very preterm children and 1720 controls born in 1975–1988, Bhutta and colleagues (2002) reported an overall weighted mean difference of 10.9 IQ points (95% confidence interval 9.2–12.5) equating to a 0.73 SD deficit. The results were not affected by age at assessment, country of birth or by hospital versus population-based data, but, as would be expected, the greatest deficits were found in studies in which children with neurosensory impairments were included.

Follow-up data from cohorts born in the 1990s onwards continue to highlight the high prevalence of cognitive impairment in middle childhood despite major advances in neonatal intensive care over this period (Anderson and Doyle 2003; Hack et al. 2005; Fily et al. 2006; Johnson et al. 2009a). A number of studies have also identified a significantly increased risk of cognitive impairment in boys compared with girls, particularly for extremely preterm survivors (Brothwood et al. 1986; Hintz et al. 2006; Johnson et al. 2009a), a finding common to functional domains.

The gestational age-related gradient in outcomes is no more evident than in the domain of cognition. In the Bavarian Longitudinal Study there was no relationship between gestational age and IQ at 33 weeks' gestation or more, but there was a progressive reduction in scores for each week from 32 to 27 weeks (Wolke et al.

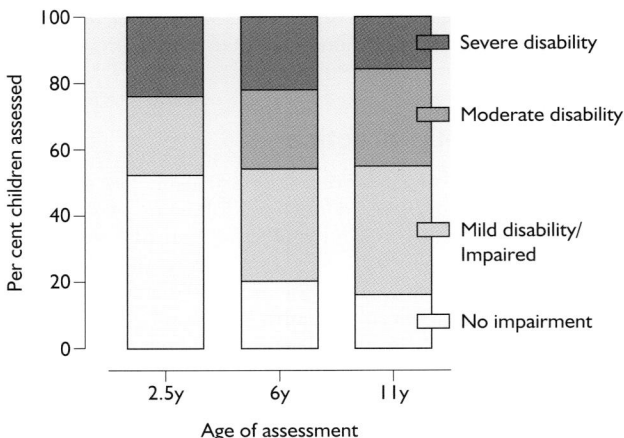

Fig. 3.8 Prevalence of disability among evaluated children born at 25 weeks of gestation or less in 1995 at 2.5, 6 and 11 years of age (the EPICure study). *(Redrawn from Johnson et al. (2009a).)*

2001). This represents an average deficit of approximately 2.5 IQ points per week ≤32 weeks and would predict a 20-point deficit for babies of 24 weeks' gestation. Consideration of the EPICure study 6-year assessment results, which used the same IQ test, confirms this prediction (Fig. 3.8). As gestational age is a major factor in defining outcome the interpretation of test scores for birthweight-defined cohorts becomes much more difficult.

Follow-up studies have become increasingly multidisciplinary in nature and it is now evident that preterm children are at particular risk for a range of neuropsychological deficits including visuospatial impairments, sensorimotor processing difficulties and deficits in a range of attention and executive functions which have been shown to confer additional functional deficit over low IQ alone (Bohm et al. 2002, 2004; Anderson and Doyle 2004; Marlow et al. 2007; Mulder et al. 2010). Executive functions may be considered an umbrella term for higher order cognitive processes required for purposeful, goal-directed behaviour and comprise skills such as working memory, inhibition, planning, shifting, fluency and processing speed. Although these skills are highly task-dependent, making comparisons between studies particularly problematic, two recent meta-analyses have shown that these are specific areas of deficit in preterm populations and that, like IQ, they are associated with gestational age (Aarnoudse-Moens et al. 2009; Mulder et al. 2009).

These skills play a key role in learning and school performance (Bull and Scerif 2001; St Clair-Thompson and Gathercole 2006). It is therefore unsurprising that, although the majority of preterm children attend mainstream schools, they have poorer academic attainment across the national curriculum than their term-born classmates, even among those who are free of neurosensory and cognitive impairment (Botting et al. 1998; Schneider et al. 2004; Litt et al. 2005; Aarnoudse-Moens et al. 2009; Johnson et al. 2009c; Johnson and Marlow 2011a). Of all the subjects studied at school, preterm children have particular difficulties with mathematics and the majority of learning difficulties observed are within this domain (Klebanov et al. 1994; Johnson et al. 2009c; Taylor et al. 2009; Johnson and Marlow 2011a). Unlike problems with reading, mathematics difficulties appear to be specific learning disabilities that are not accounted for by poor cognitive ability.

Given these learning difficulties, very preterm children have a significantly higher prevalence of SEN and a markedly greater reliance on learning support than their classmates (Saigal et al. 2003; MacKay et al. 2010). In the EPICure study, 57% of extremely preterm children in mainstream schools required SEN provision at 11 years of age and 23% had a formal statement of SEN compared with just 1% of their classmates (Johnson et al. 2009c). The need for SEN provision is not confined to those born extremely preterm. Whilst it was traditionally thought that the outcomes of babies born late and moderately preterm (32–26 weeks) were largely the same as those of their term-born counterparts, recent studies have high-lighted the increased risk for cognitive and educational deficits in this population (Chyi et al. 2008; MacKay et al. 2010; Mathiasen et al. 2010). Although the prevalence of serious impairment is far lower than in very preterm survivors, the population-attributable risk of SEN presents a greater public health burden (Fig. 3.2).

The prevalence of SEN increases throughout secondary education and thus the number already requiring support at the end of primary education is of concern. Furthermore, the educational dis-advantage persists beyond childhood: studies report a significant disadvantage in GCSE results (Pharoah et al. 2003) and a reduced earning potential and participation in higher education (Lindstrom et al. 2007; Hack et al. 2009).

As the UK adopts an age-based school entry system, preterm children born in the summer months may be entered in an aca-demic year earlier than if they had been born at term. There is concern that the effects of preterm birth on school performance are compounded by their relative social and emotional immaturity if entered an academic year earlier. In the EPICure study, we found that children who would have entered school an academic year earlier had comparable attainment with their extremely preterm counterparts but required greater SEN provision (Johnson et al. 2009c). Many parents and clinicians believe that delayed or deferred entry would be advantageous for the child, but systematic, hypothesis-driven research is needed in this area before evidence-based recommendations can be made.

In addition, research is required to understand the nature and origins of learning difficulties in order to identify the key compo-nents for population-specific interventions. It is important to rec-ognise that there is no single cognitive phenotype associated with preterm birth. The profile of strengths and limitations will differ between individual children and careful assessment is thus indi-cated for all preterm children (Aylward 2002). A routine evaluation by an educational psychologist may be beneficial for these survivors.

Behaviour and psychology

Improved multidisciplinary follow-up has also led to a greater understanding of the behavioural sequelae of prematurity. The majority of studies in this area have used screening questionnaires completed by parents and/or teachers. Most frequently cited in the literature is the Child Behavior Checklist (Fig. 3.9), which is used widely but is relatively long and can appear somewhat negative for the respondent. The Strengths and Difficulties Questionnaire (SDQ) is free to use (www.sdqinfo.org) and is gaining popularity, particu-larly in the UK, for its brevity and cross-cultural validity.

Using screening questionnaires, almost all studies have shown a significant excess of behaviour problems in very preterm and extremely preterm cohorts with prevalence estimates ranging from 13% to 46%. There is less agreement however for the risk of behav-ioural morbidity in moderate and late preterm cohorts (see Johnson and Marlow, 2011b, for a review).

When internalising and externalising problems are assessed there appears to be little consensus between studies (Bhutta et al. 2002) but at the subscale level there is far greater consistency. In a cross-cultural comparison of outcomes in four population-based cohorts (Canada, Germany, the Netherlands, USA) of children born <1001 g in 1977–1987, all four cohorts had significantly increased scores for social, thought and attention problems which were elevated by 0.5–1.2 SD relative to controls (Hille et al. 2001). In a more recent study of extremely preterm children in Sweden, a remarkably similar pattern of results was found (Fig. 3.10) (Farooqi 2009). A similar behavioural profile is also identified in studies using the SDQ (Gardner et al. 2004; Indredavik et al. 2005; Samara et al. 2008).

These questionnaires are essentially screening tools and thus they are likely to yield many overreferrals. Indeed, studies using

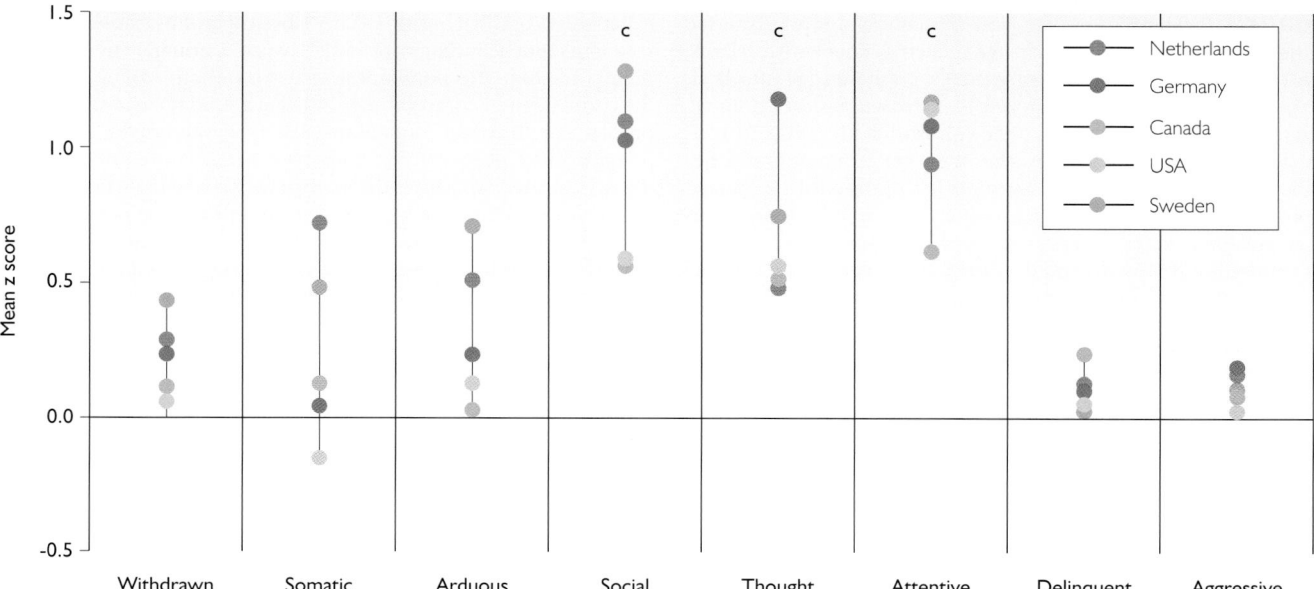

Fig. 3.9 Mean 'z' or standard deviation scores for eight subscales of the Child Behavior Checklist from five studies (higher scores denote greater impairment); the studies all demonstrate an excess of social, thought and attentional problems among extremely low-birthweight children and Swedish extremely preterm children. *(Redrawn from Farooqi (2009).)*

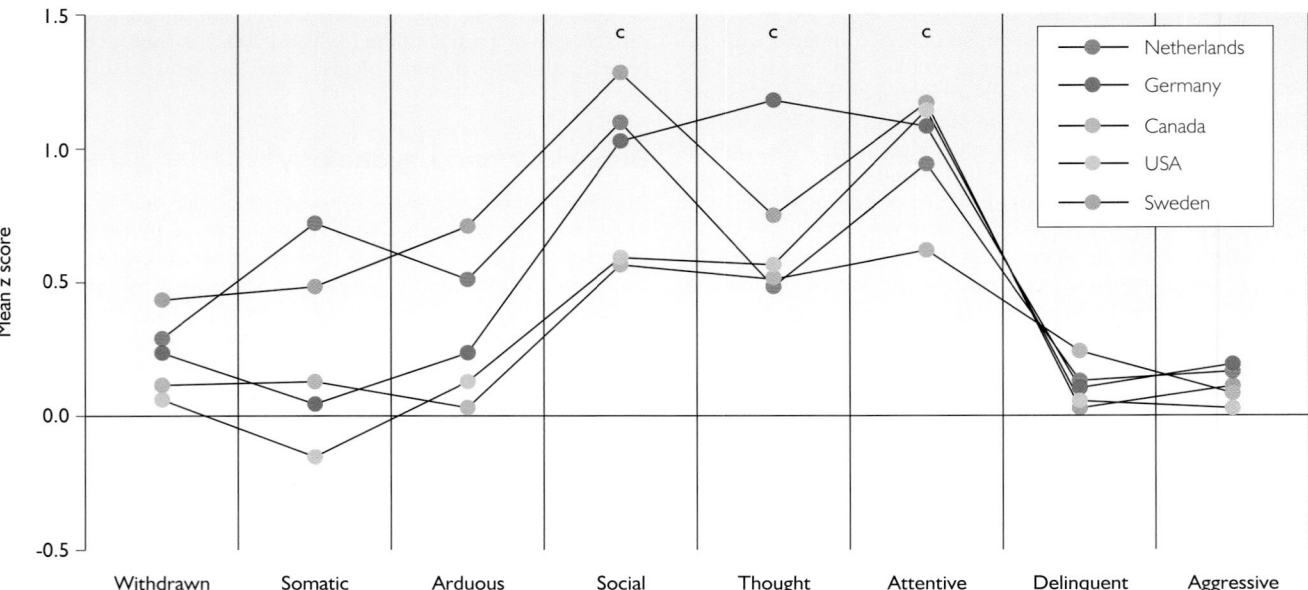

Fig. 3.10 Mean (sd) mental processing composite (MPC) of the Kaufman ABC for children in the Bavarian Longitudinal Study (births in 1985) and in the EPICure study (births in 1995). *(Data from Wolke et al. (2001).) and in the EPICure study (births in 1995; Data from Marlow et al 2006).*

diagnostic psychiatric evaluations yield lower prevalence estimates. Such studies are rare given the cost and logistics of implementing diagnostic tests, but are preferable and enable direct comparisons as outcomes are classified using a standardised nosology (e.g. DSM-IV criteria). In five diagnostic studies, prevalence estimates of 22–28% and associated odds ratios of 3–4 have been reported for psychiatric disorders despite differences in the populations studied (Johnson and Marlow 2011b). When individual disorders are considered, studies have shown an excess of ADHD, emotional disorders and autism spectrum disorders (ASD). However, the comorbidities and clinical presentation of these are different from those of the general population and are indicative of a different causative pathway (Johnson and Marlow 2011b).

ADHD is the most prevalent and frequently studied disorder. Studies have shown a gestational age-related gradient with relative risks of 2.6–2.7 for ADHD in very preterm children (Bhutta et al. 2002; Linnet et al. 2006) and a fourfold increased risk for extremely preterm survivors (Hack et al. 2009; Johnson et al. 2010). In contrast to the general population, the male predominance and frequency of comorbid conduct disorders are not typically observed in preterm populations. Furthermore, preterm children appear to be at greater risk for inattention than hyperactivity/impulsivity, both in term of symptoms and diagnoses (Botting et al. 1997; Hack et al. 2009; Johnson et al. 2010). In the EPICure study we reported that the significant excess of ADHD in extremely preterm children at 11 years was accounted for by a specific risk for ADHD/inattentive-subtype disorders. Hyperactivity in preterm children appears to be accounted for by poor general cognitive ability, but inattention may be an additional specific morbidity related to specific deficits in working memory and processing speed observed in this population (Nadeau et al. 2001).

Perhaps the greatest proliferation of recent interest has focused on the association of ASD with preterm birth. Many clinicians can provide anecdotal evidence of infants in their follow-up clinic with behavioural patterns characteristic of the autism spectrum. Indeed, recent studies using the parent-completed Modified Checklist for Autism in Toddlers (M-CHAT) have reported that up to 25% of very preterm infants screened positive for autistic features

(Limperopoulos et al. 2008; Kuban et al. 2009). This has raised concern regarding a high prevalence of ASD in preterm survivors. However, the specificity of screening in infancy is confounded by the high prevalence of neurodevelopmental delay (Johnson et al. 2009b), particularly where the recommended follow-up M-CHAT interview is not used.

The few diagnostic studies that exist have confirmed the risk for ASD but have reported 1–2% prevalence of ASD in low-birthweight children and 8% prevalence in extremely preterm children (Johnson et al. 2010a), which is remarkably higher than the 0.6% prevalence in the general population. ASD were strongly associated with cognitive impairment and we have drawn parallels with Romanian adoptees who exhibit similar behavioural profiles and who have also experienced highly abnormal early physical and psychosocial environments. Such findings are indicative of a non-genetic, environmental origin in this population. In terms of both ADHD and ASD, the correlates and comorbidities indicate a fundamental underlying problem with brain organisation and development following preterm birth (Johnson and Marlow 2011b). Furthermore, symptoms associated with both disorders have been shown to be generally increased in preterm populations and thus there may be many children with a high level of subthreshold difficulties.

Diagnostic studies have also found a four- to sixfold increased risk for emotional disorders in school-aged children (Johnson and Marlow 2011b). However, it appears that the risk is specific to anxiety and few studies have found a significant association with depression. Although emotional disorders are often associated with poor physical health and female sex in the general population, cognitive impairment was more closely associated with such difficulties in preterm children. Indeed, the majority of children with psychiatric diagnoses in the EPICure study had other associated impairments (Fig. 3.11).

The results of both screening and diagnostic studies have thus highlighted a 'preterm behavioural phenotype' that is associated with inattention, anxiety and social problems. The generally high level of these symptoms means that, even in the absence of diagnosed disorders, many preterm children may present with behavioural problems that do not fulfil diagnostic criteria yet which may

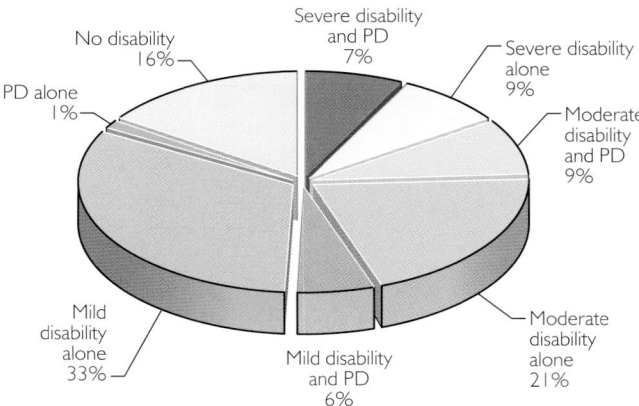

Figure 3.11 Prevalence of psychiatric diagnoses (PD) mapped on to the categories of disability among evaluated 11-year-old children from the EPICure study.

have an impact on everyday function. If these children are not identified during routine neonatal follow-up, difficulties may not be picked up until the child enters school. The preterm child, however, is less likely to be 'hyperactive' in the classroom setting, but is more likely to be anxious or withdrawn and, therefore, less likely to come to the teacher's attention. SEN may thus go unrecognised and become exacerbated throughout schooling. Routine behavioural screening and psychiatric referral if incorporated in neonatal follow-up may therefore be beneficial in reducing the burden of disability in preterm populations.

Motor/neurology

Studies of school-age very preterm children consistently demonstrate poor motor performance in terms of manipulative and gross motor skills. A range of tests can be used but the Movement ABC has been most frequently used to quantify the degree of impairment in this group. In a series of three studies from 6 to 12 years, persistence of motor difficulties was demonstrated (Marlow et al. 1993, 1989b; Powls et al. 1995) and these findings have been replicated in many other studies (Levene et al. 1992; Jongmans et al. 1993). Median scores for the preterm group tend to lie at or outside the 75th percentile for comparison groups. Although a significant disability when in infant school, these impairments are less intrusive and less obvious as teenagers, when motor skills are less prominent aspects of performance.

An alternative approach is to use detailed standardised or semistandardised neurological assessments, such as the scheme of Touwen (1984). The detection of 'minor neurological' or 'soft' signs correlates well with the more functional assessments (Marlow et al. 1989b).

The high proportion of children with impaired motor skills/minor neurological abnormalities may be considered the mild end of a spectrum of disability of which CP is the extreme expression and have been labelled as 'borderline' or 'minimal' CP (Hadders-Algra et al. 1999). One would predict some correlation with brain injuries but the relationship of either motor skills or minor neurological signs to perinatal events or neonatal ultrasound findings is not clear (Levene et al. 1992; Jongmans et al. 1993). More recent studies have failed to demonstrate a relationship between function and teenage MRI appearances, despite a high rate of abnormal scan findings (Cooke and Abernethy 1999; Stewart et al. 1999).

The motor organisational problems may also be reflected in the high frequency of non-right-handedness and less consistent

laterality seen in preterm populations, which show poor correlation with other impaired outcomes or brain injury (Marlow et al. 1989a; Powls et al. 1996a).

Growth and medical outcomes

Despite the concentration on neurological, cognitive and psychological outcomes, it is important not to forget that other aspects of somatic development are frequently disturbed by very preterm birth. VLBW and very preterm children remain smaller throughout childhood than their peers. This is very marked in extremely preterm children, in whom head growth over the first 3 years remains particularly poor and in whom a slim somatotype persists (Wood et al. 2003). Very long-term growth is only rarely reported. In one study bone age and parental heights of 91 VLBW children were integrated to predict adult height (Powls et al. 1996b). Heights for the VLBW group were lower than matched comparison children. However, TW2 RUS score was also significantly advanced over chronological age, indicating that final height would also be impaired: 17% were predicted to be below the 3rd percentile and 33% below the 10th percentile as adults.

Respiratory outcomes are discussed in Chapter 27 part 3, cardiovascular in Chapter 28 and other medical outcomes, including auditory and ocular outcomes, in Chapters 40.5 and 33.

Function and quality of life in surviving ex-preterm children

Although the literature and foregoing discussion are really concerned with the measurement of performance using narrowly focused cognitive or behavioural assessments, such results are difficult to translate into a comprehensive picture of the function of children within society. To a large extent these integrative aspects of outcome may be more important than focused measures of impairment in determining the progress of a neonatal intensive care survivor through life; indeed, the functional definition of outcome at around 2 years has been recommended as a means of defining outcomes for comparative work (Johnson 1995; Report of a BAPM/RCPCH Working Group 2008).

Once infancy is past, the development of a child progresses over multiple domains and functional performance becomes more difficult to register as a single summative measure, hence the reliance on 'medical disability' (CP, cognitive impairment, sensory loss) as an outcome. The recent revision of the World Health Organization ICF has classified outcomes in health and health-related domains (http://www.who.int/classifications/icf/en/). These domains are classified from body, individual and societal perspectives by means of two lists, a list of body functions and structure, and a list of domains of activity and participation, together with a range of environmental factors that may modify the impact of an impairment.

The issue of measuring functional outcomes in perinatal outcome studies has been reviewed by Msall and Tremont (2002). These authors develop the thesis that outcome is assessable and better described in four major domains:

1. impairment (disturbance at organ level)
2. functional limitations of personal activities (self-care, mobility, communication, social interaction)
3. disability in social roles (play, school, work)
4. societal limitations (difficulty in participating imposed by social framework).

There are now a range of measures to support such assessments in childhood, each with its own strengths and limitations (Msall and

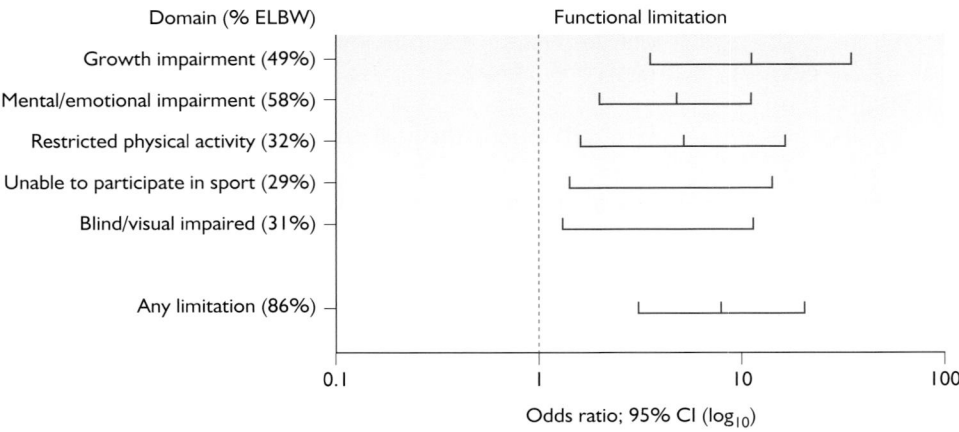

Fig. 3.12 Odds ratio for measures of functional limitation (upper panel) and service/aids use for teenage children of <750 g birthweight compared with term comparison children. CI, confidence interval; ELBW, extremely low birthweight. *(Redrawn from Hack et al. (2000).)*

Tremont 2002). Several studies have evaluated functional measures in the preschool years (<6 years) (Saigal et al. 1990; Msall et al. 1993; Msall and Tremont 2000; Palta et al. 2000). For example, in the survivors of the Cryo-ROP study at 5.5 years, all of <1251 g birthweight, 87% had normal functional skills compared with their non-disabled peers and the rates of severe functional disability (< −4 SD of peers) rose from 3.7% of those without ROP to 26% of those with threshold disease (Msall et al. 2000). Functional status was related to visual status at follow-up; in those with favourable visual status, some disability was found in the domains of self-care (25%), communication (22%), motor (5%) and continence (5%), in contrast to those with poor visual outcomes who had disability in 77%, 66%, 43% and 50% of these domains, respectively. Such a picture can demonstrate the vulnerability imposed by medical impairments and help the understanding of those factors that impart protection against disability. In the USA the concept of 'kindergarten-readiness' provides a multidimensional categorisation that can reflect the overall functioning of the child.

Although preschool and school-age children have been frequently studied, there are fewer studies that have evaluated function in adolescence. Hack and colleagues (2000) evaluated functional outcomes for a group of teenagers born <750 g birthweight, 750–1499 g or at term. For the highest risk group of extremely low-birthweight infants as teenagers, two-thirds accessed non-routine educational or medical services, three-quarters used medication, spectacles or other aids to daily living and 86% demonstrated some functional limitation (Fig. 3.12). The intermediate birthweight group still had significant functional limitation compared with terms but the differences were less marked. That use of medication and contacts with a doctor did not differ significantly between the three groups indicates that the needs of these children are generally outside medical practice. Ongoing service provision for this vulnerable group is an important health issue.

A range of quality-of-life measures is available that have been studied in very preterm children. These range from health-related measures such as the Health Utilities Index (www.healthutilities.com) (Saigal et al. 1996), through self-esteem (Saigal et al. 2002) to more subjective measures (Bjerager et al. 1995). Generally such measures seem to indicate that, whereas health and performance may be considerably worse in the preterm groups, happiness and contentment are not significantly worsened by the presence of disabilities.

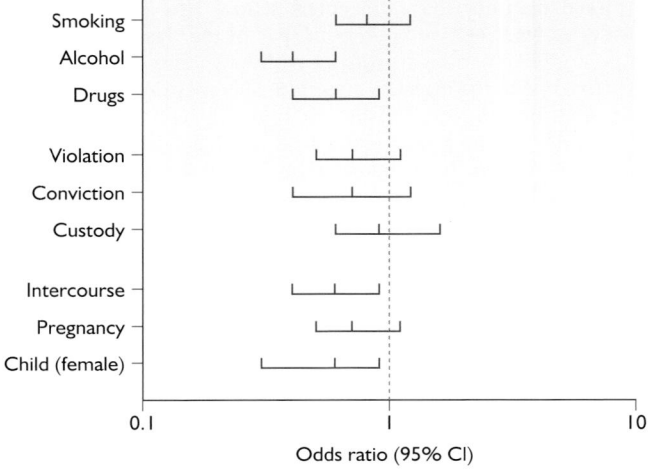

Fig. 3.13 Odds ratio for risk-taking behaviours by young adults who were of very low birthweight compared with normal birthweight comparison children. CI, confidence interval. *(Redrawn from Hack et al. (2002).)*

The ex-preterm young adult

The very first reports of outcome in young adult life are now starting to appear (Hack et al. 2002; Cooke 2004; Saigal et al. 2006). Many of the outcomes are as one might expect from the preceding discussion in terms of lower rates of achievement at school or progression into higher education and higher frequency of low IQ, although the smallest, most immature study from Hamilton, Ontario, Canada, provides the most optimistic outcome and suggests a resilience and adaptation that encourage integration. However, surprisingly, VLBW young adults were found to engage in less risk-taking behaviour, such as the use of alcohol, tobacco or drugs (Hack et al. 2002; Cooke 2004), and tended to be less likely to come into contact with the law (Fig. 3.13) (Hack 2006). Whether this represents resilience on the part of the child-cum-adult to engage socially in an appropriate manner or whether this is the end result of the introversion and attentional deficits seen in many of the studies of psychological outcome remains to be determined (Harrison 2002).

One can conclude from these studies that the subjective consideration of quality of life may rise above the objective, performance-driven consideration of impaired function, which permeates our description of outcomes. Outcome for young adults who were born very preterm may not be as subjectively bad as is anticipated by the close attention to and concentration on impaired function throughout childhood and the integration of this new generation of survivors into society may be considerably better than anticipated.

References

Aarnoudse-Moens, C.S., Smidts, D.P., Oosterlaan, J., et al., 2009. Executive function in very preterm children at early school age. J Abnorm Child Psychol 37, 981–993.

Accardo, P.J., 1982. Freud on diplegia. Commentary and translation. Am J Dis Child 136, 452–456.

Amiel-Tison, C., Grenier A., 1986. Neurological Assessment in the First Year of Life. OUP, Oxford.

Anderson, P., Doyle, L.W., 2003. Neurobehavioral outcomes of school-age children born extremely low birth weight or very preterm in the 1990s. JAMA 289, 3264–3272.

Anderson, P.J., Doyle, L.W., 2004. Executive functioning in school-aged children who were born very preterm or with extremely low birth weight in the 1990s. Pediatrics 114, 50–57.

Anderson, P.J., De Luca, C.R., Hutchinson, E., et al., 2010. Underestimation of developmental delay by the new Bayley-III Scale. Arch Pediatr Adolesc Med 164, 352–356.

Anonymous, 1990. Enhancing the outcomes of low-birth-weight, premature infants. A multisite, randomized trial. The Infant Health and Development Program. JAMA 263, 3035–3042.

Anonymous, 1995. Disability and Perinatal Care: Report of Two Working Groups. NPEU & Oxford HA, Oxford.

Anonymous, 1998. A randomised trial of parental support for families with very preterm children. The Avon Premature Infant Project. Arch Dis Child 79, F4–11.

Astbury, J., Orgill, A.A., Bajuk, B., et al., 1990. Neurodevelopmental outcome, growth and health of extremely low-birthweight survivors: how soon can we tell? Dev Med Child Neurol 32, 582–589.

Aylward, G.P., 2002. Cognitive and neuropsychological outcomes: more than IQ scores. Ment Retard Dev Disabil Res Rev 8, 234–240.

Bhutta, A.T., Cleves, M.A., Casey, P.H., et al., 2002. Cognitive and behavioral outcomes of school-aged children who were born preterm: a meta-analysis. JAMA 288, 728–737.

Bjerager, M., Steensberg, J., Greisen, G., 1995. Quality of life among young adults born with very low birthweights. Acta Paediatr 84, 1339–1343.

Blair, E., Stanley, F., 1990. Intrauterine growth and spastic cerebral palsy. I. Association with birth weight for gestational age. Am J Obstet Gynecol 162, 229–237.

Bohm, B., Katz-Salamon, M., Institute, K., et al., 2002. Developmental risks and protective factors for influencing cognitive outcome at 5 1/2 years of age in very-low-birthweight children. Dev Med Child Neurol 44, 508–516.

Bohm, B., Smedler, A.C., Forssberg, H., 2004. Impulse control, working memory and other executive functions in preterm children when starting school. Acta Paediatr 93, 1363–1371.

Botting, N., Powls, A., Cooke, R.W., et al., 1997. Attention deficit hyperactivity disorders and other psychiatric outcomes in very low birthweight children at 12 years. J Child Psychol Psychiatry 38, 931–941.

Botting, N., Powls, A., Cooke, R.W., et al., 1998. Cognitive and educational outcome of very-low-birthweight children in early adolescence. Dev Med Child Neurol 40, 652–660.

Brothwood, M., Wolke, D., Gamsu, H., et al., 1986. Prognosis of the very low birthweight baby in relation to gender. Arch Dis Child 61, 559–564.

Budin, P., 1907. The Nursling. Caxton Press, London.

Bull, R., Scerif, G., 2001. Executive functioning as a predictor of children's mathematics ability: inhibition, switching, and working memory. Dev Neuropsychol 19, 273–293.

Childs, A.M., Cornette, L., Ramenghi, L.A., et al., 2001. Magnetic resonance and cranial ultrasound characteristics of periventricular white matter abnormalities in newborn infants. Clin Radiol 56, 647–655.

Chyi, L.J., Lee, H.C., Hintz, S.R., et al., 2008. School outcomes of late preterm infants: special needs and challenges for infants born at 32 to 36 weeks gestation. J Pediatr 153, 25–31.

Coenraad, S., Goedegebure, A., Van Goudoever, J.B., et al., 2010. Risk factors for sensorineural hearing loss in NICU infants compared to normal hearing NICU controls. Int J Pediatr Otorhinolaryngol 74, 999–1002.

Cooke, R.W., 2004. Health, lifestyle, and quality of life for young adults born very preterm. Arch Dis Child 89, 201–206.

Cooke, R.W., Abernethy, L.J., 1999. Cranial magnetic resonance imaging and school performance in very low birth weight infants in adolescence. Arch Dis Child Fetal Neonatal Ed 81, F116–F121.

Cross, K.W., 1973. Cost of preventing retrolental fibroplasia? Lancet 2, 954–956.

Davies, A., 1997. A critical review of neonatal hearing screening in the detection of congenital hearing impairment. Health Technol Assess 1, 75.

de Groot, L., Hopkins, B., Touwen, B., 1995. Muscle power, sitting unsupported and trunk rotation in pre-term infants. Early Hum Dev 43, 37–46.

de Groot, L., De Groot, C.J., Hopkins, B., 1997a. An instrument to measure independent walking: are there differences between preterm and fullterm infants? J Child Neurol 12, 37–41.

de Groot, L., Hopkins, B., Touwen, B., 1997b. Motor asymmetries in preterm infants at 18 weeks corrected age and outcomes at 1 year. Early Hum Dev 48, 35–46.

de Vries, A.M., De Groot, L., 2002. Transient dystonias revisited: a comparative study of preterm and term children at 2 1/2 years of age. Dev Med Child Neurol 44, 415–421.

de Vries, L.S., Van Haastert, I.L., Rademaker, K.J., et al., 2004. Ultrasound abnormalities preceding cerebral palsy in high-risk preterm infants. J Pediatr 144, 815–820.

Downs, J.A., Edwards, A.D., Mccormick, D.C., et al., 1991. Effect of intervention on development of hip posture in very preterm babies. Arch Dis Child 66, 797–801.

Doyle, L.W., 2001. Outcome at 5 years of age of children 23 to 27 weeks' gestation: refining the prognosis. Pediatrics 108, 134–141.

Doyle, L.W., Roberts, G., Anderson, P.J., 2010. Outcomes at age 2 years of infants <28 weeks' gestational age born in Victoria in 2005. J Pediatr 156, 49–53.

Drillien, C.M., 1958. Growth and development of a group of children of very low birthweight. Arch Dis Child 33, 10–18.

Drillien, C.M., 1972. Abnormal neurologic signs in the first year of life in low-birthweight infants: possible prognostic significance. Dev Med Child Neurol 14, 575–584.

Drillien, C.M., 1980. Low-birthweight children at early school-age: a longitudinal study. Dev Med Child Neurol 22, 26–47.

Einspieler, C., Prechtl, H.F.R., 2005. Prechtl's assessment of general movements: a diagnostic tool for the functional assessment of the young nervous system. Ment Retard Dev Disabil Res Rev 11, 61–67.

Eliasson, A.C., Krumlinde-Sundholm, L., Rosblad, B., et al., 2006. The Manual

Ability Classification System (MACS) for children with cerebral palsy: scale development and evidence of validity and reliability. Dev Med Child Neurol 48, 549–554.

Farooqi, A., 2009. Pervasive behavioural problems are common in children born at less than 26 weeks of gestation. Evid Based Ment Health 12, 63.

Fily, A., Pierrat, V., Delporte, V., et al., 2006. Factors associated with neurodevelopmental outcome at 2 years after very preterm birth: the population-based Nord-Pas-de-Calais EPIPAGE cohort. Pediatrics 117, 357–366.

Flynn, J., 1999. Searching for justice: the discovery of IQ gains over time. Am Psychologist 54, 5–20.

Gardner, F., Johnson, A., Yudkin, P., et al., 2004. Behavioral and emotional adjustment of teenagers in mainstream school who were born before 29 weeks' gestation. Pediatrics 114, 676–682.

Gesell, A., Armatruda, A., 1947. Developmental Diagnosis: normal and abnormal child development, second ed. Hoeber, New York.

Haataja, L., Mercuri, E., Guzzetta, A., et al., 2001. Neurologic examination in infants with hypoxic-ischemic encephalopathy at age 9 to 14 months: use of optimality scores and correlation with magnetic resonance imaging findings. J Pediatr 138, 332–337.

Hack, M., 2006. Young adult outcomes of very-low-birth-weight children. Semin Fetal Neonatal Med 11, 127–137.

Hack, M., Taylor, H.G., Klein, N., et al., 2000. Functional limitations and special health care needs of 10- to 14-year-old children weighing less than 750 grams at birth. Pediatrics 106, 554–560.

Hack, M., Flannery, D.J., Schluchter, M., et al., 2002. Outcomes in young adulthood for very-low-birth-weight infants. N Engl J Med 346, 149–157.

Hack, M., Taylor, H.G., Drotar, D., et al., 2005. Chronic conditions, functional limitations, and special health care needs of school-aged children born with extremely low-birth-weight in the 1990s [see comment]. JAMA 294, 318–325.

Hack, M., Taylor, H.G., Schluchter, M., et al., 2009. Behavioral outcomes of extremely low birth weight children at age 8 years. J Dev Behav Pediatr 30, 122–130.

Hadders-Algra, M., Brogren, E., Katz-Salamon, M., et al., 1999. Periventricular leucomalacia and preterm birth have different detrimental effects on postural adjustments. Brain 122, 727–740.

Hagberg, B., Hagberg, G., Olow, I., et al., 1996. The changing panorama of cerebral palsy in Sweden. VII. Prevalence and origin in the birth year period 1987–90. Acta Paediatr 85, 954–960.

Harrison, H., 2002. Outcomes in young adulthood for very-low-birth-weight infants. N Engl J Med 347, 141–143.

Hess, J.H., Mohr, G.J., Bartelme, P.F., 1934. The physical and mental growth of prematurely born children. University of Chicago Press, Chicago.

Hille, E.T., Den Ouden, A.L., Saigal, S., et al., 2001. Behavioural problems in children who weigh 1000 g or less at birth in four countries. Lancet 357, 1641–1643.

Hille, E.T., Van Straaten, H.I., Verkerk, P.H., 2007. Prevalence and independent risk factors for hearing loss in NICU infants. Acta Paediatr 96, 1155–1158.

Himmelmann, K., Hagberg, G., Beckung, E., et al., 2005. The changing panorama of cerebral palsy in Sweden. IX. Prevalence and origin in the birth-year period 1995–1998. Acta Paediatr 94, 287–294.

Hintz, S.R., Kendrick, D.E., Vohr, B.R., et al., 2006. Gender differences in neurodevelopmental outcomes among extremely preterm, extremely-low-birthweight infants. Acta Paediatr 95, 1239–1248.

Indredavik, M.S., Vik, T., Heyerdahl, S., et al., 2005. Psychiatric symptoms in low birth weight adolescents, assessed by screening questionnaires. Eur Child Adolesc Psychiatry 14, 226–236.

Jarvis, S., Glinianaia, S.V., Torrioli, M.G., et al., 2003. Cerebral palsy and intrauterine growth in single births: European collaborative study. Lancet 362, 1106–1111.

Johnson, A., 1995. Disability and perinatal care. Pediatrics 95, 272–274.

Johnson, S., 2007. Cognitive and behavioural outcomes following very preterm birth. Semin Fetal Neonatal Med 12, 363–373.

Johnson, S., Marlow, N., 2011a. Educational outcomes in extremely preterm children: neurological outcomes and predictors of attainment. Dev Neuropsychol 36, 74–95.

Johnson, S., Marlow, N., 2011b. Psychiatric disorders and preterm birth. Pediatr Res, In press.

Johnson, S., Marlow, N., Wolke, D., et al., 2004. Validation of a parent report measure of cognitive development in very preterm infants. Dev Med Child Neurol 46, 389–397.

Johnson, S., Wolke, D., Marlow, N., 2008. Developmental assessment of preterm infants at 2 years: validity of parent reports. Dev Med Child Neurol 50, 58–62.

Johnson, S., Fawke, J., Hennessy, E., et al., 2009a. Neurodevelopmental disability through 11 years of age in children born before 26 weeks of gestation. Pediatrics 124, e249–57.

Johnson, S., Hennessy, E., Hollis, C., et al., 2009b. Screening for autism spectrum disorders in extremely preterm children. Acta Paediatr 98, 163–163.

Johnson, S., Hennessy, E., Smith, R., et al., 2009c. Academic attainment and special

educational needs in extremely preterm children at 11 years of age: the EPICure study. Arch Dis Child Fetal Neonatal Ed 94, F283–F289.

Johnson, S., Hollis, C., Kochhar, P., et al., 2010a. Autism spectrum disorders in extremely preterm children. J pediatr 156, 525–531.

Johnson, S., Hollis, C., Kochhar, P., et al., 2010b. Psychiatric disorders in extremely preterm children: longitudinal finding at age 11 years in the EPICure Study. J Am Acad Child Adolesc Psychiatry 49, 453–463.

Jongmans, M., Henderson, S., De Vries, L., et al., 1993. Duration of periventricular densities in preterm infants and neurological outcome at 6 years of age. Arch Dis Child 69, 9–13.

Khadilkar, V., Tudehope, D., Burns, Y., et al., 1993. The long-term neurodevelopmental outcome for very low birthweight (VLBW) infants with 'dystonic' signs at 4 months of age. J Paediatr Child Health 29, 415–417.

Kiely, J.L., Paneth, N., 1981. Follow-up studies of low-birthweight infants: suggestions for design, analysis and reporting. Dev Med Child Neurol 23, 96–100.

Klebanov, P.K., Brooks-Gunn, J., McCormick, M.C., 1994. School achievement and failure in very low birth weight children. J Dev Behav Pediatr 15, 248–256.

Koldewijn, K., Van Wassenaer, A., Wolf, M.J., et al., 2010. A neurobehavioral intervention and assessment program in very low birth weight infants: outcome at 24 months. J Pediatr 156, 359–365.

Kraemer, S., 2000. The fragile male. Br Med J 321, 1609–1612.

Kuban, K.C., O'Shea, T.M., Allred, E.N., et al., 2009. Positive screening on the Modified Checklist for Autism in Toddlers (M-CHAT) in extremely low gestational age newborns. J Pediatr 154, 535–540.

Levene, M., Dowling, S., Graham, M., et al., 1992. Impaired motor function (clumsiness) in 5 year old children: correlation with neonatal ultrasound scans. Arch Dis Child 67, 687–690.

Limperopoulos, C., Bassan, H., Sullivan, N.R., et al., 2008. Positive screening for autism in ex-preterm infants: prevalence and risk factors. Pediatrics 121, 758–765.

Lindstrom, K., Winbladh, B., Haglund, B., et al., 2007. Preterm infants as young adults: a Swedish national cohort study. Pediatrics 120, 70–77.

Linnet, K.M., Wisborg, K., Agerbo, E., et al., 2006. Gestational age, birth weight, and the risk of hyperkinetic disorder. Arch Dis Child 91, 655–660.

Litt, J., Taylor, H.G., Klein, N., et al., 2005. Learning disabilities in children with very low birthweight: prevalence, neuropsychological correlates, and educational interventions. J Learning Disabil 38, 130–141.

Lorenz, J.M., Paneth, N., Jetton, J.R., et al., 2001. Comparison of management strategies for extreme prematurity in New Jersey and the Netherlands: outcomes and resource expenditure. Pediatrics 108, 1269–1274.

MacKay, D.F., Smith, G.C., Dobbie, R., et al., 2010. Gestational age at delivery and special educational need: retrospective cohort study of 407,503 schoolchildren. PLoS Med 7, e1000289.

Marlow, N., 2006. Introduction: Neurodevelopmental follow up after preterm birth. Early Hum Dev 82, 149–150.

Marlow, N., Roberts, B.L., Cooke, R.W., 1989a. Laterality and prematurity. Arch Dis Child 64, 1713–1716.

Marlow, N., Roberts, B.L., Cooke, R.W., 1989b. Motor skills in extremely low birthweight children at the age of 6 years. Arch Dis Child 64, 839–847.

Marlow, N., Roberts, L., Cooke, R., 1993. Outcome at 8 years for children with birth weights of 1250 g or less. Arch Dis Child 68, 286–290.

Marlow, E.S., Hunt, L.P., Marlow, N., 2000. Sensorineural hearing loss and prematurity. Arch Dis Child Fetal Neonatal Ed 82, F141–F144.

Marlow, N., Hennessy, E., Bracewell, M., et al., 2007. Motor and executive function at 6 years of age following extremely preterm birth. Pediatrics 120, 793–804.

Mathiasen, R., Hansen, B.M., Andersen, A.M., et al., 2010. Gestational age and basic school achievements: a national follow-up study in Denmark. Pediatrics 126, e1553–61.

McCarton, C.M., Brooks-Gunn, J., Wallace, I.F., et al., 1997. Results at age 8 years of early intervention for low-birth-weight premature infants. The Infant Health and Development Program. JAMA 277, 126–132.

McCormick, M.C., Richardson, D.K., 2002. Premature infants grow up. N Engl J Med 346, 197–198.

Morris, C., 2007. Defintion and classification of cerebral palsy: a historical perspective. Dev Med Child Neurol 49 (Suppl.), 3–7.

Msall, M.E., Tremont, M.R., 2000. Functional outcomes in self-care, mobility, communication, and learning in extremely low-birth weight infants. Clin Perinatol 27, 381–401.

Msall, M.E., Tremont, M.R., 2002. Measuring functional outcomes after prematurity: developmental impact of very low birth weight and extremely low birth weight status on childhood disability. Mental Retard Dev Disabil Res Rev 8, 258–272.

Msall, M.E., Rogers, B.T., Buck, G.M., et al., 1993. Functional status of extremely preterm infants at kindergarten entry. Dev Med Child Neurol 35, 312–320.

Msall, M.E., Phelps, D.L., Digaudio, K.M., et al., 2000. Severity of neonatal retinopathy of prematurity is predictive of neurodevelopmental functional outcome at age 5.5 years. Behalf of the Cryotherapy for Retinopathy of Prematurity Cooperative Group. Pediatrics 106, 998–1005.

Mulder, H., Pitchford, N.J., Hagger, M.S., et al., 2009. Development of executive function and attention in preterm children: a systematic review. Dev Neuropsychol 34, 393–421.

Mulder, H., Pitchford, N.J., Marlow, N., 2010. Processing speed and working memory underlie academic attainment in very preterm children. Arch Dis Child: Fetal Neonatal Ed 95, F267–F272.

Mutch, L.M., Johnson, M.A., Morley, R., 1989. Follow up studies: design, organisation, and analysis. Arch Dis Child 64, 1394–1402.

Nadeau, L., Boivin, M., Tessier, R., et al., 2001. Mediators of behavioral problems in 7-year-old children born after 24 to 28 weeks of gestation. J Dev Behav Pediatr 22, 1–10.

Nelson, K.B., Ellenberg, J.H., 1982. Children who 'outgrew' cerebral palsy. Pediatrics 69, 529–536.

Nuffield Council on Bioethics, 2006. Critical Care Decisions in Fetal and Neonatal Medicine: Ethical Issues. Report of a Working Group. Nuffield Council on Biothethics, London.

O'Connor, A.R., Stephenson, T., Johnson, A., et al., 2002. Long-term ophthalmic outcome of low birth weight children with and without retinopathy of prematurity. Pediatrics 109, 12–18.

Palisano, R., Rosenbaum, P., Walter, S., et al., 1997. Development and reliability of a system to classify gross motor function in children with cerebral palsy. Dev Med Child Neurol 39, 214–223.

Pallas Alonso, C.R., De La Cruz Bertolo, J., Medina Lopez, M.C., et al., 2000. [Cerebral palsy and age of sitting and walking in children weighing less than 1,500 g at birth.] An Esp Pediatr 53, 48–52.

Palta, M., Sadek-Badawi, M., Evans, M., et al., 2000. Functional assessment of a multicenter very low-birth-weight cohort at age 5 years. Newborn Lung Project. Arch Pediatr Adolesc Med 154, 23–30.

Pederson, S., Sommerfelt, K., Markestad T., 2000. Early motor development of premature infants with birthweight less than 2000 grams. Acta Paediatr 89, 1456–1461.

Pennefather, P.M., Clarke, M.P., Strong, N.P., et al., 1995. Ocular outcome in children born before 32 weeks gestation. Eye 9, 26–30.

Pharoah, P.O., Platt, M.J., Cooke, T., 1996. The changing epidemiology of cerebral palsy. Arch Dis Child Fetal Neonatal Ed 75, F169–F173.

Pharoah, P.O., Stevenson, C.J., West, C.R., 2003. General Certificate of Secondary Education performance in very low birthweight infants. Arch Dis Child 88, 295–298.

Pike, A.A., Marlow, N., 2000. The role of cortical evoked responses in predicting neuromotor outcome in very preterm infants. Early Hum Dev 57, 123–135.

Platt, M.J., Cans, C., Johnson, A., et al., 2007. Trends in cerebral palsy among infants of very low birthweight (<1500 g) or born prematurely (<32 weeks) in 16 European centres: a database study. Lancet 369, 43–50.

Powls, A., Botting, N., Cooke, R.W., et al., 1995. Motor impairment in children 12 to 13 years old with a birthweight of less than 1250 g. Arch Dis Child Fetal Neonatal Ed 73, F62–F66.

Powls, A., Botting, N., Cooke, R.W., et al., 1996a. Handedness in very-low-birthweight (VLBW) children at 12 years of age: relation to perinatal and outcome variables. Dev Med Child Neurol 38, 594–602.

Powls, A., Botting, N., Cooke, R.W., et al., 1996b. Growth impairment in very low birthweight children at 12 years: correlation with perinatal and outcome variables. Arch Dis Child Fetal Neonatal Ed 75, F152–F157.

Powls, A., Botting, N., Cooke, R.W., et al., 1997. Visual impairment in very low birthweight children. Arch Dis Child Fetal Neonatal Ed 76, F82–F87.

Prechtl, H.F., Einspieler, C., Cioni, G., et al., 1997. An early marker for neurological deficits after perinatal brain lesions. Lancet 349, 1361–1363.

Report of a BAPM/RCPCH Working Group, 2008. Classification of Health Status at 2 Years as a Perinatal Outcome. British Association of Perinatal Medicine, London.

Robertson, C.M., Watt, M.J., Yasui, Y., 2007. Changes in the prevalence of cerebral palsy for children born very prematurely within a population-based program over 30 years. JAMA 297, 2733–2740.

Robertson, C.M., Howarth, T.M., Bork, D.L., et al., 2009. Permanent bilateral sensory and neural hearing loss of children after neonatal intensive care because of extreme prematurity: a thirty-year study. Pediatrics 123, e797–807.

Rosenbaum, P., Paneth, N., Goldstein, M., et al., 2007. The definition and classification of cerebral palsy April 2006. Dev Med Child Neurol 49 (Suppl.), 8–14.

Roth, S.C., Baudin, J., McCormick, D.C., et al., 1993. Relation between ultrasound appearance of the brain of very preterm infants and neurodevelopmental impairment at eight years. Dev Med Child Neurol 35, 755–768.

Saigal, S., Szatmari, P., Rosenbaum, P., et al., 1990. Intellectual and functional status at school entry of children who weighed 1000 grams or less at birth: a regional perspective of births in the 1980s. J Pediatr 116, 409–416.

Saigal, S., Feeny, D., Rosenbaum, P., et al., 1996. Self-perceived health status and health-related quality of life of extremely low-birth-weight infants at adolescence. JAMA 276, 453–459.

Saigal, S., Lambert, M., Russ, C., et al., 2002. Self-esteem of adolescents who were born prematurely. Pediatrics 109, 429–433.

Saigal, S., Den Ouden, L., Wolke, D., et al., 2003. School-age outcomes in children who were extremely low birth weight from four international population-based cohorts. Pediatrics 112, 943–950.

Saigal, S., Stoskopf, B., Streiner, D., et al., 2006. Transition of extremely low-birth-weight infants from adolescence to young adulthood: comparison with normal birth-weight controls. JAMA 295, 667–675.

Salt, A., Redshaw, M., 2006. Neurodevelopmental follow-up after preterm birth: follow up after two years. Early Hum Dev 82, 185–197.

Samara, M., Marlow, N., Wolke, D., 2008. Pervasive behavior problems at 6 years of age in a total-population sample of children born at </=25 weeks of gestation. Pediatrics 122, 562–573.

Sameroff, A., Chandler, M., 1965. Reproductive risk and the continuum of caretaking casualty. In: Horowitz, F. (Ed.), Review of Child Development Research. University of Chicago Press, Chicago, Ch 4, pp 187–244.

Saudino, K., Dale, P., Oliver, B., et al., 1998. The validity of parent-based assessment of the cognitive abilities of 2-year-olds. Br J Dev Psychol 16, 349–363.

Schneider, W., Wolke, D., Schlagmuller, M., et al., 2004. Pathways to school achievement in very preterm and full term children. Eur J Psychol Ed 19, 385–406.

Schulz, K.F., Altman, D.G., Moher, D., 2010. CONSORT 2010 statement: updated guidelines for reporting parallel group randomised trials. PLoS Med 7, e1000251.

Sheridan, M., 1962. Infants at risk of handicapping conditions. Monthly Bulletin of the Ministry of Health and the Public Health Laboratory Service, pp 238–245.

Silverman, W.A., 1979. Incubator-baby side shows (Dr. Martin A. Couney). Pediatrics 64, 127–141.

Sommerfelt, K., Pedersen, S., Ellertsen, B., et al., 1996. Transient dystonia in non-handicapped low-birthweight infants and later neurodevelopment. Acta Paediatr 85, 1445–1449.

Spittle, A.J., Orton, J., Doyle, L.W., et al., 2007. Early developmental intervention programs post hospital discharge to prevent motor and cognitive impairments in preterm infants. Cochrane Database Syst Rev (2), CD005495.

Spittle, A.J., Ferretti, C., Anderson, P.J., et al., 2009. Improving the outcome of infants born at <30 weeks' gestation – a randomized controlled trial of preventative care at home. BMC Pediatr 9, 73.

St Clair-Thompson, H.L., Gathercole, S.E., 2006. Executive functions and achievements in school: shifting, updating, inhibition, and working memory. Q J Exp Psychol (Colchester) 59, 745–759.

Stewart, A.L., Reynolds, E.O., Lipscomb, A.P., 1981. Outcome for infants of very low birthweight: survey of world literature. Lancet 1, 1038–1040.

Stewart, A., Rifkin, L., Amess, P.N., et al., 1999. Brain structure and neurocognitive and behavioural function in adolescents who were born very preterm. Lancet 353, 1653–1657.

Taylor, H.G., Espy, K.A., Anderson, P.J., 2009. Mathematics deficiencies in children with very low birth weight or very preterm birth. Dev Disabil Res Rev 15, 52–59.

Tin, W., Fritz, S., Wariyar, U., et al., 1998. Outcome of very preterm birth: children reviewed with ease at 2 years differ from those followed up with difficulty. Arch Dis Child Fetal Neonatal Ed 79, F83–F87.

Touwen, B., 1984. Examination of the child with minor neurological dysfunction. Clinics in Developmental Medicine (2nd edition) Vol 71.

Tyson, J.E., Parikh, N.A., Langer, J., et al., 2008. Intensive care for extreme prematurity – moving beyond gestational age. N Engl J Med 358, 1672–1681.

von Elm, E., Altman, D.G., Egger, M., et al., 2007. The Strengthening the Reporting of Observational Studies in Epidemiology (STROBE) statement: guidelines for reporting observational studies. Lancet 370, 1453–1457.

Wilson-Costello, D., Friedman, H., Minich, N., et al., 2005. Improved survival rates with increased neurodevelopmental disability for extremely low birth weight infants in the 1990s. Pediatrics 115, 997–1003.

Wolke, D., Ratschinski, G., Ohrt, B., et al., 1994. The cognitive outcome of very preterm infants may be poorer than often reported: an empirical investigation of how methodological issues make a big difference. Eur J Pediatr 153, 906–915.

Wolke, D., Sohne, B., Ohrt, B., et al., 1995. Follow-up of preterm children: important to document dropouts. Lancet 345, 447.

Wolke, D., Schulz, J., Meyer, R., 2001. Entwicklungslangzeitfolgen bei ehemaligen, sehr unreifen Frühgeborenen. Monatsschr Kinderheilk 149, 53–61.

Wood, N.S., Marlow, N., Costeloe, K., et al., 2000. Neurologic and developmental disability after extremely preterm birth. EPICure Study Group. N Engl J Med 343, 378–384.

Wood, N.S., Costeloe, K., Gibson, A.T., et al., 2003. The EPICure Study: growth and associated problems in children born at 25 weeks or less gestational age. Arch Dis Child, 88, F492–F500.

Yoshinaga-Itano, C., Sedey, A.L., Coulter, D.K., et al., 1998. Language of early- and later-identified children with hearing loss. Pediatrics 102, 1161–1171.

Developmental care 4

Angela Huertas-Ceballos   Gillian Kennedy

Introduction

Increasing numbers of premature infants are surviving thanks to technological advances. Mortality has been dramatically reduced but morbidity remains a challenge (Riley et al. 2008). Follow-up studies on children at school age have shown that they are more likely to have difficulties with attention, fine motor skills and interpersonal relationships (Saigal et al. 2003; Johnson et al. 2009). Developmental care (more specifically, the Newborn Individualized Developmental Care and Assessment Program (NIDCAP)) has been claimed to improve outcomes (Bhutta et al. 2002; Als et al. 2004). This chapter will describe some of the developmental care practices within the context of the developing brain and the evidence behind these approaches.

Brain development in relation to developmental care

Preterm babies are projected into an alien extrauterine setting at a time when their brains are growing more rapidly than at any other time in their life. Their experience is a contrast between the expected environment of their mother's womb and the feel of their parents' bodies after birth and the comfort of their family and community social group (Hofer 1987).

As is well known, development of the brain is influenced by predetermined genetic processing and endogenous and exogenous stimulation. The genetic processing is largely exempt from external influences as it occurs predominantly in the first 20 weeks of gestation. It is after this that the so-called critical periods of brain development occur when environmental influences shape neuronal connectivity and activity (Liu et al. 2007). In essence, during critical periods the brain requires appropriate sensory input from external influences in order to make appropriate connections.

The neonatal intensive care unit (NICU) does not provide the sensory experience that the premature infant was expecting in terms of type, timing or intensity. Consequently there is the potential for these windows of opportunity to be missed. Furthermore, studies on preterm infants have demonstrated that the dual stress for the baby of maternal separation together with frequent painful procedures or discomfort results in potentially neurotoxic brain-altering events (Anand and Scalzo 2000).

Such research findings emphasise the need to recognise that both family relationships and the care given during the preterm infant's stay in the NICU influence the infant's neurodevelopment. Current thinking is that developmental care should be implemented alongside medical interventions in order to maximise the baby's potential and achieve the best possible outcome.

© 2012 Elsevier Ltd

Developmental care

Developmental care is an umbrella term for a variety of approaches used with preterm infants whilst in NICU. The aim is to adapt the infant's sensory experience of the world positively and involve the family and care team. Developmental care includes modifications of both care-giving practices and the baby's physical environment.

The aim of developmental care is to promote the infant's neurodevelopment through increasing comfort, decreasing stress and promoting sleep. Key points related to the most commonly applied developmental care practices are outlined below.

The nursery environment

Environmental modifications to light and noise are those most commonly considered when the term 'developmental care' is used. Indeed, these aspects are important as they have significant influence on the infant's autonomic stability and have the potential to cause harm (Long et al. 1980).

Light

The development of the central visual system may be disrupted by overstimulation of the eyes. Bright light disrupts release of growth hormone and may prolong the time spent in rapid-eye movement sleep (Duffy et al. 1984). Little is known about the development of circadian rhythms in premature infants. However, it has been demonstrated that babies exposed to periods of cycled versus continuous lighting have longer periods of sleep and are more efficient feeders with improved weight gain (Mann et al. 1996).

Recommendations for modifying the nursery environment to support neurodevelopment include dimming lights whilst maintaining a safe level of accurate clinical observation as well as cycling lighting to simulate day–night patterns (White 2007). Individualised bedside lighting and shielding the infant from light with an incubator cover or blanket are recommended (Als and Mcanulty 2000). At term, the baby requires the opportunity to explore the world visually with adequate levels of lighting. This is vital for continued development of the visual system (Stanley et al. 2008).

Noise

In utero, infants are exposed to sound of 40–60 dB, yet in the NICU sound may exceed 120 db at times. Loud sound levels are known to cause stress in preterm infants. Moreover, preterm infants are unable to habituate to sound within their environment and, consequently, environmental noise interferes with sleep and creates increased distractibility which persists into childhood (Gray and Philbin 2004).

Developmental care aiming to reduce auditory environmental stimuli includes noise monitors (White 2007), lowering the volume of monitor alarms, covering incubators with thick, padded covers and conducting teaching rounds either in an unobtrusive manner or away from the cot side (Lawhon and Melzar 1988).

Guidelines with recommendations for nursery design, which encompass optimal light and sound levels, have been published in the USA (White 2007).

Family-centred care (FCC)

The family has a pivotal role within developmental care and, to reflect this, the term 'family-centred/supportive care' is used. In this model, families have unrestricted access to their infant. Different interpretations of this premise vary from providing seats for parents next to their baby's incubator to providing a 'private room' within the nursery for the family. Here, they live with their baby until discharge, fully caring for the child with support from the team, as required (Westrup 2009).

One of the key objectives of FCC is to educate and integrate parents into the newborn intensive care environment and to encourage active participation in their baby's care. Furthermore, it aims to help parents observe and interpret their baby's behavioural needs, thus enhancing relationships. This is particularly important given that preterm infants inevitably have lower levels of signalling (Minde et al. 1983).

Kangaroo mother care (KMC)

Developed 30 years ago, KMC aimed to improve infant survival in the absence of incubators. Whilst wearing only a nappy, the baby is placed between the mother's breasts in a vertical position with head and trunk aligned and limbs flexed, with supportive material binding surrounding both. Heat is transmitted from mother to baby, stabilising the baby's temperature; her breathing provides stimulation for her infant's respiration and the upright positioning helps minimise gastro-oesophageal reflux. Today, KMC involves relatives, fathers and same-sex partners as well as biological mothers (Fig. 4.1).

It has been demonstrated that KMC has a positive effect on state organisation, physiological stability, decreased arousal and increased quiet sleep and neurodevelopment. It facilitates the family's psychological healing, enhances parent–infant bonding and improves lactation (Conde Agudelo and Belizan 2003; Charpak et al. 2005). Maternal benefits include increased self-confidence, less postpartum depression and better ability to respond to and care for her baby during admission and after discharge (Tallandini and Scalembra 2006).

There are published guidelines for the implementation of KMC on ventilated and non-ventilated infants (Charpak et al. 2000).

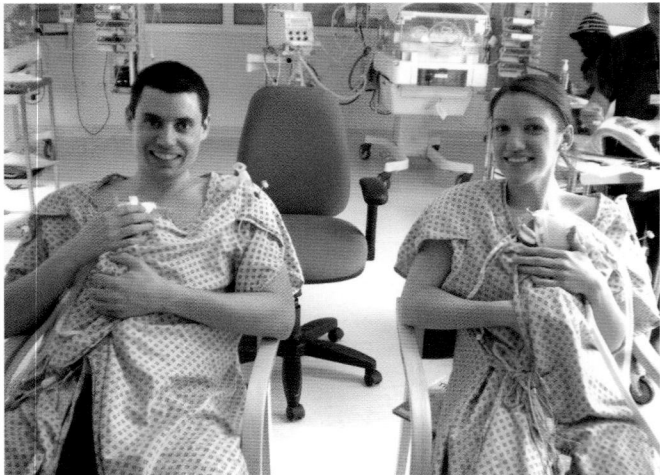

Fig. 4.1 Twins nursed in kangaroo care fashion by their parents at University College Hospital, London. Kangaroo care is an effective developmental care method that should be available for parents of babies at any gestational age admitted to neonatal units, independently of the level of care they receive.

Incubator environment

Staff can increase the baby's comfort during the lengthy periods the child is cared for in an incubator or cot by adopting relatively simple measures such as the following.

Postural support

Swaddling seems to improve sleep quality and diminish stress and pain responses in the preterm infant and it is suggested that it may also improve neuromuscular development (Short et al. 1996). Comfortable swaddling should avoid limb overextension, overheating or interference with respiratory effort. Alternatively, consideration may be given to positioning as, for example, prone or left side-lying may reduce gastro-oesophageal reflux (Ewer et al. 1999) whereas side-lying may enhance neuromuscular development. Supportive bedding materials, including nests, are used to help the infant maintain head and trunk alignment. The position facilitates the baby's efforts to bring the hands together or to the mouth; these are calming strategies that promote further development.

Chemosensory support

The sensory pathways for both taste and smell develop early in utero with the fetus exposed to the mother's diet via the amniotic fluid (Browne 2008). After birth, the infant shows preferences for these flavours, demonstrating the ability to detect and discriminate smell and taste through physiological and behavioural responsiveness. Smell has been shown to influence positively the quality of the infant's arousal and sleep states and aid the infant's recognition, hence encouraging relationships, particularly maternal. Noxious stimuli can have a negative effect (Bartocci et al. 2001).

Exposing preterm infants to the smell of their mother's amniotic fluid and/or colostrum as soon as possible after delivery may ameliorate the effect of separation and facilitate both bonding and later progression to oral feeding (Schaal et al. 1998). Tastes of expressed breast milk may be incorporated into mouth care even with very preterm infants.

Non-nutritive sucking (NNS)

Considerable research has been devoted to NNS whereby the infant is offered a pacifier most usually during tube feeds or as a comforter during painful procedures. The reported benefits related to NNS include earlier discharge, quicker transition to oral feeds and improved physiological stability during painful interventions, particularly when NNS is combined with expressed breast milk or sucrose (Pinelli and Symington 2005).

Support during cares and procedures

It is easy for parents and staff to appreciate that interventions such as blood sampling or lumbar puncture cause pain and discomfort. It is less readily appreciated that routine care procedures like weighing can also engender stress for the infant. Consideration of the following may provide developmental support.

Timing and pacing of cares

As far as possible, the baby's sleep should be respected and protected given its importance for brain development. Whilst it may be considered advantageous to 'cluster' cares and procedures and then to leave the baby undisturbed, the intensity of the interventions may tax the infant physiologically more than allowing the infant to rest for a short time between activities, ideally with carer support (Holsti et al. 2005).

Gentle handling

The unborn baby lives in a warm, fluid-filled environment, gently rocked by constant oscillations of amniotic fluid. Caregiving in the NICU can be intrusive, painful and stressful. Gentle handling, avoiding sudden changes in posture, is recommended. Supporting the infant with still hands (containment holding) which are gently enveloping can help the baby endure difficult experiences and recover more quickly, particularly when combined with appropriate pacing of caregiving (Als and Gilkerson 1995). Parental holding in this way is probably the ideal physical contact for the preterm infant. The benefit of massage is disputed and can prove overstimulating for more fragile infants.

Pain

Pain and stress are usually recognised in preterm and term babies using pain scales that include facial expressions and physiological variables like heart rate, respiratory rate, mean blood pressure and changes in skin colour (Ch. 25). Pain can be treated with medication, behavioural approaches or both. Pharmacological strategies to provide pain relief include boluses or continuous infusions of morphine, midazolam or fentanyl for ventilated babies and chloral hydrate or oral sucrose before painful procedures. Behavioural interventions include swaddling, gentle handling, NNS, breastfeeding and KMC (Chermont et al. 2009).

Newborn Individualized Developmental Care and Assessment Program

NIDCAP is a structured comprehensive approach that selects appropriate developmental care methods which are continually adapted to the baby's needs at given times in order to promote development. The family are the baby's main advocates and are integral to care.

Based on Als' synactive theory of development (Als 1982), the preterm baby is viewed as an active and competent individual who has prematurely delivered into an alien environment. The baby's developing competencies are described within the context of five subsystems that emerge and interact in response to internal and external stimuli, each system having the potential to support or disrupt the equilibrium of another. These subsystems are:

1. autonomic/physiological (i.e. heart rate, respiratory rate, colour, gastrointestinal signs)
2. motor (posture, tone, movements)
3. state organisation (sleep, wakefulness, arousal)
4. attentional and interactive (increasing periods of quiet alertness where the infant relates to the environment)
5. self-regulatory (strategies the infant uses to maintain or regain a state of equilibrium).

Signals of competence or challenge within each subsystem are reflected in the infant's behaviour.

NIDCAP aims to reduce the discrepancy between the womb and NICU environment (Als et al. 2004) by:

- taking into account the individual infant's current thresholds of behavioural organisation
- diminishing stress
- supporting each infant's strengths and competencies.

A behavioural summary is written by a highly skilled developmental specialist based on in-depth structured observation of the infant before, during and after care. This highlights the infant's avoidance and approach responses, together with a description of the efforts the baby makes to regain equilibrium when challenged. Recommendations for care are then provided that aim to minimise noxious stimuli and to support the infant's developmental agenda. Thus, the carer adjusts the timing of intervention to respect the baby's sleep/wake patterns and assists the baby during care by pacing procedures and supporting the infant's own efforts at self-regulation (Als and Butler 2008).

Discussion of evidence for developmental care

Single studies comparing preterm infants receiving NIDCAP care versus basic developmental care have shown that NIDCAP infants require significantly fewer days of assisted ventilation, are less likely to develop chronic lung disease, have fewer days on parenteral feeds, have shorter transition to full feeds and better average daily weight gain, are younger at discharge and have fewer cases of necrotising enterocolitis (Als et al. 2003; Symington and Pinelli 2006; Cooper et al. 2007; McAnulty et al. 2009; Peters et al. 2009). They also have fewer developmental problems when tested at different ages and are diagnosed with fewer visual problems. Magnetic resonance imaging (MRI) studies have shown better posterior limb of the internal capsule myelination at term age and more mature right hemisphere and frontal lobe function at 8 years of age. Additionally, higher scores have been recorded on maternal perception of her child and on measures of improved family outcome (Als et al. 2003, 2004; Symington and Pinelli 2006; Cooper et al. 2007; McAnulty et al. 2009; Peters et al. 2009).

In contrast with these studies, a Cochrane review showed evidence of no effect for some outcomes, i.e. length of stay, feeding and growth, and respiratory support when comparing NIDCAP

with controls, findings that were confirmed on an unpublished meta-analysis including the two most recent trials (Ohlsson et al. 2009).

Possible reasons for these conflicting results include methodological issues of the individual studies, short exposure to the intervention, small sample sizes, lack of blinding of outcome assessors and, most importantly, the likely contamination between the two arms under investigation.

No harmful effects from NIDCAP or developmental care interventions have been published to date.

Various issues will need to be addressed if more research is to be conducted in NIDCAP. Further studies involving imaging with functional MRI, for example, would be a good measure by proxy of further development.

Summary

The NICU environment plays a major role in the short- and long-term outcomes of preterm babies. Developmentally supportive care and, more specifically, NIDCAP have been suggested to reduce the adverse impact of this alien environment.

Despite the conflicting evidence, many units around the world have instinctively adopted a range of developmental care strategies. For many, using such approaches to provide gentler care just seems intrinsically 'right'. Whilst at present the most robust scientific evidence indicates that NIDCAP has no significant effect, it appears that there is benefit in individualising developmental care approaches to meet the needs and developmental agenda of the infant. By implementing a few simple measures it is possible to deliver care which shifts from being task-oriented to being baby-led. Adjusting the timing of care procedures to protect sleep, dimming lights, keeping noise to a minimum and promoting kangaroo care for fathers as well as mothers are worthwhile changes which even the busiest NICU can manage most of the time and which will yield rich benefits in terms of parental satisfaction and infant comfort.

References

Als, H., 1982. Towards a synactive theory of development: promise for the assessment and support of infant individuality. Infant Mental Health J 3, 229–243.

Als, H., Butler, S., 2008. Newborn individualized developmental care and assessment program: changing the future for infants and families in intensive and special care nurseries. Early Childhood Services 2, 1–22.

Als, H., Gilkerson, L., 1995. Developmentally supportive care in the neonatal intensive care unit. Zero to Three 15, 2–10.

Als, H., Mcanulty, G., 2000. Developmental care guidelines for use in the newborn intensive care unit (NICU). NIDCAP training binder. NIDCAP Federation International, Boston, MA, pp. 1–6.

Als, H., Gilkerton, L., Duffy, F., et al., 2003. A Three-center, randomized, controlled trial of individualized developmental care for very low birth weight preterm infants: medical, neurodevelopmental, parenting, and caregiving effects. J Dev Behav Pediatr 24, 399–408.

Als, H., Duffy, F.H., McAnulty, G.B., et al., 2004. Early experience alters brain function and structure. Pediatrics 113, 846–857.

Anand, K.J.S., Scalzo, F., 2000. Can adverse neonatal experiences alter brain development and subsequent behaviour? Biol Neonate 77, 69–82.

Bartocci, M., Winberg, J., Papendieck, G., et al., 2001. Cerebral hemodynamic response to unpleasant odors in the preterm newborn measured by near-infrared spectroscopy. Pediatr Res 50, 324–330.

Bhutta, A.T., Cleves, M.A., Casey, P.H., et al., 2002. Cognitive and behavioral outcomes of school-aged children who were born preterm: a meta-analysis. JAMA 288, 728–737.

Browne, J., 2008. Chemosensory development in the fetus and newborn. Newborn Infant Nurs Rev 8, 181–186.

Charpak, N., de Calume, Z.F., Ruiz, J.G., 2000. 'The Bogota Declaration on Kangaroo Mother Care': conclusions at the

second international workshop on the method. Second International Workshop of Kangaroo Mother Care. Acta Paediatr 89, 1137–1140.

Charpak, N., Ruiz, J.G., Zupan, J., et al., 2005. Kangaroo mother care: 25 years after. Acta Paediatr 94, 514–522.

Chermont, A.G., Falcao, L.F., de Souza Silva, E.H., et al., 2009. Skin-to-skin contact and/or oral 25% dextrose for procedural pain relief for term newborn infants. Pediatrics 124, e1101–e1107.

Conde Agudelo, A., Belizan, J., 2003. Kangaroo mother care to reduce morbidity and mortality in low birthweight infants. Cochrane Database Syst Rev (2), CD002771.

Cooper, L.G., Gooding, J.S., Gallagher, J., et al., 2007. Impact of a family-centered care initiative on NICU care, staff and families. J Perinatol 27 (Suppl. 2), S32–S37.

Duffy, M.G., Jensen, F., Als, H., 1984. Neural plasticity, a new frontier for infant development. In: Fitzgerald, H.E., Lester,

B.M., Yogman, M.W. (Eds.), Theory and Research in Behavioral Pediatrics. Plenum Press, New York, pp. 67–96.

Ewer, A., James, M., Tobin, J., 1999. Prone and left lateral positioning reduce gastro-esophageal reflux. Arch Dis Child Fetal Neonatal Ed 81, F201–F205.

Gray, L., Philbin, M.K., 2004. Effects of the neonatal intensive care unit on auditory attention and distraction. Clin Perinatol 31, 243–260, vi.

Hofer, M.A., 1987. Early social relationships: a psychobiologist's view. Child Dev 58, 633–647.

Holsti, L., Grunau, R.E., Oberlander, T.F., et al., 2005. Prior pain induces heightened motor responses during clustered care in preterm infants in the NICU. Early Hum Dev 81, 293–302.

Johnson, S., Fawke, J., Hennessy, E., et al., 2009. Neurodevelopmental disability through 11 years of age in children born before 26 weeks of gestation. Pediatrics 124, e249–e257.

Lawhon, G., Melzar, A., 1988. Developmental care of the very low birth weight infant. J Perinat Neonatal Nurs 2, 56–65.

Liu, W.F., Laudert, S., Perkins, B., et al., 2007. The development of potentially better practices to support the neurodevelopment of infants in the NICU. J Perinatol 27 (Suppl. 2), S48–S74.

Long, J., Lucey, J., Philip, A., 1980. Sound level in NICU. Pediatrics 65, 143–145.

Mann, N., Haddow, R., Stokes, L., et al., 1996. Effect of night and day on preterm infants in a newborn nursery: randomised trial. BMJ 293, 1265–1267.

McAnulty, G.B., Duffy, F.H., Butler, S.C., et al., 2009. Effects of the Newborn Individualized Developmental Care and Assessment Program (NIDCAP) at age 8 years: preliminary data. Clin Pediatr doi:10.1177/0009922809335668.

Minde, K., Whitelaw, A., Brown, J., et al., 1983. Effect of neonatal complications in premature infants on early parent–infant interactions. Dev Med Child Neurol 25, 763–777.

Ohlsson, A., Peters, K.L., Walther, F.J., et al., Panel discussion: Is NIDCAP effective in improving outcomes in preterm infants? Proceedings of Hot Topics Conference, Washington DC, USA, 2009.

Peters, K.L., Rosychuk, R.J., Hendson, L., et al., 2009. Improvement of short- and long-term outcomes for very low birth weight infants: Edmonton NIDCAP trial. Pediatrics 124, 1009–1020.

Pinelli, J., Symington, A., 2005. Non-nutritive sucking for promoting physiologic stability and nutrition in preterm infants. Cochrane Database Syst Rev (4), CD001071.

Riley, K., Roth, S., Sellwood, M., et al., 2008. Survival and neurodevelopmental morbidity at 1 year of age following extremely preterm delivery over a 20-year period: a single centre cohort study. Acta Paediatr 97, 159–165.

Saigal, S., den Ouden, L., Wolke, D., et al., 2003. School-age outcomes in children who were extremely low birth weight from four international population-based cohorts. Pediatrics 112, 943–950.

Schaal, B., Marlier, L., Soussignan, R., 1998. Olfactory function in the human fetus: evidence from selective neonatal responsivenesss to the odor of amniotic fluid. Behav Neurosci 112, 1438–1449.

Short, M.A., Brooks-Brunn, J.A., Reeves, D.S., et al., 1996. The effects of swaddling versus standard positioning on neuromuscular development in very low birth weight infants. Neonatal Netw 15, 25–31.

Stanley, N., Garaven, M., Browne, J.V., 2008. Visual development in the human fetus, infant and young child. Newborn Infant Nurs Rev 8 (4).

Symington, A., Pinelli, J., 2006. Developmental care for promoting development and preventing morbidity in preterm infants. Cochrane Database Syst Rev (2), CD001814.

Tallandini, M., Scalembra, C., 2006. Kangaroo mother care: maternal perception and interaction with preterm babies. Infant Mental Health J 27, 251–275.

Westrup, B., 2009. Neonatal family centred couplet care for all families. Proceedings of Symposium, Stockholm.

White, R.D., 2007. Recommended standards for the newborn ICU. J Perinatol 27 (Suppl. 2), S4–S19.

Counselling and support for parents and families

Ian A Laing   Chinthika Piyasena   Hazel E McHaffie

5

CHAPTER CONTENTS

Introduction

Having a newborn infant in a neonatal unit is an extremely stressful experience for parents. The mother is usually suffering fatigue and physical discomfort from the delivery. Both parents are anxious. Their hopes and dreams are threatened. The future is uncertain, the path unknown. The couple face a strain on their personal and combined resources and cannot know in advance if they will be equal to the challenge.

The parent's principal preoccupation is the establishment of a relationship with this new member of their family, but conditions are far from ideal. Instead of a 3.5-kg term infant on a postnatal ward, the centre of admiration and congratulations, they have an ill baby, often scrawny, distanced from them by a Perspex barrier. Their own feelings of guilt and helplessness are compounded by the fact that there seems to be no role for them; neonatal nurses and doctors are the caregivers; machines and tests replace parental caresses.

If families are to look back on these days and weeks with satisfaction and look forward constructively to the rest of their lives, the professional team must handle them with care. The aim of this chapter is to offer guidance to less experienced clinicians in order to facilitate the best service the circumstances will allow.

Nothing can substitute for personal experience. All junior staff should watch their seniors in action, and take the opportunity to attend counselling sessions with the parents where possible. These interactions depend to an extent on an intangible chemistry between parent and professional, and this chemistry is strongly influenced by the personalities of both. But much can be learned from observing closely how the discussions progress, noting the apposite phrase which crystallises a moment, the tactics which deflect anger, the way in which trust is reinforced.

Although the doctor and the parents may differ on many fronts – culture, religious belief, social class, life choices, education, expectations – these differences must not be permitted to create insuperable hurdles. The baby is our patient but is the parents' child. The decisions should be the right decisions for this family at this point in their lives. The professional's task is to share medical insight and knowledge whilst respecting parental values and beliefs, working with them to make wise choices on behalf of the child.

© 2012 Elsevier Ltd

The relationship with parents

Initial introductions

Courtesy matters. It is polite and helpful, for example, before meeting either or both of the parents, to establish what their names are and how they prefer to be addressed. Similarly the couple need to know their boundaries, and the doctor should introduce him- or herself, and state his or her role in the team. Shaking hands with both parents at first meeting is symbolic of a future trusting relationship. The overall approach should be one of mutual respect.

Establishing trust

The doctor should always bear in mind the importance of trust. Once lost, it is very hard to regain. And whatever the status or level of experience of the professional, unfounded opinions, unrealistic predictions and false hope undermine confidence.

Before the first interview, the doctor must know any relevant family history, and the details of the pregnancy, labour and delivery. The initial meeting may well take place in the delivery room, with parents who have had only the briefest introduction to their newborn baby. At this stage it is essential to keep things simple. Even for the highly educated, this is no time to be bombarded with complex diagnoses, specialist jargon or intricate pathophysiology. The following example gives basic clear information and may be enough for the first interaction: 'Your baby has come out very early and is very small. His lungs have not yet matured. We have connected him to a ventilator, and he is stable for now. We will tell you much more when you are able to visit the baby unit.'

Questions should be answered honestly. Where doubt exists, professionals should resist the impulse to declare that the baby will be 'fine'. It is much better to reply, 'He's comfortable in his incubator at the moment. But we need to see how he progresses in the next few hours before we can be sure how things will go. We'll keep you informed and I can promise you we won't hide anything from you.'

Roles and responsibilities

Every neonatal unit should have a dedicated counselling room where staff can meet families without fear of interruption. In this room, the parents can be confident that they have the undivided attention of the staff and can have all their concerns addressed. Doctors should take their cue from the family as to the amount they can absorb or tolerate at a given sitting.

Neonatal units often have written protocols about who should conduct interviews. The consultant holds overall responsibility not only for the child's care but also for the interactions with the family. Junior paediatricians should never be in the position of communicating with families beyond their level of experience, though parents appreciate informal interactions from all members of the team. Meetings of a particularly sensitive nature should be conducted by the consultant in the presence of a nurse who is looking after the baby and who has established a rapport with the parents. The junior doctor involved should be encouraged to attend for the benefit of his or her training and as he or she too has had a direct role in the baby's care. Regardless of who is present behind closed doors, the whole team needs to know what is said and decided, in order to facilitate effective teamwork. Thereafter, full and careful documentation is essential.

A primary task for the consultant is that of assessing the full clinical picture as far as it can be known. Good counselling depends on accurate facts and knowledge of the literature. There will often be areas of uncertainty, but if there have been exhaustive efforts to find

out as much as possible, the family will usually respect an honest admission from a senior member of staff of 'I don't know'. A statement such as 'I am confused' does not inspire confidence, but a frank 'There are uncertainties ahead and we can't be sure at this stage how things will go, but we'll continue to discuss everything with you' allows the parent to appreciate the evolving picture. The capacity of the parents to tolerate bad news will vary, but the truth should never be compromised. 'Truth sometimes hurts but deceit hurts more' (Fallowfield 1997).

Teamwork

Managing sick infants well is a team effort. A wise doctor will listen to the parents. They have a unique investment in their child and stand in the most privileged position in relation to the baby. With their focus on one infant, they not infrequently detect subtle but important changes in their child's condition. Staff should give proper attention to such misgivings; they are often correct.

Consent to treatment

The subject of consent is currently fraught with difficulties in the developed world. Until recent years it was assumed that babies admitted to a neonatal unit brought with them implied consent, which allowed staff to carry out any procedure on the baby without obtaining specific consent. A new tension has arisen, partly stemming from a small number of legal cases in which medical staff strayed beyond ethical boundaries to the detriment of the patient. As a result, more and more protocols are being developed demanding that written informed consent be obtained for procedures and treatments (e.g. postnatal steroids), allegedly to protect the child, the parents and the staff. Unfortunately, if genuinely informed consent is to be obtained, each interview between staff and parents must be lengthy in order to do the subject justice. Such interviews erode the time that staff can devote to the child's care, and clearly this could have an adverse effect on prognosis. Should a lumbar puncture be delayed at 03:00 hours while parents, already exhausted, are wakened at home and asked to drive to the neonatal unit for an in depth interview, or should staff be allowed to carry out the procedure and discuss this with the couple during daylight hours?

It would be best to explain to the parents at the time of admission to the unit that every effort will be made to keep them up to date and to seek their permission for procedures, but that urgent situations might, of necessity, preclude such interactions. For a procedure that carries clear risks, consent must be obtained by the practitioner designated to carry it out and who must be qualified to do so. Great care must be taken to explain the nature of the investigation or treatment, the intended benefits and the risks attached. Consent is best obtained from the mother; the father may consent if he has parental rights. (See Ch. 6.2 regarding competence for consent.)

Each neonatal unit should have written guidelines for staff to indicate which procedures require consent to be formally documented on an official form. These are usually major undertakings, such as exchange transfusions and operative procedures including laser treatment for retinopathy of prematurity. The parents should be given a copy of the signed consent form on which the benefits and risks are clearly documented.

Consent for less invasive procedures and treatments which carry minimal risks is traditionally obtained verbally, though it is prudent to document this in the case record. Examples may include immunisations, the administration of vitamin K at birth (specifying by which route), the use of breast milk fortifier, and neonatal screening investigations such as blood sampling to identify phenylketonuria, hypothyroidism and cystic fibrosis.

Consent for research is outside the scope of this chapter, but is nonetheless an important aspect of neonatal care. Parental claims around lack of informed consent for the Continuous Negative Extrathoracic Pressure (CNEP) trial led to one of the largest inquiries so far in this field in the UK (NHS Executive West Midlands Regional Office 2000). The inquiry and the subsequent report were found to be flawed (Hey and Chalmers 2000) and the report was later withdrawn.

It is known that parental recall of events in the newborn period is unreliable (Hey and Chalmers 2000). This highlights the importance of documenting informed consent for clinical trials and for invasive procedures.

Life and death decision-making

Making crucial decisions on behalf of their baby is one of the most difficult experiences parents ever face. Staff may be understandably anxious about the burden parents may carry and about the potential for guilt (McHaffie and Fowlie 1996). In reality, parents want to be given the opportunity to be active in decision-making and they do not appear to suffer adversely as a result (McHaffie 2001).

For this they require direct and open communication about the child's current condition and prognosis. Information should be provided with a good measure of compassion, avoiding euphemisms, using the words 'death' and 'dying' to help validate the situation (Williams et al. 2008). A 'guided consensus' is an effective way of handling the process (Laing 1989). One approach is for the parents to consider goals for care with the clinician, exploring those which are realistic and those which have little chance of success. In this way, the parents feel their voice is heard and they have a chance to evaluate their hopes against the child's best interest (Royal College of Paediatrics and Child Health & Ethics Advisory Committee 2004). It is critical that, before withdrawal of intensive care takes place, the parents as well as the staff are confident that this action is in the child's best interest.

In most cases, consensus is reached without dissension. However, if either the parents or the staff think that intensive care should continue, then any decision to withdraw should be put on hold pending careful review. Usually, parental uncertainty arises from a failure or reluctance to comprehend fully the gravity of the situation. Continued intensive care brings clarity in the fullness of time. The child will either deteriorate or improve, and the decision is then more straightforward.

It is not the intention of this chapter to explore the ethical issues around withdrawal of neonatal intensive care. These have been developed in previous publications (Warnock 1998; McHaffie et al. 2001a).

The dying baby

There can never be a time when high-quality communication is more important than when a baby is dying. The parents will remember professional sensitivity or insensitivity for the rest of their lives.

In the rare event that a newborn infant collapses and dies without warning, there is little time to build a relationship with the family. The consultant must take control of decision-making and communication. Major priorities are that the child should be free of all distress, with dignity respected, and the family should be encouraged to spend the last minutes holding their dying child, free from the encumbrances of intensive care. Helping them to acknowledge their own unique role, to accept the reality of the child's short life

and death and to be involved with the baby after death will facilitate the creation of memories, which can comfort and sustain them in the ensuing years (McHaffie 2001).

Much more commonly, babies die in a neonatal unit after some time and following a deliberate reorientation of care to comfort measures. The parents have had time to get to know the staff, and have been closely involved in decision-making.

Caring for an infant's death

The consultant and a senior nurse should explore with the parents what their wishes may be. Parents may need guidance as to what options are available, and here senior nursing staff may be especially sensitive. Knowing what the options are – to invite close family members and friends to 'say goodbye', organise a baptismal or blessing service, involve siblings, take photographs, collect mementoes, hold and groom the baby, even perhaps take the baby home – enables parents to decide what is right for them and minimises later regret. Tolerances and preferences as to the exact nature of their own involvement vary, but it is important for clinicians to be non-judgemental of parents (McHaffie 2001).

In times of crisis, there can be a great need for spiritual guidance. Religious figures can help parents observe specific rituals where possible, which have the potential to bring comfort to the family, including the choice of burial and funeral services available (Williams et al. 2008).

The way the death is managed will materially influence parental satisfaction and acceptance of the wisdom of the choices made. Staff should be especially careful in their preparation of parents as to what will or might happen. Protracted deaths, unpleasant sights and sounds, and conflicting advice can all undermine parental confidence and leave families with a burden of guilt and distressing memories (McHaffie 2001). In an individual case, it is difficult to predict what will happen, but parents should be reassured that every effort will be made to ensure the baby will slip peacefully into death.

Ensuring freedom from distress is a sensitive issue that has attracted much debate. According to the law, any intervention with the purpose of procuring death is illegal, but medication given to alleviate suffering which has the side-effect of hastening death is permissible (Royal College of Paediatrics and Child Health & Ethics Advisory Committee 2004). Comfort may best be assured by the intravenous administration of opiates as necessary, with appropriate reassurance to the parents about the purpose of this analgesia.

Parental reactions to death vary but will usually include a mixture of anger, denial, numbness and great sadness. Having staff supporting them with whom they have already established a relationship allows them to laugh, or cry, share anecdotes, or express their fears and hostility, without fear of misunderstanding. Such members of staff may also express their own sorrow more freely, which the parents will appreciate. Although priority must always be given to the parents' needs and privacy, junior staff may learn best from watching the experts at work.

Asking for permission to carry out an autopsy is an extremely painful part of this process. With the adverse publicity of recent years, it has become even more sensitive. But where there are unanswered questions about this child or future obstetric risk, it may be the only method of obtaining answers (Brodlie et al. 2002). A principal reason for resisting postmortem examination is the fear of mutilation, and parents may need help to acquire a balance of perspective which will enable them to make appropriate choices (McHaffie et al. 2001a). Assuring parents that their child will be handled in a dignified manner may help them make the correct choice for them.

Bereavement

Newly bereaved parents may find it difficult to leave behind the support of the neonatal team. The usual support systems such as friends and family that they now turn to are inadequate.

Parents appreciate staff attending the funeral, contacting them to check they are coping, and, if the parents wish, seeing them to talk about the baby. Commonly it is the nurse or nursing staff (with whom the parents have built a relationship) who provide these signs of caring, often in their own time. These gestures allow the parents to feel that they and their baby were valued and important to those caring for the infant.

Other sources of help, for both parents and staff, exist and should be suggested where appropriate. Self-help groups such as the Stillbirth and Neonatal Death Society or Compassionate Friends may offer solace to certain families. Other parents who have had similar experiences are trained to offer counselling via such organisations. But the difficulty parents sense in approaching strangers when they feel vulnerable and emotional should not be underestimated.

Medical follow-up

The consultant is the person who is key in the formal bereavement meeting, which takes place 4–6 weeks later (McHaffie et al. 2001b). The importance of this follow-up cannot be overemphasised. Parents value an unhurried session with the neonatologist and nurse most closely involved with their family. They have a great need to obtain information to help piece together what happened. It is also a forum to discuss the results of outstanding investigations, to discuss their implications and assess the parents' own future obstetric risks. The follow-up interview also provides an opportunity for staff to watch and listen to ensure that the couple are mutually supportive and experiencing a normal grieving process (McHaffie et al. 2001c). Such a meeting might ideally involve the appropriate consultant obstetrician and an observing paediatric trainee, but maintenance of intimacy is essential.

Other considerations

The general practitioner should monitor the mother's mood and somatic symptoms and offer advice on issues such as inhibiting breast milk production (Williams et al. 2008). Postpartum depression is common amongst mothers in the first few weeks to months following delivery. Having an ill newborn infant, prolonged neonatal intensive care and, of course, bereavement can compound feelings of guilt and inadequacy. Although postpartum psychosis is uncommon, the onset is earlier after birth than postpartum depression, and represents a psychiatric emergency (Pearlstein et al. 2009).

Conflict

In a well-managed neonatal unit, conflict between staff and families should be rare. Nevertheless, disputes do occasionally occur, and it is the duty of staff to identify the cause of any conflict and where possible anticipate and deflect it.

Anticipating trouble

Where emotions run high, there is a constant need for vigilance. Are the parents taking advice from well-meaning but ill-informed members of their family, and should these family members be interviewed too? Is there interparental conflict, and should this be acknowledged and sidelined so that both parents, despite their differences, can contribute constructively to their child's care? Is the drug abuse of one or both partners interfering with their ability to make decisions? Should other professionals be brought in to facilitate better control of tempers or hostility so that discussions can be constructive once more?

Averting trouble

Almost always, conflict arises out of uncertainty, parental fatigue, and perceived or actual poor communication. Occasionally a schism can occur on the basis of ethnic or religious differences. Neonatal staff have stressful jobs. They too are only human and personal problems may make them vulnerable. It may be advisable on occasion to allocate another member of staff to a family, where interpersonal tension exists.

In a misguided attempt to cope with all situations, doctors sometimes forget they have allies. Colleagues and peers can be extremely helpful sources of advice. Conflict may diminish simply by bringing in another professional, perhaps of a different gender or ethnic background, perhaps from another city, able to look afresh at the clinical and emotional background out of which tension has emerged. Skilled interpreters may be invaluable in cases where language barriers are the root cause of conflict.

When tension stems from a breakdown of trust, written information may help. A detailed, factual account of the child's illness and prognosis may be taken by parents and discussed with trusted advisors, family and friends. The parents may be encouraged to write down all the questions troubling them. Each can then be explored in a follow-up interview. This exchange may also be documented, even recorded in audio format, giving the parents the opportunity to consider the situation calmly and in their own time.

Sometimes, parents are helped by having chosen advocates present. Young and inexperienced parents may benefit from their own parents sharing the discussions. A member of a minority religious group may draw strength from a minister or adviser who can explain the parents' stance from a more detached point of view. A sensitive clinician will be aware of special vulnerabilities and needs, and seek to circumvent conflict.

Managing abuse

Staff should be trained in containment of aggression. Occasionally, however, parents may be gratuitously or vindictively verbally abusive. They should be told politely but firmly that this is unacceptable. If the abuse is repeated, senior staff should give serious consideration to excluding the parent(s). If there is any threat of physical violence, security officers should be summoned immediately to have the offending party removed, in order to protect the babies, the staff and other visitors to the unit. The consultant will then meet with senior management, social workers, hospital security and the police, to develop a plan which will maximise the safety of all those involved, even if it means, in extreme cases, excluding the parents on a permanent basis from the unit.

Dealing with complaints

The consultant takes ultimate responsibility for the care of the baby and family: if a complaint is made, the consultant should be involved in addressing it. It is worth noting that if complaints are not addressed quickly, then they tend to multiply.

A first task is to establish the facts. Listening to the parents is the most important aspect of dealing with such a situation and every effort should be made to adopt an unhurried and sympathetic approach. If the complaint is justified, then staff should be generous in their apology. 'I am sorry we made a mistake. I recognise you are angry. We will do everything to ensure that this does not happen to you or to any other family again.' If the complaint is not justified, then, having listened attentively to the criticisms, the consultant should express regret for the parents' distress but endeavour to give a reasonable and justifiable explanation for any misunderstanding. It may or may not be accepted, but simply being given a fair hearing may well go a long way to satisfying the parents.

Multiple complaints

Multiple complaints usually arise when an initial complaint has not been dealt with immediately. The family should be encouraged to write down each complaint and give the list to the staff beforehand. The consultant and colleagues can then explore the justification for each, obtain a full account of the events from those involved and agree upon a strategy which promises the best chance of regaining the family's confidence. In this situation, and especially where the complaints are of a serious nature, it is often helpful to have an independent chairperson to reconcile staff and family. Where this person is perceived to be autonomous and impartial, it can be easier to steer clear of personal attack, preserve a proper balance and sense of proportion and highlight areas of genuine concern.

Special situations

Some situations that are encountered in neonatal units deserve a special mention. Certain types of parents may need special nurturing.

Parents of the acutely collapsed baby

This is often the most demanding of crises. The parents have relaxed, and believe that their child is now out of danger. Suddenly there is an acute deterioration. 'It must be somebody's fault' is a very understandable reaction, but a painful one for dedicated staff to cope with. Immediate answers may not be available. The doctor in charge does not yet know whether the 4-day-old baby has developed an unexpected septicaemia or whether there is a congenital abnormality such as hypoplastic left heart syndrome that has manifested itself now that the ductus has closed. There is a rush to treat infection, and to obtain cardiology advice. The parents may be forgiven for thinking that the staff cannot even identify which organ is triggering the crisis. In such circumstances, honesty is the best policy. The clinician should be very candid but also emphasise the positive aspects of care. 'Your baby, Rosemary, is very ill. We have put her back on the ventilator. There are a number of possible reasons for her new illness and it's important we identify the cause of her problems accurately. At the moment we are treating her for infection. I've asked for a specialist, a cardiologist, to come urgently to the unit so that we can get the best advice available. I am taking responsibility for the team caring for your baby, and as soon as I have more answers I will come and discuss our plans with you.'

Parents of the baby with chronic disease

After the whirlwind of delivery, resuscitation, ventilation, replacement surfactant and the rollercoaster of the early days of life, it is very common for a baby to enter a stable phase where there is neither a perceived improvement nor deterioration. This stage can be immensely frustrating for parents. Weeks go by and nothing seems to be happening. Some days the baby looks less good than others. The parents sleep poorly. The staff may also feel discouraged.

Ongoing concern for the parents and good communication are imperative. Parents should never be made to feel they are in the way or troublesome with their frequent questions. Rather, understanding their dilemma can be supportive. 'We know you're having trouble sleeping. Don't hesitate to ring any time in the night just for reassurance. We understand how worrying this stage can be.' Provided it does not encourage false hope, it can be supportive to identify some area of progress and lift the parents' spirits by offering them a different perspective. For example, parents of a child with bronchopulmonary dysplasia may feel discouraged by his ventilator dependency. By saying, 'Yes, your baby is still in 30% oxygen, but look at his excellent growth. With every day that passes, he is making new lung', you are acknowledging the legitimacy of their concerns but giving them encouraging news too.

Long weary days cocooned in a neonatal unit can be depressing. Dedicated parents may need to be given permission to resume a life outside the hospital. Encouraging them gradually to change their visiting patterns may help them to acquire a healthier perspective.

The absent parent

Parents may feel inadequate in the intensive care setting, and may express their fear by staying away. It is the staff's duty to maintain the highest possible standard but this is much harder to achieve without parental collaboration. Every effort should be made to address the cause of their reluctance, to gain their confidence, and, with patience, to draw them into the team. Strategies might include meeting the absent parent on neutral territory; suggesting they bring a supportive friend or relative in too; identifying a specific and positive role for them to play; and perhaps contacting the family's general practitioner or health visitor to obtain insight into the home situation.

The unsupported teenage mother

Even the most junior members of staff will find themselves caring for mothers and fathers who are several years younger than they are, but their attitude should never be patronising. Though chronologically younger, such parents may be surprisingly mature in experience, outlook and ability to cope. The unsupported teenage mother, however, represents a special challenge. Her abandonment may be temporary or permanent, but efforts should be made to establish the reasons for the schism. Where the teenager's feelings will not be violated, separate interviews with her own mother may be indicated, in order to befriend her, and to persuade her that both mother and grandmother have an essential role in the child's care and future. If this is inappropriate or fails, then a close friend and/or a social worker should be brought in to support the teenage mother for the important decisions about her own and the baby's future. Patience, gentleness and understanding will all be needed.

The parent who takes control

This is a common situation. It occurs particularly where parents are intelligent, talented and challenging in their own professional lives. They are familiar with internet searches and soon become 'experts' in their baby's condition, treatment and prognosis. Such parents are used to being in control, and tend to channel their own understandable anxieties into aggression, passive or overt. Staff should be sufficiently resilient to tolerate a mild degree of challenging behaviour, but as soon as it threatens to interfere with the quality of care of the infant, then it must be addressed.

The consultant should meet with staff and listen carefully to the facts, ensuring that they are neither exaggerated nor diminished. Together with another member of staff, he or she should then meet with the parents, and appeal to them to recognise the expertise and professionalism of the staff, and not allow their strong personalities to jeopardise the care the team want to provide for the family. Regaining control is essential to good relationships, and it is a mistake to allow parents to dictate which nurses and doctors they wish to take care of their baby. It may be necessary to set up regular meetings with such a couple to ensure that they are allowing the care of the child to progress unhindered by their anxieties.

The parent with special educational needs

In law, parents have responsibility for their child. Staff have an ethical duty to ensure that the care of the child is equally good no matter the educational attainments of the parents. On rare occasions, however, neonatologists are faced with parents whose level of literacy or understanding prevents them from properly grasping what is happening. Sometimes other members of the family may be able to act in loco parentis, and it is reassuring to have supportive grandparents who can make rational suggestions in the best interests of all concerned. Occasionally, it may be necessary to formalise this arrangement. If there is any doubt about who carries parental responsibility, or competence, the child-safeguarding team must be involved.

The parent who is a healthcare professional

It can be difficult to be the parent of an imperilled infant and also a healthcare professional. Roles and expectations between the two can become confused. Staff should encourage such a person to be a parent first, and expect no more of them than from any other articulate and intelligent mother or father. 'I am going to pretend that you are not a doctor. Indeed, with your permission, I would like to call you Mr Jones while your baby is in the unit', will often produce a smile of relief from the parent.

The mother with threatened extreme preterm labour

Ideally, counselling should involve both parents. The purpose is to provide information and to guide decision-making regarding the initiation or non-initiation of resuscitation. It is not possible to establish universal practice guidelines owing to the uniqueness of every situation. Gestational age should not be used as the sole determinant of prognosis. Other relevant factors include gender, whether steroids have been administered antenatally, the presence of infection and whether there is more than one fetus (Batton 2009). It may be clear to the clinician that a fetus is too immature, and attempts at resuscitation are contraindicated. If however a good outcome is probable, resuscitation should be initiated irrespective of the parental view. The difficulty arises where it is not clear to the perinatal team whether the neonate might survive intact or with only mild deficits. Simply providing up-to-date outcome data and the intricate details about prolonged intensive care and expecting the parents to decide is unfair. Nevertheless the clinical team should be fully aware of the most relevant studies. Several meetings with the parents will be necessary to provide a clinical perspective effectively and empathetically. Parental choice must be taken into consideration but the professional team must always be primarily advocates for the child. The parents should be reassured that, in the event of non-initiation of resuscitation, the infant would receive compassionate care and that they themselves would be allowed to be involved in the dying process and its aftermath as much as they wish (Batton 2009).

Preserving your own health

Intensive care is demanding, and neonatal doctors and nurses work extremely hard for the families. We are groomed to succeed, and we feel guilty and inadequate when we do not. Every child's death and each physical deterioration can feel like failure. It is a mistake to cover up such feelings, and to look for solace in excess.

A healthy way to deal with perceived failure is to discuss troubling cases openly with peers. Reassurance may come from hearing that there was nothing further that could have been done, or from a shared sense of sorrow. Some teams favour routine debriefing after any stressful situation. These meetings, if skilfully handled, can be educational, and also beneficial for the corporate as well as individual morale. Maintaining a balance that includes an active life outside the neonatal unit is essential. Whether your interest is in the gym or theatre, climbing mountains or juggling flaming torches, it is essential for the carers to care for themselves if they are to be sufficiently restored to return to the neonatal unit and deal empathically with the next family.

Concluding thoughts

Neonatology combines the rigours of intensive care with the need to communicate openly and in detail with families. Counselling and support for parents cannot adequately be achieved in one meeting and take great patience and tact. Staff need to be articulate, thoughtful, sensitive and, above all, excellent at listening. It is hoped that this chapter has pointed the way, but excellence in practice is learned from peers, mentors and the families themselves.

References

Batton, D.G., 2009. Committee on Fetus and Newborn. Clinical report – Antenatal counselling regarding resuscitation at an extremely low gestational age. Pediatrics 124 (1), 422–427.

Brodlie, M., Laing, I.A., Keeling, J.W., et al., 2002. Ten years of neonatal autopsies in tertiary referral centre: retrospective study. BMJ (Clinical research ed.) 324, 761–763.

Fallowfield, L., 1997. Truth sometimes hurts but deceit hurts more. Ann N Y Acad Sci 809, 525–536.

Hey, E., Chalmers, I., 2000. Investigating allegations of research misconduct: the vital need for due process.

BMJ (Clinical research ed.) 321, 752–755.

Laing, I.A., 1989. Withdrawing from invasive neonatal intensive care. In: Mason J.K. (Ed.), Paediatric Forensic Medicine and Pathology. Chapman & Hall, London, pp. 131–140.

McHaffie, H.E., 2001. Crucial Decisions at the Beginning of Life. Radcliffe Medical Press, Abingdon.

McHaffie, H.E., Fowlie, P.W., 1996. Life, Death and Decisions. Hochland & Hochland, Cheshire.

McHaffie, H.E., Fowlie, P.W., Hume, R., et al., 2001a. Consent to autopsy for neonates. Arch Dis Child Fetal Neonat Ed 85, F4–F7.

McHaffie, H.E., Laing, I.A., Lloyd, D.J., 2001b. Follow up care of bereaved parents after treatment withdrawal from newborns. Arch Dis Child Fetal Neonat Ed 84, F125–F128.

McHaffie, H.E., Laing, I.A., Parker, M., et al., 2001c. Deciding for imperilled newborns: medical authority or parental autonomy? J Med Ethics 27, 104–109.

NHS Executive West Midlands Regional Office, 2000. Report of a Review of the Research Framework in North Staffordshire Hospital NHS Trust (Griffiths report). Department of Health, London.

Pearlstein, T., Howard, M., Salisbury, A., et al., 2009. Postpartum depression. Am J Obstet Gynecol 200, 357–364.

Royal College of Paediatrics and Child Health & Ethics Advisory Committee, 2004. Withholding or Withdrawal of Life-sustaining Treatment in Children: a Framework for Practice, second ed. Royal College of Paediatrics and Child Health, London.

Warnock, M., 1998. An Intelligent Person's Guide to Ethics. Gerald Duckworth, London, pp. 40–53.

Williams, C., Munson, D., Zupancic, J., et al., 2008. Supporting bereaved parents: practical steps in providing compassionate perinatal and neonatal end-of-life care. A North American perspective. Semin Fetal Neonat Med 13, 335–340.

Further reading

Gustaitis, R., Young, E.W.D., 1986. A Time to be Born, a Time to Die. Addison-Wesley, Reading, MA.

Hindmarch, C., 2000. On the Death of a Child. Radcliffe Medical Press, Oxford.

Kohner, N., Henley, A., 1995. When a Baby Dies. The Experience of Late Miscarriage, Stillbirth and Neonatal Death. Pandora Press, London.

Kohner, N., Leftwich, A., 1995. Pregnancy Loss and the Death of a Baby: a Training Pack for Professionals. National Extension College, Cambridge.

Tschudin, V., 1997. Counselling for Loss and Bereavement. Baillière Tindall, London.

6

Ethical and legal aspects of neonatology

John Wyatt   Bertie Leigh   Janet Rennie

© 2012 Elsevier Ltd

John Wyatt

Introduction

All medical care is based on a primary moral commitment – a belief in the intrinsic value of human life. In this respect the practice of neonatology is no different from any other branch of medicine. It starts from a commitment to preserve and protect the life, health and well-being of newborns. It is this commitment that has motivated and driven the remarkable advances which neonatal medicine has achieved in the last 50 years. Yet these advances have created complex, troubling and controversial dilemmas for clinicians, for parents, for healthcare institutions and for the law courts.

The aim of this chapter is to provide a brief review of some of the moral and ethical issues raised by the practice of neonatology and provide references for further study.

Plurality of moral beliefs and ethical approaches

Modern societies reflect a plurality of moral beliefs, assumptions and 'world views' and ethical discussion is inevitably controversial and contested. There is little or no consensus amongst modern moral philosophers and ethical approaches range from consequentialist (in which the consequences of an action determine its morality), deontological or duty-based approaches, and virtue ethics, in which the character of the moral agent is central.

Despite the plurality of foundational beliefs and ethical approaches, it is frequently possible to reach broad consensus about whether particular clinical actions are morally right or wrong. We are all agreed that it is right to listen to parents, to treat them with respect and to seek their consent for giving invasive treatment. We are all agreed that it is wrong to inflict painful and unpleasant medical procedures on babies unless there is a realistic prospect that they can bring some benefit. As health professionals we have a responsibility to try to come to consensus on substantive ethical issues wherever possible, even if we disagree about the reasons behind our shared conclusions.

The value of life of the newborn

A very long-standing ethical debate concerns the fundamental value of the life of an individual newborn. The infanticide of unwanted, diseased or malformed newborns has been a common and socially approved practice in many cultures (Milner 2000). Infanticide and the exposure of unwanted newborns was a common practice in the classical Greek and Roman world and the oldest extant textbook on midwifery, written by the first-century Roman physician Soranus, has a chapter entitled, 'How to recognise the newborn that is worth rearing' (Soranus and Temkin 1991).

In the history of the west, a marked change in the attitude to newborn lives can be traced to the rise of Christianity. Jewish and Christian teaching emphasised the intrinsic value of life of all human beings, and linked into the *imago dei*, the image of God which each human life carried (Wyatt 2009). The idea of the sanctity of all human life sprang from the Judaeo-Christian ethical tradition but has been incorporated into national and international codes of law and human rights.

The UN Universal Declaration of Human Rights (United Nations 1948) and the UN Convention on the Rights of the Child (United Nations 1989) both enshrine the intrinsic value of newborn life and the legal rights which every newborn holds. The latter upholds the 'inherent right to life' of every child from the moment of birth and lays a duty on member states to 'ensure to the maximum extent possible the survival and development of the child'.

It is clear that there is a stark difference in both national and international law between the legal rights of the newborn and those of the fetus. In most jurisdictions the fetus has no separate legal identity and cannot be the bearer of legal rights. But from the moment of birth, the newborn infant comes under the full protection of national and international legal conventions.

Recent philosophical challenges

The concept that a newborn life has an innate or intrinsic value equivalent to that of an older child or adult has recently come under sustained attack from a group of influential philosophers and ethicists. Although their views have gained little support amongst health and legal professionals, they are widely discussed in school and university courses on ethics, and it is important that neonatologists are aware of their existence.

Michael Tooley (Tooley 1972), Peter Singer (Singer 1995) and John Harris (Harris 1985) have argued that some form of self-awareness, the ability to see oneself as existing over time, is a necessary condition for having a right to life. Their views can be traced back to the thinking of the 17th-century English philosopher John Locke, who defined a person as 'a thinking intelligent being that has reason and reflection and can consider itself as itself, the same thinking thing, in different times and places' (Locke 1690). By this definition a newborn cannot be regarded as a 'person', and hence does not have an intrinsic right to life. Singer and others argue that the point at which human infants acquire a minimal sense of self-awareness is an empirical question which can be defined from psychological experiments but may not occur until the end of the first year of life. From this perspective a newborn infant should be regarded in the same way as the fetus as a 'potential person', a being whose life, although still of some significance, is intrinsically of less value than the life of an older child or adult.

Although logically defensible, this perspective has not gained significant currency amongst clinicians, and existing UK ethical guidelines from the General Medical Council (2007), British Medical Association (2007) and Royal College of Paediatrics and Child Health (2004) support the international consensus and argue that newborns should be treated with the same degree of respect, care and protection which we offer to all other patients. The guidance provided by the Nuffield Council on Bioethics Working Party (NCBWP) (2006) also supported the right of newborns and argued that 'a child of 6 days, months or years was worthy of equal consideration'.

Best interests

Doctors have a moral duty towards each individual patient to attempt to preserve life, restore health and prevent disease. Although the newborn's right to life is respected, all agree that there is no moral duty on doctors to provide every possible treatment in every possible clinical circumstance. Instead every action and treatment should be oriented towards the best interests of the individual child.

Although the phrase 'best interests' is intuitively attractive, it is notoriously vague and has been subjected to sustained legal and philosophical analysis. It is generally agreed that the determination of best interests involves the clinician in a difficult task of balancing and weighing a range of factors and opinions. General Medical Council guidance states that this should include the views of the parents and their cultural, religious or other beliefs and values, and the views of other healthcare professionals involved in providing care to the child. Preference should be given to treatment choices which least restrict the child's future options (General Medical Council 2007).

An assessment of best interests may also include, firstly, the current experience of the baby, especially the degree of pain and distress and the ability of the healthcare team to control this, and, secondly, the anticipated long-term outcome. The perspective, values and goals of the parents may be at variance with those of the health professionals and this may give rise to conflict and misunderstanding. In addition there may be disagreements and differing perspectives amongst the members of the health professional team, and it is important for these differences to be aired and, wherever possible, a consensus position reached. Where there is continuing disagreement and debate it is often helpful to request a second opinion from an experienced external clinician. The baby is reliant on the parents and the health professional team working in partnership, and every effort must be expended to develop and sustain a relationship of mutual understanding, respect and trust.

Both UK law and professional medical guidance seem to indicate that, where there is a conflict of interests, it is the child's interests which should, in principle, trump all others. Others have argued that the interests of the baby must not be allowed to take precedence over the interests of the parents and other siblings. The NCBWP recommended that those who make decisions in respect of a child should carefully consider the interests of all those who may be affected, especially other family members, old or young (Nuffield Council on Biothics 2006). However, national and international statutes suggest that, in the event of a direct conflict of interests, the baby's best interests should carry greater weight than those of the parents or carers.

Balancing burdens and benefits

A traditional and helpful approach to ethical decision-making in medicine is the balancing of burdens and benefits, and this balance-sheet approach has often been adopted in cases which have come before the law courts. All treatments carry potential benefits to the patient but they also incur burdens and risks. The essence of ethical practice is to ensure that the potential benefits of all treatments offered should exceed their burdens. Any proposed treatment should be assessed within this framework, considering a range of factors – physical, emotional, social – and both short-term and long-term outcomes. The balance-sheet approach provides a helpful framework for ensuring that all aspects of a treatment decision are highlighted and incorporated into the decision-making process (General Medical Council 2010).

Withholding and withdrawing life-sustaining treatment

If life-sustaining treatment is futile because death is inevitable, or the treatment is excessively burdensome relative to the likely benefits, then there is no ethical duty to commence or continue treatment. It is generally agreed that there is no fundamental moral difference between withholding life-sustaining treatment (such as resuscitation at birth) and withdrawing treatment which has already been commenced, although the psychological and emotional experience for staff and for parents may be different (British Medical Association 2007). Where there is genuine uncertainty about the likely benefit of invasive treatment, it may be appropriate to commence 'provisional' intensive support, whilst explaining to the parents that support will be withdrawn subsequently if it becomes apparent that there is no response to the treatment and that the prognosis is hopeless. On occasions parents may refuse to give consent to the withdrawal of life-sustaining treatment despite the unanimous conviction of the healthcare team that the treatment is futile or excessively burdensome. Parents need to be treated with respect, patience and empathy but, if no agreement can be reached, the primary ethical duty of the staff must be to protect the best interests of the baby, if necessary by recourse to legal proceedings.

Neonatal euthanasia

The mainstream approach to medical ethics has always drawn a sharp distinction between the withdrawal of life-sustaining treatment and an act of intentional killing or homicide. The distinction is not only one of an act of omission versus one of commission but is also based on the underlying intention of the act. When futile life-sustaining treatment is withdrawn, the intention is not to kill, but it is to limit the continuing harm and injury created by the treatment. If the infant continues to live following withdrawal of treatment, the medical goal is not to ensure that death occurs as soon as possible, but it is to provide palliative care, symptom relief, including the use of analgesic and sedative medication, and holistic care addressed to all the needs of the infant and family.

In 2005 a group of paediatricians from the Netherlands published a set of medical guidelines (known as the Groningen protocol) which supported the active ending of newborn life, using lethal drugs, under specified conditions (Verhagen and Sauer 2005). They suggested that intentional ending of life should be restricted to infants with 'a hopeless prognosis' who were likely to have a life 'full of suffering', but who were physiologically stable and not dependent on intensive support technology. The Groningen protocol has created considerable discussion and controversy but the active ending of newborn life has been explicitly rejected by professional and regulatory bodies in the UK and in most other national jurisdictions. Instead emphasis has been placed on the importance of skilled palliative care, effective symptom control and ensuring the active involvement and support of parents and other family members in end-of-life care (ACT 2009). There is a growing consensus that muscle relaxant agents have little or no role in palliative care, and their use may be positively unhelpful as they mask the clinical signs of pain and distress.

Quality of life and disability perspectives

Although it is often suggested that it is possible for health professionals and families to predict the future 'quality of life' of the critically ill newborn, there are major theoretical and practical problems with this concept. In particular it is often assumed by health professionals that a neurological or cognitive impairment translates automatically into a loss of well-being or life satisfaction. Yet empirical studies of health-related quality of life in ex-preterm survivors challenge this assumption (Saigal et al. 2006; Zwicker and Harris 2008).

Many disabled adults assert that many of the most significant factors which impair their life experiences are the social attitudes and political responses to their disability, rather than the biological impairment itself. In addition there is empirical evidence that health professionals and parents consistently undervalue the 'quality of life' of disabled adolescents and adults (Saigal and Tyson 2008). The unthinking use of 'quality of life' concepts in clinical decision-making is often unhelpful, and may be used as a cloak for prejudices and negative stereotypes about the lives of disabled people. Instead greater attention should be paid to recording and assessing the real-world subjective life experiences of babies, children and adults who have undergone neonatal intensive care.

Resuscitation of extreme preterm

Considerable attention had been paid to the ethical and practical clinical issues surrounding the resuscitation of extremely preterm infants at the limits of viability. The NCBWP guidelines use a week-by-week analysis depending on the gestational age of the infant at birth (Nuffield Council on Biothics 2006). However there are a number of other clinical variables, such as birthweight, twinning, gender and exposure to antenatal steroids, which are of great importance in influencing the prospects of survival (National Institute of Child Health and Development 2008). Hence decisions about the appropriateness of resuscitation should be carefully individualised to the unique patient and family context rather than depend on the

unthinking use of published guidelines or clinical algorithms. Wherever possible detailed discussion with parents should be carried out before delivery and neonatologists should demonstrate attentive respect for the parents' beliefs and values, with the aim of achieving a consensus on appropriate action. If no agreement can be reached, clinicians have a moral and legal duty to act in an emergency in what they perceive to be the baby's best interests. As discussed above, preference should be given to treatment choices that least restrict the child's future options. This suggests that, in the presence of genuine uncertainty, resuscitation followed by a short period of provisional intensive care to allow detailed assessment and discussion would be appropriate.

Conclusion

Neonatology enshrines a primary moral commitment to the welfare and best interests of every newborn infant. Yet within the challenging context of a pluralistic society, it may be increasingly hard to find consensus on how this translates into practical decision-making in the intensive care unit. The perspective, values and goals of the parents may be at variance with those of the health professionals and this may give rise to conflict and misunderstanding. Yet the baby is reliant on the parents and the health professional team working in partnership, and every effort must be expended to develop and sustain a relationship of mutual understanding, respect and trust.

References

ACT, 2009. A Neonatal Pathway for Babies with Palliative Care Needs. ACT (Association for Children's Palliative Care), Bristol.

British Medical Association, 2007. Withholding and Withdrawing Life-prolonging Medical Treatment: Guidance for Decision Making, third ed. BMA, London.

General Medical Council, 2007. 0–18 Years: Guidance for all Doctors. Available online at: http://www.gmc-uk.org/guidance/ethical_guidance/children_guidance_index.asp.

General Medical Council, 2010. End of Life Care. Available online at: http://www.gmc-uk.org/guidance/ethical_guidance/6858.asp.

Harris, J., 1985. The Value of Life: Introduction to Medical Ethics. Routledge, Abingdon.

Locke, J., 1690. An Essay Concerning Human Understanding. Penguin Classics, London.

Milner, L.S., 2000. Hardness of Heart/Hardness of Life: The Stain of Human Infanticide. University Press of America, Lanham.

National Institute of Child Health and Development, 2008. NICHD Neonatal Research Network (NRN): Extremely Preterm Birth Outcome Data. Available online at: http://www.nichd.nih.gov/about/org/cdbpm/pp/prog_epbo/epbo_case.cfm.

Nuffield Council on Biothics, 2006. Critical Care Decisions in Fetal and Neonatal Medicine: Ethical Issues. Available online at: http://www.nuffieldbioethics.org/neonatal-medicine.

Royal College of Paediatrics & Child Health, 2004. Witholding or Withdrawing Life Sustaining Treatment in Children: A Framework for Practice, second ed. Royal College of Paediatrics & Child Health, London.

Saigal, S., Tyson, J., 2008. Measurement of quality of life of survivors of neonatal intensive care: critique and implications. Semin Perinatol 32, 59–66.

Saigal, S., Stoskopf, B., Pinelli, J., et al., 2006. Self-perceived health-related quality of life

of former extremely low birth weight infants at young adulthood. Pediatrics 118, 1140–1148.

Singer, P., 1995. Rethinking Life and Death: The Collapse of Our Traditional Ethics. Oxford University Press, Oxford.

Soranus & Temkin, O., 1991. Gynecology. Johns Hopkins University Press, Maryland.

Tooley, M., 1972. Abortion and Infanticide. Philos Public Aff 2, 37–65.

United Nations, 1948. Universal Declaration of Human Rights. United Nations, New York.

United Nations, 1989. Convention on the Rights of the Child. United Nations, New York.

Verhagen, E., Sauer, P.J., 2005. The Groningen protocol – euthanasia in severely ill newborns. N Engl J Med 352, 959–962.

Wyatt, J.S., 2009. Matters of Life and Death, second ed. InterVarsity Press, Leicester.

Zwicker, J.G., Harris, S.R., 2008. Quality of life of formerly preterm and very low birth weight infants from preschool age to adulthood: a systematic review. Pediatrics 121, e366–e376.

Bertie Leigh   Janet M Rennie

Introduction

When neonatal medicine emerged as a distinct subspecialty, medical ethics was at a similar stage of infancy. Most decisions were assumed to be matters of 'common sense' and the law was widely regarded as another country where they did things differently. Today it is accepted that neonatologists have to take profound decisions of public importance which are likely to be subject to formal analysis in the courts. Decisions taken at the outset of a baby's life often have an impact decades later. The baby who is the subject of the decision may be unable to play any part in the discussion today, but as an adult will be able to ask pointed questions of the erstwhile clinician. In this chapter we will discuss some of these issues and give general advice as to how paediatricians should conduct themselves in those areas of their practice which are likely to bring them into contact with the law.

Clinicians and litigation

Maintaining professional standards

Neonatologists must maintain their own skills and the competence of their teams. Remaining 'in good standing' with the Royal College of Paediatrics and Child Health (RCPCH) involves participating in revalidation, appraisal and continuing professional development. Consultants must ensure that the neonatal unit has clear written guidelines and adequate staffing, that the facilities and equipment meet current standards (Ch. 2) and that outcomes are audited. Accurate, detailed contemporaneous notes must be kept: they are an intrinsic part of good care and the only part that is directly visible when the quality is called into question. Anticipation of possible litigation is not paranoia; it is good medicine to create clinical notes that record the progression of the patient in detail and make it explicit why particular decisions were taken, just as it is to obtain a second opinion in difficult cases. Intemperate remarks about colleagues and hasty judgements about areas that are not within your own competence are poor practice as well as being forensically unwise.

Handling adverse events, mistakes and complaints

Always be open and honest with the parents, but think calmly before you meet them after any adverse event. That a ventilator fails, or an intravenous infusion runs wild or a nurse makes a drug error is unfortunate, but it may not contribute to the baby's eventual problems. Do not make the mistake of thinking that because you are being candid about a complication you should be more hasty than you would be in other circumstances to give a gloomy prognosis. Think carefully about the way in which to treat the baby so as to minimise any damage and to break bad news so as to minimise parental distress.

If parents complain about your treatment or counselling, seek the advice and support of senior colleagues, including the clinical director and service manager early on, before matters get out of hand.

Appearing in court

Understanding the legal processes outlined in this chapter will help. Sometimes a decision is made not to defend a case even when the staff involved feel that they did nothing wrong and that the adverse outcome was outside their control. There are all sorts of reasons why it is decided not to defend a case in court, and the decision does not necessarily imply that the criticism advanced by the claimant is correct. In this situation, give in gracefully and remember that giving evidence in court is not a pleasant experience for any doctor. However, if it is decided to defend the case, then be prepared to spend time and energy in preparation (reading all the notes and documents in the case) and in attending court.

In a civil court, remember that the judge is the most important person in the room. Address all your answers to him or her, not to the barrister who is questioning you. Tell the truth, in simple language, think before you start talking and speak very slowly: this gives the judge time to write down what you are saying and you time to think about your answer carefully. Do not be afraid of generating silence whilst you consider your answer. The pace of a courtroom seems very slow to those used to the frenetic activity of intensive care units. Do not engage the opposing barrister in banter, or let him needle you, or try to score a point at his expense – it is his home territory, not yours; his views are not in issue, but your objectivity is. Answer the question after due thought, preferably with a straight 'yes' or 'no'; but if you feel you are being forced to answer an inappropriately closed question then do not be afraid to say 'yes, but …' with one concise, crisp sentence. Resist the temptation to embark on a mini-lecture. When you have finished your answer, stop. Do not fall into the temptation of embellishing or clarifying, simply because the cross-examiner waits and looks as if he expects you to do so.

Situations with a high risk of litigation in neonatology

General

Good notekeeping and clear protocols are vital, and it is important to keep copies of old protocols when they are updated because they establish the standard of care for that era. Never amend protocols by adding to them in manuscript so that it is impossible to tell when the old version was superseded: always redate and reissue the whole protocol. Do not 'save up' amendments or hesitate to change the protocol simply because the amendment involves only a few words. A protocol you can no longer defend in detail is a hazard to the unit and its patients. Always communicate the updated protocol to those who need to follow it and explain the reasons for the change. Cases are judged by the standards of the day, and in a rapidly advancing field like neonatal medicine it can be difficult to recall precisely when practice changed in your unit unless there is documentation.

The standards of care are those of a reasonably competent practitioner, and the courts do not expect that protocols will be changed to reflect every research finding. For a while, there was a fear that protocols would be used to drive litigation in cases where the clinical management had not followed a prescribed guideline. This is not a justification for the lack of a protocol, because in practice claimants usually succeed only when the standard of care is substandard by definitions that are common and beyond dispute. If the unit decides to deviate from a national (National Institute for Health and Clinical Excellence (NICE)) guideline the reasons for this must be clearly laid out.

Resuscitation

If a baby develops athetoid cerebral palsy as a result of damage to the deep grey matter after a short period of acute profound hypoxia in the immediate run-up to delivery, the quality and timeliness of the resuscitation will be under intense scrutiny. Minutes matter in this situation, and if the neonatal team arrive late, for whatever reason, the fact should be documented and the reason. Common problems are failure to intubate, incorrect endotracheal tube position and failure to use chest compression. It is not below a reasonable standard of care to intubate the oesophagus, but it is substandard care not to recognise it. It may not be below a reasonable standard of care for a junior doctor to be unable to intubate, but it will be if this doctor persists in the attempt too long, allowing the baby to desaturate, rather than using bag and mask and calling for help. It is substandard care to use a very small size of endotracheal tube in a term baby, or to insert it so far that it lies deep in the right main bonchus and leave it there.

A need for resuscitation does not equate to a diagnosis of 'birth asphyxia' and this cannot be stressed too often. Still less does it provide any basis for long-term prognostication. To act on the presumption that it does will not discharge a duty of candour but will cause needless and unwarranted distress. Use the term 'birth depression', for which there are a number of causes, including hypoxia–ischaemia during labour. Similarly, the term 'flat' is imprecise and means different things to different observers. We have seen this term applied to anything from stillborn babies through to babies who responded to blow-by oxygen after a few minutes. Similarly, 'shocked' should not be used to describe a baby unless there is genuine evidence of cardiovascular shock with hypotension and acidosis.

Obtain both cord blood pH results if possible and document the baby's early course very carefully with a narrative about the condition at birth and the response to resuscitation. Remember that babies who recover sufficiently quickly to remain with their mothers are sometimes at the end stage of a prolonged period of 'chronic partial' hypoxic ischaemia and develop seizures at 12–24 hours.

If resuscitation has to be abandoned make sure the decision is appropriate, be sure that the baby is not left alone and treat the body with dignity at all times. Never, ever leave a baby's body exposed and unattended on the resuscitaire and rush out of the labour ward. Initiating resuscitation in very immature babies generates a great deal of anxiety, but if stopping resuscitation appears to be the appropriate decision, supported by senior input, then fear of litigation should never inhibit clinical judgement.

Early neonatal encephalopathy and brain damage

Babies who seize in early neonatal life do not always have hypoxic–ischaemic encephalopathy, even if there was birth depression. However, there is a high risk of sequelae in this situation and the diagnosis should be pursued with vigour. Lumbar puncture and a search for infection are mandatory (Ch. 40.2). Investigations should include imaging, electroencephalogram (EEG) and metabolic screening. Do not prognosticate too early, but if it is appropriate to offer to withdraw care seek the support of a colleague, and warn the parents that the baby might not die.

The first duty of the the neonatologist is to limit any futher adverse effects by maintaining blood pressure, glucose levels and blood gases. Referral for therapeutic hypothermia should be considered where a local programme exists (Ch. 40.4).

Current litigation practice in the UK is dominated by claimants with cerebral palsy who ascribe their disability to hypoxic ischaemia

during labour, and a key plank of their causation argument is their ability to demonstrate early neonatal encephalopathy. The notes need to be careful, thorough, non-judgemental and include a daily description of the baby's neurological state. Avoid the temptation to record an absence of change without explaining what has not changed and make positive factual observations of the child's condition.

Investigation needs to be thorough and appropriate. This is not difficult (Ch. 40.1), but it is remarkable how often there is no pH, no head circumference, or no description of fontanelle tension, muscle tone or level of alertness in a baby who is being treated with several anticonvulsants and whose nursing notes suggest that she is totally obtunded. A Kleihauer test can be vitally important in establishing the diagnosis of fetomaternal haemorrhage. It is embarrassing, to say the least, if a diagnosis of congenital cytomegalovirus, CHARGE syndrome or an inborn error of metabolism is only established once legal proceedings are well underway.

There is no doubt that asphyxia can cause brain damage, but the majority of babies who suffer asphyxia at birth do not go on to develop brain damage, and 90% of cases of cerebral palsy are not attributable to birth asphyxia. Furthermore, sometimes the signs of fetal compromise in labour are associated with brain damage that has been sustained previously. This means that the association can be difficult to understand and is in part a diagnosis of exclusion. We suggest that the following list of features reflects the approach of most experts who advise the courts at the moment:

1. There must be evidence of significant fetal compromise if the fetal heart rate was being monitored at the time when it is suggested the damaging hypoxic ischaemia was sustained. Since the vast majority of children tolerate the stresses of labour without sustaining damage, there must be good evidence to pinpoint the insult to this time. Although electronic monitoring is not specific it is highly sensitive and it is unlikely that a child will suffer brain damage due to ischaemia at a time when the heart rate appears to be normal in rate and variation.
2. If it is suggested that profound damage was inflicted at the end of labour the neonate must exhibit clear evidence of this recent near-death experience. The Apgar score is not measured to predict outcome, but if the baby scores 2 for circulation at birth it is unlikely that the circulation has recently collapsed, and a 5-minute Apgar of 6 or above is not consistent with a recent acute profound hypoxic–ischaemic injury.
3. The human organism will metabolise anaerobically in response to hypoxic ischaemia. Thus a baby who does not have an acidosis is highly unlikely to have experienced significant hypoxic ischaemia recently. If the cord blood was sampled the diagnosis of acute profound hypoxic ischaemia in the immediate run-up to delivery becomes difficult to establish if the arterial pH is above 7.0 and the base deficit less than 12, and can usually be excluded if the pH is above 7.1 and the base deficit less than 8. It is always important to consider the arterial as well as the venous cord blood and this is particularly important in cases of possible cord occlusion.
4. It is unlikely that brain damage has been sustained without there being signs of temporary damage to at least one other body system, although whether this has been recorded may be a function of how ill the baby was perceived as being at the time.
5. The baby born after 34 weeks must have exhibited severe or moderate neonatal encephalopathy (Ch. 40.4), because this is the stage in the evolution of the disease process in which

permanent damage is sustained. Increasingly, this diagnosis is supported by evidence of an abnormal EEG or aEEG.

6. The child must have a disability capable of being attributed to birth asphyxia. Traditional thinking held that spastic and athetoid cerebral palsy were the only disabilities in this category, but it is now appreciated that learning difficulties can be caused by perinatal hypoxic ischaemia, although a motor disability is usually present as well.

7. Other more probable diagnoses must be excluded. This necessarily involves a careful and detailed investigation by a wide range of modern modalities, including biochemical tests and magnetic resonance imaging (MRI). Particularly important in this category is the diagnosis of stroke.

In many of the cases we are asked to assess, the fact that the baby has sustained perinatal hypoxic–ischaemic damage is not in dispute so much as the precise timing of the insult. Where the mother reports a sudden loss of fetal movements a day or two before delivery this may take on a more sinister significance in the light of subsequent events. In all these cases early cerebral imaging, EEG or Doppler studies may be decisive. In future, diffusion-weighted MRI or MR spectroscopy may shed more light on the precise timing of events.

Preterm brain injury

Preterm brain injury is usually caused by a complex sequence of interacting factors, which makes establishing causation even more difficult than at term. Further, much preterm brain injury is not preventable in the present state of the art, however meticulous the care. However, if the prematurity was the result of an inappropriate early delivery (because of miscalculated dates, for example) the child may mount a claim for iatropathic prematurity. Some disabled ex-preterm children born after the mid- to late 1990s have mounted successful claims based on the association of hypocarbia with periventricular leukomalacia. The same is true for those whose mothers were not offered antenatal steroids (when appropriate) after about 1994, when the first Royal College of Obstetricians and Gynaecologists (RCOG) guidelines were issued.

Adverse outcome after preterm birth is an area where neonatologists need all their skills in communicating with parents as well as treating their patients. The parents of a disabled child understandably seek a reason, and something to blame. If they are kept in touch with their baby's care and given an accurate prognosis and an explanation of any interacting causes as early as possible, they are less likely to ascribe the whole problem to the brief power cut on day 6, the disconnected ventilator tubing on day 33 or the possible misplaced nasogastric tube on day 40. Early and full explanations can avoid a long-drawn-out period of attrition which often ends in disappointment for all concerned. In our experience, it is very rare to go through a set of notes documenting a neonatal intensive care unit (NICU) stay of several months and find that there were absolutely no problems or errors at all, but it is rarely the case that any deficiency in care can be identified as the cause of an adverse outcome in a very preterm baby. As many studies have shown, there are simply too many hurdles for such babies to surmount for it to be clear which inflicted the lesion which will later prove disastrous.

Jaundice (Ch. 29.1)

Kernicterus is often a preventable disease, and, although it almost vanished from UK neonatal practice, it has now returned with a vengeance. The National Patient Safety Agency has made kernicterus a 'never event' in the UK. Midwives and others concerned with newborn care need to be taught that neonatal jaundice can be an emergency. Early discharge policies and the welcome move towards exclusive breastfeeding have produced a new population of vulnerable babies. There is only one way the bilirubin is going in the first few days of life, and that is up. New NICE guidelines (www.nice.org.uk) became available in 2010 regarding the management of neonatal jaundice, including advice on when to measure the bilirubin and when to start and stop phototherapy (Ch. 29.1).

Evidence shows that the following are especially high-risk groups:

- near-term babies (35–37 weeks)
- babies whose mothers exclusively breastfeed
- babies whose siblings required treatment for neonatal jaundice (often a proxy for haemolytic disease)
- preterm babies with acidosis, and/or low albumin levels, or an 'open' blood–brain barrier because of germinal matrix and intraventricular haemorrhage or sepsis, who can develop kernicterus at low levels of bilirubin.

Effective intervention in all such groups requires anticipation as well as reaction.

Example Baby W was born normally at 07.26 on a Friday after a quick and easy labour. He weighed 3.68 kg with a head circumference of 35.5 cm. The baby check was carried out in the hospital during the morning by the family general practitioner (GP) who was providing care, and mother and baby went home soon afterwards. It was the mother's second child. The father was known to suffer from spherocytosis and during the pregnancy he was admitted to the same hospital with a haemolytic crisis

On Saturday the community midwife visited at home and noted that W was jaundiced. She advised putting him outside in his pram in the 'sunlight'. By Sunday W was more markedly jaundiced and he was feeding less well; again sunlight was advised and the midwife said that a bilirubin estimation would be performed the following day.

On Monday W was irritable and arching his back, and would not feed. His mother took him to the GP, who arranged admission to the hospital, where his bilirubin was found to be 636 µmol/l. An exchange transfusion was done but was too late to prevent kernicterus, which was apparent on the late MRI. W is disabled by choreoathetoid cerebral palsy, upgaze palsy and deafness.

Hypoglycaemia

This is an area in which many claims are unsuccessful. Most experts consider that as a rule only prolonged periods of symptomatic hypoglycaemia are damaging, and there is now a typical (not pathognomonic) MR pattern described (Traill et al. 1998; Kinnala et al. 1999; Murakami et al. 1999), which has recently been extended (Burns et al. 2008) (Fig. 6.1). There can be no complacency about the management of hypoglycaemia, and appropriate protocols for screening high-risk groups must be in place and audited (Ch. 34.1). Transitional care areas are high-risk areas for this reason, and need to be recognised as such. Symptomatic hypoglycaemia is an emergency and intravenous treatment is mandatory. It is unusual for a term baby of normal weight whose mother is not diabetic to present with symptomatic hypoglycaemia, and there should be a high index of suspicion that the underlying diagnosis is hyperinsulinaemia right from the start in this situation, with the appropriate level of investigation and intervention, with early recourse to expert help.

Like hyperbilirubinaemia, it is now known that the normal healthy breastfed baby is not immune from hypoglycaemic damage

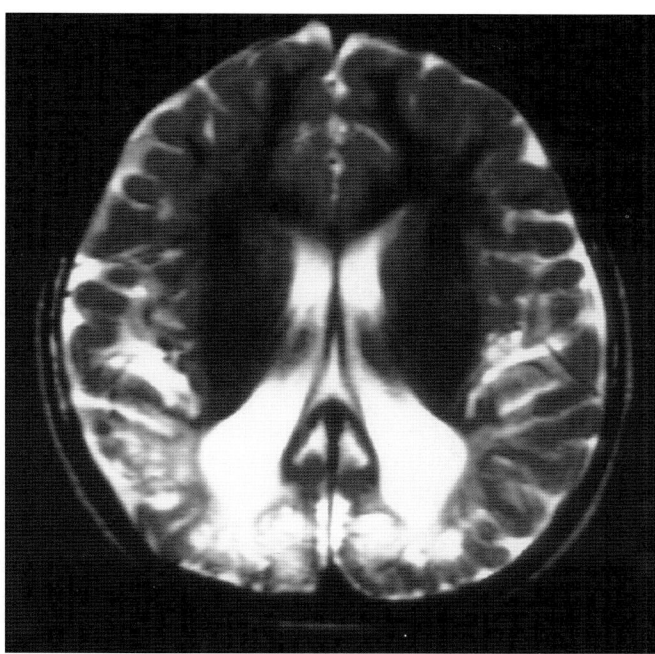

Fig. 6.1 Magnetic resonance imaging in a case of probable hypoglycaemic brain damage.

due to breast milk insufficiency, although the problem is rare. Monitoring the adequacy of breastfeeding is difficult, but must be routine midwifery practice and guidelines regarding the use of supplementary feeds need to be worked out between professionals. Babies who are small for dates or whose mothers have diabetes must have glucose screening using an appropriate method and with reasonable frequency (Table 34.3).

Retinopathy of prematurity

Children who are blinded from retinopathy of prematurity often litigate, not usually for poor management of their oxygen therapy but because the screening policy (Ch. 33) has failed them. This happens in two ways: either the recommended screen does not take place in the critical window of opportunity for treatment, or the screen takes place but the diagnosis is missed. There are clear UK (and international) guidelines that must be followed, and if a planned screening examination cannot take place at the scheduled time (for example, the baby may be too ill to tolerate the handling or even the dilating drops) the reasons should be carefully documented. The same is true if surgery has to be postponed.

Deafness

Most deafness is of genetic origin, and a careful family history and appropriate genetic testing are important. Claimants who attribute their hearing loss to gentamicin toxicity or hypoxic ischaemia occasionally succeed in proving their case. The impact of the discovery that a particular mutation enhances individual vulnerability to gentamicin toxicity has not yet been determined.

Infectious disease

Neonatal group B streptococcal disease commonly leads to litigation and deviations will be harder to defend now that there are guidelines endorsed by the RCOG and RCPCH supporting a strategy for antenatal prophylaxis based on risk factors. Neonatologists need to work with their obstetric colleagues to devise and implement local guidelines and to think carefully about what should be done, for example, if a baby who should have been exposed to intrapartum prophylaxis is born before her mother receives it.

Neonatal meningitis is hazardous for doctors as well as for babies. Although the prognosis of established disease is poor, we see cases in which there has been an alleged delay in investigation or treatment, of inadequate dosing, inappropriate antibiotic choice or short duration of treatment. Clinicians must be aware that neonatal meningitis carries a high risk of adverse sequelae and take care to optimise antibiotic and supportive treatment, investigate fully and refer on when appropriate. Increasingly, when a disease has had an adverse outcome, the fact that this was predictable will not of itself prevent those concerned on the patient's behalf from scrutinising the records in retrospect to see whether the management was in fact optimal.

'Missed' abnormalities at the neonatal examination

It is difficult for parents to understand that no one was to blame when their baby, who was checked over and passed fit, collapses with coarctation of the aorta and requires major surgery, or develops amblyopia from a cataract, or a limp from developmental dysplasia of the hip. Yet none of these conditions is reliably detected by the routine neonatal examination (Ch. 14). Biochemical screening is reliable, but there are sometimes failures in communication which result in a hypothyroid baby starting treatment late. The introduction of screening for medium-change acyl dehydrogenase deficiency is welcome, but serves to increase the need for adequate back-up to ensure that affected babies receive appropriate and timely expert advice.

Vitamin K-deficiency bleeding

There is still no agreed UK standard regarding the dose, route or frequency of vitamin K prophylaxis for vitamin K-deficiency bleeding. Parents are offered a choice in many hospitals. Parents who refuse vitamin K for their baby altogether should have their refusal documented. However, sick babies who are admitted to neonatal units should have intramuscular vitamin K. In this instance it does not matter what the mother said before the baby became ill, because by that stage vitamin K is a medically indicated treatment. It is inappropriate to wait for 7 hours for 'consent' in a baby of 28 weeks whose mother required an appendicectomy and who herself was admitted to the intensive care unit ventilated. If that baby develops intraventricular haemorrhage he may allege that the delay in vitamin K contributed to the problem. Any baby can become sick, and if he received oral vitamin K after birth (or no vitamin K) he should be given a further intramuscular dose, especially if surgery is required.

Scarring and iatropathic problems (Ch. 44)

The scars of neonatal intensive care are not usually disabling, but on occasion extravasation injury can cause tethering around a joint which inhibits movement or causes disfiguring scars. This may be unavoidable, but constant vigilance is required to avoid inflicting scars which will grow with the baby.

Since the Department of Health warned that there is an increased risk of cardiac tamponade when Silastic long lines are sited in the right atrium, neonatologists should only continue to site lines in the heart when there is no alternative. A long line which inadvertently lies in the left ascending lumbar vein can cause permanent paraplegia, via direct extravasation into the subarachnoid space or by causing a vasculitic response with venous congestion in the small veins of the epidural plexus.

Relations with parents

The therapeutic alliance with parents

Wherever possible the neonatologist and the parent should form a relationship based on profound mututal trust (Ch. 5) and close cooperation. The quality of care on the NICU is enhanced if the parent who is to look after the child exclusively in the near future is fully involved in the decisions about the treatment of the child and in the delivery of that treatment in so far as may be practical.

Maintaining this relationship requires time and effort, and time can be difficult to find in the hurly-burly of a busy intensive care unit. Continuity can help, and the 'attending' system operated by most neonatal teams may be modified to allow parents to form a relationship with one consultant.

Many parents find it advantageous to have contact with several consultants, who might put things in different ways, and sharing the emotionally draining load of counselling is valuable if senior staff are to avoid 'burnout'. If parents are to derive maximum benefit from this multiplicity of view, colleagues must have confidence in each other to communicate in their own way, not to undermine each other and to convey the same message. This demands that the doctors involved maintain a high degree of communication so that the parents are not confronted with conflicting information and inconsistent advice. Practitioners must be aware of what each other has said and such extensive sharing of information demands detailed records and regular discussions. We have found that including this as an item on the agenda at the weekly meeting between consultants and senior nurses has been invaluable in achieving better information sharing.

Informed consent

It is well established in English law that an adult patient with capacity to take a decision can refuse treatment for good reason, bad reason or no reason at all. The law respects the patient's autonomy and the doctor who operates or treats such a patient without that patient's consent is guilty of an assault. Assault may give rise to a liability to compensate without proof of damage in the civil courts, to a prosecution in the criminal courts and may be punished by the General Medical Council as professional misconduct. The same legal principles apply to babies save that the operative consent has to be given by someone with parental responsibility. Parents have the right to decide what treatment their children should receive and doctors should act in partnership with parents wherever possible. However, parental rights are not beyond the review or control of the court: they derive from the parental duty to look after the child and they exist for the benefit of the child rather than the parent. Indeed, it has been suggested that, when a doctor operated on a child with the consent of a parent but the operation was manifestly not in the best interests of the child, the doctor would commit an act of trespass as well as being liable to an action brought by, or on behalf of, the child in negligence.

Which procedures require written consent?

A consent will be equally valid whether it is given orally or by conduct, as where someone sticks out an arm to receive an injection. Similarly it does not need to be recorded in writing to provide a defence to a claim of assault. The reason why the consent to more serious interventions is recorded in writing is to provide evidence, not only that the patient consented but also that the doctor complied with the obligation to counsel the patient. When seeking consent a doctor incurs a duty to explain what is involved in the procedure, and to advise of the risks and benefits so as to put the parent in a position to take a sensible decision. In order to demonstrate that the parents' rights were respected it is increasingly necessary to record that the proper explanations were given and formalities were complied with. Just as consent to an injection is incomplete without knowing what is in the needle, there is an increasing need to record in detail the explanation that was given. In the past, written consent was only sought for major procedures such as surgery or exchange transfusion. The British Association of Perinatal Medicine (www.bapm.org) has produced a useful list of procedures for which it is proposed that consent is obtained.

Who is able to give consent?

Single mothers

Either parent has the right to consent to the treatment, providing the parents are married or the father has acquired parental responsibility. If the doctor is on notice that the parents disagree it will be wise either to try to obtain the agreement of the second parent or to suggest that they should go to court to have their differences resolved, but as the court stated in one leading case:

> *If the parents disagree, one consenting and the other refusing, the doctor will be presented with a professional and ethical dilemma but not with a legal problem because, if he has the consent of one authorised person, the treatment will not without more constitute a trespass or criminal assault.*

There are a few exceptions to this general rule: ritual circumcision should only be done with the agreement of both parents (*Re U*). There are procedures on children which should only be done with the prior authority of a court order even where both parents consent. These include non-therapeutic sterilisation and the donation of regenerative tissue such as bone marrow, or of an organ such as a kidney. Although it has not happened yet, it seems likely that progress with stem cells will lead to neonatologists being involved in such issues in the future. The court will seek to balance the degree of risk to the baby against the likely benefit to the family of which that baby is a member.

Very young mothers

Increasingly common on the NICU is the single mother aged under 15 years. Often she will be '*Gillick*-competent' – able to understand information given to her about her baby and make decisions for herself – but sometimes children are born to mothers so immature that the doctors would be reluctant to accept their consent to treatment of themselves. Nevertheless, only the mother can give a lawful consent to treatment of her child. Often the doctors will be able to involve the grandparents or the biological father in the treatment of the baby, for the same reason that it is good practice to involve the parents of the *Gillick*-competent child in her own treatment. However, it may well be that in such circumstances the hospital will feel that the Social Services department should be involved because the baby, if not the young mother, is in need of support. Social Services are the lead agency for children in need and may decide to make an application to the court.

Psychiatrically ill mothers

Women with long-standing psychoses sometimes relapse when pregnant or during the puerperium, and women without any previous psychiatric morbidity can become seriously ill for the first time after giving birth. If they are single, this can present major problems for those caring for their baby. The starting point in this situation is with the mother's consultant psychiatrist, in order to establish a perception of her ability to process information and take decisions. On occasion, we have managed withdrawal of care in this situation by involving a team of psychiatrists, social workers, family members and other therapists with a team from the neonatal unit. Where the mother is too ill to give informed consent we have had to involve Social Services or the courts: even here it is good practice to involve the mother as much as possible.

Use of interpreters

Recent National Health Service (NHS) guidelines have made it clear that the long-established practice of relying on family members (particularly children) as interpreters is no longer acceptable. The reason for this is that the mother or father of the interpreter may have information which he or she wishes to convey, but which he or she does not want the rest of the family to know – for example, a diagnosis of human immunodeficiency virus. Further, there is no way of knowing that family members are translating complex medical information accurately. If parents do not speak English well enough to understand the information they need to give consent, a suitable interpreter must be obtained. There is a scarcity of interpreters in some languages and the cost of face-to-face interpreters is a considerable financial burden for many trusts; telephone interpreters can be used for some consultations. Provision of interpreters cannot overcome the problems associated with the everyday informal contact which is essential to effective partnership between the parents and the rest of the team on the neonatal unit.

Documentation of counselling, and which risks to mention

Neonatologists are under an obligation to ensure that parents understand the nature and purpose of the procedure for which they are seeking consent. This includes making sure that they understand the expected consequences and the risks involved in the procedure. It is less often spelled out that the doctor has an obligation to make clear the consequences and risks of not undergoing the procedure. A doctor who negligently deters a patient or parent from consenting to a procedure by giving an exaggerated view of the hazards will incur a potential liability if the parents decide not to allow their baby to undergo the procedure and the baby meets with disaster as a result.

As to what risks should be mentioned, it is sometimes said that there is a 1% rule – all risks with an incidence of 1% should be mentioned. That may be a useful starting point but it certainly does not describe the risks which need to be mentioned. A much more remote risk of death or disability will usually have to be discussed. The doctor should also take account of how much real choice there is, how much time there is to take the decision and how much information the parents wish to have.

Refusal of treatment

There are some cases where the parents refuse treatment which the doctor believes is essential in the interests of the child. In those cases the courts can make orders authorising treatment and the doctor must not hesitate to take whatever step is clearly necessary in the interests of the patient. However it is much better to carry the parents with you if possible and conflict resolution can often be achieved by the use of mediation services or family advocates. Often the most effective first step is to offer to obtain a second opinion, either from a colleague in the same hospital or from another institution: it is important to stress that the opinion needs to come from a respected neonatal doctor or a subspecialist in the management of the condition in question. Both parents and doctors can benefit from such advice and most colleagues are willing to give such advice to NHS patients without making a charge.

The court has various legal bases on which it can make an order that treatment will be lawful. For example, it can simply determine a single issue as to what would be in the child's interest under section 8 of the Children's Act 1989, or it can make the child a ward of court so that all important steps in the child's life have to be sanctioned by the court. Alternatively, under what is called the 'inherent jurisdiction', it can make whatever orders seem appropriate. As Lord Woolf put it, particularly in regard to cases involving children, the last thing the court should be concerned about is whether the right procedure has been used (*e R (A Minor) (Blood Transfusion) [1993] 2 FLR 757*). The important thing is to ensure that the best interests of the child are identified.

The fact that the parents and doctors disagree to such an extent that the court has to resolve the difference of opinion increases the importance of maintaining the doctor–parent relationship. Disagreement, where it is moderately expressed with mutual understanding and respect, does not necessarily entail enmity. These cases arise when both doctor and parent want what is best for the child in a situation where neither can foresee the future or know how the child would wish them to act. Having submitted their shared dilemma to the court, the parents just as much as the doctors may be prepared to play their full role in the baby's care, whatever the decision may be. It is the doctor's professional duty to facilitate that process.

Jehovah's Witness parents

An adult Jehovah's Witness is free to refuse a blood transfusion and a doctor who forces an unwilling Jehovah's Witness to accept the treatment will be guilty of an assault. However, it is important to note that not all Jehovah's Witnesses share the same views: some will accept treatment with some blood products (such as fresh frozen plasma) and others do choose to accept blood when the alternative is death. It is vital to ascertain the wishes of the individual patient and to help the patient to stand up to pressure from co-religionists or other family members. Useful guidance on this topic is available from the Association of Anaesthetists' website (www.aagbi.org).

As with any parent, Jehovah's Witnesses have the right to take decisions as to what treatment their child should receive. However, if it is plain that the blood needs to be given, the court will make an order that it is lawful to do so, even when both parents object. If the baby's condition is so precarious that death or serious injury is likely to follow unless blood products are immediately given, again it will be lawful to do so even though there is no time to get a court order. In *Re R (A Minor)* the court had to deal with a child with B-cell lymphoblastic leukaemia who was given blood products on admission as an emergency measure without the parents' consent, and the court subsequently approved the administration of blood products in the future. However, it is important to note that the court decided that the medical consultant should not be given a blanket authority to carry out such treatment without further reference to the parents, and that the parents should still be involved as far as possible in the care of their daughter and able to draw attention to treatments alternative to the use of blood products.

In our experience the best approach in this situation is first to think hard about the indication for blood products – is there an alternative? What is standard and safe practice? Juniors must discuss the situation with a consultant, and consultants may wish to seek the support of another colleague. The reason for the transfusion and the urgency should be carefully explained to the parent (or parents), and an offer made to talk to any religious advisers the family may choose. Many hospitals have panels of on-call volunteer Jehovah's Witness ministers who are prepared to come and help. They can provide invaluable assistance in the counselling and mediation process, and in our experience have largely obviated the need for court applications in recent years. Only if such a reasoned approach fails should a court order be sought, and then only if time allows. Obtaining a court order involves the hospital's solicitors and social workers, but when required a court order can usually be obtained within hours.

Emergency situations

In an acute emergency or when the parents refuse to consent to treatment that is immediately necessary for the preservation of the life or long-term health of the child, the doctor is empowered to act. The precise basis of this agency of necessity (as it is sometimes called) is unclear, but the doctor's duty is towards the child; if it is clear that the child is about to die because some treatment is immediately necessary the doctor should act in the child's interest even if the parents forbid administration of the treatment.

Thus when a paediatrician is called to resuscitate a newborn baby with an Apgar score that indicates that any delay may result in brain damage, if not death, the doctor is not required to obtain the consent of the parents before addressing the immediate needs of the patient.

There may be cases where the parents refuse to consent to treatment that is immediately necessary to preserve the well-being of the baby, when the situation is so acute that there is no opportunity to enlist the authority of the court. Then the doctor must act in the best interests of the patient. However, it is helpful to know that the authority of the High Court can be enlisted in a telephone hearing surprisingly quickly. Once the acute emergency has passed, the situation should be explained to the parents. If the parents cannot be reconciled to the decision that has been taken and there is any significant likelihood of a recurrence or the treatment needs to be continued, then the court should be approached as as soon as possible.

Discontinuation of futile treatment

A decision to withdraw life-sustaining treatment precedes about 30% of deaths in a NICU, and an understanding of the process is an essential part of every consultant neonatologist's training. The best source of guidance remains the RCPCH Framework for Practice of September 1997, updated in 2004, and this framework has now been cited with approval by the judiciary on several occasions (www.rcpch.ac.uk). We have reviewed some of the key judgments in this area (Rennie and Leigh 2008).

The framework identifies five situations in which the decision will be considered:

1. the brain-dead child
2. the permanent vegetative state

3. the no-chance situation, when disease is so severe that life-sustaining treatment simply delays death without significant alleviation of suffering, rendering medical treatment inappropriate
4. the no-purpose situation, when there may be survival with treatment but the degree of impairment will be so great that it is unreasonable to expect the patient to bear it
5. the unbearable situation, when in the face of progressive or irreversible illness, the child or family feels that further treatment is more than can be borne.

The detailed guidance given by the RCPCH should be followed. It is vital here to stress the following:

1. The withdrawal or withholding of treatment does not imply that a baby will receive no care. The baby remains your patient and you must do your best for her just as much whilst she is dying.
2. It must be noted that there is no significant difference between withholding and withdrawing care as far as the courts are concerned. It is unlawful to take any positive act which will result directly in a person's death, but the withdrawal of treatment in hopeless circumstances is not a positive act.
3. The decision should be discussed widely within the clinical team and varying views recorded. If there is substantial dissent or if the parents do not agree, a sensible first course may well be to obtain a second opinion from another clinician with experience of the clinical problem. In the last resort the courts are there to give guidance but, as the RCPCH Framework makes clear, in most cases it will be possible to avoid an application to the court.

Many neonatologists believe that, on occasion, to continue intensive care may be inappropriate and inhumane. Many would take the same view about 'show code' or sham resuscitation, done for the benefit of the parents when most of those in the room see the situation as hopeless (Paris et al. 2010), although not all intensivists view this the same way (Truog 2010). Managing this kind of case is challenging and requires a degree of consensus in the treating team. Kant's view that 'it is immoral to use one human being as a means rather than as an end in itself' may imply that inflicting the burden of intensive care on a baby when there is no prospect of success cannot be justified. The problem lies in defining 'no prospect', or 'no chance', because there may be differences of opinion amongst the treating team, or between them and outside experts. When there is unanimity of opinion, the matter can usually be resolved either with or without the intervention of the court.

Unrealistic expectations regarding treatment

Reports of 'miracle survivors', with titles such as 'Neonatal viability: pushing the envelope' (Muraskas et al. 1998), have raised parental expectations to the level that a good outcome is assumed for every baby born after 23 weeks' gestation. Parents often request that 'everything be done' for their babies, however complex the problem and however overwhelmingly the odds are stacked against success, and they sometimes have difficulty in coming to terms with the disappointment of these hopes.

The most extreme example is probably that of baby K, an anencephalic, whose mother insisted on full intensive care support for over 2 years. Neonatologists need to be careful not to add to these unrealistic expectations, or to use the word 'miracle' themselves; the argument used by the doctor who initially resuscitated baby K was that the mother 'needed more time' to adjust to the fact that she could not live. Additional time did not lead to any more acceptance, and baby K's mother continued to believe that a miracle would happen. As Paris et al. (2000) put it: 'if parents are expecting a miracle they have come to the wrong place'.

At the other end of the spectrum are the parents who want a guarantee of success before agreeing to treatment for their child (Paris and Bell 1993). Things have moved on considerably since the 1963 Johns Hopkins case of a baby with Down syndrome and duodenal atresia who was 'allowed' to die over an 11-day period, and newborn babies are now recognised to have rights. Few would accede to a parental request for no treatment in this situation today, but the judgement regarding what is a 'reasonable' chance of success does vary between professionals and these differences need to be recognised.

There are now several documented cases in which the courts have been involved in this situation, in both the USA and the UK. The implication of the decision of the European Court in the case of Glass is that doctors should be much more willing to enlist the guidance of the courts at an early stage. We think that in future the courts are likely to be involved in a wider range of these problems than hitherto and that there can be advantages in hospital and parents going to the courts together for guidance at a time when attitudes are less entrenched. Just as we suggested when parents refuse to consent to treatment (see above), the authority of the court can be used to resolve a shared uncertainty as opposed to an established antagonism. Whatever the decision, it may be easier to implement if both sides have been through this process.

Negligence

Medical negligence consists of a breach of duty of care which causes damage. Claims in the UK are heard in civil (not criminal) courts by a judge sitting alone who has to find that it is more likely than not that there was a breach of duty and that the claimant's disability was caused by the mistake in question.

Breach of duty

The doctor will be in breach of her duty of care only if she fails to provide a reasonable standard of care. Lord Scarman described the standard which must be achieved by quoting a Scottish judge who had said (*Maynard v W Midlands 1985*):

> *In the realm of diagnosis and treatment there is ample scope for genuine difference of opinion and one man clearly is not negligent merely because his conclusion differs from that of other professional men … The true test for establishing negligence in diagnosis or treatment on the part of a doctor is whether he has been guilty of such failure as no doctor of ordinary skill would be guilty of acting with ordinary care.*

The principle that the law will respect treatment which accords with a respectable school of thought is known as the 'Bolam test' (*Bolam v Friern 1957*). It applies whether the doctor is reaching a diagnosis (*Maynard v W Midlands 1985*), giving warning of the hazards of treatment (*Sidaway v Bethlem and Maudsley 1985*) or performing a surgical procedure (*Whitehouse v Jordan 1981*). The court reserves the right to reject an opinion which it believes does not stand up to logical analysis (*Bolitho v City & Hackney 1992*). In the case of care delivered by a team, the law does not require the most junior trainee to have the skills of the consultant. However, it does require the trainee to be competent to perform the tasks allocated to her (*Wilsher v Essex Health Authority 1986*).

Where a defendant is in breach of her duty of care, the claimant will only be entitled to be compensated for damage caused by that breach of duty. This can cause additional complications; for example, when a senior registrar at a London teaching hospital failed to respond to her bleep to attend a child with croup, the evidence was that it would have made no difference to the exegesis if she had attended, unless she had decided to intubate the child as a precaution against a subsequent attack. The House of Lords held that causation could not be proved if a reasonable senior registrar in her position would have decided not to intubate (*Bolitho v City & Hackney 1992*). If the defendant is guilty of an act of negligence then the court will require that the claimant is put in the position in which he or she would have been if there had been no negligence, insofar as money can achieve this.

Standards of care

The law holds that doctors are to be judged by the state of their art at the time of treatment. They will not be negligent if they fail to anticipate a hazard which was unknown at the time (*Roe v Minister of Health 1954*). It is often said that the *Bolam* test provides a protection for the slower members of the profession, who cannot keep up with the state of their art – provided that they do not fall too far behind. However as medicine becomes more systematised at the hands of NICE and the evidence base of the Cochrane Centre expands, it is increasingly difficult to defend suboptimal care when damage has been caused. Where a case presents a powerful emotional charge it is hard to defend any adverse outcome that optimal care would hope to avoid. We were recently both involved in a case where a 5-month-old baby suffered a cardiac arrest as a result of a pneumothorax as she was being moved from the table after open-heart surgery. The facts were 27 years old, the witnesses all dead or otherwise unavailable and the records vestigial and mostly lost, yet the court was prepared to infer a breach of duty from the fact that the pneumothorax was not diagnosed before it caused an arrest (*Mugweni v NHS London 2011*).

This was not atypical of cases that come to court after many years have elapsed. Even when the notes still exist, they are vestigial by modern standards. Investigations appear to be sporadic and haphazard. The witnesses are worse: those who survive can rarely remember anything of the facts in issue, even though they may be debating the few hours in which it seems the claimant met with the catastrophe which has blighted her existence. Under the rigours of cross-examination, those involved may be hard-pressed to remember the routine practice or treatment policy of 1995 and to describe in coherent terms how it differed from that which was followed in 1985 or 2005. In many cases their grasp of the most basic elements of medicine appears to have slipped with the years: this may be unsurprising but it can be humiliating and distressing.

Limitation

Adult patients of sound mind must issue their writs in respect of personal injuries within 3 years of learning who caused their damage (Limitation Act 1980 section 11). They do not need to know that the injury was caused by negligence, but they may well be able to argue that only when they knew that their treatment was inadequate did they realise that their injury was not caused by their disease process. The court has a discretion to extend time indefinitely when the interests of justice demand it (Limitation Act 1980 section 13).

The difficulty for the paediatrician is that time does not run at all against the child under 18, or a patient under a disability. Thus, the survivor of a neonatal disaster has an unfettered right to issue a writ at any time prior to his 21st birthday. If at the age of 18 the young person does not know who or what has caused the damage, time will not start to run until he does. If he never becomes capable of managing his own affairs his 3 years does not start to run until his death. Since individuals with cerebral palsy currently enjoy a life expectancy which sometimes differs only marginally from the national average, hospitals need to keep neonatal records for a very long time. They are advised to keep all records until the child is aged 26 but records of catastrophic cases should be kept for 80 years. This creates storage problems in the present twilight years of paper records. Whenever the trial takes place, the court will judge the case on the available evidence. When a child acquired cerebral palsy because 68 minutes had elapsed between the delivery of twins, it seemed that this was in part attributable to a difficulty in finding the registrar where obstetric services were split between two sites. No satisfactory explanation could be provided 17 years after the event. The court rejected the defendant's argument that the judge should be less willing to draw an adverse inference against the defendant whom delay had deprived of a proper opportunity to rebut the claim (*Bull & Wakeham v Exeter Health Authority 1993*).

Criminal cases

The doctor enjoys no privileged position under the criminal law of the land and allegations of homicide will be judged by the same rules as apply to the rest of society.

Murder

Murder consists of unlawfully killing a person with the intention of killing or causing grievous bodily harm. It can only be committed by a positive act, unlike manslaughter, which can be committed by omitting to act where there is a duty to do so. There is scope for argument about whether certain events are omissions or positive acts: switching off a ventilator is a positive act whereas ceasing to ventilate may be an omission, depending on the circumstances.

Manslaughter

Medical manslaughter is committed when a doctor causes the death of a patient as a result of an act or omission which amounts to gross negligence. Whether negligence is gross or not is a question of fact for the jury, but the prosecution must first demonstrate a breach of duty as judged by the *Bolam* test. The doctor who causes the death of a patient in the course of bona fide treatment without deliberately killing the child will not be guilty of any crime if she is acting in accordance with a respectable school of thought.

Where a neonatologist is called and finds a baby weighing 400 g, her first duty is to assess the baby. If she decides not to attempt resuscitation, or to abandon it if the baby does not respond, she cannot be guilty of a crime if a respectable school of thought would have taken the same view, because she will not be guilty of an act of negligence. The case will be judged in all the circumstances, so that a consultant at a major teaching hospital would not be able to rely solely on the fact that a reasonable paediatrician in a peripheral unit with poor facilities would have decided the case was hopeless. However, the burden will remain on the prosecution throughout to prove, so that the jury is sure, that no respectable neonatologist would have failed to resuscitate that child in those circumstances and that the failure to resuscitate did hasten death. Furthermore the negligent failure must be gross, so that the jury is sure that the action merits a criminal sanction.

Child protection law

Neonatologists need to be aware of the law in this area, particularly with respect to babies under their care whose parents have previous children in care for neglect or who are substance-abusing. All those involved in the care of children in hospital must have undergone level III child protection training.

Weblinks

www.bapm.org: British Association of Perinatal Medicine website. Several useful documents can be downloaded from the site, including standards for neonatal intensive care and a list of procedures which require consent.

www.dh.gov.uk: UK Department of Health site. Useful documents regarding good practice in seeking consent.

www.nhsla.com: National Health Service Litigation Authority website. Includes

some practical advice on risk management and the clinical negligence scheme for trusts.

References

Bolam v Friern Hospital Management Committee [1957] 1 WLR 582.

Bolitho v City & Hackney Health Authority [1992] Lloyd's Law Reports: Medical 1998 26.

Bull & Wakeham v Exeter Health Authority [1993] 4 Med LR 117 (CA).

Burns, C.M., Rutherford, M.A., Boardman, J.P., et al., 2008. Patterns of cerebral injury and neurodevelopmental outcomes after symptomatic neonatal hypoglycemia. Pediatrics 122, 65–74.

e R (A Minor) (Blood Transfusion) [1993] 2 FLR 757

In The Matter of Re U (Child) 1999 WL 1142460.

Kinnala, A., Rikkalainen, H., Lapinleimu, H., et al., 1999. Cerebral magnetic resonance imaging and ultrasonography findings after neonatal hypoglycemia. Pediatrics 103, 724–729.

Limitation Act 1980 HMSO, London, sections 11 and 13.

Maynard v West Midlands Regional HA 1985 1 All ER 635.

Mugweni v NHS London [2011] EWHC 334 (QB).

Murakami, Y., Yamashite, Y., Matsuishi, T., et al., 1999. Cranial MRI of neurologically impaired children suffering from neonatal hypoglycaemia. Pediatr Radiol 29, 23–27.

Muraskas, J., Bhola, M., Tomich, P., et al., 1998. Neonatal viability: pushing the envelope. Pediatrics 101, 1095.

Paris, J.J., Bell, A.J., 1993. Guarantee my child will be 'normal' or stop all treatment. J Perinatol 13, 469–472.

Paris, J.J., DeLisser, H.M., Savani, R.C., 2000. Ending innovative therapy for infants at the margins of viability: case of twins. J Perinatol 4, 251–256.

Paris, J.J., Angelos, P., Schreiber, M.D., 2010. Does compassion for a family justify providing futile CPR? J Perinatol 30, 1–3.

Rennie, J.M., Leigh, B., 2008. The legal framework for end-of-life decisions in the UK. Semin Fetal Neonat Med 13, 296–3000.

Roe v Minister of Health [1954] 2 QB 66.

Sidaway v Board of Governors of the Bethlem Royal Hospital and Maudsley Hospital [1985] AC 871.

Traill, Z., Squier, M., Anslow, P., 1998. Brain imaging in neonatal hypoglycaemia. Arch Dis Child 79, F145–F147.

Truog, R.D., 2010. Is it always wrong to perform futile CPR? N Engl J Med 626, 477–479.

Whitehouse v Jordan [1981] 1 All ER 261.

Wilsher v Essex Health Authority [1986] 3 All ER 801.

Science and the emergence of neonatal medicine

Malcolm Chiswick

7

Introduction

This chapter focuses on how our understanding of certain neonatal disorders has emerged and describes the research that underpinned it. Most advances are not the result of serendipitous discovery but are due instead to the gradual accumulation of research-based knowledge over an extended timeframe. Along the way, landmark publications appear and are highlighted in this chapter, but they need to be reviewed in the context of their building blocks.

Emerging care of the premature infant

The importance of feeding and warmth to the survival of premature infants had been known for centuries but it was not until the second half of the 19th century that serious efforts were made to improve their outcome. Two obstetricians, Stéphane Tarnier and Pierre Budin, led the way in Paris, France, at the Maternité and the Hôpital de la Charité.

Tarnier introduced hygienic measures at the Maternité which substantially reduced mortality from puerperal sepsis. He developed a closed incubator, and introduced gavage feeding in 1884. His pupil, Pierre Budin, had remarkably prescient ideas that were to occupy the minds of paediatricians into the 20th century. He developed what was probably the first follow-up clinic for infants and wrote about the outcome for premature babies in his treatise, *The Nursling*, which was originally published in 1900 and included information on breastfeeding and mother–infant bonding, hygiene, hypothermia and cyanotic episodes (Budin 1907).

© 2012 Elsevier Ltd

Feeding the premature infant

The compromised ability of the feeble newborn to feed adequately, together with sepsis, were important causes of mortality before the 20th century. Methods of feeding premature babies included the trickling of milk into the infant's mouth directly from the mother's breast or from a wet nurse, and the use of spoons, small cups, droppers and quills.

Otto Heubner (1843–1926) is best known for the name of the branch of the anterior cerebral artery. An internal physician by training, he was subsequently appointed as Professor of Paediatrics in Berlin, Germany. His research with Max Rubner using indirect calorimetry to determine the caloric needs of infants promoted feeding according to requirements rather than empirical observations (Rubner and Heubner 1898, 1899; cited by Weaver 2009). The chemical composition of milk and its calorific value were known by the close of the 19th century and many felt that 100–150 cal/kg/day were optimal for growth, largely based on Rubner and Heubner's observations.

Although formula feeds based on evaporated cow's milk and approximating in composition to human milk were used by the second quarter of the 20th century, it was still widely considered that human milk was superior for premature infants. When Gordon and McNamara (1941) highlighted caloric loss in the stools resulting from the premature infant's difficulty in absorbing fat, their observations led to the increasing use of half-skimmed cow's milk preparations. In order to meet caloric needs the protein content had to be increased and the formulas also had a higher electrolyte and mineral content than human milk. Gordon et al. (1947) and later others showed that babies fed a half-skimmed milk formula gained weight more rapidly than those fed breast milk. The relatively high protein intakes were associated with raised blood urea levels (Omans et al. 1961).

However, there remained a concern that premature infants exclusively fed on expressed breast milk did not grow as well as those who received formula feeds. In a randomised trial Davies (1977) observed that babies of 28–32 weeks' gestation fed on expressed breast milk had significantly slower rates of head and linear growth in the first month of life compared with formula-fed infants.

In a review of nutritional studies Gordon and Levine (1944) commented that 'an optimum diet has been defined as one in which no change can promote greater health and well-being of the populace'. Therein lay an enigma that continues to challenge paediatric nutritional researchers. Is the aim to encourage growth in the early weeks that characterises normal fetal growth (Usher and McLean 1974); to satisfy some other concept of optimal postnatal weight gain; to permit accumulation of carbohydrate, fat and protein and minerals at a rate observed in the last trimester of pregnancy (Widdowson and Spray 1951); to influence later neurodevelopmental outcome in some way (Churchill 1963; Drillien 1964); or perhaps to minimise the risk of the infants developing adult disease such as hypertension, stroke and diabetes (Barker 1994)?

Early versus late feeding

By the late 1940s the practice of starting feeds at 24 hours or sooner ('early feeding') was causing concern because milk aspiration was considered to be a prominent cause of pneumonia and cyanotic episodes. Generalised oedema in the first week of life was also attributed to early feeding. In the USA and subsequently in the UK it became common practice to delay the first feed. For example, Gaisford and Schofield (1950) studied 231 premature babies in whom the time of the first feed was determined by the baby's vigour. The average age when babies in different birthweight categories were offered their first feed ranged from 48 to 73 hours, but in many the delay was more than 100 hours. The authors concluded that a period of starvation was safe. Similarly, Crosse et al. (1954) described that feeding began on the third day in infants who weighed 3–4 lb (1.4–1.8 kg), and on the fourth day for those under 3 lb (1.4 kg).

During the 1960s evidence accumulated suggesting that early starvation might be causally related to cerebral palsy in premature infants (Churchill 1963; Drillien 1964). There was also growing experimental evidence in animals of the harmful effects of early malnutrition (McCance and Widdowson 1962).

In what proved to be a landmark publication, Smallpiece and Davies (1964) observed that infants who weighed 1000–2000 g could safely be fed within 2 hours of birth on undiluted breast milk at 60 ml/kg/day, increasing daily to 160 ml/kg/day. They suffered less symptomatic hypoglycaemia and their bilirubin levels were lower than those of infants who were fed later. Similar beneficial effects of early feeding were subsequently reported by others but it was several years before the practice became widely adopted. An excellent historical review of changing attitudes to the first feed and the underlying scientific concepts was written by Davies (1978).

Thermoregulation and the premature infant

The vulnerability of newborn infants exposed to a cold environment has been known from ancient times. Methods used to keep small and feeble babies warm included fireside heat, hot-water bottles, animal skins and plant leaves. Probably the first device which can be considered to be an incubator was a warming tub – a double-walled metal tub with the space between the walls filled with warm water. This was developed in 1835 and used at the Foundling Hospital in St Petersburg. The subsequent history of the development of incubators was addressed by Cone (1985).

The emergence of public viewing of babies nursed in incubators at various fairs and exhibitions in Europe and the USA from around 1896 until 1940 was addressed by Silverman (1979) in a captivating account. The incubator exhibitions did at least raise the profile of small babies and provide access to warmth and nutrition and for some it was their only hope of survival. Arguably it also stimulated an interest in the science of thermoregulation in infants.

Thermoregulation

From the early 1900s animal physiologists had studied birds and mammals, establishing that there was a critical environmental temperature below which heat production was necessary to maintain a normal body temperature and above which stability of temperature was dependent on physical factors such as changes in insulation and body posture (Scholander et al. 1950). The critical temperature varied between species and habitat. Given what was known about the lability of body temperature in small infants, and that heat loss occurred by evaporation, conduction, radiation and convection, a key question was how babies might protect themselves when exposed to a cool environment.

In 1943 Day and associates published their results of a detailed study of premature infants aged 4–53 days, in which heat production (oxygen consumption) and different forms of heat loss were measured in relation to environmental temperature. They observed that in cool air vasoconstriction was active but total heat loss per unit area of skin was greater than that of adults. Although infants increased their heat production in cool air, 'the sustained muscular movement necessary to raise heat production is more difficult for these feeble subjects than for adults' (Day et al. 1943).

More than a decade later Silverman et al. (1958) in a randomised controlled trial observed that prematurely born infants nursed in incubators maintained at a temperature of 31.7 °C during the first 5 days of life had a better survival rate than those nursed at 28.9 °C (84% versus 68%). The beneficial effect was observed in all birth-weight categories.

Brück (1961) showed that infants from birth, including those of low birthweight, had a very well-developed thermoregulatory control system. They could adjust their peripheral blood flow and sweat secretion and the temperature threshold at which these controls were activated was related to body size. The increased heat production when infants were exposed to a cool environment was the result of non-shivering thermogenesis rather than shivering.

The metabolic response to a cool environment

Smith (1962) suggested that brown fat might be a source of heat production in the cold-adapted rat as oxygen consumption of the tissue was high. A major advance was a study by Dawkins and Hull (1964); these authors observed that exposure to cold was associated with a rise in temperature of brown adipose tissue. Hydrolysis of the fat was associated with a marked rise in plasma glycerol levels and a smaller increase in plasma free fatty acids, suggesting that most of the liberated free fatty acids was metabolised within the brown adipose tissue.

Silverman et al. (1964) observed that when babies were exposed to a cool environment the nape of the neck was warmer than other sites. The distribution of brown adipose tissue in the human infant at necropsy was studied by Aherne and Hull (1966), who showed that it was relatively depleted in infants who had died following a history of hypothermia or cold injury.

It is perhaps intuitive that the metabolic response of newborn babies to a cool environment might be influenced by their state of oxygenation. Cross et al. (1958) reported that oxygen consumption (metabolic rate) in premature and term babies decreased when they were exposed to 15% oxygen. They speculated that, although this might be a defence mechanism against hypoxia, it might also impair thermoregulation and that a low body temperature in the newborn might be symptomatic of hypoxia. Hill (1959) shed light on this issue in laboratory animals when she observed that it was only in a cool environment, when the metabolic rate had already increased to maintain body temperature, that induced hypoxia caused a fall in oxygen consumption and a fall in rectal temperature. In a neutral thermal environment induced hypoxia had no effect on oxygen consumption.

The neutral thermal environment for newborn babies

Additional clinical studies of thermoregulation in newborn babies emerged and closely reflected observation in animals. This culminated in defining the thermal environment for newborn babies that made minimal demands on the infant's energy reserves with core body temperature being regulated by changes in skin blood flow, posture and sweating (Hey and Katz 1970). The concept of thermal neutrality was later reviewed further by Hey (1975).

Respiratory distress syndrome

In 1903 Hochheim, reporting on a necropsy study in newborn infants, drew attention to infants whose alveolar ducts and alveoli were coated with a layer of eosinophilic material originally described as myelin. The next half-century saw intense research and debate about the origin and significance of this material, which was subsequently referred to as hyaline (from the Greek for glass). The suggested causes of the hyaline membranes included aspiration of amniotic fluid or vernix caseosa, infection, congenital or developmental anomaly, intrauterine hypoxia, oxygen poisoning, injury and necrosis of bronchiolar epithelium. The various aetiological theories put forward were based almost entirely on histochemical analysis of lung tissue with little in the way of clinicopathological correlation. Distressed breathing in premature infants was recognised but it was generally attributed to 'congenital atelectasis' or 'asphyxia'.

By the 1950s the association of hyaline membranes at necropsy with prematurity and respiratory distress was confirmed and the terms 'hyaline membrane disease' and 'idiopathic respiratory distress syndrome' became increasingly used. Gitlin and Craig (1956) concluded that the membranes were composed of fibrin formed in situ as a result of exudation of fibrinogen from pulmonary capillaries. The radiological features of the disorder were described and the reticular–granular pattern on chest X-ray was distinguished from the coarse opacities associated with amniotic fluid aspiration and pneumonia (Donald and Steiner 1953).

Pulmonary mechanics and surfactant

In 1929 von Neergaard compared the pressure–volume curves of air-filled porcine lungs with curves produced after filling the lungs with isotonic gum solution which had the potential to abolish surface tension forces at the air–tissue interface. Based on these experiments he suggested that surface tension forces were more important than elasticity in lung recoil, and that surface forces might interfere with lung expansion. The importance of this was not appreciated at a time when there was still growing preoccupation with the significance of hyaline membranes.

Gruenwald (1947) suggested that an unusually high surface tension might be responsible for the uneven pattern of expansion observed in the lungs of premature infants and for resistance to lung inflation. During the 1950s the relationship between the pressure–volume characteristics of lung and surface tension force became clarified. Pattle (1955), studying nerve gases at the Ministry of Defence at Porton Down, UK, observed that foam found in the trachea of rabbits with induced acute lung oedema had an altogether peculiar property in that it was unaffected by silicone antifoams. He concluded that the stability of the foam was due to an insoluble surface layer on the foam bubbles which originated from the original lining of the air spaces.

At the same time researchers from the Department of Physiology at the Harvard School of Public Health were studying pulmonary mechanics and the implication of surface tension forces at the air–liquid interface. Radford (1954) calculated the internal surface area of the lungs from their pressure–volume characteristics assuming that surface tension was constant and equal to that of plasma. His calculation of the surface area was much lower than data derived from morphological examination. This anomaly held a clue to the surface-active property of the lung lining.

Clements (1957) studied surface films prepared from rat, cat and dog lungs using a modified Wilhelmy balance, which compresses and expands the surface film while measuring surface tension. He showed that surface tension fell to a minimum as the surface area of the film was compressed, but, more importantly, only a 10% expansion from the compressed state restored the surface tension to its maximum value – the surface film was showing hysteresis. In the absence of the specialised surface film, which Clements referred to as pulmonary surfactant, the high surface tension would resist lung expansion, cause small air spaces at high pressure to empty into larger air spaces and promote uneven expansion and atelectasis.

The association of surfactant deficiency with hyaline membrane disease was established by Avery and Mead (1959), who measured the surface tension of lung extracts of infants using a Wilhelmy balance. The extracts from infants who weighed more than 1200 g and who had died from causes other than hyaline membrane disease achieved much lower surface tensions than lung extracts from infants who had died from hyaline membrane disease and from smaller babies.

Thus, more than half a century after Hochheim's original description of hyaline membranes, the underlying physicochemical abnormalities of the lungs were discovered. Gandy et al. (1970) revisited the histopathological changes in the lung in hyaline membrane disease and measured surface tension in lung extracts. They observed that the presence or absence of osmiophilic granules, which represent stored surfactant within type 2 pneumocytes, did indeed reflect surface tension measurements.

Antepartum glucocorticoids for the prevention of respiratory distress syndrome

Liggins et al. (1967), while studying the influence of the fetal endocrine system in promoting parturition in ewes, observed that ablation of the fetal pituitary or hypothalamus led to prolongation of gestation. Stimulation of the fetal adrenals by corticotrophin or infusion of cortisol led to premature parturition (Liggins, 1968, 1969). A striking feature was that lambs born at 117–123 days' gestation following dexamethasone infusion showed partial expansion of their lungs, a feature which is not normally apparent at this gestation and which is dependent on adequate surfactant activity. Liggins suggested that the dexamethasone-treated fetuses may have had accelerated surfactant production.

DeLemos et al. (1970) extended these observations in a novel way. They infused cortisol into one of twin fetal lambs and observed that the lungs of treated lambs were more mature than their untreated twins in terms of pressure–volume curves and surface tension measurements of lung extracts. Similar evidence for hormonal control of fetal lung development has been shown in the rabbit (Chiswick et al. 1973).

Supporting evidence for the hormonal control of pulmonary surfactant development in human fetuses was provided in an autopsy study by Naeye et al. (1971). They observed that infants who had died with hyaline membrane disease had lighter adrenal glands than those dying from other causes and infection arising before birth was correlated with the absence of hyaline membrane disease. Anencephalic infants with no adrenal fetal cortical zone had a reduced mass of osmiophilic granules in their type 2 pneumocytes compared with non-anencephalic infants.

The first controlled trial of antepartum glucocorticoid treatment for the prevention of respiratory distress syndrome (RDS) commenced in December 1969 and enrolled 282 mothers admitted in preterm labour or in whom delivery was planned before 37 weeks (Liggins and Howie 1972). RDS was seen significantly less in infants of mothers treated with betamethasone but this was confined to infants under 32 weeks' gestation whose mothers had been treated

for at least 24 hours before delivery. Neonatal mortality was significantly reduced, and there were no deaths with hyaline membrane disease or intraventricular haemorrhage among infants of mothers who had received betamethasone longer than 24 hours before delivery.

This important trial was the forerunner of many others which shed light on whether there was a true gestational age cut-off point below which antenatal glucocorticoids were ineffective, whether repeated doses of glucocorticoids were beneficial, and whether there were maternal contraindications to their use.

Treatment of respiratory distress syndrome

Before the discovery of surfactant deficiency as the underlying cause of RDS, treatment was largely supportive and relied on oxygen, intravenous fluids and the maintenance of acid–base balance. The use of supplemental oxygen suffered a setback with its restrictive use because of fears about retrolental fibroplasia. This was associated at the time with a rise in mortality from RDS (Avery and Oppenheimer 1960).

Mechanical ventilation

The experimental use of positive-pressure mechanical ventilation for newborn infants with hyaline membrane disease was reported by Donald and Lord (1953). During the 1960s, with further experience limited to a few specialist neonatal units, the practical problems became apparent, especially the challenge of prolonged mechanical ventilation including endotracheal tube instability and problems maintaining nutrition. Intuitively it was felt that the treatment carried huge risks and that it was a last resort for infants dying with hyaline membrane disease. The third child of President John F Kennedy died of RDS, having been delivered at 34 weeks weighing 2.11 kg in August 1963. His obituary in the *New York Times* stated that all that could be done was to 'monitor the infant's blood chemistry and to try to keep it near normal'. The following year, Delivoria-Papadopoulos and Swyer (1964) described their experience of mechanical ventilation of severely acidaemic and apnoeic infants with 'terminal' hyaline membrane disease and concluded that the best hope of success with this treatment was its application in the preterminal rather than the terminal state.

The growth of neonatal intensive care units and the development of regional referral centres in the UK during the 1970s led to an increasing experience of mechanical ventilation in infants with RDS. A major concern was the occurrence of pneumothoraces and bronchopulmonary dysplasia, which Northway et al. (1967) had originally described. For staff on the emerging intensive care units assisted ventilation was a steep learning curve because ventilators had hitherto been machines used by anaesthetists – not paediatricians. An important advance, certainly in the UK, were publications by Reynolds (1971) and Herman and Reynolds (1973) describing the effect of alterations of ventilator settings on pulmonary gas exchange in hyaline membrane disease and the use of strategies that might minimise high inspired concentrations of oxygen and high peak inspiratory pressures.

Gregory et al. (1971) reported the successful use of continuous positive airway pressure (CPAP) in spontaneously breathing infants with RDS. Different methods of applying CPAP emerged but the influence on clinical practice was that it drew attention to the benefits of respiratory support of some kind before the infant had reached a terminal state of respiratory failure.

During the subsequent decades advances occurred at a rapid pace. Non-invasive continuous blood gas monitoring facilitated the earlier detection of deteriorating infants. Interest grew in different

SINGLETON HOSPITAL
STAFF LIBRARY

ventilator strategies aimed at reducing the risk of barotrauma. Sedative drugs and muscle relaxants were increasingly used. However, the major advance – the one that really improved survival rates in RDS – was surfactant replacement therapy.

Surfactant replacement therapy

Based on their notion that pulmonary ischaemia was very important in the pathogenesis of RDS, Chu et al. (1967) conducted a detailed cardiorespiratory function study of infants with the disease. Intravenous acetylcholine was associated with an increase in effective pulmonary flow and appeared to have other beneficial functional effects. Administration of dipalmitoyl lecithin by aerosol was followed by an increase in lung compliance but this occurred even in infants who subsequently died and there was no apparent clinical benefit.

The effect of natural surfactant derived from rabbit and bovine lung was tested on premature animals during the 1970s with encouraging results. Fujiwara et al. (1980) treated 10 premature infants with severe hyaline membrane disease by intratracheal administration of an artificial surfactant modified from bovine lung tissue. Oxygenation improved and it was possible to reduce the ventilator settings. Eight infants survived.

During the 1980s synthetic and bovine or porcine-derived surfactants were used in many randomised controlled trials and treatment reduced mortality and pulmonary air leaks. Further trials have compared different types of surfactant, examined more critically the role of multiple versus single dosage and shown that prophylactic treatment soon after delivery is more beneficial than rescue treatment. Halliday (2008) has provided an excellent review of the development of surfactant replacement therapy.

Intraventricular haemorrhage

During the early part of the 20th century it became clear that intraventricular haemorrhage (IVH) was seen more commonly in premature infants. Browne (1922) drew attention to the association of IVH and premature birth 'even when the delivery had been easy and natural' and he attributed this to 'the great delicacy of the vessels in the premature fetus'. The early debate about the cause of IVH essentially focused on the anatomical origin of the bleeding. It was thought that the source of the bleeding was engorged veins of the choroid plexus or from the subependymal region with leakage into the ventricular cavity. Attention was focused on engorgement of the terminal vein which drains the subependymal region.

The pathological anatomy was advanced by the study of Hambleton and Wigglesworth (1976), who used a dye injection and stereomicroscopic method to examine the brains of babies who had died within 10 days of birth. Among premature infants with subependymal haemorrhage or IVH they were unable to confirm rupture of the terminal vein or germinal layer infarction. They observed a rich capillary network within the germinal layer which was supplied by Heubner's artery, a branch of the anterior cerebral artery. Injection of the carotid artery caused prominent leaks within the germinal layer capillary bed. The authors speculated that the capillaries might rupture by a rise in arterial pressure in conditions of hypercapnia or hypoxia.

Enlarging on this, Wigglesworth and Pape (1978) suggested an integrated model which might explain both haemorrhagic and ischaemic lesions in the preterm brain. The model took into account the state of development of the cerebral vessels and the effects thereon of increased or decreased perfusion pressure in precipitating haemorrhagic and ischaemic lesions.

As the use of mechanical ventilation for babies with RDS was evolving, death from IVH appeared to be an important limiting factor. A major advance was the ability to diagnose IVH in life by computed tomographic brain scanning (Papile et al. 1978) and ultrasound imaging (Pape et al. 1979). The importance of the paper by Papile and her collaborators (1978) was their grading of the extent of the IVH (grades I–IV).

Ultrasound imaging proved to be more convenient as a cot-side investigation and it became established as an important research tool. Many studies were published seeking to relate obstetric and neonatal factors with IVH. A plethora of 'risk factors' emerged which were difficult to interpret because of confounding variables but they appeared to have had their basis in altered regulation of cerebral blood flow, sudden changes in blood volume and coagulation abnormalities.

Ultrasound imaging made it possible to assess the effects of various agents for reducing the risk of IVH such as phenobarbital (Donn et al. 1981), vitamin E (Chiswick et al. 1983), etamsylate (Cooke and Morgan 1984) and indometacin (Ment et al. 1985). None of those agents became firmly established or stood the test of time, although indometacin has enjoyed a recent revival. This was possibly because the background incidence of IVH fell as a result of improvements in obstetric and neonatal care such as the use of antenatal corticosteroids, surfactant replacement and efforts to promote circulatory stability. Long-term outcome studies from the various prophylaxis regimens were few.

Periventricular leukomalacia

The pattern of pathology that we now term 'periventricular leukomalacia' (PVL) was described in the 19th century under a different name (Virchow 1867). The first comprehensive description of PVL was by Banker and Larroche (1962) and was based on postmortem examinations of infants set against a review of neuropathological observations that had been made in the 19th century. They used the term 'periventricular leukomalacia' to reflect their observation of bilateral 'necrosis of the white matter dorsal and lateral to the external angles of the lateral ventricles' and suggested a relationship with a compromised arterial supply.

The vascular anatomy and its relationship to PVL were clarified by De Reuck et al. (1972), who showed that the lesions were located in the periventricular arterial border zones between the ventriculopetal and ventriculofugal branches of the deep penetrating arteries and suggested that impaired perfusion was an aetiological factor. In a postmortem study of infants with PVL, Armstrong and Norman (1974) observed that most had suffered perinatal complications or had been born prematurely. They noted that haemorrhage occurred within infarcts in some infants and differentiated this from subependymal-related haemorrhage. They observed that cavity formation in the infarcted areas was associated with degeneration of the corticospinal tracts and speculated that this may form an anatomical basis for spastic hemiplegia or quadriplegia.

During the 1980s descriptions of the cerebral ultrasound appearance of PVL appeared. The ultrasound characteristics of haemorrhagic periventricular leukomalacia and their correlation with autopsy findings were described by Hill et al. (1982). The reported incidence of PVL ranged from less than 5% (Calvert et al. 1986) to 18% (Sinha et al. 1985). As with IVH, these studies allowed associated clinical factors to be explored. Subsequent reports suggested that neonatal cranial ultrasound expressions of white-matter damage were reasonably good predictors of neurodevelopmental outcomes (Fawer et al. 1987).

Meanwhile both experimental and clinical evidence accumulated to suggest an association between a maternal or fetal inflammatory response and white-matter injury. Gilles et al. (1976) had shown that intraperitoneal injection of lipopolysaccharides into kittens caused white-matter changes not dissimilar to that seen in humans. Elevated levels of proinflammatory cytokines in umbilical cord plasma and amniotic fluid (Yoon et al. 1996, 1997) were reported to be associated with PVL, and other studies showed that clinical markers of intra-amniotic infection preceding premature birth are linked to white-matter damage.

Necrotising enterocolitis

During the 19th century and first half of the 20th century there were many published reports of newborn infants with intestinal perforation. Most of these cases were likely to be perforations secondary to intestinal obstruction and caused by congenital bowel malformations or meconium plugs, but in others there was no evidence of obstruction.

Thelander (1939) summarised the published cases of bowel perforations that were unassociated with obstruction and considered that infection might have played a role. In 1944 Willi observed ulceration or perforation of the terminal ileum or large bowel at postmortem in infants under 3 months who had died with symptoms of severe enteritis. He called this condition 'malignant enteritis' but was unable to isolate any causative organism. Similar cases with ulcerated lesions of the gut were reported as 'enterocolitis ulcerosa necroticans'. Although the vulnerability of the preterm infant to this disorder became apparent there was continuing uncertainty about the aetiology.

Corday et al. (1962) drew attention to a syndrome in adult patients characterised by unexplained haemorrhagic and necrotic lesions of the gastrointestinal tract associated with a range of remote systemic disturbances such as myocardial infarction, shock states and severe burns. In a series of experiments, cardiac arrhythmias and haemorrhagic shock were induced in mongrel dogs and resulted in increased vascular resistance of the arteriolar bed supplying the bowel wall due to angiospasm.

Lloyd (1969) observed that 80% of the infants who suffered gastrointestinal perforations experienced a significant episode of asphyxia or shock during the perinatal period. Drawing on the research observations of physiologists who had studied the mechanisms that allow diving mammals to operate successfully in deep water and on Corday's observations in adult patients, Lloyd postulated that perforations of the gastrointestinal tract were the result of ischaemic necrosis related to an asphyxial defence mechanism characterised by selective circulatory ischaemia.

Outbreaks of necrotising enterocolitis were widely reported in the 1970s but no single organism has been consistently associated with the disease. As the decade progressed it became clear that enteral feeding including the rapid advancement of feeds was a provoking factor especially in preterm infants and the condition was seen less frequently in infants who were solely fed on human milk. More recently, attention has focused on the aetiological role of immunological defence mechanisms of the gut, especially in preterm infants.

Retinopathy of prematurity

The authoritative account of the discovery of retinopathy of prematurity (ROP) (Silverman 1980) described how Stewart Clifford, a Boston paediatrician, observed nystagmus and opacities in the eyes of a 3-month-old premature girl in 1941. Subsequent examination under anaesthesia revealed a grey membrane covered with blood vessels which appeared to be behind the lens and both eyes were affected.

Terry (1942) described five premature infants with 'fibroblastic overgrowth of a persistent vascular sheath behind each crystalline lens'. The term 'retrolental fibroplasia' (RLF) was coined shortly after. By 1946 he had seen more than 100 cases, with 75% occurring in babies who weighed $3\frac{1}{2}$ lb (1.6 kg) or less. He was aware of apparent variations in the frequency of RLF in different medical centres and suggested that individual differences in technique of premature infant care in these centres may act as an aetiological factor (Terry 1946). Sadly he would never know the fruits of his observations as he died of a heart attack in the same year.

Based on serial ophthalmoscopic examinations of premature infants from birth, Owens and Owens (1948) described the progressive vascular changes in the retina that preceded the fibrotic changes behind the lens. Numerous causes were suspected not directly related to the role of oxygen, including precocious exposure to light, vitamin E deficiency, supplemental iron and water-soluble vitamins, and blood transfusions. Reports of RLF soon appeared from England and other countries.

Role of oxygen

Kinsey and Zacharias (1949) first mooted that oxygen therapy might be related to RLF on the basis that infants who developed the disorder tended to come from nurseries where oxygen was more likely to be administered. Campbell (1951) reported her experiences of RLF in Melbourne, Australia, where the first cases appeared in 1948 and coincided with the introduction of the 'oxygen cot' which supplied oxygen in concentrations of 40–60%. The incidence of RLF in premature babies was 18.7% whereas the incidence in other premature babies who had apparently received oxygen in a more restricted way was 6.9%.

Similarly, Crosse and Evans (1952) reported from Birmingham, UK, that during 1931–1947 there had been no recorded cases of RLF, whereas a policy of liberal oxygen administration from January 1949 to June 1950 was associated with an incidence of severe RLF of 10.2%.

In the same year Jefferson (1952) reported her follow-up examination of more than 600 infants nursed at two premature baby units in Manchester, UK, from 1947 to 1951. The incidence of RLF ranged from 3% in those more than 4 lb (1.8 kg) at birth, to 41% in those less than 3 lb (1.4 kg). She observed that cases began to appear when oxygen tents were introduced and it was later confirmed that the concentration of oxygen in the tents could reach 60% even at the lowest flow rate of 0.5 l/min.

However, the debate about oxygen as a cause continued, with some arguing that it was sudden removal from an oxygen-rich environment that was causal and that relative hypoxia might have a role (Szewczyk 1952). Ashton et al. (1953) observed obliteration of the retinal vessels when young kittens were exposed to 60–80% oxygen for several days. Transfer of the animals to air led to a reopening of some vessels but many were permanently obstructed and the reformed network was grossly abnormal with revascularisation extending into the vitreous, haemorrhages and retinal detachment.

The National Cooperative Study

A multicentre study was started in the USA in 1953 to determine whether oxygen administration was implicated in RLF. The cooperative study enrolled infants who weighed 1500 g or less and had survived 48 hours (Kinsey and Hemphill 1955). Among singletons who received more than 50% oxygen for 28 days the incidence of vascular changes of RLF (70%) and of scarring RLF (17%) was significantly higher than in those whose oxygen concentration was limited to less than 50% and based on clinical needs (RLF 31%, scarring RLF 5%). Very soon after these results were published it became routine practice to limit oxygen supplementation to no more than 40–50% and as a result few cases of RLF subsequently occurred.

The curtailed use of oxygen at a time when arterial oxygen levels were not measured was associated with increased mortality from hyaline membrane disease (Avery and Oppenheimer 1960). Similarly, the restricted use of oxygen in the UK was associated with increased mortality in the first 24 hours after birth (Cross 1973) and led the author to plead for the wider use of arterial oxygen monitoring in special care baby units.

The 'new' retinopathy of prematurity

There appeared to have been a resurgence of ROP from the late 1970s affecting very premature infants and progressing to cicatricial disease and not wholly explicable by excess use of supplemental oxygen. A major landmark was the publication of the Committee for the Classification of Retinopathy of Prematurity (1984) as this facilitated research including therapeutic trials of cryotherapy and subsequently laser photocoagulation based on proper evaluation of the stage and distribution of the disease. Although our knowledge of the causes of ROP in very premature babies is still incomplete, a major step forward was our understanding of the role of vascular endothelial growth factor and insulin-like growth factor 1 in its pathogenesis.

Birth asphyxia

Animals respond to an asphyxial insult by apnoea followed by gasping, which becomes weaker and ceases in the absence of resuscitation. The time interval between the onset of the asphyxial insult and the last gasp has been used as a proxy for an animal's relative tolerance to asphyxia and it became a helpful tool in studying the physiological changes that occur in asphyxia.

Greater tolerance of the young to asphyxia

Le Gallois (1812), cited by Dawes (1968, p. 143), observed that following an asphyxial insult in animals the time to the last gasp was longer with decreasing age after birth. The greater tolerance of the newborn animal to asphyxia was subsequently confirmed by many other researchers and seemed counterintuitive to the idea that the young are less resilient.

Effect of environmental temperature

It had been known since the 19th century that a low environmental temperature prolonged the time to the last gasp in asphyxiated animals. Speculation about the mechanism of prolonged gasping in a cold environment centred on reduced metabolic demand of the brain and heart.

Westin et al. (1962) described 10 severely asphyxiated term infants who had not responded to positive-pressure ventilation. They were immersed supine in a bath of running cold water at 4.5–14°C from 4 to 39 minutes as determined by the onset of regular breathing, although all infants apparently responded promptly with an improvement in heart rate, colour and muscle tone. The lowest rectal temperatures ranged from 23 to 32°C. All but one infant survived, apparently without neurodevelopmental impairment.

Subsequent research showed that rapid cooling of asphyxiated fetal monkeys during secondary apnoea did not hasten recovery (Daniel et al. 1966) and interest waned with a better understanding of the pathophysiological sequence of events following asphyxia in newborn babies, and the crucial role of positive-pressure ventilation, and maintenance of the circulation in a thermoneutral environment.

Circulation and cardiac glycogen

Le Gallois (1812) attached importance to the maintenance of the circulation during asphyxia in newborn animals and observed that in rabbits the time to the last gasp was reduced when the circulation was interrupted by removal of the heart. Similar observations were made more than a century later across a range of newborn species.

The importance of carbohydrate as an energy source in asphyxiated young animals was shown by Himwich et al. (1941) in experiments on newborn rats asphyxiated in 100% nitrogen. Prior injection of inhibitors of anaerobic glycolysis (sodium iodoacetate or sodium fluoride) led to a reduction in gasping time. Dawes et al. (1959) showed that, following umbilical cord ligation in immature lambs, the time to the last gasp was positively related to levels of cardiac glycogen at different gestational ages.

These observations were extended by Dawes et al. (1963), who observed in lambs that, if glycolysis was maintained during asphyxia by administration of glucose and base sufficient to reduce the fall in arterial pH, the circulation was maintained longer than in untreated lambs.

Sequence of circulatory and respiratory changes following asphyxia

Dawes et al. (1960) described the sequence of events that occur when near-term fetal monkeys were asphyxiated at delivery by ligation of the cord with the head covered in a bag of saline. A brief period of respiratory activity was followed by apnoea (subsequently referred to as primary apnoea) which lasted up to 1 minute or so. Gasping then ensued and gradually became weaker, culminating in the last gasp and the onset of terminal apnoea. The average time to the last gasp was about 8 minutes, following which death ensued without resuscitation. Soon after the asphyxial insult the heart rate fell steeply and remained slow unless resuscitation occurred. Blood pressure rose transiently at first and then progressively fell. This sequence has been instrumental to our understanding of birth asphyxia and resuscitation in human babies.

Assessment of vital signs at birth and resuscitation

Virginia Apgar, commenting on resuscitation in the introduction to her landmark paper (Apgar 1953), wrote: 'Seldom have there been such imaginative ideas, such enthusiasms, and dislikes, and such unscientific observations and study about one clinical picture'. At that time there was no standardised way of describing the 'one clinical picture' she referred to – the state of the baby at birth.

The importance of her method of assessment was that it brought together in one score the circulatory, respiratory and neurological variables that were relevant to the evolving research into the pathophysiology of birth asphyxia. Her interest was driven by her wish to study the effects of caesarean section and maternal pain relief on the baby's condition at birth. The score was not used to determine when babies needed resuscitation but she subsequently recommended that the assessment should be extended beyond 1 minute in those babies who required resuscitation.

Descriptions of resuscitation of newborn babies have their origins in ancient texts and it would serve little purpose to highlight those except to promote a sense of incredulity. In 1966 Cross published an informative account of resuscitation of the asphyxiated newborn drawing on the extensive scientific literature that had accumulated by that time.

Birth asphyxia and brain damage

In a controversial presentation to the Obstetric Society, London, UK, in 1861, Little proposed an association between difficult delivery, asphyxia, prematurity and congenital spastic paralysis (Little 1862). The term 'cerebral palsy' was coined later by William Osler. Little's theories were later challenged by Freud in a series of monographs culminating in his classic book on infantile cerebral palsy (Freud 1968). Freud agreed that some cases of cerebral palsy were associated with birth complications but argued that birth complications and cerebral palsy might be the result of the same earlier developmental abnormality of the brain.

Studies of asphyxia in newborn guinea pigs had shown histological changes in the central nervous system (Windle and Becker 1942). In newborn Rhesus monkeys acutely asphyxiated by detaching the placenta at hysterotomy while keeping the fetal membranes intact for 11–16 minutes before resuscitation, a common pattern of symmetrical damage to brainstem and basal ganglia nuclei was observed with the cerebral cortex less severely affected (Ranck and Windle 1959).

Myers et al. (1969) induced partial asphyxia in fetal monkeys by oxytocin-stimulated contractions and showed that many had evidence of brain swelling and neuronal damage. Subsequently, different approaches to inducing chronic partial asphyxia were used including maternal hypotension and partial placental ablation. In an extensive review, Myers (1972) drew attention to the importance of hypotension and severe metabolic acidaemia as a prelude to brain damage, and that damage followed 30 minutes to several hours of partial asphyxia. Brain swelling was often a feature associated with damage to the cerebral cortex with less involvement of the brainstem, basal ganglia and thalamus. This contrasted with the earlier studies of Ranck and Windle (1959) where the main damage was to brainstem nuclei rather than the cerebral cortex.

Birth asphyxia and neonatal encephalopathy

By the 1960s it had become clear that babies who had abnormal neurological signs as newborns were at an increased risk of neurodevelopmental abnormalities in later months and years and some of these babies had a history of fetal distress and depressed vital signs at birth.

The importance of neonatal encephalopathy as a risk factor for a poor outcome in babies with birth asphyxia was clarified by a survey of more than 54 000 pregnant women cared for in maternity hospitals in the USA between 1959 and 1966 (Nelson and Ellenberg 1981). Among surviving children with Apgar scores of 0–3 at 10–20 minutes, 82% escaped cerebral palsy but the children with cerebral palsy were characterised by the occurrence of seizures within 24 hours of birth.

Sarnat and Sarnat (1976) characterised the clinical features of the encephalopathy in newborn infants who had a prominent history of fetal distress or a low Apgar score at 1 or 5 minutes. They were able to define three stages based mainly, but not exclusively, on their level of arousal, presence of seizures and primitive reflexes. Subsequently many studies showed the importance of the severity of the encephalopathy in determining neurodevelopmental outcome (Peliowski and Finer 1992).

Rhesus haemolytic disease

For centuries it had been observed that some babies were born severely oedematous and pale and died shortly after birth. In those who lived a little longer severe jaundice was a prominent feature. The terminology for what were thought to be separate conditions was 'universal oedema of the newborn', 'congenital anaemia of the newborn', and 'icterus gravis neonatorum'; if the liver and spleen were enlarged and there was erythroblastic activity in peripheral blood the term 'erythroblastosis fetalis' was used.

Diamond et al. (1932) concluded that universal oedema, familial icterus gravis neonatorum and anaemia of the newborn were closely related and were caused by the same underlying pathological process with haemolysis and erythroblastosis being common to all.

Darrow (1938), a pathologist who herself experienced a series of perinatal losses from erythroblastosis fetalis, suggested that the cause of the fetal haemolysis was the transplacental passage of fetal red blood cells to the mother, who produced antibodies which subsequently found their way into the fetal circulation. The discovery and naming of the Rh antigen are generally attributed to Landsteiner and Weiner (1940), who injected blood from rhesus monkeys into rabbits and guinea pigs. When the derived antisera were tested against human blood samples, 85% were Rh-positive.

Infants with erythroblastosis fetalis were often treated by simple blood transfusion. In 1943 Mollison reported that the survival time of rhesus-positive red blood cells in these babies was considerably shorter than that of transfused rhesus-negative red cells. The outcome of transfused babies remained poor until a convenient method of exchange transfusion was introduced by Diamond in 1946 which utilised catheterisation of the umbilical vein. He described his experience in an address to the American Academy of Pediatrics (Diamond 1948). The major contribution of exchange transfusion to the management of rhesus haemolytic disease was underlined by Mollison and Walker (1952), who showed that infants treated by exchange transfusion had an improved survival rate and a lower incidence of kernicterus.

The prediction of the severity of rhesus haemolytic disease before birth attracted attention because many infants were stillborn. The estimation of serum rhesus antibody titres in the mother were of limited benefit in safely timing preterm delivery. The management of affected pregnancies took a leap forwards following Liley's observations that amniotic fluid bilirubin levels measured by spectrophotometry, as described earlier by Bevis (1953), were good predictors of fetal risk (Liley 1961). The outcome for affected fetuses was improved still further by intrauterine transfusion (Liley 1963).

The successful prevention of rhesus haemolytic disease by immunisation of mothers followed a string of research findings including the introduction of the Kleihauer–Betke staining technique for the detection of fetal erythrocytes in maternal blood; the detection of fetal erythrocytes in the blood of Rh-negative mothers after delivery (Finn et al. 1961); observations that ABO incompatibility afforded protection against Rh sensitisation (Nevanlinna and Vainio 1956; Stern et al. 1956); and the finding that anti-Rh (anti-D) protected against sensitisation in Rh-negative volunteers injected with rhesus-positive blood (Finn et al. 1961). These research observations culminated in the first reports of the successful prevention of Rh immunisation in high-risk pregnant women by Clarke and Sheppard (1965) in Liverpool, UK, and Freda et al. (1965) in New York, USA.

References

Aherne, W., Hull, D., 1966. Brown adipose tissue and heat production in the newborn infant. J Pathol Bacteriol 91, 223–234.

Apgar, V., 1953. A proposal for a new method of evaluation of the newborn infant. Anesth Analg 32, 260–267.

Armstrong, D., Norman, M.G., 1974. Periventricular leukomalacia in neonates. Complications and sequelae. Arch Dis Child 49, 367–375.

Ashton, N., Ward, B., Serpell, G., 1953. Role of oxygen in the genesis of retrolental fibroplasia. A preliminary report. Br J Ophthalmol 37, 513–520.

Avery, M.E., Mead, J., 1959. Surface properties in relation to atelectasis and hyaline membrane disease. Am J Dis Child 97, 517–523.

Avery, M.E., Oppenheimer, E.H., 1960. Recent increase in mortality from hyaline membrane disease. J Pediatr 57, 553–559.

Banker, B.Q., Larroche, J.C., 1962. Periventricular leukomalacia of infancy. A form of neonatal anoxic encephalopathy. Arch Neurol 7, 386–410.

Barker, D.J.P., 1994. Mothers, Babies and Disease in Later Life. BMJ Publishing Group, London.

Bevis, D.C.A., 1953. The composition of liquor amnii in haemolytic disease of the newborn. J Obstet Gynaecol Br Emp 60, 244–251.

Browne, F.J., 1922. Neonatal death. Ninetieth Annual Meeting of the British Medical Association. Section of Obstetrics and Gynaecology. BMJ 2, 583–596.

Brück, K., 1961. Temperature regulation in the newborn infant. Biol Neonat 3, 65–119.

Budin, P., 1907 (translated by Maloney W J). The Nursling: The Feeding and Hygiene of Premature and Full-term Infants. Caxton, London.

Calvert, S.A., Hoskins, E.M., Fong, K.W., et al., 1986. Periventricular leukomalacia: Ultrasonic diagnosis and neurological outcome. Acta Paediatr Scand 75, 489–496.

Campbell, K., 1951. Intensive oxygen therapy as a possible cause of retrolental fibroplasia: A clinical approach. Med J Aust 2, 48–50.

Chiswick, M.L., Ahmed, A., Jack, P.M.J., et al., 1973. Control of foetal lung development in the rabbit. Arch Dis Child 48, 709–713.

Chiswick, M.L., Johnson, M., Woodhall, C., et al., 1983. Protective effect of vitamin E (DL-alpha-tocopherol) against intraventricular haemorrhage in premature babies. BMJ 287, 81–84.

Chu, J., Clements, J.A., Cotton, E.K., et al., 1967. Neonatal pulmonary ischemia. Part 1. Clinical and physiological studies. Pediatrics 40, 709–782.

Churchill, J.A., 1963. Weight loss in premature infants developing spastic diplegia. Obstet Gynaecol 22, 601–605.

Clarke, C.A., Sheppard, P.M., 1965. Prevention of rhesus haemolytic disease. Lancet ii, 343.

Clements, J.A., 1957. Surface tension of lung extracts. Proc Soc Exp Biol Med 95, 170–172.

Committee for the Classification of Retinopathy of Prematurity, 1984. An international classification of retinopathy of prematurity. Arch Ophthalmol 102 (8), 1130–1134.

Cone Jr, T.E., 1985. History of the Care and Feeding of the Premature Infant. Little, Brown, Boston.

Cooke, R.W., Morgan, M.E., 1984. Prophylactic ethamsylate for periventricular haemorrhage. Arch Dis Child 59, 82–83.

Corday, E., Irving, D.W., Gold, H., et al., 1962. Mesenteric vascular insufficient. Intestinal ischemia induced by remote circulatory disturbances. Am J Med 33, 365–376.

Cross, K.W., 1966. Resuscitation of the asphyxiated infant. Br Med Bull 22, 73–78.

Cross, K.W., 1973. Cost of preventing retrolental fibroplasia? Lancet ii, 954–956.

Cross, K.W., Tizard, J.P.M., Trythall, D.A.H., 1958. The gaseous metabolism of the new-born infant breathing 15% oxygen. Acta Paediatr 47, 217–237.

Crosse, V.M., Evans, P.J., 1952. Prevention of retrolental fibroplasia. Arch Ophthalmol 48 (1), 83–87.

Crosse, V.M., Hickman, E.M., Howarth, B.E., Aubrey, J., 1954. The value of human milk compared with other feeds for premature infants. Arch Dis Child 29, 178–195.

Daniel, S.S., Dawes, G.S., James, L.S., et al., 1966. Hypothermia and the resuscitation of asphyxiated fetal monkeys. J Pediatr 68, 45–53.

Darrow, R., 1938. Icterus gravis (erythroblastosis) neonatorum. Arch Pathol 25, 378–417.

Davies, D.P., 1977. Adequacy of expressed breast milk for early growth of preterm infants. Arch Dis Child 52, 296–301.

Davies, D.P., 1978. The first feed of low birth weight infants: Changing attitudes in the twentieth century. Arch Dis Child 53, 187–192.

Dawes, G.S., 1968. Foetal and Neonatal Physiology. Year Book Medical Publishers, Chicago, p. 143.

Dawes, G.S., Mott, J.C., Shelley, H.J., 1959. The importance of cardiac glycogen for the maintenance of life in foetal lambs and newborn animals during anoxia. J Physiol 146, 516–538.

Dawes, G.S., Jacobson, H.N., Mott, J.C., et al., 1960. Some observations on foetal and new-born rhesus monkeys. J Physiol 152, 271–298.

Dawes, G.S., Jacobson, H.N., Mott, J.C., et al., 1963. The treatment of asphyxiated mature fetal lambs and rhesus monkeys with intravenous glucose and sodium carbonate. J Physiol 169, 167–184.

Dawkins, M.J.R., Hull, D., 1964. Brown adipose tissue and the response of new-born rabbits to cold. J Physiol 172, 216–238.

Day, R., Curtis, J., Kelly, M., 1943. Respiratory metabolism in infancy and in childhood. XXVII. Regulation of body temperature of premature infants. Am J Dis Child 65, 376–398.

DeLemos, R.A., Shermeta, D.W., Knelson, J.H., et al., 1970. Acceleration of appearance of pulmonary surfactant in the fetal lamb by administration of corticosteroids. Am Rev Resp Dis 102, 459–561.

Delivoria-Papadopoulos, M., Swyer, P.R., 1964. Assisted ventilation in terminal hyaline membrane disease. Arch Dis Child 39, 481–484.

De Reuck, J., Chattha, A.S., Richardson, E.P., 1972. Pathogenesis and evolution of periventricular leukomalacia. Arch Neurol 27, 229–236.

Diamond, L.K., 1948. Replacement transfusion as a treatment for erythroblastosis fetalis. Pediatrics 2, 520–524.

Diamond, L.K., Blackfan, K.D., Baty, J.M., 1932. Erythroblastosis fetalis and its association with universal edema of the fetus, icterus gravis neonatorum and anaemia of the newborn. J Pediatr 1, 269–309.

Donald, I., Lord, J., 1953. Augmented respiration: Studies in atelectasis neonatorum. Lancet i, 9–17.

Donald, I., Steiner, R.E., 1953. Radiography in the diagnosis of hyaline membrane. Lancet ii, 846–849.

Donn, S.M., Roloff, D.W., Goldstein, G.W., 1981. Prevention of intraventricular haemorrhage in preterm infants by phenobarbitone. Lancet ii, 215–217.

Drillien, C.M., 1964. The Growth and Development of the Prematurely Born Infant. Livingstone, Edinburgh.

Fawer, C.L., Diebold, P., Calame, A., 1987. Periventricular leukomalacia and neurodevelopmental outcome in preterm infants. Arch Dis Child 62, 30–36.

Finn, R., Clarke, C.A., Donohoe, W.T.A., et al., 1961. Experimental studies on the prevention of Rh haemolytic disease. BMJ ii, 1486–1490.

Freda, J., Gorman, J.G., Pollack, W., 1965. Prevention of rhesus haemolytic disease. Lancet ii, 690.

Freud, S., 1968. Infantile Cerebral Paralysis (translated by Russin LA). University of Miami Press, Florida.

Fujiwara, T., Chida, S., Watabe, Y.J., et al., 1980. Artificial surfactant therapy in hyaline membrane disease. Lancet i, 55–99.

Gaisford, W., Schofield, S., 1950. Prolongation of the initial starvation period in premature infants. BMJ 1, 1404–1405.

Gandy, G., Jacobson, W., Gairdner, D., 1970. Hyaline membrane disease. I. Cellular changes. Arch Dis Child 45, 289–310.

Gilles, F.H., Leviton, A., Kerr, C.S., 1976. Endotoxin leucoencephalopathy in the telencephalon of the newborn kitten. J Neurol Sci 27, 183–191.

Gitlin, D., Craig, J.M., 1956. The nature of the hyaline membrane in asphyxia of the newborn. Pediatrics 17, 64–71.

Gordon, H.H., Levine, S.Z., 1944. The metabolic basis for the individualized feeding of infants, premature and full-term. J Pediatr 25, 464–475.

Gordon, H.H., McNamara, H., 1941. Fat excretion of premature infants. i. Effect on fecal fat of decreasing fat intake. Am J Dis Child 62, 328–345.

Gordon, H.H., Levine, S.Z., McNamara, H., 1947. Feeding of premature infants: A comparison of human and cow's milk. Am J Dis Child 73, 442–452.

Gregory, G.A., Kitterman, J.A., Phibbs, R.H., et al., 1971. Treatment of the idiopathic respiratory distress syndrome with continuous positive airway pressure. N Engl J Med 284, 1333–1340.

Gruenwald, P., 1947. Surface tension as a factor in the resistance of neonatal lungs to aeration. Am J Obstet Gynecol 53, 996–1007.

Halliday, H.L., 2008. Surfactants: past, present and future. J Perinatol 28, S47–S56.

Hambleton, G., Wigglesworth, J.S., 1976. Origin of intraventricular haemorrhage in the preterm infant. Arch Dis Child 51, 651–659.

Herman, S., Reynolds, E.O.R., 1973. Methods for improving oxygenation in infants mechanically ventilated for severe hyaline membrane disease. Arch Dis Child 48, 612–617.

Hey, E., 1975. Thermal neutrality. Br Med Bull 31, 69–74.

Hey, E.N., Katz, G., 1970. The optimum thermal environment for naked babies. Arch Dis Child 45, 328–334.

Hill, J.R., 1959. The oxygen consumption of the new-born and adult mammals. Its dependence on the oxygen tension in the inspired air and on the environmental temperature. J Physiol 149, 346–373.

Hill, A., Leland Melson, G., Brent Clark, H., et al., 1982. Hemorrhagic periventricular leukomalacia: Diagnosis by real time ultrasound and correlation with autopsy findings. Pediatrics 69, 282–284.

Himwich, H.E., Bernstein, A.O., Herrlich, H., et al., 1941. Mechanisms for the maintenance of life in the newborn during anoxia. Am J Physiol 135, 387–391.

Hochheim, K., 1903. Ueber einige Befunde in den Lugen von Neugeborenen und die Beziehung derselben zur Aspiration von Fruchtwasser. Centralbl Pathol 14, 537–538.

Jefferson, E., 1952. Retrolental fibroplasia. Arch Dis Child 27, 329–336.

Kinsey, V.E., Hemphill, F.M., 1955. Etiology of retrolental fibroplasia and preliminary report of the Cooperative Study of Retrolental Fibroplasia. Trans Am Acad Ophthalmol Otolaryngol 59, 15–24.

Kinsey, V.E., Zacharias, L., 1949. Retrolental fibroplasia. JAMA 139, 572–578.

Landsteiner, K., Weiner, A.S., 1940. An agglutinable factor in human blood recognized by immune sera in Rhesus blood. Soc Exp Biol New York 42, 223.

Le Gallois, M., 1812. Expériences sur le principe de la vie. Hautel, Paris.

Liggins, G.C., 1968. Premature parturition after infusion of corticotrophin or cortisol into foetal lambs. J Endocrinol 42, 323–329.

Liggins, G.C., 1969. Premature delivery of foetal lambs infused with corticosteroids. J Endocrinol 45, 515–523.

Liggins, G.C., Howie, R.N., 1972. A controlled trial of antepartum glucocorticoid treatment for prevention of the respiratory distress syndrome of premature infants. Pediatrics 50, 515–525.

Liggins, G.C., Kennedy, P.C., Holm, L.W., 1967. Failure of initiation of parturition after electro-coagulation of the pituitary of the foetal lamb. Am J Obstet Gynecol 98, 1080–1086.

Liley, A.W., 1961. Liquor amnii analysis in the management of the pregnancy complicated by Rhesus sensitization. Am J Obstet Gynecol 82, 1359–1370.

Liley, A.W., 1963. Intrauterine transfusion of foetus in haemolytic disease. BMJ 2, 1107–1109.

Little, W.J., 1862. On the influence of abnormal parturition, difficult labours, premature births and asphyxia neonatorum on the mental and physical condition of the child, especially in relation to deformities. Trans Obstet Soc Lond 3, 293–344.

Lloyd, J.R., 1969. The etiology of gastrointestinal perforations in the newborn. J Pediatr Surg 4, 77–84.

McCance, R.A., Widdowson, E.M., 1962. Nutrition and growth. Proc R Soc Lond B 156, 326–337.

Ment, L.R., Duncan, C.C., Ehrenkranz, R.A., et al., 1985. Randomized indomethacin trial for prevention of intraventricular

hemorrhage in very low birth weight infants. J Pediatr 107, 937–943.

Mollison, P.L., 1943. The survival of transfused erythrocytes in haemolytic disease of the newborn. Arch Dis Child 18, 161–172.

Mollison, P.L., Walker, W., 1952. Controlled trials of the treatment of haemolytic disease of the newborn. Lancet i, 429–433.

Myers, R.E., 1972. Two patterns of perinatal brain damage and their conditions of occurrence. Am J Obstet Gynecol 112, 246–276.

Myers, R.E., Beard, R., Adamsons, K., 1969. Brain swelling in the newborn rhesus monkey following prolonged partial asphyxia. Neurology 19, 1012–1018.

Naeye, R.L., Harcke Jr, H.T., Blanc, W.A., 1971. Adrenal gland structure and the development of hyaline membrane disease. Pediatrics 47, 650–657.

Nelson, K.B., Ellenberg, J.H., 1981. Apgar scores as predictors of chronic neurologic disability. Pediatrics 68, 36–44.

Nevanlinna, H.R., Vainio, T., 1956. The influence of mother–child ABO incompatibility on Rh immunization. Vox Sang 1, 26–36.

Northway Jr, W.H., Rosan, R.C., Porter, D.Y., 1967. Pulmonary disease following respirator therapy of hyaline membrane disease: Bronchopulmonary dysplasia. N Engl J Med 276, 357–368.

Omans, W.B., Barness, L.A., Rose, C.S., et al., 1961. Prolonged feeding studies in premature infants. J Pediatr 59, 951–957.

Owens, W.C., Owens, E.U., 1948. Retrolental fibroplasia in premature infants. Trans Am Acad Ophthalmol Otolaryngol 53, 18–41.

Pape, K.E., Blackwell, R.J., Cusick, G., et al., 1979. Ultrasound detection of brain damage in preterm infants. Lancet i, 1261–1264.

Papile, L.-A., Burstein, J., Burstein, R., et al., 1978. Incidence and evolution of subependymal and intraventricular hemorrhage: A study of infants with birth weights less than 1,500 gm. J Pediatr 92, 529–534.

Pattle, R.E., 1955. Properties, function and origin of the alveolar lining layer. Nature 175, 1125–1126.

Peliowski, A., Finer, N.N., 1992. Birth asphyxia in the term infant. In: Sinclair, J.C., Bracken, M.B. (Eds.), Effective Care of the Newborn Infant. Oxford University Press, Oxford, pp. 249–280.

Radford, E.J., 1954. Method for estimating respiratory surface area of mammalian lungs from their physical characteristics. Proc Soc Exp Biol Med 87, 58–61.

Ranck, J.B., Windle, W.F., 1959. Brain damage in the monkey, Macaca mulatta, by asphyxia neonatorum. Exp Neurol 1, 130–153.

Reynolds, E.O.R., 1971. Effect of alterations in mechanical ventilator settings on pulmonary gas exchange in hyaline membrane disease. Arch Dis Child 46, 152–159.

Rubner, M., Heubner, O., 1898. Die naturliche Ernährung eines Säuglings. Z Biol 36, 1–55.

Rubner, M., Heubner, O., 1899. Die kunstliche Ernährung eines Normalen und eines atrophischen Säuglings. Z Biol 38, 315–398.

Sarnat, H.B., Sarnat, M.S., 1976. Neonatal encephalopathy following fetal distress. Arch Neurol 33, 696–705.

Scholander, P.F., Hock, R., Walters, V., et al., 1950. Heat regulation in some arctic and tropical mammals and birds. Biol Bull 99, 237–258.

Silverman, W.A., 1979. Incubator-baby side shows. Pediatrics 64, 127–141.

Silverman, W.A., 1980. Retrolental Fibroplasia: A Modern Parable. Grune and Stratton, New York.

Silverman, W.A., Fertig, J.W., Berger, A.P., 1958. The influence of the thermal environment upon the survival of newly born premature infants. Pediatrics 22, 876–886.

Silverman, W.A., Zamelis, A., Sinclair, J.C., et al., 1964. Warm nape of the newborn. Pediatrics 33, 984–987.

Sinha, S., Davies, J.M., Sims, D.G., et al., 1985. Relation between periventricular haemorrhage and ischaemic brain lesions diagnosed by ultrasound in very preterm infants. Lancet ii, 1154–1156.

Smallpiece, V., Davies, P.A., 1964. Immediate feeding of premature infants with undiluted breast-milk. Lancet 2, 1349–1352.

Smith, R.E., 1962. Thermoregulation by brown adipose tissue in cold. Fed Proc 21, 221.

Stern, K., Davidson, I., Masatis, L., 1956. Experimental studies on Rh immunization. Am J Clin Pathol 26, 833–843.

Szewczyk, T.S., 1952. Retrolental fibroplasia: Etiology and prophylaxis. Am J Ophthalmol 35, 301–311.

Terry, T.L., 1942. Extreme prematurity and fibroblastic overgrowth of persistent vascular sheath behind each crystalline lens. I. Preliminary report. Am J Ophthalmol 25, 203–204.

Terry, T.L., 1946. Retrolental fibroplasia. J Pediatr 29, 770–773.

Thelander, H.E., 1939. Perforation of the gastrointestinal tract of the newborn infant. Am J Dis Child 58, 371–393.

Usher, R.H., McLean, F.H., 1974. Normal fetal growth and the significance of fetal growth retardation. In: Davis, J.A., Dobbing, J. (Eds.), Scientific Foundations of Paediatrics. Heinemann, London.

Virchow, R., 1867. Zur pathologischen Anatomie des Gehirns. I. Congenitale Encephalitis und Myelitis. Virchows Arch Pathol Anat 38, 129–142.

von Neergaard, K., 1929. Neue Auffassungen über einen Grundbegriff der Atemmechanik. Die Retraktionskraft der Lunge, abhängig von der Oberflächenspannung in den Alveolen. Z Gesamte Exp Med 66, 373–394.

Weaver, L.T., 2009. 'Growing babies': Defining the milk requirements of infants 1890–1910. Soc Hist Med 23, 320–337.

Westin, B., Nyberg, R., Miller Jr, J.A., et al., 1962. Hypothermia and transfusion with oxygenated blood in the treatment of asphyxia neonatorum. Acta Paediatr 139 (Suppl.), 1–80.

Widdowson, E.M., Spray, C.M., 1951. Chemical development in utero. Arch Dis Child 26, 205–214.

Wigglesworth, J.S., Pape, K.E., 1978. An integrated model for haemorrhagic and ischaemic lesions in the newborn brain. Early Hum Dev 2, 179–199.

Willi, H., 1944. Über eine bösartige Enteritis bei Säuglingen des ersten Trimenons. Ann Pediatr 162, 87–112.

Windle, W.F., Becker, R.F., 1942. Effect of anoxia at birth on the central nervous system of the guinea pig. Proc Soc Exp Biol Med 51, 213–219.

Yoon, B.H., Romero, R., Yang, S.H., et al., 1996. Interleukin-6 concentrations in umbilical cord plasma are elevated in neonates with white matter lesions associated with periventricular leukomalacia. Am J Obstet Gynecol 174, 1433–1440.

Yoon, B.H., Jun, J.K., Romero, R., et al., 1997. Amniotic fluid inflammatory cytokines (interleukin-6, interleukin-1β, and tumor necrosis factor-alpha), neonatal brain white matter lesions, and cerebral palsy. Am J Obstet Gynecol 177, 19–26.

section 2

Prenatal life

Basic genetics 8

Andrew Green

The nature and structure of a gene

Genetics is traditionally defined as the science of biological variation, and has been a scientific discipline for over a century. Human genetics makes up a large part of the field of genetics, but the principal laws of genetics are universal and apply equally to all species, including humans. Mendel's studies in the 19th century were originally felt to have no relevance to humans, and it is only in retrospect that their importance can be seen. Many of the principles of genetics were discovered through the study of smaller organisms, such as bacteria, yeast and fruit flies. The basic genetic mechanisms of cell division, development and differentiation happen in the same way in widely divergent species. Therefore, it is impossible to look at human genetics in isolation and there are large amounts of information from lower species which have a bearing on human disorders. The study of the genetics of small organisms has had a profound impact on our understanding of human development, and of how human diseases develop. It is likely that such basic science will continue to contribute significantly to the understanding of human genetic disease. In this chapter, I hope to outline the basic elements of genetics, and describe the types of genetic tests now available to help in neonatal diagnosis.

The basic unit of inheritance for any species is the gene. The original concept of a gene arose long before the relationship between genes and nucleic acids was ever understood. A gene was considered to be a stable heritable element which conferred a particular property or phenotype on an individual organism. This element was passed on to subsequent generations of a particular species, and the nature of the phenotype varied according to the nature of the gene. The concept of dominant and recessive traits, which will be discussed below, was derived from studies of inheritance patterns, long before the molecular basis of the gene was understood.

A gene can also be considered in another way, as a specific length of deoxyribonucleic acid (DNA) which encodes a particular function, in most cases the synthesis of a protein. This also is a stable heritable unit. Each cell in an organism, regardless of its function, has the entire set of genes for that particular organism, but only a proportion of those genes will be active. DNA is found in the nucleus of every cell of an organism, as a double helix (Fig. 8.1).

Each strand of the double helix has a backbone of alternating phosphate and deoxyribose sugar molecules, with the sugars attached to the 5' and 3' hydroxyl groups of the phosphate group. Attached to the sugar molecule, lying within the helix, is one of four nitrogen-containing nucleic acid bases. Two of these bases, adenine (A) and guanine (G), are purines, and two are the smaller pyrimidines cytosine (C) and thymine (T). The A and T bases pair together by hydrogen bonding, and the G and C bases similarly pair by hydrogen bonds (Fig. 8.2). The two strands of the double helix are held together by paired A–T or G–C bases of opposite strands of the double helix. The DNA strand can be read in only one direction, from 5' (left hand) to 3' (right hand). The two strands of DNA are complementary to each other, and the sequence of one strand can be predicted from its opposite. If one strand reads 5'-CAGCGTA-3', then the opposite strand must read 5'-TACGCTG-3'. The double-stranded sequence would then be written as below:

5'-CAGCGTA-3'
3'-GTCGCAT-5'

© 2012 Elsevier Ltd

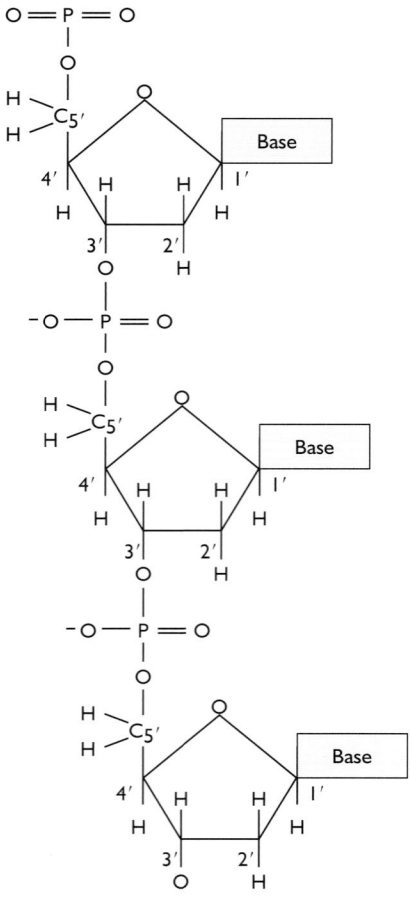

Fig. 8.1 Structure of a DNA chain. The deoxyribose and phosphate residues are linked to form the sugar–phosphate backbone.

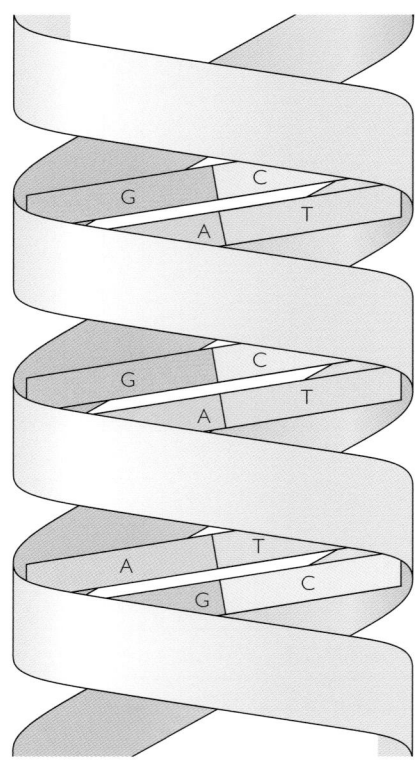

Fig. 8.2 Double-helix structure of DNA. The double helix of deoxyribose and phosphate molecules is held together by paired purine and pyrimidine bonds.

The simplicity of the double-helix structure allows for several important functions for DNA.

First, huge amounts of information can be stored in the DNA strand. If a molecule of DNA is 1 million bases long, then there are $4^{1\,000\,000}$ possible sequences for that stretch of DNA. A genome is the complete DNA sequence of an organism. In humans, the estimated genome size is 3×10^9 basepairs (bp). The draft DNA sequence of the entire human genome has been completed, which is a major milestone in human scientific development. It is estimated that the genome has between 22 000 and 25 000 genes. However, despite the DNA sequence being available, the detailed function of many of these genes remains unknown. The next step after the sequencing of the human genome is the understanding of the complexities of all the human genes. The routine practical clinical application of the knowledge of the human genome is still some way off.

Second, the double helix provides a framework for DNA replication. One strand of DNA acts as a template for the synthesis of a new strand. The double helix unwinds, allowing DNA replication enzymes access to the template strand of DNA. The replication system builds a new strand of DNA based on the template. The new double helix formed as a result will contain one original strand and a newly synthesised complementary second strand. This is the basic mechanism of DNA replication in all species.

Third, the double helix provides a basis for repair of damaged DNA. A damaged base can be replaced, knowing its complementary base is present on the opposite strand. Damage to the sugar–phosphate backbone can also be repaired using the opposite strand as a template.

Decoding the information in DNA

About 90% of the DNA in the human genome does not code for any specific property; only about 10% of the genome actually contains coding information in the form of a gene. In simple terms, the genetic code in DNA is transcribed into a molecule called messenger RNA (mRNA). The mRNA is then translated into a protein, which carries out the function encoded by the specific DNA.

A gene has several distinct elements (Fig. 8.3). The major part of the gene is divided into coding regions, called exons, and non-coding regions, called introns. Just before (5′) the first exon, there is a promoter which indicates where transcription of a gene should start. There can be several promoters for one gene, and different promoters can be used according to the tissue in which the gene is being expressed; in other words, the promoter is tissue-specific. Further 5′ of the promoter there can also be enhancers or suppressors, which can increase or decrease the level of transcription of the gene. Not all of the mRNA will code for protein, as some exons will code for mRNA that does not directly encode protein. These areas, known as untranslated regions, can be either at the start (5′) or the end (3′) of the mRNA.

To express the DNA code, mRNA is used. There are several different types of RNA, but mRNA is the most important in decoding DNA. There are three differences between RNA and DNA. First, the sugar backbone of RNA contains ribose rather than deoxyribose. Second, mRNA exists as a single strand, and remains more unstable.

Table 8.1 The genetic code

FIRST POSITION	U	AMINO ACID	C	AMINO ACID	A	AMINO ACID	G	AMINO ACID	THIRD POSITION
				SECOND POSITION					
U	UUU	Phe	UCU	Ser	UAU	Tyr	UGU	Cys	U
	UUC	Phe	UCC	Ser	UAC	Tyr	UGC	Cys	C
	UUA	Leu	UCA	Ser	UAA	Stop	UGA	Stop	A
	UUG	Leu	UCG	Ser	UAG	Stop	UGG	Trp	G
C	CUU	Leu	CCU	Pro	CAU	His	CGU	Arg	U
	CUC	Leu	CCC	Pro	CAC	His	CGC	Arg	C
	CUA	Leu	CCA	Pro	CAA	Gln	CGA	Arg	A
	CUG	Leu	CCG	Pro	CAG	Gln	CGG	Arg	G
A	AUU	Ile	ACU	Thr	AAU	Asn	AGU	Ser	U
	AUC	Ile	ACC	Thr	AAC	Asn	AGC	Ser	C
	AUA	Ile	ACA	Thr	AAA	Lys	AGA	Arg	A
	AUG	Met	ACG	Thr	AAG	Lys	AGG	Arg	G
G	GUU	Val	GCU	Ala	GAU	Asp	GGU	Gly	U
	GUC	Val	GCC	Ala	GAC	Asp	GGC	Gly	C
	GUA	Val	GCA	Ala	GAA	Glu	GGA	Gly	A
	GUG	Val	GCG	Ala	GAG	Glu	GGG	Gly	G

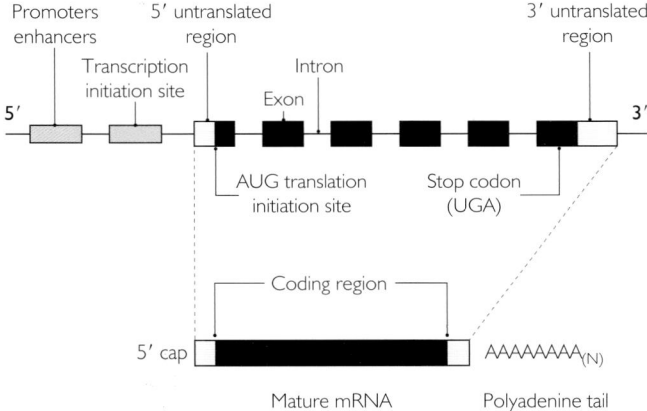

Fig. 8.3 An idealised gene.

Third, in RNA, the base uracil (U) is used instead of thymine, whereas the other three nucleic acids remain the same.

The DNA code in most genes is expressed as a protein, which is a peptide made of the building blocks of individual amino acids. Each amino acid is coded for by a sequence of three DNA bases, known as a codon. For some amino acids, there is more than one codon (Table 8.1). A long series of DNA codons in a gene will thus code for an entire protein. The mRNA codons coding for amino acids are identical to DNA codons, with the substitution of uracil (U) for thymine (T). There is a tightly controlled mechanism for the generation of protein from a DNA template.

To decode a gene into protein, the DNA is first transcribed into mRNA. A strand (the 'sense' strand) of the DNA double helix is used by the enzyme RNA polymerase to synthesise a complementary strand of mRNA. Transcription of mRNA starts from the 5′ end of the first exon of the gene, until the end of the most 3′ exon. The intervening introns are initially included, and the first molecule is known as pre-mRNA. The intronic RNA sequences are spliced out

and a 3′ polyadenine tail is added, producing mature mRNA. The mature mRNA is then transferred from the nucleus to the ribosome, to be used as a template for the production of protein. The mature mRNA has both 5′ and 3′ untranslated regions.

Protein synthesis does not begin at the 5′ end of the mRNA, but at the first 5′ AUG codon, which codes for the amino acid methionine. Protein translation stops at the first truncation codon (usually UGA) thereafter (see Fig. 8.3). In the ribosome, amino acid-specific transfer molecules, called transfer RNAs (tRNAs), bind a free molecule of their specific amino acid. The binding is carried out by an anticodon in the tRNA, which is complementary to the mRNA that codes for that specific amino acid. Using its anticodon, the tRNA binds the specific mRNA codon for its amino acid. By a complex machinery, the amino acid is then added to a growing peptide chain which will eventually form the mature protein (Fig. 8.4). The 5′ end of the mRNA corresponds to the NH_2 (amino terminus) of the protein, and the 3′ end of the mRNA corresponds to the COOH (carboxyl terminus) of the protein. Many proteins in higher species are modified after translation by the addition of phosphate or lipid groups.

Chromosomes and cell division

The first coiling of DNA is in the form of the double helix. However, there are subsequent higher orders of coiling and packaging of DNA. The first order gives a loop of about 146 bp in size, wound around a histone protein. The complex is known as a nucleosome. The highest order of coiling of a large DNA molecule, with its associated histones and other proteins, is known as a chromosome.

A chromosome consists of one very long double helix of DNA, containing very many genes in millions of basepairs. Humans are diploid; that is, they have two copies of every chromosome. The normal human chromosome complement is 46, made up of 22 pairs of autosomes (non-sex chromosomes) and two sex chromosomes, either X and Y in a male, or X and X in a female. Each member of a pair of autosomes contains the same genetic information. The pair of X chromosomes in a female will contain the same genetic information, but the X and Y chromosomes in a male only have a small number of genes in common. A normal human metaphase karyotype is shown in Figure 8.5.

When cells divide, the genetic content must also be duplicated so that the daughter cells have the correct genetic material. Most cell division occurs as mitosis, where one cell divides to give two genetically identical cells. This is the process which allows the formation of a complete human being from one fertilised embryo, and is also the process by which the cells of many organs are constantly renewed. Mitosis is one short period during a carefully programmed cell cycle (Fig. 8.6). After mitosis, the cell may enter a resting phase (G0), or go on to divide again (G1). A cell in G1 will then go on to synthesise new DNA as described above (S phase). There is then a second gap phase (G2), followed by mitosis (M).

Prior to mitosis, the cell can be said to be in interphase, during which the chromosomes are very elongated. Just before mitosis, in S phase, the chromosomes are duplicated and begin to condense as two (sister) chromatids per chromosome. This condensation phase is known as prophase. In the next phase, metaphase, the condensed chromatids line up along the plane of the cell, and spindle fibres develop between the centromeres (narrow waist of each chromatid) and the polar centrioles. Standard analysis of human chromosomes is carried out in metaphase. The chromatids separate, starting from each centromere, and pass to the new daughter cell, in the step called anaphase. By the telophase, the chromatids have reached to opposite poles of the dividing cell, and division completes.

Meiosis is the form of division required to form gametes (sperm or oocyte). Gametes are haploid, with only one of each chromosome – 23 in the case of humans. This allows the formation of a new diploid organism from two haploid gametes. Meiosis occurs in

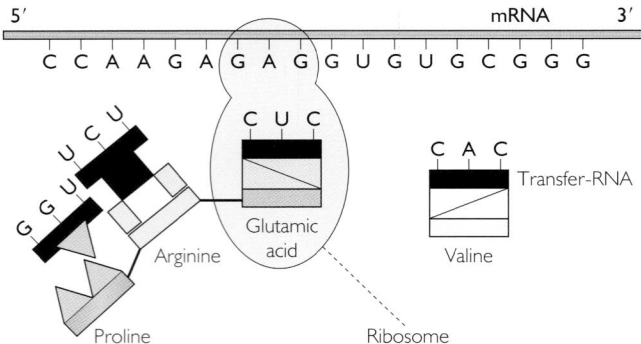

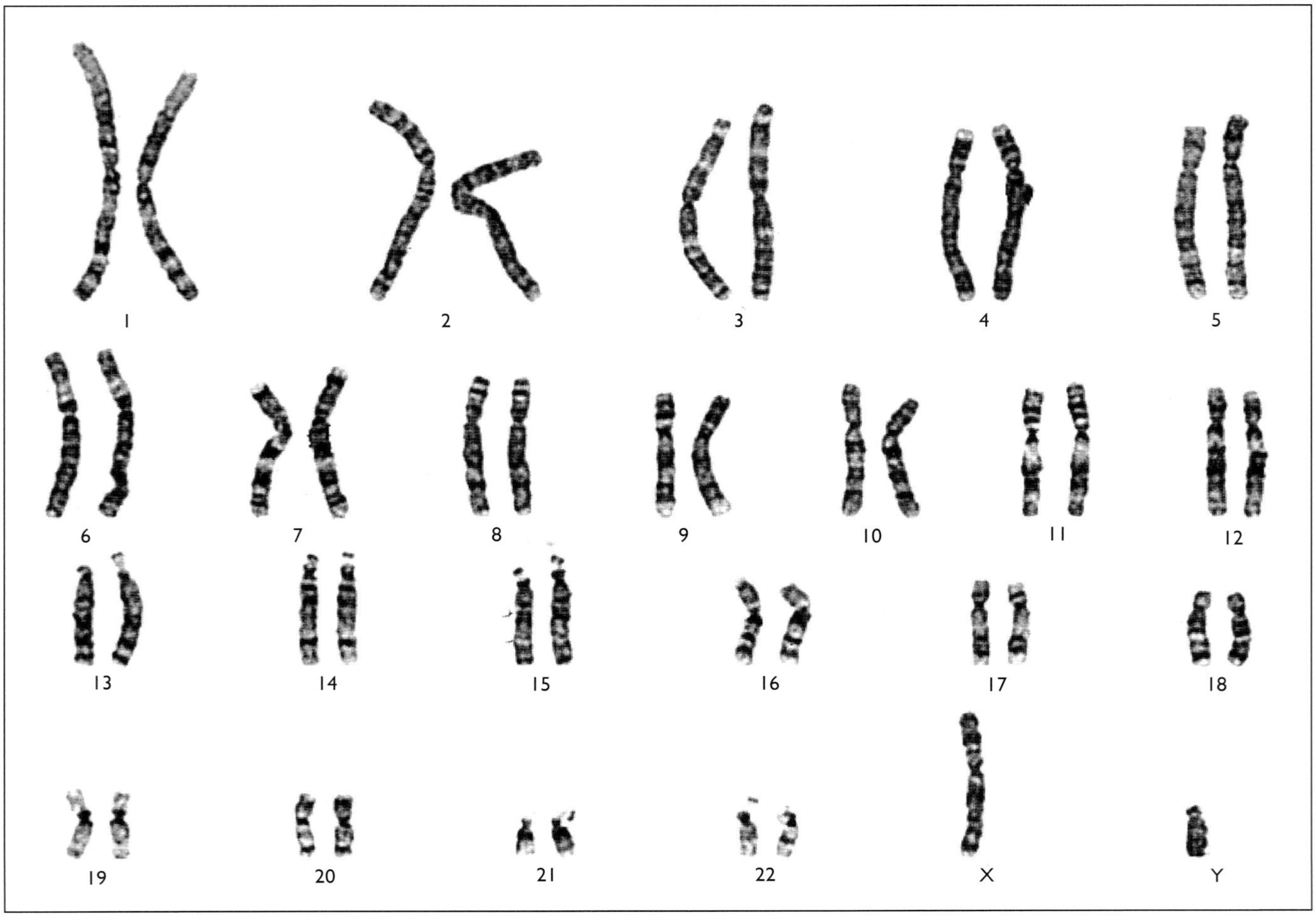

Fig. 8.4 Protein synthesis from mRNA.

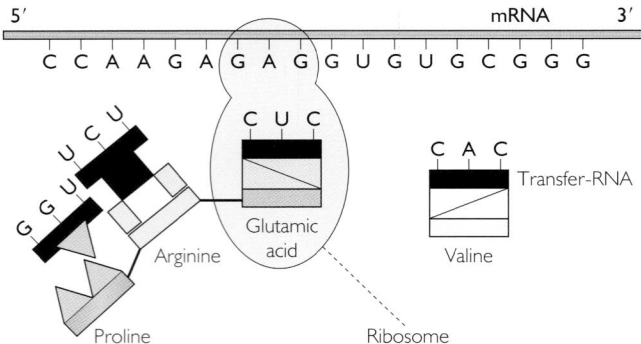

Case: Unilabs   Slide: male   Cell: I   Patient:

Fig. 8.5 A normal human metaphase karyotype.

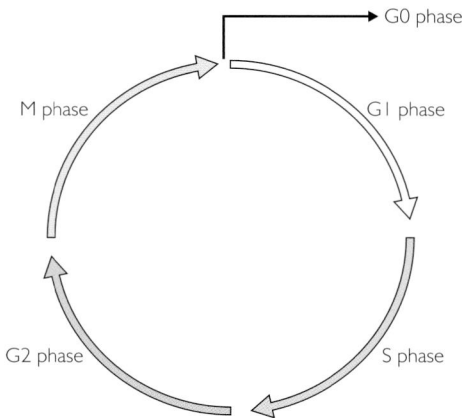

Fig. 8.6 Cell cycle.

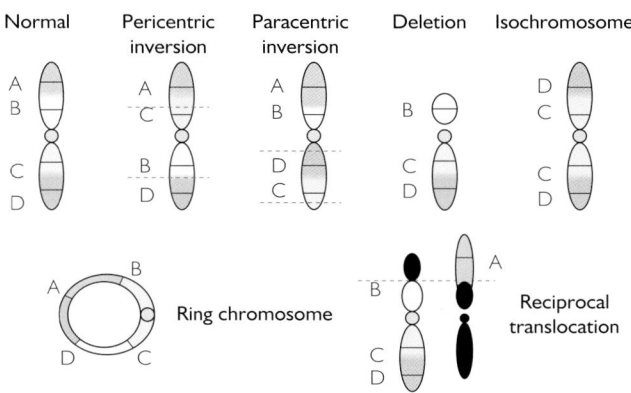

Fig. 8.7 Different types of chromosome anomaly. A–D represent notional chromosomal loci.

two stages, meiosis I and meiosis II. The first phase of meiosis I, prophase I, is similar to that in mitosis, with the appearance of two condensed chromatids which have duplicated. At this stage, crossing over of genetic material from one chromatid to another can occur. It is estimated that one or two crossovers occur per chromosome in each meiosis. This introduces further genetic diversity, ensuring that the inherited chromosomes are different from the chromosomes of the parent. Metaphase I then occurs, where chromatids do not separate but go to the opposite ends of the cell in anaphase I and telophase I. The cells at this stage are still diploid.

The second meiotic division then occurs, where chromatids condense again in prophase II, and line up along the axis of the dividing cell in metaphase II. The chromatids then separate, passing to opposite ends of the cell in anaphase II. The new cells are then haploid, with 23 chromosomes, and the chromatids elongate into thin strands in telophase II.

Chromosome analysis

To examine chromosomes from a patient (a karyotype), dividing cells in culture must be examined. These cells are usually lymphocytes, amniotic fluid cells or fibroblasts. Cells are arrested in the metaphase stage of mitosis, and stained in such a way that the chromosomes are easily visualised. The usual technique used is G-banding (using a Giemsa stain), which gives a characteristic positive and negative banding pattern to each chromosome. Each chromosome has a constriction, called a centromere, dividing the chromosome into a short arm (p) and a long arm (q). Each arm has a number of prominent bands, which can then be subdivided into smaller bands. The gene for the ABO blood group is localised to chromosome 9q34. The gene thus lies in the fourth subband from the centromere (q34) of the third band from the centromere (q34) on the long arm (q34) of chromosome 9 (9q34).

Chromosome abnormalities can be broadly classified into abnormalities of chromosome number or a rearrangement of a normal number of chromosomes. The critical issue in most cases for determining the significance of a chromosome abnormality is whether the abnormality gives rise to an excess or deficiency of the normal diploid state (aneuploidy).

Abnormalities of chromosome number are relatively common, but many are not recognised as they may result in the early loss of a pregnancy. Triploidy (69 chromosomes) and tetraploidy (92 chromosomes) are relatively common causes of early pregnancy loss. Trisomy, the presence of a single extra chromosome (47

chromosomes), is also a common cause of miscarriage. Specific trisomies can give rise to an affected neonate, the commonest being trisomy 21 (Down syndrome), trisomy 13 (Patau syndrome) and trisomy 18 (Edward syndrome). All these trisomies usually occur as a result of autosomal non-dysjunction in meiotic division of the oocyte. In non-dysjunction, the specific chromatids fail to separate, resulting in an extra chromosome in one oocyte and no chromosome in the opposite gamete. A fertilised embryo from the oocyte with an extra chromosome will therefore be trisomic. The fertilised oocyte with an absent chromosome will be monosomic, and be lost as an early miscarriage. Non-dysjunction tends to occur more frequently with increasing maternal age. Non-dysjunction can occur in the male germline, but rarely produces viable offspring.

There are numerous types of chromosome rearrangements, the commonest of which are shown in Figure 8.7. Pericentric and paracentric chromosome inversions are usually balanced, and inherited without any phenotypic effect. Paracentric inversions are usually associated with a low risk of producing a liveborn unbalanced karyotype, but pericentric inversions may carry a higher risk. Insertions, duplications, deletions, isochromosomes and ring chromosomes are all usually aneuploid and associated with significant clinical abnormalities. Reciprocal translocations occur where there is exchange of genetic material from one arm of a chromosome in return for genetic material from a different chromosome. Reciprocal translocations are usually balanced, without any clinical effect, but may carry a risk of having a child with problems due to an unbalanced karyotype.

Another type of translocation is between the acrocentric chromosomes (13–15, 21 and 22), where there is no appreciable coding material on a very small short (p) arm. This is known as a Robertsonian translocation. Robertsonian translocations are one of the commonest human chromosome translocations, and in the balanced form have no clinical effect. A Robertsonian translocation involving chromosomes 14 and 21 is shown in Figure 8.8. Those who carry a Robertsonian translocation involving chromosome 21 may be at significantly higher risk of having a child with Down syndrome as an unbalanced product of the translocation. The same applies to a lesser extent for those carrying a Robertsonian translocation involving chromosome 13, and a subsequent risk of a child with Patau syndrome.

The nomenclature for reporting a chromosome analysis is strict, and needs to be read carefully. A karyotype is reported initially as the number of chromosomes, regardless of whether or not those chromosomes are normal. The sex chromosomes are then described. If there is no further abnormality, the report is then complete. Any

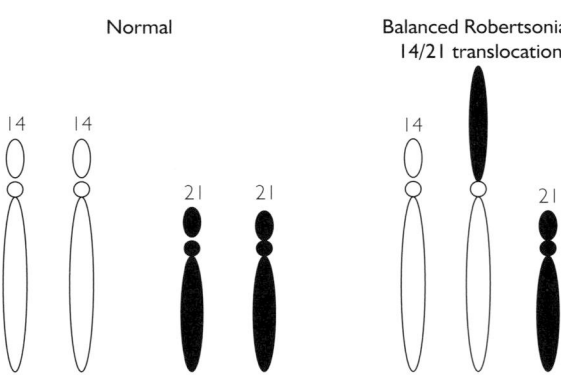

Normal

Balanced Robertsonian
14/21 translocation

Fig. 8.8 Robertsonian translocation.

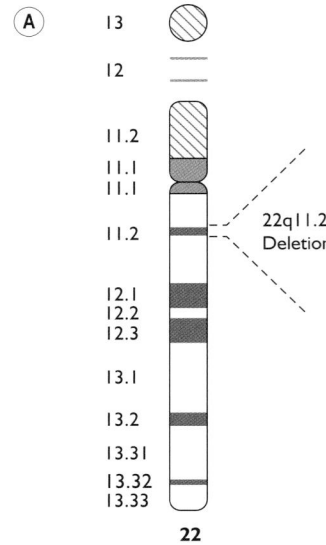

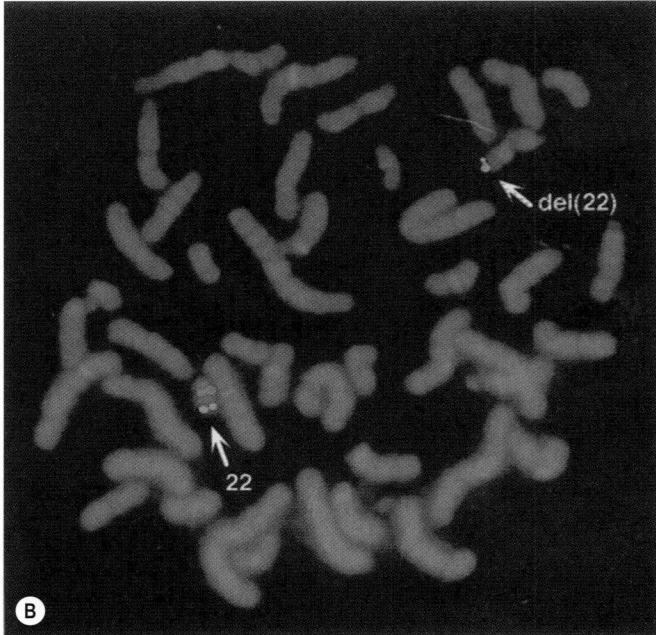

Fig. 8.9 (a) Ideogram of chromosome 22, indicating the region of 22q11.2 deleted in Di George syndrome. (b) Fluorescent in situ hybridisation (FISH) study of metaphase chromosomes from a patient with a microdeletion of chromosome 22q11.2. The normal chromosome 22 on the left (arrow) shows red signal from a FISH probe for the critical region of 22q11.2 and green signal from a control probe for the telomeric region of 22q13.3. The deleted chromosome 22 is shown on the right (arrow), with only the green signal from the control 22q13.3 visible. No red signal is seen from the critical region FISH probe on the deleted chromosome 22, as the region of that chromosome 22 corresponding to the critical region 22q11.2 probe is absent. The 22q11.2 microdeletion, usually 3 megabases in size, is too small to be seen using conventional G-banded chromosome analysis.

further abnormality is added after the sex chromosomes. A normal male karyotype is thus 46,XY. A male with non-dysjunctional Down syndrome will have the karyotype 47,XY,+21, an extra unattached chromosome 21. A male with Down syndrome due to a Robertsonian translocation between chromosomes 14 and 21 will have the karyotype 46,XY,t(14;21), and his carrier mother will have a karyotype 45,XX,t(14;21).

A standard laboratory chromosome analysis will be performed on G-banded chromosomes, which will detect many common and less common chromosome abnormalities, and in most cases no further laboratory work is required. However, recombinant DNA technology has allowed new techniques for chromosome analysis, based on the hybridisation of fluorescently labelled fragments of DNA to the DNA of chromosomes, prepared in a standard fashion, immobilised on a glass slide. The slides can then be visualised by eye using a fluorescent microscope, or indirectly by generating an image of the hybridisation on computer. This technique is known as fluorescent in situ hybridisation (FISH). The information that can be gained from this technique depends on the origin of the fragments of DNA hybridised to the chromosome preparation. Labelled whole chromosome 'paints', consisting of DNA exclusively from one chromosome, are now commercially available. For example, whole chromosome paints can be used to identify the origin of extra chromosomal material which cannot be identified using G-banding techniques. Whole chromosome paints are also helpful in determining the origin of subtle complex translocations. It is also now technically possible to use a chromosome 21 paint on uncultured cells in interphase, to look for trisomy 21. A cell would show three fluorescent nuclear dots, representing three chromosomes 21, as opposed to two in the normal situation.

Fluorescently labelled small DNA fragments, corresponding to 40–50 kb of DNA from a specific chromosomal region, can also be hybridised to metaphase chromosomes. Chromosomal deletions which cannot be detected within the resolution of conventional cytogenetic analysis can be detected by this FISH method. A normal karyotype will give two hybridisation signals, one from the same part of each chromosome. A karyotype containing a submicroscopic chromosomal deletion involving the segment of the chromosome corresponding to the 50-kb DNA fragment will give only one hybridisation signal. An example would be the submicroscopic deletion of chromosome 22q11 which occurs in most cases of the Di George spectrum (see Chapter 31), which can only be seen by FISH analysis (Fig. 8.9). FISH diagnosis of submicroscopic chromosomal deletions is likely to become available for a variety of specific clinical syndromes.

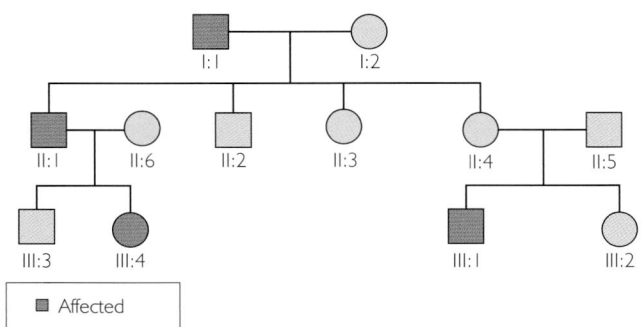

Fig. 8.10 Autosomal dominant inheritance. Note male-to-male transmission and non-penetrance in II:4.

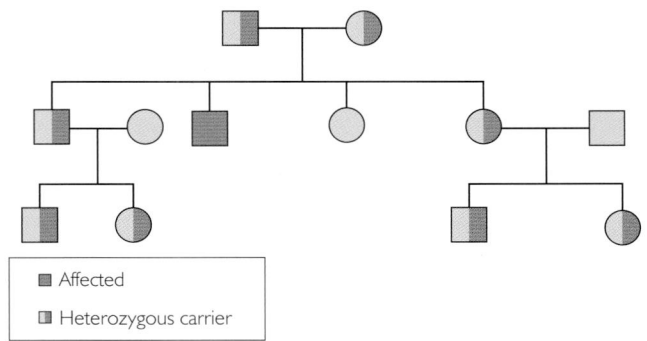

Fig. 8.11 Autosomal recessive inheritance.

Patterns of inheritance

Single gene disorders have one of three principal modes of inheritance: autosomal dominant (AD), autosomal recessive (AR) and X-linked recessive (XLR). Other rare forms of inheritance include X-linked dominant (XLD) and mitochondrial disorders, as well as disorders due to abnormalities of genetic imprinting. Disorders caused by inheritance of unstable elements of DNA are now increasingly being recognised (see below).

Autosomal dominant inheritance

AD disorders are characterised by vertical transmission from parent to child, and the hallmark of these conditions is male-to-male transmission of the disease (Fig. 8.10).

Those affected with an AD disorder have a fault in one or other copy of the two genes responsible for that condition. Each child of a person with an AD disorder has a 50:50 chance of inheriting the gene responsible for the condition from its parent. There are many examples of AD disorders, including neurofibromatosis 1 and 2, familial adenomatous polyposis coli, myotonic dystrophy and Huntington disease. There can often be variability in both expression and penetrance of AD disorders. For example, neurofibromatosis 1, an AD condition, will almost always manifest in someone who has a neurofibromatosis 1 gene fault. This means that the condition has almost complete penetrance. However, different people can manifest the condition in different ways, some showing mild skin lesions and others showing severe intracerebral complications. This means that the expression of the condition is very variable. In contrast, only 80% of those who have a single gene fault for the rare hereditary form of retinoblastoma will actually develop an eye tumour. The penetrance in this situation is 80%, but the expression of the gene fault is consistent, as manifested by a retinoblastoma.

AD disorders are not commonly seen in neonatal practice. A list of the more frequent conditions is outlined in Table 8.2.

Autosomal recessive inheritance

When a child is diagnosed with an AR disorder, then both copies of a particular gene responsible for the condition are faulty. Both the child's parents are therefore carriers for that condition, with one normal and one faulty gene. Two of the child's four grandparents are also carriers, and it is likely that many of the child's relatives are also unknowingly carriers (Fig. 8.11). In most cases, being a carrier for an AR condition has no effect on that person. When both parents are carriers for a fault in the same gene, then there is a 25% chance of each of their children being affected by the condition.

Table 8.2 Autosomal dominant disorders in neonatal practice

SYSTEM AFFECTED	CONDITION
Neurological	Congenital myotonic dystrophy Neurofibromatosis type 1
Ocular	Congenital cataract Retinoblastoma
Haematological	Spherocytosis
Skeletal	Stickler syndrome Craniosynostosis syndromes Achondroplasia Osteogenesis imperfecta
Other	Beckwith–Wiedemann syndrome Noonan syndrome

The risk of a healthy carrier sibling having a child with the same condition depends on the chances of that sibling's partner also being a carrier. A child of a person with an AR disorder will automatically be a carrier. The child's chances of being affected will depend upon whether the child's unaffected parent is a carrier for a fault in the same gene.

AR disorders are commonly encountered in neonatal practice, and the nature of the disorder depends on the population being seen. Each regional population has its own recessive disorder, where the frequency of carriers for that disorder is highest. For instance, cystic fibrosis (CF) is a very common AR disorder in western Europe, whereas sickle-cell anaemia is the commonest AR disorder in West Africa. Common examples of AR conditions include CF, sickle-cell anaemia, several of the mucopolysaccharidoses, beta-thalassaemia, spinal muscular atrophy and congenital adrenal hyperplasia (Table 8.3). Prenatal diagnosis is available for many of these conditions.

X-linked recessive inheritance

In XLR inheritance, the condition affects almost exclusively males; females can be carriers (Fig. 8.12). The classic examples of such conditions are haemophilia A and B, Duchenne's and Becker's muscular dystrophy and Hunter syndrome.

The daughters of a man with an XLR condition are all obligate carriers. The sons of a man with an XLR condition are all normal, as they inherit his Y chromosome and not his X chromosome. When a woman is a carrier of an X-linked condition, each of her

Table 8.3 Autosomal recessive disorders in neonatal practice

SYSTEM AFFECTED	CONDITION
Neurological	Spinal muscular atrophy Congenital myopathies
Ocular	Congenital cataract Congenital glaucoma Albinism
Haematological	Thalassaemia Sickle-cell anaemia
Skeletal	Short-rib polydactyly syndromes Jeune syndrome
Endocrine	Congenital adrenal hyperplasia
Metabolic	Cystic fibrosis Phenylketonuria Galactosaemia α_1-antitrypsin deficiency

Table 8.4 X-linked recessive disorders in neonatal practice

SYSTEM AFFECTED	CONDITION
Neurological	Hunter syndrome
Ocular	Lowe syndrome Ocular albinism
Haematological	Glucose-6-phosphate dehydrogenase deficiency Haemophilia
Skeletal	Amelogenesis imperfecta
Endocrine	Androgen insensitivity syndrome
Metabolic	Adrenoleukodystrophy Fabry disease Lesch–Nyhan syndrome Steroid sulphatase deficiency

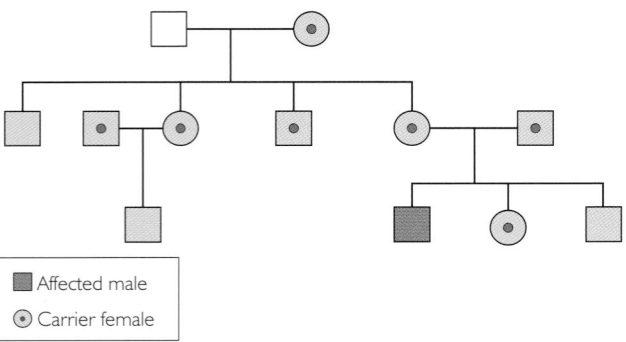

■ Affected male
⊙ Carrier female

Fig. 8.12 X-linked recessive inheritance.

sons has a 50:50 chance of being affected and each of her daughters has a 50:50 chance of being a carrier. There can be a relatively high mutation rate for some XLR conditions, and affected boys may not have a family history of the condition. About one-third of occurrences of Duchenne's muscular dystrophy are as a result of new mutations. Prenatal diagnosis is available for a wide range of XLR diseases. The more common X-linked disorders in neonatal practice are shown in Table 8.4.

Polygenic inheritance

Many congenital conditions do not have a clear mode of inheritance and can be classed as polygenic or oligogenic, where a disease may arise as a result of the effects of several genes. A good example is cleft lip and palate, which usually occurs in the absence of a family history. However, monozygotic twins have a high concordance for cleft palate, suggesting a genetic influence.

Other forms of inheritance

There are also much rarer forms of inheritance, including XLD, which can be hard to distinguish from AD, except that females will

be more mildly affected and there is no male-to-male transmission. An example of an XLD condition is hypophosphataemic rickets.

Mitochondrially inherited diseases show a very unusual pattern of inheritance. Most of the proteins in the mitochondria are encoded for by nuclear genes, but the mitochondria also contain their own small genome of 18 kb, with many copies per cell. The mitochondrial genome replicates independently and far more frequently than the nuclear genome. Several important mitochondrial proteins are encoded by the mitochondrial genome. Mitochondria are only inherited via oocytes, and not sperm. Therefore, when a gene fault is in the mitochondrial genome it will pass exclusively down the female line, but both males and females can be affected. The children of an affected male will not inherit his mitochondrial gene fault. Children with mitochondrial disorders can present with many varied symptoms, including myoclonic seizures, acute acidoses, muscle weakness, deafness or diabetes. A number of mutations or deletions in the mitochondrial genome have been described in patients with a wide variety of conditions, including myoclonic epilepsy with lactic acidosis and stroke-like episodes (MELAS) and myoclonic epilepsy with ragged red fibres on muscle biopsy (MERRF). To complicate matters further, Leber's hereditary ophthalmopathy is a mitochondrially inherited condition with a characteristic mitochondrial mutation, but the expression appears to have an XLR influence.

Some conditions show a phenomenon known as genetic imprinting. An imprinted gene has been marked during meiosis, to indicate the parent from whom it comes. For some genes it appears to be important not only to inherit two copies of that gene, but also to inherit one from each parent. Some genes may be silenced, depending upon which parent has passed on that gene. A good example is the presence of a small deletion of chromosome 15q, which has a different effect depending upon which chromosome 15 is deleted. If the deletion occurs on the chromosome inherited from a child's normal father, the child will develop Prader–Willi syndrome. If the deletion occurs on the chromosome inherited from a child's normal mother, the child will develop a completely different clinical condition, Angelman syndrome. The genes in this area of chromosome 15 are therefore imprinted. In addition, if a child has two maternal copies of chromosome 15 (maternal disomy), but no paternal copy, he or she will also develop Prader–Willi syndrome. Other conditions that show imprinting effects include Russell–Silver syndrome, Beckwith–Wiedemann syndrome and the rare condition of transient neonatal diabetes mellitus.

A new molecular mechanism for genetic disease has been described – that of inherited unstable triplet repeat expansions. At least nine different conditions are caused by this phenomenon. In one of these conditions, a normal person has a stable number of a repetitive element of three bases of DNA (for example, 20 copies of a CAG repeat) in a particular gene, that gene functions normally, and the children of that person have the same number of repeats in their gene. An affected person has an increased number of repeats (say 100 copies) in that gene, and the affected children of that person have more serious disease, with perhaps 200 repeats in the gene. The molecular genetic findings appear to be the genetic correlate of the phenomenon of anticipation, where a condition appears to worsen from generation to generation. The most extreme example is that of congenital myotonic dystrophy, where a minimally affected mother can have a profoundly affected infant. In this case, there is a small repeat expansion of, say, 150 repeats in the mother, increasing to many hundreds of repeats in her affected infant.

This molecular mechanism is responsible for fragile X syndrome, Huntington disease, Friedreich's ataxia, several forms of spinocerebellar ataxia, and probably several more conditions.

Molecular genetic analysis for single gene disorders

Laboratory tests for single gene disorders have been available for a considerable time. Haemoglobin electrophoresis for sickle-cell anaemia and thalassaemia, and enzyme assays for Tay–Sachs disease, are very effective in resolving clinical issues in individual families. However, an increasing number of specific DNA-based tests can now be used in the diagnosis and prediction of single gene disorders.

The two major techniques used in molecular genetic analysis are the polymerase chain reaction (PCR) and Southern blotting. PCR is a technique which allows amplification of a specific genetic region in large quantities from a small amount of DNA template (Fig. 8.13). The DNA sequence of the region to be amplified must be known, so that synthetic pieces of single-stranded DNA (oligonucleotide primers) corresponding to the region can be designed and manufactured. The oligonucleotide primers are added in great excess to the DNA template, along with a thermostable DNA polymerase, and free nucleotides (A, C, T, G). The mixture is heated up to cause the two strands of template DNA to separate, and then cooled. As the DNA cools, the oligonucleotides bind to the template sequence and are extended by the polymerase. A new copy of the template DNA is thus produced. The cycle is repeated 30–40 times, with an exponential increase in the amount of the target sequence.

DNA generated by PCR can be used in many different ways to detect an abnormality in the sequence. If a known genetic abnormality is being sought, then specific PCR assays for mutations have been developed, such as the amplification-resistant mutation system (ARMS) test or the use of a specific DNA restriction enzyme which recognises a known mutant DNA sequence. In searching for an unknown mutation in a PCR product, the PCR-generated product is analysed on a semiautomated fluorescent DNA analyser, read up 600–700 basepairs of DNA sequence in the PCR product. If a pathogenic DNA mutation is found, then the test can help to confirm a clinical diagnosis.

Southern blotting is a more protracted procedure involving the digestion of a relatively large amount of DNA by a restriction

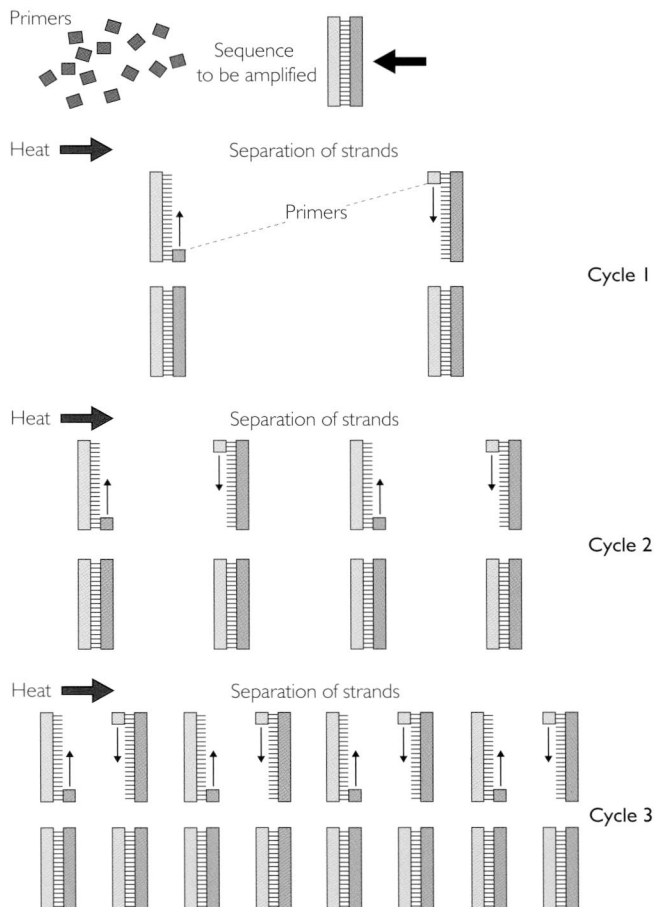

Fig. 8.13 Polymerase chain reaction.

enzyme. The digested DNA is then electrophoresed through an agarose gel, giving a smear of DNA of different sizes. The DNA is then transferred (blotted) and fixed to a membrane. The fixed DNA is then hybridised to a labelled DNA probe specific for the gene to be analysed, and the specific sizes of DNA to which the probe binds allows determination of the genotype (Fig. 8.14). This test is often superseded by PCR technology.

There are different degrees to which molecular genetic tests can contribute to clinical diagnosis. Some specific molecular genetic tests can be used to detect a known pathogenic DNA mutation and give a diagnosis, even without any knowledge of the patient's clinical status. For instance, the PCR detection of the F508del deletion in both copies of a person's CF (*CFTR*) gene immediately gives a diagnosis of CF. Such direct mutation tests are possible when both the gene responsible for a condition has been isolated and specific pathogenic mutations have been identified. Similarly, a PCR test detects a deletion of exons 7 and 8 in both alleles of a gene called *SMN* on chromosome 5q in almost all children with spinal muscular atrophy. Southern blot analysis of DNA from infants with congenital myotonic dystrophy shows a very large expansion in a triplet repeat DNA sequence in the myotonin kinase gene on chromosome 19, as described earlier.

In other cases, molecular genetic diagnosis can point towards a diagnosis without confirming it. For instance, the presence of a single F508del *CFTR* gene mutation in a child with a history suggestive of CF increases the likelihood of that child being affected.

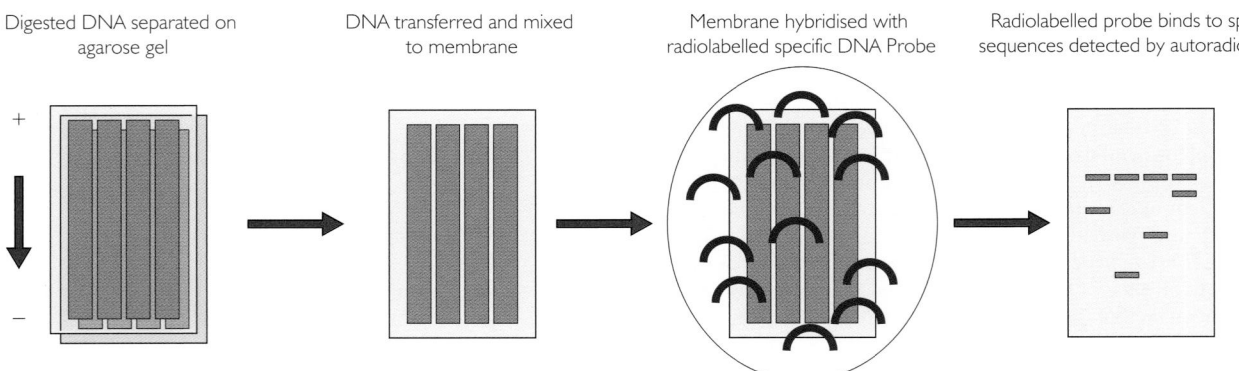

Digested DNA separated on agarose gel

DNA transferred and mixed to membrane

Membrane hybridised with radiolabelled specific DNA Probe

Radiolabelled probe binds to specific sequences detected by autoradiography

Fig. 8.14 Southern blotting and hybridisation.

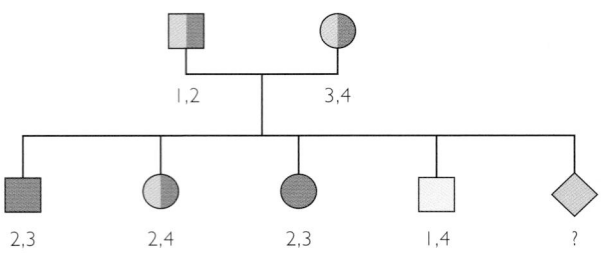

Fig. 8.15 Linkage analysis in an autosomal recessive disorder, using an intragenic polymorphic marker. Alleles 2 and 3 are associated with a gene mutation and can be used to predict the status of another sibling.

In some cases, where either a gene is not known or very few gene mutations have been identified in a known gene, gene-tracking studies can be performed in a family to predict whether a person in that family is affected. This is known as linkage analysis. Such a study requires careful clinical examination of several family members, to establish whether they are affected or unaffected. When their clinical status is clear, DNA samples are then obtained.

Gene-tracking analysis in the family uses the property of normal variations in a gene between different people. Some genetic areas show wide variation between individuals, and a DNA marker from such an area, which can detect many variations, is described as being polymorphic. Each variant of a polymorphic marker is known as an allele. There are now thousands of polymorphic markers covering most of the human genome, and such markers can be found very close to most known genes. There are several types of polymorphic DNA markers, including those characterised by different numbers of specific DNA-cutting enzyme recognition sites, or restriction fragment length polymorphisms. Other markers detect the variation in number of anonymous elements of repetitive DNA, and are called microsatellites or minisatellites.

If the two alleles of a polymorphic marker can be distinguished, to discriminate between the two copies of that particular chromosome from where the marker comes, then the marker is informative in that individual. When a gene location is known, but the actual gene has yet to be found, the alleles of informative markers lying either side of the gene will be inherited along with each copy of the gene in question. This can be used to predict a child's clinical status.

If one set of alleles is found in the affected members of the family but not in the unaffected, then the presence or absence of these alleles in the at-risk individual can be used to predict their chances of being affected. An example of linkage analysis for an AR disorder is shown in Figure 8.15. This form of linkage analysis is often used in families with XLR conditions such as Duchenne's muscular dystrophy, to predict whether a woman is a carrier. Such linkage analysis can also be used in prenatal diagnosis.

Because of its nature, linkage analysis is more prone to error than is direct mutation testing. This can be due to difficulties in assessing a person's clinical status, and because of the possibility of recombination between the polymorphic markers. However, with the rapid advances in molecular genetics, many more mutations are being found in many different genes, and linkage analysis is often superseded by direct mutation testing.

New diagnostic genetic technology

There are two new forms of genetic analysis which are being introduced into widespread clinical practice in the next 3–5 years.

Genomic arrays

A new technological development is the ability to immobilise thousands and, more recently, millions of distinct recognisable pieces of DNA on slides of silicone or glass as ordered microarrays, colloquially known as DNA microchips. This genomic array technology can permit analysis of thousands of individual loci simultaneously, and gives chromosome analysis at a resolution at least 100 times greater than conventional G-banded chromosome analysis. Genomic array technology will identify pathogenic chromosomal anomalies in 20–25% of infants in whom no underlying diagnosis had been identified previously. There is a drawback, in that genomic array technology will often find genetic variants of unknown significance, and the current understanding of the role of such variants in disease pathogenesis is limited.

Next generation DNA sequencing

Present DNA sequencing technology allows analysis of several thousand DNA bases over a period of weeks. New short oligonucleotide DNA sequencing technology, called collectively next generation sequencing, can now permit the analysis of millions of DNA bases over a much shorter period of time. With this technology many genes can be analysed in a short clinically relevant period of time at reasonable cost. Thus in children with specific sets of malformations, direct sequencing of multiple genes in a short period of time will soon be available to provide rapid clinical information for clinicians and families.

Glossary

Glossary

Further reading

Tobias, E., Connor, J.M., Ferguson-Smith, M.A., 2011. Essential medical genetics, sixth ed. Wiley-Blackwell, Oxford.

Lewin, B., 2007. Genes IX. Jones & Bartlett Publishers Inc., U.S.

Strachan, T., Read, A.P., 2010. Human molecular genetics, fourth ed. Garland Science.

Online Mendelian Inheritance in Man. A list of genetic disorders and the latest genetic developments for each condition.

Website http://www.ncbi.nlm.nih.gov/omim

Gene reviews – a website of disease specific expert clinical and genetic reviews. http://www.ncbi.nlm.nih.gov/books/NBK1116/

Glossary

3′ distal end of a gene, as indicated by the bond at the third hydroxyl group of the deoxyribose sugar

5′ proximal end of a gene, as indicated by the bond at the fifth hydroxyl group of the deoxyribose sugar

acrocentric a chromosome with effectively only a long arm – chromosomes 13, 14, 15, 21 and 22

allele a genetic variation of a gene or DNA marker

aneuploidy an excess or deficiency of chromosomal material

anticodon an element of transfer RNA which binds a specific amino acid

autosomal dominant inheritance pattern characterised by transmission through several generations, male-to-male transmission and a 50:50 risk to the children of an affected person

autosomal recessive inheritance pattern characterised by several affected members of the same generation, with carrier parents and a 1:4 recurrence risk where both parents are carriers

basepair unit of double-stranded DNA

centromere element of chromosome involved in chromosome replication, found as a constriction in the chromosome

chromatid condensed chromosome found just before mitosis

codon 3-bp element of DNA encoding an amino acid

diploid a complement of two copies of each chromosome per cell

DNA marker a piece of DNA corresponding to a specific gene or chromosomal segment

enhancers elements of DNA which are involved in increasing gene transcription

exon a part of a gene which is transcribed into mRNA

expression the way in which a gene fault manifests clinically

FISH fluorescent in situ hybridisation, a powerful technique for studying specific chromosomes or regions of chromosomes

gamete a germ cell – sperm or oocyte

genetic imprinting the marking of a gene according to which parent has passed that gene to the child

haploid a complement of one copy of each chromosome per cell (as in sperm or oocyte)

haplotype a pattern of alleles of DNA markers representing one of the two copies of a chromosomal region

histone a DNA-binding protein important in chromosomal folding

interphase phase of mitosis in which the chromosomes are very elongated

intron the part of a gene between the exons which is not transcribed into mRNA

isochromosome an abnormal chromosome made up of two long or two short arms of a normal chromosome

karyotype an analysis of the chromosome complement of a cell type

linkage analysis the use of polymorphic DNA markers to perform gene-tracking studies within a family

meiosis the process of cell division to give haploid germ cells

metaphase phase of mitosis in which the chromosomes are very condensed and easier to analyse

microsatellite marker a DNA marker which detects variation in number of an anonymous small repetitive element of DNA

minisatellite marker a DNA marker which detects variation in number of an anonymous medium repetitive element of DNA

mitosis the normal process of cell division to give two diploid copies of a cell

non-dysjunction a failure of meiosis, giving two copies of a chromosome in one gamete and no copy of a chromosome in the other gamete

nucleosome the combination of a histone and its bound DNA

oligonucleotide primers small lengths of synthetic single-stranded DNA of a specific sequence

paracentric inversion a rearrangement of chromosomal material within one arm of a chromosome

PCR polymerase chain reaction: a method of generating large amounts of specific DNA from a small amount of target sequence

penetrance the number of people known to carry a gene mutation who manifest the condition

pericentric inversion a rearrangement of chromosomal material around the centromere of a chromosome

promoter element of a gene which is necessary to activate gene transcription

prophase phase of the cell cycle where condensation of the chromosomes occurs, just before metaphase

reciprocal translocation exchange of chromosomal segments between different chromosomes

restriction enzyme an enzyme which cuts double-stranded DNA at a specific unique short DNA sequence

restriction fragment length polymorphism a genetic variation between two copies of the same gene, where one gene may have one copy of a restriction enzyme recognition site, and the other two. This variation can be detected using PCR or Southern blotting

ribosome area of the cell where mRNA is converted into protein

ring chromosome an abnormal chromosome where the tips of the long and short arms have fused

Robertsonian translocation a fusion of two acrocentric chromosomes

Southern blotting a process of immobilising DNA to nylon membrane for genetic analysis

suppressor a DNA element which reduces the expression of a gene

telomere the end of a chromosome

telophase the last phase of mitosis

transcription the process of converting DNA into mRNA

translation the production of protein from a DNA sequence

triploidy three of each chromosome, i.e. 69 chromosomes in humans

trisomy one extra chromosome, i.e. 47 chromosomes in humans

X-linked recessive inheritance characterized by affected males in several generations, and by female carriers

Antenatal diagnosis and fetal medicine

Dharmintra Pasupathy   Mark Denbow   Phillipa Kyle

© 2012 Elsevier Ltd

Introduction

The field of prenatal diagnosis and fetal medicine continues to advance at a rapid pace. Improved ultrasound imaging has enhanced the detection of fetal anomaly, and the use of other modalities, such as magnetic resonance imaging (MRI), has allowed further detailed assessment, especially of the central nervous system (CNS).

The drive for early detection of pregnancies at increased risk of aneuploidy continues, with first-trimester combined biochemical and ultrasound assessment now generally available. Molecular technologies continue to be refined, with the most notable advance being the accurate identification of free fetal deoxyribonucleic acid (DNA/RNA) in the maternal circulation, allowing non-invasive determination of fetal rhesus (Rh) status and the potential for genetic diagnoses.

The shift away from invasive procedures to assess fetal well-being continues. Fetal anaemia now is recognised by alterations in middle cerebral artery (MCA) blood flow velocity, and analysis of both the arterial and venous sides of the circulation allows improved accuracy of optimal timing of delivery in cases of fetal growth restriction (FGR).

The complications of monochorionic twin pregnancies contribute significantly to the workload of a modern fetal medicine unit. The dilemmas in management in cases of discordant fetal anomaly, and the transfusional complications, including twin-to-twin transfusion syndrome (TTTS), have led to the development of several techniques that enable the relatively safe occlusion of interfetal blood flow.

Fetal surgery continues to be developed. Most units have shifted their emphasis away from open techniques, where maternal complications are common, to endoscopic procedures, with most attention currently being directed towards the repair of neural tube defects (NTDs) and congenital diaphragmatic hernis (fetoscopic endotracheal occlusion (FETO) procedure).

Fetal physiology

Our understanding of fetal physiology has for years been based on indirect sources. Observations in preterm neonates were first assumed to apply to the fetus of comparable gestation, and then extrapolated back to the mid-trimester. Non-invasive techniques such as cardiotocography (CTG), ultrasound and Doppler have provided information on fetal circulation, growth and behaviour. Amniotic fluid, being largely dependent on fetal urination, has been the traditional source for information about fetal biochemistry and endocrinology (Dallaire and Portier 1986). Access to the fetal circulation in the 1980s allowed fetal haematology and biochemistry

to be evaluated directly in utero. Knowledge of normal values in the mid-trimester fetus is essential in the prenatal diagnosis of several fetal diseases and forms the basis for more effective treatment of maternal alloimmunisation and better management of growth retardation, and is a prerequisite for other diagnostic and therapeutic approaches in the fetus. The main topics of clinical interest are summarised below, although more detailed listings are available elsewhere (Rodeck and Nicolini 1988).

Haematology

Haemoglobin (Hb), packed cell volume (PCV) and red cell mass increase, while mean corpuscular volume (MCV), reticulocytes and nucleated red blood cells (RBCs) decrease significantly with gestation (Millar et al. 1985; Forestier et al. 1986), reflecting the increase in fetal haemopoietic tissue, and the progressive change from hepatic to myeloid erythropoiesis. The normal range for Hb increases from 9–13 g/dl at 17 weeks to 13–18 g/dl at term (Nicolaides et al. 1988b), as does haematocrit, from 29–42% at 18 weeks to 35–48% at 30 weeks (Forestier et al. 1986). The myeloid series does not change with gestation, nor do platelets, which normally exceed 150×10^9/l. Normal ranges are available for coagulation factors, which are reduced compared with the adult (Mibashan and Rodeck 1984).

Acid–base balance

In normal pregnancies, pH changes with gestational age, and ranges in the umbilical vein from 7.32 to 7.44. On the other hand, P_{O_2} decreases with gestational age, whereas P_{CO_2} and bicarbonate rise. The decrease in fetal P_{O_2} is compensated for by the rise in fetal Hb, so that total oxygen content remains unchanged at 6–7 mmol/l. Normal ranges have been established for both umbilical venous and arterial samples (Fig. 9.1) (Nicolaides et al. 1989).

Cardiovascular physiology

Mean umbilical venous pressure is 4–5 mmHg between 20 and 33 weeks' gestation (Nicolini et al. 1989e). Blood volume has been measured in vivo, on the basis of the change in fetal haematocrit produced by transfusion of a known quantity of red cells. Fetoplacental blood volume rises from 25 ml at 18 weeks to 150 ml at 31 weeks, but during the same interval it decreases when expressed as a function of fetal weight, from 117 to 93 ml/kg (Nicolaides et al. 1987b).

Biochemistry

Reference ranges are available for electrolytes and biochemical indices of renal, hepatic and bone function (Moniz et al. 1985; Forestier et al. 1987). Fetal sodium and potassium are the same as maternal levels. Fetal glucose levels are lower than in the mother, and their maternofetal gradients have been used as an index of placental transfer (Nicolini et al. 1989b). Bilirubin is three times higher in the mid-trimester fetus than in the mother, but albumin levels are considerably lower, with values rising from 16 g/l at 15 weeks to 40 g/l at term (Moniz et al. 1985).

Renal function

Urea and creatinine levels in utero reflect the excretory function of the placenta and not that of the kidneys. Urinary sodium and phosphate decrease and creatinine increases with gestational age, consistent with progressive maturation of tubular function and an

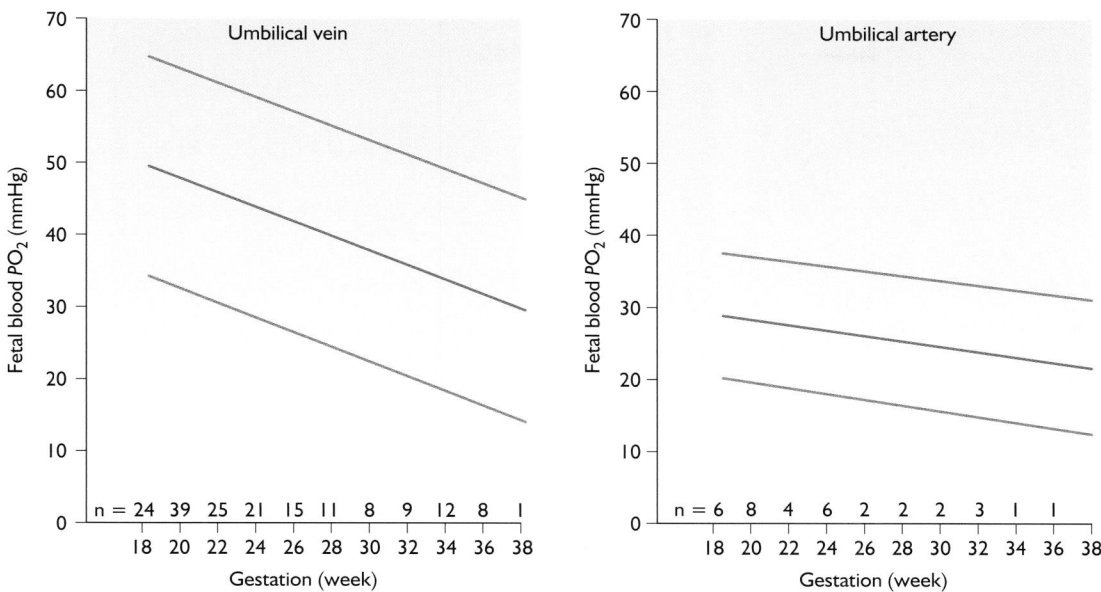

Fig. 9.1 Reference range (mean and 95% data intervals) for Po_2 in umbilical venous and arterial blood throughout gestation. *(Reproduced from Nicolaides et al. (1989).)*

increase in glomerular filtration rate. Potassium and urea, however, do not change, suggesting that the changes in tubular reabsorption occur simultaneously with those in tubular secretion and glomerular filtration. Reference ranges related to gestation are used in the assessment of renal function in fetuses with obstructive uropathies (Nicolini et al. 1992).

Fetal pain

This is a complex area but is of importance with the increasing number of in utero (and often in feto) interventions being developed in the field of fetal medicine/surgery. It is clear that the fetus mounts a stress response to painful stimuli from 18 weeks (Giannakaulopoulos et al. 1994, 1999; Teixeira et al. 1996, 1999), but whether this is perceived as pain is uncertain. Neurons first link the cortex with the rest of the brain at 16 weeks, and their activation might be associated with an unpleasant experience, if not pain itself. By 26 weeks, the system for nociception is present and functioning (Kostovic and Rakic 1990) and it seems likely that the fetus can feel pain from this stage. This evidence leads to the consideration of fetal analgesia for invasive procedures during the second and third trimesters. However, the challenge remains selecting the safest and most effective type and route of analgesic drug without increasing maternal or fetal risks.

Antenatal diagnosis

Ultrasound

Ultrasound is the chief method for detecting structural abnormalities. Since the first report of detection of a fetal anomaly leading to termination of pregnancy (Campbell et al. 1972), a wide range of major malformations have been detected. With advances in ultrasound imaging, the appearances of an increasing number of minor malformations have now been described.

The standard of ultrasound achieved in practice has continued to improve dramatically and is available to an increasing proportion of the population. Routine ultrasound screening is recommended in the UK (Royal College of Obstetricians and Gynaecologists 1984). This examination is delayed until 18–20 weeks, when cardiac and renal structure becomes discernible. Routine screening detects 60–80% of major and 35% of minor congenital malformations (Levi et al. 1989; Chitty et al. 1991; Luck 1992), in contrast to the 25% detected (Hegge et al. 1989) under the indication-based system favoured in the USA (National Institutes for Health 1984).

Only the main areas of ultrasound diagnoses are summarised below; exhaustive listings are available elsewhere (Reznikoff-Etievant 1988; Whittle and Connor 1994).

Neural tube defects (Ch. 40.8)

The diagnosis of anencephaly is straightforward: the cranial vault cannot be visualised in the standard view for biparietal diameter measurement. Detection of open myelomeningocele is more complex. Although larger defects may be suggested by gross disruption in vertebral integrity in the longitudinal plane or by soft-tissue signs, smaller defects will only be apparent in the horizontal planes of a few localised vertebrae, as subtle splaying in the lateral processes. These views can be difficult to obtain, especially if the fetal spine lies against the uterine wall, and in this context screening has been greatly facilitated by two cranial signs found in almost all fetuses with myelomeningocele. Scalloping of the frontal bones gives the head a lemon-shaped appearance ('lemon' sign), whereas the normally dumbbell-shaped cerebellum appears either absent or banana-shaped ('banana' sign: Fig. 9.2) (Nicolaides et al. 1986a; Furness et al. 1987; Pilu et al. 1988). The latter results from downward herniation of posterior fossa contents, and the former from the subsequent reduction in intracranial volume.

Ultrasound screening using the lemon and banana signs should theoretically detect 96–100% of myelomeningoceles (Campbell et al. 1987; Van den Hof et al. 1990). Ultrasound features such as head circumference greater than the 90th percentile and lesions at L3 and above have been been demonstrated in multivariate analysis to be independently associated with lower rates of survival in children born with spina bifida (Van Der Vossen et al. 2009). In a

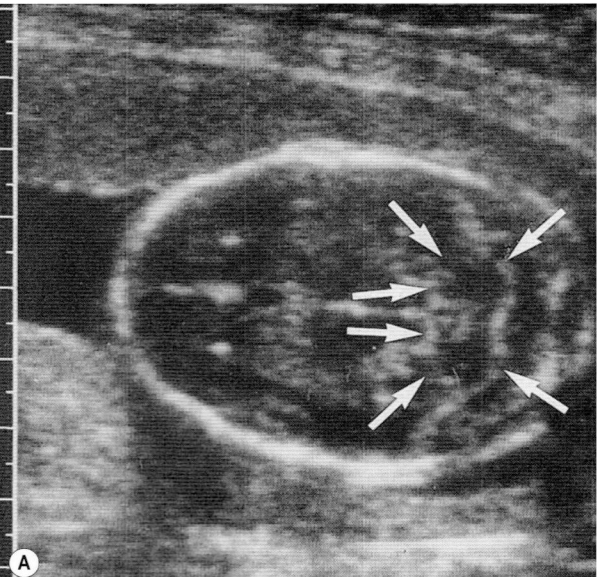 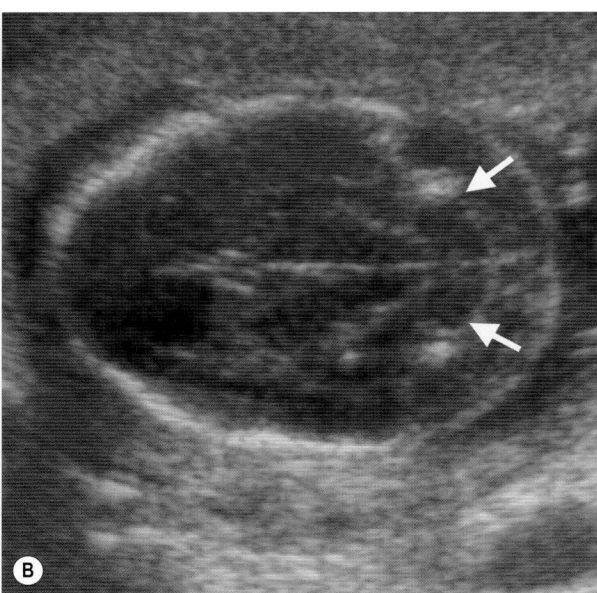

Fig. 9.2 (A) The normal dumbbell shape of the cerebellum (arrows) on ultrasound at 18 weeks. (B) Anterior curvature of the cerebellum, the 'banana' sign (arrows), in a fetus of similar gestation with open spina bifida.

long-term follow-up study of an unselected cohort of infants born with spina bifida between 1963 and 1971, by the mean age of 30 years the survival rate was approximately 50%. Only one-third of the survivors lived independently, with up to a third requiring daily care. Sensory levels recorded at infancy were correlated with rates of mortality and morbidity, with higher sensory levels associated with poorer outcome (Hunt and Oakeshott 2003; Oakeshott and Hunt 2003). See Chapter 40 part 8 for more information on neonatal aspects of spina bifida.

It is important to recognise that ultrasound is both a screening and a diagnostic test, and that small spinal lesions in fetuses with suspicious cranial signs on screening may only be detected on detailed scanning by a very experienced operator, and that the antenatal prediction of the level of the lesion may not always correspond to that found after birth. In cases of genuine uncertainty, an elevated amniotic fluid concentration of acetylcholinesterase may also be measured to confirm the presence of an open NTD (Loft et al. 1993).

Other craniospinal malformations

Ventriculomegaly is diagnosed in utero by elevated ratios of various measurements of the lateral ventricle to hemispheric width in the transverse plane (Fiske et al. 1981; Campbell and Pearce 1983) or enlargement of the atrium of the posterior horn of the lateral ventricle (Cardoza et al. 1988). Unless there is progressive or gross dilatation, caution should be exercised in the interpretation of mild ventriculomegaly, especially in the mid-trimester. In a recent review of the literature on isolated mild ventriculomegaly, defined as ventricular atrial width of 10.0–15.0 mm, there was no conclusive evidence that the width of the ventricular atria was associated with the risk of neurodevelopmental outcome (Melchiorre et al. 2009). The pooled incidence of neurodevelopmental delay in this review was 11%. Limitations in the current literature include evidence from small retrospective case series and lack of long-term follow-up studies. Important adverse prognostic indicators include progressive ventricular dilatation and other associated abnormalities.

The level of obstruction is determined by examining the third and fourth ventricles and the aqueduct of Sylvius. Hydranencephaly is distinguished from severe hydrocephalus by the absence of midline structures and the lack of a residual cortical rim, but the distinction may be difficult in extreme cases. In holoprosencephaly, the extent of midline ventricular fusion varies with the degree of failure of cleavage of the prosencephalon (Pilu et al. 1987), and there are often concomitant facial anomalies. The diagnosis of microcephaly should only be made in the presence of serial measurements of head circumference 3–4 standard deviations (SD) below the mean, so as to exclude growth retardation or incorrect dating. The ultrasonic appearances of encephalocele, and intracranial cysts, tumours and haemorrhage, are well described. Agenesis of the corpus callosum, increasingly recognised as separation of the lateral ventricles with upward displacement of the third ventricle, is more difficult to diagnose, and is often detected in association with other CNS abnormalities (Sandri et al. 1988).

The diagnosis of posterior fossa abnormalities, and most notably the Dandy–Walker malformation and its variants, is challenging. The classic appearance is of complete or partial agenesis of the cerebellar vermis with a posterior fossa cyst (Fig. 40.90). However, in one series from a tertiary unit in the UK, the correlation with postmortem was only 43% (6/14) for this abnormality (Carroll et al. 2000). This has led to evaluation of fetal MRI for complex neurological abnormalities (see below).

Cardiac defects

Following characterisation of the normal ultrasonic appearances of the fetal heart, a wide range of defects have been diagnosed. Inspection of the four-chamber view in a transverse plane during the routine 18-week scan detects approximately 20–40% of severe congenital heart disease (Fermont et al. 1985; Sharland and Allan 1992). This view is abnormal with major defects such as hypoplastic ventricles, atrioventricular canal defects and tricuspid atresia, although minor lesions such as septal defects may be missed. Visualisation of venoatrial and ventriculoarterial connections is

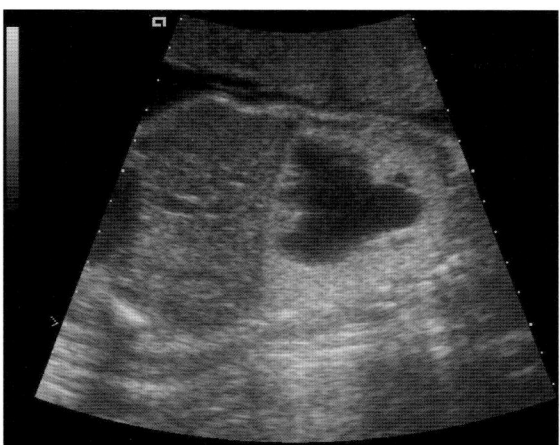

Fig. 9.3 Congenital cystic adenomatous malformation (CCAM) of the lung. A longitudinal view of a large macrocystic CCAM.

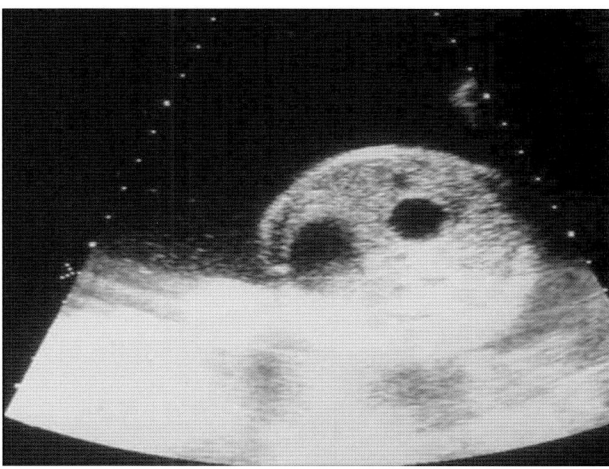

Fig. 9.4 The 'double-bubble' appearance of duodenal atresia.

more complex, but if it were introduced into routine screening it would theoretically increase the detection rate to greater than 80% (Stumpflen et al. 1996). Some cases are missed because of the evolution of the abnormality such that the heart may appear to be normal at the time of screening. The introduction of the five-chamber view, sagittal and parasagittal views has increased the detection rate of outflow tract anomalies (Allan 2004; Gardiner 2006; Jeanty et al. 2008).

Indications for fetal echocardiography include an abnormal four-chamber view or outflow tracts, an affected sibling or parental history, diabetes, exposure to cardiac teratogens, raised nuchal translucency (NT) measurement in a euploid fetus, and monochorionic twin gestations. A high degree of accuracy can then be achieved for diagnosis of major vessel lesions such as pulmonary stenosis, truncus arteriosus and transposition of the great vessels (Davis et al. 1990). Colour flow Doppler facilitates the demonstration of cardiac structure, and M-mode and pulsed-wave Doppler provide an index of cardiac function, which is particularly useful in arrhythmias.

Intrathoracic defects (for neonatal surgical management, see Ch. 29.4)

Most intrathoracic lesions identified prenatally are benign, but their significance is the association with pulmonary hypoplasia. Indirect indices of the severity of compression on the developing lung are the degree of mediastinal shift, the presence of polyhydramnios due to limited swallowing, and hydrops secondary to obstructed venous return. Left-sided diaphragmatic hernias are detected on ultrasound because of displacement of the heart to the right, fluid-filled bowel within the chest, and absence of the stomach intra-abdominally (Chinn et al. 1983; Nakayama et al. 1985). As herniated liver has the same echotexture as the lung, right-sided lesions are more difficult to detect, especially in the absence of polyhydramnios or pleural effusion. Clues include derangement in the normal intra-abdominal course of the gallbladder and intrahepatic vein, although small lesions may go undetected.

The appearances of congenital cystic adenomatoid malformation (CCAM) (now often termed congenital pulmonary airway malformation; Ch. 27.5) of the lung vary from solitary large cysts to solid echogenic lesions, with the worst prognosis (Fig. 9.3) (Adzick 1985a; Stocker et al. 1977; Adziek et al. 1985). The assessment of

prognosis is difficult, although in more recent series it appears good, other than in a small minority (6%), in which both mediastinal shift and hydrops are present (Roelofsen et al. 1994; Barrett et al. 1995). Some disappear, many get smaller, and only a few stay the same or progress. Diagnosis cannot always be certain antenatally, and differentiation between CCAM, sequestrated lung, tracheal or bronchial atresia, and congenital diaphragmatic hernia may be difficult (McCullagh et al. 1994; King et al. 1995). Mediastinal teratomas have features on ultrasound similar to solid type III or microcystic CCAM lesions (Romero et al. 1982).

Gastrointestinal defects (for neonatal surgical management, see Ch. 29.4)

Oesophageal atresia can be diagnosed when polyhydramnios occurs with non-visualisation of the fetal stomach, although these signs may not be present in the common form associated with tracheo-oesophageal fistula (Farrant 1980). Duodenal atresia produces polyhydramnios and a characteristic 'double-bubble' appearance (Fig. 9.4), which may not be apparent until the third trimester (Nelson et al. 1982). Associated anomalies are common in the above two conditions, unlike in more distal obstructions. Small-bowel obstructions are more likely to be associated with increased amniotic fluid volume than are large-bowel obstructions such as anal atresia, which may go undetected in utero. Peristalsis may be seen (Arulkumaran et al. 1990) and bowel perforations may show up as ascites or, more commonly, hyperechogenicity from meconium peritonitis (Blumenthal et al. 1982). Caution must be exercised when gut echogenicity is detected as an isolated finding, as, although this may be associated with cystic fibrosis (Muller et al. 1985) and aneuploidy, the majority occur in normal fetuses (Fakhry et al. 1986). Meconium peritonitis can also produce pseudocysts, the differential diagnosis of which includes gastrointestinal duplications and choledochal, mesenteric and ovarian cysts.

The distinction of exomphalos from gastroschisis is crucial, given the high incidence of cardiac and chromosomal abnormalities in the former (Gilbert and Nicolaides 1987). Aneuploidy seems largely confined to fetuses in which the herniated liver is not present within the exomphalos (Nyberg et al. 1989; Benacerraf et al. 1990). More severe degrees of failure of fusion of the ectomesodermic folds, such as ectopia cordis, ectopia vesicae, pentalogy of Cantrell and the body stalk anomaly, are readily apparent. In contrast, gastroschisis is rarely associated with aneuploidy or genetic conditions. Non-genetic associations include young maternal age, socioeconomic deprivation, ethnicity, maternal smoking, medication (aspirin, ibuprofen, paracetamol and decongestants), illicit drug use and maternal nutritional status (Rasmussen 2008). There are however trends in the incidence of gastroschisis which remain unexplained. These include the increasing incidence of gastroschisis in the UK and the clustered distribution of cases in the population (Tan et al. 1996; Penman et al. 1998). These patterns suggest a clustered exposure to one or more risk factors which are increasing over time (Rasmussen 2008).

Genitourinary defects (for neonatal diagnosis and management, see Ch. 35.2)

Renal and urinary tract abnormalities are common and comparatively easy to detect, largely because obstructive lesions manifest as cystic spaces, whereas those with poor urine output are characterised by oligohydramnios. Major anomalies such as renal agenesis or low obstructive uropathy will be detected on routine scan at 18–20 weeks, when urine output makes a major contribution to amniotic fluid volume, whereas more minor lesions, such as mild ureteropelvic junction obstruction, may not be obvious until later. As the lack of amniotic fluid in renal agenesis significantly impairs the ultrasound picture, it can be extremely difficult to demonstrate the absence of kidneys in the renal fossae. In these circumstances, referral for confirmation by transvaginal ultrasound and/or amnio-infusion has been recommended (Fisk et al. 1991). However, colour flow Doppler imaging of the renal arteries may be adequate to provide the diagnosis: the absence of renal artery colour image confirms no functioning tissue (Sepulveda et al. 1995).

Multicystic kidneys are distinguished from hydronephrotic kidneys by their cystic spaces being more peripheral and variable in size, and their stroma more central (Fig. 9.5) (Beretsky et al. 1984). The cysts of infantile polycystic kidneys are too small to be resolved by ultrasound, but the kidneys appear enlarged with abnormal echogenicity, associated with oligohydramnios. Occasionally with later-onset infantile polycystic kidney disease the kidneys may appear normal in utero (Romero et al. 1984).

The significance of mild pelvicalyceal dilatation remains controversial. Studies show that progressive enlargement, or an anteroposterior diameter of >10 mm in the third trimester, is more likely to be associated with pathology (Ouzounian et al. 1996). The

ultrasound picture in low obstructive uropathy depends on the severity and duration of obstruction. The bladder is variably enlarged and thick-walled, and careful scanning reveals dilatation of the upper urethra in those with posterior urethral valves (PUVs) (Hobbins et al. 1984). Oligohydramnios, upper tract dilatation and hyperechogenic fetal kidneys may also be present.

Skeletal defects (for neonatal diagnosis and management, see Ch. 31, Ch. 34.4)

Isolated malformations detected on routine scanning include kyphoscoliosis, hemivertebrae, limb reduction and shortening, sacral agenesis, polydactyly and flexion deformities. Over 100 distinct skeletal dysplasias are amenable to prenatal diagnosis, both by serial measurement of long bones and by detection of abnormal skeletal shape or mineralisation. Although severe limb shortening, abnormal head or chest shape, or polyhydramnios may alert the sonologist to their presence, determination of the exact type of skeletal dysplasia is difficult in the absence of a previous history, and requires detailed evaluation of hands and feet, thoracic dimensions, face and cranium, and measurement of all the long bones, before consulting comprehensive tables of diagnostic features (Romero et al. 1988). Even then, diagnosis may only be made postnatally, when additional investigations such as skeletal X-ray are available. In achondrogenesis, thanatophoric and diastrophic dwarfism, severe limb reduction will be obvious by 18 weeks (Filly and Golbus 1982), whereas in the heterozygous form of achondroplasia this may not be observed until almost the third trimester (Filly et al. 1981). If achondroplasia is suspected, amniocentesis can be performed for DNA testing on fibroblasts to detect or exclude the fibroblast growth receptor 3 (FGR-3) mutation known to cause achondroplasia (Bonaventure et al. 1996). Abnormal bone shape is a feature of camptomelic and thanatophoric dysplasia, whereas fractures, callus formation and hypomineralisation may be seen in osteogenesis imperfecta types II–IV (Brons et al. 1988). Hypomineralisation is also seen in hypophosphatasia and achondrogenesis. Radial aplasia may be associated with trisomy 18, but also with rare genetic syndromes such as Fanconi's anaemia and the thrombocytopenia–absent radius syndrome.

Soft-tissue abnormalities

Cleft lip, whether isolated or associated with cleft palate, can be detected by imaging the fetal face in coronal and transverse views (Salvodelli et al. 1982). Rarer midline clefts are often accompanied by other midline defects, such as holoprosencephaly, ethmocephaly or proboscis. The diagnosis of isolated cleft palate is extremely difficult prenatally (Pilu et al. 1986). These lesions are usually only detected on detailed scans of patients who have either other abnormalities or an at-risk history. Isolated unilateral clefts are rarely associated with either aneuploidy or genetic syndromes; however, these risks increase with bilateral clefts and the presence of associated anomalies.

Cystic hygromas are readily apparent as multiseptate thin-walled cystic lesions, found most commonly around the dorsolateral region of the neck (Chervenak et al. 1983). As they result from obstruction of the jugulolymphatic channels (Andres and Brace 1990), hygromas frequently progress in utero to hydrops and fetal demise (Abramowicz et al. 1989), although spontaneous resolution is possible (Chodirker et al. 1988). They have a strong association with aneuploidy (50–80%), and therefore karyotyping is advised. Hydrops is obvious as generalised skin oedema with ascites, and in many cases there will also be pericardial and pleural effusions, placentomegaly and polyhydramnios.

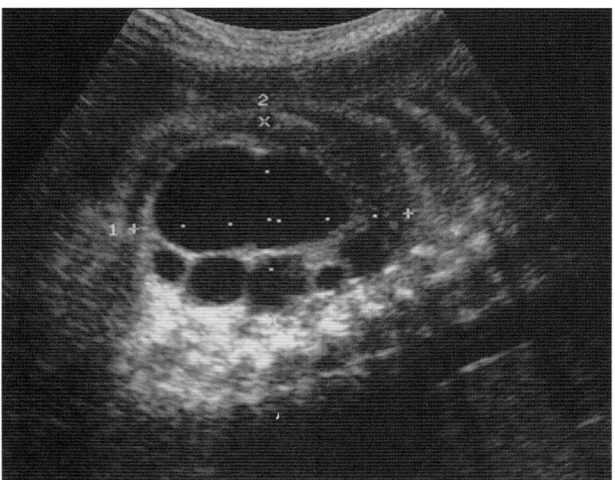

Fig. 9.5 Multicystic kidney disease.

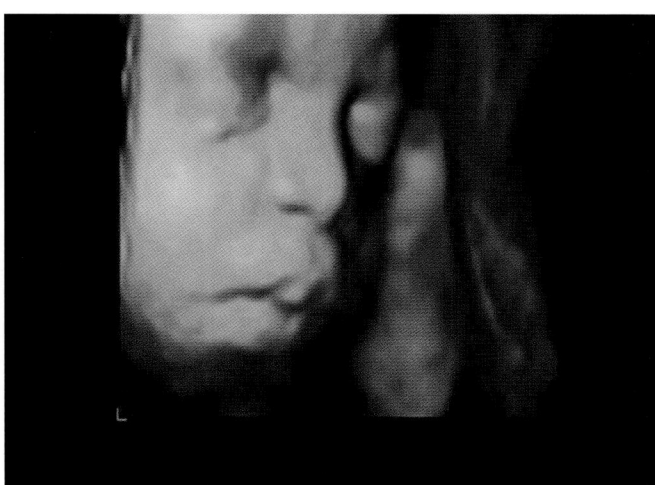

Fig. 9.6 Three-dimensional ultrasound of the face of a fetus with known cardiac abnormality and oesophageal atresia. No dysmorphic facial features were confirmed.

Other imaging modalities

3D/4D ultrasound

The use of three-dimensional (3D) ultrasound in prenatal diagnosis has increased in recent years with the development of computational technologies (Fig. 9.6). In cases of facial anomalies, the use of 3D ultrasound has improved the accuracy of detection of facial clefts (Rotten and Levaillant 2004). In CNS abnormalities, assessment of the corpus callosum is now possible using the C-plane of 3D volumes (VCI) (Fig. 9.7), and simultaneous visualisation with 3D ultrasound may improve the precise location of NTDs.

Transvaginal ultrasound and MRI

The greater resolution provided by high-frequency transvaginal transducers for structures within their 6–7-cm focal zone is ideal for visualisation of the first-trimester fetus.

MRI of the fetus was first described in the 1980s. Recently, faster capture times have helped to counter the problems created by fetal movements (Fig. 9.8). Although MRI has been used to aid the prenatal diagnosis of many conditions, its strength lies in assessing intracranial anatomy, and in particular the posterior fossa. Conditions including agenesis of the corpus callosum are reliably detected by MRI; the recognition of neuronal migration disorders depends on the severity of the disorder and the gestation at which the MRI is made. MRI has a place in prenatal diagnosis, although experience in this form of fetal imaging is still being collected.

Screening strategies for Down syndrome

In the past, standard screening policy was to offer women over the age of 35 years chorionic villus sampling (CVS) or amniocentesis for karyotyping. As only 25–30% of trisomy 21 fetuses are born to 'older' mothers, and as utilisation in this group rarely exceeds 50%, it is hardly surprising that the birth prevalence of Down syndrome fell by only 15% with this strategy (Walker and Howard 1986). Newer policies, which increase detection rates without increasing the numbers undergoing antenatal karyotyping, have been introduced into practice. The UK National Screening Committee (2008) currently recommends a screening test for Down syndrome with a detection rate greater than 75% and a false-positive rate of less than 3%, which is age-standardised and based on a cut-off of 1:250 at term. The committee also recommends that the detection rate is increased to greater than 90% with a false-positive rate of less than 2% from April 2010.

Biochemical

The average maternal serum alpha-fetoprotein (AFP) value in Down syndrome pregnancies is 0.7–0.8 multiples of the median (Wald and Cuckle 1987). As this association is largely independent of maternal age, the two were then combined to give each woman a specific age- and AFP-adjusted risk (Cuckle et al. 1987). Subsequently, raised human chorionic gonadotrophin (hCG) (Bogart et al. 1989), particularly the free β-hCG subunit, and low unconjugated oestriol (Canick et al. 1988) levels were found to be associated with trisomy 21. Again, in the absence of any relation to maternal age or each other, their levels and maternal age were next combined using an algorithm to predict fetal risk (Wald et al. 1988). The reason for these biochemical changes is not yet understood, but is thought to relate to functional immaturity, producing a delay in the normal gestational rise or fall. Cut-offs of 1:250–1:300 have shown a sensitivity of up to 70%, with a false-positive rate of 5%. The term 'false-positive' in this context describes the percentage of the population that would be given a high-risk result if the test were taken up by the entire population. Subsequent refinements using free β-hCG (Nicolaides et al. 2005) and a prior dating scan (Gardosi and Mongelli 1993), and confining the assay to 15–18 weeks' gestation, have increased the accuracy of the test. Additional biochemical measurement of unconjugated oestriol (triple test) and with inhibin (quadruple test) improves the detection rate (Driscoll and Gross 2009). The quadruple test has a sensitivity approaching 80% for trisomy 21 with a fixed false-positive rate of 5% (National Collaborating Centre for Women's and Children's Health 2008). Detection rates are greater in older mothers (i.e. over 35 years of age), but this is at the cost of higher false-positive rates (Haddow et al. 1994).

As biochemical screening takes place in the mid-trimester, it does not allow susceptible women the option of first-trimester CVS for karyotyping. The drive now is to bring screening for aneuploidy into the first and early second trimester, to allow earlier detection and easier termination procedures to be performed.

Ultrasound plus biochemistry in first and second trimesters

There have been major advances in ultrasound screening for aneuploidy. In the first trimester (10–14 weeks) the association between increased NT (Fig. 9.9) and aneuploidy has been confirmed in several studies (Szabo and Gellen 1990; Nicolaides et al. 1994a; Landwehr et al. 1996). The association is with trisomies 21, 18 and 13 in particular. A sensitivity, when related to crown–rump length and maternal age, of almost 80%, with a false-positive rate of 5%, has been reported by one group in a low-risk population cohort of 96 127 (Snijders et al. 1998).

Recently, NT measurement has been combined with two first-trimester biochemical markers to improve the efficacy of early screening for trisomy 21. Levels of free β-hCG are increased in the serum of mothers carrying a fetus with Down syndrome, while levels of pregnancy-associated plasma protein A are decreased. When this test is combined with NT, the combined test yields a detection rate of 90% for a similar false-positive rate (Stenhouse et al. 2004; Nicolaides et al. 2005). The integrated test, which combines first-trimester screening (combined test) with second-trimester

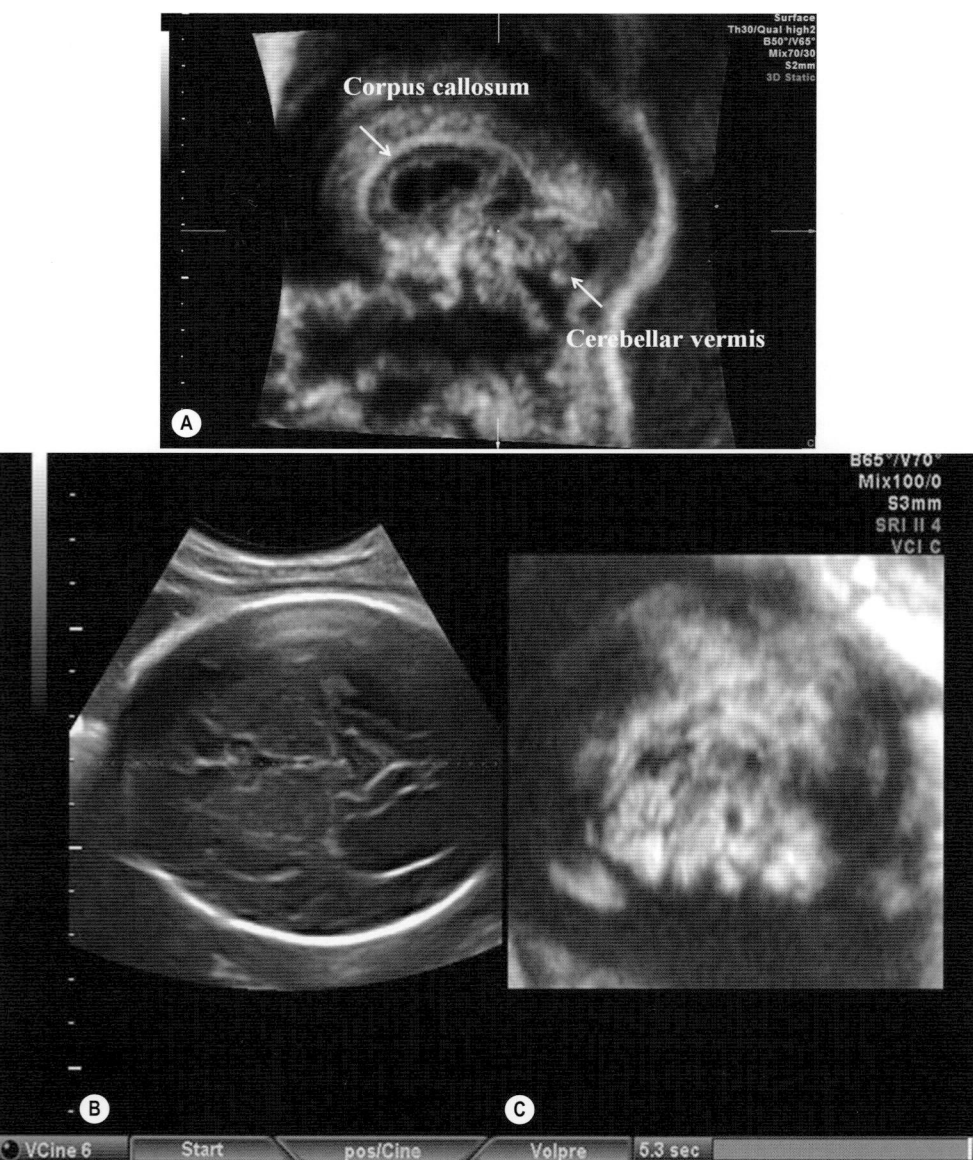

Fig. 9.7 (A) Three dimensional volume contrast imaging (3D VCI) demonstrating the C-plane to visualise the corpus callosum, cerebellum and vermis – only the C-plane image shown. (B and C) 3D VCI showing A-plane image and C-plane volume reconstruction of the sagittal midline view. In this case there was complete agenesis of the corpus callosum, which was confirmed by magnetic resonance imaging.

screening (AFP, oestriol and inhibin), further increases the detection rate of Down syndrome to 95% (Malone et al. 2005).

Recent attention has focused on the relevance of the presence/absence of the fetal nasal bone (Clark et al. 2003). In a series from King's College Hospital, London, UK, the nasal bone was absent in 43 of 59 (73%) trisomy 21 fetuses and in 3 of 603 (0.5%) chromosomally normal fetuses. The likelihood ratio, therefore, for trisomy 21 was 146 (95% confidence interval (CI) 50–434) for absent nasal bone and 0.27 (0.18–0.40) for nasal bone being present. Subsequent work by the same group (Cicero et al. 2003) has shown in a retrospective series that the integration of nasal bone screening into the OSCAR test (One-Stop Clinic for Assessment of Risk) would lead to a detection rate of 97%; alternatively, for a false-positive rate of 0.5%, the detection rate is 90.5%. There is some evidence that the detection rate increases when used in addition to the combined test (Orlandi et al. 2005), although this has not been consistently reproduced by other groups (Kozlowski et al. 2006; National Collaborating Centre for Women's and Children's Health 2008). Additional ultrasound markers to increase the sensitivity and reduce the false-positive rates are also being assessed, including the ductus venosus waveform and triscuspid regurgitation (Kagan et al. 2009; Maiz et al. 2009).

Subtle markers of aneuploidy

With advances in ultrasound resolution, many structures not previously visualised, such as the digits, feet and soft tissues of the neck, can now be demonstrated. Accordingly, the minor malformations and abnormal postures characteristic of aneuploid neonates may be seen in utero. Postaxial polydactyly is found more frequently in

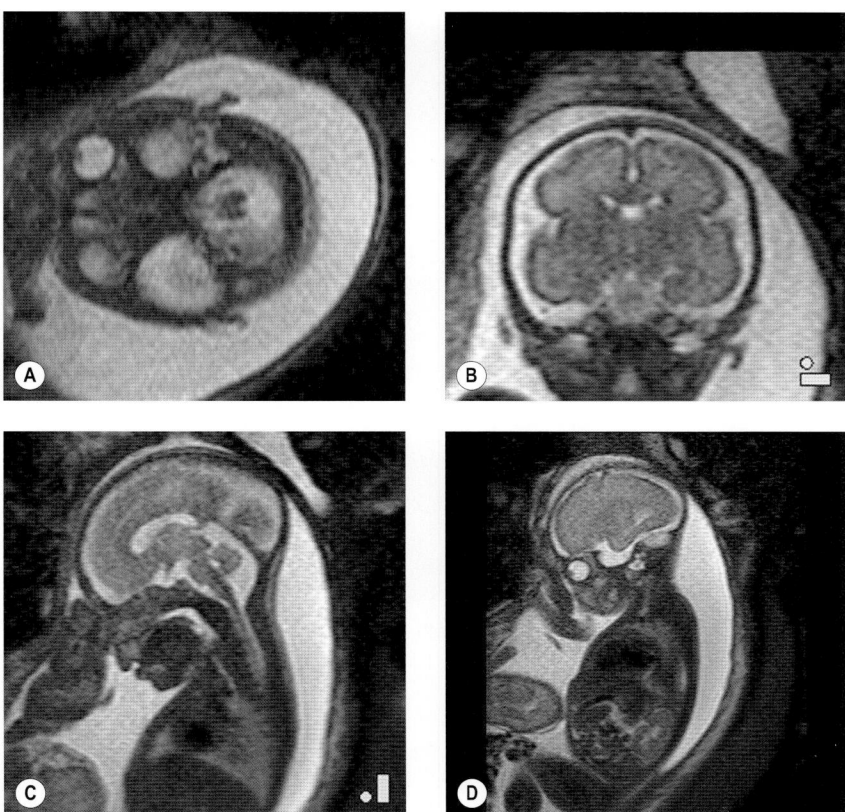

Fig. 9.8 Fetal magnetic resonance imaging. Sagittal view of a normal mid-trimester fetus.

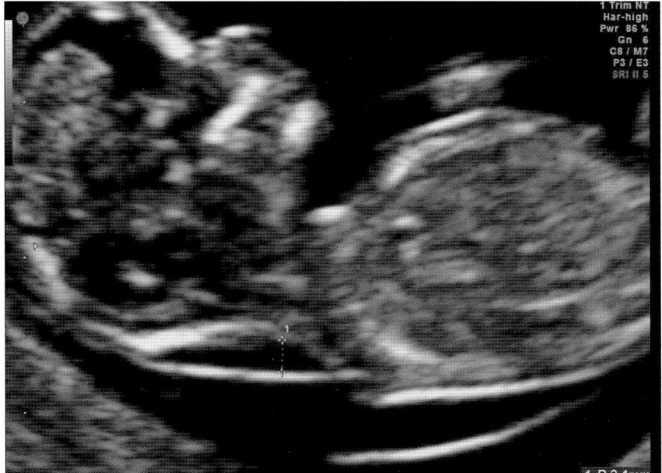

Fig. 9.9 Transabdominal ultrasound view of a nuchal translucency measurement in a fetus at 12 weeks' gestation.

trisomy 13 than in 18, but ventricular septal defects are common in both (Wladimiroff et al. 1989). The profile of the trisomy 18 fetus reveals micrognathia and a protuberant upper lip (Benacerraf et al. 1986a). The hands remain clenched in trisomy 18, with characteristic overlapping of the fingers, and the typical rocker bottom and equinovarus deformity are found in the feet. The sonographic features of trisomy 21 are more elusive. These may include increased nuchal thickness (first or second trimester), mild renal pelvic dilatation, hyperechogenic bowel, brachycephaly and hypoplasia of the middle phalanx of the fifth finger (clinodactyly).

Invasive procedures and prenatal diagnosis

Samples of fetal tissues suitable for karyotyping, biochemical analysis and DNA studies are obtained by CVS and amniocentesis. In many cases the choice of procedure is left to the patient, based on her informed perception of the relative advantages and disadvantages of each. Fetal blood sampling (FBS), a technically more difficult procedure, is performed after 18–20 weeks' gestation, not just for antenatal diagnosis but also for therapy. Each invasive procedure is associated with a small chance of procedure-related loss. In general, therefore, invasive procedures are offered rather than recommended to parents, who, after appropriate counselling, should be given time to consider the various risks of the condition being tested against those of the procedure.

Amniocentesis

Amniocentesis is the commonest invasive procedure for prenatal diagnosis. Most are done at 14–16 weeks' gestation, when the amniotic cavity contains 150–200 ml of fluid, allowing 15–20 ml to be withdrawn without complication (working rule is x ml withdrawn $= x$ weeks in gestation). A 22G needle is inserted transabdominally and guided to a pool under ultrasound control (Fig. 9.10). Simultaneous ultrasound monitoring reduces the number of dry and bloody taps (Romero et al. 1985; de Crespigny and Robinson 1986) and obviates the rare risk of severe fetal trauma. It has thus replaced the older technique of 'semiblind' insertion following ultrasound identification of a pool. Transplacental insertions have been linked

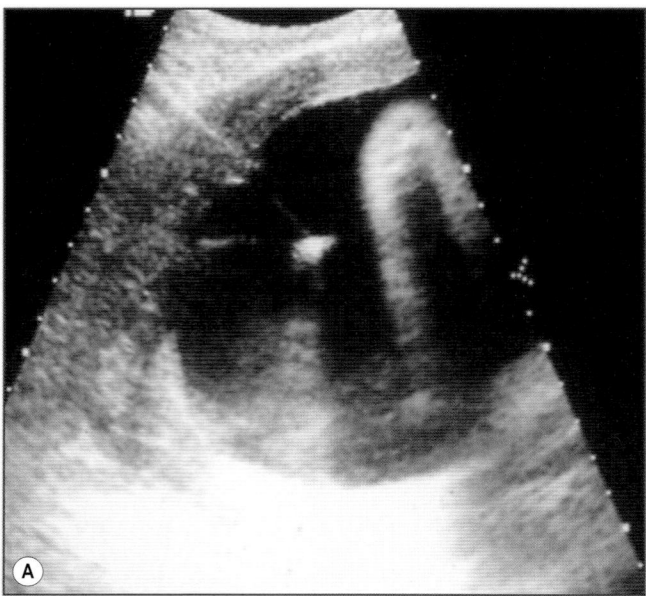

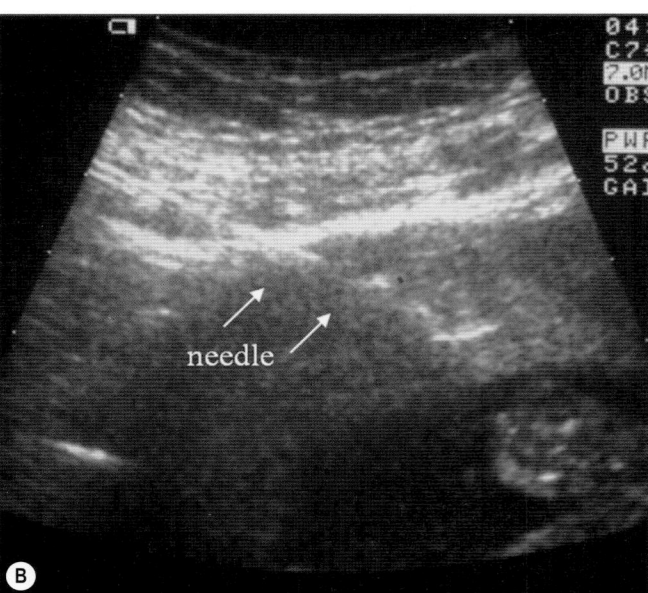

Fig. 9.10 (A) Amniocentesis: the 22G needle is introduced under ultrasound guidance (from top left). (B) Chorionic villus sampling: the 18G needle is introduced under ultrasound guidance (from top left).

with an increased miscarriage rate (Tabor et al. 1986; Kappel et al. 1987) and should be avoided. Even with an extensive anterior placenta, a small window avoiding the placenta can usually be found.

Patients are quoted a risk of spontaneous miscarriage attributable to the procedure of 1%, based on the results of the only randomised controlled trial (RCT; Tabor et al. 1986). Amniotic fluid contains cells desquamated from fetal skin, gastrointestinal, urogenital and respiratory tracts, and the amnion. In view of their small number, up to 2 weeks' cell culture is required prior to cytogenetic analysis, although with new techniques this period is shortening. A major disadvantage of amniocentesis is that termination of affected fetuses is not performed until well into the mid-trimester. Although amniotic fluid can be satisfactorily obtained and cultured at 11–13 weeks (Hanson et al. 1987; Benacerraf et al. 1988), the risks are increased with a greater miscarriage rate than with CVS (Nicolaides et al. 1994b), and therefore is not recommended.

Approximately 0.5% of amniotic cell cultures fail to grow, and maternal cell contamination leads to diagnostic difficulty in 0.2% (Thirkelsen 1979; Reid et al. 1996).

Fluorescent in situ hybridisation (FISH; Ch. 8) was introduced to allow rapid detection of trisomy 13, 18 and 21 together with sex chromosome aneuploidies. FISH allows the detection of specific DNA sequences with chromosome-specific painting probes.

Quantitative fluorescent polymerase chain reaction (QF-PCR), a more recent technique, is a rapid method of detection of trisomy 13, 18 and 21 and sex chromosomes. Compared with FISH, this technique is entirely automated, quicker, feasible on fewer cells and more cost-effective with comparable detection rates (Hultén et al. 2003; Nicolini et al. 2004; Chitty et al. 2006). Maternal cell contamination is also much more readily identified (Hultén et al. 2003). At present in the UK, the National Screening Committee advocates the use of QF-PCR for the detection of trisomy 13, 18 and 21 in women with high-risk screening results but with normal ultrasound. Full karyotope is only advocated in cases with abnormal ultrasound findings (including NT ≥3 mm) or family/previous

history of chromosomal abnormalities. Most undetected karyotype abnormalities as a result of this clinical policy are not clinically significant (Caine et al. 2005).

Chorionic villus sampling

Although obtaining chorionic tissue suitable for cytogenetic and biochemical analysis was first reported more than 30 years ago (Mohr 1968), CVS was only introduced into clinical practice in the mid-1980s. CVS was originally performed transcervically, but is now most commonly performed transabdominally (Fig. 9.10). Safety appears to be better with the transabdominal route (miscarriage rates 1% versus 4%) (Jackson et al. 1992; Smidt-Jensen et al. 1992). Initially, CVS was performed between 8 and 12 weeks. However, concern was raised following a report of limb reduction defects, some in association with the oromandibular syndrome (Firth et al. 1991, 1994). In all cases, CVS was performed before 66 days' gestation, and by single-needle transabdominal aspiration. Subsequent population and case–control studies have been unable to confirm any link (Froster and Jackson 1996), but theoretically it seems plausible that a procedure which may cause embolism, thrombosis or vasoconstriction at the time of limb bud formation may lead to such malformations. Thus, it has been recommended that CVS be performed after 10 weeks' gestation (Kuliev et al. 1993; Rodeck 1993). CVS rates remain high owing to first-trimester combined screening leading to aneuploidy testing, and for cases requiring genetic molecular testing.

The CVS-related fetal loss rate before 28 weeks above the background rate is 1–2% in centres with much experience (Nicolaides et al. 1994b). One problem with CVS is a 1.0–1.5% incidence of confined placental or pseudomosaicism, where a discrepancy exists between chorionic and fetal karyotypes, necessitating further investigation by amniocentesis (Hahnemann and Vejerslev 1997). In most cases, a bizarre aneuploid or polyploid mosaic is identified in the chorion, whereas the fetal karyotype, assessed from skin fibroblasts, is normal.

Fetal blood sampling

FBS is performed by direct ultrasound-guided needling of various fetal vessels. This is done as an outpatient procedure under local anaesthesia from 17 weeks' gestation. Sedation is rarely necessary. The most common approach, which involves inserting a 20G needle transabdominally into the umbilical vein about 1 cm from the placental cord insertion (Daffos et al. 1983), yields an adequate sample in 97% of cases (Daffos et al. 1985). Maternal contamination from inadvertent intervillous sampling is ruled out before removal of the needle by comparing the sample's MCV distribution, determined rapidly on a particle size analyser, with that of the mother (Rodeck 1980). Even at term, fetal MCV, which declines rapidly with gestation, remains significantly higher than that of healthy mothers (Fisk et al. 1989). The vein is the preferred vessel to sample, being simpler and safer (Weiner 1987); accidental sampling of the artery can be confirmed by ultrasonic observation of the direction of flow following injection of sterile saline (Nicolaides et al. 1986d). When there is difficulty approaching the cord insertion because of obesity, oligo- or polyhydramnios, or fetal position, blood may be aspirated from the intrahepatic portion of the fetal umbilical vein (Koresawa et al. 1987; Nicolini et al. 1988c). Although FBS from the intrahepatic vein is more difficult than at the cord insertion, it obviates the need for laboratory confirmation of its source, and in multiple pregnancies the operator is certain as to which fetus is sampled (Bang 1983).

Determining the loss rate attributable to FBS is difficult, as fetal demise in the weeks after the procedure may instead be due to the underlying high-risk indication. This was clearly demonstrated in one series, which showed increased loss rates in procedures performed on sicker fetuses, i.e. prenatal diagnosis (2%), fetal structural abnormality (6%), assessment of severe FGR (14%), and hydrops (25%) (Maxwell et al. 1991). A reported summation of all the published series calculated an overall loss rate in procedures performed in low-risk cases of 2.7% (Ghidini et al. 1993), although others have reported a lower loss rate of 0.9% (Weiner and Okamura 1996), and this figure has been corroborated by the US International Registry (Megerian and Ludomirsky 1994). Such results are only achieved after considerable training and experience. Most losses are due to cord haematoma, cord tamponade or haemorrhage, and, unlike losses after CVS or amniocentesis, are apparent at the time of the procedure. In late pregnancy, emergency caesarean section is performed to salvage these infants, although some may be damaged. Intra-amniotic bleeding is observed ultrasonically after 40% of samplings (Daffos et al. 1985; Weiner 1987), and a histological study of cords within 48 hours of FBS showed that a degree of extravasation occurs in all cases (Jauniaux et al. 1989). This bleeding is almost always transient, owing to the abundance of thromboplastins in amniotic fluid (Ney et al. 1989).

Skin and muscle biopsy

Prenatal diagnosis of many severe genodermatoses necessitates histological and ultrastructural examination of fetal skin, obtained at 18–22 weeks, initially by fetoscopy (Rodeck et al. 1980) but more recently by ultrasound-guided techniques (Bang 1985). The usual site chosen is the fetal buttock or leg. In a review of 269 pregnancies at risk of severe inherited skin disease the main indication for fetal skin biopsy was the risk of recurrence of epidermolysis bullosa. In such families, in over 90% of cases a prenatal diagnosis was established (Fassihi et al. 2006). Epidermolysis bullosa letalis is characterised by separation of the epidermis from dermis at the lamina lucida on light microscopy, and a paucity of hemidesmosomes on electron microscopy (Rodeck et al. 1980) (Ch. 32). The

prenatal diagnostic features of epidermolysis bullosa dystrophica, epidermolytic hyperkeratosis, harlequin ichthyosis and Sjögren–Larsson syndrome have similarly been described (Elias et al. 1980; Golbus et al. 1980; Kusseff et al. 1982). In oculocutaneous albinism, in which there is a lack of active melanin synthesis in hair bulb melanocytes, the biopsy must be taken from a hair-bearing area such as the scalp (Eady et al. 1983). In the review above, over a 25-year period the miscarriage rate for fetal skin biopsy was approximately 1% (Fassihi et al. 2006). Fetal skin scarring was observed postnatally in only 6 of the 191 cases.

Although DNA analysis is available for the diagnosis of the most common muscular dystrophies, most notably Duchenne muscular dystrophy, there are circumstances when a direct fetal muscle biopsy is required. This is usually when genetic testing has proved inconclusive. The procedure is performed under ultrasound control with the biopsy forceps guided into the outer aspect of the fetal buttock so as to avoid major structures.

Fetal medicine

With the combination of ultrasound and invasive procedures, several conditions can be managed more rationally than in the past, such as congenital malformations, maternal exposure to infectious agents and FGR. In others, the fetus can be treated; intravascular transfusion (IVT) has greatly improved the survival of alloimmunised fetuses, making it thus far the best model for fetal therapy.

Management of non-lethal malformations

Table 9.1 lists the risks of chromosomal and other structural malformations associated with common non-lethal congenital malformations. These are considerably higher for anomalies detected in utero than at birth. For example, in the literature the risk of an abnormal karyotype for infants with congenital heart disease is 5–10% and for exomphalos 10%, compared with risks of 32% and 66%, respectively, from antenatal studies (Nicolaides et al. 1986b; Copel et al. 1988a). Multiple malformations carry a 10-fold higher risk of aneuploidy than isolated malformations (Snijders et al. 1996). The demonstration of any fetal anomaly on ultrasound therefore prompts a detailed search for other abnormalities. Rapid karyotyping by FBS, amniotic fluid FISH or transabdominal CVS is offered. This is recommended not only in the mid-trimester to allow termination of aneuploid pregnancies, but also in the third trimester, where knowledge of a serious chromosomal defect may alter antenatal and intrapartum management, including mode of delivery. Furthermore, termination of pregnancy after 24 weeks' gestation is legal in the UK if there is a substantial risk that the fetus has an abnormality that would result in the birth of a child with a serious handicap. Karyotyping should also be performed for conditions where the risk of intrauterine death (IUD) is high, such as hydrops, because postmortem autolysis may jeopardise subsequent chromosomal studies and thus future genetic counselling. Indeed, postmortem karyotyping following termination for fetal abnormality has a 27% failure rate, and therefore pretermination sampling is advised (Kyle et al. 1996).

The option of termination of pregnancy is offered for severe malformations and support given to those who wish to continue through to delivery despite a poor prognosis. Other malformations are suitable for early postnatal correction, such as certain cardiac defects, duodenal atresia and gastroschisis. Intrauterine surgery may have a role in a few situations, but less so than was originally hoped. The significance of antenatal detection of some conditions, such as

Table 9.1 Reported frequencies of chromosomal and other structural abnormalities in fetuses with malformations detected in utero. The risk of aneuploidy will be lower if the malformation is isolated, and for the softer markers the risk will vary with maternal age

CONDITION	ANEUPLOIDY (%)	STRUCTURAL MALFORMATIONS (%)
Hydrocephalus	10–15	30–60
Cystic hygroma	45–80	15–65
Non-immune hydrops	3–15	25
Cleft lip/palate	1	15–50
Congenital heart disease	25–30	10–20
Diaphragmatic hernia	20–30	17–55
Tracheo-oesophageal fistula	15	50–60
Duodenal atresia	30–35	50–70
Exomphalos	50–65	60–75
Multicystic kidney	5–10	12–40
Pelviureteric junction obstruction	1–2	20–27
Posterior urethral valves	6–24	25–40

pelviureteric junction obstruction or multicystic kidney, is not so much the alteration of perinatal management as the initiation of timely investigation and follow-up in infancy.

The worse prognosis for abnormalities diagnosed in utero rather than neonatally largely reflects the increased risks of aneuploidy, multiple malformations and IUD. Whereas cystic hygroma at birth carries an excellent prognosis following surgical correction, the same-named lesion detected in utero leads to survival in less than 5% (Abramowicz et al. 1989; Langer et al. 1990). This high loss rate, which applies equally to euploid fetuses, reflects the frequency of hydrops and hypoxaemia in this condition (Tannirandorn et al. 1990).

Fetal growth restriction (Ch. 10)

The term 'small for gestational age' (SGA) describes both fetuses that are constitutionally small and those with FGR. Approximately 50–70% of fetuses with a birthweight <10th centile are constitutionally small. However, as a group, SGA fetuses are at higher risk of IUD, birth hypoxia, neonatal complications, impaired neuro-development and, according to the Barker hypothesis, potential hypertension and diabetes in later life.

While FGR may be suspected by abdominal palpation and measurement of the symphyseal–fundal height, the diagnosis is made ultrasonographically, with the abdominal circumference and/or estimated fetal weight <10th centile. Serial measurements are superior to single estimates not only in the prediction of genuine FGR but also in predicting poor outcome.

The incidence of a fetal karyotype abnormality in FGR is as high as 6–16% (Eydoux et al. 1989; Nicolaides and Economides 1990; Nicolini et al. 1990a), although this risk is based on series of referred patients in which severe FGR, often with oligohydramnios and malformations, was the indication for rapid karyotyping. With severe FGR and no structural malformations, the risk is lower, 2–3% (Snijders et al. 1996). The risk of aneuploidy remains remote in the milder forms of FGR, which complicates 5–10% of all pregnancies in the late third trimester. Karyotyping warrants consideration in severe FGR, when associated with fetal malformations, or in the

presence of normal liquor volume or uterine or umbilical Doppler studies.

While ultrasound has assisted in establishing the diagnosis of FGR, the role of Doppler ultrasound has been extensively researched in terms of: (1) prediction of risk and (2) monitoring affected pregnancies with FGR. The role of uterine artery Doppler analysis in predicting FGR appears to be limited, even in high-risk pregnancies (Chien et al. 2000), while screening a low-risk population with umbilical artery Doppler does not reduce perinatal mortality or morbidity (Bricker and Nielson 2004). However, monitoring of high-risk pregnancies with umbilical artery Doppler has been shown to reduce perinatal morbidity and mortality (Alfirevic and Neilson 1995; Neilson and Alfirevic 2003). In particular, absent end-diastolic flow (EDF) is associated with adverse perinatal outcome (Rochelson et al. 1987). Although acidaemia and hypoxaemia are unlikely in the presence of EDF, 45–80% of fetuses with absent EDF are acidaemic (pH <7.31) and 79–100% hypoxaemic (Nicolaides et al. 1988a; Nicolini et al. 1990a).

With knowledge of the fetal compensatory response to hypoxia by redistribution of blood flow, pulsed Doppler investigation of the involved fetal vessels provides more information about fetal condition. Redistribution of blood flow away from the kidneys (leading to oligohydramnios), gut (leading to hyperechogenic bowel) and skin towards the brain, adrenals and heart can be demonstrated by increased flow velocity within the MCA, and decreased flow velocity within the descending aorta. Alterations in the venous circulatory system may represent an end-stage response with cardiac decompensation, which can be measured at the level of the ductus venosus (Hecher et al. 1995a). Increased pulsatility and reversed velocity at the time of atrial contraction may be found. Decision-making regarding timing of delivery is currently based on combining the results of Doppler studies with growth velocity, amniotic fluid levels and CTG. The risk of prematurity associated with delivery is balanced against the continued exposure to in utero fetal hypoxaemia and acidaemia. In a recent multicentre study of neonates with prenatally diagnosed intrauterine growth restriction born before 33 weeks, although low Apgar score and Doppler changes were independent predictors of perinatal survival, gestational age greater than

29 weeks and 2 days and birthweight threshold of 600 grams were better predictors of survival (Baschat et al. 2007). In addition to immediate increased risk of perinatal morbidity and mortality, the risk of long-term neurodevelomental delay in surviving infants is also increased (Rijken et al. 2007; Delobel-Ayoub et al. 2009; Petrini 2009). The longer term effect of fetal compensation in response to hypoxia is difficult to disentangle from the effects of prematurity. The Truffle study is a European RCT of delivery based on either early or late changes in venous circulation compared with delivery based on CTG changes suggestive of fetal hypoxia. The primary outcome of this trial is survival without neurodevelopmental delay at 2 years of age corrected for prematurity.

Red cell alloimmunisation

Despite a dramatic decline in incidence, maternal sensitisation has not disappeared, for a variety of reasons, including antenatal sensitisation, prophylaxis failure and antibodies other than anti-D. Untreated, 45–50% of affected infants will have no or only mild anaemia, and 25–30% will have moderate anaemia posing neonatal problems only. The remaining 20–25% develop hydrops and usually die in utero or neonatally; in half, the hydrops develops prior to 30 weeks (Bowman and Pollack 1965). The aim of antenatal management is to identify severely affected fetuses, to correct their anaemia by transfusion, and then deliver them at the optimal time. At each gestational age the risks of invasive monitoring are weighed against those of conservative management and delivery. A suggested algorithm for the management of these cases is outlined in Figure 9.11.

Anti-D prophylaxis

RhD-negative women are at risk of sensitisation from fetomaternal bleeding, not only at delivery but also in other situations, such as external cephalic version and amniocentesis. Although the prevention programme has reduced neonatal deaths attributable to haemolytic disease of the newborn (HDN) from 18.4/100 000 in 1977 to 1.3/100 000 in 1992, there remains a sensitisation rate of around 1.5% among Rh-negative women. Administration of 500 IU of anti-D at 28 and 34 weeks can reduce the risk of immunisation to 0.2% (Crowther 2003). Anti-D prophylaxis is now recommended by the Royal College of Obstetricians and Gynaecologists (2003) and the National Institute for Health and Clinical Excellence (2003), with either a dose of 500 IU at 28 and 34 weeks, or a single larger dose of 1500 IU early in the third trimester. The rationale is that all Rh-negative women are at risk from hidden bleeds. The introduction of routine antenatal prophylaxis at 28 weeks in the UK has reduced the incidence of new sensitisation (Chilcott et al. 2003; Crowther 2003).

It is, however, important to note that clinically significant disease can be caused by other red cell alloantibodies such as Rh-c, Kell, Rh-E and Fy^a (Duffy). At present, immunoprophylaxis is not available for non-RhD disease and so immunisation will continue to occur.

Antenatal screening and management of RBC alloimmunisation

Routine serological testing of women is carried out:

- to identify pregnancies at risk of fetal and neonatal alloimmune disease (HDN)
- to identify RhD-negative women who require antenatal anti-D prophylaxis
- to provide compatible blood swiftly in emergencies.

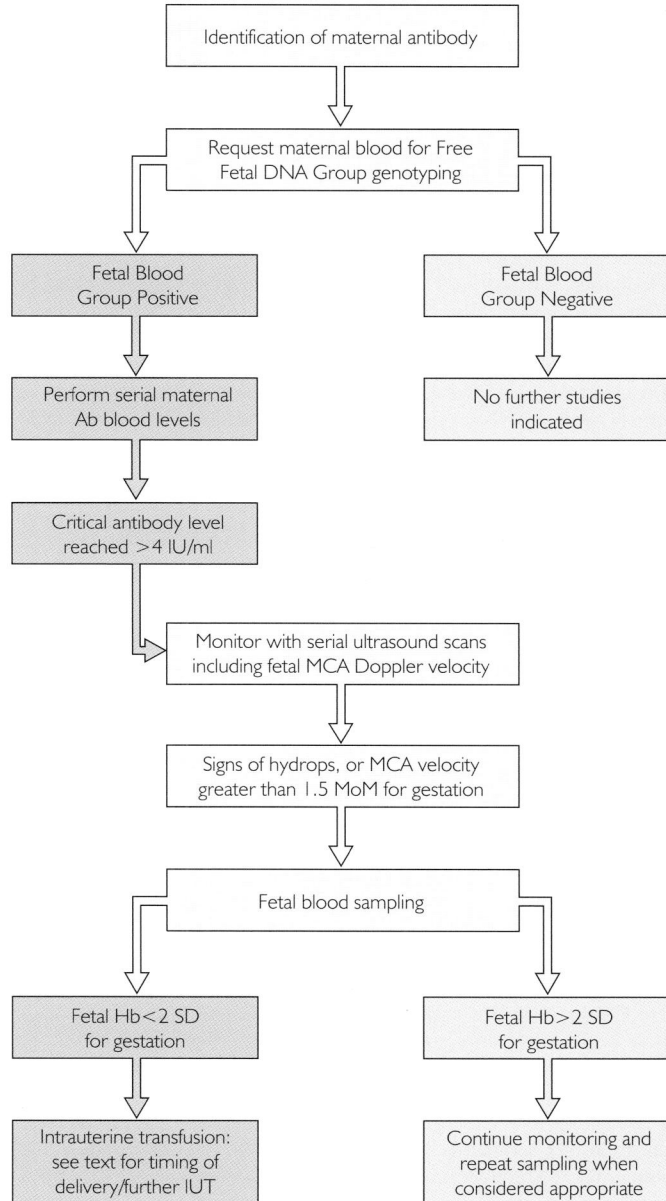

Fig. 9.11 A proposed algorithm for the management of red cell alloimmunisation.

All women who have no antibodies at 10–16 weeks' gestation should be tested once again between 28 and 36 weeks. Some workers believe that RhD-negative women should have two further tests, one at 28 weeks and one at 34–36 weeks, but sensitisation late in pregnancy is unlikely to result in HDN requiring treatment.

Quantification of the anti-D has simplified interpretation of positive antibody screens. Severe fetal anaemia is not expected at <4 IU/ml (Bowell et al. 1982) and is rare (0.25%) at <10 IU/ml. Further evaluation therefore is warranted at levels >4 IU/ml. Above this threshold, antibody levels have a limited role as they correlate poorly with the degree of fetal anaemia (Nicolaides et al. 1985b), although a rising level suggests an increase in severity. Prior to non-invasive methods of assessment, a level >15 IU/ml indicated the need for invasive assessment of fetal anaemia. No such similar cut-off levels apply to anti-c, Kell and Fy[a], and close monitoring is required in these cases, even with low titres.

When the fetus has been shown to be Rh-positive, the maternal antibody concentration should be checked every 2–4 weeks. Monitoring is now primarily with assessment of blood velocity in the MCA (see below). Additional ultrasonographic assessments include measurement of placental thickness, umbilical vein diameter, spleen and liver size (Chitkara et al. 1988; Nicolaides et al. 1988c; Roberts et al. 1989) or Doppler assessment of velocities in the descending aorta and ductus venosus (Copel et al. 1988b; Nicolaides et al. 1990; Oepkes et al. 1993, 1994), although none have been shown to be as reliable as MCA Doppler measurements in predicting the degree of anaemia. While the demonstration of fetal ascites indicates severe anaemia (PCV <15%, Hb <4 g/dl) in the mid-trimester, ascites only actually develops in two-thirds of fetuses with an Hb <4 g/dl (Nicolaides et al. 1985b). Anaemia of this degree is not associated with hypoxaemia, but is associated with increased fetal lactate levels, suggesting tissue hypoxia (Soothill et al. 1987). This is unlikely to cause developmental delay, but should be corrected as soon as possible by transfusion.

Determination of paternal zygosity and fetal genotype

Following the identification of antibodies in the maternal circulation, determination of the paternal Rh status is important. Approximately 15% of the UK population are RhD-negative, and, of the positive fathers, 56% are heterozygous for the D-gene, with a 50% chance of passing this on to the fetus. In cases of proven paternal heterozygosity, fetal antigen status should then be determined. Recent advances, since the identification of the Rh gene in 1991 (Colin et al. 1991), have allowed fetal antigen status to be determined, firstly from amniotic fluid (Bennett et al. 1993) and now from maternal blood by identification and analysis of free fetal DNA (Lo et al. 1998). This latter technique is known as non-invasive prenatal diagnosis (NIPD) and has replaced invasive testing in routine clinical service in the UK (Finning et al. 2002; Wright and Chitty 2009). At present NIPD is only offered to women with RhD antibodies who are at risk of pregnancies complicated by HDN. It has the potential use for routine screening in all RhD-negative women, and studies are currently underway to evaluate its performance as a screening test (Maddocks et al. 2009; Wright and Chitty 2009). Concerns of persistence of free fetal DNA from one pregnancy to the next have been largely discounted by the demonstration of its rapid clearance from the maternal circulation soon after birth.

Non-invasive assessment for fetal anaemia

Recent advances in Doppler imaging have resulted in a shift in practice away from early invasive assessment (and hence an avoidance of increased maternal sensitisation). Attention has focused on the Doppler velocimetric assessment of the MCA to predict fetal anaemia (Fig. 9.12). The rationale is that the MCA responds quickly to hypoxaemia owing to the strong dependence of the brain on oxygen and also reflects the hyperdynamic circulation associated with anaemia. Several groups have shown a strong negative correlation between either peak systolic velocity or mean velocity and fetal Hb or haematocrit (Mari et al. 2000; Teixeira et al. 2000; Abdel-Fattah et al. 2002). In the largest series, the peak systolic velocity in the MCA predicted moderate or severe anaemia without hydrops in 100% of cases, with a false-positive rate of 12% (Mari et al. 2000). The demonstration of increased velocity in the MCA indicates a strong likelihood of fetal anaemia. At this point, invasive testing is

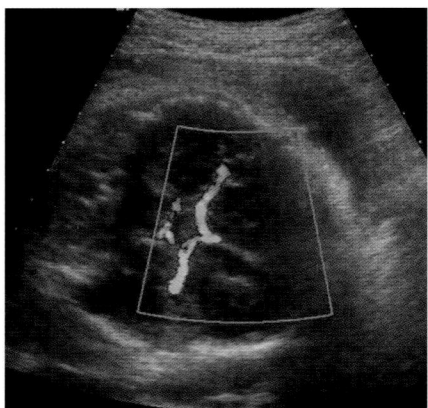

Fig. 9.12 Colour Doppler appearances of the circle of Willis and the middle cerebral arteries.

indicated. Use of MCA monitoring compared with more traditional methods of monitoring appears to allow the first invasive procedure to be performed later in gestation without compromising fetal well-being (Bartha et al. 2006).

Fetal blood transfusion

FBS allows direct assessment of fetal PCV and Hb, and permits transfusion to be performed at the same procedure if anaemia is detected. However, as FBS has a loss rate, and provokes fetomaternal haemorrhage and thus increases antibody levels in 70% of procedures in which the placenta is transgressed (Nicolini et al. 1988a), it is avoided until MCA Doppler measurements predict significant anaemia.

IVTs are now given by ultrasound-guided FBS (Bang et al. 1982; Berkowitz et al. 1986; Nicolaides et al. 1986c). The decision to administer an IVT is based on the PCV or Hb at FBS. Most use an Hb of less than 2 SD for the gestation (Nicolaides et al. 1988a, b) as an indication for transfusion; some use an absolute haematocrit below 30%. The needle tip is kept within the umbilical vein and fresh Rh-negative packed cells compatible with the mother are infused at 10–15 ml/min. The fetal heart rate and flow of infused blood are monitored on ultrasound to guard against inadvertent needle dislodgement and cord tamponade. The volume transfused is determined by consideration of the estimated fetoplacental volume and the fetal and donor PCV (Nicolaides et al. 1986c) or Hb (Nicolaides et al. 1988b), according to published nomograms. The PCV is rechecked after transfusion, and, if less than the desired 40–45%, a further increment is given.

The timing of the second transfusion should be based on the pre- and posttransfusion fetal Hb from the first transfusion, and from serial MCA Doppler velocities. After the second transfusion, the rate of fall in PCV in the fetus may be determined (when the PCV is estimated to have fallen to 20–25%) and the timing of subsequent transfusions arranged, although these again are often modified by the MCA Doppler velocities. Kleihauer testing of fetal samples indicates that erythropoiesis is usually completely suppressed after two or three transfusions (Nicolini et al. 1989c). As the donor blood in the fetal circulation is not susceptible to immune destruction, the rate of fall in PCV declines with increasing transfusions and thus the interval between procedures can be increased. The same principles are used in scheduling delivery between 36 and 38 weeks. Once an intrauterine transfusion has been performed, the timing of delivery will depend on when the last transfusion was performed and how many days it is likely to take for the Hb to fall to a level about 2 SD below the mean. Intrauterine transfusions are not usually performed after 36 weeks. In a woman with no previous history but an antibody level above 4 IU/ml (or 1 : 16 titre), the delivery can be planned at 37–38 weeks of gestation.

Survival

With serial IVTs, survival rates of 78–95% have been achieved in severely affected fetuses (Nicolaides 1986c; Poissonier et al. 1989). One series has reported that, in almost 600 IVTs, intact survival was 98% in those commenced in non-hydropic fetuses at greater than 24 weeks, and 70% in hydropic fetuses less than 24 weeks' gestation (Harman 1995). There are few follow-up studies focusing on morbidity, but one published study suggested that, when prematurity is removed, long-term morbidity secondary to intrauterine transfusion is low (Hudon et al. 1998). Therefore, the prognosis is now extremely optimistic. Fetal mortality correlates inversely with gestational age, and operator experience is undoubtedly also of importance.

Fetal thrombocytopenia

Alloimmune thrombocytopenia (Ch. 30)

Perinatal alloimmune thrombocytopenia complicates at least 1 : 3500 births, with intracranial haemorrhage (ICH) affecting 10–20% (Kamphius et al. 2010). Maternal antiplatelet antibodies cross the placenta, in a situation analogous to Rh disease. The consequent fetal thrombocytopenia may be profound, with a risk of spontaneous ICH in utero, particularly in the third trimester (Morales and Stroup 1985; de Vries et al. 1988; Friedman and Aster 1989), but it may occur as early as 18 weeks' gestation. The human platelet-specific antigens are biallelic polymorphisms which involve the platelet surface glycoproteins. Recently, a nomenclature of human platelet antigens (HPAs) has been developed (von dem Borne and Decary 1990). At present, HPAs 1–5 have been recognised. The genetic basis for these five HPAs has been identified, all involving a single point mutation in the DNA coding for the glycoproteins involved (Williamson et al. 1992). The most common is HPA 1, which has a high-frequency (85%) or a low-frequency (15%) antigen. Only 2% of women will be homozygous for the low-frequency 'b' allele, and thus at risk of developing antibodies and alloimmunisation. Fortunately, the actual occurrence of alloimmunisation is much rarer than this (0.06%) (Blanchette et al. 1990) because the development of antibodies is dependent on the human leukocyte antigen (HLA) type. HLA-Drw52a and HLA-Dr3 are most commonly associated with the development of HPA 1a antibodies. The incidence of women who were HPA 1a-negative was 2% in a screening and intervention programme of 100 000 unselected pregnant women in Norway. Anti-HPA 1A antibodies were detected in approximately 10% of women who were HPA 1a-negative. In the 161 HPA 1a-positive infants of negative mothers, there were 55 cases of severe thrombocytopenia and two cases of ICH (Kjeldsen-Kragh et al. 2007).

Management

The most reliable method of assessing likely disease severity is by inference from previous pregnancies: usually, a current pregnancy will be as severely affected as, or more affected than, previous pregnancies (Nicolini et al. 1991). This guides when investigation and treatment should begin, which may be as early as 18 weeks' gestation. Percutaneous FBS and estimation of fetal platelet count is the only way to determine whether a fetus is affected (Daffos et al. 1988b).

There are several management options available, and therefore patient care should be tailored dependent on previous history and parental preference.

Fetal platelet transfusions

These are used to cover the samplings and delivery, but may also be employed in a prophylactic manner, with weekly transfusions during the second and third trimesters and delivery once lung maturity is achieved. This prophylactic regimen was favoured in Europe until recently, but is arduous for the mother. In practice, transfusions are usually commenced at 26–28 weeks' gestation to cover the time of greatest risk (Nicolini et al. 1988b), although in cases of severe disease the first transfusion may be indicated as early as 20–22 weeks. A normal platelet count does not exclude the diagnosis, and therefore the procedure should be repeated at 28–32 weeks, unless from sampling amniotic fluid or fetal blood the fetal platelet type is found to be compatible.

Intravenous immunoglobulin

Cumulative data suggest that intravenous immunoglobulin (IVIG) is an important treatment option in this condition. Maternal infusion is less invasive and simpler than direct fetal sampling. However, it is expensive. Reports of maternal IVIG raising the fetal platelet count are variable (Bussel et al. 1988; Nicolini et al. 1990b). It may be that the IVIG has a preventive effect on ICH, other than by increasing the fetal platelet count. In a series of 54 women with thrombocytopenic fetuses due to alloimmune thrombocytopenia given IVIG weekly, in whom 10 had a previous infant with ICH, no ICH occurred and yet 20% showed no increase in the platelet count with therapy (Bussel et al. 1996). Data from observational studies suggest comparable neonatal outcomes between cases managed only using IVIG compared with those managed using IVIG and fetal sampling (Radder et al. 2001; van den Akker et al. 2007). Most centres currently advocate the use of repeated IVIG from early in the second trimester with possible fetal sampling and transfusion later in the second trimester based on previous history, followed by delivery by caesarean section 2–4 weeks before term (Kanhai et al. 2007). Other groups now rely on this treatment solely (Radder et al. 2001), or a combination of IVIG and platelet sampling, with the latter's timing and frequency dependent on the previous history and platelet count.

Conservative

The final option is to follow the fetus regularly by ultrasound and, in countries where late termination is permitted, to offer termination if ICH is found. This approach may be suitable in cases in which there is no severe history and hence the risk of ICH versus a complication from recurrent sampling or transfusion is low. Sampling may be performed prior to delivery to assess whether a transfusion is required to cover this (Kaplan et al. 1988).

There is no clear evidence to demonstrate that one treatment strategy is superior to the others. Although prophylactic platelet transfusions may be the most effective, there is a considerable procedure-related loss secondary to the serial procedures (Weiner et al. 1994), and therefore this needs to be weighed against the overall risk of ICH with untreated disease. Currently, the balance appears to be swinging to weekly maternal IVIG, and only limited FBS, with platelet transfusion if necessary.

Autoimmune thrombocytopenic purpura

Transplacental passage of antibodies in maternal immune thrombocytopenic purpura (ITP) also produces fetal thrombocytopenia. The older literature suggested that the 50% of infants with thrombocytopenia had a risk of ICH during vaginal delivery (Hegde 1985), and accordingly FBS for fetal platelet count determination prior to labour used to be performed in pregnancies complicated by ITP to decide on the mode of delivery (Moise et al. 1988; Scioscia et al. 1988). More recent studies show a low incidence of severe fetal thrombocytopenia (5–20%) or infant morbidity with maternal ITP (Kelton et al. 1982; Weiner 1990; Burrows and Kelton 1993), with no documented cases of antenatal ICH or ICH attributable to mode of delivery, even in cases of severe thrombocytopenia. There is no correlation between maternal and fetal platelet counts (Payne et al. 1997); the level of platelet-associated antibody does not correlate with fetal thrombocytopenia (Burrows and Kelton 1990; Samuels et al. 1990).

Management

Treatment for maternal thrombocytopenia includes steroids, splenectomy (outside pregnancy) and IVIG to raise the platelet count prior to delivery. There is no evidence that these treatments affect fetal platelet count. Fetal morbidity appears extremely low in this condition, so that opinion has moved away from fetal intervention unless there has been a strong history of a previously affected child with severe thrombocytopenia.

Congenital infections (Ch. 39.2)

Counselling a woman after perinatal exposure to teratogenic infectious agents previously involved quoting empirical risks. Now, direct serological investigation of the fetus and DNA analysis of fetoplacental tissues can be used to determine whether fetal infection has occurred. In rubella this may facilitate continuation of pregnancy, whereas in toxoplasmosis it determines the choice of antimicrobial therapy. FBS has no role in evaluating fetal status in maternal human immunodeficiency virus infection, as the procedure itself could infect the fetus.

Rubella

Prenatal diagnosis of rubella infection is usually indicated following maternal exposure in the early second trimester, or where doubt exists as to whether exposure in the first trimester resulted from primary infection or reinfection. Rubella-specific IgM is detected in fetal serum by radioimmunoassay (Morgan-Capner et al. 1985; Daffos et al. 1988a), provided that FBS can be delayed until 21–22 weeks, when the fetal humoral response to infection becomes detectable. Even at 23 weeks occasional false-negative IgM levels have been reported (Enders and Jonatha 1987). To improve the accuracy of prenatal testing at this late gestation, fetal blood or other tissues are also tested by hybridisation with a cDNA probe to rubella virus (Cradock-Watson et al. 1989). Earlier in pregnancy the same technique can be used on CVS specimens (Terry et al. 1986), although concern remains that placental infection may not indicate fetal infection (Alford et al. 1964).

Congenital infection leads to the classic rubella triad of cataracts, congenital heart defects (most commonly pulmonary stenosis) and deafness (Gregg 1941). With advancing gestation, transplacental passage reduces, with congenital infection rates of 50% in the first month falling to just 10% by 3 months (Enders et al. 1988). In addition, the severity of the syndrome reduces with advancing gestation.

Cytomegalovirus

The most severe congenital infections are due to primary maternal cytomegalovirus infection. Primary infection is associated with a 40% transmission rate, although only 10% of those fetuses will develop long-term sequelae, mostly hearing and learning defects (Peckham et al. 1987). Among the 5–10% who are symptomatic at birth, there will be a neonatal mortality of 30%, with long-term handicap in all survivors. Infection in earlier gestation results in higher transmission and poorer outcome.

Prenatal diagnosis is based on ultrasound findings and the detection of viral particles in the amniotic fluid (Davis et al. 1971), or, less commonly, in fetal blood. Specific IgM in fetal serum may also be diagnostic (Lange et al. 1982). Ultrasound findings include FGR, ascites or hydrops, intracranial calcification, ventriculomegaly and bowel echogenicity. Nevertheless, 90% of infants with congenital cytomegalovirus infection remain neurologically and developmentally normal. The risk of adverse outcome is increased if there is microcephaly, intracranial calcification, ventriculomegaly or evidence of a cerebral migration disorder (Ch. 40.8), and in these situations termination of pregnancy should be discussed.

Toxoplasmosis

Although, as pregnancy advances, maternal exposure leads to an increased risk of fetal infection, severity is greatest with exposure in the first trimester, with little chance of severe congenital disease after 20 weeks' gestation. Termination of an infected fetus remains an option, although fetoplacental infection is largely treatable (Desmonts and Couvreur 1974). The aim of fetal testing is to allow optimal transplacental therapy, initially with maternal spiramycin (3 g/day) to prevent transplacental transmission, with the addition of pyrimethamine and sulfadiazine if fetal testing proves positive (Daffos et al. 1988a). These two drugs are directly antiparasitic and have been shown to limit fetal damage. They are not used in the first instance when information about maternal infection is known, but rather only when fetal infection is proven, because of the potential hazards to mother and fetus. The diagnosis of fetal infection is now made with PCR analysis of amniotic fluid, which has replaced the more cumbersome multiple testing that was previously required (Hohlfield et al. 1994). If fetal infection is proven, the prognosis is still likely to be good, although vision may be affected later. However, intracranial signs of calcification and/or ventriculomegaly are poor prognostic signs (Berrebi et al. 1994), and termination would be offered.

Parvovirus

Human parvovirus (B19) infection is associated with increased risks of miscarriage, hydrops and IUD (Anand et al. 1987), with an overall fetal loss rate of 9% in infected pregnancies (Public Health Laboratory Service 1990). Parvovirus is best identified in fetal blood or other tissues by dot-blot hybridisation, electron microscopy or, most commonly, PCR of B19-specific DNA (Sheikh et al. 1992). The mainstay of diagnosis, however, remains maternal serology in women with appropriate clinical symptoms. Anti-B19 IgM appears in the serum at the onset of illness and remains detectable for up to 3 months. IgG response begins after 7 days and persists, probably to confer lifelong immunity. FBS is not routinely indicated in pregnancies with maternal infection because at least 90% will result in livebirths and parvovirus does not seem to be teratogenic.

It is the profound fetal anaemia secondary to an infective erythroid aplasia that accounts for the significant mortality rate. Following documented maternal infection, close fetal monitoring for signs of anaemia is indicated. Assessment of the MCA velocity for early detection of anaemia may be useful (as with monitoring of fetuses at risk of alloimmunisation) for 12 weeks postexposure, as fetal anaemia may occur 1–11 weeks after maternal infection (Rodis et al. 1988). FBS and IVT are indicated in the presence of suspected anaemia or hydrops. The incidence of coexisting fetal thrombocytopenia requiring platelet transfusion has been reported as high as 25% (Forestier et al. 1999; Simms et al. 2009). Hydrops without fetal anaemia has been documented and viral particles have been identified in the fetal myocardium, suggesting that a myocarditis may be contributory. It appears that profoundly anaemic fetuses which are salvaged by transfusion have a good prognosis, although more than one IVT may be necessary on occasion (Schwartz et al. 1988; Peters and Nicolaides 1990).

Tachyarrhythmias

Supraventricular tachycardia (SVT) is the most common fetal tachyarrhythmia, with rates between 200 and 300 beats/min. Atrial flutter and fibrillation often run at faster rates. As SVT is often intermittent, treatment is indicated only when SVT is sustained or associated with hydrops (Kleinman et al. 1985). In utero therapy seems preferable to delivery and neonatal treatment, as the fetus tolerates haemodynamic compromise better in utero, where gas exchange is not hindered by pulmonary oedema. Transplacental treatment by giving the mother digoxin leads to cardioversion in only 25–50% of non-hydropic cases (Stewart and Wladimiroff 1987; Maxwell et al. 1988) and is usually not effective in the presence of hydrops (Frohn-Mulder et al. 1995). These poor results partly reflect difficulties in achieving therapeutic maternal levels owing to the increased intravascular volume and glomerular filtration rate of pregnancy.

The addition of second-line drugs, such as flecainide and verapamil, results in improved eventual cardioversion, with over 90% conversion (including fetuses with hydrops) with flecainide in one series (Ebenroth et al. 2001). The same group also demonstrated that the fetuses that required second-line therapy in utero had a significantly more complex postnatal course.

Reports of sudden death in adults with antiarrhythmics such as amiodarone have slowed their incorporation into fetal treatment. Direct fetal intravascular or intraperitoneal therapy may be useful in refractory cases or those with hydrops (Flack et al. 1993). Adenosine has been reported to cause a chemical cardioversion when injected directly into the fetal circulation, and then sinus rhythm was maintained by transplacental digoxin therapy (Kohl et al. 1995). This needs to be explored further in cases resistant to initial maternal treatment. Doses required are much higher per kilogram estimated fetal bodyweight than in the neonate, presumably to allow for transplacental passage into the maternal circulation, and to account for the enhanced fetoplacental blood volume.

Congenital heart block

Complete heart block in the fetus is rare, with a reported incidence of between 1:5000 and 1:20000. The intrinsic ventricular rate is around 50–65 beats/min and the heart usually enlarges and hypertrophies to compensate for the slow rate. Hydrops may occur as congestive heart failure develops.

Congenital heart block (CHB) with a structurally abnormal heart carries a poor prognosis (85% mortality), whereas with a structurally normal heart the prognosis is good (Machado et al. 1988). In 1966, the association between isolated CHB and maternal connective tissue disease was first described (Hull et al. 1966). Anti-Ro and anti-La (SSA and SSB) antibodies are present in 60–80% of cases, often in mothers with subclinical disease. These antibodies are most frequently found in women with Sjögren syndrome, or, less often, with systemic lupus erythematosus. Various therapeutic options based on maternal transplacental therapy are available, although none have shown proven efficacy. These include sympathomimetic agents to increase fetal heart rate and function (Johnson et al. 1994)

and maternal dexamethasone to suppress fetal myocardial inflammation (Bierman et al. 1989; Chua et al. 1991). In practice, these are only used with a fetal heart rate <50 beats/min, or signs of complication, including hydrops. Recurrence rate following one fetus with CHB due to immune antibodies is approximately 18% (Izmirly et al. 2010).

Abnormalities of amniotic fluid volume

Oligohydramnios

Causes of oligohydramnios in the mid-trimester include urinary tract malformations, preterm premature rupture of membranes (PPROM) and FGR, and at these gestations survival is less than 25% whatever the cause (Barss et al. 1984; Mercer and Brown 1986). Conditions with a lethal prognosis, such as renal agenesis and aneuploidies, should be ruled out. Absence of the acoustic window makes inspection of fetal anatomy difficult. Transvaginal ultrasound facilitates visualisation of the renal fossae, as does colour Doppler of the renal arteries (Sepulveda et al. 1995). If still equivocal, invasive procedures may be required, including amnioinfusion and/or instillation of fluid into the fetal peritoneal cavity (Nicolini et al. 1989d). Amnioinfusion of a warmed physiological solution not only restores the acoustic window, but also allows confirmation of PPROM, especially when a dye is added (Fisk et al. 1991).

As 5–10% of fetuses in pregnancies with severe oligohydramnios will be chromosomally abnormal (Hackett et al. 1987), rapid karyotyping is carried out at the time of amnioinfusion. In the rare case of a euploid fetus with oligohydramnios, intact membranes and an intact renal tract, there may be a role for serial amnioinfusions in the prevention of lethal pulmonary hypoplasia (Arulkumaran et al. 1990), which otherwise complicates at least 60% of cases of severe mid-trimester oligohydramnios (Moore et al. 1989).

Polyhydramnios

The more severe the polyhydramnios, the more likely that an underlying cause will be found. Using the maximum vertical pocket, mild and severe polyhydramnios have been arbitrarily defined as a deepest pool greater than 8 cm and 15 cm, respectively (Chamberlein et al. 1984). The amniotic fluid index (AFI) definitions for mild and severe polyhydramnios are values outside the 97.5th centile for gestation and an AFI >40 cm, respectively (More and Cayle 1990).

Exclusion of maternal diabetes is essential; thereafter, a detailed fetal assessment is mandatory. In one series, 11% of neonates had a structural anomaly (most notably tracheo-oesophageal fistula, oesophageal atresia, duodenal atresia or conditions that impair fetal swallowing such as arthrogryposis), which increased with increasing severity of the polyhydramnios (Dashe et al. 2002). If sonographic evaluation was normal, the risk of a major anomaly was just 1% with mild polyhydramnios, but 11% if severe. Aneuploidy was present in 10% of fetuses with sonographic anomalies and in 1% without. Overall the fetal loss rate was 4%, of which 60% had anomalies.

The increased risks of preterm labour and PPROM in polyhydramnios seem mainly confined to those with severe polyhydramnios, i.e. an AFI >40 cm or a deepest pool >15 cm (Carlson et al. 1990; Fisk et al. 1990b). Amniotic reduction (AR) has been used with anecdotal success in severe polyhydramnios in order to prolong gestation and relieve maternal discomfort (Queenan 1970; Feingold et al. 1986). Removal of relatively small volumes of amniotic fluid can restore amniotic pressure to normal (Fisk et al. 1990b), but usually larger volumes are removed to limit the number of procedures that may be required. Nevertheless, removal of volumes greater than 6 litres at one time does carry the risk of precipitating abruption and/or preterm labour (Elliot et al. 1994).

Prostaglandin synthetase inhibitors have been used to reduce amniotic fluid in the past but are no longer recommended owing to potential fetal side-effects.

Multiple pregnancy (Ch. 23)

The incidence of twin pregnancies in the UK is 14.4 per 1000 births (National Health Service OPCS 1997), an increase of 25% compared with the early 1980s. The incidence is highest in older women (19.1 per 1000 in women aged 35–39 years in 1992), among whom a significant increase occurred owing to assisted reproductive techniques. This relatively small increase in frequency of multiple pregnancy will have a disproportionate effect on perinatal mortality and morbidity. Twin pregnancies have an eightfold increased risk of cerebral palsy, and triplet pregnancies a 47-fold increase (Patterson et al. 1993).

Up to a third of twin pregnancies are monozygotic, of which the majority share a single monochorionic placenta. For more information about zygosity, see Chapter 23. Perinatal morbidity and mortality in monochorionic twins is three- to fivefold higher than in dichorionic twins (Benirschke and Kim 1973; Neilson et al. 1989; Bejar et al. 1990); furthermore, previable losses are also significantly increased (Sebire et al. 1997). Much of the increase in risk is due to the presence of vascular anastomoses which are implicated in TTTS, and the co-twin sequelae after IUD of one twin.

Twin–twin transfusion syndrome

TTTS complicates approximately 15% of monochorionic diamniotic twin pregnancies (Sebire et al. 2000), and accounts for 15–17% of overall perinatal mortality in twins (Weir et al. 1979; Steinberg et al. 1990). It has classically been attributed to transfusion of blood via placental vascular anastomoses between the two fetal circulations. Vascular anastomoses are present in 96% of monochorionic placentas, and interfetal transfusion is a normal event in the majority of these pregnancies (Denbow et al. 2000). However, placentas from pregnancies affected by TTTS are characterised by two findings: first, an imbalance in interfetal transfusion is set up by the presence of unidirectional arteriovenous anastomoses, and, second, there is an absence of compensatory bidirectional arterioarterial anastomoses (Machin et al. 1996; Denbow et al. 1998b, 2000).

Presentation in the mid-trimester has until recently been associated with an 80–100% perinatal loss rate, either from preterm delivery secondary to polyhydramnios or from IUD following severe growth restriction or circulatory overload (Weir et al. 1979; Gonsoulin et al. 1990). The majority of cases complicated by TTTS have estimated fetal weight discordance in utero, and differences of <15% are unusual (Fisk et al. 1990a). There is some evidence that the prognosis worsens with an increasing difference in abdominal circumference measurements (Saunders et al. 1992), cumulatively reflecting the severity of overload/early hydrops in the recipient and growth restriction in the donor.

TTTS presents in the second trimester with discordant amniotic fluid volume (Fig. 9.13) (Duncan et al. 1997). The donor twin becomes oliguric, with consequent oligohydramnios, hence appearing enshrouded within its membrane and finally stuck to the uterine wall. In addition, neither the urinary bladder nor the stomach is usually visible, once anhydramnios is present. The growth velocity of the donor may follow the asymmetrical pattern seen with fetuses affected by FGR. Furthermore, it may also exhibit abnormal umbilical and MCA velocities, with absent/reversed flow in the former and redistribution in the latter (Hecher et al. 1995b).

The overloaded recipient develops polyuria and severe polyhydramnios. The degree of polyhydramnios cannot be solely explained by the transfusion of blood volume from the donor to the recipient, and there are emerging data implicating alterations in the renin–angiotensin system resulting in the polyhydramnios/oligohydramnios sequence (Mahieu-Caputo et al. 2001).

Venous Doppler studies in the recipient fetus deteriorate in accordance with the disease process. There may be evidence of pulsatile venous flow, progressing to reverse EDF within the ductus venosus (Hecher et al. 1995c). The development of tricuspid regurgitation indicates worsening of the right-sided cardiac failure. The recipient fetus may develop hydrops, the mechanism of which has been assumed to be volume overload. Doppler studies have shown that severe cases are often associated with venous waveform patterns consistent with raised central venous pressure (Rizzo et al. 1994; Hecher et al. 1995c). Typically, recipient fetuses with cardiac dysfunction develop cardiomegaly, tricuspid regurgitation, ventricular hypertrophy and, ultimately, right ventricular outflow tract obstruction (Zosmer et al. 1994).

A number of groups have attempted to 'stage' TTTS in an attempt to rationalise treatment (Quintero et al. 1999; Taylor et al. 2000). Several prognostic criteria have been used, including arterial and venous Doppler studies, fetal size discordancy, bladder dynamics and amniotic fluid volume. However, sudden unpredictable deterioration in clinical condition can still occur.

Therapeutic options for TTTS

A variety of treatments, including transplacental drug therapy, selective fetocide, AR, laser ablation (LA) of the intertwin placental anastomoses, and intrauterine venesection and exchange transfusion, have been attempted, with varying degrees of success. Current treatment mainly involves the use of AR, LA and selective fetocide, alone or in combination according to disease severity and progression.

Serial amnioreduction

Serial AR remains the simplest of treatment options, with at least one fetus surviving (at 4 weeks postnatal age) in 71% of pregnancies (Mari et al. 2001). Although AR aims primarily to control polyhydramnios to allow prolongation of gestation, there is some evidence in TTTS that it may ameliorate fetal condition and the disease process. AR was associated with a 74% median increase in uterine blood flow in one study (Bower et al. 1995), while others have demonstrated that fetal MCA pulsatility indices fell acutely with AR in both recipient and donor fetuses (Mari et al. 1992).

Until recently, serial aggressive AR was the mainstay of management of this condition. However, because of the high rates of perinatal mortality and morbidity and that no attempt was being made to affect the disease process itself, other techniques have been developed.

Laser ablation

The technique of LA of placental vessels was first developed in animals in 1985 (de Lia et al. 1985) and later applied to human pregnancies with TTTS (de Lia et al. 1995; Ville et al. 1995). The initial technique involved the photocoagulation of all surface chorionic vessels crossing the interwin septum with a neodymium:yttrium–aluminium–garnet (Nd:YAG) laser. The early results were disappointing, with perinatal survival similar to that of AR (de Lia et al. 1995; Ville et al. 1995). The high procedure-related loss rates

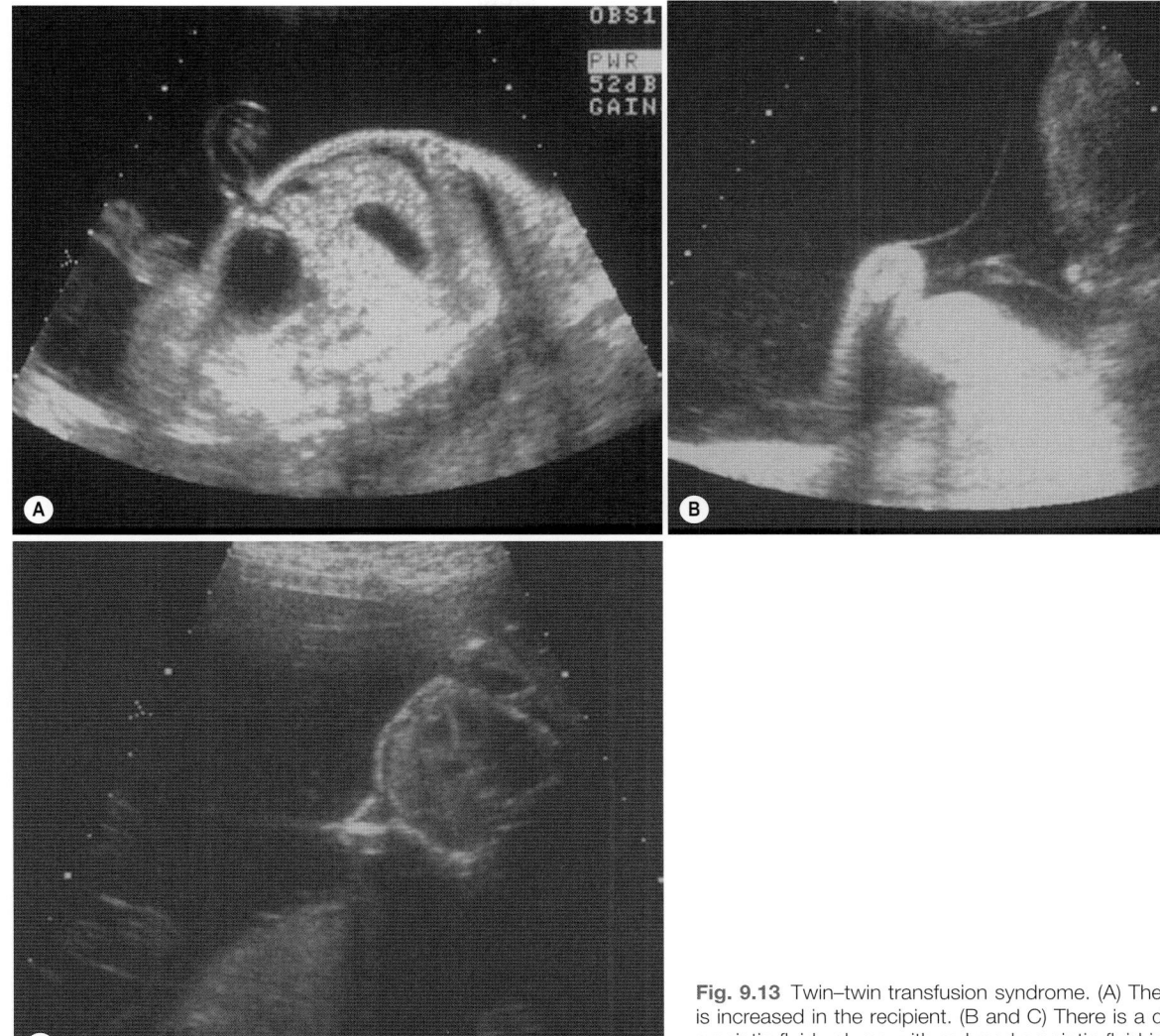

Fig. 9.13 Twin–twin transfusion syndrome. (A) The size of the bladder is increased in the recipient. (B and C) There is a discrepancy in amniotic fluid volume with reduced amniotic fluid in the donor and increased amniotic fluid in the recipient.

were attributed to the unnecessary destruction of viable placental tissue using such a non-selective technique.

However, with refinement of the technique and increased operator experience, rates for survival of at least one twin have improved to 75% (Eurofetus 2003). Now, most operators perform targeted ablation, with selection and ablation of confirmed anastomoses, while leaving viable placental tissue untouched.

Selective fetocide

Selective fetocide has been suggested to have a role in the management of TTTS by a number of groups. In its favour, the procedure may be performed once the IUD of one of the twins appears imminent, or once all other treatment options have failed. Indeed, this usually allows the parents to feel that the procedure is absolutely necessary to allow even a single twin to be saved. However, this delay may allow some degree of insult to happen to the surviving fetus, before its co-twin is terminated. Either the donor or the recipient fetus may become preterminal, and, in order to be a safe and effective procedure, the possibility of acute transfusion of the remaining twin into the terminated twin must be avoided (see below).

Management of TTTS

Most clinicians treat pregnancies complicated by TTTS on a case-by-case basis. First, disease severity is assessed by staging; thereafter, management is contentious. A Cochrane review in 2008 has provided some clarity. Perinatal outcomes were evaluated in one RCT of septostomy versus serial AR and two RCTs comparing LA with serial AR (Roberts et al. 2008). There were no differences in the incidence of one or more fetal deaths between septostomy and AR (Moise et al. 2003). LA was associated with lower rates of perinatal (relative risk 0.59, 95% CI 0.40–0.87) and neonatal (relative risk 0.29, 95% CI 0.14–0.61) death (Roberts et al. 2008). The larger of the two studies in this review, the Eurofetus study, consisted mainly of twins with moderate to severe disease. Severity of TTTS is commonly graded by the Quintero staging system (Ch. 23) (Quintero 1999). In the Eurofetus study there were only 11 twins with stage 1 TTTS. In this group there remains an equipoise on the appropriate management of these cases. Subgroup analysis suggested greater benefit of laser with earlier disease. However, this is a post hoc analysis and the results must be interpreted with caution. Some observational data suggest the majority of these mild cases do not progress and AR may be associated with higher perinatal survival rates (Fisk et al. 2009). There is a need for RCTs in the management of these mild cases.

Neurological outcome

There are emerging data regarding the longer term sequelae of TTTS. Cerebral white-matter lesions are increased in monochorionic twin pregnancies overall, both with and without TTTS, and this has been attributed to haemodynamic imbalance due to the shared circulation (Bejar et al. 1990). However, in surviving twins from pregnancies complicated by severe TTTS and managed by AR, the incidence of antenatally acquired neurological lesions was found to be 35%, although, with the exception of one case, these lesions were relatively subtle, and thus of uncertain long-term significance (Denbow et al. 1998a). Both donors and recipients were shown to be at risk, although the aetiology of the damage is uncertain. It has been speculated that in the recipient the raised haematocrit, and hence potential for intravascular sludging, leads to cortical damage, with the donor's neurological injury secondary to anaemia. However, large differences in fetal Hb concentrations in utero are uncommon (Denbow et al. 1998c). It has been shown that LA, rather than AR, reduces the incidence of cerebral palsy in survivors (4.2% versus 24.4%) because the disease process is largely arrested at the time of treatment (Quintero et al. 2003); however this has yet to be substantiated in an RCT. Follow-up data from surviving infants in the Eurofetus trial failed to demonstrate a difference in neurodevelopment at 2 years of age between twins treated by AR compared with LA (Örtqvist et al. 2008).

Acute interfetal transfusion

Following the IUD of one of a monochorionic twin pair, there is approximately a 25% incidence of necrotic brain and/or renal lesions (increasing to 50% if the pregnancy was complicated by TTTS) and a similar risk of IUD in the otherwise healthy co-twin (Fusi and Gordon 1990; van Heteren et al. 1998). The aetiology of this insult appears to be haemodynamic. An imbalance in interfetal transfusion following the death of one twin in utero gives rise to a period of hypotension, potentially resulting in ischaemia, as the initially healthy twin transfuses blood into the dead twin's circulation (Fusi et al. 1991). The phenomenon of acute interfetal transfusion also has implications in pregnancies where selective fetocide is indicated, e.g. discordant fetal anomaly, TTTS in extremis, and twin reversed arterial perfusion sequence.

Selective fetocide ideally should involve an occlusive technique, to prevent any residual possibility of the surviving twin exsanguinating into the non-viable twin's circulation. After initial reports of ultrasound-guided techniques, including vascular occlusion with absolute alcohol (Denbow et al. 1997), histoacryl gel injection (Dommergues et al. 1995) or thrombogenic coils (Bebbington et al. 1995), it subsequently became clear that success rates were poor, resulting in co-twin death or damage (Denbow et al. 1999; Nicolini et al. 2001). Now, cord occlusion is performed with bipolar diathermy, with co-twin survival (taking into account pre-existing morbidity) of 76%. Serial ultrasound or MRI on the surviving twin's brain is recommended to look for evidence of cortical damage.

Multifetal pregnancy reduction and selective fetocide in dichorionic twins

Multifetal pregnancy reduction

This procedure aims to obviate the daunting perinatal mortality in high-order multiple pregnancies (more than three fetuses) by reducing fetal numbers to a twin or triplet gestation with improved perinatal outcome. In non-reduced higher order (more than three fetuses) pregnancies, approximately one-third will miscarry prior to 24 weeks (Evans et al. 2002).

The initial approach, which involved transvaginal aspiration, has been abandoned in view of high loss rates (Itskowitz et al. 1989) and all are now done by transabdominal injection of KCl into the fetal thorax (Berkowitz et al. 1988; Evans et al. 1988). Most such pregnancies are the result of overzealous use of ovulation induction agents and are therefore usually multizygotic and multichorionic, although not always in twins (Wenstrom et al. 1993). The procedure is best delayed until 10–12 weeks, when the risks of abortion and spontaneous regression have subsided and the NT can be measured. The optimal number of fetuses to be left remains controversial, but most centres reduce to twins. The chief risk, that of complete abortion of all fetuses, varies around 4–16% and is influenced by the starting number (triplets 4.5%, quadruplets 8%, quintuplets 11%) and the finishing number after the reduction (ideally two), together with operator experience (Evans et al. 2003).

Trichorionic triplets pose the hardest decision in terms of consideration of multifetal pregnancy reduction. One series compared the outcome of reduced trichorionic triplets with that of those managed expectantly (Papageorghiou et al. 2002). Although the rate of miscarriage in the reduced group was higher (8.3% versus 3.2%), the rate of preterm delivery was considerably lower (9.8% versus 23.1%). Overall, the non-reduced pregnancies had a higher chance of survival (93.3% versus 90.3%) but at the cost of a higher estimated incidence of handicap (1.5% versus 0.6% per fetus).

Selective fetocide

In twin pregnancies discordant for fetal anomaly, selective termination of the affected fetus is an option. Intracardiac KCl injection is the recommended technique (Isada et al. 1992), except in monochorionic pregnancies because of the risk of acute interfetal transfusion. In the 20% of cases concordant for fetal sex with a single placental mass on ultrasound, determination of chorionicity will require careful evaluation of the membranous septum. This requires evaluation of the septal thickness and the presence or absence of the lambda sign (Fig. 9.14) (Finberg 1992). A septum that is 0.2 mm thick and/or contains three or four layers strongly suggests dichorionic placentation (Barss et al. 1985; D'Alton and Dudley 1989), although the reproducibility and hence the usefulness of this measurement has been shown to be poor after the first trimester (Stagiannis et al. 1995). A combination of all the signs should provide more than 90% accuracy in chorionicity determination in the second trimester (Scardo et al. 1995), but 100% accuracy in the first trimester (Monteagudo et al. 1994; Carroll et al. 2002). One series indicated an overall loss rate of 4% (2.4% in twins, 12.5% in triplets) following selective fetocide (Eddelman et al. 2002), with over 80% of deliveries occurring beyond 32 weeks' gestation. Loss rates are lower if the procedure is performed before 16 weeks (Evans et al. 1994).

Fetal surgery

In several congenital malformations, a satisfactory outcome is often achieved with postnatal surgical correction. In some, however, the uncorrected malformation results in progressive organ damage in utero, jeopardising survival. There may be a role in such conditions for in utero intervention. Initial attempts at fetal surgery took one of two forms: open surgical correction at hysterotomy, or bypassing obstructive lesions by ultrasound-guided insertion of catheter shunts (Fig. 9.15). More recently there has been increasing interest in endoscopic surgical techniques, resulting in lowered maternal morbidity.

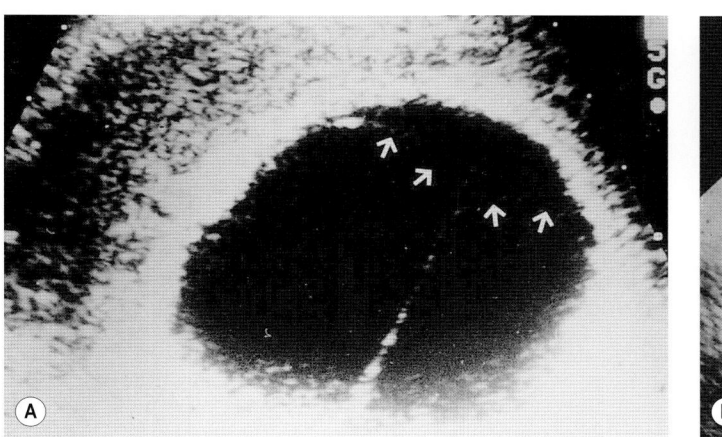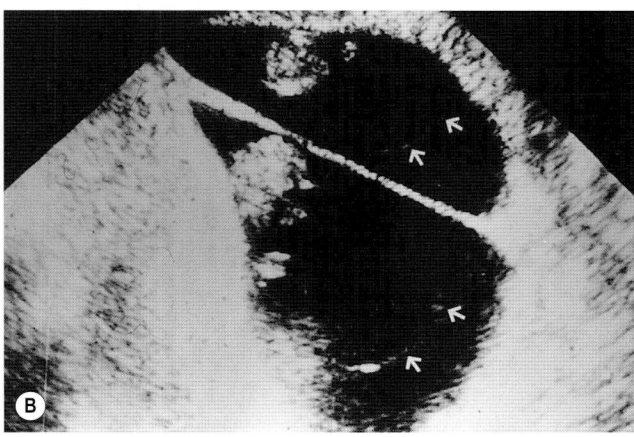

Fig. 9.14 Transvaginal ultrasound view of first-trimester (A) monochorionic and (B) dichorionic twin gestations, showing the amnions and chorions before fusion. *(Reproduced from the RCOG Press.)*

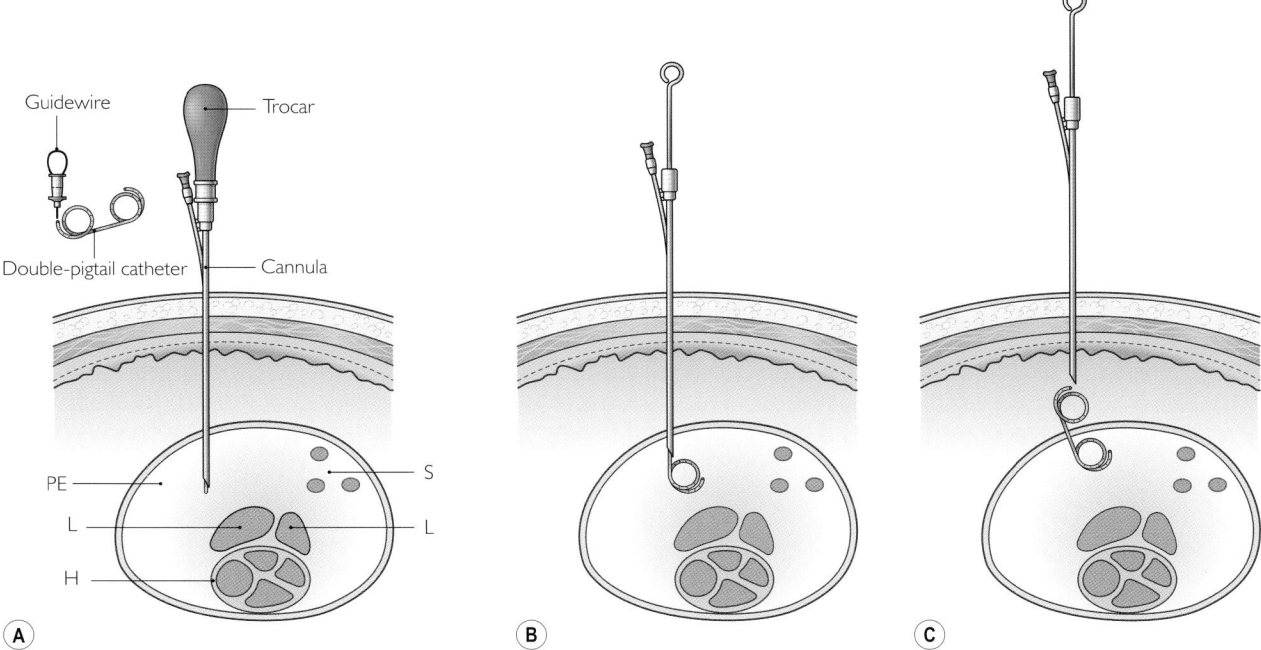

Fig. 9.15 Pleuroamniotic shunting. (A) The trocar and cannula are inserted transamniotically into the effusion. The guidewire is then straightened, the double-pigtail catheter inserted into the cannula and the wire removed. (B) A short introducer rod then deposits half the catheter within the hemithorax. (C) The cannula is then withdrawn into the amniotic cavity, and a long introducer rod is inserted to position the other half of the shunt in the amniotic cavity. H, heart; S, spine; L, lungs. *(Reproduced from Rodeck et al. (1988).)*

These techniques should only be contemplated in centres with expertise, and for conditions in which animal models have demonstrated benefit from correction in utero. Unfortunately, the overall results for open fetal surgery have been disappointing. Despite being limited to a few very specialised centres, the problem of inexorable preterm labour subsequent to surgery has limited the enthusiasm for the approach. If fetal surgery is to be considered in the future, it is essential that chromosomal and other structural malformations first be excluded. Moreover, reliable antenatal predictors are needed when selecting cases for intervention, so that fetal surgery is withheld from those which would otherwise have a satisfactory outcome, and from those in which the pathology is irreversible.

Intrathoracic lesions

Diaphragmatic hernia (Ch. 27.6)

The mortality rate from diaphragmatic hernia diagnosed in utero remains high at 75% despite optimal postnatal care (Adzick et al. 1985b; Harrison et al. 1990). The main determinant of outcome is the degree of pulmonary hypoplasia resulting from in utero lung compression, dependent on the timing and volume of visceral herniation through the diaphragm. Predictors of perinatal loss include earlier gestational age at diagnosis, lung area to head circumference ratio (LHR) of less than 1, herniation of the liver into the thoracic cavity and gestational age at delivery (Jani et al. 2007; Worley et al. 2009). Increasingly, fetal MRI is also used to quantify the volume of herniation and estimation of LHR and fetal lung volume (Jani et al. 2008; Kilian et al. 2009; Worley et al. 2009). A recent study using fetal MRI found neonatal mortality rates of 86% in cases where the fetal liver occupied more than 20% of the fetal thorax compared with 13% in cases with lower volumes of herniation (Worley et al. 2009). MRI was also found to have slightly better prognostic accuracy in the assessment of pulmonary hypolasia and the prediction of neonatal outcome than sonographic assessments (Kilian et al. 2009).

An alternative, less invasive, corrective approach to diaphragmatic hernia is tracheal ligation. The underlying theory is that preventing drainage of lung liquid will allow the lung to grow (PLUG – plug the lung until it grows), and animal experiments have confirmed this hypothesis (Harrison et al. 1993; Wilson et al. 1993). Open tracheal ligation, unfortunately, still carries the risk of preterm labour, and may also result in tracheal stenosis. The recent development of endoscopic techniques (e.g. FETO) for insertion of a temporary tracheal plug looks promising, (Flake et al. 2000; Harrison et al. 2001) but much work needs to be done on the optimal timing, duration and method for FETO before it can be introduced into clinical practice.

In a recent series of 210 cases, the success rate of tracheal occlusion was approximately 97%. The entry criteria of the study were severe congenital diaphragmatic hernia on the basis of intrathoracic herniation of the liver and LHR of less than 1 (Jani et al. 2009). The survival rate was 49% and 35% for isolated left- and right-sided congenital diaphragmatic hernias respectively. Approximately 10% of all deaths were related to the removal of the balloon used for occlusion. When compared with historical data on those managed expectantly, the survival rates increased from 24% to 49% for left-sided lesions and from 0% to 35% in right-sided lesions. However, only RCTs will provide the definitive benefit associated with this procedure. An RCT from the USA was recently abandoned because of the high rates of survival in the control arm of the trial, resulting in there being no difference in survival rates between both arms of the study (Harrison et al. 2003). Because the tracheal balloon needs to be removed or decompressed prior to delivery, ongoing perinatal management is essential; serious complications have been reported (Jani et al. 2009).

Fetal hydrothorax

Perinatal mortality in fetal hydrothorax exceeds 50%, and is higher when associated with hydrops than in isolation (Roberts et al. 1986; Castillo et al. 1987). Compression of the lung during its canalicular phase (17–24 weeks) produces pulmonary hypoplasia, whereas large effusions cause polyhydramnios by impairing swallowing, and hydrops by vena caval obstruction and cardiac compression (Benacerraf and Frigoletto 1985). Chylothorax, the commonest cause in neonates, is diagnosed after alimentation by demonstrating chylomicrons in pleural fluid (Chernick and Reed 1970). The diagnosis may also be made in the fetus by showing high lymphocyte cell counts in aspirated pleural fluid (Elser et al. 1983; Benacerraf et al. 1986b).

Ultrasound-guided aspiration of fetal hydrothoraces facilitates neonatal resuscitation if performed immediately prior to delivery (Schmidt et al. 1985). Because the fluid reaccumulates within 6–48 hours (Petres et al. 1982; Nicolaides et al. 1985a), long-term drainage is required. This is achieved by a plastic pleuroamniotic shunt, inserted under ultrasound guidance (Fig. 9.15). In three series totalling 34 patients (Rodeck et al. 1988; Longaker et al. 1989; Nicolaides and Azar 1990), resolution was achieved in 17 (50%) patients, 16 (94%) of whom survived, with no respiratory complications. Only two infants survived when hydrops persisted (12%).

A single aspiration is performed 1 week beforehand, as the effusion does not always reaccumulate (Benacerraf and Frigoletto 1985; Benacerraf et al. 1986b), especially with small or unilateral effusions. In fetal hydrothoraces unassociated with other abnormalities, shunting is indicated in the presence of hydrops or polyhydramnios, or if detected in mid-trimester. The catheters should be clamped immediately at delivery to prevent a pneumothorax; alternatively, the neonate should be electively intubated and ventilated.

Cystic adenomatoid malformation of the lung (Ch. 27.5)

This rare malformation may result in pulmonary hypoplasia, hydrops and perinatal death in a small percentage of cases (Adzick et al. 1985a). The solid type of lesion is more likely to be associated with a poor prognosis than is the macrocystic lesion, where cysts can be visualised on ultrasound. In the macrocystic type of lesion, long-term drainage of a solitary intrathoracic cyst can be performed, resulting in good outcome at birth (Nicolaides et al. 1987a). The San Francisco group has also shown that, with severe CCAM associated with hydrops, a combination that carries an extremely poor prognosis, open fetal surgical resection by lobectomy offers a good chance of survival. Lobectomy of the massively enlarged pulmonary lobe was performed between 21 and 27 weeks' gestation in eight fetuses, resulting in five survivors (Adzick et al. 1993). This is therefore one of the conditions where fetal surgery may have a role, although it should only be embarked upon in those cases which otherwise would have an extremely poor outlook.

Obstructive uropathy

Posterior urethral valves (Ch. 35.2)

In fetuses with PUVs unassociated with other anomalies, the two main factors determining perinatal outcome are pulmonary hypoplasia and renal dysplasia (Harrison et al. 1982; Nakayama et al. 1986), which seem related to the duration and severity of obstruction. Lack of a urinary contribution to amniotic fluid in the mid-trimester leads to pulmonary hypoplasia. Although its pathogenesis is not understood (Nicolini et al. 1989a), numerous animal and human studies indicate that lung hypoplasia is a consequence of oligohydramnios. Urethral obstruction has also been considered responsible for renal dysplasia, presumably mediated by raised urinary pressure (Harrison et al. 1981; Kurth et al. 1981). However, intravesical pressure seems only marginally raised in fetuses with low obstructive uropathies (Nicolini et al. 1991). There is an alternative embryological theory, which suggests that renal dysplasia is not secondary to PUVs but results from the same early defect, resulting in abnormal interaction between the urethral bud and the metanephrogenic mesenchyme (Berman and Maizels 1982; Stephens 1983).

As the surgical correction of PUVs is relatively simple postnatally, a hypothesis emerged that bypass of the obstruction in utero would minimise renal dysplasia and restore amniotic fluid, thereby preventing pulmonary hypoplasia and allowing survival at birth (Harrison et al. 1981). The basis for such intervention was rigorously tested in animals. Urinary obstruction in fetal lambs produces both renal dysplasia and lung hypoplasia (Glick et al. 1983; Harrison et al. 1983), whereas early decompression prevents these sequelae (Harrison et al. 1982; Glick et al. 1984).

The presence of a normal amniotic fluid volume indicates that lung hypoplasia will not occur, that the obstruction is incomplete and that the kidneys are producing adequate amounts of urine. Therefore, any benefit from bypass procedures needs to be restricted to those fetuses with severe oligohydramnios, in whom irreversible renal damage has not yet developed. Vesicoamniotic shunting of a fetus with severe renal dysplasia would not only fail to prevent neonatal renal failure, but would also fail to prevent pulmonary hypoplasia if the kidneys in utero were unable to restore amniotic fluid volume. Accordingly, accurate prediction of fetal renal function is important in selecting potential cases for intrauterine surgery. Although renal cysts are visualised in only 44% of dysplastic kidneys, their presence strongly suggests dysplasia (Mahoney et al. 1984). Hyperechogenicity of the renal parenchyma predicts dysplasia with a sensitivity of 73% and a specificity of 80% (Mahoney et al. 1984).

In view of the inaccuracy of ultrasound in predicting renal function, other methods have been sought. Biochemical analysis of fetal urine for the prediction of later renal function has been thought to be useful by some (Glick et al. 1985; Grannum et al. 1989) but not by others (Weiner et al. 1986; Wilkins et al. 1987). Initially, threshold values to define an isotonic urine with probable poor outcome, Na^+ 0.100 mEq/l, Cl^- 0.90 mEq/l and osmolality 0.210 mmol/l, were used. Refinements have been made by providing normal values for electrolytes (Na^+ and Cl^-) with gestation between 16 and 33 weeks (Nicolini et al. 1992) and by serial sampling, which may provide more accurate information (Johnson et al. 1994). Others have suggested that urinary microproteins may be useful indicators of renal damage, in particular urinary (Mandelbrot et al. 1991; Lipitz et al. 1993; Muller et al. 1993), and possibly fetal, serum β_2-microglobulin (Berry et al. 1995). In present practice a decision whether to shunt or not is based on a combination of urinary electrolytes, β_2-microglobulin, the appearance of the renal tract on ultrasound and on bladder and liquor volumes.

The standard method of vesicoamniotic shunting is by ultrasound-guided insertion of an indwelling plastic double-pigtail catheter (Harrison et al. 1982; Manning et al. 1986), as for pleuroamniotic shunting. The results of 73 cases of shunting procedures for low obstructive uropathy reported to the International Registry were not encouraging, with only a 41% perinatal survival rate (Manning et al. 1986). However, this included fetuses with pathologies other than PUVs, with chromosomal and other abnormalities, and with normal amniotic fluid volume, and 70% of the contributing centres had had experience of only one case. Most of the scepticism about this procedure (Elder et al. 1987; Reuss et al. 1988) may thus be attributed to poor case selection.

It appears, therefore, that inclusion criteria should be rigorously applied to restrict shunting to those few fetuses in which it may be of benefit, i.e. otherwise normal euploid fetuses with sonographically 'normal' kidneys, with severe oligohydramnios and biochemical evidence of adequate renal function.

The long-term outcome following vesicoamniotic shunting is somewhat better when all obstructive uropathies (e.g. prune-belly syndrome, urethral atresia, vesicoureteral reflux) are considered (Freedman et al. 1999). At 2-year follow-up of the 62% of fetuses that survived, one-third had undergone renal transplantation for renal failure, with a further 21% having renal impairment; the remaining 43% had normal renal function. Only 50% were acceptably continent at follow-up.

Most of the studies on fetal intervention have been observational studies. A systematic review failed to identify any RCT on fetal bladder shunting (Clark et al. 2003). Meta-analysis of the non-randomised observational studies suggests an improvement in perinatal survival associated with shunting, especially in fetuses with poor predicted outcome. However, this is an invasive procedure associated with both maternal morbidity and risk of miscarriage or preterm labour. Currently in the UK, the PLUTO trial, a multicentre RCT, aims to provide conclusive evidence on the benefit of

vesicoamniotic shunting compared with expectant management. The study outcomes include rates of perinatal survival and fetal renal function at 4–6 weeks following birth and at 12 months of life (Zaccara et al. 2005; The PLUTO Collaborative Study Group 2007). We currently await the findings of this study.

Other surgical conditions

Hydrocephalus (Ch. 40.8 and Ch. 40.5)

Obstruction of the aqueduct of Sylvius causes a rise in cerebrospinal fluid pressure, ventricular enlargement, cortical thinning and irreversible neurological damage. As ventricular shunting in the neonatal period dramatically improves outcome (Laurence and Coates 1962), and as ventriculomegaly may progress in utero, the hypothesis emerged that intrauterine decompression of fetal hydrocephalus would prevent neurological damage. Although initial work in a primate model suggested that in utero shunting improved survival and outcome (Michejda and Hodgen 1981), reports to the International Registry (Manning et al. 1986) demonstrated that in utero shunting in human fetuses resulted in increased survival of severely handicapped infants, and therefore the technique has been abandoned.

Sacrococcygeal teratoma (Ch. 36 and Ch. 29.4)

Congenital sacrococcygeal teratomas are usually benign and in the neonatal period are associated with good outcome after surgical resection. When they are diagnosed in the mid-trimester, however, hydrops frequently develops secondary to cardiac failure from arteriovenous shunting, indicating impending fetal demise (Flake et al. 1986). One group has reported success with in utero open surgical resection of the tumour (Adzick et al. 1993), although their previous more problematic experience had suggested that resection must take place before the initiation of end-stage cardiac failure in the fetus and the hydropic placenta, leading to the maternal 'mirror syndrome' (Langer et al. 1989; Adzick et al. 1997).

Alternative therapies include cytoreduction of the tumour mass by ablative techniques, thereby reducing the venous steal and hence risk of high-output cardiac failure. Several thermocoagulative techniques have been employed, with only limited success rates reported (Paek et al. 2001).

Neural tube defects (Ch. 40.8)

There is growing experience with in utero closure of NTDs. An experimental model of spina bifida in the sheep suggests that in utero correction of the spinal defect can prevent the neurological dysfunction normally seen at birth (Meuli et al. 1995). Results in humans have been less impressive, although a substantial reduction in shunt-dependent hydrocephalus was demonstrated in one series (Tulipan et al. 2003). It is also clear that in utero therapy has no benefit with lesions higher in the fetal spine (above L3) and gestations greater than 25 weeks. The Management of Myelomeningocele Study (MOMS) aims to compare in utero surgery with postnatal surgery. This RCT in the USA is currently still in the recruitment phase.

Fetal valvuloplasty

There have been several reports of treatment of valve atresia in utero. In one report, two fetuses with complete or almost complete pulmonary atresia and imminent hydrops underwent pulmonary valvuloplasty in utero at mid-gestation (Tulzer et al. 2002). Both children (one aged 18 months and one aged 12 months) now have biventricular circulation. In a larger series of cases with severe aortic stenosis at risk of hypoplastic left heart syndrome, growth of the left heart structures was maintained following fetal valvulopalsty

(Tworetzky et al. 2004). As with other fetal surgeries, further research and experience are necessary before this becomes standard practice.

Weblinks

www.eurofetus.org: Eurofetus.
www.fetalmedicine.com: The Fetal Medicine Foundation.
www.ncc-wch.org.uk: National Collaborating Centre for Women's and Children's Health.

www.nice.org.uk: National Institute for Health and Clinical Excellence.
www.pluto.bham.ac.uk: The PLUTO Trial.
www.rcog.org.uk: Royal College of Obstetricians and Gynaecologists.

www.screening.nhs.uk: UK National Screening Committee.
www.spinabifidamoms.com: MOMS trial.
www.trufflestudy.org: TRUFFLE trial.

References

Abdel-Fattah, S.A., Soothill, P.W., Carroll, S.G., et al., 2002. Middle cerebral artery Doppler for the prediction of fetal anaemia in cases without hydrops: a practical approach. Br J Radiol 75, 726–730.

Abramowicz, J.S., Warsof, S.L., Doyle, D.L., et al., 1989. Congenital cystic hygroma of the neck diagnosed prenatally: outcome with normal and abnormal karyotype. Prenat Diagn 9, 321–327.

Adzick, N.S., Harrison, M.R., Glick, P.L., et al., 1985a. Fetal cystic adenomatoid malformation: prenatal diagnosis and natural history. J Pediatr Surg 20, 483–488.

Adzick, N.S., Harrison, M.R., Glick, P.L., et al., 1985b. Diaphragmatic hernia in the fetus: prenatal diagnosis and outcome in 94 cases. J Pediatr Surg 20, 357–361.

Adzick, N.S., Harrison, M.R., Flake, A.W., 1993. Fetal surgery for cystic adenomatoid malformation of the lung. J Pediatr Surg 28, 1–6.

Adzick, N.S., Crombleholme, T.M., Morgan, M.A., et al., 1997. A rapidly growing teratoma. Lancet 349, 538.

Alfirevic, Z., Neilson J.P., 1995. Doppler ultrasonography in high-risk pregnancies: systematic review with meta-analysis. Am J Obstet Gynecol 172, 1379–1387.

Alford, C.A., Neva, F.A., Weller, T.H., 1964. Virologic and serologic studies on human products of conception after maternal rubella. N Engl J Med 271, 1275–1281.

Allan, L., 2004. Techniques of fetal echocardiography. Pediatr Cardiol 25, 223–233.

Anand, A., Gray, E.S., Brown, T., et al., 1987. Human parvovirus infection in pregnancy and hydrops fetalis. N Engl J Med 316, 183–186.

Andres, R.L., Brace R.A., 1990. The development of hydrops fetalis in the ovine fetus after lymphatic ligation or lymphatic excision. Am J Obstet Gynecol 162, 1331–1334.

Arulkumaran, S., Nicolini, U., Fisk, N.M., et al., 1990. Fetal vesicorectal fistula causing oligohydramnios in the second trimester. Br J Obstet Gynaecol 97, 449–451.

Bang, J., 1983. Ultrasound guided fetal blood sampling. In: Albertini, A., Crosignani, P.F. (Eds.), Progress in Perinatal Medicine. Excerpta Medica, Amsterdam, p. 223.

Bang, J., 1985. Intrauterine needle diagnosis. In: Holm, H.A., Kristensen, J.K. (Eds.), Interventional Ultrasound. Munksgaard, Copenhagen, pp. 122–128.

Bang, J., Bock, J.E., Trolle, D., 1982. Ultrasound guided fetal intravenous transfusion for severe rhesus haemolytic disease. Br Med J 284, 373–374.

Barrett, J., Chitayat, D., Sermer, M., et al., 1995. The prognostic factors in the prenatal diagnosis of the echogenic fetal lung. Prenat Diagn 15, 849–853.

Barss, V.A., Benacerraf, B.R., Frigoletto, F.D., 1984. Second trimester oligohydramnios, a predictor of poor fetal outcome. Obstet Gynecol 64, 608–610.

Barss, V.A., Benacerraf, B.R., Frigoletto, F.D., 1985. Ultrasonographic determination of chorion type in twin gestation. Obstet Gynecol 66, 779–783.

Bartha, J.L., Abdel-Fattah, S.A., Hunter, A., et al., 2006. Optimal interval between middle cerebral artery velocity measurements when monitoring pregnancies complicated by red cell alloimmunization. Fetal Diagn Ther 21, 22–25.

Baschat, A.A., Cosmi, E., Bilardo, C.M., et al., 2007. Predictors of neonatal outcome in early-onset placental dysfunction. Obstet Gynecol 109, 253–261.

Bebbington, M.W., Wilson, R.D., Machan, L., et al., 1995. Selective feticide in twin transfusion syndrome using ultrasound-guided insertion of thrombogenic coils. Fetal Diagn Ther 10, 32–36.

Bejar, R., Vigliocco, G., Gramajo, H., et al., 1990. Antenatal origin of neurologic damage in newborn infants. Am J Obstet Gynecol 162, 1230–1236.

Benacerraf, B.R., Frigoletto, F.D., 1985. Mid-trimester fetal thoracocentesis. J Clin Ultrasound 13, 202–204.

Benacerraf, B.R., Frigoletto, F.D., Greene, M.F., 1986a. Abnormal facial features and extremities in human trisomy syndromes: prenatal ultrasound appearances. Radiology 159, 243–246.

Benacerraf, B.R., Frigoletto, F.D., Wilson, M., 1986b. Successful mid-trimester thoracocentesis with analysis of the lymphocyte subpopulation in the pleural effusion. Obstet Gynecol 155, 398–399.

Benacerraf, B.R., Greene, M.F., Saltzman, D.H., et al., 1988. Early amniocentesis for prenatal cytogenetic evaluation. Radiology 169, 709–710.

Benacerraf, B.R., Saltzman, D.H., Estroff, J.A., et al., 1990. Abnormal karyotype of fetuses with omphalocele: prediction based on omphalocele contents. Obstet Gynecol 75, 317–319.

Benirschke, K., Kim, C., 1973. Multiple pregnancy. N Engl J Med 288, 1329–1336.

Bennett, P.R., Kim, C.L., Colin, Y., et al., 1993. Prenatal determination of fetal RhD type by DNA amplification following chorion villus biopsy or amniocentesis. N Engl J Med 329, 607–610.

Beretsky, L., Lankin, D.H., Rusoff, J.H., et al., 1984. Sonographic differentiation between the multicystic dysplastic kidney and the uretopelvic junction obstruction in utero using high resolution real time scanners employing digital detection. J Clin Ultrasound 11, 349–356.

Berkowitz, R.L., Chitkara, U., Goldberg, J.D., et al., 1986. Intrauterine intravascular transfusion for severe red blood cell iso-immunisation: ultrasound guided percutaneous approach. Am J Obstet Gynecol 60, 746–749.

Berkowitz, R.L., Lynch, L., Chitkara, U., et al., 1988. Selective reduction of multifetal pregnancies in the first trimester. N Engl J Med 318, 1043–1047.

Berman, D.J., Maizels, M., 1982. The role of urinary obstruction in the genesis of renal dysplasia. A model in the chick embryo. J Urol 128, 1091–1096.

Berry, S., Lecolier, B., Smith, R.S., et al., 1995. Predictive value of fetal serum b-microglobulin for neonatal renal function. Lancet 345, 1277–1278.

Bierman, F.Z., Baxi, L., Jaffe, I., et al., 1989. Fetal hydrops and congenital complete heart block: response to maternal steroid therapy. J Pediatr 112, 646–648.

Blanchette, V.S., Chen, L., Salmon de Freiberg, S., et al., 1990. Immunization to the Pl[A1] antigen: results of a prospective study. Br J Haematol 74, 209–215.

Blumenthal, D.H., Rushovich, A.M., Williams, R.K., et al., 1982. Prenatal sonographic findings of meconium peritonitis with pathological correlation. J Clin Ultrasound 10, 350–352.

Bonaventure, J., Rousseau, F., Legeani-Mallet, L., et al., 1996. Common mutations in fibroblast growth receptor 3 (FGR-3) gene account for achondroplasia, hypochondroplasia, and thanatophoric dwarfism. Am J Med Genet 63, 148–154.

Bowell, P., Wainscoat, J.S., Peto, T.E., et al., 1982. Maternal anti-D concentrations and outcome in rhesus haemolytic disease of the newborn. Br Med J 285, 327–329.

Bower, S.J., Flack, N.J., Sepulveda, W., et al., 1995. Uterine artery blood flow response to correction of amniotic fluid volume. Am J Obstet Gynecol 173, 502–507.

Bowman, J.M., Pollack, J.M., 1965. Amniotic fluid spectrophotometry and early delivery in the management of erythroblastosis fetalis. Pediatrics 35, 815–835.

Bricker, L., Neilson, J.P., 2004. Routine Doppler ultrasound in pregnancy. (Cochrane Review). In: The Cochrane Library, Issue 2.

Brons, J.T.J., Wladimiroff, J.W., Van Der Harten, J.J., et al., 1988. Prenatal ultrasonographic diagnosis of osteogenesis imperfecta. Am J Obstet Gynecol 159, 176–181.

Burrows, R.F., Kelton, J.G., 1990. Thrombocytopenia at delivery: a prospective survey of 6715 deliveries. Am J Obstet Gynecol 163, 731–734.

Burrows, R.F., Kelton, J.G., 1993. Fetal thrombocytopenia and its relation to maternal thrombocytopenia. N Engl J Med 329, 1463–1466.

Bussel, J.B., Berkowitz, R.L., McFarland, J.G., et al., 1988. Antenatal treatment of neonatal alloimmune thrombocytopenia. N Engl J Med 319, 1372–1378.

Bussel, J.B., Berkowitz, R.L., Lynch, L., et al., 1996. Antenatal management of alloimmune thrombocytopenia with intravenous gamma-globulin: a randomized trial of the addition of low-dose steroid to intravenous gamma-globulin. Am J Obstet Gynecol 174, 1414–1423.

Caine, A., Maltby, E.A., Parkin, C.A., et al., 2005. Prenatal detection of Down's syndrome by rapid aneuploidy testing for chromosomes 13, 18, and 21 by FISH or PCR without a full karyotype: a cytogenetic risk assessment. Lancet 366, 123–128.

Campbell, S., Pearce, J.M., 1983. Ultrasound visualization of congenital malformations. Br Med Bull 39, 322–331.

Campbell, S., Johnstone, F.D., Holt, E.M., et al., 1972. Anencephaly: early ultrasonic diagnosis and active management. Lancet ii, 1226–1227.

Campbell, J., Gilbert, W.M., Nicolaides, K.H., et al., 1987. Ultrasound screening for spina bifida: cranial and cerebellar signs in a high-risk population. Obstet Gynecol 70, 247–250.

Canick, J.A., Knight, G.J., Palomaki, G.E., et al., 1988. Maternal serum unconjugated oestriol as an antenatal screening test for Down's syndrome. Br J Obstet Gynaecol 95, 330–333.

Cardoza, J.D., Goldstein, R.B., Filly, R.A., 1988. Exclusion of fetal ventriculomegaly with a single measurement: the width of the lateral ventricular atrium. Radiology 169, 711–714.

Carlson, D.E., Platt, L.D., Medearis, A.L., et al., 1990. Quantifiable polyhydramnios: diagnosis and management. Obstet Gynecol 75, 989–993.

Carroll, S.G., Porter, H., Abdel-Fattah, S., et al., 2000. Correlation of prenatal ultrasound diagnosis and pathologic findings in fetal brain abnormalities. Ultrasound Obstet Gynaecol 16, 149–153.

Carroll, S.G., Soothill, P.W., Abdel-Fattah, S., et al., 2002. Prediction of chorionicity in twin pregnancies at 10–14 weeks of gestation. Br J Obstet Gynaecol 109, 182–186.

Castillo, R.A., Devoe, L.D., Falls, G., et al., 1987. Pleural effusions and pulmonary hypoplasia. Am J Obstet Gynecol 157, 1252–1255.

Chamberlain, P.F., Manning, F.A., Morrison, I., et al., 1984. Ultrasound evaluation of AFV. II. The relationship of increased AFV to perinatal outcome. Am J Obstet Gynecol 150, 250–254.

Chernick, V., Reed, M.H., 1970. Pneumothorax and chylothorax in the neonatal period. J Pediatr 76, 624–632.

Chervenak, F.A., Isaacson, G., Blakemore, K.J., et al., 1983. Fetal cystic hygroma. Causes and natural history. N Engl J Med 309, 822–825.

Chien, P.F., Arnott, N., Gordon, A., et al., 2000. How useful is uterine artery Doppler flow velocimetry in the prediction of pre-eclampsia, intrauterine growth retardation and perinatal death? An overview. Br J Obstet Gynaecol 107, 196–208.

Chilcott, J., Lloyd Jones, M., Wight, J., et al., 2003. A review of clinical effectiveness and cost-effectiveness of routine anti-D prophylaxis for pregnant women who are rhesus-negative. Health Technol Assess 7, iii-62.

Chinn, D.H., Filly, R.A., Callen, P.W., 1983. Congenital diaphragmatic hernia diagnosed prenatally by ultrasound. Radiology 148, 119–123.

Chitkara, U., Wilkins, I., Lynch, L., et al., 1988. The role of sonography in assessing severity of fetal anemia in Rh and Kell iso-immunised pregnancies. Obstet Gynecol 71, 393–398.

Chitty, L.S., Hunt, G.H., Moore, J., et al., 1991. Effectiveness of routine ultrasonography in detecting fetal structural abnormalities in a low risk population. Br Med J 303, 1165–1169.

Chitty, L.S., Kagan, K.O., Molina, F.S., et al., 2006. Fetal nuchal translucency scan and early prenatal diagnosis of chromosomal abnormalities by rapid aneuploidy screening: observational study. Br Med J 332, 452–456.

Chodirker, B.N., Harman, C.R., Greenburg, C.R., 1988. Spontaneous resolution of a cystic hygroma in a fetus with Turner syndrome. Prenat Diagn 8, 291–296.

Chua, S., Ostman-Smith, I., Sellers, S., et al., 1991. Congenital heart block with hydrops fetalis treated with high-dose dexamethasone: a case report. J Obstet Gynecol Reprod Biol 42, 155–158.

Cicero, S., Bindra, R., Rembouskos, G., et al., 2003. Integrated ultrasound and biochemical screening for trisomy 21 using fetal nuchal translucency, absent fetal nasal bone, free beta-hCG and PAPP-A at 11 to 14 weeks. Prenat Diagn 23, 306–310.

Clark, T.J., Martin, W.L., Divakaran, T.G., et al., 2003. Prenatal bladder drainage in the management of fetal lower urinary tract obstruction: a systematic review and meta-analysis. Obstet Gynecol 102, 367–382.

Colin, Y., Cherif Zahar, B., Le Van Kim, C., et al., 1991. Genetic basis of the RhD positive and RhD negative blood group polymorphism as determined by Southern analysis. Blood 78, 2747–2752.

Copel, J.A., Cullen, M., Green, J.J., et al., 1988a. The frequency of aneuploidy in prenatally diagnosed congenital heart disease: an indication for fetal karyotyping. Am J Obstet Gynecol 158, 409–413.

Copel, J.A., Grannum, P.A., Belanger, K., et al., 1988b. Pulsed Doppler flow–velocity waveforms before and after intrauterine intravascular transfusion for severe erythroblastosis fetalis. Am J Obstet Gynecol 158, 768–774.

Cradock-Watson, J.E., Miller, E., Ridehalgh M.K.S., et al., 1989. Detection of rubella virus in fetal and placental tissues and in the throats of neonates after serologically confirmed rubella in pregnancy. Prenat Diagn 9, 91–96.

Crowther, C.A., 2003. Anti-D administration in pregnancy for preventing Rhesus alloimmunisation (Cochrane Review). In: The Cochrane Library, Issue 2.

Cuckle, H., Wald, N.J., Thompson, N.G., 1987. Estimating a woman's risk of having a pregnancy associated with Down's syndrome using her age and maternal serum alpha-fetoprotein level. Br J Obstet Gynaecol 94, 387–402.

Daffos, F., Capella-Pavlovsky, M., Forestier, F., 1983. Fetal blood sampling via the umbilical cord using a needle guided by ultrasound. Report of 66 cases. Prenat Diagn 3, 271–277.

Daffos, F., Capella-Pavlovsky, M., Forestier, F., 1985. Fetal blood sampling during pregnancy with use of a needle guided by ultrasound: a study of 606 consecutive cases. Am J Obstet Gynecol 153, 655–660.

Daffos, F., Forestier, F., Capella-Pavlovsky, M., et al., 1988a. Prenatal management of 746 pregnancies at risk for congenital toxoplasmosis. N Engl J Med 318, 271–275.

Daffos, F., Forestier, F., Kaplan, C., et al., 1988b. Prenatal diagnosis and management of bleeding disorders with fetal blood sampling. Am J Obstet Gynecol 158, 939–946.

Dallaire, L., Potier, M., 1986. Amniotic fluid. In: Milunsky, A. (Ed.), Genetic Disorders and the Fetus. Plenum Press, New York, pp. 53–67.

D'Alton, M.E., Dudley, D.K., 1989. The ultrasonographic prediction of chorionicity in twin gestation. Am J Obstet Gynecol 160, 557–561.

Dashe, J.S., McIntire, D.D., Ramus, R.M., et al., 2002. Hydramnios: anomaly prevalence and sonographic detection. Obstet Gynecol 100, 134–139.

Davis, L.E., Tweed, G.V., Chin, T.D., et al., 1971. Intrauterine diagnosis of cytomegalovirus infection: viral recovery from amniocentesis fluid. Am J Obstet Gynecol 109, 1217–1219.

Davis, G.K., Farquhar, C.M., Allan, L.D., et al., 1990. Structural cardiac abnormalities in the fetus: reliability of prenatal diagnosis and outcome. Br J Obstet Gynaecol 97, 27–31.

de Crespigny, L., Robinson, H.P., 1986. Amniocentesis: a comparison of 'monitored' versus 'blind' needle insertion technique. Aust N Z J Obstet Gynaecol 26, 124–128.

de Lia, J.E., Rogers, J.G., Dixon, J.A., 1985. Treatment of placental vasculature with a neodymium-yttrium-aluminum-garnet laser via fetoscopy. Am J Obstet Gynecol 151, 1126–1127.

de Lia, J.E., Kuhlmann, R.S., Harstad, T.W., et al., 1995. Fetoscopic laser ablation of placental vessels in severe previable twin-twin transfusion syndrome. Am J Obstet Gynecol 172, 1202–1211.

Delobel-Ayoub, M., Arnaud, C., White-Konning, M., et al., 2009. Behavioural problems and cognitive performance at 5 years of age after very preterm birth: the EPIPAGE Study. Pediatrics 123, 1485–1492.

Denbow, M.L., Batten, M., Kyle, P., et al., 1997. Selective termination of monochorionic twin pregnancy discordant for fetal abnormality. Br J Obstet Gynaecol 104, 626–627.

Denbow, M.L., Battin, M., Cowan, F., et al., 1998a. Neonatal cranial ultrasonographic findings in preterm twins complicated by severe feto-fetal transfusion syndrome. Am J Obstet Gynecol 178, 479–483.

Denbow, M.L., Cox, P., Talbert, D., et al., 1998b. Colour Doppler energy insonation of placental vasculature in monochorionic twins: absent arterio-arterial anastomoses in association with twin-twin transfusion syndrome. Br J Obstet Gynaecol 105, 760–765.

Denbow, M.L., Fogliani, R., Kyle, P., et al., 1998c. Haematological indices at fetal blood sampling in monochorionic pregnancies complicated by feto-fetal transfusion syndrome. Prenat Diagn 18, 941–946.

Denbow, M.L., Overton, T., Duncan, K., et al., 1999. High failure rate of umbilical vessel occlusion by ultrasound guided injection of absolute alcohol or enbucrilate gel. Prenat Diagn 19, 527–532.

Denbow, M.L., Cox, P., Taylor, M., et al., 2000. Placental angioarchitecture in monochorionic twin pregnancies: relationship to fetal growth, feto-fetal transfusion syndrome and pregnancy outcome. Am J Obstet Gynecol 182, 417–426.

Desmonts, G., Couvreur, J., 1974. Congenital toxoplasmosis: a prospective study of 378 pregnancies. N Engl J Med 290, 1110–1116.

de Vries, L., Connell, J., Bydder, J.M., et al., 1988. Recurrent intracranial haemorrhages in utero in an infant with alloimmune thrombocytopenia. Br J Obstet Gynaecol 95, 299–302.

Dommergues, M., Mandelbrot, L., Delezoide, A.L., et al., 1995. Twin-to-twin transfusion syndrome: selective feticide by embolization of the hydropic fetus. Fetal Diagn Ther 10, 26–31.

Driscoll, D.A., Gross, S., 2009. Prenatal screening for aneuploidy. N Engl J Med 360, 2556–2562.

Duncan, K., Denbow, M.L., Fisk, N., 1997. The aetiology and management of twin-twin transfusion syndrome. Prenat Diagn 17, 1227–1236.

Eady, R.A.J., Gunner, D.B., Rodeck, C.H., et al., 1983. Prenatal diagnosis of oculocutaneous albinism by electron microscopy of fetal skin. J Invest Dermatol 80, 210–212.

Ebenroth, E.S., Cordes, T.M., Darragh, R.K., 2001. Second-line treatment of fetal supraventricular tachycardia using flecainide acetate. Pediatr Cardiol 22, 483–487.

Eddelman, K., Stone, J., Lynch, L., et al., 2002. Selective termination of anomalous fetuses in multifetal pregnancies: two hundred cases at a single center. Am J Obstet Gynecol 187, 1168–1172.

Elder, J.S., Duckett, J.W., Snyder, H.M., 1987. Intervention for fetal obstructive uropathy: has it been effective? Lancet ii, 1007–1010.

Elias, J., Mazur, M., Sabbhaga, R., et al., 1980. Prenatal diagnosis of harlequin ichthyosis. Clin Genet 17, 275–279.

Elliot, J.P., Sawyer, S.T., Radin, T.G., et al., 1994. Large-volume therapeutic amniocentesis in the treatment of hydramnios. Obstet Gynecol 84, 1025–1027.

Elser, H., Borutto, F., Schneider, A., et al., 1983. Chylothorax in a twin pregnancy of 34 weeks – sonographically diagnosed. Eur J Obstet Gynaecol Reprod Biol 16, 205–211.

Enders, G., Jonatha, W., 1987. Prenatal diagnosis of intrauterine rubella. Infection 15, 162–164.

Enders, G., Nickerl-Pacher, U., Miller, E., et al., 1988. Outcome of confirmed periconceptual maternal rubella. Lancet 1, 1445–1447.

Eurofetus, 2003. Endoscopic access to the fetoplacental unit. www.eurofetus.org.

Evans, M., Fletcher, J.C., Zador, I.E., et al., 1988. Selective first-trimester termination in octuplet and quadruplet pregnancies: clinical and ethical issues. Obstet Gynecol 71, 289–296.

Evans, M.I., Goldberg, J.D., Dommergues, M., et al., 1994. Efficacy of second-trimester selective termination for fetal abnormalities: international collaborative experience among the world's largest centers. Am J Obstet Gynecol 171, 90–94.

Evans, M., Wapner, R., Ayoub, M., et al., 2002. Spontaneous abortions in couples declining multifetal pregnancy reduction. Fetal Diagn Ther 17, 343–346.

Evans, M., Krivchenia, E., Gelber, S., et al., 2003. Selective reduction. Clin Perinatol 30, 103–111.

Eydoux, P., Choiset, A., Le Porrier, N., et al., 1989. Chromosomal prenatal diagnosis: study of 936 cases of intrauterine abnormalities after ultrasound assessment. Prenat Diagn 9, 255–268.

Fakhry, J., Reiser, M., Shapiro, L.R., et al., 1986. Increased echogenicity in the lower fetal abdomen: a common normal variant in the second trimester. J Ultrasound Med 5, 489–492.

Farrant, P.T., 1980. The antenatal diagnosis of oesophageal atresia by ultrasound. Br J Radiol 53, 1202–1203.

Fassihi, H., Eady, R.A.J., Mellerio, J.E., et al., 2006. Prenatal diagnosis for severe inherited skin disorders: 25 years' experience. Br J Dermatol 154, 106–113.

Feingold, M., Cetrulo, C.L., Newton, E.R., et al., 1986. Serial amniocenteses in the treatment of twin-twin transfusion with acute polyhydramnios. Acta Genet Med Gemellol 35, 107–113.

Fermont, L., de Geeter, B., Aubry, M.C., et al., 1985. A close collaboration between obstetricians and cardiologists allows antenatal detection of severe cardiac malformation by 2D echocardiography. In: Second World Congress of Paediatric Cardiology. Springer-Verlag, New York, p. 10.

Filly, R.A., Golbus, M.S., 1982. Ultrasonography of the normal and pathological fetal skeleton. Radiol Clin North Am 20, 311–323.

Filly, R.A., Golbus, M.S., Carey, J.C., et al., 1981. Short-limbed dwarfism: ultrasonic diagnosis by mensuration of the fetal femoral length. Radiology 138, 653–656.

Finberg, H.J., 1992. The 'twin-peak' sign: reliable evidence of dichorionic twinning. J Ultrasound Med 11, 571–577.

Finning, K.M., Martin, P.G., Soothill, P.W., et al., 2002. Prediction of fetal D status from maternal plasma: introduction of a new noninvasive fetal RHD genotyping service. Transfusion 42, 1079–1085.

Firth, H.V., Boyd, P.A., Chamberlain, P.F., et al., 1991. Severe limb abnormalities after chorion villus sampling at 56–66 days gestation. Lancet 337, 762–763.

Firth, H.V., Boyd, P.A., Chamberlain, P.F., et al., 1994. Analysis of limb reduction defects in babies exposed to chorion villus sampling. Lancet 343, 1069–1071.

Fisk, N.M., Tannirandorn, Y., Santolaya, J., et al., 1989. Fetal macrocytosis in association with chromosomal abnormalities. Obstet Gynecol 74, 611–616.

Fisk, N., Borrell, A., Hubinont, C., et al., 1990a. Fetofetal transfusion syndrome: do the neonatal criteria apply in utero? Arch Dis Child 65, 657–661.

Fisk, N.M., Tannirandorn, Y., Nicolini, U., et al., 1990b. Amniotic pressure in disorders of amniotic fluid volume. Obstet Gynecol 76, 210–214.

Fisk, N.M., Ronderos-Dumit, D., Soliani, A., et al., 1991. Diagnostic and therapeutic transabdominal amnioinfusion in oligohydramnios. Obstet Gynecol 78, 270–278.

Fisk, N.M., Duncombe, G.J., Sullivan, M.H.F., 2009. The basic and clinical science of twin-twin transfusion syndrome. Placenta 30, 379–390.

Fiske, C.E., Filly, R.A., Callen, P.W., 1981. Sonographic measurement of lateral ventricular width in early ventricular dilatation. J Clin Ultrasound 9, 303–307.

Flack, N.J., Zosmer, N., Bennett, P.R., et al., 1993. Amiodarone given by 3 routes to terminate fetal atrial flutter associated with severe hydrops. Obstet Gynecol 82, 714–716.

Flake, A.W., Harrison, M.R., Adzick, N.S., et al., 1986. Fetal sacrococcygeal teratoma. J Pediatr Surg 21, 563–566.

Flake, A., Crombleholme, T., Johnson, M., et al., 2000. Treatment of severe congenital diaphragmatic hernia by fetal tracheal occlusion: clinical experience with 15 cases. Am J Obstet Gynecol 183, 1059–1066.

Forestier, F., Daffos, F., Galacteros, F., et al., 1986. Hematological values of 163 normal fetuses between 18 and 30 weeks of gestation. Pediatr Res 20, 342–346.

Forestier, F., Daffos, F., Rainout, M., et al., 1987. Blood chemistry of normal human fetuses at mid-trimester of pregnancy. Pediatr Res 21, 579–583.

Forestier, F., Tissot, J.D., Vial, Y., et al., 1999. Haematological parameters of parvovirus B19 infection in 13 fetuses with hydrops fetalis. Br J Haematol 104, 925–927.

Freedman, A., Johnson, M., Smith, C., et al., 1999. Longterm outcome in children after antenatal intervention for obstructive uropathies. Lancet 354, 374–377.

Friedman, J.M., Aster, R.H., 1985. Neonatal alloimmune thrombocytopenic purpura and congenital porencephaly in two siblings associated with a 'new' maternal antiplatelet antibody. Blood 65, 1412–1415.

Frohn-Mulder, I., Stewart, P., Witsenburg, M., et al., 1995. The efficacy of flecainide versus digoxin in the management of fetal supraventricular tachycardia. Prenat Diagn 15, 1297–1302.

Froster, U.G., Jackson, L., 1996. Limb defects and chorionic villus sampling: results from an international registry, 1992–94. Lancet 347, 489–494.

Furness, M.E., Barbary, J.E., Verco, P.W., 1987. Fetal head shape in spina bifida in the second trimester. J Clin Ultrasound 15, 451–453.

Fusi, L., Gordon, H., 1990. Twin pregnancy complicated by single intrauterine death. Problems and outcome with conservative management. Br J Obstet Gynaecol 97, 511–516.

Fusi, L., McParland, P., Fisk, N., et al., 1991. Acute twin-twin transfusion: a possible mechanism for brain-damaged survivors after intrauterine death of a monochorionic twin. Obstet Gynecol 78, 517–520.

Gardiner, H.M., 2006. Keeping abreast of advances in fetal cardiology. Early Hum Dev 82, 415–419.

Gardosi, J., Mongelli, M., 1993. Risk assessment adjusted for gestational age in maternal serum screening for Down's syndrome. Br Med J 306, 1509–1511.

Ghidini, A., Sepulveda, W., Lockwood, C., et al., 1993. Complications of fetal blood sampling. Am J Obstet Gynecol 168, 1339–1344.

Giannakoulopoulos, X., Sepulveda, W., Kourtis, P., et al., 1994. Fetal plasma cortisol and beta-endorphin response to intrauterine needling. Lancet 344, 77–81.

Giannakoulopoulos, X., Teixeira, J., Fisk, N., et al., 1999. Human fetal and maternal noradrenaline responses to invasive procedures. Paediatr Res 45, 494–499.

Gilbert, W.M., Nicolaides, K.H., 1987. Fetal omphalocele: associated malformations and chromosomal defects. Obstet Gynecol 70, 633–635.

Glick, P.L., Harrison, M.R., Noall, R.A., et al., 1983. Correction of congenital hydronephrosis in utero. III. Early mid-trimester ureteral obstruction produces renal dysplasia. J Pediatr Surg 18, 681–687.

Glick, P.L., Harrison, M.R., Adzick, N.S., et al., 1984. Correction of congenital hydronephrosis in utero. IV. In utero decompression prevents renal dysplasia. J Pediatr Surg 19, 649–657.

Glick, P.L., Harrison, M.R., Golbus, M.S., et al., 1985. Management of the fetus with congenital hydronephrosis. II. Prognostic criteria and selection for treatment. J Pediatr Surg 20, 376–387.

Golbus, M.S., Sagebiel, R.W., Filly, R.A., et al., 1980. Prenatal diagnosis of bullous ichthyosiform erythroderma (epidermolysis hyperkeratosis) by fetal skin biopsy. N Engl J Med 302, 93–95.

Gonsoulin, W., Moise, K., Kirshon, B., et al., 1990. Outcome of twin-twin transfusion diagnosed before 28 weeks of gestation. Obstet Gynecol 75, 214–216.

Grannum, P.A., Ghidini, A., Scioscia, A., et al., 1989. Assessment of fetal renal reserve in low level obstructive uropathy. Lancet i, 281–282.

Gregg, N.M., 1941. Cataract following German measles in the mother. Trans Ophthalm Soc Aust 3, 34–36.

Hackett, G.A., Nicolaides, K.H., Campbell, S., 1987. Doppler ultrasound assessment of fetal and uteroplacental circulations in severe second trimester oligohydramnios. Br J Obstet Gynaecol 94, 1074–1077.

Haddow, J.E., Palomaki, G.E., Knight, G.J., et al., 1994. Reducing the need for amniocentesis in women 35 years of age or older with serum markers for screening. N Engl J Med 330, 1114–1118.

Hahnemann, J.M., Vejerslev, L.O., 1997. European Collaborative Research on mosaicism in CVS (EUCROMIC) – fetal and extrafetal cell lineages in 192 gestations with CVS mosaicism involving single autosomy trisomy. Am J Med Genet 70, 179–187.

Hanson, F.W., Zorn, E.M., Tennant, F.R., et al., 1987. Amniocentesis before 15 weeks gestation: outcome, risks and technical problems. Am J Obstet Gynecol 156, 1524–1531.

Harman, C.R., 1995. Invasive techniques in the management of alloimmune anaemia. In: Harman, C.R. (Ed.), Invasive Fetal Testing and Treatment. Blackwell Science, Boston, pp. 107–192.

Harrison, M.R., Filly, R.A., Parer, J.T., et al., 1981. Management of the fetus with a urinary tract malformation. JAMA 246, 635–639.

Harrison, M.R., Golbus, M.S., Filly, R.A., et al., 1982. Management of the fetus with congenital hydronephrosis. J Pediatr Surg 17, 728–742.

Harrison, M.R., Ross, N.A., Noall, R., et al., 1983. Correction of congenital hydronephrosis in utero. I. The model: fetal urethral obstruction produces hydronephrosis and pulmonary hypoplasia in fetal lambs. J Pediatr Surg 18, 247–256.

Harrison, M.R., Langer, J.C., Adzick, N.S., et al., 1990. Correction of congenital diaphragmatic hernia in utero. V. Initial clinical experience. J Pediatr Surg 25, 47–57.

Harrison, M., Albanese, C., Hawgood, S., et al., 2001. Fetoscopic temporary tracheal occlusion by means of detachable balloon for congenital diaphragmatic hernia. Am J Obstet Gynecol 185, 730–733.

Harrison, M.R., Keller, R.L., Hawgood, S.B., et al., 2003. A randomized trial of fetal endoscopic tracheal occlusion for severe fetal congenital diaphragmatic hernia. N Engl J Med 349, 1916–1924.

Hecher, K., Campbell, S., Doyle, P., et al., 1995a. Assessment of fetal compromise by Doppler ultrasound investigation of the fetal circulation. Arterial, intracardiac and venous blood flow studies. Circulation 91, 129–138.

Hecher, K., Ville, Y., Nicolaides, K., 1995b. Fetal arterial Doppler studies in twin-twin transfusion syndrome. J Ultrasound Med 14, 101–108.

Hecher, K., Ville, Y., Snijders, R., et al., 1995c. Doppler studies of the fetal circulation in twin-twin transfusion syndrome. Ultrasound Obstet Gynecol 5, 318–324.

Hegde, U.M., 1985. Immune thrombocytopenia in pregnancy and the newborn. Br J Obstet Gynaecol 92, 657–659.

Hegge, F.N., Franklin, R.W., Watson, P.T., et al., 1989. An evaluation of the time of discovery of fetal malformations by an indication-based system for ordering obstetric ultrasound. Obstet Gynecol 74, 21–24.

Hobbins, J.C., Romero, R., Grannum, P., et al., 1984. Antenatal diagnosis of renal anomalies with ultrasound. I. Obstructive uropathy. Am J Obstet Gynecol 148, 868–877.

Hohlfield, P., Daffos, F., Costa, J., et al., 1994. Prenatal diagnosis of congenital toxoplasmosis with a polymerase-chain-reaction test on amniotic fluid. N Engl J Med 331, 695–699.

Hudon, L., Moise, Jr, K.J., Hegemier, S.E., et al., 1998. Long-term neurodevelopmental outcome after intrauterine transfusion for the treatment of fetal hemolytic disease. Am J Obstet Gynecol 179, 858–863.

Hull, D., Binns, B.A., Joyce, D., 1966. Congenital heart block and widespread fibrosis due to maternal lupus erythematosus. Arch Dis Child 41, 688–690.

Hultén, M.A., Dhanjal, S., Pertl, B., 2003. Rapid and simple prenatal diagnosis of common chromosome disorders: advantages and disadvantages of the molecular methods FISH and QF-PCR. Reproduction 126, 279–297.

Hunt, G.M., Oakeshott, P., 2003. Outcome in people with open spina bifida at age 35, prospective community based cohort study. Br Med J 326, 1365–1366.

Isada, N.B., Pryde, P.G., Johnson, M.P., et al., 1992. Fetal intracardiac potassium chloride injection to avoid the hopeless resuscitation of an abnormal abortus. I. Clinical issues. Obstet Gynecol 80, 296–299.

Itskowitz, J., Boldes, R., Thaler, I., et al., 1989. Transvaginal ultrasonography-guided aspiration of gestational sacs for selective abortion in multiple pregnancy. Am J Obstet Gynecol 160, 215–217.

Izmirly, P.M., Llanos, C., Lee, L.A., et al., 2010. Cutaneous manifestation of neonatal lupes and risk of subsequent congenital heart block. Arthritis Rheum 62, 1153–1157.

Jackson, L.G., Zachary, J.M., Fowler, S.E., et al., 1992. A randomized comparison of transcervical and transabdominal chorionic-villus sampling. N Engl J Med 327, 594–598.

Jani, J.C., Nicolaides, K.H., Keller, R.L., et al., 2007. Observed to expected lung area to head circumference ratio in the prediction of survival in fetuses with isolated diaphragmatic hernia. Ultrasound Obstet Gynecol 30, 67–71.

Jani, J., Cannie, M., Sonigo, P., et al., 2008. Value of prenatal magnetic resonance imaging in the prediction of postnatal outcome in fetuses with diaphragmatic hernia. Ultrasound Obstet Gynecol 32, 791–799.

Jani, J.C., Nicolaides, K.H., Gratacós, E., et al., 2009. Severe diaphragmatic hernia treated by fetal endoscopic tracheal occlusion. Ultrasound Obstet Gynecol 34, 304–310.

Jauniaux, E., Donner, C., Simon, P., et al., 1989. Pathological aspects of the umbilical cord after percutaneous umbilical blood sampling. Obstet Gynecol 73, 215–218.

Jeanty, P., Chaoui, R., Grochal, F., 2008. A review of findings in fetal cardiac section drawings. Part 4. Sagittal and parasagittal views. J Ultrasound Med 27, 919–923.

Johnson, M.P., Bukowski, T.P., Reitleman, C., et al., 1994. In utero surgical treatment of fetal obstructive uropathy: a new comprehensive approach to identify appropriate candidates for vesicoamniotic shunt therapy. Am J Obstet Gynecol 170, 1770–1779.

Kagan, K.O., Valecia, C., Livanos, P., et al., 2009. Tricuspid regurgitation in screening for trisomies 21, 18 and 13 and Turner syndrome at 11+0 to 13+6 weeks of gestation. Ultrasound Obstet Gynecol 33, 18–22.

Kamphius, M.M., Paridaans, N., Porcelijn, L., et al., 2010. Screening in pregnancy for fetal or neonatal alloimmune thrombocytopenia: systematic review. Br J Obstet Gynaecol 117, 1335–1343.

Kanhai, H.H.H., Porcelijn, L., Engelfriet, C.P., et al., 2007. Management of alloimmune thrombocytopaenia. Vox Sang 93, 370–385.

Kaplan, C., Daffos, F., Forestier, F., et al., 1988. Management of alloimmune thrombocytopenia: antenatal diagnosis and in utero transfusion of maternal platelets. Blood 72, 340–343.

Kappel, B., Nielsen, J., Hansen, K.B., et al., 1987. Spontaneous abortion following mid-trimester amniocentesis. Clinical significance of placental perforation and blood stained amniotic fluid. Br J Obstet Gynaecol 94, 50–54.

Kelton, J.G., Inwood, M.J., Barr, R.M., et al., 1982. The prenatal prediction of thrombocytopenia in infants of mothers with clinically diagnosed immune thrombocytopenia. Am J Obstet Gynecol 144, 449–454.

Kilian, A.K., Schaible, T., Hofmann, V., et al., 2009. Congenital diaphragmatic hernia: predictive value of MRI relative lung-to-head ratio compared with MRI fetal lung volume and sonographic lung-to-head ratio. AJR Am J Roentgenol 192, 153–158.

King, S.J., Pilling, D.W., Walkinshaw, S., 1995. Fetal echogenic lung lesions: prenatal ultrasound diagnosisis and outcome. Pediatr Radiol 25, 208–210.

Kjeldsen-Kragh, J., Killie, M.K., Tomter, G., et al., 2007. A screening and intervention program aimed to reduce mortality and serious morbidity with severe neonatal alloimmune thrombocytopaenia. Blood 110, 833–839.

Kleinman, C.S., Copel, J.A., Weinstein, E.M., et al., 1985. In utero diagnosis and treatment of fetal supraventricular tachycardia. Semin Perinatol 9, 113–129.

Kohl, T., Tercanli, S., Kececioglu, D., et al., 1995. Direct fetal administration of adenosine for the termination of incessant supraventricular tachycardia. Obstet Gynecol 85, 873–874.

Koresawa, M., Inaba, J., Iwasaki, H., 1987. Fetal blood sampling by liver puncture. Acta Obstet Gynaecol Japon 39, 395–399.

Kostovic, I., Rakic, P., 1990. Developmental history of the transient subplate zone in the visual and somatosensory cortex of the macaque monkey and human brain. J Comp Neurol 297, 441–470.

Kozlowski, P., Knippel, A.J., Froehlich, S., et al., 2006. Additional performance of nasal bone in first trimester screening. Nasal bone in first trimester screening. Ultraschall Med 27, 336–339.

Kuliev, A.M., Modell, B., Jackson, L., et al., 1993. Risk evaluation of CVS. Prenat Diagn 13, 197–209.

Kurth, K.H., Alleman, E.R., Schroeder, F.H., 1981. Major and minor complications of posterior urethral valves. J Urol 126, 517–519.

Kusseff, B.G., Matsouka, L.Y., Stenn, K.S., et al., 1982. Prenatal diagnosis of Sjögren–Larsson syndrome. J Pediatr 101, 998–1001.

Kyle, P.M., Sepulveda, W., Blunt, S., et al., 1996. High failure rate of postmortem karyotyping after termination for fetal abnormality. Obstet Gynecol 88, 859–862.

Landwehr, J.B., Johnson, M.P., Hume, R.F., et al., 1996. Abnormal nuchal findings on screening ultrasonography: aneuploidy stratification on the basis of ultrasonographic anomaly and gestational age at detection. Am J Obstet Gynecol 175, 995–999.

Lange, I., Rodeck, C.H., Morgan-Capner, P., et al., 1982. Prenatal serological diagnosis of intrauterine cytomegalovirus infection. Br Med J 284, 1673–1674.

Langer, J.C., Harrison, M.R., Scmidt, K.G., et al., 1989. Fetal hydrops and death from sacrococcygeal teratoma: rationale for fetal surgery. Am J Obstet Gynecol 160, 1145–1150.

Langer, J.C., Fitzgerald, P.G., Desa, D., et al., 1990. Cervical cystic hygroma in the fetus: clinical spectrum and outcome. J Pediatr Surg 25, 58–62.

Laurence, K.M., Coates, S., 1962. The natural history of hydrocephalus: detailed analysis of 182 unoperated cases. Arch Dis Child 37, 345–362.

Levi, S., Crouzet, P., Schaaps, J.P., et al., 1989. Ultrasound screening for fetal malformations. Lancet i, 678.

Lipitz, S., Ryan, G., Samuell C., et al., 1993. Fetal urine analysis for the assessment of renal function in obstructive uropathy. Am J Obstet Gynecol 168, 174–179.

Lo, Y.M., Hjelm, N.M., Fidler, C., et al., 1998. Prenatal diagnosis of fetal RhD status by molecular analysis of maternal plasma. N Engl J Med 339, 1734–1738.

Loft, A.G., Hogdall, E., Larsen, S.O., et al., 1993. A comparison of amniotic fluid alpha-fetoprotein and acetylcholinesterase in the prenatal diagnosis of open neural tube defects and anterior abdominal wall defects. Prenat Diagn 13, 93–109.

Longaker, M.T., Laberge, J., Dansereau, J., et al., 1989. Primary fetal hydrothorax: natural history and management. J Pediatr Surg 24, 573–576.

Luck, C.A., 1992. Value of routine ultrasound scanning at 19 weeks: a four-year study of 8894 deliveries. Br Med J 304, 1474–1478.

Machado, M.V.L., Tynan, M.J., Curry, P.V.L., et al., 1988. Fetal complete heart block. Br Heart J 60, 512–515.

Machin, G., Still, K., Lalani, T., 1996. Correlations of placental vascular anatomy and clinical outcomes in 69 monochorionic twin pregnancies. Am J Med Genet 61, 229–236.

Maddocks, D.G., Alberry, M.S., Atitilakos, G., et al., 2009. The SAFE project: towards non-invasive prenatal diagnosis. Biochem Soc Transact 37, 460–465.

Mahieu-Caputo, D., Muller, F., Joly, D., et al., 2001. Pathogenesis of twin-twin transfusion syndrome: the renin–angiotensin system hypothesis. Fetal Diagn Ther 16, 241–244.

Mahoney, B.S., Filly, R.A., Callen, P.W., et al., 1984. Fetal renal dysplasia: sonographic evaluation. Radiology 152, 143–146.

Maiz, N., Valencia, C., Kagan, K.O., et al., 2009. Ductus venosus Doppler in screening for trisomies 21, 18 and 13 and Turner syndrome at 11–13 weeks gestation. Ultrasound Obstet Gynecol 33, 512–517.

Malone, F.D., Canick, J.A., Ball, R.H., et al., 2005. First-trimester or second-trimester screening, or both, for Down's syndrome. N Engl J Med 353, 2001–2011.

Mandelbrot, L., Dumez, Y., Muller, F., et al., 1991. Prenatal prediction of renal function in fetal obstructive uropathies. J Perinat Med 19, 283–297.

Manning, F.A., Harison, M.R., Rodeck, C.H., et al., 1986. Catheter shunts for fetal hydronephrosis and hydrocephalus. N Engl J Med 315, 336–340.

Mari, G., Wasserstrum, N., Kirshon, B., 1992. Reduction in the middle cerebral artery pulsatility index after decompression of polyhydramnios in twin gestation. Am J Perinatol 9, 381–384.

Mari, G., Deter, R.L., Carpenter, R.L., et al., 2000. Noninvasive diagnosis by Doppler ultrasonography of fetal anemia due to maternal red-cell alloimmunization. Collaborative Group for Doppler Assessment of the Blood Velocity in Anemic Fetuses. N Engl J Med 342, 9–14.

Mari, G., Roberts, A., Detti L., et al., 2001. Perinatal morbidity and mortality rates in severe twin-twin transfusion syndrome: results of the International Amnioreduction Registry. Am J Obstet Gynecol 185, 708–715.

Maxwell, D.J., Crawford, D.C., Curry, P.V., et al., 1988. Obstetric importance, diagnosis and management of fetal tachycardias. Br Med J 297, 107–110.

Maxwell, D., Johnson, P., Hurley, P., et al., 1991. Fetal blood sampling and pregnancy loss in relation to indication. Br J Obstet Gynaecol 98, 892–897.

McCullagh, M., MacConnachie, I., Garvie, D., et al., 1994. Accuracy of prenatal diagnosis in congenital cystic adenomatoid malformation. Arch Dis Child Fetal Neonat Ed 71, F111–F113.

Megerian, G., Ludomirsky, A., 1994. Role of cordocentesis in perinatal medicine. Curr Opin Obstet Gynaecol 6, 30–35.

Melchiorre, K., Bhide, A., Gika, A.D., et al., 2009. Counselling in isolated mild ventriculomegaly. Ultrasound Obstet Gynecol 34, 212–224.

Mercer, L.J., Brown, L.G., 1986. Fetal outcome with oligohydramnios in second trimester. Obstet Gynecol 67, 840–842.

Meuli, M., Meuli-Simmen, C., Hutchins, G.M., et al., 1995. In utero surgery rescues neurological function at birth in sheep with spina bifida. Nature Med 1, 342–347.

Mibashan, R.S., Rodeck, C.H., 1984. Haemophilia and other genetic defects of haemostasis. In: Rodeck, C.H., Nicolaides, K.H. (Eds.), Prenatal Diagnosis. Proceedings of the Eleventh Study Group of the Royal College of Obstetricians and Gynaecologists. RCOG, London, pp. 179–194.

Michejda, M., Hodgen, G.D., 1981. In utero diagnosis and treatment of non-human primate fetal skeletal anomalies. I. Hydrocephalus. JAMA 246, 1093–1097.

Millar, D.S., Davis, L.R., Rodeck, C.H., et al., 1985. Normal blood cell values in the early mid-trimester fetus. Prenat Diagn 5, 367–373.

Mohr, J., 1968. Foetal genetic diagnosis: development of techniques for early sampling of foetal cells. Acta Pathol Microbiol Immunol Scand 73, 73–77.

Moise, K.J., Carpenter, R.J., Cotton, D.B., et al., 1988. Percutaneous umbilical cord blood sampling in the evaluation of fetal platelet counts in pregnant patients with autoimmune thrombocytopenic purpura. Obstet Gynecol 72, 346–350.

Moise, Jr, K.J., Dorman, K., Lamvu, G., et al., 2003. A randomised trial of amnioreduction versus septostomy in the treatment of twin-twin transfusion syndrome. Am J Obstet Gynecol 193, 701–707.

Moniz, C.F., Nicolaides, K.H., Bamforth, F.J., et al., 1985. Normal ranges for biochemical substances relating to renal, hepatic and bone function in fetal and maternal plasma throughout pregnancy. J Clin Pathol 38, 468–472.

Monteagudo, A., Timor-Tritsch, I.E., Sharma, S., 1994. Early and simple determination of chorionic and amniotic type in multifetal gestations in the first fourteen weeks by high-frequency transvaginal ultrasonography. Am J Obstet Gynecol 170, 824–829.

Moore, T.R., Cayle, J.E., 1990. The amniotic fluid index in normal human pregnancy. Am J Obstet Gynecol 162, 1168–1173.

Moore, T.R., Longo, J., Leopold, G.R., et al., 1989. The reliability and predictive value of an amniotic fluid scoring system in severe second trimester oligohydramnios. Obstet Gynecol 73, 739–742.

Morales, W.J., Stroup, M., 1985. Intracranial hemorrhage in utero due to isoimmune neonatal thrombocytopenia. Obstet Gynecol 65, 20S–21S.

Morgan-Capner, P., Rodeck, C.H., Nicolaides, K.H., et al., 1985. Prenatal detection of rubella-specific IgM in fetal sera. Prenat Diagn 5, 21–26.

Muller, F., Aubry, M.C., Gasser, B., et al., 1985. Prenatal diagnosis of cystic fibrosis. II. Meconium ileus in affected fetuses. Prenat Diagn 5, 109–117.

Muller, F., Dommergues, M., Mandelbrot, L., et al., 1993. Fetal urinary biochemistry predicts postnatal renal function in children with bilateral obstructive uropathies. Obstet Gynecol 82, 813–820.

Nakayama, D.K., Harrison, M.R., de Lorimier, A.A., 1986. Prognosis of posterior urethral valves presenting at birth. J Pediatr Surg 21, 43–45.

National Collaborating Centre for Women's and Children's Health, 2008. Antenatal Routine Care for the Healthy Pregnant Woman. Available online at: rcog.org.uk.

National Health Service Fetal Anomaly Screening Programme, 2010. NHS Fetal Anomaly Screening Programme 18^{+0} to 20^{+6} Weeks Fetal Anomaly Scan National Standards and Guidance for England. Available online at: fetalanomaly. screening.nhs.uk.

National Health Service OPCS, 1997. Birth Statistics. Review of the Register General on Births and Patterns of Family Building in England and Wales. HMSO, London.

National Institute for Health and Clinical Excellence, 2003. Routine Anti-D Prophylaxis for Rhesus Negative Women. Clinical Guideline no. 41. NICE, London. Available online at: nice.org.uk.

National Institutes for Health Consensus Development Statement, 1984. United States Department of Health and Human Services (NIH publication 84–667), Washington DC.

Neilson, J.P., Alfirevic, Z., 2003. Doppler ultrasound for fetal assessment in high risk pregnancies (Cochrane Review). In: The Cochrane Library, Issue 2.

Neilson, J., Danskin, F., Hastie, S., 1989. Monozygotic twin pregnancy: diagnostic and Doppler ultrasound studies. Br J Obstet Gynaecol 96, 1413–1418.

Nelson, L.H., Clark, C.E., Fishburn, J.I., et al., 1982. Value of serial ultrasonography in the in utero detection of duodenal atresia. Obstet Gynecol 59, 657–660.

Ney, J.A., Fee, S.C., Dooley, S.L., et al., 1989. Factors influencing hemostasis after umbilical vein puncture in vitro. Am J Obstet Gynecol 160, 424–426.

Nicolaides, K.H., Azar, G.B., 1990. Thoraco-amniotic shunting. Fetal Diagn Ther 5, 153–164.

Nicolaides, K.H., Economides, D.L., 1990. Cordocentesis of small-for-gestational age fetuses. In: Chamberlain, G. (Ed.), Modern Antenatal Care of the Fetus. Blackwell Science, Oxford, pp. 127–149.

Nicolaides, K.H., Rodeck, C.H., Lange, I., et al., 1985a. Fetoscopy in the assessment of unexplained fetal hydrops. Br J Obstet Gynaecol 92, 671–679.

Nicolaides, K.H., Rodeck, C.H., Mibashan, R.S., 1985b. Obstetric management and diagnosis of haematological disease in the fetus. Clin Haematol 14, 775–805.

Nicolaides, K.H., Campbell, S., Gabbe, S.G., et al., 1986a. Ultrasound screening for spina bifida: cranial and cerebellar signs. Lancet ii, 71–74.

Nicolaides, K.H., Rodeck, C.H., Gosden, C.N., 1986b. Rapid karyotyping in non-lethal malformations. Lancet i, 283–287.

Nicolaides, K.H., Soothill, P.W., Rodeck, C.H., et al., 1986c. Ultrasound guided sampling of umbilical cord and placental blood to assess fetal well-being. Lancet i, 1065–1067.

Nicolaides, K.H., Soothill, P.W., Rodeck, C.H., et al., 1986d. Rh disease: intravascular fetal blood transfusion by cordocentesis. Fetal Ther 1, 185–192.

Nicolaides, K.H., Blott, M., Greenough, M., 1987a. Chronic drainage of fetal pulmonary cyst (letter). Lancet i, 618.

Nicolaides, K.H., Clewell, W.H., Rodeck, C.H., 1987b. Measurement of human fetoplacental blood volume in erythroblastosis fetalis. Am J Obstet Gynecol 157, 50–53.

Nicolaides, K.H., Bilardo, C.M., Soothill, P.W., et al., 1988a. Absence of end-diastolic frequencies in the umbilical artery: a sign of fetal hypoxia and acidosis. Br Med J 297, 1026–1027.

Nicolaides, K.H., Clewell, W.H., Mibashan, R.S., et al., 1988b. Fetal haemoglobin measurement in the assessment of red cell isoimmunization. Lancet i, 1073–1075.

Nicolaides, K.H., Fontanorosa, M., Gabbe, S.G., et al., 1988c. Failure of ultrasonographic parameters to predict the severity of fetal anemia in rhesus isoimmunisation. Am J Obstet Gynecol 158, 920–926.

Nicolaides, K.H., Economides, D.L., Soothill, P.W., 1989. Blood gases, pH, and lactate in appropriate- and small-for-gestational-age fetuses. Am J Obstet Gynecol 161, 996–1001.

Nicolaides, K.H., Bilardo, C.M., Campbell, S., 1990. Prediction of fetal anemia by measurement of the mean blood velocity in the fetal aorta. Am J Obstet Gynecol 162, 209–212.

Nicolaides, K.H., Brizot, M.L., Snijders, R.J.M., 1994a. Fetal nuchal translucency: ultrasound screening for fetal trisomy in the first trimester of pregnancy. Br J Obstet Gynaecol 101, 782–786.

Nicolaides, K.H., Brizot, M., Patel, F., et al., 1994b. Comparison of chorionic villus sampling and amniocentesis for fetal karyotyping at 10–13 weeks gestation. Lancet 344, 435–439.

Nicolaides, K.H., Spencer, K., Avgidou, K., et al., 2005. Multicenter study of first-trimester screening for trisomy 21 in 75 821 pregnancies: results and estimation of the potential impact of individual risk-orientated two-stage first-trimester screening. Ultrasound Obstet Gynecol 25, 221–226.

Nicolini, U., Kochenour, N.K., Greco, P., et al., 1988a. Consequences of fetomaternal haemorrhage after intrauterine transfusion. Br Med J 297, 1379–1381.

Nicolini, U., Rodeck, C.H., Kochenour, N.K., et al., 1988b. In-utero platelet transfusion for alloimmune thrombocytopenia. Lancet ii, 506.

Nicolini, U., Santolaya, J., Ojo, E., et al., 1988c. The fetal intrahepatic vein as an alternative to cord needling for prenatal diagnosis and therapy. Prenat Diagn 8, 665–671.

Nicolini, U., Fisk, N.M., Rodeck, C.H., et al., 1989a. Low amniotic pressure in oligohydramnios – is this the cause of pulmonary hypoplasia? Am J Obstet Gynecol 161, 1098–1101.

Nicolini, U., Hubinont, C., Santolaya, J., et al., 1989b. Maternal–fetal glucose gradient in normal pregnancies and in pregnancies complicated by alloimmunization and fetal growth retardation. Am J Obstet Gynecol 161, 924–927.

Nicolini, U., Kochenour, N.K., Greco, P., et al., 1989c. When to perform the next intrauterine transfusion in patients with Rh allo-immunization: combined intravascular and intraperitoneal transfusion allows longer intervals. Fetal Ther 4, 14–20.

Nicolini, U., Santolaya, J., Hubinont, C., et al., 1989d. Visualization of fetal intra-abdominal organs in second trimester severe oligohydramnios by intraperitoneal infusion. Prenat Diagn 9, 191–194.

Nicolini, U., Talbert, D.G., Fisk, N.M., et al., 1989e. Pathophysiology of pressure changes during intrauterine transfusion. Am J Obstet Gynecol 160, 1139–1145.

Nicolini, U., Nicolaidis, P., Fisk, N.M., et al., 1990a. Fetal blood sampling from the intrahepatic vein: analysis of safety and clinical experience with 214 procedures. Obstet Gynecol 76, 47–53.

Nicolini, U., Tannirandorn, Y., Gonzalez, P., et al., 1990b. Continuing controversy in alloimmune thrombocytopenia: fetal hyperimmunoglobulinemia fails to prevent thrombocytopenia. Am J Obstet Gynecol 163, 1144–1146.

Nicolini, U., Tannirandorn, Y., Vaughan, J., et al., 1991. Further predictors of renal dysplasia in fetal obstructive uropathy: bladder pressure and biochemistry of 'fresh urine'. Prenat Diagn 11, 159–166.

Nicolini, U., Fisk, N.M., Rodeck, C., 1992. Fetal urine biochemistry: an index of renal maturation and dysfunction. Br J Obstet Gynaecol 99, 46–50.

Nicolini, U., Poblete, A., Boschetto, C., et al., 2001. Complicated monochorionic twin pregnancies: experience with bipolar cord coagulation. Am J Obstet Gynecol 185, 703–707.

Nicolini, U., Lalatta, F., Natacci, F., et al., 2004. The introduction of QF-PCR in prenatal diagnosis of fetal aneuploides: time for reconsideration. Hum Reprod Update 10, 541–548.

Nyberg, D., Fitzsimmons, J., Mack, L., 1989. Chromosomal abnormalities in fetuses with omphalocele: significance of omphalocele contents. J Ultrasound Med 8, 299–308, 363.

Oakeshott, P., Hunt, G.M., 2003. Long-term outcome in open spina bifida. Br J Gen Pract 53, 632–636.

Oepkes, D., Vandenbussche, F.P., Van Bel, F., et al., 1993. Fetal ductus venosus blood flow velocities before and after treatment of red cell alloimmunised pregnancies. Obstet Gynecol 82, 237–241.

Oepkes, D., Brand, R., Vandembusschel, F.P., et al., 1994. The use of ultrasonography and Doppler in the prediction of fetal haemolytic anaemia: a multivariate study. Br J Obstet Gynaecol 101, 680–684.

Orlandi, F., Rossi, C., Orlandi, E., et al., 2005. First-trimester screening for trisomy-21 using a simplified method to assess the presence or absence of the fetal nasal bone. Am J Obstet Gynecol 192, 1107–1111.

Örtqvist, L., Laurence, B., Stephanie, S., et al., 2008. Long-term neurodevelopmental outcome in twin-to-twin transfusion syndrome (TTTS) in the Eurofetus trial. Am J Obstet Gynecol 199, S118.

Ouzounian, J.G., Castro, M.A., Fresquez, M., et al., 1996. Prognostic significance of antenatally detected fetal pyelectasis. Ultrasound Obstet Gynecol 7, 424–428.

Paek, B., Jennings, R., Harrison, M., et al., 2001. Radiofrequency ablation of human fetal sacrococcygeal teratoma. Am J Obstet Gynecol 184, 503–507.

Papageorghiou, A.T., Liao, A.W., Skentou, C., et al., 2002. Trichorionic triplet pregnancies at 10–14 weeks: outcome after embryo reduction compared to expectant management. J Maternal Fetal Neonat Med 11, 307–312.

Payne, S.D., Resnik, R., Moore, T.R., et al., 1997. Maternal characteristics and risk of severe neonatal thrombocytopenia and intracranial haemorrhage in pregnancies complicated by autoimmune thrombocytopenia. Am J Obstet Gynecol 177, 149–155.

Peckham, C.S., Johnson, C., Ades, A., et al., 1987. Early acquisition of cytomegalovirus infection. Arch Dis Child 62, 780–785.

Penman, D.G., Fisher, R.M., Noblett, H.R., et al., 1998. Increase in incidence of gastroschisis in the south west of England in 1995. Br J Obstet Gynaecol 105, 328–331.

Petterson, B., Nelson, K., Watson, L., et al., 1993. Twins, triplets, and cerebral palsy in births in Western Australia in the 1980s. Br Med J 307, 1239–1243.

Peters, M.T., Nicolaides, K.H., 1990. Cordocentesis for the diagnosis and treatment of human fetal parvovirus infection. Obstet Gynecol 75, 501–504.

Petres, R.E., Redwine, F.O., Cruickshank, D.P., 1982. Congenital bilateral hydrothorax: antepartum diagnosis and successful intrauterine surgical management. JAMA 248, 1360–1361.

Petrini, J.R., Dias, T., McCormick, M.C., et al., 2009. Increased risk of adverse neurological development for later preterm infants. J Pediatr 154, 169–176.

Petterson, B., Nelson, K., Watson, L., et al., 1993. Twins, triplets, and cerebral palsy in births in Western Australia in the 1980s. Br Med J 307, 1239–1243.

Pilu, G., Reece, E.A., Romero, R., et al., 1986. Prenatal diagnosis of craniofacial malformations by ultrasound. Am J Obstet Gynecol 155, 45–50.

Pilu, G., Romero, R., Rizzo, N., et al., 1987. Criteria for the antenatal diagnosis of holoprosencephaly. Am J Perinatol 4, 41–49.

Pilu, G., Romero, R., Reece, A., et al., 1988. Subnormal cerebellum in fetuses with spina bifida. Am J Obstet Gynecol 158, 1052–1056.

Poissonier, M.-H., Brossard, Y., Demedeiros, N., et al., 1989. Two hundred intrauterine exchange transfusions in severe blood incompatibilities. Am J Obstet Gynecol 161, 709–713.

Public Health Laboratory Service Working Party on Fifth Disease, 1990. Prospective study of human parvovirus B19 infections in pregnancy. Br Med J 300, 1166–1170.

Queenan, J.T., 1970. Recurrent acute polyhydramnios. Am J Obstet Gynecol 106, 625–626.

Quintero, R., Morales, W., Allen, M., et al., 1999. Staging of twin-twin transfusion syndrome. J Perinatol 19, 550–555.

Quintero, R.A., Dickinson, J.E., Morales, W.J., et al., 2003. Stage-based treatment of twin-twin transfusion syndrome. Am J Obstet Gynecol 188, 1333–1340.

Radder, C.M., Brand, A., Kanhai, H.H., 2001. A less invasive treatment strategy to prevent intracranial hemorrhage in fetal and neonatal alloimmune thrombocytopenia. Am J Obstet Gynecol 185, 683–688.

Rasmussen, S.A., 2008. Non-genetic risk factors for gastroschisis. Am J Med Genet C: Semin Med Genet 148C, 199–212.

Reid, R.S., Sepulveda, W., Kyle, P.M., et al., 1996. Amniotic fluid culture failure and clinical significance and association with aneuploidy. Obstet Gynecol 87, 588–592.

Reuss, A., Wladimiroff, J.W., Stewart, P.A., et al., 1988. Non-invasive management of fetal obstructive uropathy. Lancet ii, 949–951.

Reznikoff-Etievant, M.F., 1988. Management of alloimmune neonatal thrombocytopenia and antenatal thrombocytopenia. Vox Sang 55, 193–201.

Rijken, M., Wit, J.M., Le Cassle, S., et al., 2007. The effect of perinatal risk factors on growth in very preterm infants at 2 years of age: the Leiden Follow-Up Project on Prematurity. Early Hum Dev 83, 527–534.

Rizzo, G., Arduini, D., Romanini, C., 1994. Cardiac and extracardiac flows in discordant twins. Am J Obstet Gynecol 170, 1321–1327.

Roberts, A.B., Clarkson, N.S., Pattison, M.G., et al., 1986. Fetal hydrothorax in the second trimester of pregnancy: successful intrauterine treatment at 24 weeks gestation. Fetal Ther 1, 203–209.

Roberts, A.B., Mitchell, J.M., Pattison, N.S., 1989. Fetal liver length in normal and isoimmunized pregnancies. Am J Obstet Gynecol 161, 42–46.

Roberts, D., Gates, S., Kilby, M., et al., 2008. Interventions for twin-twin transfusion syndrome: a Cochrane review. Ultrasound Obstet Gynecol 31, 701–711.

Rochelson, B., Schulman, H., Farmakides, G., et al., 1987. The significance of absent end-diastolic velocity in umbilical artery velocity waveforms. Am J Obstet Gynecol 155, 1213–1218.

Rodeck, C.H., 1980. Fetoscopy guided by real time ultrasound for pure fetal blood samples, fetal skin samples, and examination of the fetus in utero. Br J Obstet Gynaecol 87, 449–456.

Rodeck, C.H., 1993. Fetal development after chorionic villus sampling. Lancet 341, 468–469.

Rodeck, C.H., Nicolini, U., 1988. Physiology of the mid-trimester fetus. Br Med Bull 44, 826–849.

Rodeck, C.H., Eady, R.A.J., Gosden, C.M., 1980. Prenatal diagnosis of epidermolysis bullosa letalis. Lancet i, 949–952.

Rodeck, C.H., Fisk, N.M., Fraser, D.I., et al., 1988. Long-term in utero drainage of fetal hydrothorax. N Engl J Med 319, 1135–1138.

Rodis, J., Hovick, T.J., Quinn, D.L., et al., 1988. Human parvovirus infection in pregnancy. Obstet Gynecol 72, 733–738.

Roelofsen, J., Oostendorp, R., Volovics, A., et al., 1994. Prenatal diagnosis and fetal outcome of cystic adenomatoid malformation of the lung: case report and historical survey. Ultrasound in Obstetrics and Gynecology 4, 78–82.

Romero, R., Chervenak, F.A., Kotzen, J., et al., 1982. Antenatal sonographic findings of extralobar pulmonary sequestration. J Ultrasound Med 1, 131–132.

Romero, R., Cullen, M., Jeanty, P., et al., 1984. The diagnosis of congenital renal anomalies with ultrasound. II. Infantile polycystic kidney disease. Am J Obstet Gynecol 150, 259–262.

Romero, R., Jeanty, P., Reece, E.A., et al., 1985. Sonographically monitored amniocentesis to decrease intraoperative complications. Obstet Gynecol 65, 426–430.

Romero, R., Pilu, G., Pilu, G., et al., 1988. Prenatal Diagnosis of Congenital Anomalies. Appleton and Lange, Connecticut.

Rotten, D., Levaillant, J.M., 2004. Two- and three-dimensional sonographic assessment of the fetal face. 2. Analysis of cleft lip, alveolus and palate. Ultrasound Obstet Gynecol 24, 402–411.

Royal College of Obstetricians and Gynaecologists, 2003. Clinical Guidelines: Use of Anti-D Immunoglobulin for Rh Prophylaxis. Available online at: www.rcog.org.uk.

Royal College of Obstetricians and Gynaecologists Working Party on Routine Ultrasound Examination in Pregnancy, 1984. RCOG, London, pp. 13–16.

Salvodelli, G., Schmid, W., Schinzel, A., 1982. Prenatal diagnosis of cleft lip and palate by ultrasound. Prenat Diagn 2, 313–317.

Samuels, P., Bussel, J.B., Braitman, L.E., et al., 1990. Estimation of the risk of thrombocytopenia in the offspring of pregnant women with presumed immune thrombocytopenic purpura. N Engl J Med 323, 229–235.

Sandri, F., Pilu, G., Cerisoli, M., et al., 1988. Sonographic diagnosis of agenesis of the corpus callosum in the fetus and newborn infant. Am J Perinatol 5, 226–231.

Saunders, N., Snijders, R., Nicolaides, K., 1992. Therapeutic amniocentesis in twin-twin transfusion syndrome appearing in the second trimester of pregnancy. Am J Obstet Gynecol 166, 820–824.

Scardo, J.A., Ellings, J.M., Newman, R.B., 1995. Prospective determination of chorionicity, amnionicity, and zygosity in twin gestations. Am J Obstet Gynecol 173, 1376–1380.

Schmidt, W., Harms, E., Wolf, D., 1985. Successful prenatal treatment of non-immune hydrops fetalis due to congenital chylothorax. Br J Obstet Gynaecol 92, 671–679.

Schwarz, T.F., Roggendorf, M., Hottentrager, B., et al., 1988. Human parvovirus B19 infection in pregnancy. Lancet ii, 566–567.

Scioscia, A.L., Grannum P.A.T., Copel, J.A., et al., 1988. The use of percutaneous umbilical blood sampling in immune thrombocytopenic purpura. Am J Obstet Gynecol 159, 1066–1068.

Sebire, N., Snijders, R., Hughes, K., et al., 1997. The hidden mortality of monochorionic twin pregnancies. Br J Obstet Gynaecol 104, 1203–1207.

Sebire, N., Souka, A., Skentou, H., et al., 2000. Early prediction of severe

twin-to-twin transfusion syndrome. Hum Reprod 15, 2008–2010.

Sepulveda, W., Stagiannis, K.D., Flack, N.J., et al., 1995. Prenatal diagnosis of renal agenesis using color flow imaging in severe second-trimester oligohydramnios. Am J Obstet Gynecol 173, 1788–1792.

Sharland, G., Allan, L., 1992. Screening for congenital heart disease prenatally. Results of a 2-year study in the South East Thames Region. Br J Obstet Gynaecol 99, 220–225.

Sheikh, A.U., Ernest, J.M., O'Shea, M., 1992. Long-term outcome in fetal hydrops from parvovirus B19 infection. Am J Obstet Gynecol 167, 337–341.

Simms, R.A., Leibling, R.E., Patel, R.R., et al., 2009. Management and outcome of pregnancies with parvovirus B19 infection over seven years in a tertiary fetal medicine unit. Fetal Diagn Ther 25, 373–378.

Smidt-Jensen, S., Permin, M., Philip, J., et al., 1992. Randomised comparison of amniocentesis and transabdominal and transcervical chorionic villus sampling. Lancet 340, 1238–1244.

Snijders, R.J.M., Farrias, M., von Kaisenberg, C., et al., 1996. Fetal abnormalities. In: Snijders, R.J.M., Nicolaides, K.H. (Eds.), Ultrasound Markers for Fetal Chromosomal Defects. Parthenon Publishing, London, pp. 1–62.

Snijders, R.J., Noble, P., Sebire, N., et al., 1998. UK multicentre project on assessment of risk of trisomy 21 by maternal age and fetal nuchal translucency thickness at 10–14 weeks gestation. Lancet 352, 343–346.

Soothill, P.W., Nicolaides, K.H., Rodeck, C.H., 1987. The effect of anaemia on fetal acid/base status. Br J Obstet Gynaecol 94, 880–883.

Stagiannis, K.D., Sepulveda, W., Southwell, D., et al., 1995. Ultrasonographic measurement of the dividing membrane during the second and third trimesters: a reproducibility study. Am J Obstet Gynecol 173, 1546–1550.

Steinberg, L., Hurley, V., Desmedt, E., et al., 1990. Acute polyhydramnios in twin pregnancies. Aust N Z J Obstet Gynaecol 30, 196–200.

Stenhouse, E.J., Crossley, J.A., Aitken, D.A., et al., 2004. First-trimester combined ultrasound and biochemical screening for Down syndrome in routine clinical practice. Prenat Diagn 24, 774–780.

Stephens, F.D., 1983. Congenital Malformations of the Urinary Tract. Praeger, New York, pp. 433–462.

Stewart, P.A., Wladimiroff, J.W., 1987. Cardiac tachyarrhythmias in the fetus: diagnosis, treatment and prognosis. Fetal Ther 2, 7–16.

Stocker, J.T., Madewell, J.E., Drake, R.M., 1977. Congenital cystic adenomatoid

malformation of the lung. Classification and morphological spectrum. Hum Pathol 8, 155–171.

Stumpflen, I., Stumpflen, A., Wimmer, M., et al., 1996. Effect of detailed fetal echocardiography as part of routine prenatal ultrasonographic screening on detection of congenital heart disease. Lancet 348, 854–857.

Szabo, J., Gellen, J., 1990. Nuchal fluid accumulation in trisomy 21 detected by vaginosonography in the first trimester. Lancet 336, 1133.

Tabor, A., Philip, J., Madsen, M., et al., 1986. Randomised controlled trial of genetic amniocentesis in 4606 low risk women. Lancet i, 1287–1293.

Tan, K.H., Kilby, M.D., Whittle, M.J., et al., 1996. Congenital anterior abdominal wall defects in England and Wales: retrospective analysis of OPCS data. Br Med J 313, 303–306.

Tannirandorn, Y., Nicolini, U., Nicolaidis, P.C., et al., 1990. Fetal cystic hygromata: insights gained from fetal blood sampling. Prenat Diagn 10, 189–193.

Taylor, M., Denbow, M.L., Duncan, K., et al., 2000. Antenatal factors at diagnosis that predict outcome in twin-twin transfusion syndrome. Am J Obstet Gynecol 183, 1023–1028.

Teixeira, J., Fogliani, R., Giannakoulopoulos, X., et al., 1996. Fetal haemodynamic stress response to invasive procedures. Lancet 347, 624.

Teixeira, J., Glover, V., Fisk, N., 1999. Acute cerebral redistribution in response to invasive procedures in the human fetus. Am J Obstet Gynecol 181, 1018–1025.

Teixeira, J.M., Duncan, K., Letsky, E., et al., 2000. Middle cerebral artery peak systolic velocity in the prediction of fetal anemia. Ultrasound Obstet Gynecol 15, 205–208.

Terry, G.M., Ho-Terry, L., Warren, R.C., et al., 1986. First trimester prenatal diagnosis of congenital rubella: a laboratory investigation. Br Med J 292, 930–933.

The PLUTO Collaborative Study Group, 2007. PLUTO trial protocol: percutaneous shunting for lower urinary tract obstruction randomised controlled trial. Br J Obstet Gynaecol 114, 904, e4.

Thirkelsen, A.J., 1979. Cell culture and cytogenetic technique. In: Murken, J.-D., Stengel-Rutkowski, S., Schwinger, E.N. (Eds.), Prenatal Diagnosis. Proceedings of the 3rd European Conference on Prenatal Diagnosis of Genetic Disorders. Ferdinand Enke, Stuttgart, pp. 258–270.

Tulipan, N., Sutton, L.N., Bruner, J.P., et al., 2003. The effect of intrauterine myelomeningocoele repair on the incidence of shunt-dependent hydrocephalus. Paediatr Neurosurg 38, 27–33.

Tulzer, G., Arzt, W., Franklin, R.C., et al., 2002. Fetal pulmonary valvuloplasty for critical pulmonary stenosis or atresia with intact septum. Lancet 360, 1567–1568.

Tworetzky, W., Wilkins-Haug, L., Jennings, R.W., et al., 2004. Balloon dilatation of severe aortic stenosis in the fetus: potential for prevention of hypoplastic left heart syndrome: candidate selection, technique and results of successful intervention. Circulation 110, L2125–L2131.

UK National Screening Committee, 2007. Antenatal Screening – Working Standards for Down's Syndrome Screening. Available online at: dh.gov.uk/publications.

UK National Screening Committee, 2008. NHS Fetal Anomaly Screening Programme – Screening for Down's Syndrome: UK NSC Policy Recommendations 2007–2010, Models of Best Practice. Gateway reference 9674. Available online at: dh.gov.uk/ publications.

van den Akker, E.S.A., Oepkes, D., Lopriore, E., et al., 2007. Noninvasive antenatal management of fetal and neonatal alloimmune thrombocytopaenia: safe and effective. Br J Obstet Gynaecol 114, 469–473.

Van den Hof, M.C., Nicolaides, K.H., Campbell, J., et al., 1990. Evaluation of the lemon and banana signs in one hundred and thirty fetuses with open spina bifida. Am J Obstet Gynecol 162, 322–327.

Van Der Vossen, S., Pistorius, L.R., Mulder, E.J.H., et al., 2009. Role of prenatal ultrasound in predicting survival and mental and motor functioning in children with spina bifida. Ultrasound Obstet Gynecol 34, 253–258.

van Heteren, C., Nijhuis, J., Semmekrot, B., et al., 1998. Risk for surviving twin after fetal death of co-twin in twin-twin transfusion syndrome. Obstet Gynecol 92, 215–219.

Ville, Y., Hyett, J., Hecher, K., et al., 1995. Preliminary experience with endoscopic laser surgery for severe twin-twin transfusion syndrome. N Engl J Med 332, 224–227.

Walker, S., Howard, P.J., 1986. Cytogenetic prenatal diagnosis and its relative effectiveness in the Mersey region and North Wales. Prenat Diagn 6, 13–23.

Wald, N.J., Cuckle, H.S., 1987. Recent advances in screening for neural tube defects and Down's syndrome. Baillière's Clin Obstet Gynaecol 1, 649–676.

Wald, N.J., Cuckle, H.S., Densem, J.W., et al., 1988. Maternal serum screening for Down's syndrome in early pregnancy. Br Med J 297, 883–887.

von dem Borne, A., Decary, F., 1990. Nomenclature of platelet-specific antigens. Hum Immunol 29, 1–2.

Weiner, C.P., 1987. Cordocentesis for diagnostic indications: two years' experience. Obstet Gynecol 70, 664–667.

Weiner, C.P., 1990. Use of cordocentesis in fetal hemolytic disease and autoimmune thrombocytopenia. Am J Obstet Gynecol 162, 1126–1127.

Weiner, C.P., Okamura, K., 1996. Diagnostic fetal blood sampling – technique related losses. Fetal Diagn Ther 11, 169–175.

Weiner, C.P., Williamson, R., Bonsib, S.M., et al., 1986. In utero bladder diversion – problems with patient selection. Fetal Ther 1, 196–202.

Weiner, E., Zosmer, N., Bajoria, R., et al., 1994. Direct fetal administration of immunoglobulins: another disappointing therapy in alloimmune thrombocytopenia. Fetal Diagn Ther 9, 159–164.

Weir, P., Ratten, G., Beischer, N., 1979. Acute polyhydramnios – a complication of monozygous twin pregnancy. Br J Obstet Gynaecol 86, 849–853.

Wenstrom, K.D., Syrop, C.H., Hammitt, D.G., et al., 1993. Increased risk of monochorionic twinning associated with assisted reproduction. Fertil Steril 60, 510–514.

Whittle, M.J., Connor, J.M., 1994. Prenatal Diagnosis in Obstetric Practice, second ed. Blackwell Science, Oxford.

Wilkins, I.A., Chitkara, U., Lynch, L., et al., 1987. The nonpredictive value of fetal urinary electrolytes: preliminary report of outcomes and correlations with pathological diagnosis. Am J Obstet Gynecol 157, 694–698.

Williamson, L.M., Bruce, D., Lubenko, A., et al., 1992. Molecular biology for platelet alloantigen typing. Transfusion Med 2, 225–264.

Wilson, J.M., Di Fiore, J.W., Peters, C.A., 1993. Experimental fetal tracheal ligation prevents the pulmonary hypoplasia associated with fetal nephrectomy: possible application for congenital diaphragmatic hernia. J Pediatr Surg 28, 1433–1440.

Wladimiroff, J.W., Stewart, P.A., Reuss, A., et al., 1989. Cardiac and extracardiac anomalies as indicators for trisomies 13 and 18, a prenatal ultrasound study. Prenat Diagn 9, 515–520.

Worley, K.C., Dashe, J.S., Barber, R.G., et al., 2009. Fetal magnetic resonance imaging in isolated diaphragmatic hernia: volume of herniated liver and neonatal outcome. Am J Obstet Gynecol 200, 318.e1–318.e6.

Wright, C.F., Chitty, L.S., 2009. Cell-free fetal DNA and RNA in maternal blood: implications for safer antenatal testing. Br Med J 339, b2451.

Zaccara, A., Giorlandino, C., Mobili, L., et al., 2005. Amniotic fluid index and fetal bladder outlet obstruction. Do we really need more? J Urol 174, 1657–1660.

Zosmer, N., Bajoria, R., Weiner, E., et al., 1994. Clinical and echographic features of in utero cardiac dysfunction in the recipient twin in twin-twin transfusion syndrome. Br Heart J 72, 74–79.

Fetal growth, intrauterine growth restriction and small-for-gestational-age babies

10

Imelda Balchin   Donald Peebles

CHAPTER CONTENTS

© 2012 Elsevier Ltd

Introduction and definitions

A fetus is defined, antenatally, as small for gestational age (SGA) when its estimated fetal weight (EFW) is below a specified percentile for its gestation, for a given population. Thus, SGA is a statistical concept, based on the distribution of EFW within a population. The World Health Organization (WHO) has chosen the 10th percentile as an arbitrary threshold for identifying SGA (WHO 1995). Another commonly used threshold is the total population mean EFW minus two standard deviations of a population-based growth curve (i.e. setting the normal range for growth as roughly between the 2.5th and the 97.5th percentile) (Marsal et al. 1996). Babies defined as SGA using the 10th percentile threshold have a higher rate of adverse outcome than average-for-gestational-age babies (De Jong et al. 1998; McIntire et al. 1999). However, not all fetuses with SGA have an abnormal pattern of growth. In reality, up to 70% of fetuses identified as SGA are 'constitutionally small' and healthy, while the remainder have intrauterine growth restriction (IUGR) with abnormal growth velocity and increased risk of adverse outcome (Manning et al. 1981; Patterson and Pouliot 1987; Lin and Santolaya-Forgas 1998).

A fetus with IUGR is one that has failed to achieve its genetically determined growth potential, owing to one or more pathological factors (Table 10.1). In comparison with a normally grown fetus with no structural or chromosomal defect, an IUGR fetus has at least a 10-fold increased risk of perinatal mortality (McIntire et al. 1999; Regev et al. 2003). In the developed world, IUGR is the commonest cause of stillbirth and the second leading cause of perinatal mortality, after preterm birth. A significant proportion of IUGR fetuses are not detected before birth and recent reports show that undiagnosed IUGR was a factor in over 50% of stillbirths in the UK (Confidential Enquiry into Maternal and Child Health 2007).

There are many reasons why IUGR poses a major challenge to clinicians and researchers. The aetiology of IUGR is heterogeneous with multiple causal pathways, and there is no proven therapy. The most effective intervention is delivery, thus many clinicians advocate early intervention for suspected IUGR. However, it is important to distinguish between a constitutionally small fetus from one that is IUGR, in order to avoid iatrogenic morbidity to the mother and baby due to unnecessary operative and/or preterm delivery. Central to this problem is the lack of standard definitions or uniform diagnostic criteria for IUGR. Consequently, many researchers have used the definitions for SGA and IUGR interchangeably, and

Table 10.1 Risk factors for intrauterine growth restriction

Fetal	**Chromosomal anomaly**: triploidy, trisomies (21,18,13), Turner syndrome, uniparental disomy, confined placental mosaicism **Structural malformation**: cardiac malformations, neural tube defects, gastroschisis, diaphragmatic hernia, renal agenesis, multiple malformations **Genetic abnormalities and syndromes**: Bloom, Brachmann–de Lange, Cornelia de Lange, De Sanctis–Cachione, Donohue, Dubowitz, Fanconi, Johanson–Blizzard, Mulibrey nanism, osteochondrodysplasias, Prader–Willi, Roberts, Russell–Silver, Rubenstein–Taybi, Seckel, Williams–Beuren **Fetal infections**: cytomegalovirus, toxoplasmosis, rubella, malaria, human immunodeficiency virus, varicella-zoster, herpes simplex, Epstein–Barr virus, congenital tertiary syphilis **Multiple pregnancies**: monochorionic gestation, twin-to-twin transfusion
Maternal	**Past obstetric history**: previous intrauterine growth restriction, stillbirth, preterm birth **Social/environmental/nutritional**: extreme reproductive age, short interpregnancy interval, poor diet, anorexia nervosa, body mass index <20, active inflammatory bowel disease, smoking, substance abuse (alcohol, cocaine, opiates, amphetamines), self-neglect and/or psychiatric illness, medication (β-blockers, overtreatment of hypertension), high altitude **Vasculopathy**: chronic hypertension, pre-eclampsia, diabetes mellitus, sickle-cell disease, antiphospholipid syndrome, systemic lupus erythematosus **Renal disease**: glomerulonephritis, lupus nephritis, chronic renal failure **Thrombophilia**: factor V Leiden G1691A, prothrombin G20210A **Hypoxia**: severe anaemia, chronic lung disease, severe asthma, cyanotic heart disease **Reduced plasma volume expansion**
Placenta	**Abnormalities of the umbilical cord**: single umbilical artery, velamentous insertion of the cord, overcoiled umbilical cord **Tumours**: chorioangiomatosis, placental mesenchymal dysplasia **Vascular**: vascular malformations, fetal thrombotic vasculopathy, placental abruption **Abnormal placental development**: abnormal trophoblast invasion, recurrent bleeding, placenta praevia, circumvallate placenta, confined placental mosaicism
Uterine	Uterine abnormality, uterine fibroids, assisted reproductive techniques
Endocrine factors	Vascular endothelial growth factor, placental growth factor, fms-like tyrosine kinase 1, pregnancy-associated plasma protein A, insulin-like growth factor

used different thresholds to identify the normal range for growth. This has led to classification bias and difficulties in interpreting findings from IUGR studies. In essence, the use of a 10th percentile threshold alone fails to identify IUGR fetuses with abnormal growth pattern but whose EFW is above the threshold value (Marconi et al. 2008).

To improve the identification of SGA fetuses with adverse outcomes, the 10th percentile threshold of a 'standard' or 'healthy obstetric population' with low-risk pregnancies and normal perinatal outcome should be used instead of a growth curve based on the entire obstetric population (Ferdynus et al. 2009). In addition, since IUGR is more common in babies born preterm, the growth standard should be ultrasound-based fetal weight reference rather than neonatal birthweight reference (Bukowski et al. 2001). The use of a growth standard that takes into account biological variation in fetal size due to fetal gender, ethnicity, maternal size and parity, or a 'customised growth standard', also improves the antenatal detection of SGA fetuses with adverse outcomes (Mongelli and Gardosi 1996; Figueras et al. 2007). Defining a fetus as SGA using both the population-based and the customised standard was associated with a fivefold increase in the detection rate of fetuses with adverse outcomes (Zhang et al. 2007). However, in reality, the use of a customised growth standard is limited by a number of factors: (1) a large pregnancy database with sufficient numbers of normal pregnancies with different biological characteristics, mentioned above, is required to create an accurate customised growth standard; (2) fetal gender cannot always be identified accurately by ultrasonography, and, even when this is correctly identified, the parents may not want

this information to be revealed; and (3) the customised growth standard may be less accurate for fetuses of mixed heritage. After birth, IUGR can be confirmed in a newborn by measuring an index of body mass or malnutrition, known as neonatal ponderal index. This is calculated as (birthweight (g)/height (cm)^3) × 100. A ponderal index below the 10th percentile is more closely associated with adverse perinatal outcome than birthweight alone (Walther and Ramaekers 1982; WHO 1995).

Incidence and recurrence rate

Using the 10th percentile threshold, at least 10% of singleton pregnancies will be labelled as SGA. The incidence of SGA is higher in multiple pregnancies, with approximately 20% of dichorionic and 30% of monochorionic twins being categorised as SGA (Klam et al. 2005). The true incidence of IUGR in the general obstetric population is likely to be underestimated since it is often undetected. For example, it is found that approximately 30% of babies born before 35 weeks of gestation were below the 10th percentile for gestational age compared with 4.5% of babies born at term (37 or more weeks of gestation) (Bukowski et al. 2001). Thus, the incidence of SGA is six times higher in babies born preterm than in those born at term. IUGR occurs in 30–40% of pregnancies affected by pre-eclampsia (Walker 2000). In women who had a previous IUGR pregnancy, the recurrence rate is about 20% (Patterson et al. 1986). However, this is increased to approximately 50% in women with previous early IUGR (before 34 weeks of gestation), with a highest recurrence risk

Table 10.2 Consequences of intrauterine growth restriction

INTRAPARTUM	NEONATAL	LONG-TERM	ADULTHOOD
Fetal death	Hypoxic–ischaemic encephalopathy	Bronchopulmonary dysplasia	Diabetes
Acute-on-chronic hypoxia	Seizures	Cognitive delay	Obesity
Metabolic acidosis	Respiratory distress syndrome	Cerebral palsy dysplasia	Hypertension
Meconium aspiration	Hypotension		Dyslipidaemia
	Heart failure		Cardiac disease
	Pulmonary haemorrhage		Stroke
	Pulmonary hypertension		Bronchitis
	Renal failure		Early menopause
	Hypoglycaemia		
	Hyperglycaemia		
	Hypothermia		
	Polycythaemia		
	Hyperviscosity		
	Renal vein thrombosis		
	Thrombocytopenia		
	Hyperbilirubinaemia		
	Feeding intolerance		
	Necrotising enterocolitis		
	Coagulopathy		
	Infection		
	Congenital abnormality		
	Adrenal insufficiency		
	Retinopathy of prematurity		
	Neonatal death		

in women with pre-existing renal disease and superimposed pre-eclampsia.

The aetiology of IUGR

The consequences of IUGR are shown in Table 10.2. Normal fetal growth requires both a normal fetus and an adequate supply of substrates (i.e. oxygen and nutrients) from the maternal circulation into the fetal circulation via the placenta. The latter depends on adequate levels of substrates within the maternal circulation, adequate maternal blood flow to the placenta, and a normally functioning placenta. It was initially thought that about 80–90% of IUGR was caused by problems with the supply of substrates while an intrinsic fetal factor is the cause of a further 15–20% of cases. However, recent investigations have shown that normal endocrine signalling also plays an important role in the control and regulation of fetal and placental growth.

Factors affecting fetal growth potential (IUGR of fetal origin)

Chromosomal abnormalities, especially triploidy and trisomies 13, 18 and 21, are responsible for about 7% of fetuses with IUGR; however this figure is as high as 19% in tertiary referral centres (Snijders et al. 1993). Structural abnormalities are responsible for about 10–20% of IUGR. Genetic abnormalities and syndromes are commonly associated with IUGR. Congenital infections account for about 5% of IUGR cases (Pearce and Robinson 1995). IUGR is more common if fetal infection occurs early in pregnancy. Common causes of fetal infection in the developed world include cytomegalovirus and toxoplasmosis, with rubella occurring less often owing to vaccination. Common causes of fetal infections in the developing world include malaria, which accounts for up to 70% of SGA babies

in endemic areas of sub-Saharan Africa (Steketee et al. 2001), and congenital human immunodeficiency virus (HIV) infection due to maternal-to-child transmission in utero.

Multiple pregnancies are associated with a high incidence of IUGR, especially in monochorionic or higher order gestations. A growth discordance of 15% or more occurs in up to 30% of twin pregnancies and this can be used as a marker for IUGR; however, both twins can be affected (Fieni and Gramelli 2004; Klam et al. 2005). This has been attributed to 'uterine overcrowding'. Chorionicity is the most important determinant of perinatal and long-term outcomes. There is a higher incidence of chromosomal and structural abnormalities associated with monochorionicity; problems specific to twinning are discussed in Chapter 23 (Fick et al. 2006).

Factors leading to substrate deprivation (IUGR of maternal origin)

Fetal deprivation of nutrition or oxygen may unusually occur as a consequence of maternal undernutrition. This is associated with anorexia nervosa, body mass index less than 20 (Naeye et al. 1973; Godfrey et al. 1996; Conti et al. 1998), substance abuse and self-neglect, including smoking, moderate to high alcohol intake, cocaine, opiates and amphetamines (Little et al. 1988; Holzman and Paneth 1994; Johnstone et al. 1996; English et al. 1997; Cnattingius 2004; Jaddoe et al. 2007). Other maternal factors associated with IUGR include extremes of reproductive age, and poor socioeconomic status (Naeye et al. 1973; Russell 1982; Wilcox et al. 1995; Ahluwalia et al. 2001; Smith et al. 2003). Severe maternal medical disorders may affect uterine artery blood flow; for example, vasculopathy associated with long-term diabetes (Haeri et al. 2008), chronic hypertension (Gilbert et al. 2007) and renal disease (Jones and Hayslett 1996; Fink et al. 1998). Maternal obesity increases the risk of developing these medical disorders and their complications in pregnancy, including IUGR. Severe maternal anaemia (Levy et al. 2005), poorly controlled asthma (Bracken et al. 2003) or cyanotic heart disease may reduce maternal oxygen supply to the placenta (Drenthen et al. 2007). Certain maternal drug treatments such as beta-adrenoreceptor antagonists, phenytoin and long-term corticosteroids have been shown to have a negative effect on fetal growth (Montan 2004).

Factors affecting the transfer of substrates (IUGR of placental origin)

Poor placental function and resulting substrate deprivation are responsible for the majority of IUGR pregnancies. Placentae of IUGR pregnancies show reduced cytotrophoblast invasion and reduced surface area, increased thickness of the exchange barrier formed by the trophoblast and the fetal capillary endothelium, reduced villous density with fewer loops and coils, atheromatous change within the maternal spiral arteries, increased placental apoptosis and piling up of trophoblast due to shedding of apoptotic cells (Sheppard and Bonnar 1976; Giles et al. 1985; Jackson et al. 1995; Krebs et al. 1996; Smith et al. 1997; Kingdom et al. 2000). Normal placental development requires successful trophoblast invasion into the inner third of the myometrium and the entire length of maternal spiral arteries. The trophoblast cells destroy the muscular and elastic walls of these vessels, resulting in large flaccid uteroplacental vessels (Brosens et al. 1967). Conversion of high-resistance spiral arteries into low-resistance uteroplacental vessels is necessary to accommodate the massive increase in uterine blood flow observed in pregnancy to meet the metabolic demands of the feto-placental unit.

To assess changes in volume blood flow within the placental circulation requires the measurement of vessel diameter, which is difficult for small vessels. However, changes in vascular resistance in the uteroplacental circulation can be assessed non-invasively using Doppler ultrasound waveform analysis of pulsatile flow in the umbilical artery (fetoplacental circulation) and uterine artery (maternoplacental circulation). The shape of the uterine or umbilical artery waveform showing high diastolic velocity with continuous diastolic flow indicates a high-flow, low-resistance uteroplacental circulation. The waveform can also be quantified by using the ratio of systolic to diastolic maximum velocity (S/D), the pulsatility index (PI; peak systolic flow minus end-diastolic flow divided by mean flow) or the resistance index (RI; peak systolic flow minus end-diastolic flow divided by peak systolic flow). The PI is the most widely studied Doppler index.

It has been shown that trophoblast invasion in early pregnancy is more extensive in pregnancies with low-resistance compared with high-resistance Doppler indices in the uterine artery (Prefumo et al. 2004). In non-pregnant women the high-resistance uteroplacental vasculature leads to a rapid rise and fall in velocity during systole, an early diastolic 'notch' in the waveform, and low end-diastolic flow velocities (Schulman et al. 1986). Spiral artery transformation results in a significant reduction in uterine artery resistance (decreased PI and RI) between 8 and 26 weeks of gestation, and a loss of the diastolic 'notch' between 20 and 26 weeks of gestation (Jauniaux et al. 1992; Thaaler et al. 1992). Diastolic flow in the umbilical artery also increases as gestation increases in a normal pregnancy, producing a fall in the PI (Hendricks et al. 1989; Reed 1997).

Placentae from pre-eclamptic pregnancies share many histological features with the placentae of IUGR pregnancies, suggesting a common pathogenesis. In addition, both pre-eclamptic and IUGR pregnancies are associated with increased resistance or impedance to uterine artery blood flow (Trudinger et al. 1985; Ducey et al. 1987). Pre-eclampsia is a pregnancy-specific systemic endothelial disorder which affects about 2% of pregnancies. Although the development of maternal hypertension in the second half of the pregnancy with the presence of significant proteinuria is diagnostic of pre-eclampsia, the aetiology is heterogeneous with variable clinical presentation (Sibai et al. 2005). Early-onset pre-eclampsia (before 34 weeks of gestation) is associated with a higher incidence of poor placental function, a more severe IUGR with a higher risk of maternal mortality and morbidity (Witlin et al. 2000). Conversely, late-onset pre-eclampsia is more prevalent but with minimal placental dysfunction.

A single umbilical artery (SUA) is associated with a 20-fold increased risk of cardiac anomalies and a threefold increased risk of renal anomalies. However, even in fetuses with isolated SUA there is a twofold increased risk of IUGR (Hua et al. 2010). Both acquired (e.g. antiphospholipid syndrome) and inherited thrombophilias predispose to IUGR, as they may increase the risk of thrombotic lesions within the placenta (Yasuda et al. 1995). It has been suggested that there is an increased frequency of the prothrombin mutation and the methyltetrahydrofolate reductase mutation in mothers of IUGR babies (Kuperminc et al. 1999). Tobacco smoking increases the risk of SGA and acts in a dose- and gestation-dependent manner to reduce birthweight, probably via adverse effects on placental blood flow (Thompson et al. 2001). A recent SCOPE study showed that the SGA rate in women who stopped smoking by 15 weeks of gestation was equivalent to that of non-smokers (McCowan et al. 2009).

Endocrine factors

Important regulators of fetal growth, differentiation and function are the insulin-like growth factors (IGF), including IGF-1 and 11, IGF-binding proteins (IGFBP) 1–6, IGF receptors 1 and 2 and IGFBP-specific proteases. IGF plays an important role in trophoblast invasion (Lawrence et al. 1999), and abnormalities in IGF signalling have been associated with IUGR (Irwin et al. 1999). A reduced fetal serum IGF-1 is associated with IUGR, while overexpression of IGF-11 is associated with fetal overgrowth, as observed in Beckwith–Wiedemann syndrome. In addition, low plasma IGFBP-1 in early pregnancy is associated with an increased risk of pre-eclampsia. Pregnancy-associated plasma protein A (PAPP-A) is a trophoblast-derived protease that cleaves IGFBP-4, thus increasing the bioavailability of IGF (Laviola et al. 2005). A low maternal serum PAPP-A in the first trimester of pregnancy is also associated with an increased risk for subsequent development of pre-eclampsia (Poon et al. 2008), and PAPP-A levels are significantly lower in women developing early-onset than late pre-eclampsia (Poon et al. 2010).

In addition, decreased levels of angiogenic proteins, such as vascular endothelial growth factor (VEGF) and placental growth factor (PlGF), and increased levels of angiogenic inhibitor, such as fms-like tyrosin kinase 1 (sFlt-1), are associated with reduced trophoblast invasion (Savvidou et al. 2006; Smith et al. 2007; Stepan et al. 2007). There is an inverse correlation between maternal PlGF and uterine artery PI (Schlembach et al. 2007). Elevated maternal sFlt-1 is associated with increased uterine artery PI, pre-eclampsia and IUGR; and higher sFlt-1 levels were observed in women with adverse pregnancy outcomes resulting in delivery before 34 weeks of gestation. An inverse correlation has been shown between birthweight and maternal corticotrophin-releasing hormone (CRH) levels at 33 weeks of gestation. An elevated CRH level is associated with a 3.6-fold increased risk of IUGR (Wadhwa et al. 2004). In addition, there is a relationship between birthweight and maternal neurokinin B and nitric oxide metabolite levels (D'Anna et al. 2004).

Physiological sequelae of IUGR

The majority of fetuses with IUGR will be substrate-deprived due to the abnormal transfer of oxygen and nutrients (glucose, amino acids, lipids) across the placenta. Insights into the fetal responses to such deprivation are important as they: (1) underpin the rationale for the techniques used to monitor fetal wellbeing; (2) often lead to improved short-term survival; and (3) can also cause some of the short- and long-term complications associated with IUGR.

Fetal heart rate

Acute fetal hypoxaemia is associated with well-described changes in fetal heart rate (FHR); these underpin the use of electronic fetal monitoring on the labour ward (Ch. 12). However, experiments in fetal sheep where the fetoplacental circulation was embolised every day for 10 days leading to chronic hypoxaemia and a 50% reduction in umbilical flow did not change baseline FHR or lead to decelerations or changes in short-term variability (Gagnon et al. 1996). These suggest that changes in FHR patterns are likely to be a late occurrence in the sequence of haemodynamic change seen in the IUGR fetus (Fig. 10.1), and agree with studies from human fetuses with absent end-diastolic flow in the umbilical artery. Here, abnormal FHR patterns were only observed when the middle cerebral artery (MCA) began to lose its compensatory maximal dilation, i.e. the fetus was entering a preterminal phase (Weiner et al. 1994).

Regional blood flow

In contrast, changes in regional blood flow with maintained, chronic fetal hypoxaemia are well described in a number of animal species. In fetal sheep blood flow to the brain, heart and adrenal

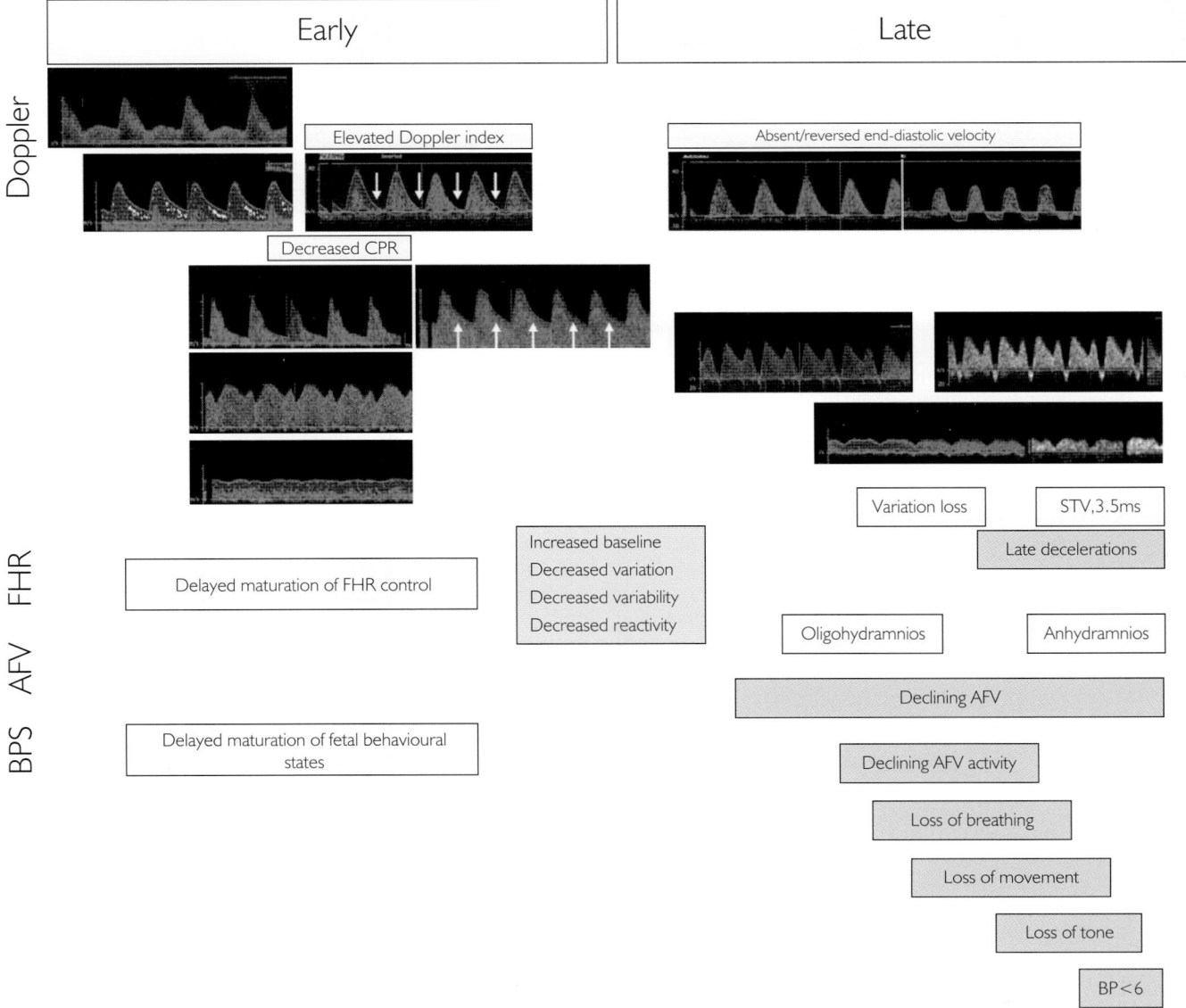

Fig. 10.1 Schematic representation of sequential changes in fetal physiological parameters observed in intrauterine growth restriction fetuses with worsening acid–base status. CPR, cardiopulmonary resuscitation; FHR, fetal heart rate; STV, short-term variability; AFV, amniotic fluid volume; BP, biophysical profile. *(Reproduced with permission from Baschat (2011).)*

glands increases rapidly with the onset of acute hypoxaemia and remains high if hypoxaemia is maintained; this effect is observed from mid- to late gestation (Bocking et al. 1988; Matsuda et al. 1992; Richardson et al. 1996). The effect of the increased blood flow is to maintain substrate delivery that is critically important for the maintenance of growth and optimal function of these key organs. Doppler studies in fetuses with IUGR suggest that vascular resistance is increased in a variety of vessels, including the splanchnic, renal and pulmonary circulations, suggesting that the reductions in blood flow to the gut, kidneys and lungs that are observed during acute hypoxia in fetal sheep are maintained during sustained hypoxaemia (Vyas et al. 1989; Mari et al. 1995; Rizzo et al. 1996). Detection of substrate deficiency occurs both locally and at central chemoreceptors and is sensitive and rapid; detection of cerebral vasodilation is therefore an early finding in IUGR.

Abnormal cerebral blood flow is an extremely sensitive test for the prediction of IUGR, but it has poor specificity in the detection of adverse perinatal outcome (Chan et al. 1996). Whilst redistribution of cardiac output optimises short-term survival with chronic hypoxaemia, there is some evidence that it is responsible for some of the immediate postnatal complications observed in growth-restricted neonates. Kempley et al. (1991) described a reduction in flow velocity, which persisted until the end of the first week of life, in both superior mesenteric artery and the coeliac axis in growth-restricted compared with normally grown neonates of similar gestational age. The increased incidence of necrotising enterocolitis (NEC) observed in IUGR fetuses may be related to ischaemic damage occurring either in utero or following delivery (Hackett et al. 1987). Oligohydramnios, a common finding in IUGR pregnancies, is probably related to reduced renal perfusion and glomerular filtration. Again, chronic reduction in lung growth might underlie the excess incidence of chronic lung disease observed in infants with severe IUGR (Lal et al. 2003). Because of the correlation between the growth of an organ and its blood supply, organ size appears to be a sensitive indicator of redistribution of cardiac output; indeed, relative shortening of the femurs in the early second trimester has been reported as an early sign of incipient growth restriction, often preceding other evidence by several weeks (Todros et al. 2004).

In addition to the redistribution of cardiac output, chronic hypoxia can also influence the venous pattern of blood flow and return of blood to the heart. Approximately 25–50% of blood returning from the placenta via the umbilical vein is shunted via the ductus venosus (DV), which connects with the inferior cava near its entrance to the heart (Behrman et al. 1970; Edelstone and Rudolp 1979). This well-oxygenated blood is preferentially streamed through the foramen ovale into the left atrium and from there towards the cardiac and cerebral circulations (Kiserud 1999). In both human and other mammalian fetuses the amount of blood flowing through the DV increases during hypoxia (Behrman et al. 1970; Tchirikov et al. 1998). A direct consequence of increased DV shunting is that the proportion of umbilical vein flow that passes via the hepatic circulation is reduced; a fall in hepatic perfusion and decreased substrate supply can impair liver function and glycogen synthesis and storage (reflected in a decrease in growth velocity in the abdominal circumference). Not surprisingly, flow velocity is maintained in the DV even with severe IUGR (Kiserud et al. 1994), because the DV and left atrium are linked by a direct column of blood. Increases in left atrial filling pressure, due mainly to impaired ventricular contractility, but also increased afterload, will lead to reduced forward flow in the DV during atrial systole. Decreased or absent flow during atrial systole is a late finding in the haemodynamic response to hypoxia and, because it indicates cardiac

compromise, correlates strongly with poor perinatal outcome (Baschat et al. 2003).

The consequences of IUGR

The short-term consequences of IUGR include the increased risk of perinatal mortality, and perinatal morbidity, including birth asphyxia, meconium aspiration and the consequences of preterm birth. About half of IUGR survivors will have significant short- or long-term morbidity (Dobson et al. 1981). The extent and severity of morbidity depend on the cause and severity of IUGR and the neonatal consequence of fetal adaptation to chronic hypoxia, complications during labour and delivery, the gestational age at birth and immaturity of function, place of birth and the presence of chromosomal or structural anomalies. The commonest causes of death are prolonged hypoxia, birth asphyxia, prematurity and congenital anomalies. It is anticipated that a preterm IUGR baby will have more complications than a term IUGR baby and would require specialist neonatal care from birth. An IUGR fetus with chronic hypoxia is at increased risk of birth asphyxia at all gestational ages (McIntire et al. 1999). In the immediate neonatal period, birth asphyxia and metabolic acidosis may lead to multiorgan dysfunction, including hypoxic–ischaemic encephalopathy, seizures, intraventricular haemorrhage, respiratory distress due to surfactant deficiency, meconium aspiration or pulmonary haemorrhage, persistent pulmonary hypertension, hypotension due to myocardial dysfunction, transient tricuspid valve insufficiency, renal failure due to acute cortical necrosis, coagulopathy and elevated aminotransferase due to liver hypoxia, hypocalcaemia, and adrenal insufficiency due to haemorrhage (Kramer et al. 1990; Villar et al. 1990; Gilbert and Danielsen 2003).

The fetal redistribution of circulation to vital organs in response to hypoxaemia and substrate deprivation may lead to problems with neonatal adaptation to extrauterine life. For example, there is an increased risk of NEC due to bowel ischaemia. The risk of NEC is higher in IUGR babies with absent or reversed end-diastolic flow in the umbilical artery before birth (Dorling et al. 2005). Since the reduced splanchnic blood flow may persist in the first week of life, oral feeding should be introduced cautiously during this time. Other complications include hypoglycaemia due to limited glycogen stores; polycythaemia due to the increased synthesis of erythropoietin in chronic hypoxia and consequently hyperviscosity, renal vein thrombosis and hyperbilirubinaemia; respiratory distress syndrome; problems with thermoregulation due to limited adipose tissue stores and a relatively large body surface area; retinopathy of prematurity; and hyperglycaemia due to low insulin secretion in very preterm neonates.

Beyond the neonatal period, there is an increased risk of developing neurological abnormalities including cognitive delay and cerebral palsy, especially in babies born preterm (Wood et al. 2000; Yanney and Marlow 2004). Magnetic resonance imaging of the brain of IUGR infants has shown reduced volume of cerebral cortical grey matter (Tolsa et al. 2004). About 90% of babies with SGA will show catch-up growth by 6 months of age, but 10% will remain below the third percentile for height at 2–3 years of age and may benefit from growth hormone therapy (Saenger et al. 2007). However, animal models have shown that IUGR is associated with reduced leptin levels, a satiety factor which controls appetite and food intake (Geary et al. 1999). Although the level of leptin increased in the adult IUGR offspring, there is a decreased anorexic response to leptin, and this is especially demonstrated in IUGR offspring with rapid catch-up growth (Desai et al. 2007). It has been suggested that altered control of appetite in the adult IUGR off-spring leads to adult obesity. Besides obesity, there is a growing body of evidence to support the concept that there are fetal origins for adult diseases such as adult hypertension, high cholesterol levels, type 2 diabetes mellitus, abnormal coagulation factors, coronary heart disease, stroke, bronchitis, premature menopause in women and Down syndrome pregnancy (Barker and Osmond 1986; Barker et al. 1989a, b, 1992, 1993, 1997; Barker 1990; Phipps et al. 1993; Martyn et al. 1995; Cresswell et al. 1997; Shaheen 1997; Van Montfrans et al. 2001). One hypothesis is that the IUGR fetus is programmed to exhibit the 'thrifty phenotype' where the metabolism is permanently reset to adapt to poor nutritional conditions, such that the extrauterine exposure to western diet predisposes the offspring to obesity and metabolic syndrome as an adult.

Primary prevention of IUGR

Prepregnancy counselling and health education, as well as optimising any pre-existing medical conditions before pregnancy, are important. Prepregnancy folic acid supplementation to prevent neural tube defects should be advocated, as well as the importance of good nutrition, the avoidance of harmful substances such as smoking, alcohol, illicit drug abuse, and reduction of caffeine intake (Ouellette et al. 1977; Lumley et al. 2006). In addition, women should be informed that smoking cessation before the third trimester will reduce the risk of IUGR (Lieberman et al. 1994). In women who have a high risk of pre-eclampsia, low-dose aspirin reduces the risk of developing pre-eclampsia by 17% and reduces the risk of SGA by 10% (Duley et al. 2007).

Since maternal obesity increases the risk of hypertensive disorders in pregnancy, which in turn increases the risk of IUGR (Callaway et al. 2006), it may be beneficial to encourage weight loss before pregnancy, or to limit weight gain during pregnancy in obese women (Cedergren 2006). Women with eating disorders should also be counselled regarding the increased risk of IUGR pregnancies. It has been shown that a pregnant woman with a body mass index of less than 20 has a higher risk of an SGA fetus when the total gestational weight gain is less than 8 kg, in comparison with a weight gain of more than 16 kg (Cedergren 2007). However, the provision of social support for women of low socioeconomic status has not been shown to reduce the incidence of SGA, as poor diet is the probable mechanism by which socioeconomic status influences growth (Hodnett and Fredericks 2003).

In order to prevent congenital infection and IUGR, all women should be vaccinated against rubella before pregnancy. In malaria-endemic areas, the routine use of antimalarial drugs and insecticide-treated nets for women in their first two pregnancies has been shown to reduce the incidence of low-birthweight babies (WHO 2005; Garner and Gulmezoglu 2006). Antiretroviral treatment in women with HIV infection can reduce in utero maternal-to-child-transmission of HIV from 25% to 2%, and thus prevent IUGR due to congenital HIV infection (WHO 2006).

Antenatal screening and diagnosis

The antenatal diagnosis of IUGR relies on a number of observations, including: (1) current fetal size, taking into account the fetal growth potential such as ethnicity, fetal gender, maternal height and parity; (2) serial ultrasound measurements of fetal size to demonstrate reduced growth velocity, where the EFW decreases in its percentile value for gestational age; (3) indicator of fetal compromise,

where fetal Doppler demonstrates redistribution of fetal circulation in response to hypoxaemia, particularly a decreased impedance to MCA blood flow; and (4) indicator of poor uteroplacental function, where uterine artery Doppler (UAD) indicates a persistent high-resistance circulation at 24 or more weeks of gestation and/or umbilical artery Doppler waveform shows increased impedance to blood flow.

However, in an unselected obstetric population, the evidence does not support the use of routine fetal biometry after 24 weeks of gestation, routine umbilical artery Doppler ultrasound, routine UAD ultrasound or routine antenatal electronic fetal heart monitoring for the prediction of IUGR (Goffinet et al. 1997; Chien et al. 2000; Royal College of Obstetricians and Gynaecologists 2002). Each screening tool will have a higher positive predictive value if there is an increased risk of IUGR based on maternal history and clinical examination. Therefore, the principle of antenatal care is the identification of pregnancies at high risk of IUGR through history, examination, and biochemical and ultrasound screening.

Ultrasound assessment of gestational age and fetal size

A reliable estimate of gestational age is a prerequisite for the early detection of IUGR, interpretation of serum screening tests and planning for elective delivery. Gestational age is the strongest determinant of fetal size and perinatal outcome. The last menstrual period (LMP) should not be used alone to date a pregnancy. Even if LMP is recalled accurately, it is not a precise indicator of the conception date (Geirsson and Busby-Earle 1991; Savitz et al. 2002; Nakling et al. 2005). This is because the timing of ovulation varies cyclically, even in women with regular menstrual cycles. In addition, errors in recall are common, with a tendency to digit preference when recalling dates, and falsely identifying non-menstrual bleeding as a menstrual period (Gjessing et al. 1999; Nakling et al. 2005).

Dating methods using ultrasonographic assessment of fetal size before 20 weeks of gestation have been shown to reduce the percentage of pregnancies classified as 'postterm' by up to 74% when compared with dating based on LMP only. In the first trimester of pregnancy (up to 14 weeks), ultrasound measurement of the fetal crown–rump length (CRL) provides a relatively accurate estimate of gestational age, with a standard deviation of approximately 7 days (Hogberg 1997; Taipale and Hiilesmaa 2001). The CRL measurement becomes less reliable beyond 13 weeks because the fetus becomes increasingly flexed with advancing gestation.

In the second trimester, the most accurate estimate of gestational age is the head circumference (HC), while the most sensitive indicator of fetal size is the abdominal circumference (AC) (Chang et al. 1993; Chitty et al. 2007). The accuracy of dating using HC is improved with the addition of AC and femur length (FL) measurements, such that fetal biometry in the second trimester also provides an accurate estimate of gestational age within 7 days (Chervenak et al. 1998). In addition, the calculation of EFW is more accurate using all three biometric measures than any one measurement alone (Hadlock et al. 1985). Using the Hadlock formula, which combines HC, AC and FL, the EFW is within 15% of the actual fetal weight when the fetus weighs between 1500 and 3999 g (Benson and Doubilet 1991). Errors as high as 25% between the predicted and actual fetal weight occur when a fetus weighs below 1500 g, with the tendency to overestimate fetal weight; or when a fetus weighs above 4000 g, with the tendency to underestimate (Manning et al. 1981).

Most obstetric units use a combination of the LMP and dating based on ultrasound fetal biometry, only favouring the ultrasound dates if the discrepancy is greater than 7, 10 or 14 days depending on gestational age at first ultrasound scan. However, it is recommended that the use of CRL measurement between 10 and 13 weeks alone should be used to determine gestational age (National Institute for Health and Clinical Excellence 2008). For women who booked late for antenatal care, the use of ultrasound for dating is less reliable beyond 24 weeks, owing to the increased variation in fetal growth rate and imprecise measurements as a result of descent of the fetal head into the pelvis, shadowing from fetal bony parts and fetal crowding (Campbell et al. 1984). The transcerebellar diameter is a useful adjunct in determining gestational age in the second and third trimester because its measurement is independent of fetal head shape and there is a tendency for cerebellar growth to be preserved in IUGR (Chavez et al. 2004, 2007). However, if pregnancy dating is performed beyond 24 weeks, serial ultrasound scans should also be performed to confirm a normal growth velocity, instead of a one-off measurement of fetal size.

Identification of high-risk pregnancy

Once the best estimate of gestational age is determined, the principle of antenatal care is the recognition of pregnancies at high risk of IUGR through history, examination, and biochemical and ultrasound screening.

Maternal history

In addition to the risk factors mentioned in the aetiology section, women with recurrent bleeding should be regarded as high-risk. A previous IUGR pregnancy increases the risk of recurrent IUGR in subsequent pregnancies (Ananth et al. 2007).

Clinical examination

The traditional screening methods for fetal growth using abdominal palpation or measurement of symphysis–fundal height (SFH) have poor detection rates for IUGR. In a low-risk population, abdominal palpation has a sensitivity of only 21% and a specificity of 96% for detecting SGA fetuses (Bais et al. 2004). After 20 weeks of gestation, the SFH in centimetres from the upper edge of the pubic symphysis to the top of the uterine fundus approximates to the number of weeks of gestation. Differences in maternal build and subjectivity of this test have led to a considerable variation in the results of studies using SFH, with the largest study showing a sensitivity of only 27%, and a specificity of 88% for detecting SGA fetuses (Persson et al. 1986). The selection of women with SFH that is below expectation for ultrasound fetal biometry reduces the false-positive rate for detecting SGA when compared with a policy of scanning all women in the third trimester, but the sensitivity is not improved with this method (Harding 1995).

Maternal serum screening

The combined test is offered to all women in the first trimester for Down syndrome screening. This involves fetal nuchal translucency scan and maternal serum PAPP-A and human chorionic gonadotrophin (hCG) levels. Women who missed the first trimester screening have the option of serum screening in the second trimester, including alpha-fetoprotein, oestriol, hCG and inhibin A. Pregnancies identified as high-risk for Down syndrome due to significantly reduced PAPP-A levels should be monitored for fetal growth, even when invasive testing showed normal fetal karyotype.

Other methods of screening which have not been adopted in clinical practice include using angiogenic markers such as PlGF or sFlt-1. These have sensitivities of 55–60% and specificities of 60–70% of predicting pre-eclampsia or IUGR (Stepan et al. 2007). In addition, sFlt-1 had a higher sensitivity of 80% and a specificity of 94% for predicting adverse outcome resulting in delivery before 34 weeks of gestation.

Ultrasound screening

Ultrasound screening for structural malformation is offered to all women between 20 and 22 weeks of gestation. In the absence of structural malformations, the markers associated with an increased risk of IUGR include bright or echogenic fetal bowel, single umbilical artery, isolated short femur (where the femur is below the fifth percentile for gestational age but the abdominal circumference measurements and the EFW are within the normal range) (Weisz et al. 2008). Beyond 24 weeks of gestation, there is no evidence that routine ultrasound scan to assess growth in a low-risk population improves perinatal outcome, and it has been suggested that this may increase the rate of caesarean section.

Screening for adverse outcome using UAD has produced variable results depending on gestational age, presence of risk factors and severity of outcome. In a study of high-risk multiparous women, abnormal UAD had a sensitivity of 80% and a positive predictive value of 70% for identifying women who subsequently developed pre-eclampsia, SGA below the fifth percentile, placental abruption, preterm birth and perinatal mortality (Harrington et al. 2004). In a recent systematic review and meta-analysis of 74 studies totalling 79 547 patients with pre-eclampsia and 61 studies of 41 141 IUGR pregnancies, it was reported that an abnormal UAD waveform had a higher predictive value for both pre-eclampsia and IUGR when performed in the second trimester (beyond 16 weeks of gestation) than in the first trimester (Cnossen et al. 2008). Screening with UAD was also more predictive of pre-eclampsia than IUGR, and increased PI with diastolic notching was the best predictor of pre-eclampsia (positive likelihood ratio of 21 for high-risk patients and 7.5 for low-risk patients). Increased PI and diastolic notching were the best predictors of IUGR in low-risk patients (positive likelihood ratio 9.1). For severe IUGR, the predictive value was higher (positive likelihood ratio 14.6).

Identifying IUGR using ultrasound fetal biometry

Ultrasound of fetal size alone has a low predictive ability and high false-positive rate for detecting IUGR. The fetal AC indicates the nutritional state of the fetus, as this is a measure of subcutaneous, intra-abdominal and extraperitoneal fat and liver size. An AC below the 10th centile was found to predict SGA with an odds ratio of 13.5 in a low-risk population and 18.4 in a high-risk population (Chang et al. 1992). A more recent study has shown that the accuracy of predicting SGA was similar when either the AC or the EFW alone was below the 10th centile. In addition, the likelihood of SGA was found to be greater when both the AC and the EFW were below the 10th centile (Chauhan et al. 2006). Although EFW calculations do not aid in the diagnosis of IUGR, they are helpful in planning delivery and neonatal care. Serial measurements of fetal biometry every 2–4 weeks should be used to identify any deviation of growth across the centiles.

Ultrasound assessment of liquor volume

Liquor volume is assessed by measuring the maximum pool depth, or, more accurately, by adding the pool depth in each quadrant of the uterus to produce the amniotic fluid index. Although oligo-hydramnios is associated with more severe IUGR, the predictive value of these measurements is limited, so they are used as an adjunct to other elements of the fetal assessment.

Management of IUGR and timing of delivery

Currently, there is no therapy for IUGR and the most effective intervention is timely delivery of the baby. Other interventions to be considered include: (1) reduction of maternal risk factors, e.g. smoking reduction; (2) maternal administration of corticosteroids if preterm birth is anticipated; and (3) delivery in a unit with appropriate neonatal intensive care facilities (Roberts and Dalziel 2006). The perinatal outcome of an IUGR pregnancy, and thus its management, depends on the aetiology, gestational age, severity of IUGR and severity of maternal disease.

Investigation of IUGR aetiology

Ultrasound scan should be performed to exclude structural malformations. The presence of sonographic soft markers in a structurally normal fetus may indicate the possibility of aneuploidy. Amniocentesis or chorionic villus sampling should be offered to identify chromosomal abnormality. Isolated karyotypic abnormalities within the placenta are also associated with IUGR. The diagnosis of maternal infection is important and maternal serology tests for toxoplasmosis, cytomegalovirus and rubella should be performed. If maternal serology is positive, amniocentesis should be considered to confirm fetal infection.

Timing of delivery

In fetuses with no chromosomal or structural abnormality, the timing and mode of delivery should take into account the risk of morbidity due to iatrogenic preterm delivery (such as respiratory distress syndrome and brain injury), the risk of continuing intra-uterine hypoxia and stillbirth, and the severity of maternal disease. Thus, antenatal fetal and maternal surveillance should be performed diligently. Fetal surveillance consists of serial ultrasound assessment of growth (usually every second week), liquor volume, Doppler assessment of the fetal circulation and maternal uterine artery and FHR monitoring. Since pre-eclampsia occurs in up to 40% of cases of IUGR, maternal surveillance for raised blood pressure, proteinuria and biochemical markers is also important.

In a large prospective study of 604 infants born before 34 weeks because of severe IUGR, gestational age was the most important determinant of overall survival before 27 weeks and intact survival before 29 weeks; if the fetus was delivered after these gestations and weighed more than 600 g then DV Doppler was the only predictor of adverse outcome (Baschat et al. 2007). Besides gestational age, the finding of an abnormal fetal umbilical artery Doppler in high-risk pregnancies is more predictive of adverse outcome than a biophysical profile or fetal heart trace (Gonzalez et al. 2007).

Increased resistance (high PI or RI) in the umbilical artery in high-risk pregnancies indicates IUGR of placental origin, and is associated with increased risk of antenatal admissions, inductions of labour, operative delivery, increased admission to neonatal units and increased perinatal mortality (Hackett et al. 1987;

Gudmundsson and Marsal 1988; Wilson et al. 1992). Meta-analyses indicate that the use of Doppler ultrasound to guide clinical decision-making is likely to improve outcomes in pregnancies with suspected IUGR and pre-eclampsia (Alfirevic and Neilson 1995; Neilson and Alfirevic 2001). When Doppler ultrasound was used to guide management, perinatal mortality was reduced by 38%.

The Growth Restriction Intervention Trial (The GRIT Study Group 2003) recruited pregnancies between 24 and 36 weeks of gestation with abnormal umbilical artery Doppler waveform when the clinicians were uncertain about the timing of delivery. These pregnancies were randomised to either immediate delivery after completion of antenatal corticosteroids or deferred delivery until there was abnormal FHR or favourable gestational age. It was found that the perinatal mortality rates were the same in both groups. Clinicians were prepared to delay delivery by about 4 days, resulting in a fivefold higher stillbirth rate. However, in the immediate-delivery group, there was a similar rate of early neonatal deaths (The GRIT Study Group 2003). The neurological outcomes at 2 years also showed no statistically significant difference in both groups in babies born after 31 weeks of gestation. However, there was a trend towards more disability in the immediate-delivery group for babies delivered before 30 weeks of gestation (Thornton et al. 2004).

Since the GRIT trial, more recent studies have investigated in more depth the phases of fetal Doppler abnormality. Doppler ultrasound of MCA showing increased diastolic velocity (reduced PI) identifies IUGR fetuses with redistribution of blood flow to the brain. These changes in SGA fetuses have been associated with the development of abnormal FHR patterns and increased admission to the neonatal unit (Mari and Deter 1992). Changes in the MCA occur relatively early in the process of hypoxia, and although it is used to confirm the diagnosis of IUGR, it is not useful in deciding the timing of delivery. However, normalisation of the PI values suggests a deteriorating fetus.

Significant predictors of adverse perinatal outcome are absent/reversed umbilical artery flow and absent/reversed α-wave in the DV Doppler waveform. Since the α-wave corresponds to end-diastolic atrial contraction, these changes reflect myocardial dysfunction and are late signs of fetal hypoxia and indicate imminent heart failure; such changes in DV flow are an indication for delivery, even at gestations less than 29 weeks (Fig. 10.1). A very late sign of fetal hypoxia which follows absent/reversed DV α-wave is the occurrence of pulsations in the umbilical vein and/or reduced short-term variability of FHR.

In IUGR fetuses at 30–34 weeks of gestation (where there is a good prospect of intact survival) the presence of absent/reversed end-diastolic flow in the umbilical artery is an indication for immediate delivery. Beyond 34 weeks of gestation, fetuses with IUGR typically have normal umbilical artery Dopplers (Chang et al. 1994), but are still at risk of poor outcome (Hershkovitz et al. 2000). Even if umbilical artery Doppler is normal, delivery should be considered if there is a decrease in growth velocity, oligohydramnios, abnormal cardiotocograph and/or evidence of cardiac redistribution (low MCA PI).

Fetal therapy for IUGR

There is insufficient evidence to support maternal bed rest, maternal oxygen administration or nutritional supplementation including routine zinc, magnesium, iron, folate or vitamin D supplementation (Crowther et al. 1990; Mahomed 2005a, b, c; Mahomed and Gulmezoglu 2005; Makrides and Crowther 2005; Say et al. 2005a, b, c). Calcium supplementation of 1 g/day during pregnancy has been shown to reduce the risk of hypertension in pregnancy and pre-eclampsia but does not appear to reduce SGA, low birthweight or admission to neonatal intensive care unit (Hofmeyr et al. 2010). In addition, antihypertensive treatment for maternal hypertension has no beneficial effect on fetal growth. The use of vasodilating agents such as L-arginine, a nitric oxide donor, has been shown to improve uterine artery blood flow; however a randomised clinical trial is needed to evaluate its use as therapy for IUGR (Sieroszewski et al. 2004). A recent study showing that sildenafil increased mortality in growth-restricted fetal sheep highlights the challenge of avoiding systemic vasodilation and uterine hypoperfusion (Miller et al. 2009). Vector-mediated delivery of VEGF to the uterine arteries has been shown to increase uterine blood flow over a period of about 5 weeks and may be a potential candidate (David et al. 2008).

Mode of delivery

While the mode of delivery for IUGR pregnancies less than 35 weeks is more likely to be caesarean section following the administration of steroids, the optimal mode of delivery at later gestations is unclear. Even at term IUGR pregnancies are more likely to be delivered by caesarean section because of fetal distress and are more likely to have low Apgar scores, hypoglycaemia, respiratory distress and be admitted to a neonatal unit than fetuses with normal growth

velocities (Owen et al. 1997; Minior and Divon 1998). The severity of fetal hypoxia, parity and cervical assessment should be considered in deciding between induction of labour and caesarean section. Continuous electronic monitoring of the FHR pattern during labour is indicated because normal uterine contractions can lead to deterioration of fetal hypoxia. A pathological cardiotocograph can be investigated using fetal blood sampling or, if this is not possible, delivery by caesarean section.

Postnatal

Histological examination of the placenta is indicated following delivery of an IUGR fetus to confirm whether placental lesions were a contributory factor. Screening the baby for infection or congenital abnormality may be indicated. Babies with severe IUGR, especially when born preterm, should be routinely followed up to detect abnormal neurological development. Postnatal counselling of the mother is important since IUGR with absent or reversed EDF in the umbilical arteries has a recurrence risk of approximately 20%. In addition to IUGR recurrence, there is an increased risk of developing pre-eclampsia or placental abruption in subsequent pregnancies (Ananth et al. 2007). Consideration should be given to thrombophilia screening.

References

Ahluwalia, I.B., Merritt, R., Beck, L.F., et al., 2001. Multiple lifestyle and psychosocial risk and delivery of small for gestational age infants. Obstet Gynecol 97, 649–656.

Alfirevic, Z., Neilson, J.P., 1995. Doppler ultrasonography in high-risk pregnancies: systematic review with meta-analysis. Am J Obstet Gynecol 172, 1379–1387.

Ananth, C.V., Peltier, M.R., Chavez, M.R., et al., 2007. Recurrence of ischemic placental disease. Obstet Gynecol 110, 128–133.

Bais, J.M., Eskes, M., Pel, M., et al., 2004. Effectiveness of detection of intrauterine growth retardation by abdominal palpation as screening test in a low risk population: an observational study. Eur J Obstet Gynecol Reprod Biol 116 (2), 164–169.

Barker, D.J.P., 1990. The fetal and infant origins of adult disease. Br Med J 301, 1111.

Barker, D.J.P., Osmond, C., 1986. Infant mortality, childhood nutrition, and ischaemic heart disease in England and Wales. Lancet 1, 1077–1081.

Barker, D.J.P., et al., 1989a. Weight in infancy and death from ischaemic heart disease. Lancet 334 (8663), 577–580.

Barker, D.J.P., Osmond, C., Law, C.M., 1989b. The intrauterine and early postnatal origins of cardiovascular disease and chronic bronchitis. J Epidemiol Commun Health 43, 237–240.

Barker, D.J.P., et al., 1992. The relation of fetal length, ponderal index and head circumference to blood pressure and the risk of hypertension in adult life. Paediatr Perinatal Epidemiol 6, 35–44.

Barker, D.J.P., et al., 1993. Growth in utero and serum cholesterol concentrations in adult life. Br Med J 307, 1524–1527.

Barker, D.J.P., et al., 1997. Intrauterine programming of coronary heart disease and stroke. Acta Paediatr Int J Paediatr Supplement 86, 178–182.

Baschat, A.A., 2011. Venous Doppler evaluation of the growth restricted fetus. Clin Perinatol 38, 103–112

Baschat, A.A., Gembruch, U., Weiner, C.P., et al., 2003. Qualitative venous Doppler waveform analysis improves prediction of critical perinatal outcomes in premature growth-restricted fetuses. Ultrasound Obstet Gynecol 22, 240–245.

Baschat, A.A., Cosmi, E., Bilardo, C.M., et al., 2007. Predictors of neonatal outcome in early-onset placental dysfunction. Obstet Gynecol 109, 253–261.

Behrman, R.E., Lees, M.H., Peterson, E.N., et al., 1970. Distribution of the circulation in the normal and asphyxiated fetal primate. Am J Obstet Gynecol 108, 956–969.

Benson, C.B., Doubilet, P.M., 1991. Fetal measurements: normal and abnormal fetal growth. In: Rumack, C.M., Wilson, S.R., Charboneau, J.W. (Eds.), Diagnostic Ultrasound. Mosby-Year Book, St Louis, MO, pp. 723–738.

Bocking, A.D., Gagnon, R., White, S.E., et al., 1988. Circulatory responses to prolonged hypoxaemia in fetal sheep. Am J Obstet Gynecol 159, 1418–1424.

Bracken, M.B., Triche, E.W., Belanger, K., et al., 2003. Asthma symptoms, severity, and drug therapy: a prospective study of effects on 2205 pregnancies. Obstet Gynecol 102, 739–752.

Brosens, I., Robertson, W.B., Dixon, H.G., 1967. The physiological response of the vessels of the placental bed to normal pregnancy. J Pathol Bacteriol 93, 569–579.

Bukowski, R., Gahn, D., Denning, J., Saade, G., 2001. Impairment of growth in fetuses destined to deliver preterm. Am J Obstet Gynecol 185, 463–467.

Callaway, L.K., Prins, J.B., Chang, A.M., et al., 2006. The prevalence and impact of overweight and obesity in an Australian obstetric population. Med J Aust 184, 56–59.

Campbell, S., Trickey, N., Whittle, M., 1984. Report of the RCOG Working Party on Routine Ultrasound Examination in Pregnancy. Chameleon, London.

Cedergren, M.I., 2006. Effects of gestational weight gain and body mass index on obstetric outcome in Sweden. Int J Gynaecol Obstet 93, 269–274.

Cedergren, M.I., 2007. Optimal gestational weight gain for body mass index categories. Obstet Gynecol 110, 759–764.

Chan, F.Y., Pun, T.C., Lam, P., et al., 1996. Fetal cerebral Doppler studies as a predictor of perinatal outcome and subsequent neurologic handicap. Obstet Gynecol 87, 981–988.

Chang, T., Robson, S., Boys, R., et al., 1992. Prediction of small for gestational age infant: which ultrasonic measurement is best? Obstet Gynecol 80, 1030–1038.

Chang, T.C., Robson, S.C., Spencer, J.A.D., et al., 1993. Identification of fetal growth retardation: comparison of Doppler waveform indices and serial ultrasound measurements of abdominal circumference and fetal weight. Obstet Gynecol 82, 230–236.

Chang, T., Robson, S., Spencer, J., et al., 1994. Prediction of perinatal morbidity at term in small fetuses: comparison of fetal growth and Doppler ultrasound. Br J Obstet Gynaecol 101, 422–427.

Chauhan, S.P., Cole, J., Sanderson, M., et al., 2006. Suspicion of intrauterine growth restriction: Use of abdominal circumference alone or estimated fetal weight below 10%. J Mat Fetal Neonatal Med 19, 557–562.

Chavez, M.R., Ananth, C.V., Smulian, J.C., et al., 2004. Fetal transcerebellar diameter measurement with particular emphasis in the third trimester: a reliable predictor of gestational age. Am J Obstet Gynecol 191, 979–984.

Chavez, M.R., Ananth, C.V., Smulian, J.C., et al., 2007. Fetal transcerebellar diameter measurement for prediction of gestational age at the extremes of fetal growth. J Ultrasound Med 26, 1167–1171.

Chervenak, F.A., Skupski, D.W., Romero, R., et al., 1998. How accurate is fetal biometry in the assessment of fetal age? Am J Obstet Gynecol 178, 678–687.

Chien, P., Arnott, N., Gordon, A., et al., 2000. How useful is uterine artery Doppler flow velocimetry in the prediction of pre-eclampsia, intrauterine growth restriction and perinatal death? An overview. Br J Obstet Gynecol 107, 196–208.

Chitty, L., Evans, T., Chudleigh, P., 2007. Fetal size and dating: Charts recommended for clinical obstetric practice. British Medical Ultrasound Society. Available at http://www.bmus.org/publications/pu-femeasure.asp.

Cnattingius, S., 2004. The epidemiology of smoking during pregnancy: smoking prevalence, maternal characteristics, and pregnancy outcomes. Nicotine Tob Res 6 (Suppl. 2), S125–S140.

Cnossen, J.S., Morris, R.K., Riet, G., et al., 2008. Use of uterine artery Doppler ultrasonography to predict pre-eclampsia and intrauterine growth restriction: a systematic review and bivariable meta-analysis. CMAJ 178 (6), 701–711.

Confidential Enquiry into Maternal and Child Health, 2007. Perinatal Mortality 2005: England, Wales and Northern Ireland. CEMACH, London.

Conti, J., Abraham, S., Taylor, A., 1998. Eating behaviour and pregnancy outcome. J Psychom Res 44, 465–477.

Cresswell, J.L., et al., 1997. Is the age of menopause determined in-utero? Early Hum Dev 49, 143–148.

Crowther, C.A., Verkuyl, D.A., Neilson, J.P., et al., 1990. The effects of hospitalization for rest on fetal growth, neonatal morbidity and length of gestation in twin pregnancy. Br J Obstet Gynaecol 97, 872–877.

D'Anna, R., Baviera, G., Corrado, F., et al., 2004. Neurokinin B and nitric oxide plasma levels in pre-eclampsia and isolated intrauterine growth restriction. Br J Obstet Gynecol 111, 1046–1050.

David, A.L., Torondel, B., Zachary, A., et al., 2008. Local delivery of adenovirus VEGF to the uterine arteries increases vessel relaxation and uterine artery blood flow in the pregnant sheep. Gene Ther 15, 1344–1350.

De Jong, C.L.D., Francis, A., vanGeijn, H.P., et al., 1998. Fetal growth rate and adverse perinatal events. Ultrasound Obstet Gynecol 13, 86–89.

Desai, M., Gayle, D., Han, G., et al., 2007. Programmed hyperphagia due to reduced anorexigenic mechanisms in intrauterine growth-restricted offspring. Reprod Sci 329–337.

Dobson, P.C., Abell, D.A., Beischer, N., 1981. Mortality and morbidity of fetal growth retardation. Aust NZ J Obstet Gynaecol 21, 69–72.

Dorling, J., Kempley, S., Leaf, A., 2005. Feeding growth restricted preterm infants with abnormal antenatal Doppler results. Arch Dis Child Fetal Neonatal Ed 90, F359–F363.

Drenthen, W., Pieper, P.G., Roos-Hesselink, J.W., et al., 2007. Outcome of pregnancy in women with congenital heart disease: a literature review. J Am Coll Cardiol 49, 2303–2311.

Ducey, J., Schulman, H., Farmakides, G., et al., 1987. A classification of hypertension in pregnancy based on Doppler velocimetry. Am J Obstet Gynecol 157, 680–685.

Duley, L., Henderson-Smart, D.J., Meher, S., et al., 2007. Antiplatelet agents for preventing pre-eclampsia and its complications. Cochrane Database Syst Rev 2, CD004659.

Edelstone, D.I., Rudolp, A.M., 1979. Preferential streaming of ductus venosus blood to the brain and heart in fetal lambs. Am J Physiol 237, H724–H729.

English, D., Hulse, G., Milne, E., et al., 1997. Maternal cannabis use and birth weight: a meta-analysis. Addiction 92, 1553–1560.

Ferdynus, C., Quantin, C., Abrahamowicz, M., et al., 2009. Can birth weight standards based on healthy populations improve the identification of small-for-gestational-age newborns at risk of adverse neonatal outcomes? Pediatrics 123, 723–730.

Fick, A.L., Feldstein, V.A., Norton, M.E., et al., 2006. Unequal placental sharing and birth weight discordance in monochorionic diamniotic twins. Am J Obstet Gynecol 195, 178–183.

Fieni, S., Gramelli, D., 2004. Very-early onset discordant growth in monochorionic twin pregnancy. Obstet Gynecol 103, 115–117.

Figueras, F., Figueras, J., Meler, E., et al., 2007. Customised birthweight standards accurately predict perinatal morbidity. Arch Dis Child Fetal Neonatal Ed 92, F277–F280.

Fink, J.C., Schwartz, S.M., Benedetti, T.J., et al., 1998. Increased risk of adverse maternal and infant outcomes among women with renal disease. Paediatr Perinatal Epidemiol 12, 277–287.

Gagnon, R., Johnston, L., Murotsuki, J., 1996. Fetal placental embolization in the late-gestation ovine fetus: alterations in umbilical blood flow and fetal heart rate patterns. Am J Obstet Gynecol 175, 63–72.

Garner, P., Gulmezoglu, A.M., 2006. Drugs for preventing malaria in pregnant women. Cochrane Database Syst Rev (4), CD000169.

Geary, M., Pringle, P.J., Persaud, M., et al., 1999. Leptin concentrations in maternal serum and cord blood: relationship to maternal anthropometry and fetal growth. Br J Obstet Gynaecol 106, 1054–1060.

Geirsson, R.T., Busby-Earle, R.M.C., 1991. Certain dates may not provide a reliable estimate of gestational age. Br J Obstet Gynaecol 98 (1), 108–109.

Gilbert, W.M., Danielsen, B., 2003. Pregnancy outcomes associated with intrauterine growth restriction. Am J Obstet Gynecol 188, 1596–1599.

Gilbert, W.M., Young, A.L., Danielson, B., 2007. Pregnancy outcomes in women with chronic hypertension: a population-based study. J Reprod Med 52, 1046–1051.

Giles, W., Trudinger, B., Baird, P., 1985. Fetal umbilical artery flow velocity waveforms and placental resistance; pathological correlation. Br J Obstet Gynaecol 92, 31–38.

Gjessing, H.K., Skjaerven, R., Wilcox, A.J., 1999. Errors in gestational age: evidence of bleeding early in pregnancy. Am J Public Health 89, 213–218.

Godfrey, K., Robinson, S., Barker, D.J.P., et al., 1996. Maternal nutrition in early and late pregnancy in relation to placental and fetal growth. Br Med J 213, 410–414

Goffinet, F., Paris-Llado, J., Nisand, I., et al., 1997. Umbilical artery Doppler velocimetry in unselected and low risk pregnancies: a review of randomised controlled trials. Br J Obstet Gynaecol 104, 425–430.

Gonzalez, J.M., Stamilio, D.M., Ural, S., et al., 2007. Relationship between abnormal fetal testing and adverse perinatal outcomes in intrauterine growth restriction. Am J Obstet Gynecol 196, e48–e51.

Gudmundsson, S., Marsal, K., 1988. Umbilical and uteroplacental blood flow velocity waveforms in pregnancies with fetal growth retardation. Eur J Obstet Gynecol Reprod Biol 27, 187–196.

Hackett, G.A., Campbell, S., Gamsu, H., et al., 1987. Doppler studies in the growth retarded fetus and prediction of neonatal necrotising enterocolitis, haemorrhage and neonatal morbidity. Br Med J 294, 13–16.

Hadlock, F.P., Deter, R.J., Sharman, R.S., et al., 1985. Estimating fetal weight with the use of head, body and femur measurements: a prospective study. Am J Obstet Gynecol 151, 333–337.

Haeri, S., Khoury, J., Kovilam, O., et al., 2008. The association of intrauterine growth abnormalities in women with type diabetes mellitus complicated by vasculopathy. Am J Obstet Gynecol 199 (278), e1–e5.

Harding, K., 1995. Screening for the small fetus: A study of the relative efficacies of ultrasound biometry and symphysiofumdal height. Aust N Z J Obstet Gynaecol 35 (2), 160–164.

Harrington, K., Fayyad, A., Thakur, V., et al., 2004. The value of uterine artery Doppler in the prediction of uteroplacental complications in multiparous women. Ultrasound Obstet Gynecol 23, 50–55.

Hendricks, S., Sorensen, T., Wang, K., et al., 1989. Doppler umbilical artery waveform indices – normal values from fourteen to forty-two weeks. Am J Obstet Gynecol 161, 761–765.

Hershkovitz, R., Kingdom, J., Geary, M., et al., 2000. Fetal cerebral blood flow redistribution in late gestation: identification of compromise in small fetuses with normal umbilical artery Doppler. Ultrasound Obstet Gynecol 15, 209–212.

Hodnett, E.D., Fredericks, S., 2003. Support during pregnancy for women at increased risk of low birthweight babies. Cochrane Database Syst Rev (3), CD000198.

Hofmeyr, G.J., Atallah, A.N., Duley, L., 2010. Calcium supplementation during pregnancy for preventing hypertensive disorders and related problems. Cochrane Database Syst Rev (8), CD001059.

Hogberg, U., 1997. Early dating by ultrasound and perinatal outcome: A cohort study. Acta Obstet Gynecol Scand 76 (10), 907–912.

Holzman, C., Paneth, N., 1994. Maternal cocaine use during pregnancy and perinatal outcomes. Epidemiol Rev 16, 315–334.

Hua, M., Odibo, A.O., Macones, G.A., et al., 2010. Single umbilical artery and its associated findings. Obstet Gynecol 115, 930–934.

Irwin, J.C., Suen, L.F., Martina, N.A., et al., 1999. Role of the IGF system in trophoblast invasion and pre-eclampsia. Hum Reprod 14 (Suppl.2), 90–96.

Jackson, M.R., Walsh, A.J., Morrow, R.J., et al., 1995. Reduced placental villous tree elaboration in small-for-gestational-age pregnancies: relationship with umbilical artery Doppler waveforms. Am J Obstet Gynecol 172, 518–525.

Jaddoe, V.W., Bakker, R., Hofman, A., et al., 2007. Moderate alcohol consumption during pregnancy and the risk of low birth weight and preterm birth. The generation R study. Ann Epidemiol 17, 834–840.

Jauniaux, E., Jurkovic, D., Campbell, S., et al., 1992. Doppler ultrasonograhic features of the developing placental circulation; correlation with anatomic findings. Am J Obstet Gynecol 166, 585–587.

Johnstone, F., Raab, G., Hamilton, B., 1996. The effect of human immunodeficiency virus infection and drug use on birth characteristics. Obstet Gynecol 88, 321–326.

Jones, D.C., Hayslett, J.P., 1996. Outcome of pregnancy in women with moderate or severe renal insufficiency. N Engl J Med 335, 226–232.

Kempley, S.T., Gamsu, H.R., Vyas, S., et al., 1991. Effects of intrauterine growth retardation on postnatal visceral and cerebral blood flow velocity. Arch Dis Child 66, 1115–1118.

Kingdom, J., Huppertz, B., Seaward, G., et al., 2000. Development of the placental villous tree and its consequences for fetal growth. Eur J Obstet Gynecol Reprod Biol 92, 35–43.

Kiserud, T., 1999. Hemodynamics of the ductus venosus. Eur J Obstet Gynecol Reprod Biol 84, 139–147.

Kiserud, T., Eik-Nes, S.H., Blaas, H.G., et al., 1994. Ductus venosus blood velocity and the umbilical circulation in the seriously growth-retarded fetus. Ultrasound Obstet Gynecol 4, 109–114.

Klam, S.L., Rinfet, D., Leduc, L., 2005. Prediction of growth discordance in twins with the use of abdominal circumference ratios. Am J Obstet Gynecol 192, 247–251.

Kramer, M.S., Olivier, M., McLean, F.H., et al., 1990. Impact of intrauterine growth retardation and body proportionality on fetal and neonatal outcome. Pediatrics 86, 707–713.

Krebs, C., Macara, L.M., Leiser, R., et al., 1996. Intrauterine growth restriction with absent end-diastolic flow velocity in the umbilical artery is associated with maldevelopment of the placental terminal villous tree. Am J Obstet Gynecol 175, 1534–1542.

Kupferminc, M.J., Eldor, A., Steinman, N., et al., 1999. Increased frequency of genetic thrombophilia in women with complications of pregnancy. N Engl J Med 340, 9–13.

Lal, M.K., Maktelow, B.N., Draper, E.S., et al., 2003. Chronic lung disease of prematurity and intrauterine growth retardation: a population – based study. Pediatrics 111, 483–487.

Laviola, L., Perrini, S., Belsanti, G., et al., 2005. Intrauterine growth restriction in humans is associated with abnormalities in in placental insulin-like growth factor signalling. Endocrinology 146, 1498–1505.

Lawrence, J.B., Oxvig, C., Overgaard, M.T., et al., 1999. The insulin-like growth factor (IGF)-dependent IGF binding protein-4 protease secreted by human fibroblasts is pregnancy-associated plasma protein-A. Proc Natl Acad Sci USA 96, 3149–3153.

Levy, A., Fraser, D., Katz, M., et al., 2005. Maternal anemia during pregnancy is an independent risk factor for low birthweight and preterm delivery. Eur J Obstet Gynaecol 122, 182–186.

Lieberman, E., Gremy, I., Lang, J., et al., 1994. Low birthweight at term and the timing of fetal exposure to maternal smoking. Am J Public Health 84, 1127–1131.

Lin, C.C., Santolaya-Forgas, J., 1998. Current concepts of fetal growth restriction. Part 1. Causes, classification, and pathophysiology. Obstet Gynecol 92, 1044–1055.

Little, B., Snell, L., Gilstrap, L.R., 1988. Metamphetamine abuse during pregnancy: outcome and fetal effects. Obstet Gynecol 72, 541–544.

Lumley, J., Oliver, S.S., Chamberlain, C., et al., 2006. Interventions for promoting smoking cessation during pregnancy. Cochrane Database Syst Rev.

Mahomed, K., 2005a. Folate supplementation in pregnancy. Cochrane Database Syst Rev.

Mahomed, K., 2005b. Iron supplementation in pregnancy. Cochrane Database Syst Rev.

Mahomed, K., 2005c. Zinc supplementation in pregnancy. Cochrane Database Syst Rev.

Mahomed, K., Gulmezoglu, A.M., 2005. Vitamin D supplementation in pregnancy. Cochrane Database Syst Rev.

Makrides, M., Crowther, C.A., 2005. Magnesium supplementation in pregnancy. Cochrane Database Syst Rev.

Manning, F.A., Hill, L.M., Platt, L.D., 1981. Qualitative amniotic fluid volume determination by ultrasound: antepartum detection of intrauterine growth retardation. Am J Obstet Gynecol 193, 254–258.

Marconi, A.M., Ronzoni, S., Bozzetti, P., et al., 2008. Comparison of fetal and neonatal growth curves in detecting growth restriction. Obstet Gynecol 112, 1227–1234.

Mari, G., Deter, R.L., 1992. Middle cerebral artery flow velocity waveforms in normal and small-for-gestational-age fetuses. Am J Obstet Gynecol 166, 1262–1270.

Mari, G., Abuhamad, A.Z., Uerpairojkit, B., et al., 1995. Blood flow velocity waveforms of the abdominal arteries in appropriate – and small for gestational age fetuses. Ultrasound Obstet Gynecol 6, 15–18.

Marsal, K., Persson, P.-H., Larsem, T., et al., 1996. Intrauterine growth curve based on ultrasonically estimated foetal weights. Acta Paediatr 85, 843–848.

Martyn, C.N., et al., 1995. Plasma concentrations of fibrinogen and factor

VII in adult life and their relation to intra-uterine growth. Br J Haematol 89, 142–146.

Matsuda, Y., Patrick, J., Carmichael, L., et al., 1992. Effects of sustained hypoxemia on the sheep fetus at midgestation: endocrine, cardiovascular, and biophysical responses. Am J Obstet Gynecol 167, 531–540.

McCowan, L.M., Dekker, G.A., Chan, E., et al., 2009. Spontaneous preterm birth and small for gestational age infants in women who stop smoking early in pregnancy: prospective cohort study. Br Med J 338, b1081.

McIntire, D.D., Bloom, S.L., Casey, B.M., et al., 1999. Birthweight in relation to morbidity and mortality among newborn infants. N Engl J Med. 340, 1234–1238.

Miller, S.L., Loose, J.M., Jenkin, G., et al., 2009. The effects of sildenafil citrate (Viagra) on uterine blood flow and well being in the intrauterine growth-restricted fetus. Am J Obstet Gynecol 200 (1), 102–107.

Minior, V.K., Divon, M.Y., 1998. Fetal growth restriction at term: Myth or reality? Obstet Gynecol 92, 57–60.

Mongelli, M., Gardosi, J., 1996. Reduction of false-positive diagnosis of fetal growth restriction by application of customised fetal growth standards. Obstet Gynecol 88, 844–848.

Montan, S., 2004. Drugs used in hypertensive diseases in pregnancy. Curr Opin Obstet Gynecol 16, 111–115.

Naeye, R.L., Blanc, W., Paul, C., 1973. Effects of maternal nutrition on human fetus. Pediatrics 52, 494–503.

Nakling, J., Buhaug, H., Backe, B., 2005. The biologic error in gestational length related to the use of the first day of last menstrual period as a proxy for the start of pregnancy. Early Hum Dev 81, 833–839.

National Institute for Health and Clinical Excellence, 2008. Antenatal Care: Routine Care for Healthy Pregnant Women. RCOG press.

Neilson, J.P., Alfirevic, Z., 2001. Doppler ultrasound for fetal assessment in high risk pregnancies. Cochrane Database Syst Rev.

Ouellette, E., Rosett, H., Rosman, N., et al., 1977. Adverse effects on offspring of maternal alcohol abuse during pregnancy. N Engl J Med 297, 528–530.

Owen, P., Harrold, A.J., Farrel, T., 1997. Fetal size and growth velocity in the prediction of intrapartum caesarean section for fetal distress. Br J Obstet Gynaecol 104, 445–449.

Patterson, R.M., Pouliot, R.N., 1987. Neonatal morphometrics and perinatal outcome: Who is growth retarded? Am J Obstet Gynecol 157, 691–693.

Patterson, R.M., Gibbs, C.E., Wood, R., 1986. Birth weight percentile and perinatal outcome: recurrence of intrauterine growth retardation. Obstet Gynecol 68, 464–468.

Pearce, M.J., Robinson, G., 1995. Fetal growth and intrauterine growth retardation. In: Chamberlain, G. (Ed.), Turnbull's Obstetrics, second ed. Churchill Livingstone, Edinburgh, pp. 299–312.

Persson, B., Stangenberg, M., Lunell, N.O., et al., 1986. Prediction of size of infants at birth by measurement of symphysis fundus height. Br J Obstet Gynaecol 93 (3), 206–211.

Phipps, K., et al., 1993. Fetal growth and impaired glucose tolerance in men and women. Diabetologia 36, 225–228.

Poon, L.C.Y., Maiz, N., Valencia, C., et al., 2008. First-trimester maternal serum PAPP-A and preeclampsia. Ultrasound Obstet Gynecol 33, 23–33.

Poon, L.C.Y., Stratieva, V., Piras, S., et al., 2010. Hypertensive disorders in pregnancy: combined screening by uterine artery Doppler, blood pressure and serum PAPP-A at 11–13 weeks. Prenat Diagn 30, 216–223.

Prefumo, F., Sebire, N.J., Thilaganathan, B., 2004. Decreased endovascular trophoblast invasion in first trimester pregnancies with high-resistance uterine artery Doppler indices. Hum Reprod 19, 206–209.

Reed, K.L., 1997. Doppler – the fetal circulation. Clinical Obstet Gynecol 40, 750–754.

Regev, R.H., Lusky, A., Dolfin, T., et al., 2003. Excess mortality and morbidity among small-for-gestational-age premature infants: a population based study. J Pediatr 143, 186–191.

Richardson, B., Korkola, S., Asano, H., et al., 1996. Regional blood flow and the endocrine response to sustained hypoxemia in the preterm fetus. Pediatr Res 40, 337–343.

Rizzo, G., Cappona, A., Chaoui, R., et al., 1996. Blood flow velocity waveforms from peripheral pulmonary arteries in normally grown and growth-retarded fetuses. Ultrasound Obstet Gynecol 8, 87–92.

Roberts, D., Dalziel, S., 2006. Antenatal corticosteroids for accelerating fetal lung maturation for women at risk of preterm birth. Cochrane Database Syst Rev (3), CD004454.

Royal College of Obstetricians and Gynaecologists, 2002. The Investigation and Management of the Small-for-gestational-age Fetus. Guideline No. 31. RCOG, London, pp. 1–16.

Russell, J.K., 1982. Early Teenage Pregnancy. Churchill Livingstone, Edinburgh.

Saenger, P., Czernichow, P., Hughes, I., et al., 2007. Small for gestational age: short stature and beyond. Endocrinol Rev 28, 219–251.

Savitz, D.A., Terry, J.W., Dole, N., et al., 2002. Comparison of pregnancy dating by last menstrual period, ultrasound scanning, and their combination. Am J Obstet Gynecol 187 (6), 1660–1666.

Savvidou, M.D., Yu, C.K., Harland, L.C., et al., 2006. Maternal serum concentration of soluble fms-like tyrosine kinase 1 and vascular endothelial growth factor in women with abnormal uterine artery Doppler and in those with fetal growth restriction. Am J Obstet Gynecol 195, 1668–1673.

Say, L., Gulmezoglu, A.M., Hofmeyr, G.J., 2005a. Bed rest in hospital for suspected impaired fetal growth. Cochrane Database Syst Rev.

Say, L., Gulmezoglu, A.M., Hofmeyr, G.J., 2005b. Maternal oxygen admnistration for suspected impaired fetal growth. Cochrane Database Syst Rev.

Say, L., Gulmezoglu, A.M., Hofmeyr, G.J., 2005c. Maternal nutrient supplementation for suspected impaired fetal growth. Cochrane Database Syst Rev.

Schlembach, D., Wallner, W., Sengenberger, R., et al., 2007. Angionenic growth factor levels in maternal and fetal blood: correlation with Doppler ultrasound parameters in pregnancies complicated by preeclampsia and intrauterine growth restriction. Ultrasound Obstet Gynecol 29, 407–413.

Schulman, H., Fleischer, A., Farmakides, G., et al., 1986. Development of uterine artery compliance in pregnancy as detected by Doppler ultrasound. Am J Obstet Gynecol 155, 1031–1036.

Shaheen, S., 1997. The beginnings of chronic airflow obstruction. Br Med Bull 53, 58–70.

Sheppard, L., Bonnar, J., 1976. The ultrastructure of the arterial supply of the human placenta in pregnancy complicated by fetal growth retardation. Br J Obstet Gynaecol 83, 948–959.

Sibai, B., Dekker, G., Kupferminc, M., 2005. Pre-eclampsia. Lancet 365, 785–799.

Sieroszewski, P., Suzin, J., Karowicz-Bilinska, A., 2004. Ultrasound evaluation of intrauterine growth restriction therapy by a nitric oxide donor (L-arginine). J Maternal Fetal Neonat Med 15, 363–366.

Smith, S.C., Baker, P.N., Symonds, E.M., 1997. Increased placental apoptosis in intrauterine growth restriction. Am J Obstet Gynecol 177, 1395–1401.

Smith, G.C.S., Pell, J.P., Dobbie, R., 2003. Interpregnancy interval and risk of preterm birth and neonatal death: retrospective cohort study. Br Med J 327, 313–318.

Smith, G.C.S., Crossley, J.A., Aitken, D.A., et al., 2007. Circulating angiogenic factors in early pregnancy and the risk of preeclampsia, intrauterine growth restriction, spontaneous preterm birth and stillbirth. Obstet Gynecol 109, 1316–1324.

Snijders, R., Sherrod, C., Gosden, C., et al., 1993. Fetal growth retardation: associated malformations and chromosomal abnormalities. Am J Obstet Gynecol 168, 547–555.

Steketee, R.W., Nahlen, B.L., Praise, M.E., et al., 2001. The burden of malaria in pregnancy in malaria-endemic areas. Am J Trop Med Hyg 64 (Suppl. 1–2), 28–35.

Stepan, H., Unversucht, A., Wessel, N., et al., 2007. Predictive value of maternal angiogenic factors in second trimester pregnancies with abnormal uterine perfusion. Hypertension 49, 818–824.

Taipale, P., Hiilesmaa, V., 2001. Predicting delivery date by ultrasound and last menstrual period in early gestation. Obstet Gynecol 97 (2), 189–194.

Tchirikov, M., Rybakowski, C., Hunecke, B., et al., 1998. Blood flow through the ductus venosus in singleton and multifetal pregnancies and in fetuses with intrauterine growth retardation. Am J Obstet Gynecol 178, 943–949.

Thaaler, I., Weiner, Z., Itskovitz, J., et al., 1992. Systolic or diastolic notch in uterine artery blood flow velocity waveforms in hypertensive pregnant patients: relationship to outcome. Obstet Gynecol 80, 277–282.

The GRIT study group, 2003. A randomised trial of timed delivery for the compromised preterm fetus: short term outcomes and Bayesian interpretation. Br J Obstet Gynaecol 110, 27–32.

Thompson, J.M., Clark, P.M., Robinson, E., et al., 2001. Risk factors for small-for-gestational-age babies: the Auckland Birthweight Collaborative Study. J Paediatr Child Health 37, 369–375.

Thornton, J.G., Hornbuckle, J., Vail, A., et al., 2004. GRIT Study Group, 2004. Infant wellbeing at 2 years of age in the Growth Restriction Intervention Trial (GRIT): multicentred randomised controlled trial. Lancet 364, 513–520.

Todros, T., Massarenti, I., Gaglioti, P., et al., 2004. Fetal short femur length in the second trimester and the outcome of pregnancy. Br J Obstet Gynaecol 111, 83–85.

Tolsa, C.B., Zimine, S., Warfield, S.K., et al., 2004. Early alteration of structural and functional brain development in premature infants born with intrauterine growth restriction. Pediatr Res 56, 132–138.

Trudinger, B.J., Giles, W.B., Cook, C.M., 1985. Uteroplacental blood flow velocity-time waveforms in normal and complicated pregnancy. Br J Obstet Gynaecol 92, 39–45.

Van Montfrans, J.M., et al., 2001. Birth weight corrected for gestational age is related to the incidence of Down's syndrome pregnancies. Twin Res 4, 318–320.

Villar, J., de Onis, M., Kestler, E., et al., 1990. The differential neonatal morbidity of the intrauterine growth retardation syndrome. Am J Obstet Gynecol 163, 151–157.

Vyas, S., Nicolaides, K.H., Campbell, S., 1989. Renal artery flow velocity waveforms in normal and hypoxemic fetuses. Am J Obstet Gynecol 161, 168–172.

Wadhwa, P.D., Garite, T.J., Porto, M., et al., 2004. Placental corticotropin-releasing hormone (CRH), spontaneous preterm birth, and fetal growth restriction: a prospective investigation. Am J Obstet Gynecol 191, 1063–1069.

Walker, J., 2000. Pre-eclampsia. Lancet 356, 1260–1265.

Walther, F., Ramaekers, L., 1982. The ponderal index as a measure of the nutritional status at birth and its relation to some aspects of neonatal morbidity. J Perinat Med 10, 42–47.

Weiner, Z., Farmakides, G., Schulman, H., et al., 1994. Central and peripheral hemodynamic changes in fetuses with absent end-diiastolic velocity in umbilical artery: correlation with computerized fetal heart rate pattern. Am J Obstet Gynecol 170, 509–515.

Weisz, B., David, A.L., Chitty, L., et al., 2008. Association of isolated short femur in the mid-trimester fetus with perinatal outcome. Ultrasound Obstet Gynecol 31, 512–516.

WHO, 1995. Expert Committee report: Physical status: the use and interpretation of anthropometry. Technical report series 854. World Health Organization, Geneva.

WHO, 2005. Protecting Vulnerable Groups in Malaria-endemic Areas in Africa Through Accelerated Deployment of Insecticide-treated Nets. WHO UNICEF Joint Statement.

WHO, 2006. Antiretroviral Drugs for Treating Pregnant Women and Preventing HIV Infection in Infants. Towards Universal Access: Recommendations for a Public Health Approach: HIV/AIDS Programme.

Wilcox, M.A., Smith, S.J., Johnson, I.R., et al., 1995. The effect of social deprivation on birth weight, excluding physiological and pathological effects. Br J Obstet Gynaecol 102, 918–924.

Wilson, D., Harper, A., McClure, G., et al., 1992. Long term predictive value of Doppler studies in high risk fetuses. Br J Obstet Gynaecol 99, 575–578.

Witlin, G.A., Saade, G.R., Mattar, F.M., et al., 2000. Predictors of neonatal outcome in women with severe pre-eclampsia or eclampsia between 24 and 33 weeks' gestation. Am J Obstet Gynecol 182, 607–611.

Wood, N., Marlow, N., Costeloe, K., et al., 2000. Neurologic and developmental disability after extremely preterm birth. EPICure Study Group. N Engl J Med 343, 378–384.

Yanney, M., Marlow, N., 2004. Paediatric consequences of fetal growth restriction. Semin Fetal Neonatal Med 9, 411–418.

Yasuda, M., Takakuwa, K., Tokunaga, A., et al., 1995. Prospective studies of the association between anticardiolipin antibody and outcome of pregnancy. Obstet Gyneco l86, 555–559.

Zhang, X., Platt, R.W., Cnattingius, S., et al., 2007. The use of customised versus population-based birthweight standards in predicting perinatal mortality. Br J Obstet Gynaecol 114, 474–477.

Maternal illness in pregnancy

David Williams   Lila Mayahi

11

© 2012 Elsevier Ltd

Good maternal health is necessary for the best pregnancy outcome. Women with chronic diseases, or those who become unwell during pregnancy, are often unable to make the optimal adaptations to pregnancy and therefore the best pregnancy outcome is compromised.

In this chapter are discussed medical conditions and illnesses which may be acquired during pregnancy, as well as chronic medical conditions and the way they may affect the health of mother and fetus.

Of most relevance to a neonatologist is the way maternal illness affects fetal development and the impact on neonatal health.

Women with chronic medical conditions should receive prepregnancy advice before embarking on pregnancy to ensure they are on safe and effective treatments and aware of the implications their condition may have on pregnancy.

The first part of this chapter will focus on serious conditions that can lead to the most unwanted outcome, maternal and perinatal death. Thereafter the focus will be on the most prevalent illnesses.

In each section are discussed the pathophysiology of the disease, its prevalence and incidence, the clinical presentation, appropriate diagnostic tools, best management and outcomes. Where appropriate the impact on breastfeeding will also be discussed.

Thromboembolic disease

Venous thromboembolic events are a leading cause of maternal morbidity and mortality in the developed countries. This is in contrast to the developing world in which haemorrhage and complications from hypertensive disorders are the leading causes of maternal death. Fatal pulmonary embolism, although a rare complication of pregnancy, continues to be the leading cause of pregnancy-related mortality in western Europe and the USA as other causes of maternal mortality (haemorrhage, sepsis) have declined. More obesity in pregnancy, as well as higher caesarean delivery rates, over the past several decades has had an impact on this increased risk of complications for venous thromboembolism.

During pregnancy, the risk for venous thromboembolism is increased sixfold over the non-pregnant state and increases to 20-fold in the immediate puerperium.

Pathogenesis of thromboembolism in pregnancy

Pregnancy evokes a physiologically hypercoagulable state that is protective against haemorrhage at the time of delivery and placental separation. The hypercoagulable state of pregnancy is provoked by thrombin-mediated fibrin generation. The procoagulant changes of pregnancy include an increase in plasma concentration of coagulation factors and fibrinolysis inhibitors, reduced venous flow and increased venous dilatation. Physiological increases in all coagulation factors occur during pregnancy, with the exception of factors XI and XIII, which are frequently decreased. In addition, free protein S levels fall and acquired resistance to activated protein C develops during pregnancy. Risk for thromboembolism is further increased by compression of the inferior vena cava and iliac veins by the gravid uterus, promoting stasis. By 25–29 weeks' gestation, venous flow velocity is reduced by approximately 50% in the legs and does not return to normal non-pregnancy flow velocity until around 6 weeks postpartum. During pregnancy, local damage to pelvic veins may occur during vaginal and especially caesarean delivery and this provides an increased risk for thrombosis. When these physiological coagulation changes combine with genetic predisposition conditions such as thrombophilias, socioenvironmental factors and other medical factors (obesity, inactivity and caesarean section), the risk for thromboembolism is increased.

Most deep venous thrombosis (DVT) occurs in the antepartum period, equally distributed across all trimesters, whereas most pulmonary embolism occurs in the postpartum period.

Thromboembolism in inherited and acquired anticoagulation deficiencies

Thrombophilias are disorders of homeostasis that predispose to thrombotic events. The prevalence of inherited thrombophilias depends on the population and/or ethnicity. Approximately 15% of the western population is affected by a thrombophilia. Approximately 50% of cases of venous thromboembolism in pregnancy are associated with inherited or acquired thrombophilias. The absolute risk of venous thromboembolism for pregnant women with antithrombin III deficiency is reported to be as high as 40–68% (Dargaud et al. 2009; Brown and Hiett 2010). Protein C, in its active form, is responsible for inactivation of factors V and VIII and activation of fibrinolysis. Protein S is a vitamin K-dependent, naturally occurring inhibitor of haemostasis that is synthesised and released from the endothelium and shows autosomal dominant inheritance. It is a cofactor for protein C in the neutralisation of activated factor V and in fibrinolysis. The incidence of thromboembolism has been reported to be 2.5% per year for protein C-deficient individuals, and 3.5% per year for those with protein S deficiency (Brown and Hiett 2010). Protein C deficiency is also autosomal dominant, and the heterozygous trait results in plasma protein C levels of 55–65% of normal. During pregnancy, an incidence of DVT up to 25% has been reported for heterozygote protein C-deficient individuals. The risk for stillbirth is also increased in women with these protein deficiencies (Nelson and Greer 2006). Activated protein C resistance results from a point mutation in the factor V gene (the factor V Leiden mutation; FVL) and is the most frequent aetiology for thrombosis. The gene mutation is inherited as an autosomal dominant trait and is particularly prevalent in the white population. Heterozygosity for the FVL gene defect confers a five- to 10-fold increased risk for thrombosis.

Acquired thrombophilias include antiphospholipid antibodies and lupus anticoagulant. These conditions are typically diagnosed in women with recurrent pregnancy loss rather than thromboembolism. However, both disorders should be considered as risk factors for thromboembolism during pregnancy, and they may also increase the risk of thromboembolic disease in the fetus. For antiphospholipid antibody syndrome, the absolute risk for thrombosis has been reported to be as high as 30% (Nelson and Greer 2006).

Clinical presentation and diagnosis of thromboembolic disease

During pregnancy, venous thromboembolism may present with symptoms of DVT, or pulmonary embolism. The most common symptoms of DVT are pain, tenderness and swelling of the lower extremity. In pregnancy, 85% of DVT cases present in the left leg. This is due to the abrupt right-angle drainage of the left iliac vein that leads to more venous stasis in the left leg.

Clinical signs of a suspected DVT include heat, redness and swelling. The signs and symptoms result from obstructed venous return and/or in combination with vascular inflammation. The risk of pulmonary embolism is greater with femoral or iliac thrombosis and can occur without obvious swelling. Symptoms of pulmonary embolus include dyspnoea, pleuritic chest pain, cough and haemoptysis. Clinical signs include tachycardia, tachypnoea, crepitations, fever, pleuritic rub, cyanosis and the development of an accentuated second heart sound and gallop rhythm. Massive pulmonary embolism, defined as obstruction of more than 50% of the pulmonary circulation, may present with syncope, representing cardiovascular collapse, and recognised with hypotension.

Diagnostic evaluation test for thromboembolism

Doppler flow studies with compression sonography are the primary non-invasive tests used in the diagnosis of DVT. Compression ultrasonography has a sensitivity of 97% and a specificity of 94% for the diagnosis of symptomatic, proximal DVT in the general population. Doppler combined with real-time ultrasound and colour flow have become the diagnostic studies of choice in cases of suspected proximal vein thrombosis (Kearon et al. 1998). Imaging provides additional information about venous compressibility.

Magnetic resonance imaging (MRI) has a sensitivity for thrombi above the knee of nearly 100% and has a place in the evaluation of the patient suspected of having a pelvic thrombus with a negative Doppler/ultrasound examination. A chest X-ray to rule out other diagnoses is a first step in investigating the breathless pregnant patient. Computed tomography (CT) scanning, unlike ultrasonography and MRI, is associated with fetal as well as maternal radiation exposure.

D-dimer is a specific degradation product of cross-linked fibrin. Levels of D-dimer are increased in the presence of thrombi, but also increase with the progression of normal pregnancy and are therefore of little positive diagnostic value. Guidelines for the evaluation of pulmonary embolism in pregnancy attempt to balance diagnostic efficacy, decreasing maternal morbidity and mortality and minimisation of fetal exposure to ionising radiation. The most commonly used non-invasive study is the ventilation–perfusion scan (V/Q scan). Ventilation–perfusion lung scanning delivers a higher fetal dose of radiation (100–370 µGy) than does CT pulmonary angiography (PA) (3–131 µGy). Perfusion scanning alone in women with a normal chest X-ray reduces radiation exposure (Groves et al. 2006). Although helical CT gives good diagnostic sensitivity for pulmonary embolus, there are concerns about the future risk of maternal breast cancer following helical CT to the chest. Pulmonary embolus is however a life-threatening condition and pregnancy must not interfere with the most appropriate investigations when a pulmonary embolism is suspected.

Management of thromboembolism during pregnancy

Anticoagulation

Anticoagulation is the treatment of established DVT or pulmonary embolism occurring during pregnancy and the puerperium, and for prophylaxis against venous thromboembolism in women with a history of earlier thromboembolic episodes. Anticoagulation is also indicated for those women considered to be at risk because of the presence of a thrombophilic state. Low-molecular-weight heparin (LMWH) is the anticoagulant of choice for treatment of thromboembolism during pregnancy, and management requires an individualised, well-planned approach. Heparin does not cross the placenta and is not excreted into breast milk, giving the advantage over warfarin, which crosses the placenta and poses teratogenic fetal risk with exposure in the first trimester. LMWH preparations have more uniform activity, predictable dose–response, dose-independent mechanisms of clearance and longer plasma half-life than unfractionated heparin. An additional advantage of LMWH is that laboratory monitoring or dose adjustment is only required for those with high-risk thrombotic conditions such as metal heart valves or newly started on therapeutic LMWH.

Therapy for acute deep vein thrombosis–thrombophlebitis

Anticoagulation during pregnancy must be tailored to meet the needs of the women, especially peripartum. The current management approach for acute DVT during pregnancy is with twice-daily weight-based dosing of LMWH. However, in most pregnant women except those who are very overweight or underweight or those with impaired renal function, dose adjustments are not necessary.

Anticoagulation for labour and delivery

Anticoagulated patients are at risk of bleeding at the time of delivery. If a therapeutically anticoagulated patient needs an emergency caesarean section, the preferred method of anaesthesia is a general anaesthetic.

During the postpartum period, anticoagulation can usually be resumed within 6 hours of delivery, but discussion with the anaesthetist is necessary regarding timing of removal of neuraxial anaesthesia.

In the postpartum period, anticoagulation with warfarin is an alternative to heparinisation. A therapeutic warfarin range is considered to be at a target international normalised ratio (INR) of 2.0–3.0 for oral anticoagulation in a patient with a first-time DVT. Warfarin is continued at a therapeutic dose for 6 months after a thromboembolic event, or until 6 weeks postpartum, whichever is the longer. No significant levels of warfarin appear in breast milk; therefore, women can breastfeed on warfarin. Warfarin is associated with a higher risk for bleeding complications than heparin, and requires close monitoring of the INR.

Postthrombotic syndrome occurs in up to 60% of patients after a DVT. Wearing a compression stocking on the affected leg after the acute event reduces the risk of this complication (McColl et al. 2000).

Therapy for pulmonary embolus

Acute treatment for pulmonary embolism during pregnancy includes prompt therapeutic anticoagulation with LMWH. Care coordination and management strategies are dictated by the critical nature of the woman's illness and her haemodynamic status.

Inferior vena cava interruption

Inferior vena cava interruption with filters to prevent recurrent thromboembolism is very rarely indicated. Difficulties retrieving filters have led to significant morbidity and therefore their insertion should be reserved for extraordinary situations when anticoagulation is required but not possible or is ineffective.

Thrombolytic therapy

Thrombolytics, such as streptokinase, urokinase and tissue plasminogen activator, have been used in the treatment of major pulmonary embolism during pregnancy. When there is haemodynamic collapse due to pulmonary embolus, the life-saving potential of thrombolytics generally exceeds the potential complications of haemorrhage (Leonhardt et al. 2006).

Management of women with a history of prior thromboembolism

Women with a history of DVT or pulmonary embolism during a prior pregnancy or while on oral contraceptives are at increased risk for recurrent thrombosis during subsequent pregnancies. Fifteen to 25% of thromboembolic events in pregnancy are recurrent events (James et al. 2007). The risk of recurrent thromboembolism in women with a prior pregnancy-related event has been reported to be 4–12%.

The usual treatment regimen for women with a prior DVT includes thromboprophylaxis with LMWH throughout pregnancy until 6 weeks postpartum. Thromboprophylaxis should be considered for those with a history of unprovoked thrombosis, morbidly obese pregnant women (body mass index >40) and those confined to bed for prolonged periods (e.g. premature rupture of membranes, placenta praevia). The use of pneumatic compression devices for the prevention of pregnancy-related thrombosis has not been well studied and the risks are primarily extrapolated from

perioperative data (ACOG Practice Bulletin 2007). Pulmonary embolism after caesarean delivery is much higher than after vaginal delivery by a factor of 2.5–20 (ACOG Practice Bulletin 2007). The duration of thromboprophylaxis after caesarean section for this high-risk group has not been studied. As the risk of peripartum DVT is highest during the first week or so postpartum, it is not unreasonable to continue mechanical means with a compression stocking or boot, or with low-dose LMWH for the first week after delivery.

Hypertension

Women can become pregnant with hypertension (chronic hypertension: 2–4% of pregnancies) or develop hypertension during pregnancy (gestational hypertension: 4%), or develop hypertension in association with proteinuria (pre-eclampsia: 4% of first-time pregnancies). Approximately 20% of women with pre-existing hypertension go on to develop pre-eclampsia. Hypertension during pregnancy is defined as a diastolic blood pressure of 90 mmHg or greater on two occasions more than 4 hours apart or a single diastolic blood pressure above 110 mmHg (Davey and MacGillivray 1988).

In normal pregnancy there is an increase in heart rate and cardiac output with a fall in total peripheral resistance. Cardiac output rises until the 24th week of pregnancy, by which time it has increased by approximately 45%. The rise in cardiac output does not keep pace with the fall in systemic vascular resistance and maternal blood pressure therefore tends to fall during the first and second trimester until about the 20th week, when it reaches its nadir. From this time total systemic vascular resistance begins to rise and so maternal blood pressure also rises gradually.

Clinical presentation

Chronic hypertension

Women with essential hypertension tend to be older, parous and likely to have a family history of hypertension. In pregnancies where pre-eclampsia does not develop, the risk of a poor outcome (intrauterine growth restriction, preterm delivery, maternal renal and vascular problems) is directly proportional to the degree of hypertension and the number of antihypertensives that need to be used to control it. Most chronic hypertension is mild or moderate (<160/110 mmHg), and a good outcome can be expected unless pre-eclampsia develops. Antihypertensive medication can sometimes be discontinued in the first and second trimester because of the fall in blood pressure secondary to the physiological changes of pregnancy. The recent UK National Institute for Health and Clinical Excellence (NICE) guideline (2010) on the management of hypertension in pregnancy suggested that women with chronic hypertension should have a target blood pressure between 130/80 and 150/100 mmHg. This pragmatic recommendation protects the mother from cardiovascular end-organ damage while preventing reduced uteroplacental perfusion pressure that may lead to reduced fetal growth. There is no robust evidence to recommend beta-blockers, calcium channel blockers, methyldopa or any other antihypertensive over another. To some extent the choice is guided by clinician familiarity and maternal tolerance.

Pre-eclampsia

Pre-eclampsia is a multisystem disorder unique to humans and exclusively associated with pregnancy (Williams and de Swiet

1997). It is defined as a syndrome developing after 20 weeks of gestation, characterised by hypertension (a diastolic pressure of at least 90 mmHg on two consecutive occasions at least 4 hours apart) and proteinuria (>300 mg/24 hours). Across the world pre-eclampsia and eclampsia probably account for up to 50 000 maternal deaths per annum, the vast majority in the developing nations.

Pre-eclampsia develops in women predisposed to cardiovascular disease and who also have poor development of their placenta. The poorly perfused placenta appears to be the source of factors that lead to maternal vascular injury. This leads to a microangiopathy, which results in hypertension, multiorgan dysfunction and, on occasion, a consumptive coagulopathy (Williams and de Swiet 1997).

At present, there is uncertainty about the most effective prophylaxis against pre-eclampsia. Little can be done effectively to prevent pre-eclampsia. A meta-analysis of trials that tested the efficacy of low-dose aspirin (LDA) to prevent pre-eclampsia revealed a 15–20% decrease in incidence in those who received aspirin prophylaxis (Duley et al. 2001). Another Cochrane publication showed that calcium supplementation approximately halves the risk of pre-eclampsia (Hofmeyr et al. 2010). There is no additional benefit from magnesium, garlic, fish oil, antioxidant vitamins or folic acid.

Once pre-eclampsia has developed, it will progress at a variable rate until the fetus and placenta have been delivered. If a woman presents at term (>37 weeks), labour should be induced to prevent serious deterioration in the maternal and/or fetal condition. At earlier gestations, antenatal management aims to be conservative in order to prolong pregnancy and improve fetal maturity while attempting to avoid the development of severe maternal complications or fetal compromise.

Maternal investigations to assess the severity of pre-eclampsia include measures of renal and liver function and a platelet count. The assessment of fetal well-being should involve growth scans, assessment of liquor volume and umbilical artery Doppler velocimetry. Some women with pre-eclampsia have no evidence of fetal compromise while others have minimal maternal symptoms or signs but significant fetal compromise. Although control of blood pressure alone will do little or nothing to prevent disease progression, there is an increased risk of stroke, cardiac failure and abruption when hypertension exceeds 170/110 mmHg. By preventing significant rises in blood pressure, antihypertensives may help to allow a clinically useful period of fetal development and thus improve neonatal outcome.

A variety of antihypertensive agents are available; all act by different mechanisms. The new NICE (2010) guideline suggests the use of labetalol or nifedipine slow-release as first-line treatments (Visintin et al. 2010). When beta-blockers are given in high dose and throughout pregnancy for the treatment of chronic hypertension, they can be associated with intrauterine growth restriction (Rubin et al. 1983). The judicious use of beta-blockers in doses more usually prescribed since 2000 has not had the same association with fetal growth restriction. Angiotensin-converting enzyme (ACE) inhibitors should not be used in pregnancy as they are teratogenic (Cooper et al. 2006). ACE inhibitors do not appear to be secreted in breast milk in a clinically significant quantity and therefore they have a role in the management of postpartum hypertension.

Intravenous hydralazine or labetalol is the mainstay for the acute control of severe hypertension prior to delivery or in the immediate postpartum period. Acute hypotension must be avoided as uteroplacental blood flow can be compromised, leading to fetal compromise. Labetalol is a risk factor for neonatal hypoglycaemia and babies should be monitored.

HELLP syndrome

In 1982, Weinstein first used the term HELLP (haemolysis, elevated liver enzymes and low platelet count) syndrome to describe a particularly severe and rapidly progressive form of pre-eclampsia. Elevated liver enzymes and low platelets are common features of pre-eclampsia, but haemolysis is unusual. The importance of recognising haemolysis rests largely on the need to place women affected by HELLP at high risk of maternal and fetal mortality.

Eclampsia

Eclampsia is the development of seizures in association with pre-eclampsia. In the UK, eclampsia occurs uncommonly, affecting 5/10 000 pregnancies. While the term 'pre-eclampsia' suggests there is a progressive deterioration in the maternal condition to the point of eclampsia, almost 40% of eclamptic seizures occur before either hypertension or proteinuria is documented. About 40% of cases of eclampsia occur antepartum, 15% intrapartum and 45% postpartum, usually within the first 24 hours. The pathophysiology of the seizures is likely to be multifactorial; cerebral vasospasm causing both ischaemia and overperfusion have been observed, leading to disruption of the blood–brain barrier and cerebral oedema. Rarely, cortical blindness can occur.

There is clear evidence that magnesium sulphate is the drug of choice to prevent recurrent eclampsia in a woman who already has had an eclamptic seizure (Duley et al. 2003). The Magpie trial (2007) demonstrated that the use of magnesium sulphate in women with pre-eclampsia halved the incidence of eclampsia. At the dosage given in the trial there appeared to be no short-term serious harmful effects on either the mother or the baby. The recommendation is to use magnesium sulphate in women with severe pre-eclampsia and in those who have had an eclamptic seizure.

Heart disease

Owing to the major physiological changes to the heart in pregnancy, symptoms and signs of healthy pregnancy are often mistaken for pathology. The commonest reason for cardiological referral during pregnancy is the detection of a murmur that proves to be an innocent flow murmur in 90% of cases, due to the 50% increase in cardiac output. The other common presentation is with palpitations. The majority are due to benign arrhythmias such as ventricular and atrial unifocal ectopics that do not require treatment. Serious dysrhythmias are rare. The principles of treatment are no different from in non-pregnant patients, with the exception of some dysrhythmic agents that may be restricted because of insufficient safety data. Adenosine and direct current cardioversion can be used safely during pregnancy and are well tolerated by the fetus. Beta-blockers are first-line treatment to prevent supraventricular arrhythmias (Trappe 2003).

Heart disease in pregnancy is the leading cause of maternal mortality in the UK (Confidential Enquiry into Maternal Death in the UK 2002). In developed countries, the incidence of heart disease in pregnancy has declined over the last 50 years owing to the dramatic reduction in the incidence of rheumatic fever that followed the introduction of penicillin (Lupton et al. 2002). In contrast, congenital heart disease in pregnancy is increasingly common because of the advances in paediatric cardiac surgery and medical therapy which have taken place over the last 30 years, which mean that more affected women are surviving into the reproductive age. The risk of a child inheriting polygenic cardiac disease is varied according to the parent's condition, being 3% in conditions such as tetralogy of

Fallot but as high as 10–18% with atrial septal defect, coarctation of the aorta and aortic stenosis (Burn et al. 1998).

Decisions about embarking on pregnancy with congenital heart disease need to balance the desire for children against the risk of mortality and morbidity. In the most serious conditions, women with Eisenmenger syndrome, primary pulmonary hypertension and inoperable cyanotic heart disease have a 30–50% risk of maternal mortality during pregnancy.

Valve disease

In general, pregnant women tolerate valvular regurgitation better than stenosis. This is because the reduced systemic vascular resistance improves forward flow and limits the effects of regurgitation. Stenosis, in contrast, creates a fixed impediment to the increase in cardiac output that accompanies pregnancy and labour, possibly precipitating pulmonary oedema and arrhythmias. In the UK, calcific degeneration of congenital bicuspid aortic valves is the leading cause of stenosis encountered in pregnancy. Pregnancy in women with artificial heart valves is a major dilemma. Most cardiologists currently recommend a tissue valve for women wanting to have children as, unlike mechanical valves, they avoid the need for anticoagulation, but they wear out more quickly.

Peripartum cardiomyopathy

Peripartum cardiomyopathy is a poorly understood condition, with an incidence of 1:1500 to 1:4000 live births. It has been defined clinically as the onset of cardiac failure with no identifiable cause in the last month of pregnancy or within 5 months after delivery, in the absence of heart disease before the last month of pregnancy (Demakis et al. 1971). It is associated with older maternal age, greater parity, black race, pre-eclampsia and multiple gestations (Veille 1984). Diagnosis rests on the echocardiographic identification of new left ventricular systolic dysfunction during a limited period around parturition, in a woman with symptoms and signs of heart failure and when other causes of cardiomyopathy have been excluded. All patients usually exhibit cardiomegaly on chest X-ray. Endomyocardial biopsy demonstrates myocarditis in up to 76% of patients, and may be necessary where the diagnosis is unclear. Treatment of peripartum cardiomyopathy includes diuretics to decrease pulmonary congestion and volume overload and vasodilators to reduce afterload. Hydralazine is the drug of choice prepartum, in addition to nitrates (Pearson et al. 2000). ACE inhibitors are the mainstay of treatment postpartum, even in mothers who are breastfeeding. The beta-blocker carvedilol has been shown to improve overall survival in pregnant women with dilated cardiomyopathy. Atrial arrhythmias should be treated with digoxin, which may also be used for its positive inotropic effect (Rahimtoola and Tak 1996). The benefits of class 3 (amiodarone) and class 4 (verapamil) agents needs to be balanced against their side-effects: fetal hypothyroidism and premature delivery, fetal bradycardia, heart block and hypotension respectively. Patients with poor cardiac function, as evidenced by an ejection fraction <35%, are at risk of thromboembolism and anticoagulation may be considered (Pearson et al. 2000).

After stabilisation of the mother's symptoms, in most cases induction and vaginal delivery can be attempted in consultation with consultant obstetrician and anaesthetic staff (George et al. 1997). The advantages of vaginal delivery are minimal blood loss, greater haemodynamic stability, avoidance of surgical stress and less chance of postoperative infection and pulmonary complications. Effective pain management is a necessity to avoid further increases in cardiac output from pain and anxiety.

Myocardial infarction

Ischaemic heart disease in pregnancy is uncommon, occurring in an estimated 1 in 10 000 deliveries (Hankins et al. 1985). Myocardial infarction is more common during the third trimester or puerperium of either the first or second pregnancies. occurs within 2 weeks of labour or delivery, mortality may be as high as 45% (Hankins et al. 1985). Patients typically present with ischaemic chest pain in the presence of an abnormal electrocardiogram (ECG) and elevated cardiac enzymes. Symptoms may often be masked or unclear during labour and delivery, and the ECG and cardiac enzymes can be insensitive. Cardiac-specific troponin I is a more sensitive indicator of myocardial infarction than creatinine kinase muscle–bone serum concentrations, which increase during normal labour (Shivvers et al. 1999).

Management of myocardial infarction must involve early coronary angiography. In the immediate postpartum period, spontaneous coronary artery dissection is the most common cause of myocardial infarction. The pathophysiological mechanisms responsible in the coronary arteries are similar to those responsible for aortic dissection, although the exact pathogenesis remains unclear. Most women with peripartum coronary artery dissection have no risk factors for coronary artery disease, but most affect the left anterior descending artery (McKechnie et al. 2001). Treatments include coronary stenting and emergency coronary artery bypass grafting.

Diabetes Mellitus (see Ch. 22 for management of the infant of a diabetic mother)

In the UK 2–5% of pregnant women have diabetes. Most of these pregnancies are due to gestational diabetes, and the rest are due to either type 1 or type 2 diabetes. The prevalence of type 2 diabetes is increasing throughout the world. Diabetes in pregnancy is associated with risks to the woman and to the developing fetus. Miscarriage, pre-eclampsia and preterm labour are more common in women with pre-existing diabetes. In addition, diabetic retinopathy can worsen rapidly during pregnancy. Stillbirth, congenital malformations, macrosomia, birth injury, perinatal mortality and neonatal hypoglycaemia are more common in offspring of women with diabetes.

Women with gestational diabetes have an increased risk of developing type 2 diabetes in later life. For this reason all women need postpartum assessment of glucose tolerance at more than 6 weeks postpartum. Advice on lifestyle and diet will reduce the future risk of diabetes.

In preconception counselling women with established diabetes should be informed that establishing good glycaemic control before conception and continuing this throughout pregnancy will reduce the risk of miscarriage, congenital malformation, stillbirth and neonatal death. These risks can be reduced, but not eliminated.

Overall the risk of congenital anomalies is three to five times greater in women with diabetes than in the general population and is related directly to the percentage of glycosylated haemoglobin at the time of conception (Stiete et al. 1995). The mechanism of this teratogenic effect is unclear, but appears to relate to glucose control and lipid levels.

Intrauterine fetal death

Despite advances in antenatal monitoring, women with poorly controlled diabetes still have an increased incidence of intrauterine fetal

	Plasma glucose	Plasma glucose
	Fasting	2 Hours
Normal	<5.4	<7.9
Glocose Intolerance	5.5–6.9mmol/l	8.0–10.9
Gestational Diabetes	>/=7.0mmol/l	>/=11.0mmol/l

Fig. 11.1 Revised World Health Organization criteria for 75 g oral glucose tolerance test during pregnancy.

death, especially beyond the due date. The underlying mechanism has not been elucidated, but relates to glucose control as reflected in the glycosylated haemoglobin.

Screening for gestational diabetes and impaired glucose tolerance

There are few conclusive data to support a screening programme for gestational diabetes in all age group mothers, as only small numbers of young and lean women will go on to develop gestational diabetes. What has been shown is that 75 g oral glucose loading is an appropriate mode of testing. If the screening test is abnormal, then the pregnant mother should go on to have an oral glucose tolerance test. The diagnostic criteria are shown in Figure 11.1.

Management of diabetic pregnancy

Just as outside pregnancy the aim is to keep to a normal blood glucose level, diet, insulin and oral hypoglycaemic agents are the key components of diabetic management. A meta-analysis into large randomised controlled trials comparing oral hypoglycaemic and insulin demonstrates that there were no differences in glycaemic control or pregnancy outcomes, including incidence of babies that were large for gestational age, caesarean sections and increased birthweight (Dhulkotia et al. 2010).

Diet

The aim is to provide sufficient energy for both mother and fetus, which amounts to 30–35 kcal/kg of non-pregnant ideal body weight. Daily carbohydrate consumption should be in the region of 220–240 g, providing at least 45% of the necessary calorie intake. Detailed and ongoing advice from an experienced dietician is important to the success of dietary management. The first line of treatment for gestational diabetes is diet; if this approach fails, then hypoglycaemic therapy is considered.

Oral hypoglycaemic agents

If diet fails to control gestational diabetes, then metformin is the next line of treatment (Rowan et al. 2008). Metformin counteracts the excessive insulin resistance of gestational diabetes without risk of hypoglycaemia. It has been shown to be as effective as insulin in the management of gestational diabetes and with regard to pregnancy outcome (Rowan et al. 2008). Metformin does cross the placenta, but does not appear to be harmful to the developing fetus. Follow-up studies of offspring exposed to metformin in utero are ongoing, but after 2 years do not show differences compared with those exposed to insulin.

Insulin

Women with gestational diabetes who are not controlled by diet or metformin may need additional insulin. Increasingly, pen-type syringes are being used to deliver insulin, typically with three doses of short-acting insulin preprandially and one dose of a long-acting insulin at night. The newer insulin analogues appear suitable for pregnancy. Continuous subcutaneous insulin infusion may provide the best glucose control of diabetic pregnant women.

Labour and the puerperium

Preterm delivery is more common in diabetic pregnancy, and, if steroids are given to promote fetal lung maturity, the hyperglycaemic effect requires extra monitoring, but not usually a sliding scale of insulin.

Women with well-controlled diabetes, no vascular disease and a normally grown fetus appear to be at no more risk than non-diabetic counterparts and may be allowed to carry at least to the due date. With a macrosomic fetus and poor glucose control, early delivery may be contemplated to reduce the risk of stillbirth.

During labour women with type 1 diabetes can be treated with an insulin sliding scale, 10% glucose solution and hourly blood glucose monitoring. Once the baby is delivered the rate of insulin infusion should be reduced, or stopped if the woman has insulin-requiring gestational diabetes or type 2 diabetes. Insulin requirements fall back to prepregnancy levels as soon as the placenta has been delivered.

Breastfeeding and effects on glycaemic control

Women with insulin-treated pre-existing diabetes are at increased risk of hypoglycaemia in the postnatal period, especially when breastfeeding. Women with gestational diabetes should discontinue hypoglycaemic treatment after birth. Women with pre-existing type 2 diabetes who are breastfeeding can resume or continue to take hypoglycaemic agents following birth.

Thyroid disease

Hypothyroidism

Hypothyroidism affects 2–5% of all pregnancies. It is unusual to diagnose hypothyroidism for the first time during pregnancy, although it may develop as part of postpartum thyroiditis. The majority of women are therefore already on thyroxine replacement therapy when they attend for their first antenatal visit. It is good practice to check thyroid-stimulating hormone (TSH) levels every trimester and adjust requirements for thyroxine accordingly. Elevated TSH levels during the first trimester of pregnancy have been associated with an increased risk of mental and cognitive disturbance in children. It has been shown that children of women with hypothyroxinaemia but normal TSH during gestation had a delayed mental and motor function at 1 and 2 years of age. Therefore, not only TSH but also free thyroxine should be monitored, especially in the first half of pregnancy (Haddow et al. 1999; Pop et al. 2003).

Taking into account the high prevalence of thyroid disorders during pregnancy and associated neonatal morbidity, an ongoing debate has developed as to the potential for routine screening of hypothyroidism in early pregnancy.

The aim of treatment for hypothyroidism is to keep TSH less than 2.5 mU/l in the first trimester and less than 3 mU/l in later pregnancy. Thyroid function should be rechecked 6 weeks after delivery (Okosieme et al. 2008).

Thyrotoxicosis

Thyrotoxicosis occurs in 0.2% of pregnancies; Graves disease accounts for 95% of these cases. Both carbimazole (which is metabolised to methimazole) and propylthiouracil are used in the management of thyrotoxicosis during pregnancy. Less propylthiouracil crosses the placenta than methimazole. Carbimazole has been associated with cutis aplasia, although this is a very rare and tenuous association. Propylthiouracil also crosses into breast milk in lower quantities than does carbimazole. However, in practice it is doubtful whether there is any material difference between these two drugs, and treatment should be at a dose that maintains free thyroxine at the upper end of the normal range (Okosieme et al. 2008).

It has been reported that, in up to 10% of women who have had Graves disease, TSH receptor-stimulating antibodies cross the placenta and produce fetal tachycardia and transient neonatal thyrotoxicosis. Although the levels of these thyroid-stimulating antibodies can be measured in maternal blood, the assays are not readily available and measuring fetal heart rate in at-risk women is likely to be more useful. Treatment of fetal thyrotoxicosis is by increasing the maternal dose of antithyroid drugs until the fetal heart rate is in the normal range. Although rare, neonatal thyrotoxicosis has a significant mortality, hence early treatment is vital. Women who have been treated and 'cured' of Graves disease still have the autoantibodies and therefore neonatal thyrotoxicosis remains a possibility.

Hyperthyroidism should be distinguished from gestational transient thyrotoxicosis, which is due to the TSH receptor-stimulating effects of human chorionic gonadotrophin (hCG). This hCG-induced hyperthyroidism does not lead to clinical thyrotoxicosis and need not be treated with antithyroid drugs.

Neurological disorders in pregnancy

Epilepsy

Approximately 1 in 200 pregnant women have epilepsy. Not all women with epilepsy take antiepileptic drugs (AEDs), but, for those who do take AEDs, important clinical issues relate to the risks of uncontrolled seizures with the potential teratogenic effects of AEDs. Women who attend for prepregnancy counselling and who have been seizure-free for 2 years should be considered for withdrawal of anticonvulsant therapy, if appropriate for the cause of epilepsy.

Seizures can result in physical trauma or even death in the mother and fetus. Uncontrolled tonic clonic grand mal seizures result in metabolic and respiratory acidosis that is transferred to the fetus and may result in fetal bradycardia and intrauterine death (Katz et al. 2006).

Most women with epilepsy have already been diagnosed and need no further investigations. Women who develop seizures for the first time during pregnancy need to be investigated. Causes of seizures include cerebral vein thrombosis, thrombotic thrombocytopenic purpura, cerebral infarction, drug and alcohol withdrawal, hypoglycaemia, hyponatraemia, eclampsia and pseudoepilepsy. The largest prospective study of pregnant patients with epilepsy has shown that 58% of epileptic women experience no change in the frequency of their seizures during their pregnancy, about 18% have an increase in their seizure rate (EURAP Study Group 2006). The physiological changes in pregnancy, such as slower gastrointestinal absorption,

increased plasma volume, decreased protein binding, lack of sleep, poor compliance or nausea and vomiting of the first trimester, may all account for this. While the fetus is relatively resistant to short episodes of hypoxia and there is no evidence of adverse effects of single seizures on the fetus, status epilepticus has been associated with a 50% risk of fetal loss or handicap.

It is best for the mother and the baby, if the woman is on the lowest effective dose of AED to control their epilepsy during pregnancy.

The mechanism by which AEDs cause congenital anomalies appears to be multifactorial, with some degree of genetic vulnerability not yet defined.

The underlying risk of malformation for any one drug is about 6–7% (i.e. about two- to threefold the background malformation rate). Unfortunately, the risk rises at least additively with each additional anticonvulsant; thus it is approaching 20% if a woman is on three anticonvulsants, and with some combinations the increase in risk is even greater.

Despite the risk of teratogenicity it is important to emphasise to women with epilepsy that uncontrolled seizures can be more hazardous to the fetus than the risks associated with anticonvulsants. The risks of congenital abnormalities may be minimised by maintaining women on the lowest possible dose of drug that keeps them seizure-free, and by the use of single rather than multiple AEDs.

Folic acid 5 mg once daily periconception and throughout pregnancy has been suggested to reduce the risk of malformations and neurodisability, but evidence is currently lacking.

Antiepileptic drugs

Carbamazepine

A total of 1% of carbamazepine-exposed infants have spina bifida (Rosa 1991). There is also an increase in the rate of craniofacial defects and fingernail hypoplasia.

Phenytoin has been associated with microencephaly, mental retardation, growth deficiency and congenital heart defect.

Sodium valproate carries a 1–2% risk of neural tube defects occurring in the fetus. It is also associated with congenital heart defects. Cognitive function is probably affected by valproate, though the size of the effect is uncertain. There is also concern that there may be a link between valproate exposure and autism (Williams and Hersh 1997). Further prospective research is needed to identify the link between maternal valproate use and neurodisability in the offspring.

Lamotrigine

Lamotrigine is the most extensively investigated of the newer AEDs. Pharmacokinetic changes are pronounced: on average, plasma concentrations decreased by 68% during pregnancy, with a wide individual variability (Pennell et al. 2004). A decline in plasma concentration of lamotrigine has been associated with breakthrough seizures in up to 75% of pregnant women on monotherapy (de Haan et al. 2004). Some authorities believe women with epilepsy on lamotrigine should have their serum levels checked and the dose of lamotrigine adjusted accordingly. A prospective pregnancy data registry has also shown that patients on lamotrigine require more frequent dose adjustment during pregnancy (Vajda et al. 2006).

Very limited or no information is available on possible changes in disposition of the other new-generation AEDs (e.g. gabapentin, vigabatrin).

Early detailed ultrasound should be offered to all mothers with epilepsy in order to exclude neural tube defects and life-threatening congenital heart anomalies.

There is a theoretical risk of vitamin K deficiency in the neonates of mothers who take anticonvulsants during pregnancy. It was formerly suggested that vitamin K supplements be given to the mother in the last few weeks of pregnancy and to the neonate at birth to prevent haemorrhagic disease of the newborn, but this recommendation is not current. Newborn babies of mothers taking anticonvulsants should receive intramuscular vitamin K.

The risk of an epileptic seizure is approximately doubled in labour because of exhaustion, pain and lack of sleep; therefore, the usual doses of anticonvulsant should be given. Caesarean section is only indicated for obstetric reasons. If the dose of anticonvulsant has been increased during the pregnancy a reduction should be made after delivery.

Breastfeeding

AEDs pass into breast milk. The concentration of drug depends on the pharmocokinetics in the mother and pharmacokinetics and pharmocodynamics in the baby. The mother should be informed about the possibility of drug effects on breastfeeding but not discouraged from breastfeeding (Tomson 2005).

Stroke

Cerebrovascular accidents (Stroke) during pregnancy or the puerperium are an important cause of maternal death and serious maternal morbidity (Kittner et al. 1996). The reported incidence of Stroke in relation to pregnancy varies from 3.8 to 26 cases per 100 000 deliveries or pregnancies, depending on the population studied (Jaigobin and Silver 2000).

The majority of Stroke events occur postpartum and therefore do not have a direct impact on neonatal health. Uncontrolled high blood pressure and pre-eclampsia place a woman at increased risk for Stroke. While strokes are rare in women of childbearing age, with gradually decreasing maternal mortality rates over the past 20 years, they now account for over 10% of the total number of maternal deaths in the UK (CEMD 2001). Strokes are defined as acute ischaemic or haemorrhagic events causing the onset of focal neurological symptoms.

Subarachnoid haemorrhage

The incidence is 1–2 per 10 000, with an overall mortality of between 27% and 40% (Treadwell et al. 2008). Most cases of subarachnoid haemorrhage are due to ruptured cerebral aneurysms, and typically present with thunderclap headache, vomiting, seizures or reduced level of consciousness. Presentation in pregnancy may be confused with eclampsia, and the diagnosis should be confirmed with neuroimaging or cerebrospinal fluid analysis. The relative risk of intracerebral haemorrhage during pregnancy and 6 weeks postpartum has been reported to be 5.6 times that of the non-pregnant patient, and 50% of all aneurysmal ruptures in women below the age of 40 years are pregnancy-related. Surgical treatment after aneurysmal subarachnoid haemorrhage during pregnancy improves both maternal and fetal outcome, and management should generally follow the same course as for the non-pregnant population (Dias 1994). The mode of delivery for women with arteriovenous malformation or aneurysms is still contentious. If the arteriovenous malformation or aneurysm is successfully operated on, then vaginal delivery is appropriate. The risk of recurrent haemorrhage during labour may be reduced by epidural anaesthesia, minimising pushing in the second stage, and by performing an instrumental delivery if required.

Cerebral venous thrombosis

Cerebral venous thrombosis (CVT) occurs most commonly during the puerperium. It has an incidence of 1 per 10 000 deliveries in the developed world but in the developing world it is the most common cause of stroke, with an incidence of 40–50 per 10 000 deliveries (Canhao et al. 2005). It is typically associated with infection and dehydration, though there are many other recognised causes. Occlusion of the cerebral cortical veins can result in venous infarction with associated focal neurological symptoms and signs. Cavernous sinus thrombosis may also lead to a painful eye and sometimes exophthalmos. The risk of peripartum CVT increases with hypertension, advancing maternal age, caesarean delivery, associated infections and excess vomiting during pregnancy (Lanska and Kryscio 2000). The diagnosis of CVT is made by CT or MRI.

The death rate from all-cause CVT is 2–10%, although mortality is significantly less for pregnancy-associated CVT (Cantu and Barinagarrementeria 1993). CVT should be treated with therapeutic LMWH with factor Xa monitoring (Bates et al. 2004).

Multiple sclerosis (MS)

This disease is relatively common, with an incidence of approximately 1:1000, and it tends to occur during the childbearing years, with a peak incidence at 30 years of age. The cause of MS is unknown and the course is unpredictable. Common symptoms include the acute onset of diplopia, vertigo, gait instability, bladder incontinence, loss of vision and fatigue. The common neuropathological lesion is a plaque demonstrating myelin loss and gliosis associated with inflammatory infiltrates. There are retrospective and prospective (Roullet et al. 1993) data that suggest improvement of MS during pregnancy and fewer relapses (Korn-Lubetzki et al. 1984); however this benefit is largely reversed during the first 3 postpartum months when there are higher reports of relapses (Confavreux et al. 1998).

Spinal and epidural anaesthesia appear to be safe in labour, despite a diagnosis of MS. There is no long-term effect of pregnancy or breastfeeding on the course of MS; however the children of women with MS have a 30-fold increased risk of developing the condition (a 3% risk compared with the background rate of 0.1% in the general population) (Sadovnick 1984).

Current MS therapy includes intravenous corticosteroids and other immunosuppressive agents (i.e. cyclophosphamide) for acute relapses and immunosuppressive drugs (azathioprine, ciclosporin A, cyclophosphamide and methotrexate – although the last two are contraindicated in pregnancy) for long-term treatment. The two immune modulator pharmacological agents which are mainly used for relapsing–remitting-type MS are interferon-beta and glatiramer (a polymer) (Janssen and Genta 2000). It is generally recommended that interferon therapy should be discontinued before conception. Available data suggest no increased risk of adverse fetal or pregnancy outcomes associated with glatiramer acetate use (Coyle 2009).

Labour and delivery

Delivery is not more complicated in MS patients than in women without MS, and the mode of delivery is decided strictly on obstetrical criteria. Maternal exhaustion seen in the second stage can be managed with operative vaginal delivery. MS patients who have recently received long-term corticosteroid therapy or who are on low-dose corticosteroid therapy at the time of delivery may have adrenal insufficiency and should be given supplemental corticosteroids.

Breastfeeding

Systemically administered steroids appear in human milk in a ratio of 1 : 10 (breast milk : maternal serum) and have not been found to affect the neonatal pituitary–adrenal axis in doses of prednisolone up to 40 mg. Azathioprine is not found in breast milk and the benefits of breastfeeding exceed potential risks associated with ciclosporin A. It is not known whether interferon-beta is secreted into breast milk. The Committee on Drugs of the American Academy of Pediatrics advises that methotrexate should be avoided during lactation owing to potential immune suppression, neutropenia, adverse effects on growth and carcinogenesis (American Academy of Pediatrics Committee on Drugs 2001). Breastfeeding is unrestricted during intravenous immunoglobulin therapy and there is no known negative effect on the developing immune system of the newborn baby.

Renal disease and pregnancy

Most women with chronic kidney disease who become pregnant have mild renal dysfunction and pregnancy usually succeeds without affecting renal prognosis. In general, women with serum creatinine (sCr) levels of less than 125 μmol/l have good obstetric outcomes and a good long-term renal prognosis. Those women with moderate (sCr > 125 < 180 μmol/l) or severe (sCr > 180 μmol/l) renal insufficiency do less well, with an increased risk of an accelerated decline in renal function and poor pregnancy outcome correlated with the level of renal impairment. When sCr is greater than 180 μmol/l, more than 50% of women develop pre-eclampsia, especially if there is associated hypertension. One in three women with sCr > 180 μmol/l develop end-stage renal failure within 1 year of delivery (Davison 2001). The main parameters that can be controlled during pregnancy and may improve pregnancy outcome are the management of associated hypertension, prevention of recurrent urinary tract infections (UTIs) with antibiotic prophylaxis and prevention of thrombosis in women with proteinuria >1 g/24 hours.

Asymptomatic bacteriuria

The incidence of asymptomatic bacteriuria is in the region of 5%. *Escherichia coli* is the most commonly isolated pathogen and is present in 80–90% of UTIs and up to 95% of acute pyelonephritis (Connolly and Thorp 1999). Up to 30% of pregnant women with untreated bacteriuria will go on to develop pyelonephritis. Under these circumstances there is a risk of preterm delivery and low birthweight (Ovalle and Levancini 2001). An association between untreated UTI in pregnancy and risk of neonatal mental retardation has also been reported (McDermott et al. 2000).

Acute pyelonephritis

Pyelonephritis has been shown to affect 1.3% of pregnancies, with *E. coli* being the most common pathogen. The diagnosis is likely if there are symptoms of a UTI together with a high fever, nausea, vomiting, rigors and renal-angle pain and tenderness. The patient should be admitted to hospital and treated with intravenous broad-spectrum antibiotics. Ceftriaxone, because of its safety and negligible side-effects, has been suggested as an effective antibiotic for acute antepartum pyelonephritis (Sharma and Thapa 2007).

Renal transplantation and pregnancy

Pregnancy is becoming increasingly common in women who have been the recipients of renal transplants. About 1 in 50 women of childbearing age with renal allografts become pregnant (Davison 2001). There is an increased incidence of maternal hypertension, preterm delivery (45–66%) and fetal growth restriction (40%) that reflects the level of renal function and coexistent complications such as hypertension, proteinuria and UTIs.

To prevent rejection of the renal allograft immunosuppressive therapy with prednisolone, ciclosporin A, azathioprine, tacrolimus, sirolimus and mycophenolate mofetil (MMF) has been used. All these drugs cross the placenta and enter the fetal circulation. MMF is teratogenic and should be replaced with azathioprine during pregnancy. The European Best Practice Guidelines (2002) also recommend avoiding sirolimus during pregnancy.

Breastfeeding

Breastfeeding for transplant-recipient mothers remains an area in which recommendations are evolving. The lack of reported adverse effects, together with the documented benefits of breastfeeding, outweigh the theoretical risks.

Haematology

Physiological changes during pregnancy

Plasma volume increases progressively throughout pregnancy so that by 36 weeks' gestation it is 50% greater than in the non-pregnant state. There is also an increase in the red cell mass, but the expansion in plasma volume is far greater than the increase in red cell mass, hence the net effect is a fall in haemoglobin concentration, haematocrit and red cell count. Despite this haemodilution, there is usually no change in mean corpuscular volume or mean corpuscular haemoglobin concentration. Pregnancy causes a two- to threefold increase in the requirement for iron, and a 10–20-fold increase in folate requirements to meet the demands of the expanding red cell mass, fetus and placenta. The lower limit of normal for haemoglobin concentration in the non-pregnant female is 11.5–12 g/dl. In pregnancy, levels below 10.5 g/dl may be abnormal, although in certain situations, such as multiple pregnancies, the physiological dilution of haemoglobin may cause even lower concentrations of haemoglobin.

Iron-deficiency anaemia

On a global basis iron-deficiency anaemia is still a leading cause of maternal morbidity and mortality. In developed countries significant iron-deficiency anaemia is uncommon, although most women are routinely prescribed supplements of iron and folic acid. There is no consensus about the value of giving prophylactic iron to a population which is well nourished. This is not the case in the developing world.

Folate-deficiency anaemia

Folic acid deficiency is the major cause of megaloblastic anaemia in pregnancy; vitamin B_{12} deficiency is very rare, except in developing countries or strict vegans. Folate deficiency is more likely if the woman is taking AEDs or if she suffers from haematological conditions such as haemolytic anaemia and thalassaemia. Diagnosis of folate deficiency should be confirmed by the measurement of serum and red cell folate levels (it should be noted that the normal range in pregnancy is lower than in non-pregnant women). All women planning pregnancy are now advised to take 400 μg/day folate periconceptionally to lower the risk of neural tube defects and other fetal abnormalities and this reduces the risk of folate deficiency still further. In addition, women who have had a previous fetus with a neural tube defect and women taking anticonvulsants or sulfasalazine and who have diabetes are advised to take 5 mg/day folate periconceptionally.

Haemoglobinopathies

The most common types of haemoglobinopathies include sickle-cell disease and thalassaemia. Their incidence varies according to ethnicity.

Sickle-cell disease

Most women with sickle-cell disease will be aware of the diagnosis before they become pregnant. Haemoglobin electrophoresis is however part of routine antenatal screening in pregnancy in the UK. Sickle-cell crises may occur in any trimester, but dehydration in early pregnancy due to hyperemesis may be an exacerbating factor. Pregnant women with sickle-cell disease are at increased risk of miscarriage, preterm labour, pre-eclampsia and intrauterine growth restriction. Prepregnancy counselling and screening of the father are vital to give the couple an accurate estimate of the risk of having an affected child.

Thalassaemias

There are two types of thalassaemia arising from abnormal globin synthesis, leading to alpha- or beta-thalassaemia. Alpha-thalassaemia major is not compatible with life, but carriers may be asymptomatic and can become anaemic during pregnancy. Beta-thalassaemia major is inherited when both parents are carriers. These individuals need lifelong transfusions and have complications as a result of iron overload. Thalassaemia trait is usually asymptomatic but may cause significant anaemia during pregnancy. Prenatal diagnosis of both parents is necessary to identify a fetus at risk of inheriting thalassaemia major.

Gestational thrombocytopenia and immune thrombocytopenic purpura

Gestational thrombocytopenia is a benign condition that requires no intervention. The platelet count falls during a normal pregnancy and in about 10% of women falls $<100 \times 10^9/l$ by term.

Idiopathic thrombocytopenic purpura is diagnosed when thrombocytopenia occurs in the absence of other haematological abnormalities or clinical features such as splenomegaly or lymphadenopathy. Antibodies against platelet surface result in destruction of the platelets. Have the facility to identify antiplatelet antibodies, but usually the diagnosis of idiopathic thrombocytopenic purpura follows exclusion of other causes of thrombocytopenia. The platelet count may increase with corticosteroids, or, in resistant cases, intravenous gamma-globulin can be infused. The risk of thrombocytopenia or haemorrhage in the fetus from transplacental passage of IgG antiplatelet antibodies is low (<5%).

Malignant disease and pregnancy

The incidence of malignant neoplasms in women of reproductive age has increased over the past decade and is still rising. Haematological malignancies, such as lymphomas, have a peak incidence in young adulthood and therefore on occasion will invariably coincide with pregnancy. During pregnancy, difficult decisions need to be made between the maternal benefits of prompt treatment of the malignancy and the adverse effects of this treatment on the developing fetus.

Care of a pregnant patient with a malignancy should be individualised and a multidisciplinary team approach should be established (Pentheroudakis and Pavlidis 2006). If chemotherapy is the treatment of choice, the interests of the fetus are best served by delaying treatment until the second trimester and also too close to delivery (Cardonick and Iacobucci 2004). In general, radiation should be avoided during pregnancy. The placenta should be sent to pathology for all patients with malignancies diagnosed during pregnancy as occasionally cancers, especially melanoma, cross the placenta.

Long-term follow-up of offspring exposed to chemotherapy is essential, especially regarding secondary malignancies and fertility. Drug metabolism of chemotherapeutic agents in pregnancy may warrant higher doses of some medications and lower doses of others. Prospective data are needed to guide such management and, given the rarity of cancers in pregnancy, international collaboration is warranted.

Respiratory disease

During pregnancy, women breathe more deeply rather than more quickly and, at some point, this physiological adaption makes most women develop a subjective feeling of breathlessness. This normal symptom of pregnancy is sometimes difficult to differentiate from pathological breathlessness.

Asthma

The most commonly encountered respiratory disease in pregnancy is asthma, which affects 3% of the childbearing population (Littlejohns et al. 1989). There is no consistent effect of pregnancy on asthma, with some individuals showing improvement, others deterioration and some no change.

The management of asthma in pregnancy is the same as in non-pregnant women. Inhaled steroids are preferable to oral treatment, but oral prednisolone should not be withheld from a pregnant patient if required to treat severe asthma. The National Institute of Child Health and Human Development Maternal Fetal Medicine Units Network Asthma Study found a trend towards an increased incidence of low birthweight among infants born to women exposed to oral steroids (Schatz et al. 2004). There is no evidence of any teratogenic effects with the conventional drugs used to treat asthma, including β-agonists, oral or inhaled steroids, sodium cromoglycate and theophyllines (Bracken et al. 2003; Schatz et al. 2004). Leukotriene receptor antagonists (montelukast and zafirlukast) have been assigned a pregnancy category B, since animal studies have not demonstrated a risk to the fetus, but to date there are no adequately powered studies in pregnant women (Spector 2001). For some women with asthma the clinical benefit of leukotriene receptor antagonists will outweigh the remote possibility of fetal harm.

Regional anaesthesia is preferable to general anaesthesia because of the increased risks of postoperative chest infection following intubation. Women who suffer with asthma should be encouraged to breastfeed, as there is some evidence that it may help to prevent atopic problems in their offspring. None of the drugs used in the management of asthma are contraindicated in breastfeeding. The 4% background risk of a child developing asthma is increased approximately two- to threefold if one parent has asthma, particularly if he or she is atopic.

Cystic fibrosis

Cystic fibrosis is an autosomal recessive disorder arising from a defect on chromosome 7. The prevalence of the abnormal gene is about 4% in many white populations, with an incidence of homozygous cystic fibrosis of one in 2500 livebirths (Dodge et al. 1997). The median survival of women with this condition has changed from the early teens to the fourth decade over the last 50 years. Thus women with cystic fibrosis are increasingly surviving into the reproductive age. The ability of the mother to carry the pregnancy to term appears to be primarily related to her prepregnancy lung function, although severe underweight is also an important risk factor. Ideally the parents should seek preconception counselling for advice on genetic and prenatal diagnosis, compliance with medical therapy, optimisation of lung function, nutritional assessment, psychological assessment, medication review, venous access for antibiotic therapy, mode of delivery and breastfeeding.

If the mother is generally fit there is little evidence to suggest that the fetus will be affected by the mother's cystic fibrosis, though there is an increased risk of preterm delivery (Odegaard et al. 2002). Patients with a low forced expiratory volume in 1 second (less than 50%) should be managed in tertiary centres by a multidisciplinary team as this level of pulmonary dysfunction carries a significant risk of maternal mortality from respiratory failure (Lau et al. 2010).

Rheumatological disorders

Rheumatoid arthritis

Pregnancy was thought to confer a favourable outcome on women with rheumatoid arthritis, but a significant minority (approximately 20%) deteriorate during pregnancy. There is an increased risk of preterm birth, pre-eclampsia and caesarean section in mothers with rheumatoid arthritis (Skomsvoll et al. 1998; Reed et al. 2006). The risk of relapse is increased in the 3 months postpartum, but the majority of women do not report a relapse.

Management with prednisolone, sulfasalazine, non-steroidal anti-inflammatory drugs (NSAIDs) and hydroxychloroquine (Costedoat-Chalumeau et al. 2003) form the mainstay of treatment of active rheumatoid arthritis. Regular use of NSAIDs should be avoided in the third trimester to prevent premature closure of the fetal ductus arteriosus. 5-Aminosalicylic acid preparations include mesalazine, olsalazine, balsalazide and sulfasalazine. They are folic acid antagonists and should be given throughout pregnancy with folic acid 5 mg daily. Methotrexate should be avoided for 3 months prior to conception. Folic acid should be continued throughout pregnancy for women who have taken methotrexate prior to pregnancy. Leflonamide also has teratogenic potential and should be avoided in pregnancy and washed out of the mother with cholestyramine prior to conception.

Biological agents like intravenous immunoglobulin, etanercept, infliximab and anakinra carry acceptable US Food and Drug Administration ratings (B) for use in pregnancy. These immunoglobulins are not transmitted to the fetus until relatively late in pregnancy (Hyrich et al. 2006; Salmon and Alpert 2006). Less information is available about adalimumab, but it probably behaves similarly to infliximab. There is no reliable information about abatacept in humans. Rituximab is potentially less safe because reversible fetal cytopenias, including B-cell depletion, have

occurred in infants of mothers who are given this drug during pregnancy.

Systemic lupus erythromatosus

Systemic lupus erythematosus (SLE) affects women of childbearing age and fertility is generally conserved, except when renal function is seriously compromised (creatinine clearance <50 ml/min), the disease is active, or when amenorrhoea has been induced by cytotoxic therapy. The risk of flare during pregnancy relates to the level of maternal disease activity in the 6–12 months before conception (Mintz et al. 1986).

SLE flares during pregnancy and postpartum are generally mild or moderate, with a predominance of cutaneous, articular and minor haematological manifestations (thrombocytopenia) (Mintz et al. 1986). Lupus affecting the kidneys and the brain presents the most challenging problems for the mother and the well-being of the offspring. Management of these complications requires specialist help from rheumatologists who are expert in the management of SLE.

Pregnancies in women with lupus nephritis, but less so with other forms of SLE, are at increased rate of pregnancy loss, premature birth, intrauterine growth restriction and pre-eclampsia.

Pregnant women with SLE who have anti-Ro/SS-A and anti-La/SSB antibodies have a 1:50 risk of offspring affected by neonatal lupus (Brucato 2008). Neonatal lupus can present as fetal heart block, cutaneous lupus or hepatic involvement. Women who have had one infant affected by neonatal lupus have a 1:20 risk of another affected offspring. In all cases where the mother carries the antibodies, fetal medicine doctors must screen for heart block (all degrees of heart block, first, second and third degree) from 16 to 32 weeks' gestation. Maternal steroids and intravenous immunoglobulin have been tried with some success to prevent progression of fetal heart block (David et al. 2010).

Antiphospholipid syndrome

Antiphospholipid syndrome (APS) is characterised by the presence of antiphospholipid antibodies in the setting of either vascular thrombosis or pregnancy complication. The pregnancy complications include repeated pregnancy losses, fetal growth restriction and pre-eclampsia. Women with APS can also be affected by infertility, and maternal thrombosis. Treatment with heparin can reduce the risk of pregnancy loss to less than 30% (Empson et al. 2002). The pathophysiology of the disease includes thrombosis and inflammation via the complement cascade that contributes to poor pregnancy outcomes.

Current recommendations, based on existing data and expert opinion, suggest that women with no history of thrombosis or pregnancy complication should receive no treatment or treatment with low dose aspirin (LDA) alone during pregnancy; women with antiphospholipid antibodies and a history of pregnancy complication should receive prophylactic-dose LMWH with LDA; women with antiphospholipid antibodies and a history of vascular thrombosis should receive full-dose LMWH and LDA. The increased risk of thrombosis in the postpartum period requires treatment with anticoagulation for up to 6 weeks postpartum and is also recommended for patients with APS (Derksen et al. 2004).

Liver disease

There are two forms of liver disease specific to pregnancy that are thought to pose a particular risk to the mother and/or baby: obstetric cholestasis and acute fatty liver of pregnancy.

Intrahepatic cholestasis of pregnancy/obstetric cholestasis

Obstetric cholestasis is a disease of pregnancy with a prevalence of <1% but more commonly seen in south American, Chinese and Scandinavian women (Milkiewicz et al. 2002). It usually presents in the third trimester of pregnancy with itching mainly of palms of the hands and soles of feet. The abnormal biochemical finding that may alert the obstetrician to this condition is a rise in the liver transaminases in >80% of patients, raised bilirubin in <25% and raised serum bile acids in the majority of affected women (Milkiewicz et al. 2002). The synthetic function of the liver remains normal.

The aetiology of the condition is not understood, but it appears to have both genetic and environmental components. It seems at least in part to be induced by high levels of oestrogen and progesterone, as symptoms may recur if an affected woman subsequently uses combined oral contraception. In one study, a third of pregnancies affected by obstetric cholestasis were complicated by 'fetal distress' (the nature of which is often not simply hypoxia – see later) and almost 2% were associated with intrauterine death (Lammert et al. 2000; Glantz et al. 2004). Jaundice is uncommon, even though liver function tests are commonly abnormal. Women affected by obstetric cholestasis should be offered ursodeoxycholic acid (URSO) to relieve their pruritus and this often corrects biochemical abnormalities. URSO makes bile acids more hydrophilic and aids their excretion. It is not licensed for use in pregnancy, but there are no reports of harm associated with its use.

It is not known why there appears to be an increased risk of stillbirth with obstetric cholestasis, but it has been suggested that if the placenta has similar difficulty with bile acid transport as the maternal liver (perhaps by inheriting the same defect), then bile acid levels in the fetus will rise to dangerously high levels. Certainly, bile acids have been shown to cause asystole in beating cardiomyocytes in tissue culture. If this in vitro model is correct, it is possible that URSO may also protect the fetus, but this has not been established. There are concerns about sudden fetal death associated with obstetric cholestasis and some centres advocate delivery around 37 weeks. Prospective trials are needed to assess whether complications associated with early delivery are justified by the decreased risk of stillbirth. Maternal liver function and pruritus usually resolve within a few days of delivery.

Acute fatty liver of pregnancy

Acute fatty liver of pregnancy (AFLP) is a rare complication of pregnancy with an estimated prevalence of around 1 per 5000 pregnancies. AFLP occurs in the second half of pregnancy, usually close to term. Presentation is typically with nausea. There are often hypertension and proteinuria and the condition is associated with pre-eclampsia, multiple pregnancy and maternal obesity. It is also more common when the fetus is male (ratio 3:1). Transaminases are elevated, as is alkaline phosphatase (above the normal upper limit for pregnancy), but the biochemical findings that generally distinguish AFLP from pre-eclampsia are a much higher elevation of uric acid and elements of liver dysfunction, e.g. hypoglycaemia, prolonged INR and hypoalbuminaemia. Jaundice is a late feature of the disease. MRI or CT scanning is unhelpful with the diagnosis. Liver biopsy is diagnostic (showing microvesicles of fat in the hepatocytes), but is risky if clotting is abnormal and under these circumstances is therefore not recommended. Precise diagnosis is less important than prompt delivery, which is usually mandated by deteriorating maternal and fetal condition.

General supportive measures include control of hypertension and correction of hypoglycaemia and deficiencies in clotting factors. The fetus should be delivered without delay. Maternal and neonatal mortality associated with AFLP is improving, due to earlier diagnosis and prompt delivery. If the mother survives, full recovery is the rule (Pereira et al. 1997). On occasion, mothers with AFLP develop the condition because the fetus they are carrying is affected with a long-chain fatty acid disorder, 3 hydroxyacyl-coenzyme-A dehydrogenase deficiency (Treem et al. 1994).

Viral hepatitis

Infection with hepatitis viruses A, B, C and D produces a clinical picture in the pregnant woman very similar to that outside pregnancy. Management of vertical transmission of hepatitis A, B and C to the neonate is described elsewhere. Hepatitis E, which is epidemic in some areas of South-east Asia, differs in that this usually mild disease carries a significant risk of maternal morbidity and mortality during pregnancy. The reasons for this change in pathogenicity are unclear.

Gasteroentrology

Inflammatory bowel diseases

Inflammatory bowel diseases (IBDs), which include ulcerative colitis and Crohn disease, are more common in younger people and women. Active IBD at the time of conception or during pregnancy significantly increases the risk of preterm delivery and low-birthweight offspring (Dominitz et al. 2002). Risk factors for a poor pregnancy outcome include a history of IBD surgery and increasing maternal age (Mahadevan et al. 2007).

There is a risk of disease flare postpartum, but not regularly enough to recommend pre-emptive immunosuppression. Breast-feeding does not influence disease activity in the postpartum period (Klement et al. 2004).

Pharmacological treatment

Pharmacological treatments that are used for treatment of IBD and include corticosteroids, 5-aminosalicylic acid preparations such as sulfasalazine, azathioprine, ciclosporin A, tacrolimus, inteferons and antitumour necrosis factor (Moffatt and Bernstein 2007).

Biliary tract disease

Weight gain and hormonal changes predispose pregnant women to biliary sludge and gallstone formation. Oestrogen increases bile lithogenicity whereas progesterone impairs gallbladder emptying. The reported incidence of biliary sludge and gallstones during pregnancy ranges from as high as 31% to 12%. Most women are asymptomatic and no therapy is indicated. However, when cholelithiasis becomes symptomatic surgical intervention may be required. Symptoms of active gallstone disease are similar to those of non-pregnant women with differential diagnoses that include hyperemesis, idiopathic pancreatitis and peptic disease.

Ultrasonography is a sensitive test for cholelithiasis but is less sensitive for the detection of common bile duct stones and dilated biliary ducts. Magnetic resonance cholangiopancreatography can be safely used during pregnancy. In the pregnant patient, therapeutic endoscopic retrograde cholangiopancreatography has become the standard of care when treating choledocholithiasis.

Common gastrointestinal symptoms in pregnancy

Gastro-oesopheageal reflux is common in pregnancy, especially in the third trimester. Peptic ulcer disease appears to be less common in pregnancy. Histamine receptor antagonists and proton pump inhibitors are safely used in pregnancy. *Helicobacter pylori* eradication therapy may be appropriate if simple measures have failed.

Nausea and vomiting affect approximately 50% of pregnant women in the first trimester. More severe and protracted vomiting occurs in a minority of women and can lead to hyperemesis with ketosis, dehydration and weight loss. Hyperemesis gravidarum occurs in <1% of pregnancies. The main risks are dehydration and thrombosis, and very rarely Wernicke's encephalopathy due to vitamin B_1 (thiamine) deficiency. The mainstay of treatment is to correct hypovolaemia, electrolyte imbalances and vitamin deficiencies. Antiemetics such as dopamine antagonists (metoclopramide, domperidone), phenothiazines (chlorpromazine, prochlorperazine), anticholinergics (dicyclomine) or antihistamine H_1-receptor antagonists (promethazine, cyclizine) can be safely used. In women with severe hyperemesis who have not responded to one of the antiemetic therapies mentioned above, there have been promising results reported with both corticosteroids and 5-hydroxytryptamine-3 receptor antagonists. Furthermore, corticosteroids appear to be effective in some women with hyperemesis gravidarum. Thromboprophylaxis with LMWH is necessary for those admitted to hospital.

Psychiatric diseases

Depression can occur both antenatally and postpartum. Postnatal depression includes a spectrum from postpartum 'blues', which affects 50% of women and is a mild, self-limiting condition. It is characterised by symptoms such as weeping, sadness, irritability and anxiety. The symptoms usually peak around the fourth day and resolve by the 10th day. In contrast, significant mental illness leading to suicide now accounts for at least 10% of all maternal deaths in the UK (Confidential Enquiry into Maternal Death in the UK 2002). This disturbing statistic is made more shocking by the violent nature of the suicides.

Postpartum depression

One in eight new mothers develop postpartum depression. Women who have had one episode of postpartum depression have a 1:4 risk of recurrence. Many of these women will suffer a severe depressive illness and 2% will see a psychiatrist during the first postpartum year. Very rarely (2:1000), puerperal psychosis will develop (Vesga-Lopez et al. 2008).

Postpartum depression usually has an insidious onset within the first 3–6 months after childbirth. The mother's depressive thoughts typically centre on feelings of inadequacy in the maternal role and concerns for neonatal well-being. The signs and symptoms include increasing sleeplessness, loss of appetite and lack of energy. Maternal thyroid function should be checked, as postpartum thyroid disease is associated with depression.

During pregnancy, untreated maternal depression has been associated with adverse effects on the fetus, including preterm labour, low birthweight, decreased Apgar scores, elevated levels of fetal stress hormones and changes in neurobehavioural function (e.g. hypotonia and motor difficulties) (Marcus 2009). One study found that the relapse rate of major depression was 68% in women who discontinued antidepressant medication, compared with 26% in women who continued medications. Depression may also affect the mother's ability to care for herself and obtain appropriate prenatal care.

An epidemiological study of more than 15 000 infants during a period of nearly 30 years found that certain birth defects occurred more frequently in mothers taking specific selective serotonin reuptake inhibitors (SSRIs; e.g. sertraline and occurrence of omphalocele and/or septal defects; paroxetine and right ventricular outflow tract obstruction defects). However, the overall absolute risk of congenital abnormality with SSRIs seems small (Cantor et al. 2009). A 1.5- to twofold increased risk of cardiac defects (particularly ventricular septal defects) was reported in infants exposed to paroxetine in the first trimester (Cantor et al. 2009). Although subsequent studies did not confirm this association, the American College of Obstetrics and Gynecology (ACOG) still recommends a fetal echocardiogram for fetuses exposed to paroxetine (ACOG Committee 2006). SSRIs taken during pregnancy increased rates of persistent pulmonary hypertension of the newborn (PPHN) to 2.4 times that of infants of mothers who were not taking an SSRI (Kallen and Olausson 2008). However, PPHN, although a serious and potentially life-threatening condition, did not occur in the majority (nearly 99%) of infants with late in utero exposure to SSRIs (Cantor et al. 2009). This is another situation where treatment of the maternal condition needs to be balanced against potential harm to the fetus.

Third-trimester exposure to SSRIs has also been associated with 'transient neonatal complications' such as increased muscle tone, irritability, jitteriness, disrupted sleep and abnormal breathing (ACOG Committee 2006). Another study found that late-term SSRI exposure was associated with increased rates of prematurity, decreased birthweight and size and other anomalies (Cantor et al. 2009).

Sertraline and paroxetine have been reported to have undetectable levels in the breastfed infant whose mother is taking these drugs (Moretti 2009). Thus, these medications may be a good choice for lactating women.

Treatment of bipolar disorders with lithium, valproate, carbamazepine, lamotrigine and oxcarbazepine has been associated with increased teratogenicity (in particular with cardiac and neural tube malformations) (Dodd and Berk 2006). Lithium is associated with a rare increased risk of Ebstein's anomaly, which affects 1:1000 infants exposed to lithium in utero. Maternal need for treatment with lithium needs to be balanced against this rare consequence. Renal excretion of lithium increases significantly during the third trimester, which usually necessitates an increase in maternal dose and a consequent reduction postpartum. Lithium is secreted into breast milk and has been associated with adverse neonatal events such as lethargy, hypotonia, cyanosis and electrocardiogram changes (Menon 2008). Breastfeeding is therefore best avoided in the mother who takes lithium (Menon 2008).

Drugs of misuse

The prevalence of illegal drug use in pregnancy is unknown, but one-third of drug users in the UK are female and 90% are of childbearing age.

Effects of drug use on the mother

Drug dependency has health implications for the mother as regards nutritional, medical and sociopsychological aspects. In cases of intravenous drug use, there are greater risks of infectious diseases such as human immunodeficiency virus, hepatitis, abscesses and endocarditis that may account for the prematurity, low birthweight and poor nutritional status observed in the offspring of these women (Fischer 2000).

Opioids

Dependence on heroin is associated with low birthweight, prematurity and fetal demise (Hulse et al. 1997). Clinical signs of neonatal abstinence include: gastrointestinal disturbances, irritability, hyperactivity, feeding and sleeping disturbances, autonomic hyperactivity and, rarely, seizures (Osborn et al. 2004). The onset, duration and severity of neonatal symptoms vary, but usually start within 24–72 hours of delivery.

Cocaine and amphetamines

Cocaine can be injected, snorted or inhaled. It is a potent vasoconstrictor and can reduce maternofetal blood flow and cause maternal hypertension. Fetal complications associated with cocaine use during pregnancy include placental abruption, intrauterine growth restriction, congenital anomalies affecting the ocular and urogenital systems and spontaneous abortion. The mother may develop pre-eclampsia, pulmonary oedema, seizures and cardiac arrhythmias (Bandstra and Burkett 1991).

How are pharmacological agents handled in pregnancy and breastfeeding?

Pharmacokinetic and pharmacodynamic changes during pregnancy have an impact on maternal drug levels and efficacy. These changes include delayed gastric emptying, increased plasma volume, decreased albumin levels (decreased drug–protein binding), enhanced hepatic metabolism and increased renal clearance. The speed of drug elimination, the lipid solubility of the drug and whether it is protein-bound will have an effect on how much passes across the placenta.

The placenta

The placenta may be a mechanical barrier which blocks the passage of large molecules between mother and fetus, but most drugs eventually pass across this lipid membrane by passive diffusion. Drugs which pass across the placenta most quickly are of high lipid solubility, low molecular weight and have reduced protein binding and slow elimination from the maternal circulation.

There are several other ways in which drugs pass across the placenta. These include passive diffusion, active transfer, facilitated diffusion, phagocytosis and pinocytosis. The placenta is also filled with enzymes that degrade drugs and hormones. For example, thyroxine is metabolised by type 3 iodothyronine deiodinase (D_3) and reduces uteroplacental passage of maternal thyroxine.

Timing and dosing of drug exposure during pregnancy

Possible toxic effects of drugs on the fetus are organised into five categories that relate to the timing of drug exposure during pregnancy: (1) miscarriage; (2) physical malformation; (3) growth impairment; (4) behavioural teratology; and (5) neonatal toxicity. Exposure to a teratogen in the 14 days postconception is likely to result in miscarriage. Drug exposure during days 14–35 of pregnancy will have the greatest effect on structural and neurochemical development. However, maternal drugs taken throughout pregnancy can have an impact on fetal neurodevelopment that only becomes evident when behavioural problems develop in childhood. Maternal medicines taken near delivery can have a directly toxic effect on the neonate, for example benzodiazepines at term occasionally cause transient sedation of the neonate and then withdrawal symptoms.

The fetus is predisposed to damage from pharmacological agents owing to low levels of drug-binding plasma proteins, immature hepatic metabolism and a permeable blood–brain barrier. Furthermore, transportation of drug metabolites back to the maternal circulation often leads to higher drug concentrations in fetal than in maternal blood (Table 11.1).

Table 11.1 US Food and Drug Administration categories for drug use in pregnancy

CATEGORY	INTERPRETATION
A	Adequate, well-controlled studies in pregnant women have not shown an increased risk of fetal abnormalities to the fetus in any trimester of pregnancy
B	Animal studies have revealed no evidence of harm to the fetus; however, there are no adequate and well-controlled studies in pregnant women or: Animal studies have shown an adverse effect, but adequate and well-controlled studies in pregnant women have failed to demonstrate a risk to the fetus in any trimester
C	Animal studies have shown an adverse effect and there are no adequate and well-controlled studies in pregnant women or No animal studies have been conducted and there are no adequate and well-controlled studies in pregnant women
D	Adequate well-controlled or observational studies in pregnant women have demonstrated a risk to the fetus; however, the benefits of therapy may outweigh the potential risk. For example, the drug may be acceptable if needed in a life-threatening situation or serious disease for which safer drugs cannot be used or are ineffective
X	Adequate well-controlled or observational studies in animals or pregnant women have demonstrated positive evidence of fetal abnormalities or risks The use of the product is contraindicated in women who are or may become pregnant

Pharmacotherapy during lactation

Apart from improved mother–child bonding, breastfed babies benefit from lower prevalence rates of infection and mortality rates and also improved later cognitive development and intellectual function (Fergusson et al. 1982; Lucas et al. 1992). Maternal benefits include facilitation of involution of the uterus and suppression of ovulation. It is therefore important that women who take medication are informed as to whether they can safely breastfeed whilst on their medication.

The passage of a drug into breast milk is influenced by many factors, including its volume of distribution, molecular weight, lipid/water solubility, relative affinity for plasma and milk proteins, the pH of blood and milk (the degree of ionisation of a drug) and blood flow to the breast. Once a drug is absorbed into the bloodstream, a proportion binds to plasma proteins. The remaining unbound (free, active) drug is able to cross membranes and enter breast milk. Lower molecular weight and higher lipid solubility facilitate passage of drugs into breast milk. The absolute dosage of drug received by a breastfed infant is also affected by milk yield, milk composition, and the degree of breast emptying during a previous feed. Breast milk has a lower pH than plasma, so the pH of the drug is important in the way it may be handled by diffusion into the alveolar ducts of the breast. Hind milk (the milk that is expressed towards the end of a feed) carries a high concentration of lipids and therefore a greater concentration of lipid-soluble drugs. In contrast, colostrum exhibits a high protein level and therefore a high concentration of protein-bound drugs.

It is prudent to monitor breastfed babies for signs of drug-related toxicity and adverse effects. The physiology of the neonate (more so the preterm baby) is immature and characterised by a limited ability to metabolise and excrete drugs. Hepatic function (oxidation and glucuronidation) is immature. Renal function too is immature, characterised by lower glomerular filtration and tubular secretion rates, with resultant higher plasma drug concentrations. Gastric pH is higher and bowel motility slower, with consequent unpredictable drug absorption. Bioavailability of medications is also different: a lower degree of plasma protein binding relative to the adult implies higher free (active) drug levels. The capacity to metabolise drugs however increases rapidly, and by the third month of life often exceeds that of the adult. The factors affecting infant exposure to drugs are therefore highly variable. Maternal drug dosages consistent with the absence of ill effects on the breastfed baby remain to be established, although an infant plasma concentration of 10% (or less) of that established as therapeutic in the mother is considered acceptable and safe (Bennett 1996).

References

ACOG Committee Opinion No. 354, 2006. Treatment with selective serotonin reuptake inhibitors during pregnancy. Obstet Gynecol 108 (6), 1601–1603.

ACOG Practice Bulletin No. 84, 2007. Prevention of deep vein thrombosis and pulmonary embolism. Obstet Gynecol 110 (2 Pt 1), 429–440.

American Academy of Pediatrics Committee on Drugs, 2001. Transfer of drugs and other chemicals into human milk. Pediatrics 108 (3), 776–789.

Bandstra, E.S., Burkett, G., 1991. Maternal-fetal and neonatal effects of in utero cocaine exposure. Semin Perinatol 15 (4), 288–301.

Bates, S.M., et al., 2004. Use of antithrombotic agents during pregnancy: the Seventh ACCP Conference on Antithrombotic and Thrombolytic Therapy. Chest 126 (3 Suppl), 627S–644S.

Bennett, P.N., 1996. Drugs and Human Lactation. Elsevier, Amsterdam, pp. 67–74.

Bracken, M.B., et al., 2003. Asthma symptoms, severity, and drug therapy: a prospective study of effects on 2205 pregnancies. Obstet Gynecol 102 (4), 739–752.

Brown, H.L., Hiett, A.K., 2010. Deep vein thrombosis and pulmonary embolism in pregnancy: diagnosis, complications, and management. Clin Obstet Gynecol 53 (2), 345–359.

Brucato, A., 2008. Prevention of congenital heart block in children of SSA-positive mothers. Rheumatology (Oxford) 47 (Suppl 3), iii35–iii37.

Burn, J., et al., 1998. Recurrence risks in offspring of adults with major heart defects: results from first cohort of British collaborative study. Lancet 351 (9099), 311–316.

Canhao, P., et al., 2005. Causes and predictors of death in cerebral venous thrombosis. Stroke 36 (8), 1720–1725.

Cantor, S.J., Weller, R.A., Weller, E.B., 2009. Selective serotonin reuptake inhibitor use during pregnancy and possible neonatal complications Curr Psychiatry Rep 11 (3), 253–257.

Cantu, C., Barinagarrementeria, F., 1993. Cerebral venous thrombosis associated with pregnancy and puerperium. Review of 67 cases. Stroke 24 (12), 1880–1884.

Cardonick, E., Iacobucci, A., 2004. Use of chemotherapy during human pregnancy. Lancet Oncol 5 (5), 283–291.

Confavreux, C., et al., 1998. Rate of pregnancy-related relapse in multiple sclerosis. Pregnancy in Multiple Sclerosis Group. N Engl J Med 339 (5), 285–291.

Confidential Enquiry into Maternal Death in the UK. 2002.

Connolly, A., Thorp Jr, J.M., 1999. Urinary tract infections in pregnancy. Urol Clin North Am 26 (4), 779–787.

Cooper, W.O., et al., 2006. Major congenital malformations after first-trimester exposure to ACE inhibitors. N Engl J Med 354 (23), 2443–2451.

Costedoat-Chalumeau, N., et al., 2003. Safety of hydroxychloroquine in pregnant patients with connective tissue diseases: a study of one hundred thirty-three cases compared with a control group. Arthritis Rheum 48 (11), 3207–3211.

Coyle, P.K., 2009. Disease-modifying agents in multiple sclerosis. Ann Indian Acad Neurol 12 (4), 273–282.

Dargaud, Y., et al., 2009. A risk score for the management of pregnant women with increased risk of venous thromboembolism: a multicentre prospective study. Br J Haematol 145 (6), 825–835.

Davey, D.A., MacGillivray, I., 1988. The classification and definition of the hypertensive disorders of pregnancy. Am J Obstet Gynecol 158 (4): 892–898.

David, A.L., et al., 2010. Congenital fetal heart block: a potential therapeutic role for intravenous immunoglobulin. Obstet Gynecol 116 (Suppl 2), 543–547.

Davison, J.M., 2001. Renal disorders in pregnancy. Curr Opin Obstet Gynecol 13 (2), 109–114.

de Haan, G.J., et al., 2004. Gestation-induced changes in lamotrigine pharmacokinetics: a monotherapy study. Neurology 63 (3), 571–573.

Demakis, J.G., et al., 1971. Natural course of peripartum cardiomyopathy. Circulation 44 (6), 1053–1061.

Derksen, R.H., Khamashta, M.A., Branch, D.W., 2004. Management of the obstetric antiphospholipid syndrome. Arthritis Rheum 50 (4), 1028–1039.

Dhulkotia, J.S., et al., 2010. Oral hypoglycemic agents vs insulin in management of gestational diabetes: a systematic review and metaanalysis. Am J Obstet Gynecol 203 (5), 457–459.

Dias, M.S., 1994. Neurovascular emergencies in pregnancy. Clin Obstet Gynecol 37 (2), 337–354.

Dodd, S., Berk, M., 2006. The safety of medications for the treatment of bipolar disorder during pregnancy and the puerperium. Curr Drug Saf 1 (1): 25–33.

Dodge, J.A., et al., 1997. Incidence, population, and survival of cystic fibrosis in the UK, 1968-95. UK Cystic Fibrosis Survey Management Committee. Arch Dis Child 77 (6), 493–496.

Dominitz, J.A., Young, J.C., Boyko, E.J., 2002. Outcomes of infants born to mothers with inflammatory bowel disease: a population-based cohort study. Am J Gastroenterol 97 (3), 641–648.

Duley, L., et al., 2001. Antiplatelet drugs for prevention of pre-eclampsia and its consequences: systematic review. Br Med J 322 (7282), 329–333.

Duley, L., Gulmezoglu, A.M., Henderson-Smart, D.J., 2003. Magnesium sulphate and other anticonvulsants for women with pre-eclampsia. Cochrane Database Syst Rev (2), CD000025.

Empson, M., et al., 2002. Recurrent pregnancy loss with antiphospholipid antibody: a systematic review of therapeutic trials. Obstet Gynecol 99 (1): 135–144.

EURAP Study Group, 2006. Seizure control and treatment in pregnancy. Observations from the EURAP epilepsy pregnancy registry. Neurology 66 (3), 354–360.

European Best Practice Guidelines for Renal Transplantation, 2002. Section IV: Long-term management of the transplant recipient. IV.10. Pregnancy in renal transplant recipients. Nephrol Dial Transplant 17 (Suppl 4), 50–55.

Fergusson, D.M., Beautrais, A.L., Silva, P.A., 1982. Breastfeeding and cognitive development in the first seven years of life. Soc Sci Med 16 (19), 1705–1708.

Fischer, G., 2000. Treatment of opioid dependence in pregnant women. Addiction 95 (8), 1141–1144.

George, L.M., Gatt, S.P., Lowe, S., 1997. Peripartum cardiomyopathy: four case histories and a commentary on anaesthetic management. Anaesth Intensive Care 25 (3), 292–296.

Glantz, A., Marschall, H.U., Mattsson, L.A., 2004. Intrahepatic cholestasis of pregnancy: Relationships between bile acid levels and fetal complication rates. Hepatology 40 (2), 467–474.

Groves, A.M., et al., 2006. CT pulmonary angiography versus ventilation-perfusion scintigraphy in pregnancy: implications from a UK survey of doctors' knowledge of radiation exposure Radiology 240 (3), 765–770.

Haddow, J.E., et al., 1999. Maternal thyroid deficiency during pregnancy and subsequent neuropsychological development of the child. N Engl J Med 341 (8), 549–555.

Hankins, G.D., et al., 1985. Myocardial infarction during pregnancy: a review. Obstet Gynecol 65 (1), 139–146.

Hofmeyr, G.J., et al., 2010. Calcium supplementation during pregnancy for preventing hypertensive disorders and related problems. Cochrane Database Syst Rev (8), CD001059.

Hulse, G.K., et al., 1997. The relationship between maternal use of heroin and methadone and infant birth weight. Addiction 92 (11), 1571–1579.

Hyrich, K.L., et al., 2006. Pregnancy outcome in women who were exposed to anti-tumor necrosis factor agents: results from a national population register. Arthritis Rheum 54 (8), 2701–2702.

Jaigobin, C., Silver, F.L., 2000. Stroke and pregnancy. Stroke 31 (12), 2948–2951.

James, A.H., et al., 2007. Thromboembolism in pregnancy: recurrence and its prevention. Semin Perinatol 31 (3), 167–175.

Janssen, N.M., Genta, M.S., 2000. The effects of immunosuppressive and anti-inflammatory medications on fertility, pregnancy, and lactation. Arch Intern Med 160 (5), 610–619.

Kallen, B., Olausson, P.O., 2008. Maternal use of selective serotonin re-uptake inhibitors and persistent pulmonary hypertension of the newborn. Pharmacoepidemiol Drug Saf 17 (8), 801–806.

Katz, O., et al., 2006. Pregnancy and perinatal outcome in epileptic women: a population-based study. J Matern Fetal Neonatal Med 19 (1): 21–25.

Kearon, C., et al., 1998. Noninvasive diagnosis of deep venous thrombosis. McMaster Diagnostic Imaging Practice Guidelines Initiative. Ann Intern Med 128 (8), 663–677.

Kittner, S.J., et al., 1996. Pregnancy and the risk of stroke. N Engl J Med 335 (11), 768–774.

Klement, E., et al., 2004. Breastfeeding and risk of inflammatory bowel disease: a systematic review with meta-analysis. Am J Clin Nutr 80 (5), 1342–1352.

Korn-Lubetzki, I., et al., 1984. Activity of multiple sclerosis during pregnancy and puerperium. Ann Neurol 16 (2), 229–231.

Lammert, F., et al., 2000. Intrahepatic cholestasis of pregnancy: molecular pathogenesis, diagnosis and management. J Hepatol 33 (6), 1012–1021.

Lanska, D.J., Kryscio, R.J., 2000. Risk factors for peripartum and postpartum stroke and intracranial venous thrombosis. Stroke 31 (6), 1274–1282.

Lau, E.M., et al., 2010. Pregnancy and cystic fibrosis. Paediatr Respir Rev 11 (2), 90–94.

Leonhardt, G., et al., 2006. Thrombolytic therapy in pregnancy. J Thromb Thrombolysis 21 (3), 271–276.

Littlejohns, P., Ebrahim, S., Anderson, R., 1989. Prevalence and diagnosis of chronic respiratory symptoms in adults. Br Med J 298 (6687), 1556–1560.

Lucas, A., et al., 1992. Breast milk and subsequent intelligence quotient in children born preterm. Lancet 339 (8788), 261–264.

Lupton, M., et al., 2002. Cardiac disease in pregnancy. Curr Opin Obstet Gynecol 14 (2), 137–143.

Mahadevan, U., et al., 2007. Pregnancy outcomes in women with inflammatory bowel disease: a large community-based study from Northern California. Gastroenterology 133 (4), 1106–1112.

Marcus, S.M., 2009. Depression during pregnancy: rates, risks and consequences–Motherisk Update 2008. Can J Clin Pharmacol 16 (1), e15–e22.

McColl, M.D., et al., 2000. Prevalence of the post-thrombotic syndrome in young women with previous venous thromboembolism. Br J Haematol 108 (2), 272–274.

McDermott, S., et al., 2000. Urinary tract infections during pregnancy and mental retardation and developmental delay. Obstet Gynecol 96 (1), 113–119.

McKechnie, R.S., et al., 2001. Spontaneous coronary artery dissection in a pregnant woman. Obstet Gynecol 98 (5 Pt 2), 899–902.

Menon, S.J., 2008. Psychotropic medication during pregnancy and lactation. Arch Gynecol Obstet 277 (1), 1–13.

Milkiewicz, P., et al., 2002. Obstetric cholestasis. Br Med J 324 (7330), 123–124.

Mintz, G., et al., 1986. Prospective study of pregnancy in systemic lupus erythematosus. Results of a multidisciplinary approach. J Rheumatol 13 (4), 732–739.

Moffatt, D.C., Bernstein, C.N., 2007. Drug therapy for inflammatory bowel disease in pregnancy and the puerperium. Best Pract Res Clin Gastroenterol 21 (5), 835–847.

Moretti, M.E., 2009. Psychotropic drugs in lactation–Motherisk Update 2008. Can J Clin Pharmacol 16 (1), e49–e57.

Nelson, S.M., Greer, I.A., 2006. Thrombophilia and the risk for venous thromboembolism during pregnancy, delivery, and puerperium. Obstet Gynecol Clin North Am 33 (3), 413–427.

Odegaard, I., et al., 2002. Maternal and fetal morbidity in pregnancies of Norwegian and Swedish women with cystic fibrosis. Acta Obstet Gynecol Scand 81 (8), 698–705.

Okosieme, O.E., Marx, H., Lazarus, J.H., 2008. Medical management of thyroid dysfunction in pregnancy and the postpartum. Expert Opin Pharmacother 9 (13), 2281–2293.

Osborn, D.A., Cole, M.J., Jeffrey, H.E., 2004. Opiate treatment for opiate withdrawal in newborn infants. [3]. Cochrane Library, Oxford.

Ovalle, A., Levancini, M., 2001. Urinary tract infections in pregnancy. Curr Opin Urol 11 (1), 55–59.

Pearson, G.D., et al., 2000. Peripartum cardiomyopathy: National Heart, Lung, and Blood Institute and Office of Rare Diseases (National Institutes of Health) workshop recommendations and review. JAMA 283 (9), 1183–1188.

Pennell, P.B., et al., 2004. The impact of pregnancy and childbirth on the metabolism of lamotrigine. Neurology 62 (2), 292–295.

Pentheroudakis, G., Pavlidis, N., 2006. Cancer and pregnancy: poena magna, not anymore. Eur J Cancer 42 (2), 126–140.

Pereira, S.P., et al., 1997. Maternal and perinatal outcome in severe pregnancy-related liver disease. Hepatology 26 (5), 1258–1262.

Pop, V.J., et al., 2003. Maternal hypothyroxinaemia during early pregnancy and subsequent child development: a 3-year follow-up study. Clin Endocrinol (Oxf) 59 (3), 282–288.

Rahimtoola, S.H., Tak, T., 1996. The use of digitalis in heart failure. Curr Probl Cardiol 21 (12), 781–853.

Reed, S.D., Vollan, T.A., Svec, M.A., 2006. Pregnancy outcomes in women with rheumatoid arthritis in Washington State. Matern Child Health J 10 (4), 361–366.

Rosa, F.W., 1991. Spina bifida in infants of women treated with carbamazepine during pregnancy. N Engl J Med 324 (10), 674–677.

Roullet, E., et al., 1993. Pregnancy and multiple sclerosis: a longitudinal study of 125 remittent patients. J Neurol Neurosurg Psychiatry 56 (10), 1062–1065.

Rowan, J.A., et al., 2008. Metformin versus insulin for the treatment of gestational diabetes. N Engl J Med 358 (19), 2003–2015.

Rubin, P.C., et al., 1983. Placebo-controlled trial of atenolol in treatment of pregnancy-associated hypertension. Lancet 1 (8322), 431–434.

Sadovnick, A.D., 1984. Empiric recurrence risks for use in the genetic counselling of multiple sclerosis patients. Am J Med Genet 17 (3), 713–714.

Salmon, J.E., Alpert, D., 2006. Are we coming to terms with tumor necrosis factor inhibition in pregnancy? Arthritis Rheum 54 (8), 2353–2355.

Schatz, M., et al., 2004. The relationship of asthma medication use to perinatal outcomes. J Allergy Clin Immunol 113 (6), 1040–1045.

Sharma, P., Thapa, L., 2007. Acute pyelonephritis in pregnancy: a retrospective study. Aust N Z J Obstet Gynaecol 47 (4), 313–315.

Shivvers, S.A., et al., 1999. Maternal cardiac troponin I levels during normal labor and delivery. Am J Obstet Gynecol 180 (1 Pt 1), 122.

Skomsvoll, J.F., et al., 1998. Obstetrical and neonatal outcome in pregnant patients with rheumatic disease. Scand J Rheumatol Suppl 107, 109–112.

Spector, S.L., 2001. Safety of antileukotriene agents in asthma management. Ann Allergy Asthma Immunol 86 (6 Suppl 1), 18–23.

Stiete, H., et al., 1995. [Risk groups of newborn infants of diabetic mothers in relation to their somatic outcome and maternal diabetic metabolic status in pregnancy.] Z Geburtshilfe Neonatol 199 (4), 156–162.

The Magpie Trial Follow-Up Study Collaborative Group, 2007.

The Magpie Trial: a randomised trial comparing magnesium sulphate with placebo for pre-eclampsia. Outcome for women at 2 years. Br J Obstet Gynaecol 114 (3), 300–309.

Tieu, J., et al., 2010. Screening and subsequent management for gestational diabetes for improving maternal and infant health. Cochrane Database Syst Rev (7), CD007222.

Tomson, T., 2005. Gender aspects of pharmacokinetics of new and old AEDs: pregnancy and breastfeeding. Ther Drug Monit 27 (6), 718–721.

Trappe, H.J., 2003. [Cardiac arrhythmias during pregnancy–what to do?] Herz 28 (3), 216–226.

Treadwell, S.D., Thanvi, B., Robinson, T.G., 2008. Stroke in pregnancy and the puerperium. Postgrad Med J 84 (991), 238–245.

Treem, W.R., et al., 1994. Acute fatty liver of pregnancy and long-chain 3-hydroxyacyl-coenzyme A dehydrogenase deficiency. Hepatology 19 (2), 339–345.

Vajda, F.J., et al., 2006. Foetal malformations and seizure control: 52 months data of the Australian Pregnancy Registry. Eur J Neurol 13 (6), 645–654.

Veille, J.C., 1984. Peripartum cardiomyopathies: a review. Am J Obstet Gynecol 148 (6), 805–818.

Vesga-Lopez, O., et al., 2008. Psychiatric disorders in pregnant and postpartum women in the United States. Arch Gen Psychiatry 65 (7), 805–815.

Visintin, C., et al., 2010. Management of hypertensive disorders during pregnancy: summary of NICE guidance. Br Med J 341, c2207.

Williams, D.J., de Swiet, M., 1997. The pathophysiology of pre-eclampsia. Intensive Care Med 23 (6), 620–629.

Williams, P.G., Hersh, J.H., 1997. A male with fetal valproate syndrome and autism. Dev Med Child Neurol 39 (9), 632–634.

Obstetrics for the neonatologist

12

Sukrutha Veerareddy   Maggie Blott

Introduction

There is increasing evidence that safe high-quality maternity services are best provided by multidisciplinary teams led by fully trained obstetricians and midwives working with neonatologists, anaesthetists and many other specialist care providers. *Safer Childbirth* (Royal College of Obstetricians and Gynaecologists (RCOG) 2007) and *Standards for Maternity Care* (RCOG 2010) have set the standards by which this care may be best achieved. The aim of modern obstetric management is the early identification of complicated pregnancies and those with abnormal placental function (National Institute for Health and Clinical Excellence (NICE) 2010), so that medical care may be focused on those women. Women with low-risk pregnancies should have their care provided by midwives (NICE 2010).

The aim of this chapter is to outline the intrapartum assessment of the fetus who is thought to be normal. Antenatal assessment of fetal well-being is also very important and is covered in detail in other chapters of this book.

Common complications that occur in labour and the management strategies will be covered in this chapter. Clearly, this account cannot be exhaustive: the intention is to concentrate on aspects of obstetric care of relevance to the neonatologist. Further reading and useful weblinks are included at the end of the chapter.

© 2012 Elsevier Ltd

Intrapartum assessment and management

This section begins by discussing the mechanism of normal labour and the use of Syntocinon to correct slow progress in labour. Fetal response to labour and ways of assessing intrapartum fetal well-being are discussed, as are the different modes of delivery and why any particular way is chosen.

Diagnosis of labour

Recognition of the onset of labour determines all subsequent management objectives. The onset of labour is a complex physiological process and cannot easily be defined by a single event. Although labour is a continuous process, it is convenient to divide it into stages in order to ensure that the woman and the staff providing her care have an accurate and shared understanding of the concepts, enabling them to communicate effectively.

Latent first stage of labour

The onset of labour is a transition period from 'not in labour' to the diagnosis of active labour; this period is called the latent phase. In a woman having her first baby this period of time can last for several days, whereas in a multiparous patient it frequently does not occur at all. During this time there are painful contractions, with gradual cervical change, including effacement (shortening) of the cervix and dilatation up to 3–4 cm. During this period women are encouraged to stay at home, mobilise and not to focus on the contractions.

Established first stage of labour

The diagnosis of labour is made when there is progressive cervical dilatation in the presence of regular painful contractions and descent of the presenting part.

Once labour has been established, regular examinations of the cervix are performed (NICE guidelines (NICE 2010) on intrapartum care suggest 4-hourly), and the rate of cervical dilatation is plotted against time on a graph described as a partogram. The average rate of cervical dilatation and the construction of a partogram against which progress could be charted were established by studying a very large number of women in normal labour (Philpott 1972); women falling behind the average rate of progress, determined as a rate of cervical dilatation at 1 cm per hour, are readily identified by charting their progress on the partogram, and following medical review they can be considered for augmentation of labour with Syntocinon.

This charting of labour progress led to 'active management of labour' (O'Driscoll et al. 1984; Sadler et al. 2000; Tabowei and Oboro 2003), whereby women falling outside 'normal' progress automatically had augmentation of labour. It is now clear, however, that the active management of labour does not reduce the rate of caesarean section (CS) or increase spontaneous vaginal birth. In addition the injudicious use of Syntocinon in the presence of fetal compromise has considerably worsened the condition of many babies at birth. It is clear that regular training and updating of midwifery and medical staff are mandatory in units where Syntocinon is routinely used to ensure that the hypoxic fetus is recognised early and timely intervention undertaken to protect the baby.

Second stage of labour

Once the cervix is fully dilated (second stage), progress is defined as descent of the presenting part through the birth canal. This is judged by hourly vaginal examinations. In the absence of an epidural, the usual limits of duration for pushing are 60–90 minutes for a woman having her first baby and 30–60 minutes for multiparous women. These recommendations have some support, in that fetal hypoxia and acidaemia increase progressively during the second stage (Humphrey et al. 1974; Aldrich et al. 1995; Honjo and Yamaguchi 2001; Nordstrom et al. 2001). However, in recent years, with the increasing use of epidural analgesia (Caliskan et al. 2010), allowing more time in the second stage before starting active pushing has been shown to improve the chance of vaginal delivery (Hoult et al. 1977; Hansen et al. 2002) without a major deterioration in fetal pH. Nevertheless, the need for operative assistance in the presence of an epidural remains significantly increased (Fraser et al. 2000), and many consider one additional hour sufficient to minimise this possibility (Maresh 1983). NICE recommends that in nulliparous women birth should be expected to occur within 3 hours of the start of the active second stage (NICE 2010). A diagnosis of delay in the active second stage should be made after 2 hours of active pushing in a primiparous and 1 hour in a multiparous woman. Unless delivery is imminent the usual action would be to ask for a medical review to assess the condition of both the mother and her baby and to determine whether an operative vaginal birth is required.

Interventions during labour

Amniotomy and augmentation of labour with an intravenous infusion of Syntocinon are interventions that are regularly undertaken when labour progress is deemed to be slow.

Amniotomy

Active management of labour includes routine amniotomy (membrane rupture) if the cervix fails to dilate 2 hours following the diagnosis of labour (O'Driscoll et al. 1984; Frigoletto et al. 1995; Rogers et al. 1997). While there is some evidence (Smyth 2007) that there may be a reduction in the length of the second stage of labour in women having their first baby, earlier amniotomy is associated with a higher incidence of caput formation and moulding of the fetal head (Caldeyro-Barcia 1974) and an increased incidence of early uniform fetal heart rate (FHR) decelerations and a significantly lower median umbilical artery pH at birth (albeit still within the normal range) (Caldeyro-Barcia 1974). These findings can be explained on the basis of increased uterine activity, greater head compression and (probably most importantly) cord compression. In the presence of an abnormal FHR pattern membrane rupture may provide additional information if meconium is present, although 20% of normal women will have meconium present in the amniotic fluid (Gibb 1992). Rupture of the membranes is also required before fetal blood sampling (FBS) or application of a fetal scalp electrode.

Meconium

The incidence of meconium in the liquor increases with advancing gestational age (Oyelese 2006) The overall reported incidence is 12%, with an incidence of less than 10% at 38 weeks to virtually 100% of pregnancies at 42 weeks complicated by meconium staining of the liquor. The prelabour passage of meconium may reflect

Table 12.1 National Institute for Health and Clinical Excellence categorisation of fetal heart rate features

FEATURE	BASELINE (bpm)	VARIABILITY (bpm)	DECELERATIONS	ACCELERATIONS
Reassuring	110–160	≥5	None	Present
Non-reassuring	100–109	<5	Typical variable decelerations with over 50% of contractions, occurring for over 90 minutes. Single prolonged deceleration for up to 3 minutes	The absence of accelerations with otherwise normal trace is of uncertain significance
Abnormal	<100 >180 Sinusoidal pattern ≥10 minutes	<5 for 90 minutes	Either atypical variable decelerations with over 50% of contractions or late decelerations, both for over 30 minutes. Single prolonged deceleration for more than 3 minutes	

a previous transient fetal stimulation, possibly hypoxia, and infection and thyrotoxicosis are rare causes. The passage of meconium in utero is associated with significant increases in perinatal morbidity and mortality (Nathan et al. 1994; Martin and Vidyasagar 2008) as the aspiration of meconium into the lungs during intrauterine gasping, or when the baby takes its first breath, can result in a life-threatening disorder known as meconium aspiration syndrome (Maresh 1983).

Occasionally green 'meconium-stained' liquor is actually bile-stained, due to fetal vomiting associated with intestinal obstruction. Thus, meconium remains an indication for continuous electronic FHR monitoring (EFM) during labour, and the presence of meconium lowers the threshold for making a diagnosis of fetal hypoxia if FHR abnormalities occur.

Effects of oxytocin

The aim of augmentation of labour with Syntocinon infusion is to achieve optimal uterine activity with a maximum contraction frequency of 4–5/10 minutes. Uterine perfusion decreases during contractions as a result of a decrease in blood flow to the intervillous space (Peebles et al. 1994; Simpson 2004). Fetal oxygenation remains unaffected, as long as there is sufficient time for relaxation between contractions to allow reperfusion of the placental bed (Simpson and James 2008). Nevertheless, in clinical practice the use of Syntocinon is associated with an increased incidence of FHR decelerations and therefore vigilance is essential, and requires continuous high-quality recording of the FHR (Bakker et al. 2007).

Electronic fetal heart rate monitoring

Several randomised controlled trials have suggested that continuous EFM confers no advantage over intermittent auscultation for normal, uncomplicated labours (MacDonald et al. 1985; Thacker 2004). When continuous monitoring is indicated the cardiotocogram (CTG) must be interpreted in the context of the clinical picture.

Recently produced evidence-based guidelines on the use and interpretation of the CTG in intrapartum fetal surveillance have been produced (NICE 2010). This guideline categorises FHR features into

Table 12.2 National Institute for Health and Clinical Excellence categorisation of fetal heart rate (FHR) traces

CATEGORY	DEFINITION
Normal	An FHR trace in which all four features are classified as reassuring
Suspicious	An FHR trace with one feature classified as non-reassuring and the remaining features classified as reassuring
Pathological	An FHR trace with two or more features classified as non-reassuring or one or more abnormal categories

'reassuring', 'non-reassuring' and 'abnormal' groups (Table 12.1), enabling classification of the CTG trace as 'normal', 'suspicious' or 'pathological' (two non-reassuring features, or one abnormal feature) (Table 12.2). 'Suspicious' traces can be managed conservatively but 'pathological' traces demand either a FBS or delivery.

Baseline rate

This is the mean FHR in beats per minute (bpm) determined over a 5–10-minute interval, when stable in the absence of accelerations and decelerations. The normal baseline FHR lies between 110 and 160 bpm at term (Table 12.1).

Fetal tachycardia

Acute rises in FHR in labour may reflect an increase in catecholamine secretion and indicate an early adaptive response to fetal hypoxia before the development of fetal acidaemia. Chorioamnionitis should always be suspected. Epidural analgesia can cause maternal fever and fetal tachycardia (Macaulay et al. 1992). Rarely a fetal tachyarrhythmia may be recognised for the first time in labour. Fetal tachycardia above 180 bpm has traditionally been regarded as a sign of fetal compromise, particularly if found in association with other abnormal FHR patterns when the likelihood of acidosis is significantly increased (Fig. 12.1). FBS or delivery then becomes a priority.

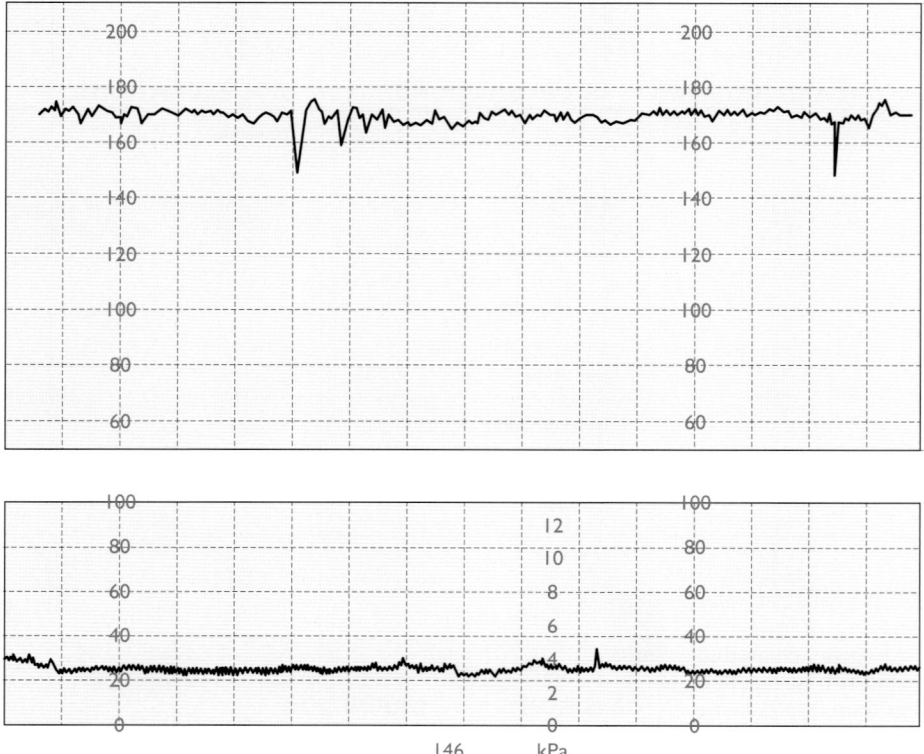

Fig. 12.1 Baseline tachycardia.

Fetal bradycardia

A persistent low baseline between 100 and 110 bpm can be seen in some postdate pregnancies and in fetuses whose mothers are taking drugs such as beta-blockers. Fetal heart block is another possibility.

Acute bradycardia below 100 bpm can occur following vaginal examination and full dilatation of the cervix and after epidural top-ups. An acute fall in FHR indicates an acute interruption of oxygen delivery, secondary to maternal hypotension/aortocaval compression, umbilical cord compression, cord prolapse, placental abruption or, rarely, a ruptured uterus (Fig. 12.2). Acidaemia develops within 10–15 minutes and will continue to progress unless the situation is corrected. If the bradycardia fails to recover after appropriate treatment, immediate delivery is necessary (Verspyck and Sentilhes 2008). However, if the baseline FHR returns to normal and there are no other abnormal FHR features, conservative management is appropriate. Fetal bradycardia in association with other FHR abnormalities can be sinister. The worst combination of FHR abnormalities described has been progressive bradycardia associated with absent FHR variability, which is regarded as a terminal response of a dying fetus (Verspyck and Sentilhes 2008) (Fig. 12.2).

Baseline variability

This refers to oscillations of the recorded baseline FHR. During periods of fetal activity, baseline variability is usually ≥5 bpm (<25 bpm) and there should be two or more accelerations in a 20-minute period (Fig. 12.3). Episodes of low variability, often less than 5 bpm, are associated with the quiet fetal behavioural state (Beard et al. 1971). Such physiological episodes do not last more

than 40 minutes. Excessive variability (>25 bpm) is an early adaptive response to fetal hypoxia, and in isolation is not found to be predictive of fetal acidaemia. Commonly, however, abnormalities of the baseline variability are seen in conjunction with other FHR abnormalities. In such cases further tests of fetal well-being are appropriate.

Accelerations

An acceleration is a transient rise in FHR of at least 15 bpm, which lasts for more than 15 seconds. If the rate remains raised then this may be considered tachycardia. It has been known for some time that acceleration is the only pattern not related to fetal acidaemia (Trochez et al. 2005).

Decelerations

A deceleration is a transient fall in FHR. Decelerations are not part of the normal CTG appearance in term fetuses. In general, decelerations should be considered transient bradycardias. Fetal acidaemia only occurs after a considerable reduction in fetal oxygen delivery.

Early decelerations

These are decelerations in which the trough of the decrease in the FHR is synchronous with the peak of the uterine contraction and does not fall below 90 bpm. They are rare, occur when the head is deeply engaged in the late first stage or early second stage and are generally benign. If the early decelerations persist in the presence of a delayed second stage or there are other abnormalities of the FHR, FBS or delivery is indicated.

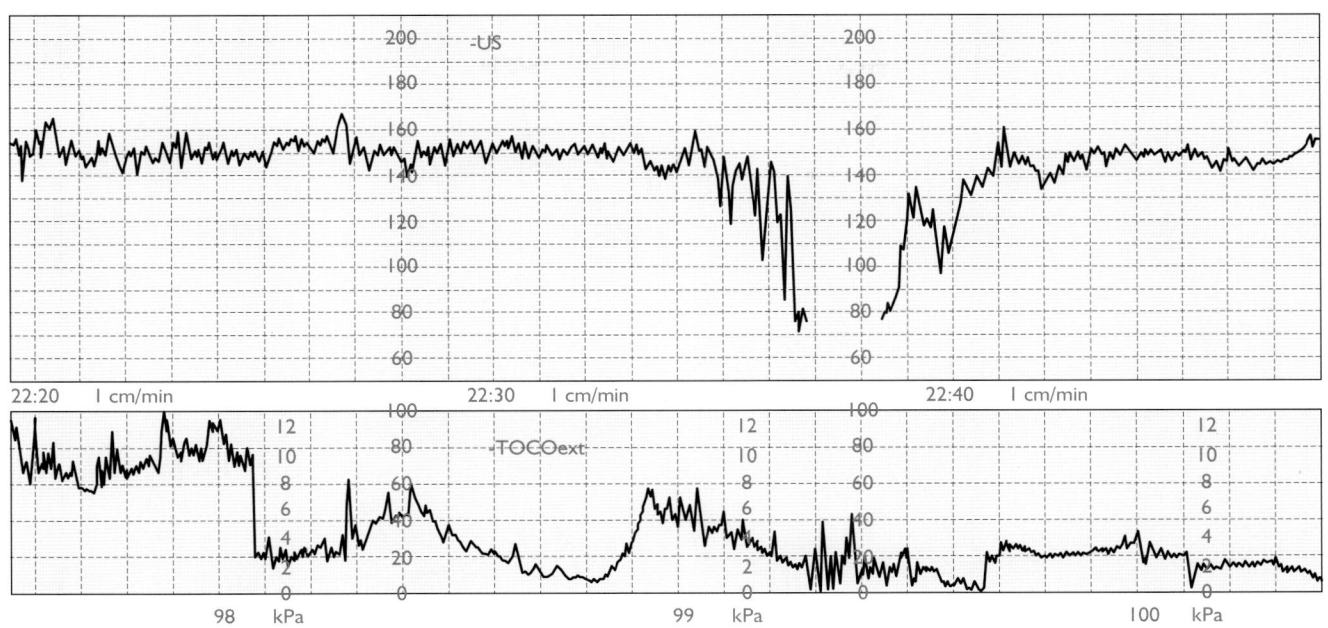

Fig. 12.2 Prolonged deceleration.

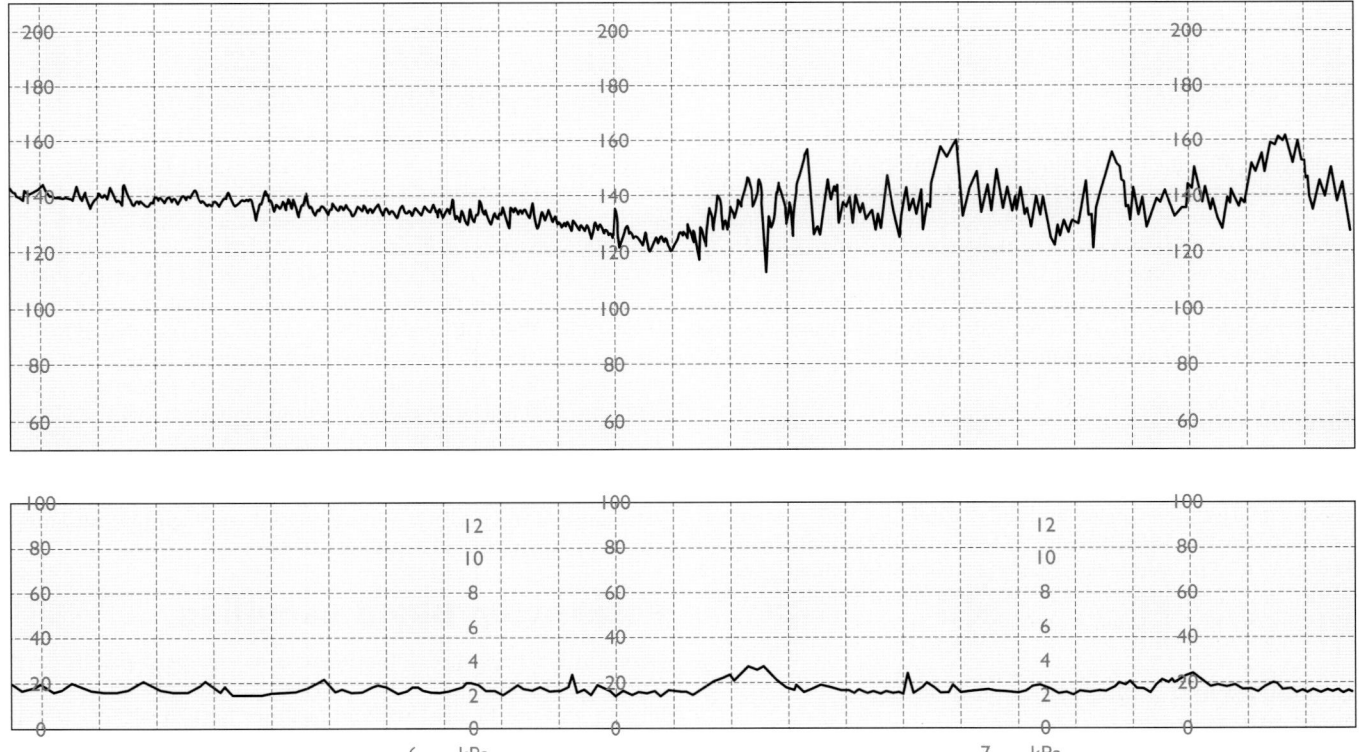

Fig. 12.3 Normal CTG.

Variable decelerations

A variable deceleration (Kazandi et al. 2003) is one where the morphology of the deceleration and/or the timing in relationship to the contraction varies (Figs 12.4 and 12.5). Typical variable decelerations are a fetal response to cord compression where the fetus is coping with labour; NICE guidance (2010) suggests that they only become a non-reassuring feature if they are present for greater than 50% of contraction over a 90-minute period. Atypical variable decelerations are an abnormal feature on a CTG and suggest fetal acidosis; if they occur for greater than 50% of contractions over a 30-minute period then either FBS or delivery is mandatory.

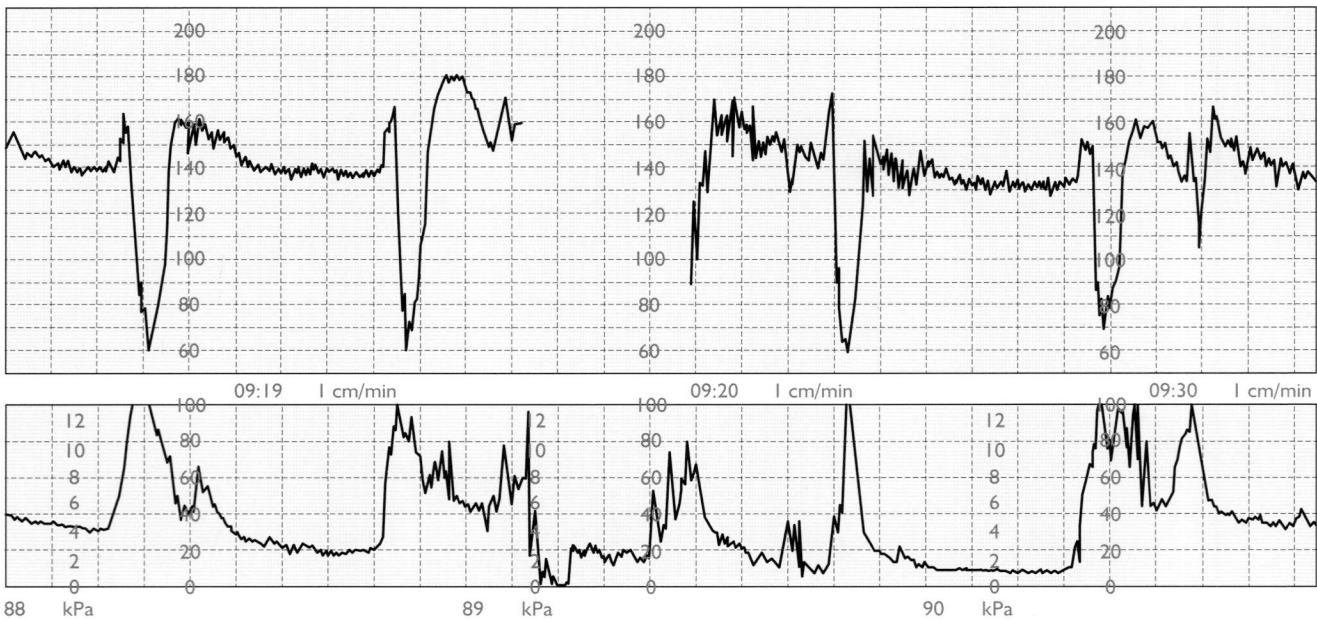

Fig. 12.4 Variable decelerations.

Late decelerations

These are decelerations in which the trough of the decrease in the FHR occurs after the peak of the uterine contraction. They are associated with fetal acidaemia and when present the fetus must either have further assessment by FBS or be delivered within 30 minutes. Late decelerations, particularly in the setting of other FHR abnormalities, suggest fetal hypoxia secondary to uteroplacental insufficiency. The characteristic changes associated with chronic placental failure include loss of accelerations, reduced baseline variability and the onset of recurrent decelerations (Fig. 12.4).

Preterm fetus

The interpretation of the FHR pattern of the preterm fetus in labour is similar to that of its term counterpart, with some subtle differences. The baseline is higher and the variability is often less. Accelerations occur less frequently and are less marked. The differentiation between quiet and active sleep patterns may not be evident until 32 weeks' gestation. Small brief (20-second) decelerations are often seen and are not considered significant.

Sinusoidal and pseudosinusoidal fetal heart rate patterns

The classical CTG pattern in severe fetal anaemia is described as 'sinusoidal' (Fig. 12.6). This is a preterminal pattern which is rarely seen. Five rigid criteria must be fulfilled to make the diagnosis (Modanlou and Murata 2004):

1. a stable baseline FHR of 120–160 bpm, with regular oscillations
2. an amplitude of 5–15 bpm
3. a frequency of 2–5 cycles/min
4. absent short-term variability
5. no areas of normal FHR variability or reactivity.

Pseudosinusoidal fetal heart rate patterns

Pseudosinusoidal FHR patterns (vaguely defined as undulatory waveforms), in contrast, are common and usually benign. They are strongly associated with the use of pethidine and epidural analgesia and are also seen with fetal sucking movements. Such patterns will generally improve with time.

From the review of FHR patterns it is clear that no single abnormal pattern reliably predicts fetal outcome. Comprehensive evaluation of all the FHR characteristics must be integrated into the clinical scenario before decisions can be made on management. Of most importance is the influence of prelabour placental insufficiency on fetal tolerance to interruptions in oxygen delivery during labour. Acidaemia develops more rapidly in cases of intrauterine growth restriction (Verspyck and Sentilhes 2008).

The future of FHR monitoring requires further understanding and acceptance of the need for a more physiological approach to interpretation (Verspyck and Sentilhes 2008).

Fetal scalp blood sampling

Clinical trials have shown that there is an increased risk of CS if CTG is used without FBS. This has led NICE to recommend that EFM should not be used without facilities for FBS (RCOG 2001). Fetal scalp sampling involves taking a small sample of blood from the fetal scalp. It is a difficult process for both the mother and the doctor as it is uncomfortable and can be technically difficult to perform, particularly if the cervix is less than 4 cm dilated. The mother is positioned in the left lateral position and an amnioscope (a specially designed speculum) is inserted into the vagina. Under direct vision the skin of the fetal scalp is punctured and a capillary tube of fetal blood is collected and then analysed in a blood gas analyser.

The normal values for pH in fetal scalp blood are shown in Table 12.3. If the pH is 7.2 or less, immediate delivery is indicated. If the

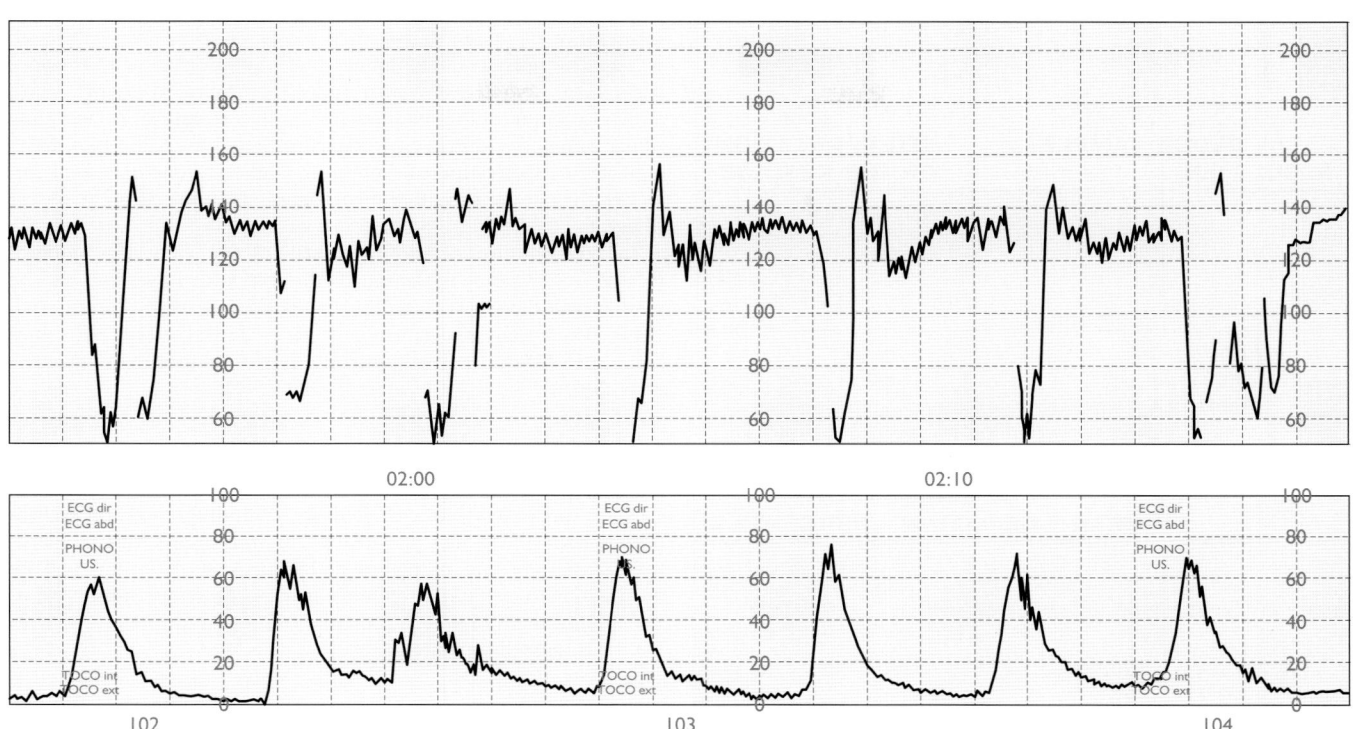

Fig. 12.5 Variable decelerations.

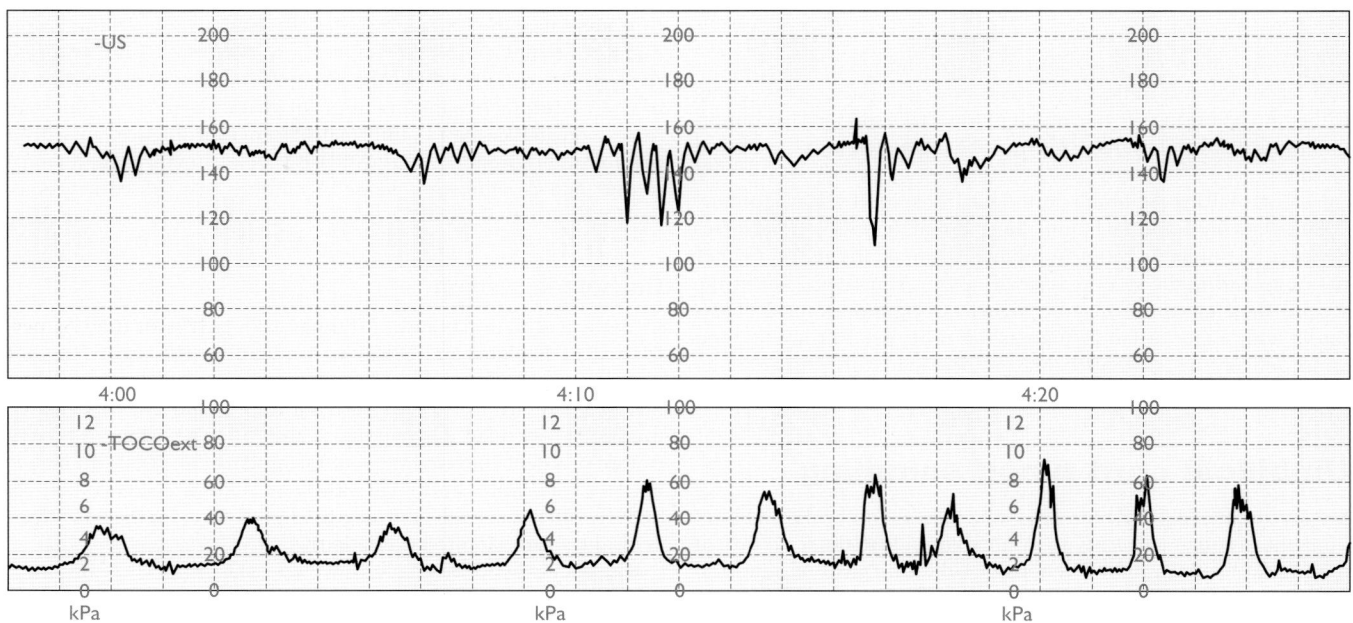

Fig. 12.6 Sinusoidal CTG.

Table 12.3 The classification of fetal blood sample (FBS) results

FETAL BLOOD SAMPLE RESULT (pH)	INTERPRETATION OF THE RESULTS
≥7.25	Normal FBS result
7.21–7.24	Borderline FBS result
≤7.20	Abnormal FBS result

Table 12.4 Normal values for umbilical cord blood gas data (in term fetuses with Apgar scores >7 at 5 minutes)

	MEAN	STANDARD DEVIATION	2.5TH PERCENTILE
UA pH	7.26	0.07	7.10
UA P_{CO_2} (mmHg)	53	10	35
UA P_{O_2} (mmHg)	17	6	6
UA BE (mEq/l)	24	3	211
UV pH	7.34	0.06	7.20
UV P_{CO_2} (mmHg)	41	7	28
UV P_{O_2} (mmHg)	29	7	16
UV BE (mEq/l)	23	3	28

UA, umbilical artery; BE, base excess; UV, umbilical vein.

pH is greater than 7.2, it is appropriate to continue with the labour and repeat the test, unless the situation deteriorates, necessitating earlier intervention. The rate of fall of the fetal scalp pH is as important as each absolute value. This must be integrated into the clinical picture.

Fetal pH falls more rapidly during active second stage (Hofmeyr 2004). Data from normal labours suggest that the scalp pH decreases by 0.016 pH units per hour in the first stage of labour and by 0.11 pH units during the second stage of labour. The rate of fall in the second stage of labour may be higher during a prolonged bradycardia with a rate of fall as high as 0.1 units per 10 minutes, and rapid delivery is essential to prevent acidaemia at birth (Sheiner et al. 2001).

Umbilical cord blood sampling

Measurement of pH and blood gas values from umbilical cord blood immediately after delivery is an invaluable guide to the condition of the fetus at birth. Umbilical venous blood values give an indication of the effects of placental gas transfer and correction of buffered arterial metabolic acids. Oxygen saturation and pH values are always higher in umbilical venous blood, which is the best representation of cerebral blood oxygen content. Umbilical arterial blood gas analysis indicates the fetal response to labour and reflects the situation in the blood supplying the lower fetal body (Spencer 1993).

The normal values for umbilical blood gas results are shown in Table 12.4. Arterial and venous cord pH are likely to be significantly different if there is an element of cord compression, hence the importance of taking paired cord blood samples (Westgate et al. 1994). The normal range defines the 'physiological acidaemia' of the normal, vigorous newborn. Indeed, umbilical artery pH values above 7.05 in term infants show no significant association with low Apgar scores or adverse neurodevelopmental outcome (Goldaber et al. 1991). Correction of even quite marked acidaemia after birth by healthy babies is rapid and correlates with a low $P_{a CO_2}$ at 1 hour of age.

The distribution of umbilical arterial pH values in preterm infants (<32 weeks) is skewed to the left, with lower values. The median value was pH 7.25, but the range was wide (Zanini et al. 1980). There is an association between umbilical arterial pH values below pH 7.0 and adverse outcome in the preterm baby (Victory et al. 2003).

Delivery of the baby

This section covers mode of delivery, including common indications for specific modes of delivery. The indications for CS, instrumental delivery and induction of labour in term infants will be outlined, with particular reference to possible fetal complications. The management of breech presentations and multiple pregnancies will be discussed separately.

Term infants

The majority of term infants will deliver normally, with or without assistance. In the UK the aim is to provide all women with 1 : 1 care in labour (RCOG 2007) and , in addition, some women will choose to have a doula with them to provide additional support. While UK operative vaginal delivery rates have remained constant at approximately 11%, CS rates are increasing. The CS rate in England and Wales was 21.5% in 2000/01 compared with 10.4% in 1985. The drive to reduce the CS rate includes encouraging vaginal birth after caesarean (VBAC) birth, and refusing to perform CS for maternal request. The concern about the rising CS rate is the increased rate of complications in subsequent pregnancies. There is a higher rate of scar pregnancies and abnormal placentation in women with a previous CS (Rosenberg et al. 2010) as well as convincing epidemiological data showing an increase in stillbirth in a subsequent pregnancy (Smith et al. 2003).

Caesarean section

In the recent national audit (Thomas 2001), 37% of the CSs performed in England and Wales were planned. The most frequent indications were previous CS and breech presentation (Thomas 2001). There are a few 'absolute' indications for elective CS, for instance major placenta praevia or abnormal lie, where the baby cannot be safely delivered vaginally (Hannah et al. 2000). In maternal HIV infection with a high viral load there is evidence that CS delivery offers a considerable degree of protection for the baby from vertical transmission (Newell 2000).

It is widely assumed that elective CS ensures good condition at birth, and certainly the incidence of neonatal seizures and encephalopathy in babies born by elective CS is very low. However, maternal hypotension due to regional anaesthesia, with or without aortocaval compression, can reduce placental perfusion and lead to acute fetal hypoxia. There is an increased incidence of fetal respiratory complications, such as transient tachypnoea of the newborn and hyaline membrane disease in the absence of the normal 'stress' of labour (Morrison et al. 1995). The risk of neonatal respiratory morbidity is related to the gestational age at which the elective CS is performed. For this reason, an elective CS should usually be undertaken at or after 39 weeks of gestation.

Emergency CS may be indicated either for fetal hypoxia or for failure to progress in labour. The urgency of the procedure will be determined by the presumed aetiology and severity of the problem. Rather than attempting vaginal delivery the data suggest that, in cases of placental abruption with evidence of fetal compromise, perinatal outcome is significantly improved by urgent CS (Okonofua and Olatunbosun 1985; Green 1989).

Instrumental vaginal delivery

This is usually indicated for fetal compromise, delay in the second stage of labour or maternal exhaustion. Instrumental vaginal delivery can be performed using either forceps or the ventouse and both of these can cause significant complications to the mother and fetus (Ezenagu et al. 1999; Gardella et al. 2001; Al-Kadri et al. 2003).

Neonatal intracranial and subgaleal haemorrhage are potentially life-threatening complications (Whitby et al. 2004). In one review the rate of subdural or cerebral haemorrhage in ventouse deliveries did not differ significantly from that associated with forceps use or CS during labour (Whitby et al. 2004). There is a clear link between the use of the ventouse and subgaleal haemorrhage, with an incidence of around 1 in 1000 normal deliveries compared with 7 per 1000 ventouse births (Towner et al. 1999).

The risk of extracranial or intracranial trauma relates to the cup application time, number of pulls, and whether or not two sets of instruments are used (Gardella et al. 2001). The risk is further increased when delivery is completed by CS following a protracted attempt at operative vaginal delivery (Ezenagu et al. 1999). CS in the second stage of labour is associated with an increased risk of major obstetric haemorrhage, prolonged hospital stay and admission of the baby to the special care baby unit compared with completed instrumental delivery.

Rotational delivery with the Kielland forceps carries additional risks and requires specific expertise and training, which is becoming scarce (Chow et al. 1987). Alternatives to rotational forceps include manual rotation followed by direct traction forceps or rotational vacuum extractor.

Shoulder dystocia

Shoulder dystocia is defined as a delivery where additional obstetric manoeuvres are required to deliver the shoulders of the baby, it occurs when the anterior shoulder impacts against the maternal symphysis or rarely the posterior shoulder against the sacral promontory. It is an obstetric emergency as delay in delivering the baby will lead to rapid hypoxia and death unless delivery is effected rapidly. The Confidential Enquiry into Stillbirths and Deaths in Infancy report noted that 47% of babies who die after a shoulder dystocia did so within 5 minutes of the head being delivered (Focus Group Shoulder Dystocia 1998). Shoulder dystocia has a reported incidence of 0.6% and is associated with a high perinatal morbidity and mortality; there are also maternal complications with a high incidence of fourth-degree tears and postpartum haemorrhage. The principal risk factor is fetal macrosomia, although the majority of cases occur in infants weighing <4500 g (Focus Group Shoulder Dystocia 1998; RCOG 2005). Additional risk factors include maternal diabetes mellitus, a history of previous shoulder dystocia, prolonged labour and delay in the second stage of labour. Obstetric brachial plexus injury complicates about 4–16% of all cases of shoulder dystocia, of which 10% of the babies will have permanent damage, usually an Erb's palsy (p >000) Unfortunately, at present

there is no reliable method for antenatal prediction of shoulder dystocia.

A number of manoeuvres can be employed to expedite delivery of the shoulders and all obstetricians and midwives should have regular training in 'shoulder dystocia drills' (Focus Group Shoulder Dystocia 1998; RCOG 2005). Rarely, deliberate fracture of the baby's clavicles is necessary.

Induction of labour

Most women will go into labour before 42 weeks. Induction of labour is generally offered between 41 and 42 weeks, to reduce the risks of postmaturity, and prolonged pregnancy is the commonest indication for induction of labour. A policy of offering routine induction of labour after 41 weeks reduces perinatal mortality without increasing the CS rate (Okonofua and Olatunbosun 1985). The insertion of vaginal prostaglandin E_2 is the preferred method of induction unless the cervix is already shortened (effaced) and starting to dilate, when artificial membrane rupture and Syntocinon stimulation should be used. Hyperstimulation is a potential complication inherent to all these methods and causes inappropriate myometrial reaction. Hyperstimulation can result in hypertonus or tachysystole (>6 contractions in 10 min). In either case, the fetus does not have long enough to recover from the acute hypoxic stress of the uterine activity and CTG abnormalities ensue. Women with prelabour rupture of the membranes at term may also require induction of labour if they do not go into labour. This group of women should be offered either conservative management or immediate stimulation of labour. If the woman chooses to wait she will normally be readmitted 24 hours after the membrane rupture. As prolonged rupture of the membranes of >18 hours is associated with an increased risk of infection with group B *Streptococcus*, women in this group should be offered intravenous antibiotics (Shipp et al. 1999).

Breech presentation

The management of term breech presentations has, until recently, been the subject of intense controversy. The interpretation of studies that compare outcome after vaginal breech birth and cephalic birth is confounded by the fact that breech presentation per se appears to be a marker for poor perinatal outcome. Thus, poor outcomes following vaginal breech birth may be the result of underlying conditions causing breech presentation rather than damage during delivery. However, the care during labour, the delivery methods used and the skill of the birth attendant may also influence outcome.

Vaginal breech delivery carries the risk of cord compression/prolapse, extended arms at delivery and difficult delivery of the aftercoming head. This risk may be approximately 1–2%. The controversy over the mode of delivery of term breech presentations was finally clarified with the publication of the Term Breech Trial (Hannah et al. 2000). This was a randomised controlled trial to compare a policy of planned CS with planned vaginal birth for selected breech presentation pregnancies. The three primary outcomes – perinatal mortality, neonatal mortality and serious neonatal morbidity – were significantly lower for the planned CS group than for the planned vaginal birth group, with no differences in serious maternal complications. Consequently, most clinicians in the UK now recommend elective CS for term breech singletons. Some vaginal breech deliveries will inevitably occur, for instance in undiagnosed breeches in the second stage of labour, or as a result of informed maternal choice. In such an event an experienced obstetrician or midwife should conduct delivery. Continuous EFM should be instituted and early CS should be performed, particularly in the event of poor progress in the second stage of labour.

The challenge for clinicians now is how to maintain and teach vaginal breech delivery skills when these deliveries occur so infrequently.

The alternative management for the breech presentation at term is to offer external cephalic version (ECV). ECV at term can reduce non-cephalic births by nearly 60% (Hofmeyr 2000) and routine tocolysis appears to be effective (Hofmeyr 2004). ECV does carry small risks of fetal bradycardia and fetomaternal haemorrhage and therefore should be performed on the labour ward with access to obstetric theatre.

Multiple pregnancy

The optimal mode of delivery in multiple pregnancies is controversial. Elective CS is frequently performed for triplets and higher order multiples, although no randomised controlled trials are available to support this practice. The planned mode of delivery of twins will be influenced by both the chorionicity and the presentations. In dichorionic diamniotic twin pregnancy with a vertex–vertex presentation, most obstetricians would currently advise vaginal delivery (Chervenak et al. 1985). When the first twin presents as a breech, delivery by CS is often recommended (Chervenak et al. 1985), based on findings from the Term Breech Trial in singletons (Hofmeyr 2000). For twins presenting as first twin vertex, second twin non-vertex, opinion is divided as to the optimal mode of delivery. Some would perform an elective CS, believing that this reduces the neonatal mortality and morbidity of the second twin (Smith et al. 2002). It has been suggested that second twins born at term are at substantially higher risk of death than first twins owing to complications of vaginal delivery (Smith et al. 2002) irrespective of the presentation of the second twin. Others would advocate that, with careful fetal monitoring and recourse to urgent CS if necessary, the risks to the second twin can be minimised. Vaginal delivery of the second, non-vertex, twin can be effected by internal podalic version followed by breech extraction.

In an attempt to clarify the situation, the group that carried out the Term Breech Trial is currently setting up the Term Twin Trial. Hopefully it will provide a definitive answer to the optimal mode of delivery of term twins.

The situation with monochorionic twins is not as clear: approximately 33% of all twins are monochorionic, i.e. they share the same placenta and vascular placental anastomoses. Complications include twin–twin transfusion syndrome, the complications that arise with the death of a co-twin and discordant malformation. Chorionicity can be reliably determined at the 12-week scan and regular ultrasound scans are the mainstay of antenatal management. The perinatal mortality rate for monochorionic twins is quoted as 11% compared with 5% in dichorionic twins and the increased risk continues after 32 weeks (Duncan 2005). The recommendations are that monochorionic twins should be delivered at 36–37 weeks. There is no clear evidence about mode of delivery, although the quoted incidence of 10% for acute twin-to-twin transfusion syndrome has led to many obstetricians delivering all monochorionic twins by planned CS (Barigye et al. 2005).

Other high-risk situations for the fetus

Cord prolapse

Cord prolapse has been defined as the descent of the umbilical cord through the cervix alongside (occult) or past the presenting part (overt) in the presence of ruptured membranes (Beard and Johnson 1972). The overall incidence of cord prolapse ranges from 0.1% to 0.6% (Macaulay et al. 1992) and is higher in breech presentation, at ~1% (Lin 2006).

The principal cause of asphyxia is cord compression and umbilical arterial vasospasm. Manual elevation is achieved by inserting a gloved hand in the vagina to displace the presenting part upwards. If the delivery is likely to be prolonged, particularly if it involves ambulance transfer, elevation through bladder filling (Foley catheter with 500–750 ml of normal saline and clamped) may be more practical. Tocolysis has been used to reduce contractions and correct bradycardia (Draycott 2008).

CS is associated with a lower perinatal mortality than spontaneous vaginal delivery in cases of cord prolapse when delivery is not imminent. However, when vaginal birth is imminent, outcomes are similar to or better than CS. The prognosis of cord prolapse managed in a hospital setting is generally good; most units will regularly run drills to practise for unexpected cord prolapse (Murphy and MacKenzie 1995).

Ruptured uterus

Ruptured uterus is another obstetric emergency in which fetal compromise can rapidly develop. It typically occurs in multiparous women with a uterine scar or with uterine stimulation with Syntocinon. The classical clinical symptoms and signs are severe pain (which will 'break through' epidural analgesia), cessation of contractions, intrapartum bleeding and haematuria. Early warning signs are often seen on the CTG. The fetal outcome from this acute hypoxic insult will be determined by the speed of delivery and the fetal condition prior to uterine rupture. The prognosis for babies delivered from the maternal peritoneal cavity, having been completely extruded from the uterus, is poor (Leung et al. 1993).

Maternal cardiac/respiratory arrest

Finally, in the rare event of maternal cardiac/respiratory arrest, fetal delivery is often essential if maternal resuscitation is to succeed. The physical effects of a third-trimester uterus on lung expansion and aortocaval compression make maternal resuscitation difficult. If the maternal condition is not dramatically improved after 5 minutes of intensive resuscitation, rapid fetal delivery by CS should be performed, Both the maternal and fetal outcomes are often poor. The potential causes for a maternal cardiorespiratory arrest can be amniotic fluid embolism, pulmonary embolism, myocardial infarction, massive cerebrovascular event and hypovolaemia.

Preterm infants

Preterm is defined as less than 37 completed weeks of gestation. The mode of delivery of preterm infants will be influenced by the gestational age, the fetal and maternal condition and whether the mother is already in spontaneous preterm labour. It is therefore difficult to make generalisations, and decisions need to be taken on an individual basis after discussion with the parents.

The optimal management of preterm breech presentations and multiple pregnancies is less well established than in the term setting. Unfortunately, the incidence of breech presentation is higher preterm. In the absence of good evidence that a preterm breech needs to be delivered by CS, the decision about the mode of delivery should be made after close consultation with the parents.

Multiple pregnancies are at increased risk of almost every pregnancy complication, including preterm labour and delivery.

The antenatal diagnosis of chronic uteroplacental insufficiency and its importance are discussed in detail in Chapter 9. If the fetus shows sign of compromise antenatally delivery should be undertaken by CS as such fetuses are less likely to compensate for the acute hypoxic stress of reduced placental perfusion with each uterine contraction for prolonged periods. In the absence of fetal compromise, expectant management with increased fetal surveillance is preferable to delivery, as the risks of prematurity are appreciable. Rapid deterioration or abnormal CTGs should prompt delivery by CS.

Severe early-onset maternal pre-eclampsia often causes chronic uteroplacental insufficiency. Recurrent episodes of minor antepartum haemorrhage due to placenta praevia can lead to intrauterine growth restriction. The main risk to the neonate, however, is from preterm delivery. Preterm placental abruption requiring delivery is also associated with growth restriction in a substantial proportion of cases. The fetal effects of a placental abruption depend on the degree of placental separation and the condition of the placenta prior to the acute event. In addition, the maternal condition in any of these situations can be the principal indication for preterm delivery, even when the fetus appears healthy.

The optimal mode of delivery for women thought to be in labour and at high risk of delivering a small baby is controversial and there is no clear evidence to guide the obstetrician. Decisions are made on a case-by-case basis and are based on the stage of the labour, the likely outcome for the baby as well as the wishes of the parents. Before 28 weeks it can be very difficult to deliver a baby through a transverse incision as the lower segment does not form until 28 weeks, so the myometrium can be very thick, making delivery very difficult and traumatic for the baby. These operations should only ever be performed by experienced obstetricians, who will make a decision at the time of the operation as to whether to make a vertical or transverse incision in the uterus. A classical CS (i.e. a vertical incision in the uterus) is associated with an increased risk of uterine rupture in the next pregnancy. There is some evidence, however, that low vertical incisions performed to deliver the very small infant may not be associated with a high risk of scar dehiscence in the next pregnancy, and there are reports of women going on to have normal births in the subsequent pregnancy (Shipp et al. 1999). Claims that elective CS reduces the chances of fetal and neonatal death and chronic morbidity have been met by counterclaims that such a policy leads to iatrogenic preterm delivery with the additional risk of serious maternal morbidity. FBS is usually avoided because of the increased risk of serious fetal trauma. For the same reason, vacuum extraction is not used below 34 weeks and forceps delivery is performed for obstetric reasons.

Preterm labour

There are numerous predisposing causes for preterm labour and often an underlying aetiology is not identifiable. Preterm prelabour rupture of the membranes (PPROM), chorioamnionitis, polyhydramnios and antepartum haemorrhage are common pathologies leading to preterm labour. The diagnosis of preterm labour can be very difficult and many obstetricians are now testing for the presence of fibronectin to help with the diagnosis. Fibronectin is a glycoprotein which is not detectable after fusion of the membranes at 22 weeks. The presence of fibronectin after 22 weeks and before 36 weeks suggests separation of the chorion from the decidua, possibly in response to chronic inflammation. The test is performed at the bedside and has a positive predictive value of 37% but a negative predictive value of 99%. Women who present with possible preterm labour who are negative for the presence of fibronectin can be discharged home, and when fibronectin is present admitted for tocolysis and steroids (Berghella et al. 2008).

Preterm prelabour rupture of the membranes

PPROM complicates ~2% of pregnancies but is associated with 40% of preterm deliveries and can result in significant neonatal morbidity and mortality (Carroll et al. 1996). The three causes of neonatal death associated with PPROM are prematurity, sepsis and pulmonary hypoplasia. Women with intrauterine infection deliver earlier and infants born with sepsis have a mortality rate four times higher than those without sepsis (Maxwell 1993). In addition, there are maternal risks associated with chorioamnionitis (RCOG 2002a).

PPROM is diagnosed on the basis of maternal history, liquor visualisation in the vagina and ultrasound evidence of oligohydramnios. Common aetiologies for early membrane rupture include polyhydramnios, infection, maternal urinary tract infection, cervical weakness and recurrent bleeding. After diagnosis and the exclusion of infection the management thereafter is usually expectant, the mother has careful monitoring to look for signs of infection and delivery is planned for after 34 weeks, as at gestations below this the risks of prematurity are greater than those of the most common complication, chorioamnionitis (Fox et al. 1992; Merenstein and Weisman 1996). If infection develops most women will go into labour, but if not then after discussion with the mother and the neonatologist, delivery will be undertaken. Cord prolapse and placental abruption can also occur (Maxwell 1993).

Chorioamnionitis can be caused by a variety of vaginal pathogens. Group B *Streptococcus* infection can result in serious neonatal morbidity and cause preterm labour. Intrapartum antibiotics are effective and decrease neonatal colonisation, sepsis and death (Anthony et al. 1978; Boyer and Gotoff 1986). Transient and intermittent carriage is common (Anthony et al. 1978) and antenatal screening is a poor predictor of the intrapartum state. Bacterial vaginosis is implicated in preterm labour (Hay et al. 1994). ORACLE (Overview of the Role of Antibiotics in Curtailing Labour and Early delivery) (Kenyon et al. 2001, 2003), a large randomised controlled trial, was set up to investigate the role of antibiotics. ORACLE I (Kenyon et al. 2001) included women with PPROM and showed that maternal administration of oral erythromycin is associated with delayed delivery and decreased respiratory, cerebral and infective morbidity. Co-amoxiclav, the other study agent, is not routinely recommended as it is associated with necrotising enterocolitis. Consequently, oral erythromycin is now routinely given to women with PPROM.

ORACLE II (Kenyon et al. 2003), which included women in threatened preterm labour without evidence of PPROM, showed no evidence of benefit from prophylactic antibiotic use. Hence antibiotics should not be routinely prescribed for women in spontaneous preterm labour without evidence of clinical infection.

Tocolysis

There are situations when urgent delivery of the preterm infant is required, such as in the presence of infection or after a placental abruption; however, for the majority of women in preterm labour it is safe to use tocolytic therapy to give time to administer antenatal steroids. When tocolytic therapy is indicated, it should be continued if possible for 48 hours to try to maximise the effects of steroids. Atosiban, an oxytocin antagonist, is effective in delaying delivery for up to 7 days and is associated with fewer maternal adverse effects (RCOG 2002b).

Antenatal steroid therapy in preterm labour

The slow uptake of maternally administered corticosteroids following the original description of benefit in 1972 (Liggins and Howie 1972) remains an important lesson in perinatal medicine. Uptake increased following a review by Crowley (2000), who demonstrated that corticosteroids reduce the occurrence of hyaline membrane disease overall, and reduce the incidence of respiratory distress syndrome, intraventricular haemorrhage, necrotising enterocolitis and neonatal death. A Cochrane review indicates that antenatal corticosteroids reduce the incidence of respiratory distress syndrome, neonatal death and intraventricular haemorrhage (Crowley 1995, 2000; NIH 1995; Penney 2004). There is evidence of benefit in all major subgroups of preterm babies, irrespective of race or gender (Elimian et al. 1999). Some still question the value of steroid therapy for those cases where preterm delivery is preceded by PPROM, especially in babies weighing ≤1000 g (Chapman et al. 1999; Harding et al. 2001). However, Crowley's original meta-analysis showed clear benefit for the use of antenatal corticosteroids after PPROM in reducing respiratory distress syndrome (Crowley et al. 1990; Vermillion et al. 2000). An analysis of 'the number needed to treat' suggests that at >34 weeks 94 women will need to be treated to prevent one case of RDS, while at <31 weeks one case of RDS is prevented for every five women treated (Crowley 2000).

There are growing concerns that repeated antenatal doses could cause decrease in birthweight, in fetal brain, and other organ size and abnormal neuronal development (Kay et al. 2000). Within Crowley's meta-analysis, betamethasone and dexamethasone were found to be equally effective in preventing RDS (Crowley 2000). However, a large study suggested that treatment with betamethasone, but not dexamethasone, is associated with a decreased risk of cystic periventricular leukomalacia among premature infants born at 24–31 weeks of gestation (Baud et al. 1999). The RCOG Scientific Advisory Committee recommends that betamethasone is the steroid of choice to enhance lung maturation (RCOG 2002a).

The effect of treatment is optimal if the baby is delivered >24 hours and <7 days after the start of treatment (Crowley 2004).

In clinical practice, elective use of steroids is often used where preterm delivery is anticipated, for instance severe intrauterine growth restriciton, severe pre-eclampsia and multiple pregnancies. The effects of steroids used for these purposes, however, have not been fully established.

Maternal diabetes mellitus is a recognised risk factor for neonatal respiratory distress syndrome (Carlson et al. 1984; Mimouni et al. 1987). The use of antenatal corticosteroids in pregnancies complicated by maternal diabetes mellitus is recommended, but a significant reduction in rates of respiratory distress syndrome has not been demonstrated.

Weblinks

www.cochrane.org/reviews: Cochrane Reviews.

www.rcog.org.uk: Royal College of Obstetricians and Gynaecologists.

www.K2ms.com: K2 Medical Systems.

www.nice.org.uk: National Institute for Health and Clinical Excellence (NICE).

References

Aldrich, C.J., D'Antona, D., Spencer, J.A., et al., 1995. The effect of maternal pushing on fetal cerebral oxygenation and blood volume during the second stage of labour. Br J Obstet Gynaecol 102, 448–453.

Al-Kadri, H., Sabr, Y., Al-Saif, S., et al., 2003. Failed individual and sequential instrumental vaginal delivery: contributing risk factors and maternal–neonatal complications. Acta Obstet Gynecol Scand 82, 642–648.

Anthony, B.F., Okada, D.M., Hobel, C.J., 1978. Epidemiology of group B Streptococcus: longitudinal observations during pregnancy. J Infect Dis 137, 524–530.

Bakker, P.C., Kurver, P.H., Kuik, D.J., et al., 2007. Elevated uterine activity increases the risk of fetal acidosis at birth. Am J Obstet Gynecol 196, 313–316.

Barigye, O., Pasquini, L., Galea, P., et al., 2005. High risk of unexpected late fetal death in monochorionic twins despite intensive ultrasound surveillance: a cohort study. PLoS Med 2, e172.

Baud, O., Foix-L'Helias, L., Kaminski, M., et al., 1999. Antenatal glucocorticoid treatment and cystic periventricular leukomalacia in very premature infants. N Engl J Med 341, 1190–1196.

Beard, R.J., Johnson, D.A., 1972. Fetal distress due to cord prolapse through a

fenestration in a lower segment uterine scar. J Obstet Gynaecol Br Commonw 79, 763.

Beard, R.W., Filshie, G.M., Knight, C.A., et al., 1971. The significance of the changes in the continuous fetal heart rate in the first stage of labour. J Obstet Gynaecol Br Commonw 78, 865–881.

Berghella, V., Hayes, E., Visintine, J., et al. 2008. Fetal fibronectin testing for reducing the risk of preterm birth. Cochrane Database Syst Rev (4), CD006843.

Boyer, K.M., Gotoff, S.P., 1986. Prevention of early-onset neonatal group B streptococcal disease with selective intrapartum chemoprophylaxis. N Engl J Med 314, 1665–1669.

Caldeyro-Barcia, R., 1974. Adverse perinatal effects of early amniotomy during labor. In: Gluck, L. (Ed.), Modern Perinatal Medicine. Mosby, Chicago, pp. 431–439.

Caliskan, E., Ozdamar, D., Doger, E., et al., 2010. Prospective case control comparison of fetal intrapartum oxygen saturations during epidural analgesia. Int J Obstet Anesth 19, 77–81.

Carlson, K.S., Smith, B.T., Post, M., 1984. Insulin acts on the fibroblast to inhibit glucocorticoid stimulation of lung maturation. J Appl Physiol 57, 1577–1579.

Carroll, S., Sebire, N., Nicolaides, K., 1996. Pre-term pre-labour amniorrhexis. Curr Opin Obstet Gynecol 8, 441–448.

Chapman, S.J., Hauth, J.C., Bottoms, S.F., et al., 1999. Benefits of maternal corticosteroid therapy in infants weighing </=1000 grams at birth after preterm rupture of the amnion. Am J Obstet Gynecol 180, 677–682.

Chervenak, F.A., Johnson, R.E., Youcha, S., et al., 1985. Intrapartum management of twin gestation. Obstet Gynecol 65, 119–124.

Chow, S.L., Johnson, C.M., Anderson, T.D., et al., 1987. Rotational delivery with Kielland's forceps. Med J Aust 146, 616–619.

Crowley, P.A., 1995. Antenatal corticosteroid therapy: a meta-analysis of the randomized trials, 1972 to 1994. Am J Obstet Gynecol 173, 322–335.

Crowley, P., 2000. Prophylactic corticosteroids for preterm birth. Cochrane Database Syst Rev (2), CD000065.

Crowley, P., 2004. Prophylactic steroids for preterm birth. Cochrane Database Syst Rev.

Crowley, P., Chalmers, I., Keirse, M.J., 1990. The effects of corticosteroid administration before preterm delivery: an overview of the evidence from controlled trials. Br J Obstet Gynaecol 97, 11–25.

Draycott, T., Winter, C., Crofts, J., Barnfield, S., 2008. Module 8. Cord Prolapse. PROMPT: PRactical Obstetric MultiProfessional Training Course Manual. RCOG Press, London.

Duncan, K.R., 2005. Twin-to-twin transfusion: update on management options and outcomes. Curr Opin Obstet Gynecol 17, 618–622.

Elimian, A., Verma, U., Canterino, J., et al., 1999. Effectiveness of antenatal steroids in obstetric subgroups. Obstet Gynecol 93, 174–179.

Ezenagu, L.C., Kakaria, R., Bofill, J.A., 1999. Sequential use of instruments at operative vaginal delivery: is it safe? Am J Obstet Gynecol 180, 1446–1449.

Focus Group Shoulder Dystocia, 1998. Confidential Enquiries into Stillbirths and Deaths in Infancy. Fifth Annual Report. Maternal and Child Health Research Consortium, London.

Fox, J.F., McCaul, R.W., M. W. E. R. W. E. M. B. M. J. C., 1992. Neonatal morbidity between 34-37 weeks gestation. Am J Obstet Gynecol 166.

Fraser, W.D., Marcoux, S., Krauss, I., et al., 2000. Multicenter, randomized, controlled trial of delayed pushing for nulliparous women in the second stage of labor with continuous epidural analgesia. The PEOPLE (Pushing Early or Pushing Late with Epidural) Study Group. Am J Obstet Gynecol 182, 1165–1172.

Frigoletto, F.D., Jr., Lieberman, E., Lang, J.M., et al., 1995. A clinical trial of active management of labor. N Engl J Med 333, 745–750.

Gardella, C., Taylor, M., Benedetti, T., et al., 2001. The effect of sequential use of vacuum and forceps for assisted vaginal delivery on neonatal and maternal outcomes. Am J Obstet Gynecol 185, 896–902.

Gibb, D., Arulkumaran, S., 1992. Cardiotocograph Interpretation: Clinical Scenarios. Meconium Stained Amniotic Fluid. Fetal Monitoring in Practice. Butterworth-Heinemann, Oxford, ch. 8.

Goldaber, K.G., Gilstrap, L.C., III, Leveno, K.J., et al., 1991. Pathologic fetal acidemia. Obstet Gynecol 78, 1103–1107.

Green, J., 1989. Placenta abnormalities: placenta praevia and abruptio placentae. Maternal-fetal medicine: principles and practice. W. B. Saunders, Philadelphia.

Hannah, M.E., Hannah, W.J., Hewson, S.A., et al., 2000. Planned caesarean section versus planned vaginal birth for breech presentation at term: a randomised multicentre trial. Term Breech Trial Collaborative Group. Lancet 356, 1375–1383.

Hansen, S.L., Clark, S.L., Foster, J.C., 2002. Active pushing versus passive fetal descent in the second stage of labor: a randomized controlled trial. Obstet Gynecol 99, 29–34.

Harding, J.E., Pang, J., Knight, D.B., et al., 2001. Do antenatal corticosteroids help in the setting of preterm rupture of membranes? Am J Obstet Gynecol 184, 131–139.

Hay, P.E., Lamont, R.F., Taylor-Robinson, D., et al., 1994. Abnormal bacterial colonisation of the genital tract and subsequent preterm delivery and late miscarriage. Br Med J 308, 295–298.

Hofmeyr, G.J., 2000. External cephalic version facilitation for breech presentation at term. Cochrane Database Syst Rev (2), CD000184.

Hofmeyr, G.J., 2004. Interventions to help external cephalic version for breech presentation at term. Cochrane Database Syst Rev (1), CD000184.

Honjo, S., Yamaguchi, M., 2001. Umbilical artery blood acid-base analysis and fetal heart rate baseline in the second stage of labor. J Obstet Gynaecol Res 27, 249–254.

Hoult, I.J., MacLennan, A.H., Carrie, L.E., 1977. Lumbar epidural analgesia in labour: relation to fetal malposition and instrumental delivery. Br Med J 1, 14–16.

Humphrey, M.D., Chang, A., Wood, E.C., et al., 1974. A decrease in fetal pH during the second stage of labour, when conducted in the dorsal position. J Obstet Gynaecol Br Commonw 81, 600–602.

Kay, H.H., Bird, I.M., Coe, C.L., et al., 2000. Antenatal steroid treatment and adverse fetal effects: what is the evidence? J Soc Gynecol Investig 7, 269–278.

Kazandi, M., Sendag, F., Akercan, F., et al., 2003. Different types of variable decelerations and their effects to neonatal outcome. Singapore Med J 44, 243–247.

Kenyon, S.L., Taylor, D.J., Tarnow-Mordi, W., 2001. Broad-spectrum antibiotics for spontaneous preterm labour: the ORACLE II randomised trial. ORACLE Collaborative Group. Lancet 357, 989–994.

Kenyon, S., Boulvain, M., Neilson, J., 2003. Antibiotics for preterm rupture of membranes. Cochrane Database Syst Rev (2), CD001058.

Leung, A.S., Leung, E.K., Paul, R.H., 1993. Uterine rupture after previous cesarean delivery: maternal and fetal consequences. Am J Obstet Gynecol 169, 945–950.

Liggins, G.C., Howie, R.N., 1972. A controlled trial of antepartum glucocorticoid treatment for prevention of the respiratory distress syndrome in premature infants. Pediatrics 50, 515–525.

Lin, M.G., 2006. Umbilical cord prolapse. Obstet Gynecol Surv 61, 269–277.

Macaulay, J.H., Randall, N.R., Bond, K., et al., 1992. Continuous monitoring of fetal temperature by noninvasive probe and its relationship to maternal temperature, fetal heart rate, and cord arterial oxygen and pH. Obstet Gynecol 79, 469–474.

MacDonald, D., Grant, A., Sheridan-Pereira, M., et al., 1985. The Dublin randomized controlled trial of intrapartum fetal heart rate monitoring. Am J Obstet Gynecol 152, 524–539.

Maresh, M., Choong, K.-H., Beard, R.W., 1983. Delayed pushing with lumbar epidural analgesia in labour. Br J Obstet Gynaecol 90, 623–627.

Martin, G.I., Vidyasagar, D., 2008. Introduction: Proceedings of the First International Conference for Meconium Aspiration Syndrome and Meconium-induced Lung Injury. J Perinatol 28 (Suppl. 3), S1–S2.

Maxwell, G.L., 1993. Preterm premature rupture of membranes. Obstet Gynecol Surv 48, 576–583.

Merenstein, G.B., Weisman, L.E., 1996. Premature rupture of the membranes: neonatal consequences. Semin Perinatol 20, 375–380.

Mimouni, F., Miodovnik, M., Whitsett, J.A., et al., 1987. Respiratory distress syndrome in infants of diabetic mothers in the 1980s: no direct adverse effect of maternal diabetes with modern management. Obstet Gynecol 69, 191–195.

Modanlou, H.D., Murata, Y., 2004. Sinusoidal heart rate pattern: Reappraisal of its definition and clinical significance. J Obstet Gynaecol Res 30, 169–180.

Morrison, J.J., Rennie, J.M., Milton, P.J., 1995. Neonatal respiratory morbidity and mode of delivery at term: influence of timing of elective caesarean section. Br J Obstet Gynaecol 102, 101–106.

Murphy, D.J., MacKenzie, I.Z., 1995. The mortality and morbidity associated with umbilical cord prolapse. Br J Obstet Gynaecol 102, 826–830.

Nathan, L., Leveno, K.J., Carmody, III, T.J., et al., 1994. Meconium: a 1990s perspective on an old obstetric hazard. Obstet Gynecol 83, 329–332.

Newell, M.L., 2000. Vertical transmission of HIV-1 infection. Trans R Soc Trop Med Hyg 94, 1–2.

NICE, 2010. Intrapartum Care of Healthy Women and Their Babies During Childbirth. Clinical Guideline no. 55 RCOG Press, London.

NIH, 1995. Consensus Development Panel on the Effect of Corticosteroids for Fetal Maturation on Perinatal Outcomes. 273.

Nordstrom, L., Achanna, S., Naka, K., et al., 2001. Fetal and maternal lactate increase during active second stage of labour. Br J Obstet Gynaecol 108, 263–268.

O'Driscoll, K., Foley, M., MacDonald, D., 1984. Active management of labor as an alternative to cesarean section for dystocia. Obstet Gynecol 63, 485–490.

Okonofua, F.E., Olatunbosun, O.A., 1985. Cesarean versus vaginal delivery in abruptio placentae associated with live fetuses. Int J Gynaecol Obstet 23, 471–474.

Oyelese, Y., Culin, A., Ananth, C.V., et al., 2006. Meconium stained amniotic fluid across gestation and neonatal acid–base status. Obstet Gynecol 2, 345–349.

Peebles, D.M., Spencer, J.A., Edwards, A.D., et al., 1994. Relation between frequency of uterine contractions and human fetal cerebral oxygen saturation studied during labour by near infrared spectroscopy. Br J Obstet Gynaecol 101, 44–48.

Penney, G.C., C. M. J., 2004. Antenatal Corticosteroids to Prevent Respiratory Distress Syndrome. Greentop Guideline no. 7. RCOG Press, London.

Philpott, R.H., 1972. Graphic records in labour. Br Med J 4, 163–165.

RCOG, 2001. The Use of Electronic Fetal Monitoring. Evidence Based Clinical Guideline no. 8, RCOG Press, London.

RCOG, 2002a. Intrauterine Infection and Perinatal Brain Injury. Scientific Advisory Committee Opinion Paper 3. RCOG, London.

RCOG, 2002b. Tocolytic Drugs for Women in Preterm Labour RCOG, London.

RCOG, 2005. Available online at: www.rcog.org.uk/files/rcog-corp/uploaded-files/GT42ShoulderDystocia.

RCOG, 2007. Safer Childbirth: Minimum Standards for the Organisation and Delivery of Care in Labour. Working Party Report. Royal College of Obstetricians and Gynaecologists, Royal College of Midwives, Royal College of Anaesthetists, Royal College of Paediatrics and Child Health, London.

RCOG, 2010. Standards for Maternity Care: Report of a Working Party. RCOG Press, London.

Rogers, R., Gilson, G.J., Miller, A.C., et al., 1997. Active management of labor: does it make a difference? Am J Obstet Gynecol 177, 599–605.

Rosenberg, T., Pariente, G., Sergienko, R., et al., 2011. Critical analysis of risk factors and outcome of placenta previa. Arch Gynecol Obstet. 284, 47–51.

Sadler, L.C., Davison, T., McCowan, L.M., 2000. A randomised controlled trial and meta-analysis of active management of labour. Br J Obstet Gynaecol 107, 909–915.

Sheiner, E., Hadar, A., Hallak, M., et al., 2001. Clinical significance of fetal heart rate tracings during the second stage of labor. Obstet Gynecol 97, 747–752.

Shipp, T.D., Zelop, C.M., Repke, J.T., et al., 1999. Intrapartum uterine rupture and dehiscence in patients with prior lower uterine segment vertical and transverse incisions. Obstet Gynecol 94, 735–740.

Simpson, K.R., 2004. Monitoring the preterm fetus during labor. Am J Matern Child Nurs 29, 380–388.

Simpson, K.R., James, D.C., 2008. Effects of oxytocin-induced uterine hyperstimulation during labor on fetal oxygen status and fetal heart rate patterns. Am J Obstet Gynecol 199, 34–35.

Smith, G.C., Pell, J.P., Dobbie, R., 2002. Birth order, gestational age, and risk of delivery related perinatal death in twins: retrospective cohort study. Br Med J 325, 1004.

Smith, G.C., Pell, J.P., Dobbie, R., 2003. Caesarean section and risk of unexplained stillbirth in subsequent pregnancy. Lancet 362, 1779–1784.

Smyth, R.M.D., Alldred, S.K., Markham, C., 2007. Amniotomy for shortening spontaneous labour. Cochrane Database Syst Rev (4), CD006167.

Spencer, J.A.D., 1993. Fetal response to labour. Intrapartum fetal surveillance.

Tabowei, T.O., Oboro, V.O., 2003. Active management of labour in a district hospital setting. J Obstet Gynaecol 23, 9–12.

Thacker, S.B., Stroup, D., Chang, M., 2004. Continuous electronic heart rate monitoring for fetal assessment during labor. Cochrane Database Syst Rev (1), CD000063.

Thomas, J., P. S., 2001. The National Sentinal Caesarean Section Audit Report. RCOG Press, London.

Towner, D., Castro, M.A., Eby-Wilkens, E., et al., 1999. Effect of mode of delivery in nulliparous women on neonatal intracranial injury. N Engl J Med 341, 1709–1714.

Trochez, R.D., Sibanda, T., Sharma, R., et al., 2005. Fetal monitoring in labor: are accelerations good enough? J Matern Fetal Neonatal Med 18, 349–352.

Vermillion, S.T., Soper, D.E., Bland, M.L., et al., 2000. Effectiveness of antenatal corticosteroid administration after preterm premature rupture of the membranes. Am J Obstet Gynecol 183, 925–929.

Verspyck, E., Sentilhes, L., 2008. [Abnormal fetal heart rate patterns associated with different labour managements and intrauterine resuscitation techniques]. J Gynecol Obstet Biol Reprod (Paris) 37 (Suppl. 1), S56–S64.

Victory, R., Penava, D., da Silva, O., et al., 2003. Umbilical cord pH and base excess values in relation to neonatal morbidity for infants delivered preterm. Am J Obstet Gynecol 189, 803–807.

Westgate, J., Garibaldi, J.M., Greene, K.R., 1994. Umbilical cord blood gas analysis at delivery: a time for quality data. Br J Obstet Gynaecol 101, 1054–1063.

Whitby, E.H., Griffiths, P.D., Rutter, S., et al., 2004. Frequency and natural history of subdural haemorrhages in babies and relation to obstetric factors. Lancet 363, 846–851.

Zanini, B., Paul, R.H., Huey, J.R., 1980. Intrapartum fetal heart rate: correlation with scalp pH in the preterm fetus. Am J Obstet Gynecol 136, 43–47.

section 3

Care around birth

Resuscitation and transport of the newborn

Colm O'Donnell   Colin J Morley
Steve Kempley   Nandiran Ratnavel

13

CHAPTER CONTENTS

Part 1: **Stabilisation and resuscitation of the newborn**

Colm O'Donnell   Colin J Morley

Many interventions, including pinching, shaking and electrocution, have been used to revive apparently lifeless newborns over the years, with claims for success made for all (Fig. 13.1; O'Donnell et al. 2006a). A series of animal experiments by a group of physiologists led by Geoffrey Dawes in the 1950s and 1960s demonstrated the importance of positive-pressure ventilation (PPV) in neonatal resuscitation (Dawes 1968). In the seminal experiment, a term rhesus monkey was delivered and subjected to an acute and total asphyxial insult (its umbilical cord was ligated and a saline-filled bag placed over its head). The monkey made initial rapid breathing efforts but

© 2012 Elsevier Ltd

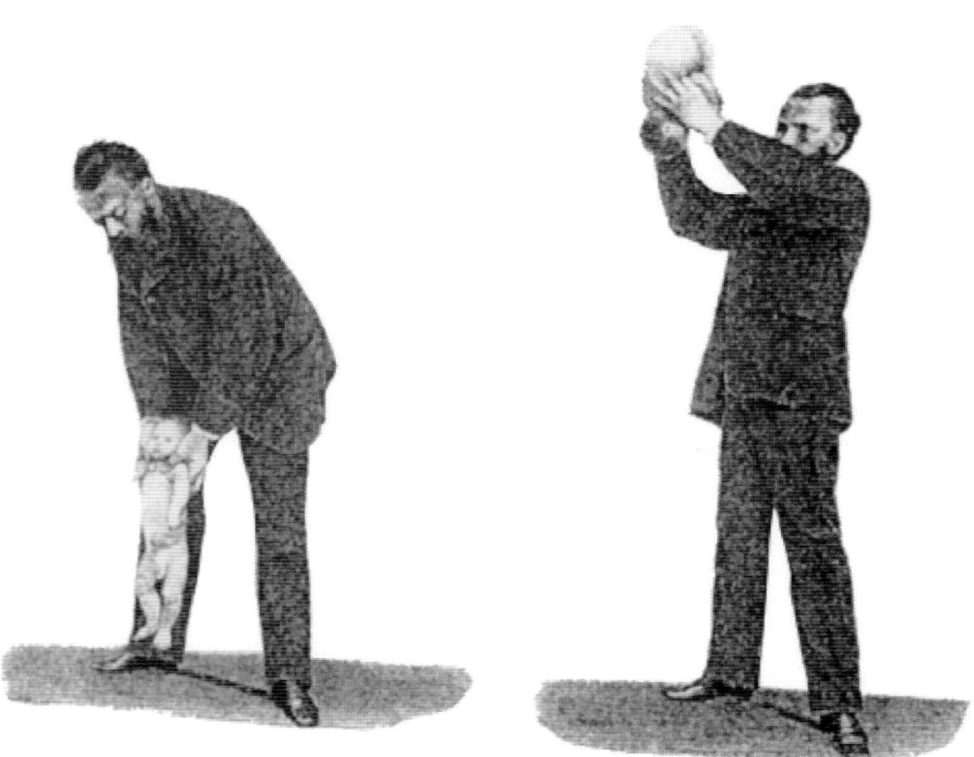

Fig. 13.1 Illustration (reputedly of Dr Bernhard Schultze himself) demonstrating the Schultze method of neonatal resuscitation. *(Reproduced from Schultze (1871).)*

these were ineffective because of the bag. Figure 13.3 is a hand-drawn representation of what was recorded. The heart rate (HR) fell, the animal became more acidaemic and hypotensive and breathing efforts ceased. The animal slid inexorably toward death unless it was revived by endotracheal PPV. This resulted in a prompt increase in HR with recovery in acid–base status and blood pressure and was followed by a return of spontaneous respiration. These studies were responsible for PPV becoming the mainstay of neonatal resuscitation and underpin neonatal resuscitation practice in the delivery room to this day.

Formal courses teaching neonatal resuscitation evolved in the 1980s, notably the Neonatal Resuscitation Program in the USA (Kattwinkel 2006) and the Newborn Life Support Course in the UK (Richmond 2006). These courses taught the causes and physiology of neonatal asphyxia and response to resuscitation described by Dawes. They taught a structured approach to assessing and assisting newborns that was agreed to be 'accepted practice' by 'experts in the field' but based on little hard evidence. Doctors, midwives and nurses have attended these courses in ever-increasing numbers, and attendance at such courses is mandatory for physician training in many countries. In 1996, the International Liaison Committee on Resuscitation (ILCOR), a body representing resuscitation societies around the world, made recommendations for resuscitation of all age groups. The first guidelines to make specific recommendations for newborns were published in 1999 (Kattwinkel et al. 1999). First convened in 2000 (Contributors and Reviewers for the Neonatal Resuscitation Guidelines 2000), the Neonatal Task Force of ILCOR has reconvened at 5-yearly intervals to assess neonatal resuscitation research and update the guidelines accordingly (The International Liaison Committee on Resuscitation 2006; Perlman et al. 2010).

Epidemiology of neonatal resuscitation

It is estimated that up to 10% of newborns receive some help to establish regular breathing at birth, making respiratory support one of the most commonly performed medical interventions (Perlman et al. 2010). The rates of late fetal death, stillbirth, birth asphyxia and perinatal sepsis are higher in developing countries than in developed countries; consequently, term infants are more frequently resuscitated in developing countries. The more immature an infant, the higher the chance that respiratory support after birth will be needed. In developed countries, preterm birth occurs more frequently than birth asphyxia; hence premature infants constitute the majority who receive respiratory support and resuscitation.

The approach to newborn resuscitation

While most babies require either no or minimal resuscitation, it is important to be prepared for babies who may need resuscitation. Ask about the history of the pregnancy and labour, as many easily identifiable features increase the risk that the baby will need help after birth (Box 13.1).

About 25% of depressed babies are undiagnosed before birth. This is why everybody who has the responsibility of caring for a neonate must be trained in basic resuscitation techniques.

Always check the equipment before the baby is born.

Newborns have problems that make respiratory support and resuscitation fundamentally different from other ages:

- Their lungs are full of 'lung liquid' and have never been aerated.

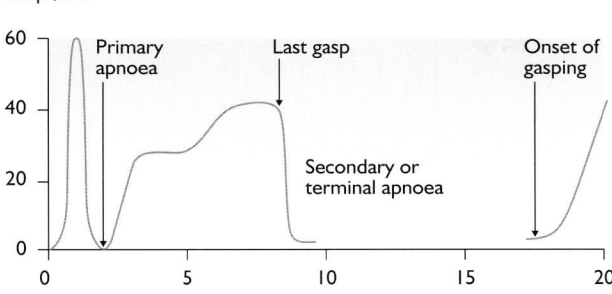

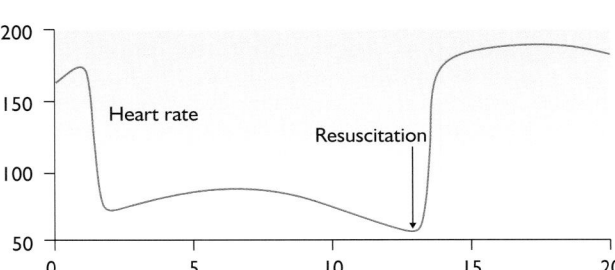

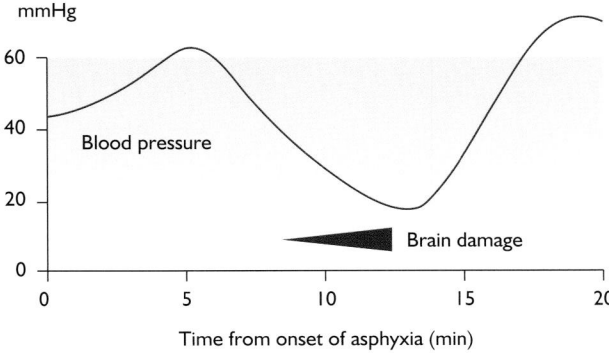

Fig. 13.2 Scheme showing the response of an asphyxiated Rhesus monkey to resuscitation. *(Reproduced from Dawes 1968.)*

Box 13.1 Factors that increase the risk that the baby will need help after birth	
Prematurity	The more immature the baby, the more likely he or she will need help
Antepartum haemorrhage	This is usually mother's blood. However, it can be baby's blood. Rarely, the baby may have exsanguinated (vasa praevia)
	Some fetal haemorrhages are concealed, e.g. fetomaternal, retroplacental or subgaleal (subaponeurotic)
Signs of fetal compromise	Oxygenation of the baby's vital organs may be compromised
Heavily meconium-stained liquor	The baby may be very hypoxic and depressed. He or she may have been gasping in utero and inhaled meconium
Very small-for-dates babies	These babies may not cope with the stress of labour
Maternal general anaesthetic	The baby may not breathe spontaneously
Congenital abnormality affecting the lungs	For example diaphragmatic hernia, cystic adenomatoid malformation. Baby may not breathe effectively
Hydrops fetalis	The chest wall may be oedematous and stiff and pleural effusions and ascites may compromise breathing
Intrauterine infection	The lungs may be stiff with congenital pneumonia
Mechanical factors	Prolapsed cord, difficult forceps delivery, cephalopelvic disproportion, breech delivery, shoulder dystocia, precipitate delivery and prolonged labour all increase the chance of oxygenation being compromised
Prolonged rupture of the membranes >3 weeks	If the membranes have been ruptured with little liquor the lungs may not develop properly and lung hypoplasia can occur
A large baby	The delivery may be difficult

- Preterm infants have a very compliant chest wall that distorts with their inspiratory efforts.
- In the first few minutes the oxygen saturation is lower and they appear cyanosed.

Many adults needing resuscitation do not have a heart beat or breathe adequately, because they have cardiac dysrhythmia caused by an acute coronary event. Circulatory support with chest compressions, cardioversion and/or drugs is the priority when resuscitating adults (Hüpfl et al. 2010). When a baby's heart beat is slow or absent it is due to progressive myocardial acidaemia and hypoxia, not an acute dysrhythmia. The acidaemia and hypoxia cannot be corrected by chest compressions, adrenaline (epinephrine) or cardioversion alone or in combination. In newborns the acidaemia and hypoxia are treated by aerating the fluid-filled lungs and establishing gas exchange. The priority in neonatal resuscitation – even when faced with an absent heart beat – is *always* to provide respiratory support.

Assessment of the newborn

In 1953, an American anaesthetist, Dr Virginia Apgar, proposed a method of evaluating newborns to 'compare the effect of obstetric and anesthetic interventions' (Fig. 13.3). The Apgar score is the sum of values 0–2 assigned for each of five items (breathing, HR, colour, tone and reflex irritability) 1 minute after birth. Later the score was routinely assessed at 5 and 10 minutes of life. At the outset, Apgar stated that each element of the score was not of equal importance, but thought that weighting the score would make it cumbersome and less likely to be applied (Apgar 1953). She believed the score

Current Researches in Anesthesia and Analgesia—July-August, 1953

A Proposal for a New Method of Evaluation of the Newborn Infant.*

Virginia Apgar, M.D., New York, N. Y.

Department of Anesthesiology, Columbia University, College of Physicians and Surgeons and the Anesthesia Service, The Presbyterian Hospital

 RESUSCITATION OF INFANTS at birth has been the subject of many articles. Seldom have there been such imaginative ideas, such enthusiasms, and dislikes, and such unscientific observations and study about one clinical picture. There are outstanding exceptions to these statements, but the poor quality and lack of precise data of the majority of papers concerned with infant resuscitation are interesting.

There are several excellent review articles[1][2] but the main emphasis in the past has been on treatment of the asphyxiated or apneic newborn infant. The purpose of this paper is the reestablishment of simple, clear classification or "grading" of newborn infants which can be used as a basis for discussion and comparison of the results of obstetric practices, types of maternal pain relief and the effects of resuscitation.

The principle of giving a "score" to a patient as a sum total of several objective findings is not new and has been used recently in judging the treatment of drug addiction.[3] The endpoints which have been used previously in the field of resuscitation are "breathing time" defined as the time from delivery of the head to the first respiration, and "crying time" the time until the establishment of a satisfactory cry.[4] Other workers have used the terms mild, moderate and severe depression[5] to signify the state of the infant. There are valid objections to these systems. When mothers receive an excessive amount of depressant drugs in the antepartum period, it is a common occurence that the infants breathe once, then become apneic for many minutes. Evaluation of the breathing time is difficult. A satisfactory cry is sometimes not established even when the infant leaves the delivery room, and in some patients with cerebral injury, the baby dies without ever having uttered a satisfactory cry. Mild, moderate and severe depression of the infant leaves a fair margin for individual interpretation.

A list was made of all the objective signs which pertained in any way to the condition of the infant at birth. Of these, five signs which could be determined easily and without interfering with the care of the infant were considered useful. A rating of zero, one or two, was given to each sign depending on whether it was absent or present. A score of ten indicated a baby in the best possible condition. The time for judging the five objective signs was varied until the most practi-

*Presented before the Twenty-Seventh Annual Congress of Anesthetists, Joint Meeting of the International Anesthesia Research Society and the International College of Anesthetists, Virginia Beach, Va., September 22-25, 1952.

Fig. 13.3 Dr Virginia Apgar's original paper describing her method for evaluating newborns. *(Reproduced from Apgar 1953.)*

would be useful for comparing populations of infants but that it would be neither sensitive nor specific enough to prognosticate in individual infants (Apgar 1966). In the early 1950s, newborns were largely ignored in the delivery room (Apgar remarked at the time that 'surely nine months' observation of the mother merits one minute's observation of the baby'; Apgar 1966). The Apgar score was hugely important in drawing attention to infants in the delivery room and, more than 50 years later, it is still universally recorded.

The Apgar score is now used for purposes for which it was not intended. Although persistently low Apgar scores are associated with poor neurological outcome in populations, the predictive value of low Apgar scores for individual infants is poor (O'Donnell et al. 2006b). It is relatively easy to calculate the Apgar score for healthy infants but there is disagreement on how to score premature infants and those receiving respiratory support (Lopiore et al. 2004). As the Apgar score is subjective there is considerable interobserver variability in how scores are assigned, which makes it somewhat inaccurate (O'Donnell et al. 2006b).

Muscle tone

In adults and older children, tone is assessed by examining passive resistance to movement of the limbs over one or more joints for a

minute or more. In contrast, a newborn's tone is assessed in seconds by observing posture and movements. Tone is the first sign that can be evaluated. Though the quality of an infant's tone is subjective and varies with gestational age, it is an important and frequently underrated sign. Healthy newborns have a flexed posture that is most notable at the hips, knees and elbows (Ch. 40.1); the degree of flexion increases with maturity. Whatever the gestation, a baby with flexed posture or who is moving the limbs has reasonable tone and is not seriously asphyxiated. Clinicians presented with a baby with a flexed posture can thus be reassured and proceed with less haste. A baby who is limp is more likely to be in poor condition and needs immediate close attention.

Spontaneous breathing

For such a fundamental act it is surprising how little is known about how babies begin to breathe after birth. Many infants, even the most immature, cry shortly after delivery. Others may not cry but breathe independently, albeit irregularly, at birth. Breathing movements in babies may be subtle and movement of the abdomen, due to diaphragmatic contraction, is often more easily seen than chest excursion. The majority of newly born very premature babies breathe at birth. MacDonald et al. (1980) reported that 72% of babies of 27–28 weeks' gestation, born in the early 1970s, had sustained breathing at 1 minute of age without PPV. Among infants <28 weeks born in the modern era, about 70% cry and 80% breathe spontaneously after birth (O'Donnell et al. 2010).

Relatively little is known about the nature of the initial breathing. Karlberg et al. (1962) reported that among 18 well term newborns the time of onset of breathing varied from 3 to 80 seconds; the inspired tidal volume varied from 12 to 67 mL (approximately 3.5–14.7 mL/kg), and they often used a negative pressure up to 70 cmH$_2$O. te Pas et al. (2009b) described patterns of breathing where preterm and term infants take quick large inspirations, followed by prolonged expiration, usually achieved by crying or laryngeal adduction, associated with contraction of the abdominal muscles causing a high intrathoracic pressure during most of expiration. The presumption is that this 'expiratory braking' helps to establish and maintain a functional residual capacity (FRC). A baby's respiratory efforts are rarely directly measured during neonatal resuscitation and the efficacy of breathing is largely judged by its effect on the infant's HR. An infant's breathing efforts must be sufficient to ensure a HR >100 beats per minute (bpm) (Contributors and Reviewers for the Neonatal Resuscitation Guidelines 2000).

Breathing difficulty may present at or shortly after birth. Many of the signs – intercostal, subcostal and sternal recession – are due to the powerful diaphragm exerting its influence on the newborn's pliable thoracic cage as it tries to draw air into relatively stiff (poorly compliant) lungs. Expiratory grunting during expiration has long been recognised as a sign of respiratory difficulty. Harrison et al. reported in 1968 that when infants who were grunting were intubated the grunting ceased; however, the oxygen in their arterial blood (Pao_2) fell. When the endotracheal tube (ETT) was removed, grunting resumed and the Pao_2 increased. This demonstrated that grunting is a mechanism infants use to preserve their lung volume and create an FRC by generating positive end-expiratory pressure (PEEP) by partially closing their larynx during a forced expiration (see PEEP below).

Heart rate

HR is the most sensitive indicator of a newborn's condition and it increases rapidly in bradycardic infants with effective resuscitation

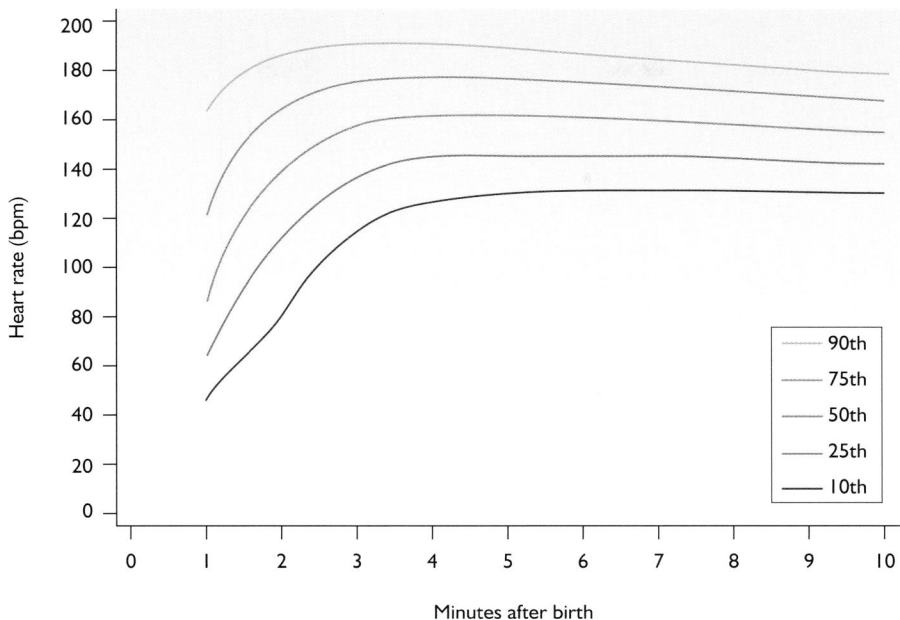

Fig. 13.4 Centiles showing heart rate measured with a pulse oximeter of infants who were not resuscitated at birth. *(Reproduced from Dawson et al. (2010a).)*

(Fig. 13.3). Clinically, HR is best determined by listening to the chest with a stethoscope (auscultation). The number of beats in 6 seconds is multiplied by 10 to give the HR in bpm (Kattwinkel 2006). A short interval – far shorter than the 15–60 seconds used to count HR in older children or adults – is thought necessary because the HR is more rapid and changes quickly in newborns. This has the disadvantage that errors are increased 10-fold and so can be inaccurate (Kamlin et al. 2006). The HR can sometimes be counted by feeling umbilical cord pulsations, but, as they are often impalpable, auscultation is superior to cord palpation, which is no longer recommended. Neither provides information readily available to the resuscitation team, leading to some advocating that the person listening to the HR 'tap it out' with a finger as a visual cue. Resuscitative efforts may be interrupted to allow the HR to be determined by auscultation, which is not ideal. It is taught that the HR should be counted every 30 seconds. However, this does not enable a dynamic assessment of the HR changes. Many of these problems may be addressed by using a pulse oximeter (see below), which is now recommended by ILCOR (Perlman et al. 2010).

It is taught that an infant's HR should be >100 bpm after birth; that respiratory support should be given if the HR is <100 bpm; and that chest compression should also be given if the HR is <60 bpm (Kattwinkel 2006). In reality, well term newborns who are not resuscitated frequently have a HR <100 bpm in the first 2 minutes after birth, which rapidly increases with time (Fig. 13.4; Dawson et al. 2010a). For babies who have reasonable tone and who are crying or making breathing efforts, HR <100 bpm on its own is not an indication for intervention. However, if a baby is limp, not breathing and the HR is <100 bpm, PPV is needed. If the HR does not increase promptly, the most likely reason is that the PPV is ineffective. Before chest compression is started, it is imperative that ventilation is optimised. If the baby remains bradycardic despite ventilation with PEEP (see later) moving the chest, then chest compressions should be given. However, the most likely reason for

continued bradycardia is that the respiratory support is inadequate (Perlman and Risser 1995).

Colour

Compared with adults, children and older infants, the fetus has low Pao_2 (~2–3 kPa) and oxygen saturation of haemoglobin in arterial blood (Sao_2, ~50%); hence newborns appear cyanosed immediately after birth. As they aerate their lungs and establish gas exchange, the peripheral oxygen saturation (Spo_2) increases over the next few minutes and they look increasingly pink. They first look pink centrally – i.e. their tongue, lips, face and torso – while their peripheries (arms and legs) become pink later. There is substantial interobserver variability in the determination of pinkness and this determination correlates poorly with zan infant's Spo_2 (O'Donnell et al. 2007). It takes normal newborns several minutes to achieve an Spo_2 >90% (Fig. 13.5; Dawson et al. 2010b). It is less important to decide whether or not an infant is pink than to determine oxygenation is improving (becoming 'pinker') with time. In the minutes after birth, the oxygenation of a baby receiving respiratory assistance is best measured using a pulse oximeter with the sensor on the right wrist (see below).

Occasionally babies are born very pale. These babies are usually also limp and bradycardic. This sickly yellowish colour signifies poor circulation and acidosis. These babies must be resuscitated without delay, and help will be required. Even more rarely, babies are born a ghostly, milky-white colour. These infants may have better tone and be more responsive than one would expect for an asphyxiated infant. Despite adequate PPV some have bradycardia that responds quickly to infusion of volume. These babies may have had an acute haemorrhage, which is usually heralded by a large antepartum haemorrhage (e.g. placental abruption, vasa praevia), but may be concealed because it was due to a fetomaternal haemorrhage. These babies may require urgent blood transfusion,

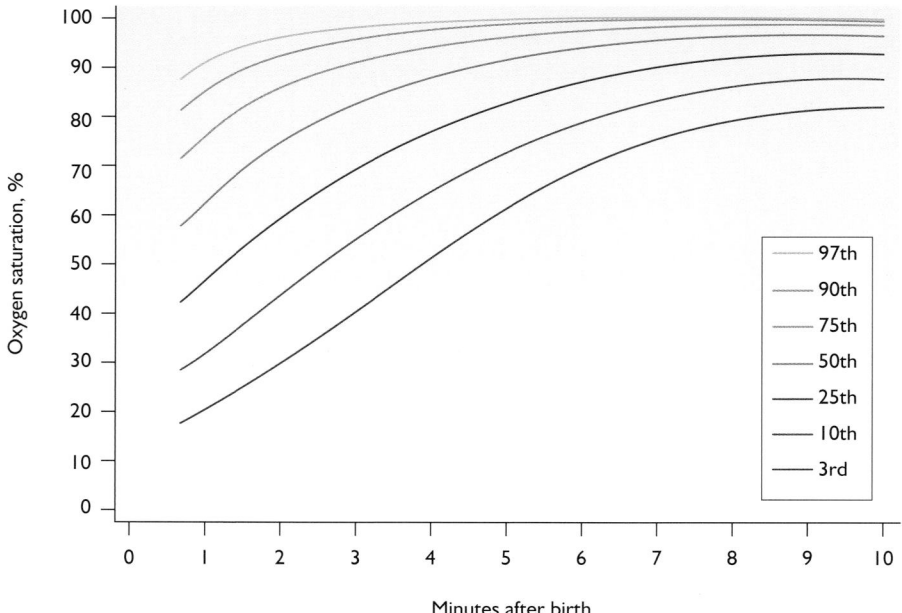

Fig. 13.5 Centiles showing oxygen saturation measured with a pulse oximeter of infants who were not resuscitated at birth. *(Reproduced from Dawson et al. 2010b.)*

and on occasion a transfusion of uncrossmatched O-negative blood in the delivery room can be life-saving.

Pulse oximetry

A pulse oximeter measures both HR and Sp_{O_2} using a sensor that has a light-emitting diode and a detector placed in opposition around a baby's hand or foot. See Chapter 19 for more information on this method of monitoring.

When placed preductally (on the right wrist) oximeters can give data about 20 seconds after the sensor has been applied correctly. If placed immediately after birth a signal can usually be obtained by 90 seconds (O'Donnell et al. 2005a). Pulse oximeters count the HR more accurately than clinicians listening with a stethoscope or feeling the umbilical cord (Kamlin et al. 2006). In addition, the HR is counted accurately (Kamlin et al. 2008) and displayed continuously, non-invasively and without the need for resuscitation to be interrupted. Fuelled by uncertainty about using oxygen during neonatal resuscitation, pulse oximeters in the delivery room are now advocated by ILCOR (Perlman et al. 2010).

Interpreting the changing Sp_{O_2} data immediately after birth requires knowledge of the normal changes with time. The preductal Sp_{O_2} of newborns who do not need resuscitation has a wide range and increases during the first 10 minutes. At 1 minute the median (10th and 90th centiles) is 66% (33%, 85%), at 5 minutes it is 89% (72%, 97%), and at 10 minutes it is 96% (87%, 99%) (Fig. 13.5; Dawson et al. 2010b). Babies born prematurely or by caesarean section (CS) have lower Sp_{O_2} than those born vaginally at term and it increases more slowly. The appropriate Sp_{O_2} for an infant at any given time – or more pertinently, the value which suggests that the Sp_{O_2} is too low and O_2 should be given – is not yet clear. The recent publication of centile charts (Fig. 13.5) has been very helpful in illustrating the normal range for babies who did not require resuscitation (Dawson et al. 2010b). The appropriate inspired oxygen for infants (particularly preterm) who receive respiratory support at birth is still being investigated. We suggest a target is to keep the Sp_{O_2} >10th centile and <90th centile targets. There is good evidence

from animal studies that hypoxia on its own does not cause brain damage. Hypoxia with hypotension and bradycardia is potentially damaging.

Techniques of resuscitation

Delivery-room stabilisation and resuscitation comprise interventions to minimise the infant's heat loss, and provide respiratory and circulation support, as determined by ongoing assessment of their clinical condition. Measures are taken to reduce heat loss for all babies. Respiratory support is the key to neonatal resuscitation and is always the priority for infants in poor condition at birth. Circulatory support is rarely needed (Wyckoff et al. 2005).

Figure 13.6 shows the ILCOR algorithm, on which most other algorithms are based.

Thermoregulation

Hypothermia can cause respiratory compromise, acidosis, circulatory collapse and death in newborns of any gestation. It is of particular concern for premature babies who have less insulation (body fat) and bulk (energy stores) and are more skinny (greater body surface area:body mass ratio) than their term counterparts. Maintaining the body temperature of preterm infants in 'the thermoneutral zone' (36–37°C, the range in which the infant's metabolic demands were least) substantially reduced mortality, and remains a key plank of neonatal care (Ch. 15) (Silverman and Sinclair 1966).

Though less common than hypothermia, there is an association between hyperthermia after birth and poor neurodevelopmental outcome. Whether this is because hyperthermia is largely due to chorioamnionitis, itself associated with adverse neurological outcomes, or because there is an independent effect of high temperature is unclear.

Therapeutic hypothermia for term babies with a recent hypoxic–ischaemic insult is an effective therapy which is discussed in

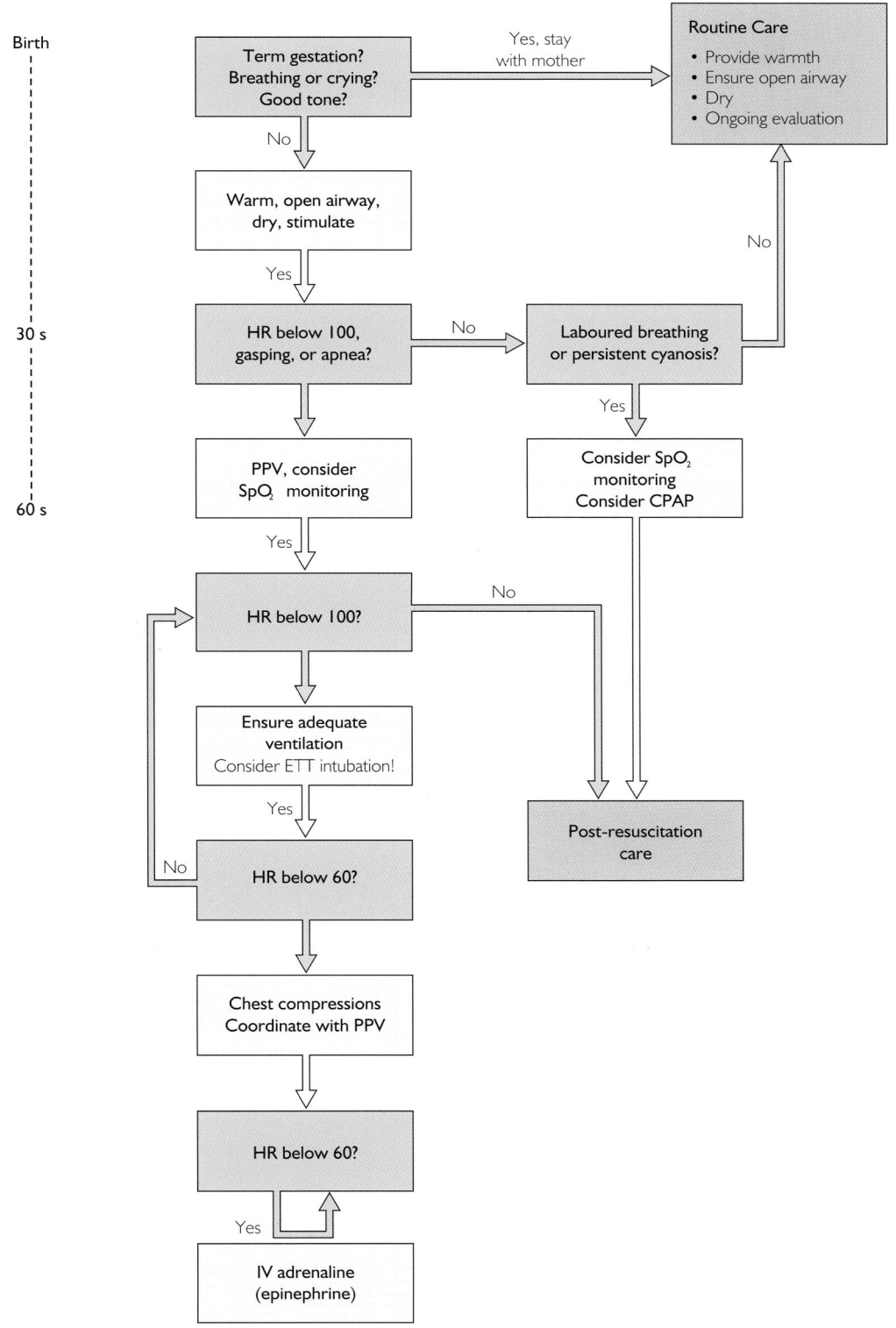

Fig. 13.6 Adapted from International Liaison Committee on Resuscitation algorithm for resuscitation. CPAP, continuous positive airway pressure; ETT, endotracheal tube; HR, heart rate; PPV, positive-pressure ventilation.

Chapter 40, part 4 (Jacobs et al. 2007). If a baby is born who is likely to fit the criteria for treatment with therapeutic hypothermia, i.e. apnoeic, requiring respiratory support through an ETT at 10 minutes, low pH of cord blood, it is reasonable to turn off external heat sources (e.g. radiant warmers) to allow the infant to cool passively. However, the baby's temperature must be closely monitored as it is surprisingly easy to cool these infants more than to the intended level of 33.5 °C.

Strategies to keep newborns in the thermoneutral range usually combine measures to provide heat and to reduce heat loss. The simplest external heat source is the mother's body. Babies may be placed directly (skin to skin) on the mother's chest and covered with a blanket or towel.

To minimise heat loss, babies should be delivered in a warm room (the World Health Organization recommends 25 °C). Evaporative heat loss is a particular concern for all newborns as they are naked and wet at birth (Ch. 15). Term babies should be dried and covered with a hat. If there is concern about keeping a baby warm, heated blankets or a radiant heat source can be used. In general these measures are adequate for term babies. However, despite these measures, hypothermia on admission to the neonatal intensive care unit (NICU) was common among extremely preterm babies in the UK in the mid-1990s (40% of infants <26 weeks <35 °C) and the risk of death and disability was increased among these infants (Costeloe et al. 2000). Several randomised trials have examined the effect of placing very premature babies, directly after birth, in clear plastic (food-grade polyethylene) bags without first drying them. These showed significant increases in temperature on admission to the NICU (Vohra et al. 1999, 2004). Polyethylene wrapping exploits a simple principle – light in the infrared spectrum (i.e. heat) is admitted through the polyethylene, while evaporative heat loss is reduced (impressive misting is seen on the inside of the wrap). Polyethylene wrapping has been recommended for reducing hypothermia among preterm infants (Perlman et al. 2010). It is worth noting, however, that overheating is possible, so it is prudent to check the baby's temperature if he or she remains under radiant heat in a plastic bag for protracted periods. More recently, Trevisanuto et al. (2010) demonstrated that a polyethylene cap was as effective as polyethylene wrapping and both were more effective than drying for preventing hypothermia in preterm infants placed under radiant heat. Exothermic mattresses are used as a heat source to prevent hypothermia in preterm infants. The effect of any of these interventions – polyethylene bags, polyethylene caps and exothermic mattresses – in combination is unclear.

Airway management

Compared with humans of other ages, newborns have relatively large heads and floppy airways. Though babies with respiratory difficulty are often placed prone in the nursery to improve their breathing, it is recommended that, immediately after birth, infants are placed supine on a firm surface (Kattwinkel 2006), although this is not evidence-based. It is recommended that the head is held in a 'neutral' (neither flexed nor extended) or 'sniffing' position; and, if the infant is not breathing, that 'jaw thrust' – gently pushing the baby's mandible forward with fingers placed behind the angles of the jaw – is used as a means of opening the airway (Kattwinkel 2006; Richmond 2006). When attempting to maintain an open airway during spontaneous breathing or respiratory support, try not to press on the soft tissues under the chin as this may predispose to airway obstruction by the tongue.

Newborns are frequently suctioned because clear fluid comes from their mouths. Fetal lungs are filled with liquid. Production of lung liquid ceases during labour and infants expel the liquid from the airways and reabsorb it from the lungs after birth. It is normal for clear fluid to well up from the trachea and appear in the oropharynx. There is no evidence that routine suction of the airways after birth aids a baby's breathing. The use of a standard suction catheter vaguely poked into a baby's mouth will not clear blood clots or pieces of meconium. Blindly suctioning the naso- and oropharynx of well infants with a suction catheter may cause harm by inducing vagally mediated bradycardia, laryngospasm or local trauma and should be avoided. If blood or meconium is thought to be obstructing the airways it should be removed under direct vision, using a laryngoscope and a large suction catheter. Complete airway obstruction is rarely a cause of collapse in newborns, and, when it does occur, the obstruction is usually due to an anatomical anomaly (e.g. large cystic hygroma, tracheal agenesis) that is not remediable by suction. Suction may be needed if fluid or meconium obscures the view when attempting endotracheal intubation.

Suction may be indicated when a non-vigorous infant is delivered through meconium-stained liquor (see Special circumstances, meconium-stained liquor, below).

Oropharyngeal (Guedel) airways have previously been recommended for use in newborns. These were developed for adults with depressed consciousness. While models for term babies are available, they are not suitable for very preterm infants. Studies of their use in newborns have not been reported. Laryngeal masks have been used for near-term infants with upper airway anomalies. Infants with the Pierre Robin sequence have very small chins (micrognathia). When these infants are placed supine, the tongue may obstruct the airway (glossoptosis). These infants should be nursed prone to help reduce the obstruction. Should this prove ineffective, a nasopharyngeal airway should be used. This may be a specifically designed device or an ETT of diameter appropriate for the infant's weight shortened to the distance from the infant's nose to the angle of the mandible. The aim of these devices is to maintain airway patency by relieving tongue obstruction.

Respiratory support

At birth, placental support is removed and the newborn must use the lungs to exchange gas. To do so effectively, the lung fluid must be rapidly cleared, air must enter the lungs and the blood flow through their lungs must increase. Gas exchange is a continuous process, with oxygen and carbon dioxide diffusing across pulmonary capillary membranes throughout the respiratory cycle, whether the baby is breathing in or out. For this to occur it is critical that the infant has an adequate volume of gas in the lungs at the end of expiration, i.e. an FRC. Mechanical stretching as gas enters and is retained within the lung and increased oxygen tension in the alveoli provoke profound vasodilation in the pulmonary vascular bed. The consequent drop in the pulmonary blood pressure results in a large increase in pulmonary blood flow, which allows gas exchange to occur. These physiological changes are most commonly achieved by spontaneous breathing. Occasionally infants are apnoeic or breathe inadequately. The key to successful stabilisation or resuscitation is to establish effective ventilation.

The aim of respiratory support is to assist spontaneous breathing with continuous positive airway pressure (CPAP) through a mask or nasal prongs, or, if the baby is apnoeic, give PPV with a face mask, through nasal prongs or an ETT.

It is critical for effective gas exchange that newborns quickly achieve and maintain an FRC. The key determinant of FRC in ventilated infants is the mean airway pressure (MAP). MAP is determined mainly by the CPAP or PEEP as it is applied for about two-thirds of the respiratory cycle. The peak inflating pressure (PIP) also affects MAP, but to a lesser extent than PEEP, as it is applied for about one-third of the respiratory cycle.

For adequate gas exchange babies need to breathe in and out a tidal volume (V_T) of gas of ~4–8 mL/kg body weight. The V_T that enters the lung is determined principally by the spontaneous inspiratory effort and to a lesser extent by the PIP during PPV. See Chapter 27 part 1 for more information on respiratory physiology.

Expired air ventilation

Mouth to mouth, or more often mouth to mouth and nose, assisted ventilation was advocated in early resuscitation guidelines. It was recommended that resuscitators placed their mouth around the mouth, or mouth and nose, of apnoeic newborns and breathe into the baby sufficient to produce a gentle rise of the baby's chest. Tonkin et al. (1995) demonstrated that most mothers' mouths are not large enough to encircle their infant's mouth and nose, and speculated that mouth to nose resuscitation may be a better alternative. No human studies of any of these techniques have been reported and they are rarely used in developed countries, where manual ventilation devices are available. In places where manual ventilation devices are not available, mouth to mask resuscitation, rather than mouth to mouth/nose, is recommended to reduce the risks of transmitting infections (Perlman et al. 2010).

Continuous positive airway pressure

Most babies, even the most immature, breathe or cry at birth (O'Donnell et al. 2010). If they are very preterm or have obvious respiratory difficulty, with marked sternal recession or irregular breathing, it is important to help them quickly aerate their lungs and facilitate early gas exchange. This is done by providing CPAP as soon as they start breathing. CPAP aids lung aeration, lung fluid clearance and the formation of an FRC and improves oxygenation. CPAP can be given through a face mask or nasal prongs attached to a T-piece device. The pressure should be no less than 5 cmH$_2$O and immediately after birth, while the lung fluid is being cleared, a pressure up to 8 cmH$_2$O may help. Self-inflating bags (SIBs) and flow-inflating bags (FIBs) cannot be used to provide consistent CPAP.

Aerating the lung and forming an FRC are the most important first steps in any resuscitation. Because this improves gas exchange it should be used before the inspired oxygen is increased. Treating a baby with supplementary oxygen will not be effective if the lung volume is very low. Several randomised controlled trials, enrolling very preterm infants, have shown that early CPAP is very effective for at least half the babies who do not require intubation ventilation or surfactant and have an outcome that is at least as good as babies who are routinely intubated at birth (Morley et al 2008; SUPPORT Study Group 2010).

Positive-pressure ventilation

PPV is indicated from birth if the infant is apnoeic. In general, PPV is started with a face mask. Mask ventilation is usually only needed for a few minutes. Most infants who receive mask ventilation subsequently breathe. Those who do not breathe should be intubated and ventilated.

Face masks

Face masks are the interface most commonly used to give PPV to newborns. While there are few studies to determine which type of mask is superior, round silicone masks with a cushioned rim are the most commonly used model (O'Donnell et al. 2004). Round masks are better than Rendell-Baker masks (solid triangular masks without a rim that were developed for inhalational anaesthesia) (Palme et al. 1985). Face masks should encircle the infant's mouth and nose, but not encroach on the eyes (Kattwinkel 2006); and different sizes are available. During inflations, in mannikin studies (O'Donnell et al. 2005b, c; Wood et al. 2008a, b; Tracy et al. 2011) and in infants during resuscitation (Schmölzer et al. 2010) there are gas leaks from face masks which are often large and variable and can interfere with effective resuscitation.

The way the mask is positioned and held is important (Wood et al. 2008b). With a round Laerdal-type face mask it is important to use the two-finger-top hold with chin lift. The mask is rolled on to the face from the chin and held in place with the thumb and first finger placed either side of the stem, exerting an even pressure vertically downwards. The second and third fingers are placed under the mandible and pull the jaw upwards with an equal pressure to the downward force on the mask. This can be learned by good education and practice (Wood et al. 2008b). The mask must not be held around the rim as this can cause it to kink and leak badly. If ventilation is still is not effective a good seal may be obtained with a two-handed technique to hold the mask in position and a second person doing the inflations (Tracy et al. 2011). While tidal volumes adequate for gas exchange are often not delivered to infants during mask PPV (Milner et al. 1984), it may be sufficient to stimulate the baby to breathe spontaneously.

Airway obstruction occurs during mask ventilation (Finer et al. 2009; Schmölzer et al. 2011). When babies do not respond to mask ventilation, measures should be taken to ensure the airway is patent (e.g. checking the mask position and hold, repositioning the head, jaw thrust, suctioning the airway) and that enough PIP is being used before continuing with mask ventilation. Infants who still do not respond to mask ventilation with a pressure of 30 cmH$_2$O should be intubated for further PPV (Perlman et al. 2010).

Nasal airways

Infants are primarily nose breathers. Though CPAP is often given to preterm infants via nasal prongs for prolonged periods in the neonatal nursery, respiratory support is less frequently given to newborns with nasal prongs in the delivery room. The use of a nasal tube (an ETT of appropriate internal diameter shortened to ~5 cm; also known as a nasopharyngeal tube, single nasal prong, short tube) in preference to a face mask for preterm infants was associated with a halving in the rate of intubation in the delivery room in a retrospective cohort study (Lindner et al. 1999) and with a reduction in the rate of mechanical ventilation within 72 hours in a randomised trial (te Pas and Walther 2007). As the nasal tube was only one of a number of differences in the treatment of the groups in both studies, it is difficult to determine the contribution of the nasal tube to the differences in outcomes observed between the groups.

If a short nasal tube is used, it is important that it is placed in the nostril at right angles to the face and angled back over the soft palate. Nasal tubes should not be pushed up the nose (caudally) as they can pierce the cribriform plate and cause brain injury. Binasal cannulae were superior to the seldom-used Rendell-Baker face mask in a randomised trial enrolling term and near-term infants (Capasso et al. 2005). Studies comparing nasal airways to face masks for respiratory support in the delivery room are ongoing.

Laryngeal mask airway

Laryngeal mask airways (LMAs) were developed as an alternative to ETTs to support the breathing of adults undergoing short periods of general anaesthesia. They are designed to fit over the laryngeal inlet and can be placed quickly without the need for a laryngoscope. Once inserted, a cushioned rim is inflated to achieve a seal. LMAs offer a more stable airway than a face mask and are easier to place correctly than ETTs, even by relatively inexperienced operators. They were designed to be used with patients with normally compliant lungs, not with the stiff lungs frequently encountered in newborns. The use of LMAs has been reported in case series of term infants (Gandini and Brimacombe 1999a) and in small numbers of moderately preterm infants (Gandini and Brimacombe 1999b). The use of LMAs in newborns is limited, at least in part owing to the lack of sizes small enough for infants weighing less than 2 kg, who constitute the majority of infants being resuscitated. Successful use of LMAs in the setting of upper airway anomalies has been reported (Gandini and Brimacombe 2003). It may thus be prudent to have a neonatal LMA available for use in exceptional circumstances and for people to be trained in its use.

Endotracheal tubes

When infants fail to respond to PPV by face mask, or are judged to need ongoing respiratory support, they should be intubated and ventilated. ETTs used in newborns are sterile, single-use plastic tubes with a uniform diameter. In contrast to those used for children and adults, ETTs for newborns do not have an inflatable cuff. 'Shouldered' Cole's ETTs – tubes with a narrow distal diameter that passes through the vocal cords, and a wider proximal diameter – are now rarely used. ETTs are sized by their internal diameter, with the appropriate size determined by the weight or gestation of the infant (2.5 mm for infants <1000g / ≤27 weeks; 3.0 mm for 1–2 kg/28–36 weeks; 3.5 mm for >2 kg/near term). They are usually marked at 1-cm intervals from the tip and have a black line that acts as a guide to insertion depth. The insertion depth is often determined by the infant's weight (depth of insertion at lips for oral ETTs (cm) = 6 + (infant's weight in kg), e.g. for a 1.5-kg baby, approximate depth of insertion = 7.5 cm at the lips); or may be more accurately estimated from the gestational age (Table 13.1; Kempley et al. 2008).

Intubation technique

ETTs are passed through an infant's vocal cords into the trachea under direct vision using the light from a laryngoscope placed in the mouth. ETTs may be introduced through either the mouth or

Table 13.1 Oral tracheal tube lengths by gestation

GESTATION (WEEKS)	TRACHEAL TUBE AT LIPS (CM)
23–24	5.5
25–26	6.0
27–29	6.5
30–32	7.0
33–34	7.5
35–37	8.0
38–40	8.5
41–43	9.0

(Reproduced from Kempley et al. (2008)).

nose (Ch. 44) but oral intubation is generally used at resuscitation. Laryngoscopes are designed to be held in the left hand (irrespective of the handedness of the user) and consist of a handle, a blade set at right angles to the handle and a light mounted on the blade. Before attempting intubation, ensure that the light is adequately bright.

The most important part of the laryngoscope is the blade. The laryngoscope blades used in newborns are usually straight (occasionally curved) and come in different sizes, with suitability determined by the size of the infant (size 00 for infants <1 kg, 0 for infants 1–3 kg, 1 for infants >3 kg). It is critical that the blade chosen is long enough. If it is too short to reach the epiglottis, you will not be able to see the vocal cords and will not successfully intubate the baby. The objective is to insert the blade into the mouth, to advance it to the epiglottis, to place the tip in the vollecula, and to lift up the epiglottis gently to see the larynx. Hold the laryngoscope towards the left side of the mouth and ensure that the tongue is out of the way to give enough room to see past it and insert the ETT. Once in position, the laryngoscope should be gently raised, i.e. lifted in the plane of the laryngoscope's handle, not pivoted backwards using the upper gum as a fulcrum (the function of the handle is to hold the batteries, not to act as a lever). Wait until the vocal cords open – do not attempt to force the tube through adducted cords – and then advance the ETT until the top of the black line is still seen. If the larynx is difficult to see, press it down with your left little finger or ask someone else to press it down. Once the ETT is in place, hold it with the thumb and index finger of the right hand and curl the other fingers round the baby's face to keep the ETT in position. *Don't let go* for any reason until it is firmly secured in position.

Once an ETT has been passed, the operator must confirm that it is correctly placed in the trachea. This has been traditionally done using clinical signs. The most sensitive indicator is the HR, which increases promptly in bradycardic infants given PPV through a correctly placed ETT. Other signs sought to confirm correct placement are air entry audible with a stethoscope over both hemithoraces; appearance of condensation on the inside of the ETT during expiration ('misting') and visible chest rise (Kattwinkel 2006). All of these signs are subjective and their sensitivity and specificity are difficult to determine. In preterm infants in particular, air movement can be heard widely throughout the chest even if the ETT is in the oesophagus. Also, if the chest of a preterm newborn can easily be seen to move with PPV, it is likely that the lungs are being overdistended.

ILCOR recommends using colorimetric exhaled CO_2 detectors after each intubation to confirm ETT placement (Perlman et al. 2010). These devices are placed between the ETT and the ventilation device and change colour from purple to yellow in the presence of exhaled CO_2. They identify correctly placed ETTs much quicker than clinical assessment alone (Aziz et al. 1999). If the detector does not change colour, the most common reason is that the ETT is not in the trachea. However, a detector may not change colour during PPV through a correctly placed ETT if the infant's lungs are poorly compliant with little/no tidal volume moving because the PIP is too low to inflate the lungs (Kamlin et al. 2005), or if there is cardiac arrest and no circulation in the lungs (Aziz et al. 1999).

Once it is confirmed that the ETT is in the trachea, an appropriate depth of insertion should be rechecked (see above). The tube should then be firmly secured. The position should be checked with a chest X-ray, the aim being to have the ETT tip beneath the vocal cords and above the carina (approximately T1–T4).

Intubation is an important skill that may be difficult to acquire. Babies are being intubated less frequently and doctors in training have shorter working hours than before. As a result trainees are getting fewer opportunities to master the skill (Leone et al. 2005). It has been recommended that infants should be intubated within 20 seconds (Kattwinkel 2006). However, it often takes considerably longer (Lane et al. 2004; O'Donnell 2006). The success rate of doctors attempting intubation in the delivery room is about 50% (O'Donnell 2006). Intubation has many unwanted effects, both in the short term (failure, bradycardia, hypoxia, raised intracranial pressure, mouth, laryngeal or tracheal injury) and longer term (subglottic stenosis, chronic lung disease). In contrast to infants in NICU, newborns in the delivery room do not receive premedication before intubation. This may make delivery room intubation more difficult and probably increases the occurrence of short-term side-effects. Plastic ETTs become pliable when warm so they should not be placed under the radiant heater. Some operators use introducers (or stylets) – sterile plastic-coated wires placed in the ETT lumen to make it more rigid – when attempting intubation. Tracheal injury has been reported from introducers and correctly placed ETTs may be accidentally dislodged when removing the introducer. A randomised trial did not show any difference in the rate of successful intubation by groups of trainees when an introducer was used (O'Connell and Kamlin). If introducers are used, they must not protrude beyond the end of the ETT. A fresh ETT should be available for each potential intubation, as ETTs that are opened and not immediately used become colonised with bacteria (Walsh et al. 2008).

Achieving an airway is of critical importance. However, intubation by itself does not save lives; it is the effectiveness of the ventilation that counts.

Ventilation devices

Mechanical ventilators are used to give infants PPV in the NICU. These give inflations with a duration (T_i), PIP, PEEP and frequency (rate) that are set and controlled by the machine. Most modern ventilators incorporate a flow sensor that measures the tidal volumes of gas entering and leaving the ETT. Mechanical ventilators are, however, rarely used in the delivery room. Instead, manual ventilation devices are generally used. Different types of devices are available, each with different characteristics. The operator controls the parameters that are usually set on a mechanical ventilator. No manual ventilation device incorporates a flow sensor.

Self-inflating bags

The SIB is the most commonly used device (O'Donnell et al. 2004). It does not need a compressed gas source to function, though one is often attached to allow supplemental oxygen to be delivered. SIBs come in a variety of sizes, including those designed for newborns (240–500 ml).

The PIP delivered with a SIB is determined by how hard the bag is squeezed. It is not usually measured, though a manometer may be added to the circuit. SIBs usually have a pressure-limiting 'pop-off' valve, designed to open when a given pressure (often 40–50 cmH$_2$O) is exceeded. These valves open at widely varying pressures in vitro (Kanter 1987) and very high pressures can be delivered by occluding the pop-off valve with a finger or thumb. The T_i is variable and can be very short. The greatest problem of the SIB is that CPAP cannot be delivered. When a PEEP valve is added, a very variable decelerating PEEP is produced only if the inflation rate is at least 40/min. This is particularly relevant when ventilating intubated babies, especially if they are premature. When the larynx is bypassed with an ETT, the baby cannot generate endogenous PEEP, which compounds the difficulty of achieving an FRC.

Anaesthestic (flow-inflating) bags

FIBs need a compressed gas source to inflate. Limiting the rate of gas escape through the 'tail' of the bag generates PEEP. Gas flows toward the infant when the bag is squeezed. The force with which the bag is squeezed determines the PIP, and very high PIP can be generated. The T_i is determined by the duration of the squeeze. FIBs require a greater degree of operator skill to deliver targeted pressures than SIBs or T-pieces (Bennett et al. 2005) and are less frequently used in Europe than in the USA (Leone et al. 2006). They cannot be used to deliver consistent CPAP.

T-piece devices

T-piece devices need a compressed gas source, which has been pressure-limited to a pressure suitable for the newborn. Tubing with gas flow forms the 'upstroke' of the 'T'. At one end of the 'crossbar' there is the patient outlet fixed to a face mask or ETT; at the other is a valve that controls the rate of gas escape from the system. CPAP or PEEP is generated by altering the rate of gas escape through this valve. PIP is generated by occluding the valve. The PIP and PEEP delivered are set by the operator and are more stable than that delivered with an SIB or FIB (Bennett et al. 2005). This stability of set pressures is considered one of the device's advantages. Sometimes it may be a disadvantage as occasionally a high PIP is needed to inflate a very stiff lung. It may take longer to increase the PIP with a T-piece than with an anaesthetic bag (Bennett et al. 2005). The T_i is determined by how long the outlet is occluded. This may be useful if a sustained inflation is desired. The valve should be occluded for about 0.5 seconds for inflation and open for about 0.5 seconds for expiration. When using a T-piece it is important that the gas flow rate is set (8–10 l/min is satisfactory) and then the PIP and PEEP set. The flow must not be changed during the resuscitation, otherwise the PEEP level will be altered and may become very high (Hawkes et al. 2009).

Pressure or volume during positive-pressure ventilation?

Traditionally in neonatology, pressure has been used as a proxy for the volume delivered during ventilation. Increasingly, however, mechanical ventilators used in NICUs incorporate flow sensors that measure the tidal volume. Many modern ventilators may be set to adjust the PIP automatically to deliver a desired tidal volume (usually 4–6 ml/kg). This volume-targeted approach confers benefit compared with pressure-limited ventilation (Wheeler et al. 2010).

A major limitation of manual ventilation is that the tidal volume is not measured. PPV in the delivery room is pressure-regulated and guided by subjective assessment, which is often inaccurate and frequently causes hypocarbia and hyperoxia in preterm infants (Tracy et al. 2004). A few inflations with a large tidal volume have been shown to cause lung injury in preterm lambs (Bjorklund et al. 1997). Resuscitation guidelines often recommended that initial inflations be given with a set PIP of 20 or 30 cmH$_2$O; there is, however, little science to support this. Term newborns generate larger negative pressures with their first breaths. The PIP is a very weak proxy for tidal volume. While there is a positive relationship in mannikins – the higher the PIP, the greater the tidal volume – the relationship is weak and highly variable (O'Donnell et al. 2005b). It is likely to be weaker still in babies owing to differences in the severity of lung disease between infants, changing compliance, variable face mask leak and spontaneous breaths. A set PIP cannot be an accurate proxy for an appropriate tidal volume for all babies at all times, especially when they are breathing. There is a mistaken belief that if a set PIP is achieved during mask PPV the leak from the face mask is minimal. In reality, leaks up to 90% may occur and the PIP may still be achieved (O'Donnell et al. 2005b). Achieving a PIP is not evidence of adequate volume delivery because the PIP used may be too low, the leak too large or the airway obstructed.

While clinicians have preferences for manual ventilation devices, no convincing benefit for any type of device has been demonstrated in randomised studies. However, giving respiratory support through an ETT without PEEP is inappropriate. PEEP is always used during ventilation in the NICU and has been shown to halve the oxygen requirements of preterm lambs in the first few minutes of life (Probyn et al. 2004). In studies of newly born preterm rabbits, te Pas et al. (2009a) showed the importance of PEEP in forming and maintaining end-expiratory lung volume (FRC) using high-resolution phase contrast X-rays (Fig. 13.7).

Oxygen

Traditionally it was taught that 100% oxygen should be given to infants receiving respiratory support at birth (Kattwinkel et al. 1999). Concerns emerged that high concentrations of oxygen might promote generation of reactive oxygen species which could exacerbate tissue injury, particularly during reperfusion in asphyxiated infants. Experimental animal work was followed by randomised

(Vento et al. 2001, 2003) and quasirandomised (Ramji et al. 1993; Saugstad et al. 1998) trials comparing air to 100% oxygen for resuscitation in term and near-term infants. Meta-analysis of these studies showed significantly reduced mortality in the infants who were initially resuscitated in air (Davis et al. 2004). ILCOR recommendations now state that term infants should be initially resuscitated with air, with oxygen considered for infants who fail to respond to effective ventilation and the use of oxygen guided by pulse oximetry (Perlman et al. 2010).

Preterm infants are more likely than term infants to have lung disease and are at greater risk of hypoxaemia. They also, however, have less well-developed antioxidant defences and so are at greater risk of oxidant injury. Controlled trials in which preterm infants have been randomised to receive higher (90–100%) or lower (21–30%) oxygen concentrations have been reported (Escrig et al. 2008; Wang et al. 2008). These studies were not large enough to measure clinically important outcomes and were designed to see which group achieved predetermined Spo_2 targets better. Most infants randomised to low Fio_2 received supplemental oxygen; however, they

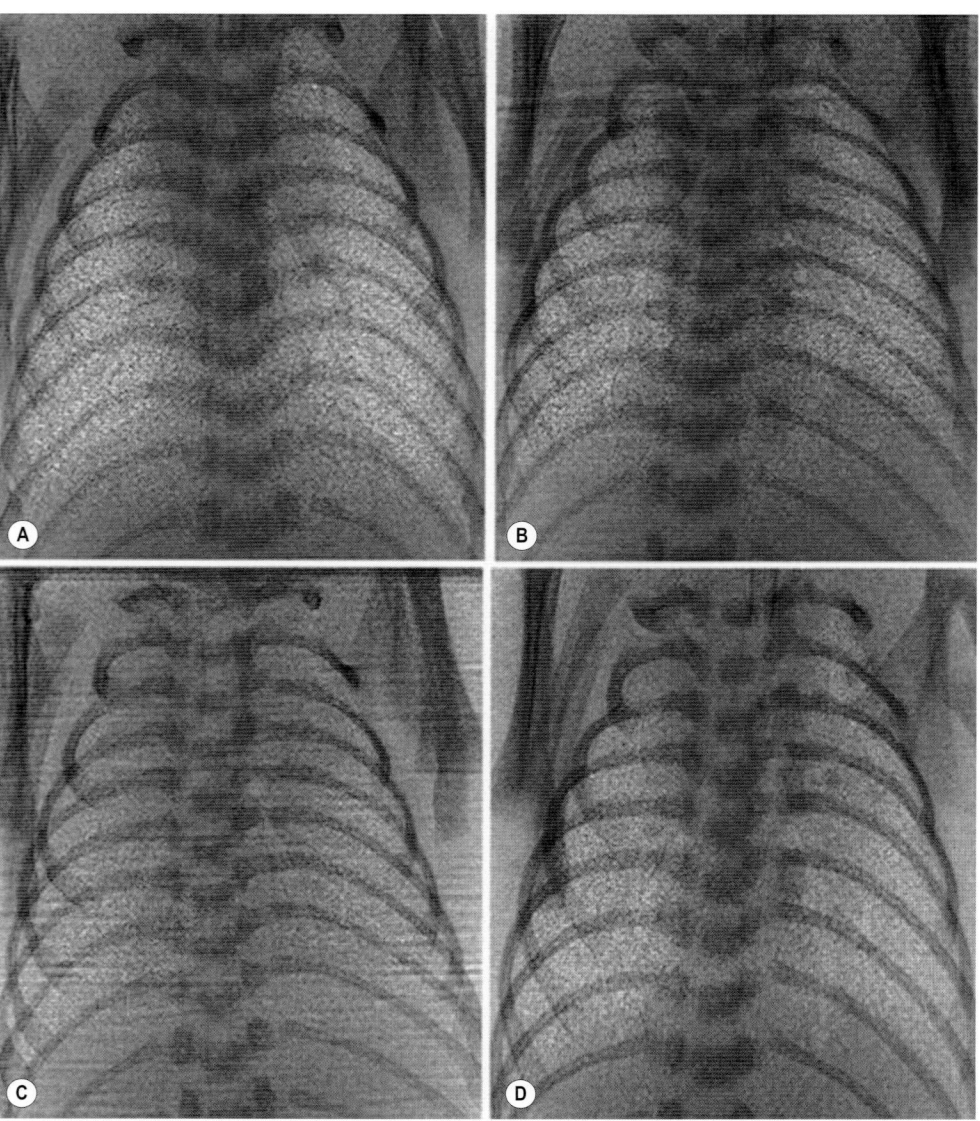

Fig. 13.7 High-resolution (phase contrast) X-rays of ventilated preterm rabbits showing the effect of positive end-expiratory pressure 5 cmH₂O (PEEP) and sustained inflations of 20 seconds (SI) on lung volume. A = SI + PEEP, B = no SI + PEEP, C = no SI + no PEEP, D = SI + no PEEP. *(Reproduced from te Pas et al. (2009b).)*

had similar SpO$_2$ after 5 minutes and received less oxygen than those randomised to high FiO$_2$. Further studies are in progress. In the meantime preterm infants should start resuscitation with air or 30% oxygen and be monitored with pulse oximetry (Perlman et al. 2010).

The gases delivered to infants in NICU are carefully warmed and humidified to reduce heat loss and to lessen drying and irritation of the airways. The gas delivered in the delivery room is neither warmed nor humidified. te Pas et al. (2010) showed a statistically significant 0.5°C difference in temperature on NICU admission among a cohort of preterm infants who received respiratory support with heated and humidified gas. It is not known whether there are other potential benefits, and this deserves further study.

Surfactant treatment

Surfactant therapy was a major advance in the care of preterm infants that reduced mortality from respiratory distress (Ch. 27.2). Randomised trials performed in an era of low antenatal steroid use demonstrated that animal-derived preparations were superior to synthetic ones, and that treatment with higher doses earlier in the infant's course seemed beneficial. More recent randomised trials have compared intubation in the delivery room and early surfactant treatment with starting infants on CPAP and reserving intubation and surfactant for those who go on to develop respiratory failure (Morley et al. 2008; SUPPORT Study Group 2010). These studies showed that these approaches were equivalent, with fewer infants randomised to CPAP being intubated and receiving surfactant and postnatal steroids (SUPPORT Study Group 2010).

Another recent randomised trial study showed that giving prophylactic surfactant to preterm infants on CPAP did not reduce the rate of mechanical ventilation in the first 5 days (Sandri et al. 2010). Preterm infants do not need to be routinely intubated in the delivery room for surfactant; the approach will probably be dictated by local preference and expertise.

Sustained inflation

Sustained (>1 second) inflations have been associated with improved outcomes in preterm babies in a retrospective cohort study and a randomised trial (Lindner et al. 1999; te Pas and Walther 2007). The sustained inflation was however only one of several differences in the way that babies were treated, so it is difficult to determine the effect of the sustained inflation alone. A 20-second inflation resulted in greater lung volume in a preterm rabbit model (te Pas et al. 2009a). It is a promising technique which deserves further study.

Supporting the circulation

A newborn infant's heart is basically healthy and usually only slows or stops due to hypoxia and acidosis. The initial management is early lung aeration and ventilation. Rarely are the hypoxia and acidosis primarily circulatory problems (e.g. fetal exsanguination or anaemia). Even in these cases respiratory support should be addressed first. The need for circulatory support – chest compressions, adrenaline and volume infusion – is rare. Wyckoff et al. (2005) reported that circulatory support was given to 0.06% (23/37 972) of infants born at a large US hospital in a 30-month period. As it is a rare event, it is very difficult to study prospectively in a systematic fashion. Therefore, studies of circulatory support in newborns are either retrospective or the information is derived from animal models. Extrapolating from animal studies is difficult as they may not match the human situation; for example, the commonest model for newborn cardiac arrest is a 2–3-day-old piglet that is hypoxic and hypotensive over a number of hours.

Chest compressions

The primary purpose of chest compressions is to perfuse the heart, thereby increasing oxygen delivery and reducing acidosis. It is recommended that chest compressions should be performed over the lower third of the sternum with two thumbs while the rest of the hands encircle the chest (Perlman et al. 2010). The sternum should be depressed approximately one-third the depth of the chest at a rate of 100 per minute. The recommended ratio of compressions to ventilation is 3:1. This ensures good respiratory support. An end-diastolic blood pressure is needed in the coronary arteries to allow perfusion. Data from a swine model of cardiac arrest demonstrate that end-diastolic pressure is increased by adrenaline and suggest that chest compressions are more effective once adrenaline has been given.

Drugs

Drugs are rarely given at resuscitation (approximately 0.04% of near-term and term deliveries) (Wyckoff et al. 2005). If drugs are to be used, it suggests that the infant has severe circulatory compromise but they may often be used because ventilation has been inadequate. In such circumstances drugs need to be given centrally. An umbilical venous catheter may be inserted much more quickly and reliably than a peripheral intravenous (IV) line in an infant with circulatory collapse, and so should always be attempted first. Intraosseous access should be used if IV access cannot be quickly achieved.

Adrenaline (epinephrine)

When an infant does not have a detectable HR or remains bradycardic (HR <60 bpm) despite effective PPV and chest compressions, adrenaline is recommended (Perlman et al. 2010). The use of IV adrenaline has been extrapolated from adult studies, which were based on studies in dogs. ETT administration seems to have evolved based on a report of its use in three newborns (Lindemann 1982). If adrenaline is to have an effect it must reach the heart. It should thus be given through an umbilical venous catheter in a dose of 0.01–0.03 mg/kg (Perlman et al. 2010). If venous access cannot be achieved, then it is reasonable to give adrenaline via the ETT. If given by this route, the dose should be increased (0.05–0.1 mg/kg; Perlman et al. 2010).

Expansion of circulating blood volume

Volume infusion is given to newborns in the delivery room more rarely than adrenaline (Wyckoff et al. 2005). Most infants are volume-replete at delivery and extra volume is unlikely to be of benefit. However, occasionally infants have had significant blood loss from fetomaternal haemorrhage or a concealed haemorrhage. This may be very difficult to diagnose but resuscitators should be aware of babies who look very pale and do not respond to adequate ventilation. A bolus of crystalloid usually in a dose of 10–20 ml/kg should be given, and, if the baby is very pale, O-negative blood.

Other drugs

Naloxone, a specific opioid antagonist, has been suggested to reverse respiratory depression in newborns whose mothers received opiate analgesics in labour. Its use is not based on any data. The priority is ventilation. Naloxone does not help emergency resuscitation and is not recommended (Perlman et al. 2010). There is no evidence that sodium bicarbonate, vasopressors or calcium improve outcomes and they may be harmful so they are not recommended (Perlman et al. 2010).

Meconium-stained liquor

Fetuses pass meconium increasingly frequently with increasing gestational age beyond term (Ch. 12). The passage of meconium in utero may be a sign of fetal hypoxia. When aspirated into the fetal/newborn lung, meconium can cause respiratory problems by a combination of airway occlusion and chemical pneumonitis, which may cause severe parenchymal lung disease complicated by pulmonary hypertension (meconium aspiration syndrome).

Large randomised controlled trials showed no benefit of intrapartum suctioning (Vain et al. 2004), and no benefit of intubation and endotracheal suction of vigorous term infants born through meconium-stained liquor (Wiswell et al. 2000). Though the benefit of intubation and endotracheal suction of non-vigorous infants born through meconium-stained liquor has not been demonstrated, suctioning the airway of an infant who requires ventilation may be useful. It is unlikely, however, to prevent meconium aspiration syndrome as most of the meconium will have been aspirated deep into the lung before birth. Meconium may very rarely block the trachea and require direct suction (see above).

A baby born under general anaesthesia

The majority of CS deliveries are performed under regional anaesthesia. Occasionally, CS deliveries are performed under general anaesthetic. Anaesthestic agents quickly cross the placenta and sedate the newborn. Therefore a person with resuscitation skills needs to be present at all CS deliveries under general anaesthesia.

Congenital anomalies

The wide availability of antenatal ultrasound has led to the increased antenatal detection of anomalies, some of which have implications for the care of the infant at birth. Despite scanning, however, some still present unexpectedly at birth.

Upper airway anomalies

A serious upper airway anomaly encountered soon after birth is the small chin (micrognathia) encountered in the Pierre Robin sequence. This small and sometimes backward-displaced chin can lead to the airway becoming obstructed by the tongue (glossoptosis). In order to relieve the obstruction, the infant should be placed prone. If this is insufficient, a nasopharyngeal airway should be used to bypass the obstruction temporarily. An LMA may be useful in an emergency as intubation can be difficult. See Chapter 27 part 7 for more detail on the management of airway anomalies.

Congenital diaphragmatic hernia

See Chapter 27 part 6. Today congenital diaphragmatic hernia (CDH) is most often diagnosed on antenatal ultrasound, though it is occasionally still diagnosed postnatally on chest X-ray in term infants with severe respiratory failure. If diagnosed before birth and the decision is made to continue with the pregnancy, the baby should be delivered at term in a tertiary centre. Most practitioners avoid mask ventilation and elect to intubate and mechanically ventilate infants shortly after birth. A wide-bore nasogastric tube is then often placed to decompress the gut.

Gastroschisis (Ch. 29.4)

Infants with gastroschisis or exomphalos rarely have problems during transition requiring resuscitation. The abdomen should be carefully loosely wrapped in polyethylene (food-grade wrap or bag) to reduce fluid and heat loss and surgical assessment should be urgently sought.

Hydrops fetalis

Newborns with hydrops fetalis have severe generalised oedema with accumulation of fluid in the chest and abdomen. They frequently need intubation, which can be difficult if the tissues are very oedematous. They may be difficult to ventilate and need a high PIP to move the chest wall. Thoracocentesis (direct aspiration of fluid from the pleural cavity) may make ventilation easier; this is, however, best performed under controlled conditions in the NICU and should not be considered in the delivery room unless the baby is in extremis. Paracentesis (aspiration of fluid from the abdomen) should not be performed blindly owing to the risk of injury to the liver and spleen, both of which are commonly enlarged in hydropic infants.

Babies still attached to the placenta

Occasionally babies are delivered in intact membranes; these infants are still attached to the placenta. It is important to remember to ligate and divide the cord as the baby may lose a significant amount of its circulating blood volume into the placenta, particularly if it is placed at a lower level than the infant.

Ethics issues

Questions about whether individual babies should be resuscitated and offered intensive care are relatively common. Much of the debate centres on what is 'the threshold of viability' for preterm infants, i.e. at what gestation does the likelihood of survival without disability outweigh the risk of death and survival with disability? Questions as to whether intensive care is appropriate may also arise for infants in whom congenital anomalies are found on antenatal ultrasound or at birth. All decisions must be guided by what is perceived to be in the child's best interests. Applying an institutional policy contrary to parental wishes is undesirable (Annas 2004). While on occasion opinions from independent ethics committees may be helpful, they are rarely available in a timely fashion. The decision should be made by parents in consultation with doctors in each individual case. If time allows, a clear plan to offer intensive care in the hope of intact survival or to offer comfort care in the expectation of death should be made before the baby delivers. Though it is tempting to wait until an extremely preterm baby is born to assess his or her condition, condition at birth does not accurately predict intact survival (Manley et al. 2010). For more discussion on ethics issues, see Chapter 6.

Teaching and training

Formal teaching of neonatal resuscitation techniques is widespread – it is estimated that 2 million people have attended a Neonatal Resuscitation Program (NRP) course in the USA alone (http://www.aap.org/nrp/intl/intl_abroad.html) – and is mandatory for training in paediatrics in many countries. While teaching the NRP has been demonstrated to improve Apgar scores in certain jurisdictions and leads to increased confidence among caregivers, it is disappointing that the introduction of widespread training in neonatal resuscitation did not reduce infant mortality in an area with high infant mortality (Carlo et al. 2010). Training has traditionally been didactic and mannikin-based. However, there are difficulties with this approach – knowledge deteriorates with time, it is difficult to acquire and maintain physical skills in this manner and there are serious concerns about how life-like the experience is. To address these issues there is increasing interest in simulation, which aims to give a more life-like experience in a controlled environment.

Research in neonatal resuscitation

Resuscitation of infants at birth has been the subject of many articles. Seldom have there been such imaginative ideas, such enthusiasms, and dislikes, and such unscientific observations and study about one *clinical picture*. There are outstanding exceptions to these statements, but the poor quality and lack of precise data of the majority of papers concerned with infant resuscitation are interesting (Apgar 1953).

The methods used to support transition and resuscitation of newborns have, until relatively recently, been subjected to little systematic study and very little in the way of randomised studies. There are likely to be many reasons for this. The need for resuscitation often arises with little or no warning. Babies cannot themselves consent to participate in research studies; instead, this decision falls to their parents. Resuscitation of a newborn is always a stressful event, in particular for families, but also for the nursing and medical staff caring for the baby and the mother. It is difficult for caregivers to acknowledge uncertainty in such situations. These factors conspire to make it difficult for caregivers to obtain prospective informed consent from stressed parents to enrol infants in studies in a short time. People correctly debate the ethics of doing research in infants who cannot give consent for themselves.

Unfortunately, the ethics of not doing research in such infants is less frequently debated. Before a new medication or device is approved for use in adults, it must be subjected to detailed studies in large numbers of adults to determine clearly that it has beneficial effects which outweigh any unwanted harmful effects. Discouraging research in babies makes it more difficult to determine that the interventions used to treat them work and are safe. This implies that a lesser standard of proof than that required for the treatment of adults is acceptable for babies. This approach is misguided, dangerous for babies and potentially infringes their human rights.

It is difficult to obtain prospective informed consent for studies of emergency interventions in all age groups; consequently, many commonly used, invasive and potentially life-saving emergency treatments are poorly studied in humans. To address these difficulties, different approaches, such as the use of deferred consent or a 'waiver of informed consent', have been used to enrol patients in studies of emergency interventions. In circumstances where it may not be possible to obtain consent prospectively, a research ethics committee may allow for patients to be enrolled without prior consent. Subsequently either the patients themselves or their next of kin or guardian are informed that they have been enrolled and their consent is sought for continued participation in the study. These have given valuable information about care of newborns and adults that has changed clinical practice. There are many areas of uncertainty in neonatal resuscitation – for example, the roles of monitoring (pulse oximetry and flow sensors), titrated oxygen, delayed cord clamping, nasal airways. These and other topics are subject to ongoing studies, including randomised clinical trials. It is critical that this research is supported, as the results of these studies will inform the body of evidence that already exists and will enable us to improve and refine the care of vulnerable newborns.

Weblinks

www.resus.org.uk: the UK Resuscitation council.

www.aap.org/nrp/intl/intl_abroad.html: the American Academy of Pediatrics neonatal resuscitation program.

References

Annas, G.J., 2004. Extremely preterm birth and parental authority to refuse treatment – the case of Sidney Miller. N Engl J Med 351, 2118–2123.

Apgar, V., 1953. A proposal for a new method of evaluation of the newborn infant. Curr Res Anesth Analg 32, 260–267.

Apgar, V., 1966. The newborn (Apgar) scoring system: reflections and advice. Pediatr Clin North Am 13, 645–650.

Aziz, H.F., Martin, J.B., Moore, J.J., 1999. The pediatric disposable end-tidal carbon dioxide detector role in endotracheal intubation in newborns. J Perinatol 19, 110–113.

Bennett, S., Finer, N.N., Rich, W., et al., 2005. A comparison of three neonatal resuscitation devices. Resuscitation 67, 113–118.

Bjorklund, L.J., Ingimarsson, J., Curstedt, T., et al., 1997. Manual ventilation with a few large breaths at birth compromises the therapeutic effect of subsequent surfactant replacement in immature lambs. Pediatr Res 42, 348–355.

Capasso, L., Capasso, A., Raimondi, F., et al., 2005. A rondomized controlled trial comparing oxygen delivery on intermittent positive pressure via nasal cannulae versus facial mask in primary neonatal resuscitation. Acta Paediatr. 94, 197–200.

Carlo, W.A., Goudar, S.S., Jihan, I., et al., 2010. Newborn-care training and perinatal mortality in developing countries. N Engl J Med 362, 614–623.

Contributors and Reviewers for the Neonatal Resuscitation Guidelines, 2000. International guidelines for neonatal resuscitation: an excerpt from the guidelines 2000 for cardiopulmonary resuscitation and emergency cardiovascular care: international consensus on science. Pediatrics 106, e29.

Costeloe, K., Hennessy, E., Gibson, A.T., et al., 2000. The EPICure study: outcomes to discharge from hospital for infants born at the threshold of viability. Pediatrics 106, 659–671.

Davis, P.G., Tan, A., O'Donnell, C.P.F., et al., 2004. Resuscitation of newborn infants with 100% oxygen or air; a systematic review and meta-analysis. Lancet 364, 1329–1333.

Dawes, G.S., 1968. Foetal and Neonatal Physiology: a Comparative Study of the Changes at Birth. Year Book Medical Publishers, Chicago IL.

Dawson, J.A., Kamlin, C.O., Wong, C., et al., 2010a. Changes in heart rate in the first minutes after birth. Arch Dis Child Fetal Neonatal Ed 95, F177–F181.

Dawson, J.A., Kamlin, C.O.F., Vento, M., et al., 2010b. Defining the reference range for oxygen saturation for infants after birth. Pediatrics 125, e1340–e1347.

Escrig, R., Arruza, L., Izquierdo, I., et al., 2008. Achievement of targeted saturation values in extremely low gestational age neonates resuscitated with low or high oxygen concentrations: a prospective randomized trial. Pediatrics 121, 875–881.

Finer, N.N., Rich, W., Wang, C., et al., 2009. Airway obstruction during mask ventilation of very low birth weight infants during neonatal resuscitation. Pediatrics 123, 865–869.

Gandini, D., Brimacombe, J., 1999a. Neonatal resuscitation with the laryngeal mask airway in normal and low birth weight infants. Anesth Analg 89, 642–643.

Gandini, D., Brimacombe, J., 1999b. Airway rescue and drug delivery in an 800 g neonate with the laryngeal mask airway. Pediatr Anaesth 9, 178.

Gandini, D., Brimacombe, J., 2003. Laryngeal mask airway for ventilatory support over a 4-day period in a neonate with Pierre Robin sequence. Pediatr Anaesth 13, 181–182.

Harrison, V.C., Heese, H.D.V., Klein, M., 1968. The significance of grunting in hyaline membrane disease. J Pediatr 41, 549.

Hawkes, C.P., Oni, O.A., Dempsey, E.M., et al., 2009. Potential hazard of the Neopuff T-piece resuscitator in the absence of flow limitation. Arch Dis Child Fetal Neonatal Ed 94, F461–F463.

Hüpfl, M., Selig, H.F., Nagele, P., 2010. Chest-compression-only versus standard cardiopulmonary resuscitation: a meta-analysis. Lancet 376, 1552–1557.

Jacobs, S.E., Hunt, R.W., Tarnow-Mordi, W.O., et al., 2007. Cooling for newborns with hypoxic-ischaemic encephalopathy. Cochrane Database Syst Rev (4), CD003311.

Kamlin, C.O.F., O'Donnell, C.P.F., Davis, P.G., et al., 2005. Colorimetric end-tidal carbon dioxide detectors: strengths and limitations. A case report. J Pediatr 147, 547–548.

Kamlin, C.O.F., O'Donnell, C.P.F., Everest, N.J., et al., 2006. Accuracy of clinical assessment of infant heart rate in the delivery room. Resuscitation 71, 319–321.

Kamlin, C.O.F., Dawson, J.A., O'Donnell, C.P.F., et al., 2008. Accuracy of pulse oximetry of measurement of heart rate of newly born infants in the delivery room. J Pediatr 152, 756–760.

Kanter, R.K., 1987. Evaluation of mask-bag ventilation in resuscitation of infants. Am J Dis Child 141, 761–763.

Karlberg, P., Cherry, R.B., Escardo, F., et al., 1962. Respiratory studies in newborn infants II. Pulmonary ventilation and mechanics of breathing in the first minutes of life, including the onset of respiration. Acta Paediatr 51, 121–136.

Kattwinkel, J. (Ed.), 2006. Textbook of Neonatal Resuscitation, fifth ed. Elk Grove, American Academy of Pediatrics and American Heart Association.

Kattwinkel, J., Niermeyer, S., Nadkarni, V., et al., 1999. ILCOR advisory statement: resuscitation of the newly born infant. An advisory statement from the Pediatric Working Group of the International Liaison Committee on Resuscitation. Pediatrics 103, e56.

Kempley, S.T., Moreiras, J.W., Petrone, F.L., 2008. Endotracheal tube length for neonatal intubation. Resuscitation 77, 369–373.

Lane, B., Finer, N.N., Rich, W., 2004. Duration of intubation attempts during neonatal resuscitation. J Pediatr 145, 67–70.

Leone, T.A., Rich, W., Finer, N.N., 2005. Neonatal intubation: success of pediatric trainees. J Pediatr 146, 638–641.

Leone, T.A., Rich, W., Finer, N.N., 2006. A survey of delivery room resuscitation practices in the United States. Pediatrics 117, 164–175.

Lindemann, L., 1982. Endotracheal administration of epinephrine during cardiopulmonary resuscitation. Am J Dis Child 136, 753–754.

Lindner, W., Vossbeck, S., Hummler, H., et al., 1999. Delivery room management of extremely low birth weight infants: spontaneous breathing or intubation? Pediatrics 103, 961–967.

Lopiore, E., van Burk, G.F., Walther, F.J., et al., 2004. Correct use of the Apgar score for resuscitated and intubated newborn babies: questionnaire study. Br Med J 329, 143–144.

MacDonald, H.M., Mulligan, J.C., Allen, A.C., et al., 1980. Neonatal asphyxia. I. Relationship of obstetric and neonatal complications to neonatal mortality in 38,405 consecutive deliveries. J Pediatr 96, 898–902.

Manley, B.J., Dawson, J.A., Kamlin, C.O.F., et al., 2010. Clinical assessment of extremely premature infants in the delivery room is a poor predictor of survival. Pediatrics 125, e559–e564.

Milner, A.D., Vyas, H., Hopkin, I.E., 1984. Efficacy of facemask resuscitation at birth. Br Med J (Clin Res Ed) 289, 1563–1565.

Morley, C.J., Davis, P.G., Doyle, L.W., et al., 2008. Nasal CPAP or intubation at birth for very preterm infants. N Engl J Med 358, 700–708.

O'Connell LAF, Kamlin COF. STINT study. PAS.

O'Donnell, C.P.F., 2006. Endotracheal intubation attempts during neonatal resuscitation: success rates, duration and adverse effects. Pediatrics 116, 16–21.

O'Donnell, C.P.F., Davis, P.G., Morley, C.J., 2004. Neonatal resuscitation: review of ventilation equipment and survey of practice in Australia and New Zealand. J Paediatr Child Health 40, 208–212.

O'Donnell, C.P.F., Kamlin, C.O.F., Davis, P.G., et al., 2005a. Feasibility of and delay in obtaining pulse oximetry at neonatal resuscitation. J Pediatr 147, 698–699.

O'Donnell, C.P.F., Davis, P.G., Lau, R., et al., 2005b. Neonatal resuscitation 2: an evaluation of manual ventilation devices and face masks. Arch Dis Child Fetal Neonatal Ed 90, F392–F396.

O'Donnell, C.P.F., Davis, P.G., Lau, R., et al., 2005c. Neonatal resuscitation 3: manometer use in a model of face mask ventilation. Arch Dis Child Fetal Neonatal Ed 90, F397–F400.

O'Donnell, C.P.F., Gibson, A.T., Davis, P.G., 2006a. Pinching, electrocution, ravens' beaks and positive pressure ventilation: a brief history of neonatal resuscitation. Arch Dis Child Fetal Neonatal Ed 91, 369–373.

O'Donnell, C.P.F., Kamlin, C.O.F., Davis, P.G., et al., 2006b. Interobserver variability of the five-minute Apgar score. J Pediatr 149, 486–489.

O'Donnell, C.P.F., Kamlin, C.O.F., Davis, P.G., et al., 2007. Clinical assessment of infant colour at delivery. Arch Dis Child Fetal Neonatal Ed 92, F465–F467.

O'Donnell, C.P.F., Kamlin, C.O.F., Davis, P.G., et al., 2010. Crying and breathing by extremely preterm infants after birth. J Pediatr 156, 846–847.

Palme, C., Nystrom, B., Tunell, R., 1985. An evaluation of the efficiency of face masks in the resuscitation of newborn infants. Lancet 1, 207–210.

Perlman, J.M., Risser, R., 1995. Cardiopulmonary resuscitation in the delivery room: associated clinical events. Arch Pediatr Adolesc Med 149, 20–25.

Perlman, J.M., Wyllie, J., Kattwinkel, J., et al., 2010. Part 11: neonatal resuscitation: 2010 International Consensus on Cardiopulmonary Resuscitation and Emergency Cardiovascular Care Science With Treatment Recommendations. Circulation 122 (suppl 2), S516–S538.

Probyn, M.E., Hooper, S.B., Dargaville, P.A., et al., 2004. PEEP during resuscitation of premature lambs rapidly improves blood gases without adversely affecting arterial pressure. Pediatr Res 56, 198–204.

Ramji, S., Ahuja, S., Thirupuram, S., et al., 1993. Resuscitation of asphyxic newborn infants with room air or 100% oxygen. Pediatr Res 34, 809–812.

Richmond, S. (Ed.), 2006. Newborn Life Support: Resuscitation at Birth, second ed. Resuscitation Council, London.

Sandri, F., Plavka, R., Ancora, S., et al., 2010. Prophylactic or early selective surfactant combined with nCPAP in very preterm infants. Pediatrics 125, e1402–e1409.

Saugstad, O.D., Rootwelt, T., Aalen, O., 1998. Resuscitation of asphyxiated newborn infants with room air or oxygen: an international controlled trial: the Resair 2 study. Pediatrics 102, e1.

Schmölzer, G.M., Kamlin, C.O.F., O'Donnell, C.P.F., et al., 2010. Assessment of tidal volume and gas leak during mask ventilation of preterm infants in the delivery room. Arch Dis Child Fetal Neonatal Ed 95, F393–F397.

Schmölzer, G.M., Kamlin, C.O.F., Dawson, J.A., et al., 2011. Airway obstruction and gas leak during mask ventilation of preterm infants in the delivery room. Arch Dis Child Fetal Neonatal Ed 96, F254–F257.

Schultze BS, 1871. Der Scheintod Neugeborener. Mauke's Verlag, Jena.

Silverman, W.A., Sinclair, J.C., 1966. Temperature regulation in the newborn infant. N Engl J Med 274, 92–94.

SUPPORT Study Group of the Eunice Kennedy Shriver NICHD Neonatal Research Network, 2010. Early CPAP versus surfactant in extremely preterm infants. N Engl J Med 362, 1970–1979.

te Pas, A.B., Walther, F., 2007. A randomized controlled trial of delivery room respiratory management in very preterm infants. Pediatrics 120, 322–329.

te Pas, A.B., Wong, C., Kamlin, C.O.F., et al., 2009a. Breathing patterns in preterm and term infants immediately after birth. Pediatr Res 65, 352–356.

te Pas, A.B., Siew, M., Wallace, M.J., et al., 2009b. Establishing functional residual capacity at birth: the effect of sustained inflation and positive end-expiratory pressure in a preterm rabbit model. Pediatr Res 65, 537–541.

te Pas, A.B., Lopiore, E., Dito, I., et al., 2010. Humidified and heated air during stabilization at birth improves temperature in preterm infants. Pediatrics 125, e1427–e1432.

The International Liaison Committee on Resuscitation, 2006. The International Liaison Committee on Resuscitation (ILCOR) Consensus on science with treatment recommendations for pediatric and neonatal patients: neonatal resuscitation. Pediatrics 117, 978–988.

Tonkin, S.L., Davis, S.L., Gunn, T.R., 1995. Nasal route for infant resuscitation by mothers. Lancet 345, 1353–1354.

Tracy, M., Downe, L., Holberton, J., 2004. How safe is intermittent positive pressure ventilation in preterm babies ventilated from delivery to newborn intensive care unit? Arch Dis Child Fetal Neonatal Ed 89, F84–F87.

Tracy, M.B., Klimek, J., Coughtrey, H., et al., 2011. Mask leak in one-person mask ventilation compared to two-person in newborn infant manikin study. Arch Dis Child Fetal Neonatal Ed 96, F195–F200.

Trevisanuto. D., Doglioni, N., Cavallin, F., et al., 2010. Heat loss prevention in very preterm infants in delivery rooms: a prospective, randomized, controlled trial of polyethylene caps. J Pediatr 156, 914–917.

Vain, N.E., Szyld, E.G., Prudent, L.M., et al., 2004. Oropharyngeal and nasopharyngeal suctioning of meconium-stained neonates before delivery of their shoulders: multicentre, randomised controlled trial. Lancet 364, 597–602.

Vento, M., Asensi, M., Sastre, J., et al., 2001. Resuscitation with room air instead of 100% oxygen prevents oxidative stress in moderately asphyxiated term neonates. Pediatrics 107, 642–647.

Vento, M., Asensi, M., Sastre, J., et al., 2003. Oxidative stress in asphyxiated term infants resuscitated with 100% oxygen. J Pediatr 142, 240–246.

Vohra, S., Frent, G., Campbell, V., et al., 1999. Effect of polyethylene occlusive skin wrapping on heat loss in very low birth weight infants at delivery: a randomized trial. J Pediatr 134, 547–551.

Vohra, S., Roberts, R.S., Zhang, B., et al., 2004. Heat loss prevention (HELP) in the delivery room: a randomized controlled trial of polyethylene occlusive skin wrapping in very preterm infants. J Pediatr 145, 750–753.

Walsh, J.A., Walsh, M., Knowles, S.J., et al., 2008. Bacterial colonisation of previously prepared endotracheal tubes in the delivery room. Arch Dis Child Fetal Neonatal Ed 93, F475–F476.

Wang, C.L., Anderson, C., Leone, T.A., et al., 2008. Resuscitation of preterm neonates by using room air or 100% oxygen. Pediatrics 121, 1083–1089.

Wheeler, K., Klingenberg, C., McCallion, N., et al, 2010. Volume-targeted versus pressure limited ventilation in the neonate. Cochrane Database Syst Rev (11), CD003666.

Wiswell, T.E., Gannon, C.M., Jacob, J., et al., 2000. Delivery room management of the apparently vigorous meconium-stained neonate: results of the multicentre international collaborative trial. Pediatrics 105, 1–7.

Wood, F.E., Morley, C.J., Dawson, J.A., et al., 2008a. Assessing the effectiveness of two round neonatal resuscitation masks: study 1. Arch Dis Child Fetal Neonatal Ed 93, F235–F237.

Wood, F.E., Morley, C.J., Dawson, J.A., et al., 2008b. Improved techniques reduce face mask leak during simulated neonatal resuscitation: study 2. Arch Dis Child Fetal Neonatal Ed 93, F230–F234.

Wyckoff, M.H., Perlman, J.M., Laptook, A.R., 2005. Use of volume expansion during delivery room resuscitation in near term and term infants. Pediatrics 115, 950–955.

Part 2: **Neonatal transport**

Steve Kempley   Nandiran Ratnavel

Transport is a vital component of any network of hospitals serving a neonatal population. Although retrieval of babies into specialist centres has been practised for over 50 years, dedicated and efficient teams able to deal with both retrieval and return are a very recent development in the National Health Service. Earlier services involved ad hoc arrangements with equipment which was adapted and secured using a variety of locally inspired methods. Retrieval was often delegated to the most junior member of the team. It is now recognised that reliable and safe equipment and vehicles are essential, not a luxury, and staff benefit from specific training and experience. Despite enormous improvements in this respect, flexibility and quick thinking remain an essential attribute for staff involved in this challenging area of neonatal medicine (Fig. 13.8).

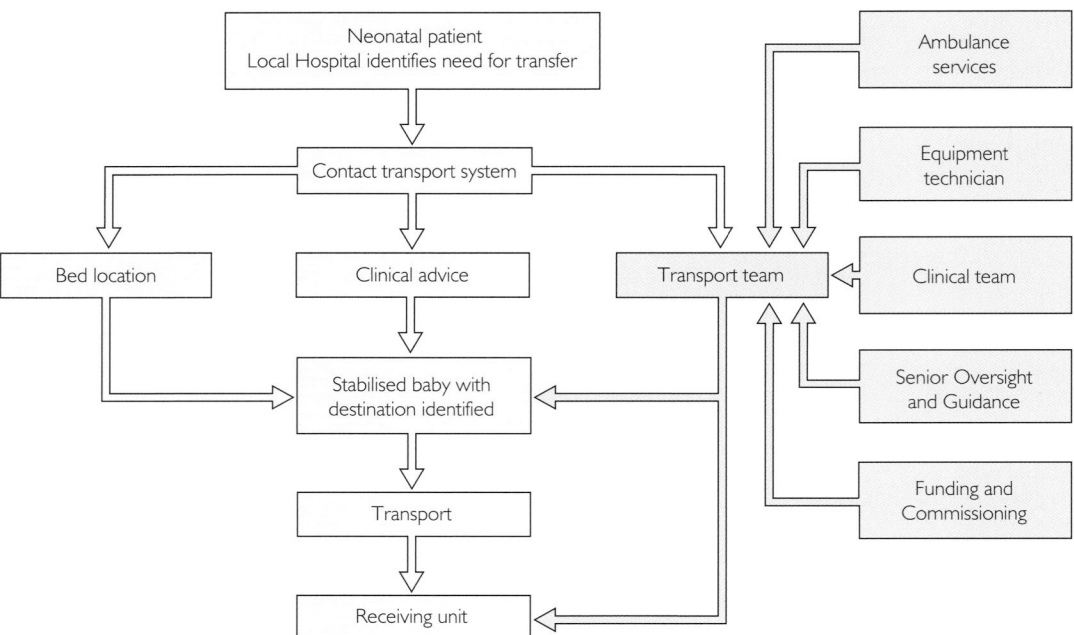

Fig. 13.8 The process of neonatal transport.

Remit of neonatal transport

Most neonatal transport services provide for any baby moving between neonatal units, although not all are 'neonates' using a strict definition (many are older than 28 days).

The requirement for neonatal transport depends on the organisation of maternity, neonatal and specialist services. In a densely populated area of the UK with large maternity units, interhospital neonatal transfers were needed for 9 per 1000 live births, of which 4–5 per 1000 were for urgent transfers of sick babies (Kempley et al. 2007). The commonest reasons for urgent transfer were medical intensive care (39%), surgery (31%), cardiac (17%) or other specialist care. However, in areas with many local, small maternity units, up to 10% of newborn babies may require transfer (Branger et al. 1994). Services must decide whether to cater only for interhospital transfer, or whether to retrieve babies from home and midwifery unit births, which may reach hospital faster using local paramedic ambulance services.

Clinical and physiological stresses and pretransport stabilisation

The clinical condition precipitating transfer may cause significant physiological dysfunction, to which will be added the effects of the transfer. Motion, vibration, noise and seasonal temperature fluctuations all act to destabilise the baby's condition (Barry and Leslie 2003). Pretransport stabilisation anticipates these effects; one should aim to optimise the infant's condition in advance rather than simply maintaining the status quo. The baby's stability should be assessed systematically, evaluating respiratory, cardiovascular, gastrointestinal, renal, metabolic, neurological, septic, haematological and biochemical parameters as well as checking fluid status and the adequacy of vascular access. The aim is to optimise the patient's ability to tolerate the transport episode.

Particular care must be taken with temperature management in premature or low-birthweight infants. The effects of skin immaturity and high surface area will be magnified by transport-specific effects such as limited incubator performance, use of unwarmed or non-humidified ventilator gases and exposure to outside environmental temperatures. Keeping a patient in the thermoneutral zone will avoid the effects of hypothermia, which increases oxygen requirement, impairs surfactant production and renders metabolic processes less efficient. Measures during stabilisation which reduce thermal stress (Advanced Life Support Group 2008) include minimising exposure for procedures, using incubator portholes, prewarming the ambulance, nursing in a prewarmed incubator and ventilation using warmed, humidified gases. The infant should wear a hat and temperature should be continuously monitored. We do not advise attempting to transfer the baby unless central temperature is at least 36.5°C. A baby that starts a journey cold will be difficult to warm up en route.

Clinical care during transport

The patient and transport equipment must be prepared and packaged prior to leaving the referring unit, with a formal checklist used for final checks of physiology and utilised equipment. A telephone call to the receiving unit gives an overview of the patient's condition, the ventilator and infusion settings and estimated time of arrival.

Once moving through the hospital the incubator system will be dependent on its own power and gases. There should be a recognised loading system into the ambulance which does not expose staff to manual handling risks and a procedure for fixation of the equipment system within the vehicle. Once in the vehicle, equipment should be connected to ambulance supplies of gas and power, to preserve those on the transport rig.

Patient monitoring must be maintained through this process and the journey. In addition to standard parameters (heart rate, oxygen saturation, blood pressure and temperature), continuous end-tidal carbon dioxide ($EtCO_2$) measurement can rapidly identify ventilation failure from endotracheal tube blockage, displacement or equipment failure. Sidestream $EtCO_2$ sampling adds little dead space; although the absolute measurement differs from arterial values, we find the qualitative waveforms very useful in a transport setting. Given the vulnerability of monitoring systems to vibration artefact, an unrestricted view of the baby is needed to assess colour, chest movement and pain.

Although incidents are minimised by pretransfer stabilisation, staff must have a rapid troubleshooting approach to solving problems. Seating should give a good vantage point to confirm that ventilator pressures are being delivered, that gas supplies are adequate, that ventilator tubing is neither disconnected nor compressed and that capnograph waveforms indicate ongoing ventilation. This can all be achieved without unfastening seatbelts. If closer inspection is needed, the ambulance should stop at the first safe opportunity; only then should staff disengage their own restraints. The majority of incidents can be readily resolved with simple adjustment of ventilation, infusions or endotracheal suction. All emergency equipment and drugs should be kept close to hand to deal with much rarer emergencies such as displaced tubes, pneumothorax or cardiac arrest.

Care at receiving hospital

On arrival in the receiving unit transport equipment must be plugged into the hospital gas and power supplies and local decontamination procedures observed. A good handover is the basis to successful ongoing management of the patient; key individuals should be identified and an efficient dialogue facilitated, with relevant staff having the opportunity to clarify information. Documentation, imaging and test results should be reviewed and the receiving unit's questions answered.

Movement of the baby from transport to unit incubator is frequently the point at which good patient preparation comes undone. Good practice ensures that all tubes and lines are secure, infusion syringes are transferred across with a minimum break in drug delivery and that lines are gathered up to prevent them becoming snagged or tangled. Tasks should be clearly delegated; following transfer the infant should be examined to ensure he or she is still being ventilated and that all tubes and lines are still in place. Only then does responsibility for the patient pass to the receiving unit staff.

Communication

Concise and efficient communication skills are required at all stages of the transfer process. This begins with an unambiguous referral to the transport service which identifies the patient, the referrer and hospital. A succinct 'sound bite' to introduce the infant's problems and to establish the need for transfer sets the scene for the subsequent referral. The transport service needs a streamlined process for collecting relevant clinical details at the initial telephone referral, encouraging important aspects of treatment to be established prior to the team's arrival.

The next level involves defining the patient's current treatment and how he or she has responded. This shapes advice given to the referring unit before the transfer team arrives. Communication failure at any stage of the transfer is associated with adverse events (Lim and Ratnavel 2008). Transport coordinators provide an interface between different agencies and need to ensure unimpeded communication with all relevant parties and collation of their input.

In addition to clinical advice, there will be a need for bed location, liaison with the receiving unit, the network centre and possibly other transfer teams. All conversations require dated and timed documentation. Many services need separate requests to the ambulance service, which needs to define the correct vehicle type. At all stages sympathetic and supportive advice to the parents will need to be maintained.

Organisation of services

Well-organised neonatal transport services must deliver appropriate clinical care with minimal delays. Critical elements include a reliable telephone contact point, specialist equipment, systems for rapidly assembling a full team, rapid access to an appropriate vehicle or aircraft and a cot-finding system. Centrally organised, integrated teams can despatch a team to a baby within 20–30 minutes, without delaying to find a cot or an ambulance, but such services involve expenses which must be justified by high usage levels. Based on rates of transfer and journey distances in England, a birth population of 80 000 per annum may be needed to justify a 24-hour neonatal transport team performing an average of two transfers per day.

Less densely populated areas may generate longer duration transfers and may need different arrangements, such as on-call teams which can be rapidly mobilised. An alternative model may involve teams which transfer both neonatal and paediatric intensive care unit (PICU) patients. Unfortunately, many healthcare systems lack medical and nursing training structures which develop high-level skills in both neonatology and PICU. The future evolution of a subspecialty of transport medicine may improve the ability of teams to cover both types of transfer.

Even with dedicated vehicles, teams will periodically require the assistance of other emergency services, so close liaison is required with local ambulance services.

Staffing

The traditional neonatal transport team consisted of a neonatal doctor and nurse, with an ambulance team who drove the vehicle. This model is progressively being replaced by integrated teams whose roles are based on competencies rather than professional designations. Neonatal transports are now being led by nurse practitioners, paramedic practitioners, nurses and doctors trained in neonatal transport.

Training

Specific neonatal transport training now constitutes part of the subspecialty training in neonatology, recognising that unit-based practice is not necessarily transferable to the transport environment. As well as clinical aspects, training involves communication skills, triage, problem-solving, equipment familiarisation and knowledge of the transport environment.

Introduction of approved transport competencies into the workplace has promoted generic competency training across professions. In addition, there are some discipline-specific competencies combining knowledge-based items and procedural/equipment competencies. With a more fluid approach to clinical work and the use of equipment, all staff members have familiarity with each other's roles and can assist more easily when circumstances are pressing. In this model it is mandatory to teach and assess the relevant competencies in a clear and structured way.

Governance

Neonatal transport is a high-risk area with the potential for adverse events, requiring a proactive approach to risk management and robust governance procedures (Ratnavel 2009). Regular case debriefs focus learning on team performance both clinically and operationally. Transport services should have their own incident-reporting system with cross-organisational mechanisms for review and feedback. Risk management structures need clear terms of reference and guidelines on criteria for serious untoward incident investigation, which must feed into the hosting organisation's reporting system. Relevant incidents should also be reported to the National Patient Safety Agency via the National Reporting and Learning System to allow a national picture of common events to be formed. This is also useful benchmarking between teams and national reviews of neonatal transfer services.

Equipment and vehicles

Equipment should only be taken on transfers if it performs an essential function. This will include a means of keeping the baby warm (usually a transport incubator), monitoring, respiratory support (including mechanical ventilation and continuous positive airway pressure), a suction system, infusion pumps, disposable items and possibly a nitric oxide system. The most important differences between equipment used on neonatal units and that used in transport are the need to minimise weight, whilst ensuring the equipment can function independently of external power sources. Transport incubator systems often lack the sophistication of unit-based equipment, but simple incubators can be supplemented by the use of active warming devices such as acetate gel mattresses.

Fixation of patient, staff, equipment and all other items in the vehicle is a basic safety requirement. All equipment, from the incubator to the syringe drivers, must be fixed to ensure they do not become lethal missiles in the event of a vehicle collision. There are different requirements for land-based and air transport which provide an absolute minimum safety standard (BS EN 13976–1 and 13718–2). Staff should be seated and secured throughout the journey; rearward-facing is safest but forward-facing reduces motion sickness. Fixation systems are now available to secure the baby safely within the incubator; the Neo-Restraint uses conformable foam wedges to prevent mass movement without causing direct pressure on delicate neonatal skin.

Dedicated neonatal vehicles provide a number of advantages over front-line ambulances. The weight of the incubator system can be markedly reduced through provision of AC power and compressed gases in the vehicle, although some independent supply will be needed for movement to or from the vehicle and to cope with emergencies (Kempley et al. 2009). Additional equipment such as a cold light source and a bigger supply of consumables can be easily accommodated on dedicated vehicles.

Air transport

Air transport is required for either long-distance transfers or to deal with local geographical issues such as islands or adverse road conditions. There are challenges involving organisation, equipment, communication, physical conditions and staff training. Air transfer often needs to link with road transfer for direct access to any hospital that does not have a landing site, needing prior plans for the compatibility of equipment in the ambulance and the aircraft. Transport services with an established airborne facility usually have a volume of work, making it reasonably cost-effective. Development of such services requires liaison between clinicians, aviation operators, ambulance managers, medical physics technicians and engineers (Skeoch et al. 2005). Ad hoc air transfers are expensive and run the risk of staff being unfamiliar with both equipment and environment.

Equipment should include the normal elements with automated loading and fully integrated gas supplies. It should be able to withstand frequent movement and vibration. Layout should allow the clinician good visibility and access; visual alarms are preferable to audio systems. Stress and electrical installation reports must be approved by the appropriate aviation safety agency. Aircraft-specific compatibility tests then need to be carried out and a servicing agreement needs to be in place.

For staff safety, clothing should be weatherproof, high-visibility and flame-retardant, with head and hearing protection provided. As air transfer increases the risk to patients and staff above and beyond the increased risk associated with road transfer, adequate insurance cover must be provided.

Air transfer imposes particular clinical considerations. Altitude reduces the partial pressure of oxygen, leading to a reduction in the infant's oxygen saturation, so that oxygen delivery may need to be increased. Expansion of gas with increasing altitude means that a small pneumothorax may expand to become dangerous; even small ones should be drained prior to transfer.

Parents

Careful consideration must be given to parents already facing distress over their baby's illness. A short detour to the labour ward may be worthwhile to allow the mother to see the baby before transfer. Parents should be given a photograph of the baby and clear directions to the destination unit. The dangerous situation where parents chase the ambulance in their own car must be avoided.

For elective journeys, parents can often accompany the baby. For acute transfers, the number of staff in the ambulance and other safety factors should be assessed. It may be unsafe to transfer a mother in a neonatal ambulance immediately after caesarean section or following intrapartum haemorrhage. Flexibility is needed; some parents prefer to stay together in the referring hospital, others prefer a parent to accompany the baby, especially if urgent surgery is imminent. An ambulance, taxi or other safe transport should be arranged for parents who follow their baby later.

References

Advanced Life Support Group, 2008. Paediatric and Neonatal Safe Transfer and Retrieval. Wiley-Blackwell, Chichester.

Barry, P., Leslie, A., 2003. Paediatric and Neonatal Critical Care Transport. BMJ Books, London.

Branger, B., Chaperon, J., Mouzard, A., et al., 1994. Hospital transfer of newborn infants in the Loire-Atlantic area (France). Rev Epidemiol Santé Publique 42, 307–314.

BS EN 13976–1: 2003, 2004. Rescue Systems. Transportation of Incubators. Interface Conditions. British Standards Institute, London.

BS EN 13718–2: 2008, 2008. Medical Vehicles and their Equipment. Air Ambulances. British Standards Institute, London.

Kempley, S.T., Baki, Y., Hayter, G., et al., 2007. Effect of a centralised transfer service on characteristics of inter-hospital neonatal transfers. Arch Dis Child Fetal Neonatal Ed 92, F185–F188.

Kempley, S.T., Ratnavel, N., Fellows, T., 2009. Vehicles and equipment for land-based neonatal transport. Early Hum Dev 85, 491–495.

Lim, M.C., Ratnavel, N., 2008. A prospective review of adverse events during interhospital transfers of neonates by a dedicated neonatal transfer service. Pediatr Crit Care Med 9, 289–293.

Ratnavel, N., 2009. Safety and governance issues for neonatal transport services. Early Hum Dev 85, 483–486.

Skeoch, C.H., Jackson, L., Wilson, A.M., et al., 2005. Fit to fly: practical challenges in neonatal transfers by air. Arch Dis Child Fetal Neonatal Ed 90, F456–F460.

section 4

General neonatal care

Examination of the newborn

Janet M Rennie

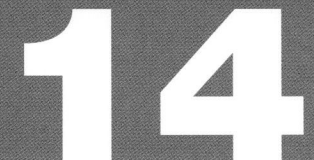

CHAPTER CONTENTS

© 2012 Elsevier Ltd

Introduction

A thorough physical examination of every neonate has long been accepted as good practice and forms a core item of the child health surveillance programme in many countries (Hall and Elliman 2003; NICE 2006). There are now agreed standards for the conduct of this examination, which forms part of the National Health Service screening programme in the UK (see Weblinks). The Newborn and Infant Physical Examination (NIPE) programme has clearly defined goals, target conditions and competency standards. The four current target conditions are hips, eyes, heart and testes. The first detailed examination should take place within 72 hours of birth and the second at 6–8 weeks. The mother should have been given information about the NIPE programme during pregnancy, and consent should be obtained. Non-consent must be recorded and followed up, and notified to the appropriate child health information department.

The aims of the routine newborn examination are:

- to review any problems arising or suspected from antenatal screening, family history or the events of labour
- to ascertain whether the family have any worries about the baby and to try to address them
- to initiate appropriate treatment and arrange for advice and follow-up where indicated (e.g. hepatitis vaccination, phototherapy for jaundice, special teat for cleft palate)
- to screen for specific target conditions, currently developmental dysplasia of the hip (DDH), cataract, undescended testes and congenital heart disease
- to diagnose congenital malformations and common neonatal problems, and give advice about management

- to detect the occasional baby who is obviously ill and requires urgent treatment
- to collect baseline information about weight and head circumference, and to check that the baby has passed urine and meconium
- to identify parents who may have problems in caring for their baby because of substance abuse, mental health problems, learning difficulties or very poor housing and to alert the appropriate professional groups
- to begin to provide health education advice, e.g. regarding breastfeeding, cot death prevention, safe transport in cars.

For some babies, early diagnosis may make all the difference to their subsequent health; examples are congenital cataract and urethral valves. For others, reassurance about minor deviations from normal (birthmarks, syndactyly of the toes, extra digits) is all that is required. The slightest variation from what the family consider to be normal may produce the most intense distress and anxiety at a stage when the mother is emotionally very labile.

The yield of abnormal findings is surprisingly high, with up to 20% of healthy newborns being found to have one minor anomaly (Adam and Hudgins 2003). Most of these are of no importance, although the number of such abnormalities matters (Table 14.1).

Table 14.1 Common minor neonatal abnormalities and their importance

Abnormalities that do not matter when isolated (three or more such abnormalities do matter)
Folded-over ears
Hyperextensibility of thumbs
Syndactyly of the second and third toes
Single palmar crease
Polydactyly, especially if familial
Umbilical hernia, especially in Afro-Caribbean babies
Single umbilical artery
Hydrocele
Fifth-finger clinodactyly
Simple dimple just above the natal cleft (see text for definition)
Undescended testes
Single café-au-lait spot
Single ash-leaf macule
Third fontanelle (5% of babies)
Capillary or strawberry haemangioma
Accessory nipples

Abnormalities that might matter even when they are isolated
Ear pits and tags
More than three café-au-lait spots in a Caucasian baby, more than five in black African babies
Multiple haemangiomas, or strawberry haemangiomas in specific places (e.g. ophthalmic division of the trigeminal nerve in Sturge–Weber syndrome, or in the midline over the spine)
Oedema of the feet – think of Turner syndrome
Asymmetric crying facies
Microcephaly
Macrocephaly
Micrognathia
Midline skin defects over the spine other than simple dimples
Scrotal swelling/discoloration (think of torsion of the testes)

Only 0.5% of babies have three such anomalies, and the risk of an accompanying major malformation then rises from 3% (with one minor anomaly) to 20%. Unfortunately, the examination is not a reliable screen for several important conditions such as DDH, cataract and congenital heart disease (see below).

Who should examine the baby?

Babies should be examined by a trained practitioner who has the time to talk and listen to the mother. In the past, all neonatal examinations were carried out by paediatricians, usually junior paediatricians with some specific basic training. Generations of paediatric residents have learnt the range of normality by performing large numbers of 'baby checks', and they have the advantage of a full medical training and a direct chain of referral. Recently, advanced neonatal nurse practitioners and trained midwives have begun to undertake the examination, and mothers are usually very satisfied with the service they provide (Lee et al. 2001; Wolke et al. 2002). In a randomised trial conducted in south-east England (Wolke et al. 2002), mothers whose baby was examined by a midwife were more satisfied than the group whose baby was examined by a paediatric senior house officer (SHO), although the general level of satisfaction was very high. The reason why the midwives' examination was preferred was that there was more provision of health education advice (related to feeding, sleeping and skin care). Once this was controlled for, the differences in satisfaction disappeared. The midwives took 5 minutes longer, on average, to conduct the examination than the SHOs. Randomisation only took place during the working day, and half of all babies born during the study period were excluded from randomisation because of problems such as maternal disease, low birthweight, operative delivery or a need for resuscitation at birth.

When should babies be examined?

Many babies are currently discharged home before 8 hours of age. The advice from the NIPE programme is that there is no optimal time to detect all abnormalities, and it is considered that the overall risk associated with babies going unscreened is greater than if babies are examined early. Hence, the conclusion is that all babies should be offered the examination before discharge even if this is at or before 6 hours. The logistics of delivering a high-quality screening examination on this timescale can be formidable in a busy maternity service, and a back-up arrangement such as a walk-in clinic or community liaison is essential to make sure that all babies are examined before 72 hours.

Examination in the delivery room

All babies should be checked soon after birth; this will generally be done by the midwife following uncomplicated full-term labour, but if the paediatrician has been called to the delivery she should make a quick appraisal of the infant after any necessary resuscitation. This examination is usually confined to ensuring that the infant looks well and that there are no major abnormalities requiring immediate attention or explanation to the parents such as hare lip/cleft palate, spina bifida, anal atresia or ambiguous genitalia. This is a most sensitive and important time for parents and they should be given the opportunity to be left alone with their baby as soon as possible. This check is not, and should not be, the full examination which forms the first NIPE screening examination.

Full routine examination

Mothers meticulously inspect their own babies, hence one of the most important functions of the examination is to answer any questions which the mother may raise. It follows that the examination should, if possible, always be done in her presence. The following general format is recommended:

1. Check the maternal medical, obstetric and social history from the notes, the mother and the nursing staff.
2. Introduce yourself to the mother with an explanation about what you are doing.
3. Fully examine the baby.
4. Give advice and information, arrange follow-up and provide reassurance where appropriate. When giving advice, remember that the neonatal examination is not a perfect screening tool.

History and background knowledge

Before approaching the mother and infant, read the baby notes to obtain basic information about the mother's previous obstetric and medical history as well as the type of delivery and the baby's condition at birth; note also the birthweight, gestational age and sex. If there are complicated medical or social problems it is helpful to discuss them with the nursing staff beforehand and also to check the mother's notes for details.

It is useful to have a mental checklist of relevant background information to obtain before starting the examination. This should include:

- The baby's sex.
- The baby's birthweight and reputed gestational age and whether these are mutually compatible.
- The mother's age and social background.
- Is there any chronic maternal disease? If so, what treatment is the mother receiving?
- Is there a history of recreational drug and/or alcohol use? Is the mother a smoker?
- Is there any possibly relevant family history?
- The outcome and dates of any previous pregnancies.
- Was the pregnancy normal? Were there any complications?
- What were the results of pregnancy screening tests, e.g. 20-week ultrasound scan?
- Were any special diagnostic procedures, e.g. amniocentesis, performed?
- Were there any signs of fetal compromise during labour?
- What drugs and/or anaesthesia were given during labour and delivery?
- How was the baby delivered?
- Was there a breech presentation after 36 weeks (an indication for a hip scan)?
- What was baby's condition at birth (Apgar scores at 1 and 5 minutes, cord pH)?
- Was any resuscitation needed?
- How long before sustained respiration was established?
- Was the baby in the neonatal unit? If so, why?
- How is the mother planning to feed the baby, and how is the feeding going?

Introductions and general 'gestalt' inspection

The doctor should introduce herself and say what she has come for. To ask the baby's name and record it helps to establish a good relationship. So many early worries are concerned with feeding that one should always enquire what method the mother is using and whether she is happy with it. Routine weighing and feed charts have been abandoned in most UK maternity units, but the incidence of readmission with hypernatraemic dehydration due to breast milk insufficiency has risen (Laing and Wong 2002). All babies lose weight after birth, 2–3% each day to a maximum of around 10%, but it is rare for a baby to lose more weight than this, or to remain more than 10% below birthweight after the 5th day (Wright and Parkinson 2004). If there is a current weight, then a quick calculation of weight lost or gained since birth should be made.

Enquire about the health of any previous children. There may have been previous stillbirths, infant deaths or adverse outcomes about which the mother may be extremely anxious. The examiner should also review and confirm any relevant items of background information gleaned from the notes. Always ask the mother whether she has any specific worries, when she is expecting to be discharged and what support she has at home. Knowledge of the father's and mother's occupation provides useful background information. By means of these preliminary pleasantries one can usually quickly establish a relationship and can gauge the level at which to discuss any problems. During these introductory minutes the examiner can try to make the mother and her partner (if present) feel like individuals, and can also do two other very important things:

1. observe the mother's attitude to her baby, and whether she is confident and happy or tense and withdrawn
2. observe the baby, noting colour, facies, breathing pattern, posture and movements.

An enormous amount can be learned by these simple observations while continuing to chat to the mother. For recording purposes it is useful to have a checklist printed or stamped in the baby's notes to serve as an aide-memoire. The examination must be appropriately documented; increasingly this involves a computerised record. The experienced observer uses 'gestalt' to assess the importance of minor dysmorphic features (Table 14.1), subtle signs of illness, or atypical behaviour patterns.

Formal examination

The baby must be undressed down to the nappy for most of the examination time; it is impossible to examine a clothed baby properly. Most parts of the examination can be performed in any behavioural state, and the order in which this is done is largely a matter of personal preference, but working from top to toe down the front and vice versa up the back is as good as any other. Full advantage should be taken of any quiet or sleeping periods to feel the anterior fontanelle, look at the eyes, auscultate the heart and palpate the abdomen. It is wise to leave the hips until nearly the end of the examination, even though this item is arguably one of the most important items on the agenda and must be done with the infant quiet and relaxed, because the Ortolani–Barlow test often makes the baby cry. Throughout the whole examination one is at first consciously, later almost subconsciously, observing such things as posture, muscle tone, movements and reaction to stimuli so that finally there is very little need for a formal evaluation of the central nervous system unless suspicious signs have come to light. A suggested order for the examination is as follows; details of what one is looking for are given in the systematic review.

Order of examination

- Remove the baby's clothes except the nappy.
- Feel the anterior fontanelle for tension (leave until later if the baby is crying!).
- Look at the face for colour or any peculiarities.

- Listen to the heart and estimate heart rate and respiratory rate. The lungs can also be auscultated but this is seldom informative.
- Palpate the abdomen.
- Return to the head and examine scalp and skull and measure head circumference and record it, together with the weight.
- Examine the eyes, ears, nose and mouth.
- Examine the neck, including the clavicles.
- Examine the arms, hands, legs and feet.
- Remove the nappy.
- Feel for the femoral pulses.
- Examine the genitalia and anus.
- Turn the baby to the prone position and examine the back and spine, and assess tone.
- Return the infant to the supine position and evaluate the central nervous system.
- Examine the hips.
- Make sure you have not omitted anything and check you have paid attention to any concerns expressed by the mother.

Systematic review

Skin

During the general examination the colour and texture of the skin should be noted as well as any birthmarks or rashes. Birthmarks are common in babies, and most are vascular or pigmentary lesions (Hernandez and Morelli 2003). Many are normal variants, but some are of great importance. Sturge–Weber syndrome occurs in 10% of those who have a port wine stain involving the ophthalmic division of the trigeminal nerve, for example.

The frequency of café-au-lait spots varies tremendously and it is common to see one spot, although more than three are rare. Some have recommended that any Caucasian baby with more than three such spots, and any African baby with more than five, be followed for the development of multisystem disease (Landau and Krafchik 1999). Many other skin lesions are described in Chapter 32, and some excellent illustrated textbooks are available (Eichenfield et al. 2008).

Skin colour

Healthy warm Caucasian babies should be reddish pink all over after the first few hours of life, but they can be covered with white cheesy vernix; this can also be stained a golden yellow in post-maturity or appear greenish if meconium has been passed before birth.

Cyanosis

Cyanosis is usually discernible when arterial blood is 80% saturated, but the ability to detect cyanosis varies between individuals and with different lighting conditions. Cyanosis can be difficult to evaluate in an infant who is very pale (anaemic or peripherally shut down) or racially pigmented. Plethoric infants (central packed-cell volume >65%) can appear cyanosed because they have more than 5 g of reduced haemoglobin per 100 ml even when adequately oxygenated. Peripheral cyanosis of the hands and feet and circumoral cyanosis (acrocyanosis) are common during the first 48 hours. It is essential to ascertain that cyanosis is not central by noting whether the tongue is blue. Traumatic cyanosis or bruising of the presenting part, sometimes associated with petechiae, is also quite common, particularly over the face if there has been a nuchal cord. If there is any doubt check arterial oxygen saturation with a pulse oximeter. Babies with confirmed central cyanosis should be admitted to the neonatal unit and investigated urgently, beginning with a blood gas estimation and a chest X-ray and proceeding to an early echocardiogram if there is no evidence of respiratory disease.

Cyanosis during crying early in postnatal life may be quite normal as a result of transient elevation of pulmonary vascular resistance with right-to-left shunting, but cyanotic attacks should always be taken seriously.

Pallor

Mature babies appear paler than preterm ones, because of their relatively thick skin. Generalised pallor may indicate anaemia, peripheral shutdown with shock, or both. The capillary filling time can be estimated by pressing on the skin and should not be longer than 3 seconds if the skin is warm.

Jaundice

This is discussed in detail elsewhere (Ch. 29.1) but is often detected first during the routine newborn examination. Icterus appearing in the first 24 hours requires urgent investigation and treatment and should at once evoke the response 'What is the mother's Rh and ABO group? Were there any antibodies and are there any other signs of congenital infection?'

Jaundice appearing between 2 and 4 days is extremely common. Jaundice in preterm (including near-term) babies requires very careful evaluation and if any jaundiced baby is ill in any way (unduly lethargic, feeding poorly, vomiting or has an unstable temperature), infection – or worse, bilirubin encephalopathy – must be excluded. The level of bilirubin is hard to judge by eye, and hence it must be measured. A transcutaneous bilirubinometer can be used (Ch. 29.1). This is particularly important in Afro-Caribbean, Oriental and Asian babies in whom clinical assessment of jaundice is fraught with hazard. Healthy term infants are not immune from kernicterus but levels of bilirubin above 500 µmol/l are probably required to produce it (Ch. 29.1). Audits have shown that common factors are lack of professional concern about jaundice, inadequate breastfeeding and a failure to recognise that the near-term baby (35–37 weeks) is particularly susceptible. These risk factors have been recognised by the National Institute for Health and Clinical Excellence (NICE), together with a family history of a sibling requiring treatment for neonatal jaundice. All babies with risk factors should be examined at around 48 hours to assess whether visible jaundice is present.

Skin texture

Note whether the skin is peeling (common in postterm infants), nice and firm (normal) or very loose (intrauterine growth retardation or dehydration). Oedema is uncommon in full-term infants and should always raise the question of hypoalbuminaemia. Pedal oedema and a low hairline should make the examiner think of Turner syndrome in a baby girl (Ch. 31).

Skin rashes

These are very common in newborn babies. Flat lesions are described as macular (by definition macules are <1 cm but the term is not always used this way). Raised lesions are described as papular when they are up to 1 cm in size and nodular up to 2 cm. Raised clear fluid-filled lesions are vesicular (<1 cm) or bullous (>1 cm). When raised lesions contain purulent fluid they are termed pustular. Diagnosis of a petechial rash, which does not blanch on pressure, should prompt a platelet count. Milia are tiny cream papules, which are inclusion cysts containing trapped keratinised stratum corneum, and which usually resolve without treatment.

The most frequent skin disorder of newborn infants is erythema toxicum neonatorum (toxic erythema; Ch. 32). There is an eosinophilic infiltrate into the dermis and there can be an associated eosinophilia in the blood. The rash usually starts between 24 and 48 hours of age and resolves by the fifth day. The appearance has been compared to a flea bite.

Transient neonatal pustular melanosis (Ch. 32) is extremely common in Afro-Caribbean babies, and is a similar reaction to erythema toxicum although the lesions are present from birth. These pustules contain neutrophils. The pustules are very fragile and easily wiped away to leave a scaly area. This area resolves into hyperpigmented brown macules. They have been termed lentigines because of their resemblance to lentils, but they are not true lentigines. The macules last for several months before fading. No treatment is needed and the main importance of recognising the condition is to avoid overtreatment on the basis that they are thought to be due to a staphylococcal infection.

Milia are papules that commonly appear on the face or scalp, although they can occur anywhere, including on the penis and inside the mouth (where they are called Epstein's pearls when they are found on the palate). They are tiny white smooth-surfaced papules. They are inclusion cysts which contain trapped keratinized stratum corneum. They usually clear up within a few months and no action other than reassurance is necessary.

Miliaria rubra, or prickly heat, is common in hot humid climates. The rash usually occurs mainly on the head and upper trunk.

Head and skull

Babies' heads can be considerably distorted and moulded during labour and delivery; there may be a marked caput succedaneum (oedema caused by pressure over the presenting part) which subsides in 2–3 days, or the soft skull bones can be greatly moulded. Either or both of these factors can produce bizarre head shapes which persist for the first few days and sometimes longer. It is important to distinguish deformation – the result of impact from mechanical forces on normal tissue – from malformation. Up to 20% of babies show effects of intrauterine constraint (Graham 1994). Babies who have been in the breech presentation for a long time in utero often have a 'breech head' with a prominent occipital shelf (Dunn 1976).

Feel the anterior fontanelle for its tension and size; it can measure up to 3 × 3 cm at its widest points, though the size is very variable. Fullness may indicate raised intracranial pressure (cerebral oedema, hydrocephalus or meningitis). The posterior fontanelle is often open at this age but is usually only fingertip size, with only 3% more than 2 cm in diameter. Examine the cranial sutures for any undue separation, which is abnormal. Overriding of the bones of the vault is common in the first 48 hours, but ridging at the suture lines, as opposed to the 'step-up' feel of overriding, implies craniosynostosis (premature fusion of the sutures). The sagittal suture is the most commonly affected. Craniosynostosis occurs in about 0.4 per 1000 births and may require a neurosurgical procedure for cosmetic correction, or to allow brain growth if several sutures are fused (Hunter and Rudd 1977). Limb defects, particularly syndactyly, are the most common associated malformations and it may be worth asking the parents if they have fused toes.

Palpate the skull bones; small areas of craniotabes caused by pressure from the maternal pelvis occur in 2% of normal newborns and are of no significance (Graham and Smith 1979). Cephalhaematomas – collections of blood between the periosteum and the skull bones – are felt as softish bumps over the affected bone, most commonly the parietal, and do not extend across the suture lines. Explain their benign nature to the mother and add that they may take 6 weeks or more to subside. A boggy swelling crossing a suture line is more sinister and can indicate subgaleal haemorrhage (Ch. 40.3). There may be a chignon from the use of a vacuum extractor. Neonatal skull fractures are rare. Elevation of the 'ping-pong' ball type of fracture where the bone is depressed but not fractured can be achieved with the application of a vacuum extractor. Linear skull fractures usually require no treatment but should be followed with a repeat X-ray because if the dura has been torn a 'growing' fracture can develop (Rothman et al. 1976; Scarfo et al. 1989).

Inspect the scalp for any injury such as forceps marks or lacerations from scalp electrodes, fetal blood sampling or instrumental delivery. Look also for any bald patches or naevi over the scalp. A small defect of the scalp, cutis aplasia, can be confused with the scar of a scalp clip electrode. Cutis aplasia (Ch. 32) is a serious congenital abnormality with a risk of infection and bleeding from the underlying dural venous sinuses, and may be a clue to an underlying diagnosis such as Adams–Oliver syndrome.

Measure the occipitofrontal head circumference (OFC) at its maximum and ensure that it falls within the normal range (approximately 33–37 cm at term). Compare the measurement with any pre-existing measurements; rapid enlargement of the head after birth with boggy swelling crossing the suture lines is due to the rare and dangerous condition of subgaleal haemorrhage (Ch. 40.3). There is a strong association with ventouse delivery. If the head is unduly small (below the second centile) consider dysmorphic syndromes, congenital infections or isolated microcephaly. If the head is unduly large from the beginning consider familial megalencephaly or hydrocephalus. A large head in the presence of widely separated sutures or a full fontanelle requires immediate ultrasound evaluation. Remember that moulding of the skull can lead to an erroneous OFC measurement which returns to normal once the moulding has subsided.

Face

Most babies' faces are unremarkable, apart from perhaps resembling one or other parent. Occasionally, however, the facial appearance is the first clue to an underlying disorder such as Down syndrome. The bloated cherubic face of infants born to mothers with diabetes is also characteristic (Ch. 22). If unusual facial features are seen this should prompt a particularly diligent search for other dysmorphic manifestations, but if the baby is asymptomatic and otherwise normal the appearance may well be familial and a glance at the parents may confirm this. Nasal septal deviation is quite common, and the nose usually straightens over the first few days. Occasionally there is a frank dislocation of the nasal septum which requires relocation (see below).

There is a difference between facial palsy and asymmetric crying facies. The latter is often due to congenital absence of the depressor anguli oris muscle (DAOM); these babies can wrinkle their foreheads and close their eyes, in contrast to babies with a facial nerve palsy. The incidence of absent DAOM is about 0.6–0.8% of the population, and there is an association with congenital heart disease (Lin et al. 1997). When the diagnosis is that of facial palsy, spontaneous recovery occurs within 4 weeks in 90% of cases (Smith et al. 1981).

Ears

Look at the general shape, size and position of the ears and feel the cartilage. Low-set ears are those in which the top of the pinna falls below a line drawn from the outer canthus of the eye at right angles to the facial profile (Fig. 14.1). Abnormally small or large floppy ears are characteristic of several syndromes, and the combination

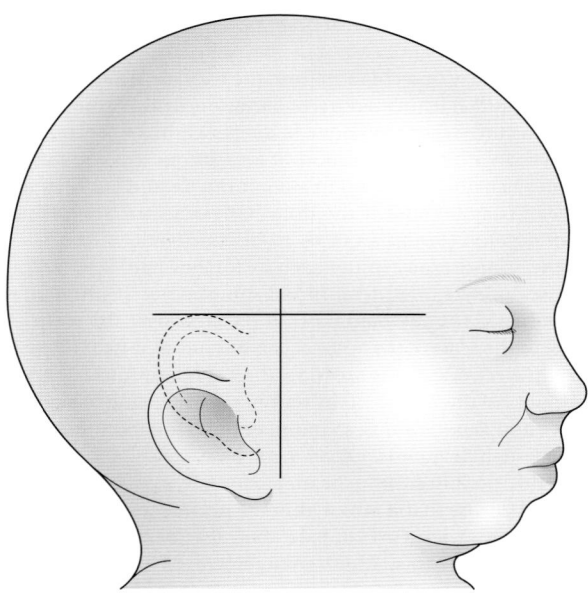

Fig. 14.1 Normal ears.

of ear anomalies and a coloboma can be a clue to CHARGE syndrome (Ch. 31). Overfolding of the helix can result from fetal constraint, and in mild cases resolves without treatment over the first weeks of life. Taping and splinting have now been shown to be remarkably successful even in cases which would previously have required surgery (Brown et al. 1986; Ruder and Graham 1996). Note any preauricular pits, skin tags or accessory auricles. Otoscopic examination does not form part of the routine examination.

The prevalence of isolated ear tags is 1.7 per 1000 with bilateral tags in 6% (Adam and Hudgins 2003). Ear pits and tags can be autosomal dominant, but it is important to assess hearing in these babies. Routine renal ultrasonography is probably unnecessary if ear pits or tags are isolated (Kugelman et al. 2002).

Hearing screening

Congenital hearing impairment in one or both ears affects about 1–2 : 1000 babies, and early aiding is associated with better language, communication, mental health and employment prospects. Much congenital deafness is now known to be genetic, with recessive mutations at the connexin locus accounting for many cases (Nance 2003). Universal hearing screening in the neonatal period is now in place in the UK.

Nose

Inspect the nose for its general shape and width of the bridge. If it appears abnormally wide, measure the distance between the inner canthi; this should not exceed about 2.5 cm in the term infant. The nose can appear quite squashed as a result of intrauterine compression. Occasionally the septal cartilage is dislocated and this can be recognised by deviation of the columella. Compression of the tip of the nose causes collapse and increased deviation of the nostrils in this condition, which requires treatment by an ear, nose and throat surgeon. Flaring of the alae nasi is not normal and its presence indicates respiratory illness. Babies are obligate nose breathers and hence complete nasal obstruction (diagnosed by failure to mist a mirror) causes intense respiratory distress which requires immediate investigation. Snuffly noses are quite common, but provided the

baby can breathe normally during feeding, serious problems are rarely present; if in doubt ensure that both nares are patent by passing a fine catheter through each nostril.

Eyes

The eyes should always be inspected for any gross abnormality, noting their size, dimensions and slant; check for any strabismus or nystagmus. A third of newborns have an intermittent exotropia but esotropia is not normal. Congenital cataract is the commonest form of preventable childhood blindness and evaluating the red reflex is an essential part of the neonatal examination (see below), although it is not feasible to perform full fundoscopy on every baby. Fundoscopy should of course be attempted if there is any question of abnormality.

Look for (and ask about) any discharge from the eyes. A slight mucoid discharge ('sticky eye') is very common in the first 2 days after birth, but later is likely to be due to failure of canalisation of the nasolacrimal duct. A membranous obstruction in this structure persists in 70% of neonates, but resolves spontaneously by 3 months of age in 70% and by a year in 96% (Young and MacEwen 1997). After a year probing may be required; earlier in life simple cleaning of crusts is the best treatment. Referral is not required, but beware photophobia or conjunctivitis, which suggests another diagnosis. Occasionally congenital obstruction of the nasolacrimal duct combines with an obstruction to retrograde flow to produce a dacrocystocele – a tense blue grey swelling just beneath the medial canthus. These often become infected (dacrocystitis). A frankly purulent discharge, particularly if accompanied by redness and swelling of the eyelids, should always be taken seriously and demands bacterial investigation and treatment. Subconjunctival haemorrhages are very common after birth (analogous to petechiae in the skin), and are harmless although the mother may need reassurance. The sclerae provide a guide to jaundice.

Iris

The iris is normally blue or grey in the newborn. Look for colobomas (keyhole-shaped pupil): if present there could also be a defect in the retina, and this should prompt a search for other congenital malformations. Babies with aniridia often have a poor visual outcome.

Cornea

Check that the cornea does not appear abnormally large, especially if the baby has prominent eyes. The corneal diameter is normally about 10 mm, and if this is greater than 13 mm (particularly if the cornea is also hazy) the baby might have congenital glaucoma (Ch. 33). The cornea should be bright and clear; corneal opacities deserve referral to an ophthalmologist as they can be due to herpetic ulceration, posterior corneal defects, endothelial dystrophies or abnormal metabolic infiltrations. Corneal haze after a forceps delivery usually resolves.

Cataracts can be occasionally seen with the naked eye using a bright light shone tangentially. The lens should always be examined through an ophthalmoscope held 15–20 cm from the eye. If the lens is clear you should be able to see a red retinal reflex. If there is any doubt an ophthalmological opinion must be sought urgently, as the baby may have a congenital cataract. The best results are obtained after early treatment, before there is any chance of stimulus deprivation amblyopia (Ch. 33). A dull red reflex can also be secondary to congenital melanoma or cytomegaloviral retinitis. Unfortunately the neonatal screen performs poorly in the detection of cataract: 83/235 (35%) of cases diagnosed in the UK between 1995 and 1996 were detected at the newborn screen with further cases being uncovered at the 6-week check (Rahi and Dezateux 1999, 2001). Two-thirds were bilateral. The prevalence was estimated as 2.5 per 10 000 children. Babies in whom cataract is diagnosed must be investigated for the cause (Ch. 33). Congenital cataract is a target condition of the current NIPE programme, with the aim that 95% of all cases detected should be seen by an ophthalmologist within 2 weeks.

Mouth

Note if the mouth is of normal size or if there is micrognathia. Observe any asymmetry of the corners of the mouth and the nasolabial folds.

Inspection of the inside of the mouth is best done either while the baby is crying lustily or by making him open it (pressing down on the chin sometimes does the trick). It is better not to use a tongue depressor. One should ensure that the palate is intact by seeing it directly; palpation is not enough. It is embarrassing, to say the least, to have missed a cleft in the soft palate which later turns up as a feeding problem or nasal regurgitation.

Minor variations of normal which may be seen include: Epstein's pearls (white patches of microkeratosis akin to milia on the palate); natal teeth (which are rare in Caucasian populations but are usually best removed, especially if loose); short frenulum or 'tongue tie' (which very rarely needs treatment, Ch. 20); and bluish swellings (ranulae) on the floor of the mouth which are mucus retention cysts and need no treatment.

Neck

The baby has a relatively short neck, which should be inspected for general shape and symmetry, palpated for any lumps or swellings and tested for its full range of movements.

A webbed neck may suggest Turner syndrome (Ch. 31). A very short webbed neck with or without torticollis may indicate underlying abnormalities of the cervical spine (Klippel–Feil syndrome). Redundant skin posteriorly is one of the characteristics of Down syndrome (Ch. 31).

Cystic hygromas are soft fluctuant swellings, usually arising in the posterior triangle, which transilluminate readily. Sternomastoid 'tumours' are lesions in the sternomastoid muscle caused by haemorrhage or ischaemia resulting in secondary fibrosis (Ch. 37).

The clavicles should be palpated for fractures, especially if there is any suggestion of Erb's palsy, or if there was shoulder dystocia.

Chest and cardiorespiratory system

In spite of advances in antenatal scanning, most congenital heart disease is still unsuspected before birth, and babies still present with cyanosis, shock or a murmur. Congenital heart disease is one of the commonest groups of congenital abnormalities, being found in 7–8 per 1000 newborns. Unfortunately the neonatal examination performs no better in the detection of congenital heart disease or DDH than it does for cataract. Even in the best hands, the neonatal check fails to detect over half of all babies who are subsequently found to have significant heart disease (Ainsworth et al. 1999; Wren et al. 1999; Lee et al. 2001). A large retrospective study of all births in the northern region of the UK revealed 1590 babies with heart disease diagnosed by the age of a year from a cohort of 300 102 births (Wren et al. 1999). As many as 33% presented with signs before the newborn examination was carried out (five died), and of the

remaining 1061 babies the examination revealed an abnormality in just under half. Even when an abnormality was suspected, the usual arrangement for discharge with a 6-week paediatric follow-up was shown to be too late for some; a further nine babies died between discharge and 6 weeks. The main causes of death are hypoplastic left heart, interruption of the aortic arch, critical aortic stenosis and coarctation of the aorta.

Start by inspecting the chest. Breast swelling is quite normal at this age and a few drops of 'witches' milk' may be expressed from them. These changes are of no significance unless there is obvious inflammation, but the mother may need reassurance.

Many deductions about the cardiorespiratory state can also be made by simple inspection. As well as noting the infant's colour, the single best clue to overall function, observe the respiratory rate and other signs of respiratory distress such as retractions and grunting. If there is any doubt about the presence of cyanosis, check with a pulse oximeter. Pulse oximetry can improve the detection of congenital heart disease (Richmond et al. 2002; Koppel et al. 2003; Reich et al. 2003). About 5% of babies had a postductal oxygen saturation <95% at more than 2 hours of age, but only 1% of babies had a low result when it was checked twice: 10% of these had cardiac disease. The American Heart Association/American Academy of Pediatrics recently reviewed the question of pulse oximetry screening after 24 hours of age in some detail (Mahle et al. 2009). Ten studies with a population of 123 846 infants were summarised, with a false-positive rate of 0.035% when screening was done after 24 hours. A UK economic evaluation of the addition of pulse oximetry concluded that, of 121 infants in every 100 000 livebirths currently undetected by antenatal screening, 39 (32%) would be detected by clinical examination alone and 82 (68%) would be detected by pulse oximetry (Knowles et al. 2005). The additional cost per timely diagnosis was £4900 for pulse oximetry. Pulse oximetry was considered a promising alternative but further evaluation was recommended. Pulse oximetry can also detect babies with systemic illness (Ewer et al 2011). Certain groups of babies are at high risk of congenital heart disease, including those with Down syndrome (40–50% have heart defects), and in these babies screening echocardiography should be performed. Pulse oximetry is not part of the standard newborn screening examination, but most hospitals now have a pulse oximeter available in the room where newborn examinations are carried out, and this is a sensible addition given the current evidence.

The respiratory rate is normally 40–60 breaths/min. A baby whose respiratory rate is persistently above 60 breaths/min needs very careful evaluation and continued observation, because this is unusual; 60 breaths/min is just above the 90th centile for the normal respiratory rate at term (Fleming et al. 2011). Remember that all infants, particularly preterm ones, can have pauses of 5–10 seconds interspersed with periods of regular breathing (periodic breathing; Ch. 27.4). True apnoeic attacks last longer than this and are extremely rare in the full-term neonate. Observe the respiratory pattern. When the infant is quiet, there should be no flaring of the alae nasi, no grunting and no retractions. On crying, some babies, especially if premature, may exhibit mild sternal or subcostal retraction.

The lungs can be auscultated at the same time as the heart, but by and large this is an unrewarding exercise if there are no respiratory symptoms.

Palpate the precordium for any thrills or a pronounced ventricular heave. The point of maximal impulse is usually found in the left fourth intercostal space inside the mid-clavicular line. Percussion of an asymptomatic infant's chest is a waste of time.

Check the peripheral pulses: a persistent ductus arteriosus with a significant left-to-right shunt produces a bounding quality. Always palpate the femoral pulses; if they are absent or difficult to feel, suspect coarctation. Four-limb blood pressure may help by confirming a differential between the upper and lower limbs; however, normal newborns can have a difference of up to 20 ± 3.5 mmHg (Piazza et al. 1985). A difference of 20 mmHg or more suggests coarctation (Ch. 28).

Innocent heart murmurs

An innocent murmur is one that does not signify cardiac disease. Sixty per cent of normal newborns have a systolic murmur at the age of 2 hours (Braudo and Rowe 1961), but the incidence falls to around 1% by the time the routine neonatal examination is performed (Ainsworth et al. 1999; Farrer and Rennie 2003). Murmur is not the only sign of significant heart disease, and currently the neonatal examination detects only about a half of all babies who eventually present in the neonatal period with significant problems. Ainsworth et al. (1999) found a high incidence of problems when a murmur was present, but all those who care for the newborn must be aware that the absence of a murmur does not guarantee a normal heart, and vice versa. It is possible to make a positive diagnosis of an innocent murmur using clinical skills alone (Farrer and Rennie 2003), and the following features were emphasised in a study from Oxford (Arlettaz et al. 1998):

- grade 1–2/6 murmur at the left sternal edge
- no clicks on auscultation
- normal pulses
- otherwise normal clinical examination.

When a positive diagnosis of an innocent murmur was made in this way, no babies with cardiac disease were identified with subsequent echocardiography. About 23% of those who were offered echocardiography had significant cardiac disease (Farrer and Rennie 2003).

The usual origin of an innocent murmur is the acute angle at the pulmonary artery bifurcation; a few cases have patent ductus arteriosus or tricuspid regurgitation which resolves rapidly. McCrindle and colleagues (1996) suggested six features to help non-cardiologists identify significant murmurs:

1. pansystolic
2. grade 3/6 or more
3. best heard in the upper left sternal border
4. harsh quality
5. abnormal second heart sound
6. early or mid-systolic click.

Clinical examination was correct 98% of the time when similar criteria were applied to childhood murmurs, albeit by paediatric cardiologists (Smythe et al. 1990; McCrindle et al. 1996). Clinical evaluation without laboratory tests was equally effective in the hands of general paediatricians in Denmark (Hansen et al. 1995). Electrocardiogram (ECG) and chest X-ray have traditionally been used to assist in the classification of murmurs as innocent, but the clinical diagnosis is rarely changed by ECG (Newburger et al. 1983; Smythe et al. 1990) or chest X-ray (Newburger et al. 1983; Temmerman et al. 1991), and these tests should be abandoned for this purpose. An examination by an experienced colleague is a better aid to the identification of genuinely innocent murmurs. The widespread availability of echocardiography now means that this investigation, with the accompanying expert consultation, should be offered early to babies whose neonatal murmur cannot confidently be classified as innocent.

Mention of 'heart murmurs' produces intense anxiety, and talking about 'holes in the heart' is guaranteed to produce a flood of tears; now that it is clear that many are due to pulmonary vessel 'kinking' in a normal heart this is perhaps a less disturbing explanation. You

Table 14.2 Action to be taken when a heart murmur is heard

Is there peripheral circulatory collapse?	If so, immediate investigation is required
Is there central cyanosis?	Confirm with pulse oximeter. Urgent investigation if saturation low
Is there any evidence of heart failure (tachycardia, tachypnoea, enlarged liver)?	If so, immediate investigation is required
Can the femoral pulses be felt easily?	If not, check four-limb blood pressure
Are there any dysmorphic features?	If so, investigation should be done
Is the murmur grade 1–2/6, systolic, not harsh, heard at the left sternal edge only in a well baby with normal pulses?	The murmur is probably innocent. Check the result of pulse oximetry. If mother and baby are about to go home, inform parents about the problem and arrange follow-up at 3–4 weeks. Some units offer echocardiography to these infants
Is the murmur grade 3+ or more, running into diastole, or pansystolic, or is there a click, abnormal second heart sound or femoral pulses which are difficult to feel?	This murmur may be pathological. Even if the baby is well, ask a more senior colleague to listen. Watch the baby for signs of heart failure. Arrange echocardiography with the accompanying expert opinion as soon as possible. Carry out pulse oximetry, a chest X-ray and electrocardiogram as a baseline and to assist in differential diagnosis

can reassure the parents that 80–90% of murmurs found in the neonatal period will disappear during the first year, most of them within the first 3 months, and that if this is the case the baby will be discharged from the outpatient department. A practical guide to the action to be taken when a murmur is discovered is given in Table 14.2.

Abdomen

Inspection

Simple observation may yield quite a lot of information. Abdominal distension is easily appreciated, and because of the poorly developed abdominal musculature and scanty subcutaneous fat the intra-abdominal organs can sometimes be seen, particularly the bowel in premature infants. Look for any discharge or reddening of the skin around the umbilicus, which is a common source of infection. The state of the cord stump will depend on the age of the baby, but the cord usually separates by 2 weeks and a delay of longer than 30 days should be investigated (Ch. 39.1). Umbilical granulomas are common, developing in the stump after the cord falls off in an area where the umbilicus has not re-epithelialised completely. They are friable and bleed easily. They are caused by a proliferation of endothelial cells. The diagnosis is a clinical one, and it is important to distinguish a granuloma from a persistent urachus (which will occasionally discharge urine) or an umbilical polyp, which is a remnant of the vitelline duct. Granulomas can be treated with topical silver nitrate; care must be taken not to burn the adjacent normal skin. Recently, application of table salt three times a day has been found to be a successful alternative (Derakhshan 1998). Polyps and urachal cysts need surgery.

Shortly after birth the three vessels are easily seen. A single umbilical artery is present in 4 per 1000 of newborns. There is an association with intrauterine growth restriction, and renal abnormalities were found in 7% of cases in one series (Bourke et al. 1993). A single umbilical artery in a baby with any other problem justifies further investigation of the renal tract. There is no need to investigate further for isolated single umbilical artery in a well term baby with no other problem (Deshpande et al. 2009). Further investigation of the renal tract will also be required for infants who were found to have abnormalities on prenatal ultrasonography (see Ch. 35.2).

Palpation

It is essential for your hands to be warm and for the infant to be quiet and relaxed; if necessary have him suck on a dummy or a clean gloved finger. Remember that a baby with a full stomach may well regurgitate milk if you press too hard, often to the distress of the mother who may have just spent a lot of time in feeding the baby!

Palpate the abdominal musculature; there is frequently a diastasis of the recti. Feel for the liver edge, which can be up to 2 cm below the right costal margin in normal infants. The kidneys are usually palpable with patience, and some observers have even gone so far as to state that failure to feel them indicates their absence. It is, however, probably much more important to detect any abnormally large renal masses. The spleen can often be 'tipped', but if more than 1 cm is palpable, investigation is needed. Feel for an enlarged bladder; if present try to express it and observe the urinary stream. Auscultation need not form part of the routine abdominal examination unless there is reason to suspect gastrointestinal abnormality (distension, bile-stained vomit, failure to pass meconium or bloody stools).

Record the time of passage of first stool and urine; 99% of term babies have passed their first stool and urine by 34 hours (Ch. 20, Fig. 20.1).

Genitalia

Male

Inspect the penis for length (normally about 3 cm); occasionally a penis looks deceptively short but palpation will usually disclose a respectable organ buried in suprapubic fat. True micropenis is rare but is an important sign of congenital hypopituitarism. Check the position of the urethral meatus, and if it is abnormally situated describe the hypospadias as glandular, coronal, midshaft or perineal; also inspect the shaft of the penis for curvature and compress it at its base to stimulate an erection which may reveal a latent chordee. Glandular hypospadias without chordee usually needs no treatment, but in more severe degrees of hypospadias the baby will need corrective surgery at some time before school age. All cases should have the benefit of specialist advice and the parents must be told not to circumcise the baby because the foreskin will be essential for the future repair.

Always ask about the urinary stream in boys. A poor stream may be present if there is meatal stenosis with hypospadias; constant dribbling of urine is nearly always abnormal and may indicate urethral valves.

Examine the scrotum for rugosity and feel for the testes. At full term both testes should be palpable even if retractile. Normally the

midpoint of the testis is at the midpoint of the scrotum. A retractile testis can be pulled into a normal position even if it does not remain there. A testis which is incompletely descended can only be brought down to the correct position under tension, or be wholly impalpable. About 4–5% of male term babies have at least one testis which is undescended at birth, and about 1% are still undescended at a year. If both testes are undescended at the neonatal examination the NIPE standard is for a review within 24 hours by a senior clinician and referral to a surgeon if the diagnosis is confirmed, with an appointment within 26 weeks. Babies with unilateral undescended testes should be reviewed in 6 weeks, with surgical referral for those with persistent failure or maldescent. The rationale for early treatment is that surgery may improve fertility and reduce the risk of testicular cancer. There is a strong association between undescended testis and inguinal hernia.

A bluish black discoloration of the scrotum suggests testicular torsion, especially now that very few baby boys acquire bruising of their genitalia during a vaginal breech delivery. Neonatal testicular torsion occurred some time before birth in almost all cases, and in this situation the testis is hard and not tender (Driver and Losty 1998). Referral to a paediatric surgeon is indicated, and these days many treat with analgesia and antibiotics in the immediate neonatal period, because the testis is usually already infarcted. However most recommend that the contralateral testis is fixed in the medium term.

Hydroceles can occur in the newborn period, but usually resolve spontaneously and do not require treatment. Examine the groins for indirect inguinal hernis; these are not uncommon, particularly in preterm infants, and can usually be reduced easily. If present, the mother should be warned about the symptoms and signs of incarceration/strangulation and an urgent surgical appointment organised so that early surgery can be arranged.

Female

Inspect the vulva. The clitoris and labia minora are relatively prominent in preterm infants, but at full term the labia majora should cover the labia minora although the clitoris may still appear relatively large. There is often a white mucoid vaginal discharge which is occasionally blood-stained; this is normal and the mother should be reassured accordingly. Small hymenal skin tags or mucoid cysts which resolve spontaneously may occur around the vaginal opening. Inguinal hernis are rare in the female and their presence should raise the question of other abnormalities in the genital tract. For further advice see Chapter 29, part 4.

At this stage in the examination, check the position of the anus and anal tone. A 'wink' can be produced by gently touching the anal margin.

Spine

With the baby prone, inspect the back for any obvious curvature and look for any midline abnormality over the spine and base of skull such as a swelling, dimple, hairy patch or naevus. Any of these may indicate an underlying abnormality of the vertebral column or spinal cord; occult spinal dysraphism is the most common spinal axis malformation by far, and early detection should prevent upper urinary tract deterioration, infection and permanent damage to the nervous system.

Simple sacrococcygeal pits are common and harmless; in a study from St George's Hospital, London, UK, no infant in a series of 75 with sacral dimple or pit alone was found to have a spinal abnormality (Gibson et al. 1995). The problem lies in defining the 'simple dimple' or 'simple pit', because any midline lesion other

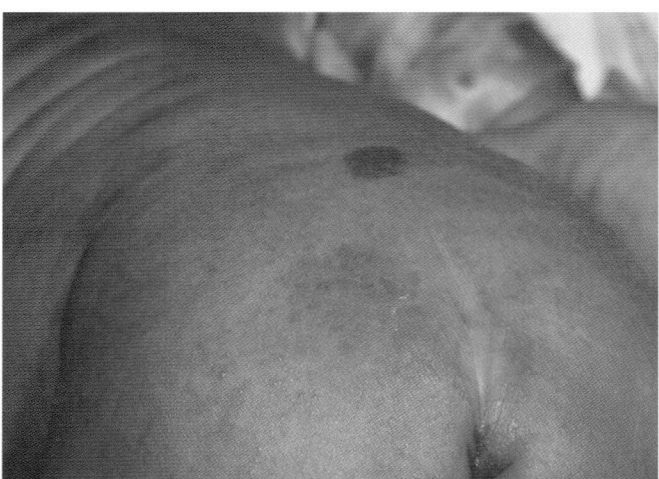

Fig. 14.2 A simple dimple above the anus, with an erythematous macule in the midline over the spine at a higher level.

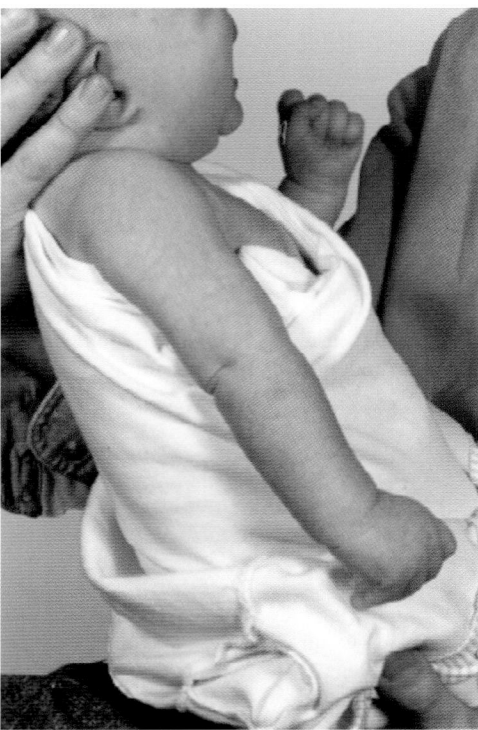

Fig. 14.3 Erb's palsy.

than those in or just above the natal cleft should be investigated. Similarly, any lesion at any level with a fatty pad, hairy patch or an area of atretic skin deserves further investigation. One helpful definition was given by Kriss and Desai (1998). These authors carefully evaluated 207 neonates with 216 dorsal cutaneous stigmata who were born in their hospital between 1993 and 1996 (the 207 were 4.8% of the births). All 207 (but not all babies) had ultrasound of the spine. Magnetic resonance imaging (MRI) was only performed if the ultrasound was abnormal. Of the 160 with 'simple' dimples – defined as being less than 2.5 cm from the anus and less than 5 mm wide, and with a midline placement and no other cutaneous stigmata – no baby had spinal dysraphism. Sixteen of the other babies were found to have abnormalities. Ultrasound was used to assess the position of the conus of the spinal cord (around L1–2 in the newborn, below L3 abnormal; Hill and Gibson 1995), and the mobility of the nerve roots, and the presence of an intrathecal mass. Figure 14.2 shows an example of a 'simple dimple' but with an associated midline erythematous macule which is a trigger for investigation. Kriss and Desai (1998) did not attempt to assess the incidence of spinal lesions in the babies without cutaneous markers: 50–80% of late-presenting cases with spinal dysraphism have a cutaneous marker.

Ultrasound can be very helpful in expert hands, and MRI may be indicated (Medina et al. 2001). Both MRI and ultrasound are better than plain radiographs.

See Chapter 40, part 8 for more information on spinal cord diastematomyelia and midline abnormalities. Always examine the back in the midline if at follow-up a baby has a limp, foot abnormalities, bladder or bowel problems or scoliosis.

Upper limbs

Inspect the arms for shape, posture and symmetry and size. In normal upper limbs the fingertips reach to midthigh when the arms are abducted to the body. Examine the hand for any flexion deformities of the fingers and inspect the palms for the arrangement of creases. Although about 45% of individuals with Down syndrome have single transverse palmar creases, this finding occurs unilaterally in 4% and bilaterally in 1% of the Caucasian population and is a normal phenotypic variant in the Chinese population (16.8%). Polydactyly (hands and feet) is sometimes a familial trait, but look

carefully for any other dysmorphic features. All digital remnants should be removed surgically. Previously some were tied off with black silk and left to separate by dry gangrene, but this left a stump which produced an unsightly lump or a painful neuroma in many cases.

Observe spontaneous arm movements; stroking the hand or forearm is sometimes necessary to elicit active motion in the shoulder, elbow, wrist and hand. Test passive movements for muscle tone and range of motion. Owing to intrauterine restriction of space and activity the newborn may lack some elbow extension. Lack of active movement and pain on passive manoeuvres suggest a fracture or infection, whereas in brachial plexus or cervical spine injury passive motion is not restricted. A brachial plexus lesion is revealed by lack of movement in the arm; initially the arm is flaccid. After 48 hours an upper palsy can be distinguished from a complete palsy. In an upper root palsy (C5, 6, sometimes C7) the arm is internally rotated and pronated, there is no active abduction or elbow flexion (Erb's palsy, the 'waiter's tip' position; Fig. 14.3). The incidence of brachial plexus palsy remains around 1.6–2.9 per 1000, although a recent UK study reported a lower incidence of 0.4 per 1000 (Evans-Jones et al. 2003; Pondaag et al. 2004; Lagerkvist et al. 2010). In a complete palsy of upper and lower roots the arm is flail; there may be a ptosis and a Horner syndrome due to damage to the stellate ganglion adjacent to C8 and T1. Phrenic palsy should be considered in these cases. The hand may become clawed (Klumpke's paralysis). Whilst the prognosis of brachial plexus lesions is generally good, with most series reporting a recovery rate of 75–95%, this may be overly optimistic. Over half the babies in the UK series still had signs at 6 months, and about 0.5 per 1000 in the Swedish series still had deficits at 18 months of age. The results of surgical repair have improved markedly and babies who have no recovery in biceps function by 3 months should be referred to a specialist (Gilbert et al. 1991).

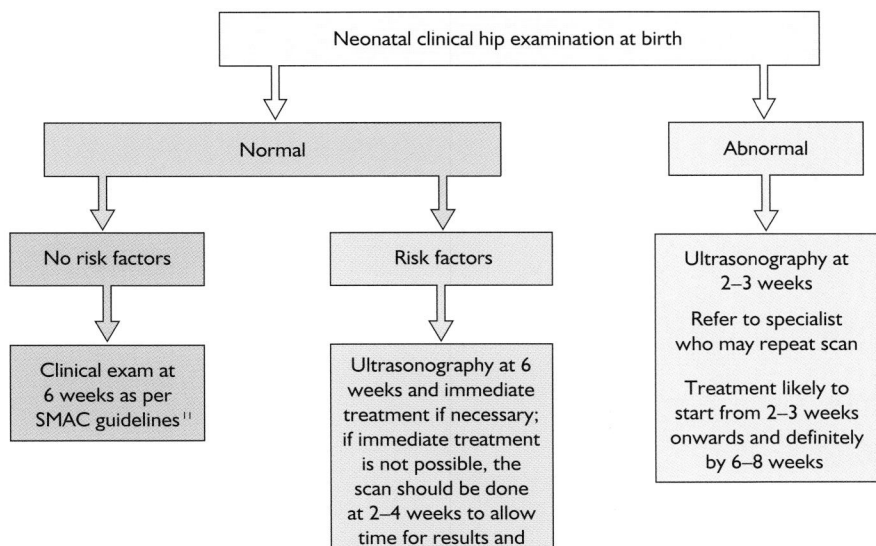

Fig. 14.4 Assessing developmental dysplasia of the hip. SMAC – Standing Medical Advisory Committee. Arch Dis Child 1986;61:921-6 *(Reproduced from Sewell et al. (2009), with permission.)*

Lower limbs

Inspect the legs and feet for posture, symmetry, general size and shape as well as for any obvious deformities. Observe spontaneous or stimulated active movements and test the range of passive movements.

The midpoint of the newborn baby's length is just above the umbilicus (compared with the symphysis pubis in the adult). Asymmetry in leg girth or length suggests one of the limb reduction defects. Some restriction of joint motion is common, secondary to limitation of intrauterine space. Babies who were vertex presentations usually have fully flexed hips and knees, but in those who were extended breech presentations the knees may remain fully extended for a few days so that the feet are somewhere near the mouth. The knees may lack up to 30° of full extension in the neonate. The tibiae are often laterally bowed and internally rotated. The feet should be inspected for their general configuration. They may provide confirmatory evidence of dysmorphic syndromes such as the 'rocker bottom' shape and short hallux in Edward syndrome. A convex 'rocker bottom' sole and a rigid foot may also indicate congenital vertical talus which will require surgery (Staheli 1993). Puffy feet and hypoplastic nails are characteristic of Turner syndrome.

The feet and ankles may be found in many positions, most of which are related to intrauterine moulding (especially if there has been oligohydramnios); much more rarely, there is an underlying neurological deficit. A calcaneovalgus position of the foot is almost invariably due to fetal position in utero and will correct in time with or without simple manipulation. If there is an equinovarus position, without using undue force an attempt should be made to overcorrect it by abduction and dorsiflexion of the foot and ankle so that the little toe touches the outside of the leg. If this manoeuvre is successful, no treatment is indicated, but deformities that cannot be so corrected (true talipes equinovarus) require urgent orthopaedic attention (Ch. 37). Simple metatarsus adductus (inturning of the forefoot) is common, and 90% resolve with no treatment.

Overriding toes are common; syndactyly is often familial; neither usually needs treatment. It is most important to explain the nature and natural history of these minor deformities to the parents.

Hips

Screening for congenital dislocation of the hip was introduced into the UK in 1966, and remains one of the most important items in the newborn examination; it is currently a NIPE target condition. This condition is now termed developmental dysplasia of the hip or DDH (Ch. 37) (Sewell et al. 2009). The incidence of DDH is around 1–3% of newborns. Expert management of DDH diagnosed in the neonatal period can be expected to produce a normal hip, while treatment initiated after the first year of life is usually followed by a worse result even after surgical treatment. Around a quarter of adult hip replacements in people aged 60 or less are associated with DDH (Furness et al. 2001). Sadly, despite initial confidence in the ability of the Ortolani and Barlow tests to detect DDH, the number of cases diagnosed late (0.2 per 1000) has not reduced and may even have increased (Sanfridson et al. 1991). The number of babies who require surgery for DDH has not much changed since the 1960s, at 0.78 per 1000 births (Godward and Dezeteux 1998).

The UK National Screening Committee recommends that an ultrasound be performed in babies with an abnormal clinical examination, those with a first-degree family history of hip problems in childhood, and those who were presenting by the breech after 36 weeks. Other risk factors such as talipes, oligohydramnios and torticollis are not considered strong enough evidence to mandate ultrasound. The target for performing the ultrasound examination is 2–3 weeks (Fig. 14.4).

The cornerstone of the screening strategy for DDH remains a careful history and clinical examination. The Ortolani–Barlow manoeuvres must be performed in every newborn. Details follow, although these tests are hard to describe in words and are much better taught by demonstration. A teaching aid, the 'baby hippy', is also available.

Procedure

The infant should be lying supine on a flat firm surface, with the legs relaxed, pacified if necessary by sucking on a dummy or finger. The examination may well make the baby cry and interpretation is difficult if the thigh muscles are actively contracting.

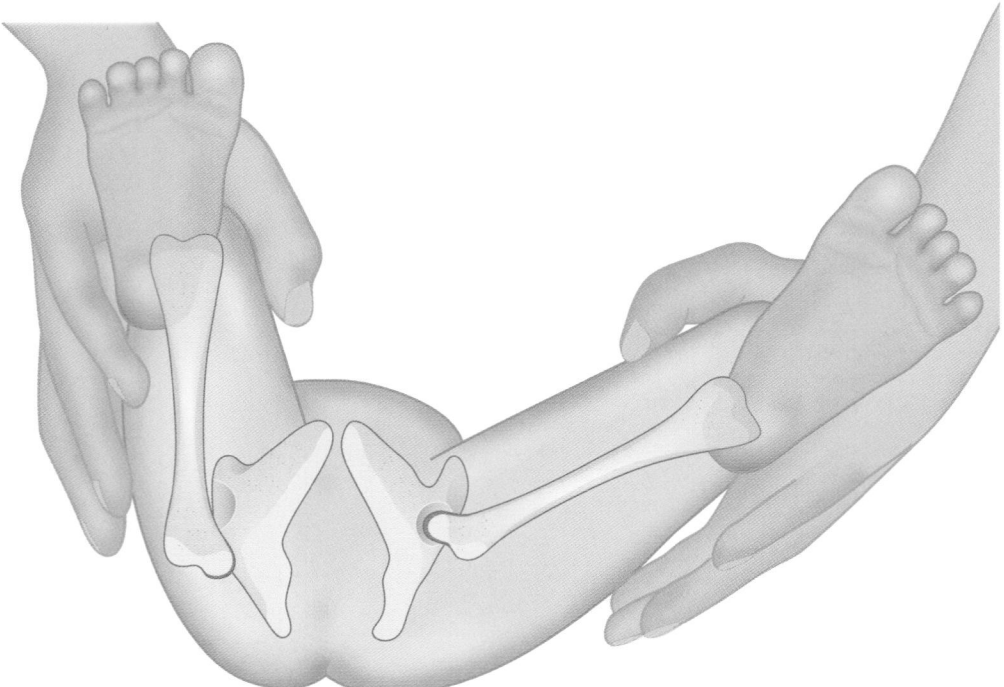

Fig. 14.5 Barlow and Ortolani test (see text for description). *(Reproduced from Sewell et al. (2009), with permission.)*

First, straighten out the legs and look for any obvious inequality in length, and asymmetric skin folds, although these are common and not a sensitive indicator of hip pathology. Fully flex the knees and flex the hips to a right angle. Look for any difference in the relative height of the knees, which can indicate a problem with one hip. Limited hip adduction (<60°) in 90° of hip flexion may be the most sensitive sign for detecting a dislocated hip in neonates. Neither the Ortolani nor Barlow test will detect a dislocated, irreducible hip or a stable hip with abnormal anatomy. In normal babies it is possible to abduct the hips fully so that the knees almost touch the couch. Inability to do so may indicate a dislocated hip that cannot be reduced and is an indication for an ultrasound scan.

Carry out Ortolani's test (Ortolani 1937). This manoeuvre is designed to return a dislocated femoral head to the acetabulum. Place the middle finger of each hand over the greater trochanters, thumbs over the internal aspect of the thighs, palms over the knees. Then, simultaneously, pull the leg away from the pelvis and slowly abduct and externally rotate the hips, pressing forwards and medially with the middle fingers (Fig. 14.5). A previously dislocated hip is indicated by a definite 'clunk' as the displaced femoral head slips forward into the acetabulum, rather like engaging the gear lever of a car. This is a quite different sensation from a ligamentous 'click' which is more common (Jones 1989). It does, however, take some experience to tell the difference, the clue being whether there is any sensation of movement.

The next stage of the examination is to do Barlow's test (Barlow 1962). This test is designed to 'dislocate' an unstable hip which is in joint. Some hips are 'loose' but cannot be completely dislocated using this clinical test. Hold the hips and knees as before. With the hips at about 70° abduction, test each hip in turn by pressing forwards and medially (i.e. towards the symphysis pubis) with the finger. Normally no movement is felt, but if the hip is dislocated the femur is felt to move, again with a 'clunk' as it slips into the acetabulum. The reverse procedure is then performed by pressing backwards and laterally with the thumb. Normally there is again no movement but a dislocatable hip will 'clunk' out of the acetabulum and will return there when the pressure is released.

Following the examination and ultrasound screening for high-risk groups it should be possible to classify the hip(s) into one of the following categories:

- normal
- a stable hip with acetabular dysplasia on ultrasound (found because of positive family history)
- a clinically unstable ('loose') hip with acetabular dysplasia on ultrasound
- a dislocatable hip (one that can be pushed out of the acetabulum and back again): Barlow-positive
- a reducible dislocated hip: Ortolani-positive
- an irreducible dislocated hip (this can be missed unless attention is paid to limited abduction; see above)
- a dislocatable or dislocated hip secondary to another problem, e.g. central nervous system disease.

For further information on the management of these types of DDH see Chapter 37.

Neurological

Although much has been written about the neurological assessment of the neonate, formal testing is seldom needed during routine examination of the newborn. More detail is contained in Chapter 40 part 1. Enough screening information can usually be gleaned from talking to the mother and from carefully watching, handling and listening to the baby throughout the examination.

The following general observations can act as a screening test, although one must take into account both gestational age (considered in more detail elsewhere) and postnatal age. The infant may be neurologically very labile during the first few days, and the most meaningful results are only obtained after this time. For a more comprehensive neurological assessment of both preterm and full-term neonates, see Dubowitz et al. (1999).

Behavioural state

Healthy term infants should move between behavioural states, spending most time in quiet and active sleep.

Posture

The undisturbed normal neonate lies predominantly in a flexed position with no lateral preference. When prone the knees are often tucked under the abdomen. The fists are clenched and the thumbs are intermittently furled. With the head in the midline the limbs are roughly symmetrical. Remember, however, that the presentation at birth can influence posture for several days.

Spontaneous motor activity

Normal infants move their limbs in an alternating fashion. Many babies may appear jittery. The prevalence of jittering was 44% in a sample of almost 1000 infants in Boston examined between 8 and 72 hours of age (Parker et al. 1990). Half were jittery solely when crying and the remainder were jittery during several behavioural states. How to distinguish jittering from fits is discussed in Chapter 40 part 2.

Muscle tone and strength

This is tested by:

1. Assessing resistance to passive movements.
2. Pull-to-sit manoeuvre. Pull the baby up from the supine position by his wrists. In term infants there should be some elbow flexion and the head should come up almost in line with the body. When held sitting the head should remain erect for 2–3 seconds. The palmar grasp reflex may be tested at the same time.
3. Ventral suspension. Hold the baby in the air with a hand under the chest – he should be able to hold his head in line with his body for a few seconds and he should be able to flex his limbs against gravity.

Other general observations

Crying will almost certainly be noted at some time during the examination. Pay particular attention if it is either high-pitched or very weak, or if the infant is reported to cry excessively.

Feeding and sucking patterns will be obvious from the history.

The eyes have already been discussed; they should lie in the midposition in the orbit and move in a conjugate fashion. Note any constant deviation, persistent strabismus and nystagmus.

Suspicious neurological signs

With practice and experience one is soon able to judge from the history and handling an infant during the examination whether he is behaving normally. The purpose of such a screening procedure is to pick out those infants who merit more detailed study and follow-up. The features which should arouse suspicion and which need careful follow-up are:

- persistent failure to suck properly
- a high-pitched cry
- extreme irritability or 'starey-eyed' appearance
- abnormal posturing, e.g. opisthotonus, excessive fisting, constantly fisted thumbs
- generalised persistent hypertonia
- 'frog' posture or generalised hypotonia
- paucity of spontaneous movements, including facial expressions

- asymmetrical movements
- a history of convulsions
- midline lesions over the spine.

Biochemical screening

The list of conditions which can be identified by screening a blood sample in the newborn period grows longer every year (Ch. 34.3), and various pressure groups have campaigned for the introduction of tests for maple syrup urine disease, congenital adrenal hyperplasia, galactosaemia, biotinidase deficiency and familial hyperlipidaemia, for example. Screening for cystic fibrosis and medium-chain acyl dehydrogenase deficiency has been introduced since the last edition of this book.

Health education

The normal newborn examination represents an opportunity to provide advice about well-baby care. Information is contained in the parent-held child health records, but a selection of leaflets on the following topics should be available, and the examining doctor needs to be prepared to give advice on a range of topics, including those following. Women who reported receiving healthcare advice were more satisfied with the consultation about their newborn than those who were not offered such advice (Wolke et al. 2002). Mothers appreciated advice on topics such as jaundice, skin care, sleeping, and stool and nappy care.

Jaundice

Kernicterus is a preventable disease, and its resurgence has been a distressing feature of the otherwise welcome early-discharge policy. Jaundice is the most common reason for readmission to the maternity unit. Leaflets are available informing parents of the importance of recognising jaundice. Health professionals should follow the NICE guideline (see Ch. 29.1); babies at increased risk of jaundice should be assessed within 48 hours.

Cot death prevention (www.sids.org.uk)

Babies should sleep alone, on their backs, parents should not smoke, infant bedrooms should be kept at a comfortable temperature of about 18°C and babies should be kept warm but not overclothed. There should be local initiatives in place for Care of the Next Infant – next siblings of infants who died of cot death.

Prevention of haemorrhagic disease of the newborn

If the parents choose oral vitamin K and the baby is to be breastfed, further oral doses of vitamin K are needed (Ch. 30). Local policies may vary as to which babies are not considered suitable for oral vitamin K prophylaxis, i.e. require intramuscular treatment because they are at high risk of vitamin K-deficiency bleeding. Examples include preterm babies, babies whose mothers are taking antituberculous or anticonvulsant drugs, and babies with evidence of liver disease.

Breastfeeding promotion

The hospital should be a 'baby-friendly' environment. The simple rules which have been shown to help promote breastfeeding (Ch. 20, Ch. 16.2) should be followed. A breastfeeding counsellor should be available to provide advice and suitable literature.

Sleeping

Advice on sleeping position, co-sleeping and bedding ties in with cot death prevention. Parents may welcome suggestions on websites or books with information about sleep routines, crying babies and colic.

Safe transport in cars

The newborn period is a good time to give advice on the purchase of safe types of car seat and to encourage their use.

Maternal depression

Those working in a maternity hospital should be aware of the maternal depression scales and how to administer them. Literature informing mothers about this common and important problem and where to get help could help prevent tragedy. Screening for depression is not advocated at present.

Gestational age

The most reliable basis for assigning gestational age is an early obstetric ultrasound, and when this agrees with the mother's menstrual dates this gives the best assessment. An evaluation of the neonatal methods of estimating gestational age revealed that even the best were only half as accurate as those based on obstetric ultrasound at 15–19 weeks of gestation (Wariyar et al. 1997). The clinical methods had 95% confidence intervals of 17 days, whereas the obstetric ultrasound had 95% confidence intervals of less than 7 days. Any maturity estimation based on ultrasound obtained only during the second half of pregnancy is unreliable, and information from uterine size and date of quickening is valueless from the neonatal point of view.

The criteria used for estimating gestational age after birth may be divided into those that are based on physical maturation and those that are dependent on development of the nervous system. Many complex scoring systems have been devised. Some criteria are more valuable than others, and little is lost by using only a few items (Parkin et al. 1976; Klimek et al. 2000). The physical items proved more robust than the items assessing tone and posture in the evaluation of Wariyar et al. and a retrospective assessment based on when the infant acquired the ability to suck and swallow reliably (34–35 weeks) was surprisingly accurate providing the infant was not oxygen-dependent (Wariyar et al. 1997). Direct ophthalmoscopy can be used to visualise the lens, although the cornea is usually too opaque for this to be possible in very preterm babies (whose eyelids may also be fused). After about 27 weeks a grading system can be applied to the vessels of the lens, which cover the entire anterior surface between 27 and 28 weeks, and reach only to the middle of the lens by 31–32 weeks and are at the periphery by 33–34 weeks (Hittner et al. 1977). This method of assessment is not much used because it requires dilatation of the pupil and is only applicable at less than 48 hours of age.

Physical characteristics

Various attempts have been made to quantify some of these changes by using scoring systems. Farr et al. (1966) used a system of 34 points derived from 11 criteria; Dubowitz et al. (1970) and Dubowitz et al (1999) used the same physical criteria with a total of 35 points. Parkin et al. (1976) produced a much simpler scheme with 13 points derived from only four of the above criteria. This simple system proved as accurate as the Dubowitz or expanded Ballard (Ballard et al. 1979, 1991) score if half-scores were allotted (Wariyar et al. 1997). The newer Ballard score (Ballard et al. 1991) is valid for very preterm infants, although the accuracy in this group has been questioned. The appearance times of four reflexes as described by Robinson (1966) are probably most useful for premature infants <34 weeks.

For details of these scoring systems, see previous editions of this book. They are little used now that most women have early ultrasound, but remain of occasional value in a baby born after a concealed pregnancy.

Weblinks

Information and guidance regarding the NHS programmes for examination and hearing screening
www.hearing.screening.nhs.uk
www.newbornphysical.screening.nhs.uk

www.nice.org.uk: National Institute for Health and Clinical Excellence – guidelines on postnatal management of the mother and baby, and neonatal jaundice.

References

Adam, M., Hudgins, L., 2003. The importance of minor anomalies in the evaluation of the newborn. Neoreviews 4, e99.

Ainsworth, S.B., Wyllie, J.P., Wren, C., 1999. Prevalence and clinical significance of cardiac murmurs in neonates. Arch Dis Child 80, F43–F45.

Arlettaz, R., Archer, L.N.J., Wilkinson, A.R., 1998. Archives of Disease in Childhood Fetal and Neonatal Edition. 78, F166–F170.

Ballard, J.L., Novak, K.K., Driver, M.A., 1979. A simplified score of fetal maturation of newly born infants. J Pediatr 95, 769–774.

Ballard, J.L., Khoury, J.C., Wedig, K., et al., 1991. New Ballard score, expanded to include extremely premature infants. J Pediatr 119, 417–423.

Barlow, T.G., 1962. Early diagnosis and treatment of congenital dislocation of the hip. J Bone Joint Surg 44, B292–BB301.

Bourke, W.G., Clarke, T.A., Mathews, T.G., et al., 1993. Isolated single umbilical artery – the case for screening. Arch Dis Child 68, 600–601.

Braudo, M., Rowe, R.D., 1961. Auscultation of the heart in the early neonatal period. Am J Dis Child 101, 575–586.

Brown, F.E,, Cohen, L.B., Addante, R.R., et al., 1986. Correction of congenital auricular deformities by splinting in the neonatal period. Pediatrics 78, 406–411.

Derakhshan, M.R., 1998. Curative effect of common salt on umbilical granuloma. Iran J Med Sci 23, 132–133.

Deshpande, S.A., Jog, S., Watson, H., et al., 2009. Do babies with isolated single umbilical artery need routine postnatal renal ultrasonography? Arch Dis Child Fetal Neonatal Ed 94, F265–F267.

Driver, C.P., Losty, P.D., 1998. Neonatal testicular torsion. Br J Urol 82, 855–858.

Dubowitz, L.M.S., Dobowitz, V., Goldberg, C., 1970. Clinical assessment of gestational age in the newborn infant. J Pediatr 77, 1–10.

Dubowitz, L., Dobowitz, V., Mercuri, E., 1999. The Neurological Assessment of the Preterm and Fulllterm Newborn Infant, second ed. Clinics in Developmental Medicine no. 148. MacKeith Press, Cambridge.

Dunn, P.M., 1976. Congenital postural deformities. Br Med Bull 32, 71–76.

Eichenfield, L.F., Frieden, I.J., Esterly, N.B., 2008. Textbook of Neonatal Dermatology, second ed. Elsevier, Philadelphia.

Evans-Jones, G., Kay, S.P.J., Weindling, A.M., et al., 2003. Congenital brachial palsy: incidence causes and outcome in the UK and republic of Ireland. Arch Dis Child 88, F185–F189.

Ewer, A.K., Middleton, L.J., Furmston, A.T., et al., 2011. Pulse oximetry screening for congenital heart defects in newborn infants (PulseOx): a test accuracy study. Lancet 378, 785–794.

Farr, V., Kerridge, D.F., Mitchell, R.G., 1966. The value of some external characteristics in the assessment of gestational age. Dev Med Child Neurol 8, 657–660.

Farrer, K.F.M., Rennie, J.M., 2003. Neonatal murmurs: are senior house officers good enough? Arch Dis Child 88, F147–F151.

Fleming, S., Thompson, M., Stevens, R., et al., 2011. Normal ranges of heart rate and respiratory rate in children from birth to 18 years: a systematic review of observational studies. Lancet 377, 1011–1018.

Furness, O., Lie, S.A., Espehaug, B., et al., 2001. Hip disease and the prognosis of total hip replacements. J Bone Joint Surg 83, 579–586.

Gibson, P., Britton, J., Hall, D.M.B., et al., 1995. Lumbosacral skin markers and identification of occult spinal dysraphism in neonates. Acta Paediatr Scand 84, 208–209.

Gilbert, A., Brockman, R., Carlioz, H., 1991. Surgical treatment of brachial plexus palsy. Clin Orthop Rel Res 264, 39–47.

Godward, S., Dezeteux, C., 1998. Surgery for congenital dislocation of the hip as a measure of outcome of screening. Lancet 351, 1149–1152.

Graham Jr, J.M., 1994. When is it best to be born? A morphological perspective – craniofacial deformation. In: Amiel-Tison, C., Stewart, A. (Eds.), The Newborn Infant: One Brain for Life. INSERM, Paris, pp. 23–38.

Graham Jr, J.M., Smith, D.W., 1979. Parietal craniotabes in the neonate: its origin and significance. J Pediatr 95, 114–116.

Hall, D.M.B., Elliman, D., 2003. Health for All Children, fourth ed. Oxford University Press, Oxford.

Hansen, L.K., Birkebaek, N.H., Oxhoj, H., 1995. Initial evaluation of children with heart murmurs by the non-specialised paediatricians. Eur J Pediatr 154, 15–17.

Hernandez, J.A., Morelli, J.G., 2003. Birthmarks of potential medical significance. NeoReviews 4, e263.

Hill, C.A., Gibson, P.J., 1995. Ultrasound determination of the normal location of the conus medullaris in neonates. Am J Neuroradiol 16, 469–472.

Hittner, H.M., Hirsch, N.J., Rudolph, A.J., 1977. Assessment of gestational age by examination of the anterior vascular capsule of the lens. J Pediatr 91, 455–458.

Hunter, A.G.W., Rudd, N.L., 1977. Craniosynostosis II: Its familial characteristics and associated clinical findings in 109 patients lacking bilateral polysyndactyly or syndactyly. Teratology 15, 301–310.

Klimek, R., Klimek, M., Rzepecka-Weglarz, B., 2000. A new score for postnatal clinical assessment of fetal maturity in newborn infants. Int J Gynecol Obstet 71, 101–105.

Knowles, I., Griebsch, I., Dezateux, C., et al., 2005. Newborn screening for congenital heart defects: a systematic review and cost-effectiveness analysis. Health Technol Assess 9, 44.

Koppel, R.I., Druschel, C.M., Carter, T., et al., 2003. Effectiveness of pulse oximetry screening for congenital heart disease in asymptomatic newborns. Pediatrics 111, 451–455.

Kriss, V.M., Desai, N.S., 1998. Occult spinal dysraphism in neonates: assessment of high risk cutaneous stigmata on sonography. Am J Radiol 171, 1687–1693.

Kugelman, A., Tubi, A., Bader, D., et al., 2002. Preauricular tags and pits in the newborn: the role of renal ultrasonography. J Pediatr 141, 388–391.

Jones, D.A., 1989. Importance of the clicking hip in screening for congenital dislocation of the hip. Lancet 1, 599–601.

Lagerkvist, A.-L., Johnansson, U., Johansson, A., et al., 2010. Obstetric brachial plexus palsy: a prospective, population-based study of incidence, recovery, and residual impairment at 18 months of age. Dev Med Child Neurol 52, 529–534.

Laing, I.A., Wong, C.M., 2002. Hypernatraemia in the first few days: is the incidence rising? Archives of Disease in Childhood Fetal and Neonatal Edition 87, F158–F162.

Landau, M., Krafchick, B.R., 1999. The diagnostic value of café au lait macules. J Am Acad Dermatol 40, 877–890.

Lee, T.W.R., Skelton, R.E., Skene, C., 2001. Routine neonatal examination: effectiveness of trainee paediatrician compared with advanced neonatal nurse practitioner. Arch Dis Child 85, f100–f104.

Lin, D.S., Huang, F.Y., Lin, S.P., et al., 1997. Frequency of associated anomalies in congenital hypoplasia of depressor anguli oris muscle: a study of 50 patients. Am J Med Genet 71, 215–218.

Mahle, W.T., Newburger, J.W., Matherne, G.P., et al., 2009. Role of pulse oximetry in examining newborns for congenital heart disease: a scientific statement from the American Heart Association and the American Academy of Pediatrics. Pediatrics 124, 823–826.

McCrindle, B.W., Shaffer, K.M., Kan, J.S., et al., 1996. Cardinal clinical signs in the differentiation of heart murmurs in children. Arch Paediatr Adolesc Med 150, 169–174.

Medina, L.S., Crone, K., Kuntz, K.M., 2001. Newborns with suspected occult spinal dysraphism: a cost effectiveness analysis of diagnostic strategies. Pediatrics 108, e101.

Nance, W.E., 2003. The genetics of deafness. Mental Retard Dev Disabil Res Rev 9, 109–119.

Newburger, J.W., Rosenthal, A., Williams, R.G., et al., 1983. Noninvasive tests in the initial evaluation of heart murmurs in children. N Engl J Med 308, 61–64.

NICE, 2006. Routine Postnatal Care of Women and their Babies. www.nice.org.uk

Ortolani, M., 1937. Un segno poco noto e sua importanza per la diagnosi precoce di prelussazione congenita dell'anca. Pediatrica (Napoli) 45, 129–136.

Parker, S., Zuckerman, B., Bauchner, H., et al., 1990. Jitteriness in full term neonates: prevalence and correlates. Pediatrics 85, 17–23.

Parkin, J.M., Hey, E.N., Clowes, J.S., 1976. Rapid assessment of gestational age at birth. Arch Dis Child 51, 259–263.

Piazza, S.F., Chandra, S., Harper, R.G., et al., 1985. Upper versus lower systolic blood pressure in full term normal newborn. Am J Dis Child 139, 797–799.

Pondaag, W., Malessy, M.J.A., Thomeer, R.T.W.M., 2004. Natural history of obstetric brachial plexus palsy: a systematic review. Dev Med Child Neurol 46, 138–144.

Rahi, J.S., Dezateux, C., 1999. National cross sectional study of detection of congenital and infantile cataract in the United Kingdom: role of childhood screening and surveillance. Br Med J 318, 362–365.

Rahi, J.S., Dezateux, C., 2001. Measuring and interpreting the incidence of congenital ocular anomalies: Lessons from a National Study of Congenital Cataract in the UK. Invest Ophthalmol Visual Sci 42, 1444–1448.

Reich, J.D., Miller, S., Brogdon, B., et al., 2003. The use of pulse oximetry to detect congenital heart disease. J Pediatr 142, 268–272.

Richmond, S., Reay, G., Abu Harb, M., 2002. Routine pulse oximetry in the asymptomatic newborn. Arch Dis Child 87, F83–F88.

Robinson, R.J., 1966. Assessment of gestational age by neurological examination. Arch Dis Child 41, 437–447.

Rothman, L., Rose, J.S., Laster, D.W., et al., 1976. The spectrum of growing skull fracture. Pediatrics 57, 26–31.

Ruder, R.O., Graham Jr, J.R., 1996. Evaluation and treatment of the deformed and malformed auricle. Clin Pediatr 35, 461–465.

Sanfridson, J., Redland-Johnell, I., Uden, A., 1991. Why is congenital dislocation of the hip still missed? Analysis of 96,891 infants screened in Malmo, 1956–1987. Acta Orthop Scand 62, 87–91.

Scarfo, G.B., Mariotti, A., Tomaccini, D., et al., 1989. Growing skull fracture. Child's Nerv Syst 5, 163–167.

Sewell, M.D., Rosendahl, K., Eastwood, D.M., 2009. Developmental dysplasia of the hip. Br Med J 339, 1242–1247.

Smith, J.D., Crumley, R.L., Lee, A.H., 1981. Facial paralysis in the newborn. Otolaryngol Head Neck Surg 89, 1021–1024.

Smythe, J.F., Teixeira, O.H., Vlad, P., et al., 1990. Initial evaluation of heart murmurs: are laboratory tests necessary. Pediatrics 86, 497–500.

Staheli, L.T., 1993. Shoes and common lower limb problems. In: David, T.J. (Ed.) Recent Advances in Paediatrics, vol. 11. Churchill Livingstone, Edinburgh, pp. 161–173.

Temmerman, A.M., Mooyaart, E.L., Taverne, P.P., 1991. The value of the routine chest roentenogram in the cardiological evaluation of infants and children: a prospective study. Eur J Pediatr 150, 623–636.

Wariyar, U., Tin, W., Hey, E., 1997. Gestational assessment assessed. Arch Dis Child 77, F216–F.

Wessex Universal Neonatal Hearing Screening Trial Group, 1998. Controlled trial of universal neonatal screening for early identification of permanent childhood hearing impairment. Lancet 352, 1957–1964.

Wolke, D., Dave, S., Hayes, J., et al., 2002. Routine examination of the newborn and maternal satisfaction: a randomised controlled trial. Arch Dis Child 86, F155–F160.

Wren, C., Richmond, S., Donaldson, L., 1999. Presentation of congenital heart disease in infancy: implications for routine examination. Arch Dis Child 80, F49–F53.

Wright, C.M., Parkinson, K.N., 2004. Postnatal weight loss in term infants: what is 'normal' and do growth charts allow for it? Arch Dis Child 89, F254–F257.

Young, J.D.H., MacEwen, C.J., 1997. Managing congenital lacrimal obstruction in general practice. Br Med J 315, 293–296.

Temperature control and disorders

Anoo Jain

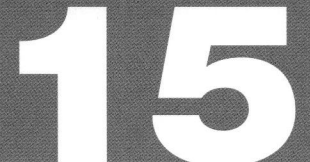

Introduction

The ability of the newborn to maintain a normal temperature is critical to his or her survival yet, even in today's neonatal intensive care units, thermal care is often given a low priority (Costeloe et al. 2000; Confidential Enquiry into Maternal and Child Health 2003). Silverman et al. (1958) demonstrated a link between poor temperature control and increased neonatal mortality and morbidity over 50 years ago. The 1995 EPICure cohort demonstrated that a low admission temperature was an independent risk factor for increased mortality in newborn infants delivered at less than 26 weeks' gestation (Costeloe et al. 2000). In this cohort mortality for newborn infants who were admitted to the neonatal intensive care unit at 23, 24 and 25 weeks' gestation was 58%, 43% and 30% respectively if the admission temperature was less than 35°C. In addition the Confidential Enquiry into Stillbirths and Deaths in Infancy (CESDI) Project 27/28 report of care for newborn infants at 27 and 28 weeks' gestation showed that mortality was 73% in babies with an admission temperature below 36°C compared with 59% in warmer babies (Confidential Enquiry into Maternal and Child Health 2003).

The newborn baby has many thermal homeostatic mechanisms, but a large surface area to body weight ratio and being born wet into a draughty, cold environment contribute to significant cold stress.

© 2012 Elsevier Ltd

Body temperature control mechanisms

The production of heat energy is central to the homeostatic repertoire of the newborn (Morrison et al. 2008). Heat is generated in most tissues from the inefficiency of mitochondrial adenosine triphosphate production and utilisation. This can occur from an increase in heart rate, shivering in skeletal muscle and nonshivering thermogenesis. The increase in heart rate response is mediated by the sympathetic nervous system. When a skeletal muscle shivers or the heart rate increases then heat is generated. However shivering is not an important feature of the newborn's cold response. Instead, nonshivering thermogenesis in brown adipose tissue (BAT) plays a critical role in temperature homeostasis in the newborn infant.

Central nervous thermoreceptive mechanisms

Environmental temperature has a direct and more rapid effect on skin temperature than on core body temperature (Morrison et al. 2008). Thermal afferents from the skin to the preoptic hypothalamus promote rapid cold defence responses before core body temperature is affected. At a molecular level the transient receptor potential family of cation channels mediates sensation across a broad range of cold and warm physiological temperatures.

Central nervous system thermoregulatory pathways to and from the preoptic hypothalamus can stimulate heat production in response to a cold environment, fall in body temperature or the presence of cytokines in BAT, the heart or skeletal muscle. Cutaneous cold afferents to the preoptic hypothalamus then generate α motor neuron activity and shivering. In addition to cutaneous receptors, the preoptic hypothalamus receives afferents from core body structures such as the brain, spinal cord and abdomen via the spinothalamocortical pathway. Cold and warm receptors are included in the splanchnic and vagus nerve abdominal afferents. Deep body structures are not as susceptible to changes in environmental temperature as the skin but play an indirect role in temperature regulation.

Brown adipose tissue

BAT has a specific heat-generating function and is found in characteristic areas of the baby, such as interscapular, axillary, perirenal, and thoracic regions and between neck muscles (Blackburn and Loper 1992). In the term newborn, BAT accounts for 2–7% of the infant's weight. BAT cells begin to differentiate at 26–30 weeks' gestation, continue to develop until approximately 5 weeks after delivery and over this timeframe can increase by up to 150% (Blackburn and Loper 1992). BAT metabolism is controlled by the sympathetic nervous system, noradrenaline (norepinephrine) release and β$_3$-adrenergic receptor binding to brown adipocytes (Morrison et al. 2008). Heat is generated by a facilitated proton leak across the mitochondrial membranes of brown adipocytes that uncouples oxidative phosphorylation. This occurs because of the high expression of uncoupling protein 1 (UCP1) in BAT mitochondria (Budge et al. 2003; Symonds et al. 2003). Dawkins and Scopes (1965) and Hey (1969) demonstrated that oxygen consumption almost doubled (4.8 versus 8.2 ml/kg/min) and plasma glycerol increased at an environmental temperature of 25–26°C compared with 34–35°C. These results strongly suggested that heat production occurred in BAT when the human newborn was exposed to cold. Although not specific to BAT, MRI studies have demonstrated that the preterm infant has significantly less adipose tissue and an altered deposition pattern compared with term newborn infants

(Uthaya et al. 2004, 2005). This might suggest that the preterm infant has limited ability to generate heat through nonshivering thermogenesis from both a lack of BAT and lower UCP1 expression.

Response to a cold environment

As the environmental temperature falls, the baby makes physiological and behavioural responses to maintain a constant deep body temperature. These are initiated by hypothalamic and cutaneous temperature receptors.

Physiological

Nonshivering thermogenesis results from metabolic activity in BAT (see above). Nonshivering thermogenesis is impaired in all newborns in the first 12 hours, particularly in those who are ill. Peripheral vasoconstriction also occurs in response to cold, diverting blood from the surface to the core. This is well developed in term babies but limited in very immature babies in the immediate neonatal period.

Behavioural

Whereas a child or adult will wake up and become restless when cold, the newborn infant may continue to sleep. Cold term and preterm babies tend to be more active, sleep less and adopt a flexed posture in an attempt to increase heat production and decrease heat loss.

Response to a warm environment

As the environmental temperature rises, the newborn baby attempts to prevent a rise in body temperature.

Physiological

Sweating in response to a warm environment occurs in term newborns from birth (Hey and Katz 1969; Harpin and Rutter 1982). The amount of water lost by sweating per unit area of skin is considerably lower than that lost by a heat-acclimatised adult, although the density of sweat glands is greater in the newborn. Sweating is most marked on the forehead, temple and occiput. The palms and soles only sweat in response to emotional stress. Sweating provides some measure of defence against overheating. In congenital hypohidrotic ectodermal dysplasia sweating is impaired and these babies are particularly susceptible to heat stress. Sweating is absent in babies born at less than 36 weeks' gestation but usually appears by about 2 weeks of age. Babies of opiate-abusing mothers have a well-developed ability to sweat at any gestational age. Vasodilatation in response to heat occurs in term and preterm babies, so that their skin is warm and red when overheated (Harpin et al. 1983).

Behavioural

As the environmental temperature increases, term and preterm babies become less active, sleep more and lie in an extended, sunbathing posture (Rutter and Hull 1979a; Harpin et al. 1983).

Normal heat transfer

The normal fetus has a temperature approximately 0.5–1°C higher than that of the mother. At birth the newborn loses heat rapidly, mainly by evaporation. This can result in a drop of 2–3°C and the

SINGLETON HOSPITAL
STAFF LIBRARY

triggering of the cold defence responses described above. Term newborns can increase their metabolic rate by 100% after birth but this response is blunted in a preterm or low birthweight baby (Bruck 1961). In addition the altered distribution and decreased quantity of adipose tissue and a surface area to volume ratio 3–5 times greater than that of an adult put the newborn at high risk of temperature loss.

Heat balance

The law of conservation of energy demands that, under equilibrium conditions, heat loss balances heat production. If production exceeds loss, the body temperature rises and vice versa until a new equilibrium is reached. The rate of production or loss of heat is dependent on the magnitude of the gradient between the baby and the external environment and flows from warm to cold.

Heat production

The baby produces heat by metabolic activity in all body tissues. Basal metabolic rate is difficult to measure since the newborn is rarely awake, quiet and starved, but resting levels can be measured. The resting metabolic rate (usually measured indirectly as the resting oxygen consumption) describes the metabolism of a baby who is lying still, asleep, more than an hour after the previous feed, and in thermal neutral surroundings. Under these conditions, the heat production of a healthy term newborn is similar to that of an adult when expressed per unit weight, but almost half that of an adult when expressed per unit surface area. Surface area determines a subject's heat loss and thus the relatively low heat production per unit area explains why the newborn requires a much warmer environment than an adult. Resting metabolic rate is similar in term and preterm newborn infants when expressed per unit weight, but considerably lower in preterm newborn infants when expressed per unit surface area (Fig. 15.1). Preterm babies thus require higher ambient temperatures than term newborn infants (Hey and Katz 1970).

Resting metabolic rate rises in the immediate newborn period (Hill and Rahimtulla 1965; Hey 1969). The maximum rate of heat production is approximately 50 kcal/m²/h reached by the age of 3–6 months and then remains constant into adult life. Many factors influence a newborn baby's heat production (Table 15.1), which is higher in rapid eye movement sleep than deep sleep, suggesting that the brain is metabolically highly active. The baby is also able to increase heat production in response to cold stress but there is considerable individual variation (see below).

Sources of heat loss

Conduction

Conductive heat loss involves transfer of heat from the body core to the body surface and then to objects that are in contact with it (mattress, scales). Conductive loss can be minimised by insulation, skin to skin contact and mattresses in incubators.

Convection

Heat is lost by convection from the exposed surface of the baby to the surrounding air, and is largely determined by the difference in temperature between the two. If the ambient temperature exceeds the surface temperature of the baby, heat will be gained by convection. Convective heat loss also depends on the air speed. If it is rapid, the insulating effect of still air close to the baby's surface is lost (forced convection) and convective heat loss increases (wind chill factor). Convection is a major source of heat loss when newborn babies are exposed in cool, draughty rooms. Convective heat loss can be minimised by swaddling, using hats, warming oxygen and minimising draughts.

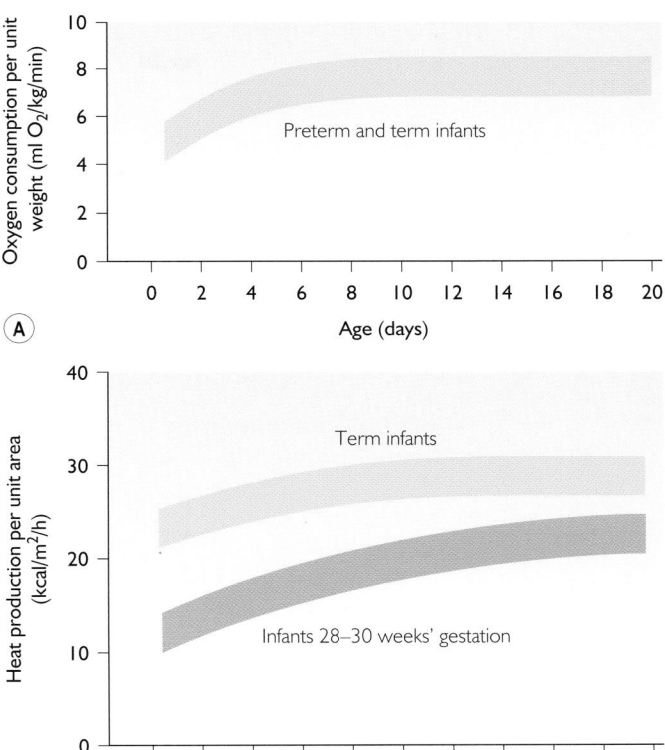

Fig. 15.1 Resting metabolic rate in the newborn period when expressed per unit weight (A) and per unit surface area (B). The ranges shown are the mean values ± 1 standard deviation. *(Derived from data of Hey (1969).)*

Table 15.1 Factors affecting a newborn infant's heat production

HEAT PRODUCTION IS INCREASED	HEAT PRODUCTION IS DECREASED
Awake	Deep sleep
Active	Ill (e.g. asphyxia or hypoxia)
Postfeeding	Starvation
Rapid growth	Malnutrition
Neonatal thyrotoxicosis	Hypothyroidism
Left-to-right cardiac shunt	Cyanotic congenital heart disease
Drugs (e.g. theophylline)	Drugs (e.g. chlorpromazine, caffeine)

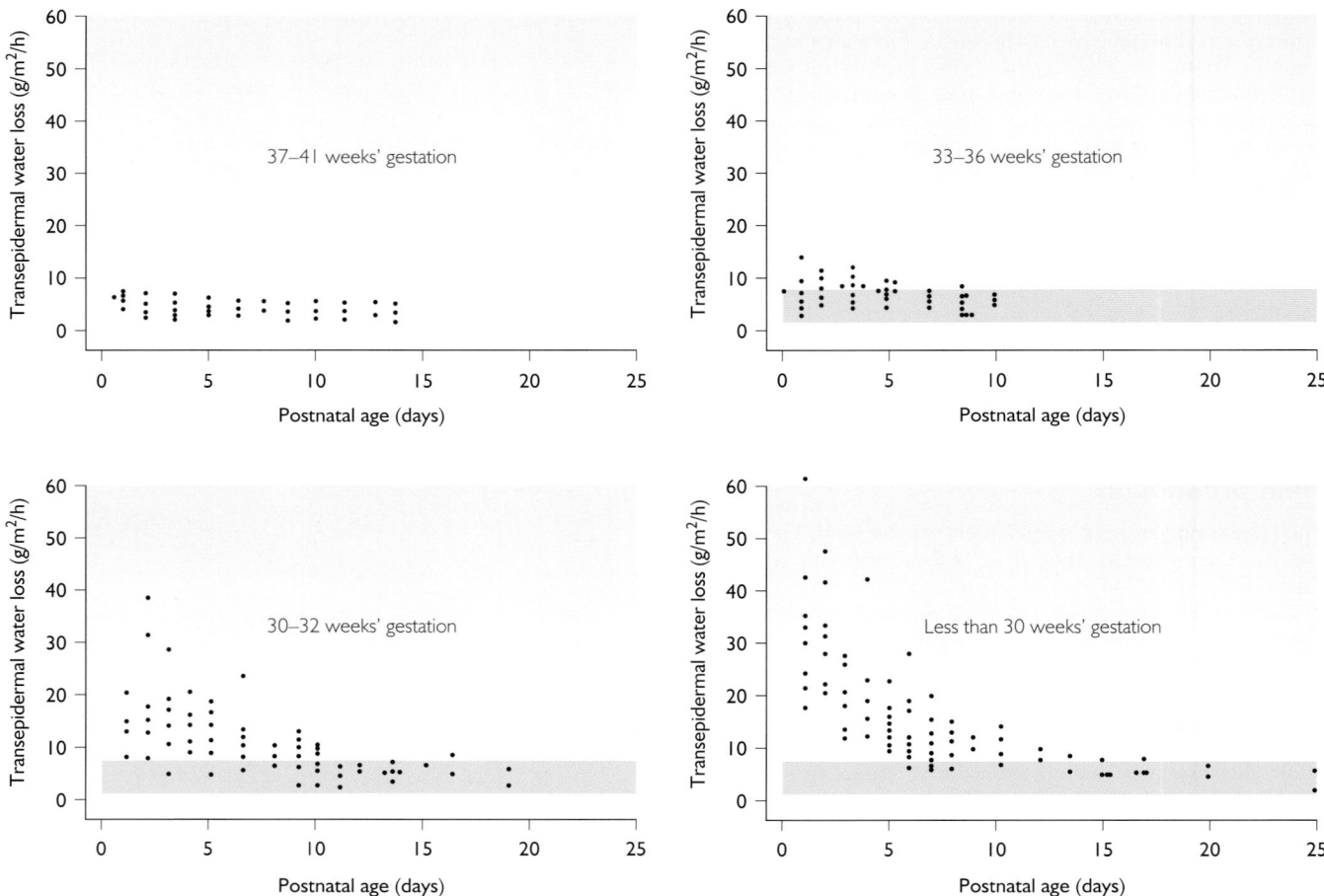

Fig. 15.2 Transepidermal water loss from the abdomen of newborn infants, showing the separate influences of gestation and postnatal age. The shaded area is the range of water loss in term infants for comparison. *(From data of Harpin and Rutter (1983).)*

Radiation

Heat is lost by radiation from the exposed skin of the baby to the surrounding surfaces. This loss is proportional to the difference between these surface temperatures but independent of the temperature and speed of the intervening air. Radiation loss is an important channel of heat loss when babies are naked in a delivery room or a single-walled incubator, but a source of heat gain when a baby is nursed under a radiant warmer.

Evaporation of water

As water evaporates from a baby's skin, heat is lost (each millilitre of water that evaporates removes 560 calories of heat). Under normal conditions in a term baby, evaporative heat loss amounts to about a quarter of the resting heat production (Hey and Katz 1969). About a quarter of this loss is by evaporation of water from the respiratory tract, the remainder occurring by passive diffusion of water through the epidermis (transepidermal water loss (TEWL)). Nevertheless evaporative heat loss is not a major source of heat loss in term babies, except at delivery, when the skin is wet with amniotic fluid. Mature babies have the ability to increase evaporative heat loss in response to a warm environment by sweating (Hey and Katz 1969; Harpin and Rutter 1982).

However, preterm babies have high evaporative heat losses compared with term babies (Fanaroff et al. 1972; Okken et al. 1979).

This is the result of a high TEWL, which is up to six times higher per unit surface area in a newborn baby of 26 weeks' gestation than in a term baby (Fig. 15.2) (Hammarlund and Sedin 1979; Rutter and Hull 1979b; Hammarlund et al. 1983; Jain et al. 2000). The high TEWL occurs because the immature baby's skin has a thin, poorly keratinised stratum corneum that offers little resistance to the diffusion of water. Postnatal existence rapidly hastens the development of an effective epidermal barrier (Evans and Rutter 1986), so that by about 2–3 weeks of age even the most prematurely born baby has a TEWL approaching that of a term newborn infant (Hammarlund and Sedin 1979; Rutter and Hull 1979b; Hammarlund et al. 1983; Jain et al. 2000). The high TEWL of preterm babies is further increased by trauma to the skin (Harpin and Rutter 1983). However the epidermal barrier is not influenced by use of antenatal corticosteroids (Jain et al. 2000).

Use of a radiant warmer increases evaporative heat loss by a factor of about 0.5–2.0; conventional phototherapy also increases TEWL, although it is claimed that light emitting diode phototherapy does not have this effect.

The high evaporative heat loss of babies of less than 30 weeks' gestation in the first week or so of life complicates management of their fluid balance; for advice on this topic, see Chapter 18. Reduction of this high evaporative loss can be achieved in a number of ways:

- Increasing the ambient humidity – evaporative heat loss decreases linearly as humidity rises (Chapter 18 of the 4th edition; Fig. 18.4), so that losses at high humidity are very low (Hey and Katz 1969; Hammarlund and Sedin 1979; Thompson et al. 1984).

- Draught exclusion – for example, an incubator with low air speeds can be used (Yeh et al. 1980; Okken et al. 1982) or the baby can be nursed under a acrylic shield closed at one end (Fanaroff et al. 1972).
- Waterproofing the baby – plastic bubble blankets or clear plastic film draped over the preterm baby will reduce insensible water loss by 75% (Marks et al. 1977). Topical emollients such as soft paraffin, Aquaphor and vegetable oil have a place in waterproofing the newborn infant so that TEWL is decreased (Wananukul and Praisuwanna 2002). However a Cochrane review suggests that their routine use should be avoided because of the added risk of coagulase-negative staphylococcal infection (risk ratio (95% confidence interval (CI)) 1.31 (1.02, 1.7) and any nosocomial infection 1.20 (1.00, 1.43) (Conner et al. 2004).

Measurement of temperature

Rectal, axilla and between skin and mattress temperatures correlate well with core temperature as recorded by an electronic thermometer inserted 5 cm beyond the anus (Mayfield et al. 1984) but in general terms the peripheral temperature will underestimate the core reading. However, for most purposes the measurement of axillary temperature should be used, except during therapeutic hypothermia or when there is concern that the baby is significantly hypothermic. The normal range of rectal temperature in the newborn is 36.5–37.5 °C. Although axillary temperature is generally lower than rectal temperature by about 0.5 °C, the current American Academy of Pediatrics guidelines recommend adopting a similar normal range, 36.5–37.4 °C (American Academy of Pediatrics, 2010). The National Institute for Health and Clinical Excellence guideline defines normal newborn axillary temperature as 'around 37 °C' (NICE clinical guideline 37, Routine postnatal care of women and their babies. Issue date June 2006). More information on temperature monitoring can also be found in Chapter 19. The World Health Organization (WHO, 1997) defines mild hypothermia as 36–36.5 °C, moderate hypothermia as 32–36 °C and severe hypothermia as <32 °C.

The goal of good thermal care is to achieve a core temperature between 36.8 °C and 37.3 °C with a core–peripheral difference of less than 1 °C.

Rectal temperature

This can be measured using a flexible thermocouple or thermistor inserted 5 cm from the anal margin. Shallower insertion gives a falsely low recording because blood from the surface of the legs may return via venous plexuses around the anus. Rectal temperature measurement is contraindicated in necrotising enterocolitis, and carries a risk of damage to the mucosa.

Axillary temperature

Because of the risk associated with rectal temperature measurement, axillary measurement is preferred. This is the current recommendation of the American Academy of Pediatrics. In this way temperature is usually measured by an electronic thermometer with the probe placed firmly in the roof of the axilla with the baby's upper arm held against the side of the chest wall. The axillary temperature can be up to 1 °C lower than rectal temperature, but the normal range is still usually defined as 36.5–37.4 °C (see above).

Skin temperature

A thermocouple or thermistor lightly taped to the newborn infant's skin can be left for repeated or continuous measurements. The upper abdomen is a convenient site, as changes with environmental temperature are not as great as at a peripheral site and the skin is conveniently flat. The normal range depends on the tissue insulation, the newborn infant's size and the time after delivery. The newborn infant below 1 kg birthweight has an abdominal skin temperature close to the rectal or axilla temperature. If the temperature probe is placed between the newborn infant's back and the underlying mattress and then allowed to equilibrate, the final measured temperature is similar to core, rectal or axillary measurements (Mayfield et al. 1984).

Other estimates of core temperature

Oesophageal temperature at the level of the heart and nasopharyngeal temperature at the brim of the internal acoustic meatus are feasible and good approximations of brain or central temperature but are invasive (Seguin and Vieth 1996; Ko et al. 2001). Dollberg et al. (1994, 2000) demonstrated that an insulated transcutaneous core temperature sensor using a method that relies on the principle of zero heat flow provides a reliable estimate of rectal temperature in preterm infants. More recently a novel earphone type infrared tympanic thermometer has been used in adult surgical patients and was within a mean (±SD) of 0.08 (0.34) °C and 0.11 (0.55) °C of respectively oesophageal or rectal temperature (Kiya et al. 2007).

Body temperature and thermal neutrality

Thermal neutral range

This is defined as the range of environmental temperatures at which a baby's heat production and oxygen consumption (as a proxy measure of metabolic rate) are minimal and there is no sweating (Chapter 18 of the 4th edition; Fig. 18.4). In the term naked newborn the range is wider and lower than in the preterm baby. An exact definition of the thermal neutral range is complicated as some of the elaborate original work was done in an era when the addition of incubator humidity was not the norm (Bruck 1961; Agate and Silverman 1963; Scopes and Ahmed 1966). However Hey studied 123 healthy naked newborns weighing between 960 and 4760 g in an incubator with 50% relative humidity and 30–35 °C temperature. The thermal neutral range at birth and 10 days of age was 34–34.5 °C and 35–35.5 °C, then 32.5–33.5 °C and 34–34.7 °C for babies with a birthweight of 2000 g or 1000 g respectively (Hey and Katz 1970). A later study based on gestation rather than birthweight determined similar ranges of the thermal neutral zone (Sauer et al. 1984). In clothed cot nursed babies an environmental temperature of 23–27 °C was necessary for thermal neutrality (Hey and O'Connell 1970; Azaz et al. 1992) compared with an environmental temperature of 29 °C for those with birthweight <1.5 kg (Hey and O'Connell 1970). Newborn babies are best nursed at an environmental temperature close to this range (Hey and O'Connell 1970; Hey 1971).

'Normal' temperature

The concept of a single 'normal' temperature for a newborn infant is erroneous. Clearly, a baby with a normal body temperature can be sweating or be markedly cold stressed, so body temperature is an insensitive guide to the suitability of the thermal environment. Doctors, nurses and parents commonly assume that if a baby has a normal body temperature the ambient temperature conditions must be satisfactory. In doing so, they fail to distinguish between being cold and feeling cold. A careful observer can recognise that a baby is feeling cold before the baby actually becomes cold, by assessing the baby's posture, activity, skin colour and peripheral skin temperature. However, the very low birthweight baby is an exception. A baby of less than 1 kg has such a low heat production per surface area, limited metabolic response to cold and poor tissue insulation that he or she appears poikilothermic (body temperature drifts up and down with the ambient temperature). Measurement of body temperature in such a baby is a convenient and reliable guide to the suitability of the thermal environment.

The WHO (1997) recommendations for thermal protection in the newborn infant do not specify a gestational age, but the broad recommendations are that a newborn infant should maintain a temperature of 36.5–37.5°C to avoid cold stress with a delivery room temperature of 25°C. A 10-step 'warm chain' prevents heat loss in the newborn infant and has been successfully field-tested in eight developing countries.

Li et al. (2004) studied the range of temperature in 200 term Chinese infants over the first 72 hours after delivery. The mean (SD) rectal temperature at delivery was 36.9°C (0.28), which dropped by a mean of 0.4°C (0.34) over the first 30 minutes, then rose by a mean of 0.24°C (0.26) over 15 hours. The core temperature stabilised at a mean of 36.7°C by 48–72 hours. Skin to skin care was the only intervention necessary to restore normal temperature. In addition there is a recognised drop in core temperature of 0.5–0.6°C in the first 2 hours of nighttime sleep that develops over the first 2–4 months of age (Azaz et al. 1992; Heraghty et al. 2008).

Practical management of the thermal environment

At delivery

The ideal temperature of a delivery room or operating theatre is about 25°C, comfortable for the mother, her attendants and the baby (WHO 1997). However most delivery rooms are cooler than this, and the wet newborn infant is delivered into a draughty room. Thus, delivery itself usually presents a significant cold stress.

The newborn baby should be given to the mother to establish bonding and breastfeeding. There is evidence that skin to skin contact facilitates breastfeeding and hence this should be encouraged, although not at the cost of thermal stress; the baby should be dried and covered if the room is not warm enough. Weighing, bathing and application of name bands can all be deferred. The baby can also be clothed appropriately later. Babies who need resuscitation should be dried (if term) and placed under the radiant warmer of a resuscitaire. Preterm babies of less than 32 weeks' gestation should be placed into a polyethylene film or bag straight from delivery and without prior drying. This has been shown to be an effective way of avoiding a fall in rectal temperature in the immediate postnatal period (Vohra et al. 1999, 2004; Bjorklund et al. 2000; Cramer et al. 2005). Wrapped babies had significantly higher admission temperatures than unwrapped infants (weighted mean difference 0.63°C, 95% CI 0.38, 0.87) although there was no significant difference in mortality. The baby should remain in the polyethylene film or bag until he or she has been weighed, transferred into a humid incubator and has a temperature of >36.5°C.

In addition phase change gel mattresses and skin to skin care in combination with polyethylene film or bag are associated with a rise in admission temperature and a reduction in hypothermia of premature newborn infants on admission to neonatal intensive care (Lyon and Stenson 2004; McCall et al. 2008; Almeida et al. 2009; Singh et al. 2010).

Nursing care of the newborn infant

Parents prefer to see their baby dressed. A clothed baby who is placed in a cot covered by blankets and nursed in a warm room is usually in a neutral thermal environment and generally appears content. Clothing more than doubles the insulation, and bedding (a sheet and two blankets) further increases it, so that the resistance to heat loss of a clothed, wrapped baby is three times greater than that of a naked one (Table 15.2) (Hey et al. 1970; Hey 1983). The head is a large part of the total surface area of the baby, has a higher surface temperature and consequently loses much heat. A hat is an effective method of increasing thermal insulation, and is especially useful in low birthweight babies, who have relatively larger heads and whose trunk may need to be exposed.

The following recommendations are made for nursing healthy babies (Hey 1971):

Table 15.2 Resistance to heat loss (insulation) in an infant weighing 2.5 kg lying on a foam mattress in a cool, draught-free room. Insulation is measured in clo units (1 clo unit = 0.155°C m²/W or 0.18°C m²/kcal)

RESISTANCE DUE TO	NAKED	HAT WRAPPED IN ONE SHEET	CLOTHED IN A COT UNDER BLANKETS
1 flannelette sheet and 2 blankets around a clothed baby			0.61
1 flannelette swaddling sheet around an unclothed baby		0.81	
Thick gauze hat		0.22	0.22
Vest, napkin and long nightdress			1.25
Boundary layer of still air around the skin	0.78	0.78	0.78
Vasoconstricted body tissues	0.29	0.29	0.29
Total resistance	1.07	2.10	3.15
Reproduced from Hey (1983).			

- 2–2.5 kg: clothed, with bedding, in a room temperature of about 24 °C
- 1.5–2 kg: clothed, with a hat and bedding, in a room temperature of about 26 °C
- 1.5 kg: clothed, with a hat, in an incubator temperature of about 30–32 °C.

Babies weighing more than about 1800 g are commonly nursed in an environment 1–2 °C cooler than this. They will have a minor and clinically unimportant increase in oxygen consumption as a result.

Incubator care

A closed incubator provides a baby with a high ambient temperature whilst allowing attendants to work at a lower, more comfortable temperature. Most incubators work by forced convection: air is heated and then circulated by a fan within the canopy of the incubator at an air speed of about 20 cm/s. There are two means of controlling the heater output:

1. Air mode. The air temperature is set to a desired level and maintained by thermostat. The heater output is proportional to the difference between the set temperature and the actual temperature. If the incubator air temperature is just below the set temperature, the heater output will be low; if it is substantially below the set temperature, the heater will be on full power. This means that fluctuations in air temperature due to cycling of the thermostat are small.
2. Servo mode. The heater output is controlled by the newborn infant's skin temperature. A temperature probe is taped to the skin, preferably the upper abdomen, and the heater cycles to keep the skin temperature at that site constant. In practice, air temperature fluctuations are greater in servo mode than air mode, especially when the newborn infant is handled (Fig. 15.3).

Air mode is probably satisfactory for nursing most babies (Bell and Rios 1983). Servo mode has the disadvantages of wide fluctuations in air temperature, particularly during nursing procedures, of providing an inappropriately low ambient temperature when the baby is febrile and of lack of control when a baby with very high insensible water loss is nursed in a dry incubator (Belgaumkar and Scott 1975a; Ducker et al. 1985; Thomas and Burr 1999; Thomas 2003). The servo probe may become detached, resulting in an inappropriate air temperature. However, a Cochrane review has determined that servo control of abdominal skin temperature at 36 °C reduced the neonatal death rate among low birthweight infants: relative risk 0.72 (95% CI 0.54, 0.97) (Sinclair 2002).

A naked baby nursed in an incubator loses heat predominantly by radiation, less by convection and evaporation (Fig. 15.4). Covering or clothing the baby or using a double walled incubator will reduce radiation heat losses (Marks et al. 1981). In practice, a higher air temperature setting can compensate for the radiant losses. Nursing and medical procedures disrupt the environmental temperature control, resulting in temperature instability (Mok et al. 1991; Thomas 2003).

Temperature settings used in incubators depend on whether the baby is clothed or naked, the birthweight and postnatal age. The values shown in Table 15.3 are estimates to provide an environmental temperature at the lower end of the neutral thermal range under conditions of low air speed (below 10 cm/s), moderate relative humidity (50%) and where the temperature of the inner wall is the same as the air temperature. When used in the servo mode, the required set skin temperatures are the same as those recommended for babies nursed under radiant warmers (Table 15.4).

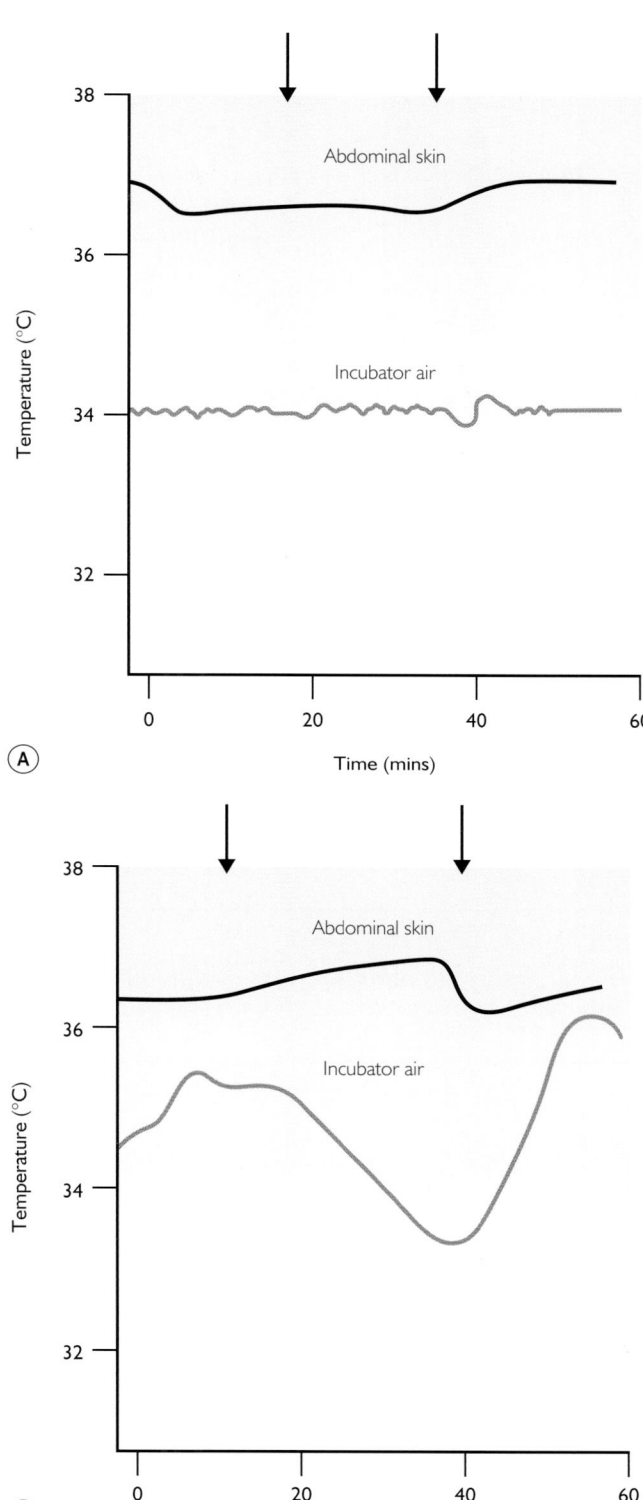

Fig. 15.3 Fluctuations in incubator air temperature when used (A) in air mode and (B) in servo mode. In air mode, the set temperature (air) is 34°C; in servo mode, the set temperature (skin) is 36.3°C. Handling for brief spells for routine nursing procedures is indicated (↓).

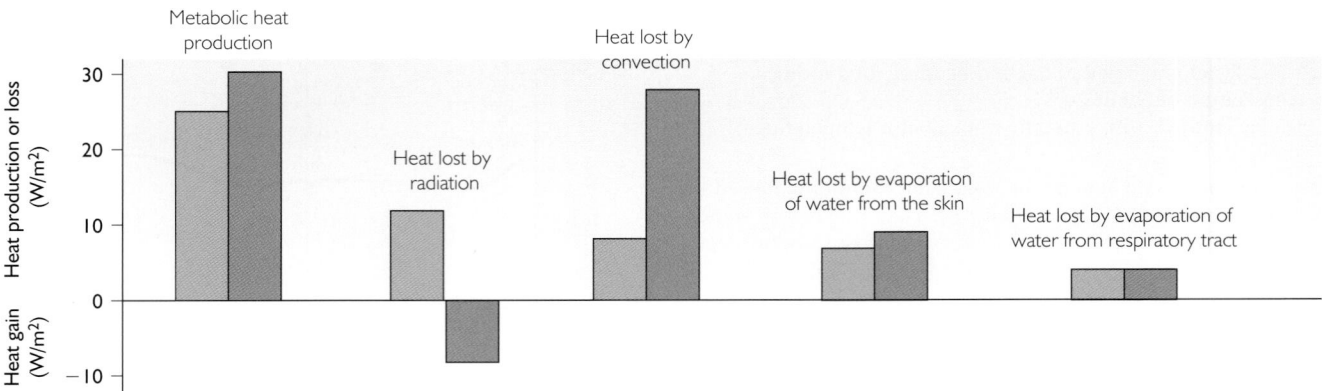

Fig. 15.4 Heat production, losses and gains of 11 preterm infants (mean birthweight 1.58 kg, gestation 32 weeks, age 7 days) nursed naked in an incubator (lighter bars) and under a radiant warmer (darker bars) in presumed neutral thermal conditions. *(Redrawn from Wheldon and Rutter (1982).)*

Table 15.3 Average incubator air temperatures needed to provide a suitable thermal environment for naked, healthy infants

BIRTHWEIGHT (KG)	ENVIRONMENTAL TEMPERATURE			
	35°C	**34°C**	**33°C**	**32°C**
1.0–1.5	For 10 days	After 10 days	After 3 weeks	After 5 weeks
1.5–2.0		For 10 days	After 10 days	After 4 weeks
2.0–2.5		For 2 days	After 2 days	After 3 weeks
>2.5			For 2 days	After 2 days

Notes:
1. In a single-walled incubator, the environmental temperature needs to be increased by 1°C for every 7°C difference between room and incubator temperature.
2. Very low birthweight infants (1 kg) need higher air temperatures and a humidified incubator in the first week (Wheldon and Hull 1983; Sauer et al. 1984).
3. The values are averages but there is considerable individual variation.
Reproduced from Hey (1975).

Table 15.4 Suggested abdominal skin temperature settings for infants nursed under radiant warmers or in servo mode incubators

BIRTHWEIGHT (kg)	ABDOMINAL SKIN TEMPERATURE (°C)
<1.0	36.9
1.0–1.5	36.7
1.5–2.0	36.5
2.0–2.5	36.3
>2.5	36.0

There is a complex relationship between the water content of the air (absolute humidity), the water content of the air expressed as a percentage of the maximum possible water content (relative humidity) and air temperature (Hey 1971). Room air at 20°C in the British Isles has a relative humidity of about 50%. In a warm neonatal intensive care unit at 30°C the same room air is only about 30% saturated, whereas in an unhumidified incubator at 37°C the relative humidity may be as low as 25%. A baby of less than 30 weeks' gestation, a day or so old, nursed in an unhumidified incubator, may have an evaporative heat loss that exceeds metabolic heat production (Fig. 15.5). The baby may therefore remain cold, even in an air temperature of 37°C. Humidification is an effective way of reducing this evaporative heat loss and maintaining a normal body temperature (Fig. 15.6). Humidity is recommended for babies below 30 weeks' gestation in the first week of life and thereafter its use depends on thermal stability (Harpin and Rutter 1985; Hammarlund et al. 1986). Modern incubator humidifiers provide good humidity control: the maximum setting is appropriate and will produce a relative humidity of 80–90% at the maximum air temperature. Humidification is probably of no advantage to the more mature baby.

Care under radiant warmers

Radiant warmers are an alternative device for nursing babies. The baby lies on an open cradle under a heat source emitting radiant energy in the frequency spectrum 700–300 000 nm. The heater is placed approximately 90 cm from the skin surface. The maximum output does not usually exceed 500 W/m (Baumgart 1984). A

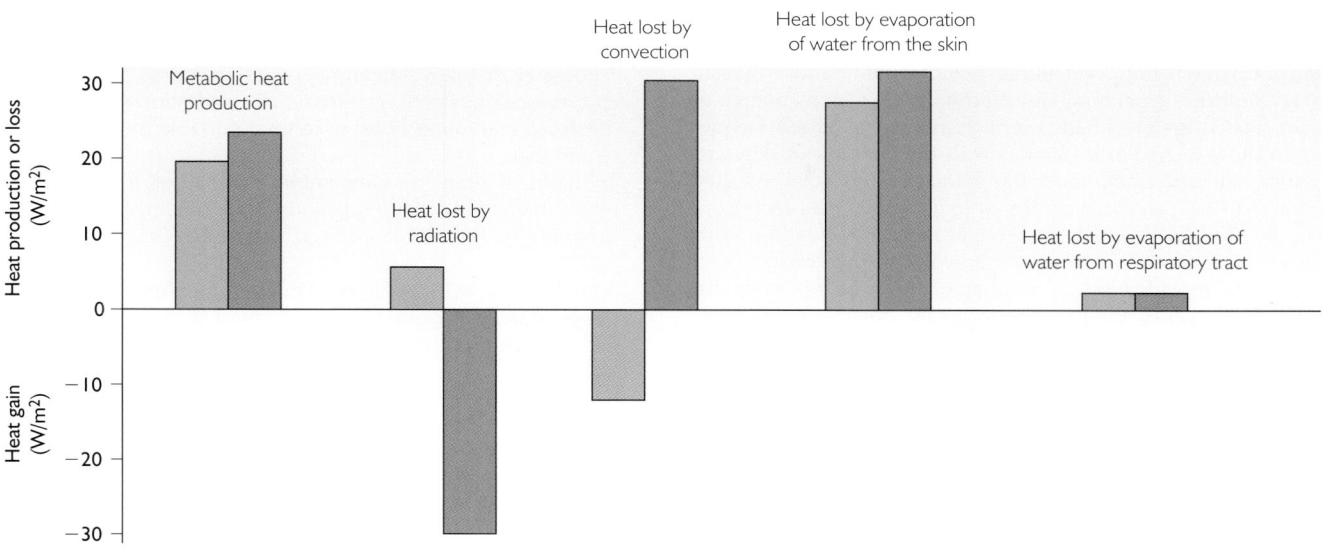

Fig. 15.5 Heat production, losses and gains of an infant of 28 weeks' gestation, birthweight 1.08 kg, on the third day. When nursed naked in a dry incubator (lighter bars), air temperature 37.7°C, rectal temperature fell to 36.4°C. This is because the infant's high skin evaporative heat loss exceeded the metabolic heat production. When nursed under a radiant warmer (darker bars), set to provide a skin temperature of 36.8°C, rectal temperature rapidly rose to 36.8°C because of the high radiant heat gain. *(Redrawn from Wheldon and Rutter (1982).)*

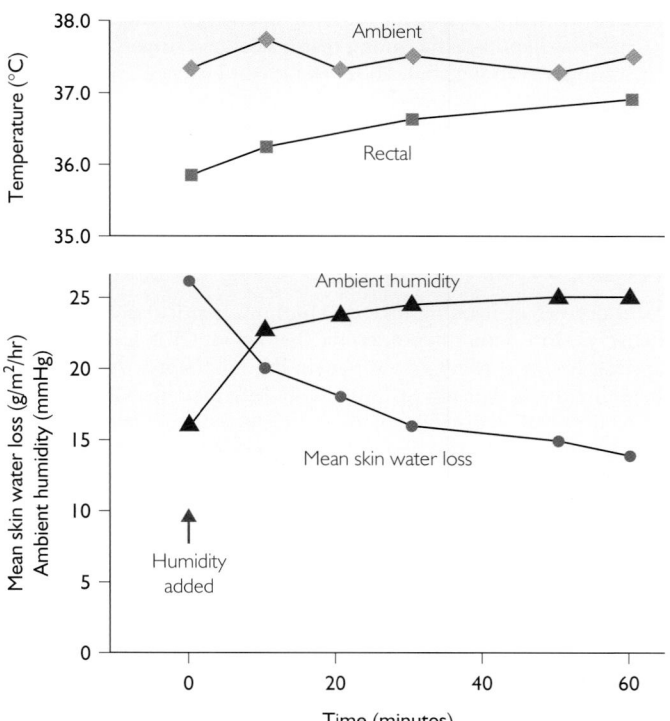

Fig. 15.6 The effect of humidifying an incubator. The baby (30 weeks' gestation, 1 day old) has a rectal temperature of 35.8°C in spite of an incubator temperature of 37.3°C. When humidity is added, skin water loss falls and the rectal temperature steadily increases to 37.0°C.

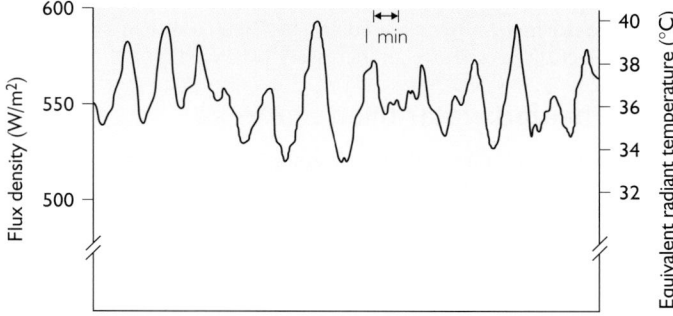

Fig. 15.7 Typical recording of radiant flux density incident on the upper abdomen of an infant nursed under a radiant warmer. The infant is 32 weeks' gestation, birthweight 1.42 kg, age 9 days: the room temperature is 28.5°C. The estimated mean radiant temperature is shown on the right hand axis. Fluctuations are due to cycling of the servo control system. *(Redrawn from Wheldon and Rutter (1982).)*

thermistor taped to the skin on the upper abdomen is set to the desired temperature and is used to control the overhead heat output. The recommended set temperatures depend on the baby's size (see Table 15.4). Fixed output low power heaters are only suitable for brief warming procedures such as resuscitation.

The thermal environment is obviously different from that provided by an incubator (Wheldon and Rutter 1982; Baumgart 1985). The baby is exposed to cool, dry, draughty air and a markedly fluctuating radiant heat source (Fig. 15.7). Heat loss by convection is high, but heat is gained by radiation (see Fig. 15.4). Several studies have shown that newborn infants nursed under radiant warmers have higher resting levels of oxygen consumption than those nursed in incubators, although the increase is not significant (weighted mean difference 0.27 ml/kg/min (95% CI 0.26, 0.63)) (Flenady and Woodgate 2003). Evaporative heat loss is consistently higher in babies nursed under radiant warmers and is due to an increase in water loss from the skin rather than from the respiratory tract and is significant (weighted mean difference 0.94 g/kg/day (95% CI 0.47, 1.41)) (Wheldon and Rutter 1982; Flenady and Woodgate 2003). Surface temperature distribution is also more uneven in babies nursed under radiant warmers: the peripheries are cooler than in those nursed in incubators with the same mean skin temperature. Skin and limb blood flow is increased by 50% and there is a small (5%) increase in cardiac output caused by an increase in heart rate. Radiant warmers therefore produce a fluctuating, asymmetrical thermal environment compared with the constant even temperature provided by an incubator. However, no study has shown that either method is superior to the other in terms of the mortality, morbidity and growth of babies nursed in them (Flenady and Woodgate 2003). Radiant warmers are potentially more dangerous than incubators. Overheating from probe detachment or interference can occur quickly, so the baby's surface or core temperature needs continuous independent monitoring. The increased evaporative water loss may result in hypernatraemic dehydration (Jones et al. 1976). Covering a baby who is under a radiant warmer with a rigid acrylic box will reduce insensible water losses (Yeh et al. 1979; Bell et al. 1980). However, this impairs the radiant heat exchange between the baby and warmer, producing a thermal environment with features of a warmer and an incubator. A more acceptable measure is to cover the newborn infant in a clear plastic film, resulting in lower oxygen consumption and less demand for radiant heat (Baumgart et al. 1981, 1982; Baumgart 1984).

The advantage of using a radiant warmer is that it can be an effective way of keeping a newborn infant warm (see Fig. 15.5), particularly in the first 24 hours after delivery, when considerable handling and practical procedures are necessary (Meyer et al. 2001).

The heated water filled mattress

This is an alternative method of keeping babies warm and is suitable for use in developing countries. Compared with the incubator or radiant warmer, it is cheap, simple and is not dependent on a continuous supply of electricity. The mattress is a polyvinyl bag filled with 10 litres of water and heated by a foil pad. This has a high thermal capacity and continues to provide warmth even if the power source fails. The water temperature is thermostatically controlled and regulated between 35°C and 38°C. It is safe to nurse a preterm baby in a cot on a heated water filled mattress if the baby is stable and does not have to be undressed for observation (Sarman and Tunell 1989). Temperature control, metabolic rate and weight gain compare favourably with similar babies nursed in incubators. The heated water filled mattress is therefore an excellent method for rewarming hypothermic babies, being safer than and superior to an incubator (Sarman et al. 1989). Preterm babies nursed on a water-filled mattress suffer less cold stress and may grow better than those nursed in a warm room (Greenabate et al. 1994).

Thermal environment during transport

Transporting babies from one hospital to another for intensive care is a considerable challenge (see Ch. 13 part 2). Such babies are often cold to start with, their heat losses are great and their heat production is small. Furthermore, the environmental temperature during transport may be below 0°C. Transport incubators are generally less satisfactory in terms of performance than nursing incubators. The essentials of keeping a baby warm during transport are:

- To reduce high radiant heat losses which occur if the baby has to be nursed naked – this can be achieved by covering, by use of a double walled incubator and by using a phase change gel mattress under the newborn infant.

- To reduce high evaporative heat loss – the baby should be covered in a plastic film, bubble blanket or a plastic bag.
- To observe the baby – heart rate, respiratory rate, temperature and transcutaneous oxygen tension or saturation should be measured continuously using secured portable monitoring equipment.
- To maintain a high air temperature – in babies of 1 kg or below, the required air temperature is close to 37°C. Prewarming the ambulance is recommended (see Ch. 13 part 2).
- Added humidity to assist maintenance of a normal body temperature in the immature baby, although few transport incubators currently allow this.

Surgery

The baby undergoing surgery is at particular risk of cold stress. The operating theatre air and wall temperatures are often low and the room is draughty. Starvation and sedation will blunt the response to cold stress. Furthermore, exposed organs lose water, and therefore heat, by evaporation.

Cold stress can be minimised by the following measures:

- Raise the air temperature in the theatre to 28–30°C.
- Insulate the baby before transporting to theatre: this is effectively achieved by wrapping the limbs, trunk and scalp with cotton-wool roll.
- Minimise the area of the baby exposed for surgery.
- Use a reusable forced air warming blanket (a 'bear hugger') to prevent hypothermia during major neonatal surgery (Kongsayreepong et al. 2002). A radiant heater is an alternative.

Disorders of temperature control

The baby with a low body temperature (below 36°C)

Mild degrees of hypothermia are common, particularly following delivery. More severe hypothermia (below 34°C) is less common and occurs as a result of overwhelming cold stress. In hospital, hypothermia is typically seen in small, sick preterm babies in the early neonatal period, when they are nursed in incubators and handled frequently. Use of a polyethylene bag to cover such babies in the delivery room has been shown to reduce early hypothermia (Vohra et al. 1999). The use of a radiant warmer also avoids this early hypothermia (Meyer et al. 2001).

Outside hospital, accidental hypothermia is liable to occur when a birth is unexpected or has been concealed. Hypothermia may occur in the first few weeks of life, particularly if the baby is nursed in an unheated room and the outside temperature drops below freezing. Infection (particularly pneumonia and septicaemia), serious congenital abnormality (particularly cyanotic heart disease or severe cardiac failure) and low birthweight are predisposing factors. Respiratory syncytial virus infection, especially pneumonia or bronchiolitis, is particularly associated with hypothermia in very young babies. Malnutrition also predisposes to hypothermia, by reducing tissue insulation and the metabolic response to cold. If accidental cold exposure and infection have been eliminated as the cause, hypothyroidism should be considered. Rapid screening for hypothermia is feasible using a simple chemical strip to record axillary or abdominal skin temperature (Kennedy et al. 2000).

Babies with moderate or severe hypothermia are lethargic, feed poorly and have a weak cry and reduced movements. Peripheral oedema is common and areas of sclerema may occur in severe cases. Marked facial erythema may give a false impression but the skin always feels strikingly cold. The diagnosis will be made when rectal temperature is measured with a low reading thermometer, but will be missed if the usual clinical thermometer with a minimum reading of 35°C is used. In very severe cases (rectal temperature below 28°C), the baby may appear virtually dead, with profound cardiorespiratory depression. There are anecdotal reports of such babies being 'left for dead' but eventually making a full recovery.

There is limited information available about the safest and most effective method of rewarming hypothermic babies. However a rapid rate of rewarming has potential adverse consequences. In sheep that had hypoxic ischaemic insult who were subjected to moderate therapeutic hypothermia (30–33°C), electrical seizure activity was significantly increased when rewarming took place over less than 1 hour with no concurrent loss of neuronal cell loss (Gerrits et al. 2005). In dogs undergoing severe hypothermia (25°C) depressed myocardial contractile function with hypotension persisted through rewarming over 6 hours (Tveita et al. 1994). There are no data to suggest an adverse long term neurocognitive outcome in newborn infants during rewarming (either following hypoxic ischaemic insult or following cold exposure). However fast rewarming rates during bypass for cardiac surgery in adults have been associated with a poor neurocognitive outcome at 6 weeks (Newman et al. 1995; Grigore et al. 2002). In light of the above the current recommendation is to rewarm babies at a rate of 0.5°C per hour following therapeutic hypothermia (Azzopardi et al. 2009). In an incubator, this can be achieved using the maximum air temperature setting, or by setting the air temperature to a level which is 1–2°C higher than body temperature, and increasing it in a step-wise fashion until the baby is warm. Radiant warmers are effective in treating hypothermic babies, using a set skin temperature of 37°C. Sarman et al. (1989) found that a heated water filled mattress was superior to an incubator in rewarming 53 hypothermic preterm newborn infants. Skin to skin contact has also been shown to be a safe and effective method of rewarming (Christensson et al. 1988; WHO 1997).

Care should be taken when interpreting blood gas results in hypothermia, as pH is temperature dependent. The pH rises by 0.016 pH units for every 1°C fall in temperature, so that blood with a pH of 6.94 at 37°C will have a pH of 7.10 at 27°C. Because pH is always measured at 37°C, it is easy to overestimate and therefore overtreat a metabolic acidosis in a hypothermic newborn infant. Abdominal distension is common and necrotising enterocolitis may occur. Feeding should not start until a normal body temperature has been achieved. Haemorrhagic pulmonary oedema is a sinister sign and a common autopsy finding in babies who die from hypothermia. The reported mortality rate in severe hypothermia is 20–50%, but this includes those with congenital abnormalities or serious infection that contributed to the hypothermia. Most survivors develop normally.

The baby with a raised body temperature (above 38°C)

There are only two explanations for a raised body temperature: the baby may have an increased set point temperature or may be overheated. In a study of a large number of term babies, a raised body temperature was found in 1% in the early neonatal period (Voora et al. 1982). Of these, 10% had a bacterial infection and 90% were overheated. Babies with a raised set point temperature behave as if they are cold. Heat production is increased, probably by nonshivering thermogenesis, and heat loss is reduced by cutaneous vasoconstriction. Pyrexia is a less reliable sign of sepsis than in older infants.

Of 371 babies aged up to 30 days, the rates of serious bacterial infection were 4.4% for those with a rectal temperature of 38.1–39.0°C, 7.6% for the range 39.1–39.9°C and 18% above 39.9°C, but only 6% had a temperature in the last range (Bonadio et al. 1990). An increased set point temperature is also seen in babies with a serious congenital abnormality of the brain, especially hydranencephaly, encephalocoele, holoprosencephaly and trisomy 13, and following severe birth asphyxia, where it is a poor prognostic sign. Such babies often have instability of thermoregulation because of hypothalamic damage (Cross et al. 1971).

Overheating is the commonest cause of a raised temperature and usually the cause of hyperpyrexia (above 41°C rectal). It is common in restless, active and overwrapped babies left in a warm room. It is also seen in babies born to a pyrexial mother. A baby's temperature at birth reflects maternal temperature and is usually about 0.5°C higher than the mother's. Epidural anaesthesia is commonly associated with an elevated maternal temperature. The baby is therefore likely to have a raised temperature and to be investigated for sepsis (Lieberman et al. 1997).

Hyperpyrexia is rare in babies and usually results from a mechanical or electrical failure of a warming device. An incubator in direct sunlight behaves like a greenhouse: short wave radiation passes directly through the acrylic canopy and long-wave radiation heats the acrylic, which in turn radiates to the baby. Serious overheating may occur if the servo probe becomes detached from the baby under a powerful radiant warmer. In early infancy, overheating occurs with excessive wrapping, during heatwaves and if babies are left in closed cars exposed to sunlight.

Hyperthermia may be associated with an increase in apnoea of prematurity (Perlstein et al. 1970; Belgaumkar and Scott 1975b). In the post hypoxic ischaemic animal model even 1–2°C hyperthermia leads to increased cerebral damage (Gunn and Bennet 2001). In addition hyperthermic piglets had worse neuropathology and behavioural scores after hypothermic cardiac arrest and newborn baboons of hyperthermic mothers had profound acidosis and hypoxia (Gunn and Bennet 2001). In light of the risks of hyperthermia the International Liaison Committee on Resuscitation (2006) newborn guidelines advocate avoidance of iatrogenic hyperthermia.

Shock, protracted fits, diarrhoea, disseminated intravascular coagulation and renal and hepatic failure occur in overheated babies (Bacon et al. 1979), but the few who have died from overheating have done so suddenly, without prior symptoms. Overheating is linked with sudden death in infancy (Guntheroth and Spiers 2001) and is described in families with a history of malignant hyperpyrexia (Denborough et al. 1982) and hypohidrotic ectodermal dysplasia (Bernstein et al. 1980).

Table 15.5 Differences between a healthy infant who is overheated and a febrile infant with a raised set-point temperature

OVERHEATED INFANT	FEBRILE INFANT
High rectal temperature	High rectal temperature
Warm hands and feet	Cold hands and feet
Core/skin difference less than 2°C	Core/skin difference greater than 3°C
Pink skin	Pale skin
Extended posture	Lethargic

The distinction between an overheated baby and one with an increased set point temperature is important (Pomerance et al. 1981; Harpin et al. 1983). The overheated baby needs a cooler environment, not a series of painful investigations to find an infective cause for the 'fever'. There are several important differences (Table 15.5). An evaluation of risk factors for sepsis is important. A useful physical sign is the degree of difference in skin temperature between the abdomen and the hand: the abdomen is always warmer than the hand; in the overheated baby the difference is less than 2°C (often less than 1°C), but in the infected baby it usually exceeds 3.5°C. The same applies to the difference between the rectal temperature and the temperature of the sole of the foot (Messaritakis et al. 1990).

Therapeutic hypothermia
(see Ch. 40.4 for further details)

Hypothermia is successfully used in conjunction with cardiopulmonary bypass in babies undergoing open heart surgery, to extend the time available for surgery. Moderate whole body hypothermia (rectal 33–34°C) and local cooling of the head using a water cooled cap are well tolerated and associated with a consistent reduction in death and neurological impairment at 18 months in babies who have been subjected to asphyxial insults during labour, and are becoming widely used treatment (see Ch. 40.4) (Thoresen and Whitelaw 2000; Edwards et al. 2010).

References

Agate Jr, F.J., Silverman, W.A., 1963. The control of body temperature in the small newborn infant by low-energy infra-red radiation. Pediatrics 31, 725–733.

Almeida, P.G., Chandley, J., Davis, J., et al., 2009. Use of the heated gel mattress and its impact on admission temperature of very low birth-weight infants. Adv Neonatal Care 9, 34–39.

American Academy of Pediatrics, Committee on Fetus and Newborn, 2010. Policy Statement, Hospital stay for Healthy Term Newborns. Pediatrics 125, 405–409.

Azaz, Y., Fleming, P.J., Levine, M., et al., 1992. The relationship between environmental temperature, metabolic rate, sleep state, and evaporative water loss in infants from birth to three months. Pediatr Res 32, 417–423.

Azzopardi, D.V., Strohm, B., Edwards, A.D., et al., 2009. Moderate hypothermia to treat perinatal asphyxial encephalopathy. N Engl J Med 361, 1349–1358.

Bacon, C., Scott, D., Jones, P., 1979. Heat stroke in well-wrapped infants. Lancet i, 422–425.

Baumgart, S., 1984. Reduction of oxygen consumption, insensible water loss and radiant heat demand with use of a plastic blanket for low birthweight infants under radiant warmers. J Pediatr 100, 787–790.

Baumgart, S., 1985. Partitioning of heat losses and gains in premature newborn infants under radiant warmers. Pediatrics 75, 89–99.

Baumgart, S., Engle, W.D., Fox, W.W., et al., 1981. Effect of heat shielding on convective and evaporative heat losses and on radiant heat transfer in the premature infant. J Pediatr 99, 948–956.

Baumgart, S., Fox, W.W., Polin, R.A., 1982. Physiologic implications of two different heat shields for infants under radiant warmers. J Pediatr 100, 787–790.

Belgaumkar, T.K., Scott, K.E., 1975a. Effects of low humidity on small premature infants in servocontrol incubators. I. Decrease in rectal temperature. Biol Neonate 26, 337–347.

Belgaumkar, T.K., Scott, K.E., 1975b. Effects of low humidity on small premature infants in servocontrol incubators. II. Increased severity of apnoea. Biol Neonate 26, 348–352.

Bell, E.F., Rios, G.R., 1983. Air versus skin temperature servo control of infant incubators. J Pediatr 103, 954–959.

Bell, E.F., Weinstein, M.R., Oh, W., 1980. Heat balance in premature infants: comparative effect of convectively incubated and radiant warmer, with and without plastic heat shield. J Pediatr 96, 460–465.

Bernstein, R., Hatchuel, I., Jenkins, T., 1980. Hypohidrotic ectodermal dysplasia and sudden infant death syndrome. Lancet ii, 1024.

Bjorklund, L.J., Hellstrom-Westas, L., Vohra, S., et al., 2000. Reducing heat loss at birth in very preterm infants (multiple letters). J Pediatr 137, 739–740.

Blackburn, S.T., Loper, D.L., 1992. Thermoregulation. In: Eoyang, T. (Ed.), Maternal, Fetal and Neonatal Physiology: A Clinical Perspective. W.B. Saunders, Philadelphia, pp. 677–697.

Bonadio, W.A., Romine, K., Gyuro, J., 1990. Relationship of fever magnitude to rate of serious bacterial infections in neonates. J Pediatr 116, 733–735.

Bruck, K., 1961. Temperature regulation in the newborn infant. Biol Neonate 3, 65.

Budge, H., Dandrea, J., Mostyn, A., et al., 2003. Differential effects of fetal number and maternal nutrition in late gestation on prolactin receptor abundance and adipose tissue development in the neonatal lamb. Pediatr 53, 302–308.

Christensson, K., Bhat, G.J., Amadi, B.C., et al., 1988. Randomised study of skin-to-skin versus incubator care for rewarming low-risk hypothermic neonates. Lancet 352, 1115.

Confidential Enquiry into Maternal and Child Health, 2003. CESDI Project 27/28: An Enquiry into Quality of Care and its Effect on the Survival of Babies Born at 27–28 Weeks. The Stationery Office, London.

Conner, J.M., Soll, R.F., Edwards, W.H., 2004. Topical ointment for preventing infection in preterm infants. Cochrane Database Syst Rev (1), CD001150.

Costeloe, K., Hennessy, E., Gibson, A.T., et al, 2000. The EPICure study: outcomes to discharge from hospital for infants born at the threshold of viability. Pediatrics 106, 659–671.

Cramer, K., Wiebe, N., Hartling, L., et al., 2005. Heat loss prevention: A systematic review of occlusive skin wrap for premature neonates. J Perinatol 25, 763–769.

Cross, K.W., Hey, E.N., Kennaird, D.L., et al., 1971. Lack of temperature control in infants with abnormalities of the central nervous system. Arch Dis Child 46, 437–443.

Dawkins, M.J., Scopes, J.W., 1965. Non-shivering thermogenesis and brown adipose tissue in the human new-born infant. Nature 206, 201–202.

Denborough, M.A., Galloway, G.J., Hopkinson, K.C., 1982. Malignant hyperpyrexia and sudden infant death. Lancet ii, 1068–1069.

Dollberg, S., Atherton, H.D., Sigda, M., et al., 1994. Effect of insulated skin probes to increase skin-to-environmental temperature gradients of preterm infants cared for in convective incubators. J Pediatr 124, 799–801.

Dollberg, S., Rimon, A., Atherton, H.D., et al., 2000. Continuous measurement of core body temperature in preterm infants. Am J Perinatol 17, 257–264.

Ducker, D.A., Lyon, A.J., Ross Russell, R., et al., 1985. Incubator temperature control: effects on the very low birthweight infant. Arch Dis Child 60, 902–907.

Edwards, A.D., Brocklehurst, P., Gunn, A.J., et al., 2010. Neurological outcomes at 18 months of age after moderate hypothermia for perinatal hypoxic ischaemic encephalopathy: synthesis and meta-analysis of trial data. BMJ 340, c363.

Evans, N.J., Rutter, N., 1986. Development of the epidermis in the newborn. Biol Neonate 49, 74–80.

Fanaroff, A.A., Wald, M., Gruber, H.S., et al., 1972. Insensible water loss in low birth weight infants. Pediatrics 50, 236–245.

Flenady, V.J., Woodgate, P.G., 2003. Radiant warmers versus incubators for regulating body temperature in newborn infants. Cochrane Database Syst Rev (4), CD000435.

Gerrits, L.C., Battin, M.R., Bennet, L., et al., 2005 Epileptiform activity during rewarming from moderate cerebral hypothermia in the near-term fetal sheep. Pediatr Res 57, 342–346.

Greenabate, C., Tafari, N., Rao, M.R., et al., 1994. Comparison of heated water-filled mattress and space-heated room with infant incubator in providing warmth to low birthweight newborns. Int J Epidemiol 23, 1226–1233.

Grigore, A.M., Grocott, H.P., Mathew, J.P., et al., 2002. The rewarming rate and increased peak temperature alter neurocognitive outcome after cardiac surgery. Anesth Analg 94, 4–10.

Gunn, A.J., Bennet, L., 2001. Is temperature important in delivery room resuscitation? Semin Neonatol 6, 241–249.

Guntheroth, W.G., Spiers, P.S., 2001. Thermal stress in sudden infant death: is there an ambiguity with the rebreathing hypothesis? Pediatrics 107, 693–698.

Hammarlund, K., Sedin, G., 1979. Transepidermal water loss in newborn infants. III. Relation to gestational age. Acta Paediatr Scand 68, 795–801.

Hammarlund, K., Sedin, G., Stromberg, B., 1983. Transepidermal water loss in newborn infants. VIII. Relation to gestational age and post-natal age in appropriate and small for gestational age infants. Acta Paediatr Scand 72, 721–728.

Hammarlund, K., Stromberg, B., Sedin, G., 1986. Heat loss from the skin of preterm and full term newborn infants during the first weeks after birth. Biol Neonate 50, 1–10.

Harpin, V.A., Rutter, N., 1982. Sweating in preterm babies. J Pediatr 100, 614–619.

Harpin, V.A., Rutter, N., 1983. Barrier properties of the newborn infant's skin. J Pediatr 102, 419–425.

Harpin, V.A., Rutter, N., 1985. Humidification of incubators. Arch Dis Child 60, 219–224.

Harpin, V.A., Chellappah, G., Rutter, N., 1983. Responses of the newborn infant to overheating. Biol Neonate 44, 65–75.

Heraghty, J.L., Hilliard, T.N., Henderson, A.J., et al., 2008. The physiology of sleep in infants. Arch Dis Child 93, 982–985.

Hey, E.N., 1969. The relation between environmental temperature and oxygen consumption in the new-born baby. J Physiol 200, 589–603.

Hey, E.N. (Ed.), 1971. The Care of Babies in Incubators. two hundred and sixteenth ed. J & A Churchill, London.

Hey, E.N., 1975. Thermal neutrality. Br Med Bull 31, 69–74.

Hey, E.N. (Ed.), 1983. Temperature Regulation in Sick Infants. Springer, Berlin.

Hey, E.N., Katz, G., 1969. Evaporative water loss in the new-born baby. J Physiol 200, 605–619.

Hey, E.N., Katz, G., 1970. The optimum thermal environment for naked babies. Arch Dis Child 45, 328–334.

Hey, E.N., O'Connell, B., 1970. Oxygen consumption and heat balance in the cot-nursed baby. Arch Dis Child 45, 335–343.

Hey, E.N., Katz, G., O'Connell, B., 1970. The total thermal insulation of the new-born baby. J Physiol 207, 683–698.

Hill, J.R., Rahimtulla, K.A., 1965. Heat balance and the metabolic rate of new-born babies in relation to environmental temperature, and the effect of age and of weight on basal metabolic rate. J Physiol 280, 239–265.

International Liaison Committee on Resuscitation, 2006. The International Liaison Committee on Resuscitation (ILCOR) consensus on science with treatment recommendations for pediatric and neonatal patients: neonatal resuscitation. Pediatrics 117, e978–e988.

Jain, A., Rutter, N., Cartlidge, P.H., 2000. Influence of antenatal steroids and sex on maturation of the epidermal barrier in the preterm infant. Arch Dis Child Fetal Neonatal Ed 83, F112–F116.

Jones, R.W.A., Rochefort, M.J., Baum, J.D., 1976. Increased insensible water loss in newborn infants nursed under radiant heaters. BMJ ii, 1347–1350.

Kennedy, N., Gondwe, L., Morley, D.C., 2000. Temperature monitoring with ThermoSpots in Malawi. Lancet 355, 1364.

Kiya, T., Yamakage, M., Hayase, T., et al., 2007. The usefulness of an earphone-type infrared tympanic thermometer for intraoperative core temperature monitoring. Anesth Analg 105, 1688–1692.

Ko, H.K., Flemmer, A., Haberl, C., et al., 2001. Methodological investigation of measuring nasopharyngeal temperature as noninvasive brain temperature analogue in the neonate. Intensive Care Med 27, 736–742.

Kongsayreepong, S., Gunnaleka, P., Suraseranivongse, S., et al., 2002. A reusable, custom-made warming blanket prevents core hypothermia during major neonatal surgery. Can J Anaesth 49, 605–609.

Li, M-x., Sun, G., Neubauer, H., 2004. Change in the body temperature of healthy term infant over the first 72 hours of life. J Zhejiang Univ Sci 5, 486–493.

Lieberman, E., Lang, J.M., Frigoletto, F., et al., 1997. Epidural analgesia, intrapartum fever and neonatal sepsis evaluation. Pediatrics 99, 415–419.

Lyon, A.J., Stenson, B., 2004. Cold comfort for babies. Arch Dis Child Fetal Neonatal Ed 89, F93–F94.

Marks, K.H., Friedman, Z., Maisels, M.J., 1977. A simple device for reducing insensible water loss in low birth weight babies. Pediatrics 60, 223–226.

Marks, K.H., Lee, C., Bolan, C.D., et al., 1981. Oxygen consumption and temperature control of premature infants in a double-wall incubator. Pediatrics 68, 93–98.

Mayfield, S.R., Bhatia, J., Nakamura, K.T., et al., 1984. Temperature measurement in term and preterm infants. J Pediatr 104, 271–275.

McCall, E.M., Alderdice, F.A., Halliday, H.L., et al., 2008. Interventions to prevent hypothermia at birth in preterm and/or low birthweight infants. Cochrane Database Syst Rev (1), CD004210.

Messaritakis, J., Anagnostakis, D., Laskari, H., et al., 1990. Rectal-skin temperature difference in septicaemic newborn infants. Arch Dis Child 65, 380–385.

Meyer, M.P., Payton, M.J., Salmon, A., et al., 2001. A clinical comparison of radiant warmer and incubator care for preterm infants from birth to 1800 grams. Pediatrics 108, 395–401.

Mok, Q., Bass, C.A., Ducker, D.A., et al., 1991. Temperature instability during nursing procedures in preterm neonates. Arch Dis Child 66, 783–786.

Morrison, S.F., Nakamura, K., Madden, C.J., 2008. Central control of thermogenesis in mammals. Exp Physiol 93, 773–797.

Newman, M.F., Kramer, D., Croughwell, N.D., et al., 1995. Differential age effects of mean arterial pressure and rewarming on cognitive dysfunction after cardiac surgery. Anesth Analg 81, 236–242.

Okken, A., Jonxis, J.H.P., Rispens, P., et al., 1979. Insensible water loss and metabolic growth rate in low birth weight newborn babies. Pediatr Res 13, 1072–1075.

Okken, A., Blijam, C., Franz, W., et al., 1982. Effects of forced convection of heated air on insensible water loss and heat loss in preterm infants in incubators. J Pediatr 101, 108–112.

Perlstein, P.H., Edwards, N.K., Sutherland, J.M., 1970. Apnoea in premature infants and incubator air temperature changes. N Engl J Med 282, 461–466.

Pomerance, J.J., Brand, R.J., Meredith, J.L., 1981. Differentiating environmental from disease-related fevers in the term newborn. Pediatrics 67, 485–487.

Rutter, N., Hull, D., 1979a. Response of term babies to a warm environment. Arch Dis Child 54, 178–183.

Rutter, N., Hull, D., 1979b. Water loss from the skin of term and preterm babies. Arch Dis Child 54, 858–868.

Sarman, I., Tunell, R., 1989. Providing warmth for preterm babies by a heated, water filled mattress. Arch Dis Child 64, 29–33.

Sarman, I., Can, G., Tunell, R., 1989. Rewarming preterm infants on a heated, water filled mattress. Arch Dis Child 64, 687–692.

Sauer, P.J., Dane, H.J., Visser, H.K., 1984. New standards for neutral thermal environment of healthy very low birthweight infants in week one of life. Arch Dis Child 59, 18–22.

Scopes, J.W., Ahmed, I., 1966. Range of critical temperatures in sick and premature newborn babies. Arch Dis Child 41, 417–419.

Seguin, J.H., Vieth, R., 1996. Thermal stability of premature infants during routine care under radiant warmers. Arch Dis Child Fetal Neonatal Ed 74, F137–F138.

Silverman, W.A., Fertig, J.W., Berger, A.P., 1958. The influence of the thermal environment upon the survival of newly born premature infants. Pediatrics 22, 876–886.

Sinclair, J.C., 2002. Servo-control for maintaining abdominal skin temperature at 36C in low birth weight infants. Cochrane Database Syst Rev (1), CD001074.

Singh, A., Duckett, J., Newton, T., et al., 2010. Improving neonatal unit admission temperatures in preterm babies: exothermic mattresses, polythene bags or a traditional approach? J Perinatol 30, 45–49.

Symonds, M.E., Mostyn, A., Pearce, S., et al., 2003. Endocrine and nutritional regulation of fetal adipose tissue development. J Endocrinol 179, 293–299.

Thomas, K.A., 2003. Preterm infant thermal responses to caregiving differ by incubator control mode. J Perinatol 23, 640–645.

Thomas, K.A., Burr, R., 1999. Preterm infant thermal care: differing thermal environments produced by air versus skin servo-control incubators. J Perinatol 19, 264–270.

Thompson, M.H., Stothers, J.K., McLellan, N.J., 1984. Weight and water loss in the neonate in natural and forced convection. Arch Dis Child 59, 951–956.

Thoresen, M., Whitelaw, A., 2000. Cardiovascular changes during mild therapeutic hypothermia and rewarming in infants with hypoxic-ischemic encephalopathy. Pediatrics 106, 92–99.

Tveita, T., Mortensen, E., Hevroy, O., et al., 1994. Experimental hypothermia: effects of core cooling and rewarming on hemodynamics, coronary blood flow, and myocardial metabolism in dogs. Anesth Analg 79, 212–218.

Uthaya, S., Bell, J., Modi, N., 2004. Adipose tissue magnetic resonance imaging in the newborn. Horm Res 62 (Suppl. 3), 143–148.

Uthaya, S., Thomas, E.L., Hamilton, G., et al., 2005. Altered adiposity after extremely preterm birth. Pediatr Res 57, 211–215.

Vohra, S., Frent, G., Campbell, V., et al., 1999. Effect of polyethylene occlusive skin wrapping on heat loss in very low birth weight infants at delivery: A randomized trial. J Pediatr 134, 547–551.

Vohra, S.S.R.R., Zhang, B., Janes, M., et al., 2004. Heat Loss Prevention (HeLP) in the delivery room: A randomized controlled trial of polyethylene occlusive skin wrapping in very preterm infants. J Pediatr 45, 750–753.

Voora, S., Srinivasan, G., Lilien, L.D., et al., 1982. Fever in full-term newborns in the first four days of life. Pediatrics 69, 40–44.

Wananukul, S., Praisuwanna, P., 2002. Clear topical ointment decreases transepidermal water loss in jaundiced preterm infants receiving phototherapy. J Med Assoc Thai 85, 102–106.

Wheldon, A.E., Hull, D., 1983. Incubation of very immature infants. Arch Dis Child 58, 504–508.

Wheldon, A.E., Rutter, N., 1982. The heat balance of small babies nursed in incubators and under radiant warmers. Early Hum Dev 6, 131–143.

WHO, 1997. Thermal Protection of the Newborn. World Health Organization, Geneva.

Yeh, T.F., Amma, P., Lilien, L.D., 1979. Reduction of insensible water loss in premature infants under the radiant warmer. J Pediatr 94, 651–653.

Yeh, R.F., Voora, S., Lilien, L.D., et al., 1980. Oxygen consumption and insensible water loss in premature infants in single-space vs double-walled incubators. J Pediatr 97, 967–997.

Infant feeding

16

Mary Fewtrell   Sirinuch Chomtho   Alan Lucas

CHAPTER CONTENTS

© 2012 Elsevier Ltd

Part 1: New perspectives in neonatal nutrition

Mary Fewtrell   Sirinuch Chomtho

Since the first edition of this textbook there have been major conceptual changes in neonatal nutrition. Previously, the main objective in feeding infants was meeting nutritional needs, preventing nutritional deficiencies and promoting growth. However, increasing evidence shows that early nutrition has biological effects on the individual with important implications for later health. Thus, the way infants are fed may influence clinical course and prognosis. For instance, in preterm infants, early nutrition may influence propensity to life-threatening diseases such as necrotising enterocolitis (NEC) (Lucas and Cole 1990) and systemic sepsis, and, in the long term, have a major impact on cognitive function (Lucas et al. 1992, 1998) and disease risk in later life – notably cardiovascular disease (Singhal et al. 2001, 2004).

Until recently, early nutritional practice was underpinned largely by observational or physiological studies, or by small clinical trials designed to test for the effects of specific products on nutritional status, growth and tolerance. Our new understanding of the importance of early nutrition has emerged with the application of the pharmaceutical trial model to nutritional interventions. Randomised trials have now produced an evidence base for many areas of nutritional practice, based on short-term and, importantly, long-term efficacy and safety testing.

Nutritional programming

The concept that there are sensitive periods in early life when insults or stimuli may have long-term or lifetime effects is known as 'programming' (Lucas 1991), and has been recognised for over a century. The evidence that nutrition could operate as a programming agent was first shown in animals in the early 1960s (McCance 1962). Animal studies have shown that nutrition during critical periods in early life can programme outcomes such as changes in metabolism, endocrine function, gut function, size, body fatness, blood pressure, insulin resistance, blood lipids, learning, behaviour and longevity (Lucas 1994). Over the past few years, the long-term findings from large-scale randomised intervention studies in human infants have been emerging, showing that human infants, like other species, are programmed by early diet to a major degree. Early diet can have long-term effects on blood pressure (Singhal et al. 2001), insulin resistance (Singhal et al. 2003), blood lipids (Singhal et al. 2003), tendency to obesity (Singhal et al. 2002), bone health (Fewtrell et al. 1999, 2009), atopy (Lucas et al. 1990), cognitive function (Lucas et al. 1992) and brain structure (Isaacs et al. 2008). The effect sizes are large; in the case of cardiovascular risk factors (blood pressure, blood lipids, insulin resistance), the programming effects of early nutrition are greater than non-pharmacological

interventions in adult life, such as exercise and weight loss. These new findings must now be factored into the design of modern nutritional practices and are considered further in the following sections.

Nutrition during fetal life

An understanding of fetal nutritional physiology is vital to clinical practice. From analysis of 'reference fetuses' of different gestational ages, it is possible to calculate daily fetal nutrient accretion rates (Widdowson and Dickerson 1964; Fomon et al. 1982) and to use these as a basis for studying postnatal nutrition and its disorders. For example, the intrauterine accretion of calcium and phosphorus is substantially higher than that which can be supplied by a standard formula or mature breast milk to premature infants. Several other nutrients are laid down late in gestation, so that the preterm infant has low body stores. One example is body fat. By mid-gestation, body fat content is less than 1% of body weight; at 28 weeks, 3.5%; at 34 weeks, 7.8%; and at term, 15%. During the last month of intrauterine life, the fetus lays down about 7 g of fat per day (Widdowson and Dickerson 1964). Carbohydrate stores are also laid down relatively late. Shelley (1964) estimated liver glycogen to be about 1 g/100 g of tissue at 31 weeks and 4 g/100 g at term. Widdowson and Dickerson (1964) calculated total body carbohydrate to be 9 g at 33 weeks and 34 g at term. These data have been used to calculate the ability of infants of different gestations to withstand starvation and maintain glucose homeostasis after birth.

Total body water falls progressively from over 95% of body weight in the first trimester to around 75% at term (Kennedy et al. 1999) and continues to fall throughout infancy.

Lipid-soluble vitamins are transferred across the placenta by simple or facilitated diffusion (Friis-Hansen 1982), hence fetal blood concentrations of such vitamins correlate well with those in the mother, with the exception of vitamin E, for which fetal blood levels are around 30% of maternal values (Mino and Nishino 1973). These vitamins accumulate in fetal tissues throughout pregnancy. Blood concentrations, and perhaps body stores, are reduced in preterm infants and those of poorly nourished mothers. Water-soluble vitamins are transported against concentration gradients, mostly by active transport: fetal blood levels of vitamins B_1, B_2, B_6, B_{12}, folate and vitamin C are two- to fourfold higher than those in maternal blood. Preterm babies and babies of undernourished mothers have lower blood levels of water-soluble vitamins at birth (Baker et al. 1975).

'Biological clock' of fetal development

Intermediary metabolism

Throughout fetal life there is a progressively changing picture of enzymatic differentiation (Greengard 1977). Certain enzymes of amino acid metabolism develop late, including those concerned with the synthesis of cysteine from methionine, taurine from cysteine and tyrosine from phenylalanine, with degradation of tyrosine and production of urea (Boehm et al. 1988). As a result, low-birthweight (LBW) infants might be expected to have increased dietary requirements for certain amino acids (such as cysteine and taurine; and be at risk for possibly deleterious accumulation of others (such as phenylalanine, tyrosine and methionine; Ch. 34.3).

Key enzymes in gluconeogenic pathways (e.g. phosphoenolpyruvate carboxykinase) may not develop until near or even just after term delivery (Greengard 1977). A constant transplacental glucose infusion renders gluconeogenesis relatively unimportant in utero, and the fetal liver is more concerned with the storage of glucose as glycogen; phosphorylase and glucose 6-phosphatase ensure immediate glucose release after birth and defer the need for gluconeogenesis until around 24–48 hours of age; in contrast, the preterm neonate, born with low stores of liver glycogen (Widdowson 1981) and reduced gluconeogenic ability, is at risk of hypoglycaemia (Ch. 34.1).

Gastrointestinal tract

See Chapter 29.

Adaptations to extrauterine nutrition

Adaptation to feeding after birth involves major postnatal changes in gut structure and function and in intermediary metabolism. Although the fetal intestine is structurally mature by 25 weeks' gestation and capable of digesting and absorbing milk feeds, motor activity develops more slowly, and may limit the tolerance to enteral feeds.

Postnatally, enteral feeding appears to play a key part in triggering gut development. Studies on piglets and rats show marked structural and functional changes in the gastrointestinal (GI) tract and its adnexae following feeding – changes not seen in unfed animals. These effects are not confined to the gut: for example, enteral feeding may cause increased responsiveness to glucose by pancreatic β cells. Enteral feeding is not a new experience for the newborn infant: by the end of pregnancy, the fetus is swallowing about 500 ml of amniotic fluid daily, providing up to 3 g of protein (Friis-Hansen 1982), a similar fluid intake and about 25–50% of the protein intake of the breastfed infant at term. Enteral feeding in utero contributes to fetal nutrition and may help to prepare the gut for extrauterine feeding.

The following factors are important in regulating the adaptation of the intestine to extrauterine nutrition:

- Endocrine secretion. Corticosteroids and thyroxine are critical triggers for gut development. Adrenalectomy, hypophysectomy and thyroidectomy in animals delay gut maturation, whereas administration of glucocorticoids or thyroxine prior to delivery causes elongation of microvilli, increases the activities of the brush-border enzymes sucrase, enteropeptidase and alkaline phosphatase, and induces pancreatic enzyme secretion postnatally.

- Intraluminal factors. These may be endogenous (secreted by the GI tract) or exogenous (dietary nutrients), and act either directly on the cells of the GI tract or indirectly via effects on hormone secretion. For example, in neonatal rats, enteral feeding with sucrose increases intestinal sucrase and isomaltase, whereas lactose increases gut lactase, a finding consistent with the observed tolerance of preterm infants to lactose despite the late development of lactase in infants born at term. Surges in plasma levels of gut hormones can be induced by small, nutritionally insignificant volumes of milk, leading to the concept of minimal enteral feeding, where small volumes of milk are used to promote intestinal maturation and adaptation even when the infant is too sick to tolerate full enteral nutrition. However, although intraluminal factors undoubtedly influence GI development, they do not provide the sole trigger for ontogenetic changes, as normal maturational patterns of enzymes may occur in surgically bypassed segments of gut (Tsuboi et al. 1986).

- Minimal enteral feeding (trophic feeding) has been demonstrated to produce more ordered patterns of gut motility (Berseth and Nordyke 1993) and more rapid gut transit times (McClure and Newell 1999). Altough some studies have suggested that minimal enteral feeding can promote intestinal maturation, enhance feeding tolerance and decrease the time taken to reach full enteral feeds, a recent systematic review and meta-analysis (Bombell and McGuire 2009) of trophic feeding in very-low-birthweight (VLBW) infants, including data on 754 infants from nine randomised controlled trials (RCTs), concluded that there was no evidence for an effect of trophic feeding on feed tolerance or growth rate in VLBW infants; nor was there a statistically significant effect on the incidence of NEC (relative risk (RR) 1.07 (95% confidence interval (CI) 0.667–1.70). The authors concluded that further large pragmatic controlled trials are required, particularly in high-risk groups such as those born growth-restricted with absent or reversed end-diastolic flow in the umbilical artery.

- Breast milk hormones and growth factors (see Chapter 16 part 2). A large number of substances present in human milk have been demonstrated to play a role in regulating the adaptive changes that accompany the transition to enteral feeding. These include bombesin, somatostatin, epidermal growth factor, insulin-like growth factors IGF-1 and IGF-2 and nucleotides. In many cases these substances undergo only limited degradation in the stomach and appear to retain bioactivity in the intestine. Although they may not be essential for survival, the higher incidence of GI disease in infants fed formula raises the possibility that these compounds may contribute to the protective effect of human milk.

- Bacteria. Studies on the GI flora of infants fed human milk or formula suggest that the indigenous microflora are an important factor in GI development and function (see later), altering the activities of various enzymes.

Biological consequences of depriving babies of enteral feeds after birth

Exclusive intravenous feeding in rats results in decreased weight of the small intestine, pancreas and oxyntic area of the stomach, associated with a significant reduction in small-intestinal DNA and a dramatic reduction in antral gastrin content; in contrast, animal studies have shown that other organs not directly concerned with nutrition, such as spleen and testes, remain unaffected (Johnson et al. 1975) and Heird (1977) demonstrated intestinal mucosal atrophy during parenteral nutrition, with concomitant reduction in brush-border enzyme activities. These effects may be related to the very low concentrations of circulating gut hormones found in human infants deprived of enteral feeding.

Although after short periods of parenteral nutrition in neonates tolerance to enteral feeds usually increases rapidly (in the absence of structural anomaly of the gut), it remains to be established whether prolonged avoidance of enteral feeding could deprive the neonate of critical signals for gut development.

Non-nutritional consequences of enteral feeding

When a neonate is fed, dynamic alterations occur in splanchnic blood flow, with a significant increase in velocity, which is 35% greater in formula-fed term infants than in breastfed infants. Fasting velocities are also higher in formula-fed infants (Coombs et al. 1992). In preterm infants, there is a significant correlation between the increase in mean superior mesenteric artery blood flow seen after a test feed and subsequent early tolerance of enteral feeds (Fang et al. 2001). Preterm infants fed hourly have higher preprandial blood flow in the superior mesenteric artery, with no significant postprandial change, whereas those fed 3-hourly show lower preprandial blood flow and significant postprandial hyperaemia, with a longer latency and smaller amplitude after expressed breast milk than after preterm formula (Lane et al. 1998). These findings suggest that both the frequency and composition of feeds influence splanchnic blood flow in preterm infants. Changes may also occur in pulmonary function, with decreased tidal volume, minute ventilation and compliance in VLBW infants randomised to intermittent versus continuous feeds (Blondheim et al. 1993).

Individual nutrients: physiology and dietary needs of term and preterm infants

Calculation of the nutrient requirements for term infants has traditionally been based on the composition of breast milk. However, the precise dietary intake of breastfed babies is unknown, and there is ongoing uncertainty over what should be regarded as an ideal pattern of growth during infancy, with data from animals and now humans increasingly suggesting that accelerated early growth may be associated with adverse effects on later health (Singhal and Lucas 2004). Thus, appropriate dietary goals continue to be disputed. The EC Directive Compositional Criteria for Infant Formulae (European Commission 2006) are shown in Table 16.1. All infant formula manufacturers in the UK are required by law to comply with these.

LBW babies are not a homogeneous population: their requirements and tolerance of individual nutrients are influenced by gestation, postnatal age and concomitant illness. Nevertheless, there is some international consensus on the advisable intakes for each nutrient. This field was comprehensively reviewed by the Committee on Nutrition of the European Society for Paediatric Gastroenterology and Nutrition (Agostoni et al. 2010), and by a panel of international experts (Tsang et al. 2005), who considered separately the needs of infants above or below 1000 g; a summary of the recommendations by these panels for intakes of individual nutrients

is shown in Table 16.2. The scientific and clinical basis for current recommendations for the desirable nutrient intakes in preterm infants is illustrated below.

Proteins and amino acids

The protein intake per kilogram bodyweight for the human infant is greater than for adults. In mammals, the protein content of milk correlates highly with postnatal growth rate. Nine amino acids are considered essential in human nutrition: arginine, lysine, leucine, isoleucine, valine, methionine, phenylalanine, threonine and tryptophan. However, because of the late development of certain enzymes of amino acid metabolism, the newborn infant may have a temporarily increased requirement for cysteine and histidine, and perhaps for taurine (see below).

Digestion and absorption

Luminal hydrolysis results in the breakdown of most large-molecular-weight proteins into peptides and amino acids. Most peptides are then hydrolysed by peptidases on the microvillus membrane prior to transport through the membrane, but some are absorbed intact. Although pepsin secretion is lower in preterm than term infants at birth, it is unaffected by the type of diet (Hamosh 1996). The activity of brush-border peptidases is also low in preterm infants at birth, but increases rapidly.

Protein requirements for term babies

These are discussed further in Chapter 16, part 2. The EC Directive guidelines recommend that formulas containing unmodified cow's milk protein should contain 1.1–2.1 g of protein per 100 ml of reconstituted feed. As growth velocity falls during infancy, there is a progressively decreased need for protein intake per kilogram of bodyweight. In recent years, there has been increasing speculation over the role of excess infant protein intake and increased risk of later obesity (Koletzo et al. 2009); hence there have been moves to lower the protein intakes of term infants.

Estimating the protein requirements for the preterm baby

That the rapid growth in preterm babies might greatly increase the need for dietary protein has been appreciated for over 40 years. The increasing survival of extremely preterm and extremely low-birthweight (ELBW) infants, and the appreciation that these infants often acquire substantial nutrient deficits accompanied by compromised growth during early postnatal life, has led to a re-evaluation of their protein requirements. Recent recommendations take account of a number of factors and serve as a model for the investigation of requirements for other nutrients.

Relation of protein intake to growth

Previous recommendations were based largely on estimated requirements to match the growth rate of a fetus of equivalent postconceptional age. Weight gain and linear growth are the traditional measures of nutritional status. Gordon et al. (1947) demonstrated that preterm infants gained weight more rapidly on high-protein-containing formulas than on human milk, and Davidson et al. (1967) showed that weight gain was greater in preterm infants fed a formula supplying 4 g/kg/24 h rather than 2 g/kg/24 h. High intakes of protein may also result in an increase in linear growth and a greater rate of increase in head circumference (Brooke et al.

Table 16.1 Composition of mature human milk and nutritional criteria for the composition of infant formula for full-term infants per 100 ml

	MEAN VALUES FOR POOLED SAMPLES OF EXPRESSED MATURE HUMAN MILK	GUIDELINES FOR INFANT FORMULAS Minimum	Maximum
Energy			
kJ	293	250	295
kcal	70	60	71
Protein (g)	1.3	1.1	2.1
Lactose (g)	7	2.8	NS
Total carbohydrate (g)		5.5	10.0
Fat (g)	4.2	2.6	4.1
Vitamins (μg)			
A	60	35	127
D	0.01	0.63	1.92
E*	0.35	0.5[†]	1.2[†]
K	0.21	2.4	NS
Thiamin	16	35	212
Riboflavin	30	48	212
Nicotinic acid	230	150	NS
Pyridoxine	6	22.5	124
B_{12}	0.01	0.06	NS
Folic acid	5.2	6.25	35
Biotin	0.76	1.0	5.3
C	3.8	6.25	22.1
Minerals			
Sodium (mg)	15	12.5	41.3
Potassium (mg)	60	37.5	112
Chloride (mg)	43	30	112
Calcium (mg)	35	30	97
Phosphorus (mg)	15	15	65
Magnesium (mg)	2.3	3.0	10.6
Iron (mg)	0.76	0.18	0.89
Iodine (μg)	7	6.25	35
Zinc (mg)	0.295	0.3	1.1
Copper (μg)	39	21	74

*mg (TE), tocopherol equivalents; NS, not specified.
[†]minimum 0.5/g polyunsaturated fatty acids (PUFA), maximum 1.2/g PUFA.
Adapted from European Commission (2006).

Table 16.2 Recommended intakes of individual nutrients for (formula-fed) stable/growing preterm infants

	ESPGHAN		TSANG ELBW		VLBW	
	per kg/day	per 100 kcal	per kg/day	per 100 kcal	per kg/day	per 100 kcal
Energy						
kcal	110–135		130–150		110–130	
kJ						
Protein (g)	4.0–4.5 <1 kg 3.5–4.0 1–1.8 kg	3.6–4.1 <1 kg 3.2–3.6	3.8–4.4	2.5–3.4	3.4–4.2	
Fat (g)	4.8–6.6	4.4–6.0 <40% MCT	6.2–8.4	4.1–6.5	5.3–7.2	
Linolenic acid (mg)	385–1540	350–1400				
Linoleic/ALA	5–15.1		5–15		5–15	
ALA (mg)*	>55 (0.9% FA)	>50				
DHA (mg)*	12–30	11–27	ge21	ge16	ge18	ge16
AA (mg)	18–42	16–39	ge28	ge22	ge24	ge22
Carbohydrate (g)	11.6–13.2	10.5–12	9–20	6.0–15.4	7–17	5.4–15.5
Lactose						
Oligomers						
Sodium (mg)	69–115	63–105	69–115	46–88	69–115	53–105
Potassium (mg)	66–132	60–120	78–117	52–90	78–117	60–106
Chloride (mg)	105–177	95–161	107–249	71–192	107–249	82–226
Calcium (mg)	120–140	110–130	100–220	67–169	100–220	77–200
Phosphate (mg)	60–90	55–80	60–140	40–108	60–140	46–127
Magnesium (mg)	8–15	7.5–13.6	7.9–15	5.3–11.5	7.9–15	6.1–13.6
Iron (mg)	2–3	1.8–2.7	2–4	1.33–3.08	2–4	1.5–3.6
Zinc (mg)	1.1–2.0	1.0–1.8	1.0–3.0	0.67–2.3	1.0–3.0	0.77–2.7
Copper (µg)	100–132	90–120	120–150	80–115	120–150	92–136
Selenium (µg)	5–10	4.5–9.0	1.3–4.5	0.9–3.5	1.3–4.5	1.0–4.1
Manganese (µg)	<27.5	6.4–2.5	0.7–7.5	0.5–5.8	0.7–7.5	0.5–6.8
Iodine (µg)	11–55	10–50	10–60	6.7–46.2	10–60	7.7–54.5
Vitamin A (IU: 1 µg RE = 33.33 IU)	400–1000	360–740	700–1500	467–1154	700–1500	538–1364
Vitamin D (IU)	800–1000		150–400	100–308	150–400	115–364
Vitamin E (mg α-TE)	2.2–11	2–10	6–12[†]	4.0–9.2	6–12[†]	4.6–10.9
Vitamin K (µg)	4.4–28	4–25	8–10	5.3–7.7	8–10	6.2–9.1
Vitamin C (mg)	11–46	10–42	18–24	12.0–18.5	18–24	13.8–21.8
Thiamin (µg)	140–300	125–275	180–240	120–185	180–240	138–218
Riboflavin (µg)	200–400	180–365	250–360	167–277	250–360	192–327
Pyridoxine (µg)	45–300	41–273	150–210	100–162	150–210	115–191
Niacin (µg)	380–5500	345–5000	3.6–4.8	2.4–3.7	3.6–4.8	2.8–4.4

Table 16.2 Continued

	ESPGHAN		TSANG ELBW		VLBW	
	per kg/day	per 100 kcal	per kg/day	per 100 kcal	per kg/day	per 100 kcal
B$_{12}$ (μg)	0.1–0.77	0.08–0.7	0.3	0.2–0.23	0.3	0.23–0.27
Folate (μg)	35–100	32–90	25–50	17–38	25–50	19–45
Taurine (mg)			4.5–9.0	3.0–6.9	4.5–9.0	3.5–8.2
Inositol (mg)	4.4–53	4–48	32–81	21–62	32–81	25–74
Choline (mg)	8–55	7–50	14.4–28	9.6–21.5	14.4–28	11.1–25.5

*Ratio of AA to DHA should be in the range of 1.0–2.0 to 1 (wt/wt) and eicosapentaenoic acid supply should not exceed 30% of DHA supply.
†Maximum = 25 IU.
ESPGHAN, European Society of Paediatric Gastroenterology and Nutrition (Agostoni 2010); Tsang ELBW, extremely low-birthweight (Tsang et al. 2005); VLBW, very-low-birthweight; MCT, medium-chain triglyceride; ALA, alpha-linolenic acid; FA, fatty acid; DHA, docosahexaenoic acid; AA, arachidonic acid; RE, retinol equivalent; α-TE, α-tocopherol equivalent.

1982; Lucas et al. 1984). Weight gain approximating to that in utero can be achieved at approximately 3 g/kg/day protein intake (Ziegler 1986; Tsang et al. 2005). Intakes of protein less than 3–3.5 g/kg/day can support intrauterine rates of weight gain, but only when accompanied by very high energy intakes, which then promote a much higher body fat than would be seen in the fetus.

Newer recommendations also recognise the need for compensation of the initial protein gap and early catch-up growth. Recent studies have highlighted the cumulative deficits in protein and energy intakes seen in preterm infants, particularly the smallest and sickest infants during early postnatal life. Even beyond this 'transition' period, actual intakes rarely match those recommended due to various clinical conditions (Embleton et al. 2001).

A factorial approach

Protein requirements may be derived using a combination of values for body composition and for nitrogen retention, obtained from balance studies. The results from a number of such studies show that protein gain increases linearly with intakes between approximately 2 and 4.5 g/kg/24 h (Ziegler 1986; Tsang et al. 2005). These calculations involve making assumptions about desirable postnatal growth performance, but the results emphasise that, in order to achieve the accretion of nitrogen at the same rate as seen in utero during the second half of gestation – estimated to be approximately 1.7g/kg/day, although this falls at the end of gestation – the preterm infant requires substantially greater intakes of protein than would be obtained by a term infant fed on breast milk. In a sick infant in whom a temporary period of reduced nutritional intake is necessary, it is important at least to prevent catabolism. Theoretically, a protein intake of 0.7 g/kg/24 h will result in a reduction of protein turnover to the point of equilibrium (that is, zero gain and zero loss), and from a pragmatic point of view this should be the minimum acceptable daily intake.

There is also increasing focus on matching the lean body mass and protein gain of the fetus rather than simply weight gain. Fetal weight gain consists predominantly of lean body mass, such that, at term, lean body mass represents about 87% of weight. In contrast, postnatal weight gain contains a much higher proportion of fat. Hence it is generally considered that lean body mass gain is preferable to weight gain in the evaluation of postnatal growth.

Assessment of protein undernutrition

A low concentration of plasma protein is a traditional index of protein malnutrition. Preterm infants fed on human milk (banked or own mother's) may develop hypoproteinaemia after the second month of postnatal life, and this is prevented by protein supplementation (Ronnholm et al. 1982). Intakes in the range 3–4.5g/kg/day will achieve acceptable plasma albumin and transthyretin concentrations (Kashyap et al. 1988).

Assessment of protein 'overload'

Schultz et al. (1980) showed that, compared with a breastfed control group of infants receiving 2.0 g protein per kilogram per day, a formula-fed group receiving 4.4 g protein per kilogram per day demonstrated azotaemia, a lower blood glucose, hyperaminoacidaemia (especially phenylalanine) and metabolic acidosis, and regained birthweight more slowly. However, balance and stable isotope studies (Young 1981) have emphasised that the amount of energy absorbed is critical for the rate of protein synthesis. If energy intake is low, high protein intakes cannot be utilised and the infant's metabolic machinery is stressed; in contrast, diets with high available energy and large protein intakes, of at least 4 g/kg/24 h, result in increased nitrogen retention and growth, without metabolic strain. For this reason, it is conventional to express protein (and indeed other nutrient requirements) in relation to energy intake (Table 16.2) as well as in absolute terms.

Short- and long-term outcome studies

Arguably the most important issue is whether early protein intake could have longer term consequences, either adverse or beneficial. A recent systematic review (Premji et al. 2006) identified five RCTs comparing different protein intakes in preterm infants and reported improved weight gain and higher nitrogen accretion in infants receiving formulas with higher protein content (>3 but <4 g/kg/day). None of the studies examined cognitive outcome. However, a study in 495 ELBW infants (Ehrenkranz et al. 2006) suggested that in-hospital growth velocity had a significant impact on neurodevelopment and growth outcomes at 18–22 months postterm. In another study, preterm infants randomised to receive a preterm formula containing 2 g/100 ml protein showed both better short-term growth than those fed a standard term formula containing

1.45 g/100 ml and improved neurodevelopment 7.5–8 years later (Lucas et al. 1992). Finally, a recent observational study reported that higher protein and energy intake during the first week of life in ELBW infants was associated with higher Bayley mental developmental index (MDI) scores at 18 months and with a lower likelihood of restricted linear growth. Each 1 g/kg/day increase in protein during week 1 was calculated to be associated with an 8.2-point increase in Bayley MDI (Stephens et al. 2009).

Despite increasing evidence supporting the clinical benefits of an adequate protein intake, a study by Goldman et al. (1974) cautioned that excessive intakes could have adverse effects. A total of 304 infants below 2000 g were randomised to 2% or 4% protein diets, providing, respectively, 3.0–3.6 and 6.0–7.2 g protein per kilogram per day. Infants below 1300 g in the high protein intake group had a markedly higher incidence of low IQs (below 90) by Stanford–Binet score at 5 years of age. The incidence of strabismus in infants below 1700 g fed on a high protein intake was also increased.

Protein quality

All protein supplies are not equal and it is recognised that net protein utilisation (N retained/N intake) differs with different feeding regimens. Whey proteins have a lower concentration of aromatic amino acids (tyrosine and phenylalanine) than are found in caseins; the studies by Goldman et al. (1974) were performed with high-casein formulas (like cow's milk), but most modern formulas are whey-predominant, reducing the possibility of hypertyrosinaemia and hyperphenylalaninaemia. Whey is also a good source of cysteine, a potentially essential amino acid in the newborn period (see above). However, there are still considerable differences in the protein composition of modern infant formulas compared with breast milk. A large part of this difference relates to the lower concentration of α-lactalbumin and higher concentration of β-lactoglubulin in bovine milk. It is now possible to make whey fractions from bovine milk with lower β-lactoglubulin and higher α-lactalbumin. These fractions contain higher concentrations of essential amino acids, particularly tryptophan and cysteine. Their addition to infant formulas may result in plasma amino acid patterns closer to those seen in breastfed infants, and allow a reduction in the total protein levels, with potential benefits for the infant's growth pattern (Lien et al. 2004; Sandstrom et al. 2008).

Amino acid composition

There is increasing focus on amino acid requirements rather than protein requirements, on the basis that infants require specific amino acids, not proteins. Little is known about the optimal intakes of specific amino acids. However, a different amino acid composition of protein may well alter the total amount required. Breastfed infants have higher plasma and urine taurine concentrations and a higher rate of synthesis of bile acids than those fed on formula; the latter may partially explain the better fat absorption of infants fed human milk rather than formulas (Gaull et al. 1977). Rhesus monkeys fed a taurine-deficient formula for the first 6 or 12 months of life show abnormal retinal structure, although the abnormalities show some degree of spontaneous regression by 12 months even when the animals remain on the deficient diet (Imaki et al. 1993). A randomised trial of taurine supplementation in formula-fed preterm infants (Tyson et al. 1989) showed no effect on growth, behaviour or electroretinograms, but some evidence of more rapid auditory maturation in the supplemented group at the equivalent of term (as assessed by brainstem-evoked response). More recently, Wharton et al. (2004) have shown that preterm infants with the

highest plasma taurine concentrations during the neonatal period have better numeracy skills during adolescence and better development of the related parietal cortical grey matter. Thus, it seems prudent to add taurine to LBW formulas to achieve concentrations similar to those of breast milk.

Glutamine is used as a fuel by the small intestine and as a precursor for the synthesis of purine and pyrimidine bases. Numerous studies in animals and adult humans have demonstrated that it has beneficial effects on the GI tract, including the maintenance of structure and function during parenteral nutrition. A systematic review that included data from 2365 preterm infants who participated in seven randomised trials of either enteral or parenteral glutamine supplementation concluded there was no evidence of a beneficial effect of supplementation on mortality or short-term morbidity. The single study that assessed longer term outcomes found no effect on neurodevelopment at 18 months' corrected age (Tubman et al. 2008).

Arginine is a precursor for the synthesis of nitric oxide, which in turn is important as a regulator of vascular perfusion. Plasma arginine concentrations have been found to be inversely related to the severity of respiratory distress syndrome, and low concentrations have been reported in infants who develop NEC. A single randomised trial of arginine supplementation (1.5 mmol/kg/day, given either enterally or parenterally) versus placebo in preterm infants found a significantly reduced incidence of NEC in supplemented infants (RR 0.24; 95% CI 0.10–0.61), with no adverse effects. However, given the high incidence of NEC in the study population, the data are insufficient at present to support a practice recommendation. A multicentre randomised controlled study of arginine supplementation in preterm neonates is needed, focusing on the incidence of NEC, particularly the more severe stages (2 or 3).

Fat

Digestion and absorption

Fat provides about half the energy for infants fed human milk, and its digestion commences in the stomach, catalysed by lingual lipase and gastric lipase (Hamosh 1996). Gastric lipolysis is quantitatively greater in the infant than in the adult, and the output and activity of lipases in the preterm infant are equal to those of adults maintained on a high-fat diet. Although gastric function and the production of lipase are unaffected by infant diet, the extent of fat digestion is greater in babies fed human milk (25%) than formula (14%), probably because of the structural differences between triglyceride in human milk fat globules and that in formula fat particles. Both lingual and gastric lipases are able to penetrate the milk fat globule membrane and digest triglyceride without disrupting its structure. The contribution of pancreatic lipases is relatively lower in infants than in adults. However, the bile salt-stimulated lipase (BSSL) present in human milk may contribute significantly to fat digestion. BSSL is present in high quantities even in the milk of mothers who deliver prematurely, and its concentration is independent of milk volume. Unlike gastric and pancreatic lipases, BSSL shows no positional or fatty acid specificity and is able to produce free fatty acids which are more easily absorbed than mono- or diglycerides at the low bile salt concentration seen in newborn infants.

The products of fat digestion are absorbed, resynthesised as triglycerides and secreted mainly into the lymphatic system as chylomicrons, and thence into the blood via the great veins. The foregoing applies to long-chain triglycerides, which are best absorbed if they are unsaturated. In contrast, medium-chain triglycerides

(MCTs: 8–10 carbon atoms to the chain) are handled quite differently: their digestion is largely independent of bile salts; they are well absorbed, hydrolysed or intact, and pass to the liver via the portal system. Faecal fat excretion in newborn infants is greater in infants fed on cow's milk than in those fed on human milk or vegetable fats.

Most modern formulas contain a mixture of animal and vegetable oils, adjusted to mimic the pattern of fatty acid saturation and chain lengths found in breast milk. When compared with human milk, such fat mixtures have a reduced content of fatty acids esterified to glycerol in the 2 position and an increase in those esterified in the 1 and 3 positions. The latter undergo hydrolysis in the gut, releasing palmitic acid, which is poorly absorbed and tends to form calcium soaps; this may be partly responsible for the harder stools seen in formula-fed infants, and could influence calcium absorption. A recent review identified nine publications in preterm or term infants in which 'standard' infant formulas containing high palmitate concentrations were compared with either low palmitate formulas or formulas containing a modified synthetic fat blend (Betapol) with a high proportion of fatty acids esterified in the 2 position to mimic that found in human milk (Koo et al. 2006). Standardised results from these studies were consistently positive in favour of the low/synthetic palmitate groups with respect to intestinal fractional absorption of fat, palmitic acid and calcium. Total body bone mass was also significantly higher in two studies (Kennedy et al. 1999; Koo et al. 2003), suggesting that increased calcium absorption results in measurable biological effects in the short term (Kennedy et al. 1999). However, follow-up of one of these cohorts at age 10 years found no persisting effect of the intervention on bone mass, suggesting that any effect may be transient (Fewtrell et al. unpublished observations).

Fat requirements

Because there are clinical and physiological ceilings on the amount of dietary energy that it is desirable to supply as carbohydrate or protein, a minimum of around 30% of dietary energy needs to be supplied as fat. Linoleic and alpha-linolenic acids are essential fatty acids for the development of the brain and for prostaglandin synthesis. Essential fatty acid deficiency is also associated with skin lesions and retarded growth.

Two other dietary factors are important for lipid metabolism. Carnitine plays a key role by facilitating transport of long-chain fatty acids across the mitochondrial membrane prior to their oxidation (Wharton 1987). Carnitine deficiency during the neonatal period has been reported in infants who experience intrapartum hypoxia and acidosis (Bayes et al. 2001). Preterm and small-for-gestational age (SGA) infants may have impaired endogenous carnitine synthesis, and if carnitine intake is deficient (as in total parenteral nutrition (TPN)) plasma and tissue concentrations fall. Nevertheless, there is currently insufficient evidence to judge whether such infants are put at clinical risk from a low-carnitine diet is uncertain. A randomised trial found that preterm infants who received supplemental carnitine in parenteral nutrition did not demonstrate any reduction in apnoea of prematurity, ventilatory requirements or need for supplemental oxygen therapy compared with those who received placebo (O'Donnell et al. 2002). Standard formulas usually contain similar concentrations of carnitine to those in breast milk, but some preterm formulas have additional carnitine.

Choline is required for phospholipid and acetylcholine synthesis (Wharton 1987). About half the choline requirement is derived from the diet. Human and cow's milk-based diets provide a sufficient intake.

Inositol, a six-carbon cyclic polyalcohol sugar, is a component of membrane phospholipids, and compounds containing inositol are important in signal transduction. Breast milk, particularly colostrum, contains high concentrations, whereas the levels in infant formulas are lower and intravenous feeding solutions have none. At present, it is recommended that all preterm infants receive supplementation based upon the level of inositol in human milk. A systematic review of three RCTs of inositol supplementation in preterm infants concluded that supplementation results in a statistically significant and clinically important reduction in the risk of chronic lung disease, retinopathy of prematurity (stage 4 or needing therapy), intraventricular haemorrhage (grade III–IV) and death (Howlett and Ohlsson 2003). The authors suggest a multicentre RCT of appropriate size is required to confirm these findings.

Essential fatty acid requirements

Two groups of long-chain polyunsaturated fatty acids (LCPUFAs, i.e. polyunsaturated fatty acids with greater than 18-carbon chain length) have received increasing interest in recent years: these are homologues of linoleic acid of the n-6 series (dihomogammalinolenic acid, arachidonic acid) and of α-linolenic acid of the n-3 series (eicosapentaenoic acid, docosahexaenoic acid (DHA)). The LCPUFAs are synthesised from the precursor essential fatty acids by a process of chain elongation and desaturation (Fig. 16.1). They are found in high concentrations in the phospholipids of cell membranes, notably in the central nervous system (O'Brien et al. 1964). In addition, arachidonic acid, dihomogammalinolenic acid and eicosapentaenoic acid are precursors for eicosanoids – important modulators and mediators of a variety of essential biological processes.

Rapid accumulation of LCPUFAs in the brain, particularly DHA, occurs from the third trimester to 18 months postpartum

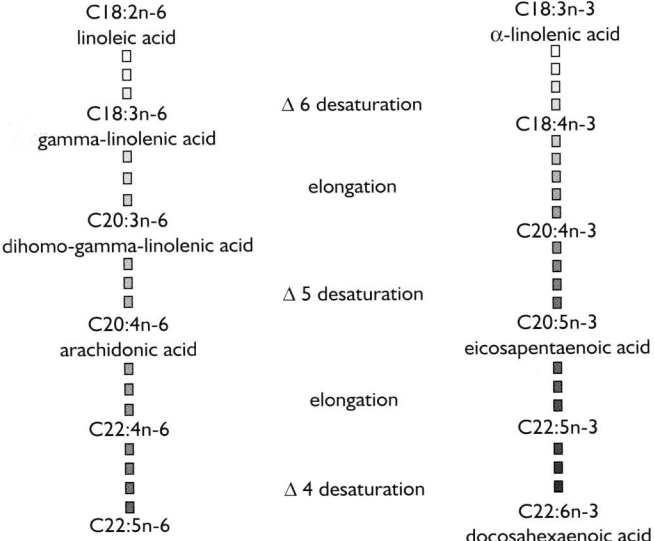

Fig. 16.1 Major steps in the formation of long-chain polyunsaturated fatty acids (LPCs) from the C:18 essential fatty acids. Unsaturated fatty acids contain at least one double bond between adjacent carbon atoms: the number of double bonds is represented by 1n, 2n, 3n, etc. LPCs are further classified by the position of the first double bond from the methyl or omega end of the hydrocarbon chain, represented as -3, -6, -9 or _-3, _-6, _-9. Linoleic acid (C18:2n-6) thus has a chain length of 18 carbons with two double bonds, the first of which is at the sixth carbon atom from the omega end.

(Clandinin et al. 1981). Human milk contains both the precursor essential fatty acids and adequate LCPUFAs for structural lipid accretion (Clandinin et al. 1980), but infant formulas traditionally contained only the parent essential fatty acids, the assumption being that the infant could synthesise LCPUFAs from these. However, term and preterm infants fed on formulas which contain minimal LCPUFAs have been shown to have lower red cell LCPUFAs and lower LCPUFAs in the phospholipids of the cerebral cortex and subcutaneous tissues than infants fed breast milk (Carlson et al. 1986; Farquharson et al. 1992, 1995; Makrides et al. 1994). Largely on the basis of the biochemical data, ESPGHAN (1987) recommended several years ago that formulas for LBW infants should be enriched with metabolites of both linoleic and linolenic acids, approximating the levels typical of human milk; indeed, the majority of preterm and term infant formulas now contain preformed LCPUFAs. However, although there is clear evidence that supplementing infant formulas with LCPUFAs results in biochemical improvement, there is less evidence of lasting clinical benefits; recently updated systematic reviews concluded there was no evidence for a clinical benefit of LCPUFA supplementation of term (Simmer et al. 2008a) or preterm (Simmer et al. 2008b) infant formula. In the most recent and largest trial conducted in this field, preterm infants (<33 weeks' gestation) were randomised to receive either high DHA (1% of total fatty acids) versus a typical current DHA intake (0.3%) achieved by a combination of supplementing mothers who were expressing milk for their infant and the use of DHA-supplemented formulas. No effect of high-dose supplementation was seen overall at 18 (Makrides et al. 2009) or 26 months' (Smithers et al. 2010) corrected age, although girls had significantly higher Bayley MDI at 18 months. Longer term follow-up studies are currently in progress, testing for effects of LCPUFAs on health outcomes, including cardiovascular risk as well as cognitive function.

Term babies

The EC Directive guidelines (European Commission 2006) recommend that the fat content of infant formulas should lie between 2.6 and 4.1 g per 100 ml of feed. The guidelines also specify levels for alpha-linoleic acid (not less than 12 mg/100 kcal) and linoleic acid (300–1200 mg/100 kcal), with the linoleic/alpha-linoleic ratio between 5 and 15, for term infant formulas. However, there is currently no requirement to add LCPUFAs, although, if added, their content shall not exceed 1% of total fat for n-3 LCP and 2% of total fat for n-6 LCP. Furthermore, the DHA content shall not exceed that of the n-6 LCP and the eicosapentaenoic acid content shall not exceed the DHA content.

Preterm babies

The main problem with dietary fat in preterm infants is the increased tendency to steatorrhoea. Reduced fat absorption in LBW infants relates to:

- reduced pancreatic lipase and carboxylic ester hydrolase activity
- reduced bile acid pool size and secretion rate: the duodenal bile acid concentration may well be below the critical level for micelle formation
- possible reduction in activity or excretion of lingual lipase.

Fat absorption from fresh breast milk is approximately 90%, but the observed range is enormous. Williamson et al. (1978) found that fat absorption from expressed breast milk fell to 55% in VLBW infants fed pasteurised milk, and to around 45% when the milk was boiled. These data may reflect loss of the bile salt-stimulated lipase found in human milk due to heat treatment.

A controversial issue is the addition of large quantities of MCTs to specially designed preterm infant formulas, largely because such babies absorb palmitic acid (n-16) poorly. The MCT content of human milk is low (less than 2% total fatty acids), whereas modern preterm formulas may contain up to 40% of the fat in this form. MCTs may spare dietary nitrogen and enhance calcium and magnesium absorption (Tantibhedyangkul and Hashim 1978). However, a review that included eight small randomised trials of MCT versus long-chain triglycerides in preterm infants concluded there was no evidence for an effect of MCT on short-term growth, GI intolerance, or NEC, although larger studies would be required to confirm these findings and to examine longer term outcomes (Klenoff-Brumberg and Genen 2003).

Carbohydrate

Physiology

The carbohydrate in human milk is almost entirely lactose, which provides 40% of ingested energy (Kien 1996). Other carbohydrates, e.g. sucrose and maltodextrins, may be hydrolysed efficiently by active brush-border sucrase, maltase and isomaltase, even in preterm infants, and starch or glucose polymers can be digested by salivary and pancreatic amylase, by amylase present in human milk, and by intestinal mucosal hydrolases.

Dietary lactose undergoes one of two processes: hydrolysis into glucose and galactose by the intestinal brush-border lactase, followed by absorption of glucose and galactose, or fermentation in the colon, with production of various gases and short-chain fatty acids. Energy from the latter can be absorbed, compensating at least in part for the inefficiency of dietary energy utilisation. Short-chain fatty acids administered into the colon have also been shown to stimulate intestinal growth following gut resection in animal models, and prevent mucosal atrophy after resection and TPN. There is controversy over the possible role of lactose fermentation in the development of NEC. However, although there are some experimental data linking excessive carbohydrate fermentation in the small intestine with an inflammatory condition resembling NEC, there is little evidence that colonic lactose fermentation is a primary factor.

Galactose and glucose are absorbed by the same carrier mechanism, and more than 90% reaches the portal vein. Most galactose is removed by the liver on first pass, and appears to be preferentially used for glycogen synthesis rather than conversion to glucose.

There is currently intense interest in the prebiotic role of oligosaccharides in human milk. Prebiotics are defined as non-digestible food ingredients that selectively stimulate the growth and/or activity of one or more bacteria in the colon, and therefore benefit the host. They promote the bifidogenic-dominant colonic microflora observed in breastfed infants, which in turn protects the infant from enteropathogenic bacteria. Human milk contains hundreds, if not thousands, of oligosaccharides; the composition is genetically determined with wide interindividual variation, making it difficult to define (and therefore to mimic) the oligosaccharide content of breast milk. Cow's milk formulas traditionally contained no oligosaccharides, but, in recent years, oligosaccharide mixtures such as GosFos (a mixture of 90% galacto-oligosaccharides with 10% fructo-oligosaccharides) have been added. Randomised trials of supplementation of formula with oligosaccharides have shown enhanced colonisation with beneficial intestinal flora in both term and preterm infants, but there is less evidence for effects on clinical outcome (Osborn and Sinn 2007).

Term infants' requirements

The EC Directive recommendation (European Commission 2006) for carbohydrate intake is that it should be between 5.5 and 10.0 g per 100 ml of reconstituted feed, and that the lactose content should be above 2.7 g/100 ml (Table 16.1). Other carbohydrate sources that are permitted in modern formulas are maltose, sucrose, glucose, maltodextrin, glucose syrup and precooked or gelatinised starch.

Preterm infants' requirements

It is difficult to infer from physiological studies which carbohydrate is optimal for LBW infants. Lactose may enhance gut absorption of calcium and magnesium and may encourage a favourable gut flora; excessive intakes may result in diarrhoea and metabolic acidosis, yet in practice a high lactose intake in preterm infants is usually well tolerated.

One approach in the design of preterm formulas is to use lactose as the principal carbohydrate source, but to replace a proportion of the carbohydrate with glucose polymers in order to prevent excess osmolality (see Table 16.2 for recommended intakes).

Energy

The fundamental energy (E) equation is:

$$E_{intake} + E_{stored} = E_{expended} + E_{excreted} \qquad (1)$$

Energy expended may be subdivided further:

$$E_{expended} = E_{BMR} + E_{activity} + E_{synthesis} + E_{thermoreg} \qquad (2)$$

where E_{stored} is the energy deposited during growth, E_{BMR} is the basal energy requirement, $E_{activity}$ is the additional cost of muscular activity, $E_{synthesis}$ is the metabolic cost of growing (excluding energy stored in new tissue) and $E_{thermoreg}$ is the energy cost of maintaining body temperature.

Traditionally, the tools used to derive these values have been energy balances and indirect calorimetry (energy expenditure calculated from oxygen consumption and carbon dioxide production) performed under different experimental conditions during rest. More recently, the 'doubly labelled water method' has been used to measure total energy expenditure over periods of several days. This non-invasive method depends on monitoring the differential disappearance from the body of two stable (non-radioactive) isotopes, ^{18}O and deuterium, both administered orally as labelled water.

There has been dispute over which conversion factors should be used for either human or cow's milk to derive the metabolisable energy content (the gross energy of the food from bomb calorimetry minus the energy lost in the stools and urine) from macronutrient concentrations. Although not entirely appropriate to the milk-fed neonate, the conventional Atwater conversion factors derived by Southgate and Durnin (1970) are commonly used.

Term infants' requirements

The EC Directive guidelines recommend that formula should contain similar energy contents to those reported in human milk, i.e. 60–71 kcal/100 ml of reconstituted feed. However, from studies employing the doubly labelled water method, Lucas et al. (1987) suggested that infants fed on human milk may receive lower energy intakes than those commonly reported and those employed in modern formulas – they obtained a value of 58 kcal/100 ml at 3 months; this may explain why modern formula-fed term infants grow faster than their breastfed counterparts.

Term SGA infants have been reported to have energy expenditures 5–10% higher than infants who are appropriate for gestational age, and may therefore benefit from increased energy to promote catch-up growth. In one study, a high-energy formula resulted in a marginal increase in weight gain and head growth (Brooke and Kinzey 1985). However, it is likely that both extra energy and protein are required simultaneously.

Preterm infants' requirements

The energy requirements for preterm infants cannot be calculated without some consideration of the desired composition of weight gain, as the deposition of different types of tissue incurs different energy costs. For example, 9 kcal are stored in each gram of fat, compared with 4 kcal per gram of protein. Thus, a weight gain high in fat will require more energy to be stored than one high in protein. As previously mentioned, the ratio of energy to protein is important in determining the relative amount of lean tissue versus fat which is deposited. These considerations are not just theoretical, as the different diets used for preterm infants do result in variations in the composition of tissue deposited (Fig. 16.2). At present it is not known whether it is best to aim for a weight gain with 15% fat (as in the fetus) or nearer 40% fat (as in a term infant) and, unless this can be shown to have implications for future health, one might argue that it is academic. The results to date have been conflicting: DeGamarra et al. (1987) and Cooper et al. (1989) both found no differences in growth at 2 or 3 years of age in preterm infants who had shown wide differences in adiposity as infants. However, Agras et al. (1990) reported that greater adiposity at birth was a predictor of greater fatness at 6 years of age. In our own randomised trial of diet in preterm infants we found major differences in growth rates between diet groups during the neonatal period, but no differences in either growth (Fewtrell et al. 1999) or body fat mass or lean mass (Fewtrell et al. 2004) between diet groups at follow-up in childhood or early adult life (Fewtrell et al. 2009a).

All the components of the energy equation have been either measured or estimated in preterm infants, in order to calculate the optimal energy intake. The daily energy cost of activity is around 10 kcal/kg; the cost of thermogenesis, 10 kcal/kg/24 h (depending on thermal environment); and, at growth rates of 15 g/kg/24 h, the cost of tissue synthesis is about 10–20 kcal/kg (Reichman et al.

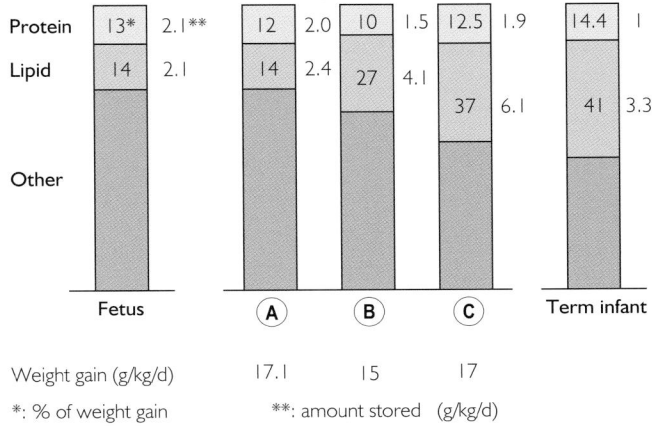

Weight gain (g/kg/d) 17.1 15 17

*: % of weight gain   **: amount stored (g/kg/d)

Fig. 16.2 Weight gain composition of the fetus (32–36 weeks) and of the term infant (0–4 months), compared with that of preterm infants fed different diets. (A) Protein-supplemented pooled human milk. (B) Pooled human milk. (C) Preterm formula. Figures represent the percentage of weight gain as protein or fat.

1982; Wharton 1987). The remaining component of energy expenditure, basal metabolic rate (BMR), cannot be measured in preterm infants as it requires at least a 12-hour fast. However, total energy expenditure, which includes all four of these components, has been measured over 5 days with both the doubly labelled water method and indirect calorimetry in four preterm infants (Roberts et al. 1986) growing at a mean rate of 15 g/kg/24 h, and was 58 kcal/kg/24 h (range 57–60). Other studies making measurements over 24-hour periods have produced similar figures, in the range 50–70 kcal/kg/24 h. If these figures are entered into equation (2):

$$E_{\text{expended}} = E_{\text{BMR}} + E_{\text{activity}} + E_{\text{synthesis}} + E_{\text{thermoreg}}$$
$$57{-}70 \qquad ? \qquad 10 \qquad 10{-}20 \qquad 10$$

a value for BMR of between 17 and 40 g/kg/24 h is obtained (Dauncey et al. 1977).

In order to estimate energy requirements, it is necessary to consider both the energy stored and energy excreted. In the study by Roberts et al. (1986), energy stored was 59 kcal/kg/24 h (which is about twice the figure for in utero energy deposition and substantially higher than ideal estimates for preterm infants, owing to the increased fat deposition seen postnatally). Energy losses in the stools have been estimated to be around 10–30 kcal/kg bodyweight, but massive losses may occur (well in excess of 50% of intake) in sick babies with an immature gut. If these figures are entered into equation (1):

$$E_{\text{intake}} = E_{\text{stored}} + E_{\text{expended}} + E_{\text{excreted}}$$
$$59 \qquad 57{-}70 \qquad 10{-}30$$

the required intake would be between 126 and 159 kcal/kg/24 h. This is slightly higher than the range recommended by ESPGHAN of 110–135 kcal/kg/24 h for healthy, growing preterm infants with adequate protein intake, and the 110–130 kcal/kg/24 h recommended by the recent international panel of experts for the stable preterm infant, although similar to their recommendations for ELBW infants (130–150 kcal/kg/24 h).

Water (see Ch. 18)

Water is a major nutrient (for review, see Wharton 1987). However, the quantity deposited in growth (around 10 ml/kg/24 h by preterm infants, for instance) is minute compared with water turnover. Clearly, in sick babies it would be impossible to allow nutrient intakes to vary in parallel with water requirement, and water must be treated as an 'independent variable'.

Nucleotides

There has been increasing interest over the last decade in the role of nucleotides in infant nutrition (Yu 2002). Breast milk contains at least 13 different nucleotides, accounting for up to 20% of non-protein nitrogen (Janas and Picciano 1982). Cow's milk has lower levels, accounting for about 5% of non-protein nitrogen, and a different nucleotide profile. Nucleotides are structural components of nucleic acids and therefore essential elements of the energy transfer system. They are assumed to play an important role in carbohydrate, lipid, protein and nucleic acid metabolism, and to act as modulators of many physiological processes, including immunity; it has been suggested that they are one of the anti-infective agents in breast milk, responsible for the lower levels of infection reported in breastfed infants. There is good evidence for the role of dietary nucleotides in animals (for example, enhancing T-cell function, and improving intestinal growth and maturation in weaning rats).

A variety of short-term effects have been reported for nucleotide-supplemented formulas in infants, including an alteration in the bowel flora following supplementation, with a predominance of lactobacilli as seen in the breastfed infant (Gil et al. 1986). There is also some evidence on the effect of nucleotide supplementation on clinical outcome in infants; a recent systematic review and meta-analysis examining the immune response to nucleotide-supplemented formulas identified 15 eligible randomised trials and concluded that infants fed nucleotide-supplemented formulas showed a better antibody response to immunisation; and fewer episodes of diarrhoea than infants fed unsupplemented formula or breast milk (Gutierrez-Castrellon et al. 2007). The EU Directive currently permits the addition of nucleotides to infant formulas for term infants up to a maximum concentration of 5 mg/100 kcal.

Macrominerals (Tables 16.1–16.3)

Sodium, potassium and chloride

Calculation of desirable intakes of sodium, potassium and chloride requires knowledge of renal function (see Ch. 18).

Preterm infants' requirements

Sodium

Major adjustments in body sodium occur in the neonatal period: massive renal losses of up to 10 mmol/kg/24 h or more can occur in the first week and may be independent of intake. It is impossible to predict accurately sodium needs in the early neonatal period, and in very small and sick infants, regardless of diet, plasma sodium should be monitored and hyponatraemia of <133 mmol/l, and certainly <130 mmol/l, should be corrected.

Preterm breast milk has a higher sodium content (>10–20 mmol/l during the early weeks of lactation) than mature donor milk (about <6 mmol/l). Hyponatraemia has been noted in preterm infants fed human milk; it is more severe in those fed donor milk. Intakes from donor milk and preterm milk, providing around 1 and 2 mmol/kg/24 h, respectively, during the first month, are often inadequate, and Aperia et al. (1982) have recommended 3 mmol/kg/24 h.

The high sodium content of modern preterm formulas is usually only required in the early neonatal period. After that, the excess sodium needs to be excreted. However, in a large randomised study (Lucas et al. 1988), preterm neonates fed on a formula providing 3.6 mmol/l did not have an increased risk of hypernatraemia, compared with those fed standard formula or breast milk (providing under half the sodium intake), and 13–16 years later did not show any elevation in blood pressure (Singhal et al. 2001).

Potassium and chloride

In general, human milk and the available adapted formulas provide adequate potassium and chloride to meet intrauterine accretion rates of 0.9 and 0.7 mmol/kg/24 h, respectively (Wharton 1987).

Calcium and phosphorus (Table 16.4)

Term infants

Calcium is less well absorbed from cow's milk than from human milk. However, in spite of the high levels of calcium and phosphorus in cow's milk, the relatively higher phosphorus intake has in the past resulted in hyperphosphataemia, hypocalcaemia with

Table 16.3 Trace metals

	PHYSIOLOGY	DEFICIENCY STATES
Iodine	Well absorbed, concentrated in thyroid gland, incorporated in thyroxine and tri-iodothyronine. Excess is excreted in urine	Endemic goitre in areas where human milk is deficient; soy formulas are iodine-deficient and are usually supplemented
Zinc	Present in a large number of metalloenzymes, including alkaline phosphatase and carbonic anhydrase. Required for insulin activity. Absorption partly by active transport. Bioavailability influenced by diet: poor absorption from diets of plant origin. Nadir in plasma zinc at around 2–3 months. Infants fed by total parenteral nutrition and those with gut disease are especially liable to clinical deficiency	Acrodermatitis syndrome. Delayed diagnosis if signs mistaken for 'nappy rash' of another aetiology NB may be inherited as a rare autosomal recessive disorder). Also mild deficiency in infancy, or later, may be associated with reduced growth, loss of appetite, impaired taste acuity and perhaps pica. Impaired immune responses, poor wound healing
Copper	Copper-containing enzymes include cytochrome oxidase, tyrosinase and uricase; required for iron utilisation, myelinisation and connective tissue formation. Absorption: stomach and small intestine. Stored in liver and muscle, attached to caeruloplasmin	See text
Manganese	Role: found in mitochondria, required for carbohydrate metabolism; actively absorbed in duodenum. Transport protein: transmanganin, a specific β-globulin. Excretion is largely biliary	No deficiency state described in human infants
Chromium	Role: potentiates insulin-induced glucose uptake. Poorly absorbed. Transported by transferring. Body stores: low	In one study, diabetic glucose tolerance tests were corrected in infants with kwashiorkor
Fluoride	Enters bone and teeth, increasing their hardness. Supplementation is not recommended currently during the first 6 months	Dental caries. Excess: fluorosis, including rotting of teeth
Molybdenum	Present in xanthine oxidase. Active transfer across the placenta	No deficiency disease clearly recognised in human infants
Selenium	Role: antioxidant – cofactor for vitamin E	Deficiency not defined in neonates but described in children and adults living in the Keshan province of China: generalised myopathy with cardiac failure and haemolytic anaemia. Possibly occurs in preterm infants on unsupplemented long-term parenteral nutrition
Cobalt	Cobalt is a component of vitamin B_{12} and may not be needed independently of B_{12} requirement	

convulsions (see below), and other complications such as dental hypoplasia (Stimmler et al. 1973). Moreover, the high phosphorus content in unmodified cow's milk may also induce hypomagnesaemia, and, in some cases of neonatal tetany, convulsions can only be alleviated by administration of magnesium. Current recommendations for calcium and phosphorus are shown in Table 16.1.

Preterm infants' requirements

Considerable attention has been focused on the calcium and phosphorus requirements of LBW infants (Wharton 1987) stimulated by the high incidence of metabolic bone disease seen in this population (see Chapter 34 part 4).

Magnesium

The recommended intake for term infants is given in Table 16.1, and the physiology outlined in Table 16.3. Body magnesium content, largely in bone, rises rapidly in the third trimester, so that

preterm infants are born with low reserves. In preterm infants, net magnesium absorption in the first week is about 50% and is largely independent of vitamin D. Magnesium deficiency may impair calcium homoeostasis. Atkinson et al. (1983) showed that infants fed on preterm milk (2.5–3.0 mg magnesium per 100 ml) failed to retain this element at intrauterine accretion rates, and showed evidence of falling reserves; in contrast, a formula-fed group receiving two to three times more magnesium retained it at a somewhat greater rate than in utero. In infants fed human milk, dietary supplementation with phosphorus improves magnesium retention by reducing urine losses.

Iron

Term infants

Iron stores at birth are influenced by gestation, birthweight and the extent of the placental transfusion at delivery. Healthy breastfed infants absorb iron well from human milk and usually maintain

Table 16.4 Digestion, physiological role and deficiency states of calcium, phosphorus and magnesium

	DIGESTION	PHYSIOLOGICAL ROLE	DEFICIENCY STATES
Calcium	Absorption by both passive and active transport: Ca, Mg-ATPase facilitates uptake into the mucosal cells, where a calcium-binding protein is induced by vitamin D. 20–60% retention, according to diet (better with human milk) but increased by vitamin D and parathormone and reduced by complexing with dietary fat, phosphate and phytates. Part bound, e.g. to protein, part free in plasma	Bones are major stores. Also required for cell membrane function, neuromuscular activity, clotting and a wide variety of cellular functions	Tetany, bone demineralisation, arrhythmias, paralytic ileus, fits
Phosphorus	70–95% absorption, increased by vitamin D, reduced by insoluble intraluminal complex formation, e.g. with phytate or if excessive calcium salts added. Commonly elevated in plasma in the neonatal period in cow's milk formula-fed term infants; nadir in preterm infants at 1–2 weeks	Bone mineralisation, ATP, DNA, RNA, phospholipids and many other biological roles	Rickets is rare in full-term newborns. Phosphate deficiency syndrome may arise, particularly in infants fed by total parenteral nutrition: listlessness, poor feeding, rapid shallow breathing, muscle weakness, impaired oxygen release from haemoglobin, bone disease, nephrocalcinosis
Magnesium	Some transport mechanisms may be shared with calcium: absorption increased by vitamin D and parathormone and decreased by steatorrhoea and phytates. High fetal plasma levels, which may fall after birth	Stored in bone. Important intracellular cation, muscle contraction, cofactor for carbohydrate, protein and energy metabolism	Weakness, poor feeding, failure to thrive, paralytic ileus, calcium-resistant tetany, fits, apnoea

normal iron stores during the first 4–6 months. However, the bioavailability of iron in cow's milk (especially) and cow's milk formulas is much less than in human milk. The EC Directive (European Commission 2006) recommended that formulas used from birth should, if iron is added, contain 0.18–0.9 mg/100 ml (Table 16.1).

Preterm infants' requirements

A 1.0-kg fetus contains 64 mg iron (Widdowson and Dickerson 1964), and this increases subsequently in utero at a rate of 1.8 mg/kg/24 h. About 25% of iron is stored in the liver as ferritin, and most of the rest is present in haemoglobin. After birth, therefore, a 1.0-kg infant only has sufficient iron to synthesise about 18.0 g haemoglobin (3.4 mg iron per gram haemoglobin), and since the iron content of human milk is 40 μg per 100 ml or less (providing 80 μg/kg/24 h fed at 200 ml/kg/24 h), preterm infants fed human milk will eventually develop an iron-deficiency anaemia without supplementation.

Iron stores usually remain adequate during the first 6–8 weeks, and iron supplementation at this stage has no influence on anaemia of prematurity. By around 12 weeks, iron stores become depleted in unsupplemented infants, and iron-deficiency anaemia develops. Intakes of 2.0–3.0 mg/kg/24 h have been shown by several groups to prevent such anaemia. However, variations in local practice regarding blood sampling, transfusion and use of erythropoietin treatment will influence iron requirements.

It is recommended that preterm infants receive a supplement of 2–3 mg/kg/24 h of iron, starting between 2 and 6 weeks of age (2–4 weeks in ELBW infants) and continuing until 12 months, or until

full mixed feeding provides an adequate iron intake. However, this should be adjusted according to blood transfusions and the use of erythropoietin in individual infants. A trial of high (20.7 mg/l) versus normal (13.4 mg/l) iron formulas in preterm infants found no difference in weight gain or development at 12 months post-term; however, the higher iron group had higher glutathione peroxidase concentrations, lower plasma zinc and copper levels and more respiratory tract infections, suggesting possible adverse effects from the higher intake (Friel et al. 2001).

Recombinant human erythropoietin (r-HuEPO) is occasionally used in preterm infants to reduce the requirement for blood transfusion. Studies have demonstrated (Shannon 1995) that infants treated with r-HuEPO require higher amounts of iron – up to 6 mg/kg/24 h – and that this should be initiated at the same time as the r-HuEPO.

Trace metals

Summaries of the physiological roles and the consequences of deficiency are shown in Table 16.3, and recommended intakes for term infants in Table 16.1.

Zinc

Zinc has been found in over 70 metalloproteins, mostly enzymes, including both DNA and RNA polymerase; it plays a critical role in cell replication and growth (Wharton 1987).

Zinc accumulates in the fetus during the last trimester at around 250 μg/kg/24 h. The amount of zinc provided by 200 ml of human milk per kilogram per day falls from 1650 µg on the first day of lactation to 160 µg after 4 months. Therefore, human milk collected during the early (but not later) months of lactation theoretically provides enough zinc to meet in utero accretion rates. Zinc in banked donor milk should be adequate, although redistribution and alterations in the zinc-binding pattern during processing in human milk banks with an increase in the fat fraction and decrease in the whey fraction might reduce zinc bioavailability. Dauncey et al. (1977) found that preterm infants fed human milk did not achieve positive zinc balance until after 40 days of age.

Zinc deficiency has been described as a late sequel (2–4 months) of preterm birth (Reifen and Zlotkin 1993). These infants develop a syndrome very similar to acrodermatitis enteropathica, with growth arrest, irritability, anorexia, alopecia, diarrhoea, vesiculopustular lesions of the hands and feet, and the characteristic perioral, facial and perineal dermatitis; plasma zinc levels, though not necessarily helpful, are usually <35 µg/100 ml (5.4 mmol/l) (normal: 70 µg/100 ml). Infants respond rapidly to oral zinc sulphate (providing 1.0–3.5 mg zinc per day).

The EC Directive guidelines recommend a zinc concentration of 300–1060 µg/100 ml formula for term infants, and the ESPGHAN (1987) Committee on Nutrition recommended a daily intake of 1.1–2.0 mg/kg for preterm infants. The value of zinc supplementation for the long-term growth and development of infants born preterm or SGA requires further study.

Copper

Copper accumulates in the fetus during the last trimester at about 50 µg/kg/24 h; similar to iron and zinc, there is a hepatic store of copper at birth which is utilised during early infancy. The copper content of human milk falls from 600 µg/l during the first week of lactation to 220 µg/l by 5 months, but there is no evidence that human milk-fed infants require additional copper.

Several cases of copper deficiency have been described in infants born prematurely and fed on cow's milk-based formulas or copper-free parenteral nutrition solutions. The features of copper deficiency include psychomotor retardation, hypotonia, pallor and hypopigmentation, hepatosplenomegaly, X-ray changes of osteoporosis, blurring and cupping of metaphyses with subperiosteal new bone formation and fractures, and sideroblastic anaemia resistant to iron therapy. Neutropenia may also be present and the bone marrow shows vacuolated erythroid and myeloid cells, with iron deposition in the vacuoles. Several of these features are liable to develop when plasma copper falls below 20 mg/100 ml and caeruloplasmin below 5 mg/100 ml. Treatment with copper 0.6–0.8 mg/kg/24 h, given as 1% copper sulphate solution, is effective. A daily copper intake of 100–132 µg/kg is recommended for preterm infants.

Iodine

Iodine is found almost entirely in the thyroid, where it is incorporated into thyroglobulin and thyroid hormones. It is possible that a syndrome of transient hypothyroidism, seen in preterm infants, could be due to lack of iodine in iodine-deficient areas. The iodine content of breast milk is affected by maternal diet but is usually sufficient. The EC Directive guidelines suggest a minimum of 6.4 µg per 100 ml of formula.

Other trace minerals

Manganese, selenium, chromium and molybdenum are all essential elements, but no definite deficiency states have been described in preterm infants fed human milk or cow's milk-based formulas (Wharton 1987); quantitative recommendations cannot be made on strong grounds. Manganese is found in very large unphysiological quantities in some formulas (especially soy-based ones), with values up to 100–1000 times those in human milk. It is not known whether these intakes are toxic, but there seems no basis for giving more than 5 µg per 100 ml of formula (human milk contains around 0.5–2.5 µg/100 ml).

Aluminium

Aluminium is not a nutrient – it has not been found in any metalloprotein, yet it has been added to drinking water (as a clarifying agent); it contaminates artificial formulas, especially soy formulas, which may contain 100 times the aluminium level of breast milk. However, the main source of exposure for infants, particularly those who are preterm, is aluminium contamination of some components of intravenous feeding solutions, notably calcium and phosphate salts, which have a high affinity for aluminium and encourage leaching from glass containers. A randomised trial in 227 preterm infants who received standard versus specially sourced low-aluminium parenteral nutrition solutions showed significant deficits in neurodevelopment at 18 months post-term of the order of a one developmental quotient point loss for each day of standard TPN received (Bishop et al. 1997). Follow-up of this cohort at age 13–15 years suggested that higher neonatal exposure to aluminium was also associated with lower bone mass (Fewtrell et al. 2009b).

It has been suggested that aluminium intake should be <5 µg/kg/day. However, Poole et al. (2008) calculated aluminium intakes of patients and found that even with the least contaminated currently available solutions it is impossible to meet the US Food and Drug Administration target of <5 µg/kg/day in patients under 50 kg; the situation is worst for those weighing <3 kg. Nevertheless, preterm and other sick infants clearly need parenteral nutrition for survival and to ensure optimal growth and development, and the risks of withholding parenteral nutrition would outweigh any possible adverse effects from aluminium exposure.

Vitamins

Clinical vitamin deficiency is rare in the neonatal period. Vitamin deficiency can occur in certain circumstances; these include maternal vitamin depletion, with reduced placental transport and low vitamin concentrations in breast milk, unsupplemented formulas, TPN, the use of unconventional non-milk-based diets, parasitic infestation, neonatal gut and biliary disease, and prematurity.

Optimal intake levels for many vitamins have not been determined in human infants. Broadly, vitamin intakes from breast milk have been taken as a guide (Table 16.1), but excess supplementation in formulas is usually employed in order to compensate for losses during preparation and storage and lower bioavailability. There is no clear evidence showing detrimental effects of excess vitamin supplementation, except for vitamins A and D, though it has been suggested that excessive vitamin E intake may interfere with wound healing and iron status.

The physiological roles of vitamins and clinical consequences of deficiency are summarised in Table 16.5.

Term infants

Current recommended levels for formula-fed infants are shown in Table 16.1.

Table 16.5 Vitamins: physiology and diseases caused by deficiency (or excess)

	PHYSIOLOGY	DEFICIENCY (OR EXCESS)
Vitamin A	Retinyl esters are the main contributor to vitamin A activity in milk, though both cow's and human milk contain the retinal precursor beta-carotene. Partly emulsified by bile salts, partly hydrolysed by lipase and re-esterified to retinyl palmitate in gut mucosa. One-sixth of dietary carotene is converted into active vitamin A. Stored in liver. Secreted by liver into the bloodstream in association with retinal-binding protein: secretion of vitamin A is tightly regulated like that of a hormone. Required for the synthesis of rhodopsin and other retinal pigments: important for the development of epithelial cells (and therefore the maintenance of epithelial membranes). Degraded by light	Xerophthalmia, susceptibility to infection, keratinisation of mucous membranes, blindness. Excess, e.g. 18 000 IU/day or above: raised intracranial pressure, dry skin, loss of hair, brittle bones, irritability
Vitamin E	Placental transfer low. Liver stores may be low. Iron may interfere with absorption and activity. Polyunsaturated fatty acids increase E requirement. Role: antioxidant, prevents oxidation of unsaturated fats thereby increasing stability of cell membranes	Clinical disease states poorly defined. Reduces postnatal red cell haemolysis
Vitamin D	Absorptive mechanisms not fully investigated in human infant: bile salts may be required – absorbed into lymphatic system. Stored in adipose tissue and muscle with small amounts in skin and liver. Sunlight-induced synthesis in the skin from 7-dehydrocholesterol will be minimal in many neonates; active metabolites are 25- and 1,25-hydroxyvitamin D (25-OHD and 1,25-$(OH)_2$D): these act as steroid hormones. Principal role: the enhancement of calcium and phosphate absorption from gut and renal conservation of these elements of bones and teeth of over 4000 IU/day	Rickets, tetany. Maternal vitamin D deficiency may rarely result in neonatal rickets. Very small amounts of vitamin D in breast milk. Maternal insufficiency increasingly recognised, especially in darker-skinned individuals and groups who cover themselves for religious reasons – increased risk of deficiency in their infants with breastfeeding if no supplement given. Also important for the normal mineralisation. Excess: intakes may result in hypercalcaemia. At intakes greater than 10 000 IU/kg per day: ectopic calcification, failure to thrive
Vitamin K	Emulsified by bile salts. Synthesis by gut flora is much debated. Stores in liver are relatively small. Maternal deficiency predisposes to neonatal deficiency. Role: manufacture of clotting factors (including II, VII, IX and X) and bone metabolism	Haemorrhagic disease of newborn. Excess: haemolytic anaemia can be caused by the water-soluble analogue
Thiamine (B_1)	Role: coenzyme in many enzyme systems: pathways involving acetyl coenzyme A	Anorexia, irritability, fatigue, oedema, heart failure, constipation, peripheral neuropathy
Riboflavin (B_2)	Component of flavoenzymes: involved in electron transport processes, e.g. in energy metabolism, fatty acid oxidation. Degraded by light	Cheilosis, angular stomatitis, impaired fatty acid oxidation and iron economy
Niacin	Part of NAD–NADP system of Krebs cycle; involved in protein and fat synthesis. Dietary tryptophan will supply niacin: 60 mg tryptophan = 1 mg niacin	Diarrhoea, dermatitis, neurological disturbance
Pyridoxine (B_6)	Role: modification of functional groups, especially in amino acid metabolism (decarboxylation, transamination, oxidation, desulphurylation)	Convulsion, dermatitis, weakness, anaemia
Vitamin B_{12}	Coenzyme for methionine synthesis and indirectly for DNA synthesis, folic acid metabolism, conversion of methylmalonic to succinic acid	Pernicious anaemia, central nervous system damage
Folic acid	Role: enzyme systems taking part in one-carbon transfers in DNA, RNA, methionine and serine synthesis, needed for histidine utilisation. Synthesised by gut flora	Megaloblastic anaemia, retarded growth, gastrointestinal disturbance
Pantothenic acid	Roles: part of coenzyme A system, involved in energy and fat metabolism. Synthesised by gut flora	No dietary deficiency state described in humans
Biotin	Role: carboxylation reactions, especially concerned with fatty acid synthesis. Produced by gut flora	Possibly skin rashes
Vitamin C	Water-soluble. Absorbed in upper intestine. Not stored: excess excreted in urine. Maternal deficiency may result in neonatal deficiency. Intake from unsupplemented pasteurised cow's milk is minimal. Role: involved in collagen synthesis and in several aspects of amino acid metabolism: protects against hypertyrosinaemia and hyperphenylalaninaemia in newborn period; promotes conversion of folic acid to folinic acid, catecholamine synthesis, carnitine synthesis, iron absorption	Biochemical deficiency may arise in newborn period – overt scurvy rare below 3 months of age

Preterm infants' requirements (Table 16.2)

Preterm infants may have special needs for some vitamins because:

- they are born with low body stores, especially of the fat-soluble vitamins which normally accumulate during the third trimester
- they may have reduced absorptive capacities for some vitamins (e.g. vitamin E)
- they might benefit from 'pharmacological doses' of certain vitamins, e.g. vitamin E.

A brief account follows, summarising information about vitamins of particular importance (Wharton 1987; Tsang et al. 2005).

Vitamin A

Vitamin A is required for the synthesis of retinal pigments and for the development and maintenance of epithelial membranes. The active form, retinol, is transported in plasma, bound to retinol-binding protein (RBP). The commonly used unit for vitamin A is μg retinol equivalent (μg RE: 1 μg RE = 3.33 IU vitamin A). Synthesis of RBP usually occurs late in gestation, and plasma retinol and RBP concentrations are lower in preterm than in term infants (Shenai et al. 1981). RBP also has a lower level of saturation in premature neonates. These data suggest that preterm infants have low body stores of vitamin A and are therefore at risk of deficiency. Low vitamin A status has been associated with an increased risk of chronic lung disease.

There is insufficient vitamin A in human milk to support the needs of the preterm infant (approximately 120–180 μg RE/l) and supplementation of human milk-fed preterm infants seems wise (see below). Vitamin A can be obtained from the diet in two forms: preformed vitamin A (largely retinol) and carotenoids (chiefly β-carotene). Although β-carotene is potentially a good, non-toxic source of vitamin A, the efficacy of retinol synthesis in preterm infants is uncertain and it is recommended that the vitamin A requirement is met by providing preformed vitamin A. The recommended intake is 400–1000 μg RE/kg/day or 1330–3330 IU vitamin A/kg/day. Vitamin A is light-degraded: 70% can be lost from human milk during a 3-hour enteral infusion into an infant under phototherapy lighting. Care must be taken to ensure that the principal source of vitamin A given to preterm infants is not light-exposed.

Several studies have been performed to assess whether large doses of vitamin A can reduce the incidence of chronic lung disease (see Chapter 27 part 3). Meta-analysis of eight eligible studies suggested that regular doses of vitamin A either intramuscularly (six studies) or orally (two studies) were associated with a reduction in death or oxygen requirement at 1 month and a reduction in oxygen requirement in survivors at 36 weeks' gestation, although the latter outcome was confined to infants with birthweight <1000 g. Meta-analysis of three studies with data on retinopathy of prematurity suggested a trend towards reduced incidence in vitamin A-supplemented infants (Darlow and Graham 2007). A single study reported no difference in neurodevelopmental outcome at 18–22 months postterm. The authors suggested that whether clinicians choose to use repeated intramuscular injections of vitamin A, which are painful, should perhaps depend on the incidence of chronic lung disease in their unit, and recommended that the benefits, safety and acceptability of delivering vitamin A in an intravenous emulsion compared with repeated intramuscular injections should be assessed in future.

Vitamin D

The term 'vitamin D' is often used to refer to both vitamin D_2, originating from the plant sterol ergosterol, and vitamin D_3, the natural vitamin synthesised in the skin from 7-dehydrocholesterol. Vitamin D_2 (or D_3) is converted to 25-hydroxyvitamin D (25-OHD, calcidiol) in the liver, and thence into the active metabolite 1,25-dihydroxyvitamin D (1,25-$(OH)_2$D, calcitriol) in the kidney. A major function of 1,25-$(OH)_2$D is to increase calcium and phosphorus absorption from the intestine, but it also conserves these two elements by its action on the kidney.

Preterm infants may have greater requirements for vitamin D than infants born at term; they have lower stores at birth and greater demands for skeletal mineralisation, and although the vitamin D pathway is intact, it may not be fully developed at very low gestation. Requirements will be greater still where maternal vitamin D status is suboptimal – an increasingly recognised scenario. The dose normally recommended for full-term infants, 400 IU/day, is probably well in excess of requirements for normal babies. However, in preterm infants, doses of up to 800–1000 IU/day have been recommended, with the aim of achieving circulating 25-OH vitamin D values >80 nmol/l (von Kries et al. 1999). These doses have been shown to increase calcium absorption; however it is important to remember that vitamin D is no substitute for calcium and phosphorus supplementation in the prevention of bone disease (see Chapter 34 part 4). The use of 1,25-OHD rather than vitamin D may seem logical, as in very small preterm infants absorption of vitamin D may be impaired by a small bile salt pool size and fat malabsorption. Nevertheless, the use of such active metabolites of vitamin D, and especially the more potent ones (for example, 1a-OHD), is experimental and potentially dangerous.

Vitamin E

Increased intakes of vitamin E, which is a powerful antioxidant, may be required to prevent haemolytic anaemia in preterm infants, especially those receiving a diet rich in PUFA or iron. (Polyunsaturated lipids in cell membranes are liable to oxidative damage, which may be enhanced by iron.) There has been much interest in the use of pharmacological doses of vitamin E in preterm infants, but a review including 26 randomised studies suggested that supplementation in preterm infants reduced the risk of intracranial haemorrhage but increased the risk of sepsis. In VLBW infants, vitamin E increased the risk of sepsis, and reduced the risk of severe retinopathy and blindness among those examined. The authors concluded that evidence does not support the routine use of vitamin E supplementation by the intravenous route at high doses or aiming at serum tocopherol levels greater than 3.5 mg/dl (Brion et al. 2003).

Human milk contains adequate vitamin E in relation to its PUFA content. The recommended intake for preterm infants is 2.2–11 mg α-TE/kg/day (1 mg α-TE = 1.49 IU), but this should be adapted in relation to the amount of PUFA in the diet.

Vitamin K

Despite recent controversy over the optimum route for administration and the dose required, vitamin K should be given routinely to all newborn babies as a prophylaxis against vitamin K-deficiency bleeding (VKDB). When given orally to breastfed infants, repeat doses are required to avoid the risk of intracranial bleeding from late VKDB. A Danish group reported that 12-weekly oral doses of 1 mg are completely effective, even in infants with liver disease (Norgaard-Hansen and Ebbesen 1996). However, von Kries et al. (1999) reported that not all cases of late-onset VKDB were prevented by three doses of oral vitamin K. The situation in sick term or preterm babies is not controversial: all such infants should receive 0.5–1.0 mg of vitamin K parenterally on the first day.

Folic acid

Folic acid dosages for preterm infants vary considerably. In a large randomised study, Stevens et al. (1979) were unable to demonstrate differences in growth between LBW infants given either a supplement of 100 μg of folic acid per day (from 3 weeks to 12 months) or a formula containing only 3.5 μg folic acid per 100 ml (similar to human milk), and no infant became anaemic. More recently, however, Worthington-White et al. (1994) showed that formula-fed preterm infants who received supplemental folate for the first 6 months (100 μg/24 h) had higher serum folate concentrations and a significantly reduced fall in haemoglobin over the study period. Haiden et al. (2006a) randomised 64 preterm infants (birthweight 801–1300 g) receiving erythropoietin and iron treatment to treatment with either vitamin B_{12} and folate (100 μg/kg/day) or a lower dose of folate (60 μg/kg/day). Infants in the treatment group showed enhanced erythropoeisis with a reduced fall in haemoglobin. In a second study, ELBW infants (birthweight <800 g) randomised to combined therapy with erythropoietin, iron, folate and vitamin B_{12} had a significantly lower requirement for transfusion than control infants (Haiden et al. 2006b). An intake of at least 100 μg folate/24 h seems prudent for all LBW infants until 40 weeks' postconceptional age.

Vitamin C and pyridoxal phosphate (B₆)

Vitamin C has been shown to prevent hypertyrosinaemia and hyperphenylalaninaemia in LBW infants, especially those on high protein intakes. In view of this and the low vitamin C levels of unsupplemented preterm infants, a supplement is recommended (see below).

Supplementary B_6 might also be expected to improve protein utilisation, in view of its role as a cofactor in amino acid metabolic pathways; B_6 intake should be related to protein intake.

Riboflavin (B₂)

Most human milk-fed preterm infants develop biochemical evidence of riboflavin deficiency if they have received no supplement after the first week (Lucas and Bates 1984). This problem is compounded by the massive destruction of riboflavin by light when milk is handled in neonatal units. Early biochemical riboflavin deficiency has been shown to be prevented using a preterm formula containing 180 μg riboflavin per 100 ml, or by using a riboflavin-containing multivitamin preparation (Lucas et al. 1987). The recommended intake for preterm infants is 200–400 μg/kg/day.

References

Agostoni, C., Buonocore, G., Carnielli, V.P., et al., 2010. Enteral nutrient supply for preterm infants: Commentary from the European Society of Paediatric Gastroenterology, Hepatology and Nutrition Committee on Nutrition. J Paediatr Gastrol Nutr 50, 85–91.

Agras, W.S., Kraemer, H.C., Berkowitz, R.I., et al., 1990. Influence of early feeding style on adiposity at 6 years of age. Journal of Pediatrics 116, 805–809.

Aperia, A., Broberger, O., Zetterstrom, R., 1982. Implications of limitation of renal function for the nutrition of low birthweight infants. Acta Paediatrica Scandinavica Supplement 296, 49–52.

Atkinson, S.A., Radde, I.C., Anderson, G.H., 1983. Macromineral balances in premature infants fed their own mother's milk or formula. Journal of Pediatrics 102, 96–106.

Baker, H., Frank, O., Thompson, A.D., et al., 1975. Vitamin profile of 174 mothers and newborn at parturition. American Journal of Clinical Nutrition 28, 59–65.

Bayes, R., Campoy, C., Goicoechea, A., et al., 2001. Role of intrapartum hypoxia in carnitine nutritional status in the early neonatal period. Early Human Development 65, S103–S110.

Berseth, C.L., Nordyke, C., 1993. Enteral nutrients promote postnatal maturation of intestinal motor activity in preterm infants. American Journal of Physiology 264, 1046–1051.

Bishop, N.J., Morley, R., Day, J.P., et al., 1997. Aluminium neurotoxicity in preterm infants receiving intravenous-feeding solutions. New England Journal of Medicine 336, 1557–1561.

Blondheim, O., Abbasi, S., Fox, W.W., et al., 1993. Effect of enteral gavage feeding rate on pulmonary functions of very low birth weight infants. Journal of Pediatrics 122, 751–755.

Boehm, G., Muller, D.M., Beyreiss, K., et al., 1988. Evidence for functional immaturity of the ornithine-urea cycle in very-low-birth-weight infants. Biology of the Neonate 54, 121–125.

Bombell, S., McGuire, W., 2009. Early trophic feeding for very low birth weight infants. Cochrane Database of Systematic Reviews (3), CD000504.

Brion, L.P., Bell, E.F., Raghuveer, T.S., 2003. Vitamin E supplementation for prevention of morbidity and mortality in preterminfants. Cochrane Database of Systematic Reviews (4), CD003665.

Brooke, O.G., Kinzey, J.M., 1985. High energy feeding in small for gestation neonates. Archives of Disease in Childhood 60, 42–46.

Brooke, O.G., Wood, C., Barley, J., 1982. Energy balance, nitrogen balance and growth in preterm infants fed expressed breast milk, a premature infant formula and two low-solute adapted formulae. Archives of Disease in Childhood 57, 898–904.

Carlson, S.E., Rhodes, P.G., Ferguson, M.G., 1986. Docosahexaenoic acid status of preterm infants at birth and following feeding with milk or formula. American Journal of Clinical Nutrition 44, 798–804.

Clandinin, M.T., Chappell, J.E., Leong, S., et al., 1980. Extrauterine fatty acid accretion in infant brain: implications for fatty acid requirements. Early Human Development 4, 131–138.

Clandinin, M.T., Chappell, J.E., Heim, T., et al., 1981. Fatty acid utilization in perinatal de novo synthesis of tissues. Early Human Development 5, 355–366.

Coombs, R.C., Morgan, M.E., Durbin, G.M., et al., 1992. Doppler assessment of human neonatal gut blood flow velocities: postnatal adaptation and response to feeds. Journal of Pediatric Gastroenterology and Nutrition 15, 6–12.

Cooper, P.A., Rothberg, A., Davies, V.A., et al., 1989. Three-year growth and developmental follow-up of very low birth weight infants fed own mother's milk, a premature formula, or one of two standard formulas. Journal of Paediatric Gastroenterology and Nutrition 8, 348–354.

Darlow, B.A., Graham, P.J., 2007. Vitamin A supplementation to prevent mortality and short and long-term morbidity in very low birth weight infants (Cochrane Review). Cochrane Database of Systematic Reviews (4), CD000501.

Dauncey, M.J., Shaw, J.C., Urman, J., 1977. The absorption and retention of magnesium, zinc and copper by low birthweight infants fed pasteurized human breast milk. Pediatric Research 11, 1033–1039.

Davidson, M., Levine, S., Bauer, C., et al., 1967. Feeding studies in low birthweight infants. Journal of Pediatrics 70, 695–713.

De Gamarra, M.E., Schutz, Y., Catzeflis, C., et al., 1987. Composition of weight gain during the neonatal period and longitudinal growth follow-up in premature babies. Biology of the Neonate 52, 181–187.

Ehrenkranz, R.A., Dusick, A.M., Vohr, B.R., et al., 2006. Growth in the neonatal intensive care unit influences neurodevelopmental and growth outcomes of extremely low birthweight infants. Pediatrics 117, 1253–1261.

Embleton, N., Pang, N., Cooke, R.J., 2001. Postnatal malnutrition and growth retardation: An inevitable consequence of current recommendations in preterm infants? Pediatrics 107, 270–273.

ESPGHAN. 1987. Nutrition and feeding of preterm infants. Committee on Nutrition of the Preterm Infant, European Society of Paediatric Gastroenterology and Nutrition. Acta Paediatrica Scandinavica Supplement 336, 1–14.

European Commission. 2006. Commission Directive 2006/141/EC of 22 December 2006 on infant formula and follow-on formulae. Official Journal of the European Union. Available online at: http://eur-lex.europa.eu/LexUriServ/LexUriServ.do?uri=OJ:L:2006:401:0001:0033:EN:PDF.

Fang, S., Kempley, S.T., Gamsu, H.R., 2001. Prediction of early tolerance to enteral feeding in preterm infants by measurement of superior mesenteric artery blood flow velocity. Archives of Disease in Childhood. Fetal and Neonatal Edition 85, F42–F45.

Farquharson, J., Cockburn, F., Patrick, W.A., et al., 1992. Infant cerebral cortex phospholipid fatty acid composition and diet. Lancet 340, 810–813.

Farquharson, J., Jamieson, E.C., Abbasi, K.A., et al., 1995. Effect of diet on the fatty acid composition of the major phospholipids of infant cerebral cortex. Archives of Disease in Childhood 72, 198–203.

Fewtrell, M.S., Prentice, A., Jones, S.C., et al., 1999. Bone mineralization and turnover in preterm infants at 8–12 years of age: the effect of early diet. Journal of Bone and Mineral Research 14, 810–820.

Fewtrell, M.S., Lucas, A., Cole, T.J., et al., 2004. Prematurity and reduced body fatness at 8–12y of age. American Journal of Clinical Nutrition 80, 436–440.

Fewtrell, M.S., Williams, J.E., Singhal, A., et al., 2009a. Early diet and peak bone mass: 20 year follow-up of a randomized trial of early diet in infants born preterm. Bone 45, 142–149.

Fewtrell, M.S., Bishop, N.J., Edmonds, C.J., et al., 2009b. Aluminum exposure from intravenous feeding solutions and later bone health: 15-year follow-up of a randomized trial of preterm infants. Pediatrics 124, 1372–1379.

Fomon, S.J., Kaschke, F., Ziegler, E.E., et al., 1982. Body composition of reference children from birth to age 10 years. American Journal of Clinical Nutrition 35, 1169–1175.

Friel, J.K., Andrews, W.I., Aziz, K., et al., 2001. A randomized trial of two levels of iron supplementation and developmental outcome in low birth weight infants. Journal of Pediatrics 139, 254–260.

Friis-Hansen, B., 1982. Body water metabolism in early infancy. Acta Paediatrica Scandinavica Supplement 296, 44–48.

Gaull, G.E., Rassin, D.K., Raiha, N.C.R., et al., 1977. Milk protein quantity and quality in low-birth-infants. III. Effects on sulfur amino acids in plasma and urine. Journal of Pediatrics 90, 348–355.

Gil, A., Corral, E., Martinez, A., et al., 1986. Effects of the addition of dietary nucleotides to an adapted milk formula on the microbial pattern of faeces in term newborn infants. Journal of Clinical Nutrition and Gastroenterology 1, 127–131.

Goldman, H.I., Goldman, J.S., Kaufman, I., 1974. Late effects of early dietary protein intake on low birthweight infants. Journal of Pediatrics 84, 764–769.

Gordon, H., Levine, S., McNamara, H., 1947. Feeding of premature infants. American Journal of Diseases of Children 73, 442–452.

Greengard, O., 1977. Enzymic differentiation of human liver: comparison with the rat model. Pediatric Research 11, 669–676.

Gutierrez-Castrellon, P., Mora-Magana, I., Diaz-Garcia, L., et al., 2007. Immune response to nucleotide-supplemented infant formulae: systematic review and meta-analysis. Br J Nutr 98, S64–S67.

Haiden, N., Klebermass, K., Cardona, F., et al., 2006a. A randomized, controlled trial of the effects of adding vitamin B12 and folate to erythropoietin for the treatment of anemia of prematurity. Pediatrics 118, 180–188.

Haiden, N., Schwindt, J., Cardona, F., et al., 2006b. A randomized, controlled trial of erythropoietin, iron, folate and vitamin B12 on the transfusion requirements of extremely low birth weight infants. Pediatrics 118, 2004–2013.

Hamosh, M., 1996. Digestion in the newborn. Clinics in Perinatology 23, 191–210.

Heird, W.C., 1977. Effects of total parenteral alimentation on intestinal function. In: Sunshine, P. (Ed.), Gastrointestinal Function and Neonatal Nutrition. Ross Laboratories, Columbus, OH, p. 16.

Howlett, A., Ohlsson, A., 2003. Inositol for respiratory distress syndrome in preterm infants. Cochrane Database of Systematic Reviews (4), CD000366.

Imaki, H., Jacobson, S.G., Kemp, C.M., et al., 1993. Retinal morphology and visual pigment levels in 6- and 12-month-old rhesus monkeys fed a taurine-free human infant formula. Journal of Neuroscience Research 36, 290–304.

Isaacs, E.B., Gadian, D.G., Sabatini, S., et al., 2008. The effect of early human diet on caudate volumes and IQ. Pediatr Res 63, 308–314.

Janas, L.M., Picciano, M.F., 1982. The nucleotide profile of human milk. Pediatric Research 16, 659–662.

Johnson, L.R., Copeland, E., Dudrick, S.J., et al., 1975. Structural and hormonal alterations in the gastrointestinal tract of parenterally fed rats. Gastroenterology 68, 1177–1183.

Kashyap, S., Schultze, K., Forsyth, M., et al., 1988. Growth, nutrient retention, and metabolic response in low birth weight infants fed varying intakes of protein and energy. J Pediatr 113, 713–721.

Kennedy, K., Fewtrell, M.S., Morley, R., et al., 1999. Double-blind randomised trial of a synthetic triglyceride (betapol) in formula fed term infants: effects on stool biochemistry, stool characteristics and bone mineralisation. American Journal of Clinical Nutrition 70, 920–927.

Kien, C.L., 1996. Digestion, absorption and fermentation of carbohydrates in the newborn. Clinics in Perinatology 23, 211–228.

Klenoff-Brumberg, H.L., Genen, L.H., 2003. High versus low medium chain triglyceride content of formula for promoting short term growth of preterm infants. Cochrane Database Syst Rev (1), CD002777.

Koletzko, B., von Kries, R., Closa, R., et al., 2009. Lower protein in infant formula is associated with lower weight up to age 2 y: a randomized clinical trial. Am J Clin Nutr 89, 1836–1845.

Koo, W.W., Hammami, M., Margeson, D.P., et al., 2003. Reduced bone mineralization in infants fed palm olein-containing formula: a randomized, double-blinded, prospective trial. Pediatrics 111, 1017–1023.

Koo, W.K.K., Hockman, E.M., Dow, M., 2006. Palm olein in the fat blend of infant formulas: Effect on the intestinal absorption of calcium and fat, and bone mineralization. J Am Coll Nutr 25, 117–122.

Lane, A.J., Coombs, R.C., Evans, D.H., et al., 1998. Effect of feed interval and feed type on splanchnic haemodynamics. Archives of Disease in Childhood. Fetal and Neonatal Edition 79, F49–F53.

Lien, E.L., Davis, A.M., Euler, A.R., et al., 2004. Growth and safety in term infants fed reduced-protein formula with added bovine lactalbumin. J Paediatr Gastroenterol Nutr 38, 170–176.

Lucas, A., 1991. Programming by early nutrition in man. Ciba Foundation Symposium 156, 38–50.

Lucas, A., 1994. Role of nutritional programming in determining adult morbidity. Archives of Disease in Childhood 71, 288–290.

Lucas, A., Bates, C., 1984. Transient riboflavin depletion in preterm infants. Archives of Disease in Childhood 59, 837–841.

Lucas, A., Cole, T.J., 1990. Breast milk and neonatal necrotising enterocolitis. Lancet 336, 1519–1523.

Lucas, A., Gore, S.M., Cole, T.J., et al., 1984. A multicentre trial on the feeding of low birthweight infants: effects of diet on early growth. Archives of Disease in Childhood 59, 722–730.

Lucas, A., Ewing, E., Roberts, S.B., et al., 1987. How much energy does the breast-fed infant consume and expend? British Medical Journal 295, 75–77.

Lucas, A., Morley, R., Hudson, G.J., et al., 1988. Early sodium intake and later blood pressure in preterm infants. Archives of Disease in Childhood 63, 656–657.

Lucas, A., Brooke, O.G., Morley, R., et al., 1990. Early diet of preterm infants and development of allergic or atopic disease: randomised prospective study. British Medical Journal 300, 837–840.

Lucas, A., Morley, R., Cole, T.J., et al., 1992. Breast milk and subsequent intelligence quotient in children born preterm. Lancet 339, 261–264.

Lucas, A., Morley, R., Cole, T.J., 1998. Randomised trial of early diet in preterm babies and later intelligence quotient. British Medical Journal 317, 1481–1487.

Makrides, M., Neumann, M.A., Byard, R.W., et al., 1994. Fatty acid composition of brain, retina and erythrocytes in breast- and formula-fed infants. American Journal of Clinical Nutrition 60, 189–194.

Makrides, M., Gibson, R.A., McPhee, A.J., et al., 2009. Neurodevelopmental outcome of preterm infants fed high-dose docosahexaenoic acid. A randomized controlled trial. JAMA 301, 175–182.

McCance, R., 1962. Food, growth, and time. Lancet 2, 271–272.

McClure, R.J., Newell, S.J., 1999. Randomised controlled trial of trophic feeding and gut motility. Archives of Disease in Childhood. Fetal and Neonatal Edition 80, F54–F58.

Mino, M., Nishino, H., 1973. Fetal and maternal relationship in serum vitamin E level. Journal of Nutritional Science and Vitaminology 19, 475–482.

Norgaard-Hansen, K., Ebbesen, F., 1996. Neonatal vitamin K prophylaxis in Denmark: three years' experience with oral administration during the first three months of life compared with one oral administration at birth. Acta Paediatrica 85, 1137–1139.

O'Brien, J.S., Fillerup, D.L., Mead, J.F., 1964. Quantification and fatty acid and fatty aldehyde composition of ethanolamine, choline, and serine glycerophosphatides in human cerebral grey and white matter. Journal of Lipid Research 5, 329–338.

O'Donnell, J., Finer, N.N., Rich, W., et al., 2002. Role of L-carnitine in apnea of prematurity: a randomized, controlled trial. Pediatrics 109, 622–626.

Osborn, D.A., Sinn, J.K.H., 2007. Prebiotics in infants for prevention of allergic disease and food hypersensitivity. Cochrane database of Syst Rev (4), CD 006474.

Poole, R.L., Hintz, S.R., Mackenzie, N.I., et al., 2008. Aluminum exposure from pediatric parenteral nutrition: meeting the new FDA regulation. JPEN J Parenter Enteral Nutr 32, 242–246.

Premji, S.S., Fenton, T.R., Sauve, R.S., 2006. Higher versus lower protein intake in formula-fed low birth weight infants. Cochrane Database Syst Rev (1), CD003959.

Reichman, B.L., Chessex, P., Putet, G., et al., 1982. Partition of energy metabolism and energy cost of growth in the very low-birthweight infant. Pediatrics 69, 443–451.

Reifen, R.M., Zlotkin, S., 1993. In: Tsang, R.C., Lucas, A., Uauy, R., et al. (Eds.), Nutritional Needs of the Preterm Infant. Scientific Basis and Practical Guidelines. Caduceus Medical Publishers, New York, p. 198.

Roberts, S.B., Coward, W.A., Schlingenseipen, K.-H., et al., 1986. Comparison of doubly labelled water method with calorimetry and a nutrient balance study for assessing energy expenditure, water intake and metabolizable energy intake in preterm infants. American Journal of Clinical Nutrition 44, 315–322.

Ronnholm, K.A.R., Sipila, I., Siimes, M.A., 1982. Human milk protein supplementation for the prevention of hypoproteinemia without metabolic imbalance in breast milk fed very low birthweight infants. Journal of Pediatrics 101, 243–247.

Sandstrom, O., Lonnerdal, B., Graverholt, G., et al., 2008. Effects of alpha-lactalbumin-enriched formula containing different concentrations of glycomacropeptide on infant nutrition. Am J Clin Nutr 87, 921–928.

Schultz, K., Soltesz, G., Mestyan, J., 1980. The metabolic consequences of human milk and formula feeding in premature infants. Acta Paediatrica Scandinavica 69, 647–652.

Shannon, K., 1995. Recombinant human erythropoetin in neonatal anaemia. Clinics in Perinatology 22, 627–640.

Shelley, H.J., 1964. Carbohydrate reserves in the newborn infant. British Medical Journal i, 273–275.

Shenai, J.P., Chytil, F., Jhaveri, A., et al., 1981. Plasma vitamin A and retinol binding protein in premature and term neonates. Journal of Pediatrics 99, 302–305.

Simmer, K., Patole, S., Rao, S.C., 2008a. Longchain polyunsaturated fatty acid supplementation in infants born at term. Cochrane Database of Systematic Reviews (1), CD000376.

Simmer, K., Schulzke, S.M., Patole, S., 2008b. Long-chain polyunsaturated fatty acid supplementation in preterm infants. Cochrane Database of Systematic Reviews (1), CD000375.

Singhal, A., Lucas, A., 2004. Early origins of cardiovascular disease: is there a unifying hypothesis? Lancet 363, 1642–1645.

Singhal, A., Cole, T.J., Lucas, A., 2001. Early nutrition in preterm infants and later blood pressure: two cohorts after randomised trials. Lancet 357, 413–419.

Singhal, A., Farooqi, I.S., O'Rahilly, S., et al., 2002. Early nutrition and leptin concentrations in later life. American Journal of Clinical Nutrition 75, 993–999.

Singhal, A., Fewtrell, M., Cole, T.J., et al., 2003. Low nutrient intake and early growth for later insulin resistance in adolescents born preterm. Lancet 361, 1089–1097.

Singhal, A., Cole, T., Fewtrell, M., et al., 2004. Breast milk feeding and the lipoprotein profile in adolescents born preterm. Lancet 363, 1571–1578.

Smithers, L.G., Collins, C.T., Simmonds, L.A., et al., 2010. Feeding preterm infants milk with a higher dose of docosahexaenoic acid than that used in current practice does not influence language or behaviour in early childhood: a follow-up study of a randomized controlled trial. Am J Clin Nutr 91, 628–634.

Southgate, D.A.T., Durnin, J.V.G.A., 1970. Calorie conversion factors. An experimental reassessment of the factors used in the calculation of the energy values of human diets. British Journal of Nutrition 24, 517–535.

Stephens, B.E., Walden, R.V., Gargus, R.A., et al., 2009. First-week protein and energy intakes are associated with 18-month developmental outcomes in extremely low birth weight infants. Pediatrics 123, 1337–1343.

Stevens, D., Burman, D., Strelling, K., et al., 1979. Folic acid supplementation in low birthweight infants. Pediatrics 64, 333–335.

Stimmler, L., Snodgrass, G.J.A.I., Jaffe, E., 1973. Enamel hypoplasia of the teeth associated with neonatal tetany. Lancet i, 1085–1086.

Tantibhedyangkul, P., Hashim, S.A., 1978. Medium chain triglyceride feeding in premature infants: effects on calcium and magnesium absorption. Pediatrics 61, 537–545.

Tsang, R.C., Uauy, R., Koletzko, B., et al., 2005. Nutrition of the Preterm Infant: Scientific Basis and Practical Guidelines, second ed. Digital Educational Publishing, Cincinatti, OH, USA.

Tsuboi, K.K., Kwon, L.K., Ford, W.D.A., et al., 1986. Delayed ontological development in the bypassed ileum of the infant rat. Gastroenterology 80, 1550–1556.

Tubman, R.T.R.J., Thompson, S., McGuire, W., 2008. Glutamine supplementation to prevent morbidity and mortality in preterm infants. Cochrane Database Syst Rev (1), CD001457.

Tyson, J.E., Lasky, R., Flood, D., et al., 1989. Randomized trial of taurine supplementation for infants <1300 gram birth weight: effect on auditory brainstem-evoked responses. Pediatrics 83, 406–415.

von Kries, R., Hachmeister, A., Gobel, U., 1999. Can 3 oral 2 mg doses of vitamin K effectively prevent late vitamin K deficiency bleeding? European Journal of Pediatrics 158, S183–S186.

Wharton, B.A., 1987. Nutrition and Feeding of Preterm Infants. Blackwell Scientific. Oxford.

Wharton, B., Morley, R., Isaacs, E.B., et al., 2004. Low plasma taurine and later neurodevelopment. Arch Dis Child Fetal Neonatal Ed 89, F497–F498.

Widdowson, E.M., 1981. Nutrition. In: Davis, J.A., Dobbing, J. (Eds.), Scientific Foundations of Pediatrics, second ed. Heinemann, London, pp. 41–43.

Widdowson, E.M., Dickerson, J.W.T., 1964. Chemical composition of the body. In: Comar, C.L., Bronner, F. (Eds.), Mineral Metabolism, vol. II, Part A. Academic Press, New York, pp. 1–247.

Williamson, S., Finucaine, E., Elliott, J., et al., 1978. Effect of heat treatment of human milk on absorption of nitrogen, fat, sodium, calcium and phosphorus by preterm infants. Archives of Disease in Childhood 53, 555–563.

Worthington-White, D.A., Behnke, M., Gross, S., 1994. Preterm infants require additional folate to reduce the severity of the anemia of prematurity. American Journal of Clinical Nutrition 60, 930–935.

Young, V.R., 1981. Protein-energy interrelationships in the newborn: a brief consideration of some basic aspects. In: Lebenthal, E. (Ed.), Textbook of Gastroenterology and Nutrition in Infancy, vol. 1. Raven Press, New York, pp. 257–263.

Yu, V.Y.H., 2002. Scientific rationale and benefits of nucleotide supplementation of infant formula. Journal of Paediatrics and Child Health 38, 543–549.

Ziegler, E.E., 1986. Protein requirements of preterm infants. In: Fomon, S.J., Heird, W.C. (Eds.), Energy and Protein Needs During Infancy. Academic Press, Orlando.

Part 2: Feeding the full-term baby

Mary Fewtrell   Alan Lucas

Breastfeeding

Breastfeeding is a complex physiological event: indeed, the term itself could be regarded as a misnomer, since 'feeding' is only one of several physiological processes that occur when a newborn infant is put to the breast. These processes can be summarised as follows:

- provision of nutrients
- provision of immunological and antimicrobial protection
- induction of adaptive events that equip the infant for extrauterine nutrition
- the passage of non-nutritive factors (other than antimicrobial ones) from mother to infant, e.g. breast milk hormones and growth factors
- provision of digestive enzymes, e.g. milk lipases
- effects on the mother, e.g. contraceptive role
- facilitation of mother–infant bonding
- 'programming' effects on long-term health.

Nutritive aspects of human milk

Human milk does not have a constant composition, and significant changes take place during the course of lactation, diurnally and during each feed. Uncertainty over the precise dietary intake of breastfed infants poses a major problem for nutritional science. In Tables 16.6 and 16.7, the composition of average mature human milk is tabulated (DHSS 1977) together with the composition of unmodified cow's milk.

Protein

The protein content of milks of mammalian species appears to be related to the postnatal growth rate of the infant (Bernhart 1961). Human infants have especially slow postnatal growth rates compared with many other mammals, and the protein content of human milk is correspondingly very low. Previously, the protein content of mature human milk may have been overestimated, because of its high content of non-protein nitrogen: a realistic figure is 1.0 g/100 ml, compared with 3.5 g/100 ml in cow's milk.

The two main classes of protein in milk are whey and casein. Human milk is whey-predominant (around 60% of total protein). Cow's milk, however, is casein-predominant, with only 20% whey. In human whey, α-lactalbumin is the dominant protein, followed by lactoferrin. In contrast, the major whey protein in cow's milk is β-lactoglobulin, which is absent from human milk and may be antigenic when fed to human infants. α-lactalbumin is present in cow's milk, but lactoferrin occurs in only small amounts. Whey proteins have a high nutritive value for human infants; their essential amino acid content is high. It is now possible to prepare bovine milk whey fractions high in α-lactalbumin and lower in β-lactoglobulin, and there is some evidence that their addition to infant formulas may allow the total protein content to be lowered, resulting in a slower pattern of weight gain, more like that of a breastfed infant (see Ch. 16.1). Caseins may precipitate at low pH, forming a 'curd' in the infant's stomach, and this has led to the widespread belief that casein-dominant formulas may be more satisfying for hungry infants. Human milk casein yields a softer, more flocculent curd than cow's milk casein.

Human milk has a cysteine content about twice that of cow's milk and a methionine/cysteine ratio that is seven times less than cow's milk. In view of the late development of cystathionase (which converts methionine to cysteine), cysteine may be an essential amino acid in the newborn, and it has been suggested that the high cysteine content of human milk is biologically advantageous. In addition, the relatively low content of tyrosine and phenylalanine in human milk may be related to the newborn infant's limited capacity to metabolise these amino acids.

The non-protein nitrogen content in human milk is unusually high – about 25% of the total, compared with 6% in cow's milk. It consists of free amino acids, urea, creatinine, creatine, uric acid and ammonia. Clearly, free amino acids must be included with protein from a nutritional point of view; it is unknown whether other

Table 16.6 Nutrient content of some baby milks available in the UK (per 100 ml*)

COMPOSITION PER 100 ml	MATURE HUMAN MILK		DEMINERALISED WHEY-BASED FORMULAS			MODIFIED MILK FORMULAS (CASEIN-DOMINANT)		
	DHSS[†]	Macy[‡]	Milupa Aptamil Newborn	Cow & Gate First Infant Milk	SMA First	Milupa Extra Hungry Infant Milk	Cow & Gate Infant Milk for Hungrier Babies	SMA Extra Hungry Baby
Macronutrients								
Protein[§] (g)	1.34	1.45	1.3	1.3	1.3	1.6	1.6	1.6
Casein (%)	2	32	40	40	40	80	80	80
Whey (%)	2	68	60	60	60	20	20	20
Fat (g)	4.2	3.8	3.5	3.5	3.6	3.2	3.2	3.6
Total LCPUFA (mg)			23	18	19	21		19
Arachidonic acid (mg)			12	7	12	21		19
Docosahexaenoic acid (mg)			7	7	7	6		7
Carbohydrate	7.0		7.3	7.3	7.3	7.7	7.7	7
Sugars (g)	7.0	7.0	7.2	7.2	7.3	7.6	7.6	7
Energy								
kcal	70	68	66	66	67	66	66	67
kJ	293	285	275	275	280	275	275	280
Minerals								
Calcium	35	33	50	50	42	70	70	56
Chloride	43	43	41	41	43	55	54	55
Magnesium	2.8	4.0	5	5	4.5	5	5.2	5.3
Phosphorus	15	15	28	28	24	44	44	44
Potassium	60	55	63	63	65	80	82	80
Sodium	15	15	18	17	16	20	20	20
Trace elements								
Copper (µg)	39	40	40	40	33	40	40	33
Iodine (µg)	76	150	12	12	10	12	12	10
Iron (µg)	76	150	530	530	640	530	50	640
Manganese (µg)	ND	0.7	7.5	7.5	5	7.5	7.5	5
Zinc (µg)	295	530	500	500	600	500	500	600
Vitamins								
A retinol (µg RE)	60	53	55	55	66	55	55	75
B₁ thiamin (µg)	0.16	0.16	0.05	0.05	0.1	0.05	0.05	0.11
B₂ riboflavin (µg)	31	42.6	100	110	110	100	110	110
B₆ pyridoxine (µg)	6	11	40	40	60	40	40	60
B₁₂ (µg)	0.01	Trace	0.18	0.18	0.18	0.18	0.18	0.18
Biotin (µg)	0.76	0.4	1.5	1.5	2	1.9	1.6	2
Folic acid (µg)	5.2	0.18	12	12	11	12	19	13
Niacin (µg)	230	172	790	430	500	430	440	500

Table 16.6 Continued

COMPOSITION PER 100 ml	MATURE HUMAN MILK		DEMINERALISED WHEY-BASED FORMULAS			MODIFIED MILK FORMULAS (CASEIN-DOMINANT)		
	DHSS[†]	Macy[‡]	Milupa Aptamil Newborn	Cow & Gate First Infant Milk	SMA First	Milupa Extra Hungry Infant Milk	Cow & Gate Infant Milk for Hungrier Babies	SMA Extra Hungry Baby
C ascorbic acid (mg)	3.8	4.3	8.6	8.3	9	8.3	9.1	9
D (μg)	0.01	0.01	1.2	1.2	1.2	1.2	1.2	1.1
E (mg)	0.35	0.56	1.2	1	0.74	1.1	1	0.74
K (μg)	ND	1.7	4.5	4.5	6.7	4.4	4.4	6.7
Others								
Nucleotides (mg)			2.8	3.2	2.6	3.2	3.2	
Choline (mg)			10	10	10	10	10	6.7
Taurine (mg)			6.7	5.3	4.7	5.3	5.3	4.7

*Manufacturer's information.
[†]DHSS (1977, 1980, 1981).
[‡]Macy et al. (1953).
[§]Total nitrogen × 6.38.
LCPUFA, long-chain polyunsaturated fatty acid; ND, not determined; RE, retinol equivalent.

Table 16.7 Nutrient content of follow-on baby milks available in the UK (per 100 ml*)

COMPOSITION PER 100 ml	FOLLOW-ON MILK				
	Cow's milk	Milupa Aptamil follow-on milk	Cow & Gate follow-on milk	Heinz Nurture Growing Baby follow-on milk	SMA Nutrition follow-on milk
Macronutrients					
Protein[†] (g)	3.4	1.4	1,4	1.8	1.5
Casein (%)	77	80	80	80	80
Whey (%)	23	20	20	20	20
Fat (g)	3.9	3.2	3.2	3.5	3.6
Saturated (%)	63.2	1.4	1.4	0.8	1.4
LCPUFA (mg)			27		19
Arachidonic acid (mg)			15		12
Docosahexaenoic acid (mg)			8.5		7.1
Carbohydrate (g)	4.6	8.6	8.6	7.3	7.2
Energy					
kcal	67	68	68	68	67
kJ	280	285	285	285	281
Minerals					
Calcium (mg)	124	62	62	75	50
Chloride (mg)	98	43	43	65	43

Table 16.7 Continued

COMPOSITION PER 100 ml	FOLLOW-ON MILK				
	Cow's milk	Milupa Aptamil follow-on milk	Cow & Gate follow-on milk	Heinz Nurture Growing Baby follow-on milk	SMA Nutrition follow-on milk
Magnesium (mg)	12	4.8	4.8	8	6.4
Phosphorus (mg)	98	34	34	50	33
Potassium (mg)	155	61	61	94	70
Sodium (mg)	52	20	20	30	16
Trace elements					
Copper (μg)	20	41	41	43	33
Iodine (μg)	ND	12	12	20	10
Iron (μg)	50	1000	1000	1200	1200
Manganese (μg)	ND	7.7	7.7	3.9	5
Zinc (μg)	360	520	520	700	800
Vitamins					
A retinol (μg RE)	40	6566	66	79	75
B_1 thiamin (μg)	40	50	50	120	100
B_2 riboflavin (μg)	200	110	110	150	110
B_6 pyridoxine (μg)	40	40	40	40	60
B_{12} cyanocobalamin (μg)	0.3	0.17	0.17	0.2	0.18
Biotin (μg)	2.1	1.5	1.5	3	2
Folic acid (μg)	5	12	12	18	11
Niacin (μg)	80	440	440	650	500
C ascorbic acid (mg)	1.5	9.4	9.4	10	12
D (μg)	0.02	1.4	1.4	1.1	1.5
E (mg)	0.09	1.2	1.2	0.5	0.74
K (μg)	ND	5.1	5.1	7.4	6.7
Others					
Nucleotides (mg)		3.2	3.2	3.1	2.6
Choline (mg)		10	10	14.1	20
Taurine (mg)		5.5	5.5	6.8	4.7

*Manufacturer's information.
†Total nitrogen × 6.38.
LCPUFA, long-chain polyunsaturated fatty acid; ND, not determined; RE, retinol equivalent.

non-protein nitrogen fractions have nutritional value (Carlson 1985). The free amino acids in human milk include taurine, which is present in significantly higher amounts than in cow's milk. During early lactation, milk protein content is much higher than in mature milk (Fig. 16.3). The falling protein content could represent an adaptation to the infant's decreasing protein requirements, or simply reflect the maturation of the mammary gland.

Energy

Published values for the energy content of breast milk (obtained unphysiologically as expressed breast milk) of around 70 kcal/100 ml have been challenged. Using the doubly labelled water method, which avoids milk sampling, Lucas et al. (1987) suggest that a figure close to 60 kcal/100 ml is realistic. Most formulas still have significantly higher energy contents than this (see below).

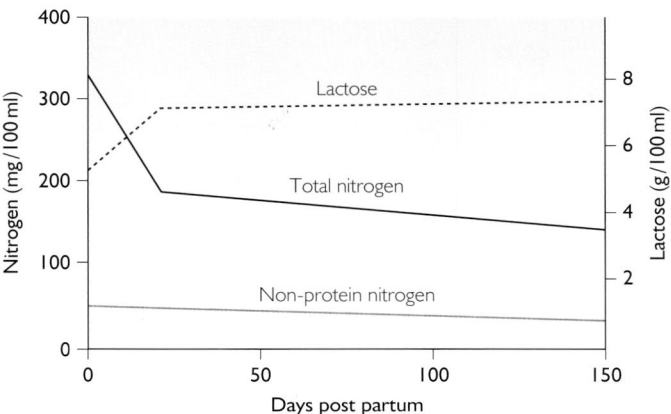

Fig. 16.3 Concentration of lactose, total nitrogen and non-protein nitrogen in human milk during the course of lactation.

Table 16.8 Fatty acid composition of mature human and cow's milk lipids (%, w/w)

FATTY ACID	HUMAN MILK	COW'S MILK
4:0	–	3.0
6:0	Trace	1.6
8:0	Trace	1.3
10:0	1.3	3.0
12:0	3.1	3.1
14:0	5.1	14.2
15:0	0.4	1.3
16:0	20.2	49.9
16:1	5.7	3.7
18:0	5.9	5.7
18:1	46.4	6.7
18:2	13.0	1.6
18:3	1.4	1.8

Fat

The fat content of milk from different mothers is very variable, and in an individual usually increases during early lactation (1–2 weeks) and later declines. (Indeed, with the exception of lactose and lysozyme, most breast milk nutrients, including minerals and vitamins, decline after the first 2–3 months of lactation.) The fat concentration rises markedly during a feed, from around 2.1 g/100 ml to 4.1 g/100 ml (Lucas et al. 1980).

Cow's milk and human milk have similar fat contents and most of the lipid is triglyceride (98%); the principal difference is the pattern of fatty acids (Table 16.8). Human milk fatty acid profiles are, however, markedly influenced by diet. Vegetarians, for instance, consume more long-chain fatty acids than those on a mixed diet, and the amount of certain long-chain polyunsaturated fatty acids, notably docosahexaenoic acid, is markedly affected by the amount of fish and marine products in the maternal diet. Human milk has a higher proportion of unsaturated fatty acids than cow's milk and a greater concentration of the essential fatty acids. Unlike cow's milk, fatty acids in human milk are esterified to glycerol predominantly in the 1 position, which improves their absorption.

Breast milk lipids occur as globules ranging in size from 1 to 10 microns, emulsified in the aqueous phase of milk (Jensen 1996). These globules consist of non-polar core lipids (such as triglycerides and cholesterol esters) covered with bipolar materials (including protein and phospholipids) which constitute the milk lipid globule membrane. The latter prevents the globules from coalescing and presents a large surface area for the action of lipolytic enzymes.

Carbohydrate

Lactose is present in higher concentrations in human milk (7 g/100 ml) than in cow's milk (4.7 g/100 ml). Lactose enhances calcium absorption from the gut, promotes the growth of lactobacilli and may help to create a favourable gut flora that protects against gastroenteritis.

Minerals

All major minerals are present in higher concentrations in cow's milk than in human milk (Table 16.7); with the higher protein content of cow's milk, they account for its high renal solute load. The amount of sodium in cow's milk is regarded as excessive for the human infant. However, early human milk has a high sodium content which may be 10 times that seen in mature milk. The raised phosphate/calcium ratio in cow's milk has been implicated in neonatal hypocalcaemia (see below).

Trace metals

The major trace metal concentrations in mature human and cow's milk are shown in Table 16.8. Zinc concentrations in mature human milk are rather less than those in cow's milk, whereas the reverse is the case for copper; cow's milk has substantially greater magnesium content. Copper, iron and zinc are present in higher concentrations in human colostrum than in later milk. However, the comparison of levels of trace nutrients in different milks is of less relevance than the bioavailability of these elements. There is good bioavailability of iron and other minerals from human milk. In cow's milk, iron and zinc are less available, the latter being bound to high-molecular-weight fractions.

Vitamins

In the west, vitamin deficiencies are generally rare in fully breastfed infants when the mother is well nourished. Vitamins K and D, however, require special consideration.

Vitamin K

Levels are low in breast milk (0.4–2.8 µg/ml), though they are higher in colostrum (0.8–4.8 µg/ml). In contrast, non-supplemented formulas usually contain around 6–11 µg/ml and supplemented formulas up to 100 µg/ml. Parenteral prophylaxis at birth with 1 mg vitamin K is effective against vitamin K-deficiency bleeding in breastfed infants (Ch. 30). There is still debate about the most suitable oral regimen, although repeated doses are considered necessary (Ch. 30).

Vitamin D

In the human infant, cholecalciferol (vitamin D) is derived mainly from the skin, synthesised from 7-dehydrocholesterol under the influence of sunlight. Breast milk provides only about 10 IU of vitamin D daily in winter and 20 IU daily in the summer, and water-soluble vitamin D is present only in trace amounts that have negligible activity. Healthy, exclusively breastfed (EBF) infants have adequate bone mineralisation in the first 16 weeks of life (Roberts et al. 1981) and maintain satisfactory serum levels of 25-hydroxycholecalciferol for at least 6 months (Birkbeck and Scott 1980), suggesting that vitamin D supplements during this period are unnecessary, at least in mothers who are themselves vitamin D-sufficient. However, rickets has been reported in association with prolonged breastfeeding (Mughal et al. 1999). Over the past few years there have also been reports of an increase in the incidence of rickets in children of South East Asian origin living in the UK, particularly those living at higher latitudes; many women in this group are themselves vitamin D-insufficient or deficient (Ashraf and Mughal 2002). Although it is recommended that all breastfed infants receive 280–400 IU vitamin D daily from the age of 6 months if consuming <500 ml/day of infant formula, and that 'at-risk' groups should start supplements before 6 months, this frequently does not happen in practice, and there have been calls for a renewed campaign to raise awareness (Bolling et al. 2005; Leaf 2007). The situation regarding maternal supplementation was somewhat confused following the recent guidance from the National Institute for Health and Clinical Excellence that there is insufficient evidence to support routine provision of vitamin D to pregnant women (National Collaborating Centre for Women's and Children's Health 2003), whilst the Department of Health highlights pregnancy and lactation as high-risk periods and recommends a vitamin D intake of 10 μg (400 IU) per day; this is very unlikely to be met by diet alone since the average daily intake is around 3 μg/day.

Multivitamins

It has been recommended that in the UK children receive daily vitamin A (233 μg; 770 IU), vitamin C (20 mg) and vitamin D (7 μg) as a combined preparation from 6 months to 5 years (DHSS 1988) (available under the Healthy Start Scheme, although there have been problems with supply of these drops). However, in the most recent UK Infant Feeding Survey, conducted in 2005 (Bolling et al. 2005), only a tiny proportion of mothers were giving their babies vitamin supplements, increasing slightly by the age of 8–10 months. The proportion of babies receiving vitamins had also decreased since 2000, suggesting that mothers are not aware of the recommendations, and their importance for the health of their babies (Bolling et al. 2005). The American Academy of Pediatrics recommends that breastfed infants and those receiving <500 ml/day of infant formula should start vitamin D (5 μg/day) within the first 2 months of life (American Academy of Pediatrics 2003). This seems sensible, especially when there is doubt about the mother's dietary status.

Iron

The newborn term infant has an iron content of about 250–300 mg (75 mg/kg body weight). This iron will cover the needs of the term infant during the first 4–6 months of life and is why the iron requirements of healthy term infants during this period can be provided by human milk, which contains very little iron. Because iron stores are proportional to body mass at birth, babies who are small for gestational age may become iron-depleted well before 6 months. In the term infant, iron requirements rise markedly after age 4–6 months and amount to about 0.7–0.9 mg/day during the remaining part of the first year. These requirements are very high, especially in relation to body size and energy intake. In the first year of life, the term infant almost doubles its total iron stores and triples its body weight. The increase in body iron during this period occurs mainly during the latter 6 months.

The breastfed infant's requirement for supplemental iron is controversial. The low levels of iron in breast milk (compared with those in supplemented modern formulas) are very well absorbed (around 80%, compared with about 4–6% from fortified formulas). Nevertheless, a small proportion of breastfed infants have lower iron stores at 6 months, and a greater proportion appear deficient at 9 months or later, than those fed iron-supplemented formula (Saarinen and Siimes 1979; Garry et al. 1981; Haschke et al. 1993). Iron status is influenced by several factors, including birthweight, maternal iron status during pregnancy and the placental transfusion received at delivery; indeed, a randomised trial showed that delayed clamping of the umbilical cord resulted in improved iron status at age 6 months (Chaparro et al. 2006).

Iron-deficiency anaemia is common in infancy and childhood. Although often asymptomatic, iron deficiency may be associated with adverse effects on cognitive outcome, although it remains uncertain whether the poor development of iron-deficient infants is due to poor social background or iron deficiency or a combination of the two factors (Grantham-McGregor and Ani 2001). In formula-fed babies, continued use of iron- and vitamin C-fortified formulas during infancy is effective in preventing iron-deficiency anaemia, but, in babies receiving breast milk plus weaning foods beyond 6 months, good nutritional advice is required with an emphasis on the provision of foods that are either rich in iron (for example, red meat) or iron-supplemented. Recommended intakes of iron between 6 and 12 months vary. The American Academy of Pediatrics recommends 11 mg/day, whilst the World Health Organization (WHO)/Food and Agriculture Organization give different figures depending on bioavailability: 6.2 mg/day for 15%, up to 9.3 mg/day for 10% and 18.6 mg/day for 5% (Joint FAO/WHO Expert Consultation on Human Vitamin and Mineral Requirements 1998).

Fluoride

Fluoride is not a nutrient, although epidemiological studies show its role in preventing dental caries. It has both systemic and topical actions. Systemically it acts on the teeth prior to eruption, being built into the structure of the enamel and making it resistant to decay. It also limits enamel demineralisation. Fluoride also acts topically by promoting remineralisation, possibly through antibacterial effects. The relative roles of systemic versus topical fluoride are still being debated. In areas where the water supply is fluoridated, infants consuming reconstituted formulas will have adequate intake, but in breastfed babies intake will inevitably be low. The British Dental Association (Dowell and Joyston-Bechal 1981) and the American Academy of Pediatrics have recommended that an intake of 0.25 mg fluoride should be achieved from 2 weeks to 2 years of age (available as drops), but emphasise the dangers (fluorosis) of exceeding this dosage from all sources combined. When water becomes the principal part of the breastfed infant's fluid intake, supplementation is no longer required if the water supply is fluoridated.

Nutritional adequacy of breast milk as the sole diet for healthy term babies

Maternal breast milk production rises to a peak in the third and fourth months after delivery, providing a mean of around 750–850 ml/24 h (more in boys than girls). The majority of EBF babies consume between 500 ml and 1200 ml per 24 h. By the end of this period, at intakes of 150 ml/kg the infant would consume 1.5 g/kg/24 h of protein and 85–105 kcal/kg/24 h (according to which values for milk energy are accepted: see Lucas et al. 1987). Beyond 4–6 months, protein and energy intakes per kilogram body weight will fall as the infant grows, and eventually, without the introduction of complementary (weaning) foods, breast milk alone will no longer meet the infant's needs and complementary foods are required. However, the point at which this occurs is variable and difficult to define, even for populations (Reilly et al. 2005).

Data on the adequacy of 6 months' exclusive breastfeeding for meeting iron requirements have also been published. Consistent with findings from a randomised trial in Honduras, Chantry et al. (2007) reported that American infants EBF for 6 months are more likely to have a history of anaemia (adjusted odds ratio (OR) 0.20, 95% confidence interval (CI) 0.06–0.63) and low serum ferritin (OR 0.19, 95% CI 0.06–0.57) than those with full breastfeeding for 4–5 months. This finding is of concern given the risk of non-reversible long-term cognitive deficits associated with iron deficiency. Although the risk may be reduced by measures such as improving maternal iron status during pregnancy, delayed umbilical cord clamping and supplementing at-risk infants such as those born with low birthweight, in the absence of a screening policy it is likely that iron deficiency, which is usually asymptomatic, will be missed.

Optimal duration of exclusive breastfeeding

A systematic review of the optimal duration of exclusive breastfeeding was commissioned by the WHO in 2001, primarily to assess the effects on growth and health of exclusive breastfeeding for 6 months versus 3–4 months, with mixed breastfeeding (with complementary foods) thereafter (Kramer and Kakuma 2002). Sixteen studies meeting the specified inclusion criteria for the review were included: seven from developing countries and nine from developed countries. With the exception of two randomised trials conducted in Honduras, all studies were observational. The conclusions were as follows:

- Infants exclusive breastfeeding for 6 months show no evidence of weight or length deficits compared with those exclusive breastfeeding until 3–4 months, although larger sample sizes would be required to rule out small increases in the risk of undernutrition.
- Infants with suboptimal iron stores at birth who receive exclusive breastfeeding for 6 months without iron supplementation may be at risk of inadequate iron stores during infancy. This is more likely to occur in a developing country.
- Infants exclusive breastfeeding until 6 months have a significantly reduced incidence of one or more episodes of gastrointestinal (GI) infection during the first year. This finding is based primarily on an observational analysis of data from a large randomised trial of a breastfeeding promotion intervention in Belarus (Kramer et al. 2003). Because of its healthcare system and clean water supply, Belarus is regarded as a developed country in the context of infection risk. The incidence of GI infection during the first year was 7.4% (213/2862) in infants exclusive breastfeeding to 3–4 months, compared with 5.0% (31/621) in those exclusive breastfeeding to 6 months (OR 0.61, 95% CI 0.41–0.93). However, the difference in the proportion of infants hospitalised with GI infection did not differ significantly between groups (2.2% versus 1.8%, OR 0.75, 95% CI 0.38–1.04).

Following the WHO recommendation, in 2003 the UK Department of Health altered the advice for England and Wales in line with WHO recommendations, and suggested that mothers should exclusively breastfeed for the first 6 months before introducing solids. The advice to delay the introduction of solids until 6 months was subsequently extended to formula-fed infants. Since 2001, four further studies from developed countries have suggested that more prolonged exclusive breastfeeding is associated with a reduced risk of GI or respiratory infection (Chantry et al. 2006; Paricio Talayero et al. 2006; Quigley et al. 2007; Rebhan et al. 2009); however, one UK study suggested that the increased risk associated with not being EBF was due to the introduction of infant formula rather than solid foods (Quigley et al. 2009). Against this, and of particular relevance for populations at risk of food allergy and coeliac disease, are emerging data suggesting that delaying the introduction of certain allergenic foods may actually increase the risk of subsequent disease (Prescott et al. 2008); this hypothesis is currently being tested in two UK randomised trials. With regard to gluten, the current consensus is that gluten is best introduced gradually alongside continued breastfeeding, and that the timing itself may not be so critical in determining the risk of disease (Agostoni et al. 2008).

Antibacterial aspects of human milk

Grulee's studies in Chicago in the 1930s, based on a 9-month period of supervised follow-up of 20 061 babies, provided convincing evidence of the anti-infective advantages of breastfeeding in the pre-antibiotic era (Grulee et al. 1935). With overall improvements in public health and obstetric and paediatric care in western countries, these major differences in infection rates have diminished dramatically, though much less so in developing countries. In developed countries, an increased morbidity (but not mortality) due to infection in bottle-fed babies is supported by recent evidence (Howie et al. 1990; Quigley et al. 2009), even when account has been taken of class differences in feeding preferences. Human milk may also have a protective effect against diarrhoea, respiratory tract infections and otitis media beyond the period of breastfeeding (Hanson 1998).

Immunoglobulins

The principal immunoglobulin in milk, secretory IgA, is present in the highest concentrations in the first few days postpartum. There is little evidence that absorption of the relatively low concentrations of IgG in human milk occurs. Secretory IgA is relatively resistant to low pH and proteolytic enzymes, and can be recovered from the stools of breastfed infants. It is likely that its protective effects are confined to the gut and perhaps to the respiratory tract. A wide variety of antibodies against viruses and bacteria and their toxins have been described in human milk, but their actions within the gut are not fully understood.

Other antimicrobial factors

Although all complement components have been demonstrated in human milk, their relatively low concentration, and the observation that heating milk up to 56°C for 30 minutes does not decrease its bacteriostatic action against *Escherichia coli*, has cast doubt on the anti-infective role of milk complement. Human milk is one of the richest sources of lysozyme, which is present in about 3000 times the concentration reported in cow's milk. In vitro, it acts with IgA to lyse *E. coli* and some salmonellae, but its role in vivo is not established.

The iron-binding protein lactoferrin may deprive gut organisms of free iron as a growth factor, and has been shown to be bacteriostatic and bacteriocidal in vitro, although its protective role in vivo is uncertain. Lactoferrin increases markedly in milk during lactation, and has received recent attention as a possible growth factor.

Other factors present in human milk, for example oligonucleotides and glycoconjugates, may act as receptors and divert pathogens or toxins away from binding to the infant's pharynx or gut. Breast milk also contains nucleotides that may promote cell-mediated immunity (see Chapter 16 part 1), and prebiotic oligosaccharides that may promote the growth of a bifidogenic-dominant colonic microflora, which in turn protects the infant from enteropathogenic bacteria.

Nutritive aspects of antimicrobial factors

Previously it was believed that antimicrobial proteins, including IgA and lactoferrin, which constitute a significant proportion (30–40%) of milk protein, were not available for nutrition. Prentice et al. (1987) have challenged this view, suggesting that the great majority of these proteins are digested: by 6 weeks, only 1% of lactoferrin and 17% of secretory IgA is detected in the stools and 95% of total dietary protein could be regarded as nutritionally available.

Effects on gut flora

Recent work suggests that the factors that influence postnatal colonisation of the gut are complex, including delivery mode and environmental factors. However, studies performed since 1980 show relatively few differences in gut microbiota between breastfed and formula-fed infants. The most consistent differences are that clostridia, *Bacteroides* and Enterobacteriaceae tend to be more prevalent in formula-fed infants, whilst staphylococci tend to be more numerous in breastfed infants (Adlerberth and Wold 2009).

Cells in milk

Human milk is populated with macrophages, polymorphonuclear leukocytes and T and B lymphocytes; it has been calculated that the breastfed infant ingests as many viable leukocytes each day as he or she has circulating at any one time. The B lymphocytes contain cell lines that have synthesised IgA in the breast, but whether these cells survive for long enough in the infant's gut to carry out any further useful biological role is unknown. There is evidence that T cells in milk may transfer tuberculin sensitivity from mother to infant (Schlesinger and Covelli 1977), presumably mediated through lymphokines, which might have been secreted before the infant ingested the milk. There is no evidence that T lymphocytes are transferred across the gut in humans or participate in graft-versus-host disease. However, cells transferred from mother to infant may induce tolerance of maternal human leukocyte antigen status; previously breastfed infants who receive a renal allograft from their mother have less organ rejection (Flores et al. 1993).

Breast milk hormones

Possible 'messenger' substances in human milk

In recent years a wide variety of hormones and growth factors have been described in human milk (Sack 1980; Savino and Liguori 2008). These include steroids, prolactin, thyroxine, gonadotrophins, melatonin, epidermal growth factor, prostaglandins and a number of adipokines and hormones known to be involved in appetite regulation and energy metabolism. It is an important question whether or not the lactating mother, in addition to providing nutrients and anti-infective factors, might also exert some control over neonatal metabolism, appetite and development through the mediation of chemical messengers and trophic factors secreted into her milk. More research is required in humans to confirm this hypothesis and determine whether interventions with these substances might be useful.

Enzymes in human milk

The bile salt-stimulated lipase in human milk may play a significant part in intestinal lipolysis (Hamosh 1996). Its presence may partly account for improved fat absorption from human milk compared with cow's milk, and for the observation that pasteurisation results in lower fat absorption from breast milk in preterm infants. Bile salt-stimulated lipase also has esterase activity, which may assist the digestion of breast milk retinyl esters.

Several other enzymes have been described in human milk. Breast milk amylase is identical in structure to the salivary enzyme, and probably compensates for the relatively slow postnatal development of the latter. Several proteases are also present, including trypsin, elastase and plasmin. However, it is doubtful whether they play an important role in the neonatal period because of the high antiprotease activity of human milk.

Other factors in breast milk

Babies may consume from breast milk a variety of substances which have no physiological value to them. Addictive drugs cause increasing concern. Some evidence suggests a need for caution over the regular use of alcohol by breastfeeding mothers: Little et al. (1989) initially showed that 1 unit of alcohol or more each day for the first 3 months was associated with reduced motor development scores in the infant at 1 year. However, in a more recent study of 915 infants from the Avon Longitudinal Study of Parents and Children (ALSPAC) cohort, alcohol use during lactation was not associated with a deficit in motor skills at 18 months (Little et al. 2002).

Pesticide residues are officially monitored. Organohalogens such as dioxins and polychlorinated biphenyls (PCBs) in breast milk are of current concern. These lipophilic chemicals are excreted in breast milk in 10–50 times the concentration in cow's milk or formulas, frequently exceeding accepted safety limits for cow's milk. They accumulate in fat over long periods, and some are highly toxic to skin, liver, and immune and nervous systems. They are also suspected carcinogens. Studies in infants to date have suggested that prenatal exposure to these substances may be associated with decreased psychomotor function, abnormal thyroid function tests (decreased triiodothyronine and thyroxine with elevated thyroid-stimulating hormone), and effects on immune status. However, despite relatively high levels of PCBs in breast milk, reflected in a threefold level of plasma PCBs in children at 2.5 years of age compared with formula-fed infants, no significant negative effects on outcome have been found. Indeed, a study of Dutch infants followed up to 6 years of age suggested that breastfeeding itself counteracts the adverse developmental effects of dioxins and PCBs (Boersma and Lanting 2000), whilst a more recent Dutch study of infants born in 2000 concluded that the current decreased exposure to polychlorinated dibenzo-p-dioxins/dibenzofurans and PCBs does not impair thyroid function of newborns and neurodevelopment of infants up to 24 months of age (Wilhelm et al. 2008).

Human immunodeficiency virus and other viruses in breast milk

Human immunodeficiency virus (HIV) has been found in breast milk in HIV-positive mothers, and there is good evidence that transmission to the breastfed baby occurs in up to 15% of cases (Ch. 39). It is known that exclusive breastfeeding is protective against postnatal transmission of HIV, compared with mixed breastfeeding; several studies have confirmed the increased risk of transmission of

HIV when solids are combined with breastfeeding during the first 6 months. Accordingly, exclusive breastfeeding for 6 months is the World Health Organization's (2008) recommendation to HIV-infected mothers for whom exclusive replacement feeding (that is, with infant formula) is not acceptable, feasible, affordable, safe or sustainable. In countries where formula-feeding is safe, including the UK, it is recommended that such mothers do not breastfeed.

Both hepatitis B virus (HBV) and hepatitis C virus (HCV) may be found in the breast milk of seropositive mothers, and transmission to the infant has been reported. However, most evidence suggests that breast milk is an uncommon route of infection (Uehara et al. 1993; Moriya et al. 1995). Mothers who wish to donate breast milk are now routinely screened for HBV, HCV and HIV, and excluded if positive.

Cytomegalovirus is found in the milk of between 32% and 96% of seropositive mothers when polymerase chain reaction is used (Hamprecht et al. 2001), and breastfed babies of seropositive mothers show a higher rate of seropositivity at 1 year of age (70%) than those who are bottle-fed (30%) (Minamishima et al. 1994). This does not generally pose a problem for healthy term babies, but may do in those born preterm (see Ch. 39).

Maternal aspects of breastfeeding

Advice and assistance

The UK Baby Friendly Initiative (BFI) under the umbrella of UNICEF was set up in 1994 and aims to increase the incidence and duration of breastfeeding. The BFI has produced '10 steps to successful breastfeeding' for maternity services and a 'seven-point plan for the protection, promotion and support of breastfeeding' in community healthcare settings (see Weblinks). The BFI has also recently produced best practice standards for breastfeeding on neonatal units (see Ch. 21 regarding storage and expression of breast milk). There are numerous documents about breastfeeding and other aspects of infant feeding aimed at parents and/or health professionals such as those produced by the Department of Health, the National Childbirth Trust, La Lèche League, and Bliss (the premature baby society). In 2008, Best Beginnings launched the DVD 'From bump to breastfeeding', which is being distributed to all pregnant women in the UK (see Weblinks).

Despite greater focus on increasing the incidence and exclusivity of breastfeeding in the UK, rates remain among the lowest in Europe. In the 2005 Infant Feeding Survey (Bolling et al. 2005), breastfeeding initiation rates were 78% in England, 70% in Scotland, 67% in Wales and 63% in Northern Ireland: an increase of about 5% since 2000. However, the rates fell sharply to 63% at 1 week, 48% at 6 weeks and 25% at 6 months. The prevalence of exclusive breastfeeding had not increased, with 65% of mothers exclusively breastfeeding at birth but only 21% at 6 weeks and <2% at 6 months. Nine out of 10 mothers who gave up breastfeeding within 6 months stated that they would have preferred to breastfeed for longer. Overall, among all mothers ceasing to breastfeed, the single largest factor behind cessation of breastfeeding was 'insufficient milk', with 39% giving this as a reason.

A recent review commissioned by the former Health Development Agency concluded that, when implementing interventions to increase breastfeeding initiation and continuation rates, each locality should consider the best package of interventions to address the diverse needs of its local population group(s) (Dyson et al. 2009). Effective evidence-based interventions included routine implementation of the UNICEF UK BFI across NHS hospital trusts; an appropriate mix of education and support programmes routinely delivered by both health professionals/practitioners and peer supporters in accordance with local population needs; and changes to policy and practice within the community and hospital settings to support effective positioning and attachment, using a predominantly 'hands-off' approach, encouraging unrestricted baby-led breastfeeding, which helps prevent engorgement; and encouraging the combination of supportive care, teaching breastfeeding technique, sound information and reassurance for breastfeeding women with 'insufficient milk'.

Artificial feeding for the normal term infant

General considerations

The purpose of artificial feeding is to provide a satisfactory food for infants in situations where a substitute for breast milk is required. The 'ideal' artificial diet should:

- meet the nutrient needs of healthy infants
- be well tolerated without inducing metabolic stress or biochemical disturbance
- not result in short- or long-term morbidity.

In the early days of artificial milks, they frequently failed to meet any of these criteria – sometimes with serious consequences. Modern formulas come much closer to attaining these goals (Table 16.6).

Recommended dietary allowances for formula-fed infants

From a teleological point of view, breast milk should be the nutritional standard for formula-fed infants. Many of the current recommended daily allowances are based on the concentrations of nutrients in human milk. However, in constructing a formula from non-human milk components, account must be taken of: (1) the bioavailability; (2) the digestibility; and (3) the biological value of the nutrients, all of which may differ from those in human milk. Rather than attempting to replicate human milk, which in most respects is an impossible goal, there is increasing focus on aiming to achieve the outcomes seen in the breastfed infant.

Milk volume

Based on human lactational studies, fluid intakes of around 150 ml/kg/24 h are satisfactory for the first 3–4 months in formula-fed infants. However, this is only an approximate guideline: healthy infants fed on formula ad libitum (as with breastfed infants) will show considerable variations in intake in association with normal growth. There is increasing recognition that the milk intake of breastfed infants during the first few days of life is considerably lower than that of infants fed formula ad libitum during this period (Casey et al. 1986; Dollberg et al. 2001). It is important that lactating mothers are aware of this if they are to have confidence in their ability to provide 'sufficient' milk for their infants. The role of these early differences in milk intake and growth, and potential consequences for later health, are under investigation.

Artificial formula

Unmodified cow's milk

'Doorstep' milk is not recommended for infants in the first 12 months in the UK. Problems that may be encountered with cow's milk, or unmodified cow's milk formulas, include hyperosmolar dehydration associated with high renal solute load, hypocalcaemic fits associated with phosphate overload, casein curd obstruction, vitamin deficiency (e.g. rickets, scurvy) and iron-deficiency anaemia. These problems are rarely seen in infants fed modern formulas. Skimmed and semiskimmed milk should not be used because of their low energy and vitamin A contents. Indeed, the UK Department of Health recommends that fully skimmed milk should not be given before the age of 5 years (DHSS 1988).

Goat's milk

Goat's milk is not suitable for infant feeding because of its high solute load and low vitamin content. It is particularly deficient in folate, and severe megaloblastic anaemia may result if goat's milk is the sole feed.

Modern cow's milk-based formulas

Modern milk formulas have been extensively modified from their predecessors in their protein, lipid, electrolyte and trace nutrient composition. Table 16.7 shows the composition of the standard infant formulas available in the UK, and Table 16.8 the composition of follow-on formulas. There is no information on whether or not the more recent finer degrees of modification have resulted in significant benefits, but it seems reasonable on empirical grounds to manufacture products resembling human milk as closely as possible. The need for further 'humanisation' of infant formulas is still actively under investigation. Topical issues include lowering total protein content to, say, 1.2–1.4 g/100 ml (cf. 1.5 g/100 ml currently; Table 16.6); the addition of sources of long-chain polyunsaturated fatty acid (C20 or greater); and the addition of other factors found in human milk, including nucleotides (Ch. 39.1), oligosaccharides, probiotics, α-lactalbumin and bile salt-stimulated lipase.

Soya formulas

The problems encountered with earlier soya-based formulas have been largely overcome; formulas are now supplemented with methionine, taurine and carnitine, and contain adequate minerals to allow for losses due to phytate binding in the gut. They are able to support normal growth and bone mineralisation when used as the sole diet. However, some issues remain unresolved. Attention has been drawn to the potentially large amounts of plant oestrogen (phyto-oestrogen) that may be ingested by infants who are fully fed on soya formulas: studies have shown that infants fed soya formula have plasma concentrations of phyto-oestrogens hundreds of times higher than those fed breast milk or cow's milk formula (Setchell et al. 1997). However, a follow-up study of adults who had received either soya formula or cow's milk formula in infancy found no evidence of long-term effects of early soya exposure on either general or reproductive health (Strom et al. 2001).

Although many infants receive soya formulas because of suspected cow's milk allergy, it should be recognised that soya protein is itself potentially allergenic. Double-blind placebo-controlled challenges with soya milk in infants with proven allergy to cow's milk protein have suggested that around 5% of these infants are also intolerant of soya protein (Dean et al. 1993). In the UK, it is recommended that soya formulas should only be used following advice from a health professional.

Practical aspects of formula feeding
(see Weblinks)

The following points need emphasising.

1. Attention to sterility is vital, since powdered infant formulas are not sterile products. The European Food Safety Authority's Scientific Panel on Biological Hazards concluded that *Enterobacter sakazakii* and *Salmonella* are the microorganisms of greatest concern. Although infections with these microorganisms from formula milks are rare in healthy infants, the risks can be reduced by following the guidelines which recommend using freshly boiled water, cooled to no less than 70°C, and making up formula fresh for each feed. The poor microbiological standards of drinking water that may be found in developing countries, among other factors, make formula feeding highly undesirable in this situation. Bottled water should be the same standard as water from the public supply, but some marketed waters are unsuitable for infants; for example, 'natural mineral water' may contain unacceptable levels of carbon dioxide, sodium, nitrate and fluoride (DHSS 1988).

2. For high-risk infants (preterm, low-birthweight and immunocompromised), ready-to-feed liquid formulas are recommended as these are sterile.

3. Correct reconstitution of feeds with accurate use of the scoops provided by manufacturers is vital. A systematic review concluded that errors in the reconstitution of infant formulas are widespread, with a tendency to overconcentrate, although underconcentration also occurred. This review also highlighted the range of different scoop sizes produced by manufacturers (Renfrew et al. 2003).

Breast versus formula

The relevant question for the medical profession is whether or not there are clinical grounds for wishing to influence parental choice. In the developing world, the evidence that breastfeeding has a major influence on infant mortality and morbidity is well established and the case for medical intervention is strong. In the developed world, the situation is rather different: in spite of considerable speculation on the benefits of breastfeeding, it has been harder to prove major detrimental effects of bottle-feeding. Comparisons between breast- and bottle-fed infants are almost exclusively epidemiological, as it is not possible to randomise infants to one feeding regimen or another, and potential confounding by factors that differ between breast and formula-fed infants, such as social class and circumstances, has made it difficult to evaluate published data on the differences between breast- and bottle-fed babies in their subsequent health and development. Data from both randomised and observational studies are summarised below.

Experimental studies

The Promotion of Breastfeeding Intervention Trial (PROBIT) (Kramer et al. 2001), a cluster-randomised study conducted in Belarus, involved more than 17 000 mother and term-infant pairs from clinics assigned either to standard practice or to an intervention modelled on the UNICEF BFI, which increased the incidence and exclusivity of breastfeeding. Infants from the intervention group had a significantly lower risk of developing both gastroenteritis and eczema during the first year of life. Further follow-up of this cohort at age 6 years has reported significantly higher cognitive scores with the intervention (Kramer et al. 2008), but no effect on height, adiposity, blood pressure or child behaviour (Kramer et al. 2007).

Evidence for the benefits of breast milk has also come from a large randomised trial of diet during the neonatal period in preterm infants. Those who received human milk, whether mother's own or banked, were significantly less likely to develop necrotising entero-colitis or systemic infection, and showed better feed tolerance. More recently, longer term benefits have become apparent. The use of human milk was associated with lower blood pressure (Singhal et al. 2001), reduced insulin resistance (Singhal et al. 2004), a more favourable plasma lipid profile during adolescence (Singhal et al. 2003) and higher bone mass (Fewtrell et al. 2009).

Observational studies

Two recent systematic reviews and meta-analyses have examined data on the health effects of breastfeeding. Ip et al. (2009) concluded:

- A history of breastfeeding was associated with a reduction in the risk of acute otitis media, non-specific gastroenteritis, severe lower respiratory tract infections, atopic dermatitis, asthma (in young children), obesity, type 1 and 2 diabetes, childhood leukaemia and sudden infant death syndrome.
- There was no relationship between breastfeeding in term infants and cognitive performance after including studies that had measurements of maternal IQ.
- There were insufficient good-quality data to address the relationship between breastfeeding and cardiovascular diseases and infant mortality.
- A history of lactation was associated with a reduced risk of type 2 diabetes, breast and ovarian cancer in the mother.
- Early cessation of breastfeeding or no breastfeeding was also associated with an increased risk of maternal postpartum depression.

In a second review examining data on the long-term health effects of breastfeeding for the WHO, Horta et al. (2009) concluded that subjects who were breastfed experienced:

- lower mean blood pressure and total cholesterol
- higher performance in intelligence tests
- lower prevalence of overweight/obesity and type 2 diabetes.

Overall, these data suggest that there is sufficient evidence of clinical benefit to promote breastfeeding as the 'ideal' for term infants in developed countries. To help achieve this goal, better health education (starting at school) is required in order to promote a culture in which breastfeeding is regarded as the normal way to feed infants (see above). Nevertheless, while it is important to promote and protect breastfeeding, it is also necessary to ensure that the needs of bottle-feeding mothers are met, particularly as the majority of infants in countries such as the UK, even if exclusively breastfed initially, will receive some infant formula during the first year of life. A recent systematic review of the literature on parents' experiences of bottle-feeding found several consistent themes (Lakshman et al. 2009):

- Mothers who bottle-fed their babies experienced negative emotions such as guilt, anger, worry, uncertainty and a sense of failure.
- Mothers reported receiving little information on bottle-feeding and did not feel empowered to make decisions.
- Mistakes in preparation of bottle-feeds were common.

The reviewers concluded that inadequate information and support for mothers who decide to bottle-feed may put the health of their babies at risk. A variety of emotional benefits to the mother have been put forward for breastfeeding, but these may cease to be benefits if the mother has set her mind against feeding her baby this way.

Weblinks

http://www.babyfriendly.org.uk: UNICEF UK Baby Friendly Inititiative.

http://www.bestbeginnings.org.uk/from-bump-to-breastfeeding: Best Beginnings: DVD 'From bump to breastfeeding'.

http://www.dh.gov.uk/prod_consum_dh/groups/dh_digitalassets/documents/digitalasset/dh_100127.pdf: information for parents.

http://www.food.gov.uk/multimedia/pdfs/formulaguidance.pdf: detailed instructions

for the reconstitution of artificial feeds and the hygienic use of feeding utensils.

http://www.nice.org.uk/niceMedia/pdf/EAB_Breastfeeding_final_version.pdf: interventions to improve breastfeeding rates.

References

Adlerberth, I., Wold, A.E., 2009. Establishment of the gut microbiota in Western infants. Acta Paediatrica 98, 229–238.

Agostoni, C., Decsi, T., Fewtrell, M.S., et al., 2008. ESPGHAN Committee on Nutrition 2008 Complementary feeding: a commentary by the ESPGHAN Committee on Nutrition. J Paediatr Gastroenterol Nutr 46, 99–110.

American Academy of Pediatrics. 2003. Committee on Nutrition, Section of Breast-feeding Medicine 2003 Clinical report. Prevention of rickets and vitamin D deficiency: new guidelines for vitamin D intake. Pediatrics 111, 908–910.

Ashraf, S., Mughal, M.Z., 2002. The prevalence of rickets among

non-Caucasian children. Arch Dis Child 87, 263–264.

Bernhart, F.W., 1961. Correlation between growth-rate of the suckling of various species and the percentage of total calories from protein in the milk. Nature 191, 358–360.

Birkbeck, J.A., Scott, H.F., 1980. 25-Hydroxycholecalciferol serum levels in breastfed infants. Archives of Disease in Childhood 55, 691–695.

Boersma, E.R., Lanting, C.I., 2000. Environmental exposure to polychlorinated biphenyls (PCBs) and dioxins. Consequences for longterm neurological and cognitive development of the child. Advances in Experimental Medicine and Biology 478, 271–287.

Bolling, K., Grant, C., Hamlyn, B., et al., 2005. Infant Feeding Survey 2005. The Information Centre. Available online at: http://www.ic.nhs.uk/statistics-and-data-collections/health-and-lifestyles-related-surveys/infant-feeding-survey/infant-feeding-survey-2005.

Carlson, S.E., 1985. Human milk non-protein nitrogen: occurrence and possible functions. Advances in Pediatrics 32, 43–70.

Casey, C.E., Neifert, M.R., Seacat, J.M., et al., 1986. Nutrient intake by breast-fed infants during the first five days after birth. Am J Dis Child 140, 933–936.

Chantry, C.J., Howard, C.R., Auinger, P., 2006. Full breastfeeding duration and associated decrease in respiratory tract infection in US children. Pediatrics 117, 425–432.

Chantry, C.J., Howard, C.R., Auinger, P., 2007. Full breastfeeding duration and risk for iron deficiency in US infants. Breastfeed Med 2, 63–73.

Chaparro, C.M., Neufeld, L.M., Tena Alavez, G., et al., 2006. Effect of timing of umbilical cord clamping on iron status in Mexican infants: a randomised controlled trial. Lancet 367, 1997–2004.

Dean, T.P., Adler, B.R., Ruge, F., et al., 1993. In vitro allergenicity of cow's milk substitutes. Clinical and Experimental Allergy 23, 205–210.

DHSS. 1977. The Composition of Mature Human Milk. Report on Health and Social Subjects No. 12. HMSO, London.

DHSS. 1980. Artificial Feeds for the Young Infant: Report on Health and Social Subjects No. 18. Report of the Committee on Medical Aspects of Food Policy. HMSO, London.

DHSS. 1981. Present Day Practice in Infant Feeding, 1980. Reports on Health and Social Subjects, No 20. HMSO, London.

DHSS. 1988. Present Day Practice in Infant Feeding, third report. Report on Health and Social Subjects No. 32. HMSO, London.

Dollberg, S., Lahav, S., Mimouni, F.B., 2001. A comparison of intakes of breast-fed and bottle fed infants during the first two days of life. J Am Coll Nutr 20, 209–211.

Dowell, T.B., Joyston-Bechal, S., 1981. Fluoride supplements – age related dosage. British Dental Journal 150, 273–275.

Dyson, L., Renfrew, M., McFadden, A., et al., 2009. Promotion of Breastfeeding Initiation and Duration. Evidence into Practice Briefing. Available online at: http://www.nice.org.uk/aboutnice/ whoweare/aboutthehda/hdapublications/ promotion_of_breastfeeding_initiation_ and_duration_evidence_into_practice_ briefing.jsp.

Fewtrell, M.S., Williams, J.E., Singhal, A., et al., 2009. Early diet and peak bone mass: 20 year follow-up of a randomized trial of early diet in infants born preterm. Bone 45, 142–149.

Flores, H.C., Cromwell, J.W., Leventhal, J.R., et al., 1993. Does previous breast feeding affect maternal donor renal allograft outcome? A single-institution experience. Transplantation Proceedings 25, 212.

Garry, P., Owen, G.M., Hooper, E.M., et al., 1981. Iron absorption from human milk and formula with and without iron supplementation. Pediatric Research 15, 822–828.

Grantham-McGregor, S., Ani, C., 2001. A review of studies on the effect of iron deficiency on cognitive development in children. Journal of Nutrition 131, 649S–668S.

Grulee, C.G., Sanford, H.N., Herron, P.H., 1935. Breast and artificial feeding. Journal of the American Medical Association 104, 1986–1988.

Hamosh, M., 1996. Digestion in the newborn. Clinics in Perinatology 23, 191–210.

Hamprecht, K., Maschmann, J., Vochem, M., et al., 2001. Epidemiology of transmission of cytomegalovirus from mother to preterm infant by breastfeeding. Lancet 357, 513–518.

Hanson, L.A., 1998. Breastfeeding provides passive and likely long-lasting active immunity. Annals of Allergy, Asthma, and Immunology 81, 523–533.

Haschke, F., Vanura, H., Male, C., et al., 1993. Iron nutrition and growth of breast- and formula-fed infants during the first 9 months of life. Journal of Pediatric Gastroenterology and Nutrition 16, 151–156.

Horta, B.L., Bahl, R., Martinés, J.C., et al., 2009. Evidence on the Long-term Effects of Breastfeeding: Systematic Review and Meta-analyses. World Health Organization, Geneva.

Howie, P.W., Forsyth, J.S., Ogston, S.A., et al., 1990. Protective effect of breast feeding against infection. British Medical Journal 300, 11–16.

Ip, S., Chung, M., Raman, G., et al., 2009. A summary of the Agency for Healthcare Research and Quality's evidence report on breastfeeding in developed countries. Breastfeed Med (Suppl 1), S17–S30.

Jensen, R.G., 1996. The lipids in human milk. Progress in Lipid Research 35, 53–92.

Joint FAO/WHO Expert Consultation on Human Vitamin and Mineral Requirements. 1998. Iron Vitamin and Mineral Requirements in Human Nutrition, second ed. WHO Library Cataloguing-in-Publication Data. World Health Organization, Bangkok.

Kramer, M.S., Kakuma, R., 2002. Optimal duration of exclusive breastfeeding. Cochrane Database of Systematic Reviews (1), CD003517.

Kramer, M., Chalmers, B., Hodnett, E., et al., 2001. Promotion of breastfeeding intervention trial (PROBIT): a randomized trial in the Republic of Belarus. Journal of the American Medical Association 285, 413–420.

Kramer, M.S., Guo, T., Platt, R.W., et al., 2003. Infant growth and health outcomes associated with 3 compared with 6 mo of exclusive breastfeeding. American Journal of Clinical Nutrition 78, 291–295.

Kramer, M.S., Matush, L., Vanilovich, I., et al., 2007. Effects of prolonged and exclusive breastfeeding on child height, weight, adiposity, and blood pressure at age 6.5 y: evidence from a large randomized trial. Am J Clin Nutr 86, 1717–1721.

Kramer, M.S., Aboud, F., Minorova, E., et al., 2008. Breastfeeding and child cognitive development: new evidence from a large randomized trial. Arch Gen Psychiatry 65, 578–584.

Lakshman, R., Ogilvie, D., Ong, K.K., 2009. Mothers' experiences of bottle-feeding: a systematic review of qualitative and quantitative studies. Arch Dis Child 94, 596–601.

Leaf, A.A., 2007. Vitamins for babies and young children. Arch Dis Child 92, 160–164.

Little, R.E., Anderson, K.W., Ervin, C.H., et al., 1989. Maternal alcohol use during breast-feeding and infant mental and motor development at one year. New England Journal of Medicine 321, 425–430.

Little, R.E., Northstone, K., Golding, J., et al., 2002. Alcohol, breastfeeding and development at 18 months. Pediatrics 109, E72.

Lucas, A., Lucas, P.J., Baum, J.D., 1980. The Nipple Shield Sampling System: a device for measuring the dietary intake of breast fed infants. Early Human Development 4, 365–372.

Lucas, A., Ewing, E., Roberts, S.B., et al., 1987. How much energy does the breast fed baby consume and expend? British Medical Journal 295, 75–77.

Macy, I.G., Kelly, H.J., Sloan, R.E., 1953. The Composition of Milks. Publication 254. National Academy of Science, National Research Council, Washington, DC.

Minamishima, I., Ueda, K., Minematsu, T., et al., 1994. Role of breast milk in acquisition of cytomegalovirus infection. Microbiology and Immunology 38, 549–552.

Moriya, T., Sasaki, F., Mizui, M., et al., 1995. Transmission of hepatitis C virus from mothers to infants: its frequency and risk factors revisited. Biomedicine and Pharmacotherapy 49, 59–64.

Mughal, M.Z., Salama, H., Greenaway, T., et al., 1999. Florid rickets associated with prolonged breast feeding without vitamin D supplementation. British Medical Journal 318, 39–40.

National Collaborating Centre for Women's and Children's Health. 2003. Antenatal Care: Routine Care for the Healthy Pregnant Woman. RCOG, London.

Paricio Talayero, J.M., Lizan-Garcia, M., Otero Puime, A., et al., 2006. Full breastfeeding and hospitalization as a result of infections in the first year of life. Pediatrics 118, e92–e99.

Prentice, A., Ewing, G., Roberts, S.B., et al., 1987. The nutrition role of breast-milk IgA and lactoferrin. Acta Paediatrica Scandinavica 76, 592–598.

Prescott, S.L., Smith, P., Tang, M., et al., 2008. The importance of early complementary feeding in the development of oral tolerance: Concerns and controversies. Pediatr Allerg Immunol 19, 375.

Quigley, M.A., Kelly, Y.J., Sacker, A., 2007. Breastfeeding and hospitalization for diarrheal and respiratory infection in the United Kingdom Millenium Cohort Study. Pediatrics 119, e837–e842.

Quigley, M.A., Kelly, Y.J., Sacker, A., 2009. Infant feeding, solid foods and hospitalisation in the first 8 months after birth. Arch Dis Child 94, 148–150.

Rebhan, B., Kohlhuber, M., Fromme, H., et al., 2009. Breastfeeding duration and exclusivity associated with infants' health and growth: data from a prospective cohort study in Bavaria, Germany. Acta Paediatrica 98, 974.

Reilly, J.J., Ashworth, S., Wells, J.C.K., 2005. Metabolisable energy consumption in the exclusively breastfed infant aged 3–6 months from the developed world: a systematic review. Br J Nutr 94, 56–63.

Renfrew, M., Ansell, P., Macleod, K.L., 2003. Formula feed preparation: helping reduce the risks; a systematic review. Archives of Disease in Childhood 88, 855–858.

Roberts, C.C., Chan, G.M., Follard, D., et al., 1981. Adequate bone mineralization in breast fed infants. Journal of Pediatrics 99, 192–196.

Saarinen, U.M., Siimes, M.A., 1979. Iron absorption from breast milk, cow's milk and iron supplemented formula. Pediatric Research 13, 143–147.

Sack, J., 1980. Hormones in milk. In: Firer, S., Eidelman, A.I. (Eds.), Human Milk, Its Biological and Social Value. Excerpta Medica, Amsterdam, pp. 56–61.

Savino, F., Liguori, S.A., 2008. Update on breast milk hormones: leptin, ghrelin and adiponectin. Clinical Nutrition 27, 42–47.

Schlesinger, J.J., Covelli, H.D., 1977. Evidence for transmission of lymphocyte responses to tuberculin by breast-feeding. Lancet 2, 529–532.

Setchell, K.D., Zimmer-Nechemias, L., Cai, J., et al., 1997. Exposure of infants to phyto-oestrogens from soy-based infant formula. Lancet 350, 23–27.

Singhal, A., Cole, T.J., Lucas, A., 2001. Early nutrition in preterm infants and later blood pressure: two cohorts after randomised trials. Lancet 357, 413–419.

Singhal, A., Fewtrell, M., Cole, T.J., et al., 2003. Low nutrient intake and early growth for later insulin resistance in adolescents born preterm. Lancet 361, 1089–1097.

Singhal, A., Cole, T., Fewtrell, M., et al., 2004. Breast milk feeding and the lipoprotein profile in adolescents born preterm. Lancet 363, 1571–1578.

Strom, B.L., Schinnar, R., Ziegler, E.E., et al., 2001. Exposure to soy-based formula in infancy and endocrinological and reproductive outcomes in young adulthood. Journal of the American Medical Association 286, 2402–2403.

Uehara, S., Abe, Y., Saito, T., et al., 1993. The incidence of vertical transmission of hepatitis C virus. Tohoku Journal of Experimental Medicine 171, 195–202.

Wilhelm, M., Wittsiepe, J., Lemm, F., et al., 2008. The Duisburg birth cohort study: influence of the prenatal exposure to PCDD/Fs and dioxin-like PCBs on thyroid hormone status in newborns and neurodevelopment of infants until the age of 24 months. Mutat Res 659, 83–92.

World Health Organization. 2008. HIV transmission through Breastfeeding: A Review of Available Evidence, 2007 Update. WHO Library Cataloguing-in-Publication Data. Available online at: http://whqlibdoc.who.int/publications/2008/9789241596596_eng.pdf (HIV and breastfeeding).

Part 3: **Feeding low-birthweight infants**

Mary Fewtrell   Sirinuch Chomtho   Alan Lucas

General considerations

The principal matters to be decided when planning enteral feeding in low-birthweight (LBW) infants are which diet, which route of administration and what feeding schedule should be selected. Valuable short-term studies have been performed on preterm infant feeding, but only more recently have data become available on the longer term effects of early nutrition for later health and development. Information of this nature is critical in order to assess the value of current practice.

Choice of diet

A wide range of diets have been used for feeding LBW infants, including the following:

- human milk:
  - mother's own: 'preterm milk' (PTM)
  - banked donor milk (expressed breast milk or drip breast milk)
  - fortified human milk
  - human milk formulas (separated and reconstituted human milk)
- 'term' infant formulas:
  - cow's milk-based
  - soya-based
- special 'preterm' infant formulas
- parenteral feeding (see Ch. 17):
  - partial
  - total.

Human milk

There is major interest in human milk for feeding LBW infants, and the practice of encouraging mothers to provide milk for their own preterm infants has become widespread. The value of breast milk in neonatal intensive care needs critical appraisal.

Nutritional considerations

Unmodified human milk may not always meet the theoretical requirements of LBW infants for several nutrients, including:

- protein (especially when 'mature' donor milk is used)
- energy (especially donor drip breast milk)
- sodium
- calcium, phosphorus and magnesium
- trace elements, e.g. iron, zinc and copper
- certain vitamins (e.g. B_2, B_6, folic acid, C, D, E and K).

However, human milk does have theoretical nutritional advantages compared with formulas, including the composition and easier absorption of its fats and the bioavailability of certain trace metals. Formulas designed to meet the calculated nutrient needs of preterm infants impose a greater renal solute load on the baby than that of human milk.

Infection and necrotising enterocolitis

In a large study, with randomised dietary assignments, Lucas and Cole (1990b) showed that preterm babies fed exclusively on formula had six times more confirmed necrotising enterocolitis (NEC) than infants fed exclusively on breast milk (fresh or pasteurised – but without the use of breast milk fortifiers) and three times the NEC rate of those fed formula in conjunction with breast milk. The authors suggested that using either raw maternal milk or pasteurised donor milk in the early diet of preterm infants might prevent about 500 cases of NEC each year in the UK. This finding was supported by a recent Cochrane systematic review of five randomised controlled trials (RCTs) comparing formula and donor breast milk (DBM) (Quigley et al. 2007). In a non-randomised analysis, Schanler (2005) reported that, compared with groups of infants fed DBM or preterm formula (PTF), those who received maternal breast milk had fewer episodes of late-onset sepsis and/or NEC and total infection-related events, a shorter duration of hospital stay and fewer Gram-negative organisms isolated from blood cultures than did the other groups. Most recently, Sullivan et al. (2010) reported the results of a randomised trial in which preterm babies receiving mother's own breast milk (MBM) were randomised to receive either a completely human milk-based diet, using pasteurised donor human milk-based fortifiers and/or DBM if there was insufficient MBM, or a conventional bovine milk fortifier and/or preterm infant formula. Babies who received the human milk-based diet had significantly lower rates of NEC ($p < 0.02$) and, especially, NEC requiring surgical intervention ($p = 0.007$). There was no difference between groups in growth or rates of late-onset sepsis. An RCT of feeding methods in babies at high risk of NEC because they had absent or reversed end-diastolic blood flow in the umbilical artery (the ADEPT trial) showed no difference in outcome whether feeds were initiated early or were delayed (Leaf et al. in press). Some babies took over a month to establish full feeds.

Allergy

There is a theoretical possibility that feeding the preterm infant with cow's milk proteins at a time when gut permeability may be increased (Zachariassen et al. 2010) could raise the chance of later cow's milk allergy. Indeed, Lucas et al. (1984b) showed that preterm neonates rapidly developed latent sensitisation to cow's milk. The feeding of human milk (versus formula) was associated with decreased intestinal permeability of preterm infants at 28 days of age (Shulman et al. 1998a). Many of the bioactive factors in human milk function at the level of the gastrointestinal tract to protect the infant from foreign antigens. At the 18-month follow-up of a randomised trial of early nutrition, Lucas et al. (1990a) found no overall difference in allergic reactions between infants fed formula or DBM, but in the subgroup of infants with atopy in one or more first-degree relatives, early formula feeding was associated with twice the incidence of subsequent allergic reactions compared with those in the exclusively human milk-fed group (for eczema the respective incidences were 41% and 16%).

Gastrointestinal 'tolerance'

Gastrointestinal 'tolerance' of human milk is greater than that of formulas. Cavell (1982) has shown that human milk passes through

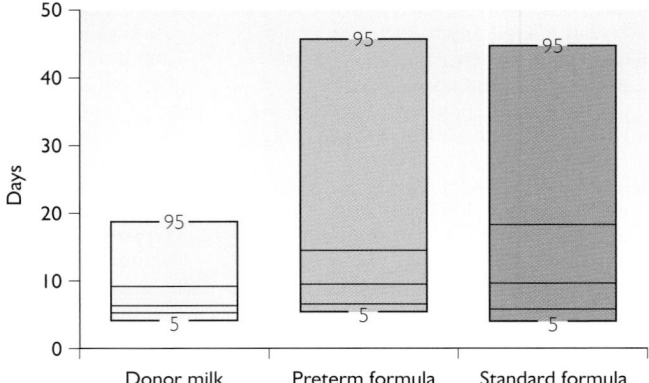

Fig. 16.4 Days to attain full enteral feeds according to diet in over 300 preterm infants under 1850 g birthweight. Data are represented in centiles; the horizontal lines in the data bar for each diet represent, from bottom to top, the 5th, 25th, 50th, 75th and 95th centiles for the number of postnatal days to reach an enteral intake of 150 mg/kg/24 h.

the stomach faster than formula in preterm infants, and intestinal lactase activity (a marker of intestinal maturity) is greater in infants fed human milk compared with formula and greater in those fed early in life (Shulman et al. 1998a, b). It often takes substantially longer to establish full enteral feeding in infants fed formula: in a five-centre study, 95% of infants fed breast milk were on full feeds by 18 days, whereas the 95th centile for formula-fed babies was more than 40 days, owing to a proportion of infants in whom it was difficult to achieve feed tolerance (Fig. 16.4). These data have implications for the design of feeding regimens (see below).

Developmental scores

Preterm babies fed on their own MBM have been shown to have higher developmental scores at 18 months and higher IQs at 7.5–8 years than those fed on other diets, even after adjusting for a range of demographic, social and clinical factors that might confound this comparison (Morley et al. 1988; Lucas et al. 1992b). At 15–16-year follow-up, the percentage of expressed breast milk in the neonatal diet correlated significantly with verbal IQ and white-matter volume (from magnetic resonance imaging) in males (Isaacs et al. 2009). Whether these findings reflect a failure to adjust for further (unknown) confounding factors, or whether fresh human milk has a beneficial effect on development, is an important question for investigation. The latter explanation is favoured by the observation that infants fed banked breast milk had higher developmental scores at 18 months than those fed term formulas, despite the lower macronutrient content of banked breast milk (Lucas et al. 1994). Developmental outcome in term small-for-gestational-age infants at 18 months was also better among those breastfed than among those fed 'term' or 'nutrient-enriched' formula (Morley et al. 2004).

Long-term cardiovascular health

Follow-up of adolescents born preterm and randomised to receive banked breast milk or PTF during the neonatal period has shown significantly lower blood pressure and a more favourable lipid profile in those who received human milk (Singhal et al. 2001, 2004). Breast milk-fed children had a low-density lipoprotein : high-density lipoprotein cholesterol ratio that was 14% lower than formula-fed children, an effect size very similar to the 10–16% benefit in this ratio associated with breastfeeding reported in subjects born at term. The lower mean blood pressure seen in children who had received human milk (81.9 (SD 7.8) mmHg versus 86.1 (SD 6.5) mmHg) was seen whether fresh MBM or banked DBM was used. The average effect size seen in this study is larger than that produced by any non-pharmacological method of reducing blood pressure during adult life (weight loss, exercise, diet). Moreover, this magnitude of reduction in blood pressure in an adult population would be expected to reduce the prevalence of hypertension by 17%, the risk of cardiovascular disease by 6% and the risk of strokes and transient ischaemic attacks by 15%.

Interestingly, children who received human milk also had evidence of both lower insulin resistance (Singhal et al. 2003) and better arterial distensibility (an early marker of vascular disease) than children from the PTF group. These effects seemed to be mediated by growth predominantly during the first 2 weeks of postnatal life, and led to the growth acceleration hypothesis – that promoting growth early in the neonatal period may not be optimal for certain aspects of longer term cardiovascular health (Singhal and Lucas 2004) (see below).

Types of breast milk

The composition of breast milk depends on its source, the mode of its collection and on the postnatal and postconceptional age of the donor; it can be further modified by its subsequent treatment.

Preterm milk

The milk of mothers who have delivered preterm infants – so-called preterm milk or PTM – has a different composition from that of mothers delivered at term, with higher total nitrogen, protein nitrogen, immune proteins, total lipid, medium-chain fatty acids, energy, vitamins, some minerals (e.g. calcium, sodium), and trace elements (e.g. zinc, copper) and with a raised IgA content in early lactation (Schanler and Atkinson 2005). The reasons for these differences remain speculative but may relate to the low volume often produced by PTM donors (Lucas and Hudson 1984). Preterm colostrum may also have greater potential for preventing infection than term colostrum owing to its higher IgA, lysozyme, lactoferrin and living cells (Lawrence and Lawrence 2005). PTM is thus more suitable than term donor milk for feeding preterm infants, particularly in view of its higher concentration of protein. However, protein intakes from PTM are very variable, and by the second month of PTM production protein concentrations often fall to values at which theoretical needs would be met only by very high-volume intakes. PTM may be given raw to the mother's own infant, in which case antimicrobial components will remain intact. Neither microbiological examination nor pasteurisation is necessary in this situation, provided that the collected milk is refrigerated adequately and fed to the infant within 48 hours, or at most 72 hours, or if it is frozen.

Many mothers who elect at the outset to provide milk for their own infants, either totally or partially, fail to do so. In over 600 MBM-fed infants from several centres studied between 1982 and 1985, maternal milk constituted less than 50% of total enteral intake. A more recent study of 243 extremely low-birthweight (ELBW: gestational age 23–29 weeks, recruited from 1997 to 2001) babies from the USA found that around 27% of the mothers were able to sustain lactation to meet the needs of their extremely premature infants (Schanler and Atkinson 2005). Factors contributing to lack of success in producing sufficient PTM include physical separation of mother and child, inadequate support, the inherent difficulty of maintaining the milk supply by manual or mechanical expression, lack of motivation and, not least, poor advice.

The difficulties faced by mothers trying to provide milk for their preterm infant must not be underestimated. They may need to express milk for a period of weeks or months in the absence of significant suckling stimulus and in the presence of a great deal of stress, a potent inhibitor of the milk ejection reflex. Simple measures have been shown to improve milk volume. These include increasing the frequency of expression (around six to eight times a day as a minimum), kangaroo care or skin-to-skin contact, relaxation tapes and avoidance of smoking. There is strong evidence that short periods of kangaroo skin-to-skin contact increase the duration of any breastfeeding for 1 month after discharge (risk ratio (RR) 4.76, 95% confidence interval (CI) 1.19–19.10) and for more than 6 weeks (RR 1.95, 95% CI 1.03–3.70) among clinically stable infants in industrialised settings (Renfrew et al. 2009).

The type of breast pump and mode of expression may also be important. Jones et al. (2001) showed that the use of breast massage prior to pumping and the use of simultaneous as opposed to sequential pumping both increased milk volumes in mothers using the Ameda electric breast pump, and that there was an additive effect of massage and simultaneous pumping. Recently, there has been some interest in the design of more physiological breast pumps – that is, using alternative strategies to simple suction, which is inherently unphysiological in human lactation (Fewtrell et al. 2001a). Pharmacological interventions have also been investigated. Some data suggest that use of dopamine antagonists to increase prolactin concentrations may improve milk production of preterm mothers experiencing lactation failure at or beyond 3 weeks postpartum, without substantially altering the nutrient composition (Campbell-Yeo et al. 2010). Oxytocin can theoretically enhance the let-down reflex, although a recent RCT did not show significant advantages over placebo in final milk production in preterm mothers when used early in the postnatal period (Fewtrell et al. 2006).

Expressed donor milk

Expressed DBM can be fore milk or hind milk, obtained either before or after the donor's own infant has fed from the breast; these two types of milk will have, respectively, lower or higher fat and energy contents than milk received by the breastfed infant. Mature donor milk will have a lower protein, sodium, zinc and copper content than that of milk produced in early lactation. A Cochrane systematic review (Quigley et al. 2007) compared outcomes in preterm infants fed DBM or formula and identified only eight studies, five of them RCTs. Meta-analysis of data from five trials suggested that infants fed DBM had a significantly reduced risk of developing NEC (typical relative risk 2.5), although feeding DBM was also associated with slower neonatal growth. Most of the studies considered were 20–30 years old and from an era when DBM was fed without fortification or mineral supplements, often as the sole diet. It is not clear whether similar effects would be seen when DBM is used in a more 'modern' context – as a supplement to MBM and supplemented with minerals and/or fortifiers. Only one trial (Schanler et al. 2005) compared nutrient-fortified DBM versus PTF as supplement to MBM. The study was unable to establish any short-term benefit for DBM over PTF. More recently, a human milk-based fortifier and PTF have become available and use of these products was associated with lower rates of NEC in a randomised trial when compared with bovine fortifiers and formulas (Sullivan et al. 2010).

Drip breast milk

This is the milk that drips spontaneously from the contralateral breast during feeding in a proportion of lactating mothers – about 20% produce significant quantities. Although previously used to feed preterm infants, including in older clinical studies, drip breast milk has a similar composition to fore milk, with very low fat and energy content (often around 50 kcal/100 ml in pooled milk); this method of collecting DBM is now not recommended and donor mothers are advised to express milk by hand or using a mechanical breast pump.

Fortified human milk

One solution to overcome the nutrient deficits in human milk for the preterm infant is to add a fortifier containing protein, energy, macrominerals, trace minerals and a comprehensive range of vitamins. Several are now commercially available (Table 16.9), usually in the form of a powder which is added to a fixed volume of milk. However, the addition of nutrients to a complex biological medium such as milk poses theoretical problems. In particular, breast milk varies greatly in composition, and the addition of a fixed supplement may result in some infants exceeding the upper recommended limit for certain nutrients while others remain below desirable intake levels. Fortification may also influence nutrient availability or alter the biological properties of human milk.

Table 16.9 Major nutrient composition of breast milk fortifiers available in the UK (amounts given are what would be added to 100 ml of human milk)*

	COW & GATE NUTRIPREM	SMA BREAST MILK FORTIFIER
Energy		
kJ	65	62
kcal	15	14.6
Protein (g)	0.8	1.0
Carbohydrate (g)	3	2.73
Fat (g)	Nil	0.16
Sodium (mg)	20	18
Potassium (mg)	40	28
Calcium (mg)	65	90
Phosphorus (mg)	46	46
Magnesium (mg)	6	3
Vitamin A (μg)	130	270
Vitamin D (μg)	5.0	7.6
Vitamin E (mg)	2.6	3.0
Vitamin K (μg)	6.3	11.0
Osmolarity (mOsmol/l)	375	182

*Manufacturers' data.

A review for the Cochrane collaboration, last updated in 2003, concluded that the use of multinutrient fortifiers is associated with short-term improvements in weight gain, linear growth, head growth, nitrogen retention and blood urea levels but that there is currently no evidence of long-term benefit, and insufficient evidence to be reassured that there are no deleterious effects (Kuschel and Harding 2004). It remains to be established whether overall outcome in infants fed fortified breast milk is better than that in infants fed a PTF when both diets provide similar nutrient intakes.

A small RCT (Arslanoglu et al. 2006) showed that adjustable fortification of human milk (based on the infant's blood urea concentration) resulted in greater weight and head circumference gains, which were significantly correlated with protein intake, than standard fortification. More recently, a 'humanised' milk fortifier, produced from pooled DBM processed to ensure the highest safety standards, has been developed. Clinical trials of the new fortifier, which avoids any exposure to cow's milk, have shown a significantly reduced risk of NEC, although this product is not yet commercially available (Sullivan et al. 2010).

Human milk banking

The National Institute for Health and Clinical Excellence (2010) has recently issued guidance on DBM banks and further advice can be obtained from the UK Association for Milk Banking (see Weblink). It is important to appreciate that, once milk has been collected, bacterially decontaminated, stored, frozen and thawed, pasteurised, exposed to light, aliquoted and instilled into feeding apparatus, it may have undergone qualitative alterations that render it significantly different from milk obtained by an infant during normal suckling.

Screening of breast milk donors for human immunodeficiency virus (HIV 1 and 2), human T-lymphotropic virus (HTLV type I and II), hepatitis B and C virus, and syphilis is advised (National Institute for Health and Clinical Excellence 2010). The risk of acquiring HIV from DBM is unknown, but there have been no reported cases of preterm infants infected in this way. Published evidence suggests that pasteurisation destroys HIV (Eglin and Wilkinson 1987). More recent studies reported that 'flash-heat' treatment of breast milk (similar to high-temperature, short-time pasteurisation) can be used to inactivate HIV-1 in resource-poor settings (Volk et al. 2010).

There are some concerns about cytomegalovirus (CMV) seroconversion in preterm infants receiving breast milk from seropositive mothers. However, the relative incidence of human milk-associated CMV infection and the severity of disease in premature infants are very low with no developmental abnormality at 24-month follow-up (Miron et al. 2005). Differences in CMV acquisition from fresh or frozen milk have been suggested and short-term high-temperature pasteurisation techniques were found to prevent CMV transmission more effectively than freezing (Schanler 2005). Different strategies to inactivate CMV and preserve non-nutritive benefits of breast milk are under investigation (Goelz et al. 2009).

'Term' infant formulas

For many years, formulas designed for full-term infants were used to feed LBW infants. Such formulas (Table 16.7) contain around 1.5 of protein/100 ml and 65–70 kcal/100 ml. Fed at 180–200 ml/kg, they provide only 2.7–3.0 g protein/kg/24 h – below the limit recommended for preterm infants (Table 16.2). Sodium, calcium and phosphorus intakes, together with those of several trace nutrients, do not meet the calculated needs of LBW infants. Data from a large multicentre trial show that infants fed standard formulas grow more slowly in the short term than those fed PTF, and have substantially lower motor and mental development scores at 18 months and lower IQs at 7.5–8 years (Lucas et al. 1990c, 1998). In our view, standard formulas have no place in the future management of preterm infants under 2 kg body weight, and PTF should be used in their place. Soya formula should not be used for feeding LBW infants.

Special preterm infant formulas

In recent years, a variety of formulas have been designed to meet the theoretical nutrient needs of LBW infants (see Chapter 16 part 1). These formulas (Table 16.10) vary significantly in their detailed composition, and continue to evolve. Clinical trials have shown

that such formulas may carry a number of short-term advantages over unsupplemented human milk: they promote faster weight, length and head circumference gain (see below), reduce hospital stay and reduce the incidence of hyponatraemia, bone disease of prematurity, hypophosphataemia, hyperbilirubinaemia and some vitamin deficiencies. More importantly, at follow-up, infants previously fed PTF have an advantage over those fed standard term formula in linear growth, developmental scores and IQ (Lucas et al. 1998).

Diets for preterm infants: overview

In summary, the available evidence suggests that human milk has an important place in neonatal intensive care. Many infants tolerate human milk better than formula, and enteral feeds can be

Table 16.10 Nutrient content of low-birthweight formulas available in the UK (per 100 ml)

COMPOSITION PER 100 ml	MATURE HUMAN MILK DHSS*	MACY et al.[†]	APTAMIL (MILUPA)	NUTRIPREM 1 PRETERM[‡] (COW & GATE)	SMA GOLD PREM 1[‡] (WYETH)
Macronutrients					
Protein[§] (g)	1.34	1.45	2.5	2.5	2.2
Fat (g)	4.2	3.8	4.4	4.4	4.4
Saturates (g)	50.1	52	1.8	1.8	2.2
Total LCP (mg)			41	41	43
DHA (mg)			20	20	17
AA (mg)			15	15	26
Carbohydrate (g)					
Total	7.0	7.0	7.6	7.6	8.4
Sugars	7.0	7.0	6.8	6.8	4.5
Energy					
kcal	70	68	80	80	82
kJ	293	285	335	335	343
Minerals (mg)					
Calcium	35	33	120	100	101
Chloride	43	43	68	68	67
Magnesium	2.8	4.0	7.9	7.9	8.2
Phosphorus	15	15	66	66	61
Potassium	60	55	82	82	74
Sodium	15	15	50	50	44
Trace elements (µg)					
Copper	39	40	80	80	90
Iodine	7	7	25	25	10
Iron	76	150	1400	1400	1400
Manganese	ND	0.7	10	10	4.8
Zinc	295	530	900	900	800
Osmolarity (mosmol/l)	88	91	315	315	202

Table 16.10 Continued

COMPOSITION PER 100 ml	MATURE HUMAN MILK DHSS*	MACY et al.[†]	APTAMIL (MILUPA)	NUTRIPREM 1 PRETERM[‡] (COW & GATE)	SMA GOLD PREM 1[‡] (WYETH)
Vitamins					
A retinol (µg)	60	53	180	180	185
B₁ thiamin (µg)	16	16	140	140	140
B₂ riboflavin (µg)	31	42.6	200	200	200
B₆ pyridoxine (µg)	6	11	120	120	120
B₁₂ cyanocobalamin (µg)	0.01	Trace	0.27	0.27	0.19
Biotin (µg)	0.76	0.4	3.0	3.0	2.4
Folic acid (µg)	5.2	0.18	28	28	29
Niacin (µg)	230	172	2400	2400	2400
C ascorbic acid (mg)	3.8	4.3	13	13	15
D cholecalciferol (µg)	0.01	0.01	3.0	3.0	3.4
E α-tocopherol (mg)	0.35	0.56	3.0	3.0	3.3
K phytomenadione (µg)	ND	1.7	6.0	6.0	6.3
Other (mg)					
Carnitine	ND	ND	1.8	1.8	2.6
Choline	ND	9	13	13	15
Inositol	ND	39	40	40	30
Taurine	4.8	ND	5.5	5.5	5.7
Nucleotides			3.2	3.2	

*DHSS (1977, 1980, 1983).
[†]Macy et al. (1983) and Mettler (1976).
[‡]Manufacturer's information.
[§]Total nitrogen × 6.38.
ND, not determined; LCP, long-chain polyunsaturated fatty acids; DHA, docosahexaenoic acid; AA, arachidonic acid.

established faster, reducing the requirement for parenteral nutrition (with its known hazards: see Ch. 17). The use of breast milk is likely to be associated with a reduction in the incidence of NEC and systemic infection, and is associated with improved cognitive outcome, lower blood pressure, more favourable plasma lipid profile and higher bone mass during childhood and adolescence. In addition, the slower initial growth rates seen in infants receiving human milk may be beneficial for later insulin resistance and arterial distensibility. However, in the preterm population, the risks and benefits of promoting growth must be balanced; poor early growth may have adverse consequences for short-term survival and for later cognitive development (Ehrenkranz et al. 2006) and bone health, whereas promoting growth (particularly during very early postnatal life) may be bad for later cardiovascular risk. On balance, in this group of infants current data clearly support the promotion of growth, since the later cardiovascular outcome of infants who grow well is no worse than that of infants born at term.

Our recommendation is to use breast milk, preferably the mother's own, but donor milk if it is not available, to establish enteral feeds (up to 150 ml/kg) in infants of 28 weeks' gestation or less and in infants who have had prolonged intravenous feeding (when the gut may be atrophic) or prolonged respiratory disease. When mothers do not provide breast milk, PTF should be used as a sole diet from birth in larger, well babies and after the establishment of human milk feeds in smaller or ill babies. If no breast milk is available, either maternal or banked, PTF should be cautiously introduced. Although term formula is sometimes used to establish enteral feeds in infants who appear not to tolerate PTF, there is no scientific evidence to support this. If term formula is used in this situation, it should be replaced by PTF as soon as possible. PTF may also be used as a supplement when mothers elect to provide their milk but do not have sufficient for the infant's requirements. Breast milk should be supplemented with phosphorus as a minimum to prevent metabolic bone disease. A multinutrient breast milk fortifier may be added if growth is unsatisfactory once the infant is tolerating full enteral feeds with breast milk. Human milk-based formulas and fortifiers may become more widely available in the future.

However, preterm infants are not a homogeneous population, and with the survival of ELBW babies any single diet is now unlikely to be optimal from birth to discharge. For instance, both the ESPGHAN Committee on Nutrition panel (Agostoni et al. 2010) and International Consensus Recommendations (Tsang et al. 2005) have recommended different protein intakes for infants weighing less than or more than 1kg. Furthermore, certain groups of babies appear more vulnerable than others to the effects of suboptimal nutrition. Lucas et al. (1990c) showed that small-for-gestational-age (SGA) preterm babies and males particularly were disadvantaged in terms of developmental scores in infancy if they were fed on mature pasteurised milk or standard term formula rather than a nutrient-enriched PTF. Further work is required to explore how diets can be tailored to individual patients' needs.

Route of administration of feeds

Infants less than 34 weeks' gestation seldom have adequately developed reflexes to suck, so that feeding has to be intragastric, transpyloric or intravenous (Ch. 17). Short-term partial parenteral nutrition, accompanied by gradually increasing enteral feeding, often needs to be employed in immature infants.

Intragastric feeding

Nasogastric or orogastric gavage feeding is the most commonly practised method of enteral feeding for preterm infants. An important pitfall to remember when giving human milk by tube is that significant loss of energy may occur from the adherence of fat to the feeding vessels. This process may be accentuated by the change in physical characteristics of the fat induced by freezing for long periods. Fat loss during continuous milk infusion can be reduced by using eccentric nozzle syringes with the nozzle in an uppermost position and set at an angle so that the open end of the syringe is higher than its plunger end (Narayanan et al. 1984). In addition, when a syringe pump is used to infuse human milk continuously the syringe should be positioned below the baby, otherwise the fat rises up the connecting tube towards the syringe and may never be received by the baby. Feeds should never be syringed in using pressure on the plunger. For advice on checking tube position and complications of tube feeding, see Chapter 21.

Transpyloric feeding

Transpyloric feeding (into the duodenum or jejunum) has been widely used in the past. There is no convincing evidence that it improves feed tolerance and growth, or reduces aspiration. Moreover, from a systematic review of nine randomised trials, transpyloric feeding was associated with a greater incidence of gastrointestinal disturbance (RR 1.45, 95% CI 1.05–2.09). There was some evidence that feeding via the transpyloric route increased mortality (RR 2.46, 95% CI 1.36–4.46). However, the outcomes of the study that contributed most to this finding were likely to have been affected by selective allocation of the less mature and sicker infants to transpyloric feeding (McGuire and McEwan 2007).

Cup feeding

Cup feeding can be a short-term adjunct to other feed methods in babies who are establishing breastfeeding, but requires careful supervision because of the risk of aspiration and is associated with significant losses from spillage. See Chapter 21 for more information.

Feeding schedules

Large, well, preterm infants

It is neither possible nor desirable to adhere to rigid feeding policies for LBW infants: gastrointestinal tolerance of enteral feeding is variable and concomitant illness may impose additional constraints, and therefore feeding must be managed on an individual basis.

The following guidelines are suggested for infants who are well enough to start full enteral feeds from the start. Feeding, by nasogastric tube if necessary, should start early to prevent hypoglycaemia, at about 2 hours of age. A commonly employed schedule for increasing feed volumes is to give, on the first four successive days, 60, 90, 120 and 150 ml/kg/24 h, and, for babies who require greater feed volumes than this, to make further daily increments to 180 ml/kg/24 h by day 10, and 200 ml/kg/24 h by day 14. There are few data on the rate at which bolus feeds should be instilled down a tube: most units favour gravity feeding over 10–20 minutes, rather than continuous infusion via a syringe pump. A systematic review of seven trials comparing continuous versus intermittent bolus feeding, involving 511 infants weighing less than 1500 g found no differences in time to achieve full enteral feeds and also no significant difference in somatic growth and incidence of NEC between feeding methods (Premji and Chessell 2003).

Most babies weighing more than 1500 g will tolerate 3-hourly feeds; smaller babies will need to be fed every 1–2 hours. Initially, the nasogastric tube should be aspirated at least 4–6-hourly, just before a feed. If the volume of aspirate is small, it may be replaced without altering the feed schedule; if it is significantly more than this or is 'dirty' rather than milky, it is advisable to reduce the feed intake accordingly, especially in infants showing increased abdominal girth. In infants who develop increasing abdominal distension, constipation or loose stools, with or without blood in the stools, enteral feeds should be stopped temporarily and NEC (Ch. 29.3) considered. If feed volumes need to be reduced below the required total fluid for more than a few hours, an intravenous infusion must be considered.

Sick and very immature preterm infants

In babies who are sick or very immature it is both undesirable and often impossible to commence full enteral feeds after birth, and an intravenous infusion must be commenced. There are theoretical and clinical trial data to support the idea of using small, subnutritional quantities of enteral food in babies who will not tolerate full feeds (see Ch. 29.3). In extremely immature infants (<27 weeks), however, even minimal enteral feeds may not be tolerated initially. A recent Cochrane review (Bombell and McGuire 2008) comparing delayed versus early initiation of enteral feeds included data from three small trials with a total of 115 very-LBW (VLBW) infants. These trials provided no evidence that delayed (>96 hours' postnatal age) introduction of progressive enteral feeds affected the incidence of NEC, mortality or other neonatal morbidities. However, with the small number of participants, important beneficial or harmful effects cannot be excluded. The timing of introduction of enteral feeds in preterm infants with severe intrauterine growth retardation, particularly when accompanied by absent or reversed end-diastolic blood flow, remains particularly controversial. Such infants may be at greater risk of NEC if they are fed, but they may also benefit more from the effects of minimal enteral feeding, in terms of adapting to enteral feeds. At present the best approach is probably to attempt minimal enteral feeding as soon as possible with human milk, being prepared for the fact that some of these babies are very slow to establish full enteral feeds.

A systematic review (McGuire and Bombell 2008) assessing the effect of slow (up to 24 ml/kg/day) versus faster rates of advancement of enteral feed volumes found three RCTs with a total of 396 VLBW infants. The authors concluded that there was no evidence that slow advancement of enteral feed volumes reduced the risk of NEC or all-cause mortality. Moreover, increasing the volume of enteral feeds at slow rates resulted in several days' delay in regaining birthweight and establishing full enteral feeds. When enteral feeding is commenced in very immature or sick infants, it may be advisable to use either a continuous infusion pump suitable for administering volumes to the nearest 0.5 ml/h or less, or slowly infused hourly boluses. Subsequent increments in feed frequency are a matter for clinical judgement, together with careful monitoring of enteral tolerance.

Psychosocial aspects

Practical involvement of parents in infant feeding during the period when suckling is not possible has considerable psychological benefits. Parents (under supervision) should be encouraged to measure out and give nasogastric tube feeds. Mothers who wish ultimately to breastfeed may start to put their baby to the breast from an early stage, provided the baby is well. A systematic review (Pinelli and Symington 2005) of 21 studies, 15 of which were RCTs, looking at the effects of non-nutritive sucking (NNS) during the administration of tube feeds found a significant decrease in length of stay in preterm babies receiving an NNS intervention. The review did not reveal a consistent benefit of NNS with respect to other major clinical variables (weight gain, energy intake, heart rate, oxygen saturation, intestinal transit time, age at full oral feeds and behavioural state). The difficulties encountered by mothers trying to express their own breast milk for their preterm infants are discussed on Ch. 21.

Postdischarge nutrition
(Fewtrell 2003)

Preterm babies frequently leave hospital severely growth-retarded and fulfilling the criteria for 'failure to thrive', yet until recently little attention has been paid to their subsequent nutrition. Although there may be a considerable degree of catch-up during childhood, particularly for weight, in our cohort of 926 preterm infants, the mean height standard deviation score (SDS) in early adult life was significantly less than the population mean (mean SDS –0.41 (SD 1.05)). The height deficit was even greater for infants weighing less than 1250 g at birth and SGA (–0.81 (SD 0.95)) (Fewtrell et al. 2009).

The small size of preterm infants at discharge is likely to be associated with deficits of a variety of nutrients, including calcium, phosphorus, iron, zinc and copper. A study of nutrient intakes in hospitalised preterm infants found cumulative energy and protein deficits of 406 kcal/kg and 14 g/kg at 1 week and 813 kcal/kg and 23 g/kg at 6 weeks of age in infants less than 31 weeks' gestation (Embleton et al. 2001). Such deficits would inevitably increase in infants fed term formula or unsupplemented breast milk after discharge.

Four main dietary options are available for use in preterm infants after hospital discharge:

1. human milk
2. term infant formula
3. preterm infant formula
4. nutrient-enriched postdischarge formula (PDF).

Formula feeding postdischarge

A study of formula-fed preterm infants after discharge from hospital demonstrated that, when fed ad libitum, these infants frequently consume volumes far in excess of those usually recommended by paediatricians: 16% took more than 350 ml/kg/24 h, 50% consumed more than 165 kcal/kg/24 h and 35% more than 4 g/kg/24 h protein (Lucas et al. 1992a). Cooke et al. (1998, 2001) studied 129 preterm infants randomised to receive PTF or term formula up to 6 months postterm. Boys (but not girls) fed PTF after discharge showed significantly greater weight and length gain and larger head circumference by 6 months postterm than those fed term formula throughout. At 18 months postterm, boys previously fed PTF were, on average, 1 kg heavier, 1 cm longer and had 1 cm greater head circumference than those fed term formula. Body composition measurements made using dual X-ray absorptiometry suggested that the additional weight gain was composed predominantly of lean tissue rather than fat. There were no significant differences in neurodevelopment measured using the Bayley scales of infant development at 18 months.

Although the use of PTF after hospital discharge is associated with growth benefits, particularly in boys, infants fed on demand may consume high volumes of PTF, and this could result in potentially toxic intakes of certain nutrients such as vitamin D. Such considerations, together with the desire to promote catch-up growth and replenishment of nutrient stores after discharge, led to the development of special postdischarge formulas. These formulas were designed such that all nutrient levels are within the range set for a standard term formula, although towards the upper end of this range for a number of nutrients (Table 16.11). Compared with a term formula, PDFs have higher protein content to promote catch-up growth, accompanied by a modest increase in energy to allow utilisation of the additional protein, additional calcium and phosphorus to permit adequate bone mineralisation and additional zinc, trace elements and vitamins to support the projected increase in growth rates.

A Cochrane review comparing outcomes in preterm infants randomised to term formula or postdischarge formula identified seven RCTs including 631 infants and concluded that there was no strong evidence for beneficial effects of postdischarge formula on growth or developmental outcome (Henderson et al. 2007). However, the review did not include a gender subgroup analysis; in two large RCTs of postdischarge versus term formula, beneficial effects on growth were seen predominantly in boys (Carver et al. 2001; Lucas et al. 2001), consistent with the beneficial effects of preterm infant formula after discharge reported in boys but not girls (Cooke et al. 1998, 2001).

Breastfeeding postdischarge

Breast milk is strongly promoted as the optimum diet for preterm infants in hospital in view of its proven benefits. However, it is not clear whether unsupplemented breast milk meets the nutritional requirements of preterm infants after discharge. Whilst the number of mothers providing breast milk for their infant for at least part of the hospital stay has increased, the proportion of mothers fully breastfeeding their infant after discharge is variable. A recent survey in Denmark reported an exclusive breastfeeding rate of 60% among 478 preterm infants of gestational age <32 weeks after hospital discharge (Zachariassen et al. 2010), but the figure was around 20% in an American study (Furman et al. 1998). However, a greater proportion of infants receive some breast milk, along with an infant formula, for at least the first few weeks after discharge.

Table 16.11 Nutrient content of postdischarge formulas available in the UK (per 100 ml)

COMPOSITION PER 100 ml	POSTDISCHARGE FORMULAS		COMPOSITION PER 100 ml	POSTDISCHARGE FORMULAS	
	Nutriprem 2* (C&G)	SMA Gold Prem 2*		Nutriprem 2* (C&G)	SMA Gold Prem 2*
Macronutrients			Iron	1200	1200
Protein[†] (g)	2.0	1.9	Manganese	7	5
Casein (%)	40	40	Zinc	900	730
Whey (%)	60	60	**Vitamins**		
Fat (g)	4.1	3.9	A retinol (μg)	100	100
Total LCP (mg)	38	21	B_1 thiamin (μg)	90	110
AA (mg)	18	13	B_2 riboflavin (μg)	150	160
DHA (mg)	14	8	B_6 pyridoxine (μg)	80	80
Carbohydrate (g)			B_{12} cyanocobalamin (μg)	0.22	0.22
Sugars (g)	6.3	6.4	Biotin (μg)	3	2.1
Total	7.5	7.5	Folic acid (μg)	20	15
Energy			Niacin (μg)	1800	1000
kcal	75	73	C ascorbic acid (mg)	12	11
kJ	315	305	D cholecalciferol (μg)	1.7	1.5
Minerals (mg)			E α-tocopherol (mg)	2.1	1.5
Calcium	94	75	K phytomenadione (μg)	5.9	6.3
Chloride	55	58	**Others**		
Magnesium	7	6.6	Choline (mg)	13	13
Phosphorus	50	42	Inositol (mg)	22	26
Potassium	77	71	Taurine (mg)	4.9	5
Sodium	28	27	Carnitine (mg)	0.9	1.1
Trace elements (μg)			Nucleotides (mg)	3.2	2.8
Copper	60	58	**Osmolality (mOsmol/kg)**	375	250
Iodine	20	10			

*Manufacturer's information.
[†]Total nitrogen $\times$ 6.38.
LCP, long-chain polyunsaturated fatty acid; AA, arachidonic acid; DHA, docosahexaenoic acid.

A number of studies have reported slower growth rates and lower bone mass in human milk-fed infants, at least in the short term. Lucas et al. (2001) studied 65 preterm infants who were breastfed (but allowed up to 2 oz of formula daily) for at least 6 weeks after discharge. Although similar in size to formula-fed infants at discharge, by 6 weeks postterm breastfed infants were significantly lighter and shorter than formula-fed infants (on average 513 g lighter and 1.6 cm shorter than infants fed PDF). Deficits persisted up to 9 months postterm, by which time all the breastfed infants were receiving term formula and solids. Collectively, these data suggest that preterm infants who are breastfed after discharge grow more slowly and have lower bone mass than formula-fed infants.

Whether the differences persist or indeed have any consequences for later outcome is under investigation.

Introduction of solid foods

There are no published data to guide either the optimal timing of weaning or the nature of solid foods for preterm infants. A recent document compiled by a group of experts in the UK and endorsed by the Neonatal Nurses' Association, community nurses and the Paediatric Group of the British Dietetic Association (King et al., 2008) recommended that weaning should start when the infant is between 5 and 7 months old actual age from birth, but also emphasises the importance of looking for signs of readiness in the individual infant; these included the infant showing interest in other people eating, putting things into his/her mouth, seeming less satisfied with milk alone and ready for something new, and the ability to be easily supported in a sitting position.

On a practical level, preterm infants are at risk of developing feeding difficulties that may have a significant impact on their post-discharge nutrition and growth. Infants who require prolonged respiratory support, have delayed introduction and establishment of oral feeds or who develop chronic lung disease are particularly vulnerable, and are more likely to have feeding problems, especially cough and vomit during feeds, throughout the first year of life (Hawdon et al. 2000). Early intervention in such infants, before oral feeding is introduced, may help minimise the potential for aversion to oral feeding and maximise the development of oromotor skills.

The term growth-retarded infant

Growth-retarded term infants are known to be at risk of continued growth failure as well as learning and behavioural problems. However, until recently, relatively little attention has been paid to the nutritional management of such infants.

de Rooy and Hawdon (2002) studied metabolic adaptation in 65 SGA infants with birthweights below the second centile over the first week of life, in relation to their mode of feeding. Exclusively breastfed infants showed a significantly greater production of ketone bodies, with no increase in the incidence of hypoglycaemia,

suggesting better metabolic adaptation. Ketone body production was lowest in formula-fed infants and intermediate in partially breastfed infants. These data strongly support breastfeeding in healthy term SGA infants, although adequate maternal support is clearly required to achieve this.

Most data suggest that catch-up growth in SGA infants, if it occurs, is largely completed during the first 9 months of life. It is not clear at present why a minority of growth-retarded infants fail to catch up, and to what extent this reflects their genetic potential.

Findings from a randomised trial (Singhal et al. 2007) and several observational studies suggest that early growth acceleration (generally defined as upward centile crossing for weight) may have adverse consequences, increasing the risk of later obesity, insulin resistance and higher blood pressure. Thus, the short-term benefits of promoting catch-up growth in SGA infants (Fewtrell et al. 2001b) must be weighed against potential adverse consequences for later health. The balance of risks and benefits of promoting early growth is likely to vary depending on the environment (for example, developing versus developed world settings). For healthy term SGA infants in a developed country setting with low risk of infectious morbidity or mortality, current consensus is that it is not advisable actively to promote rapid catch-up growth. Available data suggest that breastfeeding should be encouraged as the optimal source of nutrition for these infants, since on average it produces more gradual catch-up growth, with better developmental outcome (Morley et al. 2004).

Weblink

http://www.ukamb.org/: United Kingdom Association for Milk Banking.

References

Agostoni, C., Buonocore, G., Carnielli, V.P., et al., 2010. Enteral nutrient supply for preterm infants: commentary from the European Society of Paediatric Gastroenterology, Hepatology and Nutrition Committee on Nutrition. J Pediatr Gastroenterol Nutr 50, 85–91.

Arslanoglu, S., Moro, G.E., Ziegler, E.E., 2006. Adjustable fortification of human milk fed to preterm infants: does it make a difference? J Perinatol 26, 614–621.

Bombell, S., McGuire, W., 2008. Delayed introduction of progressive enteral feeds to prevent necrotising enterocolitis in very low birth weight infants. Cochrane Database Syst Rev CD001970.

Campbell-Yeo, M.L., Allen, A.C., Joseph, K.S., et al., 2010. Effect of domperidone on the composition of preterm human breast milk. Pediatrics 125, e107–e114.

Carver, J.D., Wu, P.Y., Hall, R.T., et al., 2001. Growth of preterm infants fed nutrient-enriched or term formula after hospital discharge. Pediatrics 107, 683–689.

Cavell, B., 1982. Reservoir and emptying function of the stomach of the premature infant. Acta Paediatrica Scandinavica Supplement 296, 60–61.

Cooke, R.J., Griffin, I.J., McCormick, K., et al., 1998. Feeding preterm infants after hospital discharge: effect of dietary manipulation on nutrient intake and growth. Pediatric Research 43, 355–360.

Cooke, R.J., Embleton, N.D., Griffin, I.J., et al., 2001. Feeding preterm infants after hospital discharge: growth and development at 18 months of age. Pediatric Research 49, 719–722.

de Rooy, L., Hawdon, J., 2002. Nutritional factors that affect the postnatal metabolic adaptation of full-term small- and large-for-gestational-age infants. Pediatrics 109, E42.

DHSS. 1977. The Composition of Mature Human Milk. Report on Health and Social Subjects No. 12, HMSO, London.

DHSS. 1980. Artificial Feeds for the Young Infant. Report on Health and Social Subjects No. 12. Report of the Committee on Medical Aspects of Food Policy. HMSO, London.

DHSS. 1983. Present Day Practice in Infant Feeding. Report on Health and Social Subjects No. 20, HMSO, London.

Eglin, R.-P., Wilkinson, A.R., 1987. HIV infection and pasteurisation of breast milk. Lancet i, 1093.

Ehrenkranz, R.A., Dusick, A.M., Vohr, B.R., et al., 2006. Growth in the neonatal intensive care unit influences neurodevelopmental and growth outcomes of extremely low birth weight infants. Pediatrics 117, 1253–1261.

Embleton, N., Pang, N., Cooke, R.J., 2001. Postnatal malnutrition and growth retardation: an inevitable problem in preterm infants? Pediatrics 107, 270–273.

Fewtrell, M.S., 2003. Growth and nutrition after discharge. Seminars in Perinatology 8, 169–176.

Fewtrell, M.S., Lucas, P., Collier, S., et al., 2001a. Randomized trial comparing the efficacy of a novel manual breast pump with a standard electric breast pump in mothers who delivered preterm infants. Pediatrics 107, 1291–1297.

Fewtrell, M.S., Morley, R., Abbott, R.A., et al., 2001b. Catch-up growth in small for gestational age term infants: a randomized trial. American Journal of Clinical Nutrition 74, 516–523.

Fewtrell, M.S., Loh, K.L., Blake, A., et al., 2006. Randomised, double blind trial of oxytocin nasal spray in mothers expressing breast milk for preterm infants. Arch Dis Child Fetal Neonatal Ed 91, F169–F174.

Fewtrell, M.S., Williams, J.E., Singhal, A., et al., 2009. Early diet and peak bone mass: 20 year follow-up of a randomized trial of early diet in infants born preterm. Bone 45, 142–149.

Furman, L., Minich, N.M., Hack, M., 1998. Breastfeeding of very low birth weight infants. Journal of Human Lactation 14, 29–34.

Goelz, R., Hihn, E., Hamprecht, K., et al., 2009. Effects of different CMV-heat-inactivation-methods on growth factors in human breast milk. Pediatr Res 65, 458–461.

Hawdon, J.M., Beauregard, N., Slattery, J., et al., 2000. Identification of neonates at risk of developing feeding problems in infancy. Developmental Medicine and Child Neurology 42, 235–239.

Henderson, G., Fahey, T., McGuire, W., 2007. Nutrient-enriched formula versus standard term formula for preterm infants following hospital discharge. Cochrane Database of Systematic Reviews (4), CD004696.

Isaacs, E.B., Fischl, B.R., Quinn, B.T., et al., 2009. Impact of breast milk on IQ, brain size and white matter development. Pediatr Res.

Jones, E., Dimmock, P.W., Spencer, S.A., 2001. A randomised controlled trial to compare methods of milk expression after preterm delivery. Archives of Disease in Childhood. Fetal and Neonatal Edition 85, F91–F95.

King, C., Mariott, L., Foote, K.D., 2008. Weaning your Premature Baby, fifth ed. BLISS, London.

Kuschel, C.A., Harding, J.E., 2004. Multicomponent fortified human milk for promoting growth in preterm infants. Cochrane Database Syst Rev CD000343.

Lawrence, R.A., Lawrence, R.M., 2005. Breastfeeding the premature infant. In: Lawrence, R.A., Lawrence, R.M. (Eds.), Breastfeeding: A Guide for the Medical Profession. Elsevier Mosby, Philadelphia, pp. 479–514.

Leaf, et al. in press.

Lucas, A., Cole, T.J., 1990. Breast milk and neonatal necrotising enterocolitis. Lancet 336, 1519–1523.

Lucas, A., Hudson, G., 1984. Preterm milk as a source of protein for low birthweight infants. Archives of Disease in Childhood 59, 831–836.

Lucas, A., McLaughlan, P., Coombs, R.R.A., 1984. Latent anaphylactic sensitisation of infants of low birthweight to cow's milk proteins. British Medical Journal 289, 1254–1256.

Lucas, A., Brooke, O.G., Morley, R., et al., 1990a. A randomised prospective study of early diet and later allergic or atopic disease. British Medical Journal 300, 837–840.

Lucas, A., Morley, R., Cole, T.J., et al., 1990c. Early diet in preterm babies and developmental status at 18 months. Lancet 335, 1477–1481.

Lucas, A., King, F.J., Bishop, N.J., 1992a. Postdischarge formula consumption in infants born preterm. Archives of Disease in Childhood 67, 691–692.

Lucas, A., Morley, R., Cole, T.J., et al., 1992b. Breast milk and subsequent intelligence quotient in children born preterm. Lancet 339, 261–264.

Lucas, A., Morley, R., Cole, T.J., et al., 1994. A randomised multicentre study of human milk versus formula and later development in preterm infants. Archives of Disease in Childhood. Fetal and Neonatal Edition 70, F141–F146.

Lucas, A., Morley, R., Cole, T.J., 1998. Randomised trial of early diet in preterm babies and later intelligence quotient. British Medical Journal 317, 1481–1487.

Lucas, A., Fewtrell, M.S., Morley, R., et al., 2001. Randomized trial of nutrient enriched formula versus standard formula for post-discharge preterm infants. Pediatrics 108, 703–711.

Macy, I.G., Kelly, H.J., Sloan, H.E., 1983. The Composition of Milks. Publication 254. National Academy of Science, National Research Council, Washington DC.

McGuire, W., Bombell, S., 2008. Slow advancement of enteral feed volumes to prevent necrotising enterocolitis in very low birth weight infants. Cochrane Database Syst Rev CD001241.

McGuire, W., McEwan, P., 2007. Transpyloric versus gastric tube feeding for preterm infants. Cochrane Database Syst Rev CD003487.

Mettler, A.E., 1976. Infant milk powder feeds compared on a common basis. Postgraduate Medical Journal 52 (suppl. 8), 3–20.

Miron, D., Brosilow, S., Felszer, K., et al., 2005. Incidence and clinical manifestations of breast milk-acquired cytomegalovirus infection in low birth weight infants. J Perinatol 25, 299–303.

Morley, R., Cole, T.J., Lucas, P.J., et al., 1988. Mothers' choice to provide breast milk and developmental outcome. Archives of Disease in Childhood 63, 1382–1385.

Morley, R., Fewtrell, M.S., Abbott, R.A., et al., 2004. Neurodevelopment in children born small for gestational age: a randomized trial of nutrient-enriched versus standard formula and comparison with a reference breastfed group. Pediatrics 113, 515–521.

Narayanan, I., Singh, B., Harvey, D., 1984. Fat loss during feeding of human milk. Arch Dis Child 59, 475–477.

National Institute for Health and Clinical Excellence. 2010. Donor Breast Milk Banks. NICE Clinical Guideline 93. NICE, London, pp. 1–16.

Pinelli, J., Symington, A., 2005. Non-nutritive sucking for promoting physiologic stability and nutrition in preterm infants. Cochrane Database Syst Rev CD001071.

Premji, S., Chessell, L., 2003. Continuous nasogastric milk feeding versus intermittent bolus milk feeding for premature infants less than 1500 grams. Cochrane Database Syst Rev CD001819.

Quigley, M.A., Henderson, G., Anthony, M.Y., et al., 2007. Formula milk versus donor breast milk for feeding preterm or low birth weight infants. Cochrane Database Syst Rev CD002971.

Renfrew, M.J., Craig, D., Dyson, L., et al. 2009. Breastfeeding promotion for infants in neonatal units: a systematic review and economic analysis. Health Technol Assess 13, 1–iv.

Schanler, R.J., 2005. CMV acquisition in premature infants fed human milk: reason to worry? J Perinatol 25, 297–298.

Schanler, R.J., Atkinson, S.A., 2005. Human milk. In: Tsang, R.C., Uauy, R., Koletzko, B., et al. (Eds.), Nutrition of the Preterm Infant: Scientific Basis and Practical Guidelines. Digital Educational Publishing, Cincinnati, 333–356.

Schanler, R.J., Lau, C., Hurst, N.M., et al., 2005. Randomized trial of donor human milk versus preterm formula as substitutes for mothers' own milk in the feeding of extremely premature infants. Pediatrics 116, 400–406.

Shulman, R.J., Schanler, R.J., Lau, C., et al., 1998a. Early feeding, antenatal glucocorticoids, and human milk decrease intestinal permeability in preterm infants. Pediatr Res 44, 519–523.

Shulman, R.J., Schanler, R.J., Lau, C., et al., 1998b. Early feeding, feeding tolerance, and lactase activity in preterm infants. J Pediatr 133, 645–649.

Singhal, A., Lucas, A., 2004. Early origins of cardiovascular disease: is there a unifying hypothesis? Lancet 363, 1642–1645.

Singhal, A., Cole, T.J., Lucas, A., 2001. Early nutrition in preterm infants and later blood pressure: two cohorts after randomised trials. Lancet 357, 413–419.

Singhal, A., Fewtrell, M., Cole, T.J., et al., 2003. Low nutrient intake and early growth for later insulin resistance in adolescents born preterm. Lancet 361, 1089–109776.

Singhal, A., Cole, T., Fewtrell, M., et al., 2004. Breast milk feeding and the lipoprotein profile in adolescents born preterm. Lancet 363, 1571–1578.

Singhal, A., Cole, T.J., Fewtrell, M., et al., 2007. Promotion of faster weight gain in infants born small for gestational age: is there an adverse effect on later blood pressure? Circulation 115, 213–220.

Sullivan, S., Schanler, R.J., Kim, J.H., et al., 2010. an exclusively human milk-based diet is associated with a lower rate of necrotizing enterocolitis than a diet of human milk and bovine milk-based

319

products. Journal of Pediatrics 156, 562–567.

Tsang, R.C., Uauy, R., Koletzko, B., et al., 2005. Nutrition of the Preterm Infant: Scientific Basis and Practical Guidelines. Digital Educational Publishing, Cincinnati, Ohio.

Volk, M.L., Hanson, C.V., Israel-Ballard, K., et al., 2010. Inactivation of cell-associated and cell-free HIV-1 by flash-heat treatment of breast milk. J Acquir Immune Defic Syndr 53, 665–666.

Zachariassen, G., Faerk, J., Grytter, C., et al., 2010. Factors associated with successful establishment of breastfeeding in very preterm infants. Acta Paediatr 99, 1000–1004.

Parenteral nutrition

Pamela Cairns

17

The fetus is nourished parenterally during pregnancy via the placenta. This is abruptly discontinued at birth and the vast majority of babies then make a successful transition to enteral feeding. Parenteral nutrition (PN) is indicated in the infant for whom feeding via the enteral route is impossible, inadequate or hazardous, because of malformation, disease or immaturity. Babies with congenital anomalies of the gut require PN until normal gut function has returned. In babies with necrotising enterocolitis or a chylothorax, resting the gastrointestinal (GI) tract for a prolonged period may be curative, and some babies with short gut require total or partial parenteral feeding for many months to allow gut adaptation. PN is essential for extremely preterm babies prior to enteral feeding or to supplement milk feeds, which can then be increased slowly while continuing to satisfy nutritional requirements.

The long-term impact of inadequate nutrition during the neonatal period is now becoming clearer. The third trimester is a critical period for neuronal development. Work in the rodent model has demonstrated permanent impairment in dendritic arborisation and axonal myelination if early nutrition is inadequate (Escobar and Salas 1995). Clinical trials of enteral nutrition in preterm human infants have suggested that nutrition during the same period may have an impact on long-term neurodevelopmental outcome (Lucas et al. 1998). Postnatal growth failure in preterm infants is associated with an increased incidence of cerebral palsy, developmental delay and abnormal neurology (Ehrenkranz et al. 2006). It is common in our neonatal units despite widespread use of PN (Cooke et al. 2004). A significant proportion of this postnatal growth failure occurs in the first few weeks of life, with subsequent inability to meet the demands of catch-up growth on top of the requirements for normal growth (Embleton et al. 2001). A recent observation study was carried out on a random sample of all hospital patients in the UK who were given PN. Neonatal cases from a total of 74 hospitals providing all levels of neonatal care were reviewed. This revealed wide variation in practice with significant delays in starting PN and inadequate nutritional content in approximately 40% of cases reviewed (National Confidential Enquiry into Patient Outcome and Death 2010). As PN is an expensive and potentially hazardous intervention (Table 17.1), it is important that it is prescribed carefully and effectively.

Composition of infusates

Fluids (see Ch. 18)

Preterm infants adapt poorly to inadequate or excessive fluid intake compared with term infants. They have increased amounts of extracellular fluid, their kidneys have poor concentrating and diluting ability (Ch. 18), they have a large surface area in relation to weight and their insensible water loss through the skin, especially in the first week, is high (Ch. 15).

Energy

The estimation of energy requirement takes into account the components of total heat production (basal metabolic rate, physical activity, specific dynamic action of food, thermoregulatory heat

© 2012 Elsevier Ltd

Table 17.1 Risks associated with total parenteral nutrition

Metabolic
Hyperglycaemia
Hyperchloraemic acidosis
Metabolic bone disease of prematurity
Abnormal aminogram
Hyperlipidaemia

Line-related

Infection
Atrial or superior venocaval thrombus
Pleural effusions
Pericardial tamponade, peritoneal extravasation
Tissue necrosis from extravasation injury

General
Cholestasis
Gut mucosal atrophy

production) and the energy cost of growth. In preterm infants, the basal metabolic rate is about 40 kcal/kg/day (Reichman et al. 1982). The energy cost of activity is 4 kcal/kg/day with minimal handling (Reichman et al. 1982) and the specific dynamic action of PN is 13% of the basal heat production or 10% of the calories infused (Rubecz and Mestyan 1973). If a baby is nursed in a thermoneutral environment, an input of 50 kcal/kg/day is generally sufficient to match ongoing expenditure but it does not meet additional requirements of growth (see Ch. 16) (Heimler et al. 1993).

Growth failure will result unless additional energy is provided. The energy cost of gaining 1 g of new tissue is 5 kcal (Reichman et al. 1982). To achieve the equivalent of third-trimester intrauterine weight gain of 14–15 g/kg/day, an additional 70 kcal/kg/day is required. Parenterally fed infants, compared with those enterally fed, begin to grow at a lower energy intake because of smaller faecal energy losses and reduced energy expenditure. Nevertheless, the goal energy intake for a rapidly growing preterm infant is about 120 kcal/kg/day (see Ch. 16 part 1), or even higher in long-term ventilated infants with chronic lung disease, whose energy requirements are increased by 25–30% (Wahlig and Georgieff 1995).

Protein

The goal of supplying protein to the neonate is to achieve nitrogen retention at in utero rates without causing metabolic disturbance. Preterm infants will lose approximately 1% of their total protein stores each day if they are given glucose alone (Rivera et al. 1993). Amino acids therefore need to be started in the first 24 hours of life. A minimum of 1.5 g/kg/day is recommended in order to prevent catabolism, although this is insufficient to support growth (Rivera et al. 1993; Thureen and Hay 2001). Commonly the amino acid intake is then increased slowly over the next few days because of concerns about the ability of the preterm infant to metabolise protein. However a number of investigators have examined higher early amino acid infusion rates, ranging from 2.4 to 3.5 g/kg/day (Thureen et al. 2003; Ibrahim et al. 2004; Te Braake et al. 2005). All reported improved nitrogen retention without any adverse

effects in the short term. It may be that starting amino acids at full rates, or at least increasing rapidly, will go some way to minimising the time to regain birthweight.

Optimal parenteral protein requirements for growth, as determined by a variety of methods, are in the range 3.5–4.0 g/kg/day for extremely low birthweight infants and 3.2–3.8 g/kg/day for very low birthweight infants (Tsang 2005). The amount of amino acids required to achieve adequate catch-up growth, if there has been a period of poor early weight gain, is likely to be higher than this (Thureen and Heird 2005). The recommended requirements for term infants are somewhat lower at 2.0–3.0 g/kg/day (Koletzko et al. 2005).

Preterm infants require not only more amino acids than term infants but also qualitatively different amino acids. Cysteine, taurine, tyrosine and histidine have been considered as semiessential amino acids in preterm infants (Laidlaw and Kopple 1987). Conversion of methionine to cysteine and taurine, and of phenylalanine to tyrosine, is affected by enzyme immaturity. However, the addition of cysteine (Malloy et al. 1984) and taurine (Thornton and Griffin 1991) to PN solutions in preterm infants did not improve nitrogen retention or weight gain. Taurine is important in the conjugation of bile acids, although humans can also conjugate bile acids with glycine. Some investigators consider that the addition of taurine to total PN (TPN) reduces the incidence of cholestasis (Heird et al. 1987). Comparison of amino acid solutions based on the composition of egg protein and breast milk has shown that the latter results in a lower risk of high plasma phenylalanine levels but a higher risk of low tyrosine levels (Puntis et al. 1989; Mitton et al. 1993). No adverse neurodevelopmental outcome has been observed after hyperphenylalaninaemia induced by PN (Lucas et al. 1993). If adequate non-protein energy is provided, the risk of hyperphenylalaninaemia is reduced (intravenous energy intake of >34 kcal/g protein). Amino acid solutions designed for paediatric patients have been shown to result in a more favourable plasma aminogram, higher nitrogen retention and better weight gain in preterm infants (Helms et al. 1987; Mitton et al. 1993). Current amino acid preparations available for neonates are based on the plasma aminograms of either cord blood or breastfed term infants.

In order to utilise the amino acids efficiently, sufficient non-nitrogen energy must be provided. Energy intake should be at least 40–50 kcal/kg/day for optimal amino acid utilisation, because, with lower energy intakes, more of the infused amino acids are oxidised to meet endogenous energy needs and less remain for tissue synthesis. Zlotkin et al. (1981) found that, when energy intakes of more than 70 kcal/kg/day were given to preterm infants, the major determinant of nitrogen retention was the protein intake. Whether this non-protein energy is derived from glucose or fat makes no difference to the nitrogen-sparing effect.

Ammonia, plasma amino acid profiles and urea levels have all been used to monitor the tolerance and adequacy of amino acid intake in the clinical setting. Current neonatal preparations are well tolerated and thus monitoring ammonia and amino acid levels is no longer required routinely. Urea levels are monitored regularly and some clinicians will limit amino acid intakes in the presence of rising urea. However urea levels reflect hydration status, renal function and illness severity and have been shown not to correlate with protein intake (Ridout et al. 2005). In contrast a low urea may reflect inadequate intake.

Carbohydrate

The goal of carbohydrate provision for the neonate is to maintain euglycaemia and promote optimal growth and body composition.

The consensus interpretation of the neurophysiological and neurodevelopmental outcome data is currently that neonatal blood glucose concentration should be maintained above 2.6 mmol/l (Ch. 34.1). The risks of hyperglycaemia and glycosuria increase with decreasing gestation and birthweight (Louik et al. 1985).

The rate of endogenous glucose metabolism in well, fasting neonates has been estimated to be 4–6 mg/kg/min (Denne 1998). Some premature infants will require more than this to maintain a satisfactory blood glucose. Glucose infusions should be commenced at 4 mg/kg/min (10% dextrose at 60 ml/kg/day will provide an infusion rate of 4 mg/kg/min) and increased as required. If a concentration of more than 12.5% dextrose is required, this should be given centrally owing to the risks of subcutaneous tissue infiltration. Since glucose tolerance improves with increasing postnatal age the glucose infusion rate can usually be progressively increased. Excessive carbohydrate will theoretically increase CO_2 production, although it is uncertain whether this is ever of clinical relevance. It may also impair liver function by inducing the storage of triglycerides and other fatty acids within the liver cells. The European Society of Paediatric Gastroenterology, Hepatology and Nutrition recommends that preterm infants' maximum glucose intake should be 8.3 mg/kg/min while term infants may tolerate up to 13 mg/kg/min (18 g/kg/day) (Koletzko et al. 2005).

If hyperglycaemia occurs, the baby should be carefully assessed. Hyperglycaemia occurring in a previously metabolically stable baby may be the first sign of infection, although immature infants may have limited tolerance of intravenous glucose even when infused at physiological rates. Hyperglycaemia during glucose infusion appears to be due primarily to persistent endogenous hepatic glucose production secondary to an insensitivity of hepatocytes to insulin (Cowett et al. 1988). Insulin can be infused in infants who remain hyperglycaemic at a glucose infusion rate of 8 g/kg/day (6 mg/kg/min) (Ostertag et al. 1986), commencing at 0.05 units/kg/h. A randomised controlled trial in infants of below 1000 g birthweight with glucose intolerance has shown that insulin therapy improves glucose intake and weight gain (Collins et al. 1991). However the practice of prescribing early insulin replacement therapy in order to increase the glucose intake in very low birthweight infants appears to offer little clinical benefit and may be associated with increased risk (Beardsall et al. 2008) and is not currently recommended (Sinclair et al. 2009).

Lipid

The goals of providing fat to neonates are to prevent fatty acid deficiency, facilitate provision of lipid soluble vitamins and promote optimal growth and body composition.

Nitrogen sparing effects of carbohydrate and fat are similar in parenterally fed infants, although lipid has the benefit of being calorie-dense (Pineault et al. 1988; Van Aerde et al. 1994). Abnormal plasma fatty acid patterns have been noted within 2–3 days of lipid free alimentation, with a deficiency state in 10 days (Lee et al. 1993). Essential fatty acid deficiency can be prevented by as little as 0.5 g/kg/day of Intralipid (Lee et al. 1993), a fat emulsion derived from soybean oil containing 54% linoleic acid and 8% linolenic acid. While soybean-based emulsions have been the gold standard for many years, the balance of ω-3 and ω-6 fatty acids is probably not ideal for the preterm infant. Linoleic acid (an ω-6 polyunsaturated fatty acid (PUFA)) is the dominant fatty acid in soy-based emulsions. However there is concern that this has the potential to inhibit the production of ω-3 PUFAs, such as docosahexaenoic acid (needed for retinal and brain development). As the metabolites of the ω-3 and ω-6 fatty acids are anti-inflammatory and proinflammatory respectively, an imbalance may have an impact on the

infant's immune response. Olive oil-based emulsions contain oleic acid (ω-9 long-chain monounsaturated) as the main fatty acid and therefore may provide a more appropriate balance between ω-6 and ω-3 fatty acids. However studies have not shown any clinically significant effect to date (Webb et al. 2008). Fat emulsions containing equal proportions of long- and medium-chain triglycerides (LCT/MCT) have been used in infants, and one study showed greater nitrogen retention with LCT/MCT than with LCT emulsions (Unger et al. 1986).

Phytosterols found in soybean oils are thought to contribute to PN-associated liver disease. This, in addition to the proinflammatory effects of linoleic acid, has led to discontinuation of soy lipid emulsion as the mainstay of treatment. Fish oil has a high concentration of eicosapentaenoic acid, docosahexaenoic acid and ω-3 fatty acids. Recent experience has suggested that fish oil monotherapy has a potentially beneficial effect in infants with PN-related liver disease (Gura et al. 2008). The development of lipid emulsions combining soy, olive and fish oils and MCTs offers a potentially beneficial product which is currently being evaluated in the preterm population.

Lipid utilisation is limited and often unpredictable in preterm and in small-for-gestational-age infants, owing to deficient cellular uptake and utilisation of free fatty acids rather than low lipoprotein lipase activity (Rovamo et al. 1988). Carnitine plays an important role in the oxidation of fatty acids by facilitating their transport across mitochondrial membranes. Preterm infants fed parenterally with carnitine-free solutions develop low blood and tissue carnitine concentrations because of their small carnitine depots and limited capacity for carnitine biosynthesis. Carnitine supplementation, however, does not improve growth or lipid tolerance and is not recommended (Cairns and Stalker 2000).

There have been a number of concerns over the early use of lipid; however, randomised controlled trials have established the benefits and safety of parenteral fat commenced on the day of birth (Gilbertson et al. 1991; Sosenko et al. 1993; Ibrahim et al. 2004). Concern had been expressed about the effects of lipid infusion on respiratory function. However oxygenation and pulmonary haemodynamics in infants with severe respiratory distress syndrome were not affected when parenteral fat was infused at a dose of 1–4 g/kg/day (Brans et al. 1986; Gilbertson et al. 1991) but deteriorated when the infusion rate exceeded an equivalent of 6–7 g/kg/day (Pereira et al. 1980). An association between parenteral fat administration and coagulase-negative staphylococcal bacteraemia in infants has been found (Freeman et al. 1990) but there is no evidence that it impairs immune function in infants (English et al. 1981; Strunk et al. 1985). An increase in circulating free fatty acid levels can theoretically compete with bilirubin for binding to albumin. However, fat emulsion is also capable of binding unconjugated bilirubin (Thaler and Wennberg 1977) and infusions of 2–4 g/kg/day have been found to have no effect on total or unbound serum bilirubin (Brans et al. 1987). At levels of free fatty acids, bilirubin and albumin usually occurring in this population, significant displacement does not occur (Adamkin et al. 1992).

Free radicals generated when soy lipid emulsion undergoes peroxidation could be potentially damaging. Light-induced formation of triglyceride hydroperoxides can be prevented by covering the lipid emulsion with aluminium foil, although this has largely fallen out of fashion (Neuzil et al. 1995). There is also evidence suggesting that failure to photoprotect PN contributes to high blood glucose and triglyceride levels (Khasu et al. 2009). Lipid tolerance can be improved by using a continual infusion over 24 hours and by using a 20% rather than 10% concentration. Compared with 10% Intralipid, 20% Intralipid has a lower phospholipid/triglyceride ratio and liposomal content, and thus results in lower plasma triglyceride, cholesterol and phospholipid concentrations (Haumont et al. 1989).

A 20% lipid emulsion should be started at 1 g/kg/24 h and increased daily by 1 g/kg to 3 g/kg/24 h as tolerated (Hilliard et al. 1983). Plasma triglyceride levels should be monitored (see Table 17.4, below), as plasma turbidity assessed by visual inspection or nephelometry does not reliably predict serum concentration (Schreiner et al. 1979). If the baby has poor growth but is tolerating lipids, the total dose can be increased to 3.5 g/kg/day. When triglyceride levels exceed 2.0 mmol/l, it is necessary to reduce or interrupt fat infusion until normal values are regained. The lipid infusion should be reduced or interrupted for 24–48 hours during acute sepsis, because of the reduced fat oxidation rate (Park et al. 1986).

Minerals

Early hypernatraemia in preterm infants is caused mainly by their high insensible water loss (Ch. 18, Ch. 15), while early hyponatraemia is caused mainly by water overload. Late hyponatraemia in preterm infants is due to limited tubular sodium reabsorption, and diuretic therapy may contribute (Al-Dahhan et al. 1983). No sodium should be added to intravenous fluids or PN until postnatal natriuresis has occurred (Ch. 18). Thereafter, 3–5 mmol/kg/day is recommended, to prevent late hyponatraemia, and further increased if the infant is receiving furosemide for chronic lung disease or has significant ongoing renal losses. Although a potassium intake of 1–2 mmol/kg/day is required for the growing preterm infant, it should be withheld in the first 3 days after birth in those who are extremely preterm, because they are at risk of developing non-oliguric hyperkalaemia from immature distal tubular function. Hypochloraemic alkalosis is prevented by a chloride intake of 2 mmol/kg/day. Chloride intakes in excess of 6 mmol/kg/day are inadvisable because of the risk of hyperchloraemic metabolic acidosis (Groh-Wargo et al. 1988). Hyperchloraemic acidosis can be avoided by replacing part of the sodium chloride load with sodium acetate (Olunfunmi et al. 1997).

Parenteral administration of calcium at 1 mmol/kg/day from birth can reduce early neonatal hypocalcaemia in preterm infants (Salle et al. 1977). Requirements calculated to match intrauterine accretion rates in a rapidly growing preterm infant are, however, higher than those used to maintain short-term homeostasis. PN solutions should contain 1.3–1.5 mmol/100 ml of calcium and phosphorus (molar ratio of 1:1 or a ratio of 1.3:1 by weight) and 0.2–0.3 mmol/100 ml of magnesium. Factors that affect solubility of calcium and phosphorus are discussed below (see Techniques, below). High intakes of calcium and phosphorus should only be given through a central venous line.

Trace elements and vitamins

Table 17.2 summarises the recommendations on parenteral minerals and trace elements for preterm infants based on expert consensus published by Tsang (2005). Trace elements are added routinely to the aqueous component of PN. Zinc and selenium levels should be monitored after the first month of prolonged PN, particularly in infants with underlying GI pathology. Because selenium and chromium are excreted mainly through the kidneys, intake may need to be reduced when renal function is impaired. The aluminium content of PN infusates may be up to 1 μmol/dl as a result of aluminium contamination of the components used, such as calcium gluconate, which can contribute up to 80% of the total aluminium load. As it has been suggested that this will adversely affect neurodevelopment, aluminium contamination should be reduced as far as possible (Bishop et al. 1997).

Table 17.2 Recommendations for intravenous mineral, trace elements and vitamins in very low birthweight infants (amount per kilogram per day)

Sodium	3–5 mmol
Chloride	3–7 mmol
Potassium	2–3 mmol
Calcium	1.5–2.0 mmol
Phosphorus	1.5–1.9 mmol
Magnesium	0.2–0.3 mmol
Zinc	6.1 μmol
Copper	0.3 μmol
Selenium	19–57 nmol
Manganese	18.2 nmol
Iodine	7.9 nmol
Chromium	1–5.8 nmol
Molybdenum	2.6 nmol

Table 17.3 Vitamins

RECOMMENDATIONS		COMPOSITION of VITLIPID (per ml)
Vitamin A	700–1500 IU	230 units
Vitamin D	40–160 IU	40 units
Vitamin E	2.8–3.5 IU	0.7 units
Vitamin K	10 μg	20 μg

Paediatric multivitamin preparations are available (Moore et al. 1986). Water-soluble vitamins can be added to either the aqueous or the lipid component. Fat-soluble vitamins should be added to the lipid component. If they are added to the amino acid solution as part of a multivitamin preparation, about 80% of vitamin A and 30% of vitamins D and E is lost during administration owing to adherence to tubing and photodegradation, especially during phototherapy (Gilles et al. 1983; Smith et al. 1988). By adding the vitamin preparation into the fat emulsion instead of the amino acid–glucose mixture, vitamin losses can be reduced and the risk of deficiency minimised (Baeckert et al. 1988; Dahl et al. 1994). A dose of 4 ml/kg Vitlipid (Fresenius Kabi) will give an adequate amount of vitamin A (Table 17.3). Fat-soluble vitamin levels should be monitored in all babies requiring more than 1 month's PN.

Techniques

All preparations should be carried out under strict aseptic conditions using a laminar flow hood and terminal filtration with a 0.22-μm filter prior to delivery to the ward. PN should never be made up at ward level, neither should additions be made to the bag.

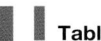

The solubility of calcium and phosphorus depends on other components within the infusate and the order in which they are mixed. The higher amino acid concentrations recommended for use in preterm infants help to enhance their solubility by decreasing the pH of the solution. Phosphorus should be added before calcium to avoid the high concentrations of phosphorus causing immediate precipitation with calcium. Precipitation with phosphates is more likely with calcium chloride than with the gluconate salt. Glycerophosphates may allow greater delivery of calcium and phosphorus because they are stable in solution and have equivalent retention rates to standard salts (Hanning et al. 1991; Raupp et al. 1991).

Administration

An infusion pump is required to maintain a constant rate of delivering the PN solution. A 0.22-μm bacterial filter is commonly used. Distal to the filter, a second infusion pump delivers the fat emulsion close to the intravascular catheter. It is important to minimise mixing of the fat emulsion with calcium and heparin as this increases the risks of formation of calcium–phosphorus crystals and flocculation of the lipid due to the destabilising effect of divalent cations (Raupp et al. 1988).

Although PN can be given peripherally it is preferable to use a centrally placed line. Fine Silastic lines inserted percutaneously or umbilical venous lines are the preferred central venous catheters in neonates (Ch. 44). These should provide secure central access for the duration of PN for the majority of neonates. In infants with a requirement for long term PN, insertion of a surgically placed central line and the addition of heparin (1 unit/ml) to the infusate further reduce significantly the incidence of phlebitis and thrombosis of both peripheral (Alpan et al. 1984) and central (Bailey 1979) venous catheters. PN has been administered routinely through umbilical arterial catheters. This has been found to be comparable to central venous catheters in efficacy and safety (Kanarek et al. 1991).

The importance of careful monitoring of the baby receiving TPN cannot be overemphasised (Table 17.4). Frequent monitoring is necessary when the PN is being increased and adjusted or the baby is clinically unstable. As the baby's condition stabilises and electrolyte requirements are unchanged for several days the frequency of monitoring can be reduced.

Hazards

Infections and technical complications

Infants on PN have an increased risk of bacterial sepsis caused by *Staphylococcus epidermidis* or *S. aureus* (Beganovic et al. 1988) and fungal sepsis caused by *Candida* (Weese-Mayer et al. 1987). The prevalence of catheter-related sepsis in infants ranges from 8% to 45%, with staff training playing a key role in its prevention (Puntis et al. 1989, 1991). The risk of polymicrobial bacteraemia is increased by manipulations of the parenteral infusate at the bedside (Fleer et al. 1983; Jarvis et al. 1983). Precautions which should be taken to minimise the risk of sepsis are listed in Table 17.5.

Complications of central venous catheterisation are discussed in Chapter 44.

Metabolic complications

The risks of abnormal plasma aminograms, hyperammonaemia, hyperchloraemic metabolic acidosis, metabolic bone disease and trace element deficiencies are minimised with the careful choice of

---

 Table 17.4 Monitoring during parenteral nutrition

- ☐ Daily body weight and weekly body length and head circumference
- ☐ Initially during grading-up of parenteral nutrients or during periods of metabolic instability:
  - – Strict fluid balance
  - – 6–12-hourly blood glucose
  - – Daily plasma sodium, potassium, calcium, urea and acid–base
  - – Twice-weekly triglycerides
- ☐ When on full parenteral nutrition and during metabolic steady state:
  - – Strict fluid balance
  - – 12–24-hourly blood glucose
  - – Twice-weekly plasma sodium, potassium, calcium, urea and acid–base
- ☐ Plasma magnesium, phosphorus, alkaline phosphatase, albumin, transaminases, triglycerides and bilirubin (total and conjugated) weekly
- ☐ Plasma amino acids and ammonia not usually routinely monitored
- ☐ Trace elements and fat-soluble vitamins should be monitored monthly

Table 17.5 Precautions to minimise the risk of sepsis

Preparation and manipulation of parenteral nutrition solutions should only take place in the pharmacy

Avoid carrying out manipulations in the ward

Central venous catheters must be placed under strict aseptic conditions

Skin exit site for catheter placed in area which can be meticulously cleansed

Proper care of the site and all the connectors and tubings is essential

The total parenteral nutrition line should not be broken for the administration of drugs

The requirement for a central line should be considered daily and the line removed at the first opportunity

---

amino acid solutions and appropriate additives to the infusate. Cholestatic jaundice occurs in 10–40% of infants on PN (Ch. 29.1); it is very uncommon in those who receive it for less than 2 weeks, but up to 80% of those who require TPN for more than 2 months develop cholestasis (Beale et al. 1979). Likely mechanisms include immaturity of the hepatobiliary system (Merritt 1986), prolonged fasting (Rager and Finegold 1975), impaired bile secretion and bile salt formation (Sondheimer et al. 1978), coexisting sepsis (Kubota et al. 1988) and underlying medical conditions associated with hypoxia or GI conditions requiring surgery (Bell et al. 1986). In the vast majority, cholestasis resolves when enteral feeding is initiated, but progression to biliary cirrhosis (Pereira et al. 1981) can occur. Discontinuing the TPN for 1–2 weeks may allow significant recovery, as may discontinuing the lipids alone. The use of a fish oil-containing lipid emulsion in this situation offers a potential therapeutic approach (Gura et al. 2008). Minimisation of sepsis, in particular line-related sepsis, and commencement of enteral nutrition at the first possible opportunity will reduce the likelihood of PN-associated liver disease.

In view of the potential metabolic complications, parenteral lipids should be used with caution initially in infants with fulminating sepsis, prior to adequate clinical stabilisation with antibiotic therapy. Amino acids and electrolyte solutions should be monitored with great care in infants with severely impaired renal function. The total nitrogen intake may be limited, but should not be discontinued completely, as this will result in catabolism.

Transition to enteral nutrition

In spite of the adequacy of PN in meeting nutritional requirements for postnatal growth, enteral feeding itself is vital for adaptation to extrauterine nutrition through its trophic effects on the GI tract and its physiological effects on GI exocrine and endocrine secretion and motility (Lucas et al. 1983). Milk feeds result in surges of secretion, glucagon, gastrin and motilin, all of which have trophic effects and mediate GI secretion and motility. It has been shown in human infants that enteral feeding is necessary for normal gastric acid secretion (Hyman et al. 1983). Enteral feeding is associated with increases in blood gastrin and motilin levels (Shulman and Kanarek 1993) and intestinal motor activity (Berseth and Nordyke 1993). Glucagon, in addition to its role in GI motility, stimulates bile flow (Aynsley-Green 1983). Infants on TPN with no enteral intake secrete extremely dilute bile, a finding which may explain some of the adverse hepatobiliary changes associated with TPN (Al-Rabeeah et al. 1986). Those who are parenterally fed also have significantly fewer immunoglobulin-containing intestinal plasma cells than those who are enterally fed (Knox 1986). The early introduction of milk feeds prescribed even in subnutritional quantities is therefore beneficial for growth, development and maintenance of normal structure and function in the GI and hepatobiliary systems (Berseth 1995). Once enteral feeds are being absorbed the PN should be reduced proportionally in the majority of infants. Once the infant has tolerated 100–120 ml/kg/day enterally consideration should be given to removing the central line and discontinuing PN, in order to minimise the infection risk. In a small number of neonates with evidence of malabsorption it may be necessary to provide concentrated PN in addition to substantial amounts of enteral feed. Paediatric dietetic involvement with these infants is essential.

Conclusion

Despite the many unanswered questions, PN remains an essential part of the care of many preterm and sick neonates. The optimal nutritional input for long-term health remains unknown. But it is becoming clear that many babies suffer extrauterine growth restriction in our neonatal intensive care units because of excessive caution with both PN and introduction of enteral feeds. Because of the potential complications PN should only be used in neonatal units where there are appropriate facilities and staff. Access to an appropriately skilled dietician and pharmacist is essential. PN is life-saving in many instances of neonatal GI failure, benefits long-term health and is an essential facet of modern neonatal intensive care.

References

Adamkin, D.H., Radmacher, P.G., Klingbeil, R.L., 1992. Use of intravenous lipid and hyperbilirubinemia in the first week. J Pediatr Gastroenterol Nutr 14, 135–139.

Al-Dahhan, J., Haycock, G.B., Chantler, C., et al., 1983. Sodium homeostasis in mature and immature neonates. I. Renal aspects. Arch Dis Child 58, 335–342.

Alpan, G., Eyal, F., Springer, C., et al., 1984. Heparinization of alimentation solutions administered through peripheral veins in premature infants: a controlled study. Pediatrics 74, 374–378.

Al-Rabeeah, A., Thurston, O.G., Walker, K., 1986. Effect of total parenteral nutrition on biliary lipids in neonates. Can J Surg 29, 289–291.

Aynsley-Green, A., 1983. Plasma hormone concentrations during enteral and parenteral nutrition in the human newborn. J Pediatr Gastroenterol Nutr 2, 108–112.

Baeckert, P.A., Greene, H.L., Fritz, I., et al., 1988. Vitamin concentrations in very low birth weight infants given vitamins intravenously in a lipid emulsion: measurement of vitamins A, D and E and riboflavin. J Pediatr 113, 1057–1063.

Bailey, M.J., 1979. Reduction of catheter-associated sepsis in parenteral nutrition using low-dose intravenous heparin. BMJ 1, 1671–1673.

Beale, E.F., Nelson, R.M., Bucciarelli, R.L., et al., 1979. Intrahepatic cholestasis associated with parenteral nutrition in premature infants. Pediatrics 64, 342–347.

Beardsall, K., Vanhaesebrouck, S., Ogilvie-Stuart, A., et al., 2008. Early insulin therapy in very- low-birth-weight-infants. N Engl J Med 359, 1873–1884.

Beganovic, N., Verloove-Vanhorick, S.P., Brand, R., et al., 1988. Total parenteral nutrition and sepsis. Arch Dis Child 63, 66–69.

Bell, R.L., Ferry, G.D., Smith, E.O., et al., 1986. Total parenteral nutrition related cholestasis in infants. JPEN J Parenter Enteral Nutr 10, 356–359.

Berseth, C.L., 1995. Minimal enteral feedings. Clin Perinatol 22, 195–204.

Berseth, C.L., Nordyke, C., 1993. Enteral nutrients promote postnatal maturation of intestinal motor activity in preterm infants. Am J Physiol 264, G1046–G1051.

Bishop, N.J., Morley, R., Day, J.P., et al., 1997. Aluminum neurotoxicity in preterm infants receiving intravenous-feeding solutions. N Engl J Med 336, 1557–1561.

Brans, Y.W., Dutton, E.B., Andrew, D.S., et al., 1986. Fat emulsion tolerance in very low birth weight neonates: effect on diffusion of oxygen in the lungs and on blood pH. Pediatrics 78, 79–84.

Brans, Y.W., Ritter, D.A., Kenny, J.D., et al., 1987. Influence of intravenous fat emulsion on serum bilirubin in very low birthweight infants. Arch Dis Child 62, 156–160.

Cairns, P.A., Stalker, D.J., 2000. Carnitine supplementation of parenterally fed neonates (Cochrane Review). Cochrane Database Syst Rev (4), CD000950.

Collins Jr, J.W., Hoppe, M., Brown, K., et al., 1991. A controlled trial of insulin infusion and parenteral nutrition in extremely low birth weight infants with glucose intolerance. J Pediatr 118, 921–927.

Cooke, R.J., Ainsworth, S.B., Fenton, A.C., 2004. Postnatal growth retardation: a universal problem in preterm infants. Arch Dis Child Fetal Neonatal Ed 89, F428–F430.

Cowett, R.M., Anderson, G.E., Maguire, C.A., et al., 1988. Ontogeny of glucose homeostasis in low birth weight infants. J Pediatr 112, 462–465.

Dahl, G.B., Svensson, L., Kinnander, N.J.G., et al., 1994. Stability of vitamins in soybean oil fat emulsion under conditions simulating intravenous feeding of neonates and children. JPEN J Parenter Enteral Nutr 18, 234–239.

Denne, S.C., 1998. Carbohydrate requirements. In: Polin, R.A., Fox, W.W. (Eds.), Fetal and Neonatal Physiology, second ed. W.B. Saunders, Philadelphia, pp. 325–327.

Ehrenkranz, R.A., Dusick, A.M., Vohr, B.R., et al., 2006. Growth in the neonatal intensive care unit influences neurodevelopmental and growth outcomes of extremely low birth weight infants. Pediatrics 117, 1253–1261.

Embleton, N.E., Pang, N., Cooke, R.J., 2001. Postnatal malnutrition: an inevitable consequence of current recommendations in preterm infants? Pediatrics 107, 270–273.

English, D., Roloff, J.S., Lukens, J.N., et al., 1981. Intravenous lipid emulsions and human neutrophil function. J Pediatr 99, 913–916.

Escobar, C., Salas, M., 1995. Dendritic branching of claustral neurons in neonatally undernourished rats. Biol Neonate 68, 47–54.

Fleer, A., Senders, R.C., Visser, M.R., et al., 1983. Septicemia due to coagulase-negative staphylococci in a neonatal intensive care unit: clinical and bacteriological features and contaminated parenteral fluids as a source of sepsis. Pediatr Infect Dis 2, 426–431.

Freeman, J., Goldman, D.A., Smith, N.E., et al., 1990. Association of intravenous lipid emulsion and coagulase-negative staphylococcal bacteria in neonatal intensive care units. N Engl J Med 323, 301–308.

Gilbertson, N., Kovar, I.Z., Cox, D.J., et al., 1991. Introduction of intravenous lipid administration on the first day of life in the low birth weight neonate. J Pediatr 119, 615–623.

Gilles, J., Jones, G., Pencharz, P., 1983. Delivery of vitamins A, D and E in parenteral nutrition solutions. JPEN J Parenter Enteral Nutr 7, 11–14.

Groh-Wargo, S., Ciaccia, A., Moore, J., 1988. Neonatal metabolic acidosis: effect of chloride from normal saline flushes. JPEN J Parenter Enteral Nutr 12, 159–161.

Gura, K.M., Lee, S., Valim, C., et al., 2008. Safety and efficacy of a fish oil based fat emulsion in the treatment of parenteral nutrition associated liver disease. Pediatrics 121, e678–e686.

Hanning, R.M., Atkinson, S.A., Whyte, R.K., 1991. Efficacy of calcium glycerophosphate vs conventional mineral salts for total parenteral nutrition in low-birth-weight infants: a randomized clinical trial. Am J Clin Nutr 54, 903–908.

Haumont, D., Deckelbaum, R.J., Richelle, M., et al., 1989. Plasma lipid and plasma lipoprotein concentrations in low birth weight infants given parenteral nutrition with twenty or ten percent lipid emulsion. J Pediatr 115, 787–793.

Heimler, R., Doumas, B.T., Jendrzejczak, B.M., et al., 1993. Relationship between nutrition, weight change, and fluid compartments in preterm infants during the first week of life. J Pediatr 122, 110–114.

Heird, W.C., Dell, R.B., Helms, R.A., et al., 1987. Amino acid mixture designed to maintain normal plasma amino acid patterns in infants and children requiring parenteral nutrition. Pediatrics 80, 401–408.

Helms, R.A., Christensen, M.L., Mauer, E.C., et al., 1987. Comparison of a pediatric versus standard amino acid formulation in preterm neonates requiring parenteral nutrition. J Pediatr 110, 466–470.

Hilliard, J.L., Shannon, D.L., Hunter, M.A., et al., 1983. Plasma lipid levels in preterm neonates receiving parenteral nutrition. Arch Dis Child 58, 29–33.

Hyman, P.E., Feldman, E.J., Ament, M.E., et al., 1983. Effect of enteral feeding on the maintenance of gastric acid secretory function. Gastroenterology 84, 341–345.

Ibrahim, H.M., Jeroudi, M.A., Baier, R.J., et al., 2004. Aggressive early total parental nutrition in low birth weight infants. J Perinatol 24, 482–486.

Jarvis, W.R., Highsmith, A.K., Allen, J.R., et al., 1983. Polymicrobial bacteremia associated with lipid emulsion in a neonatal intensive care unit. Pediatr Infect Dis 2, 203–208.

Kanarek, K.S., Kuznicki, M.B., Blair, R.C., 1991. Infusion of total parenteral nutrition via the umbilical artery. JPEN J Parenter Enteral Nutr 15, 71–74.

Khasu, M., Harrison, A., Lalari, V., et al., 2009. Impact of shielding parenteral nutrition from light on routine monitoring of blood glucose and triglyceride levels in preterm neonates. Arch Dis Child Fetal Neonatal Ed 94, F111–F115.

Knox, W.F., 1986. Restricted feeding and human intestinal plasma cell development. Arch Dis Child 61, 744–749.

Koletzko, B., Goulet, O., Hunt, J., et al., 2005. Guidelines on paediatric parenteral nutrition of the European Society of Paediatric Gastroenterology, Hepatology and Nutrition (ESPGHAN) and the European Society for Clinical Nutrition and Metabolism (ESPEN), supported by the European Society of Paediatric Research (ESPR). J Pediatr Gastroenterol Nutr 41, S1–87.

Kubota, A., Okada, A., Nezu, R., et al., 1988. Hyperbilirubinemia in neonates associated with total parenteral nutrition. JPEN J Parenter Enteral Nutr 12, 602–606.

Laidlaw, S.A., Kopple, J.D., 1987. Newer concepts of the indispensable amino acids. Am J Clin Nutr 46, 593–605.

Lee, E.J., Simmer, K., Gibson, R.A., 1993. Essential fatty acid deficiency in parenterally fed preterm infants. J Paediatr Child Health 29, 51–55.

Louik, C., Mitchell, A.A., Epstein, M.F., et al., 1985. Risk factors for neonatal hyperglycemia associated with 10% dextrose infusion. Am J Dis Child 139, 783–786.

Lucas, A., Bloom, S.R., Aynsley-Green, A., 1983. Metabolic and endocrine effects of depriving preterm infants of enteral nutrition. Acta Paediatr Scand 72, 245–249.

Lucas, A., Baker, B.A., Morley, R.M., 1993. Hyperphenylalaninaemia and outcome in intravenously fed preterm infants. Arch Dis Child 68, 579–583.

Lucas, A., Morley, R., Cole, T.J., 1998. Randomised trial of early diet in preterm babies and later intelligence quotient. BMJ 317, 1481–1487.

Malloy, M.H., Rassin, D.K., Richardson, C.J., 1984. Total parenteral nutrition in sick preterm infants: effects of cysteine supplementation with nitrogen intakes of 240 and 400 mg/kg/day. J Pediatr Gastroenterol Nutr 3, 239–244.

Merritt, R.J., 1986. Cholestasis associated with total parenteral nutrition. J Pediatr Gastroenterol Nutr 5, 9–22.

Mitton, S.G., Burston, D., Brueton, M.J., et al., 1993. Plasma amino acid profiles in preterm infants receiving Vamin 9 glucose or Vamin Infant. Early Hum Dev 32, 71–78.

Moore, M.C., Greene, H.L., Phillips, B., et al., 1986. Evaluation of a pediatric multiple vitamin preparation for total parenteral nutrition in infants and children. Pediatrics 77, 530–538.

National Confidential Enquiry into Patient Outcome and Death, 2010. A Mixed Bag: an Enquiry into the Care of Hospital Patients Receiving Parenteral Nutrition. Available online at: http//www.ncepod.org.uk.

Neuzil, J., Darlow, B.A., Inder, T.E., et al., 1995. Oxidation of parenteral lipid emulsion by ambient and phototherapy lights: potential toxicity of routine parenteral feeding. J Pediatr 126, 785–790.

Olunfunmi, P., Ryan, S., Matthew, L., et al., 1997. Randomised controlled trial of acetate in preterm neonates receiving parenteral nutrition. Arch Dis Child Fetal Neonatal Ed 77, F12–F15.

Ostertag, S.G., Jovanovic, L., Lewis, B., et al., 1986. Insulin pump therapy in the very low birth weight infant. Pediatrics 78, 625–630.

Park, W., Paust, H., Brosicke, H., et al., 1986. Impaired fat utilization in parenterally fed low birth weight infants suffering from sepsis. JPEN J Parenter Enteral Nutr 10, 627–630.

Pereira, G.R., Fox, W.W., Stanley, C.A., et al., 1980. Decreased oxygenation and hyperlipemia during intravenous fat infusions in premature infants. Pediatrics 66, 26–30.

Pereira, G.R., Sherman, M.S., DiGiacomo, J., et al., 1981. Hyperalimentation induced cholestasis. Am J Dis Child 135, 842–845.

Pineault, M., Chessex, P., Bisaillon, S., et al., 1988. Total parenteral nutrition in the newborn: impact of the quality of infused energy on nitrogen metabolism. Am J Clin Nutr 47, 298–304.

Puntis, J.W., Ball, P.A., Preece, M.A., et al., 1989. Egg and breast milk based nitrogen sources compared. Arch Dis Child 64, 1472–1477.

Puntis, J.W., Holden, C.E., Smallman, S., et al., 1991. Staff training: a key factor in reducing intravascular catheter sepsis. Arch Dis Child 66, 335–337.

Rager, R., Finegold, M.J., 1975. Cholestasis in immature newborn infants: is parenteral alimentation responsible? J Pediatr 86, 264–269.

Raupp, P., von Kries, R., Schmidt, E., et al., 1988. Incompatibility between fat emulsion and calcium plus heparin in parenteral nutrition of premature babies. Lancet I, 700.

Raupp, P., von Kries, R., Pfahl, H., et al., 1991. Glycero- vs glucose phosphate in parenteral nutrition of premature infants: a comparative in vitro evaluation of calcium/phosphorus compatibility. JPEN J Parenter Enteral Nutr 15, 469–473.

Reichman, B.L., Chessex, P., Putet, G., et al., 1982. Partition of energy metabolism and energy cost of growth in the very low birth weight infant. Pediatrics 69, 446–451.

Ridout, E., Melara, D., Rottinghaus, S., et al., 2005. Blood urea nitrogen concentration as a marker of amino acid intolerance in neonates with birth weight less than 1250 g. J Perinatol 25, 130–133.

Rivera Jr, A., Bell, E.F., Bier, D.M., 1993. Effect of intravenous amino acids on protein metabolism of preterm infants during the first three days of life. Pediatr Res 33, 106–111.

Rovamo, L.M., Nikkila, E.A., Raivio, K.O., 1988. Lipoprotein lipase, hepatic lipase, and carnitine in premature infants. Arch Dis Child 63, 140–147.

Rubecz, I., Mestyan, J., 1973. Energy metabolism and intravenous nutrition of premature infants. Biol Neonate 23, 45–58.

Salle, B.L., David, L., Chopard, J.P., et al., 1977. Prevention of early neonatal hypocalcemia in low birth weight infants with continuous calcium infusion: effect on serum calcium, phosphorus, magnesium, and circulating immunoactive parathyroid hormone and calcitonin. Pediatr Res 11, 1180–1185.

Schreiner, R.L., Glick, M.R., Nordschow, C.D., et al., 1979. An evaluation of methods to monitor infants receiving intravenous lipids. J Pediatr 94, 197–200.

Shulman, D.I., Kanarek, K., 1993. Gastrin, motilin, insulin, and insulin-like growth factor-I concentrations in very low birth weight infants receiving enteral or parenteral nutrition. JPEN J Parenter Enteral Nutr 17, 130–133.

Sinclair, J.C., Bottino, M., Cowett, R.M., 2009. Interventions for prevention of hyperglycemia in very low birth weight infants. Cochrane Database Syst Rev (3), CD007615.

Smith, J.L., Canham, J.E., Wells, P.A., 1988. Effect of phototherapy light, sodium bisulfite, and pH on vitamin stability in total parenteral nutrition and mixtures. JPEN J Parenter Enteral Nutr 12, 394–402.

Sondheimer, J.M., Bryan, H., Andrews, W., et al., 1978. Cholestatic tendencies in premature infants on and off parenteral nutrition. Pediatrics 62, 984–989.

Sosenko, I.R.S., Rodriguez-Pierce, M., Bancalari, E., 1993. Effect of early initiation of intravenous lipid administration on the incidence and severity of chronic lung disease in premature infants. J Pediatr 123, 975–982.

Strunk, R.C., Murrow, B.W., Thilo, E., et al., 1985. Normal macrophage function in infants receiving Intralipid by low-dose intermittent administration. J Pediatr 106, 640–645.

Te Braake, F.W., van den Aker, C.H., Wattimena, D.J., et al., 2005. Amino acid administration to premature infants immediately after birth. J Pediatr 147, 457–461.

Thaler, M.M., Wennberg, R.P., 1977. Influence of intravenous nutrients on bilirubin transport. II. Emulsified lipid solutions. Pediatr Res 11, 167–171.

Thornton, L., Griffin, E., 1991. Evaluation of a taurine containing amino acid solution in parenteral nutrition. Arch Dis Child 66, 21–25.

Thureen, P.J., Hay Jr, W.W., 2001. Early aggressive nutrition in preterm infants. Semin Neonatal 6, 403–415.

Thureen, P., Heird, W., 2005. Protein and energy requirements of the preterm/low birth weight infant. Pediatr Res 57, 95–98R.

Thureen, P.J., Melara, D., Fennessey, P.V., et al., 2003. Effect of low vs high intravenous amino acid intake on very low birth weight infants in the early neonatal period. Pediatr Res 53, 24–32.

Tsang, R.C., 2005. Summary of reasonable nutritional intakes for preterm infants. In: Tsang, R.C., Uauy, R., Koletzko, B., et al. (Eds.), Nutrition of the Preterm Infant, second ed. Digital Educational Publishing, Ohio, pp. 417–418.

Unger, A., Goetzman, B.W., Chan, C., et al., 1986. Nutritional practices and outcome of extremely premature infants. Am J Dis Child 140, 1027–1033.

Van Aerde, J.E., Sauer, P.J., Pencharz, P.B., et al., 1994. Metabolic consequences of increasing energy intake by adding lipid to parenteral nutrition in full-term infants. Am J Clin Nutr 59, 659–662.

Wahlig, T.M., Georgieff, M.K., 1995. The effects of illness on neonatal metabolism and nutritional management. Clin Perinatol 22, 77–96.

Webb, A.N., Hardy, P., Peterkin, M., et al., 2008. Tolerability and safety of olive oil-based lipid emulsion in critically ill neonates: a blinded randomized trial. Nutrition 24, 1057–1064.

Weese-Mayer, D.E., Fondriest, D.W., Brouilette, R.T., et al., 1987. Risk factors associated with candidemia in the neonatal intensive care unit: a case control study. Pediatr Infect Dis J 6, 190–196.

Zlotkin, S.H., Bryan, M.H., Anderson, G.H., 1981. Intravenous nitrogen and energy intakes required to duplicate in utero nitrogen accretion in prematurely born human infants. J Pediatr 99, 115–120.

Appendix: How to write a total parenteral nutrition (TPN) prescription

There are two approaches to the provision of neonatal TPN. The first is to use standard bags, that is, bags containing the desired quantity of amino acids, dextrose and electrolytes for a preterm infant receiving 150 ml/kg/day TPN. Therefore the nutrients are increased proportionately as the fluid volume is increased over the first week. These have the advantage of cost and convenience and are suitable for the majority of preterm infants. They also have the advantage of minimising prescriber error and can be useful in units with limited access to specialist paediatric dietetic and pharmacy services. Those infants with high electrolyte requirements, a significant volume of non-nutritional infusates or prolonged fluid restriction may benefit from individualised prescriptions. Some units use individualised prescriptions for all their patients for this reason; others have agreed a small number of standard bags with varying concentrations of nutrients. Many units use a mixture of standard bags to enable PN to be commenced outside working hours, with individualised PN commencing the next working day.

The method of prescribing TPN also varies widely across units. The precise volume and concentrations of amino acid, dextrose and electrolyte solutions may be calculated in the neonatal intensive care unit or in the pharmacy, with or without the aid of a computer program. It is important for each hospital to assess its processes for all sources of potential human error and minimise this. In St Michael's Hospital, Bristol, we prescribe the desired quantity of nutrients for each individual baby and the calculations are carried out in the pharmacy. It is important to be familiar with the exact process in each hospital as 15% dextrose in one hospital may refer to an overall concentration of 15% while in another it may mean that 15% dextrose has been added to the solution, resulting in a significantly more dilute product.

General guidelines

- Decide the total daily fluid intake for the baby.
- Subtract all other intravenous infusion volumes (such as arterial line fluid or inotropes).
- Order parenteral nutrition (PN) for the remaining volume. As the enteral input increases, the intravenous protein, lipid and carbohydrate intake will reduce proportionately.
- When calculating the desired sodium intake, remember to take into consideration any saline or sodium bicarbonate infusions.

Protein

- Start early (within the first 24 hours if possible for all preterm infants).
- Start at 1.5 g/kg/day.
- Use a neonatal formulation.
- Increase by 1 g/kg/day to a total of 3.5 g/kg/day.
- Use with caution in babies with renal impairment (may need restriction to 2.5 g/kg/day) or with suspected inborn errors of metabolism (stop while investigations are awaited).

Dextrose

- Prescribe as mg/kg/min, starting at 6 mg/kg/min.
- Increase by daily increments of 2 mg/kg/min if tolerated to a maximum of 8.3 mg/kg/min.
- If using a peripheral cannula, note that the maximum overall dextrose concentration of the solution should be 12.5%.

Lipid

- Start at 1 g/kg/day on day 1 of PN. Use 20% emulsion.
- Increase by 1 g/kg/day to a maximum of 3.5 g/kg/day.
- Check triglyceride levels after a 4-hour lipid-free period twice weekly.
- Use with caution in babies with acute sepsis (temporary lipid intolerance), labile pulmonary hypertension (altered prostaglandin synthesis) or severe jaundice (fatty acid displacement of bilirubin from albumin).

Electrolytes and minerals

- Add sodium when the plasma sodium starts to fall, and titrate. The usual maintenance dose is a total of 2–4 mmol/kg/day. Allow for sodium content of other infusions. Once sodium intake is greater than 3 mmol/kg/day, use sodium acetate.
- Start potassium at 1–2 mmol/kg/day on day 3 and titrate.
- Start calcium and phosphate at 1–1.5 mmol/kg/day on day 1. Discuss with pharmacist if higher concentrations are desired.
- Start magnesium at 0.2 mmol/kg/day and titrate.
- Add maintenance trace elements, such as Peditrace (Fresenius Kabi) 1 ml/kg/day.

Vitamins

- Add water-soluble vitamins to amino acid solution from day 1, such as Solvito N (Fresenius Kabi) 1 ml/kg/day.
- Add fat-soluble vitamins to lipid emulsions from day 1, such as Vitlipid N Infant (Fresenius Kabi) 4 ml/kg/day to a maximum of 10 ml.

Fluid and electrolyte balance

Neena Modi

18

Introduction

This chapter will discuss the principles of newborn electrolyte and water balance and present a practical approach to clinical management. Renal function, clinical monitoring and renal disease are discussed in Chapter 35 part 1.

Postnatal alterations in body water distribution

The newborn baby's body is largely composed of water. The extracellular compartment forms around 65% of bodyweight at 26 weeks' gestation, reducing to 40% at term and 20% by the age of 10 years (Fig. 18.1) (Friis-Hansen 1961, 1983). Superimposed on this gradual reduction with age is a more abrupt contraction that occurs shortly after birth (Shaffer et al. 1986; Bauer and Versmold 1989; Shaffer and Meade 1989; Bauer et al. 1991; Heimler et al. 1993; Singhi et al. 1995). This is due to loss of the interstitial fluid component of the extracellular fluid (ECF) compartment and is closely related to cardiopulmonary adaptation. The contraction of ECF accounts, at least in part, for early postnatal weight loss and occurs rapidly in healthy babies, but is delayed in babies with respiratory distress syndrome (RDS) (Modi and Hutton 1990).

Several studies suggest that the contraction of the ECF is triggered by atrial natriuretic peptide released in response to increased atrial stretch as pulmonary vascular pressure falls (Kojima et al. 1987; Tulassay et al. 1987; Rozycki and Baumgart 1991; Bétrémieux et al. 1995) and left atrial venous return increases. The intravascular compartment may also be acutely expanded during birth by the reabsorption of lung liquid and the effect of a variable placental transfusion. As the timing of the diuresis/natriuresis is to some extent related to the fall in pulmonary vascular pressure, it is not surprising that attempts to improve the course of RDS with diuretics have not shown benefit (Brion and Soll 2001).

A corollary of the isotonic loss of ECF is that net water and sodium balance in the first days after birth is negative (Fig. 18.2) (Shaffer and Weismann 1992). This is borne out by the observation that in newborn babies an increase in sodium intake leads to an increase in excretion (Rees et al. 1984b; Shaffer and Meade 1989; Lambert et al. 1990) until contraction of the extracellular compartment occurs. Sodium balance then becomes positive, commensurate with growth. However, preterm babies have a limited capacity to excrete a sodium load (see Ch. 35 part 1), so that, despite increasing excretion in response to an increase in intake, sodium retention readily occurs (Costarino et al. 1992; Bétrémieux et al. 1995). If there is concurrent restriction in the intake of water, these babies readily become hypernatraemic (Shaffer and Meade 1989). If a more liberal intake of water accompanies the intake of sodium, isotonic expansion of the extracellular compartment is the result, evidenced by weight gain at a time when weight loss is to be expected. In most babies, this cumulative positive balance is lost later, so that the normal postnatal change in body water distribution occurs but is delayed (Bétrémieux et al. 1995). Delayed loss of extracellular water increases the risks and severity of respiratory

© 2012 Elsevier Ltd

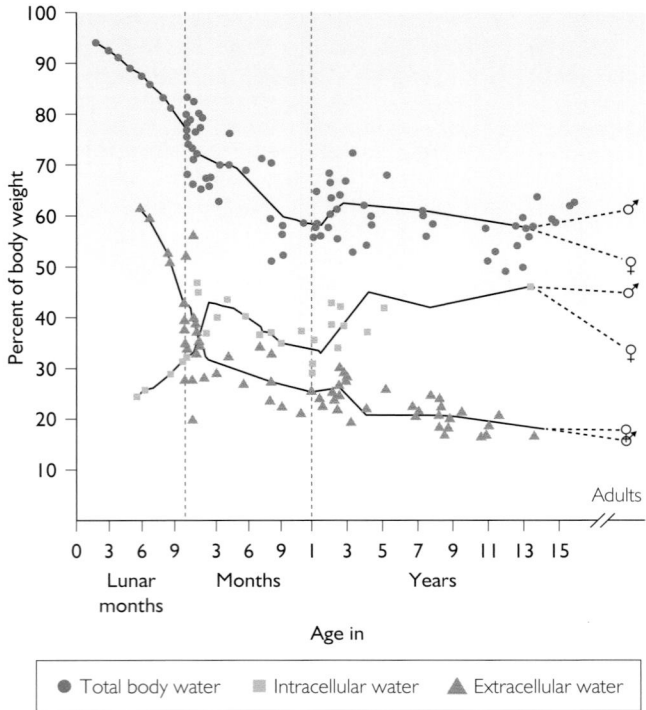

Fig. 18.1 Body water compartments as percentages of bodyweight from early fetal life to adult life. *(Adapted from Friis-Hansen (1961).)*

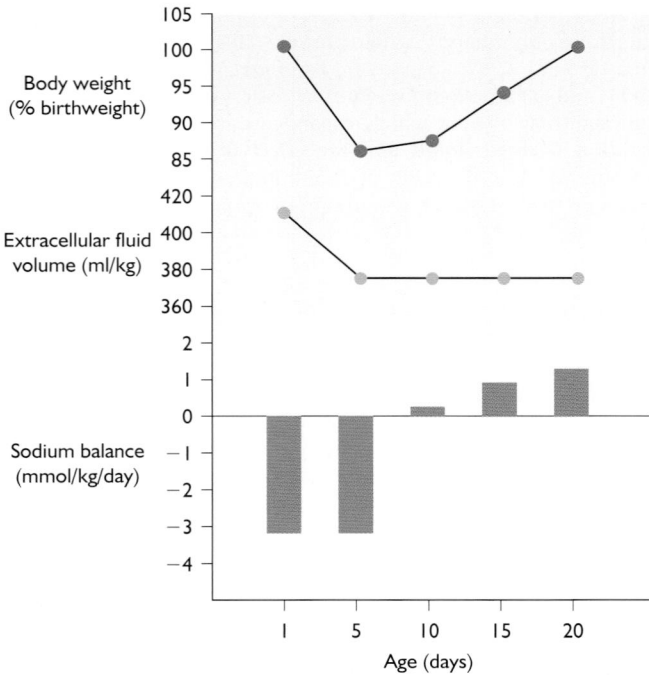

Fig. 18.2 Postnatal changes in bodyweight, extracellular volume and sodium balance. *(Adapted from Shaffer and Weismann (1992).)*

illness in the newborn (Mohan et al. 1984; Rojas et al. 1984; Singhi and Chookang 1984; Singhi et al. 1985; Hartnoll et al. 2000b) and weight gain in the first days after birth, in babies with RDS, is associated with an increased risk of developing chronic lung disease (Van Marter et al. 1990).

Present-day management involving antenatal steroid therapy, postnatal surfactant, good intrapartum care and immediate postnatal stabilisation has modified the natural history of RDS so that cardiopulmonary adaptation generally occurs rapidly and the postnatal loss of ECF occurs imperceptibly, as in a full-term baby. In the pre-surfactant era, the abrupt onset of diuresis/natriuresis (Modi and Hutton 1990) heralded the improvement in respiratory function.

Non-renal influences on water balance

Insensible water loss occurs through the skin, respiratory tract and in stool. Stool water loss is usually small and usually less than 5 ml/kg/24 h in the first days after birth. The upper respiratory tract warms and humidifies inspired gases, and full saturation (44 mg/l) is achieved by the mid-trachea. If the upper respiratory tract is bypassed with an endotracheal tube, respiratory water loss must be reduced by adequate humidification of inspired gases. Humidification is also advisable when delivering low-flow oxygen and during continuous positive airway pressure.

The skin is an important regulator of water balance in extremely preterm babies. Transepidermal water loss reflects skin immaturity and may be considerable, even exceeding urine volume. Sodium is not lost through the skin, because babies born below 36 weeks' gestation do not sweat, though this develops within the first 2 weeks after birth (Harpin and Rutter 1982).

The stratum corneum of the skin consists of overlapping dead epidermal cells filled with keratin that form a barrier to water loss. Keratinisation begins at around 18 weeks' gestation, but the fetal epidermis is still very thin at 26 weeks and the stratum corneum is barely visible. During the last trimester, the epidermis and stratum corneum thicken and keratinisation becomes more marked (Evans and Rutter 1986). Each millilitre of water that evaporates from the skin is accompanied by the loss of 560 calories of heat, and so it is difficult to keep a baby with a high transepidermal water loss warm. This is the principle underlying the practice of placing extremely preterm babies in a plastic bag at delivery for thermal protection (see Ch. 15).

Skin maturation, unlike the maturation of renal function, is accelerated by birth, but not by antenatal steroid therapy (Jain et al. 2000). Transepidermal loss falls exponentially with increasing gestational and postnatal age (Fig. 18.3) (Hammarlund and Sedin 1979; Hammarlund et al. 1982, 1983; Sedin et al. 1985). After 32 weeks' gestation, water loss through the skin is around 12 ml/kg/day (Rutter 1989). Transepidermal loss is influenced by ambient humidity, skin integrity, environmental and skin temperature, air speed and radiant heat sources, including phototherapy (Tables 18.1 and 18.2). Radiant heat sources can increase transepidermal water loss by a factor of up to 0.5–2 (Rutter 1989). A high environmental humidity reduces transepidermal water loss, an effect that is most marked in the most immature infants (Fig. 18.4) (Hammarlund and Sedin 1979). Insensible water loss can be reduced to less than 40 ml/kg/day in infants weighing less than 1000 g if ambient humidity is maintained above 90% (Takahashi et al. 1994). Humidification is easier with an incubator, particularly if double-walled, but a low-cost stratagem is to use bubblewrap or other plastic sheeting and a humidified body box to achieve a high

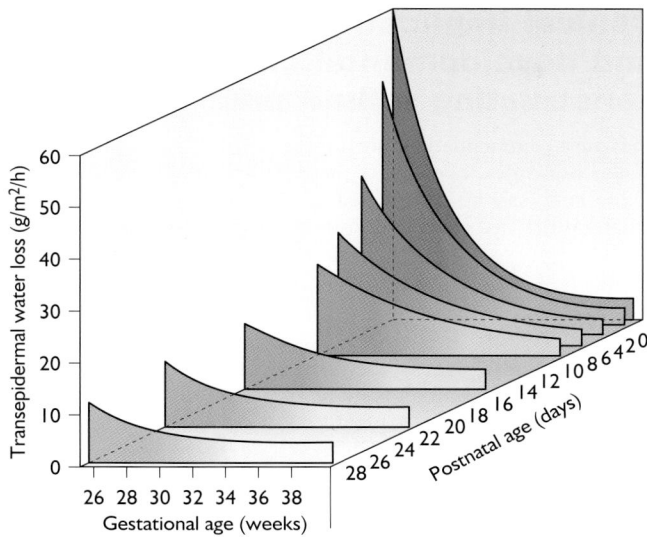

Fig. 18.3 Transepidermal water loss in relation to gestational age at birth at different postnatal ages in appropriate-for-gestational-age infants. *(Adapted from Sedin et al. (1985).)*

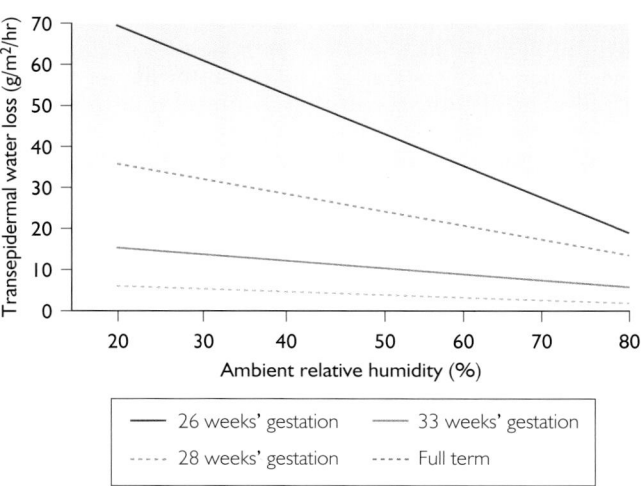

Fig. 18.4 The effect of ambient relative humidity on transepidermal water loss (based on the data of Hammarlund and Sedin 1979). *(Reproduced from Rutter (1989).)*

Table 18.1 Factors influencing insensible water loss

INCREASED LOSS	DECREASED LOSS	INCUBATOR
Lower gestational age	Clothing	Body box
Lower postnatal age	High humidity	Plastic blanket
Denuded/broken skin		Good skin care
Increased skin temperature		Topical ointments and emollients
Increased activity		Humidification of inspired gases
Increased environmental temperature		High humidity
Radiant heat sources		
Radiant warmers		
Phototherapy units		
Draughts		
Excessive crying		

Table 18.2 Transepidermal water loss at an ambient humidity of 50% (mean ± SD)

GESTATIONAL AGE (weeks)	n	POSTNATAL AGE (days)					
		0–1	3	7	14	21	28
25–27	9	129 ± 39	71 ± 9	43 ± 9	32 ± 10	28 ± 10	24 ± 10
28–30	13	42 ± 13	32 ± 9	24 ± 7	18 ± 6	15 ± 6	15 ± 6
31–36	22	12 ± 5	12 ± 4	12 ± 4	9 ± 3	8 ± 2	7 ± 1
37–41	24	7 ± 2	6 ± 1	6 ± 1	6 ± 1	6 ± 0	7 ± 1

Reproduced from Hammarlund et al. (1983).

humidity microenvironment immediately around the baby. The degree of humidification that can be achieved without causing condensation ('rain-out') on the inner wall of the incubator is dependent on the temperature gradient across the incubator wall. Condensation predisposes to skin maceration and should be avoided. Draughts should be eliminated. Stripping of the stratum corneum and deeper abrasions of the skin can be reduced by using non-abrasive tape such as Micropore, neonatal electrodes and skin protectants, prior to affixing urine bags and electrodes. Water-impermeable barriers, such as soft paraffin, or topical ointments reduce transepidermal water loss (Pabst et al. 1999; Wananukul and Praisuwanna 2002) but concern about increased infection and difficulty in fixing electrodes have limited their use. Adequate provision of fluid is also necessary, using a system that allows the intravenous glucose delivery rate to be altered independently of fluid volume in order to avoid hyperglycaemia (Al Rubeyi et al. 1994), osmotic diuresis and worsening of the situation. The extent to which transepidermal water loss is reduced, hypernatraemic dehydration and hyperglycaemia avoided and temperature stability maintained is an index of the quality of nursing and medical care and a useful measure for audit.

Clinical implications of postnatal and developmental changes: constructing a fluid prescription

Didactic recommendations are unnecessary. With an understanding of the principles involved, a prescription tailored to the needs of the baby can be constructed. Fluid management in common situations in neonatal intensive care is summarised in Tables 18.3–18.5.

The first days after birth

The goal of fluid management during the period of postnatal adaptation is to permit an isotonic contraction of the extracellular compartment and a brief period of negative sodium and water balance.

Water should be provided in an intake sufficient to allow the excretion of a relatively small initial renal solute load (Ziegler and Fomon 1971) and, in very preterm babies, to maintain tonicity in the face of initially high, but rapidly falling, transepidermal losses.

Table 18.3 Estimated starting intravenous intake, at an ambient humidity of 50%*

GESTATIONAL AGE (weeks)	BIRTHWEIGHT (kg)	APPROXIMATE TRANSEPIDERMAL WATER LOSS (ml/kg/24 h)	ALLOWANCE FOR URINE OUTPUT (ml/kg/24 h)	ESTIMATED INTAKE RANGE (ml/kg/24 h)	SUGGESTED STARTING VOLUME (ml/kg/24 h)[†]
<27	<1.0	120	30–60	150–180	150[‡]
27–30	1.0–1.5	40	30–60	70–100	90
31–36	1.5–2.5	15	30–60	45–75	60
>36	>2.5	10	30–60	40–70	60

*At higher ambient humidities, transepidermal water losses will be reduced and requirements will be lower.
[†]Once sustained weight loss of at least 5% is achieved, proceed to the intravenous volume necessary to support nutritional goals without stepwise increments.
[‡]A cautious approach, commencing at the lower end of the estimated requirement, is recommended.

Table 18.4 Goals of immediate fluid management in extremely preterm babies

GOAL	MEANS OF ACCOMPLISHING GOAL
Minimise insensible water loss	Provide high humidity around infant using incubator or body box and plastic sheeting; minimum handling; meticulous skin care; eliminate draughts
Facilitate loss of extracellular fluid	Minimise intravenous sodium administration until postnatal diuresis/natriuresis marked by weight loss is underway
Maintain glucose homeostasis	Use a variable glucose delivery system if glucose tolerance is unstable (Al Rubeyi et al. 1994)
Optimise nutritional support	Commence parenteral and minimal enteral nutrition on day 1; stepwise increments are unnecessary in stable infants
Maintain renal perfusion	Monitor blood pressure, core–peripheral temperature gap, capillary refill time, urine output, cardiac function and central venous pressure; use volume and inotropic support as necessary

Table 18.5 Common clinical problems in fluid balance management

PROBLEM	ACTION
Respiratory distress syndrome	Initial infusion volume determined by anticipated insensible water loss; delay maintenance intravenous sodium administration until postnatal diuresis/natriuresis marked by weight loss is underway
Patent ductus arteriosus	Routine fluid restriction inappropriate as this will compromise nutrition; fluid-restrict if there is evidence of heart failure; indometacin/ibuprofen toxicity is exacerbated by dehydration
Severe birth asphyxia at term	Anticipate possibility of renal failure; 0.9% NaCl may be necessary for initial resuscitation and restoration of renal perfusion; restrict maintenance intake to 20–30 ml/kg/day until renal function can be assessed; central vascular access likely to be necessary for infusion of hypertonic glucose
Chronic lung disease	Avoid prolonged periods of fluid restriction; poor nutrition will worsen prognosis; diuretic-induced chronic sodium depletion will further compromise growth
Necrotising enterocolitis	Intestinal fluid loss may be considerable; interpretation of changes in body weight is difficult; profound intravascular volume depletion may be present without weight loss; monitor toe–core temperature gap; provide isotonic volume replacement (0.9% NaCl) if temperature gap exceeds 3°C
Preoperative	Fluid intake should not be reduced preoperatively; the infant should be well hydrated
Intraoperative	Minimise transepidermal water loss; administer glucose 5% or 10% in 0.9% NaCl during surgery
Postoperative	Unrecognised hypovolaemia is common and may contribute to postoperative hyponatraemia; infuse glucose 5% or 10% in 0.9% NaCl for at least 12 hours following surgery

Estimate the likely magnitude of insensible water loss using the information presented in Figures 18.3 and 18.4 and Table 18.2. A rational initial intravenous fluid volume would be the sum of an allowance for urinary water of 30–60 ml/kg/day plus estimated insensible water loss (Table 18.3) (Modi 1997). Given present-day care and an ambient humidity in excess of 50%, this usually equates to around 100 ml/kg/day for babies below 1500 g. If insensible water losses are predicted to be high, for example during the period immediately after delivery when the baby is being stabilised, start with a high intake but reduce this once a high-humidity environment is established. As it is not possible to predict precisely transepidermal water loss, the integrity of renal function or the timing of the postnatal natriuresis/diuresis, the adequacy of the estimate must be assessed within 6–8 hours.

The immediate administration of maintenance sodium in parenteral fluid is unwarranted and adversely affects respiratory outcome even in infants exposed to antenatal steroids. Costarino et al. (1992) compared sodium restriction for 5 days after birth with immediate administration of 3–4 mmol/kg/day in a blind trial. Water was prescribed independently. In the latter group sodium balance was positive on the first day after birth and there was a significantly higher incidence of bronchopulmonary dysplasia (BPD). Hartnoll et al. (2000a), in a blind, controlled trial, randomised infants born at 25–30 weeks' gestation to receive a parenteral sodium intake of 4 mmol/kg/day from the first day after birth or when a weight loss of 6% had occurred. ECF volume was measured at birth and on day 14. A significant reduction in ECF volume was observed in the group who received the delayed sodium intake, in contrast to the early-intake group, in whom no reduction was seen. By the end of the first week, 35% of babies in the delayed-intake group and 8.7% of the early-intake group, and by 28 days after birth 40% of the delayed-intake group compared with 18% of the early-intake group, no longer required additional oxygen. There was no difference between the groups in the rate of reduction in pulmonary artery pressure (Hartnoll et al. 2001), suggesting that the poorer respiratory outcome in the early-intake group was not attributable to delayed cardiopulmonary adaptation but rather to persistent expansion of the extracellular compartment and delayed clearance of pulmonary interstitial fluid.

Intravenous sodium in maintenance fluid should be avoided until the physiological postnatal diuresis/natriuresis (Modi and Hutton 1990; Bétrémieux et al. 1995) is underway, marked clinically by the onset of weight loss (Bauer et al. 1991; Singhi et al. 1995; Tang et al. 1997). There is no 'correct' figure for postnatal weight loss, as hydration at birth is variable (Tang et al. 1993) and birthweight does not correlate closely with extracellular water volume (Shaffer et al. 1986). Early postnatal weight loss reflects both the loss of body water and the loss of body solids. With improved nutritional support for preterm babies, early postnatal weight loss is diminished, though body water loss remains the same. In a study comparing healthy preterm babies with a group with RDS, during the first week after birth, both groups lost an identical amount of body water, namely 10% of the total body water content at birth. However, the healthy babies lost a maximum of 5.9% of birthweight, in contrast to a loss of 8.6% in the RDS group. This was because the healthy babies received a higher energy intake and gained solids to a significantly greater extent (Fig. 18.5) (Tang et al. 1997).

Glucose delivery should commence at around 7 mg/kg/min. Increasingly this is delivered with amino acids as parenteral nutrition immediately after birth. When glucose requirements are unstable the use of 5% and 50% glucose solutions delivered through a Y connection allows the glucose delivery rate and the volume infused to be readily altered independently (Barr et al. 1977) (Table 18.6).

Fluid 'restriction'

Neonatal paediatricians have long been concerned about 'excessive' fluid intake. Associations have been described between 'high' fluid intakes and increased risk of symptomatic patent ductus arteriosus (Stevenson 1977; Bell et al. 1980), necrotising enterocolitis (Bell

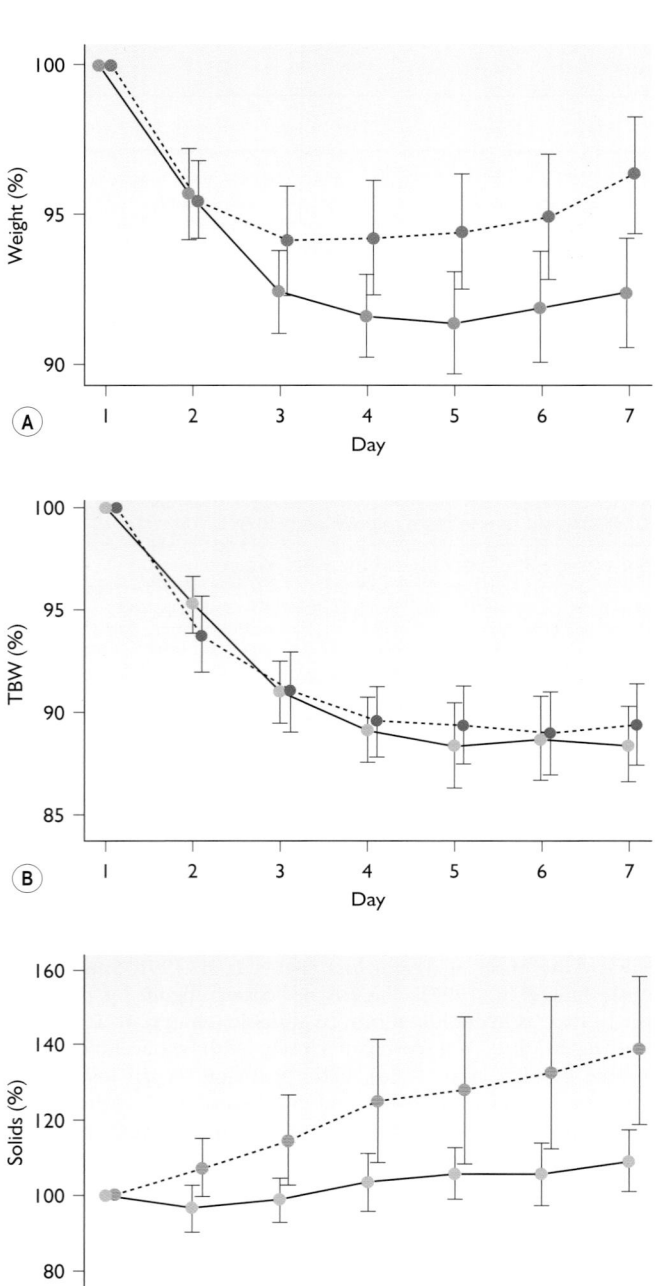

Fig. 18.5 Weight, total body water (TBW) and body solids during the first week after birth in healthy preterm babies (dotted line) and babies with respiratory distress syndrome (solid line). Values (mean ± 95% confidence interval) are expressed as a percentage of the value at birth. *(Adapted from Tang et al. (1997).)*

et al. 1979) and BPD (Brown et al. 1978; Van Marter et al. 1990; Costarino et al. 1992). On the basis of a systematic review of four randomised trials (Bell et al. 1980; von Stockhausen and Struve 1980; Lorenz et al. 1982; Tammela and Koivisto 1992), only one of which found a significant reduction in the subsequent diagnosis of a patent ductus arteriosus and no overall difference in BPD, 'careful restriction' of fluid intake has been recommended (Bell and

Acarregui 2001). However the term 'fluid restriction' is imprecise, and covers a wide range of water and sodium intake. Sodium intake was not controlled in these studies, so that increased 'fluid' meant an increased intake of both sodium and water. It is primarily the increased intake of sodium and resulting expansion of the extracellular compartment that appears responsible for the increase in morbidity.

The growing infant

Once the phase of immediate postnatal adaptation is over, the management of fluid and electrolyte balance must be tailored to the paramount demands of growth. It is questionable whether stepwise increments in parenteral nutrition are necessary once postnatal weight loss has been achieved as stable preterm babies are capable of excreting large volumes of water (Coulthard and Hey 1985; Modi 1997) and tolerating the metabolic load of immediate total parenteral nutrition. Milk feeds should be commenced concurrently providing enteral feeding is indicated (Ch. 16, Ch. 29.3). The energy density of parenteral nutrition should determine the volume prescribed, with the target a nutritional intake in excess of 100 kcal/kg/day. Once fully enterally fed, preterm babies may require in excess of 200 ml/kg/day of breast milk to achieve satisfactory growth, though non-renal, not renal, factors may limit tolerance.

Sodium is essential for growth, and a deficiency inhibits DNA synthesis in the most immature cells (Ostlund et al. 1993). Chronic limitation of intake is associated not only with extracellular volume contraction and poor weight gain, but also with poor skeletal and tissue growth (Chance et al. 1977; Haycock and Aperia 1991; Wassner 1991; Haycock 1993) and adverse neurodevelopmental outcome (Haycock 1993). In babies below 32 weeks' gestation fed intravenously, commence sodium administration at 4 mmol/kg/day once 5% weight loss has been achieved. Human milk provides about 1 mmol/kg sodium daily in a volume of about 150 ml/kg (Ch. 16, Table 16.1, 15 mg/100 ml). If retained, this is sufficient for normal growth. The full-term baby has efficient renal tubular and intestinal reabsorption but extremely immature babies require around 4 mmol/kg/day, or more if, for example, they are on treatment with diuretics (Haycock and Aperia 1991). The earliest sign of chronic sodium depletion will be poor weight gain, and not hyponatraemia, which is a late occurrence. A sodium intake of around 4 mmol/kg/day should continue until at least 32 weeks' postmenstrual age, by which time maturation of sodium conservation is likely to have occurred (Roy et al. 1976; Al-Dahhan et al. 1984).

Monitoring fluid balance

Fluid balance should be monitored carefully and is the responsibility of both medical and nursing staff. All too often, a failure to detect a problem in its early stages leads to a potentially reversible situation becoming irreversible. If a baby is unwell and requiring intensive care, or is largely dependent on intravenous fluids, the serum sodium, potassium, creatinine and bodyweight should be measured daily, and urine output monitored continuously (Table 18.7). Nursing charts should be designed so that hourly intake and output volumes can be recorded if required. Accurate weighing is important, taking the weights of attachments into account and recording net weight. Isotonic expansion of the extracellular compartment will be missed if changes in bodyweight are not considered in conjunction with the serum sodium concentration. Satisfactory fluid management is marked by a urine flow rate of at least 0.5–1 ml/kg/h on the first day, rising to 2–3 ml/kg/h

Table 18.6 Example of variable glucose delivery utilising simultaneous 5% and 50% solutions delivered through a Y connection (Al Rubeyi et al. 1994)

GLUCOSE DELIVERY RATE (mg/kg/min)	5% GLUCOSE INFUSION RATE (ml/kg/h)	50% GLUCOSE INFUSION RATE (ml/kg/h)	TOTAL VOLUME (ml/kg/24 h)
7	2.3	0.6	70
	5.5	0.3	140
5	2.6	0.3	70
	5.8		140

Table 18.7 Monitoring fluid balance in acutely ill infants

VARIABLE	FREQUENCY	COMMENTS
Weight	Daily	Steady initial loss of 1–2% daily; maximum weight loss variable but usually in the range of 5–10%; weight gain should have commenced by 7–10 days
Urine output	Continuously	Review 4–8-hourly; should exceed 0.5 ml/kg/h on day 1 in extremely preterm infants; thereafter, 2–3 ml/kg/h in all infants; less than 1 ml/kg/h requires investigation
Serum sodium	Daily or twice daily	132–144 mmol/l
Serum potassium	Daily or twice daily	3.8–5.7 mmol/l; spurious elevation due to haemolysis common
Serum creatinine	Daily	Usually a steady decline after birth, although a rise is not unusual in very preterm babies (Miall et al 1999).

thereafter, daily weight loss of the order of 1–2%, followed by weight gain of the order of 14–16 g/kg/day once a balanced energy intake greater than 100 kcal/kg/day has been achieved, a steady fall in serum creatinine and Na and K concentrations within the normal range (Table 18.7). The interpretation of urinary indices, urine flow rate and serum creatinine are discussed in Chapter 35 part 1.

Common clinical problems

Hypernatraemia and hyponatraemia

Changes in the serum sodium concentration reflect both sodium and water balance. In hypernatraemia (serum sodium >145 mmol/l) there is an absolute or relative deficit of water in relation to body sodium. In hyponatraemia (serum sodium <135 mmol/l), there is relative or absolute excess of body water. In both hypernatraemia and hyponatraemia, total body sodium may be increased, decreased or unchanged. It is a reasonable assumption that hyponatraemia and hypernatraemia contribute to neurological morbidity in sick newborn babies, though quantification of the effect, particularly in preterm babies, is difficult. Brain cell volume is affected by acute changes in extracellular tonicity. The regulation of cell volume following cell swelling or shrinkage in response to changes in extracellular tonicity is brought about by the accumulation or loss of inorganic ions and organic solutes. Compensatory changes in electrolyte content occur rapidly, so that, during acute exposure to hypertonicity, there is a rapid movement of electrolytes into the cell, in favour of water retention. Adaptation to chronic hyperosmolar states occurs by increasing the concentration of intracellular organic osmolytes (Strange 1993). These include polyols (sorbitol, myoinositol), certain amino acids (taurine, alanine, proline) and methylamines (betaine, glycerylphosphorylcholine).

Loss of organic osmolytes occurs more slowly than movement of electrolytes. If chronic hyperosmolality is corrected rapidly, the influx of water into the cell continues, resulting in cell swelling and cerebral oedema. Cell swelling can lead to occlusion of blood flow, hypoxia and release of cytotoxic neuroexcitatory amino acids. Conversely, an acute fall in serum sodium concentration will first lead to the movement of water into cells and the development of intracellular oedema and brain swelling. Over a period of time, the concentration of intracellular osmolytes decreases, so as to favour the movement of water out of the cell. If extracellular hypotonicity is then corrected rapidly, the continued movement of water out of the cell will result in brain shrinkage.

Although the timescale over which the human brain adapts to alterations in tonicity by increasing or decreasing intracellular organic osmolytes is not clearly established, a chronic imbalance in tonicity should probably be corrected slowly, over at least 48–72 hours. The management of acute imbalance may be quicker. If hypernatraemia has developed rapidly, over a period of hours, reducing the serum sodium by 1 mmol/l/h appears safe. If hypernatraemia develops slowly, over a period of days, the rate of reduction in serum sodium should not exceed 0.5 mmol/l/h.

Proton magnetic resonance spectroscopy provides a non-invasive direct means of quantifying the organic osmolyte response to disturbances in osmolality. Lee et al. (1994) reported a 44% increase in cerebral osmolyte content in a child with chronic hypernatraemia (serum Na 195 mmol/l) that returned to normal 36 days after start of therapy. We have found a normal cerebral myoinositol 8 days after the start of therapy in a term neonate in whom hypernatraemia (serum Na 173 mmol/l) developed over a period of 8 days (unpublished data).

When attempting to establish the cause of hyponatraemia or hypernatraemia, assess the change in bodyweight in conjunction with the clinical context. If a baby gains weight in the first days after birth at a time when weight loss would be anticipated and the serum sodium concentration is normal, isotonic expansion of the extracellular compartment has occurred and sodium and water balance is positive, at a time when it should be negative (Bétrémieux et al. 1995). Hyponatraemia with weight loss or inadequate weight gain suggests sodium depletion. Hypernatraemia with weight loss suggests dehydration; hypernatraemia with weight gain suggests sodium and water overload. Hyponatraemia due to water excess responds to water restriction but should not detract from treatment of the underlying cause. Hyponatraemia due to sodium deficit requires an increase in sodium intake, but, once body stores have been replenished, this should be reduced to maintenance requirements.

Hypernatraemia

In extremely preterm babies, hypernatraemia occurring in the first few days of postnatal life is usually due to excessive transepidermal water loss, possibly compounded by sodium administration in excess of excretory capacity. As this is a situation in which hypernatraemia may escalate rapidly, it should be treated promptly by increasing the volume of infused fluid, avoiding an excessive sodium intake, avoiding or treating hyperglycaemia and redoubling efforts to reduce insensible water loss.

Hypernatraemia arising in otherwise healthy, breastfed, full-term neonates is well described. The incidence has been variably reported because of differences in methods of ascertainment. Oddie et al. (2001) in a large population-based survey describe an occurrence of 7.1/10 000 breastfed infants. Laing and Wong (2002) report an occurrence of 14.4/10 000 infants in a single large centre, and Manganaro et al. (2001) 276/10 000 breastfed hospital admissions. Some authors cite the finding of a high urinary sodium concentration in the infant and a high breast milk sodium concentration as evidence that the condition is due to an excessive sodium intake (Bajpai et al. 2002). In fact, breast milk sodium is inversely related to breast milk volume (Neville et al. 1988). The term neonate who has had an inadequate intake of breast milk is usually both dehydrated and sodium-depleted. Volume depletion, by stimulating the renin–angiotensin–aldosterone system (RAAS), would normally reduce the urinary loss of sodium. The explanation for the seemingly paradoxical occurrence of a high urinary sodium concentration is that severe dehydration initiates a compensatory natriuresis in many mammalian species, including humans, and is a homeostatic response that serves to protect against hypernatraemia and hyperosmolality (McKinley et al. 2000). This dehydration-induced natriuresis is a physiological response that occurs even in the sodium-restricted state and appears to be mediated by osmoreceptor-stimulated oxytocin release (Huang et al. 1996). Hypernatraemia secondary to salt poisoning is distinguished by a high fractional excretion of sodium and absence of weight loss (Coulthard and Haycock 2003).

Management of hypernatraemic dehydration

Mild hypernatraemic dehydration may be corrected by enteral feeding. If intravenous rehydration is necessary 0.9% saline with glucose 5% or 10%, followed by 0.45% saline with glucose 5% or 10%, should be used (Laing and Wong 2002), and not hypo-osmolar salt-poor fluid. Milk feeds should be continued except where a specific contraindication exists. If there are signs of circulatory compromise administer an initial resuscitation volume of 20–30 ml/kg of normal (0.9%) saline over 30–60 minutes. Then calculate the initial infusion rate as follows:

1. Estimate daily maintenance fluid volume (M) in ml.
2. Estimate the total deficit (D) in ml. If the serum sodium is 149–169 mmol/l, aim to administer the deficit over 2 days ($T = 2$); if the serum sodium is 170 mmol/l or above, aim to administer the deficit over 3 days or more ($T = 3$ or more).
3. Calculate the initial infusion rate in ml/h as $[M + D/T]/24$.

Check serum electrolytes and blood glucose 1 hour after starting therapy, and then 4-hourly for 12 hours. If the serum sodium is falling at a rate greater than 0.5 mmol/l/h, reduce the rate of infusion. Aim to reduce the serum sodium at a rate not exceeding 12 mmol/l/day (see above). Too rapid correction of hypernatraemia can cause cerebral oedema, convulsions and permanent brain injury. Extremely severe hypernatraemia (serum sodium greater than 200 mmol/l) requires correction by peritoneal dialysis.

Hyponatraemia

The serum sodium concentration at birth reflects the maternal value. Often, a low serum sodium concentration at birth suggests that the mother has received a large volume of salt-poor intravenous fluid during labour, or consumed large volumes of water, resulting in an excess transfer of water to the baby. Labour ward policies should avoid the use of fixed-concentration solutions for intrapartum drug administration, as an increase in dose will result in increased infusion volume. Newborn hyponatraemia has also been described following maternal diuretic and laxative abuse and in pre-eclampsia. Dilutional hyponatraemia is more common than sodium depletion in neonatal intensive care (see following section). Sodium loss may be renal (e.g. secondary to diuretic use, polyuric phase of recovery from renal failure) or gastrointestinal. Chronic sodium loss will first be accompanied by extracellular volume contraction, poor weight gain and a normal serum sodium concentration. Hyponatraemia is a late sign. Common causes of neonatal hyponatraemia are listed in Table 18.8. Endocrine causes of hyponatraemia are discussed in Chapter 34 part 2.

Management of hyponatraemia

In acute severe hyponatraemia (serum sodium <120 mmol/l), particularly if associated with neurological signs, the intravenous infusion of 3% sodium chloride may be justified. The rate of correction should not exceed 1 mmol/l/h and the infusion of 3% sodium chloride should be stopped before a normal serum sodium is reached. As 3% sodium chloride contains approximately 0.5 mmol/ml, the infusion of 1 ml/kg will raise the serum sodium by 1 mmol/l (if ECF volume is 50% of body weight; in extremely preterm babies ECF volume may be higher). Hence the rate of infusion of 3% sodium chloride should never exceed 1 ml/kg/h.

Hyponatraemia due to sodium depletion should be managed with an increased sodium intake until the deficit is corrected. Dilutional hyponatraemia requires a reduction in fluid intake (see section below and Table 18.5).

Appropriate and inappropriate antidiuretic hormone secretion

The release of antidiuretic hormone (ADH) (arginine vasopressor (AVP)) is stimulated by a rise in osmolality and by baroreceptors located in the cardiac atria, aorta and carotid sinus. ADH has two principal actions: to increase the reabsorption of water, and vasoconstriction, contributing to the maintenance of blood pressure (BP). The pressor effect of ADH is one of the mediators through which central arterial BP is maintained, and both hypovolaemia and hypotension will result in a rise in circulating ADH (Dunn et al.

Table 18.8 Causes of hyponatraemia in the newborn

Primary water excess

Excess intake

To mother: large intrapartum infusion of sodium-free fluid
To baby: excessive intravenous intake

Impaired excretion

Intrinsic renal failure
Indometacin/ibuprofen
Appropriate or inappropriate antidiuretic hormone secretion
Adrenocortical failure

Primary sodium depletion

Insufficient intake

Maternal laxative or diuretic abuse
Use of non-sodium-supplemented donor breast milk for preterm
 babies

Excessive loss

Renal

Diuretics, including xanthines

Tubular dysfunction

Pyelonephritis
Nephrotoxic agents
Obstructive uropathies

Endocrine

Salt-losing forms of congenital adrenal hyperplasia
Hypoaldosteronism

Gastrointestinal

External

Vomiting
Stoma losses

Central nervous system

External drainage of cerebrospinal fluid in posthaemorrhagic
 hydrocephalus
Cerebral salt wasting

Mixed

Water excess and sodium depletion

Sodium and water depletion treated with continued infusion of
 sodium-free fluid
Chronic lung disease treated with long-term diuretic therapy

Water excess disproportionate to whole-body sodium excess

Congestive cardiac failure
Liver failure

Nephrotic syndrome

1976). Under experimental conditions, a rise in ADH occurs when intravascular volume falls by about 10% (Dunn et al. 1976). Little is known of setting of baroreceptor responses in the human preterm newborn, though a doubling of urinary AVP has been described after 10% blood loss in a 26-week, 800-g infant (Rees et al. 1984a).

It has been suggested that the syndrome of inappropriate ADH (SIADH) secretion occurs frequently in the newborn (Rees et al. 1984a). Elevated ADH and hyponatraemia are certainly common in acutely ill infants. However, the maintenance of central BP overrides the defence of tonicity, as shown in experiments on human volunteers in whom progressive salt depletion was induced by a salt-free diet and vigorous sweating (McCance 1936) but water intake was unrestricted. Whole-body sodium depletion was initially accompanied by isotonic contraction of the extracellular compartment and rapid weight loss. With increasing depletion of the intravascular compartment, baroreceptor-stimulated ADH-induced water reabsorption slowed the rate of weight loss but at the cost of a fall in plasma osmolality. In such a situation, the release of ADH is not inappropriate for volume status. This effect, namely an ADH response appropriate to intravascular volume status, probably underlies the impaired water excretion seen in ill infants.

In a large prospective study, Gerigk et al. (1996) found that, although plasma osmolality was lower in acutely ill infants and children, compared with a control group, both ADH and plasma renin activity were raised, indicating activation of the RAAS. The intravenous infusion of isotonic saline resulted in a better reduction in ADH and plasma renin activity when compared with hypotonic saline and oral fluid, suggesting that ADH was appropriately elevated in response to a reduced intravascular volume.

The recognition of an inadequate intravascular volume can be difficult. In the study described above (Gerigk et al. 1996), only a third of infants and children had overt signs of dehydration. Newborn babies are at risk of intravascular volume depletion (Wardrop and Holland 1995) from immediate cord clamping, which may lead to a reduction in blood volume by as much as 50% when compared with late clamping (Linderkamp et al. 1992) and subsequently from frequent blood sampling. As the normal range for BP in the newborn is wide and BP correlates poorly with blood volume (Barr et al. 1977; Bauer et al. 1993), BP measurements cannot be relied upon to detect hypovolaemia. Careful attention should be paid to assessment of the circulation using central venous pressure monitoring (Skinner et al. 1992), capillary refill time, the core–peripheral temperature difference and Doppler echocardiographic assessments (Pladys et al. 1994; Evans 2003). The core–peripheral temperature difference correlates with circulating AVP (Lambert et al. 1990).

Postoperative hyponatraemia is similarly a consequence of unrecognised intravascular volume depletion and continuing provision of salt-poor fluid, with ADH-driven water retention. Glucose in 0.9% NaCl (Judd et al. 1987) (Table 18.5), not colloid, is the preferred fluid (So et al. 1997) for intraoperative and postoperative support. Once water retention and hyponatraemia have occurred, water restriction is necessary to correct the hyponatraemia safely.

True inappropriate ADH secretion is probably rare in the newborn (Haycock 1995). This diagnosis should be made only in accordance with the classic criteria of Bartter and Schwartz (1967) when hyponatraemia exists with normovolaemia, normal BP, normal renal and cardiac function, evidence of continuing sodium excretion and urine that is not maximally dilute. In the newborn, SIADH has been described in acute brain injury and central nervous system infection and following maternal substance abuse (Winrow et al. 1992).

In pathological circumstances such as heart or liver failure, hypotension occurs together with an expanded extracellular compartment and there is whole-body sodium excess despite hyponatraemia. Myocardial dysfunction may contribute to impaired water excretion. The pathophysiology of disordered salt and water balance in severe chronic lung disease is complex. Hyponatraemia with clinical signs suggestive of an expanded extracellular compartment may reflect whole-body sodium depletion by chronic diuretic therapy and suboptimal nutrition together with impaired free water clearance (Hazinski et al. 1988) driven by abnormal transmural pressure gradients leading to effective central hypotension and increased AVP release. During acute exacerbations of respiratory failure associated with air trapping, a decrease in central venous return, pulmonary blood flow and left atrial filling will lead to a similar situation (Rao et al. 1986). A degree of pulmonary hypertension is an almost invariable accompaniment of chronic lung disease, and fluid retention may be attributable to poor cardiac function. Steroid therapy is another possible cause of compromised cardiac function (Brand et al. 1993; Haney et al. 1995), though now rarely used in chronic lung disease.

Common pharmacological influences on fluid balance

Indometacin and ibuprofen

Indometacin and ibuprofen are non-selective cyclo-oxygenase (COX) inhibitors that promote patent ductus arteriosus closure through inhibition of prostaglandin synthetase. Indometacin is also administered antenatally as a tocolytic, and to reduce liquor volume in polyhydramnios. These substances reduce sodium excretion by enhancing tubular reabsorption. In the preterm infant COX inhibition appears to lower glomerular filtration rate, an effect that may reflect dependence on renal prostaglandins to maintain an adequate renal blood flow in the face of high RAAS activity (Oliver et al. 1980). As amelioration of the oliguric response to indometacin has been described in the presence of an AVP V_2-receptor antagonist (Walker et al. 1994), AVP stimulation may be another mode of action.

A temporary reduction of sodium and water excretion is described in all reports of babies given indometacin. Ibuprofen, a licensed product, has largely replaced indometacin for pharmacological duct closure. Although meta-analyses suggest that ibuprofen has fewer side-effects than indometacin (Ohlsson et al. 2010), oligohydramnios and neonatal renal failure have been described after maternal exposure (Bavoux 1992; Kaplan et al. 1994). Suggestions that the simultaneous administration of furosemide or dopamine

eliminates the renal side-effects of indometacin without reducing efficacy of duct closure (Yeh et al. 1982) have not been substantiated (Fajardo et al. 1992; Barrington and Brion 2002).

With careful management salt and water retention and dilutional hyponatraemia can be avoided. If indometacin is to be used in a dose of 0.2 mg/kg 12-hourly, or if the baby is extremely immature, restrict sodium and water intake by 30%. Indometacin, 0.1 mg/kg 24-hourly (Rennie and Cooke 1991), and ibuprofen are less likely to result in adverse renal effects. Careful monitoring of urine output, serum sodium and weight gain are advisable whenever COX inhibitors are used.

Glucocorticoid steroids

The synthetic glucocorticoids dexamethasone and betamethasone, widely used in perinatal medicine, have a number of potent actions. They are gene transducers as well as having direct effects at the level of the cell membrane. They increase β_2-receptor density, antioxidant levels and the density of Na^+/K^+-ATPase, affect a variety of cytokines and growth factors, enhance surfactant production, increase clearance of lung liquid, suppress inducible nitric oxide synthase and are catabolic. A temporary inhibition in growth is well documented during therapy and this often results in a rise in blood urea.

The abundance of Na^+/K^+-ATPase is regulated by glucocorticoids (Celsi et al. 1991) in an age-dependent manner (Celsi et al. 1993). In rats, betamethasone will increase Na^+/K^+-ATPase mRNA in the kidney during infancy, but not during fetal life, nor in adults. In contrast, lung tissue Na^+/K^+-ATPase is maximally induced by glucocorticoids during the perinatal period. The inference is that glucocorticoids interact with other transcriptional factors, expressed in an age-dependent fashion, to activate the genes for Na^+/K^+-ATPase so that different tissues have different periods of sensitivity to glucocorticoid regulation. Glucocorticoids enhance renal tubular regulation of sodium balance, potentiate atrial natriuretic peptide stimulation of cGMP production (Hayamizu et al. 1994) and enhance the maturation of renal acidification (Baum and Quigley 1993). In addition to the well-known effects on the lungs, antenatal exposure to dexamethasone accelerates the maturation of renal function in human preterm newborns (Al-Dahan et al. 1987) and induces both Na^+/K^+-ATPase and Na^+ channels in lung epithelial cells, thus facilitating the clearance of lung liquid (O'Brodovich et al. 1993). This may underlie the seemingly paradoxical effect of glucocorticoids in triggering a diuresis in the fluid-retaining baby with chronic lung disease (Schrod et al. 1991; Greenough et al. 1993).

References

Al-Dahan, J., Stimmler, L., Chantler, C., et al., 1987. The effect of antenatal dexamethasone administration on glomerular filtration rate and renal sodium excretion in premature infants. Pediatr Nephrol 1, 131–135.

Al-Dahhan, J., Haycock, G.B., Nichol, B., et al., 1984. Sodium homeostasis in term and preterm neonates. III. Effect of salt supplementation. Arch Dis Child 59, 945–950.

Al Rubeyi, B., Murray, N., Modi, N., 1994. A variable dextrose delivery system for neonatal intensive care. Arch Dis Child Fetal Neonatal Ed 70, F79.

Bajpai, A., Aggarwal, R., Deorari, A.K., et al., 2002. Neonatal hypernatremia due to

high breast milk sodium. Indian Pediatr 39, 193–196.

Barr, P.A., Bailey, P.E., Sumners, J., et al., 1977. Relation between arterial blood pressure and blood volume and effect of infused albumin in sick preterm infants. Pediatrics 60, 282–289.

Barrington, K., Brion, L.P., 2002. Dopamine versus no treatment to prevent renal dysfunction in indomethacin-treated preterm newborn infants (Cochrane Review). Cochrane Database Syst Rev (3), CD003213.

Bartter, F.C., Schwartz, W.B., 1967. The syndrome of inappropriate secretion of antidiuretic hormone. Am J Med 42, 790–806.

Bauer, K., Versmold, H., 1989. Postnatal weight loss in preterm neonates less than 1500 g is due to isotonic dehydration of the extracellular volume. Acta Paediatr Scand Suppl 360, 37–42.

Bauer, K., Bovermann, G., Roithmaier, A., et al., 1991. Body composition, nutrition, and fluid balance during the first two weeks of life in preterm neonates weighing less than 1500 grams. J Pediatr 118, 615–620.

Bauer, K., Linderkamp, O., Versmold, H.T., 1993. Systolic blood pressure and blood volume in preterm infants. Arch Dis Child 69, 521–522.

Baum, M., Quigley, R., 1993. Glucocorticoids stimulate rabbit proximal convoluted tubule acidification. J Clin Invest 91, 110–114.

Bavoux, F., 1992. Fetal toxicity of non-steroidal anti-inflammatory agents. Presse Med 21, 1909–1912 (in French).

Bell, E.F., Acarregui, M.J., 2001. Restricted versus liberal water intake for preventing morbidity and mortality in preterm infants. Cochrane Database Syst Rev CD000503.

Bell, E.F., Warburton, D., Stonestreet, B.S., et al., 1979. High-volume fluid intake predisposes premature infants to necrotising enterocolitis. Lancet 2, 90.

Bell, E.F., Warburton, D., Stonestreet, B.S., et al., 1980. Effect of fluid administration on the development of symptomatic patent ductus arteriosus and congestive heart failure in premature infants. N Engl J Med 302, 598–604.

Bétrémieux, P., Modi, N., Hartnoll, G., et al., 1995. Longitudinal changes in extracellular fluid volume, sodium excretion and atrial natriuretic peptide, in preterm neonates with hyaline membrane disease. Early Hum Dev 41, 221–222.

Brand, P.L., Van Lingen, R.A., Brus, F., et al., 1993. Hypertrophic obstructive cardiomyopathy as a side effect of dexamethasone treatment for bronchopulmonary dysplasia. Acta Paediatr 82, 614–617.

Brion, L.P., Soll, R.F., 2001. Diuretics for respiratory distress syndrome in preterm infants. Cochrane Database Syst Rev CD001454.

Brown, E.R., Stark, A., Sosneko, I., et al., 1978. Bronchopulmonary dysplasia: possible relationship to pulmonary oedema. J Pediatr 92, 982–984.

Celsi, G., Nishi, A., Akusjärvi, G., et al., 1991. Abundance of Na+, K+-ATPase mRNA is regulated by glucocorticoid hormones in infant rat kidneys. Am J Physiol 260, F192–F197.

Celsi, G., Wang, Z.M., Akusjarvi, G., et al., 1993. Sensitive periods for glucocorticoid regulation of Na+, K+-ATPase mRNA in the developing lung and kidney. Pediatr Res 33, 5–9.

Chance, G.W., Radde, I.C., Willis, D.M., et al., 1977. Postnatal growth of infants of 1.3 kg birth weight; effects of metabolic acidosis, of caloric intake and of calcium, sodium and phosphate supplementation. J Pediatr 91, 787–793.

Costarino Jr, A.T., Gruskay, J.A., Corcoran, L., et al., 1992. Sodium restriction versus daily maintenance replacement in very low birth weight premature neonates: a randomized, blind therapeutic trial. J Pediatr 120, 99–106.

Coulthard, M.G., Haycock, G.B., 2003. Distinguishing between salt poisoning and hypernatraemic dehydration in children. BMJ 326, 157–160.

Coulthard, M.G., Hey, E.N., 1985. Effect of varying water intake on renal function in healthy preterm babies. Arch Dis Child 60, 614–620.

Dunn, F.L., Brennan, T.J., Neelson, A.E., et al., 1976. The role of blood osmolality and volume in regulating vasopressin secretion by the rat. J Clin Invest 52, 3212–3219.

Evans, N., 2003. Volume expansion during neonatal intensive care: do we know what we are doing? Semin Neonatol 8, 315–323.

Evans, N.J., Rutter, N., 1986. Development of the epidermis in the newborn. Biol Neonate 49, 74–80.

Fajardo, C.A., Whyte, R.K., Steele, B.T., 1992. Effect of dopamine on failure of indomethacin to close the patent ductus arteriosus. J Pediatr 121, 771–775.

Friis-Hansen, B., 1961. Body water compartments in children: changes during growth and related changes in body composition. Pediatrics 28, 169–181.

Friis-Hansen, B., 1983. Water distribution in the fetus and newborn infant. Acta Paediatr Scand Suppl 305, 7–11.

Gerigk, M., Gnehm, H.E., Rascher, W., 1996. Arginine vasopressin and renin in acutely ill children: implication for fluid therapy. Acta Paediatr 85, 550–553.

Greenough, A., Chan, V., Emery, E.F., et al., 1993. Respiratory status and diuresis following treatment with dexamethasone. Early Hum Dev 32, 87–91.

Hammarlund, K., Sedin, G., 1979. Transepidermal water loss in newborn infants. III. Relation to gestational age. Acta Paediatr Scand 68, 795–801.

Hammarlund, K., Sedin, G., Stromberg, B., 1982. Transepidermal water loss in newborn infants. VII. Relation to post-natal age in very pre-term and full-term appropriate for gestational age infants. Acta Paediatr Scand 71, 369–374.

Hammarlund, K., Sedin, G., Stromberg, B., 1983. Transepidermal water loss in newborn infants. VIII. Relation to gestational age and post-natal age in appropriate and small for gestational age infants. Acta Paediatr Scand 72, 721–728.

Haney, I., Lachance, C., Van Doesburg, N.H., et al., 1995. Reversible steroid-induced hypertrophic cardiomyopathy with left ventricular outflow tract obstruction in two newborns. Am J Perinatol 12, 271–274.

Harpin, V.A., Rutter, N., 1982. Sweating in preterm babies. J Pediatr 100, 614–619.

Hartnoll, G., Betremieux, P., Modi, N., 2000a. Randomised controlled trial of postnatal sodium supplementation on body composition in 25 to 30 week gestational age infants. Arch Dis Child Fetal Neonatal Ed 82, F24–F28.

Hartnoll, G., Betrémieux, P., Modi, N., 2000b. Randomised controlled trial of postnatal sodium supplementation on body composition in 25–30 weeks gestational age infants. Arch Dis Child Fetal Neonatal Ed 82, F24–F28.

Hartnoll, G., Betremieux, P., Modi, N., 2001. Randomised controlled trial of postnatal sodium supplementation in infants of 25–30 weeks gestational age: effects on cardiopulmonary adaptation. Arch Dis Child Fetal Neonatal Ed 85, F29–F32.

Hayamizu, S., Kanda, K., Ohmori, S., et al., 1994. Glucocorticoids potentiate the action of atrial natriuretic polypeptide in adrenalectomized rats. Endocrinology 135, 2459–2464.

Haycock, G.B., 1993. The influence of sodium on growth in infancy. Pediatr Nephrol 7, 871–875.

Haycock, G.B., 1995. The syndrome of inappropriate secretion of antidiuretic hormone. Pediatr Nephrol 9, 375–381.

Haycock, G.B., Aperia, A., 1991. Salt and the newborn kidney. Pediatr Nephrol 5, 65–70.

Hazinski, T.A., Blalock, W.A., Engelhardt, B., 1988. Control of water balance in infants with bronchopulmonary dysplasia: role of endogenous vasopressin. Pediatr Res 23, 86–88.

Heimler, R., Doumas, B.T., Jendrzejczak, B.M., et al., 1993. Relationship between nutrition, weight change and fluid compartments in preterm infants during the first week of life. J Pediatr 122, 110–114.

Huang, W., Lee, S.L., Arnason, S.S., Sjoquist, M., 1996. Dehydration natriuresis in male rats is mediated by oxytocin. Am J Physiol 270, R427–R433.

Jain, A., Rutter, N., Cartlidge, P.H., 2000. Influence of antenatal steroids and sex on maturation of the epidermal barrier in the preterm infant. Arch Dis Child Fetal Neonatal Ed 83, F112–F116.

Judd, B.A., Haycock, G.B., Dalton, N., et al., 1987. Hyponatraemia in premature babies and following surgery in older children. Acta Paediatr Scand 76, 385–393.

Kaplan, B.S., Restaino, I., Raval, D.S., et al., 1994. Renal failure in the neonate associated with in utero exposure to non-steroidal anti-inflammatory agents. Pediatr Nephrol 8, 700–704.

Kojima, T., Hirata, Y., Fukuda, Y., et al., 1987. Plasma atrial natriuretic peptide and spontaneous diuresis in sick neonates. Arch Dis Child 62, 667–670.

Laing, I.A., Wong, C.M., 2002. Hypernatraemia in the first few days: is the incidence rising? Arch Dis Child Fetal Neonatal Ed 87, F158–F162.

Lambert, H.J., Coulthard, M.G., Palmer, J.M., et al., 1990. Control of sodium and water balance in the preterm neonate. Pediatr Nephrol 4, C53.

Lee, J.H., Arcinue, E., Ross, B.D., 1994. Brief report: organic osmolytes in the brain of an infant with hypernatremia. N Engl J Med 331, 439–442.

Linderkamp, O., Nelle, M., Kraus, M., et al., 1992. The effect of early and late cord-clamping on blood viscosity and other hemorheological parameters in full-term neonates. Acta Paediatr 81, 745–750.

Lorenz, J.M., Kleinman, L.I., Kotagal, U.R., et al., 1982. Water balance in very low-birth-weight infants: relationship to water and sodium intake and effect on outcome. J Pediatr 101, 423–432.

Manganaro, R., Mami, C., Marrone, T., et al., 2001. Incidence of dehydration and hypernatremia in exclusively breast-fed infants. J Pediatr 139, 673–675.

McCance, R.A., 1936. Experimental sodium chloride deficiency in man. Proc R Soc Lond (Biol) 119, 245–268.

McKinley, M.J., Evered, M.D., Mathai, M.L., 2000. Renal Na excretion in dehydrated and rehydrated adrenalectomized sheep maintained with aldosterone. Am J Physiol Regul Integr Comp Physiol 279, R17–R24.

Miall, L.S., Henderson, M.J., Turner, A.J., et al., 1999. Plasma creatinine rises dramatically in the first 48 hours of life in preterm infants. Pediatrics 104, e76.

Modi, N., 1997. Management of postnatal disorders of fluid balance. In: Brace, R. (Ed.), Fetus and Neonate. Vol. IV. Body Fluids and Kidney. Cambridge University Press, Cambridge.

Modi, N., Hutton, J.L., 1990. The influence of postnatal respiratory adaptation on sodium handling in preterm neonates. Early Hum Dev 21, 11–20.

Mohan, P., Rojas, J., Davidson, K.K., et al., 1984. Pulmonary air leak associated with neonatal hyponatremia in premature infants. J Pediatr 105, 153–157.

Neville, M.C., Keller, R., Seacat, J., et al., 1988. Studies in human lactation: milk volumes in lactating women during the onset of lactation and full lactation. Am J Clin Nutr 48, 1375–1386.

O'Brodovich, H., Canessa, C., Ueda, J., et al., 1993. Expression of the epithelial Na+ channel in the developing rat lung. Am J Physiol 265, C491–C496.

Oddie, S., Richmond, S., Coulthard, M., 2001. Hypernatraemic dehydration and breast feeding: a population study. Arch Dis Child 85, 318–320.

Ohlsson, A., Walia, R., Shah, S.S., 2010. Ibuprofen for the treatment of patent ductus arteriosus in preterm and/or low birth weight infants. Cochrane Database Syst Rev (4), CD003481.

Oliver, J.A., Pinto, J., Sciacca, R.R., et al., 1980. Increased renal secretion of norepinephrine and prostaglandin E_2 during sodium depletion in the dog. J Clin Invest 66, 748–756.

Ostlund, E.V., Eklof, A.C., Aperia, A., 1993. Salt-deficient diet and early weaning inhibit DNA synthesis in immature rat proximal tubular cells. Pediatr Nephrol 7, 41–44.

Pabst, R.C., Starr, K.P., Qaiyumi, S., et al., 1999. The effect of application of

aquaphor on skin condition, fluid requirements, and bacterial colonization in very low birth weight infants. J Perinatol 19, 278–283.

Pladys, P., Betremieux, P., Lefrancois, C., et al., 1994. [Doppler echocardiography in the evaluation of volume expansion effects in newborn infants.] Arch Pediatr 1, 470–476.

Rao, M., Eid, N., Herrod, L., et al., 1986. Antidiuretic hormone response in children with bronchopulmonary dysplasia during episodes of acute respiratory distress. Am J Dis Child 140, 825–828.

Rees, L., Brook, C.G., Shaw, J.C., et al., 1984a Hyponatraemia in the first week of life in preterm infants. Part I. Arginine vasopressin secretion. Arch Dis Child 59, 414–422.

Rees, L., Shaw, J.C., Brook, C.G., et al., 1984b Hyponatraemia in the first week of life in preterm infants. Part II. Sodium and water balance. Arch Dis Child 59, 423–429.

Rennie, J.M., Cooke, R.W., 1991. Prolonged low dose indomethacin for persistent ductus arteriosus of prematurity. Arch Dis Child 66, 55–58.

Rojas, J., Mohan, P., Davidson, K.K., 1984. Increased extracellular water volume associated with hyponatremia at birth in premature infants. J Pediatr 105, 158–161.

Roy, R.N., Chance, G.W., Radde, I.C., et al., 1976. Late hyponatremia in very low birthweight infants (less than 1.3 kilograms). Pediatr Res 10, 526–531.

Rozycki, H.J., Baumgart, S., 1991. Atrial natriuretic factor and postnatal diuresis in respiratory distress syndrome. Arch Dis Child 66, 43–47.

Rutter, N., 1989. The hazards of an immature skin. In: Harvey, D.R.H., Cooke, R.W.I., Levitt, G.A. (Eds.), The Baby Under 1000g. Butterworth, London.

Schrod, L., Frauendienst-Egger, G., Forgber, I., et al., 1991. Dexamethasone in the treatment of bronchopulmonary dysplasia. Pneumologie 45, 892–896 (in German).

Sedin, G., Hammarlund, K., Nilsson, G.E., et al., 1985. Measurements of transepidermal water loss in newborn infants. Clin Perinatol 12, 79–99.

Shaffer, S.G., Meade, V.M., 1989. Sodium balance and extracellular volume regulation in very low birth weight infants. J Pediatr 115, 285–290.

Shaffer, S.G., Weismann, D.N., 1992. Fluid requirements in the preterm infant. Clin Perinatol 19, 233–250.

Shaffer, S.G., Bradt, S.K., Hall, R.T., 1986. Postnatal changes in total body water and extracellular volume in the preterm infant with respiratory distress syndrome. J Pediatr 109, 509–514.

Singhi, S.C., Chookang, E., 1984. Maternal fluid overload during labour; transplacental hyponatraemia and risk of transient neonatal tachypnoea in term

infants. Arch Dis Child 59, 1155–1158.

Singhi, S., Chookang, E., Hall, J.S., et al., 1985. Iatrogenic neonatal and maternal hyponatraemia following oxytocin and aqueous glucose infusion during labour. Br J Obstet Gynaecol 92, 356–363.

Singhi, S., Sood, V., Bhakoo, O.N., et al., 1995. Composition of postnatal weight loss & subsequent weight gain in preterm infants. Indian J Med Res 101, 157–162.

Skinner, J.R., Milligan, D.W., Hunter, S., et al., 1992. Central venous pressure in the ventilated neonate. Arch Dis Child 67, 374–377.

So, K.W., Fok, T.F., Ng, P.C., et al., 1997. Randomised controlled trial of colloid or crystalloid in hypotensive preterm infants. Arch Dis Child Fetal Neonatal Ed 76, F43–F46.

Stevenson, J.G., 1977. Fluid administration in the association of patent ductus arteriosus complicating respiratory distress syndrome. J Pediatr 90, 257–261.

Strange, K., 1993. Maintenance of cell volume in the central nervous system. Pediatr Nephrol 7, 689–697.

Takahashi, N., Hoshi, J., Nishida, H., 1994. Water balance, electrolytes and acid–base balance in extremely premature infants. Acta Paediatr Jpn 36, 250–255.

Tammela, O.K., Koivisto, M.E., 1992. Fluid restriction for preventing bronchopulmonary dysplasia? Reduced fluid intake during the first weeks of life improves the outcome of low-birth-weight infants. Acta Paediatr 81, 207–212.

Tang, W., Modi, N., Clark, P., 1993. Dilution kinetics of H(2)18O for the measurement of total body water in preterm babies in the first week after birth. Arch Dis Child 69, 28–31.

Tang, W., Ridout, D., Modi, N., 1997. Influence of respiratory distress syndrome on body composition after preterm birth. Arch Dis Child Fetal Neonatal Ed 77, F28–F31.

Tulassay, T., Seri, I., Rascher, W., 1987. Atrial natriuretic peptide and extracellular volume contraction after birth. Acta Paediatr Scand 76, 444–446.

Van Marter, L.J., Leviton, A., Allred, E.N., et al., 1990. Hydration during the first days of life and the risk of bronchopulmonary dysplasia in low birth weight infants. J Pediatr 116, 942–949.

Von Stockhausen, H.B., Struve, M., 1980. [Effects of highly varying parenteral fluid intakes in premature and newborn infants during the first three days of life.] Klin Padiatr 192, 539–546 (in German)

Walker, M.P., Moore, T.R., Brace, R.A., 1994. Indomethacin and arginine vasopressin interaction in the fetal kidney: a mechanism of oliguria. Am J Obstet Gynecol 171, 1234–1241.

Wananukul, S., Praisuwanna, P., 2002. Clear topical ointment decreases transepidermal water loss in jaundiced preterm infants receiving phototherapy. J Med Assoc Thai 85, 102–106.

Wardrop, C.A., Holland, B.M., 1995. The roles and vital importance of placental blood to the newborn infant. J Perinat Med 23, 139–143.

Wassner, S.J., 1991. The effect of sodium repletion on growth and protein turnover in sodium-depleted rats. Pediatr Nephrol 5, 501–504.

Winrow, A.P., Kovar, I.Z., Jani, B.R., et al., 1992. Early hyponatraemia and neonatal drug withdrawal. Acta Paediatr 81, 847–848.

Yeh, T.F., Wilks, A., Singh, J., et al., 1982. Furosemide prevents the renal side effects of indomethacin therapy in premature infants with patent ductus arteriosus. J Pediatr 101, 433–437.

Ziegler, E.E., Fomon, S.J., 1971. Fluid intake, renal solute load, and water balance in infancy. J Pediatr 78, 561–568.

Intensive care monitoring and data handling

Andrew Lyon

19

Introduction

Successful care of the newborn depends on understanding the pathophysiology of the conditions affecting the baby. To follow changes in clinical condition, and the effects of treatment, it is essential that we are able to monitor the progress of the baby.

There are many devices used in the monitoring of the newborn baby. Many are well established and considered standard in all cases, e.g. heart rate, while others are still finding their place in routine clinical care of certain groups of babies, e.g. cerebral

© 2012 Elsevier Ltd

function monitors. There are several areas of debate, e.g. whether transcutaneous partial pressure of oxygen (Po_2) or saturation gives the better information, and also about when invasive monitoring, such as intra-arterial blood pressure (BP), should be used.

If information is collected from monitors it must be interpreted and then acted upon. This requires not only knowledge of the underlying physiology, but also at least a basic understanding of how the monitors work. In particular it is important to know the limitations of the devices and the circumstances in which they become unreliable.

Electrical safety

With the large number of devices attached to babies, electrical safety is of paramount importance and all equipment must conform to strict regulations.

The Medicines and Healthcare products Regulatory Agency (MHRA) is a government body with a responsibility to ensure safety of all medical devices. This body ensures that all European Union Directives on safety of medical equipment are implemented. In essence all devices must carry a CE mark as a sign of conformity, which includes assurance that the device meets the general requirements for safety of medical electrical equipment. This also applies to any equipment used for research. Current standards for medical equipment are available on the MHRA website.

There has been debate about whether mobile phones, and other equipment capable of transmission, can interfere with medical devices and monitoring equipment in particular. The MHRA has included recommendations on the use of transmitting devices close to patient monitors (Table 19.1).

The British Association of Perinatal Medicine has published recommendations for units carrying out intensive and high-dependency care of the newborn (BAPM 2001). Units must have an agreed policy for the purchase and maintenance of all equipment, as well as for staff support and training. This must be done in consultation with a department of medical physics and be supported by an adequate budget.

Cardiovascular monitoring

Heart rate and ECG

The electrodes used to obtain the electrocardiogram (ECG) should be placed lateral enough on the chest to minimise any shadow on X-ray. Correct positioning is important if these leads are also used to produce a respiratory trace by impedance changes.

The displayed trace is not of diagnostic quality and a full 12-lead ECG must be requested if an arrhythmia is suspected (Ch. 28, Appendix 3).

Changes in the ECG pattern can indicate conditions such as hyperkalaemia and myocardial ischaemia. A reduction in the size of the complexes may be an early sign of pulmonary air leak or cardiac tamponade (Merenstein et al. 1972).

Heart rate can be derived and displayed from the ECG. With many multiparameter monitors, the heart rate can also be obtained from the BP trace, removing the need to stick electrodes on to fragile skin. Access to the ECG signal does have the advantage that it is possible to check artefacts such as an artificially high heart rate due to 'double counting' of the QRS and T waves.

Tachycardia is associated with haemorrhage, hypovolaemia or inadequate analgesia. Bradycardia in the ventilated infant is often a sign of a blocked endotracheal tube, while in the self-breathing baby it is usually an indicator of apnoeic episodes.

Echocardiography

Echocardiography is used for the assessment of structural heart defects as well as helping to detect, and determine management of, the patent ductus arteriosus. It can also help in the assessment of ventricular function following asphyxia and in chronic lung disease. Although echocardiography may help guide the use of volume replacement or inotrope support in a baby with hypotension, there is, as yet, no evidence that its routine use in monitoring the newborn baby has any impact on long-term outcome.

Table 19.1 Medicines and Healthcare products Regulatory Agency recommendations on use of transmitting equipment in hospitals

RISK OF INTERFERENCE	TYPE OF COMMUNICATION SYSTEM	RECOMMENDATION
High	Analogue emergency service radios	Use in hospitals only in an emergency, never for routine communication
	Private business radios (PBRs) and PMR446, e.g. porters' and maintenance staff radios (two-way radios)	Minimise risks by changing to alternative lower risk technologies
Medium	Cellphones (mobile phones)	A total ban on these systems is not required and is impossible to enforce effectively
	Terrestrial trunked radio system (TETRA)	Should be switched off near critical care or life support medical equipment
	Laptop computers, palmtops and gaming devices fitted with higher power wireless networks such as GPRS and 3G	Should be used only in designated areas
	HIPERLAN	Authorised health and social care staff and external service personnel should always comply with local rules regarding use
Low	Cordless telephones (including DECT) Low-power computer wireless networks such as RLAN systems and Bluetooth	These systems are very unlikely to cause interference under most circumstances and need not be restricted

Perfusion

Tissue survival depends on both oxygenation and the blood flow (perfusion) through the capillary bed. Monitoring tissue perfusion is important for early recognition of circulatory failure and in assessing response to therapy.

Blood pressure

Normal values for BP in the neonate are shown in Appendix 4. Perfusion is dependent on the systemic BP but, particularly in the first 48 hours of postnatal life, there is no good correlation between level of BP and tissue perfusion (Groves et al. 2008). During the first days of life many aim to maintain a mean arterial BP around a value equal to the gestational age in weeks. Use of gestational age criteria may lead to overtreatment, which has been associated with adverse outcome. In any particular baby, the level used to diagnose significant, and symptomatic, hypotension will depend on other clinical features of perfusion including renal function, acid–base state and oxygenation. There is no indication to treat low BP where there is clinical evidence of good perfusion (Dempsey et al. 2009).

BP can be monitored directly with transducers attached to arterial lines. These need calibrating to zero and changes in position of the transducer relative to the heart may alter the reading. The calibration and position should be checked if there has been a sudden change in BP. Visual display of the waveform is important in assessing reliability, as damping of the arterial trace affects systolic and diastolic BP. Mean pressure remains more reliable but even this can become unreliable when the trace is damped (Cunningham et al. 1994a).

Non-invasive oscillometric methods significantly overestimate BP at the lower end and are poor at detecting hypotension. They should not be used to verify low readings from arterial lines. Mean BP is taken as the point where the oscillations in the cuff are maximum and, although related to the true mean BP, this value will differ from that obtained from an intra-arterial line (Diprose et al. 1986).

As changes in BP are not always a good indication other methods are needed to help assess tissue perfusion.

Skin perfusion

In low-flow states, blood supply in the skin is reduced to protect perfusion of vital organs. Skin blood flow is used as a marker of overall perfusion but it is also affected by the thermal environment (Gorelick et al. 1993).

Capillary refill time correlates poorly with hypovolaemia in children (Leonard and Beattie 2004). Normal values for neonates, nursed in different thermal environments, have been published (Strozik et al. 1997), and, in general, the skin reperfuses in less than 3 seconds. Capillary refill is better estimated on the skin of the forehead or chest rather than the toes, but it is an unreliable indicator of cardiovascular status in neonates (LeFlore and Engle 2005).

Decreasing skin blood flow results in a widening of the central–peripheral temperature gap. This can indicate hypovolaemia, or a decrease in venous return, before the BP falls (Lambert et al. 1998). Delay in establishing vasomotor tone makes these changes an unreliable measure of tissue perfusion in the very-low-birthweight infant immediately after birth (Osborn et al. 2004). In the absence of other indicators of hypovolaemia, such as a rising heart rate, a widening temperature gap is more likely to be due to cold stress (Lyon et al. 1997).

Central venous pressure

Central venous pressure (CVP) can be measured with an umbilical venous catheter in the right atrium. Close attention to maintaining the position of the transducer relative to the heart is essential, and the monitor must be calibrated to zero frequently. There is little information on the use of CVP in the newborn baby. A value of zero in the ventilated neonate is usually associated with other signs of hypovolaemia (Skinner et al. 1992).

Lactate

Measurement of lactate can be incorporated into blood gas or glucose analysers. Accumulation of lactate, implying increasing anaerobic metabolism, occurs in sepsis and with a reduction in tissue perfusion. There is poor correlation with arterial pH and, in the absence of a raised lactate, a metabolic acidosis is unlikely to be due to hypoperfusion. Values above 3 mmol/l soon after birth are abnormal and serial measurements can provide important prognostic information in ill, ventilated neonates (Deshpande and Ward Platt 1997).

Lactate levels are elevated following asphyxia. Levels below 5 mmol/l at 30 minutes of age have been followed by a good outcome (da Silva et al. 2000), while those above 7.5 mmol/l have been associated with moderate or severe encephalopathy with a sensitivity of 94% and specificity of 67% (Shah et al. 2004). Persistently high lactate levels, above 10–15 mmol/l, suggest an inborn error of metabolism (Ch. 34.3).

Other measures of perfusion

Change in urine output, monitored using pre-weighed nappies or cotton wool balls, is an insensitive marker of tissue perfusion, with volumes decreasing only after a fall in BP. Normal urine output is discussed on Ch. 35.1.

Venous oxygen tension or saturation, measured in blood taken from a catheter passed through the foramen ovale into the left atrium, may be a better indicator of oxygen delivery but is not in routine use (O'Connor and Hart 1994). Near-infrared spectroscopy (NIRS) (Yoxall and Weindling 1996) and gastric intramucosal pH measured by tonometry (Campbell and Costeloe 2001) are techniques not yet applicable to everyday clinical use. Using echocardiography to measure flow in the superior vena cava (SVC) gives a better reflection of cerebral blood flow than does cerebral artery Doppler measures or mean BP (Evans et al. 2002). Low SVC flow has been associated with early neonatal death and/or severe intraventricular haemorrhage (Miletin and Dempsey 2008).

Taking low SVC flow as the indicator of poor perfusion, there was poor correlation between capillary refill time, mean BP and urine output with SVC flow. However combining a capillary refill time of >4 seconds with a serum lactate concentration of >4 mmol/l increased the specificity of detecting a low SVC flow state to 97% as well as improving the positive and negative predictive values (Miletin et al. 2009).

Respiratory system monitoring

Respiration

There are several methods used for respiratory monitoring, and these are discussed in Ch. 27.4. Respiration monitors are used routinely to detect apnoea. They add little extra benefit to the monitoring of the ventilated baby, where more useful information is obtained from the ventilator.

The relationship between apnoea, bradycardia and desaturation is complex. In the majority of episodes, apnoea or hypoventilation is the initiating event, causing a fall in oxygen saturation, which in turn triggers a reflex bradycardia (Adams et al. 1997).

Apnoea monitors alone have been shown to miss significant episodes of both apnoea and bradycardia (Southall et al. 1983). In the absence of monitors that measure airflow, mixed or obstructive apnoea will only be identified by the accompanying bradycardia and desaturation.

An apnoea monitor should be attached to all spontaneously breathing babies who have either apnoeic attacks or respiratory disease likely to be complicated by apnoea. However, if there are true concerns, then respiratory monitoring should always include a measure of heart rate and oxygen saturation.

Oxygen

Knowledge of the partial pressure of oxygen in arterial blood (Pao_2) is essential in intensive care. This can be measured intermittently, by arterial puncture or sampling from an indwelling catheter, or continuously, by use of an intravascular transducer. The frequency of sampling depends on the clinical condition of the baby and on the reliability placed on values obtained from continuous oxygen monitors.

Arterial puncture

This is painful, and crying alters the Pao_2 (Dinwiddie et al. 1979). A patent ductus arteriosus may result in a higher Pao_2 in the right arm and head/neck compared with other areas of the body.

Capillary and venous samples

Results from arterialised capillary samples can be misleading if the baby is poorly perfused or the blood not free-flowing. They should not be used in the assessment of the acutely ill baby. Capillary and venous samples underestimate Pao_2 significantly and should not be used to predict arterial values in neonates (Courtney et al. 1990). Neither should be used in the assessment of the acutely ill neonate but both show a good correlation with acid–base state and Pco_2 in the stable baby (Yildizdaş et al. 2004).

Indwelling arterial lines

Indwelling arterial lines allow repeated sampling without disturbing the infant and can be used for continuous BP monitoring. Further information on the techniques used to insert arterial lines, and their complications, can be found in Chapter 44.

Umbilical artery catheter

The tip of the umbilical artery catheter is positioned in the descending aorta (Ch. 44). High catheters (above the diaphragm) have fewer complications (Ch. 44) than those positioned low (just above the aortic bifurcation), and can remain in situ for longer (Barrington 2000a). Low-dose heparin (1 unit/ml) added to the infusion fluid reduces the risk of catheter blockage (Barrington 2000b).

X-ray is needed to confirm the site of the tip (Ch. 43) but accuracy of initial positioning has been shown to be improved, reducing significantly the need for further manipulation of the line, using the formula (Wright et al. 2008):

$$\text{insertion length (cm)} = (4 \times \text{birthweight (kg)}) + 7$$

Peripheral artery catheters

The radial or posterior tibial arteries are commonly used, but the ulnar, dorsalis pedis and axillary arteries are alternatives (Ch. 44). The brachial and femoral arteries should be avoided.

Complications are rare, but vasospasm and thrombus formation can cause major problems, even when collateral circulations are intact. Low-dose heparin must be added to the infusion.

The Allen test is used to test the integrity of the palmar arches before either the radial or ulnar artery is cannulated but, even in adults, this has not been shown to be accurate in predicting post-cannulation hand ischaemia (Barone and Madlinger 2006). This test is even less reliable in the newborn, mainly because of technical difficulties. It is essential that the limb is observed closely, and the catheter removed at the first sign of impaired perfusion.

Total occlusion of the artery may persist after the catheter is removed. For this reason, the ulnar artery should not be used if the radial artery in that hand has been cannulated previously.

Continuous intravascular blood gas monitoring

With intermittent sampling, major fluctuations in condition may be difficult to follow. Increasing the frequency of sampling introduces significant blood loss in small infants.

Continuous intravascular Pao_2, Pco_2, pH and temperature monitoring are possible (Goddard et al. 1974; Morgan et al. 1999). Although reliable, the accuracy of these electrodes deteriorates with time as a result of fibrin deposition. The use of indwelling blood gas monitoring electrodes is now very limited; most units use non-invasive monitors for oxygen and carbon dioxide monitoring, with arterial catheters for BP measurement and sampling.

Transcutaneous monitoring

These probes contain a heater that arterialises the blood in the skin. Oxygen diffuses through a membrane into the electrode, where it is reduced, setting up an electric current, the size of which is related to the partial pressure of the gas being monitored. This is displayed as the transcutaneous value, e.g. transcutaneous Po_2 (Tco_2).

Calibration takes several minutes and, once sited, the electrode takes around 15 minutes to equilibrate. The heat from the probe will burn the skin if not moved every 2–4 hours (Golden 1981; Poets et al. 1991). The combination of resiting and recalibration can mean that the sensor is not recording on the baby for substantial periods of time.

Falsely low readings are obtained if the probe is placed over poorly perfused skin, e.g. a bony surface (Takiwaki et al. 1991), if the infant lies on the electrode or if there is poor peripheral circulation (Vyas et al. 1988). Falsely high readings occur when there is poor contact with the skin, allowing air to get under the electrode.

There is a larger difference between Tco_2 and Pao_2 in older infants (Poets and Southall 1994), but within infants the ratio between Tco_2 and Pao_2 remains constant. Although absolute values may not be accurate, the trend in Tco_2 can still give useful information.

The sensitivity and specificity of transcutaneous monitors at detecting hypoxia (Pao_2 <6.6 kPa) have been estimated at 85% and 97%, respectively. For hyperoxia (Pao_2 >13.3 kPa), the sensitivity is 87% and specificity 89%. This means that the monitors will miss approximately 15% of both hypoxic and hyperoxic events, defined by these limits (Poets and Southall 1994).

Target values for Tco_2 depend on maturity, severity of illness and underlying diagnosis. It is common practice in preterm infants to aim for Tco_2 between 6 and 10 kPa.

Saturation monitoring

Pulse oximetry is now the standard method of oxygen monitoring. It is based on the principle that oxygenated haemoglobin absorbs light in the infrared region of the spectrum (850–1000 nm) while deoxygenated haemoglobin absorbs light in the visible red band (600–750 nm). The ratio of the light absorbed at two different wavelengths correlates with the proportions of oxygenated and deoxygenated haemoglobin in the tissues. The oximeter detects pulsation, which ensures that it is measuring only light absorbed by the haemoglobin in the blood vessels.

Pulse oximeters are easy to use, require no calibration and give immediate information. They are prone to artefact, and users must be aware of the many problems that can result in incorrect readings.

Strong ambient light and light bypassing the tissues cause an optical shunt, which is a common cause of artefact. Poor perfusion will affect the function of the oximeter, with most needing a pulse pressure of >20 mmHg (Morris et al. 1989; Falconer and Robinson 1990) or a systolic BP >30 mmHg (Severinghaus and Spellman 1990). Tight tape around the probe can affect the signal by impairing arterial pulsation, and can cause scarring and deformation of the hand or foot.

On the same baby, two oximeters may give different readings (Grieve et al. 1997). Some display functional saturation and others fractional saturation. The latter allows for levels of carboxyhaemoglobin and methaemoglobin, and is, in general, 2% lower.

Movement artefact is common and often makes interpretation of readings difficult, as well as being the most common cause of false alarms. It is important to check that the light plethysmography waveform shows a good-quality signal (Poets and Southall 1994). Another method of validation is to compare the pulse rate measured by the oximeter with that from an ECG monitor (Poets and Stebbens 1997). The readings are reliable only when the two heart rates are the same. In practice this usually means that the rates are within 5–10 beats of each other.

Figure 19.1 shows a typical trace with both heart rates. There is initially a period of poor agreement between the rates, and the dips in the saturation are caused by artefact. There then follows a period of good agreement, with reliable saturation readings.

Recent developments in pulse oximetry have reduced the false-alarm rates. In particular, instruments using the Masimo Signal extraction technology have been shown to identify true desaturations and bradycardias at least as reliably as a conventional oximeter but with 93% fewer false alarms (Bohnhorst et al. 2000). There is also a reported improvement in performance in clinical situations in which extreme motion artefact is likely (Sahni et al. 2003).

Detection of hypoxia

Oximeters use 'look-up' tables based on data from healthy adults to convert light absorption to saturation. Low levels have been derived by extrapolation from higher values and as a consequence these monitors underestimate the true degree of hypoxaemia.

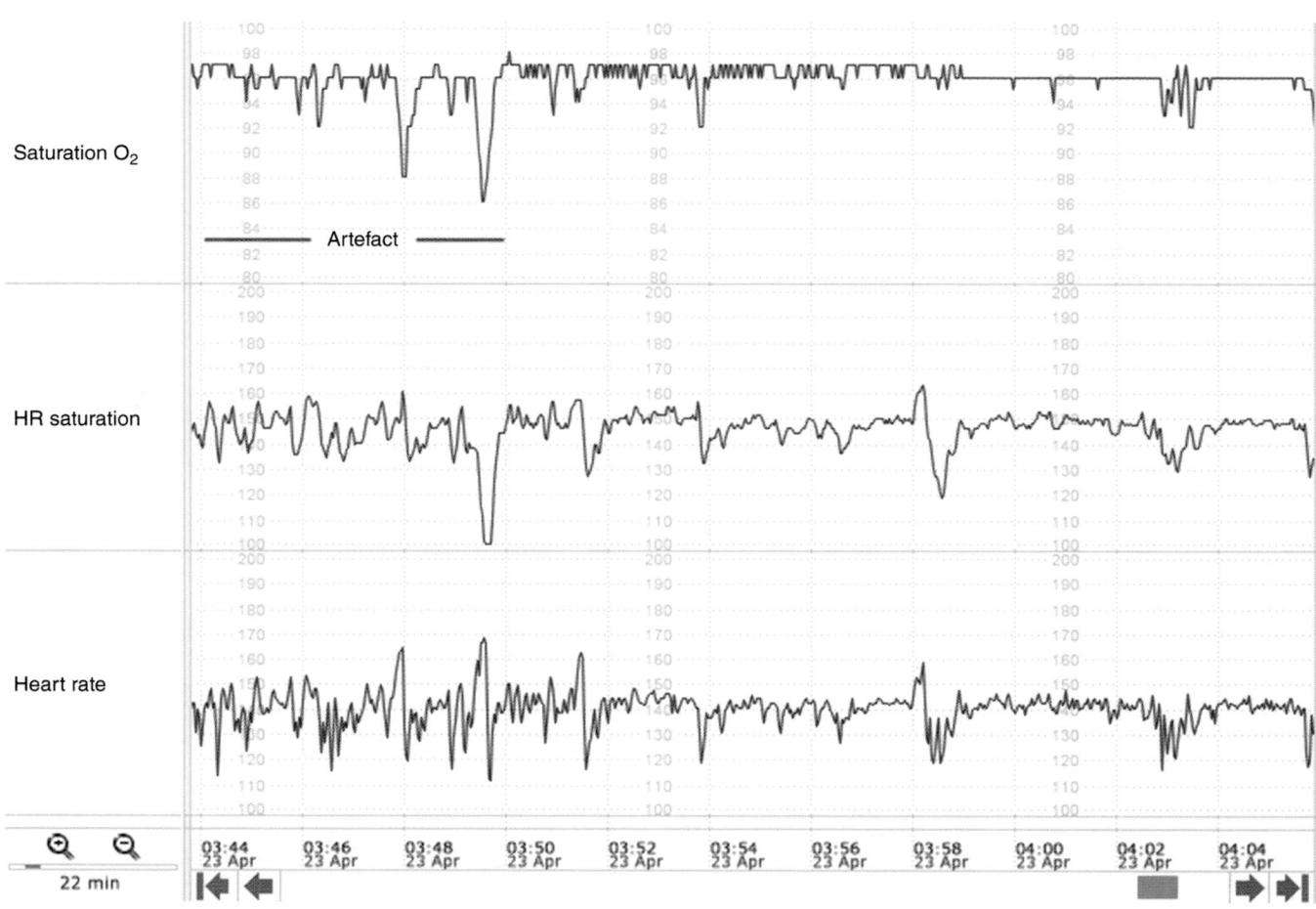

Fig. 19.1 Artefact on oxygen saturation recording shown by lack of agreement of heart rate traces.

Sensitivity and specificity for the detection of hypoxaemia have been estimated at 92% and 97%, respectively (Poets and Southall 1994).

Hyperoxia

The shape of the haemoglobin dissociation curve means that oximeters have a low sensitivity to hyperoxia, with small shifts in saturation reflecting large changes in Po_2. With an upper alarm limit set at 95%, newer instruments detect hyperoxia (>10.6 kPa) with a sensitivity of around 95% but a specificity of only 26–45%. Lowering the alarm limits improves the sensitivity but decreases the specificity even further (Bohnhorst et al. 2002).

Normal values for oxygen saturation

A functional saturation below 95%, obtained repeatedly while the infant is breathing regularly, should be regarded as abnormal, irrespective of age. Occasional falls in saturation below 80% are probably normal during the first 6 months of life (Poets 1999). However, there are no data that tell us at what baseline saturation level intervention should be considered or how often, or for how long, and to what nadir saturation may be allowed to fall. We know a lot about saturation monitoring in normal babies but remain uncertain about how to apply this technology to infants with respiratory disease.

It is difficult to recommend limits for oxygen saturation in babies with lung disease (see Monitoring the sick baby, below). Applying data from normal babies may increase their exposure to inspired oxygen, which in itself may be damaging (Anonymous 2000a; Saugstad 2001; Tin et al. 2001), while low saturations in infants have been associated with acute life-threatening events (Iles and Edmunds 1996).

Data from the SUPPORT study in infants under 28 weeks' gestation randomised to a low (85–89%) or high (91–95%) target range of oxygen saturation has shown no difference in the composite outcome of severe retinopathy or death. However there was an increase in mortality and a substantial decrease in severe retinopathy among survivors in the low target range (SUPPORT study group 2010). BOOST-II was an MRC funded randomised controlled trial comparing the effects of targeting arterial oxygen saturations in babies less than 28 weeks' gestation at the same levels as in the SUPPORT study. The composite primary outcome was mortality and major disability at 2 years corrected age. This study ceased recruitment following publication of the SUPPORT trial (SUPPORT 2010) showing a lower mortality in babies whose target oxygen saturation was 91–95%. A preliminary safety meta-analysis of data from SUPPORT and the BOOST trials recruiting in the UK, Australia and New Zealand confirmed this result and hence current recommendation is to target oxygen saturation at 91–95% (Stenson et al. 2011).

The higher mortality found in the SUPPORT study is of concern and until data are available from trials such as BOOST-II, many recommend that oxygen therapy be considered when baseline saturation is less than 93% (Poets 1998). The safe upper limit is uncertain but recent outcome data suggest around 95%. Infants in hospital are commonly allowed lower saturations, but, if being discharged home in oxygen, they should be maintained with a saturation above 93% (Poets 1998).

Carbon dioxide

The partial pressure of carbon dioxide (Pco_2) is important in determining the adequacy of alveolar ventilation and interpreting the acid–base balance. Pco_2 is affected by crying, which commonly occurs during intermittent sampling. Capillary samples are useful for monitoring stable infants with chronic respiratory problems, but care must be exercised in their interpretation (Courtney et al. 1990). Venous samples may be an acceptable alternative when monitoring trends in Pco_2, but the literature is limited and even greater care should be taken in interpreting the values obtained. In the particular situation of a baby with cardiac arrest, the difference between arterial and venous PCO2 is very large.

Transcutaneous CO$_2$ monitoring

Transcutaneous CO_2 ($TcCO_2$) is commonly combined with oxygen monitoring in the same probe. Most $TcCO_2$ electrodes work by measuring the change in pH of an electrolyte solution, separated from the skin by a hydrophobic membrane, which is permeable to carbon dioxide but not to hydrogen ions.

$TcCO_2$ is in general 27% higher than the corresponding arterial measurement, due partly to local tissue production of carbon dioxide as well as to the heating coefficient of blood. The electrodes need calibration against a known concentration of carbon dioxide every 4 hours. This can take 10 minutes, adding to the time that the probe is not in use monitoring the baby.

Over a 4-hour period, there is an upward drift in the $TcCO_2$ but overall there remains a good correlation between transcutaneous and arterial CO_2, making it a useful trend monitor. Repeated blood gas estimations are still required, but changes in $TcCO_2$ can give early warning of developing problems, such as a blocking endotracheal tube (Fig. 19.2). In transport, $TcCO_2$ monitoring has resulted in babies arriving with lower ventilator pressures and better blood gases (O'Connor and Grueber 1998).

There are no data on normal values for $TcCO_2$. Experience with these monitors has been that each baby has an individual relationship between arterial and $Tcco_2$. These probes are more useful as a means of following trends than as a measurement of true arterial Pco_2.

End-tidal CO$_2$ monitoring

Capnography measures the concentration of CO_2 in exhaled gas and has been used extensively in patients under general anaesthesia and in adult intensive care. Small tidal volumes, rapid respiratory rates and inhomogeneous alveolar ventilation/perfusion in neonates with lung disease have limited the use in the newborn (Hand et al. 1989). $Tcco_2$ monitoring provides a more accurate estimation of $Paco_2$ (Tobias and Meyer 1997) and remains the preferred method of monitoring CO_2 during transport (Tingay et al. 2005).

The problem of inhomogeneous lung disease has been diminished by replacement surfactant. Studies using newer mainstream monitors, with low dead space and resistance, have shown capnography to have some place in monitoring trends in carbon dioxide (Rozycki et al. 1998). Colorimetric CO_2 detectors are useful adjuncts for airway management, especially for checking endotracheal tube placement during resuscitation (Molloy and Deakins 2006).

Acid–base balance

Monitoring of the pH, bicarbonate and base excess is important in the assessment of respiratory status. Capillary and venous samples can be used to monitor changes in acid–base state in the stable baby (Yildizdaş et al. 2004) but arterial blood should be used in the assessment of the ill neonate.

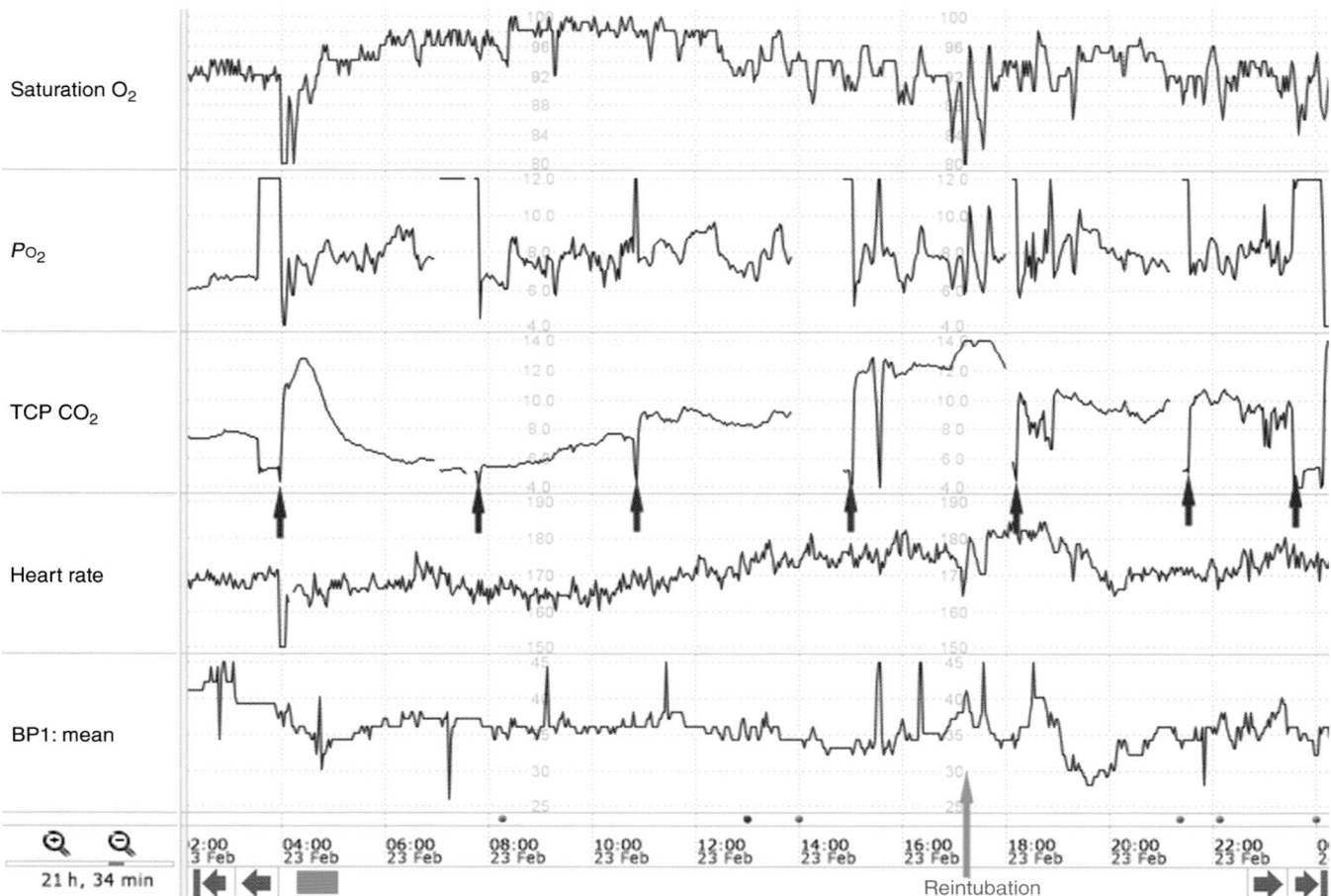

Fig. 19.2 Trend graphs of an infant showing a rise in transcutaneous CO_2 for several hours before a blocked tube was diagnosed. Black arrows show times when the probe was off the baby for recalibration.

Continuous online respiratory function monitoring

This is now available on most ventilators. Data are presented as numerical values, time-based waveforms of flow, volume and airway pressures, and flow/volume and pressure/volume loops. The interpretation of this information requires knowledge of how the data are obtained as well as an understanding of the underlying pathophysiology.

These monitors have been shown to reduce mortality in adults with acute respiratory distress syndrome (Anonymous 2000b). In infants, their use has reduced ventilator time (Stenson et al. 1998) and short-term morbidity (Rosen et al. 1993), although as yet there is little evidence that overall outcome is improved. Further critical evaluation is required, as not all the information used in adult trials can be obtained reliably in newborn infants.

A flow sensor, usually a hot-wire anemometer, needs to be connected directly to the endotracheal tube and this adds 1 ml to the respiratory dead space. In the smallest infants this could necessitate increased minute ventilation to maintain CO_2 elimination (Stokes et al. 1986). Data from different devices may not be comparable. Changes in gas composition affect the measurements. Pure oxygen is 12% more viscous than room air, so reducing the fraction of inspired oxygen (Fio_2) may result in an apparent increase in tidal volume (Yeh et al. 1984).

Functional residual capacity

Measurements of tidal volume and functional residual capacity (FRC) can be used to avoid high end-inspiratory and low end-expiratory lung volumes. FRC varies considerably over the course of an illness and can change rapidly with treatments such as surfactant or high-frequency oscillatory ventilation. There is presently no readily applicable method for repeated measurements of FRC that would be suitable for routine clinical use. FRC is inferred from the chest X-ray appearances and the Fio_2 required to achieve adequate oxygenation, although the relationship between the radiographic and measured lung volumes is inconsistent (Thome et al. 1998).

Leaks

There is generally some leak around the uncuffed endotracheal tubes used in newborn infants. The mean leak has been estimated at around 15% (Bernstein et al. 1995). A leak makes some of the derived data, such as compliance and resistance, unreliable (Mahmoud et al. 2009) and also complicates the interpretation of loops and waveforms. Most of the leak occurs in inspiration and is calculated as inspired minus expired volume, expressed as a percentage of the inspired volume. The displayed expired tidal volume has usually taken the leak into account and further correction is not needed.

The size of the leak only becomes important if there is a problem with ventilation. Flow-triggered ventilators are susceptible to autocycling in the presence of an airway leak, the rate of autocycling being proportional to the size of the leak (Bernstein et al. 1995).

Tidal volume

A healthy, spontaneously breathing term baby with no lung disease has a tidal volume of around 7–9 ml/kg bodyweight (Anonymous 1993). The ventilated infant with respiratory disease has fewer functional airspaces, and there may be regional inhomogeneity of pressure/volume characteristics within the lungs. 'Normal' tidal volumes may therefore expose parts of the lungs to excess end-inspiratory volume. Because of this, target tidal volumes are generally set around the 4–6 ml/kg range, depending on the CO_2 elimination. When there is pulmonary hypoplasia, target tidal volumes may need to be lower, as the inspiratory capacity of the lungs per unit bodyweight will be less than normal.

Some devices display tidal volume breath by breath, while others give a rolling average. Spontaneous breaths are generally smaller than ventilator breaths, so if averaging is used it will not give a true impression of the ventilator tidal volumes, if there is significant spontaneous breathing. Displayed values are not weight-corrected.

Minute ventilation

A rolling average of expired minute ventilation can be calculated and subdivided into the relative proportions attributable to ventilator and spontaneous breaths. Whether this is any more useful than looking at tidal volumes is unclear. There is no evidence that measuring minute ventilation is any more useful than monitoring transcutaneous P_{CO_2}.

Compliance and resistance

There are a variety of methods for deriving these data from continuous dynamic pressure/volume traces, but they are unlikely to be useful in everyday clinical practice. The values are affected by lung volume at the time of measurement and are unreliable if inappropriately short inspiratory or expiratory times are used. They are made inaccurate by leaks around the endotracheal tube. The variable nature of infant–ventilator interactions complicates their interpretation in real time.

The C20:C ratio is a derived index of lung overdistension which compares the compliance during the last 20% of inflation with that of the whole breath (Fisher et al. 1988). This index is unreliable in newborn infants because it requires a ventilator which generates a slow rise in inflation pressure, or a constant flow of gas into the lungs during inflation, and little or no air leak (Neve et al. 2000), conditions seldom met in neonatal ventilation.

Waveforms

Simultaneous time-based traces of flow, volume and pressure are the most commonly used graphical representation of respiratory function and provide the most readily interpretable information. The scaling of the graphs is important. Autoscaling should be used with caution, as changes in the size of the waveforms, due to variation in respiratory function, may be obscured by the system redrawing them on a new scale.

The time-based waveforms help in determining appropriate inspiratory and expiratory times. Figure 19.3 shows simultaneous traces of flow, volume and pressure over time from a ventilated

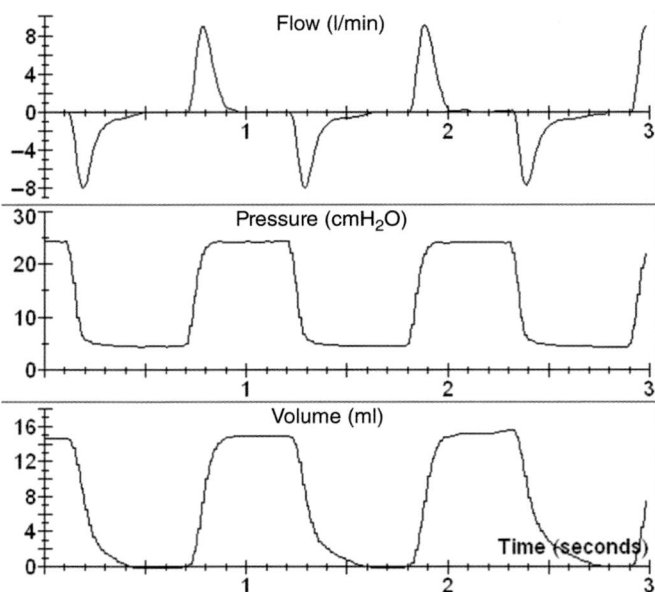

Fig. 19.3 Simultaneous time-based waveforms of flow, pressure and volume from a ventilated infant.

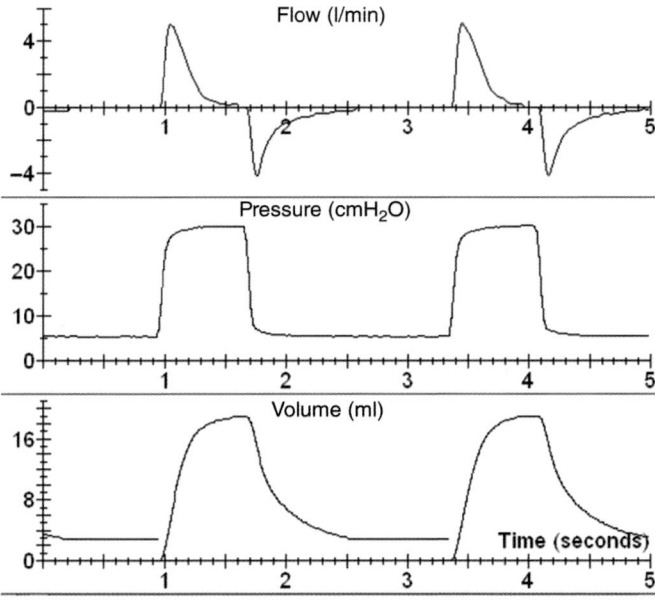

Fig. 19.4 Time-based waveforms from an infant with a modest leak around the endotracheal tube.

infant. With the onset of inflation, pressure rises to a peak and is maintained at this level for the duration of inspiration. As the pressure has risen, gas flows into the lungs and inspiratory flow (shown above the line) rises rapidly to a peak before falling to zero. No further volume passes into the lungs for the remainder of the set inspiratory time. The volume trace rises rapidly to a peak and then plateaus, with the inspired tidal volume held in the lungs until the onset of expiration. If there is an air leak around the endotracheal tube, the volume plateau is not horizontal but slopes upward from left to right (Fig. 19.4). The gradient of the slope reflects the size of the leak. Under these circumstances, the flow trace does not return

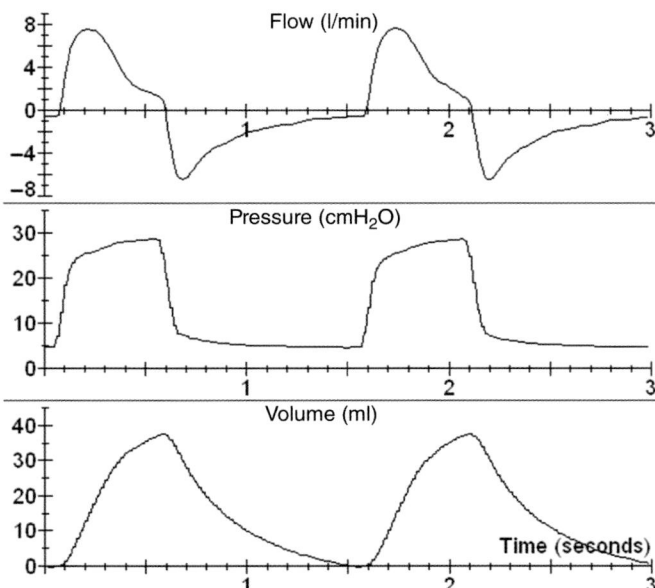

Fig. 19.5 Simultaneous waveforms from an infant with a long expiratory phase. After 1 second in expiration, expiratory flow has not quite reached zero before the onset of the next inspiration.

to zero but continues at a low level after the initial rapid rise and fall (Fig. 19.4). In the case of a very large leak, or when the endotracheal tube has slipped out of the trachea, the volume trace continues to rise steeply until it goes off the screen and the flow remains high throughout inspiration. Under these circumstances, little or no expiratory flow is seen at the onset of expiration.

At the onset of expiration, the pressure in the ventilator circuit falls to the set positive end-expiratory pressure (PEEP) level. Gas flows out of the lungs and expiratory flow (conventionally displayed below the baseline) accelerates to a peak and then falls to zero (Fig. 19.3). The volume trace falls from the inspiratory volume peak to zero. If there is an air leak around the endotracheal tube, the volume trace does not return to zero because the gas that leaked around the tube in inspiration cannot be exhaled (Fig. 19.4). Monitoring devices are usually set to re-zero the volume baseline at the onset of the next inspiratory flow. If the next inflation begins before the expiratory flow has returned to zero, gas is trapped in the lungs. This phenomenon is called occult or inadvertent PEEP (Simbruner 1986). It will impair gas exchange and occasionally may be life-threatening (Stenson et al. 1995). Inspection of the expired flow waveform allows the clinician to ensure that expiratory flow has returned to zero before the onset of the next inflation and prevent this complication. In Figure 19.5, expiratory flow has not quite returned to zero when the next inflation arrives, despite an expiration time of around 1 second.

With an obstructing endotracheal tube, the height of the peak flow on the inspiratory and expiratory flow waveforms lessens, and the width of the expiratory flow pattern broadens because the increase in airway resistance makes gas movements take longer. Excessive rain-out of humidity in the tubing can partially obstruct the bias flow in the circuit. This causes fluctuations in airway pressure, resulting in small flow oscillations at the airway, which are seen in the flow baseline at times when there should be no flow. They can result in autocycling of the ventilator, and the presence of an oscillating flow baseline should prompt inspection of the circuit for trapped water.

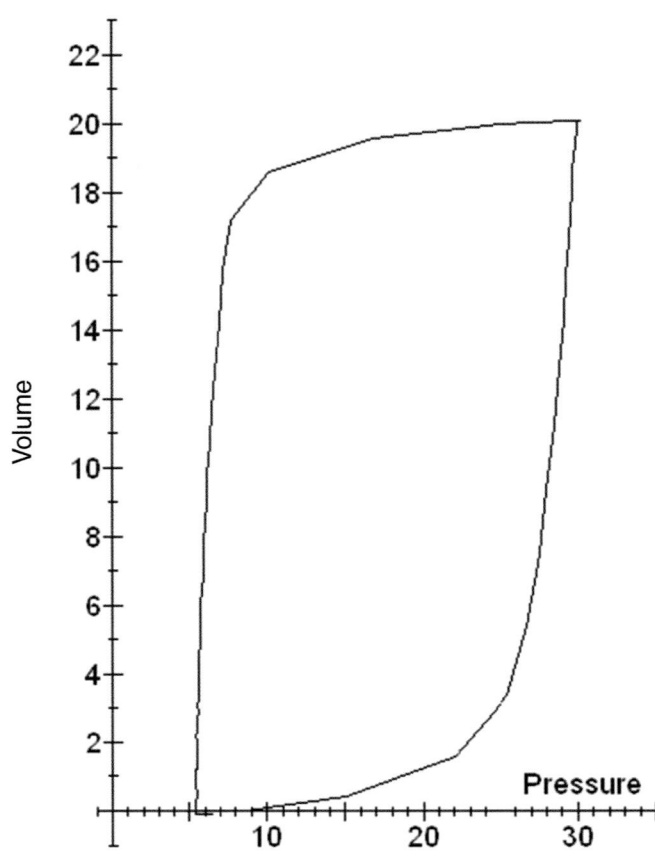

Fig. 19.6 Pressure/volume loop from an infant on pressure-limited ventilation.

Loops

Pressure/volume and flow/volume are the commonest displayed loops. They are distorted by infant–ventilator interactions. If the screen is watched in real time, breaths that are relatively free from interaction can be identified when the infant is settled. Pressure/volume loops can be inspected to determine the critical opening pressure of the airspaces and the upper inflection point where the slope of the pressure/volume relationship begins to flatten because of overdistension. This has been used in adults to facilitate less damaging ventilation strategies (Ranieri et al. 1999). However, in order to plot the progressive change in lung volume that occurs for a given change in pressure, the pressure has to rise slowly enough to allow changes in volume to keep pace. Pressure-limited neonatal ventilators generate relatively square pressure waves with a rapid rise to peak inspiratory pressure and an equally rapid fall to the PEEP level in expiration. This means that the changes in lung volume during inspiration are mostly plotted against the peak inspiratory pressure and during expiration against the end pressure, giving the loops a rectangular appearance which bears little relationship to the underlying pressure/volume characteristics of the lung (Fig. 19.6). Significant leaks around the endotracheal tube make interpretation even more difficult.

Inspection of flow/volume loops can give information about airway resistance. If resistance is increased, flow is slower. This can be observed from the time-based waveforms without the need to look at flow/volume loops. If there are secretions in the endotracheal tube, the expiratory limb of the loop can show a saw-tooth pattern, indicating the need for endotracheal suction (Jubran and Tobin 1994).

Neurological system monitoring

Compared with the respiratory and cardiovascular systems, there is little available for continuous neurological monitoring. Examination of the nervous system is often intermittent and assessment subjective. It is more difficult when sedative drugs and neuromuscular paralysis agents are given.

EEG, aEEG and cerebral function monitors

Continuous electroencephalography (EEG) recording is now feasible and clinically useful. EEG is the best method for detecting seizure activity. Changes in the background give important prognostic information following hypoxic–ischaemic injury (Ch. 40.4).

Interpretation of the full EEG can be difficult and techniques to simplify the data have been introduced. Amplitude-integrated EEG (aEEG) monitoring is a compressed and rectified signal from one or more channels of EEG. The original 'cerebral function' monitors produced only one channel of aEEG with no access to the raw signal, but digital technology now allows multiple channels with access to the underlying EEG signal, which helps with artefact rejection. The aEEG has been shown to be helpful in monitoring cerebroelectrical background activity in sick neonates and in detection of subclinical seizures (Toet et al. 2008). It has a predictive value in the first hours of life following asphyxial injury (Spitzmiller et al. 2007). The interpretation of the aEEG trace, and its prognostic value, in babies undergoing therapeutic hypothermia still needs further evaluation. There are some preliminary data to show that cooling delays return of sleep-wake cycling in babies who will have a good outcome (Thoresen et al 2010). Its use in the preterm baby has been less clearly defined although reference values have been published (Olishar et al. 2004) and there are some data on its use in predicting outcome in preterm infants with large intraventricular haemorrhages (Hellstrom-Westas et al. 2001).

Although aEEG can be used for long periods, it must be remembered that it is a simplified method for monitoring electrocortical background activity and has limitations. Its simplicity is an advantage but can result in difficulties in interpreting whether a pattern represents seizure or other activity. At least one standard EEG should be recorded in monitored infants.

Cerebral ultrasound

Ultrasound offers an easy method of imaging the neonatal brain. Repeated scans allow progress to be monitored and give prognostic information. Abnormalities that persist are more likely to be genuine, and most conditions evolve over time, allowing more certain diagnosis. Ultrasound changes must be interpreted with care.

Intracranial pressure monitoring

Indirect measurements of intracranial pressure taken across the anterior fontanelle have been found to be unreliable and inaccurate. Invasive intracranial pressure monitoring may have its place in specialist units, but has not been shown to improve outcome in the baby with neonatal encephalopathy secondary to a hypoxic–ischaemic insult.

Near-infrared spectroscopy

NIRS is capable of providing information on cerebral haemoglobin oxygen saturation, cerebral blood volume, cerebral blood flow, cerebral oxygen delivery, cerebral venous saturation and cerebral oxygen availability/utilisation. Compared with aEEG, NIRS as a monitoring device is less well integrated in neonatal intensive care but this is changing. Particularly in cardiac surgery cerebral monitoring, together with aEEG, is becoming more commonly used not only during cardiopulmonary bypass but also before and in the hours and days after surgery (Toet and Lemmers 2009).

Temperature monitoring

Measuring central temperature is important. The rectum should not be used as there is a small risk of damage to the mucosa. Rectal temperature is unreliable and is affected by the depth of insertion of the thermometer, whether the baby has just passed a stool and by the temperature of the blood returning from the lower limbs.

The temperature of the skin over the liver or in the axilla reflects central temperature. A more accurate measurement can be obtained by placing the probe between the scapulae and a non-conducting mattress. No tape is needed on the skin since the baby lies on the probe, holding it in place. This so-called zero heat flux temperature has been shown to be very close to the central temperature (Dollberg et al. 1993).

The measure of a single temperature tells us how well the baby is maintaining that temperature but nothing about how much energy is being used to achieve thermal balance. The continuous measurement and display of a central (abdominal, axillary or zero heat flux) and a peripheral (foot) temperature detects cold stress. Figure 19.7 shows an increasing temperature gap during a procedure. The baby is exposed to cold stress, but if the central temperature alone was being measured, then this would not have been apparent. Central measures of temperature vary, but the baby is

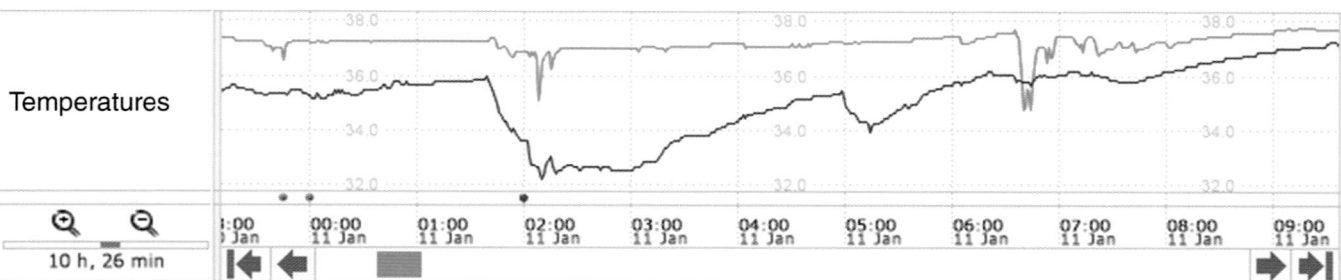

Fig. 19.7 Trend in central (top trace) and peripheral (bottom trace) temperatures, showing widening of the gap during handling, with slow recovery after the procedure.

usually between 36.8°C and 37.3°C with a central–peripheral temperature gap of around 1°C.

A high central temperature, particularly if unstable, along with a wide central–peripheral gap is seen in septic babies (Messaritakis et al. 1990).

Monitoring the sick baby

What needs to be monitored will always depend on the clinical condition of the baby. Invasive devices carry risks but continuous intra-arterial BP monitoring is important in the sick or unstable baby, including the ventilated preterm newborn. Continuous measurement and display of a central and a peripheral (foot) temperature give important information on thermal balance as well as some indication of tissue perfusion.

Monitoring oxygen, carbon dioxide and acid–base state is essential in intensive care. There must be a method of continuous oxygen monitoring, although there will still be a need for intermittent blood sampling. This is usually done every 4–6 hours but may need to be more frequent if there are repeated changes in ventilation or the clinical condition fluctuates. All ventilators must display online respiratory function parameters as well as waveforms and loops. Close monitoring of tidal volume is important in preventing lung overdistension.

Although continuous oxygen monitoring is considered a standard of care for the sick neonate with lung disease there has been a failure to show its effect on clinically meaningful outcomes. Despite the lack of comparative literature, saturation is now the most widely used method but this is subject to artefact and can underestimate both hypoxia and hyperoxia.

The use of oxygen has been closely linked to retinopathy of prematurity (ROP) and brain damage (Tin et al. 2001). There is evidence that fluctuations in oxygen levels within the baby may be important in the pathogenesis of ROP (Cunningham et al. 1995) and the use of saturation monitors has been associated with significantly more variable oxygenation than with transcutaneous monitors (Quine and Stenson 2008).

Before deciding on the best technique for oxygen monitoring we need more data on how to prevent ROP and other oxygen-related disorders. We need to know the relative importance of the absolute level of oxygen and the degree of fluctuation in P_{O_2} before we can decide on the optimum method of continuous monitoring (Poets and Bassler 2008). There is a conflict between trying to reduce mortality while preventing conditions such as severe retinopathy (SUPPORT study group 2010). Further randomised trials (BOOST-II) are underway to try and help answer the question as to the best baseline level for saturation in the preterm baby but fluctuations in oxygen may be equally important.

At this time the upper limit for a preterm baby receiving oxygen should be set at 95% to try and avoid significant periods of hyperoxia. Setting tight limits will result in very frequent alarms. Using an alarm range of 86–95%, while aiming to keep the baby around 90%, is reasonable but this recommendation may well change once the current trials are complete. If the preterm baby is breathing air then it may be reasonable to set the upper alarm to 100% but it is important to lower this again if oxygen is given.

There is less anxiety about the upper level of oxygen saturation in the term baby and this should be set at 98% with a lower limit of 92%.

In babies with persistent pulmonary hypertension the upper limit should be set to 100%. The lower limit may have to be lowered if there are frequent alarms due to the condition of the baby. This must be an individual clinical decision.

These limits may be unsuitable for babies with cyanotic heart disease; in this group levels need to be decided clinically for each baby and are often around 75–85%.

Clinical and laboratory monitoring

Infection

Infection is an important cause of morbidity and mortality. Babies must be screened whenever there is a clinical indication of suspected sepsis. The screen should include culture of blood, cerebrospinal fluid, urine, secretions and swabs, although which are needed in each case will depend on the clinical picture and policy of the individual unit.

The coagulase-negative *Staphylococcus* is commonly grown in cultures and the differentiation of infection from colonisation can be difficult. In all situations the result of cultures must be interpreted in the light of the clinical features and other supportive laboratory tests, particularly differential white count, platelet count and C-reactive protein. There are many studies looking at the best predictors of infection in the neonate but none have come up with any method that has acceptable values for sensitivity and specificity.

In the ventilated baby there is debate about the usefulness of routine culture of endotracheal aspirates. These cultures have a very poor predictive value (Lau and Hey 1991) and have not been found to be predictive of pathogens that are subsequently isolated during an infective episode (Slagel et al. 1989). The organisms isolated usually reflect colonisation and this practice can lead to overdiagnosis and antibiotic overuse with the risk of increased resistance developing. Many false negatives may also lead to undertreatment. There is a need for a robust definition of ventilator-associated pneumonia in the newborn which will allow better surveillance and targeting of infections associated with this invasive therapy. Until this time the routine cultures of tracheal aspirates offer little of diagnostic value.

Fluid balance (see Ch. 18)

Input/output charts should be used to help assess fluid balance, but it is important to measure all fluids given to the baby, including drugs and flushes for catheters (Noble-Jamieson et al. 1986).

Allowance must be made for evaporative fluid losses unless the baby is nursed in high humidity. Respiratory fluid losses can be high if there is inadequate humidification of the ventilator gases.

Urine output can be assessed by using pre-weighed nappies or cotton wool balls, but these must be weighed as soon as possible after voiding, to avoid evaporative loss (Cooke et al. 1989).

Fluid shifts in the baby are reflected in weight changes, but it is difficult in clinical practice to get good reproducible measurements, even when using within-incubator scales.

In the first days of life, changes in plasma sodium reflect hydration, with hyponatraemia being due to fluid overload and hypernatraemia to dehydration. Analysers now measure sodium along with the blood gases. Several measurements of plasma sodium throughout the day, along with the input/output and weight chart, give a good estimate of fluid balance in the sick neonate.

Biochemistry

As well as repeated estimations of plasma sodium, to help assess fluid balance, other electrolytes, glucose, creatinine, bilirubin and calcium should be measured once daily, and more often if clinically indicated. Laboratory methods are discussed in Chapter 42 and normal values are given in Appendix 6. If parenteral nutrition is being used, then appropriate biochemical monitoring is essential (Ch. 17).

Haematology

Blood losses from sampling should be recorded and the sick ventilated baby must have a haemoglobin and/or haematocrit measured at least daily. Deciding on the optimum time for transfusion with red cells is difficult and there are no good data in the literature to help. Individual units need to develop their own guidelines.

Thrombocytopenia is often seen in sepsis, particularly if there is a consumptive coagulopathy or where central intravenous lines have been infected with coagulase-negative staphylococci. In ill babies, the platelet count, clotting studies and fibrinogen should be monitored regularly. Heparin in arterial lines can contaminate the samples for clotting studies and care must be taken in the interpretation of the results.

Daily total white counts, and the differential, can give an indication of developing sepsis. Absolute values are very varied, but changes, either up or down, can be indicative of infection.

Flow charts and plotting results on graphs are useful as they show trends in biochemical and haematological data.

Point-of-care testing

Point-of-care (near-patient) testing is expanding with the development of highly accurate instruments.

Blood gas analysers on the nursery are a mandatory part of the equipment of any intensive care unit. Glucose should always be measured using whole blood glucose analysers such as the Yellow Springs, although most blood gas analysers will also measure blood glucose. Cotside stick methods (Dextrostix, BM-glycaemie, or Reflostix) are no longer considered sufficiently accurate for neonatal use (Ch. 34.1).

New generations of analysers allow the measurement of a whole range of parameters without sending blood to the laboratory. Each unit must determine which bedside tests are indicated based on an analysis of test accuracy, clinical importance and cost–benefit ratio. There are major issues about maintenance of appropriate standards and quality control that also need to be addressed.

X-ray monitoring (Chs 43 and 44)

Although routine radiographs have been shown to be safe and not expose the extremely-low-birthweight infant to any excessive radiation risk (Sutton et al. 1998), the use of X-rays should be limited and determined by clinical need.

The chest X-ray is vital in the initial assessment of all babies with respiratory disease. Further X-rays, throughout the course of the respiratory illness, should be done as clinically indicated.

Abdominal X-rays help in the diagnosis of necrotising enterocolitis (NEC) and in detecting intestinal perforation. There is debate as to how often these X-rays should be repeated in infants with NEC, but in a very sick baby X-rays are indicated at least daily (sometimes more often) because perforation can be difficult to detect clinically.

There are many other indications for X-rays, including checking the position of endotracheal tubes and the tips of central arterial and venous lines.

Intravenous pumps

All pumps used to deliver intravenous fluids must have in-line pressure alarms. These detect occlusion in the line distal to the pump. Many have adjustable limits and can be set to detect small changes in pressure, which could give an early warning of fluid extravasation into the tissues.

Unfortunately there is no evidence that any of the currently marketed infusion devices are capable of predicting or detecting infiltration in any patient population. Pressure changes caused by patient movement are far greater than those found in the early stages of fluid extravasation (Phelps et al. 1990).

Close observation of the infusion site at regular intervals, stopping the infusion at the first sign of swelling or redness, is all that is available to detect fluid extravasation and hopefully prevent or minimise subsequent tissue damage. Scarring from tissue infiltration is now a common cause of complaint and litigation. It is important that all units have a policy for the observation of intravenous infusions and that there is a record of the sites being observed at least hourly.

Data handling

Technical advances have increased the amount and complexity of data from monitors, but more is not necessarily better. For example, although there are theoretical reasons why the large number of parameters available from ventilator monitors should be helpful, there is, for many, little evidence that in routine clinical care they make any difference. Inexperienced doctors and nurses, who may be responsible for much of the day-to-day care, are faced with increasingly complex, and potentially useless, information, before they have even grasped the basic principles. There is a serious danger of data overload. An increasing multitude of alarms, often indicating minor technical problems only, result in the 'crying wolf' situation, with staff less likely to react appropriately to correct alarms (Tsien and Facklet 1997). There is a need to assess critically what is essential for the care of the baby, and the introduction of new monitoring parameters should be resisted without assessment of their usefulness by rigorous clinical trials.

Monitoring is not just about reading values from machines. It is the ability to integrate a whole range of data, including observation of the whole baby, into meaningful information. 'Experience' and 'gut feeling' are really recognition of patterns, although the process may occur subconsciously. Experienced nursing staff are an essential part of the monitoring of the baby and they often raise concerns about potential problems. However, even the most experienced clinical staff can be slow at recognising developing problems even when the patterns, on retrospective review, have been obvious for some time (Alberdi et al. 2001).

Continuous trend monitoring

Monitors and blood tests give information on the condition of the baby at a single moment. Displaying data as a continuous graph allows trends to be visualised, hopefully facilitating detection of abnormalities and allowing earlier intervention. The typical patterns in the trends of central–peripheral temperature differences shown in Figure 19.7 are a good example.

Plotted trends can show that a parameter is changing significantly, even before the values are outside the set alarm ranges. They may also make it clearer which readings are due to artefact.

Figure 19.2 shows the high P_{CO_2} associated with a blocked endotracheal tube, necessitating an emergency reintubation. Although the clinical deterioration was sudden, it can be seen that the P_{CO_2} had been rising slowly for several hours. Earlier assessment may well have avoided the subsequent collapse. Trend monitoring of Tc_{CO_2} may also facilitate earlier diagnosis of pulmonary air leak (McIntosh et al. 2000).

A randomised controlled trial of trend monitoring in neonatal intensive care failed to show that it improved outcome (Cunningham et al. 1998). Data overload, an inability to ascertain which data were important, a failure to include enough relevant information, or simply that staff were ignorant of the patterns that existed may be the reasons why trend monitoring did not make any difference to outcome. Also, it is often the change in a number of parameters that is important and it can be difficult to visualise these all at once. Computers can be used to recognise complex trends and what is needed are computerised decision support systems if the full potential of continuous trend data is to be recognised (Alberdi et al. 2000). In such systems, artefact detection and removal remain a challenge, but this has been shown to be feasible (Cunningham et al. 1994b).

Weblinks

http://www.bapm.org/media/documents/publications/hosp_standards.pdf: British Association of Perinatal Medicine. Standards for hospitals providing neonatal intensive and high-dependency care.

http://www.mhra.gov.uk/Howweregulate/Devices/index.htm: Medicines and Healthcare products Regulatory Agency. Information regarding government standards for medical equipment in the UK.

http://www.npeu.ox.ac.uk/boost: BOOST II. Information on Benefits of Oxygen Saturation Targeting (BOOST II) study. Funded by the Medical Research Countil, BOOST II UK is a double-blind randomised controlled trial to compare the effects of targeting arterial oxygen saturations at levels of 85–89% versus 91–95% in babies born at less than 28 weeks' gestation.

References

Adams, J.A., Zabaleta, I.A., Sackner, M.A., 1997. Hypoxemic events in spontaneously breathing premature infants: etiologic basis. Pediatr Res 42, 463–471.

Alberdi, E., Gilhooly, K., Hunter, J., et al., 2000. Computerisation and decision making in neonatal intensive care: a cognitive engineering investigation. J Clin Monit 16, 85–94.

Alberdi, E., Becher, J.C., Gilhooly, K., et al., 2001. Expertise and the interpretation of computerised physiological data: implications for the design of computerised physiological monitoring in neonatal intensive care. Int J Hum Comput Stud 55, 191–216.

Anonymous, 1993. Respiratory mechanics in infants: physiologic evaluation in health and disease. American Thoracic Society/European Respiratory Society. Am Rev Respir Dis 147, 474–496.

Anonymous, 2000a. Supplemental Therapeutic Oxygen for Prethreshold Retinopathy Of Prematurity (STOP-ROP), a randomized, controlled trial. I. Primary outcomes. Pediatrics 105, 295–310.

Anonymous, 2000b. Ventilation with lower tidal volumes as compared with traditional tidal volumes for acute lung injury and the acute respiratory distress syndrome. The Acute Respiratory Distress Syndrome Network. N Engl J Med 342, 1301–1308.

Barone, J.E., Madlinger, R.V., 2006. Should the Allen test be performed before radial artery cannulation? J Trauma 61, 468–470.

Barrington, K.J., 2000a. Umbilical artery catheters in the newborn: effects of position of the catheter tip (Cochrane Review). Cochrane Database Syst Rev (2), CD000505.

Barrington, K.J., 2000b Umbilical artery catheters in the newborn: effects of heparin (Cochrane Review). Cochrane Database Syst Rev (2), CD000507.

Bernstein, G., Knodel, E., Heldt, G.P., 1995. Airway leak size and autocycling of three flow-triggered ventilators. Crit Care Med 23, 1739–1744.

Bohnhorst, B., Poets, C.F., 1998. Major reduction in alarm frequency with a new pulse oximeter. Intensive Care Med 24, 277–278.

Bohnhorst, B., Peter, C.S., Poets, C.F., 2000. Pulse oximeters' reliability in detecting hypoxemia and bradycardia: comparison between a conventional and two new generation oximeters. Crit Care Med 28, 1565–1568.

Bohnhorst, B., Peter, C.S., Poets, C.F., 2002. Detection of hyperoxaemia in neonates: data from three new pulse oximeters. Arch Dis Child Fetal Neonatal Ed 87, F217–F219.

British Association of Perinatal Medicine, 2001. Standards for Hospitals Providing Neonatal Intensive and High Dependency Care, second edition. British Association of Perinatal Medicine, London.

Campbell, M.E., Costeloe, K.L., 2001. Measuring intramucosal pH in very low birthweight infants. Pediatr Res 50, 398–404.

Cooke, R.J., Werkman, S., Watson, D., 1989. Urine output measurements in premature infants. Pediatrics 83, 116–118.

Courtney, S.E., Weber, K.R., Breakie, L.A., et al., 1990. Capillary blood gases in the neonate. A reassessment and review of the literature. Am J Dis Child 144, 168–172.

Cunningham, S., Symon, A.G., McIntosh, N., 1994a. Changes in mean blood pressure caused by damping of the arterial pressure waveform. Early Hum Dev 36, 27–30.

Cunningham, S., Symon, A.G., McIntosh N., 1994b. The practical management of artifact in computerised physiological data. Int J Clin Monit Comput 11, 211–216.

Cunningham, S., Fleck, B.W., Elton, R.A., et al., 1995. Transcutaneous oxygen levels in retinopathy of prematurity. Lancet 346, 1464–1465.

Cunningham, S., Deere, S., Symon, A., et al., 1998. A randomized, controlled trial of computerized physiologic trend monitoring in an intensive care unit. Crit Care Med 26, 2053–2060.

da Silva, S., Hennebert, N., Denis, R., et al., 2000. Clinical value of a single postnatal lactate measurement after intrapartum asphyxia. Acta Paediatr 89, 320–323.

Dempsey, E.M., Al Hazzani, F., Barrington K.J., 2009. Permissive hypotension in the extremely low birthweight infant with signs of good perfusion. Arch Dis Child Fetal Neonatal Ed 94, F241-F244.

Deshpande, S.A., Ward Platt, M.P., 1997. Association between blood lactate and acid–base status and mortality in ventilated babies. Arch Dis Child Fetal Neonatal Ed 76, F15–F20.

Dinwiddie, R., Patel, B.D., Kumar, S.P., et al., 1979. The effects of crying on arterial oxygen tension in infants recovering from respiratory distress. Crit Care Med 7, 50–53.

Diprose, G.K., Evans, D.H., Archer, L.N.J., et al., 1986. Dinamap fails to detect hypotension in very low birth weight infants. Arch Dis Child 61, 771–773.

Dollberg, S., Xi, Y., Donnelly, M.M., 1993. A noninvasive transcutaneous alternative to rectal thermometry for continuous measurement of core temperature in the piglet. Pediatr Res 34, 512–517.

Evans, N., Klucklow, M., Simmons, M., et al., 2002. Which to measure, systemic or organ blood flow? Middle cerebral artery and superior vena cava flow in very preterm infants. Arch Dis Child Fetal Neonatal Ed 87, F181–F184.

Falconer, R.J., Robinson, B.J., 1990. Comparison of pulse oximeters: accuracy at low arterial pressure in volunteers. Br J Anaesth 65, 552–557.

Fisher, J.B., Mammel, M.C., Coleman, J.M., et al., 1988. Identifying lung overdistension during mechanical ventilation by using volume-pressure loops. Pediatr Pulmonol 5, 10–14.

Goddard, P., Keith, I., Marcovitch, H., et al., 1974. Use of a continuously recording intravascular oxygen electrode in the newborn. Arch Dis Child 49, 853–860.

Golden, S.M., 1981. Skin craters – a complication of transcutaneous oxygen monitoring. Pediatrics 67, 514–516.

Gorelick, M.H., Shaw, K.N., Baker, M.D., 1993. Effect of ambient temperature on capillary refill in healthy children. Pediatrics 92, 699–702.

Grieve, S.H., McIntosh, N., Laing, I.A., 1997. Comparison of two different pulse oximeters in monitoring preterm infants. Crit Care Med 25, 2051–2054.

Groves, A.M., Kuschel, C.A., Knight, D.B., et al., 2008. Relationship between blood pressure and blood flow in newborn preterm infants. Arch Dis Child Fetal Neonatal Ed 93, F29-F32.

Hand, I.L., Shepard, E.K., Krauss, A.N., et al., 1989. Discrepancies between transcutaneous and end-tidal carbon dioxide monitoring in the critically ill neonate with respiratory distress syndrome. Crit Care Med 17, 556–559.

Hellstrom-Westas, L., Klette, H., Thorngren-Jerneck, K., et al., 2001. Early prediction of outcome with aEEG in preterm infants with large intraventricular haemorrhages. Neuropediatrics 32, 319–324.

Iles, R., Edmunds, A.T., 1996. Prediction of early outcome in resolving chronic lung disease of prematurity after discharge from hospital. Arch Dis Child 74, 304–308.

Jubran, A., Tobin, M.J., 1994. Use of flow–volume curves in detecting secretions in ventilator-dependent patients. Am J Respir Crit Care Med 150, 766–769.

Lambert, H.J., Baylis, P.H., Coulthard, M.G., 1998. Central–peripheral temperature difference, blood pressure, and arginine vasopressin in preterm neonates undergoing volume expansion. Arch Dis Child Fetal Neonatal Ed 78, F43–F45.

Lau, Y.L., Hey, E.N., 1991. Sensitivity and specificity of daily tracheal aspirate cultures in providing organisms causing bacteremia in ventilated neonates. Pediatr Infect Dis J 10, 290–294.

LeFlore, J.L., Engle, W.D., 2005. Capillary refill time is an unreliable indicator of cardiovascular status in term neonates. Adv Neonatal Care 5, 147–154.

Leonard, P.A., Beattie, T.F., 2004. Is measurement of capillary refill time useful as part of the initial assessment of children? Eur J Emerg Med 11, 158–163.

Lyon, A.J., Pikaar, M.E., Badger, P., et al., 1997. Temperature control in very low birthweight infants during the first five days of life. Arch Dis Child Fetal Neonatal Ed 76, F47–F50.

Mahmoud, R.A., Fischer, H.S., Proquitté, H., et al., 2009. Relationship between endotracheal tube leakage and under-reading of tidal volume in neonatal ventilators. Acta Paediatr 98, 1116–1122.

McIntosh, N., Becher, J.C., Cunningham, S., et al., 2000. Clinical diagnosis of pneumothorax is late: use of trend data and decision support might allow preclinical detection. Pediatr Res 48, 408–415.

Merenstein, G.B., Dougherty, K., Lewis, A., 1972. Early detection of pneumothorax by oscilloscope monitor in the newborn infant. J Pediatr 80, 98–101.

Messaritakis, J., Anagnostakis, D., Laskari, H., et al., 1990. Rectal–skin temperature difference in septicaemic newborn infants. Arch Dis Child 65, 380–382.

Miletin, J., Dempsey, E.M., 2008. Low superior vena cava flow on day 1 and adverse outcome in the very low birthweight infant. Arch Dis Child Fetal Neonatal Ed 93, F368–F371.

Miletin, J., Pichova, K., Dempsey, E.M., 2009. Bedside detection of low systemic flow in the very low birth weight infant on day 1 of life. Eur J Pediatr 168, 809–813.

Molloy, E.J., Deakins, K., 2006. Are carbon dioxide detectors useful in neonates? Arch Dis Child Fetal Neonatal Ed 91, F295–F298.

Morgan, C., Newell, S.J., Ducker, D.A., et al., 1999. Continuous neonatal blood gas monitoring using a multiparameter intra-arterial sensor. Arch Dis Child Fetal Neonatal Ed 80, F93–F98.

Morris, R.W., Nairn, M., Torda, T.A., 1989. A comparison of fifteen pulse oximeters. Part I: A clinical comparison; Part II: A test of performance under conditions of poor perfusion. Anaesth Intensive Care 17, 62–73.

Neve, V., de la Roque, E.D., Leclerc, F., et al., 2000. Ventilator-induced overdistension in children: dynamic versus low-flow inflation volume-pressure curves. Am J Respir Crit Care Med 162, 139–147.

Noble-Jamieson, C.M., Kuzmin, P., Airede, K.I., 1986. Hidden sources of fluid and sodium intake in ill newborn infants. Arch Dis Child 61, 695–696.

O'Connor, T.A., Grueber, R., 1998. Transcutaneous measurement of carbon dioxide tension during long-distance transport of neonates receiving mechanical ventilation. J Perinatol 18, 189–192.

O'Connor, T.A., Hart, R.T., 1994. Mixed venous oxygenation in critically ill neonates. Crit Care Med 22, 343–346.

Olishar, M., Klebermass, K., Kuhle, S., et al., 2004. Reference values for amplitude integrated electroencephalographic activity in preterm infants younger than 30 weeks' gestational age. Pediatrics 112, e61–e66.

Osborn, D.A., Evans, N., Kluckow, M., 2004. Clinical detection of low upper body blood flow in very premature infants using blood pressure, capillary refill time, and central–peripheral temperature difference. Arch Dis Child Fetal Neonatal Ed 89, F168–F173.

Phelps, S.J., Tolley, E.A., Cochran, E.B., 1990. Inability of inline pressure monitoring to predict or detect infiltration of peripheral intravenous catheters in infants. Clin Pharm 9, 286–292.

Poets, C.F., 1998. When do infants need additional inspired oxygen? A review of the current literature. Pediatr Pulmonol 26, 424–428.

Poets, C.F., 1999. Assessing oxygenation in healthy infants. J Pediatr 135, 541–543.

Poets, C.F., Bassler, D., 2008. Providing stability in oxygenation for preterm infants: is transcutaneous oxygen really better than pulse oximetry? Arch Dis Child Fetal Neonatal Ed 93, F330–F331.

Poets, C.F., Southall, D.P., 1994. Noninvasive monitoring of oxygenation in infants and children: practical considerations and areas of concern. Pediatrics 93, 737–746.

Poets, C.F., Stebbens, V.A., 1997. Detection of movement artifact in recorded pulse oximeter saturation. Eur J Pediatr 156, 808–811.

Poets, C.F., Samuels, M.P., Noyes, J.P., et al., 1991. Home monitoring of transcutaneous oxygen tension in the early detection of hypoxaemia in infants and young children. Arch Dis Child 66, 676–682.

Quine, D., Stenson, B.J., 2008. Does the monitoring method influence stability of oxygenation in preterm infants? A randomised crossover study of saturation versus transcutaneous monitoring. Arch Dis Child Fetal Neonatal Ed 93, F347–F350.

Ranieri, V.M., Suter, P.M., Tortorella, C., et al., 1999. Effect of mechanical ventilation on inflammatory mediators in patients with acute respiratory distress syndrome: a randomized controlled trial. JAMA 282, 54–61.

Rosen, W.C., Mammel, M.C., Fisher, J.B. et al., 1993. The effects of bedside pulmonary mechanics testing during infant mechanical ventilation: a retrospective analysis. Pediatr Pulmonol 16, 147–152.

Rozycki, H.J., Sysyn, G.D., Marshall, M.K., et al., 1998. Mainstream end-tidal carbon dioxide monitoring in the neonatal intensive care unit. Pediatrics 101, 648–653.

Sahni, R., Gupta, A., Ohira-Kist, K., et al., 2003. Motion resistant pulse oximetry in neonates. Arch Dis Child Fetal Neonatal Ed 88, F505–F508.

Saugstad, O.D., 2001. Update on oxygen radical disease in neonatology. Curr Opin Obstet Gynecol 13, 147–153.

Severinghaus, J.W., Spellman, M.J.J., 1990. Pulse oximeter failure thresholds in hypotension and vasoconstriction. Anesthesiology 73, 532–537.

Shah, S., Tracy, M., Smyth, J., 2004. Postnatal lactate as an early predictor of short-term outcome after intrapartum asphyxia. J Perinatol 24, 16–20.

Simbruner, G., 1986. Inadvertent positive end-expiratory pressure in mechanically ventilated newborn infants: detection and effect on lung mechanics and gas exchange. J Pediatr 108, 589–595.

Skinner, J.R., Milligan, D.W.A., Hunter, S., et al., 1992. Central venous pressure in the ventilated neonate. Arch Dis Child 67, 374–377.

Slagel, T.A., Bifano, E.M., Wolf, J.W., et al., 1989. Routine endotracheal cultures for the prediction of sepsis in ventilated babies. Arch Dis Child 64, 34–38.

Southall, D.P., Levitt, G.A., Richards, J.M., et al., 1983. Undetected episodes of prolonged apnea and severe bradycardia in preterm infants. Pediatrics 72, 541–551.

Spitzmiller, E., Phillips, T., Meinzen-Derr, J., et al., 2007. Amplitude-integrated EEG is useful in predicting neurodevelopmental outcome in full-term infants with hypoxic–ischaemic encephalopathy: a meta-analysis. J Child Neurol 22, 1069–1078.

Stenson, B.J., Glover, R.M., Wilkie, R.A., et al., 1995. Life-threatening inadvertent positive end-expiratory pressure. Am J Perinatol 12, 336–338.

Stenson, B.J., Glover, R.M., Wilkie, R.A., et al., 1998. Randomised controlled trial of respiratory system compliance measurements in mechanically ventilated neonates. Arch Dis Child Fetal Neonatal Ed 78, F15–F19.

Stenson, B., Brocklehurst, P., Tarnow-Mordi, W., 2011. Increased 36 week survival with high oxygen saturation target in extremely preterm infants. N Engl J Med 364, 1680–1683.

Stokes, G.M., Milner, A.D., Wilson, A.J., et al., 1986. Ventilatory response to increased dead spaces in the first week of life. Pediatr Pulmonol 2, 89–93.

Strozik, J.R., Pieper, C.H, Roller, J., 1997. Capillary refilling time in newborn babies: normal values. Arch Dis Child 67, 374–377.

SUPPORT Study Group of the Eunice Kennedy Shriver NICHD Neonatal Research Network. 2010. Target ranges of oxygen saturation in extremely preterm infants. N Engl J Med 362, 1959–1969.

Sutton, P.M., Arthur, R.J., Taylor, C., et al., 1998. Ionising radiation from diagnostic x rays in very low birthweight babies. Arch Dis Child Fetal Neonatal Ed 78, F227–F229.

Takiwaki, H., Nakanishi, H., Shono, Y., et al., 1991. The influence of cutaneous factors on the transcutaneous pO_2 and pCO_2 at various body sites. Br J Dermatol 125, 243–247.

Thome, U., Topfer, A., Schaller, P., et al., 1998. Comparison of lung volume measurements by antero-posterior chest X-ray and the SF6 washout technique in mechanically ventilated infants. Pediatr Pulmonol 26, 265–272.

Thoresen, M., Hellstrom-Westas, L., Liu, X., De Vries, L.S., 2010. Effect of hypothermia on amplitude-integrated Electroencephalogram in infants with asphyxia. Pediatrics 126, e131–e139.

Tin, W., Milligan, D.W., Pennefather, P., et al., 2001. Pulse oximetry, severe retinopathy, and outcome at one year in babies of less than 28 weeks gestation. Arch Dis Child Fetal Neonatal Ed 84, F106–F110.

Tingay, D.G., Stewart, M.J., Morley, C.J., 2005. Monitoring of end tidal carbon dioxide and transcutaeous carbon dioxide during neonatal transport. Arch Dis Child Fetal Neonatal Ed 90, F523–F526.

Tobias, J.D., Meyer, D.J., 1997. Noninvasive monitoring of carbon dioxide during respiratory failure in toddlers and infants: end-tidal versus transcutaneous carbon dioxide. Anesth Analg 85, 55–58.

Toet, M.C., Lemmers, P.M., 2009. Brain monitoring in neonates. Early Hum Dev 85, 77–84.

Toet, M.C., van Rooij, L.G.M., de Vries, L.S., 2008. The use of amplitude integrated EEG for assessing neonatal neurological injury. Clin Perinatol 35, 665–678.

Tsien, C.L., Facklet, J., 1997. Poor prognosis for existing monitors in the intensive care unit. Crit Care Med 25, 614–619.

Vyas, H., Helms, P., Cheriyan, G., 1988. Transcutaneous oxygen monitoring beyond the neonatal period. Crit Care Med 16, 844–847.

Wright, I.M., Owers, M., Wagner, M., 2008. The umbilical arterial catheter: a formula for improved positioning in the very low birth weight infant. Pediatr Crit Care Med 9, 498–501.

Yeh, M.P., Adams, T.D., Gardner, R.M. et al., 1984. Effect of O_2, N_2, and CO_2 composition on nonlinearity of Fleisch pneumotachograph characteristics. J Appl Physiol 56, 1423–1425.

Yildizdaş, D., Yapicioğlu, H., Yilmaz, H.L., et al., 2004. Correlation of simultaneously obtained capillary, venous, and arterial blood gases of patients in a paediatric intensive care unit. Arch Dis Child 89, 176–180.

Yoxall, C.W., Weindling, A.M., 1996. The measurement of peripheral venous oxyhaemoglobin saturation in newborn infants by near infrared spectroscopy with venous occlusion. Pediatr Res 39, 1103–1106.

Care of the normal term newborn baby

Patrick H T Cartlidge   Divyen K Shah   Janet M Rennie

20

Healthy term newborn babies are most appropriately cared for by their mothers, supervised by midwives. The National Institute for Health and Clinical Excellence (NICE) has produced two documents, *Intrapartum Care* (2007) and *Postnatal Care* (2006), which contain helpful advice (see Weblinks, below). Clear protocols and guidelines are needed to manage the baby who develops a problem such as symptomatic hypoglycaemia, jaundice, sepsis or hypernatraemic dehydration. Minor problems are common and often cause considerable parental anxiety, but they are rarely of clinical importance.

The information in this chapter aims to guide those who are responsible for well term newborns, highlighting common problems and areas where local protocols need to be developed. The normal newborn examination is detailed in Chapter 14.

Anticipatory care

Most maternal illnesses have no serious effects on the baby (Ch. 11 and Table 20.1). Nevertheless, awareness of such illnesses is essential so that appropriate and prompt action can be taken to prevent unnecessary sequelae, such as severe jaundice in babies with a family history of hereditary spherocytosis. Fetal medicine has had a dramatic impact in this area, often providing prior warning of diverse problems such as ambiguous genitalia, cardiac disease and intrathoracic masses (Ch. 9).

© 2012 Elsevier Ltd

Table 20.1 Maternal illness: effect on the baby and neonatal management

MATERNAL ILLNESS	EFFECT ON BABY	NEONATAL MANAGEMENT
Cardiovascular disease		
Ischaemic heart disease	–	–
Rheumatic heart disease	–	–
Congenital heart disease		
Acyanotic	Increased risk of congenital heart disease	Echocardiogram
Cyanotic	IUGR Increased risk of congenital heart disease	Echocardiogram
Hypertension	IUGR, may need to be delivered preterm Neonatal hypotension from drug therapy; hypoglycaemia from labetalol	Check blood pressure if unwell Check glucose in babies whose mothers were given labetalol (Ch. 34.1)
Respiratory disease		
Asthma	IUGR if severe Increased incidence of asthma	No neonatal intervention proven to reduce the risk of asthma
Chronic bronchitis	IUGR	–
Cystic fibrosis	–	No hazard from maternal lung pathogens. Breastfeeding is safe
Endocrine and metabolic disease		
Diabetes*	Infant of a diabetic mother (Ch. 22)	Needs careful neonatal evaluation
Thyrotoxicosis*	Neonatal thyrotoxicosis (Ch. 34.2)	Needs careful neonatal evaluation
Hyperparathyroidism	Neonatal hypocalcaemia (Ch. 34.2)	Monitor serum calcium during first 7 days
Other endocrine disease, e.g. Addison disease, hypothyroidism	–	–
Phenylketonuria*	Impaired development and microcephaly. Congenital heart disease	Nothing can be done in the neonatal period
Gastrointestinal disease		
Coeliac disease	–	–
Crohn disease	Prematurity or IUGR if severe	–
Ulcerative colitis	Prematurity or IUGR if severe	–
Peptic ulceration	–	–
Stomas, colostomy	–	–
Renal disease		
Chronic renal disease (nephrotic, renal failure)	IUGR Some forms of renal disease are hereditary, e.g. polycystic disease, Alport syndrome	Depends on aetiology and inheritance risk
Urinary infection	IUGR	Usually none Investigate if mother has vesicoureteric reflux
Neurological disease		
Epilepsy: effect of anticonvulsants	Teratogenic drug effects, but rare with common anticonvulsants Sedation from maternal drugs Occasional withdrawal symptoms Sedation from maternal drugs in breast milk (rare)	Extra maternal vitamin K no longer recommended Monitor Monitor Monitor, breastfeeding rarely interrupted

Table 20.1 Continued

MATERNAL ILLNESS	EFFECT ON BABY	NEONATAL MANAGEMENT
Dystrophia myotonica*	Infant affected (usually more severely) May be seriously ill in respiratory failure	See Ch. 40.7
Myasthenia*	Neonatal myasthenia (Ch. 40.7)	Monitor, usually no problems
Degenerative disease	–	–
Multiple sclerosis	–	–
Motor neurone disease	–	–
Infection in the mother		
Pyrexia of unknown origin	–	Monitor for infection
Recognisable acute infection	Usually nil Risk greatest for viral infections (Ch. 39.2)	See Ch. 39.2
Chronic maternal infection and carrier state*	Can be serious, e.g. human immunodeficiency virus, tuberculosis	See Chs. 11, 39.2
Allergic disorders		
Hayfever, eczema	Inherited atopic tendency	Avoid early allergen exposure (e.g. cow's milk), particularly if mother has severe atopic disease
Haematological disorders		
Anaemia (iron, folate deficiency)	–	–
Autoimmune haemolytic anaemia	IgG transmitted to fetus causing haemolysis	Monitor for jaundice and anaemia
Haemoglobinopathies	Neonatal problems uncommon since most are β-chain defects (Ch. 30)	–
Hereditary spherocytosis	Neonatal haemolysis and jaundice in the 50% of infants affected	Monitor for jaundice and anaemia
Idiopathic thrombocytopenic purpura	Fetal haemorrhage can occur but is rare Neonatal haemorrhage also rare	Check platelet count and observe for bleeding. May need treating (Ch. 30)
Glucose-6-phosphate dehydrogenase deficiency	Neonatal jaundice Increased risk of infection (Ch. 29.1)	Monitor for jaundice and sepsis
Inherited thrombophilic disorders (e.g. factor V Leiden)	Increased risk of stroke or CSVT (Ch. 40.3) in baby, if also affected	
Autoimmune disease		
Systemic lupus erythematosus*	Congenital heart block	Cardiac pacing if heart block (Ch. 28). No treatment if heart rate normal
Psychiatric disorders		
Bipolar disorders	Lithium treatment associated with congenital heart disease, arrhythmias	Balance risk of treatment according to maternal mental state; consider withdrawing lithium in first trimester and 7–10 days before term
Drug dependency	IUGR Drug withdrawal Drug effects (occasionally)	Monitor and treat drug withdrawal (Ch. 26)

Table 20.1 Continued

MATERNAL ILLNESS	EFFECT ON BABY	NEONATAL MANAGEMENT
Malignant disease		
Ongoing malignancy	May need preterm delivery	–
Previously treated malignancy	Reduced fertility but no neonatal effects except IUGR after Wilms' tumour	–
Miscellaneous		
Abdominal trauma	Rare	–
Malnutrition	IUGR (Ch. 10)	–
Smoking	IUGR Increased respiratory morbidity and sudden infant death syndrome in infancy	–

*Maternal illnesses that may seriously affect the baby.
CSVT, cerebral sinus venous thrombosis; IUGR, intrauterine growth restriction.

Care immediately after birth

Neonatal resuscitation (Ch. 13.1)

Umbilical cord clamping

Umbilical blood flow decreases rapidly after delivery to less than 20% of the fetal value by 40–60 seconds of age (Gill et al. 1981). Physiological cord closure usually occurs within 3–5 minutes of birth but some cords pulsate for more than 15 minutes. There is no need to rush immediately to clamp the cord, since there are few risks associated with delayed clamping and there may be some benefits. Delayed clamping increases the risk of the neonate developing jaundice requiring treatment (McDonald and Middleton 2008). One randomised trial comparing time to cord clamping of 30 seconds versus 3 minutes showed benefit in haemoglobin levels both at 1 hour and 10 weeks in a group of 34–36-week gestation babies (Ultee et al. 2008). It is essential that there is a foolproof routine for clamping or ligating the umbilical cord, otherwise a fatal neonatal haemorrhage can ensue.

Umbilical cord care

Correct umbilical care during the first week significantly reduces the incidence of infection, not only in the neonate but also in the mother. Necrotic Wharton's jelly is readily colonised by organisms from the environment, which may spread to cause skin, conjunctival or systemic infection in the baby, or breast abscess in the mother.

Umbilical cord colonisation can be reduced by using topical antibiotics (Elias-Jones 1986). Yet, in developed countries, there is no evidence that topical antibiotics or antiseptics reduce systemic infection, and moreover they delay cord separation. Simply keeping the cord clean and dry is a reasonable and safe mode of care (Zupan and Garner 2000) and is the method adopted in the UK at present.

Prevention of eye infection

In many countries, it was routine to administer one drop of 0.5–1.0% silver nitrate into each eye immediately after delivery, to prevent gonococcal ophthalmia. Silver nitrate is effective, reduces the incidence of other types of conjunctivitis and is largely free from side-effects (Bell et al. 1993), although babies find it uncomfortable and some studies have reported a chemical conjunctivitis in up to 90% of recipients (Nishida and Risenberg 1975). A 2.5% solution of povidone-iodine is more effective (Isenberg et al. 1995) and protects against chlamydial conjunctivitis, which is otherwise more difficult to prevent even with the use of erythromycin ointment. Whether or not prophylaxis is justified depends on the incidence and severity of neonatal conjunctivitis in the local population; it is not used in the UK. Many US states have now changed from silver nitrate to erythromycin.

Vitamin K

Haemorrhagic disease of the newborn is potentially fatal. It exists in an early and late form, and is primarily a risk in breastfed babies and those with liver disease (Ch. 29.2). The condition can be prevented by giving 1 mg of vitamin K intramuscularly (i.m.) after delivery to all babies (McNinch and Tripp 1991). A study that suggested an increased risk of leukaemia in later childhood generated considerable anxiety about the practice of universal i.m. vitamin K administration (Golding et al. 1992), but subsequent studies from different parts of the world – Sweden (Ekelund et al. 1993), the USA (Klebanoff et al. 1993), Denmark (Olsen et al. 1994), Germany (Von Kries et al. 1996) and the UK (Ansell et al. 1996) – have failed to confirm these findings.

Various oral regimens have been used, either to avoid giving injections or to avoid the putative risk of malignancy. From these studies it is clear that a single oral dose at birth does not eliminate the risk of haemorrhagic disease, particularly late-onset disease (Hanson and Ebbesen 1996), which in one series was 13 times more common after oral than after i.m. vitamin K prophylaxis (McNinch and Tripp 1991). Repeated doses of oral vitamin K have been suggested as an alternative to a single dose of i.m. vitamin K. Local practice in Britain varies, but the following are commonly used regimens. Konakion MM is the only licensed preparation currently available for prophylaxis against haemorrhagic disease of the newborn in the UK.

- i.m. Konakion MM – a single 1-mg dose at or soon after birth or

- oral Konakion MM Paediatric – 2 mg at birth and at 4–7 days for all babies, and a third dose at 1 month of age for exclusively breastfed babies.

Infants at increased risk of haemorrhagic disease because of maternal liver disease or maternal anticonvulsant or antituberculosis drugs, should receive i.m. or intravenous Konakion (Royal College of Paediatrics and Child Health 1999). In addition, there remains a concern that the oral regimen may not prevent late haemorrhagic disease, particularly in breastfed babies. This is only in part because of the failure to administer a complete course (Von Kries et al. 1995). This concern can be probably ameliorated by giving an oral dose of 2 mg at birth followed by 1 mg weekly for 3 months (Hanson and Ebbesen 1996; McNinch et al. 2007).

Thermal care (Ch. 15)

The normal axillary temperature is 36.5–37.5 °C (Chs. 15, 19).

The risk of developing hypothermia is greatest immediately after delivery. It is not uncommon for the body temperature of a normal full-term baby to drop to 35–35.5 °C by 15–30 minutes of age. The adverse effects of hypothermia are detailed in Chapter 15 and include hypoglycaemia, acidosis, pulmonary hypertension and impaired surfactant production.

In order to prevent hypothermia the underlying mechanisms of heat exchange, namely evaporation, conduction, convection and radiation, must be considered (Ch. 15). Evaporative heat loss, even from babies born into a water pool, is almost eliminated by prompt drying. Conductive heat loss is lessened by prewarming the towels and any other equipment that will be in contact with the baby. Convective heat loss is ameliorated by having a warm and draught-free delivery room and covering the baby. All doors and windows should be closed, air circulation systems likely to cool the baby should be turned off (or the baby placed away from the air vent) and the room temperature should be at least 20 °C. Radiant heat is lost from the exposed skin of the baby to any surrounding surfaces that directly overlook the infant, and is proportional to the difference in temperature between these surfaces and to the distance between the surfaces. This problem is readily overcome by avoiding leaving the baby exposed and staying away from cold (external) windows and walls. Radiant heaters and heated blankets achieve a reversal of some of these processes and can allow the infant to gain heat.

Many mothers wish to have early skin-to-skin contact with their baby and this should be encouraged. Because the baby will be naked, it is sensible to increase the temperature of the room to a level comfortable for a naked and resting person (23–25 °C) and/or use an overhead heat source. The baby should be dry and covered with a warm towel or sheet, and draughts should be excluded. These are all wise precautions that do not distract from an intensely personal experience. Babies cared for like this maintain their body temperature, cry less, have better blood glucose control and base-excess values than do cot-nursed babies (Christensson et al. 1992). They are also more likely to establish successful long-term breast-feeding (Righard and Alade 1990).

Bathing babies shortly after birth may cause neonatal hypothermia and should be avoided. Most blood, meconium and vernix is quickly and effectively removed during the initial drying in warm towels, and thereafter any surplus can be wiped clear with a tissue.

Measurement

Babies should be weighed shortly after birth. The head circumference should also be recorded at this stage.

Labelling and security

In hospital, as opposed to home confinements, it is essential to attach a nametag immediately after delivery to prevent incidents of confused identity. There seems to be little benefit, however, from the more complex procedure of footprinting the baby (Thompson et al. 1981).

Bonding

Developmental care is outlined in detail in Chapter 4. In simple practical terms, both parents should be left alone with their baby immediately after birth, when babies are particularly bright-eyed and attractive. Putting the baby to the breast early is one of the most important determinants of successful lactation (Christensson et al. 1992) and, by releasing oxytocin, promotes uterine contraction, the milk ejection reflex, and complex maternal behavioural responses (Unvas-Moberg and Eriksson 1996). Moreover, simple skin contact at this stage has been shown to stimulate release of maternal oxytocin and prolactin and aid the first breastfeed (Righard and Alade 1990).

The normal neonate

Cardiorespiratory function

The normal term infant has a pulse rate of 110–150 beats/min and a blood pressure of 50–55/30 to 80/50 mmHg (Appendix 4). Occasional ectopic beats are quite common. The respiratory rate should be less than 60 breaths/min and is usually 35–45 breaths/min. Periodic breathing, with bursts of respiratory activity separated by apnoeic pauses of 3–10 seconds, is normal in preterm babies but is rare at term (Ch. 27.4).

Temperature

The term baby maintains a core temperature very close to 37 °C, so that any departure from this always requires careful evaluation, in particular to exclude sepsis. For the healthy clothed term baby who is in a cot, keeping the room temperature at 20–22 °C is adequate. If the room temperature falls below 20 °C, the baby should be covered with a blanket and may need to wear a bonnet. It is very important, however, to avoid overheating by lying the baby by a radiator, in direct sunlight, overwrapping or putting an external heat source inside the cot.

Weight changes

All babies should be weighed shortly after birth. Normal infants lose up to 10% of birthweight by the fifth day, primarily as a result of extracellular water loss. Only 3% of the babies in the Millennium Baby Study failed to regain their birth weight by the 12th day (Wright and Parkinson 2004). Most babies who are discharged early are currently not weighed again, but a re-evaluation of the practice has recently been suggested, and seems sensible (Laing and Wong 2002).

Weight loss in the first few days averages 4–7% and should not exceed 10% of the birthweight. Weight loss should always be assessed in relative terms, even though it means that a 4500-g baby may lose up to 450 g. In general, breastfed babies lose more weight (5–10%) than bottle-fed ones (2–6%) (Maisels et al. 1988), but this difference may be less if the baby breastfeeds more frequently (Avoa and Fischer 1990). From 1 week of age, the normal baby should gain weight at about 10–15 g/kg/day until the age of 6 months.

Urine output and staining of nappies

Many babies pass urine immediately after birth, and then, particularly if breastfed, may pass very little urine in the next 24–36 hours. It is very unusual for any illness to present in an otherwise normal baby solely with anuria or oliguria. Normal neonatal urine is virtually colourless. Pink staining of the nappy is commonly due to harmless urate crystals.

Bowel activity

Many babies open their bowels in the first few minutes, and usually regularly thereafter. There was no difference in the time to first stool (7–8 hours) between breast- and formula-fed babies in one study of 1000 babies in Buffalo, and 99.7% had passed at least one stool

by 36 hours (Metaj et al. 2003) (Fig. 20.1). Initially babies pass meconium, a dark-greenish substance composed of intestinal secretions, bile, swallowed amniotic debris and the remains of desquamated intestinal mucosal cells. By 2–3 days, 'changing' stools, a mixture of meconium and more normal stools, are passed. Once feeding is established, breastfed babies pass very soft mustard-yellow stools, often with every feed. Their stools are acid (Kleessem et al. 1995). Bottle-fed babies pass a less acid, firmer and paler stool, only once or twice a day.

Neurological activity

The neurological capabilities of the neonate are outlined on Ch. 40.1. Newborn babies can see, and prefer a face to 'scrambled'

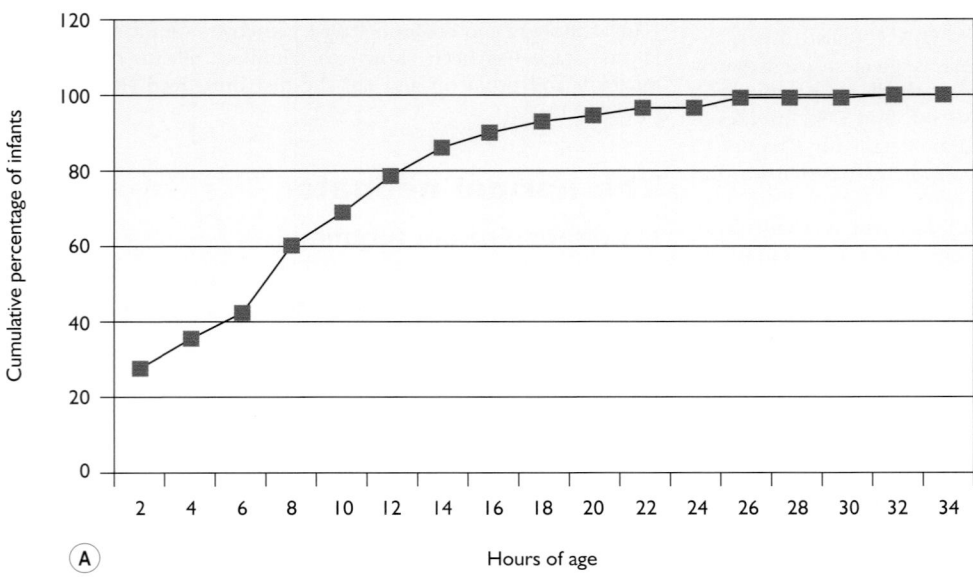

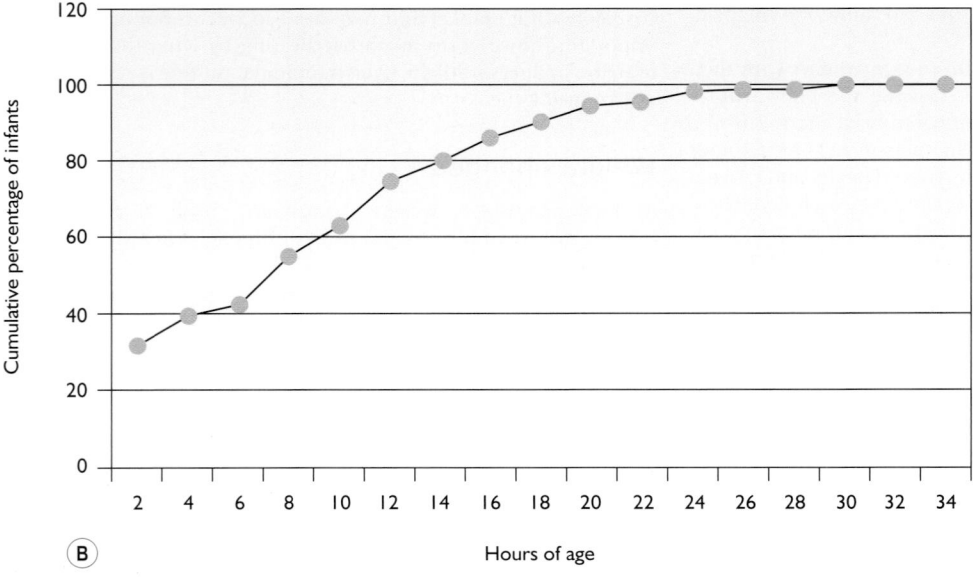

Fig. 20.1 Time to first stool (A) and urine (B) in 1000 healthy babies of >34 weeks' gestation; 99% had passed their first stool and first urine by 34 hours' postnatal age. *(Redrawn from Metaj et al. (2003).)*

shapes, they can hear and smell, and within the first few days and weeks of life they learn to recognise their mother by these senses (Trevarthen et al. 1981; Varendi et al. 1994).

In the neonatal period, babies have irregular sleep–waking cycles. In the first few days they spend up to 18 hours asleep, with 50–60% of the sleep being rapid-eye movement (Schulte 1981). They wake to feed or when uncomfortable, usually because the nappy is wet or soiled, but the sleep–wake pattern gradually becomes more regular. Circadian rhythmicity in heart rate and body temperature is detectable by 1 month of age (Glotzbach et al. 1994).

Postnatal care

Routine observation

At about 4 hours after birth, it is desirable to make a check of general well-being and to measure the baby's temperature, pulse and respiration. In hospital, this is often conveniently done on admission to the postnatal ward. In this situation, the baby's identity should also be verified, the security of the cord clamp confirmed and a check made to ensure that vitamin K has been given. There is no need routinely to check the blood pressure, haematocrit or blood glucose (American Academy of Pediatrics 1993). Thereafter, temperature, pulse and respiration should be recorded if the baby becomes unwell. Temperature instability, tachycardia and tachypnoea are important signs of neonatal sepsis (Ch. 39.2; Mifsud et al. 1988). Feed charts have largely been abandoned, but an observation chart should be used when appropriate (for example, see Fig. 21.1).

Rooming-in

Standard management should be that the mother and her baby remain together all the time. This helps to prevent cross-infection and promote successful breastfeeding. It also facilitates the mother's desire to learn how to recognise, respond and manage every demand and need of her baby. If the mother is ill or exhausted, or if she requests it, help may be needed to settle her baby.

Sleeping position

The risk of sudden infant death syndrome (SIDS) is reduced if babies are placed to lie on their back (Oyen et al. 1997). Side-sleeping is less safe and sleeping on the front is associated with the highest risk (Mitchell et al. 1997). Occasionally, babies are placed to sleep on their front for medical reasons, but this is the exception. The risk of SIDS is also reduced by the avoidance of cigarette smoking during pregnancy, avoiding exposure of the baby to cigarette smoking after birth, and by precautions to avoid overheating.

Prevention of infection on a postnatal ward

Handwashing

The major risk to the normal baby is from organisms carried by medical and nursing staff, who must be meticulous in washing their hands before they touch any baby. The extended family should do the same. The parents (particularly the mother) and baby quickly share commensal organisms, but, even so, good hygiene is important. Gowns are not required for staff or family (Birenbaum et al. 1990).

Baby washing

If the cross-infection techniques are good, and the baby rooms in, so that he is colonised from the mother, all that is required is a wash with baby soap. If there is an outbreak of skin infection, then chlorhexidine washing can be instituted. The use of hexachlorophene to wash babies should be avoided because it can be toxic (Martin-Bouyer et al. 1982).

Visitors

Healthy visitors are not generally an infectious hazard, and the number allowed should be decided on a common-sense basis. There are rarely justifiable medical reasons why fathers, siblings and grandparents should not be allowed free access to the new family member. The exception to this has been the recent swine flu epidemic; young children are 'super-shedders' of flu virus and many maternity hospitals have justifiably excluded them from visiting on these grounds.

Cord care

The early care of the cord with simple cleaning is described above. A 'healthy' cord is dry. The cord usually drops off naturally within 2 weeks, but this may be delayed if antibiotics or antiseptics are applied (Zupan and Garner 2000).

Well-baby care

The hazards of hypothermia lessen once the baby has adapted to extrauterine life, and so it is not necessary to delay washing beyond the second or third day of life. At this time the mother can participate fully. This first wash can be just 'topping and tailing', that is, washing the face and hair and cleaning up the groin and perineum. For inexperienced mothers, this first bath may need to be supervised or even demonstrated.

The foreskin

At birth the foreskin is adherent to the surface of the glans penis, and is not meant to be retractile. Indeed, the foreskin remains non-retractile in most boys until about 2 years of age. Forcible retraction during infancy tears the prepuce and may cause later scarring and phimosis. There is some evidence that urinary infections are less common in circumcised boys (Schoen 1993; Craig et al. 1996), but this is not sufficient justification for routine neonatal circumcision (Winberg et al. 1989). Parents who elect to have their son circumcised usually do so for cultural or religious reasons. The operation should always be performed by a trained anaesthetic and surgical team.

Immunisations

Hepatitis B

In the UK, hepatitis B immunisation is offered to infants of mothers who are HBsAg-positive. Babies born to highly infectious mothers should also receive hepatitis B immunoglobulin. The first dose of the immunoglobulin should be given within 24 hours of birth, and ideally should be ordered in advance. Repeat doses of the active immunisation should be given at 1, 2 and 12 months of age. See the UK government 'Green Book' on immunisation for helpful advice (see Weblinks, below).

Tuberculosis (TB)

The recent rise in TB in the UK has led to a recommendation for universal TB vaccination in many inner-city areas. The 'Green Book' recommendation is for vaccination of infants living in areas of the UK where the annual incidence of TB is 40/100 000 or greater, or with a parent or grandparent who was born in a country with such an incidence (see Weblinks, below).

Routine neonatal clinical examination (Ch. 14)

Timing and personnel

All newborn babies should be examined carefully at least once in the first few days. The examination should be carried out by an appropriately trained individual.

It is essential for those carrying out the examination to have a clear understanding of what they are trying to achieve. There are four main functions to the examination:

1. Detecting serious problems which would otherwise not have been detected and which merit early assessment and treatment. Basically there are only three common ones: congenital heart disease, developmental dysplasia of the hip, and eye defects.
2. Checking for many very rare but serious conditions, e.g. the enlarged bladder of posterior urethral valves, the posterior abdominal mass of a congenital tumour or a dermal sinus.
3. Noting and explaining to the parents the multitude of normal variations and minor anomalies that may be present (Table 20.2).
4. Health promotion: give advice on nutrition, reducing the risk of SIDS, parental smoking, transport in cars. It also gives the

Table 20.2 Minor abnormalities and normal variations that may cause parental anxiety

Skin lesions
  'Stork bite'
  Milia
  Erythema toxicum
  Strawberry naevi (rarely present at birth)
  Cutis marmorata
  Miliaria
  Mongolian patches
  Innocent pigmented naevi
  Epithelial pearls in the mouth
Cephalhaematoma
Subconjunctival haemorrhage
Peripheral and traumatic cyanosis
Tongue tie
Diastasis recti
Protuberant xiphisternum
Hydroceles
Sacral dimple
Umbilical anomalies, e.g. hernia
Physiological jaundice
Snuffles
Talipes calcaneovalgus
Vulval mucosal tag
Breast enlargement

parents a chance to ask about any aspects of the healthcare of their baby.

The examination has a low specificity and sensitivity, so findings must be interpreted with caution. On the one hand, the clinician has to be careful not to overinterpret signs found on the first day in such a way that the infant is subjected to unnecessary investigations and treatment, and the parents to unnecessary anxiety. On the other hand, most congenital heart disease is not detected at this examination and false reassurance should be avoided (Abu-Harb et al. 1994). The details of the examination are given in Chapters 14, 28.

Gestational age assessment

Gestational age is most accurately calculated using early antenatal ultrasound data and the menstrual history. Knowledge of whether a baby is preterm and/or small for dates may alter management, and so it is important to know such a baby's gestational age. Smaller babies may require more support in establishing sucking feeds and may take longer in making the transition to the extrauterine environment.

Biochemical screening

Currently in the UK, newborn screening is recommended for phenylketonuria (PKU), congenital hypothyroidism, cystic fibrosis (CF), sickle-cell disease and medium-chain acyl-CoA dehydrogenase deficiency (MCADD).

Phenylketonuria

At 5–9 days of age, all babies have a heelprick blood sample analysed for phenylalanine: a raised level may indicate PKU. The baby should only be tested for PKU if milk intake is normal. The blood is collected onto an absorbent card, taking care to fill each of the circles with blood. Approximately 1:2000 infants are positive on screening, about five times more than the prevalence of the disease (1:10 000). Those with positive tests are recalled and their plasma phenylalanine remeasured to determine whether or not they have PKU. If PKU or a variant is confirmed by a second raised phenylalanine level, the baby should be referred to a specialist centre for full investigation and ongoing care.

Congenital hypothyroidism

Using another of the blood spots, a radioimmunoassay is done for thyroid-stimulating hormone (TSH): those with a high TSH are then recalled for further evaluation. This is required in about 0.2–0.3% of all infants tested. The incidence of congenital hypothyroidism detected in this way is about 1:4000 (Ch. 34.2). All infants identified should be treated as quickly as possible.

Cystic fibrosis

The original blood spot screening test for CF was based upon the work by Crossley et al. (1979), which showed that immunoreactive trypsinogen (IRT) was significantly increased in neonates with CF (incidence 1:2000). The blood spot test as used at present first identifies samples with IRT values above the 99.5th percentile and subjects these to a two-stage mutation analysis for the CF transmembrane conductance regulator (CFTR) gene. Babies with CFTR mutations detected in both genes (either a homozygote or compound heterozygote) have a presumptive positive diagnosis of CF.

Most babies with only one mutation detected will be unaffected carriers but there is a risk that they carry a second abnormal allele not detected by the mutation panel used. They are therefore tested again on a repeat dried blood spot specimen taken between day 21 and day 28 of life and assayed for IRT.

Sickle-cell disease

In areas of the UK where there are significant numbers of babies of ethnic groups known to be at high risk of sickle-cell disease (e.g. south-east London), neonatal screening is offered.

Medium-chain acyl-CoA dehydrogenase deficiency

About 1:10 000 babies born in the UK has MCADD. Screening allows most babies with MCADD to be recognised early so that dietary changes can be made to minimise the risk of serious illness.

Hearing screening

In the UK, 1–2:1000 babies are born with a hearing loss in one or both ears. Neonatal hearing screening is now offered to all newborn infants (http://hearing.screening.nhs.uk/).

Feeding the normal term baby

Human milk is undoubtedly the preferred food for term infants, and every effort should be made to encourage a mother to breast-feed. In the developing world, breastfeeding dramatically improves survival and so bottle-feeding should be avoided if at all possible. Schemes that give mothers accurate, evidence-based information about breastfeeding to enable informed choice of feeding method (such as the UNICEF Baby Friendly Initiative) demonstrate improvements in breastfeeding rates (Kramer et al. 2001; Tappin et al. 2001).

Breastfeeding

There have been numerous initiatives, through UNICEF, the Department of Health and the Royal College of Midwives. The 2005 Infant Feeding Survey (see Weblinks) showed that 78% of mothers initiate breastfeeding in England. Forty-eight per cent of all mothers in the UK were breastfeeding at 6 weeks, while 25% were still breastfeeding at 6 months. Between 2000 and 2005 there was a small increase in the prevalence of breastfeeding at all ages up to 9 months in England and Wales and Northern Ireland.

Preparation

Ideally, breastfeeding education should start in the antenatal period, with advice on what constitutes normal breastfeeding behaviour. Practical help should be available in the immediate postnatal period to assist in the proper initiation of lactation (Table 20.3).

Lactation

Following the expulsion of the placenta, the anterior pituitary gland releases large amounts of prolactin, a hormone essential for lactation. Frequent breastfeeds in the early postnatal period stimulate the development of prolactin receptors in the mammary gland. It is thought that breast milk output is related more to the number of prolactin receptors than to levels in the blood. Delayed suckling

Table 20.3 Policies to promote breastfeeding

Antenatal education
Baby put skin to skin soon after birth
Baby put to breast as soon after birth as possible
Establish rooming-in
Feed at least 8 times per day, up to 12 times if necessary
Do not have specific duration of feeds at the breast
Finish the first breast, going to the second if hungry
No supplementary/complementary feeds
No dummies
No discharge gift packs
Regular assessment of the mother's breasts

results in reduced levels of prolactin and thus fewer prolactin receptors stimulated. When the baby suckles, nerve impulses are sent from the breast to the posterior pituitary and oxytocin is released. Oxytocin causes the myoepithelial cells to contract and milk is squeezed from the alveoli towards the nipple and into the mouth of the suckling infant. This is the milk ejection reflex or let-down reflex. At first an unconditional reflex, it quickly becomes conditional and readily inhibited by anxiety and pain.

Initially, lactation is hormonally driven, and colostrum will be produced whether or not suckling takes place. Colostrum is thick, viscous and small in volume, with intakes of 4–14 ml each feed. Over the next 48–96 hours, milk production increases markedly and the volumes produced start to be governed by suckling and milk removal, activities that are essential for the continuation of lactation (Prentice et al. 1989). After 1–2 weeks, on average 700–800 ml/day of milk is produced, with a wide range from 450 to 1200 ml. At the end of each feed, about 100 ml of milk is left in the breasts (Dewey et al. 1991). Babies seem able to judge their own intake such that they grow normally, so an assessment of intake should only be attempted if weight gain is unsatisfactory.

Milk is produced for as long as it is removed from the breast. The rate of milk secretion may differ between breasts if the duration or frequency of suckling is not equal. This suggests autocrine regulation of milk secretion by the production of a local factor within each breast that controls lactation. This factor has been identified and is termed the feedback inhibitor of lactation (Wilde et al. 1995).

Attachment and positioning

Correct attachment and positioning are of fundamental importance to successful breastfeeding, so the mother should be taught these skills at the first feed. A helpful DVD is From Bump to Breastfeeding, produced by Best Beginnings (see Weblinks section). Correct technique ensures effective milk drainage and a satiated baby (Woolridge 1986), thereby minimising problems such as sore and cracked nipples, breast engorgement and mastitis. The baby will feed frequently until the milk supply is abundant. If incorrectly positioned, the stimulus for an increase in yield will be compromised and lactation will decrease. Resulting breast pain or anxiety about sufficiency of milk supply will inhibit the milk ejection reflex, a demoralising experience for the mother.

With the baby positioned for breastfeeding, the head and body must be in alignment, with the baby well supported in a position that is sustainable for mother and baby and brought in close to the mother's body. Correct attachment is vital for the lips to form a seal with the breast. The mouth is open wide against the breast and the tongue protrudes beyond the lower gum. The baby's nose is aimed

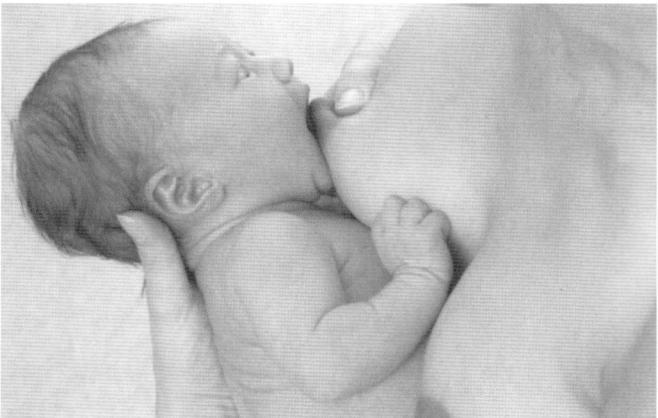

Fig. 20.2 Positioning for breastfeeding. The head and body must be in alignment, with baby well supported in a position that is sustainable for mother and baby and brought in close to the mother's body. The mouth is open wide against the breast and the tongue protrudes beyond the lower gum. The baby's nose is aimed toward the nipple to facilitate extension of the lower jaw. *(Courtesy of Mother and Baby Picture Library/Ruth Jenkinson.)*

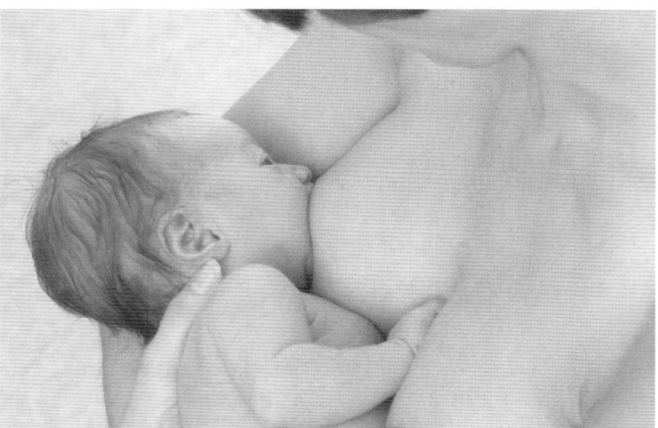

Fig. 20.3 A correctly attached baby. *(Courtesy of Mother and Baby Picture Library/Ruth Jenkinson.)*

toward the nipple to facilitate extension of the lower jaw (Fig. 20.2). The baby is attached with the nipple adjacent to the junction of the hard and soft palate in the roof of the mouth. A significant amount of breast is drawn into the mouth, enabling the baby's jaw and tongue to compress and strip or milk the lactiferous sinuses. The nipple only forms one-third of the 'teat' in baby's mouth; the rest is breast tissue.

A correctly attached baby is shown in Figure 20.3. The baby's head is slightly extended and both nostrils are clear of the breast. The mouth is wide open and lips flanged backwards. The chin must be touching the breast. If the areola is visible, more should be seen above than below the mouth, indicating that the nipple is in the roof of the mouth. A correctly attached baby takes long deep sucks with pauses.

Frequency and duration

The optimum time to initiate breastfeeding is shortly after delivery, ideally during the period of skin contact, since for the first 2 hours of life babies are usually alert and the sucking reflex intense. It is important not to miss this phase since thereafter babies enter a deep sleep before periods of wakefulness ensue, which are accompanied by the desire for frequent short feeds. Healthy infants may feed 10 or more times a day in the first few days and this should not be limited. At this time, when only colostrum is being produced, the baby should suckle both breasts during a feed. The duration of each feed is variable; in general, the endpoint is when the baby loses interest in sucking or the breast is empty, usually 7–10 minutes.

After the first few days, most breastfed babies will gradually settle into a 2–3-hourly feeding pattern. Most of the milk will come in the first 4–6 minutes, although many babies will continue to suck intermittently thereafter for comfort. At this time there is some evidence to show that prolonged feeding at one breast, ensuring that it is empty, reduces complications (Evans et al. 1995). Also, the fat content of breast milk increases during the feed, and so it is important not to limit the length of time a baby suckles (Woolridge and Fisher 1988). After this breast is empty, if the baby has gone to sleep, then the feed is over; however, if he is still hungry, some milk should be given from the other breast. To ensure that one breast at a time is completely emptied, the mother should alternate which breast she offers first.

Complementary and supplementary feeds

Complementary feeds are those offered after a baby has breastfed. Supplementary feeds are those that replace the entire breastfeed. They may be given from a bottle or cup. The additional feed of choice is mother's expressed milk. The decision to give additional feeds to a breastfeeding baby is a major one, since it frequently inhibits the establishment of successful breastfeeding (Kurinij and Shiono 1991; Blomquist et al. 1994; Michaelsen et al. 1994). Probably the only genuine justifications for complementary or supplementary feeds are hypoglycaemia and dehydration with a weight loss more than 10–12% of birthweight. Whatever the reason for using complementary or supplementary feeds, the mother should, if at all possible, continue to express milk on a regular basis until breastfeeding is established. Topping up with water or a glucose solution is a major cause of lactation failure and should be avoided.

Monitoring breastfeeding

Whilst breastfeeding is being established, it is wise to monitor the frequency of feeds and the number of wet nappies, which should become heavier with urine. Weighing the baby should be done only when there is concern; if weight gain is poor or persistent weight loss occurs, examine the baby carefully for signs of ill health and take a urine sample to exclude infection. If there are no signs of illness, the problem is usually that of poor intake; in such babies, urine output is low and hypernatraemia is common.

Bottle-feeding

Starting feeds

Tables of composition of currently available formula milks compared with breast milk can be found in Chapter 16. The first feed should be offered at about 4 hours of age. Thereafter, the baby is fed on demand, which in most cases is about every 4 hours, less frequent than most breastfed babies. As with breastfed babies, there is no justification for offering water or a glucose solution.

Technique of feeding

The baby should be swaddled and held closely and comfortably to the mother so that she can hold the bottle with her free hand. Touching the baby's mouth or lips with the teat will usually evoke the rooting reflex. The mouth will open, the teat can be popped in, and he will begin to suck. The sucking mechanism is different from breastfeeding (Mathew 1991) since there is not the equivalent of the milk ejection reflex, so that, in addition to compressing the teat with the gums and squeezing milk into the mouth as in breastfeeding, the baby has to generate a vacuum in his or her mouth to suck the milk out of the bottle. The amount obtained per suck can be altered by varying the size of the hole in the teat, but, in general, large holes should be used only in babies with sucking problems.

Temperature

Traditionally, bottle milk is warmed to body temperature before feeding, but there is no need to do this. Babies take room temperature milk perfectly satisfactorily.

Frequency of feeds

Demand feeding should be the norm, and bottle-fed babies usually settle into a 3–4-hourly schedule, taking about six feeds per day.

Volume of feeds

Healthy term infants should be demand-fed and allowed to take what they want. Most babies who take the volumes outlined settle down to an intake of 150–180 ml/kg/24 h. As with breastfed babies, if weight gain is satisfactory, a relaxed attitude should be adopted towards individual variation.

Feeding problems

Feeding problems must be sorted out with the mother and baby together, and this may require readmission of both to the postnatal wards. Feeding problems are emphatically not an indication for transferring an otherwise normal baby to a neonatal unit.

Excellent advice on maternal problems can be found in the publication *Successful Breastfeeding*, third edition, Royal College of Midwives (2003).

Newborn feeding problems are common. Typical symptoms include poor feeding, crying, poor weight gain and vomiting.

Reluctant feeding

Babies feed at variable intervals and durations, and if a baby is gaining weight normally, he is getting enough nutrition regardless of his habit. The average number of feeds and wet and dirty nappies is six in 24 hours. The time to be concerned is if feeding lasts for only 2–3 minutes, if weight gain is poor or if a baby deviates from a previously established pattern of feeding. The first thing to do is to ensure that the baby has a normal oropharynx and is not ill. The examination should be focused on the detection of a cleft palate (clefts of the soft palate are unfortunately often missed by routine neonatal examinations), thrush or the rare occurrence of significant tongue tie. Also assess for signs of respiratory distress, congenital heart disease, infection, a dysmorphic syndrome (e.g. Down syndrome) or a primary neuromuscular disorder. Check for hypoglycaemia as a consequence (or even a cause) of a poor intake. Investigations will depend on the clinical circumstances.

If all these are normal but the baby still feeds poorly, the commonest causes are:

1. preterm
2. large for dates
3. the aftermath of a difficult delivery, e.g. vacuum extraction
4. sedation from intrapartum or antenatal drug therapy (e.g. maternal pethidine)
5. sedation from drugs in the breast milk (uncommon).

Prolonged sedation from drugs in breast milk is very unusual, and is rarely a contraindication to breastfeeding. If babies continue to be floppy and feed poorly, consider investigations along the lines suggested for hypotonia (Ch. 40.7).

Tongue tie (ankyloglossia)

Tongue tie is characterised by an abnormally short lingual frenulum. It varies in degree, from a mild form in which the tongue is bound only by a thin mucous membrane to a severe form in which the tongue is anchored to the floor of the mouth. Breastfeeding may be difficult because of an inability to suck effectively, causing sore nipples and poor weight gain.

Most tongue ties are asymptomatic and do not require treatment and others resolve spontaneously over time. If the condition is thought to be causing feeding problems, conservative treatment includes breastfeeding advice and massaging the frenulum. Some practitioners believe that if a baby with tongue tie has difficulty breastfeeding, surgical division of the lingual frenulum should be carried out as early as possible. However a systematic review by Suter and Bornstein (2009) suggests that at the moment there is no evidence for the best method of surgical management.

If division of the tongue tie is performed in early infancy, it is usually performed without anaesthesia, although local anaesthetic is sometimes used. The baby is swaddled and supported at the shoulders to stabilise the head and sharp, blunt-ended scissors are used to divide the lingual frenulum. There should be little or no blood loss and feeding may be resumed immediately. Many paediatricians are troubled by the use of surgical treatment without an anaesthetic.

Crying

Persistent crying in the neonate is usually due to hunger. There are many other causes for babies crying, notably pain. If the diagnosis is hunger, the appropriate treatment is milk, even if the baby was fed only 2 hours previously. If the crying baby shows no enthusiasm for feeding and is clean and dry, then he probably just needs a cuddle; skin contact can be particularly comforting. If this does not work, one must exclude occult but painful conditions such as otitis media, urinary tract infection, intussusception, bone and joint sepsis and incarcerated hernia. It is commonly believed that crying in a baby is due to wind, but this should be assumed only when other causes have been excluded. Infantile colic is discussed below.

Wind

The bottle-fed baby will usually swallow some air with a feed. This may be because the hole in the teat is too small to let milk into the mouth as quickly as a hungry baby wishes, and so he sucks air around the teat. A large hole may also result in air swallowing because the milk comes into the mouth too rapidly and the baby splutters. Poor parental feeding technique may allow the level of the milk in the teat to go below the hole in the teat, or the baby may continue to suck on an empty teat and swallow air. The breastfed baby usually swallows less air during a feed. Air swallowing is most common in the first 2 weeks whilst supply and demand are being established. With insufficient milk, the baby may suck in air; with an abundance of milk, the baby may splutter at an over-vigorous milk ejection reflex.

Regardless of the type of feed, afterwards it is traditional to sit the baby upright in the hope that the stomach gas bubble will lie under the oesophageal hiatus and then, by rubbing or patting the back, the bubble will be induced to burst upwards – very satisfying for all. 'Winding' the baby in this way is supposed to prevent excess gas being propelled through the infant's small intestine, where, by analogy with older patients, it is believed to cause abdominal pain and/or infantile colic. This may not be evidence-based but it has a long tradition and appears harmless. Nevertheless, it should be considered the cause of crying only once an alternative explanation has been excluded.

Colic

Infantile colic can occur in the late neonatal period. Its aetiology remains a mystery, although food and lactose intolerance in the mother and baby have been investigated, with equivocal results (Jakobsson and Linberg 1983; Illingworth 1985; Moore et al. 1988). Stressful psychosocial factors may play a part (Rautava et al. 1993). The treatment includes reassurance about the benign nature of the symptoms. Massage of the abdomen, and patting the baby's back whilst he lies prone with the abdomen supported, appear to help, as do antispasmodic drugs (Weissbluth et al. 1984). Feeding technique should be checked, but giving up breastfeeding or changing the type of milk in bottle-fed babies is not justified without a clear reason.

Poor weight gain/persisting hunger

Bottle-fed babies receive ad libitum calories and fluid in measurable quantities, so this problem is much more common in breastfed infants, who, if denied adequate liquid and/or calories, will present with poor weight gain, persistent crying or both. If no other cause for these features is found, inadequate intake can be confirmed by careful test weighing. Checking the serum electrolytes may uncover hypernatraemic dehydration. If, despite implementing all the tricks outlined above to improve milk intake, the breastfed baby still fails to thrive, there comes a time when some extra source of liquid and/or calories is indicated. This time has come when:

- there is persistent failure to settle a crying and fractious breastfed baby over a short period of time

- the initial weight loss exceeds 10–12%
- there is dehydration, hypoglycaemia, hypernatraemia or severe jaundice (see Ch. 29.1)
- the baby has not regained birthweight by 10 days of age
- the mother has sore nipples or engorgement, only one breast is being used and the baby is hungry
- the mother is demoralised by a crying baby – calming the baby and offering help to correct poor positioning and attachment, with expression of milk, which can be given by cup, may transform the situation and allow normal lactation to be established.

One of the purported advantages of breastfeeding is a reduction in the incidence of cow's milk protein allergy (Host et al. 1988). There is the possibility that this syndrome may be induced even by one or two cow's milk formula feeds in the neonatal period. However, the evidence for this is weak, and the giving of glucose solution when breast milk is insufficient has little to recommend it. Moreover, there is no evidence that this practice decreases atopic disease in general (Gustafsson et al. 1992).

One may be forced into trying complementary and/or supplementary feeds in term babies with feeding problems, although the use of such feeds can make matters worse and cause lactation to fail completely. It may be, however, that the use of such feeds is the first objective marker of lactation that, for some reason or another, is unfortunately going to prove inadequate.

Dehydration fever

If a baby in the first week of life develops a fever, two likely and important causes are infection (Ch. 39.2) and overheating due to some defect in the environmental control (Ch. 15). If these are excluded in a febrile baby who appears well but has an inadequate intake and has lost 10% or more of his birthweight, he may be suffering from dehydration. This can be confirmed clinically, and by measuring the plasma osmolality, which in dehydration fever will usually exceed 310 mOsmol/l. Such a baby drinks clear fluids (or bottle milk) avidly, whereupon his temperature falls and he gains weight.

Gastroenterological symptoms

Vomiting (Ch. 29.4), diarrhoea (Ch. 29.3), abdominal distension (Ch. 29.3) and jaundice (Ch. 29.1) all require evaluation in their own right: they are rarely due to feeding problems, although jaundice is associated with breastfeeding.

Weblinks

From Bump to Breastfeeding: www.bestbeginnings.org.uk.
'Green Book' on immunisation: www.dh.gov.uk.

National Institute for Health and Clinical Excellence (NICE): www.nice.org.uk.
CG 37 Postnatal Care.
CG 55 Intrapartum Care.
Newborn bloodspot screening: www.newbornbloodspot.screening.nhs.uk.

2005 Infant feeding survey: www.ic.nhs.uk/ statistics-and-data-collections/health-and-lifestyles-related-surveys/infant-feeding-survey/infant-feeding-survey-2005.

References

Abu-Harb, M., Hey, E., Wren, C., 1994. Death in infancy from unrecognised congenital heart disease. Arch Dis Child 71, 3–7.

American Academy of Pediatrics, 1993. Routine evaluation of blood pressure, hematocrit and glucose in newborns. Pediatrics 92, 474–476.

Ansell, P., Bull, D., Roman, E., 1996. Childhood leukaemia and intramuscular vitamin K: findings from a case-control study. Br Med J 313, 204–205.

Avoa, A., Fischer, P.R., 1990. The influence of prenatal instruction about breast feeding on neonatal weight loss. Pediatrics 86, 313–315.

Bell, T.A., Grayson, T.J., Krohn, M.A., et al., 1993. Randomized trial of silver nitrate, erythromycin and no eye prophylaxis for the prevention of conjunctivitis among newborns not at risk for gonococcal ophthalmitis. Pediatrics 92, 755–760.

Birenbaum, H.J., Glorioso, L., Rosenberger, C., et al., 1990. Gowning on a postpartum ward fails to decrease colonization in the newborn infant. Am J Dis Child 144, 1031–1033.

Blomquist, H.K., Jonsbo, F., Serenius, F., et al., 1994. Supplementary feeding in the maternity ward shortens the duration of breast feeding. Acta Paediatr 83, 1122–1126.

Christensson, K., Siles, C., Moreno, L., 1992. Temperature, metabolic adaptation and crying in healthy full term newborns cared for skin to skin or in a cot. Acta Paediatr 81, 488–493.

Craig, J.C., Knight, J.F., Sureshkumar, P., et al., 1996. Effect of circumcision on the incidence of urinary tract infection in pre-school boys. J Pediatr 128, 23–27.

Crossley, J.R., Elliott, R.B., Smith, P.A., 1979. Dried blood spot screening for cystic fibrosis in the newborn. Lancet 1, 472–474.

Dewey, K.G., Heinig, M.J., Nonunsen, L.A., et al., 1991. Maternal versus infant factors related to breast milk intake and a residual milk volume: the DARLING Study. Pediatrics 87, 829–837.

Ekelund, H., Finnstrom, O., Gunnarskog, J., et al., 1993. Administration of vitamin K to newborn infants and childhood cancer. Br Med J 307, 89–91.

Elias-Jones, A.C., 1986. Triple antibiotic spray application to umbilical cord. Early Hum Dev 13, 299–302.

Evans, K., Evans, R., Simmer, K., 1995. Effect of the method of breast feeding on breast engorgement, mastitis and infantile colic. Acta Paediatr 84, 849–852.

Gill, R.W., Trudinger, B.J., Garrett, W.J., et al., 1981. Fetal umbilical venous flow measured in utero by pulsed Doppler and B-mode ultrasound. I. Normal pregnancies. Am J Obstet Gynecol 139, 720.

Glotzbach, S.F., Edgar, D., Boeddiker, M., et al., 1994. Biological rhythmicity in normal infants during the first 3 months of life. Pediatrics 94, 482–488.

Golding, J., Greenwood, R., Birmingham, K., et al., 1992. Childhood cancer, intramuscular vitamin K and pethidine given during labour. Br Med J 305, 341–346.

Gustafsson, D., Lowhagen, T., Andersson, K., 1992. Risk of developing atopic disease after early feeding with cow's milk based formula. Arch Dis Child 67, 1008–1010.

Hanson, K.N., Ebbesen, F., 1996. Neonatal vitamin K prophylaxis in Denmark: three years experience with oral administration during the first 3 months of life compared with one oral administration at birth. Acta Paediatr 85, 1137–1139.

Host, A., Husby, S., Osterballe, O., 1988. A prospective study of cows milk allergy in exclusively breast fed infants. Acta Paediatr Scand 77, 663–670.

Illingworth, R.S., 1985. Infantile colic revisited. Arch Dis Child 60, 981–985.

Isenberg, S.J., Apt, L., Wood, M., 1995. A controlled trial of povidone iodine as prophylaxis against ophthalmia neonatorum. N Engl J Med 332, 562–566.

Jakobsson, I., Linberg, T., 1983. Cow's milk proteins cause infantile colic in breast fed infants: a double blind crossover study. Pediatrics 71, 268–271.

Klebanoff, M.A., Read, J.S., Mills, J.L., et al., 1993. The risk of childhood cancer after neonatal exposure to vitamin K. N Engl J Med 329, 905–908.

Kleessem, B., Bunke, H., Tovar, K., et al., 1995. Influence of two infant formulas and human milk on the development of the fecal flora in newborn infants. Acta Paediatr 84, 1347–1356.

Kramer, M.S., Chalmers, B., Hodnett, E.D., et al., 2001. Promotion of breastfeeding intervention trial (PROBIT). JAMA 285, 413–420.

Kurinij, N., Shiono, P.H., 1991. Early formula supplementation of breast feeding. Pediatrics 88, 745–750.

Laing, I.A., Wong, C.M., 2002. Hypernatraemia in the first few days: is the incidence rising? Arch Dis Child 87, 158–162.

Maisels, M.J., Gifford, K., Antle, C.E., et al., 1988. Jaundice in the healthy newborn: a new approach to an old problem. Pediatrics 81, 505–511.

Martin-Bouyer, G., Lebreton, R., Toga, M., et al., 1982. Outbreak of hexachlorophene poisoning in France. Lancet 1, 91.

Mathew, O.P., 1991. Science of bottle feeding. J Pediatr 119, 511–519.

McDonald SJ, Middleton P, 2008. Effect of timing of umbilical cord clamping on maternal and neonatal outcomes. Cochrane Database Syst Rev (2), CD004074.

McNinch, A.W., Tripp, J.H., 1991. Haemorrhagic disease of the newborn in the British Isles: 2 year prospective study. Br Med J 303, 1105–1109.

McNinch A.W., Busfield, A., Tripp, J., 2007. Vitamin K deficiency bleeding in Great Britain and Ireland: BPSU surveys 1993–4 and 2001–2. Arch Dis Child 92, 759–766.

Metaj, M., Laroia, N., Lawrence, R.A., et al., 2003. Comparison of breast- and formula-fed normal newborns in time to first stool and urine. J Perinatol 23, 624–628.

Michaelsen, K.F., Larsen, P.S., Thomsen, B.L., et al., 1994. The Copenhagen cohort study on infant nutrition and growth: duration of breast feeding and influencing factors. Acta Paediatr 83, 565–571.

Mifsud, A., Seal, D., Wall, R., et al., 1988. Reduced neonatal mortality from infection after introduction of respiratory monitoring. Br Med J 296, 17–18.

Mitchell, E.A., Tuohy, P.G., Brunt, J.M., et al., 1997. Risk factors for sudden infant death syndrome following the prevention campaign in New Zealand: a prospective study. Pediatrics 100, 835–840.

Moore, D.J., Robb, T.A., Davidson, G.P., 1988. Breath hydrogen response to milk containing lactose in colicky and non-colicky infants. J Pediatr 113, 979–984.

Nishida, H., Risenberg, H.M., 1975. Silver nitrate ophthalmic solution and chemical conjunctivitis. Pediatrics 56, 368–373.

Olsen, J.H., Hertz, H., Blinkengerg, K., et al., 1994. Vitamin K regimens and incidence of childhood cancer in Denmark. Br Med J 308, 895–896.

Oyen, N., Markestad, T., Skjaerven, R., et al., 1997. Combined effects of sleeping position and prenatal risk factors in sudden infant death syndrome: the Nordic Epidemiological SIDS Study. Pediatrics 100, 613–621.

Prentice, A., Addey, C.V.P., Wilde, C.J., 1989. Evidence for local feedback control of human milk secretion. Biochem Soc Transact 17, 122.

Rautava, P., Helenius, H., Lehtonen, L., 1993. Psychosocial predisposing factors for infantile colic. Br Med J 307, 600–604.

Righard, L., Alade, M.O., 1990. Effect of delivery room routines on success of first breastfeed. Lancet 336, 1105–1107.

Royal College of Paediatrics and Child Health, 1999. Medicines for Children. RCPCH, London.

Royal College of Midwives, 2003. Successful Breastfeeding, third ed. Churchill Livingstone, Edinburgh.

Schoen, E.J., 1993. Circumcision updated – indicated? Pediatrics 92, 860–861.

Schulte, F.J., 1981. Developmental neurophysiology. In: Davis, J.A., Dobbing, J. (Eds.), Scientific Foundation of Paediatrics, second ed. Heinemann, London, pp. 785–829.

Suter, V.G., Bornstein, M.M., 2009. Ankyloglossia: facts and myths in diagnosis and treatment. J Periodontol 80, 1204–1219.

Tappin, D.M., Mackenzie, J.M., Brown, A.J., et al., 2001. Breastfeeding rates are increasing in Scotland. Health Bull 59, 102–113.

Thompson, J.E., Clark, D.A., Salisbury, B., et al., 1981. Footprinting the newborn infant: not cost effective. J Pediatr 99, 797–798.

Trevarthen, C., Murray, L., Hubley, P., 1981. Psychology of infants. In: Davis, J.A., Dobbing, J. (Eds.), Scientific Foundation of Paediatrics, second ed. Heinemann, London, pp. 211–274.

Ultee, C.A., van der Deure, J., Swart, J., et al., 2008. Delayed cord clamping in preterm infants delivered at 34–36 weeks gestation: a randomised trial. Arch Dis Child Fetal Neonatal Ed 93, F20–F23.

Unvas-Moberg, K., Eriksson, M., 1996. Breast feeding: physiological endocrine and behavioural adaptations caused by oxytocin and local neurogenic activity in the nipple and mammary gland. Acta Paediatr 85, 525–530.

Varendi, H., Porter, R.H., Winberg, J., 1994. Does the newborn baby find the nipple by smell? Lancet 344, 989–990.

Von Kries, R., Hachmeister, A., Gobel, U., 1995. Repeated oral vitamin K prophylaxis in West Germany: acceptance and efficacy. Br Med J 310, 1097–1098.

Von Kries, R., Gobel, U., Hachmeister, A., et al., 1996. Vitamin K and childhood cancer: a population based case-control study in Lower Saxony, Germany. Br Med J 313, 199–203.

Weissbluth, M.D., Christoffel, K.K., Todd-Davis, A., 1984. Treatment of infantile colic with dicyclomine hydrochloride. J Pediatr 104, 951–955.

Wilcken, B., Wiley, V., Sherry, G., et al., 1995. Neonatal screening for cystic fibrosis: a comparison of two strategies for case detection in 1.2 million babies. J Pediatr 127, 965–970.

Wilde, C.J., Addey, C.V.P., Boddy, L.M., et al., 1995. Autocrine regulation of milk secretion by a protein in milk. Biochem J 305, 51.

Winberg, J., Bollgren, I., Gothefors, L., et al., 1989. The prepuce: a mistake of nature. Lancet i, 598–599.

Woolridge, M.W., 1986. The 'anatomy' of infant sucking. Midwifery 2, 164–171.

Woolridge, M.W., Fisher, C., 1988. Colic, 'overfeeding' and symptoms of lactose malabsorption in the breast-fed baby: a possible artifact of feed management? Lancet 2, 382–384.

Wright, C.N., Parkinson, K.N., 2004. Postnatal weight loss in term infants: what is 'normal' and do growth charts allow for it? Arch Dis Child 89, 254–257.

Zupan, J., Garner, P., 2000. Topical umbilical cord care at birth (Cochrane Review). Cochrane Database Syst Rev (2), CD001057.

Care of the normal small baby and convalescent NICU graduate

21

Kate Farrer

Introduction

This chapter focuses on the care of well, small babies who are suitable for nursing on the special care baby unit (SCBU) or transitional care unit (TCU), including the convalescing neonatal intensive care unit (NICU) graduates.

The normal small baby

Traditionally babies weighing below the 10th centile have been regarded as small for dates, although babies with birthweights between the 3rd and 10th centile rarely pose a problem if clinically well and feeding adequately. Modern antenatal care usually distinguishes genuine intrauterine growth retardation (IUGR) from the normal small baby. IUGR babies are more susceptible than normal small babies to some of the complications of prematurity and are discussed in greater detail in Chapter 10.

© 2012 Elsevier Ltd

Special care baby units and transitional care units

Whenever possible small, well babies should be cared for on post-natal wards with their mothers. Babies separated from their mother at birth display separation distress calls which cease at reunion (Christensson et al. 1995) and separation from the mother on the first night may increase the risk of allergy in later life (Montgomery et al. 2000). The weight, gestation and other criteria which determine admission to the neonatal unit or TCU should be agreed locally between neonatal and postnatal ward staff. Typically, new-borns less than 34 weeks' gestation or below 1.7 kg require NICU admission. Any baby who needs continuous monitoring and oxygen, or who meets other high-dependency criteria, will require SCBU admission.

Unfortunately, in recent years the availability of TCUs has declined, owing to lack of funds or appropriately trained staff. However, they remain popular with staff and parents (Simpson 2000) and may decrease the risks of mother–child separation and the risk of nosocomial infection. Nutritive sucking develops from around 32 weeks but regular sucking feeds are not usually established until 35 weeks, thus the necessity for tube-feeding is often the main factor requiring TCU admission and preventing discharge home (Table 21.1). The organisation of neonatal care is further discussed in Chapter 2.

Observations and monitoring on the transitional care unit

Routines, including clinical examination, cord care, screening, weighing and administration of vitamin K, are as for term babies – remembering that low-birthweight (LBW) babies should have intramuscular (not oral) vitamin K (Ch. 30). TCUs should be maintained at a stable temperature and contain essential equipment, including a fully equipped resuscitation area with piped oxygen, air and suction. The usual strict precautions to minimise nosocomial infection should apply (Ch. 39.2); each baby should have his or her own equipment, e.g. stethoscope, cotton wool and alcohol for hand rubbing.

Small and preterm babies have a greater risk of developing illnesses in the neonatal period (Engle et al. 2007) than mature well-grown babies. The TCU is often the ideal place to monitor babies who are at risk of conditions which could make them unwell, e.g. meconium aspiration, sepsis (group B *Streptococcus* exposure or after prolonged rupture of the membranes), narcotic withdrawal and hypoglycaemia. The length and nature of observations for such conditions vary and are rarely standardised between units. Historically 'sepsis observations' or 'meconium observations' have been recorded for up to 48 hours, which may be undesirable for staff and families and are probably unnecessary. The current National Institute for Health and Clinical Excellence guideline on intrapartum care (2007, section 1.11.8) recommends observations of well-being, feeding, skin colour, perfusion, temperature, pulse and respiration at 1 and 2 hours of age and then 2-hourly intervals for 12 hours in well babies born through meconium-stained liquor. A suitable chart is reproduced in Figure 21.1. The modified Finnegan chart (Ch. 26) is used in many units to monitor babies at risk of narcotic abstinence syndrome (Ch. 26). All units need to adhere to strict guidelines for monitoring babies at risk of hypoglycaemia (see below and Ch. 34.1).

Temperature control

Small babies, with a larger surface area to body mass ratio than term babies, are prone to hypothermia. If the baby is in an ambient temperature below 22–23°C, he or she may be using the thermoregulatory mechanisms described in Chapter 15, which will place a metabolic demand on the baby (Azaz et al. 1992).

If a small baby has a temperature of 36.0°C or less on admission to the TCU, examine him or her and check that the baby is otherwise well. Check the baby is dry then fully clothe him or her, including a hat, before swaddling in a sheet and blankets. Extra heat can be provided from a radiant heater or heated mattress. If, despite adequate warming attempts, the baby remains hypothermic, or if a stable baby develops hypothermia, an evaluation is required to exclude sepsis and measurement of glucose levels. The baby's temperature should be rechecked after removing from a source of additional heat.

Hypoglycaemia (see Ch. 34.1)

The definition and pathophysiology of hypoglycaemia are discussed in more detail in Chapter 34 part 1. Preterm, small and IUGR babies are more likely to develop hypoglycaemia than term or appropriately grown babies. For healthy LBW and IUGR term or near-term babies, detection and prevention of hypoglycaemia by adequate feeding can be safely supervised in the TCU.

The blood glucose level at which adverse sequelae might arise is still uncertain. Some small babies have low glycogen stores and poor ketone body responses to hypoglycaemia. If the caloric intake is poor, then the baby is at risk of developing prolonged hypoglycaemia with a risk of adverse neurological sequelae. For an IUGR baby the risk of symptomatic hypoglycaemia is greatest between 24 and 48 hours of age, hence the importance of accurate and continued monitoring in this group, who are not generally suitable for transfer from hospital to community care before this vulnerable period has passed. Whole-blood glucometer readings, not reagent sticks, should be used for monitoring. Hypoglycaemia diagnosed on the ward using a glucometer should always be confirmed with a laboratory glucose level. Attempts should be made to keep the blood glucose above 2.0 mmol/l; this minimises the risk of developing severe hypoglycaemia (<1.0 mmol/l). There is no evidence that transient low levels of glucose, which are not associated with signs, cause any adverse long-term sequelae.

Table 21.1 Categories of babies suitable for transitional care

Low-birthweight babies and babies with intrauterine growth retardation
Convalescent neonatal intensive care unit graduates
Babies requiring close observation
    Potential to develop symptoms of meconium aspiration, hypoglycaemia, drug withdrawal or sepsis
    At risk of hypoxic–ischaemic encephalopathy, e.g. with poor cord gas but well following delivery
    Infants of diabetic mothers
Babies with specific feeding difficulties
    Cleft lip or palate
    Requiring tube feeds (>3-hourly)
Babies requiring phototherapy
Twins and triplets of appropriate weight and gestation
Babies posing infection risk (if isolation cubicle available), e.g. gonococcal ophthalmia, *Listeria*

SINGLETON HOSPITAL
STAFF LIBRARY

Baby hospital details		Mother hospital details

Date and time of birth ....

Time observations due to finish ....

Meconium observations	(at 1 and 2 hours, then 2 hourly for 12 hours)
Group B *Streptococcus* observations	(4-hourly for 24 hours)
Prolonged rupture of membranes	(4-hourly for 24 hours)

Date					
Time					
General well-being/ interest in feeding					
Chest movements and nasal flaring					
Skin colour and perfusion, CRT					
Heart rate					
Respiratory rate					
Temperature					
Muscle tone					
Feeding (volume, type, method)					
Blood sugar if required					

Fig. 21.1 Observation chart for meconium/group B *Streptococcus*/prolonged rupture of the membranes (PROM). CRT, capillary refill time.
(Adapted from the neonatal meconium/group B streptococcus/PROM observations table, with kind permission of Dr David Long and East Kent Hospital Trust.)

Hypoglycaemia: monitoring, prevention and treatment

For those at risk, feeds should be started as soon as possible after birth. The mother should be encouraged to hold her baby skin to skin and put the baby to her breast in the labour ward. In general, within the first 24 hours, every endeavour should be made to keep the blood glucose >2.0 mmol/l and thereafter above 2.5 mmol/l. Blood glucose monitoring should start at 4 hours of age (earlier if there is IUGR) and then every 4–6 hours until two consecutive levels are above 2.5 mmol/l. Monitoring should recommence if feeding is reduced or the baby is unwell. If there is difficulty keeping the blood glucose level above 2.0 mmol/l, an extra feed should be given by cup, bottle or tube and further investigations performed. A baby who cannot cope with breast, cup or bottle feeds should be tube-fed; syringe-/cup-feeding carries a high risk of aspiration (see below). If the glucose level remains low, or the baby has clinical signs or cannot tolerate feeds, then he or she should be admitted to the NICU.

Feeding on the transitional care unit

The following sections discuss the various methods of feeding. The route, type, frequency, volume and rate of increment of feeds vary widely and few good quality data exist to help inform practice. The mother should be involved as much as possible with the feeding of her baby and the ultimate method of feeding should be her preferred choice. The merits and nutritional aspects of the different types of milk are discussed in Chapter 16.

Non-nutritive sucking

The sucking reflex develops from 28 weeks with effective suck, coordinated with breathing and swallowing, developing from 32 weeks and maturing fully by 35–37 weeks. Promoting non-nutritive sucking, using a pacifier or finger during tube-feeding, may help develop or maintain an effective sucking mechanism and decrease the length of hospital stay by easing the transition from tube to sucking feeds (Symington and Pinelli 2006).

Breastfeeding

If the mother intends to breastfeed the baby should, when possible, go to the breast in the delivery room soon after birth. Subsequently, regular breastfeeds help to stimulate colostrum and establish lactation. Preterm and LBW babies may need complementary feeds by cup, tube or bottle, until effective suckling feeds and weight gain are achieved. Monitoring for hypoglycaemia is often necessary for at least the first 48 hours or longer if the feeding is poor. Skin-to-skin contact, peer support, simultaneous breast milk pumping, multidisciplinary staff training and the Baby Friendly accreditation have been shown to improve successful breastfeeding (Renfrew et al. 2009).

Bottle-feeding

Breastfeeding should be encouraged when possible but if bottle-feeding is the desired, or required, method of feeding, ideally the baby should be demand-fed, aiming for a 3–4-hourly schedule and 6–8 feeds per day. If most of the required volume is taken and the baby is not hypoglycaemic, no further 'top-up' feed is necessary. One of the few advantages of bottle-feeding is that the exact volume of feed is known; if the baby is not taking enough, particularly if there are concurrent problems with hypoglycaemia or weight gain,

he or she should be topped up 3-hourly using a nasogastric tube. There is no firm evidence to support that using a teat causes 'nipple confusion' and the use of dummies has not been shown to affect breastfeeding.

Tube-feeding

Indications

The most common indication for tube-feeding is that a preterm or LBW baby is unable to suck the required amount of milk from the breast or bottle effectively. The decision to tube feed a baby is usually based on several factors, including:

- gestation at birth
- blood glucose levels
- frequency of waking for feed
- efficiency of sucking
- unsafe swallow
- inadequate volume taken
- dehydration, weight loss or paucity of weight gain.

Tube feeds can usually be administered on the TCU if they are not required more frequently than every 3–4 hours. Enteral feeding tubes may be placed via the nose or mouth. Evidence is lacking for superiority of either route (Hawes et al. 2004). Oral tubes are easier to pass but more prone to displacement, local irritation and vagal stimulation. Nasal placement may compromise respiration but the tubes remain in place more reliably. Breast- and bottle-feeding are both still possible with an indwelling nasogastric tube. Finger-feeding involves attaching a feeding tube to the side of a finger which is then inserted into the mouth in order to stimulate sucking. A breast supplementer is a similar device which may be attached to the breast whilst the baby sucks at the nipple and is another method that may encourage the baby to suck and swallow whilst breastfeeding is being established.

Complications of tube-feeding

Complications of tube-feeding in adults prompted the National Patient Safety Agency (NPSA), in consultation with the British Association of Perinatal Medicine, the Neonatal Nurses Association and the Royal College of Paediatrics and Child Health, to release guidance recommending that gastric tube position be confirmed by pH indicator strips, not litmus paper (National Patient Safety Agency 2005). Other methods, including X-ray, auscultation, the presence of respiratory distress and the appearance of aspirate, or bubbling, are not to be used to confirm position. Reported complications from tube-feeding in neonates are rare but include pharyngeal, oesophageal, gastric, duodenal and bladder perforation with pneumomediastinum and peritonitis (Bell 1985; Sands et al. 1989; Mattar et al. 1997). Soft silicone tubes have been passed into the bronchus (Laing et al. 1986). Gastro-oesophageal reflux has been shown to be almost universal in tube-fed preterm infants, increasing the risk of aspiration pneumonia (Peter et al. 2002).

Frequency and volume

In general, for preterm and small-for-gestational-age babies the volume given should be divided into a 3-hourly feeding schedule if there is normoglycaemia. Three-hourly feeds can usually be given on the TCU but if needed more frequently admission to SCBU is usually necessary. If the tube feed is complementing a bottle feed, the deficit should be made up. If the tube feed is complementing a breastfeed, in the first few days when only colostrum is likely to have been taken, the full volume should be given. Thereafter, a smaller proportion can be given based on clinical assessment.

Cup-feeding

Cup-feeding was reintroduced into the UK in the late 1980s by Sandra Lang. The technique involves swaddling the baby and sitting him or her in a semiupright position. The rim of a cup half-full of milk is then gently placed on the baby's lower lip, directing the rim towards the corners of the upper lip, tipping the milk to touch the baby's lip as he or she swallows it. Milk should not be poured into the baby's mouth. The method appears safe if carefully monitored, and breathing and oxygen saturation remained stable during one study of 15 cup-feeding sessions (Dowling et al. 2002). Cup-feeding involves sipping and lapping rather than sucking, thus breastfeeding should continue in order to enhance the sucking experience. Cup-feeding improves the likelihood of exclusive breastfeeding by discharge but increases the length of stay (Collins et al. 2008). Cup-feeding prolongs breastfeeding if frequent supplementary feeds are needed initially and following caesarean section (Becker et al. 2008). Cup-feeding is a useful adjunct to other methods of feeding, but is a short-term solution which carries a risk of aspiration if not carefully supervised. Milk spillage is a real problem, particularly when expressed breast milk is in short supply.

Milk expression and storage

For babies unable to suckle at the breast successfully, mothers should be encouraged and supported to start milk expression as early as possible. Physical and emotional stress to the mother may inhibit adequate milk production. Skin-to-skin nursing, multidisciplinary support and Baby Friendly accreditation have been shown to improve the chances of successful breastfeeding (Renfrew et al. 2009). Double pumping, skin-to-skin care and non-nutritive sucking at the breast can all help increase milk volume. Neonatal and maternity teams, with the help of lactation consultants, should support mothers to achieve this. Early (within 6 hours if possible), frequent (up to 10 times a day) and effective milk expression encourages maximum milk production. Adequately draining the breast is important as this stimulates further milk production and 'hind milk' has greater calorific value. If, despite frequent, effective expression, milk supply is inadequate, domperidone can increase maternal supply. Expressed breast milk can be safely stored in a refrigerator at less than 10 °C for 3 days. It can be deep-frozen for 3 months and, once thawed, should be used within 24–48 hours.

Weight

All babies lose weight after birth – up to 10% of their bodyweight in the first 4–5 days – before gaining weight at 10–15 g/kg/day. It may take 6–10 days before the 32-week gestation, or 1.5–1.8-kg, baby shows steady weight gain.

Infection

Babies born at 32–35 weeks have physiological immunodeficiency (Ch. 39.1). They are born before the transplacental transfer of maternal immunoglobulin is complete and developmental maturity of lymphocyte function. Babies nursed in TCUs are susceptible to infection and strict nosocomial precautions should apply. If the baby has been delivered after prolonged rupture of the membranes, or other risk factors for neonatal infection are present (e.g. maternal factors, including pyrexia), then the baby requires evaluation with consideration of a full infection screen plus antibiotic treatment pending results (Ch. 39.2).

Skin

Skin integrity is an important barrier against infection. Tape should be thoughtfully applied and its use minimised as it is the primary cause of skin breakdown in LBW babies (Lund et al. 2001).

Jaundice

Small and preterm babies are more likely to develop jaundice, particularly if they are not feeding well or have been polycythaemic. If jaundice becomes apparent the bilirubin level and maternal blood group should be checked. Phototherapy should be instituted at bilirubin levels appropriate for gestation (Ch. 29.1), and a BiliBlanket can be chosen as first-line treatment in the preterm group. When assessing whether a jaundiced baby is fit for discharge many variables need to considered, including postnatal age, gestation, weight gain/loss, feeding, bilirubin trend, rate of rise/fall and time since cessation of phototherapy. The bilirubin level should be checked for rebound 12–18 hours after ceasing phototherapy but the baby does not necessarily have to remain in hospital for this to be done.

Care of the intensive-care graduate

Babies who have required neonatal intensive care usually have a phase when they are well but still not ready for discharge. Satisfactory feeding and growth, maintenance of temperature at ambient room temperature and maintenance of adequate oxygen saturation levels without supplementary oxygen all need to be achieved before discharge, although a small number of NICU graduates with chronic lung disease (CLD) will be discharged still needing supplementary oxygen (Ch. 27.3). Convalescing NICU graduates in general remain well but routines should be in place to detect any new problems. Serious complications of prematurity, such as CLD (Ch. 27.3), retinopathy of prematurity (ROP: Ch. 33) and hydrocephalus (Ch. 40.5) are dealt with elsewhere in this book.

Routine surveillance

The NICU graduate needs a full examination once or twice a week. The routine should include the details listed in Table 21.2. Each week, full blood and reticulocyte count plus electrolyte, urea, calcium, phosphate and alkaline phosphatase levels should be assessed. The baby's bodyweight and head circumference should be plotted weekly on an appropriate chart to ensure normal progression. Cranial ultrasound follow-up assessments should continue at appropriate intervals (Ch. 40.5). New clinical findings which might arise during this time include hernia, anaemia, metabolic bone disease, murmurs, poor weight gain and cavernous haemangiomas.

Emotional, developmental and environmental needs, NIDCAP

The emotional and psychological needs of the baby and family continue to be important. Developmental programmes such as the Newborn Individualized Developmental Care and Assessment Program (NIDCAP) are increasingly popular and important, despite conflicting evidence of benefit (Pinelli and Symington 2005; Peters et al. 2009). The ethos of NIDCAP is to deliver individualised, developmentally supportive, family-centred care to optimise health and developmental outcome. Overall it would seem appropriate to

Table 21.2 Routine surveillance for the neonatal intensive care unit graduate

NAME	DATE	GESTATION AGE AT BIRTH	CORRECTED GESTATION
Weight		Head circumference	
Current problems			
Medication			
Feeding			
Cardiovascular system	Pulse	Heart sounds	
Respiratory			
Abdomen			
Genitalia			
Neurological		Cranial ultrasound	
Eye check			
Laboratory tests	Haemoglobin	Electrolytes	Alkaline phosphatase

adopt a less 'chaotic, non-circadian environmental approach' in the modern neonatal nursery (Mirmiran and Ariagno 2000). Developmental care is further discussed in Chapter 4.

Feeding the convalescent premature baby

Many advantages result from the early introduction of minimal enteral feeding to very-low-birthweight (VLBW) babies even while they are still quite ill (Chs. 16, 29.3). Full enteral nutrition is achieved earlier, and the complications of long-term total parenteral nutrition are reduced (Ch. 17). By the time the baby is convalescent from the acute neonatal illness, he or she will usually be tolerating hourly feeds at a total daily volume of 150–180 ml/kg.

A large body of experience shows that, when introducing feeds, breast milk is better tolerated than formula (Ch. 16.3). Non-nutritive sucking using a pacifier during tube-feeding may have benefits (Symington and Pinelli 2006) and help train the baby in the techniques of sucking, although excessive pacifier use in the neonatal period may be detrimental to exclusive and overall breast-feeding duration (Becker et al. 2008). If well, once a baby is 30–32 weeks' gestation, he or she can be put to the mother's breast if she intends to breastfeed. Kangaroo mother care (Ch. 4), involving skin-to-skin contact, can help milk production. Once the baby is 33–34 weeks' gestation he or she should make a reasonable attempt at sucking feeds, and by 35 weeks most neurologically normal convalescent ex-premature babies should be able to suck and swallow safely. For those mothers who have maintained their lactation by expression, every attempt should be made to encourage the baby to go to the breast, and if possible to have the mother rooming in or on the TCU.

Nutritional supplements

Sodium

Hyponatraemia is common, particularly in breastfed babies, as breast milk lacks adequate amounts of sodium for the needs of the preterm baby (Ch. 16.3). In addition the fractional excretion of sodium is relatively high (Chs. 18, 35.1). Sodium supplements should be given; some babies need up to 10 mmol/kg/day.

Phosphate and vitamin D

Extremely low-birthweight (ELBW) babies are at risk of metabolic bone disease (see Ch. 35.4), which manifests biochemically as hypophosphataemia, elevated alkaline phosphatase and occasionally, in severe cases, hypercalcaemia. Vitamin D supplementation, 4–800 units daily often given as part of a multinutrient supplement, with appropriate phosphate supplements (approximately 0.5 mmol/100 ml breast milk), reduce the risk of metabolic bone disease (Ch. 34.4).

Iron and folic acid

VLBW babies are born before most of the body's stores of iron are laid down in the third trimester of pregnancy. Supplements of enteral iron 2–3 mg/kg/day should be started at 2–6 weeks of age (ESPGHAN Committee on Nutrition 2010) but delayed until 4–6 weeks in infants who receive multiple blood transfusions as excessive iron has been associated with increased risk of infection and poor growth (Domellof 2007). Preterm babies receiving entirely breast milk may become folate-deficient and develop megaloblastic anaemia (Strelling et al. 1979). Most NICUs give 100 µg folic acid daily until term corrected for gestational age, or until discharge.

Growth and weight gain

The standard rules of neonatal weight gain apply. Babies should gain weight at roughly 15 g/kg/day. The baby may feed voraciously, particularly towards the end of the convalescent phase in the neonatal unit and may take more than 180–200 ml/kg/day. This sort of catch-up growth is frequently seen once the baby goes home and the parents are much less rigid than the nursing staff, feeding volumes of up to 300 ml/kg/day (Lucas et al. 1992). Not uncommonly peripheral, rather firm, oedema may develop, which can cause concern but no diuretics or other treatment is required.

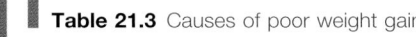

Table 21.3 Causes of poor weight gain

Inadequate caloric intake
Expressed breast milk
Vomiting
Low-volume feeds

Insufficient supply of essentials other than energy
Sodium deficiency
Anaemia (inadequate oxygen-carrying capacity)

Increased energy expenditure
Bronchopulmonary dysplasia
Sepsis
Hyperactivity
Thyrotoxicosis
Cerebral irritability
Seizures
Drug withdrawal

Drug therapy
Diuretic

Cold stress
Bathing, handling, inadequate clothing

Misery
Lack of non-nutritive sucking
Discomfort

Excessive nutrient losses
Short-bowel syndrome
Gastro-oesophageal reflux
Hypertrophic pyloric stenosis
Necrotising enterocolitis
Gastroenteritis
Protein-energy malnutrition
Milk lactose and protein intolerance
Congenital enteropathies

Poor weight gain (Table 21.3)

The commonest cause of poor weight gain is inadequate caloric intake. Intake should be increased to a volume of 180–200 ml/kg/day of breast milk if tolerated, and if the mother is producing large volumes of milk the hind milk may contain more fat than the fore milk. If weight gain remains poor, then appropriate supplements should be considered, usually breast milk fortifier but occasionally supplementary feeds (Ch. 16.3). CLD, anaemia and hyponatraemia also cause poor weight gain. If, despite adequate calorie, sodium and nutrient intake, weight gain remains poor, other causes of failure to thrive should be considered (Table 21.3).

Head growth and shape

Weekly occipitofrontal circumference measurement is important. Accelerated growth might be due to hydrocephalus (Ch. 40.5) and slow growth may indicate cerebral atrophy. Preterm babies may develop a long thin dolichocephalic head shape as the relatively immobile baby with soft skull bones lies predominantly on one side (Cartlidge and Rutter 1988). This can be minimised by appropriate positioning but even without intervention the head shape

normalises spontaneously (Rutter et al. 1993). Since supine sleeping has been advocated to decrease the risk of sudden infant death syndrome (SIDS), plagiocephaly, particularly brachycephaly to the right, and torticollis have increased (Hummel and Fortado 2005).

Anaemia of prematurity

The preterm baby often becomes anaemic, with a haemoglobin nadir of 7–9 g/dl at 6–8 weeks of age. The aetiology of the condition is multifactorial (Ch. 30) including iatrogenic blood loss at a time when the rapidly expanding intravascular volume may outstrip the bone marrow's capacity to produce sufficient red cells. If the baby is well and breathing air, a haemoglobin can be allowed to remain as low as 7 g/dl without transfusion, particularly if the reticulocyte count (3–10%) is reassuring. If symptoms of anaemia such as poor feeding, lethargy or congestive heart failure (Alvarson 1995) occur, the baby may benefit from 15 ml/kg transfusion of packed red cells.

Data reporting the effects of transfusion on apnoea are conflicting. Some authors conclude that transfusion decreases the frequency of apnoea (Stute et al. 1995). However, others suggest that transfusion has little effect on apnoea but tachycardia and tachypnoea may be significantly improved (Westkamp et al. 2002).

VLBW babies may have a marked eosinophilia by the age of 3–4 weeks. This often follows an episode of proven sepsis (Manoura et al. 2002) but is otherwise a benign finding

Murmurs

During the convalescent period, a heart murmur may be noted for the first time. Murmurs associated with cardiac failure, cyanosis or decreased femoral pulses need prompt investigation. Mild pulmonary artery stenosis may be noted as a soft ejection systolic murmur. Once confirmed, this benign murmur does not require further investigation and resolves as the baby grows (Arlettaz et al. 2001).

Hernias and testes

Inguinal hernias occur in 11% of babies under 1500 g and 17% under 1000 g, and they are more likely to occur in boys and in babies with CLD (Kumar et al. 2002). Hernias should ideally be repaired prior to discharge but the timing of surgery is a matter of clinical judgement. Repairing large hernias in babies with severe CLD can result in serious deterioration; other babies with CLD may have improved respiratory status following repair (Emberton et al. 1996). There is no need to rush into surgery for cosmetic reasons. Spinal anaesthetic may decrease the risk of postoperative events (Libby 2009).

Delayed descent of the testes is very common in ELBW babies. No specific treatment is indicated, but, if the testes are still not descended by the time of discharge, appropriate follow-up should be arranged with a paediatric surgeon.

Umbilical hernias are common, especially in babies with Down syndrome, Afro-Caribbean babies and those with CLD. They invariably resolve but may become large; if still present at 1 year of age, referral should be made to a paediatric surgeon.

Retinopathy of prematurity (see Ch. 33)

All babies less than 32 weeks' gestation and below 1500 g birthweight require assessment to exclude ROP (Royal College of Paediatrics and Child Health, Royal College of Ophthalmologists, British Association of Perinatal Medicine and Bliss 2008). Many units perform this at 4–5 weeks of age for all eligible babies. The examination can destabilise the sick baby and care should be taken when giving a mydriatic with systemic side-effects, e.g. bradycardia and arrhythmias.

Hearing

Since 2003 the Newborn Hearing Screening Programme ensures parents of all newborns are offered hearing screening in the first weeks of life. These tests are very important for NICU graduates who are at increased risk of hearing deficit owing to either illness, e.g. hypoxia and sepsis, or drug treatment. Deafness due to aminoglycoside or furosemide toxicity is very rare in clinical practice and there has been recent discovery of genetic susceptibility to aminoglycosides. A mitochondrial mutation (the m.1555A>G mutation) renders individuals susceptible to gentamicin ototoxicity, and in this situation the high sensitivity to gentamicin means that exposure to levels which are well within the therapeutic range can result in hearing loss; some affected individuals become deaf without any gentamicin exposure at all.

Discharging small babies

Traditionally there has been a focus on the need to attain a particular weight before discharge but the advent of neonatal community nurses has made such rules more flexible (Merritt et al. 2003; Rose et al. 2008). The process of discharge planning should start soon after admission. Coordinated individualised discharge planning programmes involving the family, including plans for structured home visiting, are successful and popular (Bliss 2009; POPPY Steering Group 2009). The recommendations of the American Academy of Pediatrics (2008) are helpful:

- a sustained pattern of weight gain rather than a specific achieved weight
- physiological stability
- the ability to suck some feeds and maintain normal body temperature in an open environment
- parental involvement and preparation prior to discharge
- home support post discharge
- outpatient follow-up to ensure adequate weight gain and to monitor development.

Apnoeic episodes may occur up to 8 days apart in otherwise well babies, thus an interval of this length from the last apnoea is recommended before discharge (Darnall et al. 1997). The British Thoracic Society advocates discharge for infants with CLD when their oxygen requirement is stable with mean saturation of 93% or above and without frequent episodes of desaturation (Balfour-Lynn et al. 2009). Further management of the baby requiring home oxygen for CLD is discussed on Ch. 27.3.

Prior to discharge, each baby should have a complete neonatal examination, including visualisation of the normal red light reflex and examination of the hips to assess stability (Ch. 37). Hearing screening plus ROP checks for those who qualify should be performed and follow-up arranged if indicated.

Advice to parents

Written information and useful website addresses can help parental understanding and preparation prior to discharge (Bliss 2009; POPPY Steering Group 2009). Preterm infants have 8–10 times the risk of SIDS compared with low-risk term babies and advice aimed at decreasing the risk of SIDS should include recommendations for the baby to sleep on his or her back in a cigarette-free environment and not to be overwrapped (Fleming et al. 1996). Parents are advised not to sleep in the same bed as the baby, especially if they smoke, have recently drunk alcohol, are very tired or are taking drugs which make them sleepy. A baby under 8 weeks old sharing a bed with parents has a twofold increased risk of SIDS if the parents are non-smokers and 11-fold if the parents smoke (Carpenter et al. 2004). The baby's cot should probably be in the parents' bedroom until 6 months of age (Fleming et al. 1996).

Monitors

Although preterm babies are more likely than term babies to have adverse cardiorespiratory events until 43 weeks' corrected gestational age, there is no evidence that these events are precursors to SIDS, and after 43 weeks' corrected gestational age, the frequency of cardiorespiratory events in preterm babies is the same as for healthy term babies (Rangasamy et al. 2001). There is no evidence that the incidence of SIDS or acute life-threatening events is reduced by home apnoea alarms and it is possible that many cardiorespiratory events are missed by standard monitors.

Flying

Parents often want to know if their baby is 'fit to fly'. Infants under 1 year are more susceptible to hypoxia resulting from flight cabin pressurisation, especially if they were born preterm or have CLD. It is generally believed flying is safe in the first year of life for most healthy infants but for those at risk preflight testing with a 'fitness to fly' test, available in some tertiary centres, can help guide the need for in-flight supplemental oxygen (Bossley and Balfour-Lynn 2007).

Car seat testing

Infants under 2 kg are at increased risk of altered breathing pattern, desaturation or bradycardia in a car seat, which improves when the infant is supine; thus car seat testing may be wise for this group of babies (Ojadi et al. 2005).

Resuscitation training

Teaching parents resuscitation procedures helps alleviate anxiety and increase parental confidence (Dracup et al. 2000); however, there is no evidence that resuscitation training reduces post discharge mortality or morbidity. Additional video instruction, as produced by the charity Bliss and the American Heart Association, is associated with improved performance (Brannon et al. 2009).

Feeding and supplements

Breastfeeding should be the preferred option and discharge planning should include plans to achieve full breastfeeding, with an adequate support network. Exclusive breastfeeding to 6 months of age is safe and beneficial (Kramer and Kakuma 2002). Breast milk or hydrolysed formula in preference to intact cow's milk protein formulas may delay the onset of childhood atopic disease (Frank et al. 2008). Post discharge nutrition and follow-on formulas for the NICU graduate are discussed in Ch. 16.3.

The NICU graduate should receive iron and vitamin D supplementation from the time of discharge until at least 6 months of age. For the breastfed preterm TCU graduate, similar supplementation should be given but, as all formulas are now supplemented, it is doubtful whether additional vitamins and iron are required for bottle-fed babies.

Immunisations

Premature babies are at increased risk of vaccine-preventable infections and should be vaccinated according to the recommended schedule without correction for prematurity (Department of Health 2006). In addition after 6 months of age, but before the 1st winter influenza season starts, infants with oxygen dependent CLD should receive two doses of the influenza vaccine, 1 month apart. Annual repeats are only necessary if the infant remains oxygen dependent. Also babies with CLD, particularly those going home on oxygen, should receive palivizumab respiratory syncytial virus prophylaxis during their first winter and, if they remain on oxygen, prophylaxis until 2 years of age is advised (Department of Health 2005).

The evidence base for immunisation of preterm infants is limited; however, the available data support early immunisation without correction for gestational age (Bonhoeffer et al. 2006). For a number of antigens the antibody response to initial doses may be lower than that of term infants, but protective concentrations are often achieved and memory successfully induced. The 2–3–4-month schedule may be preferable for immunisation of preterm infants in order to achieve protection as early as possible. There is no evidence that delaying vaccination for babies who have received steroids is beneficial. An additional dose may be required to achieve persistence of protection, particularly for babies who have received steroids for CLD.

Adverse events following immunisation are increased in premature infants, particularly if there is a pre-existing tendency to episodes of cardiorespiratory instability such as apnoea or desaturations (Pfister et al. 2004), thus delaying immunisation until stability is sensible. Adverse incidents do not appear to be related to gestational age and are unlikely after 48 hours following immunisation. Warning parents about possible adverse events can help to alleviate parental anxiety. Minor adverse events include low-grade fever, soreness at the injection site and malaise. Vaccination also causes a rise in the C-reactive protein (Balkundi et al. 1994). Prophylactic paracetamol decreases the risk of fever but should not be routinely administered as it reduces antibody responses to several antigens (Prymula et al. 2009).

Post discharge support and follow-up

Parents of babies with significant ongoing medical concerns, including oxygen-dependent CLD, are often given 'open access' letters or

Table 21.4 Criteria for outpatient follow-up of neonatal intensive care unit graduates

≤30 weeks' gestation
<1.50 kg birthweight
Neonatal encephalopathy
Seizures
Meningitis
Septicaemia
Necrotising enterocolitis
Significant hyperbilirubinaemia (including those requiring exchange transfusion)
Abnormalities on cranial ultrasound scan
Persisting murmurs
Persisting structural abnormalities, e.g. hernia, vesicoureteric reflux, undescended testicles
Babies with chronic lung disease at discharge
Babies whose families have social problems, e.g. narcotic abuse
Infants of human immunodeficiency virus-positive mothers

'parents' passports' to allow direct admission to the paediatric services should the need arise. Appropriate telephone numbers for the community support team plus access to 24-hour advice are needed. Initially this advice might be given from the neonatal team who are familiar to the family and every effort should be made to document the calls and advice given. NICU wards rarely have the facility to record incoming calls but some community teams may have recordable phones, especially if messages need to be left. Responsibility for supporting the families of infants with long-term needs is often transferred to the paediatric community nurses at or soon after discharge.

A baby discharged from the TCU who had an uncomplicated course may not need hospital follow-up. The routine child health surveillance system is adequate for the needs of many of these babies. Most NICU graduates require follow-up, but it is important to be selective (Table 21.4). Careful multidisciplinary follow-up is necessary for babies with potential or actual complex problems so that motor delay, spasticity and poor weight gain are detected and managed promptly. Long-term follow-up of babies who have been very sick or premature, with accurate data collection, helps consolidate epidemiological information about outcome. The current UK recommendations are for all babies born at <32 weeks gestation to be assessed at 2 years (Lyon 2007).

Weblinks

http://www.breastfeeding.nhs.uk

http://www.breastfeedingnetwork.org.uk

http://www.immunisation.nhs.uk

References

Alvarson, D.C., 1995. The physiologic impact of anemia in the neonate. Clin Perinatol 22, 609–625.

American Academy of Pediatrics, 2008. Hospital discharge of the high-risk neonate. Pediatrics 122, 1119–1126.

Arlettaz, R., Archer, N., Wilkinson, A.R., 2001. Closure of the ductus arteriosus and development of pulmonary branch stenosis in babies of less than 32 weeks gestation. Arch Dis Child Fetal Neonatal Ed 85, 197–200.

Azaz, Y., Fleming, P.J., Levine, M., et al. 1992. The relationship between environmental temperature, metabolic rate, and evaporative water loss in infants from birth to three months. Pediatr Res 32, 417–423.

Balfour-Lynn, I.M., Field, D.J., Gringras P., et al. 2009. British Thoracic Society guidelines for home oxygen in children. Thorax 64, ii1–ii26.

Balkundi, D.R., Nycyk, J.A., Cooke, R.W.I., 1994. Immunization and C reactive protein in infants on neonatal intensive care units. Arch Dis Child Fetal Neonatal Ed 71, 149.

Becker GE, McCormick FM, Renfrew MJ, 2008. Methods of milk expression for lactating women. Cochrane Database Syst Rev (4), CD006170.pub2.

Bell, M.J., 1985. Perforation of the gastrointestinal tract and peritonitis in the neonate. Surg Gynecol Obstet 160, 20–26.

Bliss, 2009. The Bliss Baby Charter Standards. Bliss, London.

Bonhoeffer, J., Siegrist, C-A., Heath, P.T., 2006. Immunisation of premature infants. Arch Dis Child 91, 929–935.

Bossley, C., Balfour-Lynn, I.M., 2007. Is this baby fit to fly? Hypoxia in aeroplanes. Early Hum Dev 83, 755–759.

Brannon, T.S., White, L.A., Kilcrease, J.N., et al. 2009. Use of instructional video to prepare parents for learning infant cardiopulmonary resuscitation. Proc (Bayl Univ Med Cent) 22, 133–137.

Carpenter, R.G., Irgens, L.M., Blair, P., et al. 2004. Sudden unexplained infant death in 20 regions in Europe: case control study. Lancet 363, 185–191.

Cartlidge, P.H.T., Rutter, N., 1988. Reduction of head flattening in preterm infants. Arch Dis Child 63, 755–757.

Christensson, K., Cabrera, T., Christensson, E., et al., 1995. Separation distress call in the human neonate in the absence of maternal contact. Acta Paediatr 84, 468–473.

Collins, C.T., Makrides, M., Gillis, J., et al., 2008. Avoidance of bottles during the establishment of breast feeds in preterm infants. Cochrane Database Syst Rev (4), CD005252.pub2.

Darnall, R., Kattwinkel, J., Nattie, C., et al., 1997. Margin of safety for discharge after apnoea in preterm infants. Pediatrics 100, 795–801.

Department of Health, 2005. Joint Committee on Vaccination and Immunisation. Available online at: http://www.advisorybodies.doh.gov.uk/jcvi/mins220605.htm.

Department of Health, 2006. The Green Book – Immunisation against infectious diseases. DoH, London, pp. 78–82.

Domellof, M., 2007. Iron requirements, absorption and metabolism in infancy and childhood. Curr Opin Clin Nutr Metab Care 10, 329–335.

Dowling, D.A., Meier, P.P., DiFiore, J., et al., 2002. Cup-feeding for preterm infants: mechanics and safety. J Hum Lact 18, 13–20.

Dracup, K., Moser, D.K., Doering, L.V., et al., 2000. A controlled trial of cardiopulmonary resuscitation training for ethnically diverse parents of infants at high risk for cardiopulmonary arrest. Crit Care Med 28, 3289–3295.

Emberton, M., Patel, L., Zideman, D.A., et al., 1996. Early repair of inguinal hernia in preterm infants with oxygen dependent bronchopulmonary dysplasia. Acta Paediatr 85, 96–99.

Engle, W.A., Tomashek, K.M., Wallman, C., et al., 2007. 'Late-preterm' infants: a population at risk. Pediatrics 120, 1390–1401.

ESPGHAN Committee on Nutrition, 2010. Enteral nutrient supply for preterm infants: commentary from the European Society for Paediatric Gastroenterology, Hepatology, and Nutrition Committee on Nutrition. J Pediatr Gastroenterol 50, 1–934.

Fleming, P.J., Blair, P.S., Bacon, C., et al., 1996. Environment of infants during sleep and risk for SIDS: results of 1993–1995 case control study for CESDI. BMJ 313, 191–195.

Frank, R., Greer, M.D., Scott, H., et al., 2008. Effects of early nutritional interventions on the development of atopic disease in infants and children: the role of maternal dietary restriction, breastfeeding, timing of introduction of complementary foods, and hydrolyzed formulas. Pediatrics 121, 183–191.

Hawes, J., McEwan, P., McGuire, W., 2004. Nasal versus oral route for placing feeding tubes in preterm or low birth weight infants. Cochrane Database Syst Rev (3), CD003952.pub2.

Hummel, P., Fortado, D., 2005. Impacting infant head shapes. Adv Neonatal Care 5, 329–340. Intrapartum Care: care of healthy women and their babies during childbirth. Available from www.nice.org.uk/CG055.

Kramer, M.S., Kakuma, R., 2002. Optimal duration of exclusive breastfeeding. Syst Rev (1), CD003517.

Kumar, V.H., Clive, J., Rosenbrantz, T.S., et al., 2002. Inguinal hernia in preterm infants (<32-week gestation). Pediatr Surg Int 18, 147–152.

Laing, I.A., Lang, M.A., Callaghan, O., et al., 1986. Nasogastric compared with nasoduodenal feeding in low birthweight infants. Arch Dis Child 61, 138–141.

Libby, A., 2009. Spinal anesthesia in preterm infant undergoing herniorraphy. J Am Assoc Nurse Anesth 77, 199–206.

Lucas, A., King, F., Bishop, N.R., 1992. Post-discharge formula consumption in infants born preterm. Arch Dis Child 67, 691–692.

Lund, C., Osbourne, J., Kuller, J., et al., 2001. Neonatal skin care: clinical outcomes of the AWHONN/NANN evidence-based clinical practice guideline. J Obstet Gynaecol Neonatal Nurs 30, 41.

Lyon, A., 2007. How should we report neonatal outcomes? Semin Fetal Neonatal Med 12, 332–336.

Manoura, A., Hatzidaki, E., Karakaki, E., 2002. Eosinophilia in sick neonates. Haematologica 32, 31–37.

Mattar, M.S., Dahniya, M.H., Al-Marzouk, N.F., 1997. Urinary bladder perforation: an unusual complication of neonatal nasogastric tube feeding. Pediatr Radiol 27, 858–859.

Merritt, T.A., Pillers, D., Prows, S.L., 2003. Early NICU discharge of very low birth weight infants: a critical review and analysis. Semin Neonatol 8, 95–115.

Mirmiran, M., Ariagno, R.L., 2000. Influence of light in the NICU on the development of circadian rhythms in preterm infants. Semin Perinatol 24, 247–257.

Montgomery, S.M., Wakefield, A.J., Morris, D.L., et al., 2000. The initial care of newborn infants and subsequent hayfever. Allergy 55, 916–922.

National Patient Safety Agency, 2009. Reducing the harm caused by misplaced naso and orogastric feeding tubes in babies under the care of neonatal units. National Patient Safety Agency, London.

Ojadi, V., Petrova, A., Mehta, R., et al. 2005. Risk of cardio-respiratory abnormalities in preterm infants placed in car seats: a cross-sectional study. BMC Pediatr 5, 28.

Peter, C.S., Wiechers, C., Bohnhorst, B., et al., 2002. Influence of nasogastric tubes on gastroesophageal reflux in preterm infants: a multiple intraluminal impedance study. J Pediatr 141, 277–279.

Peters, K.L., Rosychuk, R.J., Hendson, L., et al., 2009. Improvement of short- and long-term outcomes for very low birth weight infants: Edmonton NIDCAP trial. Pediatrics 124, 1009–1020.

Pfister, R.E., Aeschbach, V., Niksic-Stuber, V., et al., 2004. Safety of DTaP-based combined immunization in very-low-birth-weight premature infants: frequent but mostly benign cardiorespiratory events. J Pediatr 145, 58–66.

Pinelli, J., Symington, A.J., 2005. Non-nutritive sucking for promoting physiologic stability and nutrition in preterm infants. Cochrane Database Syst Rev (4), CD001071.pub2.

POPPY Steering Group, 2009. Family-centred care in neonatal units. A summary of research results and recommendations from the POPPY project. National Childbirth Trust, London.

Prymula, R., Siegrist, C-A., Chlibek, R., et al., 2009. Effect of prophylactic paracetamol administration at time of vaccination on febrile reactions and antibody responses in children: two open-label, randomised controlled trials. Lancet, 374, 1339–1350.

Rangasamy, R., Corwin, M., Hunt, C., et al., 2001. Cardiorespiratory events recorded on home monitors; comparison of healthy infants with those at increased risk for SIDS. JAMA 285, 2199–2207.

Renfrew, M.J., Craig, D., Dyson, L., et al., 2009. Breastfeeding promotion for infants in neonatal units: a systematic review and economic analysis. Health Technol Assess 40, 1–146.

Rose, C., Ramsay, L., Leaf, A., 2008. Strategies for getting preterm babies home earlier. Arch Dis Child 93, 271–273.

Royal College of Paediatrics and Child Health, Royal College of Ophthalmologists, British Association of Perinatal Medicine and Bliss, 2008. UK Retinopathy of screening Guidelines.

Rutter, N., Hinchcliffe, W., Cartlidge, P.H.T., 1993. Do preterm infants always have flattened heads? Arch Dis Child 68, 606–607.

Sands, T., Glasson, M., Berry, A., 1989. Hazards of nasogastric tube insertion in the newborn infant. Lancet 334, 680.

Simpson, D., 2000. Transitional care for neonates. Pract Midwife 3, 13–15.

Strelling, M.K., Blackledge, D.G., Goodall, H.B., 1979. Diagnosis and management of folate deficiency in low birthweight infants. Arch Dis Child 54, 271–277.

Stute, H., Greiner, B., Linderkamp, O., 1995. Effect of blood transfusion on cardiorespiratory abnormalities in preterm infants. Arch Dis Child Fetal Neonatal Ed 72, F194–F196.

Symington, A.J., Pinelli, J., 2006. Developmental care for promoting development and preventing morbidity in preterm infants. Cochrane Database Syst Rev (2), CD001814.pub2.

Westkamp, E., Soditt, V., Adrian, S., et al., 2002. Blood transfusion in anemic infants with apnea of prematurity. Biol Neonate 82, 228–232.

Further reading

Jones, E., King, C., 2005. Feeding and Nutrition in the Preterm Infant. Elsevier, Oxford.

Lang, S., 2002. Breastfeeding Special Care Babies, second ed. Elsevier.

Neonatal complications following diabetes in pregnancy

Jane M Hawdon

22

CHAPTER CONTENTS

Diabetes may predate pregnancy or a woman may develop transient or permanent diabetes during pregnancy. The fertility and well-being of women with diabetes dramatically improved with the availability of insulin, but a high perinatal mortality rate of 20–25% persisted until the 1960s. In the last three decades perinatal mortality rates have fallen, but these vary between countries and regions and progress against aspirations has been disappointing, with a neonatal death rate in the UK of 9.3 per 1000 births, 3.8 times the national rate (Table 22.1) (Roversi et al. 1979; Hunter 1992; Casson et al. 1997; Hawthorne et al. 1997; Confidential Enquiry into Maternal and Child Health 2005; Hawdon 2010).

When there is good preconceptional care and control of diabetes and in the absence of congenital abnormalities or other complications, babies should be managed as any other healthy term baby (National Collaborating Centre for Primary Care 2006). There is no indication for routine attendance of paediatricians at the delivery or routine admission to a neonatal unit (Confidential Enquiry into Maternal and Child Health 2005, 2007a, b; National Institute for Health and Clinical Excellence 2008).

However, there may be complications for the fetus and in the newborn. Some neonatal complications are not specific to diabetes in pregnancy, but relate to being born preterm or by caesarean section (Confidential Enquiry into Maternal and Child Health 2005; Hawdon 2010) and are covered elswhere in this book. These will be minimised by careful consideration of timing of delivery, maternal steroid administration prior to preterm delivery and reduced rate of unnecessary caesarean sections. Other complications are secondary to the abnormal metabolic environment of the fetus and ongoing disturbances postnatally and are more specific to diabetes in pregnancy (Table 22.1). Of women who have prepregnancy diabetes, approximately one-third have type 2 diabetes, and the incidence and nature of complications do not vary according to type of diabetes (Confidential Enquiry into Maternal and Child Health 2005; Bell et al. 2008). Adequate antenatal screening and assessment should identify the pregnancies at greatest risk so that a management plan may be made, and the baby should be born in a centre where there are staff trained to manage unexpected complications.

Before discussing the aetiology and management of the fetal and neonatal complications of maternal diabetes, it is appropriate to be reminded of Farquhar's vivid and classic description of babies born after diabetes in pregnancy (Farquhar 1959):

> They emerge at least alive from within the fiery metabolic furnace of diabetes mellitus, but they resemble one another so closely that they might well be related. They are plump, sleek, liberally coated with vernix caseosa, full-faced and plethoric. During their first two or more extrauterine hours they lie on their backs, bloated and flushed, their legs flexed and abducted, their lightly closed hands on each side of the head, the abdomen prominent and their respiration sighing. They convey a distinct impression of having such a surfeit of both food and fluid pressed upon them by an insistent hostess that they desire only peace so that they may recover from their excesses.

© 2012 Elsevier Ltd

Table 22.1 Neonatal outcomes in the UK

	CEMACH COHORT	UK	RATE RATIO
Neonatal death	9.3/1000	3.6/1000	2.6
Preterm delivery	37%	7.3%	5
Congenital anomaly	5.5%	2.1%	2.6
Birthweight >90th centile	52%	10%	5.2
Shoulder dystocia	7.9%	3%	2.6
Erb's palsy	4.5/1000	0.42/1000	11
Apgar <7 at 5 min	2.6%	0.76%	3.4
Admission NNU	56%	10%	5.6
Term admission SC	33%	10%	3.3

NNU, any admission to a neonatal unit, all levels of care; SC, admission of a term baby to a neonatal unit, special care only: 67.1% of these were assessed to be avoidable.
Data from Confidential Enquiry into Maternal and Child Health (CEMACH) survey (2005).

Congenital abnormalities

Despite major improvements in the care of diabetes in pregnancy, there has been little overall change in the incidence of congenital anomalies (Molsted-Pedersen et al. 1964; Casson et al. 1997; Confidential Enquiry into Maternal and Child Health 2005; Hawdon 2010). Congenital anomalies in the offspring of women with diabetes occur with a frequency up to 10 times that observed in the general population. Congenital anomalies (along with intrapartum causes) now account for a large proportion of perinatal losses and have replaced respiratory distress syndrome (RDS) as the leading cause of perinatal loss (Damm and Molsted-Pedersen 1989; Casson et al. 1997; Confidential Enquiry into Maternal and Child Health 2005, 2007a).

The cause of diabetic embryopathy is not fully understood. Genetic factors (diabetes-related genes) are unlikely to play a role, as the incidence of birth defects is not increased in babies of fathers with diabetes (Comess et al. 1969). Also, insulin cannot be teratogenic, because the human placenta is impermeable to insulin at early gestation (Adam et al. 1969) and fetal pancreatic β cells are not present before the 10th week (Like and Orci 1972). It is likely that congenital anomalies are related to the diabetic intrauterine environment during the period of organogenesis, before the seventh week of gestation (Mills et al. 1979). Therefore, most occur before the pregnancy is recognised and the intensified diabetes treatment is initiated. Possible contributory factors are hyperglycaemia (Freinkel 1988; Miodovnik et al. 1988), hyperketonaemia (Horton and Sadler 1983; Sadler et al. 1989), increased levels of somatomedin-inhibiting factors (Sadler et al. 1986), decreased myoinositol concentration in the neuroectoderm (Sussman and Matschinsky 1988) and disturbances in the secretion of relaxin, an insulin homologue (Edwards and Newall 1988). Finally, hypoglycaemia can also be embryotoxic in experimental animals (Buchanan et al. 1986) but data from human studies are reassuring (Miodovnik et al. 1988).

Anomalies overrepresented in pregnancies complicated by diabetes are caudal regression syndrome (Passarge and Lenz 1966;

Coombs and Kitzmuiller 1991), neural tube defects, holoprosencephaly (Barr et al. 1983), vertebral dysplasia, congenital heart disease, ventricular septal defect, transposition of the great vessels and small left colon syndrome (Philippart et al. 1975; Confidential Enquiry into Maternal and Child Health 2005).

It is clear that efforts to prevent birth defects should start before conception, with contraceptive advice offered so that every pregnancy can be planned in advance with optimum periconceptual metabolic control. Some reports suggest that early first-trimester improvement in glycaemic control (Fuhrmann et al. 1983; Edwards and Newall 1988; Diabetes Control and Complications Trial Research Group 1993) combined with prenatal diagnosis of anomalies using serum α-fetoprotein determinations and ultrasound scanning (Molsted-Pedersen and Pedersen 1985) could reduce the impact of congenital anomalies.

Obstetricians and neonatologists must ensure that there has been adequate counselling of parents, involving the specialist team who will care for the baby postnatally, and that delivery takes place at an appropriate centre (dependent on the nature of the anomaly) to enable early access to specialist care. Routine postnatal echocardiography to screen for congenital heart anomalies is not indicated, unless an abnormality has been suspected on antenatal scanning or the baby presents with clinical signs of congenital heart disease (National Institute for Health and Clinical Excellence 2008).

Macrosomia

'Macrosomic' and 'large-for-gestational-age' are not interchangeable terms. Macrosomia describes a baby who is heavier than his or her genetically determined birthweight and the clinical appearance of a baby who has had somatic growth in excess over head growth, and thus may be present in a baby of 'normal' birthweight.

Macrosomia and organomegaly attributed to fetal hyperinsulinaemia are well-known characteristics of pregnancy complicated by diabetes (Confidential Enquiry into Maternal and Child Health 2005; Hawdon 2010). Glucose crosses the placenta by facilitated diffusion, therefore maternal hyperglycaemia imposes a carbohydrate surplus on the fetus. The fetus responds with increased secretion of insulin. Because insulin is an anabolic hormone the fetal hyperinsulinaemia stimulates protein, lipid and glycogen synthesis to cause macrosomia. Although this classic maternal hyperglycaemia–fetal hyperinsulinism theory of Pedersen (1954) is widely accepted, the metabolic and endocrine disturbances are much more complex. For example, free amino acids also have a stimulatory effect on the development of the β cell, and the anabolic actions of insulin, in utero at least, could in part be mediated through the insulin-induced release of insulin-like growth factors (Milner 1988). In addition, birthweight is positively correlated with maternal concentrations of triglycerides and free fatty acids (Knopp et al. 1992).

Rates of macrosomia vary between centres; for example, from only 8% with birthweights above the 90th centile in an Italian study of strict maternal diabetic control to 52% with birthweights above the 90th centile in the recent UK cohort (Roversi et al. 1979; Hawthorne et al. 1997; Confidential Enquiry into Maternal and Child Health 2005). There is no direct relationship between overall maternal diabetes control and macrosomia (Bradley et al. 1988) – some babies are born with macrosomia after a pregnancy in which maternal blood glucose levels were well controlled. The reason for this may include the fact that glucose level is not the only parameter describing optimal diabetic control in pregnancy. However associations of birthweight with maternal glucose levels (even when not excessively raised) and cord blood C peptide levels have been

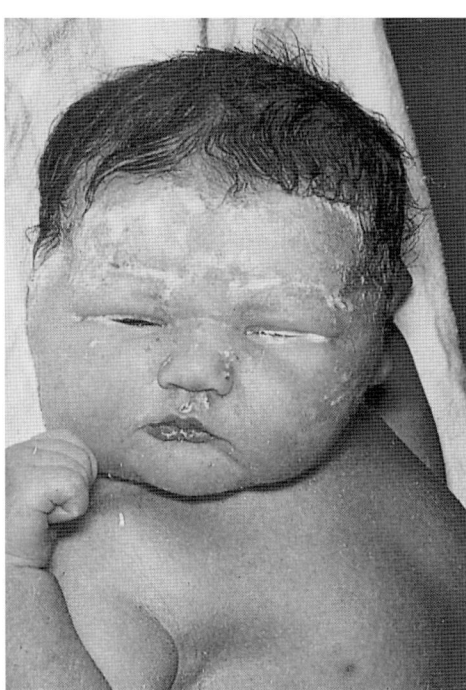

Fig. 22.1 An infant born after poor control of maternal diabetes. There is increased adiposity and facial plethora, together with respiratory distress.

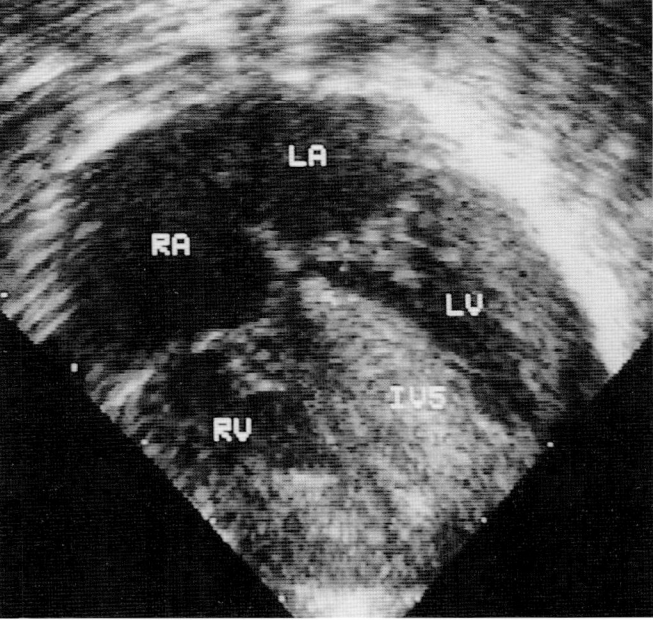

Fig. 22.2 Echocardiographic image of a four-chamber view of a neonatal heart, demonstrating hypertrophy of the intraventricular septum (IVS) secondary to fetal hyperinsulinism. RA, right atrium; LA, left atrium; RV, right ventricle; LV, left ventricle.

reported. Enhanced control of even mild gestational diabetes is associated with reduced fetal overgrowth and risk of shoulder dystocia (Hod et al. 1996; Mello et al. 2000; HAPO Study Cooperative Research Group 2008; Landon et al. 2009).

The striking physical appearance (Fig. 22.1) of macrosomic infants has already been described. Much of the increased mass is fat (Whitelaw 1977). The organomegaly is selective, the liver and heart are often enlarged and skeletal length is increased in proportion to weight, but the brain size is not increased relative to gestational age and so the head may appear disproportionately small (Naeye 1965).

The clinical significance of macrosomia is the risk of the complications of delivery of a large infant, such as shoulder dystocia, obstructed labour, perinatal asphyxia and birth injury (e.g. brachial plexus injury or fractured clavicle or humerus) (Acker et al. 1985; Mimouni et al. 1988; Confidential Enquiry into Maternal and Child Health 2005).

Finally, parents and health professionals must be prepared for 'catch-down' in postnatal growth of macrosomic babies, especially when breastfed. This is a normal and healthy adaptation and, provided the baby appears to be feeding well and is healthy, there should be no concern if there is an initial period of slow weight gain such that weight crosses down centile lines (Owen et al. 2006, 2008).

Hypertrophic cardiomyopathy

Cardiac enlargement and hypertrophy in babies of diabetic mothers were reported as early as 1944 (Miller et al. 1944). The condition has now been studied more extensively (Soltész et al. 1978). Improved echocardiographic techniques have shown a generalized myocardial hypertrophy with a disproportionate thickening of the septum (Mace et al. 1979; Reller and Kaplan 1988; Veille et al.

1992). Symptomatic infants generally have severe hypertrophy with hypertrophied septal muscles bulging into the left ventricle, thereby narrowing the left ventricular outflow tract (Fig. 22.2). Although the condition is transient it may cause fetal or neonatal death (McMahon et al. 1990; Sardesai et al. 2001). The cardiomyopathy has been related to maternal diabetes control (Mace et al. 1979; Reller and Kaplan 1988) and to fetal and neonatal hyperinsulinaemia (Breitweser et al. 1980). Resolution of the signs can be expected in 2–4 weeks, and the septal hypertrophy regresses within 2–12 months (Way et al. 1979; Reller and Kaplan 1988) (see also Ch. 28).

If clinical signs occur, the presentation is usually within the first weeks of postnatal life with cardiorespiratory distress and congestive heart failure. Systolic ejection murmurs can be heard in most affected infants, and chest radiography reveals cardiomegaly (Way et al. 1979). The majority of the infants need supportive care only. If congestive heart failure develops, propranolol is recommended. (Way et al. 1979). Digitalis and other positive inotropic agents are generally contraindicated because they increase systolic contraction and may exacerbate the outflow tract obstruction (Way et al. 1979).

Intrauterine growth restriction

Maternal vascular disease may complicate diabetes and lead to placental insufficiency and impaired fetal growth, so some infants will be born small-for-gestational-age (Cordero and Landon 1993). Overzealous diabetic control and maternal hypoglycaemia may have the same result (Langer et al. 1989). The small-for-gestational-age infant of the diabetic mother appears to be at even greater risk of adverse outcome, especially neurodevelopmental sequelae (Petersen et al. 1998), because the perinatal problems associated with diabetes in pregnancy are compounded by those of intrauterine malnutrition (see Ch. 10).

Effects of antenatal and intrapartum hypoxia–ischaemia

Stillbirth, encephalopathy, hyperviscosity, polycythaemia, jaundice

The mechanism for increased risk of significant fetal hypoxia–ischaemia during diabetes in pregnancy is not fully understood. In the UK cohort of diabetes in pregnancy, 10% of perinatal deaths were related to intrapartum causes (Confidential Enquiry into Maternal and Child Health 2005, 2007a). In addition, there will be many babies affected by intrapartum hypoxia–ischaemia born alive and requiring expert resuscitation. This is one of the reasons why delivery after diabetes in pregnancy must occur in units where expert advanced neonatal life support is available. If a neonate has unexpected and severe complications of hypoxia–ischaemia the baby will require transfer to a neonatal unit which provides intensive care, if this is not available in the hospital of birth. As total body cooling becomes an established treatment for hypoxic-ischaemic encephalopathy, transfer for this treatment at a specialist centre should be considered (Jacobs et al. 2007).

Infants born after diabetes in pregnancy have an increased risk of being polycythaemic and developing neonatal hyperviscosity syndrome (Mimouni et al. 1986). Normoblastaemia and extensive extramedullary erythropoiesis were observed as early as 1944 (Miller et al. 1944) and the aetiology of the increased erythropoiesis has since been described (Phillips et al. 1982). Elevated umbilical plasma erythropoietin concentrations have been correlated directly with plasma insulin levels in both infants of diabetic mothers (IDMs) and controls (Widness et al. 1981). The raised erythropoietin levels are thought to be secondary to relative cellular hypoxia, which is the result of insulin-induced high glucose uptake and high metabolic rate. A more direct effect of insulin was shown in another study in which insulin stimulated growth in culture of late erythroid progenitors in cord blood from premature infants, term infants and IDM (Perrine et al. 1986).

Lysis of this red cell load contributes to the prolonged unconjugated hyperbilirubinaemia often found in IDMs. There may also be functional immaturity of hepatic enzymes (Stevenson et al. 1981).

Renal vein thrombosis and thrombosis in other vessels, which has been reported to occur with increased frequency in IDMs, is probably related to polycythaemia and hyperviscosity (Avery et al. 1957).

Polycythaemia and hyperbilirubinaemia should be managed as described elsewhere in this book.

Respiratory complications

Although the incidence of RDS was previously reported to be 5–6 times higher after diabetes in pregnancy than in the normal population, this incidence is falling in line with improved control of diabetes and prevention of preterm delivery (Hanson and Persson 1993). Rarely, babies born after diabetes in pregnancy have typical RDS despite a normal lecithin–sphingomyelin ratio in the amniotic fluid. This may be because RDS is secondary to the retarded maturation of the pulmonary surfactant system, including surfactant proteins (Carlson et al. 1984; Nogee et al. 1988; Gewolb 1993), rather than simply to the reduced production of phospholipids. Animal studies have demonstrated that insulin inhibits cortisol-induced lecithin synthesis by pneumocytes, probably by inhibiting the production of fibroblast–pneumocyte factor, which promotes phosphatidylcholine synthesis (Smith et al. 1975). It has also been

demonstrated that butyrate inhibits the transcription of mRNA for surfactant proteins (Peterec et al. 1994).

There is also an increased risk for transient tachypnoea of the newborn (Hanson and Persson 1993) or respiratory distress associated with cardiac abnormalities. Finally, many babies are delivered before term and/or by caesarean section, and the contribution of these factors to increased respiratory morbidity from RDS or transient tachypnoea of the newborn must be considered (Morrison et al. 1995). The management of these respiratory complications, should they occur, should be as recommended elsewhere in this book.

Hypocalcaemia and hypomagnesaemia

Neonatal hypocalcaemia has been reported in up to 50% of babies born after diabetes in pregnancy (Tsang et al. 1972; Mimouni et al. 1986) and both its incidence and severity appear to be related to diabetes control (Tsang et al. 1972; Demaini et al. 1994). Hypocalcaemia is usually associated with hyperphosphataemia and occasionally with hypomagnesaemia. The aetiology is not entirely clear, but neonatal hypoparathyroidism has been demonstrated and may in part be secondary to maternal magnesium loss (Mimouni et al. 1989; Demaini et al. 1994; Martinez et al. 1994). Perinatal hypoxia–ischaemia may also exacerbate hypocalcaemia.

No published study has commented upon the clinical significance of hypocalcaemia or hypomagnasenia. Usually no clinical signs are seen and no treatment is necessary.

Disordered postnatal metabolic adaptation (see Ch. 34.1)

Almost all babies, regardless of circumstances of pregnancy, manifest a period (of some hours postnatally) of asymptomatic hypoglycaemia before a spontaneous increase in blood glucose level occurs. This is more prolonged or becomes clinically significant for some babies born after diabetes in pregnancy (Persson 2009). However, all regain normal blood glucose control within the first few days after birth. For the full definition and symptoms of hypoglycaemia, see Ch. 34.1. It is likely that plasma insulin levels fall to normal within 12–24 hours of birth in all infants except those whose mothers' diabetes was poorly controlled (Hawdon and Aynsley-Green 1996). Where maternal blood glucose levels are raised but below the diagnostic level for diabetes, there is only a marginal and barely significant relationship between maternal fasting blood glucose levels and incidence of neonatal hypoglycaemia (HAPO Study Cooperative Research Group 2008).

Hyperinsulinism at birth is the result of increased placental transfer of glucose and other nutrients stimulating increased fetal insulin secretion (see above) (Block et al. 1974). The pancreas shows hyperplasia and hypertrophy of the islets of Langerhans (Miller et al. 1944; Cardell 1953) without evidence of pancreatic pathology. An increase of the glucagon and pancreatic polypeptide cell fractions in the pancreas has also been shown by immunocytochemical methods (Miller et al. 1944) and a counterregulatory hormone response has been demonstrated which is likely to curtail the period of hypoglycaemia (Milner et al. 1981; Broberger et al. 1984; Hertel and Kuhl 1986). However, it has been reported that some infants fail to develop the normal increase in plasma glucagon at 2–4 hours of age (Bloom and Johnston 1972).

The effect of hyperinsulinism on the liver has been confirmed using stable isotope methods (Kalhan et al. 1977) which demonstrated decreased glucose production. If raised insulin levels persist beyond the first postnatal day, other metabolic fuels may be affected. For example, in theory plasma free fatty acid and blood ketone body concentrations may be lower than in normal term infants, although clinical studies have not confirmed this (Patel and Kalhan 1992). Plasma amino acid concentrations are less affected than in organic hyperinsulinism secondary to congenital pancreatic disorders. The characteristic low blood levels of branched-chain amino acids are a not invariable finding (Vejtorp et al. 1977; Soltész et al. 1978), possibly because of other transient disturbances in postnatal metabolic adaptation, including the effects of concurrent asphyxia or hypoxia.

Management must be with the aim of balancing the risks of prolonged and severe hypoglycaemia against the effects of over-intrusive practices, such as unnnecessary separation of mother and baby or formula supplementation (Confidential Enquiry into Maternal and Child Health 2007b; National Institute for Health and Clinical Excellence 2008; Hawdon 2010).

Those caring for the baby must regularly monitor the baby for abnormal feeding behaviour and neurological signs, and must document their findings. If at any stage there are abnormal clinical signs, the blood glucose level must be measured and an urgent paediatric review arranged. It is UK national guidance that IDMs should have regular blood glucose monitoring (National Institute for Health and Clinical Excellence 2008). Blood glucose screening may be discontinued when at least two consecutive prefeed blood glucose levels are satisfactory and the baby remains well (see Ch. 34.1).

In the healthy baby, blood glucose monitoring should not commence before 3–4 hours of age in order to avoid 'false positives' associated with the physiological fall in blood glucose. Measurements should be prefeed. It should be noted that test strip reagents are inaccurate, especially at high packed cell volume (Dacombe et al. 1981). Measurement using an accurate method only occurred in 25% of cases in the UK cohort (Confidential Enquiry into Maternal and Child Health 2005).

Hypoglycaemia is usually prevented by supporting early (within 1–2 hours after birth) and frequent breastfeeding, as it has been shown that a feed of 10 ml/kg human milk can cause an increase of blood glucose of the order of 1 mmol/l at this time (Aynsley-Green and Soltesz 1985). Additional breast milk or formula supplementation should only occur when indicated by clinical signs and low blood glucose levels. There is evidence in other groups of babies that excessive formula supplementation may impair counterregulatory responses so volumes of formula should be kept to the minimum required (de Rooy and Hawdon 2002).

Sick infants unable to tolerate enteral feeding, or those who remain hypoglycaemic despite full enteral feeds, should receive an intravenous infusion of glucose at an initial rate of 5 mg/kg/min (3 ml/kg/h of 10% dextrose) but increasing rapidly if indicated by repeat blood glucose monitoring. Glucose should not be administered at a rate higher than that required to maintain normoglycaemia, in order to avoid continued stimulation of insulin secretion. Rarely, babies with severe and persistent hyperinsulinism require glucose infusions in excess of 10 mg/kg/min. If enteral feeds have been tolerated these should not be reduced when intravenous glucose is commenced. Neurological signs of hypoglycaemia in any infant warrant immediate correction by a bolus injection of 200–400 mg/kg glucose followed by glucose infusion or increased rate of glucose infusion, the rate being adjusted as necessary to maintain normoglycaemia. In other circumstances, boluses should be avoided as increased insulin secretion and rebound hypoglycaemia will result.

A single injection of glucagon (0.03–0.1 mg/kg), which has a temporary hyperglycaemic effect by releasing glucose from glycogen stores, is a useful measure in the event of delay in siting intravenous lines.

Intravenous glucose should be weaned gradually as indicated by blood glucose monitoring. Rebound hypoglycaemia may occur if the glucose infusion is decreased too quickly.

Iatrogenic complications

Preterm delivery or delivery by caesarean section when there is no clear clinical indication places the baby at risk of unnecessary harm (Hawdon 2010). In addition, frequent failings in postnatal care have been reported to have an impact on the baby's course (Confidential Enquiry into Maternal and Child Health 2005, 2007a, b). These included 'routine' admission of babies to neonatal units, 'routine' supplementation or replacement of breastfeeds with formula, delayed 'skin-to-skin' contact and first feed, poor management of temperature control and testing of blood glucose too soon after birth.

Outcome

According to some studies, infants born after pregnancy complicated by diabetes are at greater risk of brain injury, psychomotor delay, subtle neurological abnormalities and electroencephalogram changes. There are a number of risk factors – placental dysfunction, hypoxia–ischaemia, episodes of maternal ketosis or hypoglycaemia during pregnancy and neonatal hypoglycaemia (Haworth et al. 1976; Rizzo et al. 1995; Stenninger et al. 1998). As these are all interdependent variables it is impossible to determine which is the most important factor. For example, both neonatal hypoglycaemia and adverse neurodevelopmental outcome may be comorbidities following aberrant antenatal metabolic control (Stenninger et al. 1997; Silverman et al. 1998; Ornoy et al. 2001). Studies of well-controlled diabetes in pregnancy show a favourable neurodevelopmental outcome (Persson and Gentz 1984; Rizzo et al. 1994; Sells et al. 1994).

Although many studies have shown that on follow-up the majority of children of mothers with diabetes have normal weight for height and normal height for age, in some cases poor antenatal diabetic control and the presence of neonatal macrosomia (and possibly overfeeding in infancy) increase the risk of obesity in later life (Cummins and Norrish 1980; Vohr et al. 1980; Anonymous 1990; Silverman et al. 1998).

The risk of insulin-dependent diabetes developing by the age of 20 years in the offspring of women with diabetes is at least seven times that for non-diabetic parents, and later impaired glucose tolerance is associated with aberrant diabetic control during pregnancy (Persson and Gentz 1984; Silverman et al. 1998). Interestingly, this is only one-third of the risk reported for the offspring of fathers with insulin-dependent diabetes (Warram et al. 1984) and this is possibly because of a lower rate of DR4 allele transmission from mothers or an effect of programming by the intrauterine environment (Field 1988).

Avoiding harm

Careful medical and obstetric care to achieve strict glycaemic control throughout pregnancy, in combination with appropriate neonatal care, greatly reduces the risk of the many complications discussed in this chapter. The vast majority of infants of mothers who achieved good diabetic control are of normal size and postnatal metabolic adaptation is normal (King et al. 1982). Therefore it is important to avoid iatrogenic problems such as needless separation of mothers and babies, or practices which impede successful breastfeeding. All hospitals must have written protocols for the prevention and management of potential neonatal complications, including

hypoglycaemia, and for admission to the neonatal unit (National Institute for Health and Clinical Excellence 2008). Unless there are risk factors for other complications (e.g. infection) and as long as the baby appears well, it is not necessary to monitor vital signs (temperature, pulse, respiration rate) or to screen for other potential complications, e.g. polycythaemia (National Institute for Health and Clinical Excellence 2008).

References

Acker, D.B., Sachs, B.P., Friedman, E.A., 1985. Risk factors for shoulder dystocia. Obstet Gynecol 66, 762–768.

Adam, P.A.J., Teramo, K., Raiha, N., et al., 1969. Human fetal insulin metabolism early in gestation. Response to acute elevation of the fetal glucose concentration and placental transfer of human insulin. Diabetes 18, 403–416.

Anonymous, 1990. Hyperinsulinaemia and macrosomia. N Engl J Med 323, 340–342.

Avery, M.E., Oppenheimer, E.H., Gordon, H.H., 1957. Renal vein thrombosis in newborn infants of diabetic mothers. N Engl J Med 256, 1134–1138.

Aynsley-Green, A., Soltesz, G., 1985. Hypoglycaemia in infancy and childhood. Curr Rev Paediatr 1, 54–58.

Barr, M., Hanson, J.W., Currey, K., et al., 1983. Holoprosencephaly in infants of diabetic mothers. J Pediatr 102, 565–568.

Bell, R., Bailey, K., Cresswell, T., et al., 2008. Trends in prevalence and outcomes of pregnancy in women with pre-existing type I and type II diabetes. Br J Obstet Gynaecol 115, 445–452.

Block, M.B., Pildes, R.S., Mossabhoy, N.A., et al., 1974. C-peptide immunoreactivity: a new method for studying infants of insulin-treated diabetic mothers. Pediatrics 53, 923–928.

Bloom, S.R., Johnston, D.F., 1972. Failure of glucagon release in infants of diabetic mothers. BMJ iv, 453–454.

Bradley, R.J., Nicolaides, K.H., Brudenell, J.M., 1988. Are all infants of diabetic mothers 'macrosomic'? BMJ 297, 1583–1584.

Breitweser, J.A., Meyer, R.A., Sperling, M.A., et al., 1980. Cardiac septal hypertrophy in hyperinsulinaemic infants. J Pediatr 96, 535–539.

Broberger, U., Hansson, U., Largercrantz, H., et al., 1984. Sympathoadrenal activity and metabolic adjustment during the first 12 hours after birth in infants of diabetic mothers. Acta Paediatr Scand 73, 620–625.

Buchanan, T.A., Schemmer, J.K., Freinkel, N., 1986. Embryotoxic effects of brief maternal insulin hypoglycaemia during organogenesis in the rat. J Clin Invest 78, 643–649.

Cardell, B.S., 1953. Hypertrophy and hyperplasia of the pancreatic islets in newborn infants. Pathology 66, 335–341.

Carlson, K.S., Smith, B.T., Post, M., 1984. Insulin acts on the fibroblast to inhibit glucocorticoid stimulation of lung maturation. J Appl Physiol 57, 1577–1579.

Casson, I.F., Clarke, C.A., Howard, C.V., et al., 1997. Outcomes of pregnancy in insulin dependent diabetic women: results of a five year population cohort study. BMJ 315, 275–278.

Comess, L.J., Bennett, P.H., Man, M.B., et al., 1969. Congenital anomalies and diabetes in the Pima Indians of Arizona. Diabetes 18, 471–477.

Confidential Enquiry into Maternal and Child Health, 2005. Pregnancy in Women with Type 1 and Type 2 Diabetes in 2002–2003. CEMACH, London.

Confidential Enquiry into Maternal and Child Health, 2007a. Diabetes in Pregnancy: Are We Providing the Best Care? Findings of a National Enquiry. CEMACH, London.

Confidential Enquiry into Maternal and Child Health, 2007b. Diabetes in Pregnancy: Caring for the Baby after Birth. Findings of a National Enquiry. CEMACH, London.

Coombs, C.A., Kitzmuiller, J.C., 1991. Spontaneous abortion and congenital malformation in diabetes. Clin Obstet Gynecol 5, 315–331.

Cordero, L., Landon, M.B., 1993. Infant of the diabetic mother. Clin Perinatol 20, 635–648.

Cummins, M., Norrish, M., 1980. Follow-up of children of diabetic mothers. Arch Dis Child 55, 259–264.

Dacombe, C.M., Dalton, R.G., Goldie, D.F., et al., 1981. Effect of packed cell volume on blood glucose estimations. Arch Dis Child 56, 789–791.

Damm, P., Molsted-Pedersen, L., 1989. Significant decrease in congenital malformations in newborn infants of an unselected population of diabetic mothers. Am J Obstet Gynecol 161, 1163–1167.

Demaini, S., Mimouni, F., Tsang, R.C., et al., 1994. Impact of metabolic control of diabetes during pregnancy on neonatal hypocalcaemia: a randomized study. Obstet Gynecol 83, 918–922.

de Rooy, L.J., Hawdon, J.M., 2002. Nutritional factors that affect the postnatal metabolic adaptation of full-term

small- and large-for-gestational-age infants. Pediatrics 109 (3), E42.

Diabetes Control and Complications Trial Research Group, 1993. The effect of intensive treatment of diabetes on the development and progression of long term complications in insulin dependent diabetes mellitus. N Engl J Med 329, 977–986.

Edwards, J.R.G., Newall, D.R., 1988. Relaxin as an aetiological factor in diabetic embryopathy. Lancet i, 1428–1430.

Farquhar, J.W., 1959. The child of a diabetic woman. Arch Dis Child 34, 76–96.

Field, L.L., 1988. Insulin-dependent diabetes mellitus: a model for the study of multifactorial disorders. Am J Hum Genet 43, 793–798.

Freinkel, N., 1988. Diabetic embryopathy and fuel-mediated organ teratogenesis: lessons from animal models. Horm Metab Res 20, 463–475.

Fuhrmann, K., Reicher, H., Semmler, K., et al., 1983. Prevention of congenital malformations in infants of insulin-dependent diabetic mothers. Diabetes Care 6, 213–223.

Gewolb, I.H., 1993. High glucose causes delayed fetal lung maturation in vitro. Exp Lung Res 19, 619–630.

Hanson, U., Persson, B., 1993. Outcome of pregnancies complicated by type I insulin dependent diabetes in Sweden: acute pregnancy complications, neonatal mortality and morbidity. Am J Perinatol 10, 330–333.

HAPO Study Cooperative Research Group, 2008. Hyperglycemia and adverse pregnancy outcomes. N Engl J Med 358, 1991–2002.

Hawdon, J.M., 2010. Care of the neonate. In: McCance, D.R., Maresh, M., Sacks, D.A., (Eds.), Practical Management of Diabetes. Wiley-Blackwell, Oxford.

Hawdon, J.M., Aynsley-Green, A., 1996. Neonatal complications, including hypoglycaemia. In: Dornhorst, A., Hadden D., (Eds.), Diabetes and Pregnancy: An International Approach to Diagnosis and Management. Wiley, Chichester, pp. 303–318.

Haworth, J.C., McRae, K.N., Dilling, L.A., 1976. Prognosis of infants of diabetic mothers in relation to neonatal hypoglycaemia. Dev Med Child Neurol 18, 471–479.

Hawthorne, G., Robson, S., Ryall, E.A., et al., 1997. Prospective population based survey of outcome of pregnancy in diabetic women: results of the Northern Diabetic Pregnancy Audit, 1994. BMJ 315, 279–281.

Hertel, J., Kuhl, C., 1986. Metabolic adaptation during the neonatal period in infants of diabetic mothers. Acta Endocrinol 277 (suppl), 136–140.

Hod, M., Rabinerson, D., Kaplan, B., et al., 1996. Perinatal complications following gestational diabetes mellitus how 'sweet' is ill? Acta Obstet Gynecol Scand 75, 809–815.

Horton, Jr., W.E., Sadler, T.W., 1983. Effects of maternal diabetes on early embryogenesis: alterations in morphogenesis produced by ketone body, beta-hydroxybutrate. Diabetes 32, 610–616.

Hunter, D.J.S., 1992. Diabetes in pregnancy. In: Chalmers, I., Enkin, M., Keirse, M.J.N.C. (Eds.), Effective Care in Pregnancy and Childbirth. Oxford University Press, Oxford, pp 579–594.

Jacobs, S., Hunt, R., Tarnow-Mordi, W., et al., 2007. Cooling for newborns with hypoxic ischaemic encephalopathy (review). Cochrane Database Syst Rev (4), CD003311.

Kalhan, S.C., Savin, S.M., Adam, P.A.F., 1977. Attenuated glucose production rate in newborn infants of insulin dependent diabetic mothers. N Engl J Med 296, 375–376.

King, C.K., Tserng, K., Kalhan, S.C., 1982. Regulation of glucose production in newborn infants of diabetic mothers. Pediatr Res 16, 608–612.

Knopp, R.H., Magee, M.S., Walden, C.E., et al., 1992. Prediction of infant birth weight by GDM screening tests. Importance of plasma triglyceride. Diabetes Care 15, 1605–1613.

Landon, M.B., Spong, C.Y., et al., 2009. A multicenter, randomized trial of treatment for mild getstational diabetes. N Engl J Med 361, 1339–1348.

Langer, O., Levy, J., Brustman, C., 1989. Glycemic control in gestational diabetes mellitus – how tight is tight enough: small for gestational age versus large for gestational age? Am J Obstet Gynecol 161, 646–653.

Like, A., Orci, L., 1972. Embryogenesis of the human pancreatic islets. A light and electron microscopic study. Diabetes 21, 511–534.

Mace, S., Hirschfeld, S.S., Riggs, T., et al., 1979. Echocardiographic abnormalities in infants of diabetic mothers. J Pediatr 95, 1013–1019.

Martinez, M.E., Catalan, P., Lisbona, A., et al., 1994. Serum osteocalcin concentrations in diabetic pregnant women and their newborns. Horm Metab Res 26, 338–342.

McMahon, J.N., Berry, P.J., Joffe, H.S., 1990. Fatal hypertrophic cardiomyopathy in an infant of a diabetic mother. Pediatr Cardiol 11, 211–212.

Mello, G., Parretti, E., Mecacci, F., et al., 2000. What degree of maternal metabolic control in women with type 2 diabetes is associated with normal body soze and proportins in full term infants? Diabetes Care 23, 1494–1498.

Miller, H.C., Johnson, R.D., Durlacher, S.H., 1944. A comparison of newborn infants with erythroblastosis fetalis with those born to diabetic mothers. J Pediatr 24, 603–615.

Mills, J.L., Baker, L., Goldman, A.S., 1979. Malformations in infants of diabetic mothers occur before the seventh gestational week. Diabetes 28, 292–293.

Milner, R.D.G., 1988. Endocrine control of fetal growth. In: Linblad, B.S. (Ed.), Perinatal Nutrition. Academic Press, New York, pp 45–62.

Milner, R.D.G., Wirdham, P.K., Tsanakas, J., 1981. Quantatitive morphology of B, A, D and PP cells in infants of diabetic mothers. Diabetes 30, 271–274.

Mimouni, F., Tsang, R.C., Hertzberg, V.S., et al., 1986. Polycythemia, hypomagnesemia and hypocalcemia in infants of diabetic mothers. Am J Dis Child 140, 798–800.

Mimouni, F., Miodovnik, M., Siddiqi, T.A., et al., 1988. Perinatal asphyxia in infants of insulin-dependent diabetic mothers. J Pediatr 113, 345–353.

Mimouni, F., Tsang, R.C., Hertzberg, V.S., et al., 1989. Parathyroid hormone and calcitriol changes in normal and insulin dependent diabetic pregnancies. Obstet Gynecol 74, 49–54.

Miodovnik, M., Mimouni, F., Dignan, P.S.J., et al., 1988. Major malformations in infants of IDDM women. Vasculopathy and early first-trimester poor glycemic control. Diabetes Care 11, 713–718.

Molsted-Pedersen, L., Pedersen, J.F., 1985. Congenital malformations in diabetic pregnancies. Acta Paediatr Scand suppl. 320, 79–84.

Molsted-Pedersen, L., Tygstrup, I., Pedersen, J., 1964. Congenital malformations in newborn infants of diabetic women. Lancet i, 1124–1126.

Morrison, J.J., Rennie, J.M., Milton, P.J.D., 1995. Neonatal respiratory morbidity and timing of elective caesarean section at term. Br J Obstet Gynaecol 102, 101–106.

Naeye, R.L., 1965. Infants of diabetic mothers: a quantitive, morphologic study. Pediatrics 35, 980–988.

National Collaborating Centre for Primary Care, 2006. Postnatal Care: Routine Postnatal Care of Women and their Babies. NICE, London, http://www.nice.org.uk/Guidance/CG37.

National Institute for Health and Clinical Excellence. 2008. Diabetes in Pregnancy. NICE, London.

Nogee, L., McMahan, M., Whitsett, J.A., 1988. Hyaline membrane disease and surfactant protein, SAP-35, in diabetes in pregnancy. Am J Perinatol 5, 374–377.

Ornoy, A., Ratzon, N., Greenbaum, C., et al., 2001. School-age children born to diabetic mothers and to mothers with gestational diabetes exhibit a high rate of inattention and fine gross motor impairment. J Paediatr Endocrinol Metab 14 (suppl 1), 681–689.

Owen, C.G., Martin, R.M., Whincup, R.H., et al., 2006. Does breastfeeding influence risk of type 2 diabetes in later life? A quantitative analysis of published evidence. Am J Clin Nutr 84, 1043–1054.

Owen, C.G., Whincup, P.H., Kaye, S.J., et al., 2008. Does initial breastfeeding lead to lower blood cholesterol in adult life? A quantitative review of the evidence. Am J Clin Nutr 88, 305–314.

Passarge, E., Lenz, W., 1966. Syndrome of caudal regression in infants of diabetic mothers: observation of further cases. Pediatrics 37, 672–675.

Patel, D., Kalhan, S., 1992. Glycerol metabolism and triglyceride–fatty acid cycling in the human newborn: effect of maternal diabetes and intrauterine growth retardation. Pediatr Res 31, 52–58.

Pedersen, J., 1954. Weight and length at birth of infants of diabetic mothers. Acta Endocrinol 16, 330–341.

Perrine, S.P., Greene, M.F., Lee, P.D.K., et al., 1986. Insulin stimulates cord blood erythroid progenitor growth: Evidence for an aetiological role in neonatal polycythemia. Br J Haematol 64, 503–511.

Persson, B., 2009. Neonatal glucose metabolism in offspring of mothers with varying degrees of hyperglycaemia during pregnancy. Semin Fetal Neonatal Med 14, 106–110.

Persson, B., Gentz, J., 1984. Follow-up of children of insulin-dependent and gestational diabetic mothers. Neuropsychological outcome. Acta Paediatr Scand 73, 343–358.

Peterec, S.M., Nichols, K.V., Dynia, D.W., et al., 1994. Butyrate modulates surfactant protein m RNA in fetal rat lung by altering mRNA transcription and stability. Am J Physiol 267, L9–15.

Petersen, M.B., Pedersen, S.A., Greisen, G., et al., 1998. Early growth delay in diabetic pregnancy: relation to psychomotor development at age 4. BMJ 296, 598–600.

Philippart, A.J., Reed, O.J., Georgeson, K.E., 1975. Neonatal small left colon syndrome: intramural not intraluminal obstruction. J Pediatr Surg 10, 733–739.

Phillips, A.F., Dubin, J.W., Malty, P.J., et al., 1982. Antenatal hypoxaemia and hyperinsulinaemia in the chronically hyperglycaemic fetal lamb. Pediatr Res 16, 653–658.

Reller, M.D., Kaplan, S., 1988. Hypertrophic cardiomyopathy in infants of diabetic mothers: an update. Am J Perinatol 5, 353–358.

Rizzo, T.A., Ogata, E.S., Dolley, S.L., et al., 1994. Perinatal complications and cognitive developemnt in 2 to 5-year-old children of diabetic mothers. Am J Obstet Gynecol 171, 706–713.

Rizzo, T.A., Dooley, S.L., Metzger, B.E., et al., 1995. Prenatal and perinatal influences on longterm psychomotor development in offspring of diabetic mothers. Am J Obstet Gynecol 173, 1753–1758.

Roversi, G.D., Garguilo, M., Nicolini, U., et al., 1979. A new approach to the treatment of diabetic pregnant women. Am J Obstet Gynecol 135, 567–576.

Sadler, T.W., Phillips, L.S., Balkan, W., et al., 1986. Somatostatin inhibitors from diabetic rat serum after birth and development of mouse embryos in culture. Diabetes 35, 861–865.

Sadler, T.W., Hunter, II, E.S., Wynn, R.E., et al., 1989. Evidence for multifactorial origin of diabetes-induced embryopathies. Diabetes 38, 70–74.

Sardesai, M.G., Gray, A.A., McGrath, M.M., et al., 2001. Fatal hypertrophic cardiomyopathy in the fetus of a woman with diabetes. Obstet Gynecol 98, 925–927.

Sells, C.J., Robinson, N.M., Brown, Z., et al., 1994. Longterm developmental follow up of infants of diabetic mothers. J Pediatr 125, s9–s17.

Silverman, B.L., Rizzo, T.A., Cho, N.H., et al., 1998. Long term effects of the intrauterine environment. The Northwestern University Diabetes in Pregnancy Center. Diabetes Care 21 (suppl 2), b142–b149.

Smith, B.T., Giroud, C.J.P., Robert, M., et al., 1975. Insulin antagonism of cortisol action on lecithin synthesis by cultured fetal lung cells. J Pediatr 87, 953–955.

Soltész, G., Schultz, K., Mestyan, G., et al., 1978. Blood glucose and plasma free amino acid concentrations in infants of diabetic mothers. Pediatrics 61, 77–82.

Stenninger, E., Schollin, J., Aman, J., 1997. Early postnatal hypoglycaemia in newborn infants of diabetic mothers. Acta Paediatr 86, 1374–1376.

Stenninger, E., Flink, R., Eriksson, B., et al., 1998. Long-term neurological dysfunction and neonatal hypoglycaemia after diabetic pregnancy. Arch Dis Child 79, F174–F179.

Stevenson, D.K., Ostrander, C.R., Hopper, A.O., et al., 1981. Pulmonary excretion of carbon monoxide as an index of bilirubin production. II a. Evidence for possible delayed clearance of bilirubin in infants of diabetic mothers. J Pediatr 98, 822–824.

Sussman, I., Matschinsky, F.M., 1988. Diabetes affects sorbitol and myoinositol levels of neuroectodermal tissue during embryogenesis in rats. Diabetes 37, 974–981.

Tsang, R.C., Kleinman, L.I., Sutherland, J.M., et al., 1972. Hypocalcaemia in infants of diabetic mothers: studies in calcium, phosphorus and magnesium metabolism and parathormone responsiveness. J Pediatr 80, 384–395.

Veille, J.C., Sivakoff, M., Hanson, R., et al., 1992. Interventricular septal thickness in fetuses of diabetic mothers. Obstet Gynecol 79, 51–54.

Vejtorp, M., Pedersen, F., Klebbe, F.G., et al., 1977. Low concentration of plasma amino acids in newborn babies of diabetic mothers. Acta Paediatr Scand 66, 53–58.

Vohr, B.R., Lipsitt, L.P., Oh, W., 1980. Somatic growth of children of diabetic mothers with reference to birth size. J Pediatr 97, 196–199.

Warram, J.H., Krolewski, A.S., Gottlieb, M.S., et al., 1984. Differences in risk of insulin dependent diabetes in offspring of diabetic mothers and diabetic fathers. N Engl J Med 311, 149–152.

Way, G.L., Wolfe, R.R., Eshaghpour, E., et al., 1979. The natural history of hypertrophic cardiomyopathy in infants of diabetic mothers. J Pediatr 95, 1020–1026.

Whitelaw, A., 1977. Subcutaneous fat in newborn infants of diabetic mothers: an indication of quality of diabetic control. Lancet i, 15–18.

Widness, J.A., Susa, J.B., Garcia, J.F., et al., 1981. Increased erythropoiesis and elevated erythropoietin in infants born to diabetic mothers and in hyperinsulinemic rhesus fetuses. J Clin Invest 67, 637–642.

Twins 23

Edile Murdoch   Gordon Smith

CHAPTER CONTENTS

Epidemiology

Estimates of the incidence of twin conceptions are hampered by the unknown number of abortions and early fetal deaths that occur in multiple pregnancies. Ultrasound studies in early pregnancy sometimes reveal the death and later reabsorption of one fetus in the first trimester – the vanishing twin syndrome (Landy et al. 1986; Pharoah et al. 2001). Thus, the prevalence of twins at a certain time is all that can be accurately estimated. Furthermore, some multiple births may not be recorded if a pair, one stillborn and one liveborn, are delivered before 24 weeks' gestation. The stillborn would be registered as an abortion and the liveborn baby appears in the records as a single birth.

The incidence of multiple births has steadily increased in the developing countries since the early 1980s (Imaizumi 1997; Kiely and Kiely 2001). In England and Wales it rose from 9.0/1000 births in 1980 to 14.8/1000 in 2001. The incidence has been stable since then, although it has markedly increased among women aged 45 and above (Fig. 23.1). The incidence of triplets rose much faster still until 1998, quadrupling in 15 years. It subsequently declined and in 2008 the rate in England and Wales was 2.4 per 10 000 maternities (Office for National Statistics, Birth Statistics 2008).

The increase in multiple births is partly due to assisted reproductive technology (ART), such as ovulation induction and multiple embryo transfer in vitro fertilisation (IVF), in the treatment of subfertility (Loos et al. 1998). However, there is also a contribution from the rise in average maternal age (Kiely and Kiely 2001), which is strongly associated with twinning (Fig. 23.1). The rate of twinning associated with ART depends on many aspects of practice, including ultrasonic monitoring of the response to ovulation induction, the number of embryos transferred and the use of selective reduction. There is significant international variation in practice which is mirrored by variation in multiple rates associated with ART, and rates of multiple births are higher in the USA (Kappor and Pal 2009).

Most of the international and temporal variation in twinning is explained by variation in dizygotic (DZ) twinning (see below). This is partly explained by varying use of ART methods, but is also explained by racial variation in the frequency of DZ twinning. In general, black Africans have the highest rates; the Far Eastern, mongolian, races the lowest; the rates for Asian Indians and Caucasians lie between these. The prevalence of monozygotic (MZ) twin births had been constant worldwide at 3.5/1000 maternities until recently. A small increase in the MZ twinning rate has been noted since the 1980s (Allen and Parisi 1990) and this may also reflect increased use of ART as separation of an embryo into MZ twins is more common with IVF conceptions.

© 2012 Elsevier Ltd

Perinatal mortality

The perinatal mortality rate is over four times higher in twins and four to nine times higher in triplets. The increased rate of loss in multiples is explained by an increased risk of both stillbirth and neonatal death. In an annual review of all births and perinatal deaths in Scotland in 2007, the risk of stillbirth in multiple births was 16.1 per 1000, compared with the risk in singletons of 5.3 per 1000 (Information Services Division, NHS Scotland 2008). The risk of neonatal death in multiples was 18.0 per 1000, compared with the risk in singletons of 2.8 per 1000. The majority of the stillbirths lacked a clear explanation for the death, whereas the majority of the neonatal deaths were related to prematurity. The risk of stillbirth is strongly associated with chorionicity and this is discussed below. There is also an increased risk of death of the second twin as a result of anoxia, arising from complications following vaginal birth of the second twin, which is apparent in term births following vaginal delivery of twin one but is not apparent among infants delivered by elective caesarean section (Smith et al. 2005). Twins conceived as a result of infertility treatment tend to be delivered earlier and to be of lower birthweight than spontaneously conceived twins (Lambalk and van Hooff 2001), and babies from these pregnancies have a higher perinatal mortality rate than those spontaneously conceived (Hurst and Lancaster 2001). The explanation is uncertain but the cause of the parental subfertility may be a contributory factor.

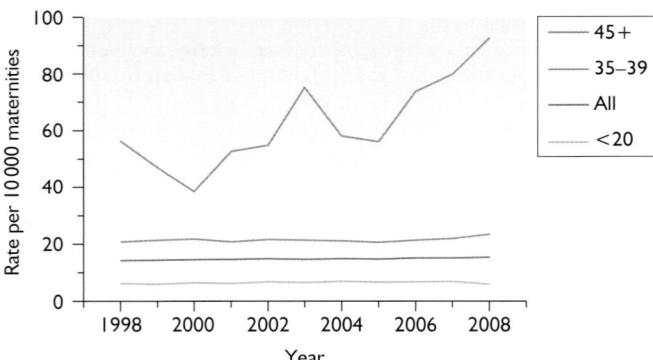

Fig. 23.1 Trends between 1998 and 2008 in twin births (per 10 000 maternities), with illustration of rates within some age categories. *(Data from Office for National Statistics, Birth Statistics (2008).)*

Zygosity

DZ twins arise when two ova are released and fertilised in one menstrual cycle, whereas MZ twins arise when one ovum is fertilised and the resulting zygote divides into two. The ratio of MZ to DZ twins varies in different populations. In the UK approximately two-thirds are DZ, so, in all, about one-third of the pairs will be of unlike sex, one-third both girls and one-third both boys. MZ splitting appears to be 6–12 times more common following ovulation stimulation, whether or not fertilisation took place in vitro (Derom et al. 2000; Blickstein et al. 2003). There also appear to be some extremely rare examples of MZ twinning occurring as an autosomal-dominant trait (Segreti et al. 1979). DZ twinning is known to be affected by a number of factors in addition to race, many of which appear to be related to differing maternal gonadotrophin levels. The rates are known to increase with maternal age, height, parity and frequency of intercourse (MacGillivray et al. 1988).

Chorionicity

Given that there are two fetal membranes, the amnion and chorion, there are three possible combinations of sacs in twin pregnancy:

1. both twins may have completely independent membranes: dichorionic and diamniotic (DCDA)
2. both twins may have separate amnions but share the chorion: monochorionic, diamniotic (MCDA)
3. both twins may share both membranes: monoamniotic (MA).

The relationship between chorionicity and zygosity is complex (Fig. 23.2). For practical purposes, MCDA and MA twins are invariably MZ. However, DCDA can follow both MZ and DZ twinning and further tests are required postnatally to determine zygosity in non-sex-discordant twins. Chorionicity is best determined by ultrasound in the first trimester of pregnancy (see Ch. 9 and Fig. 9.14) when the presence of the lambda sign (DCDA) or T sign (MCDA) has an accuracy close to 100% (Shetty and Smith 2005). However, even in the third trimester, chorionicity can be determined with reasonable accuracy. Diagnosis of MA twinning requires detailed and expert assessment as a thin dividing membrane can easily be missed with suboptimal ultrasound.

Monoamniotic twins

MA twins arise when the splitting of the single zygote is delayed until the end of the second week after fertilisation and account for approximately 1% of MZ twin pregnancies. Earlier studies have

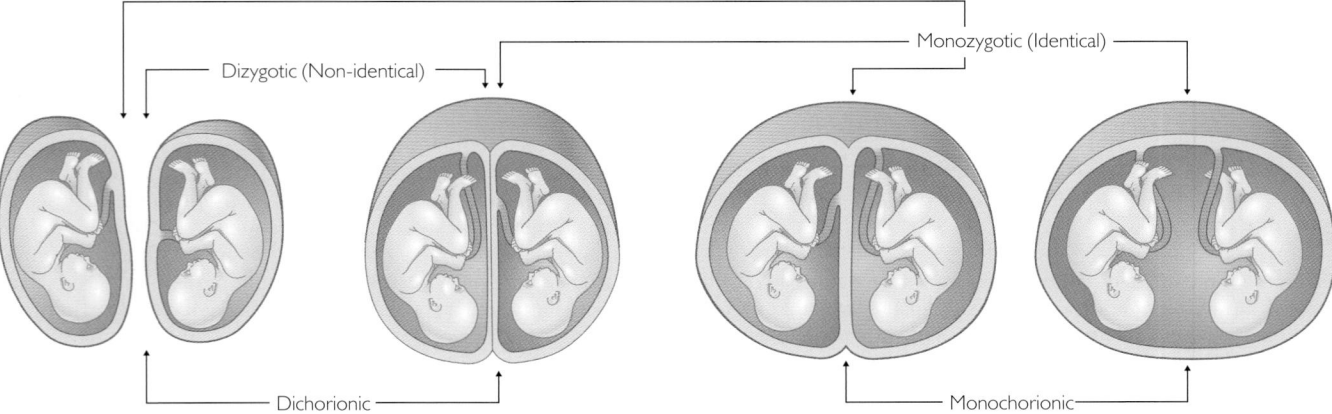

Fig. 23.2 Relationship between zygosity and chorionicity. *(Reproduced with permission from Multiple Births Foundation (1997).)*

reported perinatal mortality rates as high as 30–70% (Allen et al. 2001) but in cases diagnosed during the second trimester the mortality rate is probably much lower – about 10%. Nevertheless, MA twins represent a serious and shared challenge to obstetricians and neonatologists in balancing the risk of intrauterine death against the complications associated with preterm delivery. The primary cause of fetal death is cord compression as a result of cord entanglement. There have been no randomised trials on the management of MA pregnancies but protocols include intensive ultrasound surveillance, sulindac to reduce amniotic fluid volume and delivery by planned caesarean delivery at 32 weeks' gestational age (Pasquini et al. 2006). Superficial vascular anastomoses are common in MA pregnancies (Bajoria 1998) and twin–twin transfusion syndrome (TTTS) is rare.

Conjoined twins

Conjoined twins occur in approximately 1/50 000 pregnancies (Zake 1984). They are a form of MZ twinning in which the division of the zygote is incomplete. The increased incidence of additional unrelated malformations suggests that conjoined twinning may be associated with a fundamental disturbance of embryogenesis (Edmonds and Layde 1982). The factors associated with conjoined twinning are female sex (Milham 1966; Benirschke and Kim 1973; Zake 1984), triplet sets with an MA pair (Schinzel et al. 1979) and it may be more common in parts of Africa (Zake 1984). Seasonal clustering has also been reported (Milham 1966). The site and extent of the fusion are highly variable. Thoracopagus is the commonest form and accounts for about 70% of cases (Rudolph et al. 1967; Edmonds and Layde 1982). Inevitably ethical dilemmas arise with conjoined twins, particularly when surgical separation means that preserving the life of one is likely to be at the expense of the other (Reijal et al. 1992).

Monochorionic, diamniotic twins

MCDA twins have an additional risk to other twin pregnancies, namely the complication of TTTS (Ch. 9). All monochorionic placentas have vascular anastomoses between the two fetal circulations: intertwin transfusion is therefore a normal event. It is only when this transfusion becomes unbalanced, i.e. with net transfer of blood from one twin (donor) to the other (recipient), that TTTS occurs. This haemodynamic imbalance in the parenchymatous arteriovenous network is associated with an absence of superficial anastomoses (Bajoria et al. 1995). Acute TTTS results from an acute haemodynamic imbalance across the superficial arterioarterial or venovenous anastomoses. It is less common than chronic TTTS and tends to occur during labour, when it can cause severe hypovolaemia in the donor and hypervolaemia in the recipient (Fig. 23.4). However, the most common presentation of TTTS is chronic. It complicates, to a varying degree, up to a third of monochorionic pregnancies and is the cause of up to 20% of perinatal mortality in twins. In the past, the diagnosis was made on the neonatal criteria of an intrapair cord blood haemoglobin difference of 5 g/l and birthweight discrepancy. It is now recognised that, in the more severe cases, presenting in the second trimester, these differences are usually absent and the main problems for the recipient fetus are severe polyhydramnios, cardiac hypertrophy, tricuspid regurgitation, venous overload and hydrops and, for the donor, oligohydramnios, sometimes resulting in a 'stuck' twin (Wee and Fisk 2002).

The diagnosis of TTTS is based on amniotic fluid discrepancy measured as the maximum vertical cord free pool using ultrasound.

The criteria for diagnosis are that the deepest pool in the recipient sac is greater than 8 cm and less than 2 cm in the donor sac. Thereafter, the condition is staged based on further ultrasonic criteria and the system described by Quintero et al. (1999) is in widespread use:

stage I: bladder of donor visible
stage II: bladder of donor is not visualised for 1 hour but the
    Doppler is normal
stage III: Doppler abnormalities
stage IV: hydrops is present
stage V: demise of one or both twins.

In the newborn, the recipient twin is characteristically heavier and polycythaemic and faces the complications of high blood viscosity, such as cardiac failure, hyperbilirubinaemia and intravascular thromboses, whereas the donor shows signs of intrauterine growth retardation, anaemia and hypoproteinaemia. Renal failure and/or renal tubular dysgenesis due to chronic renal hypoperfusion in utero may also occur (Kriegsmann et al. 2000). When anaemia is the presenting feature, care must be taken to distinguish from other causes of anaemia such as fetomaternal haemorrhage. Hypovolaemia in the donor leads to activation of the renin–angiontensin system, which has trophic effects on vascular smooth muscle. Postnatally, the treatment of the polycythaemic or anaemic twin is similar to singletons with the same problems (Ch. 30). In addition, the recipient may have short- and long-term cardiovascular problems (Karatza et al. 2002). The risk of congenital heart disease is 15–23 times higher in twins affected by TTTS, typically pulmonary stenosis and atrioventricular defects. With the vascular and blood volume changes in TTTS the recipient twin is at risk of increased blood pressure and right heart disease (ventricular hypertrophy/ cardiomyopathy, atrioventricular valvar regurgitation and right ventricular outflow obstruction) (Bahatiar et al. 2007). Right ventricular outflow obstruction may become severe enough to require valvotomy in infancy.

There is a relatively high risk of brain damage, often due to periventricular leukomalacia, in TTTS whether or not the donor twin dies, although the risk is undoubtedly increased when there is intrauterine death of one twin. The risk of necrotising enterocolitis is also increased (Hack et al. 2008).

The obstetric management of TTTS is discussed in detail in Chapter 9 (El and Ville 2008).

Postnatal determination of zygosity

Like-sex DZ twins can only be distinguished reliably from the one-third of MZ twins who have dichorionic placentas by DNA analysis. The minisatellite probe test is a highly reliable tool (Hill and Jeffreys 1985), requiring only small quantities of blood or other tissues. Tests are most practically done on placental samples at delivery or on cheek swabs taken from infants or children. Cord blood is frequently used but great care is required to avoid contamination with maternal blood. Blood groups or other genetic markers such as red cell enzymes, serum proteins and tissue enzymes (in particular from the placenta) have all been used for determining zygosity but DNA analysis has now become the standard method. The steps to determine zygosity in newborn twins are shown in Figure 23.3 (Multiple Births Foundation 1997).

Fetal growth in multiple pregnancy

The growth and development of the twin fetus are affected not only by the same intrauterine factors as the singleton fetus but also by the interaction with the second fetus. At best one fetus must

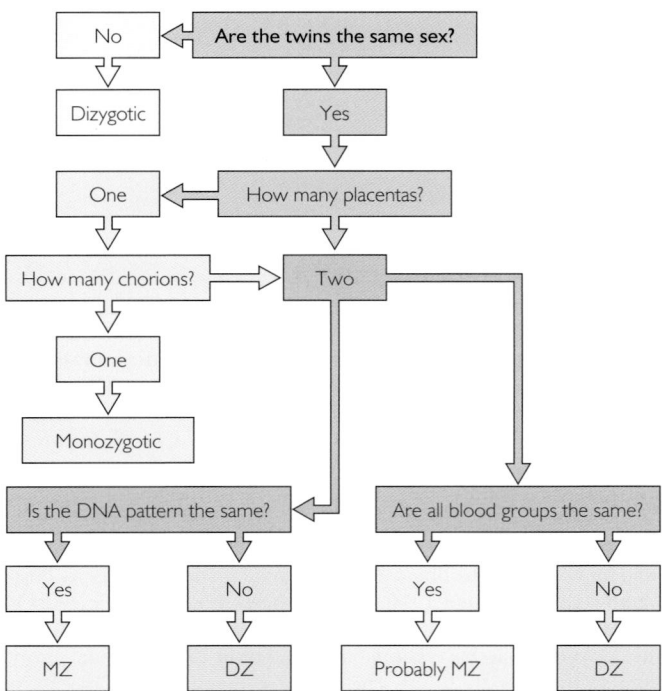

Fig. 23.3 Flow chart for determining zygosity. MZ, monozygotic; DZ, dizygotic.

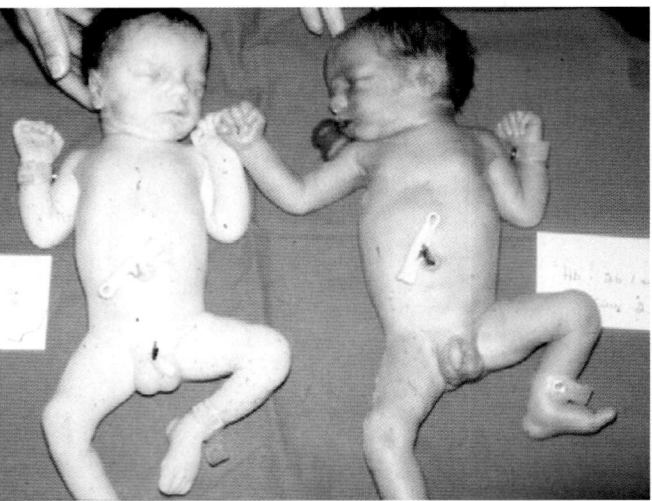

Fig. 23.4 The fetofetal transfusion syndrome, showing intrauterine growth retardation and pallor of the donor (left) and plethora of the recipient.

compete for nutrition, and at worst one twin may be severely, even lethally, damaged by the co-twin (Bryan 1986). Intrauterine growth rates differ between singletons and twins from about 26 weeks, with the divergences then increasing with increasing gestational age (Alexander et al. 1998; Min et al. 2000; Liu and Blair 2002; Hack et al. 2008). As with singletons, primiparous pairs grow more slowly than multiparous (Liu and Blair 2002). The typical pattern of intrauterine growth of twins is similar to that of a growth-retarded singleton in that the weight falls disproportionately more than the occipitofrontal circumference. Birthweight and occipitofrontal circumference centile charts for English twins are now available (Buckler and Green 1994). Some 52% of twins and 92% of triplets are of low birthweight (<2500 g) compared with 6% of singletons, and as many as 10% of twins and 32% of triplets are of very low birthweight (VLBW; <1500 g) (Blickstein 2002). Indeed, twins and triplets contributed at least 35% of the VLBW infants in a population-based study (Blickstein 2002). The average weight of a newborn twin is about 800 g less than a singleton (Liu and Blair 2002) but if allowance is made for differences in gestational age the discrepancy is reduced to 500 g. Opposite-sex twins tend to be heavier than like-sex twins (Liu and Blair 2002), and boys are heavier than girls in both like- and opposite-sex pairs (Liu and Blair 2002). Dichorionic twins tend to be heavier than monochorionic (Ananth et al. 1998) but DZ twins are heavier than both di- and monochorionic MZ twins (Corney et al. 1972). Discordant growth refers to interfetal differences in birthweight between the large and small infant, expressed as a percentage of the large twin's weight: its defining value varies from 10% to 25% in different reports. Birthweight discordance may be due to the different sites of implantation of the two placentas or of the umbilical cords, but the commonest cause of large discrepancies in fetal growth is probably haemodynamic imbalance in the chronic form of TTTS (Fig. 23.4). Discordant size during the first half of gestation is likely to be associated with an intrinsic factor such as a malformation (Weissman et al. 1994).

However, twin pregnancies where the babies are ultimately discrepant for birth weight exhibit difference in growth even as early as 11 weeks' gestational age (Kalish et al. 2003).

Antenatal management

A scheme for the typical antenatal management is outlined in Figure 23.5. When twins are identified, a scan should be requested at around 12 weeks' gestational age by a sonographer who is certified for both determination of chorionicity and measurement of nuchal translucency. Chorionicity is most accurately determined at this gestational age. Moreover, this is within the window for measurement of nuchal translucency to estimate Down syndrome risk. This is important as the serum measurements used to assess Down syndrome risk cannot generally be applied in twin pregnancies. Routine scans are generally scheduled to assess fetal growth and well-being at 4-weekly intervals in DCDA twin pregnancies and 2-weekly intervals in MCDA and MA twin pregnancies. Moreover, many units would offer an earlier anomaly scan in these cases because of the higher frequency of congenital abnormality in MZ twins (see below).

Chromosomal anomalies

These are usually discordant in DZ twins and, surprisingly, also occasionally in MZ twins (Riekhof et al. 1972). The twins are then known as heterokaryotypes and it is assumed that the maldistribution of chromosomes occurred at about the same time as the twinning process. Heterokaryotypes XY/XO are the explanation for the occasional pair of MZ twins of different sexes (Riekhof et al. 1972).

Klinefelter syndrome appears to be more common in twins and in their relatives (Soltan 1968). There also appears to be an increased incidence of Turner syndrome in twins (Carothers et al. 1980) and of twinning among the (normal) family members of patients with Turner syndrome (Nielsen and Dahl 1976). Carothers et al. (1980) suggest that there may be a postzygotic mechanism common to twinning and X-chromosome loss. Genotypic discordance in MZ twins may be caused by a variety of mechanisms (Machin 1996; Gringras and Chen 2001). X inactivation is likely to be the cause of

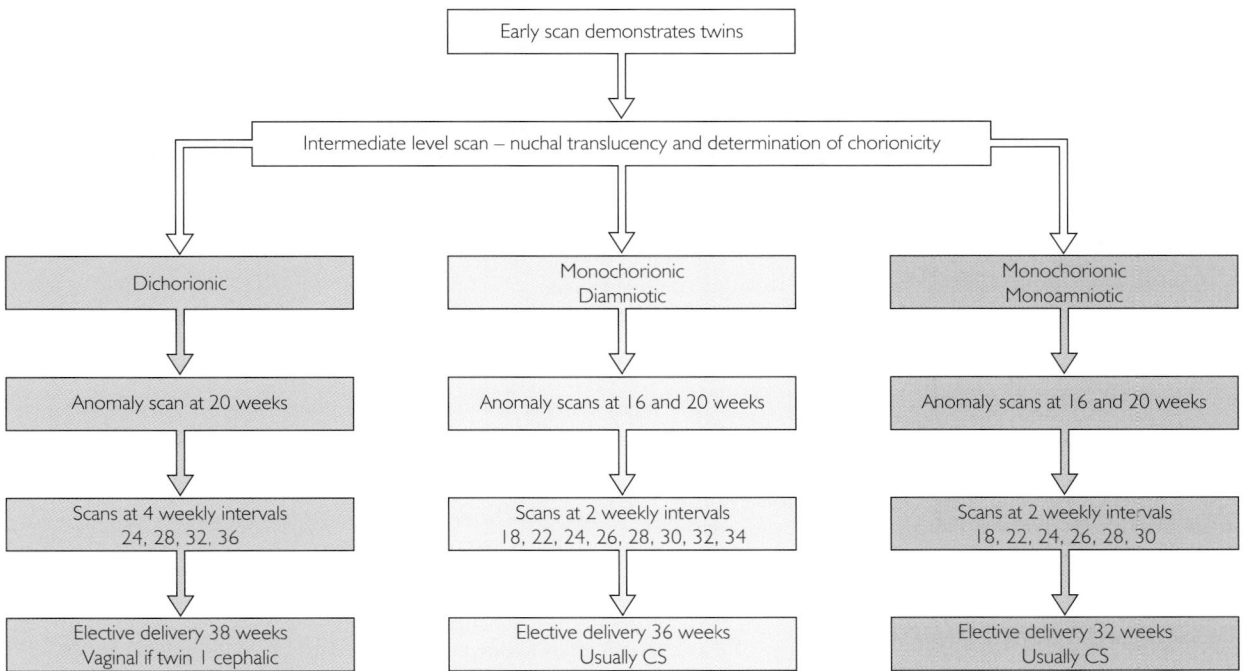

Fig. 23.5 Overview of antenatal management of twins. CS, caesarean section.

some cases of discordancy for genetic disorders such as Duchenne's muscular dystrophy in MZ twins.

Some anomalies, such as oesophageal atresia (Van Staey et al. 1984) and some cardiac malformations (Burn and Corney 1984), occur more commonly in twins. Cardiac malformations are usually discordant in MZ twins, suggesting that the malformation develops as a result of some process peculiar to MZ twins.

The teratogenic effects of both drugs and intrauterine infections may have intrapair differences in expression (Bryan et al. 1987). This may be because of a difference in fetal susceptibility. In other instances where the teratogenic effect of the drug is sharply limited, as in the case of thalidomide, the discordance could be due to the insult acting at the very beginning or end of the sensitive period. As DZ twins can be conceived several days apart, one embryo may be a few days retarded or accelerated in development and therefore escape unscathed.

Congenital anomalies

In most, though not all, studies a higher prevalence of anomalies has been found among multiple births than among singletons (Little and Bryan 1988). Factors that may cause this apparent variation include the gestational criterion used for defining stillbirth, the range of anomalies studied, opportunities for and thoroughness of examination, twinship itself, maternal age and zygosity distribution.

The increase is limited to MZ twins (Corney et al. 1983). Concordance rates vary considerably by type of anomaly but in general discordance is more common even among MZ twins (Little and Bryan 1988). The less favourable environment of a monochorial placentation accounts for some, but not all, of the increase seen in MZ twins (Melnick and Myrianthopoulos 1979; Corney et al. 1983).

Congenital anomalies in twins pose additional dilemmas. Not only may some conditions be treated antenatally but the possibility of selective feticide, when one twin has an irremediable anomaly, provides a new and difficult choice for both obstetricians and parents (Bryan 2004).

Anomalies unique to multiple conception

Anomalies unique to the twinning process include conjoined twinning, fetus in fetu, acardia and fetus papyraceus.

Twin reversed arterial perfusion

Twin reversed arterial perfusion, previously known as acardia or chorioangiopagus parasiticus, occurs in about 1/30 000–35 000 deliveries (Gringras and Chen 2001). It varies in its manifestations from a mass of amorphous tissues to an incomplete but otherwise well-formed fetus. An imbalance in the interfetal circulation resulting in atrophy of the heart or a primary failure of cardiac development has been suggested as the aetiological mechanism. As survival of the acardiac fetus is dependent on a shared circulation with the (usually normal) co-twin, twin reversed arterial perfusion occurs only in monochorionic, and therefore MZ, pregnancies. Relatively little attention has been paid to the pump twin. They appear to have a surprisingly high incidence of malformations (Schinzel et al. 1979) but, even when potentially normal, these babies have a high mortality rate of up to 50%, usually as a result of the combination of intrauterine cardiac failure and prematurity (Van Allen et al. 1983). The size of the acardiac twin relative to the pump twin appears strongly to influence the perinatal outcome, with a significantly higher rate of prematurity and therefore mortality among those with a higher birthweight ratio (Moore et al. 1990). Their perinatal management should be greatly improved now that the problems can be foreseen by routine ultrasonic examination. Various methods, including embolisation and laser coagulation, have been used to cause feticide of the acardiac twin (Ch. 9).

Death of one fetus

The possible dangers of an intrauterine death to a surviving mono-chorionic twin are now well recognised. Many types of anomaly have been reported in the surviving twin (Little and Bryan 1988) and the nature of these anomalies probably depends on the stage of gestation at which the co-twin dies (Hoyme et al. 1981). Review of pooled data on 53 cases suggests that disruptions of the central nervous system are the most common complication (72%), followed by the gastrointestinal system (19%), kidneys (15%) and lungs (8%) (Szymonowicz et al. 1986). Cardiac malformations have also been reported (Corney et al. 1983), as have cases of aplasia cutis (Mannino et al. 1977). These diverse lesions are probably all the result of a damaging, if not lethal, hypoxic episode resulting from the severe transient hypotension that may occur as the vascular resistance falls in the dying fetus (Fusi et al. 1991). A systematic review reported the risks following death of a co-twin. For dichorionic twin pregnancies, there was a 57% risk of preterm birth, a 1% risk of neurological abnormality and a 4% risk of death. The equivalent risks for monochorionic twin pregnancies were 68%, 18% and 12% (Ong et al. 2006).

Intrapartum management

In view of the increased risks of intrauterine death, many obstetricians recommend earlier elective delivery of twins. Given the effects of chorionicity, this is also used in informing the time of delivery. Many units will deliver MCDA twins at 36 weeks and DCDA twins at 38 weeks. However, this approach is probably associated with an increased risk of respiratory complications, such as transient tachypnoea of the newborn.

Conventional practice has been to aim for vaginal delivery where the first twin is in a cephalic presentation. More recently, there has been a trend for elective caesarean delivery for MCDA twins in view of the risk of acute intrapartum TTTS. Vaginal delivery of the second twin has for some time been recognised as a time of particular risk. Following delivery of the first twin, there is a risk of cord prolapse, abruption and malpresentation. Studies of nationally collected data from the UK have demonstrated increased rates of perinatal death of the second twin at term (Smith et al. 2005). A multicentre randomised controlled trial of elective caesarean versus attempting vaginal birth is currently in progress and should provide clear evidence for or against the routine use of caesarean delivery. When vaginal birth is attempted, this is usually done with continuous electronic fetal monitoring. Epidural anaesthesia is recommended as it facilitates manipulations to deliver the second twin, such as internal podalic version and breech extraction.

Postnatal management: routine

Examination of the newborn should focus on risks identified: congenital anomalies, deformities from intrauterine crowding, dislocated hips, cardiac examination. It is helpful to examine twins side by side when assessing discordance (Samanich 2009).

It is enormously important for a mother of twins to establish the easiest and most satisfactory feeding routine for both herself and her babies as soon as possible (Leonard 2003). For far too many, the feeding of twins is remembered as a period of frustration, exhaustion and failure. Many who planned to breastfeed have been bitterly disappointed.

For some, the advantages of bottle feeding so that others can feed their babies outweigh other considerations. But any mother who would like to breastfeed should be given every encouragement and practical help. Most mothers can fully breastfeed two babies but they will need informed prenatal preparation (Flidel-Rimon and Shinwell 2002; Leonard 2003), including demonstrations by mothers, as well as a lot of help during the neonatal period. No mother should be expected to feed her newborn twins simultaneously without an attendant.

Whether the babies are fed together or separately is entirely up to the mother's preference and practicality. There have been no studies that compare milk production in the two methods. Many find it easier to feed separately initially until breastfeeding is well established.

Co-bedding

Many parents now choose to co-bed their twins in the neonatal period and early months. Preliminary studies suggest that the babies may have more settled sleep and more synchronous waking (Nyqvist and Lutes 1998). In preterm twins, more rapid weight gain and earlier discharge from hospital have been reported (Corney et al. 1972). A recent study found that there was no significant increase in core temperature or lowering of oxygen saturation in co-bedded infants (Ball et al. personal communication). There is currently no evidence of an increase in sudden infant death syndrome in co-bedded twins and there is anecdotal evidence that such physical contact with each other can reduce the frequency of apnoeic episodes in some preterm pairs. Furthermore, babies in one cot have the advantage of being more likely to remain longer in the parents' bedroom.

Postnatal management: high-risk care

The risks identified for both monochorionic and dichorionic twins should determine our planning of postnatal assessment and clinical care. TTTS is a major cause of morbidity, mortality and preterm delivery. Growth discordance >20% increases early perinatal morbidity and mortality when associated with fetal growth restriction and/or low birth weight (Alam et al. 2009). Acute and long-term assessment of cardiac structure and function, renal function, neurological damage and outcome, necrotising enterocolitis, growth and genetic risks should be part of routine postnatal assessment and planning. If there is risk of TTTS, early identification of birthweight, haemoglobin and bilirubin helps identify the donor and recipient twin. Early assessment of cardiac structure and function should be considered for both twins, including blood pressure assessment. Renal function and fluid management require careful consideration for both the recipient and donor twin in conjunction with the results of cardiac and blood pressure assessments. Enteral feeding should be planned to minimise the risk of necrotising enterocolitis. Cranial ultrasound and magnetic resonance imaging can help identify the development of periventricular leukomalacia. Long-term outpatient follow-up should in particular consider neuro-development assessment as well as cardiac and blood pressure assessment.

Bereavement

Parents who lose one twin face particular problems (Lewis and Bryan 1988; Bryan 1995). They have to experience the joy of a new baby and the tragedy of bereavement simultaneously. Because they still have a live infant their loss is usually greatly underestimated.

The parents are too often discouraged from talking about their dead baby. Yet concentration on the healthy baby to the exclusion of the stillbirth or neonatal death may encourage the mother to idealise the dead child (her angel baby) and hence alienate her from the survivor, especially if the surviving twin is difficult to handle because of illness or disturbed behaviour.

The pride involved in expecting twins is enormous, and failure is therefore deeply felt. Mothers inevitably feel shame and often some guilt. This guilt may be increased by any implication from friends or medical staff that the death was all for the best, even if logically this may seem so. Twinship is also important to the survivor and this continues into adulthood. This has implications for the care of the surviving twin and parents from birth onwards (Woodward 1998).

Some parents have difficulty in distinguishing the two babies in their own minds. Some may feel that the dead one never existed – a fantasy baby. Substantive mementos, such as photographs or even an ultrasound scan showing the two babies together, can help to clear the emotional confusion. Naming the dead baby not only helps to distinguish the babies but later makes it much easier to talk to the survivor (who should always be told) about the twin.

Blood or placental samples should always be taken for zygosity determination. Even if one baby dies, parents usually want to know whether or not their twins were identical. The zygosity may also be important for reliable genetic counselling about congenital anomalies and the chances of further twin conceptions.

Where both babies are born alive but one baby is likely to die, the family should be encouraged to spend extra time with this one so that precious memories can be created and the parents may later find comfort in knowing that they gave this baby as much love and care as they could. A photograph of the two babies (together with their parents if they so wish) should be taken as quickly as possible.

If a twin is born dead before 24 completed weeks of the pregnancy (a miscarriage) and a sibling is liveborn, the legal paradox and ambiguity add to the parents' difficulties.

Most, if not all, mothers continue to think of their surviving child as a twin even if the other baby was stillborn. Many parents welcome the opportunity to reminisce about their lost baby, particularly with the medical staff, who may be the only people who knew the baby. Many years later they still appreciate an enquiry about their feelings towards the dead baby and any concerns about the survivor's feelings about the dead twin.

An increasing number of parents are likely to face bereavement by choosing to lose a malformed twin fetus through selective feticide. Their grief can be powerful but may be delayed until the delivery of the healthy baby. It is important that the fetus is respected and its loss recognised (Bryan 2004).

Parents' responses to the loss of normal fetuses in a multifetal pregnancy reduction vary (Bryan 2002). Some are just relieved to have two (or one) healthy babies. Others will value support in coping with their guilt and grief over the death of one or more potentially healthy children. Some will not wish the subject to be mentioned, especially if they have not told their family.

Social

Parents of multiples need particular understanding. Few are prepared for the emotional as well as practical and financial stresses involved in caring for more than one baby at once (Taylor and Emery 1988; Botting et al. 1990; Spillman 1992; Garel et al. 1997). They are often faced not only with the problem of caring for and relating to two babies at once but also with two babies, each of whom is more difficult because of the prematurity, low birthweight and other neonatal problems already described.

A mother's relationship with her babies will be further impeded if she finds it difficult to tell them apart. The babies should always be clearly identifiable and called by their names. The cot should be made recognisable at a distance so that the parents can start relating to the particular baby as they approach. Similarly, parents should be encouraged to dress the babies differently from the start despite pressure from friends and relatives. Twin names such as Joy and Jay or Robert and Roberta are also best avoided if the children's individuality is to be respected.

The long-term effects of early mother–twin relationships have yet to be established. Mothers of preterm twins have been found to show fewer initiatives and responses to their babies than mothers of preterm singletons and to be less responsive to both positive signals and to crying. They also had less physical contact with, and talked less to, them. At 18 months, the cognitive development of the twins was less advanced than that of the single-born controls and maternal behaviour in the newborn period was predictive of the level of development of the children at 18 months (Ostfeld et al. 2000).

One twin may be ready to go home before the other, but most units now try to discharge the babies together; otherwise, the baby left behind may suffer in his or her relationship with the mother. Moreover, it has been shown that earlier discharge from hospital is the most important factor affecting the self-esteem of a school-age twin (Hay and O'Brien 1987). If discharge together is not practicable, because one baby needs a much longer stay, parents should be encouraged and helped to visit the remaining baby. Facilities for the healthy child to attend with the parents must always be provided.

Acknowledgement

The authors and editor acknowledge the contribution of the late Dr Elizabeth Bryan, author of this chapter in the first four editions of this textbook.

References

Alam, M.R.C., Brizot, M.L., Liao, A.W., et al., 2009. Early neonatal morbidity and mortality in growth-discordant twins. Acta Obstet Gynecol Scand 88, 167–171.

Alexander, G.R., Kogan, M., Martin, J., et al., 1998. What are the fetal growth patterns of singletons, twins and triplets in the United States? Clin Obstet Gynecol 41, 114–125.

Allen, G, Parisi, P., 1990. Trends in monozygotic and dizygotic twinning rates by maternal age and parity. Further analysis of Italian data, 1949–1985, and rediscussion of US data, 1964–1985. Acta Genet Med Gemellol (Roma) 39, 317–328.

Allen, V.M., Windrim, R., Barrett, J., et al., 2001. Management of monoamniotic twin pregnancies: a case series and systematic review of the literature. Br J Obstet Gynaecol 108, 931–936.

Ananth, C.V., Vintzileos, A.M., Shen-Schwarz, S., et al., 1998. Standards of birthweight in twin gestations stratified by placental chorionicity. Obstet Gynecol 91, 917–924.

Bahatiar, M.O., Dulay, A.T., Weeks, B.P., et al., 2007. Prevalence of congenital heart defects in monochorionic/diamniotic twin gestations a systematic literature review. J Ultrasound Med 26, 1491–1498.

Bajoria, R., 1998. Abundant vascular anastomoses in monoamniotic versus diamniotic monochorionic placentas. Am J Obstet Gynecol 179, 788–793.

Bajoria, R., Wigglesworth, J., Fisk, N., 1995. Angioarchitecture of monochorionic placentas in relation to the twin–twin transfusion syndrome. Am J Obstet Gynecol 172, 856–863.

Benirschke, K., Kim, C.K., 1973. Multiple pregnancy. N Engl J Med 288, 1329–1336.

Bieber, F.R., Nance, W.E., Morton, C.C., et al., 1981. Genetic studies of anacardiac monster: evidence of polar body twinning in man. Science 214, 775–777.

Blickstein, I., 2002. Normal and abnormal growth in multiples. Seminars in Neonatology 7, 177–185.

Blickstein, I., Jones, C., Keith, L.G., 2003. Zygotic splitting rates following single embryo transfers in in-vitro fertilization. N Engl J Med 348, 2366–2367.

Botting, B.J., Macfarlane, A.J., Price, F.V. (Eds.), 1990. Three, Four and More. A Study of Triplets and Higher Order Births. HMSO, London.

Bryan, E.M., 1986. The intrauterine hazards of twins. Arch Dis Child 61, 1044–1045.

Bryan, E.M., 1995. Perinatal bereavement after the loss of a twin. In: Ward, H., Whittle, M. (Eds.), Multiple Pregnancy. RCOG Press, London, pp. 186–195.

Bryan, E., 2002. Loss in higher multiple pregnancy and multifetal pregnancy reduction. Twin Res 5, 169–174.

Bryan, E., 2004. Problems surrounding selective feticide. In: Abramsky, L., Chapple, J. (Eds.), Prenatal Diagnosis. The Human Side. Chapman & Hall, London.

Bryan, E.M., Little, J., Burn, J., 1987. Congenital anomalies in twins. Baillieres Clin Obstet Gynaecol 1, 697–721.

Buckler, J.M.H., Green, M., 1994. Birth weight and head circumference standards for English twins. Arch Dis Child 71, 516–521.

Burn, J., Corney, G., 1984. Congenital heart defects and twinning. Acta Genet Med Gemellol (Roma) 33, 61–69.

Carothers, A.D., Frackiewicz, A., deMey, R., et al., 1980. A collaborative study of the aetiology of Turner syndrome. Ann Hum Genet 43, 355–368.

Corney, G., Robson, E.B., Strong, S.J., 1972. The effects of zygosity on the birthweight of twins. Ann Hum Genet 36, 45–59.

Corney, G., MacGillivray, I., Campbell, D.M., et al., 1983. Congenital anomalies in twins in Aberdeen and North-East Scotland. Acta Genet Med Gemellol (Roma) 28, 353–360.

Daw, E., 1983. Fetus papyraceus – 11 cases. Postgrad Med J 59, 598–600.

DellaPorta, K., Aforismo, D., Butler-O'Hara, M., 1998. Co-bedding of twins in the neonatal intensive care unit. Pediatr Nurs 24, 529–531.

Derom, R., Derom, C., Vlietinck, R., 2000. The risk of monozygotic twinning. In: Blickstein, I., Keith, L.G. (Eds.), Iatrogenic Multiple Pregnancy. Parthenon Press, London, pp. 9–19.

Edmonds, D.E., Layde, P.M., 1982. Conjoined twins in the United States 1970–1977. Teratology 25, 301–308.

El, K.A., Ville, Y., 2008. Update on twin-to-twin transfusion syndrome. Best Pract Res Clin Obstet Gynaecol 22, 63–75.

Flidel-Rimon, O., Shinwell, E.S., 2002. Breast-feeding multiples. Semin Neonatol 7, 231–239.

Frutiger, P., 1969. Zum Problem der Akardie. Acta Anat 74, 505–531.

Fusi, L., McParland, P., Fisk, N., et al., 1991. Acute twin–twin transfusion: a possible mechanism for brain-damaged survivors after intrauterine death of a monochorionic twins. Obstet Gynecol 78, 517–520.

Garel, M., Salobir, C., Blondel, B., 1997. Psychological consequences of having triplets: a 4-year follow-up study. Fertil Steril 67, 1162–1165.

Gillim, D.L., Hendricks, C.H., 1953. Holoacardius: review of the literature and a case report. Obstet Gynecol 2, 647–653.

Gliniania, S.V., Skjaerven, R., Magnus, P., 2000. Birthweight percentiles by gestation age in multiple births – a population-based study of Norwegian twins and triplets. Acta Obstet Gynecol Scand 79, 450–458.

Gringras, P., Chen, W., 2001. Mechanisms for differences in monozygous twins. Early Hum Dev 64, 105–117.

Hack, K.E., Derks, J.B., Elias, S.G., et al., 2008. Increased perinatal mortality and morbidity in monochorionic versus dichorionic twin pregnancies: Clinical implications of a large Dutch cohort study. Br J Obstet Gynaecol 115, 58–67.

Hay, D.A., O'Brien, P.J., 1987. Early influences on the school social adjustment of twins. Acta Genet Med Gemellol (Roma) 36, 239–248.

Hill, A.V.S., Jeffreys, A.J., 1985. Use of minisatellite DNA probes for determination of twin zygosity at birth. Lancet 2, 1394–1395.

Hoyme, H.E., Higginbottom, M.C., Jones, K.L., 1981. Vascular etiology of disruptive structural defects in monozygotic twins. Pediatrics 67, 288–291.

Hurst, Y., Lancaster, P., 2001. Assisted Conception in Australia and New Zealand, 1999 and 2000. Assisted Conception Series no. 6. AIHW, Sydney.

Imaizumi, Y., 1997. Trends of twinning rates in ten countries, 1972–1996. Acta Genet Med Gemellol (Roma) 46, 209–218.

Information Services Division, NHS Scotland, 2008. Scottish Perinatal and Infant Mortality Report. ISD Publications, Common Services Agency, Edinburgh.

James, W.H., 1978. A note on the epidemiology of acardiac monsters. Teratology 16, 211–216.

Kalish, R.B., Chasen, S.T., Gupta, M., et al., 2003. First trimester prediction of growth discordance in twin gestations. Am J Obstet Gynecol 189, 706–709.

Kappor, M., Pal, L., 2009. Epidemic of plurality and contributions of assisted reproductive technology therein. Am J Med Genet C Semin Med Genet 151C, 128–135.

Karatza, A.A., Wolfenden, J.L., Taylor, M.J.O., et al., 2002. The influence of twin–twin transfusion syndrome on fetal cardiovascular structure and function: prospective study of 136 monochorionic twins. Heart 88, 271–277.

Kiely, J.L., Kiely, M., 2001. Epidemiological trends in multiple births in the United States, 1971–1998. Twin Res 3, 131–133.

Kriegsmann, J., Coerdt, W., Kommoss, F., et al., 2000. Renal tubular dysgenesis (RTD) – an important cause of the oligohydramnion-sequence. Report of 3 cases and review of the literature. Pathol Res Pract 196, 861–865.

Lambalk, C.B., van Hooff, M., 2001. Natural versus induced twinning and pregnancy outcome: a Dutch nationwide survey of primiparous dizygotic twin deliveries. Fertil Steril 75, 731–736.

Landy, H.J., Weiner, S., Corson, S.L., et al., 1986. The 'vanishing twin': ultrasonic assessment of fetal disappearance in the first trimester. Am J Obstet Gynecol 155, 14–19.

Leonard, L.G., 2003. Breastfeeding rights of multiple birth families and guidelines for health professionals. Twin Res 6, 34–45.

Lewis, E., Bryan, E.M., 1988. Management of perinatal loss of a twin. BMJ 297, 1321–1323.

Little, J., Bryan, E.M., 1988. Congenital anomalies in twins. In: MacGillivray, I., Campbell, D., Thompson, B. (Eds.), Twinning and Twins. John Wiley, Chichester, pp. 207–240.

Liu, Y.C., Blair, E., 2002. Predicted birthweight for singletons and twins. Twin Res 5, 529–537.

Loos, R., Derom, C., Vlietinck, R., et al., 1998. The East Flanders Prospective Twin Survey (Belgium): a population-based register. Twin Res 1, 167–175.

MacGillivray, I., Samphier, M., Little, J., 1988. Factors affecting twinning. In: MacGillivray, I., Campbell, D.M., Thompson, B. (Eds.), Twinning and Twins. John Wiley, Chichester, pp. 67–93.

Machin, G.A., 1996. Some causes of genotypic and phenotypic discordance in monozygotic twin pairs. Am J Med Genet 61, 216–228.

Mannino, F.L., Jones, K.L., Benirschke, K., 1977. Congenital skin defects and fetus papyraceus. J Pediatr 91, 559–564.

Melnick, M., Myrianthopoulos, N.C., 1979. The effects of chorion type on normal and abnormal developmental variation in monozygous twins. Am J Med Genet 4, 147–156.

SINGLETON HOSPITAL
STAFF LIBRARY

Milham, S., 1966. Symmetrical conjoined twins: an analysis of the birth records of 22 sets. J Pediatr 69, 643–647.

Min, S.J., Luke, B., Gillespie, B., et al., 2000. Birthweight references for twins. Am J Obstet Gynecol 182, 1250–1257.

Moore, T.R., Gale, S., Benirschke, K., 1990. Perinatal outcome of forty-nine pregnancies complicated by acardiac twinning. Am J Obstet Gynecol 163, 907–912.

Multiple Births Foundation, 1997. Are They Identical? Zygosity Determination for Twins, Triplets and More. MBF, London.

Nielsen, J., Dahl, G., 1976. Twins in the sibships and parental sibships of women with Turner's syndrome. Clin Genet 10, 93–96.

Nyqvist, K.H., Lutes, L.M., 1998. Co-bedding twins: a developmentally supportive care strategy. J Obstet Gynecol Neonatal Nurs 27, 450–456.

Office for National Statistics, Birth Statistics 2008. Review of the National Statistician on Births and Patterns of Family Building in England and Wales 2008. ONS, London, Series FM1 No. 37: 1–110.

Ong, S.S., Zamora, J., Khan, K.S., et al., 2006. Prognosis for the co-twin following single-twin death: a systematic review. Br J Obstet Gynaecol 113, 992–998.

Ostfeld, B.M., Smith, R.H., Hiatt, M., et al., 2000. Maternal behaviour toward premature twins: implications for development. Twin Res 3, 234–241.

Pasquini, L., Wimalasundera, R.C., Fichera, A., et al., 2006. High perinatal survival in monoamniotic twins managed by prophylactic sulindac, intensive ultrasound surveillance, and Cesarean delivery at 32 weeks' gestation. Ultrasound Obstet Gynecol 28, 681–687.

Pharoah, P.O.D., Anand, D., Platt, M.J., et al., 2001. Epidemiology of the vanishing twins. Twin Res 4, 202.

Quintero, R.A., Morales, W.J., Allen, M.H., et al., 1999. Staging of twin–twin transfusion syndrome. J Perinatol 19, 550–555.

Reijal, A-L.R., Nazer, H.M., Abu-Osba, Y.K., et al., 1992. Conjoined twins: medical, surgical and ethical challenges. Aust N Z J Surg 62, 287–291.

Riekhof, P.L., Horton, W.A., Harris, D.J., et al., 1972. Monozygotic twins with the Turner syndrome. Am J Obstet Gynecol 112, 59–61.

Rudolph, A.J., Michaels, J.P., Nichols, B.L., 1967. Obstetric management of conjoined twins. In: Bergsme, D. (Ed.), Conjoined Twins. D. Birth Defects Original Article Series III. National Foundation March of Dimes, New York.

Samanich, J., 2009. Health care supervision for twin pairs. Am J Med Genet C Semin Med Genet 151C, 162–166.

Schinzel, A.A.G.L., Smith, D.W., Miller, J.R., 1979. Monozygotic twinning and structural defects. J Pediatr 95, 921–930.

Segreti, W.D., Winter, P.M., Nance, W.E., 1979. Familial studies of monozygotic twinning. In: Nance, W.E., Allens, G., Parisi, P. (Eds.), Twin Research. Biology and Epidemiology. Allan R Liss, New York, pp. 55–60.

Shetty, A., Smith, A.P., 2005. The sonographic diagnosis of chorionicity. Prenat Diagn 25, 735–739.

Smith, G.C.S., Shah, I., White, I.R., et al., 2005. Mode of delivery and the risk of delivery-related perinatal death among twins at term: a retrospective cohort study of 8073 births. Br J Obstet Gynaecol 112, 1139–1144.

Soltan, H.C., 1968. Genetic characteristics of families of XO and XXY patients, including evidence of source of X chromosomes in 7 aneuploid patients. J Med Genet 5, 173–180.

Spillman, J.R., 1992. A study of maternity provision in the UK in response to the needs of families who have a multiple birth. Acta Genet Med Gemellol (Roma) 41, 353–364.

Szymonowicz, W., Preston, H., Yu, V.Y.H., 1986. The surviving monozygotic twin. Arch Dis Child 61, 454–458.

Taylor, E.M., Emery, J.L., 1988. Maternal stress, family and health care of twins. Children Soc 4, 351–366.

Van Allen, M.I., Smith, D.W., Shepard, T.H., 1983. Twin reversed arterial perfusion (TRAP) sequence: a study of 14 twin pregnancies with acardius. Semin Perinatol 7, 285–293.

Van Staey, M., De Bie, S., Matton, M.T., et al., 1984. Familial congenital esophageal atresia. Personal case report and review of the literature. Hum Genet 66, 260–266.

Wee, L.Y., Fisk, N.M., 2002. The twin–twin transfusion syndrome. Semin Neonatol 7, 187–202.

Weissman, A., Achiron, R., Lipitz, S., et al., 1994. The first trimester growth-discordant twin: an ominous prenatal finding. Obstet Gynecol 84, 110–11470.

Woodward, J., 1998. The Lone Twin. Understanding Twin Bereavement and Loss. Free Association Books, London.

Zake, E.Z.N., 1984. Case reports of 16 sets of conjoined twins from a Uganda hospital. Acta Genet Med Gemellol (Roma) 33, 75–80.

Further reading

Bryan, E., Denton, J., Hallett, F., 2001. Guidelines for Professionals: Multiple Births and their Impact on Families. Multiple Births Foundation, London.

Pharmacology

24

Imti Choonara   John McIntyre   Sharon Conroy

Introduction

Medicines have made a significant contribution to reducing both mortality and morbidity in neonates. The benefits of antibiotics, analgesics, surfactant and anticonvulsants are discussed in detail in other sections of this textbook.

The practising neonatologist does not need to be an expert in clinical pharmacology. There are, however, advantages in understanding basic facts regarding how neonates handle medicines and

© 2012 Elsevier Ltd

the practical problems associated with the administration of medicines to neonates of different weights and gestation.

History of drug toxicity in neonates

Some of the most important examples of drug toxicity in humans have occurred in newborn infants or the developing fetus. These cases illustrate the difference between neonates and adults in relation to drug absorption, distribution, metabolism and toxicity, as well as formulation issues (Table 24.1).

Percutaneous toxicity

One of the earliest recognised drug toxicities in humans was methaemoglobinaemia, due to the effects of aniline dye, which was reported in 1886. The dye had been used to stamp the name of the institution on nappies for newborn babies. Ten newborn infants developed cyanosis after percutaneous absorption of the dye. Several months later another outbreak was observed and the connection to the dye was noted (Choonara and Rieder 2002). Subsequently there have been other cases of newborn infants developing cyanosis following percutaneous absorption of aniline dye.

The absorption of compounds is enhanced by prolonged contact of a wet nappy with the perineum. The greater surface area to weight ratio of newborn infants in comparison with children and adults results in greater relative exposure of topical medicines/chemicals. Also the relative increase in the water content of the dermis and the thinner stratum corneum facilitate transcutaneous diffusion of small molecules. There have been other examples of percutaneous toxicity occurring in the newborn infant, including neurotoxicity in association with hexachlorophane and hypothyroidism following the use of topical iodine (Choonara and Rieder 2002).

Protein binding and sulphonamides

In 1956, Silverman and colleagues reported a difference in mortality rate and kernicterus among premature infants who received two different antibiotic regimens (Choonara and Rieder 2002). Neonates who received a combination of penicillin and sulphisoxazole had a significantly higher mortality than those who received oxytetracycline. It was almost 10 years before laboratory studies showed that the sulphonamide had displaced bilirubin from albumin by nature

of its higher binding affinity. This marked increase in the free bilirubin concentration resulted in kernicterus. This unfortunate adverse drug reaction shows the importance of considering protein binding of drugs in the neonate. This is especially so in sick preterm infants where there are high plasma concentrations of bilirubin together with an impaired capacity to metabolise and excrete bilirubin due to the reduced activity of glucuronosyltransferase.

Impaired metabolism and chloramphenicol

In 1959, the grey-baby syndrome was reported with the antibiotic chloramphenicol. Newborn infants developed abdominal distension, vomiting, cyanosis, cardiovascular collapse, irregular respiration and eventually death (Choonara and Rieder 2002). The following year, pharmacokinetic studies showed that neonates were unable to metabolise chloramphenicol to the same extent as children and adults. This was due to impaired glucuronidation of chloramphenicol, and a halving of the dose of chloramphenicol prevented the development of the grey-baby syndrome. Recognition of the limited capacity for drug metabolism in the neonate has led to more appropriate dosage regimens for other medicines.

Thalidomide and teratogenicity

Only 2 years after the death of several newborn infants in association with the use of chloramphenicol, a short letter to *The Lancet* reported the possible association between the administration of thalidomide, given as an antiemetic or sedative during pregnancy, and multiple congenital abnormalities in the newborn infant, in particular phocomelia (McBride 1961). Thalidomide was an exceptionally safe antiemetic when studied in healthy adult volunteers. Animal studies involving thalidomide in pregnant rats initially showed no evidence of teratogenicity. Careful retrospective analysis showed that the effect of thalidomide on the human fetus was time-specific (Table 24.2). Subsequent studies in rats showed that the species was sensitive but only at 12 days' gestation. It is important to remember the difference between the human fetus and animal models and to be aware of the potential teratogenic effect of medicines that are otherwise exceptionally safe.

Thalidomide itself is not teratogenic. It is the metabolites of thalidomide, in particular the monocarboxylic and dicarboxylic metabolites, that are teratogenic. These metabolites, however, do not cross over from maternal plasma into the fetus. Thalidomide

Table 24.1 Important examples of drug toxicity in the neonate

YEAR	DRUG/COMPOUND	TOXICITY	MECHANISM
1886	Aniline dye	Methaemoglobinaemia	Percutaneous absorption
1956	Sulphisoxazole	Kernicterus	Bilirubin displacement from plasma proteins
1959	Chloramphenicol	Grey-baby syndrome	Impaired metabolism
1961	Thalidomide	Phocomelia	Fetal production of teratogenic metabolite
1982	Sodium chloride/water	Alcohol poisoning	Formulation
1984	Vitamin E and renal failure	Coagulopathy, hepatic	Formulation?
1998	Cisapride	Arrhythmia	Drug interaction
2006	Ceftriaxone	Calcium precipitation in heart and lungs	Drug interaction

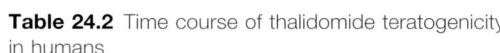

Table 24.2 Time course of thalidomide teratogenicity in humans

DAYS' GESTATION ON EXPOSURE	EFFECT
21–22	Absence of external ears and paralysis of central nerves
24–27	Phocomelia of arms
26–29	Phocomelia of legs
34–36	Hypoplastic thumbs and anorectal stenosis

itself crosses over into the fetus and is then metabolised to produce the toxic metabolites. It is unfortunate that the fetus with limited capacity to metabolise medicines can, in this case, metabolise the drug with the subsequent formation of a potent teratogen.

Formulation problems

In the early 1980s there were two major tragedies involving premature infants that were thought to be related to the constituents of the medicinal products rather than the drug itself. Ten ventilated preterm infants developed central nervous system depression with associated hypotonia, apnoea and seizures (Gershanik et al. 1982). This was followed by a severe metabolic acidosis and multiorgan failure and was described as the gasping syndrome. These infants all had umbilical arterial catheters and were receiving multiple injections of heparinised bacteriostatic sodium chloride, used for flushing the catheters, and also medications reconstituted with bacteriostatic water. Both the sodium chloride and the water contained 0.9% benzylalcohol. The infants who died had significant levels of benzylalcohol in their serum.

The unit that described this inadvertent poisoning stopped using bacteriostatic saline and water and subsequently no further cases were noted. The healthy adult can tolerate up to 30 ml of 0.9% benzylalcohol as a single dose (approximately 0.5 ml/kg). The newborn infants who developed the gasping syndrome were receiving between 20 and 50 times this amount on a daily basis.

In 1983, an intravenous (IV) form of vitamin E was marketed as a prevention for the retinopathy of prematurity. Seven months later, E-ferol was withdrawn from the market following the deaths of 38 infants who had received the drug (Phelps 1984). The affected infants showed signs of hepatic, renal and haematopoietic toxicity. It has been postulated that the emulsifiers used to solubilise vitamin E were responsible.

Ceftriaxone and calcium drug interaction

Ceftriaxone is a widely used cephalosporin. It is a highly protein-bound antibiotic and may displace bilirubin. Despite these concerns it has, however, been extensively used in neonates. In 2002 a fatality was reported following co-administration of ceftriaxone and calcium-containing solutions to a neonate in France. This report resulted in a national pharmacovigilance investigation and in 2006 the French Health Products Safety Agency issued a warning letter regarding the risk of precipitation of ceftriaxone–calcium salt in neonates. There have been seven reported deaths worldwide (Bradley et al. 2009). Ceftriaxone is therefore no

longer recommended in the neonatal period (World Health Organization 2008).

Licensing

The Medicines Act of 1968 requires that all medicines manufactured or marketed in the UK have been authorised and examined for efficacy, safety and quality. The Medicines Act was introduced in response to significant cases of drug toxicity that occurred in the late 1950s and early 1960s. Two of these involved the developing fetus (thalidomide) and the newborn infant (chloramphenicol). It is ironic that legislation that was introduced to protect all humans has failed to protect those who are at the greatest risk – newborn infants. This is despite the fact that tragedies in the newborn infant precipitated the legislation.

Unlicensed and off-label use

Unlicensed medicines involve modifications to a licensed medicine (e.g. tablets that are crushed and prepared into suspensions), using chemicals as medicines, the manufacture of formulations under a 'specials' licence and using medicines licensed in other countries. A particular problem in neonates and children is the off-label use of medicines. This includes the use of licensed medicines: at doses outside that stated in the product licence; for different indications; outside the licensed age range; and by an alternative route, e.g. the use of an IV formulation orally.

Over 50% of drug prescriptions on a British neonatal intensive care unit were off-label and 90% of babies received a drug that was either unlicensed or used in an off-label way (Conroy et al. 1999). Such results do not imply that current prescribing is inappropriate but reflect the lack of scientific evidence and appropriate formulations for drug therapy in the neonate. In children there is a greater risk associated with the use of unlicensed and off-label medicines (Turner et al. 1999). This is not to say that clinicians should restrict themselves to the use of licensed products. However, neonates deserve the same high standards in drug treatment as adults. This can only be achieved by the scientific study of clinically needed medicines in newborn infants in a controlled setting. Such clinical trials would not only provide evidence of efficacy but also reduce the number of deaths associated with the use of new medicines in a non-controlled manner. If there are deaths in a clinical trial, the investigators and regulatory authorities have a responsibility to review the reasons for any deaths at an early stage and to consider whether the experimental drug may be responsible. A review of published paediatric clinical trials over a 7 year period identified 99 randomised controlled clinical trials in neonates (Sammons et al. 2008). Three of the trials involving neonates were then terminated prematurely by independent safety monitoring committees because of drug toxicity. In nine other neonatal clinical trials, patients experienced severe drug toxicity.

Furthermore, licensing should provide appropriate formulations. Many ampoules of off-label drugs contain amounts such that 10-fold errors can occur with the use of a single vial, e.g. morphine.

Legislative changes

In Europe and the USA, new legislation has been introduced that provides a financial incentive for the pharmaceutical industry to study appropriate medicines in newborn infants. It is essential that any clinical trials in neonates involve medicines that are likely to be of significant clinical benefit to neonates and are not simply

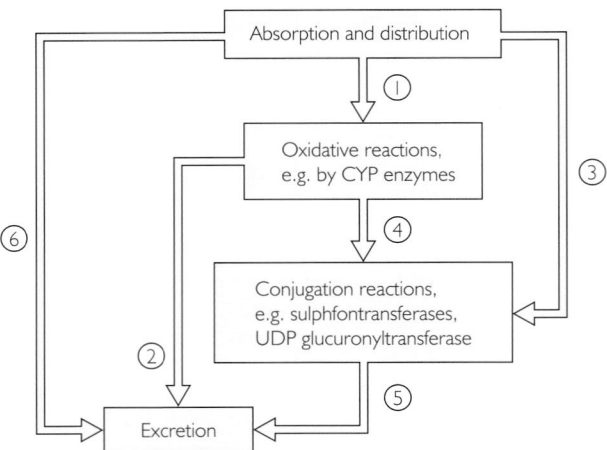

Fig. 24.1 Biotransformation of drugs. 1, Transformation of hydrophobic compounds to more soluble compounds by adding a functional group (oxygen, sulphur or carbon). The cytochrome P450 is the largest group of these enzymes. 2, Direct excretion via bile or urine. 3, 4, The substrates are conjugated to increase their water solubility and excretion. 5, Excretion of the conjugated compound. 6, Some drugs are excreted unchanged in the urine or bile. *(Adapted from de Wildt et al. (1999a).)*

Box 24.1 Factors affecting drug absorption

Drug properties

Molecular weight
Lipid solubility
Degree of ionisation
Drug release characteristics
Drug-induced alterations in gut motility

Patient characteristics

Surface area available for absorption
pH of stomach and duodenum
Gastric emptying rate
Gastrointestinal microflora
Enzyme activity in gut wall
Gastrointestinal blood flow

studied to increase the considerable profits that can be obtained by such a patent extension.

Drug handling

Large variations in gestation, size and disease states, combined with rapid maturational changes, make optimising drug therapy in the neonatal period more challenging than at any other time. This section focuses on what the body might do to drugs, using specific examples relevant to clinical practice to illustrate key principles. An overview of the major components involved in drug handling is given in Figure 24.1.

Absorption

Many drugs in neonatal practice are administered IV and bypass the need for absorption. All the drug delivered can be assumed to be available to the body. However, for drugs administered extravascularly, the body compartment to which the drug is delivered is usually separated from the intended site of action and absorption is an important first step in making the drug available. The fraction of drugs absorbed by a given route compared with an IV dose is called the bioavailability. Absorption characteristics are relevant to drugs given orally, intramuscularly, rectally or transcutaneously. In practice, oral administration is the only one commonly used, as the variability from the other sites is usually too great for predictable drug therapy.

Clinical implications

Absorption from the gastrointestinal tract will depend on the physicochemical properties of the drug and individual patient factors and may be significantly different in newborns (Box 24.1).

In the immediate newborn period, gastric pH may be neutral. With increasing maturity and postnatal age, there is a decrease in intragastric pH (Kelly et al. 1993). There is a rapid fall within hours

to between 1.5 and 3.5 in preterm and term infants. However, other factors such as feeds make it difficult to maintain an acid pH consistently in the neonatal period. Acid-labile drugs, such as oral penicillin, may have enhanced absorption. Acidic drugs, such as phenobarbital, may have reduced absorption, owing to their increased degree of ionisation in the more neutral environment.

The gastric emptying time will affect the absorption time profile. Gut motility is influenced by gestational age, postnatal age and the type of feeding used (Riezzo et al. 2001). Another variable that alters absorption is the colonisation of the gastrointestinal tract with microflora. This is influenced by maternal flora, type of feed and antibiotic use. The metabolic capacity of microflora may influence absorption of drugs, but the clinical importance of this is far from clear.

Nevertheless, some drugs are given orally with good effect. Caffeine to treat apnoea of prematurity is often administered by an oral route, and effective, therapeutic concentrations of caffeine are achieved rapidly (Giacoia et al. 1989).

Key message

Absorption of drugs given by the extravascular route will depend on the physicochemical properties of the drug and patient characteristics. Extreme variability in patient characteristics means that extrapolating bioavailability data from adult studies is flawed. Furthermore, other issues such as administration difficulties, losses due to vomiting and spillage may be far more important determinants of drug effect than absorption characteristics. Oral administration cannot guarantee predictable drug delivery in the critical situation.

Drug distribution

In an optimum drug dosage regimen, a desired target concentration is achieved. This requires consideration of the distribution volume of the drug, usually referred to as the apparent volume of distribution (V_d). This is not a real physiological volume but relates the amount of drug in the body to the blood concentration. Distribution of the drug depends on:

- the size of the body water and fat compartments
- protein-binding capacity
- haemodynamic factors such as cardiac output and regional blood flow.

Clinical implications

The age-related changes in body compartments and protein binding are particularly relevant in the neonatal period. In adults, total body water is 50–55% of bodyweight. In an extremely premature infant, total body water constitutes approximately 92% of bodyweight and body fat less than 1%. At term, total body water is around 75% of bodyweight and body fat has increased to 15%. The intracellular volume increases from 25% bodyweight in the preterm infant to around 33% at term. Selecting a drug dose is made more difficult by rapid postnatal changes. There is a rapid contraction in the extracellular volume shortly after birth, with interstitial fluid loss (Hartnoll et al. 2000).

For water-soluble drugs, the differences in body composition tend to result in a V_d that is greater in newborns, especially preterms. Therefore, at equal doses per bodyweight, peak concentrations in blood will be lower (although mean concentration at steady state is unaffected by V_d). For drugs distributed mainly in the extracellular fluid space, the dose required on a milligram per kilogram basis would be significantly greater, because of the larger extracellular fluid compartment. However, for highly lipophilic drugs, very premature infants may have a reduced V_d.

Aminoglycosides, such as gentamicin, bind minimally to proteins and are mainly distributed in body water. Therefore, in preterm infants, the V_d is greater (0.35–0.75 l/kg) (Vervelde et al. 1999; Rocha et al. 2000) and a higher loading dose is required.

By contrast, benzodiazepines are lipophilic and highly protein-bound. The median V_d of midazolam in preterm neonates is 1.1 l/kg, which is similar to that seen in children or adults (de Wildt et al. 2001). Recommended loading doses per bodyweight are similar in neonates and children.

Protein binding

The pharmacological effect of a drug is related to the unbound fraction in the blood. The degree of binding to plasma proteins is a major factor in determining drug distribution. The age-related quantitative and qualitative changes in plasma proteins are crucial to the likely clinical effects. Acidic and neutral drugs are largely bound to albumin, whereas basic drugs bind to albumin, α_1-acid glycoprotein and lipoprotein.

Clinical implications

With increasing prematurity, the total plasma protein and plasma albumin are lower (Pacifici et al. 1986) and the binding affinity less. The consequence is increased concentrations of unbound drug. Protein binding is also affected by endogenous substances, most notably bilirubin. Because of competitive binding, increased bilirubin levels may displace and therefore increase the free drug levels. Conversely, certain drugs may displace bilirubin from albumin-binding sites and so increase the risk of bilirubin toxicity. In practice, it is only when plasma protein binding is high (90% or more) that clinically important displacement of bilirubin will occur. Table 24.3 shows examples of where this may happen.

The in vitro binding studies alert us to potential risks of drugs displacing bilirubin. The affinity for albumin binding by bilirubin exceeds the affinity for most drugs and the clinical risk is likely to be very small. Clinical problems are likely to occur with drugs such as indometacin, other non-steroidal anti-inflammatory drugs, ceftriaxone and X-ray contrast media.

Table 24.3 Protein binding of drugs

DRUG	% BOUND TO PROTEIN	POTENTIAL PROBLEM
Aspirin	95	Yes
Caffeine	25	No
Ceftriaxone	83–96	Yes
Diazepam	75–90	Possible
Digoxin	16–30	No
Furosemide	95	Yes
Indometacin	95	Yes
Penicillin	65	No
Phenobarbital	20–35	No
Phenytoin	90	Yes
Theophylline	35–55	No

Key message

The neonate has a very different body composition and protein-binding capacity. Rapid changes occur in the context of a unique set of circumstances for each individual, altering the V_d and protein binding. Predicting drug levels, both blood and tissue, is difficult, and standard pharmacokinetic data from adults are of little practical help.

Biotransformation

The process of removing the drug from the body is called clearance, and the total body clearance is a summation of all the clearance mechanisms involved. There are a number of pathways that can lead to the elimination of drugs from the body (see Fig. 24.1) but the two principal mechanisms in the newborn are the hepatic and renal pathways. The ontogeny of these clearance mechanisms is crucial to the pharmacological response of the newborn (Alcorn and McNamara 2002; Bartelink et al. 2006; Anderson and Lynn 2009).

For many drugs, elimination requires a chemical alteration of the drug molecule: biotransformation. Most drugs are lipophilic and transformation to more water-soluble metabolites is a key step. Biotransformation reactions are conventionally grouped into two main types, phase 1 and phase 2 reactions. Phase 1 reactions, by adding or revealing a functional group (oxygen, sulphur or carbon), make a compound more water-soluble. This may then be directly excreted or act as a substrate for the phase 2 reaction.

The primary organ for drug biotransformation is the liver, where a variety of enzymes are involved in modifying both endogenous and exogenous substances. Other organs such as the kidney, gut, lung and skin may also have some biotransforming capacity. These are probably of little clinical relevance.

Phase 1 reactions

Phase 1 reactions include oxidation, reduction, hydrolysis and hydroxylation reactions. Most of these are carried out by the hepatic cytochrome P-450 (CYP) oxidase system, involving haem-containing

Table 24.4 Major cytochromes involved in drug metabolism

CYP	ACTIVITY IN NEONATES	DRUG SUBSTRATES OF THE ENZYME	DRUG INHIBITORS OF THE ENZYME
1A2	↓	Caffeine Theophylline	Amiodarone Cimetidine
2C9	↓	Ibuprofen Phenytoin	Amiodarone Fluconazole
2C19	↓	Diazepam	Cimetidine Indometacin
2D6	↓?	Codeine Metoclopramide	Amiodarone Cimetidine Ranitidine
2E1	↓	Paracetamol	
3A4/7	↓ (3A4) ↑ (3A7)	Cisapride Erythromycin Fentanyl Lidocaine Midazolam	Amiodarone Cimetidine Ciprofloxacin Erythromycin Fluconazole

CYP, cytochrome P-450.

proteins. The nomenclature for CYP uses a three-tier classification based on the genes: the family (at least 40% homology, e.g. CYP3), a subfamily (highly related genes, e.g. CYP3A) and the individual gene (e.g. CYP3A4). The isoforms of the 3A subfamily (CYP3A4, CYP3A5, CYP3A7) account for the majority of drug-metabolising enzymes. They are responsible for the metabolism of about 50% of drugs (Alcorn and McNamara 2002). The activity of most enzymes is significantly reduced in the neonate (Table 24.4). The neonate compensates for reduced activity in the major pathways by utilising alternative pathways. Enzyme activity may increase rapidly after birth (CYP2D and CYP2E1) or slowly during infancy (CYP1A2).

Phase 2 reactions

In these reactions, excretion of the drug is enhanced by conjugation of endogenous molecules to drug substrate. The important reactions in the newborn are glucuronidation, sulphation, acetylation, glutathione conjugation, methylation and amino acid conjugation. Compared with phase 1 enzymes, the ontogeny of these phase 2 reactions is less well established.

Clinical implications

The rapidly changing balance of different enzymes explains many of the noticeable differences in drug clearance during the newborn period. Each enzyme has an independent developmental pattern. Fetal CYP enzymes such as CYP3A7 decline rapidly after birth and activities of neonatal ones such as CYP3A4 rise within a few weeks of birth and continue to do so in the first year (de Wildt et al. 1999a). Such changes have been used to generate models to predict clearance of drugs but such models still lack accuracy (Björkman 2006).

Glucuronidation is most deficient in the immediate neonatal period, and other conjugation pathways, such as sulphation, have to compensate. Methylation reactions are often insignificant in adults but may have a prominent role in the neonate. However, as a review of the glucuronosyl transferase (UGT) isoforms indicated,

clinically useful generalisations are hard to make (de Wildt et al. 1999b). In practice, there is large interindividual variability to glucuronidation activity. The various disease states and environmental factors, as well as changes in UGT, contribute to this (Allegaert et al. 2009).

Examples

Midazolam clearance reflects hepatic CYP3A, and, in adults, clearance correlates with hepatic CYP3A4/5 activity. Plasma clearance is reduced in the newborn period, particularly in the preterm infant (Jacqz-Aigrain et al. 1990).

Theophylline is a CYP1A2 substrate. Clearance is low in the first few days after birth. CYP1A2 activity increases over the first 6 months of life. The clearance and metabolite pattern reaches adult values by 55 weeks of age and is mainly related to post-conceptional age.

Propofol clearance involves both phase 1 (hydroxylation, mainly CYP2B6) and phase 2 (glucuronidation) reactions. Clearance in preterm and term neonates is reduced and shows significant inter-individual variation (Allegaert et al. 2007). Propofol may be useful in neonates but should be used cautiously because of the risks of accumulation and the large interindividual variability (Allegaert et al. 2007).

Paracetamol is metabolised by glucuronidation and sulphation. These combined account for 82% and 68% of paracetamol metabolites excreted in the urine in adults and children, respectively. There are significant changes in the elimination pathway with increasing maturity. The sulphation pathway is relatively well developed compared with glucuronidation in the fetal/early neonatal period, as demonstrated by a low glucuronide to sulphate ratio in the preterm infant (0.1–0.2) (van Lingen et al. 1999). This changes over time to 0.3, 0.75, 1.6 and 1.8 in the term infant, young child, adolescent and adult, respectively (Levy et al. 1975; Miller et al. 1976). The clearance increases with postconceptional age and therefore dose regimens that achieve a target concentration must be adapted accordingly (Table 24.5) (Anderson et al. 2002).

Table 24.5 Clearance and dose for paracetamol

POSTCONCEPTIONAL AGE (weeks)	CLEARANCE (ml/min/kg)	SUGGESTED DOSE (mg/kg/day)
30	1.33	25
34	2.33	45
40	3.50	60
60	4.50	90

Morphine is conjugated in the liver to morphine-3-glucuronide (M3G) and morphine-6-glucuronide (M6G). The analgesic properties are thought to come from morphine and M6G. Glucuronidation of morphine is reduced in premature infants and morphine clearance in the neonate (range 0.8–7.8 ml/min/kg) closely correlates with increasing postconceptional age (Saarenmaa et al. 2000). As would be predicted, clearance in children (25 ml/min/kg) is considerably greater.

Key message

Biotransformation in the liver is a key step in the effective clearance of many drugs. Although understanding of the processes involved is incomplete, appreciation of those maturational factors already known can help in rational drug selection and dosing regimes.

Excretion

Most drugs or their metabolites are ultimately eliminated from the body via the kidney. Renal excretion depends on glomerular filtration, tubular reabsorption and tubular secretion. The dynamics of this system change with advancing maturity and postnatal age.

The elimination half-life ($t_{1/2}$) describes the disappearance of a drug from the blood and is the time taken for the concentration of a drug to fall by one-half. It is helpful in determining drug dose intervals. Many drugs follow first-order kinetics and are eliminated by the kidneys in proportion to the glomerular filtration rate (GFR). Knowledge of the $t_{1/2}$ for the drug will then allow dose adjustment when renal function is impaired, a common problem in the neonatal period.

Clinical implications

The amount of drug filtered by the glomerulus depends on its functional capacity and the blood flow. The amount of drug–protein binding is also a determinant, as the amount of drug filtered is inversely related to the degree of protein binding.

During fetal life, GFR is low. It rises with increasing gestational age but is constant when corrected for fetal bodyweight. At birth, the GFR in preterm infants is 0.6–0.8 ml/min and in term infants 2–4 ml/min (van den Anker 1996). Increases in cardiac output, changes in vascular resistance that increase renal blood flow and increased permeability of the glomerular membrane result in significant increases in GFR in the first few days of life. These changes occur in both term and preterm infants. The implication for many drugs in the immediate newborn period, particularly for preterm infants, is a longer $t_{1/2}$ and extended dosing interval. However, this then changes during the first week of life. Changes in serum creatinine after the first 48 hours of life may give an approximate measure of the newborn's GFR (Drukker and Guignard 2002).

Tubular reabsorption and secretory function may be functionally immature in the neonate. The rate of maturation is slower than for GFR. This is an additional modulator in renal elimination to consider for some drugs, such as penicillins, where tubular secretion is the main mechanism of excretion. Furthermore, concomitant drugs that alter renal function or maturation, such as indometacin, can also profoundly alter excretion.

Examples

Vancomycin is eliminated by glomerular filtration and therefore gestational and postnatal age would be expected to affect the pharmacokinetics. The elimination $t_{1/2}$ in neonates ranges from 3.5 to 10 hours and there is a positive correlation with serum creatinine (James et al. 1987). Dosage schedules based on bodyweight and serum creatinine have been shown to be clinically useful (Grimsley and Thomson 1999). However, neonates rarely receive vancomycin in the first week of life when renal function is most likely to be impaired and a dosing regimen based on weight alone can be effective (de Hoog et al. 2000). Furthermore, exposure to antenatal corticosteroids diminishes the gestational age-dependent difference in the renal excretion of antibiotics.

Ceftazidime is also predominantly eliminated through glomerular filtration. With increasing gestational age and GFR, clearance increases and $t_{1/2}$ decreases; dosage recommendations should be based on gestational age and GFR.

Key message

Renal function is crucial to clearance of a drug from the serum and elimination from the body. Gestational age and postnatal age are important determinants of renal function. Dosing schedules that allow for this are required, to achieve a therapeutic drug concentration.

Drug prescribing and administration

Safe and accurate drug prescribing and administration in the neonatal patient can present complex challenges. Some of the risks involved can be minimised by applying common sense to prescribing practice. For example, there is no point in prescribing doses based on bodyweight such that it is impractical to measure the dose safely and accurately from the drug formulations available. Additionally, this may increase the risk of medication errors. It is difficult to measure volumes less than 0.05 ml accurately even with a 1-ml syringe. This applies to both IV and oral drug therapy.

Prescribing protocols should be agreed by medical, pharmacy and nursing staff which include rounding up or down doses to an acceptable number of whole numbers or decimal places, depending on the drug and the preparations available for administration.

Oral or nasogastric route of administration

Liquid or powder formulations of medicines are necessary for oral or nasogastric administration. They should not be mixed with large volumes of milk or other feeds as interactions can occur with the feed. If the feed is not completed an inadequate dose will be administered.

Medicines contain excipients to enhance the flavour and acceptability of the formulation, or to improve solubility of the drug or to stabilise or preserve the final product. Excipients do not contribute to the pharmacological activity of the drug but may cause toxicity, e.g. phenobarbital elixir containing 38% alcohol (Whittaker et al. 2009).

Liquid medicines should always be measured in an oral syringe or suitable dropper device in order to ensure accurate measurement. Hypodermic syringes should never be used for oral or nasogastric administration as they may result in inadvertent IV administration (Cousins and Upton 1998). Many liquid medicines can be administered down a nasogastric tube when necessary, provided that adequate care is taken to prevent blockage of the tube. All doses should be flushed through using sterile water. The National Patient Safety Agency makes clear recommendations on the choice and use of equipment to ensure safe administration of liquid medicines through nasogastric and gastrostomy tubes.

Delivery of oral liquid medicines via a dropper device may be useful in babies. Accuracy of dosing depends on factors such as the angle at which the dropper is held and the viscosity and density of the product, so may not be accurate.

Topical administration

The skin of a neonate, especially if premature, offers an immature protective barrier to substances applied topically, particularly in the first week of life. The skin is well hydrated due to the high total body and extracellular fluid content in a newborn baby, and offers a large surface area for absorption in proportion to bodyweight. This has resulted in instances of drug toxicity (see above). This route of drug delivery may overcome the problems of oral or IV therapy but further work is necessary to develop reliable drug delivery systems.

Intravenous administration (Box 24.2)

Many drugs need to be diluted before they can be given intravenously in neonates. Products containing benzyl alcohol or high levels of propylene glycol should not be used in neonates because of the risk of toxicity.

Injections presented as dry powders in vials for reconstitution are likely to have a displacement volume, which must be taken into account if the correct dose is to be drawn from the vial. Caution must be exercised when drawing up the neonatal dose from proportions of vials or ampoules designed for older children or adults, in order to prevent 10-fold errors (Chappell and Newman 2004).

The hub of a syringe contains a 'dead space' that may be more than 0.1 ml (Koren 1997). Because of this, care must be taken in drawing up drugs requiring dilution. If the active drug is drawn up first, followed by the diluent, the syringe will contain around 0.1 ml extra of the concentrated drug solution. This may be clinically significant. It is therefore safer to draw up some of the diluent first into the syringe, add the required amount of drug solution from

---

> **Box 24.2** Administration of intravenous drugs
>
> Administer the drug at an access point close to the patient
> Be aware of the fluid volume and/or electrolytes administered with the drug and flush solutions
> Give slowly over 3–5 minutes or as an infusion
> Be aware of the danger of bolus and flushes into infusions containing maintenance drugs
> Ensure that drugs and fluids are compatible before allowing them to mix together
> Use a central line where possible, especially for irritant drugs, inotropes and if drugs will be required for a long time

another syringe and follow with the rest of the diluent to the required final volume.

If drugs are being given as a bolus into an IV infusion line, then they should be given at an access point as close to the patient as possible. If the infusion is running, then it is not normally necessary to flush the drug. In fluid-restricted babies, these flush volumes should be taken into account. Many drugs contain considerable amounts of sodium or potassium, e.g. benzylpenicillin injection contains 1.68 mmol sodium per 600 mg vial. This needs to be considered in babies undergoing strict fluid balance and electrolyte monitoring, or babies with unexplained electrolyte disturbances.

With drugs required to reach the patient quickly, a flush will be needed to deliver the drug to the patient in the required timeframe. Similarly, with drugs undergoing monitoring, such as aminoglycoside antibiotics, it is important that the time the drug is delivered to the patient is known for results to be interpretable; hence a flush is advisable.

Entry sites should be carefully observed for signs of thrombophlebitis or 'tissuing'. They should not be bandaged in a manner that obscures a good view of the tissues surrounding the point of cannula entry. Peripheral veins with comparatively slow blood flow will be irritated by a high osmotic load, extremes of pH and some chemical substances and excipients. Central venous access should be used for irritant or inotropic drugs, and for administration of medicines over long periods of time. Preterm infants are particularly vulnerable to extravasation and tissue damage because of the fragility of their vascular system and skin.

In-line filters (0.22 μm) have been suggested to be effective in removing air, particulate matter, microbial contaminants and endotoxins. Some of the available products are appropriate for neonatal use as they are of low volume and therefore do not require large flush volumes to push drugs through them. There is insufficient evidence to recommend the use of IV in-line filters to prevent morbidity or mortality in neonates (Foster et al. 2006). However, intravenous administration sets and lines only required changing every 4 days when a 0.2-μm filter removing endotoxins was used, therefore saving time and money without an increase in adverse outcomes.

Intramuscular administration

The intramuscular (IM) route of administration should be avoided if possible, as it is a painful route of administration, especially in the neonate who has very little muscle mass. It is also an unreliable route of drug administration, as absorption from the IM site can be slow and erratic. This is due to poor blood supply to the site, reduced muscular contractions and vasomotor instability, which can result in an exaggerated vasoconstriction reflex, further reducing blood flow to the site (Barrett and Rutter 1994). The IM route should never be used if there is a bleeding problem, e.g. thrombocytopenia or in a patient on anticoagulants.

Rectal administration

This can be a useful route of administration for some drugs if the oral and IV routes are not available, though, in the neonate, absorption may be less complete and slower than if drugs are given orally or IV. Suppositories containing appropriate neonatal doses, however, are not always available. Suppositories are often cut in half or quarters. The drug content is not necessarily distributed evenly through the suppository and therefore the actual dose administered may differ from that intended. Consequently, this is a practice that should not be encouraged.

Drug interactions

Serious drug interactions are fortunately uncommon. They are preventable by the involvement of clinical pharmacists in reviewing drug prescription charts. Some of the major types of drug interactions and their mechanisms are described below (Table 24.6). The most important recent drug interaction in neonates has been the formation and precipitation of ceftriaxone–calcium salts in neonates who have received intravenous ceftriaxone alongside solutions containing intravenous calcium (World Health Organization 2008). This drug interaction has resulted in the death of at least seven neonates (Bradley et al. 2009). As different health professionals at different time points may separately prescribe ceftriaxone and calcium-containing intravenous solutions, including parenteral nutrition, it is best to avoid the use of ceftriaxone entirely in the neonatal period.

Pharmacodynamic interactions

These occur when drugs given together have similar or antagonistic pharmacological effects or side-effects. Such interactions are usually predictable from a knowledge of the pharmacology of both drugs and may be caused by competition at receptor sites or occur when both drugs act on the same physiological system.

When morphine and midazolam are administered together to provide analgesia and sedation for ventilation, the two drugs interact. Their similar adverse effect profile causes increased sedation (in this case the desired effect) and respiratory depression. However, they can be given safely together, provided that adequate monitoring of the patient is assured, appropriate respiratory support is available and dose adjustment is performed in relation to the clinical response of the patient.

Pharmacokinetic interactions

If the administration of one drug changes the absorption, distribution, metabolism or excretion of another drug, resulting in an increased or decreased amount of drug becoming available to produce an effect, then this is a pharmacokinetic interaction. They can be divided into several types.

Drug absorption interactions

The rate of absorption of a drug, or the total amount finally absorbed, may be altered by such an interaction. Delayed absorption is unlikely to be a major clinical problem, unless the drug involved requires a high peak plasma concentration to be rapidly achieved, e.g. a sedative or an analgesic agent. However, if the interaction results in a reduction in the total amount of drug absorbed, the result may be ineffective therapy.

Protein-binding alterations

Most drugs are bound loosely to plasma proteins. Drugs can displace each other from such protein-binding sites, and the displaced drug will therefore be available for effect or toxicity in its free form in the plasma. This is only likely to be significant if the drug is normally extensively protein-bound, i.e. to an extent greater than 90%, and is not normally widely distributed throughout the body. In most patients, such displacement interactions rarely produce more than a short-lived effect. However, for the neonate with reduced renal and hepatic excretion, it may be relevant in a small number of drugs.

Enzyme induction

Many drugs are metabolised in the liver. Induction of the hepatic microsomal enzyme system by one drug may increase the rate of metabolism of another drug. This may result in lowered plasma concentrations of the second drug and potentially a reduced effect.

An example is the increase in the metabolism of corticosteroids such as dexamethasone by phenobarbital. This results in a reduction of the steroid plasma concentration and consequently reduced clinical effectiveness. The steroid dose will need to be increased to produce the desired clinical response.

Discontinuation of a drug known to induce hepatic enzymes may result in increased serum concentrations of a second drug, with toxicity as a result. Care must therefore be taken when discontinuing enzyme-inducing agents, as dose reduction of interacting drugs may be necessary. Phenobarbital, phenytoin, carbamazepine and rifampicin are examples of important enzyme-inducing agents.

Table 24.6 Major drug interactions

DRUGS	TYPE OF INTERACTION	EFFECT
Midazolam + morphine	Pharmacodynamic	Increased sedation
Indometacin + gentamicin	Renal excretion	Increased risk of nephrotoxicity
Erythromycin + cisapride	Enzyme inhibition	Decreased metabolism of cisapride → ↑ risk of toxicity
Erythromycin + midazolam	Enzyme inhibition	Decreased metabolism of midazolam → ↑ sedation
Ceftriaxone + calcium salts	Precipitation	Death. Precipitation in heart and lungs of ceftriaxone–calcium salts

Enzyme inhibition

Drugs that inhibit hepatic microsomal enzymes may result in reduced metabolism of other drugs and therefore raised serum concentrations, with potential for increased effect and toxicity. These are usually the most dangerous type of drug interactions. Erythromycin, cimetidine, ciprofloxacin and fluconazole are examples of common enzyme inhibitors.

Erythromycin inhibits the metabolism of midazolam, resulting in markedly increased plasma midazolam concentrations with accompanying profound sedation. Dose reductions are necessary to avoid toxicity and may need to be of the order of 50–75%.

Cimetidine inhibits the metabolism of phenytoin, with a resulting increase in plasma concentrations of the anticonvulsant and the potential for toxicity. Metronidazole may also have the same effect on phenytoin levels in some patients. It is necessary to monitor the phenytoin levels carefully and make careful dose adjustments as needed.

Renal excretion

Many drugs are renally excreted through glomerular filtration and active tubular secretion. Some drugs are actively transported across the kidney tubules and competition for such active transport mechanisms may occur. This can result in delayed excretion of competing drugs. Similarly, the concomitant administration of indometacin and aminoglycoside antibiotics, such as gentamicin, may result in drug toxicity. Indometacin reduces glomerular filtration in the kidney, the main route of elimination for these antibiotics. This may result in retention of the antibiotic, with consequential high levels and the potential for both renal toxicity and ototoxicity.

Drug therapy for the fetus

Improved diagnostic methods during pregnancy have led to the development of drug interventions for fetal disorders diagnosed in utero.

Corticosteroids in preterm labour

A frequently seen example is the use of corticosteroid therapy in mothers threatening preterm labour. The Cochrane review in 2006, of trials using corticosteroid drugs for women expected to deliver prematurely, showed that a single course of corticosteroid significantly reduces neonatal death and morbidity (Roberts and Dalziel 2006). Weekly courses do not confer a benefit over a single course (Guinn et al. 2001).

Antiarrhythmic agents in fetal tachycardia

Intrauterine development of sustained fetal tachycardia and congestive heart failure is a life-threatening condition requiring urgent treatment. Treatment of the fetal arrhythmias by giving drugs to the mother can be successful. Drugs used include digoxin, quinidine, verapamil, flecainide, propafenone, propranolol, procainamide, amiodarone and sotalol. This wide range of drugs suggests that the search for optimal therapy of this condition is still ongoing. Digoxin and flecainide have been the most commonly used agents, but sotalol may also be a valuable treatment option in some circumstances (Oudijk et al. 2000).

Antiretroviral therapy to prevent vertical transmission of HIV

There is an increasing prevalence of women infected with human immunodeficiency virus (HIV) and they now account for almost half the annual incidence of infections. Most of these women are of childbearing age and it has been estimated that they transmit the infection to their babies at a rate of around 1500 cases per day worldwide.

Complex regimens combining antepartum, intrapartum and postpartum administration of antiretroviral therapy together with prudent use of caesarean section can reduce transmission of infection from mother to baby to 0–2.8% (Ch. 39.2) (Grosch-Wörner et al. 2000). Zidovudine has been the drug used in most of the studies. Nevirapine and lamivudine have also been studied.

Unfortunately, expensive and complicated drug therapy is unlikely to be practical in many parts of the world where the rates of HIV infection are at their highest. Work is ongoing to evaluate the benefit of simpler, cheaper and more practical methods of drug delivery in these areas.

Endocrine disorders

Other conditions such as congenital adrenal hyperplasia and fetal thyroid disorders have also been treated by maternal administration of drugs. This field of therapeutics is an exciting and developing area, which requires more research in the future.

Drugs in breast milk

Breastfeeding has significant advantages for both the infant and the mother. It is associated with a significant reduction in both morbidity and mortality in the infant and is therefore to be encouraged. Decisions to limit a mother's breastfeeding must be justified by the fact that the risk to the baby clearly outweighs the benefits (Ito 2000). Consideration must be given to how much drug is excreted into the milk, and the risk of this amount to the baby.

Risk of drug toxicity in breastfed infants

The risk of an adverse drug reaction following breastfeeding by a mother taking medicines is small. A prospective study of over 800 infants who were being breastfed by women taking regular medicines detected no major adverse drug reactions (Ito et al. 1993). Just over 10% of mothers reported a minor adverse drug reaction in the infant (diarrhoea, drowsiness or irritability were the most frequent). This important study emphasises the safety of breastfeeding in mothers requiring medicines, although a note of caution is required regarding over-the-counter codeine-containing analgesia. One mother who was an ultrarapid metaboliser of codeine to morphine had high levels of morphine in her breast milk, which may have contributed to the cot death of her baby (Koren et al. 2006).

The following drugs – cytotoxics, ergotamine, immunosuppressants, lithium and phenindione – are contraindications for breastfeeding. Additionally, there are a group of medicines that may potentially cause problems during breastfeeding (Table 24.7). It is advisable to discuss management with the local paediatric clinical pharmacist or the local drug information centre for a risk/benefit assessment.

Breast milk is produced while the infant is suckling. The breast stores only a small amount of milk between feeds. Because of this, the timing of drug doses in relation to feeds is important in determining how much drug will pass to the baby. If it is possible for the mother to time taking the dose immediately after a feed, then her drug serum concentration will be at the lowest when the baby next feeds, which means that the minimal amount will be transferred to the milk and the baby. It is however clearly difficult to control this completely if a baby is suckling every couple of hours. See Weblink section for the website of the UK Drugs in Lactation Advisory Service.

Therapeutic drug monitoring

Therapeutic drug monitoring (TDM) has been defined as 'the measurement of drug concentrations in biologic fluids to assess whether they correlate with the patient's clinical condition and whether the dosage or dosage intervals need to be changed' (Soldin and Soldin

Table 24.7 Drugs that may cause problems during breastfeeding

GROUP	DRUGS
Anticonvulsants	Ethosuximide, lamotrigine, phenobarbital, primidone
Antidepressants	Doxepin, fluoxetine
Antibiotics	Chloramphenicol, metronidazole
Anxiolytics	Alprazolam, diazepam
Antihypertensives	Acebutolol, atenolol, nadolol, sotalol
Antiarrhythmics	Amiodarone
Antipsychotics	Chlorpromazine, haloperidol
Bronchodilators	Theophylline
Radioisotopes	–
Non-medicinal	Alcohol, amphetamine, cocaine, coffee, heroin, marijuana, phencyclidine

2002). The purpose is to optimise the management of patients receiving drug therapy for the treatment or prevention of disease.

For TDM to aid in drug therapy, the following criteria must be satisfied (Soldin and Soldin 2002):

- clinically interpretable correlation between serum drug concentration and pharmacodynamic effect
- narrow margin (therapeutic index) between serum concentrations causing toxic effects and those producing therapeutic effect
- serum concentration produced by a given dose is unpredictable because of inter- and intrapatient pharmacokinetic differences
- pharmacodynamic effects of the drug are not easily measurable
- a rapid and reliable method for drug serum concentration analysis must be available.

The drugs that require TDM in neonates are shown in Table 24.8. The timing of blood sampling for analysis is important. Steady state should be reached before levels are taken, unless, of course, toxicity is suspected before this time. It takes three to four half-lives of the drug to reach steady state. For a drug such as phenobarbital that has a $t_{1/2}$ of around 2–4 days in the neonate, steady state will not be achieved until after 1–2 weeks of treatment. Steady state can be achieved more quickly using a loading dose. A further complicating factor in neonates is the rapidly changing pharmacokinetic capacity of these patients. The significant improvements in renal and hepatic elimination mechanisms after birth may mean steady state is never achieved for drugs given in the neonatal period.

Therapeutic ranges

Recommended therapeutic ranges for drugs are usually based on adult data. Hospital laboratories tend to quote the same reference ranges irrespective of the age of the patient. This leads to the assumption that patients of all ages respond in the same way to similar blood levels. This is unlikely to be the case, as receptor numbers and sensitivities may be different, and the drug concentration reaching the receptor sites in patients of different ages is also likely to vary, owing to altered pharmacokinetic handling. The therapeutic range for phenobarbital has been shown to be higher in the neonate than in older children and adults.

Table 24.8 Neonatal drugs that require monitoring

DRUG	WHEN TO SAMPLE	THERAPEUTIC RANGE
Amikacin	Predose (trough): just prior to next dose Postdose (peak): 1 hour after an IV dose	Trough level < 8 mg/l Peak level 20 mg/l
Digoxin	At least 6 hours after dose	0.8–2.2 µg/l
Gentamicin/tobramycin	Predose (trough): just prior to next dose Postdose (peak): 1 hour after an IV dose	Trough level <2 mg/l (preferably <1 mg/l) Peak level 5–10 mg/l
Phenobarbital	Immediately prior to next dose	20–40 mg/l
Phenytoin	Immediately prior to next dose	6–15 mg/l
Vancomycin*	Predose (trough): immediately prior to next dose	Trough level 5–15 mg/l (15–20 mg/l for less sensitive strains of MRSA)

*There is controversy regarding the value of measuring peak levels of vancomycin, as there is no evidence that transiently high peak levels cause toxicity. MRSA, meticillin-resistant *Staphylococcus aureus*.

Neonates have reduced levels of plasma proteins, and those plasma proteins have a reduced affinity and capacity to bind drugs. This means that drugs which are normally highly protein-bound will be less so in the neonate, resulting in a higher free – and, therefore, active – fraction of drug. Levels are usually reported in terms of total concentration; hence the same level in a neonate and an adult may produce very different effects in terms of efficacy and toxicity.

Difficulties in relation to TDM in the neonate also occur with the presence of interfering endogenous compounds that may not be present in adult patients. Digoxin-like immunoreactive substances may be present in neonates. These cross-react with many digoxin assay methods, falsely elevating total serum drug concentrations (Soldin and Soldin 2002). It is possible that other compounds interfering with other drug assays may be found in the future.

Weblink

http://www.ukmicentral.nhs.uk/drugpreg/guide.htm: UK Drugs in Lactation Advisory Service. Useful information regarding prescribing for breastfeeding mothers.

References

Alcorn, J., McNamara, P.J., 2002. Ontogeny of hepatic and renal systemic clearance pathways in infants: part 1. Clin Pharmacokinet 41, 959–998.

Allegaert, K., Peeters, M.Y., Verbesselt, R., et al., 2007. Inter-individual variability in propofol pharmacokinetics in preterm and term neonates. Br J Anaesth 99, 864–870.

Allegaert, K., Vanhaesebrouck, S., Verbesselt, R., et al., 2009. In vivo glucuronidation activity of drugs in neonates: extensive interindividual variability despite their young age. Ther Drug Monit 31, 411–415.

Anderson, G.D., Lynn, A.M., 2009. Optimizing pediatric dosing: a developmental pharmacologic approach. Pharmacotherapy 29, 680–690.

Anderson, B.J., van Lingen, R.A., Hansen, T.G., et al., 2002. Acetaminophen developmental pharmacokinetics in premature neonates and infants: a pooled population analysis. Anesthesiology 96, 1336–1345.

Barrett, D.A., Rutter, N.,1994. Transdermal delivery and the premature neonate. Crit Rev Ther Drug Carrier Syst 11, 1–30.

Bartelink, I.H., Rademaker, C.M., Schobben, A.F., et al., 2006. Guidelines on paediatric dosing on the basis of developmental physiology and pharmacokinetic considerations. Clin Pharmacokinet 45, 1077–1097.

Björkman, S., 2006. Prediction of cytochrome p450-mediated hepatic drug clearance in neonates, infants and children: how accurate are available scaling methods? Clin Pharmacokinet 45, 1–11.

Bradley, J.S., Wassel, R.T., Lee, L., et al., 2009. Intravenous ceftriaxone and calcium in the neonate: assessing the risk for cardiopulmonary adverse events. Pediatrics 123, e609–e613.

Chappell, K., Newman, C., 2004. Potential tenfold drug overdoses on a neonatal unit. Arch Dis Child Fetal Neonatal Ed 89, F483–F484.

Choonara, I., Rieder, M.J., 2002. Drug toxicity and adverse drug reactions in children – a brief historical review. Paediatric and Perinatal Drug Therapy 5, 12–18.

Conroy, S., McIntyre, J., Choonara, I., 1999. Unlicensed and off label drug use in neonates. Arch Dis Child Fetal Neonatal Ed 80, F142–F145.

Cousins, D., Upton, D., 1998. Inappropriate syringe use leads to fatalities. Pharm Pract 8, 209–210.

de Hoog, M., Schoemaker, R.C., Mouton, J.W., et al., 2000. Vancomycin population pharmacokinetics in neonates. Clin Pharmacol Ther 67, 360–367.

de Wildt, S.N., Kearns, G.L., Leeder, J.S., et al., 1999a. Cytochrome P450 3A: ontogeny and drug disposition. Clin Pharmacokinet 37, 485–505.

de Wildt, S.N., Kearns, G.L., Leeder, J.S., et al., 1999b. Glucuronidation in humans. Pharmacogenetic and developmental aspects. Clin Pharmacokinet 36, 439–452.

de Wildt, S.N., Kearns, G.L., Hop, W.C., et al., 2001. Pharmacokinetics and metabolism of intravenous midazolam in preterm infants. Clin Pharmacol Ther 70, 525–531.

Drukker, A., Guignard, J.P., 2002. Renal aspects of the term and preterm infant: a selective update. Curr Opin Pediatr 14, 175–182.

Foster, J.P., Richards, R., Showell, M.G., 2006. Intravenous in-line filters for preventing morbidity and mortality in neonates. Cochrane Database Syst Rev (2), CD005248.

Gershanik, J., Boecler, B., Ensley, H., et al., 1982. The gasping syndrome and benzyl alcohol poisoning. N Engl J Med 307, 1384–1388.

Giacoia, G.P., Jungbluth, G.L., Jusko, W.J., 1989. Effect of formula feeding on oral absorption of caffeine in premature infants. Dev Pharmacol Ther 12, 205–210.

Grimsley, C., Thomson, A.H., 1999. Pharmacokinetics and dose requirements of vancomycin in neonates. Arch Dis Child Fetal Neonatal Ed 81, F221–F227.

Grosch-Wörner, I., Schäfer, A., Obladen, M., et al., 2000. An effective and safe protocol involving zidovudine and caesarean section to reduce vertical transmission of HIV-1 infection. AIDS 14, 2903–2911.

Guinn, D.A., Atkinson, M.W., Sullivan, L., et al., 2001. Single vs weekly courses of antenatal corticosteroids for women at risk of preterm delivery: a randomised controlled trial. JAMA 286, 1581–1587.

Hartnoll, G., Betremieux, P., Modi, N., 2000. Body water content of extremely preterm infants at birth. Arch Dis Child Fetal Neonatal Ed 83, F56–F59.

Ito, S., 2000. Drug therapy for breast-feeding women. N Engl J Med 343, 118–126.

Ito, S., Blajchman, A., Stephenson, M., et al., 1993. Prospective follow-up of adverse reactions in breast-fed infants exposed to maternal medication. Am J Obstet Gynecol 168, 1393–1399.

Jacqz-Aigrain, E., Wood, C., Robieux, I., 1990. Pharmacokinetics of midazolam in critically ill neonates. Eur J Clin Pharmacol 39, 191–192.

James, A., Koren, G., Milliken, J., et al., 1987. Vancomycin pharmacokinetics and dose recommendations for preterm infants. Antimicrob Agents Chemother 31, 52–54.

Kelly, E.J., Newell, S.J., Brownlee, K.G., et al., 1993. Gastric acid secretion in preterm infants. Early Hum Dev 35, 215–220.

Koren, G., 1997. Therapeutic drug monitoring principles in the neonate. Clin Chem 43, 222–227.

Koren, G., Cairns, J., Chitayat, D., et al., 2006. Pharmacogenetics of morphine poisoning in a breastfed neonate of a codeine-prescribed mother. Lancet 368, 704.

Levy, G., Khanna, N.N., Soda, D.M., et al., 1975. Pharmacokinetics of acetaminophen in the human neonate: formation of acetaminophen glucuronide and sulfate in relation to plasma bilirubin concentration and D-glucaric acid excretion. Pediatrics 55, 818–825.

McBride, W.G., 1961. Thalidomide and congenital abnormalities. Lancet ii, 1358.

Miller, R.P., Roberts, R.J., Fischer, L.J., 1976. Acetaminophen elimination kinetics in neonates, children and adults. Clin Pharmacol Ther 19, 284–294.

Oudijk, M.A., Michon, M.M., Kleinman, C.S., et al., 2000. Sotalol in the treatment of fetal dysrhythmias. Circulation 101, 2721–2726.

Pacifici, G.M., Viani, A., Taddeucci-Brunelli, G., et al., 1986. Effects of development, ageing, and renal and hepatic insufficiency as well as hemodialysis on the plasma concentrations of albumin and alpha 1-acid glycoprotein: implications for binding of drugs. Ther Drug Monit 8, 259–263.

Phelps, D.L., 1984. E-Ferol: What happened and what now? Pediatrics 74, 1114–1116.

Riezzo, G., Indrio, F., Montagna, O., et al., 2001. Gastric electrical activity and gastric emptying in preterm newborns fed standard and hydrolysate formulas. J Pediatr Gastroenterol Nutr 33, 290–295.

Roberts, D., Dalziel, S.R., 2006. Antenatal corticosteroids for accelerating fetal lung maturation for women at risk of preterm birth. Cochrane Database Syst Rev (3), CD004454.

Rocha, M.J., Almeida, A.M., Afonso, E., et al., 2000. The kinetic profile of gentamicin in premature neonates. J Pharm Pharmacol 52, 1091–1097.

Saarenmaa, E., Neuvonen, P.J., Rosenberg, P., et al., 2000. Morphine clearance and effects in newborn infants in relation to gestational age. Clin Pharmacol Ther 68, 160–166.

Sammons, H.M., Gray, C., Hudson, H., et al., 2008. Safety in paediatric clinical trials – a 7-year review. Acta Paediatr 97, 474–477.

Soldin, O.P., Soldin, S.J., 2002. Review: therapeutic drug monitoring in pediatrics. Ther Drug Monit 24, 1–8.

Turner, S., Nunn, A.J., Fielding, K., et al., 1999. Adverse drug reactions to unlicensed and off-label drugs on paediatric wards: a prospective study. Acta Paediatr 88, 965–968.

van den Anker, J.N., 1996. Pharmacokinetics and renal function in preterm infants. Acta Paediatr 85, 1393–1399.

van Lingen, R.A., Deinum, J.T., Quak, J.M., et al., 1999. Pharmacokinetics and metabolism of rectally administered paracetamol in preterm neonates. Arch Dis Child Fetal Neonatal Ed 80, F59–F63.

Vervelde, M.L., Rademaker, C.M., Krediet, T.G., et al., 1999. Population pharmacokinetics of gentamicin in preterm neonates: evaluation of a once daily dosage regimen. Ther Drug Monit 21, 514–519.

Whittaker, A., Currie, A.E., Turner, M.A., et al., 2009. Toxic additives in medication for preterm infants. Arch Dis Child Fetal Neonatal Ed 94, F236–F240.

World Health Organization, 2008. Ceftriaxone: fatal outcome with calcium-containing solutions. WHO Drug Information 22, 193–194.

Neonatal analgesia

25

Steven M Sale   Anoo Jain   Judith Meek

CHAPTER CONTENTS

Introduction

Pain has been described as 'an unpleasant sensory and emotional experience which is usually associated with tissue damage or described in terms of such damage'. While neonates have a broadly similar type of response to painful stimuli as adults, the presence or absence of pain as a conscious event can never be proven. Infants and neonates have only a limited ability to communicate compared with adults, and their responses can be inconsistent or absent (Marshall et al. 1980). Much depends on the nature of self-awareness, consciousness and the development of 'self' in fetal life (Glover and Fisk 1996; Lloyd-Thomas and Fitzgerald 1996; Szawarski 1996). Given the impossible task of making judgements on the nature of pain perception in the fetus and neonate, the term 'nociception' (the anatomical and physiological system of pain sensation) has been felt to be more appropriate.

© 2012 Elsevier Ltd

Despite increasing interest in provision of analgesia to the neonatal population there is evidence that procedural pain is poorly managed (Johnston et al. 1997). Moreover, this is not a small problem: neonates, particularly those who are unwell, are subjected to a large number of nociceptive stimuli. A total of 500 invasive procedures were recorded in one neonate during a single hospital stay, and this is not unusual (Barker and Rutter 1995). The American Academy of Pediatrics has produced a policy statement on the prevention and management of neonatal pain which emphasises that painful procedures are a very common part of routine neonatal care (Batton et al. 2006).

Nociception in the infant

Nociceptive pathways begin to develop as early as 6 weeks' gestation when dorsal horn cells in the spinal cord have formed synapses with the developing sensory neurons (Okado 1981). These sensory neurons grow peripherally to reach the skin and mucosal surfaces by 20 weeks (Humphrey 1964; Valman and Pearson 1980). At full term the density of cutaneous nociceptive nerve endings is at least as great as that of the adult (Gleiss and Stuttgen 1970). Organisation of the laminar structure of the cells in the dorsal horn, and their synapses, and the appearance of specific neurotransmitter vesicles begins at 13 weeks and is completed by 30 weeks (Rizvi et al. 1986). By this time, nerve tracts associated with nociception are fully myelinated up to the thalamic level (Gilles et al. 1983). Synaptic connections of the thalamocortical tracts occur at 24 weeks' gestation (Kostovic and Rakic 1984), and myelination of the nociceptive thalamocortical radiations is complete by 37 weeks (Gilles et al. 1983). Other nociceptive tracts may not be fully myelinated until much later (Anand and Carr 1989), but lack of myelination does not imply lack of function. Synaptic connections of C-fibres do not appear to mature functionally until the third trimester but noxious stimuli can still be transmitted via A-β fibres (Fitzgerald et al. 1994). Descending inhibitory tracts, which act via inputs into spinal cord cells to suppress the transmission of noxious stimuli, are also not fully functional at term. The lack of descending inhibition from higher centres will tend to increase afferent nociceptive transmission in the spinal cord.

Few neurophysiological or cytochemical studies have been attempted in the human infant. Positron emission tomography has shown that glucose utilisation, and by inference cerebral metabolism, is maximal in sensory areas of the neonatal brain (Chugani and Phelps 1986) and that auditory and visual evoked potentials have developed by 30 weeks' gestation (Henderson-Smart et al. 1983). These data, along with electroencephalograph data (Torres and Anderson 1985), imply a very complex level of integration and maturity within the cerebral cortex by this time. Somatosensory evoked responses are present from 28 weeks' gestation, although the latency is long, owing to slow peripheral and central transmission. Studies using functional near-infrared spectroscopy (fNIRS) have demonstrated haemodynamic changes related to clinical noxious stimuli (heel lance (Slater et al. 2006) and venesection (Bartocci et al. 2006)) in the sensory cortex of newborns as young as 25 weeks' gestation. These responses are diminished during sleep (Slater et al. 2006). Slater et al. (2009a) have also used event-related evoked potentials to demonstrate cortical responses to heel lance.

While nociceptive connections remain immature in the preterm neonate, the larger receptive fields, the immaturity of the descending inhibitory pathways, and the ability of non-C-fibres to transmit nociceptive inputs into the dorsal horn facilitated by subthreshold C-fibre effects give the impression of an underdamped, poorly discriminative system with a potential for much exaggerated responses. This is borne out in the observations of Fitzgerald et al. (1989) and Andrews and Fitzgerald's (1994) on the cutaneous withdrawal reflex and other studies which have shown that newborn reactions to painful stimuli can be diffuse, unlocalised or sometimes completely absent (Marshall et al. 1980). This failure to respond consistently to a standard noxious stimulus can confound attempts to quantify pain using behavioural measurement.

Effects of nociception

The initial effects of nociception can be categorised under physiological, stress and behavioural responses. All of these responses can compromise the physiological stability of a neonate receiving intensive care.

Haemodynamic responses to noxious stimuli occur as early as 18 weeks' gestation in the human fetus (Teixeira and Fogliani 1996). Neonates undergoing awake nasotracheal intubation have a rise in mean arterial pressure of 57% with a similar rise in intracranial pressure during the procedure (Kelly and Finer 1984). Age-related differences in cardiovascular responses to noxious stimuli have been reported (Porter et al. 1991). In a study on lumbar puncture in preterm infants, the less mature babies (<32 weeks' gestational age) showed the greatest rise in blood pressure during the handling phase rather than during the actual procedure. This was in contrast to the more mature babies, who displayed maximum response during the procedure itself. Other physiological responses that have been investigated in the context of nociception are R-to-R interval and frequency analysis on electrocardiogram (Porter et al. 1988), transcutaneous oxygen tension, ventilatory patterns and sweating.

Hormonal responses to noxious stimuli can also be identified in the human fetus and the response obtunded by opioids (Fisk et al. 2001). Neonatal stress responses to surgery appear to be greater in magnitude and shorter-lived than in older infants (Anand 1990; Okur et al. 1995) and the subsequent nitrogen loss appears to be greater in the younger age groups. Inadequate suppression of these responses during major surgery affects postoperative recovery (Anand et al. 1987), but it remains unclear if complete elimination of the responses is desirable either. Some measure of stress response during surgery can be achieved by real-time analysis of blood sugar provided glucose-containing solutions are avoided (Wolf et al. 1998).

Preterm infants exhibit hypersensitivity and postinjury hyperalgesia following heel lancing, which can be prevented by the application of local anaesthetic (Fitzgerald et al. 1989). There is also evidence that early tissue injury can cause hyperinnervation (increased branching of nociceptive nerve endings), which persists and may lead to hyperalgesia and allodynia (Constantinou et al. 1994).

The impression that emerges is that even the very preterm infant has complex interneuronal connections capable of integrated responses to tactile or nociceptive input. They have inconsistent responses to external stimuli, which may reflect the late functional connections of sensory afferents (particularly C-fibres) within the spinal cord. However, the combination of larger receptive fields, recruitment of non-nociceptive afferents and reduced inhibitory controls results in 'underdamped' responses (long-lasting, exaggerated and poorly localised) once afferent stimuli have achieved central activation above a threshold level. Inconsistency of response may reflect the profound effects that conscious state (Grunau and Craig 1987) and other external responses (Haouari et al. 1995) have on behaviour.

Secondary effects of nociception

Neonates who experience repeated noxious stimuli can show both short-term hypersensitivity (Fitzgerald et al. 1989) and longer term persistence of immature pain responses (Johnston and Stevens 1996). Preterm infants have been shown to have increased cortical responses to heel lancing than term born controls (Slater et al. 2010a). At 18 months they have been reported to respond less than normal infants to everyday painful experiences (Grunau et al. 1994), and at 4–5 years show increased somatisation (an inappropriate expression of psychosocial distress as physical symptomatology). Awake circumcision without analgesia causes irritability, reduced attentiveness and poor orientation that can last longer than the expected duration of pain (Dixon et al. 1984), and 3–6 months later circumcised infants have exaggerated responses to painful stimuli compared with a matched group who have not been circumcised (Taddio et al. 1997).

Comforting strategies that reduce the stress of interventional procedures in preterm infants are associated with improved developmental and clinical outcomes (Als et al. 1986). The results of the multicentre NOPAIN trial evaluated the risks and benefits of providing analgesia to ventilated neonates. A low-dose morphine infusion was found to reduce the incidence of neurological complications (intraventricular haemorrhage and periventricular leukomalacia) in ventilated infants when compared with midazolam or dextrose (Anand et al. 1999). The subsequent larger NEOPAIN trial raised concerns about the risk of severe intraventricular haemorrhage, periventricular leukomalacia and death in those who received boluses of morphine (Anand et al. 2004). Although later analysis of these data demonstrated that the risk of intraventricular haemorrhage was associated with morphine rather than causal (Hall et al. 2005), there have been ongoing concerns about the liberal use of opioids and induction of apoptosis in the developing brain (Hu et al. 2002), increase of longer term responses to painful stimuli (McRae et al. 1997) and an association with self-destructive behaviour in adolescence (Jacobson et al. 1987).

Measurement of pain/nociception in the neonate

Most of the early studies on infant pain measurement were based on a single noxious stimulus such as heel prick (procedural pain)

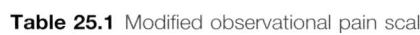

Table 25.1 Modified observational pain scale

AGITATION	FACIAL EXPRESSION	MOVEMENT	VENTILATION
2 = Major	2 = Grimace/ nasal flare	2 = Flexed/tense	2 = Fighting ventilator
1 = Responds to comforting	1 = Movement	1 = Appropriate	1 = Comfortable
0 = No movement	0 = No movement	0 = No movement	0 = Apnoea
A modified observational pain scale used on the paediatric intensive care unit in the Bristol Royal Hospital for Children. Hourly observations are recorded. A total score of 2 or less implies oversedation, 3–5 is ideal and 6 or more implies undersedation.			

and were primarily developed for research purposes. This was a useful model because it provided a relatively consistent stimulus from which to identify and grade responses. However, the behavioural tools derived from studies on procedural pain have limited applicability to other situations such as postoperative pain and the discomfort from prolonged immobility in the neonatal intensive care unit. There are few validated tools for prolonged pain or discomfort, they require training to increase reliability and are labour-intensive with a low degree of clinical utility. The Bristol Royal Hospital for Children uses a modified observational pain scale that is simple to use, requires minimal training and is feasible in a clinical setting (Table 25.1). The tools available are either unidimensional, using behavioural responses to pain, or multidimensional, using a combination of behavioural, physiological and contextual indicators. Behavioural indicators are more specific than physiological changes in all age groups. Many of these tools are developed from validated techniques used in older children and infants, such as the Children's Hospital of Eastern Ontario Scale. Scales such as the Premature Infant Pain Profile (PIPP) have adjustments for gestational age and sleep state, as an acknowledgement that these alter the measurable responses to pain (Stevens et al. 1996). In the paralysed neonate behavioural tools cannot be used and physiological measures such as cardiovascular responses to handling have to be used.

Table 25.2 shows some of the commonly used pain-scoring systems as described by Anand et al. (2006). The Royal College of Nursing (UK) has published an algorithm for selecting the most appropriate pain scale for specific clinical situations, as well as guidelines for recognition and assessment of acute pain in children (see Weblinks).

There is no 'gold-standard' pain scale, as it is not possible to correlate scores with preverbal infants' pain experience. However Slater et al. (2008) have demonstrated a positive correlation of the cortical response measured by fNIRS in term neonates with the PIPP score. The correlation is strongest with the facial (behavioural) rather than the physiological components. However, there are several occasions when the newborns had zero PIPP scores when subjected to heel lances, but had measurable cortical responses. Therefore while pain scoring is the best clinical tool available at the present time, it may underestimate the cortical response, especially in the most preterm (Slater et al. 2009b) and sick infants.

Pharmacological considerations

Classically, neonates are regarded as highly susceptible to drugs, particularly opioids, in terms of both pharmacodynamics (physiological effects of the drug on the body) and pharmacokinetics (how the body handles the drug). However, the limited studies available have shown that there is large individual variability in this population associated with maturity, previous exposure to drugs and organ function. Individual drug effects from dosing regimens are therefore poorly predictive and can only be described in general terms.

Pharmacodynamics

Opioid receptors change both in numbers and in receptor type during development and in the rat this is associated with a large change in sensitivity (Pasternak et al. 1980). It has been suggested from human studies that have compared plasma concentrations of opioid drugs that human neonates could be relatively resistant to the ventilatory effects of opioids, and that the sensitivity observed after opioid administration is due to selective distribution of the drug to the brain after administration. Lipid-soluble drugs, such as fentanyl, are preferentially redistributed into the neonatal brain after a bolus injection and attain high initial peak concentrations at the effect site (biophase). In contrast, elimination of the drug from biophase is slow because of the limitations on peripheral uptake and drug elimination. Fat-soluble opioids such as fentanyl will therefore have a more rapid onset of effect, greater potency and slower offset than can be predicted by simply analysing pharmacokinetic data. Delivery of morphine into biophase may also be enhanced in the neonate and young infant owing to immaturity of the blood–brain barrier (Kupfererberg and Way 1963).

Pharmacokinetics

Neonates have a high percentage of body water and less fat than older infants. Consequently, relatively large loading doses of water-soluble drugs such as morphine may need to be given over the first few hours of an infusion to achieve adequate plasma concentrations and effect. Subsequent drug elimination in the 'drug-naïve' neonate is delayed due to immaturity of hepatic and renal function. Therefore, once steady state has been achieved infusion rates need to be reduced substantially to prevent accumulation.

A fourfold reduction in the elimination half-life of morphine takes place in the first few years of life, with mean values of 7.2 hours below 1 month, compared with 1.7 hours in adults (McRorie et al. 1992). This is due primarily to the prolonged clearance of the drug. However there is wide individual variability between subjects, particularly in the neonate. The mean elimination half-life in the newborn was measured at 13.9 hours with a standard deviation of 6.4 hours (Olkkolo et al. 1988). Pharmacokinetic data for fentanyl show a similar pattern with even greater variability in the premature infant (Collins et al. 1985; Koehntop et al. 1986; Gauntlett et al. 1988). Hepatic clearance of fentanyl may be drastically reduced in neonates undergoing intra-abdominal surgery or those with raised intra-abdominal pressure (Koehntop et al. 1986).

Table 25.2 Commonly used measures of pain in neonates

MEASURE	VARIABLES INCLUDED	TYPE OF PAIN	PSYCHOMETRIC TESTING
Premature Infant Pain Profile (PIPP) (Slater et al. 2009b)	Heart rate Oxygen saturation Facial actions Takes state and gestational age into account	Procedural Postoperative (minor)	Reliability, validity, clinical utility well established
Neonatal Infant Pain Score (NIPS) (Anand et al. 2006)	Facial expression Crying Breathing patterns Arm and leg movements Arousal	Procedural	Reliability Validity
Neonatal Facial Coding System (NFCS) (Anand et al. 1987)	Facial actions	Procedural	Reliability, validity, clinical utility, high degree of sensitivity to analgesia
Neonatal Pain, Agitation and Sedation Sale (N-PASS)	Crying Irritability Behavioural state Facial expression Extremity tone Vital signs	Postoperative Procedural Ventilated	Reliability, validity, includes sedation end of scale, does not distinguish pain from agitation
Cry, Requires oxygen, Increased vital signs, Expression, Sleeplessness (CRIES) (Slater et al. 2008)	Crying Facial expression Sleeplessness Requires oxygen to stay at >96% saturation Increased vital signs	Postoperative	Reliability Validity
COMFORT scale (Stevens et al. 1996)	Movement Calmness Facial tension Alertness Respiration rate Muscle tone Heart rate Blood pressure	Postoperative Critical care Developed for sedation Recently validated for postoperative pain in 0–3-year-old infants	Reliability Validity Clinical utility

(Modified from Anand et al. (2006).)

This has been attributed to the effects of raised intra-abdominal pressure on liver blood flow (Masey et al. 1985). The implications for infants undergoing abdominal surgery are clear: some infants will have a sustained effect from doses of opioid that would normally be expected to have a limited duration of action.

Clinical analgesia

Opioids and paracetamol remain the most commonly used analgesics but there is increasing use of ketamine (an N-methyl-D-aspartate (NMDA) antagonist), clonidine (α_2 agonist), local anaesthetics and non-steroidal anti-inflammatory drugs (NSAIDs).

Opioids

Morphine, fentanyl and codeine are the most commonly used opioids in the UK. All can cause ventilatory depression, hypotension, urinary retention and decreased intestinal motility leading to delayed feeding after abdominal surgery.

Morphine remains the historical gold standard with which other analgesics are compared. Morphine has both slower onset and offset than fentanyl after a single dose, but after long-term infusion this effect is reversed because of the shorter terminal elimination half-life of morphine. In the ventilated neonate, an intravenous loading dose (50–150 µg/kg) is required to achieve effective analgesia, followed by an infusion rate between 5 and 20 µg/kg/h. However as tolerance develops, the infusion rate may need to be further increased. Nurse-controlled analgesia (NCA) is a useful technique for control of infant pain. The baby receives a background morphine infusion (2.5–10 µg/kg/h) topped up at appropriate intervals by 'nurse-controlled' doses (varying from about 2.5 to 10 µg/kg) according to formal pain assessment.

Morphine should be used with caution in the spontaneously breathing postoperative neonate. Loading doses of 10–50 µg/kg morphine can be given by slow infusion over 15 minutes in conjunction with sedation scores at 5-minute intervals. Once the desired level of comfort has been achieved, the infusion is discontinued, even if the full dose has not been delivered. Additional

SINGLETON HOSPITAL
STAFF LIBRARY

doses are then given in the same fashion according to regular documented pain scores, thereby maintaining a therapeutic level on an individual titrated basis. NCA can also be used with a low background morphine infusion (1–5 µg/kg/h). All infants under 6 months receiving opioids need to stay in a high-dependency unit for continual monitoring with direct observation, pulse oximetry and ventilatory monitoring.

Fentanyl provides intense analgesia and relative cardiovascular stability. At high doses (50–150 µg/kg as a single injection), it can control pulmonary hypertension (Hickey 1985). These doses are well above analgesic doses (0.5–10 µg/kg). Fahnenstich and colleagues (2000) observed chest wall rigidity in 8 out of 89 neonates following relatively small doses of 3–5 µg/kg fentanyl, all cases responded quickly to either naloxone or neuromuscular blockade. The high lipid solubility of fentanyl and increased skin permeability of the preterm neonate make transdermal administration a feasible route of administration, which is currently being evaluated. Transtracheal fentanyl provides rapid absorption in rabbits but awaits clinical trials in humans (Irazuzta et al. 1996).

Remifentanil is eliminated by the action of plasma esterases and consequently is not dependent on immature hepatic metabolic processes. It is cleared rapidly and predictably, thereby making it an attractive drug for short neonatal surgery when rapid recovery is needed (Berde et al. 2005). It has been used to good effect for sedation during mechanical ventilation – doses of up to 0.1 µg/kg/min provided adequate sedation in most infants (Giannantonio et al. 2009) – and provides good conditions when used with suxamethonium for tracheal intubation. There is emerging evidence of its efficacy and safety when used to provide intraoperative analgesia in major neonatal surgery (Michel et al. 2008; Marsh and Hodgkinson 2009).

Codeine has, reputedly, a lower incidence of opioid-related side-effects. It has been advocated for use in neonatal practice at a dose of 1 mg/kg orally/intramuscularly/rectally. Single-dose administration appears safe but with repeated doses unwanted side-effects do occur (Reisime and Pasternak 1996). Codeine is metabolised to morphine, but there is considerable variability, and in a small genetic subgroup of 'poor metabolisers' (9% in UK, 30% in Hong Kong Chinese) codeine has virtually no analgesic effect (Williams et al. 2001). This large interpatient variability necessitates caution when using codeine for long-term use in neonates.

Tolerance and withdrawal

While initial doses of opioid infusions needed for analgesia and sedation are low, the dose requirements increase rapidly. Neonates undergoing extracorporeal membrane oxygenation require five times the initial opioid infusion rate by day 6 to achieve the same level of sedation due to a combination of enhanced elimination (Arnold et al. 1991) and true tolerance (Greeley and Debruijn 1998). The use of long-term infusions of morphine for sedation alone is debatable: it is better to reserve analgesic drugs for pain relief or use low-dose infusions of morphine in conjunction with other long-acting sedatives such as chloral hydrate or promethazine.

Opioid antagonists (naloxone 4–10 µg/kg) easily reverse opioid side-effects but must be used with caution with neonates receiving opioid infusions as acute antagonism may trigger a syndrome of withdrawal. Withdrawal is characterised by an excitation of the central nervous system, the gastrointestinal system and the autonomic nervous system (Suresh and Anand 1998). Opioid abstinence syndrome can occur after 48 hours of morphine infusion but is more usually observed after 4–5 days. Management includes the use of a reducing opioid regimen (with morphine or methadone), α_2 antagonists (clonidine 3–5 µg/kg 8–12-hourly) and benzodiazepines for anxiolysis. Weaning schedules can last weeks. Preventive methods include the judicious use of opioids combined with formal comfort scores to optimise the rate of opioid withdrawal.

Non-opioids

Paracetamol (acetaminophen) is primarily metabolised by glucuronidation in older children but by sulphation in neonates (van Lingen et al. 1999). Once the main metabolic pathways are saturated paracetamol is oxidated by the cytochrome P450 system to a reactive intermediary compound which is bound to glutathione, but can react with hepatocyte macromolecules in the absence of glutathione. Neonates may have some protection from the hepatic toxicity effects of paracetamol by having greater glutathione stores and slower oxidative metabolism (Truog and Anand 1989). Paracetamol is a widely accepted treatment for moderate pain in neonates. Current data suggest that its short-term use in term and preterm neonates is safe and efficacious (Anand et al. 2000). It has additive effects when combined with opioids thereby allowing lower doses and subsequently lower incidence of side-effects (Menon et al. 1998). Loading doses of paracetamol are similar for premature and term neonates (25 mg/kg orally or 35 mg/kg by triglyceride suppository). Subsequent maintenance regimens must be tailored to the maturity of the infant. Anderson et al. (2002) found that adequate plasma concentrations can be achieved by an oral dose of 25 mg/kg/day in premature neonates at 30 weeks post-conception, 45 mg/kg/day at 34 weeks' gestation, 60 mg/kg/day at term, and 90 mg/kg/day at 6 months of age. Rectal doses must be increased by a third the oral dose to account for the decreased absorption by this route. These regimens may cause hepatotoxicity in some individuals if used for longer than 2–3 days.

Intravenous paracetamol is available but there is much international discussion as to the safe and most efficacious dose when used in the neonatal population. In the UK it is currently licensed for use in infants aged over 10 days, and less than 10 kg, at a dose of 7.5 mg/kg, not exceeding 30 mg/kg/day; however many paediatric anaesthetists are using higher doses (Wilson-Smith and Morton 2009). This dosing does not take into consideration maturational changes in paracetamol metabolism or the evidence that intravenous paracetamol can be given to premature infants and those under 10 days if an appropriately reduced dose is administered. In Australia 15 mg/kg 6-hourly is administered to term infants over 10 days' age with a reduced dose of 7.5 mg/kg 6-hourly in term infants under 10 days (Anderson and Allegaert 2009). Further investigation is needed to establish the safety of intravenous paracetamol in premature neonates.

NSAIDs have antipyretic and anti-inflammatory properties with no respiratory depressant or sedative side-effects. As with paracetamol, they have an opioid-sparing effect in older children. Concern over potentially serious side-effects has limited NSAID use for analgesia. Current knowledge of their neonatal effect results almost entirely from their use in the treatment of patent ductus arteriosus (PDA). Side-effects of indometacin include oliguria from decreased renal perfusion; necrotising enterocolitis and gut perforation from decreased splanchnic perfusion (Shorter et al. 1999); and gastrointestinal bleeding from reduced platelet function. Decreased cerebral blood flow may have a preventive effect on intraventricular haemorrhage in preterm neonates (Ment et al. 1996). Ibuprofen has been used as an oral analgesic in term neonates and has a lower incidence of side-effects than indometacin when used for treatment of PDA (Van Overmeire et al. 2000). It should be used with caution in jaundiced patients as it may displace bilirubin from albumin and, at a dose of 5–10 mg/kg, ibuprofen need only be repeated every 12–24 hours as its half-life is prolonged compared with that in adults (Aranda et al. 1997).

Over the last decade there has been a resurgence of interest in ketamine and clonidine. Ketamine is a centrally acting NMDA receptor antagonist and potent analgesic. It has been used with proven efficacy and safety for the anaesthesia of neonates for some years. It can be given intravenously (0.5–2 mg/kg), rectally (3–8 mg/kg), intramuscularly (2–5 mg/kg) and via the neuroaxial route (Pellier et al. 1999). It has the advantage of promoting cardiovascular stability, especially in hypovolaemic patients; it maintains respiratory drive and is a bronchodilator. It increases salivation and respiratory secretions and is usually given with an anticholinergic agent (e.g. atropine 10 μg/kg iv) and is often combined with midazolam (e.g. 25 μg/kg) to provide procedural analgesia and sedation. Intravenous doses of 2 mg and intramuscular doses of 3 mg/kg have been found to induce sedation in 45 seconds and 4 minutes respectively (Cotsen et al. 1997). S(+)-ketamine, one of the two enantiomers of ketamine, has threefold greater analgesic potency than racemic ketamine and may prove to have fewer side-effects. It has been used effectively in caudal anaesthesia (Marhofer et al. 2000) but further clinical trials are needed to evaluate its parenteral use in neonates.

Clonidine is an α_2 agonist that is commonly used via the caudal route (1–2 μg/kg) in combination with local anaesthetic drugs. It provides dose-dependent analgesia following oral and intravenous administration. It has the advantage of having less respiratory depression than opioids, although there are case reports of postoperative apnoea in term and preterm infants (Breschan et al. 1999; Bouchut et al. 2001). Oral doses of up to 4 μg/kg 8-hourly have been used in the treatment of neonatal opioid withdrawal (Suresh and Anand 1998).

Pure sedative drugs have an adjuvant role in the treatment of neonatal pain. In combination with analgesics, they may reduce anxiety and stress by promoting sleep. Of the benzodiazepines, lorazepam (20–100 μg/kg) has a longer duration, resulting in a smoother sedative effect (McDermott et al. 1992). Benzodiazepines have an additive effect on the respiratory depression of opioids. Chloral hydrate, promethazine and triclofos sodium are other popular sedative drugs.

Local anaesthetics

The use of local and regional anaesthesia/analgesic techniques has a significant, albeit specialised, role in the treatment of neonatal pain (Table 25.3). High-dose opioid techniques may be beneficial to the sick neonate by suppressing nociceptive processing

Table 25.3 Analgesic doses

	POPULATION	DOSE	NOTES
Morphine	Ventilated neonate Unventilated neonate	50–150 μg/kg iv 5–20 μg/kg/h iv 2.5–10 μg/kg iv 2.5–10 μg/kg/h iv 10–50 μg/kg iv	Loading dose Infusion NCA (bolus every 30 min) NCA (background infusion) Slow loading dose
Fentanyl	For ventilated neonates only	0.5–10 μg/kg iv	
Alfentanil	For ventilated neonates only	5–10 μg/kg iv 0.5–1 μg/kg/h iv	Loading dose Infusion
Codeine		1 mg/kg po/pr	
Paracetamol	All ages 30 weeks PCA 34 weeks PCA 40 weeks PCA 60 weeks PCA	25 mg/kg po, 35 mg/kg pr 25 mg/kg po, 30 mg/kg pr 45 mg/kg po, 60 mg/kg pr 60 mg/kg po, 80 mg/kg pr 90 mg/kg po, 120 mg/kg pr	Loading dose Maximum daily dose Maximum daily dose Maximum daily dose Maximum daily dose
Paracetamol	Term neonates <10 days Term neonates >10 days	30 mg/kg iv 60 mg/kg iv	Maximum daily dose Maximum daily dose
Ibuprofen		5–10 mg/kg po	Every 12–24 hours
Ketamine		0.5–2 mg/kg iv* 3–8 mg/kg pr	Coadministration with an anticholinergic advised due to increased respiratory secretions
Clonidine		2–4 μg/kg po	For opioid withdrawal
Lorazepam		20–100 μg/kg iv	
Chloral hydrate/ triclofos sodium		30–50 mg/kg po/pr	
Promethazine		0.5 mg/kg iv/po	

Doses of commonly used analgesic and sedative drugs. These dosing regimens are guides only and care must be taken as there is considerable variation in effect.
NCA, nurse-controlled analgesia; iv, intravenous; po, orally; pr, per rectum; PCA, postconceptual age.
*2 mg/kg ketamine is an anaesthetic dose and may cause apnoea.

and the neural–humoral responses to pain but are complicated by respiratory depression. Conversely, regional analgesia has been shown to be as effective as morphine infusions without causing sedation or ventilatory depression (Armitage 1988; Wolf and Hughes 1993), leading to faster recovery times. There are many recent studies to suggest that in experienced hands regional anaesthesia/analgesia is safe and easy with few side-effects (Strafford et al. 1995; Giaufre et al. 1996; Martinez-Telleria et al. 1997; Uguralp et al. 2002). Local anaesthetics can block nociceptive transmission at various sites – topically and by local infiltration to the skin, regionally by nerve blocks or neuroaxially via the caudal, lumbar or thoracic epidural route. Single-shot administration can provide up to 12 hours of analgesia or indwelling catheters can be used for local anaesthetic infusions or repeat bolus.

Newborns are at a higher risk for local anaesthetic toxicity, which had previously led to concern over the use of local anaesthetics in this age group. Lower alpha-1-glycoprotein levels (Lerman et al.

1989) and reduced clearance of amide local anaesthetics result in potentially higher plasma levels, which can cause seizures and cardiovascular collapse (Berde 1993). This is further exacerbated by acidosis, hypoxia, hypercapnia, hyponatraemia and hyperkalaemia – and the neonate is at a greater risk for developing many of these. Care should be taken when calculating the safe maximum doses of lidocaine (3 mg/kg) and bupivicaine (2 mg/kg bolus). Epidural infusions of bupivicaine (0.2 mg/kg/h, 1.25 mg/ml) can be given safely for up to 48 hours but Larsson et al. (1997) found a significant number of neonates had a still rising plasma bupivicaine level at 48 hours, suggesting that accumulation may occur with prolonged epidural infusions.

Eutectic mixture of local anaesthetics (EMLA) contains 2.5% lidocaine and 2.5% prilocaine. Prilocaine has a metabolite o-toluidine which can cause methaemoglobinaemia. Taddio et al. (1998), in a meta-analysis of 11 trials, showed the incidence of clinically relevant methaemaglobinaemia to be zero, allaying previous concerns over the use of EMLA in those under 3 months. However, the risk of

---

Table 25.4 A suggested plan for provision of analgesia in the neonatal unit for various common scenarios

Postoperative analgesia	

Non-ventilated baby	1. Determine opioid history
	   e.g. loading dose in theatre or long-term administration
	2. Inadequate analgesia
	   10–50 µg/kg iv morphine* bolus over 15 minutes with formal pain/comfort scoring at 5-minute intervals until analgesia is optimal
	3. Analgesia maintenance
	   0–20 µg/kg/h iv morphine*
	4. Regular paracetamol (caution after 48 hours: see text)
	5. Transfer to enteral analgesics, e.g. codeine, as soon as possible

Ventilated baby	1. Inadequate analgesia
	   50–150 µg/kg iv morphine* bolus as required
	2. Analgesia maintenance
	   0–40 µg/kg/h iv morphine*
	3. Regular paracetamol (caution after 48 hours: see text)
	4. Fentanyl* with critically ill babies (conveys haemodynamic stability)
	   0.5–10 µg/kg iv bolus if analgesia inadequate
	   2.5–10 µg/kg/h for iv maintenance

Background sedation	

Ventilated baby	1. Opioid infusion
	   Critically ill baby: use fentanyl* 2.5–10 µg/kg/h iv
	   Otherwise morphine* 0–20 µg/kg/h
	2. Optimise opioid infusion with pain/comfort scoring
	   Limit dose to reduce tolerance (kinetic and dynamic)
	   Ensure adequate analgesia to avoid stress response
	3. Consider secondary agents to reduce opioid requirements
	   Sedatives, e.g. triclofos or lorazepam
	   Clonidine
	4. Non-pharmacological strategies (see text)

Procedural analgesia	

e.g. venepuncture or chest drain insertion	1. Use local anaesthesia where possible; first establish appropriate safe dose for patient then consider:
	   Local infiltration
	   EMLA (allow skin contact of at least 60 minutes)
	   Ametop (allow skin contact of 45 minutes)
	2. Non-pharmacological strategies (see text)
	3. Consider single iv opioid bolus (as above)

*Infants receiving opioid infusions must be fully monitored with regular formal pain/comfort scoring in a high-dependency or intensive care unit.
EMLA, eutectic mixture of local anaesthetics.

significant methaemoglobinaemia increases if excess doses are used too frequently and if other methaemoglobin-inducers are used. Amethocaine is an alternative topical anaesthetic that is being increasingly used in the UK; further studies are needed to establish its safety for the newborn but early work suggests it to be a safe and effective anaesthetic for venepuncture after 40–60-minutes' application in newborn infants from 27 weeks' gestation and lasting 4–6 hours (Jain and Rutter 2000). Both EMLA and Ametop have been found to be not particularly effective for heel-lancing pain. Venepuncture by an experienced practitioner causes less pain than heel-lancing and should be the method of choice (Shah and Ohlsson 1999). Neonatal circumcision is still widely performed without anaesthesia and has been shown to have long-term effects on pain perception 6 months after the procedure (Taddio et al. 1997). In a Cochrane review EMLA was found to attenuate the physiological effects of pain following circumcision (Taddio et al. 2000). However the authors concluded that, while EMLA was more effective than placebo and should be used in place of nothing, there are more effective analgesic methods such as penile dorsal nerve blocks and ring blocks which need further evaluation – initial reports suggest dorsal nerve blocks to be safe with a low incidence of complications (Fontaine et al. 1994).

Environmental and behavioural interventions

There is a growing body of evidence that environmental, behavioural and non-pharmacological strategies can reduce the behavioural and physiological indicators of pain and stress in the newborn. These principles are encompassed in the concept of developmental care which leads to improved neurobehavioural organisation, lower morbidity and earlier discharge (Als et al. 1986, 1994). Minimising painful procedures to those absolutely necessary and clustering them together can reduce the frequency of noxious stimuli. Other techniques thought to be beneficial include decreasing handling, reducing ambient noise and light, and establishing day–night cycles (Franck and Lawhon 1998).

Behavioural strategies useful in reducing pain scores during painful procedures include gentle sensory stimulation of the visual, tactile (Gray et al. 2000), auditory (Locsin 1981) and taste senses. Oral sucrose and sweet compounds are safe and effective at reducing pain scores during invasive procedures. There is a dose-dependent effect from 5% to 50% but the optimal dose is not known (Stevens and Ohlsson 2000). Bellieni et al. (2001) combined oral 10% glucose, non-nutritive sucking and multisensorial stimulation into a process of 'sensorial saturation'. They found that this was more effective at reducing pain scores than any of these techniques alone (Bellieni et al. 2001). A Cochrane review has recommended oral sucrose as analgesia for procedural pain in newborns, based on its effect in reducing pain scores (Stevens et al. 2010), but a recent randomised controlled trial has demonstrated that, while reducing the PIPP score, oral sucrose does not reduce the cortical response (Slater et al. 2010b). Proprioceptive, vestibular and thermal stimulation occurs through swaddling, rocking and maintaining a flexed position (facilitated tucking) (Franck and Lawhon 1998). The use of melatonin is still in the research domain but it may prove useful to regulate the circadian rhythm (Seron-Ferre et al .2001). An overview of general strategy is shown in Table 25.4.

Weblink

Royal College of Nursing: www.rcn.org.uk/development/practice/pain/downloads.

References

Als, H., Lawhon, G., Brown, E., et al., 1986. Individualized behavioral and environmental care for the very low birth weight preterm infant at high risk for bronchopulmonary dysplasia: neonatal intensive care unit and developmental outcome. Pediatrics 78, 1123–1132.

Als, H., Lawhon, G., Duffy, F.H., et al., 1994. Individualized developmental care for the very low-birth-weight preterm infant. Medical and neurofunctional effects. JAMA 272, 853–858.

Anand, K.J., 1990. Neonatal stress responses to anesthesia and surgery. Clin Perinatol 17, 207–214.

Anand, K.J., Carr, D.B., 1989. The neuroanatomy, neurophysiology, and neurochemistry of pain, stress, and analgesia in newborns and children. Pediatr Clin North Am 36, 795–822.

Anand, K.J., Sippell, W.G., Aynsley-Green, A., 1987. Randomised trial of fentanyl anaesthesia in preterm babies undergoing surgery: effects on the stress response. Lancet 1, 62–66.

Anand, K.J., Barton, B.A., McIntosh, N., et al., 1999. Analgesia and sedation in preterm neonates who require ventilatory support: results from the NOPAIN trial. Neonatal Outcome and Prolonged Analgesia in Neonates. [erratum appears in Arch Pediatr Adolesc Med 1999 Aug; 153(8):895.]. Arch Pediatr Adolesc Med 153, 331–898.

Anand, K.J., Menon, G., Narsinghani, U., et al., 2000. Systemic analgesic therapy. In: Anand, K.J., Stevens, B., McGrath, P. (Eds.), Pain in Neonates, second ed. Elsevier, Amsterdam, pp. 159–188.

Anand, K.J.S., Whit Hall, R., Desai, N., et al., 2004. Effects of morphine in ventilated preterm infants: primary outcomes from NEOPAIN randomised trial. Lancet 363:167.

Anand, K.J.S., Aranda, J.V., Berde, C.B., et al., 2006. Summary proceedings from the Neonatal Pain Control Group. Pediatrics 117, S9–S22.

Anderson, B.J., Allegaert, K., 2009. Intravenous neonatal paracetamol dosing: the magic of 10 days. Paediatr Anaesth 19, 289–295.

Anderson, B.J., van Lingen, R.A., Hansen, T.G., et al., 2002. Acetaminophen developmental pharmacokinetics in premature neonates and infants: a pooled population analysis. Anesthesiology 96, 1336–1345.

Andrews, K., Fitzgerald, M., 1994. The cutaneous withdrawal reflex in human neonates: sensitization, receptive fields, and the effects of contralateral stimulation. Pain 56, 95–101.

Aranda, J.V., Varvarigou, A., Beharry, K., et al., 1997. Pharmacokinetics and protein binding of intravenous ibuprofen in the premature newborn infant. Acta Paediatr 86, 289–293.

Armitage, E.N., 1988. Is there a place for regional anesthesia in pediatrics?–Yes! Acta Anaesthesiol Belg 39, 191–195.

Arnold, J.H., Truog, R.D., Scavone, J.M., et al., 1991. Changes in the pharmacodynamic response to fentanyl in neonates during continuous infusion. J Pediatr 119, 639–643.

Barker, D.P., Rutter, N., 1995. Exposure to invasive procedures in neonatal intensive care unit admissions. Arch Dis Child Fetal Neonatal Ed 72, F47–F48.

Bartocci, M., Bergqvist, L.L., Lagercrantz, H., et al., 2006. Pain activates cortical areas in the preterm newborn brain. Pain 122, 109–117.

Batton, D.G., Barrington, K.J., Wallman, C., 2006. Prevention and management of pain in the neonate: an update. Pediatrics 118, 2231–2241.

Bellieni, C.V., Buonocore, G., Nenci, A., et al., 2001. Sensorial saturation: an effective analgesic tool for heel-prick in preterm infants: a prospective randomized trial. Biol Neonate 80, 15–18.

Berde, C.B., 1993. Toxicity of local anesthetics in infants and children. J Pediatr 122, S14–S20.

Berde, C.B., Jaksic, T., Lynn, A.M., et al., 2005. Anesthesia and analgesia during and after surgery in neonates. Clin Ther 27, 900–921.

Bouchut, J.C., Dubois, R., Godard, J., 2001. Clonidine in preterm-infant caudal anesthesia may be responsible for postoperative apnea. Reg Anesth Pain Med 26, 83–85.

Breschan, C., Krumpholz, R., Likar, R., et al., 1999. Can a dose of 2microg.kg(-1) caudal clonidine cause respiratory depression in neonates? Paediatr Anaesth 9, 81–83.

Chugani, H.T., Phelps, M.E., 1986. Maturational changes in cerebral function in infants determined by 18-FDG positron emission tomography. Science 231, 840–844.

Collins, C., Koren, G., Crean, P., et al., 1985. Fentanyl pharmacokinetics and hemodynamic effects in preterm infants during ligation of patent ductus arteriosus. Anesth Analg 64, 1078–1080.

Constantinou, J., Reynolds, M.L., Woolf, C.J., et al., 1994. Nerve growth factor levels in developing rat skin: upregulation following skin wounding. Neuroreport 5, 2281–2284.

Cotsen, M.R., Donaldson, J.S., Uejima, T., Morello, F.P., 1997. Efficacy of ketamine hydrochloride sedation in children for interventional radiologic procedures. AJR Am J Roentgenol 169, 1019–1022.

Dixon, S., Snyder, J., Holve, R., Bromberger, P., 1984. Behavioral effects of circumcision with and without anesthesia. J Dev Behav Pediatr 5, 246–250.

Fahnenstich, H., Steffan, J., Kau, N., et al., 2000. Fentanyl-induced chest wall rigidity and laryngospasm in preterm and term infants. Crit Care Med 28, 836–839.

Fisk, N.M., Gitau, R., Teixeira, J.M., et al., 2001. Effect of direct fetal opioid analgesia on fetal hormonal and hemodynamic stress response to intrauterine needling. Anesthesiology 95, 828–835.

Fitzgerald, M., Millard, C., McIntosh, N., 1989. Cutaneous hypersensitivity following peripheral tissue damage in newborn infants and its reversal with topical anaesthesia. Pain 39, 31–36.

Fitzgerald, M., Butcher, T., Shortland, P., 1994. Developmental changes in the laminar termination of A fibre cutaneous sensory afferents in the rat spinal cord dorsal horn. J Comp Neurol 348, 225–233.

Fontaine, P., Dittberner, D., Scheltema, K., 1994. The safety of dorsal penile nerve block for neonatal circumcision. J Fam Pract 39, 243–248.

Franck, L.S., Lawhon, G., 1998. Environmental and behavioral strategies to prevent and manage neonatal pain. Semin Perinatol 22, 434–443.

Gauntlett, I.S., Fisher, D.M., Hertzka, R.E., et al., 1988. Pharmacokinetics of fentanyl in neonatal humans and lambs: effects of age. Anesthesiology 69, 683–687.

Giannantonio, C., Sammartino, M., Valente, E., et al., 2009. Remifentanil analgosedation in preterm newborns during mechanical ventilation. Acta Paediatr 98, 1111–1115.

Giaufre, E., Dalens, B., Gombert, A., 1996. Epidemiology and morbidity of regional anesthesia in children: a one-year prospective survey of the French-Language Society of Pediatric Anesthesiologists. Anesth Analg 83, 904–912.

Gilles, F.J., Shankle, W., Dooling, E.C., 1983. Myelinated tracts: growth patterns. In: Gilles, F.J., Leviton, A., Dooling, E.C. (Eds.), The Developing Human Brain: Growth and Epidemiologic Neuropathy. John Wright, Boston, pp. 117–183.

Gleiss, J., Stuttgen, G., 1970. Morphologic and functional development of the skin. In: Stave, U. (Ed.), Physiology of the Perinatal Period. Appleton-Century-Crofts, New York, pp. 889–906.

Glover, V., Fisk, N., 1996. We don't know; better to err on the safe side from mid-gestation. Br Med J Clin Res Ed 313, 796.

Gray, L., Watt, L., Blass, E.M., 2000. Skin-to-skin contact is analgesic in healthy newborns. Pediatrics 105, e14.

Greeley, W.J., Debruijn, N.P., 1998. Changes in sufentanil pharmacokinetics within the neonatal period. Anesth Analg 67, 86–90.

Grunau, R.V., Craig, K.D., 1987. Pain expression in neonates: facial action and cry. Pain 28, 395–410.

Grunau, R.V., Whitfield, M.F., Petrie, J.H., 1994. Pain sensitivity and temperament in extremely low-birth-weight premature toddlers and preterm and full-term controls. Pain 58, 341–346.

Hall, R.W., Kronsberg, S.S., Barton, B.A., et al., 2005. Morphine, hypotension, and adverse outcomes among preterm neonates: who's to blame? Secondary results from the NEOPAIN trial. Pediatrics 115, 1351–1359.

Haouari, N., Wood, C., Griffiths, G., et al., 1995. The analgesic effect of sucrose in full term infants: a randomised controlled trial. Br Med J 310, 1498–1500.

Henderson-Smart, D.J., Pettigrew, A.G., Campbell, D.J., 1983. Clinical apnea and brain-stem neural function in preterm neonates. N Engl J Med 308, 353–357.

Hickey, P.R., 1985. Blunting of the stress response in the pulmonary circulation of infants with fentanyl. Anesth Analg 64, 1137–1141.

Hu, S., Sheng, W., Lokensgard, J., et al., 2002. Morphine induces apoptosis of human microglia and neurons. Neuropharmacology 42, 829–836.

Humphrey, T., 1964. Some correlations between the appearance of human fetal reflexes and the development of the nervous system. Prog Brain Res 4, 93–135.

Irazuzta, J.E., Ahmed, U., Gancayco, A., et al., 1996. Intratracheal administration of fentanyl: pharmacokinetics and local tissue effects. Intens Care Med 22, 129–133.

Jacobson, B., Eklund, G., Hamberger, L., et al., 1987. Perinatal origin of adult self-destructive behaviour. Acta Psychiatr Scand 76, 364–371.

Jain, A., Rutter, N., 2000. Does topical amethocaine gel reduce the pain of venepuncture in newborn infants? A randomised double blind controlled trial. Arch Dis Child Fetal Neonatal Ed 83, F207–F210.

Johnston, C.C., Stevens, B.J., 1996. Experience in a neonatal intensive care unit affects pain response. Pediatrics 98, 925–930.

Johnston, C.C., Collinge, J.M., Henderson, S.J., et al., 1997. A cross-sectional survey of pain and pharmacological analgesia in Canadian neonatal intensive care units. Clin J Pain 13, 308–312.

Kelly, M.A., Finer, N.H., 1984. Nasotracheal intubation in the neonate: Physiological responses and the effects of atropine and pancuronium. J Pediatr 105, 303–309.

Koehntop, D.E., Rodman, J.H., Brundage, D.M., et al., 1986. Pharmacokinetics of fentanyl in neonates. Anesth Analg 65, 227–232.

Kostovic, I., Rakie, P., 1984. Development of prestriate visual projections in the monkey and human fetal cerebrum revealed by transient cholinesterase staining. J Neurosci 4, 25–42.

Kupfererberg, H.J., Way, E.L., 1963. Pharmacologic basis for increased sensitivity of the newborn rat to morphine. J Pharmacol Exp Ther 141, 105–112.

Larsson, B.A., Lonnqvist, P.A., Olsson, G.L., 1997. Plasma concentrations of bupivacaine in neonates after continuous epidural infusion. Anesth Analg 84, 501–505.

Lerman, J., Strong, H.A., LeDez, K.M., et al., 1989. Effects of age on the serum concentration of alpha 1-acid glycoprotein and the binding of lidocaine in pediatric patients. Clin Pharmacol Ther 46, 219–225.

Lloyd-Thomas, A.R., Fitzgerald, M., 1996. Reflex responses do not necessarily signify pain. Br Med J Clin Res Ed 313, 797–798.

Locsin, R.G., 1981. The effect of music on the pain of selected post-operative patients. J Adv Nurs 6, 19–25.

Marhofer, P., Krenn, C.G., Plochl, W., et al., 2000. S(+)-ketamine for caudal block in paediatric anaesthesia. Br J Anaesth 84, 341–345.

Marsh, D.F., Hodkinson, B., 2009. Remifentanil in paediatric anaesthetic practice. Anaesthesia 64, 301–308.

Marshall, R.E., Stratton, W.C., Moore, J.A., et al., 1980. Circumcision 1. Effects upon newborn behavior. Infant Behav Dev 3, 1–9.

Martinez-Telleria, A., Cano Serrano, M.E., Martinez-Telleria, M.J., et al., 1997. [Analysis of regional anesthetic efficacy in pediatric postop pain.] Cirugia Pediatr 10, 18–20.

Masey, S.A., Koehler, R.C., Buck, J.R., et al., 1985. Effect of abdominal distention on central and regional hemodynamics in neonatal lambs. Pediatr Res 19, 1244–1249.

McDermott, C.A., Kowalczyk, A.L., Schnitzler, E.R., et al., 1992. Pharmacokinetics of lorazepam in critically ill neonates with seizures. J Pediatr 120, 479–483.

McRae, M.E., Rourke, D.A., Imperial-Perez, F.A., et al., 1997. Development of a research-based standard for assessment, intervention, and evaluation of pain after neonatal and pediatric cardiac surgery. Pediatr Nurs 23, 263–271.

McRorie, T.I., Lynn, A.M., Nespeca, M.K., et al., 1992. The maturation of morphine clearance and metabolism. Am J Dis Child 146, 972–976.

Menon, G., Anand, K.J., McIntosh, N., 1998. Practical approach to analgesia and sedation in the neonatal intensive care unit. Semin Perinatol 22, 417–424.

Ment, L.R., Vohr, B., Oh, W., et al., 1996. Neurodevelopmental outcome at 36 months' corrected age of preterm infants in the Multicenter Indomethacin Intraventricular Hemorrhage Prevention Trial. Pediatrics 98, 714–718.

Michel, F., Lando, A., Aubry, C., et al., 2008. Experience with remifentanil-sevoflurane balanced anesthesia for abdominal surgery in neonates and children less than 2 years. Paediatr Anaesth 18, 532–538.

Okado, N., 1981. Onset of synapse formation in the human spinal cord. J Comp Neurol 201, 211–219.

Okur, H., Kucukaydin, M., Ustdal, K.M., 1995. The endocrine and metabolic response to surgical stress in the neonate. J Pediatr Surg 30, 626–630.

Olkkolo, K.T., Maunuksela, E.L., Korpela, R., et al., 1988. Kinetics and dynamics of postoperative morphine in children. Clin Pharmacol Ther 44, 123–136.

Pasternak, G.W., Zhang, A.Z., Tecoff, L., 1980. Developmental differences between high and low affinity opioid binding sites: their relationship to analgesia and ventilatory depression. Life Sci 27, 1185–1190.

Pellier, I., Monrigal, J.P., Le Moine, P., et al., 1999. Use of intravenous ketamine-midazolam association for pain procedures in children with cancer. A prospective study. Paediatr Anaesth 9, 61–68.

Porter, F.L., Porges, S.W., Marshall, R.E., 1988. Neonatal pain cries and vagal tone: parallel changes in response to circumcision. Child Dev 59, 495–496.

Porter, F.L., Blackwell, M., Miller, J.P., 1991. Differences in developmental blood pressure (BP) regulation during lumbar puncture (Lps) in newborns. Pediatr Res 29, 230.

Reisime, T., Pasternak, G., 1996. Opioid analgesics and antagonists. In: Hardman, J.G., Limbird, L.E., Mounoff, P.B., et al. (Eds.), Goodman and Gilman's: The Pharmacological Basis of Therapeutics, ninth ed. McGraw-Hill, New York, pp. 521–555.

Rizvi, T.A., Wadhwa, S., Mehra, R.D., et al., 1986. Ultrastructure of marginal zone during prenatal development of human spinal cord. Exp Brain Res 64, 483–490.

Seron-Ferre, M., Torres-Farfan, C., Forcelledo, M.L., et al., 2001. The development of circadian rhythms in the fetus and neonate. Semin Perinatol 25, 363–370.

Shah, V., Ohlsson, A., 1999. Venepuncture versus heel lance for blood sampling in term neonates. Cochrane Database Syst Rev (2), CD001452.

Shorter, N.A., Liu, J.Y., Mooney, D.P., et al., 1999. Indomethacin-associated bowel perforations: a study of possible risk factors. J Pediatr Surg 34, 442–444.

Slater, R., Cantarella, A., Galllella, S., et al., 2006. Cortical pain responses in human infants. J Neurosci 26(14), 3662–3666.

Slater, R., Cantarella, A., Franck, L., et al., 2008. How well do clinical pain assessment tools reflect pain in infants? PLoS Med 5:e129.

Slater, R., Worley, A., Fabrizi, L., et al., 2009a. Evoked potentials generated by noxious stimulation in the human infant brain. Eur J Pain 14, 321–326.

Slater, R., Cantarella, A., Yoxen, J., et al., 2009b. Latency to facial expression change following noxious stimulation in infants is dependent on postmenstrual age. Pain 146:177–182.

Slater, R., Cornelissen, L., Fabrizi, L., et al., 2010a. Oral sucrose as an analgesic drug for procedural pain in newborn infants; a randomised controlled trial. Lancet 376:1225–1232.

Slater, R., Fabrizi, L., Worley, A., et al., 2010b. Premature infants display increased noxious-evoked neuronal activity in the brain compared to healthy age-matched term-born infants. Neuroimage 52, 583–589.

Stevens, B., Ohlsson, A., 2000. Sucrose for analgesia in newborn infants undergoing painful procedures. Cochrane Database Syst Rev (2), CD001069.

Stevens, B., Johnston, C., Petryshen, P., et al., 1996. Premature Infant Pain Profile: development and initial validation. Clin J Pain 12, 13–22.

Stevens, B., Yamada, J., Ohlsson, A., 2010. Sucrose for analgesia in newborn infants undergoing painful procedures. Cochrane Database Syst Rev (1), CD001069.

Strafford, M.A., Wilder, R.T., Berde, C.B., 1995. The risk of infection from epidural analgesia in children: a review of 1620 cases. Anesth Analg 80, 234–238.

Suresh, S., Anand, K.J., 1998. Opioid tolerance in neonates: mechanisms, diagnosis, assessment, and management. Semin Perinatol 22, 425–433.

Szawarski, Z., 1996. Probably no pain in the absence of self. Br Med J Clin Res Ed 313, 796–797.

Taddio, A., Katz, J., Ileersich, A.L., et al., 1997. Effects of neonatal circumcision on pain response during subsequent routine vaccination. Lancet 349, 599–603.

Taddio, A., Ohlsson, A., Einarson, T.R., et al., 1998. A systematic review of lidocaine-prilocaine cream (EMLA) in the treatment of acute pain in neonates. Pediatrics 101, E1.

Taddio, A., Ohlsson, K., Ohlsson, A., 2000. Lidocaine-prilocaine cream for analgesia during circumcision in newborn boys. Cochrane Database Syst Rev (2), CD000496.

Teixeira, J., Fogliani, R., 1996. Fetal haemodynamic stress response to invasive procedures. Lancet 347, 524.

Torres, F., Anderson, C., 1985. The normal EEG of the human newborn. J Clin Neurophysiol 2, 89–103.

Truog, R., Anand, K.J., 1989. Management of pain in the postoperative neonate. Clin Perinatol 16, 61–78.

Uguralp, S., Mutus, M., Koroglu, A., et al., 2002. Regional anesthesia is a good alternative to general anesthesia in pediatric surgery: Experience in 1,554 children. J Pediatr Surg 37, 610–613.

Valman, H.B., Pearson, J.F., 1980. What the fetus feels. Br Med J Clin Res Ed 280, 233–234.

van Lingen, R.A., Deinum, J.T., Quak, J.M., et al., 1999. Pharmacokinetics and metabolism of rectally administered paracetamol in preterm neonates. Arch Dis Child Fetal Neonatal Ed 80, F59–F63.

Van Overmeire, B., Smets, K., Lecoutere, D., et al., 2000. A comparison of ibuprofen and indomethacin for closure of patent ductus arteriosus. N Engl J Med 343, 674–681.

Williams, D.G., Hatch, D.J., Howard, R.F., 2001. Codeine phosphate in paediatric medicine. Br J Anaesth 86, 413–421.

Wilson-Smith, E.M., Morton, N.S., 2009. Survey of i.v. paracetamol (acetaminophen) use in neonates and infants under 1 year of age by UK anesthetists. Paediatr Anaesth 19, 329–337.

Wolf, A.R., Hughes, D., 1993. Pain relief for infants undergoing abdominal surgery: comparison of infusions of i.v. morphine and extradural bupivacaine. Br J Anaesth 70, 10–16.

Wolf, A.R., Doyle, E., Thomas, E., 1998. Modifying infant stress responses to major surgery: spinal vs extradural vs opioid analgesia. Paediatr Anaesth 8, 305–311.

The baby of a substance-abusing mother

Cassie Lawn   Neil Aiton

26

© 2012 Elsevier Ltd

Introduction

Substance abuse in pregnancy poses serious health risks to mothers and the developing baby, as well as potentially hindering parents' ability to care adequately for their children. Babies can suffer from consequences of congenital malformations and the adverse effects of drugs on pregnancy, or develop acute drug withdrawal after birth.

Drug abuse is common in women of childbearing age: the European Monitoring Centre for Drugs and Drug Addiction annual report for 2008 (EMCDDA 2008) states that, in the 16–34-year age group in England and Wales, 13.8% of individuals have used cannabis, 4.5% cocaine, 3.1% ecstasy and 1.8% amphetamines during the preceding year. Rates are slightly higher for all drugs in Scotland and lower in Northern Ireland. Drug use is even higher in the 16–24-year age group and 0.2% of all adults surveyed in England and Wales admitted to opiate use in the preceding year. Accurate figures for fetal exposure to substance abuse are difficult to obtain because of the illegal status of most drugs of abuse. In pregnancy rates of abuse of 0.4–31% have been reported (Khalsa and Gfroerer 1991). Although drug abuse occurs in all races and social classes, there is an increased risk in women who are younger, unmarried or who have lower educational achievements. In the USA, the National Survey on Drug Use and Health of 2008 revealed 5.2% of pregnant women admitted using illicit drugs in the previous month; however underreporting is very likely (Substance Abuse and Mental Health Services Administration 2008).

A study of 3000 babies born in a high-risk obstetric population in the USA revealed 44% were positive for morphine, cocaine or cannabis using meconium immunoassay, although only 11% of mothers admitted using illegal drugs (Ostrea et al. 1992). A study of 30 000 maternal urine samples at delivery in 1992 in California showed 5% of samples contained one or more illicit drugs (Vega et al. 1993). Meconium analysis from 400 infants in a study in Glasgow in 2001 revealed that approximately 13% of samples were positive for cannabinoids, 2.75% for cocaine and 1.75% for amphetamines (Williamson et al. 2006). Testing of 807 consecutive positive pregnancy tests in an urban UK population revealed approximately 17% (one in six women) were positive for illegal substances: 14.5% for cannabinoids, 1.4% for opiates, 0.5% for benzodiazepines, 0.4%, ethanol 0.2% for cocaine, 0.1% for amphetamines and 0.1% for methadone (Sherwood et al. 1999).

General effects of substance abuse in pregnancy

Substance abuse during pregnancy can have adverse effects on the health of the mother, the pregnancy itself, the fetus and the newborn infant after birth. Poverty, poor nutrition and lack of antenatal care also independently have a detrimental effect on pregnancy outcome. There is also a high risk of acquiring human immunodeficiency virus (HIV), hepatitis B and hepatitis C infection with intravenous drug use. Intrauterine growth restriction and preterm birth are more common (Messinger et al. 2004).

The effects of substance abuse on the fetus can be divided into drugs that have a direct teratogenic effect during the first trimester of pregnancy (e.g. cocaine; see Table 26.1), those which influence ongoing fetal growth or development through continued exposure (e.g. alcohol and barbiturates) and those which can have an adverse effect in the neonatal period by causing sedation, fits or withdrawal (e.g. benzodiazepines or opioids).

Providing appropriate care to this group is often challenging. Flexible care from experienced multidisciplinary teams is required, with child safeguarding a priority.

Approach to management of substance abuse in pregnancy

If a mother is suspected of abusing drugs a careful history should be taken regarding the quantity, duration, frequency and route of drug use, and counselling and support should be offered, along with multidisciplinary antenatal care. A careful search should be made for comorbid conditions such as psychiatric disorders, domestic violence, sexual or emotional abuse, the presence of sexually transmitted diseases and blood-borne virus infection (hepatitis B, hepatitis C and HIV infection). Frequent antenatal visits with serial ultrasound scans should be offered to confirm gestation and monitor fetal growth and well-being. If there has been high-risk behaviour such as sex-working or intravenous drug abuse continuing during the pregnancy, repeated virology testing is indicated (see Ch. 39.2).

The precise model of care will vary depending on local circumstances, but an example of a care pathway is given in Figure 26.1. A multidisciplinary open-access service may improve engagement by reducing the burden of appointments and improve continuity and consistency of care. Such a service might involve a specialist midwife, obstetrician, liaison heath visitor, neonatologist, neonatal nurse and social worker. In general, the initial approach should be to deal with the elements of substance abuse that contribute the greatest risk to the mother and fetus, such as injecting or regular alcohol abuse. The aim is then to reduce chaotic drug use, eventually achieving a stable period without use of illegal drugs before considering detoxification. Moving to detoxification too quickly can increase the chances of relapse.

General management of infants of substance-abusing mothers

Assessment following birth should include careful physical examination for evidence of malformation (Tables 26.1 and 26.2). Further investigations may be indicated, such as cranial ultrasound and eye examination. Toxicology screening (see Methods of testing, below) should be considered, particularly if there was no toxicology monitoring in pregnancy. Assessment for signs of neonatal withdrawal – also called neonatal abstinence syndrome – should be made (see Assessment of withdrawal, below). The most common drugs likely to result in withdrawal are opioids, benzodiazepines, antidepressants and alcohol. The timing of onset of symptoms depends on the drug(s) taken (Table 26.3), and there may be more than one phase in polydrug abuse. The signs and symptoms of withdrawal from different drugs are broadly similar and largely non-specific with central nervous system irritability and autonomic system dysfunction. Opioids are more likely to cause significant autonomic dysfunction (Table 26.4) than substances such as cocaine, amphetamines or benzodiazepines that cause predominantly central nervous system symptoms (see Table 26.2) (Oei and Lui 2007). Differential diagnoses include hypoglycaemia, hypocalcaemia, hypomagnesaemia, hyperthyroidism and causes of neonatal encephalopathy, such as central nervous system haemorrhage, sepsis and hypoxia. Drugs that are associated with neonatal seizures include opioids, shorter acting barbiturates, tricyclic antidepressants, alcohol, selective serotonin reuptake inhibitors (SSRIs) and serotonin noradrenaline reuptake inhibitors (SNRIs).

Supportive therapy should be offered with minimal stimulation and with swaddling or skin-to-skin care, the use of a dummy and frequent feeding. If pharmacological therapy is required a drug from the same class as that which is causing withdrawal may be preferable where possible. There are few comparative studies of different drugs used in the treatment of withdrawal. The most commonly used treatments, their main components and their mechanism of action are outlined in Table 26.5. A survey of the management of withdrawal in the UK and Ireland (O'Grady et al. 2009) showed morphine sulphate was the most commonly used first-line agent for opiate withdrawal by 92% of units, and in polysubstance

Table 26.1 Maternal drugs associated with teratogenic effects

DRUG	MALFORMATION
Alcohol	Fetal alcohol spectrum disorder (Volpe 2008)
Anticonvulsants Barbiturates Phenobarbital*	Fetal hydantoin syndrome: abnormal pre- and postnatal growth, central nervous system function, craniofacial appearance and distal limbs Neural tube defects, cardiac anomalies, facial clefts, hypospadias, other genitourinary anomalies, gastrointestinal anomalies and skeletal defects (Holmes et al. 2001; Volpe 2008)
Cocaine	Central nervous system: microcephaly, agenesis of the corpus callosum or septum pellucidum, septo-optic dysplasia, lissencephaly and schizencephaly (Volpe 2008) Possible increase in urogenital anomalies (Chasnoff et al. 1988; Chávez et al. 1989)
Selective serotonin reuptake inhibitors	Increased risk of septal heart defects with first-trimester use of sertraline and citalopram (Pedersen et al. 2009)

*Teratogenic effects are more common with multiple anticonvulsant therapy in pregnant women.

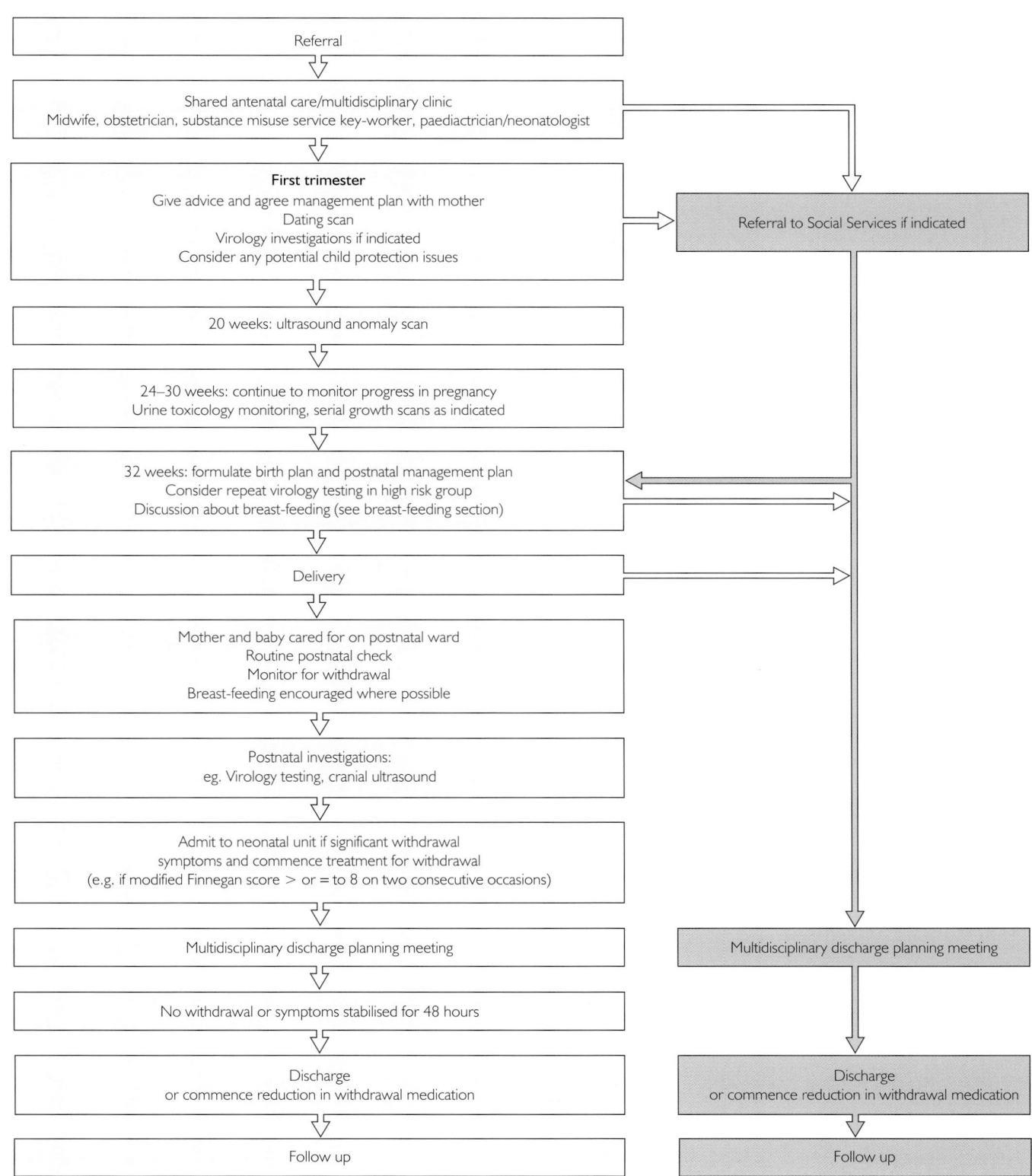

Fig. 26.1 Model care plan.

Table 26.2 Effects of cocaine on the fetus and newborn

OBSERVATION	PUTATIVE MECHANISMS
Uterine stimulation	Catecholamines
Placental abruption	Direct effect on myometrium
Preterm birth	
Fetal hypoxia, death	Catecholamine-induced vasoconstriction of maternofetal unit
Intrauterine growth retardation: reduced weight, length and head circumference	Increased fetal metabolic rate
Central nervous system malformation (see Table 26.1)	Direct effect on neuronal migration and differentiation
Intraventricular haemorrhage/infarction	Disturbed autoregulation/hypertensive episodes/vasoconstriction
Meconium-stained liquor	Sympathetic activation
Necrotising enterocolitis	Sympathetic activation
Limb reduction defects	Vasoconstrictive episodes
Retinal infarction	Vasoconstrictive episodes
Gut atresias	Vasoconstrictive episodes
Myocardial ischaemia	
Genitourinary anomalies	
Increased sudden infant death syndrome	Secondary to abnormal sleep patterns and arousal

Table 26.3 Drugs described as being associated with neonatal withdrawal

DRUG	TIME OF ONSET OF WITHDRAWAL
Opiates/opioids	
Heroin	0–48 hours, peak 12–24 hours
Methadone	1–5 days, peak 2–3 days
Codeine	<48 hours
Dihydrocodeine (DF118)	<48 hours
Oxycodone (Percocet/OxyContin)	<24 hours
Pentazocine	<24 hours
Alcohol	<24 hours
Benzodiazepines	
Diazepam (Valium)	2–6 weeks
Chlordiazepoxide (Librium)	3 weeks
Tricyclic antidepressants	0–72 hours
SSRIs/SNRIs	0–72 hours
Cocaine*	48–72 hours
Barbiturates	
Shorter acting	0–24 hours
Long acting	2–4 months
Amphetamines	–
Phencyclidine hydrochloride (PCP/angel dust)	24–72 hours

*Direct effect of the drug, not withdrawal.
SSRIs, selective serotonin reuptake inhibitors; SNRIs, serotonin noradrenaline reuptake inhibitors.

Table 26.4 Signs of opiate withdrawal

CENTRAL NERVOUS SYSTEM	GASTROINTESTINAL	AUTONOMIC AND OTHER
Tremors	Poor feeding	Yawning
Irritability	Uncoordinated suck	Sweating
High-pitched cry	Vomiting	Fever
Hypertonicity	Diarrhoea	Hiccups
Hyperactivity	Dehydration	Tachypnoea
Increased wakefulness		Fever/temperature instability
Excess sucking		Poor weight gain
Poor feeding		Excoriation of skin due to rubbing
Exaggerated Moro reflex		Skin mottling
Seizures		Nasal congestion
		Salivation

Table 26.5 Agents used for treating neonatal withdrawal

DRUG	MAIN COMPONENTS/MECHANISM OF ACTION/INDICATIONS FOR USE	DOSE
Opiates		
Morphine	Opiate replacement Opiate/opioid withdrawal Treatment of withdrawal seizures	50–100 µg/kg 6-hourly increasing by 25–50% every 24–48 hours until symptoms are controlled.
Methadone	Opiate replacement Opiate/opioid withdrawal Treatment of withdrawal seizures	Can be increased to 4-hourly (Osbourne et al. 2005)
Tincture of opium* Paregoric[†]	Opiate replacement Opiate/opioid withdrawal Treatment of withdrawal seizures	Methadone 100 µg/kg 6-hourly increased by 50 µg/kg until symptoms controlled (British National Formulary for Children 2010–2011)
Chlorpromazine	A phenothiazine antipsychotic which can cause sedation, reduce seizure threshold and cause cerebellar dysfunction Controls CNS and gastrointestinal signs of opiate/opioid withdrawal (Kahn et al. 1969). High risk of seizures if used as sole agent in opioid withdrawal May be useful in the treatment of SSRI withdrawal (Nordeng et al. 2001) and in benzodiazepine withdrawal	0.5–1 mg/kg every 6 hours intramuscularly or orally (maximum 6 mg/kg daily). When stable wean dose by maximum 2 mg/kg daily every third day
Phenobarbital	A barbiturate anticonvulsant. Sedative Long half-life: monitor blood levels Most commonly used treatment for opiate/opioid withdrawal seizures May be a useful second-line treatment of opioid withdrawal but does not alleviate gastrointestinal symptoms; however reduces duration of care needed (Osborn et al. 2005) Reported to be effective in withdrawal from volatile inhalant substance abuse (Tenenbein et al. 1996)	Loading dose 20 mg/kg intravenously then maintenance 2.5–5 mg/kg once daily intravenously or orally. (Check trough levels: aim for 20–40 mcg/ml)
Diazepam	A benzodiazepine Widely used in adults to control symptoms of alcohol withdrawal Replacement in benzodiazepine withdrawal As an anticonvulsant	For seizures 1.25–2.5 mg per rectum 300–400 µg/kg intravenously
Clonidine	A non-narcotic alpha 2 stimulant which decreases symptoms of withdrawal in opiate-addicted adults and children (Gold et al. 1978; Baumgartner and Rowen 1991) May be useful adjunct therapy to decrease hypertension and tachycardia in alcohol withdrawal Reduces duration of drug treatment in opioid withdrawal when used with opiate replacement (Agthe et al. 2009) 6 out of 7 infants with opiate withdrawal treated successfully with clonidine (Hoder et al. 1984)	3–5 µg/kg/day, divided into 4–8-hourly doses (test dose–1mcg/kg watch for hypotension)

*Tincture of opium (used in the USA but not widely used in the UK) (Anonymous 1998).
[†]Paregoric, a mixture of opium, camphor, alcohol and anise oil, is no longer in use due to toxicity of additives.
CNS, central nervous system; SSRIs, selective serotonin reuptake inhibitors.

withdrawal by 69% of units. Phenobarbital was the first choice for treatment of seizures from opiate withdrawal and polydrug withdrawal in 73% and 81% of units respectively. A similar survey in the USA revealed that 63% of neonatal units used opioids (either tincture of opium or morphine sulphate) to treat opioid withdrawal and 52% used opioids to treat polydrug withdrawal. In the USA, 70% of units used phenobarbital and 25% used morphine to control opioid seizures; 81% used phenobarbital to control seizures secondary to polydrug withdrawal (Sarkar and Donn 2006).

Urgent infant HIV and hepatitis B testing is indicated at birth if mothers are untested or there has been continuing high-risk behaviour since previous tests to enable commencement of appropriate treatment to reduce the possibility of perinatal viral transmission. Consideration should also be given to routine hepatitis B immunisation.

Methods of testing

Urinalysis is the most commonly used method to detect and monitor substance abuse in the mother and newborn infant. Intermittent drug use can be missed as many drugs of abuse are present in the blood and urine for just a few hours (with the notable exception of marijuana, with which the urine can remain positive for weeks). Rapid urine dipstick testing is available, but full laboratory analysis can give more information on persisting drug metabolites. Mouth swabbing of mothers can detect recent use of many illicit substances, but is more likely to produce false-negative results than urine testing. Breathalyser testing is easy to perform and useful where there have been problems with alcohol abuse. Maternal or infant hair, meconium (Ostrea et al. 2001) and homogenised cord tissue testing (Montgomery et al. 2006) reflect historical drug use several months prior to delivery, but are not routinely available.

Assessment of withdrawal

A variety of scoring charts for monitoring symptoms of neonatal withdrawal are in use. The modified Finnegan chart is the most widely used (Fig. 26.2) – by 52% of units in the UK and 65% of neonatal units in the USA (Finnegan et al. 1975; Lipsitz 1975).

There are a number of problems with using this scoring system in clinical practice. These include an overemphasis on minor symptoms, interobserver variability and a tendency to 'score' infants at the time the chart is completed rather than reflecting the status of a baby over the preceding hours. In addition, the scoring for length of sleep following a feed is less appropriate for babies who are in the early stages of establishing breastfeeding than it is for those who are bottle-feeding. A total derived from the scoring chart is often used as a threshold for commencing pharmacological treatment, and will vary depending upon the type of scoring system used. A modified Finnegan score of ≥8 on two consecutive assessments 4 hours apart is a commonly used threshold for treatment. Scoring can help to assess changes over time but it should not replace the use of clinical judgement. The key indications for treatment are significant feeding problems (including vomiting and need for nasogastric feeding), watery diarrhoea or the baby remaining very unsettled despite feeds, swaddling and the use of a dummy.

Breastfeeding

The benefits of breastfeeding mean that it should be encouraged whenever it is safe to do so. However, many drugs of abuse such as heroin, amphetamine, cocaine and phencyclidine pass readily into breast milk and breastfeeding is not advised if the mother continues to abuse these substances or is HIV-positive. Methadone by contrast is highly protein-bound in maternal plasma; therefore, only very small amounts pass into breast milk, but this is poorly correlated with maternal dose. There is now a growing amount of evidence to support its safe use in women who are breastfeeding (Philipp et al. 2003). Breastfeeding with the abuse of any drug depends upon a careful assessment of the risks and benefits. For example, breastfeeding with low doses of maternal diazepam could be considered if the baby is monitored for any evidence of the potential consequences of sedation such as difficulty sucking or poor weight gain.

Outcome

When examining pregnancy outcome it is difficult to prove a causal relationship between drug abuse in pregnancy and adverse outcome. This is because of the difficulties in controlling for pregnancy complications, poor maternal health and social circumstances, maternal malnutrition, poverty and maternal chronic infections such as HIV or hepatitis B or C. Low birthweight and prematurity, which are also more common, themselves contribute to increased risk of poor outcome. Unrecognised or untreated withdrawal can cause

significant morbidity and mortality in the newborn. There are also reports of increased risk of sudden infant death syndrome in infants of opioid-abusing mothers (Hunt and Hauck 2006). The largest longitudinal cohort study ($n = 1227$) looking at outcome with cocaine and opiate exposure found that, after controlling for birthweight and environmental risks, there was no association with developmental, motor or behavioural deficits (Messinger et al. 2004).

Specific drugs of abuse

Opiates/opioids

Opioids are natural and synthetic substances with morphine-like activity. Opiates are a subclass of opioids extracted from opium, including morphine, codeine, heroin and methadone. Heroin still accounts for the greatest share of morbidity and mortality related to drug use in the European Union. However in the last decade its use may have declined slightly in favour of synthetic opioids such as fentanyl (EMCDDA 2009). Between 1 and 6 per 1000 15–64-year-olds in Europe have a significant opiate addiction (EMCDDA 2009). Continued abuse of illegal opioids during pregnancy increases the risks of miscarriage, premature delivery and low birthweight, and the risk of blood-borne infections is high for those who inject (Lam et al. 1992). Sudden cessation of a regular drug habit can result in pregnancy loss and therefore mothers should seek specialist advice before discontinuing their drug use abruptly. Methadone replacement therapy can be used to manage opioid abuse safely in pregnancy (Jones et al. 2008) and there is no evidence of an increase in fetal malformations. Appropriate doses of methadone eliminate the pharmacological symptoms of withdrawal in the mother. This can lead to a reduction or cessation in illegal opioid abuse that reduces the ongoing risks to the mother and fetus, increasing the chance of a favourable outcome. More recently, other types of opioid substitution treatment are being used, in particular buprenorphine (Jones et al. 2008), the use of which may increase as the subsequent neonatal withdrawal is shorter than that of methadone.

The risk of withdrawal is greatest with heavy opiate abuse in the 3 months prior to delivery. Naloxone should be avoided at resuscitation because of the high risk of precipitating acute withdrawal. Withdrawal from methadone varies depending on dose (<20 mg/day, 10%; 20–40 mg/day, 40–50%; 60 mg/day or greater, 90%) (Dashe et al. 2002). Preterm infants <35 weeks seem to manifest less severe symptoms than term infants (Doberczak et al. 1991), which may be secondary to developmental immaturity of the central nervous system or less prolonged fetal exposure. Most opiates (see Table 26.3) have short half-lives and therefore cause withdrawal symptoms within 48 hours of delivery. Methadone, which has a longer half-life, causes a more gradual onset of symptoms and infants usually present around 2–3 days of age. Presentation of withdrawal after 5 days is very unlikely (Shaw and McIvor 1994); however if withdrawal symptoms are already present these can increase and worsen over the first 10 days as methadone is excreted by the baby and the proportion of occupied opiate receptors decreases. This explains why the dose of medication required to treat opiate withdrawal sometimes needs to be increased during this period. Withdrawal from opioids is characterised by marked central nervous system symptoms and autonomic disturbance with gastrointestinal upset (see Table 26.4). Significant withdrawal (see Assessment of withdrawal, above) not responding to supportive care will require drug treatment (see Table 26.5). The treatment of choice is morphine sulphate (Osbourne et al. 2005), although other opiate-based treatments have been used successfully,

	SYMPTOMS		SCORE		
CNS	Excessive high-pitched cry <5 mins	2			
	Continuous high-pitched cry >5 mins	3			
	Sleeps <1 hour after feeding	3			
	Sleeps <2 hours after feeding	2			
	Sleeps <3 hours after feeding	1			
	Hyperactive Moro reflex	2			
	Markedly hyperactive Moro reflex	1			
	Mild tremors when disturbed	1			
	Moderate to severe tremors when disturbed	2			
	Increased muscle tone	1			
	Excoriation	1			
	Myoclonic jerks (twitching/jerking of limbs)	3			
	Generalised convulsions	5			
Respiratory	Sweating	1			
Vasometer	Hyperthermia (37.5 –38C)	1			
Metabolic	Hyperthermia (>38.2C)	2			
	Frequent yawning (>3 –4 / interval)	1			
	Mottling	1			
	Nasal stuffiness	1			
	Frequent sneezing (>3 –4 / interval)	1			
	Nasal flaring	2			
	Respiratory rate >60/min	1			
	Respiratory rate > 60/min with recession	2			
Gastrointestinal	Excessive sucking	1			
	Poor feeding (infrequent/incoordinate suck)	2			
	Regurgitation (during post-feed)	2			
	Projectile vomiting	3			
	Loose stools (curdy/seedy appearance)	2			
	Watery stools (water ring on nappy around stool)	3			
	TOTAL SCORE				
	Date/time				

Fig. 26.2 Modified Finnegan chart. *(Modified from Finnegan LP, Connaughton JF Jr, Kron RE, Emich JP. Neonatal abstinence syndrome: assessment and management. Addict Dis. 1975;2(1-2):141-58.)*

particularly in the USA. Morphine is widely available and has a short half-life that achieves stable drug levels and symptom control relatively quickly. Treatment should be aimed at normalisation of infant behaviour without oversedation. Cardiorespiratory monitoring is recommended until this is achieved.

Adjunct therapy with clonidine reduces the duration of drug treatment in opioid withdrawal when used with opiate replacement. Phenobarbital may also be useful in reducing the duration of care needed but does not alleviate gastrointestinal symptoms. If seizures are present despite opiate treatment, the usual anticonvulsants are indicated (diazepam, clonazepam, phenobarbital). Phenobarbital is the anticonvulsant most commonly used for withdrawal in the UK and USA (Sarkar and Donn 2006; O'Grady et al. 2009).

Control of opioid withdrawal is usually possible by 10–14 days. After stability is achieved for at least 48 hours, a reduction of morphine can be commenced either in hospital or in the community when the parents or carers feel confident to assess their baby and administer the medication. Reduction should be in 10% increments or less at intervals of 2–3 days or more according to initial response. The relationship between opioid exposure in pregnancy and neurodevelopmental outcome is inconsistent because of difficulty in controlling for confounding variables such as low birthweight, prematurity, multiple drug exposure and quality of home environment. Severity of withdrawal has not been shown to alter the long-term outcome (Messinger et al. 2004).

Cocaine

Cocaine abuse in pregnancy is a major concern. Infant meconium and early pregnancy maternal urine testing in the UK suggests that approximately 3% of pregnant women use cocaine whilst pregnant. Cocaine can be taken by inhalation of the powder or by intravenous injection. Other derivatives such as its freebase (crack) can be smoked (often mixed with cannabis or tobacco). Cocaine creates prolonged sympathetic nervous stimulation, causing vasoconstriction and hypertension. It freely crosses the placenta and fetal blood–brain barrier. Vasoconstriction is the main mechanism for fetal damage. Exposure to cocaine in pregnancy is associated with clear drug-induced effects (Table 26.2) (Plessinger and Woods 1993; Ogunyemi and Hernández-Loera 2004; Bauer et al. 2005). Higher early-pregnancy loss and third-trimester complications and an increased risk of stillbirth, sudden infant death syndrome and neonatal death are more common with cocaine abuse in pregnancy. Teratogenic effects on the central nervous system are well recognised secondary to the effect of cocaine on neuronal migration and differentiation (see Table 26.1) (Volpe 2008). Other teratogenic effects of cocaine have not been definitively established but there is likely to be an increase in urogenital anomalies (Chasnoff et al. 1988; Chávez et al. 1989). Cardiovascular toxicity in women causes hypertension, which can mimic the effects of pre-eclampsia. Exposure in utero to cocaine may lead to fetal cerebral infarction, intracranial haemorrhage or retinal vascular damage (McGlone et al. 2009).

Cocaine abuse close to the time of delivery may present between 48 and 72 hours of age with tremor, hypertonia, high-pitched cry, irritability, excess suck, hyperalertness and tachycardia; these are thought to be the direct effect of cocaine rather than of withdrawal (Anonymous 1998).

Deficits have been found in neurobehavioural features such as attention, emotional control, aggressiveness and emotional expressivity and in higher motor functions, which can be ameliorated by a high-quality home environment (Singer et al. 2004; Volpe 2008). Supportive therapy is usually sufficient for withdrawal symptoms.

Careful examination for congenital anomaly, including cranial ultrasound and ophthalmological review, should be undertaken. Breastfeeding should be avoided with cocaine use as it transfers readily to breast milk and there have been reports of seizures following breastfeeding (Chasnoff et al. 1987).

Alcohol

'Fetal alcohol spectrum disorder (FASD) is an umbrella term used to describe a continuum of alcohol-related disorders, with fetal alcohol syndrome (FAS) the most severe form. At the other end of the continuum, the neurological and behavioural features of FASD may occur later without apparent dysmorphic features. A safe level of alcohol use in pregnancy has not been established. FAS is the most common identifiable cause of mental retardation in the world, with prevalence rates of 0.18–1.5 per 1000 live births (National Task Force on Fetal Alcohol Syndrome and Fetal Alcohol Effect 2004; Elliott et al. 2008). The prevalence of FASD is unknown, but is possibly as high as 1% of all live births in the USA (Sampson et al. 1997).

The diagnosis of FAS requires a history of alcohol ingestion associated with abnormal growth, neurological abnormality and the characteristic facial findings (short palpable fissures, smooth philtrum and thin vermilion border of the upper lip), as illustrated in Figure 26.3. Numerous additional features can occur and may add weight to the diagnosis, including feeding difficulties, mandibular hypoplasia, abnormal palmar creases, abnormal ear creases, nail hypoplasia, clinodactyly, cardiac defects, poor hearing and optic disc hypoplasia. Poor growth may manifest itself in antenatal and postnatal periods (<10th centile). Neurological abnormalities may be structural or functional and include microcephaly, structural brain abnormalities (in the corpus callosum, brainstem or basal ganglia) or seizures. Charts of lip and philtrum appearances such

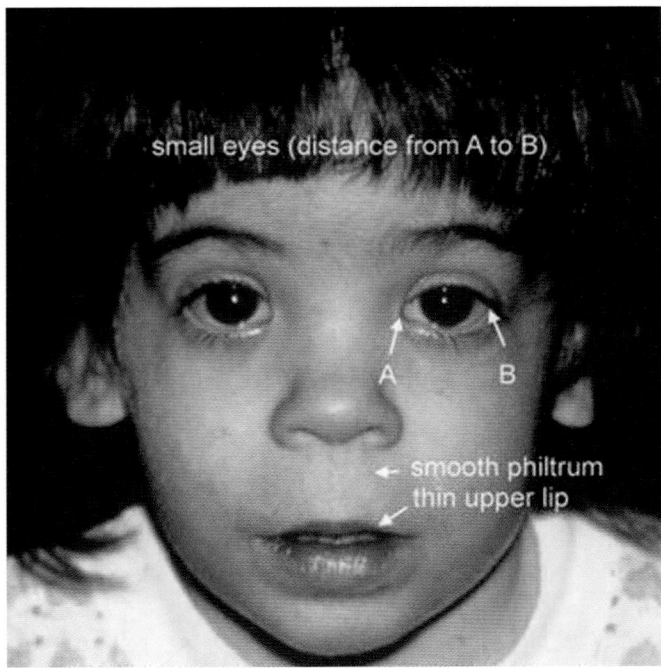

Fig. 26.3 Child with fetal alcohol syndrome. *(Courtesy of Professor Susan Astley.)*

as that shown in Figure 26.4 offer a systematic approach to aid facial diagnosis (National Task Force on Fetal Alcohol Syndrome and Fetal Alcohol Effect 2004; Astley 2006). Careful clinical postnatal assessment for features of FASD should include an early cranial ultrasound and a low threshold for ophthalmological referral. Functional deficits may not be apparent in the neonatal period and follow-up is required by child health services if there is significant alcohol exposure during pregnancy. Following birth, infants exposed to alcohol can suffer acute withdrawal associated with hypoglycaemia and acidosis. Acute withdrawal usually only requires supportive measures with frequent small feeds. If seizures are present benzodiazepines or phenobarbital are the treatments of choice.

Prevention of FASD is the aim. Short screening questionnaires to identify alcohol abuse have been validated (Reinert and Allen 2007) and consideration should be given to their routine use at pregnancy booking to allow effective intervention.

Selective serotonin reuptake inhibitors/ serotonin noradrenaline reuptake inhibitors

Although SSRIs and SNRIs are not recreational drugs, they are widely used antidepressants which are known to cause significant symptoms in the newborn infants of mothers who take them in the third trimester of pregnancy. Depression and anxiety are common in pregnant women and SSRIs (e.g. fluoxetine, sertraline, citalopram and paroxetine) and SNRIs (e.g. venlafaxine, duloxetene) have been used increasingly during pregnancy and breastfeeding. It is likely that SSRIs and SNRIs only represent a very low risk of teratogenicity even if used in the first trimester. Fluoxetine, sertraline and paroxetine use in the third trimester carries an increased risk of low birthweight and growth restriction (Oberlander et al. 2006). Infants who are exposed to third-trimester SSRIs or SNRIs may suffer withdrawal, with predominantly central nervous system symptoms (Moses-Kolko et al. 2005; Nordeng and Spigset 2005; Sanz et al. 2005). Up to 60% of infants may show symptoms within 24 hours of birth which usually resolve spontaneously within a few days and are rarely serious, although seizures have been reported (Ferreira et al. 2007). There is an increased risk of developing persistent pulmonary hypertension of the newborn with paroxetine, sertraline or fluoxetine (Chambers et al. 2006). Chlorpromazine has been reported to be effective for symptom relief (Nordeng et al. 2001).

Other drugs of abuse

Marijuana

Marijuana is detectable in the neonatal urine days to weeks after exposure. It is the most commonly abused illicit substance. The impact of prenatal abuse on outcome is not clear. There is no evidence to support birth defects or increased mortality in the first 2 years of life in exposed infants (Ostrea et al. 1997). There may however be later effects on functioning, which may include cognitive defects, impulsivity, hyperactivity, depressive symptoms and substance use disorders (Gray et al. 2005; Huizink and Mulder 2006).

Cigarette smoking

Cigarette smoking in pregnancy has been associated with placental abruption, premature rupture of the membranes, placenta praevia, prematurity, low birthweight and increased early and late neonatal mortality (Cnattingius et al. 1988; Malloy et al. 1988; Mitchell et al.

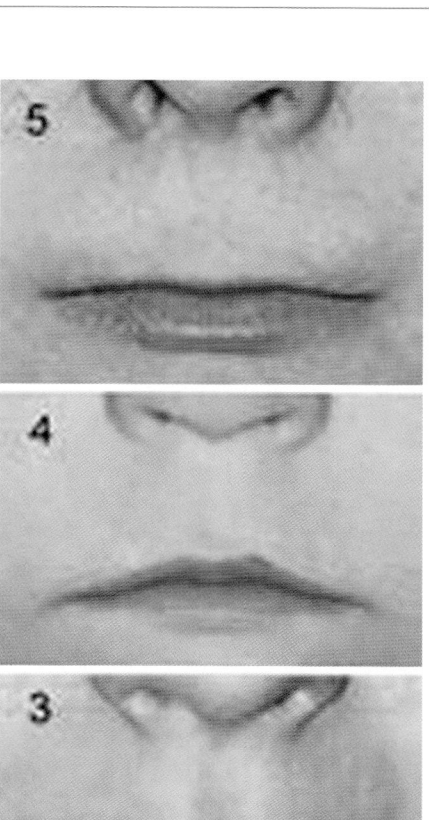
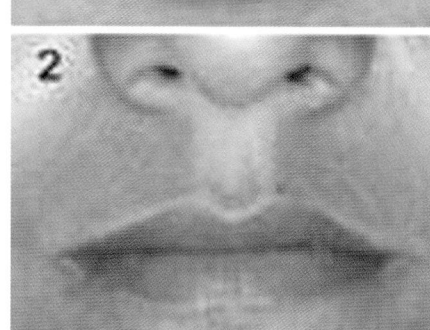
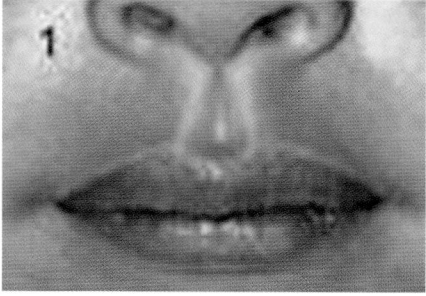

Fig. 26.4 Lip–philtrum guide for fetal alcohol syndrome. *(Reproduced from http://depts.washington.edu/fasdpn/htmls/fas-face.htm: accessed 22 June 2010.)*

1997). There is a 2–4 times increased risk in sudden infant death syndrome in infants of mothers who smoke compared with infants of non-smoking mothers. Asthma is more common in children of mothers who smoked in pregnancy (Jouni et al. 2004).

Benzodiazepines

Benzodiazepines can be legally prescribed or abused. Higher doses in the last trimester can cause sedation, floppiness, apnoea, poor feeding and reduced weight gain in the early neonatal period secondary to the direct effect of the drug and metabolites. The onset of benzodiazepine withdrawal is often delayed, appearing slowly 1–4 weeks after delivery. Chlorpromazine can be effective in treating the symptoms but replacement therapy with a benzodiazepine (see Table 26.5) may also be considered: this then requires a staged reduction. No long-term detrimental effect on neurodevelopmental outcome has been shown (McElhatton 1994).

Amphetamines

Methamphetamine (speed, meth, ice, crystal) is a very addictive stimulant. It is estimated that 5% of pregnant women in the US population have used it during their pregnancy (Arria et al. 2006). Prenatal amphetamine exposure is likely to be associated with prematurity (Oei et al. 2010) and intrauterine growth restriction, although study confounders such as multiple drug use prevent a definitive conclusion (NTP-CERHR 2005; Smith et al. 2006). It remains uncertain whether there is an increased risk of congenital anomaly or negative impact on neurodevelopmental outcome.

Phencyclidine hydrochloride (PCP/angel dust)

There is limited evidence from small studies, which show hypertonicity, irritability, sleep problems and temperature instability in newborns with prenatal exposure (Chasnoff et al. 1983; Golden et al. 1987; Wachsman et al. 1989).

Barbiturates

These freely cross the placenta and are known teratogenic agents (see Table 26.1) which can cause acute or delayed withdrawal. Delayed withdrawal presents between 2 and 4 months. Treatment is usually supportive, but phenobarbital replacements may be indicated (see Table 26.5), and these require staged withdrawal.

3,4-methylenedioxymethamphetamine (MDMA), ecstasy

There are conflicting studies on the teratogenic effects of ecstasy, which include increased risk of talipes and congenital heart disease, but small patient numbers cannot confirm a causal relationship (McElhatton et al. 1999). Withdrawal is recognised in adults and paediatricians should be aware of a possible neonatal counterpart.

Inhalants

These are volatile compounds (hydrocarbons or nitrites) which produce effects of intoxication via direct inhalation. Abuse in pregnancy may increase the risk of miscarriage, prematurity or fetal malformation (Jones and Balster 1998). There is an association with cardiac arrhythmia and sudden death. Infants exposed in pregnancy may show symptoms of withdrawal after delivery. Phenobarbital has been used to control symptoms (see Table 26.5) (Tenenbein et al. 1996).

Ketamine

Ketamine is an anaesthetic induction agent which has a recognised withdrawal syndrome in adults characterised by poor attention span and restlessness. Similar symptoms may be possible in the neonatal period secondary to maternal abuse.

Tricyclic antidepressants

Tricyclic antidepressants are commonly prescribed antidepressants rather than drugs of abuse but infants can suffer withdrawal (including seizures) in the neonatal period within the first 72 hours following delivery. There is no evidence of increased congenital malformations or long-term adverse effects on development outcome (Simon et al. 2002).

Polydrug use

Polydrug use is common and it is often difficult to separate out the effects of individual drugs. Timing of withdrawal depends on which drugs are involved (Table 26.3). New symptoms developing in the second week of life are unlikely to be related to opioid withdrawal and other causes should be sought (e.g. benzodiazepines). It is difficult to make clear recommendations regarding drug treatment. Morphine sulphate or tincture of opium is the most commonly used treatment in the UK and USA for polydrug withdrawal (Sarkar and Donn 2006; O'Grady et al. 2009); however more than one drug may be required.

Summary

Substance abuse is common in women of childbearing age. Infants of substance-abusing mothers are at significant risk from the teratogenic effects of the drug, are more likely to suffer from preterm birth and growth restriction and are at risk of neonatal withdrawal. They also suffer significant social disadvantage if drug-seeking behaviour continues after delivery and interferes with normal parenting. Untreated or unrecognised withdrawal has significant morbidity and mortality. A multidisciplinary approach to mothers combined with careful antenatal planning and postnatal management can reduce the risk of harm and improve the outcome for mothers and their newborn infants.

References

Agthe, A.G., Kim, G.R., Mathias, K.B., et al., 2009. Clonidine as an adjunct therapy to opioids for neonatal abstinence syndrome: a randomized, controlled trial. Pediatrics 123, e849–e856.

Anonymous, 1998. Neonatal drug withdrawal. American Academy of

Pediatrics Committee on Drugs. Pediatrics 101, 1079–1088. Erratum in: Pediatrics 102, 660.

Arria, A.M., Derauf, C., Lagasse, L.L., et al., 2006. Methamphetamine and other substance use during pregnancy: preliminary estimates from the Infant

Development, Environment, and Lifestyle (IDEAL) study. Matern Child Health J 10, 293–302.

Astley, S.J., 2006. Comparison of the 4-digit diagnostic code and the Hoyme diagnostic guidelines for fetal alcohol spectrum disorders. Pediatrics 118, 1532–1545.

Bauer, C.R., Langer, J.C., Shankaran, S., et al., 2005. Acute neonatal effects of cocaine exposure during pregnancy. Arch Pediatr Adolesc Med 159, 824–834.

Baumgartner, G.R., Rowen, R.C., 1991. Transdermal clonidine versus chlordiazepoxide in alcohol withdrawal: a randomized, controlled clinical trial. South Med J 84, 312–321.

British National Formulary for Children, 2010–2011. BMJ Group, London, pp. 262.

Chambers, C.D., Hernandez-Diaz, S., Van Marter, L.J., et al., 2006. Selective serotonin-reuptake inhibitors and risk of persistent pulmonary hypertension of the newborn. N Engl J Med 354 (6), 579–587.

Chasnoff, I.J., Burns, W.J., Hatcher, R.P., et al., 1983. Phencyclidine: effects on the fetus and neonate. Dev Pharmacol Ther 6, 404–408.

Chasnoff, I.J., Lewis, D.E., Squires, L., 1987. Cocaine intoxication in a breast-fed infant. Pediatrics 80, 836–838.

Chasnoff, I.J., Chisum, G.M., Kaplan, W.E., 1988. Maternal cocaine use and genitourinary tract malformations. Teratology 37, 201–204.

Chávez, G.F., Mulinare, J., Cordero, J.F., 1989. Maternal cocaine use during early pregnancy as a risk factor for congenital urogenital anomalies. JAMA 262, 795–798.

Cnattingius, S., Haglund, B., Meirik, O., 1988. Cigarette smoking as risk factor for late fetal and early neonatal death. BMJ 297, 258–261.

Dashe, J.S., Sheffield, J.S., Olscher, D.A., et al., 2002. Relationship between maternal methadone dosage and neonatal withdrawal. Obstet Gynecol 100, 1244–1249.

Doberczak, T.M., Kandall, S.R., Wilets, I., 1991. Neonatal opiate abstinence syndrome in term and preterm infants. J Pediatr 118, 933–937.

Elliott, E.J., Payne, J., Morris, A., et al., 2008. Fetal alcohol syndrome: a prospective national surveillance study. Arch Dis Child 93, 732–737.

EMCDDA, 2008. A Cannabis Reader: Global Issues and Local Experiences. Monograph series 8, Volume 1. European Monitoring Centre for Drugs and Drug Addiction, Lisbon.

EMCDDA, 2009. A Cannabis Reader: Global Issues and Local Experiences. Monograph series 8, Volume 1. European Monitoring Centre for Drugs and Drug Addiction, Lisbon.

Ferreira, E., Carceller, A.M., Agogué, C., et al., 2007. Effects of selective serotonin reuptake inhibitors and venlafaxine during pregnancy in term and preterm neonates. Pediatrics 119, 52–59.

Finnegan, L.P., Connaughton Jr, J.F., Kron, R.E., et al., 1975. Neonatal abstinence syndrome: assessment and management. Addict Dis 2, 141–158.

Gold, M.S., Redmond Jr, D.E., Kleber, H.D., 1978. Clonidine blocks acute opiate-withdrawal symptoms. Lancet 2, 599–602.

Golden, N.L., Kuhnert, B.R., Sokol, R.J., et al., 1987. Neonatal manifestations of maternal phencyclidine exposure. J Perinat Med 15, 185–191.

Gray, K.A., Day, N.L., Leech, S., et al., 2005. Prenatal marijuana exposure: effect on child depressive symptoms at ten years of age. Neurotoxicol Teratol 27, 439–448.

Hoder, E.L., Leckman, J.F., Poulsen, J., et al., 1984. Clonidine treatment of neonatal narcotic abstinence syndrome. Psychiatry Res 13, 243–251.

Holmes, L.B., Harvey, E.A., Coull, B.A., et al., 2001. The teratogenicity of anticonvulsant drugs. N Engl J Med 344, 1132–1138.

Huizink, A.C., Mulder, E.J., 2006. Maternal smoking, drinking or cannabis use during pregnancy and neurobehavioral and cognitive functioning in human offspring. Neurosci Biobehav Rev 30, 24–41.

Hunt, C.E., Hauck, F.R., 2006. Sudden infant death syndrome. CMAJ 174, 1861–1869.

Jones, H.E., Balster, R.L., 1998. Inhalant abuse in pregnancy. Obstet Gynecol Clin North Am 25, 153–167.

Jones, H.E., Martin, P.R., Heil, S.H., et al., 2008. Treatment of opioid-dependent pregnant women: clinical and research issues. J Subst Abuse Treat 35, 245–259.

Jouni, J.K., Gissler, J., Gissler, M., 2004. Maternal smoking in pregnancy, fetal development, and childhood asthma. Am J Public Health 94, 136–140.

Kahn, E.J., Neumann, L.L., Polk, G.A., 1969. The course of the heroin withdrawal syndrome in newborn infants treated with phenobarbital or chlorpromazine. J Pediatr 75, 495–500.

Khalsa, J.H., Gfroerer, J., 1991. Epidemiology and health consequences of drug abuse among pregnant women. Semin Perinatol 15, 265–270.

Lam, S.K., To, W.K., Duthie, S.J., et al., 1992. Narcotic addiction in pregnancy with adverse maternal and perinatal outcome. Aust N Z J Obstet Gynaecol 32, 216–221.

Lipsitz, P.J., 1975. A proposed narcotic withdrawal score for use with newborn infants. A pragmatic evaluation of its efficacy. Clin Pediatr (Phila) 14, 592–594.

Malloy, M.H., Kleinman, J.C., Land, G.H., et al., 1988. The association of maternal smoking with age and cause of infant death. Am J Epidemiol 128, 46–55.

McElhatton, P.R., 1994. The effects of benzodiazepine use during pregnancy and lactation. Reprod Toxicol 8, 461–475.

McElhatton, P.R., Bateman, D.N., Evans, C., et al., 1999. Congenital anomalies after prenatal ecstasy exposure. Lancet 354, 1441–1442.

McGlone, L., Mactier, H., Weaver, L.T., 2009. Drug misuse in pregnancy: losing sight of the baby? Arch Dis Child 94, 708–712.

Messinger, D.S., Bauer, C.R., Das, A., et al., 2004. The maternal lifestyle study: cognitive, motor, and behavioral outcomes of cocaine-exposed and opiate-exposed infants through three years of age. Pediatrics 113, 1677–1685.

Mitchell, E.A., Tuohy, P.G., Brunt, J.M., et al., 1997. Risk factors for sudden infant death syndrome following the prevention campaign in New Zealand: a prospective study. Pediatrics 100, 835–840.

Montgomery, D., Plate, C., Alder, S.C., et al., 2006. Testing for fetal exposure to illicit drugs using umbilical cord tissue vs meconium. J Perinatol 26, 11–14.

Moses-Kolko, E.L., Bogen, D., Perel, J., et al., 2005. Neonatal signs after late in utero exposure to serotonin reuptake inhibitors: literature review and implications for clinical applications. JAMA 293, 2372–2383.

National Task Force on Fetal Alcohol Syndrome and Fetal Alcohol Effect, 2004. Fetal Alcohol Syndrome: Guidelines for Referral and Diagnosis. CDC Centers for Disease Control and Prevention, Atlanta, GA.

Nordeng, H., Spigset, O., 2005. Treatment with selective serotonin reuptake inhibitors in the third trimester of pregnancy: effects on the infant. Drug Saf 28, 565–581.

Nordeng, H., Lindemann, R., Perminov, K.V., et al., 2001. Neonatal withdrawal syndrome after in utero exposure to selective serotonin reuptake inhibitors. Acta Paediatr 90, 288–291.

NTP-CERHR, 2005. Monograph on the potential human reproductive and developmental effects of amphetamines. NTP CERHR MON 16, vii–III1.

Oberlander, T.F., Warburton, W., Misri, S., et al., 2006. Neonatal outcomes after prenatal exposure to selective serotonin reuptake inhibitor antidepressants and maternal depression using population-based linked health data. Arch Gen Psychiatry 63, 898–906.

Oei, J., Lui, K., 2007. Management of the newborn infant affected by maternal opiates and other drugs of dependency. J Paediatr Child Health 43, 9–18.

Oei, J., Abdel-Latif, M.E., Clark, R., et al., 2010. Short-term outcomes of mothers and infants exposed to antenatal amphetamines. Arch Dis Child Fetal Neonatal Ed 95, F36–F41.

O'Grady, M.J., Hopewell, J., White, M.J., 2009. Management of neonatal abstinence syndrome: a national survey and review of practice. Arch Dis Child Fetal Neonatal Ed 94, F249–F252.

Ogunyemi, D., Hernández-Loera, G.E., 2004. The impact of antenatal cocaine use on maternal characteristics and neonatal outcomes. J Matern Fetal Neonatal Med 15, 253–259.

Osborn, D.A., Jeffery, H.E., Cole, M.J., 2005. Sedatives for opiate withdrawal in newborn infants. Cochrane Database Syst Rev (3), CD002053.

Osbourne, D.A., Jeffery, H.E., Cole, M.J., 2005. Opiate treatment for opiate withdrawal in newborn infants. Cochrane Database Syst Rev (3), CD002059.

Ostrea Jr, E.M., Brady, M., Gause, S., et al., 1992. Drug screening of newborns by meconium analysis: a large-scale, prospective, epidemiologic study. Pediatrics 89, 107–113.

Ostrea Jr, E.M., Ostrea, A.R., Simpson, P.M., 1997. Mortality within the first 2 years in infants exposed to cocaine, opiate, or cannabinoid during gestation. Pediatrics 100, 79–83.

Ostrea Jr, E.M., Knapp, D.K., Tannenbaum, L., et al., 2001. Estimates of illicit drug use during pregnancy by maternal interview, hair analysis, and meconium analysis. J Pediatr 138, 344–348.

Pedersen, L.H., Henriksen, T.B., Vestergaard, M., et al., 2009. Selective serotonin reuptake inhibitors in pregnancy and congenital malformations: population based cohort study. BMJ 339, b3569.

Philipp, B.L., Merewood, A., O'Brien, S., 2003. Methadone and breastfeeding: new horizons. Pediatrics 111, 1429–1430.

Plessinger, M.A., Woods Jr, J.R., 1993. Maternal, placental, and fetal pathophysiology of cocaine exposure during pregnancy. Clin Obstet Gynecol 36, 267–278.

Reinert, D.F., Allen, J.P., 2007. The alcohol use disorders identification test: an update of research findings. Alcohol Clin Exp Res 31, 185–199.

Sampson, P.D., Streissguth, A.P., Bookstein, F.L., et al., 1997. Incidence of fetal alcohol syndrome and prevalence of alcohol-related neurodevelopmental disorder. Teratology 56, 317–326.

Sanz, E.J., De-las-Cuevas, C., Kiuru, A., et al., 2005. Selective serotonin reuptake inhibitors in pregnant women and neonatal withdrawal syndrome: a database analysis. Lancet 365, 482–487.

Sarkar, S., Donn, S.M., 2006. Management of neonatal abstinence syndrome in neonatal intensive care units: a national survey. J Perinatol 26, 15–17.

Shaw, N.J., McIvor, L., 1994. Neonatal abstinence syndrome after maternal methadone treatment. Arch Dis Child Fetal Neonatal Ed 71, F203–F205.

Sherwood, R.A., Keating, J., Kavvadia, V., et al., 1999. Substance misuse in early pregnancy and relationship to fetal outcome. Eur J Pediatr 158 (6), 488–492.

Simon, G.E., Cunningham, M.L., David, R.L., 2002. Outcomes of prenatal antidepressant exposure. Am J Psychiatry 159, 2055–2061.

Singer, L.T., Minnes, S., Short, E., et al., 2004. Cognitive outcomes of preschool children with prenatal cocaine exposure. JAMA 291, 2448–2456.

Smith, L.M., LaGasse, L.L., Derauf, C., et al., 2006. The infant development, environment, and lifestyle study: effects of prenatal methamphetamine exposure, polydrug exposure, and poverty on intrauterine growth. Pediatrics 118, 1149–1156.

Substance Abuse and Mental Health Services Administration, 2008. Results from the 2008 National Survey on Drug Use and Health: National Findings. Office of Applied Studies, Rockville, MD.

Tenenbein, M., Casiro, O.G., Seshia, M.M., et al., 1996. Neonatal withdrawal from maternal volatile substance abuse. Arch Dis Child Fetal Neonatal Ed 74, F204.

Vega, W.A., Kolody, B., Hwang, J., et al., 1993. Prevalence and magnitude of perinatal substance exposures in California. N Engl J Med 329, 850–854.

Volpe, J.J., 2008. Teratogenic effects of drugs and passive addiction. In: Neurology of the Newborn, fifth ed. WB Saunders, Philadelphia, pp. 1011–1031.

Wachsman, L., Schuetz, S., Chan, L.S., et al., 1989. What happens to babies exposed to phencyclidine (PCP) in utero? Am J Drug Alcohol Abuse 15, 31–39.

Williamson, S., Jackson, L., Skeoch, C., et al., 2006. Determination of the prevalence of drug misuse by meconium analysis. Arch Dis Child Fetal Neonatal Ed 91, F291–F292.

section 5

Disorders of the newborn

Pulmonary disease of the newborn

Anne Greenough   Anthony D Milner   Simon Hannam
Grenville F Fox   Carmen Turowski   Mark Davenport   Gavin Morrison

27

CHAPTER CONTENTS

© 2012 Elsevier Ltd

Part 1: Physiology

Anne Greenough   Anthony D Milner

Introduction

This chapter reviews the growth of the respiratory system before and after birth, the mechanisms responsible for the production and clearance of lung fluid, how the healthy infant achieves an expanded air-filled lung, the fetal and postnatal development of respiratory control and the development and function of surfactant and the surfactant proteins.

Morphological development of the lung

The primary goal of lung development is to create a large gas exchange area with a thin air–blood barrier. This is achieved by branching of the airways to form the conducting and proximal respiratory airways and by septation to subdivide the airspaces into alveoli (Roth-Kleiner and Post 2005).

There are four major stages of lung development:

1. 3–6 weeks
2. 6–17 weeks: pseudoglandular
3. 17–26 weeks: canalicular
4. 27 weeks to term: alveolar.

The nerves of the lung develop from neural crest cells and migrate via the vagus nerve to the future trachea and lung; there is then progressive extension of the nerve supply (Sparrow et al. 1999). The human fetal lung originates in the 3-week-old embryo as a ventral diverticulum that arises from the caudal end of the laryngo-tracheal groove of the foregut. The commitment of the foregut endoderm cell to form the lung bud is dependent on the transcription factor, hepatocyte nuclear factor 3-beta (Ang and Rossan 1994). The lung primordium divides into the right and left lung buds and then there is a repetitive process of invasion of the new buds into the surrounding mesenchyme, formation and elongation of the airway tubes and their division to form new airway buds (Roth-Kleiner and Post 2005). Fibroblast growth factor-10 (FGF-10)-stimulated sonic hedgehog (Shh) production in the epithelium of the lung bud and increasing expression of Shh and bone morphogenetic protein 4 (BMP4) lateralises FGF-10 activity, which induces outgrowth of new end buds (Roth-Kleiner and Post 2005). The bronchial tree is developed by the 16th week of gestation. Gli proteins are essential for lung-branching morphogenesis (Motoyama et al. 1998). During the canalicular stage of development, there is continued branching of respiratory bronchioles, vascularisation of the terminal tubules and thinning of the airway epithelium. Arteries and veins develop alongside the respiratory airways. Towards the end of the canalicular stage (24 weeks), pulmonary gas exchange becomes theoretically possible. By 20–22 weeks of gestation, both type I and type II pneumocytes can be identified. Type I cells are flattened and form over 90% of the gas-exchanging surface of the mature lung. The cuboidal type II cells have a secretory function, and, from 24 weeks, osmiophilic lamellar bodies containing surfactant can be identified.

From 24 weeks to term, further terminal branching occurs, with the development of saccules. New tissue ridges are lifted off the existing primary septa and grow in a centripetal direction into the airspaces. These secondary septa subdivide the sacculi into smaller units, the alveoli (Roth-Kleiner and Post 2005). During this period, a capillary network forms around each saccule. A variety of growth factors and their receptors as well as extracellular matrix proteins are involved in the angiogenic process and may also be involved in branching and septation (Table 27.1) (Roth-Kleiner and Post 2005). For example, vascular endothelial growth factor (VEGF-α) is expressed by respiratory epithelial cells, stimulating pulmonary vasculogenesis mediated via paracrine signalling to receptors expressed by progenitor cells in the mesenchyme (Whitsett and Wert 2006); inhibition of VEGF signalling using a blocker Su-5416, either before or after birth, resulted in reduced vascularisation and alveolarisation (Le Cras et al. 2002).

Although alveoli begin to appear as shallow indentations at about 32 weeks of gestation, most alveolar development occurs postterm. The lung grows postnatally mainly by an increase in alveolar number, and, by 4 years of age, the adult number of alveoli is present (Thurlbeck 1982). The subsequent increase in lung volume and surface area is due to an increase in alveolar size. In the first 5 years, there is little elastin in the alveolar walls, which only extends around the alveolar walls by 18 years (Loosli and Potter 1959); the early 'relative' deficiency of elastin may facilitate the increase in size of the alveoli in the growing lung. There is a two- to threefold increase in diameter and length of airways between birth and adulthood (Hislop and Haworth 1989). The amount of bronchial smooth muscle relative to airway size increases between birth and adulthood; the increase in the first weeks after birth is particularly rapid.

Factors influencing lung growth and development

Abnormal lung growth can be the result of inadequate space, or reduction in either fetal breathing or amniotic fluid volume. The time of onset of the insult determines which structures are affected.

Table 27.1 Effect of growth factor activity on branching and septation

	BRANCHING	SEPTATION
FGF-7	↓ Branching	
FGF-10	↓ Branching	
FGF-3/FGF-4	–	↓ Alveolarisation
Shh	↓ Branching	
PDGF-A	↓ Branching	↓ Alveolarisation
PDGF-B	Branching normal but ↓ lung growth	
VEGF	↓ Branching	↓ Alveolarisation
TGF-β	↑ Branching	Emphysema in adults
Bmp-4	Mice die before branching	
EGF/TGF-α	↓ Branching	
Wnt2	–	↓ Alveolarisation
Wnt5a	↑ Branching	
Wnt7b	↓ Branching	

Modified from Roth-Kleiner and Post (2005).
FGF, fibroblast growth factor; Shh, sonic hedgehog; PDGF, platelet-derived growth factor; VEGF, vascular endothelial growth factor; TGF, transforming growth factor; Bmp, bone morphogenetic protein; EGF, epidermal growth factor; Wnt, signalling pathway which describes a network of proteins.

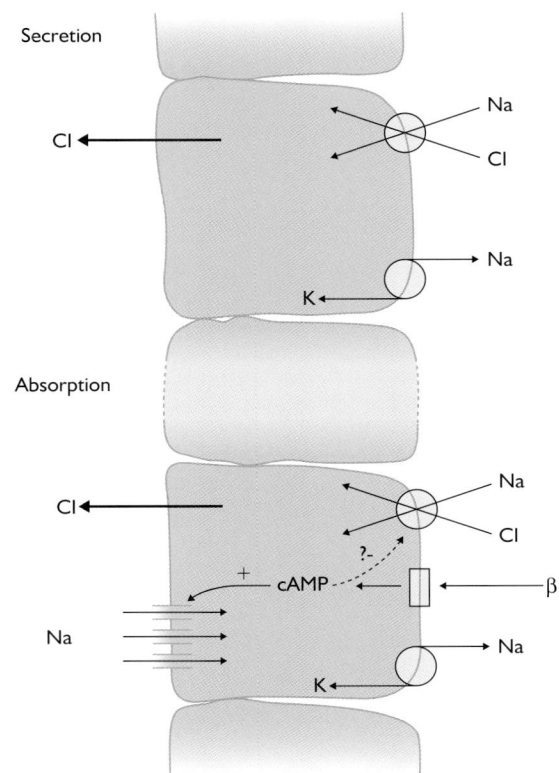

Fig. 27.1 Schematic model to explain the secretory and absorptive states of the lung. Na^+/K^+-ATPase (K^{Na}) generates a gradient for Na^+ which enters the intracellular space across the basolateral membrane linked to Cl^2 (≑). β (⏛) receptor; (Na, ⊗) sodium channel in apical membrane; cAMP, cyclic AMP. *(Reproduced from Walters & Ramsden (1985).)*

Prior to 16 weeks of gestation, branching of the airways is impaired permanently, which will also reduce the potential for the number of alveoli. An insult occurring later affects the number of alveoli. Space restriction can be due to an abnormality extrinsic to the lung, for example congenital diaphragmatic hernia, pleural effusion or asphyxiating thoracic dystrophy, or intrinsic to the lung, for example cystic adenomatoid malformation. Other factors influencing lung growth and development include malnutrition, particularly vitamin A deficiency (Massaro and Massaro 1996, 2000), maternal smoking (Milner et al. 1999) and glucocorticoid administration (Burri and Hislop 1998).

Fetal breathing movements

Phrenic nerve or cervical cord resections which abolish fetal breathing movements (FBMs) are associated with arrest of lung growth. Fetal breathing is dependent on normal diaphragmatic function and pulmonary hypoplasia in newborns occurs with generalised neuromuscular disorders, isolated phrenic nerve agenesis and diaphragmatic amyoplasia. During periods of FBM, rhythmical contractions of the diaphragm slow the loss of lung liquid and help to maintain lung expansion when the upper airway resistance is reduced; this may be the mechanism by which FBMs preserve lung growth.

Fetal lung liquid

In fetal life, work in animal models has demonstrated that the lung is filled with liquid, increasing from 4–6 ml/kg bodyweight at midgestation to about 20 ml/kg near term. The hourly rate of production is initially 2 ml/kg, increasing to 5 ml/kg at term. Fetal lung liquid contributes one-third to one-half to the daily turnover of amniotic fluid. Compared with either amniotic fluid or plasma, lung liquid has a high chloride but low bicarbonate and protein concentration. The dominant force mediating lung liquid secretion is the secondary active transport of chloride ions from the interstitial space into the lung lumen (Fig. 27.1) (Olver and Strang 1974). Sodium ions and water follow passively down electrical and osmotic gradients. A pressure in the lumen of the lung approximately 1 cmH₂O greater than that in the amniotic cavity is generated, which is essential for lung growth. The presence of lung liquid is important for normal lung development; chronic drainage results in pulmonary hypoplasia (Fewell et al. 1983), and lung fluid restriction in the embryonic rat lung affects growth but not airway branching (Souza et al. 1995). Tracheal ligation increases fetal intrathoracic pressure and causes lung hyperplasia; experimentally this can reverse the pulmonary hypoplasia associated with oligohydramnios and congenital diaphragmatic hernia (DiFiore and Wilson 1994; Harrison et al. 1996). There is, however, concern that although tracheal ligation results in increased cell proliferation and normal-sized lungs, it may be associated with decreased surfactant production (Bullard et al. 1997) and altered alveolar structure (Davey et al. 2001).

During labour and delivery, the concentration of adrenaline (epinephrine) increases and, as a consequence, lung liquid secretion ceases and resorption begins. Fetal lung liquid absorption is via activation or opening of sodium channels on the apical surface of the pulmonary epithelium (Hummler et al. 1996). Thyroid hormone and cortisol are necessary for maturation of the normal response of the fetal lung to adrenaline (Barker et al. 1991). Exposure to postnatal oxygen tensions increases sodium transport across the pulmonary epithelium (Ramminger et al. 2000).

Amniotic fluid volume

Pulmonary hypoplasia is associated with oligohydramnios following prolonged rupture of the membranes or chronic drainage following amniocentesis. It appears to be due to the increased efflux of lung liquid from the intrapulmonary space and not the result of external compression of the fetal thorax squeezing out lung liquid, as the amniotic fluid pressure under such circumstances is at or below the normal range (Nicolini et al. 1989). Prolonged oligohydramnios is associated with a decrease in lung liquid volume and a reduction in both the rate of lung liquid secretion and tracheal fluid flow rate (Dickinson and Harding 1987).

Pulmonary circulation

The pulmonary blood vessels and lymphatics develop from the mesenchyme of the splanchnic mesoderm of the foregut; this surrounds the lung buds as they push out from the laryngeal floor. Adjacent blood vessels fuse to form a rudimentary vasculature. The vascular plexus within each lung bud becomes supported by paired segmental arteries, which arise from the dorsal aorta. At 32 days of gestation, the sixth branchial arches appear, which give off the pulmonary arteries, hence the segmental arteries cease to supply the lung. By 50 days of fetal age, the adult blood supply pattern is achieved. Occasionally, an early segmental artery persists, captured within a lobe or lung segment (see sequestered lobe, p. 587) (Haworth 1992). There is progressive dichotomous branching of the pulmonary arteries during lung growth; 70% of the preacinar arteries are formed between the 10th and 14th week of gestation. Additional branching in the canalicular phase and in the last trimester around the developing saccules greatly increases the vascular supply to the area of gas exchange.

During fetal as compared with adult life, the arterial walls contain a greater proportion of smooth muscle. Postnatally, there is rapid thinning – in the first 2 weeks, due to distension, and over the next year, due to a slow reduction in the number of muscle fibres (Hislop and Reid 1981). If such remodelling does not occur, the pulmonary vascular resistance (PVR) remains high, leading to persistent pulmonary hypertension (p. 495). Abnormal remodelling alters the pulmonary vascular reactivity and the response to pharmacological agents. Normal postnatal development can be divided into three overlapping phases (Hall and Haworth 1986; Haworth 1992). Stage 1 starts from birth and lasts for about 4 days, and represents adaptation to extrauterine life. The vessel walls become thinner (Haworth et al. 1987). Initially, the endothelial cells are squat, have a low surface-to-volume ratio and have many surface projections, but, within 5 minutes after birth, the endothelial cells become thinner with less cell-to-cell contact; fewer projections are evident as their surface membrane material is donated to allow the cells to spread rapidly (Fig. 27.2). During stage 2, when the cells have taken up their definitive position, they deposit connective tissue and fix the wall structure. In stage 3, there is growth of the pulmonary vasculature, which lasts until adulthood. At birth, almost the entire pulmonary vasculature is innervated. The majority of nerves contain the vasoconstrictor neuropeptides tyrosine and tyrosine hydroxylase (Haworth 1992). Both nerve density and the immunoreactive

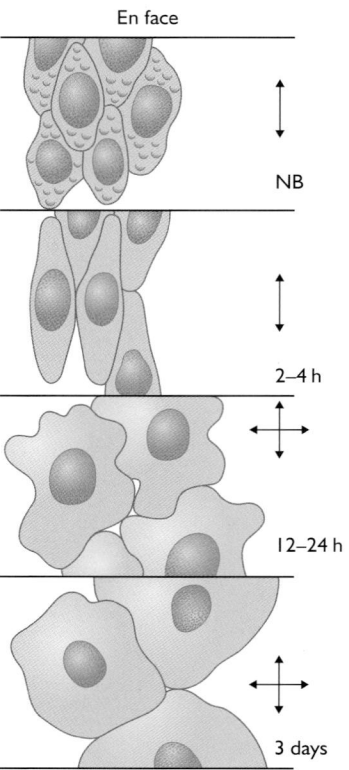

Fig. 27.2 Illustration of en face shape changes – the spreading of endothelial cells from birth to 3 days. *(Reproduced from Haworth (1992).)*

expression of the neurotransmitters increase particularly rapidly in the first 2 weeks (Wharton et al. 1988).

Cardiorespiratory adaptation at birth

Aeration of the lungs at birth

In fetal life, the respiratory system is fluid-filled. The replacement of lung liquid by air is largely accomplished within a few minutes of birth. Lung liquid production ceases during labour; that effect is mediated by catecholamines (Walters and Olver 1978) and arginine vasopressin (Hooper et al. 1993). Some liquid is squeezed out under the high vaginal pressure during the second stage of delivery (Karlberg et al. 1962), while the majority is absorbed into the pulmonary lymphatics and capillaries (Strang 1977). The transpulmonary pressure, which inflates the lungs, displaces liquid from the terminal respiratory units into the perivascular spaces. Air entry into the lung displaces liquid and reduces the hydraulic pressure in the pulmonary circulation, increasing blood flow. This increases the effective vascular surface area for fluid exchange, facilitating water absorption into the pulmonary vascular bed.

Stimulus for the first breath

Fetal breathing activity ceases during labour. Following birth, one of the most important stimuli to the onset of breathing is cooling. Audiovisual, proprioceptive and touch stimuli recruit central neurons and increase central arousal (Condorelli and Scarpelli 1975; Hasan and Rigaux 1992). Hypoxia mediated by central chemoreceptors is important, but peripheral chemoreceptor activity is not critical to the onset of respiration (pp. 454–455). The median time for the onset of respiratory activity is 10 seconds (Vyas et al. 1981).

A high negative pressure is required to overcome the high flow resistance and inertia of liquid in the airways, as well as the surface tension at the air–liquid interface (Karlberg et al. 1962). Both Karlberg et al. (1962) and Milner and Saunders (1977) recorded inspiratory pressures during the first breath of greater than 20 cmH$_2$O, but not in all infants. Subsequently, using a dual-pressure tip transducer, Vyas et al. (1986) demonstrated that pressures of greater than 20 cmH$_2$O were the norm. Expiration is active for the first few breaths, with pressures ranging from 18 to 115 cmH$_2$O; this may aid the distribution of ventilation and facilitate further fluid clearance from the lungs.

Changes in lung mechanics after birth

There is a fall in airways resistance and rise in functional residual capacity (FRC), which is most rapid in the first 2 hours. Compliance, however, progressively increases over the 24-hour period as lung liquid is gradually absorbed. The changes in lung mechanics occur at a slower rate following elective caesarean section, when there is a delay in lung fluid absorption.

Circulatory changes at birth

In the fetus, only about 12% of the right ventricular output enters the pulmonary circulation (Friedman and Fahey 1993), because of the high PVR, the presence of a patent ductus arteriosus and the low-resistance placental component of the systemic circulation. At birth, clamping of the umbilical cord and removal of the placenta from the circulation reduce venous return through the inferior vena cava to the right atrium. The foramen ovale closes because of the resultant lower right atrial pressure and the increase in left atrial pressure that occurs with the increased pulmonary venous return. The loss of the umbilical venous return also means diminished flow through the ductus venosus and passive closure occurs usually within 3–7 days of birth.

PVR falls rapidly in the first minutes after birth, then more gradually over the next days and weeks of life. This fall in PVR, which is associated with a structural reorganisation and thinning of the vessel walls, allows for an eightfold increase in pulmonary blood flow. There are several mechanisms responsible for the fall in PVR. Lung aeration results in opening up the pulmonary capillary bed, acute lowering of PVR and an increase in pulmonary blood flow. This is due to both a mechanical effect and oxygenated blood passing through the pulmonary circulation. In fetal lambs, mechanical expansion of the lungs with a non-oxygenated gas caused a decrease in PVR and a fourfold increase in pulmonary blood flow; a further increase resulted when oxygen was used as the ventilatory gas (Tietel et al. 1987). Inflation of the lungs also stimulates pulmonary stretch receptors, which leads to reflex vasodilation of the pulmonary vascular bed. Mechanical expansion additionally creates surface forces at the gas–liquid interface within the alveoli, which physically expand small blood vessels and decrease perivascular pressure (Walther et al. 1993).

Prostaglandins and endothelial-derived products (endothelin-1 and nitric oxide (NO)) are important in regulating fetal and transitional pulmonary vascular tone (Table 27.2) (Shaul 1995; Zenge et al. 2001). The fetal PVR is high because of the low oxygen tensions and low prostaglandin (PG) I$_2$ and NO levels and the presence of vasoconstrictor substances such as endothelin-1. In healthy infants, the majority of measurable changes in cardiopulmonary haemodynamics occur by 8 hours, although some degree of

Table 27.2 Factors that modulate pulmonary vascular resistance (PVR) in the near-term and term transitional and neonatal pulmonary circulation

LOWERS PVR	INCREASES PVR
Endogenous mediators and mechanisms	
Oxygen	Hypoxia
Nitric oxide	Acidosis
PGI$_2$, E$_2$, D$_2$	Endothelin-1
Adenosine, ATP, magnesium	Leukotrienes
Bradykinin	Thromboxanes
Atrial natriuretic factor	Platelet-activating factor
Alkalosis	Ca^{2+} channel activation
K$^+$ channel activation	α-adrenergic stimulation
Histamine	PGF$_{2\alpha}$
Vagal nerve stimulation	
Acetylcholine	
β-adrenergic stimulation	
Mechanical factors	
	Overinflation or underinflation
	Excessive muscularisation, vascular remodeling
Lung inflation	Altered mechanical properties of smooth muscle
Vascular cell structural changes	Pulmonary hypoplasia
Interstitial fluid and pressure changes	Alveolar capillary dysplasia Pulmonary thromboemboli
Shear stress	Main pulmonary artery distension Ventricular dysfunction, venous hypertension

From Kinsella and Abman (1995).
PG, prostaglandin; ATP, adenosine triphosphate.

right-to-left ductal shunting may be found up to 12 hours after birth (Walther et al. 1993). In most infants the ductus has closed or is closing by 24 hours of age, but there is a significant delay in ductal closure in infants with respiratory failure and pulmonary hypertension. During early neonatal life, the pulmonary circulation remains unstable, and in certain disease states, particularly those associated with asphyxia or chronic hypoxia, the PVR increases or remains at the high fetal levels – persistent pulmonary hypertension (pp. 495–500).

Postnatal function

The airways

The nasal portion of the airway is supported by its larger bony and smaller cartilaginous portions. Nasal resistance to airflow, which constitutes approximately one-third of the total pulmonary resistance, is determined by the physical dimensions in a given individual, which are related to ethnic origin (Ohki et al. 1991), and the state of the mucous membranes lining the airway. The prime function of the nose is to act as an entry port for respiration, humidifying and warming inspired gas and trapping extraneous particles. Infants are not necessarily obligate nose breathers and full-term infants can establish oral breathing in the presence of nasal occlusion (Rodenstein et al. 1985). The pharyngeal portion of the airway is very compliant.

Chemoreceptors in the larynx serve to prevent the entry of foreign material by triggering reflex apnoea. Changes in laryngeal diameter modulate airway resistance and lung volume can be maintained by expiratory adduction of the vocal cords (Duara 1992). Laryngeal resistance can be varied by active abduction of the vocal cords during inspiration and by passive as well as active adduction during expiration. Inspiratory abduction and expiratory adduction of the vocal cords occur during FBMs.

The trachea and main bronchi are supported by cartilaginous rings; nevertheless, smooth-muscle contraction can cause narrowing and markedly increase resistance, at least in the adult. In the newborn, the small airways are more compliant than in the adult and expiratory collapse tends to lead to air trapping.

The thorax

In the newborn, compared with the adult, the thorax is round rather than dorsoventrally flattened and the rib orientation is horizontal rather than caudal, thus the expansion potential of the thorax is limited. The neonatal thoracic cage has relatively soft and flexible bony elements, which makes the chest wall subject to collapse during increased inspiratory efforts and the lungs rather collapsed at rest. To compensate, the infant attempts to elevate lung volume at end expiration by a rapid breathing rate, a short expiratory time, intercostal activity and grunting (expiratory laryngeal adduction). Grunting disappears in rapid eye movement (REM) sleep (Harding 1986). Instability of end-expiratory lung volume, particularly in the premature neonate, may explain fluctuations in arterial oxygen levels (Asonye and Vidyasagar 1981).

The respiratory muscles (Fig. 27.3)

The main inspiratory muscle is the diaphragm, a dome-shaped muscle attached to the ribs. Diaphragmatic contraction results in the abdominal contents moving downwards, increasing the vertical dimension of the thoracic cavity. If the dome's descent is impeded by abdominal pressure, then the lower ribs are pulled up. This increases the ribcage diameter by virtue of the linkages between ribs provided by the intercostal muscles and by the articulations of the ribs that lead to the 'pump and bucket handle action'. The configurations of the adult and neonatal diaphragm differ, the latter being relatively flat following birth, the dome shape developing with the physical growth of the thorax and internal organs (Devlieger 1987). There is an exaggerated asymmetrical movement of the newborn diaphragm during respiration. These differences mean the diaphragm is less efficient in the neonate than in the adult. The number of skeletal muscle fibres in the diaphragm is, however, fixed at the time of birth and the subsequent increase in muscle weight is due to hypertrophy. The diaphragm consists of: (1) type I fibres, which are oxidative with a slow twitch and fatigue-resistant; (2) type IIa fibres, which are oxidative–glycolytic with a fast twitch but also fatigue-resistant; and (3) type IIb fibres, which are glycolytic with a fast twitch and are fatigable (Woodrum 1992).

The proportion of type I fibres is low at birth and increases until 6 months of age; there is an associated increase in type IIb, but a decrease in type IIa fibres. Type IIc fibres, which are present at birth, disappear completely by 6 months (Mayock et al. 1987). This means that at birth the diaphragm has a relatively high percentage of oxidative fibres (type I, IIa and IIc) which are fatigue-resistant. The proportion of type I fibres, however, may be low in the preterm infant, putting the baby at risk of diaphragmatic muscle fatigue. Optimal function of the diaphragm is dependent on ribcage stability and adequate abdominal muscle tone. This is particularly important when the system is loaded, as with stiff lungs or obstructed airways.

Upper airway muscles

Patency of the upper airway is dependent on the upper airway muscles and the diaphragm. There is active contraction of the laryngeal muscles, particularly in early expiration, and there is relatively late relaxation of the inspiratory muscles. That activity reduces the flow rate and is modified by carbon dioxide levels; high levels result in a reduced resistance to flow. If the FRC is reduced, the above muscle activity is increased, such that the airway is almost completely occluded in expiration and gas has to be forced out by contraction of the abdominal muscles, producing a grunt.

Gas exchange in the neonatal lung

At rest, oxygen consumption in the newborn (7 ml/min/kg) is approximately twice that of adults. Minute ventilation is proportionally increased and is achieved largely by an increased breathing rate. The rate is increased because there are constraints on increasing tidal volume imposed by the relatively stiff lungs and unstable ribcage. The disadvantage, however, of increasing rate is that this increases the amount of dead-space ventilation, although the proximal airways have a relatively low volume (Mortola 1983). Overventilation or underperfusion of some lung units contributes to the wasted ventilation. The contribution of ventilation–perfusion mismatch, as estimated from the arterial–alveolar differences for oxygen (a-ADo$_2$), is most marked in preterm infants in the first hours after birth.

A major difference between the blood gases of newborn and older infants is the lower Pao$_2$ in relation to the inspired oxygen tension. This is largely because of right-to-left shunting of blood either through areas of the lung with very low ventilation–perfusion ratios or, less commonly, through persisting fetal vascular channels (foramen ovale and ductus arteriosus). Estimates of the total shunt in healthy infants are 24% of the cardiac output in the first hour after birth and 10% at 1 week of age. Shunting through fetal vascular channels is important immediately after birth in immature infants or in sick infants with raised PVR. The low Pao$_2$ due to right-to-left shunting (through cardiac shunts and perfused but non-ventilated lung units) cannot be overcome by administering 100% oxygen, because the blood that is being ventilated soon becomes fully saturated and increasing the oxygen tension adds little further oxygen. On the other hand, carbon dioxide accumulation from partial right-to-left shunting can be compensated for by increased ventilation of functioning lung units. Thus, provided respiratory efforts are maintained, Paco$_2$ will be normal or even low, despite right-to-left shunting.

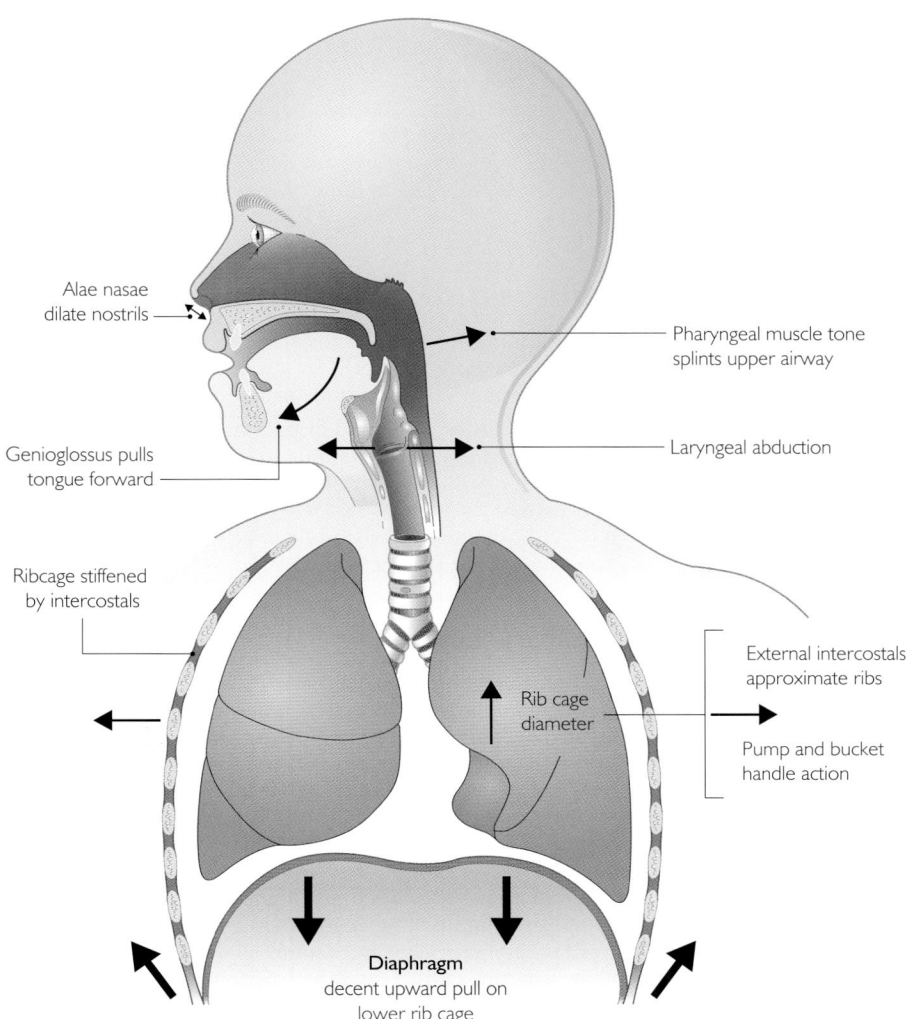

Alae nasae
dilate nostrils

Genioglossus pulls
tongue forward

Ribcage stiffened
by intercostals

Pharyngeal muscle tone
splints upper airway

Laryngeal abduction

External intercostals
approximate ribs

Rib cage
diameter

Pump and bucket
handle action

Diaphragm
decent upward pull on
lower rib cage

Fig. 27.3 Diagrammatic representation of the respiratory pump showing the various muscles and actions that make up inspiration. Although the diaphragm is the main muscle, many others act to optimise its function by opening the airways and splinting the floppy ribcage.

Gas transport in the blood (Delivoria-Papadopoulos and Di Giacomo 1992)

Oxygen

Haemoglobin increases the oxygen transport capacity of the blood 70-fold over that of plasma. As a consequence, the majority of oxygen in whole blood is transported as oxyhaemoglobin (HbO_2) and only a small proportion is dissolved in solution. The haemoglobin concentration is regulated by a renal sensing mechanism, which operates to maintain a balance between the oxygen supply and requirement of the renal tissues. A decrease in concentration or arterial oxygen saturation of haemoglobin or an increase in haemoglobin affinity for oxygen increases erythropoietin production. Haemoglobin is a tetramer: each of the four subunits contains a haem moiety (porphyrin and one atom of ferrous iron) attached to a polypeptide (globin) chain. The four iron atoms can each combine with an oxygen molecule; they remain in the ferrous state, that is, the reaction is oxygenation rather than oxidation. In adult haemoglobin, the four globin chains are predominantly $\alpha_2\beta_2$ (HbA), whereas in the fetus they are $\alpha_2\gamma_2$ (HbF). The quarternary structure of haemoglobin determines its affinity for oxygen: uptake

of oxygen by haemoglobin results in a change of position of the haem moieties, facilitating further oxygen binding. The result is that the oxygen–haemoglobin dissociation curve (the relationship of the percentage oxygen saturation of haemoglobin to the Po_2) has a characteristic sigmoid shape. The oxygen–haemoglobin disssociation curve is affected by the pH, temperature and concentration of 2,3-diphosphoglycerate (2,3-DPG). A rise in temperature or fall in pH (Bohr shift) shifts the curve to the right, which means that a higher Po_2 is required for haemoglobin to bind to a given amount of oxygen. This is quantified as the P_{50}, the Po_2 at which the haemoglobin is half saturated with oxygen. The higher the P_{50}, the lower the affinity of haemoglobin for oxygen. 2,3-DPG is formed from a product of glycolysis and thus its concentration falls when the pH is low. 2,3-DPG binds preferentially to the β chains of deoxygenated haemoglobin. An increase in 2,3-DPG causes more oxygen to be liberated, that is, the oxygen dissociation curve is shifted to the right.

The fetus and newborn

Compared with in the adult, fetal red blood cells (RBCs) are larger, have a shorter half-life and differ in ultrastructure. They also differ with regard to their mechanical, osmotic, thermal and acidic fragility, and contain haemoglobin F (HbF), which is less easily denatured in alkaline or acidic solutions than is adult haemoglobin. The γ chains of HbF have the same number of amino acids as the β chains, but differ in sequence by 39 amino acids. The γ chains of HbF have poorer binding to 2,3-DPG. The effect of 2,3-DPG on the P_{50} of fetal haemoglobin is approximately 40% of the effect on the P_{50} of adult haemoglobin. The oxygen tension of fetal blood is one-fifth to one-quarter that of the adult, but the fetal arterial blood oxygen content and oxyhaemoglobin saturation are similar to those of the adult. This results from the high oxygen-carrying capacity and the increased oxygen affinity of HbF. The latter facilitates the movement of oxygen from mother to fetus. Oxygen delivery to the fetal tissues is sustained because the steep fetal oxygen dissociation curve means that a small decrease in oxygen tension results in a major change in oxyhaemoglobin saturation and unloading of oxygen.

In the term newborn, 70–80% of the haemoglobin is HbF: in preterm babies, about 90% of haemoglobin is HbF. Birth, intrauterine hypoxia and haemolytic disease of the newborn do not cause a change in the proportions of HbA and HbF at any given gestational age. Near term, however, the demand for accelerated erythropoeisis leads preferentially to synthesis of HbA. During the first year, HbF decreases from 70% to less than 2% of the total haemoglobin.

The high oxygen affinity of HbF has disadvantages in postnatal life. In particular, the low P_{50} decreases the driving potential for oxygen diffusion, limiting the rate at which oxygen can be unloaded (Altura and Chand 1981). The oxygen consumption of the newborn at minimal activity, even in a thermally neutral environment, increases by 100–150% in the first few days. To meet these demands, the baby's blood oxygen affinity decreases rapidly over the first 5 days and then more gradually, reaching adult values by 6 months (Delivoria-Papadopoulos et al. 1971). During the first 5 days, the 2,3-DPG levels rise to above those found in the adult; this decreases blood oxygen affinity by lowering intercellular pH. Prematurely born babies have a lower 2,3-DPG content, lower P_{50} and higher fetal haemoglobin concentration. They have a smaller oxygen unloading capacity and do not catch up until 3 months of age (Guyton 1971).

Carbon dioxide

Carbon dioxide is 20 times more soluble in water than is oxygen. Carbon dioxide is carried in the blood by three mechanisms: the majority as bicarbonate (85%), but also dissolved and in combination with proteins as carbamino compounds. Bicarbonate is formed very rapidly in RBCs, because of the presence of carbonic anhydrase, which catalyses the first part of the following reaction:

$$CO_2 + H_2O \rightarrow H_2CO_3 \rightarrow HCO_3^- + H^+$$

Ionic dissociation of H_2CO_3 is fast. HCO_3^- then diffuses out of the RBC down a concentration gradient, but H^+ cannot follow and binds to haemoglobin. This is facilitated in the presence of reduced haemoglobin, which is a weaker acid than oxyhaemoglobin, and thus deoxygenation of the blood increases its ability to carry carbon dioxide (the Haldane effect). To maintain electrical neutrality, as HCO_3^- diffuses out, Cl^- diffuses into the RBC (the chloride shift). These events increase the osmolar content of the RBC, thus the packed cell volume is higher on the venous than on the arterial side of the circulation. Carbon dioxide also combines with the N terminals of amino acids of proteins, particularly haemoglobin, to form carbamino compounds:

$$CO_2 + R_2 + NH_2 \rightarrow RNHCOO^- + H^+$$

The newborn's blood has a greater carbon dioxide transport capacity. This is because of the high haemoglobin level. In addition, carbon dioxide competes with 2,3-DPG for the haemoglobin binding site, and, since 2,3-DPG binds less avidly with HbF than with adult haemoglobin, more carbon dioxide can be taken up. RBC carbonic anhydrase levels, however, are 25% lower in the neonate and even more so in those born prematurely (Kleinmann et al. 1967).

Regulation of breathing

The rhythmic transition from the inspiratory to the expiratory phase of the respiratory cycle is ordered by a centrally generated respiratory rhythm, which consists of three neural phases:

1. inspiration, corresponding to inspiratory muscle contraction
2. phase 1 expiration, corresponding to postinspiration or passive expiration, when inspiratory muscles cease to contract progressively
3. phase 2 expiration, corresponding to active exhalation with expiratory muscle contraction.

Respiratory 'centre'

The respiratory rhythm (described above) is generated by a loose complex of respiratory neurons, which lie within the ventrolateral region of the brainstem. The respiratory rhythm generator also produces sighs and gasps. A variety of models of the central respiratory rhythm generator have been proposed, but a common assumption is that chemical neurotransmission is required to mediate the synaptic interactions which play a role in generation of transmission and expression of the respiratory rhythm. Respiratory rhythm-generating areas, such as the pre-Boetzinger complex, receive multiple inputs from many areas outside and within the vicinity of the complex (Doi and Ramirez 2008). Afferents from the forebrain, hypothalamus, central and peripheral chemoreceptors, muscles, joints and pain receptors are integrated into the 'centre'. The number of intersynaptic connections reaches a peak towards the end of fetal life. The complex projects to various respiratory-related areas that contain neuromodulators which are in turn modulated by multiple other areas. Most areas contain multiple neuromodulators that are partly released from the same neurons, thus neuromodulation occurs at all levels of integration (Doi and Ramirez 2008).

Neurotransmitters

Excitatory

The excitatory neurotransmitters include glutamate, which excites NMDA and non-NMDA receptors; the latter are involved in generating and transmitting respiratory rhythms to spinal and cranial respiratory neurons (Funk et al. 1993). The transmission of inspiratory drive is further fine-tuned by presynaptic glutaminergic modulation at the level of the spinal cord. Serotonin (5-hydroxytryptamine (5-HT)) neurons in the medulla oblongata constitute a critical system in the modulation of autonomic and respiratory effector neurons (Paterson and Darnall 2009). 5-HT has diverse effects on respiratory neuronal activity, but the most consistent effect is to restore a normal breathing pattern in metabolic states such as hypoxia or ischaemia, which cause apneustic breathing (Lalley et al. 1994). The developmental profile of $5-HT_{2A}$ receptors changes over the first year after birth in the hypoglossal nucleus critical to airway patency (Paterson and Darnall 2009).

STAFF LIBRARY

Inhibitory

Both gamma-aminobutyric acid (GABA) and glycine are essential for generating respiratory rhythm in the primary network. GABA and glycine are released by late and postinspiratory neurons to turn off inspiratory neurons and so facilitate the transition from inspiration to expiration. Adenosine is ubiquitously formed in the body and has both central and peripheral effects. When administered centrally, it depresses ventilation; this effect is most pronounced in young full-term and preterm animal models. If adenosine is given systemically, however, it stimulates breathing, probably by stimulating peripheral chemoreceptors; this effect may be more important in the adult. Adenosine antagonists (theophylline and caffeine) stimulate breathing and also block – but not in humans – hypoxia-induced respiratory depression (Runold et al. 1989).

Chemoreceptors

Both central and peripheral chemoreceptors are involved in modification of respiratory activity in response to changes in blood gases. The central chemoreceptors are situated near the ventral surface of the medulla and respond to changes in carbon dioxide/pH and oxygen supply. The peripheral chemoreceptors are situated at the bifurcation of the common carotid arteries (carotid bodies) and in the aortic bodies above and below the aortic arch, the former being more important in humans.

In the fetus, the arterial chemoreceptors are active in utero, but have reduced sensitivity. They are virtually silenced when the arterial P_{O_2} rises at birth (Blanco et al. 1984). Resetting of the carotid chemoreceptors to hypoxia then occurs. This is probably triggered by the rise in blood oxygen levels. The resetting of the chemoreceptors to hypoxia is essentially complete within 24–48 hours of birth (Calder et al. 1994) and may be due to a change in dopamine levels. Dopamine inhibits chemoreceptor discharge in both the newborn and adult. If rat pups are delivered into a hypoxic environment (12%), they maintain both their low sensitivity to hypoxia, with persistence of the immature inhibitory response to hypoxia (Eden and Hanson 1987), and a high dopamine turnover. In the lamb, hyperoxia induced by mechanical ventilation of the fetus for a few days before birth causes premature resetting (Blanco et al. 1987).

Responses to changes in oxygen tension (Fig. 27.4)

The fetus

Fetuses respond to hypoxia with a suppression of ventilation, which is most marked in growth-retarded fetuses (Bekedam and Visser 1985); the hypoxic suppression of ventilation is mediated by the lateral part of the lower pons. In response to hypoxia there are also cardiovascular reflexes; these include bradycardia and redistribution of the circulation to favour the heart, brain and adrenals, which minimise oxygen consumption and conserve oxygen supplies for vital organs. Hyperoxia stimulates continuous fetal breathing.

The newborn

The newborn's response to hypoxia in the perinatal period is a biphasic response: a transient increase in minute ventilation followed by a decrease to or below baseline levels. The initial increase in ventilation is probably due to activation of peripheral chemoreceptors, as it is abolished by carotid sinus nerve section. The subsequent reduction in ventilation may result from a fall in Pa_{CO_2}

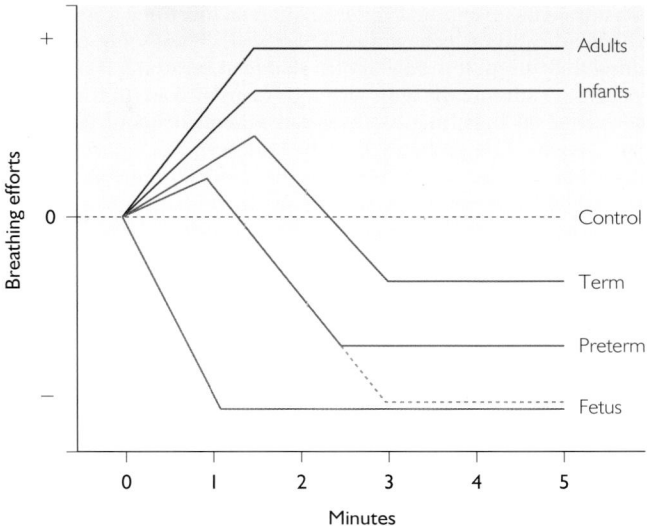

Fig. 27.4 Diagrammatic representation of the age-related responses to hypoxia, induced by breathing hypoxic gases for 5 minutes (solid lines). Breathing efforts assessed by diaphragmatic electromyogram in the fetus and by ventilatory responses in others. The dashed line indicates that apnoea may occur in preterm infants, resembling a fetal response. (*Reproduced from Henderson-Smart (1983).*)

following the initial hyperventilation and may be due to a depression of central respiratory neurons (Rigatto et al. 1988). It may also be explained by the suppressant effect of hypoxia in the fetal state persisting into the neonatal period. The biphasic response to hypoxia disappears at 12–14 days and the adult pattern is then seen, that is, stimulation without depression (Fig. 27.4). Very immature infants respond to hypoxia in a similar fashion to fetuses, that is, with apnoea. This inhibition of breathing is at a suprapontine level. More mature preterm infants have an initial increase (but less than in term infants) and then a more dramatic fall in ventilation in response to hypoxia (Rigatto 1992). In non-REM sleep, the decrease in ventilation is the predominating response. The response to hypoxia is also modified by the temperature of the environment in which the infant is nursed; transient hyperventilation on exposure to 12% O_2 is not seen if the infant is in a cold rather than a warm environment (Ceruti 1966).

A hyperoxic gas causes a temporary suppression of breathing; this is attributed to the withdrawal of peripheral chemoreceptor drive. During the first few days, the reduction in ventilation with 100% oxygen is less, consistent with inactivity of the carotid afferents during this resetting period. After a few minutes of hyperoxia, ventilation increases to above control levels. In adults, a similar but less marked hyperventilation has been attributed to hyperoxic cerebral vasoconstriction, which leads to increased brain tissue carbon dioxide. The response to hyperoxia is slower in more immature infants. Prolonged exposure to supplemental oxygen also reduces the response to hyperoxia.

Response to carbon dioxide/acidosis

The fetus

Fetal breathing can be detected as early as 14 weeks of gestation in the human. The amount of time the fetus spends breathing increases with advancing gestational age. Initially, fetal breathing was thought to depend only on behavioural reflexes, as it was only observed during REM sleep. It is now known that fetal breathing is modified by chemical stimuli; the fetus responds to an increase in Pa_{CO_2} with an increase in breathing, both elevated frequency and diaphragmatic activity. It is probably that the hydrogen ion concentration, rather than carbon dioxide per se, is the major stimulus to respiratory activity, although there is some evidence that carbon dioxide may have an effect independent of pH (Millhorn and Eldridge 1986). During non-REM sleep, however, only very high Pa_{CO_2} levels (>100 mmHg) can initiate breathing activity (Rigatto et al. 1988). Hypoxia inhibits fetal breathing. Lesions in the ventrolateral pons eliminate the hypoxic inhibition of breathing and are associated with a lower threshold for carbon dioxide drive-augmented breathing through all states (Johnston et al. 1989). Fetal breathing is also suppressed during labour.

The newborn

Inhalation of CO_2 increases ventilation in the newborn in both REM and quiet sleep. The slope of minute ventilation versus Pa_{CO_2} levels in the newborn is similar to that of adults, but the response is shifted to the left because of lower resting carbon dioxide levels (Rigatto 1984). The tidal volume component of the ventilatory response assumes greater importance with postnatal development. The percentage of inhaled CO_2 influences the pattern of breathing. A low percentage of CO_2 (2%) primarily stimulates an increase in tidal volume (Kalapesi et al. 1981), whereas a higher percentage provokes an increase in respiratory frequency and tidal volume (Moriette et al. 1985). Periodic breathing is abolished with a small increase in inhaled CO_2 (Kalapesi et al. 1981). Sleep state also influences the response to carbon dioxide, both in adults (Phillipson and Bowes 1986) and in the newborn. In term infants, the slope of ventilatory response is less during active than quiet sleep (Fig. 27.5). This may be due to mechanical instability associated with ribcage distortion in active sleep, since the diaphragmatic response is intact. In preterm infants (Rigatto et al. 1991), the slope of the ventilatory response is less, but increases with postnatal growth. As diaphragm electromyogram responses to CO_2 inhalation are also reduced in the preterm infant, this is probably due to the immaturity of the central chemoreceptors rather than mechanical differences in the respiratory pump (Rigatto 1984).

Respiratory reflexes

The Hering–Breuer reflexes

Hering and Breuer (1868) described three respiratory reflexes. The Hering–Breuer inflation reflex is stimulated by lung inflation and results in cessation of respiratory activity. This reflex is generated by stretch receptors within the airway and has an afferent pathway lying within the vagi. In the newborn, the reflex produces a pattern of rapid, shallow tidal breathing and operates within the tidal volume range. The reflex is active from FRC and is maximal after an inspiration of approximately 4 ml/kg above FRC (Hassan et al. 2001).

The Hering–Breuer expiratory reflex is stimulated if inhalation is prolonged. The active expiration seen in infants ventilated at slow rates and long inflation times may be a manifestation of this reflex (Greenough 1988).

In animal models, the Hering–Breuer deflation reflex is evidenced by a prolonged inspiration generated in response to deflating the lung rapidly, either by attaching the endotracheal tube to a suction source or creating a pneumothorax, or following an unusually vigorous expiratory effort which takes the lung below its end-expiratory level. This response does occur in the newborn (Marsh et al. 1994) and may have a role in maintaining the FRC. The strength of the reflex is increased if rapid lung volume reduction is commenced at FRC rather than end inspiration (Hannam et al. 2001).

Head's paradoxical reflex

Head (1889) noted that, if vagal conduction was blocked, rapid inflation, instead of producing apnoea, resulted in a stronger and more pronounced diaphragmatic contraction; this was named Head's paradoxical reflex. It has subsequently been termed the inspiratory augmenting reflex or provoked augmented inspiration and is the underlying mechanism of the first breath and sighing. This reflex improves compliance and reopens partially collapsed airways. It has an important role in promoting lung expansion during resuscitation. Its frequency is increased by low compliance, hypercapnia and hypoxia (Cherniack et al. 1981).

The intercostal phrenic inhibitory reflex

Rapid chest wall distortion results in a shortening of inspiratory efforts. This reflex response is inhibited by an increase in FRC or

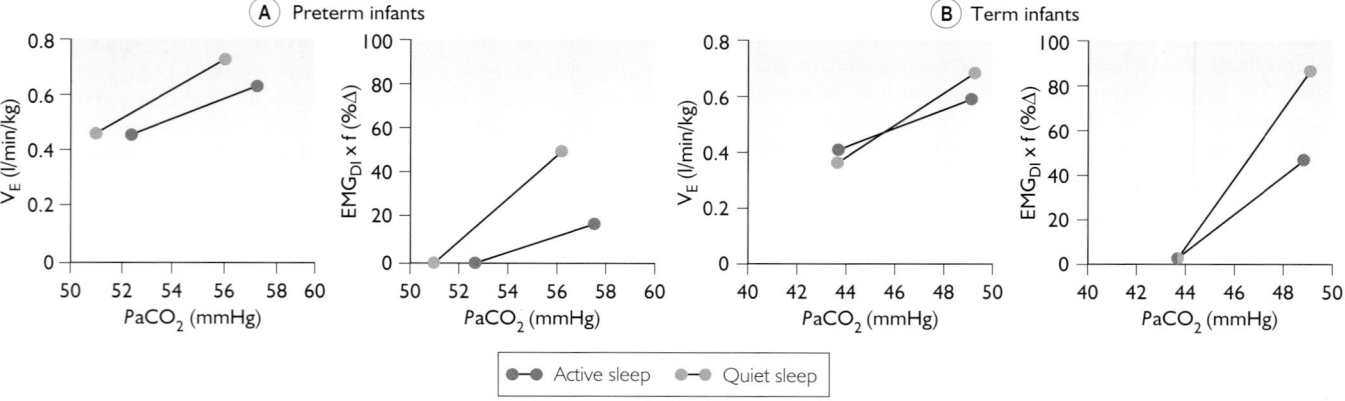

Fig. 27.5 The ventilatory response to CO_2 rebreathing in neonates. Note that (A) preterm and (B) term infants showed a decreased response to CO_2 in 'phasic' rapid eye movement sleep as compared with quiet sleep. The vertical axis on the figures in (B) is a measure of electromyogram (EMG) activity multiplied by the change in respiratory rate. *(Reproduced from Rigatto (1992).)*

applying continuous positive airway pressure; the mechanism may be improved chest wall stability (Martin et al. 1977).

Irritant reflexes

Subepithelial chemoreceptors in the trachea, bronchi and bronchioles detect insults to the epithelial surfaces; thus, inhalation of toxic gases causes a change in frequency and depth of respiration. The response is less in REM sleep and in the premature infant (Fleming et al. 1978), who has a smaller number of small myelinated vagal fibres and poorly developed receptors.

Upper airway reflexes

Breathing is stimulated by cold via the trigeminal afferents of the facial skin, whereas irritant stimuli to the nasal mucosa cause inhibition of breathing and cardiovascular reflex responses resembling those in diving mammals. The latter response is enhanced under anaesthesia and in the newborn (Wealthall 1975), when cortical dampening of the responses is reduced. Vigorous suctioning of the nasopharynx can stimulate apnoea and bradycardia via these reflexes (Cordero and Hon 1971).

The laryngeal chemoreceptors defend the lower airway from inhalation. Introduction of water into the interarytenoid notch induces apnoea (Pickens et al. 1989). In active sleep, laryngeal stimulation is more likely to induce apnoea and less likely to cause arousal (Phillipson and Bowes 1986). This is of potential clinical significance since gastro-oesophageal reflux is more common during active sleep (Jeffery et al. 1980). Maturation of the laryngeal chemoreflex is characterised by an increase in coughing and a decrease in swallowing and apnoea (Thach 2007). Those changes are probably

the result of central processing of afferent stimuli rather than of a reduction in sensitivity or change in receptor distribution in the larynx (Thach 2007).

Lung mechanics (Table 27.3)

Lung volumes

The tidal volume is the amount of gas entering or leaving the lung with each breath. Minute volume is calculated by multiplying the tidal volume by the respiratory rate over 1 minute. The volume exchanged following a maximum inspiratory and expiratory effort is called the vital capacity and in the infant can be measured during crying (crying vital capacity), or more accurately by pressurising a face mask to 20–25 cmH$_2$O and then inflating a rigid walled jacket with pressures of 40–60 cmH$_2$O (Turner et al. 1995). The residual volume remains after a maximum expiratory effort; residual volume plus vital capacity gives the total lung capacity. At end expiration, the volume of gas remaining in the lung is referred to as the FRC and can be estimated by rebreathing an inert gas, such as helium (FRC$_{he}$). Only areas of the lung in communication with the airways will be measured by such a method. Alternatively, the patient can be placed in a body plethysmograph and the FRC$_{pleth}$ estimated by applying Boyle's law during airway occlusion; FRC$_{pleth}$ is FRC$_{he}$ plus trapped gas. The dead space is the part of the respiratory system which does not take part in ventilation and is made up of the anatomical dead space (the conducting airways) and the physiological dead space, which includes non-functioning alveoli. Alveolar ventilation can be estimated from the tidal volume minus the dead space. In infants with respiratory distress, particularly transient

Table 27.3 Lung mechanics in healthy babies

Measurements	NO. OF INFANTS STUDIED	MEAN	STANDARD DEVIATION	RANGE
Tidal volume (ml/kg)	266	4.8	1.0	2.9–7.9
Respiratory rate (breaths/min)	266	50.9	13.1	25–104
Minute volume (ml/min/kg)	266	232	3.6	78–444
Dynamic compliance (ml/cmH$_2$O/kg)	266	1.72	0.5	0.9–3.7
Total pulmonary resistance (cmH$_2$O/l/s)	266	42.5	1.6	3.1–171
Work of breathing (G.cm)	266	11.9	7.4	1.1–52.6
Expiratory time (s)	291	0.57	0.17	0.27–1.28
Inspiratory time (s)	291	0.51	0.10	0.28–0.87
Time to maximum expiratory flow/total expiratory time (s)	291	0.51	0.12	0.18–0.83
Static compliance (ml/cmH$_2$O/kg)	299	3.70	1.45	2.0–14.8
Respiratory system resistance (cmH$_2$O/l/s)	299	63.4	16.6	34.9–153.3
Time constant of respiratory system (s)	299	0.24	0.10	0.08–1.1
Thoracic gas volume (ml/kg)	271	29.8	6.2	14.5–45.6

Data of Milner and Marsh, reproduced with their permission (1999).
The tidal flow and volume were measured by a type 00 Fleisch pneumotachograph, and intrathoracic pressure with a 4-cm oesophageal balloon. Babies supine and in quiet sleep. Dead space eliminated by a bias flow of air.

tachypnoea of the newborn, the respiratory rate is increased and the tidal volume may be decreased. In respiratory distress syndrome (RDS) and pneumonia, the FRC is low and the physiological dead space increased.

Compliance

Compliance is a measure of the distensibility of the lungs and chest wall, the change in volume per unit pressure. Dynamic compliance is assessed during tidal breathing by measurement of the change in volume (usually using the integrated signal of a flow-measuring device, a pneumotachograph) divided by the change in pleural pressure (which under certain conditions is similar to the change in oesophageal pressure) between points of zero airflow (Fig. 27.6). In situations with a rapid respiratory rate and chest wall distortion, dynamic compliance measurements can be inaccurate. Dynamic compliance is measured in ventilated infants by relating the volume change from a positive pressure inflation to the pressure drop (that is, positive inflation pressure – positive end-expiratory pressure), providing that the infant is not making spontaneous respiratory efforts, as these might interfere with volume delivery during inflation.

Static compliance requires the measurement of changes in lung volume over a larger range than the tidal volume or an assumption has to be made that the end-expiratory transpulmonary pressure represents a static value, which is unlikely to be true in infants with lung disease (Silverman 1983). Static compliance is usually measured in spontaneously breathing infants using an occlusion technique, which relies on occlusion at end inspiration causing a transient inhibition of breathing by stimulation of the Hering–Breuer reflex. The airway pressure during the occlusion is related to the volume above end expiration at which the occlusion was made. This technique requires temporary cessation of breathing, which may be difficult to provoke in an infant with a rapid respiratory rate or a weak Hering–Breuer reflex. Static compliance measurements assess the compliance of both the lung and chest wall. In the newborn, the chest wall compliance is very high, so, essentially, dynamic and static compliance values are similar. Compliance is reduced in infants with RDS.

Resistance

Resistance is a measure of the pressure necessary to generate airflow. Airway resistance can be assessed in a body plethysmograph, but after the first week the infant will usually require sedation and this technique is not applicable to oxygen-dependent patients. Pulmonary resistance (Fig. 27.7), however, can be measured on the neonatal intensive care unit, using an oesophageal balloon and pneumotachograph; the pressure difference corresponding to the flow change between points of equal lung volume is measured. Resistance is increased in infants with meconium aspiration syndrome and, at follow-up, in those who required neonatal ventilation (Yüksel and Greenough 1992). Resistance can also be calculated from the volume and flow traces obtained after the release of the occlusion discussed above. The time constant, the time for 63% of the volume to leave the lungs, can be measured; thus, the resistance can be calculated, as the time constant equals the product of the compliance and the resistance (Lesouef et al. 1984).

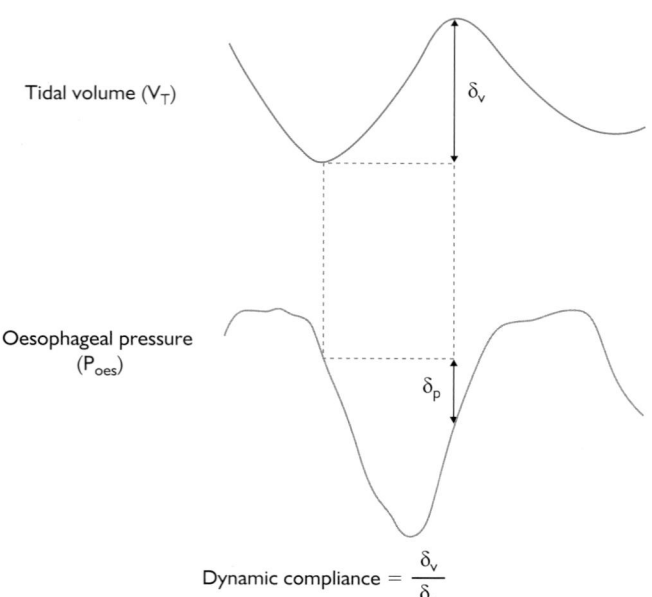

Fig. 27.6 Volume and oesophageal pressure traces during spontaneous breathing. The dynamic compliance is calculated by dividing the tidal volume (δ_v) by the pressure gradient between the beginning and end of inspiration (δ_p). *(Reproduced from Greenough et al. (1995).)*

Dynamic compliance $= \dfrac{\delta_v}{\delta_p}$

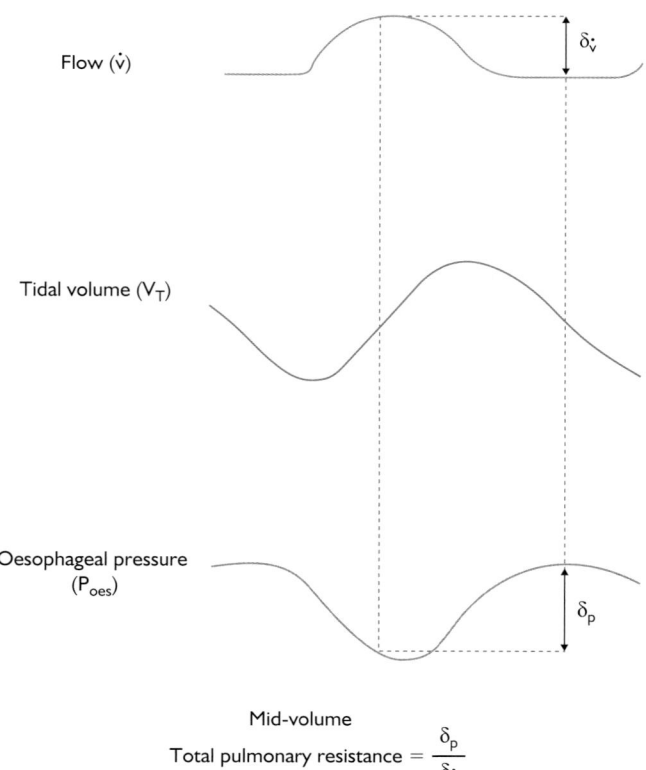

Total pulmonary resistance $= \dfrac{\delta_p}{\delta_{\dot{v}}}$

Fig. 27.7 Flow, volume and pressure traces during tidal breathing. The total pulmonary resistance is calculated by dividing the pressure gradient between midinspiration and midexpiration (δ_p) by the simultaneous flow difference ($\delta_{\dot{v}}$). *(Reproduced from Greenough et al. (1995).)*

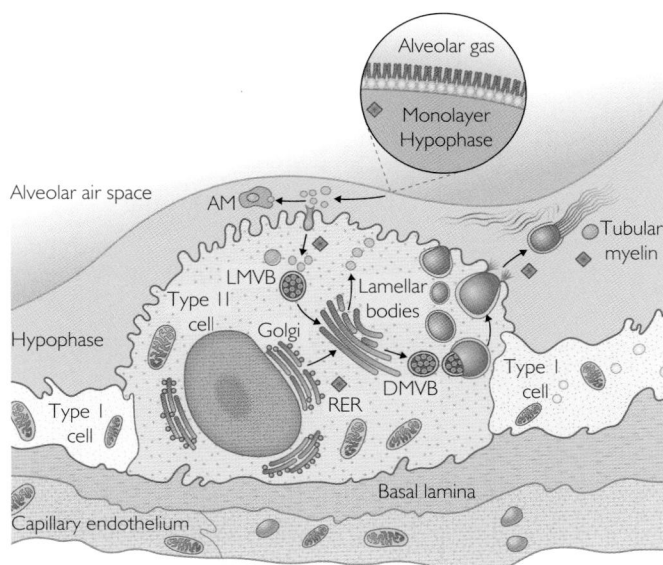

Fig. 27.8 An alveolar type II cell showing two surfactant release mechanisms: lamellar bodies and the constitutive release of surfactant protein A. Surfactant is shown both being phagocytosed by an alveolar macrophage (AM) and being taken back into the cell and reutilised. The inset shows a monolayer which, in the gel phase, is able to withstand very large lateral forces, literally splinting open the alveolus. RER, rough endoplasmic reticulum; LMVB, light multivesicular body; DMVB, dense multivesicular body. *(Reproduced from Nicholas et al. (1997).)*

Surfactant

Origins of surfactant

Alveolar type II cells

Alveolar type II cells produce surfactant (Fig. 27.8) (Post and van Golde 1988). They are compact cuboidal cells, occurring most often at the corners of the air spaces. They cover about 2% of the alveolar surface and account for about 15% of the cell numbers. They differentiate from the columnar epithelium during the canalicular phase of development (p. 448), but are not prominent until about 24 weeks' gestation, when they can be identified by their osmiophilic lamellar inclusion bodies (Kuhn 1982). The biosynthesis of surfactant phosphatidylcholine occurs in the endoplasmic reticulum of the type II cell. The phospholipid then moves via intracellular pathways towards the lamellar bodies, for secretion into the alveolus. The characteristic feature of the alveolar type II cell is the lamellar body, storage granules of surfactant (Hallman et al. 1976).

Lamellar bodies

A mature lamellar body is about 1.5 μm in diameter. They consist of a limiting membrane surrounding about 20–70 close-packed phospholipid bilayers, or lamellae, each with a width of 66 Å, arranged in a hemisphere. The ends of these lamellae abut on to a baseplate, which is probably an extension of the limiting membrane. In the centre is a matrix core of proteinaceous material (Stratton 1976a, b). Lamellar bodies, isolated from lung tissue by density gradient centrifugation, contain surfactant lipids and the surfactant proteins A, B and C (SP-A, SP-B, SP-C).

Recycling of surfactant

Surfactant may be degraded locally in the alveoli and small airways, the breakdown products being absorbed and recycled by the alveolar cells (Fig. 27.9). More than 90% of the phosphatidylcholine on the alveolar surface is reprocessed; this conserves surfactant components as well as reactivating them to regenerate surfactant. The turnover time is approximately 10 hours (Stevens et al. 1989). The contribution, therefore, to the alveolar surfactant pool from de novo synthesis is modest.

There is negative-feedback regulation of surfactant production mediated by SP-A binding to type II cells (Tino and Wright 1998). Surfactant secretion is controlled by stretch receptors and stimulated by gas entering the lung, causing alveolar distension (Rooney et al. 1977). Other factors controlling secretion (Rooney 2001) include β-adrenergic receptors on alveolar type II cells, which increase in number towards the end of gestation.

Composition

Surfactant is a complex mixture of substances including phospholipids, neutral lipids and proteins.

Phosphatidylcholine and phosphatidylglycerol

Lipids are the major constituent of surfactant and the most important are phosphatidylcholine (PC) and phosphatidylglycerol (PG), representing 70–80% and 5–10% of the lipids, respectively. Another 10% of the lipids is made up of phosphatidylinositol (PI), phosphatidylserine (PS) and phosphatidylethanolamine (PE). Approximately 60% of the PC has both fatty acids saturated (i.e. disaturated) and, as the primary saturated fatty acid is palmitic acid, the major compound in surfactant is dipalmitoyl phosphatidycholine (DPPC). The palmitic acid residues are non-polar and hydrophobic and orient towards the air, whereas the PC is polar and hydrophilic and associates with the liquid phase (Ikegami and Jobe 1993). The shape and orientation of the DPPC mean that it generates a stable monolayer and is able to maintain low surface pressures: during expiration the molecules become very closely packed, as the palmitoyl moieties lack the C–C bonds that produce the kinks in the acyl chains (Wright and Clements 1987). DPPC is relatively rigid at body temperature and cannot adsorb to a surface (Goerke 1998); its phase transition (melt) is approximately at 41°C. At body temperature, DPPC cannot move rapidly enough to maintain a surface monolayer during the respiratory cycle and a 'spreading' agent such as PG is required for normal surfactant function.

PC is synthesised in the endoplasmic reticulum of the type II pneumocytes. There is an increase in surfactant production towards the end of gestation. From 27 to 31 days (term) in rabbits, there is a 10-fold increase in surfactant; during a similar time period, PC increases from 30% to 70% of the total phospholipids, whereas sphingomyelin decreases from 40% to 10%. This change is due to increased synthesis, whereas after birth there is increased secretion. In surfactant from human term and preterm infants, the fractional concentrations of not only DPPC (PC16:0/16:0), but also palmitoylmyristoyl PC (PC16:0/14:0) and palmitoylpalmitoleoyl PC (PC16:0/16:1) increase with maturation (Bernhard et al. 2001); in animal models, the concentrations of the last two phospholipids correlate significantly with respiratory rate.

The proportions of the acidic phospholipids PG and PI change with lung development. Initially PI is the primary acidic phospholipid, but with increasing maturation it is replaced by PG. Patients with RDS have low levels of DPPC and absent PG (Hallman et al. 1976). In poorly controlled diabetic pregnancies, the fetuses have low levels of PG even near term. If RDS progresses to chronic lung

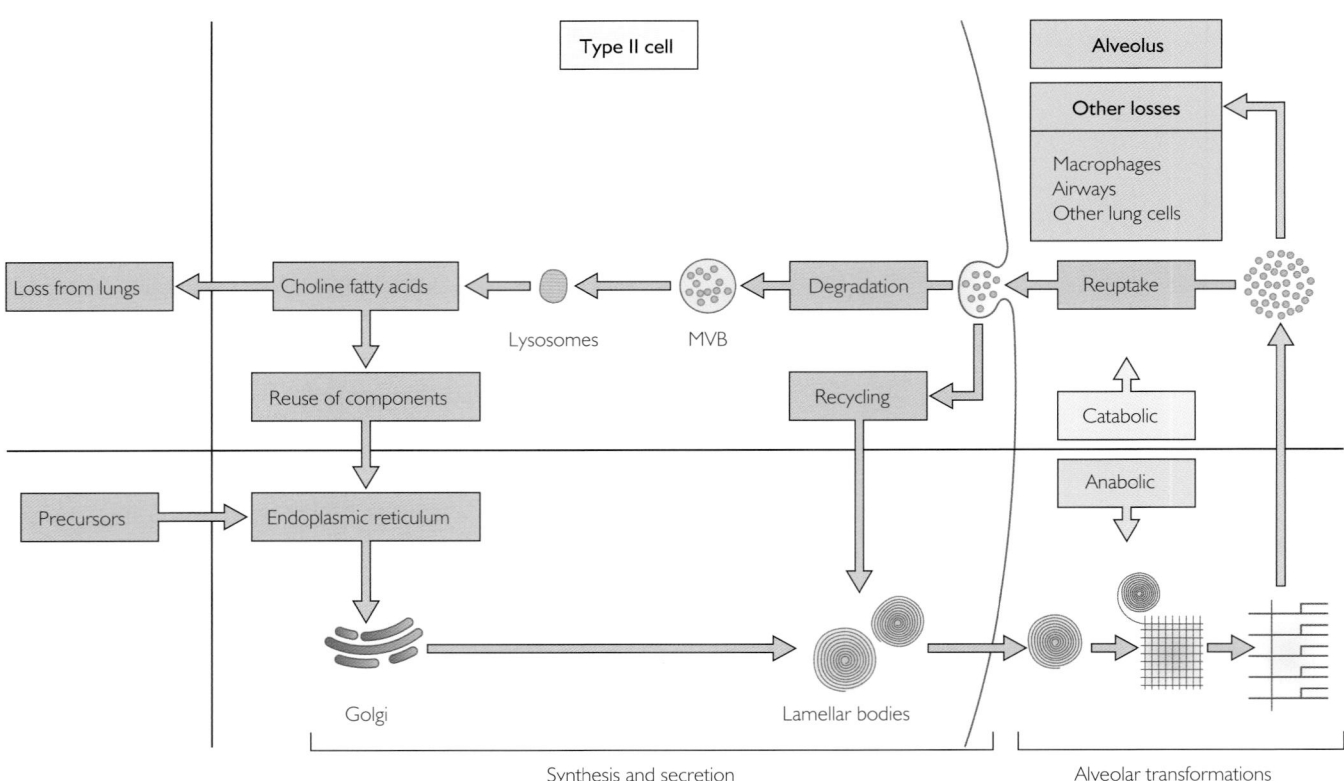

Fig. 27.9 Illustration of surfactant metabolism based on the saturated phosphatidylcholine component of surfactant. The anabolic pathway for synthesis and secretion links with alveolar transformations of the lamellar surfactant to tubular myelin and the monolayer. Catabolic pathways for phospholipid vesicles are minor pathways in the newborn lung but active in the adult lung. The majority of the surfactant is taken back into type II cells for recycling during the newborn period. MVB, multivesicular body. *(Reproduced from Jobe and Ikegami (2001).)*

disease, the appearance of PG is delayed; PI also predominated with acute lung.

Other lipids

About 10% of the total lipids in surfactant are neutral lipids. These are cholesterol, triacylglycerols and free fatty acids (Post et al. 1982). They appear to be an integral part of the surfactant in lamellar bodies and on the alveolar surface. Cholesterol alters the fluidity and organisation of lipid-rich membranes. Sphingomyelin represents less than 2% of surfactant lipid, and glycolipids and carbohydrates a very small fraction of the surfactant mass. The amount of sphingomyelin, a minor component of surfactant, remains unchanged through gestation and thus the change in the amount of DPPC or lecithin can be assessed by comparing it with the amount of sphingomyelin. Thus, lung maturity can be assessed by measurement of the ratio of lecithin to sphingomyelin, the L:S ratio (p. 464).

Surfactant proteins

Four surfactant-associated proteins – SP-A, SP-B, SP-C and SP-D – have been identified and constitute 5–10% of surfactant by weight (Dobbs 1989).

Surfactant protein A

SP-A is composed of approximately 248 amino acids (Benson et al. 1985). It is a large glycoprotein belonging to the calcium-dependent

collectin family of proteins. It constitutes approximately 5% of surfactant by weight. There is considerable heterogeneity in its structure because of extensive posttranslational modification. The human gene is located on chromosome 10; gene expression occurs exclusively in type II pneumocytes (Bruns et al. 1987), which appear to be the main site of synthesis (Williams and Benson 1981). Lamellar bodies are enriched with SP-A compared with lung homogenates (O'Reilly et al. 1988).

Synthesis of SP-A increases after 28 weeks of gestation (Batenburg and Hallman 1990). SP-A binds to and confers calcium-dependent aggregation on surfactant phospholipids (Hawgood et al. 1985). SP-A has an essential role in determining the structure of tubular myelin, and the stability and rapidity of spreading and recycling of phospholipids (Veldhuizen et al. 1996). It regulates the synthesis and secretion of phospholipids, and enhances their uptake by type II cells by binding to specific high-affinity receptors on the apical surface of the type II cells. SP-A partially inhibits surfactant secretion from type II cells (Dobbs et al. 1987) and may prevent the accumulation of surfactant on the alveolar surface. SP-A genetic variants have been reported to predispose to or protect from the development of RDS (Bhandari and Gruen 2006). SP-A polymorphisms have been associated with severe RSV infection (Lofgren and Ramet 2002) and an increased risk of bronchopulmonary dysplasia (Weber and Borkhardt 2000).

Surfactant protein B

The active 79-amino-acid SP-B peptide (molecular weight (MW) 7500–9000) is produced by the proteolytic cleavage of pro-SP-B, a 25 000–33 000 MW precursor protein (Curstedt et al. 1988). SP-B constitutes 1–2% of surfactant by weight (Weaver 1998). The active SP-B peptide contains highly positively charged amino acids that form an amphipathic helix with the hydrophilic amino acid residues positioned near the phospholipid head groups at the membrane surface. It is composed of two identical polypeptide chains, held together by a disulphide bond (Johansson and Cursted 1997). SP-B is encoded by a single-copy gene located on chromosome 2 (Emrie et al. 1988). The mRNA for SP-B is detectable in human fetal lung tissue as early as 12–14 weeks of gestation, localised in the epithelial cells of bronchi and bronchioles. After 25 weeks it is localised in the type II cells. Glucocorticoids increase expression of SP-B in fetal lung. Expression is restricted to type II pneumocytes and Clara cells. The active SP-B peptide is stored in lamellar bodies and secreted with phospholipids into the airway lumen.

SP-B is required for the formation of tubular myelin and increases the spreading of surfactant phospholipids on to an air–water interface (Chang et al. 1998). SP-B disrupts phospholipid vesicles and alters the ordering and packing of the PC molecules. SP-B combined with lipid mixtures constitutes most of the surface activity of natural surfactant in vitro and increases lung compliance in vivo; SP-C and SP-B together are even more effective. SP-C and SP-B both stimulate lipid uptake in isolated cells. SP-B can also protect the pulmonary surfactant film from inactivation by serum proteins (Friedrich et al. 2000).

Absence of SP-B influences the composition of pulmonary surfactants. It is associated with absence of or markedly decreased PG and an additional aberrant SP-C peptide (Vorbroker et al. 1995). DPPC synthesis is preserved in SP-B deficiency but SP-C cannot be processed to its active peptide and no secretion of normal surfactant occurs (Beers et al. 2000). In SP-B knockout mice, both lamellar bodies and tubular myelin structures are absent. SP-B deficiency, with complete absence of SP-B, is an autosomal recessively inherited disorder (Andersen et al. 2000). SP-B deficiency causes hypoxaemic respiratory failure and leads to lethal respiratory failure within the first year of life and is refractory to mechanical ventilation, surfactant therapy, glucocorticoids and extracorporeal membrane oxygenation (Chetcuti and Ball 1995; Hamvas et al. 1995). It can present as a congenital form of alveolar proteinosis, but not all cases have this feature; pulmonary hypertension is a prominent clinical finding. Lung transplantation is currently the only successful intervention. More than 27 loss-of-function mutations have been identified in the SP-B gene, resulting in lethal neonatal failure. The most frequent mutation is a 121ins2 frameshift mutation, accounting for 60–70% of cases (Bhandari and Gruen 2006). The gene frequency of this mutation is 1 per 1000–3000 (Cole et al. 2000) and the condition is rare – an extimated disease incidence of 1 in 1.5 million births (Clark and Side Clark 2005). Partial deficiencies of SP-B with less severe clinical courses have now been reported (Thompson 2001).

Surfactant protein C

This small hydrophobic protein has a MW of 3000–6000 depending on the separation system used. It constitutes 1–2% of surfactant by weight and is unique to surfactant. The mRNA for SP-C is present from early lung morphogenesis at the distal tips of the branching airways (Wert et al. 1993), but subsequently SP-C expression occurs only in the type II cells. The SP-C gene is located on chromosome 8 (Glasser et al. 1988). SP-C contains 35 amino acids and is likely to be a transmembranous peptide. It has a hydrophobic valine-rich region, which may be required for its function. SP-C can impart

surface-like properties to phospholipids (Revak et al. 1988). Concentrations as low as 1% can dramatically enhance surface adsorption and spreading of phospholipids in vitro. It may play a role in enhancing the reuptake of phospholipids. Surprisingly, SP-C knockout mice have normal respiratory function and lung development (Glasser et al. 2001); it is possible that SP-B replaces SP-C. In humans, however, SP-C deficiency has been associated with an interstitial lung disease (Nogee et al. 2000; Guilot et al. 2009), and, in a Finnish population, SP-C polymorphisms were associated with RDS and premature birth (Lahti et al. 2004).

Surfactant protein D

SP-D has a MW of 46 000 and is produced by type II and bronchiolar epithelial cells. Its expression increases with advancing gestation in association with differentiation of terminal airway cells (Crouch et al. 1991); SP-D production begins in the bronchiolar and terminal epithelium from about 21 weeks of gestation (Mori et al. 2002). SP-D expression is widely distributed in epithelial cells in the body; in the lung, SP-D expression occurs in the type II cells, Clara cells and other airway cells and glands. Glucocorticoids increase SP-D expression. SP-D does not have significant surfactant-like activities when mixed with phospholipids. It is, however, involved in the immune function of the lung (Kuan et al. 1992). SP-D polymorphisms have not been associated with RDS (Clark and Side Clark 2005). Indeed, an association has been found between one variant of the SP-D gene and a lower prevalence RDS; the polymorphism was associated with a lower number of repetitive surfactant doses and a lower requirement for supplementary oxygen on day 28 (Hilgendorff et al. 2009).

Synthesis

Phosphatidylcholine synthesis

PC is produced by the cytidine diphosphate (CDP) choline pathway (Fig. 27.10) (Rooney 1985). Choline is taken up by the cell by facilitated transport and is then phosphorylated by choline kinase to phosphocholine, which in turn is converted to CDP choline (the rate-limiting step), which is then transferred to diacylglycerol to give PC. This produces molecules containing one saturated fatty acid, palmitic acid, and one unsaturated fatty acid, usually oleic acid. This molecule is then remodelled by deacylation to lysophosphatidylcholine, followed by reacylation with a palmitic acid derived from either palmitoyl CoA or a second molecule of lysophosphatidylcholine (Batenburg 1982) to give DPPC. It has been suggested that only 50% of the DPPC is synthesised directly from saturated diacylglycerols as precursors (Paterson and Darnall 2009) and the rest by remodelling. Two remodelling mechanisms exist: both involve deacylation of de novo synthesised 1-saturated-2-unsaturated PC to acyl-2-lysophosphatidylcholine. The latter is then either reacylated by reaction with a saturated acylCoA or transacylated in a reaction involving two molecules of lysophosphatidylcholine (Rooney 1992). Only the former mechanism is quantitatively important. Cholinephosphate cytidylyltransferase (CT), which catalyses phosphocholine to CDP choline, is essentially inactive without lipids; CT activity is activated during fetal lung development and after corticosteroid administration. Several other hormones, including thyroid hormones and insulin, and epidermal growth factor (EGF) influence this sequence of events. PC synthesis via the methylation of PE is of minor importance, except in conditions of choline deficiency (Yost et al. 1986).

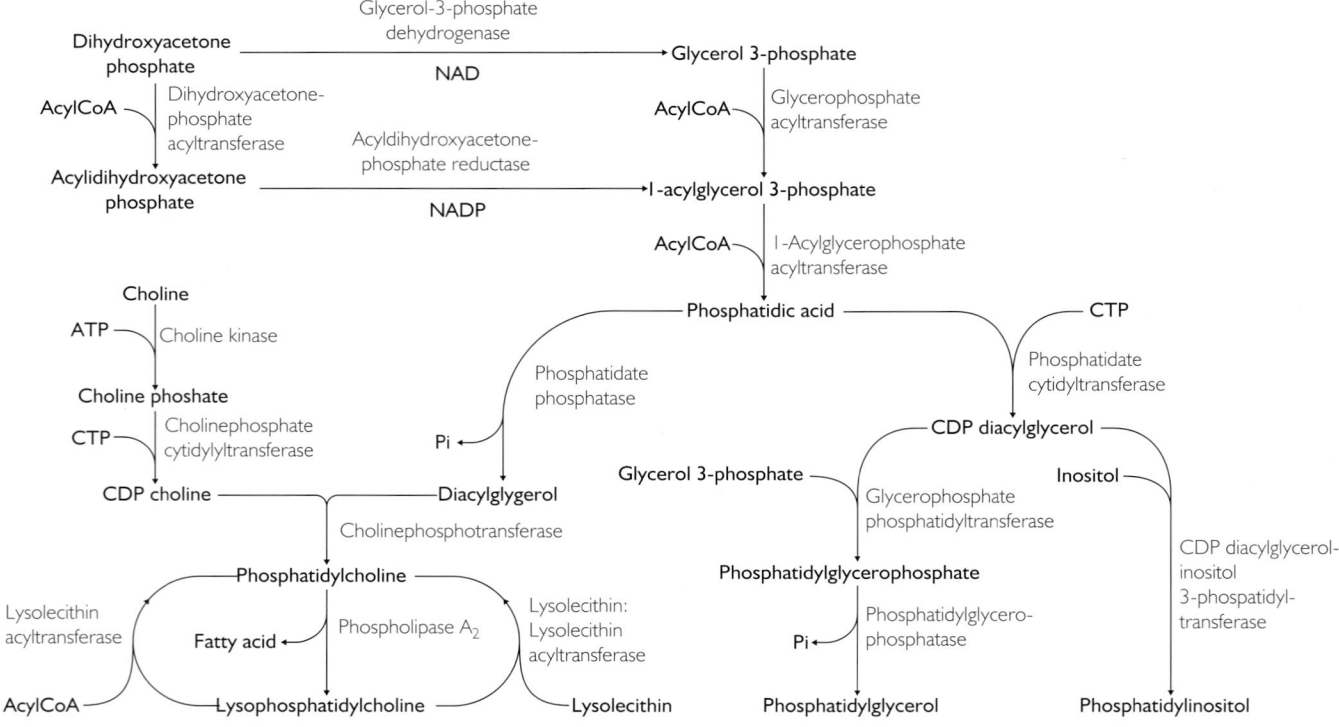

Fig. 27.10 Pathways in the biosynthesis of phosphatidylcholine, phosphatidylglycerol and phosphatidylinositol. *(Reproduced from Rooney (1985).)*

Phosphatidylglycerol synthesis

PG is synthesised together with the other acidic phospholipids, PI and PS, from CDP-diacylglycerol, which is in turn derived from phosphatidic acid (Fig. 27.10).

Factors affecting surfactant maturation

Glucocorticoids

Endogenous cortisol is an important physiological stimulus to fetal lung maturation. In the fetal sheep, there is a marked increase in plasma cortisol concentration at the end of gestation and this is associated with an increase in DPPC in lung tissue and lung lavage fluid (DiFiore and Wilson 1994). Administration of betamethasone to pregnant rabbits results in an increase in the total amount of phospholipid, as well as an increase in the percentage of PC in the total phospholipids (Rooney et al. 1979). Cortisol induces fetal lung fibroblasts to produce fibroblast pneumocyte factor, which then stimulates surfactant production by the fetal type II pneumocytes (Smith 1978). In animal experiments, glucocorticoids increase lung aeration, decrease the surface tension of the lung extract and increase synthesis of both surfactant phospholipids and proteins (Kari et al. 1995). In preterm infants, antenatal treatment with dexamethasone increases the surface activity of surfactant isolated from airway specimens and the ratio of SP-A to PC, but not in offspring of mothers with severe hypertension (Kari et al. 1995). Dexamethasone increases pulmonary surfactant secretion through an enhancement of β_2-adrenoreceptor gene expression (Isohama et al. 1997). In a primary culture of rat alveolar cells, while dexamethasone had no effect on the basal secretion rate of PC, it augmented both the PC secretion and the cAMP formation increased by terbutaline, and increased the mRNA expression of β_2 receptors in type II cells (Isohama et al. 1997).

Beta-adrenergic drugs

Beta-adrenergic drugs stimulate adenylcyclase and inhibit phosphodiesterases, thereby increasing the amount of intracellular cAMP, which in turn increases the production (Lawson et al. 1978) and secretion of surfactant. cAMP stimulates the synthesis of disaturated phospholipids and SP-A; in addition, it mediates the effect of a number of hormones.

Thyroid hormones

Thyroxine (T_4) increases surfactant production and lung maturation. Infants who develop RDS have lower cord blood levels of T_4 than those who do not. T_4 does not easily cross the placenta, but triiodothyronine (T_3) given to pregnant rats is associated with an increase in T_3 in the fetal serum. T_3 increases the type II cell receptors' response to fibroblast pneumocyte factor, which is necessary for appropriate surfactant production. TRH, unlike T_4 and T_3, readily crosses the placenta; it increases the amount of surfactant phospholipid. The effects of TRH are not entirely mediated by thyroid hormone. TRH stimulates prolactin production and functions as a neurotransmitter in the central nervous system.

Prolactin

Prolactin levels are lower in infants who develop RDS than in those who do not; they are also lower in immature than in mature infants and lower in males than in females (Dhanireddy et al. 1983). The effect of prolactin both in vivo and in cultured lung systems, however, is variable and the role of prolactin in surfactant production regulation remains speculative.

Epidermal growth factor

EGF may be important in the development of the pulmonary epithelium. Infusion of this substance into lambs prevents the development of hyaline membrane disease (Catterton et al. 1979) and increases lung distensibility. There is a reduced amount of SP-A in the offspring of rats with EGF autoantibodies (Raaberg et al. 1995). Müllerian-inhibiting substance inhibits lung maturation by blocking phosphorylation of EGF receptors (Catlin et al. 1991); this may be an explanation for the higher incidence of RDS in males. In non-human primate fetuses delivered at 78% of term, in utero treatment with EGF resulted in higher SP-A levels and L:S ratios in treated than in untreated fetuses (Goetzman et al. 1994).

Fibroblast pneumocyte factor

Alveolar cells need the presence of fibroblasts and their pneumocyte factor to produce surfactant (Smith 1979). Glucocorticoids act on the fetal lung fibroblasts to induce the production of fibroblast pneumocyte factor, which in turn stimulates rapid surfactant synthesis by the alveolar type II cell.

Insulin

Insulin delays the maturation of alveolar type II cells and decreases the proportion of saturated PC (Gross et al. 1980). In addition, infants of diabetic mothers have delayed appearance of PG (Ojomo and Coustan 1990). Hyperglycaemia also plays a role in the delay in lung maturation seen in these babies (Gewolb et al. 1985). Insulin inhibits SP-A gene expression (Miakotina et al. 2002).

Testosterone

Premature male infants are more prone to RDS than are similarly immature female infants (Perelman et al. 1986). Male lungs are approximately 1 week more immature as determined by the disaturated PC content. These differences may be due to inhibition of surfactant production in males by androgens (Torday 1985); lipid concentration in the lung appears to be at least partly directly or indirectly regulated by androgens (Ojeda et al. 1997). In addition, androgens delay lung maturation through their action on lung fibroblasts (Provost et al. 2002).

Surfactant physical properties and functions

Surfactant prevents atelectasis and thus reduces the work of breathing. This is achieved by reduction of surface tension and by surfactant becoming a 'solid' monolayer, promoting stability of the alveoli, in expiration. Surfactant also prevents the transudation of fluid: in conditions of high surface tension, fluid is sucked into the alveolar spaces from the capillaries.

The presence of an insoluble surface film capable of maintaining a very low surface tension (or high surface pressure) in the air spaces was first inferred by Pattle (1955). A small bubble will normally diminish in size and disappear; the smaller it becomes, the more rapidly its diameter decreases. This follows from the relationship described by the Laplace equation:

$$P = 2\gamma/r$$

where P = internal pressure, γ = surface tension and r = radius, that is, the pressure difference across the bubble's wall is given by twice the tension in the wall divided by the radius. Thus, in the presence of a high surface tension and small radius, the high pressure difference causes gas to diffuse from the bubble into the surrounding liquid. In the lung, however, the presence of an insoluble surface film means that the surface tension is reduced as the radius decreases.

The contribution of surface tension to the pressure volume behaviour of the lung was demonstrated by von Neergaard (1929), who showed that lungs inflated with saline have a higher compliance than if filled with air. Saline abolishes the surface tension forces, which are an important component of the static recoil force of the lung.

Surfactant lowers surface tension by forming an insoluble surface film. This opposes the surface tension of the underlying liquid by exerting surface pressure. The surface properties of surfactant result from its composition, that is, molecules with both a hydrophobic and hydrophilic chain. When forming a film on water, the polar group is attracted to the water, whereas the non-polar group is turned towards the gas phase. DPPC is a symmetrical molecule and the two straight hydrophobic fatty acid chains allow close packing of the monolayer. Compression of such a monolayer results in it being changed from a liquid to a condensed gel or solid state (Clements 1977; Morley and Bangham 1981); this is because the transition temperature of the refined mixture rises to above 37°C, so that in vivo the refined monolayer may be solid (Clements 1977). In RDS, the PC is relatively unsaturated and of lower quantity than in the mature species. This means an unstable monolayer is formed on compression in expiration, which buckles and does not reduce surface tension effectively. Even when the monolayer has been refined, there is so little DPPC available the alveoli are of small size. Thus, infants with RDS have a low FRC and an increased work of breathing.

Inhibition of surface activity of surfactant by proteins

The alveolar surfactant system may be altered by an inhibitory effect of proteins leaked from the intravascular or interstitial space, owing to an increased permeability of the capillary endothelial and/or alveolar–epithelial barrier (Seeger et al. 1985). In RDS, the alveolar capillary membrane permeability is increased, and the hyaline membranes are a massive aggregation of fibrin. In addition, proteinaceous material may be inhaled, for example as in meconium aspiration syndrome. There is a marked rank order of potency of proteins in interfering with surfactant function – fibrin monomer > fibrinogen > albumin > elastin > IgG > IgM – such that fibrin has 50 times greater effectiveness than albumin. Once the proteins are present in the surface monolayer, they inhibit the ability of the compressed surfactant to lower surface tension. The leakage of protein on to the alveolar surface, at least in premature rabbits, can be inhibited by surfactant treatment and treatment with antenatal steroids or thryotrophin-releasing hormone. In other conditions, such as meconium aspiration syndrome, the inhibitory effect of the proteins can be overcome by increasing the dose of surfactant. Exogenous surfactants differ with regard to their inhibition by proteins; calf lung surfactant extract and Alveofact are only moderately inhibited by fibrinogen (Barr et al. 1975). KL$_4$ surfactant, which has a synthetic peptide in lieu of SP-B, resists inhibition to serum proteins more than a natural surfactant (beractant) (Manalo et al. 1996).

Assessment of surfactant maturity

The fluid which is secreted by the fetal lung moves out into the amniotic fluid, carrying surfactant with it. As the lung matures, so the composition of the surfactant in the amniotic fluid changes. The proportion of surfactant (lecithin) in the amniotic fluid can be compared with that of sphingomyelin (L:S ratio). An L:S ratio greater than 2.0 is usually associated with lung maturity and in 95% of cases will predict the absence of RDS. A mature L:S ratio, however, can be associated with RDS in the infants of diabetic mothers or in those with rhesus disease; in these cases, the abnormality is deficiency of PG rather than a lack of DPPC. Relating the amniotic fluid surfactant to the albumin level provides a more reliable predictor of the absence of RDS in infants of diabetic mothers than assessing the amount of DPPC (Tanasijevic et al. 1996). Unfortunately, an L:S ratio <2.0 predicts RDS with an accuracy of only 54%. The lower the L:S ratio, the more likely the baby is to develop RDS: 21% of babies with an L:S ratio of 1.5–2.0 are affected, compared with 80% with an L:S ratio below 1.5.

Identification of PG in the amniotic fluid is helpful, as babies with PG rarely develop RDS. A combination of a low L:S ratio with absence of PG from amniotic fluid samples obtained within 3 days of delivery is a better predictor of the duration of respiratory support than is either gestational age or birthweight, but only in pregnancies not complicated by premature rupture of the membranes (Harper and Lorentz 1993). In diabetic pregnancies, the presence of PG correlated to an L:S ratio of >3.0 and a lamellar body count of at least 50 000 (Ghidini et al. 2002).

The L:S ratio can also be assessed in fluid from the pharynx (Barr et al. 1975; Hill 1976; Weller et al. 1976) or stomach (Motoyama et al. 1976). This can give retrospective demonstration that a baby had mature lungs at birth or provide further documentation on the course of a baby's illness (Kanto et al. 1976).

The level of serum SP-A in the first 24 hours has been shown to increase with advancing gestational age and differs significantly between infants with and without RDS (Kaneko et al. 2001). SP-A can also be measured in cord blood using an enzyme-linked immunosorbent assay system, so has been suggested to be a useful serum marker to predict the development of RDS (Kaneko et al. 2001). Tests of surfactant maturity, however, are now rarely employed, as many clinicians have the policy of giving exogenous surfactant very soon after birth to all infants born below a certain gestational age, because of the proven efficacy of prophylactic surfactant administration. Such tests may, however, be useful in developing countries (Denavit-Saubié et al. 1978).

References

Altura, B.M., Chand, N., 1981. Bradykinin-induced relaxation of renal and pulmonary arteries is dependent upon intact endothelial cell. Br J Pharmacol 74, 10–11.

Andersen, C., Ramsay, J.A., Nogee, L.M., et al., 2000. Recurrent familial neonatal deaths: hereditary surfactant protein B deficiency. Am J Perinatol 17, 219–224.

Ang, S.L., Rossan, J., 1994. HNF-3beta is essential for node and notocord development in mouse development. Cell 78, 561–574.

Asonye, U.O., Vidyasagar, D., 1981. Clinical applications of continuous transcutaneous PO$_2$ monitoring. In: Lauersen, N.H., Hochberg, H.M. (Eds.), Clinical Perinatal Biochemical Monitoring. Williams & Wilkins, Baltimore, pp. 205–219.

Barker, P.M., Walters, D.V., Markiewicz, M., et al., 1991. Development of the lung liquid reabsorptive mechanism in fetal sheep: synergism of triiodothyronine and hydrocortisone. J Physiol 433, 435–449.

Barr, P.A., Jenkins, P.A., Baum, J.D., 1975. L/S ratio in hypopharyngeal aspirate of newborn infants. Arch Dis Child 50, 856–861.

Batenburg, J.J., 1982. The phosphatidylcholine-lysophosphatidylcholine cycle. In: Farrell, P.M. (Ed.), Lung Development: Biological and Clinical Perspectives. Academic Press, New York, p. 36.

Batenburg, J.J., Hallman, M., 1990. Developmental biochemistry of alveoli. In: Scarpelli, E.M. (Ed.), Pulmonary Physiology: Fetus, Newborn, Child and Adolescent. Lea & Febiger, Philadelphia, pp. 106–139.

Beers, M.F., Hamvas, A., Moxley, M.A., et al., 2000. Pulmonary surfactant metabolism in infants lacking surfactant B. Am J Respir Cell Mol Biol 22, 380–391.

Bekedam, D.J., Visser, G.H.A., 1985. Effects of hypoxemic events on breathing, body movements and heart rate variation: a study in growth retarded human fetuses. Am J Obstet Gynecol 153, 52–56.

Benson, B., Hawgood, S., Schilling, J., et al., 1985. Structure of canine pulmonary surfactant apoprotein: cDNA and complete amino acid sequence. Proc Natl Acad Sci U S A 82, 6379–6383.

Bernhard, W., Hoffman, S., Dombrowsky, H., et al., 2001. Phosphatidylcholine molecular species in lung surfactant: composition in relation to respiratory rate and lung development. Am J Respir Cell Mol Biol 25, 725–731.

Bhandari, V., Gruen, J.R., 2006. The genetics of bronchopulmonary dysplasia. Semin Perinatol 30, 185–191.

Blanco, C.E., Dawes, G.S., Hanson, M.A., et al., 1984. The response to hypoxia of arterial chemoreceptors in fetal sheep and newborn lambs. J Physiol 351, 25–37.

Blanco, C.E., Hanson, M.A., McCooke, H.B., et al., 1987. Studies of chemoreceptor resetting after hyperoxic ventilation of the fetus in utero. In: Ribero, J.A., Pallot, D.J. (Eds.), Chemoreceptors in Respiratory Control. Croom Helm, London, pp. 221–227.

Bruns, G.S.H., Veldman, G.M., Latt, S.A., et al., 1987. The 35 kd pulmonary surfactant associated protein is encoded on chromosome 10. Hum Genet 76, 58–62.

Bullard, K.M., Sonne, J., Hawgood, S., et al., 1997. Tracheal ligation increases cell proliferation but decreases surfactant protein in fetal murine lungs in vitro. J Pediatr Surg 32, 207–213.

Burri, P.H., Hislop, A.A., 1998. Structural considerations. Eur Respir J 12 (suppl. 27), 59s–65s.

Calder, N.A., Williams, B.A., Kumar, P., et al., 1994. The respiratory response of healthy term infants to breath-by-breath alternations in inspired oxygen at two postnatal ages. Pediatr Res 35, 321–324.

Catlin, E.A., Uitvlugt, N.D., Donahoe, P.K., et al., 1991. Muellerian inhibiting substance blocks epidermal growth factor receptor phosphorylation in fetal rat lung membranes. Metabolism 40, 1178–1184.

Catterton, W.Z., Escobedo, M.B., Sexson, W.R., et al., 1979. Effect of epidermal growth factor on lung maturation in fetal rabbits. Pediatr Res 13, 104–110.

Ceruti, E., 1966. Chemoreceptor reflexes in the newborn infant: effect of cooling on the response to hypoxia. Pediatrics 37, 556–564.

Chang, R., Nir, S., Poulain, F.R., 1998. Analysis of binding and membrane destabilisation of phospholipid membranes by surfactant apoprotein B. Biochemica et Biophysica Acta 1371, 254–264.

Cherniack, N.S., von Euler, C., Glogowska, M., et al., 1981. Characteristics and rate of occurrence of spontaneous and provoked augmented breaths. Acta Paediatr Scand 111, 349–360.

Chetcuti, P.A.J., Ball, R.J., 1995. Surfactant aproprotein B deficiency. Archives of Disease in Childhood. Fetal and Neonatal Edition 73, F125–F127.

Clark, H., Side Clark, L., 2005. The genetics of neonatal respiratory disease. Semin Fetal Neonatal Med 10, 271–282.

Clements, J.A., 1977. Functions of the alveolar lining layer. Am Rev Respir Dis 115, 67–71.

Cole, F.S., Hamvas, A., Rubenstein, P., et al., 2000. Population based estimates of surfactant protein B deficiency. Pediatrics 105, 538–541.

Condorelli, S., Scarpelli, E.M., 1975. Somatic-respiratory reflex and onset of regular breathing movements in the lamb foetus in utero. Pediatr Res 9, 879–884.

Cordero, L., Hon, E., 1971. Neonatal bradycardia following nasopharyngeal stimulation. Journal of Pediatrics 78, 441–447.

Crouch, E., Rust, K., Mariencheck, W., et al., 1991. Developmental expression of pulmonary surfactant protein D (SP-D). Am J Respir Cell Mol Biol 5, 13–18.

Curstedt, T., Johansson, J., Barros-Soderling, J., 1988. Low molecular mass surfactant protein type 1. The primary structure of hydrophobic 8-Kda polypeptide with eight half cysteine residues. Eur J Biochem 172, 521–525.

Davey, M.G., Hooper, S.B., Cock, M.L., et al., 2001. Stimulation of lung growth in fetuses with lung hypoplasia leads to altered postnatal lung structure in sheep. Pediatr Pulmonol 32, 267–276.

Delivoria-Papadopoulos, M., DiGiacomo, J.E., 1992. Oxygen transport and delivery. In: Polin, R.A., Fox, W.W. (Eds.), Fetal and Neonatal Physiology. W B Saunders, Philadelphia, pp. 801–813.

Delivoria-Papadopoulos, M., Roncevic, N.P., Oski, F.A., 1971. Postnatal changes in oxygen transport of term, premature and sick infants: the role of red cell 2,3-diphosphoglycerate and adult hemoglobin. Pediatr Res 5, 235–245.

Denavit-Saubié, M., Champagnat, J., Zieglgaensberger, W., 1978. Effects of opiates and methionine-enkephalin on pontine and bulbar respiratory neurones of the cat. Brain Res 155, 55–67.

Devlieger, H., 1987. The chest wall in the preterm infant. MD Thesis. Université Catholique de Louvain, Louvain, pp. 136–140.

Dhanireddy, R., Smith, Y.F., Hamosh, M., et al., 1983. Respiratory distress syndrome in the newborn: relationship to serum prolactin, thyroxine and sex. Biol Neonate 43, 9–15.

Dickinson, K.A., Harding, R., 1987. Decline in lung liquid volume and secretion and tracheal flow rate in lambs. J Appl Physiol 62, 24–38.

DiFiore, J.W., Wilson, J.M., 1994. Lung development. Semin Pediatr Surg 3, 221–232.

Dobbs, L.G., 1989. Pulmonary surfactant. Annu Rev Med 40, 431–446.

Dobbs, D.L., Wright, J.R., Hawgood, S., et al., 1987. Pulmonary surfactant and its components inhibit secretion of phosphatidylcholine from cultured rat alveolar type II cells. Proc Natl Acad Sci U S A 84, 1010–1014.

Doi, A., Ramirez, J.M., 2008. Neuromodulation and the orchestration of the respiratory rhythm. Respir Physiol Neurobiol 164, 96–104.

Duara, S., 1992. Structure and function of the upper airway in neonates. In: Polin, R.A., Fox, W.W. (Eds.), Fetal and Neonatal Physiology. W B Saunders, Philadelphia, pp. 823–828.

Eden, G.J., Hanson, M.A., 1987. Effects of chronic hypoxia on chemoreceptor function in the newborn. In: Ribero, J.A., Pallot, D.J. (Eds.), Chemoreceptors in Respiratory Control. Croom Helm, London, pp. 369–377.

Emrie, P.A., Jones, C., Hofmann, T., 1988. The coding sequence for the human 18 000 dalton hydrophobic pulmonary surfactant protein is located on chromosome 2 and identifies a restriction fragment length polymorphism. Somatic and Cellular Molecular Genetics 14, 105–110.

Fewell, J.E., Hislop, A.A., Kitterman, J.A., et al., 1983. Effect of tracheostomy on lung development in fetal lambs. J Appl Physiol 55, 1103–1108.

Fleming, P.J., Bryan, A.C., Bryan, M.H., 1978. Functional immaturity of pulmonary irritant receptors and apnea in newborn preterm infants. Pediatrics 61, 515–518.

Friedman, A.H., Fahey, J.T., 1993. The transition from fetal to neonatal circulation: normal responses and implications for infants with heart disease. Semin Perinatol 17, 106–121.

Friedrich, W., Schmalisch, G., Stevens, P.A., et al., 2000. Surfactant protein SP-B counteracts inhibition of pulmonary surfactant by serum proteins. Eur J Med Res 5, 277–282.

Funk, G.D., Smith, J.C., Feldman, J.L., 1993. Generation and transmission of respiratory oscillations in medullary slices: role of excitatory amino acids. J Neurophysiol 70, 1497–1515.

Gewolb, I.H., Rooney, S.A., Barrett, C., 1985. Delayed pulmonary maturation in the fetus of the streptozotocin-diabetic rat. Exp Lung Res 8, 141–151.

Ghidini, A., Spong, C.Y., Goodwin, K., et al., 2002. Optimal thresholds of the lecithin/sphingomyelin ratio and lamellar body count for the prediction of the presence of phosphatidylglycerol in diabetic women. J Matern Fetal Neonatal Med 12, 95–98.

Glasser, S.W., Korfhagen, T.R., Perne, C.M., 1988. Two genes encoding human pulmonary surfactant proteolipid SPL (pVal). Journal of Biological Chemistry 263, 10326–10331.

Glasser, S.W., Burhans, M.S., Korfhagen, T.R., et al., 2001. Altered stability of pulmonary surfactant in SP-C deficient mice. Proc Natl Acad Sci U S A 98, 6366–6371.

Goerke, J., 1998. Pulmonary surfactant: functions and molecular composition. Biochim Biophys Acta 1408, 79–89.

Goetzman, B.W., Read, L.C., Plopper, C.G., et al., 1994. Prenatal exposure to epidermal growth factor attenuates respiratory distress syndrome in rhesus infants. Pediatr Res 35, 30–36.

Greenough, A., 1988. The premature infant's respiratory response to mechanical ventilation. Early Hum Dev 17, 1–5.

Greenough, A., Roberton, N.R.C., Milner, A.D., 1995. Neonatal Respiratory Disorders. Edward Arnold, London, p. 105.

Gross, I., Smith, G.J., Wilson, C.M., et al., 1980. The influence of hormones on the biochemical development of fetal rat lung in organ culture: II insulin. Pediatr Res 14, 834–838.

Guillot, L., Epaud, R., Thouvenin, G., et al., 2009. New surfactant protein C gene mutations associated with diffuse lung disease. J Med Genet 46, 490–494.

Guyton, A.C., 1971. Regulation of cardiac output. Anaesthesiology 29, 314–326.

Hall, S.M., Haworth, S.G., 1986. Conducting pulmonary arteries structural adaptation to extrauterine life. Cardiovasc Res 21, 208–216.

Hallman, M., Miyai, K., Wagner, R.M., 1976. Isolated lamellar bodies from rat lung; correlated ultrastructural and biochemical studies. Laboratory Investigation 35, 79–86.

Hamvas, A., Nogee, L.M., deMello, D.E., et al., 1995. Pathophysiology and treatment of surfactant protein-B deficiency. Biol Neonate 67 (suppl. 1), 18–32.

Hannam, S., Ingram, D.M., Rabe-Hesketh, S., et al., 2001. Characterisation of the Hering Breuer deflation reflex in the human neonate. Respir Physiol 124, 51–64.

Harding, R., 1986. The upper respiratory tract in perinatal life. In: Johnston, B.M., Gluckman, P.D. (Eds.), Reproductive and Perinatal Medicine. Respiratory Control and Lung Development in the Fetus and Newborn. Perinatology Press, Ithaca, pp. 331–376.

Harper, M.A., Lorentz, W.B., 1993. Immature lecithin:sphingomyelin ratios and neonatal respiratory course. Am J Obstet Gynecol 168, 495–498.

Harrison, M.R., Adzick, N.S., Flake, A.W., et al., 1996. Correction of congenital diaphramgatic hernia in utero VIII: Response of the hypoplastic lung to tracheal occlusion. J Pediatr Surg 31, 1339–1348.

Hasan, S.J., Rigaux, A., 1992. Effect of bilateral vagotomy on oxygenation, arousal and healthy movements in fetal sheep. J Appl Physiol 73, 1402–1412.

Hassan, A., Gossage, J., Ingram, D., et al., 2001. Volume of activation of the Hering Breuer inflation reflex in the newborn infant. J Appl Physiol 90, 763–769.

Hawgood, S., Benson, B.J., Hamilton, R.L., 1985. Effects of surfactant associated protein and calcium ions on the structure and surface activity of lung surfactant lipids. Biochemistry 24, 185–190.

Haworth, S.G., 1992. Development of the pulmonary circulation. In: Polin, R.A., Fox, W.W. (Eds.), Fetal and Neonatal

Physiology. W B Saunders, Philadelphia, pp. 671–682.

Haworth, S.G., Hall, S.M., Chew, M., et al., 1987. Thinning of fetal pulmonary arterial wall and postnatal remodelling: ultrastructural studies on the respiratory unit arteries of the pig. Virchows Arch A Pathol Anat Histopathol 411, 161–171.

Head, H., 1889. On the regulation of respiration. J Physiol 10, 1–70.

Henderson-Smart, D.J., 1983. Regulation of breathing in the perinatal period. In: Saunders, N.A., Sulivan, C.E. (Eds.), Sleeping and Breathing: Lung Biology in Health and Disease. Marcel Dekker, New York.

Hering, E., Breuer, J., 1868. Die selbsteurung der Amnung durch den nevus vagus sitzber. Sitzungsbericht der Kaiserlichen Akademie der Wissenschaften in Wien 57, 672–677.

Hilgendorff, A., Heidinger, K., Bohnert, A., et al., 2009. Association of polymorphisms in the human surfactant protein-D (SFTPD) gene and postnatal pulmonary adaptation in the preterm infant. Acta Paediatr 98, 112–117.

Hill, C.M., 1976. The determination of the fatty acid profile of lecithin from human amniotic fluid and the pharyngeal aspirate of the newborn. J Physiol 257, 15–17P.

Hislop, A., Haworth, S.G., 1989. Airway size and structure in the normal fetal and infant lung and the effect of premature delivery and artificial ventilation. Am Rev Respir Dis 140, 1717–1726.

Hislop, A., Reid, L., 1981. Growth and development of the respiratory system. Anatomical development. In: Davis, J.A., Dobbing, J. (Eds.), Scientific Foundations of Paediatrics. Heinemann, London, pp. 390–432.

Hooper, S.B., Wallace, M.J., Harding, R., 1993. Amiloride blocks the inhibition of fetal lung liquid secretion caused by AVP but not by asphyxia. J Appl Physiol 74, 111–115.

Hummler, E., Barker, P., Gatzy, J., et al., 1996. Early death due to defective neonatal lung fluid clearance in alpha-EnaC-deficient mice. Nat Genet 12, 325–328.

Ikegami, M., Jobe, A.H., 1993. Surfactant metabolism. Semin Perinatol 17, 233–240.

Isohama, Y., Kumanda, Y., Tanaka, K., et al., 1997. Dexamethasone increases beta 2-adrenoreceptor-regulated phosphatidylcholine secretion in rat alveolar type II cells. Jpn J Pharmacol 73, 163–169.

Jeffery, H.E., Reid, I., Rahilly, P., et al., 1980. Gastro-esophageal reflux in "near-miss" sudden infant death infants in active but not quiet sleep. Sleep 3, 393–399.

Jobe, A.H., Ikegami, M., 2001. Biology of surfactant. Clin Perinatol 28, 655–669.

Johansson, J., Curstedt, 1997. Molecular structures and interactions of pulmonary surfactant. Eur J Biochem 244, 675–693.

Johnston, B.M., Bennet, L., Gluckman, P.D., 1989. In: Gluckman, P.D., Johnston, B.M., Nathanielsz, P.W. (Eds.), Research in Perinatal Medicine, Vol. VIII. Advances in Fetal Physiology. Perinatology Press, Ithaca, pp. 77–193.

Kalapesi, Z., Durand, M., Leahy, F.N., et al., 1981. Effect of periodic or regular respiratory pattern on the ventilatory response to low inhaled CO_2 in preterm infants during sleep. Am Rev Respir Dis 123, 8–11.

Kaneko, K., Shimizu, H., Arakawa, H., et al., 2001. Pulmonary surfactant protein A in sera for assessing neonatal lung maturation. Early Hum Dev 62, 11–21.

Kanto, W.P., Borer, R.C., Barr, M., et al., 1976. Tracheal aspirate lecithin:sphingomyelin ratios as predictors of recovery from respiratory distress syndrome. Journal of Pediatrics 89, 612–616.

Kari, M.A., Akino, T., Hallman, M., 1995. Prenatal dexamethasone and exogenous surfactant therapy: surface activity and surfactant components in airway specimens. Pediatr Res 38, 678–684.

Karlberg, P., Cherry, R.B., Escardo, F.E., et al., 1962. Respiratory studies in newborn infants. II. Pulmonary mechanics of breathing in the first minutes of life, including the onset of respiration. Acta Paediatr Scand 51, 121–136.

Kinsella, J.P., Abman, S.H., 1995. Recent developments in the pathophysiology and treatment of persistent pulmonary hypertension of the newborn. Journal of Pediatrics 126, 853–864.

Kleinmann, L.I., Petering, H.G., Sutherland, J.M., 1967. Blood carbonic anhydrase activity and zinc concentration in infants with respiratory distress syndrome. NEJM 227, 1157–1161.

Kuan, S.F., Rust, K., Crouch, E., 1992. Interactions of surfactant protein D with bacterial lipopolysaccharides. Surfactant protein D is an *Escherichia coli*-binding protein in bronchoalveolar lavage. J Clin Invest 90, 97–106.

Kuhn, C., 1982. The cytology of the lung: ultrastructure of the respiratory epithelium and extracellular lining layers. In: Farrell, P.M. (Ed.), Lung Development: Biological and Clinical Perspectives. Academic Press, New York, p. 27.

Lahti, M., Marttila, R., Hallman, M., 2004. Surfactant protein C gene variation in the Finnish population – association with perinatal respiratory disease. Eur J Hum Genet 12, 312–320.

Lalley, P.M., Bischoff, A.M., Richter, D.W., 1994. Serotonin 1-alpha-receptor activation suppresses respiratory apneusis in the cat. Neurosci Lett 172, 59–62.

Lawson, E.E., Brown, E.R., Torday, J.S., et al., 1978. The effect of epinephrine on tracheal fluid flow and surfactant flux in

fetal sheep. Am Rev Respir Dis 118, 1023–1026.

Le Cras, T.D., Markham, N.E., Tuder, R.M., et al., 2002. Treatment of newborn rats with a FEGF receptor inhibitor causes pulmonary hypertension and abnormal lung structure. Am J Physiol Lung Cell Mol Physiol 283, 555–562.

Lesouef, P.N., England, S.J., Bryan, A.C., 1984. Passive respiratory mechanics in newborns and children. Am Rev Respir Dis 129, 552–556.

Lofgren, J., Ramet, M., 2002. Association between surfactant protein A gene locus and severe respiratory syncytial virus infection in infants. J Infect Dis 185, 283–289.

Loosli, C.G., Potter, E.L., 1959. Pre and postnatal development of the respiratory portion of the human lung. Am Rev Respir Dis 80, 5–20.

Manalo, E., Merritt, T.A., Kheiter, A., et al., 1996. Comparative effects of some serum components and proteolytic products of fibrinogen on surface tension-lowering abilities of beractant and a synthetic peptide containing surfactant KL_4. Pediatr Res 39, 947–952.

Marsh, M., Fox, G., Hoskyns, E.W., et al., 1994. The Hering Breuer deflationary reflex in the newborn infant. Pediatr Pulmonol 18, 163–169.

Martin, R.J., Nearman, H.S., Katona, P.G., et al., 1977. The effect of a low continuous positive airway pressure on the reflex control of respiration in the preterm infant. Journal of Pediatrics 90, 976–981.

Massaro, G.D., Massaro, D., 1996. Formation of pulmonary alveoli and gas exchange surface area: quantitation and regulation. Annu Rev Physiol 58, 73–92.

Massaro, G.D., Massaro, D., 2000. Retinoic acid treatment partially rescues failed septation in rats and in mice. Am J Physiol 278, L955–L960.

Mayock, D.E., Hall, J., Watchko, J.F., et al., 1987. Diaphragmatic muscle fiber type development in swine. Pediatr Res 22, 449–454.

Miakotina, O.L., Goss, K.L., Snyder, J.M., 2002. Insulin utilises the PI 3-kinase pathway to inhibit SP-A gene expression in lung epithelial cells. Respir Res 3, 27.

Millhorn, D.E., Eldridge, F.L., 1986. Role of ventrolateral medulla in regulation of respiratory and cardiovascular systems. J Appl Physiol 61, 1249–1263.

Milner, A.D., Saunders, R.A., 1977. Pressure and volume changes during the first breath of human neonates. Arch Dis Child 52, 918–924.

Milner, A.D., Marsh, M.J., Ingram, D.M., et al., 1999. Effects of smoking in pregnancy on neonatal lung function. Arch Dis Child Fetal Neonatal Ed 80, F8–F14.

Mori, K., Kurihara, N., Hayashida, S., et al., 2002. The intrauterine expression of surfactant protein D in terminal airways of human fetuses compared with surfactant protein A. Eur J Pediatr 161, 431–434.

Moriette, G., van Reempts, P., Moore, M., et al., 1985. The effect of rebreathing CO_2 on ventilation and diaphragmatic electromyography in newborn infants. Respir Physiol 62, 387–397.

Morley, C.J., Bangham, A.D., 1981. Physical properties of surfactant under compression. In: Wichert, V. (Ed.), Progress in Respiratory Research 15. Clinical Importance of Surfactant Defects. Karger, Basle, p. 188.

Mortola, J.P., 1983. Some functional mechanical implications of the structural design of the respiratory system in newborn mammals. Am Rev Respir Dis 128, S69–S72.

Motoyama, E.K., Namba, Y., Rooney, S.A., 1976. Phosphatidylcholine content and fatty acid composition of tracheal and gastric liquids from premature and full term newborn infants. Clin Chim Acta 70, 449–454.

Motoyoma, J., Liu, J., Mo, R., et al., 1998. Essential function of Gli2 and Gli3 in the formation of the lung, trachea and oesophagus. Nat Genet 20, 54–57.

Nicholas, T.E., Doyle, I.R., Bersten, A.D., 1997. Surfactant replacement therapy in ARDS: white knight or noise in the system? Thorax 52, 195–197.

Nicolini, U., Fisk, N.M., Talbert, D.G., et al., 1989. Intrauterine manometry: technique and application to fetal pathology. Prenat Diagn 9, 243–254.

Nogee, L.M., Wert, S.E., Profitt, S.A., et al., 2000. Allelic heterogeneity in hereditary SP-B deficiency. Am J Respir Crit Care Med 161, 973–981.

Ohki, M., Naito, K., Cole, P., 1991. Dimensions and resistances of the human nose: racial differences. Laryngoscope 101, 276–278.

Ojeda, M.S., Gomez, N., Giminez, M.S., 1997. Androgen regulation of lung lipids in the male rat. Lipids 32, 57–62.

Ojomo, E.O., Coustan, D.R., 1990. Absence of evidence of pulmonary maturity at amniocentesis in term infants of diabetic mothers. Am J Obstet Gynecol 163, 954–957.

Olver, R.E., Strang, L.B., 1974. Ion fluxes across the pulmonary epithelium and the secretion of lung liquid in the foetal lamb. J Physiol 241, 327–357.

O'Reilly, M.A., Nogee, L., Whitsett, J.A., 1988. Requirement of the collagenous domain for carbohydrate processing and secretion of surfactant protein of Mr 5 35 000. Biochim Biophys Acta 969, 176–184.

Paterson, D.S., Darnall, R., 2009. 5-HT_{2A} receptors are concentrated in regions of the human infant medulla involved in respiratory and autonomic control. Auton Neurosci 147, 48–55.

Pattle, R.E., 1955. Properties, function and origin of the alveolar lining layer. Nature 175, 1125–1126.

Perelman, R.H., Palta, M., Kirby, R., et al., 1986. Discordance between male and female deaths due to the respiratory distress syndrome. Pediatrics 78, 238–244.

Phillipson, E.A., Bowes, G., 1986. Control of breathing during sleep. In: Cherniack, N.S., Widdicombe, J.G. (Eds.), Handbook of Physiology – the Respiratory System. American Physiological Society, Bethesda, pp. 649–690.

Pickens, D.L., Schefft, G.L., Thach, B.T., 1989. Pharyngeal fluid clearance and aspiration preventive mechanisms in sleeping infants. J Appl Physiol 66, 1164–1171.

Post, M., van Golde, L.M.G., 1988. Metabolic and developmental aspects of the pulmonary surfactant system. Biochim Biophys Acta 947, 249–286.

Post, M., Batenburg, J., Schuurmans, E., et al., 1982. Lamellar bodies isolated from adult human lung tissue. Exp Lung Res 3, 17–28.

Provost, P.R., Blomquist, C.H., Drolet, R., et al., 2002. Androgen inactivation in human lung fibroblasts: variations in levels of 17 beta-hydroxysteroid dehydrogenase type 2 and 5 alpha-reductase activity compatible with androgen inactivation. JCEM 87, 3883–3892.

Raaberg, L., Nexo, E., Jorgensen, P.E., et al., 1995. Fetal effects of epidermal growth factor deficiency induced in rats by autoantibodies against epidermal growth factor. Pediatr Res 37, 175–181.

Ramminger, S.J., Baines, D.L., Olver, R.E., et al., 2000. The effects of PO_2 upon transepithelial ion transport in fetal rat distal lung epithelial cells. J Physiol 524, 539–547.

Revak, S.D., Merritt, T.A., Degryse, E., et al., 1988. Use of human surfactant low molecular weight apoproteins in the reconstitution of surfactant biological activity. J Clin Invest 81, 826–833.

Rigatto, H., 1984. Control of ventilation in the newborn. Annu Rev Physiol 46, 661–674.

Rigatto, H., 1992. Control of breathing in fetal life and onset and control of breathing in the neonate. In: Polin, R.A., Fox, W.W. (Eds.), Fetal and Neonatal Physiology. W B Saunders, Philadelphia, pp. 790–801.

Rigatto, H., Lee, D., Davi, M., et al., 1988. Effect of increased arterial $PaCO_2$ on fetal breathing and behavior in sheep. J Appl Physiol 64, 982–987.

Rigatto, H., Kwiat Kouski, K.A., Hansan, S.U., et al., 1991. The ventilatory response to endogenous CO_2 in preterm infants. Am Rev Respir Dis 143, 101–104.

Rodenstein, D.O., Perlmutter, N., Stanescu, D.C., 1985. Infants are not obligatory

nasal breathers. Am Rev Respir Dis 131, 343–347.

Rooney, S.A., 1985. The surfactant system and lung phospholipid biochemistry. Am Rev Respir Dis 131, 439–460.

Rooney, S.A., 1992. Regulation of surfactant-associated phospholipid synthesis and secretion. In: Polin, R.A., Fox, W.W. (Eds.), Fetal and Neonatal Physiology. W B Saunders, Philadelphia, pp. 971–985.

Rooney, S.A., 2001. Regulation of surfactant secretion. Comp Biochem Physiol 129, 233–243.

Rooney, S.A., Gobran, L.I., Wai-Lee, T.S., 1977. Stimulation of surfactant production by oxytocin-induced labour in the rabbit. J Clin Invest 60, 754–759.

Rooney, S.A., Gobran, L.I., Marino, P.A., et al., 1979. Effects of betamethasone on phospholipid content, composition and biosynthesis in fetal rabbit lung. Biochim Biophys Acta 572, 64–76.

Roth-Kleiner, M., Post, M., 2005. Similarities and dissimilarities of branching and septation during lung development. Pediatr Pulmonol 40, 113–114.

Runold, M., Lagercrantz, H., Prabhakar, M.R., et al., 1989. Role of adenosine in hypoxic ventilatory depression. J Appl Physiol 67, 541–546.

Seeger, W., Stohr, G., Neuhof, H., 1985. Surfactant inhibitory plasma-derived proteins. In: Walters, D.V., Strang, L.B., Geubelle, F. (Eds.), Physiology of the Fetal and Neonatal Lung. Kluwer Academic Press, Lancaster, pp. 225–240.

Shaul, P.W., 1995. Nitric oxide in the developing lung. Adv Pediatr 42, 367–414.

Silverman, M., 1983. Respiratory function testing in infancy and childhood. In: Laszlo, G., Sudlow, M.F. (Eds.), Measurement in Clinical Respiratory Physiology. Academic Press, London, pp. 293–328.

Smith, B.T., 1978. Fibroplast pneumocyte factor: intercellular mediator of glucocorticoid effect on fetal lung. In: Stern, L. (Ed.), Neonatal Intensive Care. Mason, New York, pp. 25–32.

Smith, B.T., 1979. Lung maturation in the fetal rat: acceleration by injection of fibroblast pneumocyte factor. Science 204, 1094–1095.

Souza, P., O'Brodovich, H., Post, M., 1995. Lung fluid restriction affects growth but not airway branching of embryonic rat lung. Int J Dev Biol 39, 629–637.

Sparrow, M.P., Weichselbaum, M., McCray, P.B., 1999. Development of the innervation and airway smooth muscle in human fetal lung. Am J Respir Cell Mol Biol 20, 550–560.

Stevens, P.A., Wright, J.R., Clements, J.A., 1989. Surfactant secretion and clearance in the newborn. J Appl Physiol 67, 1595–1605.

Strang, L.B., 1977. Neonatal Respiration. Blackwell Scientific, Oxford.

Stratton, C.J., 1976a. The high resolution ultrastructure of the periodicity and architecture of the lipid-retained and extracted lung multilamellar body laminations. Tissue Cell 8, 713–728.

Stratton, C.J., 1976b. The three dimensional aspect of mammalian lung lamellar bodies. Tissue Cell 8, 693–712.

Tanasijevic, M.K., Winkelman, J.W., Wybenga, D.R., et al., 1996. Prediction of fetal lung maturity in infants of diabetic mothers using the FLM S/A and disaturated phosphatidylcholine tests. Am J Clin Pathol 105, 17–22.

Thach, B.T., 2007. Maturation of cough and other reflexes that protect the fetal and neonatal airway. Pulm Pharmacol Ther 20, 365–370.

Thompson, M.W., 2001. Surfactant protein B deficiency: insights into surfactant function through clinical surfactant protein deficiency. Am J Med Sci 321, 26–32.

Thurlbeck, W.M., 1982. Postnatal human lung growth. Thorax 37, 564–571.

Tietel, D.F., Iwamoto, H.S., Rudolph, A.M., 1987. Effects of birth related events on central blood flow patterns. Pediatr Res 22, 557–566.

Tino, M.J., Wright, J.R., 1998. Interactions of surfactant protein A with epithelial cells and phagocytes. Biochim Biophys Acta 1408, 241–263.

Torday, J.S., 1985. Dihydrotesterone inhibits fibroblast pneumocyte factor-mediated synthesis of saturated phosphatidylcholine by fetal rat lung cells. Biochim Biophys Acta 835, 23–28.

Turner, D.J., Stick, S.M., Lesouef, K.L., et al., 1995. A new technique to generate and assess forced expiration from raised lung volume in infants. Am J Respir Crit Care Med 151, 1441–1450.

Veldhuizen, R.A.W., Yao, L.-J., Hearn, S.A., et al., 1996. Surfactant-associated protein A is important for maintaining surfactant large-aggregate forms during surface-area cycling. Biochem J 313, 835–840.

von Neergaard, K., 1929. Neue auffassungen uber einen grundbegriff der Atemmechanik. Die Retraktionskraft der Lunge abhaengig von der Oberflaechenspannung in den Alveolen. Z Gesamte Exp Med 66, 373–394.

Vorbroker, D.K., Profitt, S.A., Nogee, L.M., et al., 1995. Aberrant processing of surfactant protein C in hereditary SP-B deficiency. Am J Physiol 268, L647–L656.

Vyas, H., Milner, A.D., Hopkin, I.E., 1981. Comparison of intrathoracic pressure and volume changes during the spontaneous onset of respiration in babies born by caesarean section and by vaginal delivery. Journal of Pediatrics 99, 787–791.

Vyas, H., Field, D., Hopkin, I.E., et al., 1986. Determinants of the first inspiratory volume and functional residual capacity at birth. Pediatr Pulmonol 2, 189–193.

Walters, D.V., Olver, R.E., 1978. The role of catecholamines in lung liquid absorption at birth. Pediatr Res 12, 239–242.

Walters, D.V., Ramsden, C.A., 1985. The secretion and absorption of fetal lung liquid. In: Walters, D.V., Strang, L.B., Geubelle, F. (Eds.), Physiology of the Fetal and Neonatal Lung. Kluwer Academic Press, Lancaster, pp. 61–74.

Walther, F.J., Benders, M.J., Leighton, J.O., 1993. Early changes in the neonatal circulatory transition. Journal of Pediatrics 123, 625–632.

Wealthall, S.R., 1975. Factors resulting in a failure to interrupt apnea. In: Bosma, J.F., Showacre, J. (Eds.), Development of Upper Respiratory Anatomy and Function. US Government Printing Office, Washington, DC, pp. 212–225.

Weaver, T.E., 1998. Synthesis, processing and secretion of surfactant proteins B and C. Biochim Biophys Acta 1408, 173–179.

Weber, B., Borkhardt, A., 2000. Polymorphisms of surfactant protein A genes and the risk of bronchopulmonary dysplasia in preterm infants. Turkish Journal of Pediatrics 41, 181–185.

Weller, P.H., Jenkins, P.A., Gupta, J., et al., 1976. Pharyngeal lecithin:sphingomyelin ratio in newborn infants. Lancet i, 12–14.

Wert, S.E., Glasser, S.W., Korfhagen, T.R., et al., 1993. Transcriptional elements from the human SP-C gene direct expression in the primordial respiratory epithelium of transgenic mice. Dev Biol 156, 426–443.

Wharton, J., Haworth, S.G., Polak, J.M., 1988. Postnatal development of the innervation and paraganglia in the porcine pulmonary arterial bed. J Pathol 154, 19–27.

Whitsett, J.A., Wert, S.E., 2006. Milecular determinants of lung morphogenesis. In: Cherniack, V., Boat, T.F. (Eds.), Kendig's Disorders of the Respiratory Tract in Children. W B Saunders, Philadelphia, pp. 3–18.

Williams, M.C., Benson, B.J., 1981. Immunocytochemical localization and identification of the major surfactant protein in adult rat lung. J Histochem Cytochem 29, 291–305.

Woodrum, D., 1992. Respiratory muscles. In: Polin, R.A., Fox, W.W. (Eds.), Fetal and Neonatal Physiology. W B Saunders, Philadelphia, pp. 829–841.

Wright, J.R., Clements, J.A., 1987. Metabolism and turnover of lung surfactant. Am Rev Respir Dis 135, 426–444.

Yost, R.W., Chander, A., Dodia, C., et al., 1986. Stimulation of the methylation pathway for phosphatidylcholine synthesis in rat lungs by choline deficiency. Biochim Biophys Acta 875, 122–125.

Yüksel, B., Greenough, A., 1992. Neonatal respiratory support and lung function abnormalities at follow-up. Respir Med 86, 97–100.

Zenge, J.P., Rairigh, R.L., Grover, T.R., et al., 2001. NO and prostaglandins modulate the pulmonary vascular response to hemodynamic stress in the late gestation fetus. Am J Physiol Lung Cell Mol Physiol 281, 1157–1163.

Part 2: **Acute respiratory disease**

Anne Greenough   Anthony D Milner

Respiratory distress syndrome

Respiratory distress syndrome (RDS), in non-intubated babies who have not received exogenous surfactant therapy or been exposed to antenatal corticosteroids, is characterised by a respiratory rate >60/min, dyspnoea (intercostal, subcostal indrawing, sternal retraction) with a predominantly diaphragmatic breathing pattern and characteristic expiratory grunt, all presenting within 4–6 hours of delivery. Oxygen administration is required to prevent cyanosis and there is a reticulogranular chest X-ray (CXR) appearance as a result of widespread atelectasis. Nowadays, that presentation is very unusual; antenatal corticosteroids are routinely given and very prematurely born babies are intubated and given surfactant usually within the first hour after birth. The diagnosis in such babies then is based on their premature birth and CXR appearance. Pathophysiologically, the condition is characterised by non-compliant (stiff) lungs, which contain less surfactant than normal and become atelectatic at end-expiration. Histologically, hyaline membranes line the terminal airways. These membranes give the condition its alternative name, hyaline membrane disease (HMD), which, to be semantically correct, should be used only in the presence of histological confirmation; thus, the term RDS is preferred.

Incidence

In the modern era of neonatal intensive care, approximately 1% of infants develop RDS (Rubatelli et al. 1998).

Aetiology

RDS results from immaturity of the lungs, particularly the surfactant-synthesising systems. Various factors contribute to the immaturity and others interact with it to increase or decrease the incidence of the disorder.

Predisposing factors

Prematurity

The risk of RDS is inversely proportional to gestational age: 50% of babies less than 30 weeks of gestational age, as compared with 2% of those between 35 and 36 weeks, develop RDS (Rubatelli et al. 1998). RDS is almost invariable in infants of less than 28 weeks of gestation, but it does remain a significant problem up to 34 weeks' gestation (Lewis et al. 1996). The maturation of surfactant synthesis is a mirror image of the incidence of RDS at different gestations. Some of the dyspnoea and hypoxaemia in very preterm babies is due to their immature lung structure, with increased connective tissue and poorly developed alveoli. Other factors make the preterm neonate inherently susceptible to RDS. Their lung epithelia are more leaky than those of a baby born at term, increasing the likelihood of protein passing on to the alveolar surface, where it will inhibit surfactant function (see below). They are more prone to asphyxia, hypoxia, hypotension and hypothermia, all of which are likely to impair surfactant synthesis or increase alveolar capillary leakiness.

Gender

Boys are much more likely to develop RDS than girls, with a male-to-female ratio of 1.7 : 1, and are more likely to die from the disease (Farrell and Avery 1975). In male fetuses, the delayed maturation of the lecithin-to-sphingomyelin (L : S) ratio and late appearance of phosphatidylglycerol (PG) (Fleisher et al. 1985) are androgen-induced (Kotas and Avery 1971; Torday 1992).

Race

Black babies have a lower incidence of RDS – 60–70% of that of white babies of the same gestational age (Hulsey et al. 1993). This is evident even in very immature babies: in one series only 40% of African infants <32 weeks' gestational age developed RDS, compared with 75% of Caucasian infants (Kavvadia and Greenough 1998). No black baby with an L : S ratio >1.2 developed RDS, but white babies did develop the disease at those low ratios (Richardson and Torday 1994). Allelic variation in the surfactant protein A gene has been reported between American whites and Nigerian blacks (Rishi et al. 1992).

Caesarean section

Caesarean section carried out before the mother went into labour was reported to increase the risk of her baby developing RDS (Fedrick and Butler 1970; Usher et al. 1971), although this was not a consistent finding. Data from infants born at gestations above 32–34 weeks confirm the association of caesarean section before labour with both RDS and transient tachypnoea of the newborn (TTN) (Annibale et al. 1995; Morrison et al. 1995). The timing of the caesarean section is also important: the need for mechanical ventilation is 120 times greater after elective caesarean section at 37–38 weeks as compared with 39–41 weeks in babies with surfactant deficiency (Madar et al. 1999). Review of 24 077 repeat caesarean deliveries at term demonstrated that births at 37 and 38 weeks compared with 39 weeks were associated with an increased risk of a composite outcome of neonatal death, respiratory complications, hypoglycaemia, newborn sepsis and admission to the neonal unit (Tita et al. 2009). A review of nine studies comparing the outcome by mode of delivery of at or near-term infants demonstrated that all studies reported elective caesarean section was associated with an excess of respiratory morbidities with an average increased risk of two- to threefold (Hansen et al. 2007).

Birth depression

Babies who are depressed at birth are at increased risk of RDS. The incidence of RDS in babies less than 32 weeks of gestation was 54% in those with an Apgar <4 compared with 42% in babies with Apgars >4 (p < 0.005) (Beeby et al. 1994). During fetal asphyxia, lung perfusion falls, resulting in ischaemic damage to pulmonary capillaries. When the fetus recovers from the acute asphyxia, pulmonary hyperperfusion occurs and, if delivery occurs shortly afterwards, a protein-rich fluid leaks out of the damaged pulmonary capillaries. This leakage of proteins inhibits surfactant activity on the alveolar surface (Ikegami 1994). The protein leak can be prevented by exogenous surfactant (Ikegami et al. 1992), but in babies who respond poorly to surfactant administration, this benefit is probably overwhelmed by a large alveolar protein leak (Kobayashi et al. 1991). The surfactant protein (SP)-A (p. 460) is of specific benefit in minimising the inhibitory effect of protein on either endogenous or exogenous surfactant (Yukitake et al. 1995). One of the beneficial effects of antenatal steroids (p. 462) is that they reduce this capillary leakiness (Ikegami et al. 1987). The association between asphyxia and RDS is also influenced by hypoxia and acidaemia, predisposing to pulmonary hypertension and hypoperfusion with a right-to-left shunt (p. 498) and reducing surfactant synthesis by inhibiting the synthetic enzymes. RDS following birth depression blends into a spectrum with acute RDS (ARDS).

Maternal diabetes

Fetuses of diabetic mothers have abnormal surfactant synthesis, in particular a delay in the appearance of PG (Ojomo and Coustan 1990). Insulin delays the maturation of alveolar type II cells and decreases the proportion of saturated phosphatidylcholine in the surfactant (Gross et al. 1980). There are decreased levels of SP-A in amniotic fluid from diabetic pregnancies as compared with fluid from non-diabetic women (Snyder and Mendelson 1987). In cultured human lung tissue, insulin inhibits accumulation of SP-A and its mRNA (Snyder and Mendelson 1987; Dekowski and Snyder 1992). The incidence of RDS in infants of diabetic mothers (IDM) is increased by elective caesarean section before labour at 36–37 weeks. Improvements in maternal diabetic control during pregnancy have now facilitated delay in delivery until the 39th–40th week of gestation and RDS now occurs in fewer than 1% of patients (Kjos et al. 1990), even though in some the surfactant pattern at amniocentesis remains immature (Ojomo and Coustan 1990).

Hypothyroidism

Thyroid activity is important in the prenatal development of the surfactant system (p. 459). Preterm babies who develop RDS have lower levels of thyroid hormones in their cord blood than controls (Cuestas et al. 1976; Dhanireddy et al. 1983). The postnatal nadir in serum thyroxine concentration (seen in preterm infants) is very low in neonates with RDS (Vulsma and Kok 1996). Most term babies with congenital hypothyroidism detected by screening do not develop RDS, but some cases do occur (Cohen et al. 1991).

Genetic predisposition

There are reports of families in which several relatively mature babies have developed RDS. At preterm gestations, if a woman has one baby with RDS, the relative risk of RDS in a subsequent low-birthweight (LBW) baby may be increased threefold (Nagourney et al. 1996). SP-B deficiency results in lethal respiratory failure (Nogee et al. 1994), which is associated with histopathological features of congenital alveolar proteinosis (Nogee et al. 1993). This abnormality has been described in families (Nogee et al. 1994) and the inheritance is autosomal recessive. Partial deficiency of SP-B, which may be compatible with survival, has been reported (Cole et al. 2000). Polymorphisms in intron 4 of the SP-B gene have been found to modify the course of RDS independently, as indicated by the frequency of severe RDS and the occurrence of bronchopulmonary dysplasia (BPD) (Makri et al. 2002). Specific alleles of the SP-A and SP-B genes associate interactively with susceptibility to RDS and dominant mutations of SP-C associate with BPD (Hallman and Haataja 2003).

Twins

The second twin is more likely to develop RDS (Hacking et al. 2001), although this is not a consistent finding and others have reported no difference between twins and singletons (Winn et al. 1992). There is similarity of L:S ratios in twins, which is greater in monozygotic than dizygotic pairs (Leslie et al. 1991).

Hypothermia

Surfactant function is defective in cold babies and the concomitant hypoxia and acidaemia impair surfactant synthesis (Merritt and Farrell 1976). In addition, below $34\,^{\circ}C$, even in the presence of adequate amounts of PG, dipalmitoyl phosphatidycholine (DPPC) cannot spread to form an adequately functioning monolayer. Hypothermia in animals induces pulmonary hypertension and a fall in Pa_{O_2} (Will et al. 1978); similar mechanisms may occur in neonates. Coagulation disorders are more common in hypothermic infants.

Nutrition

In animal studies, maternal malnutrition compromises fetal surfactant synthesis as well as lung growth (Lin and Lechner 1991). Postnatally, although calorie deprivation does not appear to be important (Farrell 1986), specific deficiencies of fatty acids or inositol may be relevant (Hallman et al. 1987). Inositol supplementation in babies with RDS improves outcome (Hallman et al. 1992), reducing the risk of BPD or death, and severe retinopathy of prematurity (ROP) (Howlett and Ohlsson 2003).

Intrauterine growth retardation

An appropriately grown infant of 28 weeks' gestational age is much more likely to develop severe RDS than a growth-retarded 32-week-gestation infant of similar birthweight (Piper et al. 1996). Severely growth-retarded infants, however, have a higher incidence of RDS and it is more severe (Thompson et al. 1992; Piper et al. 1996).

Haemolytic disease of the newborn

The development of pulmonary maturity may be delayed in severely affected infants with haemolytic disease of the newborn with or without hydrops (Quinlan et al. 1984). A possible mechanism is the increased levels of insulin due to beta-islet cell hypertrophy, as occurs in IDM (Ch. 22). The presence of heart failure with

proteinaceous pulmonary oedema fluid aggravates any pre-existing surfactant deficiency due to prematurity.

Time of cord clamping

Preterm neonates who had undergone early cord clamping and had a low red cell mass, particularly when combined with some degree of birth depression, were more prone to develop RDS. As a consequence, it was recommended that following preterm delivery the cord should not be clamped until 1–2 minutes after delivery (Usher et al. 1975). A small prospective study of babies less than 33 weeks' gestation showed that a 30-second delay in cord clamping had no effect on mortality, but that the late-clamped babies were easier to ventilate in the first few days and required fewer blood transfusions (Kinmond et al. 1993).

Factors with equivocal effects on the incidence of RDS

Maternal hypertension

Some have reported a higher incidence of RDS in preterm infants of hypertensive mothers (Troche et al. 1995), perhaps due to delivery by caesarean section before labour. In contrast, no effect of pre-eclampsia with or without growth retardation was demonstrated on the results of lung maturity tests, neonatal morbidity including RDS or mortality (Schiff et al. 1993; Friedman et al. 1995). In another study, RDS occurred in 15% of infants of mothers with hypertensive pre-eclampsia but in 38% of non-hypertensive controls of similar weight and gestation (Shah et al. 1995).

Prolonged rupture of membranes

There is no consensus regarding the impact of prolonged rupture of membranes (Hallak and Bottoms 1993; Wolf et al. 1993). An apparent benefit may be explained by greater use of antenatal steroids in affected pregnancies (Thompson and Greenough 1993).

Factors reducing the incidence of RDS (see prevention of RDS, pp. 473–475)

Maternal addiction

Maternal narcotic addiction and smoking (Lieberman et al. 1992) reduce the incidence of RDS. Heroin can mature the surfactant-synthesising systems. The effect of cocaine is unclear (Beeram et al. 1995; Hanlon-Lundberg et al. 1996), although in animal models it induces surfactant synthesis (Sosenko 1993).

Pathology

The initial histological finding (Gandy et al. 1970) in non-surfactant-treated infants with RDS is alveolar epithelial cell necrosis developing within half an hour of birth. The epithelial cells become detached from the basement membrane and small patches of hyaline membranes form on the denuded areas. At the same time, there is diffuse interstitial oedema. The lymphatics are dilated by the delayed clearance of fetal lung fluid and the capillaries next to the membranes have a sludged appearance. There are very few osmiophilic granules in the type II cells, which in places contain vacuoles, suggesting that all the lamellar bodies have been discharged. In the early stages, all these changes are rather patchy, but, by 24 hours, more extensive generalised membrane formation in the transitional ducts and respiratory bronchioles occurs. Hyaline membranes line the overdistended terminal and respiratory bronchioles (Fig. 27.11), particularly where the airways branch, and may

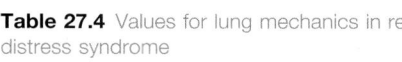

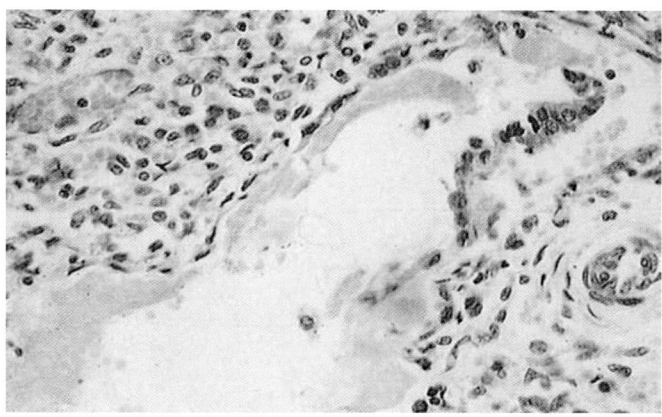

Fig. 27.11 Histology of respiratory distress syndrome, showing pink-staining hyaline membranes lining a terminal bronchiole with surrounding atelectasis.

Table 27.4 Values for lung mechanics in respiratory distress syndrome

Tidal volume (V_T)	4–6 ml/kg
Minute volume (V_E)	250–400 ml/kg/min
Alveolar ventilation (V_A)	50–90 ml/kg/min
Physiological dead space (V_D/V_T)	60–75%
Functional residual capacity (FRC)	3–20 ml/kg
Crying vital capacity	20–30 ml
Dynamic compliance (C_L)	0.0003–0.0005 l/cmH₂O/kg
Inspiratory resistance ($R_{aw\ Insp}$)	55–95 cmH₂O/l/s
Expiratory resistance ($R_{aw\ Exp}$)	140–200 cmH₂O/l/s
Work of breathing	800–3000 g.cm/min/kg
From various sources quoted in the text.	

extend into the putative alveolar ducts. The most distal component of the respiratory unit, the terminal sacs, although collapsed, are not lined by membranes. The hyaline membranes are eosinophilic on staining with haematoxylin and eosin, and contain nuclear debris from necrotic pneumocytes. Occasionally, when the infant has hyperbilirubinaemia, the membranes are yellow, reflecting the presence of unconjugated bilirubin. The hyaline membranes are formed by coagulation of plasma proteins, which have leaked on to the lung surface through damaged capillaries and epithelial cells; the fibrillary component of the membranes is derived from exuded fibrin. After 24 hours, a few inflammatory cells appear within the airway lumen; macrophages are usually the most prominent cell, although some polymorphs may also be present. Ingestion of the membrane by macrophages takes place over the next 2 or 3 days as the membrane separates. Macrophages are also present beneath the membrane within the interstitium, which is usually oedematous and where there may be a mild fibroblastic response. Epithelial regeneration is detectable after 48 hours, usually beneath the separating membranes. Cuboidal cells from the unaffected transitional ducts become large and mitotic; they flatten out and spread beneath the hyaline membranes. Other cells produce lamellar bodies. Many of these reparative cells form abnormally thick epithelial squames and, with damaged capillaries, can present a considerable barrier to efficient gas exchange. During this stage of repair, surfactant can be detected in increasing quantities on the alveolar surface (Gandy et al. 1970). By 7 days of age, the hyaline membranes will have disappeared in an infant with uncomplicated RDS. In ventilated babies, however, the healing process is markedly altered and delayed. There is a hyperplastic healing process, with massive shedding of bronchiolar epithelial cells and type II pneumocytes. Hyaline membranes remain prominent. The terminal airways may be plugged with secretions and there is progressive scarring and fibrosis of the alveoli and airways, leading to the picture of BPD (p. 552).

Pathophysiology

Lung function

The lungs are stiff, with compliance values of approximately 0.3–0.5 ml/cmH₂O/kg, when the disease is at its worst (Bhutani et al. 1988a) (Table 27.4). As surfactant begins to appear, the compliance improves and has usually returned to values of 1–2 ml/cmH₂O/kg

(Migdal et al. 1987) by 6–7 days of age. In severe disease, the functional residual capacity (FRC) may be as low as 3 ml/kg (Dimitriou and Greenough 1995a), whereas the FRC is at a normal level of 25–30 ml/kg in recovering babies (Richardson et al. 1986). Babies with RDS have a low tidal volume and a large physiological dead space. Minute ventilation, however, may be increased by an elevated respiratory rate in an attempt to sustain alveolar ventilation, but this is usually unsuccessful, resulting in alveolar underventilation and carbon dioxide retention. Pressure–volume loops on lungs excised at postmortem from babies dying of HMD have a characteristic pattern (Fig. 27.12). During inflation, the volume change for a given increase in pressure is very small, and, during deflation, the change in volume follows a track almost similar to that seen during inflation, whereas, in the normal lung, air is retained until low pressures are reached (hysteresis). As the pressure drops to zero, very little or no air is retained within the surfactant-less alveoli, corresponding to the very small FRC measured in vivo. Inspiratory resistance is usually normal in RDS (Hjalmarson and Olsson 1974) but expiratory resistance is increased, probably as a result of the closure of the airway prior to the expiratory grunt (Strang 1977). It is also increased by the presence of an endotracheal tube (ETT) (Edberg et al. 1991). An inevitable sequela of the abnormal lung mechanics is that the work of breathing is increased in neonates with RDS to twice that seen in those without RDS (Hjalmarson and Olsson 1974; McCann et al. 1987).

The time constant gives a measure of the time available for gas to leave the lung during expiration, which is normally accepted to take three time constants. The time constant is the compliance (l/cmH₂O) multiplied by the airways resistance (in cmH₂O/l/s). It is very short in neonates with severe RDS:

$$\underset{\text{(compliance)}}{0.001\ \text{l/cmH}_2\text{O}} \times \underset{\text{(resistance)}}{100\ \text{cmH}_2\text{O/l/s}} = \underset{\text{(time constant)}}{0.1\ \text{seconds}}$$

In babies with less stiff lungs, however, the time constant will be longer, and if the baby breathes rapidly (at 80/min), this will result in gas being retained in the lungs when the next inspiration starts (Strang 1977). Clinical studies (South and Morley 1986b; Hird and Greenough 1991) have shown the respiratory rate of infants with RDS to be about 80–90/min, with an average inspiratory time of 0.25–0.35 seconds. This pattern of respiration may be adopted so

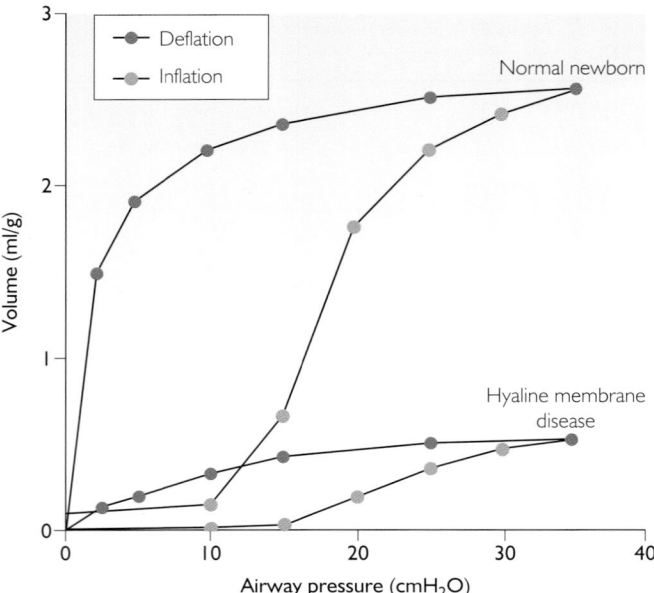

Fig. 27.12 Pressure–volume loops in excised lungs of neonates dying with and without hyaline membrane disease (HMD). In HMD, the deflation curve closely follows the inflation curve and little air is retained at zero pressure. In normal lungs, much more air is retained on the deflation limb of the loop (the phenomenon of hysteresis). *(Reproduced from Gribetz et al. (1959).)*

that the neonate retains gas within the lungs and some level of FRC is maintained.

A characteristic feature of RDS is the expiratory grunt. This is the result of the baby attempting to sustain an FRC by delaying the escape of air from the lungs during expiration. The baby tries to do this in two ways: firstly, during expiration, the diaphragm continues to contract, trying to delay or brake the reduction in thoracic volume and thus retain gas within the alveoli (Davis and Bureau 1987); secondly, by contracting the constrictor muscles of the larynx, an attempt is made to close the upper airway, as in the Valsalva manouevre. Since the abdominal muscles contract at the same time as the laryngeal muscles relax, there is an explosive exhalation of air, which is the characteristic 'grunt'. Bypassing this laryngeal component of expiratory braking by putting an ETT through the cords results in a fall in the Pao_2 in babies with RDS (Harrison et al. 1968).

Surfactant

The preterm baby is born with poor reserves of surfactant (p. 459). Most babies, however, have some present in the first few hours after birth. The deterioration seen in babies with non-surfactant-treated RDS is due in part to the disappearance of these small quantities of surfactant, compounded by fatigue as the neonate struggles to sustain ventilation in stiff, surfactant-deficient lungs. The disappearance of surfactant is primarily due to the inhibitory effect of proteins on surfactant (see above) (Ikegami et al. 1983), which leak on to the alveolar surface in the early oedematous stage of lung damage. The deleterious effect of hypoxia and acidaemia on surfactant synthesis (p. 462) may also play a part, but patency of the ductus is not relevant (Alpan et al. 1989). The levels of surfactant proteins are also low in the first few hours in babies with RDS and rise as the babies recover. The lungs remain non-compliant and atelectatic

until surfactant begins to reappear from 36 to 48 hours of age, as demonstrated by measurement of L : S ratios of pharyngeal aspirates (Kanto et al. 1976).

Pulmonary hypertension

Pulmonary artery pressure (PAP) remains high throughout the first week and even longer in some cases of RDS (Evans and Archer 1991b; Skinner et al. 1992a). The more severe the RDS, the higher the PAP, which may remain close to systemic levels in fatal cases (Walther et al. 1992). At least during systole, PAP can be higher than systemic pressure, at which time there is likely to be right-to-left ductal shunting. In diastole, the systemic pressure is likely to be higher than the pulmonary pressure and the overall effect is bidirectional ductal shunting, and this is frequently detected echocardiographically in RDS (Evans and Archer 1991a, b; Skinner et al. 1992b).

Mechanisms of hypoxia: right-to-left shunt with ventilation–perfusion imbalance

Hypoxaemia in RDS is due to a large right-to-left shunt. There are four main sites of right-to-left shunts:

1. Obligatory shunts present due to drainage of the veins of the myocardium directly into the left side of the heart and anastomoses between the bronchial and pulmonary circulation. These are small and of no haemodynamic or clinical significance.
2. Shunting through the foramen ovale occurs if right atrial pressure is higher than left atrial pressure. Interatrial right-to-left shunting is rare in neonates with RDS (Stahlman et al. 1972; Evans and Iyer 1994).
3. Shunting through a patent ductus arteriosus (PDA): the ductus arteriosus is patent in most babies with RDS during the first 48–72 hours (Dudell and Gersony 1984; Rigby et al. 1984). If the PAP exceeds the aortic pressure, there will be a significant right-to-left shunt. Right-to-left shunts at ductal level are common in persistent pulmonary hypertension of the newborn (PPHN; p. 495) but in uncomplicated RDS are small and constitute <10% of the total right-to-left shunt (Seppänen et al. 1994). Right-to-left ductal shunting means that blood taken from an umbilical artery catheter (UAC) can have a much lower Pao_2 than blood passing up the carotid arteries to the eyes. Colour Doppler studies in babies with RDS have demonstrated that intravascular shunting at the ductal or foramen ovale level is relatively unusual and the shunts through these channels are predominantly bidirectional or left-to-right in the first few days after birth. This has little effect on blood gas values, but increases the cardiac output and the load on the right ventricle (Evans and Archer 1991b; Evans and Iyer 1994; Seppänen et al. 1994).
4. The true intrapulmonary right-to-left shunt, when pulmonary capillary blood passes through the lung without coming into contact with a ventilated alveolus.

The combination of the above is the true right-to-left shunt. There is another right-to-left shunt which contributes to the total shunt or venous admixture seen in babies with RDS, and it is the result of pulmonary blood flow passing partially ventilated alveoli, that is, ventilation–perfusion imbalance. This large component of the right-to-left shunt in RDS can be eliminated by giving the baby 100% oxygen to breathe for 15 minutes (the hyperoxia or nitrogen washout test). This eliminates shunting resulting from partially oxygenated alveoli, and a shunt calculated at the end of a period breathing 100% oxygen is the true shunt outlined above. In most babies with RDS, the majority of the right-to-left shunt is the fourth component of the true shunt plus the shunt from ventilation–perfusion imbalance.

Carbon dioxide retention

The increased $P\text{aco}_2$ in RDS is due to hypoventilation secondary to atelectasis, decreased tidal volume and increased dead space. Ventilation is also non-homogeneous, so whereas end-tidal $PA\text{co}_2$ is a good measure of $P\text{aco}_2$ in patients with normal lungs, in babies with RDS there is a risk that measurement of $PA\text{co}_2$ will seriously underestimate $P\text{aco}_2$. Since the mixed venous $P\text{co}_2$ (normally 6.13 kPa, 46 mmHg) is usually only a fraction of a kilopascal above arterial or alveolar $P\text{co}_2$ (normally 5.33 kPa, 40 mmHg), the right-to-left shunt has to be enormous before the admixture of venous blood significantly contributes to hypercapnia in RDS.

Prevention of respiratory distress syndrome

Prevention of prematurity

Tocolytic drugs to prevent preterm labour have proved disappointing (King et al. 1988; Leonardi and Hankins 1992), prolonging pregnancy for not more than 48 hours (Keirse 1995). Genital tract infection is associated with preterm labour, and in women with preterm rupture of the membranes (PROM) there is evidence that treatment with antibiotics reduces the prematurity rate (Gomez et al. 1995).

Antenatal steroid therapy

Not all steroids cross the placenta; cortisol is largely inactivated, but degradation is resisted by synthetic steroids such as betamethasone and dexamethasone. Antenatal administration of dexamethasone or betamethasone to pregnant women in preterm labour significantly reduces the incidence of RDS and neonatal death (Roberts and Dalziel 2010). Several other serious complications of prematurity, including germinal matrix/intraventricular haemorrhage (GMH/IVH) and necrotising enterocolitis (NEC), are also reduced (Ward 1994; Crowley 1995; Eriksson et al. 2009). No long-term adverse effects were demonstrated from a single course of antenatal corticosteroids (Dessens et al. 2000). In a population-based cohort of 79 395 infants, antental steroid therapy was found to be an independent risk factor for asthma between 36 and 72 months of age (odds ratio 1.23) (Pole et al. 2009), but antenatal exposure to a single course of betamethasone did not alter lung function or the prevalence of wheeze and asthma at age 30 (Dalziel et al. 2006). Follow-up of antenatally steroid-treated babies shows no excess of handicap compared with controls (MacArthur et al. 1981; Doyle et al. 1989).

Some of the beneficial effects of corticosteroids are the consequence of reducing the incidence and severity of RDS, whereas others represent the maturing effect of steroids on many body systems. The interaction with the benefits of postnatal exogenous surfactant therapy is of particular importance. The effects of antenatal steroids (Table 27.5) include inducing the enzymes for surfactant synthesis and the genes for the production of the surfactant proteins A, B, C and D (Mendelson et al. 1993), and improving the quality of the surfactant produced (Ueda et al. 1995). Glucocorticoids, such as dexamethasone, can cause substantial stimulation of SP-B gene expression to two to three times adult levels in fetal lung explants (Benson 1993). They mature the non-surfactant-producing

Table 27.5 Benefits of antenatal steroids

Improved Apgar scores	Gardner et al. (1995)
Maturation of lung structure	Bunton and Plopper (1984) Lanteri et al. (1994)
Initiation of surfactant protein synthesis	Mendelson et al. (1993)
Improved NO-mediated pulmonary venous relaxation	Zhou et al. (1996)
Reduced pulmonary capillary leakiness	Ikegami et al. (1997)
Interaction with postnatal exogenous surfactant therapy	p. 475
Increased resistance to high oxygen exposure	Frank (1992)
Better blood pressure in early neonatal period	Moise et al. (1995)
Higher neonatal white cell counts	Barak et al. (1992)
Less patent ductus arteriosus	Eronen et al. (1993); Ward (1994)
Less GMH/IVH	Crowley (1995); Garland et al. (1995)
Less NEC	Ward (1994)

NO, nitric oxide; GMH/IVH, germinal matrix/intraventricular haemorrhage; NEC, necrotising enterocolitis.

tissues of the lung (Bunton and Plopper 1984; Lanteri et al. 1994); the septa become longer, thinner and less cellular, with larger air spaces and increased numbers of alveolar divisions. In addition, antenatal steroids increase antioxidant enzyme activity and reduce oxidative stress (Vento et al. 2009); the maximum effect was seen with steroids administered 2–4 days before delivery and females benefited more.

Timing of treatment

Results from randomised trials have demonstrated that the benefit is maximal in babies delivered between 24 and 168 hours after starting the maternal therapy (Crowley 1995). A smaller but useful benefit is also seen in women receiving less than 24 hours of therapy.

Number of courses

There are doubts about the safety of multiple courses of corticosteroids (Ikegami et al. 1997; French et al. 1999), which cannot be recommended as routine treatment. Repeated courses of therapy may suppress the maternal and fetal hypothalamic–pituitary–adrenal axis (Ballard et al. 1980), as well as increasing the risk of maternal hyperglycaemia and infection. Neonatal Cushing syndrome as been reported after repeated antenatal courses of steroids (Bradley et al. 1994). Steroids, however, may depress the neonatal adrenal gland when used in conventional doses (Kari et al. 1996). Evidence from eight randomised controlled trials in animal models highlighted that, although repeated doses of antenatal corticosteroids have beneficial effects in terms of lung function, they can have adverse effects on brain function and fetal growth (Aghajafari et al.

2002). Similar effects have been seen in infants following repeated courses. In one study (Wapner et al. 2006), infants exposed to more than four courses had significant weight reductions. In a large randomised study (Crowther et al. 2006), although repeated courses of steroids (weekly) reduced both the risk of RDS and need for supplementary oxygen and shortened the duration of mechanical ventilation, z scores for weight and head circumference were lower at hospital discharge. In another large randomised study (Murphy et al. 2008), infants exposed to repeated courses (fortnightly) had similar morbidity and mortality, but weighed less, were shorter and had a smaller head circumference (Murphy et al. 2008). Data regarding the efficacy of rescue steroids after only one standard administration are mixed. A single rescue course of antenatal corticosteroids before 33 weeks in women who had completed a single course before 30 weeks of gestation was associated with a lower rate of neonatal morbidity and significantly decreased RDS and surfactant use (Garite et al. 2009), but in another study the requirement for surfactant was increased in infants exposed to a single repeated dose of betamethasone (Peltoniemi et al. 2007). A single repeated dose of antenatal betamethasone given for imminent preterm birth at least 1 week after standard betamethasone treatment, however, was not shown to influence neurodevelopmental outcome and had no signifcant effect on growth at 2 years of age (Peltoniemi et al. 2009).

Gestational age

In the original study by Liggins and Howie (1972), the greatest benefit was seen at gestations of 30–34 weeks, with a much smaller, although statistically significant, benefit below 30 weeks. Crowley's meta-analysis (Crowley 1995) demonstrated a benefit in neonates less than 31 weeks, but evidence for benefit in babies of less than 28 weeks is less strong (Doyle et al. 1986; Garite et al. 1992).

Preterm rupture of membranes

Although there has been concern that, in PROM, antenatal steroids may increase risk of infection, with appropriate clinical surveillance this was not a problem in the studies reviewed by Crowley (1995); indeed, a beneficial effect of antenatal steroids in pregnancies complicated by PROM was demonstrated.

Maternal hypertension

Liggins and Howie (1972) reported that steroid-treated hypertensive women had a significantly increased stillbirth rate and perinatal mortality; as a consequence, such women were excluded from trials (Crowley 1995). Clinical experience and observational studies, however, suggest that steroids can be used safely in this situation (Lamont et al. 1983).

Diabetes

In the past, glucocorticoids were avoided in diabetic pregnancies because of their potential for causing hyperglycaemia; however, they should be given, as the insulin regimen can be altered during the brief period of hyperglycaemia. Steroids switch on the surfactant protein-synthesising systems in experimental diabetic rats (Moglia and Phelps 1996).

Twins

Multiple pregnancies have often been excluded from trials of antenatal corticosteroids.

Guidelines for antenatal steroid usage

Guidelines have been produced by the Royal College of Obstetricians and Gynaecologists (1996), the British Association of Perinatal Medicine (Sweet et al. 2007), and the National Institutes of Health of the USA (NIH Consensus Panel Development 1995). Their recommendations include:

- Antenatal treatment with corticosteroids should be considered for all women at risk of preterm labour between 24 and 36 weeks. Treatment should consist of two doses of betamethasone given intramuscularly 24 hours apart or four doses of dexamethasone given 12 hours apart. Betamethasone, however, is now preferred, as in an observational study (Baud et al. 1999) it was associated with a lower risk of periventricular leukomalacia (PVL). In a non-randomised comparison, betamethasone compared with dexamethasone was associated with lower rates of RDS and BPD (Feldman et al. 2007).
- Treatment for less than 24 hours is associated with significant improvement in outcome; thus, corticosteroids should be given unless immediate delivery is anticipated.
- In the absence of chorioamnionitis, antenatal corticosteroids are recommended in pregnancies complicated by preterm PROM.
- Unless there is evidence that corticosteroids will have an adverse effect on the mother, they are also recommended in other complicated pregnancies.

Thyroid preparations

Thyroid hormones are involved in the induction of surfactant synthesis (Ballard 1984; Gonzales et al. 1986). There are reports of apparent success with intra-amniotic therapy (Romaguera et al. 1993), as thyroid hormones and thyroid-stimulating hormone do not cross the placenta, but most researchers have studied the administration of thyrotrophin-releasing hormone (TRH) to the mother, usually in combination with dexamethasone. There is a consistent synergism between TRH and steroids in animal studies (Moraga et al. 1994; Polk et al. 1995). Although the results of early clinical studies were promising, in the ACTOBAT study (ACTOBAT Study Group 1995), the TRH group suffered increased morbidity, as they delivered at significantly earlier gestations. Meta-analysis of the results of 11 trials, which included 4500 women, has demonstrated that prenatal administration of TRH in addition to corticosteroids did not reduce the risk of neonatal respiratory distress or BPD. Indeed, the data showed there were adverse effects: an increase in requirement for ventilation and more likelihood of having a low Apgar score at 5 minutes (Crowther et al. 2000). Antenatally administered TRH can also produce transient suppression of the pituitary–thyroid axis and transient complications in the mother, including nausea, vomiting and increased blood pressure (BP) (Gross and Moya 2001).

Other antenatal drugs

Various drugs have been used in animal experiments to mature the surfactant synthetic pathways. These include opiates, aminophylline (Karotkin et al. 1976) and ambroxol (Robertson 1981). Benefit from ambroxol has been reported (Wauer et al. 1992), but this is not a consistent finding (Dani et al. 1997). Some (Wyszogrodski et al. 1974) but not all (Fiascone et al. 1992) animal experiments suggest that antenatal beta-mimetics may improve neonatal lung function. Their effect in the human neonate appears to be small (Laros et al. 1991), although, in a randomised controlled trial (Eisler et al. 1999), infants whose mothers had received an infusion of terbutaline prior to elective delivery had significantly better lung function.

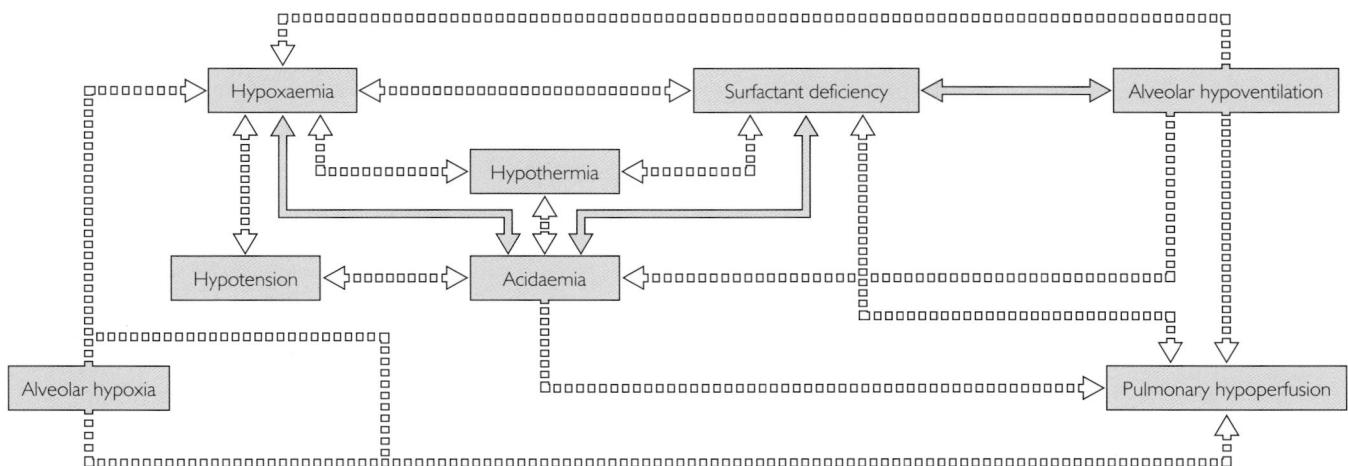

Fig. 27.13 Interrelationship of factors affecting surfactant and other components of lung function; solid lines indicate major effects. *(Reproduced from Roberton (1992).)*

Prevention of intrapartum asphyxia

Asphyxia worsens RDS and predisposes to pulmonary haemorrhage. If asphyxia is absent and the preterm neonate is presenting by the vertex, there is no need to proceed to caesarean section on a routine basis (Ahn et al. 1992), but if fetal compromise develops, delivery by caesarean section should be considered even at early gestations.

Prevention of postnatal asphyxia

It is important to prevent postnatal hypoxic damage to lung capillaries and minimise the risk of haemorrhagic pulmonary oedema, by rapidly establishing normal blood gases and normal pulmonary perfusion and ensuring maximum surfactant release from the type II pneumocytes by adequate expansion of the lungs. Inadequate ventilation leads to poor surfactant release, resulting in hypoxia and acidaemia, leading to a vicious cycle (Fig. 27.13). As a consequence, it had been argued that, unless a baby of <30 weeks of gestation is in excellent condition at 30 seconds of age, crying and vigorous, the baby should be actively resuscitated by intubation and intermittent positive-pressure ventilation (IPPV). The studies (Drew 1982; Robson and Hey 1982) which demonstrated such an approach, reducing morbidity and mortality from RDS, however, were performed before the modern era of neonatal intensive care and a less aggressive approach using continuous positive airway pressure (CPAP) rather than IPPV is now preferred in many centres (p. 231). Prevention of asphyxia, however, remains important, and appropriate resuscitation may require endotracheal intubation (Linder et al. 1999).

Avoiding drug depression

Many drugs given to the mother in preterm labour – including opiate analgesics and anaesthetic agents – can result in marked hypotonia and respiratory depression in the infant. In general, as well as using the specific opiate antagonist naloxone (except in infants of drug-addicted mothers, in whom naloxone will precipitate drug withdrawal signs), affected babies may require ventilation from birth until the drugs are excreted or metabolised.

Avoidance of maternal fluid overload

Excessive fluid administration to the mother in labour may result in neonatal hyponatraemia (Tarnow-Mordi et al. 1981).

Prophylactic surfactant

All trials of surfactant therapy have shown a reduction in oxygen requirements and the ventilator pressures required. Problems with the measurement techniques resulted in confusion regarding the effect of surfactant on compliance, as the early improvements may not be detected by dynamic compliance measurements. Surfactant also results in elevation of lung volume (Cotton et al. 1993), in association with increased oxygenation (Dimitriou et al. 1997).

A large number of studies have been carried out assessing the impact of prophylactic surfactant, i.e. administering surfactant within the first few minutes after birth. Many varieties of surfactant have been used (Table 27.6). Meta-analyses of the results have been performed (Soll 1996; Soll and Blanco 2009; Soll and Morley 2009) demonstrating positive effects of both synthetic and natural surfactants. Prophylactic use of natural surfactant results in a significant reduction in pneumothorax, mortality, and the combined outcome of mortality and BPD, but not BPD alone (Soll 2000a). In a randomised trial, Lucinactant, a synthetic surfactant containing a functional SP-B mimic that is leucine and lysine repeating units (KL4), was associated with significantly lower incidence of RDS at 24 hours than a non-protein-containing synthetic surfactant and lower RDS-related mortality at 14 days than either the non-protein-containing surfactant or a bovine-derived surfactant (Moya et al. 2005). In another study (Sinha et al. 2005), however, Lucinactant was not more effective and meta-analysis of the results of the two randomised trials does not demonstrate that Lucinactant was associated with significant benefits at 36 weeks' postmaturational age compared with an animal-derived surfactant (Pfister et al. 2007).

Meta-analyses of the results of trials comparing administering surfactant prophylactically or selectively, or early versus late, have demonstrated prophylactic/early administration is more effective. Prophylactic versus selective surfactant administration has been associated with a significant reduction in neonatal mortality, BPD/death and pneumothorax (Stevens et al. 2007) and early versus late administration a reduction in neonatal mortality and pneumothorax (Yost and Soll 2000). Early surfactant replacement with extubation to nasal CPAP (nCPAP), as compared with later, selective surfactant replacement and continued mechanical ventilation, was associated with an increased utilisation of exogenous surfactant replacement therapy (Stevens et al. 2007). In a subsequent trial (Sandri et al. 2010) prophylactic surfactant followed by extubation to nCPAP was not superior to early selective surfactant in terms of

Table 27.6 Surfactants which have been used in clinical studies

TYPE OF SURFACTANT	ANIMAL SOURCE	COMPOSITION (OR ADDITIVES IF ANIMAL-DERIVED)
Protein-containing animal surfactants		
Surfactant TA	Cow	DPPC, palmitic acid triglyceride
Survanta	Cow	Similar to Surfactant TA
Infasurf (CLSE)	Cow	
Curosurf	Pig	
BLES	Cow	
Alveofact SF-RI 1	Cow	
Human surfactant	Liquor amnii	
Artificial surfactant		
Non-protein surfactants		
ALEC (Pumactant)		70% DPPC, 30% PG
Exosurf		DPPC + tyloxapol and hexadecanol
Peptide-containing synthetic surfactants		
Venticute		DPPC, POPG, PA, rSP-C
Lucinactant		Synthetic SP-B analogue made of lysine–leucine (KL4)

DPPC, dipalmitoyl phosphatidylcholine; PG, phosphatidylglycerol; POPG, palmitoyloleoylphosphatidylglycerol; PA, palmitic acid; rSP-C, recombinant surfactant protein C.

requirement for mechanical ventilation in the first 5 days after birth in infants born between 25 and 28 + 6 weeks' gestation. In a study of 1316 infants (SUPPORT study group 2010), infants randomised to intubation and surfactant treatment within 1 hour of birth compared with those randomised to CPAP in the delivery room had similar outcomes with respect to the primary outcome of death or BPD. Infants who received CPAP, however, less frequently required postnatal stertoids ($p < 0.001$), required fewer days of mechanical ventilation ($p = 0.03$) and were more likely to be alive and free from the need for mechanical ventilation by day 7 ($p = 0.01$). Those results suggest that when nasal CPAP is used in the labour ward administration of surfactant can be delayed until the infant has displayed signs of respiratory distress.

Clinical features of respiratory distress syndrome

The diagnostic criteria for RDS were laid down before use of prophylactic surfactant. These comprised: a respiratory rate above 60/min; grunting expiration; indrawing of the sternum, intercostal spaces and lower ribs during inspiration; and cyanosis without added oxygen (Rudolph and Smith 1960).

Natural history

The disease is present within the first 4 hours after birth. In the absence of treatment with exogenous surfactant, over the next 24–36 hours the baby tires, dyspnoea worsens and the baby becomes oedematous. As surfactant synthesis commences, the severity of the disease begins to abate from 36–48 hours of age, and this is associated with a spontaneous diuresis (Kavvadia et al. 1998).

Respiratory signs

The more mature baby with RDS may breathe at a fast respiratory rate, exceeding 100/min. This faster rate is more efficient in terms of work of breathing. Some babies may alternate a breathing pattern of shallow tachypnoea up to 100–120/min with one in which they breathe comparatively slowly (40–60/min) with marked recession and grunting. The slow-breathing baby often has episodes of apnoea, and this is a sign that respiration is beginning to fail (Davis and Bureau 1987). In addition to tachypnoea, there is marked intercostal and sternal recession, and flaring of the alae nasi. The main respiratory muscle is the diaphragm. In the presence of a compliant ribcage, diaphragmatic contraction results in a marked seesaw pattern, the chest moving inwards and the abdomen moving outwards during inspiration and vice versa on expiration. On auscultation there is a reduction in air entry. An expiratory grunt is a feature of most forms of neonatal respiratory disease and results from the baby trying to sustain FRC (p. 457). In uncomplicated RDS, these clinical features gradually return to normal by 7 days at the latest.

Cardiovascular signs

The heart rate in mild to moderate cases of RDS is 140–160/min and shows normal variability. In infants with severe RDS, the heart rate tends to be slower (120/min) with little beat-to-beat variation. The heart sounds are normal. Murmurs are not normally present; if heard in the first 24–48 hours, they suggest congenital heart disease or ischaemic myocardial injury and require further investigation. A murmur appearing after 3–4 days is usually due to a PDA. Heart failure is not a feature of RDS; if present, it suggests cardiac disease.

Neonates with RDS are often hypotensive and this is associated with a worse prognosis (Hallman et al. 1993). Hypotension is less common in babies who receive antenatal steroids (Moise et al. 1995). There are many causes for the hypotension, including hypoxia and acidaemia depressing the myocardium and reducing cardiac output, a low blood volume and high-pressure ventilation compromising venous return and reducing cardiac output. Hypotension predisposes to acidaemia, which increases pulmonary vascular resistance, GMH/IVH (Ch. 40.5), renal failure (Ch. 35.1) and NEC (Ch. 29.3). It is essential, therefore, to measure the BP and correct symptomatic hypotension.

Central nervous system

The preterm baby even without RDS is hypotonic, inactive and lies in the frog position, spending most of the day asleep. Abnormal neurological signs are often subtle (Ch. 40.1), but if present they are ominous, suggesting development of a GMH/IVH.

Abdominal examination

Examination of the abdomen is usually unremarkable; the liver, spleen and kidneys are often palpable but are rarely significantly enlarged. Hepatosplenomegaly suggests heart failure or sepsis and should be dealt with accordingly, and an easily felt liver in a baby with severe respiratory failure suggests a right tension pneumothorax (p. 484).

Most babies with severe RDS have an ileus (Dunn 1963), and do not pass meconium. Improvement in their general condition is often heralded by the appearance of bowel sounds and the passage of meconium, although gastric emptying may still be delayed. Jaundice is not uncommon; phototherapy and exchange transfusion are indicated in preterm infants at much lower bilirubin levels than in the full-term neonate (Ch. 29.1).

Differential diagnosis (Table 27.7)

The differential diagnosis in the first 6 hours can usually be made on the basis of the history (including the gestation), the clinical examination, the blood gases and the CXR. It is impossible, however, to exclude infection as the cause of the baby's symptoms. Furthermore, infection with group B streptococcus (GBS; *Streptococcus agalactiae*) can coexist with RDS. As a consequence, it is important to treat all infants presenting with respiratory distress with antibiotics until the results of cultures are available. PPHN (p. 495) can be differentiated by the absence of significant parenchymal lung disease and the relevant echocardiographic findings. Infants with RDS, however, may also have marked pulmonary hypertension (Walther et al. 1992). Such infants will have an oxygen requirement that is out of proportion to their CXR appearance and a poor response to surfactant therapy. Respiratory distress presenting after 4–6 hours of age in an infant who has been adequately observed is usually due to pneumonia or heart failure secondary to heart disease. Other conditions, such as aspiration and inhalation of the feed, some malformations and, occasionally, a small pneumothorax can present after 6 hours of age, but these are less common.

Investigations

Haematological

There are no unique haematological findings in RDS. The haemoglobin will vary with the local practice regarding cord clamping (Yao and Lind 1974). Anaemia may develop later due to GMH/IVH (Ch. 40.5) or iatrogenic losses (Ch. 30). Results of measurements of the coagulation system are often prolonged owing to prematurity in infants with RDS, although disseminated intravascular coagulation (DIC) is rare. The presence of a coagulopathy can be due to complications such as birth asphyxia, septicaemia or a GMH/IVH. Infants who have suffered intrauterine growth retardation are also at increased risk of coagulation abnormalities (Hannam et al. 2003). The white blood count is normal for the baby's birthweight and gestation (Manroe et al. 1979). Thrombocytopenia is not a feature of RDS unless there is DIC (Ch. 30).

Biochemical

The plasma electrolyte pattern is usually normal, although marked early hyponatraemia can be seen if the mother has been fluid-overloaded during labour (Tarnow-Mordi et al. 1981). The plasma calcium is frequently low (1.5–1.7 mmol/l) in the first 48–72 hours in ill LBW babies. Although infants of very-low-birthweight (VLBW) are prone to hypoglycaemia, when sick they are also susceptible to hyperglycaemia (Ch. 34.1). Infection should be considered in a baby with hyperglycaemia. Babies with RDS may have impaired renal function, with a reduced glomerular filtration rate and renal plasma flow and a correspondingly raised urea and creatinine (Guignard et al. 1976); they are also poor at excreting hydrogen ions (Allen and Usher 1971). Fluid restriction has been advocated to improve lung function, but no such effect was seen in a randomised trial (Kavvadia et al. 1998).

Serum albumin levels are often below 25–30 g/l in preterm infants (Cartlidge and Rutter 1986) and are lower in the cord blood of babies who develop RDS than in controls (Bland 1972). The albumin may remain below 25 g/l for days or even weeks in critically ill babies; this is the result of albumin leaking into the subcutaneous tissues, poor protein intake and impaired albumin synthesis. Administration of albumin, however, does not improve lung function (Greenough 1998) and may increase the risk of BPD development (Dimitriou et al. 2002c); hence it should be avoided.

Blood gas measurements

Hypoxaemia occurs and can be used to assess the severity of the lung disease. A mixed metabolic and respiratory acidaemia is found in most cases of RDS, with the Pa_{CO_2} being raised in all but the mildest cases; indeed, the absence of hypercapnia or the presence of a low Pa_{CO_2} should suggest a diagnosis other than RDS in a dyspnoeic neonate (p. 478).

Hormone levels

Cortisol levels of ill 26-week babies are lower than those of healthy preterm babies; they remain low for several days after birth and are further depressed by prenatal therapy with dexamethasone (Kari et al. 1996). Levels of thyroid-stimulating hormone, thyroxine and triiodothyronine, although initially normal in cord blood (Klein et al. 1981), drop below normal during the first week (Franklin et al. 1986).

Echocardiography

Echocardiographic studies in neonates with RDS confirm the presence of a PDA in most cases (Ch. 28), but are otherwise normal in the absence of PPHN or severe depression of myocardial function. Doppler echocardiography is used to investigate the degree of pulmonary hypertension (p. 495).

Measurement of surfactant status

This has limited applicability, as apparently typical RDS can develop in the presence of L:S ratios greater than 2.0, even when PG is present (Wigton et al. 1993), and surfactant-deficient RDS and congenital pneumonia due, in particular, to GBS can coexist. In addition, although assessment of surfactant proteins can be used to determine pulmonary maturity, the tests are expensive and time-consuming. There may, however, be a role for rapid early assessments of neonatal surfactant levels (Chida et al. 1993; Bhuta et al. 1997) if supplies of surfactant are limited.

Chest X-ray

The CXR appearance contributes to the establishment of the diagnosis. In addition, thymic (Fig. 27.14), cardiac and skeletal abnormalities can be identified and the positions of the ETT and indwelling cannulae checked. Classically, in RDS the CXR shows diffuse, fine granular opacification in both lung fields with an air bronchogram where the air-filled bronchi stand out against the atelectatic lungs. In reality, the appearance can be very variable,

Table 27.7 Differential diagnosis of dyspnoea in the neonate

CONDITION	GESTATIONAL AGE	HISTORY	EXAMINATION*	GASES†	PRESENTATION‡ <6 h	PRESENTATION‡ >6 h	CHEST RADIOGRAPH	COMMENTS
Respiratory distress syndrome (RDS)	Premature				+++	N	Diagnostic, but see p. 480	Working diagnosis in all preterm neonates unless chest radiograph suggests alternative. Always consider infection (Ch. 39.2)
Transient tachypnoea	FT > premature§	Often caesarean delivery	Mild hypoxaemia needing 40% O_2		+++	R	Diagnostic, but see p. 485	Commonest cause of breathlessness in term babies. By definition, a mild disease (pp. 485–486)
Meconium aspiration	FT‖	Meconium-stained liquor at resuscitation. Postmaturity	Meconium-stained baby. Meconium in larynx		+++	N	Streaky	Diagnosis obvious on history. Infection may coexist
Pneumothorax or pneumomediastinum	FT > premature	May be excessive resuscitation at birth			++	R¶	Diagnostic	
Massive pulmonary haemorrhage	Premature > FT	Asphyxia or other cause of heart failure, bleeding tendency. Use of artificial surfactant	Crepitations; usually marked pallor. Blood up larynx or in endotracheal tube. PDA after presentation		+	++	Unhelpful; usually a white-out	Diagnosis based on clinical findings
After severe asphyxia	FT**	Severe asphyxia Low Apgar	Other features of asphyxia (Ch. 40.4)	Marked metabolic acidaemia	++	N	Unhelpful	Tachypnoea driven by acidaemia
Infection (pneumonia)	Any	May be helpful	Rarely differentiates this from other causes of dyspnoea	Often severe acidaemia and easy to reduce CO_2 without increasing PaO_2	++	+++	Unhelpful in most cases, though may show patchy changes	Impossible to exclude in any baby (Ch. 39.2). This is the working diagnosis in the absence of specific chest radiograph findings in neonates >6 hours old with respiratory disease. WBC. CRP may be helpful
Congenital malformations	FT > premature	Usually normal delivery. May have been detected on antenatal ultrasound	Rarely helpful	May be profound hypoxaemia with raised CO_2	+++	+	Virtually always diagnostic	Diaphragmatic hernia, cysts, effusions, agenesis all present this way. TOF should not present this way (Ch. 29.4)

Condition	Gestation	History	Examination	Blood gases			Chest X-ray	Comments
Congenital heart disease	FT > premature		Murmurs, heart size, signs of heart failure	CO_2 normal or reduced. In cyanotic CHD PaO_2 rarely >6–7 kPa even in oxygen with IPPV	R	++	May be helpful or diagnostic	The alternative common diagnosis in infants presenting after 6 hours and particularly after 24 hours of age. ECG and echocardiogram usually diagnostic
Pulmonary hypoplasia	Any	Prolonged rupture of membranes	No kidneys palpable, amnion nodosum. Dwarf (p. 581)	Profound hypoxaemia and hypercapnia	+++	N	Diagnostic; very small lungs	Virtually always rapidly fatal
Persistent pulmonary hypertension	FT > premature	May have had mild asphyxia	May hear soft murmur of TI	Gases like cyanotic CHD, i.e. marked hypoxaemia with normal or reduced CO_2	+++	+	Usually normal or nearly so	Can be difficult to exclude cyanotic CHD unless echocardiogram available
Inhalation of feed	Any	Obvious			R	+++	Unhelpful	Should not happen in well-run units. Normal term babies rarely inhale, so always seek alternative diagnosis, especially infection
Inborn errors of metabolism	FT > premature	May be positive family history or history of unexplained neonatal death in the past	No evidence of lung disease. Tachypnoea driven by acidaemia	Severe metabolic acidaemia, normal PaO_2; low $PaCO_2$	R	+++	Often normal	Diagnosis based on blood changes plus ketonaemia in many cases (Ch. 34.3)
Primary neurological or muscle disease	FT > premature	May be positive family history or history of unexplained neonatal death or infant death. Polyhydramnios may occur	Marked hypotonia. Areflexia, odd face, deformities. No evidence of lung disease	Gases normal (unless apnoeic)	++	+	Often normal	Usually easy to identify as a group
Upper airway obstruction	FT > premature	May be typical in choanal atresia (p. 604)	Stridor present. Problems resolve on intubation. Laryngoscopy may be diagnostic	Gases normal when intubated; CO_2 may be raised beforehand	+	+	Often normal	

*Mentioning features other than cardinal features of respiratory disease (pp. 476–477).

†Most conditions cause hypoxaemia and hypercarbia; only if the blood gas patterns differ from this is it noted here.

‡Frequency of presentation graded + to +++; N, never, R, rarely.

§Full-term (FT) greater than premature. This means that the condition can occur at any gestation, but since full-term babies are more common than preterm ones, there are more cases in full-term neonates.

¶If preterm, consider Listeria.

¶Usually as a complication of pre-existing severe lung disease, especially hyaline membrane disease.

**Severely asphyxiated premature babies will get RDS.

PDA, patent ductus arteriosus; WBC, white blood cells; CRP, C-reactive protein; TOF, tracheo-oesophageal fistula; CHD, coronary heart disease; IPPV, intermittent positive-pressure ventilation; ECG, electrocardiogram; TI, inspiratory time; CHS, central hypoventilation syndrome.

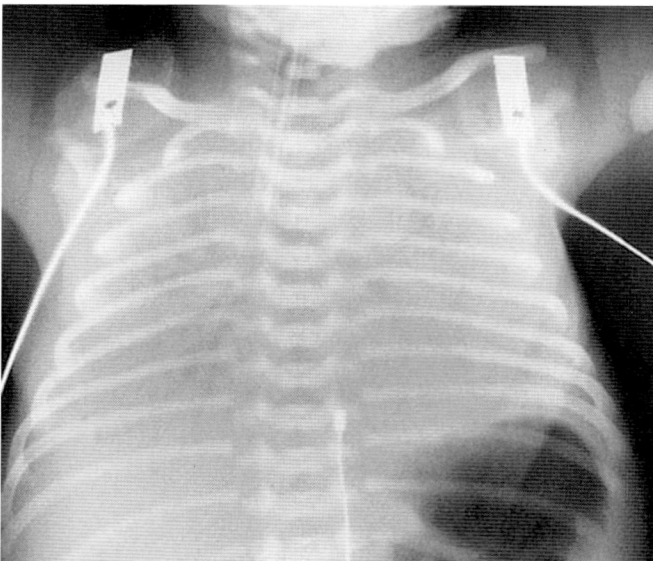

Fig. 27.14 Severe respiratory distress syndrome. The lungs are totally opaque and cannot be separated from the heart border because of widespread atelectasis. An air bronchogram can be seen in the right lung.

from a slight granularity to lungs that are so opaque that it is impossible to distinguish between the lung field and the cardiac silhouette. A 'whiteout' on an X-ray taken at 1 hour of age, however, may be due to retained fetal lung fluid. By 4 hours of age, as a result of clearance of the fluid, the CXR appearance may show marked improvement. The CXR appearance also depends on the phase of the respiratory cycle, the appearance being much worse on an expiratory rather than an inspiratory one. Positive-pressure support with both CPAP and IPPV can improve the CXR appearance in a baby who had marked X-ray changes while breathing spontaneously; surfactant treatment has the same effect (Edwards et al. 1985).

Treatment

Initial care

Transportation from the labour ward to the neonatal intensive care unit (NICU)

It is essential to ensure that there is no deterioration in a baby's lung disease during transfer. All VLBW neonates who require intubation for resuscitation should be ventilated in the transport incubator. Ventilator settings during transport are based on the oxygen saturation and the clinical assessment of the baby, in particular whether there is adequate chest wall expansion. Practice differs regarding whether babies who have been intubated to be given surfactant should be extubated on to nCPAP or remain intubated for transfer and assessment can take place on the NICU. Others do not intubate infants routinely in the labour ward, but transfer babies on nCPAP.

Initial management in the NICU

As soon as the baby arrives in the NICU, he or she must be put into an incubator prewarmed to 35–36°C or placed under a radiant heater. In the next 30–60 minutes, the following procedures should be carried out in all neonates with RDS:

- Weigh the infant.
- Examine carefully.
- Measure the head circumference to facilitate diagnosis of the rare infant with a subgaleal haemorrhage and subsequently rapidly enlarging head circumference (Ch. 40.3).
- Connect to electrocardiogram (ECG) and respiration monitors (Ch. 19).
- Measure the baby's temperature.
- Measure Pao_2, $Paco_2$ and pH. Consider inserting an indwelling arterial line in babies requiring high oxygen concentrations.
- Measure the BP using a continuously recording device once an arterial cannula is in situ, and Dinamap if no cannula is in place.
- Treat abnormalities of blood gases (p. 521).
- Draw blood for haemoglobin and white cell count. Crossmatch all ill neonates, as most eventually need transfusion.
- Take a set of cultures, including a blood culture; a lumbar puncture is not required for all infants (Ch. 39.2). A blood sample for culture can be taken from the UAC during the sterile insertion routine.
- Send blood for electrolyte measurement: this establishes a baseline and identifies early abnormalities due to problems with maternal fluid balance.
- Measure coagulation levels in ill and bruised babies and those less than 30 weeks' gestation.
- Insert a peripheral cannula for the administration of antibiotics.
- In critically ill infants or those with extremely low birthweight (ELBW), insert umbilical arterial and venous catheters.
- Obtain a CXR, preferably after inserting the UAC.
- Give surfactant, if it has not been given prophylactically in the labour ward (Ch. 13.1).
- Update the parents.

General management of the baby with RDS

Minimal handling

If hypoxic babies are disturbed and handled, their respiration may become very irregular or stop altogether, their right-to-left shunt increases and their Pao_2 falls rapidly. Major disturbances, such as sucking out an ETT, performing a lumbar puncture or taking a CXR, can cause catastrophic falls in Pao_2. The 'minimal handling' maxim dominates the whole approach to managing all sick babies with RDS.

Physiotherapy

In the first 24–48 hours, secretions are not a problem unless infection develops. As a consequence, chest physiotherapy and routine suctioning of the ETT are contraindicated.

Temperature control

The baby's thermal environment should be controlled and, if babies are exposed during any procedure, they should be under a radiant heat source, with as much of their surface as possible covered in order to minimise heat losses.

Blood gas management

Abnormalities of Pao_2, $Paco_2$ and acid–base metabolism are characteristic of RDS, and keeping the blood gases within a reasonably normal range is the single most important component of the treatment. The detailed management of oxygen administration, CPAP and IPPV are covered on pages 517–523.

Pao₂

The Pa_{O_2} drawn from a UAC distal to the ductus should be maintained in the range 7–10 kPa (50–75 mmHg). Nowadays many units use pulse oximetry to monitor preterm infants, but the success of maintaining pulse oximeter saturation levels varies between and within centres (Hagadorn et al. 2005) and this is not a method of monitoring for very prematurely born infants at high risk of ROP.

Paco₂

The Pa_{CO_2} in a normal newborn baby is in the range 4.6–5.4 kPa (35–40 mmHg). Cerebral blood flow increases about 30% with each 1 kPa increase in Pa_{CO_2}. A degree of permissive hypercarbia has been associated with a reduced incidence of BPD (Garland et al. 1995) but comparison, however, of Pa_{CO_2} target levels of 55–65 mmHg (minimal ventilation) and 35–45 mmHg revealed the latter was associated with a trend towards a higher mortality and neurodevelopmental impairment at 22 months of age (Thome et al. 2006). Hypercarbia in the early days of life remains a risk factor for IVH and we advise caution in the use of this approach during the acute phase of RDS (Thome and Carlow 2002; Kaiser et al. 2006). Higher Pa_{CO_2} levels in more mature neonates with RDS and in <1.50-kg infants more than a week old who are being weaned off IPPV are acceptable, providing the baby is clinically stable with satisfactory pH and base excess levels. Hypocapnia (Pa_{CO_2} <3.3 kPa) should be avoided because of its role in the genesis of PVL (Ch. 40.5). A rapidly rising Pa_{CO_2} is a sign of impending respiratory failure, usually associated with a fall in pH, and therefore indicates that the baby should be intubated and ventilated irrespective of postnatal age. More gradual changes with an acceptable pH (>7.25) can be managed conservatively, particularly when the baby is not in the acute phase of illness.

pH

Metabolic alkalaemia is rare and almost always iatrogenic as a result of excessive amounts of intravenous bicarbonate having been given. It requires no therapy. Respiratory alkalaemia is usually due to excessive ventilator pressures.

Acidaemia is common in neonates with RDS. It is always essential to establish whether the acidaemia is respiratory with a raised Pa_{CO_2}, or metabolic with a normal Pa_{CO_2} and a negative base excess, or a combination of a metabolic and respiratory acidosis, which is more usual. The commonest cause of a metabolic acidaemia in a baby with RDS is a raised lactate from anaerobic metabolism. This in turn can be secondary to hypoxaemia, hypotension, anaemia or infection. When a metabolic acidaemia does develop, it is essential to identify the cause, so direct treatment can be instituted – for example, oxygen for hypoxia, antibiotics for infection, transfusion for anaemia or IPPV for exhaustion.

Acidaemia inhibits surfactant synthesis (p. 462) and increases pulmonary vascular resistance (Rudolph and Yuan 1966). Once the pH falls below 7.15, other physiological functions such as myocardial contractility (Beierholm et al. 1975) and diaphragmatic activity (Howell et al. 1985) begin to deteriorate. The sick neonate has difficulty in excreting an acid load (Allen and Usher 1971). Ill VLBW neonates should have their pH kept >7.25 at all times. If the pH is <7.25 with a base deficit <10 mmol/l, intravenous alkali therapy is appropriate, if other therapies are not immediately successful. Inappropriately large or fast infusions of base to correct metabolic acidaemia, however, may cause hypernatraemia or cerebral haemorrhage. Two alkalis have been used in neonatal therapy, sodium bicarbonate and trishydroxymethylaminomethane (THAM); both are effective. The theoretical risk that, following infusion of bicarbonate, the cerebrospinal fluid might become even more acidotic does not seem to apply to the neonate. THAM administration does not give a sodium load or increase the Pa_{CO_2} and is preferable to bicarbonate if the neonate has a high Pa_{CO_2} but apnoea may result and thus THAM should only be given to ventilated neonates. The dose of base to be given is calculated as:

$$\text{Dose (mmol)} = \text{base deficit (mmol/l)} \times \text{body weight (kg)} \times 0.4$$

The rate of infusion should never exceed 0.5 mmol/min. Seven per cent THAM solution contains approximately 0.5 mmol/ml of base.

Blood pressure

All neonates suffering from RDS must have their BP monitored regularly (Ch. 19). It is important to determine whether a baby is hypotensive because he or she is anaemic. In general, the first transfusion should be 15 ml/kg given by infusion over 10–15 minutes if the hypotension is severe in the first hours after birth; thereafter, transfusions of blood or albumin are better given more slowly, at a rate guided by the condition of the neonate, clinical response and the BP rise during the transfusion. Transfusions should also be given to babies who are not hypotensive but have features suggesting hypovolaemia, such as poor capillary filling, peripheral vasoconstriction and a falling pH, coupled with the record of large volumes of blood having been removed for analysis. There is, however, no place for routine plasma expanders soon after delivery (NNNI Trial Group 1996). If the neonate's haemoglobin is not low, saline should be given rather than albumin, because the response to albumin is small and rarely sustained (Emery et al. 1992) and it has adverse effects. If the hypotensive neonate is severely hypoxic or acidaemic, cardiac function may be impaired and the baby will tolerate volume expansion badly, in which case dopamine is the preferred treatment (Gill and Weindling 1993). Dopamine should also be used in those in whom volume expansion has failed to increase BP; trials have shown it to be more effective than dobutamine (Emery and Greenough 1993; Klarr et al. 1994). The actions of dopamine are complex (Seri 1995). At 0.5–2.0 µg/kg/min, dopaminergic actions dilate renal, mesenteric and coronary arteries; from 2 to 10 µg/kg/min, myocardial contractility is increased directly by both α- and β-receptor-mediated actions and also by the release of noradrenaline (norepinephrine) from cardiac adrenergic nerves. At doses above 10–15 µg/kg/min, dopamine begins to show α-adrenergic activity and is a vasoconstrictor of all vascular beds. Initially, therefore, 2–4 µg/kg/min should be given (Seri et al. 1993), increasing the dosage until the BP is acceptable.

If plasma volume expansion plus dopamine does not reverse hypotension, other agents can be tried:

- Dobutamine. This is an isoprenaline analogue with a primarily β-adrenergic inotropic effect on the myocardium, with little peripheral vascular effect, and no specific effect on the renal vascular bed.
- Isoprenaline. This beta-mimetic drug has a chronotropic and inotropic effect and is therefore of greatest benefit if hypotension is accompanied by bradycardia. It is not useful in shock because of its peripheral vasodilator effects.
- Adrenaline (epinephrine). This increases BP by peripheral vasoconstriction plus increased myocardial contractility. Its vasoconstrictor effects on the renal vasculature are clearly undesirable.
- Dopexamine hydrochloride. This is a synthetic catecholamine with predominant β₂-adrenergic and dopaminergic activity. In low doses (2–4 µg/kg/min) it can improve BP and urine

output (Kawczynski and Piotrowski 1996), but at higher doses it reduces systemic vascular resistance.

* Hydrocortisone 1–2 mg may be successful (Helbock et al. 1993).

Maintenance of haemoglobin

There are many reasons for a preterm neonate being anaemic (Ch. 30). There may have been an intrapartum haemorrhage, defective placental transfusion or a twin-to-twin or fetomaternal haemorrhage. Blood loss after birth is iatrogenic, but a sudden drop in the haematocrit/haemoglobin level in a baby with RDS suggests the development of a GMH/IVH (Ch. 40.5). Ill neonates, in particular those who are premature, tolerate haemoglobin levels <13 g/dl (packed cell volume (PCV) <40) poorly (Strauss 1995). This is presumably because of the increase in cardiac output required to meet the oxygen demands of the tissues when there is reduced blood oxygen-carrying capacity. One policy, therefore, is to transfuse all ill neonates when their haemoglobin has fallen below 13 g/dl (PCV <40) (James et al. 1997). Blood for transfusion should be from a cytomegalovirus-negative donor and be partially packed to a haemoglobin level appropriate for a premature baby (PCV 40–45%), but it does not need to be fresh blood, as the adverse metabolic features of 2–3-week-old donor blood are of no clinical significance when given as a 15 ml/kg transfusion over 30–120 minutes. The blood should be irradiated to avoid the risk of graft-versus-host disease (Ch. 30). If the baby has a clinically important patent ductus, he or she should receive furosemide 1.0 mg/kg during the transfusion; otherwise, there is no need to give diuretic cover. Transfusions may be needed several times a week during the acute phase of the illness and should be continued for as long as the baby is ventilated or has BPD requiring more than 30–40% oxygen. With modern transfusion practice, donor exposure can be reduced to a minimum (Ch. 30).

Coagulation abnormalities

Routine administration of fresh frozen plasma soon after birth is of no benefit (NNNI Trial Group 1996), but it is important to check for coagulation disorders, as these may be of sufficient magnitude to require treatment, particularly in a baby who is small for gestational age (Hannam et al. 2003).

If an overt coagulation disturbance occurs, such as DIC or thrombocytopenia, this should be treated by appropriate factor replacement (Ch. 30), but it is also essential to control and reverse the underlying problem, such as hypoxaemia or sepsis, which caused the coagulopathy in the first place.

Fluid and electrolyte balance (see Ch. 18)

Renal function is often impaired in RDS. Urine production may be no more than 1.0–1.5 ml/kg/h, close to the definition of oliguric renal failure (1 ml/kg/h) (Ch. 35.1); however, peripheral oedema is usually due to leaky capillaries. Sodium and potassium do not usually need to be added to the fluid intake for the first 36–48 hours, though the frequent presence of hypocalcaemia in such babies (Chs. 34.3 and 34.4) means that calcium should usually be given (Ch. 17).

Antidiuretic hormone (ADH) levels are raised in babies with RDS, particularly when they are very ill (Rees et al. 1980) or after they develop a pneumothorax (Paxson et al. 1977; Wiriyathan et al. 1986). Babies who develop BPD have particularly raised ADH levels in the first few days after birth (Kavvadia et al. 2000b). Plasma levels of atrial natriuretic peptide are also high in the first few days in babies with RDS (Shaffer et al. 1986). There is a complex interrelationship between atrial natriuretic peptide levels, ductal

shunting with atrial distension in RDS and the postnatal natriuresis that appears to be an integral part of the recovery phase of RDS (Ch. 18) (Kääpä et al. 1995). The increased capillary permeability in RDS results in fluid loss into all tissues, including the lungs.

Analysis of randomised trials demonstrates that restricted water intake significantly increases postnatal water loss and significantly reduces the risk of PDA and NEC (Bell and Acarregui 2008). We therefore recommend that infants with RDS should start on 40–60 ml/kg/24 h of a 10% dextrose solution or a suitable 'standard bag' of total parenteral nutrition (TPN) to avoid catabolism. For further advice on fluid balance, see Chapter 18.

Characteristically, diuresis occurs around the time the baby's lung function improves (Kavvadia et al. 1998). Once this happens, previous constraints on the fluid balance to 40–60 ml/kg/24 h need to be relaxed to prevent dehydration, haemoconcentration and worsening jaundice.

Albumin

Hypoalbuminaemia, with a low colloid osmotic pressure predisposing to tissue oedema, is common in RDS. Infusions of albumin, however, do not improve respiratory function (Gonzales et al. 1986); indeed, they may impair it (Kavvadia et al. 1998) and increase the risk of BPD (Dimitriou et al. 2002c).

Nutrition in RDS

Since the protein and caloric reserves of the VLBW neonate are small, it is essential that some form of nutrition, including protein, is given as soon after birth as possible. Neonates with severe respiratory illness may have an ileus and delayed gastric emptying; bowel sounds are absent and meconium is not passed. Enteral feeding initially may not be feasible in some ventilated babies <1.5 kg or some larger sick neonates. Parenteral nutrition, initially amino acids and glucose, should be given (see Ch. 17). There have been anxieties regarding the use of intralipid in neonates with severe lung disease, in whom it may cause a fall in PaO_2 by increasing pulmonary vascular resistance (Prasertsom et al. 1996).

Milk in the stomach may compromise ventilation, increase the work of breathing (Heldt 1988), lower the PaO_2 and even cause apnoea. In spontaneously breathing babies, respiratory problems may be aggravated by the presence of a nasogastric tube obliterating one-half of the upper airway (Greenspan et al. 1990). However, gastro-oesophageal reflux (GOR), NEC and the physiological changes mentioned do not appear to be a major problem in VLBW neonates (Newell et al. 1989b), even in those who are ventilated and with an indwelling UAC, provided that milk (ideally breast milk; see Ch. 16) is only given to babies with clear evidence of bowel activity. Furthermore, there are powerful reasons for attempting to introduce enteral feeds as soon as possible; the prolonged absence of enteral feeding compromises gut growth, the development of enzymes and normal peristaltic activity, and limits early weight gain. The sooner enteral feeding is attempted in VLBW neonates, the sooner full enteral feeding is established (Lucas et al. 1986; Troche et al. 1995). Thus, once bowel sounds are present in a ventilated neonate who is appropriately grown and has passed meconium, irrespective of whether or not there is an indwelling UAC (Troche et al. 1995), enteral feeding should be started, using if possible the mother's milk (Ch. 16).

Drug therapy in RDS

Antibiotics

It can be difficult to differentiate severe early-onset septicaemia from severe RDS and both conditions may coexist. Without antibiotic treatment, early-onset septicaemia can be fatal within hours (Ch. 39.2). For this reason, all dyspnoeic newborn babies, irrespective of their gestation or CXR appearance, should have appropriate bacterial cultures taken and be treated with antibiotics from the earliest signs of respiratory illness. Penicillin and gentamicin are appropriate therapy as they act synergistically against GBS and are also effective against many of the other organisms that cause early-onset septicaemia and pneumonia. In babies with RDS who are stable or who are improving, antibiotics should be stopped when negative culture results are notified at 48–72 hours.

Diuretics

There have been several trials of diuretics in preterm infants with RDS; no long-term benefits were reported (Brion and Soll 2008). Diuretics should be reserved for infants who are oliguric and have obvious signs of fluid retention and deteriorating lung function. The response to a dose of 1 mg/kg furosemide should be evaluated. If a diuresis does not result, a combination of furosemide and dopamine may be effective.

Vitamins

Vitamin K should be given to all neonates (Ch. 30).

Pulmonary vasodilators

Pulmonary hypertension should be suspected in infants whose hypoxia is more severe than would be anticipated from their CXR appearance. Administration of pulmonary vasodilators can result in an improvement in oxygenation, but all have side-effects (p. 498). Randomised trials have not demonstrated any long-term benefits of administering inhaled nitric oxide (iNO) to prematurely born infants (p. 499) (Finer and Barrington 2009).

Analgesia/sedation

Appropriate analgesia/sedation should be given to ventilated infants (see below and Ch. 25) and analgesia administered prior to a painful procedure being undertaken. Sedation is contraindicated in infants with RDS who are breathing spontaneously. Infants who are electively intubated should receive premedication; effective regimes are a combination of atropine, an analgesic (such as fentanyl) and a muscle relaxant (such as mivacurium or succinylcholine) (Dempsey et al. 2006; Lemyre et al. 2009).

Methylxanthines

Methylxanthines are of proven benefit in apnoea of prematurity (p. 571) and in weaning babies less than 30 days old from IPPV (p. 528). Caffeine with its wider therapeutic margin is the agent of choice. In a large randomised trial, caffeine administration was associated with a lower incidence of BPD and better neurodevelopmental outcome (Schmidt et al. 2006, 2007). In spontaneously breathing babies with RDS, apnoeic attacks are usually a sign of impending ventilatory exhaustion (Davis and Bureau 1987) and are then an indication for IPPV.

Indometacin

The use of indometacin in preventing or treating a patent ductus is discussed in detail in Chapter 28.

Surfactant therapy

Surfactant given as 'rescue' therapy improves the outcome in babies with established RDS, resulting in a reduction in pneumothorax, mortality and the combined outcome of mortality and BPD (Seger and Soll 2009; Soll 2009b).

Method of administration

The surfactant preparation is delivered over a period of a few seconds down the ETT. The surfactant usually disseminates homogeneously (Davis and Whitin 1992), particularly if large rather than small doses are used (van der Bleek et al. 1993). As might be expected, deposition is influenced by gravity, with dependent parts of the lung receiving more of the dose (Broadbent et al. 1995). There seems, however, to be no benefit from manoeuvres aimed at trying to improve the distribution to different lobes (Yukitake et al. 1995).

To avoid mechanical ventilation, surfactant has been given via a thin ETT to spontaneously breating infants receiving CPAP (Kribs et al. 2007). In a subsequent observational study, the same centre reported that technique of administration was associated with increases in the use of CPAP and survival without BPD (Kribs et al. 2008). Appropriately designed trials are required to determine whether such a technique offers long-term advantages.

Mechanism of action

Exogenous surfactant works in two ways: firstly, by coating the alveolar surface and elevating lung volume, thus improving oxygenation and pulmonary perfusion. A fall in PAP and a rise in pulmonary blood flow and left-to-right ductal shunting have been reported in most studies (Seppänen et al. 1994; Hamdan and Shaw 1995), but not all (Bloom et al. 1995). Secondly, exogenous surfactant administration is incorporated into the type II cells and can provide substrate for, or even stimulate, surfactant production (Oetomo et al. 1990; Pinkerton et al. 1994).

Size and number of doses

Although beneficial effects, both clinically and physiologically, are seen after a single dose of surfactant, usually in the range of 100 mg/kg (Corbet et al. 1991; de Winter et al. 1994), most studies show that better results are obtained with more than one dose. The Osiris trial (Osiris Collaborative Group 1992), however, showed no benefit of three or four doses of Exosurf compared with two doses. Meta-analysis has demonstrated that multiple doses give a better outcome than a single dose, with a significant reduction in the pneumothorax rate (Soll 2000b). Meta-analysis of trials of animal-derived surfactants (Soll and Ozek 2009) demonstrated that multiple doses improved oxygenation and decreased the risk of pneumothorax.

Variation in response

Not all babies respond to surfactant. Factors that lead to an unsatisfactory response include the presence of a PDA, cardiogenic shock or PPHN and airleaks, which in some cases will lead to protein leaking on to the alveolar surface, impairing surfactant function (Frantz and Close 1985; Kinsella and Abman 1995). Infants who have been exposed to chorioamnionitis may have a poorer response to surfactant (Been et al. 2010). Failure to respond to surfactant marks out a group of babies with a worse prognosis (Skelton and Jeffrey 1996). Very premature infants may suffer a postsurfactant slump: in an uncontrolled study 70% of affected infants responded to a repeat course after day 6 of life (Katz and Klein 2006).

Different types of surfactant

Natural surfactants, as they more closely mimic the 'physiological' mixture of lipids and proteins (SP-B and SP-C), have a more rapid effect on oxygenation than do synthetic surfactants. Meta-analysis of randomised trials comparing natural and synthetic surfactants demonstrated that the natural surfactant was associated with significant reductions in mortality and pneumothorax and a marginal increase in IVH, but not in grade 3 or 4 IVH (Soll and Blanco 2009). The synthetic surfactant (Lucinactant) containing a polypeptide KL4 composed of lysine and leucine (Cochrane et al. 1996) appears to be as resistant as natural surfactants to the inhibitory effects of proteins on the alveolar surface (Manalo et al. 1996).

Side-effects during the administration of the surfactant

There may be transient hypoxaemia and bradycardia. There were initial anxieties that, following surfactant instillation, there was either a fall (Cowan et al. 1991) or a rise in cerebral blood flow velocity (van Bel et al. 1992) and even an increase in GMH/IVH (Collaborative European Multicentre Study Group 1991). Systemic hypotension and a transient flattening of the electroencephalogram (EEG) were also reported (Cowan et al. 1991; Hellstrom-Westas et al. 1992). More detailed studies have shown little more than a transient perturbation in cerebral haemodynamics, without evidence of cerebral ischaemia, if care is taken with the surfactant instillation (Edwards et al. 1992; Bell et al. 1994; Lundstrom and Greisen 1996) and the pooled data show either no effect or even a slight reduction in the incidence of GMH/IVH following surfactant administration.

Swamping alveolar macrophages with instilled surfactant could, in theory, increase the baby's susceptibility to infection (Schrod et al. 1996), but no clinical evidence has been found of such an association. Anxiety has been expressed that immune responses to exogenous surfactant proteins instilled into the lung would cause short- or long-term problems, but none has been reported. Surprisingly, antibodies to surfactant proteins have been found in both surfactant- and placebo-treated infants (Chida et al. 1991).

Pulmonary haemorrhage (MPH), particularly in ELBW neonates, has been noted following surfactant administration, this was increased (doubled) with the use of a synthetic surfactant (Exosurf) (Stevenson et al. 1992; Raju and Langenberg 1993).

Follow-up studies have not demonstrated any additional neurological deficits in surfactant-treated survivors (Morley and Morley 1990; Long et al. 1995) nor any increase in severe ROP (Termote et al. 1994). Surfactant-treated infants may have improved long-term lung function compared with untreated controls (Abbasi et al. 1993; Yuksel et al. 1993b).

Monitoring

The general principles of monitoring the ill preterm neonate are laid out in Chapter 19.

Complications

Many of the complications are dealt with in detail elsewhere and will be only briefly summarised below.

Airleaks, pneumothorax, pulmonary interstitial emphysema (p. 490)

In the past, some form of airleak was reported in about 5% of babies with RDS who were breathing spontaneously; the incidence doubled with CPAP and rose to as high as 35–40% in babies treated with IPPV plus positive end-expiratory pressure (PEEP) and inspiratory times exceeding 1 second. Nowadays, with the use of synchronised IPPV (p. 517) and surfactant (p. 459), the overall incidence of airleaks is less than 10% in ventilated infants.

Patent ductus arteriosus

The incidence of symptomatic PDA is increased by fluid overload (Bell et al. 1980). A clinically significant ductus in a ventilated preterm baby presents as signs of heart failure and a loud precordial murmur filling systole, frequently extending into diastole. The oxygen and ventilatory requirements increase and affected babies may develop massive pulmonary haemorrhange (p. 509). Management is outlined on pages 511–512.

Germinal matrix/intraventricular haemorrhage (see Ch. 41, part 5)

The development of a large GMH/IVH is usually associated with clinical deterioration characterised by anaemia, increased ventilatory requirements and abnormal neurological signs, which can be subtle (Ch. 40.1). In many cases, smaller GMH/IVHs are asymptomatic and detected only on routine ultrasound. Many aspects of the management of respiratory failure in the neonate are directed towards preventing GMH/IVHs, for example avoiding procedures which might provoke surges in cerebral blood flow, including the avoidance of hypercarbia and wide swings in $Paco_2$ and correcting coagulation disturbances.

Bronchopulmonary dysplasia

This is a most important complication of RDS in terms of morbidity, duration of therapy and associated costs. It is described in detail in Chapter 27, part 3.

Renal failure

One of the purposes of attempting early correction and maintenance of BP, using dopamine to preserve renal perfusion and paying meticulous attention to the fluid balance in babies with RDS, is to sustain renal function. In some cases this is not successful, and in others an acute episode of collapse, such as may occur with bilateral tension pneumothoraces, results in acute tubular necrosis (Ch. 35.1). If renal failure develops, it should be treated as outlined in Chapter 35, part 1. If biochemical control cannot be achieved, then either peritoneal dialysis or haemofiltration may be used. Haemofiltration avoids the major problem with peritoneal dialysis, which is that the intraperitoneal fluid splints the diaphragm and makes oxygenation difficult in ventilated neonates.

Outcome

Survival

Death from RDS in a baby weighing more than 1.5 kg is now exceptionally rare and the overall mortality from the condition has been reduced to between 5% and 10%.

Sequelae

Readmission to a general paediatric ward in the first 2 years after birth is common, but after that age readmissions are infrequent (Greenough et al. 2004). Amongst VLBW infants, infants with birthweight <750 g and gestational age of less than 28 weeks require the greatest number of admissions and longest duration of stay. In the first year, the duration of stay is inversely related to birthweight (Yuksel and Greenough 1994). Readmissions are particularly likely in infants who developed BPD and subsequently suffered a respiratory syncytial virus infection (Greenough et al. 2001). Other causes of readmission include sequelae of surgery for NEC, failure to thrive and repair of an inguinal hernia, which is common in males with a birthweight of less than 1.00 kg.

Respiratory

The most important respiratory sequel of RDS is BPD (Ch. 27.3). Airway problems secondary to prolonged intubation may also occur (p. 610). After discharge, babies who have survived RDS in the neonatal period are more likely to have respiratory illness, particularly in the first year after birth, than are infants born at term or prematurely without respiratory problems. Preterm babies have lung function abnormalities at follow-up: an increased airways resistance and air trapping. These sequelae are more common in neonates who required prolonged ventilation and they are particularly severe in those who developed BPD (Ch. 37.3).

Long-term neurological sequelae

See Chapter 3.

Transient tachypnoea of the newborn

Incidence

This is between 4 and 5.7 (Morrison et al. 1995) per 1000 infants delivered between 37 and 42 weeks of gestation. TTN does occur in prematurely born infants, although coexisting problems such as RDS may mask the presentation; an incidence of 10 per 1000 has been reported in all babies born in 65 hospitals (Dani et al. 1999), which is higher than in term infants.

Aetiology

TTN is due to a delay in fetal lung fluid clearance (Avery et al. 1966a). It is more common in infants who are born by caesarean section without labour (Morrison et al. 1995). In babies who develop TTN, noradrenaline (norepinephrine) levels are lower than in those delivered following labour (Greenough and Lagercrantz 1992). In the absence of labour, anticipatory lung fluid clearance has not occurred (p. 449) (Walters and Olver 1978).

The relative risk for respiratory distress after birth by caesarean section without labour has been reported to be 1.74 if delivery occurs at 37 rather than 38 weeks of gestation (Morrison et al. 1995). Similarly, TTN and RDS were found to be more common in twins delivered by caesarean section if this was performed prior to 38 weeks of gestation (Chasen et al. 1999). Others (Lewis et al. 1996), however, have suggested that respiratory morbidity may only be increased by delivery by caesarean section if this occurs prior to the 36th week of gestation.

Respiratory distress after elective caesarean section in babies born at term may be due to surfactant deficiency per se (Madar et al. 1999), but surfactant deficiency may also be important in the pathogenesis of TTN (James et al. 1984). Other risk factors for TTN include male sex (Dani et al. 1999; Webb and Shaw 2001) and a family history of asthma (Schatz et al. 1991; Demissie et al. 1998; Schatz 1999). The proposed mechanism for the association of TTN and maternal asthma is that infants of asthmatic mothers have a genetic predisposition to β-adrenergic hyporesponsiveness (Schatz et al. 1991). Resorption of fetal lung fluid is a catecholamine-dependent process; it has been reported (Currie et al. 2010) that beta 1 and 2 adrenoreceptor polymorphisms, known to alter catecholamines, are operative in TTN. NO polymorphisms were not detected in the second transmembrane-spanning domain of the epithelial sodium channel (Landmann et al. 2005).

Presentation

The classical presentation is isolated tachypnoea with respiratory rates up to 100–120/min. The infants rarely grunt, which is a sign indicating atelectasis. Retraction, indicating non-compliant lungs, is minimal. The chest may be barrel-shaped as a result of hyperinflation, and the liver and spleen are palpable because of downward displacement of the diaphragm. Peripheral oedema is often present and affected babies lose weight more slowly than controls (Rawlings et al. 1984). On auscultation, there may be added moist sounds, similar to those heard in heart failure. Tachycardia is common, but the BP is usually normal. TTN usually settles within 24 hours, but may persist for several days. Some infants with TTN have been reported to require high concentrations of supplementary oxygen (Halliday et al. 1981), even 100% oxygen for several days (Bucciarelli et al. 1976) or IPPV (Tudehope and Smyth 1979), but whether such patients had TTN is arguable.

Investigations

Affected infants usually have a mild hypoxia; a marked respiratory or metabolic acidosis is unusual, and, if present, makes a review of the diagnosis mandatory. The CXR shows hyperinflation, prominent perihilar vascular markings, oedema of the interlobar septa and fluid present in the fissures (Dani et al. 1999) (Fig. 27.15). The prominent perihilar streaking is due to engorgement of the periarterial lymphatics, which participate in the clearance of lung fluid; fluid may also be present in the costophrenic angles. The CXR usually clears by the next day, although complete resolution may take 3–7 days. Lung ultrasonography shows a difference in lung echogenicity between the upper and lower lung areas in infants with TTN; comet-like tails have been seen in the inferior fields, which were not seen in the healthy controls (Copetti and Cattarossi 2007; Aslan et al. 2008). Infants with TTN have a reduced tidal volume, but a raised minute volume due to the increased respiratory rate. Compliance is reduced; airways resistance and FRC are raised (Sandberg et al. 1987b).

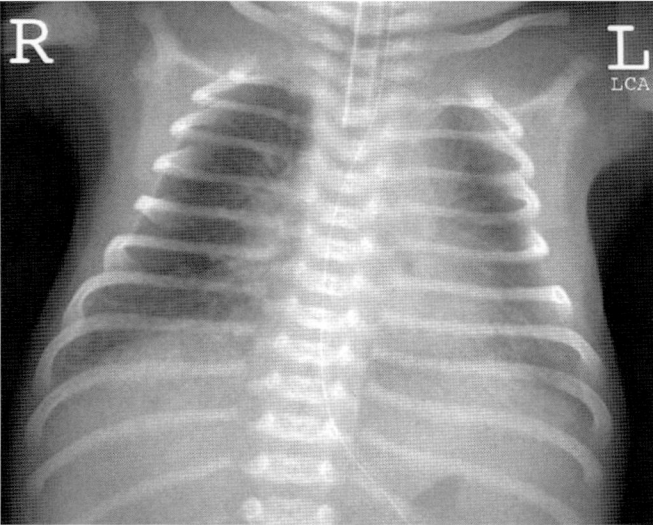

Fig. 27.15 Transient tachypnoea of the newborn. There is fluid in the right horizontal fissure and pulmonary venous congestion.

Differential diagnosis

A rapid respiratory rate may be due to cerebral irritation from sub-arachnoid blood or perinatal hypoxic ischaemia (Ch. 40.3), but these infants are distinguished by their history and the presence of a respiratory alkalaemia. The CXR appearance of TTN may be mimicked by heart failure. If the heart failure is due to asphyxia, there will be a positive history and the heart will usually be enlarged; if it is due to congenital heart disease, a murmur may be present. It is not possible to differentiate TTN from early-onset sepsis (Ch. 39.2) and this needs to be considered when planning the initial treatment.

Prevention

Continuous infusion of terbutaline given to mothers prior to elective caesarean section was associated with improved lung function in their offspring (Eisler et al. 1999), but the mothers who received terbutaline had significantly higher levels of bleeding.

Treatment

Most infants with TTN require no form of respiratory support other than added oxygen and rarely require an inspired oxygen concentration greater than 40% or support for more than 3 days. Intravenous penicillin and gentamicin should be administered until infection has been excluded (Ch. 39.2). Hydration should be maintained with intravenous glucose electrolyte solutions, and nasogastric tube feeds withheld until the respiratory rate settles. Diuretics are of no proven benefit (Wiswell et al. 1985; Lewis and Whitelaw 2002). In a randomised trial, although infants who were given oral furosemide 2 mg/kg followed by 1 mg/kg 12 hours later lost more weight than the placebo group, there were no significant differences between the two groups with regard to the durations of tachypnoea or hospitalisation or the severity of symptoms (Lewis and Whitelaw 2002).

Monitoring

The standard monitoring outlined in Chapter 19 should be applied. A UAC should be inserted if the baby has a persisting requirement for more than 40% oxygen.

Complications

These are rare, though airleaks may occur, particularly if the baby requires CPAP or IPPV.

Prognosis

The condition is self-limiting, although the symptoms may last throughout the perinatal period. There is debate whether babies who have had TTN are more likely to wheeze at follow-up (Shohat et al. 1989; Schatz et al. 1991).

Minimal respiratory disease

Minimal respiratory distress is usually diagnosed if transient respiratory signs persist for less than 4 hours (Hjalmarson 1981).

Aetiology

Some babies are hypothermic, with a temperature of less than 35°C. Surfactant function is temperature-dependent (Gluck et al.

1972) and the babies often improve within an hour or two when their temperature returns to normal. Some babies have a moderately low pH at 7.20–7.25, which may transiently compromise surfactant synthesis (Merritt and Farrell 1976). The tachypnoea may be the result of mild intrapartum asphyxia with or without minor degrees of aspiration of meconium or amniotic squames. In most cases, the condition probably represents the very mild end of the spectrum of delayed clearance of lung liquid, which in the more marked form is diagnosed as TTN.

Clinical features

The baby, near or at term, presents within the first 2–3 hours, commonly after being transferred to the postnatal ward with the mother. The infant usually has an expiratory grunt, which may be quite loud; there is mild sternal or intercostal recession and a respiratory rate of up to 80–100/min. Cyanosis, if present, is relieved by administering 25–30% oxygen. There are no added sounds in the chest and the rest of the clinical examination is normal.

Differential diagnosis

This is always a retrospective diagnosis, made once the baby has recovered and shows no signs of infection or more serious pulmonary disease. The major anxiety when the baby first presents is whether the diagnosis is early-onset sepsis (Ch. 39.2). In some infants with mild pulmonary hypoplasia tachypnoea is the only presenting feature (Aiton et al. 1996); such cases, however, can be distinguished by the persistence of the tachypnoea, small-volume lungs on CXR and abnormal lung function tests.

Investigations

It is advisable to check the infant's blood gas, take a CXR to exclude other diagnoses and undertake a blood count and blood culture. Hypoglycaemia should be excluded, particularly if the baby's mother has diabetes or the baby is small for dates. The blood gas analyses will usually show mild hypoxaemia in air ($Pa{o_2}$ 6–8 kPa, 45–60 mmHg), which rapidly becomes normal in 25–30% oxygen; $Pa{co_2}$ and the pH will usually be normal or there will be a mild metabolic acidaemia, with a pH of 7.20–7.25 and a base deficit of 10 mmol/l. The haemoglobin and white cell count will be normal. The CXR, particularly if taken within 1–2 hours of birth, often shows some streakiness or a rather non-specific haziness, both of which probably represent delayed clearing of the fetal lung liquid, but this is not an indication for an early CXR, i.e. before 4 hours (p. 480).

Treatment

Antibiotics should be given to all infants with respiratory distress, as infection cannot be excluded until the results of the cultures are available at 48 hours after birth.

Prognosis

The prognosis is excellent. Most babies are asymptomatic by 12 hours of age.

Pulmonary airleaks

Pneumothorax and pulmonary interstitial emphysema (PIE) are the most common forms of airleaks in the newborn;

pneumomediastinum, pneumopericardium and pneumoperitoneum also occur. Rarely, multiple airleaks may be complicated by
subcutaneous emphysema and systemic air embolism.

Pathophysiology

Pulmonary airleaks occur when there is uneven alveolar ventilation,
air trapping and high transpulmonary pressure swings; the final
common pathway is alveolar overdistension and rupture. Uneven
ventilation is compounded by a lack of redistribution of pressure
through the alveolar connecting channels, the pores of Kohn, which
are reduced in number in the immature lung (Macklin 1936). The
rupture is thought to occur at the alveolar bases, in apposition to
blood vessels. The gas tracks along the sheaths of pulmonary blood
vessels to the mediastinum, where it accumulates in the roots of the
lungs; air may then rupture into the pleura, mediastinum, pericardium or extrathoracic areas. The existence of PIE supports this
hypothesis, as, after alveolar rupture, gas is trapped in the parenchyma by the extensive connective tissue matrix and increased interstitial water in the preterm lung. This prevents decompression into
the mediastinum, thereby splinting the lung and compressing the
blood vessels. An alternative hypothesis is that interstitial air directly
enters the pleural cavity after rupture of a subpleural bleb (Plenat
et al. 1978).

Pneumothorax

Incidence

An early study (Steele et al. 1971), which involved X-raying the
chest of all newborns, demonstrated that 1% had airleaks, although
only 10% of those with airleaks were symptomatic. The incidence
was reported to be higher if there was associated lung disease or
the neonate was receiving assisted ventilation; 4% of infants with
lung disease developed airleaks, compared with 16% in infants
receiving CPAP and 34% in those requiring mechanical ventilation
(MacFarlane and Heaf 1988). In the last two decades, the incidence
of pneumothorax has decreased in response to the use of surfactant
therapy (p. 459), pancuronium (p. 488) and fast ventilator rates
(p. 519), with most units reporting airleak rates of less than 10% in
ventilated babies.

Aetiology

Spontaneous pneumothoraces may occur immediately after
birth owing to the high transpulmonary pressure swings generated
by the newborn during his or her first breaths (Vyas et al. 1986)
or because of active resuscitation. Familial spontaneous pneumothoraces occurring in neonates are very rare (Engdahl and Gershan
1998). Pneumothoraces in one series (Zanardo et al. 2007) were
commoner following elective than emergency caesarean section
or vaginal births. There was a significant progressive reduction in
the incidence of pneumothorax when the elective caesarean
sections were performed from 37 weeks onwards (Zanardo et al.
2007). Pneumothorax is usually a complication of respiratory
disease, for example RDS or meconium aspiration syndrome
(MAS) or congenital malformations, in which there is uneven ventilation, alveolar overdistension and air trapping, made worse in
many cases by IPPV. Pneumothorax may occasionally result
from direct injury to the lung, for example direct perforation by
suction catheters or introducers passed through the ETT (Anderson
and Chandra 1976; Vaughan et al. 1978) or by central venous
catheter placement (Gabwell et al. 2000). Malposition of the ETT

is associated with an increased risk of pneumothorax (Niwas
et al. 2007).

Components of ventilatory support have been incriminated in
increasing the incidence of airleak. These include high levels of
PEEP (Berg et al. 1975), but the data were not from a randomised
study. A prolonged inflation time was also noted to be a risk factor
(Primhak 1983), perhaps because of provocation of active expiration against the ventilator (Greenough 1988). The higher (50%
versus 16%) incidence of airleak with an inspiratory : expiratory
(I : E) ratio of >1.0 : 1 compared with an I : E ratio of <0.7 : 1 (Tarnow-
Mordi et al. 1985) might also be explained by a similar mechanism.
Both high peak inspiratory (Oh and Stern 1977; Greenough et al.
1984a) and mean airway pressures (MAPs) increased the incidence
of airleaks (Tarnow-Mordi and Wilkinson 1985). Airleaks occur
in babies who have started to exhale while the ventilator is still
trying to inflate their lungs (active expiratory reflex) (Greenough
et al. 1983).

Clinical features

Small pneumothoraces may be asymptomatic, but, when a large
pneumothorax develops, all of the clinical features of respiratory
distress may be present. In addition, with very large or tension
pneumothoraces, the infant's overall condition usually deteriorates,
often dramatically, with pallor, shock and deterioration in oxygenation. An increased resonance on percussion may be detected and
there is a decrease in air entry on the affected side. A tension pneumothorax will result in a shift of the mediastinum and the position
of the cardiac impulse; there is also abdominal distension due to
displacement of the diaphragm and, with a right-sided pneumothorax, downward displacement of the liver. At the time of a pneumothorax, there is a marked increase in cerebral blood flow velocity,
which correlates closely with the systemic haemodynamic changes
(Hill et al. 1982). Pneumothorax is associated with haemorrhage
into the germinal layer and ventricles of preterm infants. Increased
levels of arginine vasopressin may also occur, resulting in fluid
retention (Ch. 35.1).

Diagnosis

Continuous monitoring of the heart rate, BP and $Paco_2$ will give
warning of the baby's deterioration. Transillumination with an
intense beam from a fibreoptic light is of considerable help in the
preterm baby with a thin chest wall: abnormal air collections cause
increased transmission of light on the involved side; however, PIE
can give a similar appearance. The CXR remains the gold standard
for diagnosing pneumothorax and should be done unless the
infant's clinical condition makes emergency drainage mandatory.
The diagnosis of a pneumothorax on the CXR is usually obvious,
but rarely the appearance of either lobar emphysema or cystic adenomatoid malformation of the lung may resemble a pneumothorax
(Liang et al. 2000). A small pneumothorax may only be recognised
by a difference in radiolucency between the two lung fields (Fig.
27.16). A large pneumothorax will be associated with absent lung
markings and a collapsed lung on the ipsilateral side (Fig. 27.17).
A tension pneumothorax will be demonstrated by eversion of
the diaphragm, bulging intercostal spaces and mediastinal shift
(Fig. 27.18).

Ill, ventilated infants are usually nursed in the supine position
and intrapleural air rises to lie retrosternally. Retrosternal air is best
demonstrated by a horizontal-beam, lateral-view CXR (Fig. 27.19),
which is also useful in demonstrating the position of the chest drain
tip (see below; Fig. 27.20).

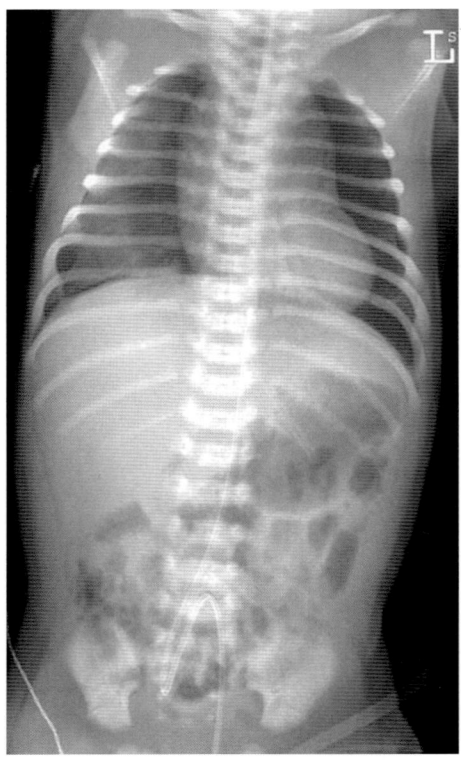

Fig. 27.16 Bilateral pneumothoraces. Note bulging at the intercostals' margins. The difference in the translucency of the two sides indicates that there is more free air on the left.

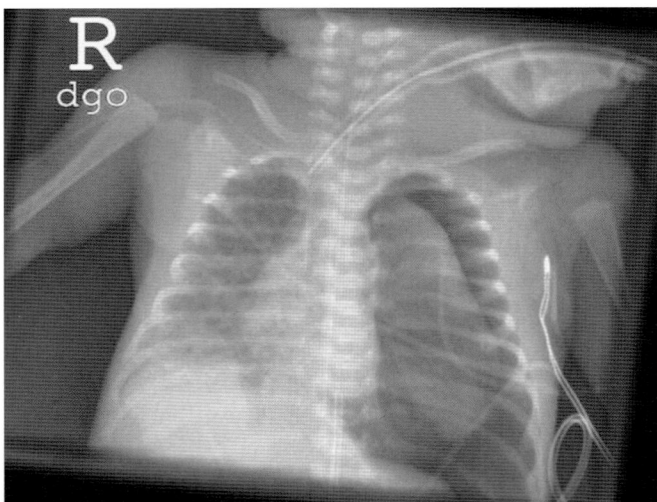

Fig. 27.17 Large left-sided tension pneumothorax. Note that the non-compliant lung has only partially collapsed.

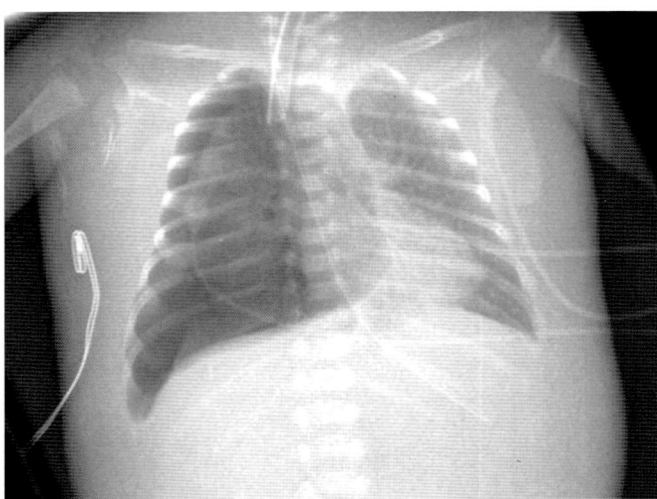

Fig. 27.18 Large right-sided tension pneumothorax with bulging over the midline and compression of the left lung.

Prevention

The risk of pneumothorax can be reduced by administering surfactant (p. 459), by using the minimum ventilator pressure required (p. 517) and by abolishing the baby's active expiratory efforts.

Paralysis/sedation

Breathing out of phase with the ventilator during IPPV increases the incidence of pneumothorax (see above). Neuromuscular blocking agents should only be given selectively, that is, to infants who are actively expiring against the ventilator (Greenough et al. 1984b). Meta-analysis of six trials in which routine neuromuscular paralysis was compared with no routine paralysis demonstrated that no significant difference was found in airleak, mortality or BPD, but there was a signicant reduction in IVH (Cools and Offringa 2009). In subgroup analysis of trials in which a selected group of infants with evidence of asynchronous respiratory effort were studied, there was a significant reduction in IVH of all grades and a trend towards less airleak (Cools and Offringa 2009). It was concluded, therefore, that for ventilated preterm infants with evidence of asynchronous respiratory effort, neuromuscular paralysis with pancuronium seems to have a favourable effect on IVH and possibly on pneumothorax. Active expiration may be difficult to detect clinically at slow rates; however, if a neonate's oxygenation fails to improve and obvious respiratory efforts continue as the ventilator rate is increased to 60–80/min, this identifies the majority of neonates with a persisting active respiratory pattern who are likely to benefit from paralysis (Greenough and Greenall 1988). Infants who receive neuromuscular blocking agents, such as pancuronium, require higher peak pressures when the first dose is given, to maintain oxygenation; ventilator rates should be reduced to <60/min to avoid gas trapping

(Hird et al. 1990). Other neuromuscular blocking agents include vecuronium, atracurium and cistracurium. A single dose of vecuronium has been shown to reduce hypoxaemic episodes without impairing lung function (McEvoy et al. 2007).

Many clinicians prefer to avoid use of neuromuscular blocking agents and administer analgesics and/or sedatives to try and suppress respiratory activity, but also to minimise any discomfort felt by a ventilated baby (Ch. 25). Stress hormone levels have been demonstrated to be significantly related to the severity of illness and to fall with sedation (Barker and Rutter 1996). Administration of analgesics and/or sedatives, although having benefits, has not been demonstrated in randomised trials to reduce the pneumothorax rate (Lago et al. 1998) and they have side-effects. In a randomised trial (Orsini et al. 1996), fentanyl administration was associated with a reduction in stress markers, but no improvements in long-term outcome. Fentanyl can cause muscle rigidity and precipitate movement disorders, and withdrawal symptoms can occur. Plasma fentanyl clearance increases with maturity; thus gestational age should be

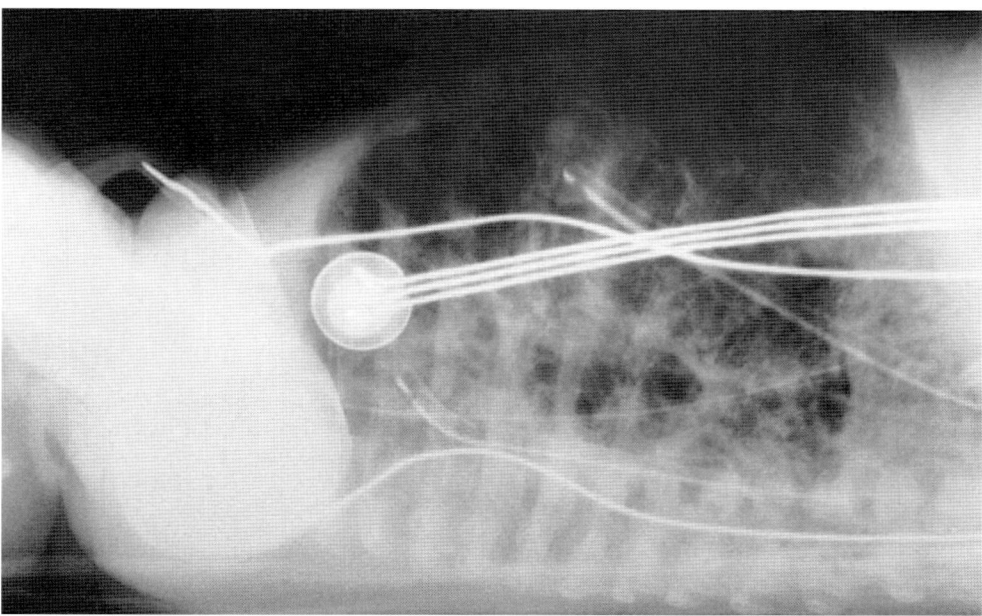

Fig. 27.19 Lateral chest X-ray with anterior collection of air. Only one chest drain is positioned to lie anteriorly; the other tip lies posteriorly and the pneumothorax has been inadequately drained.

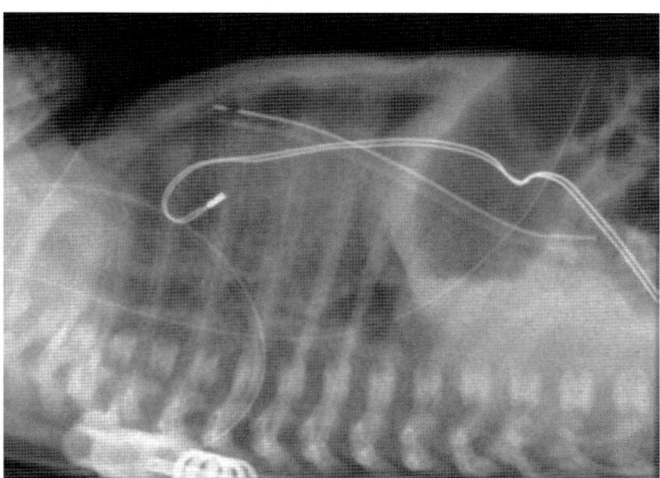

Fig. 27.20 Lateral chest X-ray demonstrating a correctly anteriorly placed tip of a chest drain.

taken into account when prescribing fentanyl (Saarenmaa et al. 2000). Naloxone is an effective antidote to fentanyl. Morphine, compared with placebo, significantly reduced adrenaline (epinephrine) concentrations in ventilated neonates, but did not influence the occurrence of airleak (Quinn et al. 1993). Morphine does not appear to be associated with adverse effects on intelligence, motor function or behaviour at follow-up (MacGregor et al. 1998), but should be used with caution in prematurely born infants, because of its low clearance, which correlates with gestational age (Saarenmaa et al. 2000). In a large ($n = 898$) randomised trial (Bhandari et al. 2005), morphine infusion did not improve short-term pulmonary outcomes amongst ventilated infants and additional analgesia with morphine was associated with more airleaks and longer durations of high-frequency ventilation, nasal CPAP and oxygen therapy. In addition, secondary data analysis from that randomised trial demonstrated that use of morphine delayed the attainment of full feeds, partly by delaying the start of feeding, although its use did not increase gastrointestinal complications (Menon et al. 2008). Diamorphine may be preferable to morphine, as in a randomised trial (Wood et al. 1998) both agents reduced the stress response to ventilation, but diamorphine had a more rapid onset of sedation and did not have morphine's tendency to increase hypotension. Midazolam is sedative in ventilated babies (Jacqz-Aigrain et al. 1994), but it does not influence the course of RDS and in high doses it causes respiratory suppression, hypotension and reduced cerebral blood flow. Long-term use can result in accumulation and an encephalopathic illness has been described. Midazolam is reversed by flumazenil. Midazolam is not as effective a sedative as chloral (Northern Neonatal Network 2000), but chloral can cause gastric irritation and its metabolite is hepatotoxic.

Modes of ventilation

High-frequency positive-pressure ventilation

Ventilating babies at rates of >60/min rather than at 30–40/min reduced the incidence of airleaks (Bland et al. 1980; Heicher et al. 1981). Those data were subsequently confirmed by the results of two multicentre randomised studies (Octave Study Group 1991; Pohlandt et al. 1992). Meta-analysis of the results of the randomised trials (Greenough et al. 2008) demonstrated that the risk for airleak at the faster compared with the slower rate was significantly reduced. The most likely explanation for the reduction in airleak at the faster frequency was that spontaneous respiration synchronises with the ventilator at fast rates (Greenough et al. 1984a), whereas infants actively expire at slow rates. There have, however, been no randomised trials comparing different ventilator rates in infants routinely exposed to antenatal steroids and postnatal surfactant; whether fast rates are more effective than slow rates in preventing pneumothoraces in such a population remains unknown.

Patient-triggered ventilation

Meta-analysis of the results of randomised trials demonstrated that the incidence of airleak was not reduced by use of patient-triggered ventilation (PTV) (Greenough et al. 2008). During pressure support ventilation (PSV), both the initiation and termination of ventilator inflation are determined by the infant's respiratory efforts. PSV does reduce the rate of asynchrony (Dimitriou et al. 1998a), but a reduction in the incidence of pneumothorax has not been reported.

High-frequency oscillation

Meta-analysis of the results of randomised trials has demonstrated that high-frequency oscillation (HFO) does not reduce the incidence of pneumothorax in preterm infants (Henderson-Smart et al. 2007). In a randomised trial (HiFO Study Group 1993), use of HFO was associated with a reduction in the incidence of pneumothorax, but this was at the expense of an increase in intracerebral haemorrhage (ICH).

Treatment

Asymptomatic pneumothoraces need no treatment, other than careful observation of the infant. In term infants with mild symptoms, a pneumothorax may respond to increasing the inspired oxygen concentration to 100%, which will favour resorption of the extra-alveolar gas; but this strategy should not be used in prematurely born infants at risk of ROP. Expectant management can be successful in infants who have relatively mild disease, i.e. on lower ventilatory settings and better blood gases (Litmanovitz and Carlo 2008). However, there is always a risk of the pneumothorax becoming a tension pneumothorax and there should be a low threshold for inserting a chest drain in a ventilated baby.

A pneumothorax must always be drained using a chest drain in symptomatic infants and those with tension pneumothoraces. If the infant is in extremis and there is no time for formal insertion of a chest drain, emergency drainage of a pneumothorax can be done by needle aspiration. A butterfly needle (18 G) should be used. This is then attached to a three-way tap, which is held under water in a small sterile container. The needle is inserted through the skin in the second intercostal space anteriorly, and then the skin and needle are moved sideways before advancing the needle through the underlying muscle; this reduces the likelihood of leaving an open needle track for entry of air once the needle has been removed. Care must be taken not to remove too much air by needle aspiration, as the needle might then tear the expanding lung. Following emergency drainage, a chest tube should be inserted (Ch. 44).

Insertion of a chest tube (10–14 FG) should be performed under local anaesthesia through either the second intercostal space just lateral to the midclavicular line or the sixth space in the midaxillary line (see Ch. 44). The tip of the chest tube should lie retrosternally to achieve the most effective drainage. A retrospective review of 149 cases of chest drain placement (Allen et al. 1981) revealed that inserting the chest drain through the anterior chest wall achieved retrosternal positioning in 85% of occasions compared with only 47% inserted through the lateral chest wall. The lateral site, however, is preferred for cosmetic reasons, as any resultant scar is less obvious. Retrosternal placement of the chest tube tip should be confirmed by CXR (Chs. 43, 44); a second drain is only infrequently required to ensure complete drainage if the first drain has been appropriately sited.

Complications of malpositioned chest tubes include traumatisation of the thoracic duct resulting in a chylothorax, cardiac tamponade due to a haemorrhagic pericardial effusion and phrenic nerve injury; the latter complication is more likely if the drainage tube is positioned deep in the chest (Williams et al. 2003). Once inserted, the tube should be connected to an underwater seal drain with suction applied at a level of 5–10 cmH$_2$O. Heimlich valves are useful during transport, but can become blocked and so fail to operate if left in situ for any length of time. Once a chest drain has been inserted, it should be left in situ for at least a further 24 hours after it has ceased bubbling. The chest tube should then be clamped for a further few hours and only removed if no pleural air accumulates. Pneumothoraces persisting for an average of 10 days may respond to fibrin glue, but this treatment has been reported to have significant risks (Sarkar et al. 2003).

After drainage of an uncomplicated pneumothorax, a baby not on IPPV usually improves rapidly. In a ventilated, very prematurely born baby, a pneumothorax often precipitates a serious deterioration in condition, with the development of a large intracerebral bleed.

Bronchopleural fistula

A large tear in the pleural surface of the lung, a bronchopleural fistula, may not close with conventional tube drainage of the pneumothorax. Alternative strategies are surgical closure at thoracotomy (Grosfeld et al. 1980), selective bronchial intubation (see below) (Al-Nishi et al. 1994) or instillation of fibrin glue into the pleural space (Berger and Gilhooly 1993).

Prognosis

The mortality, although not the incidence, varies with birthweight and is in general double that of babies who have RDS but no airleak. If a parenchymal haemorrhage occurs in association with a pneumothorax (Ch. 40.5), this has a detrimental effect on neurological outcome.

Pulmonary interstitial emphysema

Aetiology

PIE is gas trapped within the perivascular sheaths of the lung. In the surfactant-deficient lung of the preterm infant (Plenat et al. 1978), rupture of the small airways occurs distal to the termination of their fascial sheath, and air dissects into the interstitium. PIE occurs mainly in neonates with RDS (Campbell 1970), but has been less frequently reported in infants with aspiration syndromes or sepsis. PIE is associated with positive-pressure ventilation, high peak inspiratory pressures and malpositioned ETTs (Hart et al. 1983; Greenough et al. 1984a). It has rarely been described in spontaneously breathing infants (Dembinski et al. 2002). PIE may be lobar in distribution, but more commonly involves both lungs. It frequently occurs with either a pneumothorax or pneumomediastinum.

Incidence

There is an inverse relationship between the incidence of PIE and birthweight (Hart et al. 1983).

Pathophysiology

In infants with PIE, the trapped gas reduces pulmonary perfusion by compressing the vessels and interferes with ventilation. As a result, there is profound hypoxaemia combined with carbon dioxide retention.

Presentation

PIE is found on the CXR of a severely ill neonate carried out either on a routine basis or because the baby's condition was deteriorating.

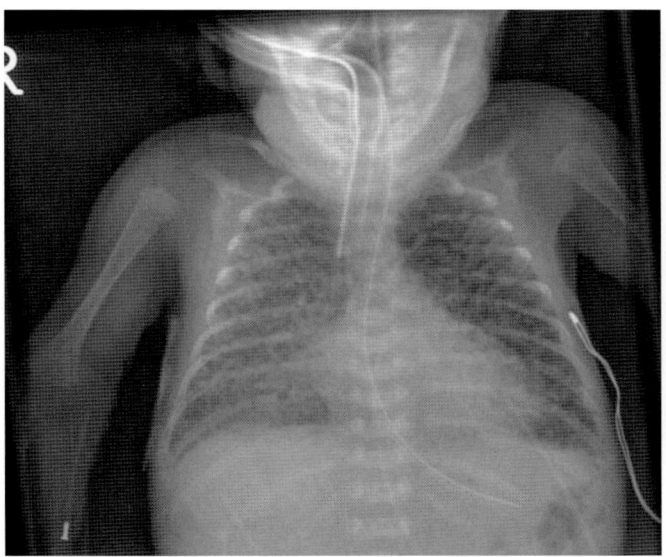

Fig. 27.21 Bilateral pulmonary interstitial emphysema.

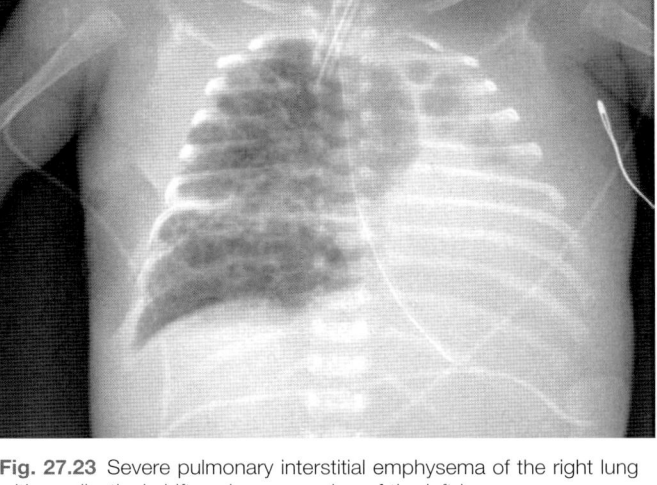

Fig. 27.23 Severe pulmonary interstitial emphysema of the right lung with mediastinal shift and compression of the left lung.

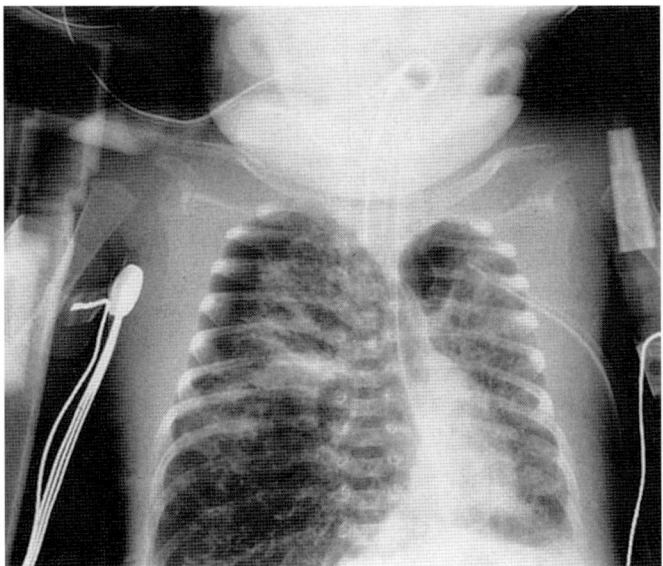

Fig. 27.22 Gross pulmonary interstitial emphysema (PIE) of the right lung with overdistension and downward displacement of the diaphragm and moderately severe PIE of the left lung.

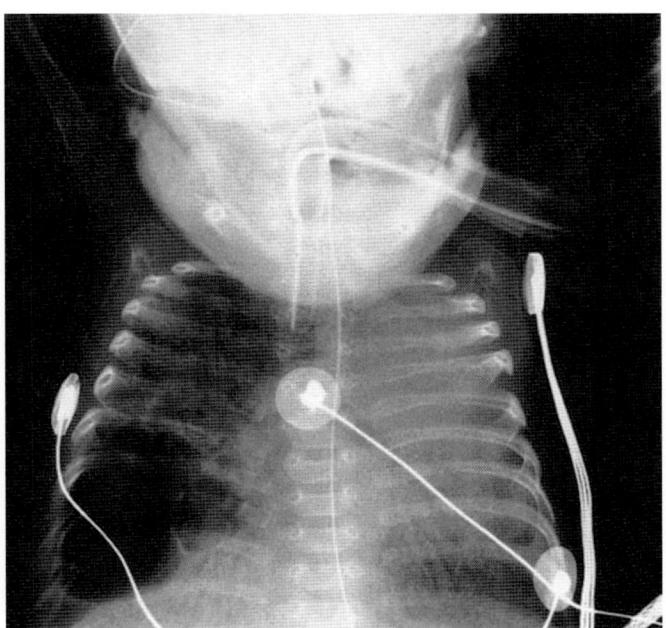

Fig. 27.24 Pulmonary interstitial emphysema of the right lung with gross cystic changes in the right middle lobe compressing the right lower lobe and left lung.

Diagnosis

Transillumination of the chest with diffuse PIE will give the same appearance as a large pneumothorax. The CXR, however, is diagnostic, demonstrating hyperinflation and a characteristic cystic appearance, which may be diffuse, multiple, small, non-confluent, cystic radiolucencies (Figs 27.21 and 27.22), which may be unilateral (Fig. 27.23); at a later stage, large bullae may appear (Fig. 27.24). The appearance may be confused with lobar emphysema or with cystic adenomatoid malformation of the lung.

Treatment

Affected babies usually have severe RDS and/or sepsis; their ventilator management is particularly difficult. For both generalised and localised disease, ventilator pressures should be kept at the minimum compatible with acceptable gases (Pao_2 <6–7 kPa (45–52 mmHg), pH >7.25); the baby should be paralysed to minimise the risk of extension of the airleaks. Withdrawal of PEEP may result in disappearance of the PIE (Leonidas et al. 1975).

Generalised PIE may respond to increasing the ventilator rate to 100–120/min (Ng and Easa 1979), in that the number of babies who progress to pneumothorax may be reduced, but there were no other advantages. Indeed, in one series (Greenough et al. 1984a), the severity of the PIE increased, possibly because of the absence of a pneumothorax decompressing the interstitial emphysema. Transfer from conventional ventilators to high-frequency jet ventilation (HFJV) (Pokora et al. 1983; Boros et al. 1985), high-frequency flow interruption (Frantz et al. 1983) or oscillation (Clark et al. 1986)

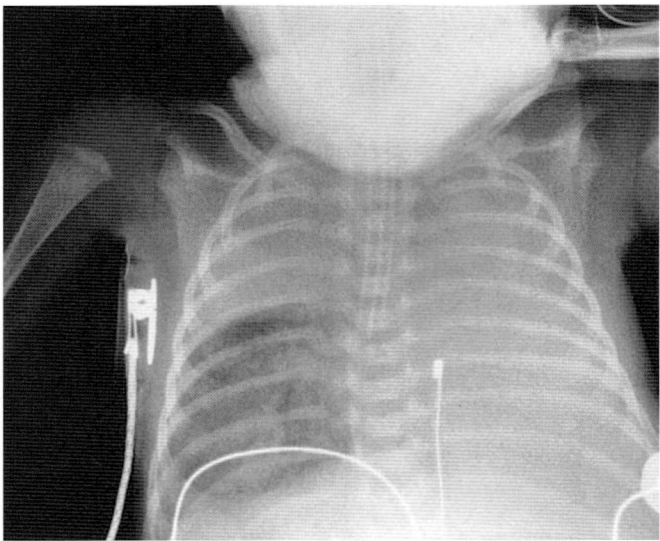

Fig. 27.25 Endotracheal tube inserted into the right main bronchus with resultant collapse of the left lung and right upper lobe.

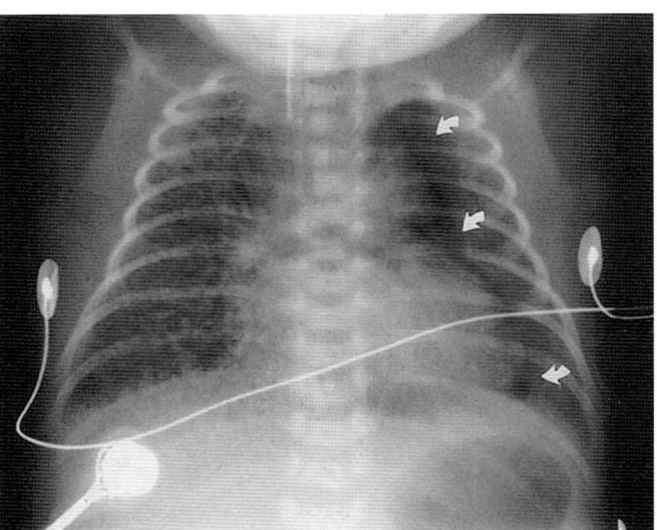

Fig. 27.26 Left-sided pneumomediastinum (between the arrows and the heart border).

has improved oxygenation in some infants with severe respiratory failure due to PIE, but a randomised controlled trial failed to show that HFO had benefit in PIE (HiFO Study Group 1993). HFJV has been reported in a randomised trial to be more successful support than rapid-rate conventional ventilation (Keszler et al. 1991); survival and the incidence of BPD, GMH/IVH, PDA, airway obstruction and airleak, however, were similar in the two groups.

The conservative ventilatory management outlined above for generalised PIE should also be tried for localised disease and is often successful. In addition, in localised PIE, placing the infant with the hyperinflated lung dependent in the lateral decubitus position at all times can result in partial or complete atelectasis of the desired segments (Cohen et al. 1984; Swingle et al. 1984). In this position, the upper 'good' lung receives a greater proportion of the ventilation (Heaf et al. 1983); the affected dependent lung is underventilated and hence decompresses. Selective bronchial intubation may also be useful. As soon as the affected lung is bypassed, it becomes atelectactic (Fig. 27.25). If selective intubation is maintained for 24–48 hours, when the affected lung is reventilated the PIE does not usually recur (Brooks et al. 1977; Chan and Greenough 1992; Al-Nishi et al. 1994). This technique is more useful if the left lung is affected, as selective intubation of the right main bronchus is easier to perform. It may be necessary to support the infant on high-frequency oscillatory ventilation (HFOV) to maintain adequate blood gases during selective intubation (Rettwitz-Volk et al. 1993). The collections may persist and compress the adjacent normal lung parenchyma, causing a sudden deterioration in the infant's condition. Resection of the affected area may be required to alleviate the respiratory distress.

Prognosis

The incidence of BPD is greatly increased following diffuse PIE (p. 490) (Stahlman et al. 1979; Yu et al. 1983) and radiologically the changes of PIE may merge imperceptibly into those of BPD. The mortality from diffuse PIE is high, but studies reporting outcome generally predate routine use of antenatal steroids and postnatal surfactant (Hart et al. 1983; Greenough et al. 1984a; Morisot et al. 1990).

Pneumomediastinum

Pneumomediastinum occurs in approximately 2.5 per 1000 live-births, in those babies with gas trapping associated with RDS, pneumonia, MAS and mechanical ventilation.

Presentation

An isolated pneumomediastinum may be asymptomatic or the infant may have mild respiratory distress; it only rarely causes severe symptoms. The sternum may appear bowed and the heart sounds muffled. Mediastinal shift rarely occurs. Air may track up into the soft tissues of the neck, but this is uncommon. Pneumomediastinum often coexists with multiple airleaks, including PIE and pneumothorax, in severely ill, ventilated babies (Fig. 27.26).

Diagnosis

This is made on the CXR (Fig. 27.26), as a halo of air adjacent to the borders of the heart, and on lateral view it produces marked retrosternal hyperlucency. The mediastinal gas may elevate the thymus away from the pericardium, resulting in a cresentic configuration resembling a spinnaker sail (Moseley 1960).

Treatment

An isolated pneumomediastinum is often asymptomatic and in general requires no treatment. It is very difficult to drain a pneumomediastinum, as the gas is collected in multiple independent lobules. Relatively successful attempts have been made, however, with multiple needling and tube drainage (Taylor et al. 1993). In term infants, use of a high inspired oxygen concentration will be associated with resorption of the extra-alveolar air, but this should not be attempted in preterm infants at risk from ROP.

Pneumopericardium

A pneumopericardium usually causes cardiac tamponade with sudden hypotension, bradycardia and cyanosis. The heart sounds are muffled, but a friction rub is rarely audible. The signs may be

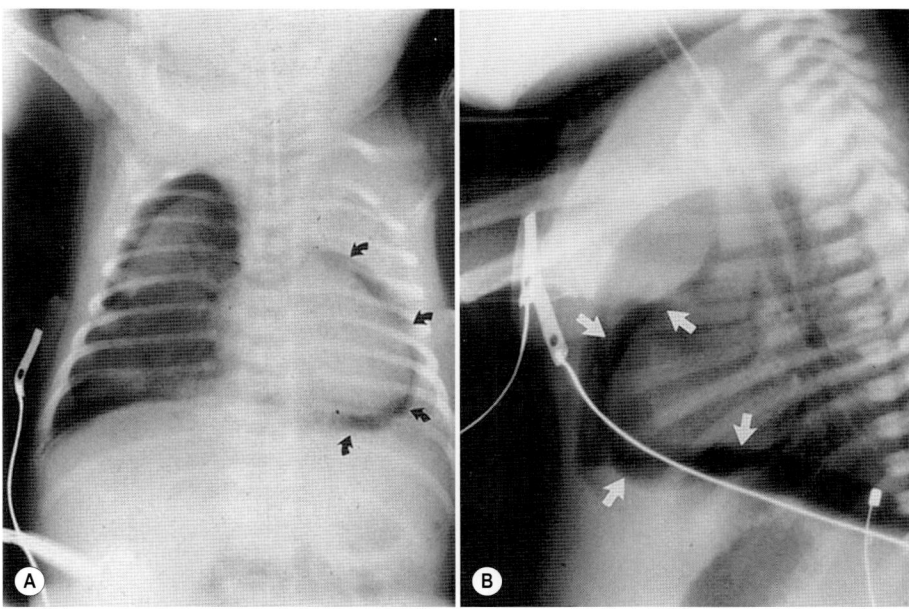

Fig. 27.27 Pneumopericardium: (A) anteroposterior view; (B) lateral view. There is also a right pneumothorax.

confused with those of a tension pneumothorax, but the CXR is diagnostic (Fig. 27.27). It is usually accompanied by other major airleaks such as pneumomediastinum, widespread PIE or tension pneumothorax.

Aetiology

Pneumopericardium rarely occurs spontaneously (Itani and Mikati 1998) or in babies supported by CPAP (Heckman et al. 1998). The majority of cases occur in ventilated, prematurely born babies. Its frequent association with PIE and pneumomediastinum suggests that the gas enters the pericardium through a defect in the pericardial sac, probably at the pericardial reflection near the ostia of the pulmonary veins.

Diagnosis

The CXR demonstrates gas completely surrounding the heart (Fig. 27.27), outlining the base of the great vessels and contained within the pericardium. Gas can be seen inferior to the diaphragmatic surface of the heart, differentiating this abnormality from a pneumomediastinum in which the mediastinal gas is limited inferiorly by the attachment of the mediastinal pleura to the central tendon of the diaphragm. In a haemodynamically significant pneumopericardium, the transverse diameter of the heart is significantly reduced.

Treatment

A conservative approach can be adopted for small asymptomatic lesions. All symptomatic pneumopericardia should be drained immediately by direct pericardial tap via the subxiphoid route. The BP should be monitored continuously, and the tap repeated if bradycardia or hypotension recurs. Catheter drainage may be necessary if the pericardial air reaccumulates.

Prognosis

The mortality rate for symptomatic pneumopericardium is between 80% and 90% (Hook et al. 1995) and many survivors have neurological sequelae.

Pneumoperitoneum

This may result from perforation of the gut, but may also be caused by air dissecting from the chest through the diaphragmatic foramina into the peritoneum (Aranda et al. 1972) (Fig. 27.28), particularly in ventilated babies who already have a pneumothorax and a pneumomediastinum. In some cases, the gas localises in the connective tissue on the posterior wall of the abdomen, a pneumoretroperitoneum (Karlowicz 1994).

Diagnosis

If the pneumoperitoneum is large, the diagnosis can be made from the anteroposterior X-ray (Fig. 27.29). For smaller leaks, a horizontal-beam lateral or right lateral X-ray is required (Fig. 27.30). Rupture of the bowel, usually due to NEC, can generally be excluded by the absence of a history of gastrointestinal disease, in particular bloody stools or intestinal obstruction, and a normal gut gas pattern on erect abdominal X-ray. If there is still doubt, differentiating a pneumoperitoneum caused by transdiaphragmatic air dissection from one due to perforated bowel can be made by measuring the Po_2 of aspirated intraperitoneal gas (Vanhaesebrouck et al. 1989). In ventilator-induced pneumoperitoneum, the intraperitoneal Po_2 is very high, reflecting the PAo_2, whereas the Po_2 of a surgical pneumoperitoneum is similar to that of room air or lower.

Treatment

If the abdomen is not under sufficient tension to cause respiratory embarassment, then no treatment is necessary. If there is tension,

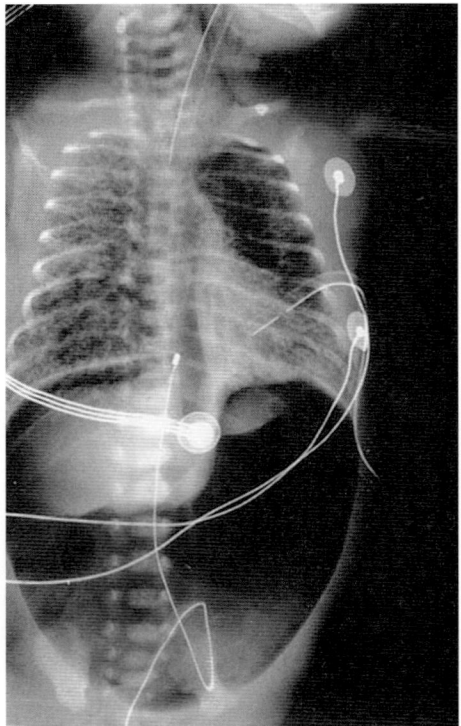

Fig. 27.28 Pneumoperitoneum associated with gross pulmonary interstitial emphysema.

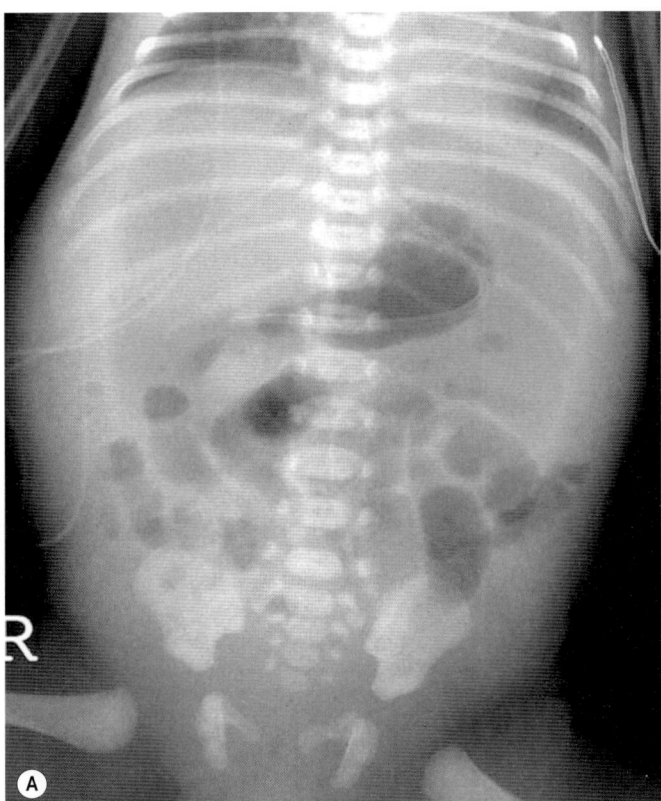

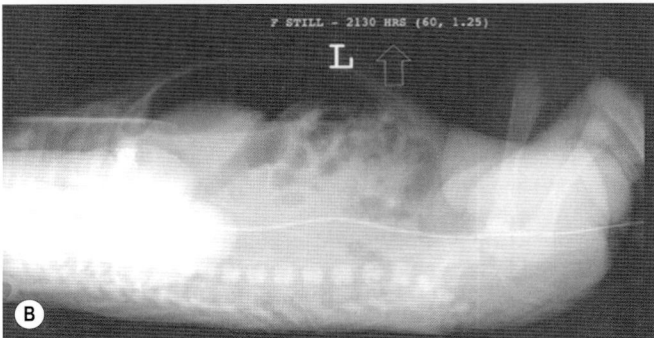

Fig. 27.29 Pneumoperitoneum due to gastrointestinal perforation. (A) Anteroposterior view shows the classic 'football' sign. (B) The lateral X-ray of the same infant shows a large collection of free air above the liver.

the peritoneum should be drained either by needle aspiration or by inserting a drainage tube.

Systemic air embolism

This is a rare complication of IPPV. Affected infants are usually premature, have severe pulmonary insufficiency necessitating very high ventilator pressures (>40 cmH$_2$O) and the majority (94%) have other airleaks (Lee and Tanswell 1989). This condition has, however, been reported in infants supported by CPAP (Wong et al. 1997). It is associated with a sudden and catastrophic deterioration in the baby's condition, with pallor or cyanosis, hypotension and bizarre ECG irregularities.

Pathogenesis

Gas embolism results from alveolar–capillary or bronchovenous fistulae, which have been demonstrated by barium studies at autopsy. Such communications are more likely to occur in airleak syndromes, but may also follow trauma to the lung. Laceration of lung tissue favours reversal of the intrabronchial pressure–pulmonary venous pressure gradient, thereby increasing the risk of pulmonary vascular air embolism.

Diagnosis

On the CXR, gas can be seen in the systemic and pulmonary arteries and veins (Fig. 27.31). Gas can be withdrawn from the umbilical venous or arterial catheters, and this has been observed in over half the reported cases.

Treatment

Early withdrawal of air from the UAC may be of benefit, particularly if the leak is small or has been introduced through an intravascular line.

Prognosis

This condition is usually fatal (Lee and Tanswell 1989).

Subcutaneous emphysema

This condition, with air tracking into the neck or other subcutaneous tissues, is usually associated with a pneumomediastinum. It requires no treatment. A localised subcutaneous collection of air

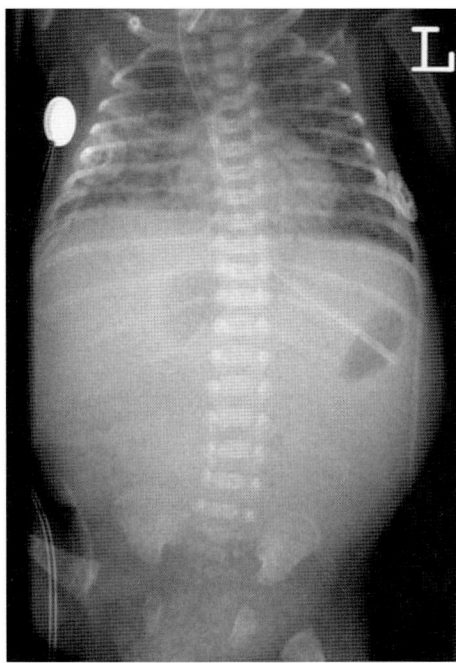

Fig. 27.30 Pneumoperitoneum indicated on the anteroposterior view by a small amount of non-anatomical air to the right of the vertebral column.

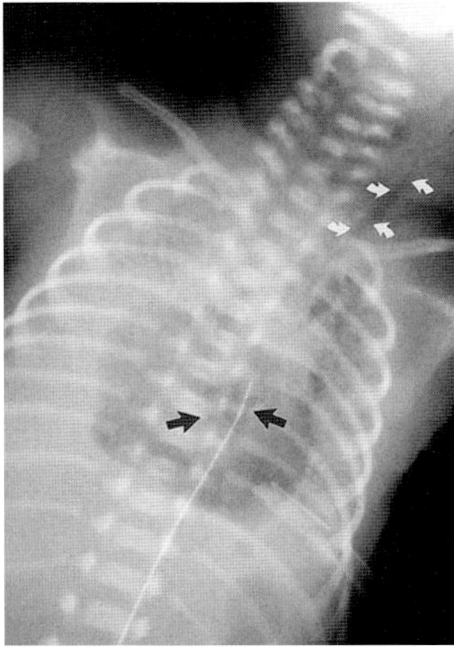

Fig. 27.31 Postmortem X-ray of a baby who died from systemic air embolism. Gas can be seen (black arrows) within the heart and in the great vessels in the neck (white arrows).

under tension – a bronchocutaneous fistula – has been described (Baildam et al. 1993).

Persistent pulmonary hypertension of the newborn

The dominant pathophysiological feature of PPHN is a high PAP. This condition has been called persistent fetal circulation, but this term should be avoided, as one of the characteristic features of the fetal circulation, the high-flow, low-resistance circuit through the placenta, is missing.

Definition and classification

Persistent fetal circulation syndrome was first used by Gersony et al. (1969) to describe babies who had a structurally normal heart, but large right-to-left shunts at atrial and ductal levels secondary to pulmonary hypertension. It is now understood that PPHN is the common endpoint of several different pathophysiological mechanisms. PPHN is present when an infant with an echocardiographically confirmed structurally normal heart has:

- severe hypoxaemia, usually a Pao_2 5–6 kPa (37.5–45 mmHg) in an F_1o_2 of 1.0 and IPPV if necessary
- mild lung disease, but the hypoxaemia is disproportionately severe for the radiological, clinical and acid–base abnormalities
- evidence of a right-to-left ductal shunt (usually a Pao_2 in the distal aortic (UAC) blood 1–2 kPa (7.5–15 mmHg) lower than simultaneous preductal (right radial artery) Pao_2 estimation); in the absence of a ductal shunt; a large shunt may be demonstrated echocardiographically at the foramen ovale (Valdes-Cruz et al. 1981).

There are a number of distinct syndromes which can result in a baby developing PPHN:

- Primary PPHN or PPHN in the presence of mild neonatal lung disease. Those with primary disease are the babies originally described by Gersony et al. (1969) who are profoundly hypoxic but have no clinical or autopsy evidence of lung disease. This entity merges into PPHN in babies who have disproportionately severe hypoxaemia from what appears clinically, radiologically and on $Paco_2$ measurements to be mild parenchymal lung disease. There is now considerable evidence to suggest that this entity is due to excessive muscularisation of the pulmonary arterial system starting in the antenatal period (see below), perhaps aggravated by perinatal asphyxia (Reece et al. 1987).
- PPHN secondary to severe perinatal asphyxia. In these babies, hypoxia and acidaemia, both of which are powerful pulmonary artery constrictors (Lyrene and Philips 1984), prevent the normal postnatal changes in circulation. The tendency to PPHN may be increased in such neonates by similar structural changes in the vasculature to those outlined above and the large right-to-left shunt may be aggravated by systemic hypotension secondary to postasphyxial myocardial damage (Cabal et al. 1980).
- PPHN secondary to infection. This particularly severe form of the disease, characteristically associated with GBS sepsis, is probably due to the release of vasoactive substances.
- PPHN secondary to pulmonary hypoplasia. This is characteristic of neonates with diaphragmatic hernia, and is due to the abnormal development and reduced cross-sectional area of the pulmonary vasculature (Geggel and Reid 1984).

- PPHN secondary to drug therapy. This has been reported after the use of prostaglandin synthetase inhibitors before delivery. One survey demonstrated that mothers of inborn term babies with PPHN were 9.6 times more likely to have taken aspirin in pregnancy and 17.5 times more likely to have taken other prostaglandin synthetase inhibitor drugs (van Marter et al. 1996). These drugs, either by a direct effect on the pulmonary vasculature or by closing the fetal ductus, cause fetal pulmonary hypertension which persists postnatally (Levin et al. 1979; Turner and Levin 1984). It is probably the result of changes in the pulmonary arterial musculature similar to those reported in primary PPHN (Levin et al. 1978) (Fig. 27.32). Administration of ibuprofen, a cyclo-oxygenase inhibitor, in the first 6 hours after birth has been associated with the development of pulmonary hypertension (Gournay et al. 2002).
- PPHN secondary to alveolar capillary dysplasia. Several reports have appeared of babies with clinical PPHN in whom, at postmortem, there appeared to be misalignment of the pulmonary vessels and poor apposition of the vessels to the alveoli (Cater et al. 1989). This condition is fatal and does not respond to extracorporeal membrane oxygenation (ECMO) (Chelliah et al. 1995).
- PPHN secondary to congenital heart disease. Conditions that obstruct the venous outflow from the lungs or cause myocardial failure can cause pulmonary hypertension and/or marked right-to-left shunting with hypoxaemia. They are considered in detail in Chapter 28.
- Iatrogenic PPHN secondary to overventilation (p. 517).

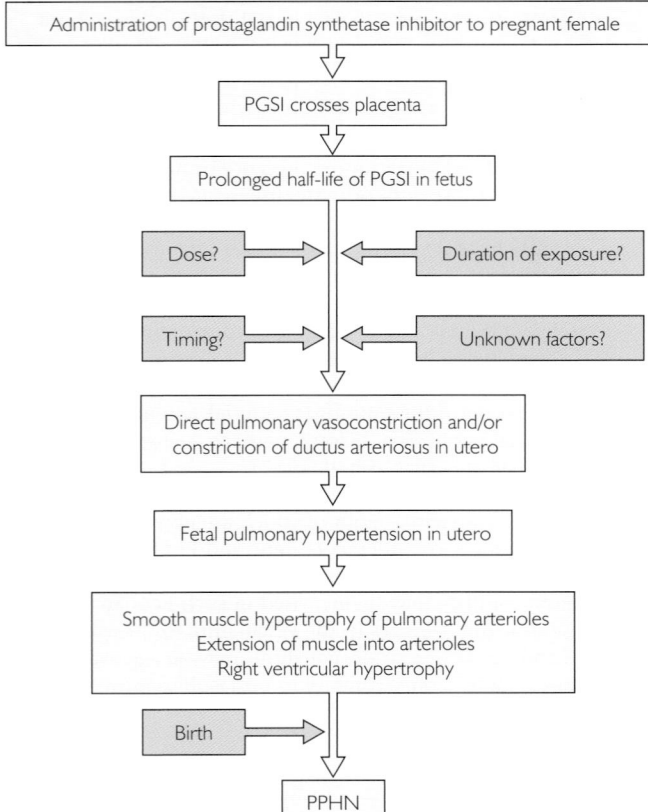

Fig. 27.32 Mechanism of drug-induced persistent pulmonary hypertension of the newborn. PGSI, prostaglandin synthetase inhibitor. *(Reproduced from Turner and Levin (1984).)*

Pathophysiology

The pathognomonic feature of this condition is the presence of pulmonary hypertension, producing right-to-left shunts at the level of the ductus arteriosus and the foramen ovale (Duara and Fox 1986; Skinner et al. 1996). The comparatively small difference between pre- and postductal Pa_{O_2} levels, rarely greater than 2–3 kPa (15–21 mmHg), however, suggests that only a small component of the shunt occurs at duct level and the majority is through the foramen ovale (Valdes-Cruz et al. 1981). PAP is at or above systemic levels. Skinner et al. (1996) have shown that a marked reduction in left ventricular function is a significant marker of severe disease.

Abnormal pulmonary vasculature

Infants with PPHN have abnormal pulmonary vascular reactivity, structure and/or growth. In postmortem studies on babies with PPHN, virtually all secondary to meconium inhalation, the muscularity of the pulmonary arteries is markedly increased (Murphy et al. 1981, 1984). Not only is the amount of muscle in the vessel wall increased, but also the muscle extends to vessels surrounding the alveoli, whereas in the normal baby muscular pulmonary arteries rarely extend past the terminal bronchiole. The exact intrauterine events that increase pulmonary vascular reactivity and impair structure are poorly understood. Impaired vascular epidermal growth factor (VEGF) signalling, however, can cause fetal pulmonary hypertension with structural remodelling, right ventricular hypertrophy and impaired pulmonary vasodilation in experimental models (Grover et al. 2003). Chronic intrauterine pulmonary hypertension can markedly decrease lung VEGF expression; selective inhibition of VEGF mimics the structural and physiological changes of experimental PPHN (Grover et al. 2003). Babies with PPHN have lower blood VEGF levels than controls (Lassus et al. 2001). Postnatally, sustained pulmonary hypertension rapidly accelerates pulmonary vascular injury, with aggressive smooth-muscle proliferation and remodelling. Initially the effects of hypertension are at least partially offset by release of endogenous vasodilators, but this may not be sustained (Abman et al. 1996).

Vasoactive agents

NO is a potent pulmonary vasodilator, active in the transition of the circulation at birth (p. 450). A significant rise in pulmonary blood flow at birth is related to the acute release of NO; vasodilation occurs through cGMP kinase-mediated stimulation of K^+ channels (Cornfield et al. 1996). Other vasodilator products, including prostaglandin (PG) I_2, also modulate changes in pulmonary vascular tone at birth. NO modulates PGI_2 activity in the perinatal lung (Zenge et al. 2001). Adenosine release may also contribute to the fall in pulmonary vascular resistance; this may be through enhanced production of NO (Konduri and Mital 2000).

Endothelin-1 is a potent pulmonary vasoconstrictor; the plasma level is raised in neonates with hypoxia (Kourembanas et al. 1991) and severe PPHN (Rosenberg et al. 1993; Kumar et al. 1996). Increased circulating levels of endothelin-1 mediate in part GBS-induced pulmonary hypertension (Navarrete et al. 2003). Raised levels of the constrictor leukotrienes LTC4 and LTD4 have been found in the blood of some, but not all, neonates with PPHN when compared with ventilated neonates without this complication; the levels fall with successful therapy (Stenmark et al. 1983; Hammerman et al. 1987; Kühl et al. 1989; Dobyns et al. 1994). In the PPHN accompanying sepsis due to GBS or other organisms (Shankran et al. 1982; Gibson et al. 1988; Waites et al. 1989), including viruses (Toce and Keenan 1988), there is initial severe arterial spasm followed by increased vascular permeability and an increased lung fluid content and lymph flow (Rojas et al. 1983; Sandberg et al. 1987a; Philips et al. 1988). In these babies it is thought that thromboxane A_2 (Runkle et al. 1984; Hammerman et al. 1987; Gibson et al. 1988) is responsible and that it has its effect without affecting the morphometry of the pulmonary vasculature (Barefield et al. 1994). In animal models, PPHN, but not the haematological features of GBS sepsis, can be prevented by treatment with drugs which inhibit thromboxane A_2 synthesis, such as indometacin (Runkle et al. 1984), and reversed by intravenous infusion of the vasodilator prostaglandin PGE_2 or isoprenaline (Brigham et al. 1988; Crowley et al. 1991). The increased capillary permeability in sepsis-induced PPHN appears to be due to the action of bacterial endotoxins sequestering white cells in the lungs (Rojas and Stahlman 1984; Sandberg et al. 1987a), where they release vasoactive agents such as tumour necrosis factor. There is an additional effect of thromboxane A_2 since, as with the short-term effects on the pulmonary vasculature, long-term effects can be mitigated by the use of indometacin.

Vascular hypoplasia

The PPHN of diaphragmatic hernia and other conditions associated with pulmonary hypoplasia is due to a reduction in the number of intralobar arteries and their increased muscularity (Geggel et al. 1985).

Blood gas changes/asphyxia

A fall in pH causes pulmonary vasoconstriction in experimental animals (Rudolph and Yuan 1966; Rudolph 1977), and hypoxia is a potent vasoconstrictor (Lyrene and Philips 1984). Neonatal pulmonary vasculature is extremely sensitive to changes in pH, Pao_2 and $Paco_2$ (Cassin et al. 1964). Therefore, perinatal and postnatal hypoxaemia and metabolic or respiratory acidaemia can cause marked pulmonary arterial spasm, pulmonary hypertension, a large right-to-left shunt and PPHN, particularly in babies with prenatal pulmonary arterial muscular hypertrophy.

Polycythaemia

A rise in haematocrit in experimental animals causes pulmonary hypertension. The factors involved, however, are not clear, since a rise in pulmonary vascular resistance is not seen if fetal blood as opposed to adult blood is used to raise the haematocrit (Fouron et al. 1985) and polycythaemia is not a consistent feature of neonates with PPHN (Fox and Duara 1983).

Heredity

Familial cases have been reported.

Clinical features

In babies with primary PPHN, the presentation is often subtle and may mimic that of cyanotic congenital heart disease. Babies with primary PPHN virtually always present within 12 hours of birth and very rarely after 24 hours. In PPHN which is secondary to pre-existing lung disease, the clinical features will be those of GBS sepsis (Ch. 39.2), RDS (p. 476) or MAS (p. 503), together with the cyanosis of severe PPHN. Secondary effects from the hypoxia, such as acidaemia and hypotension, may be present. The age at diagnosis still depends on the underlying problem and its severity. In GBS infection (Ch. 39.2), severe asphyxia (Ch. 40.4) and congenital diaphragmatic hernia (CDH; p. 593), PPHN will appear within 6 hours of birth in a critically ill neonate.

The baby remains cyanosed even when high oxygen concentrations are administered by IPPV. Respiratory distress, however, is often mild. The respiratory rate is usually increased to 60–100/min; the higher rates are seen in term babies. Retraction is mild, grunting rare and the air entry is normal. The heart rate is normal or slightly increased. All pulses, including the femorals, are normal. The first heart sound is normal, but the second is commonly single and loud because of the rise in PAP. There is a right parasternal heave and a soft systolic murmur may be heard, signifying tricuspid incompetence or, occasionally, mitral incompetence. Heart failure is not usually present, but the infant may be hypotensive. Examination of the abdomen, genitourinary system and the central nervous system is usually normal in the absence of predisposing factors such as sepsis or asphyxia.

Differential diagnosis

Cyanotic congenital heart disease, which presents in the first 12 hours, is usually a severe form, with heart failure, distinctive murmurs and obvious changes on the CXR and ECG. In PPHN, however, the CXR and ECG are often within the normal limits, and the findings on examination of the cardiovascular system are comparatively subtle (see above).

Echocardiography will establish the normal cardiac anatomy in PPHN. The response to ventilation with 100% oxygen may differentiate PPHN from cyanotic congenital heart disease (Fox and Duara 1983). In the former, the Pao_2 will usually increase to >13 kPa (100 mmHg), whereas in cyanotic heart disease it will not rise above 5–6 kPa (37.5–45 mmHg). Not all neonates with PPHN, especially those with sepsis and CDH, however, respond in this way.

Investigations

Haematological and biochemical

Thrombocytopenia has been reported in severe cases (Segal et al. 1980); it may be a manifestation of abnormal prostaglandin activation.

Blood gases

In both primary and secondary PPHN, maximal Pao_2 values of 6 kPa (45 mmHg) are characteristic, often with a difference of at least 1–2 kPa (7.5–15 mmHg) between preductal and postductal Pao_2 (Ch. 19). At diagnosis there may be a metabolic acidaemia, but respiratory acidaemia, by definition, is unusual. Metabolic acidaemia can be controlled by an initial infusion of base, followed by BP support and maintaining the haematocrit above 40%. A resistant acidosis is a feature of either the terminal stages of PPHN or some other underlying problem – in particular, overwhelming sepsis.

Chest X-ray

In secondary PPHN, the X-ray will be that of the underlying lung disease, although, by definition, the appearance will be less severe than anticipated for the severity of the hypoxaemia. In primary PPHN, the CXR changes are often minimal (Fig. 27.33); there may be a mild non-specific increase in lung markings, but little else is noted.

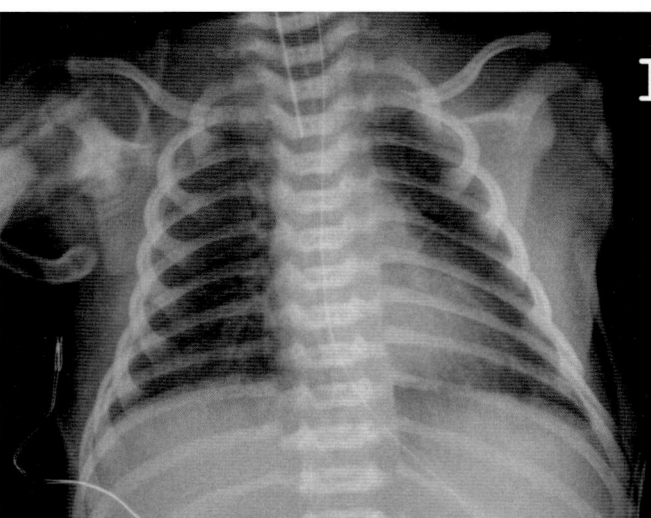

Fig. 27.33 Chest X-ray of an infant with primary persistent pulmonary hypertension of the newborn with absence of lung field markings.

Electrocardiogram

Various ECG changes have been reported in neonates with PPHN. The ECG may be normal, or more typically shows changes of right axis deviation, right atrial enlargement and right ventricular hypertrophy and overload (Henry 1984). In babies who develop PPHN following severe asphyxia, the ECG may show the changes of sub-endocardial ischaemia (Appendix 3).

Echocardiography

Echocardiography is an essential investigation in suspected PPHN, and if the skill is not available a cyanosed baby requires transfer to a centre where this can be done. Firstly, and most importantly, it will exclude the various forms of cyanotic congenital heart disease by showing a normal cardiac anatomy. Secondly, pulmonary hypertension, right-to-left shunting at the ductal and foramen ovale level and ventricular function can be assessed (Skinner et al. 1996).

Bacteriology

PPHN can be secondary to sepsis; thus it is important that the infant is screened for infection (Ch. 39.2).

Treatment

The treatment of PPHN can be divided into two components: that of the hypoxaemia and PPHN and that of the coexisting lung disease, which is covered elsewhere.

Minimal handling

It is important to adhere to the 'minimal handling' maxim. Slight disturbance, for example turning the baby or taking the baby's temperature, may precipitate severe hypoxaemia, and interventions such as ETT suctioning or physiotherapy can have devastating effects. Monitoring must therefore be continuous and interference with the baby reduced to an absolute minimum. ETT suctioning should be carried out only when essential to maintain ETT patency; chest physiotherapy is contraindicated.

Blood pressure and blood volume

The size of the right-to-left shunt is in part dependent on the systemic BP (see above); thus, in babies born at term, the systemic BP should be maintained at a mean of at least 40 mmHg, with a systolic of 50 mmHg. Aggressive therapy should be used to achieve an appropriate systemic BP, including volume challenges and, particularly, administration of inotropes. The haemoglobin level should be kept greater than 13 g/dl (PCV 40%) in order to maximise oxygen transport to the tissues. If polycythaemia (central PCV <70–75%) is present, the existence of PPHN is one of the situations in which a dilutional exchange transfusion is justified.

Coagulation disorders

If present, these should be corrected by appropriate factor replacement.

Fluid and electrolyte balance

Electrolyte abnormalities and hypoglycaemia must be corrected and pH and base deficit kept within normal limits by use of THAM or bicarbonate as appropriate. Urine output must be carefully monitored.

Antibiotics

Broad-spectrum antibiotic cover should be given to all babies with PPHN.

Respiratory support

Once a baby's Pao_2 falls below 5–6 kPa (37–45 mmHg) in 70% oxygen, the baby should be ventilated. Sufficient peak pressure should be used to achieve a $Paco_2$ of not greater than 4.8–5.5 kPa (35–40 mmHg) and a pH <7.30. The inspired oxygen concentration should be increased as necessary to achieve a Pao_2 of at least 8–9 kPa (56–63 mmHg). For the full-term baby prone to fight the ventilator, neuromuscular blocking agents should be used; in this situation there are theoretical reasons for preferring D-tubocurarine to pancuronium (Hutchinson and Yu 1980).

PPHN unresponsive to conservative treatment

Alkalinisation

This was described first by Peckham and Fox (1978). Reduction of the $Paco_2$ to 2.5–3.5 kPa (19–26 mmHg) and elevation of the pH to 7.55–7.60 resulted in a rise in Pao_2. Hyperventilation is no longer advocated, because a $Paco_2$ of 2.5–3.5 kPa (19–26 mmHg) results in a 50% reduction of cerebral blood flow, which could cause cerebral ischaemia. Although in babies born at term no long-term adverse sequaelae have been described, hypocapnia in preterm babies has been linked to PVL (Griesen et al. 1987; Ikonen et al. 1992) and marked hypocapnia (2.5 kPa (19 mmHg)) may reduce cardiac output (Cartwright et al. 1984). Hyperventilation, via barotrauma, may also result in airleaks (Fox 1982) and BPD (Fox and Duara 1983; Beck 1985). In addition, persisting hypocapnic alkalaemia markedly increases the hypoxic reactivity of the pulmonary vasculature, thus tending to perpetuate the pathophysiology of PPHN (Gordon et al. 1993).

High-frequency oscillation: jet ventilation

Anecdotally, these forms of respiratory support have been associated with improvements in oxygenation (Kohelet et al. 1988; Spitzer et al. 1988; Varnholt et al. 1992).

Extracorporeal membrane oxygenation

ECMO is an effective rescue therapy for infants with PPHN (UK Collaborative ECMO Trial Group 1996) (see p. 525).

Vasodilator drugs

Tolazoline

Tolazoline is no longer the drug of choice for PPHN. Between 25% and 50% of babies with primary PPHN or PPHN secondary to RDS or MAS respond to this agent, but the effects on the systemic circulation are at least as great as those on the pulmonary vasculature, and side-effects, including significant hypotension, are common. Other side-effects have been reported and include renal failure and gastrointestinal haemorrhage (Ward 1984). Side-effects may be minimised by a dilute, slow infusion (Nuntnarumit et al. 2002), but we recommend that iNO be considered first.

Prostacyclin

Prostacyclin (PGI_2) affects vascular tone by increasing cAMP levels. This agent, in doses of 5–40 ng/kg/min, is an effective pulmonary vasodilator, but has a wide list of side-effects (Petros 1995).

Endotracheal administration of tolazoline (Curtis et al. 1993) or PGI_2 (Kelly et al. 2002) can cause selective vasodilation. Inhalation of PGI_2 in animals and babies has been shown to be at least as effective as the parenteral preparation, with fewer side-effects, and to cause an equivalent response to iNO (Bindl et al. 1994; Zobel et al. 1995). High doses of aerosolised PGI_2, however, could spill over into the systemic circulation, and thus the magnitude of the dose administered is critical if this therapy is to be a selective pulmonary vasodilator.

Iloprost is a PGI_2 analogue; it has advantages over PGI_2 in that it has a longer half-life and does not need to be dissolved in an alkaline solution, which is potentially damaging to the lung. There are case reports of it improving oxygenation in infants poorly responsive to iNO (de Luca et al. 2007).

Magnesium sulphate

As a loading dose of 200 mg/kg followed by an infusion of 20–100 mg/kg/h, it is effective (Tolsa et al. 1995; Wu et al. 1995) but less so and with more side-effects than iNO (Ryan et al. 1994). During magnesium therapy, levels must be carefully monitored, as hypermagnesaemia can cause sedation, muscle relaxation, hyporeflexia, and calcium and potassium disturbances. Magnesium sulphate has not been assessed in appropriately designed randomised trials; its use cannot therefore be recommended (Ho and Rasa 2007).

Inhaled nitric oxide

NO is a vasodilator substance that relaxes vascular smooth muscle. It is synthesised in the endothelial cells from L-arginine and oxygen (Edwards 1995). Neonates who suffer from PPHN may have low levels of arginine (Vosatka et al. 1994), but this is not a universal finding (Kavvadia et al. 1999). NO diffuses into the smooth-muscle cells, where it activates guanylate cyclase to increase 3,5-GMP and hence produces relaxation of the smooth muscles. When NO is inhaled, it diffuses across the alveolar capillary membrane and activates guanylate cyclase in the pulmonary arteriolar smooth muscle. The resulting increase in cGMP causes smooth-muscle relaxation. NO then binds rapidly to haemoglobin; once bound, it is inactivated and therefore produces no systemic effects.

Clinical studies. Since the preliminary studies of Kinsella et al. (1992) and Roberts et al. (1992), there have been many reports of the benefit of NO in PPHN. The efficacy of iNO is improved if it is combined with a strategy to improve lung volume (Wilcox et al. 1994; Kinsella and Abman 1995). iNO can be delivered with either HFJV or HFOV (Coates et al. 2008). In infants with PPHN and severe lung disease, the combination of HFOV and iNO is better than iNO or HFOV alone (Kinsella et al. 1997). Even in patients with moderate PPHN, iNO can increase arterial oxygenation and reduce the amount of ventilatory support required (Sadiq et al. 2003). Not all term babies, however, respond: a poor response has been seen in those with severe parenchymal disease, systemic hypotension and myocardial dysfunction, as well as in those with structural pulmonary abnormalities, for example infants with pulmonary hypoplasia or dysplasia, who can develop a sustained dependence on iNO (Goldman et al. 1996).

In term-born babies, meta-analysis of the results of nine randomised trials demonstrated that use of iNO was associated with an improvement in oxygenation and a reduction in the combined outcome of death or need for ECMO; the effect was due to a reduction in the need for ECMO (Soll 2009a). No excess of adverse neurodevelopmental outcomes has been demonstrated in babies exposed to iNO in randomised trials (Neonatal Inhaled Nitric Oxide Study Group 2000; Field et al. 2007; Konduri et al. 2007). No significant long-term benefits of iNO have been demonstrated in babies with CDH and they have a higher incidence of sensorineural hearing loss (Neonatal Inhaled Nitric Oxide Study Group 1997).

Meta-analysis of 11 randomised trials demonstrated that the effect of iNO in preterm babies depends on the timing of administration and the population (Barrington and Finer 2007). Early rescue treatment based on oxygenation criteria did not affect mortality or BPD rates and there was a trend towards an increase in ICH. Early, routine use for intubated infants, however, was associated with a just significant reduction in the combined outcome of death or BPD (relative risk (RR) 0.91, 95% confidence interval (CI) 0.84–0.99) and a reduction in the incidences of severe ICH and PVL (RR 0.70, 95% CI 0.53–0.91). One study, however, was from a single centre (Schreiber et al. 2003) and in the other (Kinsella et al. 2006) the positive effects were only in infants with a birthweight between 1000 and 1250 g. In a subsequent large trial ($n = 800$), in which preterm infants were randomised to early, prolonged, low-dose iNO therapy, no significant differences were demonstrated in any important outcomes (Mercier et al. 2010). In the meta-analysis, overall use of iNO after 3 days based on an elevated risk of BPD showed no effect on BPD (Barrington and Finer 2007). In one trial (Ballard et al. 2006), however, the rate of survival without BPD at 36 weeks' postmaturational age was higher in the iNO group, who were also discharged home sooner and received supplementary oxygen for a shorter time (Ballard et al. 2006). At follow-up of that trial, the iNO-treated infants received significantly less bronchodilators, inhaled and systemic steroids, diuretics and supplemental oxygen after discharge, but there were no significant differences in the rates of rehospitalisation or wheezing (Hibbs et al. 2008).

iNO delivery. Studies in term infants have demonstrated that levels of 5 ppm may be equally as effective as higher doses (Davidson et al. 1998; Wood et al. 1999), but lower doses (2 ppm) are not (Cornfield et al. 1999). Indeed, initial treatment with a subtherapeutic dose of iNO may diminish the clinical response to higher doses and have adverse sequelae (Cornfield et al. 1999). It has been recommended to start at 20 ppm in term newborns with PPHN; increasing to 40 ppm does not generally improve oxygenation in infants who have failed to respond to 20 ppm (Kinsella 2008). iNO can be delivered during transport; the method of delivery is influenced by the mode of transport either by road or by air (Lutman and Petros 2008).

NO has a very short duration of action; thus, rebound vasoconstriction and hypoxaemia can result if the NO is suddenly withdrawn. Therefore, to prevent sudden withdrawal of NO during routine nursing procedures, in-line suction devices are recommended to prevent interrupting the circuit and handbagging circuits should contain an additional iNO source. It is important to wean iNO as soon as oxygenation has improved and the baby has stabilised, otherwise tolerance may occur. During weaning from iNO, the level should be gradually reduced; decreasing to 1 ppm minimises the deterioration in oxygenation (Davidson et al. 1999). Increasing the inspired oxygen concentration by 10–20% immediately prior to cessation of iNO may also be helpful. Scavenging is not necessary in a well-ventilated environment (8–12 air changes per hour) but, even so, environmental checks are recommended to reassure staff that accidental macrocontamination has not occurred. See above: it is essential to exclude congenital heart disease in neonates being considered for iNO.

Infants at or near term with hypoxic respiratory failure (an oxygenation index of at least 25) should be considered for iNO, but only after their lung volume has been optimised and their cardiovascular status stabilised. Neonates who are hypoxaemic secondary to congenital heart disease, right ventricular-dependent circulation, severe left ventricular dysfunction, duct-dependent circulation or methaemoglobinaemia should not be given iNO. There is currently insufficient evidence to recommend routine use of iNO in prematurely born babies or in term babies with CDH.

Side-effects. NO should be administered only if continuous NO and nitrogen dioxide (NO_2) monitoring are available and there is immediate access to methaemoglobin analysis (Young and Dyar 1996). NO reacts rapidly with O_2 to form NO_2, which is toxic to the lung. The nitrosylhaemoglobin produced by NO binding to haemoglobin is rapidly converted to methaemoglobin, which is then reduced by methaemoglobin reductase in erythrocytes. Unfortunately, immature infants and those of certain ethnic groups have low levels of methaemoglobin reductase. Particularly in VLBW babies with RDS (Mupanemunda and Edwards 1995), care needs to be taken that NO_2 is not being formed (Miller et al. 1994), and that the baby is not developing methaemoglobinaemia (Walsh-Sukys 1993; Kinsella and Abman 1995). These problems are more likely if high concentrations of NO (Ahluwalia et al. 1994) are used for prolonged periods in high inspired oxygen concentrations (Miller et al. 1994). Inhaled NO administration has been associated with an increased bleeding time (George et al. 1998). It seems prudent to try to avoid iNO therapy in babies with a low platelet count or a bleeding diathesis, until these have been treated.

Phosphodiesterase inhibitors

Phosphodiesterases (PDEs) are enzymes which catalyse the hydrolytic cleavage of the 3′ PDE bond of the cyclic nucleotides (cGMP and AMP), which play a central role in pulmonary vascular smooth-muscle relaxation. PDE inhibitors which have been used to treat neonates with pulmonary hypertension include dipyridamole (a non-specific PDE_5 inhibitor), milrinone (a PDE_3 inhibitor) and sildenafil (a PDE_5 inhibitor). Milrinone administration has been associated with improvement in oxygenation in neonates unresponsive to iNO (Bassler et al. 2006; McNamara et al. 2006), but some of the infants developed severe ICH (Bassler et al. 2006). In animal models of pulmonary hypertension, sildenafil (a PDE_5 inhibitor) was more effective than iNO in the treatment of pulmonary hypertension (Shekerdemian et al. 2002). Sidenafil has been shown selectively to reduce pulmonary vascular resistance in both animal models and humans. It produces vasodilation by increasing cGMP by inhibiting the PDE involved in degradation of cGMP to guanosine monophosphate (McNamara et al. 2006). In a small trial, infants with oxygen index (OI) >25 were randomised to receive oral sildenafil (1 mg/kg 6-hourly) or placebo; the infants who received sildenafil experienced an improvement in oxygenation. Six of seven sidenafil-treated infants survived compared with only one of the six controls (McNamara et al. 2006). Despite the limited evidence available, sildenafil is being increasingly used (Hunter et al. 2009). Sildenafil has been used to support infants as they are being weaned off iNO (Konig 2009).

Calcium channel antagonists

Diltiazem has reduced right ventricular pressure in neonates with PPHN (Islam et al. 1999).

Endothelin receptor antagonists

Bosentan is an orally active dual endothelin receptor antagonist (ETA and ETB) and has been shown to reduce PVR and pulmonary arterial pressure in pulmonary hypertension in adults. Successful use in infants is limited to a few case reports (Nakwan et al. 2009).

Inhaled ethyl nitrite gas

Inhaled O-nitrosoethanol gas administered to seven babies with PPHN produced sustained improvements in oxygenation, without adverse effects (Moya et al. 2002).

Monitoring babies with persistent pulmonary hypertension of the newborn

This has to be meticulous and continuous. An indwelling continuously recording PaO_2 cannula should be placed in the aorta, but the umbilical artery PaO_2 measurements should be supplemented by a measure of the preductal PaO_2, using either a right radial artery catheter or a transcutaneous monitor placed on the right upper chest. Preductal (right hand) and postductal (either foot) SpO_2 measurements give useful additional information.

Weaning the baby with persistent pulmonary hypertension of the newborn off therapy

Once the baby has acceptable blood gases weaning can begin. This should be done cautiously as, for some days afterwards, a fall in PAP and a decrease in the right-to-left shunt can result in the pulmonary arteries once more going into spasm, perhaps due to the sensitising effects of alkalaemia (Gordon et al. 1993). The ventilator pressure should be reduced to <30 cmH_2O first, and then the rate of infusion of the vasodilator drugs reduced. In PPHN, the ventilator pressures should never be reduced by more than 1–2 cmH_2O increments and the oxygen concentration by no more than 3–5% increments.

Complications

If a pneumothorax occurs, it must be drained; the hypoxaemia caused by a pneumothorax may so aggravate the pulmonary arterial vasocontriction that it pushes the baby into irreversible hypoxaemia, hypotension and bradycardia. PIE is particularly difficult to manage, as a reduction in ventilator pressure will almost inevitably result in a rise in $PaCO_2$ and a reduction in pH and PaO_2, with worsening of the PPHN. The preterm baby with PPHN who is severely hypoxaemic, acidotic and/or hypotensive is at risk of brain injury, particularly if hypocapnia is used as treatment.

Natural history and prognosis

This varies with the aetiology. Many neonates respond promptly to treatment and the resulting mortality is low, in the 10–20% range, with most of the deaths being due to complications of prematurity or the neurological sequelae of severe birth asphyxia. For those requiring ECMO with primary PPHN or PPHN complicating RDS or MAS, survival figures of 80–90% are reported (p. 525). Most babies die either from irreversible hypoxia secondary to the PPHN or from myocardial failure as bacterial toxins cause arrhythmias or profound hypotension. The results in diaphragmatic hernia are given in Chapter 27, part 6.

Sequelae

Whether or not sequelae occur in survivors depends on whether the intensity of respiratory support caused BPD and whether any neurological damage resulted from severe hypoxia.

Meconium aspiration syndrome

MAS results from the inhalation of meconium before, during or immediately after delivery.

Incidence

In Europe the incidence is between 1:1000 and 1:5000, whereas in North America rates of 2–5:1000 have been reported. In Australia and New Zealand, the rate of MAS was 0.43:1000, with a decrease in incidence between 1995 and 2002 (Dargaville and Copnell 2006). Five per cent of babies born through meconium-stained liquor develop MAS (Cleary and Wiswell 1998).

Aetiology

Meconium inhalation

To develop MAS, an infant must pass meconium, inhale it and the inhaled material must damage the lungs. All these factors are inextricably interlinked with the presence of fetal asphyxia.

Passage of meconium

An overall prevalence of 8–22% for the presence of meconium in liquor is quoted (Gregory et al. 1974; Ramin et al. 1996; Cleary and Wiswell 1998). Meconium aspiration is a disease of term or postterm babies (Ch. 12). Meconium staining of the liquor occurs in 5% or less of preterm pregnancies (Mazor et al. 1995), when it suggests chorioamnionitis, but the prevalence increases to 10% or more after 38 weeks, reaching 22% in patients at a gestational age of 42 weeks, and 44% in babies who deliver 1–2 weeks later.

The fetal passage of meconium may be due to a vagal reflex, but more convincing are the data showing that motilin, which is produced mainly by the jejunum and stimulates peristalsis, is very low in preterm infants and non-asphyxiated term infants, but is raised in asphyxiated term babies who pass meconium intrapartum (Mahmoud et al. 1988).

Inhalation of meconium

Meconium inhalation can occur before the onset of labour, as meconium has been found in the lungs of stillborn babies (Brown and Gleicher 1981) and in babies who die in the early neonatal period, who could not have inhaled meconium intrapartum (Manning et al. 1978; Byrne and Gau 1987; Sunoo et al. 1989). Prolonged severe fetal hypoxia can stimulate fetal breathing, to the extent that amniotic fluid is inhaled (Hooper and Harding 1990), and fetal gasping movements also draw intra-amniotic material into the alveoli (Boddy and Dawes 1975; Manning et al. 1979). Perinatally, meconium inhalation can occur if the baby breathes or gasps with the mouth, pharynx or larynx full of meconium-stained liquor. This may occur late in the second stage of labour, particularly if there is a severe mixed acidaemia with a fetal pH <7.0 (Ramin et al. 1996), when the raised $Paco_2$ may have provoked intrapartum gasping. Postnatally, any meconium in the upper airway potentially can cause MAS. If meconium is inhaled, development of severe MAS depends in part on whether there is coexisting asphyxia (Katz and Bowes 1992; Hernandez et al. 1993).

Effect of meconium on the lungs

Meconium is a sticky material composed of inspissated fetal intestinal secretions. When inhaled, it probably has at least four interacting deleterious effects on a neonatal lung (Fig. 27.34):

1. It creates a ball valve mechanism in the airways whereby air can be sucked in past the plug but cannot be exhaled. This increases airways resistance, mainly in expiration, causing gas trapping, lung overdistension and pneumothorax.
2. It acts as a chemical irritant. Inflammatory cells and mediators are released, which affect vessel contractility, lead to capillary leakage and injure the lung parenchyma. The cytokines cause airway and alveolar epithelial necrosis (Zagariya et al. 2000). Cell injury and apoptosis may also result from the high concentrations of phospholipase A_2 found in meconium (Holopainen et al. 1999). Thus, 24–48 hours after inhalation there is an exudative and inflammatory pneumonitis with alveolar collapse and cellular necrosis.
3. The organic nature of inhaled material, although initially sterile, may predispose the baby to pulmonary infection, particularly with *Escherichia coli*. Meconium may inhibit phagocytosis and the neutrophil oxidative burst (Clark and Duff 1995), hence bacteria can grow in meconium-stained amniotic fluid. Meconium staining of the liquor may be a marker of chorioamnionitis, predisposing the baby to congenital pneumonia (Wen et al. 1993; Mazor et al. 1995) and meconium inhibits polymorph function (Clark and Duff 1995).
4. Meconium inhibits surfactant function and production (Clark et al. 1987; Moses et al. 1991; Dargaville et al. 2001); the inhibition is in a concentration-dependent manner (Sun et al. 1993). The water/methanol-soluble phase (bilirubin and proteins) and, particularly, the chloroform-soluble phase (free fatty acids, triglycerides and cholesterol) of meconium inhibit surfactant (Sun et al. 1993). In addition, phospholipase A_2 degrades surfactant (Schiff et al. 1993) and lysophosphatidylcholine can inhibit surfactant secretion (Grossman et al. 1999). Meconium alters the morphological ultrastructure of surfactant and hence decreases its surface tension-lowering ability (Bae et al. 1998). Infants with severe MAS, i.e. requiring ECMO, have been shown to have lower levels of phosphatidylcholine (Janssen et al. 2006).

These four factors combine to cause the severe airway and alveolar disease which is more likely to occur if there is coexisting asphyxial lung damage (Jovanovic and Nguyen 1989; Katz and Bowes 1992; Ramin et al. 1996).

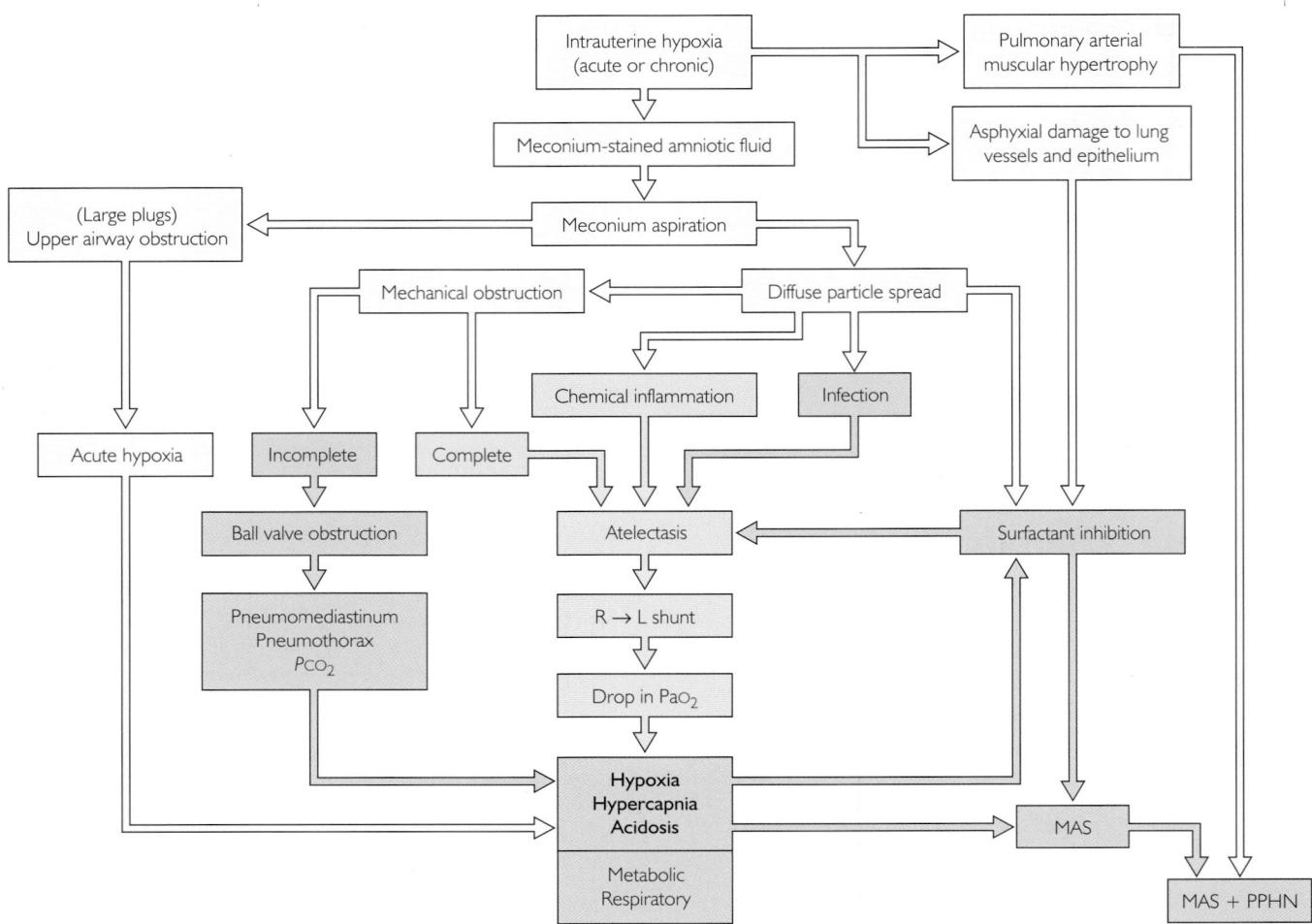

Fig. 27.34 Aetiology of meconium aspiration syndrome (MAS) and its associated clinical syndromes. PPHN, persistent pulmonary hypertension of the newborn.

Effect on pulmonary vasculature

A rise in PAP occurs in all babies with hypoxia and acidaemia (p. 455). Meconium in the lung increases PAP, even if the blood gases are normal (Tyler et al. 1978). The inflammatory response (see above) results in release of vasoactive substances, which cause vasoconstriction; in addition, there may be maldevelopment of the pulmonary vessels secondary to chronic hypoxia (p. 450).

Pathology

Petechial haemorrhages may be present on the lung surfaces due to acute hypoxaemia, particularly if death has occurred rapidly after birth. The lungs may be greenish yellow in colour and the cut surface can show congestion and haemorrhage and meconium can be expressed from the cut ends of the smaller bronchi. The pathognomonic histological feature is the presence of amniotic squames, together with meconium in the terminal airways. Meconium itself appears as a granular eosinophilic material, often containing small yellow meconium bodies. Aspirated material will stimulate a macrophage reaction, but, in the absence of an infective process, acute inflammation with neutrophils is not a feature. In addition to the meconium, hyaline membranes are frequently present. There may also be non-specific changes of an asphyxial insult to the lung,

which include interstitial oedema and haemorrhage. The changes of PPHN may be seen in the pulmonary vascular tree. Infants who die of MAS will have been ventilated at high pressures and thus the histological changes merge into those of BPD. In babies with MAS who die early in the neonatal period, severe asphyxial damage may be seen in other organs, in particular the brain, kidney and myocardium.

Prevention

Antenatal

Attempts to prevent MAS have largely proved unsuccessful. In a large randomised trial (Fraser et al. 2005) which included 1998 pregnant women in labour at 36 weeks or more of gestation who had thick meconium staining of the amniotic fluid, those randomised to amnioinfusion did not have a reduced risk of moderate or severe MAS, perinatal death or other major maternal or neonatal disorders. Suppression of fetal breathing movements by maternal narcotic administration, although successful in a baboon model (Block et al. 1981), did not reduce the incidence of MAS in two clinical series (Dooley et al. 1985; Byrne and Gau 1987).

Intrapartum/postpartum

Timing and mode of delivery

A prospective study (Yoder et al. 2002) demonstrated that reduction in postterm delivery was the most important factor in decreasing the incidence of MAS. MAS is frequently reported to be higher in infants born by caesarean section rather than vaginal delivery; caesarean sections are usually performed on infants with fetal distress, a risk factor for MAS, which may explain the association.

Airway suctioning

Although it is clear that some meconium can be inhaled prelabour, it is assumed that many cases of MAS arise due to inhalation of meconium during the few minutes before birth. In uncontrolled studies, meticulous clearing of the airway at delivery was reported to reduce the incidence of MAS (Gregory et al. 1974; Ting and Brady 1975; Carson et al. 1976). The results of several subsequent studies, however, suggested that routine suctioning through the cords or intubation with endotracheal toilet was not justified, as the manoeuvres not only failed to reduce the incidence of MAS but also were associated with increased morbidity (Falciglia 1988; Linder et al. 1988; Falciglia et al. 1992). Randomised trials have now been reported which have addressed whether intrapartum intubation and tracheal suctioning are necessary. No significant differences in the incidence of MAS or in other major outcomes were demonstrated between babies randomised to receive either naso- or oropharyngeal suctioning prior to delivery of the shoulders or no suctioning (Vain et al. 2002). Similarly, no significant differences were demonstrated in the incidence of MAS or other respiratory complications between apparently vigorous infants who were randomised to intubation and tracheal suctioning or routine delivery room care (Wiswell et al. 2000). In addition, meta-analysis of the results of four randomised trials which included vigorous term meconium-stained babies (Halliday 2000) did not demonstrate significant benefit with regard to mortality, MAS or hypoxic–ischaemic encephalopathy (HIE) from routine endotracheal intubation at birth as compared with routine resuscitation, including oropharyngeal suction. The event rates for the outcomes, however, were low, thus making reliable estimates of treatment effect impossible. Nevertheless, on the evidence to date, intubation and suctioning should be restricted to newborns who are depressed (Bhutani 2008) – that is, they have a heart rate of less than 100 beats/min, poor respiratory effort and poor tone. As soon as possible after delivery, affected babies should be handed to the paediatrician, who should gently insert a laryngoscope and carefully clear the upper airway of any meconium-stained material. If no meconium is seen below the cords, it is not worth proceeding (Linder et al. 1988). If, however, meconium is seen, direct tracheal suction is indicated. Studies in animal models have demonstrated that inhaled meconium stayed in the trachea and major bronchial divisions for several minutes after the onset of respiration and was, therefore, still in a site from which it could be aspirated (Pfenninger et al. 1984).

IPPV

The indications for resuscitation by IPPV (Ch. 13.1) are not affected by the presence of meconium, other than it is always important to clear as much meconium from the airway as possible before applying positive-pressure ventilation .

Compression of the neonatal thorax

This is no longer recommended, as it seems unlikely to prevent gasping, which has a large diaphragmatic component, and compression of the thorax can stimulate respiratory efforts.

Bronchial lavage

Instilling water or saline into the lower respiratory tract is controversial; an increase in wet lung has been noted following this procedure (Carson et al. 1976) and repeated bronchial lavage can do harm. Once on IPPV, tracheal suction with saline lavage, however, resulted in a 35% improvement in airway resistance in one study (Beeram and Dhanireddy 1992). Surfactant lavage can be beneficial (see below).

Postnatal gastric aspiration

Many clinicians routinely aspirate the stomach of a baby who has inhaled meconium at delivery, assuming the baby will have also swallowed meconium and gastric aspiration will prevent subsequent meconium inhalation following vomiting or reflux. Routine gastric lavage prior to feeding, however, did not decrease the incidence of MAS in babies born through meconium-stained liquor (Narchi and Kulaylat 1999).

Clinical signs

The baby is usually mature, or postmature, with long fingernails and a dry skin which soon starts to flake. The skin, nails and umbilical cord are often stained greenish yellow. The baby is not usually febrile, unless secondarily infected. Peripheral oedema is not a feature, and, if present, suggests either renal damage or iatrogenic fluid overload.

Respiratory

The baby has tachypnoea, which may exceed 120/min. Intercostal and subcostal recession occurs and there is use of accessory muscles and flaring of the nostrils. An expiratory grunt may be heard. The meconium in the airways causes widespread sticky crepitations and occasional rhonchi, air trapping and an overdistended chest with an increased anteroposterior diameter. The baby may remain symptomatic for only 24 hours or be very dyspnoeic for 7–10 days before recovery. In patients who required ventilation, the respiratory disease has usually abated to a resting tachypnoea of 50–70/min in room air by 14 days of age.

Cardiovascular

In the absence of asphyxial damage to the myocardium, there are no specific cardiovascular features of MAS. Hypotension suggests myocardial damage, as do signs of congestive heart failure. In uncomplicated MAS, the heart rate tends to be around 110–125/min, and the BP is maintained within the normal range. If PPHN (pp. 495–504) develops, S2 may remain single, and there may be the murmur of tricuspid incompetence (Ch. 28).

Abdominal examination

The liver and spleen are often palpable because of downward displacement of the diaphragm caused by air trapping. In a severely affected infant, bowel sounds may be absent, with delayed passage of meconium. There may be urinary retention and bladder distension in babies with severe neurological problems or those who receive pancuronium.

Central nervous system

Depending on the severity of the coexisting neurological insult, the baby may behave normally or show features of HIE (Ch. 40.4).

Differential diagnosis

Apparently faeculent liquor may be due to yellow-green bilious vomiting secondary to upper gastrointestinal tract obstruction (Wynn and Schreiner 1979). It is important to exclude concurrent illness, especially infection and PPHN.

Pathophysiology

The respiratory failure and hypoxaemia in babies with MAS are due to stiff lungs, marked ventilation–perfusion imbalance and pulmonary hypertension precipitating extrapulmonary right-to-left shunts. Babies with MAS have a reduced compliance and tidal volume and an increased airways resistance, but the tachypnoea increases the minute volume to twice normal (Bancalari and Berlin 1978). In the early stages of the disease, when the airways are plugged by meconium, there is a marked ventilation–perfusion abnormality, which lessens as the lungs recover. In those who develop PPHN, the PAP will be higher than the systemic, with right-to-left shunting through the ductus arteriosus and/or the foramen ovale.

Investigations

Haematological

The nucleated red blood cell (Dollberg et al. 2001) and the white cell (Manroe et al. 1979; Merlob et al. 1980) counts are often raised. White cell function is reduced (Clark and Duff 1995). Thrombocytopenia often occurs in neonates with meconium aspiration who have PPHN (Segal et al. 1980), are ventilated (Ballin et al. 1987) or develop DIC secondary to severe asphyxia (Ch. 30).

Biochemical

If coexisting asphyxia is severe, there may be inappropriate ADH production and hyponatraemia (Ch. 35.2). Renal failure secondary to acute tubular necrosis may cause hyperkalaemia and a raised urea. Hypocalcaemia may also occur, as in any critically ill neonate (Ch. 34.2).

Blood gases

Hypoxia is common, but in mature infants with mild to moderate disease and an efficient respiratory pump, ventilation is not a problem and the Pa_{CO_2} may even be low, normal or only slightly raised. A Pa_{CO_2} >8 kPa (60 mmHg) is unusual and is seen only in patients with severe lung disease who eventually need ventilation.

Changes in pH initially reflect the metabolic acidaemia of intrapartum asphyxia; mature babies commonly correct their acidaemia spontaneously from pH levels in the 7.10–7.15 range and base deficit values of 10–15 mmol/l (Spencer et al. 1993). After the first hour or two, persisting metabolic acidaemia indicates an underlying problem such as sepsis, hypotension and/or renal failure, which should be sought and remedied.

Urine analysis

Many babies with MAS, although not in overt renal failure, have a raised urinary β_2-microglobulin, indicating they have incurred some renal damage (Cole et al. 1985). The urine may be greenish-brown in colour as a result of the absorption of meconium pigments across the pulmonary epithelium and their excretion in the urine (Dehan et al. 1978).

Echocardiography

In uncomplicated MAS, the ECG and echocardiogram will be normal. If there has been severe intrapartum asphyxia, there may be ECG changes suggesting subendocardial ischaemia, and the echocardiogram will show reduced cardiac contractility. In those with PPHN, echocardiography demonstrates right-to-left shunting at ductal and atrial levels and a jet of tricuspid insufficiency, indicating raised right ventricular pressures.

Chest X-ray

The common early changes are widespread patchy infiltration and, in 20–30% of patients, small pleural effusions. Overexpansion is also common in the early stage. In mild to moderate cases, the changes resolve within 48 hours. In severe cases, as the disease progresses, by 72 hours of age with or without ventilation the appearance is often changed to that of diffuse and homogeneous opacification of both lung fields, as a result of a pneumonitis and interstitial oedema secondary to the irritant effect of the inhaled meconium (Fig. 27.35). These changes gradually resolve over the next week, but in severe cases the X-ray may still be abnormal at 14 days, and may merge into the pattern seen in BPD, although this is uncommon. Airleaks, in particular pneumothorax and pneumomediastinum, are very common in MAS (p. 486).

Microbiology

All babies suffering from MAS should have an infection screen as soon as possible after admission to the NICU.

Monitoring

There is a temptation to undermonitor full-term babies with MAS because, despite marked tachypnoea and a very abnormal CXR appearance, they often look surprisingly pink and vigorous. This temptation should be resisted, not only because of the importance of early detection of blood gas abnormalities, electrolyte disturbance or hypotension before secondary effects develop, but also because the baby with MAS has a major risk of sudden deterioration due to a tension pneumothorax.

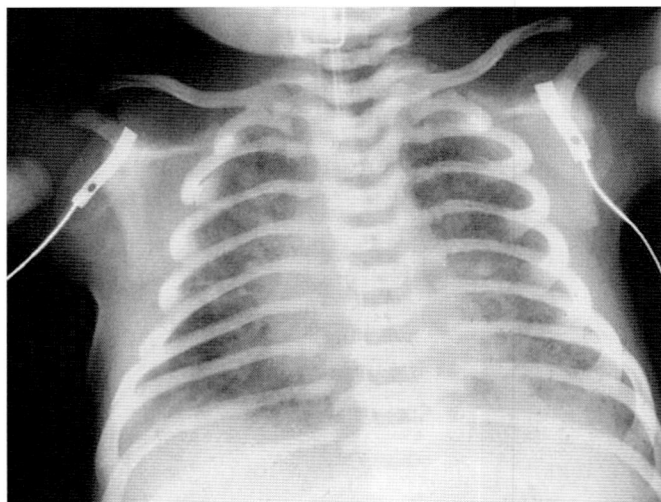

Fig. 27.35 Severe confluent pneumonitis in meconium aspiration syndrome.

Treatment

The aim is to support the baby until alveolar macrophages clear the debris and lung function returns to normal.

Oxygen therapy

Many babies with MAS can be managed by giving an appropriate concentration, up to 80–90%, of warmed humidified oxygen. The oxygen saturation should be maintained at 95% or the Pa_{O_2} greater than 10 kPa during the acute stage of the illness. In many mild cases, oxygen therapy at 40% or less for 24–48 hours is all that is required and Pa_{O_2} in room air is normal by 48 hours of age.

Acid–base homeostasis

Carbon dioxide retention is only a problem in severe cases. A Pa_{CO_2} of 7.5–8 kPa (55–60 mmHg) is acceptable, providing the pH is sustained above 7.25. Intubation and ventilation are indicated if the Pa_{CO_2} rises above 8 kPa (60 mmHg), particularly in the presence of a Pa_{O_2} <6 kPa (45 mmHg) early in the disease.

The first blood gas analysis taken after birth may show a marked metabolic acidaemia. Provided that the baby is otherwise stable, with a normal Pa_{O_2} and Pa_{CO_2}, and is passing urine, base deficits of 10–15 can be left to correct spontaneously (Ch. 35.2). The acidaemia should be corrected, however, if the base deficit is greater than 15 or the pH below 7.10.

In babies who show features of HIE, more rigid control of the blood gases is required (Ch. 40.4); hypoxia, hypercapnia and acidaemia are all undesirable. This indication for intubation and ventilation takes priority over the more conservative management of the blood gases outlined for babies with uncomplicated lung disease.

Continuous positive airways pressure

CPAP can improve oxygenation, but is likely to increase the risk of pneumothorax. In addition, use of nasal prongs in term neonates usually makes them irritable and restless, with a fall in Pa_{O_2}.

Intermittent positive-pressure ventilation

Babies with MAS can be very difficult to ventilate; a long expiratory time and a low level of PEEP are theoretically best in MAS; elevation of PEEP can improve oxygenation, but increases the risk of pneumothorax. Administration of a neuromuscular blocking agent is virtually always required. When the blood gases start to improve, weaning can usually be rapid. Once the infant is in <50–60% oxygen and has peak pressures of 20 cmH$_2$O, neuromuscular blockade can be stopped. We then prefer to transfer infants to PTV and wean by a reduction in peak pressures, extubating infants into headbox oxygen without a period on CPAP.

High-frequency ventilation

HFJV used with surfactant, but not alone, has been reported to improve oxygenation in MAS (Davis et al. 1992). A retrospective review, however, reported no significant difference in the outcome of infants with MAS supported by HFJV (Baumgart et al. 1992). HFOV, particularly when used with NO, improved oxygenation and outcome in infants with PPHN and MAS (Kinsella et al. 1997).

Extracorporeal membrane oxygenation

In a randomised trial, ECMO improved survival of MAS infants with an oxygenation index >40 by 50% (UK Collaborative ECMO Trial Group 1996). Approximately 94% of babies with MAS who are managed with ECMO survive; this does not appear to be at an increased risk of disability or adverse neurological outcome (UK Collaborative ECMO Trial Group 1998).

Pulmonary vasodilators (p. 498)

Drugs used to treat pulmonary hypertension can be effective in babies with MAS (Goetzman et al. 1976; Stevenson et al. 1979; Kinsella et al. 1992; Finer et al. 1994; Tolsa et al. 1995). Inhaled NO improves oxygenation and decreases the need for ECMO (Neonatal Inhaled Nitric Oxide Study Group 1997; Clark et al. 2000) but in these trials no other significant differences in major outcomes were noted.

Surfactant

Exogenous surfactant therapy has been used with anecdotal success (Auten et al. 1991; Khammash et al. 1993). In a randomised prospective study, babies who received surfactant within 6 hours of birth had fewer airleaks, were on IPPV and oxygen for a shorter period and were much less likely to require ECMO (Findlay et al. 1996). The maximum effect on oxygenation was after three doses or more, suggesting that larger doses are required in MAS. Once on ECMO, the use of surfactant speeds recovery and the rate of weaning from ECMO (Lotze et al. 1993). In a randomised trial, up to four doses of surfactant reduced the need for ECMO in term infants with respiratory failure, half of whom had MAS (Lotze et al. 1998); however, there were no other significant differences in outcome. Meta-analysis of the results of four randomised trials demonstrated that surfactant administration reduced the risk of requiring ECMO, but not mortality (El Shahed et al. 2007).

Lavage with surfactant may be a particularly effective method of improving gas exchange by washing out meconium and the products of inflammation (Ohama et al. 1994), as well as diluting the meconium. Multiple small-volume dilute surfactant lavages have been reported to improve oxygenation (Lam and Yeung 1999). Large aliquots (15 ml/kg) have also been used without adverse acute effects and a trend to improvement in oxygenation at 48 hours compared with controls (Dargaville et al. 2007). In a randomised trial, no advantages of lavage compared with bolus were found with regard to length of hospitalisation or complications, but the sample size was small and the lavage group had improvements in oxygenation, decreases in MAP and A–a gradients (Gadzinowski et al. 2008). In a randomised trial, lavage with the protein-containing synthetic surfactant Surfaxin (KL-4 surfactant) improved lung function (Wiswell et al. 2002).

Antibiotics

The presence of organic and potentially infected material in the liquor and in the lung may predispose to pneumonia. Neonates with MAS should be put on broad-spectrum antibiotics, penicillin and gentamicin. The antibiotics should be discontinued when the culture results are known to be negative or after 7 days, when the baby is in the convalescent stage of the illness and requiring less than 30–40% oxygen.

Blood volume and blood pressure

If the haemoglobin falls below 13 g/dl or the PCV below 40%, the baby should be transfused. BP control is essential in all neonates with MAS, aiming to keep the pressure within the normal range (Appendix 4). Hypotension is usually only a problem in babies who have suffered severe intrapartum asphyxia with coexisting myocardial injury or after vasodilators. If hypotension occurs, it is managed in the usual way with volume expansion and/or inotropes, depending on the neonate's myocardial and renal function (Ch. 35.2).

Physiotherapy

In neonates with mild to moderate disease who are not ventilated and require less than 60% inspired oxygen concentration, chest physiotherapy is rarely necessary. In the severely affected baby who is intubated and paralysed, chest percussion and ETT suction may be helpful, but should be continued only as long as this produces significant amounts of greenish material and abandoned if the neonate becomes hypoxaemic.

Steroids

In an animal model, although steroids reduced respiratory symptoms due to MAS, the mortality rate was higher (Fox and Duara 1983). In a randomised trial involving 35 infants (Yeh et al. 1977), steroid treatment in the first 6 hours after birth resulted in no significant differences in the duration of ventilation or survival and the steroid-treated group experienced an increased time to wean. In a subsequent small trial (Wu et al. 1999), major outcomes (mortality and BPD) were not influenced by steroid therapy. More recently, steroid administration resulted in more rapid improvement in ventilated infants with MAS and PPHN (Da Costa et al. 2001). Further studies are required to determine if steroid administration influences long-term outcomes.

Complications

Babies with MAS may suffer from HIE (Ch. 40.4) and renal failure (Ch. 35.2), which are dealt with elsewhere.

Pneumothorax, airleaks

Pneumothorax, pneumomediastinum, pneumopericardium and pneumoperitoneum can all occur; approximately 50% of ventilated MAS babies suffer some form of airleak, but PIE is unusual.

Persistent pulmonary hypertension

This is a common complication of severe MAS, and appears to be particularly frequent in fatal cases (Wiswell et al. 1990).

Bronchopulmonary dysplasia

This is a rare complication of MAS, although it may occur in any baby who survives after long-term high-pressure IPPV.

Mortality

Mortality rates are between 4% and 12% (Cleary and Wiswell 1998). The majority of deaths are from respiratory failure, PPHN or airleaks (Wiswell et al. 1990), but some die from the associated neurological or renal sequelae of severe asphyxia.

Morbidity

Neurological

The neurological sequelae in these babies are those of the coexisting HIE (Ch. 40.4).

Pulmonary

MAS predisposes to long-term respiratory morbidity (MacFarlane and Heaf 1988; Swaminathan et al. 1989; Yuksel et al. 1993a). In a single-centre study (Beligere and Rao 2008), infants with MAS had later neurodevelopmental delay, even if they responded to conventional treatment. At school age, although the majority of neonates who survived MAS were completely asymptomatic, 30–40% had problems with asthma and less than half had completely normal lung function tests (MacFarlane and Heaf 1988; Swaminathan et al. 1989). Other data (Koumbourlis et al. 1995) also suggest that meconium aspiration predisposes to increased bronchial hyperreactivity. The lung function abnormalities at follow-up relate to the severity of MAS (Wilcox et al. 1994). At 6–9 years of age, evidence of residual airways disease was seen in patients who had moderate to severe MAS (Cordier et al. 1984), whereas 12 children who had had mild MAS had normal lung function (Stevens et al. 1988).

Aspiration of amniotic fluid

Postmortem studies of stillbirths have revealed that amniotic squames can be inhaled by the fetus in utero, presumably as a result of 'terminal' gasping activity preceding intrauterine death (Wigglesworth 1984). The importance of less severe manifestations of this entity, in the absence of meconium staining of the amniotic fluid, is speculative, but there is a postnatal lung disease attributed to the inhalation of non-meconium-stained amniotic squames (Schaffer and Avery 1977).

Aspiration of fluid at delivery

Aspiration of blood can result in early-onset respiratory distress and a radiographic appearance of aspiration syndrome (Gordon et al. 2003). It occurs during birth by caesarean section or a vaginal birth complicated by abruptio placentae. Aspiration of 'pool' fluid during a water birth may also cause respiratory distress (Fig. 27.36).

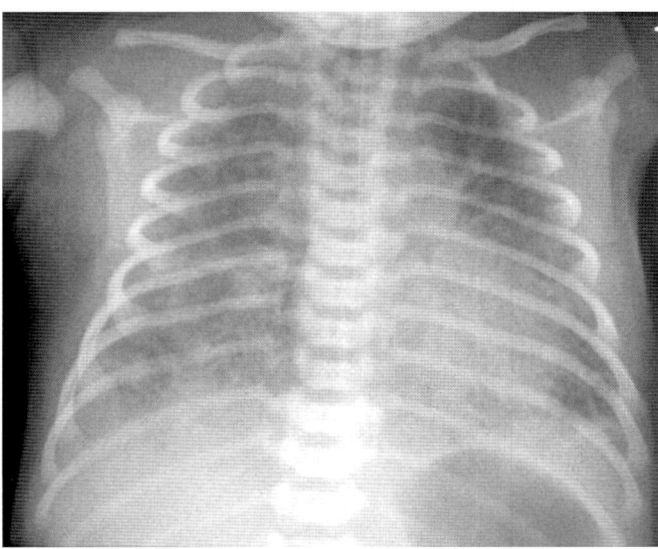

Fig. 27.36 Bilateral changes due to aspiration of pool fluid at an underwater birth.

Table 27.8 Types of aspiration syndrome in the newborn

1. Sucking/swallowing incoordination
   a. Prematurity
   b. Secondary to structural malformation or neurological disorders:
      Cleft palate, Pierre Robin syndrome
      Tracheo-oesophageal fistula, laryngeal cleft
      Hypoxic–ischaemic encephalopathy
   c. Syndromes with poor sucking, e.g. Prader–Willi
2. Syndromes attributed to gastro-oesophageal reflux
   a. In babies on intermittent positive-pressure ventilation – right upper lobe collapse
   b. Wilson–Mikity syndrome
   c. Apnoeic attacks
3. Massive regurgitation and inhalation of a feed

Other aspiration syndromes
(Table 27.8)

In the neonatal period, aspiration can occur due to malfunction of coordination of sucking, swallowing and breathing.

Swallowing incoordination

Pathophysiology

The anatomical structure of the pharynx and larynx protects the airway from inhalation (Ch. 7.7) (Lund 1976) and there are defensive reflexes. The presence of any material in the pharynx initiates swallowing and reflex breath-holding (Wilson et al. 1981). If the airway remains threatened, additional reflexes, including more prolonged apnoea, choking, laryngospasm and coughing, are provoked (Pickens et al. 1988; Davies et al. 1989). These mechanisms provide a less effective shield over the airway in the neonatal period than they do in older children and adults. During sucking, the term neonate may have a reduction in ventilation (Al-Sayed et al. 1994), Pao_2 and heart rate (Mathew 1991), progressing in some infants to apnoea (Steinschneider et al. 1982; Guilleminault and Coons 1984; Mathew et al. 1985; Itani et al. 1988). This may be because of poor breathing/swallowing coordination or additional problems such as velopalatine insufficiency with reflux into the nasopharynx (Plexico and Loughlin 1981). The preterm neonate additionally has immature sucking/swallowing coordination (Shoemaker et al. 2007), which may be overwhelmed by oral feeding, and a high incidence of GOR (Newell et al. 1989a). If there has been brain damage, the neurological control of swallowing may be compromised. Preterm babies can protect their airway as well as those born at term, but these frequent challenges mean that its integrity may eventually be breached (Itani et al. 1988) and inhalation of stomach contents results. Even if the defence mechanisms are effective in preventing intrapulmonary inhalation, significant symptoms, especially apnoea (Newell et al. 1989a; Marino et al. 1995), may still result.

Coordinating sucking, swallowing and breathing becomes more difficult at all gestations if the neonate is sedated, for example by the transplacental passage of opiates, or if the neonate is tachypnoeic with RDS or TTN (Timms et al. 1993).

Other common causes of breathing/swallowing incoordination in both preterm and term babies are structural malformations in the upper airway or gastrointestinal tract, or neurological problems interfering with normal swallowing. Biochemical problems such as hypoglycaemia or hyponatraemia may occasionally have the same effect. Most causes of dysphagia and sucking/swallowing incoordination are extremely rare and usually present with the primary disorder rather than with dysphagia.

Clinical features

The commonest manifestation of swallowing/breathing incoordination in the term baby is choking, spluttering and becoming transiently apnoeic and blue during a feed. The baby thereafter usually remains asymptomatic. Many of these babies are at the extreme end of the normal spectrum of the response to feeding (Mathew 1991). More serious examples are seen in babies who have brain damage or have abnormalities such as a cleft palate. In these, even saliva may continually collect in the pharynx and the baby will be 'mucousy'. In severe cases, babies have saliva dribbling from their mouths and may cough and splutter when trying to clear their airways: cyanosis and bradycardia can occur (Guilleminault and Coons 1984; Itani et al. 1988). Persisting retention of secretions in the pharynx and larynx, in addition to causing noisy breathing and upper respiratory tract symptoms, may result in tachypnoea and retraction, and, on auscultation, widespread conducted sounds are heard. Affected babies can have reflex apnoea caused by the presence of foreign materials in the larynx (Bartlett 1985).

Investigation and differential diagnosis

On the basis of the history and clinical examination, it should be possible to distinguish babies who have had a single or at most two or three episodes due to immature mechanisms being overwhelmed, from those with GOR or a chronic neurological or structural problem (Table 27.9). The clinical presentation of oesophageal atresia, with maternal polyhydramnios, followed by the baby having major problems with secretions in the first 2–3 hours, is sufficiently classical that it should not be missed. Other babies may have covert GOR, or may be refluxing into the nasopharynx during a feed, with subsequent reflex apnoea (Plexico and Loughlin 1981). Appropriate oesophageal pH (Newell et al. 1989a; Khalaf et al. 2001) or contrast studies will demonstrate the abnormality.

Treatment

If no clinical abnormality is found (which is usually the case) in a term baby who has been admitted to the neonatal unit following such an episode on the postnatal ward, breast- or bottle-feeding can be continued under careful supervision, proceeding to further investigation only if choking persists. In convalescent LBW neonates, or those with recognised neurological or structural problems, all that is usually necessary in the absence of signs of aspiration pneumonia is to omit one or two feeds, before carefully restarting them, by nasogastric tube if necessary.

Babies with a tracheo-oesophageal fistula or laryngeal cleft should have surgical repair as soon as possible (Ch. 29.4). Problems associated with palatal defects may be considerably improved by the use of a palatal prosthesis (Ch. 27.7). In babies with Pierre Robin syndrome, laryngomalacia or other surgical problems in which there is not only tongue/palate incoordination but also a structural predisposition to inhalation, and, in addition, no prospect of immediate surgical correction, the airways should be meticulously suctioned and the baby nursed prone. It may, however, occasionally be necessary to resort to tracheostomy in order to protect the lungs.

A small group of babies, typically those with severe neurological damage secondary to HIE or with a primary problem such as dystrophia myotonica, may have prolonged difficulties. Frequent

Table 27.9 Dysphagia in the newborn

Gross anatomical defects	
Palate	Cleft palate, submucous cleft
Tongue	Macroglossia, cysts, tumours, lymphangioma, ankyloglossia superior
Nose	Choanal atresia
Mandible	Micrognathia, Pierre Robin syndrome
Temporomandibular joint	Ankylosis (congenital or infective), hypoplasia
Pharynx	Cyst, diverticulum, tumour
Larynx	Cleft, cyst
Oesophagus	Atresia, stenosis, short oesophagus, web, diverticulum, duplication, lung buds, tracheo-oesophageal fistula
Thorax	Vascular rings
Neuromuscular incoordination	
Delayed maturation	Prematurity, normal variant
Cerebral palsy	All types
Brain damage	Postasphyxial, postinfection (prenatal or postnatal)
Abnormalities of the cranial nerve nuclei and their tracts	Bulbar and suprabulbar palsy
	Moebius syndrome
	Pharyngeal, cricopharyngeal incoordination (idiopathic, secondary to brain damage)
Congenital laryngeal stridor	
Myopathies	Myotonic dystrophy, myasthenia gravis
Hypotonia from any cause	Brain damage, Werdnig–Hoffman syndrome
Infections	Tetanus, polio, stomatitis, oesophagitis

Modified from Illingworth (1969).

suctioning of the mouth and pharynx will be required and it may help to keep the baby lying prone or semiprone, allowing the baby's mouth to empty by gravity. Persistence of problems is an ominous prognostic feature; despite suctioning and positioning and meticulous nursing care, inhalation of secretions will eventually result, progressing to aspiration pneumonia, which is a common terminal event in such cases.

Gastro-oesophageal reflux (Ch. 29.3)

GOR should be suspected in neonates with apparently inexplicable and recurrent respiratory problems, especially if there is recurrent apnoea unresponsive to theophylline (Newell et al. 1989a), a history suggesting reflux or recurrent vomiting, or right upper lobe collapse or consolidation on X-ray. The diagnosis should be confirmed by radiological or pH probe demonstration of reflux (Orenstein and Orenstein 1988; Newell et al. 1989a; Holopainen et al. 1999).

Treatment

If episodes of apnoea or recurrent pulmonary disease in a neonate are confirmed to be due to reflux, small frequent feeds or continuous milk infusion are advocated; nasojejunal feeds or thickened feeds may also be beneficial (Newell et al. 1989a). Antacids should be given if there is evidence of oesophagitis. Cisapride is no longer prescribed, because of the reports of toxicity and apparent lack of efficacy. Consequently, if the above measures fail, some clinicians prescribe another prokinetic agent, domperidone. Whether neonates benefit from any form of medical therapy for reflux has been questioned (Hrabovsky and Mullett 1986) and fundoplication may be necessary if problems from GOR persist. In our experience, this is rarely necessary, except in babies with chronic severe reflux and BPD.

Aspiration pneumonia

This may occur following one of the episodes of sucking/swallowing incoordination or reflux described above and is most likely to occur in babies with neurological defects or structural malformations. It may be covert due to reflux, or can follow an episode of massive regurgitation and vomiting, which usually only occurs in ill and convalescent babies of all gestations on the NICU. The baby, often still tube-fed, is found covered in vomit, and is usually cyanosed, apnoeic or gasping, and bradycardic.

Prevention

Most cases of aspiration pneumonia can and should be prevented by prompt clinical recognition and appropriate management of the disorders in which they are likely to occur (Table 27.8) and by careful attention to the feeding technique. Professional speech and language therapy input is essential for safe oral feeding in many of these babies.

Pathophysiology

The foreign material aspirated into the airway can have three effects: physical obstruction, chemical irritation and promotion of infection. All fluids, including water, are damaging, but gastric contents are particularly damaging because of their acidic pH (James et al. 1984). In the first few days after birth, the pH of a neonate's stomach contents can be 2.5 or less if the infant is unfed (Avery et al. 1966b) or fed only clear fluids with no buffering capacity. Inhaled curd is particulate and can obstruct airways, leading to lung collapse and/or consolidation, and may predispose to infection.

Clinical findings

In babies with sucking/swallowing incoordination, the features of their primary diagnosis will be present (Table 27.9). In addition, if such infants have chronic pooling of secretions in their upper airway, they will be mucousy with rattling, noisy respiration, often coupled with respiratory distress due to obstruction of the airway by secretions. Widespread conducted sounds, therefore, are often heard on auscultation of the chest.

After a massive regurgitation or vomit which triggers an episode of apnoea, cyanosis and bradycardia, but which has been promptly and efficiently dealt with (see below), many neonates show no abnormal physical signs 10–15 minutes later. In these babies, the clinical features suggesting that inhalation pneumonia has actually occurred are the non-specific ones of respiratory distress (p. 476). In a neonate with pre-existing lung disease, respiratory function deteriorates. In both groups, crepitations and rhonchi may be heard on auscultation.

Investigations

In the baby who rapidly reverts to normal and shows no signs of respiratory compromise 15–30 minutes after the episode, it is still advisable to do a CXR. A new area of consolidation, particularly in the right upper lobe, is very suggestive of inhalation, but more generalised and non-specific changes may occur. In either the chronic situation or following a single severe episode, if the baby has the signs of respiratory disease he or she should be investigated for infection (Ch. 39.2). Measuring the electrolytes, blood sugar and calcium is indicated in all babies and may identify a cause for a convulsion.

Treatment

The vomiting episode

When the baby is found, the mouth, nose and pharynx should be quickly and effectively sucked out. If the infant has become cyanosed, oxygen should be given by mask. Most babies respond briskly at this stage and no further treatment is required other than the evaluation outlined above. If the baby does not respond promptly, the airway should be cleared using a laryngoscope and inhaled material aspirated under direct vision. This should always be done if the episode is so severe that the baby remains apnoeic or intubation is required for resuscitation.

General management

Oxygen

Sufficient oxygen should be given to keep the PaO_2 in the normal range. If the aspiration has been severe, or it complicates pre-existing lung disease in a small preterm baby, the episode may trigger apnoea or cause such severe pneumonitis that the baby will require IPPV.

Physiotherapy

If there are copious secretions following inhalation, or if the CXR shows an area of consolidation, then 4-hourly physiotherapy should be given to encourage drainage from the affected region. The baby should also be nursed in the position that optimises drainage from the affected lobe.

Feeding

In most babies it is wise to stop oral feeds for 24–48 hours after an episode of aspiration/inhalation. In the preterm neonate, recourse to intravenous feeding may be necessary. In the term baby, once the tachypnoea has settled, oral feeding can be restarted unless there is some chronic problem, in which case a period of nasogastric feeds will need to be used.

Antibiotics

Until the cultures are negative, it is impossible to be sure that the whole episode was not triggered by infection. As a consequence, broad-spectrum antibiotic cover should be given, usually flucloxacillin and an aminoglycoside (Ch. 39.2). Antibiotics should be continued for at least 5–7 days or until the baby is clinically much improved if there are marked CXR changes or the neonate required IPPV, even if the cultures are negative.

Morbidity and mortality of aspiration pneumonia

This is dependent on the underlying pathology, since the lung disease following inhalation per se is rarely, if ever, fatal. Babies with persistent failure to suck or swallow secretions after severe birth asphyxia and those with congenital neurological problems have a guarded prognosis on the basis of their underlying defects. Most babies with a structural defect do well with appropriate surgery, but there remains an appreciable mortality with laryngotracheo-oesophageal cleft (p. 610) or Pierre Robin syndrome (p. 605). For the baby whose problems are due to immaturity, the outlook is excellent, since it can be anticipated that the lung disease will respond to the therapy outlined, although some infants may develop BPD and have a prolonged convalescence.

Pulmonary haemorrhage

This condition is a form of fulminant lung oedema with leakage of red cells and capillary filtrate into the lungs. It must be differentiated from the common occurrence of a small amount of blood-stained material aspirated from the ETT of a ventilated baby as a result of trauma. Pulmonary haemorrhage occurs most commonly in babies weighing <1500 g, who often have a PDA (Garland et al. 1994).

Incidence

The incidence of pulmonary haemorrhage in infants with a birth-weight less than 1500 g, treated with surfactant, was reported to be 11.9% (Pandit et al. 1999).

Aetiology

Massive pulmonary haemorrhage (MPH) represents the extreme end of the spectrum of pulmonary oedema in the neonate. This has four main causes (Bland 1982) (Table 27.10), which all increase fluid leak into the pulmonary interstitium and thus elevate pulmonary lymphatic flow. Although intra-alveolar fluid may appear at an early stage of interstitial oedema (Snashall 1980), pulmonary oedema usually occurs as lung interstitial fluid rises and fluid leaks into the alveoli because the alveolar epithelium either has been damaged or becomes leaky owing to distension by the interstitial fluid. The first change is a rise in pulmonary capillary pressure; this causes an increase in interstitial fluid, which eventually leaks into the alveoli through holes in the epithelium. Initially these holes are large enough to allow passage of molecules such as albumin, but small enough to retain molecules such as IgG, IgM, and fibrinogen, and the majority of red cells. As the changes become more marked, the holes in the endothelium and epithelium increase in size and larger molecules leak through. In most cases, the amount of blood lost is small and the haematocrit of the lung effluent is less than 10%. MPH can occur following severe birth depression and in infants with hydrops due to rhesus haemolytic disease, left heart failure, congenital heart disease, sepsis, hypothermia, fluid overload, oxygen toxicity and haemostatic failure. Infants who are small for gestational age are more likely to suffer a pulmonary haemorrhage (De Carolis et al. 1998), the association being independent of other factors (Finlay and Subhedar 2000). In

Table 27.10 Causes of pulmonary oedema in the neonate

INCREASED PULMONARY MICROVASCULAR PRESSURE	REDUCED INTRAVASCULAR ONCOTIC PRESSURE	REDUCED LYMPHATIC DRAINAGE	INCREASED MICROVASCULAR PERMEABILITY
Heart failure	Prematurity	Pulmonary interstitial emphysema	Sepsis
Hypoxia	Hydrops	Pulmonary fibrosis	Endotoxaemia
Transfusions	Fluid overload	Raised central venous pressure	Emboli
Intravenous fat	Hypoproteinaemia		Oxygen toxicity
Increased pulmonary blood flow	Loss in gut		
Pulmonary hyperplasia	Loss from kidneys Malnutrition		

Reproduced with permission from Bland (1992).

addition, the neonate with severe RDS on IPPV in a high oxygen concentration and heart failure secondary to a large pulmonary blood flow from a PDA may suffer an MPH (Garland et al. 1994; Evans and Kluckow 1999). Meta-analysis of the results of 29 trials (Raju and Langenberg 1993) demonstrated an association of MPH with synthetic, but not natural, surfactant use. Rescue surfactant therapy was not demonstrated to have a significant effect on MPH (Soll and Morley 2009), but prophylactic surfactant increased the risk (RR 3.28; 95% CI 1.5–9.2) (Soll 2000b). MPH is seen in babies with DIC, albeit rarely, but does not usually occur in babies with thrombocytopenia, haemorrhagic disease of the newborn or haemophilia. Following the marked clinical deterioration with MPH, however, it is not uncommon for secondary DIC to develop (Cole et al. 1973).

Pathology

The changes present in the lungs are dependent on the stage of the illness reached by the time of death. In deaths before 48 hours of age and in stillbirths, interstitial haemorrhage is common, but in deaths after 48 hours and following surfactant administration (Pappin et al. 1994), intra-alveolar bleeding dominates the clinical picture. The lungs are solid at postmortem and usually a deep reddish-purple colour; they are gasless and sink in water. Their pressure/volume characteristics will be those of low-compliance, surfactant-less lungs (p. 457). Hyaline membranes will often be present, since MPH frequently complicates primary RDS. As in RDS, there will be necrosis and desquamation of the alveolar lining cells. In cases which come to autopsy more than 48 hours after the haemorrhage, and particularly if the neonate survives for several days on IPPV, usually in a high oxygen concentration and at high pressures, the changes merge into those seen in severe BPD (p. 555).

Clinical features

The two striking clinical features of MPH are a sudden deterioration and usually the simultaneous appearance of copious bloody secretions from the baby's airway, either up the ETT or from the larynx and mouth in a non-intubated infant. The baby usually is hypotensive, pale and frequently limp and unresponsive, although term babies may occasionally be active and restless secondary to hypoxaemia, and 'fight' the ventilator.

Cardiac

The condition is commonly secondary to heart failure, hence the infant may have a tachycardia greater than 160/min and the murmur of a PDA is frequently heard (Garland et al. 1994). Other signs of heart failure, including hepatosplenomegaly and a triple rhythm, can occur. The presence of peripheral oedema may indicate heart failure, hydrops, hypoalbuminaemia or fluid overload. Hypotension is virtually always present, because of a combination of blood and fluid loss, heart failure and coexisting hypoxaemia and acidaemia.

Respiratory

Infants are dyspnoeic and cyanotic and auscultation of the chest reveals widespread crepitations with a reduction in air entry.

Differential diagnosis

Small amounts of blood coming up the ETT are usually due to trauma. A few babies may deteriorate clinically without apparent cause for an hour or two before the haemorrhage develops, but once copious blood-stained fluid appears from the airway, the diagnosis is self-evident. The underlying cause, however, should be established, since this will influence subsequent treatment.

Investigations

Haematological

Although the haematocrit of the oedema fluid is usually <10%, considerable quantities of blood may be lost, and the haemoglobin may fall to 10 g/dl or even lower. Cole et al. (1973) found that coagulation disturbances were not a regular feature of their patients prior to the haemorrhage, but DIC is not uncommon afterwards.

Biochemical

Affected preterm babies usually have the same problems as those with severe RDS. In particular, hypoglycaemia, hypocalcaemia, hypoalbuminaemia and renal failure should be sought and remedied.

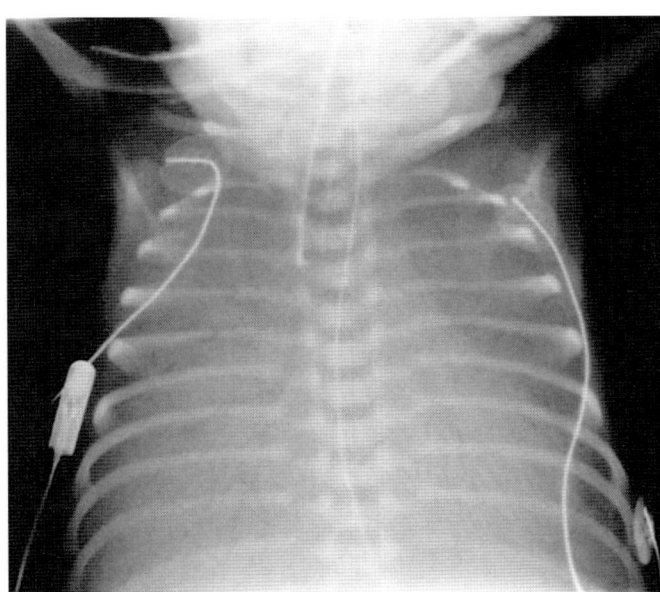

Fig. 27.37 Widespread homogeneous opacification of the lungs in a baby with massive pulmonary haemorrhage. *(Reproduced from Greenough et al. (1996).)*

Chest X-ray

The CXR in the baby who has had a large MPH shows a virtual 'whiteout' (Fig. 27.37) with just an air bronchogram visible. This appearance is indistinguishable from severe surfactant deficiency and may be a reflection of the secondary surfactant deficiency that occurs following pulmonary haemorrhage. As the condition improves on IPPV, the changes may clear or merge into those of BPD. Rarely, a lobar pattern of consolidation is found, suggesting that the haemorrhage has occurred in just a part of the lung.

Bacteriology

The haemorrhage may be precipitated by sepsis. For this reason, an infection screen must always be taken immediately after the event. The baby's condition, however, will usually preclude performing a lumbar puncture (Ch. 39.2).

Blood gases

All components of arterial blood gas analysis deteriorate rapidly after the bleed. Hypoxia is severe, the $Paco_2$ may increase to 10 kPa (75 mmHg) or more and there is usually a marked metabolic acidosis with a base deficit of at least 10 mmol/l. The combined respiratory and metabolic acidaemia may result in a pH of 7.10 or less.

Monitoring

The blood gases should be meticulously supervised. Clotting studies should be done daily until they normalise. A daily CXR should be performed because of the high ventilator pressures that are frequently required and the potential complications.

Treatment

Particular attention must be paid to maintaining the BP with blood transfusion, progressing to inotropes as necessary (Ch. 28). The severe acidaemia should be corrected with intravenous base if IPPV and correction of the hypoxia and hypotension do not promptly return the pH and base deficit to an acceptable level. Underlying disorders must be treated. Heart failure due to anaemia in, for example, haemolytic disease should be treated by exchange transfusion with packed cells, aiming for a haemoglobin level of 13–14 g/dl. Asphyxial myocardial damage may need inotrope support (see below), and sepsis should be treated as outlined on Ch. 39.2.

Control of pulmonary oedema and heart failure

Fluid balance

Fluid input should be restricted to 60–80 ml/kg/24 h, particularly if there is a coexisting patent ductus. The BP can be sustained by judicious infusion of blood, but mainly by the use of inotropes.

Diuretics

These babies have left ventricular failure and pulmonary oedema. Furosemide (1 mg/kg) should be given as soon as possible after the haemorrhage and repeated as necessary, to treat fluid overload.

Intermittent positive-pressure ventilation

All babies with MPH should be intubated and ventilated. They usually have severe lung disease, and peak inflating pressures above 30 cmH$_2$O may be necessary. For this reason, and since mature babies in particular become very restless, neuromuscular blockade and sedation should be used routinely until the haemorrhage is controlled. During IPPV, a high PEEP (up to 6–7 cmH$_2$O) should be employed; in experimental studies this does not reduce the total lung water, but redistributes it back into the interstitial space, improving oxygenation and ventilation–perfusion balance (Pare et al. 1983; Malo et al. 1984).

Surfactant

Paradoxically, although surfactant may precipitate MPH (p. 459), after stabilising the baby on IPPV after the haemorrhage, a single dose of surfactant has been suggested to improve oxygenation (Pandit et al. 1995).

Patent ductus arteriosus

PDA is common in preterm neonates who develop MPH; use of prophylactic indometacin may reduce both complications (Clyman 1996). While the baby is critically ill, the use of indometacin or equivalent is contraindicated, but this should be reconsidered 24–48 hours later, once the coagulopathy is controlled and the hypoxia and acid–base disorders corrected.

Physiotherapy/suction

In the first few hours after the haemorrhage, there may be copious bloody secretions. Suction is required every 10–15 minutes in extreme cases, as there is a significant risk of the secretions clotting and blocking the airway or ETT. Physiotherapy, however, is not of proven value, and, as these neonates are extremely fragile, it should not be used as a routine in the early stages, instead relying on adequate humidification to keep the secretions sufficiently liquid that they can be sucked up the ETT.

Coagulopathy

The features of DIC are frequently present. Transfusion of platelets, however, is rarely required, but infusions of fresh frozen plasma are indicated and usually successful in promptly correcting the clotting deficiencies. After the first 24–48 hours when the baby has become stable on IPPV, the acid–base disturbances have been corrected and septicaemia (if present) treated, the coagulation problems usually remit and further factor replacement is not usually necessary.

Antibiotics

Sepsis is a recognised cause of MPH; thus, antibiotics should be started after taking cultures. If the baby is already receiving antibiotics, it is recommended to broaden the spectrum to cover infection by staphylococci and *Pseudomonas* species.

Complications

These babies are susceptible to all the major complications of respiratory failure. High-pressure ventilation predisposes them to airleaks, and BPD is a common sequela (Pandit et al. 1999). At the time of their sudden collapse, they are susceptible to neurological damage and GMH/IVH (Ch. 40.5); the occurrence of cerebral bleeds may be doubled in babies who suffer pulmonary haemorrhage (Finlay and Subhedar 2000). The occurrence of seizures is increased in infants with pulmonary haemorrhage (Tomaszcwska et al. 1998).

Mortality

For many years this was regarded as a universally fatal condition (Garland et al. 1994). In the modern era of intensive care, survival is improved; but affected infants are the sickest and most immature and their mortality rate is of the order of 38% (Pandit et al. 1999).

Asphyxial lung disease/acute respiratory distress syndrome

Intrapartum asphyxia or severe lung injury may result in severe respiratory distress ARDS.

Aetiology

ARDS results from lung injury from a number of causes, including asphyxia, shock, sepsis, MAS and DIC.

Pathophysiology

Asphyxia damages pulmonary blood vessels, making them leaky, and this, plus the pulmonary oedema secondary to heart failure occurring as a result of asphyxial damage to the myocardium (Burnard and James 1961; Bucciarelli et al. 1977; Walther et al. 1985), may compromise surfactant function (p. 459). Severe metabolic acidaemia can also depress myocardial contractility, again leading to heart failure, pulmonary oedema and tachypnoea (Beierholm et al. 1975; Watters et al. 1987). If the leak of protein-rich fluid on to the alveoli becomes large enough, ARDS develops, with epithelial degeneration, surfactant inhibition, interstitial cellular infiltration, pulmonary hypertension and eventually alveolar fibrosis (Royall and Levin 1988).

Metabolic acidaemia stimulates hyperventilation (Javaheri et al. 1979). In the neonate, the chemoreceptors are sensitive to pH (Walker 1984; Navarrete et al. 2003); the increase in respiration is more likely to be due to stimulation of peripheral chemoreceptors than medullary centres (Bureau et al. 1979).

Damage to the central nervous system may stimulate tachypnoea by two mechanisms. Firstly, the neural control of respiration may be damaged, resulting in hyperventilation. This is well recognised in older patients (Leigh and Shaw 1976). Neurologically damaged babies may hyperventilate to $Paco_2$ levels of 2.5–3.0 kPa (19–23 mmHg) in the first few days after birth. Secondly, neurogenic pulmonary oedema may occur following any rise in intracranial pressure (ICP) or brain injury. It is primarily due to an increased pulmonary vascular permeability leading to interstitial pulmonary oedema, hypoxia and tachypnoea (Colice et al. 1984; Maron 1987). The mechanism is probably active in the newborn, and explains, for example, the sudden deterioration in respiratory function following a GMH/IVH, but may also be of importance in babies with HIE or subdural haemorrhage following birth asphyxia.

Asphyxia caused by cord occlusion with blood trapped in the placenta causing fetal anaemia (Shepherd et al. 1985; Vanhaesebrouck et al. 1987) and acute fetal haemorrhage from ruptured vasa praevia or following a large fetomaternal haemorrhage will result in the birth of a baby who is anaemic, shocked and acidotic (Raye et al. 1970). Chronic fetal anaemia due to rhesus disease or fetomaternal haemorrhage also produces babies with acidaemia, anaemia and tachypnoea (Phibbs et al. 1972). The lowered buffering capacity of blood with a low haemoglobin will also potentiate the effect of metabolic acidaemia on respiration (see above).

Clinical features

Some babies who suffer intrapartum asphyxia remain tachypnoeic for 24–48 hours after delivery (Thiebeault et al. 1984); less commonly, severe lung disease, ARDS (Faix et al. 1989), occurs.

Infants with ARDS are severely hypoxaemic. This is primarily a disease of term babies, who, within the first hour or two, usually present with tachypnoea of 100/min or more, rather than with retraction and grunting, although in some babies the clinical picture may be dominated by the neurological sequelae of asphyxia, and apnoea may occur (Thiebeault et al. 1984). The baby may be tachycardic and hypotensive with a triple rhythm, or have the systolic murmurs of tricuspid or mitral incompetence (Bucciarelli et al. 1977; Finley et al. 1979); if there has been severe myocardial damage, other signs of heart failure, crepitations and hepatomegaly may be found (Cabal et al. 1980).

Differential diagnosis

This is a diagnosis of exclusion in the neonate who has suffered intrapartum asphyxia. The CXR excludes complications such as pneumothorax and does not show the features of 'wet lung' seen in transient tachypnoea. Excluding sepsis, as always, is important, as GBS infection may masquerade as asphyxia (Peevy and Chalhub 1983).

Investigations

The blood gases should be measured on an arterial sample; babies with ARDS are severely hypoxaemic. Respiration is stimulated by the metabolic acidaemia (base deficit >20 mmol/l, with a corresponding low pH), damage to the central nervous system or by lung receptors stimulated by pulmonary oedema; the $Paco_2$ is usually <4 kPa (30 mmHg). Hypoglycaemia is common after asphyxia, as is DIC (Ch. 30); both should be remedied promptly if found.

A CXR is essential and will demonstrate diffuse pulmonary infiltrates. In severe cases there will be a 'whiteout' as in severe RDS.

Evidence of myocardial damage should be sought by performing an echocardiograph to assess ventricular function and an ECG should be obtained. The ECG may show changes of ST-segment depression and T-wave inversion if there is severe asphyxia (Cabal et al. 1980; Setzer et al. 1980) but in lesser degrees of asphyxia there may only be slight flattening of the T-wave (Jedeikin et al. 1983). The level of the myocardial isoenzyme of creatine kinase may be raised (Primhak et al. 1985). If myocardial damage is present, much greater care has to be taken regarding use of bolus infusions.

Monitoring

A UAC is the preferred site for monitoring blood gases and BP. Affected babies are peripherally shut down, making clinical assessment of oxygenation impossible and arterial puncture difficult; frequent samples may be needed until the pH returns to normal.

Management

Surfactant administration can improve oxygenation in ARDS. It is most effective if given early and in larger doses than in RDS (Ogawa et al. 1999). In adults and children with ARDS, prone positioning has been shown to improve oxygenation (Curley et al. 2000).

Blood gases

The baby should receive sufficient warmed humidified oxygen to keep the Pao_2 above 8 kPa (60 mmHg). Prolonged high-pressure ventilation similar to that used for neonatal RDS (pp. 517–519) may be necessary (Faix et al. 1989). A high level of PEEP should be used to try and restore the FRC to more normal values; this will also increase the MAP level and hence oxygenation. An excessive amount of PEEP, however, will impair gas exchange by causing alveolar overdistension. High-volume strategy HFO can also improve oxygenation (Giffin and Greenough 1994), particularly in those patients who had a positive response to PEEP elevation (p. 521). HFJV has also been used with anecdotal success (Pfenninger et al. 1991). Inhaled NO has been used in patients with ARDS to improve oxygenation (Demirakca et al. 1996).

Metabolic acidaemia

Term neonates can recover spontaneously and quickly from pH levels of 7.10–7.15 and base deficits of >15 mmol/l (Daniel et al. 1966; Sykes et al. 1982; Spencer et al. 1993). For this reason, immediately after delivery, expectant treatment of uncomplicated metabolic acidaemia is justified if the pH is above 7.10, but an arterial gas should be checked 30–60 minutes later to ensure that spontaneous correction is taking place. If the pH is below this value, or the infant has heart failure attributed to acidaemia, then the pH should be corrected to 7.30–7.40 using the standard formula (Ch. 35.2).

Hypotension and heart failure

These are two of the most serious complications of severe asphyxia, as they are associated with secondary ischaemic injury to the central nervous system, myocardium (endocardial ischaemia), kidneys (renal failure) and intestine (NEC). They must, therefore, be corrected urgently. The general approach to hypotension outlined in Chapter 28 should be followed, taking great care with fluid balance if the myocardium is compromised. In general, the fluid intake should initially be restricted to 40 ml/kg/24 h. If heart failure is present, furosemide should be given. IPPV with PEEP helps to control pulmonary oedema.

Anaemia

A haemoglobin <13 g/dl (PCV <40%) is an indication for transfusion in asphyxial lung disease. If there is coexisting myocardial asphyxial injury, the transfusion should be given slowly and carefully with a diuretic. In such a situation, if the haemoglobin level is <8–9 g/dl, the safest way of increasing it is with a single-volume exchange transfusion using packed red blood cells.

Hypoxic–ischaemic encephalopathy

The management of this is outlined in detail in Chapter 40, part 4.

Antibiotics

After collecting the appropriate samples to assess if the baby is infected, including a blood culture, broad-spectrum antibiotics, usually penicillin plus an aminoglycoside (Ch. 39.2), should be administered. Aminoglycoside levels must be carefully monitored, as these infants are at risk of renal dysfunction.

Prognosis

The mortality of ARDS is high (Pfenninger et al. 1991), particularly in those infants who develop secondary infection or do not respond to elevation of their PEEP level. Airleaks and infection are commonly seen in infants with ARDS.

Pleural effusions
Isolated

These are uncommon in the neonatal period. The incidence of primary fetal hydrothorax is estimated at one case per 15 000 pregnancies (Linder et al. 1988).

Aetiology

Pleural effusions diagnosed antenatally are frequently associated with chromosomal or congenital abnormalities (Nicolaides and Azar 1990). Intrauterine (cytomegalovirus, toxoplasmosis, rubella, adenovirus), perinatal (GBS and *Staphylococcus*) and postnatal (*Staphylococcus*) infection can all result in pleural effusions. Isolated effusions are usually a chylothorax (p. 515). Approximately 9% of infants with MAS have pleural effusions; rarer associations are TTN, PPHN, heart failure and congenital myotonic dystrophy. Right-sided diaphragmatic hernia can be associated with a hydrothorax, which results from a fluid-filled peritoneal sac in the right side of the chest (Whittle et al. 1989). An effusion will develop following repair of CDH (Ch. 29.6). Trauma, for example by direct erosion of the inferior vena cava by a TPN catheter into the pleural space, can result in a pleural effusion (Leipala et al. 2001). A unilateral hydrothorax may also occur if a central venous catheter migrates into the pulmonary vasculature (Madhavi et al. 2000). Pleural effusions are usually part of a generalised oedematous state (hydrops fetalis); an isolated fetal pleural effusion can progress to generalised hydrops.

Clinical signs

Infants with large effusions are frequently difficult to resuscitate as, antenatally, the pleural effusion may have prevented normal lung growth. In infants with underlying pulmonary hypoplasia, there will be a reduced pulmonary vascular bed and the babies will have PPHN. On examination, the trachea and mediastinum will be

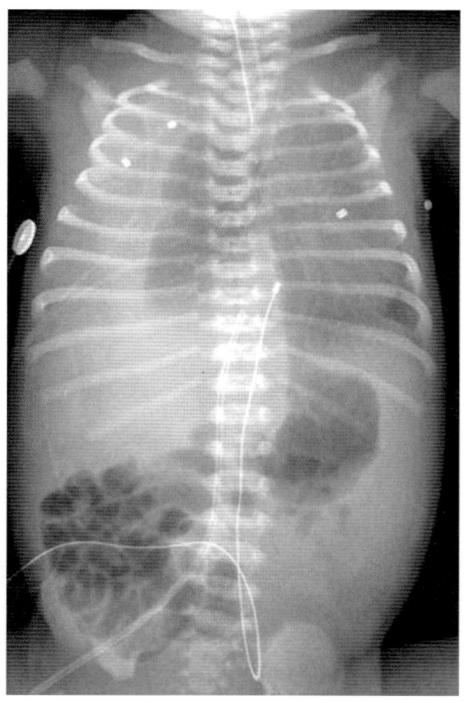

Fig. 27.38 Chest X-ray demonstrates a right pleural effusion. Antenatally, the infant was hydropic with bilateral pleural effusions; pigtail catheters were inserted bilaterally (with successful drainage on the right) and are still in situ, shown by the two radiopaque dots on each side of the chest.

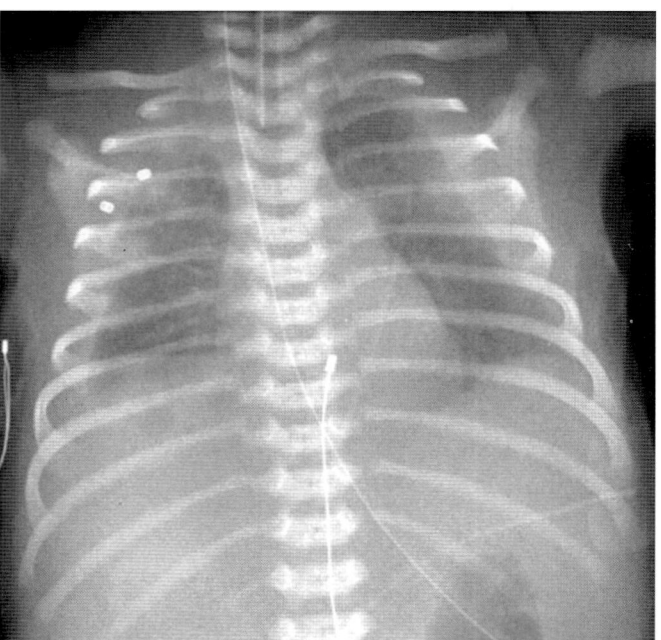

Fig. 27.39 Bilateral pleural effusions. Note the presence of a pigtailed catheter on the right side of the chest; this was placed antenatally.

shifted to the contralateral side and the ipsilateral lung will be dull to percussion with absent breath sounds. Small effusions may be asymptomatic and diagnosed incidentally on a chest radiograph.

Diagnosis

Antenatally, pleural effusions are detected by ultrasonography and should be suspected in fetuses whose mothers have polyhydramnios (Pijpers et al. 1989). Postnatally, on the CXR there may be a 'whiteout' on the affected site (Figs 27.38 and 27.39), but if the pleural effusion is small, it is important to remember that fluid will collect in the most dependent parts of the chest, around the lateral chest wall or the diaphragm (Figs 27.40 and 27.41).

Differential diagnosis

At birth, the presentation of a large effusion is similar to that of CDH (Ch. 27.6), but there are no bowel sounds in the chest. The CXR appearance may be confused with an eventration or atelectasis.

Treatment

Antenatally, pleural effusions are drained either intermittently by thoracocentesis (Petres et al. 1982) or continuously by a thoraco-amniotic shunt (Booth et al. 1987). Indications for antenatal drainage include the development of hydrops and mediastinal shift with a unilateral effusion. At birth, infants with large pleural effusions require active resuscitation by intubation and positive-pressure ventilation (Pijpers et al. 1989). Thoracocentesis may also be required to achieve effective ventilation and this may also be necessary later in the postnatal period. See Chapter 44 for details of the technique.

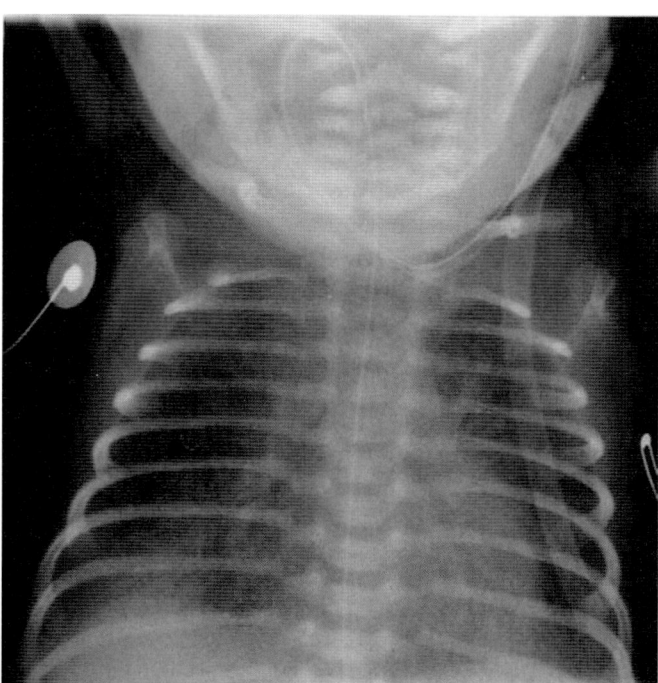

Fig. 27.40 Small pleural effusion. Chest X-ray in the erect position: note obliteration of the right hemidiaphragm. *(Reproduced from Greenough et al. 1996.)*

Aspirated fluid should always be sent for cytology to determine the lymphocyte count, and for biochemical and microbiological analysis. If the effusion is due to infection, the fluid will have a high protein content, with neutrophils present, and organisms may be isolated. The fluid should also be sent for cytological examination; a high lymphocyte count indicates a chylothorax. If a chest tube is

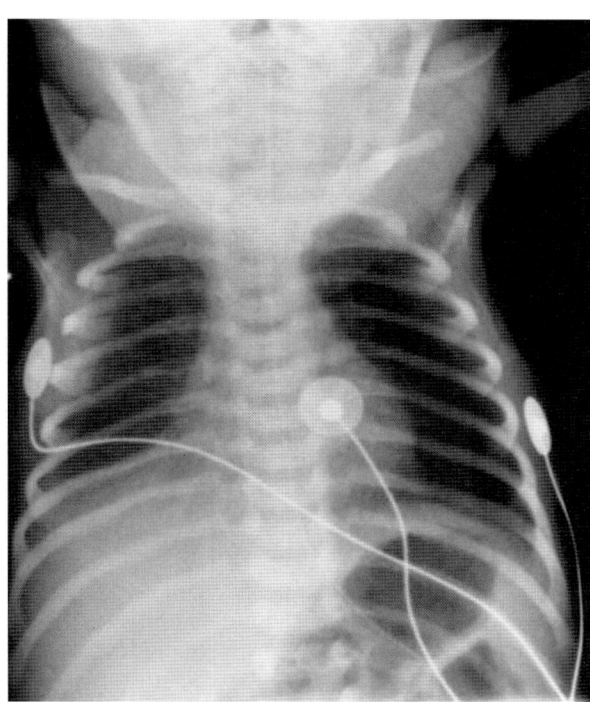

Fig. 27.41 Small pleural effusion. Supine X-ray showing a rim of fluid. *(Reproduced from Greenough et al. (1996).)*

used to drain a pleural effusion, it is important to ensure that the tip does not abut the mediastinum, as this increases the risk of phrenic nerve injury (Williams et al. 2003).

Prognosis

Antenatally diagnosed pleural effusions, particularly if present prior to 32 weeks of gestation, have a mortality rate as high as 55% (Hagay et al. 1993). Bilateral fetal pleural effusions are frequently associated with pulmonary hypoplasia. Postnatally, effusions persisting for more than 3 days increase the risk of chronic oxygen dependency (Long et al. 1984).

Chylothorax

Incidence

One in 10 000 deliveries and one in 2000 neonatal intensive care admissions were reported to have a chylothorax (Van Aerde et al. 1984).

Aetiology

Chylothorax may occur spontaneously or be associated with lymphoedema due to congenitally abnormal lymph vessels in conditions such as Turner or Noonan syndrome or congenital lymphangiectasia. In the last condition, there is diffuse dilatation of the interlobular and subpleural lymphatics. A congenital abnormality in the lymphatic system at the level of the thoracic duct below or above the fifth thoracic vertebra leads to a right- or left-sided chylothorax (Van Aerde et al. 1984). It can be associated with foregut malformations and extralobar sequestration. Rarely, trauma to the thoracic duct at delivery by hyperexpansion of the spinal column in association with increased venous pressure during birth results

in a chylothorax, but more commonly it is a complication of certain types of cardiac surgery (repair of coarctation of the aorta or ligation of a PDA) or repair of a congenital posterolateral diaphragmatic hernia (Mercer 1986). Another iatrogenic cause is superior vena caval (SVC) obstruction in patients who have had venous catheterisation for TPN (Amodio et al. 1987).

Clinical signs

Unusually, chylothoraces result in hydrops, owing to impairment of venous return by cardiac and vena caval compression and/or loss of protein into the pleural space. In 50% of cases, chylothoraces present in the first week with symptoms as described under isolated pleural effusion. Typically, the lesion is right-sided. Chronic chylothorax may be associated with hypovolaemia, hypoalbuminaemia, hyponatraemia and weight loss. Such patients are immunocompromised owing to loss of lymphocytes and humoral antibodies.

Diagnosis

In an unfed infant, the fluid obtained at thoracocentesis is clear, yellow and contains large numbers of lymphocytes (20–50 per high-power field). Lipoprotein electrophoresis demonstrates a high triglyceride and a low cholesterol level. Once the infant is milk-fed, the fluid will become chylous, clearing once a medium-chain triglyceride formula is introduced. Chylothorax associated with SVC obstruction should be suspected in infants with swelling of the face, neck and upper extremities; ultrasonography will confirm the presence of fluid in the chest and the position of the catheter tip. Doppler ultrasonography will identify the SVC obstruction.

Treatment

Chylothoraces may need to be drained antenatally (see above). Postnatally, many cases respond to a single thoracocentesis, as this results in lung expansion tamponading the defect and preventing further pleural fluid formation. If the fluid reaccumulates, drainage is required and the baby should be fed with a milk containing fat only in the form of medium-chain triglycerides. In the gut, long-chain fatty acids pass into the lymph as chylomicrons after being re-esterified to triglycerides, before entering the venous network, whereas medium-chain fatty acids pass directly into the portal venous blood. Pregestemil or Pepti-Junior can be tried, but a semi-elemental milk may be required and should be continued for at least 2 weeks after the effusion has disappeared (Hashim et al. 1964; Brodman et al. 1974; Puntis et al. 1987). Rarely, in non-responsive cases, TPN should be used. Pleural abrasion, ligation of the thoracic duct and pleurodesis are possible options for those chylothoraces that fail to respond to medical management (Andersen et al. 1984; Puntis et al. 1987).

Prognosis

This condition usually resolves, but the mortality rate has been suggested to be as high as 60% for bilateral chylothoraces (Carmant and Le Guennec 1989).

Haemothorax

Aetiology

Trauma with damage to the arteries alongside the ribs from misplacement of a chest drain to drain a pneumothorax is the commonest cause of a neonatal haemothorax; it can also occur at thoracic surgery. Rare causes include clotting abnormalities (Grausz and Harvey 1967), penetration of the fetal thorax at amniocentesis (Achiron and Zakut 1986), spontaneous rupture of a PDA and arteriovenous malformations.

Diagnosis

The CXR will demonstrate a 'whiteout', and a radioisotope lung scan can identify an underlying arteriovenous fistula.

Treatment

Resuscitation by urgent transfusion of blood and clotting factors may be required. Surgical intervention should be considered if a large blood vessel has been traumatised.

Management of neonatal respiratory failure

Oxygen therapy

Supplementary oxygen therapy

In mild to moderate respiratory disease, all that is usually required to keep the baby's Pa_{O_2} at 8–12 kPa (60–90 mmHg) (Appendix 7) is the administration of warmed humidified supplementary oxygen. Additional support by CPAP or IPPV is indicated only if a satisfactory Pa_{O_2} cannot be achieved in 60–80% oxygen in a headbox, or at lower inspired oxygen concentrations if there are other features of respiratory failure. To avoid sudden changes in the inspired oxygen concentration such as when the incubator doors are opened, the oxygen should be given into a Perspex box placed over the baby's head and shoulders (headbox). The concentration of oxygen administered should be measured by an analyser placed near the baby's mouth. This form of therapy is frequently sufficient for preterm babies more than 30 weeks of gestational age with RDS, all babies with minimal respiratory disease and most with TTN (p. 485). The occasional mature baby with RDS and most cases of meconium aspiration can also be managed with headbox oxygen, even though they may require concentrations of up to 80% for 72 hours or more, providing they do not develop other signs of respiratory failure.

A system for automated adjustments in the fraction of the inspired oxygen concentration to maintain the oxygen saturation level within the intended range has been shown to reduce hyperoxaemia (Claure et al. 2009).

Nasal cannula-administered oxygen

In babies requiring prolonged oxygen therapy for BPD, administration of oxygen by nasal cannula allows the baby to be picked up and cuddled and bottle- or breastfed. It is, however, difficult to assess the concentration of oxygen administered to such babies. Purpose-built double cannulae or an 8 FG feeding catheter cut to length and inserted 2–3 cm into one nostril can be used. Correct fixation of the catheter to the nostril is important to prevent restricting the flow rate, accidental displacement and excessive advancement of the catheter, which has been associated with gastric rupture (Cigada et al. 2001). A humidifed high-flow nasal cannula (HFNC) is now used in some centres as an alternative to CPAP; usually flow rates of less than 2 l/min are used (see below). The potential reasons for the increased use are ease of administration, perceived improved tolerance and minimal nasal trauma compared with nCPAP (Shoemaker et al. 2007).

Oxygen toxicity

Oxygen is toxic to tissues because it forms free radicals, such as superoxide (O_2^-) and hydroxyl (OH^-) (Kelly and Lubec 1995). The neonate is exposed to complex physiological and pharmacological stresses from these agents (Smith et al. 1993; Saugstad 1996). If adults are exposed to even a few hours of pure oxygen, they develop tracheitis and reduced tracheal mucus velocity. After about 16–24 hours, they experience chest discomfort and cough. During the first 24 hours, there is a significant alveolar–capillary leak of protein (Davis et al. 1983). Dyspnoea develops after a further 24–48 hours (Jackson 1985). If pure oxygen exposure is continued for 3–4 days, animals develop a fatal lung disease with oedematous alveolar walls, interstitial haemorrhage, atelectasis (Clark and Lambertsen 1971) and type II cell hyperplasia (De Los Santos et al. 1987). Surfactant is depleted in the early stages of oxygen exposure, with a reduction in both DPPC and PG levels (King et al. 1989), which continue to fall after the animal is removed from 100% oxygen (Holm et al. 1987; Demirakca et al. 1996). Another deleterious effect of breathing pure oxygen is that all the nitrogen is washed out of the alveoli; as oxygen is much more rapidly taken up by pulmonary capillary blood than is nitrogen, this predisposes to atelectasis. Pulmonary alveolar macrophage function is significantly reduced in animals by exposure to more than 80% oxygen for at least 3 days (Sherman et al. 1988).

Exposure of the neonatal lung to a high inspired oxygen concentration in the presence of lung disease also causes damage, probably because the oxygen free radicals interact with lung cell lipids. Neonates, however, seem to be more resistant to pulmonary oxygen toxicity than are adults (Clark and Lambertsen 1971). This resistance is dependent on the presence in the tissues of antioxidant enzymes such as superoxide dismutase, catalase and glutathione peroxidase. In the term lung, the cells, including type II pneumocytes, are able rapidly to switch on antioxidant enzymes after birth (Frank et al. 1978; Keeney et al. 1992), an effect that may be stimulated by epidermal growth factor (Price et al. 1993), but this is less efficient in the preterm lung (Loo et al. 1989; Frank and Sosenko 1991; Keeney et al. 1993). The level of antioxidant enzymes and the resistance of the lung to hyperoxia are increased at term by prenatal maternal and postnatal treatment with dexamethasone (Davis and Whitin 1992; Frank 1992). In preterm animals, the postnatal increase in enzymes and oxygen resistance may be absent (Keeney et al. 1993; Sosenko et al. 1995). Administration of surfactant protects against oxygen toxicity (Huang et al. 1995; Piantadosi et al. 1995).

Although 100% oxygen clearly damages the lungs, the danger of lower oxygen concentrations to the human neonate is much less clear. In adult humans, oxygen concentrations less than 60% rarely do harm, and exposure to between 50% and 90% resulted in limited damage (Klein 1990). In mature rabbits, exposure to 60% oxygen for 3 weeks caused alveolar interstitial oedema, but increased surfactant production (Holm et al. 1987). Rats kept in 60% oxygen for 2 weeks had small lungs with parenchymal thickening (Han et al. 1996). Studies in neonatal baboons suggest that exposure to a high oxygen concentration even without IPPV is damaging (DeLemos et al. 1987a).

Administration of 100% oxygen to babies is never justified, as, with large shunts, the increase in Pa_{O_2} achieved by increasing from 90% oxygen to 100% oxygen is trivial and is not worth the risks of both oxygen toxicity to the lung and the atelectasis that results from nitrogen washout.

Assisted ventilation in the newborn

Continuous positive airway pressure

CPAP is a positive distending pressure applied continuously. The aim of CPAP is to hold the alveoli and airways open and prevent them collapsing during expiration. The major benefit of CPAP is that it stabilises the ribcage, reducing chest wall distortion during inspiration and consequently increases the efficiency of the diaphragm (Shaffer et al. 1978). It regularises the respiratory rate, which usually falls because of stimulation of the Hering–Breuer reflex, and results in an increase in inspiratory time and tidal volume. There is an increase in the FRC in proportion to the level of applied pressure; some alveoli, however, will be overdistended, resulting in a fall in dynamic compliance (Moomjian et al. 1981). If too small a diameter tube is used to administer the CPAP, the work of breathing may increase as a result of the increased effort required to overcome the resistance of the tube (Le Souef et al. 1984).

Continuous positive airways pressure delivery

CPAP was initially given through an ETT (Gregory et al. 1971), but, in an attempt to avoid the hazards of intubation, many other devices have been used, including Gregory's original headbox, face chambers and negative-pressure chambers. These devices have mostly been abandoned. Facemask CPAP has a high complication rate (Gregory 1986) and thus is not recommended. The mask must be applied firmly to the face to prevent gas leaks and maintain the pressure and this can distort the baby's face; furthermore, the apparatus holding the mask in place must be strapped tightly around the back of the head, which can distort its shape. In early series, pressure necrosis and even GMH/IVH or cerebellar haemorrhage were reported (Pape et al. 1976). It is difficult to use a nasogastric tube with facemask CPAP because this breaks the seal; yet, without the nasogastric tube, the stomach cannot be easily aspirated and gaseous abdominal distension results. The presence of the facemask also makes it difficult to tend to the baby's mouth and nose. CPAP is now usually delivered to the baby through either a pair of tubes inserted into both nostrils or a single tube into one nostril. An alternative device, described by Benveniste et al. (1976), applies a jet of gas near to the exit of the curved attachment for the prongs in a way that mimics the actions of an expiratory valve and thus applies CPAP. This device has been widely used in the Scandinavian studies of CPAP in RDS (Jacobsen et al. 1993; Kamper et al. 1993). The method of nCPAP delivery used influences outcome. For example, there is a variation in the resistance to flow with the different nCPAP devices; the resistance is lowest in devices with short double prongs. That finding may explain why meta-analysis of the results of two studies demonstrated that short binasal prongs were more effective at preventing reintubation than were single nasal or nasopharyngeal prongs (De Paoli et al. 2002).

CPAP can be delivered using an underwater seal (de Klerk and de Klerck 2001); if the bubbling is vigorous, the baby experiences vibration of the chest at frequencies similar to those experienced during HFOV (p. 523). During 'bubble' CPAP, the column of water in the expiratory limb generates CPAP equal to the length of the tube that is immersed under water. In a small randomised trial of infants ready for extubation, gas exchange was maintained despite a significant reduction in minute volume during 'bubble' CPAP, suggesting that the chest vibrations may have contributed to gas exchange. In comparison with historical controls, however, ROP (grades I and II) was commoner in infants supported by bubble CPAP (Nowadzky et al. 2009). In a crossover trial (Morley et al. 2005) of high- versus slow-amplitude bubbling, no differences were found with regard to oxygen saturation or transcutaneous carbon dioxide levels. Variable-flow nCPAP has been reported to be associated with better lung recruitment than with either continuous flow nCPAP via nasal prongs or continuous flow nCPAP via modified nasal cannulae (Courtney et al. 2001) and the work of breathing was lower with variable flow CPAP (Pandit et al. 2001). Those beneficial effects may be due to gas entrainment by the high-velocity jet flows; lung overdistension, however, may occur in infants with mild disease if CPAP levels greater than 6 cmH2O are used with variable flow CPAP. In one trial (Gupta et al. 2009b), however, bubble CPAP was equally as effective as variable flow CPAP delivered by the Infant Flow Driver and, indeed, the extubation failure rate was significantly lower with bubble CPAP in infants ventilated for less than 14 days (Gupta et al. 2009b).

During bi-level CPAP two alternating levels of CPAP are delivered; the theoretical benefits are that the switching between CPAP levels might recruit unstable alveoli, the delta pressure generates a tidal volume and some of the respiratory work is unloaded. In a small randomised trial, bi-level nCPAP compared with nCPAP was associated with better respiratory outcomes and shorter duration of respiratory support (Lista et al. 2010).

HFNC delivers CPAP, usually at low levels. It is attractive in that trauma to the nose may be reduced by the use of smaller nasal cannulae than are used during CPAP, but there may be desiccation of the nasal mucosa with associated bleeding and airway obstruction if non-humidified HFNC is employed (Finer and Mannino 2009). The current delivery systems may not prevent excessive pressure delivery to the infant's airway and this may result in lung overexpansion (Finer and Mannino 2009), and the presence of a leak of 30% can reduce the delivered pressures to less than 3 cmH2O (Lampland et al. 2009). Appropriately powered randomised trials with long-term outcomes are required to determine if HFNC with known pressure delivery is more or less efficacious than current methods of delivering continuous positive airways pressure.

Continuous positive airways pressure settings

In relatively mature infants with acute RDS who have not received treatment with surfactant, CPAP pressures of 5–8 cmH2O may be required; however, in immature infants in the recovery stage of their illness who have more compliant lungs, levels in excess of 2–3 cmH2O may not be tolerated. It is important not to use too high a CPAP level, as this will cause lung overdistension, resulting in impairment of ventilation and carbon dioxide retention. CPAP and F_IO_2 levels should be adjusted on the basis of blood gas analyses. If the neonate still has unsatisfactory oxygenation in 50–60% oxygen, he or she should be intubated and ventilated.

Hazards of continuous positive airways pressure

Traumatic injuries to the nose and face from the prong(s) can occur (Robertson et al. 1996), including distortion of the nose, flaring of the nose, circular distortion and columella nasal necrosis. Although these can be minimised by good nursing technique, they are not completely avoidable. Randomised comparisons have demonstrated similar rates of injury with binasal prongs, nasopharyngeal tube and mask CPAP (Buettiker et al. 2004; Yong et al. 2005) and the only significant risk factor for nasal trauma was the duration of CPAP (Yong et al. 2005). Nasal CPAP support at 24 hours of age was an independent predictive factor for early-onset septicaemia in a prospective study of 462 ELBW infants (Rønnestad et al. 2005). In addition, in a case–control study (Graham et al. 2006), nasal CPAP was significantly associated with Gram-negative blood stream infections. The increased risk of infection was suggested to be due to trauma to the nares, increasing ports of entry for bacteria

(Kopelman and Holbert 2003). These adverse effects emphasise the importance of remembering that use of nCPAP requires meticulous attention to the airway and frequent suctioning may be necessary. Rigorous training is required for success; the correct size prongs should be used and the neonate's neck should be properly positioned (de Klerk and de Klerck 2001).

Airleaks do occur in infants supported by CPAP (De Bie et al. 2002; Gurakan et al. 2002). In a non-randomised study (Makhoul et al. 2002), pneumothoraces developed more often in infants supported by nCPAP than in those supported by synchronised intermittent mandatory ventilation (sIMV). In the COIN trial (Morley et al. 2008), the incidence of pneumothorax was three times higher in the CPAP arm; there was no excess of severe ICH or PVL, but pneumothoraces with normal cranial ultrasound findings have been associated with increased adverse neurodevelopmental outcome (Laptook et al. 2005). nCPAP, then, should never be used in units without facilities for both the rapid recognition and drainage of a tension pneumothorax and the subsequent use of IPPV.

Clinical studies

When first introduced, CPAP was applied to babies requiring 50–60% oxygen to keep their PaO_2 >8 kPa (60 mmHg). With increased familiarity, the technique was used earlier in babies with RDS, often when they needed no more than 35–40% oxygen to maintain an acceptable PaO_2. Used in this way, it improved blood gases and seemed to cause more rapid recovery (Gregory et al. 1971; Baum and Roberton 1974; Boros and Reynolds 1975; Durbin et al. 1976; Allen et al. 1977). In early randomised controlled trials, however, the benefits of CPAP seemed to be small (Roberton 1976a, b) and problems were experienced, and the results of prospective trials of CPAP in babies with relatively mild lung disease suggested that treated babies did less well than controls (Han et al. 1987; Hauer et al. 1996).

Early CPAP is now used in many centres in preference to early intubation and IPPV (Avery et al. 1987; Jacobsen et al. 1993; Kamper et al. 1993; Gitterman et al. 1997; Linder et al. 1999). In non-randomised trials, its use has been associated with a reduction in the requirement for mechanical ventilation and in the incidence of BPD. Comparison with a historical control group demonstrated that use of CPAP rather than intubation and ventilation was associated with fewer procedures related to respiratory support and the amount of pain medication was significantly lower (Axelin et al. 2009). However, in a large randomised (COIN) trial, which included 610 infants born at 25–28 weeks of gestation, although infants randomised to CPAP had a lower risk of death or need for oxygen therapy at 28 days, there was no significant difference in the rates of oxygen dependency at 36 weeks postmaturational age and the pneumothorax rate was significantly greater in the CPAP group (Morley et al. 2008). The higher pneumothorax rate might be explained by use of 8 cmH$_2$O CPAP and/or the lower use of surfactant in the CPAP group (Morley et al. 2008). If early CPAP is used, many centres termporarily intubate the baby so that surfactant can be given (Verder et al. 1994), and administer the surfactant early rather than late (Verder et al. 1999). The INSURE (intubation–surfactant–treatment–extubation) method is a combination of early surfactant treatment and early extubation on to CPAP (Blennow et al. 1999). In one study (van den Berg et al. 2010), the INSURE procedure did not induce any perturbation of cerebral oxygen delivery and extraction, but electrical brain activity decreased for a prolonged time. Meta-analysis of six trials demonstrated that the INSURE approach compared with selective surfactant with continued ventilation in infants with RDS was associated with a significant reduction in BPD, need for mechanical ventilation and airleaks

(Stevens et al. 2007). A larger proportion of the infants in the early compared with the selective surfactant group, however, received surfactant and it is well documented that prophylactic/early surfactant versus selective/rescue surfactant once RDS is established reduces the incidences of BPD/death and airleaks and improves survival (see above). Subsequent studies (Sandri et al. 2010; SUPPORT Study Group 2010) suggest that use of surfactant in the delivery room and selective use of surfactant are as effective as prophylactic surfactant.

In a randomised trial (te Pas and Walther 2007), which included 207 prematurely born infants, early versus rescue nCPAP (i.e. if necessary after arrival on the NICU) was associated with a reduction in BPD. The early nCPAP group, however, additionally received a sustained inflation of 20 cmH$_2$O for 10 seconds using a nasopharyngeal tube and T-piece ventilator, whereas bag and mask inflation was used in the other group with inflation pressures of 30–40 cmH$_2$O. In a lamb model, six manual inflations of 35–40 ml/kg compared with no bagging resulted in poorer lung function (Björklund et al. 1997). Thus, it is possible that early nCPAP did not reduce BPD, but rather volutrauma in the delivery suite increased BPD in the other group.

CPAP is frequently used during the recovery stage of RDS to support neonates following extubation from the ventilator (p. 529) (Dimitriou et al. 2000). It is also helpful in the management of infants with recurrent apnoeic attacks (Ch. 27.4); nCPAP dilates the upper airway, which may explain its selective beneficial effects on mixed and obstructive apnoea (Gaon et al. 1999). CPAP may be beneficial in upper airway obstruction due to Pierre Robin syndrome or congenital laryngeal stridor, when nasopharyngeal CPAP may be preferable, with the tip of the nasal cannula passing through the posterior choanae into the upper pharynx (Heaf et al. 1982). nCPAP has been used effectively and with an acceptable safety margin during transportation of term and preterm neonates (Murray and Stewart 2008).

Nasal-delivered ventilatory modes

Experience of ventilatory modes delivered by nasal prongs is limited and there have been no large randomised trials to determine whether these techniques offer long-term advantages for neonates.

Nasal prong-delivered IPPV (nIPPV) appears to augment the beneficial effects of nCPAP in prematurely born infants with apnoea (Lemyre et al. 2002); but there were case reports of gastrointestinal perforation with this mode of respiratory support. Meta-analysis of three trials highlighted that use of nIPPV is associated with a significant reduction in extubation failure (Carlo 2008).

Synchronised nIPPV (snIPPV) has generally been delivered by the Infant Star with a synchronised intermittent mandatory ventilation box (StarSync, Infrasonics, San Diego, CA). The StarSync module provides thoracoabdominal synchronisation via the Graesby capsule placed on the abdomen (Bhandari et al. 2009). In a retrospective non-randomised study, involving analysis of data from 471 infants (242 supported by snIPPV), snIPPV was associated with a reduction in BPD in infants with birthweight 500–750 g, but not overall (Bhandari et al. 2009); there was no excess of gastrointestinal problems (Bhandari et al. 2009). In a smaller ($n = 41$) randomised study, post surfactant extubation to snIPPV compared with ongoing ventilation was associated with a lower rate of BPD/death, but no other differences in outcomes (Bhandari et al. 2007). Others (Kugelman et al. 2008), however, have reported that nIPPV in stable premature infants resulted in increased BP and discomfort.

HFOV has been delivered by nasal prongs in case series only (Van der Hoeven et al. 1998; Colaizy et al. 2008). One series resulted in a reduction in carbon dioxide levels in some infants with a moderate respiratory acidosis on nCPAP (Van der Hoeven et al. 1998). In another, carbon dioxide levels were lower and pH was higher after 2 hours of nasal HFOV compared with CPAP support in preterm infants older than 7 days (Colaizy et al. 2008).

Continuous negative expanding pressure

This is an alternative way of providing distending pressure in which the infant's body is placed in a negative-pressure box from which the head protrudes and continuous negative external pressure (CNEP) in the range –4 to –10 cmH$_2$O is applied (Samuels and Southall 1989). In patients already ventilated, the peak and PEEPs are reduced by the level of negative pressure applied. Early attempts at CNEP were poorly tolerated, particularly in ELBW infants, because of difficulties in securing the infant and hypothermia. These problems have been overcome by specially designed neck seals (Samuels and Southall 1989) and providing a circulation of warm air. CNEP can, however, overdistend the lung and impair lung function in infants with BPD. The considerable technical challenges have meant that CNEP is not widely used in the UK.

Early studies (Outerbridge 1979) demonstrated that CNEP was associated with improvements in oxygenation; the best results were experienced in infants with severe RDS. In addition, respiratory rate decreased and, in infants with stiff lungs, compliance improved on CNEP (Gappa et al. 1994). In a randomised trial (Samuels et al. 1996), use of CNEP (–4 to –6 cmH$_2$O) was associated with a lower duration of oxygen therapy (18.3 versus 33.6 days), but there were trends towards an increase in mortality and cranial ultrasound abnormalities in the CNEP group. Follow-up at school age demonstrated no important differences in respiratory outcomes for those who had been treated with CNEP as infants, but the trial was not powered to detect such differences (Telford et al. 2007).

Intermittent positive-pressure ventilation

Indications

There are two absolute indications for starting IPPV:

1. sudden collapse with apnoea, bradycardia and failure to establish satisfactory ventilation after a short period of bag and mask ventilation
2. failure to establish adequate spontaneous ventilation in the labour ward after prompt and active resuscitation (Ch. 13.1).

The relative indications for intubation and IPPV apply to babies who are breathing spontaneously, but are clinically, or on the basis of blood gas results, showing signs of impending respiratory failure. These indications vary with the gestational age of the baby, the nature of the underlying disease and whether the major feature of the respiratory failure is carbon dioxide retention, hypoxaemia or recurrent apnoeic spells.

Most babies in impending respiratory failure fall into one of three clearly separate groups, which require different plans of action:

1. VLBW neonates <28 weeks of gestation and <1.00 kg. These babies may be ventilated from the time of resuscitation in the labour ward (Ch. 13.1). A small number of these infants establish adequate regular respiration after birth but subsequently develop signs of RDS. To prevent sudden collapse with its attendant complications and to give surfactant, such babies should be ventilated once they need more than 40% oxygen on CPAP to keep their PaO$_2$ <7–8 kPa (52–60 mmHg) or have a PaCO$_2$ >6–6.5 kPa (45–50 mmHg) with a pH <7.25.

2. Babies 1.00–1.50 kg at 28–32 weeks of gestation with RDS. Nasal CPAP may be sufficient support for infants whose PaCO$_2$ is 6.5–7.0 kPa (50–55 mmHg) but who maintain their pH >7.25 and have an oxygen requirement of less than 60%. If, however, CPAP does not result in a prompt improvement, that is, a reduction in supplementary oxygen requirement to less than 40%, such babies should be ventilated.

3. Relatively mature babies 1.50–2.50 kg and 33–36 weeks' gestation. These babies have a more rigid ribcage and better developed respiratory muscles than very immature babies, so are more able to sustain vigorous respiratory efforts and tachypnoea for some days. They may, however, tolerate CPAP badly, becoming distressed and irritable when the device is attached.

Other indications for IPPV in the neonatal period include:

- PPHN: for the neonate with primary PPHN or secondary pulmonary hypertension, intubation and control of the PaCO$_2$ within defined limits can be beneficial (p. 498)
- severe early-onset sepsis (Ch. 39.2)
- MAS
- MPH
- diaphragmatic hernia: these babies should be ventilated from birth (Ch. 27.6)
- HIE: hyperventilation to prevent cerebral oedema by keeping the PaCO$_2$ in the 3.0–3.5 kPa (22–25 mmHg) range (Ch. 40.4) is no longer justified, but sedation due to anticonvulsant drug administration often necessitates intubation and ventilation
- apnoea: the small preterm baby with recurrent apnoeas, not controlled by methylxanthines or CPAP, requires IPPV (Ch. 27.4).

Delivery

A continuous flow of gas is delivered and this distends the lung for a preset inflation time to a predetermined pressure. During expiration, the ventilator gas flow continues to deliver PEEP if required. Gas enters the lungs during the inspiratory time; the amount entering is determined by the set peak pressure and the gas flow rate. The latter should always be large enough to ensure that the preset peak pressure can be reached during the available inflation time. At a fast flow, the lungs are distended more quickly and the peak pressure is reached sooner, thereby creating a relatively square-wave inspiratory gas flow. When the desired pressure has been reached, the pressure-limiting valve opens and prevents any further rise. The longer the inflation time, the longer the lungs are held distended at this pressure. The higher the pressure is set, depending on the compliance of the lungs, the larger the volume of gas which enters the lungs, though this is limited in non-compliant lungs by the size of the leak around the ETT.

Peak inflating pressures. When starting a baby on IPPV, the peak inflating pressure should be adjusted to ensure adequate, but not excessive, chest wall expansion; in practice this usually equates to a delivered volume of approximately 6 ml/kg (Dimitriou and Greenough 1995b). Sufficient pressure must be used to achieve acceptable blood gases. Since high pressures/volumes are likely to cause a pneumothorax (p. 487) or lead to BPD (p. 552), the lowest possible peak pressure compatible with normal blood gases should be employed. In general, the starting pressures for a baby with respiratory distress should be about 16–18 cmH$_2$O. The peak pressure is then adjusted according to the blood gas results, which should be determined within 15 minutes of commencing mechanical ventilation. Underventilation produces a high PaCO$_2$ and a low

Pa_{O_2}, and overventilation a low Pa_{CO_2} and sometimes an excessively high Pa_{O_2}.

PEEP. This acts like CPAP to hold the peripheral airways open during expiration. PEEP should always be used during ventilation, as it conserves surfactant on the alveolar surface, except in severe PIE or certain cases of overinflation (Wyszogrodski et al. 1975). If too high a PEEP level is applied, particularly if combined with a short expiratory time, the lung cannot deflate properly. This causes hyperinflation, a reduced tidal volume and compromised gas exchange, and the Pa_{CO_2} rises accompanied by a fall in Pa_{O_2}. Early studies demonstrated that a PEEP of about 5 cmH_2O, rather than no PEEP or much higher levels, improved oxygenation (Herman and Reynolds 1973; Memon et al. 1979); the mechanism was via the effects of MAP on lung volume and oxygenation. The results of subsequent studies suggested that babies with acute RDS or apnoea do not require more than 3 cmH_2O of PEEP (Fiascone et al. 1992; Greenough et al. 1992). Babies who have severe RDS which does not respond to surfactant can require higher PEEP levels to optimise lung volume (da Silva et al. 1994). Infants ventilated beyond the first week without cystic chronic lung disease have improved oxygenation at 6 cmH_2O (Greenough et al. 1992).

Mean airway pressure. There is a good correlation between the MAP level and oxygenation (Herman and Reynolds 1973; Boros et al. 1977), such that Pa_{O_2} may be improved by increasing the inspiratory time, the level of PEEP or the peak inflating pressure, all three manoeuvres elevating MAP. Elevation of the PEEP level, however, is the most effective method of increasing lung volume and hence oxygenation. At a critical level, determined by the infant's lung function, further elevation of the MAP level can impair oxygenation. The MAP level can be calculated from various formulae, but they assume a square-wave inflating pressure and therefore overestimate the MAP. Such calculations are now rarely necessary as the MAP level is displayed on most currently available ventilators.

Ventilator rates. Historically, babies with RDS were ventilated at a ventilator rate that matched their respiratory rate, about 80–100/ min, but this resulted in a high incidence of BPD (Reynolds and Taghizadeh 1974). Studies (Herman and Reynolds 1973; Boros and Campbell 1980; Reyes et al. 2006) then showed that if an I:E ratio of 1:2 was used, the Pa_{O_2} was higher at ventilator rates of 30/min compared with 80/min. At a rate of 30/min, the Pa_{O_2} was found to be higher if the inspiratory time was longer than the expiratory time (a reverse I:E ratio) and 5 cmH_2O of PEEP was employed. Those data were restricted to neonates with severe RDS. Nevertheless, by the late 1970s, ventilator rates of 20–40/min with long inspiratory times were being widely used in infants with all types of lung disease, with an incidence of pneumothorax and other forms of airleak of 35–40% (p. 486). Subsequently, faster rates were preferred. Heicher et al. (1981) found that they could ventilate babies at 60/min with inspiratory times of 0.5 seconds at lower peak inspiratory pressures and with better blood gases and fewer pneumothoraces than when rates of 30/min and inspiratory times of 1 second were used. Subsequently, it was demonstrated (Greenough et al. 1987b) that, when babies with RDS were kept at the same MAP, rates of 120/min produced an improvement in Pa_{O_2} compared with rates of 30 and 60/min; the improvement resulted from the neonates breathing in synchrony with the ventilator. By increasing the ventilator rate as necessary up to 100/min, most neonates were induced to breathe in synchrony (Greenough et al. 1986; South and Morley 1986a) and thus had better blood gases (Greenough et al. 1987a), but whether synchrony decreased the pneumothorax rate was not investigated. Meta-analysis of randomised trials (Greenough et al. 2008) has demonstrated that high-frequency positive-pressure ventilation compared with conventional

mechanical ventilation (CMV) significantly reduced the incidence of airleaks. No advantages of rates in excess of 20–40/min have been demonstrated in infants born at term and in paralysed infants; it is important in such infants to keep the ventilator rate at 60/min or less to reduce the likelihood of gas trapping (Hird et al. 1990).

Inspiratory and expiratory times, I:E ratios. In the 1970s, I:E ratios of 2:1 or even 3:1 were applied, giving inspiratory times as long as 1.5 seconds. This increased the MAP and improved oxygenation, but the reverse I:E ratio, with a concomitant prolongation of the inflation time, was one of the factors that correlated with the high pneumothorax rate (Primhak 1983; Tarnow-Mordi et al. 1985). Subsequently, the average inspiratory and expiratory times in ventilated babies with RDS were demonstrated to be 0.31 seconds (SD 0.06 seconds) and 0.42 seconds (SD 0.13 seconds), respectively (South and Morley 1986b), i.e. an I:E ratio of approximately 1:1.3. Employing such a ratio with an appropriate rate for gestational age (Greenough et al. 1987b) resulted in many babies with RDS breathing in synchrony with the ventilator, with an attendant improvement in oxygenation. Similar studies have not been undertaken in very immature infants with mild lung disease who have received both antenatal steroids and postnatal surfactant therapy; but it is likely that such infants, if they have vigorous respiratory efforts, would be best ventilated with a physiological I:E ratio (i.e. a longer expiratory to inspiratory time) and a rate similar to their spontaneous respiratory frequency. An I:E ratio of 1:1 results in best gas exchange for babies ventilated beyond the first week after birth (Chan and Greenough 1994b).

Ventilator settings with pressure-limited ventilators (Table 27.11)

Babies with abnormal lungs

Initially guided by the baby's colour and chest expansion, the following initial ventilator settings are appropriate, providing the chest wall moves adequately, until the result of blood gas analyses is available (Table 27.12):

Pressure: 18–20/3 cmH_2O
Rate: 60/min
Inspiratory time: 0.3–0.4 seconds
Oxygen concentration: 60–80%

Table 27.11 Adjustments to conventional ventilation according to disease

RESPIRATORY DISEASE	VENTILATORY SETTINGS
Respiratory distress syndrome	Low positive end-expiratory pressure Rates 60–80/min
Meconium aspiration syndrome	Low positive end-expiratory pressure Long expiratory time
Pulmonary hypoplasia	Low positive end-expiratory pressure
Pulmonary airleak	Minimise peak inspiratory pressure
Pulmonary haemorrhage	High positive end-expiratory pressure
Pulmonary oedema	Long inspiratory times

Table 27.12 Adjustments to ventilator settings on the basis of blood gas changes

Low PaO_2	High $PaCO_2$	Increase peak pressure, which will also increase mean airway pressure: in spontaneously breathing babies ↑ rates may also work
Low PaO_2	Normal $PaCO_2$	↑ F_{IO_2}; ↑ MAP but maintain PIP (i.e. ↑ PEEP or ↑ T_I)
Low PaO_2	Low $PaCO_2$	Consider alternative diagnosis, e.g. PPHN, sepsis, overventilation. ↑ F_{IO_2}; ↑ MAP; use vasodilators
PaO_2 normal	High $PaCO_2$	↓ PEEP, ↑ rate; keep MAP constant
PaO_2 normal	Low $PaCO_2$	↓ rate: maintain MAP
PaO_2 high	$PaCO_2$ high	Rare: check for mechanical problems, e.g. blocked tube, ↓ PEEP, ↓ T_I: ↑ rate ↓ F_{IO_2}
PaO_2 high	$PaCO_2$ normal	↓ MAP (usually ↓ PIP): ↓ F_{IO_2}
PaO_2 high	$PaCO_2$ low	↓ pressure, ↓ rate, ↓ F_{IO_2} (see text)
PaO_2 normal	$PaCO_2$ normal	Sit tight! Unless plan to wean

MAP, mean arterial pressure; PIP, peak inspiratory pressure; PEEP, positive end-expiratory pressure; PPHN, persistent pulmonary hypertension of the newborn.

Babies with normal lungs

For babies with primary neurological or myopathic problems, e.g. congenital myopathy (Ch. 40.7), fractured cervical spine, severe neurological depression due to birth asphyxia (Ch. 40.4), drugs (Ch. 26) or preterm babies with recurrent apnoea (Ch. 27.4), the initial ventilator settings should be:

Pressure: 15/3 cmH$_2$O
Rate: 20–30/min
Inspiratory time: 0.35–0.40 seconds
Oxygen concentration: 21–30%

Volume-targeted ventilation

During volume-targeted ventilation (VTV), a set tidal volume is delivered despite changes in the infant's respiratory function; this is achieved by servo-controlled changes in the inflating pressure. There are different forms of VTV (Sharma et al. 2007). During volume-controlled or volume-supported ventilation, the desired tidal volume is selected and the duration of inflation depends on the time taken for the volume to be delivered. During volume guarantee ventilation, a preset expiratory tidal volume is selected, but the preset inspiratory time determines the duration of inflation and the maximum pressure set by the clinician limits the maximum inflation pressure. There is also volume-limited ventilation, during which the pressure support for any inflation is aborted if the measured inspired tidal volume exceeds a preset upper limit. During volume control ventilation, there is a breath-by-breath servo-controlled flow, which is constant during inspiration so that the required volume is delivered over the set inspiratory time. At the same preset ventilator settings, the Stephanie and VIP Bird ventilators deliver signifantly lower peak pressures and tend to deliver lower MAPs than the Draeger and SLE. At a VTV level of 5 ml, the SLE and the VIP Bird deliver significantly shorter inflation times. The above differences relate to differences in the airway pressure waveforms delivered by the four ventilators. The VIP Bird had a less variable volume delivery, but this was always significantly lower than the preset volume guarantee level, but higher than the volume displayed by the ventilator (Sharma et al. 2007).

Clinical studies have demonstrated that the combination of volume guarantee and pressure support compared with sIMV improve infant–ventilator synchrony (El-Moneim et al. 2005) and reduce breath-to-breath variability (Bhandari et al. 2007). Meta-analysis of four randomised trials demonstrated that VTV was associated with lower rates of severe ICH and pneumothorax and the duration of ventilation (McCallion et al. 2005); the trial designs and the ventilators used, however, differed considerably. Subsequent trials have not shown such striking differences. In one (Cheema et al. 2007), volume guarantee halved the occurrence of hypocarbia but only in infants over 25 weeks of gestation; all the infants between 23 and 25 weeks of gestation had out-of-range PCO_2 results. In another trial, infants randomised to volume control ventilation met predefined success criteria sooner and had a shorter duration of mechanical ventilation, but there were no significant differences in other outcomes (Sinha et al. 1997). At follow-up, less of the volume control ventilation group in the latter trial (Sinha et al. 1997) required inhaled steroids/bronchodilators but neurodevelopmental outcome was similar (Singh et al. 2009). Comparison with HFOV demonstrated that volume guarantee was associated with both lower levels of lung inflammation and duration of oxygen dependency (Lista et al. 2008).

A problem with volume ventilation is that not all the tidal volume is delivered to the baby's lungs, as, with the onset of inflation, the pressure rises, compressing the gas in the ventilator circuit as well as in the baby. Furthermore, unless cuffed ETTs are used, as the pressure rises, there is a variable leak of gas around the ETT. As a consequence, the volume required to ventilate the baby cannot be calculated with accuracy. In addition, in an vitro study, the tidal volume displayed by the ventilator underestimated that delivered due to endotracheal leakage depending on ventilator pressures (Mahmoud et al. 2009).

Levels of volume-targeted ventilation

Results from physiological studies have demonstrated that, within the tidal volume range, higher rather than lower levels of tidal volume are likely to be more beneficial. Higher levels of lung inflammatory markers were experienced at VTV levels of 3 rather than 5 ml/kg (Lista et al. 2006), 6 rather than 3 ml/kg reduced the duration of hypoxaemic episodes (Polimeni et al. 2006) and the work of breathing as assessed by the pressure–time product was lower in infants ventilated at 6 rather than 4 ml/kg in infants with acute (Patel et al. 2010a) or recovering from (Patel et al. 2009b) respiratory distress. The most appropriate tidal volume level will probably vary with postnatal age and disease type, as, despite use of permissive hypercapnia, tidal volume requirements increase with advancing postnatal age over the first 3 weeks after birth, probably reflecting the increase in alveolar dead space (Keszler et al. 2009).

Patient-triggered ventilation

PTV is a mode in which the patient's inspiratory efforts 'trigger' positive-pressure inflations.

Assist/control and synchronous intermittent mandatory ventilation

The initial triggered ventilation modes used in the 1980s were assist/control (A/C), otherwise known as synchronous IPPV (sIPPV) or now assist control ventilation (ACV), during which all of the infant's respiratory efforts could trigger positive-pressure inflations, and sIMV, during which the maximum number of breaths that could be triggered was determined by the preset sIMV rate.

Various triggering systems have been used. Their performance can be evaluated by their susceptibility to autotrigger, their sensitivity (the number of the baby's inspiratory efforts that are detected) and their trigger delay or response time (the delay between the sensor being activated and the ventilator inflating the baby). Autotriggering occurs if there is excessive condensation in the ventilator circuit, which can cause changes in flow or pressure, and if there is a large leak around the ETT.

During A/C or sIMV, it is important to limit the ventilator inflation time, or it may extend into the spontaneous expiration of the baby, resulting in asynchrony or even active expiration (Hird and Greenough 1990). In addition, a prolonged inflation time has been shown to reduce the triggering rate by stimulating the Hering–Breuer reflex (Upton et al. 1990). If, however, the inflation time is too short (0.2 second), the volume delivered by the ventilator is compromised (Field et al. 1985; Dimitriou and Greenough 2000). The optimum inflation time, therefore, appears to be between 0.3 and 0.4 seconds.

Clinical studies

ACV or sIMV, compared with conventional ventilation, in a series of physiological studies was associated with a lower rate of asynchrony (Bernstein et al. 1993), higher tidal volume and improved blood gases (Cleary et al. 1995); additional advantages were reduced fluctuations of both BP (Hummler et al. 1994) and cerebral blood flow velocity (Gournay et al. 2002). Meta-analysis (Greenough et al. 2008) of the results of randomised trials, however, demonstrated that the only advantage of ACV or sIMV was a significantly shorter duration of weaning, as the incidences of BPD, severe ICH and airleaks and the mortality rate were similar. Thus, on current evidence, use of ACV or sIMV cannot be recommended for infants with acute RDS. ACV, however, is useful in infants recovering from RDS; in a randomised trial it was shown to shorten the duration of weaning significantly (Chan and Greenough 1993b).

There have been no randomised comparisons of ACV and sIMV in RDS, but the results of three randomised trials suggest that ACV rather than sIMV is the more efficacious weaning mode (Chan and Greenough 1993a, 1994a; Dimitriou et al. 1995). Weaning involving reducing the sIMV rate below 20/min, compared with a reduction in the peak inflating pressures during ACV, was associated with a significantly longer duration of weaning (p. 529). In a randomised short-term physiological study, the work of breathing was higher when volume guarantee was combined with sIMV compared with ACV (Abubakar and Keszler 2005).

Pressure support ventilation

During PSV, the patient's inspiratory effort triggers the onset of a positive-pressure inflation and the end of the spontaneous inspiration dictates the termination of the inflation. PSV has been demonstrated (Dimitriou et al. 1998a) to reduce the asynchrony rate; it is important to determine whether this translates into a lower incidence of airleak. Pressure support increases total minute ventilation and stabilises breathing in proportion to the level of support provided between partial and full-pressure support (Gupta et al. 2009a). In a randomised trial of 107 ELBW infants, pressure support compared with sIMV reduced the number of infants still ventilated at 28 days, and amongst those infants with a birthweight of 700–1000 g it was associated with fewer days of supplementary oxygen (Reyes et al. 2006). In a physiological study (Patel et al. 2009a), addition of PSV to sIMV using the same criteria as in the randomised trial (Reyes et al. 2006) was associated with a significant reduction in the work of breathing as assessed by the measurement of the transdiaphragmatic pressure time product. Those results further support the concept that weaning is best achieved by modes providing pressure support to every breath.

Proportional assist ventilation

During proportional assist ventilation (PAV), the applied ventilator pressure is servo-controlled throughout each respiratory cycle, based on a continuous input from the patient, such that the baby controls the timing, depth and airflow contour of the entire ventilator breath. In addition, negative ventilator resistance and elastance can be applied (unloading), to relieve the resistive and elastic work of breathing, respectively (Schulze et al. 1998). The clinician sets the level of unloading and this enhances the effect of respiratory muscle effort.

During PAV, it is essential that there is adequate back-up ventilation should the baby develop hypoventilation or apnoea. Other possible adverse effects include excessive resistive and elastic unloading, which result, respectively, in resonant oscillations and runaway ventilator pressures. It is also important to avoid using PAV with a major leak around the ETT, as the leak flow mimics inspiration and hence may cause the ventilator repeatedly to deliver inflations to the set upper pressure limit. In an in vitro study (Patel et al. 2010b), increasing unloading was matched by an inspiratory load reduction but, during unloading, delivered pressures were between 1 and 4 cmH_2O above those expected. Oscillations appeared in the airway pressure when the elastic unloading was greater than 0.5 cmH_2O/ml with a low-resistance model and 1.5 cmH_2O/ml with a high-resistance model and when the resistive unloading was greater than 100 cmH_2O/l/s. There was a time lag in the delivery of airway pressure of at least 60 ms. The impact of these problems needs careful evaluation in the clinical setting.

Clinical studies

In preterm infants, PAV compared with A/C and IMV, in a short-term physiological study (Schulze et al. 1998), allowed adequate gas exchange at lower MAPs. It is important to determine if PAV offers long-term advantages over other modes of ventilation in appropriately designed trials (Schulze et al. 1999).

Neurally adjusted ventilatory assist

During neurally adjusted ventilatory assist (NAVA), partial ventilatory assist is controlled by the electrical activity of the diaphragm (EAdi) (Sinderby et al. 1999), which represents the final neural output of the respiratory centres to the diaphragm. The pressure during inspiration during NAVA is delivered in proportion to the EAdi and this proportionality can be adjusted by the clinician. There is limited information regarding NAVA in infants; data from animal models suggest that, in comparison with PSV, NAVA was associated with better synchrony and a lower work of breathing (Beck et al. 2007).

High-frequency jet ventilation

HFJV is a modification of the technique initially developed to provide respiratory support during bronchoscopy. Frequencies between 60 and 600/min may be used. During HFJV, a

SINGLETON HOSPITAL
STAFF LIBRARY

high-pressure source delivers gas in short bursts down a small-bore injector cannula; the tip of the cannula usually lies within the ETT, pointing towards the lung (Froese and Bryan 1987). The bursts of gas entrain additional gas from areas surrounding the jet cannula down the ETT; expiration is passive. In most studies, rates of 100–200/min have been used. In an animal model (Weisberger et al. 1986), a relatively narrow range of inspiratory and expiratory times was demonstrated to provide optimum HFJV. A significantly higher airway pressure gradient is necessary to maintain a constant tidal volume if the inspiratory time is shortened, and reduction in expiratory time below 170 ms results in air trapping. Most jet ventilators operate like constant-flow time-cycled ventilators and the pressure waveform is typically triangular, although pressure servo-controlled jet ventilators are available and produce a square pressure waveform. Keszler and Durand (2001) have described jet ventilators in detail. On HFJV, the PEEP is increased to optimise lung volume and a background IMV rate of 2–5/min employed to open up the alveoli on inspiration (Keszler and Durand 2001). During weaning, it is also important to maintain lung volume; thus, as with HFO, the F_IO_2 is reduced before the MAP.

Clinical studies

HFJV has been used as a rescue mode of support to improve blood gas tensions in infants with respiratory failure unresponsive to conventional ventilation (Pokora et al. 1983); adequate blood gas tensions were achieved with lower peak inflation pressures (Carlo et al. 1984). It was also used with good results in babies with airleaks, in particular bronchopleural fistulae (Boros et al. 1985; Gonzales et al. 1987), PPHN (Carlo et al. 1989) and diaphragmatic hernia (Boros et al. 1985). The results of randomised trials, however, have been conflicting. In a small trial of 42 infants, no improvement in outcome with HFJV was demonstrated (Carlo et al. 1987), and in another study (Engle et al. 1997), although oxygenation improved in infants with PPHN, no long-term benefits were ascribed to HFJV use. Keszler et al. (1991, 1997) reported two positive trials: HFJV use was associated in the first (Keszler et al. 1991) with more rapid resolution of PIE, and in the second (Keszler et al. 1997) with a reduction in the incidence of BPD at 36 weeks and need for home oxygen. Another trial (Wiswell et al. 1996), however, was halted for safety reasons, as infants exposed to HFJV as opposed to CMV had higher rates of severe ICH (41% versus 22%) and PVL (31% versus 6%). Meta-analysis of three trials demonstrated that HFJV use was associated with a significant reduction in BPD, but a non-significant trend towards an increase in PVL (Bhuta and Henderson-Smart 2000).

Complications

HFJV use has been associated with a high incidence of necrotising tracheobronchitis (Mammel and Boros 1987), an ischaemic lesion resulting from intraluminal tracheal pressure compromising mucosal and submucosal blood flow. In HFJV, the lesions range from moderate erythema of the airway to severe necrotising tracheobronchitis with total tracheal obstruction (Boros et al. 1985). The high mean pressure and near-constant intraluminal pressure may be important factors in the pathogenesis of this problem (DeLemos et al. 1987b). Not all workers, however, have found a high incidence of necrotising tracheobronchitis, perhaps because of meticulous humidification (Carlo et al. 1987), but others have reported that HFJV causes more tracheal damage than IPPV (McEvoy et al. 1982; Ophoven et al. 1984) and that the longer the technique is applied, the more likely that necrotising tracheobronchitis will develop (Boros et al. 1977; Fox et al. 1984).

High-frequency flow interrupters

High-frequency flow interrupters (HFFIs) deliver small volumes of gas at high frequencies. A high-pressure gas source fed into a CPAP circuit immediately opposite the ETT connector is interupted. These devices can be used at frequencies of up to 20 Hz (1200/min).

Clinical studies

HFFI use has been associated with improvements in blood gases in babies with PIE, and radiological resolution of the PIE (Fox et al. 1978; Gaylor et al. 1987). No long-term benefits of HFFI have been reported from randomised trials (Pardou et al. 1993; Craft et al. 2003).

Complications

Unlike HFOV (see below), neither HFJV nor HFFI incorporates an active expiratory phase and thus gas trapping may be experienced, particularly at fast frequencies. Tracheal necrosis has been experienced with HFFI.

High-frequency oscillatory ventilation

During HFOV, frequencies between 180 and 3000/min (3–50 Hz) may be used; however, in practice, frequencies of 10–15 Hz are most commonly employed. Unlike other forms of respiratory support, there is an active expiratory phase as well as an active inspiratory phase; this means that gas trapping is unlikely, even though very fast frequencies are employed. During HFOV, a volume generator feeds into a CPAP circuit close to the patient. The generator can be a piston, bellows or a loudspeaker driven by a generator and audio amplifier. Continuous flow is necessary to add fresh gas to the circuit and remove expired gas. HFOV may also be given at the same time as conventional ventilation (Murthy and Petros 1996), but there are no data to suggest such an approach has long-term benefit.

During HFOV, two volume strategies have been pursued: a low-volume strategy, in which MAP is limited with the aim of preventing damage due to barotrauma, and a high-volume strategy, in which MAP is elevated to promote optimum alveolar expansion and hence improve oxygenation. Comparison of the two strategies in animal models demonstrated that the high-volume strategy is less damaging to the lungs (McCulloch et al. 1988). An escalating recruitment manoeuvre, i.e. stepwise increases in MAP, was the most effective method of volume recruitment on initiation of HFOV in a piglet model (Pellicano et al. 2009). Volume delivery during HFOV is proportional to the product of the frequency and the square of the oscillatory amplitude (Slutsky et al. 1981). Early studies suggested that HFOV provided a tidal exchange considerably less than the baby's anatomical dead space (Froese and Bryan 1987). It was suggested that gas exchange occurred additionally by mechanisms distinct from those operating during conventional ventilation; these included bulk flow by convection, convective mixing between lung units (Pendelluft) and augmented diffusion (Chang 1984). It has more recently been demonstrated that infants are oscillated at a tidal volume similar to their anatomical dead space (Dimitriou et al. 1998b).

Management during high-frequency oscillatory ventilation

Oxygenation is influenced by the inspired oxygen concentration and the MAP, the latter controlling lung volume. If a high-volume strategy is used as a rescue support, then the infants should be transferred to HFOV at a MAP 2 cmH_2O higher than that on CMV (Chan and Greenough 1993c). The MAP is then gradually increased to optimise oxygenation. Infants with severe respiratory failure on conventional ventilation often have very low lung volumes and an increase in MAP on HFOV of up to 10 cmH$_2$O may be necessary to maximise oxygenation (Dimitriou and Greenough 1995). The optimum MAP and the change in MAP necessary to optimise oxygenation are dependent on the severity of the infant's lung disease and lung volume. If too high a level of MAP is used, this will result in lung overdistension and deterioration in blood gases. It is thus important to increase the MAP in incremental stages, leaving sufficient time at each step for the lung volume to equilibrate; this usually happens within 10 minutes, but may take up to 20 minutes (Thome et al. 1998). Continuous monitoring of oxygenation should be employed; in an infant with atelectasis this will demonstrate an improvement in oxygenation when the MAP is increased. The MAP should then only be further increased once the monitoring demonstrates no further change in oxygenation, i.e. the lung volume has stabilised; such an approach will minimise the risk of overdistension. Closed endotracheal suctioning is usually performed without disconnection from the ventilator with the hope of maintaining lung volume. However, an in vitro study has demonstrated that airway pressures and tidal volumes were not maintained during closed suctioning with either HFOV or CMV (Kiraly et al. 2009).

Carbon dioxide elimination is dependent on the delivered volume, which is influenced primarily by the oscillatory amplitude, but also by the frequency and I:E ratio. On commencing HFOV, the oscillatory amplitude is increased until chest wall vibration is apparent, and then adjusted as needed to correct hypocapnia or hypercapnia. If an oscillator capable of delivering a constant volume is employed, oscillating at the resonant frequency of the respiratory system in RDS (between 12 and 24 Hz, 720–1440/min), this is associated with an increased volume delivery to the infant (Hoskyns et al. 1991).

The resonant frequency of the respiratory system in preterm infants with RDS remains remarkably constant in the early stages of their illness, despite large changes in static compliance (Lee and Milner 2000). Unfortunately, this does not apply to the majority of commercially available oscillators, whose performance is impaired at increased frequencies (Laubscher et al. 1996). Thus, altering the frequency from 10 to 15 Hz using such oscillators has very little impact on carbon dioxide elimination (Chan and Greenough 1994c). Reducing the frequency below 10 Hz, particularly with the Sensor Medics oscillator, however, results in a greater volume delivery (Laubscher et al. 1996) and thus this manoeuvre can be very useful to improve carbon dioxide elimination in a mature infant with severe respiratory failure. Increasing the I:E ratio from 1:2 to 1:1 on the Sensor Medics increases the delivered volume and hence carbon dioxide elimination (Dimitriou et al. 1999) and has not been associated with gas trapping in infants with respiratory failure (Alexander et al. 1993).

HFOV in animals suppresses spontaneous respiration; although this in part is explained by changes in blood gas tensions, this effect also appears to be related to stimulation of pulmonary mechanoreceptors; vagal fibres are stimulated continuously and to a greater extent during HFOV than with static lung inflation (Man et al. 1983). In humans, spontaneous respiration is reduced, but not usually inhibited (Chan et al. 1995); however, this rarely interferes with the effectiveness of respiratory support (HIFI Study Group 1989; Chan et al. 1995). Hence, we do not recommend routine neuromuscular blockade for infants supported by HFOV.

Early versus selective delayed surfactant administration resulted in a better outcome for infants supported by high-volume strategy HFOV (Plavka et al. 2002). In a randomised trial involving 43 infants, a smaller proportion of infants given early rather than delayed surfactant suffered the combined outcome of death

or supplementary oxygen requirement at 36 weeks' PCA (29% versus 64%) or had had an ICH (43% versus 82%) (Plavka et al. 2002).

Clinical studies

There have been many anecdotal reports of benefit using HFOV (Marchak et al. 1981) in babies with severe RDS (Chan et al. 1994), hypoplastic lungs, pneumonia, PPHN (Boynton et al. 1984), PIE (Clark et al. 1986) and diaphragmatic hernia (Karl et al. 1983). Use of HFOV enabled blood gas tensions to be maintained, with a lowering of MAP and resolution of PIE (Clark et al. 1986), and may be applied only to the affected side if selective intubation is employed (Rettwitz-Volk et al. 1993). Severe lobar emphysema may resolve on HFOV if a low-volume strategy is pursued (Kohlhauser et al. 1995). HFOV, however, is not a successful form of rescue respiratory support in all babies. Failure to improve oxygenation after 6 hours of treatment identifies those babies most likely to die (Chan et al. 1994; Paranka et al. 1995) or survive with disability (Cheung et al. 1997).

There have been two randomised trials of HFOV in infants with severe respiratory failure (Henderson-Smart et al. 2009). In term-born infants (Clark et al. 1992), HFOV was a more effective rescue support than CMV, but there were no significant differences in the requirement for ECMO or duration of ventilator or oxygen dependency between the two groups. In preterm infants (HiFO Study Group 1993), use of HFOV was associated with a significant reduction in new pulmonary airleak (RR 0.73, 95% CI 0.55–0.96), but a significant increase in ICH (RR 1.77, 95% CI 1.06–2.96).

Prophylactic trials in which infants have been randomised to receive HFOV or CMV in the first 24 hours after birth have been performed. The trials have differed with respect to administration of antenatal corticosteroids and postnatal surfactant, and the types of oscillator and conventional ventilator used. Meta-analysis of the results of those trials (Henderson-Smart et al. 2007) has demonstrated that HFOV had no significant effect on mortality, but was associated with a modest but significant reduction in BPD at term.

Complications

In an initial prospective randomised study (HIFI Study Group 1989), prophylactic use of HFOV in infants of birthweight between 750 g and 2000 g with respiratory failure due to RDS, pneumonia or PPHN was associated, worryingly, with a significant increase in the incidence of complicated GMH/IVH. The study design, however, has been criticised, as, in particular, a low-volume strategy was pursued. In one trial (Moriette et al. 2001), even though a high-volume strategy was used, a trend towards an increase in severe ICH was also noted, although this did not reach statistical significance when adjusted for differences in pregnancy-related hypertension rates between the two groups. Follow-up of that study, however, demonstrated that neurodevelopmental outcome at 2 years of age was not worse in the HFOV arm than in the conventionally treated infants (Truffert et al. 2007). Meta-analysis of the results of all prophylactic studies (Henderson-Smart et al. 2007) did not find a statistically significant effect overall on short-term neurological abnormality and no significant excess of ICH or PVL was noted in the HFOV arm of the largest trial to date, which only included very immature infants (Johnson et al. 2002).

During HFOV, very effective carbon dioxide elimination can be achieved. Rapid, large changes in carbon dioxide tensions can occur and are associated with changes in cerebral blood flow velocity (Kavvadia et al. 2001). In a case–control study (Dimitriou et al. 2002a), rescue HFOV was associated with worse neurodevelopmental status at 2 years; this adverse outcome was commoner in very immature babies and could not be predicted by their initial response to HFOV.

Extracorporeal membrane oxygenation

ECMO, a form of cardiopulmonary bypass, provides a method of gas exchange in patients with respiratory failure without resorting to damaging patterns of ventilatory support and allows the lungs a chance to recover. ECMO has been used as a method of respiratory support in newborns suffering from RDS, MAS, sepsis, primary PPHN, congenital heart disease and diaphragmatic hernia. Introduction of the new techniques of respiratory support for term infants has been associated with a reduction in the number of infants being referred for ECMO (Hintz et al. 2000). A greater proportion of infants now receive HFOV, iNO and/or surfactant prior to being referred for ECMO. Delay in the institution of ECMO in infants with severe MAS, however, has been associated with longer post-ECMO ventilation and a higher mortality rate (Gill et al. 2002). Delay in referral may reflect an inappropriately pessimistic view of the survival rate of MAS infants supported by ECMO (Walker et al. 2003). Early discussion with an ECMO centre is advocated to ensure appropriate timing of referral and it has been recommended that ECMO be thought of as an extension of conventional treatment in severe MAS, rather than as a last resort (Davis and Skekerdemian 2001).

Criteria for instituting extracorporeal membrane oxygenation

These have included (Bartlett et al. 1982; Andrews et al. 1984; Loe et al. 1985; Beck et al. 1986):

- severe but reversible cardiac or pulmonary disease unresponsive to optimal ventilation and pharmacological therapy; there should be no ventilator-induced damage or chronic lung disease and the baby must have had less than 10 days of aggressive IPPV
- estimated mortality risk greater than 80%; an OI (MAP × F_IO_2/PaO_2 postductal × 100) >40 historically had been associated with 90% mortality, but in the UK ECMO trial (UK Collaborative ECMO Trial Group 1996, 1998), an OI >40 was associated with a 41% mortality rate
- birthweight >2.0 kg
- gestational age greater than 34 weeks
- no bleeding disorder
- absence of prolonged perinatal hypoxic ischaemia predicted to produce brain damage
- no chromosomal or congenital abnormality incompatible with quality of life.

Technique

Cannulation for ECMO is either venoarterial (VA) or venovenous (VV) (Andrews et al. 1983). Venous blood is usually drained from the right jugular vein; oxygen is then added and carbon dioxide removed by the membrane lung; oxygenated blood is then returned to the patient. For VA bypass, the right common carotid artery and right internal jugular vein are used. Approximately 80% cardiopulmonary bypass is achieved and the level of respiratory support can be reduced, limiting further barotrauma. In VV bypass, oxygenated blood is returned via the right femoral vein or umbilical vein and the carotid artery is spared. VV ECMO can also be undertaken through a double-lumen catheter. A disadvantage of VV ECMO is that cardiopulmonary bypass is not attained and thus the infant must have good myocardial function. There have been no

head-to-head trials comparing VA and VV ECMO, but data from the ELSO registry suggest that mortality may be lower with VV ECMO (8.5% versus 16.2%) (Gauger et al. 1995).

Total respiratory support is provided by an extracorporeal blood flow of approximately 100 ml/kg/min, increasing up to 120 ml/kg/min (Bartlett et al. 1982; Loe et al. 1985). To allow the lung to rest, during VA ECMO, inspired oxygen concentrations of 21–40% and ventilator rates of 10–20/min at pressures of 16–20 cmH$_2$O are used. In both VA and VV ECMO, venous blood is pumped to an oxygenator, which has blood and gas compartments separated by a semipermeable membrane, where diffusion of oxygen and carbon dioxide occurs. Oxygen transfer is controlled by the membrane's surface area, pump flow and the degree of saturation of the venous blood. Carbon dioxide elimination is adjusted by altering the flow rate. Infants are heparinised to achieve whole-blood activated clotting times (ACT) two to three times normal (an ACT of 160–200 s). Haematocrit and platelet count are maintained with transfusion of saline-washed, packed red blood cells and platelet concentrates as necessary.

When the baby starts to improve, as indicated by improving oxygenation, the ECMO circuit flow is gradually reduced to 50 ml/min. When stable vital signs, adequate urine output and acceptable arterial blood gases are achieved on this minimal flow for 4–5 hours, the ECMO cannulae are clamped, and the baby excluded from the ECMO circuit, which can be restarted if necessary.

Results

A multicentre UK trial involving 185 infants demonstrated that, compared with CMV, ECMO reduced mortality by 50% in infants with PPHN or MAS (UK Collaborative ECMO Trial Group 1996). Survival rates are highest in infants with MAS (90%), 76% in BPD infants but only 50% in CDH infants (Table 27.13).

Complications

Local vascular complications occur, including haemorrhage, vessel thrombosis and problems with wound healing. The babies can suffer from anaemia and thrombocytopenia as the result of consumption of blood products at the oxygenator's membrane surface. Mechanical problems occur in up to 20% of patients.

Sequelae

The results of anecdotal follow-up studies need to be interpreted with caution, as the infants were extremely ill prior to receiving ECMO and their original illness may be at least partially responsible

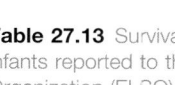

Table 27.13 Survival related to disease of the first 7647 infants reported to the Extracorporeal Life Support Organization (ELSO) registry

DIAGNOSIS	SURVIVAL RATE
Meconium aspiration syndrome	93
Severe respiratory distress syndrome	83
Persistent pulmonary hypertension of the newborn	83
Sepsis	77
Congenital diaphragmatic hernia	59
From Kanto (1994) with permission.	

for any chronic morbidity. Follow-up at 1 year of infants entered into the UK multicentre randomised trial did not demonstrate any excess of severe disability. At 4 years of age, one in four survivors had evidence of impairment with or without disability; the ECMO group had higher survival rates (Bennett et al. 2001).

There have been few studies reported on the long-term respiratory status of ECMO survivors. Short et al. (1987) found a 15% prevalence of BPD, the risk factors being culture-proven streptococcal sepsis and late placement (7–8 days of age) on ECMO. Other risk factors for BPD are lung hypoplasia and failure to respond to a trial of HFOV (Schwendeman et al. 1992). Comparison of non-randomised infants suggested that conventionally treated patients, compared with those supported by ECMO with similar illness severity, have a higher rate of BPD (Walsh-Sukys 1993). Examination at 1 year of 77 infants from the UK randomised trial demonstrated that the ECMO-treated infants had slightly better lung function, with higher inspiratory conductance and V_{max} FRC (Beardsmore et al. 2000). At 7 years, there were no significant differences in the learning problems of the two groups, but there were higher respiratory morbidity and an increased risk of behavioural problems in children in the control group (McNally et al. 2006).

Liquid ventilation

Liquid ventilation (Clark and Gollan 1966) is performed using perfluorocarbons (PFCs), which have a low surface tension (25% of that of water) and a high solubility for respiratory gases, particularly oxygen. PFCs contain carbon and fluorine bonds, which are extremely strong, making them pharmacologically and chemically inert; in addition, they are radiopaque.

Liquid ventilation may be total, in which the PFC is preoxygenated and warmed as it is circulated to fill the lungs to the expected FRC (Hirschl et al. 1995a). The PFC is then moved backwards and forwards at a relatively slow rate and high tidal volume because of the high viscosity of PFC (Hirschl et al. 1995a). Total liquid ventilation requires different circuitry from that used in current clinical practice. Partial liquid ventilation (PLV) or PFC-associated gas exchange has been used to support patients. During PLV, PFC again fills the lungs to FRC, but the patient is then gas-ventilated 'on top'. If no further PFC is given, the PFC in the lung simply evaporates away. Throughout the period of PLV, usually less than 7 days, the PFC is topped up via a side port in the ETT so that a meniscus remains visible there (Hirschl et al. 1995a; Leach et al. 1995a).

In animal models, liquid, as compared with gas, ventilation has been demonstrated to reduce ventilation–perfusion mismatch and improve compliance and oxygenation (Tütüncü et al. 1993). It also appears to be a less damaging form of respiratory support, particularly in very immature animals (Wolfson et al. 1992; Hirschl et al. 1995a). It is compatible with both NO (Wilcox et al. 1995) and surfactant (Leach et al. 1995a). Indeed, it appears to have several advantages over surfactant therapy, as it is not inactivated by proteins and has better spreading capability (Leach et al. 1995b).

Clinical studies

Experience to date is limited to small series; the majority of patients receive PLV while on ECMO. Under such circumstances, in adults (Hirschl et al. 1995b), children and neonates (Gross et al. 1995; Leach et al. 1995b; Greenspan et al. 1997), PLV has been demonstrated to improve oxygenation and compliance. PLV has also improved oxygenation in premature infants with severe respiratory failure (Leach et al. 1996). It has been suggested that PLV can enhance pulmonary function (Pranikoff et al. 1996) and that lung growth can apparently be induced by distension of the lung with PFC in neonates with CDH (Hirschl et al. 2003). In a small randomised trial, however, no statistically significant differences in the number of ventilator-free days or survival rate were found between CDH infants supported by ECMO who did or did not additionally receive PLV (Hirschl et al. 2003).

Care of babies on ventilators

Intubation

The technique of intubating babies and the choice of tubes are described on Ch. 44. Intubating small, sick babies can be difficult; babies may become hypoxaemic, acidaemic and bradycardic during the procedure. During intubation, stress hormones are released (Lehtinen et al. 1984; Shribman et al. 1987), BP and ICP rise (Raju et al. 1980), and this, together with the blood gas changes, predisposes the neonate to GMH/IVH (Ch. 40.5) (Kelly and Finer 1984; Marshall et al. 1984; Friesen et al. 1987). For this reason, it is recommended (Kelly and Finer 1984) that infants who are electively intubated should receive premedication; effective regimes are a combination of atropine, an analgesic (such as fentanyl) and a muscle relaxant (such as mivacurium or succinylcholine) (Dempsey et al. 2006; Lemyre et al. 2009). Atropine abolishes the bradycardia and muscle relaxants attenuate the rise in ICP. In addition, use of suxamethonium, a rapidly acting muscle relaxant, shortens the duration of intubation and hence reduces the duration of hypoxaemia that commonly occurs during intubation. Suxamethonium should, however, be given with a vagolytic drug to pre-empt the potential profound bradycardia that can occur with its administration. Sedation analgesia should also be administered with the muscle relaxant. Morphine commonly has been used, often on its own (Whyte et al. 2000), but fentanyl and alfentanil have a more rapid onset and shorter duration of action. Fentanyl can cause chest wall rigidity, but this resolves promptly with administration of suxamethonium and can be minimised by slow bolus administration.

It is important to use an appropriate-sized tube (Ch. 44). If too small a tube is used, suctioning becomes difficult. In addition, if there is a large leak around the tube, high peak inflating pressures cannot be achieved. Tube size also influences the inspiratory and expiratory resistance; the calculated mean difference in expiratory resistance between tubes of 2.5 mm and 3.5 mm internal diameter was 93 cmH$_2$O/l/s (Farstad and Bratlid 1991). Shortening an ETT to an appropriate length also reduces its resistance. Changing an oral ETT used for labour ward resuscitation to a nasal ETT on a routine basis is not necessary. There is no evidence that nasal tubes are superior to oral tubes for routine use (McMillan et al. 1986). Nasal ETTs can be easily fixed at the nose, which might reduce laryngeal trauma, but ulceration and excoriation of the nostrils can occur. Oral tubes are generally thought to be easier to insert, but infants may suck on an oral ETT and, at follow-up, high palatal arches, pressure-induced grooves and even clefts in the palate have been described.

Humidification

Inadequate warming and humidification of inspired gases will cool the baby and lead to dehydration of the bronchial secretions with airway plugging and obstruction of the ETT. The gas from the ventilator should reach the ETT adequately warmed and humidified. The British Standards Institution (1970) recommends that the minimal accepted humidity is 33 mgH$_2$O per litre inspired gas, which is 75% of that obtained during normal breathing.

Fixation

Many techniques for immobilising ETTs have been described. These include purpose-made devices such as a flange sewn to the ETT and then tied to either side of a bonnet or simply using adhesive tape stuck around the tube and then to the infant's face. It is important to use a system which minimises accidental extubation and avoids causing cosmetic deformity (Ch. 44).

Suctioning

Suctioning can cause bradycardia, hypoxia, bacteraemia and pneumothorax, and an increase in cerebral blood flow and ICP but a fall in cerebral oxygenation (Simbruner et al. 1981; Perlman and Volpe 1983; Murdoch and Darlow 1984; Tarnow-Mordi 1991; Skov et al. 1992), though these effects are less in the paralysed baby (Fanconi and Duc 1987). The technique of ETT suction must allow oxygen administration throughout the procedure, and if the baby becomes bradycardic or the tcPo$_2$, continuous Pao$_2$ monitoring or oximetry demonstrates the oxygenation to have fallen below 6 kPa or the Spo$_2$ below 80%, suction should be discontinued and the infant reconnected to the ventilator.

Inserting the suction catheter until a resistance is felt (when the catheter hits the carina) should be avoided. The suction tube should only be inserted far enough to reach just beyond the tip of the ETT (Bailey et al. 1988).

Both saline and water can damage the lungs and/or the surfactant system (Lachman 1987), particularly if the fluid is not adequately warmed (John et al. 1980). If some form of lubrication is deemed essential to enable the suction catheter to pass down the ETT, the smallest amount of fluid necessary, probably 0.3–0.5 ml, should be used.

Endotracheal suctioning during the acute respiratory illness should be minimised and tailored to the need of the individual neonate. There is no evidence that suctioning is needed more often than every 12 hours in the routine care of babies ventilated for RDS (Wilson et al. 1991).

Complications of intubation

The mucosa of the larynx and trachea shows deciliation, necrosis and desquamation within hours of intubation (Joshi et al. 1972; Gau et al. 1987) and metaplastic change in the trachea occurs (Rasche and Kuhns 1972). Nevertheless, remarkably few long-term sequelae are seen. Many neonates have some hoarseness and/or mild stridor, but only in the 24–48 hours after extubation, and although tracheomegaly can occur after prolonged intubation (Bhutani et al. 1986), it seems to cause little functional problem. Serious damage to the larynx and trachea, such as granulomata or subglottic stenosis or cysts, is uncommon. These sequelae occur in babies who have had prolonged and/or repeated intubations (Sherman et al. 1986) and can be minimised by meticulous attention to ETT immobilisation and by skilled and judicious timing of extubation.

Tracheostomy

See Chapter 27 part 7.

Paralysing babies during ventilation

Administration of neuromuscular blocking agents can reduce the incidence of airleaks if given to preterm babies who are actively expiring against the ventilator (Greenough et al. 1984a). Such agents, however, do have adverse effects. In babies with active respiration, albeit out of phase with ventilator inflation, abolition of spontaneous respiratory activity is associated with a fall in Pao$_2$ and a rise in Paco$_2$ (Runkle et al. 1984) following pancuronium or morphine administration. Lung function may deteriorate, with a fall in compliance and FRC and a rise in airways resistance, leading to a fall in oxygenation (Bhutani et al. 1988b). This deterioration in oxygenation can usually be overcome by increasing the peak inspiratory pressure by 4–6 cmH$_2$O immediately prior to giving the first dose of pancuronium. The use of a neuromuscular blocker results in neonates being ventilated for a longer period of time and developing oedema (Greenough et al. 1987), although this is not associated with a fall in plasma volume (Buckner et al. 1991). Prolonged use has been suggested to cause contractures or muscle atrophy (Sinha and Levene 1984; Rutledge et al. 1986), but this can be avoided by appropriate passive physiotherapy.

Paralysis should also be considered for:

- the mature term baby with MAS, PPHN or GBS sepsis who is chronically restless, hypoxic and impossible to maintain in synchrony with the ventilator, despite sedation and rate and inspiratory time manipulation; infants with CDH should all be paralysed from birth (Ch. 27.6)
- any neonate, irrespective of gestation, who shows the 'active expiratory reflex' pattern and in whom this is not abolished by synchronous ventilation and sedation
- any neonate who develops severe PIE and infants who remain restless despite sedation following drainage of a pneumothorax.

Pancuronium is the most commonly used drug in this situation, given at intervals to suppress all respiratory activity, as it has fewer side-effects than curare. Strict attention to fluid balance is mandatory, as fluid retention during paralysis is common. The excretion of pancuronium in the neonate with kidney and liver problems is variable and this agent interacts with other drugs, in particular the aminoglycosides (Nugent et al. 1979); in consequence, very high plasma levels and prolonged paralysis may occur with infusions of the drug. This may worsen pulmonary mechanics (Bhutani et al. 1988). Hence, infusions should be avoided and the drug given by boluses as required, although this does not necessarily avoid all the side-effects. Other neuromuscular blocking agents include vecuronium, atracurium and cistracurium, the last is a potent isomer of atracurium, but is devoid of histamine-releasing properties in clinical doses and has no breakdown neuromuscular products associated with neuromuscular blocking activity (Reich et al. 2004). In contrast, vecuronium has an active metabolite and is dependent on hepatobiliary and renal excretion (Reich et al. 2004). In neonates and infants, there is a markedly shorter recovery of neuromuscular transmission after cisatracurium than after vecuronium (Reich et al. 2004). Variation in sensitivity of the neuromuscular junction in neonates also means that the inital dose of vecuronium given should be small (10–20 µg) and, as the duration of action and recovery time is longer in babies, maintenance doses should also be low. If 'paralysis' is required for a prolonged period, infants become oedematous, and this is only partially responsive to fluid restriction. It is important to restrict use of neuromuscular blocking agents, as a high daily dose in association with loop diuretics has been associated with an increased risk of senorineural hearing loss (Robertson et al. 2006).

Analgesia/sedation (Ch. 25)

Physiotherapy in ventilated neonates

Meta-analysis of the results of 13 studies, however, demonstrated no significant differences in long-term outcomes amongst ventilated infants who were or were not given opioids, but those receiving morphine took significantly longer to reach full enteral feeding (Bellu et al. 2010). Amongst infants supported by CPAP, a single low dose of morphine (0.01 mg/kg) was associated with significant reductions in heart and respiratory rates; although the overall incidence of apnoea did not differ compared with the pre-morphine period, six infants experienced delayed apnoea (Enders et al. 2008). Remifentanil is an ultra-short-acting opioid with a half-life of 10–35 minutes. In a randomised trial (Silva et al. 2008), the length of time to awaken and extubate was 18 and 12 times longer, respectively, with morphine than with remifentanil. It has been shown to provide adequate analgesia in ventilated infants at an infusion rate of 0.094 μg/kg/min (Giannantonio et al. 2009) and has been used as an induction agent for the INSURE procedure (Welzing et al. 2009).

Physiotherapy in ventilated neonates

Problems with retained sticky secretions or ETT blockage are rare in the first 3–4 days of IPPV if adequate humidification of the ventilator gases is undertaken. Chest physiotherapy on ventilated babies with RDS may cause serious hypoxia and release of stress hormones (Griesen et al. 1985); physiotherapy is, therefore, not warranted as a routine (Fox et al. 1978; Simbruner et al. 1981; Wilson et al. 1991). Frequent endotracheal suction and/or regular chest physiotherapy may be needed, however, in babies with:

- pneumonia and increased secretions (Ch. 39.2)
- meconium aspiration (p. 501)
- MPH (p. 509)
- bronchorrhoea as BPD develops (p. 552).

Posture

The position of ventilated neonates should be changed 2–3-hourly from the back to the right and then the left side, to aid movement of airway secretions. The prone position (except in babies with UACs) with the baby's head turned to one side should also be used, since this will facilitate drainage of secretions and improvement of blood gases (Wagaman et al. 1979; Dimitriou et al. 1996). The neonate with severe PIE should lie on the affected side, since this hastens the disappearance of interstitial gas.

Deterioration on intermittent positive pressure ventilation

Not all babies who are stable on IPPV remain so: their condition may, and often does, worsen, and this can be a sudden collapse or a gradual deterioration.

Sudden collapse

Sudden spontaneous episodes of hypoxaemia are not uncommon in ventilated preterm babies. These may be due to episodes of active exhalation (Bolivar et al. 1995) and usually respond to short-term increases in F_IO_2 or pressure; infants who continue to expire actively should be paralysed. More prolonged deterioration is usually due to one of three things: a blocked or displaced ETT, an acute airleak, usually a pneumothorax, or the sudden development of a large GMH/IVH. If the third possibility is not present, prompt and efficient management of the other two is essential to prevent it developing. It is important to establish that the ETT is in situ and patent by observing whether there is adequate chest wall excursion and auscultating the chest. A capnometer, which detects exhaled carbon, may facilitate detection of extubation (Sutherland and Quinn 1993) by demonstrating the absence of intermittent changes in

carbon dioxide in time with ventilation. The development of a pneumothorax, by either transillumination or CXR, must then be excluded; if the infant's condition is critical, emergency chest aspiration should be considered (Ch. 44).

Gradual deterioration

The respiratory condition of infants with RDS who have not received surfactant will worsen over the first 24–48 hours. Other reasons for a ventilated baby to deteriorate gradually include the development of pneumonia, a GMH/IVH, anaemia, hypotension, an airleak or pulmonary oedema. In addition, partial blockage of the ETT and progression to BPD will be associated with worsening blood gases.

The severely hypoxic neonate

Hypoxia with normocapnia or hypocapnia

In the absence of severe lung disease and in infants with mild RDS or MAS, the blood gas abnormalities should be managed as outlined for PPHN. In infants with severe lung disease who remain severely hypoxic (Pao_2, 5 kPa in 95% oxygen) despite treatment of coexisting problems, the options are to increase the level of ventilatory support, use vasodilator drugs (p. 498) and, in an infant born at or near term, consider use of ECMO (pp. 525–526). The MAP should be increased because, by causing an improvement in lung volume, this can increase oxygenation. MAP can be increased by elevating either the peak inflating pressure or PEEP level or by prolonging the inflation time (with a reversed I:E ratio); the most effective manoeuvre, however, is to increase the PEEP level. Infants who are actively expiring against the ventilator and/or are receiving a peak inflating pressure >25 cmH₂O should be paralysed. If these manoeuvres fail and the infant has an adequate BP (Appendix 4), pulmonary vasodilator drugs (p. 498) should be given.

It is essential to check that the baby has not been overventilated to such an extent that the MAP is compromising pulmonary artery perfusion and causing iatrogenic PPHN. The diagnostic clues are a low Pao_2 and a very low $Paco_2$, often less than 3–3.5 kPa (23–26 mmHg), a raised pH (<7.45–7.50) and a CXR showing dark overexpanded lungs. A similar situation may be seen with inadvertent PEEP in older babies with BPD and an increased airways resistance; reducing the ventilator rate and hence increasing the expiratory time will dramatically improve ventilation (Stenson et al. 1995).

Profound hypoxaemia with carbon dioxide retention

If severe hypoxaemia is combined with hypercapnia, particularly if this is 7–8 kPa (52–60 mmHg), and technical problems with the ventilator circuit and tube have been excluded, the ventilator pressure and/or rate should be increased. If very high inflation pressures (35 cmH₂O) are being used, in a neonate who is clinically stable with an acceptable BP, less than perfect blood gases can be tolerated, provided that the Pao_2 is 5.5–6.0 kPa (41–45 mmHg), the $Paco_2$ 8 kPa (60 mmHg) and the pH 7.25.

Weaning

It is important to wean an infant from mechanical ventilation and extubate as soon as possible, as complications of IPPV such as infection, BPD and airleak are related to the duration of IPPV. There are, however, dangers in trying to get a baby off IPPV too quickly, particularly in the very preterm baby in whom too rapid a weaning process may result in a recurrence of severe atelectasis and the need for more intensive ventilator support than before.

Once satisfactory blood gases have been achieved (Pa_{O_2} 8–12 kPa (60–90 mmHg), Pa_{CO_2} >5.5–6.5 kPa (40–50 mmHg), pH >7.25) and the baby has been stable at these levels for 6 hours, weaning should begin. During weaning, the most damaging modality of ventilation should be reduced first, i.e. the peak inspiratory pressure, as this is a factor in the aetiology of pneumothorax and BPD (Ch. 27.3). After reducing the peak pressures down to 25 cmH$_2$O and the inspired oxygen concentration to less than 60%, if the Pa_{O_2} is >8–9 kPa (60–70 mmHg) and the Pa_{CO_2} is well controlled or if there is a respiratory alkalaemia, the oxygen concentration and peak pressures can then be reduced simultaneously. In general, the settings should be reduced in small increments: 5–10% for oxygen and 2–3 cmH$_2$O for peak inspiratory pressure; too rapid or too large changes can result in the baby becoming hypercapnic and/or hypoxic. After each change, it is important to check the blood gases within 30–60 minutes to ensure that they are still satisfactory. If the blood gases are acceptable (Pa_{O_2} >8 kPa (60 mmHg), pH >7.25) and the baby is breathing spontaneously, the settings should be reduced every 4–6 hours.

Pancuronium should not be discontinued until problems due to airleaks (severe PIE or pneumothorax) have been controlled and the ventilator settings have been reduced to 22–25 cmH$_2$O and 50–60% oxygen.

Once the baby is making spontaneous respiratory efforts and the peak pressures have been reduced to 14–18/3 cmH$_2$O (depending on the size of the baby), the inflation time should be reduced to 0.3–0.4 seconds. The infant should be transferred to ACV and the inflating pressures reduced still further depending on the size of the infant, before considering extubation. This approach has been shown to shorten the duration of weaning significantly (Chan and Greenough 1993a). ACV rather than sIMV is preferred as reducing the ventilator rate below 20/min, regardless of whether a patient-triggered mode is used, increases the work of breathing (Roze et al. 1997). Other triggered modes, for example PSV with or without volume guarantee (p. 522), can be used to wean babies; whether these modes are more effective than ACV requires investigation in appropriately designed randomised trials.

Once the neonate is in 30% oxygen and the peak inflating pressures reduced to 10–16 cmH$_2$O, the baby will usually be ready to extubate. Delay in extubation following 36 hours of optimised mechanical ventilation does not improve the rate of successful extubation (Danan et al. 2008). Some prefer to extubate babies only after they have been able to maintain their blood gases on endotracheal CPAP (etCPAP). The period on etCPAP should, however, be limited to an hour or less (Kim and Boutwell 1987), as breathing through a narrow ETT increases the work of breathing (p. 457), so the baby can tire easily. Indeed, in randomised trials, direct extubation from a low IMV rate rather than after a period of etCPAP was associated with an increased chance of successful extubation (Davis and Henderson-Smart 2001).

Infants with a birthweight less than 1.0 kg should be extubated on to nCPAP rather than directly into supplementary oxygen delivered into a headbox. Randomised trials have demonstrated that use of nCPAP postextubation reduces the need for increased respiratory support (Dimitriou et al. 2000). If nCPAP is used, after 24–48 hours the baby should then be nursed in a headbox in the same inspired oxygen concentration, restarting nCPAP if the baby develops apnoeas or shows signs of increasing respiratory distress. Time-cycling babies on and off CPAP, with increasingly longer periods off CPAP on successive days if tolerated, is not advantageous and indeed prolongs the duration of CPAP, compared with reducing the CPAP pressures (Soe 2007).

In babies >1.50 kg birthweight, weaning can often be rapid, over a period of 12–24 hours, with no need for prolonged periods on nCPAP. Conversely, in neonates <1.00 kg birthweight, the later stages of weaning may take weeks (see below). Infants older than 1 week may benefit from extubation on to higher levels of CPAP than preterm infants less than 1 week old (6 rather than 3 cmH$_2$O) (Chan and Greenough 1993a).

In babies <1.5 kg and <32 weeks of gestational age, methylxanthines should be adminstered at least 12 hours prior to extubation. In prospective randomised controlled trials, administration of methylxanthines has been demonstrated to reduce the failure in extubation in preterm infants within 1 week of age (Henderson-Smart and Davis 2003). Theophylline, however, has side-effects, including tachycardia, vomiting, diuresis and hyperglycaemia; these are dose-related, hence it is important to monitor levels carefully. Theophylline also increases energy expenditure and augments carbohydrate utilisation, which could be detrimental to growth (Carnielli et al. 2000). A further disadvantage is that theophylline has to be given three times a day. Caffeine, then, is the weaning agent of choice, as it is administered once daily, has a lower toxicity level and fewer side-effects and in a randomised trial (Sims et al. 1989) was demonstrated to be equally effective as theophylline. Doxapram has been used in infants who appear resistant to methylxanthines, but even in low dose may cause elevation of BP and result in high plasma levels of doxapram (Huon et al. 1998); thus, we do not recommend its use.

Weaning problems

After any step in weaning, the baby may deteriorate or the blood gases at the new setting may be unacceptable. One finding which is common in VLBW neonates and which suggests that the weaning procedure is not progressing smoothly is the development over 6–12 hours of a metabolic acidaemia, a sign that the work of breathing at the new ventilator setting is excessive. In this situation, after ensuring that the baby has not suffered some unrelated adverse event such as a blocked ETT or a pneumothorax, all that is usually required is to revert to the previous ventilator setting. In some babies, however, following the deterioration, much more vigorous ventilation may be necessary for 24–48 hours before the weaning process can once more be resumed.

Extubation

Extubation carries the risk of severe hypoxia leading to GMH/IVH, inhalation of gastric contents and the need for reintubation, with a possibility of laryngeal trauma. It is essential, therefore, only to attempt extubation with the baby in the best possible condition, including normal electrolytes, a haemoglobin >13 g/dl and normal acid–base status. Feeding should be discontinued 6–12 hours before extubation and not restarted for a further 12 hours, so that the risks of regurgitation and inhalation of milk are reduced to a minimum.

After extubation, the neonate often has considerable difficulty clearing secretions as airway ciliary function has been compromised by the damage caused by the ETT. The inspired oxygen must, therefore, be humidified and warmed. No clear benefit has been demonstrated in routine, periextubation active chest physiotherapy (Flenady and Gray 2002; Hough et al. 2008) and thus physiotherapy and suction should be adapted on the basis of clinical findings or the CXR.

Prediction of successful extubation

A variety of univariate indices have been assessed in an attempt to improve prediction of extubation success, including minute ventilation (Wilson et al. 1998; Vento et al. 2004; Kamlin et al. 2006) and compliance (Kavvadia et al. 2000a; Dimitriou et al. 2002b) and resistance (Veness-Meeham et al. 1990) of the respiratory system, but none has been found to be a consistently reliable predictor. In one study (Kavvadia et al. 2000a), a low lung volume (FRC <26 ml/kg) was more predictive of extubation failure (need for reintubation) than compliance, tidal volume or respiratory rate results, but only if the lung volumes post- rather than pre-extubation were considered. In addition, although respiratory muscle strength, as measured by the maximal inspiratory pressure (Pi_{max}), has been reported to differ significantly according to extubation outcome (Shoults et al. 1979; Belani et al. 1980), in another study (Kamlin et al. 2006) the significant difference in Pi_{max} results according to extubation outcome disappeared when the Pi_{max} results were corrected for weight. Extubation success depends on the adequacy of respiratory drive, the capacity of the respiratory muscles and the load imposed upon them and hence composite indices are likely to be more predictive than univariate indices. The tension time index of the diaphragm (TT_{di}) (Bellemare and Grassino 1982a, b) is a measure of the load on and the capacity of the diaphragm; it requires measurement of intrathoracic and intra-abdominal pressure to obtain transdiaphragmatic pressure. A non-invasive tension time index (TT_{mus}) based on airway pressure measurements, however, has been developed and was 100% sensitive and specific in predicting extubation failure in children (Harikumar et al. 2009). A TT_{di} of >0.15 and a TT_{mus} of >0.18 were 100% sensitive and 100% specific in predicting extubation failure, but only 20 infants were included in the study (Currie et al. 2010).

Extubation problems

Stridor

Minor degrees of stridor are not uncommon and usually only last for an hour or two or at most 24 hours. If persistent, the infant may benefit from high-pressure nasopharyngeal CPAP, using pressures up to 6–8 to 10 cmH_2O; whether or not this will work can only be assessed on a trial-and-error basis. Nebulised adrenaline (epinephrine) can also be administered. If the stridor is marked and unresponsive with severe respiratory distress and there is progressive deterioration of the blood gases, there is no alternative but to reintubate. In such patients, the ETT should be left in place with the baby on minimal ventilation for at least 2–3 days before a further attempt at extubation is made after pretreating the baby with dexamethasone (0.5 mg/kg) for 24 hours and continuing the drug for 24–48 hours after extubation (Corbet et al. 1991). The management of the baby in whom this does not work and in whom some more serious laryngeal damage has occurred is outlined on Chapter 27 part 7.

Lobar collapse

Despite careful physiotherapy and suction postextubation, up to 20% of neonates develop collapse consolidation of one lung or just one lobe, particularly the right upper, because of plugging of the bronchi with secretions (Wyman and Kuhns 1977) (Fig. 27.42). This complication seems to be more common after nasal intubation (Spitzer and Fox 1982). It may cause such severe

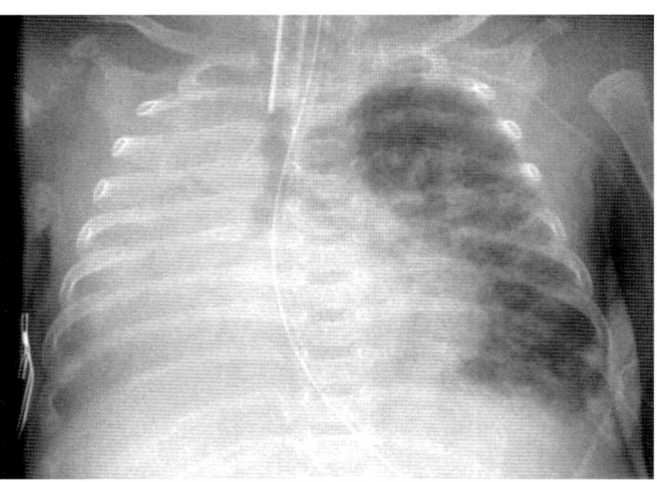

Fig. 27.42 Atelectasis of the right lung. The infant required reintubation and ventilation prior to the chest radiograph because of poor blood gases postextubation.

deterioration that reintubation and IPPV are necessary, but other infants may be virtually asymptomatic. Milder cases can be treated by vigorous physiotherapy. Occasionally it is worth sucking out the airway of more severely affected neonates under direct vision at laryngoscopy. By turning the head away from the affected lung, the suction catheter can usually be directed into the appropriate main stem bronchus.

In order to detect areas of asymptomatic collapse, particularly in the right upper lobe, before they progress to total lung collapse, neonates should be X-rayed within 24 hours of extubation and whenever there is any deterioration in their clinical condition or blood gases. The development of significant intercostal/subcostal retractions and an increase in the inspired oxygen concentration of at least 7% has been suggested to be a sensitive indicator of radiological deterioration (Fok et al. 1998).

Recurrent failure to wean or extubate

Repeated unsuccessful attempts to extubate a neonate over a period of a week is usually only a problem in ELBW neonates whose weight is not increasing and in whom the repeated episodes of extubation and deterioration make adequate nutrition even more difficult to achieve. Rarely it is due to laryngeal damage. Poor lung function is not usually responsible (Veness-Meeham et al. 1990). Affected infants should be reintubated and restarted on IPPV at the minimal settings necessary to achieve normal blood gases and kept there until they are in a better condition and gaining weight consistently. Repeated failure to wean a neonate off IPPV is very suggestive of a neurological problem, secondary to either GMH/IVH or some primary muscular or neurological disorder, including, particularly in term babies, the congenital hypoventilation syndrome (Ondine's curse).

References

Abbasi, S., Bhutani, V.K., Gerdes, J.S., 1993. Long term pulmonary consequences of respiratory distress syndrome in preterm infants treated with exogenous surfactant. Journal of Pediatrics 122, 446–452.

Abman, S.H., Ivy, D., Ziegler, J.W., et al., 1996. Mechanisms of abnormal vasoreactivity in persistent pulmonary hypertension of the newborn infant. J Perinatol 16, S18–S23.

Abubakar, K., Keszler, M., 2005. Effect of volume guarantee combined with assist/control vs synchronized intermitten ventilation. J Perinatol 25, 638–642.

Achiron, R., Zakut, H., 1986. Fetal haemothorax complicating amniocentesis. Acta Obstetrica Gynaecologica Scandinavica 65, 869–870.

ACTOBAT Study Group, 1995. Australian collaborative trial of antenatal thyrotropin releasing hormone (ACTOBAT) for prevention of neonatal respiratory disease. Lancet 345, 877–882.

Aghajafari, F., Murphy, K., Matthews, S., et al., 2002. Repeated doses of antenatal corticosteroids in animals: a systematic review. Am J Obstet Gynecol 186, 843–849.

Ahluwalia, J.S., Kelsall, A.W.R., Raine, J., et al., 1994. Safety of inhaled nitric oxide in premature neonates. Acta Paediatr 83, 347–348.

Ahn, M.O., Cha, K.Y., Phelan, J.P., 1992. The low birthweight infant: is there a preferred route of delivery? Clin Perinatol 19, 411–423.

Aiton, N.R., Fox, G.R., Hannam, S., et al., 1996. Pulmonary hypoplasia presenting as persistent tachypnoea in the first few months of life. Br Med J 312, 1149–1150.

Alexander, J., Blowes, R., Ingram, D., et al., 1993. Determination of the resonant frequency of the respiratory system during high frequency oscillatory ventilation. Early Hum Dev 35, 234.

Allen, A.C., Usher, R.H., 1971. Renal acid excretion in infants with respiratory distress syndrome. Pediatr Res 5, 345–355.

Allen, L.P., Reynolds, E.O.R., Rivers, R.P.A., et al., 1977. Controlled trial of continuous positive airway pressure given by face mask for hyaline membrane disease. Arch Dis Child 52, 373–378.

Allen, R.W., Jung, A.L., Lester, P.D., 1981. Effectiveness of chest tube evacuation of pneumothorax in neonates. Journal of Pediatrics 99, 629–634.

Al-Nishi, N., Dyer, D., Sharief, N., et al., 1994. Selective bronchial occlusion for treatment of bullous interstitial emphysema and bronchopleural fistula. J Pediatr Surg 29, 1545–1547.

Alpan, G., Mauray, F., Clyman, R.I., 1989. Effect of patent ductus arteriosus on water accumulation and protein permeability in the lungs of mechanically ventilated premature lambs. Pediatr Res 26, 570–575.

Al-Sayed, L., Schrank, W., Thach, B.T., 1994. Ventilatory sparing strategies and swallowing pattern during bottle feeding in human infants. J Appl Physiol 77, 78–83.

Amodio, J., Abramson, S., Berdon, W., et al., 1987. Iatrogenic causes of large pleural fluid collections in the premature infant: ultrasonic and radiographic findings. Pediatr Radiol 17, 104–108.

Andersen, E.A., Hertel, J., Pedersen, S.A., et al., 1984. Congenital chylothorax: management by ligature of the thoracic duct. Scand J Thorac Cardiovasc Surg 18, 193–194.

Anderson, K.D., Chandra, R., 1976. Pneumothorax secondary to perforation of segmental bronchi by suction catheters. J Pediatr Surg 11, 687–693.

Andrews, A.F., Klein, M.D., Tommasian, J.M., 1983. Venovenous ECMO in neonates with respiratory failure. J Pediatr Surg 18, 339–346.

Andrews, A.F., Roloff, D., Bartlett, R.H., 1984. Use of extracorporeal membrane oxygenation in persistent pulmonary hypertension of the newborn. Clin Perinatol 11, 729–735.

Annibale, D.J., Hulsey, T.C., Wagner, C.L., et al., 1995. Comparative neonatal morbidity of abdominal and vaginal deliveries after uncomplicated pregnancies. Arch Pediatr Adolesc Med 149, 862–867.

Aranda, J.V., Stern, L., Dunbar, J.S., 1972. Pneumothorax with pneumoperitoneum in a newborn infant. Am J Dis Child 123, 163–166.

Aslan, E., Tutdibi, E., Martens, S., et al., 2008. Transient tachypnoa of the newborn: a role for polymorphisms in the β adrenergic receptor encoding genes? Acta Pediatrica 97, 1346–1350.

Auten, R.L., Notter, R.H., Kendis, J.W., et al., 1991. Surfactant treatment of full term newborns with respiratory failure. Pediatrics 87, 101–107.

Avery, G.B., Randolph, J.G., Weaver, T., 1966a. Gastric acidity in the first day of life. Pediatrics 37, 1005–1007.

Avery, M.E., Gatewood, O.B., Brumley, G., 1966b. Transient tachypnea of the newborn. Am J Dis Child 111, 380–385.

Avery, M.E., Tooley, W.H., Keller, J.B., et al., 1987. Is chronic lung disease in low birthweight infants preventable? A survey of eight centers. Pediatrics 79, 26–30.

Axelin, A., Ojajarvi, U., Vitanen, J., et al., 2009. Promoting shorter duration of ventilator treatment decreases the number of painful procedures in preterm infants. Acta Pediatrica 98, 1751–1755.

Bae, C.W., Takahasi, A., Chida, S., et al., 1998. Morphology and function of pulmonary surfactant inhibited by meconium. Pediatr Res 44, 187.

Baildam, E.M., Dady, I.M., Chiswick, M.L., 1993. Bronchocutaneous fistula associated with mechanical ventilation. Arch Dis Child 69, 525–526.

Bailey, C., Kattwinkel, J., Teja, K., et al., 1988. Shallow versus deep endotracheal suctioning in young rabbits: pathological effects on the tracheal and bronchial wall. Pediatrics 82, 746–751.

Ballard, P.L., 1984. Combined hormonal treatment and lung maturation. Semin Perinatol 8, 283–292.

Ballard, P.L., Gluckman, P.D., Liggins, G.C., et al., 1980. Steroid and growth hormone levels in premature infants after prenatal betamethasone therapy to prevent respiratory distress syndrome. Pediatr Res 14, 122–127.

Ballard, R.A., Troug, W.E., Cnaan, A., et al., 2006. Inhaled nitric oxide in preterm infants undergoing mechanical ventilation. NEJM 355, 343–353.

Ballin, A., Koren, G., Kohelet, D., et al., 1987. Reduction in platelet counts induced by mechanical ventilation in newborn infants. Journal of Pediatrics 111, 445–449.

Bancalari, E., Berlin, J.A., 1978. Meconium aspiration and other asphyxial disorders. Clin Perinatol 5, 317–334.

Barak, M., Cohen, A., Herschikowitz, S., 1992. Total leukocyte and neutrophil count changes associated with antenatal betamethasone administration in premature infants. Acta Paediatr 81, 760–763.

Barefield, E.S., Hicks, T.P., Phillips, J.B., 1994. Thromboxane and pulmonary morphometry in the development of the pulmonary hypertensive response to group B streptococcus. Crit Care Med 22, 506–514.

Barker, D.P., Rutter, N., 1996. Stress, severity of illness, and outcome in ventilated preterm infants. Arch Dis Child Fetal Neonatal Ed 75, F187–F190.

Barrington, K.J., Finer, N.N., 2007. Inhaled nitric oxide for preterm infants: a systematic review. Pediatrics 120, 1088–1099.

Bartlett, D., 1985. Ventilatory and protective mechanisms of the infant larynx. Am Rev Respir Dis 131 (suppl.), 49–50.

Bartlett, R.H., Andrews, A.F., Toomasian, J.M., et al., 1982. ECMO for newborn respiratory failure, 45 cases. Surgery 92, 425–433.

Bassler, D., Choon, G., McNamara, P., et al., 2006. Neonatal persistent pulmonary hypertension treated with milinone: four case reports. Biol Neonate 89, 1–5.

Baud, O., Foix-L'Helias, L., Kaminski, M., et al., 1999. Antenatal glucocorticoid treatment and cystic periventricular leukomalacia in very premature infants. NEJM 341, 1190–1196.

Baum, J.D., Roberton, N.R.C., 1974. Distending pressure in infants with respiratory distress syndrome. Arch Dis Child 49, 771–781.

Baumgart, S., Hirsch, R.B., Butler, S.Z., et al., 1992. Diagnosis related criteria in the consideration of extracorporeal membrane oxygenation in neonates previously breathed with high frequency jet ventilation. Pediatrics 89, 491–494.

Beardsmore, C., Dundas, I., Poole, K., et al., 2000. Respiratory function in survivors of the United Kingdom Extra Corporeal Membrane Oxygenation Trial. Am J Respir Crit Care Med 161, 1129–1135.

Beck, R., 1985. Chronic lung disease following hypocapnic alkalosis for persistent pulmonary hypertension. Journal of Pediatrics 106, 527–528.

Beck, R., Anderson, K.D., Pearson, G.D., et al., 1986. Criteria for extracorporeal membrane oxygenation in a population of infants with persistent pulmonary hypertension of the newborn. J Pediatr Surg 21, 297–302.

Beck, J., Campoccia, F., Allo, J.C., et al., 2007. Improved synchrony and respiratory unloading by neurally adjusted ventilatory assist (NAVA) in lung-injured rabbits. Pediatr Res 61, 289–294.

Beeby, P.J., Elliott, E.J., Henderson-Smart, D.J., et al., 1994. Predictive value of umbilical artery pH in preterm infants. Arch Dis Child Fetal Neonatal Ed 71, F93–F96.

Been, J.V., Rours, I.G., Kornelisse, R.F., et al., 2010. Chorioamnionitis alters the response to surfactant inpreterm infants. Journal of Pediatrics 156, 10–15.

Beeram, M.R., Dhanireddy, R., 1992. Effects of saline instillation during tracheal suction on lung mechanics in newborn infants. J Perinatol 12, 120–123.

Beeram, M.R., Young, M., Abedin, M., 1995. Effect of maternal illicit drug use on the mortality of very low birth weight infants. J Perinatol 15, 456–460.

Beierholm, E.A., Grantham, N., O' Keefe, D.D., et al., 1975. Effects of acid–base changes, hypoxia and catecholamines on ventricular performance. Am J Physiol 228, 1555–1561.

Belani, K.G., Gilmour, I.J., McComb, C., et al., 1980. Preextubation ventilatory measurements in newborns and infants. Anesth Analg 59, 467–472.

Beligere, N., Rao, R., 2008. Neurodevelopmental outcome of infants with meconium aspiration syndrome: report of a study and literature review. J Perinatol 28, S93-S101.

Bell, E.F., Acarregui, M.J., 2008. Restricted versus liberal water intake for preventing morbidity and mortality in preterm infants. Cochrane Database for Systematic Reviews (1), CD000503.

Bell, E.F., Warburton, D., Stonestreet, B.S., et al., 1980. Effect of fluid administration on the development of symptomatic patent ductus arteriosus and congestive heart failure in premature infants. NEJM 303, 598–604.

Bell, A.H., Skov, L., Lundstrom, K.E., et al., 1994. Cerebral blood flow and plasma hypoxanthine in relation to surfactant treatment. Acta Paediatr 83, 910–914.

Bellemare, F., Grassino, A., 1982a. Effect of pressure and timing of contraction on human diaphragm fatigue. J Appl Physiol 53, 1190–1195.

Bellemare, F., Grassino, A., 1982b. Evaluation of human diaphragm fatigue. J Appl Physiol 53, 1196–1206.

Bellu, R., de Waal, K., Zanini, R., 2010. Opioids for neonates receiving mechanical ventilation: a systematic review and meta-analysis. Archives of Disease in Childhood Fetal Neonatal Edition 95, 241–251.

Bennett, C.C., Johnson, A., Field, D.J., et al., 2001. UK collaborative randomised trial of neonatal extracorporeal membrane oxygenation: follow-up to age 4 years. Lancet 357, 1094–1096.

Benson, B.J., 1993. Genetically engineered human pulmonary surfactant. Clin Perinatol 20, 791–811.

Benveniste, D., Berg, O., Pederson, J.E.P., 1976. A technique for delivery of continuous positive pressure to the neonate. Journal of Pediatrics 88, 1015–1019.

Berg, T.J., Pagtakhan, T.D., Reed, M.H., et al., 1975. Bronchopulmonary dysplasia and lung rupture in hyaline membrane disease: influence of continuous distending pressure. Pediatrics 55, 51–53.

Berger, J.T., Gilhooly, J., 1993. Fibrin glue treatment of persistent pneumothorax in a premature infant. Journal of Pediatrics 122, 958–960.

Bernstein, G., Cleary, J.P., Heldt, G.P., et al., 1993. Response time and reliability of three neonatal patient triggered ventilators. Am Rev Respir Dis 148, 358–364.

Bhandari, V., Bergqvist, L.L., Kronsberg, S.S., et al., 2005. Morphine administration and short term pulmonary outcomes among ventilated preterm infants. Pediatrics 116, 352–359.

Bhandari, V., Gavino, R.G., Nedrelow, J.H., et al., 2007. A randomised controlled trial of synchronized nasal intermittent positive pressure ventilation in RDS. J Perinatol 27, 697–703.

Bhandari, V., Finer, N.N., Ehrenkranz, R.A., et al., 2009. Synchronized nasal intermittent positive-pressure ventilation and neonatal outcomes. Pediatrics 124, 517–526.

Bhuta, T., Henderson-Smart, D.J., 2000. Elective high frequency jet ventilation versus conventional ventilation for respiratory distress syndrome in preterm infants. Cochrane Database Syst Rev (2), CD000328.

Bhuta, T., Kent-Biggs, J., Jeffrey, H.E., 1997. Prediction of surfactant dysfunction in term infants by click test. Pediatr Pulmonol 23, 287–291.

Bhutani, V.K., 2008. Developing a systems approach to prevent meconium aspiration syndrome: lessons from multinational trials. J Perinatol 28, S30-S35.

Bhutani, V.K., Ritchie, W.G., Shaffer, T.H., 1986. Acquired tracheomegaly in very preterm neonates. Am J Dis Child 140, 449–452.

Bhutani, V.K., Abbasi, S., Silvieri, E.M., 1988a. Continuous skeletal muscle paralysis: effect on neonatal pulmonary mechanics. Pediatrics 81, 419–422.

Bhutani, V.K., Sivieri, E.M., Abbasi, S., Shaffer, T.H., 1988b. Evaluation of neonatal pulmonary mechanics and energetics. Pediatr Pulmonol 4, 150–158.

Bindl, L., Fahnenstich, H., Peukert, U., 1994. Aerosolized prostacyclin for pulmonary hypertension in neonates. Arch Dis Child Fetal Neonatal Ed 71, F214–F216.

Björklund, L.J., Ingimarsson, J., Curstedt, T., et al., 1997. Manual ventilation with a few large breaths at birth compromises the therapeutic effect of subsequent surfactant replacement in immature lambs. Pediatr Res 42, 348–355.

Bland, R.D., 1972. Cord blood total protein level as a screening aid for the idiopathic respiratory distress syndrome. NEJM 287, 9–13.

Bland, R.D., 1982. Edema formation in the newborn lung. Clin Perinatol 9, 593–611.

Bland, R.D., 1992. Formation of fetal liquid and its removal near birth. In: Polin, R.A., Fox, W.W. (Eds.), Fetal and Neonatal Physiology. W B Saunders, Philadelphia, pp. 782–789.

Bland, R.D., Kim, M.H., Light, M.J., et al., 1980. High frequency ventilation in severe hyaline membrane disease: an alternative therapy. Crit Care Med 8, 275–280.

Blennow, M., Jonsson, B., Dahlstrom, A., et al., 1999. Lungfunktionen kan forbattras hos for tidigt fodda barn. Surfactant behandling och CPAP minskar behovet av respiratorvard. Lakartidningen 96, 1571–1576.

Block, M.R., Kallenberger, D.A., Kern, J.D., et al., 1981. In utero meconium aspiration by the baboon fetus. Obstet Gynecol 57, 37–40.

Bloom, M.C., Roques-Gineste, M., Fries, F., et al., 1995. Pulmonary haemodynamics after surfactant replacement in severe neonatal respiratory distress syndrome. Archives of Disease in Childhood Fetal and Neonatal Edition 73, F95–F98.

Boddy, K., Dawes, G.S., 1975. Fetal breathing. Br Med Bull 31, 3–7.

Bolivar, J.M., Gerhardt, T., Gonzalez, A., et al., 1995. Mechanism for episodes of hypoxemia in preterm infants undergoing mechanical ventilation. Journal of Pediatrics 127, 767–773.

Booth, P., Nicolaides, K.H., Greenough, A., et al., 1987. Pleuroamniotic shunting for fetal chylothorax. Early Hum Dev 15, 365–367.

Boros, S.J., Campbell, K., 1980. A comparison of the effects of high frequency–low tidal volume and low frequency–high tidal volume mechanical ventilation. Journal of Pediatrics 97, 108–112.

Boros, S.J., Reynolds, J.W., 1975. Hyaline membrane disease treated with early nasal end expiratory pressure: one year's experience. Pediatrics 56, 218–223.

Boros, S.J., Matalon, S., Ewald, R., et al., 1977. The effect of independent variations in inspiratory:expiratory ratio and expiratory pressure during mechanical ventilation in hyaline membrane disease. The significance of mean airway pressure. Journal of Pediatrics 91, 794–798.

Boros, S.J., Mammel, M.C., Coleman, J.M., et al., 1985. Neonatal high frequency jet ventilation: four years' experience. Pediatrics 75, 657–663.

Boynton, B.R., Mannino, F.L., Davis, R.F., et al., 1984. Combined high-frequency oscillatory ventilation and intermittent mandatory ventilation in critically ill neonates. Journal of Pediatrics 105, 297–302.

Bradley, B.S., Kumar, S.P., Mehta, P.N., et al., 1994. Neonatal cushingoid syndrome resulting from serial courses of antenatal betamethasone. Am J Obstet Gynecol 83, 869–872.

Brigham, K.L., Serafin, W., Zadoff, A., et al., 1988. Prostaglandin E_2 attenuation of sheep lung responses to endotoxin. J Appl Physiol 64, 2568–2574.

Brion, L.P., Soll, R., 2008. Diuretics for respiratory distress syndrome in preterm infants. Cochrane Database for Systematic Reviews (1), CD001454.

British Standards Institution, 1970. Specifications for Humidifiers for Use with Breathing Machines. BS4494. British Standards Institution, London.

Broadbent, R., Fox, T.F., Dolovich, M., et al., 1995. Chest position and pulmonary deposition of surfactant in surfactant depleted rabbits. Archives of Disease in Childhood Fetal and Neonatal Edition 72, F84–F89.

Brodman, R.F., Zarelson, T.M., Schiebler, G.L., 1974. Treatment of congenital chylothorax. Journal of Pediatrics 85, 516–520.

Brooks, J.G., Bustamente, S.A., Koops, B.L., 1977. Selective bronchial intubation for the treatment of severe localised pulmonary interstitial emphysema in newborn infants. Journal of Pediatrics 91, 648–652.

Brown, B.L., Gleicher, N., 1981. Intrauterine meconium aspiration. Obstet Gynecol 57, 26–29.

Bucciarelli, R.L., Egan, E.A., Gressner, I.H., et al., 1976. Persistence of fetal cardiopulmonary circulation. Manifestation of transient tachypnea of the newborn. Pediatrics 58, 192–197.

Bucciarelli, R.L., Nelson, R.M., Egan, E.A., et al., 1977. Transient tricuspid insufficiency of the newborn. A form of myocardial dysfunction in stressed newborns. Pediatrics 59, 330–337.

Buckner, P.S., Todd, D.A., Lui, K., et al., 1991. Effect of short-term muscle relaxation on neonatal plasma volume. Crit Care Med 19, 1357–1360.

Buettiker, V., Hug, M.I., Baenziger, O., et al., 2004. Advantages and disadvantages of different nasal CPAP systems in newborns. Intensive Care Med 30, 926–930.

Bunton, T.E., Plopper, C.G., 1984. Triamcinolone induced structural alterations in the development of the lung of the fetal rhesus Macaque. Am J Obstet Gynecol 148, 203–215.

Bureau, M.A., Begin, R., Berthiaume, Y., 1979. Central chemical regulation of respiration in term newborn. J Appl Physiol 47, 1212–1217.

Burnard, E.D., James, L.S., 1961. Failure of the heart after undue asphyxia at birth. Pediatrics 28, 545–565.

Byrne, D.L., Gau, G., 1987. In utero meconium aspiration: an unpreventable cause of neonatal death. Br J Obstet Gynaecol 94, 813–814.

Cabal, L.A., Devaskar, U., Siassi, B., et al., 1980. Cardiogenic shock associated with perinatal asphyxia in preterm infants. Journal of Pediatrics 96, 705–710.

Campbell, R.E., 1970. Intrapulmonary interstitial emphysema. A complication of hyaline membrane disease. American Journal of Radiology 110, 449–456.

Carlo, W.A., 2008. Should nasal high frequency ventilation be used in preterm infants? Acta Paediatr 97, 1484–1485.

Carlo, W.A., Chatburn, R.L., Martin, R.J., 1984. Decrease in airway pressure during high frequency jet ventilation versus conventional ventilation in infants with respiratory distress syndrome. Journal of Pediatrics 104, 101–107.

Carlo, W.A., Chatburn, R.L., Martin, R.J., 1987. Randomized trial of high frequency jet ventilation in respiratory distress syndrome. Journal of Pediatrics 110, 275–278.

Carlo, W.A., Beoglos, A., Chatburn, R.L., et al., 1989. High frequency jet ventilation in neonatal pulmonary hypertension. Am J Dis Child 143, 233–238.

Carmant, L., Le Guennec, J.-C., 1989. Congenital chylothorax and persistent pulmonary hypertension of the newborn. Acta Paediatr Scand 78, 789–792.

Carnielli, V.P., Verlato, G., Benini, F., et al., 2000. Metabolic and respiratory effects of theophylline in the preterm infant. Arch Dis Child Fetal Neonatal Ed 83, F39–F43.

Carson, B.S., Losey, R.W., Bowes, W.W., et al., 1976. Combined obstetric and pediatric approach to prevent meconium aspiration syndrome. Am J Obstet Gynecol 126, 712–715.

Cartlidge, P.H.T., Rutter, N., 1986. Serum albumin concentrations and oedema in the newborn. Arch Dis Child 61, 657–660.

Cartwright, D., Gregory, G.A., Lou, H., et al., 1984. The effect of hypocarbia on the cardiovascular system of puppies. Pediatr Res 18, 685–690.

Cassin, S., Dawes, G.S., Mott, J.C., et al., 1964. The vascular resistance of the fetal and newly ventilated lung of the lamb. J Physiol 171, 61–79.

Cater, G., Thibeault, D.W., Beatty, E.C., et al., 1989. Misalignment of lung vessels and alveolar capillary dysplasia: a cause of persistent pulmonary hypertension. Journal of Pediatrics 114, 293–300.

Chan, V., Greenough, A., 1992. Severe localized pulmonary interstitial emphysema – decompression by selective bronchial intubation. J Perinat Med 20, 313–316.

Chan, V., Greenough, A., 1993a. Randomized trial of methods of extubation in acute and chronic respiratory distress. Arch Dis Child 68, 570–572.

Chan, V., Greenough, A., 1993b. Randomised controlled trial of weaning by patient triggered ventilation or conventional ventilation. Eur J Pediatr 152, 51–54.

Chan, V., Greenough, A., 1993c. Determinants of oxygenation during high frequency oscillation. Eur J Pediatr 152, 350–353.

Chan, V., Greenough, A., 1994a. Comparison of weaning by patient triggered ventilation or synchronous intermittent mandatory ventilation in preterm infants. Acta Paediatr 83, 335–337.

Chan, V., Greenough, A., 1994b. Inspiratory and expiratory times for infants ventilator-dependent beyond the first week of life. Acta Paediatr 83, 1022–1024.

Chan, V., Greenough, A., 1994c. The effect of frequency on carbon dioxide levels during high frequency oscillation. J Perinat Med 22, 103–106.

Chan, V., Greenough, A., Gamsu, H.R., 1994. High frequency oscillation for preterm infants with severe respiratory failure. Arch Dis Child Fetal Neonatal Ed 70, F44–F46.

Chan, V., Greenough, A., Dimitriou, G., 1995. High frequency oscillation, respiratory activity and changes in blood gases. Early Hum Dev 40, 87–94.

Chang, H.K., 1984. Mechanisms of gas transport during ventilation by high frequency oscillation. J Appl Physiol 56, 553–563.

Chasen, S.T., Madden, A., Chervenak, F.A., 1999. Cesarian delivery of twins and neonatal respiratory disorders. Am J Obstet Gynecol 181, 1052–1056.

Cheema, I.U., Sinha, A.K., Kempley, S.T., et al., 2007. Impact of volume guarantee ventilation on arterial carbon dioxide in newborn infants: a ranomised controlled trial. Early Hum Dev 83, 183–189.

Chelliah, B.P., Brown, D., Cohen, M., et al., 1995. Alveolar capillary dysplasia – a cause of persistent pulmonary hypertension unresponsive to a second course of extracorporeal membrane oxygenation. Pediatrics 96, 1159–1161.

Cheung, P.Y., Prasertsom, W., Finer, N.N., et al., 1997. Rescue high frequency oscillatory ventilation for preterm infants: neurodevelopmental outcome and its prediction. Biol Neonate 71, 282–291.

Chida, S., Phelps, D.S., Soll, R.F., et al., 1991. Surfactant proteins and anti-surfactant antibodies in sera from infants with respiratory distress syndrome with and without surfactant treatment. Pediatrics 88, 84–89.

Chida, S., Tujiwara, T., Konishi, M., et al., 1993. Stable microbubble test for predicting the risk of respiratory distress syndrome. Eur J Pediatr 152, 152–156.

Cigada, M., Gavazzi, A., Assi, E., et al., 2001. Gastric rupture after nasopharyngeal oxygen administration. Intensive Care Med 27, 939.

Clark, P., Duff, P., 1995. Inhibition of neutrophil oxidative burst and phagocytosis by meconium. Am J Obstet Gynecol 173, 1301–1305.

Clark, L.C., Gollan, F., 1966. Survival of mammals breathing organic liquids equilibrated with oxygen at atmospheric pressure. Science 152, 1756.

Clark, J.M., Lambertsen, C.J., 1971. Pulmonary oxygen toxicity. Pharmacology Review 23, 37–133.

Clark, R.H., Gerstmann, D.R., Null, D.N., et al., 1986. Pulmonary interstitial emphysema treated by high frequency oscillatory ventilation. Crit Care Med 14, 926–930.

Clark, D.A., Nieman, G.F., Thompson, J.E., et al., 1987. Surfactant displacement by meconium free fatty acids: an alternative explanation for atelectasis in meconium aspiration syndrome. Journal of Pediatrics 110, 765–770.

Clark, R.H., Gertsman, D.R., Null, D.M., et al., 1992. Prospective randomized comparison of high frequency oscillatory and conventional ventilation in respiratory distress syndrome. Pediatrics 89, 5–12.

Clark, R.H., Kueser, T.J., Walker, M.W., et al., 2000. Low-dose nitric oxide therapy for persistent pulmonary hypertension of the newborn. Clinical Inhaled Nitric Oxide Research Group. NEJM 342, 469–474.

Claure, N., D'Ugard, C., Bancalari, E., 2009. Automated adjustment of inspired oxygen in preterm infants with frequent fluctuations in oxygenation: a pilot clinical trial. Journal of Pediatrics 155, 640–645.

Cleary, J.M., Wiswell, T.E., 1998. Meconium-stained amniotic fluid and the meconium aspiration syndrome: an update. Pediatr Clin North Am 45, 511–529.

Cleary, J.P., Bernstein, G., Mannino, F.L., et al., 1995. Improved oxygenation during synchronized intermittent mandatory ventilation in neonates with respiratory distress syndrome: a randomized crossover study. Journal of Pediatrics 126, 407–411.

Clyman, R.I., 1996. Recommendations for the postnatal use of indomethacin: an analysis of four separate treatment strategies. Journal of Pediatrics 128, 601–607.

Coates, E.W., Klinepeter, M.E., O'Shea, T.M., 2008. Neonatal pulmonary hypertension treated with inhaled nitric oxide and high frequency ventilation. J Perinatol 28, 675–679.

Cochrane, C.G., Revak, D.S., Merritt, T.A., et al., 1996. The efficacy and safety of KL_4 surfactant in preterm infants with respiratory distress syndrome. Am J Respir Crit Care Med 153, 404–410.

Cohen, R.S., Smith, D.W., Stevenson, D.K., et al., 1984. Lateral decubitus position as therapy for persistent pulmonary interstitial emphysema in neonates: a preliminary report. Journal of Pediatrics 104, 441–443.

Cohen, G.R., Thorp, J., Yeast, J.D., et al., 1991. A markedly immature lecithin:sphingomyelin ratio at term and congenital hypothyroidism. Am J Dis Child 145, 1227–1228.

Colaizy, T.T., Younis, U., Bell, E.F., et al., 2008. Nasal high frequency ventilation for premature infants. Acta Paediatr 97, 1518–1522.

Cole, V.A., Normand, I.C.S., Reynolds, E.O.R., et al., 1973. Pathogenesis of hemorrhagic pulmonary edema and massive pulmonary hemorrhage in the newborn. Pediatrics 51, 175–187.

Cole, J.W., Portman, R.J., Lim, Y., et al., 1985. Urinary β_2-microglobulin in full term newborns: evidence for proximal tubular dysfunction in infants with meconium stained amniotic fluid. Pediatrics 76, 958–964.

Cole, F.S., Hamvas, A., Rubenstein, P., et al., 2000. Population based estimates of surfactant protein deficiency. Pediatrics 105, 538–541.

Colice, G.L., Matthay, M.A., Bass, E., et al., 1984. Neurogenic pulmonary edema. Am Rev Respir Dis 130, 941–948.

Collaborative European Multicentre Study Group, 1991. Factors influencing the clinical response to surfactant replacement therapy in babies with severe respiratory distress syndrome. Eur J Pediatr 150, 433–439.

Cools, F., Offringa, M., 2009. Neuromuscular paralysis for newborn infants receiving mechanical ventilation. Cochrane Database Systematic Reviews (4), CD002773.

Copetti, R., Cattarossi, L., 2007. The double lung point: an ultrasound sign diagnostic of transient tachypnoea of the newborn. Neonatology 91, 203–209.

Corbet, A., Bucciarelli, R., Goldman, S., et al., 1991. Decreased mortality rate among small premature infants treated at birth with a single dose of synthetic surfactant. A multicenter controlled trial. Journal of Pediatrics 118, 277–284.

Cordier, M.P., Gaultier, C.L., Boule, M., 1984. Infants with meconium aspiration syndrome: follow-up study (abstract). Am Rev Respir Dis 129, 218.

Cornfield, D.N., Reeve, H.L., Tolarova, S., et al., 1996. Oxygen causes fetal pulmonary vasodilation through activation of a calcium-dependent potassium channel. Proceedings of the National Academy of Sciences of the the United States of America 93, 8089–8094.

Cornfield, D.N., Maynard, R.C., de-Regnier, R.-A.O., et al., 1999. Randomized controlled trial of low dose inhaled nitric oxide in the treatment of term and near

term infants with respiratory failure and pulmonary hypertension. Pediatrics 104, 1089–1094.

Cotton, R.B., Olsson, T., Law, A.B., et al., 1993. The physiological effects of surfactant treatment on gas exchange in newborn premature infants with hyaline membrane disease. Pediatr Res 34, 495–501.

Courtney, S.E., Pyon, K.H., Saslow, J.G., et al., 2001. Lung recruitment and breathing pattern during variable versus continuous positive airway pressure in premature infants: an evaluation of three devices. Pediatrics 107, 304–308.

Cowan, F., Whitelaw, A., Wertheim, D., et al., 1991. Cerebral blood flow velocity changes after rapid administration of surfactant. Arch Dis Child 66, 1105–1109.

Craft, A.P., Bhandari, V., Finer, N.N., 2003. The sy-fi study: a randomized prospective trial of synchronized intermittent mandatory ventilation versus a high-frequency flow interrupter technique in infants less than 1000 g. J Perinatol 23, 14–19.

Crowley, P.A., 1995. Antenatal corticosteroid therapy. A meta-analysis of the randomized trials 1972–1994. Am J Obstet Gynecol 173, 322–335.

Crowley, M.R., Fineman, J.R., Soier, S.J., 1991. Effect of vasoactive drugs on thromboxane A_2 mimetic-induced pulmonary hypertension in newborn lambs. Pediatr Res 29, 167–172.

Crowther, C.A., Alfirevic, Z., Haslam, R.R., 2000. Prenatal thyrotropin-releasing hormone for preterm birth. Cochrane Database Syst Rev (2), CD000019.

Crowther, C.A., Haslam, R.R., Hiller, J.E., et al., 2006. Neonatal respiratory distress syndrome after repeat exposure to antenatal corticosteroids: a randomised controlled trial. Lancet 366, 1913–1919.

Cuestas, R.A., Lindall, A., Engel, R.R., 1976. Low thyroid hormones and respiratory distress syndrome of the newborn. NEJM 295, 297–302.

Curley, M.A., Thompson, J.E., Arnold, J.H., 2000. The effects of early and repeated positioning in paediatric patients with acute lung injury. Chest 118, 156–163.

Currie, A., Patel, D.S., Rafferty, G.F., et al., 2010. Prediction of extubation outcome in neonates using tension time index. Arch Dis Child Nov 20.

Curtis, J., O'Nell, J.T., Pettett, G., 1993. Endotracheal administration of tolazoline in hypoxia induced pulmonary hypertension. Pediatrics 92, 403–408.

Da Costa, D.E., Nair, A.K., Pai, M.G., et al., 2001. Steroids in full term infants with respiratory failure and pulmonary hypertension due to meconium aspiration syndrome. Eur J Pediatr 138, 113–115.

da Silva, W.J., Abbasi, S., Pereira, G., et al., 1994. Role of positive end expiratory pressure changes on functional residual capacity in surfactant treated preterm infants. Pediatr Pulmonol 18, 89–92.

Dalziel, S.R., Rea, H.H., Walker, N.K., et al., 2006. Long term effects of antenatal betamethasone on lung function 30 year follow up of a randomised controlled trial. Thorax 61, 678–683.

Danan, C., Durrmeyer, X., Brochard, L., 2008. A randomised trial of delayed extubation for the reduction of reintubation in extremely preterm infants. Pediatr Pulmonol 43, 117–124.

Dani, C., Grella, P.V., Lazzarin, L., et al., 1997. Antenatal ambroxol treatment does not prevent the respiratory distress syndrome in premature infants. Eur J Pediatr 156, 392–393.

Dani, C., Reali, M.F., Bertini, G., et al., 1999. Risk factors for the development of respiratory distress syndrome and transient tachypnoea in newborn infants. Italian Group of Neonatal Pneumology. Eur Respir J 14, 155–159.

Daniel, S.S., Adamsons, K., James, L.S., 1966. Lactate and pyruvate as an index of prenatal oxygen deprivation. Pediatrics 37, 942–953.

Dargaville, P.A., Copnell, B., 2006. The epidemiology of meconium aspiration syndrome: incidence, risk factors, therapies and outcome. Pediatrics 117, 1712–1721.

Dargaville, P.A., South, M., McDougall, P.N., 2001. Surfactant and surfactant inhibitors in meconium aspiration syndrome. Journal of Pediatrics 138, 113–115.

Dargaville, P.A., Mills, J.H., Copnell, B., et al., 2007. Therapeutic lung lavage in meconium aspiration syndrome: a preliminary report. Journal of Pediatrics and Child Health 43, 539–545.

Davidson, D., Barefield, E.S., Kattwinkel, J., et al., 1998. Inhaled nitric oxide for the early treatment of persistent pulmonary hypertension of the term newborn: a randomized double-masked, placebo-controlled, dose–response multicenter study. The I-NO/PPHN Study Group. Pediatrics 101, 325–334.

Davidson, D., Barefield, E.S., Kattwinkel, J., et al., 1999. Safety of withdrawing inhaled nitric oxide therapy in persistent pulmonary hypertension of the newborn. Pediatrics 104, 231–236.

Davies, A.M., Koenig, J.S., Thach, B.T., 1989. Characteristics of upper airway chemoreflex prolonged apnea in human infants. Am Rev Respir Dis 139, 668–673.

Davis, G.M., Bureau, M.A., 1987. Pulmonary and chest wall mechanics in the control of respiration in the newborn. Clin Perinatol 14, 551–579.

Davis, P.G., Henderson-Smart, D.J., 2001. Extubation from low rate intermittent positive airways pressure versus extubation after a trial of endotracheal continuous positive airways pressure in intubated preterm infants. Cochrane Database Syst Rev (4), CD0001078.

Davis, P.J., Skekerdemian, L.S., 2001. Meconium aspiration syndrome and extracorporeal membrane oxygenation. Archives of Disease in Childhood Fetal and Neonatal Edition 84, F1–F3.

Davis, J.M., Whitin, J., 1992. Prophylactic effects of dexamethasone in lung injury caused by hyperoxia and hyperventilation. J Appl Physiol 72, 1320–1325.

Davis, W.B., Rennard, S.I., Bitterman, P.B., et al., 1983. Early reversible changes in human alveolar structures induced by hyperoxia. NEJM 309, 878–883.

Davis, J.M., Russ, G.A., Metlay, L., et al., 1992. Short-term distribution kinetics of intratracheally administered exogenous lung surfactant. Pediatr Res 31, 445–450.

De Bie, H.M., van Toledo-Eppinga, L., et al., 2002. Neonatal pneumatocele as a complication of nasal continuous positive airway pressure. Arch Dis Child Fetal Neonatal Ed 86, F202–F203.

De Carolis, M.P., Romagnoli, C., Cafforio, C., et al., 1998. Pulmonary haemorrhage in infants with gestational age of less than 30 weeks. Eur J Pediatr 157, 1037–1038.

Dehan, M., Francoual, J., Lindenbaum, A., 1978. Diagnosis of meconium aspiration by spectrophotometric analysis of urine. Arch Dis Child 53, 74–76.

Dekowski, S.A., Snyder, J.M., 1992. Insulin regulation of messenger ribonucleic acid for the surfactant-associated protein in human fetal lung in vitro. Endocrinology 131, 669–676.

de Klerk, A.M., de Klerck, R.K., 2001. Use of continuous positive airway pressure in preterm infants: comments and experience from New Zealand. Pediatrics 108, 761–763.

De Los Santos, R., Seidenfeld, J.J., Anzueto, A., et al., 1987. One hundred percent oxygen lung injury in adult baboons. Am Rev Respir Dis 136, 657–661.

DeLemos, R.A., Coalson, J.J., Gerstmann, D.R.,et al., 1987a. Oxygen toxicity in the premature baboon with hyaline membrane disease. Am Rev Respir Dis 136, 677–682.

DeLemos, R.A., Gerstmann, D.R., Clark, R.H., et al., 1987b. High frequency ventilation – the relationship between the ventilator design and clinical strategy in the treatment of hyaline membrane disease and its complications: a brief review. Pediatr Pulmonol 3, 370–372.

De Luca, D., Zecca, E., Piastra, M., et al., 2007. Iloprost as rescue therapy for pulmonary hypertension of the neonate. Pediatric Anaesthesia 17, 394–395.

Dembinski, J., Herep, A., Kan, N., et al., 2002. CT imaging of pulmonary lobar interstitial emphysema in spontaneously breathing preterm infant. Am J Perinatol 19, 285–290.

Demirakca, S., Dortsch, J., Knotlie, C., et al., 1996. Inhaled nitric oxide in neonatal and paediatric acute respiratory distress syndrome: dose response, prolonged inhalation and weaning. Crit Care Med 24, 1913–1919.

Demissie, K., Marcella, S.W., Breckenridge, M.B., et al., 1998. Maternal asthma and transient tachypnea of the newborn. Pediatrics 102, 84–90.

Dempsey, E.M., Hazzani, F.A., Faucher, D., et al., 2006. Facilitation of neonatal endotracheal intubation with mivacurium and fentanyl in the neonatal intensive care unit. Archives of Disease in Childhood Fetal Neonatal Edition 91, F279–F282.

De Paoli, A.G., Morley, C.J., Davis, P.G., et al., 2002. In vitro comparison of nasal continuous positive airway pressure devices for neonates. Archive of Disease in Childhood. Fetal and Neonatal Edition 87, F42–F45.

Dessens, A.B., Smolders-de Haas, H., Koppe, J.G., 2000. Twenty-year follow-up of antenatal corticosteroid treatment. Pediatrics 105, E77.

de Winter, J.P., Merth, I.T., van Bel, F., et al., 1994. Changes in respiratory system mechanics in ventilated lungs of preterm infants with two different schedules of treatment. Pediatr Res 35, 541–549.

Dhanireddy, R., Smith, Y.F., Hamosh, M., et al., 1983. Respiratory distress syndrome in the newborn: relationship to serum prolactin, thyroxine and sex. Biol Neonate 43, 9–15.

Dimitriou, G., Greenough, A., 1995a. Volume delivery during positive pressure inflation – relationship to spontaneous tidal volume of neonates. Early Hum Dev 41, 61–68.

Dimitriou, G., Greenough, A., 1995b. Measurement of lung volume and optimization of oxygenation during high frequency oscillation. Arch Dis Child Fetal Neonatal Ed 72, F180–F183.

Dimitriou, G., Greenough, A., 2000. Performance of neonatal ventilators. British Journal of Intensive Care 10, 186–188.

Dimitriou, G., Greenough, A., Giffin, F., et al., 1995. Synchronous intermittent mandatory ventilation modes versus patient triggered ventilation during weaning. Arch Dis Child Fetal Neonatal Ed 72, F188–F190.

Dimitriou, G., Greenough, A., Castling, D., et al., 1996. A comparison of supine and prone positioning in oxygen-dependent and convalescent premature infants. British Journal of Intensive Care 6, 254–259.

Dimitriou, G., Greenough, A., Kavadia, V., 1997. Changes in lung volume, compliance and oxygenation in the first 48 hours of life in infants given surfactant. J Perinat Med 25, 49–54.

Dimitriou, G., Greenough, A., Kavvadia, V., et al., 1998a. Volume delivery during high frequency oscillation. Arch Dis Child Fetal Neonatal Ed 78, F148–F150.

Dimitriou, G., Greenough, A., Laubscher, B., et al., 1998b. Comparison of airway pressure triggered and airflow triggered ventilation in very immature infants. Acta Paediatr 87, 1256–1260.

Dimitriou, G., Greenough, A., Kavvadia, V., Milner, A.D., 1999. Comparison of two inspiratory:expiratory ratios during high frequency oscillation. Eur J Pediatr 158, 796–799.

Dimitriou, G., Greenough, A., Kavvadia, V., et al., 2000. Elective use of nasal continuous positive airways pressure following extubation of preterm infants. Eur J Pediatr 159, 434–439.

Dimitriou, G., Greenough, A., Broomfield, D., et al., 2002a. Rescue high frequency oscillation and predictors of adverse neurodevelopmental outcome in preterm infants. Early Hum Dev 66, 133–141.

Dimitriou, G., Greenough, A., Endo, A., et al., 2002b. Prediction of extubation failure in preterm infants. Archives of Disease in Childhood Fetal Neonatal Edition 86, F32–F35.

Dimitriou, G., Greenough, A., Kavvadia, V., 2002c. Fluid restriction, colloid infusion and chronic lung disease development in very low birth weight infants. Neonatal Intensive Care 15, 13–18.

Dobyns, E.L., Wescott, J.Y., Kennaugh, J.M., et al., 1994. Eicosanoids decrease with successful extracorporeal membrane oxygenation therapy in neonatal pulmonary hypertension. Am J Respir Crit Care Med 149, 873–880.

Dollberg, S., Livny, S., Mordecheyev, N., et al., 2001. Nucleated red blood cell counts in meconium aspiration syndrome. Obstet Gynecol 97, 593–596.

Dooley, S.L., Pesavento, D.J., Depp, R., et al., 1985. Meconium below vocal cords at delivery; correlation with intrapartum events. Am J Obstet Gynecol 153, 761–770.

Doyle, L.W., Kitchen, W.H., Ford, G.W., et al., 1986. Effects of antenatal steroid therapy on mortality and morbidity in very low birthweight infants. Journal of Pediatrics 108, 287–292.

Doyle, L.W., Kitchen, W.H., Ford, G.W., et al., 1989. Antenatal steroid therapy and 5 year outcome of extremely low birthweight infants. Obstet Gynecol 73, 743–746.

Drew, J.H., 1982. Immediate intubation at birth of the very low birthweight infant. Am J Dis Child 136, 207–210.

Duara, S., Fox, W.W., 1986. Persistent pulmonary hypertension of the neonate. In: Thibeault, D.W., Gregory, G.A. (Eds.), Neonatal Pulmonary Care, second ed. Appleton Century Crofts, Norwalk, CT, pp. 461–481.

Dudell, G.G., Gersony, W.M., 1984. Patent ductus arteriosus in neonates with severe respiratory disease. Journal of Pediatrics 104, 915–920.

Dunn, P.M., 1963. Intestinal obstruction in the newborn with special reference to transient functional ileus associated with

respiratory distress syndrome. Arch Dis Child 38, 459–467.

Durbin, G.M., Hunter, N.J., McIntosh, N., et al., 1976. Controlled trial of continuous inflating pressure for hyaline membrane disease. Arch Dis Child 51, 163–169.

Edberg, K.E., Sandberg, K., Silberberg, A., 1991. Lung volumes, gas mixing and mechanics of breathing in mechanically ventilated very low birth weight infants with idiopathic respiratory distress syndrome. Pediatr Res 30, 496–500.

Edwards, A.D., 1995. The pharmacology of inhaled nitric oxide. Arch Dis Child Fetal Neonatal Ed 72, F127–F130.

Edwards, D.K., Hilton, S.V.W., Merritt, T.A., et al., 1985. Respiratory distress syndrome treated with human surfactant. Radiographic findings. Radiology 157, 329–334.

Edwards, A.D., McCormick, D.C., Roth, S.C., et al., 1992. Cerebral hemodynamic effects of treatment with modified natural surfactant investigated by near infrared spectroscopy. Pediatr Res 32, 532–536.

Eisler, G., Hjertberg, R., Lagercrantz, H., 1999. Randomised controlled trial of effect of terbutaline before elective caesarian section on postnatal respiration and glucose homeostasis. Arch Dis Child Fetal Neonatal Ed 80, F88–F92.

El-Moneim, E.S.A., Fuerste, H.O., Krueger, M., et al., 2005. Pressure support ventilation combined with volume guarantee versus synchronized intermittent mandatory ventilation: a pilot crossover trial in premature infants in their weaning phase. Pediatric Critical Care Medicine 6, 286–292.

El Shahed, A.I., Dargaville, P.E., Ohlsson, A., et al., 2007. Surfactant for meconium aspiration syndrome in full term/near term infants. Cochrane Database Systematic Reviews (3), CD002054.

Emery, E.F., Greenough, A., 1993. Randomized trial of two inotropes in preterm infants. Eur J Pediatr 152, 1–3.

Emery, E.F., Greenough, A., Gamsu, H.R., 1992. Randomized controlled trial of colloid infusions in hypotensive preterm infants. Arch Dis Child 67, 1185–1188.

Enders, J., Gebauer, C., Pulzer, F., et al., 2008. Analgosedation with low dose morphine for preterm infants with CPAP: risks and benefits. Acta Pediatrica 97, 880–883.

Engdahl, M.S., Gershan, W.M., 1998. Familial spontaneous pneumothorax in neonates. Pediatr Pulmonol 25, 398–400.

Engle, W.D., Yoder, M.C., Andreoli, S.P., et al., 1997. Controlled prospective randomised comparison of high frequency jet ventilation and conventional ventilation in neonates with respiratory failure and persistent pulmonary hypertension. J Perinatol 17, 3–9.

Eriksson, L., Haglund, B., Ewald, U., et al., 2009. Short and long term effects of antenatal corticosteroids assessed in a

cohort of 7827 children born preterm. Acta Obstetric Gynecology Scandinavica 88, 933–938.

Eronen, M., Kari, A., Pesonen, E., et al., 1993. The effect of antenatal dexamethasone administration on the fetal and neonatal ductus arteriosus. Am J Dis Child 147, 187–192.

Evans, N.J., Archer, L.N.J., 1991a. Doppler measurement of pulmonary artery pressure and extrapulmonary shunting in the acute phase of hyaline membrane disease. Arch Dis Child 66, 6–11.

Evans, N.J., Archer, L.N.J., 1991b. Doppler assessment of pulmonary artery pressure during recovery from hyaline membrane disease. Arch Dis Child 66, 802–804.

Evans, N.J., Iyer, P., 1994. Incompetence of the foramen ovale in preterm infants supported by mechanical ventilation. Journal of Pediatrics 125, 786–792.

Evans, N., Kluckow, M., 1999. High pulmonary blood flow and pulmonary hemorrhage. Pediatr Res 45, 195a.

Faix, R.G., Viscardi, R.M., Dipietro, M.A., et al., 1989. Adult respiratory distress syndrome in full term newborns. Pediatrics 83, 171–176.

Falciglia, H.S., 1988. Failure to prevent meconium aspiration syndrome. Obstet Gynecol 71, 249–253.

Falciglia, H.S., Henderschott, C., Potter, P., et al., 1992. Does DeLee suction at the perineum prevent meconium aspiration syndrome? Am J Obstet Gynecol 167, 1243–1249.

Fanconi, S., Duc, G., 1987. Intratracheal suction in sick preterm infants: prevention of intracranial hypertension and cerebral hypoperfusion by muscle paralysis. Pediatrics 79, 538–543.

Farrell, P.M., 1986. Nutrition and infant lung function. Pediatr Pulmonol 2, 44–59.

Farrell, P.M., Avery, M.E., 1975. State of the art. HMD. Am Rev Respir Dis 111, 657–688.

Farstad, T., Bratlid, D., 1991. Effect of endotracheal tube size and ventilator settings on the mechanics of a test system during intermittent flow ventilation. Pediatr Pulmonol 11, 15–21.

Fedrick, J., Butler, N.R., 1970. Certain causes of neonatal death. I. Hyaline membranes. Biol Neonate 15, 229–255.

Feldman, D.M., Carbone, J., Belden, L., et al., 2007. Betamethasone vs dexamethasone for the prevention of morbidity in very low birthweight neonates. Am J Obstet Gynecol 197, 284.

Fiascone, J.M., Hu, L.-M., Vreeland, P.N., 1992. Terbutaline does not improve lung function in preterm infants. Am J Obstet Gynecol 167, 847–853.

Field, D.J., Milner, A.D., Hopkin, I., 1985. Inspiratory time and tidal volume during high frequency positive pressure ventilation. Arch Dis Child 60, 259–261.

Field, D., Elbourne, E., Hardy, P., et al., 2007. Neonatal ventilation with inhaled nitric oxide vs ventilatory support without inhaled nitric oxide for infants with severe respiratory failure born at or near term: The INNOVO multicentre randomised controlled trial. Neonatology 91, 73–82.

Findlay, R.D., Taeusch, H.W., Walther, F.J., 1996. Surfactant replacement therapy for meconium aspiration syndrome. Pediatrics 97, 48–52.

Finer, N., Barrington, K.J., 2009. Nitric oxide for respiratory failure ini infants born at or near term. Cochrane Database Syst Rev (1), CD000399.

Finer, N.N., Mannino, F.L., 2009. High-flow nasal cannula: a kinder, gentler CPAP? Journal of Pediatrics 154, 160–162.

Finer, N.N., Etches, P.C., Kamstra, B., et al., 1994. Inhaled nitric oxide in infants referred for extracorporeal membrane oxygenation: dose response. Journal of Pediatrics 124, 302–308.

Finlay, E.R., Subhedar, N.V., 2000. Pulmonary haemorrhage in preterm infants. Eur J Pediatr 159, 870–871.

Finley, J.P., Howwman-Giles, R.B., Gilday, D.L., et al., 1979. Transient myocardial ischemia of the newborn infant demonstrated by thallium myocardial imaging. Journal of Pediatrics 94, 263–270.

Fleisher, B., Kulovich, M.V., Hallman, M., et al., 1985. Lung profile: sex difference in normal pregnancy. Obstet Gynecol 66, 327–330.

Flenady, V., Gray, P.H., 2002. Chest physiotherapy for preventing morbidity in babies being extubation from mechanical ventilation. Cochrane Database for Systematic Reviews (2), CD000283.

Fok, T.F., Kew, J., Loftus, W.K., et al., 1998. Clinical predictors of post-extubation radiological changes of the chest in newborn infants. Acta Paediatr 87, 88–92.

Fouron, J.C., Bard, H., Riopel, L., et al., 1985. Circulatory changes in newborn lambs with experimental polycythemia: comparison between fetal and adult type blood. Pediatrics 75, 1054–1060.

Fox, W.W., 1982. Mechanical ventilation in the management of persistent pulmonary hypertension of the neonate (PPHN). 83rd Ross Conference on Pediatric Research: Cardiovascular Sequelae of Asphyxia in the Newborn. Ross Laboratories, Columbus, OH, p. 102.

Fox, W.W., Duara, S., 1983. Persistent pulmonary hypertension in the neonate. Diagnosis and management. Journal of Pediatrics 103, 505–514.

Fox, W.W., Schwartz, J.G., Shaffer, T.H., 1978. Pulmonary physiotherapy in neonates: physiologic changes and respiratory management. Journal of Pediatrics 92, 977–981.

Fox, W.W., Spiker, A.R., Musci, M., 1984. Tracheal secretion impaction during hyperventilation for persistent pulmonary hypertension of the neonate (abstract). Pediatr Res 18, 323.

Frank, L., 1992. Prenatal dexamethasone treatment improves survival of newborn rats during prolonged high oxygen exposure. Pediatr Res 32, 215–221.

Frank, L., Sosenko, I.R.S., 1991. Failure of premature rabbits to increase antioxidant enzymes during hyperoxic exposure: increased susceptibility to pulmonary oxygen toxicity compared with term rabbits. Pediatr Res 29, 292–296.

Frank, L., Bucher, J.R., Roberts, R.J., 1978. Oxygen toxicity in neonatal and adult animals of various species. J Appl Physiol 45, 699–704.

Franklin, R.C., Purdie, G.L., O'Grady, C.M., 1986. Neonatal thyroid function: prematurity, prenatal steroids and respiratory distress syndrome. Arch Dis Child 61, 589–592.

Frantz, I.D., Close, R.H., 1985. Elevated lung volume and alveolar pressure during jet ventilation of rabbits. Am Rev Respir Dis 131, 134–138.

Frantz, I.D., Werthammer, J., Stark, A.R., 1983. High frequency ventilation in premature infants with lung disease: adequate gas exchange at low tracheal pressure. Pediatrics 71, 483–488.

Fraser, W.D., Hofmeyr, J., Lede, R., et al., 2005. Amnioinfusion for the prevention of the meconium aspiration syndrome. NEJM 353, 909–917.

French, N.P., Hagan, R., Evans, S.F., et al., 1999. Repeated antenatal corticosteroids: size at birth and subsequent development. Am J Obstet Gynecol 180, 114–121.

Friedman, S.A., Schiff, E., Kao, L., et al., 1995. Neonatal outcome after preterm delivery for pre-eclampsia. Am J Obstet Gynecol 172, 1785–1792.

Friesen, R.H., Honda, A.T., Thieme, R.E., 1987. Changes in anterior fontanelle pressure in preterm neonates during tracheal intubation. Anesth Analg 66, 874–878.

Froese, A.B., Bryan, A.C., 1987. High frequency ventilation. Am Rev Respir Dis 135, 1363–1374.

Gabwell, C.E., Salzberg, A.M., Sonnino, R.E., et al., 2000. Potentially lethal complications of central venous catheter placement. J Pediatr Surg 35, 709–713.

Gadzinowski, J., Kowalska, K., Vidyasagar, D., 2008. Treatment of MAS with PPHN using combined therapy: SLL, bolus surfactant and iNO. Journal of Pernatology 28, S56–S66.

Gandy, G., Jacobson, W., Gairdner, D., 1970. Hyaline membrane disease. I. Cellular changes. Arch Dis Child 45, 289–310.

Gaon, P., Lee, S., Hannam, S., et al., 1999. Assessment of effect of nasal continuous positive pressure on laryngeal opening using fibreoptic laryngoscopy. Archives of Disease in Childhood Fetal and Neonatal Edition 80, F230–F232.

Gappa, M., Costeloe, K., Southall, D.P., et al., 1994. Effect of continuous negative extrathoracic pressure on respiratory mechanics and timing in infants recovering from neonatal respiratory distress syndrome. Pediatr Res 36, 364–372.

Gardner, M.O., Goldenberg, R.L., Gaudier, F.L., et al., 1995. Predicting low Apgar scores of infants weighing less than 1000 grams: the effect of corticosteroids. Obstet Gynecol 85, 170–174.

Garite, J.J., Rumney, P.J., Briggs, G.G., et al., 1992. A randomized placebo-controlled trial of betamethasone for the prevention of respiratory distress syndrome at 24–28 weeks' gestation. Am J Obstet Gynecol 166, 646–651.

Garite, T.J., Kurtzman, J., Maurel, K., et al., 2009. Impact of rescue course of antenatal corticosteroids: a multicenter randomised placebo controlled trial. Am J Obstet Gynecol 200, 248e1–248e9.

Garland, J., Buck, R., Weinberg, M., 1994. Pulmonary hemorrhage risk in infants with a clinically diagnosed patent ductus arteriosus. A retrospective cohort study. Pediatrics 94, 719–723.

Garland, J., Buck, R.K., Allred, E.N., et al., 1995. Hypocarbia before surfactant therapy appears to increase bronchopulmonary dysplasia risk in infants with respiratory distress syndrome. Arch Pediatr Adolesc Med 149, 617–622.

Gau, G.S., Ryder, T.A., Mobberley, M.A., 1987. Iatrogenic epithelial change caused by endotracheal intubation of neonates. Early Hum Dev 15, 221–229.

Gauger, P.G., Hirschl, R.B., Delosh, T.N., et al., 1995. A matched pairs analysis of venoarterial and venovenous extracorporeal life support in neonatal respiratory failure. ASAIO Journal 41, M573–M579.

Gaylor, M.S., Quissell, B.J., Lair, M.E., 1987. High frequency ventilation in the treatment of infants weighing less than 1500 grams with pulmonary interstitial emphysema. Pediatrics 79, 915–921.

Geggel, R.L., Reid, L.M., 1984. The structural basis for persistent pulmonary hypertension of the newborn. Clin Perinatol 11, 525–549.

Geggel, R.L., Murphy, J.D., Langleben, D., et al., 1985. Congenital diaphragmatic hernia: arterial structural changes and persistent pulmonary hypertension after surgical repair. Journal of Pediatrics 107, 457–464.

George, T.N., Johnson, K.J., Bates, J.N., et al., 1998. The effect of inhaled nitric oxide therapy on bleeding time and platelet aggregation in neonates. Journal of Pediatrics 132, 731–734.

Gersony, W.M., Duc, G.V., Sinclair, J.C., 1969. 'PFC' syndrome (abstract). Circulation 40 (suppl. III), 87.

Giannantonio, C., Sammartino, M., Valente, E., et al., 2009. Remifentanil analgosedation in preterm newborns during mechanical ventilation. Acta Pediatrica 98, 1111–1115.

Gibson, R.L., Truog, W.E., Redding, G.J., 1988. Thromboxane associated pulmonary hypertension during three types of Gram positive bacteremia in piglets. Pediatr Res 23, 553–556.

Giffin, F., Greenough, A., 1994. ARDS type disease in children: modern respiratory management. Intensive Care Britain, third ed. Greycoat Publishing, London, pp. 28–31.

Gill, A.B., Weindling, A.M., 1993. Randomized controlled trial of plasma protein fraction versus dopamine in hypotensive very low birthweight infants. Arch Dis Child 69, 284–287.

Gill, B.S., Neville, H.L., Khan, A.M., et al., 2002. Delayed institution of extracorporeal membrane oxygenation is associated with increased mortality rate and prolonged hospital stay. J Pediatr Surg 37, 7–10.

Gitterman, M.K., Fusch, C., Gitterman, A.R., et al., 1997. Early nasal continuous positive airway pressure treatment reduces the need for intubation in very low birthweight infants. Eur J Pediatr 156, 384–388.

Gluck, L., Kulovich, M.V., Eidelman, A.I., et al., 1972. Biochemical development of surfactant activity in mammalian lung. IV. Pulmonary lecithin synthesis in the human fetus and newborn and etiology of the respiratory distress syndrome. Pediatr Res 6, 81–99.

Goetzman, B.W., Sunshine, P., Johnson, J.D., et al., 1976. Neonatal hypoxia and pulmonary vasospasm: response to tolazoline. Journal of Pediatrics 89, 617–621.

Goldman, A.P., Tasker, R.C., Haworth, S.G., et al., 1996. Four patterns of response to inhaled nitric oxide for persistent pulmonary hypertension of the newborn. Pediatrics 98, 708–713.

Gomez, R., Ghezzi, F., Romero, R., et al., 1995. Premature labor and intra-amniotic infection. Clinical aspects and role of the cytokines in diagnosis and pathophysiology. Clin Perinatol 22, 281–342.

Gonzales, L.W., Ballard, P.L., Ertsey, R., et al., 1986. Glucocorticoids and thyroid hormones stimulate biochemical and morphological differentiation of human fetal lung in organ culture. JCEM 62, 678–691.

Gonzales, F., Harris, T., Black, P., et al., 1987. Decreased gas flow through pneumothoraces in neonates receiving high frequency jet ventilation versus conventional ventilation. Pediatrics 110, 464–466.

Gordon, J.B., Martinez, F.R., Keller, P.A., et al., 1993. Differing effects of acute and prolonged alkalosis on hypoxic pulmonary vasoconstriction. Am Rev Respir Dis 148, 1651–1656.

Gordon, E., South, M., McDougall, P.N., et al., 2003. Blood aspiration syndrome as a cause of respiratory distress in the newborn infant. Journal of Pediatrics 142, 200–202.

Gournay, V., Savagner, C., Thiriez, G., et al., 2002. Pulmonary hypertension after ibuprofen prophylaxis in very preterm infants. Lancet 359, 1486–1488.

Graham, P.L., Begg, M.D., Larson, E., et al., 2006. Risk factors for late onset Gram-negative sepsis in low birth weight infants hospitalized in the neonatal intensive care unit. Pediatr Infect Dis J 25, 113–117.

Grausz, J.P., Harvey, D.R., 1967. Neonatal haemothorax: a report of two cases. Arch Dis Child 42, 675–676.

Greenough, A., 1988. The premature infant's respiratory response to mechanical ventilation. Early Hum Dev 17, 1–5.

Greenough, A., 1998. Use and misuse of albumin infusions in neonatal care. Eur J Pediatr 157, 699–702.

Greenough, A., Greenall, F., 1988. Observation of spontaneous respiratory interaction with artificial ventilation. Arch Dis Child 63, 168–171.

Greenough, A., Lagercrantz, H., 1992. Catecholamine abnormalities in transient tachypnoea of the premature newborn. J Perinat Med 20, 223–226.

Greenough, A., Morley, C.J., Davis, J.A., 1983. The interaction of spontaneous respiration with artificial ventilation in preterm babies. Journal of Pediatrics 103, 769–773.

Greenough, A., Dixon, A.D., Roberton, N.R.C., 1984a. Pulmonary interstitial emphysema. Arch Dis Child 59, 1046–1051.

Greenough, A., Morley, C.J., Wood, S., Davis, J.A., 1984b. Pancuronium prevents pneumothoraces in ventilated premature babies who actively expire against positive pressure ventilation. Lancet i, 1–3.

Greenough, A., Morley, C.J., Pool, J., 1986. Fighting the ventilator: are fast rates an effective alternative to paralysis? Early Hum Dev 13, 189–194.

Greenough, A., Greenall, F., Gamsu, H.R., 1987a. Synchronous respiration – which ventilator rate is best? Acta Paediatr Scand 76, 713–718.

Greenough, A., Pool, J., Greenall, F., et al., 1987b. Comparison of different rates of artificial ventilation in premature neonates with respiratory distress syndrome. Acta Paediatr Scand 76, 706–712.

Greenough, A., Chan, V., Hird, M.F., 1992. Positive end expiratory pressure in acute and chronic neonatal respiratory distress. Arch Dis Child 67, 320–323.

Greenough, A., Milner, A.D., Roberton, N.R.C., 1996. Neonatal Respiratory Disorders. Edward Arnold, London.

Greenough, A., Cox, S., Alexander, J., et al., 2001. Healthcare utilisation of infants with chronic lung disease related to hospitalisation for RSV infection. Arch Dis Child 85, 463–468.

Greenough, A., Alexander, J., Burgess, S., et al., 2004. Health care utilization of prematurely born, preschool children related to hospitalization for RSV infection. Arch Dis Child 89, 673–678.

Greenough, A., Dimitriou, G., Prendergast, M., et al., 2008. Synchronised mechanical ventilation for respiratory support in newborn infants. Cochrane Database for Systematic Reviews (1), CD000456.

Greenspan, J.S., Wolfson, M.R., Holt, W.J., et al., 1990. Neonatal gastric intubation: differential respiratory effects between nasogastric and orogastric tubes. Pediatr Pulmonol 8, 254–258.

Greenspan, J.S., Wolfson, M.R., Rubenstein, D., et al., 1997. Partial liquid ventilation of human preterm neonates. Journal of Pediatrics 117, 106–111.

Gregory, G.A., 1986. Devices for applying continuous positive airway pressure. In: Thibeault, D.W., Gregory, G.A. (Eds.), Neonatal Pulmonary Care, second ed. Appleton Century Crofts, Norwalk, CT, pp. 307–320.

Gregory, G.A., Kitterman, J.A., Phibbs, R.H., et al., 1971. Treatment of idiopathic respiratory distress syndrome with continuous positive pressure. NEJM 284, 1333–1340.

Gregory, G.A., Gooding, C.A., Phibbs, R.H., et al., 1974. Meconium aspiration in infants: a prospective study. Journal of Pediatrics 85, 848–852.

Gribetz, I., Frank, N.R., Avery, M.E., 1959. Static volume pressure relations of excised lungs of infants with hyaline membrane disease; newborn and stillborn infants. J Clin Invest 38, 2168–2175.

Griesen, G., Frederiksen, P.S., Hertel, J., et al., 1985. Catecholamine response to chest physiotherapy and endotracheal suctioning in preterm infants. Acta Paediatr Scand 74, 525–529.

Griesen, G., Munck, H., Lou, H., 1987. Severe hypocarbia in preterm infants and neurodevelopmental deficit. Acta Paediatr Scand 76, 401–404.

Grosfeld, J., Lemons, J., Ballantine, T.V., et al., 1980. Emergency thoracotomy for acquired bronchopleural fistula in the premature infant with respiratory distress. J Pediatr Surg 15, 416–421.

Gross, I., Moya, F.R., 2001. Is there a role for antenatal TRH therapy for the prevention of neonatal lung disease? Semin Perinatol 25, 406–416.

Gross, I., Smith, G.J., Wilson, C.M., et al., 1980. The influence of hormones on the biochemical development of the fetal rat lung in organ culture. Pediatr Res 14, 834–838.

Gross, G.W., Greenspan, J.S., Fox, W.W., et al., 1995. Use of liquid ventilation with perflubron during extracorporeal membrane oxygenation: chest radiographic appearances. Pediatr Radiol 194, 717–720.

Grossman, G., Tashiro, K., Kobayaski, T., et al., 1999. Experimental neonatal respiratory failure induced by lysophosphatidyl choline: effect of surfactant treatment. J Appl Physiol 86, 633–640.

Grover, T.R., Parker, T.A., Zenge, J.P., et al., 2003. Intrauterine hypertension decreases lung VEGF expression and VEGF inhibition causes pulmonary hypertension in the ovine fetus. Am J Physiol Lung Cell Mol Physiol 284, L508–L517.

Guignard, J.-P., Torrado, A., Mazouni, S.M., et al., 1976. Renal function in respiratory distress syndrome. Journal of Pediatrics 88, 845–850.

Guilleminault, C., Coons, S., 1984. Apnea and bradycardia during feeding in infants weighing <2000 gm. Journal of Pediatrics 104, 932–935.

Gupta, S., Sinha, S.K., Donn, S.M., 2009a. The effect of two levels of pressure support ventilation on tidal volume delivery and minute ventilation in preterm infants. Arch Dis Child Fetal Neonatal Ed 94, F80-F83.

Gupta, S., Sinha, S.K., Tin, W., et al., 2009b. A randomized controlled trial of post-extubation bubble continuous positive airway pressure versus Infant Flow Driver continuous positive airway pressure in preterm infants with respiratory distress syndrome. Journal of Pediatrics 154, 645–650.

Gurakan, B., Tarcan, A., Arda, I.S., et al., 2002. Persistent pulmonary interstitial emphysema in an unventilated neonate. Pediatr Pulmonol 34, 409–411.

Hacking, D., Warkins, A., Fraser, S., et al., 2001. Respiratory distress syndrome and birth order in premature twins. Arch Dis Child Fetal Neonatal Ed 84, F117–F121.

Hagadorn, J.I., Furey, A.M., Nghiem, T.H., et al., 2005. Achieved versus intended pulse oximeter saturation in infants born less than 28 weeks gestation: the AVIOx Study. Pediatrics 18, 1574–1582.

Hagay, Z., Reece, A., Roberts, A., et al., 1993. Isolated fetal pleural effusion: a prenatal management dilemma. Obstet Gynecol 81, 147–152.

Hallak, M., Bottoms, S.F., 1993. Accelerated pulmonary maturation from preterm premature rupture of membranes: a myth. Am J Obstet Gynecol 169, 1045–1049.

Halliday, H.L., 2000. Endotracheal intubation at birth for preventing morbidity stained infants born at term. Cochrane Database Syst Rev (2), CD000500.

Halliday, H.L., McClure, G., Reid, M., 1981. Transient tachypnoea of the newborn: two distinct clinical entities? Arch Dis Child 56, 322–325.

Hallman, M., Haataja, K., 2003. Genetic influences and neonatal lung disease. Seminars in Neonatalogy 8, 19–27.

Hallman, M., Arjomaa, P., Hoppu, K., 1987. Inositol supplementation in respiratory distress syndrome: relationship between serum concentration, renal excretion and lung effluent phospholipids. Journal of Pediatrics 110, 604–610.

Hallman, M., Bry, K., Hoppu, K., et al., 1992. Inositol supplementation in premature infants with respiratory distress syndrome. NEJM 326, 1233–1239.

Hallman, M., Merritt, T.A., Bry, K., et al., 1993. Association between neonatal care practices and efficacy of exogenous human surfactant: results of a bi-center randomized trial. Pediatrics 91, 552–560.

Hamdan, A.H., Shaw, N.J., 1995. Changes in pulmonary artery pressure in infants with respiratory distress syndrome following treatment with Exosurf. Arch Dis Child Fetal Neonatal Ed 72, F176–F179.

Hammerman, C., Lass, N., Strates, E., et al., 1987. Prostanoids in neonates with persistent pulmonary hypertension. Journal of Pediatrics 110, 470–472.

Han, V.K.M., Beverly, D.W., Clarson, C., et al., 1987. Randomized controlled trial of very early continuous distending pressure in the management of preterm infants. Early Hum Dev 15, 21–32.

Han, R.N.N., Buch, S., Tseu, I., et al., 1996. Changes in structure, mechanics and insulin-like growth factor related gene expression in the lungs of newborn rats exposed to air or 60% oxygen. Pediatr Res 39, 921–929.

Hanlon-Lundberg, K., Williams, M., Rhim, T., et al., 1996. Accelerated fetal lung maturity profiles and maternal cocaine exposure. Obstet Gynecol 87, 128–132.

Hannam, S., Lees, C., Edwards, R.J., et al., 2003. Neonatal coagulopathy in preterm, small-for-gestational-age infants. Biol Neonate 83, 177–181.

Hansen, A.K., Wisborg, K., Uldbjerg, N., et al., 2007. Elective caesarean section and respiratory morbidity in the term and near term neonate. Acta Obstetrics and Gynaecology Scandinavica 86, 389–394.

Harikumar, G., Egberongbe, Y., Nadel, S., et al., 2009. Tension time index as a predictor of extubation outcome in ventilated children. American Journal for Respiratory and Critical Care Medicine 180, 982–988.

Harrison, V.C., Heese, H., de, V., Klein, M., 1968. The significance of grunting in hyaline membrane disease. Pediatrics 41, 549–559.

Hart, S.M., McNair, M., Gamsu, H.R., et al., 1983. Pulmonary interstitial emphysema in very low birthweight infants. Arch Dis Child 58, 612–615.

Hashim, S.A., Roholt, H.B., Babayan, V.K., et al., 1964. Treatment of chyluria and

chylothorax with medium chain triglyceride. NEJM 270, 756–761.

Hauer, A.C., Rosegger, H., Haas, J., et al., 1996. Reaction of term newborns with prolonged postnatal dyspnoea to early oxygen, mask CPAP and volume expansion: a prospective randomized clinical trial. Eur J Pediatr 155, 805–810.

Heaf, D.P., Helms, P.J., Dinwiddie, R., 1982. Nasopharyngeal airways in Pierre Robin syndrome. Journal of Pediatrics 100, 698–703.

Heaf, D.P., Helms, P., Gordon, I., et al., 1983. Postural effects on gas exchange in infants. NEJM 308, 1505–1508.

Heckman. M., Linder, W., Pohlandt, F., 1998. Tension pneumopericardium in a preterm infant without mechanical ventilation; a rare cause of cardiac arrest. Acta Paediatr 87, 346–348.

Heicher, D.A., Kasting, D.S., Richards, J.R., 1981. Prospective clinical comparison of two methods of mechanical ventilation of neonates: rapid rate and short inspiratory time versus slow rate and long inspiratory time. Journal of Pediatrics 98, 957–961.

Helbock, H.J., Insoft, R.M., Conte, F.A., 1993. Glucocorticoid responsive hypotension in extremely low birthweight newborns. Pediatrics 92, 715–717.

Heldt, G.P., 1988. The effect of gavage feeding on the mechanics of the lung, chest wall and diaphragm in preterm infants. Pediatr Res 24, 55–58.

Hellstrom-Westas, L., Bell, A.H., Skov, L., et al., 1992. Cerebro-electrical depression following surfactant treatment in preterm neonates. Pediatrics 89, 643–647.

Henderson-Smart, D.J., Davis, P.G., 2003. Prophylactic methlxanthines for extubation in preterm infants. Cochrane Database for Systematic Reviews (1), CD000139.

Henderson-Smart, D.J., Bhuta, T., Cools, F., et al., 2007. Elective high frequency oscillatory ventilation versus conventional ventilation for acute pulmonary dysfunction in preterm infants. Cochrane Database Syst Rev (1), CD000104.

Henderson-Smart, D.J., De Paoli, A.G., Clark, R.H., et al., 2009. High frequency oscillatory ventilation versus conventional ventilation for infants with severe pulmonary dysfunction born at or near term. Cochrane Database for Systematic Reviews (3), CD002974.

Henry, G.W., 1984. Non-invasive assessment of cardiac function and pulmonary hypertension in persistent pulmonary hypertension of the newborn. Clin Perinatol 11, 627–640.

Herman, S., Reynolds, E.O.R., 1973. Methods for improving oxygenation in infants mechanically ventilated for severe HMD. Arch Dis Child 48, 612–617.

Hernandez, C., Little, B.B., Dax, J.S., et al., 1993. Prediction of the severity of meconium aspiration syndrome. Am J Obstet Gynecol 169, 61–70.

Hibbs, A.M., Walsh, M.C., Martin, R.J., et al., 2008. One year respiratory outcomes of preterm infants enrolled in the nitric oxide to prevent chronic lung disease trial. J Pediatr 153, 525–529.

HIFI Study Group, 1989. High-frequency oscillatory ventilation compared with conventional mechanical ventilation in the treatment of respiratory failure in preterm infants. NEJM 320, 88–93.

HiFO Study Group, 1993. Randomized study of high-frequency oscillatory ventilation in infants with severe respiratory distress syndrome. Journal of Pediatrics 122, 609–619.

Hill, A., Perlman, J.M., Volpe, J.J., 1982. Relationship of pneumothorax to occurrence of intraventricular hemorrhage in the premature newborn. Pediatrics 69, 144–149.

Hintz, S.R., Suttner, D.M., Sheehan, A.M., et al., 2000. Decreased use of neonatal extracorporeal membrane oxygenation (ECMO): how new treatment modalities have affected ECMO utilization. Pediatrics 106, 1339–1343.

Hird, M.F., Greenough, 1990. Causes of failure of neonatal patient triggered ventilation. Early Hum Dev 23, 101–108.

Hird, M.F., Greenough, A., 1991. Inflation time in mechanical ventilation of preterm neonates. Eur J Pediatr 150, 440–443.

Hird, M., Greenough, A., Gamsu, H.R., 1990. Gas trapping during high frequency positive pressure ventilation using conventional ventilators. Early Hum Dev 22, 51–56.

Hirschl, R.B., Merz, S.I., Montoya, J.P., et al., 1995a. Development and application of a simplified liquid ventilator. Crit Care Med 23, 157–163.

Hirschl, R.B., Pranikoff, T., Gauger, P., et al., 1995b. Liquid ventilation in adults, children and full term neonates. Lancet 346, 1201–1202.

Hirschl, R.B., Philip, W.F., Glick, V., 2003. A prospective randomized trial of perfluorocarbon-induced lung growth in newborns with congenital diaphragmatic hernia. J Pediatr Surg 38, 283–289.

Hjalmarson, O., 1981. Epidemiology and classification of acute neonatal respiratory disorders. Acta Paediatr Scand 70, 773–783.

Hjalmarson, O., Olsson, T., 1974. Mechanical and ventilatory parameters in healthy and diseased newborn infants. Acta Paediatrica Scandinavica Supplement 247, 26–48.

Ho, J.J., Rasa, G., 2007. Magnesium sulphate for persistent pulmonary hypertension of the newborn. Cochrane Database Syst Rev (3), CD005588.

Holm, B.A., Notter, R.H., Leary, J.F., et al., 1987. Alveolar epithelial changes in rabbits after a 21 day exposure to 60% oxygen. J Appl Physiol 62, 2230–2236.

Holopainen, R.L., Aho, H., Laine, D.J., et al., 1999. Human meconium has high phospholipase A$_2$ activity and induces cell injury and apoptosis in piglet lungs. Pediatr Res 46, 626–632.

Hook, B., Hack, M., Morrison, S., et al., 1995. Pneumopericardium in very low birthweight infants. J Perinatol 15, 27–31.

Hooper, S.B., Harding, R., 1990. Changes in lung liquid dynamics induced by prolonged fetal hypoxemia. J Appl Physiol 69, 127–135.

Hoskyns, E.N., Milner, A.D., Hopkin, I.E., 1991. Combined conventional ventilation with high frequency oscillation in neonates. Eur J Pediatr 150, 357–361.

Hough, J.L., Flenady, V., Johnston, L., et al., 2008. Chest physiotherapy for reducing respiratory morbidity in infants requiring ventilatory support. Cochrane Database for Systematic Reviews (3), CD006445.

Howell, S., Fitzgerald, R.S., Roussos, C., 1985. Effects of uncompensated and compensated metabolic acidosis on canine diaphragms. J Appl Physiol 59, 1376–1382.

Howlett, A., Ohlsson, A., 2003. Inositol for respiratory distress syndrome in preterm infants. Cochrane Database Syst Rev (4), CD000366.

Hrabovsky, E.E., Mullett, M.D., 1986. Gastroesophageal reflux and the premature infant. J Pediatr Surg 21, 583–587.

Huang, Y.-C.T., Sane, A.C., Simonson, S.G., 1995. Artificial surfactant attenuates hyperoxic lung injury in primates. I: Physiology and biochemistry. J Appl Physiol 78, 1816–1822.

Hulsey, T.C., Alexander, G.R., Robillard, P.Y., et al., 1993. Hyaline membrane disease: the role of ethnicity and maternal risk characteristics. Am J Obstet Gynecol 168, 572–576.

Hummler, H., Gerhardt, T., Claure, N., et al., 1994. Influence of patient triggered ventilation (PTV) on ventilation and blood pressure fluctuations in neonates. Pediatr Res 35, 338A.

Hunter, L., Richens, T., Davis, C., et al., 2009. Sildenafil use in congenital diaphragmatic hernia. Archives of Disease in Childhood Fetal Neonatal Edition 94, F467.

Huon, C., Rey, E., Mussat, P., et al., 1998. Low-dose doxapram for treatment of apnoea following early weaning in very low birthweight infants: a randomized, double-blind study. Acta Paediatr 87, 1180–1184.

Hutchinson, A.A., Yu, V.Y.H., 1980. Curare in the treatment of pulmonary hypertension as it occurs in the idiopathic respiratory distress syndrome. Australian Journal of Paediatrics 16, 94–100.

Ikegami, M., 1994. Surfactant inactivation. In: Boynton, B.R., Carlo, W.A., Jobe, A.H. (Eds.), New Therapies for Neonatal Respiratory Failure. Cambridge University Press, Cambridge, pp. 36–48.

Ikegami, M., Jacobs, H., Jobe, A., 1983. Surfactant function in respiratory distress syndrome. Journal of Pediatrics 102, 443–447.

Ikegami, M., Berry, D., Elkady, T., et al., 1987. Corticosteroids and surfactant change lung function and protein leaks in the lungs of ventilated premature rabbits. J Clin Invest 79, 1371–1378.

Ikegami, M., Jobe, A.H., Tabor, B.L., et al., 1992. Lung albumin recovery in surfactant treated preterm ventilated lambs. Am Rev Respir Dis 145, 1005–1008.

Ikegami, M., Jobe, A.H., Newnham, J., et al., 1997. Repetitive prenatal glucocorticoids improve lung function and decrease growth in preterm lambs. Am J Respir Crit Care Med 156, 178–184.

Ikonen, R.S., Janas, M.O., Koivikko, M.J., et al., 1992. Hyperbilirubinaemia, hypocarbia and periventricular leukomalacia in preterm infants: relationship to cerebral palsy. Acta Paediatr 81, 802–809.

Illingworth, R.S., 1969. Sucking and swallowing difficulties in infancy. Diagnostic problems of dysphagia. Arch Dis Child 44, 655–665.

Islam, S., Masiakos, P., Schnitzer, J.J., et al., 1999. Diltiazem reduces pulmonary arterial pressures in recurrent pulmonary hypertension associated with pulmonary hypoplasia. J Pediatr Surg 34, 712–714.

Itani, M.H., Mikati, M.A., 1998. Early onset neonatal spontaneous pneumopericardium. Lebanese Medical Journal 46, 165–167.

Itani, Y., Fujioka, M., Nishimura, G., et al., 1988. Upper GI examination in older premature infants with persistent apnea: correlation with simultaneous cardiorespiratory monitoring. Pediatr Radiol 18, 464–467.

Jackson, R.M., 1985. Pulmonary oxygen toxicity. Chest 88, 900–905.

Jacobsen, T., Gronvall, J., Petersen, S., et al., 1993. Minitouch treatment of very low birthweight infants. Acta Paediatr 82, 934–938.

Jacqz-Aigrain, E., Daoud, P., Burtin, P., et al., 1994. Placebo-controlled trial of midazolam sedation in mechanically ventilated newborn babies. Lancet 334, 640–650.

James, D.K., Chiswick, M.L., Harkes, A., et al., 1984. Non-specificity of surfactant deficiency in neonatal respiratory disorders. Br Med J (Clin Res Ed) 288, 1635–1638.

James, L., Greenough, A., Naik, S., 1997. The effect of blood transfusion on oxygenation in premature ventilated neonates. Eur J Pediatr 156, 139–141.

Janssen, D.J., Carnielli, V.P., Cogo, P., et al., 2006. Surfactant phosphatidylcholine metabolism in neonates with meconium aspiraton syndrome. Journal of Pediatrics 149, 634–639.

Javaheri, S., Herrera, L., Kazemi, H., 1979. Ventilatory drive in acute metabolic acidosis. J Appl Physiol 45, 913–918.

Jedeikin, R., Primhak, A., Shennan, A.T., et al., 1983. Serial electrocardiographic changes in healthy and stressed neonates. Arch Dis Child 58, 605–611.

John, E., Ermocilla, R., Golden, J., et al., 1980. Effects of gas temperature and particulate water on rabbit lung during ventilation. Pediatr Res 14, 1186–1191.

Johnson, A.H., Peacock, J.C., Greenough, A., et al., 2002. High frequency oscillation ventilation for the prevention of chronic lung disease of prematurity. NEJM 347, 633–642.

Joshi, V.V., Mandavia, S.G., Stern, L., et al., 1972. Acute lesions induced by endotracheal intubation. Am J Dis Child 124, 646–649.

Jovanovic, R., Nguyen, H.T., 1989. Experimental meconium aspiration in guinea pigs. Obstet Gynecol 73, 652–656.

Kääpä, P., Seppänen, M., Kero, P., et al., 1995. Haemodynamic control of atrial natriuretic peptide plasma levels in neonatal respiratory distress syndrome. Am J Perinatol 12, 235–239.

Kaiser, J.R., Gauss, C.H., Pont, M.M., et al., 2006. Hypercapnia during the first 3 days of life is associated with severe intraventricular haemorrhage in very low birth weight infants. J Perinatol 26, 279–285.

Kamlin, C.O., Davis, P.G., Morley, C.J., et al., 2006. Predicting successful extubation of very low birthweight infants. Archives of Disease in Childhood Fetal Neonatal Edition 91, F180–F183.

Kamper, J., Wulff, K., Larsen, C., et al., 1993. Early treatment with nasal continuous positive airway pressure in very low birthweight infants. Acta Paediatr 82, 193–197.

Kanto, W.P., 1994. A decade of experience with neonatal extracorporeal membrane oxygenation. Journal of Pediatrics 124, 335–347.

Kanto, W.P., Borer, R.C., Barr, M., et al., 1976. Tracheal aspirate lecithin-sphingomyelin ratios as predictors of recovery from respiratory distress syndrome. Journal of Pediatrics 89, 612–616.

Kari, M.A., Raivio, K.O., Stenman, U.H., et al., 1996. Serum cortisol, dehydroepiandrosterone sulphate and steroid-binding globulins in preterm neonates: effect of gestational age and dexamethasone therapy. Pediatr Res 40, 319–324.

Karl, S.R., Ballantine, T.V.N., Schnides, M.T., 1983. High frequency ventilation at rates of 375–1800 cycles/minute in 4 neonates with congenital diaphragmatic hernia. J Pediatr Surg 18, 822–828.

Karlowicz, M.G., 1994. Pneumoretroperitoneum and perirenal air associated with tension pneumothorax. Am J Perinatol 11, 63–64.

Karotkin, E.H., Kido, M., Cashore, W.J., et al., 1976. Acceleration of fetal lung maturation by aminophylline in fetal rabbits. Pediatr Res 10, 722–724.

Katz, V.L., Bowes, W.A., 1992. Meconium aspiration syndrome: reflections on a murky subject. Am J Obstet Gynecol 166, 171–183.

Katz, L.A., Klein, J.M., 2006. Repeat surfactant therapy for postsurfactant slump. J Perinatol 26, 414–422.

Kavvadia, V., Greenough, A., 1998. Influence of ethnic origin on respiratory distress syndrome in very premature infants. Arch Dis Child Fetal Neonatal Ed 78, F25–F28.

Kavvadia, V., Greenough, A., Dimitriou, G., et al., 1998. Comparison of respiratory function and fluid balance in very low birthweight infants given artificial or natural surfactant or no surfactant. J Perinat Med 26, 469–474.

Kavvadia, V., Greenough, A., Lilley, J., et al., 1999. Plasma arginine levels and the response to inhaled nitric oxide in neonates. Biol Neonate 76, 340–347.

Kavvadia, V., Greenough, A., Dimitriou, G., 2000a. Prediction of extubation failure in preterm neonates. Eur J Pediatr 159, 227–231.

Kavvadia, V., Greenough, A., Dimitriou, G., et al., 2000b. A comparison of arginine vasopressin levels and fluid balance in the perinatal period in infants who did and did not develop chronic oxygen dependency. Biol Neonate 78, 86–91.

Kavvadia, V., Greenough, A., Boylan, G., et al., 2001. Effect of a high volume strategy high frequency oscillation on cerebral haemodynamics. Eur J Pediatr 160, 140–141.

Kawczynski, P., Piotrowski, A., 1996. Circulatory and diuretic effects of dopexamine infusion in low birthweight infants with respiratory failure. Intensive Care Med 22, 65–70.

Keeney, S.E., Cress, S.E., Brocon, S.E., et al., 1992. The effect of hyperoxic exposure on antioxidant enzyme activities of the alveolar type II cells in neonatal and adult rats. Pediatr Res 31, 441–444.

Keeney, S.E., Mathews, M.J., Rassin, D.K., 1993. Antioxidant enzyme responses to hyperoxia in preterm and term rats after prenatal dexamethasone administration. Pediatr Res 33, 177–180.

Keirse, M.J.N.C., 1995. Betamimetic tocolytics in preterm labour. In: Enkin, M.N., Kierse, M.J.N.C., Renfrew, M.J., et al. (Eds.), Pregnancy and Childbirth Module of the Cochrane Collaboration; Issue 2. Update Software, Oxford.

Kelly, M.A., Finer, N.N., 1984. Nasotracheal intubation in the neonate: physiologic responses and effects of atropine and pancuronium. Journal of Pediatrics 105, 303–309.

Kelly, F.J., Lubec, G., 1995. Hyperoxic injury of immature guinea pig lung is mediated via hydroxyl radicals. Pediatr Res 38, 286–291.

Kelly, L.K., Porta, N.F., Goodman, D.M., et al., 2002. Inhaled prostacyclin for term infants with persistent pulmonary hypertension refractory to inhaled nitric oxide. Journal of Pediatrics 141, 830–832.

Keszler, M., Durand, D.J., 2001. Neonatal high-frequency ventilation. Past, present and future. Clin Perinatol 28, 579–607.

Keszler, M., Donn, S.M., Bucciarelli, R.L., et al., 1991. Multicenter controlled trial comparing high frequency jet ventilation and conventional mechanical ventilation in patients with pulmonary interstitial emphysema. Journal of Pediatrics 119, 85–93.

Keszler, M., Modanlou, H.D., Brudno, S., et al., 1997. Multicenter controlled clinical trial of high frequency jet ventilation in preterm infants with uncomplicated respiratory distress syndrome. Pediatrics 120, 107–113.

Keszler, M., Nassabeh-Montazami, S., Abubakar, K., 2009. Evolution of tidal volume requirement during the first 3 weeks of life in infants < 800 g ventilated with volume guarantee. Archives of Disease in Childhood Fetal Neonatal Edition 94, F279–F282.

Khalaf, M.N., Porat, R., Brodsky, N.L., et al., 2001. Clinical correlations in infants in the neonatal intensive care unit with varying severity of gastroesophageal reflux. Journal of Gastroenterology and Nutrition 32, 45–49.

Khammash, H., Perlman, M., Wojtulewicz, J., et al., 1993. Surfactant therapy in full term neonates with severe respiratory failure. Pediatrics 92, 135–139.

Kim, E.H., Boutwell, W.C., 1987. Successful direct extubation of very low birthweight infants from low intermittent mandatory ventilation rate. Pediatrics 80, 409–414.

King, J.F., Grant, A., Keirse, M.J.N.C., et al., 1988. Betamimetics in preterm labour: an overview of the randomised controlled trials. Br J Obstet Gynaecol 95, 211–222.

King, R.J., Coalson, J.J., Seidenfeld, J., et al., 1989. Oxygen and pneumonia induced lung injury. II. Properties of surfactant. J Appl Physiol 67, 357–365.

Kinmond, S., Aitchison, T.C., Holland, B.M., et al., 1993. Umbilical cord clamping and preterm infants: a randomized trial. Br Med J 306, 172–175.

Kinsella, J.P., 2008. Inaheld nitric oxide in the term newborn. Early Hum Dev 84, 709–716.

Kinsella, J.P., Abman, S.H., 1995. Recent developments in the pathophysiology and treatment of persistent pulmonary hypertension of the newborn. Journal of Pediatrics 126, 853–864.

Kinsella, J.P., Neish, S.R., Shaffer, E., et al., 1992. Low dose inhalational nitric oxide in persistent pulmonary hypertension of the newborn. Lancet 340, 819–820.

Kinsella, J.P., Truog, W.E., Walsh, W.F., et al., 1997. Randomised multicentre trial of inhaled nitric oxide and high frequency oscillatory ventilation in severe persistent pulmonary hypertension of the newborn. Journal of Pediatrics 131, 55–62.

Kinsella, J.P., Cutter, G.R., Walsh, W.F., et al., 2006. Early inhaled nitric oxide therapy in premature newborns with respiratory failure. NEJM 355, 354–364.

Kiraly, N.J., Tingay, D.G., Mills, J.F., et al., 2009. The effects of closed endotracheal suction on ventilation during conventional and high frequency oscillatory ventilation. Pediaric Research 66, 400–404.

Kjos, S.L., Walter, F.J., Montorom, M., et al., 1990. Prevalence and etiology of respiratory distress in infants of diabetic mothers: predictive value of lung maturation tests. Am J Obstet Gynecol 163, 898–903.

Klarr, J.M., Faix, R.G., Pryce, C.J.E., et al., 1994. Randomized trial of dopamine versus dobutamine for treatment of hypotension in preterm infants with respiratory distress syndrome. Journal of Pediatrics 125, 117–122.

Klein, J., 1990. Normobaric pulmonary oxygen toxicity. Anesth Analg 70, 195–207.

Klein, A.H., Foley, B., Foley, T.P., et al., 1981. Thyroid function studies in cord blood from premature infants with and without RDS. Journal of Pediatrics 98, 818–820.

Kobayashi, T., Nitta, K., Ganzuka, M., et al., 1991. Inactivation of exogenous surfactant by pulmonary edema fluid. Pediatr Res 29, 353–356.

Kohelet, D., Perlman, M., Kirpalani, H., et al., 1988. High frequency oscillation in the rescue of infants with persistent pulmonary hypertension. Crit Care Med 16, 510–516.

Kohlhauser, C., Popow, C., Helbich, T., et al., 1995. Successful treatment of severe neonatal lobar emphysema by high frequency oscillatory ventilation. Pediatr Pulmonol 19, 52–55.

Konduri, G.G., Mital, S., 2000. Adenosine and ATP cause NO-dependent pulmonary vasodilation in fetal lambs. Biol Neonate 78, 220–229.

Konduri, G.G., Vohr, B., Robertson, C., et al., 2007. Early inhaled nitric oxide therapy for term and near term newborn infants with hypoxic respiratory failure: neurodevelopmental follow up. Journal of Pediatrics 150, 235–240.

Konig, K., 2009. Successful weaning of nitric oxide facilitated by a single dose of sildenafil in a baby with persistent pulmonary hypertension of the newborn. Pedriatr Pulmonol 44, 837.

Kopelman, A.E., Holbert, D., 2003. Use of oxygen cannulas in extremely low birthweight infants is associated with mucosal trauma and bleeding, and possibly with coagulase-negative staphylococcal sepsis. J Perinatol 23, 94–97.

Kotas, R.V., Avery, M.E., 1971. Accelerated appearance of pulmonary surfactant in the fetal rabbit. J Appl Physiol 30, 358–361.

Koumbourlis, A.C., Mutich, R.L., Motoyama, E.S., 1995. Contribution of airway hyperresponsiveness to lower airway obstruction after extracorporeal membrane oxygenation for meconium aspiration syndrome. Crit Care Med 23, 749–754.

Kourembanas, S., Marsden, P.A., McQuillan, L.P., et al., 1991. Hypoxia induces endothelin gene expression and secretion in cultured human endothelium. J Clin Invest 88, 1054–1057.

Kribs, A., Pillekamp, F., Hunseler, C., et al., 2007. Early administration of surfactant in spontaneous breathing with nCPAP: feasibility and outcome in extremely premature infants (postmenstrual age ≤27 weeks). Paediatrics Anaesthesia 17, 364–369.

Kribs, A., Vierzig, A., Hünseler, C., et al., 2008. Early surfactant in spontaneously breathing with nCPAP in ELBW infants – a single centre four year experience. Acta Paediatr 97, 293–298.

Kugelman, A., Bar, A., Riskin, A., et al., 2008. Nasal respiratory support in premature infants: short-term physiological effects and comfort assessment. Acta Paediatr 97, 557–561.

Kühl, P.G., Cotton, R.B., Schweer, H., et al., 1989. Endogenous formation of prostanoids in neonates with persistent pulmonary hypertension. Arch Dis Child 64, 949–952.

Kumar, P., Kazzi, N.J., Shankaran, S., 1996. Plasma immunoreactive endothelin-1 concentrations in infants with persistent pulmonary hypertension of the newborn. Am J Perinatol 13, 335–341.

Lachman, B., 1987. Combination of saline instillation with artificial ventilation damages bronchial surfactant. Lancet i, 1375.

Lago, P., Benini, F., Agosto, C., et al., 1998. Randomised controlled trial of low dose fentanyl infusion in preterm infants with hyaline membrane disease. Arch Dis Child 79, 194–197.

Lam, B.C., Yeung, C.Y., 1999. Surfactant lavage for meconium aspiration syndrome: a pilot study. Pediatrics 103, 1014–1018.

Lamont, R.F., Dunlop, P.D.M., Levene, M.I., et al., 1983. Use of glucocorticoids in pregnancies complicated by severe hypertension and proteinuria. Br J Obstet Gynaecol 90, 199–202.

Lampland, A.L., Plumm, B., Meyers, P.A., et al., 2009. Observational study of humidified high-flow nasal cannula compared with nasal continuous positive airway pressure. Pediatrics 154, 177–182.

Landmann, E., Schmidtpott, M., Tutdibi, E., et al., 2005. Is transient tachypnoea of the newborn associated with polymorphisms in the epithelial sodium channel encoding gene? Investigation of the second transmembrane spanning domain of the α subunit. Acta Pediatrica 94, 317–323.

Lanteri, C.J., Willet, K.E., Kano, S., et al., 1994. Time course in lung mechanics following fetal steroid treatment. Am J Respir Crit Care Med 150, 759–765.

Laptook, A.R., O'Shea, T.M., Shankaran, S., et al., 2005. Adverse neurodevelopmental qoutcomes among extremely low birth weight infants with a normal head ultrasound: prevalence and antecedents. Pediatrics 115, 673–680.

Laros, R.K., Kitterman, J.A., Heilbron, D.C., 1991. Outcome of very low birthweight infants exposed to beta sympathomimetics in utero. Am J Obstet Gynecol 164, 1657–1665.

Lassus, P., Turanlati, M., Heikkala, P., et al., 2001. Pulmonary vascular endothelial growth factor and Ftt-1 in fetuses in acute and chronic lug disease and in PPHN. Am J Respir Crit Care Med 164, 1961–1967.

Laubscher, B., Greenough, A., Costeloe, K., 1996. Performance of four neonatal high frequency oscillators. British Journal of Intensive Care 6, 148–152.

Leach, C.L., Greenspan, J.S., Rubenstin, S.D., et al., 1995a. Partial liquid ventilation with Liquivent: a pilot and safety and efficacy study in premature newborns with severe respiratory distress syndrome (abstract). Pediatr Res 37, 220.

Leach, C.L., Holm, B., Morin, F.C., et al., 1995b. Partial liquid ventilation in premature lambs with respiratory distress syndrome: efficacy and compatibility with exogenous surfactant. Journal of Pediatrics 126, 412–420.

Leach, C.L., Greenspan, J.S., Rubenstein, S.D., et al., 1996. Partial liquid ventilation with perfluorocarbon in premature infants with severe respiratory distress syndrome. NEJM 335, 761–767.

Lee, S., Milner, A.D., 2000. Resonance frequency in respiratory distress syndrome. Arch Dis Child Fetal Neonatal Ed 83, F203–F206.

Lee, S.K., Tanswell, A.K., 1989. Pulmonary vascular air embolism in the newborn. Arch Dis Child 64, 507–510.

Lehtinen, A.-M., Hovorka, J., Widholm, O., 1984. Modification of aspects of the endocrine response to tracheal intubation by lignocaine, halothane and thiopentone. Br J Anaesth 56, 239–246.

Leigh, R.J., Shaw, D.A., 1976. Rapid regular respiration in unconscious patients. Arch Neurol 33, 356–361.

Leipala, J.A., Petaja, J., Fellman, V., 2001. Perforation complications of percutaneous central venous catheters in very low birthweight infants. J Paediatr Child Health 37, 168–171.

Lemyre, B., Davis, P.G., de Paoli, A.G., 2002. Nasal intermittent positive pressure ventilation (NIPPV) versus nasal continuous positive airway pressue (NCPAP) for apnea of prematurity. Cochrane Database Syst Rev (1), CD002272.

Lemyre, B., Cheng, R., Gaboury, I., 2009. Atropine, fentanyl and succinylcholine for non urgent intubations in newborns. Archives of Disease in Childhood Fetal Neonatal Edition 94, F439–F442.

Leonardi, M.R., Hankins, G.D.V., 1992. What's new in tocolytics. Clin Perinatol 19, 367–384.

Leonidas, J.C., Hall, R.T., Rhodes, P.G., 1975. Conservative management of unilateral pulmonary interstitial emphysema under tension. Journal of Pediatrics 87, 776–778.

Leslie, G.I., Gallery, E.D.M., Arnold, J.D., et al., 1991. Hyaline membrane disease and early neonatal aldosterone metabolism in infants of less than 33 weeks gestation. Acta Paediatr Scand 80, 628–633.

Le Souef, P., England, S.J., Bryan, A.C., 1984. Total resistance of the respiratory system in preterm infants with and without an endotracheal tube. Journal of Pediatrics 104, 108–111.

Levin, D.L., Fixler, D.E., Morriss, F.C., et al., 1978. Morphologic analysis of the pulmonary vascular bed in infants exposed in utero to prostaglandin synthetase inhibitors. Journal of Pediatrics 92, 478–483.

Levin, D.L., Mills, L.J., Parkey, M., et al., 1979. Constriction of the fetal ductus arteriosus after administration of indomethacin to the pregnant ewe. Journal of Pediatrics 94, 647–650.

Lewis, V., Whitelaw, A., 2002. Furosemide for transient tachypnoea of the newborn. Cochrane Database Syst Rev (1), CD000366.

Lewis, D.F., Futayyeh, S., Towers, C.V., et al., 1996. Preterm delivery from 34 to 37 weeks of gestation: is respiratory distress syndrome a problem? Am J Obstet Gynecol 174, 525–528.

Liang, J.S., Lu, F.L., Tang, J.R., et al., 2000. Congenital diaphragmatic hernia misdiagnosed as pneumothorax in a newborn. Taiwan Erch Koi Hseh Hui Tsa Chih 41, 221–223.

Lieberman, E., Torday, J., Barbieri, R., et al., 1992. Association of intrauterine cigarette smoke exposure with indices of fetal lung maturation. Obstet Gynecol 79, 564–570.

Liggins, G.C., Howie, R.N., 1972. A controlled trial of antepartum glucocorticoid treatment for prevention of the respiratory distress syndrome in premature infants. Pediatrics 50, 515–525.

Lin, Y., Lechner, A.J., 1991. Surfactant content and type II cell development in fetal guinea pig lungs during prenatal starvation. Pediatr Res 29, 288–291.

Linder, N., Aranda, J.V., Tsur, M., et al., 1988. Need for endotracheal intubation and suction in meconium stained neonates. Journal of Pediatrics 112, 613–615.

Linder, W., Vossbeck, S., Hummler, H., et al., 1999. Delivery room management of extremely low birthweight infants: spontaneous breathing or intubation? Pediatrics 103, 961–967.

Lista, G., Castoldi, F., Fontana, P., et al., 2006. Lung inflammation in preterm infants with respiratory distress syndrome: effects of ventilation with different tidal volumes. Pediatr Pulmonol 41, 357–363.

Lista, G., Castolid, F., Bianchi, S., et al., 2008. Volume guarantee versus high frequency ventilation: lung inflammation in preterm infants. Archives of Disease in Childhood Neonatal Fetal Edition 93, F252-F256.

Lista, G., Castoldi, F., Fontana, P., et al., 2010. Nasal continuous positive airway pressure (CPAP) versus bi-level nasal CPAP in preterm babies with respiratory distress syndrome: a randomised control trial. Archives of Disease in Childhood Fetal Neonatal Edition 95, F85-F89.

Litmanovitz, I., Carlo, W.A., 2008. Expectant management of pneumothorax in ventilated neonates. Pediatrics 122, e975–979.

Loe, E.A., Graves, E.D., Ochsner, J.L., et al., 1985. ECMO for newborn respiratory failure. J Pediatr Surg 20, 684–688.

Long, W.A., Lawson, E.E., Harned, H.S., et al., 1984. Pleural effusion in the first days of life. Am J Perinatol 1, 190–194.

Long, W., Zucker, J.A., Kraybill, E.N., 1995. Symposium in synthetic surfactant. II. Health and developmental outcomes at one year. Journal of Pediatrics 126, S1–S80.

Loo, C.K., Smith, G.J., Lykke, A.W.J., 1989. Effects of hyperoxia on surfactant morphology and cell viability in organotypic cultures of fetal rat lungs. Exp Lung Res 15, 597–617.

Lotze, A., Knight, G., Martin, G.R., 1993. Improved pulmonary outcome after exogenous surfactant for respiratory failure in term infants requiring extracorporeal membrane oxygenation. Journal of Pediatrics 121, 261–268.

Lotze, A., Mitchell, B.R., Short, B.L., et al., 1998. Multicenter study of surfactant (Beractant) use in the treatment of term infants with severe respiratory failure. Journal of Pediatrics 132, 40–47.

Lucas, A., Bloom, S.R., Aynsley-Green, A., 1986. Gut hormones and minimal enteral feeding. Acta Paediatr Scand 75, 719–723.

Lund, W.S., 1976. Deglutition. In: Hinchcliffe, R., Harrison, D. (Eds.), Scientific Foundations of Otolaryngology. Heinemann, London, pp. 591–598.

Lundstrom, K.E., Greisen, G., 1996. Changes in EEG, systemic circulation and blood gas parameters following two or six aliquots of porcine surfactant. Acta Paediatr 85, 708–712.

Lutman, D., Petros, A., 2008. Inhaled nitric oxide in neonatal and paediatric transport. Early Hum Dev 84, 725–729.

Lyrene, R.K., Philips, J.B., 1984. Control of pulmonary vascular resistance in the fetus and newborn. Clin Perinatol 11, 551–564.

MacArthur, B.A., Howie, R.N., Dezcete, J.A., et al., 1981. Cognitive and psychosocial development of 4-year-old children whose mothers were treated antenatally with betamethasone. Pediatrics 68, 638–643.

Madar, J., Richmond, S., Hey, E., 1999. Surfactant deficient respiratory distress after elective delivery at 'term'. Acta Paediatr 88, 1244–1248.

Madhavi, P., Jameson, R., Robinson, M.J., 2000. Unilateral pleural effusion complicating central venous catheterisation. Arch Dis Child Fetal Neonatal Ed 82, F248–F249.

Mahmoud, E.L., Benirschke, K., Vaucher, Y.E., et al., 1988. Motilin levels in term neonates who have passed meconium prior to birth. Journal of Paediatric Gastroenterology and Nutrition 7, 95–99.

Mahmoud, R.A., Fischer, H.S., Proguitte, H., et al., 2009. Relationship beteen endotracheal tube leakage and under reading of tidal volume in neonatal ventilators. Acta Paediatr 98, 1116–1122.

Makhoul, I.R., Smolkin, T., Sujov, P., 2002. Pneumothorax and nasal continuous positive airway pressure ventilation in premature neonates: a note of caution. ASAIO Journal 48, 476–479.

Makri, V., Hospes, B., Stoll-Becker, S., et al., 2002. Polymorphisms of surfactant protein B encoding gene: modifiers of the course of neonatal respiratory distress. Eur J Pediatr 161, 604–608.

Malo, J., Ali, J., Wood, L.D.H., 1984. How does positive end expiratory pressure reduce intrapulmonary shunt in canine pulmonary edema? J Appl Physiol 57, 1002–1010.

Mammel, M.C., Boros, S.J., 1987. Airway damage and mechanical ventilation. Pediatr Pulmonol 3, 443–447.

Man, G.C.W., Man, S.F.P., Kappagoda, C.T., 1983. Effects of high frequency oscillatory ventilation on vagal and phrenic nerve activity. J Appl Physiol 54, 502–507.

Manalo, E., Merritt, T.A., Kheiter, A., et al., 1996. Comparative effects of some serum components and proteolytic products of fibrinogen in surface tension-lowering abilities of Beractant and a synthetic peptide containing surfactant KL$_4$. Pediatr Res 39, 947–952.

Manning, F.A., Schreiber, F.A., Turkel, S.B., 1978. Fatal meconium aspiration 'in utero'. A case report. Am J Obstet Gynecol 132, 111–113.

Manning, F.A., Martin, C.B., Murata, Y., et al., 1979. Breathing movements before death in the primate fetus. Am J Obstet Gynecol 135, 71–76.

Manroe, B.L., Weinberg, A.G., Rosenfield, C.R., et al., 1979. The neonatal blood count in health and disease. I. Reference value for neutrophil cells. Journal of Pediatrics 95, 89–98.

Marchak, B.E., Thompson, W.K., Duffty, P., 1981. Treatment of RDS by high frequency oscillatory ventilator. A preliminary report. Journal of Pediatrics 99, 287–292.

Marino, A.J., Assing, E., Carbone, M.T., et al., 1995. The incidence of gastroesophageal reflux in preterm infants. J Perinatol 15, 369–371.

Maron, M.B., 1987. Analysis of airway fluid protein concentration in neurogenic pulmonary edema. J Appl Physiol 62, 470–476.

Marshall, T.A., Deeder, R., Pai, S., et al., 1984. Physiological changes associated with endotracheal intubation in preterm infants. Crit Care Med 12, 501–503.

Mathew, O.P., 1991. The science of bottle feeding. Journal of Pediatrics 119, 511–519.

Mathew, O.P., Clark, M.L., Pronske, M.L., et al., 1985. Breathing pattern and ventilation during oral feeding in term newborn infants. Journal of Pediatrics 106, 810–813.

Mazor, M., Furman, B., Wiznitzer, A., et al., 1995. Maternal and perinatal outcome of patients with preterm labour and meconium stained amniotic fluid. Obstet Gynecol 86, 830–833.

MacFarlane, P.I., Heaf, D.P., 1988. Pulmonary function in children after neonatal meconium aspiration syndrome. Arch Dis Child 63, 368–372.

MacGregor, R., Evans, D., Sugden, D., et al., 1998. Outcome at 5–6 years of prematurely born children who received morphine as neonates. Arch Dis Child Fetal Neonatal Ed 79, F40–F43.

Macklin, C.C., 1936. Alveolar pores and their significance in the human lung. Arch Pathol 21, 202–210.

McCallion, N., Davis, P.G., Morley, C.J., 2005. Volume targeted versus pressure limited ventilation in the neonate. Cochrane Database Systematic Reviews (3), CD003666.

McCann, E.M., Goldman, S.L., Brady, J.P., 1987. Pulmonary function in the sick newborn infant. Pediatr Res 21, 313–325.

McCulloch, P.R., Fokert, P.G., Froese, A.B., 1988. Lung volume maintenance prevents lung injury during high frequency oscillatory ventilation in surfactant deficient rabbits. Am Rev Respir Dis 137, 1185–1192.

McEvoy, R.D., Davies, N.J., Hedenstierna, G., et al., 1982. Lung mucociliary transport during high frequency ventilation. Am Rev Respir Dis 126, 452–456.

McEvoy, C., Sardesai, S., Schilling, D., et al., 2007. Acute effects of vecuronium on pulmonary function and hypoxemic episodes in preterm infants. Pediatr Int 49, 631–636.

McMillan, D.D., Rademaker, A.W., Buchan, K.A., et al., 1986. Benefits of orotracheal and nasotracheal intubation in neonates requiring ventilatory assistance. Pediatrics 7, 39–44.

McNally, H., Bennett, C.C., Elbourne, D., et al., 2006. United Kingdom collaborative randomised trial of neonatal extracorporeal membrane oxygenation: follow up to age 7 years. Pediatrics 117, e845.

McNamara, P.J., Laique, F., Muang-In, S., et al., 2006. Milrinone improves oxygenation in neonates with severe persistent pulmonary hypertension in the newborn. J Crit Care 21, 217–223.

Memon, A., Dave, R., Branca, P.A., et al., 1979. Improved method of gas exchange in HMD (abstract). Am Rev Respir Dis 119 (suppl.), 275.

Mendelson, C.R., Alcorn, J.L., Gao, E., 1993. The pulmonary surfactant protein genes and their regulation in fetal lung. Semin Perinatol 17, 223–232.

Menon, G., Boyle, E.M., Bergqvist, L.L., et al., 2008. Morphine analgesia and gastrointestinal morbidity in preterm infants: secondary results from the NEOPAIN trial. Archives of Disease in Childhood Fetal Neonatal Edition 93, F362–F367.

Mercer, S., 1986. Factors involved in chylothorax following repair of congenital posterolateral diaphragmatic hernia. J Pediatr Surg 21, 9–11.

Mercier, J.C., Hummler, H., Durrymeyer, X., et al., 2010. Inhaled nitric oxide for the prevention of bronchopulmonary dysplasia in premature babies: The EU Nitric Oxide Trial. Lancet 376, 346–354.

Merlob, P., Amir, J., Zaizov, R., et al., 1980. The differential leukocyte count in full term newborn infants with meconium aspiration and neonatal asphyxia. Acta Paediatr Scand 69, 779–780.

Merritt, T.A., Farrell, P.M., 1976. Diminished pulmonary lecithin synthesis in acidosis: experimental findings as related to the RDS. Pediatrics 57, 32–40.

Migdal, M., Dreizzen, E., Praud, J.P., et al., 1987. Compliance of the total respiratory system in healthy preterm and fullterm newborns. Pediatr Pulmonol 3, 214–218.

Miller, O.I., Celermajer, D.S., Deanfield, J.E., et al., 1994. Guidelines for the safe administration of inhaled nitric oxide. Arch Dis Child Fetal Neonatal Ed 70, F47–F49.

Moglia, B.B., Phelps, D.S., 1996. Changes in surfactant protein A mRNA levels in a rat model of insulin-treated diabetic pregnancy. Pediatr Res 39, 241–247.

Moise, A.A., Wearden, M.E., Kozinetz, C.A., et al., 1995. Antenatal steroids are associated with less need for blood pressure support in extremely premature infants. Pediatrics 95, 845–850.

Moomjian, A.S., Schwartz, J.G., Shutack, J.-G., et al., 1981. Use of external expiratory resistance in intubated neonates to increase lung volume. Arch Dis Child 56, 869–873.

Moraga, F.A., Riquelme, R.A., Lopez, A.A., et al., 1994. Maternal administration of glucocorticoid and thyrotropin-releasing hormone enhances fetal lung maturation in undisturbed preterm lambs. Am J Obstet Gynecol 171, 729–734.

Moriette, G., Pars-Uado, J., Walt, H., et al., 2001. Prospective randomized multicenter comparison of high frequency oscillatory ventilation and conventional ventilation in preterm infants less than 30 weeks with respiratory distress syndrome. Pediatrics 107, 365–372.

Morisot, C., Kacet, N., Bouchez, M.C., et al., 1990. Risk factors for fatal pulmonary interstitial emphysema in neonates. Eur J Pediatr 149, 493–495.

Morley, C.J., Morley, R., 1990. Follow-up of premature babies treated with artificial surfactant (ALEC). Arch Dis Child 65, 667–669.

Morley, C.J., Lau, R., De Paoli, A., et al., 2005. Nasal continuous positive airway pressure: does bubbling improve gas exchange? Archives of Disease in Childhood Fetal Neonatal Edition 90, F343–F344.

Morley, C.J., Davis, P.G., Doyle, L.W., et al., 2008. Nasal CPAP or intubation at birth for very preterm infants. NEJM 358, 700–708.

Morrison, J.J., Rennie, J.M., Milton, P.J., 1995. Neonatal respiratory morbidity and mode of delivery at term: influence of timing of elective caesarean section. Br J Obstet Gynaecol 102, 101–106.

Moseley, J.E., 1960. Loculated pneumomediastinum in the newborn. A thymic 'spinnaker' sign. Radiology 75, 788–790.

Moses, D., Holm, B.A., Spitale, P., et al., 1991. Inhibition of pulmonary surfactant function by meconium. Am J Obstet Gynecol 164, 477–481.

Moya, M.P., Gow, A.J., Califf, R.M., et al., 2002. Inhaled ethyl nitrite gas for persistent pulmonary hypertension of the newborn. Lancet 360, 141–143.

Moya, F.R., Gadzinowski, J., Bancalari, E., 2005. A multicenter randomised masked comparison trial of lucinactant, colfosceril palmitate, and beractant for the prevention of respiratory distress syndrome among very preterm infants. Pediatrics 115, 1018–1029.

Mupanemunda, R.H., Edwards, A.D., 1995. Treatment of newborn infants with inhaled nitric oxide. Arch Dis Child Fetal Neonatal Ed 72, F131–F134.

Murdoch, D.R., Darlow, B.A., 1984. Handling during neonatal intensive care. Arch Dis Child 59, 957–961.

Murphy, J.D., Rabinowitz, M., Goldstein, J.D., et al., 1981. Structural basis of persistent pulmonary hypertension of the newborn infant. Journal of Pediatrics 98, 962–967.

Murphy, J.D., Vawter, G.F., Reid, L.M., 1984. Pulmonary vascular disease in fatal meconium aspiration. Journal of Pediatrics 104, 758–762.

Murphy, K.E., Hannah, M.E., Willan, A.R., et al., 2008. Multiple courses of antenatal corticosteroids for preterm birth (MACS): a randomised controlled trial. Lancet 372, 2143–2151.

Murray, P.G., Stewart, M.J., 2008. Use of nasal continuous positive airway pressure during retrieval of neonates with acute respiratory distress. Pediatrics 121, e754–e758.

Murthy, B.V., Petros, A.J., 1996. High-frequency oscillatory ventilation combined with intermittent mandatory ventilation in critically ill neonates and infants. Acta Anaesthesiologica Scandinavica 40, 679–683.

Nagourney, B.A., Kramer, M.S., Klebanoff, M.A., et al., 1996. Recurrent respiratory distress syndrome in successive preterm pregnancies. Journal of Pediatrics 129, 591–596.

Nakwan, N., Choksuchat, D., Saksawad, R., et al., 2009. Successful treatment of persistent pulmonary hypertension of the newborn with bosentan. Acta Pediatrica 98, 1683–1685.

Narchi, H., Kulaylat, N., 1999. Is gastric lavage needed in neonates with meconium-stained amniotic fluid? Eur J Pediatr 158, 315–317.

Navarrete, C.T., Devia, C., Lessa, A.C., et al., 2003. The role of endothelin converting enzyme inhibition during group B streptococcus-induced pulmonary hypertension in newborn piglets. Pediatr Res 54, 387–392.

Neonatal Inhaled Nitric Oxide Study Group (NINOS), 1997. Inhaled nitric oxide in full-term and nearly full-term infants with hypoxic respiratory failure. New Engl J Med 336, 597–604.

Neonatal Inhaled Nitric Oxide Study Group (NINOS), 2000. Inhaled nitric oxide in term and near term infants: neurodevelopmental follow-up of the Neonatal Inhaled Nitric Oxide Study Group (NINOS). Journal of Pediatrics 136, 611–617.

Newell, S.J., Booth, I.W., Morgan, M.E.I., et al., 1989a. Gastro-oesophageal reflux in preterm infants. Arch Dis Child 64, 780–786.

Newell, S.J., Morgan, M.E.I., Durbin, G.M., et al., 1989b. Does mechanical ventilation precipitate gastro-oesophageal reflux during enteral feeding? Arch Dis Child 64, 1352–1355.

Ng, K.P.K., Easa, D., 1979. Management of interstitial emphysema by high frequency low positive pressure hand ventilation in the neonate. Journal of Pediatrics 95, 117–118.

Nicolaides, K.H., Azar, G.B., 1990. Thoracoamniotic shunting. Fetal Diagn Ther 5, 153–164.

NIH Consensus Panel Development, 1995. Effect of corticosteroids on fetal maturation and perinatal outcomes. J Am Med Assoc 273, 413–418.

Niwas, R., Nadroo, A.M., Sutija, V.G., et al., 2007. Malposition of endotracheal tube: association with pneumothorax in ventilated neonates. Archives of Disease in Childhood Fetal Neonatal Edition 92, F233–F234.

NNNI Trial Group (Northern Neonatal Nursing Initiative), 1996. A randomized trial comparing the effect of prophylactic intravenous fresh frozen plasma, gelatin or glucose on early mortality and morbidity in preterm babies. Eur J Pediatr 155, 580–588.

Nogee, L., de Mello, D., Dehner, L., et al., 1993. Pulmonary surfactant protein B deficiency in congenital pulmonary alveolar proteinosis. NEJM 328, 406–410.

Nogee, L., Garnier, G., Singer, L., et al., 1994. A mutation in the surfactant protein B gene responsible for fatal neonatal respiratory disease in multiple kindreds. J Clin Invest 93, 1860–1863.

Northern Neonatal Network, 2000. Neonatal Formulary. BMJ Books, London.

Nowadzky, T., Pantoja, A., Britton, J.R., 2009. Bubble continuous positive airway pressure, a potentially better practice, reduces the use of mechanical ventilation among very low birth weight infants with respiratory distress syndrome. Pediatrics 123, 1534–1540.

Nugent, S.K., Laravuso, R., Rogers, M.C., 1979. Pharmacology and use of muscle relaxants in infants and children. Journal of Pediatrics 94, 481–487.

Nuntnarumit, P., Korones, S.B., Yang, W., et al., 2002. Efficacy and safety of tolazoline for treatment of severe hypoxemia in extremely preterm infants. Pediatrics 109, 852–856.

Octave Study Group, 1991. Multicentre randomised controlled trial of high against low frequency positive pressure ventilation. Oxford Region Controlled Trial of Artificial Ventilation. Arch Dis Child 66, 770–775.

Oetomo, S.B., Lewis, J., Ikegami, M., et al., 1990. Surfactant treatments alter endogenous surfactant metabolism in rabbit lungs. J Appl Physiol 68, 1590–1596.

Ogawa, Y., Shimizu, H., Ikatura, Y., et al., 1999. Functional pulmonary surfactant deficiency and neonatal respiratory disorders. Pediatr Pulmonol 18, 175–177.

Oh, W., Stern, L., 1977. Diseases of the respiratory system. In: Behrman, R.E. (Ed.), Neonatal and Perinatal Medicine: Disease of the Fetus and Infant. C V Mosby, St Louis, p. 558.

Ohama, Y., Itakura, Y., Koyama, N., et al., 1994. Effect of surfactant lavage in a rabbit model of meconium aspiration syndrome. Acta Paediatrica Japonica 36, 236–238.

Ojomo, E.O., Coustan, D.R., 1990. Absence of evidence of pulmonary maturity at amniocentesis in term infants of diabetic mothers. Am J Obstet Gynecol 163, 954–957.

Ophoven, J.P., Mammel, M.C., Gardon, M.J., 1984. Tracheobronchial histopathology associated with high frequency ventilation. Crit Care Med 12, 829–832.

Orenstein, S.R., Orenstein, D.M., 1988. Gastroesophageal reflux and respiratory disease in children. Journal of Pediatrics 112, 847–858.

Orsini, A.G., Leef, K.H., Costarino, A., et al., 1996. Routine use of fentanyl infusions for pain and stress reduction in infants with respiratory distress syndrome. Journal of Pediatrics 129, 140–145.

Osiris Collaborative Group, 1992. Early versus delayed neonatal administration of a synthetic surfactant – the judgement of Osiris. Lancet ii, 1363–1369.

Outerbridge, E., 1979. The negative pressure ventilator. In: Thibeault, G.W., Gregory, G.A. (Eds.), Neonatal Pulmonary Care. Addison-Wesley, Menlo Park, CA, pp. 168–177.

Pandit, P.B., Dunn, M.S., Colucci, E.A., 1995. Surfactant therapy in neonates with respiratory deterioration due to pulmonary hemorrhage. Pediatrics 95, 32–35.

Pandit, B.P., O'Brien, K., Aztalos, E., et al., 1999. Outcome following pulmonary haemorrhage in infants dying after surfactant therapy. Journal of Pediatrics 124, 521–626.

Pandit, P.B., Courtney, S.E., Pyon, K.H., et al., 2001. Work of breathing during constant- and variable-flow nasal continuous positive airway pressure in preterm neonates. Pediatrics 108, 682–685.

Pape, K.E., Armstrong, D.L., Fitzhardinge, P.M., 1976. Central nervous system pathology associated with mask ventilation in the very low birthweight infant: a new etiology for intracerebellar hemorrhages. Pediatrics 58, 473–483.

Pappin, A., Shenker, N., Hack, M., et al., 1994. Extensive intraalveolar pulmonary hemorrhage in infants dying after surfactant therapy. Journal of Pediatrics 124, 521–626.

Paranka, M.S., Clark, R.H., Yoder, B.A., et al., 1995. Predictors of failure of high frequency oscillatory ventilation in term infants with severe respiratory failure. Pediatrics 95, 400–404.

Pardou, A., Vermeylen, D., Muller, M.F., et al., 1993. High frequency ventilation and conventional mechanical ventilation in newborn babies with respiratory distress syndrome: a prospective randomized trial. Intensive Care Med 19, 406–410.

Pare, P.D., Warriner, B., Baile, E.M., et al., 1983. Reduction of pulmonary extravascular water with positive end expiratory pressure in canine pulmonary edema. Am Rev Respir Dis 127, 590–593.

Patel, D.S., Rafferty, G.F., Lee, S., et al., 2009a. Work of breathing during SIMV with and without pressure support. Arch Dis Child 94, 434–436.

Patel, D.S., Sharma, A., Prendergast, M., et al., 2009b. Work of breathing and different levels of volume-targeted ventilation. Pediatrics 123, e679–e684.

Patel, D., Rafferty, G.F., Lee, S., et al., 2010a. Work of breathing and volume targeting in prematurely born infants with acute respiratory distress syndrome. Arch Dis Child 95, F443–F446.

Patel, D.S., Rafferty, G.F., Hannam, S., et al., 2010b. In vitro assessment of proportional assist ventilation. Archives of Disease in Childhood Fetal Neonatal Edition 95, F331–F337.

Paxson, C.L., Stoerner, J.W., Denson, S.E., et al., 1977. Syndrome of inappropriate antidiuretic hormone secretion in neonates with pneumothorax or atelectasis. Journal of Pediatrics 91, 459–463.

Peckham, G.J., Fox, W.W., 1978. Physiologic factors affecting pulmonary artery pressure in infants with persistent pulmonary hypertension. Journal of Pediatrics 93, 1005–1010.

Peevy, K.J., Chalhub, E.G., 1983. Occult group B streptococcal infection: an important cause of intrauterine asphyxia. Am J Obstet Gynecol 146, 989–990.

Pellicano, A., Tingay, D.G., Mills, J.F., et al., 2009. Comparison of four methods of lung volume recruitment during high frequency oscillatory ventilation. Intensive Care Med 35, 1990–1998.

Peltoniemi, O.M., Anneli Kari, M., Tammela, O., et al., 2007. Randomized trial of a single repeat dose of prenatal betamethasone treatment in imminent preterm birth. Pediatrics 119, 290–298.

Peltoniemi, O.M., Anneli Kari, M., Lano, A., et al., 2009. Two year follow up of a randomised trial with repeated antenatal betamethasone. Archives of Disease in Childhood Fetal Neonatal Edition 94, F402–F406.

Perlman, J.M., Volpe, J.J., 1983. Suctioning in the preterm infant: effects on cerebral blood flow velocity, intracranial pressure and arterial blood pressure. Pediatrics 72, 329–334.

Petres, R.E., Redwine, F.O., Cruikshank, D.P., 1982. Congenital bilateral chylothorax: antepartum diagnosis and successful intrauterine surgical management. J Am Med Assoc 248, 1360–1365.

Petros, A.J., 1995. Epoprostenol (Prostacyclin) for the Treatment of Pulmonary Hypertension. BPA Medicines Standing Committee, London.

Pfenninger, E., Dick, W., Brecht-Krauss, D., et al., 1984. Investigation of intrapartum clearance of the upper airway in the presence of meconium contaminated amniotic fluid using an animal model. J Perinat Med 12, 57–68.

Pfenninger, J., Tschappler, M., Wagner, B.P., et al., 1991. The paradox of the adult respiratory distress syndrome in neonates. Pediatr Pulmonol 10, 18–24.

Pfister, R.H., Soll, R., Wiswell, T.E., 2007. Protein containing synthetic surfactant versus animal derived surfactant extract for the prevention and treatment of respiratory distress syndrome. Cochrane Database Systematic Reviews (4), CD006069.

Phibbs, R.H., Johnson, P., Kitterman, J.A., et al., 1972. Cardiorespiratory status of erythroblastotic infants. Pediatrics 49, 5–14.

Philips, J.B. III, Lyrene, R.K., Godoy, G., et al., 1988. Hemodynamic responses of chronically instrumented piglets to bolus injections of group B streptococcus. Pediatr Res 23, 81–85.

Piantadosi, C.A., Fracicia, P.J., Duhaylongsod, F.G., et al., 1995. Artificial surfactant attenuates hyperoxic lung injury in primates. II. Morphometric analysis. J Appl Physiol 78, 1823–1831.

Pickens, D.L., Scheft, G., Thach, B.T., 1988. Prolonged apnea associated with upper airway protective reflexes in apnea of prematurity. Am Rev Respir Dis 137, 113–118.

Pijpers, L., Reuss, A., Stewart, P.A., et al., 1989. Non-invasive management of isolated bilateral fetal hydrothorax. Am J Obstet Gynecol 161, 330–332.

Pinkerton, K.E., Lewis, J.E., Rider, E.D., et al., 1994. Lung parenchyma and type II cell morphometrics: effect of surfactant treatment on preterm ventilated lamb lungs. J Appl Physiol 77, 1953–1960.

Piper, J.M., Xenakis, E.M.-J., McFarland, M., 1996. Do growth retarded premature infants have different rates of perinatal morbidity and mortality than appropriately grown premature infants? Obstet Gynecol 87, 169–174.

Plavka, R., Kopecky, P., Sebron, V., et al., 2002. Early versus delayed surfactant administration in extremely premature neonates with respiratory distress syndrome ventilated by high-frequency oscillatory ventilation. Intensive Care Med 28, 1483–1490.

Plenat, F., Vert, P., Didier, F., et al., 1978. Pulmonary interstitial emphysema. Clin Perinatol 5, 351–375.

Plexico, D.T., Loughlin, G.M., 1981. Nasopharyngeal reflux and neonatal apnea. Am J Dis Child 135, 793–794.

Pohlandt, F., Sayle, H., Schroeder, H., et al., 1992. Decreased incidence of extra-alveolar air leakage or death prior to air leakage in high versus low rate positive pressure ventilation: results of a seven centre randomized trial in preterm infants. Eur J Pediatr 151, 904–909.

Pokora, T., Bing, D., Mammel, M., et al., 1983. Neonatal high frequency jet ventilation. Pediatrics 72, 27–32.

Pole, J.D., Mustard, C.A.M., To, T., et al., 2009. Antenatal steroid thereapy for fetal lung maturation: is there an association with childhood asthma? J Asthma 46, 47–52.

Polimeni, V., Claure, N., D'Ugard, C., et al., 2006. Effects of volume-targeted synchronized intermittent mandatory ventilation on spontaneous episodes of hypoxemia in preterm infants. Biol Neonate 89, 50–55.

Polk, D.H., Ikegami, M., Jobe, A.H., et al., 1995. Postnatal lung function in preterm lambs: effects of a single exposure to betamethasone and thyroid hormones. Am J Obstet Gynecol 172, 872–881.

Pranikoff, T., Gauger, P.G., Hirschl, R.B., 1996. Partial liquid ventilation in newborn patients with congenital diaphragmatic hernia. J Pediatr Surg 31, 613–618.

Prasertsom, W., Phillipos, E.Z., van Aerde, J.E., et al., 1996. Pulmonary vascular resistance during lipid infusion in neonates. Arch Dis Child Fetal Neonatal Ed 74, F95–F98.

Price, L.T., Chen, Y., Frank, L., 1993. Epidermal growth factor increases antioxidant enzyme and surfactant system development during hyperoxia and protects fetal rat lungs in vitro from hyperoxic toxicity. Pediatr Res 34, 577–585.

Primhak, R.A., 1983. Factors associated with pulmonary airleak in premature infants receiving mechanical ventilation. Journal of Pediatrics 102, 764–767.

Primhak, R.A., Jedeikin, R., Ellis, G., et al., 1985. Myocardial ischaemia in asphyxia neonatorum. Acta Paediatr Scand 74, 595–600.

Puntis, J.W.L., Roberts, K.D., Handy, D., 1987. How should chlyothorax be managed? Arch Dis Child 62, 593–596.

Quinlan, R.W., Buhi, W.C., Cruz, A.C., 1984. Fetal pulmonary maturity in isoimmunized pregnancies. Am J Obstet Gynecol 148, 787–789.

Quinn, M.W., Wild, J., Dean, H.G., et al., 1993. Randomized double-blind controlled trial of effect of morphine on catecholamine concentrations in ventilated preterm babies. Lancet 342, 324–327.

Raju, T.N.K., Langenberg, P., 1993. Pulmonary hemorrhage and exogenous surfactant therapy: a meta-analysis. Journal of Pediatrics 123, 603–610.

Raju, T.N.K., Vidyasagar, D., Torres, C., et al., 1980. Intracranial pressure during intubation and anesthesia in infants. Journal of Pediatrics 96, 860–862.

Ramin, K.D., Leveno, K.J., Kelly, M.A., et al., 1996. Amniotic fluid meconium: a fetal environmental hazard. Obstet Gynecol 87, 181–184.

Rasche, R.F.H., Kuhns, L.P., 1972. Histopathologic changes in airway mucosa of infants after endotracheal intubation. Pediatrics 50, 632–637.

Rawlings, J.S., Smith, F.R., Wiswell, T.E., 1984. Transient tachypnea of the newborn. An analysis of neonatal and obstetric risk factors. Am J Dis Child 138, 869–871.

Raye, J.R., Gutberlet, R.L., Stahlman, M., 1970. Symptomatic posthemorrhagic anemia in the newborn. Pediatr Clin North Am 17, 402–413.

Reece, E.A., Moya, F., Yakigi, R., et al., 1987. Persistent pulmonary hypertension: assessment of perinatal risk factors. Obstet Gynecol 70, 696–700.

Rees, L., Forsling, M.L., Brook, C.D.G., 1980. Vasopressin concentrations in the neonatal period. Clin Endocrinol (Oxf) 12, 357–362.

Reich, D.L., Hollinger, I., Harrington, D.J., et al., 2004. Comparison of cisatracurium and vecuronium by infusion in neonates and small infants after congenital heart surgery. Anesthesiology 101, 1122–1127.

Rettwitz-Volk, W., Schloesser, R., von Loewenich, V., 1993. One-sided high frequency oscillating ventilation in the treatment of unilateral pulmonary emphysema. Acta Paediatr 82, 190–192.

Reyes, Z.C., Claure, N., Tauscher, M.K., et al., 2006. Randomized, controlled trial comparing synchronized intermittent mandatory ventilation and synchronized intermittent mandatory ventilation plus pressure support in preterm infants. Pediatrics 118, 1409–1417.

Reynolds, E.O.R., Taghizadeh, A., 1974. Improved prognosis of infants mechanically ventilated for hyaline membrane disease. Arch Dis Child 49, 505–515.

Richardson, D.K., Torday, J.S., 1994. Racial differences in predictive value of the lecithin/sphingomyelin ratio. Am J Obstet Gynecol 170, 1273–1278.

Richardson, P., Bowes, C.L., Carlstrom, J.R., 1986. The functional residual capacity of infants with respiratory distress syndrome. Acta Paediatr Scand 75, 267–271.

Rigby, M.L., Pickering, D., Wilkinson, A., 1984. Cross sectional echocardiography in determining persistent patency of the ductus arteriosus in preterm infants. Arch Dis Child 59, 341–345.

Rishi, A., Hatzis, D., McAlmon, F., et al., 1992. An allelic variant of the 6A gene for surfactant protein A. Am J Physiol 262, 2566–2573.

Roberton, N.R.C., 1976a. Treatment of cystic ventilator lung disease. Proc R Soc Med 69, 344–347.

Roberton, N.R.C., 1976b. CPAP or not CPAP? Arch Dis Child 51, 161–162.

Roberton, N.R.C., 1992. A Manual of Neonatal Intensive Care, third ed. Edward Arnold, London, pp. 128–129.

Roberts, D., Dalziel, S.R., 2010. Antenatal corticosteroids for accelerating fetal lung maturation for women at risk of preterm birth. Cochrane Database Syst Rev (9), CD004454.

Roberts, J.D., Polaner, D.M., Lang, P., et al., 1992. Inhaled nitric oxide in persistent pulmonary hypertension of the newborn. Lancet 340, 818–819.

Robertson, B., 1981. Neonatal pulmonary mechanics and morphology after experimental therapeutic regimes. In: Scarpelli, E.M., Cosmi, E.V. (Eds.), Reviews in Perinatal Medicine, vol. 4. Raven Press, New York, pp. 337–379.

Robertson, N.J., McCarthy, L.S., Hamilton, P.A., et al., 1996. Nasal deformities resulting from flow driver continuous positive airway pressure. Arch Dis Child Fetal Neonatal Ed 75, F209–F212.

Robertson, C.M., Tyebkhan, J.M., Peliowski, A., et al., 2006. Ototoxic drugs and sensorineural hearing loss following severe neonatal respiratory failure. Acta Paediatr 95, 214–223.

Robson, E., Hey, E., 1982. Resuscitation of preterm babies at birth reduces the risk of death from hyaline membrane disease. Arch Dis Child 57, 184–186.

Rojas, J., Stahlman, M., 1984. The effects of group B streptoccocus and other organisms on the pulmonary vasculature. Clin Perinatol 11, 591–599.

Rojas, J., Larsson, L.E., Hellerqvist, C.G., et al., 1983. Pulmonary hemodynamic and ultrastructural changes associated with group B streptococcal toxemia in adult sheep and newborn lambs. Pediatr Res 70, 1002–1008.

Romaguera, J., Ramirez, M., Adamsons, K., 1993. Intra-amniotic thyroxine to accelerate fetal maturation. Semin Perinatol 17, 260–266.

Rønnestad, A., Abrahamsen, T.G., Medbø, S., et al., 2005. Septicemia in the first week of life in a Norwegian national cohort of extremely premature infants. Pediatrics 115, e262–e268.

Rosenberg, A.A., Kennaugh, J., Koppenhafer, S.L., et al., 1993. Elevated immunoreactive endothelin I levels in newborn infants with persistent pulmonary hypertension. Journal of Pediatrics 123, 109–114.

Royal College of Obstetricians and Gynaecologists, 1996. Antenatal corticosteroids to prevent respiratory distress syndrome. Available online at: www.rcog.org.uk/guidelines/corticosteroids.

Royall, J.A., Levin, D.L., 1988. Adult respiratory distress syndrome in pediatric patients. I. Clinical aspects, pathophysiology, pathology and mechanisms of lung injury. Journal of Pediatrics 112, 169–180.

Roze, J.C., Liet, J.M., Gournay, V., et al., 1997. Oxygen cost of breathing and weaning process in newborn infants. Eur Respir J 10, 2583–2585.

Rubatelli, F.F., Bonale, L., Tangucci, M., et al., 1998. Epidemiology of neonatal acute respiratory disorders. Biol Neonate 74, 7–15.

Rudolph, A.M., 1977. Fetal and neonatal pulmonary circulation. Am Rev Respir Dis 115 (suppl.), 11–18.

Rudolph, A.J., Smith, C.A., 1960. Idiopathic respiratory distress syndrome of the newborn. Journal of Pediatrics 57, 905–921.

Rudolph, A.M., Yuan, S., 1966. Response of the pulmonary vasculature to hypoxia and hydrogen ion changes. J Clin Invest 45, 399–411.

Runkle, B., Goldberg, R.N., Streitfeld, M.M., et al., 1984. Cardiovascular changes in group B streptococcal sepsis in the piglet: response to indomethacin and the relationship to prostacyclin and thromboxane A$_2$. Pediatr Res 18, 874–878.

Rutledge, M., Hawkins, E., Langston, C., 1986. Skeletal muscle atrophy induced in infants by chronic pancuronium treatment. Journal of Pediatrics 109, 883–886.

Ryan, C.A., Finer, N.N., Barrington, K.J., 1994. Effects of magnesium sulphate and nitric oxide in pulmonary hypertension induced by hypoxia in newborn piglets. Archives of Disease in Childhood Fetal and Neonatal Edition 71, F151–F155.

Saarenmaa, E., Neuvonen, P.J., Fellman, V., 2000. Gestational age and birthweight effects on plasma clearance of fentanyl in newborn infants. Journal of Pediatrics 136, 767–770.

Sadiq, H.F., Mantych, G., Benawra, R.S., et al., 2003. Inhaled nitric oxide in the treatment of moderate persistent pulmonary hypertension of the newborn: a randomized controlled multicenter trial. J Perinatol 23, 98–103.

Samuels, M.P., Southall, D.P., 1989. Negative extrathoracic pressure in treatment of respiratory failure in infants and young children. Br Med J 299, 1253–1257.

Samuels, M.P., Raine, J., Wright, T., et al., 1996. Continuous negative extrathoracic pressure in neonatal respiratory failure. Pediatrics 98, 1154–1160.

Sandberg, K., Engelhardt, B., Hellerqvist, C., et al., 1987a. Pulmonary response to group B streptococcal toxin in young lambs. J Appl Physiol 63, 2024–2030.

Sandberg, K., Sjoqvist, B.A., Hjalmarson, O., et al., 1987b. Lung function in newborn infants with tachypnea of unknown cause. Pediatr Res 22, 581–586.

Sandri, F., Plavka, R., Ancora, G., et al., 2010. Prophylactic or early selective surfactant combined with nCPAP in very preterm infants. Pediatrics 125, e1402–e1409.

Sarkar, S., Hussain, N., Herson, V., 2003. Fibrin glue for persistent pneumothroax in neonates. J Perinatol 23, 82–84.

Saugstad, O.D., 1996. Mechanisms of tissue injury by oxygen radicals: implications for neonatal disease. Acta Paediatr 85, 1–4.

Schaffer, A.J., Avery, M.E., 1977. Aspiration pneumonia. In: Schaffer, A.J., Avery, M.E. (Eds.), Disease of the Newborn, third ed. W B Saunders, Philadelphia, pp. 116–126.

Schatz, M., 1999. Asthma and pregnancy. Lancet 350, 1202–1204.

Schatz, M., Zeiger, R.S., Hoffman, C.P., et al., 1991. Increased transient tachypnea of the newborn in infants of asthmatic mothers. Am J Dis Child 145, 156–158.

Schiff, E., Friedman, S.A., Mercer, B.M., et al., 1993. Fetal lung maturity is not accelerated in pre-eclamptic pregnancies. Am J Obstet Gynecol 169, 1096–1101.

Schmidt, B., Roberts, R.S., Davis, P., et al., 2006. Caffeine therapy for apnea of prematurity. NEJM 354, 2112–2121.

Schmidt, B., Roberts, R.S., Davis, P., et al., 2007. Long term effects of caffeine therapy for apnea of prematurity. NEJM 357, 1893–1902.

Schreiber, M.D., Gin-Mestan, K., Marks, J.D., et al., 2003. Inhaled nitric oxide in premature infants with the respiratory distress syndrome. NEJM 349, 2099–2107.

Schrod, L., Hornemann, F., von Stockhausen, H.B., 1996. Chemiluminescence activity of phagocytes from tracheal aspirates of premature infants after surfactant therapy. Acta Paediatr 85, 719–723.

Schulze, A., Rich, W., Schellenberg, L., et al., 1998. Effects of different gain settings during assisted mechanical ventilation using respiratory unloading in rabbits. Pediatr Res 44, 132–138.

Schulze, A., Gerhardt, T., Musante, G., et al., 1999. Proportional assist ventilation in low birthweight infants with acute respiratory disease. A comparison to assist/control and conventional mechanical ventilation. Journal of Pediatrics 135, 339–344.

Schwendeman, C.A., Clark, R.H., Yoder, B.A., et al., 1992. Frequency of chronic lung disease in infants with severe respiratory failure treated with high frequency ventilation and/or extracorporeal membrane oxygenation. Crit Care Med 20, 372–377.

Segal, M.L., Goetzman, B.W., Schick, J.B., 1980. Thrombocytopenia and pulmonary hypertension in the perinatal aspiration syndrome. Journal of Pediatrics 96, 727–730.

Seger, N., Soll, R., 2009. Animal derived surfactant extract for treatment of respiratory distress syndrome. Cochrane Database Syst Rev (2), CD007836.

Seppänen, M.P., Kääpä, P.O., Kero, P.O., et al., 1994. Doppler derived systolicpulmonary artery pressure in acute neonatal respiratory distress syndrome. Pediatrics 93, 769–773.

Seri, I., 1995. Cardiovascular, renal and endocrine actions of dopamine in neonates and children. Journal of Pediatrics 126, 333–344.

Seri, I., Rudas, G., Bors, Z., et al., 1993. Effects of low dose dopamine infusion on cardiovascular and renal functions, cerebral blood flow and plasma catecholamine levels in sick preterm neonates. Pediatr Res 34, 742–749.

Setzer, E., Ermocilla, R., Tonkin, I., et al., 1980. Papillary muscle necrosis in a neonatal autopsy population. Incidence and associated clinical manifestations. Journal of Pediatrics 96, 289–294.

Shaffer, T.H., Koen, P.A., Moskowitz, G.D., et al., 1978. Positive end expiratory pressure: effects on lung mechanics of premature lambs. Biol Neonate 34, 1–10.

Shaffer, S.G., Bradt, S.K., Hall, R.T., 1986. Postnatal changes in total body water and extracellular volume in the preterm infant with respiratory distress syndrome. Journal of Pediatrics 109, 509–514.

Shah, D.M., Shenai, J.P., Vaughn, W.K., 1995. Neonatal outcome of mothers with pre-eclampsia. J Perinatol 15, 264–267.

Shankran, S., Farooki, Z.Q., Desai, R., 1982. Hemolytic streptococcal infection appearing as persistent fetal circulation. Am J Dis Child 136, 725–727.

Sharma, A., Milner, A.D., Greenough, A., 2007. Performance of neonatal ventilators in volume targeted ventilation mode. Acta Pediatrica 96, 176–180.

Shekerdemian, L.S., Ravn, H.B., Penny, D.J., 2002. Intravenous sildenafil lowers pulmonary vascular resistance in a model of neonatal pulmonary hypertension. Am J Respir Crit Care Med 165, 1098–1102.

Shepherd, A.J., Richardson, C.J., Brown, J.P., 1985. Nuchal cord as a cause of neonatal anemia. Am J Dis Child 139, 71–73.

Sherman, J.M., Lowitt, S., Stephenson, C., et al., 1986. Factors influencing aquired subglottic stenosis in infants. Journal of Pediatrics 109, 322–327.

Sherman, M.P., Evans, M.J., Campbell, L.A., 1988. Prevention of pulmonary alveolar macrophage proliferation in newborn rabbits by hyperoxia. Journal of Pediatrics 112, 782–786.

Shoemaker, M.T., Pierce, M.R., Yoder, B.A., et al., 2007. High flow nasal cannula versus nasal CPAP for neonatal respiratory disease: a retrospective study. J Perinatol 27, 85–91.

Shohat, M., Levy, G., Levy, I., et al., 1989. Transient tachypnoea of the newborn and asthma. Arch Dis Child 64, 277–279.

Short, B.L., Miller, M.K., Anderson, K.D., 1987. Extracorporeal membrane oxygenation in the management of respiratory failure in the newborn. Clin Perinatol 14, 737–748.

Shoults, D., Clark, T.A., Benumof, J.L., et al., 1979. Maximum inspiratory force in predicting successful neonatal tracheal extubation. Crit Care Med 7, 485–486.

Shribman, A.J., Smith, G., Achola, K.J., 1987. Cardiovascular and catecholamine responses to laryngoscopy with and without intubation. Br J Anaesth 59, 295–299.

Silva, Y.P.E., Gomez, R.S., Marcatto, J., et al., 2008. Early awakening and extubation with remifentanil in ventilated premature neonates. Pediatric Anesthesia 18, 176–183.

Simbruner, G., Coradello, H., Foder, M., et al., 1981. Effects of tracheal suction on oxygenation, circulation and lung mechanics in newborn infants. Arch Dis Child 54, 326–330.

Sims, M.E., Rangasamy, R., Lee, S., et al., 1989. Comparative evaluation of caffeine and theophylline for weaning premature infants from the ventilator. Am J Perinatol 6, 72–75.

Sinderby, C., Navalesi, P., Beck, J., et al., 1999. Neural control of mechanical ventilation in respiratory failure. Natural Medicine 5, 1433–1436.

Singh, J., Sinha, S.K., Alsop, E., et al., 2009. Long term follow up of very low birthweight infants from a neonatal volume versus pressure mechanical ventilation trial. Arch Dis Child Fetal Neonatal Ed 94, F360-F362.

Sinha, S.K., Levene, M.I., 1984. Pancuronium bromide induced joint contractions in the newborn. Arch Dis Child 59, 73–75.

Sinha, S.K., Donn, S.M., Gavey, J., 1997. Randomised trial of volume controlled versus time cycled, pressure limited ventilation in preterm infants with respiratory distress syndrome. Arch Dis Child 77, F202-F205.

Sinha, S.K., Lacaze-Masmonteil, T., Valls, I., et al., 2005. A multicenter randomised controlled trial of lucinactant versus poractant alfa among very premature infants at high risk for respiratoary distress syndrome. Pediatrics 115, 1030–1038.

Skelton, R., Jeffery, H.E., 1996. Factors affecting the neonatal response to artificial surfactant. J Paediatr Child Health 32, 236–241.

Skinner, J.R., Boys, R.J., Hunter, S., et al., 1992a. Pulmonary and systemic arterial pressure in hyaline membrane disease. Arch Dis Child 67, 366–373.

Skinner, J.R., Milligan, D.W.A., Hunter, S., et al., 1992b. Central venous pressure in the ventilated neonate. Arch Dis Child 67, 374–377.

Skinner, J.R., Hunter, S., Hey, E.N., 1996. Haemodynamic features at presentation in persistent pulmonary hypertension of the newborn and outcome. Arch Dis Child Fetal Neonatal Ed 74, F26–F32.

Skov, L., Ryding, J., Pryds, D., et al., 1992. Changes in cerebral oxygenation and cerebral blood volume during endotracheal suctioning in ventilated neonates. Acta Paediatr 81, 389–393.

Slutsky, A.S., Brown, R., Lehr, J., et al., 1981. High frequency ventilation: a promising new approach to mechanical ventilation. Med Instrum 15, 228–233.

Smith, C.V., Hansen, T.N., Martin, N.E., et al., 1993. Oxidant stress responses in premature infants during exposure to hyperoxia. Pediatr Res 34, 360–365.

Snashall, P.D., 1980. Pulmonary oedema. Br J Dis Chest 74, 2–22.

Snyder, J.M., Mendelson, C.R., 1987. Insulin inhibits the accumulation of the major lung surfactant apoprotein in human fetal lung explants maintained in vitro. Endocrinology 120, 1250–1257.

Soe, A., 2007. Weaning from nasal CPAP in premature infants. Inspire 5, 8–10.

Soll, R.F., 1996. Appropriate surfactant usage. Eur J Pediatr 155, S8–S13.

Soll, R.F., 2000a. Multiple versus single dose natural surfactant extract for severe neonatal respiratory distress syndrome. Cochrane Database Syst Rev (2), CD000141.

Soll, R.F., 2000b. Prophylactic synthetic surfactant for preventing mortality and morbidity in preterm infants. Cochrane Database Syst Rev (2), CD001079.

Soll, R.F., 2009a. Inhaled nitric oxide in the neonate. J Perinatol 29, S63–S67.

Soll, R.F., 2009b. Synthetic surfactant for respiratory distress syndrome in preterm infants. Cochrane Database Syst Rev (1), CD001149.

Soll, R.F., Blanco, F., 2009. Natural surfactant extract versus synthetic surfactant for neonatal respiratory distress syndrome. Cochrane Database Syst Rev (1), CD000144.

Soll, R.F., Morley, C.J., 2009. Prophylactic versus selective use of surfactant for preventing morbidity and mortality in preterm infants. Cochrane Database Syst Rev (2), CD000510.

Soll, R.F., Ozek, 2009. Multiple versus single doses of exogenous surfactant for the prevention or treatment of neonatal respiratory distress syndrome. Cochrane Database Syst Rev (1), CD000141.

Sosenko, I.R., 1993. Antenatal cocaine exposure produces accelerated surfactant maturation without stimulation of antioxidant enzyme development in the late gestation rat. Pediatr Res 33, 327–331.

Sosenko, I.R.S., Chen, Y., Price, L., et al., 1995. Failure of premature rabbits to increase lung antioxidant enzyme activities after hyperoxic exposure: antioxidant enzyme gene expression and pharmacologic intervention with endotoxin and dexamethasone. Pediatr Res 37, 469–475.

South, M., Morley, C.J., 1986a. Synchronous mechanical ventilation of the neonate. Arch Dis Child 61, 1190–1195.

South, M., Morley, C.J., 1986b. Spontaneous respiratory timing in intubated neonates with RDS (abstract). Early Hum Dev 14, 147–148.

Spencer, J.A.D., Robson, S.C., Farkas, A., 1993. Spontaneous recovery after severe metabolic acidaemia at birth. Early Hum Dev 32, 103–112.

Spitzer, A.R., Fox, W.W., 1982. Post-extubation atelectasis – the role of oral versus nasal endotracheal tubes. Journal of Pediatrics 100, 806–811.

Spitzer, A.R., Davis, J., Clarke, W.T., et al., 1988. Pulmonary hypertension and persistent fetal circulation in the newborn. Clin Perinatol 15, 389–413.

Stahlman, M., Blankenship, W.J., Shepard, F.M., et al., 1972. Circulatory studies in clinical hyaline membrane disease. Biol Neonate 20, 300–320.

Stahlman, M.T., Cheatham, W., Gray, M.E., 1979. The role of air dissection in bronchopulmonary dysplasia. Journal of Pediatrics 95, 878–885.

Steele, R.W., Metz, J.R., Bass, J.W., et al., 1971. Pneumothorax and pneumomediastinum in the newborn. Radiology 98, 629–632.

Steinschneider, A., Weinstein, S.L., Diamond, E., 1982. The sudden infant death syndrome and apnea/obstruction during neonatal sleep and feeding. Pediatrics 70, 858–863.

Stenmark, K.R., James, S.L., Voelkel, N.F., et al., 1983. Leukotriene C_4 and D_4 in neonates with hypoxia and pulmonary hypertension. NEJM 309, 77–80.

Stenson, B.J., Glover, R.M., Wilkie, R.A., et al., 1995. Life-threatening inadvertent positive end expiratory pressure. Am J Perinatol 12, 336–338.

Stevens, J.C., Eigen, H., Wysomierski, D., 1988. Absence of long term pulmonary sequelae after mild meconium aspiration syndrome. Pediatr Pulmonol 5, 74–81.

Stevens, T.P., Blennow, M., Myers, E.H., et al., 2007. Early surfactant administration with brief ventilation vs selective surfactant and continued mechanical ventilation for preterm infants with or at risk for respiratory distress syndrome. Cochrane Database Syst Rev (4), CD003063.

Stevenson, D.K., Kasting, D.S., Darnall, R.A., et al., 1979. Refractory hypoxemia associated with neonatal pulmonary disease. Journal of Pediatrics 95, 595–599.

Stevenson, D., Walther, F., Long, W., et al., 1992. Controlled trial of a single dose of synthetic surfactant at birth in premature infants weighing 500–699 grams. Journal of Pediatrics 120, S3–S12.

Strang, L.B. (Ed.), 1977. Neonatal Respiration. Blackwell Scientific, Oxford, p. 207.

Strauss, R.G., 1995. Red blood cell transfusion practices in the neonate. Clin Perinatol 22, 641–655.

Sun, B., Curstedt, T., Robertson, B., 1993. Surfactant inhibition in experimental meconium aspiration. Acta Paediatr 82, 182–189.

Sunoo, C., Kosasa, T.S., Hale, R.W., 1989. Meconium aspiration syndrome without evidence of fetal distress in early labour before elective caesarean delivery. Obstet Gynecol 73, 707–709.

SUPPORT Study Group of the Eunice Kennedy Shriver NICHD Neonatal Research Network, 2010. Early CPAP versus surfactant in extremely preterm infants. NEJM 362, 1970–1979.

Sutherland, P.D., Quinn, M., 1993. Nellcor Stat Cap differentiates oesophageal from tracheal intubation. Arch Dis Child Fetal Neonatal Ed 73, F184–F186.

Swaminathan, S., Quinn, J., Stabile, M.W., et al., 1989. Long term pulmonary sequelae of meconium aspiration syndrome. Journal of Pediatrics 114, 356–361.

Sweet, D., Bevilacqua, G., Carniellli, V., et al., 2007. European consensus guidelines on the management of neonatal respiratory distress syndrome. J Perinat Med 35, 175–186.

Swingle, H.M., Eggert, L.D., Bucciarelli, R.L., 1984. New approach to management of unilateral tension pulmonary interstitial emphysema in premature infants. Pediatrics 74, 354–357.

Sykes, G.S., Molloy, P.M., Johnson, P., et al., 1982. Do Apgar scores indicate asphyxia? Lancet i, 494–496.

Tarnow-Mordi, W., 1991. Is routine endotracheal suction justified? Arch Dis Child 66, 374–375.

Tarnow-Mordi, W.O., Wilkinson, A.R., 1985. Inspiratory: expiratory ratio and pulmonary interstitial emphysema. Arch Dis Child 60, 496–497.

Tarnow-Mordi, W.O., Shaw, J.C.L., Liu, D., et al., 1981. Iatrogenic hyponatraemia of the newborn due to maternal fluid overload – a prospective study. Br Med J 283, 639–642.

Tarnow-Mordi, W.O., Narang, A., Wilkinson, A.R., 1985. Lack of association of barotrauma and airleak in hyaline membrane disease. Arch Dis Child 60, 555–560.

Taylor, J., Dibbins, A., Sobel, D.B., 1993. Neonatal pneumomediastinum: indications for and complications of treatment. Crit Care Med 21, 296–298.

Telford, K., Walters, L., Vyas, H., et al., 2007. Respiratory outcome in late childhood after neonatal continuous negative pressure ventilation. Archives of Disease in Childhood Fetal Neonatal Edition 92, F19–F24.

te Pas, A.B., Walther, F.J., 2007. A randomized, controlled trial of delivery-room respiratory management in very preterm infants. Pediatrics 120, 322–329.

Termote, J.U.M., Schalij-Delfos, N.E., Wittebol-Post, D., et al., 1994. Surfactant replacement therapy: a new risk factor in developing retinopathy of prematurity? Eur J Pediatr 153, 113–116.

Thibeault, D.W., Hall, F.K., Sheehan, M.B., et al., 1984. Postasphyxial lung disease in newborn infants with severe perinatal acidosis. Am J Obstet Gynecol 150, 393–399.

Thome, U.H., Carlow, W.A., 2002. Permissive hypercapnia. Semin Neonatol 5, 409–419.

Thome, U., Toepfer, A., Schaller, P., et al., 1998. Effect of mean airway pressure on lung volume during high-frequency oscillatory ventilation of preterm infants.

Am J Respir Crit Care Med 157, 1213–1218.

Thome, U., Carroll, W., Wu, T.J., et al., 2006. Outcome of extremely preterm infants randomised at birth to different $PaCO_2$ targets during the first seven days of life. Biol Neonate 90, 18–225.

Thompson, P.J., Greenough, A., 1993. Steroid usage in pregnancies complicated by premature rupture of the membranes. J Perinat Med 21, 219–224.

Thompson, P.J., Greenough, A., Gamsu, H.R., et al., 1992. Ventilatory requirements for respiratory distress syndrome in small for gestational age infants. Eur J Pediatr 151, 528–531.

Timms, B.J.M., Di Fiore, J.M., Martin, R.J., et al., 1993. Increased respiratory drive as an inhibitor of oral feeding of preterm infants. Journal of Pediatrics 123, 127–131.

Ting, P., Brady, J.P., 1975. Tracheal suction in meconium aspiration. Am J Obstet Gynecol 122, 767–770.

Tita, A.T.N., Landon, M.B., Spong, C.Y., et al., 2009. Timing of elective repeat caesarean delivery at term and neonatal outcomes. NEJM 360, 111–120.

Toce, S.S., Keenan, W.J., 1988. Congenital echovirus 11 pneumonia with pulmonary hypertension. Pediatr Infect Dis 7, 360–361.

Tolsa, J.F., Cotting, J., Sekarski, N., et al., 1995. Magnesium sulphate as an alternative and safe treatment for severe persistent pulmonary hypertension of the newborn. Arch Dis Child Fetal Neonatal Ed 72, F184–F187.

Tomaszcwska, M., Stork, E.K., Friedman, H.G., et al., 1998. Pulmonary haemorrhage in VLBW (<1.5 kg) infants: correlates of death and neonatal and neurodevelopmental outcomes. Pediatr Res 43, 230A.

Torday, J., 1992. Cellular timing of fetal lung development. Semin Perinatol 16, 130–139.

Troche, B., Harvey-Wilkes, K., Engle, W.D., et al., 1995. Early minimal feedings promote growth in critically ill premature infants. Biol Neonate 67, 172–181.

Truffert, P., Paris-Liado, J., Escande, B., et al., 2007. Neuromotor outcome at two years of very preterm infants who were treated with high frequency oscillatory ventilatioin or conventional ventilation for neonatal respiratory distress syndrome. Pediatrics 119, e860–865.

Tudehope, D.I., Smyth, M.H., 1979. Is transient tachypnoea of the newborn always a benign condition? Aust Paediatr J 15, 160–165.

Turner, G.R., Levin, D.L., 1984. Prostaglandin synthesis inhibition in persistent pulmonary hypertension of the newborn. Clin Perinatol 11, 581–589.

Tütüncü, A.S., Faithfull, N.S., Lachmann, B., 1993. Comparison of ventilatory support with intratracheal perfluorocarbon administration and conventional mechanical ventilation in animals with acute respiratory failure. Am Rev Respir Dis 148, 785–792.

Tyler, D.C., Murphy, J., Cheney, F.W., 1978. Mechanical and chemical damage to lung tissue caused by meconium aspiration. Pediatrics 62, 454–459.

Ueda, T., Ikegami, M., Polk, D., 1995. Effects of fetal corticosteroid treatment on postnatal surfactant function in preterm lambs. J Appl Physiol 79, 846–851.

UK Collaborative ECMO Trial Group, 1996. UK collaborative randomised trial of neonatal extracorporeal membrane oxygenation. Lancet 348, 75–82.

UK Collaborative ECMO Trial Group, 1998. UK collaborative ECMO trial; follow up to 1 year of age. Pediatrics 101, E1.

Upton, C.J., Milner, A.D., Stokes, G.M., 1990. The effect of changes in inspiratory time on neonatal triggered ventilation. Eur J Pediatr 149, 668–670.

Usher, R.H., Allen, A.C., McLean, F.H., 1971. Risk of respiratory distress syndrome related to gestational age, route of delivery and maternal diabetes. Am J Obstet Gynecol 111, 826–832.

Usher, R.H., Saigal, S., O'Neill, A., et al., 1975. Estimation of RBC volume in premature infants with and without respiratory distress syndrome. Biol Neonate 26, 241–248.

Vain, N., Sozyld, E., Prudent, L., et al., 2002. Oro-and nasopharyngeal suction of meconium stained neonates before delivery of their shoulders does not prevent meconium aspiration syndrome: results of the international, multicenter, randomized controlled trial. Pediatr Res 51, 379A.

Valdes-Cruz, L.M., Dudell, G.G., Ferrara, A., 1981. Utility of M-mode echocardiography for early identification of infants with persistent pulmonary hypertension of the newborn. Pediatrics 68, 515–525.

Van Aerde, J., Campbell, A., Smyth, J., et al., 1984. Spontaneous chylothorax in newborns. Am J Dis Child 138, 961–964.

van Bel, F., de Winter, P.J., Wijnands, H.B., et al., 1992. Cerebral and aortic blood flow velocity patterns in preterm infants receiving prophylactic surfactant treatment. Acta Paediatr 81, 504–510.

van den Berg, E., Lemmers, P.M.A., Toet, M.C., et al., 2010. Effect of the Insure procedure on cerebral oxygenation and electrical brain activity of the preterm infant. Archives of Disease in Childhood Fetal Neonatal Edition 95, F53-F58.

van der Bleek, J., Plötz, F.B., van Overbeek, F.M., et al., 1993. Distribution of exogenous surfactant in rabbits with severe respiratory failure: the effect of volume. Pediatr Res 34, 154–158.

Van der Hoeven, M., Brouwer, E., Blanco, C.E., 1998. Nasal high frequency ventilation in infants with moderate respiratory insufficiency. Arch Dis Child Fetal Neonatal Ed 79, F61–F63.

Vanhaesebrouck, P., Vanneste, K., de Praeter, C., et al., 1987. Tight nuchal cord and neonatal hypovolaemic shock. Arch Dis Child 62, 1276–1277.

Vanhaesebrouck, P., Leroy, J.G., Depraeter, C., et al., 1989. Simple test to distinguish between surgical and non-surgical pneumoperitoneum in ventilated neonates. Arch Dis Child 64, 48–49.

van Marter, L.J., Leviton, A., Allred, E.N., et al., 1996. Persistent pulmonary hypertension of the newborn and smoking and aspirin and nonsteroidal antiinflammatory drug consumption during pregnancy. Pediatrics 97, 658–663.

Varnholt, V., Lasch, P., Suske, G., et al., 1992. High frequency oscillatory ventilation and extracorporeal membrane oxygenation in severe persistent pulmonary hypertension of the newborn. Eur J Pediatr 151, 769–774.

Vaughan, R.S., Menke, J.A., Giacoia, G.P., 1978. Pneumothorax: a complication of endotracheal tube suctioning. Journal of Pediatrics 92, 633–635.

Veness-Meeham, K.A., Richter, S., Davis, J.M., 1990. Pulmonary function testing prior to extubation in infants with respiratory distress syndrome. Pediatr Pulmonol 9, 2–6.

Vento, G., Tortorolo, L., Zecca, E., et al., 2004. Spontaneous minute ventilation is a predictor of extubation failure in extremely low birth weight infants. Journal of Maternal and Fetal Neonatal Medicine 15, 147–154.

Vento, M., Aguar, M., Escobar, J., et al., 2009. Antenatal steroids and antioxidant enzyme activity in preterm infants: influence of gender and timing. Antioxid Redox Signal 11, 2945–2955.

Verder, H., Robertson, B., Greisen, G., et al., 1994. Surfactant therapy and nasal continuous positive airway pressure for newborns with respiratory distress syndrome. NEJM 331, 1051–1055.

Verder, H., Albertsen, P., Ebbesen, F., et al., 1999. Nasal continuous positive airway pressure and early surfactant therapy for respiratory distress syndrome in newborns of less than 30 weeks gestation. Pediatrics 103, E24.

Vosatka, R.J., Kashjap, S., Trifiletti, R.R., 1994. Arginine deficiency accompanies persistent pulmonary hypertension of the newborn. Biol Neonate 66, 65–70.

Vulsma, T., Kok, J.H., 1996. Prematurity-associated neurologic and developmental abnormalities and neonatal thyroid function. NEJM 334, 857–858.

Vyas, H., Field, D., Hopkin, I.E., et al., 1986. Determinants of the first inspiratory volume and functional residual capacity at birth. Pediatr Pulmonol 2, 189–193.

Wagaman, M.J., Shutack, J.G., Moomjian, A.S., et al., 1979. Improved oxygenation and lung compliance with prone positioning of the neonates. Journal of Pediatrics 94, 789–791.

Waites, K.B., Grouse, D.T., Philips, J.B., et al., 1989. Ureaplasmal pneumonia and sepsis associated with persistent pulmonary hypertension of the newborn. Pediatrics 83, 79–85.

Walker, D.W., 1984. Peripheral and central chemoreceptors in the fetus and newborn. Annu Rev Physiol 46, 687–703.

Walker, G.M., Coutts, J.A., Skeoch, C., et al., 2003. Paediatrician's perception of the use of extracorporeal membrane oxygenation to treat meconium aspiration syndrome. Arch Dis Child Fetal Neonatal Ed 88, F70–F71.

Walsh-Sukys, M.C., 1993. Persistent pulmonary hypertension of the newborn. Clin Perinatol 20, 127–143.

Walters, D.V., Olver, R.E., 1978. The role of catecholamines in lung liquid absorption at birth. Pediatr Res 12, 239–242.

Walther, F.J., Siassi, B., Ramadan, N.A., et al., 1985. Cardiac output in newborn infants with transient myocardial dysfunction. Journal of Pediatrics 107, 781–785.

Walther, F.J., Benders, M.J., Leighton, J.O., 1992. Persistent pulmonary hypertension in premature neonates with severe respiratory distress syndrome. Pediatrics 90, 899–904.

Wapner, R.J., Sorokin, Y., Thom, E.A., et al., 2006. Single versus weekly courses of antenatal corticosteroids: evaluation of safety and efficacy. Am J Obstet Gynecol 195, 633–642.

Ward, R.M., 1984. Pharmacology of tolazoline. Clin Perinatol 11, 703–713.

Ward, R.M., 1994. Pharmacologic enhancement of fetal lung maturation. Clin Perinatol 21, 523–542.

Watters, T.A., Weydland, M.F., Parmley, W.W., et al., 1987. Factors influencing myocardial response to metabolic acidosis in isolated rat hearts. Am J Physiol 253, H1261–H1270.

Wauer, R.R., Schmalisch, G., Bohme, B., et al., 1992. Randomized double blind trial of ambroxol for the treatment of respiratory distress syndrome. Eur J Pediatr 151, 357–363.

Webb, R.D., Shaw, R.J., 2001. Respiratory distress in heavier versus lighter twins. Journal of Pediatric Medicine 29, 60–63.

Weisberger, S.A., Carlo, W.A., Chatburn, R.L., et al., 1986. Effect of varying inspiratory and expiratory times during high-frequency jet ventilation. Journal of Pediatrics 108, 596–600.

Welzing, L., Kribs, A., Huenseler, C., et al., 2009. Remifentanil for Insure in preterm infants: a pilot study for evalatuion of efficacy and safety aspects. Acta Pediatrica 98, 1416–1420.

Wen, T.S., Eirksen, N.L., Blanco, J.D., et al., 1993. Association of clinical intra-amniotic infection and meconium. Am J Perinatol 10, 438–440.

Whittle, M.J., Gilmore, D.H., McNay, M.B., et al., 1989. Diaphragmatic hernia presenting in utero as a unilateral hydrothorax. Perinatal Diagnosis 9, 115–118.

Whyte, S., Birrell, G., Wyllie, J., 2000. Premedication before intubation in UK neonatal units. Arch Dis Child Fetal Neonatal Ed 82, F38–F41.

Wigglesworth, J.S., 1984. Perinatal Pathology. W B Saunders, Philadelphia, pp. 106–107.

Wigton, T.R., Tamura, R.K., Wickstrom, E., et al., 1993. Neonatal morbidity after preterm delivery in the presence of documented lung maturity. Am J Obstet Gynecol 169, 951–955.

Wilcox, D.T., Glick, P.L., Karamanoukian, H.L., et al., 1994. Perfluorocarbon associated gas exchange (PAGE) and nitric oxide in the lamb congenital diaphragmatic hernia model. Pediatr Res 35, 260A.

Wilcox, D.T., Glick, P.L., Karamanoukian, H.L., et al., 1995. Perfluorocarbon-associated gas exchange improves pulmonary mechanics, oxygenation, ventilation, and allows nitric oxide delivery in the hypoplastic lung congenital diaphragmatic hernia lamb model. Crit Care Med 23, 1858–1863.

Will, D.H., McMurtry, I.F., Reeves, J.T., et al., 1978. Cold induced pulmonary hypertension in cattle. J Appl Physiol 45, 469–473.

Williams, O., Greenough, A., Mustafa, N., et al., 2003. Extubation failure due to phrenic nerve injury. Arch Dis Child Fetal Neonatal Ed 88, F72–F73.

Wilson, S.L., Thach, B.T., Brouilette, R.T., et al., 1981. Coordination of breathing and swallowing in human infants. J Appl Physiol 50, 851–858.

Wilson, G., Hughes, G., Rennie, J., et al., 1991. Evaluation of two endotracheal suction regimes in babies ventilated for respiratory distress syndrome. Early Hum Dev 25, 87–90.

Wilson, B.J., Becker, M.A., Linton, M.E., et al., 1998. Spontaneous minute ventilation predicts readiness for extubation in mechanically ventilated preterm infants. J Perinatol 18, 436–439.

Winn, H.N., Romero, R., Roberts, A., et al., 1992. Comparison of fetal lung maturation in preterm singleton and twin pregnancies. Am J Perinatol 9, 326–328.

Wiriyathan, S., Rosenfield, C.R., Arant, B.S., et al., 1986. Urinary arginine-vasopressin in the neonatal period. Pediatr Res 20, 103–108.

Wiswell, M.T., Rawlings, J.S., Smith, F.R., et al., 1985. Effects of frusemide on the clinical course of transient tachypnoea of the newborn. Pediatrics 75, 908–910.

Wiswell, T.E., Tuggle, J.M., Turner, B.S., 1990. Meconium aspiration syndrome: have we made a difference? Pediatrics 85, 715–721.

Wiswell, T.E., Graziani, L.J., Kornhauser, M.S., et al., 1996. High-frequency jet ventilation in the early management of respiratory distress syndrome is associated with a greater risk for adverse outcomes. Pediatrics 98, 1035–1043.

Wiswell, T.E., Gannon, C.M., Jacob, J., et al., 2000. Delivery room management of the apparently vigorous meconium stained neonate: results of the multicenter international collaborative trial. Pediatrics 105, 1–7.

Wiswell, T.E., Knight, G.R., Finer, N.N., et al., 2002. A multicenter, randomized controlled trial comparing surfaxin (lucinactant) lavage with standard care for treatment of meconium aspiration syndrome (MAS). Pediatrics 109, 1081–1087.

Wolf, E.J., Vintzileos, A.M., Rosenkrantz, T.S., et al., 1993. Do survival and morbidity of very low birthweight infants vary according to the primary pregnancy complication that results in preterm delivery? Am J Obstet Gynecol 169, 1233–1239.

Wolfson, M.R., Greenspan, J.S., Deoras, K.S., et al., 1992. Comparison of gas and liquid ventilation: clinical, physiological and histological correlates. J Appl Physiol 72, 1024–1031.

Wong, W., Tok, T.F., Ng, P.C., et al., 1997. Vascular air embolism: a rare complication of nasal CPAP. J Paediatr Child Health 33, 444–445.

Wood, C.M., Rushforth, J.A., Hartley, R., et al., 1998. Randomised double blind trial of morphine versus diamorphine for sedation of preterm infants. Arch Dis Child Fetal Neonatal Ed 79, F34–F39.

Wood, K.S., McCaffery, M.J., Donovan, J.C., et al., 1999. The effect of nitric oxide concentration on outcome in infants with persistent hypertension of the newborn. Biol Neonate 75, 215–224.

Wu, T.J., Teng, R.J., Yau, K.I.T., 1995. Persistent pulmonary hypertension of the newborn treated with magnesium sulphate in premature neonates. Pediatrics 96, 472–474.

Wu, J.M., Yeh, T.F., Wang, J.Y., et al., 1999. The role of pulmonary inflammation in the development of pulmonary hypertension in the newborn with meconium aspiration syndrome (MAS). Pediatric Pulmonology Supplement 18, 205–208.

Wyman, M.L., Kuhns, L.R., 1977. Lobar opacification of the lung after tracheal extubation in neonates. Journal of Pediatrics 91, 109–112.

Wynn, R.J., Schreiner, R.L., 1979. Spurious elevation of amniotic fluid bilirubin in acute hydramnios with fetal intestinal obstruction. Am J Obstet Gynecol 134, 105–106.

Wyszogrodski, J., Taeusch, H.W. Jr, Avery, M.E., 1974. Isoxuprine induced alterations of pulmonary pressure volume relationship in premature rabbits. Am J Obstet Gynecol 119, 1107–1111.

Wyszogrodski, J., Kyei-Aboagye, N., Taeusch, H.W. Jr, 1975. Surfactant inactivation by hyperventilation: conservation by end-expiratory pressure. J Appl Physiol 38, 461–466.

Yao, A.C., Lind, J., 1974. Placental transfusion. Am J Dis Child 127, 128–141.

Yeh, T.F., Srinivasan, G., Harris, V., et al., 1977. Hydrocortisone therapy in meconium aspiration syndrome: a controlled trial. Journal of Pediatrics 90, 140–143.

Yoder, B.A., Kirsch, E.A., Barth, W.H., et al., 2002. Changing obstetric practices associated with decreasing incidence of meconium aspiration syndrome. Obstet Gynecol 99, 731–739.

Yong, S.C., Chen, S.J., Boo, N.Y., 2005. Incidence of nasal trauma associated with nasal prong versus nasal mask during continuous positive airway pressure treatment in very low birthweight infants: a randomised

control study. Archives of Disease in Childhood Fetal Neonatal Edition 90, F480–F483.

Yost, C.C., Soll, R.F., 2000. Early versus delayed slective surfactant treatment for neonatal respiratory distress syndrome. Cochrane Database Syst Rev (2), CD001456.

Young, J.D., Dyar, O.J., 1996. Delivery and monitoring of inhaled nitric oxide. Intensive Care Med 22, 77–86.

Yu, V.Y.K., Orgill, A.A., Lim, S.B., et al., 1983. Bronchopulmonary dysplasia in very low birthweight infants. Aust Paediatr J 19, 233–236.

Yukitake, K., Brown, C.L., Schlueter, M.A., 1995. Surfactant apoprotein A modifies the inhibitory effect of plasma proteins on surfactant activity in vivo. Pediatr Res 37, 21–25.

Yuksel, B., Greenough, A., 1994. Birth weight and hospital readmission of infants born prematurely. Arch Pediatr Adolesc Med 148, 384–388.

Yuksel, B., Greenough, A., Gamsu, H.R., 1993a. Neonatal meconium aspiration syndrome and respiratory morbidity during infancy. Pediatr Pulmonol 16, 358–361.

Yuksel, B., Greenough, A., Gamsu, H.R., 1993b. Respiratory function at follow-up after neonatal surfactant replacement therapy. Respir Med 87, 217–221.

Zagariya, A., Bhat, R., Uhal, B., et al., 2000. Cell death and lung cell histology in meconium aspirated newborn rabbit lung. Eur J Pediatr 59, 819–826.

Zanardo, V., Padovani, E., Pittini, C., et al., 2007. The influence of timing of elective cesarian section on risk of neonatal pneumothorax. Journal of Pediatrics 150, 252–255.

Zenge, J.P., Rairigh, R.L., Grover, T.R., et al., 2001. NO and prostaglandins modulate the pulmonary vascular response to hemodynamic stress in the late gestation fetus. Am J Respir Cell Mol Biol 281, 1157–1163.

Zhou, H., Gao, Y., Raj, J.U., 1996. Antenatal betamethasone therapy augments nitric oxide mediated relaxation of preterm ovine pulmonary veins. J Appl Physiol 80, 390–396.

Zobel, G., Dacar, D., Rodl, S., et al., 1995. Inhaled nitric oxide versus inhaled prostacyclin and intravenous versus inhaled prostacyclin in acute respiratory failure in pulmonary hypertension in piglets. Pediatr Res 38, 198–204.

Part 3: **Chronic lung disease**

Anne Greenough   Anthony D Milner

Chronic lung disease (CLD) has been used as the diagnosis for all babies who are oxygen-dependent beyond 28 days of age with an abnormal chest X-ray (CXR) appearance. On the basis of the clinical course and/or CXR appearance some identify distinct forms of CLD, such as Wilson–Mikity syndrome. Nowadays, following the consensus at a US National Institutes of Health (NIH)-sponsored workshop, the term bronchopulmonary dysplasia (BPD) rather than CLD is used as the 'umbrella' term for all oxygen-dependent babies, as it better distinguishes the neonatal lung process from the CLDs seen in later life (Jobe and Bancalari 2001). As a consequence, the term BPD as defined in the NIH consensus (Jobe and Bancalari 2001) will be used throughout this chapter, except to describe the Wilson–Mikity syndrome.

Bronchopulmonary dysplasia

The four stages of BPD were originally based on a sequence of CXR changes (Northway et al. 1967). In the present population of babies, particularly those born at very early gestations, those stages do not occur consistently. Indeed, babies may develop BPD even though they had mild or absent initial respiratory distress (Rojas et al. 1995). At an NIH-sponsored workshop, it was recommended that babies be considered to have BPD if they had been oxygen-dependent for at least 28 days and then classified as suffering from mild, moderate or severe BPD according to their respiratory support requirement at a later date. It was recommended that babies born at less than 32 weeks of gestational age be assessed at 36 weeks' postmenstrual age (PMA) or at discharge home, whichever came first. They were diagnosed as having mild BPD if at that time they

were breathing air, moderate BPD if they required less than 30% supplementary oxygen, and severe BPD if they needed more than 30% oxygen and/or positive-pressure ventilation or nasal continuous positive airway pressure (CPAP). It was recommended that infants born at 32 weeks of gestation or greater be assessed at 56 days' postnatal age or discharge home, whichever came first, and at that time the severity of their BPD be graded, as for the more immature babies, according to their respiratory support requirement (Jobe and Bancalari 2001). The consensus BPD definition has been shown to identify a spectrum of risk for adverse pulmonary and neurodevelopmental outcomes in early infancy more accurately than other definitions (Ehrenkranz et al. 2005).

Incidence

The incidence of BPD in very-low-birthweight (VLBW) babies has been reported to vary from 15% to 50%. This is partially explained by differences in the proportions of very immature babies in the populations considered, as the incidence of BPD is inversely related to gestational age. In some centres, the number of BPD infants is increasing. A survey of a geographically defined population in the Trent Health Region demonstrated that the incidence of BPD had increased from 25% in 1987 to 42% in 1997 when defined as oxygen dependency at 28 days and from 11% to 29% over the same time period when defined as oxygen dependency at 36 weeks' PMA. It was noted that this increase was associated with a greater number of babies of less than 33 weeks' gestational age being admitted to the neonatal units (Manktelow et al. 2001). The increase in the number of cases of BPD has been suggested to be due to the

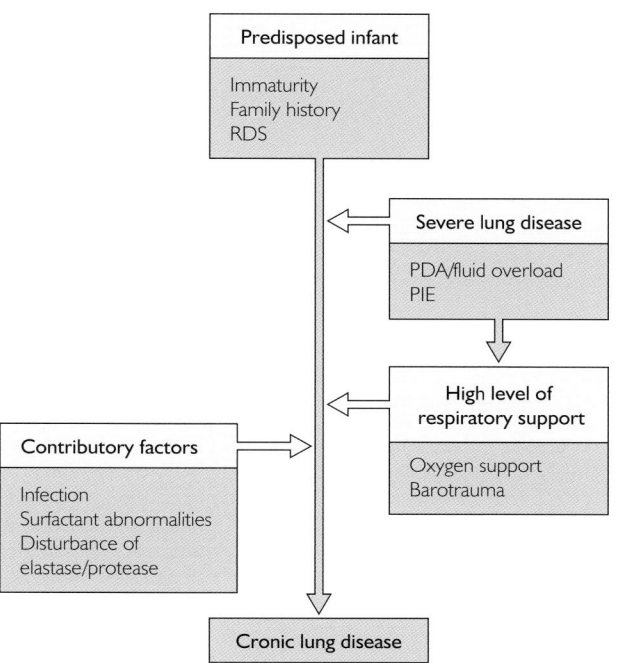

Fig. 27.43 Aetiological associations of bronchopulmonary dysplasia. PDA, patent ductus arteriosus; PIE, pulmonary interstitial emphysema; RDS, respiratory distress syndrome. *(Redrawn from Greenough et al.)*

improved survival of very immature babies. Another factor that influences the incidence of BPD is the criterion for the use of supplementary oxygen: the higher the oxygen saturation level to be maintained, the greater the number of infants who will require supplementary oxygen. A survey of members of the Vermont Oxford Network highlighted that pulse oximetry saturation thresholds varied from 84% to 96%, with only 41% of the respondents using the same criteria (90%) (Ellsbury et al. 2002). It is recommended that, at least at 36 weeks' PMA, a room air oxygen saturation test is undertaken to determine if the infant requires supplementary oxygen to maintain saturation level at 90% or above (Walsh et al. 2004).

Aetiology (Fig. 27.43)

BPD commonly occurs in prematurely born babies who have had respiratory distress syndrome (RDS), but also occurs in immature infants who had no initial lung disease (Rojas et al. 1995). Babies born at term may also develop BPD (Barnes et al. 1969; Rhodes et al. 1975), particularly if they suffer severe initial lung disease, as evidenced by a requirement for extracorporeal membrane oxygenation (Kornhauser et al. 1994).

Many factors increase the risk of BPD development, including those listed below.

Immaturity

There is an inverse relationship between the incidence of BPD and gestational age. Agents prolonging pregnancy, however, may not reduce BPD. Antenatal administration of indometacin significantly prolonged the gestation of women with threatened preterm labour between 24 and 34 weeks. There was, however, an increased BPD rate, particularly in babies delivering within 120 hours of their mothers starting treatment (Eronen et al. 1994). Administration of

indometacin may have delayed development of lamellar bodies and surfactant components (Eronen et al. 1994).

Oxygen toxicity

Northway et al. (1967) originally ascribed BPD to oxygen toxicity, as the chronic phase was invariably associated with high oxygen concentrations for more than 150 hours. Prolonged exposure to high oxygen concentrations has complex biochemical, microscopic and gross anatomical effects on lung tissues (Bonikos et al. 1976; Crapo et al. 1978; Escobedo and Gonzalez 1982). Oxygen toxicity is caused by the increased production of cytotoxic oxygen free radicals, which overwhelm the antioxidant defences. Prematurely born infants are particularly vulnerable; they have incomplete development of their pulmonary antioxidant enzyme systems and low levels of antioxidants such as vitamins C and E.

Baro- or volutrauma

BPD was first reported in babies who received oxygen concentrations of less than 60%, when used in association with CPAP (Tooley 1979) or mechanical ventilation (Ballard et al. 1992). Intermittent positive-pressure ventilation seemed particularly damaging if peak inflating pressures above 35 cmH$_2$O were used (Berg et al. 1975; Taghizadeh and Reynolds 1976). Baro- or volutrauma was further incriminated by the demonstration of an inverse relationship between hypocarbia and BPD development (Kraybill et al. 1989; Garland et al. 1995). Infants with Paco$_2$ levels <29 mmHg before surfactant therapy had an odds ratio of 5.6 for developing BPD as compared with babies who had a Paco$_2$ of at least 40 mmHg (Garland et al. 1995). Volutrauma may occur at resuscitation if rapid lung expansion is attempted. Prematurely born lambs given six manual inflations of 35–40 ml/kg, compared with those not 'bagged' at birth, had poorer lung function at 4 hours of age, as indicated by lower inspiratory capacities (Bjorklund et al. 1997). Use of high tidal volumes at resuscitation can also compromise the response to surfactant therapy in preterm lambs (Wada et al. 1997).

Patent ductus arteriosus and fluid balance

The association of patent ductus arteriosus (PDA) and an increased risk of BPD has frequently been reported. The effect is potentiated by infection, particularly if temporally related (Gonzalez et al. 1996). Prophylactic use of low-dose indometacin, initiated in the first 24 hours after birth, however, did not significantly reduce the incidence of BPD, even though it decreased the incidence of symptomatic PDA (Couser et al. 1996; Fowlie 1996). Fluid overload may explain the association of PDA and BPD, as it causes congestive heart failure and hence deterioration in lung function. Multivariate assessment of the traditional risk factors for BPD in babies with birthweight less than 1200 g also highlighted that oxygen dependency was associated with high fluid intake, as well as with PDA and high ventilator pressures at 96 hours (Palta et al. 1991). Amongst extremely-low-birthweight (ELBW) infants, daily fluid intakes were higher and there was weight loss delay in those who developed BPD or died (Oh et al. 2005).

Airleak

Pulmonary interstitial emphysema has been associated with a high incidence of BPD (Cochran et al. 1994). Respiratory function is compromised by air dissection into false air spaces, which creates a large dead space for ventilation; these spaces then increase in size with time and compress lung tissue.

Infection

Antenatal

It has been suggested that chorioamnionitis may predispose to BPD. In one series (Watterberg et al. 1996), 63% of babies with BPD but 21% of babies without BPD had exposure to chorioamnionitis. The chorioamnionitis group, however, were of significantly lower gestational age and the data were not adjusted for that difference. In a case–control study (van Marter et al. 2002), histological chorioamnionitis was only associated with an increased risk of BPD if the infant subsequently developed postnatal infection or required mechanical ventilation for longer than 7 days. An increased incidence of BPD associated with chorioamnionitis has been reported in only six of 18 subsequent studies (Been and Zimmerman 2009); gestational age adjustment was performed in only one of those studies. In the remaining studies, multivariate adjustment generally showed no difference in BPD risk (Been and Zimmerman 2009). It has been suggested that the inability of many later studies to demonstrate an increased risk of BPD following chorioamnionitis may be attributed to the increased use of antenatal steroids (Been and Zimmerman 2009). In a study of 120 prematurely born infants, 90% of whom had been exposed to antenatal steroids, no excess of BPD was demonstrated in infants exposed to chorioamnionitis, nor were there any differences in lung function at follow-up between those with or without chorioamnionitis exposure (Prendergast et al. 2010).

Postnatal

BPD is twice as common in babies who develop postnatal infection with cytomegalovirus than in non-infected babies (Sawyer et al. 1987). Review of 17 studies demonstrated that the relative risk for BPD development in babies colonised with *Ureaplasma urealyticum* was 1.72 (95% confidence interval 1.5–1.96) (Wang et al. 1995). The effect may be greatest in babies with a birthweight less than 1250 g (Wang et al. 1993) and in those who did not receive surfactant (Wang et al. 1995). Only those with persistent colonisation (which accounted for 45% of *U. urealyticum*-positive VLBW babies in one series), however, might be at increased risk of BPD (Castro-Alcaraz et al. 2002).

Surfactant abnormalities

BPD has been associated with persisting surfactant abnormalities (Obladen 1988). The lecithin:sphingomyelin ratio increased slowly in BPD babies (Hallman et al. 1987) and phosphatidylglycerol was noted to appear several months later in BPD babies who died rather than survived. Proliferative changes in BPD may reduce the number of type II cells, explaining the above findings. Abnormalities related to surfactant proteins, particularly SP-A, have also been associated with BPD (Strayer et al. 1986). Deficiency of SP-A mRNA expression persisted following RDS in a model of chronic lung injury (Coalson et al. 1995). SP-A is important in blocking the surfactant-inactivating effects of serum proteins during oedema formation (p. 460).

Chronic aspiration

The concentration of pepsin has been reported to be increased in the tracheal aspirates of ventilated preterm infants who developed BPD or died before 36 weeks PMA (Farhath et al. 2008). Those results (Farhath et al. 2008) suggest that chronic aspiration of gastric contents may contribute to the pathogenesis of BPD.

Predisposition to bronchopulmonary dysplasia

The role of a family history of asthma is controversial (Nickerson and Taussig 1980; Chan et al. 1988). Babies unable to secrete adequate amounts of cortisol in settings of increased stress injury may be at risk of continuing lung injury. Low cord and first-day serum cortisol and dehydroepiandosterone sulphate concentrations were associated with death or BPD (Nykanen et al. 2007). Similarly, at the end of the first week, babies who subsequently developed BPD had significantly lower cortisol secretion in response to adrenocorticotrophic hormone than babies who recovered without BPD (Watterberg and Scott 1995).

Genetic predisposition

Twin studies have shown that the BPD status of one twin, even after correcting for contributing factors, is a highly significant predictor of BPD in the second twin (Bhandari and Gruen 2006). Variations in candidate genes have been interrogated in a variety of sample sizes and positive associations tend to come from the smaller samples, only to be abolished in larger follow-up studies (Bhandari and Gruen 2006).

Clinical presentation

The majority of babies with BPD are born very prematurely and at 2–3 months of age remain dyspnoeic and require oxygen supplementation; some will still be ventilator-dependent. Others may have had minimal or no initial respiratory distress, but then deteriorate and become chronically oxygen-dependent; in one series (Streubel et al. 2008), 15% of ELBW infants followed this atypical pattern. A minority who have severe BPD are oedematous and have signs of right heart failure. In addition, they have chest wall retractions and other abnormalities related to a chronic increased work of breathing, such as a Harrison's sulcus. Those patients, despite increasing postnatal age, frequently fail to thrive and are at high risk of deterioration related to recurrent respiratory infections. Cor pulmonale develops in those who are chronically hypoxaemic. Copious endotracheal secretions, persistent atelectasis, lobar hyperinflation, aspiration and abnormalities of the trachea and/or bronchus are common. Bronchoscopy can reveal tracheomalacia and/or bronchomalacia. Large airway collapse can be seen on the CXR as thinning or tapering of the airways, or demonstrated by cine-computed tomography (cine-CT) (Manktelow et al. 2001). Tracheo- and bronchomalacia usually improve as the infant grows, but in severe cases surgery may be necessary. Increasing oxygen requirements, hypoxic and hypercapnic episodes in association with radiological changes of fixed lobar emphysema or recurrent atelectasis may be associated with tracheobronchial stenosis. In some affected patients, endoscopy and balloon dilation may be successful (Betremieux et al. 1995). Extubation may be complicated by inspiratory stridor secondary to tracheal scarring (Ch. 27.7).

Feeding difficulties and aspiration are common, owing to bulbar dysfunction or gastro-oesophageal reflux. They may suckle with weak pressures to maintain breathing during feeding (Mizuno et al. 2007). Parenteral nutrition may be needed, although excessive infusions of lipid solutions have been implicated in increasing the risk of BPD (Cooke 1991; Sosenko et al. 1993). Growth failure is common. Osteopenia occurs in infants with BPD and fractures can occur owing to severe metabolic bone disease in BPD babies (Fig. 27.44).

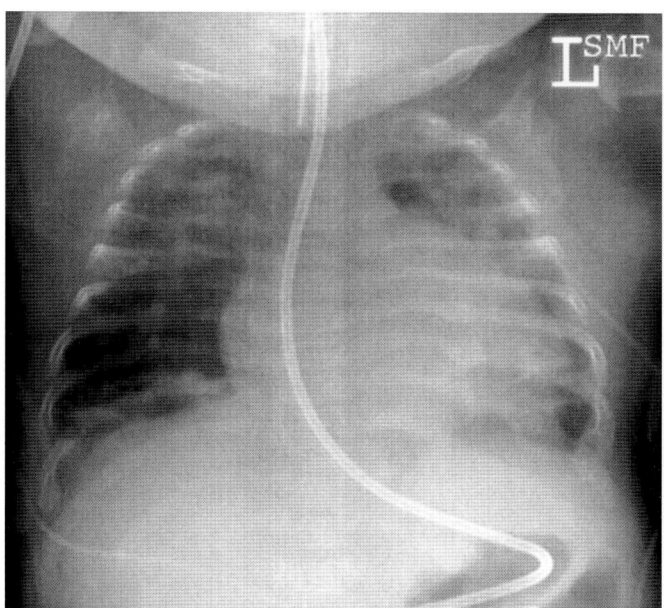

Fig. 27.44 Chest radiograph of baby with bronchopulmonary dysplasia and rib fractures due to metabolic bone disease.

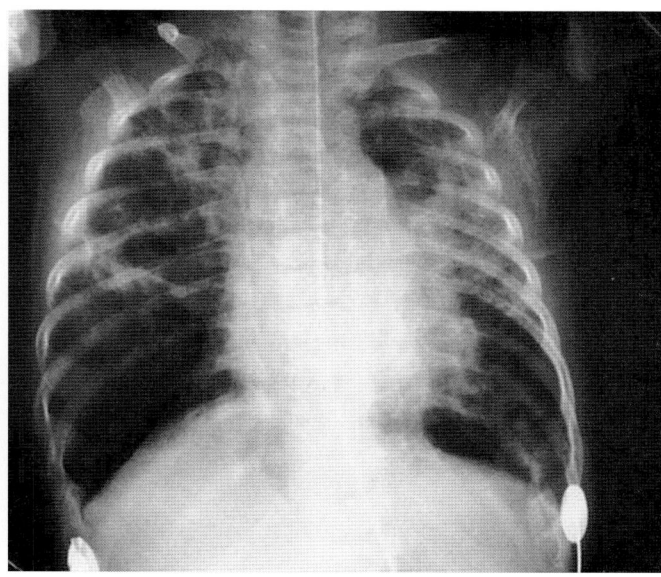

Fig. 27.46 Late stage 4 bronchopulmonary dysplasia with gross cystic overexpansion with compression of the mediastinum.

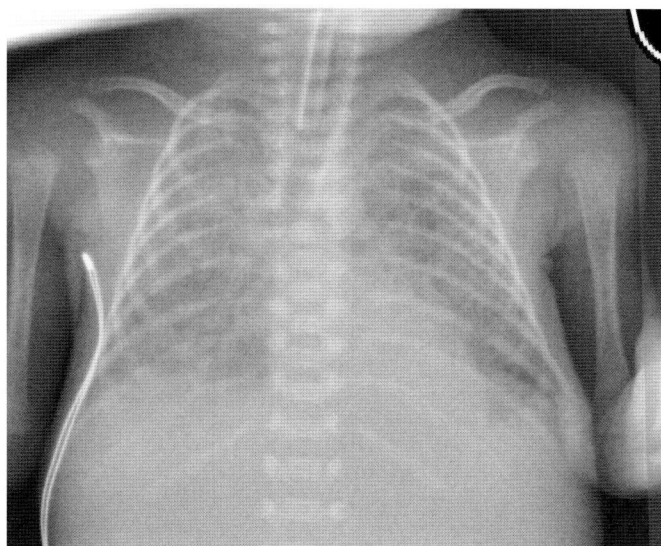

Fig. 27.45 Chest X-ray of an infant with bronchopulmonary dysplasia and a patent ductus arteriosus. Note the widespread lung changes.

Imaging

Northway et al. (1967) described four distinct radiographic appearances:

stage 1: radiographically indistinguishable from severe RDS (1–3 days)

stage 2: marked radiopacity of the lungs (4–10 days)

stage 3: clearing of the radiopacity into a cystic, bubbly pattern (10–20 days) (Fig. 27.45)

stage 4: hyperexpansion, streaks of abnormal density and areas of emphysema with variable cardiomegaly (from 1 month) (Fig. 27.46).

A variety of scoring systems to quantify the CXR appearance abnormalities have been developed. One system scored the volume of the lungs, the degree of hyperinflation and the presence and severity of interstitial changes and cysts (Yüksel et al. 1991a). Using that scoring system, it was possible to predict from the appearance of the CXR at 1 month the most severe lung function abnormalities at 6 months of age (Yüksel et al. 1991a). It was noted that the babies with the highest CXR scores and lung function abnormalities were those who had cystic elements and/or interstitial changes. As a consequence, a simplified CXR score was subsequently developed, in which only the lung volume and the presence of interstitial shadows and cysts were scored (Greenough et al. 1999). The CXR appearance so assessed differed significantly between babies who were and were not oxygen-dependent at 36 weeks' PMA (Greenough et al. 2000) and those who were and were not symptomatic in the first 6 months (Thomas et al. 2003a).

In older babies with BPD, CT scans, rather than CXR, give more detailed information. Common findings on CT scan of such patients are multifocal areas of hyperaeration, linear and triangular subpleural opacities, but not bronchiectasis (Oppenheim et al. 1994). At a median age of 19 years (Wong et al. 2008), 85% of survivors of BPD had emphysema on CT examination. High-resolution CT examination may also be helpful in predicting outcome in infancy; using a scoring system for hyperexpansion, emphysema and fibrosis/ interstitial abnormalities in BPD infants at approximately term those discharged home on oxygen had significantly higher scores (Ochiai et al. 2008).

Pathology

In babies who develop 'traditional' BPD, there is progression from the initial exudative stage of diffuse alveolar damage in RDS to a regenerative and fibroproliferative reparative stage. This can be divided into three phases: an early reparative stage, a subacute proliferative stage and a chronic fibroproliferative stage (Askin 1991). In early BPD, the lungs have a grossly abnormal appearance, being firm, heavy and darker than normal; the surface is irregular, with emphysematous areas alternating with areas of collapse.

Histological examination demonstrates areas of emphysema, which may coalesce into larger cystic areas, surrounded by areas of atelectasis. Florid obliterative bronchiolitis occurs, particularly if high peak inflating pressures have been used (Taghizadeh and Reynolds 1976), and results in occlusion of the airway lumen and distal pulmonary collapse. In older babies, airway injury is marked by smooth-muscle hypertrophy, squamous metaplasia of the respiratory epithelium and glandular hyperplasia (Margraf et al. 1991) and fibrosis alternating with areas of emphysema. Hypertrophy of the pulmonary arterial smooth muscle in the media and adventitial fibrous tissue is increased (Hislop and Haworth 1990). Later, normal conducting bronchi may be found, with marked uniform expansion of distal air spaces with little or no interstitial fibrosis. In long-standing, healed BPD, seen in babies aged between 2 and 40 months, there is alveolar septal fibrosis, cardiomegaly and evidence of pulmonary hypertensive vascular disease (Stocker 1986).

The pathology of BPD is now very heterogeneous, influenced by the age at death and severity of the initial illness, and can include a combination of airway, interstitial and blood vessel abnormalities (van Lierde et al. 1991). Babies with a predominantly bronchiolar pattern rather than interstitial damage usually have had more severe acute lung disease, required a greater degree of ventilatory support and died at a younger age (van Lierde et al. 1991). There are few reports describing the pathology of 'new' BPD: they highlight less interstitial fibrosis but an arrest in acinar development resulting in fewer, larger and simplified alveolar structures, a dysmorphic capillary configuration and variable interstitial cellularity and/or fibroproliferation (Husain et al. 1998; Coalson 2006). As a consequence, it has been proposed that the 'new' BPD is not primarily the injury/repair paradigm of traditional BPD, but rather a maldevelopment sequence resulting from interference/interruption of normal developmental signalling for terminal maturation and alveolarisation of the lungs of very preterm infants (Jobe and Ikegami 1998).

Pathophysiology

Alveolar hypoplasia and dysmorphic changes in the lung vasculature are consistent findings in BPD (Thébaud 2007). Various animal models of impaired alveolar development also display abnormal lung vascular development (Thébaud 2007). Vascular endothelial growth factor (VEGF) is required not only for the formation but also the maintenance of the pulmonary vasculature and alveolar structures throughout adulthood (Thébaud 2007). In lung tissue from infants who died from BPD, the typical patterns of alveolar simplification with dysmorphic microvasculature are associated with reduced lung VEGF and VEGFR-1 mRNA and protein exposure (Lassos et al. 2001). Babies with RDS, compared with healthy subjects, have an excess of neutrophils and alveolar macrophages in their lung effluent.

Baro/volutrauma and oxygen toxicity induce an inflammatory reaction, which persists in babies who develop BPD; 95% of 11–15-day-old babies with BPD have neutrophils in their aspirates. The activated neutrophils mediate endothelial cytotoxicity and inhibit phosphatidylcholine synthesis (Zimmerman 1995). During the acute phase of lung injury, a host response is initiated (Odezmir et al. 1997). Proinflammatory cytokines (interleukin (IL)-1β, IL-6) (Kotecha et al. 1996) and soluble intercellular adhesion molecule 1 (ICAM-1) are demonstrated in the lung lavage from day 1, reaching a peak in the second week. IL-1β activity also increases during the first week, inducing the release of inflammatory mediators, activating inflammatory cells and upregulating adhesion molecules on endothelial cells. There is release of chemokines, including the α-chemokine IL-8, which induces neutrophil chemotaxis, and the

β-chemokine macrophage inflammatory protein (MIP)-1-α, which is chemotactic for monocytes and macrophages. High concentrations of MIP-1-α have been associated with the later development of fibrosis (Murch et al. 1996b). The anti-inflammatory cytokine IL-10 partly regulates the production of tumour necrosis factor-α, IL-6 and IL-8. Sequential bronchoalveolar lavage (BAL) samples over the first 96 hours demonstrated that IL-10 mRNA was absent, possibly predisposing to chronic lung inflammation (Jones et al. 1996).

Inflammatory mediators can induce an isoform of haemoxygenase (HO), an enzyme that catalyses the rate-limited oxidative cleavage of haemoglobin. Carbon monoxide (CO) is produced endogenously as a byproduct of that reaction. Oxidative stress also significantly increases HO-1 expression in several pulmonary cell types, including macrophages, epithelial, endothelial and fibroblast cells. End-tidal CO levels were higher on days 7, 14, 21 and 28 in infants developing BPD and an end-tidal CO level >2.15 ppm on day 14 had 80% sensitivity and 92% specificity in predicting oxygen dependency at 36 weeks' PMA (May et al. 2007).

Mediator release from the neutrophils may increase airway hyperreactivity, as the BAL fluid contains elevated levels of lipid mediators, including leukotrienes (Mirro et al. 1990; Groneck et al. 1993), which cause bronchoconstriction, vasoconstriction, oedema, neutrophil chemotaxis and mucus production in the lung. Leukotriene B_4 (LTB$_4$), the anaphylatoxin C5a and IL-8 have been detected in the BAL fluid of BPD infants (Groneck et al. 1994).

There are increased concentrations of the soluble form of ICAM-1, a glycoprotein that allows cell-to-cell contact, in the tracheal aspirates of babies with early BPD (Kojima et al. 1993). Levels of soluble E-selectin, another cell adhesion molecule, are also increased in the perinatal period in babies developing BPD (Ramsay et al. 1998). Direct contact between activated cells leads to further production of proinflammatory cytokines and other mediators. The inflammatory infiltrate is associated with striking loss of endothelial, basement membrane and interstitial sulphated glycoaminoglycans (Murch et al. 1996a). Glycoaminoglycans are important in restricting albumin and ion flux, inhibiting fibrosis in fetal animals and controlling cellular proliferation and differentiation.

Differential diagnosis of bronchopulmonary dysplasia

Viral pneumonia, aspiration problems and lung infections due to immune deficiency can usually be differentiated from BPD on the history. The changes in the CXR appearance due to either total anomalous pulmonary venous return or pulmonary lymphangiectasia are present from birth.

Management

General

The aim is to keep the baby free from infection, while gradually weaning the baby off the ventilator and into progressively lower concentrations of oxygen. It is important to ensure that older babies have a comprehensive care plan, which includes attention to appropriate auditory, tactile and visual experiences and the opportunity to suckle. The provision of sleep–wake rhythms is also important. Parental support is essential through these prolonged admissions. Home oxygen therapy allows early discharge, except in those babies who require intermittent positive-pressure support or are failing to gain weight. Babies who remain chronically ventilator-dependent should be transferred to a ward more suited to dealing with older infants.

Ventilator management

The peak inspiratory pressures and inspired oxygen concentrations should be kept at the minimum compatible with achieving a Pao_2 of 6.7–9.3 kPa (50–70 mmHg) and oxygen saturations of at least 92% (Ch. 19). In infants with evidence of pulmonary hypertension, the oxygen saturation level should be maintained at least at 95%. Ventilator rates over 60 breaths/min using a conventional ventilator offer no advantage to babies developing BPD (Chan et al. 1991). After the first week, increasing the positive end-expiratory pressure level to 6 cmH₂O can improve oxygenation without adversely affecting CO_2 elimination (Greenough et al. 1992a), but this strategy may not be successful in babies with severe cystic BPD. CO_2 levels can be allowed to rise, provided that there is no evidence of a respiratory acidosis (that is, a pH less than 7.25). Sedation should be kept to the minimum, as the aim is to promote the infant's respiratory efforts so that the baby can become independent of the ventilator. Certain babies, despite appropriate respiratory support, suddenly become grey, pale, sweaty and cyanosed, frequently associated with poor chest wall expansion (BPD spells). Affected babies are difficult to ventilate by bag and mask and may take many minutes to resuscitate. These episodes seem to occur in agitated babies. Simultaneous measurements of tidal flow, airway and oesophageal pressure and oxygen saturation demonstrated that the hypoxaemic episodes were preceded by an active exhalation and a decrease in end-expiratory lung volume, which could lead to small-airway closure and the development of intrapulmonary shunts (Bolivar et al. 1995). Sedation can help to reduce the number of episodes, but if they are very frequent and troublesome it may be necessary to paralyse affected babies. High-volume strategy, high-frequency oscillation (HFO) can improve oxygenation in babies who deteriorate acutely, but may cause overexpansion in those who have cystic BPD.

Babies with BPD may require prolonged ventilation. Chronic use of either an oral or nasal endotracheal tube can result in cosmetic defects (Ch. 44). Tracheostomy avoids those problems and eases nursing of an increasingly active infant. Tracheostomies, however, may be difficult to close in this population (Ch. 27.7); thus, their use should be restricted to babies who remain fully ventilated after 3 months of age.

Weaning

Frequent attempts should be made to wean the baby from the ventilator. During weaning, a rise in $Paco_2$ should be ignored, unless the pH falls below 7.25. Methylxanthines may be useful to hasten weaning. Corticosteroids facilitate extubation (Halliday and Ehrenkranz 2003), but their short-term beneficial effects have to be weighed against possible long-term adverse effects. Extubation initially should be attempted after a short period for up to an hour on endotracheal CPAP, to ensure that the infant has adequate respiratory drive (p. 529). Nasal CPAP may be poorly tolerated in relatively mature babies (Chan and Greenough 1993), but is useful for those who have acquired tracheobronchomalacia (Panitch et al. 1994). If nasal CPAP is required for prolonged periods, it is important that an appropriate method of fixation is used (Ch. 44). Reintubation and ventilation should be avoided, unless the baby suffers frequent troublesome or a major apnoea, severe metabolic acidosis indicating respiratory fatigue or a marked deterioration in blood gases. Physiotherapy and increasing the inspired oxygen concentration should be the first-line treatment for worsening blood gases, which will usually be due to atelectasis associated with secretions.

Oxygen therapy and monitoring

Administration of supplementary oxygen via nasal cannulae has advantages regarding ease of nursing care, but the exact oxygen concentration is difficult to monitor and, as a consequence, this mode of delivery should not be used in babies at risk of retinopathy.

Transcutaneous oxygen monitoring significantly underestimates arterial Po_2 in babies with BPD. Oxygen saturation monitoring is preferred, as, over a wide range of Pao_2, $Paco_2$, pH, heart rate, blood pressure, haematocrit and fetal haemoglobin levels, a close correlation between pulse oximeter values and arterial Sao_2 at saturations greater than 78% has been demonstrated (Ramanathan et al. 1987). Chronic intermittent hypoxia may result in increased pulmonary vascular resistance, pulmonary hypertension and right heart failure and, in non-randomised studies, administering supplementary oxygen to keep the oxygen saturation at >92% was associated with a better growth rate and a reduction in hospital admissions. Aiming for higher saturations in the majority of babies with BPD, however, has apparent disadvantages. In a trial examining the efficacy and safety of supplemental therapeutic oxygen for babies with pre-threshold retinopathy of prematurity, those maintained at saturations of 96–99% rather than 89–94%, had an increased risk of adverse pulmonary events, including pneumonia and/or exacerbations of BPD (STOP-ROP Multicenter Study Group 2000); the trial, however, was not designed to assess pulmonary outcomes. In a subsequent multicentre double-blind randomised trial, 358 infants were allocated to oxygen saturations of 91–94% or 95–98% (Askie et al. 2003); no significant differences were found in weight, length, head circumference or major developmental abnormalities at 12 months of corrected age. The high saturation group, not surprisingly, required supplementary oxygen for a longer period after randomisation and had a higher rate of dependence on supplementary oxygen at 36 weeks' PMA and a significantly higher frequency of home-based oxygen therapy (Askie et al. 2003). There is an ongoing study assessing the outcome of infants randomised to 85–90% and 91–95% oxygen saturations (BOOST II). Our policy is for babies with BPD who are more than 1 month old to have an echocardiograph to determine whether they have pulmonary hypertension. If detected, then their oxygen saturations are maintained at least at 95%; if pulmonary hypertension is not present, then the oxygen saturation is maintained at least at 90%.

Cardiovascular status

BPD babies can develop pulmonary hypertension, thus a routine echocardiographic examination is recommended. Pulmonary hypertension can be indicated clinically by a single heart sound and the murmur of tricuspid regurgitation, but an easily palpable liver may simply reflect hyperexpanded lungs. Although cardiac catheterisation of babies with BPD is not routinely indicated, it can be used to assess the responsiveness of the pulmonary vascular bed to changes in the oxygen tension (Abman et al. 1985). If the pulmonary artery pressure falls with a rise in oxygenation, continuous oxygen therapy by nasal cannula should be used. Pulmonary hypertension may also be detected non-invasively by echocardiography.

Systemic hypertension is common in BPD babies and can appear after discharge. Hypertension may result from renal damage following prolonged umbilical artery catheter usage or nephrocalcinosis due to chronic diuretic therapy. In addition, certain medications, including corticosteroids (Greenough et al. 1992b), elevate the blood pressure. Although the hypertension is frequently transient and responds to antihypertensive medication (Emery and Greenough 1992), it can result in left ventricular hypertrophy.

Infection

Chest infections occur frequently in babies with BPD (Yüksel and Greenough 1992a) and should be treated with physiotherapy, antibiotics or antiviral therapy, as appropriate. The respiratory tract of a baby with BPD is frequently colonised with potentially pathogenic bacteria and it is important to differentiate this from true infection. If there is a deterioration in respiratory status or radiological appearance (Fig. 27.47), endotracheal or nasopharyngeal secretions should be cultured. In addition, nasopharyngeal secretions should be sent to determine if the infant has a viral infection. If a respiratory syncytial virus (RSV) infection is identified and other causes of a respiratory deterioration have been excluded (for example a PDA; Fig. 27.48) treatment with ribavirin should be considered (Giffin et al. 1995).

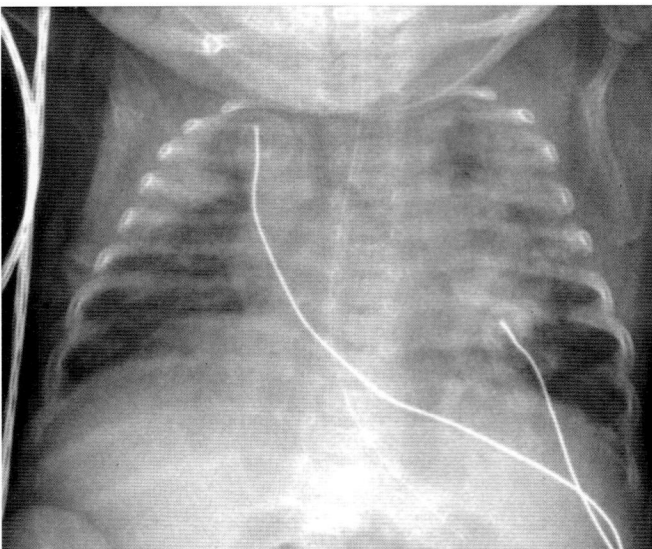

Fig. 27.47 Deterioration due to *Staphylococcus epidermidis* infection; note the left upper lobe consolidation. The baby has metabolic bone disease.

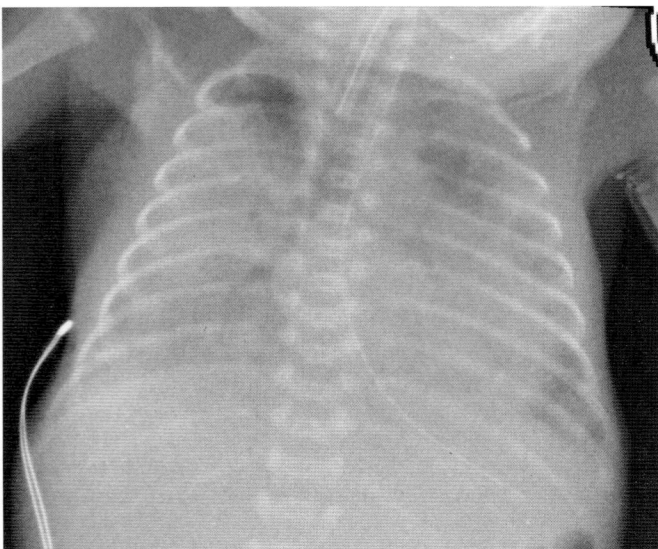

Fig. 27.48 Chest X-ray of an infant with bronchopulmonary dysplasia and a patent ductus arteriosus. Note the widespread lung changes.

Routine immunisations, but a killed polio vaccine, should be given once BPD babies reach 2 months of age, even though they remain on the neonatal intensive care unit. Immunisation against influenza should also be considered, especially for babies receiving home oxygen therapy. Immunoprophylaxis with palivizumab against RSV should be given for babies discharged home on supplementary oxygen.

Haematology

Babies who require an inspired oxygen concentration of greater than 30% should have regular packed cell volume (PCV) estimations and a transfusion (15 ml/kg) given if their PCV falls below 40%. Once respiratory support is no longer required, it is sufficient to check the haemoglobin level on a weekly basis and to transfuse only those babies who have symptomatic anaemia with a poor reticulocyte response (Ch. 30).

Fluid and electrolytes

Excessive fluid intake should be avoided. Babies with severe BPD usually will not tolerate more than 150 ml/kg/24 h. If their weight gain is greater than 20 g/kg/24 h on such a regimen, this may indicate heart failure and regular diuretics should be considered. If chronic diuretic therapy is given, acid–base balance, chloride and calcium levels must be carefully monitored and appropriate supplements administered if these become abnormal. Regular renal ultrasounds should be performed to check for the development of nephrocalcinosis.

Nutrition

Babies with BPD require a calorie intake approximately 20–40% greater than age-matched infants without respiratory embarrassment. Energy requirements, however, above 150 kcal/kg are rare and usually associated with malabsorption (Reimers et al. 1992). For further general advice on nutrition, see Chapter 16.

Feeding problems depend on the severity of BPD; infants with BPD have poor feeding coordination, feeding endurance and performance (Mizuno et al. 2007). Babies with BPD can suffer from aspiration and gastro-oesophageal reflux. This can be difficult to manage. The osmolality should be checked if thickeners are used with a concentrated feed. Other feeding problems are common and include tiring on feeding and vomiting. Oral hypersensitivity can occur and results from repeated negative stimuli to the oral area and lack of development of appropriate feeding behaviour.

Drug therapy

Diuretics

Administration of furosemide can acutely increase lung compliance and reduce airway resistance (Kao et al. 1983; Najak et al. 1983), facilitating a reduction in ventilator requirements (McCann et al. 1985) and transient improvements in blood gases in both ventilated and non-ventilated babies (Kao et al. 1984a, 1994). Systematic review of studies, however, demonstrated that, in preterm babies less than 3 weeks of age with BPD, furosemide administration had either inconsistent or no detectable effects (Brion et al. 2006). In babies older than 3 weeks, a single dose of 1 mg/kg of furosemide improved lung compliance and airway resistance for 1 hour. Chronic administration of furosemide also improved both oxygenation and lung compliance, but the positive effects were limited to the duration of the treatment. Prolonged therapy with hydrochlorothiazide and spironolactone had been suggested to be useful in hypertensive BPD babies (Abman et al. 1984) and to improve the outcome of babies with severe BPD (Albersheim et al. 1989). Unfortunately, those results were not confirmed in randomised trials (Brion et al. 2008), lung mechanics were improved and the need for furosemide was reduced, but no long-term benefits were demonstrated in infants receiving current therapy.

Diuretics have many side-effects. Furosemide increases the urinary excretion of sodium, chloride and potassium and consequently may cause hypochloraemia, hyponatraemia and hypokalaemia, in addition to hypocalcaemia (McCann et al. 1985). It may also cause a metabolic alkalosis (De Rubertis et al. 1970), and compensatory hypoventilation and hypercarbia have been described (Hazinski 1985). Other side-effects include secondary hyperparathyroidism, rickets and ototoxicity (Rybak 1982). In adults, the ototoxicity of furosemide is related to its plasma concentration and there is a synergistic effect with aminoglycosides. Chronic diuretic therapy may cause hypercalciuria, renal calcification and nephrolithiasis (Hufnagle et al. 1982). Nephrocalcinosis is commonest in the most immature babies and those receiving the longest course of therapy or given furosemide by the intravenous route (Short and Cooke 1991). Other risk factors for nephrocalcinosis include a family history, fluid restriction, total parenteral nutrition or methylxanthine administration, and renal candidiasis. Nephrocalcinosis is associated with urinary tract infection and haematuria and, at follow-up, chronic glomerular and tubular dysfunction.

Aerosolised furosemide has been given to babies with or developing BPD (Kugelman et al. 1997), the rationale being that lung mechanics in patients with lung oedema might be improved by diuresis-independent lung fluid reabsorption and/or there may be alleviation of reactive airway disease, as occurs in adults and children. Systematic review of results of studies in which a single dose of aerosolised furosemide was given demonstrated significant improvement in tidal volume after 1 and 2 hours, but no improvement in compliance or resistance at either time point (Brion et al. 2006). A dose of 1 mg/kg appears more effective than lower doses (Rastogi et al. 1994). The review concluded that in infants both less than and older than 3 weeks of age there is insufficient information to determine whether a single dose of aerosolised furosemide improves outcome or lung function.

Methylxanthines

Intravenous aminophylline therapy can improve lung function and hasten weaning from the ventilator in babies with BPD, but only in those less than 30 days old (Rooklin et al. 1979). The lack of response in the older age group might be explained by extensive pulmonary fibrosis resulting in irreversible airways obstruction. Oral theophylline can improve lung function in BPD babies; the addition of a diuretic is synergistic (Kao et al. 1987).

Bronchodilator therapy

Inhaled bronchodilator can reduce airways resistance in babies with BPD at term (Kao et al. 1984b; Motoyama et al. 1987; Wilkie and Bryan 1987) and improve pulmonary resistance, dynamic compliance, tidal volume and transcutaneous blood gases when administered to ventilated babies with BPD at approximately 1 month of age (Cabal et al. 1987). Salbutamol administration results in a dose-related improvement in lung mechanics in ventilator-dependent babies; the beneficial effects of 200 µg salbutamol last 3 hours (Denjean et al. 1992). Inhaled ipratropium bromide gives similar short-term improvements (Wilkie and Bryan 1987). Synergism occurs between ipratropium bromide and salbutamol in improving respiratory mechanics in ventilated babies for up to 1–2 hours after administration (Brundage et al. 1990). No synergy,

however, was shown between metaproterenol and atropine, and with both treatments lung function returned to baseline values within 3 hours (Kao et al. 1989). There are no randomised trials with long-term outcomes in which treatment with bronchodilator had been initiated before discharge from the neonatal unit (Ng et al. 2001).

After discharge, inhaled bronchodilators administered via a spacer device can improve lung function and reduce symptoms in wheezy VLBW survivors (Yüksel et al. 1990; Yüksel and Greenough 1991). Nebulised bronchodilator, however, may cause a deterioration in lung function, as evidenced by an increase in airways resistance (Yüksel et al. 1991b); this can be avoided by administering the bronchodilator by inhaler and spacer device (Yüksel and Greenough 1991). Although individual BPD babies may benefit from bronchodilator administration, routine treatment is not warranted in stable patients. In such patients with a corrected age of 1 year, neither salbutamol nor ipatropium bromide resulted in a significant reduction in pulmonary resistance (De Boeck et al. 1998).

Disodium cromoglycate

Disodium cromoglycate both has an anti-inflammatory effect and reduces non-specific bronchial hyperreactivity. At follow-up, disodium cromoglycate can reduce symptoms and bronchodilator usage in VLBW infants (Yüksel and Greenough 1992b).

Corticosteroids

Steroids have a number of beneficial actions, including stabilising membranes and reducing pulmonary oedema, enhancing surfactant synthesis, suppressing collagen synthesis and reducing bronchospasm and inflammation in small airways and leukotriene production. Dexamethasone given to ventilated babies reduces the pulmonary inflammatory response, microvascular permeability and release of inflammatory mediators and neutrophil influx into the airways (Groneck et al. 1993). If corticosteroids are started after 3 weeks of age, the positive effects are a significant reduction in BPD at 36 weeks' PMA and a reduction in failure to extubate by 28 days, need for late rescue dexamethasone and home oxygen therapy (Halliday and Ehrenkranz 2001).

Numerous side-effects of steroid therapy have been reported. These include sepsis, necrotising enterocolitis, hyperglycaemia, hypertension, diabetic ketoacidosis, hypertrophic cardiomyopathy and greater weight loss (Pomerance and Puri 1980; Gunn et al. 1981; Regev et al. 1987; Noble-Jamieson et al. 1989; Israel et al. 1993; Spear et al. 1993; Rastogi et al. 1996). Nosocomial infection may be more likely to occur in babies in whom treatment is commenced at 2 rather than 4 weeks of age (Papile et al. 1998). In addition, dexamethasone used prior to 14 days of age has been associated with an increased risk of candidal sepsis (Pera et al. 2002). It is important, therefore, to exclude sepsis before embarking on steroid therapy, but a policy of prophylactic antibiotics or antifungal agents to run concurrently is not evidence-based. Dexamethasone can cause secondary adrenal suppression at the hypothalmic–pituitary level (Cronin et al. 1993).

The possible long-term effects of corticosteroids are of concern. In animal models, corticosteroids significantly impair cell multiplication in the lung and central nervous system. Dexamethasone given to rats at a critical period after birth (4–14 days) resulted in increased lung volumes, enlarged air spaces and reduced alveolar surface area and total DNA content. After the drug was withdrawn, the trend towards precocious puberty was reversed, but late sequelae were described, that is, emphysematous lungs with larger and fewer air spaces (Tschanz et al. 1995). In animal models, decreased brain weight and DNA content have also been reported, with a delay in cortical dendritic branching and disrupted postnatal glial cell for-mation. There have, however, been concerns regarding the possible adverse long-term neurodevelopmental effects of systemically administered corticosteroids (Ch. 3). The risk may be related to the timing of administration: meta-analysis of 20 randomised trials demonstrated that only early and not late treatment was associated with a significant excess of cerebral palsy (Doyle et al. 2010). No significant effect was seen on the incidence of cerebral palsy when corticosteroids were administered after 3 weeks (Halliday et al. 2003). In the trials, however, when corticosteroids were adminis-tered late, greater crossover occurred, and this may have obscured any effect (Doyle et al. 2010).

Another factor which increases adverse outcome is the steroid dosage. In one study (Wilson-Costello et al. 2009) each 1 mg/kg of corticosteroid was associated with a 2.0-point reduction in the Mental Development Index and a 40% increase in disabling cerebral palsy. In that study, older PMA was not found to mitigate the adverse effect and treatment after 33 weeks' PMA was associated with the greatest harm. High-risk compared with low-risk BPD babies, however, experienced less harm (Wilson-Costello et al. 2009). Spastic diplegia appears to be the most common form of cerebral palsy following dexamethasone administration. Concerns regarding the side-effects of corticosteroids have resulted in a decline in their use over the last 10 years; this has been associated with an increase in BPD (Yoder et al. 2009). It has been suggested (Eichenwald and Stark 2007) that it is reasonable to consider a therapeutic trial of corticosteroids in infants with life-threatening respiratory disease who require substantial ventilatory support and supplemental oxygen (FIo$_2$ >0.8). Before treatment, parents should be informed of the potential benefits and the uncertain additional risk of neurologi-cal injury (Eichenwald and Stark 2007). The respiratory status of an infant who is responsive to corticosteroids will usually improve over the first 2–3 days of treatment, thus we would not continue the therapy if there had been no response after 72 hours. If they do respond, a 7–10-day course is recommended (Eichenwald and Stark 2007). The optimum dosage is uncertain, although 0.15 mg/kg/day has been suggested (Eichenwald and Stark 2007).

In view of the concerns regarding systemically administering cor-ticosteroids, the efficacy of this therapy by the inhaled route has been investigated. Meta-analysis of four trials in which inhaled steroids were given to infants older than 14 days demonstrated improved extubation success, with no increase in sepsis (Lister et al. 2010). In one randomised trial, which included infants with moder-ate BPD, fluticasone inhalation versus placebo did not reduce the duration of ventilation or supplementary oxygen dependency; however, the trial was only powered to detect a difference of at least 21 days (Dugas et al. 2005). Meta-analysis of five randomised trials comparing inhaled versus systemic steroids administered to ventilator-dependent infants with evolving BPD after 2 weeks of age demonstrated no significant differences in the incidence of BPD at 36 weeks' PMA or the duration of intubation or oxygen dependency (Shah, S.S. et al. 2007).

Surfactant

Surfactant dysfunction may persist and contribute to the continuing respiratory support required by neonates with BPD. In a pilot study, a single dose of a natural surfactant reduced the inspired oxygen concentration requirement in babies aged between 7 and 30 days (Pandit et al. 1995).

Inhaled nitric oxide

Inhaled nitric oxide (iNO) may be useful in infants with or develop-ing BPD to reduce their oxygenation index, but the magnitude of the

response can be variable and the optimum dose ranges from 6 to 60 ppm (Lonnqvist et al. 1995). In the absence of a demonstrated well-defined risk-to-benefit ratio for the use of long-term pulmo-nary vasodilators, it has been suggested that their administration should be restricted to patients with pulmonary arterial pressure at or near systemic levels with evidence of right ventricular dysfunc-tion (Kulik et al. 2010).

Recommendations regarding drug therapy

A single dose of furosemide should be given to treat acute fluid overload, and regular chlorothiazide and spironolactone adminis-tered to infants who have signs of incipient right heart failure or are poorly tolerant of a modest fluid volume regimen (120 ml/kg/day). Caffeine, commenced to facilitate extubation, should be continued until at least 36 weeks' PMA and only stopped before if sympto-matic gastro-oesophageal reflux develops. On the neonatal inten-sive care unit, bronchodilators are rarely necessary and should be administered only to those BPD infants who have symptomatic wheeze and their respiratory support requirements are reduced as a consequence of bronchodilator administration. We consider cor-ticosteroids only for infants who are at least 2 weeks of age and have severe lung disease, remaining ventilator-dependent and in high oxygen concentrations. Systemic corticosteroids are prescribed for 3 days and only continued, for a further 7 days in a reducing dose, if there has been an obvious clinical response (i.e. a significant reduction in respiratory support requirements). Research is required to determine if there is a dosage regimen with a positive risk-to-benefit ratio. Other drug therapies, discussed above, are used only on an individual basis or in the context of a randomised trial.

Home respiratory support

Home oxygen therapy should be considered for babies who have no medical problem other than their increased inspired oxygen requirement. Some parents, however, will also cope with tube feeding their baby. This facilitates earlier discharge from the neona-tal unit and, if there is appropriate support in the community, does not lead to increased readmissions (Greenough et al. 2004). Sup-plementary oxygen can be delivered via either a single feeding catheter inserted into one nostril or twin nasal cannulae. Oxygen concentrators should be used, unless the baby requires only low amounts of oxygen. Small portable oxygen cylinders should also be provided, whichever system is used, as they are necessary for trans-porting the baby. At regular intervals, the baby should be seen at home or in hospital and progress and weight checked. The baby's oxygen saturation needs to be monitored preferably for at least 24-hour periods on a regular basis, aiming to maintain saturation levels of above 92% unless there is pulmonary hypertension. Weaning from supplementary oxygen should be gradual; if the inspired oxygen concentration is abruptly reduced, resulting in hypoxaemia, this can lead to worsening pulmonary hypertension and an increased incidence of apnoea, which responds to improv-ing arterial oxygen saturation (Sekar and Duke 1991). It is essential to ensure that patients maintain their oxygen saturation levels at all times; desaturation occurs particularly after feeding (Singer et al. 1992) and lower oxygen saturation levels may be recorded when the baby is asleep.

For the first month after oxygen is no longer needed, parents should keep the equipment at home in case of increased oxygen need associated with even minor respiratory infections. Home oxygen facilitates earlier discharge from the neonatal unit and cor-responding financial savings, but can have an adverse impact on the family's quality of life (McLean et al. 2000). It is important to be aware that some infants may require months or up to 2 years of supplementary oxygen at home (Greenough et al. 2006). Even after they no longer require home oxygen, such patients still are more symptomatic and require more treatment (Greenough et al. 2006).

Only a small number of babies with BPD have been discharged on home ventilation (Fauroux et al. 1995). The babies must have a tracheostomy. Home ventilation requires an enormous investment in equipment, community services and education for parents (Panitch et al. 1996).

Prophylaxis

Antenatal therapy

Corticosteroid treatment given to women at high risk of preterm delivery reduces the incidence of neonatal death and RDS by approximately 50% (Crowley et al. 1990), but, even in combination with postnatal surfactant, fails to have a favourable impact on the incidence of BPD (Jobe et al. 1993). The positive effects of thyrotrophin-releasing hormone seen in early studies (Ballard et al. 1992) have not been confirmed in large randomised trials.

Fluid management

Promotion of an early diuresis with a diuretic (Savage et al. 1975) or an albumin infusion (Greenough et al. 1993) does not significantly improve perinatal respiratory status. Fluid restriction in the first weeks after birth does not reduce BPD (Bell and Acarregui 2008), but does reduce the risks of PDA and necrotising enterocolitis and, in the largest study (Kavvadia et al. 2000) included in the meta-analysis, fluid restriction was associated with a significant reduction in the use of postnatal steroids. In a retrospective analysis (Oh et al. 2005) of 1382 infants, higher fluid intake and less weight loss during the first 10 days after birth were associated with an increased risk of BPD. Limiting colloid administration and avoiding early sodium supplementation might reduce the incidence of BPD. Inverse relationships between the amount of colloid received and perinatal lung function (Kavvadia et al. 1999) and the risk of BPD development (Dimitriou et al. 2002) have been demonstrated. A lower rate of BPD was noted in infants in whom sodium supplementation was not given in the first 3–5 days compared with those receiving daily maintenance sodium (Costarino et al. 1992). In addition, in a randomised trial, withholding sodium supplementation until there was evidence of weight loss equalling 6% of birth weight, rather than giving routine maintenance, was associated with a reduction in the proportion of babies who required supplementary oxygen at 7 days (Hartnoll et al. 2000).

Indometacin

In the randomised trial including 1202 ELBW infants, indometacin prophylaxis, although reducing the incidence of symptomatic PDA by 50%, did not reduce the incidence of BPD, defined as the need for supplementary oxygen at 36 weeks' PMA (Schmidt et al. 2001). Subsequent analysis demonstrated that prophylactic use of indometacin was associated with higher supplementary oxygen requirement and less weight loss by the end of the first week after birth (Schmidt et al. 2006b).

Corticosteroids

Commenced in the first 96 hours after birth, corticosteroids reduce the risk of BPD at both 28 days' and 36 weeks' PMA, lower the risk of PDA and pulmonary airleak and promote earlier extubation (Halliday and Ehrenkranz 2003). Seven trials have examined the efficacy of administration between 7 and 14 days; the overall result was a reduction in BPD and facilitation of extubation (Halliday et al. 2003). Recent studies have focused on determining the efficacy of low-dose dexamethasone; dexamethasone administered as 0.89 mg/kg over 10 days facilitated extubation without obviously increasing side-effects, but did not reduce the incidence of BPD (Doyle et al. 2006). No difference was demonstrated in death or major disability at 2 years, but the number of infants included in the study was small (Doyle et al. 2007) and further studies are required to assess this approach.

An alternative approach has been to use the inhaled route. Review of randomised trials assessing the efficacy of inhaled steroid therapy initiated in the first 2 weeks after birth demonstrated no statistically significant effects on BPD at 28 days' or 36 weeks' PMA or on mortality (Shah, V. et al. 2007). There was, however, a reduction in the requirement for rescue systemic steroids. Meta-analysis of randomised trials demonstrated that early inhaled steroids did not confer any important advantage over systemic steroids in the management of ventilator-dependent preterm infants (Shah, V. et al. 2007). In a pilot study, early intratracheal instillation of budesonide using surfactant as a vehicle was associated with a significant reduction in the combined outcome of death or BPD (Yeh et al. 2008). Side-effects are less common with inhaled steroids (Halliday and Ehrenkranz 2001); they include tongue hypertrophy but this resolves after cessation of treatment (Linder et al. 1995).

Hydrocortisone

No reduction in BPD has been demonstrated in randomised trials (Doyle et al. 2010) and one trial was halted prematurely as the hydrocortisone-treated infants had an increased rate of gastrointestinal perforation (Watterberg et al. 2004).

Methylxanthines

Caffeine

In a large randomised trial, caffeine administration to infants at risk for or having apnoea of prematurity or to facilitate removal of an endotracheal tube was associated with a significant reduction in BPD (36% versus 47%) (Schmidt et al. 2006a). In addition, in the caffeine group, positive airway pressure was discontinued 1 week earlier and a significantly lower proportion required treatment for a PDA. Caffeine administration was associated with a reduction in the risk of PDA deemed to need either pharmacological or surgical closure. Follow-up demonstrated that the caffeine-treated group had a higher rate of survival without neurodevelopmental disability at 18–21 months (Schmidt et al. 2007).

Pentoxifylline

This is a methylxanthine derivative and non-selective phophodiesterase inhibitor with anti-inflammatory effects. In a randomised trial of 150 VLBW infants, pentoxifylline administration was associated with a 27% reduction in BPD (Lauterbach et al. 2006).

Azithromycin

Azithromycin is a newer generation macrolide and has fewer side-effects and increased anti-inflammatory properties than erythromycin. Azithromycin significantly reduced IL-6 and IL-8 production by tracheal cells obtained from prematurely born infants. BPD, however, was not significantly reduced by azithromycin given for a maximum of 6 weeks in a double-blind placebo-controlled trial which included 43 infants of birthweight less than 1001 g, but postnatal steroid use was lower in the treatment group (31% versus 62%, $p = 0.05$) (Hazinski et al. 1989). Potential side-effects include late-onset infections, particularly fungal sepsis, hepatotoxicity and hearing impairment.

Vitamin E

Vitamin E is a scavenger of free radicals. The toxic effects of oxygen upon the lung are enhanced by vitamin E deficiency and can be prevented by vitamin E treatment (Taylor 1956). Healthy term and premature babies have mean plasma vitamin E levels of less than 0.25 mg/dl in the first 24 hours after birth (Moyer 1950); a level of less than 0.5 mg/dl indicates vitamin E inadequacy in adults. Daily vitamin E administration to infants requiring an inspired oxygen concentration of greater than 40% was associated with a reduction in the number of babies with a CXR appearance compatible with BPD (Ehrenkranz et al. 1978). Meta-analysis of 26 randomised trials demonstrated that vitamin E supplementation does not reduce the risk of BPD and high-dose intravenous vitamin E supplementation increased the rate of sepsis (Brion et al. 2003). Vitamin E decreases the oxygen-dependent intracellular killing ability of neutrophils, resulting in a decreased resistance to infection in preterm babies (Johnson et al. 1985). Infants whose mothers had received high-dose vitamins E and C during pregnancy in a large multicentre randomised trial did not have an improved respiratory outcome; indeed they had higher healthcare utilisation in the first 2 years after birth (Greenough et al. 2010).

Vitamin A

Vitamin A supplementation influences the normal differentiation of regenerating airways. VLBW infants are frequently deficient in vitamin A because of deprivation of transplacental acquisition. In addition, parenteral administration of vitamin A is inefficient (Chan et al. 1993) because of photodegradation and absorption of the vitamin to the intravenous tubing. VLBW neonates with BPD may have suboptimal plasma concentrations of vitamin A for extended periods (Shenai et al. 1985). In a randomised study (Shenai et al. 1987), vitamin A (retinyl palmitate 2000 IU), given by the intramuscular route on postnatal day 4 and every other day thereafter for a total of 14 injections over 28 days to oxygen-dependent babies, resulted in significantly higher mean plasma concentrations of vitamin A and a reduction in BPD and the need for supplementary oxygen, mechanical ventilation and intensive care. The results of subsequent trials have been conflicting (Pearson et al. 1992; Shenai 1999; Tyson et al. 1999), but meta-analysis of the results of eight randomised trials (Darlow and Graham 2008) highlighted that vitamin A supplementation reduced death or oxygen requirement at 1 month of age and oxygen requirement at 36 weeks' PMA. In six of the studies, vitamin A was given by intramuscular injection and neurodevelopmental outcome was only available for one of the studies. Vitamin A administration must be carefully monitored if side-effects, such as non-specific neurological signs secondary to raised intracranial pressure caused by toxic levels, are to be avoided. The optimal dosage, mode and duration of administration of vitamin A in VLBW babies need further investigation.

Superoxide dismutase

Superoxide dismutase (SOD) is a naturally occurring intracellular enzyme which converts the toxic superoxide radical into the potentially less toxic hydrogen peroxide. Pretreatment of rats with SOD prevented toxic changes in lung macrophages (Simon 1980) and damage to lung cells (Block and Fisher 1977) when exposed to hyperoxia. Human neonates are deficient in SOD (Northway 1979; Yoshioka et al. 1979). The efficacy of prophylactic SOD has been tested in a randomised trial (Suresh and Soll 2002); no favourable effect on oxygen dependency at 28 days' or 36 weeks' PMA was noted. In one study, however, treated babies, compared with those who received placebo, had a 36% reduction in repeated episodes of wheeze severe enough to require antiasthma medication in infancy (Davis et al. 2003). Toxicity has not been reported, but antioxidant therapy may affect the bactericidal activity of polymorphonuclear cells.

N-acetyl cysteine

The immature lung is deficient in glutathionine synthesis (Jain et al. 1995), which is limited by the availability of cysteine. N-acetylcysteine (NAC) is a stable precursor of cysteine. Glutathionine is an endogenous scavenger of free radicals and hence has a major role in the antioxidant defence system of the lung. In a multicentre double-blind placebo-controlled trial (Ahola et al. 2003) which included 391 infants of birthweight less than 1 kg, no significant differences were found in the incidence or severity of BPD between those who received NAC for 6 days and those who received the placebo.

Allopurinol

Allopurinol is a synthetic competitive inhibitor of xanthine oxidase and a free radical scavenger. Enteral administration of 20 mg/ml for 7 days, in a randomised placebo-controlled trial, however, failed to reduce the incidence of BPD significantly (Russell and Cooke 1995).

Melatonin

Melatonin is a potent free radical scavenger. In a randomised study, infants with RDS who received 10 intravenous injections of melatonin had significantly lower levels of proinflammatory cytokines and reduced ventilatory requirements during the prenatal period (Gitto et al. 2005).

Surfactant

Overall, exogenous surfactant replacement therapy, although significantly reducing the combined outcome of BPD and death, does not reduce the incidence of BPD alone. Early surfactant therapy with extubation on to nasal CPAP compared with selective rescue surfactant therapy and continued mechanical ventilation was associated with a lower rate of BPD (Stevens et al. 2007).

Inositol

Inositol promotes maturation of surfactant phospholipids and the synthesis of phosphatidyl inositol. Meta-analysis of two randomised trials demonstrated that inositol supplementation, although reducing the combined outcome of BPD and death, did not reduce BPD (Howlett and Ohlsson 2003).

Bronchodilators

Prophylaxis with salbutamol, started in the first 2 weeks after birth, was not associated with a significant reduction in the duration of ventilatory support, incidence of BPD or mortality (Ng et al. 2001).

Cromolyn sodium

Cromolyn sodium inhibits neutrophil activation and neutrophil chemotaxis and thus can modulate the inflammatory process in the lung (Ng and Ohlsson 2002). In a randomised trial (Watterberg and Murphy 1993), however, prophylactic cromolyn sodium failed to reduce significantly the incidence of BPD or any other clinically important outcome.

Ambroxol

In one study, ambroxol given over the first 5 days was associated with a 50% reduction in the incidence of BPD, without adverse effect (Wauer et al. 1992).

Triiodothyronine

In a randomised, placebo-controlled trial, administration of triiodothyronine and hydrocortisone for 7 days after birth to infants of less than 30 weeks' gestation was not associated with a reduction in BPD (Biswas et al. 2003).

Respiratory support

In non-randomised studies, use of CPAP rather than intubation and ventilation was associated with a lower rate of BPD. In a large randomised trial (COIN), which included 610 infants born at 25–28 weeks of gestation, although infants randomised to CPAP had a lower risk of death or need for oxygen therapy at 28 days, there was no significant difference in the rates of oxygen dependency at 36 weeks' PMA and the pneumothorax rate was significantly greater (threefold) in the CPAP group (Morley et al. 2008). The INSURE (intubation–surfactant–treatment–extubation) method is a combination of early surfactant treatment and early extubation on to CPAP. Meta-analysis of six trials demonstrated that such an approach compared with selective surfactant with continued ventilation in infants with RDS was associated with a significant reduction in BPD, need for mechanical ventilation and airleaks (Stevens et al. 2007). A larger proportion of the infants in the early compared with the selective surfactant group received surfactant. It is well documented that prophylactic/early surfactant versus selective/rescue surfactant once RDS is established reduced the incidence of BPD/death and airleaks and improved survival in 208 infants born between 25 and 28 weeks' gestational age and this questions whether the effects seen were due to early surfactant, early CPAP or both. In a randomised study (Sandri et al. 2010), prophylactic surfactant (200 mg/kg Curosurf) and extubation within 1 hour if possible was associated with similar results with regard to need for mechanical ventilation in the first 5 days (31.4% versus 33%) as nCPAP (6–7 cmH$_2$O) to selective surfactant given if there was CPAP failure (48.5% required surfactant at median 240 minutes). In addition, there were no significant differences in other outcomes (Sandri et al. 2010). In another trial, amongst infants born before 28 weeks of gestation, intubation and surfactant within 1 hour and extubation within 24 hours compared with CPAP (5 cmH$_2$O) and rescue surfactant in the first 48 hours resulted in no significant differences in BPD or death (54.1% versus 48.7%), although less of the latter group received surfactant (SUPPORT Study Group 2010). Those studies suggest that, if CPAP is used from birth, the short-term advantages of early versus delayed administration of surfactant become less apparent, but whether the long-term outcomes are similar needs to be investigated.

Permissive hypercapnia reduces ventilatory requirements, but infants randomised to target Pco$_2$ ranges of 55–65 versus 35–45 mmHg had a higher incidence of BPD or death and significantly increased combined outcome of mental impairment at 18–22 months or death (Thome et al. 2006). Meta-analysis of the results of randomised trials has demonstrated that patient-triggered ventilation does not reduce the incidence of BPD (Greenough et al. 2008). Meta-analysis of the results of randomised prophylactic trials of HFO ventilation (HFOV) in which infants were randomised to receive HFOV or conventional mechanical ventilation in the first 12 hours after birth demonstrated that HFOV was associated with a modest but significant reduction in BPD (Henderson-Smart et al. 2007). The trials, however, differed with respect to administration of antenatal corticosteroids and postnatal surfactant and the types of oscillator and conventional ventilator used. The results of a non-randomised study suggested that HFOV may protect small-airway function (Hofhuis et al. 2010). Follow-up at school age, when comprehensive respiratory and neurodevelopmental assessments can be undertaken, is needed to determine whether HFOV may have long-term benefits.

Nitric oxide

Inhaled nitric oxide (iNO) selectively decreases pulmonary vascular resistance and improves oxygenation. In addition it has anti-inflammatory effects and promotes cell and vessel growth in the immature lung (Kinsella et al. 1997). Infants dying with BPD have been noted to have disrupted pulmonary vasculature, hence a vascular hypothesis for the development of BPD has been proposed (Abman 2001) and that modulation of angiogenic growth factors might reduce BPD (Thébaud et al. 2005). Indeed, in an animal model (Tang et al. 2004), inhaled NO stimulated angiogenesis and alveolarisation. Meta-analysis of 11 randomised trials demonstrated that the effect of iNO in prematurely born babies depends on the timing of administration and the population (Barrington and Finer 2007). Early rescue treatment based on oxygenation criteria did not affect mortality or BPD rates and there was a trend towards an increase in intracerebral haemorrhage. Early, routine use for intubated infants, however, was associated with a just significant reduction in the combined outcome of death or BPD and a reduction in the incidence of severe intracerebral haemorrhage and periventricular leukomalacia. In a subsequent large trial, in which preterm infants were randomised to early, prolonged, low-dose iNO therapy, no significant differences were demonstrated in any important outcomes (Mercier et al. 2010). Use of iNO after 3 days based on an elevated risk of BPD showed no effect on BPD (Barrington and Finer 2007).

Prognosis

Mortality

Predischarge mortality is usually caused by intercurrent infection, cor pulmonale or respiratory failure. Predictors of death in hospital include male gender and length of ventilatory support and supplementary oxygen (Shaw et al. 1993). Sudden infant death syndrome was reported to be higher in babies with BPD (Werthammer et al. 1982), but this has not been subsequently confirmed (Sauve and Singhal 1985; Gray and Rogers 1994).

Morbidity

Infants with BPD require a prolonged hospital stay and have delayed discharge home; in one population-based observational study, the adjusted lengths of stay for infants with and without BPD were 84 and 58 days respectively (Klinger et al. 2006). Prematurely born infants with BPD can require supplementary oxygen for many months or even years (Greenough et al. 2002), although few remain oxygen-dependent beyond 2 years of age (Greenough et al. 2006). Infants requiring supplementary oxygen at home have the most severe lung disease, as evidenced by their requirement for hospital readmission in the first 2 years after birth being twice that of non-home oxygen-dependent BPD infants (Greenough et al. 2002) and, even when they are no longer home oxygen-dependent, they still have more outpatient attendances and are more likely to wheeze and require an inhaler between 2 and 5 years of age (Greenough et al. 2006). BPD infants require a median of two (range 0–20) rehospitalisations in the first 2 years (Greenough et al. 2001). Rehospitalisations are significantly more common in BPD babies requiring supplementary oxygen at home (Greenough et al. 2002) and those who develop RSV infections (Greenough et al. 2001). The hospitalisation rate, however, declines after the second year, such that hospitalisation was infrequent in prematurely born children at 14 years of age, regardless of BPD status (Doyle et al. 2001).

Morbidity relating to growth

The average weight and height at term of babies with severe BPD are frequently at or below the third centile; growth failure is partially the result of increased metabolic demands from increased work of breathing. Growth accelerates as respiratory symptoms improve. At school age, children who had had BPD did not have poorer growth than controls (Vrlenich et al. 1995).

Central nervous system morbidity

Delays in development have been reported to be common, with poor developmental outcome correlating positively with prolonged hospitalisation and requirement for oxygen in babies with severe BPD. Developmental delay was reported to be commoner in BPD babies oxygen-dependent beyond 36 weeks' PMA than in those oxygen-dependent only beyond 28 days or less (Gregoire et al. 1998). Ventilation for longer than 28 days has been associated with intact survival, but not in VLBW babies with evidence of significant brain injury (Thomas et al. 2003b). Amongst children without severe gross motor delays, risk factors for BPD accounted for the association of BPD and developmental delay (Laughon et al. 2009). Significant abnormalities in brainstem auditory evoked responses have been reported in infants with BPD, indicating that both myelination and synaptic function in the auditory brainstem were impaired (Wilkinson et al. 2007).

Pulmonary morbidity

Recurrent respiratory symptoms requiring treatment are common in prematurely born children, particularly in those who had BPD (Greenough et al. 2006). In a cohort of 7–8-year-olds, whereas 30% of BPD children and 24% of prematurely born children without BPD were wheezing, only 7% of term controls were so affected (Gross et al. 1999). The most severely affected remain symptomatic in adulthood (Northway et al. 1990; Vrijlandt et al. 2005). Pulmonary function abnormalities in the first year after birth in BPD babies include high airways resistance, low dynamic pulmonary compliance, reduced functional residual capacity, abnormal gas exchange (hypercarbia, low oxygen saturation), elevated minute volume and lower gas-mixing index. The most consistent finding in BPD infants has been an increased pulmonary or airway resistance (Northway et al. 1967; Stocks et al. 1978; Morray et al. 1982; Yüksel et al. 1991b). In prematurely born infants, the number of days of wheeze significantly correlated with the degree of gas trapping (Broughton et al. 2007). Lung function usually improves with age (Morray et al. 1982; Wong et al. 1982; Gerhardt et al. 1987). Nevertheless, pulmonary function tests may still be abnormal, with reduced exercise tolerance, in school-age children (Smith et al. 2008). School-age children with BPD were demonstrated to have reduced absolute and size-corrected flow rates compared with controls matched for age and size (Filippone et al. 2003). A strong correlation was demonstrated between the maximum flow at functional residual capacity at 2 years of age and forced expiratory volume in 1 second (FEV_1) at school age, which suggests persistent airflow limitation in some patients with BPD. In adolescents, evidence of airways obstruction and hyperreactivity and an increased responsiveness to histamine (Doyle et al. 2001; Allen et al. 2003) and apparently asymptomatic BPD patients desaturating on exercise have been demonstrated (Santuz et al. 1995). Amongst the most severely affected, lung function abnormalities have been reported even in adolescents and young adults. A BPD cohort born between 1964 and 1973, as adolescents and young adults were significantly shorter and weighed less than term-born controls and a matched prematurely born cohort without BPD; 68% of the BPD cohort had airways obstruction and 52% had evidence of reactive airways disease (Northway et al. 1990). In a nationwide follow-up study in the Netherlands, the prevalence of doctor-diagnosed asthma was significantly higher in prematurely born 19-year-olds than in age-matched controls. There was, however, an effect of gender; whereas the 19-year-old women who had had BPD had more asthma (24% versus 5%, $p = 0.001$) and shortness of breath during exercise (43% versus 16%, $p = 0.008$) than controls, the prevalence of reported symptoms by men with BPD was comparable with the controls (Vrijlandt et al. 2005), probably reflecting the different patterns of thoracic growth between the sexes, which at the end of puberty results in approximately 25% higher lung function in males than females.

Numerous chronic complications may be seen on the CXRs of BPD infants at follow-up, including cor pulmonale, right ventricular hypertrophy and enlargement of the main pulmonary artery, reflecting pulmonary hypertension. Atelectasis and subsegmental or segmental collapse may occur, frequently affecting the left lower lobe. Rickets, due to dietary or parenteral nutritional deficiency of calcium and vitamin D or to the calciuric effect of furosemide, may manifest by rib fractures together with generalised demineralisation and metaphyseal fraying, widening and cupping. The CXR abnormalities of severe BPD may persist for some years. Most patients, however, remain either radiologically stable or show a trend towards improvement. High-resolution CT scanning demonstrated that adult survivors of 'traditional' BPD, compared with similar-aged young adults, had multifocal areas of reduced attenuation and perfusion, bronchial thickening and decreased bronchus-to-pulmonary artery diameter ratios (Howling et al. 2000). In one series, all young adults who had required supplementary oxygen at 36 weeks' PMA had abnormal CT findings: the most common finding (84% of cases) was emphysema, which inversely correlated with the FEV_1 z-score (Wong et al. 2008) and in another (Aukland et al. 2009) 86% of ELBW infants at 10 or 18 years had lung parenchymal abnormalities detected on high-resolution CT examination, which again correlated with impairment of lung function (FEV_1).

Cardiovascular morbidity

Pulmonary hypertension can be detected non-invasively by Doppler echocardiographic demonstration of tricuspid regurgitation or estimation of the pulmonary systolic time interval. Such measurements can be used to identify a response to elevation of the inspired oxygen concentration (Benatar et al. 1995). Infants with BPD and severe pulmonary hypertension are at high risk of death, particularly in the first 6 months after diagnosis (Khemani et al. 2007). Systemic hypertension is also common in babies with severe BPD, affecting 13% of 87 patients who required home oxygen therapy. In the survivors, however, it resolved prior to weaning from supplementary oxygen (Anderson et al. 1993).

Other forms of chronic lung disease

Wilson–Mikity syndrome

Prematurely born babies, classically who have had no respiratory problems in the first week after birth, are affected. The diagnosis is made when progressive respiratory failure develops during the second week, in association with diffuse small bilateral cystic translucencies on the CXR (Wilson and Mikity 1960). The babies have intrapulmonary shunting and maldistribution of ventilation and perfusion (Krauss et al. 1970); pulmonary hypertension can be detected at cardiac catheterisation. Nowadays, this condition is rare and predominantly affects infants with a birthweight of less than 1500 g (Hoepker et al. 2008).

Clinical signs

There is an insidious onset of tachypnoea and cyanosis, and dyspnoea, especially on effort. The infant frequently has an overexpanded chest, wheezing and coughing.

Aetiology

The syndrome usually occurs in babies of less than 32 weeks' gestational age (Burnard 1966); it thus may represent a functional and anatomical immaturity of the airways (Saunders et al. 1978). Intrauterine infection may also be responsible, as babies with Wilson–Mikity syndrome have been found to have high plasma immunoglobulin M (IgM) levels on the first day after birth (Fujimura et al. 1983). In addition, the mothers of affected babies have been noted to have a high incidence of chorioamnionitis, in association with a raised cord blood IgM (Fujimura et al. 1989). Babies with a condition resembling Wilson–Mikity syndrome have been reported to have increased leukocyte elastase in tracheal aspirates at birth, indicating antenatal leukocyte migration to the lungs (Fujimura et al. 1993).

Diagnosis

A diffuse fine reticular pattern infiltrating both lung fields, interspersed with areas of emphysematous cysts, is seen on the CXR of

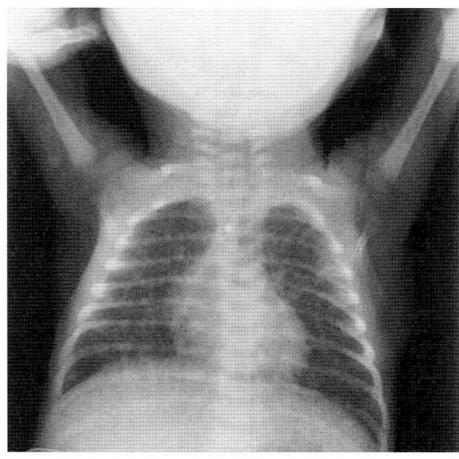

Fig. 27.49 Wilson–Mikity syndrome.

affected babies (Fig. 27.49). The changes initially, unlike in BPD, are more marked in the upper zones. As the disease progresses, the cysts coalesce and marked hyperinflation is a prominent feature.

Prognosis

Symptoms may persist for many months and respiratory infections are common during infancy. Abnormal lung function, suggesting persistent small-airway damage, has been found in survivors even at 8–10 years of age, but usually the pulmonary disease resolves. Death may occur as a result of cardiac failure, respiratory failure, infection or pulmonary hypertension.

References

Abman, S.H., 2001. Bronchopulmonary dysplasia: 'a vascular hypothesis'. Am J Respir Crit Care Med 164, 1755–1756.

Abman, S.H., Accurso, F.J., Koops, B.L., 1984. Experience with home oxygen in the management of infants with bronchopulmonary dysplasia. Clin Pediatr (Phila) 23, 471–476.

Abman, S.H., Wolfe, R.R., Accurso, F.J., et al., 1985. Pulmonary vascular response to oxygen in infants with severe bronchopulmonary dysplasia. Pediatrics 75, 80–84.

Ahola, T., Lapatto, R., Raivio, K.O., et al., 2003. N-acetylcyteine does not prevent bronchopulmonary dysplasia in immature infants: a randomised controlled trial. Journal of Pediatrics 143, 713–719.

Albersheim, S.G., Solimano, A.J., Sharma, A.K., et al., 1989. Randomized double blind controlled trial of long term diuretic therapy for bronchopulmonary dysplasia. Journal of Pediatrics 115, 615–620.

Allen, J., Zwerdling, R., Ehrenkranz, R., et al., 2003. Statement on the care of the child with chronic lung disease of infancy and childhood. Am J Respir Crit Care Med 168, 356–396.

Anderson, A.H., Warady, B.A., Daily, D.K., et al., 1993. Systemic hypertension in infants with severe bronchopulmonary

dysplasia: associated clinical factors. Am J Perinatol 10, 190–193.

Askie, L.M., Henderson-Smart, D.J., Irwig, L., et al., 2003. Oxygen saturation targets and outcomes in extremely preterm infants. NEJM 349, 959–967.

Askin, F., 1991. Respiratory tract disorders in the fetus and neonate. In: Wigglesworth, J.S., Singer, D.B. (Eds.), Textbook of Fetal and Perinatal Pathology. Blackwell Scientific, Oxford, pp. 643–688.

Aukland, S.M., Rosendahl, K., Owens, C.M., et al., 2009. Neonatal bronchopulmonary dysplasia predicts abnormal pulmonary HRCT scans in long term survivors of extreme preterm birth. Thorax 64, 405–410.

Ballard, R.A., Ballard, P.L., Creasy, R.K., et al., 1992. Respiratory disease in very low birthweight infants after prenatal thyrotropin-releasing hormone and glucocorticoids. Lancet 339, 510–515.

Barnes, N.D., Glover, W.J., Hull, D., et al., 1969. Effects of prolonged positive pressure ventilation in infancy. Lancet ii, 1096–1099.

Barrington, K.J., Finer, N.N., 2007. Inhaled nitric oxide for preterm infants: a systematic review. Pediatrics 120, 1088–1099.

Been, J.V., Zimmerman, L.J.I., 2009. Histological chorioamnionitis and respiratory outcome in preterm infants. Archives of Disease in Childhood Fetal Neonatal Edition 94, 218–225.

Bell, E.F., Acarregui, M.J., 2008. Restricted versus liberal water intake for preventing morbidity and mortality in preterm infants. Cochrane Database Systemic Reviews (1), CD000503.

Benatar, A., Clarke, J., Silverman, M., 1995. Pulmonary hypertension in infants with chronic lung disease: non-invasive evaluation and short term effect of oxygen treatment. Arch Dis Child Fetal Neonatal Ed 72, F14–F19.

Berg, T.J., Pagtakhan, T.D., Reed, M.H., et al., 1975. Bronchopulmonary dysplasia and lung rupture in hyaline membrane disease: influence of continuous distending pressure. Pediatrics 55, 51–53.

Betremieux, P., Treguier, C., Pladys, P., et al., 1995. Tracheobronchography and balloon dilatation in acquired neonatal tracheal stenosis. Arch Dis Child Fetal Neonatal Ed 72, F3–F7.

Bhandari, V., Gruen, J.R., 2006. The genetics of bronchopulmonary dysplasia. Semin Perinatol 30, 185–191.

Biswas, S., Buffery, J., Enoch, H., et al., 2003. Pulmonary effects of triiodothyronine (T_3)

and hydrocortisone (HC) supplementation in preterm infants less than 30 weeks gestation: THORN trial – thyroid hormone replacement in neonates. Pediatr Res 53, 48–57.

Bjorklund, L.L., Ingimarsson, J., Curstedt, T., et al., 1997. Manual ventilation with a few large breaths at birth compromises the therapeutic effect of subsequent surfactant replacement in immature lambs. Pediatr Res 42, 348–355.

Block, E.R., Fisher, A.B., 1977. Protection of hyperoxic induced depression of pulmonary serotonin by pre-treatment with superoxide dismutase. Am Rev Respir Dis 116, 441–446.

Bolivar, J.M., Gerhardt, T., Gonzalez, A., et al., 1995. Mechanisms for episodes of hypoxemia in preterm infants undergoing mechanical ventilation. Journal of Pediatrics 127, 767–773.

Bonikos, D.S., Benson, K.G., Northway, W.H.J., 1976. Oxygen toxicity in the newborn. The effect of chronic continuous 100 per cent oxygen exposure on the lung of newborn mice. Am J Pathol 85, 623–650.

Brion, L.P., Bell, E.F., Raghuveer, T.S., 2003. Vitamin E supplementation for prevention of morbidity and mortality in preterm infants. Cochrane Database Systemic Reviews (4), CD003665.

Brion, L.P., Primhak, R.A., Yong, W., 2006. Aerosolized diuretics for preterm infants with (or developing) chronic lung disease. Cochrane Database Syst Rev.

Brion L P, Primhak R A, Ambrosio-Perez I, 2008. Diuretics acting on the distal renal tubule for preterm infants with (or developing) chronic lung disease. Cochrane Database Syst Rev.

Broughton, S., Thomas, M.R., Marston, L., et al., 2007. Very prematurely born infants wheezing at follow up – lung function and risk factors. Arch Dis Child 92, 776–780.

Brundage, K.L., Mohsini, K.G., Froese, A.B., et al., 1990. Bronchodilator response to ipratropium bromide in infants with bronchopulmonary dysplasia. Am Rev Respir Dis 142, 1137–1142.

Burnard, E.D., 1966. The pulmonary syndrome of Wilson and Mikity and respiratory function in very small premature infants. Pediatr Clin North Am 13, 999–1016.

Cabal, L.A., Larrazabal, C., Ramanathan, R., et al., 1987. Effects of metaproterenol on pulmonary mechanics, oxygenation and ventilation in infants with chronic lung disease. Journal of Pediatrics 110, 116–119.

Castro-Alcaraz, S., Greenberg, E.M., Bateman, D.A., et al., 2002. Patterns of colonisation with *Ureaplasma urealyticum* during neonatal intensive care unit hospitalisations of very low birthweight infants and the development of chronic lung disease. Pediatrics 110, e45.

Chan, V., Greenough, A., 1993. Randomized trial of methods of extubation in acute and chronic respiratory distress. Arch Dis Child 68, 570–572.

Chan, K.N., Noble-Jamieson, C.M., Elliman, A., et al., 1988. Airway responsiveness in low birthweight children and their mothers. Arch Dis Child 63, 905–910.

Chan, V., Greenough, A., Hird, M.F., 1991. Comparison of different rates of artificial ventilation for preterm infants ventilated beyond the first week of life. Early Hum Dev 26, 177–183.

Chan, V., Greenough, A., Cheeseman, P., et al., 1993. Vitamin A levels and feeding practice of neonates with and without chronic lung disease. J Perinat Med 21, 205–210.

Coalson, J.J., 2006. Pathology of bronchopulmonary dysplasia. Semin Perinatol 30, 179–184.

Coalson, J.J., King, R.J., Yang, F., et al., 1995. SP-A deficiency in primate model of bronchopulmonary dysplasia with infection. In situ mRNA and immunostains. Am J Respir Crit Care Med 151, 854–866.

Cochran, D.P., Pilling, D.W., Shaw, N.J., 1994. The relationship of pulmonary interstitial emphysema to subsequent type of chronic lung disease. Br J Radiol 76, 1155–1157.

Cooke, R., 1991. Factors associated with chronic lung disease in preterm infants. Arch Dis Child 66, 776–779.

Costarino, A.T.J., Gruskay, J.A., Corcoran, L., et al., 1992. Sodium restriction versus daily maintenance replacement in very low birth weight premature neonates: a randomized, blind therapeutic trial. Journal of Pediatrics 120, 99–106.

Couser, R.J., Ferrara, B., Wright, G.B., et al., 1996. Prophylactic indomethacin therapy in the first 24 hours of life for the prevention of patent ductus arteriosus in preterm infants treated prophylactically in the delivery room. Journal of Pediatrics 128, 631–637.

Crapo, J.D., Peters-Golden, M., Marsh-Salin, J., et al., 1978. Pathologic changes in the lungs of oxygen-adapted rats. A morphometric analysis. Laboratory Investigation 39, 640–653.

Cronin, C.M.G., Dean, H., MacDonald, N.T., et al., 1993. Basal and post-ACTH cortisol levels in preterm infants following treatment with dexamethasone. Clinical and Investigative Medicine 16, 8–14.

Crowley, P., Chalmers, I., Keirse, M., 1990. The effects of corticosteroid administration before preterm delivery: an overview of the evidence from controlled trials. Br J Obstet Gynaecol 97, 11–25.

Darlow, B.A., Graham, P.J., 2008. Vitamin A supplementation for preventing morbidity and mortality in very low birthweight infants. Cochrane Database Syst Rev.

Davis, J.M., Parad, R.B., Michele, T., et al., 2003. Recombinant human CuZnSOD

Study Group. Pulmonary outcome at one year corrected age in premature infants treated at birth with recombinant human CuZn superoxide dismutase. Pediatrics 111, 469–476.

De Boeck, K., Smith, J., van Lierde, S., et al., 1998. Response to bronchodilators in clinically stable 1-year-old patients with bronchopulmonary dysplasia. Eur J Pediatr 157, 75–79.

Denjean, A., Gulmaraes, H., Migdal, M., et al., 1992. Dose-related bronchodilator response to aerosolized salbutamol (albuterol) in ventilator-dependent premature infants. Journal of Pediatrics 120, 974–979.

De Rubertis, F.R., Michelis, M.F., Beck, N., et al., 1970. Complications of diuretic therapy: severe alkalosis and syndrome resembling inappropriate secretion of anti-diuretic hormone. Metabolism 19, 709–719.

Dimitriou, G., Greenough, A., Kavvadia, K., 2002. Fluid retention, colloid infusion and chronic lung disease development in very low birthweight infants. Neonatal Intensive Care 15, 13–18.

Doyle, L.W., Cheun, M.M., Ford, G.W., et al., 2001. Birth weight <1501 g and respiratory health at age 14. Arch Dis Child 84, 40–44.

Doyle, L.W., Davis, P.G. , Morley, C.J., et al., 2006. Low dose dexamethasone facilitates extubation among chronically ventilator dependent infants: a multicenter, international, randomized controlled trial. Pediatrics 117, 75–83.

Doyle, L.W., Davis, P.G., Morley, C.J., et al., 2007. Outcome at two years of age of infants from the DART study: a multicentre, international, randomized controlled trial of low dose dexamethasone. Pediatrics 119, 716–721.

Doyle, L.W., Ehrenkranz, R.A., Halliday, H.L., 2010. Postnatal hydrocortisone for preventing or treating bronchopulmonary dysplasia in preterm infants: a systematic review. Neonatology 98, 111–117.

Dugas, M.A., Nguyen, D., Frenette, L., et al., 2005. Fluticasone inhalation in moderate cases of bronchopulmonary dysplasia. Pediatrics 115, e566–e572.

Ehrenkranz, R.A., Bonta, B.W., Ablow, R.C., et al., 1978. Amelioration of bronchopulmonary dysplasia following vitamin E administration. A preliminary report. NEJM 299, 564–568.

Ehrenkranz, R.A., Walsh, M.C., Vohr, B.R., et al. National Institutes of Child Health and Human Development Neonatal Research Network, 2005. Validation of the National Institutes of Health consensus definition of bronchopulmonary dysplasia. Pediatrics 116, 1353–1360.

Eichenwald, E.C., Stark, A.R., 2007. Are postnatal steroids ever justified to treat severe bronchopulmonary dysplasia? Arch Dis Child Fetal Neonatal Ed 92, F334–F337.

Ellsbury, D.L., Acarregui, M.J., McGuiness, G.A., et al., 2002. Variability in the use of supplemental oxygen for bronchopulmonary dysplasia. Journal of Pediatrics 140, 247–249.

Emery, E.F., Greenough, A., 1992. Effect of dexamethasone on blood pressure: relationship to postnatal age. Eur J Pediatr 151, 364–366.

Eronen, M., Pesonen, E., Kurki, T., et al., 1994. Increased incidence of bronchopulmonary dysplasia after antenatal administration of indomethacin to prevent preterm labor. Journal of Pediatrics 124, 782–788.

Escobedo, M.B., Gonzalez, A., 1982. A baboon model of bronchopulmonary dysplasia. Exp Mol Pathol 37, 323–334.

Farhath, S., He, Z., Nakhla, T., et al., 2008. Pepsin, a marker of gastric contents, is increased in tracheal aspirates from preterm infants who develop bronchopulmonary dysplasia. Pediatrics 121, e253–e259.

Fauroux, B., Sardet, A., Foret, D., 1995. Home treatment for chronic respiratory failure in children: a prospective study. Eur Respir J 8, 2062–2066.

Filippone, M., Artov, M., Azchello, F., et al., 2003. Flow limitation in infants with BPD and respiratory function at school age. Lancet 361, 743–754.

Fowlie, P.W., 1996. Prophylactic indomethacin: systematic review and meta-analysis. Arch Dis Child Fetal Neonatal Ed 74, F81–F87.

Fujimura, M., Takeuchi, T., Ando, M., et al., 1983. Elevated immunoglobulin M levels in low birthweight neonates with chronic respiratory insufficiency. Early Hum Dev 9, 27–32.

Fujimura, M., Takeuchi, T., Kitajima, H., et al., 1989. Chorioamnionitis and serum IgM in Wilson-Mikity.

Fujimura, M., Kitajima, H., Nakayama, M., 1993. Increased leukocyte elastase of the tracheal aspirate at birth and neonatal pulmonary emphysema. Pediatrics 92, 564–569.

Garland, J.S., Buck, R.K., Allred, E.N., et al., 1995. Hypocarbia before surfactant therapy appears to increase bronchopulmonary dysplasia risk in infants with respiratory distress syndrome. Arch Pediatr Adolesc Med 149, 617–622.

Gerhardt, T., Hehre, D., Feller, R., et al., 1987. Serial determination of pulmonary function in infants with chronic lung disease. Journal of Pediatrics 110, 448–456.

Giffin, F., Greenough, A., Yuksel, B., 1995. Antiviral therapy in neonatal chronic lung disease. Early Hum Dev 42, 97–109.

Gitto, E., Reiter, R.J., Sabatino, G., et al., 2005. Correlation among cytokines, bronchopulmonary dysplasia and modality of ventilation in preterm newborns: improvements with melatonin treatment. J Pineal Res 39, 287–293.

Gonzalez, A., Sosenko, I.R.S., Chandar, J., et al., 1996. Influence of infection on patent ductus arteriosus and chronic lung disease in premature infants weighing 1000 g or less. Journal of Pediatrics 128, 470–478.

Gray, P.H., Rogers, Y., 1994. Are infants with bronchopulmonary dysplasia at risk for sudden infant death syndrome? Pediatrics 93, 774–777.

Greenough, A., Chan, V., Hird, M.F., 1992a. Positive end expiratory pressure in acute and chronic neonatal respiratory distress. Arch Dis Child 67, 320–323.

Greenough, A., Emery, E.F., Gamsu, H.R., 1992b. Dexamethasone and hypertension in chronic lung disease of preterm infants. Eur J Pediatr 152, 134–135.

Greenough, A., Emery, E.F., Hird, M.F., et al., 1993. Randomized controlled trial of albumin infusion in ill preterm infants. Eur J Pediatr 152, 157–159.

Greenough, A., Kavvadia, K., Johnson, A.H., et al., 1999. A simple chest radiograph score to predict chronic lung disease in prematurely born infants. Br J Radiol 72, 530–533.

Greenough, A., Dimitriou, G., Johnson, A.H., et al., 2000. The chest radiograph appearances of very premature infants at 36 weeks post conceptional age. Br J Radiol 73, 366–369.

Greenough, A., Boorman, J., Alexander, J., et al., 2001. Health care utilisation of CLD infants related to hospitalisation for RSV infection. Arch Dis Child 85, 463–468.

Greenough, A., Alexander, J., Burgess, S., et al., 2002. Home oxygen status on rehospitalisation and primary care requirements of chronic lung disease infants. Archives of Diseases in Childhood 86, 40–43.

Greenough, A., Alexander, J., Burgess, S., et al., 2004. High versus restricted use of home oxygen therapy, health care utilisation and the cost of care in CLD infants. Eur J Pediatr 163, 292–296.

Greenough, A., Alexander, J., Burgess, S., et al., 2006. Preschool health care utilisation related to home oxygen status. Archives of Disease in Childhood Fetal Neonatal Edition 91, F337–F341.

Greenough, A., Milner, A.D., Dimitriou, G., 2008. Synchronized mechanical ventilation for respiratory support in newborn infants. Cochrane Database Syst Rev.

Greenough, A., Shaheen, S.O., Shennan, A., et al., 2010. Respiratory outcomes in early childhood following antenatal vitamin C and E supplementation. Thorax 65, 998–1003.

Gregoire, M.-C., Lefebvre, F., Glorieux, J., 1998. Health and developmental outcomes at 18 months in very preterm infants with bronchopulmonary dysplasia. Pediatrics 101, 856–860.

Groneck, P., Reuss, D., Goetze-Speer, B., et al., 1993. Effects of dexamethasone on chemotactic activity and inflammatory mediators in tracheobronchial aspirates of preterm infants at risk for chronic lung disease. Journal of Pediatrics 122, 938–944.

Groneck, P., Goetze-Speer, B., Oppermann, M., et al., 1994. Association of pulmonary inflammation and increased microvascular permeability during the development of bronchopulmonary dysplasia: a sequential analysis of inflammatory mediators in respiratory fluids of high risk preterm neonates. Pediatrics 93, 712–718.

Gross, S.J., Iannuzzi, D.M., Kveselis, D.A., et al., 1999. Effect of preterm birth on pulmonary function at school age: a prospective controlled study. Journal of Pediatrics 133, 188–192.

Gunn, T., Reece, E.R., Metrakos, K., et al., 1981. Depressed T cells following neonatal steroid treatment. Pediatrics 67, 61–67.

Halliday, H., Ehrenkranz, R.A., 2001. Early postnatal (<96 hours) corticosteroids for preventing chronic lung disease in preterm infants. Cochrane Database Syst Rev.

Halliday, H., Ehrenkranz, R.A., 2003. Delayed (>3 weeks) postnatal corticosteroids for chronic lung disease in preterm infants. Cochrane Database Syst Rev.

Halliday, H., Ehrenkranz, R.A., Doyle, L.W., 2003. Moderately early (7–14 days) postnatal corticosteroids for preventing chronic lung disease in preterm infants. Cochrane Database Syst Rev.

Hallman, M., Pitkainen, O., Rauvala, H., et al., 1987. Glycolipid accumulation in lung effluent in bronchopulmonary dysplasia. Pediatr Res 21, 454A.

Hartnoll, G., Betremieux, P., Modi, N., 2000. Randomised controlled trial of postnatal sodium supplementation on oxygen dependency and body weight in 25–30 week gestational age infants. Arch Dis Child Fetal Neonatal Ed 82, F19–F23.

Hazinski, T.A., 1985. Furosemide decreases ventilation in young rabbits. Journal of Pediatrics 106, 81–85.

Hazinski, T.A., France, M., Kennedy, K.A., et al., 1989. Cimetidine reduces hyperoxic lung injury in lambs. J Appl Physiol 67, 2586–2592.

Henderson-Smart, D.J., Bhuta, T., Cools, F., et al., 2007. Elective high frequency oscillatory ventilation versus conventional ventilation for acute pulmonary dysfunction in preterm infants. Cochrane Database Syst Rev (1), CD000104.

Hislop, A.A., Haworth, S.G., 1990. Pulmonary vascular damage and the development of cor pulmonale following hyaline membrane disease. Pediatr Pulmonol 9, 152–156.

Hoepker, A., Seear, M., Petrocheilou, A., et al., 2008. Wilson–Mikity syndrome: updated diagnostic criteria based on nine cases and a review of the literature. Pediatr Pulmonol 43, 1004–1012.

Hofhuis, W., Hanekamp, M.N., Ijsselstijn, H., et al., 2011. Prospective longitudinal evaluation of lung function during the first year of life after extracorporeal membrane oxygenation. Pediatr Crit Care Med 12, 159–164.

Howlett, A., Ohlsson, A., 2003. Inositol for respiratory distress syndrome in preterm infants. Cochrane Database Systemic Reviews (4), CD000366.

Howling, S.J., Northway, W.H., Hansell, D.M., et al., 2000. Pulmonary sequelae of bronchopulmonary dysplasia survivors: high-resolution CT findings. American Journal of Roentgenology 174, 1323–1326.

Hufnagle, K.G., Khan, S.N., Penn, D., et al., 1982. Renal calcification: a complication of long term frusemide therapy in premature infants. Pediatrics 70, 360–363.

Husain, A.N., Siddiqui, N.H., Stocker, J.T., 1998. Pathology of arrested acinar development in postsurfactant bronchopulmonary dysplasia. Hum Pathol 29, 710–717.

Israel, B.A., Sherman, F.S., Guthrie, R.D., 1993. Hypertrophic cardiomyopathy associated with dexamethasone therapy for chronic lung disease in preterm infants. Am J Perinatol 10, 307–310.

Jain, A., Madsen, D.C., Auld, P.A., et al., 1995. L2 oxothiazolidine-4-carboxylate, a cysteine precursor stimulates growth and normalises tissue glutathione concentrations in rats fed a sulphur amino acid deficient diet. J Nutr 125, 851–856.

Jobe, A.H., Bancalari, E., 2001. Bronchopulmonary dysplasia. NICHD-NHLBI-ORD Workshop. Am J Respir Crit Care Med 163, 1723–1729.

Jobe, A.H., Ikegami, M., 1998. Mechanisms initiating lung injury in the preterm. Early Hum Dev 53, 81–94.

Jobe, A.H., Michell, B.R., Gunkel, J.H., 1993. Beneficial effects of the combined use of prenatal corticosteroids and postnatal surfactant on preterm infants. Am J Obstet Gynecol 168, 508–513.

Johnson, L., Bowen, F.W.J., Abbasi, S., et al., 1985. Relationship of prolonged pharmacologic serum levels of vitamin E to the incidence of sepsis and necrotizing enterocolitis in infants with birthweight ,1500 g or less. Pediatrics 75, 619–638.

Jones, C.A., Cayabyab, R.G., Kwong, K.Y.C., et al., 1996. Undetectable interleukin (IL)-10 and persistent IL-8 expression early in hyaline membrane disease: a possible developmental basis for the predisposition to chronic lung inflammation in preterm newborns. Pediatr Res 39, 966–975.

Kao, L.C., Warburton, D., Sargent, C.W., et al., 1983. Furosemide acutely decreases airway resistance in chronic bronchopulmonary dysplasia. Journal of Pediatrics 103, 624–629.

Kao, L.C., Warburton, D., Cheng, M.H., et al., 1984a. Effect of oral diuretics on pulmonary mechanics in infants with chronic bronchopulmonary dysplasia: results of a double-blind crossover sequential trial. Pediatrics 74, 37–44.

Kao, L.C., Warburton, D., Platzker, A.C.G., et al., 1984b. Effect of isoproterenol inhalation on airways resistance in chronic bronchopulmonary dysplasia. Pediatrics 73, 509–514.

Kao, L.C., Durand, D.J., Dhillias, B.L., et al., 1987. Oral theophylline and diuretics improve pulmonary mechanics in infants with bronchopulmonary dysplasia. Journal of Pediatrics 111, 439–444.

Kao, L.C., Durand, D.J., Nickerson, B.G., 1989. Effects of inhaled metaproterenol and atropine on the pulmonary mechanics of infants with bronchopulmonary dysplasia. Pediatr Pulmonol 6, 74–80.

Kao, L.C., Durand, D.J., McCrea, R.C., et al., 1994. Randomized trial of long-term diuretic therapy for infants with oxygen-dependent bronchopulmonary dysplasia. Journal of Pediatrics 124, 772–781.

Kavvadia, V., Greenough, A., Dimitriou, G., et al., 1999. Comparison of the effect of two fluid input regimes on perinatal lung function in ventilated infants of very low birthweight. Eur J Pediatr 158, 917–922.

Kavvadia, V., Greenough, A., Dimitriou, G., et al., 2000. Randomized trial of fluid restriction in ventilated very low birthweight infants. Arch Dis Child Fetal Neonatal Ed 83, F91–F96.

Khemani, E., McElhinney, D.B., Rhein, L., et al., 2007. Pulmonary artery hypertension in formerly premature infants with bronchopulmonary dysplasia: clinical features and outcomes in the surfactant era. Pediatrics 120, 1260–1269.

Kinsella, J.P., Parker, T.A., Galan, H., et al., 1997. Effects of inhaled nitric oxide on pulmonary edema and lung neutrophil accumulation in severe experimental hyaline membrane disease. Pediatr Res 41, 457–463.

Klinger, G., Sirota, L., Lusky, A., et al., 2006. Bronchopulmonary dysplasia in very low birth weight infants is associated with prolonged hospital stay. J Perinatol 10, 640–644.

Kojima, T., Sasai, M., Kobayashi, Y., 1993. Increased soluble ICAM-1 in tracheal aspirates of infants with bronchopulmonary dysplasia. Lancet 342, 1023–1024.

Kornhauser, M.S., Cullen, J.A., Baumgart, S., et al., 1994. Risk factors for bronchopulmonary dysplasia after extracorporeal membrane oxygenation. Arch Pediatr Adolesc Med 148, 820–825.

Kotecha, S., Wilson, L., Wangoo, A., et al., 1996. Increase in interleukin (IL)-1b and IL-6 in bronchoalveolar lavage fluid obtained from infants with chronic lung disease of prematurity. Pediatr Res 40, 250–256.

Krauss, A.N., Levin, A.R., Grossman, H., et al., 1970. Physiologic studies on infants with Wilson–Mikity syndrome. Journal of Pediatrics 77, 27–36.

Kraybill, E.N., Runyan, D.K., Bose, C.L., et al., 1989. Risk factors for chronic lung disease in infants with birth weights of 751 to 1000 grams. Journal of Pediatrics 115, 115–120.

Kugelman, A., Durand, M., Garg, M., 1997. Pulmonary effect of inhaled furosemide in ventilated infants with severe bronchopulmonary dysplasia. Pediatrics 99, 71–75.

Kulik, T.J., Rhein, L.M., Mullen, M.P., 2010. Pulmonary arterial hypertension in infants with chronic lung disease: will we ever understand it? Journal of Pediatrics 157, 186–190.

Lassos, P., Turanlahti, M., Heikkila, P., et al., 2001. Pulmonary vascular endothelial growth factor and Flt-1 in fetuses in acute and chronic lung disease and in persistent pulmonary hypertension of the newborn. Am J Respir Crit Care Med 164, 1981–1987.

Laughon, M., O'Shea, M.T., Allred, E.N., et al., 2009. Chronic lung disease and developmental delay at 2 years of age in children born before 28 weeks' gestation. Pediatrics 124, 637–648.

Lauterbach, R., Szymura-Oleksiak, J., Pawlik, D., et al., 2006. Nebulised pentoxifylline for prevention of bronchopulmonary dysplasia in very low birthweight infants: a pilot clinical study. Journal of Maternal and Fetal Neonatal Medicine 19, 433–448.

Linder, N., Kuint, J., German, B., et al., 1995. Hypertrophy of the tongue associated with inhaled corticosteroid therapy in premature infants. Journal of Pediatrics 127, 651–653.

Lister, P., Iles, R., Shaw, B., et al., 2010. Inhaled steroids for neonatal chronic lung disease. Cochrane Database Syst Rev.

Lonnqvist, P.A., Jonsson, B., Winberg, P., et al., 1995. Inhaled nitric oxide in infants with developing or established chronic lung disease. Acta Paediatr 84, 1188–1192.

Manktelow, B.N., Draper, E.S., Annamalai, S., et al., 2001. Factors affecting the incidence of chronic lung disease of prematurity in 1987, 1992 and 1997. Archives of Disease in Childhood. Fetal and Neonatal Edition 85, F33–F35.

Margraf, L.R., Tomashefski, J.F., Bruce, M.C., et al., 1991. Morphometric analysis of the lung in bronchopulmonary dysplasia. Am Rev Respir Dis 143, 391–400.

May, C., Patel, S., Peacock, J., et al., 2007. End tidal carbon monoxide levels in prematurely born infants developing bronchopulmonary dysplasia. Pediatr Res 61, 474–478.

McCann, E.M., Lewis, K., Demin, D.D., et al., 1985. Controlled trial of furosemide therapy in infants with chronic lung disease. Journal of Pediatrics 106, 957–962.

McLean, A., Townsend, A., Clark, J., et al., 2000. Quality of life of mothers and families caring for preterm infants requiring home oxygen therapy: a brief report. J Paediatr Child Health 36, 440–444.

Mercier, J.C., Hummler, H., Durrmeyer, H., et al., 2010. Inhaled nitric oxide for the prevention of bronchopulmonary dysplasia in premature babies. Lancet 375, 346–354.

Mirro, R., Armstead, W., Leffler, C., 1990. Increased airway leukotriene levels in infants with severe bronchopulmonary dysplasia. Am J Dis Child 144, 160–161.

Mizuno, K., Nishida, Y., Taki, M., et al., 2007. Infants with bronchopulmonary dysplasia suckle with weak pressures to maintain breathing during feeding. Pediatrics 120, e1035–e1042.

Morley, C.J., Davis, P.G., Doyle, L.B., et al., 2008. Nasal CPAP or intubation at birth for very preterm infants. NEJM 358, 700–708.

Morray, J.P., Fox, W.W., Kettrick, R.G., et al., 1982. Improvement in lung mechanics as a function of age in the infant with severe bronchopulmonary dysplasia. Pediatr Res 16, 290–294.

Motoyama, E.K., Fort, M.D., Klesh, K.W., et al., 1987. Early onset of airway reactivity in premature infants with bronchopulmonary dysplasia. Am Rev Respir Dis 136, 50–57.

Moyer, W.J., 1950. Vitamin E levels in term and premature newborn infants. Pediatrics 6, 893–896.

Murch, S.H., Costeloe, K., Klein, N.J., et al., 1996a. Mucosal tumour necrosis factor – a production and extensive disruption of sulfated glycosaminoglycans begin within hours of birth in neonatal respiratory distress syndrome. Pediatr Res 40, 484–489.

Murch, S.H., Costeloe, K., Klein, N.J., et al., 1996b. Early production of macrophage inflammatory protein-1-alpha occurs in respiratory distress syndrome and is associated with poor outcome. Pediatr Res 40, 490–497.

Najak, Z.D., Harris, E.M., Lazzara, A., et al., 1983. Pulmonary effects of furosemide in preterm infants with lung disease. Journal of Pediatrics 102, 758–763.

Ng, G.Y., Ohlsson, A., 2002. Cromolyn sodium for the prevention of chronic lung disease in preterm infants. Cochrane Database of Syst Rev.

Ng, G.Y., Da, S., Ohlsson, A., 2001. Bronchodilators for the prevention and treatment of chronic lung disease in preterm infants. Cochrane Database Syst Rev (3), CD003214.

Nickerson, B.G., Taussig, L.M., 1980. Family history of asthma in infants with bronchopulmonary dysplasia. Pediatrics 65, 1140–1144.

Noble-Jamieson, C.M., Regev, R., Silverman, M., 1989. Dexamethasone in neonatal chronic lung disease: Pulmonary effects and intracranial complications. Eur J Pediatr 148, 365–367.

Northway, W.H., 1979. Observations on bronchopulmonary dysplasia. Journal of Pediatrics 95, 815–818.

Northway, W.H.J., Rosan, R.C., Porter, D.Y., 1967. Pulmonary disease following respiratory therapy of hyaline membrane disease: bronchopulmonary dysplasia. NEJM 276, 357–368.

Northway, W.H. Jr, Moss, R.B., Carlisle, K.B., et al., 1990. Late pulmonary sequelae of bronchopulmonary dysplasia. NEJM 323, 1793–1799.

Nykanen, P., Anttila, E., Heinonen, K., et al., 2007. Early hypoadrenalism in premature infants at risk for bronchopulmonary dysplasia or death. Acta Paediatr 96, 1600–1605.

Obladen, M., 1988. Alterations in surfactant composition. In: Merritt, A., Northway, W.H., Boynton, B.R. (Eds.), Bronchopulmonary Dysplasia. Blackwell Scientific, Boston, pp. 131–141.

Ochiai, M., Hikino, S., Yabuuchi, H., et al., 2008. A new scoring system for computed tomography of the chest for assessing the clinical status of bronchopulmonary dysplasia. Journal of Pediatrics 152, 90–95.

Odezmir, A., Brown, M.A., Morgan, W.J., 1997. Markers and mediators of inflammation in neonatal lung disease Pediatr Pulmonol 23, 292–306.

Oh, W., Poindexter, B.B., Perritt, R., et al., 2005. Association between fluid intake and weight loss during the first ten days of life and risk of bronchopulmonary dysplasia in extremely low birth weight infants. Journal of Pediatrics 147, 786–790.

Oppenheim, C., Marmou-Mani, T., Sayegh, N., et al., 1994. Bronchopulmonary dysplasia: value of CT in identifying pulmonary sequelae. American Journal of Roentgenology 163, 169–172.

Palta, M., Gabbert, D., Weinstein, M.R., et al., 1991. Multivariate assessment of traditional risk factors for chronic lung disease in very low birth weight neonates. The Newborn Lung Project. Journal of Pediatrics 119, 285–292.

Pandit, P.B., Dunn, M.S., Kelly, E.N., et al., 1995. Surfactant replacement in neonates with early chronic lung disease. Pediatrics 95, 851–854.

Panitch, H.B., Allen, J.L., Alpert, B.E., et al., 1994. Effects of CPAP on lung mechanics in infants with acquired tracheobronchomalacia. Am J Respir Crit Care Med 150, 1341–1346.

Panitch, H.B., Downes, J.J., Kennedy, J.S., et al., 1996. Guidelines for home care of children with chronic respiratory insufficiency. Pediatr Pulmonol 21, 52–56.

Papile, L.-A., Tyson, J.E., Stoll, B.J., et al., 1998. A multicenter trial of two dexamethasone regimens in ventilator-dependent premature infants. NEJM 338, 1112–1118.

Pearson, E., Bose, C., Snidow, T., et al., 1992. Trial of vitamin A supplementation in very low birth weight infants at risk for bronchopulmonary dysplasia. Journal of Pediatrics 121, 420–427.

Pera, A., Byun, A., Gribar, S., et al., 2002. Dexamethasone therapy and Candida sepsis in neonates less than 1250 grams. J Perinatol 22, 204–208.

Pomerance, J.J., Puri, A.P., 1980. Treatment of neonatal bronchopulmonary dysplasia with steroids. Pediatr Res 14, 649A.

Prendergast, M., May, C., Broughton, S., et al., 2011. Chorioamnionitis, lung function and bronchopulmonary dysplasia in prematurely born infants. Arch Dis Child Fetal Neonatal Ed 96, F270–F274.

Ramanathan, R., Durand, M., Larrazabal, C., 1987. Pulse oximetry in very low birth weight infants with acute and chronic lung disease. Pediatrics 79, 612–617.

Ramsay, P.L., O'Brien Smith, E., Hegemier, S., et al., 1998. Early markers for the development of bronchopulmonary dysplasia: soluble E-selectin and ICAM-1. Pediatrics 102, 927–932.

Rastogi, A., Luayon, M., Ajayi, O.A., et al., 1994. Nebulized furosemide in infants with bronchopulmonarydysplasia. Journal of Pediatrics 125, 976–979.

Rastogi, A., Akintorin, S.M., Bez, M.L., et al., 1996. A controlled trial of dexamethasone to prevent bronchopulmonary dysplasia in surfactant-treated infants. Pediatrics 98, 204–210.

Regev, R., DeVries, L.S., Noble-Jamieson, C.M., et al., 1987. Dexamethasone and increased intracranial echogenicity. Lancet i, 632–633.

Reimers, K.J., Carlson, S.J., Lombard, K.A., 1992. Nutritional managementof infants with bronchopulmonary dysplasia. Nutr Clin Pract 7, 127–132.

Rhodes, P.G., Hall, R.T., Leonidas, J.C., 1975. Chronic pulmonary disease in neonates with assisted ventilation. Pediatrics 55, 788–795.

Rojas, M.A., Gonzalez, A., Bancalari, E., et al., 1995. Changing trends in the epidemiology and pathogenesis of neonatal chronic lung disease. Journal of Pediatrics 126, 605–610.

Rooklin, A.R., Moomjian, A.S., Shutack, J.G., et al., 1979. Theophylline therapy in bronchopulmonary dysplasia. Journal of Pediatrics 95, 882–888.

Russell, G.A.B., Cooke, R.W.I., 1995. Randomised controlled trial of allopurinol prophylaxis in very preterm infants. Arch Dis Child Fetal Neonatal Ed 73, F27–F31.

Rybak, L.P., 1982. Pathophysiology of frusemide toxicity. J Otolaryngol 11, 127–133.

Sandri, F., Plavka, R., Ancora, G., et al., 2010. Prophylactic or early selective surfactant combined with nCPAP in very preterm infants. Pediatrics 125, e1402–e1409.

Santuz, P., Baraldi, E., Zaramella, P., et al., 1995. Factors limiting exercise performance in long term survivors of bronchopulmonary dysplasia. Am J Respir Crit Care Med 152, 1284–1289.

Saunders, R.A., Milner, A.D., Hopkin, I.E., 1978. Longitudinal studies of infants with the Wilson–Mikity syndrome. Biol Neonate 33, 90–99.

Sauve, R.S., Singhal, N., 1985. Long term morbidity of infants with bronchopulmonary dysplasia. Pediatrics 76, 725–733.

Savage, M.O., Wilkinson, A.R., Baum, J.D., et al., 1975. Frusemide in respiratory distress syndrome.Arch Dis Child 50, 709–713.

Sawyer, M.H., Edwards, D.K., Spector, S.A., 1987. Cytomegalovirus infection and bronchopulmary dysplasia in premature infants. Am J Dis Child 141, 303–305.

Schmidt, B., Davis, P., Moddemann, D., et al., 2001. Long term effects of indomethacin prophylaxis in extremely low birth weight infants. NEJM 344, 1966–1972.

Schmidt, B., Roberts, R.S., Davis, P., et al., 2006a, Caffeine therapy for apnea of prematurity. NEJM 354, 2112–2121.

Schmidt, B., Roberts, R.S., Fanaroff, A., et al., 2006b. Indomethacin prophylaxis, patent ductus arteriosus and the risk of bronchopulmonary dysplasia: further analysis from the trial of indomethacin prophylaxis in preterms (TIPP). Journal of Pediatrics 148, 730–734.

Schmidt, B., Roberts, R.S., Davis, P., et al., 2007. Long term effects of caffeine therapy for apnea of prematurity. NEJM 357, 1893–1902.

Sekar, K.C., Duke, J.C., 1991. Sleep apnea and hypoxemia in recently weaned premature infants with and without bronchopulmonary dysplasia. Pediatr Pulmonol 10, 112–116.

Shah, S.S., Ohlsson, A., Halliday, H.L., et al., 2007. Inhaled versus systemic corticosteroid for the treatment of chronic lung disease in ventilated very low birth weight preterm infants. Cochrane Database Systemic Review CD002057.

Shah, V., Ohlsson, A., Halliday, H.L., et al., 2007. Early administration of inhaled corticosteroids for preventing chronic lung disease in ventilated very low birth weight preterm neonates. Cochrane Database Syst Rev (2), CD001969.

Shaw, N.J., Ruggins, N., Cooke, R.W.I., 1993. Infants with chronic lung disease: predictors of mortality at day 28. J Perinatol 13, 464–467.

Shenai, J.P., 1999. Vitamin A supplementation in very low birth weight neonates: rationale and evidence. Pediatrics 104, 1369–1374.

Shenai, J.P., Chytil, F., Stahlman, M.T., 1985. Vitamin A status of neonates with bronchopulmonary dysplasia. Pediatr Res 19, 185–188.

Shenai, J.P., Kennedy, K.A., Chytil, F., et al., 1987. Clinical trial of vitamin A supplementation in infants susceptible to bronchopulmonary dysplasia. Journal of Pediatrics 111, 269–277.

Short, A., Cooke, R.W.I., 1991. The incidence of renal calcification in preterm infants. Arch Dis Child 66, 412–417.

Simon, L., 1980. Protection against toxic effect of sustained hyperoxia on lung macrophages by superoxide dismutase. Clin Res 28, 432A.

Singer, L., Martin, R.J., Hawkins, S.W., et al., 1992. Oxygen desaturation complicates feeding in infants with bronchopulmonary dysplasia after discharge. Pediatrics 90, 380–384.

Smith, L.J., van Asperen, P.P., McKay, K.O., et al., 2008. Reduced exercise capacity in children born very preterm. Pediatrics 122, e287–e293.

Sosenko, I.R.S., Rodriguez-Pierce, M., Bancalari, E., 1993. Effects of early initiation of intravenous lipid administration on the incidence and severity of chronic lung disease in premature infants. Journal of Pediatrics 123, 975–982.

Spear, M.L., Reeves, G., Pearlman, S.A., 1993. Diabetic ketoacidosis after steroid administration for bronchopulmonary dysplasia: a case report. J Perinatol 13, 232–234.

Stevens, T., Harrington, E., Blennow, M., et al., 2007. Early surfactant administration with brief ventilation vs selective surfactant and continued mechanical ventilation for preterm infants with or at risk for respiratory distress syndrome. Cochrane Database Systemic Reviews (4), CD003063.

Stocker, J.T., 1986. Pathologic features of long standing 'healed' bronchopulmonary dysplasia: a study of 28 3- to 40-month old infants. Hum Pathol 17, 943–961.

Stocks, J., Godfrey, S., Reynolds, E.O.R., 1978. Airway resistance in infants after various treatments for hyaline membrane disease: special emphasis on prolonged high levels of inspired oxygen. Pediatrics 61, 178–183.

STOP-ROP Multicenter Study Group, 2000. Supplemental Therapeutic Oxygen for Prethreshold Retinopathy Of Prematurity (STOP-ROP), a randomized, controlled trial. I: Primary outcomes. Pediatrics 105, 295–310.

Strayer, D.S., Merritt, T.A., Lwebuga-Mukasa, J., et al., 1986. Surfactant–antisurfactant immune complexesin infants with respiratory distress syndrome. Am J Pathol 122, 353–362.

Streubel, A.H., Donohue, P.K., Aucott, S.W., 2008. The epidemiology of atypical chronic lung disease in extremely low birth weight infants. J Perinatol 28, 141–148.

SUPPORT Study Group of the Eunice Kennedy Shriver NICHD Research Network, 2010. Early CPAP versus surfactant in extremely preterm infants. NEJM 362, 1970–1979.

Suresh, G.K., Soll, R.F., 2002. Superoxide dismutase for preventing chronic lung disease in mechanically ventilated preterm infants. Cochrane Database Syst Rev.

Taghizadeh, A., Reynolds, E.O.R., 1976. Pathogenesis of bronchopulmonary dysplasia following hyaline membrane disease. Am J Pathol 82, 241–264.

Tang, J.R., Markham, N.E., Lin, Y.J., et al., 2004. Inhaled nitric oxide attenuates pulmonary hypertension and improves lung growth in infant rats after neonatal treatment with a VEGF receptor inhibitor. Am J Physiol Lung Cell Mol Physiol 287, L344–L351.

Taylor, D.W., 1956. The effects of vitamin E and of methylene blue on the manifestations of oxygen poisoning in the rat. J Physiol 131, 200–210.

Thébaud, B., 2007. Angiogenesis in lung development, injury and repair: implications for chronic lung disease of prematurity. Neonatology 91, 291–297.

Thébaud, B., Ladha, F., Michelakis, E.D., 2005. Vascular endothelial growth factor gene therapy increases survival, promotes lung angiogenesis, and prevents alveolar damage in hyperoxia-induced lung injury: evidence that angiogenesis participates in alveolarization, Circulation 112, 2477–2486.

Thomas, M., Greenough, A., Johnson, A., et al., 2003a. Frequent wheeze at follow-up of very preterm infants: which factors are predictive? Arch Dis Child Fetal Neonatal Ed 88, F329–F332.

Thomas, M., Greenough, A., Morton, M., 2003b. Prolonged ventilation and intact survival in very low birth weight infants. Eur J Pediatr 162, 65–67.

Thome, U.H., Carroll, W., Wu, T.J., et al., 2006. Outcome of extremely preterm infants randomized at birth to different PaCO$_2$ targets during the first seven days of life. Biol Neonate 90, 218–225.

Tooley, W., 1979. Epidemiology of bronchopulmonary dysplasia. Journal of Pediatrics 95, 851–858.

Tschanz, S.A., Damke, B.M., Burri, P.H., 1995. Influence of postnatally administered glucocorticoids on rat lung growth. Biol Neonate 68, 229–245.

Tyson, J.E., Wright, L.L., Oh, W., et al., 1999. Vitamin A supplementation for extremely-low-birth-weight infants. National Institute of Child Health and Human Development Neonatal Research Network 340, 1962–1968.

van Lierde, S., Cornelis, A., Devlieger, H., et al., 1991. Different patterns of pulmonary sequelae after hyaline membrane disease: heterogeneity of bronchopulmonary dysplasia. Biol Neonate 60, 152–162.

van Marter, L.J., Ammann, O., Allred, E.N., et al., 2002. Chorioamnionitis, mechanical ventilation and postnatal sepsis as modulators of chronic lung disease in preterm infants. Journal of Pediatrics 140, 171–176.

Vrijlandt, E.J., Gerritsen, J., Marike Boezen, H., et al., 19 Collaborative Study Group, 2005. Gender differences in respiratory symptoms in 19 year old adults born preterm. Respir Res 6, 117.

Vrlenich, L.A., Bozynski, M.E.A., Shyr, Y., et al., 1995. The effect of bronchopulmonary dysplasia on growth at school age. Pediatrics 95, 855–859.

Wada, K., Jobe, A.H., Ikegami, M., 1997. Tidal volume effects on surfactant treatment responses with the initiation of ventilation in preterm lambs. J Appl Physiol 83, 1054–1061.

Walsh, M.C., Yao, O., Gettner, P., et al., 2004. Impact of a physiological definition on bronchopulmonary dysplasia rates. Pediatrics 114, 1305–1311.

Wang, E.E.L., Cassell, G.H., Sanchez, P.J., et al., 1993. Ureaplasma urealyticum and chronic lung disease of prematurity: critical appraisal of the literature on causation. Clin Infect Dis 17, S112–S116.

Wang, E.E., Ohlasson, A., Kellner, J.D., 1995. Association of Ureaplasma urealyticum colonization with chronic lung disease of prematurity: result of meta-analysis. Journal of Pediatrics 127, 640–644.

Watterberg, K.L., Murphy, S., 1993. Failure of cromolyn sodium to reduce the incidence of bronchopulmonary dysplasia: a pilot study. The Neonatal Cromolyn Study Group. Pediatrics 91, 803–806.

Watterberg, K.L., Scott, S.M., 1995. Evidence of early adrenal insufficiency in babies who develop bronchopulmonary dysplasia. Pediatrics 95, 120–125.

Watterberg, K.L., Demers, L.M., Scott, S.M., et al., 1996. Chorioamnionitis and early lung inflammation in infants in whom bronchopulmonary dysplasia develops. Pediatrics 97, 210–215.

Watterberg, K.L., Gerdes, J.S., Cole, C.H., et al., 2004. Prophylaxis of early adrenal insufficiency to prevent bronchopulmonary dysplasia: a multicenter trial. Pediatrics 114, 1649–1657.

Wauer, R.R., Schmatisch, G., Bohne, B., et al., 1992. Randomized double blind trial of ambroxol in the treatment of respiratory distress syndrome. Eur J Pediatr 151, 357–363.

Werthammer, J., Brown, E.R., Neff, R.K., et al., 1982. Sudden infant death syndrome in infants with bronchopulmonary dysplasia. Pediatrics 69, 301–304.

Wilkie, R.A., Bryan, M.H., 1987. Effect of bronchodilators on airway resistance in ventilator-dependent neonates with chronic lung disease. Journal of Pediatrics 111, 278–282.

Wilkinson, A.R., Bros, D.M., Ziang, Z.D., 2007. Functional impairmen of the brainstem in infants with bronchopulmonary dysplasia. Pediatrics 120, 362–371.

Wilson, M.G., Mikity, V.G., 1960. A new form of respiratory disease in premature infants. Am J Dis Child 99, 489–499.

Wilson-Costello, D., Walsh, M.C., Langer, J.C., et al., 2009. Impact of postnatal corticosteroid (PNS). Use on neurodevelopment at 18–22 months adjusted age: effects of dose, timing and risk of bronchopulmonary dysplasia in extremely low birthweight infants (ELBW). Pediatrics 123, e430–e437.

Wong, Y.C., Beardsmore, C.S., Silverman, M., 1982. Pulmonary sequelae of neonatal respiratory distress in very low birthweight infants: a clinical and physiological study. Arch Dis Child 57, 418–424.

Wong, P.M., Lees, A.N., Louw, J., et al., 2008. Emphysema in young adult survivors of moderate to severe bronchopulmonary dysplasia. Eur Respir J 32, 321–328.

Yeh, T.F., Lin, H.C., Chang, C.H., et al., 2008. Early intratracheal instillation of budesonide using surfactant as a vehicle to prevent chronic lung disease in preterm infants: a pilot study. Pediatrics 121, e1310–e1318.

Yoder, B.A., Harrison, M., Clark, R.H., 2009. Time-related changes in steroid use and bronchopulmonary dysplasia in preterm infants. Pediatrics 124, 673–679.

Yoshioka, T., Sugive, A., Shimaola, T., 1979. Superoxide dismutase activity in the maternal and cord blood. Biol Neonate 36, 173–180.

Yüksel, B., Greenough, A., 1991. Ipratropium bromide for symptomatic preterm infants. Eur J Pediatr 150, 854–857.

Yüksel, B., Greenough, A., 1992a. Acute deteriorations in neonatal chronic lung disease. Eur J Pediatr 151, 697–700.

Yüksel, B., Greenough, A., 1992b. Inhaled sodium cromoglycate for preterm infants with respiratory symptoms at follow-up. Respir Med 86, 131–134.

Yüksel, B., Greenough, A., Maconochie, I., 1990. Effective bronchodilator therapy by a simple spacer device for wheezy premature infants in the first two years of life. Arch Dis Child 65, 782–785.

Yüksel, B., Greenough, A., Green, S., 1991a. Paradoxical response to nebulized ipratropium bromide in preterm infants asymptomatic at follow-up. Respir Med 85, 189–194.

Yüksel, B., Greenough, A., Karani, J., et al., 1991b. Chest radiograph scoring system for use in preterm infants. Br J Radiol 64, 1015–1018.

Zimmerman, J.J., 1995. Bronchoalveolar inflammatory pathophysiology of bronchopulmonary dysplasia. Clin Perinatol 22, 429–456.

Part 4: **Apnoea and bradycardia**

Simon Hannam

Introduction

Apnoea is a commonly encountered phenomenon on the neonatal unit, particularly in preterm babies. Episodes of cessation of breathing can lead to hypoxaemia and bradycardia requiring resuscitation. As there are many different causes of apnoea, the treatment of the condition depends on the results of investigation into, and diagnosis of, the underlying pathology.

Definition

The American Academy of Pediatrics defines apnoea as a pause in breathing of greater than 20 seconds or one of less than 20 seconds and associated with bradycardia and/or cyanosis (American Academy of Pediatrics Taskforce on Prolonged Apnea 1978). A wide range of apnoea durations have been studied, varying from 2 (Hannam et al. 1998) to >15 seconds (Barrington and Finer 1990; Hodgman et al. 1990). In practice most apnoea alarms on neonatal units are set up to detect those apnoeas lasting for greater than 20 seconds. Apnoea must be distinguished from periodic breathing (see below), which is common in preterm infants and in which there are bursts of respiratory activity separated with apnoeic pauses lasting at least 3 seconds (Glotzbach et al. 1989).

Incidence of clinical apnoea

There is an inverse correlation between the frequency of apnoea and gestational age. Apnoea occurs in over 80% of babies born at less than 30 weeks of gestation, about 50% of those born at 30–31 weeks, 14% born at 32–33 weeks and 7% born at 34–35 weeks (Henderson-Smart 1981).

Types of apnoea

There are three types of apnoea: central, obstructive and mixed. In central apnoea, there is a cessation of both respiratory effort and nasal airflow (Fig. 27.50A). With obstructive apnoea, nasal airflow ceases as the infant makes increasing respiratory effort in an attempt to overcome partial or total upper airway obstruction (Fig. 27.50B). The third type of apnoea is described as mixed and has both central and obstructive components. During central apnoeas, upper airway obstruction can occur, as reflected by the loss of cardiac artefact in the airflow trace (Milner et al. 1980). A reclassification of apnoea has been proposed using the presence or absence of amplified cardiac airflow artefact in the respiratory airflow trace to define whether an apnoea is central or obstructive (Lemke et al. 1996). Central apnoeas are those with the cardiac artefact present, obstructive where it is absent, and mixed where the artefact is absent during part of the apnoea (Lemke et al. 1998). The distribution of apnoea type has been demonstrated to vary with the length of apnoea in preterm infants (Butcher-Puech et al. 1985). Butcher-Puech et al. (1985) analysed 1520 episodes of apnoea of over 10 seconds' duration. With increasing length of apnoea, the proportion of central apnoea decreased from 69% to 29%, whilst that of mixed apnoeas increased from 20% to 60%. Pure obstructive apnoeas in preterm babies make up between 6% and 10% of the total number of apnoeas (Upton et al. 1991; Finer et al. 1992).

Mechanisms of apnoea

Central apnoea

Signals for the involuntary control of breathing which maintain rhythmic ventilation originate in the brainstem in the area of the medulla oblongata in the pre-Bolzinger complex. Input into the respiratory centre arises from three primary sources: chemoreceptors, mechanoreceptors of the lung and upper airway, and input from the cerebral cortex. Delayed maturation of any of these sites could potentially result in apnoea.

Brainstem generator

There is evidence for immaturity of the brainstem generator in the aetiology of apnoea of prematurity. In the preterm brain it has been demonstrated that, on histological examination, there were fewer synaptic connections, a reduced number of dendritic arborisations and a generalised reduction in myelinisation (Kattwinkel 1977). Functionally, brainstem conduction times, as detected by auditory evoked responses, have been shown to be faster with increasing gestational age (Henderson-Smart et al. 1983). Of interest, this slowing improves after treatment with aminophylline (Abu-Shaweesh and Martin 2008).

Chemoreceptors

Further evidence for dysfunction of the brainstem in apnoea has been reported in studies investigating the response of preterm infants to hypercarbia. Preterm infants who were having apnoeas had a depressed ventilatory response to CO_2 compared with those not having apnoeas (Gerhardt and Bancalari 1984a).

Hypoxic respiratory depression may play a role in apnoea of prematurity. Peripheral chemoreceptors located outside the brainstem in the carotid bodies near the bifurcation of the common carotid arteries receptors are primarily responsible for the ventilatory response to hypoxia. Preterm and newborn infants have been shown to exhibit an unusual pattern in their response to hypoxia in that they have an initial rapid increase in minute ventilation followed by respiratory depression (Martin et al. 1998). Several neurotransmitters have been implicated in the development of hypoxic respiratory depression. These include γ-aminobutyric acid (GABA), adenosine and endorphins (Martin and Abu-Shaweesh 2005). When the receptors for these neurotransmitters were blocked in animal models using bicuculline, methylxanthines or naloxone, respectively, the hypoxic respiratory depressive response was reduced. Experimental evidence suggests that adenosine and the inhibitory neurotransmitter GABA might interact with each other to cause apnoea (Abu-Shaweesh and Martin 2008). Blockading $GABA_A$ receptors in piglets resulted in the reduction of an adenosine A_{2A} agonist-induced inhibition of phrenic nerve activity (Wilson et al. 2004). When the same adenosine agonist was administered directly into the cisternal system, there was inhibition of the phrenic nerve and stimulation of the laryngeal chemoreflex (LCR) (Abu-Shaweesh 2007).

A strong Hering–Breuer inflation reflex, as assessed by the prolongation of expiration following occlusion of the airway at end inspiration, has been demonstrated in preterm infants (Stocks et al. 1996). In contrast, the reflex has been shown to be significantly reduced in strength in preterm infants experiencing apnoea (Gerhardt and Bancalari 1984b). It is difficult to explain the increase in the strength of the Hering–Breuer inflation reflex in the preterm infants at term postmenstrual age as the newborn vagus nerve has a relatively few number of myelinated fibres and a smaller percentage of active slowly adapting receptors (Sachis et al. 1982; Fedorko et al. 1988). Alternatively, the inspiratory shortening might have been a reflection of a functional immaturity of the reflex arc responsible for the Hering–Breuer deflation reflex. The exact site of any defect in the reflex arc was not possible to identify. The effect of prematurity on the number and discharge properties of rapidly adapting receptors is not known. Fleming et al. (1978), however, demonstrated that preterm infants responded in an immature manner compared with term infants when they had gentle probing of the lower airway with a catheter. The Hering–Breuer deflation reflex (p. 456), which terminates expiration and promotes inspiration, has also been demonstrated to be immature in preterm babies having apnoeas (Fleming et al. 1978; Hannam et al. 1998).

Obstructive apnoea

Using the new classification of apnoea, many apnoeas previously described as being central are in fact obstructive or mixed in nature. Mechanisms leading to obstructed breaths include instability of the upper airway in preterm infants, asynchrony of the musculature of the upper airway and diaphragm, pathological changes in the upper airway and central nervous system pathologies. Obstruction of the upper airway may be a result of decreased tone in preterm infants, leading to collapse and obstruction of the upper airway (Idiong et al. 1998). Using an ultrafine fibreoptic scope, the site of upper airway obstruction in preterm babies has been shown to be at the laryngeal level (Ruggins and Milner 1991). It is not clear whether airway closure is a reflection of hypoxia associated with apnoea, whether it is due to asynchrony between the alae nasi and diaphragm sucking in the upper airway (Carlo et al. 1983) or whether it is due to passive airway narrowing due to reduced tone. Spontaneous neck flexion can also lead to obstruction in healthy preterm

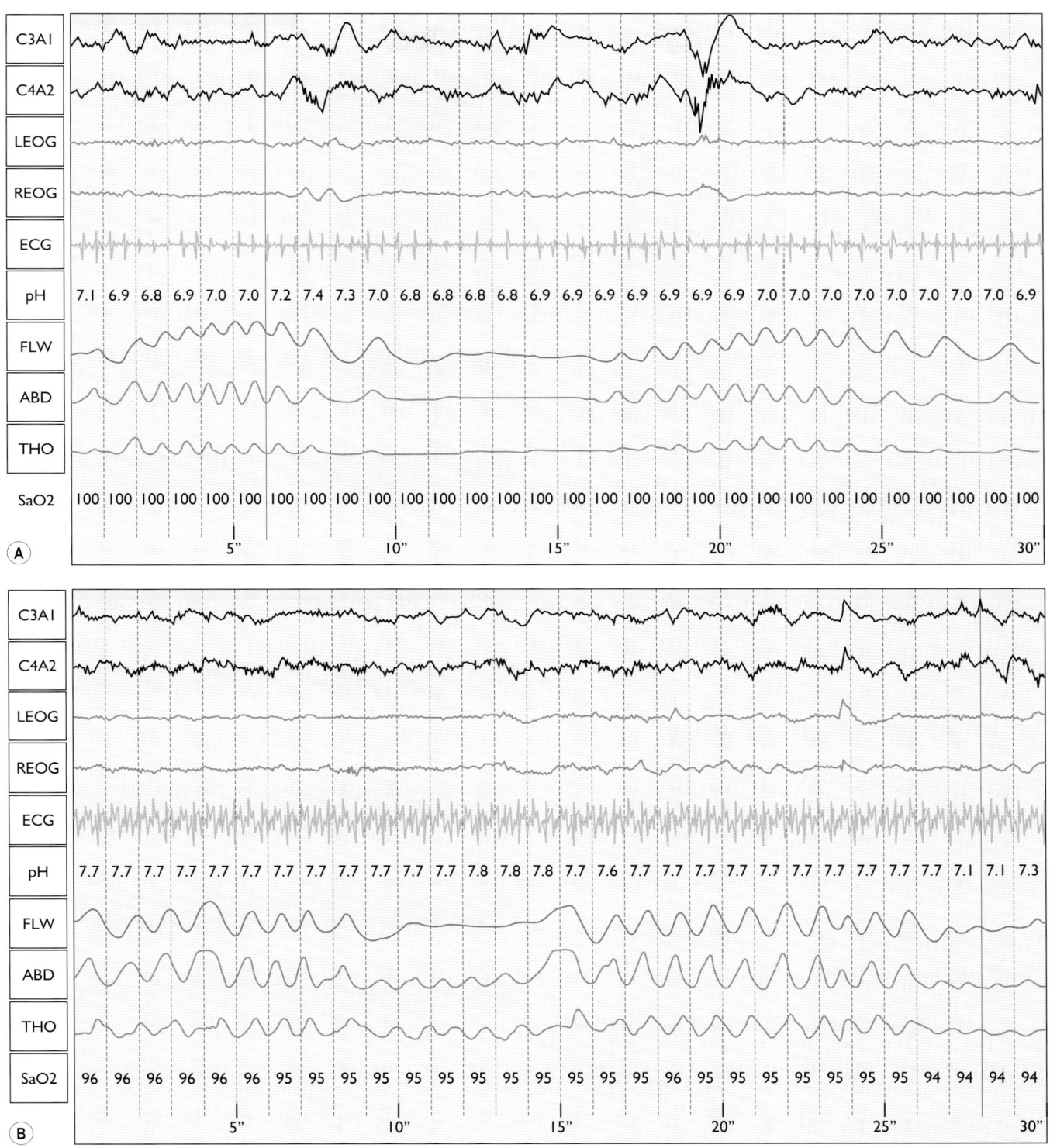

Fig. 27.50 (A) Apnoea in a preterm infant born at 28 weeks of gestation recorded at 35 weeks' corrected gestational age. The recording was made using the Alice 4 sleep study system. In order from the top down, the traces represent: two scalp electroencephalograms (C3A1 and C4A2), two electro-oculograms (LEOG, REOG), electrocardiogram (ECG), oesophageal pH, nasal flow (FLW), abdominal movement (ABD), thoracic movement (THO) and oxygen saturation (SaO_2). Time in 5-second intervals is indicated at the bottom of the trace. As can be seen, there is a central apnoea lasting 6 seconds where there is cessation of nasal airflow movement and an absence of chest and abdominal wall movements. No desaturation or bradycardia was associated with this apnoea. (B) Obstructive apnoea in a different preterm infant, again born at 28 weeks of gestation with the recording made at 35 weeks' corrected gestational age. In this apnoea, lasting 5 seconds, chest wall movements continue in the absence of nasal airflow.

babies (Thach and Stark 1979) as well as in situations where there are anatomical abnormalities of the upper airway, such as Pierre Robin sequence and Down syndrome.

Mixed apnoea

With mixed apnoea, most apnoeas commence with central apnoea followed by airway occlusion (Idiong et al. 1998). Narrowing of the airway occurs about 1 second into a central apnoea (Lemke et al. 1998). This appears to be due to the loss of tone of the muscles of the upper airway. Clearly, this could then lead to the development of airway obstruction and evolve into a mixed apnoea. All apnoeas persisting for more than 20 seconds fall into the category of mixed apnoea (Upton et al. 1992a). Obstructing the airway can also lead to central apnoea. Upton et al. (1992b) investigated the response of preterm infants to airway obstruction. There was an increased frequency of central apnoea following relief of the obstruction, raising the possibility that obstruction itself might have a role in the development of the central apnoea (Upton et al. 1992b). Apnoea may represent an immaturity of the multiple mechanisms that determine the rate and depth of respiration (Waggener et al. 1984). A relationship between cycle time and length of apnoeic episodes has been demonstrated, reflecting a 'hunting' form of ventilation whereby respiration was first stimulated then suppressed. The fact that short respiratory pauses, periodic breathing and prolonged apnoeas all occur at the nadir of spontaneous breathing cycles (Waggener et al. 1989) supports the idea of a common aetiology of apnoea. In the light of recent studies, it appears that central, mixed and obstructive apnoeas are part of a spectrum of apnoea rather than forming distinct entities and that all may have a common underlying mechanism (Poets 2003).

Factors involved in apnoea

Most apnoeic episodes in preterm babies occur in preterm babies who are otherwise healthy. These are called primary apnoeas, can be attributed to prematurity and are a diagnosis of exclusion. There are many conditions that cause or accentuate apnoea (Table 27.14). It is therefore essential to investigate infants appropriately, with a high index of clinical suspicion, when apnoeas suddenly appear in a previously well baby.

Periodic breathing, sleep state and diaphragmatic fatigue

Periodic breathing can be defined as bursts of respiratory activity of 20 seconds or less, separated by central apnoeic pauses lasting from 3 to 10 seconds (Glotzbach et al. 1989). Periodic breathing is present in almost all preterm babies, but is relatively uncommon in term babies (Glotzbach and Ariagno 1992). The aetiology of periodic breathing remains obscure, although the finding that it is absent until 48 hours of age suggests that inactivity of peripheral chemoreceptors at this time might play a role (Barrington and Finer 1990). There is disagreement as to whether periodic breathing is a benign or harmful phenomenon. Desaturation during periodic breathing has been reported (Razi et al. 2002; Rigatto 2003), although whether this is of long-term significance is unclear. Previous research suggested that periodic breathing was not linked to prolonged apnoea in preterm babies (Barrington and Finer 1990). More recent studies have contradicted this finding and have proposed a causal link between periodic breathing and prolonged apnoea (Al-Saedi et al. 1997; Rigatto 2003). In both term and

Table 27.14 Conditions exacerbating or causing apnoea in the neonatal period

Hypoxia
Central nervous system
Primary apnoea of prematurity
Intracranial haemorrhage
Seizures
Drugs
Sedatives, narcotics Postanaesthesia Prostaglandin E_2
Sepsis
Necrotising enterocolitis Meningitis Bronchiolitis
Metabolic abnormalities
Hypoglycaemia Hyponatraemia Hypocalcaemia Inborn errors of metabolism
Environmental
Hyperthermia Hypothermia
Upper airway obstruction
Choanal atresia Micrognathia (Pierre Robin sequence) Macroglossia Hypotonia of Down syndrome
Circulatory
Patent ductus arteriosus Heart failure Anaemia
Vasovagal reflex
Siting of nasogastric tube Upper airway suctioning
Immunisation

preterm babies, periodic breathing and apnoeas are more common in rapid eye movement (REM) sleep than in non-REM sleep (Schulte et al. 1977). It has been suggested that the reason for this may be chest wall distortion stimulating the costophrenic inhibitory reflex (Knill and Bryan 1976), despite this distortion being present in both REM and non-REM sleep (Davi et al. 1979).

An alternative mechanism has been suggested in a study demonstrating that arterial oxygen levels were significantly lower in REM than in quiet sleep (Martin et al. 1979). It has also been demonstrated that sleeping position, but not type of sleep, was associated with central and obstructive apnoeas in preterm infants with central apnoeas being more common in the prone position (Bhat et al. 2006). Arousals and awakenings, as well as length of sleep, were greater in the supine position. This suggested a connection between depth of sleep, sleeping position and apnoea.

Genetic predisposition

There is evidence that some infants may have a genetic predisposition towards experiencing apnoea of prematurity. A higher incidence of apnoea of prematurity in infants born to first-degree consanguineous parents has been demonstrated (Tamin et al. 2003). A genetic basis for apnoea of prematurity has also been suggested in a recent twin study (Bloch-Salisbury et al. 2010).

Hypoxia

As discussed previously, hypoxia tends to lead to respiratory depression in very immature babies. It therefore follows that any condition causing respiratory or neurological problems that lead to hypoxia can cause or accentuate apnoea in these babies. It has been demonstrated that preterm babies, with increasing levels of inspired oxygen, have decreasing apnoea frequency (Weintraub et al. 1992).

Infection

Apnoea is more likely to occur in an infected baby. The mechanism by which infection causes apnoea is unclear (Mathew 2003). Preterm infants infected with respiratory syncytial virus (RSV) are particularly prone to develop apnoea (Church et al. 1984).

Central nervous system disorders

Trauma, germinal matrix/intraventricular haemorrhage and meningitis are all associated with apnoea. Apnoea can also be a result of seizure activity (Watanabe et al. 1983). Apnoea can be associated with the Arnold–Chiari malformation. The rare condition of congenital central alveolar hypoventilation syndrome (Ondine's curse) is thought to be due to an abnormality of the neural crest cells involved in respiration, although a mutation in the *PHOX2B* gene in patients with this condition has been reported (Gaultier et al. 2004). Babies with this condition have absent ventilation sensitivity to hypoxia and hypercarbia even when they are awake. Their breathing pattern is normal when they are awake, but they become cyanosed when asleep. Prolonged respiratory support is required.

Environmental temperature

Preterm infants respond to an increase in environmental temperature beyond the thermoneutral range with a rise in apnoea frequency and periodic respiration (Perlstein et al. 1970). The mechanism for this is unclear.

Gastro-oesophageal reflux

Upper airway chemoreceptors may have a role in the development of apnoea. Instillation of saline into the airway of a sleeping infant induces apnoea, swallowing and arousal (Thach 1992). This response has been ascribed to the LCR being stimulated and, in preterm infants, an exaggerated LCR has been demonstrated (Pickens et al. 1988). Some authors feel that stimulation of the LCR plays an important role in apnoea of prematurity (Thach 2005). Of interest, the apnoea related to an exaggerated LCR might be connected to a predominance of $GABA_A$-related inhibitory pathways (Abu-Shaweesh and Martin 2008). These responses could be relevant when considering the role of gastro-oesophageal reflux (GOR) as a cause of apnoea. The association between GOR and apnoea of prematurity has been difficult to prove and recent studies have failed to demonstrate a temporal relationship between episodes of reflux and apnoea (Peter et al. 2002; DiFiore et al. 2005; Bhat et al. 2007). In support of this finding, treatment of GOR has not been shown to reduce the frequency of apnoea of prematurity (Kimball and Carlton 2001).

Apnoea and bottle feeding

Some infants, especially those with chronic lung disease, become hypoxaemic during and after bottle feeds (Rosen et al. 1984). It has not been possible to demonstrate an increased frequency of apnoea when comparing bottle, milk boluses via nasogastric tube, and continuous tube feeds (Poets et al. 1997).

Anaemia

If low levels of haemoglobin predispose infants to apnoea, blood transfusion should reduce the incidence of apnoea. A reduction in the incidence of apnoea following transfusion has been reported (Joshi et al. 1987). Other groups have not seen this response (Westkamp et al. 2002), and doubt remains regarding the efficacy of using transfusions to treat symptomatic apnoea.

Anaesthesia

Following a general anaesthetic, preterm infants are at risk of developing apnoea (Kurth et al. 1987). This problem worsens in preterm infants of increasing immaturity (Cote et al. 1995). As a result, postoperative monitoring in a high-dependency cot is essential for all preterm babies who are recovering from surgery, until they are at least a month postterm-equivalent postnatal age.

Patent ductus arteriosus

Infants who develop pulmonary oedema as a consequence of a patent ductus arteriosus are at risk of apnoea. Stimulation of pulmonary C fibres occurs in response to pulmonary oedema (Schertel et al. 1986), possibly leading to apnoea in a vagally mediated response.

Immunisation

Apnoea in preterm infants following immunisation with diphtheria, pertussis and tetanus (DPT) has been reported (Sanchez et al. 1997). For this reason, infants receiving immunisations on neonatal units need to be carefully monitored in the period following administration of vaccines.

Drugs

Analgesics such as morphine can depress neonatal respiration.

Bradycardia

As with apnoea, varying definitions of bradycardia in the preterm infant have been used by investigators. A fall in heart rate to less than 100 beats/min in a preterm infant for over 5 seconds is generally considered to constitute a bradycardia (Dransfield et al. 1983). Alternatively, a fall in heart rate of more than 30% below baseline has been used as the criterion for bradycardia (Henderson-Smart et al. 1986; Poets et al. 1993). Whatever method of calculating a bradycardia is employed, a crucial factor to take into consideration is whether or not a bradycardia is clinically significant. Brief falls in heart rate unaccompanied by apnoea or desaturation are unlikely to be of importance. Bradycardias are more common in apnoeas of longer duration (Henderson-Smart et al. 1986).

A series of complex physiological interactions leads to the scenario of apnoea, bradycardia and desaturation (Martin and Fanaroff 1998). In the majority of cases, there is an apnoea or period of hypoventilation closely followed by a fall in oxygen saturation and then bradycardia (Adams et al. 1997). Initially it was thought that this bradycardia was the direct result of myocardial hypoxia. It is now clear that the bradycardia occurs too early in apnoea to be due to this effect (Vyas et al. 1981). Almost all bradycardias commence after the onset of apnoea and after the onset of the fall in oxygen saturation (Poets et al. 1993). This would support the theory that the bradycardia occurs via the carotid chemoreceptors. Upper airway closure may also have a role in the development of the bradycardia, perhaps due to the lack of stimulation of a pulmonary inflation reflex (Upton et al. 1992c). This has been shown by the heart rate not recovering in mixed apnoea until airflow had been restored (Henderson-Smart et al. 1986).

A different scenario exists whereby bradycardia occurs simultaneously with apnoea. This presumably represents a vagally mediated, rather than hypoxic, response. It has been proposed that enhanced vagal tone might have a role in predisposing preterm infants to apnoeas and bradycardias (Mathew 2003). The diving reflex could be the reflex pathway for this type of bradycardia (Daly 1986). This reflex can be initiated by immersing the face in ice-cold water, which causes stimulation of the trigeminal nerve (Scholander 1963) and results in apnoea, bradycardia and peripheral vasoconstriction. This dramatic reflex can be harnessed clinically to terminate episodes of supraventricular tachycardia (Ch. 8).

Monitoring

Monitoring is essential in babies who have conditions that predispose them to having apnoea. This includes all infants of less than 35 weeks of gestation and those more mature infants with other serious illnesses. There is some controversy as to the type of monitoring that is most appropriate in such babies. Based on the current evidence, we use a combination of a pressure-sensitive apnoea mattress, heart rate monitoring and oxygen saturation monitoring in our special-care nursery.

Cardiorespiratory monitoring (Ch. 19)

Owing to the close association between bradycardia and apnoea, all babies who are at risk of apnoea should have monitoring of heart rate as well as respiratory effort. This can be achieved using standard electrocardiogram monitors using three electrodes, two of which can be in common with impedance equipment. There can be problems with false alarms due to either detachment of one of the electrodes or body movement. The heart rate signal from a pulse oximeter is even more prone to false alarms.

There are several devices available that monitor the movement of the chest or abdominal wall. Techniques for assessing chest wall movement include: air-filled apnoea mattresses (Lewin 1969), pressure-sensitive devices which lie under the infant (Smith and Scopes 1972), pressure-sensitive capsules attached to the abdominal wall (Valman et al. 1983) and sensors that detect changes in abdominal circumference (impedance monitor and respiratory

inductance plethysmography). The first three types of devices are bedevilled by problems with false-positive alarms, which increase the stress placed on nursing staff and parents. Also, none is able to discriminate between obstructive/mixed apnoea and central apnoea. For this to be possible, a means of measuring nasal airflow, such as a nasal thermistor (Dransfield and Fox 1980) or an end-tidal CO_2 monitor, needs to be used. Impedance monitoring involves measuring the current that passes between two low-voltage electrodes placed on opposite sides of the chest. As the infant inspires, there is an increase in the air/tissue ratio and the voltage falls. This system does have the disadvantage of picking up changes in cardiac output during an apnoea and preventing the triggering of the alarm (Southall et al. 1998).

Respiratory inductance plethysmography consists of light-weight bands placed around the chest and the abdomen. Within the bands are coils of copper wire that act as a one-turn transducer. As the cross-sectional area of the chest and abdomen vary with respiration, so does the inductance of the bands. These variations can then be displayed. Paradoxical movements of the chest and abdomen, where the chest and abdomen move out of phase, can be used to diagnose obstructive apnoea accurately. Transthoracic impedance measurements cannot be used for this purpose (Brouillette et al. 1987).

Oxygenation

Babies who are receiving oxygen treatment must have the concentration measured, and their response to oxygen treatment must be assessed. This may be achieved using direct blood gas estimations, transcutaneous (tc) oxygen measurements or pulse oximetry. Pulse oximeters are easy to site, although care has to be taken not to attach the device too tightly. There is a faster response time than with $tcPo_2$ measurements, with the oximeter signal averaged over 3–5 seconds (Hay et al. 1989). The monitors are susceptible to both movement artefact and poor cardiac output, which can lead to false alarms. Pulse oximetry is of additional value as preterm infants can have episodes of profound desaturation in the absence of apnoea or bradycardia (Poets et al. 1995). In our view, a pulse oximeter is probably the most helpful single device to use when monitoring for apnoea on the neonatal unit. A combination of a cardiorespiratory monitor and pulse oximeter should be used in infants who are having symptomatic apnoeas (Upton et al. 1991).

Investigation of apnoea

Investigating a preterm baby who is developing apnoea depends to a great extent on the overall clinical picture. Most apnoeas in preterm babies will be related to immaturity and be primary apnoea. This is, however, a diagnosis of exclusion and apnoea can herald the onset of serious disease. Therefore, the following investigations should be considered: infection screen (including lumbar puncture and urinalysis), serum glucose, serum calcium, haemoglobin, chest X-ray, cranial ultrasound scan, arterial blood gas and viral screen (especially RSV). If the apnoeas remain resistant despite treatment, the presence of a convulsive disorder should be considered and an electroencephalogram obtained.

Treatment of apnoea of prematurity

Once a preterm baby has been investigated and appropriately treated for conditions aggravating apnoea, other therapies to decrease the frequency of apnoea need to be initiated.

Treatment of individual episodes of apnoea

Most babies respond to conservative treatment of an apnoea. Once an apnoea or bradycardic episode has been detected, usually by a monitor alarming, the baby needs to be assessed urgently. Many of these episodes are self-limiting and no action needs to be taken. If the baby is still apnoeic or bradycardic when examined, a gentle stimulus such as flicking the foot may be sufficient to restore breathing. If it is suspected that the baby might have aspirated a feed, the head should be gently extended and gentle suctioning of the upper airway should be attempted. If, despite these interventions, the baby remains apnoeic or the heart rate is not restored, the baby should be ventilated using either a bag and mask or a mask and T-piece using the baby's usual F_1O_2. This resuscitation should never be done using 100% oxygen, owing to the risk of retinopathy of prematurity with hyperoxaemia. Careful monitoring of the baby's oxygen saturations should be maintained throughout. Occasionally, intubation is required despite these manoeuvres.

Pharmacotherapy

Methylxanthines (caffeine and aminophylline/theophylline) form the mainstay of the treatment of apnoea of prematurity. The exact mechanism by which these drugs exert their effect is not known, although there is competitive antagonism at the adenosine receptor between xanthines and adenosine (Herlenius et al. 1997). A possible central mechanism of action for methylxanthines in preventing apnoea via blockade of the adenosine A_{2A} receptors on GABAergic neurons has been proposed (Abu-Shaweesh and Martin 2008). This would effectively decrease the release of GABA and reduce its inhibitory effect on breathing (Abu-Shaweesh and Martin 2008). As well as their effects on apnoea, methylxanthines act by increasing minute ventilation, improve CO_2 sensitivity, decrease hypoxic depression of breathing (Abu-Shaweesh and Martin 2008) and increase the strength of diaphragmatic contractility (Aubier et al. 1981). Levels need to be monitored closely. Theophylline is methylated to form caffeine in preterm babies and it may be necessary to monitor levels of both methylxanthines in order to assess the total drug load (Bory et al. 1979).

The most commonly encountered side-effect of theophylline is tachycardia. Less frequent side-effects include seizures, abdominal distension, vomiting, diarrhoea, jitteriness and worsening of GOR. Many units are now using caffeine as their first-line therapy instead of theophylline. This is partly due to caffeine having a wider therapeutic range with fewer toxic side-effects, although significant tachycardia can still be a problem. Routine blood levels are not required, providing the infant shows a satisfactory response to treatment. Caffeine treatment is associated with a significant reduction in apnoeas in preterm infants experiencing symptomatic apnoea (Erenberg et al. 2000; Henderson-Smart and Steer 2002). Although caffeine treatment of apnoea has a similar clinical response rate to theophylline, fewer infants experience adverse effects when caffeine is used (Henderson-Smart and Steer 2010).

A recently completed randomised controlled multicentre trial investigated the short- and long-term effects of caffeine versus placebo in a large group of preterm infants with birthweights between 500 and 1250 g (Schmidt et al. 2006, 2007). The benefits of caffeine therapy were demonstrated in that those treated had reduced incidences of bronchopulmonary dysplasia, cerebral palsy and developmental delay. The main side-effect was that of poorer weight gain in the treatment group.

Doxapram, which acts as a non-specific stimulant of the central nervous system, has been used as a second-line treatment in preterm babies who failed to respond to aminophylline (Barrington et al.

1986). Side-effects include abdominal distension, irritability, jitteriness, vomiting, increased blood pressure and feed intolerance. Although doxapram reduces the number of apnoeas in the first 48 hours of its administration, there is no evidence to support its use as a first-line agent in the treatment of apnoea of prematurity above methylxanthines in current-day practice (Henderson-Smart and Steer 2004).

Ventilation

If, despite treatment with methylxanthines, an infant continues to have frequent apnoeas, continuous positive airway pressure (CPAP) needs to be considered. CPAP reduces the incidence of apnoea by around 50% (Speidel and Dunn 1976). The effect of CPAP is selective – it reduces the incidence of mixed or obstructive apnoea but has no effect on central apnoeas (Miller et al. 1985). It is possible that CPAP exerts its effect through mechanically splinting the upper airway (Miller et al. 1990). On direct visualisation of the upper airway, CPAP has been demonstrated to dilate the laryngeal opening significantly (Gaon et al. 1999). Nasal intermittent positive-pressure ventilation (nIPPV) shows promise as a treatment of apnoea of prematurity and there is some suggestion that this method of ventilation might be more effective in preventing apnoeas than conventional CPAP (Lemyre et al. 2002). Further studies are required to investigate whether synchronising nIPPV will be of additional benefit. Occasionally, apnoeas are resistant to treatment and the infant has to be intubated and ventilated. In these infants, the lowest possible oxygen concentration and ventilatory pressures need to be used, as they are often relatively easy to ventilate.

Other therapeutic options

A variety of kinaesthetic stimulations to prevent apnoeas in preterm infants have been employed. These range from rocking beds to oscillating mattresses. There is little evidence that these methods are of any therapeutic value (Osborn and Henderson-Smart 2002). A recent trial was unable to demonstrate any benefit between altering the tilt of the infant versus applying kinaesthetic infant-handling techniques (Reher et al. 2008). Other measures, such as changing the position from supine to prone (Heimler et al. 1992; Kurlak et al. 1994), altering environmental temperature (Perlstein et al. 1970) and correcting hypoxia (Weintraub et al. 1992), can decrease the incidence of apnoea.

Stopping treatment, predischarge monitoring and discharge home

Babies who have had apnoeas treated with methylxanthines tend to have had treatment discontinued by 35 weeks' postconceptional age (PCA) (Eichenwald et al. 1997). Despite this, significant apnoeas can persist up to 43 weeks' PCA (Eichenwald et al. 1997; Ramanathan et al. 2001). Most neonatalogists agree that, after stopping methylxanthines, babies who have experienced problematic apnoea of prematurity should have an event-free period of 5–7 days before discharge from the neonatal unit (Darnall et al. 1997). On the neonatal unit, preterm babies are usually nursed in the prone position to improve oxygenation and reduce apnoea frequency (Heimler et al. 1992). Because of the increased risk of sudden infant death syndrome (SIDS) in the prone position, babies should spend a period of a week or more in the supine position prior to discharge, unless there are other factors that preclude this being done (Bhat et al. 2003).

Home monitoring

Infants who are born prematurely are at much greater risk of SIDS, with an almost sixfold increase in relative risk compared with term infants (Oyen et al. 1997). It was also shown that, if the preterm infant was nursed prone, there was a 50-fold increase in the risk for SIDS. It has been recommended that preterm infants who are experiencing symptomatic apnoeas should be discharged on home cardiorespiratory monitors (Little et al. 1987), although there is no evidence that those who have had troublesome apnoea on the neonatal unit are at additional risk of SIDS (Hoppenbrouwers et al. 2008). Most home cardiorespiratory monitors are unable to detect episodes of obstructive apnoea, due to their reliance on transthoracic impedance measurements. Obstructive apnoeas were the most commonly observed event detected in a series investigating the role of home monitoring in preterm infants (Ramanathan et al. 2001). However, even these apnoeas did not seem to be precursors to SIDS. At present, therefore, there seems little justification for using home monitoring in preterm infants.

Advice regarding SIDS and acute life-threatening events

Prospective cardiorespiratory monitoring carried out on preterm infants did not identify prolonged apnoea as a risk factor for SIDS (Southall et al. 1983). Despite this, prior to discharge of their baby from the neonatal unit, parents need to be advised of the measures that can be taken to reduce the risk of SIDS. These include placing the baby to sleep in the supine position, avoiding hyperthermia, stopping smoking (Oyen et al. 1997) and not co-sleeping (Blair et al. 1999). Following discharge, a baby can occasionally experience an acute life-threatening event (ALTE). An ALTE is said to have occurred when a baby has been found apnoeic, with a change in colour (cyanosis or pallor) and tone (limpness or stiffness), and has required mouth-to-mouth resuscitation or vigorous stimulation. Ex-preterm babies are at increased risk of experiencing an ALTE (Ramanathan et al. 2001). For this reason, parents need to be taught basic infant life support prior to their baby being discharged.

Prognosis

A higher incidence of retinopathy of prematurity has been reported in preterm infants who have had troublesome apnoea (Purohit et al. 1985). It has, however, been difficult to prove that apnoeic episodes have a deleterious effect on neurological development. This is due to the presence of many confounding variables that might affect neurological outcome following intensive care on a neonatal unit. Some studies have found that apnoeas have an adverse effect on neurological development (Jones and Lukeman 1982; Butcher-Puech et al. 1985; Cheung et al. 1999) whilst others have not been able to demonstrate this association (Tudehope et al. 1986; Koons et al. 1993). There is an increasing body of evidence, however, that preterm infants who experience a high incidence of apnoea or have delayed resolution of apnoea have a worsened developmental outcome (Hunt et al. 2004; Janvier et al. 2004; Pillekamp et al. 2007).

References

Abu-Shaweesh, J., 2007. Activation of central adenosine A_{2A} receptors enhances superior laryngeal nerve stimulation-induced apnea in piglets via a GABAergic pathway. J Appl Physiol 103, 1205–1211.

Abu-Shaweesh, J.M., Martin, R.J., 2008. Neonatal apnea: What's new? Pediatr Pulmonol 43, 937–944.

Adams, J.A., Zabaleta, I.A., Sackner, M.A., 1997. Hypoxemic events inspontaneously breathing premature infants: etiologic basis. Pediatr Res 42, 463–471.

Al-Saedi, S.A., Lemke, R.P., Haider, A.Z., et al., 1997. Prolonged apnea in the preterm infant is not a random event. Am J Perinatol 14, 195–200.

American Academy of Pediatrics Taskforce on Prolonged Apnea, 1978. Prolonged apnea. Pediatrics 61, 651–652.

Aubier, M., De Troyer, A., Sampson, M., et al., 1981. Aminophylline improves diaphragmatic contractility. NEJM 305, 249–252.

Barrington, K.J., Finer, N.N., 1990. Periodic breathing and apnea in preterm infants. Pediatr Res 27, 118–121.

Barrington, K.J., Finer, N.N., Peters, K.L., et al., 1986. Physiologic effects of doxapram in idiopathic apnea of prematurity. Journal of Pediatrics 108, 124–129.

Bhat, R.Y., Leipala, J.A., Rafferty, G.F., et al., 2003. Survey of sleeping position recommendations for prematurely born infants on neonatal intensive care unit discharge. Eur J Pediatr 162, 426–427.

Bhat, R.Y., Hannam, S., Pressler, R., et al., 2006. Effect of prone and supine position on sleep, apneas and arousal in preterm infants. Pediatrics 118, 101–107.

Bhat, R.Y., Rafferty, G.F., Hannam, S., et al., 2007. Acid gastrooesophageal reflux in convalescent preterm infants: effect of posture and relationship to apnoea. Pediatr Res 62, 620–623.

Blair, P.S., Fleming, P.J., Smith, I.J., et al., 1999. Babies sleeping with parents: case-control study of factors influencing the risk of the sudden infant death syndrome. CESDI SUDI Research Group. Br Med J 319, 1457–1461.

Bloch-Salisbury, E., Hall, M.H., Sharma, P., et al., 2010. Heritability of apnea of prematurity: a retrospective twin study. Pediatrics 126, e779–787.

Bory, C., Baltassat, P., Porthault, M., et al., 1979. Metabolism of theophylline to caffeine in premature newborn infants. Journal of Pediatrics 94, 988–993.

Brouillette, R.T., Morrow, A.S., Weese-Mayer, D.E., et al., 1987. Comparison of respiratory inductive plethysmography and thoracic impedance for apnea monitoring. Journal of Pediatrics 111, 377–383.

Butcher-Puech, M.C., Henderson-Smart, D.J., Holley, D., et al., 1985. Relation between apnoea duration and type and neurological status of preterm infants. Arch Dis Child 60, 953–958.

Carlo, W.A., Martin, R.J., Bruce, E.N., et al., 1983. Alae nasi activation (nasal flaring) decreases nasal resistance in preterm infants. Pediatrics 72, 338–343.

Cheung, P.Y., Barrington, K.J., Finer, N.N., et al., 1999. Early childhood neurodevelopment in very low birth weight infants with predischarge apnea. Pediatr Pulmonol 27, 14–20.

Church, N.R., Anas, N.G., Hall, C.B., et al., 1984. Respiratory syncytial virus-related apnea in infants. Demographics and outcome. Am J Dis Child 138, 247–250.

Cote, C.J., Zaslavsky, A., Downes, J.J., et al., 1995. Postoperative apnea in former preterm infants after inguinal herniorrhaphy. A combined analysis. Anesthesiology 82, 809–822.

Daly, M.D.B., 1986. Handbook of Physiology: the Respiratory System, vol. II. American Physiological Society, Bethesda, pp. 529–579.

Darnall, R.A., Kattwinkel, J., Nattie, C., et al., 1997. Margin of safety for discharge after apnea in preterm infants. Pediatrics 100, 795–801.

Davi, M., Sankaran, K., Maccallum, M., et al., 1979. Effect of sleep state on chest distortion and on the ventilatory response to CO_2 in neonates. Pediatr Res 13, 982–986.

DiFiore, J.M., Arko, M., Whitehouse, M., et al., 2005. Apnea is not prolonged by gastrooesophageal reflux in preterm infants. Pediatrics 116, 1059–1063.

Dransfield, D.A., Fox, W.W., 1980. A noninvasive method for recording central and obstructive apnea with bradycardia in infants. Crit Care Med 8, 663–666.

Dransfield, D.A., Spitzer, A.R., Fox, W.W., 1983. Episodic airway obstruction in premature infants. Am J Dis Child 137, 441–443.

Eichenwald, E.C., Aina, A., Stark, A.R., 1997. Apnea frequently persists beyond term gestation in infants delivered at 24 to 28 weeks. Pediatrics 100, 354–359.

Erenberg, A., Leff, R.D., Haack, D.G., et al., 2000. Caffeine citrate for the treatment of apnea of prematurity: a double-blind, placebo-controlled study. Pharmacotherapy 20, 644–652.

Fedorko, L., Kelly, E., England, S., 1988. Importance of vagal afferents in determining ventilation in newborn rats. J Appl Physiol 65, 1033–1039.

Finer, N.N., Barrington, K.J., Hayes, B.J., et al., 1992. Obstructive, mixed, and central apnea in the neonate: physiologic correlates. Journal of Pediatrics 121, 943–950.

Fleming, P.J., Bryan, A.C., Bryan, M.H., 1978. Functional immaturity of pulmonary irritant receptors and apnea in newborn preterm infants. Pediatrics 61, 515–518.

Gaon, P., Lee, S., Hannam, S., et al., 1999. Assessment of effect of nasal continuous positive pressure on laryngeal opening using fibre optic laryngoscopy. Arch Dis Child Fetal Neonatal Ed 80, F230–F232.

Gaultier, C., Amiel, J., Dauger, S., et al., 2004. Genetics and early disturbances of breathing control. Pediatr Res 55, 729–733.

Gerhardt, T., Bancalari, E., 1984a. Apnea of prematurity: I. Lung function and regulation of breathing. Pediatrics 74, 58–62.

Gerhardt, T., Bancalari, E., 1984b. Apnea of prematurity: II. Respiratory reflexes. Pediatrics 74, 63–66.

Glotzbach, S.F., Ariagno, R.L., 1992. Periodic breathing. In: Beckerman, R.C., Broillette, R.T., Hunt, C.E. (Eds.), Respiratory Control Disorders in Infants and Children. Lippincott Williams & Wilkins, Baltimore, pp. 142–160.

Glotzbach, S.F., Tansey, P.A., Baldwin, R.B., et al., 1989. Periodic breathing cycle duration in preterm infants. Pediatr Res 25, 258–261.

Hannam, S., Ingram, D.M., Milner, A.D., 1998. A possible role for the Hering–Breuer deflation reflex in apnea of prematurity. Journal of Pediatrics 132, 35–39.

Hay, W.W., Brockway, J.M., Eyzaguirre, M., 1989. Neonatal pulse oximetry: accuracy and reliability. Pediatrics 83, 717–722.

Heimler, R., Langlois, J., Hodel, D.J., et al., 1992. Effect of positioning on the breathing pattern of preterm infants. Arch Dis Child 67, 312–314.

Henderson-Smart, D.J., 1981. The effect of gestational age on the incidence and duration of recurrent apnoea in newborn babies. Australian Paediatrics Journal 17, 273–276.

Henderson-Smart, D.J., Steer, P.A., 2002. Prophylactic methylxanthine for prevention of apnea in preterm infants. Cochrane Database Syst Rev (2), CD000432.

Henderson-Smart, D.J., Steer, P., 2004. Doxapram treatment for apnea in preterm infants. Cochrane Database Syst Rev (4), CD000074.

Henderson-Smart, D.J., Steer, P.A., 2010. Caffeine versus theophylline for apnea in preterm infants. Cochrane Database of Systemic Reviews (1), CDCD000273.

Henderson-Smart, D.J., Pettigrew, A.G., Campbell, D.J., 1983. Clinical apnea and brain-stem neural function in preterm infants. NEJM 308, 353–357.

Henderson-Smart, D.J., Butcher-Puech, M.C., Edwards, D.A., 1986. Incidence and mechanism of bradycardia during apnoea in preterm infants. Arch Dis Child 61, 227–232.

Herlenius, E., Lagercrantz, H., Yamamoto, Y., 1997. Adenosine modulates inspiratory neurons and the respiratory pattern in the brainstem of neonatal rats. Pediatr Res 42, 46–53.

Hodgman, J.E., Gonzalez, F., Hoppenbrouwers, T., et al., 1990. Apnea, transient episodes of bradycardia, and periodic breathing in preterm infants. Am J Dis Child 144, 54–57.

Hoppenbrouwers, T., Hodgman, J.E., Ramanathan, A., et al., 2008. Extreme and conventional cardiorespiratory events and epidemiologic risk factors for SIDS. Journal of Pediatrics 152, 636–641.

Hunt, C.E., Corwin, M.J., Baird, T., et al., 2004. Cardiorespiratory events detected by home memory monitoring and one year neurodevelopmental outcome. Journal of Pediatrics 145, 465–471.

Idiong, N., Lemke, R.P., Lin, Y.J., et al., 1998. Airway closure during mixed apneas in preterm infants: is respiratory effort necessary? Journal of Pediatrics 133, 509–512.

Janvier, A., Khairy, M., Kokkotis, A., et al., 2004. Apnea is associated with neurodevelopmental impairment in very low birth weight babies. J Perinatol 24, 763–768.

Jones, R.A., Lukeman, D., 1982. Apnoea of immaturity. 2. Mortality and handicap. Arch Dis Child 57, 766–768.

Joshi, A., Gerhardt, T., Shandloff, P., et al., 1987. Blood transfusion effect on the respiratory pattern of preterm infants. Pediatrics 80, 79–84.

Kattwinkel, J., 1977. Neonatal apnea: Pathogenesis and therapy. Journal of Pediatrics 90, 342–347.

Kimball, A.L., Carlton, D.P., 2001. Gastroesophageal reflux medications in the treatment of apnea in premature infants. Journal of Pediatrics 138, 355–360.

Knill, R., Bryan, A.C., 1976. An intercostal-phrenic inhibitory reflex in human newborn infants. J Appl Physiol 40, 352–356.

Koons, A.H., Mojica, N., Jadeja, N., et al., 1993. Neurodevelopmental outcome of infants with apnea of infancy. Am J Perinatol 10, 208–211.

Kurlak, L.O., Ruggins, N.R., Stephenson, T.J., 1994. Effect of nursing position on incidence, type, and duration of clinically significant apnoea in preterm infants. Arch Dis Child Fetal Neonatal Ed 71, F16–F19.

Kurth, C.D., Spitzer, A.R., Broennle, A.M., et al., 1987. Postoperative apnea in preterm infants. Anesthesiology 66, 483–488.

Lemke, R.P., Al-Saedi, S.A., Alvaro, R.E., et al., 1996. Use of a magnified cardiac airflow oscillation to classify neonatal apnea. Am J Respir Crit Care Med 154, 1537–1542.

Lemke, R.P., Idiong, N., Al-Saedi, S., et al., 1998. Evidence of a critical period of airway instability during central apneas in preterm infants. Am J Respir Crit Care Med 157, 470–474.

Lemyre, B., Davis, P.G., de Paoli, A.G., 2002. Nasal intermittent positive pressure ventilation (NIPPV) versus nasal continuous positive airway pressure (NCPAP) for apnea of prematurity. Cochrane Database Syst Rev.

Lewin, J.E., 1969. An apnoea-alarm mattress. Lancet 2, 667–668.

Little, G.A., Ballard, R.A., Brooks, J.R., et al., 1987. National Institutes of Health Consensus Development Conference on Infantile Apnea and Home Monitoring, Sept 29 to Oct 1, 1986. Pediatrics 79, 292–299.

Martin, R., Abu-Shaweesh, J., 2005. Control of breathing and apnea. Biol Neonate 87, 288–295.

Martin, R.J., Fanaroff, A.A., 1998. Neonatal apnea, bradycardia, or desaturation: does it matter? Journal of Pediatrics 132, 758–759.

Martin, R.J., Okken, A., Rubin, D., 1979. Arterial oxygen tension during active and quiet sleep in the normal neonate. Journal of Pediatrics 94, 271–274.

Martin, R.J., DiFiore, J.M., Jana, L., et al., 1998. Persistence of the biphasic ventilatory response to hypoxia in preterm infants. Journal of Pediatrics 132, 960–964.

Mathew, O.P., 2003. Apnea, bradycardia and desaturation. In: Mathew, O.P. (ed.) Respiratory Control and Disorders in the

Newborn. Marcel Dekker, New York, pp. 273–293.

Miller, M.J., Carlo, W.A., Martin, R.J., 1985. Continuous positive airway pressure selectively reduces obstructive apnea in preterm infants. Journal of Pediatrics 106, 91–94.

Miller, M.J., DiFiore, J.M., Strohl, K.P., et al., 1990. Effects of nasal CPAP on supraglottic and total pulmonary resistance in preterm infants. J Appl Physiol 68, 141–146.

Milner, A.D., Boon, A.W., Saunders, R.A., et al., 1980. Upper airway obstruction and apnoea in preterm babies. Arch Dis Child 55, 22–25.

Osborn, D.A., Henderson-Smart, D.J., 2002. Kinesthetic stimulation for treating apnea in preterm infants. Cochrane Database Syst Rev (4).

Oyen, N., Markestad, T., Skaerven, R., et al., 1997. Combined effects of sleeping position and prenatal risk factors in sudden infant death syndrome: the Nordic Epidemiological SIDS Study. Pediatrics 100, 613–621.

Perlstein, P.H., Edwards, N.K., Sutherland, J.M., 1970. Apnea in premature infants and incubator-air-temperature changes. NEJM 282, 461–466.

Peter, C.S., Sprodowski, N., Bohnhorst, B., et al., 2002. Gastro-esophageal reflux and apnea of prematurity: no temporal relationship. Pediatrics 109, 8–11.

Pickens, D., Schefft, D., Thach, B., 1988. Prolonged apnea associated with upper airway protective reflexes in apnea of prematurity. American Review of Respiratory Diseases 137, 113–118.

Pillekamp, F., Hermann, C., Keller, T., et al., 2007. Factors influencing apnea and bradycardia of prematurity – implications for neurodevelopment. Neonatology 91, 155–161.

Poets, C.F., 2003. Pathophysiology of apnea of prematurity. In: Mathew, O.P. (Ed.), Respiratory Control and Disorders in the Newborn. Marcel Dekker, New York, pp. 295–316.

Poets, C.F., Stebbens, V.A., Samuels, M.P., et al., 1993. The relationship between bradycardia, apnea, and hypoxemia in preterm infants. Pediatr Res 34, 144–147.

Poets, C.F., Stebbens, V.A., Richard, D., et al., 1995. Prolonged episodes of hypoxemia in preterm infants undetectable by cardiorespiratory monitors. Pediatrics 95, 860–863.

Poets, C.F., Langner, M.U., Bohnhorst, B., 1997. Effects of bottle feeding and two different methods of gavage feeding on oxygenation and breathing patterns in preterm infants. Acta Paediatr 86, 419–423.

Purohit, D.M., Ellison, R.C., Zierler, S., et al., 1985. Risk factors for retrolental fibroplasia: experience with 3025 premature infants. National Collaborative Study on Patent Ductus Arteriosus in Premature Infants. Pediatrics 76, 339–344.

Ramanathan, R., Corwin, M.J., Hunt, C.E., et al., 2001. Cardiorespiratory events recorded on home monitors: comparison of healthy infants with those at increased risk for SIDS. J Am Med Assoc 285, 2199–2207.

Razi, N.M., Delauter, M., Pandit, P.B., 2002. Periodic breathing and oxygen saturation in preterm infants at discharge. J Perinatol 22, 442–444.

Reher, C., Kuny, K.D., Pantalitschka, T., et al., 2008. Randomised crossover trial of different postural interventions on bradycardia and intermittent hypoxia in preterm infants. Arch Dis Child 93, F289–F291.

Rigatto, H., 2003. Periodic breathing. In: Mathew, O.P. (Ed.). Respiratory Control and Disorders in the Newborn. Marcel Dekker, New York, pp. 237–272.

Rosen, C.L., Glaze, D.G., Frost, J.D., 1984. Hypoxemia associated with feeding in the preterm infant and full-term neonate. Am J Dis Child 138, 623–628.

Ruggins, N.R., Milner, A.D., 1991. Site of upper airway obstruction in preterm infants with problematic apnoea. Arch Dis Child 66, 787–792.

Sachis, P., Armstrong, D., Becker, L., et al., 1982. Myelination of the human vagus nerve from 24 weeks postconceptional age to adolescence. J Neuropathol Exp Neurol 41, 466–472.

Sanchez, P.J., Laptook, A.R., Fisher, L., et al., 1997. Apnea after immunization of preterm infants. Journal of Pediatrics 130, 746–751.

Schertel, E.R., Adams, L., Schneider, D.A., et al., 1986. Rapid shallow breathing evoked by capsaicin from isolated pulmonary circulation. J Appl Physiol 61, 1237–1240.

Schmidt, B., Roberts, R.S., Davis, P., et al., 2006. Caffeine therapy for apnea of prematurity. NEJM 354, 2112–2121.

Schmidt, B., Roberts, R.S., Davis, P., et al., 2007. Long term effects of caffeine therapy for apnea of prematurity. NEJM 357, 1893–1902.

Scholander, P.F., 1963. The master switch of life. Sci Am 209, 92–106.

Schulte, F.J., Busse, C., Eichhorn, W., 1977. Rapid eye movement sleep, moto-neurone inhibition, and apneic spells in preterm infants. Pediatr Res 11, 709–713.

Smith, J.E., Scopes, J.W., 1972. A new apnoea alarm for babies. Lancet 2, 545–546.

Southall, D.P., Richards, J.M., Lau, K.C., et al., 1980. An explanation for failure of impedance apnoea alarm systems. Arch Dis Child 55, 63–65.

Southall, D.P., Richards, J.M., de Swiet, M., et al., 1983. Identification of infants destined to die unexpectedly during infancy: evaluation of predictive importance of prolonged apnoea and disorders of cardiac rhythm or conduction. Br Med J (Clin Res Ed) 286, 1092–1096.

Speidel, B.D., Dunn, P.M., 1976. Use of nasal continuous positive airway pressure to treat severe recurrent apnoea in very preterm infants. Lancet 2, 658–660.

Stocks, J., Dezateux, C., Hoo, A., et al., 1996. Delayed maturation of Hering–Breuer inflation reflex activity in preterm infants. Am J Respir Crit Care Med 154, 1411–1417.

Tamin, H., Kholagi, M., Beydoun, H., et al., 2003. National collaborative perinatal neonatal network. Consanguinity and apnea of prematurity. Am J Epidemiol 158, 942–946.

Thach, B.T., 1992. Neuromuscular control of the upper airway. In: Beckerman, R.C., Broillette, R.T., Hunt, C.E. (Eds.), Respiratory Control Disorders in Infants and Children. Lippincott Williams & Wilkins, Baltimore, pp. 47–61.

Thach, B.T., 2005. The role of respiratory control disorders in SIDS. Respiratory Physiology 149, 343–353.

Thach, B.T., Stark, A.R., 1979. Spontaneous neck flexion and airway obstruction during apneic spells in preterm infants. Journal of Pediatrics 94, 275–281.

Tudehope, D.I., Rogers, Y.M., Burns, Y.R., et al., 1986. Apnoea in very low birthweight infants: outcome at 2 years. Australian Paediatrics Journal 22, 131–134.

Upton, C.J., Milner, A.D., Stokes, G.M., 1991. Apnoea, bradycardia, and oxygen saturation in preterm infants. Arch Dis Child 66, 381–385.

Upton, C.J., Milner, A.D., Stokes, G.M., 1992a. Response to tube breathing in preterm infants with apnea. Pediatr Pulmonol 12, 23–28.

Upton, C.J., Milner, A.D., Stokes, G.M., 1992b. Response to external obstruction in preterm infants with apnea. Pediatr Pulmonol 14, 233–238.

Upton, C.J., Milner, A.D., Stokes, G.M., 1992c. Episodic bradycardia in preterm infants. Arch Dis Child 67, 831–834.

Valman, H.B., Wright, B.M., Lawrence, C., 1983. Measurement of respiratory rate in the newborn. Br Med J (Clin Res Ed) 4 (286), 1783–1784.

Vyas, H., Milner, A.D., Hopkin, I.E., 1981. Relationship between apnoea and bradycardia in preterm infants. Acta Paediatr Scand 70, 785–790.

Waggener, T.B., Stark, A.R., Cohlan, B.A., et al., 1984. Apnea duration is related to ventilatory oscillation characteristics in newborn infants. J Appl Physiol 57, 536–544.

Waggener, T.B., Frantz, I.D., Cohlan, B.A., et al., 1989. Mixed and obstructive apneas are related to ventilatory oscillations in premature infants. J Appl Physiol 66, 2818–2826.

Watanabe, K., Hakamada, S., Kuroyanagi, M., et al., 1983. Electroencephalographic study of intraventricular hemorrhage in the preterm newborn. Neuropediatrics 14, 225–230.

Weintraub, Z., Alvaro, R., Kwiatkowski, K., et al., 1992. Effects of inhaled oxygen (up to 40%) on periodic breathing and apnea

in preterm infants. J Appl Physiol 72, 116–120.

Westkamp, E., Soditt, V., Adrian, S., et al., 2002. Blood transfusion in anemic infants with apnea of prematurity. Biol Neonate 82, 228–232.

Wilson, C., Martin, R., Jaber, M., et al., 2004. Adenosine A$_{2A}$ receptors interact with GABAergic pathways to modulate respiration in neonatal piglets. Respiration Physiology and Neurobiology 141, 201–206.

Part 5: Malformations of the lower respiratory tract

Grenville F Fox

Pulmonary agenesis

Bilateral pulmonary agenesis is an extremely rare abnormality and is not compatible with postnatal life. It has been described in association with anencephaly and other congenital anomalies (Potter 1952).

Approximately 70% of cases of pulmonary agenesis are unilateral, occurring in association with other congenital anomalies, including congenital heart disease (CHD), oesophageal atresia, and vertebral and facial anomalies (Knowles et al. 1988; Osborne et al. 1989). Antenatal ultrasound diagnosis has been reported (Maymon et al. 2001), although most cases present with respiratory distress in the early neonatal period. Others may present with recurrent respiratory symptoms in early childhood or be discovered incidentally (Thomas et al. 1998).

Diagnosis is usually confirmed on a chest X-ray (CXR), which shows absence of aeration on the affected side, with marked mediastinal shift and herniation of the unaffected lung, which often shows compensatory hyperinflation.

Management is supportive, with treatment of other congenital malformations when possible. The mortality rate is high and often depends on coexisting CHD.

Pulmonary hypoplasia

Primary pulmonary hypoplasia

In this rare form of pulmonary hypoplasia, there is no apparent underlying cause. Familial cases have been described (Cregg and Casey 1997), although the disorder is usually sporadic. Acinar dysplasia has been found in some cases of primary pulmonary hypoplasia, with abnormal development occurring distal to the bronchi. There are no alveoli and the terminal bronchioles have multiple cystic branches lined by bronchial epithelium, equivalent to failure of lung development beyond the pseudoglandular phase (Rutledge and Jensen 1986).

Secondary pulmonary hypoplasia

A normal-sized thoracic cavity, normal amniotic fluid volume and normal fetal breathing movements are all required for optimal lung growth in utero. Causes of secondary pulmonary hypoplasia therefore include intrathoracic space-occupying lesions, small-chest syndromes, oligohydramnios and congenital neuromuscular disorders (Table 27.15).

Reduction in intrathoracic space

Conditions that restrict thoracic volume are frequently associated with pulmonary hypoplasia. Of these, congenital diaphragmatic hernia (CDH) has been extensively researched (Ch. 27.6), and histological studies show that this is associated with decreased bronchial and vascular branching with reduced alveolar number (Dibbins and Weiner 1974).

Reduction in amniotic fluid volume

Oligohydramnios from any cause can result in pulmonary hypoplasia, particularly if it develops before 26 weeks' gestation (Table 27.15). Attempting to restore normal amniotic fluid volume by amnioinfusion in some cases has been associated with less pulmonary hypoplasia, suggesting that adequate amniotic fluid volume is necessary for normal lung growth (Tranquilli et al. 2005).

Postmortem examination shows that pulmonary hypoplasia caused by oligohydramnios secondary to fetal renal disease results in a reduction in bronchial branching and decreased alveolar number and size. This indicates maldevelopment with onset prior to 16 weeks of fetal life, which continues into the third trimester (Hislop et al. 1979; Harrison et al. 1983).

Although not associated with severe pulmonary hypoplasia, amniocentesis in the first and second trimester may affect lung growth, leading to an increased incidence of respiratory problems and reduced lung volume and function in newborn infants (Anonymous 1978; Vyas et al. 1982; Thompson et al. 1992).

The mechanism for decreased lung growth due to oligohydramnios is uncertain and several mechanisms have been suggested, including thoracic compression (Tranquilli et al. 2005), decrease in fetal breathing movements (Adzick et al. 1984) and reduced stretching of the developing respiratory tract by fluid.

Reduction in fetal breathing movements

Pulmonary hypoplasia is associated with a number of congenital neuromuscular diseases. There is a reduction in bronchial branching, suggesting that lung growth and development are affected before the 16th week of fetal life. Fetal breathing movements are frequently seen with ultrasound scanning (USS) several weeks prior to this, and the amplitude of pressure changes during breaths has been shown to be an important determinant of normal lung growth (Liggins et al. 1981).

Clinical features

Bilateral pulmonary hypoplasia varies widely in severity. Those with mild disease may have minimal symptoms of respiratory distress, which resolve over the first few weeks of life without intervention (Aiton et al. 1996).

Severe bilateral pulmonary hypoplasia leads to significant respiratory failure, which is frequently complicated by pneumothorax and persistent pulmonary hypertension of the newborn (PPHN). When neuromuscular disease such as congenital myotonic dystrophy is present, there may be a history of reduced fetal movements and polyhydramnios due to poor fetal swallowing. Postnatally, there may be profoundly decreased muscle tone with myopathic

Table 27.15 Causes of secondary pulmonary hypoplasia

PATHOPHYSIOLOGY	CONDITION/AETIOLOGY
Reduction in intrathoracic space	Congenital diaphragmatic hernia (Areechon and Reid 1963) Congenital cystic adenomatoid malformation (Ostor and Fortune 1978) Congenital lung cysts Pleural effusions (Castillo et al. 1987) Small-chest syndromes (Table 27.15)
Reduction in fetal breathing movements	Congenital myotonic dystrophy (Vilos et al. 1984) Spinal muscular atrophy (Moerman et al. 1983) Phrenic nerve agenesis (Goldstein and Reid 1980) Cervical spinal cord lesions (Rotschild et al. 1994)

Reduction in amniotic fluid volume	Fetal renal abnormalities
	  Bilateral renal agenesis (Potter syndrome) (Potter 1946)
	  Multicystic dysplastic kidneys (Newbould et al. 1994)
	  Polycystic kidney disease (Kaariainen et al. 1988; Newbould et al. 1994)
	  Obstructive uropathy (Harrison et al. 1983)
	  Renal tubular dysgenesis (Newbould et al. 1994; Kriegsmann et al. 2000)
	Prolonged premature rupture of membranes (Bain et al. 1964)
	Uteroplacental insufficiency
	Amniocentesis

Other	Rhesus disease (Chamberlain et al. 1977)
	Trisomies 21 (Cooney and Thurlbeck 1982) and 18
	Maternal drugs
	  Angiotensin-converting enzyme inhibitors (Hanssens et al. 1991)
	  Sodium valproate (Janas et al. 1998)
	Anterior abdominal wall defects (Thompson et al. 1993a)

facies, talipes equinovarus, joint contractures and rib hypoplasia. Respiratory function is further compromised by diaphragmatic hypoplasia.

Congenital myotonic dystrophy is usually inherited in an autosomal dominant pattern via the mother, who is only mildly affected and often undiagnosed until presentation of her more severely affected baby. There may be a history of previous stillbirth or neonatal death (Ch. 41). The molecular basis of the condition is an expansion in the number of trinucleotide repeats at chromosome 19q13.3 (Brook et al. 1992).

Severe oligohydramnios due to renal disease or very early chronic leakage of amniotic fluid often causes severe pulmonary hypoplasia, resulting in early neonatal death. Affected neonates may be small for gestational age and have limb contractures and typical 'Potter's' facies with abnormal ears, flattened nose and epicanthic folds.

Diagnosis

Antenatal history and ultrasound may identify factors associated with pulmonary hypoplasia such as CDH and other causes of reduced intrathoracic space, bilateral renal anomalies and oligohydramnios or features of congenital neuromuscular disease (Table 27.15). Three-dimensional fetal ultrasonography and Doppler blood flow velocities of pulmonary arteries have been used to estimate lung volume (Lee et al. 1996; Yoshimura et al. 1999).

Severe bilateral pulmonary hypoplasia presents immediately after birth. Affected neonates are difficult to resuscitate, requiring high-pressure positive-pressure ventilation with F_IO_2 1.0. Despite this, death often occurs within minutes of birth. The CXR shows small-volume lungs with a bell-shaped chest. Lung volumes can be estimated by measuring functional residual capacity using gas dilution or plethysmographic techniques (Thompson et al. 1992, 1993a; Aiton et al. 1996), although this is not routinely necessary as the diagnosis is usually established clinically with supporting radiological evidence.

Management

Antenatal

Antenatal diagnosis of conditions leading to pulmonary hypoplasia is often possible as early as the second trimester. This may provide an opportunity for antenatal fetal intervention in some cases. If polyhydramnios is present, drainage may prolong the pregnancy and reduce the risk and consequences of preterm birth.

Drainage of large fluid-filled congenital cystic adenomatoid malformations (CCAMs), bronchogenic cysts or hydrothoraces with a pigtail intercostal catheter used to create a thoracoamniotic shunt has been shown to be associated with resolution of hydrops and may allow normal subsequent lung growth (Thompson et al. 1993b; Lopoo et al. 1999).

Antenatal intervention for severe pulmonary hypoplasia by tracheal occlusion, usually with an inflated balloon, leads to entrapment of lung fluid which causes stretching of airways, with subsequent improved airway and pulmonary vascular growth (Ch. 27.6) (Harrison et al. 2001, 2003). Outcome from three centres following percutaneous fetoscopic endoluminal tracheal occlusion in 210 cases of severe pulmonary hypoplasia secondary to CDH, some with other associated anomalies, showed survival to hospital discharge of 48% (Jani et al. 2009). More information is given in Chapter 27, part 6.

Fetal tracheal occlusion has also been successful in preventing adverse neonatal outcome due to severe pulmonary hypoplasia in a small number of cases of oligohydramnios secondary to early second-trimester rupture of membranes (Kohl et al. 2009). Transabdominal amnioinfusion has also been used for this indication, and evidence from one randomised controlled trial with intervention between 24 and 33 weeks' gestation suggested improved survival and less pulmonary hypoplasia following amnioinfusion (Tranquilli et al. 2005).

Fetal bladder catheterisation has been carried out successfully in a number of cases of obstructive uropathy diagnosed prior to 24 weeks' gestation, thus avoiding pulmonary hypoplasia, due to resolution of severe oligohydramnios (Szaflik et al. 1998).

Postnatal

The degree of respiratory support required for infants with bilateral pulmonary hypoplasia depends on the severity of underdevelopment of the lungs. In many cases, particularly when there has been anhydramnios or severe oligohydramnios noted from early in the second trimester with other severe congenital anomalies such as bilateral cystic dysplastic kidneys, continued intensive care is usually futile and hence inappropriate. In cases of mild bilateral pulmonary hypoplasia, no respiratory support may be required and close monitoring is recommended over a period of several weeks or months while the lungs grow to a normal size (Aiton et al. 1996).

Many babies with bilateral pulmonary hypoplasia require prolonged mechanical ventilation. Ventilatory requirements may be high, particularly initially. Following prolonged rupture of membranes in the second trimester, some infants require very high-pressure ventilation initially, but recover rapidly over the first 24 hours of life to enable complete weaning from any respiratory support within a few days. This has been attributed to severe atelectasis due to oligohydramnios and is referred to as 'dry-lung syndrome' (McIntosh 1988). The lung growth in these cases is likely to be normal, but initial CXR appearance and antenatal history may suggest pulmonary hypoplasia (Losa and Kind 1998).

Owing to the increased risk of infection following prolonged rupture of membranes, broad-spectrum antibiotics should be given following appropriate investigations.

Pulmonary hypertension is a common problem. Inhaled nitric oxide, high-frequency oscillation, calcium antagonists and extracorporeal membrane oxygenation (ECMO) have been advocated, with successful outcome in some cases (Islam et al. 1999; Geary and Whitsett 2002). At 34 weeks, preterm delivery is low risk and may avoid joint contractures.

Prognosis

Survival with bilateral pulmonary hypoplasia is dependent on the degree of lung underdevelopment and other associated anomalies.

Resolution of symptoms due to mild to moderate pulmonary hypoplasia may take weeks to months (Aiton et al. 1996). Long-term ventilatory support may be required for those with more severe problems, with resolution likely to occur with growth; good nutrition is essential. Lung volume measurements using several different techniques in infants with a number of different underlying diagnoses have suggested that normal lung size is likely by 6 years of age in the vast majority who survive the early neonatal period (Chatrath et al. 1971; Thompson et al. 1990; Aiton et al. 1996).

Premature rupture of membranes prior to 26 weeks' gestation is associated with pulmonary hypoplasia in approximately 25% of cases (Everest et al. 2008). The gestational age at the time of membrane rupture was found to be most predictive of outcome, with duration of rupture (longer than 14 days) and severity of oligohydramnios also identified as risk factors for pulmonary hypoplasia in a meta-analysis of relevant studies (van Teeffelen et al. 2010). Previous reports suggested that premature rupture of membranes at less than 25 weeks' gestation resulted in neonatal mortality greater than 90% due to pulmonary hypoplasia (Kilbride et al. 1996). However, more recently published case series, in which antenatal steroids, postnatal surfactant, high-frequency oscillatory ventilation and inhaled nitric oxide were used, suggest that survival has improved to approximately 70% (Everest et al. 2008; Williams et al. 2009).

Small-chest syndromes

Table 27.16 shows conditions that have congenital chest wall abnormalities leading to respiratory symptoms in the neonatal period. The ribs are usually short and many are associated with vertebral anomalies resulting in kyphoscoliosis, which may further reduce thoracic volume. Pulmonary hypoplasia may also occur in some of these conditions, but lung growth and development have been documented as being normal in many cases (Williams et al. 1984).

Antenatal diagnosis using USS is able to detect many of these conditions before 24 weeks' gestation. In one series, accuracy of diagnosis was only 65%, but prediction of mortality had 100% sensitivity and specificity (Parilla et al. 2003).

Table 27.16 Congenital chest wall abnormalities causing neonatal respiratory symptoms

CONDITION	INHERITANCE/GENETICS	CLINICAL FEATURES	PROGNOSIS
Asphyxiating thoracic dystrophy (Jeune's syndrome)	Autosomal recessive – mutation in chromosome 15q13	Short ribs, bell-shaped chest, +/– short limbs, hypoplastic iliac wings, renal abnormalities	Variable severity ranging from mild neonatal respiratory distress and long-term survival, to early severe respiratory failure and death
Chondroectodermal dysplasia (Ellis van Creveld syndrome)	Autosomal recessive – mutation in chromosome 4p16	Short ribs, polydactyly (medial), congenital heart disease, cleft lip and palate, hypoplastic nails	Neonatal respiratory distress with good outcome
Short rib–polydactyly syndromes	Autosomal recessive	Short ribs, polydactyly, vertebral and pelvic defects, short limbs, congenital heart disease, renal, genital and intestinal abnormalities	Severe neonatal respiratory failure with early death
Achondroplasia	Autosomal dominant (80% new mutations)	Small chest, short limbs, macrocephaly with frontal bossing	Mild neonatal respiratory distress, upper airway obstruction and apnoea, mild hypotonia. Good prognosis

Table 27.16 Continued

CONDITION	INHERITANCE/GENETICS	CLINICAL FEATURES	PROGNOSIS
Achondrogenesis	Autosomal recessive	Type 1 (Parenti–Fraccaro syndrome) – short limbs, large head, small barrel-shaped chest with thin ribs with fractures, unossified vertebral bodies Type 2 (Langer–Saldino syndrome) – short limbs and ribs with more ossification of skull and vertebral bodies	Stillborn or die in early neonatal period
Thanatophoric dysplasia	Sporadic – fibroblast growth factor receptor 3 gene mutation	Very short limbs with 'telephone handle' femurs; very small, pear-shaped chest; clover-leaf skull; occasional other congenital anomalies (congenital heart disease, hydronephrosis, imperforate anus, hydrocephalus)	Severe neonatal respiratory failure usually leading to death within hours. Some may survive several weeks (O'Malley et al. 1972)
Camptomelic dysplasia	Autosomal recessive	Short limbs, bowed long bones, narrow thorax, occasionally with 11 ribs. May have female phenotype with male karyotype, hydrocephalus and hypoplasia of larynx and tracheal rings	Usually severe neonatal respiratory failure and early death within weeks. Survival to 17 years noted in one case (Spranger et al. 1970)
Osteogenesis imperfecta	Type II – usually autosomal recessive, but may be dominant. Mutation in type 1 procollagen genes	Severe deformity of the chest wall and limbs due to mutiple, healed in utero fractures; soft skull, thin skin	Approximately 50% stillborn. Others usually die immediately after birth. Antenatal diagnosis by ultrasound scan (Morin et al. 1991) or chorionic villus biopsy possible
	Type III – autosomal recessive. Mutation in type 1 collagen genes	As above but less severe	Mild respiratory problems may occur in the neonatal period. Chest wall deformity is often progressive, resulting in death later in childhood in many cases
Hypophosphatasia (perinatal form)	Autosomal recessive – mutation in tissue non-specific alkaline phosphatase gene found in some cases (Gehring et al. 1999)	Poorly mineralised bones with multiple pathological fractures, short ribs and long bones, hypercalcaemia, low alkaline phosphatase	Death from respiratory failure in early neonatal period. Antenatal diagnosis possible by alkaline phosphatase assay from chorionic villus biopsy
Cleidocranial dysostosis	Autosomal dominant	Hypoplasia of clavicle, short ribs, delayed closure of anterior fontanelle and delayed eruption of teeth	Variable degree of neonatal respiratory distress may occur
Spondyloepiphyseal dysplasias	Autosomal dominant	Delayed ossification of vertebrae with kyphoscoliosis, small chest and cleft palate	May present with neonatal respiratory distress
Spondylothoracic dysostoses	Autosomal recessive	Vertebral anomalies resulting in severe chest wall deformity due to crowding of the ribs	Severe neonatal respiratory distress resulting in death within first few months (Karnes et al. 1991)
Spondylocostal dysostoses	Autosomal recessive or dominant	Vertebral and rib abnormalities resulting in some chest wall abnormality	Autosomal recessive type more likely to present with severe neonatal respiratory distress. Dominant form may present with mild symptoms only (Karnes et al. 1991)

Signs of respiratory distress may develop early in many of these conditions. The thorax often appears bell-shaped and the abdomen large. CXR shows the same, with short, horizontal ribs as well as apparent cardiomegaly and clear lung fields. Close examination of the vertebrae and other bones on a skeletal survey, along with detailed family history, may help establish the underlying diagnosis.

Four subtypes of short rib–polydactyly syndromes have been described (Saldino–Noonan, Majewski, Verma–Naumoff and Beemer–Langer syndromes), but these, along with asphyxiating thoracic dystrophy and Ellis van Creveld syndrome, are likely to represent variants of a single disorder (Martinez-Frias et al. 1993). This is supported by recent identification of the *DYNC2H1* gene mutation in both Verma–Naumoff and Ellis van Creveld syndrome (Dagoneau et al. 2009).

In many of these conditions, mechanical ventilation is often required immediately after birth and for a variable time, depending on the underlying diagnosis. Prognosis is often poor, but those surviving the first year may have a good long-term outlook (Oberklaid et al. 1977). Surgical reconstruction of the chest wall with bone grafts or synthetic prostheses has been described in cases of asphyxiating thoracic dystrophy and other similar conditions (Todd et al. 1986), with good long-term outcome being reported if this is limited to milder cases able to survive to 1 year of age before surgery is contemplated (Davis et al. 2001).

Congenital cystic adenomatoid malformation

CCAM is a rare condition, predominantly affecting the lower lobes of the lungs. These lesions have also been referred to as congenital pulmonary airway malformations and also, along with other variants, congenital lung and airway cysts and pulmonary sequestration, congenital thoracic malformations.

Unilateral CCAM is more common, more often affecting the left lung (Savic et al. 1979). Bilateral cases have also been reported (Sapin et al. 1997; Banerjea et al. 2002). The affected areas consist of a mass of cysts lined by bronchial or cuboidal epithelium, which may contain cystic and adenomatoid portions with intervening normal lung tissue. Stocker et al. (1978) described three pathological variations of CCAM. Type 1 is the most common of these, accounting for approximately 50% of cases. It consists of multiple, thin-walled cysts, lined with pseudostratified epithelium, which may contain mucus-secreting glands. The cysts are large and may be confused with congenital lobar emphysema. Type 2 CCAM accounts for approximately 40% of cases and consists of multiple, smaller cysts (less than 1–2 cm diameter), which are lined by ciliated cuboidal or columnar epithelium without glandular tissue. Type 3 lesions are rarer (less than 10% of CCAMs) and relatively solid lesions, which have very small cysts lined with ciliated cuboidal epithelium. Subsequently, a fourth type has been described which has acinar–alveolar epithelium, rather than the bronchiolar epithelium found in types 1, 2, and 3 CCAM (Morotti et al. 1999). This suggests that there are two subtypes of CCAM arising at different stages of the branching morphogenesis of lung development. The first arises at the pseudoglandular stage (types 1, 2 and 3), whilst type 4 lesions arise at the saccular stage. A simpler classification describing microcystic (cysts <5 mm) and macrocystic (cysts >5 mm) lesions has been suggested and also has prognostic value (Thorpe-Beeston and Nicolaides 1994).

The aetiology of CCAM remains obscure, although it has been suggested that it is the result of dysregulation of lung epithelial cell turnover, with both increased cell proliferation and decreased apoptosis (Cass et al. 1998). Glial cell-derived neurotropic factor is a growth factor involved in the development of fetal lung and other organs, and increased expression of this has been found in the epithelial cells of CCAM tissue compared with normal lung (Fromont-Hankard et al. 2002). Platelet-derived growth factor-BB (PDGF-BB) stimulates normal lung growth and is maximal during the canalicular stage. Increased levels of PDGF-BB have been found in rapidly growing CCAMs which were associated with hydrops (Fromont-Hankard et al. 2002).

The incidence of CCAM has been estimated at 1 in 25 000–30 000 pregnancies. Males and females are equally affected and there are no recognised patterns of inheritance. Trisomy 18 has been noted in a very small number of cases (Laberge et al. 2001). Associated congenital anomalies only occur in approximately 20% of cases (Stocker et al. 1978). Other congenital malformations of the lung such as bronchogenic cysts and pulmonary sequestration may also coexist (Cass et al. 1997; MacKenzie et al. 2001).

Clinical features

The majority of cases of CCAM are diagnosed by antenatal USS, usually at around 20 weeks' gestation. Most have a good prognosis, if not associated with the development of hydrops. The lesion may grow initially, reaching a maximum size at around 25 weeks' gestation (Kunisaki et al. 2007). About half of these regress, so that postnatal detection is not possible with either plain chest radiography or computed tomography (CT) scanning in approximately 60% of these (Cavoretto et al. 2008).

Hydrops occurs in a small number of cases and this is likely to be the result of raised central venous pressure due to vascular compression from the lesion. Oesophageal compression leading to reduced swallowing may cause polyhydramnios. This partly accounts for the increased risk of preterm birth, which has been noted in up to 50% of cases in some series, although the wide range for this may be reflective of differing approaches to antenatal intervention (Thorpe-Beeston and Nicolaides 1994; Miller et al. 1996; Duncombe et al. 2002).

Postnatal presentation is variable and ranges from absence of symptoms in up to 50% of cases (Neilson et al. 1991) to severe respiratory distress requiring artificial ventilation and other forms of respiratory support. Pneumothorax (Gardikis et al. 2002) and PPHN (Rescorla et al. 1990) have also been noted in association with CCAM in the early neonatal period. Late presentation in children and adults, most commonly with recurrent lower respiratory tract infection, is now unusual, owing to widespread routine antenatal USS (Lujan et al. 2002). However, some recently reported cases presenting from infancy to adulthood describe lung abscess (Dahabreh et al. 2000), pneumothorax (Lejeune et al. 1999), haemoptysis (Chen 1985) and incidental finding on a CXR (Avitabile et al. 1984).

A number of case reports suggest an association between CCAM and various intrathoracic neoplasms. Bronchoalveolar carcinoma has developed both in children as young as 11 years old as well as in adult patients (Granata et al. 1998). Pulmonary rhabdomyosarcoma has also been reported in a number of cases (Ozcan et al. 2001), the youngest being 13 months old. Bronchopulmonary blastoma may develop from CCAM and has been found after initial surgical resection (Papagiannopoulos et al. 2001).

Diagnosis

Antenatal USS may detect CCAM as early as 16 weeks' gestation, when the lesions appear as a hyperechogenic mass in microcystic

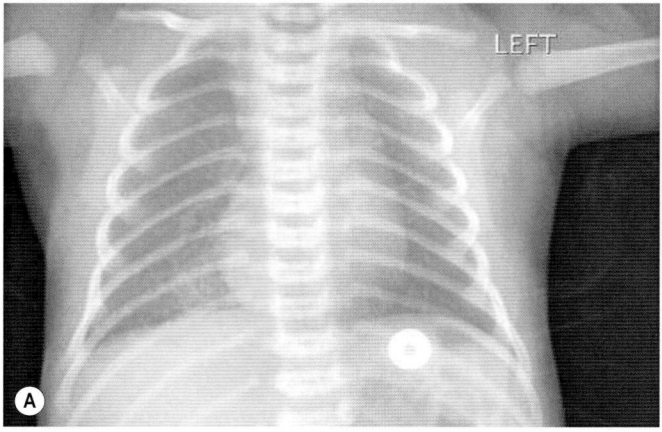

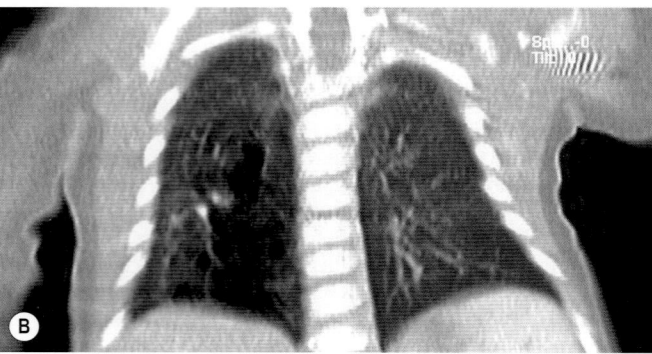

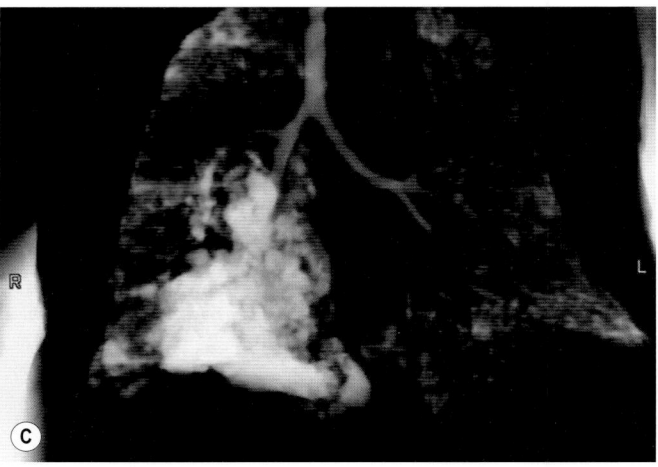

Fig. 27.51 (A) Frontal chest radiograph showing mixed increased density and subtle overinflation with lucency in the right mid- and lower zone. (B) Coronal computed tomography (CT) of chest (lung window settings), showing a multicystic lesion within the right lung. (c) Minimum-intensity projection) image of the CT dataset, demonstrating the extent of the lesion.

lesions or as larger cysts (Thorpe-Beeston and Nicolaides 1994). Serial ultrasound scans are recommended so that regression, progression and development of complications such as hydrops can be detected. Ultrasound estimation of the volume of CCAM has been used to predict the development of hydrops (Crombleholme et al. 2002), and Doppler blood flow waveforms of fetal pulmonary arteries have been found to predict pulmonary hypoplasia accurately (Fuke et al. 2003). More recently, fetal magnetic resonance imaging (MRI) has been evaluated and may be useful in distinguishing between CCAM and other anomalies such as CDH (Hubbard et al. 1999).

Initial postnatal imaging with plain CXR usually shows a cystic, solid or mixed lesion in the affected lobes, depending on the underlying type of CCAM. Mediastinal shift is common. Further evaluation with CT scanning is usually recommended in order to detect small lesions that may be difficult to visualise on a CXR (Fig. 27.51). This is important in order to establish that a lesion seen antenatally has completely involuted and to distinguish between CCAM and CDH, as well as to depict anatomical location accurately (Kim et al. 1997). The CT scan should be performed as early as possible in symptomatic cases or at a later stage within the first few weeks of life if there are no initial symptoms. Colour flow Doppler studies may be useful to exclude systemic arterial blood supply that has been noted in some cases of CCAM, although this may not be apparent until found during surgical resection (Cass et al. 1997).

Management

Termination of pregnancy may be considered in pregnancies with poor prognostic features such as bilateral CCAM, early hydrops or associated severe congenital anomalies (Thorpe-Beeston and

Nicolaides 1994; Lee et al. 1996; Golaszewski et al. 1998). Amniotic fluid reduction by amniocentesis may reduce the risk of preterm birth, although there is no direct evidence supporting this in cases of CCAM. If there is marked mediastinal shift associated with large fluid-filled cysts, thoracoamniotic shunting has led to high survival rates (Adzick et al. 1998; Crombleholme et al. 2002; Cavoretto et al. 2008) but such intervention is indicated only if there is polyhydramnios or hydrops (Dommergues et al. 1997). For massive multicystic or predominantly solid CCAM associated with hydrops, fetal lobectomy may provide an alternative therapeutic option. This was performed in 13 cases between 21 and 29 weeks' gestation, resulting in eight healthy survivors at 1–7 years' follow-up (Adzick et al. 1998).

Early postnatal surgical resection with lobectomy or segmentectomy is required in symptomatic cases. Mediastinal shift, pulmonary hypoplasia and pulmonary hypertension may be problematic in the initial postnatal period and high-frequency oscillatory ventilation (Waszak et al. 1999), inhaled nitric oxide (Banerjea et al. 2002), selective intubation of the contralateral lung (Castillo et al. 1994) and ECMO (Njinimbam et al. 1999) have been used to stabilise infants with CCAM perioperatively. The risk of recurrent infection and malignant change suggests that surgery should also be considered in asymptomatic cases, and is often recommended towards the end of the second year of life, allowing the baby to grow before the onset of symptoms, which are rare before this time in cases asymptomatic during the fetal and neonatal period (Sueyoshi et al. 2008).

Prognosis

Outcome is excellent in most cases of antenatally diagnosed CCAM in the absence of hydrops, with approximately 95% survival to hospital discharge (Cavoretto et al. 2008). Hydrops is associated with approximately 95% fetal or early neonatal mortality. Polyhydramnios, mediastinal shift, type 3 disease, presence of other congenital malformations and preterm birth are also associated with a worse outcome (Thorpe-Beeston and Nicolaides 1994; Miller et al. 1996).

Recurrence rates in partially resected CCAM are low (Mentzer et al. 1992).

Congenital lung cysts

Congenital lung cysts may be extrapulmonary (mostly arising from bronchi or trachea) or intrapulmonary (mostly arising from alveoli). They are usually single, confined to one lung and are not associated with cystic changes in other organs. The commonest site is in the carinal region, but they may occur at the periphery of the lung, below the diaphragm or in the mediastinum (Maier 1948).

Signs of respiratory distress due to congenital lung cysts are extremely unusual in the neonatal period, with only 10% diagnosed at this stage, a further 14% during the first year and over 50% in adults, many being discovered incidentally by routine CXR (Ribet et al. 1996). Symptoms and timing of presentation depend on the size and site of congenital lung cysts.

Diagnosis is usually from CXR appearance. CT, MRI or USS may be useful in differentiating large congenital lung cysts from CCAM and congenital lobar emphysema.

Surgical resection is recommended for all congenital lung cysts. More recently, thoracoscopic surgical techniques have been described for these lesions (Rothenberg 2000).

Pulmonary sequestration

Pulmonary sequestration is a congenital abnormality consisting of intrathoracic or intra-abdominal lung tissue with arterial blood supply from the thoracic or abdominal aorta. There is usually no connection to the tracheobronchial tree. Traditionally, classification has been according to the position of the lesion, as intra- or extralobular, with intralobular lesions lying adjacent to normal lung tissue within the pleura and extralobular lesions being within their own pleura. Subsequently, a classification based on the airway connection, the arterial supply, venous drainage and lung parenchyma has been advocated (Clements and Warner 1987).

It was initially suggested that pulmonary sequestrations are likely to arise as a result of an accessory lung diverticulum from the primitive foregut, with extralobular lesions being more distal. A further explanation of aetiology is that of the haphazard branching theory, in which there are abnormal connections or malinosculations between the primitive foregut and aortic–pulmonary arch system (Lee et al. 2002).

Pathophysiology

Intralobular pulmonary sequestrations usually consist of a mass of airless alveoli, which may have a cystic appearance. They are usually left-sided and involve the lower zone in 85% of cases (Weinbaum et al. 1989). Arterial supply is directly from the aorta in most cases, with venous drainage into a pulmonary vein. Extralobular lesions may be intrathoracic or abdominal, and venous drainage is into systemic veins, usually the vena cava or azygous veins (Gamillscheg et al. 1996). One variation involves sequestration in the right lung with resultant right-lung hypoplasia, with infradiaphragmatic venous drainage to the vena cava from the sequestered lobe and surrounding otherwise normal lung. This is known as scimitar

syndrome, owing to the characteristic appearance of the CXR and angiogram (Gao et al. 1993).

Clinical features

Antenatal diagnosis may be by USS, showing an echogenic intrathoracic or intra-abdominal mass. Polyhydramnios is common and fetal pleural effusions and hydrops may also occur. More recently, fetal MRI has been used to obtain further detail (Dhingsa et al. 2003).

Intralobular lesions may lead to symptoms of respiratory distress in the neonatal period owing to compression of adjacent normal lung or heart failure due to a large arteriovenous shunt. However, up to 80% of babies may remain symptom-free initially but present later in childhood or adulthood with recurrent pulmonary infection, pleural effusion or haemoptysis. The diagnosis may be made on CXR as an incidental finding. Scimitar syndrome can present in the neonatal period with massive haemorrhage from the affected lung (Alivizatos et al. 1985).

Other congenital malformations are rarely found in intralobular pulmonary sequestration. However, in two series, more than 50% of pulmonary sequestrations were associated with type 2 CCAM (Conran et al. 1999; Bratu et al. 2001). These differed from those without CCAM, with earlier presentation, usually within the first 3 months of life.

Extralobular pulmonary sequestration often remains asymptomatic and is usually found incidentally. Other congenital malformations such as CDH and CHD occur in nearly 60% of cases (Savic et al. 1979).

Diagnosis

CXR shows pulmonary sequestration as a radiodensity, usually in the posteromedial part of the left lung. Doppler ultrasonography, spiral CT scanning or MR angiography may be used to determine arterial supply and venous drainage (Hang et al. 1996) (Fig. 44.13).

Management

Antenatal drainage of polyhydramnios and insertion of thoracoabdominal shunts for associated hydrothorax may improve outcome after antenatal presentation of pulmonary sequestration (Lopoo et al. 1999).

Early surgical resection by segmentectomy or lobectomy for intralobar sequestrations, and mass excision for extralobar sequestrations, have generally been recommended in order to alleviate the mass effect of large lesions and prevent other possible short-term complications such as haemorrhage and heart failure, as well as avoiding later infection (Becmeur et al. 1998; Halkic et al. 1998; Van Raemdonck et al. 2001). Successful minimally invasive surgery using thoracoscopy or laparoscopy has also been described (Mezzetti et al. 1996; Danielson and Sherman 2001).

Transumbilical arterial embolization has been reported, with some success and minimal complications. However, complete regression occurred in only 53% of cases (Lee et al. 2008).

Prognosis

Antenatal regression and resolution of pulmonary sequestration may occur in approximately 50% of cases (Becmeur et al. 1998). Polyhydramnios and hydrops are likely to be associated with a worse outcome. Postnatal regression has also been described but appears to occur less frequently (Garcia-Pena et al. 1998).

Surgical resection in the neonatal period or later generally leads to excellent results, with favourable long-term outcome (Halkic et al. 1998; Lopoo et al. 1999). Metaplasia or neoplastic change has not been noted from histological examination of resected pulmonary sequestrations.

Congenital pulmonary lymphangiectasis

Congenital pulmonary lymphangiectasis (CPL) is a rare condition in which there is cystic dilatation of the pulmonary lymphatics with obstruction to their drainage. It is usually bilateral and associated with severe respiratory failure, although unilateral and localised lesions have been described (Rettwitz-Volk et al. 1999). It is more common in males and may be associated with other abnormalities of the lymphatics. Noonan et al. (1970) described three groups of patients with CPL:

1. CPL associated with generalised lymphangiectasis. Presentation is often antenatal with hydrops. Generalised lymphangiectasis develops with malabsorption and hemihypertrophy.
2. CPL associated with CHD. Total anomalous venous drainage, hypoplastic left heart, pulmonary stenosis, and atrial and ventricular septal defects have all been described in association with CPL.
3. CPL as a primary developmental defect of the lung. This may occur in Noonan, Turner and Down syndrome.

Pathophysiology

CPL may arise as a result of failure of fusion of embryonic lymphatic channels, which initially develop as spaces within the lung bud. It has also been suggested that it may be part of a generalised developmental anomaly of lymphatics, rather than an intrinsic lung defect. Lymphatic obstruction results in large, firm and heavy lungs which are poorly expanded.

Clinical features

Presentation is usually antenatal, with hydrops or severe respiratory distress in a term infant. Exogenous surfactant therapy may lead to temporary resolution of respiratory failure.

Diagnosis

In generalised bilateral CPL, lung fields usually have a ground-glass appearance on CXR, but are usually well inflated or even over-inflated, and have prominent interstitial lymphatics radiating from the hilar areas. Chylous pleural infusions may be present. The diagnosis is only confirmed by lung biopsy.

Localised lesions may present with a cystic mass, which appears similar to a cystic adenomatoid malformation on antenatal USS or postnatal CXR (Rettwitz-Volk et al. 1999).

Management

Surgical excision may be possible for localised CPL (Rettwitz-Volk et al. 1999). Bilateral disease presenting with severe respiratory failure has a poor prognosis.

Pulmonary alveolar proteinosis (congenital alveolar proteinosis)

Pulmonary alveolar proteinosis (PAP) is a rare condition characterised by accumulation of lipoproteinaceous material in the alveolar space, which impedes gas exchange. Presentation is usually in older children and adults but severe neonatal respiratory failure has been described. Familial recurrence has been reported, suggesting autosomal recessive inheritance in some cases (Ball et al. 1995).

Pathology

The lipoproteinaceous material found distending the alveoli stains positive for periodic acid–Schiff and represents surfactant, which accumulates owing to defective alveolar macrophage function. Changes are usually generalised in the neonatal form of the disease, although a focal distribution has also been noted (Mildenberger et al. 2001). Histological evidence from some reported cases of PAP has suggested that the underlying aetiology is a congenital deficiency of surfactant protein B (SP-B) (Nogee et al. 1993). Several mutations in the SP-B gene have been described, with the 121ins2 mutation occurring in approximately two-thirds of cases (de Mello and Lin 2001). A mutation of the granulocyte–macrophage colony-stimulating factor/interleukin (IL)-3/IL-5 receptor common beta chain has also been reported (Dirksen et al. 1997).

Clinical features and diagnosis

Presentation is usually with severe, prolonged respiratory failure in a term infant. The CXR appearance is suggestive of surfactant deficiency, with diffuse ground-glass opacification of the lung fields. CT also shows generalised opacification, with prominent interlobular septa (Newman et al. 2001).

Diagnosis is confirmed by demonstration of decreased or absent SP-B by enzyme-linked immunosorbent assay in aspirates obtained by alveolar lavage or immunostaining of lung tissue from biopsy (Ball et al. 1995).

Management

Ventilatory support is required from birth in congenital alveolar proteinosis. Temporary improvement may result from alveolar lavage and exogenous surfactant therapy, but the condition is usually fatal within a few weeks (Ball et al. 1995). Long-term survival has only been reported after lung transplantation (Huddleston et al. 2002).

Congenital lobar emphysema

This is a rare condition in which the affected lobe is hyperinflated and therefore also referred to as congenital large hyperlucent lung. The incidence in babies has been estimated as 1 in 90 000, although it may present in older children and adults (Man et al. 1983; Critchley et al. 1995). Congenital lobar emphysema is more common in males (Karnak et al. 1999) and familial cases have been described, but with no common pattern of inheritance (Thompson et al. 2000; Roberts et al. 2002). CHD occurs in 10–15% of cases (Karnak et al. 1999).

Pathophysiology

The hyperinflated lobe or lobes occurs as a result of a 'ball-valve' mechanism for which a number of aetiologies have been implicated. These include defects in bronchial cartilage, resulting in bronchomalacia (Doull et al. 1996), partial large-airway obstruction due to excessive mucus or inflammatory exudates (Thompson and Forfar 1958) and extraluminal compression of large airways by bronchogenic cysts (Gerami et al. 1969) or aberrant blood vessels (Raynor et al. 1967).

The affected lobe or lobes are distended and pale in colour, with absent ventilation and perfusion. Compression resulting in atelectasis of unaffected lobes occurs, along with mediastinal shift.

Clinical features

Presentation in the early neonatal period, with signs of respiratory distress, occurs in 50–60% of cases, with others being asymptomatic. Late presentation with recurrent lower respiratory tract infection is unusual (Karnak et al. 1999). On examination, the affected side may be hyperinflated, with reduced breath sounds, an increased percussion note and expiratory wheeze.

In case series, the left upper lobe was affected in 65% of cases, the right middle lobe in 24% and the right upper lobe in 11% (Senyuz et al. 1989; Dogan et al. 1997; Karnak et al. 1999; Thakral et al. 2001). One case series suggested that symptoms were worse when congenital lobar emphysema occurred in either upper lobe (Thakral et al. 2001).

Diagnosis

Antenatal diagnosis with USS and MRI has been reported in very few cases (Olutoye et al. 2000; Babu et al. 2001). Like other congenital lung lesions diagnosed on antenatal USS, some appear to decrease in size or even disappear altogether as the pregnancy progresses, but signs may still occur soon after birth.

Postnatally, most cases of congenital lobar emphysema can be diagnosed by a plain CXR, which typically shows hyperinflation of the affected lobe, mediastinal shift and compression of other parts of both lungs. Delayed resorption of lung fluid is commonly seen within the affected lobe as increased opacity. Ventilation perfusion scintigraphy, showing decreased ventilation and perfusion, and CT scans may also aid diagnosis (Stigers et al. 1992; Karnak et al. 1999). Echocardiography is necessary to exclude CHD, and barium swallow, bronchoscopy and cardiac catheterisation with angiography may be required to exclude a vascular ring (Roguin et al. 1980).

Management

Most cases of congenital lobar emphysema presenting with symptoms in the neonatal period require surgical lobectomy. Asymptomatic cases or those with minimal symptoms can usually be managed conservatively (Karnak et al. 1999). Successful treatment with flexible bronchoscopy (Phillipos and Libsekal 1998) and selective bronchial intubation has also been described in a small number of cases (Glenski et al. 1986).

Ciliary abnormalities

Primary ciliary dyskinesia (PCD), also known as the immotile cilia syndrome, is an autosomal recessive condition with an incidence of approximately 1 in 15 000.

Pathophysiology

PCD occurs most commonly due to absence of the dynein arms on the outer microtubular doublets (Afzelius 1976). Other abnormalities of cilial ultrastructure, recognised by electron microscopy, have also been described, along with cilial aplasia (Fonzi et al. 1982; Sturgess et al. 1986). Patients with typical symptoms and decreased ciliary beat frequency but normal cilial ultrastructure have also been described (Greenstone et al. 1983).

Clinical features

Ciliary dysfunction leads to poor clearance of respiratory tract secretions, which predisposes patients to recurrent upper and lower respiratory tract infections, sinusitis and otitis media. Bronchiectasis may develop by mid- to late childhood or during adult life as a result of chronic respiratory infection. The incidence of dextrocardia and situs inversus (Kartagener syndrome) varies from 50% to 67% in large case series (Nadel et al. 1985; Coren et al. 2002). Male infertility is common, due to reduction of sperm motility or abnormal cilial function in the vas deferens. There is also an increased risk of female infertility due to dyskinetic cilia in the fallopian tubes (Afzelius and Eliasson 1983).

Presentation in the neonatal period occurs in more than two-thirds of cases and may be with otherwise unexplained persistent signs of respiratory distress, pneumonia or mucoid nasal secretions (Whitelaw et al. 1981; Buchdahl et al. 1988). Diagnosis may also be suspected in cases of dextrocardia or with a positive family history.

Diagnosis

Diagnosis of PCD is established by analysis of a superficial brush biopsy sample of epithelial cells from the nasopharynx. This is examined under light microscopy to assess cilial function. An electronic counting device or photometric methods are used to measure ciliary beat frequency, which is reduced in PCD. Electron microscopic examination is performed to assess specific structural defects of cilia. There is considerable genetic heterogeneity in PCD, therefore genetic testing is not carried out routinely (Blouin et al. 2000).

Management

Antibiotics for respiratory tract and other infections and chest physiotherapy may delay the onset of bronchiectasis. Surgical treatment for bronchiectasis is not normally required but lobectomy and successful lung transplantation have been reported in the most severe cases (Macchiarini et al. 1994). Successful intracytoplasmic sperm injection and in vitro fertilisation have been described in male patients (Cayan et al. 2001).

Prognosis

Bronchiectasis occurs in approximately one-third of cases by late childhood, but the severity is variable and prognosis is usually better than with cystic fibrosis or other causes of childhood bronchiectasis. Life expectancy can be normal but depends on the severity of bronchiectasis (Kollberg et al. 1978).

References

Adzick, N.S., Harrison, M.R., Glick, P.L., et al., 1984. Experimental pulmonary hypoplasia and oligohydramnios; relative contributions of lung fluid and fetal breathing movements. J Pediatr Surg 19, 658–665.

Adzick, N.S., Harrison, M.R., Crombleholme, T.M., et al., 1998. Fetal lung lesions: management and outcome. Am J Obstet Gynecol 179, 884–889.

Afzelius, B.A., 1976. A human syndrome caused by immotile cilia. Science 193, 317–319.

Afzelius, B.A., Eliasson, R., 1983. Male and female infertility problems in the immotile-cilia syndrome. Eur J Respir Dis Suppl. 127, 144–147.

Aiton, N.R., Fox, G.F., Hannam, S., et al., 1996. Pulmonary hypoplasia presenting as persistent tachypnoea in the first few months of life. Br Med J 312, 1149–1150.

Alivizatos, P., Cheatle, T., de Leval, M., et al., 1985. Pulmonary sequestration complicated by anomalies of pulmonary venous return. J Pediatr Surg 20, 76–99.

Anonymous, 1978. An assessment of the hazards of amniocentesis. Report to the Medical Research Council by their Working Party on Amniocentesis. Br J Obstet Gynaecol 85 (suppl. 2), 1–41.

Areechon, W., Reid, L., 1963. Hypoplasia of lung with congenital diaphragmatic hernia. Br Med J i, 230–233.

Avitabile, A.M., Greco, M.A., Hulnick, D.H., et al., 1984. Congenital cystic adenomatoid malformation of the lung in adults. Am J Surg Pathol 8, 193–202.

Babu, R., Kyle, P., Spicer, R.D., 2001. Prenatal sonographic features of congenital lobar emphysema. Fetal Diagn Ther 16, 200–202.

Bain, A.D., Smith, I.I., Gauld, I.K., 1964. Newborn born after prolonged leakage of liquor amnii. Br Med J ii, 598–599.

Ball, R., Chetcuti, P.A., Beverley, D., 1995. Fatal familial surfactant protein B deficiency. Arch Dis Child Fetal Neonatal Ed 73, F53.

Banerjea, M.C., Wirbelauer, J., Adam, P., et al., 2002. Bilateral cystic adenomatoid lung malformation type III – a rare differential diagnosis of pulmonary hypertension in neonates. J Perinat Med 30, 429–436.

Becmeur, F., Horta-Geraud, P., Donato, L., et al., 1998. Pulmonary sequestrations: prenatal ultrasound diagnosis, treatment and outcome. J Pediatr Surg 33, 492–496.

Blouin, J.-L., Meeks, M., Radhakrishna, U., et al., 2000. Primary ciliary dyskinesia: a genome wide linkage analysis reveals extensive locus heterogeneity. Eur J Hum Genet 8, 109–118.

Bratu, I., Flageole, H., Chen, M.F., et al., 2001. The multiple facets of pulmonary sequestration. J Pediatr Surg 36, 784–790.

Brook, J.D., McCurrach, M.E., Harley, H.G., et al., 1992. Molecular basis of myotonic dystrophy: expansion of a trinucleotide (CTG) repeat at the 39 end of a transcript encoding a protein kinase family member. Cell 68, 799–808.

Buchdahl, R.M., Reiser, J., Ingram, D., et al., 1988. Ciliary abnormalities in respiratory disease. Arch Dis Child 63, 238–243.

Cass, D.L., Crombleholme, T.M., Howell, L.J., et al., 1997. Cystic lung lesions with systemic arterial blood supply: a hybrid of congenital cystic adenomatoid malformation and bronchopulmonary sequestration. J Pediatr Surg 32, 986–990.

Cass, D.L., Quinn, T.M., Yang, E.Y., et al., 1998. Increased cell proliferation and decreased apoptosis characterize congenital cystic adenomatoid malformation of the lung. J Pediatr Surg 33, 1043–1046.

Castillo, R.A., Devoe, L.D., Falls, G., et al., 1987. Pleural effusions and pulmonary hypoplasia. Am J Obstet Gynecol 157, 1252–1255.

Castillo, F., Lucaya, J., Tokashiki, N., et al., 1994. Selective intubation in a case of cystic adenomatoid malformation. Arch Dis Child Fetal Neonatal Ed 70, F70–F71.

Cavoretto, P., Molina, F., Poggi, S., et al., 2008. Prenatal diagnosis and outcome of echogenic fetal lung lesions. Ultrasound Obstet Gynecol 32, 769–783.

Cayan, S., Conaghan, J., Schriock, E.D., et al., 2001. Birth after intracytoplasmic sperm injection with use of testicular sperm from men with Kartagener/immotile cilia syndrome. Fertil Steril 76, 612–614.

Chamberlain, D., Hislop, A., Hey, E., et al., 1977. Pulmonary hypoplasia in babies with severe rhesus isoimmunisation: a quantitative study. J Pathol 122, 43–52.

Chatrath, R.R., el Shafie, M., Jones, R.S., 1971. Fate of hypoplastic lungs after repair of congenital diaphragmatic hernia. Arch Dis Child 46, 633–635.

Chen, K.T., 1985. Congenital cystic adenomatoid malformation of the lung and pulmonary tumorlets in an adult. J Surg Oncol 30, 106–108.

Clements, B.S., Warner, J.O., 1987. Pulmonary sequestration and related congenital bronchopulmonary-vascular malformations: nomenclature and classification based on anatomical and embryological considerations. Thorax 42, 401–408.

Conran, R.M., Stocker, J.T., 1999. Extralobular sequestration with frequently associated cystic adenomatoid malformation, type 2: report of 50 cases. Pediatr Dev Pathol 2, 454–463.

Cooney, T.P., Thurlbeck, W.M., 1982. Pulmonary hypoplasia in Down's syndrome. N Engl J Med. 307, 1170–1173.

Coren, M.E., Meeks, M., Morrison, I., et al., 2002. Primary ciliary dyskinesia: age at diagnosis and symptom history. Acta Paediatr 91, 667–669.

Cregg, N., Casey, W., 1997. Primary congenital pulmonary hypoplasia – a genetic component to aetiology. Paediatr Anaesth 7, 329–333.

Critchley, P.S., Forrester-Wood, C.P., Ridley, P.D., 1995. Adult congenital lobar emphysema in pregnancy. Thorax 50, 909–910.

Crombleholme, T.M., Coleman, B., Hedrick, H., et al., 2002. Cystic adenomatoid malformation volume ratio predicts outcome in prenatally diagnosed cystic adenomatoid malformation of the lung. J Pediatr Surg 37, 331–338.

Dagoneau, N., Goulet, M., Geneviève, D., et al., 2009. DYNC2H1 mutations cause asphyxiating thoracic dystrophy and short rib-polydactyly syndrome, type III. Am J Hum Genet 84, 706–711.

Dahabreh, J., Zisis, C., Vassiliou, M., et al., 2000. Congenital cystic adenomatoid malformation in an adult presenting as lung abscess. Eur J Cardio-thorac Surg 18, 720–723.

Danielson, P.D., Sherman, N.J., 2001. Laparoscopic removal of an abdominal extralobar pulmonary sequestration. J Pediatr Surg 36, 1653–1655.

Davis, J.T., Heistein, J.B., Castile, R.G., et al., 2001. Lateral thoracic expansion for Jeune's syndrome: midterm results. Ann Thorac Surg 72, 872–877.

de Mello, D.E., Lin, Z., 2001. Pulmonary alveolar proteinosis: a review. Pediatr Pathol Mol Med 20, 413–432.

Dhingsa, R., Coakley, F.V., Albanese, C.T., et al., 2003. Prenatal sonography and MR imaging of pulmonary sequestration. Am J Roentgenol 180, 433–437.

Dibbins, A.W., Weiner, E.S., 1974. Mortality from neonatal diaphragmatic hernia. J Pediatr Surg 9, 653–662.

Dirksen, U., Nishinakamura, R., Groneck, P., et al., 1997. Human pulmonary alveolar proteinosis associated with a defect in GM-CSF/IL-3/IL-5 receptor common beta chain expression. J Clin Invest 100, 2211e7.

Dogan, R., Demiricin, M., Sarigul, A., et al., 1997. Surgical management of congenital lobar emphysema. Turkish J Paediatr 39, 35–44.

Dommergues, M., Louis-Sylvestre, C., Mandelbrot, L., et al., 1997. Congenital adenomatoid malformation of the lung: is active fetal therapy indicated? Am J Obstet Gynecol 177, 953–958.

Doull, I.J., Connett, G.J., Warner, J.O., 1996. Bronchoscopic appearances of congenital lobar emphysema. Pediatr Pulmonol 21, 195–197.

Duncombe, G.J., Dichinson, J.E., Kikiros, C.S., 2002. Prenatal diagnosis and management of congenital cystic adenomatoid malformation of the lung. Am J Obstet Gynecol 187, 950–954.

Everest, N.J., Jacobs, S.E., Davis, P.G., et al., 2008. Outcomes following prolonged preterm premature rupture of the membranes. Arch Dis Child Fetal Neonatal Ed 93, F207–F211.

Fonzi, L., Lungarella, G., Palatresi, R., 1982. Lack of kinocilia in the nasal mucosa in the immotile cilia syndrome. Eur J Resp Dis 63, 558–563.

Fromont-Hankard, G., Philippe-Chomette, P., Delezoide, A.L., et al., 2002. Glial cell-derived neurotropic factor expression in normal human lung and congenital cystic adenomatoid malformation. Arch Pathol Lab Med 126, 432–436.

Fuke, S., Kanzaki, T., Mu, J., et al., 2003. Antenatal prediction of pulmonary hypoplasia by acceleration time/ejection time ratio of fetal pulmonary arteries by Doppler blood flow velocimetry. Am J Obstet Gynecol 188, 228–233.

Gamillscheg, A., Beitzke, A., Smolle-Juttner, F.M., et al., 1996. Extralobular sequestration with unusual arterial supply and venous drainage. Pediatr Cardiol 17, 57–59.

Gao, Y.A., Burrows, P.E., Benson, L.N., et al., 1993. Scimitar syndrome in infancy. J Am Coll Cardiol 22, 873–882.

Garcia-Pena, P., Lucaya, J., Hendry, G.M., et al., 1998. Spontaneous involution of pulmonary sequestration in children: a report of two cases and review of the literature. Pediatr Radiol 28, 266–270.

Gardikis, S., Didilis, V., Polychronidis, A., et al., 2002. Spontaneous pneumothorax resulting from congenital cystic adenomatoid malformation in a pre-term infant: case report and literature review. Eur J Pediatr Surg 12, 195–198.

Geary, C., Whitsett, J., 2002. Inhaled nitric oxide for oligohydramnios-induced pulmonary hypoplasia: a report of two cases and review of the literature. J Perinatol 22, 82–85.

Gehring, B., Mornet, E., Plath, H., et al., 1999. Perinatal hypophosphatasia: diagnosis and detection of heterozygote carriers within the family. Clin Genet 56, 313–317.

Gerami, S., Richardson, R., Harrington, B., et al., 1969. Obstructive emphysema due to mediastinal bronchogenic cysts in infancy. Case report and brief review of literature. J Thorac Cardiovasc Surg 58, 432–436.

Glenski, J.A., Thibeault, D.W., Hall, F.K., et al., 1986. Selective bronchial intubation in infants with lobar emphysema: indications, complications, and long-term outcome. Am J Perinatol 3, 199–204.

Golaszewski, T., Bettelheim, D., Eppel, W., et al., 1998. Cystic adenomatoid malformation of the lung: prenatal diagnosis, prognostic factors and fetal outcome. Gynecol Obstet Invest 46, 241–246.

Goldstein, J.D., Reid, L.M., 1980. Pulmonary hypoplasia resulting from phrenic nerve agenesis and diaphragmatic amyoplasia. J Pediatr 97, 282–287.

Granata, C., Gambini, C., Balducci, T., et al., 1998. Bronchioalveolar carcinoma arising in congenital cystic adenomatoid malformation in a child: a case report and review on malignancies originating in congenital cystic adenomatoid malformation. Pediatr Pulmonol 25, 62–66.

Greenstone, M.A., Dewar, A., Cole, P.J., 1983. Ciliary dyskinesia with normal ultrastructure. Thorax 38, 875–876.

Halkic, N., Cuenoud, P.F., Corthesy, M.E., et al., 1998. Pulmonary sequestration: a review of 26 cases. Eur J Cardio-thorac Surg 14, 127–133.

Hang, J.D., Guo, Q.Y., Chen, C.X., et al., 1996. Imaging approach to the diagnosis of pulmonary sequestration. Acta Radiol 37, 883–888.

Hanssens, M., Keirse, M.J., Vankelecom, F., et al., 1991. Fetal and neonatal effects of treatment with angiotensin-converting enzyme inhibitors in pregnancy. Obstet Gynecol 78, 128–135.

Harrison, M.R., Ross, N., Noall, R., et al., 1983. Correction of congenital hydronephrosis in utero. I. The model: fetal urethral obstruction produces hydronephrosis and pulmonary hypoplasia in lambs. J Pediatr Surg 18, 247–256.

Harrison, M.R., Albanese, C.T., Hawgood, S.B., et al., 2001. Fetoscopic temporary tracheal occlusion by means of detachable balloon for congenital diaphragmatic hernia. Am J Obstet Gynecol 185, 730–733.

Harrison, M.R., Keller, R.L., Hawgood, S.B., et al., 2003. A randomized trial of fetal endoscopic tracheal occlusion for severe fetal congenital diaphragmatic hernia. N Engl J Med 349, 1916–1924.

Hislop, A., Hey, E., Reid, L., 1979. The lungs in congenital bilateral renal agenesis and dysplasia. Arch Dis Child 54, 32–38.

Hubbard, A.M., Adzick, N.S., Crombleholme, T.M., et al., 1999. Congenital chest lesions: diagnosis and characterization with prenatal MR imaging. Radiology 212, 43–48.

Huddleston, C.B., Bloch, J.B., Sweet, S.C., et al., 2002. Lung transplantation in children. Ann Surg 236, 270–276.

Islam, S., Masiakos, P., Schnitzer, J.J., et al., 1999. Diltiazem reduces pulmonary arterial pressures in recurrent pulmonary hypertension associated with pulmonary hypoplasia. J Pediatr Surg 34, 712–714.

Janas, M.S., Arroe, M., Hansen, S.H., et al., 1998. Lung hypoplasia – a possible teratogenic effect of valproate. Case report. APMIS: Acta Pathol Microbiol Immunol Scand 106, 300–304.

Jani, J.C., Nicolaides, K.H., Gratacós, E., et al., 2009. Severe diaphragmatic hernia treated by fetal endoscopic tracheal occlusion. Ultrasound Obstet Gynecol. 34, 304–310.

Kaariainen, H., Koskimies, O., Norio, R., 1988. Dominant and recessive polycystic kidney disease in children: evaluation of clinical features and laboratory data. Pediatr Nephrol 2, 296–302.

Karnak, I., Senocak, M.E., Ciftci, A.O., et al., 1999. Congenital lobar emphysema: diagnostic and therapeutic considerations. J Pediatr Surg 34, 1347–1351.

Karnes, P.S., Day, D., Berry, S.A., et al., 1991. Jarcho-Levin syndrome: four new cases and classification of subtypes. Am J Med Genet 40, 264–270.

Kilbride, H.W., Yeast, J., Thibeault, D.W., 1996. Defining limits of survival: lethal pulmonary hypoplasia after midtrimester premature rupture of membranes. Am J Obstet Gynecol 175, 675–681.

Kim, W.S., Lee, K.S., Kim, I.O., et al., 1997. Congenital cystic adenomatoid malformation of the lung: CT-pathologic correlation. AJR Am J Roentgenol 168, 47–53.

Knowles, S., Thomas, R.M., Lindenbaum, R.H., et al., 1988. Pulmonary agenesis as part of the VACTERL sequence. Arch Dis Child 63, 723–726.

Kohl, T., Geipel, A., Tchatcheva, K., et al., 2009. Life-saving effects of fetal tracheal occlusion on pulmonary hypoplasia from preterm premature rupture of membranes. Obstet Gynecol 113, 480–483.

Kollberg, H., Mossberg, B., Afzelius, B., et al., 1978. Cystic fibrosis compared with the immotile-cilia syndrome. A study of mucociliary clearance, ciliary ultrastructure, clinical picture and ventilatory function. Scand J Resp Dis 59, 297–306.

Kriegsmann, J., Coerdt, W., Kommoss, F., et al., 2000. Renal tubular dysgenesis (RTD) – an important cause of the oligohydramnion-sequence. Report of 3 cases and review of the literature. Pathol Res Pract 196, 861–865.

Kunisaki, S.M., Barnewolt, C.E., Estroff, J.A., et al., 2007. Large fetal congenital cystic adenomatoid malformations: growth trends and patient survival. J Pediatr Surg 42, 404–410.

Laberge, J.M., Flageole, H., Pugash, D., et al., 2001. Outcome of prenatally diagnosed congenital cystic adenomatoid lung malformation: a Canadian experience. Fetal Diagn Ther 16, 178–186.

Lee, A., Kratochwil, A., Stumpflen, I., et al., 1996. Fetal lung volume determination by three-dimensional ultrasonography. Am J Obstet Gynecol 175, 588–592.

Lee, M.L., Tsao, L.Y., Chaou, W.T., et al., 2002. Revisit on congenital bronchopulmonary vascular malformations: a haphazard branching theory of malinosculations and its clinical classification and implication. Pediatr Pulmonol 33, 1–11.

Lee, B.S., Kim, J.T., Kim, E.A., et al., 2008. Neonatal pulmonary sequestration: clinical experience with transumbilical arterial embolization. Pediatr Pulmonol 43, 404–413.

Lejeune, C., Deschildre, A., Thumerelle, C., et al., 1999. [Pneumothorax revealing cystic adenomatoid malformation of the lung in a 13 year old child.] Arch Pediatrie 6, 863–866.

Liechty, K.W., Crombleholme, T.M., Quinn, T.M., et al., 1999. Elevated platelet-derived growth factor-B in congenital cystic adenomatoid malformations requiring fetal resection. J Pediatr Surg 34, 805–809.

Liggins, G.C., Vilos, G.A., Campos, G.A., et al., 1981. The effect of bilateral thoracoplasty on lung development in fetal sheep. J Dev Physiol 3, 275–282.

Lopoo, J.B., Goldstein, R.B., Lipshutz, G.S., et al., 1999. Fetal pulmonary sequestration: a favourable congenital lung lesion. Obstet Gynaecol 94, 567–571.

Losa, M., Kind, C., 1998. Dry lung syndrome: complete airway collapse mimicking pulmonary hypoplasia? Eur J Pediatr 157, 935–938.

Lujan, M., Bosque, M., Mirapeix, R.M., 2002. Late-onset congenital cystic adenomatoid malformation of the lung. Embryology, clinical symptomatology, diagnostic procedures, therapeutic approach and clinical follow-up. Respiration 69, 148–155.

Macchiarini, P., Chapelier, A., Vouhe, P., et al., 1994. Double lung transplantation in situs inversus with Kartagener's syndrome. J Thorac Cardiovasc Surg 108, 86–91.

MacKenzie, T.C., Guttenberg, M.E., Nisenbaum, H.L., et al., 2001. A fetal lung lesion consisting of bronchogenic cyst, bronchopulmonary sequestration and congenital cystic adenomatoid malformation: the missing link? Fetal Diagn Ther 16, 193–195.

Maier, H.C., 1948. Bronchogenic cysts of mediastinum. Ann Surg 127, 476–502.

Man, D.W., Hamdy, M.H., Hendry, G.M., et al., 1983. Congenital lobar emphysema: problems in diagnosis and management. Arch Dis Child 58, 709–712.

Martinez-Frias, M.L., Bermejo, E., Urioste, M., et al., 1993. Lethal short rib-polydactyly syndromes: further evidence for their overlapping in a continuous spectrum. J Med Genet 30, 937–941.

Maymon, R., Schneider, D., Hegesh, J., et al., 2001. Antenatal sonographic findings of right pulmonary agenesis with ipsilateral microtia: a possible new laterality association. Prenat Diagn 21, 125–128.

McIntosh, N., 1988. Dry lung syndrome after oligohydramnios. Arch Dis Child 63, 190–193.

Mentzer, S.J., Filler, R.M., Phillips, J., 1992. Limited pulmonary resections for congenital cystic adenomatoid malformation of the lung. J Pediatr Surg 27, 1410–1413.

Mezzetti, M., Dell'Agnola, C.A., Bedoni, M., et al., 1996. Video-assisted thoracoscopic resection of pulmonary sequestration in an infant. Ann Thorac Surg 61, 1836–1837.

Mildenberger, E., de Mello, D.E., Lin, Z., et al., 2001. Focal congenital alveolar proteinosis associated with abnormal surfactant protein B messenger RNA. Chest 119, 645–647.

Miller, K.E., Corteville, J.E., Langer, J.C., 1996. Congenital cystic adenomatoid malformation in the fetus: natural history and predictors of outcome. J Pediatr Surg 31, 805–808.

Moerman, P., Fryns, J.P., Goddeeris, P., et al., 1983. Multiple ankyloses, facial anomalies, and pulmonary hypoplasia associated with severe antenatal spinal muscular atrophy. J Pediatr 103, 238–241.

Morin, L.R., Herlicoviez, M., Loisel, J.C., et al., 1991. Prenatal diagnosis of lethal osteogenesis imperfecta in twin pregnancy. Clin Genet 39, 467–470.

Morotti, R.A., Cangiarella, J., Gutierrez, M.C., et al., 1999. Congenital cystic adenomatoid malformation of the lung (CCAM): evaluation of the cellular components. Hum Pathol 30, 618–625.

Nadel, H.R., Stringer, D.A., Levinson, H., et al., 1985. The immotile cilia syndrome: radiological manifestations. Radiology 154, 651–655.

Neilson, I.R., Russo, P., Laberge, J.M., et al., 1991. Congenital adenomatoid malformation of the lung: current management and prognosis. J Pediatr Surg 26, 975–980.

Newbould, M.J., Lendon, M., Barson, A.J., 1994. Oligohydramnios sequence: the spectrum of renal malformations. Br J Obstet Gynaecol 101, 598–604.

Newman, B., Kuhn, J.P., Kramer, S.S., et al., 2001. Congenital surfactant protein B deficiency – emphasis on imaging. Pediatr Radiol 31, 327–331.

Njinimbam, C.G., Hebra, A., Kicklighter, S.D., et al., 1999. Persistent pulmonary hypertension in a neonate with cystic adenomatoid malformation of the lung following lobectomy: survival with prolonged extracorporeal membrane oxygenation therapy. J Perinatol 19, 64–67.

Nogee, L.M., de Mello, D.E., Dehner, L.P., et al., 1993. Brief report: deficiency of pulmonary surfactant protein B in congenital alveolar proteinosis. N Engl J Med 328, 406–410.

Noonan, J.A., Walters, L.R., Reeves, J.T., 1970. Congenital pulmonary lymphangiectasis. Am J Dis Child 120, 314–319.

Oberklaid, F., Danks, D.M., Mayne, V., et al., 1977. Asphyxiating thoracic dysplasia. Clinical, radiological and pathological information on 10 patients. Arch Dis Child 52, 758–765.

Olutoye, O.O., Coleman, B.G., Hubbard, A.M., et al., 2000. Prenatal diagnosis and management of congenital lobar emphysema. J Pediatr Surg 35, 792–795.

O'Malley, B.P., Parker, R., Saphyakhajon, P., et al., 1972. Thanatophoric dwarfism. J Can Assoc Radiologists 23, 62–68.

Osborne, J., Masel, J., McCredie, J., 1989. A spectrum of skeletal anomalies associated with pulmonary agenesis: possible neural crest injuries. Pediatr Radiol 19, 425–432.

Ostor, A.G., Fortune, D.W., 1978. Congenital cystic adenomatoid malformation of the lung. Am J Clin Pathol 70, 595–604.

Ozcan, C., Celik, A., Ural, Z., et al., 2001. Primary pulmonary rhabdomyosarcoma arising within cystic adenomatoid malformation: a case report and review of the literature. J Pediatr Surg 36, 1062–1065.

Papagiannopoulos, K.A., Sheppard, M., Bush, A.P., et al., 2001. Pleuropulmonary blastoma: is prophylactic resection of congenital lung cysts effective? Ann Thorac Surg 72, 604–605.

Parilla, B.V., Leeth, E.A., Kambich, M.P., et al., 2003. Antenatal detection of skeletal dysplasias. J Ultrasound Med 22, 255–258.

Phillipos, E.Z., Libsekal, K., 1998. Flexible bronchoscopy in the management of congenital lobar emphysema in the neonate. Can Resp J 5, 219–221.

Potter, E.L., 1946. Bilateral renal agenesis. J Pediatr 29, 68–76.

Potter, E.L., 1952. Pulmonary pathology of the fetus and the newborn. In: Adv Pediatr, Vol. IV. Year Book Medical Publishers, Chicago.

Raynor, A.C., Capp, M.P., Sealy, W.C., 1967. Lobar emphysema of infancy: diagnosis, treatment and etiological aspects. Ann Thorac Surg 4, 374–385.

Rescorla, F.J., West, K.W., Vane, D.W., et al., 1990. Pulmonary hypertension in neonatal cystic lung disease: survival following lobectomy and ECMO in two cases. J Pediatr Surg 25, 1054–1056.

Rettwitz-Volk, W., Schlosser, R., Ahrens, P., et al., 1999. Congenital unilobar pulmonary lymphangiectasis. Pediatr Pulmonol 27, 290–292.

Ribet, M.E., Copin, M.C., Gosselin, B.H., 1996. Bronchogenic cysts of the lung. Ann Thorac Surg 61, 1636–1640.

Roberts, P.A., Holland, A.J., Halliday, R.J., et al., 2002. Congenital lobar emphysema: like father, like son. J Pediatr Surg 37, 799–801.

Roguin, N., Peleg, H., Lemer, J., et al., 1980. The value of cardiac catheterization and cineangiography in infantile lobar emphysema. Pediatr Radiol 10, 71–74.

Rothenberg, S.S., 2000. Thoracoscopic lung resection in children. J Pediatr Surg 35, 271–274.

Rotschild, A., Ling, E.W., Wensley, D.F., et al., 1994. Unilateral cervical spinal cord lesion in a term newborn associated with ipsilateral diaphragmatic atrophy and pulmonary hypoplasia. Pediatr Pulmonol 18, 53–57.

Rutledge, J.C., Jensen, P., 1986. Acinar dysplasia: a new form of pulmonary maldevelopment. Hum Pathol 17, 1290–1293.

Sapin, E., Lejeune, V., Barbet, J.P., et al., 1997. Congenital adenomatoid disease of the lung: prenatal diagnosis and perinatal management. Pediatr Surg Int 12, 126–129.

Savic, B., Birtel, F.J., Tholen, W., et al., 1979. Lung sequestration: report of seven cases and review of 540 published cases. Thorax 34, 96–101.

Senyuz, O.F., Danismend, N., Erdogan, E., et al., 1989. Congenital lobar emphysema – a report of 5 cases. Jpn J Surg 19, 764–767.

Spranger, J., Langen, L.O., Maroteaux, P., 1970. Increasing frequency of a syndrome of multiple osseous defects? Lancet 2, 716.

Stigers, K.B., Woodring, J.H., Kanga, J.F., 1992. The clinical and imaging spectrum of findings in patients with congenital lobar emphysema. Pediatr Pulmonol 14, 160–170.

Stocker, J.T., Drake, R.M., Madewell, J.E., 1978. Cystic and congenital lung disease in the newborn. Perspect Pediatr Pathol 4, 93–154.

Sturgess, J.M., Thompson, M.W., Czegledy-Nady, E., et al., 1986. Genetic aspects of immotile cilia syndrome. Am J Med Genet 25, 149–160.

Sueyoshi, R., Okazaki, T., Uroshihara, N., et al., 2008. Managing prenatally diagnosed asymptomatic congenital cystic adenomatoid malformation. Pediatr Surg Int 24, 1111–1115.

Szaflik, K., Kozarzewski, M., Adamczewski, D., 1998. Fetal bladder catheterization in severe obstructive uropathy before the 24th week of pregnancy. Fetal Diagn Ther 13, 133–135.

Thakral, C.L., Maji, D.C., Sajwani, M.J., 2001. Congenital lobar emphysema: experience with 21 cases. Pediatr Surg Int 17, 88–91.

Thomas, R.J., Lathif, H.C., Sen, S., et al., 1998. Varied presentations of unilateral lung hypoplasia and agenesis: a report of four cases. Pediatr Surg Int 14, 94–95.

Thompson, J., Forfar, J.O., 1958. Regional obstructive emphysema in infancy. Arch Dis Child 33, 97–102.

Thompson, P.J., Greenough, A., Blott, M., et al., 1990. Chronic respiratory morbidity following PROM. Arch Dis Child 65, 878–880.

Thompson, P.J., Greenough, A., Nicolaides, K.H., 1992. Lung volume measured by functional residual capacity in infants following first trimester amniocentesis or chorion villus sampling. Br J Obstet Gynaecol 99, 479–482.

Thompson, P.J., Greenough, A., Dykes, E., et al., 1993a. Impaired respiratory function in infants with anterior abdominal wall defects. J Pediatr Surg 28, 664–666.

Thompson, P.J., Greenough, A., Nicolaides, K.H., 1993b. Respiratory function in infancy following pleuro-amniotic shunting. Fetal Diagn Ther 8, 79–83.

Thompson, A.J., Reid, A.J., Reid, M., 2000. Congenital lobar emphysema occurring in twins. J Perinat Med 28, 155–157.

Thorpe-Beeston, J.G., Nicolaides, K.H., 1994. Cystic adenomatoid malformation of the lung: prenatal diagnosis and outcome. Prenat Diagn 14, 677–688.

Todd, D.W., Tinguely, S.J., Norberg, W.J., 1986. A thoracic expansion technique for Jeune's asphyxiating thoracic dystrophy. J Pediatr Surg 21, 161–163.

Tranquilli, A.L., Giannubilo, S.R., Bezzeccheri, V., et al., 2005. Transabdominal amnioinfusion in preterm premature rupture of membranes: a randomised controlled trial. Br J Obstet Gynaecol 112, 759–763.

van Leeuwen, K., Teitelbaum, D.H., Hirschl, R.B., et al., 1999. Prenatal diagnosis of congenital cystic adenomatoid malformation and its postnatal presentation, surgical indications, and natural history. J Pediatr Surg 34, 794–798.

Van Raemdonck, D., De Boeck, K., Devlieger, H., et al., 2001. Pulmonary sequestration: a comparison between pediatric and adult patients. Eur J Cardio-thorac Surg 19, 388–395.

van Teeffelen, A.S., van der Ham, D.P., Oei, S.G., et al., 2010. The accuracy of clinical parameters in the prediction of perinatal pulmonary hypoplasia secondary to midtrimester prelabour rupture of fetal membranes: a meta-analysis. Eur J Obstet Gynecol Reprod Biol 148, 3–12.

Vilos, G.A., McLeod, W.J., Carmichael, L., et al., 1984. Absence or impaired response of fetal breathing to intravenous glucose is associated with pulmonary hypoplasia in congenital myotonic dystrophy. Am J Obstet Gynecol 148, 558–562.

Vyas, H., Milner, A.D., Hopkin, I.E., 1982. Amniocentesis and fetal lung development. Arch Dis Child 57, 627–628.

Waszak, P., Claris, O., Lapillonne, A., et al., 1999. Cystic adenomatoid malformation of the lung: neonatal management of 21 cases. Pediatr Surg Int 15, 326–331.

Weinbaum, P.J., Bors-Koefoed, R., Green, K.W., et al., 1989. Antenatal sonographic findings in a case of intra-abdominal pulmonary sequestration. Obstet Gynecol 73, 860–862.

Whitelaw, A., Evans, A., Corrin, B., 1981. Immotile cilia syndrome: a new cause of neonatal respiratory distress. Arch Dis Child 56, 432–435.

Williams, A.J., Vawter, G., Reid, L.M., 1984. Lung structure in asphyxiating thoracic dystrophy. Arch Pathol Lab Med 108, 658–661.

Williams, O., Hutchings, G., Debieve, F., et al., 2009. Contemporary neonatal outcome following rupture of membranes prior to 25 weeks with prolonged oligohydramnios. Early Hum Dev 85, 273–277.

Yoshimura, S., Masuzaki, H., Miura, K., et al., 1999. Diagnosis of fetal pulmonary hypoplasia by measurement of blood flow velocity waveforms of pulmonary arteries with Doppler ultrasonography. Am J Obstet Gynecol 180, 441–446.

Part 6: **Diaphragmatic hernia**

Carmen Turowski   Mark Davenport

Introduction

A number of diaphragmatic abnormalities may present with respiratory problems during infancy, the most common being a posterolateral congenital diaphragmatic hernia (CDH). This is usually associated with severe lung hypoplasia, and, despite many advances in its management, still has a high mortality. Anterior diaphragmatic hernias are smaller and tend to present later in infancy, often with gastrointestinal symptoms alone. Eventration of the diaphragm is a condition in which the cupola becomes thinned, stretched and immobile but yet is still intact. Some degree of respiratory impairment is seen in most of these cases.

Congenital posterolateral diaphragmatic hernia

In 1848, the Czech anatomist Vincent Bochdalek described bowel herniation through the posterior part of the diaphragm, attributing it to the effects of an inverted fetus and rupture of the lumbocostal membrane. Although such posterolateral hernias are still widely known by the eponym Bochdalek's hernia, he was certainly not the first to describe this type of diaphragmatic defect as detailed reports of CDH in both children (Holt 1701) and adults (Bonet 1679) had been published previously.

The embryological development of the diaphragm is complex: its mesenchyme is derived from the septum transversum and the dorsal mesentery of the oesophagus, and its muscular component from the innermost muscle layer of the thoracic cage and descending cervical myoblasts (Kluth et al. 1996). The nerve supply to this muscle is via the phrenic nerve (C3–5). There is a communication between the pleural and the peritoneal cavities (the pleuroperitoneal canal) up to the 8th week of gestation.

The orthodox hypothesis of the aetiology of CDH ascribes intestinal herniation to a failure to close the initially patent pleuroperitoneal canal. There is then visceral migration into the hemithorax and interference with the developing lung bud. This herniation would therefore occur during the late embryonic period at 8–10 weeks' gestation. More recent work has suggested that CDH occurs because of failure of normal apposition of the septum transversum and pleuroperitoneal folds (PPFs) arising from the posterior body wall between 6 and 10 weeks' gestation. PPFs are transient structures which form early in diaphragm development and are the target for migratory muscle precursor cells and the phrenic nerve (Clugston and Greer 2007).

There is an important alternative hypothesis which suggests that the primary defect is that of lung hypoplasia. Thus it has been suggested that the pleuroperitoneal canals are too small to accommodate even a single loop of bowel (Kluth et al. 1996) and that the diaphragmatic defect occurs in the posterior mesenchymal part of the nascent diaphragm rather than the pleuroperitoneal canal (Iritani 1984). Such studies also suggest that the defect therefore occurs earlier and equivalent to about 5 weeks' gestation, i.e. within the early embryonic period.

Most recent studies investigating causative factors in CDH have used animal models. These can be divided into surgically created diaphragmatic hernias in large animals (typically sheep) during the latter stages of gestation (Karamanoukian et al. 1995; Papadakis et al. 1998) and those resulting from exposure of small animals (typically rats and mice) to teratogens, such as the pesticide nitrofen, during the early stages of gestation (Iritani 1984; Leinwald et al. 2002).

In a typical CDH mouse model, it can be shown that nitrofen-exposed early embryonic lungs are both hypoplastic and developmentally immature before the presence of a diaphragmatic hernia (Leinwald et al. 2002). Various candidate gene defects (e.g. *HoxA4*, *TGF*, *N-myc*, *Slit*, *COUP-TFII*, *FOG2* and *GATA4m*) (Leinwald et al. 2002; Doi et al. 2009a, b) have been suggested as possible causes and there is a plausible hypothesis concerning inhibition of the retinoid signalling pathway. Thus, *COUP-TFII*, *FOG2* and *GATA4* genes are all regulated by the retinoid signalling pathway, and located on chromosomes 15q26, 8q23 and 8p23.1 respectively – regions reported to be deleted in some individuals with CDH (Doi et al. 2009b). Prenatal treatment with retinoic acid, an active metabolite of vitamin A, can upregulate pulmonary gene expression levels of *COUP-TFII*, *FOG2* and *GATA4* in the nitrofen model and prevent CDH formation. Other genes, such as *Slit-2* and *Slit-3*, may also have a role in pathogenesis as they seem to direct the functional organisation and differentiation of fetal lung mesenchyme and pulmonary bronchiolar development (Doi et al. 2009a).

Anatomy and pathophysiology (Fig. 27.52)

The diaphragmatic defect occurs in the posterolateral segment, although it may range from a simple muscular slit to complete

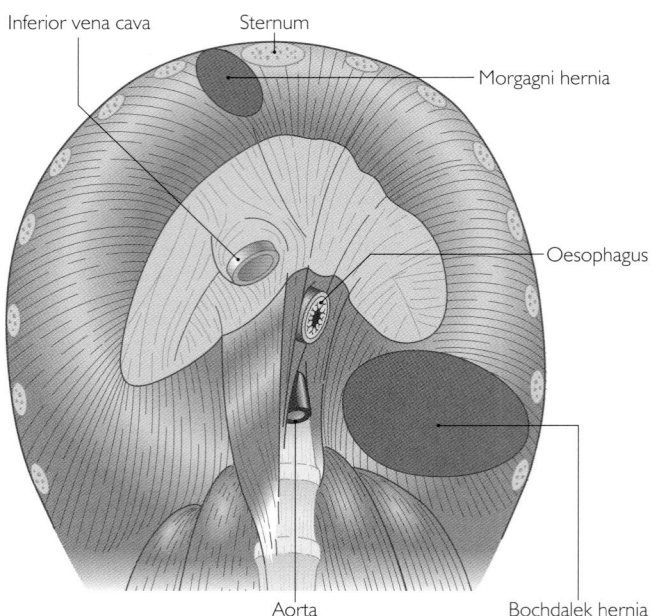

Fig. 27.52 Schematic illustration of the anatomy of congenital diaphragmatic hernia: posterolateral hernia of Bochdalek and anterior hernia of Morgagni.

agenesis. Left-sided hernias account for about 80% of most series (Charlton et al. 1991; Sweed and Puri 1993). Bilateral CDHs occur rarely and are associated with a much worse prognosis (Benjamin et al. 1988; Neville et al. 2003). In left-sided hernias, the hemithorax contains herniated bowel, stomach, spleen and often part of the left lobe of the liver. The herniated bowel is inevitably malrotated because of its abnormal development, although consequent duodenal obstruction is uncommon. A thin, almost translucent hernial sac occurs in about 20% of cases. Right-sided hernias usually contain the right lobe of the liver, and, because of its volume, this tends to plug the defect and may minimise herniation of other viscera.

Some degree of lung hypoplasia occurs with virtually all diaphragmatic hernias. This is most obvious on the ipsilateral side, where perhaps only a nubbin of tissue might remain, but is also seen on the contralateral side. Compared with normal term lungs, there is an absolute decrease in lung weight and volume and a decrease in compliance. The number of bronchial generations is reduced and true alveoli, which should start to be seen by 34 weeks' gestation, are uncommon. Most terminal air spaces are therefore still in the saccular phase of development. Along with an absolute decrease in lung tissue, there is a reduction in the total number of preacinar pulmonary vessels, although the ratio of capillaries per alveolus is retained. The pulmonary and intra-acinar arteries have an abnormally high smooth-muscle content, although it is unclear why this should be so. There is increased expression of endothelin-1 (ET-1), a potent vasoconstrictor, and its receptors (ET_A and ET_B) in such arterioles and this may be one molecular explanation for the frequency of persistent pulmonary hypertension of the newborn (PPHN) in CDH (Okazaki et al. 1998). There may also be changes in the developing cardiovascular system. For instance, the left ventricle and interventricular septum have been shown to be smaller both in CDH cases compared with age-matched human controls (Siebert et al. 1984) and in the experimental CDH lamb model (Karamanoukian et al. 1995). However, cardiac anomalies may

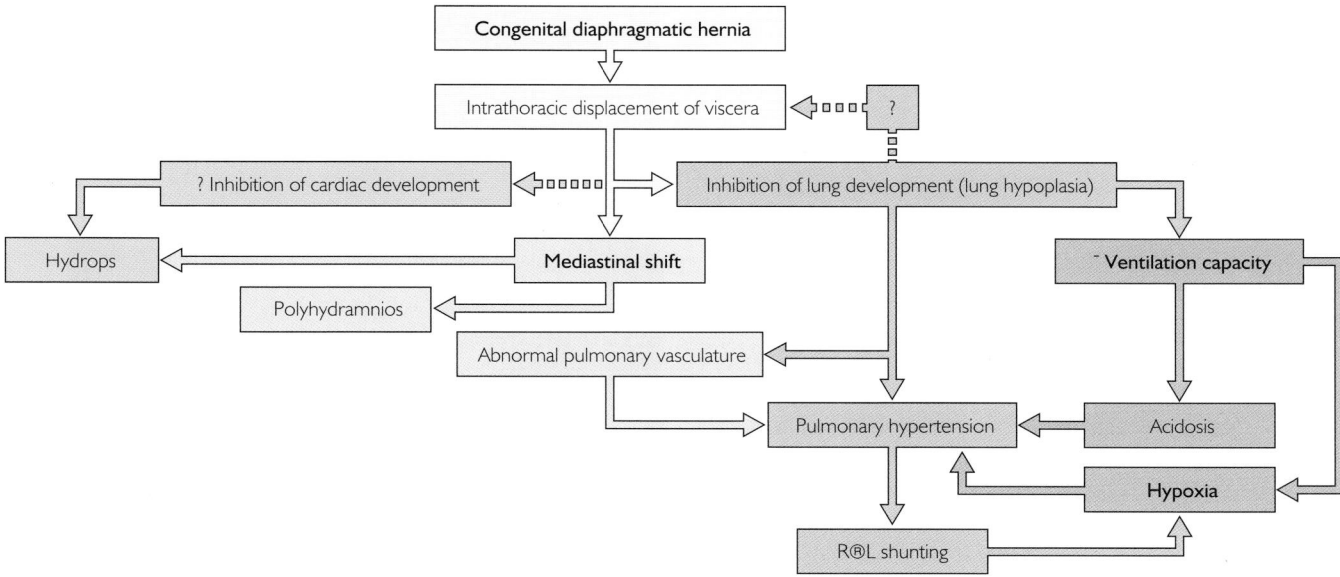

Fig. 27.53 Pathophysiology of congenital diaphragmatic hernia. Pulmonary hypertension, right–left shunting and hypoxia are the characteristic features of persistent pulmonary hypertension of the newborn.

simply be due to direct compression by herniated viscera, as right-sided hernias have been shown to cause diminution of the right rather than the left ventricle.

The pathophysiological sequence that explains some of the clinical features of a CDH is illustrated in Figure 27.53. There is also an exaggerated response of the abnormally muscularised arterial resistance vessels to hypoxia, acidosis and hypercarbia, which causes in turn pulmonary hypertension and shunting of blood at several different levels from the right to the left side of the heart – PPHN.

Demography

The prevalence of CDH at birth has been estimated to be from 1 in 2000 to 1 in 5000, and does not appear to have any predilection for race or geographical area (Wenstrom et al. 1991). The sex ratio is equal, although right-sided defects may be more common in males (Benjamin et al. 1988). Although most CDHs are sporadic, with no known cause, there may be a genetic component in a small number, as there are reports of CDH in twins and families (Crane 1979; Mishalany and Gordo 1986).

Associations

Although CDH was once thought of as an isolated anomaly, more accurate studies (including stillbirths and intrauterine deaths) and the advent of widespread prenatal ultrasound have shown this to be incorrect (Adzick et al. 1985; Benjamin et al. 1988; Sharland et al. 1992; Sweed and Puri 1993; Harrison et al. 1994). About 30–50% of diagnosed fetuses will have a further anomaly (Sweed and Puri 1993), although, because of intrauterine deaths, terminations and stillbirths, this falls to about 20–30% in live-born infants.

Various anomalies may be found, including chromosomal anomalies (e.g. Turner syndrome and trisomies 13, 18 and 21), major central nervous system malformations (e.g. anencephaly, neural tube defects) and most types of congenital cardiac defects (e.g. ventricular septal defect, aortic coarctation, tetralogy of Fallot, hypoplastic left heart and transposition of the great vessels) (Benjamin et al. 1988; Sweed and Puri 1993; Harrison et al. 1994). Similarly,

there is also a wide range of renal anomalies (e.g. agenesis and hydronephrosis) and, in males, undescended testes (Benjamin et al. 1988). Other anomalies less easy to classify include foregut duplication cysts and pulmonary sequestrations.

Fryns syndrome is characterised by a diaphragmatic hernia in an infant with an abnormal facies, distal limb anomalies, undescended testes in males and various gut and genitourinary anomalies (Fryns et al. 1979).

Clinical features

Antenatal ultrasound diagnosis of a diaphragmatic hernia has been possible for well over three decades now. The specific features include bowel loops, and liver or, more usually, stomach seen in the transverse four-chamber view within the thorax. Secondary features include mediastinal shift, hydrops fetalis and, most commonly, polyhydramnios. Right-sided defects are more difficult to diagnose, as the herniated fetal liver has a similar echogenicity to fetal lung.

The typical postnatal presentation is of increasing respiratory distress and cyanosis shortly after birth in a term infant. There are decreased breath sounds and air entry on the side of the hernia, with a shift of the trachea and cardiac impulse to the opposite side. The abdomen has a flat or even scaphoid appearance, as much of the viscera have already been displaced to the chest cavity.

A chest X-ray is diagnostic in most infants and will show air-filled loops of bowel within the hemithorax, often with severe mediastinal displacement (Fig. 27.54). Occasionally there may be confusion with the radiographic appearance of a cystic adenomatoid malformation of the lung, which may also present with respiratory distress. This can be distinguished on the plain film by noting the normal abdominal gas pattern and diaphragmatic integrity, or more accurately by introducing radiopaque contrast material into the stomach and proximal gastrointestinal tract (Fig. 27.55). An ultrasound scan can also differentiate these conditions. Occasionally, air does not enter the proximal bowel because of rapid intubation and resuscitation in the delivery room, especially if there has been an antenatal diagnosis. The usual radiographic appearance is then of

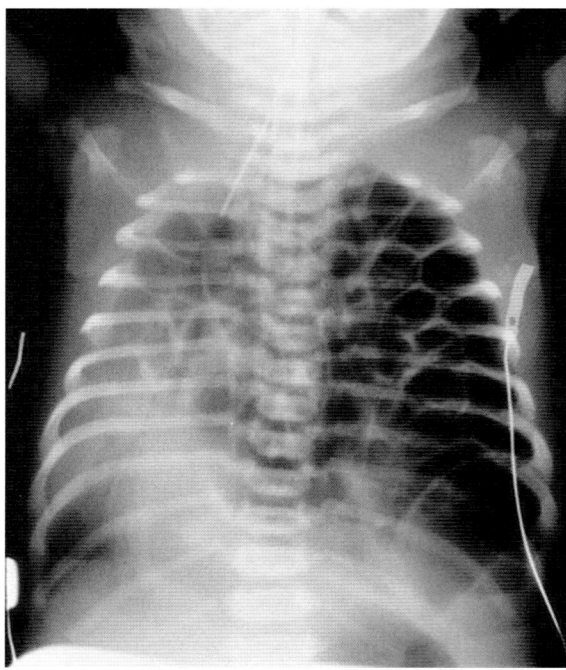

Fig. 27.54 Chest radiograph of infant at 1 hour of life, showing left diaphragmatic hernia, displacement of air-filled viscera into the hemithorax and a marked shift of mediastinum and heart.

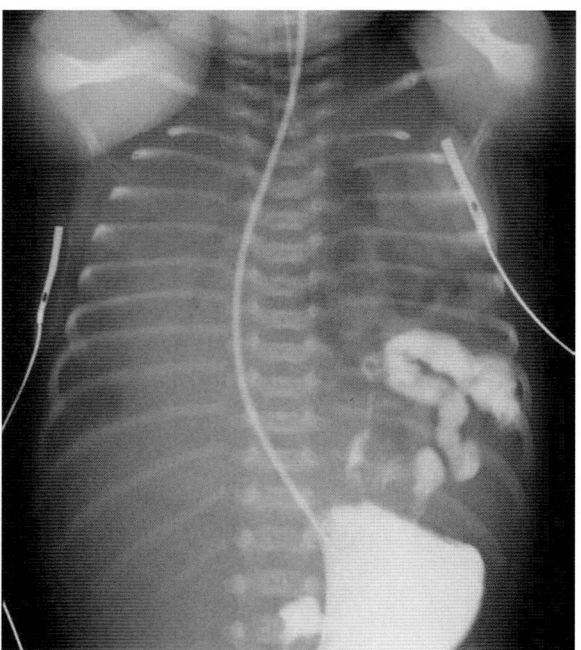

Fig. 27.55 Chest radiograph of an infant with contrast medium in the stomach and small intestine, the latter lying within the left hemithorax.

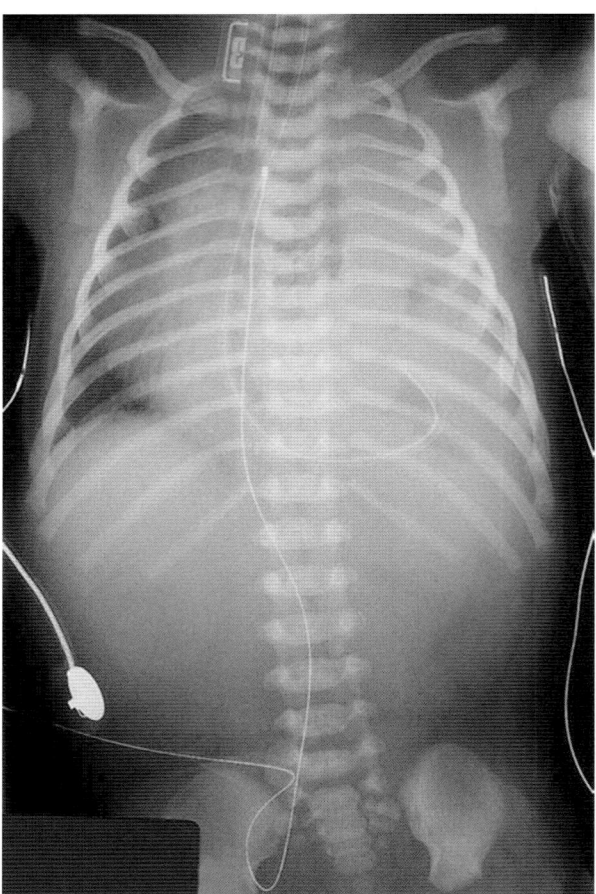

Fig. 27.56 Chest radiograph of the early appearance of a diaphragmatic hernia, with a 'white-out' on the left side.

complete opacification on the side of the hernia – a 'white-out' (Fig. 27.56).

About 5% of infants with CDH will present beyond the first 24 hours of life, with failure to thrive, recurrent chest infections, a pleural effusion, or even as an incidental finding on chest X-ray.

Management

Antenatal

An increasing proportion of infants with CDH are diagnosed in utero by screening ultrasound during the second trimester. Amniocentesis should be offered on diagnosis – if a chromosomal anomaly is found, most obstetricians would recommend termination, as this is an invariably lethal combination.

It is important that these infants are delivered in regional centres where there are the necessary obstetric, neonatal intensive care and surgical facilities. In our centre, we tend to induce vaginal delivery at about 38 weeks' gestation to minimise the risks of unintended early labour and delivery in a peripheral unit.

Fetal intervention

A number of innovative antenatal techniques have been developed to try and influence the life-threatening lung hypoplasia only evident at the time of birth. The underlying theme of initial efforts was open fetal surgery during the second trimester to restore the viscera to its correct abdominal habitus, repair the defect and allow the hypoplastic lung to self-correct during the remaining period of intrauterine life. The Fetal Medicine Center in San Francisco was a pioneer with this approach but ultimately admitted failure because of the high rates of intrauterine death and preterm labour and lack of real effect on lung growth (Harrison et al. 1993; Adzick and Harrison 1994). In one report of its experience between 1989 and 1991, 61 antenatally diagnosed fetuses were referred for consideration of surgery (Harrison et al. 1993). Second-trimester surgery was attempted in 14 fetuses. Of these, five died during the operation; a further three died in utero shortly after closure of the hysterotomy, and two were born prematurely but died. Only four survived to term and eventually to leave hospital.

A different and perhaps more elegant approach arose from the clinical observation that conditions causing congenital high-airways obstruction syndrome such as congenital laryngeal atresia resulted in lungs which were hyperplastic as fetal lungs are net fluid exporters, and obstruction caused intrabronchial hypertension and growth stimulation (Wigglesworth and Hislop 1987). In experimental animal models, tracheal occlusion replicated this and was associated with accelerated lung growth (Wilson et al. 1993; Bratu et al. 2001). In humans, the first attempts at this were relatively crude, involving open hysterotomy and tracheal clipping (Hedrick et al. 1994; Harrison et al. 2003). Latterly this has evolved into a true minimally invasive technique whereby, via a single port, a fetal tracheoscope is inserted and a detachable balloon located, inflated and then left in the fetal trachea (Papadakis et al. 1998; Harrison et al. 2003). The acronym FETO (fetal endoscopic tracheal occlusion) has been widely used for this intervention.

Currently, the technique is offered to high-risk fetuses (defined as having a 'liver-up' position and a lung-to-head ratio of ≤1.0) with an estimated survival without intervention of <10%. The aim is to insert the tracheal balloon at 26–28 weeks' gestation with removal at about 34 weeks (Keller et al. 2004; Deprest et al. 2009). A number of methods of balloon removal are now used (e.g. ultrasound-guided puncture or fetoscopy) (Deprest et al. 2006, 2009; Sinha et al. 2009), although initially the technique of ex utero intrapartum treatment was needed to remove the balloon at the time of birth (Mychaliska et al. 1996). Although no maternal complications have been reported, iatrogenic preterm rupture of the membranes may still occur (Deprest et al. 2006).

This technique, without doubt, increases ipsilateral lung growth (Danzer et al. 2008) evident on serial ultrasonography and survival rates of >50% have now been reported (Deprest et al. 2009; Doi et al. 2009a; Sinha et al. 2009). It may not, however, alter more qualitative aspects of lung parenchyma or pulmonary arteriolar anomalies (Danzer et al. 2008). One possible side-effect of a fetal tracheal balloon is postnatal tracheomegaly, although its contribution to often complex symptoms remains to be elucidated (McHugh et al. 2009).

Medical

Infants with CDH presenting within 24 hours of birth are at considerable risk of death and should be endotracheally intubated, probably paralysed and ventilated. Prolonged attempts at bagging using a facemask can be dangerous and should be avoided, specifically because of the detrimental effects of intestinal distension. A large-bore nasogastric tube (e.g. 8 FG) should also be passed to decompress the stomach and small bowel. Neonatal resuscitation should then proceed on conventional lines.

Initially, the main problem is hypoventilation due to lung hypoplasia, and there will be a proportion of infants in whom this is so extreme as to be incompatible with life, and who will die

in the delivery room. Initial peak inflation pressures should be limited to 25 cmH$_2$O (to reduce barotrauma in small, stiff lungs), with rates of 60–80 per minute. Positive end-expiratory pressure is kept low to achieve maximum alveolar ventilation and achieve a preductal arterial saturation (Sao$_2$) of >85% with an acceptable degree of hypercarbia if necessary (Paco$_2$ 45–60 mmHg and a pH of >7.3). This concept has been termed 'gentle ventilation' and the accompanying consequence 'permissive hypercapnea' and by reducing the risks of secondary barotrauma is felt to improve outcome.

In our institution, infants are paralysed (e.g. vecuronium 0.1–1.3 µg/kg/h) and have analgesia (e.g. fentanyl 2–8 µg/kg/h), although others argue that spontaneous breathing without relaxants may be preferable (Boloker et al. 2002).

Most infants will respond to medical measures and achieve acceptable blood gases. This has been described as the 'honeymoon' phase, as these infants can be deceptively well for a period before becoming increasingly unstable, often with severe hypoxic episodes, hypercarbia and an uncorrectable acidosis. The dominant pathophysiological problem in this phase is pulmonary hypertension and right-to-left shunting. Such PPHN can be diagnosed clinically by the typical rapid swings in oxygenation, and confirmed by measuring pre- and postductal arterial oxygen levels. Echocardiography during this period will show an enlarged right heart with pulmonary and tricuspid regurgitation and a right-to-left shunt at the foramen ovale and ductus arteriosus.

Newer ventilation techniques, such as high-frequency oscillatory ventilation and high-frequency jet ventilation, have been used in infants with diaphragmatic hernia and the former is used increasingly as a primary ventilation strategy permitting ventilation at lower mean airway pressures (e.g. no greater than 14–16 cmH$_2$O) (Reyes et al. 1998).

There is also a range of pharmacological agents which have been used to treat the PPHN associated with CDH, including tolazoline, prostacycline, prostaglandin E$_1$ (Shiyanagi et al. 2008), nitroprusside, diltiazem (Islam et al. 1999) and nitric oxide (Kinsella et al. 1993; Finer et al. 1994). There is a functional surfactant deficit in infants with CDH, and some benefit had been shown from using first-breath exogenous surfactant in experimental models (Glick et al. 1992) and patients. However, a more recent review of 448 CDH infants treated with extracorporeal membrane oxygenation (ECMO) showed no advantage of additional exogenous surfactant (Colby et al. 2004).

Surgical

Nowadays there is no role for early (within 24 hours of birth) surgical repair. Abdominal replacement of the viscera and repair of the hernial defect cause a marked reduction in lung compliance and detrimental fluid shifts (Sakai et al. 1987), and should therefore be carried out only when the infant has achieved a period of cardiorespiratory stability (of at least 24 hours) with acceptable blood gases on conventional ventilation (e.g. F$_i$O$_2$ 0.5, Po$_2$ 8 kPa (60 mmHg)) (Charlton et al. 1991).

European paediatric surgical centres during the early 1980s were the first to delay surgical repair (Cartlidge et al. 1986; Charlton et al. 1991), and this now seems to be the new orthodoxy (Lally et al. 1992; Nio et al. 1994). Nonetheless small randomised controlled clinical trials (Lally et al. 1992; de la Hunt et al. 1996) have not shown a clear survival advantage, probably because of the small numbers involved. During this period the largest single-centre experience with delayed surgery was reported from Manchester, where 86 high-risk infants had a survival rate of just over 70% (Charlton et al. 1991).

The surgical repair of CDH is performed through a subcostal incision. The displaced viscera are removed from the hemithorax and returned to the abdomen. A hernial sac, if found, should be excised to allow a tension-free musculoaponeurotic closure. The posterior margin of the defect may not be apparent initially and most have to be developed from the posterior abdominal wall. Primary closure is possible in about 75% of cases, but in those where this is impossible because of excessive tension or agenesis, other techniques have to be used. A patch of artificial material (e.g. GoreTex, Marlex, Permacol) remains the commonest strategy (Mitchell et al. 2008) but a muscle rotation flap (e.g. latissimus dorsi, internal oblique abdominis) can also be used to repair the defect (Bianchi et al. 1983). A chest tube left in the empty hemithorax is not necessary, and may be dangerous if used with suction, as the hypoplastic lung may overexpand and rupture. Abdominal wall closure can be problematic in a few infants owing to a small abdominal cavity and it is safer to insert a prosthetic patch to allow staged closure rather than risk compartment syndrome (Kyzer et al. 2004).

Minimally invasive repair of congenital diaphragmatic hernia

CDH repair can be accomplished using minimally invasive techniques, via either the abdomen or the chest, and this option has been increasingly available in larger centres. For instance, Gomes Ferreira et al. (2009) report a European multicentre series of 30 infants (down to 1.8 kg). Two-thirds were attempted thoracoscopically and overall about one-third were converted. Normally CO_2 is the gas used to create the pneumothorax and in these infants with long operating times and in the confined space of an infant's chest, hypercarbia can be an issue. The largest single-centre experience so far reported is from Oregon, USA, by Cho et al. (2009). Fifty-seven infants with CDH were reported, 29 of them having a thoracoscopic approach (one conversion). Postoperatively, although there were no significant differences in length of stay or postoperative mortality, there did seem to be an increased risk of hernial recurrence in the minimally invasive group (7% versus 20%). A theoretical problem with the thoracoscopic approach is that the reduction of the invariably malrotated bowel is left to chance, there being no opportunity of examining either the duodenum or the final position of the midgut. Nonetheless, it is likely that minimally invasive techniques will become a more widespread method of diaphragm repair, but pragmatically it should probably be reserved for the older more stable infant with better lung reserve.

The role of extracorporeal membrane oxygenation

ECMO is an option for infants with CDH if conventional methods of medical therapy are failing. The concept is simple: near-total cardiopulmonary support for a prolonged period of time (in practice, up to 10–14 days). ECMO was developed in the USA in the 1970s (Bartlett et al. 1977, 1985) and became available in the UK during the 1990s (albeit it is still restricted to supraregional centres). Early trials suggested benefit (Bartlett et al. 1985; O'Rourke et al. 1989a,b), but even in North America debate over its real role persisted (Azarow et al. 1997; Wilson et al. 1997; Congenital Diaphragmatic Hernia Study Group 1999) and there seems to have been a reduction in its application in CDH over time (Brown et al. 2009). The UK Collaborative ECMO Trial reported in 1996 failed to recruit enough infants in the CDH subgroup for the differences in survival to be statistically significant, but the only survivors were in the ECMO arm. The North American ECMO experience suggests that a survival rate of about 50% will be found in infants with CDH

(Guner et al. 2009), which is significantly worse than that achieved when ECMO is offered for other indications in neonates (e.g. meconium aspiration syndrome) (Heiss et al. 1989; Lally et al. 1992; UK Collaborative ECMO Trial Group 1996).

The indications, technique and morbidity associated with ECMO are fully discussed elsewhere (pp. 525–526). Surgical repair of the hernia may be performed while on ECMO but should probably be deferred until the infant has improved enough to be almost ready for decannulation and cessation of heparinisation (Wilson et al. 1994), if not following cessation itself.

Prediction of prognosis

It is logical to try and find specific or measurable features which will predict outcome in diaphragmatic hernia, because of the high mortality of this disease and the range of possible treatment options. A number of studies have assessed various factors as being of prognostic value, and can be divided into antenatal and postnatal.

Antenatal

Sebire et al. (1997) reported a difference in outcome of CDH detectable as early as 10–14 weeks' gestation, on the basis of the ultrasound-measured nuchal translucency, with higher values predicting a poor prognosis. It seems that the earlier the diagnosis is made antenatally, the worse the outcome. For instance, only 42% survived from a cohort of 83 fetuses with isolated CDH diagnosed before 24 weeks' gestation, compared with all of a cohort of 10 fetuses diagnosed after 24 weeks (Harrison et al. 1994). Polyhydramnios has also been a poor prognostic feature in some series (Albanese et al. 1998), although not in others (Sinha et al. 2009). The fetal stomach is found in the chest in most cases, but if it is found within the abdomen this seems to be a good prognostic feature. The position of the fetal liver seems to be important, with a significant (i.e. ultrasonically detectable) portion within the hemithorax having a poorer prognosis (Albanese et al. 1998; Sinha et al. 2009).

Various attempts have been made to estimate lung hypoplasia antenatally. Over the past decade this has been refined into the calculation of a single measurement – the lung-to-head ratio, where a ratio of ≤1 has an extremely poor prognosis (Lipshutz et al. 1997) and, by implication, requires antenatal intervention. In those centres able to offer FETO, then this, together with a 'liver-up' position, is the key criterion for its use (Deprest et al. 2006, 2009; Sinha et al. 2009). Nonetheless this is still a controversial area and far from being accepted universally (Yang et al. 2007).

Associated congenital cardiac anomalies are, of course, indicative of a poor outcome (Sweed and Puri 1993), but a number of groups have also looked at echocardiographic features of the fetal heart as a measure of lung hypoplasia or pulmonary vascular anomalies. UK investigators have suggested that both the ratio of left-to-right ventricular internal measurements (Crawford et al. 1989; Sharland et al. 1992) and the ratio of aortic-to-pulmonary artery diameters (Crawford et al. 1989) are valuable as prognostic features in isolated diaphragmatic hernias, both reflecting left ventricular underdevelopment.

Postnatal

For those infants who are not diagnosed antenatally, the age at presentation is important. The minority who present after 24 hours of life should have a survival prospect approaching 100%. Poor outcome is associated with early symptoms, prematurity and low birthweight.

Table 27.17 Derived predictive indices in congenital diaphragmatic hernia

Oxygenation index (OI)

$$OI = \frac{mean\ airway\ pressure\ (cmH_2O) \times F_IO\ (\%)}{PaO\ (KPa)}$$

(NB: if PaO is more familiar in mmHg then divide result by 7.5)

Ventilation index (VI)

VI = respiratory rate (breaths/min) × mean airway pressure (cmH$_2$C

Wilford Hall/Santa Rosa prediction formula

WHSR$_{PF}$ = highest Po_2 – highest Pco_2

(N.B. measured on first day)

Achieving normal arterial blood gases is the final result of an effective pulmonary system, and the degree to which this is successful has been used as a prognostic factor. Initially, this is apparent clinically in the Apgar score, but is relatively crude. However, if a postductal $Paco_2$ of 5.5 kPa (40 mmHg) or a postductal Pao_2 of 13 kPa (100 mmHg) (Bohn et al. 1987; O'Rourke et al. 1989a,b) can be achieved with conventional ventilation, this suggests adequate lung tissue for survival. The degree of ventilatory support required to achieve such blood gases can also be incorporated into a variety of indices (Table 27.17), and of these the best is probably the oxygenation index (OI). In our series, the best OI (day 1) had a sensitivity (for good outcome) and specificity of 85% and 94% respectively (Sinha et al. 2009).

At present it is not possible to measure the critical lung mass in neonates directly, although there have been attempts to measure some indirect indices of lung function (e.g. compliance and functional residual capacity (FRC)) early in the postnatal period in these infants (Sakai et al. 1987; Dimitriou et al. 1995; Kavvadia et al. 1997). Such studies have shown that day 1 compliance rather than FRC has a predictive relationship to outcome. Serial studies showed that, in survivors, only compliance increased over the first 2 weeks, FRC remaining constant (Kavvadia et al. 1997). Of course, measurement of lung volumes remains confined to specialist centres, but there is even predictive value derived from the measured lung area on the postoperative chest X-ray (Dimitriou et al. 2000).

Echocardiography has been used to assess the degree of PPHN (Haugen et al. 1991; Hasegawa et al. 1994). Some echocardiographic variables (e.g. McGoon and pulmonary artery indices) may also have value when performed sequentially, to show the improvement in pulmonary vascular stability and, perhaps, the most appropriate physiological time for surgery (Takahashi et al. 2009).

The size of the diaphragm defect itself has been related to prognosis. Diaphragmatic agenesis (Lally et al. 1992) particularly, and all those where a patch is needed to repair the defect (West et al. 1992; Sinha et al. 2009), have been associated with a poorer outcome.

Outcome in congenital diaphragmatic hernia

No surgical series of diaphragmatic hernias has ever been able to emulate Robert Gross's first report of 100% survival in seven infants and children in 1946. This paradox is, of course, entirely due to preselection, as only the least affected infants used to survive to reach paediatric surgical centres. Table 27.18 illustrates recent survival statistics from a number of different centres throughout the world.

Recurrence may occur and indeed appears to be increasing in frequency in line with increased use of prosthetic patches, ECMO and increased survival of marginal infants (Moss et al. 2001; Fisher et al. 2009). The incidence varies but with assiduous follow-up and repeated chest X-rays may be identified in up to 20% of children (Nobuhara et al. 1996; Moss et al. 2001; Fisher et al. 2009). Recurrence can present with respiratory or gastrointestinal symptoms, and is usually confirmed on a chest X-ray. Surgical repair is advised in most.

Chest wall deformity can be obvious in some older children, and can manifest as pectus excavatum or scoliosis. It is presumed to be due to a reflection of underlying lung hypoplasia but untoward neodiaphragmatic tension may play a role. Consideration should be given to surgical correction, but is probably best deferred until adolescence.

Surviving infants have usually required a prolonged stay in intensive care, often with periods of hypoxia, hypercarbia and acidosis. Although early studies suggested that long-term complications in survivors were minimal, this was probably because of selection of a smaller but 'better quality' cohort. Currently, more marginal survival is possible and the incidence of long-term problems is higher (Mychaliska et al. 1996).

Pulmonary function

Dramatic changes occur in lung structure after surgical repair, although not immediately. Lung weight and volumes do increase measurably after about 3 weeks. Sakai et al. (1987) suggested that there was a decrease in compliance in the early postoperative period, although this has been disputed by later studies (Kavvadia et al. 1997), perhaps because of variation in the timing of surgery. Histologically there is an increase in the number of alveoli, and a decrease in muscularisation of the interacinar arteries, although there is no change in bronchiolar airway generation.

In one study of long-term symptoms in CDH survivors, at discharge 16% still required oxygen, 43% required diuretics and 17% required regular bronchodilator therapy, rising to about 50% with a transient need during the first year (Muratore et al. 2001). The radiographic appearance of the chest returns to normal in most, although there are persisting anomalies in tested lung function (typically forced expiratory volume in 1 second and forced vital capacity) (Muratore et al. 2001). The progressive improvement in ventilation can be assessed using ventilation–perfusion scans, and such studies show specifically a long-term persistence of ipsilateral perfusion defects (Jeandot et al. 1989).

Gastrointestinal function

The principal gastrointestinal problem is one of acid reflux caused by distortion of the gastro-oesophageal junction and crura; this may occur in up to 50% of survivors (Kamiyama et al. 2002). This may be manifest by vomiting and feeding difficulties, and can prolong respiratory morbidity, presumably due to recurrent aspiration. Twenty-four-hour intraoesophgeal pH measurement should be performed in all survivors where reflux is thought possible. Intensive medical treatment (e.g. antacids, H$_2$ receptor blockers, proton pump blockers and prokinetic agents) should be tried, although, because of the anatomical basis for reflux, surgical correction (e.g. a Nissen antireflux procedure) may be necessary.

Neurological

There is a long-term worry of neurological impairment in survivors, which is presumed to be due to neonatal hypoxia and periods

Table 27.18 Surgical outcome in infants with high-risk congenital diaphragmatic hernia

SERIES	N	PERIOD	TREATMENT	SURVIVAL (%)
Heiss et al. (1989)	16	1974–1981	–	50
(Ann Arbor, USA)	34	1982–1987	ECMO	76
Charlton et al. (1991)	56	1976–1983	Immediate repair	55
(Manchester, UK)	86	1983–1989	Delayed repair	71
West et al. (1992)	65	1975–1987	–	43
(Indianapolis, USA)	46	1987–1992	ECMO and delayed repair	67
Skari et al. (2002) (Scandinavian Multicentre)	157	1995–1998	Delayed repair and ECMO	65
Congenital Diaphragmatic Hernia Study Group (1999) (USA multicentre)	632	1995–1997	ECMO	53 (with ECMO) 77 (no ECMO)
Boloker et al. (2002) (New York, USA)	120	1992–2000	Delayed repair, ECMO (13%), 'gentle ventilation'	76 overall (62 with ECMO)
Jaillard et al. (2003) (Lille, France)	85	1991–1998	ECMO (30%)	60 overall
Migliazza et al. (2007) (Bergamo, Italy)	111	1994–2005	Delayed repair, HFOV, 'gentle ventilation'	70 overall
Yang et al. (2007) (San Francisco, USA)	107	1995–2004	Delayed repair, ECMO (fetal medicine centre)	59
Sinha et al. (2009) (London, UK)	86	1994–2007	Delayed repair (fetal medicine centre)	52 (FETO) 64 (non-FETO)

ECMO, extracorporeal membrane oxygenation; HFOV, high-frequency oscillatory ventilation; FETO, fetal endoscopic tracheal occlusion.

of cardiovascular instability. One UK study of selected high-risk long-term survivors found a major neurological handicap in two of 23 children, although there was no clear relationship between poor outcome and measured indices of hypoxia and acidosis during the neonatal period (Davenport et al. 1992). Sensorineural hearing loss has been recently described in up to 50% of CDH survivors, although why is not really known (Morini et al. 2008). Certainly, potential audiotoxic drugs, including pancuronium, aminoglycosides and furosemide, are used during their neonatal care. Neurological follow-up in ECMO survivors is described on pages 525–526.

Anterior diaphragmatic hernias

The Italian anatomist Giovanni Battista Morgagni first described a hernia occurring between the costal and the sternal muscle origins of the diaphragm in a series published in 1769. There is usually a hernial sac, and over 90% occur on the right side (Fig. 27.57). Compared with posterolateral defects, there is seldom any associated lung hypoplasia, and, consequently, symptoms are mild. There may be other anomalies in a minority of cases, including extralobar lung sequestrations and congenital cardiac defects. Morgagni hernias have also been described in Down syndrome (Iritani 1984).

Most of the clinical features are due to incarceration of part of the bowel (commonly the transverse colon) and include vomiting, failure to thrive and intestinal obstruction. Some may be found incidentally on chest X-ray. Surgical repair is performed through an

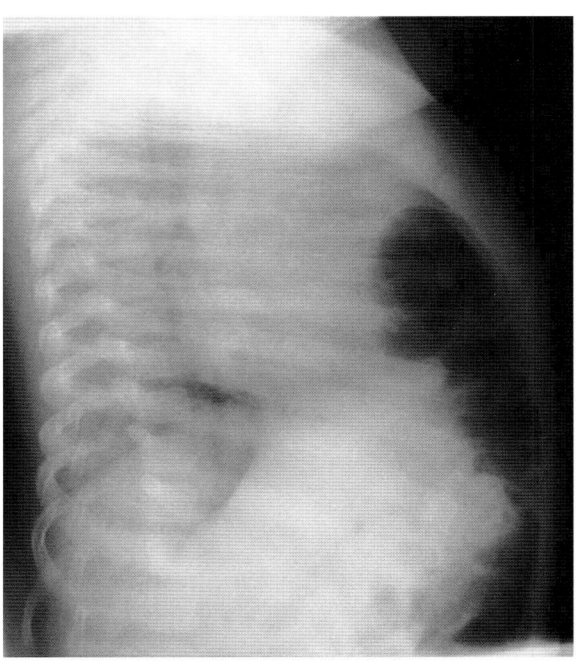

Fig. 27.57 Lateral chest radiograph of an infant who presented with intermittent vomiting, showing an anterior Morgagni hernia.

upper abdominal approach and is usually straightforward. Transabdominal laparoscopic repair is also feasible and safe (Ponsky et al. 2002).

The pentalogy of Cantrell is a syndrome of an anterior diaphragmatic defect with pericardial defects, a short sternum, exomphalos and major intracardiac anomalies (Cantrell et al. 1958). While the full-blown pentalogy is rare, incomplete manifestations may not be and this syndrome should be suspected in infants where the exomphalos defect is sited higher on the body wall than usual. Van Hoorn et al. (2008) reviewed the literature between 1987 and 2007 and identified 58 examples of pentalogy of Cantrell, of which 37 died or were terminated in utero, illustrating its poor prognosis. The defect differs anatomically from a Morgagni hernia (right or left of xiphisternum), in being a symmetrical central defect exposing the heart, and this has been attributed to a defective formation of the septum transversum.

Diaphragmatic eventration

Eventration can be congenital or acquired. Congenital absence of anterior horn cells may be responsible (Werdnig–Hoffmann disease), with others being due to intrauterine infection (e.g. rubella, cytomegalovirus) or as part of a more generalised chromosomal anomaly (e.g. trisomies 13–15 or 18). These anomalies are usually left-sided and may even be bilateral (Rodgers and Hawks 1986). Diaphragmatic denervation due to phrenic nerve injury may be related to birth injury (when it is often associated with brachial plexus injury) or thoracic surgery (e.g. patent ductus arteriosus ligation).

Eventration may be asymptomatic, but most present in infancy with respiratory distress, recurrent chest infections or bronchiectasis. Paradoxical movement of the hemidiaphragm causes mediastinal shift, basal atelectasis and futile movement of air from the ipsilateral to the contralateral lung.

Chest X-ray (posteroanterior and lateral views) and fluoroscopic screening should establish the diagnosis, and radionuclide ventilation scans may allow assessment of the degree of ventilatory impairment. The management of eventration depends on the symptoms: if asymptomatic, an expectant course should be pursued; if there is respiratory distress, however, a more aggressive approach should be followed. Positive-pressure endotracheal ventilation overcomes any immediate problems, and once the infant is stable he or she should undergo definitive surgical correction. This is achieved by radial plication of the diaphragm, approached from either the chest or abdomen. The taut plicated diaphragm increases breathing capacity and tidal volume, allowing safe ventilator weaning.

References

Adzick, N.S., Harrison, M.R., 1994. Fetal surgical therapy. Lancet 343, 897–901.

Adzick, N.S., Harrison, M.R., Glick, P.L., et al., 1985. Diaphragmatic hernia in the fetus: prenatal diagnosis and outcome in 94 cases. J Pediatr Surg 20, 357–361.

Albanese, C.T., Lopoo, J., Goldstein, R.B., et al., 1998. Fetal liver position and perinatal outcome for congenital diaphragmatic hernia. Prenat Diagn 18, 1138–1142.

Azarow, K., Messineo, A., Pearl, R., et al., 1997. Congenital diaphragmatic hernia – a tale of two cities: the Toronto experience. J Pediatr Surg 32, 395–400.

Bartlett, R.H., Gazzaniga, A.B., Huxtable, R.F., et al., 1977. Extracorporeal circulation (ECMO) in neonatal respiratory failure. J Thorac Cardiovasc Surg 74, 826–833.

Bartlett, R.H., Roloff, D.W., Cornell, R.G., et al., 1985. Extracorporeal circulation in neonatal respiratory failure: a prospective randomized study. Pediatrics 76, 479–487.

Benjamin, D.R., Juul, S., Siebert, J.R., 1988. Congenital posterolateral diaphragmatic hernia: associated malformations. J Pediatr Surg 23, 899–903.

Bianchi, A., Doig, C.M., Cohen, S.J., 1983. The reverse latissimus dorsi flap for congenital diaphragmatic hernia. J Pediatr Surg 18, 560–563.

Bochdalek, V.A., 1848. Einige Betrachtungen uber die Entstehung des angeborenen Zwerchfellbruches. Als Betrag zur pathologischen Anatomie der Hernien. Vierteljahrschrift fur die praktische Heilkunde 19, 89.

Bohn, D., Tamura, M., Perrin, D., et al., 1987. Ventilatory predictors of pulmonary hypoplasia in congenital diaphragmatic hernia, confirmed by morphological assessment. Journal of Pediatrics 111, 423–431.

Boloker, J., Bateman, D.A., Wung, J.-T., et al., 2002. Congenital diaphragmatic hernia in 120 infants treated consecutively with permissive hypercapnea/spontaneous respiration/elective repair. J Pediatr Surg 37, 357–366.

Bonet, T., 1679. De Suffocatione Observatio XLI. Suffocatio excitata a tenium intestorum vulnus diaphragmatis, in thoracem ingrestu. Sepuhuchretum sive anatomia procteia et cadaveribus morbo denatus. Geneva.

Bratu, I., Flageole, H., Laberge, J.-M., et al., 2001. Pulmonary structural maturation and pulmonary artery remodeling after reversible fetal ovine tracheal occlusion in diaphragmatic hernia. J Pediatr Surg 36, 739–744.

Brown, K.L., Sriram, S., Ridout, D., et al., 2009. Extracorporeal membrane oxygenation and term neonatal respiratory failure deaths in the United Kingdom compared with the United States: 1999 to 2005. Pediatric Critical Care Medicine.

Cantrell, J.R., Haller, J.A., Ravitch, M.M., 1958. A syndrome of congenital defects involving the abdominal wall, sternum, diaphragm, pericardium and heart. Surg Gynecol Obstet 107, 602–614.

Cartlidge, P.H.T., Mann, N.P., Kapilla, L., 1986. Preoperative stabilisation in congenital diaphragmatic hernia. Arch Dis Child 61, 1226–1228.

Charlton, A., Bruce, J.B., Davenport, M., 1991. Timing of surgery in congenital diaphragmatic hernia: low mortality after pre-operative stabilisation. Anaesthesia 46, 820–823.

Cho, S.D., Krishnaswami, S., Mckee, J.C., et al., 2009. Analysis of 29 consecutive thoracoscopic repairs of congenital diaphragmatic hernia in neonates compared to historical controls. J Pediatr Surg 44, 80–86.

Clugston, R.D., Greer, J.J., 2007. Diaphragm development and congenital diaphragmatic hernia. Semin Pediatr Surg 16, 94–100.

Colby, C.E., Lally, K.P., Hintz, S.R., et al., 2004. Surfactant replacement therapy on ECMO does not improve outcome in neonates with congenital diaphragmatic hernia. J Pediatr Surg 39, 1632–1637.

Congenital Diaphragmatic Hernia Study Group, 1999. Does extracorporeal membrane oxygenation improve survival in neonates with congenital diaphragmatic hernia? J Pediatr Surg 34, 720–725.

Crane, J.P., 1979. Familial diaphragmatic hernia: prenatal diagnostic approach and analysis of twelve families. Clin Genet 16, 244–252.

Crawford, D.C., Wright, V.M., Drake, D.P., et al., 1989. Fetal diaphragmatic hernia: the value of fetal echocardiography in the prediction of postnatal outcome. Br J Obstet Gynaecol 96, 705–710.

Danzer, E., Davey, M.G., Kreiger, P.A., et al., 2008. Fetal tracheal occlusion for severe congenital diaphragmatic hernia in humans: a morphometric study of lung parenchyma and muscularization of pulmonary arterioles. J Pediatr Surg 43, 1767–1775.

Davenport, M., Rivlin, E., D'Souza, S.W., et al., 1992. Neurodevelopmental outcome following delayed surgery for congenital diaphragmatic hernia. Arch Dis Child 67, 1353–1356.

de la Hunt, M.N., Madden, N., Scott, J.E., et al., 1996. Is delayed surgery really better for congenital diaphragmatic hernia?: a prospective randomized clinical trial. J Pediatr Surg 31, 1554–1556.

Deprest, J., Jani, J., Van Schoubroeck, D., et al., 2006. Current consequences of prenatal diagnosis of congenital diaphragmatic hernia. J Pediatr Surg 41, 423–430.

Deprest, J.A., Hyett, J.A., Flake, A.W., et al., 2009. Current controversies in prenatal diagnosis 4: Should fetal surgery be done in all cases of severe diaphragmatic hernia? Prenat Diagn 29, 15–19.

Dimitriou, G., Greenough, A., Chan, V., et al., 1995. Prognostic indicators in congenital diaphragmatic hernia. J Pediatr Surg 30, 1694–1697.

Dimitriou, G., Greenough, A., Davenport, M., 2000. Prediction of outcome in infants with congenital diaphragmatic hernia from computer assisted analysis. J Pediatr Surg 35, 489–493.

Doi, T., Hajduk, P., Puri, P., 2009a. Upregulation of Slit-2 and Slit-3 gene expressions in the nitrofen-induced hypoplastic lung. J Pediatr Surg 44, 2092–2095.

Doi, T., Sugimoto, K., Puri, P., 2009b. Prenatal retinoic acid up-regulates pulmonary gene expression of COUP-TFII, FOG2, and GATA4 in pulmonary hypoplasia. J Pediatr Surg 44, 1933–1937.

Finer, N.N., Etches, P.C., Kamstra, B., et al., 1994. Inhaled nitric oxide in infants referred for extracorporeal membrane oxygenation: dose response. Journal of Pediatrics 124, 302–308.

Fisher, J.C., Haley, M.J., Ruiz-Elizalde, A., et al., 2009. Multivariate model for predicting recurrence in congenital diaphragmatic hernia. J Pediatr Surg 44, 1173–1179.

Fryns, J.P., Moerman, F., Goddeeris, P., et al., 1979. A new lethal syndrome with cloudy corneae, diaphragmatic defects and distal limb deformities. Hum Genet 50, 65–70.

Glick, P.L., Leach, C.L., Besner, G.E., et al., 1992. Pathophysiology of congenital diaphragmatic hernia. III: Exogenous surfactant therapy for the high-risk neonate with CDH. J Pediatr Surg 27, 866–869.

Gomes Ferreira, C., Reinberg, O., Becmeur, F., 2009. Neonatal minimally invasive surgery for congenital diaphragmatic hernias: a multicenter study using thoracoscopy or laparoscopy. Surg Endosc.

Gross, R.E., 1946. Congenital hernia of the diaphragm. Am J Dis Child 71, 580–592.

Guner, Y.S., Khemani, R.G., Qureshi, F.G., et al., 2009. Outcome analysis of neonates with congenital diaphragmatic hernia treated with venovenous vs venoarterial extracorporeal membrane oxygenation. J Pediatr Surg 44, 1691–1701.

Harris, G.J., Soper, R.T., Kimura, K.K., 1993. Foramen of Morgagni hernia in identical twins: is this an inheritable defect? J Pediatr Surg 28, 177–178.

Harrison, M.R., Adzick, N.S., Flake, A.W., et al., 1993. Correction of congenital diaphragmatic hernia in utero: VI. Hard-earned lessons. J Pediatr Surg 28, 1411–1418.

Harrison, M.R., Adzick, N.S., Estes, J.M., et al., 1994. A prospective study of the outcome for fetuses with diaphragmatic hernia. J Am Med Assoc 271, 382–384.

Harrison, M.R., Mychaliska, G.B., Albanese, C.T., et al., 1998. Correction of congenital diaphragmatic hernia in utero. IX: Fetuses with poor prognosis (liver herniation and low lung-to-head ratio) can be saved by fetoscopic temporary tracheal occlusion. J Pediatr Surg 33, 1017–1022.

Harrison, M.R., Keller, R.L., Hawgood, S.B., et al., 2003. A randomized trial of fetal endoscopic tracheal occlusion for severe fetal congenital diaphragmatic hernia. NEJM 349, 1916–1924.

Hasegawa, S., Kohno, S., Sugiyama, T., et al., 1994. Usefulness of echocardiographic measurement of bilateral pulmonary artery dimensions in congenital diaphragmatic hernia. J Pediatr Surg 29, 622–624.

Haugen, S., Linker, D., Eik-Nes, S., et al., 1991. Congenital diaphragmatic hernia: determination of the optimal time for operation by echocardiographic monitoring of the pulmonary artery pressure. J Pediatr Surg 26, 560–562.

Hedrick, M.H., Estes, K.M., Sullivan, K.M., et al., 1994. Plug the Lung Until it Grows (PLUG): a new method to treat congenital diaphragmatic hernia in utero. J Pediatr Surg 29, 612–617.

Heiss, K., Manning, P., Oldham, K.T., et al., 1989. Reversal of mortality for congenital diaphragmatic hernia. Ann Surg 209, 225–230.

Holt, C., 1701. Child that lived two months with congenital diaphragmatic hernia. Philosophical Transactions 22, 992.

Iritani, I., 1984. Experimental study on pathogenesis and embryogenesis of congenital diaphragmatic hernia. Anat Embryol (Berl) 169, 133–139.

Islam, S., Masiakos, P., Schnitzer, P., et al., 1999. Diltiazem reduces pulmonary arterial pressures in recurrent pulmonary hypertension associated with pulmonary hypoplasia. J Pediatr Surg 34, 712–714.

Jaillard, S.M., Pierrat, V., Dubois, A., et al., 2003. Outcome at 2 years of infants with congenital diaphragmatic hernia: a population-based study. Ann Thorac Surg 75, 250–256.

Jeandot, R., Lambert, B., Brendel, A.J., et al., 1989. Lung ventilation and perfusion scintigraphy in the follow up of repaired congenital diaphragmatic hernia. Eur J Nucl Med 15, 591–596.

Kamiyama, M., Kawahara, H., Okuyama, H., et al., 2002. Gastroesophageal reflux after repair of congenital diaphragmatic hernia. J Pediatr Surg 37, 1681–1684.

Karamanoukian, H.L., Glick, P.L., Wilcox, D., et al., 1995. Pathophysiology of congenital diaphragmatic hernia XI: anatomic and biochemical characterisation of the heart in the fetal lamb CDH model. J Pediatr Surg 30, 925–929.

Kavvadia, V., Greenough, A., Laubscher, B., et al., 1997. Perioperative assessment of respiratory compliance and lung volume in infants with congenital diaphragmatic hernia: prediction of outcome. J Pediatr Surg 32, 1665–1669.

Keller, R.L., Hawgood, S., Neuhaus, J.M., et al., 2004. Infant pulmonary function in a randomized trial of fetal tracheal occlusion for severe congenital diaphragmatic hernia. Pediatr Res 56, 818–825.

Kinsella, J.P., Neish, S.R., Ivy, D., et al., 1993. Clinical responses to prolonged treatment of persistent pulmonary hypertension of the newborn with low doses of inhaled nitric oxide. Journal of Pediatrics 123, 103–108.

Kitano, Y., Kanai, M., von Allmen, D., et al., 2001. Lung growth induced by prenatal tracheal occlusion and its modifying factors: a study in the rat model of congenital diaphragmatic hernia. J Pediatr Surg 36, 251–259.

Kluth, D., Keijzer, R., Hertl, M., et al., 1996. Embryology of congenital diaphragmatic hernia. Semin Pediatr Surg 5, 224–233.

Kyzer, S., Sirota, L., Chaimoff, C., 2004. Abdominal wall closure with a Silastic patch after repair of congenital diaphragmatic hernia. Arch Surg 139, :296–298.

Lally, K.P., Paranka, M.S., Roden, J., et al., 1992. Congenital diaphragmatic hernia, stabilisation and repair on ECMO. Ann Surg 216, 569–573.

Langer, J.C., Winthrop, A.L., Whelan, D., 1994. Fryns syndrome: a rare familial cause of congenital diaphragmatic hernia. J Pediatr Surg 29, 1266–1267.

Leinwald, M.J., Tefft, J.D., Zhao, J., et al., 2002. Nitrofen inhibition of pulmonary growth and development occurs in the early embryonic mouse. J Pediatr Surg 37, 1263–1268.

Lipshutz, G.S., Albanese, C.T., Feldstein, V., et al., 1997. Lung-to-head ratio predicts survival in fetal diaphragmatic hernia. J Pediatr Surg 32, 1634–1636.

McHugh, K., Afaq, A., Broderick, N., et al., 2009. Tracheomegaly: a complication of fetal endoscopic tracheal occlusion in the treatment of congenital diaphragmatic hernia. Pediatr Radiol., Nov 6. [Epub ahead of print]: 19894042.

Migliazza, L., Bellan, C., Alberti, D., et al., 2007. Retrospective study of 111 cases of congenital diaphragmatic hernia treated with early high-frequency oscillatory ventilation and presurgical stabilization. J Pediatr Surg 42, 1526–1532.

Milne, L.W., Moroson, A.M., Campbell, J.R., et al., 1984. Pars sternalis diaphragmatic hernia with omphalocele: a report of 2 cases. J Pediatr Surg 19, 394–397.

Mishalany, H., Gordo, J., 1986. Congenital diaphragmatic hernia in monozygotic twins. J Pediatr Surg 21, 372–374.

Mitchell, I.C., Garcia, N.M., Barber, R., et al., 2008. Permacol: a potential biologic patch alternative in congenital diaphragmatic hernia repair. J Pediatr Surg 43, 2161–2164.

Morgagni, G.B., 1769. Seats and Causes of Disease Investigated by Anatomy, Vol 3. Translated by B Alexander. Millere and Cadell, London, p. 205.

Morini, F., Capolupo, I., Masi, R., et al., 2008. Hearing impairment in congenital diaphragmatic hernia: the inaudible and noiseless foot of time. J Pediatr Surg 43, 380–384.

Moss, R.L., Chen, C.M., Harrison, M.R., 2001. Prosthetic patch durability in congenital diaphragmatic hernia: a long-term follow-up study. J Pediatr Surg 36, 152–154.

Muratore, C.S., Kharasch, V., Lund, D.P., et al., 2001. Pulmonary morbidity in 100 survivors of congenital diaphragmatic hernia monitored in a multidisciplinary clinic. J Pediatr Surg 36, 133–140.

Mychaliska, G.B., Bealer, J.F., Graf, J.L., et al., 1996. Operating on placental support: the Ex-utero intrapartum treatment (EXIT) procedure. J Pediatr Surg 32, 227–231.

Naik, S., Greenough, A., Zhang, Y.-X., et al., 1996. Prediction of morbidity following congenital diaphragmatic hernia repair. J Pediatr Surg 31, 1651–1654.

Neville, H.L., Jaksic, T., Wilson, J.M., et al., 2003. Bilateral congenital diaphragmatic hernia. J Pediatr Surg 38, 522–524.

Nio, M., Haase, G., Kennaugh, J., et al., 1994. A prospective randomised trial of delayed versus immediate repair of congenital diaphragmatic hernia. J Pediatr Surg 29, 618–621.

Nobuhara, K.K., Lund, D.P., Mitchell, J., et al., 1996. Long-term outlook for survivors of congenital diaphragmatic hernia. Clin Perinatol 23, 873–887.

Okazaki, T., Sharma, H.S., McCune, S.K., et al., 1998. Pulmonary vascular balance in congenital diaphragmatic hernia: enhanced endothelin-1 gene expression as a possible cause of pulmonary vasoconstriction. J Pediatr Surg 33, 81–84.

O'Rourke, P.P., Crone, R.K., Vacanti, J.P., et al., 1989a. Extracorporeal membrane oxygenation and conventional medical therapy in neonates with persistent pulmonary hypertension of the newborn: a prospective randomized study. Pediatrics 84, 957–963.

O'Rourke, P.P., Vacanti, J.P., Crone, R.K., et al., 1989b. Use of postductal $PaO2$ as a predictor of pulmonary vascular hypoplasia in infants with congenital diaphragmatic hernia. J Pediatr Surg 23, 904–907.

Papadakis, K., De Paepe, M.E., Tackett, L.D., et al., 1998. Temporary tracheal occlusion causes catch-up lung maturation in a fetal model of diaphragmatic hernia. J Pediatr Surg 33, 1030–1037.

Ponsky, T.A., Lukish, J.R., Nobuhara, K., et al., 2002. Laparoscopy is useful in the diagnosis and management of foramen of Morgagni hernia in children. Surg Laparosc Endosc Percutan Tech 12, 375–377.

Reyes, C., Chang, L.K., Waffarn, F., et al., 1998. Delayed repair of congenital diaphragmatic hernia with early high-frequency oscillatory ventilation during preoperative stabilization. J Pediatr Surg 33, 1010–1014; discussion 1014–1016.

Rodgers, B.M., Hawks, P., 1986. Bilateral congenital eventration of the diaphragm. Successful management. J Pediatr Surg 21, 858–864.

Sakai, H., Tamura, M., Hosokawa, Y., et al., 1987. The effect of surgical repair on respiratory mechanics in congenital diaphragmatic hernia. Journal of Pediatrics 111, 432–458.

Sebire, N.J., Snijders, R.J., Davenport, M., et al., 1997. Fetal nuchal translucency thickness at 10–14 weeks' gestation and congenital diaphragmatic hernia. Obstet Gynecol 90, 943–946.

Sharland, G.K., Lochhart, S.M., Heward, A.J., et al., 1992. Prognosis in fetal diaphragmatic hernia. Am J Obstet Gynecol 166, 9–13.

Shiyanagi, S., Okazaki, T., Shoji, H., et al., 2008. Management of pulmonary hypertension in congenital diaphragmatic hernia: nitric oxide with prostaglandin-E1 versus nitric oxide alone. Pediatr Surg Int 24, 1101–1104.

Siebert, J.R., Haas, J.E., Beckwith, J.B., 1984. Left ventricular hypoplasia in congenital diaphragmatic hernia. J Pediatr Surg 19, 567–571.

Sinha, C.K., Islam, S., Patel, S., et al., 2009. Congenital diaphragmatic hernia: prognostic indices in the fetal endoluminal tracheal occlusion era. J Pediatr Surg 44, 312–316.

Skari, H., Bjornland, K., Frencker, B., et al., 2002. Congenital diaphragmatic hernia in Scandinavia from 1995 to 1998: predictors of mortality. J Pediatr Surg 37, 1269–1275.

Sweed, Y., Puri, P., 1993. Congenital diaphragmatic hernia: influence of associated malformations on survival. Arch Dis Child 69, 68–70.

Takahashi, S., Oishi, Y., Ito, N., et al., 2009. Evaluating mortality and disease severity in congenital diaphragmatic hernia using the McGoon and pulmonary artery indices. J Pediatr Surg 44, 2101–2106.

UK Collaborative ECMO Trial Group, 1996. UK collaborative randomised trial of neonatal extracorporeal membrane oxygenation. Lancet 248, 75–82.

van Hoorn, J.H., Moonen, R.M., Huysentruyt, C.J., 2008. Pentalogy of Cantrell: two patients and a review to determine prognostic factors for optimal approach. Eur J Pediatr 167, 29–35.

Wenstrom, K.D., Weiner, C.P., Hanson, J.W., 1991. A five year statewide experience with congenital diaphragmatic hernia. Am J Obstet Gynecol 165, 838–842.

West, K.W., Bengstrom, K., Rescorla, F.J., et al., 1992. Delayed surgical repair and ECMO improves survival in congenital diaphragmatic hernia. Ann Surg 216, 454–462.

Wigglesworth, J., Hislop, A., 1987. Fetal lung growth in congenital larnygeal atresia. Pediatr Pathol 7, 515–525.

Wilson, J.M., DiFiore, J.W., Peters, C.A., 1993. Experimental fetal tracheal ligation prevents the pulmonary hypoplasia associated with fetal nephrectomy: possible application for congenital diaphragmatic hernia. J Pediatr Surg 28, 1433–1440.

Wilson, J.M., Bower, L.K., Lund, D.P., 1994. Evolution of the technique of congenital diaphragmatic hernia repair on ECMO. J Pediatr Surg 29, 1109–1112.

Wilson, J.M., Lund, D.P., Lillehei, C.W., et al., 1997. Congenital diaphragmatic hernia–a tale of two cities: the Boston experience. J Pediatr Surg 32, 401–405.

Yang, S.H., Nobuhara, K.K., Keller, R.L., et al., 2007. Reliability of the lung-to-head ratio as a predictor of outcome in fetuses with isolated left congenital diaphragmatic hernia at gestation outside 24–26 weeks. Am J Obstet Gynecol 197, 110–111.

Gavin Morrison

Introduction

Continuing advances in neonatology present the paediatric otolaryngologist with an increasing range of baby and infant airway problems. This chapter attempts to review the causes, investigations and management of the compromised airway from the specialist paediatric airway surgeon's viewpoint. Investigation, management and prognosis are discussed. Although this chapter is entitled Pulmonary disease of the newborn, airway obstruction in the newborn can involve any site from the nostrils to the alveoli. Higher upper airway obstruction (UAO), from the nose downwards, is therefore discussed, in addition to laryngotracheobronchial airway disease.

Tracheostomy, at one time the mainstay surgical procedure for airway obstruction, has seen changing trends over the years. Immunisation programmes against diphtheria, polio and *Haemophilus influenzae* (acute epiglottitis) have dramatically reduced infective indications. The increased survival of very-low-birthweight (VLBW) babies and babies with multiple congenital abnormalities has led to a continued need for long-term tracheostomy in some infants and children. There is significant morbidity and mortality associated with tracheostomy, and newer developments now facilitate a trend away from tracheostomy, even for severe airway obstruction. Congenital and acquired subglottic stenosis (SGS) can often be successfully treated by single-stage laryngotracheal reconstruction (SS-LTR), thereby avoiding tracheostomy. The ex utero intrapartum treatment (EXIT) procedure can also now be used in difficult cases with antenatally diagnosed airway obstruction. This part looks at the assessment and management of the range of airway problems from a practical viewpoint.

Development of the nose, larynx and trachea and lungs

At 4 weeks, a median laryngotracheal groove appears in the ventral wall of the developing primitive pharynx. This groove deepens and its edges fuse to create a tube, the laryngotracheal tube. At the cranial end of this tube, the lips do not fuse, remaining open into the pharynx with a slit-like aperture. This cranial end forms the larynx, the trachea lies below this and caudally two lung buds arise and grow outward, forming the bronchi and bronchioles. The laryngotracheal tube is lined with endoderm, which becomes the respiratory epithelium. The epiglottis arises from the hypobranchial eminence at the tongue base and two arytenoid swellings appear, one on each side of the laryngotracheal groove. These develop from 6 weeks, into the epiglottis and arytenoids, creating a T-shaped laryngeal cleft. Soon after its formation, the epithelial walls of this cleft adhere to each other, and the aperture of the larynx remains occluded until the third month, when the lumen reappears. With further growth, this new definitive aperture forms above the initial primitive one and the detailed features of the larynx are created. The thyroid cartilage is developed from the ventral ends of the fourth and/or fifth branchial arches and appears as two lateral plates, while the cricoid cartilage develops from two sixth-arch cartilaginous centres, which fuse ventrally and gradually extend and fuse on the dorsal side as well.

The right and left lung buds commence before the laryngotracheal groove becomes a tube and develop out into the pleural passages. The lungs migrate caudally and at birth the bifurcation of the trachea (carina) is at the level of the fourth thoracic vertebra.

The primitive foregut is in continuity with the pharynx and elongates to form the oesophagus. The continuity between the oesophagus and the laryngotracheal groove is not maintained and the separation between these structures proceeds cranially to achieve complete separation of the lung buds and trachea from the oesophagus (Fig. 27.58).

Laryngeal webs result from incomplete separation of the arytenoid regions. Laryngeal clefts are posteriorly sited and can result in notching of the posterior cricoid or complete failure of fusion of this ring. Incomplete fusion of the tracheo-oesophageal wall can result in a laryngeal cleft superiorly and a tracheo-oesophageal fistula (TOF) more inferiorly. Congenital anomalies of the larynx and trachea are rare, estimated at between 1 in 10 000 and 1 in 50 000 (Van der Broek and Brinkman 1979). Laryngeal atresia results from failure of canalisation of the cricoid and/or separation of the arytenoids. If there is failure of development of the tracheo-oesophageal groove, then the lungs may arise from a common oesophagus or type 4 laryngeal cleft. Such infants can occasionally be resuscitated with oesophageal ventilation, but most will not survive the immediate neonatal period.

Higher upper airway obstruction

Choanal atresia

One in 7000 babies are born with choanal atresia (Lazar and Younis 1995). It can be unilateral or bilateral. This congenital anomaly occurs where there has been failure of the opening at the back of the nose. The obstruction can be membranous or bony and membranous. It is most common to find a bony stenosis with a thin central bony atretic plate or membranous closure.

Choanal atresia can occur as an isolated anomaly or as part of the CHARGE syndrome (coloboma of the eye, heart defects, atresia of the nasal choanae, retardation of growth and/or development, genital and/or urinary abnormalities and ear abnormalities and deafness) (Samadi et al. 2003). It is also sometimes found in association with other craniofacial conditions such as Treacher Collins syndrome. The atresia can be unilateral or bilateral in any of these conditions.

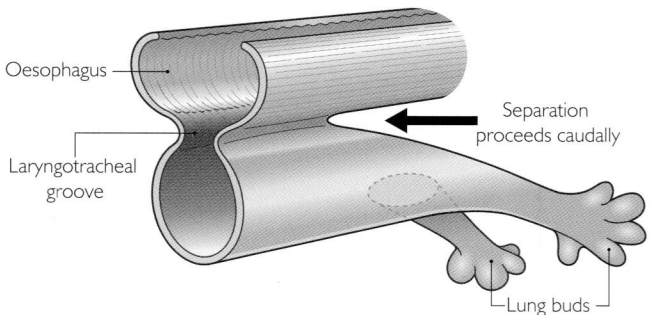

Fig. 27.58 The development of the trachea, bronchi and oesophagus.

Oesophagus

Laryngotracheal groove

Separation proceeds caudally

Lung buds

Diagnosis and management

The diagnosis of unilateral choanal atresia may only become apparent when it proves impossible to pass a fine flexible catheter through each nostril into the pharynx, and there is a lack of mirror misting at the anterior nares. There is frequently no clinical airway obstruction, or just snuffly breathing. The diagnosis may therefore be delayed until later childhood. Bilateral choanal atresia, however, presents at birth, with severe UAO. This will usually require either intubation and ventilation, or maintenance of the upper airway by placing a Guedel airway orally, securely taped to prevent displacement, prior to definitive correction. Frequent oropharyngeal suctioning will then be required.

A high-resolution computed tomography (CT) scan in the axial plane, with bone and soft-tissue windows, should be undertaken. It is important for the paediatrician to attend the scan in order to decongest the nose with a few 0.5% ephedrine nose drops and then nasal suctioning to remove mucus immediately prior to imaging. Otherwise, mucus can be interpreted radiologically as a membranous atresia.

Surgery and postoperative care

Surgical correction of bilateral choanal atresia should be undertaken as soon as this is practicable, usually within the first 14 days of life. Unilateral atresia, unless there is unusually severe airway obstruction, is better corrected electively at any time from 6 months of age or even as a toddler. The surgical outcome will tend to be better in an older child. Either a transnasal or a transpalatal surgical approach is adopted. The bony atresia is drilled away under endoscopic control, and many surgeons then insert nasal stents fashioned from endotracheal tubing. These nasal tubes need to be kept clear by regular suctioning and irrigation with a few drops of saline or bicarbonate solution, as required. The baby's parent or carer should be taught this process prior to discharge home. The nasal stents are usually removed after 2–6 weeks and subsequent anaesthetics for endoscopic examination, dilatation and sometimes laser treatments are required. If stenting is not employed then steroid nose drops are used and early serial endoscopies are required in the first month after initial choanal correction. There is a relatively high incidence of restenosis following this surgery, regardless of the technique employed. Samadi et al. (2003) reported that about five surgical procedures were required to achieve maintained patency. Holland and McGuirt (2001) report improved outcomes using topical mitomycin C application at the time of surgery.

Oropharyngeal airway obstruction and stertor

Stertor describes the low-tone breathing noise resulting from turbulent airflow in an obstructed pharynx. It is almost a snoring, and typically arises from the level of the tonsils, adenoids or tongue base. It is usually quite easily distinguishable from the higher pitched, almost musical, wheezy quality of stridor, which signifies airway obstruction at the laryngeal level or below. There will often be associated chest recession with stertor or stridor.

In the neonate, stertor is unlikely to be caused by obstructive adenoid or tonsillar tissue which has yet to hypertrophy, but it will be seen in any condition in which there are rattly oropharyngeal secretions, or with altered muscular tone in the pharynx, associated with neurological disorders, and where the tongue base and epiglottic morphology is unusual or hypotonic, causing these structures to prolapse over the laryngeal opening on attempted respiration

Table 27.19 Causes of high upper airway obstruction

Nasal agenesis
Congenital nasal septal deflection
Nasal tumour (e.g. meningomyelocele)
Choanal stenosis
Choanal atresia
Craniofacial syndromes with midface hypoplasia
Macroglossia
Oropharyngeal lymphangioma or haemangiomata
Micrognathia (e.g. Pierre Robin sequence)
Glossoptosis, prolapsing tongue base
Abnormally high or posterior larynx
Vallecular or supraglottic cysts
Pharyngeal hypotonia (neurological disease)
Excessive oropharyngeal secretions
Foreign bodies
Adenotonsillar hypertrophy

(glossoptosis). Pharyngeal UAO and stertor are common in infants with congenital abnormalities of the region, such as Treacher Collins syndrome, Pierre Robin sequence and in other conditions with an associated cleft palate. It will be seen with macroglossia (e.g. Beckwith–Wiedemann syndrome). Other common conditions include lymphangioma (cystic hygroma) involving the tongue, pharynx and neck.

Progressive UAO in the infant may indicate an enlarging mucus retention cyst, usually found in the vallecula, at the tongue base. It may be seen on a soft-tissue lateral X-ray of the neck and should be diagnosed at endoscopic laryngoscopy. Undiagnosed, this simple condition can be fatal. It requires drainage and excision or marsupialisation. Table 27.19 lists the causes of high UAO.

Management of oropharyngeal upper airway obstruction

Clinical assessment remains important, checking the patency of both nostrils, examining the oral cavity and oropharynx and studying the baby for dysmorphic features. The degree of stertor, recession and the pulse oximetry monitoring will give a good indication of the severity. A lateral soft-tissue X-ray of the neck can be helpful. Referral to a paediatric ear, nose and throat (ENT) surgeon should be made.

Initial treatment, with general supportive measures such as oxygen and perhaps humidification, will be helpful. Even inhaled or nebulised mixtures of helium and oxygen (heliox, BOC Medical) can be considered. Continuous positive airway pressure (CPAP) delivered by nasal oxygen cannulae may stent the upper airway open and avoid the need for intubation. Sometimes the airway can be maintained by the insertion of a unilateral nasopharyngeal airway (prong), which will bypass the airway obstruction and can also allow better delivery of CPAP, if required. The presence of the prong, however, stimulates increased secretions and causes feeding difficulty; regular suctioning will be required.

Where there is a removable obstructive cause, such as enlarged adenoids or tonsils or a retention cyst, ENT surgery will be corrective. Cystic hygroma in the airway may be reduced in a number of ways, such as surgical debulking, laser treatments or sclerosing agents (OK-432 or doxycycline) (Molitch et al. 1995; Wimmershoff et al. 2000; Giguere et al. 2002). If pharyngeal airway surgery and/or supportive measures are not successful in the long term, then tracheostomy surgery becomes indicated. Many causes of congenital

UAO will slowly self-correct with growth, over a number of years, and allow much later decannulation of the tracheostomy.

Where the posterior tongue is bulky and prolapses, compressing the laryngeal inlet (glossoptosis), it may occasionally be possible to perform a posterior third midline wedge resection and lead to airway improvement. Maxillofacial techniques such as mandibular distraction surgery can also have a place in promoting earlier correction of the obstructed upper airway in association with the micrognathic mandible and even the hypoplastic midface in toddlers or children with craniofacial syndromes.

Prognosis of high upper airway obstruction

Acute inflammatory conditions associated with airway obstruction and surgically correctable conditions will hold a good prognosis. The baby requiring a tracheostomy because of congenitally compromised upper airway anatomy, however, may require a tracheostomy for 18 months to 4 years of life, before there has been adequate resolution with growth.

Laryngotracheal airway obstruction

Assessment of airway obstruction and stridor

Stridor, a high-pitched audible noisy breathing, indicates airway obstruction within the larynx, trachea or bronchi. The history may help to diagnose the cause and localise the obstruction. Inspiratory stridor frequently arises from the supraglottis or the vocal cords. Laryngomalacia is the most common cause. Biphasic stridor usually indicates a vocal cord, or subglottic, level of obstruction. A biphasic vocalisation noise is often found to be caused by bilateral congenital vocal cord paralysis in the newborn. Expiratory stridor progressing to wheeze indicates lower tracheal or bronchial obstruction. Exacerbating features and whether the stridor is constant or progressive can be helpful. If the cry is absent or abnormal, there may be a congenital laryngeal lesion (e.g. web); a unilateral vocal cord paralysis can give a husky cry. An associated cough may indicate laryngitis and subglottic inflammation with laryngotracheobronchitis (LTB) or croup, while a harsh or barking cough is seen with tracheomalacia.

Stridor is frequently exacerbated by feeding. Stridor from laryngomalacia is often seen when the baby is asleep and lying supine. Stridor that is exacerbated by increased activity or upset tends to indicate a fixed, narrowed airway such as SGS.

Babies can adapt to slowly developing subglottic or tracheal stenosis, resulting in a prolonged expiratory phase which reduces recession and stridor, masking the severity of the obstruction. Acute-onset airway obstruction, in contrast, will tend to produce much more marked signs of obstruction, with tracheal tug, subcostal and intercostal recession, use of accessory respiratory muscles, increased respiratory rate and sweating. It is noteworthy, however, that recession is not specifically a sign of airway obstruction, but of airway effort, and is therefore also seen in babies with respiratory distress in the absence of significant obstruction (p. 476).

Auscultation of the stridor over the sternum is helpful, especially in a noisy ward, and can give a good indication of the volume of airflow and severity of the obstruction.

The small newborn baby, even with airway obstruction, may initially show relatively little stridor, perhaps because of the small-volume, lower speed airflow. With increasing age, stridor will tend to become more marked. Laryngomalacia, for example, will often develop only after the first few weeks of life, or even later.

The overall assessment of the baby with stridor should include oropharyngeal and chest examination and attention to the rest of the history, including an assessment of likely neurological and cardiac status.

Pulse oximetry readings and capillary blood gases, taken in the context of other associated conditions, will be helpful. To rely solely on a pulse oximeter can be misleading. Clinical evaluation of the baby remains important.

Investigations for stridor

Investigation of the baby or infant with stridor should include a chest X-ray (CXR). A lateral X-ray of the neck may yield helpful information. Some institutions undertake the so-called Cincinnati view – a coned high-kilovolt anteroposterior X-ray of the mediastinum, which can delineate the trachea and main bronchi. A barium swallow may demonstrate an abnormal swallowing reflex, aspiration or TOF, as well as compression from a vascular ring or sling. A pH study, CT scan and magnetic resonance imaging (MRI) scans, as well as an echocardiogram of the great vessels, are all additional investigations.

Investigations should be tailored to the individual baby, but the minimum investigations for a baby with stridor should include a CXR and referral to the paediatric ENT airway surgeons for diagnostic endoscopy.

Management of stridor and laryngotracheal airway obstruction

Universal supportive measures can be applied. Oxygen, humidification and nebulisers or even heliox may be helpful. Adrenaline nebuliser (1 ml of 1:1000 adrenaline mixed with 2 ml of normal saline) can be administered every few hours to most babies. Nebulised steroids may be helpful (Durward et al. 1998), and salbutamol is worth trying. Systemic steroids such as dexamethasone will reduce any acute inflammation, oedema or haemangioma. When there is respiratory failure despite these measures, CPAP or intubation and ventilation will be required.

Airway endoscopy

While the supportive measures and investigations described are helpful, almost all babies and infants with stridor and airway obstruction require endoscopy to confirm a diagnosis and, if possible, to treat the condition endoscopically. Flexible laryngoscopy with a 2–4-mm diameter flexible rhinolaryngoscope (passed through the baby's mouth whilst awake on the ward) may allow a diagnosis of a supraglottic obstruction such as a vallecular cyst or laryngomalacia and might confirm vocal cord lesions or paralysis. The subglottic airway will not be readily assessed with a flexible endoscope. If the baby is intubated, the more distal tracheobronchial tree can be visualised with a very fine flexible fibreoptic endoscope passed down the endotracheal tube (ETT). Flexible endoscopes therefore have an increasing diagnostic role in the neonatal unit, but do not allow as accurate an assessment as rigid microlaryngoscopy and bronchoscopy (MLB) and generally do not allow correction of the problem (therapeutic endoscopy).

A formal MLB in the operating theatre, under light spontaneous respiration general anaesthesia, will allow full assessment of airway obstruction and the possibility of endoscopic therapeutic procedures. The technique requires no neuromuscular blockade and only minimal sedation, so that spontaneous respiration allows a dynamic endoscopic assessment of the entire airway without the presence of an ETT. Oxygen and inhalational agents, such as isoflurane, can be

SINGLETON HOSPITAL
STAFF LIBRARY

delivered through a nasal prong. The technique relies heavily upon the use of lidocaine spray to the larynx (7 mg/kg stat). Intravenous anaesthesia such as propofol is also employed. Views are obtained using the microscope and/or rigid endoscopes. Storz ventilating bronchoscopes allow ventilation when assessing the tracheobronchial tree, if needed. These techniques allow coaxial instrumentation and laser treatments.

Care of the intubated baby

Airway obstruction and prematurity require babies to be intubated with speed and skill. Many factors appear to be associated with endotracheal airway damage leading to acquired SGS. Choice of an appropriately sized tube, movement, infection (Suzumura et al. 2000), the length of time intubated and the number of reintubations are all factors. Downing and Kilbride (1995) reported that variables more commonly found in patients with SGS included greater number of intubations, use of an inappropriately large ETT and longer durations of intubation. Contencin and Narcy (1993) believe the size of the ETT to be a major risk factor for acquired laryngotracheal stenosis in the neonate, recommending use of a size 2.5 ETT in babies under 2500 g weight. Supraglottic laryngeal damage from intubation, which will increase the likelihood of failed extubation, is significantly more common in active neonates than in those who are relatively immobile (Albert et al. 1990). Pashley (1982) reviewed the risk factors and predictors of SGS, proposing a figure of the number of intubations × the number of days intubated × the number of days ventilated. A child with a risk factor figure of greater than 3000 was at high risk.

A small leak past the ETT is desirable. A tube smaller than size 3.0 will be more difficult to manage regarding patency and ventilation. Table 27.20 gives a guide to the expected diameter of the subglottis and trachea for age with appropriate endotracheal and tracheostomy tube sizes.

Tube design may be another important feature. The Cole shouldered tube provides easier and safer intubation because of the rigidity of the fatter oropharyngeal component, but positioning is important as the shoulder can prolapse through the glottis, and its increased diameter will then cause trauma or even malacia (Brewis et al. 1999). Tube fixation techniques and the preferences for oral or nasal intubation remain debated. There is no strong evidence to support any particular method.

There is a strong clinical suspicion that an intubated baby who is very active and mobile is at greatly increased risk of developing glottic laryngeal granulations and subglottic ulceration, leading to failed extubation and stenosis. There is a difficult balance to be struck in the very immature baby (who often requires ventilation for several weeks) between the desire to avoid too much movement of the ETT and the need for 'developmental care' and periods of interaction with carers and parents (Ch. 4). Occult or overt acid reflux is considered to be a detrimental factor in laryngeal and subglottic trauma, leading to failed extubation.

Deep suctioning through an ETT will also cause mechanical trauma with ulcerations and granulations. Suction techniques should involve introducing the suction tip just beyond the end of the ETT and then applying the suction with rotation and a gradual withdrawal (Fig. 27.59).

Extubation

For the baby deemed fit for a trial of extubation, different weaning protocols have been studied. Randolph et al. (2002) found extubation failure rates are not significantly different from one another. Barrington et al. (2001) showed that nasal synchronised intermittent mandatory ventilation was effective in preventing extubation failure compared with CPAP. The use of respiratory stimulants such as doxapram or methylxanthines to facilitate successful extubation has been studied, with mixed results. Most neonatal units use caffeine prior to extubation in babies of less than 32 weeks' gestation (p. 529).

When there is initial failure of extubation, and an airway-obstructive cause seems probable, then reintubation for 48 hours with heavy sedation to reduce tube movement and the use of systemic steroids as well as ranitidine or a proton-pump inhibitor may allow subsequent successful extubation.

Failed extubation

Where there is repeated failure of extubation, referral should be made to a paediatric ENT surgeon. These babies tend to fall into

Table 27.20 Approximate neonatal and infant airway parameters

	PRE-30 WEEKS	30 WEEKS TO TERM	1 MONTH	6 MONTHS	12 MONTHS
Expected cricoid AP diameter	3.6 mm	4.4 mm	5.0 mm	5.8 mm	6.2 mm
Appropriate Portex blue line ETT size	2.5 (OD 3.4 mm)	3.0 (OD 4.3 mm)	3.0 (OD 4.3 mm)	3.5 (OD 4.8 mm)	4.0 (OD 5.4 mm)
ETT size without air leak indicating significant Cotton 1 subglottic stenosis	–	2.5	2.5	3.0	3.5
Expected transverse tracheal diameter	4.6 mm	4.75 mm	5.3 mm	6.0 mm	6.5 mm
Appropriate size of Shiley neonatal tracheostomy tube	3.0 (OD 4.5 mm)	3.0 (OD 4.5 mm)	3.0 (OD 4.5 mm)	3.5 (OD 5.2 mm)	4.0 (OD 5.9 mm)

AP, anteroposterior; ETT, endotracheal tube; OD, outer diameter.

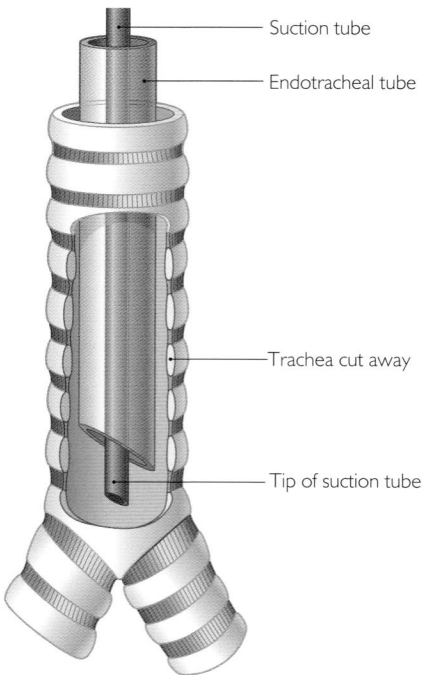

Fig. 27.59 The suction tip should usually be passed just beyond the endotracheal tube tip.

Labels in figure:
- Suction tube
- Endotracheal tube
- Trachea cut away
- Tip of suction tube

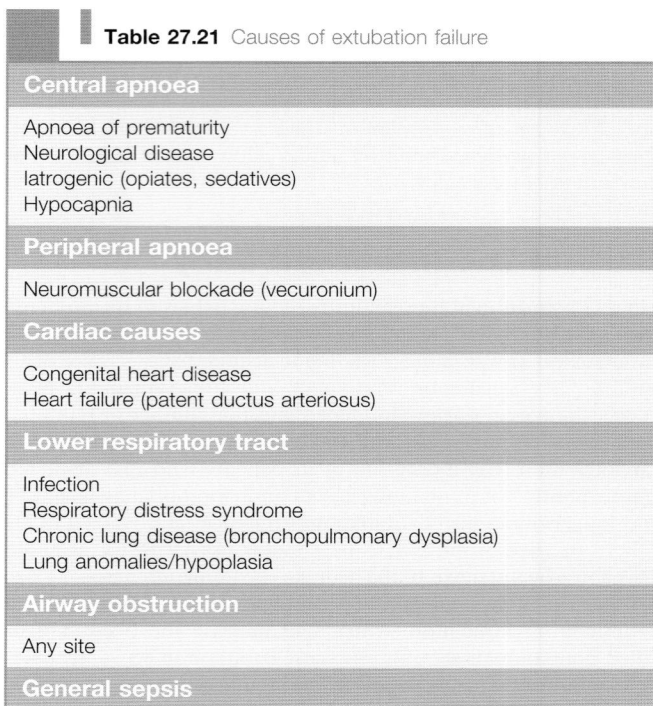

Table 27.21 Causes of extubation failure

Central apnoea
Apnoea of prematurity
Neurological disease
Iatrogenic (opiates, sedatives)
Hypocapnia
Peripheral apnoea
Neuromuscular blockade (vecuronium)
Cardiac causes
Congenital heart disease
Heart failure (patent ductus arteriosus)
Lower respiratory tract
Infection
Respiratory distress syndrome
Chronic lung disease (bronchopulmonary dysplasia)
Lung anomalies/hypoplasia
Airway obstruction
Any site
General sepsis

three distinct categories: firstly, the premature neonate who has been ventilator-dependent since birth and repeatedly fails attempts at extubation; secondly, the infant or baby who has breathed spontaneously but then fails extubation after a subsequent surgical procedure; lastly, the infant or older baby who has been readmitted and intubated for LTB or croup, pneumonia, epilepsy control or asthma, subsequently failing extubation. This last category may include children with neurological impairment, such as children with cerebral palsy.

Extubation failure implies that the baby is unable to maintain adequate arterial oxygenation and/or that the Pa_{CO_2} has become unsustainably high. Table 27.21 lists possible causes for such failed extubation. Airway obstruction is only one of the important factors and each of the causes should be excluded. In simple terms, successful extubation requires:

1. respiratory drive
2. neuromuscular function
3. adequate cardiac function and pulmonary gaseous exchange
4. clear unobstructed airways
5. no significant sepsis.

In our experience, the most common causes for neonatal intensive care extubation failure are chronic lung disease, apnoea of prematurity, sepsis, airway obstruction or multifactorial causes. Laryngomalacia is probably more common than we think (see below).

Assessing a preterm baby prior to first extubation involves consideration of all these factors. As a broad guideline, a successful outcome is likely if the infant weighs over 1000 g, if there is an air leak around an age-appropriate ETT at less than 20 cmH$_2$O peak ventilator pressure, if oxygen saturations are being maintained in 35% oxygen or less and if the ventilator requirements have been weaned to satisfactory rates. A rate of 10–15 per minute with peak inspiratory pressure of 12 mmH$_2$O for a baby under 1 kg, and less than 18 mmH$_2$O for a baby over 1 kg, is a very rough guide.

Management of extubation failure

If extubation fails because of airway obstruction, a retrial after a period of 2–4 days on systemic dexamethasone, an acid-blocking agent, and heavy sedation or paralysis to reduce tube movement may be successful.

Where there have been repeated failures of extubation, the paediatric ENT surgeon should assess the airway at MLB. The treatment of choice will depend upon the endoscopic findings. If there is relatively little airway trauma but some generalised oedema reducing the laryngeal or subglottic airway, then a further period of therapeutic reintubation may be successful. Sometimes the airway obstruction can be corrected endoscopically, for example by vaporising acquired subglottic cysts or prominent laryngeal granulations with a CO$_2$ laser. Extubation will then become possible 48–72 hours later. Where there is incipient or early SGS with oedema but a near-normal and clear airway at the level of the vocal cords and above, an anterior cricoid split operation can be undertaken. If the SGS is more severe and the fibrous tissue more mature, then an SS-LTR, employing a costochondral graft to augment the airway, may be chosen if the baby's weight is sufficient. The reconstruction is supported by an ETT for 1–2 weeks, and, if successful, subsequent extubation allows avoidance of a tracheostomy.

Where there is severe transglottic inflammation with granulations or oedema in the supraglottis as well as the subglottis, then a tracheostomy is advised, as the entire larynx cannot settle with the continued presence of an ETT. Figure 27.60 shows laryngeal granulations and exposed cartilage following prolonged complicated intubation. Very early reassessment of the larynx at endoscopy is advisable in such a situation. If after 3 weeks the inflammation has settled and the airway is adequate, tracheostomy decannulation should proceed. Unnecessary prolongation of the duration the tracheostomy is left in situ may otherwise exacerbate the development of progressive SGS.

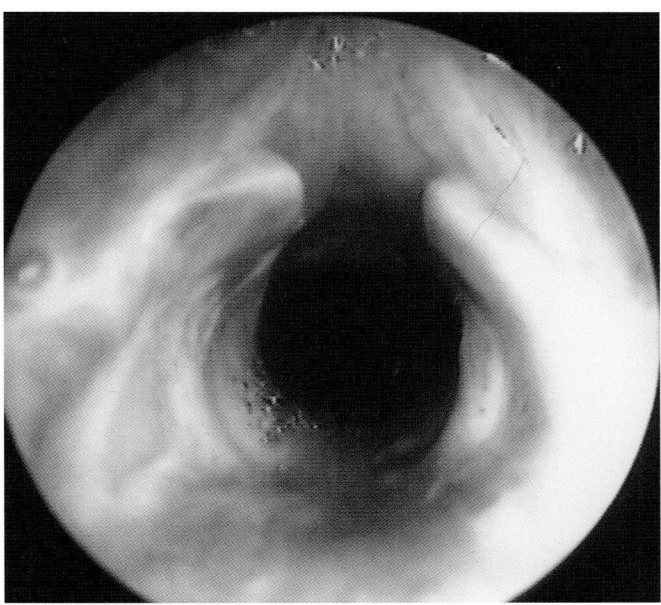

Fig. 27.60 Laryngeal granulomas and exposed cartilage following prolonged complicated intubation.

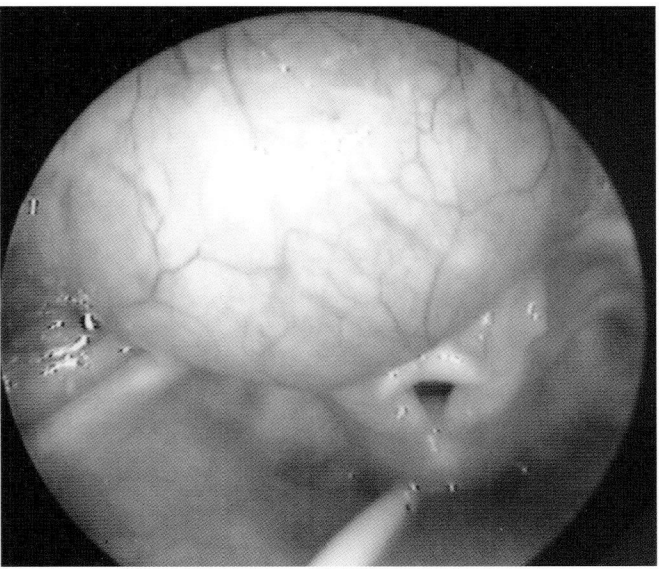

Fig. 27.61 Vallecular mucus retention cyst obstructing the airway at the tongue base.

Laryngotracheal airway obstruction: conditions and management

Laryngomalacia

Laryngomalacia is the most common cause of infant stridor. It results from laxity of the supraglottic structures: the epiglottis and the mucosa over the cuneiform and arytenoid cartilages can be sucked into the airway on inspiration. The epiglottis is usually curled and omega-shaped and there are both short and tall aryepiglottic folds tethering the arytenoid mucosa to the epiglottis. Laryngomalacia is seen with associated reflux. The airway obstruction and increased intrathoracic negative pressure will increase acid reflux. Typically it presents with inspiratory stridor after the first few weeks (sometimes days) of life. It tends to increase in severity and is often worse on feeding and sleeping supine. The cry will be normal. It is twice as common in boys. The natural history is for self-correction with growth over a 12–24-month period, but it can persist. The diagnosis should usually be confirmed with endoscopy. Treatment is often expectant; however, when there is progressive or continuing stridor with marked recession and respiratory effort, the baby will fail to thrive. If the weight charts show a consistent fall-off down the percentiles, then surgical correction should be undertaken. The endoscopic operation of aryepiglottoplasty (or supraglottoplasty) involves trimming the redundant mucosa and cuneiform cartilages away, and freeing the tethered aryepiglottic folds with microscissors. It is usually highly successful for posterior laryngomalacia, but there is a risk of supraglottic stenosis from scarring. When the laryngomalacia is of an anterior type, involving the epiglottis prolapsing back or into the laryngeal introitus, surgery may not be successful. Some paediatric ENT surgeons advocate an extended supraglottoplasty, resecting the lateral free edges of the curled epiglottis as well. Severe cases of laryngomalacia, not suitable for this endoscopic surgery, may require a tracheostomy, but this is rare.

Airway cysts and webs

Congenital laryngeal (mucus retention) cysts, laryngeal saccule cysts and supraglottic cysts can present in very early life or at a few months with stridor. A mucus cyst of the vallecula at the tongue base can present early with UAO and stridor or stertor. Lateral soft-tissue X-rays may be helpful, but these cysts are definitively diagnosed and treated endoscopically (Fig. 27.61).

Acquired subglottic cysts are commonly found in previously intubated infants, most frequently arising on the left-hand side. They will present with stridor sometimes at the time of a respiratory infection. They can be cured by laser vaporisation at endoscopy (Tierney et al. 1997).

Congenital webbing of the larynx, in which the vocal cords are fused together anteriorly, is rare, and will present with stridor and a posterior laryngeal airway. Open surgery and stenting with a keel are usually required and there is frequently an associated congenital subglottic stenosis requiring a cartilage graft reconstruction as well.

Vocal cord paralysis

Vocal cord paralysis can be unilateral or bilateral, and congenital or acquired. Congenital causes include Arnold–Chiari malformation, other neurological disease and birth trauma, while acquired causes may be from neck trauma or open-heart surgery. Even congenital cases can show spontaneous recovery of movement with development and age. Unilateral cord palsy will present with a weak or husky cry and sometimes feeding difficulty. Stridor is often present only if there is coexistent airway swelling. Swallowing difficulties with aspiration over the long term are sometimes seen. Bilateral cord paralyses, by comparison, will present with inspiratory or biphasic stridor with a vocal quality to the inspiratory noise. The cords lie very close to the midline, restricting the airway. Diagnosis is made at a dynamic microlaryngoscopy. Unilateral cases require no intervention, but bilateral cord paralysis often requires a tracheostomy.

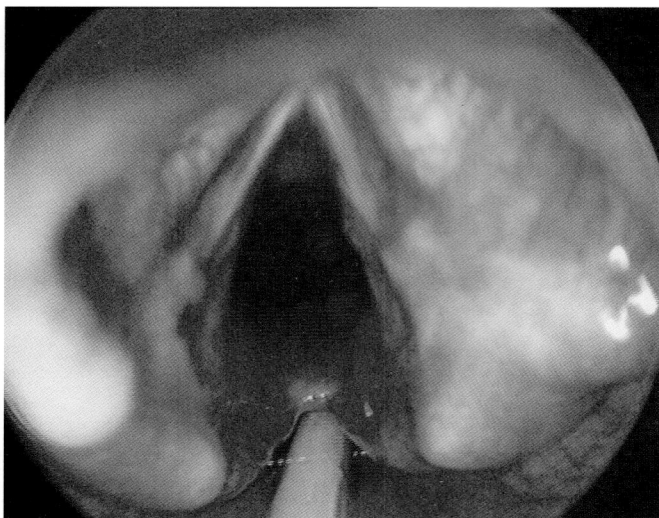

Fig. 27.62 Type 1 congenital posterior laryngeal cleft.

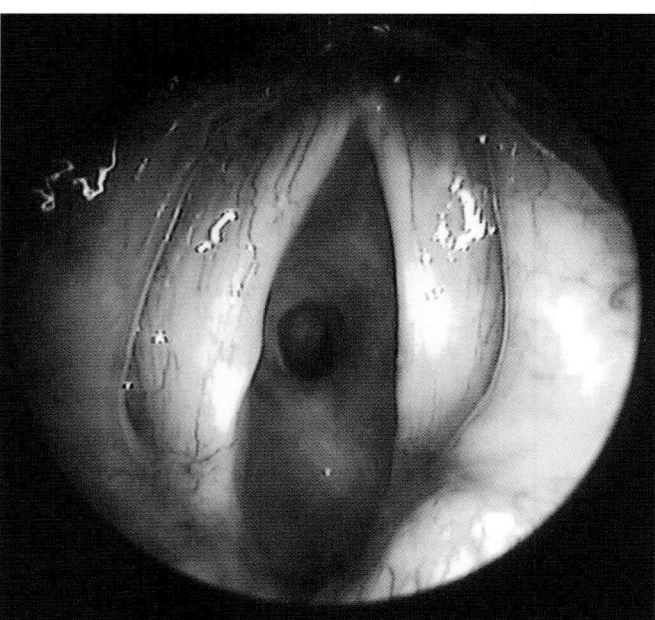

Fig. 27.63 Severe subglottic stenosis.

Croup

LTB or croup is usually managed by paediatricians and only involves the ENT surgeons when there have been multiple failures of extubation (see above). Then, endoscopy (MLB) is indicated for diagnosis, and occasionally laser reduction of laryngeal granulations. The ex-premature baby requiring intubation for subsequent croup, however, is at increased risk of developing SGS.

Congenital posterior laryngeal cleft

A congenital laryngeal cleft occurs in the posterior larynx when there is failure of closure of the tracheo-oesophageal groove as high as the interarytenoid level, and a degree of failure of fusion of the posterior cricoid cartilage lamina. There are numerous classifications described (Moungthong and Holinger 1997), but the most commonly accepted one is that of Benjamin and Inglis (1989). A type 1 cleft represents a failure of mucosal fusion in the posterior larynx, with the open notch reaching the level of the vocal cords but not affecting the posterior cricoid plate (Fig. 27.62). A type 2 cleft notches into the cricoid cartilage below the cords. In a type 3 cleft there is complete cleft of the posterior cricoid cartilage and mucosa extending into the cervical trachea. The type 4 cleft extends down into the thoracic trachea (laryngotracheo-oesophageal cleft), even to the carina or beyond.

Type 1 clefts may present late, with repeated aspiration pneumonias and maybe inspiratory stridor similar to that of laryngomalacia. Type 2 and 3 clefts are more likely to present in early life, with airway embarrassment requiring ventilation and with failed extubations. The type 4 cleft may be an immediate neonatal emergency, with great difficulty maintaining an adequate ETT position to ventilate the baby, as the tube tends to prolapse into the oesophagus. Such severe type 4 laryngeal clefts are often incompatible with long-term survival. The diagnosis is always confirmed by MLB.

Management of posterior laryngeal clefts

The type 1 clefts and some type 2 clefts can be repaired surgically from an endoscopic approach. Deeper type 2 clefts and worse will require an open neck or neck and median sternotomy approach. The cleft is repaired in layers, inserting a tibial periosteal graft in the trachealis region and perhaps a cartilage graft at the posterior cricoid level. The baby usually needs a tracheostomy as well. Tracheomalacia of the airway remains a significant problem in these challenging conditions and type 4 clefts still carry a very high mortality rate.

Subglottic stenosis

In over 95% of babies, SGS is considered acquired (Cotton et al. 1989), following prolonged intubation of low-birthweight premature infants, many of whom also develop chronic lung disease. The incidence varies but in our institution it occurs in approximately 2.5% of intubated, severely preterm babies. SGS can be congenital, when the unintubated baby is born with stridor. In these cases, endoscopy shows a narrowed, sometimes pear-shaped cricoid region or underriding of the first tracheal cartilage ring. If infants with a congenitally narrow subglottis do require intubation, the use of a standard-sized tube in this situation will cause trauma and may lead to a combined congenital and acquired SGS. The Cotton classification describes the severity of the stenosis, grade I representing up to 50% reduction in lumen cross-section, grade II 50–70%, grade III 70–99%, and grade IV complete stenosis with no lumen. The percentage can be read off a chart according to the size of ETT in relation to age (Myer et al. 1994). Figure 27.63 shows a mature severe SGS.

Factors influencing the development of SGS have been studied (Sherman et al. 1986) and are similar to those for failed extubations. The duration of intubation, the number of ETTs inserted, the duration of mechanical ventilation, the presence of postextubation stridor and the size of the ETT in relation to gestational age are significantly correlated with the development of SGS.

The management of SGS will depend upon its severity and evolution. The mildest cases may be managed conservatively, and, with growth, the condition can improve. Early oedematous SGS may be treated by the cricoid split operation and more severe mature stenoses are likely to require laryngotracheal reconstruction surgery or cricotracheal resection. A tracheostomy is frequently required for a number of years in these difficult cases.

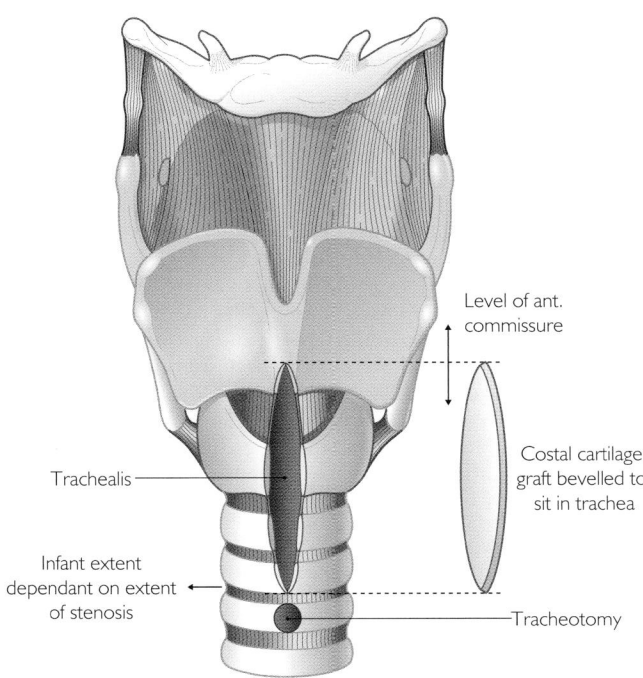

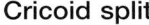

Level of ant.
commissure

Trachealis

Costal cartilage
graft bevelled to
sit in trachea

Infant extent
dependant on extent
of stenosis

Tracheotomy

Fig. 27.64 Technique of laryngotracheal reconstruction.

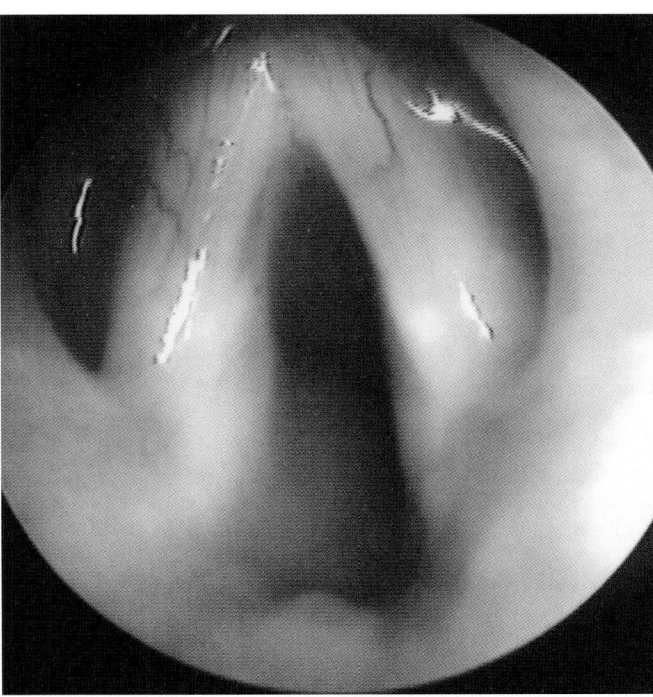

Fig. 27.65 Unilateral subglottic haemangioma.

Cricoid split

When there is failure of extubation caused by persistent isolated subglottic oedema, granulations or early soft or incipient SGS, then an open anterior cricoid split operation will often allow subsequent successful extubation. The neck is approached from a horizontal skin crease incision, the cricoid ring and adjacent airway are divided vertically, preserving the vocal cords at the anterior commissure and the baby is then reintubated with a large-sized ETT. This procedure allows oedema fluid to escape from the subglottic region, and the enlarged subglottis will usually heal quickly with an anterior fibrous union. Extubation is attempted, despite an absence of air leak, after 2–7 days following the use of systemic steroids and ranitidine. Tube movement should be kept to a minimum.

If there is accidental extubation, the risk of creating a false passage into the neck on reintubation can be reduced by rotating the ETT through 180° as it is passed through the cords and asking an assistant to apply light digital pressure to the anterior neck wound. The use of a neck drain to avoid surgical emphysema is advised until well after successful extubation.

The reported success rate for cricoid split surgery is between 69% and 75% (Grundfast et al. 1985); however, this procedure is not without potential complications, and failures will require a tracheostomy. In our own experience, the success rate was over 80%, but this was in a highly selected population (Morrison and Wareing 1999). VLBW neonates with a higher oxygen requirement are less likely to have a successful outcome.

Alternative procedures are laryngeal reconstruction, or cricotracheal resection (Fig. 27.64).

Subglottic haemangioma

Subglottic haemangiomas usually present after 6 weeks of age, with progressive stridor and recession. They can be unilateral or bilateral and are seen as a soft smooth red swelling in the subglottis (Fig. 27.65). The haemangioma enlarges over the first year or so, and the airway may become compromised, requiring tracheostomy in about 60% of cases (Chatrath et al. 2002). The presence of a cutaneous haemangioma may be a clue to the subglottic diagnosis. The natural history will be of spontaneous resolution over a few years.

MLB under general anaesthesia is required to make the diagnosis. The subglottis shows a smooth dark red swelling on one or both sides, more bulbous in the posterior airway.

Management of subglottic haemangioma

Small haemangiomata can be monitored endoscopically until they regress. If the airway is more significantly compromised, the choice is between a tracheostomy or an attempt to reduce the haemangioma and avoid or reverse a tracheostomy. Episodes on systemic steroids (prednisolone) or intralesional steroids can be beneficial and avoid a tracheostomy, but long-term systemic steroid therapy is not advised because of adverse side-effects. Laser vaporisation of some of the haemangioma may improve the airway and allow avoidance of tracheostomy. Formerly, the CO_2 laser was employed, but results were disappointing. In one large series, the time to resolution of subglottic haemangiomas did not appear to be reduced by CO_2 laser therapy (Chatrath et al. 2002). The physical characteristics of the KTP laser, with deeper penetration into the red spectrum of the haemangioma, may prove a better choice in the future.

A medical therapy for haemangioma has proved successful recently: the administration of propranolol has promoted involution of the haemangioma. In our institution we have employed a regime using 1 mg/kg/day in three divided doses for week 1, increased to 2 mg/kg/day after that for 9–12 months. Careful blood monitoring is important, including glucose, and weight charts may influence dosing. Initially pulse and blood pressure are recorded every 30 minutes then weekly over the whole treatment period. The resolution has been gradual so for subglottic haemangioma surgery might still be required as prolonged intubation, whilst awaiting involution, has led to airway damage and stenosis.

For those patients who required a tracheostomy, the mean time from diagnosis to decannulation was 30 months (Chatrath et al. 2002). In order to avoid a prolonged period with a tracheostomy, thereby reducing morbidity and enhancing language development, open single-stage excision of the haemangioma by a cricoid split approach and submucosal dissection, with or without a costal graft insertion, has achieved good results, with 80% successful extubation at the first open operation (Froehlich et al. 1995; G Morrison unpublished data 2003).

Vascular compression (rings and slings)

Investigation

The baby or infant with stridor always requires investigation. Particularly where there is evidence of a cardiac condition or associated swallowing difficulty (dysphagia lusoria), a barium swallow X-ray can be helpful. This may demonstrate a congenitally abnormal vascular ring or sling compressing the oesophagus, the trachea or both structures.

Echocardiography can also demonstrate abnormal vessels in the chest, but as ultrasonography expertise is mostly focused on the heart itself, this investigation can miss some mediastinal vessels.

A diagnostic MLB remains the most important investigation and will visualise any pulsatile vascular compression with secondary tracheomalacia or bronchomalacia.

An MRI or CT scan of the thorax will allow clarification of the configuration of the great vessels and detect compression of the trachea or main bronchi by an aberrant vessel such as a double aortic arch (Fig. 27.66) or an aberrant left pulmonary artery. Three-dimensional image reconstructions are very helpful.

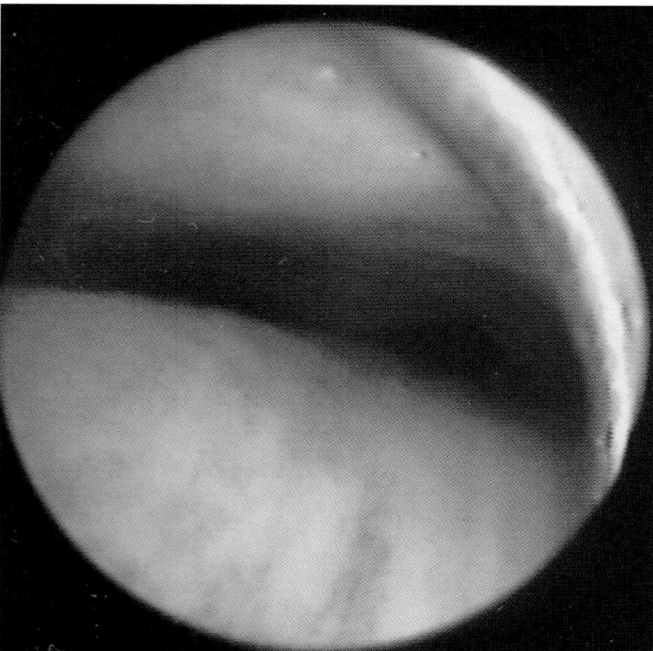

Fig. 27.66 Bronchoscopic view of double aortic arch, above the carina.

Management of vascular anomalies

Once the diagnosis has been confirmed with MLB, echocardiography and scanning, the treatment of the condition is surgical correction by paediatric cardiac surgeons. Even after this, soft-tissue swelling will frequently compromise the tracheal or bronchial airway for many months. When necessary, a tracheostomy will treat this by stenting the distal trachea open until natural resolution occurs. If one main bronchus is occluded, then intraluminal bronchial stenting can be undertaken. This is not without complications, however. Palmaz metal expandable mesh stents (Johnson and Johnson Interventional Systems, Warren, NJ) are inserted at bronchoscopy or under radiological screening and are well accepted but become incorporated into the mucosal wall and cannot be easily removed at a future date. Silastic 'hood' stents can be changed and removed, but may lead to more troublesome granulations in the airway. Stenting is advised only when the condition remains life-threatening and other measures have failed.

Congenital microtrachea

This condition, also known as long-segment congenital tracheal stenosis and as stove-pipe trachea, occurs when some or all of the trachea forms with complete tracheal cartilage rings, rather than an open D configuration. There is a large range of severity, but, as the rings are smaller in diameter than normal and do not enlarge at a normal rate, stridor tends to become progressively worse, with increased oxygen needs, over early life. Presentation may be from birth for severe stenoses or only later in childhood for the less severe cases. The microtrachea can be an isolated anomaly, but it is commonly associated with a vascular anomaly, typically an aberrant left pulmonary artery, which passes to the right before looping around the back of the stenotic trachea to reach the left side of the mediastinum (Fig. 27.67).

Management of congenital tracheal stenosis

The mildest cases can be treated conservatively with serial endoscopy. Where there is an associated vascular anomaly, this will require correction surgically. Numerous surgical techniques have been described to correct the microtrachea itself. Short-segment stenoses can be managed by resection and end-to-end anastomosis of the trachea. Longer segments can be treated by a slide tracheoplasty operation, which widens the diameter at the same time as shortening it (Cunningham et al. 1998; Lang et al. 1999). Pericardial patching to a split open trachea has also been employed, but collapse and lack of rigidity are problems with this technique (Backer et al. 2001). All of these surgical treatments are carried out under cardiac bypass. Finally, the most severe stenoses have been treated by transplant of cadaveric tracheas (Herberhold et al. 1999). This involves many months of intraluminal stenting with treatment of troublesome granulations.

Tracheomalacia, bronchomalacia

Tracheomalacia or bronchomalacia can be primary or secondary. When primary, there is generalised lack of support of the airway, with weak collapsing cartilage, causing a flattening of the normal D-shape cartilages on respiration and excessive collapse of the trachealis soft tissue into the lumen on respiration. This may involve one or both of the trachea and bronchi. The generalised tracheomalacia is likely to be self-correcting with growth. Secondary malacia occurs where there is extrinsic compression of the airway from an abnormal vessel, an unusually overriding aorta, or from a

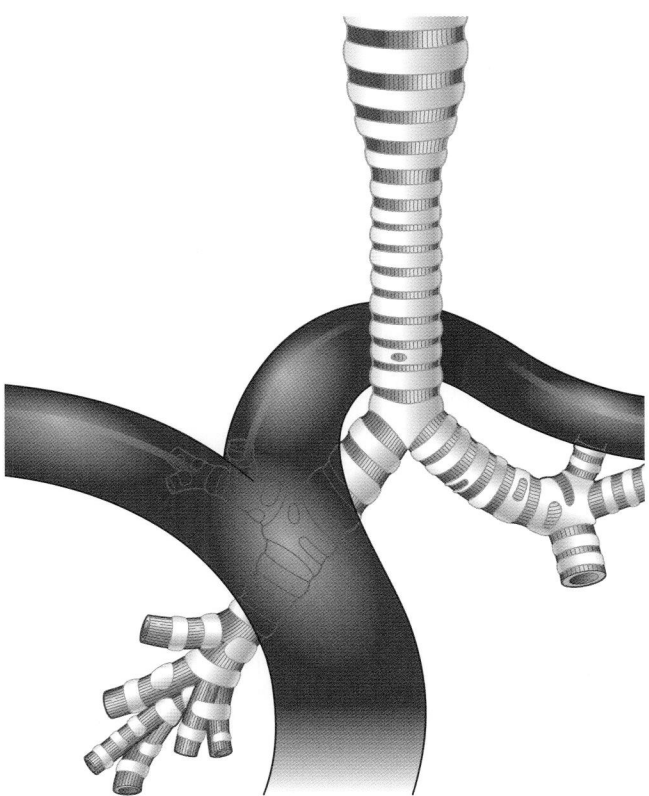

Fig. 27.67 Congenital long-segment tracheal stenosis with aberrant left pulmonary artery.

mediastinal tumour. It can also occur as localised tracheomalacia following cartilage resorption at the site of a tracheostomy or other airway surgery. Tracheomalacia will present with biphasic or primarily expiratory stridor, recession and a gruff barking cough. It is made worse by increased activity or respiratory effort, or concurrent infection.

Investigations for tracheobronchomalacia

Diagnostic MLB will confirm the tracheomalacia or bronchomalacia, so long as the study is dynamic, with the baby breathing spontaneously under a light general anaesthetic without CPAP from the anaesthetic circuit. Flexible bronchoscopy on a neonatal intensive care unit, through an ETT, will also allow this assessment if there is no positive airway pressure. Such an assessment, however, can exaggerate the degree of malacia and in a flexible assessment of any normal infant making significant respiratory effort there will be some airway collapse and bulging in of the trachealis with respiration, because of the negative intrathoracic pressure. Radiology using a contrast bronchogram under screening or video recording will also demonstrate a malacic airway and help to localise the area of obstruction or image the tree distal to an endoscopically unpassable stenosis.

Management of tracheobronchomalacia

Primary malacia can be treated by positive-pressure ventilation or CPAP until there is sufficient improvement. This conservative approach may not always be possible, however, in which case

tracheostomy or intraluminal stenting is considered. Localised tracheomalacia, if severe, may require a tracheostomy, the tube stenting the airway open. Sometimes, customised longer tubes are required. Secondary tracheomalacia will tend to self-correct once the causative external compression is rectified, but airway stenting or tracheostomy can still be required for a period. Furman et al. (1999) reviewed six cases employing a Palmaz expandable stent, reporting two deaths and three long-term successes. Granulation formation within the airway was encountered. Aortic compression of the trachea can sometimes be improved by aortopexy surgery, in which the aorta is hitched anteriorly towards the sternum. The approach can be through an anterolateral thoracotomy, a stenotomy or at transthoracic endoscopy.

Cartilage malacia following localised surgery such as tracheostomy can require tracheal reconstruction with costal cartilage grafting or excision and end-to-end anastomosis.

Bronchoscopy for atelectasis and air trapping

Infantile pneumonias are usually treated medically, with mechanical ventilation, endotracheal suctioning and physiotherapy where necessary. Bronchoscopy is not generally considered as a first-line adjunctive treatment. However, on occasions, rigid bronchoscopy under light general anaesthesia will lead to an improvement in the condition. Firstly, if the segmental or main bronchi are obstinately plugged with mucus casts, it may be possible to clear these at bronchoscopy by bronchial saline lavage and aspiration. The topical irrigation at bronchoscopy of a mucolytic agent such as rhDNase therapy (Durward et al. 2000) has been highly effective in this regard in a small number of cases. Bronchoscopy can also allow accurate collection of a tenacious mucopurulent specimen for microbiology.

Finally, unilateral air trapping and emphysema with secondary mediastinal shift in neonates can be compromising; if the problem persists, a rigid bronchoscopy to clear the segmental bronchi and inflate the collapsed regions can restore a more symmetrical ventilation.

Tracheostomy

In the 19th century, indications for tracheostomy included inhaled foreign bodies, diphtheria and croup, but the mortality was very high. In recent years, indications have changed. Infective indications, especially bacterial, are much reduced, although intubation trauma to the laryngotracheal airway following ventilation for croup (LTB) remains a common problem. Increasing survival of VLBW babies and babies with multiple congenital abnormalities has led to a lowering of the average age of patients undergoing paediatric tracheostomy, more than half of which procedures are carried out in babies under 1 year old (Ward et al. 1995). There is often continued need for long-term tracheostomy in these infants. Also, more paediatric tracheostomies are carried out for surviving babies with congenital UAOs as well as for those with neuromuscular diseases.

Broadly, there are three categories of indication for a tracheostomy: (1) for airway obstruction; (2) for assisted prolonged ventilation (especially if there is evidence of airway trauma); and (3) to provide pulmonary toilet and/or non-ventilatory support. This last category will include infants with neurological impairment or immaturity who are ventilator-dependent using an ETT but can be weaned to spontaneous respiration with a tracheostomy and supportive airway toilet. This process allows rehabilitation away from an intensive care setting. When long-term ventilation is required, the continued use of endotracheal intubation rather than

Table 27.22 Airway indications for tracheostomy

Airway obstructed above larynx (e.g. lymphangioma, Pierre Robin)
Tongue base collapse, glossoptosis
Severe laryngomalacia
Laryngeal granulations and airway trauma (postintubation)
Subglottic stenosis
Subglottic haemangioma
Respiratory papillomatosis
Bilateral vocal cord palsy
Bilateral cricoarytenoid joint fixation
Vascular compression – aberrant pulmonary artery, double aortic arch
Primary tracheomalacia
Microtrachea and congenital bronchopulmonary deformity

tracheostomy is appropriate so long as the intubation is not causing airway trauma or stenosis.

In our institution, in a series of 65 cases over 3 years, almost half the paediatric tracheostomies performed were for airway obstruction; only 8.7% were for an acute airway infection and 12.3% were required for a congenital airway anomaly. The remainder of patients in this series required a tracheostomy for long-term ventilation, airway toilet or non-ventilatory respiratory support. Table 27.22 summarises the common causes of airway obstruction requiring tracheostomy.

Posttracheostomy ward care

Postoperatively, a chest X-ray is routine to confirm the tracheostomy tube position and that there are no complications such as consolidation or pneumothorax. The tracheostomy tapes and the tube should not be changed or removed for the first week, except in airway distress, in order to allow a good tract to develop. A member of the medical staff should perform the first tube change; thereafter, weekly changes, or more frequently if there is a need, are advised. Velcro tracheostomy tapes can be used after the first tube change. The tube must be kept patent at all times. Constant humidification of the ventilated or inspired air is recommended, to stop drying of obstructive secretions. If the baby is self-ventilating, formal humidification or the application of a 'Swedish nose' (Portex Thermovent T attachment) will achieve this.

Regular tracheostomy suctioning will be required to keep the airway free of mucus secretions. A flexible catheter is inserted just to the level of the tracheostomy tube tip, and then the suction is activated by occluding its vent with a thumb while the suction tube is gently swivelled between finger and thumb as it is withdrawn. Only occasionally is it necessary to run the suction tube significantly beyond the distal tube tip, to or beyond the carina. Overzealous suctioning of this type can lead to tracheal trauma with bleeding, and granulation formation.

When a tracheostomy is inserted for long-term airway ventilation in a neonate with chronic lung disease (bronchopulmonary dysplasia), initial ventilation may be unexpectedly difficult owing to there being a much larger air leak around the tracheostomy tube up through the larynx than was possible when the long, snugger ETT was employed. Higher ventilator pressures may therefore be needed, and relatively larger tracheostomy tubes are often required, which may damage the trachea. This is one reason why tracheostomy is not necessarily a helpful procedure for the baby with severe lung disease who still requires long-term ventilatory support.

Complications and mortality of tracheostomy

Accidental decannulation and tube obstruction remain the most life-threatening complications. If the attempt to reinsert the tube results in a false passage, the attempts at ventilation will fail and can lead to pneumomediastinum and pneumothorax. Other complications include bleeding, surgical emphysema, wound infection, chest infection, airway trauma from overly vigorous suctioning and cardiorespiratory arrest.

Late sequelae of tracheostomy include the frequent formation of a suprastomal granuloma within the trachea, tracheomalacia, deglutition difficulties, language delay, chest infections and subsequent persistence of a tracheocutaneous fistula after decannulation. The most serious late complications remain tube obstruction and accidental displacement. Massive haemorrhage is rare, as is tracheal stenosis.

Mortality from tracheostomy is difficult to define. The range for paediatric published series is an overall raw mortality of 11–40% (Dutton et al. 1995). In our most recent series, the overall mortality is 19%. Tracheostomy tube-related deaths, however, are rare, ranging from 0.5% to 3.4% in different reported series (Dutton et al. 1995). Ward et al. (1995) reported a tracheostomy-related mortality rate of 2.9%, with mucus plugging of the tracheostomy being the most common cause of death.

There is a strong association between prematurity and mortality in infants with a tracheostomy, and higher comorbidity scores correlate with higher mortality rates. In one series (Gianoli et al. 1990), 80% of deaths were in preterm infants, and among those who were under 3000 g weight at the time of tracheostomy the mortality rate was 64%. The tube-related mortality rate, however, was low, at 1.6%. In our institution, the raw mortality rate among infants requiring a tracheostomy at under 1 year of (uncorrected) age was 25.6% and that among severe preterm infants requiring long-term ventilation was very much higher. Tracheostomy is not a cure-all treatment for these high-risk infants, and must be undertaken only after careful evaluation.

Home tracheostomy care

Home tracheostomy care will need to be arranged and will include local support services as well as guardians learning to care for the tracheostomy, change the tubes, and acquire appropriate resuscitation expertise. Special precautions are required for the baby with a tracheostomy, and include care with baths, refraining from swimming, and avoiding foreign bodies such as sand, dirt, talc or aerosols from entering the stoma. Care is also required with clothes and bibs and sleeping positions, to ensure that these items or the chin does not occlude the tracheostomy tube. A tube extension and 'Swedish nose' help avoid chin dipping as a cause of occlusion.

Decannulation from tracheostomy

The earliest possible decannulation is desirable. Prolonged placement of a tracheostomy tube, even in developmentally normal children, results in language delay (Jiang and Morrison 2003). The tracheostomy can be removed after definitive correction or spontaneous resolution of the underlying condition for which the tracheostomy was required and after the airway has been assessed at dynamic endoscopy. Prior to successful tracheostomy decannulation, there should be no serious aspiration or recurrent chest infections, no need for regular tracheal toilet and no need for assisted ventilation. The upper airway must be adequate and assessed at MLB, which should include removal of any obstructing suprastomal granuloma, and assessment of vocal cord mobility and airway collapse on respiration.

Once the infant is considered fit for decannulation, the usual practice would be to try a ward decannulation procedure. The tracheostomy tube is downsized to the smallest available (usually a size 3 Shiley) and the tube is then occluded with a bung or tape for short periods, by day, with observation and saturation monitoring. The tube is then occluded for progressively longer periods if tolerated; when 24 hours of occlusion is achieved, the tube can be removed and an occlusive dressing applied to the fistula site. If this ward decannulation protocol fails, the airway will require reassessment. Sometimes a surgical decannulation is required. In this case, the tracheostomy is formally reversed and closed at surgery, usually with removal of an obstructive granuloma or repair of a suprastomal tracheal collapse. The baby is then managed on an intensive care unit, intubated and ventilated with relatively little tube movement for 2–7 days prior to elective extubation (Al-Saati et al. 1993).

Antenatal airway obstruction and EXIT

Increasing sophistication of antenatal diagnosis, initially with ultrasound, increasingly allows the detection of potential airway problems that will become apparent at birth or even beforehand. Fetal MRI is helpful to define the pathology further. When a prenatal diagnosis of airway obstruction is made, a multidisciplinary approach to the pregnancy and birth is important. If long-term survival seems possible, it is feasible to plan a special delivery by the EXIT procedure (Ward et al. 2000). This procedure involves delivering the head and upper torso of the baby through a caesarean section approach while maintaining the uteroplacental blood flow and maternofetal gas exchange. This allows time for the airway obstruction to be corrected and an airway secured, prior to full delivery and ligation of the umbilical cord.

Mass lesions obstructing the fetal airway will be detected on ultrasound. Cystic hygromas are common, but only those hygromas which seem to involve the pharynx or cause airway compression are likely to cause neonatal airway obstruction. Once an obstructing lesion is detected on ultrasound, rapid-sequence fetal MRI is recommended, where transverse, sagittal and coronal planes can be studied.

In a complete laryngeal atresia it may be difficult to see the larynx fully on fetal ultrasound, but the secondary changes in the trachea and lungs are apparent. Because there is total obstruction, the liquor produced in the lungs builds up, causing gross tracheal dilatation and hypoechogenic lungs. There is often polyhydramnios, an inverted diaphragm and ascites. This is described as congenital high airway obstruction syndrome and it represents complete airway obstruction (DeCou et al. 1998). If the fetus can be brought to maturity, the EXIT procedure with tracheostomy is the management of choice.

References

Albert, D.M., Mills, R.P., Fysh, J., et al., 1990. Endoscopic examination of the neonatal larynx at extubation: a prospective study of variables associated with laryngeal damage. Int J Pediatr Otorhinolaryngol 20, 203–212.

Al-Saati, A., Morrison, G.A.J., Clary, R.A., et al., 1993. Surgical decannulation of children with tracheostomy. J Laryngol Otol 107, 217–221.

Backer, C.L., Mavroudis, C., Gerber, M.E., et al., 2001. Tracheal surgery in children: an 18-year review of four techniques. Eur J Cardiothorac Surg 19, 777–784.

Barrington, K.J., Bull, D., Finer, N.N., 2001. Randomized trial of nasal synchronized intermittent mandatory ventilation compared with continuous positive airway pressure after extubation of very low birth weight infants. Pediatrics 107, 638–641.

Benjamin, B., Inglis, A., 1989. Minor congenital laryngeal clefts: diagnosis and classification. Ann Otol Rhinol Laryngol 98, 417–420.

Brewis, C., Pracy, J.P., Albert, D.M., 1999. Localized tracheomalacia as a complication of the Cole tracheal tube. Paediatr Anaesth 9, 531–533.

Chatrath, P., Black, M., Jani, P., et al., 2002. A review of the current management of infantile subglottic haemangioma, including a comparison of CO_2 laser therapy versus tracheostomy. Int J Pediatr Otorhinolaryngol 64, 143–157.

Contencin, P., Narcy, P., 1993. Size of endotracheal tube and neonatal acquired subglottic stenosis. Study Group for Neonatology and Pediatric Emergencies in the Parisian Area. Arch Otolaryngol Head Neck Surg 119, 815–819.

Cotton, R.T., Gray, S.D., Miller, R.P., 1989. Update of the Cincinnati experience in pediatric laryngotracheal reconstruction. Laryngoscope 99, 1111–1116.

Cunningham, M.J., Eavey, R.D., Vlahakes, G.J., et al., 1998. Slide tracheoplasty for long-segment tracheal stenosis. Archives of Otolaryngology – Head and Neck Surgery 124, 98–103.

DeCou, J.M., Jones, D.C., Jacobs, H.D., et al., 1998. Successful ex-utero intrapartum treatment (EXIT) procedure for congenital high airway obstruction syndrome (CHAOS) owing to laryngeal atresia. J Pediatr Surg 33, 1563–1565.

Downing, G.J., Kilbride, H.W., 1995. Evaluation of airway complications in high-risk preterm infants: application of flexible fiberoptic airway endoscopy. Pediatrics 95, 567–572.

Durward, A.D., Nicoll, S.J., Oliver, J., et al., 1998. The outcome of patients with upper airway obstruction transported to a regional pediatric intensive care unit. Eur J Pediatr 157, 907–911.

Durward, A., Forte, V., Shemie, S., 2000. Resolution of mucus plugging and atelectasis after intratracheal rhDNase therapy in a mechanically ventilated child with refractory status asthmaticus. Crit Care Med 28, 560–562.

Dutton, J.M., Palmer, P.M., McCulloch, T.M., et al., 1995. Mortality in the pediatric patient with tracheotomy. Head Neck 17, 403–408.

Froehlich, P., Stamm, D., Floret, D., et al., 1995. Management of subglottic haemangioma. Clin Otolaryngol Allied Sci 20, 336–339.

Furman, R.H., Backer, C.L., Dunham, M.E., et al., 1999. The use of balloon-expandable metallic stents in the treatment of pediatric tracheomalacia and bronchomalacia. Archives of Otolaryngology – Head and Neck Surgery 125, 203–207.

Gianoli, G.J., Miller, R.H., Guarisco, J.L., 1990. Tracheostomy in the first year of life. Ann Otol Rhinol Laryngol 99, 896–901.

Giguere, C.M., Bauman, N.M., Sato, Y., et al., 2002. Treatment of lymphangiomas with OK-432 (Picibanil) sclerotherapy: a prospective multi-institutional trial. Archives of Otolaryngology – Head and Neck Surgery 128, 1137–1144.

Grundfast, K.M., Coffman, A.C., Milmoe, G., 1985. Anterior cricoid split: a 'simple' surgical procedure and a potentially complicated care problem. Annals of Otology, Rhinology and Laryngology 94, 445–449.

Herberhold, C., Stein, M., von Falkenhausen, M., 1999. [Long-term results of homograft reconstruction of the trachea in childhood] (in German). Laryngo-Rhino-Otologie 78, 692–696.

Holland, B.W., McGuirt, W.F. Jr, 2001. Surgical management of choanal atresia: improved outcome using mitomycin. Archives of Otolaryngology – Head and Neck Surgery 127, 1375–1380.

Jiang, D., Morrison, G.A.J., 2003. The influence of long-term tracheostomy on speech and language development in children. Int J Pediatr Otorhinolaryngol 67 (suppl. 1), S217–S220.

Lang, F.J., Hurni, M., Monnier, P., 1999. Long-segment congenital tracheal stenosis:

treatment by slide-tracheoplasty. J Pediatr Surg 34, 1216–1222.

Lazar, R.H., Younis, R.T., 1995. Transnasal repair of choanal atresia using telescopes. Archives of Otolaryngology – Head and Neck Surgery 121, 517–520.

Molitch, H.I., Unger, E.C., Witte, C.L., et al., 1995. Percutaneous sclerotherapy of lymphangiomas. Radiology 194, 343–347.

Morrison, G.A.J., Wareing, M., 1999. Defining boundaries in cricoid split and single stage laryngotracheal reconstruction. J Laryngol Otol 113 (suppl. 23), 49.

Moungthong, G., Holinger, L.D., 1997. Laryngotracheoesophageal clefts. Ann Otol Rhinol Laryngol 106, 1002–1011.

Myer, C.M. 3rd, O'Connor, D.M., Cotton, R.T., 1994. Proposed grading system for subglottic stenosis based on endotracheal tube sizes. Ann Otol Rhinol Laryngol 103, 319–323.

Pashley, N.R.T., 1982. Risk factors and the prediction of outcome in acquired subglottic stenosis in children. Int J Pediatr Otorhinolaryngol 4, 1–6.

Randolph, A.G., Wypij, D., Venkataraman, S.T., et al., 2002. Effect of mechanical ventilator weaning protocols on respiratory outcomes in infants and children: a randomized controlled trial. Pediatric Acute Lung Injury and Sepsis Investigators (PALISI) Network. J Am Med Assoc 288, 2561–2568.

Samadi, D.S., Shah, U.K., Handler, S.D., 2003. Choanal atresia: a twenty-year review of medical comorbidities and surgical outcomes. Laryngoscope 113, 254–258.

Sherman, J.M., Lowitt, S., Stephenson, C., et al., 1986. Factors influencing acquired subglottic stenosis in infants. Journal of Pediatrics 109, 322–327.

Suzumura, H., Nitta, A., Tanaka, G., et al., 2000. Role of infection in the development of acquired subglottic stenosis in neonates with prolonged intubation. Pediatr Int 42, 508–513.

Tierney, P., Francis, I., Morrison, G.A.J., 1997. Acquired subglottic cysts in low birth weight pre-term infants. J Laryngol Otol 111, 487–481.

Van der Broek, P., Brinkman, W.F.B., 1979. Congenital laryngeal defects. Int J Pediatr Otorhinolaryngol 1, 71–78.

Ward, R.F., Jones, J., Carew, J.F., 1995. Current trends in pediatric tracheotomy Int J Pediatr Otorhinolaryngol 32, 233–239.

Ward, V.M.M., Langford, K., Morrison, G., 2000. Prenatal diagnosis of airway compromise: EXIT (ex utero intra-partum treatment) and foetal airway surgery. Int J Pediatr Otorhinolaryngol 53, 137–141.

Wimmershoff, M.B., Schreyer, A., Glaessl, A., et al., 2000. Mixed capillary/lymphatic malformation with coexisting port-wine stain: treatment utilizing 3D MRI and CT-guided sclerotherapy. Dermatol Surg 26, 584–587.

Cardiovascular disease 28

Robert W M Yates

CHAPTER CONTENTS

© 2012 Elsevier Ltd

Introduction

Neonatal cardiovascular disease can be primary or secondary, congenital or acquired, structural or functional. Whatever categories of abnormality are concerned, a similar systematic approach to history, examination and investigation is required to allow correct management. In many situations, an understanding of fetal as well as of neonatal cardiovascular physiology is necessary. In this chapter the approach is pathophysiological, with particular conditions being considered in the most appropriate category.

Fetal circulation

Much of the information about the fetal circulation has been derived from animal studies. Increasingly sophisticated, non-invasive, ultrasound assessment of the human fetal circulation has demonstrated important differences in the human fetus.

Fetal circulatory pathways

The fetal circulation consists of parallel systemic and pulmonary pathways in contrast to the normal postnatal circulation, in which the systemic and pulmonary circulations exist in series (Fig. 28.1). For the most part, prenatal survival is possible with even major structural cardiovascular malformations, provided that either the right or left ventricle is able to pump blood derived from the great veins into the fetal aorta. It is this remarkably adaptive nature of the fetal circulation which enables fetuses with complex malformations such as those with atresia of either of the semilunar valves to survive throughout pregnancy. In the fetus, oxygenated blood returns from the placenta via the umbilical vein into the inferior caval vein, either through the portal system or through the venous duct. The proportion of blood channelled through these different routes changes as pregnancy progresses and will adapt continuously to the metabolic demands of the fetus by flow regulation in the venous duct. The stream of inferior caval blood entering the right atrium is divided as it hits the superior rim of the oval foramen and the majority of the blood enters the left atrium through the foramen. As pregnancy advances, the proportion crossing into the left atrium falls. Superior caval vein blood enters the right atrium and the majority will enter into the right ventricle via the tricuspid valve. Almost all of the right ventricular (RV) output will be directed through the arterial duct into the systemic circulation, bypassing the high-resistance pulmonary circulation. The proportion of pulmonary blood flow also changes with gestation, increasing during the third trimester. Just as in postnatal life, the fetal pulmonary vascular bed is reactive. Fetal pulmonary blood flow can be increased by manipulation of the pulmonary vasculature bed with pulmonary vasodilator agents (such as oxygen) administered to the mother (Rasanen et al. 1998). As pregnancy progresses, the effective cardiac output increases to a maximum of approximately 250 ml/kg/min by term, with the right ventricle contributing 55% and the left

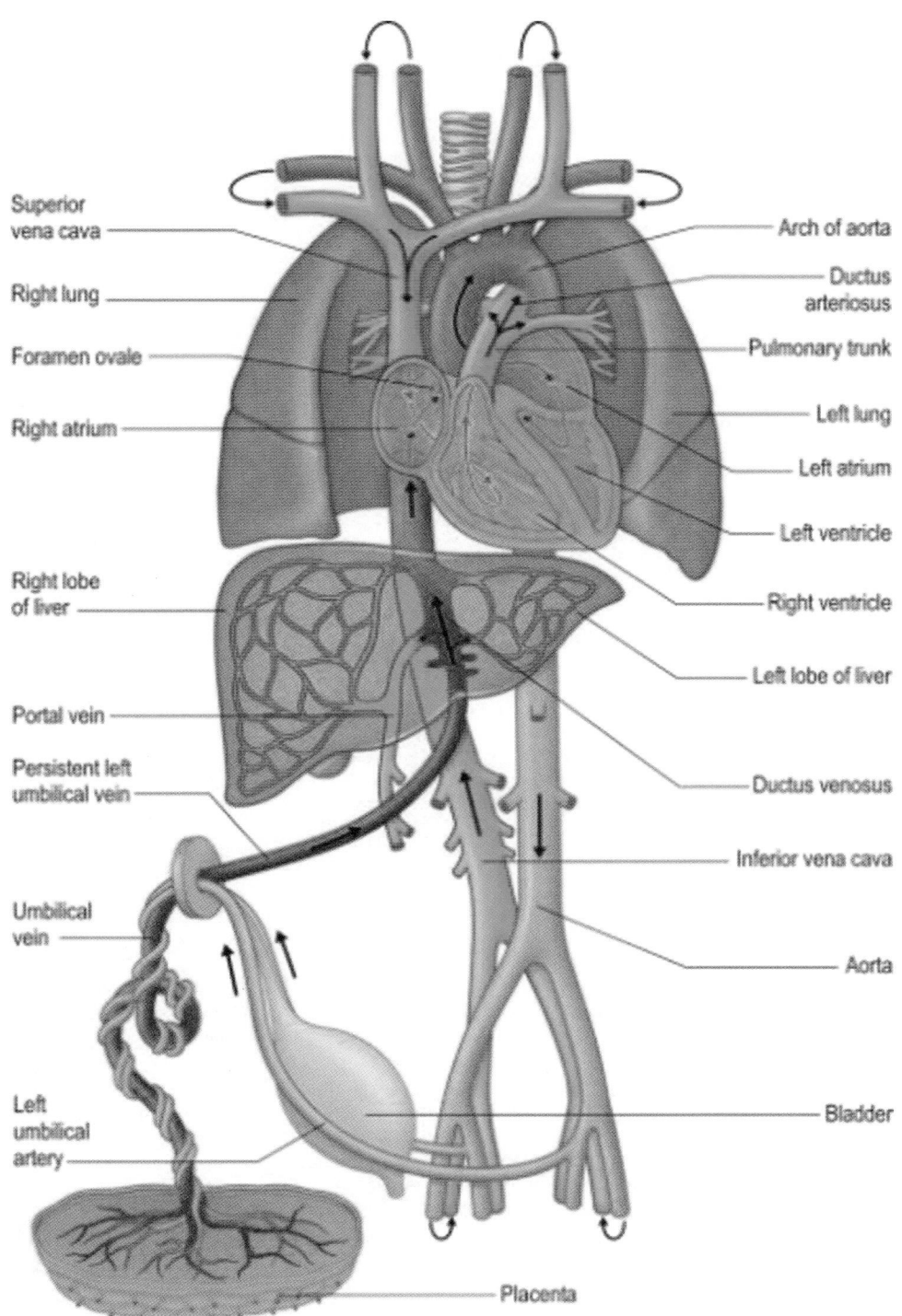

Superior vena cava

Right lung

Foramen ovale

Right atrium

Right lobe of liver

Portal vein

Persistent left umbilical vein

Umbilical vein

Left umbilical artery

Arch of aorta

Ductus arteriosus

Pulmonary trunk

Left lung

Left atrium

Left ventricle

Right ventricle

Left lobe of liver

Ductus venosus

Inferior vena cava

Aorta

Bladder

Placenta

Fig. 28.1 Schematic representation of the fetal circulatory pathways. The placenta is drawn to a greatly reduced scale. *(Reproduced with permission from Gray's Anatomy, 40th ed. Elsevier Inc. Fig 59.17.)*

ventricle 45% of the fetal cardiac output. Of the combined output, 65% returns to the placenta and 35% to the fetal organs and tissues (Rudolph 1974).

Function of the fetal heart

Compared with the normal adult heart, there are a number of differences both within the fetal heart itself as well as between the physiological environment during fetal and postnatal life which explain many of the observations of fetal cardiac function. In early fetal life, the expression of contractile proteins is different from the postnatal pattern (Hunkeler et al. 1991). In addition, the expression of different types of collagen within fetal heart muscle results in reduced compliance of the fetal heart compared with the postnatal heart (Marijianowski et al. 1994). With advancing gestation, there is continuing maturation of excitation–contraction coupling as well as increasing autonomic innervation (Grant 1999). As a result, the immature fetal heart is much less compliant and less able to generate contractile force than its adult counterpart, for the same degree of stretch. However, the observation that the Starling curve in the fetus is blunted should not be attributed to the differences in the fetal myocardium alone. It is significantly influenced by the external constraints existing around the heart in the fetus, including the fluid-filled lungs and rigid chest wall.

Changes at birth

The most dramatic events that occur with birth are a shift from a circulation in parallel to one in series, as well as a marked increase in cardiac output from both ventricles. At term, the cardiac output from each ventricle approximately equals the combined cardiac output from both ventricles in the immediately preterm fetus. With inspiration, there is a rapid fall in pulmonary vascular resistance (PVR), as lung expansion allows new vessels to open and existing vessels to enlarge. Reduced resistance and decreased pulmonary artery pressures increase pulmonary blood flow. Simultaneously, the lower resistance placental circulation is removed from the systemic circulation as the cord is cut. The increased preload occurring from placental return can now be converted into useful increased cardiac output, once the external constraints of fluid-filled lungs around the heart are replaced by more compliant air-filled lungs. The sudden increase in oxygen tension produced by breathing alters local prostaglandin synthesis, resulting in a constriction of both the arterial and venous ducts. For most neonates, functional closure of the arterial duct will have occurred within 24–72 hours and anatomical closure is complete within 1–2 weeks. The oval foramen and venous duct may remain patent for some time after birth, with the potential to allow shunting. This can mask the signs of underlying structural congenital cardiovascular malformations, such as infracardiac total anomalous pulmonary venous drainage or, occasionally, transposition of the great arteries (TGA). The oval foramen is functionally closed in the majority of cases by the third month of life. Continued patency may contribute to clinical problems in some conditions (Table 28.1).

Fetal cardiology

Diagnosis

Fetal cardiac anatomy, function and rhythm have been determined by transabdominal scanning from 18 weeks' gestation for the last two decades (Allan et al. 1985). An approach using both abdominal and (when necessary) transvaginal scanning in high-risk cases at 10–13 weeks allowed interpretable images in over 80% of cases

Table 28.1 Clinical problems associated with failure of closure of the foramen ovale, ductus venosus and ductus arteriosus after birth

Foramen ovale	Allows right-to-left shunting in persistent pulmonary hypertension of the newborn and other cardiac/respiratory conditions with increased right heart pressures
Ductus venosus	No definite problem identified (except in obstructed total anomalous pulmonary venous connection: see text)
Ductus arteriosus	Associated with major respiratory and other problems in preterm infants. Important left-to-right shunting only rarely seen in the newborn period in term infants with patent ductus arteriosus

Table 28.2 Indications for detailed fetal echocardiography

Autosomal dominant condition with cardiac implications in either parent
Structural heart disease in parent or previous sibling
Structural heart disease in two or more family members
Maternal disease with increased risk of fetal cardiac problem, e.g. diabetes mellitus, collagen vascular disease
Maternal teratogen exposure, e.g.:
 – infection: rubella
 – medication: anticonvulsants, lithium, warfarin
 – alcohol
Abnormal nuchal translucency in the first trimester with normal karyotype or karyotype declined
Abnormal four-chamber view or suspected congenital heart disease on routine midtrimester scan
Extracardiac abnormalities in the fetus
Suspected syndrome in the fetus
Maternal prostaglandin synthetase inhibitor therapy
Abnormal heart rate/rhythm in the fetus
Hydropic fetus
 – Consider in in vitro fertilisation pregnancies

(Huggon et al. 2002), with a probable low false-positive rate, although verification was incomplete. Screening fetal cardiac anatomy with a four-chamber view at 18 weeks is a routine part of the general anomaly scan, but this will pick up under 50% of cases of structural heart lesions, even in experienced hands (Stümpflen et al. 1996; Bull 1999). Heart lesions picked up by a four-chamber screening scan are generally the more complex ones with a poorer outlook both prenatally and after delivery. If views of the outflow tracts are obtained in addition to the four-chamber view, the range of abnormalities detectable is increased (Carvalho et al. 2002). In particular, transposition, tetralogy of Fallot and similar lesions should be detected.

Detailed evaluation of fetal cardiac anatomy by ultrasound is much more time-consuming and is usually reserved for women with an increased risk of having a fetus with a cardiac problem (Table 28.2). However, when detailed echocardiography was used on all pregnancies, Stümpflen and colleagues (1996) reported 86% sensitivity and 100% specificity. The conditions missed were mainly atrial septal defects (ASDs) and small ventricular septal defects (VSDs). Other workers have pointed out the difficulty in diagnosing coarctation and total anomalous pulmonary venous connection (TAPVC) in the fetus (Allan 1995). Abnormalities of fetal heart rhythm can be determined by M-mode and Doppler studies.

There are ethical aspects to fetal diagnosis and practitioners in this field need to be sensitive to parental views. Fetal cardiac scanning should be carried out in the context of expertise in all aspects of fetal medicine, including the provision of support to families. The association with non-cardiac abnormalities is strong and these are often major influences in the natural history in utero and after birth, as well as in decisions about continuation of pregnancy. For example, in one study in which cardiac scans were performed for a variety of indications, 70% of fetuses with a cardiac anomaly had an underlying chromosome abnormality (Huggon et al. 2002).

Treatment

Accurate diagnosis of structural heart disease in a fetus allows information to be given to families and provides for greater choice. Some parents will opt for termination of pregnancy and about 5% of fetuses with structural cardiac abnormalities will die in utero (Yates 2004). Cardiac diagnosis and prognosis must be considered in the context of full fetal assessment, as non-cardiac abnormalities may well be more important in determining the overall prognosis. The combination of a structural cardiac abnormality and an extracardiac abnormality will often influence outcome more adversely than anticipated for either lesion alone.

In pregnancies progressing to viability, a cardiac diagnosis will, in a minority of cases, influence place, time or mode of delivery, but non-cardiac factors also need to be taken into account. The most important point with respect to early postnatal management of heart disease is whether or not the lesion is likely to be duct-dependent, thereby allowing prostaglandin to be used before symptoms develop. Progressive underdevelopment of the ventricle in the fetus with severe arterial valve stenosis is well recognised (Simpson and Sharland 1997; Tulzer et al. 2002) and prenatal arterial valve balloon valvuloplasty has been performed with limited proven efficacy (Kohl et al. 2000; Tulzer et al. 2002). Some structural lesions do not progress with advancing gestation and, in those that do, only a tiny minority are suitable for any form of prenatal intervention. There is evidence that fetal diagnosis of severe duct-dependent congenital heart disease (CHD) results in babies reaching a cardiac centre in better condition than those not diagnosed until after delivery (Yates 2004). Benefit from fetal diagnosis in terms of improved survival and morbidity has been shown for coarctation (Franklin et al. 2002), and in improved mortality in transposition (Bonnet et al. 1999) and hypoplastic left heart (Tworetzky et al. 2001), although, in the last two conditions, the benefit from prenatal diagnosis has been difficult to demonstrate (Yates 2004). Reassurance of normality or the chance to prepare for the arrival of an abnormal baby is valued by many parents but has not been formally quantified.

Accurate diagnosis of fetal dysrhythmias is essential to avoid unnecessary intervention and to allow appropriate treatment which can almost always improve the outlook for the fetus with a haemodynamically compromising rhythm disturbance. Diagnosis and management of abnormal fetal rhythms are discussed in the section on neonatal rhythm disturbances (p. 661).

Incidence and aetiology of fetal and neonatal heart disease

Structural CHD occurs in approximately 8 per 1000 live births (Anderson et al. 2002). In populations uninfluenced by fetal

Table 28.3 Distribution of congenital cardiac lesions in newborn infants, median and interquartile (%), obtained from 34 studies involving 26 904 infants

LESION/GROUP	MEDIAN	25TH–75TH
Ventricular septal defect	32.0	27–42
Patent arterial duct	6.8	5–11
Atrial septal defect	7.5	6–11
Atrioventricular septal defect	3.8	3–5
Pulmonary stenosis	7.0	5–9
Aortic stenosis	3.9	3–6
Coarctation of aorta	4.8	4–6
Transposition of great arteries	4.4	4–5
Tetralogy of Fallot	5.2	4–8
Common arterial trunk	1.4	1–2
Hypoplastic left heart	2.8	2–3
Hypoplastic right heart	2.2	2–3
Double-inlet ventricle	1.5	1–2
Double-outlet right ventricle	1.8	1–3
Total anomalous pulmonary venous drainage	1.0	1–2
Others	10.0	8–15

(Adapted with permission from Hoffman (2002).)

diagnosis, between 30% and 40% of these children will be symptomatic in early infancy and about two-thirds of them will have been diagnosed by the end of the first year of life. There are various studies on the prevalence of CHD: diagnostic methods and criteria vary, but Table 28.3 gives figures for those presenting in the neonatal period. The true prevalence may be higher than this, because some lesions such as a bicuspid aortic valve are usually excluded. Bicuspid aortic valve occurs in 10–20 per 1000 live births and may be associated with significant morbidity in later life (Ward 2000). An increased prevalence of CHD is also supported by fetal echocardiography data, which have shown that some severe cardiac lesions will result in death in utero (Yates 2004). Furthermore, the effect of prenatal diagnosis on postnatal prevalence and spectrum of disease may be considerable (Bull 1999).

Acquired heart disease, such as endocarditis and myocarditis, may present in the newborn period. Metabolic disorders, which may involve heart muscle, can produce symptoms in the newborn period. There are no reliable data for the incidence of these problems or for the incidence of fetal and neonatal arrhythmias.

Although there have been major advances in the diagnosis and treatment of CHD, understanding of its causes remains limited. Advances in cytogenetics have provided a greater understanding of the role of inherited and environmental factors and their interaction on the development of CHD. Environmental factors such as maternal diabetes, alcohol/drug ingestion and, less commonly, some congenital infections are known to affect cardiac development adversely. The major chromosomal abnormalities such as trisomies 21, 18 and 13 cause syndromes, part of which can include structural cardiac malformations, and these have been well documented (Table 28.4). Before the advent of fluorescence in situ hybridisation (FISH), standard chromosome analysis revealed chromosomal abnormalities in about 10% of newborns with CHD (Ferencz et al. 1989). Improved genetic techniques, including FISH, cytogenetic techniques and DNA mutation analysis, have confirmed that this prevalence is much higher. An explanation of the genetic techniques and their uses is beyond the scope of this chapter but readers are referred to the American Heart Association statement on the genetic basis for congenital heart defects (Pierpont et al. 2007). Therefore, chromosomal and genetic analysis in neonates with various types of CHD is an important part of their evaluation, particularly because, in some syndromes, the extracardiac manifestations are often less evident and the cardiac abnormalities provide the clue to the diagnosis in the newborn period.

Syndromes associated with CHD, such as 22q11 deletion, Noonan's, Williams, Alagille's, Holt–Oram and others, have been shown to be associated with subtle chromosomal or genetic abnormalities such as deletions or point mutations (Tables 28.4 and 28.5). In some defects there are no associated syndromes but specific genes have been identified in association with particular defects (Tables 28.4 and 28.5). For individuals with CHD or their families, the identification of a genetic cause for the CHD is beneficial. It helps the clinician to explain the mechanism to the family and broadens the context of the diagnosis to other family members.

Such advances have altered the traditional view of a multifactorial basis for the aetiology of CHD shifting towards a genetic aetiology for an increasing number of lesions. Associated with this is the potential to provide more accurate data about recurrence risk in siblings and offspring of affected parents: this has been shown to be higher when the affected parent is female (Burn et al. 1998).

Clinical implications of adaptation to birth

Normal adaptation

Normal adaptation of the fetal circulation at birth may have adverse haemodynamic effects in some congenital cardiac malformations just as failure of normal changes to occur may be disadvantageous under certain circumstances.

Foramen ovale

If exit of blood from the left atrium through the mitral valve is impaired, the presence of a foramen ovale is important in allowing decompression of the left atrium as it is forced open by abnormally high pressure in the left atrium. Failure of this mechanism by virtue of a small foramen ovale results in pulmonary venous hypertension and respiratory distress. This problem is an important part of the pathophysiology of mitral atresia or hypoplasia. A restrictive foramen ovale is also important in obstructive lesions in the right heart, such as tricuspid atresia, pulmonary atresia with intact ventricular septum and critical pulmonary stenosis. In such

Table 28.4 Representative chromosomal disorders associated with congenital heart disease (CHD)

CHROMOSOMAL DISORDER	MAIN FEATURES	PERCENTAGE WITH CHD	HEART ANOMALY
Deletion 4p (Wolf–Hirschhorn syndrome)	Pronounced microcephaly, widely spaced eyes, broad nasal bridge (Greek helmet appearance), downturned mouth, micrognathia, preauricular skin tags, elongated trunk and fingers, severe mental retardation and seizures; one-third die in infancy	50–65	ASD, VSD, PDA, LSVC, aortic atresia, dextrocardia, TOF, tricuspid atresia
Deletion 5p (cri du chat)	Cat-like cry, prenatal and postnatal growth retardation, round face, widely spaced eyes, epicanthal fold, simian crease, severe mental retardation, long survival	30–60	VSD, ASD, PDA
Deletion 7q11.23 (Williams–Beuren syndrome)	Infantile hypercalcaemia, skeletal and renal anomalies, cognitive deficits, 'social' personality, elfin facies	53–85	Supravalvar AS and PS, PPS
Trisomy 8 mosaicism	Skeletal/vertebral anomalies, widely spaced eyes, broad nasal bridge, small jaw, high arched palate, cryptorchidism, renal anomalies (50%), long survival	25	VSD, PDA, CoA, PS, TAPVR, truncus arteriosus
Deletion 8p syndrome	Microcephaly, growth retardation, mental retardation, deep-set eyes, malformed eyes, small chin, genital anomalies in males, long survival	50–75	AVSD, PS, VSD, TOF
Trisomy 9	Severe prenatal and postnatal growth retardation, marked microcephaly, deep-set eyes, low-set ears, severe mental retardation; two-thirds die in infancy	65–80	PDA, LSVC, VSD, TOF/PA, DORV

Table 28.4 Continued

CHROMOSOMAL DISORDER	MAIN FEATURES	PERCENTAGE WITH CHD	HEART ANOMALY
Deletion 10p	Frontal bossing, short down-slanting palpebral fissures, small low-set ears, micrognathia, cleft palate, short neck, urinary/genital, upper limb anomalies	50	BAV, ASD, VSD, PDA, PS, CoA, truncus arteriosus
Deletion 11q (Jacobsen syndrome)	Growth retardation, developmental delay, mental retardation, thrombocytopenia, platelet dysfunction, widely spaced eyes, strabismus, broad nasal bridge, thin upper lip, prominent forehead	56	HLHS, valvar AS, VSD, CoA, Shone's complex
Trisomy 13 (Patau syndrome)	Polydactyly, cleft lip and palate, scalp defects, hypotelorism, micro-ophthalmia or anophthalmia, colobomata of irides, holoprosencephaly, microcephaly, deafness, profound mental retardation, rib abnormalities, omphalocele, renal abnormalities, hypospadias, cryptorchidism, uterine abnormalities; 80% die in first year	80	ASD, VSD, PDA, HLHS, laterality defects, atrial isomerism
Trisomy 18 (Edwards syndrome)	IUGR, polyhydramnios, micrognathia, short sternum, hypertonia, rocker-bottom feet, overlapping fingers and toes, TEF, CDH, omphalocele, renal anomalies, biliary atresia, profound mental retardation; 90% die in first year	90–100	ASD, VSD, PDA, TOF, DORV, D-TGA, CoA, BAV, BPV, polyvalvular nodular dysplasia
Deletion 20p12 (Alagille syndrome)	Bile duct paucity, cholestasis, skeletal or ocular anomalies, broad forehead, widely spaced eyes, underdeveloped mandible	85–94	Peripheral PA, hypoplasia, TOF, PS (left-sided heart lesions and septal defects less common)
Trisomy 21 (Down syndrome)	Hypotonia, hyperextensibility, epicanthal fold, simian crease, clinodactyly of fifth finger, brachydactyly, variable mental retardation, premature ageing	40–50	AVSD, VSD, ASD (TOF, D-TGA less common)
Deletion 22q11 (DiGeorge, velocardiofacial and conotruncal anomaly face syndrome)	Hypertelorism, micrognathia, low-set posteriorly rotated ears, 'fish mouth', thymic and parathyroid hypoplasia, hypocalcaemia, feeding/speech/learning/behavioural disorders, immunodeficiency, palate/skeletal/renal anomalies	75	IAA-B, truncus arteriosus, isolated aortic arch anomalies, TOF, conoventricular VSD
Monosomy X (Turner syndrome, 45,X)	Lymphoedema of hands and feet, widely spaced hypoplastic nipples, webbed neck, primary amenorrhoea, short stature, normal intelligence	25–35	CoA, BAV, valvar AS, HLHS, aortic dissection
Klinefelter syndrome (47,XXY)	Usually normal-appearing, tall stature, small testes, delayed puberty, emotional and behavioural problems common, variable mental retardation	50	MVP, venous thromboembolic disease, PDA, ASD

ASD, atrial septal defect; VSD, ventricular septal defect; PDA, patent ductus arteriosus; LSVC, left superior vena cava; TOF, tetralogy of Fallot; AS, aortic stenosis; PS, pulmonary stenosis; PPS, peripheral pulmonary stenosis; CoA, coarctation of the aorta; TAPVR, total anomalous pulmonary venous return; AVSD, atrioventricular septal defect; TOF/PA, tetralogy of Fallot with pulmonary atresia; DORV, double-outlet right ventricle; BAV, bicuspid aortic valve; HLHS, hypoplastic left-heart syndrome; IUGR, intrauterine growth retardation; TEF, tracheo-oesophageal fistula; CDH, congenital diaphragmatic hernia; D-TGA, D-transposition of the great arteries; BPV, bicuspid pulmonary valve; PA, pulmonary artery; IAA-B, interrupted aortic arch type B; MVP, mitral valve prolapse. (Reproduced from Pierpont et al. (2007), with permission.)

Table 28.5 Single-gene mutations associated with genetic syndromes and congenital heart defects (see Table 28.4)

CONDITION	DEFECT	CHROMOSOME LOCATION	GENE
Syndrome			
Noonan	PS, ASD, HCM	12q24 12p1.21 2p21 8q12	PTPN11 KRAS SOS1 CHD7
Holt–Oram	ASD	12q24	TBX5
Marfan	MVP, Ao root dilatation	15q21.1	FBN1
Alagille	PS, peripheral PS, PA	20p12	JAG1
CHARGE association	VSD, AVSD, IAA	8q12	CHD7
Ellis van Creveld	ASD, VSD, AVSD	4p16	EVC, EVC2
Costello	HOCM	11p15.5	HRAS
Defect			
Fallot		8q23	ZFPM2/FOG2
AVSD		3p21	CRELD1
TGA		12q24	PROSIT240
ASD/VSD		8p23	GATA4
Supravalvar AS		7q11	ELN
Atrial isomerism		Xq26 2q21 3p21.3p22 1q42.1	ZIC3 CFC1 ACVR28 LEFTYA

PS, pulmonary stenosis; ASD, atrial septal defect; HCM, hypertrophic cardiomyopathy; MVP, mitral valve prolapse; Ao, aortic; PA, pulmonary artery; VSD, ventricular septal defect; AVSD, atrioventricular septal defect; TOF/PA, tetralogy of Fallot with pulmonary atresia; IAA, interrupted aortic arch; HOCM, hypertrophic obstructive cardiomyopathy; TGA, transposition of the great arches; AS, aortic stenosis.
(Adapted from Pierpont et al. (2007).)

circumstances, right atrial enlargement and hydops fetalis may occur in utero, but, even if this does not occur, there may be post-natal problems from systemic venous engorgement and poor cardiac output. In the context of TGA, a small foramen ovale results in poor mixing of oxygenated and deoxygenated blood. In many of these conditions, particularly TGA, enlargement of a small foramen ovale by balloon atrial septostomy is an important part of the initial management. In some circumstances, surgical septostomy or sep-tectomy may be indicated, as in mitral atresia. Failure of the foramen ovale to close has the same consequences as the presence of an ASD; indeed, distinguishing between patent foramen ovale (PFO) and ASD in newborn infants can be difficult. The consequences are right-to-left shunting in the presence of structural or functional obstruction to right heart flow and left-to-right shunting otherwise. The balance between favourable and deleterious effects is different for different lesions. In general, left-to-right shunting at atrial level in early infancy is rarely a major disadvantage, whereas right-to-left shunting will worsen systemic arterial desaturation – but this may be less of a disadvantage than very high venous pressures or poor left ventricular filling resulting from poor forward flow through the right heart.

Ductus venosus

Closure of the ductus venosus is of importance in that it removes the possibility of central venous access being obtained via the umbilical vein for monitoring, balloon septostomy or cardiac catheterisation. It will also result in marked deterioration in cases of TAPVC to the portal vein as it will cause severe pulmonary venous obstruction with pulmonary congestion (Fig. 28.2). In this condition, closure of the ductus venosus may not occur until some days after birth. Delay in or failure of closure of the ductus venosus is probably rare and never of significance.

Ductus arteriosus

Closure of the DA will cause marked deterioration in duct-dependent pulmonary and duct-dependent systemic circulations, in the first instance causing worsening cyanosis, and, in the latter, shock and heart failure. Systemic arterial oxygenation in TGA will also deteriorate when the DA closes. These conditions are all discussed in more detail below (see sections on cyanosis and collapse).

Pulmonary vascular resistance

Pulmonary blood flow increases rapidly at birth as PVR falls. This normal process will have adverse effects if an increase in pulmonary venous return is disadvantageous. As discussed above, this can happen in the presence of pulmonary venous obstruction from any cause or if exit of blood from the left atrium is impeded. Increased pulmonary blood flow secondary to lesions allowing left-to-right shunting will cause respiratory distress and heart failure as PVR falls. This usually is not a problem in the early newborn phase and often is not apparent until 2 or 3 months of age. A common exception to this statement is patent ductus arteriosus (PDA) in the preterm infant (see below). Any shunt lesion may become symptomatic at an earlier postnatal age in preterm infants than in term ones; this is attributed to less well-developed pulmonary vascular musculature in the premature infant (Heymann 1995). It is also probable that widespread use of more effective mechanical ventilation and the use of surfactant may improve oxygenation, facilitating the decrease in PVR and contributing to the pathophysiological effects of a patent arterial duct in premature newborns.

Delay in the normal fall in PVR may quickly result in a clinical problem (persistent pulmonary hypertension of the newborn, PPHN). It may also play a role in the pathophysiology of chronic lung disease (CLD) and in the development of pulmonary vascular disease (PVD) in structural heart lesions, owing to unrestricted transmission of systemic pressures into the pulmonary circulation, as occurs in a large VSD or a complete atrioventricular septal defect (AVSD).

PPHN may also be seen when there has been underdevelopment of the pulmonary vascular tree in utero (such as in diaphragmatic hernia) or if there has been in utero exposure to prostaglandin synthetase inhibitors as a result of maternal therapy. Hypoxaemia in PPHN is due to right-to-left shunting, which can be either within the lungs or extrapulmonary, in which case it can be at ductal level or intracardiac through the foramen ovale.

History and examination

These are basic in the evaluation of a newborn infant with suspected cardiac disease. History-taking involves details of the current problems as well as obtaining information about pregnancy, the perinatal period, the family and social circumstances. Examination of the newborn is dealt with in Chapter 14; a number of additional points with specific reference to the cardiovascular system will be considered here.

Dysmorphic features and non-cardiac malformations

These must be carefully sought and described in detail in relation to all body systems. They are clearly important if a syndrome is to be diagnosed and may influence treatment plans and prognostic information given to families. It may be relevant to investigate other systems on the basis of certain cardiac diagnoses, for example chromosome analysis or immunological assessment. In some circumstances, recognition of an abnormality in an infant will result in a diagnosis being made in a parent, for example 22q11 deletion or Noonan syndrome. When certain non-cardiac structural abnormalities are recognised, a detailed cardiac evaluation is appropriate, as in Down syndrome and many gastrointestinal abnormalities (Tulloh et al. 1994). Of all children with chromosomal abnormalities, at least 30% have a congenital cardiac defect (Pierpoint and Moller 1987).

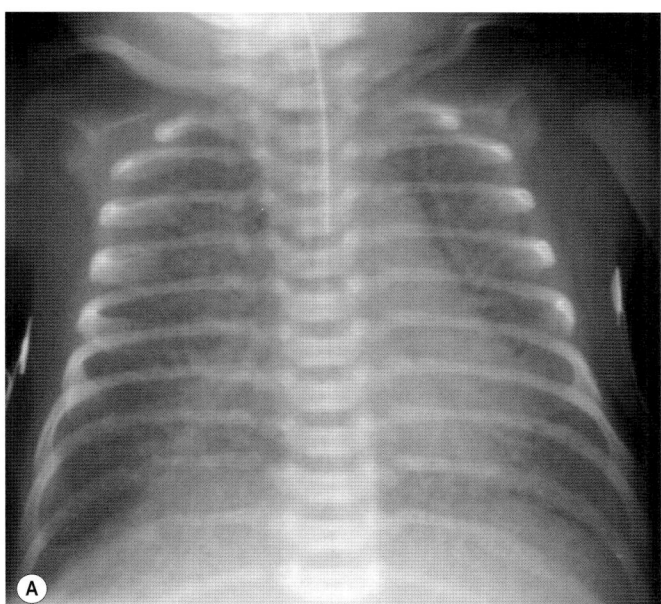
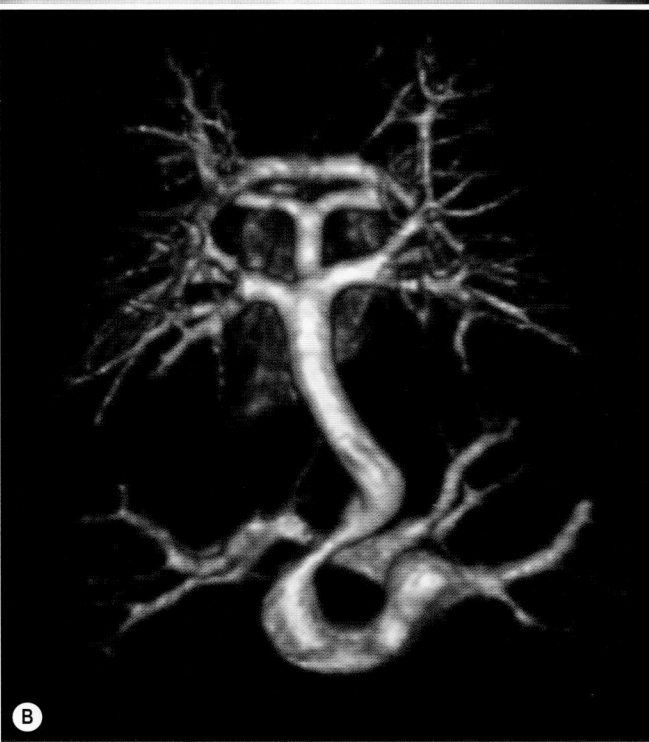

Fig. 28.2 (A) Anteroposterior chest X-ray in a neonate with obstructed total anomalous pulmonary venous connection showing pulmonary venous congestion and normal heart size. (B) Volume-rendered three-dimensional magnetic resonance imaging reconstruction in the same patient viewed from behind showing four pulmonary veins entering into a vertical confluence behind the left atrium, which is drained by a large descending vein entering into the hepatic venous system. The descending vein is narrowed as it crosses the diaphragm and the hepatic veins, with which it communicates, are dilated.

Pulses

Impalpable or weak femoral pulses in the presence of good-volume upper limb pulses suggest coarctation of the aorta, in which case other signs may well be present and might include upper limb hypertension, systolic pressure difference between arms and legs, evidence of aortic valve abnormality (ejection click), a bruit between the scapulae and signs of heart failure. If all pulses are weak, then left ventricular outflow obstruction, hypovolaemia or left ventricular dysfunction should be considered. Hypoplastic left heart may be associated with stronger femoral than right brachial pulses before the DA closes. A preterm infant severely compromised by PDA may have very weak femoral pulses. A baby with interrupted aortic arch usually collapses in the first week of life; the diagnosis and the site of interruption can sometimes be deduced by comparing arm and neck pulses as they will be much stronger proximal to the interruption.

Blood pressure

Blood pressure (BP) should be measured in both arms and in one leg in any newborn infant with cardiac symptoms and in an asymptomatic infant if other signs raise the possibility of coarctation. A difference in systolic BP of 20 mmHg or more between arm and leg is strongly suggestive of coarctation, although smaller gradients in term babies can be normal and the absence of such a difference may not rule out the diagnosis of coarctation if the DA is still patent. BP should also be measured in any unwell baby, as well as in those with urinary tract abnormalities, those on steroids, in CLD and in the infants of drug-addicted mothers. It is essential that the baby is settled; results on crying babies are misleading. Monitoring BP is part of the management of severely ill babies and this should be carried out invasively wherever possible. Obtaining a definitive non-invasive BP requires patience and attention to detail. The arterial pulse can be detected by palpation or with a Doppler probe. Both methods will only give a systolic value. Auscultation is very difficult and the flush method is rarely used. Oscillometric monitors may be useful in sequential BP monitoring of immobile babies but even then are subject to error at low pressures in infants with extremely low birthweight. Cuff size is important and for the arm it should cover 75% of the distance from axilla to elbow or have a width that is 40–50% of the arm circumference (National Institutes of Health 1987). The bladder should virtually encircle the arm. Leg BP can be measured using the same cuff around the calf with detection of a dorsalis pedis or posterior tibial pulse. Normal BP values are given in Appendix 4.

Cyanosis

Peripheral cyanosis is very common in normal newborn babies. Central cyanosis in the presence of structural cardiac disease is caused by three main mechanisms, which may coexist. The commonest is obstruction to pulmonary blood flow with a right-to-left shunt. Cyanosis is also evident when there are discordant ventriculo-arterial connections (as in transposition) with adverse streaming of blood within the heart. Thirdly, cyanosis will also occur where there is common mixing of blood, which can occur at atrial, ventricular or great artery level, allowing the mixed systemic and pulmonary venous return to be distributed to both the aorta and the pulmonary arteries.

Central cyanosis in the neonate may have a respiratory cause but can also be mimicked by facial petechiae (traumatic cyanosis) and can be seen in markedly polycythaemic infants. Plethoric infants with a low normal oxygen saturation may have enough

Table 28.6 Features of neonatal heart failure

Acute cardiorespiratory collapse
Respiratory distress, added sounds in chest
Tachycardia (unless cause of failure is heart block)
Hepatomegaly
Poor peripheral perfusion, clammy mottled skin, cold sweatiness
Oedema – usually late but characteristic of fetal heart failure (hydrops) often with pericardial, pleural and peritoneal fluid
Excess or unexpected weight gain
Poor feeding and slow weight gain in compensated heart failure
Specific signs of causative lesion

deoxygenated haemoglobin to give true central cyanosis. Pigmentation of the lips can also confuse the observer and it is important to look at the tongue to get the best possible assessment of saturation. Anaemia and desaturation make a baby look pale grey rather than really blue, and methaemoglobinaemia gives babies a slate black or grey colour which is often mistaken for cyanosis. Cyanotic, often termed 'dusky', episodes are very common and are only occasionally a presenting feature for structural heart disease; persistent cyanosis is far more likely to be cardiac, although it may vary in intensity. Cyanosis whilst crying is rarely pathological if colour and behaviour return to normal rapidly when the infant stops crying. Hypercyanotic episodes, as seen in tetralogy of Fallot and related conditions, are rare in the newborn period.

Heart failure

Fetal echo has shown that prenatal cardiac failure can be caused by myocardial dysfunction, structural abnormalities and arrhythmias. In newborns, early heart failure usually results from myocardial dysfunction, left-heart obstructive lesions, tachyarrhythmias and large arteriovenous malformations (AVMs). These result in tachycardia, tachypnoea with recession, liver enlargement and cardiomegaly. These conditions are a medical emergency. With advancing age, lesions that cause a large left-to-right shunt are the most frequent cause of heart failure (large VSD or big PDA). They manifest as PVR falls and signs appear more quickly when there are combinations of lesions. The signs of heart failure in the older neonate are subtly different, with poor feeding, slow weight gain and tachypnoea being the most common. Common features of neonatal heart failure are listed in Table 28.6.

Heart murmur

Heart murmurs in the newborn are common, occurring in up to 0.6% of newborns (Ainsworth et al. 1999). They may be associated with both major and minor cardiac lesions but also can be a normal physiological finding. Many serious cardiac conditions have unimpressive or even no murmurs in the newborn period. Other auscultatory and general cardiovascular signs are therefore very important in assessing the significance of a murmur. The absence of any other features of cardiac disease as well as the presence of certain positive murmur characteristics are required to diagnose innocent heart murmurs. The typical heart murmur in newborn babies comes from the pulmonary artery branches and disappears before 6 months of age in term infants. In practice, cardiac murmurs in the newborn that are associated with additional cardiac symptoms or signs justify prompt echocardiographic assessment unless the diagnosis has been documented prenatally, in which case knowledge of the diagnosis and clinical assessment should determine the timing of investigation. Asymptomatic murmurs will almost always need formal investigation with echocardiography but this can usually be undertaken on an elective basis.

Airway obstruction

This uncommon presentation is usually associated with inspiratory stridor. When associated with a structural cardiac abnormality, the manifestations are usually caused by a vascular ring such as a pulmonary artery sling or a double aortic arch. Major airway obstruction can occur as part of the absent pulmonary valve syndrome in association with tetralogy of Fallot.

Investigations

History and examination often allow cardiac disease to be suspected or ruled out. Investigations range from those readily available in any neonatal nursery (chest X-ray (CXR; Ch. 27 part 2), electrocardiogram (ECG), pulse oximetry and hyperoxia test) to those only available at cardiac centres (cardiac catheterisation and magnetic resonance imaging (MRI)). Echocardiography is being increasingly used outside cardiac centres and, with suitable equipment and trained operators, is very valuable in the care of the newborn, particularly to confirm or rule out a cardiac abnormality in those cases where clinical assessment, ECG and CXR have been inconclusive. The value of ECG and CXR in differentiating normal from abnormal murmurs in the newborn has not been systematically examined, and they are less often used now. The role of pulse oximetry as a screening test is also discussed below.

Chest radiography

CXR is less valuable in the newborn period in the evaluation of CHD because the appearance can be normal even in the presence of a severe congenital cardiac malformation. Its value lies in its availability, cost and the additional information it provides. Visceral situs, cardiac position, cardiac size and bony abnormalities of the chest are all well seen on the CXR. Features to look for in this context are listed in Table 28.7; examples are shown in Figures 28.3–28.6 and see Ch. 43. The role of the CXR has diminished with the more widespread use of transthoracic echocardiography.

Electrocardiogram

The ECG provides useful information in a number of areas (Table 28.8), providing attention is paid to technical aspects of obtaining a good recording, which can be difficult in a neonatal nursery. Systematic reading of the ECG will optimise the information obtained and reference should be made to normal values (Appendix 3) and to a standard text for detailed interpretation of ECGs (Park and Guntheroth 1992).

Heart rhythm

Abnormal heart rate can be confirmed on the ECG and heart rhythm can usually be ascertained. Sinus rhythm is characterised by normal P waves (frontal plane axis 0–190°) preceding every QRS complex. Sinus rate varies between 70 and 180 beats/min in healthy babies, reaching as much as 220 beats/min in sick babies. In these circumstances, P waves can be hard to see but all leads should be examined and paper run at a faster speed (50 mm/s) if necessary. First-degree heart block (prolonged PR interval) is rarely of importance in its own right in the newborn but may be a marker for structural heart

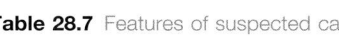

Table 28.7 Features of suspected cardiac disease

FEATURE	COMMENT
Quality of film	Adequate inspiration Normal penetration Centred on midchest Not rotated
Abdominal situs	
Bronchial situs	Normal/inverted/ambiguous
Aortic arch side	Left or right
Heart	Side Direction of apex Size Contour
Lung vasculature	Plethora Oligaemia Pulmonary venous engorgement
Diaphragm	Distinct Side of apex should be more caudal
Lung fields	Any pathology
Musculoskeletal	Vertebral/rib abnormalities Fractures

Table 28.8 Information obtainable from the electrocardiogram

Rhythm
Atrial:
  – Position
  – Enlargement
Ventricular:
  – Position
  – Hypertrophy
  – Strain/ischaemia

disease such as ASD or Ebstein's anomaly. A short PR interval is a marker for an increased tendency to supraventricular tachycardia (SVT), although delta waves in the QRS complex may easily be overlooked in neonates. A short PR interval also accompanies some structural heart lesions (Ebstein's anomaly) and may be seen in glycogen storage disease. Partial atrioventricular (AV) dissociation (second-degree heart block) and complete heart block (CHB) are considered below, as are SVT and ventricular tachycardia (VT).

Information on the atria

Inverted P waves in lead I may be a sign of an incorrectly wired ECG (right arm/left arm reversed). This can be checked by looking at lead V_6. If I and V_6 look similar, the ECG is wired up correctly and negative P waves in I then suggest one of the following:

- not sinus rhythm (Fig. 28.7)
- heart in abnormal position
- heart in normal position but atria in abnormal spatial relationship to each other.

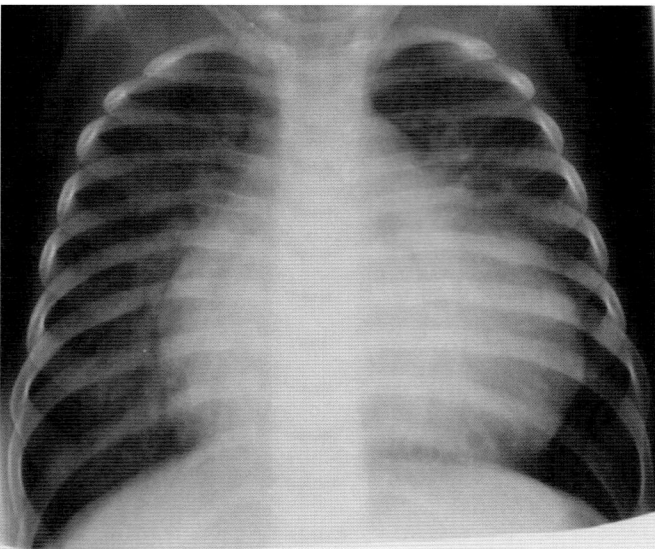

Fig. 28.3 Posteroanterior chest X-ray showing marked cardiomegaly with pulmonary plethora in association with congestive cardiac failure.

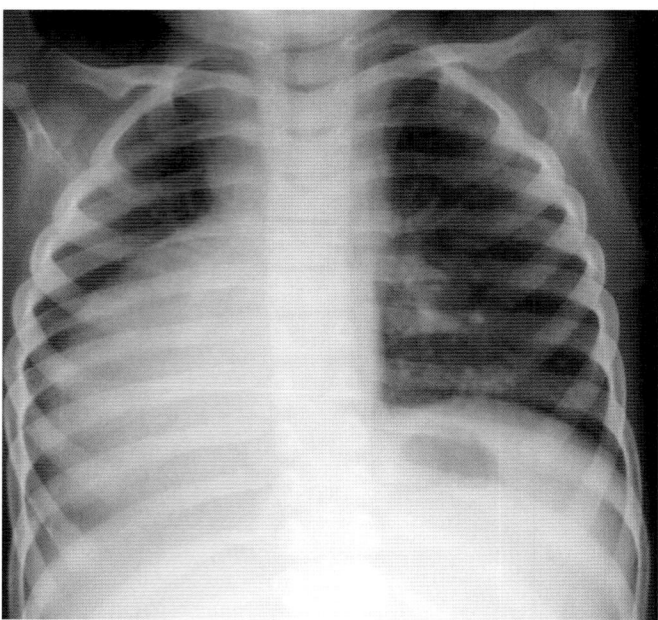

Fig. 28.4 Posteroanterior chest X-ray showing normal abdominal situs with dextrocardia.

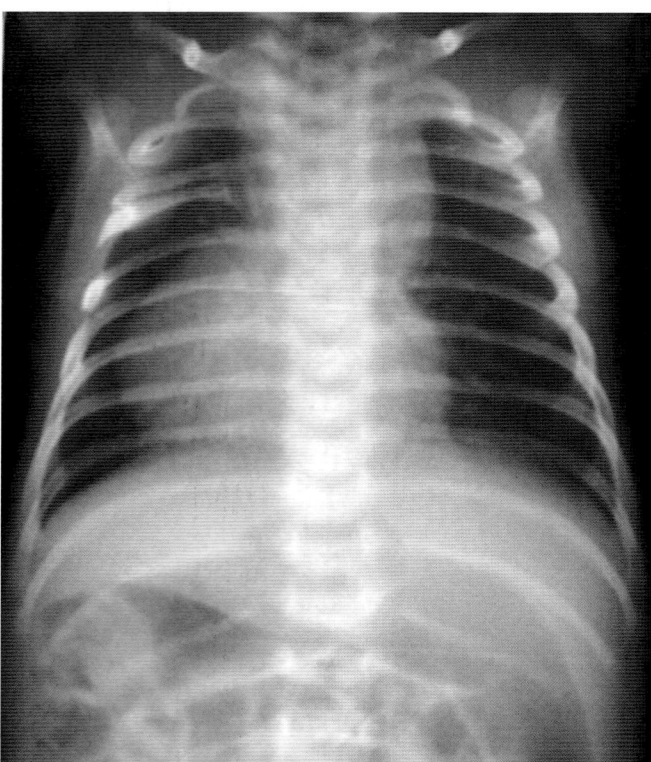

Fig. 28.5 Posteroanterior chest X-ray showing abdominal situs inversus with a midline liver and dextrocardia.

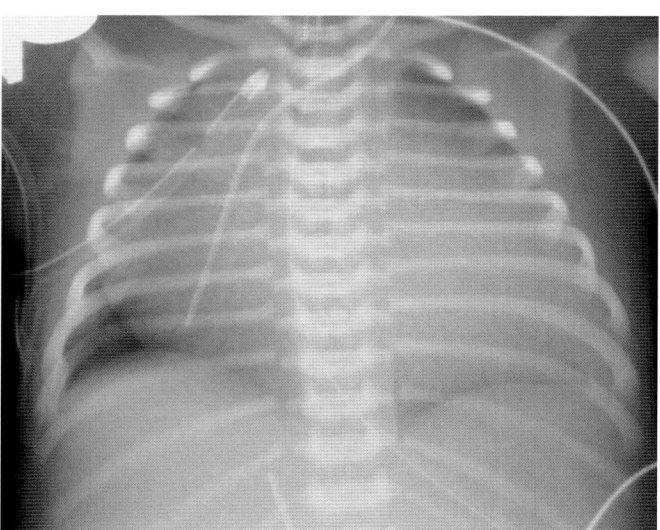

Fig. 28.6 Posteroanterior chest X-ray showing massive cardiomegaly in a neonate with severe Ebstein's anomaly.

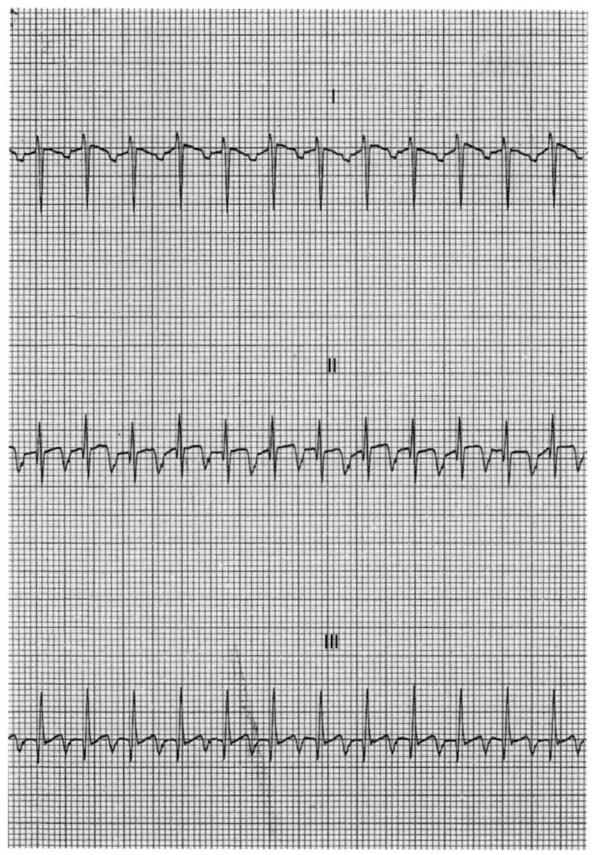

Fig. 28.7 Electrocardiogram leads I, II and III, showing inverted P wave in I. Supraventricular tachycardia at 190 beats/min.

Right atrial enlargement is indicated by tall (>2.5 mV) P waves and left atrial enlargement shown by broad (<3 mm) P waves at standard paper speed (25 mm/s).

Information on the ventricles

Abnormal ventricular positions within the chest, as in dextrocardia, or in relationship to each other, as in congenitally corrected transposition, can be suspected from abnormalities in QRS progression across the chest leads. In dextrocardia, complexes do not evolve between V_1 and V_6 but simply get progressively smaller. Q waves in V_1 mean one of the following:

- abnormal intraventricular conduction (as in left bundle branch block or some cases of pre-excitation)
- severe RV hypertrophy (RVH)
- spatial relationship between right and left ventricles abnormal (as in congenitally corrected transposition).

RVH is suggested by one or more of the following:

- right axis deviation
- Q in V_1
- large RV_1 or SV_6 (Appendix 3)
- upright T in V_1 after day 3 (Fig. 28.8).

It is important to note that conditions causing marked RVH in later infancy may cause no ECG abnormality in the immediate newborn period and only an upright T wave in V_1 in the later newborn period.

Left ventricular hypertrophy is suggested by one or more of the following:

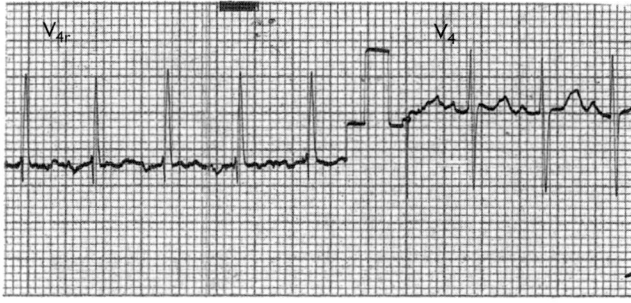

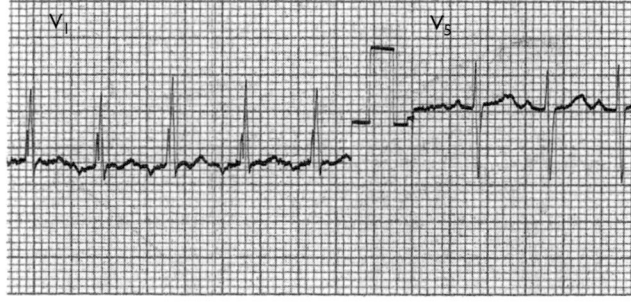

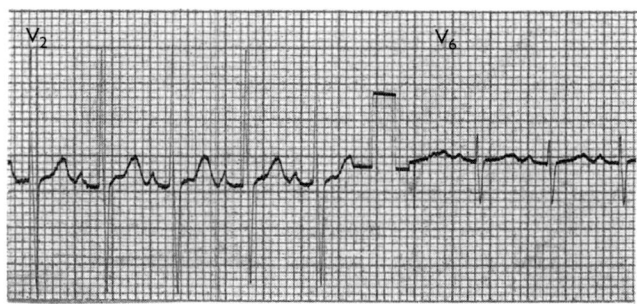

Fig. 28.8 Electrocardiogram chest leads in a 6-day-old infant. Neonatal R→S progression (normal) but upright T-wave V_1 indicating right ventricular hypertrophy.

- adult R/S progression V_1 to V_6 (dominant SV_1 dominant RV_6)
- large SV_1 or RV_6 (Appendix 3).

Biventricular hypertrophy is indicated by a combination of these findings.

Ventricular strain or ischaemia is indicted by ST depression or T-wave inversion in left chest leads (II, aVL, V_{5-6}) and may point to a primary cardiac muscle disorder or be secondary to a severe structural abnormality causing pressure or volume load on the heart. T-wave changes are seen after perinatal stress and resolve in under a week. Pericarditis is rare in the newborn period but ST segment and T-wave changes are seen.

QRS axis

The frontal QRS axis can be calculated as shown in Figure 28.9. An abnormal QRS axis may be an important diagnostic clue in a number of conditions, including AVSD (Fig. 28.10) and tricuspid atresia (QRS usually −30°); in the former case it makes the ECG a valuable screening investigation in newborn infants with Down syndrome, in whom clinical features of AVSD may be absent or very subtle.

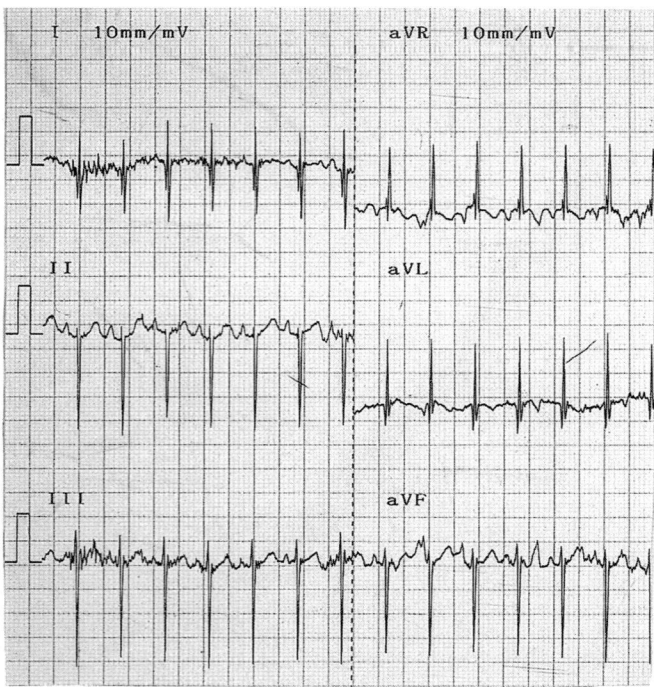

Fig. 28.9 Electrocardiogram standard leads, superior QRS axis (–90°), newborn with complete atrioventricular septal defect.

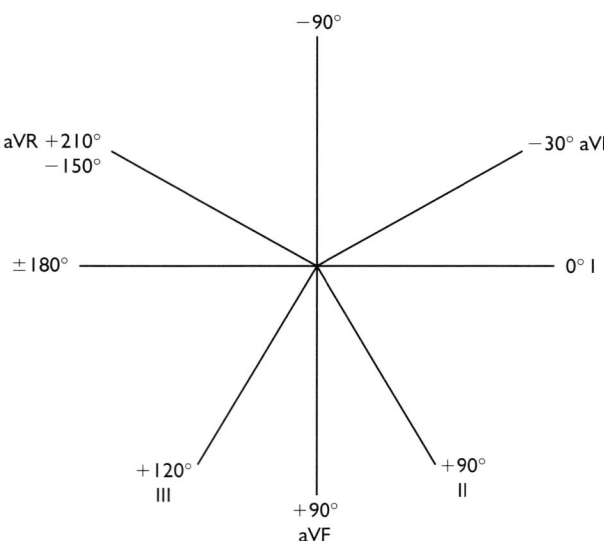

Fig. 28.10 Hexaxial reference system for calculating the frontal plane axis of the QRS complex (and of P and T waves if required). The frontal axis of the QRS complex can be estimated from the diagram showing polarity of electrocardiogram leads I, II, III, aVL, aVF and aVR. To obtain the frontal axis of a QRS complex:

1. Identify the lead in which the R and S waves are most nearly of equal size.
2. Look at right angles (190° and 290°) to the lead identified in step 1.
3. One of the leads identified in step 2 will be predominantly positive, the other predominantly negative.
4. The predominantly positive lead identified by step 3 is approximately the QRS axis (depolarisation towards a lead produces a positive deflection).
5. The approximate QRS axis obtained from step 4 can be made more accurate by estimating the equiphasic lead (step 2) more accurately by 'imagining' it between actual leads.

If all leads appear equiphasic, the QRS axis is described as indeterminate; this is rarely normal.

Pulse oximetry

Pulse oximetry has been advocated as a screening tool for CHD in newborns. Because newborns with complex CHD will often deteriorate within 48 hours of age, oximetry would be performed ideally within 24 hours of birth. However, saturations in newborns vary considerably during the first 24 hours, which can increase the false-positive rate. Most healthy newborns are now discharged before 24 hours of age, which limits the use of this technique. Oximetry should be performed on the foot of a baby breathing air. A value of less than 95% is found in about 5% of apparently well infants (Richmond et al. 2002). If these infants are further evaluated (by repeating the test initially), few cases of important structural heart disease are overlooked and some other potentially unwell infants are also detected. The American Heart Association and American Academy of Pediatrics have recently reviewed the question of pulse oximetry screening after 24 hours of age in some detail (Mahle et al. 2009). Ten studies with a population of 123 846 infants were summarised, with a false-positive rate of 0.035% when screening was done after 24 hours. Most studies used a cut-off of 95%. The detection rate for many conditions was good, but the authors conclude that additional studies are needed to determine whether this practice should become a standard of care.

Hyperoxia test and blood gas analysis

The hyperoxia (or nitrogen washout) test was described in the era before echocardiography was available and was designed to help distinguish cardiac from respiratory cyanosis without resorting to cardiac catheterisation. Babies with cyanotic heart disease usually show little rise in arterial oxygen tension in response to increased inspired oxygen. A rise of Pao_2 to a value below 20 kPa after 10 minutes in 85% or more inspired oxygen makes heart disease likely, whereas an increase in Pao_2 above 20 kPa makes respiratory disease

likely. There are some exceptions to this pattern in that babies with desaturating cardiac disease with high lung blood flow (as in unobstructed TAPVC and double-inlet ventricle, for example) will pass, whereas those with very severe respiratory disease and with PPHN may fail.

When it is essential to have an accurate measurement of arterial oxygen content, an arterial blood sample must be obtained, and further information of importance in the management of ill infants will also be available from a blood gas analysis. Transcutaneous oxygen tension monitors placed on the right upper chest (that is, preductal) can be used instead of arterial sampling as a screening test if other information is not required. Oxygen pulse saturation monitors will not provide the same assurance of a pass, as an infant will show 100% saturation at a Pao_2 value well below 20 kPa. The role of the hyperoxia test has therefore changed since its inception, but it is still helpful in two circumstances:

1. When a well baby seems dusky and there is uncertainty as to whether a cyanotic cardiac condition is present. A failed transcutaneous or pulse oximeter hyperoxia test strongly points to cyanotic heart disease.
2. A well baby with signs of heart disease who looks pink may fail the hyperoxia test, thus alerting the physician to the presence of a more complex lesion.

Echocardiography

Transthoracic echocardiography has revolutionised the diagnosis and management of neonatal heart disease. The non-invasive, immediate and portable nature makes this modality ideally suited to the investigation of even the smallest babies. It can define structure and function and has resulted in a dramatic reduction in the need for diagnostic cardiac catheterisation. It is now widely used to guide interventions such as balloon atrial septostomy on the intensive care unit.

The sequential and segmental approach forms the basis of diagnosis of all CHD. A detailed description of this is beyond the scope of this chapter but can be found in Anderson et al. (2002). This systematic approach ensures that subtle complex problems are not overlooked even in the most complex malformations. All examinations should begin with indirect evaluation of atrial situs using the great vessels at the level of the diaphragm (Figs 28.11 and 28.12). This is followed by establishing the position of the cardiac apex in the chest from a subcostal view. The same echocardiographic window allows identification of the systemic and pulmonary venous drainage and evaluation of the atrial septum. This is followed by establishing the AV connection and assessment of the AV valves. Next, the position and morphology of the ventricles are established and the ventricular septum is assessed; this is most easily viewed from the cardiac apex. Following this, the ventriculoatrial connections are documented together with the relationship of the great arteries. Assessment of the semilunar valves is followed by documentation of the coronary arteries. From the parasternal views, the branch pulmonary arteries are identified and the aortic arch with the head and neck vessels seen from the suprasternal position. Finally, assessment of function is evaluated using m-mode from a parasternal long-axis view.

Table 28.9 Uses of different ultrasound modalities

MODALITY	USES
Two-dimensional imaging	Defining anatomy Chamber size, wall thickness Function (qualitative)
Doppler	Assessment of direction and velocity of flow, turbulence and flow patterns
Colour flow	Rapid identification of site of abnormal flow patterns and flow direction Detection of regurgitation and small shunts
Pulsed wave	Sampling flow patterns in a localised region May be inaccurate with high velocities Calculation of cardiac output
Continuous wave	Excellent for high velocities Abnormal flow patterns not precisely localised
M mode	Dimensions and function

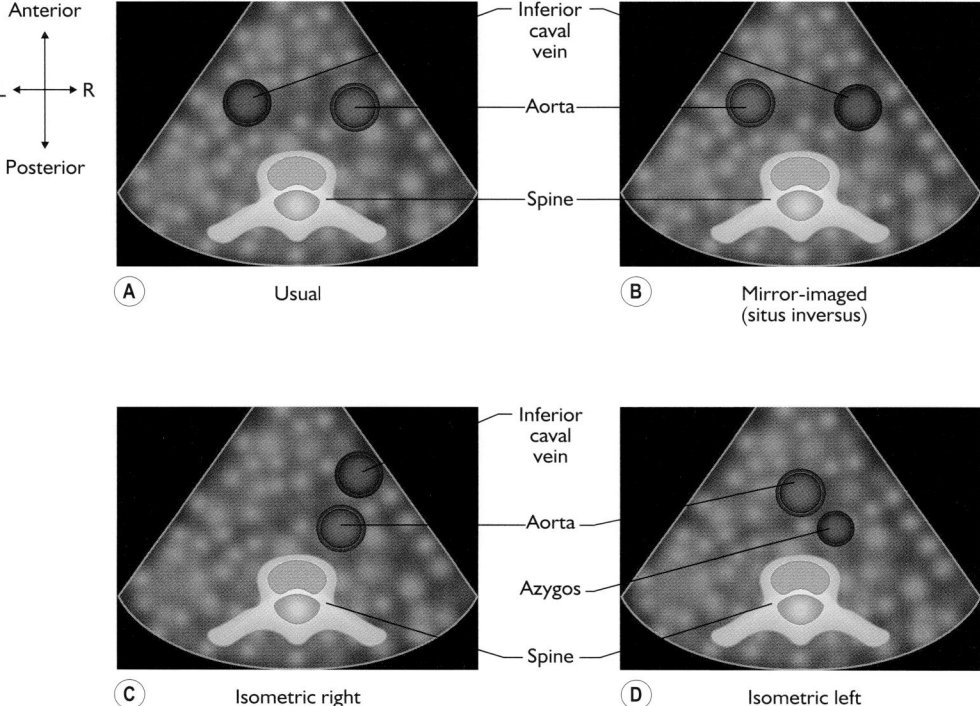

Fig. 28.11 Diagrammatic representation of echocardiographic images of arrangement of great vessels at the level of the diaphragm in: (A) normal atrial situs, (B) mirror-imaged arrangement, (C) right and (D) left atrial isomerism.

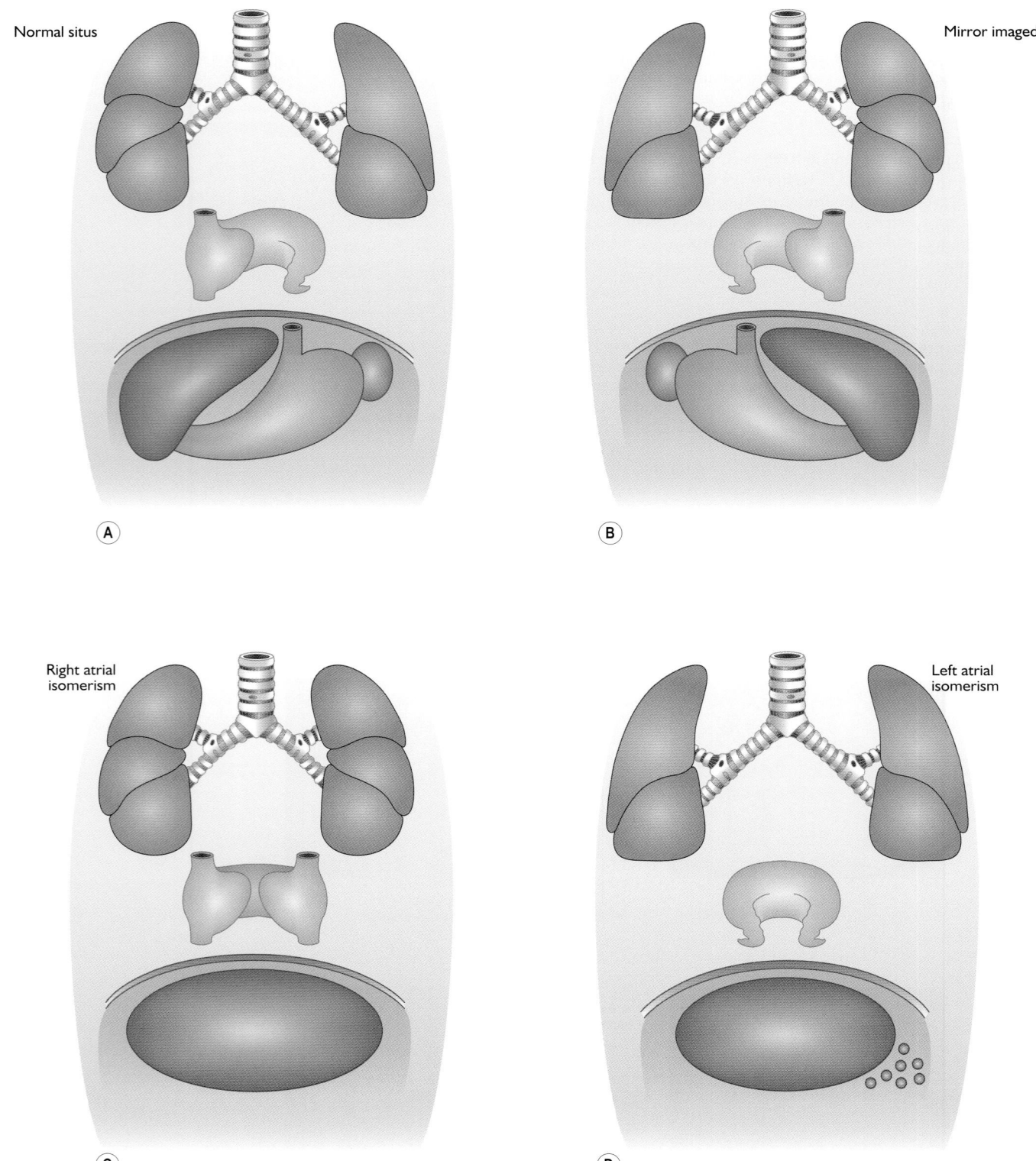

Normal situs

Mirror imaged

(A)

(B)

Right atrial
isomerism

Left atrial
isomerism

(C)

(D)

Fig. 28.12 Schematic representation of: (A) normal situs, (B) mirror-imaged arrangement, (C) right and (D) left atrial isomerism.

All ultrasound modalities have a role in evaluating the cardiovascular system (Table 28.9). Newer ultrasound modalities such as three-dimensional and four-dimensional imaging as well as new Doppler techniques including Doppler tissue imaging and strain imaging are becoming more widely used in the management of CHD but have limited applications in routine neonatal practice at present. More detailed descriptions of these techniques are found in other sources (Mertens et al. 2008).

Standard two-dimensional imaging gives anatomical detail. Doppler identifies or clarifies shunt lesions and regions of turbulent flow and allows quantification of stenosis by measuring blood velocity. This enables calculation of a pressure difference across a valve or between ventricles through a VSD using the modified Bernoulli equation ($P = 4V^2$, where P = instantaneous peak systolic pressure gradient in mmHg, V = velocity distal to the site of obstruction in m/s).

Standard echocardiographic windows and images of the heart are shown in Figure 28.13; examples of clinical scans are given in Figures 28.14–28.16. Transthoracic echocardiograms may be technically difficult in babies with severe respiratory disease on assisted ventilation. Many of these infants are premature and of low birthweight. As echocardiographic skills become more widespread, telemedicine provides the means whereby neonatal units can collaborate with cardiac centres to analyse recorded echocardiographic studies, helping in the decision-making about whether a baby needs transfer to a tertiary cardiac unit (Casey 1999).

Cardiac catheterisation

Cardiac catheterisation and angiography was once the principal means of investigating babies with CHD. It may be diagnostic for anatomical or haemodynamic information or may be therapeutic. Diagnostic catheterisation is now rarely required in the newborn baby with present-day ultrasound capability and other non-invasive imaging modalities. When it is, usually only a small amount of information is required in order to complement that already obtained by echocardiography. Cardiac catheterisation in small children carries a small but definite risk and almost inevitably requires general anaesthesia. This will influence cardiac physiology and the relevance of the information obtained.

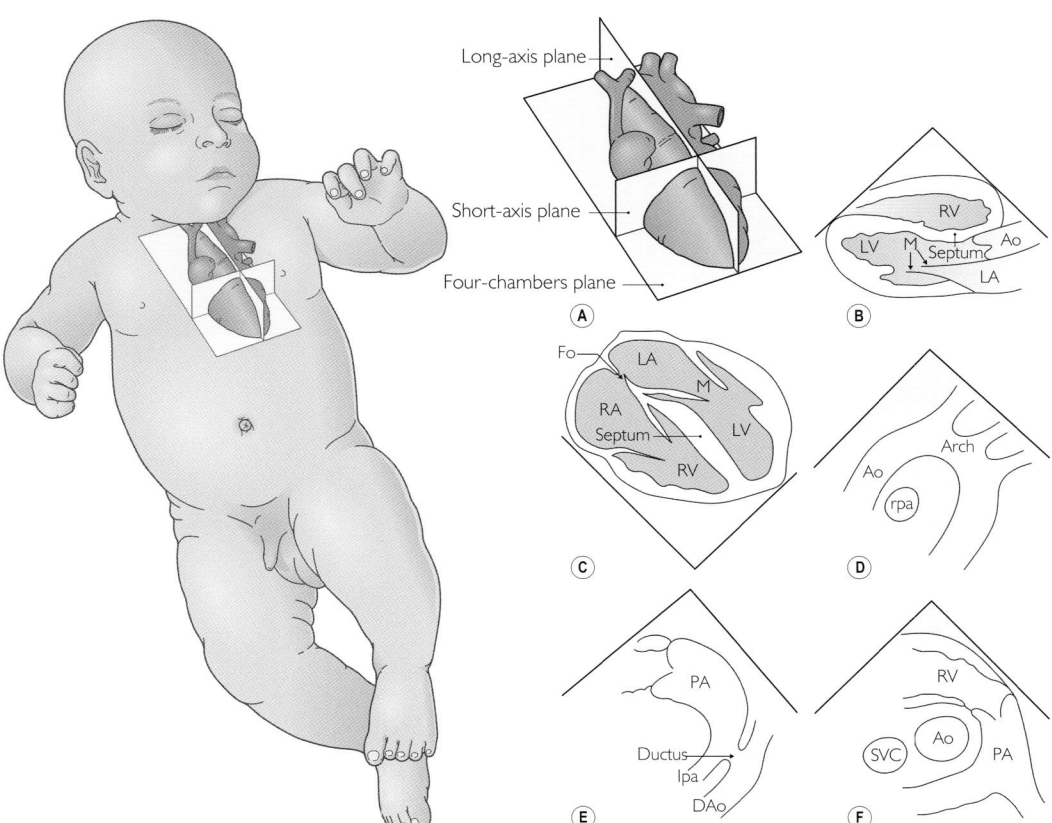

Fig. 28.13 (A) Diagram illustrating echocardiographic cross-sectional planes (two-dimensional). The long-axis plane is approximately sagittal; the four-chambers plane is approximately frontal; the short-axis plane is approximately transverse. (B–F) Diagrammatic representations of normal, cross-sectional views. (B) Long-axis cut as seen with the transducer in the parasternal position. (C) Four-chambers cut as seen from the subxiphoid site. (D) Semi-long-axis cut of the aortic arch as obtained from the suprasternal view. (E) High long-axis cut (parasagittal) to show the ductus arteriosus. (F) Short-axis cut through the great arteries just above the heart. Ao, aorta; Dao, descending aorta; Fo, foramen ovale; LA, left atrium; lpa, left pulmonary artery; LV, left ventricle; m, mitral valve leaflets; PA, pulmonary artery; RA, right atrium; rpa, right pulmonary artery; RV, right ventricle; svc, superior vena cava; t, tricuspid valve leaflets. *(Reproduced from Wilkinson and Cooke 1992.)*

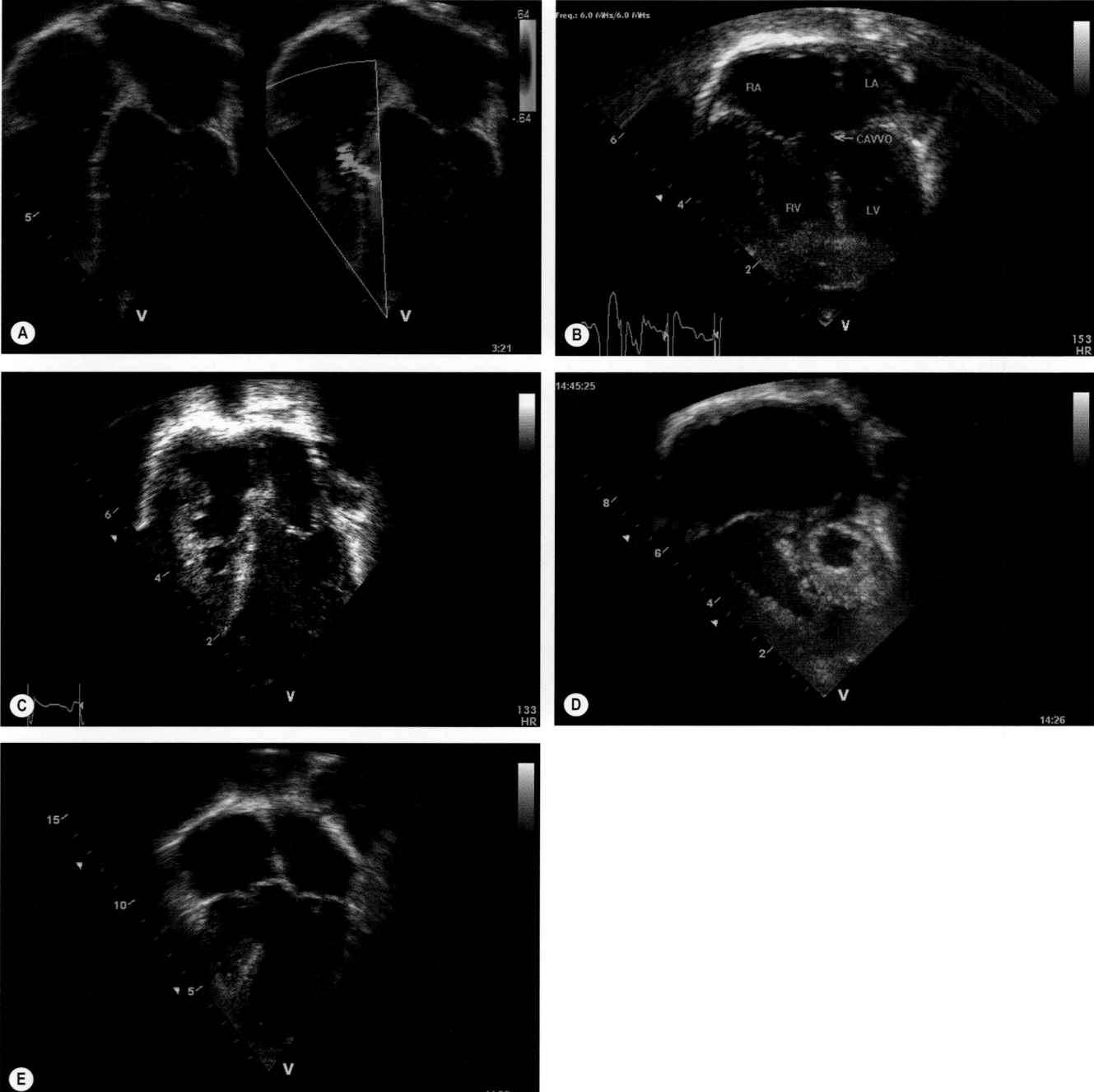

Fig. 28.14 (A) Apical four-chamber view with colour flow showing small mid-muscular ventricular septal defect (VSD). (B) Apical four-chamber view of an atrioventricular septal defect with a common atrioventricular valve orifice (CAVVO) and moderate atrial and ventricular components. The ventricles are balanced. LA, left atrium; LV, left ventricle; RA, right atrium; RV, right ventricle. (C) Apical four-chamber view showing small hypertrophied right ventricle with small tricuspid valve in a patient with pulmonary atresia and intact ventricular septum (hypoplastic right heart). (D) Apical four-chamber view showing hypoplastic left-heart syndrome with small hypertrophied left ventricle (see Fig. 28.20). (E) Apical four-chamber view of double-inlet left ventricle with VSD and hypoplastic right ventricle.

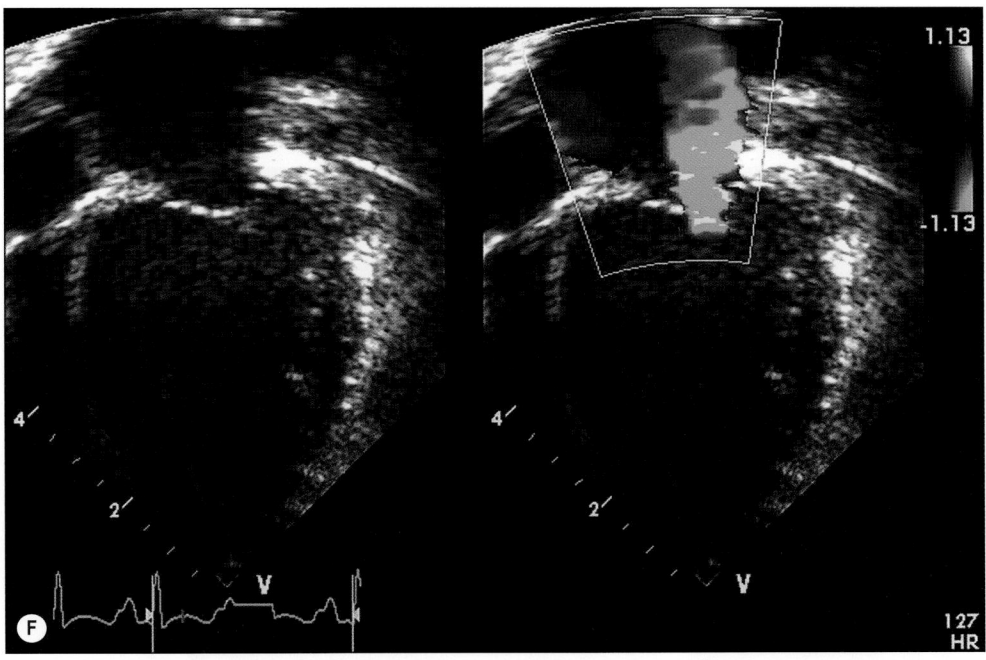

Fig. 28.14, cont'd (F) Apical four-chamber view of dilated cardiomyopathy with severe left atrial and left ventricular dilatation. Mitral regurgitation is seen on colour flow mapping.

Magnetic resonance and computed tomographic imaging

MRI provides excellent anatomical images, but, in the newborn, echocardiography often provides adequate information. The range of uses for cardiac MRI scanning in the newborn is continuing to expand as greater experience is obtained in older children and scanning technology improves. It can provide useful non-invasive anatomical information about pulmonary arterial abnormalities previously only obtainable from angiography. MRI involves no radiation hazard, but does require sedation or general anaesthesia in an environment where detailed monitoring is rather more complicated to achieve. In contrast, computed tomographic (CT) imaging, which requires shorter acquisition times and can frequently be performed with sedation alone, does have a role as a non-invasive imaging technique in neonates. It provides excellent information about aortic arch anatomy and other vascular structures (Fig. 28.17) and the relationship of the vascular structures to the airways but its drawback is the radiation dose required to acquire such images.

Treatment

General principles

In principle, medical management for CHD is largely supportive (e.g. heart failure) whereas significant structural abnormalities usually require intervention. Continued improvement in surgical results for congenital cardiac malformations has been one of the triumphs of modern paediatric cardiology. Surgical mortality for malformations, which were, up to recently, considered untreatable (e.g. hypoplastic left-heart syndrome (HLHS)) is now very acceptable. In addition, improvements in surgical results have meant a major shift in surgical emphasis away from surgical palliation towards primary neonatal correction of structural abnormalities with restoration of normal physiology wherever possible. This has been further facilitated by the advances occurring in neonatal intensive care both pre- and postoperatively.

Attention to the general aspects of medical care to achieve stability and optimise condition prior to transfer and intervention of any kind is a very important aspect of minimising morbidity and mortality for any cardiac condition. There are some specific areas related to the care of neonates with cardiac disease that require further mention.

Ductal manipulation

Establishing and maintaining an open DA is a crucial part of the resuscitation of babies with duct-dependent pulmonary or systemic circulations and usually greatly improves oxygenation in TGA. Prostaglandin E_1 and E_2 will both dilate the DA. Dosage regimens for both drugs are given in Table 28.10. Acute side-effects of prostaglandin include apnoea, jitteriness, convulsions, diarrhoea, flushing and fever and are dose-dependent. These are usually manageable without loss of therapeutic effect by stopping the infusion for a few minutes and restarting it at a lower dose. Long-term oral or nasogastric use is described (Silove et al. 1985) but of limited value. Manipulation of the DA in order to close it is considered on pages 645–647.

Heart failure

Management of heart failure is outlined in Table 28.11. Treatment of acute heart failure is considered under collapse, below. On a more chronic basis, minimising fluid restriction is necessary to achieve as good a nutritional state as possible. It is usually possible

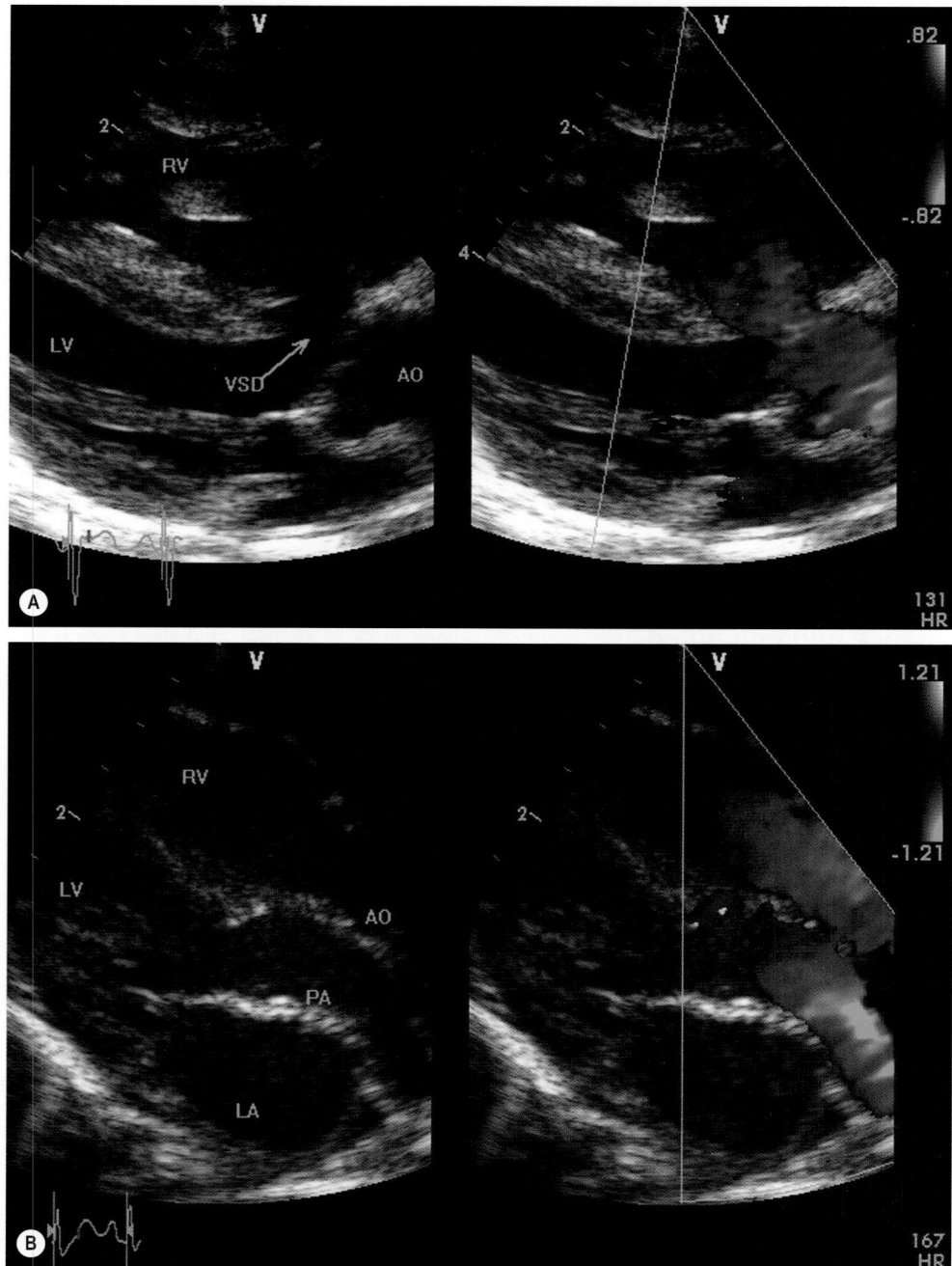

Fig. 28.15 (A) Parasternal long-axis view of a patient with tetralogy of Fallot showing subaortic ventricular septal defect. Note the flow from right ventricle to aorta seen on the colour flow mapping. Ao, aorta; LV, left ventricle; RV, right ventricle; VSD, ventricular septal defect. (B) Parasternal long-axis view showing diagnostic arrangement of the great vessels in transposition of the great arteries, which have a parallel arrangement as they arise from their respective ventricles. Ao, aorta; LA, left atrium; LV, left ventricle; PA, pulmonary artery; RV, right ventricle.

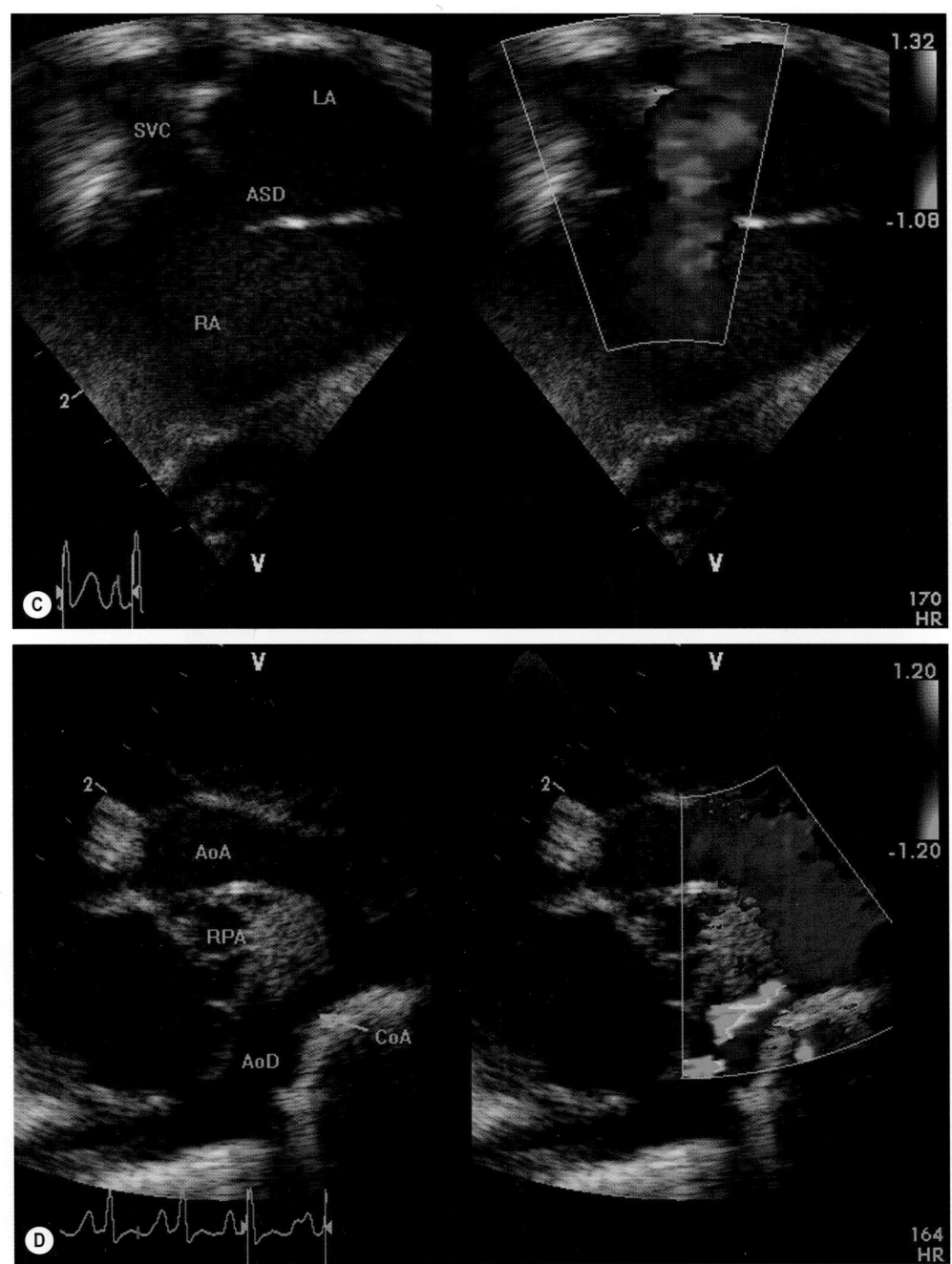

Fig. 28.15, cont'd (C) Subcostal four-chamber view of the atrial septum showing large secundum atrial septal defect with left-to-right flow seen on colour flow mapping. ASD, atrial septal defect; LA, left atrium; RA, right atrium; SVC, superior vena cava. (D) Suprasternal view showing aortic arch with coarctation. Narrowed area of aortic arch highlighted with flow disturbance seen on colour flow mapping.

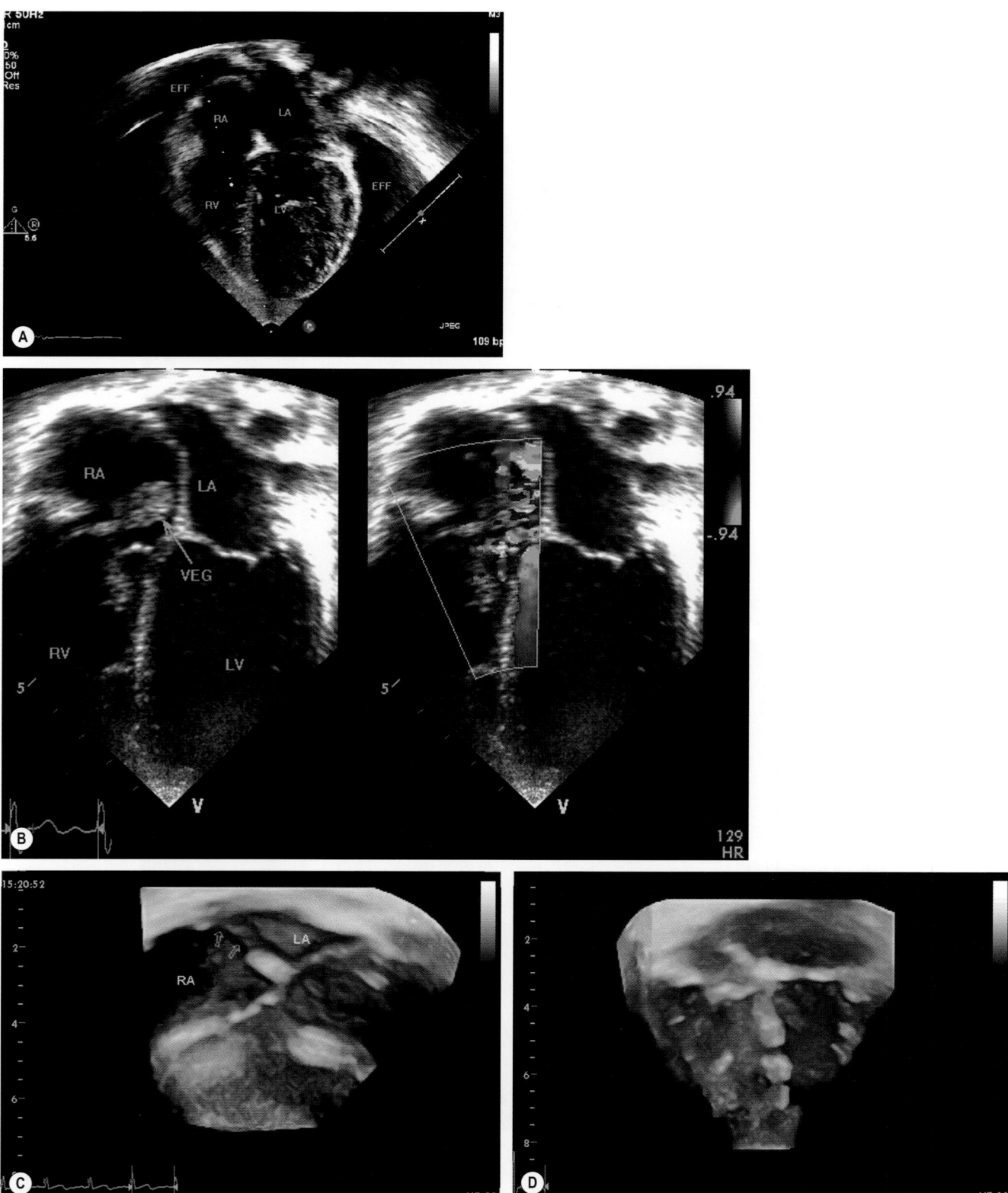

Fig. 28.16 (A) Apical four-chamber view showing global pericardial effusion (EFF, effusion). (B) Apical four-chamber view showing tricuspid valve vegetation in bacterial endocarditis (VEG, vegetation). Colour flow mapping shows moderate tricuspid regurgitation associated with the vegetation. (C) Volume-rendered three-dimensional echo image of a secundum atrial septal defect seen from the subcostal projection. (D) Volume-rendered three-dimensional echo image of multiple apical muscular ventricular septal defects seen in a four-chamber projection. LA, left atrium; LV, left ventricle; RA, right atrium; RV, right ventricle.

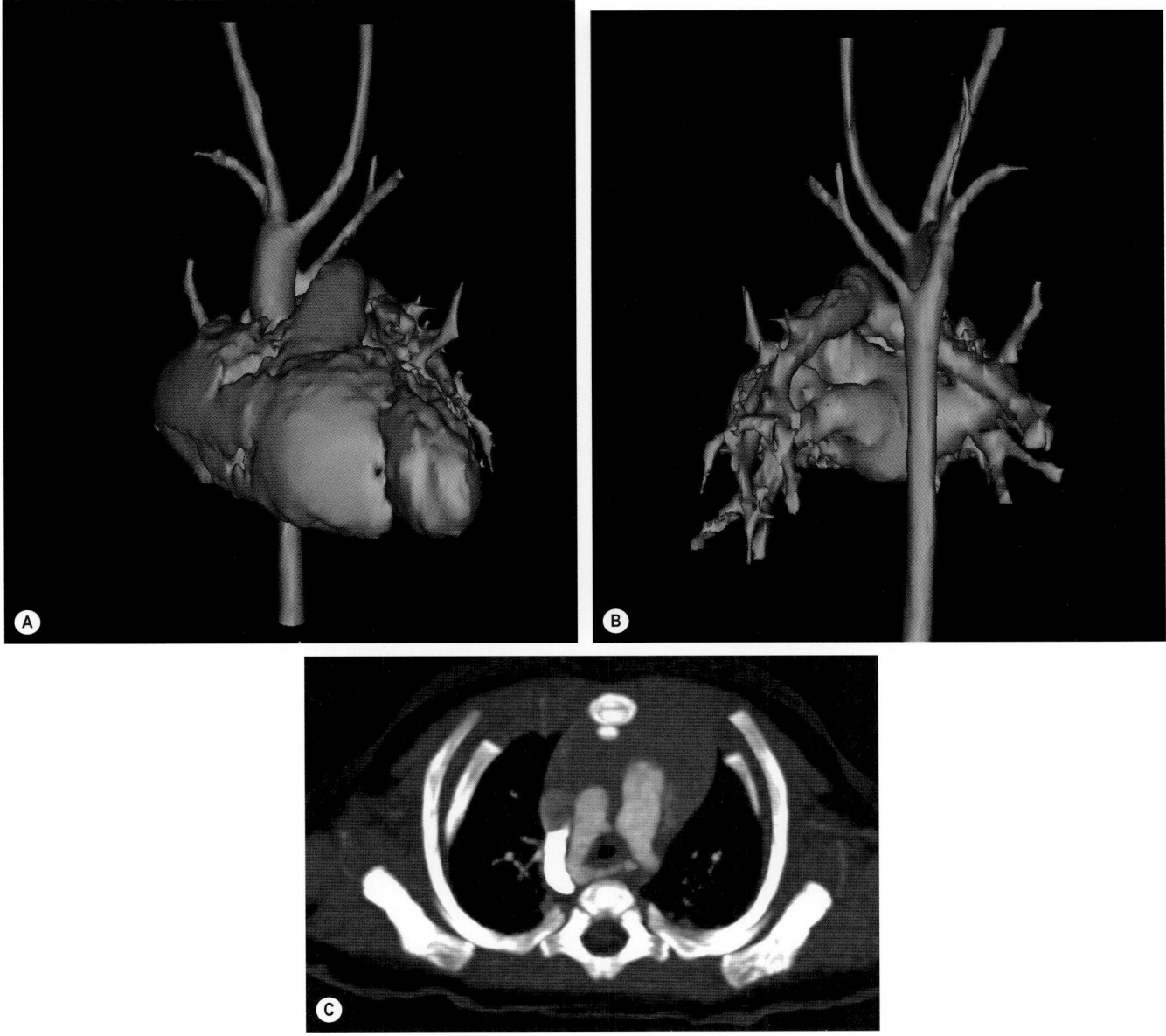

Fig. 28.17 (A) Volume-rendered computed tomography angiogram (anterior view) showing a right-sided aortic arch with aberrant left subclavian artery (LSCA). (B) Same image (posterior view). This aortic arch anatomy is usually associated with a left-sided arterial duct arising adjacent to the origin of the aberrant left subclavian artery creating a loose vascular ring. (C) Axial contrast-enhanced image, in the same patient, showing a right-sided arch with the origin of LSCA arising posterior to the trachea.

to regulate fluid status with diuretics and allow a good volume intake. Additives to increase the calorific value of milk are almost invariably needed and nasogastric feeding may be required. Loop diuretics may cause hyponatraemia, necessitating a reduction of dose with modest fluid restriction if necessary or changing to thiazide diuretics. Moitoring of serum sodium is an important part of managing heart failure in neonates on diuretics but increasing sodium supplements in this context is to be avoided if possible, as this will also cause fluid retention. There is considerable experience of angiotensin-converting enzyme (ACE) inhibitor usage in infancy (Montigny et al. 1989). There are greater risks in the use of ACE inhibitors in newborns (Lee et al. 2010) and preterm newborns appear to tolerate ACE inhibition poorly. If an ACE inhibitor is to be used, it is important to ensure that renal function is normal, avoid dehydration with diuretics before commencing the drug and increase the dosage gradually to therapeutic levels. Digoxin may be of value in chronic heart failure associated with poor muscle function, but neither drug should be used when dynamic left ventricular outflow obstruction is present.

Antiarrhythmic drugs

Arrhythmias and their management are considered on pages 661–663. Doses of commonly used antiarrhythmic agents are given in Table 28.28.

Table 28.10 Prostaglandin (PG) dosage regimens

DRUG AND ROUTE	DOSE	COMMENT
PGE$_1$ i.v.	0.005–0.1 µg/kg/min	For severe cyanosis or shock, start at higher dose range for both drugs and increase at 15–30-minute intervals to maximum if no response. More than threefold increase in dose rarely needed. Side-effects increase with higher doses
PGE$_2$ i.v.	0.005–0.05 µg/kg/min	

NB. In antenatally diagnosed duct-dependent congenital heart disease, elective prostaglandin infusion should be started at the lowest dose (5–10 ng/kg/min) as this will minimise side-effects whilst maintaining ductal patency.

Table 28.11 Heart failure management

ACUTE	CHRONIC
Resuscitate as needed for collapse/shock with ventilation, colloids and inotropic support	Avoid fluid restriction if possible, in order to maximise calorie intake
Restrict fluid to approximately two-thirds maintenance	Optimise calorie intake (high-calorie formula/supplements, nasogastric feeding)
Furosemide i.v. 1 mg/kg 6–12-hourly	Oral diuretic: furosemide 2–6 mg/kg/day (in two or three doses) and potassium-sparing diuretic or potassium supplement
Optimise oxygenation, avoid hyperoxia	If heart muscle dysfunction, consider angiotensin-converting enzyme inhibitor and/or digoxin
Treat anaemia	Treat anaemia if present

Interventional catheterisation

There has been a spectacular increase in the range of interventional catheter techniques for the management of congenital cardiac malformations. Therapeutic catheterisation for some procedures can be performed under ultrasound control, such as for balloon septostomy, but more complex therapeutic interventions usually require X-ray screening. Conditions treated in the newborn period by interventional cardiac catheterisation are listed in Table 28.12. The range of conditions amenable to interventional cardiac catheterisation in the newborn continues to expand (e.g. stenting of PDA or RV outflow in pulmonary atresia or severe tetralogy of Fallot), complementing surgical advances and sometimes avoiding the need for surgery in low-birthweight infants. Development of hybrid interventional catheter and surgical procedures is also increasing, with first-stage palliation of HLHS being the most well-developed example (Galantowicz et al. 2008).

Vascular access can be obtained via the umbilicus or percutaneously in the femoral region. Babies will invariably require general anaesthesia, and extra attention to body temperature, blood glucose, circulating volume, acid–base balance and ventilation is necessary to ensure that risk of the procedure is minimised. Mortality in diagnostic and interventional catheterisation in the newborn is less than 1%, but acute morbidity may occur in up to 25% of interventional procedures. This area is changing all the time and choosing between surgical and catheter interventions for the same condition is influenced by many factors (Andrews and Tulloh 2004).

Surgery

Cardiac surgery can be subdivided into two major groups according to whether the operation requires the use of the cardiopulmonary bypass machine. Open cardiac surgery requiring cardiopulmonary bypass is used for intracardiac repairs (e.g. arterial switch operation for repair of transposition, repair of TAPVC) and also for staged palliative surgery for complex cardiac lesions (e.g. HLHS). Closed operations do not require cardiopulmonary bypass (as in coarctation repair, clipping of the DA, Blalock–Taussig systemic-to-pulmonary anastomoses and pulmonary artery banding) and the surgery is shorter and, for the most part, lower risk than open cardiac surgery. Open operations are generally performed through a median sternotomy whereas closed operations are more commonly performed through a posterolateral thoracotomy. Practice will vary from centre to centre but, in most centres, neonatal primary correction is the treatment of choice in simple and complex TGA, TAPVC, interrupted aortic arch and common arterial trunk. Operative mortalities are given in the discussion of particular conditions. As surgical mortality rates improve, there has been increasing awareness of the morbidity associated with complex CHD (Limperopoulos et al. 2000). Attributing such problems to individual surgical techniques (such as low-flow bypass versus deep hypothermic circulatory arrest) has failed to yield consistent results. There is increasing evidence to support a multifactorial aetiology for brain injury occurring in association with complex CHD with a significant proportion of the damage occurring preoperatively, as evidenced by detailed MRI scanning undertaken before surgery (Miller and McQuillen 2007).

Persistent pulmonary hypertension of the newborn

Therapy is considered in Chapter 27, part 2.

Cardiovascular problems in the preterm infant

General considerations

The combination of CHD and prematurity adversely affects the outcome for the baby in relation to both the prematurity and for any given structural cardiac malformation. Improvements in the care of preterm infants and increased detection of fetal cardiac disease have meant an increasing number of premature, low-birthweight infants are surviving with congenital heart defects. A discussion about the patent arterial duct in the preterm infant

Table 28.12 Interventional cardiac catheterisation in newborn infants

TECHNIQUE	COMMENT
Balloon septostomy	TGA and restrictive PFO in mitral restriction or hypoplastic right heart
Balloon dilatation	
Pulmonary valve	Procedure of choice for stenosis
Aortic valve	First choice in most centres for stenosis
Coarctation	Lower success and higher complication rates than surgery
Infundibulum	Occasionally in TOF with severe RVOTO (±RVOT stenting)
Pulmonary atresia	Becoming widespread if no VSD Occasionally used if VSD present Radiofrequency-assisted perforation and valvuloplasty
Stent techniques	
Ductus arteriosus	As an alternative to systemic to PA shunt in some duct-dependent lesions Being explored as part of initial palliation of hypoplastic left heart
Embolisation/occlusion techniques	
Cerebral AVM	Treatment of choice for neonates in heart failure
Scimitar syndrome	For aberrant arterial supply to right or left lung
Patent arterial duct	Coil occlusion device: closure of PDA occasionally appropriate

TGA, transposition of the great arteries; PFO, patent foramen ovale; TOF, tetralogy of Fallot; RVOTO, RVOT, right ventricular outflow tract; VSD, ventricular septal defect; PA, pulmonary atresia; AVM, arteriovenous malformation; PDA, patent ductus arteriosus.

follows but other types of structural cardiac disease deserve mention. Persisting atrial communications are common in preterm infants but do not usually cause problems unless associated with additional defects such as a large patent arterial duct. Reducing the shunt by closing the duct is often enough to avoid problems. In other defects, the baby is often too small to be considered for corrective or even palliative surgery. In babies with a large left-to-right shunt through a VSD the effects of the left-to-right shunt will frequently worsen the lung disease associated with prematurity, increasing both mortality and morbidity. Early pulmonary artery banding to reduce pulmonary blood flow is useful provided the baby is of sufficient size and is well enough to tolerate the procedure. In duct-dependent lesions, it has been possible to maintain ductal patency with prostaglandin whilst the baby grows big enough to be considered for surgical or catheter intervention (Barker et al. 2005). This is better tolerated when the pulmonary blood supply is duct-dependent rather than the systemic circulation, probably because the duct is smaller and more restrictive in the former group of patients. When the systemic circulation is duct-dependent, the duct is large and, as

PVR falls, there is steal from the systemic circulation to the pulmonary circulation. This increases the risks of necrotising enterocolitis and exacerbates the pulmonary problems associated with prematurity. Published data confirm the poor outlook in premature babies with CHD (Andrews et al. 2006).

Patent ductus arteriosus

Closure of the DA in term babies occurs in two phases. First, the increased Pao_2 which occurs within a few hours of birth, together with the decreased circulating prostaglandins, allows the smooth muscle of the DA to constrict. Constriction causes the inner muscular wall of the DA to become ischaemic and hypoxic, promoting formation of vascular endothelial growth factor, which in turn results in production of other growth factors, transforming the DA into a non-contractile ligament (Clyman et al. 1999). In preterm infants the DA will often fail to constrict, and, in those in whom constriction occurs, complete occlusion does not occur as the profound hypoxia required to achieve this fails to develop. It is the profound hypoxia that drives the inflammatory cascade that results in cell death and remodelling. In the term baby the vasa vasorum are occluded during ductal constriction, causing the hypoxia. In the preterm infant the ductus is so thin-walled that the vasa vasorum are not required for transport of oxygen and nutrients to the vessel wall. These are derived from the lumen of the ductus instead and therefore the wall of the ductus is unable to develop the hypoxia required to achieve remodelling (Clyman et al. 1999). This enables the DA to reopen with its associated haemodynamic consequences.

A persistent DA is diagnosed when the DA fails to close after 72 hours. Symptoms will develop in 50–70% of infants at <28 weeks' gestation or with a birthweight of less than 1000 g (Hammerman and Kaplan 1990). Clinical complications will depend on the degree of left-to-right shunting through the DA, which causes increased left ventricular output and a redistribution of blood flow that can result in metabolic acidosis, intracranial haemorrhage, necrotising enterocolitis and pulmonary oedema or haemorrhage (Clyman 1996). In those babies with a persistent DA, prophylactic closure of the DA would seem attractive but has been, and remains, one of the most hotly debated topics in neonatal medicine (Benitz 2010). Concern remains about administration of a drug known to have deleterious side-effects on cerebral, renal and splanchnic blood flow. Yet there is strong clinical and experimental evidence to support the fact that the efficacy of indometacin decreases with advancing postnatal age (Hermes-DeSantos and Clyman 2006). This dilemma is worsened by the fact that it is very difficult to predict which babies will go on to develop clinical complications as a result of a persistent DA. There is evidence that a DA minimum diameter on colour flow Doppler of 1.5 mm or greater in babies less than 1500 g birthweight and postnatal age less than 10 days is strongly predictive of the development of symptoms (Kluckow and Evans 1995). A left atrial to aortic root ratio of greater than 1.5 after the first day of age also helps predict problems (Iyer et al. 1994). The Doppler waveform across the ductus (Fig. 28.18B, D, F) has been used to predict development of a symptomatic DA in a similar group of babies under 5 days old (Su et al. 1997) and in managing drug treatment (Su et al. 1999). Su and colleagues (1999) identified low-velocity (not above 1.5 m/s) left-to-right shunting through the DA (termed a pulsatile pattern: Fig. 28.14D) in the first 4 days after birth in ventilated babies under 1500 g birthweight as indicating a high risk of developing symptomatic DA (sensitivity 93.5%, specificity 100%) as opposed to a closing pattern (Fig. 28.18B), which was not associated with the development of symptoms.

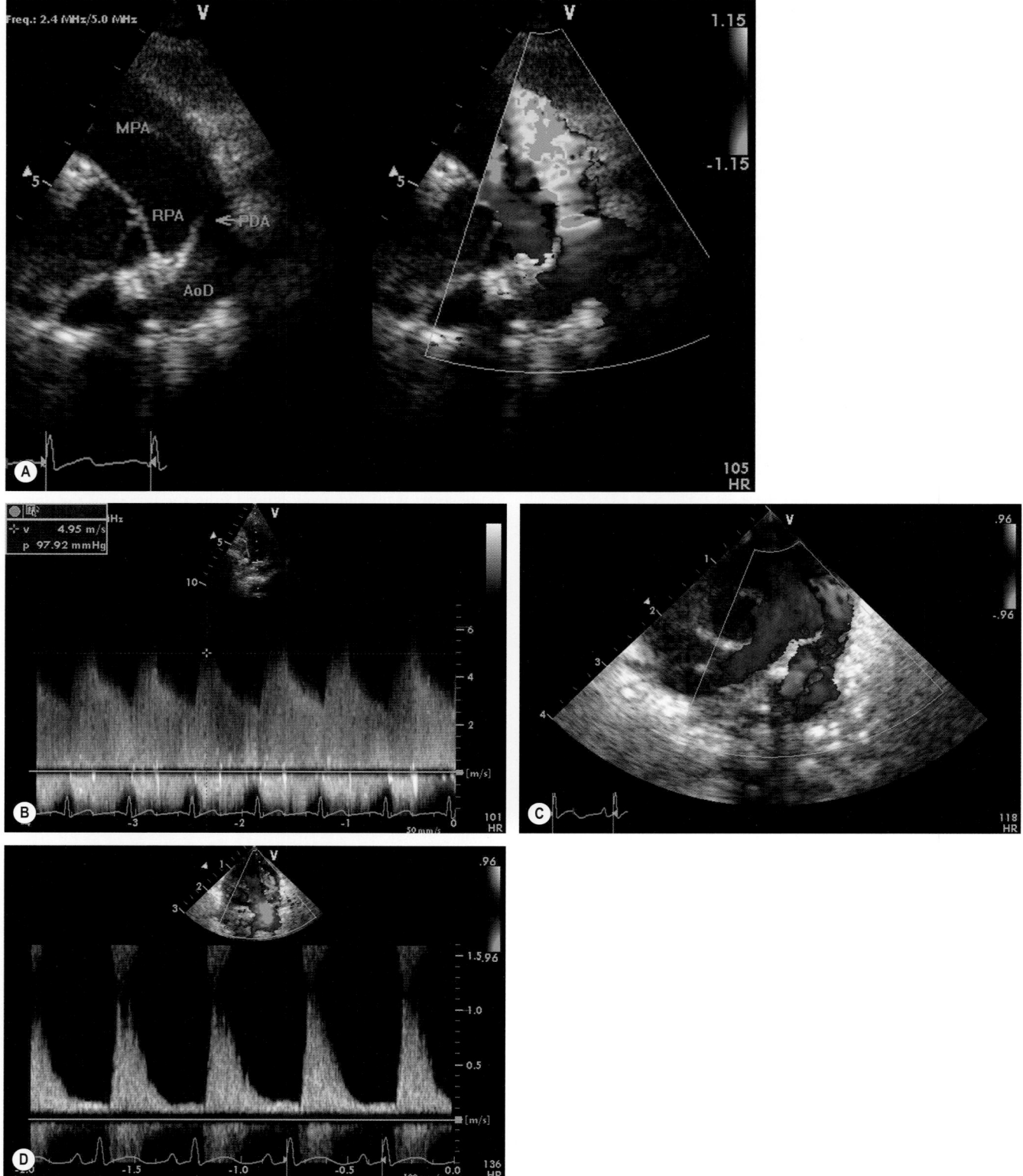

Fig. 28.18 (A) High parasternal short-axis view showing the arterial duct (patent ductus arteriosus: PDA) and the relationship with the main pulmonary artery (MPA) and descending aorta (AoD). Adjacent colour flow mapping image shows turbulent flow through a modest-sized PDA. (B) Spectral Doppler trace from the same patient shows high-velocity left-to-right flow (closing pattern). (C) Similar view to (A), with colour flow mapping showing laminar left-to-right flow through the PDA. (D) Spectral Doppler trace from same patient as in (C) with low-velocity left-to-right flow through the PDA (pulsatile pattern).

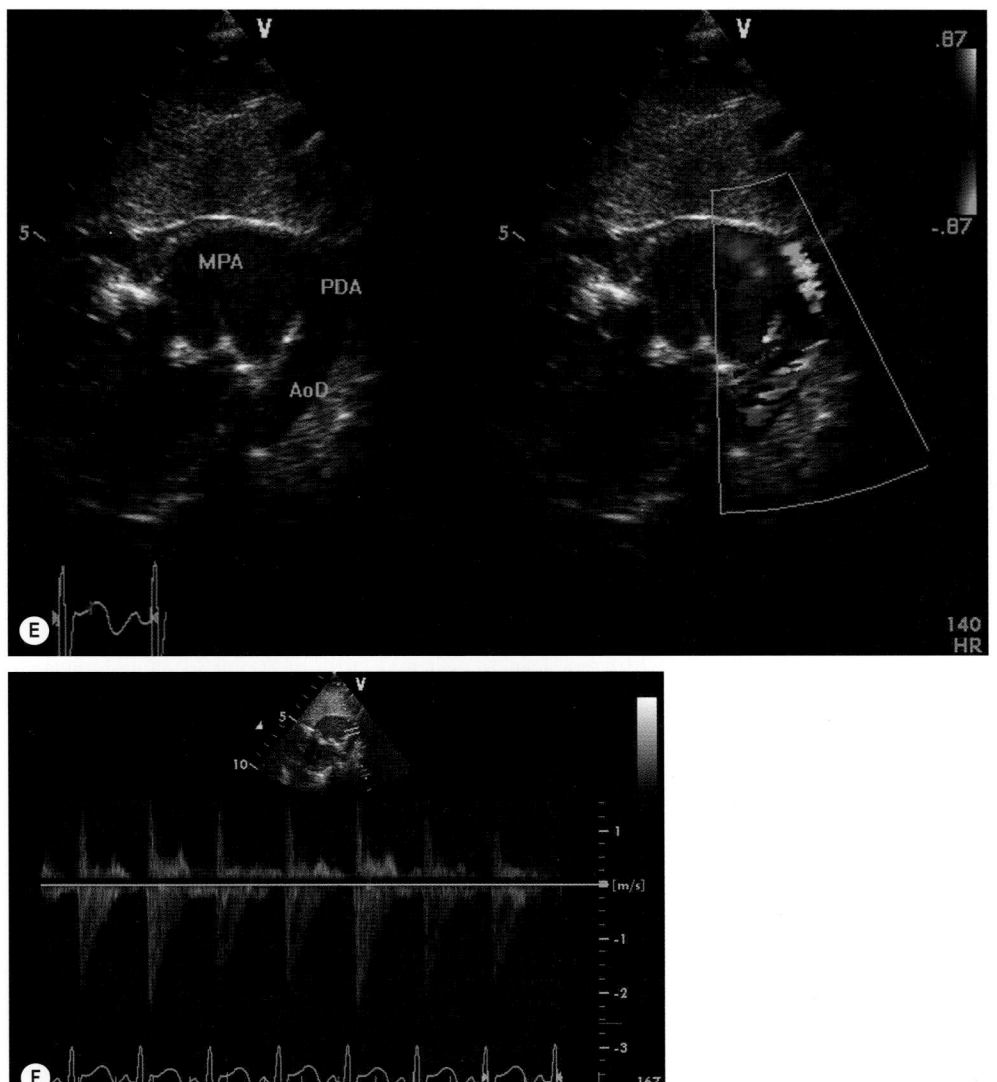

Fig. 28.18, cont'd (E) Similar view to (A) with a large PDA and right-to-left flow seen on colour flow mapping suggestive of pulmonary hypertension. (F) Spectral Doppler trace from same patient as in (E) confirming right-to-left flow associated with hypertension and, in this case, aortic coarctation.

Many thousands of babies have been enrolled in large numbers of trials to evaluate the benefit of prophylactic treatment of persistent DA. The largest of these (TIPP study; Schmidt et al. 2001) compared the effects of three daily doses of indometacin (100 μg/kg) with placebo in 1200 babies (birthweight <1000 g) given from day 1 of life. Their conclusions were that early prophylactic indometacin was associated with:

- significant reduction in PDA in the treated group (reduced need for further indometacin/surgery)
- significant reduction in intraventricular haemorrhage in the treated group
- no difference in mortality or long-term neurological outcome
- no difference in the incidence of necrotising enterocolitis or CLD.

The lack of clear benefit in neurodevelopmental outcome when indometacin is given prophylactically does not support the prophylactic use of non-steroidal anti-inflammatory drugs. Furthermore,

there is little convincing evidence to suggest improved short-term morbidity when indometacin is used prophylactically compared with its early administration once a PDA has started to cause symptoms. Use of another prostaglandin synthetase inhibitor, ibuprofen, within 3 hours of birth has been reported to reduce short-term mordidity and length of hospital stay (Fowlie and Davis 2008).

Clinical features and diagnosis

The picture of a baby with respiratory distress syndrome who is failing to improve or starts to deteriorate between 5 and 10 days of age, and who has some or all of bounding pulses, an active precordium and a continuous murmur in the pulmonary area, is easy to recognise. Progressive cardiomegaly and worsening lung shadowing on X-ray may be seen. Less gross physical signs in the clinical context may still allow a diagnosis to be made, even in the absence of a murmur. PDA can cause symptoms well before 5 days of age, particularly in infants who have received exogenous surfactant

(Couser et al. 1996); indeed, PDA may be important in the pathogenesis of pulmonary haemorrhage occurring after surfactant administration (Raju and Langenberg 1993). Apnoea in a non-ventilated baby is sometimes a manifestation of PDA and necrotising enterocolitis may be secondary to a widely patent duct. Echocardiography is more sensitive and specific than clinical signs (Evans and Archer 1990) and provides further information about the haemodynamic significance of the PDA. Echocardiographic evaluation includes visualisation of the ductus itself and Doppler evaluation of the pulmonary artery, the ductus and the descending aorta (Fig. 28.18). Additional features include volume loading of the left heart (unless there is a significant atrial communication which will unload the left heart and mask this finding). A continuous murmur in a preterm infant is far more likely to be due to PDA than to any structural lesion, but, if doubt exists, echocardiography must be performed. The little-understood systemic-to-pulmonary collateral arteries detected in preterm infants appear to be a transitory finding (Acherman et al. 2000) in most cases but cause a continuous murmur and can confuse in the diagnosis of PDA. The contribution of these vessels to CLD and the indications for intervention are unclear.

Treatment of PDA

As indicated above, this area remains very controversial (Benitz 2010). Medical and surgical interventions are used for closure of the DA in symptomatic premature infants but objective evidence on long-term outcomes to support such practice is very difficult to demonstrate. In the past, the DA was shown to close spontaneously in time in nearly all preterm infants without specific therapy (Hallidie-Smith 1972; Clarkson and Orgill 1974) but was associated with significant morbidity. By the mid-1970s surgical ligation was being performed on smaller infants and indometacin became available, which resulted in aggressive management of babies with a symptomatic PDA on the assumption that morbidity would be reduced. As a consequence of this, the natural history of the DA in extremely low-birthweight premature infants remains relatively unknown as these babies are almost invariably treated in current neonatal practice. However, the fact that some preterm infants with PDA will develop congestive heart failure, respiratory failure with pulmonary oedema and signs of other organ ischaemia is universally accepted. Some will improve rapidly after interventions to achieve ductal closure, suggesting that an active approach to the management of symptomatic PDA is likely to continue in most neonatal units.

First-line treatment involves optimising oxygen delivery by treating anaemia and achieving adequate arterial oxygen tension, as well as employing fluid restriction and diuretics. Loop diuretics such as furosemide are the most commonly used, although there are theoretical reasons as well as modest clinical evidence to suggest that furosemide may promote ductal patency by its effect on renal prostaglandin synthesis (Green et al. 1983). However, a short trial of fluid restriction and diuretic treatment is sometimes associated with clinical improvement. If there is no improvement, ductal closure is almost invariably recommended, either pharmacologically or by surgery.

Drug treatment is usually tried first unless a specific contraindication exists. Contraindications include:

- documented gastrointestinal tract or renal anomaly
- suspected CHD
- suspected or active necrotising endocarditis
- active bleeding or platelet count <50 000/mm^3
- urine output <0.6 ml/kg/h or raised creatinine
- active infection (Narayanis et al. 2000).

Indometacin is the most widely used drug. In a multicentre trial of babies under 1750 g birthweight, 21% developed sPDA and indometacin closed the ductus within 48 hours of administration in 79% of the 135 infants who received it. Spontaneous closure occurred in only 28% of controls in the same timescale. One-third of responders relapsed but many of these did not require further intervention. Many of those who did have further intervention responded to additional indometacin administration. Overall, indometacin had a 70% success rate, which was not influenced by the application of prior fluid restriction and diuretic therapy (Gersony et al. 1983). Many other studies have demonstrated similar results. Gestation under 28 weeks and postnatal age beyond 2 weeks are associated with lower success rates, as is antenatal indometacin exposure (Norton et al. 1993). Indometacin is usually given intravenously in a dose of 0.2 mg/kg on three occasions, with 8–12 hours between each dose. If a response is seen initially, but with later relapse, it is reasonable to give a further course. Some advocate an escalating stepwise dose schedule.

As well as constricting the DA, indometacin causes renal vasoconstriction, resulting in oliguria, fluid retention, hyponatraemia and elevation of blood urea and creatinine concentrations. These effects are transitory and rarely serious if fluid restriction is applied during treatment. The effect on gastrointestinal blood flow may be the explanation for gastrointestinal haemorrhage and perforation, which are seen in less than 10% of recipients of indometacin. Cranial Doppler ultrasound demonstrates significant falls in cerebral blood flow velocity after rapid intravenous administration of indometacin (Evans et al. 1987) but not if the drug is given more slowly over 30 minutes. However, near-infrared spectroscopy shows marked and prolonged reduction in cerebral blood flow and volume, cerebral oxygen delivery and cerebral vascular responsiveness, regardless of the speed of administration of the drug (Edwards et al. 1990). The evidence that indometacin reduces cerebral blood flow is countered by clear evidence that it reduces the incidence of intraventricular haemorrhage (Wells and Ment 1995) and that PDA has adverse effects on cerebral haemodynamics (Shortland et al. 1990; Evans and Kluckow 1996). A 5-day course of indometacin (Hammerman and Kaplan 1990) has been shown to reduce the relapse rate, and a 6-day lower dose (0.1 mg/kg/day) course (Rennie and Cook 1991) is associated with lower relapse rates and less biochemical disturbance.

It is not known what cerebral haemodynamic disturbances accompany these longer courses of indometacin. Ductal Doppler waveforms referred to above (Su et al. 1997) have been used to reduce the number of doses of indometacin used if evolution in the pattern from growing or pulsatile to closing (high-velocity left-to-right, Fig. 28.18) is documented before a standard course of the drug is completed. Side-effects would also appear to be reduced by this approach (Su et al. 1999). Ibuprofen has been shown to be as effective at closing the ductus in extremely preterm infants but without disturbances of cerebral haemodynamics, as demonstrated by near-infrared spectroscopy (Patel et al. 1995, 2000) and also to cause less disturbance of renal function (Van Overmeire et al. 2000) than three doses of indometacin 0.2 mg/kg administered 12 hours apart. There are current problems with availability of a suitable intravenous preparation of ibuprofen, and intravenous indometacin, in many countries.

Surgery

Surgical occlusion of sPDA is indicated if a clear contraindication to indometacin administration exists, or if the drug is ineffective. Relapse after a second short course of indometacin or after a single 6-day course is also an indication for surgery. Surgery can be

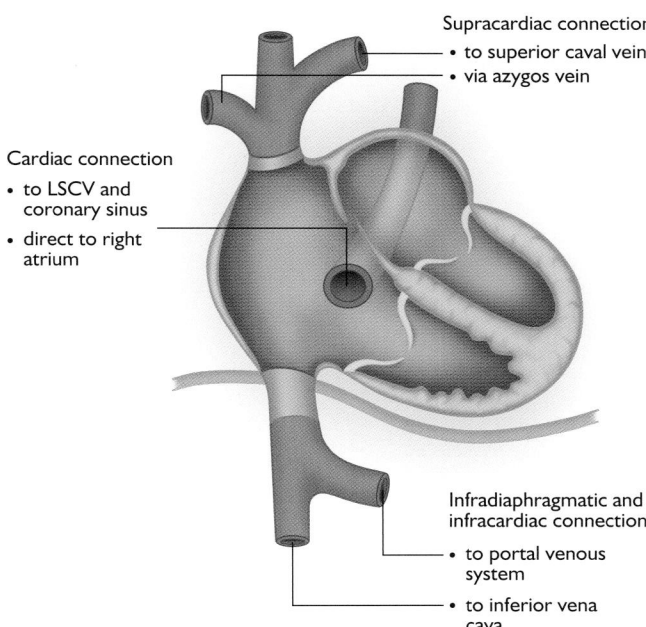

Supracardiac connection
- to superior caval vein
- via azygos vein

Cardiac connection
- to LSCV and coronary sinus
- direct to right atrium

Infradiaphragmatic and infracardiac connection
- to portal venous system
- to inferior vena cava

Fig. 28.19 Schematic representation of the potential sites of anomalous pulmonary venous connection (see Fig. 28.2).

performed in the neonatal intensive care nursery with acceptable morbidity and low short-term mortality, although this group of patients has been reported to have a 10% mortality before discharge from hospital (Robie et al. 1996).

Chronic lung disease

The pathogenesis of CLD is complex (Ch. 27, part 3) and a contribution from a PDA seems likely, although early intervention to close a PDA has not been shown to reduce its incidence. Other left-to-right shunt lesions may contribute to or be masked by chronic respiratory problems. Sustained or recurrent hypoxaemia secondary to CLD results in elevation of PVR with consequent pulmonary hypertension and right-heart enlargement. Steroid administration for treatment of CLD may cause cardiac hypertrophy with or without systemic hypertension, which may result in dynamic left ventricular outflow obstruction (Evans 1994). These changes are rarely of clinical significance and resolve with cessation of steroid therapy. Electrocardiographic and echocardiographic assessment of infants with CLD is appropriate to judge RVH and to get non-invasive (Doppler) evaluation of right heart pressures. Diuretics are of value if pulmonary oedema occurs and are also indicated if systemic venous engorgement occurs secondary to elevated right-heart pressures. There are anecdotal reports of successful use of pulmonary vasodilator therapy in the treatment of elevated right-heart pressures in association with CLD but consistent data are lacking. Reduced ventricular function or atrial dysrhythmias are late and very serious findings.

Endocarditis

Infective and non-infective thrombotic endocarditis occurs in critically ill newborn infants with structurally normal hearts, particularly the preterm (Opie et al. 1999). Clinical features are non-specific, but recurrent or relapsing bacteraemia or the presence of multiple infected sites should raise suspicion of infective endocarditis. Splenomegaly and microscopic haematuria are often present, but these have many other possible causes. Indwelling arterial or central venous cannulae are major risk factors for thromboembolic phenomena and infection. Echocardiography is helpful in diagnosis by recognition of intracardiac vegetations (Fig. 28.16B). Treatment involves removal of infected or potentially infected lines and culture-guided antibiotic therapy, which may need to be prolonged.

Arrhythmias

The same types of arrhythmia may occur in preterm infants as in term babies and are dealt with in pages 661–663. In general, tachyarrhythmias are less well tolerated in preterm infants than in term babies and require prompt intervention to restore sinus rhythm using pharmacological or electrical cardioversion. CHB is difficult to manage in premature babies because of the technical difficulties associated with trying to implant pacemakers into very small infants.

Structural heart disease in the preterm infant

Structural heart disease may occur in the preterm infant and is becoming more prevalent with the rapid improvements in neonatal care of preterm infants. Frequently, the respiratory problems associated with prematurity will mask the cardiac pathology. Diagnosis may also be delayed because of more pressing clinical concerns and because of the tendency towards delayed ductal closure in premature newborns. If the baby is being considered for ductal intervention because of sPDA, then a full echocardiographic examination is indicated. The identification of structural CHD in preterm infants will invariably complicate their management whilst on the neonatal unit. Long periods of prostaglandin administration whilst waiting for weight gain sufficient to consider surgical intervention bring their own hazards in duct-dependent lesions. Lesions with left-to-right shunts will exacerbate acute respiratory problems as well as increasing the risk of CLD and early-onset PVD. Palliative surgical interventions such as pulmonary artery banding for VSDs may improve outcome but such surgery is associated with significant morbidity in low-birthweight infants. Overall prognosis for the same lesion is significantly worse when occurring in premature versus term infants (Andrews et al. 2006).

Structural heart disease in the newborn

Heart disease in the newborn presents in one of four main ways:

1. cyanosis
2. collapse
3. heart failure
4. murmurs.

Cyanosis

The causes of cyanosis are listed in Table 28.13. In practice, it is often possible to distinguish respiratory and cardiac causes on clinical grounds; Table 28.14 gives details of helpful discriminating features. If cardiac disease is thought definite or likely, an approach to management is given in Table 28.15. Clinical features, ECG and CXR often allow an approximate cardiac diagnosis to be made. Echocardiography allows very precise diagnosis in the vast majority of cases. It is more important to stabilise an infant before transfer

Table 28.13 Conditions presenting with neonatal cyanosis

CATEGORY	DETAIL	COMMENT
Respiratory	Any respiratory disease	
Cardiac	**Inadequate pulmonary blood flow with right-to-left shunt**	
	Pulmonary atresia with intact ventricular septum Pulmonary atresia, ventricular septal defect Tricuspid atresia Tetralogy of Fallot Ebstein's anomaly	20% cyanosed as newborn
	Adverse mixing	
	Transposition of the great arteries	
	Common mixing	
	TAPVC DIV DOV Truncus arteriosus	Especially if obstructed Degree of cyanosis reflects severity of PS Heart failure common Heart failure common
Persistent pulmonary hypertension	See Ch. 27, Part 2	
Haematological	Methaemoglobinaemia	Grey/black rather than blue, arterial oxygen tension normal

TAPVC, total anomalous pulmonary venous connection; DIV, double-inlet ventricle; PS, pulmonary stenosis; DOV, double-outlet ventricle.

Table 28.14 Clinical features helpful in distinguishing respiratory from cardiac cyanosis. Note all categories have overlap between respiratory and cardiac causes

	RESPIRATORY CYANOSIS	CARDIAC CYANOSIS
History	Prematurity, meconium liquor/below cords, risk of infection	Family history of congenital heart disease
Respiration	Marked respiratory distress	Little or no respiratory distress unless shocked or metabolic acidosis
Cardiovascular examination	Normal	May have clear signs
Response to oxygen	Cyanosis likely to improve	Cyanosis unlikely to improve dramatically
Chest X-ray	Obvious respiratory pathology Normal CTR (cardio thoracic ratio)	No respiratory pathology, abnormal heart shadow or lung vasculature may be seen
Electrocardiogram	Normal	May be normal, may be helpful
Blood gases	Hypercapnia	Hypo- or normocapnia

to a cardiac centre than to get a precise diagnosis by ultrasound. Differentiating cardiac disease from PPHN may require echocardiography and the two may coexist (Table 28.16). Specific cyanotic conditions are discussed below. As previously discussed, cardiac cyanosis occurs as a result of obstruction to pulmonary blood flow with a right-to-left shunt, adverse streaming of blood on the heart or in association with common mixing of blood at atrial, ventricular or great artery level.

Pulmonary atresia

In all forms of this condition, the pulmonary valve and sometimes the subvalvar ventricular outflow tract are completely blocked, so there can be no forward flow from the right ventricle into the pulmonary artery. Valve morphology varies and may consist of two or three thin cusps which are fused, or the cusps may be extremely thick, dysplastic and immobile. Whatever cusp morphology exists,

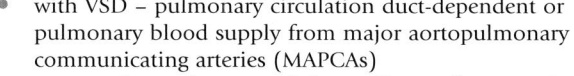

the valve ring itself is usually small in addition. Hearts with pulmonary atresia can be further subdivided as follows:

- with intact ventricular septum – pulmonary circulation always duct-dependent (includes neonates with critical pulmonary valve stenosis)

- with VSD – pulmonary circulation duct-dependent or pulmonary blood supply from major aortopulmonary communicating arteries (MAPCAs)
- as part of complex cyanotic heart disease, for example as in univentricular heart with pulmonary atresia.

Pulmonary atresia with intact ventricular septum

This condition always presents with severe cyanosis in the early newborn period, thereby making up 2.5% of symptomatic newborns with CHD but <1% of all lesions. The main pulmonary artery and its branches are usually confluent and of reasonable size, whereas the right ventricle and tricuspid valve are underdeveloped, sometimes severely so with severe RVH. The tricuspid valve is frequently malformed by tethering of its septal leaflet or displacement toward the apex (Ebstein's malformation), resulting in significant tricuspid regurgitation. Anomalies of the coronary supply to the right ventricle are common and may affect outcome. There is right-to-left shunting at atrial level. If the foramen ovale is or becomes restrictive, marked right atrial enlargement and systemic venous engorgement occur. Pulmonary blood flow is duct-dependent, and extreme cyanosis with metabolic acidosis develops as duct closure progresses. Resuscitation includes prostaglandin and, sometimes, balloon atrial septostomy. Interventional catheterisation can be used as initial treatment (Weber 2002) to perforate and dilate the pulmonary valve if appropriate and/or to stent the arterial duct, but many centres use a surgical approach, the exact sequence depending on echocardiographic assessment of the RV cavity and tricuspid valve sizes. Evaluation of coronary abnormalities using echocardiography, and angiography if needed, may influence management. Primary opening up of the RV outflow tract (RVOT) is desirable if at all possible; systemic-to-pulmonary arterial anastomosis (modified Blalock–Taussig shunt) may be required in addition. These approaches give survival to school age in the region of 80%. If RV hypoplasia is so severe that, even in the neonatal period, it is clear that a biventricular circulation cannot ultimately be established, a systemic-to-pulmonary shunt is performed in the newborn period with the eventual aim of achieving a Fontan-type circulation. In this type of circulation, systemic veins are connected to the pulmonary

Table 28.15 Management of newborn infant with suspected cyanotic congenital heart disease

1. General measures should be directed to reducing stress:
   Maintain temperature
   Avoid hypoglycaemia
   If well, proceed to 3
2. If unwell:
   Arterial blood gas
   - Treat respiratory failure; ventilate if necessary
   - Hypoxaemia alone not reason to ventilate
   - Treat metabolic acidosis
   - Consider hyperoxia test
   Consider prostaglandin (use if in doubt)
3. Chest X-ray:
   Diagnostic clues may be present
   Aid in management
   - Oligaemia: start prostaglandin
   - Plethora: start prostaglandin if very hypoxaemic or metabolic acidosis
4. Electrocardiogram: may point to specific diagnosis
5. Review:
   Drugs
   - Prostaglandin as above
   - Bicarbonate
   - Diuretic if heart failure/pulmonary congestion
   Antibiotics (infection should always be considered as differential diagnosis)
6. Echocardiography:
   If infant requires transfer, stabilise first
   Usually gives precise cardiac diagnosis

Table 28.16 Features helpful in differentiating persistent pulmonary hypertension of the newborn (PPHN) from cyanotic heart disease

	PPHN	CYANOTIC HEART DISEASE
History	Maternal prostaglandin synthetase inhibitor therapy	May have positive family history
Delivery	Fetal distress, birth asphyxia	Uneventful
Examination	Respiratory and/or neurological signs	May have clear cardiac signs
Chest X-ray	May have respiratory pathology	May have diagnostic cardiac/vascular features Often non-specific
Electrocardiogram	May have RAH, ischaemic changes	May have clear abnormality
Hyperoxia test	Variable response, may pass, not if severe fluctuating arterial oxygen tensions seen	Usually poor response
Upper/lower limb saturations	Lower limb often lower (if DA patent)	Occasionally marked discrepancy
Echocardiography	Usually can exclude heart abnormality but can be difficult	Usually diagnostic but cardiac defects may be overlooked

Note: There can be marked overlap and both can coexist.
RAH, right atrial hypertrophy; DA, ductus arteriosus.

arteries without passage of systemic venous blood through a ventricle.

Critical pulmonary valve stenosis has many features in common with this situation except that there is forward flow through the pulmonary valve and the right heart is rarely markedly hypoplastic. Infants with critical pulmonary stenosis should be treated with primary balloon dilatation, usually with a good result, even if further intervention in the form of repeat pulmonary balloon dilatation is needed in later infancy.

Pulmonary atresia with VSD

In contrast to PA with intact ventricular septum, where the anatomical problem is associated with underdevelopment of the right ventricle and associated structures, if there is a VSD present, it is the pulmonary arterial supply that is the major determinant of outcome. The spectrum of disease varies from mild tetralogy of Fallot with confluent and adequate-sized pulmonary arteries to those infants who have non-confluent and severely underdeveloped pulmonary arteries. Pulmonary blood supply may come entirely via the DA (when the pulmonary arteries are cofluent) or it may come partly or entirely from other vessels arising from the aorta (MAPCAs) or head and neck branches. The degree of cyanosis and other physical signs will depend on the amount of flow into the pulmonary circulation. If MAPCAs are large or plentiful, cyanosis is milder, continuous murmurs are heard all over the chest and heart failure may develop. This group of conditions has a significant association with extracardiac malformations, syndromes and chromosomal abnormalities. 22q11 deletion must be remembered as this syndrome has important implications for management, with increased risk of symptomatic hypocalcaemia, immunodeficiency and, if transfused non-irradiated cellular blood products, of graft-versus-host disease. If pulmonary blood flow is duct-dependent, prostaglandin will be needed and early palliative surgery is indicated. If sources of lung blood supply are complex, detailed evaluation with angiography or alternative imaging is required in early infancy in order to assess surgical options. Long-term outcome is variable, but is dependent on the pulmonary arterial supply. With confluent central pulmonary arteries a survival of 80% or more is likely, even if multiple surgical procedures are required. When the pulmonary arterial supply is derived from MAPCAs then outcome is much less favourable with significant morbidity.

Pulmonary atresia as part of a complex lesion

These infants usually have duct-dependent pulmonary blood flow and their condition will be improved by prostaglandin. Obstruction to the systemic arterial outflow of the heart exceedingly rarely coexists, just as complex lesions with systemic outflow obstruction very rarely have significant pulmonary outflow obstruction. However, almost any other cardiac structural abnormality can coexist. Thus, clinical features in addition to cyanosis vary, as do appropriate treatments. In the newborn period, surgical interventions, when appropriate, are likely to be only palliative. Extracardiac abnormalities are common and long-term outcome is often poor for both cardiac and non-cardiac reasons, particularly in those with right atrial isomerism, in whom asplenia with an increased risk of serious bacterial infection is usually present amongst other non-cardiac complications.

Tetralogy of Fallot

This constitutes 10% of all cases of structural heart disease, but only 20% of patients with tetralogy of Fallot are cyanotic in the newborn

period. RV outflow obstruction is always subvalvar (infundibular) but may be valvar and supravalvar in addition. RV outflow obstruction and a large VSD cause RVH. The VSD is subaortic with the aorta arising in part from the right ventricle (overriding aorta); it is rarely restrictive and additional significant VSDs are occasionally found. PFO or ASD commonly coexists; rarely, the pulmonary valve is absent (see below) and tetralogy of Fallot can coexist with complete AVSD. Patients presenting with cyanosis as newborns may have pulmonary atresia or a very narrow but patent RVOT. Those with pulmonary atresia will be duct-dependent. Tetralogy of Fallot without cyanosis in the newborn period is associated with a pulmonary outflow murmur, although it is frequently mistaken for a VSD murmur. Cyanosis is progressive during the first year of life as subvalvar muscular RVOT obstruction increases. Hypercyanotic spells due to infundibular constriction are rare in the newborn period but are an indication for palliative or corrective surgery. Emergency management of spells includes:

- facial oxygen (although whilst the spell occurs it is unlikely to improve oxygenation)
- morphine (50–100 μg/kg s.c., i.m. or i.v.)
- phenylephrine 20 μg/kg i.v.
- propranolol 20 μg/kg slowly i.v., may be repeated once
- heavy sedation/anaesthesia and assisted ventilation
- administration of intravenous fluids to increase circulating volume.

It is rare to need to progress beyond morphine in this protocol. Intravenous drugs should only be used in a setting where ventilation and full cardiopulmonary resuscitation can be given. Spells are usually mild initially and get progressively more frequent, severe and prolonged. Oral propranolol (1–2 mg/kg) three times daily usually prevents recurrent spells in the short and medium term whilst surgical strategies are decided.

Tetralogy of Fallot with absent pulmonary valve

This rare variant of tetralogy (<5% of cases) has small dysplastic pulmonary valve leaflets resulting in marked pulmonary regurgitation and dilatation, often massive, of the pulmonary arteries. The large pulmonary arteries compress the bronchi so that bronchomalacia develops in utero. Presentation in the newborn period is often with airway obstruction causing pulmonary collapse or over-inflation. Cyanosis is not usually marked in early infancy. Impressive systolic and diastolic murmurs from the RVOT with a single S2 in the context of airway obstruction strongly suggest the diagnosis. The dilated pulmonary arteries are seen on CXR; RVH is apparent on ECG. Severe bronchomalacia and pulmonary hypoplasia often cause death even if technically satisfactory cardiac surgical repair is achieved. Surgical mortality in those presenting early with severe pulmonary problems may be as high as 50%.

Tricuspid atresia

Tricuspid atresia represents about 2% of structural heart lesions. Associated abnormalities include VSD and TGA. Those without TGA will frequently have pulmonary stenosis whereas those with TGA may have coarctation. Blood leaves the right atrium via the foramen ovale or an ASD. If the VSD is large or there is TGA, pulmonary blood flow will be high and cyanosis mild, with the possibility of heart failure developing. A restrictive VSD and/or severe pulmonary stenosis will produce duct-dependent pulmonary circulation. A number of patients will be haemodynamically well balanced and will not require intervention until the second half of infancy. Coarctation with TGA in this setting may result in collapse from

Table 28.17 Cardiac conditions which may present with collapse

Arrhythmias – primary or secondary
Duct-dependent circulation
Transposition – ASD, VSD, PDA Pulmonary Pulmonary atresia with intact ventricular septum Tricuspid atresia – with restrictive VSD
Systemic
Hypoplastic left heart Aortic atresia Critical aortic stenosis Interrupted arch Coarctation
Duct-dependent cardiac conditions often present with other signs (cyanosis or respiratory distress) before collapse occurs. ASD, atrial septal defect; VSD, ventricular septal defect; PDA, patent ductus arteriosus.

duct-dependent systemic circulation. Clinical features are given in Table 28.17. The long-term goal is a Fontan circulation, and either systemic-to-pulmonary anastomosis or pulmonary artery banding is usually required in infancy as palliation and, if the VSD is large, to ensure undamaged pulmonary vasculature. Tricuspid atresia is the lesion with the best univentricular long-term outlook with a Fontan circulation, with an operative mortality in childhood of under 10% and a 75% 15-year good-quality survival thereafter.

Transposition

TGA represents approximately 5% of cases of structural CHD; it is rarely found in preterm infants and is rarely associated with extra-cardiac abnormalities or syndromes. It is commoner in males by a factor of 3. Associated cardiac conditions include ASD, VSD, PDA, valvar and subvalvar pulmonary stenosis, and aortic coarctation. Clinical signs will be determined by the associated abnormalities; in principle, the fewer and smaller the shunt lesions, the less mixing of blood occurs and the more severe the cyanosis will be. Presentation is occasionally delayed beyond the first week of life but in those with no shunts is usually within a few hours of birth, occasionally with severe acute cyanosis and shock. Marked pulmonary outflow obstruction will result in worse cyanosis as well as a loud murmur with pulmonary oligaemia on CXR, whereas in the absence of pulmonary stenosis, pulmonary plethora is the more usual finding. Cases with large shunt lesions will not require immediate intervention to improve oxygenation; those without large shunt lesions will usually improve oxygenation enough to avoid metabolic acidosis if the DA is opened with prostaglandin. In some cases, enlargement of the foramen ovale by balloon septostomy will be necessary to obtain adequate entry of well-saturated blood into the right ventricle, even if the DA has been reopened. Balloon septostomy can be done in the neonatal nursery under ultrasound control.

Coexistent coarctation must be repaired and the arterial switch operation is performed in the newborn period unless there is marked fixed pulmonary outflow obstruction, in which case the switch operation is not appropriate and a systemic-to-pulmonary anastomosis will be needed, with definitive surgery being deferred for some years. In TGA with intact ventricular septum the arterial switch operation is ideally performed before left ventricular muscle has involuted in response to serving the lower resistance pulmonary circulation. The timescale in which this happens is unclear, but surgery under 3 weeks of age is within a safe margin but has been successfully undertaken in babies of up to 3 months. If there is a large VSD that does not reduce in size spontaneously, the timescale is not as pressing but there is no particular advantage in delaying surgery beyond 2 months. A baby with TGA who presents beyond the early newborn period needs careful assessment to be sure that the left ventricular pressure remains high.

Coronary artery anatomy is clearly important to the surgeon and can often be delineated by echocardiography. Neonatal arterial switch operative mortality is <5% for simple TGA. Repair of transposition by intra-atrial repair (Mustard or Senning operations) is uncommonly performed now because of long-term problems with arrhythmias and RV failure.

Total anomalous pulmonary venous connection

Entry of pulmonary veins into systemic venous pathways can be at one site or several (mixed TAPVC). Most commonly, the pulmonary veins all enter a confluence behind, but separate from, the left atrium. The confluence then drains directly or indirectly into the right atrium. Drainage can be classified as in Figure 28.19. Obstruction to the pulmonary venous return can occur at a number of sites, including the pulmonary vein orifices, on entry of the confluence to the systemic veins, in the ascending vein as it courses upwards to join the inominate vein in supracardiac TAPVC, on passage through the diaphragm and on passage through the liver after the ductus venosus closes in infradiaphragmatic TAPVC. Obstruction to the pulmonary veins will cause worse cyanosis, marked respiratory distress and less cardiomegaly than unobstructed TAPVC and may prove difficult to distinguish from PPHN even with echocardiography. There is always a PFO and often an ASD (providing mixing at atrial level), with entry of blood to the left heart only through these means; thus, varying degrees of left ventricular underdevelopment are common. Coarctation and even severe hypoplasia of the left heart are very occasionally present.

TAPVC forms part of the complex abnormalities associated with left and right isomerism. In general, the more severe the pulmonary venous obstruction, the earlier the infant is symptomatic. Infradiaphragmatic TAPVC to the portal vein is associated with marked cyanosis and respiratory distress, which gets dramatically worse when the ductus venosus shuts. As they sometimes present early and very blue, infants with obstructed TAPVC often receive prostaglandin, sometimes with benefit to their general state. This improvement is presumably due either to opening of the DA and decompression of the right heart or to opening of the ductus venosus and ameliorating pulmonary venous hypertension in TAPVC to the portal vein. Infants with completely unobstructed TAPVC are sometimes not recognised until after the newborn period when recurrent respiratory tract infections and failure to thrive occur. Management is by corrective surgery, with mortality below 10% and, usually, an excellent long-term outlook. Recurrent pulmonary vein stenosis may occur after surgical repair and is more common in neonates presenting with severe disease early in the neonatal period.

Complex structural cyanotic congenital heart disease

These conditions often include more than one of the above abnormalities as well as shunt lesions and obstruction to either systemic or pulmonary arterial outflow tracts. Important pulmonary and systemic outflow obstruction very rarely coexists. Mixing of blood may occur at atrial, ventricular or at great artery level (or at more than one site). Most complex cyanotic lesions have a univentricular arrangement or have significant imbalance between the sizes of the two ventricles. Association with extracardiac abnormalities is common and, in addition to specific system abnormalities, the possibility of atrial isomerism must be considered. Atrial isomerism (sometimes termed situs ambiguus or heterotaxy) exists when abdominal, bronchial and atrial anatomy is neither the usual arrangement (situs solitus) nor a mirror image of the usual arrangement (situs inversus). The usual arrangement of viscera involves spleen and stomach being on the left-hand side and liver on the right, a morphologically left lung being on the left and a morphologically right lung (three-lobed) being on the right with a morphologically left atrium being to the left of the morphologically right atrium. Situs inversus is a mirror image of this arrangement and atrial isomerism exists when both lungs are of the same morphology (right or left) and both atria are of the same morphology (right or left). When this situation exists, the liver tends to be midline, stomach position is variable and there is either asplenia (in right isomerism) or polysplenia (in left isomerism). Very rarely the situation is less clear-cut and there are some features of right and left isomerism in the same patient.

Generally, right isomerism is associated with severe cyanotic CHD comprising TAPVC, complete AVSD and pulmonary atresia or severe pulmonary stenosis with or without transposition. The cardiac abnormalities associated with left isomerism are more variable in range and severity, but abnormalities of the systemic and pulmonary venous drainage are frequent. Cardiac lesions with left isomerism are not always cyanotic, are more commonly associated with obstruction to the systemic outflow and will invariably have an arrhythmia which varies from 'sinus' with an abnormal atrial pacemaker to CHB associated with a very poor prognosis. Clues to the presence of this type of complex abnormality include a midline liver and dextrocardia. Immediate management principles include deciding whether prostaglandin is indicated: the same criteria apply in these circumstances as in any other.

Common arterial trunk or truncus arteriosus

This malformation constitutes >1% of congenital heart lesions; it is associated with 22q11 deletion in 30% of cases. A single outlet arises from the heart, giving rise to coronary and pulmonary arteries as well as to the aortic arch, which is right-sided in 30% of cases and interrupted in 5–10%, in which case the association with 22q11 deletion is very high. This is an example of cyanosis caused by common mixing predominantly at great artery level. The VSD is usually large and the common arterial trunk overrides it; the truncal valve is abnormal and may be regurgitant or stenosed or a combination of both. Pulmonary arteries arise either laterally from the truncus, adjacent and posteriorly, or from a short main pulmonary artery. Absence of one pulmonary artery occasionally occurs.

Stenosis at the origin of a pulmonary artery if present is rarely severe; thus, high pulmonary blood flow and pressure result in early-onset PVD if the baby survives infancy without surgery. Clinical presentation is cyanosis, tachypnoea or a cardiac murmur. Heart failure occurs later in the newborn period as PVR falls. Severity of cyanosis varies but is usually only mild; other features are listed in Table 28.21. The severity and haemodynamic effect of the truncal valve abnormality influence the signs detected, as does the PVR. Definitive diagnosis is by ultrasound, and, providing both pulmonary arteries can be demonstrated, further cardiac investigation is not normally required before surgery. Corrective surgery is indicated in early infancy to avoid irreversible progressive PVD.

Chromosome 22q11 deletion and immune status should be investigated preoperatively.

The long-term outlook is determined not only by the cardiac state but also by neurodevelopmental and immunological aspects of 22q11 deletion. Corrective surgery is undertaken in the neonatal period or in early infancy and involves closure of the VSD, detachment of the pulmonary arteries from the trunk and placement of a right ventricle to pulmonary artery conduit. If present, the interrupted aortic arch is also repaired. Surgical repair has a mortality of 10% or less but further surgery in the form of replacement of the RV to pulmonary artery conduit will be required in later childhood. In addition, many patients will need truncal valve surgery at some stage, although not usually at initial intervention. If truncal valve replacement is required as part of neonatal correction, surgical mortality increases significantly.

Ebstein's anomaly of the tricuspid valve

This abnormality is characterised by downward displacement of the tricuspid valve towards the apex of the right ventricle. It accounts for 0.5% of all congenital heart defects and, in most cases, it occurs in the setting of laevocardia with concordant AV and ventriculoarterial connections. Ebstein's anomaly has a variable clinical course depending on the degree of tricuspid valve abnormality. The abnormal tricuspid valve is almost always regurgitant and may be stenotic, both problems contributing to reduced forward flow through the right ventricle. When presenting in the newborn period, it is likely that the severity of tricuspid valve abnormality and associated lesions is significant. Neonates will usually present with severe congestive cardiac failure and cyanosis because of a combination of mixing at atrial level and inadequate pulmonary blood flow. The cardiac problems are often compounded by respiratory difficulties caused by pulmonary hypoplasia secondary to severe cardiomegaly. Survival is likely to be poor if symptoms are severe in the neonatal period largely because of limited available surgical options. Therefore, management tends to be conservative with the hope that, as PVR falls, there will be improved forward flow through the right ventricle and, with it, symptomatic improvement. A prostaglandin infusion to maintain ductal patency with simultaneous pulmonary vasodilator therapy may help until PVR has fallen sufficiently to facilitate antegrade flow across the pulmonary outflow. When there is associated pulmonary atresia, a neonatal systemic to pulmonary artery shunt might be appropriate but it should be remembered that these patients are likely to represent the worst end of the disease spectrum of this condition and will often have a poor medium to long-term outlook even if a neonatal shunt is successful. Occasionally, undiagnosed neonates may present with supraventricular arrhythmias because of the associated right atrial dilatation. Increasingly sophisticated repairs of the tricuspid valve in this condition are becoming more popular with improving results but are not appropriate until later in childhood (da Silva et al. 2007).

Congenitally corrected transposition of the great arteries

Congenitally corrected transposition is included in this section as it is frequently associated with additional intracardiac lesions and, in the neonatal period, most patients present with cyanosis because of associated pulmonary outflow tract obstruction. It is a very uncommon abnormality (<1% of structural heart lesions) and involves not only ventriculoarterial discordance (as in TGA) but also AV discordance. Thus, pulmonary venous blood passes from the left atrium through the tricuspid valve into the morphological right ventricle and then is ejected into the aorta. Desaturated systemic venous blood passes through the right atrium and morphological left ventricle into the pulmonary artery. There may be dextrocardia and sometimes situs inversus. If there are no associated defects, infants are pink and the condition may not be suspected until long after the newborn period. VSDs occur in 75–80% of patients and will often cause heart failure in infancy unless important pulmonary stenosis coexists. Systemic AV valve regurgitation develops in about 30% of patients in later life and arrhythmias can develop at any age from fetal life onwards, including all degrees of AV block and SVT. Murmurs depend on associated lesions. The ECG may have heart block of any degree or a pre-excitation pattern. There are Q waves in V_1 and none in V_{5-6}.

CXR will be affected by associated lesions; it may show an abnormal heart position and often has a prominent left upper heart border due to the ascending aorta. Palliative surgery in the form of a systemic-to-pulmonary artery shunt is indicated in symptomatic infants with cyanosis. In infants with a VSD and no obstuction to pulmonary outflow, pulmonary artery banding is almost always the initial surgical intervention performed with further management dependent on the specific anatomical details in individual patients.

Collapse

Conditions that commonly present with collapse are listed in Table 28.17. Differentiating cardiac from non-cardiac causes is usually not difficult although conditions with duct-dependent circulation can, when the duct closes, mimic septicaemia and primary metabolic disorders. A cardiac cause should always be considered as part of the differential diagnosis in all cases of neonatal collapse. It is often necessary to start a prostaglandin infusion before a definitive cardiac diagnosis has been made. On the assumption that the cardiac collapse has occurred secondary to closure of the DA, it is necessary to start prostaglandin at high dosage to try and reopen the DA (Table 28.15). This increases the risk of apnoeic episodes but, usually, neonates who have collapsed will need intubation and ventilation and may require inotropic support as well.

Arrhythmias

These are discussed in a separate section. In the newborn period, arrhythmias that cause sudden unexpected collapse with no signs and a normal ECG between episodes are very rare.

Duct-dependent pulmonary circulation and transposition

These infants will normally be recognised as cyanosed and are discussed under that heading. Duct-dependent pulmonary circulation will result in extreme cyanosis and metabolic acidosis when ductal closure occurs, as will TGA if there is no mixing between systemic and pulmonary circulations via a VSD or an ASD.

Duct-dependent systemic circulation

These lesions are listed in Table 28.17, with clinical features being given in Table 28.18. They are all likely to have at least mild respiratory distress and some physical signs prior to collapse, but those features may have been unrecognised, especially if early discharge home occurred. Resuscitation must not be delayed awaiting echocardiography if the clinical picture is at all suggestive of duct-dependent systemic circulation.

Hypoplastic left-heart syndrome

This term is loosely used to describe a group of closely associated abnormalities whose common morphological feature is severe hypoplasia of the left-heart structures (of insufficient size to support the systemic circulation). It accounts for 2–3% of all CHD but a significantly higher proportion of antenatally detected and neonatal CHD. Extracardiac abnormalities are only occasionally encountered in liveborn infants with HLHS but subtle dysmorphism has been noted in up to 10% of cases (Wernovsky and Newburger 2003). Developmental abnormalities of the brain occur in up to 30% of

Table 28.18 Structural heart lesions presenting with respiratory distress or collapse in the early newborn period. All may have cyanosis if persistent pulmonary hypertension of the newborn or shocked; all have cardiomegaly with congested lung fields on chest X-ray

CONDITION	PULSES	CYANOSIS	PRECORDIUM	AUSCULTATION	ELECTRO-CARDIOGRAM	EXTRACARDIAC ASSOCIATIONS
Hypoplastic left heart	Weak, femoral stronger if DA open	Mild	Active	Gallop	Small LV voltages	Uncommon
Aortic arch interruption	Strong promixal to lesion	None	Active	Gallop, LVOT, systolic murmur	LV/RV1 T↓V_{5-6}	Common (DiGeorge)
Coarctation	Weak femoral	None	Active	Gallop, EC, LVOT, systolic murmur Murmur between scapulae	RA1 RV1 T↓V_{5-6}	Uncommon (Turner)
Critical aortic stenosis	Weak	None	Active	Gallop, EC, LVOT, systolic murmur	LV1 ST↓ T↓V_{5-6}	Uncommon

DA, ductus arteriosus; LV, left ventricular; LVOT, left ventricular outflow tract; RV, right ventricular; EC, ejection click; RA, right atrial.

patients with delayed maturation and decreased head circumference documented on preoperative MRI scanning (Licht et al. 2009). The condition consists of a small left atrium, stenosis or atresia of mitral and aortic valves and hypoplasia of the left ventricle and aorta proximal to the DA (Fig. 28.20A). There is coarctation in 60–70% of cases. The right heart is dilated and hypertrophied with a large pulmonary artery. Head and coronary arterial flow is usually through retrograde filling of the transverse and ascending aorta via the DA.

Clinical features are given in Table 28.18. Before ductal closure occurs, femoral pulses may be stronger than upper limb pulses. The natural history is for collapse and subsequent demise to occur rapidly after ductal closure, usually between 5 and 10 days after birth. Occasional survival to a few months can occur with the systemic circulation dependent on continued patency of the arterial duct. The advent of prostaglandin and ultrasound and, more recently, fetal diagnosis has meant that most liveborn infants with HLHS can be stabilised whilst treatment options for this condition are considered.

Management of HLHS can involve staged palliative surgery (Norwood approach), transplantation or alternatively compassionate care if postnatal intervention is inappropriate for social or medical reasons. Transplantation in the UK and continental Europe is a limited treatment option because of a lack of donors. Staged palliation is now widely adopted as the most effective management with improving survival rates in many units (Edwards et al. 2007). Initial surgery is performed in the neonatal period and requires transection of the pulmonary trunk, which is then anatamosed to the hypoplastic aorta, which in turn is augmented with a homograft patch. Supply to the detached pulmonary arteries is derived by placement of a systemic-to-pulmonary artery shunt (Fig. 28.20B) or a small RV to PA conduit. The first stage is followed by a superior cavopulmonary anastomosis at 4–6 months and completion of the cavopulmonary anastomosis at about 3 years to achieve a Fontan type of circulation (Fig. 28.20C, D). Survival for stage 1 is 80–90% in most specialist centres and is higher for the second and third stages. There is frequently a need for reintervention between stages and a continuing attrition in patients with this condition, as in all patients with a single-ventricle circulation. Furthermore, there is evidence to suggest that neurological outcome in patients managed with a Norwood protocol is not normal in a high percentage of cases (Wernovsky and Newburger 2003).

A number of centres have adopted a hybrid approach to first-stage management using a combination of catheter-based intervention with simultaneous surgery. This involves placement of a stent into the arterial duct to maintain patency and balloon atrial septostomy to ensure adequate-sized atrial communication. At the same time, bilateral branch pulmonary artery banding is performed to restrict pulmonary blood flow (Fig. 28.21). This avoids the need for cardiopulmonary bypass and circulatory arrest in the neonatal period when the immature brain is most susceptible to damage. Reported survival is good (Galantowicz et al. 2008), but it complicates the second-stage operation, which requires major aortic arch reconstruction as well as a superior cavopulmonary anastomosis. It has yet to be determined whether this approach will improve both survival and neurological outcome for patients with HLHS.

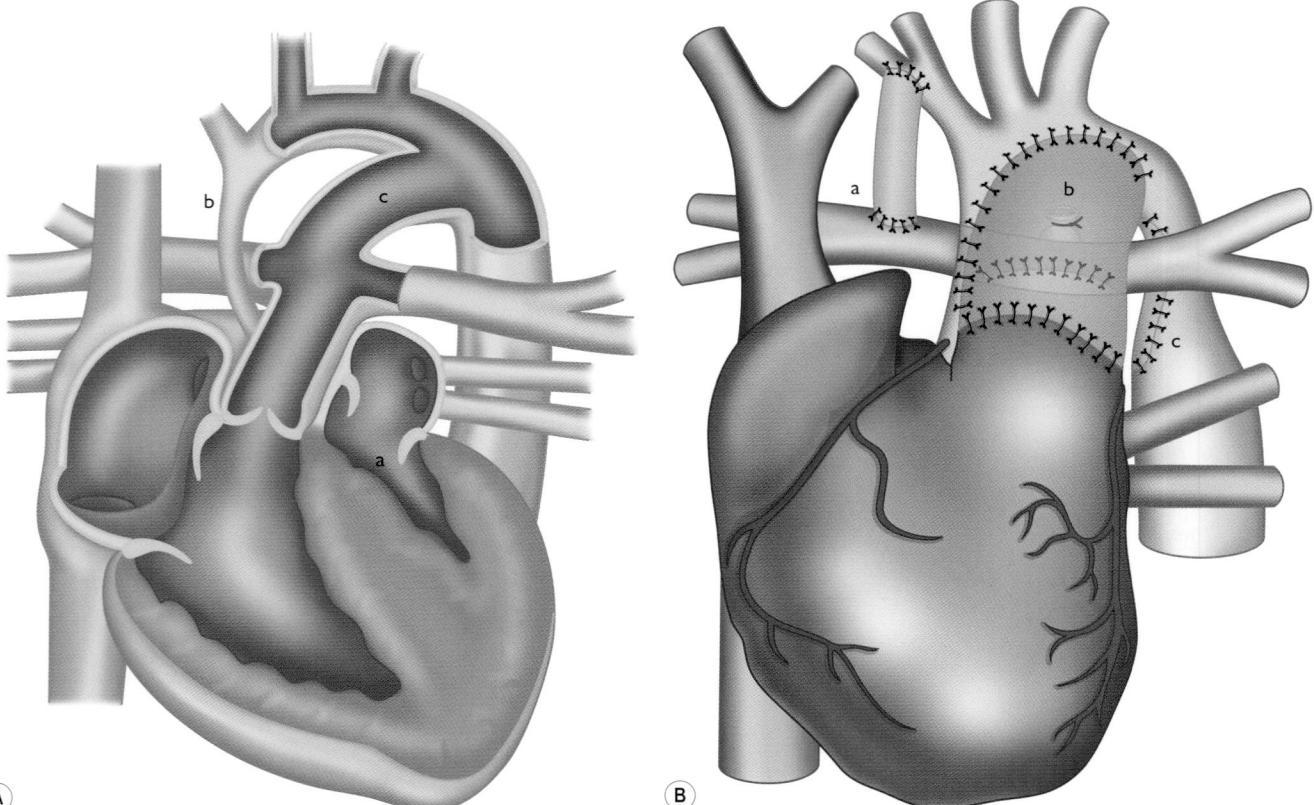

Fig. 28.20 Schematic representation of hypoplastic left-heart syndrome and the stages of surgical palliation. (A) The anatomy of hypoplastic left-heart syndrome (a, left ventricle; b, hypoplastic ascending aorta; c, large patent ductus arteriosus). (B) Norwood stage 1 operation (a, modified right Blalock–Taussig shunt; b, patch joining pulmonary artery with small aorta; c, patch to enlarge distal aortic arch).

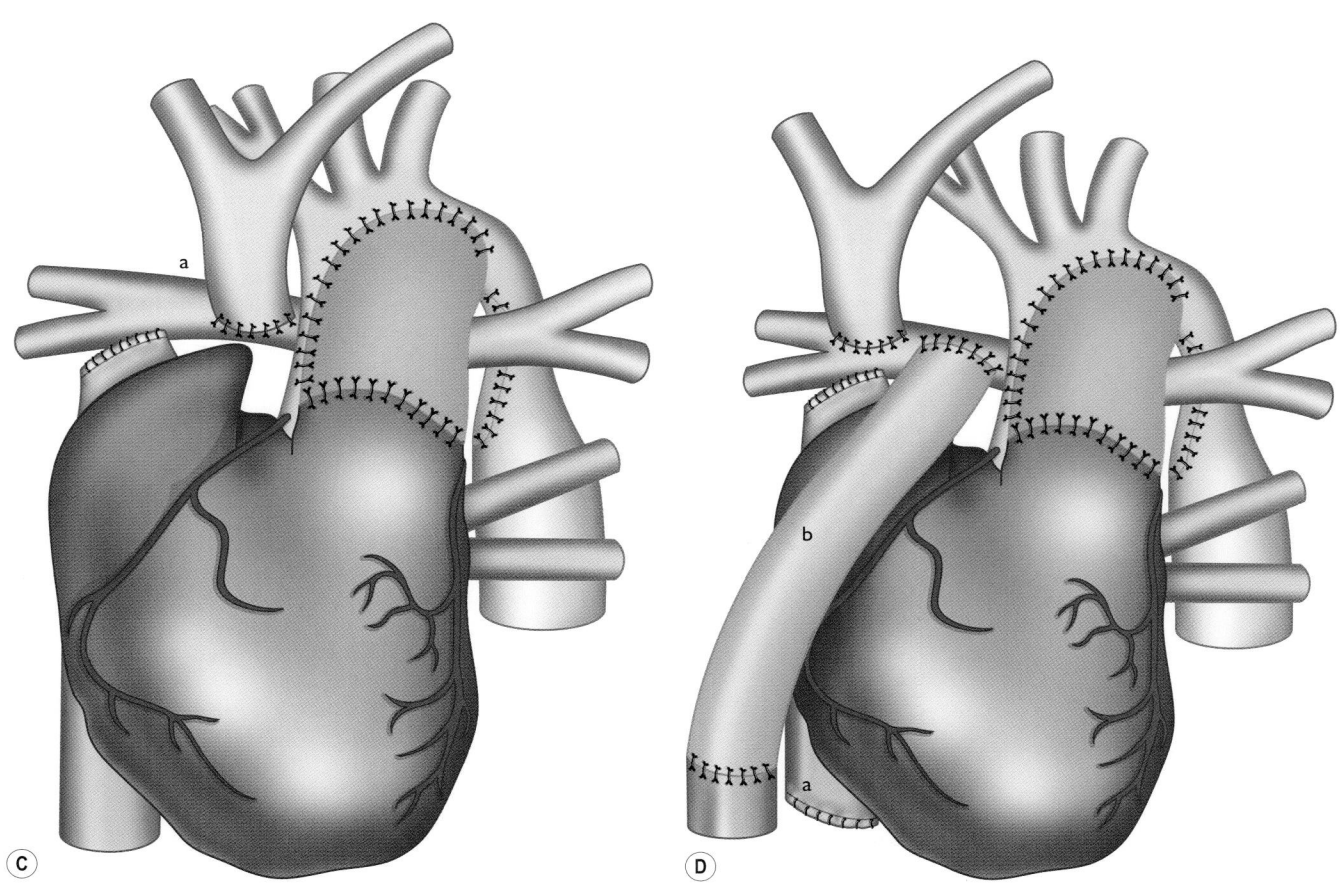

Fig. 28.20, cont'd (C) Bicavopulmonary connection (BCPC) (a, superior caval vein anastomosed to right pulmonary artery after disconnection from the heart). (D) Total cavopulmonary connection (TCPC) using an extracardiac conduit between the inferior caval vein and pulmonary artery (a, oversewn inferior caval vein stump; b, Gortex tube anastomosed between detached inferior caval vein and pulmonary artery).

Critical aortic stenosis

This lesion lies at one end of a spectrum of severity of aortic valve abnormalities, the mildest of which may cause no symptoms even in adult life. It is commoner in males and the possibility of Turner syndrome must be considered in affected females. The aortic valve may have one, two or three cusps and there is often poststenotic dilatation of the ascending aorta. Aortic stenosis of any degree may be associated with some aortic regurgitation, mitral stenosis, VSD and coarctation. Symptomatic aortic stenosis at sub- or supravalvar levels is rare in the newborn, but subvalvar aortic stenosis may develop in treated or untreated valvar aortic stenosis and in association with VSD and aortic coarctation or interruption. Progression of aortic stenosis and its unfavourable effect on the left ventricle in fetal life has been documented by ultrasound (Simpson and Sharland 1997). The evolution of fetal aortic valve disease has led to the use of prenatal cardiac interventional catheterisation to dilate the aortic valve in an attempt to promote left ventricular growth (Marshall et al. 2005). Success is limited, with the majority of patients ending up with a single-ventricle circulation despite what may be considered a successful intervention. Postnatally, the clinical picture depends on severity (Table 28.18) and ranges from an asymptomatic murmur with heart failure developing in early infancy to pulseless collapse when the DA shuts.

Angiography is not required for diagnosis, but cardiac catheterisation for balloon dilatation would be the treatment of choice in most centres, with surgical valvotomy reserved for failed valvuloplasty.

Survival is mainly determined by the state of the left ventricle, which may be dilated or severely hypertrophied. It is a matter of debate as to whether the most severe forms should be subject to Norwood-type surgery (see HLHS, above). The results after surgery and balloon dilatation are similar but recovery from dilatation is usually quicker (McCrindle et al. 2001). All infants requiring intervention in the newborn period will ultimately have further interventions for residual or recurrent stenosis or for aortic regurgitation.

Aortic arch interruption

This abnormality is present in 1% of congenital heart lesions. The DA supplies the descending aorta distal to the site of interruption, which is distal to the left subclavian artery in 30% (type A), between the left carotid and left subclavian arteries in 45% (type B) and between the innominate and left carotid in the remainder (type C). Approximately 50% of type A interruptions are associated with 22q11 deletion. Associated cardiac lesions always include VSD, often valvar or subvalvar aortic stenosis, sometimes mitral valve abnormalities, and very occasionally truncus arteriosus or aorto-pulmonary window. Clinical features are given in Table 28.18. Diagnosis can be strongly suspected clinically by careful attention to the pulses and is confirmed with clarification of associated lesions by ultrasound. Corrective surgery is usually performed through a median sternotomy with concurrent repair of intracardiac abnormalities, with up to 90% survival. Left ventricular outflow

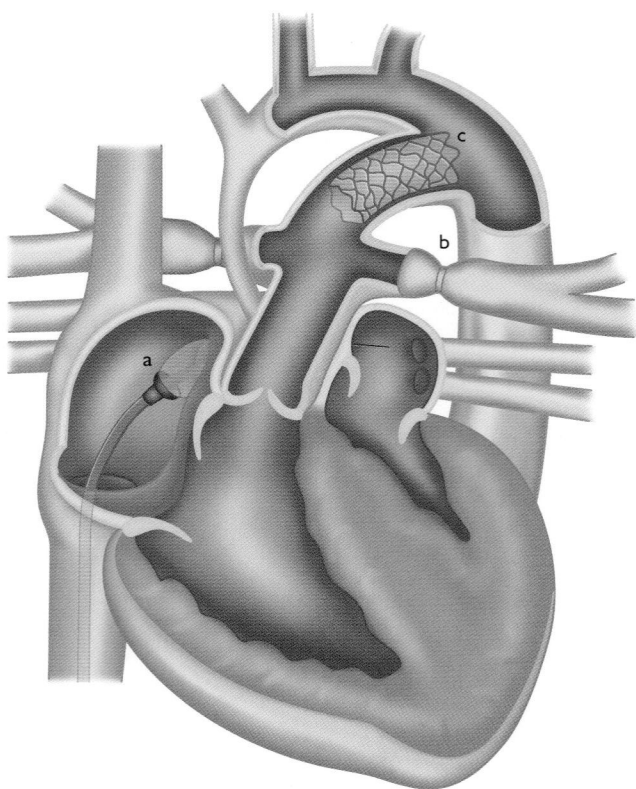

Fig. 28.21 Schematic representation of a hybrid Norwood stage 1 procedure for hypoplastic left-heart syndrome with balloon atrial septostomy (a), bilateral branch pulmonary artery banding (b) and stenting of the arterial duct (c).

obstruction may progress even after successful neonatal surgery and often requires repeat surgical intervention; further intervention to the repaired aortic arch may also be required.

Coarctation

This makes up 10% of CHD, being more common in males but having a strong association with Turner syndrome, 15% or more of whom have the condition. The position of the discrete narrowing of the aorta is distal to the left subclavian artery, opposite the point of entry to the aorta of the DA (Fig. 28.15D). The exact position varies and may evolve in relation to ductal closure and postnatal growth. The terms pre-, juxta- and postductal are used to describe the site of coarctation and bear some relationship to the age of presentation and clinical picture.

Not all cases of coarctation cause symptoms in the newborn period or infancy; some remain asymptomatic for years or occasionally decades. When coarctation presents in neonates it is commonly associated with varying degrees of aortic arch hypoplasia, which may have implications for repair. Other lesions in the left heart are very commonly associated (mitral and aortic valve abnormalities), as are VSDs. Transposition and more complex cyanotic conditions may have accompanying coarctation. In the newborn with coarctation and PDA, there is systemic pressure in the right ventricle, although, until the DA starts to close, shunting is predominantly left to right at ductal and atrial levels. Thus, as heart failure develops, the infant is pink with RVH on ECG. When the duct shuts, some constriction of the descending aorta probably occurs, but is more critical in those babies who collapse. In others, duct closure is

tolerated, although heart failure and hypertension may occur in the early weeks of life. Those infants who remain asymptomatic in the newborn period may develop heart failure in later infancy with LVH on ECG. The time and mode of presentation of infants with associated intracardiac lesions are influenced by the nature of the associated lesion.

If the coexistent lesion presents early, great care must be taken not to overlook coarctation. Coarctation can be difficult to diagnose clinically (Table 28.18) in the newborn. Pulses and upper/lower limb BPs may be normal while the ductus is open, and, if collapse occurs, all pulses can be weak because of associated left ventricular dysfunction. Similarly, echocardiography imaging and Doppler assessment can sometimes be inconclusive whilst the ductus is wide open; even angiography and direct pressure measurements can be inconclusive. If there is doubt, careful observation and serial echocardiography over a period of a few days are required until the DA constricts and the characteristic features develop. Coarctation causing collapse is resuscitated with prostaglandin and heart failure is treated with diuretics.

Inotropic support is needed in critically ill infants and renal function must be watched carefully as occasionally renal failure develops. Infants who collapse or who are in heart failure should undergo surgical repair when stabilised. Coarctation as part of a more complicated lesion must be repaired before or at the same time as the intracardiac abnormality. In some circumstances, pulmonary artery banding is performed with coarctation repair if there is a cardiac lesion which will cause pulmonary plethora and which is not to be corrected in the newborn period, for example multiple muscular VSDs. There are disadvantages to pulmonary artery banding that mean it is desirable to avoid it if possible.

Coarctation in the newborn period may be repaired using the left subclavian artery (subclavian flap repair). This results in an absent brachial pulse in the left arm but very rarely leads to ischaemic problems there. Most surgeons prefer excision of the coarctation and end-to-end repair in newborns, as is the case after infancy. Mortality of coarctation repair without major intracardiac lesions is 5%. The recurrence rate may be as high as 20% in those repaired in the newborn period.

Conclusion

Any of the causes of collapse considered above may present less dramatically, usually with evidence of heart failure, which often precedes collapse. The precise diagnosis of which duct-dependent condition exists is not important at the resuscitation stage and, if a collapsed infant could have structural heart disease as the cause, prostaglandin should be given. This is likely to be rapidly therapeutic as well as helpful in confirming a cardiac cause for the collapse. Absence of response to prostaglandin at doses at the top of the range (Table 28.10) makes duct-dependent systemic circulation unlikely but not impossible. Risks of surgery are increased if renal or multiorgan failure is present.

Heart failure

Cardiac conditions presenting with heart failure are listed in Table 28.19 and clinical details given in Tables 28.20 and 28.21. Some of these conditions may present with collapse and in retrospect a period of respiratory distress may have been present prior to collapse. Cardiac conditions causing cardiac failure are invariably associated with respiratory distress (Table 28.17). Cardiac disease will also cause respiratory distress if there is marked pulmonary venous engorgement or metabolic acidosis has developed; these two occurrences can be associated with cyanotic cardiac conditions. Some

Table 28.19 Cardiac conditions presenting with neonatal respiratory distress

CATEGORY	COMMENTS
Heart muscle disease	
Ischaemia	With birth asphyxia
Myocarditis	Any cause
Cardiomyopathy	Hypertrophic or dilated
Arrhythmias	
Arteriovenous	Cranial or other with PPHN malformation
Structural heart disease	
Week 1	
Hypoplastic left heart	May also present with collapse
Interrupted arch	
Aortic atresia/critical stenosis	
Coarctation	
Obstructed TAPVC	
Tetralogy of Fallot with absent pulmonary valve	Symptoms due to airway obstruction by large PAs
Week 2–3	
Truncus	May also present with cyanosis
DOV, DIV, TAPVC	
TGA 1 VSD	
Week 3	
Left-to-right shunt lesions	Worse when multiple defects
VSD, AVSD, PDA etc.	

PPHN, persistent pulmonary hypertension of the newborn; TAPVC, total anomalous pulmonary venous connection; PA, pulmonary atresia; DOV, double-outlet ventricle; DIV, double-inlet ventricle; TGA, transposition of the great arteries; VSD, ventricular septal defect; AVSD, atrioventricular septal defect; PDA, patent ductus arteriosus.

conditions characteristically cause both heart failure and cyanosis (Table 28.22). Signs of cardiac disease will be absent in respiratory causes of respiratory distress and a CXR usually allows the distinction to be made with confidence.

Arrhythmias (Table 28.20)

These are considered in detail on pages 661–663.

Heart muscle disease (Table 28.20)

There is little information on the incidence of heart muscle disease in the newborn, but cardiomyopathy is much more frequent under 1 year of age (about 8 per 100 000 per year) than in childhood overall (about 1 per 100 000 per year) (Lipshultz et al. 2003; Nugent et al. 2003).

Myocardial ischaemia

Subclinical myocardial ischaemia in asphyxiated and otherwise stressed infants is quite common (Barberi et al. 1999). Involvement severe enough to cause hypotension is less common, although a transient murmur from tricuspid or mitral regurgitation in association with ST depression and T-wave inversion in the left chest leads is a common finding. Specific therapy for heart failure is sometimes required; such infants usually have neurological and renal impairment in addition. Myocardial infarction in neonates may cause heart failure or sudden collapse. ECG changes include deep and wide Q waves and initial elevation of the ST segment, followed by T-wave inversion some days later. Q waves persist indefinitely but ST segment changes resolve in a week or so and T waves return to normal over a much longer timescale. Enzyme studies can be difficult to interpret in the early newborn period as other tissues may be the source of the enzymes and cardiac-specific isoenzymes need to be measured. Myocardial infarction can occur as part of generalised perinatal asphyxia or secondary to thromboembolic events (Tillett et al. 2001) and has a high mortality. Anomalous origin of the left coronary artery from the pulmonary artery is rarely symptomatic in the early weeks of life, as it is well tolerated whilst the pulmonary artery pressure remains high. It is a cause of pale sweating episodes (presumably angina), heart failure from dilated cardiomyopathy (DCM) and myocardial infarction after the newborn period. Ischaemia secondary to birth asphyxia usually recovers fully without any apparent long-term sequelae, even if intravenous inotrope support is required acutely. Long-term outlook after neonatal myocardial infarction is less well documented.

Myocarditis

Myocarditis is usually presumed and only occasionally definitely proven to be viral in origin, often in the context of a generalised viraemic illness (Kaski and Burch 2007). Heart failure and either tachy- or bradyarrhythmias can occur. Detection of a pericardial rub is rare in the newborn; pericardial effusion and even tamponade can occur. There is no specific therapy other than supportive measures: heart failure should be treated in the usual way, but digoxin used cautiously because of the risk of arrhythmias. The possible benefit in the use of steroids and immunoglobulin therapy for such cases remains unproven. Symptomatic, large or increasing pericardial effusions should be drained. Usually this is possible percutaneously. In some cases, neonates with suspected myocarditis have required extracorporeal membrane oxygenation support. Recovery of cardiac function occurs reasonably quickly if it is going to occur and there is an overlap between this group of patients and those who progress to DCM. Precise outcome figures are difficult to obtain because of this,

Dilated cardiomyopathy

This usually presents after the newborn period but fetal and neonatal presentation with heart failure does occur. Tachyarrhythmia must be excluded as a cause, as must anomalous origin of the left coronary artery, which is unlikely to present this young (see above). Detailed investigations for infective and metabolic causes are appropriate (Burch and Runciman 1996) (Table 28.23) if ischaemia or infarction is not clearly responsible.

If any of the screening investigations reveals possible aetiologies, enzyme studies on lymphocytes, fibroblasts or other tissue biopsies are indicated. If a metabolic cause is suspected from investigations or other clinical features such as skeletal myopathy, the question of blind treatment needs to be considered if the infant is critically ill.

Table 28.20 Clinical features of cardiovascular conditions not involving intracardiac structural abnormalities presenting with respiratory distress in the newborn

CONDITION	PULSES	PRECORDIUM	AUSCULTATION	ELECTROCARDIOGRAM	EXTRACARDIAC ASSOCATIONS
Arrhythmia	Normal or weak	Normal	Gallop	Diagnostic	Rare
Heart muscle disease					
Myocarditis	Normal or weak	Normal	Gallop, MR murmur, rub	Small QRS ST↑, T↓	Common (e.g. hepatitis)
Ischaemia	Normal or weak	Normal	Gallop, MR murmur, TR murmur	ST↑, T↓	Features of perinatal asphyxia
DCM	Normal or weak	Normal	Gallop, MR murmur	LV+, ST↓↓, T↓↓	Rare
EFE	Weak	Normal or active	Gallop, MR murmur	LV+, ST↓↓, T↓↓ V₅₋₆	Rare
HCM	Normal or jerky	Normal or active	Gallop, LVOT or RVOT	LV/RV+ ST↑ or T↓	Common (macrosomia, usually maternal diabetes)
Arteriovenous malformation					
Cranial	Normal or weak femorals	Active	Gallop, MR murmur, cranial bruit	LV/RV+ ST↓ or T↓	Neurological signs
Coronary	Full	Active	Gallop, continuous murmur	LV/RV+ ST↓ or T↓	

Note: Cyanosis is not present in any condition unless persistent pulmonary hypertension of the newborn occurs and all have cardiomegaly and pulmonary congestion on chest X-ray.
DCM, dilated cardiomyopathy; LV, left ventricular; EFE, endocardial fibroelastosis; HCM, hypertrophic cardiomyopathy; LVOT, left ventricular outflow tract; RVOT, right ventricular outflow tract; AVM, arteriovenous malformation.

This may be appropriate if one of the carnitine deficiency states is suspected (Ino et al. 1988). First-degree relatives of infants with DCM should be evaluated clinically by ECG and echocardiography, as familial occurrence is recognised, even when precise metabolic diagnoses are lacking.

Endocardial fibroelastosis

This can be primary, in which case it has close clinical similarities to DCM, with marked left ventricular hypertrophy on ECG. The endocardium is echogenic on ultrasound. Endocardial fibroelastosis is often secondary to obstructive left-heart lesions, in which case the clinical picture and prognosis are influenced by the nature and severity of the accompanying pathology.

Hypertrophic cardiomyopathy

This can be primary, as a manifestation of an autosomal dominant genetic disease, or secondary, for example in association with Noonan syndrome (also autosomal dominant). Most common is hypertrophic cardiomyopathy (HCM) secondary to hyperinsulinism, usually maternal diabetes mellitus (Ch. 22). Infants receiving corticosteroids for CLD may develop reversible cardiac hypertrophy out of proportion to the degree of hypertension but they rarely show symptoms (Evans 1994). The majority of infants born to mothers with diabetes or gestational diabetes have no clinical

effects from HCM. Some have a left ventricular outflow murmur and a few develop respiratory distress attributed more often to impaired left ventricular filling than to outflow obstruction. It is often possible to demonstrate some tricuspid or pulmonary regurgitation in such infants, confirming a degree of pulmonary hypertension secondary to reduced left ventricular compliance in association with hypertrophy. Symptomatic infants may benefit from cautious beta-blocker therapy (because of the possibility of associated hypoglycaemia) and the hypertrophy will almost always resolve over a period of 1–2 months (Way et al. 1979). Inotropes are contraindicated in the cardiomyopathy of infants of diabetic mothers. Hypertrophy can be global or localised and this is reflected in the ECG and echocardiographic findings. Infants of diabetic mothers also have an increased incidence of structural heart disease (5%), making detailed assessment including echocardiography important if there are any cardiac symptoms or signs in such infants. If maternal glucose intolerance cannot be confirmed, a search for metabolic causes of cardiac hypertrophy is indicated (Table 28.23) (Way et al. 1979; Burch 1994; Guenthard et al. 1995).

Isolated left ventricular non-compaction

This form of left ventricular abnormality is now well recognised in children (about 10% of childhood cases of cardiomyopathy) and has been described in the fetus (Karatza et al. 2003).

Table 28.21 Structural heart lesions presenting with respiratory distress (heart failure) after the first week of life

CONDITION	PULSES	CYANOSIS	PRECORDIUM	AUSCULTATION	ELECTROCARDIOGRAM	EXTRACARDIAC ASSOCIATIONS
Truncus arteriosus	Normal or full	Mild	Active	S2 single, EC systolic	RV+ ± LV+ ST↓, T↓ V$_{5-6}$	Common (DiGeorge)
TGA + VSD	Normal	Mild/moderate	RV+	S2 single ± VSD murmur	LV+ or RV+	Rare
TAPVC (unobstructed)	Normal or weak	Mild/moderate	RV+	S2 wide, P2 loud ± RVOT murmur	RV+ RsRVI	Rare
DIV/DOV without PS	Normal	Mild	Active	P2 loud VSD murmur	Variable	Rare
PDA	Full	None	Active	Continuous murmur at base	LV+ ± RV+	Occasional
VSD	Normal	None	Active	P2 loud PSM LLSE	LV1 ± RV+	Occasional
Complete AVSD	Normal	None	Active	P2 loud VSD murmur LLSE MR murmur apex	RA+ RV+ Superior QRS axis	Very common (Down syndrome)
AP window	Normal or full	None	Active	P2 loud, continuous murmur at midsternal edge	LV+ RV+	Rare

RV, right ventricular; LV, left ventricular; TGA, transposition of the great arteries; VSD, ventricular septal defect; TAPVC, total anomalous pulmonary venous connection; RVOT, right ventricular outflow tract; DIV, double-inlet ventricle; DOV, double-outlet ventricle; PS, pulmonary stenosis; PDA, patent ductus arteriosus; AVSD, atrioventricular septal defect.

Left-to-right shunt lesions (Table 28.21)

These include both cardiac and extracardiac malformations. Traditionally, left-to-right shunts occur within the heart or great arteries but they can also develop outside the heart as AVMs. The left-to-right shunt associated with a significant-sized AVM can cause severe cardiac failure. In contrast to the left-to-right shunts that occur in the heart, the shunting through an AVM is not dependent on PVR and therefore symptoms of cardiac failure can develop early and in some cases are seen prenatally (see below).

Symptoms from significant intracardiac shunts do not develop until PVR falls enough to permit excessive pulmonary blood flow. This may happen slightly more quickly in preterm infants, related to the relative paucity of muscle in immature lung arterioles, but, even in premature babies, symptoms do not develop in the immediate perinatal period but may only become apparent after the first or second week of life. The most common site for intracardiac shunting is across the ventricular septum due to a VSD (Fig. 28.22).

In some circumstances, when the defect is large, PVR may not fall sufficiently to result in excessive lung blood flow. These infants remain relatively well and pass into the phase of progressive vascular damage without heart failure occurring. Whether or not a period of heart failure occurs, the development of pulmonary vascular changes is universal and rapid in some lesions (e.g. complete AVSD) but unusual and not until adult life in secundum-type ASD. Other lesions lie between these extremes in both frequency and rapidity of progression to PVD. Extracardiac factors may influence the risk and hasten the development of PVD. These include extreme prematurity, CLD, airway obstruction, life at high altitude and Down syndrome.

Arteriovenous malformation (Table 28.20)

Arteriovenous fistulae may present in the newborn period with heart failure; there may be associated PPHN. Intracranial fistulae

Table 28.22 Structural cardiac conditions in which cyanosis and heart failure commonly coexist in the newborn

Transposition
- with coarctation
- with large VSD
Truncus arteriosus
Tricuspid atresia
- with large VSD
- with TGA and coarctation
Double-inlet ventricle
Total anomalous pulmonary venous connection
- with obstructed pulmonary veins
Hypoplastic left-heart syndrome with continued ductal patency
Arteriovenous malformation – usually intracerebral, often have PPHN

If significant pulmonary stenosis coexists, heart failure is unlikely and cyanosis is more marked.
VSD, ventricular septal defect; TGA, transposition of the great arteries; PPHN, persistent pulmonary hypertension of the newborn.

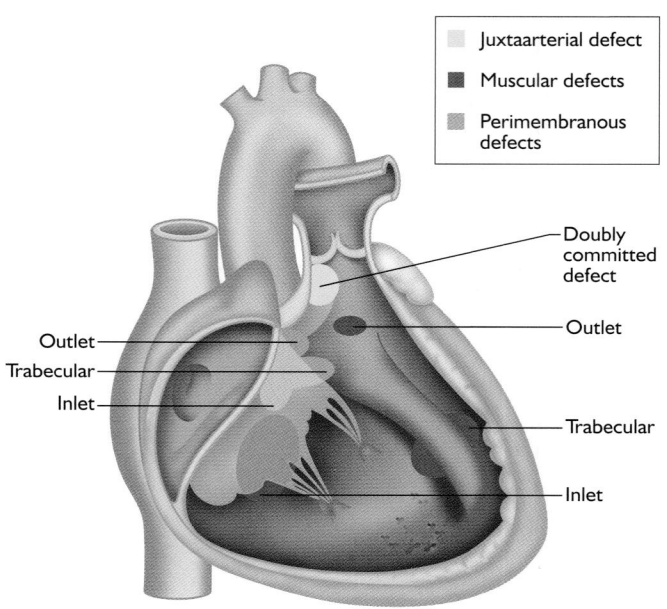

Fig. 28.22 Schematic representation of the classification of ventricular septal defects seen from the right ventricular aspect.

Table 28.23 Blood and urine screening tests for hypertrophic and dilated cardiomyopathy in infants if no clinical diagnosis apparent. Abnormal findings need detailed investigation

BLOOD FOR	URINE FOR	NASOPHARYNGEAL ASPIRATE FOR
Vacuolated lymphocytes	Amino and organic acids	Virology
Carnitine and acyl carnitine	Glycosaminoglycans	
Lactate and pyruvate (fasting)	Virology	
Creatine kinase (MM fraction)		
Thyroid function		
Autoimmune screen		
Amino acids		
Virology (especially entero-, adeno- and parvoviruses)		

are the most common (aneurysm of the vein of Galen). Intrahepatic fistulae are occasionally encountered and may coexist with intracranial shunts. As well as heart failure, signs include a bruit over the affected site. Management consists of medical support for the circulation and intervention to stop or at least reduce the shunt through the AVM. This involves catheter embolisation for intracranial abnormalities, which are most commonly vein of Galen aneurysms. The outcome is determined by the ability to achieve a marked reduction in or abolition of the arteriovenous shunt and by the severity of secondary hydrocephalus and cerebral ischaemic lesions. Babies with an in utero diagnosis of AVM who have hydrops fare particularly badly.

Intracardiac left-to-right shunts

Patent ductus arteriosus

Prematurity and PDA are considered on pages 645–647. As an isolated lesion outside the context of respiratory distress syndrome and prematurity, PDA accounts for nearly 10% of congenital heart lesions. Clinical features are given in Table 28.21; diagnosis is often clinical and confirmed by echocardiography. PDA causing symptoms in term infants is an indication for closure. If the infant is asymptomatic without evidence of pulmonary hypertension, intervention is often delayed until later in infancy, when occlusion by catheter-delivered device or surgery is performed. The size at which catheter closure can be performed is being reduced all the time. Surgery and transcatheter closure both have high success rates and excellent long-term prognosis. The factors influencing which method is chosen are many and are evolving.

Atrial septal defect

Isolated ostium secundum ASDs very rarely, if ever, cause symptoms in newborn infants, but are occasionally suspected on auscultation. Left-to-right shunting at atrial level is often found on echocardiography either as an isolated finding or in conjunction with physiological pulmonary artery branch stenosis, PDA or more complex lesions. It is not always clear whether the shunt is through an ASD or merely through a PFO. Approximately 85–90% of atrial shunts detected by ultrasound in the newborn period disappear and defects sized <3 mm almost always do (Radzik et al. 1993).

Ventricular septal defect

VSDs without associated abnormalities account for at least 15% of structural heart lesions; up to 65% of them resolve spontaneously. They may be single or multiple and can occur in any part of the ventricular septum (Fig. 28.21). The site is of importance with respect to associated lesions, likely natural history and surgical approaches. Symptoms may never occur and, if heart failure does develop, it frequently does not do so until after the newborn period; indeed, there may be no murmur until several weeks of age. This is because there is little flow across a VSD whilst PVR is high. Diagnosis is usually clinical (Table 28.21) with echocardiographic confirmation and identification of precise location. Heart failure is treated as necessary (Table 28.12). Surgery is rarely needed in the newborn period unless there are associated lesions such as coarctation. Surgery is indicated for cases in which heart failure cannot be controlled to permit satisfactory weight gain. Surgical repair of VSD has a low mortality (<3%) even in the newborn period. Palliative pulmonary artery banding is only considered when there are multiple VSDs or if surgery is indicated for another lesion such as coarctation. When VSD is part of a more complex lesion, strategies are different; in some circumstances a sizeable VSD is essential for satisfactory haemodynamics, for example in double inlet left ventricle with TGA.

Atrioventricular septal defect

The basic abnormality in this condition is in the AV septum, which in a normal heart separates the left ventricle from the right atrium. A defect here will always be associated with an abnormality of the AV valves. There may be an intra-atrial defect only (ostium primum ASD, termed partial AVSD), or additionally an intraventricular defect may also exist, in which case a complete AVSD is present and the AV valve has a single large orifice rather than two separate ones. In both forms there can be AV regurgitation, including left ventricular to right atrial shunting. Partial AVSD constitutes >2% of CHD and complete AVSD accounts for 2% of CHD. Either lesion can be part of the complex cardiac abnormalities found in left isomerism (partial AVSD) or right isomerism (complete AVSD), as described above. Partial AVSD is frequently undetected in the newborn period and may not cause heart failure in infancy, although surgical correction is required in childhood to prevent right-heart failure or PVD in adult life; cases with heart failure in infancy often have left AV valve regurgitation as well as left-to-right shunting at atrial level and require valve repair as well as surgical closure of the shunt.

Eighty per cent of cases of isolated complete AVSD are associated with Down syndrome; in the region of 35% of infants with Down syndrome and CHD have complete AVSD. Occasionally, tetralogy of Fallot coexists with AVSD, as may PDA or coarctation. In some cases of complete AVSD, one ventricle is much larger than the other (unbalanced AVSD); usually they are approximately equal sizes with volume overloading of the right ventricle. Clinical features of complete AVSD are given in Table 28.21. Symptoms of heart failure may never develop as PVD can occasionally develop rapidly, particularly in Down syndrome. Therefore, it is desirable to make the diagnosis in the newborn period. It is for this reason and because signs can be subtle that at least an ECG (which is associated with a superior axis in AVSD) is useful and routine echocardiographic screening of all newborns with Down syndrome is indicated. Adequate information is obtained by echocardiography; angiography is not usually needed. Survival without surgery is not always beyond infancy, because of heart failure. However, of those alive at 1 year, survival into the late teens or twenties is common. Corrective surgery for cases detected in infancy improves outlook, with a surgical mortality of under 5%.

Aortopulmonary window

This rare abnormality involves a connection between the ascending aorta and the main pulmonary artery. It has haemodynamic and clinical features similar to large PDA and truncus arteriosus; it may coexist with PDA and with aortic arch interruption (Table 28.21). It can easily be overlooked on echocardiography, especially if a coexistent lesion is recognised. Surgical treatment at diagnosis is appropriate and has a high success rate.

Coronary arteriovenous fistula

This is another rare shunting lesion which presents with systolic and diastolic murmurs with or without bounding pulses and heart failure depending on the size of the shunt. The coronary fistula can be into any heart chamber or to the pulmonary artery. Ultrasound usually delineates the anatomy but angiography may be needed. Surgery or transcatheter occlusion is indicated for cases causing symptoms or signs in the newborn period. In many cases the fistula will become smaller or close spontaneously.

Conclusion

All the diseases and conditions discussed above may present in other ways such as asymptomatic murmurs and coincidental findings in investigations done for other reasons. In such circumstances, management will need to be tailored in the light of the clinical picture and likely natural history.

Cardiac conditions likely to present in the asymptomatic newborn
(Table 28.24)

The commonest asymptomatic presentation of heart disease in the newborn period is the detection of a heart murmur, which may be a feature at an early stage of the natural history of many of the conditions discussed above.

Innocent heart murmurs

Detailed history and other features on physical examination are an important part of the evaluation of a heart murmur. The features of innocent murmurs in the newborn are given in Chapter 14. It is important to note that innocent murmurs have positive characteristics as well as being associated with no other clinical evidence of cardiovascular disease. It is unclear whether ECG and CXR help the experienced or trained observer distinguish innocent from pathological murmurs (Farrer and Rennie 2003). Their widespread availability perpetuates their continued use. A practical approach following the detection of a heart murmur is given below.

Pathological asymptomatic heart murmurs

The likely causes for such murmurs detected in the newborn are given in Table 28.24. The conditions listed are considered elsewhere in the chapter. As a general rule, obstructive lesions cause a murmur from birth, although the murmur associated with mild pulmonary stenosis, trivial aortic stenosis or simple bicuspid aortic valve may

not be heard. Pulmonary and particularly aortic stenosis may progress in severity. Lesions associated with left-to-right shunts frequently cause no murmur in the immediate newborn period and may not be detected until a 6- or 8-week routine check. If a pansystolic murmur suggesting VSD is heard in the newborn period, it may be due to tricuspid regurgitation, which will resolve over a matter of a few weeks. A VSD detected immediately after birth is likely to be small. If a structural abnormality is suspected as the cause of an asymptomatic murmur, an ECG and CXR should be performed. These investigations may have diagnostic features and are of some help in deciding the severity of the lesion and therefore timescale in which cardiology review and echocardiography are indicated.

Practical approach to neonatal heart murmurs

When a heart murmur is detected in the early newborn period, a number of options are open which will be influenced by local considerations, particularly availability of specialist cardiological services and echocardiography. The following are common approaches:

- If symptoms or other signs of cardiac disease exist, an ECG and CXR should be performed and cardiology referral made; this can involve the use of telemedicine to have the cardiac ultrasound assessed by a paediatric cardiologist prior to or instead of transferring the infant (Casey 1999).
- If no symptoms or other signs are present, but the murmur has features suggesting a structural lesion, an ECG and CXR should be performed and cardiology referral made.
- If no symptoms or other signs of cardiac disease are present and the murmur has features compatible with an innocent one, discharge from hospital is reasonable. Pulse oximetry should be performed (see above) in these babies prior to discharge from hospital. The family should be warned about important signs and follow-up arranged for 4–6 weeks. It has not been shown that ECG and CXR aid in this decision.

Table 28.24 Cardiac disease presenting in an asymptomatic newborn infant

CATEGORY	DETAIL	COMMENTS
Fetal diagnosis	Any cardiac condition	Diagnosis known/suspected before birth can be confirmed before symptomatic
Murmur	Causes include: Ventricular septal defect Tricuspid regurgitation Aortic stenosis Pulmonary stenosis Patent ductus arteriosus Atrial septal defect Arteriovenous septal defect Tetralogy of Fallot Innocent	
Weak femoral pulses	Coarctation	Many non-cardiac causes of weak pulses
Rhythm or rate abnormality	Fast/slow/irregular	Some are normal variants See arrhythmia section

Some cardiac conditions are diagnosed when cardiac assessment is requested following a non-cardiac diagnosis (e.g. neonatal surgical conditions or certain syndromes).

Table 28.25 Features in an infant with a murmur which suggest the possibility of a serious (duct-dependent) lesion

FEATURE	COMMENT
No weight loss after birth or excessive weight gain, especially if feeding poorly	May suggest incipient heart failure
Any suggestion of symptoms problems	If 'dusky', a transcutaneous hyperoxia test may help or pulse oximetry
Any doubt about quality of femoral pulses	Suggests coarctation
Right arm systolic blood pressure <20 mmHg above leg pressure	
Murmur loudest between scapulae	Suggests coarctation; innocent pulmonary murmur well heard front and sides
Cardiomegaly on chest X-ray	
Ventricular hypertrophy on electrocardiogram	

Table 28.26 Approach to electrocardiogram interpretation of an arrhythmia

QRS complexes	Rate	Slow/norm/fast
	Rhythm	Regular/irregular
		If irregular: premature/delayed
	Configuration	Normal/abnormal
P waves	Seen/not seen	
	Rate	Slow/normal/fast
	Rhythm	Regular/irregular
		If irregular: premature/delayed
	Axis	Normal/abnormal
	Relationship to QRS complexes	None/constant/variable
		If constant: before/within/after
		If before, PR interval:
		Normal/long
		Fixed/changing

Arrhythmias can be classified in a number of ways. They will now be considered under the headings either supraventricular or ventricular. There are important normal variations in rhythm and rate (Southall et al. 1980), which are mentioned at appropriate points below.

Sinus bradycardia

When asleep or when straining, the interval between QRS complexes can lengthen transiently up to 1.5 s, but sustained rates, even during sleep, below 80 beats/min in term or 100 beats/min in preterm infants are not normal. Sinus bradycardia is associated with normal P waves before every QRS complex; the complexes are normal unless the cause of the bradycardia has other effects on the myocardium. Sinus bradycardia is seen most commonly in association with apnoeic episodes. It may also be a manifestation of hypoxaemia, raised intracranial pressure of any cause and hyperkalaemia. It is seen in association with stress from handling and interventions in critically ill infants. Drugs may cause sinus bradycardia, for example heavy sedation administered to the infant or before birth to the mother, digoxin, propranolol and corticosteroids. Sustained sinus bradycardia in a relatively well infant is a feature of hypothyroidism.

Sinus arrhythmia and sinus arrest

These result in variable slowing of the heart rate. Neither is common in the newborn infant. Sinus arrhythmia is an increase in the heart rate during inspiration and results in a regular irregularity of heart rate in time with the respiratory cycle. Sinus arrest or pauses result in an occasional abnormally long pause (<1.6 s) between P waves, producing an irregular irregularity of the heart rate. These two variations of normal are of no significance of themselves. If they are very pronounced, they can be a marker of sinoatrial dysfunction, which may be associated with symptomatic bradycardia or tachycardia.

Atrial ectopics

These are due to premature depolarisation of a site in an atrium earlier than the sinus node discharge so that either a premature QRS complex follows or, if the ectopic is so early as to occur whilst the ventricle is in its refractory period, there is no QRS complex (blocked

- In some centres, all babies with heart murmurs are referred for echocardiography (Ainsworth et al. 1999). This is not practicable in most UK services, and if the above approaches are adopted consistently, the likelihood of a baby with serious cardiac disease coming to harm through delayed diagnosis is small (Farrer and Rennie 2003).

A baby with an asymptomatic murmur should not be allowed home until it is clear that no form of duct-dependent CHD is present; this is usually apparent on clinical grounds (Table 28.25). If there is any doubt, either a further period of observation in hospital is indicated or, preferably, echocardiography should be arranged.

Arrhythmias

In the newborn, primary cardiac arrhythmias requiring treatment are uncommon. Tachy- or bradyarrhythmias are much more likely to be secondary to extracardiac pathology, which must be identified and treated. Occasionally sustained tachyarrhythmias can present with cardiac failure or collapse secondary to impaired cardiac function caused by the arrhythmia. Gaining control of the arrhythmia will usually result in gradual return of normal cardiac function.

Recognition of arrhythmias

Infants with an arrhythmia may be asymptomatic or present with heart failure or very rarely with collapse. Some will have been recognised in utero. An ECG will usually allow precise diagnosis, although occasionally this will not be possible either because the abnormal rhythm is intermittent or because the ECG is difficult to interpret. Sinus rhythm exists if each QRS complex is preceded by a P wave with an axis of 0–190° and with a normal PR interval (90–120 ms). An approach to assessing the ECG in a possible arrhythmia involves answering the questions given in Table 28.26.

atrial ectopics; Fig. 28.23). Intermediate between these two timings for the atrial ectopic, a QRS complex will be conducted aberrantly and be broad. If non-conducted atrial ectopics occur regularly alternating with normally conducted sinus impulses, there will be bradycardia in the region of 60–80 beats/min. If ectopics are frequent or non-conducted but not alternating with sinus beats, the heart rate will be irregular (Fig. 28.23). Atrial ectopics are harmless but may cause confusion when detected in the fetus, causing bradycardia with or without an irregular rhythm. They can be correctly diagnosed by fetal ultrasound and thereby prevent unnecessary concern about fetal wellbeing being engendered. They are markers for an increased incidence of SVT, which may not necessarily be symptomatic. Atrial ectopics resolve within 3 months in 90% of cases.

Sinus tachycardia

Sinus tachycardia is a heart rate above 160 beats/min in term and above 180 beats/min in preterm infants. P waves have a normal axis and precede every QRS complex. Sinus tachycardia is always secondary, usually to a non-cardiac cause. Causes to be considered include fever, hypovolaemia, pain, respiratory failure, anaemia, fluid overload, drugs (in particular, methylxanthines and inotropes) and septicaemia. Structural heart disease or heart muscle disease may cause sinus tachycardia. The cause should be identified and treated; therapy for sinus tachycardia itself is not indicated. In the newborn, sinus tachycardia can reach 230 beats/min, so that at its higher rates it can be difficult to distinguish from the pathological types of SVT.

Supraventricular tachycardia

A simple classification of SVT is given in Table 28.27.

Atrial flutter

This is a rare rhythm in the newborn. It may be diagnosed in utero, in which case maternal digoxin and/or flecainide therapy is indicated. There is an association with myocarditis, myocardial ischaemia and structural heart disease, although the heart is often structurally normal in neonates. Atrial rates usually exceed 300 beats/min and ventricular rate and rhythm will vary with the degree and constancy of AV block. Consistent 2:1 AV block can make the rhythm hard to recognise as the characteristic flutter waves are

hidden by QRS complexes. They may become apparent when the degree of block varies spontaneously or with adenosine administration. Fetal or neonatal heart failure often develops. The rhythm can be well tolerated for short periods but attempts to restore sinus rhythm or at least to control ventricular rate are appropriate to prevent deterioration in heart muscle function. Adenosine will not restore sinus rhythm but may transiently increase AV block, allowing a diagnosis to be made if the rhythm has not been recognised prior to its use (Fig. 28.24). Shocked infants and those in heart failure warrant direct-current (DC) cardioversion to establish sinus rhythm; this should not be carried out without sedating the infant. Recurrence after cardioversion by either of these techniques may occur but is less likely in the newborn than in older children. Digoxin is used to slow ventricular rate and to help maintain sinus rhythm when achieved. Propranolol may be added to digoxin therapy to achieve further control of ventricular rate. If immediate restoration to and maintenance of sinus rhythm cannot be achieved, the outlook is still good, with spontaneous recovery, if ventricular rate and therefore symptoms can be controlled. Preventive antiarrhythmic therapy after early infancy is not required. A minority of patients have an underlying pre-excitation ECG and in many there is probably an underlying accessory pathway. The arrhythmia carries a small mortality in the newborn either from intractable heart failure or from progression to more malignant arrhythmias, spontaneously or in response to electrical or pharmacological intervention.

Atrioventricular re-entry tachycardia

This is the commonest form of SVT in the fetus and newborn and is associated with the presence of an accessory AV conduction pathway. Fetal SVT can be treated by administration of digoxin, flecainide or verapamil to the mother (Allan et al. 1991; Simpson and Sharland 1998) in specialist centres. Administration of antiarrhythmics directly to the fetus is occasionally used. It is preferable to bring the arrhythmia under control before delivery, but in some circumstances this will not be possible. It is almost always possible to achieve rate control prior to delivery. An attempt to gain control of the arrhythmia or achieve rate control is always indicated prior to considering premature delivery. Premature infants tolerate arrhythmias significantly less well than their term counterparts.

The ECG in sinus rhythm may have a pre-excitation pattern (short PR interval and delta wave on QRS upstroke), allowing Wolff–Parkinson–White syndrome to be diagnosed. Even if present, a pre-excitation pattern may be intermittent or disappear with age. The QRS complexes are narrow when SVT occurs unless aberrant conduction occurs, which is very unusual in the newborn. P waves may be visible between QRS complexes, but, if they are, they have an abnormal axis. QRS rates vary from 180 to 300 beats/min (Fig. 28.7). Distinction from sinus tachycardia is occasionally difficult but the overall clinical picture usually allows this, as well as careful examination of the ECG for features mentioned above. Infants can be asymptomatic or have episodes of pallor and breathlessness or be in heart failure. Any form of structural heart disease, myocardial tumours, myocarditis, electrolyte disturbances or indwelling right atrial lines should be considered as causes, but the heart is usually normal. Myocardial dysfunction and mitral regurgitation develop secondary to the arrhythmia and can be expected to resolve once rhythm control is achieved. If the clinical condition allows, facial immersion in cold water until conversion or for a maximum of 10 seconds is associated with an 85–90% cardioversion rate (Sreeram and Wren 1990). If this fails or is impracticable, application of ice to the face may be tried but has a lower success rate, and adenosine

Table 28.27 Simple classification of supraventricular tachycardia

SITE	RHYTHM	COMMENT
Sinus node	Sinus tachycardia	Always secondary
Atrium	Atrial flutter	Rare
	Atrial fibrillation	Very rare
	Atrial tachycardia	Uncommon
AV junction	AV re-entry tachycardia	Common
	AV nodal re-entry Tachycardia	Rare
Below AV node	His bundle tachycardia (junctional ectopic tachycardia)	Very rare Usually postoperative
AV, atrioventricular.		

intravenously should be used. Adenosine also has an 85% success rate in restoring sinus rhythm and it may unmask atrial flutter if present.

Contraindications to adenosine in the newborn are few. Dipyridamole will potentiate its effects. Side-effects include transient profound bradycardia. If these measures fail and the baby is collapsed, synchronised DC shock should be given, starting at 1 J/kg and increasing to a maximum of 3 J/kg. If rhythm control is not achieved, then starting an amiodarone infusion will usually reduce the rate over time and further attempts to cardiovert the baby using adenosine or DC shock 4–8 hours after starting amiodarone can be undertaken. Verapamil is not recommended for intravenous administration in the newborn period or infancy because of the incidence of bradycardia and hypotension associated with its use. In summary, acute treatment of SVT is as follows (drug doses are given in Table 28.28):

- DC cardioversion if collapsed (sedate unless unconscious).
- Facial immersion/icebag.
- Intravenous adenosine if vagotonic manoeuvre fails.
- Review need for cardioversion. Retry facial immersion and intravenous adenosine if DC cardioversion still not indicated.
- If in heart failure, observation is not appropriate and amiodarone should be considered in conjunction with discussion with cardiology service.
- When sinus rhythm is established, decide on appropriate maintenance–preventive treatment (see text).

Once sinus rhythm is restored, maintenance therapy with whatever agent(s) restored is usually given for about 3–6 months. Drug doses are given in Table 28.28. SVT which presents prenatally or in the neonatal period will resolve spontaneously during the first year of life in the majority of cases.

Ventricular arrhythmias

Ventricular arrhythmias have QRS–T complexes which are always different in configuration and polarity from those in sinus rhythm; the QRS complexes are usually, but not necessarily, broad. Broad complexes can be hard to recognise in the newborn as the upper limit of normal for QRS duration is only 70 ms. Associated and causative conditions for ventricular arrhythmias include any type of cardiomyopathy, myocarditis, intracardiac tumours, electrolyte disturbances, hypoxaemia and acidosis, and only rarely structural CHD. Familial long-QT syndromes (Schwartz et al. 1993) may be detected in the newborn if the family history is known or if ventricular arrhythmias occur.

Premature ventricular complexes

These are recognised by being abnormal premature QRS complexes without a preceding P wave. They are followed by a compensatory pause. Sometimes, complexes with features of both the ventricular ectopic (VE) and the normal QRS complex are seen (fusion complexes). VEs have been found in up to 33% of healthy newborn infants (Southall et al. 1980). They are rarely a sign of cardiac disease but the conditions listed above must be considered. Occasional unifocal VEs with normal clinical examination and ECG require no action in the newborn period, merely review at 6–8 weeks. Very frequent VEs, the presence of a family history suggesting a long-QT syndrome, cardiac physical signs or ECG abnormalities – particularly a long QT (Villain et al. 1992) or evidence of heart muscle disease – are an indication for echocardiography and 24-hour ECG monitoring (looking for VT). Isolated VEs with a

normal heart require no treatment and will resolve within 2 months; if they do not, echocardiography and 24-hour ECG monitoring should be performed or repeated.

Ventricular tachycardia

This is rare in the newborn and consists of a series of VEs occurring sequentially with a rate of 150–250 beats/min. Close examination reveals that there are almost always minor irregularities in rate and that the P waves, if recognised, are either dissociated from the QRS complexes or conducted retrogradely. The rhythm may be paroxysmal or sustained; if paroxysmal, fusion beats may be seen. Neonates with VT may have underlying diseases as listed above but may have normal hearts. A well infant with no underlying disease may be asymptomatic; most cardiologists would still advocate preventive treatment in such cases initially. Collapsed infants should receive synchronised DC shock; less severely symptomatic infants should be treated with lidocaine or amiodarone intravenously. Pulseless VT should be treated with full cardiopulmonary resuscitation and DC shock (1–2 J/kg). If the rhythm reflects underlying electrolyte disturbance, this should be rapidly corrected. Propranolol is the traditional oral preventive; amiodarone may be used in certain cases (Table 28.28).

Idioventricular rhythm

This has the morphology of VT but is slower (110–120 beats/min), being around the same speed as sinus rhythm. It is rarely a sign of heart disease, is usually well tolerated and has a benign natural history.

Ventricular fibrillation

The QRS complexes are fast, bizarre and irregular. Full cardiopulmonary resuscitation should be instituted if the underlying pathology is unknown or considered remediable. Ventricular fibrillation is very rare in neonates and is usually terminal whatever the cause. If controlled, long-QT syndrome must be excluded.

Atrioventricular conduction disturbances (heart block)

There are three degrees of AV conduction block.

First-degree heart block

This is present when the PR interval exceeds the upper limit of normal for age and heart rate; the maximum is 110 ms in the newborn. It is never symptomatic but may reflect underlying structural heart disease such as ASD, heart muscle disease or drug effect (for example, digoxin). It can occur in families and may progress to more severe degrees of block.

Second-degree heart block

This is present when not every P wave is followed by a QRS complex. There are two forms. Mobitz type I second-degree AV block shows the Wenckebach phenomenon in which the PR interval progressively increases until, after three to six cycles, the P wave is not conducted; the sequence then commences again. This phenomenon may be normal and is seen in sleep or under anaesthesia at any age and does not necessarily reflect underlying heart disease. Mobitz type II block has a fixed normal or long PR interval with intermittent non-conduction of the P wave. Failure to conduct the P wave

Table 28.28 Antiarrhythmic drug doses

DRUG	DOSE AND ROUTE	COMMENT
Adenosine	0.05–0.25 mg/kg rapid i.v.	Start low and increase at 2-minute intervals
Digoxin	10 μg/kg i.v. over 15 minutes, then 5 μg/kg i.v. after 6 hours; repeat after a further 6 hours After digitalisation regimen start maintenance at: 4 μg/kg/dose oral 12-hourly (give 60% of this if using i.v. route)	Acute loading doses. Ensure infant is not hypokalaemic
Propranolol	0.05 mg/kg i.v. over 2 minutes 1–2 mg/kg/dose oral 8-hourly	Acute, may repeat once. Avoid in severe heart failure Beware hypoglycaemia Never use after verapamil
Amiodarone	i.v. load with 25 μg/kg/min and titrate dose to heart rate Oral 5 mg/kg t.d.s. and decrease to b.d. then o.d. at 7 and 14 days Respectively (maintain on o.d.)	Ideally via central access Oral not suitable for acute prescription
Verapamil		Better avoided in newborns Never use after propranolol
Lidocaine	1 mg/kg i.v., then 1 mg/kg/h i.v.	
DC shock	SVT (synchronised) 0.5–1 J/kg VT/VF 1–2 J/kg	Sedation/anaesthesia required unless infant unconscious

Note: Other drugs used vary with local expertise. Advice should be sought.
DC, direct current; SVT, supraventricular tachycardia; VT, ventricular tachycardia; VF, ventricular fibrillation.

is often at regular intervals such as 2 : 1, 3 : 1 and so on. Mobitz type II block is much more likely to reflect underlying cardiac disease and frequently progresses to CHB.

Third-degree heart block

This is also termed CHB. The P waves and QRS complexes in CHB are totally dissociated. The atrial rate and responsiveness are usually normal and the ventricular rate is usually between 40 and 80 beats/min with limited variation (Fig. 28.19). Fetal and neonatal CHB may be associated with a variety of usually complex structural heart lesions, in which case heart failure is the norm and outlook is frequently poor.

Another group of patients with congenital CHB have structurally normal hearts. A high proportion of these infants have His bundle fibrosis secondary to maternal antibodies, termed anti-Ro or -La antibodies. Mothers with these antibodies may have connective tissue disorders but more usually are well with serological markers for connective tissue disease. Many neonates with normal hearts and CHB are asymptomatic. Heart failure may occur pre- or postnatally; Stokes–Adams attacks are rare. A number of factors identify infants likely to have a poor outlook without intervention; these include structural heart disease, symptoms, resting heart rate below 55 beats/min, little increase in heart rate in response to stress and broad QRS complexes. If necessary, specific emergency management should include inotropes and diuretics and, if possible, temporary transvenous pacing. Permanent pacemaker insertion is invariably epicardial in newborn infants. CHB in the fetus is usually well tolerated with a structurally normal heart; if hydrops starts to develop, thought should be given to delivery. However, the complications of transvenous pacing in premature and low-birthweight infants should not be underestimated. Evidence that the fetal heart rate can be significantly increased by drug administration to the mother is unclear; maternal steroid administration to prevent His bundle damage has been advocated but is not universally accepted. Fetal pacemaker insertion has yet to be successful.

Hypertension

Hypertension in newborn infants is primarily of renal origin, although cardiac, endocrine and pulmonary causes have been described (see Table 28.29). The incidence of hypertension in newborns is low – 0.2–3%. BP in newborn infants is influenced by gestational age, birthweight and postconceptual age. Data from Zubrow et al. (1995) are the most widely used measures with the BP considered elevated if it falls above the 95% confidence limits for infants of similar age and size (Appendix 4). As a useful rule of thumb, a systolic BP above 90 mmHg and certainly above 100 mmHg in a term baby should be evaluated carefully. In most newborns, hypertension is discovered on monitoring of vital signs. Measurement of neonatal BP is discussed on page 630.

Critically unwell infants are likely to have direct invasive BP measurements. Causes of hypertension are given in Table 28.29. Hypertension is rarely symptomatic but may cause heart failure, tachypnoea, poor feeding, irritability and other neurological signs. In premature babies, a history of CLD and indwelling umbilical arterial or venous catheters may be relevant. Thromboembolism causing renovascular hypertension is surprisingly common after umbilical arterial catheterisation and is thought to be related more to umbilical arterial endothelial damage at the time of line placement than the position of the catheter (high versus low). CLD with bronchopulmonary dysplasia may cause hypertension in 40% of infants (Abman et al. 2002) but the hypertension does not usually present until after discharge from the neonatal units.

Table 28.29 Causes of neonatal hypertension

SYSTEM	EXAMPLES	COMMENT
Renal	Renal artery emboli/thrombosis	May be UAC-related May be acutely symptomatic Often improves over 12 months Hypertension may be delayed-onset
	Renal vein thrombosis	
	Dysplastic renal disease	
	Urinary tract obstruction	
	Renal infection	
	Renal failure	Any cause
Cardiovascular	Coarctation	
Endocrine	Congenital adrenal hyperplasia	
	Hyperaldosteronism	
	Hyperthyroidism	
	Phaeochromocytoma	
	Neuroblastoma	
Respiratory disease	Acute hypercapnia	Any cause
	Chronic lung disease	Often steroid-induced
Neurological disease	Raised intracranial pressure	Any cause Treating blood pressure alone will reduce cerebral perfusion pressure
	Convulsions	Probably mediated via intracranial pressure, convulsion may be subtle or masked by drugs
Drugs	Neonatal exposure: Corticosteroids Methylxanthines Phenylephrine Inotropes Fetal exposure: Maternal cocaine	 In eye drops Overdose

Examination should look for dysmorphic features to exclude genetic syndromes and move on to four-limb BP measurements to look for aortic coarctation. After cardiovascular examination, abdominal assessment to exclude obvious renal abnormalities (e.g. large polycystic kidneys) and genital examination to exclude congenital adrenal hyperplasia are important. Routine investigation should include standard serum biochemistry with thyroid function tests, plasma cortisol, aldosterone and rennin levels. Ultrasound imaging to exclude coarctation and evaluation of the kidneys and renal blood vessels is essential. Renal angiography is not usually required in the neonatal period. Renal perfusion imaging is also less accurate in neonates because of immature renal function and needs to be interpreted with caution.

Specific treatment is appropriate if there are symptoms; in their absence, therapy should be aimed at the underlying disease and hypotensive therapy only commenced if there is severe hypertension or evidence of progressive left ventricular hypertrophy. Some drugs and dosages commonly used to treat neonatal hypertension are listed in Tables 28.30 and 28.31. In the rare circumstances where intravenous antihypertensive therapy is required, intravenous infusions of diazoxide, hydralazine, sodium nitroprusside, labetalol, esmolol or nicardipine can be used. Rapid reduction of BP can also be achieved using oral ACE inhibitors (captopril) or oral nifedipine. There are concerns about possible adverse effects of captopril on renal development in neonates and oral nifedipine is difficult to

administer in small doses. Long-term beta-blockers may not be suitable in patients with bronchopulmonary dysplasia but, often, both hypertension and pulmonary compliance are improved with long-term diuretic therapy. Alternative drugs used for longer term therapy include minoxidil, clonidine and amilodipine amongst others.

The prognosis in hypertension is that of the underlying cause, providing malignant hypertension is avoided or treated rapidly and effectively. Encephalopathic infants may need sedation or anticonvulsant medication as well as hypotensive therapy, but hypertensive encephalopathy is remarkably rare in the newborn.

Cardiac tumours

Symptomatic cardiac tumours are extremely rare in the newborn but are found more commonly since the widespread use of ultrasound scanning. So-called golfball tumours or echogenic foci, usually in the left ventricle, are isolated fetal echocardiographic findings which have usually resolved by term and are of no functional significance. They do not significantly increase the risk of a syndrome even if found in both ventricles (Simpson 1999). Postnatal follow-up is not required.

Cardiac tumours in the newborn may cause arrhythmias (Muhler et al. 1994) or, less commonly, physical obstruction within the

Table 28.30 Intravenous drugs for treating systemic hypertension

DRUG	CLASS	INTRAVENOUS (I.V.) DOSAGE	COMMENTS
Diazoxide	Vasodilator (arteriolar)	2–5 mg/kg/dose rapid i.v. bolus	Slow i.v. injection ineffective; duration unpredictable; use with caution, may cause rapid hypotension; increases blood glucose
Esmolol	Beta-blocker	100–300 µg/kg/min i.v. infusion	Very short-acting; constant i.v. infusion necessary
Hydralazine	Vasodilator (arteriolar)	0.15–0.6 mg/kg/dose i.v. bolus or 0.75–5 µg/kg/min i.v. constant infusion	Tachycardia is frequent adverse effect; must administer over 4 hours when administered as i.v. bolus
Labetalol	Alpha-blocker and beta-blocker	0.2–1 mg/kg/dose i.v. bolus or 0.25–3 mg/kg/h i.v. constant infusion	Heart failure, bronchopulmonary dysplasia, relative contraindications
Nicardipine	Calcium channel blocker	1–5 µg/kg/min i.v. constant infusion	May cause reflex tachycardia
Sodium nitroprusside	Vasodilator (arteriolar and venous)	0.5–10 µg/kg/min i.v. constant infusion	Thiocyanate toxicity can occur with prolonged use (>72 hours) or in renal failure; usual maintenance dose <2 µg/kg/min, may use 10 µg/kg/min for short duration (i.e. <10–15 min)

Table 28.31 Drugs for treating systemic hypertension

DRUG	CLASS	ORAL DOSAGE	COMMENTS
Captopril	ACE inhibitor	<3 months: 0.01–0.5 mg/kg/dose three times daily; not to exceed 2 mg/kg/day ≥3 months: 0.15–0.3 mg/kg/dose three times daily; not to exceed 6 mg/kg/day	Monitor serum creatinine and potassium levels
Clonidine	Central agonist	0.05–0.1 mg/dose 2–3 times daily	Adverse effects include dry mouth and sedation; rebound hypertension with abrupt discontinuation
Hydralazine	Vasodilator (arteriolar)	0.25–1 mg/kg/dose t.i.d. q.i.d.; not to exceed 7.5 mg/kg/day	Suspension stable up to 1 week; tachycardia and fluid retention are common adverse effects; lupus-like syndrome may develop in slow acetylators
Amlodipine	Calcium channel blocker	0.1–0.3 mg/kg/dose b.i.d.; not to exceed 0.6 mg/kg/day or 20 mg/day	Less likely to cause sudden hypotension than isradipine
Minoxidil	Vasodilator (arteriolar)	0.1–0.2 mg/kg/dose 2–3 times daily	Most potent oral vasodilator; excellent for refractory hypertension
Propranolol	Beta-blocker	0.5–1 mg/kg/dose three times daily	Maximal dose depends on heart rate; may administer as much as 8–10 mg/kg/day if no bradycardia; avoid in infants with bronchopulmonary dysplasia
Labetalol	Alpha- and beta-blocker	1 mg/kg/dose 2–3 times daily, up to 12 mg/kg/day	Monitor heart rate; avoid in infants with bronchopulmonary dysplasia
Spironolactone	Aldosterone antagonist	0.5–1.5 mg/kg/dose twice daily	Potassium-sparing diuretic; monitor electrolytes; several days necessary to observe maximum effectiveness
Hydrochlorothiazide	Thiazide diuretic	2–3 mg/kg/day orally every day or divided twice daily	Monitor electrolytes
Chlorothiazide	Thiazide diuretic	5–15 mg/kg/dose twice daily	Monitor electrolytes

ACE, angiotensin-converting enzyme.

heart. Over 95% of intracardiac tumours in the newborn are benign and at least 75% of them are rhabdomyomata. Rhabdomyomata are often multiple and may resolve, which is a reason for being cautious about surgical intervention even if symptoms are present (Muhler et al. 1994). Multiple intracardiac tumours strongly suggest the possibility of tuberous sclerosis; 50% of individuals with tuberous sclerosis will have cardiac tumours detected by echocardiography if looked for in infancy (Wallace et al. 1990). Pericardial tumours may present with pericardial effusion and tamponade in the newborn period.

Acknowledgement

The author and editor would like to acknowledge the contribution of Dr Nick Archer, author of this chapter in previous editions, for his excellent foundation.

References

Abman S.H., 2002. Monitoring cardiovascular function in infants with chronic lung disease of prematurity. Arch Dis Child 87, F15–F18.

Acherman, R.J., Siassi, B., Pratti-Madrid, G., et al., 2000. Systemic to pulmonary collaterals in very low birth weight infants: color Doppler detection of systemic to pulmonary connections during neonatal and early infancy period. Pediatrics 105, 528–532.

Ainsworth, S.B., Wyllie, J.P., Wren, C., 1999. Prevalence and clinical significance of cardiac murmurs in neonates. Arch Dis Child Fetal Neonatal Ed 80, F43–F45.

Allan, L.D., 1995. Echocardiographic detection of congenital heart disease in the fetus: present and future. Br Heart J 74, 103–106.

Allan, L.D., Crawford, D.C., Anderson, R.H., et al., 1985. Spectrum of congenital heart disease detected echocardiographically in prenatal life. Br Heart J 54, 523–526.

Allan, L.D., Chita, S.K., Sharland, G.K., et al., 1991. Flecainide in the treatment of fetal tachycardias. Br Heart J 65, 46–48.

Anderson, R.H., Baker, E.J., Macartney, F.J., et al., 2002. Paediatric Cardiology, second ed. Churchill Livingstone, London.

Andrews, R., Tulloh, R., 2004. Interventional cardiac catheterization in congenital heart disease. Arch Dis Child 89, 1168–1173.

Andrews, R.E., Simpson, J.M., Sharland, G.K., et al., 2006. Outcome after preterm delivery of infants antenatally diagnosed with congenital heart disease. J Pediatr 148, 213–216.

Barberi, I., Calabro, M.P., Cordaro, S., et al., 1999. Myocardial ischaemia in neonates with perinatal asphyxia. Electrocardiographic, echocardiographic and enzymatic correlations. Eur J Pediatr 158, 742–747.

Barker, C., Kelsall, A.W., Yates, R.W., 2005. Prolonged treatment with prostaglandin in an infant born with extremely low birthweight. Cardiol Young 15, 425–426.

Benitz, W.E., 2010. Treatment of the persistent ductus arteriosus in preterm infants: time to accept the null hypothesis? J Perinatol 30, 241–252.

Bonnet, D., Coltri, A., Butera, G., et al., 1999. Detection of transposition of the great arteries in fetuses reduces neonatal morbidity and mortality. Circulation 99, 916–918.

Bull, C., 1999. Current and potential impact of fetal diagnosis on prevalence and spectrum of serious congenital heart disease at term in the UK. Lancet 354, 1242–1247.

Burch, M., 1994. Hypertrophic cardiomyopathy. Arch Dis Child 71, 488–489.

Burch, M., Runciman, M., 1996. Dilated cardiomyopathy. Arch Dis Child 74, 479–481.

Burn, J., Brennan, P., Little, J., et al., 1998. Recurrence risks in offspring of adults with major heart defects: results from first cohort of British collaborative study. Lancet 351, 311–316.

Carvalho, J.S., Mavrides, E., Shinebourne, E., et al., 2002. Improving the effectiveness of routine prenatal screening for major congenital heart defects. Heart 88, 387–391.

Casey, F.A., 1999. Telemedicine in paediatric cardiology. Arch Dis Child 80, 497–499.

Clarkson, P.M., Orgill, A.A., 1974. Continuous murmurs in infants of low birthweight. J Pediatr 84, 208–211.

Clyman, R.I., 1996. Recommendations for the postnatal use of indomethacin: an analysis of four separate treatment strategies. J Pediatr 128, 601–607.

Clyman, R.I., Chan, C.Y., Mauray, F., et al., 1999. Permanent anatomic closure of the ductus in newborn baboons: the roles of postnatal constriction, hypoxia and gestation. Pediatr Res 45, 19–29.

Couser, R.J., Ferrata, B., Wright, G.B., et al., 1996. Prophylactic indomethacin therapy in the first twenty-four hours of life for the prevention of patent ductus arteriosus in preterm infants treated prophylactically with surfactant in the delivery room. J Pediatr 128, 631–637.

Da Silva, J.P., Baumgratz, J.F., da Fonseca, L., et al., 2007. The cone reconstruction of the tricuspid valve in Ebstein's anomaly: the operation: early and midterm results. Thoracic Cardiovasc Surg 133, 215–223.

Edwards, A.D., Wyatt, J.S., Richardson, C., et al., 1990. Effects of indomethacin on cerebral haemodynamics in very preterm infants. Lancet 335, 1491–1495.

Edwards, L., Morris, K.P., Siddiqui, A., et al., 2007. Norwood procedure for hypoplastic left heart syndrome: Blalock–Taussig shunt or right ventricle to pulmonary artery conduit? Arch Dis Child Fetal Neonatal Ed 92, F210–F214.

Evans, N., 1994. Cardiovascular effects of dexamethasone in the preterm infant. Arch Dis Child Fetal Neonatal Ed 70, F25–F30.

Evans, N.J., Archer, L.N.J., 1990. Postnatal circulatory adaptation in healthy term and preterm neonates. Arch Dis Child 65, 24–26.

Evans, N., Kluckow, M., 1996. Early ductal shunting and intraventricular haemorrhage in ventilated preterm infants. Arch Dis Child Fetal Neonatal Ed 75, F183–F186.

Evans, D.H., Levene, M.I., Archer, L.N.J., 1987. The effect of indomethacin on cerebral blood flow velocity in premature infants. Dev Med Child Neurol 29, 776–782.

Farrer, K.F., Rennie, J.M., 2003. Neonatal murmurs: are senior house officers good enough? Arch Dis Child Fetal Neonatal Ed 88, F147–F151.

Ferencz, C., Neill, C.A., Boughman, J.A., et al., 1989. Congenital cardiac malformations associated with chromosome abnormalities: an epidemiologic study. J Pediatr 114, 79–86.

Fowlie, P.W., Davis, P.G., 2008. Prophylactic intravenous indomethacin for preventing mortality an morbidity in preterm infants. Cochrane Collab Syst Rev 3.

Franklin, O., Burch, M., Manning, N., et al., 2002. Prenatal diagnosis of coarctation of the aorta improves survival and reduces morbidity. Heart 87, 67–69.

Galantowicz, M., Cheatham, J.P., Phillips, A., et al., 2008. Hybrid approach for hypopastic lft heart syndrome: intermediate results after the learning curve. Ann Thorac Surg 85, 2063–2071.

Gersony, W.M., Peckham, G.J., Ellison, R.C., et al., 1983. Effects of indomethacin in premature infants with patent ductus arteriosus: results of a national collaborative study. J Pediatr 102, 895–906.

Grant, D., 1999. Ventricular constraint in the fetus and newborn. Can J Cardiol 15, 95–104.

Green, T.P., Thompson, T.R., Johnson, D.E., et al., 1983. Furosemide promotes patent ductus arteriosus in premature infants with respiratory distress syndrome. N Engl J Med 308, 743–748.

Guenthard, J., Wylie, F., Fowler, B., et al., 1995. Cardiomyopathy in respiratory chain disorders. Arch Dis Child 72, 223–226.

Hallidie-Smith, K.A., 1972. Murmur of patent ductus arteriosus in premature infants. Arch Dis Child 47, 725–730.

Hammerman, C., Kaplan, M., 1990. Patent ductus arteriosus in the premature neonate: current concepts in pharmacologic management. Pediatr Drugs 1, 81–92.

Hermes-DeSantos, E.R., Clyman, R.I., 2006. Patent arterial duct: pathopyhsiology and management. J Perinatol 26, 514–518.

Heymann, M.A., 1995. Fetal and postnatal circulations, pulmonary circulation. In: Emmanouilides, E.C., Riemens-Schneider, T.A., Allen, H.D., et al. (Eds.), Heart Disease in Infants, Children and Adolescents, fifth ed. Williams & Wilkins, Baltimore, pp. 41–47.

Hoffman, J., 2002. Incidence mortality and natural history. In: Anderson, R.H., Baker, E.J., Macartney, F., et al., (Eds.), Paediatric Cardiology. Churchill Livingstone, London, pp. 111–139.

Huggon, I.C., Ghi, T., Cook, A.C., et al., 2002. Fetal cardiac abnormalities identified prior to 14 weeks' gestation. Ultrasound Obstet Gynecol 20, 22–29.

Hunkeler, N.M., Kullman, J., Murphy, A.M., 1991. Troponin I isoform expression in human heart. Circ Res 69, 1409–1414.

Ino, T., Sherwood, G., Benson, L.N., et al., 1988. Cardiac manifestations in disorders of fat and carnitine metabolism in infancy. J Am Coll Cardiol 11, 1301–1308.

Iyer, P., Evans, N., 1994. Re-evaluation of the left atrial to aortic root ratio as a marker of patent ductus arteriosus. Arch Dis Child Fetal Neonatal Ed 70, F112–F117.

Karatza, A.A., Holder, S.E., Gardiner, H.M., 2003. Isolated non-compaction of the ventricular myocardium: prenatal diagnosis and natural history. Ultrasound in Obstetrics and Gynaecology 21, 75–80.

Kaski. J.P., Burch, M., 2007. Viral myocarditis in childhood. Paediatr Child Health 17, 11–18.

Kluckow, M., Evans, N., 1995. Early echocardiographic prediction of symptomatic patent ductus arteriosus in preterm infants undergoing mechanical ventilation. J Pediatr 127, 174–179.

Kohl, T., Sharland, G., Allan, L., et al., 2000. World experience of percutaneous ultrasound-guided balloon valvuloplasty in human fetuses with severe aortic valve obstruction. Am J Cardiol 85, 1230–1233.

Lee, G.J., Cohen, R., Chang, A.L., 2010. ACE (1) induced acute renal failure in premature newborns with congenital heart disease. J Pediatr Pharmacol Ther 15, 290–296.

Licht, D.J., Shera, D.M., Clancy, N.R., et al., 2009. Brain maturation is delayed in patients with complex congenital heart defects. J Thorac Cardiovasc Surg 137, 529–536.

Limperopoulos, C., Majnemer, A., Shevell, M.I., et al., 2000. Neurodevelopmental status of newborns and infants with congenital heart defects before and after open heart surgery. J Pediatr 137, 638–645.

Lipshultz, S.E., Sleeper, L.A., Towbin, J.A., et al., 2003. The incidence of pediatric cardiomyopathy in two regions of the United States. N Engl J Med 348, 1647–1655.

Mahle, W.T., Newburger, J.W., Matherne, G.P., et al., 2009. Role of pulse oximetry in examining newborns for congenital heart disease: a scientific statement from the AHA and AHP. Pediatrics 124, 823–836.

Marijianowski, M.M., der Loos, C.M., Mohrschladt, M.F., et al., 1994. The neonatal heart has a relatively high content of total collagen and type I collagen, a condition that may explain the less compliant state. J Am Coll Cardiol 23, 1204–1208.

Marshall, A.C., Tworetsky, W., Bergersen, L., et al., 2005. Aortic valvuloplasty in the fetus: technical characteristics of a successful balloon dilatation. J Pediatr 147, 535–539.

McCrindle, B.W., Blackstone, E.H., Williams, W.G., et al., 2001. Are outcomes of surgical versus transcatheter balloon valvotomy equivalent in neonatal critical aortic stenosis? Circulation 104 (Suppl. l), 152–158.

Mertens, L., Ganame, J., Eyskens, B., 2008. What's new in pediatric cardiac imaging? Eur J Pediatr 167, 1–8.

Miller, S.P., McQuillen, P.S., 2007. Neurology of congenital heart disease: insight from brain imaging. Arch Dis Child 92, F435–F437.

Montigny, M., Biron, P., Fournier, A., et al., 1989. Captopril in infants for congestive heart failure secondary to a large ventricular left to right shunt. Am J Cardiol 63, 631–633.

Muhler, E.G., Kienas, W., Turniski-Harder, V., et al., 1994. Arrhythmias in infants and children with primary cardiac tumours. Eur Heart J 15, 915–921.

Narayan, M., Cooper, B., Weiss, et al., 2000. Prophylactic indomethacin: factors determining permanent patent ductus arteriosus closure. J Pediatr 136, 330–337.

National Institutes of Health, 1987. Report of the Second Task Force on Blood Pressure Control in Children. Pediatrics 79, 1–25.

Norton, M.E., Merrill, J., Cooper, B.A.B., et al., 1993. Neonatal complications after the administration of indomethacin for preterm labor. N Engl J Med 329, 1602–1607.

Nugent, A.W., Daubeney, P.E.F., Chondros, P., et al., 2003. The epidemiology of childhood cardiomyopathy in Australia. N Engl J Med 348, 1639–1646.

Opie, G.F., Fraser, S.H., Drew, J.H., et al., 1999. Bacterial endocarditis in neonatal intensive care. J Pediatr Child Health 35, 545–548.

Park, M., Guntheroth, W.G., 1992. How to Read Pediatric ECGs, third ed. Year Book, Chicago.

Patel, J., Marks, K.A., Roberts, I., et al., 1995. Ibuprofen treatment for patent ductus arteriosus. Lancet 346, 255.

Patel, J., Roberts, I., Azzopardi, D., et al., 2000. Randomized double blind controlled trial comparing the effects of ibuprofen with indomethacin on cerebral hemodynamics in preterm infants with patent ductus arteriosus. Pediatr Res 47, 36–42.

Pierpont, M.E.M., Moller, J.H., 1987. Chromosomal abnormalities. In: Pierpont, M.E.M., Moller, J.H., (Eds.), The Genetics of Cardiovascular Disease. Boston, Massachusetts, Nijhoff, pp. 13–24.

Pierpont, M.A., Basson, C.T., Benson, D.W., et al., 2007. Genetic basis for congenital heart defects: Current knowledge: A scientific statement from the American Heart Association congenital cardiac defects committee, council on cardiovascular disease in the young: Endorsed by the American academy of pediatrics. Circulation 115, 3015–3038.

Radzik, D., Davignon, A., van Doesburg, N., et al., 1993. Predictive factors for spontaneous closure of atrial septal defect diagnosed in the first 3 months of life. J Am Coll Cardiol 22, 851–853.

Raju, T.N.K., Langenberg, P., 1993. Pulmonary hemorrhage and exogenous surfactant therapy: a meta analysis. J Pediatr 123, 606–610.

Rasanen, J., Wood, D.C., Debbs, R.H., et al., 1998. Reactivity of the human fetal pulmonary circulation to maternal hyperoxygenation increases during the second half of pregnancy: a randomized study. Circulation 97, 257–262.

Rennie, J.M., Cooke, R.W.I., 1991. Prolonged low dose indomethacin for persistent ductus arteriosus of prematurity. Arch Dis Child 66, 55–58.

Richmond, S., Reay, G., Abu Harb, M., 2002. Routine pulse oximetry in the asymptomatic newborn. Arch Dis Child Fetal Neonatal Ed 87, F83–F88.

Robie, D.K., Waltrip, T., Garcia-Prats, J.A., et al., 1996. Is surgical ligation of a patent ductus arteriosus the preferred initial approach for the neonate with extremely low birth weight? J Pediatr Surg 8, 1134–1137.

Rudolph, A.M., 1974. Congenital Diseases of the Heart. Year Book Medical Publishers, Chicago.

Schmidt, B., Davis, P., Moddemann, D., et al., 2001. Long term effects of indomethacin prophylaxis in extremely low birth weight infants. N Engl J Med 344, 1966–1972.

Schwartz, P.J., Locati, E.H., Moss, A.J., et al., 1993. Diagnostic criteria for the long QT syndrome: an update. Circulation 88, 782–784.

Shortland, D.B., Gibson, N.A., Levene, M.I., et al., 1990. Patent ductus arteriosus and cerebral circulation in preterm infants. Dev Med Child Neurol 32, 386–393.

Silove, E.D., Roberts, D.G.U., De Giovanni, J.V., 1985. Evaluation of oral and low dose intravenous prostaglandin E$_2$ in management of ductus dependent congenital heart disease. Arch Dis Child 60, 1025–1030.

Simpson, J.M., 1999. The cardiac echogenic focus. Prenat Diagn 19, 972–975.

Simpson, J.M., Sharland, G.K., 1997. Natural history and outcome of aortic stenosis diagnosed prenatally. Heart 77, 205–210.

Simpson, J.M., Sharland, G.K., 1998. Fetal tachycardias: management and outcome of 127 consecutive cases. Heart 79, 576–581.

Southall, D.P., Richard, J., Mitchell, P., et al., 1980. Study of cardiac rhythm in healthy newborn infants. Br Heart J 43, 14–20.

Sreeram, N., Wren, C., 1990. Supraventricular tachycardia in infants: response to initial treatment. Arch Dis Child 65, 127–129.

Stümpflen, I., Stümpflen, A., Wimmer, M., et al., 1996. Effect of detailed fetal echocardiography as part of routine prenatal ultrasonographic screening on detection of congenital heart disease. Lancet 348, 854–857.

Su, B.H., Watanabe, T., Shimizu, M., et al., 1997. Echocardiographic assessment of patent ductus arteriosus shunt flow pattern in premature infants. Arch Dis Child Fetal Neonatal Ed 77, F36–F40.

Su, B.H., Peng, C.T., Tsai, C.H., 1999. Echocardiographic flow pattern of patent ductus arteriosus: a guide to indomethacin treatment in premature infants. Arch Dis Child Fetal Neonatal Ed 81, F197–F200.

Tillett, A., Hartley, B., Simpson, J., 2001. Paradoxical embolism causing fatal myocardial infarction in a newborn infant. Arch Dis Child Fetal Neonatal Ed 85, F137–F138.

Tulloh, R.M.R., Tansey, S.P., Parashar, K., et al., 1994. Echocardiographic screening in neonates undergoing surgery for selected gastrointestinal malformations. Arch Dis Child Fetal Neonatal Ed 70, F206–F208.

Tulzer, G., Artz, W., Franklin, R.C.G., et al., 2002. Fetal pulmonary valvuloplasty for critical pulmonary stenosis or atresia with intact ventricular septum. Lancet 360, 1567–1568.

Tworetzky, W., McElhinney, D.B., Reddy, M., et al., 2001. Improved surgical outcome after fetal diagnosis of hypoplastic left heart syndrome. Circulation 103, 1269–1273.

Van Overmeire, B., Smets, K., Lecouterie, D., et al., 2000. A comparison of ibuprofen and indomethacin for closure of patent ductus arteriosus. N Engl J Med 343, 674–681.

Villain, E., Levy, M., Kachaner, J., et al., 1992. Prolonged QT interval in neonates: benign, transient or prolonged risk of sudden death. Am Heart J 124, 194–197.

Wallace, G., Smith, H.C., Watson, G.H., et al., 1990. Tuberous sclerosis presenting with fetal and neonatal cardiac tumours. Arch Dis Child 65, 377–379.

Ward, C., 2000. Clinical significance of the bicuspid aortic valve. Heart 83, 81–85.

Way, G.L., Woolfe, R.R., Eshaghpour, E., et al., 1979. The natural history of hypertrophic cardiomyopathy in infants of diabetic mothers. J Pediatr 95, 1020–1025.

Weber, H.S., 2002. Initial and late results after catheter intervention for neonatal critical pulmonary valve stenosis and atresia with intact ventricular septum: a technique in continual evolution. Cathet Cardiovasc Interv 56, 394–399.

Wells, J.T., Ment, L.R., 1995. Prevention of intraventricular hemorrhage in preterm infants. Early Hum Dev 42, 209–233.

Wernovsky, G., Newburger, J.W., 2003. Neurological and developmental morbidity in children with complex congenital heart disease. J Pediatr 142, 6–8.

Wilkinson, J.L., Cooke R.W.I., 1992. Cardiovascular disorders. In: Roberton's textbook of Neonatology, second ed. Churchill Livingstone, Edinburgh.

Yates, R., 2004. The influence of prenatal diagnosis on postnatal outcome in patients with structural congenital heart disease. Prenat Diagn 24, 1143–1149.

Zubrow, A.B., Hulman, S., Kushner, H., et al., 1995. Determinants of blood pressure in infants admitted to neonatal intensive care units: a prospective multicenter study. Philadelphia neonatal blood pressure study group. J Perinatol 15, 470–479.

Gastroenterology

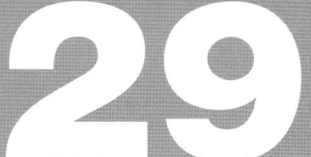

N Kevin Ives   Giorgina Mieli-Vergani   Nedim Hadžić   Simon Newell
Ian Sugarman   Mark D Stringer   Alistair G Smyth

CHAPTER CONTENTS

© 2012 Elsevier Ltd

Part 1: **Neonatal jaundice**

N Kevin Ives

Introduction

Jaundice is the most common clinical sign in neonatal medicine. Approximately 60% of healthy term infants and 80% of premature infants develop clinically visible jaundice in the first week of life, but only rarely is it the harbinger of significant disease or associated with bilirubin neurotoxicity. In the majority of cases jaundice is mild and transient, resulting from an immaturity of the liver's excretory pathway for bilirubin at a time of its heightened production. Neonatal jaundice remains one of the most common reasons for readmission to hospital in the first week of life. Prolonged jaundice, beyond 2 weeks of life in the term infant, is common and usually innocent, but may be a warning sign of underlying disease.

Up to a third of breastfed babies are clinically jaundiced at 2 weeks of age. Screening for significant jaundice in the first days and weeks of life needs to be in place so that pathological causes are diagnosed promptly and treated appropriately. The importance of identifying conjugated hyperbilirubinaemia at an early stage cannot be overstressed.

With relaxation of treatment thresholds for jaundice over the past two decades a 'kinder, gentler approach' to clinical management in healthy full-term newborns has evolved (Newman and Maisels 1992). This spared a large number of babies and their families the stress of blood tests, phototherapy, exchange transfusion and prolonged hospitalisation (Seidman et al. 2001), but a less vigilant approach to the jaundiced infant may have been engendered. Earlier postnatal discharge, inadequate community surveillance and translation of the more relaxed approach to therapy in the term baby to that in the late preterm or near-term infant led to a resurgence of kernicterus, as noted in Europe and the USA (Newman and Maisels 2000; Watchko 2001; Ives 2007; Manning et al. 2007).

Our ability to identify which babies are at greatest risk of developing levels of significant jaundice remains imprecise. The American approach has been to focus on the predictive value of an hour-specific predischarge bilirubin measurement (Bhutani et al. 1999; Maisels et al. 2009a). Recent national guidance in the UK, where discharge at less than 24 hours is becoming the norm, mandates review within 48 hours of birth of babies with risk factors, and recommends measurement of the bilirubin level in all babies presenting with clinical jaundice (National Institute for Health and Clinical Excellence 2010).

Phototherapy remains the mainstay of treatment of significant unconjugated hyperbilirubinaemia, and its optimal use will usually keep the level of jaundice below the threshold for a potentially hazardous exchange blood transfusion. In cases of isoimmune haemolysis high-dose immunoglobulin is indicated if the serum bilirubin is continuing to rise despite optimal phototherapy (Gottstein and Cooke 2003; National Institute for Health and Clinical Excellence 2010). The use of metalloporphyrins to suppress haem catabolism and modify the pattern of neonatal jaundice has not yet entered routine clinical practice.

Bilirubin biochemistry

Bilirubin is produced by a two-stage catabolism of haem in the reticuloendothelial system (Fig. 29.1). The majority of haem arises from the turnover of haemoglobin released from naturally decommissioned or pathologically destroyed erythrocytes. Haem (ferroprotoporphyrin IX) has a porphyrin ring structure which is opened preferentially at its α-methene bridge by haem oxygenase. The intermediate pigment, biliverdin IXα, is water-soluble, non-toxic and serves as the excretory product of haem in amphibians, reptiles and birds. In mammals, reduction of biliverdin IXα by biliverdin reductase results in the production of bilirubin IXα.

Bilirubin IXα is the only toxic isomer of bilirubin. The small amounts of the IXβ and IXδ isomers produced are non-toxic. Why mammalian species should expend energy producing and excreting a potentially neurotoxic haem byproduct remains unclear. One possible explanation stems from the fact that bilirubin is an antioxidant, prompting the question: 'Is bilirubin good for you?' (McDonagh 1990). Whatever the reason, we are left with the responsibility of ensuring that serum levels of free bilirubin IXα fail to reach neurotoxic levels.

Diagrammatic representation of the bilirubin molecule gives the impression of a tetrapyrrole aligned in a single plane (Fig. 29.2), but the preferred conformation of the molecule is partially folded

at its mid-methylene bridge (Fig. 29.3). This shape facilitates intramolecular hydrogen bonding, saturating the hydrophilic polar groupings, and rendering bilirubin virtually insoluble in water at physiological pH. In this form, bilirubin has lipophilic properties, enabling it to cross cell membranes and biological boundaries, such as the placenta and blood–brain barrier.

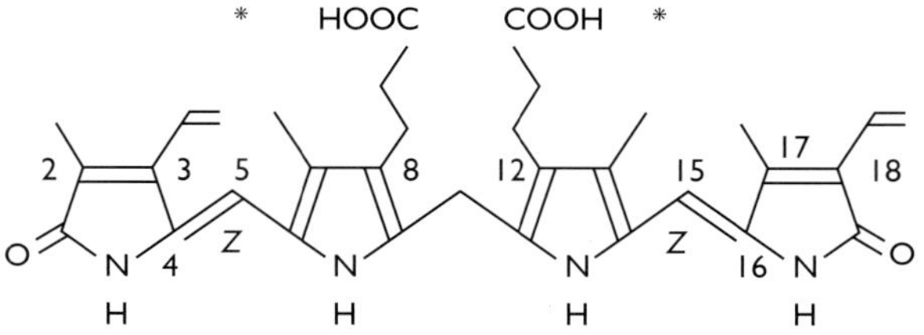

Fig. 29.2 Linear representation of bilirubin IXα with central propionic acid groups (**).

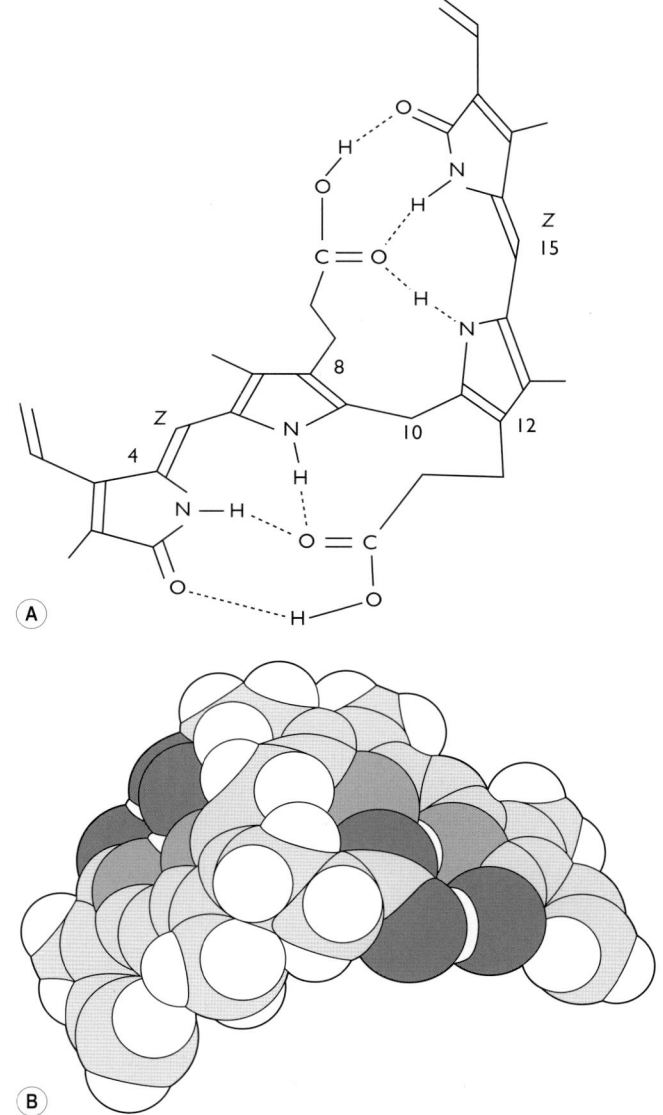

(A)

(B)

Fig. 29.3 (A) Preferred confirmation of bilirubin. (B) Atomic representation of the bilirubin-IXa ZZ molecule (nitrogen, mid-grey; oxygen, dark grey; carbon, light grey; hydrogen, white).

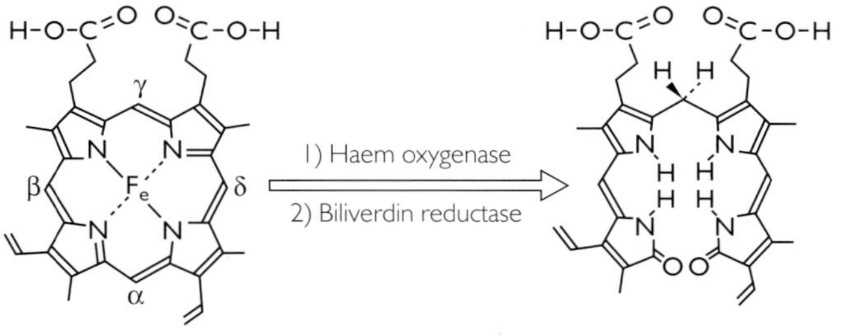

Haem **Bilirubin**

Fig. 29.1 Production of bilirubin from haem degradation.

The propionic acid groups attached to the inner two pyrrole rings of the bilirubin molecule are the site of conjugation with glucuronic acid. The mono- and diglucuronides of bilirubin so formed retain the more open, water-soluble conformation by reducing or preventing intramolecular hydrogen bonding. Polar groupings remain similarly exposed in the naturally occurring β and δ isomers of bilirubin and in the isomers produced by phototherapy, enabling them to be freely excreted in bile (Ennever 1992).

Bilirubin metabolism and excretion

In the newborn baby bilirubin arises mainly from the breakdown of red cells, with up to a quarter resulting from ineffective erythropoiesis and other haem-containing compounds, such as myoglobin and cytochromes. Bilirubin is transported in the blood bound reversibly to serum albumin on high- and low-affinity sites, with a potential molar bilirubin to albumin ratio up to 3 : 1. Under normal circumstances, the proportion of free bilirubin circulating in the jaundiced newborn is very low (<5 nmol/l).

Conjugation of bilirubin with glucuronic acid occurs in the smooth endoplasmic reticulum to form water-soluble mono- and diglucuronides of bilirubin. These reactions are catalysed by the microsomal enzyme hepatic uridine diphosphoglucuronosyl transferase (UDPGT). Conjugated bilirubin (chiefly the monoglucuronide in the newborn) is actively transported out of the liver cell and enters the biliary canaliculi as a component of bile.

In adults, most of the conjugated bilirubin is converted by colonic flora to urobilinogen before elimination in the stool. In the newborn, a significant proportion is hydrolysed by β-glucuronidase in the small gut to yield unconjugated bilirubin, which can re-enter the circulating pool via the enterohepatic circulation.

Biochemical basis of phototherapy

Phototherapy detoxifies bilirubin and facilitates its excretion from the body via routes other than conjugation in the liver (McDonagh and Lightner 1985; Ennever 1992). When bilirubin interacts with a photon of light, three photochemical reactions can occur. They are photo-oxidation, configurational isomerisation and structural isomerisation. Photo-oxidation causes disruption of the bilirubin molecule to form colourless polar fragments that are readily excreted in urine. Although this process reminds us of the need to avoid exposure of serum samples to direct sunlight (Cremer et al. 1958), it plays only a minor role in bilirubin excretion during phototherapy.

Configurational isomerisation results from molecular reorientation around the double bonds between carbon atoms 4–5 and 15–16 (Fig. 29.2). In the natural form, the arrangement of these double bonds, and hence the alignment of the end pyrrole rings, is classified as bilirubin-4Z,15Z (Z = *zusammen*, together). A photon of light striking the bilirubin molecule can temporarily disrupt the double bonds and initiate a 180° rotation of one or both end pyrrole rings to produce three isomeric forms, designated: 4Z,15E; 4E,15Z; and 4E,15E (E = *entgegen*, apart).

Formation of bilirubin-Z,E is favoured during phototherapy and its conformation (as shown in Fig. 29.4) maintains exposure of polar groups at one end of the molecule, facilitating its excretion, unconjugated, in bile. Whilst bound to albumin, the configurational isomers remain stable for a number of hours. Once in bile, a rapid deconfiguration occurs, and unconjugated bilirubin-Z,Z entering the gut is available for reuptake into the bloodstream via the enterohepatic circulation.

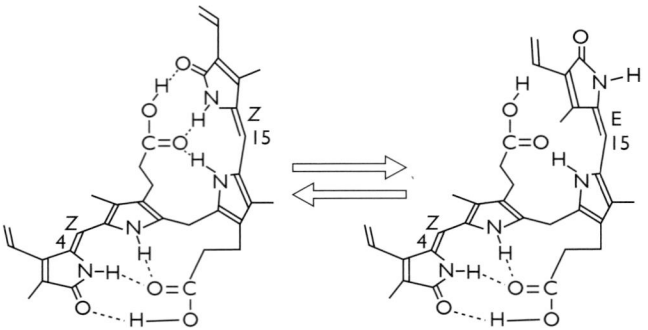

Fig. 29.4 Configurational photoisomerisation of bilirubin.

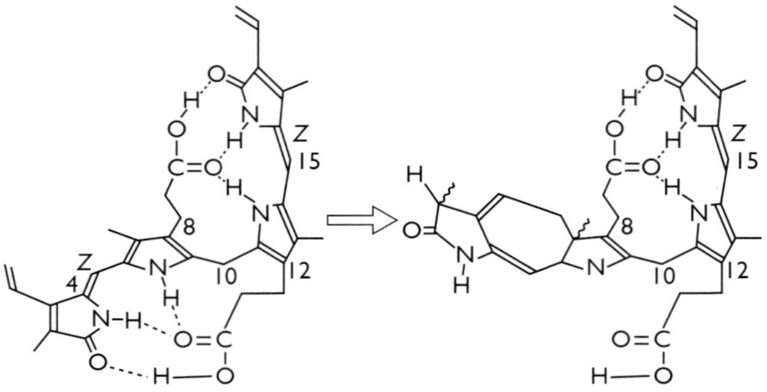

Fig. 29.5 Structural photoisomerisation of bilirubin to form lumirubin.

It was originally thought that phototherapy acted mainly through configurational isomerisation. Although rapidly produced, these isomers are slowly cleared in humans. The serum half-life of bilirubin-Z,E is about 15 hours, and after some 6–12 hours of phototherapy a steady state is achieved with approximately 20% of the total serum bilirubin in the form of the configurational isomers. Importantly, this is likely to mean that up to one-fifth of the circulating bilirubin is detoxified, despite not being in a form that is readily excreted. This fraction may reach one-quarter in combination with other isomers mentioned below.

The main contributor to bilirubin excretion during phototherapy is thought to be the formation of the structural isomer lumirubin, which is formed by 'cyclisation' of one end of the bilirubin molecule, as shown in Figure 29.5. This structural change is irreversible and allows the more polar product to be excreted in bile and urine. More efficient elimination is reflected by lumirubin's half-life of less than 2 hours and steady-state level during phototherapy of 2–6% of the total serum bilirubin. Unlike the configurational isomer, production of lumirubin follows a dose–response relationship with the irradiance of phototherapy applied. Its production is favoured by the use of light of a longer wavelength than that of conventional phototherapy, but there are few advocates for the use of green lights.

The normal pattern of neonatal jaundice

The fetus excretes unconjugated bilirubin via the placenta and maternal liver. In the absence of fetal hyperbilirubinaemia or maternal liver disease, the mean bilirubin level in umbilical cord blood at birth is 20–35 μmol/l (Knudsen and Lebech 1989). Most newborn babies have an increase in serum bilirubin in the first week of life, reaching clinically detectable levels in about 60% of term

Table 29.1 Factors that exacerbate jaundice in the newborn

Polycythaemia
    Delayed cord clamping
    Maternofetal transfusion
    Recipient of twin–twin transfusion
Extravasated blood
    Bruising (e.g. cephalhaematoma)
    Birth trauma
    Internal haemorrhage
Delayed passage of meconium
Swallowed blood
Hypocaloric feed intake
Dehydration
Breastfeeding
Prematurity

and 80% of preterm infants. This has been referred to as physiological jaundice. In healthy term formula-fed babies, the serum bilirubin peaks on the third to fourth day of life, becoming clinically detectable at levels above 80 μmol/l. Following this phase I peak, serum bilirubin levels fall rapidly for 2–3 days and then more gradually, reaching normal adult values between 1 and 2 weeks of age (phase II). Exclusively breastfed babies often have a delayed serum bilirubin peak and a more prolonged course to their jaundice. This pattern of jaundice is the result of increased bilirubin production at a time when the mechanisms for liver uptake, transport and conjugation of bilirubin are immature. At higher serum bilirubin levels, the excretion of bilirubin into bile may be rate-limiting. The biphasic pattern of normal neonatal jaundice results from a deficiency of UDPGT activity in the first phase and low intrahepatic binding protein levels in the second.

The pattern of neonatal jaundice in prematurely born babies is characterised by a higher peak serum bilirubin level, occurring on days 5–7, and a longer phase II, persisting for 2–4 weeks. This potential for heightened jaundice also applies to the late preterm infant (gestational age 34^{+0}–36^{+6} weeks). Bilirubin production during the first weeks of life is more than double that of the adult. This excess bilirubin load in the newborn results from factors that include a higher haematocrit, increased red cell turnover and a greater contribution from sources of haem other than senescent erythrocytes. In addition, the 10-fold higher level of β-glucuronidase in the small bowel brush border of the newborn reverses the conjugation process, liberating more unconjugated bilirubin to join the enterohepatic circulation. Other risk factors that exacerbate neonatal jaundice are listed in Table 29.1. It must be appreciated that in such circumstances, and despite the lack of an underlying pathology, the serum bilirubin may attain levels causal of transient auditory derangement (Tan et al. 1992) or permanent neurological damage (Maisels and Newman 1995). For this reason the confusing old terms 'physiological' and 'pathological jaundice' are best avoided (Maisels 2006).

Epidemiology and genetics

Developments in human genomics are providing explanations for the epidemiological variation in neonatal hyperbilirubinaemia and susceptibility to bilirubin encephalopathy (Watchko et al. 2002). Gilbert syndrome is a contributory factor in some pronounced and prolonged unconjugated jaundice (Monaghan 1999). A variant in the promoter for the gene encoding UDPGT results in

a reduction of the enzyme's activity by as much as two-thirds. The syndrome is common, affecting 5–10% of the population in the homozygous state. The heterozygous Gilbert's state, present in 42% of the population, has also been shown to contribute to hyperbilirubinaemia (Kadakol et al. 2001). A combination of Gilbert syndrome and glucose-6-phosphate dehydrogenase (G6PD) deficiency has been responsible for severe cases of hyperbilirubinaemia (Kaplan 2001).

In babies with pathology underlying their jaundice blood group incompatibility, G6PD deficiency and infection are the conditions most commonly associated with significant hyperbilirubinaemia and kernicterus. They vary in prevalence in different parts of the world, as reflected in the meta-analysis conducted as part of a literature review for the UK National Institute for Health and Clinical Excellence (NICE) guideline on neonatal jaundice (National Institute for Health and Clinical Excellence 2010). In Africa G6PD deficiency accounted for over 35% of cases of significant hyperbilirubinaemia and kernicterus, and for infection this figure was more than 14%. In the Middle East, infection was found in 50% of cases of kernicterus. In Europe and North America G6PD deficiency was implicated in 5% of babies with a serum bilirubin >400 μmol/l or receiving exchange transfusions, and 20% of cases of kernicterus. Infection was implicated in 2% of babies with a serum bilirubin >400 μmol/l or receiving exchange transfusions, and in 14% of cases of kernicterus. Among jaundiced babies in Europe and North America blood group incompatibility was the most prevalent underlying factor leading to higher bilirubin levels (>400 μmol/l), whereas G6PD deficiency was more common in cases of kernicterus. In all geographical settings no cause is ever found for significant hyperbilirubinaemia in an appreciable percentage of cases.

Jaundice in the healthy breastfed infant

Breastfed babies develop more marked and prolonged jaundice than those who are formula-fed. The peak bilirubin level in the formula-fed infant usually occurs on day 3 or 4, whereas in the breastfed baby it may not be reached until the end of the first week or entering the second week of life. This influence of exclusive breastfeeding is also seen in babies born prematurely (Lucas and Baker 1986). The neonatal jaundice commonly seen in the breastfed baby during the first week of life relates to lower calorie intake, and the slower passage of meconium. When associated with marked weight loss, this pattern of jaundice in the breastfed newborn has been referred to as 'lack-of-breast-milk jaundice' (Hansen 1995).

Up to one-third of breastfed babies remain clinically jaundiced beyond 2 weeks of age, and they represent the overwhelming majority of infants presenting for a prolonged jaundice screen. A reliable diagnosis of breast milk jaundice can only be made on exclusion of pathological causes. Once the diagnosis is made, parents should be warned that resolution of jaundice might take several weeks. They should be advised to report back if the nature of the jaundice changes, there is failure to thrive or their baby develops pale chalky stools and dark urine. Although interruption of breast milk feeds and supplementation with formula for 24 hours may be associated with a marked decline in serum bilirubin and lower rebound level on reintroduction, the practice is rarely justified. Also to be discouraged is the vogue for supplementing breastfed infants with water, regardless of their state of hydration. Newborns managed in this way have been shown to have higher maximum serum bilirubin levels (De Carvalho et al. 1981).

The prolonged form of jaundice seen in the breastfed baby beyond the second week of life is thought to be related to enhanced enterohepatic circulation of bilirubin. The presence in breast milk of β-glucuronidase – which unconjugates bilirubin in the infant gut, enabling it to re-enter the circulation – is thought to be contributory. Altered bacterial colonisation of the gut in the breastfed baby with a resultant decrease in the conversion of bilirubin glucuronides to urobilinoids may also play a role.

Pathophysiology of bilirubin encephalopathy

Kernicterus

Kernicterus is the name given to the characteristic pattern of yellow staining of parts of the brainstem, hippocampus, cerebellum and certain brainstem nuclei (particularly the globus pallidus and subthalamic nucleus) seen at autopsy in infants dying with acute bilirubin toxicity (Fig. 29.6). The clinical manifestations of bilirubin encephalopathy arise from the susceptibility to damage of the basal ganglia, brainstem auditory pathways and oculomotor nuclei (Volpe 2008; Shapiro 2010). This anatomical preference for bilirubin deposition and vulnerability to toxicity has not been fully explained, but may be a consequence of increased blood flow and metabolic activity in these areas (Burgess et al. 1985). Regional variation in bilirubin influx, detoxification and clearance and the variance in neuronal cell inflammatory response are also likely to be implicated (Brites et al. 2009).

The blood–brain barrier is anatomically derived from tight junctions between the endothelial cells of cerebral blood vessels. This barrier remains permeable to lipid-soluble substances, but, whilst intact, excludes water-soluble substances and large molecules, such as proteins. Free bilirubin influxes and effluxes across the intact blood–brain barrier. Disruption of the blood–brain barrier will allow an influx of albumin-bound bilirubin as well as free bilirubin into the brain, and the distribution of bilirubin staining may suggest kernicterus. There was a lack of correlation between bilirubin staining and histological evidence of neuronal injury observed in the brains of premature infants dying from other causes in the so-called low-bilirubin kernicterus era (Turkel et al. 1982).

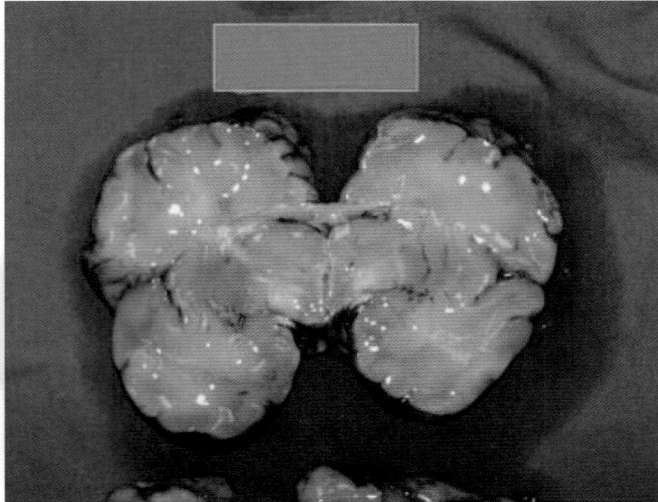

Fig. 29.6 Macroscopic appearance of brain in a term infant with kernicterus.

Bilirubin toxicity

Bilirubin's toxicity is that of a generalised cellular poison. Disruption of membrane function, lowering of action potentials, compromise of energy metabolism and disturbance of neurotransmitter synthesis and neurotransmission are some of the mechanisms implicated (Volpe 2008; Brites et al. 2009). Advances in human genomics are identifying factors that predispose to hyperbilirubinaemia and bilirubin encephalopathy (Kaplan et al. 2003). There is evidence that bilirubin is a substrate for P-glycoprotein, a plasma membrane efflux pump found on the luminal surface of brain capillary endothelial cells and considered responsible for limiting entry of certain lipophilic substrates into the central nervous system (Watchko et al. 2002; Wennberg et al. 2006). P-glycoprotein function may be inhibited by drugs. Its expression is also related to gestational maturity, and this may be a factor contributing to the greater vulnerability of the premature brain to bilirubin neurotoxicity. Also implicated is the maturational state of nerve cells exposed to bilirubin, with a greater tendency to apoptosis seen in the less well-differentiated astrocytes and neurons (Brites et al. 2009).

Attempts to reproduce bilirubin neurotoxicity experimentally point to the importance of coexisting risk factors, such as acidosis, hypoxia, hypercarbia and blood–brain barrier disruption, as being prerequisites for bilirubin's toxicity (Wennberg et al. 2006). Hypercarbia should not be underestimated as a risk factor, through disruption of the blood–brain barrier.

Agents that interfere with the binding of bilirubin to serum albumin may also promote neurotoxicity. The devastating effect in the 1960s of sulphisoxazole causing kernicterus (Silverman et al. 1956) serves as a reminder that all drugs used in neonatology should be assessed in terms of their potential to displace bilirubin from albumin (Robertson et al. 1991). Free fatty acids, if they reach a molar ratio with albumin in excess of 4 : 1, interfere with bilirubin binding. Such ratios may be attained in sick immature newborns receiving high-dose intravenous lipid preparations.

Insight into bilirubin encephalopathy can be gained from case reports of infants who experience very high levels of bilirubin but escape neurological sequelae. Hanko et al. (2001) describe a baby with ABO incompatibility developing a peak serum bilirubin of 636 µmol/l at 19 hours of age who made normal progress after the bilirubin level was reduced to <400 µmol/l by 35 hours of age. By contrast, the authors report two babies who went on to develop kernicterus from jaundice peaking at 650 and 717 µmol/l, and in whom the bilirubin was not reduced to <400 µmol/l until 60 and 68 hours. It is suggested that it may be the duration of significant hyperbilirubinaemia or 'area under the curve' that is as important in neurotoxicity. This factor has been implicated in a number of the cases studied from the Pilot USA Kernicterus Registry for term and near-term infants, as has the rate of rise in serum bilirubin (Johnson et al. 2009).

Other factors influence the passage of bilirubin into the brain and hence increase the risk of acute bilirubin encephalopathy. These include sepsis, hypoxia, seizures, hypercarbia, acidosis and hypoalbuminaemia. A healthy term baby with none of these risk factors is most unlikely to develop kernicterus below a serum bilirubin concentration of 425 µmol/l, but that risk increases significantly at bilirubin levels in excess of 515 µmol/l (Manning et al. 2007; Johnson et al. 2009).

Clinical bilirubin encephalopathy

The word 'kernicterus' originates from a description of yellow nuclear staining of the brain, but has become synonymous with the acute and chronic neurological features of what are more correctly termed bilirubin encephalopathy and its sequelae. Descriptions of classic kernicterus arise from observations of markedly jaundiced infants with erythroblastosis fetalis before the advent of effective phototherapy and exchange transfusion. At that time three clinical phases were identified (Connolly and Volpe 1990; Volpe 2008). The first few days were characterised by lethargy, hypotonia and poor suck. Towards the end of the first week, a second phase was heralded by hypertonia, often with opisthotonus. At this stage, the baby commonly exhibited a high-pitched cry, fever and seizures. The third phase was entered as the hypertonia subsided, to be replaced by hypotonia. Current-day intervention during phase 1 with feeding support, phototherapy and, if necessary, exchange transfusion can prevent evolution of long-term damage. The onset of hypertonia and opisthotonus, often coincident with peak serum bilirubin level, remain poor prognostic signs predictive of neurological sequelae. The preterm infant may exhibit little in the way of acute signs in the neonatal period, yet may go on to develop clinical kernicterus. Isolated sensorineural hearing loss may become apparent in both term and preterm infants exposed to significant hyperbilirubinaemia. Dental enamel dysplasia may be another consequence of levels of bilirubin that result in kernicterus.

The long-term features of bilirubin encephalopathy include extrapyramidal disturbances, auditory impairment and upward-gaze palsies. The resulting cerebral palsy typically has an element of athetosis, which can develop as early as 18 months of age or be delayed for several years. High-frequency sensorineural deafness frequently accompanies the cerebral palsy, but may evolve in isolation. Cognitive impairment can result from bilirubin encephalopathy, but is commonly absent. A characteristic brain magnetic resonance imaging (MRI) pattern has been described in cases of kernicterus. The presence of high-intensity areas in the posteromedial border of the globus pallidus on T_2-weighted imaging is considered the most sensitive finding (Yokochi 1995; Govaert et al. 2003). Kernicteric brain MRI changes are illustrated in Figure 29.7. It should be appreciated that chronic neurological features of clinical kernicterus can be seen in the absence of any abnormality on brain MRI (Katar et al. 2008).

Lessons from the past and present

The 'kinder, gentler approach' towards the healthy jaundiced term infant

Up until the last two decades, treatment thresholds for phototherapy and exchange transfusion tended to reflect clinical experience gained by early exponents of exchange transfusion in severe erythroblastosis fetalis. They determined that kernicterus was unlikely to occur if serum bilirubin levels were kept below 20 mg/dl (342 µmol/l). The impact was such that an 'irrational fear of 20 mg/dl' or 'vigintiphobia' (Watchko and Oski 1983) led to adoption of this exchange threshold for all infants, regardless of the cause of jaundice or their gestation. A campaign for 'a kinder, gentler approach' to the treatment of jaundice in healthy, non-haemolysing term infants was started by Newman and Maisels (1992), who carried out an extensive review of the existing literature before proposing their less interventional management regimens. It remains uncertain as to whether there are significant or long-term effects of moderate hyperbilirubinaemia (Maisels and Newman 2001).

Premature infants

Premature infants are more prone to bilirubin encephalopathy than their full-term counterparts. The greater risk to the preterm brain may have been overstated in the past following incorrect

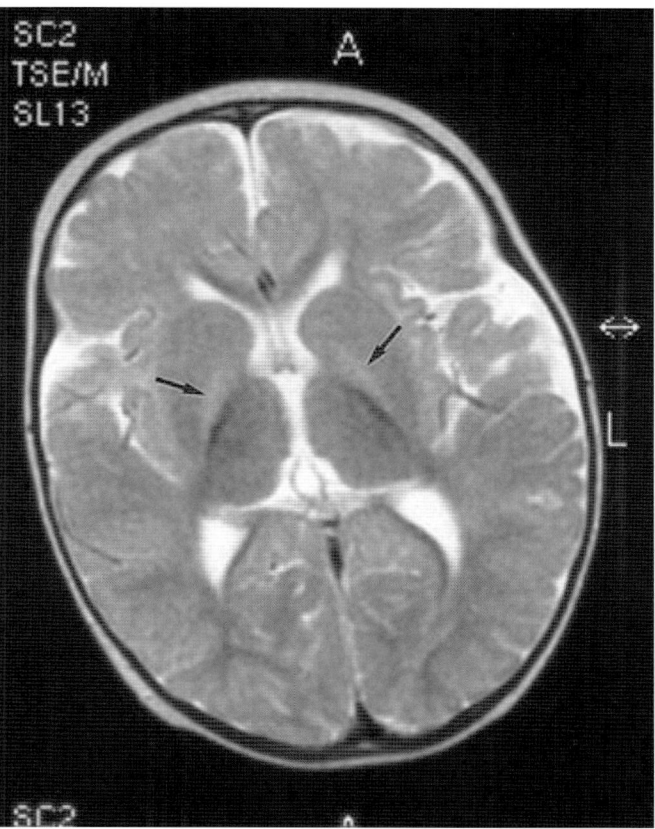

Fig. 29.7 T_2-weighted axial section of the brain imaged with magnetic resonance imaging, showing characteristic changes of kernicterus in the globus pallidus (arrowed).

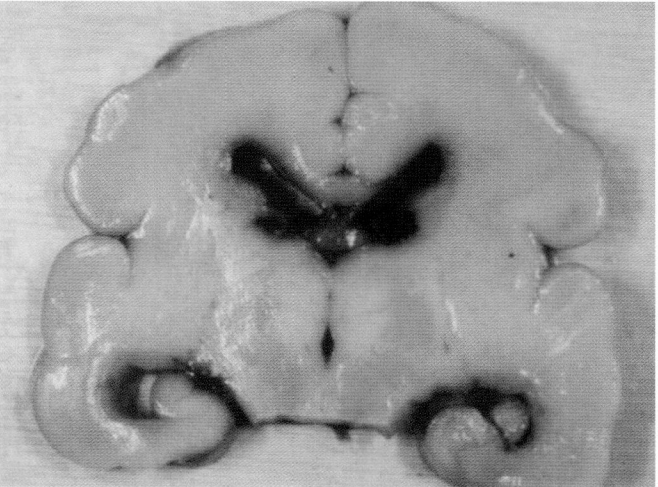

Fig. 29.8 Macroscopic appearance of brain in an extremely low-birthweight infant with low-bilirubin 'kernicterus'.

interpretation of autopsy findings in the so-called 'low-bilirubin kernicterus era' (1965–82). This was a time when all yellow staining of the basal ganglia merited the description kernicterus, regardless of histological confirmation. Agonal changes in blood–brain barrier permeability to albumin-bound as well as free bilirubin in infants dying from other causes have been implicated in this pattern of staining (Fig. 29.8). This is not to be confused with our more recent understanding of kernicterus occurring in extreme preterm infants at low pretreatment threshold bilirubin levels, as demonstrated on brain MRI (Govaert et al. 2003).

Elevated serum bilirubin levels appear in some studies to be a risk factor for hearing loss in premature babies. The high incidence of bilateral sensorineural deafness in a population of sick very-low-birthweight infants with serum bilirubin levels >240 μmol/l was dramatically reduced when lower thresholds for intervention were adopted (DeVries et al. 1985, 1987). Deafness in this population was also shown to correlate with the mean duration of hyperbilirubinaemia.

There have been calls for relaxation of the more interventional treatment regimens applied to the jaundiced preterm population (Watchko and Oski 1992), and counterarguments raised against (Ives 1992). The proponents based their argument on experience gained in a pre-intensive care era (1950–65) with relatively more mature (28–36 weeks' gestation) infants, very few of whom were exposed to serum bilirubin levels in excess of 340 μmol/l. False reassurance was also gained from trials conducted against the backdrop of the recent more interventionalist therapeutic regimens. The large National Institute of Child Health and Human Development phototherapy trial failed to demonstrate an association between maximal serum bilirubin level and neurodevelopmental outcome in term or preterm infants (Scheidt et al. 1991), but threshold criteria used for exchange transfusion had kept serum bilirubin levels low. The pre-emptive treatment of jaundice with phototherapy in low-birthweight infants has reduced dramatically the requirement for exchange transfusion, but we remain uncertain as to the appropriate thresholds for treatment (Maisels and Watchko 2003; Morris et al. 2008; Watchko and Maisels 2010).

Lessons from reports of babies with kernicterus

What is the evidence that an otherwise healthy, non-haemolysing term baby can develop kernicterus? Six cases have been reported in which apparent 'exaggerated physiological jaundice' was associated with signs of acute bilirubin encephalopathy and typical neurological sequelae (Maisels and Newman 1995). Peak recorded bilirubin levels with a range of 663–845 μmol/l occurred between days 4 and 10. Four of the babies were 37 weeks' gestation and four had significant weight loss. The largest proportion of babies reported to the Pilot USA Kernicterus Registry has idiopathic jaundice.

A prospective 2-year surveillance study of hyperbilirubinaemia (unconjugated serum bilirubin >510 μmol/l in the first month of life) in the UK and Ireland has highlighted the prevalence and risk to the baby of such levels of jaundice (Manning et al. 2007). The mean peak serum bilirubin level was 580 (range 510–802) μmol/l, and the mean gestational age was 38.2 (range 35–42) weeks. The 108 patients identified provide an incidence of this level of jaundice of 7.1/100 000 live births. Of this group, 14 (13%) had features consistent with acute bilirubin encephalopathy. From this study the UK incidence of acute bilirubin encephalopathy was 0.9/100 000 live births, although not all affected babies went on to develop chronic kernicterus. It should also be noted that this surveillance study did not take into account the more preterm population, cases of bilirubin encephalopathy that may have occurred at lower serum bilirubin levels and instances of kernicterus where there was a high conjugated component to the jaundice but the unconjugated value did not exceed 510 μmol/l. As in the case reports mentioned above (Maisels and Newman 1995), failure to establish breastfeeding ('lack-of-breast-milk jaundice') and being born near term featured amongst the patients. The pitfall of treating late preterm infants as healthy term infants has been emphasised (Bhutani and Johnson 2006). There were also similarities between the affected patient

profile in this UK and Ireland survey and the USA-based Kernicterus Registry (Johnson et al. 2009) in terms of breastfeeding predominance, darker skin tones that may mask jaundice and G6PD deficiency.

The Pilot USA Kernicterus Registry

As long as kernicterus continues to occur, better understanding of the circumstances leading to individual cases and a collective strategy of prevention will best be achieved by maintaining national registries. A pilot kernicterus registry for term and near-term infants was established in the USA in 1992 (Bhutani and Johnson 2009a; Johnson et al. 2009). The level of case ascertainment and state coverage of this registry does not allow the authors to generate information on the national incidence of kernicterus, but they are able to derive important clinical lessons. Haemolysis (19%) and G6PD deficiency (22%) feature highly as underlying causes, whilst other pathologies (23%) and idiopathic cases (36%) make up the remainder. Lactation failure with suboptimal lactation support was a feature in more than 90% of the infants who had been discharged home exclusively breastfeeding. No specific serum bilirubin threshold emerges as the trigger for bilirubin encephalopathy, but a narrow margin of safety appears to exist between levels of 425 and 595 μmol/l. Kernicterus stands out as a preventable disorder in the majority of cases reported in the registry.

The case emerges for a 'crash-cart' approach to commencing multiple phototherapy and securing blood for an urgent exchange transfusion for babies presenting with significant hyperbilirubinaemia or symptomatic bilirubin encephalopathy. Of babies managed in this manner, 73% avoided chronic sequelae. The latest report from the registry concludes: 'The major underlying root cause for kernicterus was systems failure of services by multiple providers at multiple sites and inability to identify the at-risk infant and manage severe hyperbilirubinaemia in a timely manner' (Johnson et al. 2009).

Identifying the newborn at risk of bilirubin encephalopathy

Predischarge prediction of the severity of jaundice

In the context of early postnatal discharge and a varying degree of community support, American authors have turned to a predischarge serum bilirubin estimation in an attempt to categorise the risk of subsequent significant hyperbilirubinaemia based on an hour-specific bilirubin nomogram (Bhutani et al. 1999). The nomogram was generated from measurements of total serum bilirubin in 2840 term and near-term infants eligible for discharge between 24 and 72 hours of age. The predischarge bilirubin assay was performed with the routine metabolic screen at a mean age of 33.7 ± 14.6 SD hours. Postdischarge values were obtained to determine whether the initial measurement was predictive of the natural history of jaundice. Just over 60% of the study population fell into a low-risk category and did not progress to significant jaundice. The remaining patients were in risk zones that were either high risk or they had the potential to move to the high-risk zone from an intermediate-risk zone. If applying the nomogram to other populations of newborn infants it should be remembered that this was a selected group that excluded many first-day discharges, babies with evidence of rhesus or ABO sensitisation, babies admitted to a special care baby unit/neonatal intensive care unit, and newborns who required phototherapy before the age of 60 hours for a rapidly rising serum bilirubin. A recent study has shown that an assessment that combines timed transcutaneous bilirubin levels above the 95th percentile on the Bhutani nomogram with risk factors for significant hyperbilirubinaemia is effective at preventing later significant hyperbilirubinaemia (Maisels et al. 2009a).

New UK national guidelines

Recent national guidance in the UK has emphasised review within 48 hours of birth of babies with known risk factors for significant hyperbilirubinaemia, and recommends measurement as opposed to estimating the bilirubin level in all babies presenting with clinical jaundice (National Institute for Health and Clinical Excellence 2010). The NICE guideline on neonatal jaundice aims to improve recognition of infants who have an increased risk of developing significant jaundice. Studies show that four factors are independently associated with an increased risk of hyperbilirubinaemia (Khoury et al. 1988; Newman et al. 2002; Keren et al. 2005; Maisels et al. 2009a). They are: (1) gestational age <38 weeks; (2) jaundice within 24 hours of life; (3) mother's intention to breastfeed exclusively; and (4) a family history of neonatal jaundice. The UK NICE guideline has used these four risk factors to highlight babies at risk of significant hyperbilirubinaemia (that is, requiring treatment) and to promote their earlier surveillance, and produced a care pathway (Fig. 29.9). Factors such as bruising, cephalhaematoma, vacuum delivery, male sex and race were not added to this risk assessment as studies have not shown a consistent causal association between them and hyperbilirubinaemia.

Risk factors in babies more likely to develop significant hyperbilirubinaemia include:

- gestational age under 38 weeks
- a previous sibling with neonatal jaundice requiring phototherapy
- mother's intention to breastfeed exclusively
- visible jaundice in the first 24 hours of life

For babies with any or all of the four risk factors, an additional clinical examination for clinical jaundice is to be conducted in the period up to 48 hours of age.

Clinical jaundice is more difficult to recognise in babies with dark skin tones and can be missed without close examination of the sclerae, gums and blanched skin. This explains why kernicterus registries (Johnson et al. 2009) and population studies of hyperbilirubinaemia (Manning et al. 2007) report overrepresentation of babies from ethnic groups with dark skin tones. These babies fall into the heightened risk group if they are not examined properly. In cases of doubt, a low threshold should be adopted for checking the transcutaneous or serum bilirubin.

Markers of bilirubin toxicity

The imprecise relationship between total serum bilirubin levels and adverse neurological outcome has encouraged research seeking to identify more accurate markers of bilirubin toxicity. Assessments of free bilirubin levels, bilirubin-binding capacity and brainstem auditory evoked responses have been proposed (Funato et al. 1994). These markers may prove of value in research environments, but they are not universally available in the acute clinical situation. Clinicians have traditionally focused on the total serum bilirubin as the arbiter of treatment thresholds for jaundice. An assay of free bilirubin may be the more relevant marker (Wennberg et al. 2006). Correlation of abnormal auditory brainstem responses in infants of 28–32 weeks' gestation has been demonstrated with peak free bilirubin level but not the total bilirubin value in a range of moderate jaundice (Amin et al. 2001).

More accessible than free bilirubin measurement is the bilirubin/albumin ratio, which is related indirectly to the free bilirubin level. The bilirubin/albumin ratio has also been shown to correlate with abnormal auditory brainstem responses when the total bilirubin failed to do so (Amin et al. 2001). On the basis of unbound bilirubin estimations, an exchange transfusion threshold has been proposed at a bilirubin/albumin ratio of 0.8 in the healthy term newborn, 0.72 in a sick term infant and as low as 0.4 for the sick premature infant of <1250 g (Ahlfors 1994). Although this ratio has not gained widespread clinical acceptance, it may help to inform the decision as to whether or not to perform an exchange transfusion in borderline cases (AAP 2004; Maisels et al. 2009b). (Note that, when calculating the bilirubin/albumin ratio, values for serum albumin concentration in g/l should be converted to SI units of μmol/l using the factor 15.15.)

A systematic review has examined the usefulness of the bilirubin/albumin ratio for predicting bilirubin-induced neurotoxicity in premature infants (Hulzebos et al. 2008). The authors identified six studies that suggest that there is a link between the bilirubin/albumin ratio and various indices of bilirubin encephalopathy, including abnormal auditory brainstem responses. The same authors are due to publish the results of a randomised controlled trial (Bilirubin Albumin Ratio Trial (BARTrial), http://www.controlled-trials.com/isrctn/pf/74465643) which has looked at the use of the bilirubin/albumin ratio as an adjunct to decision-making on thresholds for phototherapy and exchange transfusion in preterm infants born at less than 32 weeks' gestation. Neurodevelopmental outcome is being assessed at 18–24 months of age.

Assessing the level of serum bilirubin

Visual inspection

Clinical jaundice becomes visually apparent at serum bilirubin levels of 80–90 μmol/l, and can be observed in the majority of newborns during the first week of life. Examination for jaundice should be conducted in a well-lit room. Jaundice may be more difficult to detect in preterm infants and missed in babies with darker skin tones, in whom examination of the sclerae, gums and blanched skin may be more informative. Visual assessment can be unreliable under artificial light, and once phototherapy has been commenced. Healthcare professionals and parents can be taught to recognise clinical jaundice, but studies show that they are unable to assess its severity. Accuracy is not enhanced by the use of icterometers or assessment of the cephalocaudal progression of dermal jaundice (Kramer 1969). For these reasons, whenever a parent or healthcare professional considers that a baby is visibly jaundiced, the bilirubin level must be measured to inform appropriate clinical management and the timing of repeat assessment.

Transcutaneous bilirubinometry

Over the past decade the use of non-invasive transcutaneous bilirubinometry has become well established in the USA and is currently entering UK practice. Transcutaneous bilirubin measurement has evolved to a range of accuracy that it can be used with confidence in the assessment of the degree of jaundice up to levels of 250 μmol/l in babies of 35 weeks' gestation and above. Machines available in the UK are the Minolta JM-103 (Konica Minolta/Air-Shields) and the BiliChek (Respironics). They have been subjected to numerous trials but there are currently no published studies directly comparing the two.

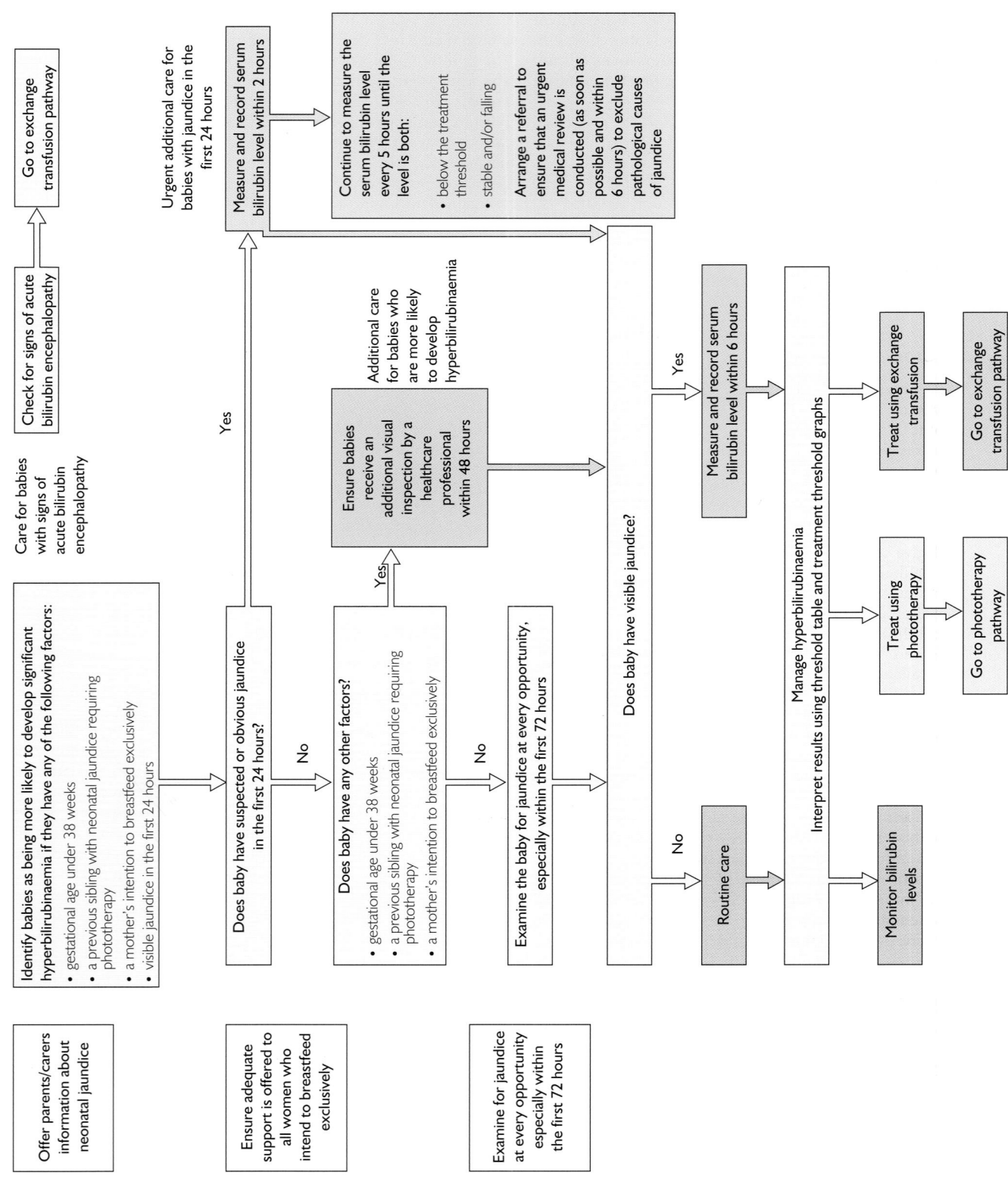

Fig. 29.9 National Institute for Health and Clinical Excellence investigation pathways.

These devices measure yellow pigments including bilirubin in blanched skin by sampling from the forehead or anterior chest wall over the sternum. They provide a significant positive correlation with serum bilirubin levels in moderately jaundiced infants and reduce the requirement for blood sampling. The difference between transcutaneous bilirubin and serum bilirubin widens at levels above 250 μmol/l, and validation of the accuracy of transcutaneous bilirubinometry in preterm babies born at <35 weeks' gestation is limited. The current UK NICE guidance recommends that, if a transcutaneous bilirubinometer records a bilirubin level above 250 μmol/l, a serum sample should be taken to check the bilirubin level more accurately. Phototherapy, through its bleaching effect on the skin, precludes the use of transcutaneous bilirubinometry to monitor the progress of treatment once phototherapy is in progress.

Invasive blood sampling

For practical purposes, a bench bilirubinometer employing direct spectrometry is used in many neonatal units to provide near-patient estimation of total serum bilirubin. It should be remembered that such instruments reflect the sum value of all species of bilirubin, conjugated and unconjugated, including photoisomers. Significant errors can arise from incorrect spectrometer use and poor maintenance. Failure by the operator to note that serum specimens are grossly lipaemic, or that the outside of the capillary tube or cuvette is dirty, will give misleading results. Regular instrument quality control and calibration are necessary. The bilirubinometer used should be accurate to within ±20–30 μmol/l, and the limitations of the machine should be known when measuring very high values. Whole-blood bilirubin assay is available on some modern blood gas analysers and may be used as an alternative. If near-patient testing is unavailable a laboratory service must be in place with a reliable and timely method of communicating results back to the nursery. It is customary to confirm pre-exchange transfusion values of total serum bilirubin with a laboratory measurement, but the procedure should not be delayed if this service is slow.

There are no clear-cut levels of total serum bilirubin that predict the risk of bilirubin encephalopathy and this has encouraged research into the measurement of free bilirubin, unbound to albumin (Wennberg et al. 2006). After several hours of phototherapy as much as 25% of the circulating unconjugated bilirubin pool may be in the form of isomers. These are probably measured within the total value for most serum bilirubin assays but may hinder the precision of attempts to use the free bilirubin level to guide management of jaundice (McDonagh 2006).

Identifying different types of jaundice

Jaundice with a pathological cause

Every jaundiced infant should be clinically evaluated to identify underlying pathology and to assess the risk potential for bilirubin encephalopathy. Family, maternal and infant history should be reviewed and the baby examined. Appropriate early investigation aims to identify treatable disease states, such as isoimmunisation (most commonly rhesus or ABO incompatibility), infection, hypothyroidism, biliary atresia and galactosaemia. Clinical features that suggest a pathological cause of jaundice and prompt further investigation are listed in Table 29.2. Many of the more commonly recognised causes of unconjugated hyperbilirubinaemia are listed in Table 29.3. Unless there are diagnostic pointers to the more rarely

Table 29.2 Clinical features that suggest a pathological cause of jaundice in the newborn

Jaundice appearing in the first 24 hours of life
Jaundice in a sick neonate
Total serum bilirubin level
    >250 μmol/l by 48 hours of life
    >300 μmol/l by 72 hours of life
Rapidly rising serum bilirubin >100 μmol/l/24 h
Jaundice that fails to respond to phototherapy
Prolonged jaundice
    >14 days in term infants
    >21 days in preterm infants
Conjugated serum bilirubin >25 μmol/l
Pale or acholuric stools and dark urine

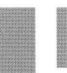

Table 29.3 Causes of unconjugated jaundice in the newborn

Haemolysis

Isoimmunisation
    Rhesus
    ABO
    Minor blood groups
Other
    Spherocytosis*
    Glucose-6-phosphate dehydrogenase deficiency
    Pyruvate kinase deficiency[†]
    Sepsis[‡]
    Disseminated intravascular coagulation
    α-thalassaemia

Polycythaemia

Small for dates
Twin–twin transfusion
Delayed cord clamping
Maternofetal transfusion
Infant of diabetic mother

Extravasated blood

Bruising, e.g. cephalhaematoma
Pulmonary haemorrhage
Cerebral haemorrhage
Intra-abdominal haemorrhage

Increased enterohepatic circulation

Pyloric stenosis
Bowel obstruction
Swallowed blood

Endocrine/metabolic

Hypothyroidism
Hypopituitarism[‡]
Hypoadrenalism[‡]
Glucuronosyl transferase deficiency
Galactosaemia[‡]
Tyrosinaemia[‡]
Hypermethioninaemia[‡]

*And other red cell morphological abnormalities.
[†]And other red cell enzyme defects.
[‡]Conjugated jaundice often coexists.

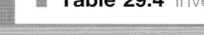

Table 29.4 Investigation of jaundice in the newborn

Early-onset jaundice
Blood group and Direct Coombs' Test
Haematocrit and full blood count
Blood film and reticulocyte count
Infection screen if indicated
Serology for congenital infections
Urine for cytomegalovirus culture
Stool for virology
Glucose-6-phosphate dehydrogenase screen
Red cell enzyme assays

Prolonged jaundice
Total and conjugated serum bilirubin
Thyroid function tests
Urine culture
Urine Clinitest for reducing substances
Liver function tests
α_1-antitrypsin assay and phenotype
Cystic fibrosis DNA screen
Immunoreactive trypsin
Plasma cortisol level
Serum amino acid screen

encountered causes of neonatal jaundice, stepwise investigation should aim to identify the common ones first (Table 29.4).

Defining the severity of jaundice

The ambiguity of the redundant terms 'physiological' and 'pathological jaundice' has been matched by attempts to describe and define the severity of jaundice. There is no consensus as to the meaning of hyperbilirubinaemia, or versions thereof with various adjectives attached. Levels of bilirubin >510 µmol/l have been described recently as 'severe', 'extreme', 'hazardous' or 'catastrophic' hyperbilirubinaemia by different authors (Bhutani et al. 1999; Maisels 2006; Manning et al. 2007; Bhutani and Johnson 2009b). If we are destined to categorise levels of jaundice, numerical ranges should suffice. The simplest use of terminology is to use 'hyperbilirubinaemia' to denote a raised level of bilirubin in the blood, 'clinical jaundice' to mean visually detectable jaundice and 'significant hyperbilirubinaemia' to describe a level of jaundice requiring treatment. Regardless of the level, jaundice in the first 24 hours of life and rates of rise in serum bilirubin consistent with haemolysis take on their own significance.

Early-onset jaundice

Jaundice within the first 24 hours of life is likely to be the result of isoimmunisation or other cause of significant haemolysis. In the absence of haemolysis, the rare Crigler–Najjar syndromes should be considered. Urgent investigation is essential (Table 29.4). Maternal rhesus status and blood group should be sought. Infants of known rhesus-negative mothers may have had cord or postnatal blood sent for a direct antiglobulin test (DAT). Antenatal anti-D prophylaxis in rhesus-negative women can result in passive transfer of antibody, resulting in a weakly positive DAT in the absence of haemolysis (Maayan-Metzger et al. 2001). Routine DAT testing on umbilical cord blood of all babies has not been shown to predict subsequent hyperbilirubinaemia accurately in the newborn. Despite

an ABO incompatibility set-up in 10–15% of pregnancies, the number of cases that result in significant haemolysis is small. The finding of a positive DAT is not predictive of the severity of jaundice, and nor does a negative result rule out the condition. Maternal anti-A or anti-B immunoglobulin G titre greater than 1 in 512 is likely to be associated with significant hyperbilirubinaemia (Bakkeheim et al. 2009).

Other blood group incompatibilities will usually be known from the maternal history. The Kell group can cause severe haemolytic disease of the newborn, whereas complications of the Duffy, Kidd and other rare blood group systems are usually less severe. A reticulocyte count of more than 6% after 3 days is suggestive of a haemolytic process, but reticulocyte counts and blood films carry a low sensitivity and specificity for diagnosing haemolysis in the newborn (Newman and Easterling 1994). Screening for G6PD deficiency should be considered in babies of relevant ethnic origin, although this condition more usually presents from day 3 onwards. Carbon monoxide is produced in equimolar quantities with bilirubin during haem catabolism, and it had been hoped that heightened end-tidal carbon monoxide concentration would serve as a useful marker of the rate of bilirubin production (Stevenson 2001). Measuring this parameter has not proved to be a reliable predictor of significant hyperbilirubinaemia.

Early-onset visible jaundice within the first 24 hours of life may be associated with a pathological cause of jaundice and is an important risk factor for subsequent significant hyperbilirubinaemia. The bilirubin level should be interpreted urgently. This should be done taking into account the baby's postnatal age in hours, and not by rounding up or down in days (or becoming confused as to whether the baby is day 0 or day 1). The UK NICE guideline provides a treatment threshold table (Fig. 29.9) and a graph for babies of greater than 38 weeks' gestation. An implementation tool (Biliwheel) is being developed to display the same thresholds and to assist in precise measurement of a baby's age in hours (Table 29.5). For the preterm babies between 23 and 37 weeks' gestation there are specific graphs by week of gestation (Fig. 29.10) providing guidance on thresholds for phototherapy and exchange transfusion (National Institute for Health and Clinical Excellence 2010).

The differential diagnosis of unconjugated jaundice

The maternal records should be checked for documentation of syphilis and hepatitis serology as well as any history suggesting congenital infection. Specific red cell morphological abnormalities, such as spherocytosis, or inborn errors of metabolism, such as galactosaemia or Crigler–Najjar syndrome types I and II, may be implicated from the family history. The jaundice associated with galactosaemia is likely to be predominantly unconjugated in the first week of life. Diagnostic pointers such as hepatomegaly, poor feeding and vomiting should prompt early screening for galactosaemia with urinalysis for non-glucose-reducing substances (Clinitest) and assessment of erythrocyte galactose-1-phosphate uridyl transferase activity.

The Crigler–Najjar syndromes present characteristically in the first few days of life with a rapidly evolving, non-haemolytic, unconjugated hyperbilirubinaemia. The type I disorder results from a complete absence of UDPGT within the hepatocyte and is inherited in an autosomal recessive manner. Affected individuals frequently require exchange transfusions in the newborn period and nocturnal phototherapy in early childhood. Definitive treatment involves liver transplantation. Crigler–Najjar syndrome type II is a less severe condition in that there is partial UDPGT activity. Inheritance is

Table 29.5 Consensus-based bilirubin thresholds for management of hyperbilirubinaemia in babies of gestational age 38 weeks or more

AGE (hours)	BILIRUBIN LEVEL (µmol/litre)			
0			>100	>100
6	>100	>112	>125	>150
12	>100	>125	>150	>200
18	>100	>137	>175	>250
24	>100	>150	>200	>300
30	>112	>162	>212	>350
36	>125	>175	>225	>400
42	>137	>187	>237	>450
48	>150	>200	>250	>450
54	>162	>212	>262	>450
60	>175	>225	>275	>450
66	>187	>237	>287	>450
72	>200	>250	>300	>450
78		>262	>312	>450
84		>275	>325	>450
90		>287	>337	>450
96+		>300	>350	>450
Action	Repeat bilirubin (6–12 hours)	Consider phototherapy (repeat bilirubin in 6 hours)	Start phototherapy	Perform an exchange transfusion unless the bilirubin level falls below threshold while the treatment is being prepared

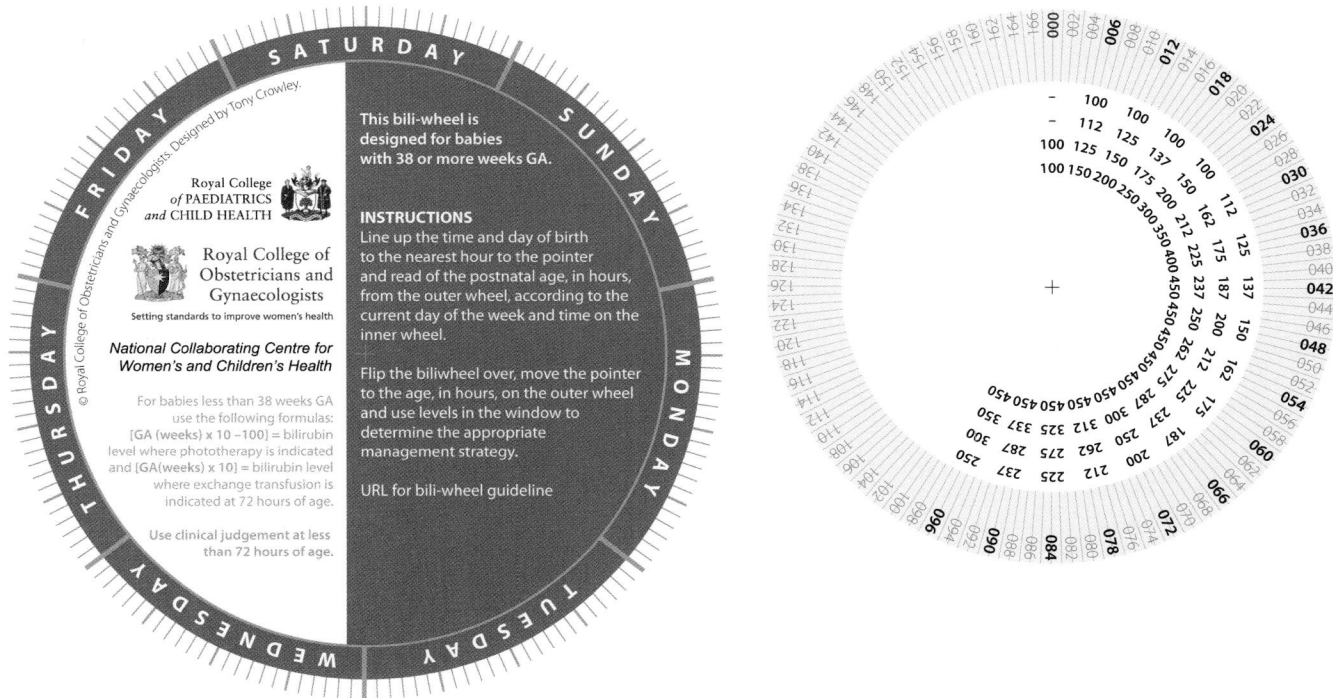

Fig. 29.10 Biliwheel.

thought to be autosomal dominant with variable expression, and serum bilirubin levels can be adequately controlled with a UDPGT inducer such as phenobarbital.

With parents of Mediterranean, Asian and African ethnicity, the increased likelihood of G6PD deficiency, especially in males, needs to be considered. Screening cord blood for evidence of G6PD deficiency may be appropriate in populations with a high incidence of this condition. It should be remembered that G6PD levels can be falsely elevated in the context of a high reticulocyte count, and so may need to be repeated at 2–3 months of age. The jaundice in affected babies usually evolves at 3–5 days of age. The differing severity of jaundice probably reflects the variety of isoenzyme deficiencies. The pronounced jaundice in neonates with G6PD deficiency may also result from an associated partial defect in bilirubin conjugation (Kaplan and Hammerman 2002). This would be in keeping with the fact that end-tidal carbon monoxide measurements have failed to demonstrate appreciable early haemolysis in such infants (Seidman et al. 1995). An affected individual is at risk of haemolytic episodes triggered by a number of common drugs. Parents and family practitioners should be given a list of medications to avoid Table 30.6 (in Haematology chapter).

Details of gestational age and evidence of birth asphyxia and trauma may explain heightened or prolonged jaundice. The mode and success of feeding should be noted and assessment made of the infant's state of hydration and weight trend since birth. Examination of the newborn should confirm gestational age and identify growth retardation. Polycythaemia, anaemia, hydrops, purpura and frank bruising should be looked for, along with general signs of infection.

A full infection screen is not an automatic requirement for cases of hyperbilirubinaemia in otherwise well newborns, but a low threshold for performing a full infection screen should be adopted. No instance of bacterial septicaemia was identified from a study reporting the investigation of over 300 newborns readmitted with a mean peak serum bilirubin level of 316 μmol/l (range 217–498 μmol/l) (Maisels and Kring 1992). Failure of unconjugated hyperbilirubinaemia to respond to phototherapy should alert the clinician to the possibility of infection (Linder et al. 1988).

Prolonged jaundice

Visibly detectable jaundice beyond 2 weeks of age in the term infant and 3 weeks in the preterm is classified as 'prolonged jaundice'. The majority of term infants presenting with prolonged jaundice have an unconjugated hyperbilirubinaemia and will be breastfeeding. Providing there are no features in the history or on clinical examination that suggest a pathological cause (in particular, the urine is not dark, stool colour is not pale and chalky, there is no hepatomegaly and the baby is thriving), screening investigations can be delayed until 3 weeks of age. Some babies will have cleared their jaundice by then but if it persists the total and conjugated serum bilirubin must be determined. Some or all of the following tests may be appropriate:

- full blood count
- examination of blood film if haemolysis is suspected
- blood group and DAT (mother's group and antibody status should be known)
- thyroid function tests if result of heelprick thyroid-stimulating hormone screen is not known
- urinalysis for reducing sugars (Clinitest)
- urinalysis for evidence of infection.

Further tests (Table 29.4 and see Chapter 29, part 2) will be indicated according to the outcome of this initial screen. A conjugated

Table 29.6 Causes of conjugated jaundice in the newborn

Prolonged parenteral nutrition
Idiopathic neonatal cholestasis
Perinatal asphyxia
Severe haemolysis, e.g. erythroblastosis
Bacterial sepsis
Intrauterine infections
    Toxoplasmosis
    Rubella
    Cytomegalovirus
    Herpes simplex
    Coxsackie and other viruses
Biliary atresia
Choledochal cyst
Spontaneous bile duct perforation
Intrahepatic biliary hypoplasia (Alagille's)
α_1-antitrypsin deficiency
Cystic fibrosis
Progressive familial intrahepatic cholestasis
Inspissated bile plug syndrome
Galactosaemia
Tyrosinaemia

bilirubin level >25 μmol/l is abnormal and merits urgent further investigation to exclude serious liver disease, such as biliary atresia.

Cholestatic or conjugated jaundice

Definitions of conjugated hyperbilirubinaemia vary. A serum conjugated bilirubin level of above 25 μmol/l is a commonly adopted cut-off. A threshold level definition of up to 10% or 20% of the total serum bilirubin may provide false reassurance in the case of total levels in excess of 250 μmol/l, and should be avoided. Pale chalky (acholuric) stools and dark bile-stained urine are the clinical markers of established conjugated jaundice, but neither may be present in the first weeks of many hepatic disease states, including biliary atresia.

Diagnosis of any associated clotting abnormality and its correction are urgent considerations in the infant with conjugated jaundice. Several conditions present with a mixture of raised unconjugated and conjugated bilirubin. Notable amongst these are the intrauterine infections, bacterial sepsis, galactosaemia, aminoacidaemias and congenital hypopituitarism. Some of the causes of conjugated hyperbilirubinaemia are listed in Table 29.6, and the initial investigations are found in Table 29.4.

If an obstructive aetiology is suspected, liver ultrasound and a hepatobiliary excretion study will be indicated. Visualisation of the gallbladder on ultrasound does not rule out biliary atresia. The importance of making an early diagnosis of biliary atresia and its prompt referral to a centre specialising in the medical and surgical management of childhood liver disorders cannot be overstated. Conjugated hyperbilirubinaemia is further described in Chapter 29, part 2.

Clinical management of the jaundiced infant

Management of neonatal jaundice should commence with prevention. Adequate support should be provided to all mothers as they

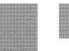

Table 29.7 Unconjugated jaundice: modes of treatment

Phototherapy
Exchange transfusion
Pharmacological agents
    Suppression of isoimmune haemolysis with intravenous
        immunoglobulin
    Competitive inhibition of haem oxygenase
    Induction of hepatic conjugation
    Inhibition of enterohepatic circulation

establish their baby's early feeding pattern. In the case of breastfeeding mothers, support in establishing successful lactation and feeding will reduce the likelihood of jaundice reaching levels requiring treatment. The importance of this practical assistance is reinforced in the NICE clinical guideline Routine Postnatal Care of Women and their Babies (National Institute of Health and Clinical Excellence 2006).

The different potential modes of treatment of unconjugated jaundice that have been advocated are shown in Table 29.7. The established treatments are phototherapy, exchange transfusion and high-dose intravenous immunoglobulin (IVIG) to suppress isoimmune haemolysis. Unconjugated hyperbilirubinaemia that is judged to be above treatment thresholds, but below those that prompt immediate exchange transfusion, can usually be controlled using phototherapy. A lack of response to optimal phototherapy may imply significant underlying haemolysis, necessitating exchange transfusion. Any infant undergoing treatment for jaundice should be adequately investigated for the cause. An infant with a total serum bilirubin level that is rising towards or has already reached or exceeded an exchange transfusion threshold should have blood urgently cross-matched for the procedure. This is a neonatal emergency and an appropriate response time from the local transfusion service should be established and audited.

Phototherapy

Observation of the effect of sunlight on the serum bilirubin level of premature infants nursed outdoors prompted the first use of a 'cradle illumination machine' (Cremer et al. 1958). It took a decade for phototherapy to gain clinical acceptance throughout the world, and a further 12 years before its mode of action started to be unravelled (McDonagh et al. 1980). Phototherapy of itself has not influenced neurodevelopmental outcome or cognitive performance in recipients (Seidman et al. 1994; Scheidt 1991), but it remains a convenient and safe means of lowering serum bilirubin. Most importantly, phototherapy reduces the need for the more hazardous alternative, namely exchange transfusion. Optimal use of phototherapy in preterm neonatal jaundice has made the need to resort to exchange transfusion in that context a rarity (Maisels and Watchko 2003).

The ease of use of phototherapy has encouraged its overuse. Many infants are 'placed under the lights' unnecessarily or treated for too long. The vogue for 'prophylactic' phototherapy from birth in very-low-birthweight infants has been shown to neither reduce the peak nor shorten the duration of their jaundice (Curtis-Cohen et al. 1985). Phototherapy would only appear to be effective as bilirubin enters the skin at serum levels >80 µmol/l (Tan 1982). The maximal effect of phototherapy is during the first 24–48 hours of its use. It is to be anticipated that, in the absence of haemolysis, phototherapy will reduce the serum bilirubin level by 25–50% during this initial phase. It has been suggested that the enterohepatic circulation of

bilirubin-Z,Z, reconstituted from configurational photoisomers in bile, causes the subsequent decay in response.

Phototherapy has a benign reputation but it is not without side-effects. The more commonly encountered are:

- diarrhoea
- increased fluid loss via the skin
- temperature instability
- erythematous rashes
- tanning
- bronze-baby syndrome.

The diarrhoea associated with phototherapy is thought to result from an irritant effect of photoisomers on the bowel. This and increased insensible water loss from the skin require attention to fluid balance. Individualised assessment of fluid requirements, especially in the premature or sicker infant, rather than a general prescription of additional fluid is to be advised. The NICE guideline on routine postnatal care recommends that 'breastfed babies should not be routinely supplemented with formula, water or dextrose water for the treatment of jaundice' (National Institute of Health and Clinical Excellence 2006). Close attention to thermoregulation is important, with the risks of cooling from surface exposure and overheating from standard phototherapy lamps. Nursing care should include regular monitoring of the infant's temperature, documentation of stool frequency and urine output, and a daily assessment of weight. The eyes of an infant receiving lamp phototherapy should be shielded to prevent potential retinal damage.

In vitro evidence of light-induced DNA damage, particularly in the presence of bilirubin, has not been mirrored by a consistent increase in melanocytic naevi in recipients of phototherapy, including children receiving long-term treatment for Crigler–Najjar syndrome. The bronze-baby syndrome results from an interaction between cholestatic jaundice and phototherapy (Onishi et al. 1982). The brown pigment produced (bilifuscin) stains the infant's skin and lingers for some weeks after phototherapy has been discontinued. There are case reports of the rare complication of bullous skin lesions resulting from transient porphyrinaemia in such cases (Mallon 1995).

The recently developed fibreoptic systems for delivering phototherapy via a body pad or wrap have made its application more versatile. Earlier trials have shown fibreoptic phototherapy to be as effective as conventional phototherapy in preterm infants, but less so in term infants (Mills and Tudehope 2003). Larger fibreoptic pads or nests designed for term infants are currently in use and should be subjected to comparative trials. A new generation of phototherapy unit has evolved using the technology of multiple light-emitting diodes. These have the advantage of not emitting infrared or ultraviolet radiation, and so can be used closer to the infant's skin for maximal efficacy (Seidman et al. 2000). Placing halogen lights closer to the baby's skin than the manufacturer's guidance may cause skin burns.

Optimal use of phototherapy

The efficacy of phototherapy depends on the dose and wavelength of light used and the proportion of the infant's surface area to which it is applied. The dose of phototherapy administered is expressed in terms of spectral irradiance (µW/cm²/nm) in the 430–490-nm band. Before the mode of action of phototherapy was better understood, it was thought that saturation of dose–response occurred within the blue light range at a spectral irradiance of 4 µW/cm²/nm. This is true of the configurational isomer bilirubin-Z,E, but production of what is thought to be the more important photoisomer, lumirubin, has a dose–response relationship that does not attain saturation until a spectral irradiance of 25–30 μW/cm²/nm is achieved (Ennever 1992).

Early phototherapy lights were designed to emit blue light at a wavelength of around 450 nm, in keeping with the maximal absorbance pattern of bilirubin. Pure blue light is poorly tolerated by staff and can mask cyanosis in an infant. Combinations of broad-spectrum white light and blue light have proved more acceptable. There are theoretical reasons why green light delivered at high irradiance would be the most efficient choice. Compared with blue light, green preferentially favours formation of lumirubin, the main excretory photoisomer, and its longer wavelength enhances skin penetration (Ennever 1990, 1992).

When single-lamp phototherapy is used, parents can be reassured that in taking their baby out of the lights briefly for feeds and cuddles they are not jeopardising treatment. The efficiency of treatment can be improved by using more than one phototherapy lamp or by combining conventional overhead lamps with a fibreoptic system beneath the baby. This multiple phototherapy, applied to a greater proportion of the body surface area, should be adopted in cases of jaundice if the serum bilirubin fails to respond to single phototherapy, is less than 50 μmol/l below the threshold for exchange transfusion or is rising rapidly (>8.5 μmol/l/h). It may prove necessary for the baby to be naked with the exception of eye pads. The American Academy of Pediatrics (AAP) defines intensive phototherapy as a spectral irradiance of at least 30 μW/cm²/nm over the relevant bandwidth (American Academy of Pediatrics 2004). Increasing the dose of phototherapy is most readily achieved by operating the light sources at the minimum safe distance from the infant placed on an overhead cot. Other measures, such as reflecting light back on to the baby with aluminium foil or white drapes, have been recommended, but care should be taken not to obscure the baby from observation.

Pharmacological agents

Synthetic metalloporphyrins have the potential to reduce bilirubin production through competitive inhibition of haem oxygenase. Tin protoporphyrin has been shown to modify the course of hyperbilirubinaemia and to avoid the need for phototherapy in term and near-term newborns (Kappas et al. 1995). Despite its early promise this approach to therapy is currently not advocated.

A preventive therapy that has entered practice is administration of high-dose IVIG to newborns presenting with severe rhesus or ABO isoimmunisation. Treatment of these conditions with IVIG has been shown to reduce significantly the need for exchange transfusion, the duration of phototherapy and the length of hospital stay (Gottstein and Cooke 2003). Babies treated in this way are more likely to require top-up red cell transfusions for late anaemia. As a precaution against overuse of a pooled human blood product it is recommended that a 0.5 g/kg dose of IVIG should be given over 4 hours to babies with a serum bilirubin that continues to climb at a rate >8.5 μmol/l/h despite multiple phototherapy (National Institute for Health and Clinical Excellence 2010). The majority of cases of ABO incompatibility are amenable to multiple phototherapy if delivered optimally. A more pre-emptive use of IVIG may be called for in cases of severe rhesus disease where there has been little or no in utero management, or cases of ABO incompatibility readmitted with a serum bilirubin level approaching exchange values.

Inducers of hepatic conjugation and agents that decrease the enterohepatic recirculation of bilirubin have been studied extensively for their ability to influence the severity and time course of neonatal jaundice significantly. These and other therapies such as traditional Chinese medicine, acupuncture and homeopathy have been considered during compilation of the UK NICE neonatal jaundice guideline and are currently not recommended (National Institute for Health and Clinical Excellence 2010).

Exchange transfusion

The practicalities of performing an exchange transfusion are covered elsewhere (Ch. 30). The need for exchange transfusion has reduced, as a result of improved in utero management and more effective phototherapy. In cases where there has been severe in utero haemolysis, early exchange may be required to correct anaemia and to remove sensitised red cells and circulating antibodies. Previous guidelines based on cord blood values now rarely apply, as most infants with severe rhesus disease will have received in utero transfusion, although a cord blood bilirubin level of more than 90 mmol/l and/or a cord blood haemoglobin level of less than 10 g/dl are still important indications that an early exchange transfusion is required. In babies who received multiple fetal transfusions information regarding how recent the transfusion was and an estimation of the proportion of fetal red cells in the baby's circulation (Kleihauer test) will govern the need for an early exchange. Many such infants respond to intensive phototherapy followed by a later top-up transfusion. If, despite multiple phototherapy, the serum bilirubin continues to rise by >8.5 μmol/l/h, high-dose IVIG is indicated, as discussed above. Exchange transfusion will be indicated if these measures fail and cross-matched blood should be made available for this eventuality. Whilst it would appear logical to keep the serum albumin level of a jaundiced infant within the normal range (Ahlfors 1994), there is no evidence that the practice of giving albumin routinely before or during an exchange transfusion confers benefit (Dennery 2002). Similarly, there is no evidence to support the routine giving of intravenous calcium during an exchange transfusion (National Institute for Health and Clinical Excellence 2010).

In addition to a small risk of blood-borne infection, exchange transfusion carries a significant risk of morbidity and mortality from vascular accidents, cardiac complications, biochemical and haematological disturbance (Keenan et al. 1985). The overall mortality rate from the procedure is quoted as being 0.3% and morbidity 5%. These figures originate from a well-conducted trial performed during an era when exchange transfusion was more commonly performed (Scheidt et al. 1990). The rate of complications is higher in sick premature newborns and lower in otherwise well term or near-term infants (Jackson 1997). Exchange transfusions are now rarely required, and so, with dwindling practical expertise, the procedure is likely to have become more hazardous. Simulation training can be usefully applied to rehearsal of the technique and familiarisation with the equipment and desired monitoring.

Exchange transfusion will remain necessary for infants who fail to respond to optimal phototherapy or who present late with bilirubin levels in excess of a given exchange value. In the latter case, the infant should be placed under multiple phototherapy, and cross-matched blood should be sought as a matter of urgency for an anticipated exchange transfusion. Attention should be paid to correcting disturbances of hydration or acid–base balance, and to the treatment of any underlying infection. Should the serum bilirubin fall below the exchange transfusion level by the time the blood is available a decision as to whether to go ahead with the exchange or not has to be made. This may be informed by the peak serum bilirubin, the duration of jaundice, the bilirubin/albumin ratio and the clinical status of the baby. Signs and symptoms of acute bilirubin encephalopathy are an absolute indication to proceed with an exchange transfusion.

Guidelines for the use of phototherapy and exchange transfusion

Premature infants

Formerly, no distinction was made between the thresholds for treatment of jaundiced term and preterm babies. Kernicterus is known to occur at lower levels of bilirubin in those born prematurely. This is not related to immaturity of the blood–brain barrier, as was once thought, but is more likely to reflect lower levels of albumin with altered binding properties in the sick infant. Recognition that preterm newborns are at higher risk of bilirubin toxicity has given rise to sliding scales prompting earlier intervention on the basis of lower birthweight or gestational age. It would appear prudent to maintain a greater safety margin in the smaller, less mature infant, but a counterargument holds that it may be beneficial to allow a premature infant to have a moderate degree of jaundice to take advantage of bilirubin's antioxidant properties (Yeo et al. 1998). A trial comparing 'aggressive' and 'conservative' phototherapy regimes for infants weighing 1000 g or less (extremely low birthweight) did not show a significant difference in the primary outcome measure of death or neurodevelopmental impairment (Morris et al. 2008). The 'aggressive' phototherapy commenced at a threshold of 85 µmol/l. Outcome in terms of rates of necrotising enterocolitis and retinopathy of prematurity were not different, but subgroup analysis suggested that 'aggressive' phototherapy was associated with a reduction in neurodevelopmental impairment in infants with birthweights of 751–1000 g. An increase in mortality observed in those with a birthweight of 501–750 g treated with 'aggressive' phototherapy raises a note of caution.

Practice in the USA has tended to adopt birthweight categories for the sliding scale of treatment thresholds for jaundice in the premature infant (Maisels and Watchko 2003; Watchko and Maisels 2010). In the UK gestational age categories for treatment are more readily used, but hitherto this has been haphazard with no national consensus (Rennie et al. 2009). The UK NICE guideline on neonatal jaundice (National Institute for Health and Clinical Excellence 2010) recommends treatment thresholds that are specific by week of gestational age for babies of less than 38 weeks' gestation. For the purpose it provides a novel adjustable Excel spreadsheet (Fig. 29.11). A rule of thumb that has been in use for some years in many UK hospitals has been adopted to determine the thresholds for phototherapy and exchange transfusion, using the simple formulae:

- for phototherapy: bilirubin in µmol/l = (gestational age × 10) − 100
- for exchange transfusion: bilirubin in µmol/l = (gestational age × 10).

It is recommended that these should be used as the treatment level for babies aged 72 hours or older. Use of these simple formulae produces thresholds for phototherapy and exchange transfusion that do not represent a significant departure from mainstream practice in the UK (Rennie et al. 2009), or from values described as 'conservative' in the USA (Morris et al. 2008). The threshold levels for the first 72 hours of life were determined by drawing straight lines from 40 and 80 µmol/l at birth to the formula-based level at 72 hours. The start values were chosen to reflect the upper limit of

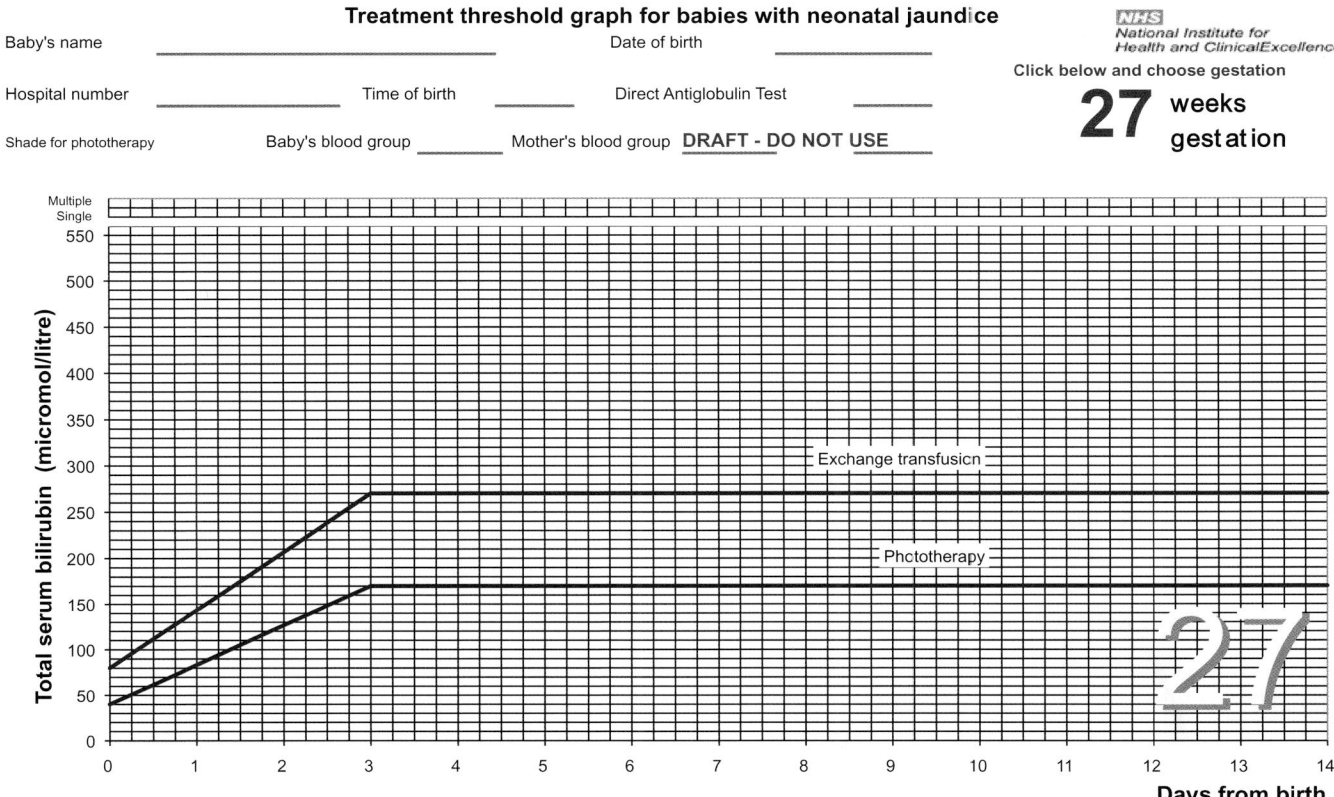

Fig. 29.11 Example of Excel spreadsheet: 27 weeks' gestation (National Institute for Health and Clinical Excellence or University College London (UCL) version) (devised by Dr Giles Kendall, Dr Janet Rennie and Professor T J Cole at UCL).

normal for the umbilical cord blood bilirubin in the absence of haemolysis and a level that is likely to be associated with significant in utero haemolysis.

There is currently insufficient evidence to support a further reduction in thresholds based on risk factors. The outcome of a recently completed trial looking at the use of the bilirubin/albumin ratio as an adjunct to decision-making on thresholds for phototherapy and exchange transfusion in preterm infants of less than 32 weeks' gestation may guide practice in this area (BARTrial: http://www.controlled-trials.com/isrctn/pf/74465643). The NICE guideline also provides advice on monitoring, intensifying and stopping phototherapy treatment (Fig. 29.12).

Term infants

Over the past 15–20 years, there has been a relaxation in the UK of the threshold for phototherapy for healthy jaundiced term new-borns from 250 to 300–350 µmol/l, and for exchange transfusion from 340 to 400–450 µmol/l. The fact that healthy term babies appear to tolerate higher levels of bilirubin than their haemolysing or sick contemporaries has prompted calls for a more relaxed approach to the management of their jaundice. The so-called 'kinder, gentler approach' to the jaundiced term infant proposed by Newman and Maisels (1992) was further developed in a 'practice parameter' issued by a subcommittee of the AAP (American

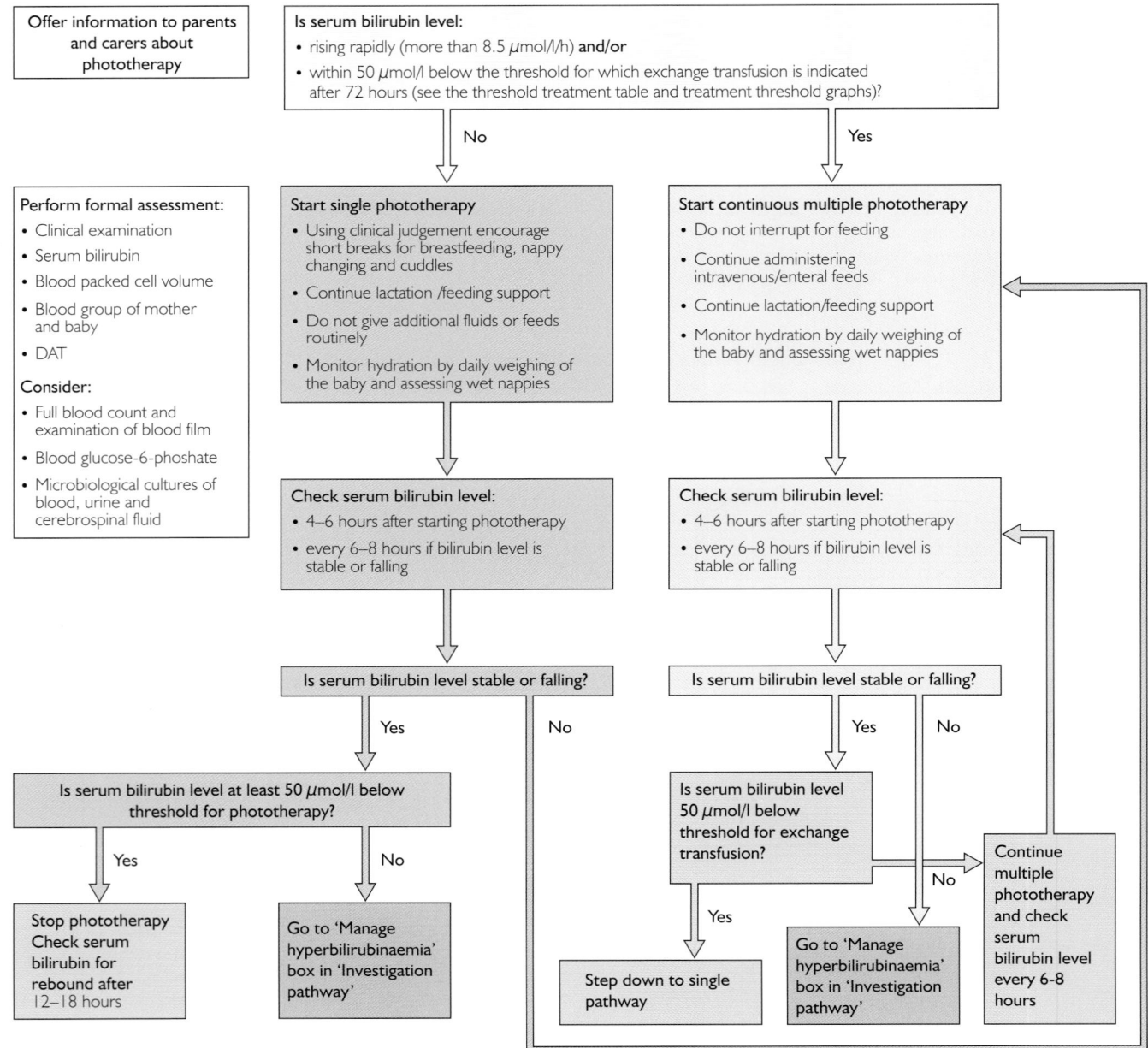

Fig. 29.12 National Institute for Health and Clinical Excellence phototherapy pathway pathway.

Academy of Pediatrics 1994). When this was applied to otherwise healthy full-term infants in the USA it was associated with a decrease in the use of phototherapy by more than 50% and of exchange transfusion by 87% (Seidman et al. 2001), and may have saved as many as 200 lives each year in the USA from procedural complications (Watchko 2001). Subsequently there was evidence that the 1994 guidelines were being 'stretched' to apply to treatment in near-term infants with gestational ages of 35 weeks and above (Seidman et al. 2001; Bhutani and Johnson 2006) and amongst term infants the recommended phototherapy thresholds were not being adhered to (Atkinson et al. 2003). The AAP subcommittee on hyperbilirubinaemia revised its practice parameter by issuing warnings on risk factors for severe jaundice and the clinical pitfalls that may result in kernicterus (American Academy of Pediatrics 2001), and went on to issue a further clinical practice guideline on the management of hyperbilirubinaemia in newborn infants of 35 or more weeks' gestation (American Academy of Pediatrics 2004). This document in turn has been updated with clarification that places emphasis on lowering treatment thresholds in the presence of listed risk factors (Maisels et al. 2009b). Cases of kernicterus have not been reported in infant populations managed with adherence to the AAP guidelines (Newman 2003), and there does not appear to have been a significant change in the reporting of kernicterus cases in the USA across this era of adopting the 'kinder, gentler approach' (Burke et al. 2009).

For babies born at 38 or more weeks' gestation, the UK NICE guideline on neonatal jaundice recommends consensus-derived thresholds for initiation of phototherapy from 96 hours of age of 350 µmol/l and for exchange transfusion of 450 µmol/l (National Institute of Health and Clinical Excellence 2010). For the period from birth to 96 hours of age a series of bilirubin levels with 6-hourly stepwise increases at which phototherapy and exchange transfusion are recommended has been tabulated (Fig. 29.9); in addition to the phototherapy pathway there is also a pathway for exchange transfusion (Fig. 29.13). These phototherapy and exchange transfusion thresholds are comparable to the most commonly reported values in a recent survey of practice in the UK (Rennie et al. 2009) and with the thresholds adopted by the AAP (American Academy of Pediatrics 2004).

Most treatment guidelines rely on total bilirubin level, but, faced with the decision as to whether or not to perform an exchange transfusion, some paediatricians have adopted the practice of subtracting the conjugated component. This should be avoided as there are unnerving case reports of kernicterus occurring in such circumstances (Bertini et al. 2005), as well as the possibility that conjugated bilirubin can displace unconjugated bilirubin from albumin. The current national guidelines in the USA (American Academy of Pediatrics 2004) and the UK (National Institute for Health and Clinical Excellence 2010) recommend adherence to treatment thresholds based on the total serum bilirubin. Specialist advice

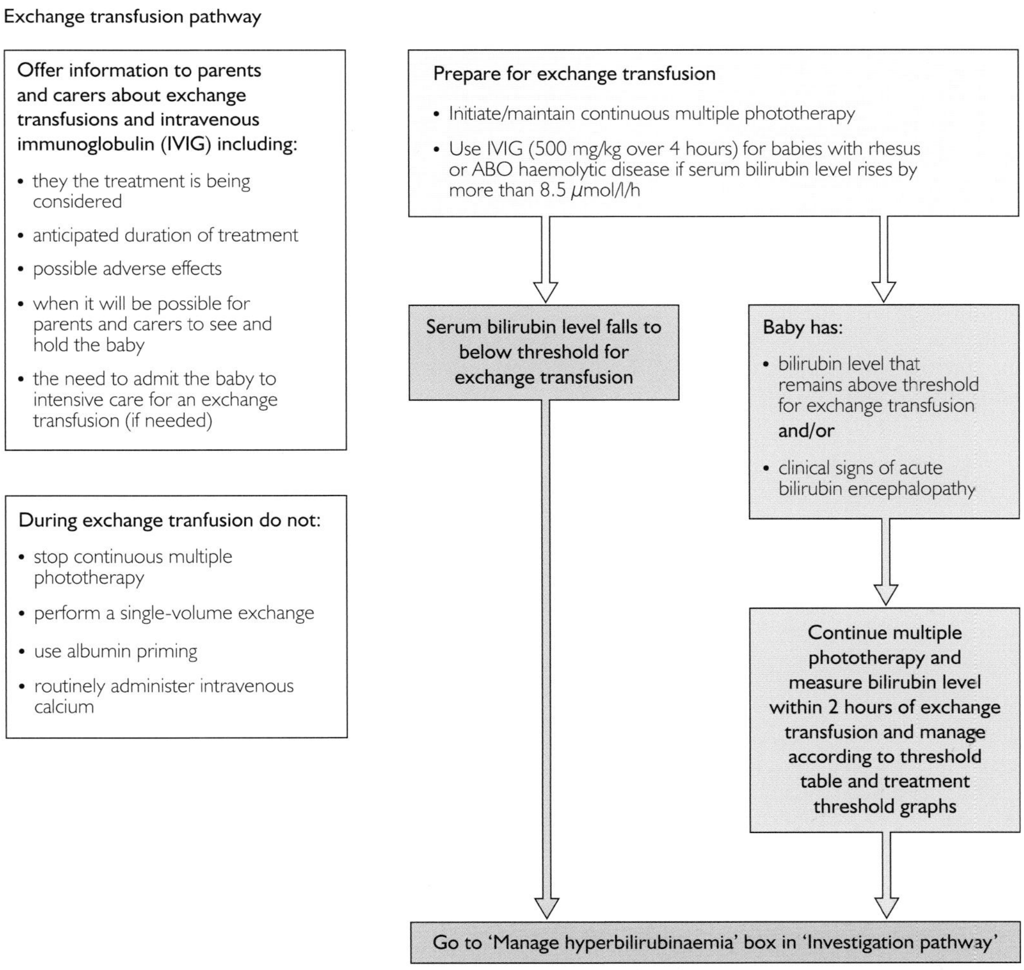

Exchange transfusion pathway

Fig. 29.13 National Institute for Health and Clinical Excellence exchange transfusion pathway.

should be sought for the exceptional cases in which the conjugated bilirubin is more than 50% of the total.

The latest American guidelines (American Academy of Pediatrics 2004; Maisels et al. 2009b) recommend reducing the thresholds for phototherapy and exchange transfusion by 40–50 μmol/l in cases where there are additional risk factors, defined as isoimmune haemolytic disease, G6PD deficiency, asphyxia, significant lethargy, temperature instability, sepsis, acidosis and hypoalbuminaemia (<30 g/l). They also suggest that 'bilirubin/albumin ratios can be used together with but not in lieu of the total serum bilirubin level as an additional factor in determining the need for exchange transfusion'.

It is also important to heed the recommendations made on the mode of phototherapy and the intervals between monitoring the serum bilirubin laid out in the recent guidelines. The UK NICE guideline recommends that, after starting phototherapy, the serum bilirubin is checked 4–6-hourly until the bilirubin level is stable or falling and every 6–12 hours thereafter. Multiple phototherapy, using more than one overhead source or in combination with a fibreoptic device of appropriate size for the baby, is recommended if the serum bilirubin is within 50 μmol/l below the threshold for which exchange transfusion is indicated. Multiple phototherapy should also be adopted when the bilirubin is rising rapidly (more than 8.5 μmol/l/h) despite single phototherapy. When the serum bilirubin has fallen to more than 50 μmol/l below the exchange transfusion threshold a stepdown from multiple phototherapy to single phototherapy should be considered. This should be performed with caution in the presence of known or suspected haemolysis, and monitored with a repeat serum bilirubin within 4–6 hours. When the serum bilirubin has fallen to more than 50 μmol/l below the phototherapy threshold, single phototherapy can be stopped. A serum bilirubin should be checked for rebound after 12–18 hours (National Institute for Health and Clinical Excellence 2010).

Population surveillance and future monitoring of best practice

In the USA a case is being made for universal hour-specific predischarge bilirubin screening to identify babies at risk of significant hyperbilirubinaemia (Maisels et al. 2009b). The accuracy of this prediction will be enhanced by taking into account the additional risk factors of prematurity and intention to breastfeed exclusively (Maisels et al. 2009a). Given that such an approach has been shown to reduce the incidence of a total serum bilirubin level of >427 μmol/l (>25 mg/dl), it may be anticipated that a reduction in the incidence of kernicterus can be achieved (Kuzniewicz et al. 2009).

In the UK the responsibility for detecting significant postdischarge jaundice rests with the primary healthcare team of midwives, health visitors, general practitioners and, of course, informed parents. The NICE guideline (National Institute for Health and Clinical Excellence 2010) seeks to inform parents better, and to alert the primary healthcare team to babies at heightened risk of significant hyperbilirubinaemia. These babies will have an additional assessment in the period leading up to 48 hours of age with inspection for signs of jaundice and attention to feeding support. A clear directive has been made to test, rather than guess, the level of bilirubin in all babies presenting with neonatal jaundice. This approach is reliant on our ability to recognise better clinical jaundice in babies with darker skin tone, who are currently overrepresented in registries of kernicterus and surveys of hyperbilirubinaemia.

Clinical kernicterus is an irreversible tragedy that should be considered a preventable condition in the term and near-term infant. National registries of cases of acute bilirubin encephalopathy and chronic kernicterus should be established to monitor adherence to national guidelines and to benchmark their impact. There are calls in the USA to designate a total serum bilirubin level >427 μmol/l (>25 mg/dl) as a reportable condition (Bhutani and Johnson 2009b). In the UK it is being proposed that kernicterus be added to the list of 'never events' incurring contractual penalties within the quality goals and sanctions of the present-day National Health Service (http//neverevents.dh.gov.uk). It could be argued that the 'never event' trigger should be an unconjugated serum bilirubin value in excess of 510 μmol/l, a level above which one in eight babies are at risk of developing signs of acute bilirubin encephalopathy, of whom as many as half may go on to develop chronic kernicterus (Manning et al. 2007). In the UK a repeat national survey of hyperbilirubinaemia >510 μmol/l and treatment threshold practice should be conducted after implementation of the 2010 NICE guidance. If preventable cases of kernicterus continue to occur the alternative approach of universal screening may need to be considered.

Weblinks

www.aap.org/jaundice: American Academy of Pediatrics.

www.cdc.gov/jaundice: American Centers for Disease Control and Prevention: links to the BiliTool, an hour-specific risk predictor and management indicator for babies of greater than 35 weeks' gestation and between 18 and 168 hours of age.

www.nice.org.uk/CG98: National Institute for Health and Clinical Excellence Clinical Guideline on Neonatal Jaundice.

www.pickonline.org/parentsinfo.html: parents of infants and children with kernicterus resource centre: has useful information and links, with videos of affected children.

References

Ahlfors, C.E., 1994. Criteria for exchange transfusion in jaundiced newborns. Pediatrics 93, 488–494.

American Academy of Pediatrics Provisional Committee for Quality Improvement and Subcommittee on Hyperbilirubinemia, 1994. Practice parameter: management of hyperbilirubinemia in the healthy term newborn. Pediatrics 94, 558–565.

American Academy of Pediatrics Subcommittee on Hyperbilirubinemia, 2001. Neonatal jaundice and kernicterus. Pediatrics 108, 763–765.

American Academy of Pediatrics Subcommittee on Hyperbilirubinemia, 2004. Management of hyperbilirubinemia in the newborn infant 35 or more weeks of gestation. [erratum appears in Pediatrics;114(4):1138]. Pediatrics 114, 297–316.

Amin, S.B., Ahlfors, C., Orlando, M.S., et al., 2001. Auditory brainstem response and bilirubin binding in premature infants. Pediatrics 107, 664–670.

Atkinson, L.R., Escobar, G.J., Takayama, J.I., et al., 2003. Phototherapy use in jaundiced newborns in a large managed care organization: do clinicians adhere to the guideline? Pediatrics 111, e555–e561.

Bakkeheim, E., Bergerud, U., Schmidt-Melbye, A.-C., et al., 2009. Maternal IgG anti-A and anti-B titres predict outcome in

ABO-incompatibility in the neonate. Acta Paediatr 1896–1901.

Bertini, G., Dani, C., Fonda, C., et al., 2005. Bronze baby syndrome and the risk of kernicterus. Acta Paediatr 94, 968–971.

Bhutani, V.K., Johnson, L., 2006. Kernicterus in late preterm infants cared for as term healthy infants. Semin Perinatol 30, 89–97.

Bhutani, V.K., Johnson, L., 2009a. Synopsis report from the pilot USA kernicterus registry. J Perinatol 29, S4–S7.

Bhutani, V.K., Johnson, L., 2009b. A proposal to prevent severe neonatal hyperbilirubinemia and kernicterus. J Perinatol 29, S61–S67.

Bhutani, V.K., Johnson, L., Sivieri, E.M., 1999. Predictive ability of a predischarge hour-specific serum bilirubin for subsequent significant hyperbilirubinaemia in healthy term and near-term newborns. Pediatrics 103, 6–14.

Brites, D., Fernandes, A., Falcao, A.S., et al., 2009. Biological risks for neurological abnormalities associated with hyperbilirubinaemia. J Perinatol 29, S8–S13.

Burgess, G.H., Oh, W., Bratlid, D., et al., 1985. The effects of brain blood flow on brain bilirubin deposition in newborn piglets. Pediatr Res 19, 691–696.

Burke, B.L., Robbins, J.M., Bird, T.M., et al., 2009. Trends in hospitalizations for neonatal jaundice and kernicterus in the United States, 1988–2005. Pediatrics 123, 524–532.

Connolly, A.M., Volpe, J.J., 1990. Clinical features of bilirubin encephalopathy. Clin Perinatol 17, 371–379.

Cremer, R.J., Perryman, P.W., Richards, D.H., 1958. Influence of light on the hyperbilirubinaemia of infants. Lancet 1, 1094–1097.

Curtis-Cohen, M., Stahl, G.E., Costarino, A.T., et al., 1985. Randomized trial of prophylactic phototherapy in the infant with very low birth weight. J Pediatr 107, 121–124.

De Carvalho, M., Hall, M., Harvey, D., 1981. Effects of water supplementation on physiological jaundice in breast-fed babies. Arch Dis Child 56, 568–569.

Dennery, P.A., 2002. Pharmacological interventions for the treatment of neonatal jaundice. Semin Neonatol 7, 111–119.

DeVries, L.S., Lary, S., Dubowitz, L.M.S., 1985. Relationship of serum bilirubin levels to ototoxicity and deafness in high-risk low birth-weight infants. Pediatrics 76, 351–354.

DeVries, L.S., Lary, S., Whitelaw, A.G., et al., 1987. Relationship of serum bilirubin levels and hearing impairment in newborn infants. Early Hum Dev 15, 269–277.

Ennever, J.F., 1990. Blue light, green light, white light, more light: treatment of neonatal jaundice. Clin Perinatol 17, 467–481.

Ennever, J.F., 1992. Phototherapy for neonatal jaundice. In: Polin, R.A., Fox, W.W. (Eds.), Fetal and Neonatal Physiology. W B Saunders, Philadelphia, pp. 1165–1173.

Funato, M., Tamai, H., Shimada, S., et al., 1994. Vigintiphobia, unbound bilirubin, and auditory brainstem responses. Pediatrics 93, 50–53.

Gottstein, R., Cooke, R.W.I., 2003. Systematic review of intravenous immunoglobulin in haemolytic disease of the newborn. Arch Dis Child Fetal Neonatal Ed 88, F6–F10.

Govaert, P., Lequin, M., Swarte, R., et al., 2003. Changes in the globus pallidus with pre(term) kernicterus. Pediatrics 112, 1256–1263.

Hanko, E., Lindemann, R., Hansen, T.W.R., 2001. Spectrum of outcome in infants with extreme neonatal jaundice. Acta Paediatr 90, 782–785.

Hansen, T.W.R., 1995. Kernicterus in a full-term infant: the need for increased vigilance (letter). Pediatrics 95, 798–799.

Hulzebos, C.V., van Imhoff, D.E., Bos, A.F., et al., 2008. Usefulness of the bilirubin/albumin ratio for predicting bilirubin-induced neurotoxicity in premature infants. Arch Dis Child Fetal Neonatal Ed 93, F384–F388.

Ives, N.K., 1992. Kernicterus in preterm infants: lest we forget (to turn on the lights). Pediatrics 90, 757–759.

Ives, N.K., 2007. Preventing kernicterus: a wake up call. Arch Dis Child 92, F330–F331.

Jackson, J.C., 1997. Adverse events associated with exchange transfusion in healthy and ill newborns. Pediatrics 99, E7.

Johnson, L., Bhutani, V.K., Karp, K., et al., 2009. Clinical report from the pilot USA Kernicterus Registry (1992 to 2004). J Perinatol 29, S4–S7.

Kadakol, A., Sappal, B.S., Ghosh, S.S., et al., 2001. Interaction of coding region mutations and the Gilbert-type promoter abnormality of the UGT1A1 gene causes moderate degrees of unconjugated hyperbilirubinaemia and may lead to neonatal kernicterus. J Med Genet 38, 244–249.

Kaplan, M., 2001. Genetic interactions in the pathogenesis of neonatal hyperbilirubinaemia: Gilbert's syndrome and glucose-6-phosphate dehydrogenase deficiency. J Perinatol 21 (suppl.1), S30–S34.

Kaplan, M., Hammerman, C., 2002. Glucose-6-phosphate dehydrogenase deficiency: a potential source of severe neonatal hyperbilirubinaemia and kernicterus. Semin Neonatol 7, 121–128.

Kaplan, M., Hammerman, C., Maisels, M.J., 2003. Bilirubin genetics for the nongeneticist: hereditary defects of neonatal bilirubin conjugation. Pediatrics 111, 886–893.

Kappas, A., Drummond, G.S., Henschke, C., et al., 1995. Direct comparison of Sn-mesoporphyrin, an inhibitor of bilirubin production, and phototherapy in controlling hyperbilirubinemia in term and near-term newborns. Pediatrics 95, 468–474.

Katar, S., Akay, H.O., Taskesen, M., et al., 2008. Clinical and cranial magnetic resonance imaging (MRI) findings of 21 patients with serious hyperbilirubinaemia. J Child Neurol 23 (4), 415–417.

Keenan, W.J., Novak, K.K., Sutherland, J.M., et al., 1985. Morbidity and mortality associated with exchange transfusion. Pediatrics 75, 417–421.

Keren, R., Bhutani, V.K., Luan, X., et al., 2005. Identifying newborns at risk of significant hyperbilirubinaemia: a comparison of two recommended approaches. Arch Dis Child 90, 415–421.

Khoury, M.J., Calle, E.E., Joesoef, R.M., 1988. Recurrence risk of neonatal hyperbilirubinemia in siblings. Am J Dis Child 142, 1065–1069.

Knudsen, A., Lebech, M., 1989. Maternal bilirubin, cord bilirubin and placental function at delivery in the development of neonatal jaundice in mature newborns. Acta Obstet Gynecol Scand 68, 719–724.

Kramer, L.I., 1969. Advancement of dermal icterus in the jaundiced newborn. Am J Dis Child 118, 454–458.

Kuzniewicz, M.W., Escobar, G.J., Newman, T.B., 2009. The impact of universal bilirubin screening on severe hyperbilirubinaemia and phototherapy use in a managed care organization. Pediatrics 124, 1031–1039.

Linder, N., Yatsiv, I., Tsur, M., et al., 1988. Unexplained neonatal jaundice as an early diagnostic sign of septicaemia in the newborn. J Perinatol 8, 325–327.

Lucas, A., Baker, B.A., 1986. Breast milk jaundice in premature infants. Arch Dis Child 61, 1063–1067.

Maayan-Metzger, A., Schwartz, T., Sulkes, J., et al., 2001. Maternal anti-D prophylaxis during pregnancy does not cause neonatal haemolysis. Arch Dis Child Fetal Neonatal Ed 84, F60–F62.

Maisels, M., 2006. What's in a name? Physiologic and pathologic jaundice: the conundrum of defining normal bilirubin levels in the newborn. Pediatrics 118, 805–807.

Maisels, M.J., Kring, E., 1992. Risk of sepsis in newborns with severe hyperbilirubinemia. Pediatrics 90, 741–743.

Maisels, M.J., Newman, T.B., 1995. Kernicterus occurs in otherwise healthy, breast-fed term newborns. Pediatrics 96, 730–733.

Maisels, M.J., Newman, T.B., 2001. Bilirubin and neurological dysfunction – do we need to change what we are doing? Pediatr Res 50, 677–678.

Maisels, M.J., Watchko, J.F., 2003. Treatment of jaundice in low birthweight infants. Arch Dis Child Fetal Neonatal Ed 88, F459–F463.

Maisels, M.J., DeRidder, J.M., Kring, E.A., 2009a. Routine transcutaneous bilirubin measurements combined with clinical risk factors improve the prediction of subsequent hyperbilirubinemia. J Perinatol 29, 612–617.

Maisels, M.J., Bhutani, V.K., Bogen, D., et al., 2009b. Hyperbilirubinaemia in the newborn infant >35 week's gestation: an update with clarifications. Pediatrics 124, 1193–1198.

Mallon, E., Wojnarowska, F., Hope, P., Elder, G., 1995. Neonatal bullous eruption as a result of transient porphyrinemia in a premature infant with hemolytic disease of the newborn. J Am Acad Dermatol 33, 333–336.

Manning, D., Todd, P., Maxwel, M., et al., 2007. Prospective surveillance study of severe hyperbilirubinaemia in the newborn in the UK and Ireland. Arch Dis Child Fetal Neonatal Ed 92, 342–346.

McDonagh, A.F., 1990. Is bilirubin good for you? Clin Perinatol 17, 359–369.

McDonagh, A.F., 2006. Ex uno plures: the concealed complexity of bilirubin species in neonatal blood samples. Pediatrics 118, 1185–1187.

McDonagh, A.F., Lightner, D.A., 1985. 'Like a shrivelled blood orange': bilirubin, jaundice and phototherapy. Pediatrics 75, 443–455.

McDonagh, A.F., Palma, L.A., Lightner, D.A., 1980. Blue light and bilirubin excretion. Science 208, 145–151.

Mills, J.F., Tudehope, D., 2003. Fibreoptic phototherapy for neonatal jaundice. Cochrane Database Syst Rev (3).

Monaghan, G., McLellan, A., McGeehan, A., et al., 1999. Gilbert's syndrome is a contributory factor in prolonged unconjugated hyperbilirubinaemia of the newborn. J Pediatr 134, 441–446.

Morris, B.H., Oh, W., Tyson, J.E., et al., 2008. Aggressive vs. conservative phototherapy for infants with extremely low birth weight. N Engl J Med 359, 1885–1896.

National Institute for Health and Clinical Excellence, 2006. Routine Postnatal Care of Women and their Babies. Clinical Guideline 37. Available online at: www.nice.org.uk/CG37 2006.

National Institute for Health and Clinical Excellence, 2010. Neonatal Jaundice. Clinical Guideline 98. Available online at: www.nice.org.uk/CG98.

Newman, T.B., Easterling, M.J., 1994. Yield of reticulocyte counts and blood smears in term infants. Clin Pediatr 33, 71–76.

Newman, T.B., Maisels, M.J., 1992. Evaluation of jaundice in the term newborn: a kinder, gentler approach. Pediatrics 89, 809–818.

Newman, T.B., Maisels, M.J., 2000. Less aggressive treatment of neonatal jaundice and reports of kernicterus: lessons about practice guidelines. Pediatrics 105, 242–245.

Newman, T.B., Liljestrand, P., Escobar, G.J., 2002. Jaundice noted in the first 24 hours after birth in a managed care organization. Arch Pediatr Adolesc Med 156, 1244–1250.

Newman, T.B., Liljestrand, P., Escobar, G.J., 2003. Infants with bilirubin levels of 30 mg/dL or more in a large managed care organization. Pediatrcs 111, 1303–1311.

Onishi, I., Itoh, S., Isobe, K., et al., 1982. Mechanism of development of the bronze baby syndrome in neonates treated with phototherapy. Pediatrics 69, 273–276.

Rennie, J.M., Seghal, A., De, A., et al., 2009. Range of UK practice regarding thresholds for phototherapy and exchange transfusion in neonatal hyperbilirubinaemia. Arch Dis Child Fetal Neonatal Ed 94, F323–F327.

Robertson, A., Carp, W., Brodersen, R., 1991. Bilirubin displacing effect of drugs used in neonatology. Acta Paediatr Scand 80, 1119–1127.

Scheidt, P.C., Bryla, D.A., Nelson, K.B., et al., 1990. Phototherapy for neonatal hyperbilirubinemia: six year follow-up of the NICHD clinical trial. Pediatrics 85, 455–463.

Scheidt, P.C., Graubard, B.I., Nelson, K.B., et al., 1991. Intelligence at six years in relation to neonatal bilirubin level: follow-up of the National Institute of Child Health and Human Development Clinical Trial of Phototherapy. Pediatrics 87, 797–805.

Seidman, D.S., Paz, I., Stevenson, D.K., et al., 1994. Effects of phototherapy for neonatal jaundice on cognitive performance. J Perinatol 14, 23–28.

Seidman, D.S., Shiloh, M., Stevenson, D.K., et al., 1995. Role of hemolysis in neonatal jaundice associated with glucose-6-phosphate dehydrogenase deficiency. J Pediatr 127, 804–806.

Seidman, D.S., Moise, J., Ergaz, Z., et al., 2000. A new blue light-emitting phototherapy device: a prospective randomized controlled study. J Pediatr 136, 771–774.

Seidman, D.S., Paz, I., Armon, Y., et al., 2001. The effect of the publication of the 'Practice parameter for the management of hyperbilirubinaemia' on treatment of neonatal jaundice. Acta Paediatr 190, 292–295.

Shapiro, S.M., 2010. Chronic bilirubin encephalopathy: diagnosis and outcome. Semin Fetal Neonatal Med 15.3, 157–163.

Silverman, W.A., Andersen, D.H., Blanc, W.A., et al., 1956. A difference in mortality rate and incidence of kernicterus among premature infants allotted to two prophylactic antibacterial regimens. Pediatrics 18614–18625.

Stevenson, D.K., Fanaroff, A.A., Maisels, M.J., et al., 2001. Prediction of hyperbilirubinaemia in near-term and term infants. J Perinatol 21, S63–S72.

Tan, K.L., 1982. The pattern of bilirubin response to phototherapy for neonatal hyperbilirubinemia. Pediatr Res 16, 670–674.

Tan, K.L., Skurr, B.A., Yip, Y.Y., 1992. Phototherapy and the brain-stem auditory evoked response in neonatal hyperbilirubinemia. J Pediatr 120, 306–308.

Turkel, S.B., Miller, C.A., Guttenberg, M.E., et al., 1982. A clinical pathologic reappraisal of kernicterus. Pediatrics 69, 267–272.

Volpe, J.J., 2008. Neurology of the Newborn, fifth ed. W B Saunders, Philadelphia, pp. 619–651.

Watchko, J.F., 2001. Recurrence of kernicterus in term and near-term infants in Denmark. Acta Paediatr 90, 1080.

Watchko, J.F., Maisels, M.J., 2010. Enduring controversies in the management of hyperbilirubinaemia in preterm neonates. Semin Fetal Neonatal Med 15, 136–140.

Watchko, J., Oski, F., 1983. Bilirubin 20 mg/dL = vigintiphobia. Pediatrics 71, 660–663.

Watchko, J.F., Oski, F.A., 1992. Kernicterus in preterm newborns: past, present, and future. Pediatrics 90, 707–715.

Watchko, J.F., Daood, M.J., Biniwale, M., 2002. Understanding neonatal hyperbilirubinaemia in the era of genomics. Semin Neonatol 7, 143–152.

Wennberg, R.P., Ahlfors, C.E., Bhutani, V.K., et al., 2006. Toward understanding kernicterus: a challenge to improve the management of jaundiced newborns. Pediatrics 117, 474–485.

Yeo, K.L., Perlman, M., Hao, Y.M.P., 1998. Outcomes of extremely premature infants related to their peak serum bilirubin concentrations and exposure to phototherapy. Pediatrics 102, 1426–1431.

Yokochi, K., 1995. Magnetic resonance imaging in children with kernicterus. Acta Paediatr 84, 937–939.

Giorgina Mieli-Vergani   Nedim Hadžić

Introduction

Liver disease in infancy is rare but represents a serious cause of morbidity and mortality. A better awareness of the causes of liver disease in this age group and their mode of presentation has led to earlier diagnosis of treatable conditions, with considerable improvement in outcome, and facilitated genetic counselling for those families with hereditary disorders.

Jaundice is usually the first sign of liver dysfunction, but its importance is often underestimated because of the frequent occurrence of physiological jaundice in the neonatal period (see Ch. 29 part 1). A raised serum bilirubin with a conjugated component of >20% and urine which contains bile pigment is always pathological. The notion that jaundice could be due to liver disease should prompt health workers to assess the colour of the urine and the stools to ascertain whether the jaundice is due to cholestasis. A neonate's urine is usually pale yellow and often colourless. Dark yellow urine (unless during phototherapy) and pale stools which are not yellow or green in an infant of any age should suggest liver disease and should prompt medical review and appropriate investigation (National Institute for Health and Clinical Excellence 2010). A persistently elevated unconjugated bilirubin, not explained by haemolysis or other neonatal problems, suggests the possibility of liver-based inherited disorders of bilirubin metabolism.

Hepatitis syndrome of infancy

Hepatitis syndrome of infancy is characterised by clinical and laboratory features of liver dysfunction, of which the most distinct is conjugated hyperbilirubinaemia. Babies usually have inflammatory changes in the liver histology – hence the name hepatitis – but the cause is only rarely infective. In most cases the baby presents with conjugated jaundice, which follows physiological jaundice; the urine becomes dark and the stools pale. Less commonly, babies may present with complications of liver dysfunction such as a bleeding diathesis, hypoglycaemia or fluid retention. The bleeding diathesis is usually due to vitamin K deficiency associated with fat malabsorption, which may also cause failure to thrive. Unless parenteral vitamin K is given, these babies may bleed catastrophically. Hepatomegaly is almost universal. Palpable splenomegaly occurs in 40–60% of cases.

Hepatitis syndrome of infancy most commonly is due to intrahepatic disease, for which there are many associated disorders. It may also be due to lesions of the biliary system. All babies require urgent investigation to identify disorders for which there is specific treatment and to prevent complications of cholestasis. If the stools contain no yellow or green pigment, cholestasis is complete and surgical conditions, including biliary atresia, must be suspected. It is essential to arrange urgent referral to a specialist centre which has the experience and skills to confirm the diagnosis and provide corrective surgery as early as possible (Mieli-Vergani et al. 1989).

Pathology

Four main pathological entities cause the syndrome:

1. hepatocellular disease (hepatitis)
2. inflammation and bile duct damage, leading in some instances to paucity of interlobular bile ducts
3. disorders of the main intrahepatic bile ducts, leading to sclerosing cholangitis
4. disorders of the extrahepatic bile ducts, most commonly biliary atresia.

Hepatocellular disease may be associated with a wide range of infective, genetic, endocrine, vascular, toxic, familial, genetic or chromosomal disorders (Vara and Dhawan 2007). Often there are no associated factors and the disorder is cryptogenic. Chronic liver disease rarely follows in infective or endocrine disorders, but occurs in at least 50% of genetic or familial disorders. Pathological categories 2–4 are invariably associated with chronic liver disease unless surgery (for some disorders in category 4) is effective. Infants with a normal serum gamma-glutamyl transpeptidase (GGT) activity or cholesterol concentration in the presence of jaundice and abnormal biochemical tests of liver function are likely to have a form of progressive familial intrahepatic cholestasis or primary bile acid synthesis abnormality (Clayton et al. 1987, 1995; Maggiore et al. 1987; Thompson and Jansen 2000; Subramaniam et al. 2010). Together with babies with sclerosing cholangitis (Amedee-Manesme et al. 1987; Baker et al. 1993), this group often develops severe chronic liver disease.

For all pathological entities, in the acute stages, the intrahepatic pathology, as revealed by liver biopsy, is dominated by cholestasis, with variable degrees of giant-cell transformation of hepatocytes and inflammatory cell infiltrate in the portal tracts (Clayton et al. 1987, 1995). In metabolic disorders, abnormal accumulation of microvesicular or macrovesicular fat, glycogen or other storage material may be found in hepatocytes or Kupffer cells. Portal tract widening with oedema, accumulation of fibrous tissue and bile duct proliferation is characteristic of disorders of the major bile ducts, the most common of which is biliary atresia. It may occur in genetic disorders such as α_1-antitrypsin deficiency (α_1ATD) and could be a harbinger of chronic liver disease.

Clinical features

The majority of babies with hepatitis syndrome present with conjugated hyperbilirubinaemia starting in the first 4 weeks of life, but may occasionally present as late as 4 months of age. The second most common presentation is spontaneous bleeding, usually secondary to vitamin K malabsorption; the jaundice may be mild or ignored because it is considered physiological by parents and their healthcare advisers. Rarely, babies present with features of hypoglycaemia or hypoalbuminaemia. Review of the perinatal case records and past medical history may reveal features suggesting intrauterine infection, exposure to toxins, drugs or intravenous nutrition, familial, genetic or metabolic disease, or consanguinity (Vara and Dhawan 2007).

Clinical examination is likely to show mild hepatomegaly and splenomegaly. Neonates with intrahepatic disease may show failure to thrive, but babies with biliary atresia typically are well nourished and have no stigmata of chronic liver disease in the first 2 months of life. Rarely, there are clinical signs of diagnostic importance (Table 29.8). If the stools are white or grey, there may be complete cholestasis, strongly pointing to surgical conditions such as biliary atresia. Standard tests of liver function, such as serum bilirubin, alkaline phosphatase, aspartate transaminase, GGT, albumin and prothrombin time, do not help to distinguish between the four main groups of disorders. Serum triglycerides and cholesterol are usually normal in the first 4 months of life but may increase

Table 29.8 Clinical signs of diagnostic importance in conjugated hyperbilirubinaemia

ABNORMAL SIGNS	DISORDERS
Skin lesions, purpura, chorioretinitis, myocarditis	Generalised viral infection
Cataract	Galactosaemia or intrauterine infection, hypoparathyroidism
Multiple congenital anomalies	Trisomy 21, 13 or 18
Cystic mass below the liver	Choledochal cyst
Ascites and bile-stained hernias	Spontaneous perforation of the bile ducts
Systolic murmur, abnormal facies, posterior embryotoxon	Arteriohepatic dysplasia (Alagille syndrome)
Cutaneous haemangiomata	Hepatic haemangioma
Situs inversus with or without polysplenia	Extrahepatic biliary atresia
Optic nerve hypoplasia and/or micropenis	Septo-optic dysplasia

Table 29.9 Investigations in conjugated hyperbilirubinaemia

Immediate investigations in all cases

Bacterial culture of blood and urine
Urine microscopy and analysis for reducing substances
Prothrombin time
Full blood count and reticulocyte count
Blood sugar, creatinine and urea
Serum sodium, potassium, bicarbonate and calcium
Blood group and cross-match

Investigations when full laboratory service is available

Biochemical tests of liver function, including split bilirubin and gamma-glutamyl transpeptidase
IgM/IgG to *Toxoplasma*, *Listeria*, cytomegalovirus, herpes virus, rubella, hepatitis A and C, HIV and syphilis serology
Hepatitis B surface antigen
α_1-antitrypsin phenotype or genotype
Red blood cell galactose-1-phosphate uridyl transferase
Sweat electrolytes and immunoreactive trypsin
Serum and urine amino acids
Serum lactate and pyruvate
Mass spectrometry for plasma or urine bile acids
Urine succinyl acetone and organic acids
Direct Coombs' test (if appropriate)
Thyroxine, TSH, cortisol
Chest X-ray/echocardiogram for cardiac lesions
Wrist X-ray for rickets
In the presence of ascites: tap for cytology, biochemical testing and culture
Ultrasound of liver to detect focal lesions and dilated bile ducts
Radionuclide scan (methyl-brom-iminodiacetic acid) scan following phenobarbital (in selected cases)

Tissue diagnosis

Percutaneous liver biopsy
Skin biopsy for fibroblast culture and enzyme analysis (in selected cases)
Bone marrow aspirate for Niemann–Pick disease
Laparotomy, intraoperative cholangiography

Ig, immunoglobulin; HIV, human immunodeficiency virus; TSH, thyroid-stimulating hormone.

thereafter, particularly in infants with bile duct hypoplasia. Serum α-fetoprotein values are physiologically elevated in young babies, especially if born praematurely, but are usually much higher in liver disease, particularly in tyrosinaemia (Lindstedt et al. 1992).

Management (Table 29.9)

The first priority on admission to hospital is to identify the causes and complications for which urgent treatment is required. These are septicaemia, urinary tract infection, toxoplasmosis, syphilis, malaria, herpes simplex and metabolic disorders like galactosaemia and fructosaemia. The most dangerous complication is spontaneous haemorrhage due to vitamin K deficiency. Such haemorrhage may well be intracranial. The initial investigations must include prothrombin time, full blood count, blood cultures, urine culture and urine analysis for non-glucose-reducing substances. Galactose and fructose must be excluded from the diet until it is shown that there is no metabolic abnormality primarily affecting their metabolism (Henriksen et al. 1981). After these tests, diagnostic investigations such as α_1-antitrypsin (α_1AT) phenotyping and galactose-1-phosphate uridyl transferase activity in red cells should be carried out. If the baby has received a blood transfusion, the parents should be investigated for a possible heterozygote status.

If septicaemia is suspected, broad-spectrum antibiotics and aciclovir must be given. Even if septicaemia is confirmed, there may still be a serious underlying disease, such as galactosaemia, haemophagocytic lymphohistiocytosis (HLH), tyrosinaemia type 1, α_1ATD or biliary atresia. The finding of non-glucose-reducing substances in the urine does not necessarily indicate galactosaemia, as they may occur in normal babies in the first 2 weeks of life and are common in all forms of liver damage due to secondary proximal tubular damage (Henriksen et al. 1981). Conversely, the absence of non-glucose-reducing substances does not exclude galactosaemia, as very ill babies may feed poorly or vomit. If the prothrombin time is found to be prolonged, vitamin K (1 mg intravenously) should be given immediately and, if bleeding is still occurring or the coagulation times are still significantly prolonged, fresh-frozen plasma

infused or exchange transfusion performed. The next priority is to identify those babies who require surgical correction of bile duct obstruction (Table 29.10). Ultrasound examination should be undertaken to exclude a choledochal cyst or focal intrahepatic lesions.

In all infants, infective (Table 29.11), metabolic (Table 29.12) and endocrine (Table 29.13) causes of liver damage affecting this age group must be excluded. With regard to infective conditions, it must be remembered that cytomegalovirus (CMV), rubella and hepatitis B virus have been found to occur in all types of hepatobiliary disease (Henriksen et al. 1981). Seropositivity for these viruses should not preclude investigation of other causes of liver damage. Galactosaemia, fructosaemia and tyrosinaemia must be diagnosed promptly because dietary intervention in the first two conditions and treatment with 2-(2-nitro-4-trifluoro-methyl-benzoyl)-1-3-cyclohexanedione (NTBC) in the last (Lindstedt et al. 1992), need to be instituted urgently to avoid severe deterioration. α_1ATD, cystic

Table 29.10 Surgically correctable disorders causing bile duct obstruction

Extrahepatic biliary atresia
Choledochal cyst
Spontaneous perforation of the bile ducts
Duodenal and low bile duct atresia
Gallstones
Haemangiomata
Extrinsic compression
Bile plugs in extrahepatic bile ducts

Table 29.11 Infections associated with conjugated hyperbilirubinaemia (see Ch. 40 part 2)

Cytomegalovirus
Rubella virus
Hepatitis A
Hepatitis B
Hepatitis C
Non-A–C hepatitis
Herpes simplex virus 1 and 2
Coxsackie A9, B
Echovirus 9, 11, 14, 19
Adenovirus
Reovirus type 3
Epstein–Barr virus
Varicella-zoster virus
Psittacosis
Bacterial infections
Listeria
Treponema pallidum
Toxoplasma gondii
Malaria
Tuberculosis
HIV

HIV, human immunodeficiency virus.

Table 29.12 Inherited metabolic disorders associated with hepatitis syndrome in infancy (see Ch. 35 part 3)

Galactosaemia
Fructosaemia
Tyrosinaemia
α_1-antitrypsin deficiency
Progressive familial intrahepatic cholestasis
Mytochondrial cytopathies
Cystic fibrosis
Niemann–Pick type C
Gaucher disease
Wolman disease
Zellweger syndrome
Infantile polycystic disease
Haemophagocytic lymphohistiocytosis
Neonatal iron storage disease (perinatal haemochromatosis)
Carbohydrate glycoprotein deficiency
Defects in synthesis of primary bile acids

Table 29.13 Endocrine disorders associated with hepatitis syndrome in infancy (see Ch. 35 part 2)

Hypopituitarism
Diabetes insipidus
Hypoadrenalism
Hypothyroidism
Hypoparathyroidism

fibrosis and Niemann–Pick disease type C should also to be sought in all infants because these are relatively common genetic conditions, presently lacking effective treatment but for which antenatal diagnosis is possible. α_1ATD must be excluded in all cases by determining the α_1AT phenotype, rather than by means of the serum α_1AT concentration, which can be within the normal range in the presence of hepatitis or infection, as α_1AT is an acute-phase reactant (Sifers et al. 1992). This is perhaps the most important investigation in distinguishing severe hepatitis with complete cholestasis from biliary atresia, as the liver disease associated with homozygous PiZ phenotype α_1ATD (see later) has many clinical and pathological similarities to biliary atresia (Psacharopoulos et al. 1983; Dick and Mowat 1985; Hadzic et al. 2005). Investigation for rarer metabolic diseases should be performed only if suggested by the family history or findings on percutaneous liver biopsy. The frequency with which infective, genetic, pharmacological and toxic causes of hyperbilirubinaemia or structural biliary abnormalities can be identified depends not only on their prevalence in the local community, but also on referral patterns and the sophistication of investigation facilities (Vara and Dhawan 2007).

Figure 29.14 summarises the aetiology of liver disease in infants referred to our tertiary referral centre for management of liver disease during an observation period of 13 years (Vara and Dhawan 2007). Despite improvement of diagnostic tests and discovery of new pathological conditions, such as progressive familial intrahepatic cholestasis syndromes or mitochondrial cytopathies (Thompson and Jansen 2000; Gillis and Kaye 2002), 40% remain undiagnosed.

Identifying bile duct obstruction

Observation of stool colour is vital. Because of photosensitivity of bile pigments in the stool, all stools passed should be saved in the dark (e.g. in a black bag or in a container) and examined for yellow or green pigment; if absent, cholestasis is complete and biliary atresia must be excluded (Fig. 29.15). Referral to a specialist centre is essential (McClement et al. 1985; Mieli-Vergani et al. 1989; McKiernan et al. 2000). A skilfully interpreted percutaneous liver biopsy performed under local anaesthesia using the Menghini technique is diagnostic in up to 90% of cases. If all portal tracts show increased oedema, fibrosis and bile duct reduplication, this strongly suggests major bile duct disease, of which the most common is biliary atresia. This appearance can also be found in genetic disorders such as PiZ α_1ATD (Schwarzenberg and Sharp 1990; Hadzic et al. 2005), cystic fibrosis, Alagille syndrome (Deprettere et al. 1987), total parenteral nutrition induced-liver injury (Pereira et al. 1981; Quigley et al. 1993) and endocrine disorders associated with septo-optic dysplasia. It also occurs in some infants who will ultimately develop bile duct hypoplasia and in disorders of the intrahepatic bile ducts (Deprettere et al. 1987). All of these disorders can cause complete cholestasis. It is essential that some of the material obtained is snap-frozen in liquid nitrogen or at −80°C for

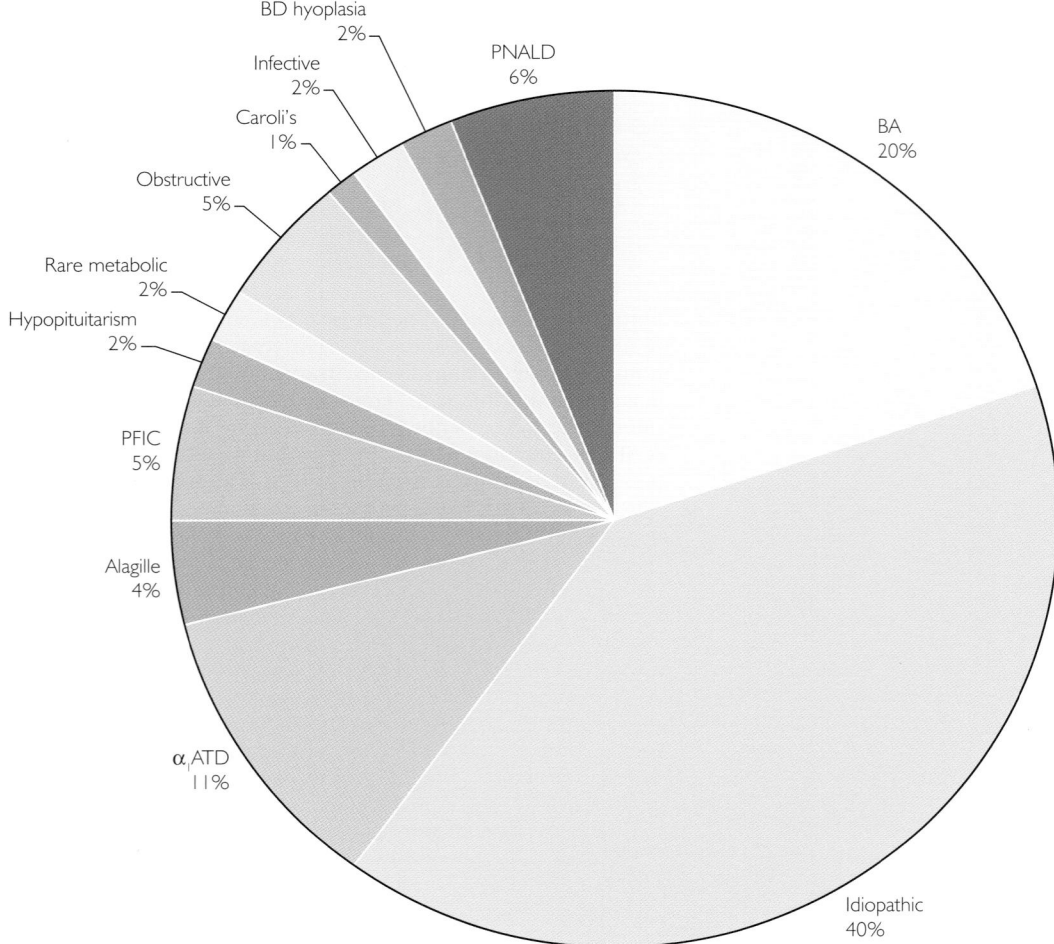

Fig. 29.14 Final diagnosis in infants with liver disease referred to King's College Hospital Paediatric Liver Centre, London, UK, over a period of 13 years (total number of patients 1625). BA, biliary atresia; α_1ATD, α_1-antitrypsin deficiency; PFIC, progressive familial intrahepatic cholestasis; BD, bile duct; PNALD, parenteral nutrition-associated liver disease.

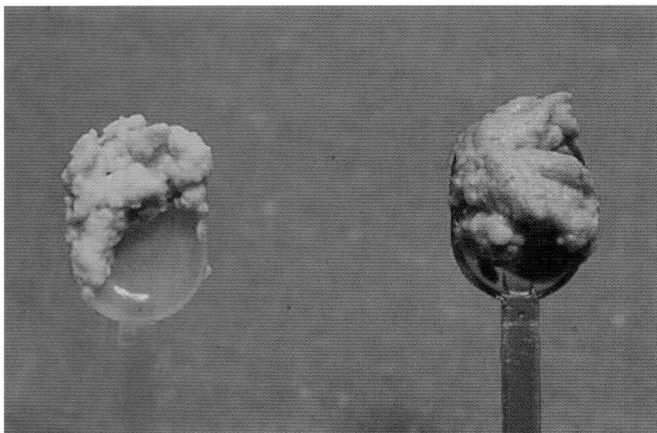

Fig. 29.15 Appearances of normal (right) and acholic baby stool (left) suggestive of biliary obstruction.

subsequent enzymatic analysis for inherited disorders (Table 29.12) if indicated by the liver histology or other investigations.

A scan with ^{99m}Tc-tagged iminodiacetic acid derivatives, such as methyl-brom-IDA, which have good hepatic uptake and relatively poor renal uptake, can be used in prolonged neonatal cholestasis. Discrimination from intrahepatic cholestasis is enhanced if the infant is pretreated with phenobarbital (5 mg/kg/day for at least 3 days). Repeated imaging up to 24 hours after intravenous injection may be required. Equally effective discrimination may be achieved by computer analysis of distribution between the liver and heart within 10 minutes of intravenous injection (El Tumi et al. 1987). Radionucleotide studies, however, are only useful if isotope is demonstrated in the gut, thereby excluding biliary atresia and avoiding an unnecessary and potentially dangerous laparotomy. Absence of excretion in the gut does not equate with biliary atresia. Daily observation of the stool colour and trends in serum bilirubin levels are essential even if patency of the bile ducts is demonstrated. If the stools remain acholic, the liver biopsy should be repeated, and further investigations may be necessary to identify the rare instances of late-onset biliary atresia.

The real difficulty arises if there is no excretion, the biopsy is not indicative of atresia and no genetic or endocrine disorder causing complete cholestasis has been identified. At specialised centres,

STAFF LIBRARY

endoscopic retrograde cholangiopancreatography (ERCP) is an important diagnostic tool in such ambiguous cases (Wilkinson et al. 1991; Shanmugam et al. 2009). In expert hands ERCP is a safe and feasible procedure, even in small babies (Shanmugam et al. 2009). A study has shown that it has a positive predictive value of 87% and negative predictive value of 100% regarding a diagnosis of biliary atresia (Shanmugam et al. 2009). Unless filling of the intrahepatic ducts can be demonstrated by ERCP, such patients should have a laparotomy. It is essential that this is undertaken by an experienced surgeon who can correctly assess the macroscopical changes in the porta hepatis and, being confident of the diagnosis, proceed to portoenterostomy (McClement et al. 1985; Davenport et al. 2008). Final confirmation of the diagnosis comes from histological examination of the excised biliary remnants, by which time an irreversible operation has been performed. Even with intraoperative cholangiography, extrahepatic ducts which are hypoplastic as a result of severe intrahepatic cholestasis may be considered atretic, leading to an unnecessary destructive operation (Davenport et al. 1997).

Surgically correctable disorders

Biliary atresia

Biliary atresia is the most frequent surgically correctable liver condition in infancy, affecting 1 : 17 000 liveborns (Livesey et al. 2009). It is unique to early infancy and is characterised by complete obstruction of the bile flow secondary to obliteration or destruction of part or all of the extrahepatic biliary tree. Study of bile duct remnants removed at surgery, and from liver specimens, indicates that biliary atresia arises from a sclerosing inflammatory process affecting previously formed bile ducts (Fig. 29.16) (Gautier and Elliot 1981). Recently, comparative anatomical studies have suggested that, in at least some cases, biliary atresia may be caused by failure of the intrauterine remodelling process at the hepatic hilum, with persistence of fetal bile ducts poorly supported by mesenchyme. As bile flow increases perinatally, bile leakage from these abnormal ducts may trigger an intense inflammatory reaction, with consequent obliteration of the biliary tree (Tan et al. 1994). The extrahepatic ducts are primarily damaged, whereas the intrahepatic bile ducts remain patent in early infancy but then also become affected and obliterated and eventually disappear. Cirrhosis with complications such as portal hypertension may appear at any time

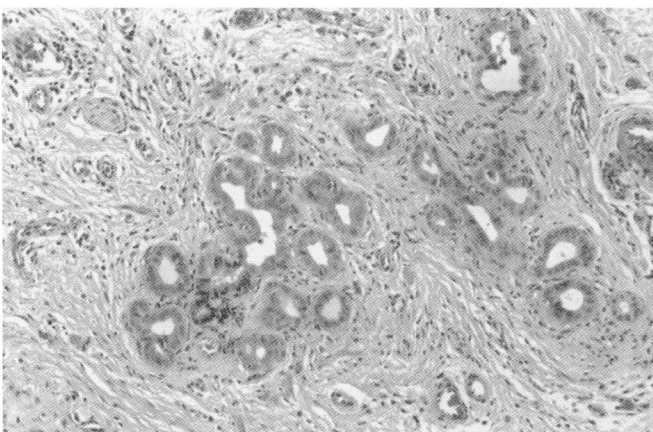

Fig. 29.16 Liver histology demonstrating expansion of the portal tract, bile duct proliferation and cholestasis, suggestive of extrahepatic biliary atresia (haematoxylin and eosin).

from 2 months of age, and death by 2 years of age is usual if the disease is not treated (Francavilla and Mieli-Vergani 2002).

The cause of biliary atresia is unknown. Familial cases are extremely rare and, of 17 cases occurring in twins, in only two instances were both affected (Silveira et al. 1991). At our centre we have seen several twin pregnancies and one triplet pregnancy where only one baby was affected. Human leukocyte antigen (HLA) phenotype appears not to play a role (Donaldson et al. 2002). Up to 25% of infants have minor or major abnormalities outside the biliary system, with a particularly high frequency of abnormalities of the vasculature below the diaphragm. Children with splenic malformations, including polysplenia and asplenia, with or without laterality defects (complete or partial situs inversus) may represent a separate aetiological subgroup – biliary atresia splenic malformation (BASM) syndrome (Davenport et al. 2006). It has also been suggested that the precarious blood supply to the biliary tree may be further jeopardised by such abnormalities. An increased incidence of maternal diabetes mellitus has been associated with the BASM syndrome (Davenport et al. 2006). Another suggested aetiological factor is a long common channel for the pancreatic and biliary ducts as they enter the duodenum, with the suggestion that pancreatic juice may reflux into the biliary system and initiate mucosal damage and subsequent inflammatory response. There have been many suggestions that perinatal infection may initiate biliary atresia, but none of the candidate viruses, e.g. reovirus type 3 (Tyler et al. 1998), has been found to infect atresia patients any more frequently than healthy babies (Brown et al. 1988; Morecki and Glaser 1989; Rauschenfels et al. 2009). Other viruses suggested to be implicated in the aetiology of biliary atresia include CMV (Fishler et al. 1998) and rotavirus (Riepenhoff-Talty et al. 1996; Rauschenfels et al. 2009). The rhesus rotavirus-infected neonatal Balb/c mouse is a widely used experimental model of biliary atresia (Barnes et al. 2009) and it will be interesting to see whether recently introduced routine rotavirus immunisation in some developed countries will affect the incidence of biliary atresia in humans.

A specific problem in the diagnosis of biliary atresia is that, as mentioned above, in most cases it results from an obliterative disorder starting in formed extrahepatic ducts which eventually leads to their destruction (Gautier and Elliot 1981). The extrahepatic and intrahepatic bile ducts may be patent in the first weeks of life, but become atretic later. Thus, in up to 30% of infants with atresia, stools are pigmented in the first weeks after birth, before bile flow is completely obstructed. All too frequently the infant's apparent well-being causes paediatricians and other health workers to dismiss consideration of this disorder in early infancy, when the chances of successful surgery are high (Mieli-Vergani et al. 1989). The longer biliary atresia has been present, the greater the likelihood that the intrahepatic bile ducts will have been obliterated and that portoenterostomy will be less likely to be successful. This is particularly true in BASM syndrome (Davenport et al. 2008). As discussed, it is essential to refer infants with acholic stools to units with experience in the interpretation of the diagnostic investigations outlined above, and in the surgical and postoperative management of biliary atresia (Table 29.14) (McKiernan et al. 2000).

At laparotomy, the surgeon must first confirm that the bile ducts are absent or atretic. This is not a simple task, and narrow but patent bile ducts in infants with intrahepatic disease and complete cholestasis have been removed by experienced surgeons (Markowitz et al. 1983). In 5–10% of babies, the surgeon can identify a patent common bile duct containing bile and in continuity with intrahepatic bile ducts (McClement et al. 1985). In these babies, a biliary–intestinal anastomosis via a long Roux-en-Y loop may allow bile to

Table 29.14 Requirements to improve the management of biliary atresia

All babies jaundiced after 14 days of age should have urine
analysis and total and direct serum bilirubin determination
If conjugated bilirubin >25 micromol/L is present, the baby should
be referred to a paediatrician for urgent investigation
If the stools have no yellow or green pigment, the baby should be
referred to a specialist centre to exclude or treat biliary atresia
'Well baby' clinics should be at 4 rather than 6 weeks of age to
identify jaundice sufficiently early to increase the chances of
successful treatment

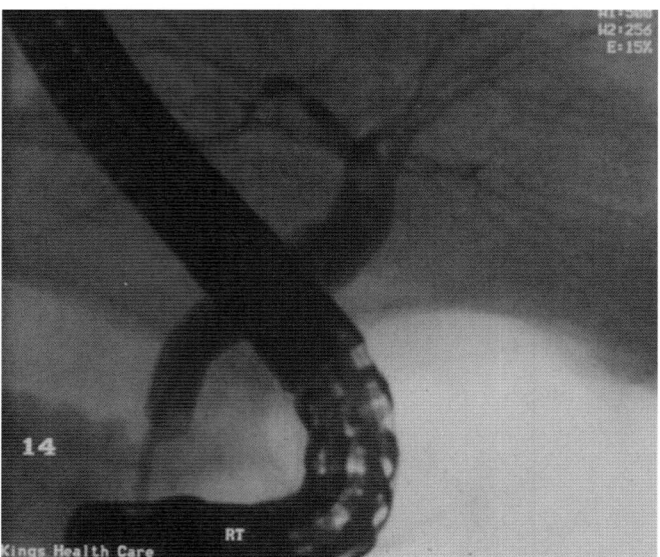

Fig. 29.17 Endoscopic retrograde cholangiopancreatography demonstrating a non-obstructive saccular dilatation of extrahepatic bile duct, strongly suggestive of a choledochal cyst.

drain satisfactorily. In the majority of patients, however, the proximal common hepatic duct is completely obliterated or absent up to where it enters the liver, and at the porta hepatis it is replaced by fibrous tissue. This tissue is transected flush with the liver and a Roux-en-Y loop of jejunum is anastomosed around the fibrous edges of the transected tissue, forming a portoenterostomy (Kasai procedure). For surgery to be effective, the intrahepatic bile ducts must be patent to the porta hepatis (McClement et al. 1985). Modifications of the Kasai procedure undertaken to reduce the risks of cholangitis fail to do so and increase the risks of liver transplantation if this becomes subsequently necessary.

In our centre, babies are started on phenobarbital preoperatively at a dose of 5–7 mg/kg/day to promote bile flow, and a dose of 45 mg/day is used postoperatively as maintenance in our unit (Davenport et al. 1997). If the jaundice reappears, the dose could be increased to 60–90 mg/day. Other centres use ursodeoxycholic acid (UDCA: 20–30 mg/kg/day) in an attempt to improve bile flow (Willot et al. 2008). With a skilful surgeon, good bile flow with normal serum bilirubin values can be achieved in more than 80% of children operated on by 60 days of age, but in only 20–70% with later surgery (Mieli-Vergani et al. 1989; Ohi et al. 1990; Davenport et al. 1997). If bilirubin returns to normal, a 90% 15-year survival has been reported (Ohi et al. 1990), with a good quality of life into the fourth decade (Chiba et al. 1992). Up to 11% of children are free of clinical and biochemical signs of liver disease after 10-year follow-up (Hadzic et al. 2003). If the bilirubin is not reduced, the rate of progression of cirrhosis is not slowed and survival beyond the second birthday is unusual without further intervention. If bile drainage is partially effective, end-stage chronic liver disease may be delayed to 6 or 7 years of age.

An important postoperative complication is cholangitis. Portal hypertension is present in almost all cases at the time of initial surgery. Approximately 50% of all survivors aged 5 years, even those with normal bilirubin levels, have oesophageal varices, but only 10–15% have gastrointestinal bleeding. For these, variceal banding or injection sclerotherapy is the treatment of choice. In approximately 10% of cases in which the serum bilirubin returns to normal, intrahepatic cholangiopathy progresses and complications of biliary cirrhosis ultimately develop (Nietgen et al. 1992). For these patients, and those for whom surgery has not been effective, liver transplantation should be considered (Nagral et al. 1997). With 1-year survival rates approaching 90% (Nietgen et al. 1992), and 5-year survival rates over 80% (Ozawa et al. 1992), liver transplantation is now a standard therapeutic option, but it remains a formidable procedure. The recipient is likely to have one or more life-threatening complications in the perioperative or postoperative period. Lifelong immunosuppressive therapy is required, with a high risk of opportunistic and community-acquired infections, requiring close medical and surgical supervision. Most of the survivors have a good quality of life and attend school, although the long-term medical

and psychological effects of liver transplantation in childhood are as yet unknown. The supply of donors of suitable size and blood group, even with an increased use of split grafts, where one donor liver is used for two recipients – usually one child and one adult – remains a major limiting factor in liver transplantation. Segmental graft transplant from living relatives has given survival rates of 90% in infants in whom Kasai portoenterostomy had been unsuccessful (Ozawa et al. 1992). The precise indications and timing, and the optimal management of some of the intraoperative and postoperative problems, including the control of rejection, remain the subject of ongoing assessment and research. Although an important mode of management for end-stage liver disease, the role of liver transplantation in biliary atresia is complementary to that of portoenterostomy (Davenport et al. 1997), except for infants in whom decompensated cirrhosis has developed because of delayed diagnosis.

Choledochal cysts

Choledochal cysts are dilatations of the biliary ducts which can be associated with intermittent biliary obstruction. If uncorrected, they lead to progressive biliary fibrosis and ultimately cirrhosis. In the newborn period, the presentation is indistinguishable from neonatal hepatitis or biliary atresia. They are increasingly diagnosed prenatally on routine ultrasound (Stringer et al. 1995; Redkar et al. 1998). Children in whom a prenatal diagnosis of choledochal cyst is made should be referred promptly to a specialised paediatric hepatology centre, since this could also be the mode of presentation of biliary atresia (Redkar et al. 1998). Cholangitis, rupture, pancreatitis and gallstones are important complications of choledochal cyst which can occur even in early infancy, while chronic cholangitis and carcinoma of the cyst wall may be long-term complications.

A cystic echo-free mass demonstrated in the biliary tree by ultrasound is strong evidence for this diagnosis. The intrahepatic bile ducts may be dilated owing to the distal stasis. The cyst can be diagnosed by magnetic resonance cholangiopancreatography, but often ERCP or percutaneous transhepatic cholangiography is needed (Fig. 29.17). The definitive treatment is surgical removal with biliary drainage via a Roux-en-Y loop (Howard 1989). With adequate surgery, the long-term prognosis is good (Stringer et al. 1995).

Spontaneous perforation of the bile duct

Spontaneous perforation of the bile duct at the junction of the cystic duct and common hepatic duct occurs when, for some unexplained reason, the common bile duct becomes blocked, usually at its distal end. Affected infants have mild jaundice, failure to gain weight and abdominal distension due to ascites, which classically causes the development of bile-stained hernias. The stools are white or cream in colour and the urine is dark. Paracentesis confirms the presence of bile-stained ascites (Howard et al. 1976).

If operative cholangiography shows free drainage of contrast into the duodenum, the ruptured duct may be sutured, but more commonly it is necessary to establish cholecystojejunostomy drainage via a Roux-en-Y loop. With effective surgery, the prognosis is excellent (Howard et al. 1976). Delay in instituting surgery may lead to severe malnutrition, peritonitis and septicaemia.

Miscellaneous conditions

The remaining surgical conditions listed in Table 29.10 are rare, and are usually dealt with either by flushing out the obstruction with a percutaneous or operative cholangiogram or by a biliary reconstruction.

Paucity of interlobular bile ducts (intrahepatic biliary hypoplasia)

This is a pathological diagnosis in which there is a decrease in the number of interlobular bile ducts seen in the portal tracts. It can be found in many conditions causing hepatitis in infancy. If it occurs with cardiovascular, skeletal and ocular anomalies, it is called Alagille syndrome (syndromic paucity of the intrahepatic bile ducts; arteriohepatic dysplasia) (Alagille et al. 1987) and is inherited in an autosomal dominant fashion with variable expression. The estimated incidence is 1 : 100 000 live births. It is caused by mutations in the human *Jagged-1* gene on chromosome 20p12 (Rand 1998). However, mutations in this gene can also be present in asymptomatic individuals and in other liver conditions, including biliary atresia (Kohsaka et al. 2002). Typically, there is a long-standing cholestasis causing jaundice, pruritus, hypercholesterolaemia and xanthomas. The severity of the cholestasis varies. Mild cases may have pruritus only. The majority have jaundice from the neonatal period, which in severe cases persists, but in others clears in late childhood or early adult life. The long-term prognosis is uncertain, but some 15% may go on to develop cirrhosis and 5–10% die from liver disease (Lykavieris et al. 2001). In one series, 25% died from cardiac involvement, classically a peripheral pulmonary stenosis or infection (Alagille et al. 1987). Diagnosis is supported by the finding of the typical facies: deep-set eyes, mild hypertelorism, overhanging forehead, a straight nose which in profile is in the same plane as the forehead, a small pointed chin, posterior embryotoxon (a remnant of an embryonic membrane between iris and cornea, seen by slit lamp) and vertebral arch defects on spinal radiographs (Fig. 29.18). A high serum cholesterol and failure to thrive support the diagnosis (Deprettere et al. 1987). The treatment is that of chronic cholestasis, with particular emphasis on adequacy of vitamin D, E, K and A supplements and the control of pruritus (Deprettere et al. 1987).

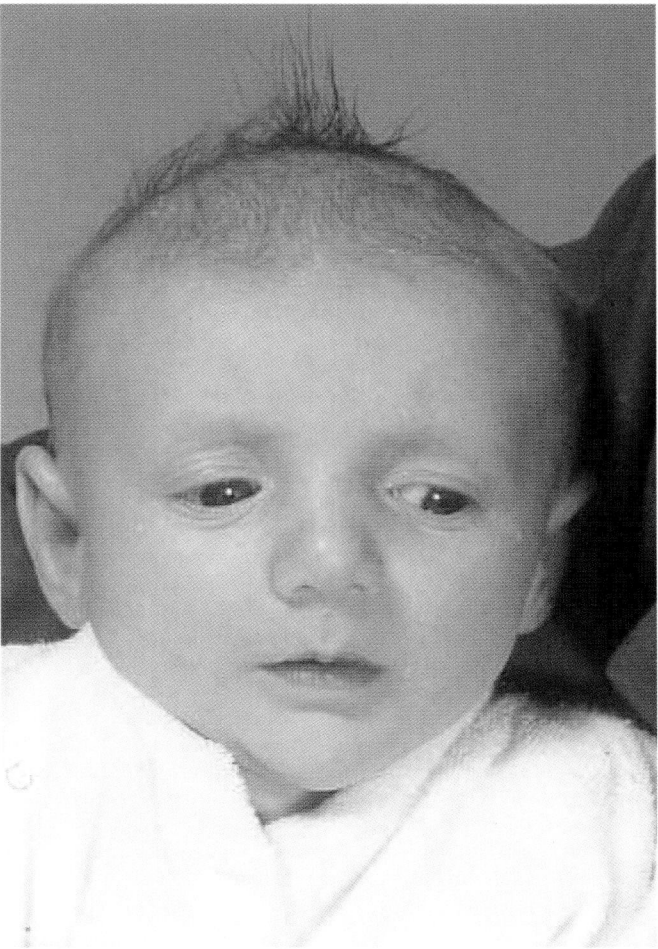

Fig. 29.18 Facial appearances of a baby with Alagille syndrome. *(Reproduced from Francavilla and Mieli-Vergani (2002).)*

Liver damage associated with parenteral nutrition

Prolonged intravenous nutrition, particularly in early infancy, causes cholestasis and hepatocellular damage, which may progress to cirrhosis if intravenous feeding continues with no enteral intake. Prevalence increases with the degree of prematurity, the duration of intravenous feeding and in the presence of associated medical and surgical conditions. Cholestatic jaundice, defined as a direct-reacting bilirubin concentration of greater than 34 μmol/l, occurred in 8.6% of 267 infants receiving intravenous nutrition (Pereira et al. 1981). The incidence was inversely proportional to the gestation, being 13.7% in babies of less than 32 weeks', 5.3% in babies of 32–36 weeks' and 1.4% in babies of greater than 36 weeks' gestation. In each gestational age group, the duration of parenteral therapy in babies with cholestasis was significantly longer than in those who remained free from this complication. The babies with cholestasis also tended to be without oral feeding for longer – 23 days as opposed to 15 days (Pereira et al. 1981). Sepsis, hypoxia, shock, blood transfusion, intra-abdominal surgery and potentially hepatotoxic drugs may aggravate the liver damage.

Pathologically, there is a distinct cholestatic hepatitis, with bilirubinostasis within the hepatocytes, the bile canaliculi and Kupffer cells. These cells also contain marked accumulation of periodic acid–Schiff-positive pigment. The hepatocytes are oedematous and may have increased numbers of nuclei. There is a lobular disarray with distension of portal tracts by inflammatory cell infiltrate, bile duct proliferation and fibrosis. A fine panlobular sinusoidal or pericellular fibrosis may be noted in up to 50% of cases. Severe fibrosis and cirrhosis may develop if total intravenous feeding cannot be stopped. Acute acalculous cholecystitis, biliary sludge and cholelithiasis are frequent complications. Follow-up biopsies 5–9 months after the height of the illness still show mild hepatocellular cholestasis, lobular disarray with ballooning of hepatocytes and increased fibrosis.

The first clinical indication of hepatic involvement is usually the appearance of conjugated hyperbilirubinaemia. Hepatomegaly may be noted. Biochemical tests of liver function are abnormal. It is important to consider other causes of cholestasis in this age group before concluding that the disorder is due to intravenous nutrition. If total parenteral nutrition (TPN) can be withdrawn, the jaundice settles within 4–6 weeks, although liver function tests may remain abnormal for several months and the liver biopsy changes can persist even longer. Tests of liver function should be carried out at least weekly during intravenous feeding.

The prognosis of TPN-associated jaundice is more serious in children with anatomical anomalies or functional intestinal failure (necrotising enterocolitis, gastroschisis, microcolon), who are TPN-dependent and prone to intermittent septic episodes for longer. They may progress to end-stage chronic liver disease, requiring isolated liver transplantation or combined liver and small bowel transplantation (Muiesan et al. 2000).

Treatment of the liver dysfunction associated with parenteral nutrition aims at improving bile flow with the use of UDCA (20–25 mg/kg/day) or phenobarbital (5 mg/kg/day). The most effective treatment, however, is early reintroduction of total or partial enteral nutrition, if tolerated.

Recently, fish oil-based intravenous lipid emulsion has been shown to reduce the risk of parenteral nutrition-associated liver disease in babies with short bowel syndrome (Puder et al. 2009).

Liver disease associated with α_1-antitrypsin deficiency

α_1AT is a glycoprotein synthesised largely in the liver. In vitro and probably in vivo it acts as an inhibitor of inflammatory response. Over 90 different alleles, controlled by a single gene, located on chromosome 14q32.1, have been isolated and identified as protease inhibitors (Pi). The alleles of α_1AT are inherited in an autosomal co-dominant fashion, the most common phenotype being homozygous PiM. α_1ATD is among the most common single-gene defects, occurring in about 1 : 2000–1 : 7000 newborns of European origin (Lomas et al. 1992; Sifers et al. 1992). Liver disease in children is associated with the homozygous PiZ variant, while PiSZ and homozygous PiS phenotypes do not cause liver injury in childhood (Schwarzenberg and Sharp 1990; Hadzic et al. 2005). The plasma deficiency of the glycoprotein is associated with a defect in secretion from the endoplasmic reticulum rather than a defect in the synthesis of the Z polypeptide (Sifers et al. 1992).

The clinical features associated with the deficiency state are very variable, with some having no overt disease, up to 20% developing liver disease of variable severity and up to 60% developing emphysema (Sveger and Eriksson 1995; Francavilla et al. 2000). Cigarette smoking is closely associated with the development of emphysema, but the cause of the liver disease is still not fully elucidated (Schwarzenberg and Sharp 1990; Lomas et al. 1992).

The putative pathogenic mechanism for the liver disease in homozygous PiZ α_1AT is abnormal 'loop sheet' polymerisation of the mutant α_1AT protein, leading to abnormal folding and inefficient export from the rough endoplasmic reticulum of the hepatocytes (Lomas et al. 1992; Sifers et al. 1992). It is likely that genetic and environmental modifiers play a role in the development of liver disease and its severity. Within a family with a PiZ child with liver disease, there is a 70% occurrence of liver disease among homozygous PiZ siblings, but the severity of liver disease is highly variable (Hinds et al. 2006). Suggested additional pathogenic factors include possession of HLA DR3, absence of breastfeeding and male sex, defects in chemotaxis, liver-specific autoimmune reactions, complement activation and the increase in the synthesis of acute-phase reactants during febrile episodes in infection (Lomas et al. 1992). The mechanisms of liver and lung disease in homozygous PiZ α_1ATD are completely different ('gain of function' as opposed to 'loss of function') (Lomas et al. 1992) and it has been reported that specific single nucleotide polymorphisms in the gene controlling α_1AT synthesis are likely to be associated with liver injury (Chappell et al. 2008).

Although over 50% of infants with the deficiency state have abnormal biochemical tests of liver function, and these remain abnormal in over 30% throughout the first 12 years of life, only 10–15% develop symptomatic liver disease (Sveger and Eriksson 1995). In 90% of deficient children the liver involvement takes the form of a conjugated hyperbilirubinaemia with hepatosplenomegaly and disturbed biochemical tests of liver function presenting in the first 4 months of life (Psacharopoulos et al. 1983; Francavilla et al. 2000). In 10% of these infants a serious bleeding diathesis due to vitamin K malabsorption is an important component of their illness, potentially leading to intracranial bleeding and permanent neurological abnormality; 1–2% present in later childhood or adult life with cirrhosis with no history of prior jaundice in infancy (Psacharopoulos et al. 1983). Emphysema usually has its onset in early adult life.

The identification of liver disease associated with α_1ATD in the individual baby is important for diagnostic, genetic and prognostic reasons. Such babies could be considered on clinical, biochemical and histological evidence to have extrahepatic biliary atresia and be subjected to the risks of unnecessary laparotomy. Infants with liver disease associated with α_1ATD have a significantly worse prognosis than those with hepatitis of unknown cause. In an epidemiological study in south-east England, seven cases of hepatitis in infants were associated with α_1ATD (Dick and Mowat 1985). By 3 years of age, four had died of cirrhosis, and cirrhosis was present in one of two reviewed at 10 years of age. In contrast, only two of 28 with idiopathic hepatitis in this study died, and none had cirrhosis at 10 years (Dick and Mowat 1985). Our experience with 82 children with the PiZ phenotype and liver disease was that approximately 25% died of cirrhosis by adolescence, a further 25% had histologically proven cirrhosis, 25% had persisting liver disease with possible cirrhosis and 25% apparently recovered from liver disease showing no clinical or biochemical abnormality (Psacharopoulos et al. 1983).

The prognosis of liver disease associated with homozygous PiZ α_1ATD is correlated with the presence of fibrosis and the severity and duration of the acute hepatitis in early infancy (Francavilla et al. 2000). In the individual baby, the liver biopsy is the most helpful guide to prognosis. In those who die or have persistent hepatic abnormality, there is a marked increase in portal tract oedema and fibrosis in the first 6 months of life (Francavilla et al. 2000). Unfortunately, there is no specific treatment for this form of liver disease, apart from liver transplantation.

Patients with α_1ATD may have renal involvement with a variety of glomerulonephropathies (Strife et al. 1983). Renal involvement may cause haematuria and/or proteinuria and contribute to hypoalbuminaemia. Subclinical renal complications may manifest as arterial hypertension after liver transplantation.

Reliable methods of genotyping from chorionic villus sampling at 8–10 weeks of gestation are available. Genetic counselling is difficult because of the varying severity of the clinical associations and difficulties in predicting the prognosis (Hinds et al. 2006). Affected families should be carefully counselled and offered the option of sibling testing and prenatal diagnosis for future pregnancies.

Cryptogenic (idiopathic) hepatitis in infancy

Despite an increasing number of specific disorders associated with hepatitis syndrome in infancy, in a high proportion of children the cause still remains unidentified (Fig. 29.14). These children are often born after an abnormal pregnancy and sometimes have a low birthweight. Frequently, they come to medical attention for complications of prematurity or intrauterine growth retardation, and subsequently develop evidence of liver disease. Although the liver disease may be severe, the mortality in such cases is usually less than 15% and long-term hepatic problems occur in less than 10%. The histological features are often non-specific, with portal and lobular inflammation, giant-cell transformation of hepatocytes and variable degree of cholestasis. The indicators of poor prognosis are severe cholestasis with proliferation and/or damage of the intralobular bile ducts and presence of fibrosis, cholangiography showing sclerosing cholangitis (Amedee-Manesme et al. 1987), family history of liver disease in childhood, or consanguinity (Deutsch et al. 1985; Baker et al. 1993), and normal serum GGT in the presence of abnormality of other liver function tests indicating persistent liver disease (Maggiore et al. 1987). This last finding suggests either a primary abnormality of bile acid formation, which must be promptly excluded, as treatment with oral primary bile salts reverses liver damage (Clayton et al. 1995; Subramaniam et al. 2010), or a progressive familial intrahepatic cholestatic (PFIC) syndrome (Thompson and Jansen 2000) due to FIC1 disease (see below; Carlton et al. 1995), or bile salt export pump (BSEP) deficiency (see below), which typically present as non-specific neonatal hepatitis with normal or low GGT (Strautnieks et al. 1997). In this context it is important to remember that the normal values for serum GGT in premature infants, neonates and infants younger than 6 months are severalfold higher than in older children and adults (Cabrera-Abreu and Green 2002).

Progressive familial intrahepatic cholestasis syndromes

Over the last decade, different types of PFIC syndromes, associated with a low or a high GGT phenotype, have been characterised (Thompson and Jansen 2000). These autosomal recessive conditions can present in infancy with prolonged conjugated jaundice (Odievre et al. 1981). GGT in the liver is normally bound to the canalicular membrane and to the cholangiocyte biliary epithelium. Under cholestatic conditions, the detergent effect of the bile acids liberates GGT from the membrane. When this is combined with a poor bile flow, GGT leaks back into the circulation, where elevated levels can be detected. In the absence of bile acids in the bile, even when there is poor bile flow, GGT is not released and the serum levels remain normal. Therefore, in the presence of cholestasis, a normal serum level of GGT correlates very well with low levels of biliary bile acids. These patients usually have low biliary but high serum levels of bile acids, in the absence of a defect in bile acid synthesis.

The original patients described with this phenotype were amongst the Old Order Amish in Pennsylvania, USA (Clayton et al. 1969). One of the original families was called Byler, and this condition has become widely known as Byler disease. Byler disease, or FIC1, represents approximately one-third of the patients with low-GGT

PFIC and maps to chromosome 18 (Carlton et al. 1995). These patients may present with neonatal hepatitis of variable severity. The FIC1 gene is widely expressed, with only relatively low-level expression in the liver. Thus, some patients with FIC1 disease have extrahepatic manifestations. Expression of FIC1 is particularly high in the small intestine and pancreas. FIC1 patients may have pancreatitis and many have significant malabsorption, which is not improved by liver transplantation. A proportion of them will have abnormal sweat test, renal tubular dysfunction and conductive deafness.

A further third of patients with low-GGT PFIC have an isolated defect in bile acid transport due to deficiency of the BSEP. The condition maps to chromosome 2 and is due to mutations of the ABCB11 gene (Strautnieks et al. 1997). These patients mostly present in the first few months of life with a mild neonatal hepatitis. Histologically, the features cannot be discriminated from 'idiopathic' giant-cell hepatitis, which typically has a good prognosis. Immunohistochemically, absence of expression of BSEP and GGT staining can be demonstrated. The disease progresses and pruritus usually becomes a prominent problem towards the end of the first year. The rate of progression is variable, resulting in end-stage liver disease between 2 and 10 years of age, or possibly even later. No treatment apart from transplantation has been shown to be of benefit, and it is particularly noteworthy that these patients appear to be incapable of excreting UDCA (Jansen et al. 1999). Treatment with modest doses of UDCA, however, may have a beneficial effect by further suppressing endogenous bile acid production. As expression of the gene appears to be entirely limited to the liver, liver transplantation is generally an excellent treatment for BSEP deficiency, but there have now been reports of disease recurrence mediated by alloantibody – anti BSEP – formation in patients homozygous for the deficiency after exposure to the BSEP present in the donor liver (Jara et al. 2009; Keitel et al, 2009).

The genetic basis of the remaining third of the low-GGT PFIC spectrum has not yet been clarified.

A form of high-GGT PFIC is associated with multidrug resistance protein (MDR) 3 deficiency, due to mutations of the ABCB4 gene (de Vree et al. 1998). It is believed that the MDR3 gene product plays a critical role in the flipping of phosphatidyl choline, the major lipid component of human bile, from the inner to the outer leaflet of the canalicular membrane. A defect in phosphatidylcholine excretion is likely to result in the production of highly detergent bile, which can cause considerable tissue damage. Indeed, children with MDR3 deficiency have low phospholipids in the bile and marked portal inflammation and bile duct proliferation in the liver biopsies (de Vree et al. 1998). Two recently described additional clinical manifestations of MDR3 deficiency are cholestasis of pregnancy and cholelithiasis syndrome, characterised by cholesterol gallstones and intrahepatic microlithiasis (Sundaram and Sokol 2007). Some patients, particularly those who have some residual protein function, show a clinical response to UDCA, which reduces the hydrophobicity of the bile. Preliminary data from a murine model show that transplanted hepatocytes are capable of ameliorating the phenotype, suggesting that such transport defects in humans are good candidates for hepatocyte transplantation or gene therapy.

Neonatal haemochromatosis

Neonatal haemochromatosis (NH), or neonatal iron storage disorder, is a rare and often fatal disorder which causes either death in utero or acute liver failure in the neonatal period. The pathogenesis is uncertain. It may represent a single phenotypic expression of different aetiologies (Collins and Goldfischer 1990). NH has been observed in siblings and it has been suggested to have an autosomal recessive mode of inheritance (Kelly et al. 2001). However, we (Rodrigues et al. 2005) and others (Verloes et al. 1996) have observed NH in neonates conceived by different fathers, suggesting a specific role for maternal factors, possibly mitochondrial (Verloes et al. 1996) or related to pregnancy, including autoimmune reactions or positive systemic lupus erythematosus serology occasionally observed in mothers of affected children (Knisely 1992; Rodrigues et al. 2005). Often the pregnancy is complicated by oligohydramnios and/or megaplacenta. Histologically, the condition is characterised by intense deposition of stainable iron in the liver, hepatocellular necrosis and diffuse hepatic fibrosis with nodular regeneration. Other organs are also typically iron-overloaded, including the pancreas, heart, thyroid and salivary glands, with a characteristic sparing of the reticuloendothelial system (Knisely 1992). Serum ferritin is usually elevated, but its levels do not allow differentiation of neonatal liver failure due to haemochromatosis from that due to other causes (Lee et al. 2001). The diagnosis should be confirmed by lip biopsy to demonstrate stainable iron in the salivary glands (Knisely 1992), although false-positive and false-negative results have been seen (personal observation).

Severe NH, if untreated, is usually fatal. The efficacy of antioxidant-chelating treatment is controversial. After reports of successful use of the cocktail including prostaglandin E_1, selenium, desferrioxamine, N-acetyl-cysteine and vitamin E (Shamieh et al. 1993; Roberts et al. 1999; Rodrigues et al. 2005), further reports have failed to show its beneficial effects (Sigurdsson et al. 1998). The treatment was largely ineffective in our own series of 19 severe cases (Rodrigues et al. 2005). Recently, it has been suggested that immune therapy with exchange transfusion and intravenous immunoglobulin may improve the outcome and reduce the need for liver transplantation in patients with NH (Rand et al. 2009). Liver transplantation is at the moment the only procedure able to divert the natural course of the disease. Liver transplantation therefore remains the only real therapeutic option in the presence of severe liver failure (Bonatti et al. 1997).

Prevention of NH is important. The recurrence of NH is high in subsequent pregnancies. Although placental abnormalities have been described in NH, they are not sufficiently specific for antenatal diagnosis. High-dose intravenous immunoglobulin therapy during gestation, on the assumption that the condition may be due to some immune dysregulation, though not preventing NH, dramatically reduces its severity (Whitington and Kelly 2008).

Haemophagocytic lymphohistiocytosis

A primary (familial) form of HLH is an established, but probably still underdiagnosed, cause of liver and multiorgan failure in early infancy. It is thought that an underlying defect in function of cytotoxic/natural killer (NK) lymphocytes, linked to perforin deficiency in about one-third of patients, is responsible for an uninhibited response of the immune system to infection (Kogawa et al. 2002). Perforin is pivotal for translocation of granzyme B from cytotoxic cells into invading microorganisms in order to initiate apoptosis. Primary HLH due to perforin deficiency has an autosomal recessive inheritance and mutations have been mapped to 10q22 (Stepp et al. 1999). Also, at least three additional genetic loci encoding proteins involved in activation of cytotoxic/NK lymphocytes, Munc 13-4 (*UNC13D*), syntaxin-11 (*STX11*) and Munc 18-2 (*STXBP2*), have been described (Zur Stadt et al. 2006), with possible phenotypical differences resulting in early-onset or delayed clinical presentations of HLH (Ohadi et al. 1999; Côte et al. 2009). Secondary forms of HLH are often infection-driven, but typically present at a later age and may have a better prognosis.

Clinically, the condition presents acutely with fever, hepatosplenomegaly, pancytopenia, skin rash, and renal and respiratory failure. Laboratory investigations demonstrate hypertriglyceridaemia, hypofibrinogenaemia and hyperferritinaemia. The affected babies become seriously ill over a matter of hours, often requiring assisted ventilation, inotropes and renal support. The diagnosis is confirmed by cytological demonstration of haemophagocytosis in the bone marrow, ascitic fluid or cerebrospinal fluid. Severe coagulopathy often precludes liver biopsy or lumbar puncture. Despite heroic supportive measures, the mortality in the presence of liver failure is more than 90%. Cytotoxic treatment with etoposide or lymphocyte ablation and ciclosporin A has been suggested for milder forms (Hirst et al. 1994). If remission is achieved, the condition can be corrected by stem-cell transplantation (Jabado et al. 1997). There is some early anecdotal evidence that anticytokine treatment (anti-interleukin-2 and antitumour necrosis factor antibodies) could be used as a temporising treatment in severely affected patients with HLH (Verbsky and Grossman 2006).

Mitochondrial cytopathies

An increasing number of infants with hypoglycaemia, sepsis, biochemical signs of liver failure and lactic acidosis are diagnosed with various mitochondrial disorders. These include respiratory chain complex (I–V) deficiency, mitochondrial DNA depletion syndrome (Alpers syndrome), Pearson marrow–pancreas syndrome and primary fatty acid oxidation defects. Most of them do not follow a mendelian mode of inheritance since mitochondrial DNA is inherited maternally and does not recombine. More than 90% of mitochondrial cytopathies are caused by mutations in nuclear genes, only a few of which have been identified (Gillis and Kaye 2002).

Multiorgan involvement is often present since mitochondria provide energy for intracellular processes of oxidative phosphorylation throughout the body. The clinical suspicion of a mitochondrial disorder should be raised in the presence of hypoglycaemia, feeding difficulties, multiorgan and liver failure, neurological impairment, pancreatic insufficiency and failure to thrive. These children are usually not dysmorphic. Elevated serum and cerebrospinal fluid lactate are frequently detected. Magnetic resonance imaging or computed tomography imaging of the head could reveal various anatomical and myelinisation defects (Ch. 40.6). Treatment is of limited help and includes prevention of hypoglycaemia, ubiquinone (coenzyme Q10), thiamine, riboflavine and dichloroacetate. The major management difficulty is consideration for liver transplantation of those children who present with liver failure but have not developed, as yet, signs of neurological impairment or respiratory failure. Whether or not these children should be offered transplantation in view of the possibility of later neurological or respiratory complications is still under debate (Dubern et al. 2001). Recent introduction of rapid testing for the commonest mutations in the DNA polymerase-gamma (*POLG*) gene, responsible for a considerable number of cases of acute liver failure in infancy, including those following exposure to the antiepileptic drug sodium valproate, could assist in the appropriate clinical selection of candidates likely to benefit long term from liver transplantation (Blok et al. 2009).

Management of disorders causing hepatitis syndrome in infancy

The essence of management is to define the site of the main pathological involvement and to identify any associated disorder, particularly those for which there is specific therapy. Infections must be treated with appropriate anti-infective agents. Fructose and galactose are omitted from the diet until fructosaemia and galactosaemia have been excluded by specific tests. Fat-soluble vitamin deficiencies must be prevented by oral or parenteral supplements (Francavilla and Mieli-Vergani 2002). The exact vitamin requirements depend on the degree of malabsorption and metabolic demands. It is mandatory to monitor the prothrombin time (vitamin K), serum calcium, phosphate and wrist X-rays, together with serum vitamin D, E and A concentrations, to assess adequacy of supplementation. Vitamin K deficiency is an immediate risk of bleeding and a parenteral dose of vitamin K (3–5 mg) is recommended at the time of initial referral of any baby with suspected liver disease, followed by oral supplementation (1 mg/day).

If cholestasis persists for more than 3 months, laboratory or radiological signs of vitamin D deficiency are likely to appear, with pathological evidence of vitamin E deficiency occurring after 5 months. Clinical evidence of vitamin A deficiency develops after some years, but biochemical evidence may be present earlier (Amedee-Manesme et al. 1988). Oral supplements are given in doses of three to five times normal requirements if cholestasis is incomplete. In complete cholestasis, doses of vitamin K 1 mg orally per day, vitamin D 50 000 units intramuscularly at 4-weekly intervals and vitamin A 5000 units intramuscularly at 4-weekly intervals will usually prevent laboratory evidence of deficiency. Vitamin E parenterally in a dose of 10 mg/kg at 2-weekly intervals is required to maintain the serum vitamin E level (Francavilla and Mieli-Vergani 2002). In infants with failure to thrive, dietary supplements of carbohydrate polymers and medium-chain triglycerides (if defects of fat oxidation have been excluded) are required.

Colestyramine (cholestyramine) with or without phenobarbital, UDCA or rifampicin may be required for pruritus. There is no medical treatment that influences the progression of idiopathic disorders.

Inherited disorders of bilirubin metabolism

Gilbert syndrome

A chronic, mild, variable unconjugated hyperbilirubinaemia, with serum bilirubin levels around 34–85 µmol/l (2–5 mg/dl), in the absence of significant haemolysis or abnormality of liver function, is the characteristic feature of this condition. The pathogenesis is undetermined. Impaired hepatic uptake of bilirubin, deficient uridine diphosphate glucuronyl transferase (UDPGT) activity and a mild excretory defect have been suggested (Monaghan et al. 1996). An abnormality of the promoter region of the *UDPGT1* gene, inherited in an autosomal recessive fashion, has been demonstrated

(Bosma et al. 1995). The frequency of the abnormal promoter among the normal population is 40%. Because clinically manifested Gilbert syndrome occurs in 3–10% of the population, other factors, such as an increased bilirubin production, must be present to bring this disease to expression. The diagnosis is rarely made with confidence before 10 years of age and is based on exclusion of other causes of unconjugated hyperbilirubinaemia. Treatment is unnecessary. Gilbert syndrome may aggravate physiologic hyperbilirubinaemia in the newborn (Bancroft et al. 1998).

Crigler–Najjar disease

This rare disorder is characterised by significant unconjugated hyperbilirubinaemia from birth. Crigler–Najjar disease type 1 results from a complete deficiency of UDPGT, and type 2 from a partial deficiency. In Crigler–Najjar disease type 1, serum bilirubin values are in excess of 350 µmol/l and the bile contains only traces of bilirubin conjugates. Crigler–Najjar disease type 2 is clinically less severe, with serum bilirubin values not exceeding 350 µmol/l. The bile of these patients contains bilirubin mono- and diglucuronides in low concentration. Genetically, both diseases result from mutations of the *UDPGT1* gene (Ritter et al. 1992; Aono et al. 1993). Both Crigler–Najjar type 1 and type 2 are inherited in an autosomal recessive fashion (Kadakol et al. 2000). The diagnosis is suspected on the basis of the clinical features and needs to be confirmed by mutation analysis, assessing bilirubin conjugates in the bile collected at endoscopy, or by measuring UDPGT activity in a percutaneous liver biopsy specimen. In Crigler–Najjar type 2, serum bilirubin levels decrease by at least 30% with phenobarbital treatment. Patients with Crigler–Najjar type 1 are at risk of developing neurological damage and kernicterus throughout their life, but particularly in early infancy. Most patients require exchange transfusions to control hyperbilirubinaemia in the newborn period, and thereafter require continuous phototherapy of sufficient intensity to keep the serum bilirubin below 300 µmol/l. This is most conveniently achieved by sleeping undressed for up to 12–15 hours under a specially built phototherapy device incorporating as many as 32 phototherapy tubes (Yohannan et al. 1983). Oral colestyramine may reduce the phototherapy requirement by binding bilirubin in the gut. After 4 years of age, phototherapy gradually becomes less effective and liver transplantation becomes necessary to prevent kernicterus (Pett and Mowat 1987). Auxiliary liver transplant, where the left lateral segment of the recipient is removed and substituted with the donor's left lateral segment, has proved successful in correcting the enzymatic defect. Hepatocyte transplantation is a therapeutic option which may offer non-surgical correction of the enzymatic defect, but a sustained medium- to long-term effect has not been achieved as yet (Fox et al. 1998).

Weblinks

www.alagille.org: Alagille's help group.
www.alpha1.org.uk: α_1-antitrypsin deficiency help group (mainly lung disease-driven).

www.childliverdisease.org: children's liver disease foundation.

References

Alagille, D., Estrada, A., Hadchouel, M., et al., 1987. Syndromic paucity of interlobular bile ducts (Alagille's syndrome or arteriohepatic dysplasia): review of eighty cases. J Pediatr 110, 195–200.

Amedee-Manesme, O., Bernard, O., Brunelle, F., et al., 1987. Sclerosing cholangitis with neonatal onset. J Pediatr 111, 225–229.

Amedee-Manesme, O., Mourey, M.S., Courturier, M., et al., 1988. Short- and long-term vitamin A treatment in children with cholestasis. Am J Clin Nutr 47, 690–693.

Aono, S., Yamada, Y., Keino, H., et al., 1993. Identification of defect in the genes for bilirubin UDP-glucuronosyl-transferase in a patient with Crigler–Najjar syndrome type II. Biochem Biophys Res Commun 197, 1239–1244.

Baker, A., Portmann, B., Westaby, D., et al., 1993. Neonatal sclerosing cholangitis in two siblings: a category of progressive intrahepatic cholestasis. J Pediatr Gastroenterol Nutr 17, 317–322.

Bancroft, J.D., Kreamer, B.S., & Gourley, G.R., 1998. Gilbert syndrome accelerates development of neonatal jaundice. J Pediat 132, 656–660.

Barnes, B.H., Tucker, R.M., Wehrmann, F., et al., 2009. Cholangiocytes as immune modulators in rotavirus-induced murine biliary atresia. Liver Int 29, 1253–1261.

Blok, M.J., van den Bosch, B.J., Jongen, E., et al., 2009. The unfolding clinical spectrum of POLG mutations. J Med Genet 46, 776–785.

Bonatti, H., Muiesan, P., Connelly, S., et al., 1997. Hepatic transplantation in children under 3 months of age: single centre's experience. J Pediatr Surg 32, 486–488.

Bosma, P.J., Chowdhury, J.R., Bakker, C., et al., 1995. The genetic basis of the reduced expression of bilirubin UDP-glucuronosyl-transferase 1 in Gilbert's syndrome. NEJM 333, 1171–1175.

Brown, W.R., Sokol, R.J., Levin, M.J., et al., 1988. Lack of correlation between infection with reovirus 3 and extrahepatic biliary atresia or neonatal hepatitis. J Pediatr 113, 670–676.

Cabrera-Abreu, J.C., Green, A., 2002. Gamma-glutamyl-transferase: value of its measurement in paediatrics. Ann Clin Biochem 39, 22–25.

Carlton, V.E., Knisely, A.S., Freimer, N.B., 1995. Mapping of a locus for progressive familial intrahepatic cholestasis (Byler disease) to 18q21-q22, the benign recurrent intrahepatic cholestasis region. Hum Mol Genet 4, 1049–1053.

Chappell, S., Hadzic, N., Stockley, R., et al., 2008. A polymorphism of the alpha-1 antitrypsin gene represents a risk factor for liver disease. Hepatology 47, 127–132.

Chiba, T., Ohi, R., Nio, M., et al., 1992. Late complications in long term survivors of bilary atresia. Eur J Pediatr Surg 2, 22–25.

Clayton, R.J., Iber, F.L., Reubner, B.H., et al., 1969. Fatal familialintrahepatic cholestasis in an Amish kindred. Am J Dis Child 117, 112–124.

Clayton, P.T., Leonard, J.V., Lawson, A.M., et al., 1987. Familial giant cell hepatitis associated with synthesis of 3β,7α-dihydroxy- and 3β,7α,12α-trihydroxy-5-cholenoic acids. J Clin Invest 79, 1031–1038.

Clayton, P.T., Casteels, M., Mieli-Vergani, G., et al., 1995. Familial giant cell hepatitis associated with greatly increased urinary excretion of bile alcohols: a new inborn error of bile acid synthesis? Pediatr Res 37, 424–431.

Collins, J., Goldfischer, S., 1990. Perinatal hemochromatosis: one disease, several diseases or a spectrum? Hepatology 12, 176–177.

Côte, M., Ménager, M.M., Burgess, A., et al., 2009. Munc 18-2 deficiency causes familial hemophagocytic lymphohistiocytosis type 5 and impairs cytotoxic granule exocytosis in patient NK cells. J Clin Invest 119, 3765–3773.

Davenport, M., Kerkar, N., Mieli-Vergani, G., et al., 1997. Biliary atresia: the King's College Hospital experience, 1974–1995. J Pediatr Surg 32, 479–485.

Davenport, M., Tizzard, S.A., Mieli-Vergani, G., et al., 2006. Biliary atresia splenic malformation syndrome: a 28 year single center experience. J Pediatr 149, 393–400.

Davenport, M., Caponcelli, E., Livesey, E., et al., 2008. Surgical outcome in biliary atresia: etiology affects the influence of age at surgery. Ann Surg 247, 694–698.

Deprettere, A., Portmann, B., Mowat, A.P., 1987. Syndromic paucity of the intrahepatic bile ducts: diagnostic difficulty; severe morbidity throughout childhood. J Pediatr Gastroenterol Nutr 6, 865–871.

Deutsch, J., Smith, A.L., Danks, D., et al., 1985. Long-term prognosis for babies with neonatal liver disease. Archives of Diseases in Childhood 60, 447–451.

de Vree, J.M., Jacquemin, E., Sturm, E., et al., 1998. Mutations in the MDR3 gene cause progressive familial intrahepatic cholestasis. Proceedings of National Academy of Sciences of the United States of America 95, 282–287.

Dick, M.C., Mowat, A.P., 1985. Hepatitis syndrome in infancy – an epidemiological study with 10-year follow-up. Arch Dis Child 60, 512–515.

Donaldson, P.T., Clare, M., Constantini, P.K., et al., 2002. HLA and cytokine gene polymorphisms in biliary atresia. Liver 22, 213–219.

Dubern, B., Broue, P., Dubuisson, C., et al., 2001. Orthotopic liver transplantation for mitochondrial respiratory chain disorders: a study of 5 children. Transplantation 71, 633–637.

El Tumi, M.A., Clark, M.D., Barrett, J.J., et al., 1987. A ten minute radiopharmaceutical test in suspected biliary atresia. Arch Dis Child 62, 180–184.

Fishler, B., Ehrnst, A., Forsgren, M., et al., 1998. The viral association of neonatal cholestasis in Sweden: a possible link between cytomegalovirus infection and biliary atresia. J Pediatr Gastroenterol Nutr 27, 57–64.

Fox, I.J., Chowdhury, J.R., Kaufman, S.S., et al., 1998. Treatment of the Crigler–Najjar syndrome type I with hepatocyte transplantation. NEJM 338, 1463–1465.

Francavilla, R., Mieli-Vergani, G., 2002. Liver and biliary disease in infancy. Medicine 30, 45–47.

Francavilla, R., Castellaneta, S.P., Hadzic, N., et al., 2000. Prognosis of alpha-1-antitrypsin deficiency-related liver disease in the era of paediatric liver transplantation. J Hepatol 32, 986–992.

Gautier, M., Elliot, N., 1981. Extrahepatic biliary atresia: morphological study of 94 biliary remnants. Arch Pathol Lab Med 105, 397–402.

Gillis, L., Kaye, E., 2002. Diagnosis and management of mitochondrial diseases. Pediatr Clin North Am 49, 203–219.

Hadzic, N., Davenport, M., Tizzard, S., et al., 2003. Long-term survival following Kasai portoenterostomy: is chronic liver disease inevitable? J Pediatr Gastroenterol Nutr 37, 430–433.

Hadzic, N., Francavilla, R., Chambers, S.M., et al., 2005. Outcome of PiSS and PiSZ alpha-1-antitrypsin deficiency presenting with liver involvement. Eur J Pediatr 164, 250–252.

Henriksen, N.T., Drablos, P.A., Aagenaes, O., 1981. Cholestatic jaundice in infancy. The importance of familial and genetic factors in the aetiology and prognosis. Arch Dis Child 56, 622–627.

Hinds, R., Hadchouel, A., Shanmungham, N.P., et al., 2006. Variable degree of liver involvement in siblings with PiZZ alpha-1-antitrypsin deficiency-related liver disease. J Pediatr Gastroenterol Nutr 43, 136–138.

Hirst, W.J., Layton, D.M., Singh, S., et al., 1994. Haemophagocytic lymphohistiocytosis – experience at two UK centres. Br J Haematol 88, 731–739.

Howard, E.R., 1989. Choledochal cysts. In: Schwarz, C., Ellis, H. (Eds.), Maingot's Abdominal Operations, ninth ed. Appleton-Century-Crofts, New York, p. 1366.

Howard, E.R., Johnstone, D.I., Mowat, A.P., 1976. Spontaneous perforation of the common bile duct in infants. Arch Dis Child 51, 883–886.

Jabado, N., de Graeff-Meeder, E.R., Cavazzana-Calvo, M., et al., 1997. Treatment of familial hemophagocytic lymphohistiocytosis with bone marrow transplantation from HLA genetically nonidentical donors. Blood 90, 4743–4748.

Jansen, P.L., Strautnieks, S.S., Jacquemin, E., et al., 1999. Hepatocanalicular bile salt export pump deficiency in patients with progressive familial intrahepatic cholestasis. Gastroenterology 117, 1370–1379.

Jara, P., Hierro, L., Martinez-Fernandez, P., et al., 2009. Recurrence of bile salt export pump deficiency after liver transplantation. N Engl J Med 361, 1359–1367.

Kadakol, A., Ghosh, S.S., Sappal, B.S., et al., 2000. Genetic lesions of bilirubin uridine-diphosphoglucuronate glucuronosyl-transferase (UGT1A1) causing Crigler–Najjar and Gilbert syndromes: correlation of genotype to phenotype. Hum Mutat 16, 297–306.

Keitel, V., Burdelski, M., Vojnisek, Z., et al., 2009. De novo bile salt transporter antibodies as a possible cause of recurrent graft failure after liver transplantation: A novel mechanism of cholestasis. Hepatology 50, 510–517.

Kelly, A.L., Lunt, P.W., Rodrigues, F., et al., 2001. Classification and genetic features neonatal haemochromatosis: a study of twenty-seven affected pedigrees and molecular analysis of genes implicated in iron metabolism. J Med Genet 38, 599–610.

Knisely, A.S., 1992. Neonatal hemochromatosis. Adv Pediatr 39, 383–403.

Kogawa, K., Lee, S.M., Villanueva, J., et al., 2002. Perforin expression in cytotoxic lymphocytes from patients with hemophagocytic lymphohistiocytosis and their family members. Blood 99, 61–66.

Kohsaka, T., Yuan, Z.R., Guo, S.X., et al., 2002. The significance of human jagged 1 mutations detected in severe cases of extrahepatic biliary atresia. Hepatology 36, 904–912.

Lee, W.S., McKiernan, P.J., Kelly, D.A., 2001. Serum ferritin level in neonatal fulminant liver failure. Arch Dis Child Fetal Neonatal Ed 85, F226.

Lindstedt, S., Holme, E., Lock, E.A., et al., 1992. Treatment of hereditary tyrosinaemia type I by inhibition of 4-hydroxyphenylpyruvate dioxygenase. Lancet 340, 813–817.

Livesey, E., Cortina Borja, M., Sharif, K., et al., 2009. Epidemiology of biliary atresia in England and Wales (1999–2006). Arch Dis Child Fetal Neonatal Ed 94, F451–F455.

Lomas, D.A., Evans, D.L., Finch, J.T., et al., 1992. The mechanism of Z alpha$_1$-antitrypsin accumulation in the liver. Nature 357, 605–607.

Lykavieris, P., Hadchouel, M., Chardot, C., et al., 2001. Outcome of liver disease in children with Alagille syndrome: a study of 163 patients. Gut 49, 431–435.

Maggiore, G., Bernard, O., Riely, C.A., et al., 1987. Normal serum gamma-glutamyl-transpeptidase activity identifies groups of infants with idiopathic cholestasis with poor prognosis. J Pediatr 111, 251–252.

Markowitz, J., Daum, F., Kahn, E.I., et al., 1983. Arteriohepatic dysplasia. I. Pitfalls in diagnosis and management. Hepatology 3, 74–76.

McClement, J.W., Howard, E.R., Mowat, A.P., 1985. Results of surgical treatment of extrahepatic biliary atresia in the United Kingdom. Br Med J 290, 345–349.

McKiernan, P.J., Baker, A.J., Kelly, D.A., 2000. The frequency and outcome of biliary atresia in the UK and Ireland. Lancet 355, 4–5.

Mieli-Vergani, G., Howard, E.R., Portmann, B., et al., 1989. Late referral for biliary atresia: missed opportunities for effective surgery. Lancet I, 421–423.

Monaghan, G., Ryan, M., Seddon, R., et al., 1996. Genetic variation in bilirubin-UDP-glucuronosyltransferase gene promoter and Gilbert's syndrome. Lancet 347, 578–581.

Morecki, R., Glaser, J., 1989. Reovirus 3 and neonatal biliary disease: discussion of divergent results. Hepatology 10, 515–517.

Muiesan, P., Dhawan, A., Novelli, M., et al., 2000. Isolated liver transplant and sequential small bowel transplantation for intestinal failure and related liver disease in children. Transplantation 69, 2323–2326.

Nagral, S., Muiesan, P., Vilca-Melendez, H., et al., 1997. Liver transplantation for extrahepatic biliary atresia. Tohoku J Exp Med 181, 117–127.

National Institute for Health and Clinical Excellence (NICE), 2010. Neonatal jaundice (Clinical guideline 98). Available online at: www.nice.org.uk/CG98.

Nietgen, G.W., Vacanti, J.P., Perez-Atayade, A., 1992. Intrahepatic bile duct loss in biliary atresia despite portoenterostomy: a consequence of ongoing obstruction. Gastroenterology 102, 2126–2133.

Odievre, M., Hadchouel, M., Landrieu, C., et al., 1981. Long-term prognosis for infants with intrahepatic cholestasis and patent extrahepatic biliary tract. Arch Dis Child 56, 373–376.

Ohadi, M., Lalloz, M.R., Sham, P., et al., 1999. Localisation of a gene for familial hemophagocytic lymphohistiocytosis at chromosome 9q21.3-22 by homozygosity mapping. Am J Hum Genet 64, 165–171.

Ohi, R., Nio, M., Chiba, T., et al., 1990. Long-term follow-up after surgery for patients with biliary atresia. J Pediatr Surg 25, 442–445.

Ozawa, K., Uemoto, S., Tanaka, K., et al., 1992. An appraisal of pediatric liver transplantation from living relatives. Initial clinical experience in 20 pediatric liver transplantations from living relatives as donors. Ann Surg 216, 547–553.

Pereira, G.R., Sherman, M.S., Digiacimo, J., 1981. Hyper-alimentation induced cholestasis. Am J Dis Child 135, 842–845.

Pett, S., Mowat, A.P., 1987. Crigler–Najjar syndrome types I and II. Clinical experience – King's College Hospital 1972–1987. Phenobarbitone, phototherapy and liver transplantation. Mol Aspects Med 9, 473–482.

Psacharopoulos, H.T., Mowat, A.P., Cook, P.J.L., et al., 1983. Outcome of liver disease associated with alpha 1-antitrypsin deficiency (PiZ); implications for genetic counselling and antenatal diagnosis. Arch Dis Child 58, 882–887.

Puder, M., Valim, C., Meisel, J.A., et al., 2009. Parenteral fish oil improves outcomes in patients with parenteral nutrition-associated liver injury. Ann Surg 250, 395–402.

Quigley, E.M., Marsh, M.N., Shaffer, J.L., et al., 1993. Hepatobiliary complications of total parenteral nutrition. Gastroenterology 104, 1583–1584.

Rand, E.B., 1998. The genetic basis of the Alagille syndrome. J Pediatr Gastroenterol Nutr 26, 234–236.

Rand, E.B., Karpen, S.J., Kelly, S., et al., 2009. Treatment of neonatal hemochromatosis with exchange transfusion and intravenous immunoglobulin. J Pediatr 155, 566–567.

Rauschenfels, S., Krassmann, M., Al-Masri, A.N., et al., 2009. Incidence of hepatotropic viruses in biliary atresia. Eur J Pediatr 168, 469–476.

Redkar, R., Davenport, M., Howard, E.R., 1998. Antenatal diagnosis of congenital anomalies of the biliary tract. J Pediatr Surg 33, 700–704.

Riepenhoff-Talty, M., Gouvea, V., Evans, M.J., et al., 1996. Detection of group C rotavirus in infants with extrahepatic biliary atresia. J Infect Dis 174, 8–15.

Ritter, J.K., Yeatman, M.T., Ferreira, P., et al., 1992. Identification of a genetic alteration in the code for bilirubin UDP-glucuronosyltransferase in the UGT1 gene complex of a Crigler–Najjar type I patient. J Clin Invest 90, 150–155.

Roberts, E.A., James, A., Chitayat, D., et al., 1999. Prenatal surveillance, rapid diagnosis and prompt institution of medical treatment in perinatal hemochromatosis (abstract). J Pediatr Gastroenterol Nutr 29, 511A.

Rodrigues, F., Kallas, M., Nash, R., et al., 2005. Neonatal hemochromatosis – medical treatment vs. transplantation: the King's experience. Liver Transpl 11, 1417–1424.

Schwarzenberg, S.J., Sharp, H.L., 1990. Pathogenesis of alpha 1-antitrypsin deficiency-associated liver disease. J Pediatr Gastroenterol Nutr 10, 5–12.

Shamieh, I., Kibort, P.K., Suchy, F.J., et al., 1993. Antioxidant therapy for neonatal iron storage disease. Pediatr Res 33, 109A.

Shanmugam, N., Harrison, P.M., Devlin, J., et al., 2009. Selective use of endoscopic retrograde cholangiopancreatography in diagnosis of biliary atresia in infants younger than 100 days. J Pediatr Gastroenterol Nutr 49, 435–441.

Sifers, R.N., Finegold, M.J., Woo, S.L.C., 1992. Molecular biology and genetics of alpha-1-antitrypsin deficiency. Seminars in Liver Diseases 12, 301–310.

Sigurdsson, L., Reyes, J., Kocoshis, S.A., et al., 1998. Neonatal hemochromatosis; outcomes of pharmacological and surgical therapies. J Pediatr Gastroenterol Nutr 26, 85–89.

Silveira, T.R., Salzano, F.M., Howard, E.R., et al., 1991. Extrahepatic biliary atresia and twinning. Braz J Med Biol Res 24, 67–71.

Stepp, S.E., Dufourcq-Lagelouse, R., Le Deist, F., et al., 1999. Perforin gene defects in familial hemophagocytic lymphohistiocytosis. Science 286, 1957–1959.

Strautnieks, S.S., Kagalwalla, A.F., Tanner, M.S., et al., 1997. Identification of a locus for progressive familial intrahepatic cholestasis PFIC2 on chromosome 2q24. Am J Hum Genet 61, 630–633.

Strife, C.F., Hug, G., Chuck, G., et al., 1983. Membranoproliferative glomerulonephritis and alpha 1-antitrypsin deficiency in children. Pediatrics 71, 88–92.

Stringer, M.D., Dhawan, A., Davenport, M., et al., 1995. Choledochal cysts: lessons from a 20-year experience. Arch Dis Child 73, 528–531.

Subramaniam, P., Clayton, P., Portmann, B., et al., 2010. Variable clinical spectrum of the commonest inborn error of bile acid metabolism – 3-beta-hydroxy-delta5-C27-steroid dehydrogenase deficiency. J Pediatr Gastroenterol Nutr 50, 61–66.

Sundaram, S.S., Sokol, R.J., 2007. The multiple facets of ABCB4 (MDR3) deficiency. Curr Treat Options Gastroenterol 10, 495–503.

Sveger, T., Eriksson, S., 1995. The liver in adolescents with alpha-1-antitrypsin deficiency. Hepatology 22, 514–517.

Tan, C.E., Driver, M., Howard, E.R., et al., 1994. Extrahepatic biliary atresia: a first trimester event? Clues from light microscopy and immunohistochemistry. J Pediatr Surg 29, 808–814.

Thompson, R.J., Jansen, P.L., 2000. Genetic defects in hepatocanalicular transport. Semin Liver Dis 20, 365–372.

Tyler, K.L., Sokol, R.J., Oberhaus, S.M., et al., 1998. Detection of reovirus RNA in hepatobiliary tissues from patients with extrahepatic biliary atresia and choledochal cysts. Hepatology 27, 1475–1482.

Vara, R., Dhawan, A., 2007. A study of the aetiological trend of infantile cholestasis over a 13 year period in a tertiary paediatric liver centre in the UK (abstract). J Pediatr Gastroenterol Nutr 44 (Suppl 1), 186.

Verbsky, J.W., Grossman, W.J., 2006. Hemophagocytic lymphohistiocytosis: diagnosis, pathophysiology, treatment, and future perspectives. Ann Med 38, 20–31.

Verloes, A., Temple, I.K., Hubert, A.F., et al., 1996. Recurrence of neonatal haemochromatosis in half sibs born of unaffected mothers. J Med Genet 33, 444–449.

Whitington, P.F., Kelly, S., 2008. Outcome of pregnancies at risk for neonatal hemochromatosis is improved by treatment with high-dose intravenous immunoglobulin. Pediatrics 121, e1615–e1621.

Wilkinson, M.L., Mieli-Vergani, G., Ball, C., et al., 1991. Endoscopic retrograde cholangiopancreatography (ERCP) in infantile cholestasis. Arch Dis Child 66, 121–123.

Willot, S., Uhlen, S., Michaud, L., et al., 2008. Effect of ursodeoxycholic acid on liver function in children after successful surgery for biliary atresia. Pediatrics 122, e1236–e1241.

Yohannan, M.D., Perry, M.J., Littlewood, J.M., 1983. Long-term phototherapy in Crigler–Najjar syndrome. Arch Dis Child 58, 460–462.

Zur Stadt, U., Beutel, K., Kolberg, S., et al., 2006. Mutation spectrum in children with primary hemophagocytic lymphohistiocytosis: molecular and functional analyses of PRF1, UNC13D, STX11, and RAB27A. Hum Mutat 27, 62–68.

Part 3: **Gastrointestinal disorders**

Simon Newell

Structure and function of the developing gastrointestinal tract

Neonatal gastrointestinal function

Digestion and absorption

This is dealt with in detail in Chapter 16 part 1.

Motility

The ontogeny of motility lags behind digestive and absorptive function (Fig. 29.19). Disordered motor function presents clinically as 'poor tolerance of feeds'. Symptoms include vomiting, high gastric residual volume, bile staining of the gastric aspirate, abdominal distension and reduced stool frequency.

The oesophagus has two complementary functions: swallowing and the prevention of gastro-oesophageal reflux. Nutritive swallowing is seldom present in the infant of less than 34 weeks' gestation, and 75% of healthy preterm infants require tube feeding until this postconceptional age. The fetus begins to swallow liquor at around 16 weeks' gestation. Initially small volumes are swallowed, increasing to around 500 ml/day by term. Fetal swallowing is an important mechanism in the regulation of liquor volume, and reduced swallowing explains the polyhydramnios seen in oesophageal atresia or in fetuses with neuromuscular conditions (Pritchard 1966).

In the term infant, the complex mechanism of swallowing with movement of the bolus of milk into the stomach, protection of the airway, inhibition of respiration and appropriate relaxation of the oesophageal sphincter and gastric fundus is achieved within a day or two of birth.

The mature suck–swallow pattern has bursts of sucks at a rate of 2 per second, with oesophageal transit on a few occasions during each burst (Papaila et al. 1989). In the preterm infant, uncoordinated motor activity explains the problems with milk tolerance and gastro-oesophageal reflux (Newell et al. 1989).

Gastric emptying is slow in the preterm infant, presenting as failure to tolerate milk feeds. Half emptying time for breast milk

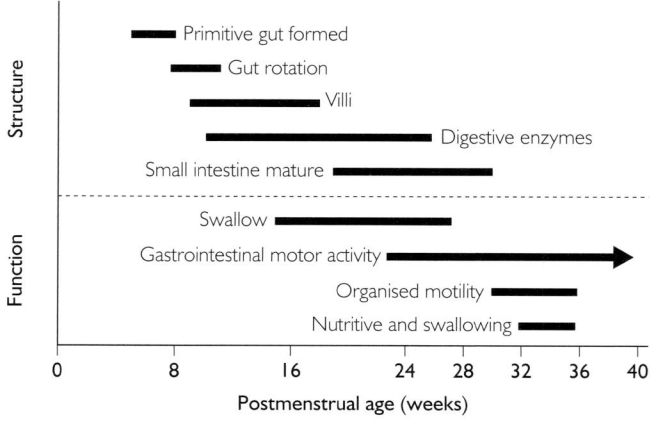

Fig. 29.19 Ontogenic timetable of gut structural and functional development. (*Redrawn from Newell et al. (1993).*)

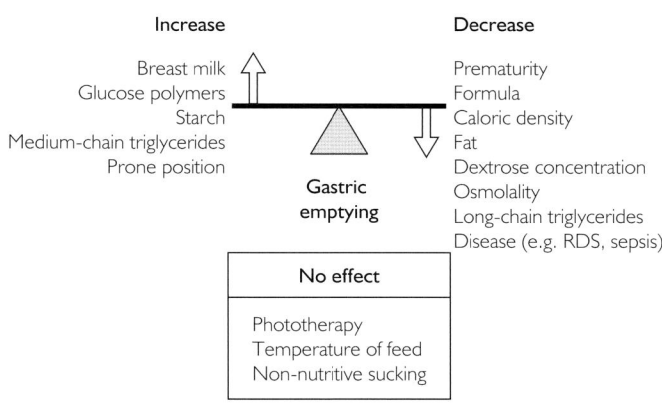

Fig. 29.20 Factors affecting gastric emptying. RDS, respiratory distress syndrome. *(Redrawn from Newell (1996).)*

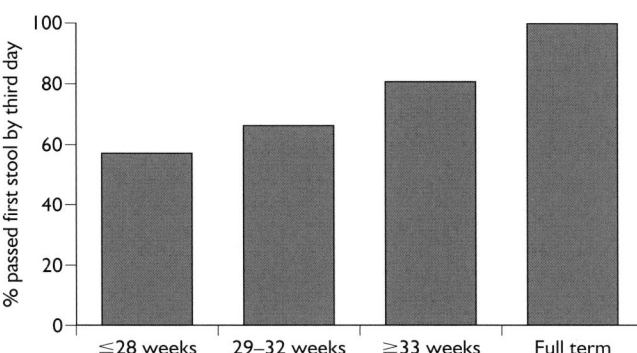

Fig. 29.21 Time of passage of first stool after birth (Clark 1977; Weaver and Lucas 1990).

Table 29.15 The gastrointestinal barrier: factors that may protect against intestinal pathogens, toxins and antigens

Non-immune
Intraluminal
– Gastric acid
– Motility
– Pancreaticobiliary secretions
– Breast milk factors
– Lysozyme
– Lactoferrin
– Oligosaccharides
Mucosal
– Mucus, bicarbonate and glycocalyx
– Microvillous membrane
Immune
– Secretory IgA
– Cellular immunity (gut-associated lymphoid tissue and milk)
– Macrophages
– Lymphocytes
– Leukocytes
– Complement

Intact absorption of large molecules occurs across the neonatal gut. Macromolecular absorption is higher in preterm and small-for-gestational-age infants and diminishes over the first months of life. This process of gut closure may occur more rapidly if breast milk is given rather than cow's milk formula.

Signs of gastrointestinal disease

Vomiting

Vomiting is a common sign and assessment should take account of volume, frequency and content of the vomitus and associated symptoms. Effortless regurgitation may represent gastro-oesophageal reflux (see below). Vomiting is often a sign of disease outside the gastrointestinal tract, notably infection (meningitis, pyelonephritis, hepatitis), disease of the central nervous system (intracranial haemorrhage, hydrocephalus), metabolic disorders (galactosaemia, congenital adrenal hyperplasia, thyrotoxicosis) and heart disease (cardiac failure).

Persistent vomiting may indicate obstruction. Upper gastrointestinal obstruction leads to vomiting shortly after birth while incomplete or lower obstruction presents later. Polyhydramnios during pregnancy or the 'mucusy' baby at delivery demands exclusion of oesophageal atresia before a feed is given. Fetal ultrasound reliably detects most cases of diaphragmatic hernia and duodenal atresia but malrotation, upper gut atresia, partial obstruction or web and duplication cysts are less often diagnosed antenatally. Most obstruction occurs distal to the ampulla of Vater, including the vast majority of duodenal atresias. Bile-stained vomiting indicates a surgical problem until proved otherwise. Hernias are an important site of obstruction at all ages.

Vomiting later in the neonatal period is less specific to obstruction. Functional obstruction occurs in necrotising enterocolitis (NEC) and ileus. Luminal obstruction may occur and is seen in meconium ileus, meconium plug syndrome and, rarely,

has been estimated as 20–40 minutes (Newell et al. 1993; Ewer et al. 1994). Emptying is faster with breast milk than formula. A number of other factors affect gastric emptying (Fig. 29.20). Breast milk fortifier does not affect gastric emptying during the introduction of milk feeds (McClure and Newell 1996), although emptying is slower with full-volume, 3-hourly feeds (Ewer and Yu 1996).

In the preterm infant, propagative small intestinal motility is poorly organised, with short bursts of motor activity before 30 weeks' gestation, which subsequently become coordinated, coincident with the timing of nutritive sucking. Small intestinal motility and tolerance of feeds are enhanced by previous exposure to enteral nutrition (Berseth and Nordyke 1993; McClure and Newell 1999).

Total gut transit time varies between 1 and 5 days (McClure and Newell 1999; Berseth et al. 2003). Passage of stool occurs within 24 hours of birth in 94–98% of healthy term infants. The passage of stools is slower in the preterm infant and frequency is inversely related to gestation (Fig. 29.21) (Clark 1977; Weaver and Lucas 1990). Around half of infants under 28 weeks' gestation have not passed their first stool within the first 3 days.

Barrier function

Mucosal protection is afforded by luminal, mucosal and systemic mechanisms (Table 29.15). Gastric acid, the first-line defence, reduces gastric pH below 4 within hours of birth in all but the most immature infants, in whom this occurs within the first week (Kelly and Newell 1994). Enteral feeds buffer gastric acidity.

lactobezoar. In malrotation, initial symptoms may be intermittent. Hirschsprung disease may not present with typical features of abdominal distension and vomiting and this diagnosis should be considered following delayed passage of meconium. Hypertrophic pyloric stenosis is a difficult diagnosis to make when signs begin – we have all been caught out by a preterm infant developing hypertrophic pyloric stenosis in front of our eyes!

Upper gastrointestinal bleeding

The appearance of small amounts of fresh blood or 'coffee grounds' in vomitus is not rare. In most infants a cause is not found and the prognosis is good. Swallowed maternal blood during birth or breastfeeding may lead to haematemesis or melaena. If blood is fresh, differentiation between adult and fetal haemoglobin is helpful.

Gastrointestinal bleeding may mark a bleeding diathesis. Classical haemorrhagic disease of the newborn still occurs if adequate vitamin K prophylaxis is not given. Late vitamin K deficiency bleeding is more common in babies with liver disease. Assessment of coagulation status is imperative if there is significant gastrointestinal bleeding, in order to rule out disseminated intravascular coagulation (DIC) or an inherited bleeding tendency.

Upper gastrointestinal ulceration occurs in the fetus (Bedu et al. 1994), the newborn after perinatal stress (De Boissieu et al. 1994) and babies receiving intensive care (Maki et al. 1993). At endoscopy, an oesophagogastritis of unknown aetiology occurs in a large proportion of infants presenting with haematemesis, frequent regurgitation or poor growth (De Boissieu et al. 1994). Rarely, haematemesis indicates congenital varices, true peptic ulcer, gastric or intestinal volvulus, duplications or haemangioma (Vinton 1994). The administration of dexamethasone or tolazoline may be associated with bleeding or perforation. We routinely use ranitidine as prophylaxis in infants receiving dexamethasone (Kelly and Newell 1994). H_2 blockade or proton pump inhibition is used for stress bleeding and other upper gastrointestinal bleeding (Bedu et al. 1994). Routine inhibition of gastric acid secretion is not recommended, and predisposes to NEC (Guillet et al. 2006).

Rectal bleeding

Rapid intestinal transit may allow upper gastrointestinal bleeding to appear as fresh blood per rectum. A small amount of fresh rectal bleeding is commonly due to an anorectal fissure. This is usually obvious on inspection or can be seen by inserting a lubricated auriscope speculum into the anal canal. A wide variety of intestinal conditions may lead to rectal bleeding, including malrotation, volvulus, intussusception and Hirschsprung disease. Meckel's diverticulum, haemangiomata and bowel telangiectasia most commonly present after the neonatal period (De La Torre et al. 2002). Rectal bleeding may denote NEC, particularly in the preterm baby (see below).

Dietary protein intolerance is an important cause of bleeding and colitis, with blood and mucus per rectum (see below).

Diarrhoea

The immediate and universal consequence of diarrhoea is loss of water and electrolytes. Dehydration may be rapid because of low body mass and the relative importance of colonic water and electrolyte conservation. Infective causes are common and a history of contact and stool culture is important. Loose, abnormal stools may indicate NEC (see below) or even Hirschsprung disease. In persistent diarrhoea, rare disorders of mucosal function should be considered (see below) which may lead to diarrhoea in utero and polyhydramnios. Pancreatic malabsorption occurs in cystic fibrosis, Schwachman syndrome and pancreatic hypoplasia but does not usually present with diarrhoea in the neonatal period.

Constipation

Delayed passage of meconium may indicate obstruction or Hirschsprung disease. Meconium ileus, with thick, inspissated stools and abdominal distension often associated with palpable faecal masses, is almost pathognomonic of cystic fibrosis (see below). In meconium plug syndrome, symptoms usually resolve after the first passage of meconium. Hypothyroidism, hypercalcaemia, diabetes insipidus and renal tubular acidosis may all present with constipation.

In very-low-birthweight (VLBW) infants, infrequent or delayed passage of meconium or stool may be associated with poor tolerance of feeds, particularly in the preterm infant with intrauterine growth restriction. Suppositories may be helpful in inducing defecation.

Necrotising enterocolitis

Epidemiology

The incidence of NEC lies between one and three cases per 1000 live births. NEC occurs in 2–5% of VLBW infants, and in 1–8% of admissions to neonatal intensive care (Beeby and Jeffrey 1992; Kliegman et al. 1993; Fitzgibbons et al. 2009; Rees et al. 2010). This equates with 500–1500 cases each year in England and Wales. The mortality of NEC was 22% in 1998 (Lucas and Morley 1998), but has now fallen to around 13% (Rees et al. 2010). Most affected infants are preterm, but 12% of infants with NEC are born at term (Fig. 29.22) (Beeby and Jeffrey 1992; Kliegman et al. 1993; Clark and Miller 1996). NEC occurs in 14% of infants under 26 weeks' gestation and in less than 1% after 32 weeks. Mortality ranges from 42% to 16% across a birthweight range of 500–1500 g (Fitzgibbons et al. 2009). The onset of signs is most commonly in the second week (Fig. 29.23). There are no reliable seasonal, sexual or geographical patterns with NEC.

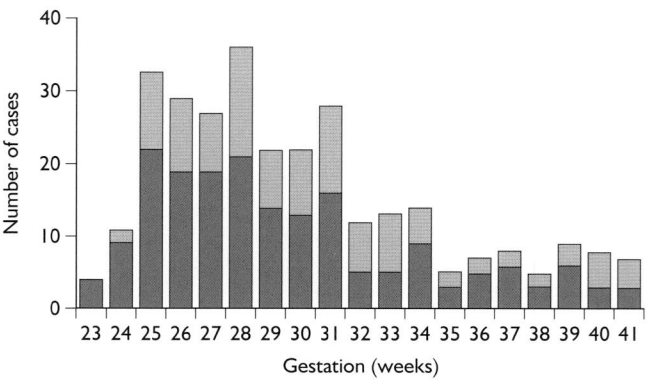

Fig. 29.22 Gestation at diagnosis of necrotising enterocolitis: results of a survey in the UK over a period of 1 year. All cases are shown by the open bars. Cases confirmed at surgery, with gas in the portal tract, or free gas in the abdomen are shaded. *(Redrawn from Lucas A. Abbott R in collaboration with the Royal College of Paediatrics and Child Health Research Unit.)*

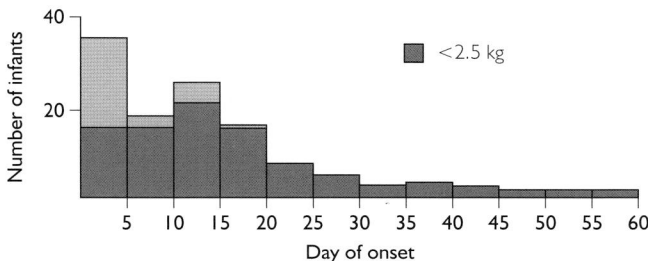

Fig. 29.23 Age at onset of necrotising enterocolitis in 129 cases notified to the Communicable Diseases Surveillance Centre, July 1980 to June 1981. *(Redrawn from Communicable Disease Report (1982).)*

 Table 29.16 Risk factors incriminated in the aetiology of necrotising enterocolitis

- Prematurity
- Intrauterine growth restriction
- Abruptio placentae
- Premature rupture of membranes
- Perinatal asphyxia
- Low Apgar score
- Umbilical catheterisation
- Hypoxia and shock
- Hypothermia
- Patent ductus arteriosus
- Non-human milk
- Hypertonic feeds
- Rapid introduction of enteral feeds
- Fluid overload
- Pathogenic bacteria
- Polycythaemia
- Thrombocytosis
- Anaemia
- Exchange transfusion
- Cyanotic congenital heart disease

NEC is a common end point precipitated by a number of different circumstances (Table 29.16). Babies with NEC may be divided broadly into three groups (Beeby and Jeffrey 1992). In the term baby, NEC is almost universally associated with major risk factors for gut ischaemia, principally perinatal asphyxia, and often occurs in the first days. NEC may occur at term in Hirschsprung disease (Beeby and Jeffrey 1992). Preterm infants under 30 weeks' gestation who develop NEC usually have no risk factors other than prematurity. In contrast, preterm infants of 30–36 weeks' gestation have greater evidence of perinatal asphyxia than case controls and a higher rate of intrauterine growth restriction (Beeby and Jeffrey 1992). In most preterm infants, NEC develops in the second or third weeks, after the introduction of enteral feeds (Fig. 29.23) (Communicable Disease Report 1982).

Pathology

NEC may affect any part of the gastrointestinal tract. In babies who come to surgery, or in those who die, the commonest sites of disease are the terminal ileum, caecum and ascending colon. NEC is a transmural disease. The bowel appears purple and discoloured, and is often distended with areas of serosal damage. Pneumatosis, the presence of submucosal and subserosal gas within the bowel wall, is the most characteristic appearance of the gut at laparotomy,

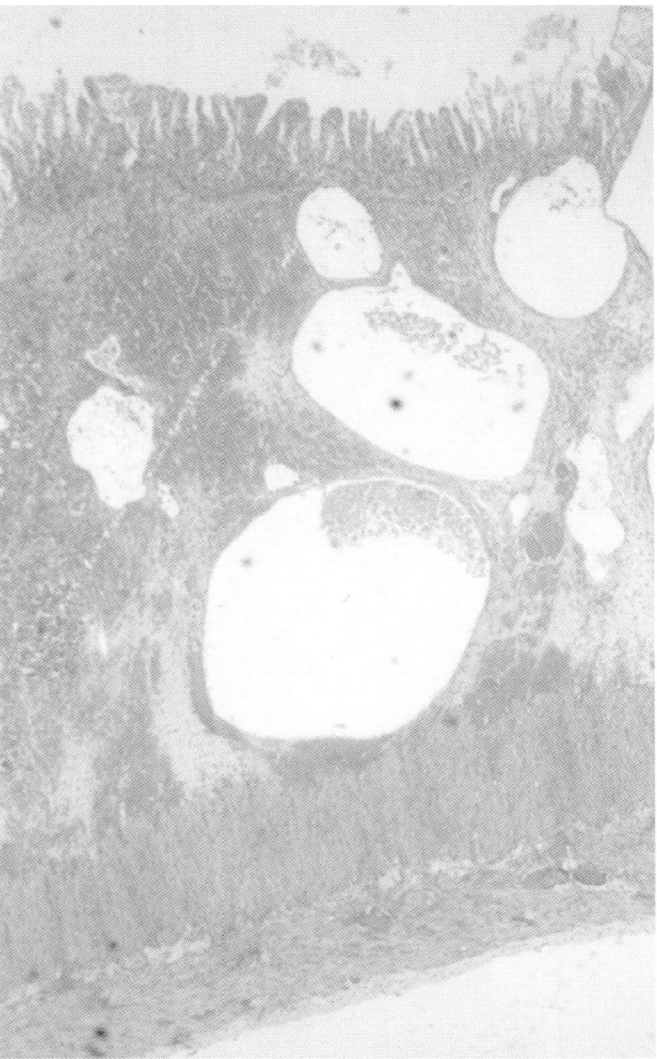

Fig. 29.24 Pathological specimen showing necrotising enterocolitis. Pneumatosis is evident with gas bubbles within the bowel wall.

histologically and radiographically (Fig. 29.24). This gas is largely nitrogen and hydrogen and is produced by gas-forming bacteria.

Histologically the earliest signs are a coagulative necrosis of the mucosa with microthrombus formation, leading to patchy mucosal ulceration, oedema and haemorrhage. In focal intestinal perforation, haemorrhagic necrosis is a feature that distinguishes this condition from classical NEC (Pumberger et al. 2002).

Cytokines have an important role in modulating intestinal inflammation and damage in NEC (Kliegman et al. 1993; Claud 2009). Raised levels of interleukins-1, -3 and -6, tumour necrosis factor-α and platelet-activating factor (PAF) relate to severity of the disease. PAF, the lipid-derived, proinflammatory cytokine, has a central role (Ewer 2002). Human infants with NEC have high levels of PAF and low levels of PAF-acetylhydrolase, an enzyme important in PAF degradation (Kliegman et al. 1993). Enterocyte death is induced by imbalance in the pro- and anti-inflammatory balance with increased proapoptotic protease activity (Jilling et al. 2004; Claud 2009). This understanding moves on rapidly, offering the potential of prophylaxis or novel treatment in the future.

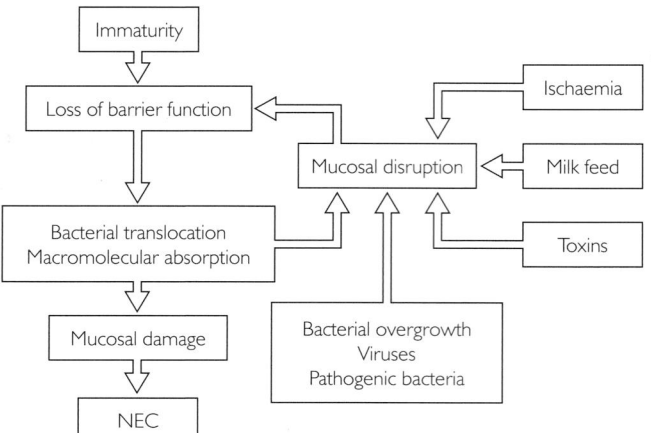

Fig. 29.25 Interaction of the main factors involved in the pathogenesis of necrotising enterocolitis (NEC).

Table 29.17 Organisms associated with epidemics of necrotising enterocolitis (Rotbart and Levin 1983; Clark and Miller 1996)

- *Klebsiella* spp.
- Non-pathogenic *Escherichia coli*
- Enterotoxigenic *Escherichia coli*
- *Enterobacter* spp.
- *Clostridium difficile*
- *Clostridium butyricum*
- *Clostridium perfringens*
- *Salmonella* spp.
- *Pseudomonas aeruginosa*
- Rotavirus
- Coronavirus

Aetiology

Numerous potential risk factors have been explored (Table 29.16). It is clear that none is in itself necessary or sufficient to produce NEC. The major candidate factors include hypoxia, prematurity and poor mucosal integrity, the bacterial flora and the presence of a metabolic substrate – milk – in the intestinal lumen (Fig. 29.25). These subjects will be discussed individually and have been reviewed extensively (Kliegman et al. 1993; Clark and Miller 1996; Claud 2009).

Gut hypoxia

The pathology of NEC is that of vascular congestion, haemorrhage and ulceration, supporting underlying hypoxic ischaemia. In the term infant with NEC, risk factors for gut hypoxia are almost invariably present. NEC may follow severe generalised hypoxia, maternal cocaine abuse and exchange transfusion (Beeby and Jeffrey 1992; Ozek et al. 2010). In lambs, polycythaemia reduces oxygen delivery to the gut and produces NEC, although the previously reported association in the human is not borne out in more recent literature.

An adverse intrauterine environment leads to chronic fetal hypoxia and intrauterine growth restriction, and diversion of cardiac output away from the gut with reduced blood flow through the superior mesenteric artery.

Studies have shown that absent or reversed end-diastolic flow on fetal Doppler studies predispose to NEC (odds ratio for NEC 2.13 (1.49–3.03)) (Dorling et al. 2005). In such infants reduction of gut blood flow is still evident after birth. The result is the consensus that infants with abnormal fetal Doppler studies, often associated with intrauterine growth restriction, are considered at high risk of NEC. In such fetuses, oligohydramnios and fetal echogenic bowel predict difficulties in the introduction of milk (Ewer et al. 1993). Intrauterine growth restriction is an important risk factor for NEC in infants over 29 weeks' gestation (Beeby and Jeffrey 1992).

The preterm infant is at particular risk of intestinal hypoxia during intensive care. In the animal model, bacterial colonisation and excessive formula feeding do not precipitate NEC unless hypoxia is also present (Caplan et al. 1994). In the newborn, after feeds, intestinal oxygen use is increased but not blood flow, predisposing to tissue hypoxia. Patent ductus arteriosus diminishes superior mesenteric artery blood flow and is more common in infants

with NEC (Rowe et al. 1994). Indometacin has long been said to predispose to NEC, although this is not borne out in meta-analysis (Jones et al. 2011). Perhaps the reason for this is that indometacin causes a focal intestinal perforation rather than true NEC; the combination of indometacin and steroids appears to be particularly potent in this regard.

Some of the earliest reports of NEC were in infants after exchange transfusion for rhesus haemolytic disease through an umbilical venous catheter. Umbilical arterial cannulation has been held to reduce gut blood supply and provoke embolisation or thrombus formation, predisposing to NEC. The studies confirming this relationship were all published prior to 1980. Most neonatologists avoid full milk feeds with an umbilical catheter in place, but early or late introduction of small volume feeds with a high or low umbilical artery catheter does not predispose to NEC (Kempley et al. 1993; Davey et al. 1994). The umbilical venous catheter does not predispose to NEC (Raval et al. 1995).

Mucosal integrity

Loss of mucosal integrity disrupts barrier function, allowing macromolecular absorption and bacterial translocation, and interferes with digestion. The preterm gut has an immature microvillous membrane with relative deficiency of mucus and secretory IgA, with increased permeability to small and large molecules (Rouwet et al. 2002). Further mucosal damage increases permeability to microorganisms and toxins. This process may initiate NEC (Clark and Miller 1996; Claud 2009). Antenatal corticosteroid administration induces intestinal maturation, decreases permeability and protects against NEC.

Microbial infection

Most NEC is not infectious. In sporadic disease, the presence of bacteria is probably necessary for NEC to occur but is not sufficient without other risk factors. In epidemic NEC there may be an identified infectious agent (Table 29.17) (Rotbart and Levin 1983; Clark and Miller 1996). Infection with clostridia, which produce a potent toxin, occurs in epidemics and in Hirschsprung's enterocolitis. Infants with NEC during epidemics fare better than infants with sporadic disease, although this may be related to heightened awareness and earlier detection of NEC on the neonatal unit (Clark and Miller 1996).

In sporadic disease, a large variety of microorganisms are associated with the pathogenesis of NEC (Table 29.18) (Communicable Disease Report 1982; Clark and Miller 1996). Positive blood

Table 29.18 Organisms isolated from blood cultures in infants with necrotising enterocolitis

	REFERENCE				
	Kliegman and Fanaroff (1981)	Communicable Disease Report (1982)	Beeby and Jeffrey (1992)	McKeown et al. (1992)	Chan et al. (1994)
Coagulase-negative staphylococci	–	10	6	11	2
Staphylococcus aureus	1	4	–	2	2
Escherichia coli	24	3	8	3	3
Klebsiella	6	1	7	5	–
Enterobacter spp.	–	–	1	4	4
Proteus mirabilis	1	1	–	1	–
Clostridium spp.	1	5	2	–	–
Streptococcus faecalis	2	1	1	–	–
Pseudomonas aeruginosa	2	–	–	–	1
Candida albicans	1	–	–	–	–
Miscellaneous	4	2	–	5	–

cultures are found in 10–50% and correlate with isolates from stool or peritoneal fluid (Beeby and Jeffrey 1992; McKeown et al. 1992; Chan et al. 1994). Overall, the microbiological picture is dominated by *Escherichia coli*, *Klebsiella*, *Enterobacter* and coagulase-negative staphylococci. In surgical patients, peritoneal culture shows a wider variety of microorganisms in extremely low-birthweight infants (under 1000 g) than in larger preterm infants (Rowe et al. 1994).

Unhindered proliferation of potentially pathogenic species may occur, promoting bacterial translocation and absorption toxic products, explaining the increased risk of NEC in infants whose mothers were treated with co-amoxiclav after preterm rupture of membranes (Kenyon et al. 2001). Among klebsiellas, rapid carbohydrate fermenters are more pathogenic.

Enteral nutrition

The choice of milk and the management of enteral nutrition are crucial to the prevention of NEC. All studies have demonstrated that most infants with NEC have received milk (Kliegman and Fanaroff 1981; Rowe et al. 1994; Lucas and Morley 1998; Llanos et al. 2002). In unfed infants with NEC, symptoms present early, often following an asphyxial insult (Clark and Miller 1996). Intraluminal milk may simply promote bacterial proliferation or increase bacterial endotoxin production by Gram-negative bacteria (Kliegman et al. 1993). Bacterial action upon unabsorbed nutrients results in gas formation and the production of short-chain fatty acids, which can be toxic to intestinal epithelium. Long-chain fats and undigested casein may contribute to inflammation and injury (Kliegman et al. 1993) and the lipid in milk increases mucosal permeability. Immature patterns of motility and decreased digestive capacity predispose the preterm infant to NEC (Berseth 1994; Newell 2000). In healthy infants who do not develop NEC, milk induces a cellular and humoral inflammatory mucosal reaction with an increase in circulating cytokines (Kliegman et al. 1993).

The method of enteral feedings influences incidence of NEC (Uauy et al. 1991) but prolonged delay of oral feeding is not recommended. The evidence that aggressive enteral feeding with rapid increase in feed volume is causative is more compelling (McKeown et al. 1992), although there is an absence of good randomised controlled trial data (Kennedy et al. 2000). Hyperosmolar feeds, as may occur when multiple additives are given, promote mucosal damage and NEC (Book et al. 1975).

Breast milk protects against NEC (Lucas and Cole 1990; McGuire and Anthony 2003; Meinzen-Derr et al. 2009). Infants given breast milk are seven to 10 times less likely to suffer from NEC, a benefit that is attenuated when breast milk is given with formula. Putative important factors in breast milk include immunoglobulins, lysozyme, complement, macrophages, growth factors, PAF-acetylhydrolase (Kliegman et al. 1993) and production of anti-inflammatory cytokines (Dvorak et al. 2003). Prebiotic oligosaccharides in breast milk are bifidogenic, promoting a gut flora which may protect against NEC (Coppa et al. 2006).

Trophic feeding – the use of minimal enteral feeds with parenteral nutrition – does not increase the risk of NEC (McClure and Newell 2000; Bombell and McGuire 2009). Trophic feeding prior to standard milk advancement may protect against NEC (Berseth et al. 2003).

Clinical features

Presentation may vary from insidious deterioration with non-specific signs, lethargy, temperature instability and apnoeic episodes to a rapidly progressive illness with shock, peritonitis and death. In the infant without gastrointestinal symptoms, early recognition of NEC requires a high index of suspicion. The baby's general condition is similar to that seen in sepsis with pallor, skin mottling and often jaundice. Bleeding may be due to DIC. Some infants have initial mild feed intolerance exhibited by increased volume of gastric residuals or emesis and then go on to demonstrate the classic

Table 29.19 Presenting features of necrotising enterocolitis (%)

	REFERENCE		
	Kliegman and Fanaroff (1981)	Communicable Disease Report (1982)	Lucas and Morley (1998)
Abdominal distension	78	75	77
Lethargy	9	71	64
Visible blood in stool	28	70	39
Hypotonia	–	63	64
Vomiting/aspirates (bile)	28	52	–
Abdominal tenderness	21	43	58
Apnoea	27	41	64
Bleeding diathesis	–	20	–
Abdominal wall oedema	–	19	–
Shock/sepsis	24	–	–

triad of abdominal distension, bloody, mucusy stools and bile-stained vomit or aspirates. There is little information on the 'normal' gastric residual in a preterm baby, but, in general, residuals of up to 2–3 ml are well tolerated. Clinical experience supports the common practice of careful review of a baby who consistently has more than 50% of feed volume as a 'residual'.

The commonest abdominal sign is distension (Table 29.19). Careful assessment should be made for tenderness: often, distended loops are palpable and an intra-abdominal mass may represent localised perforation. Blue abdominal discoloration suggests disease progression and occasionally the abdominal wall becomes indurated and red, a sign of underlying peritonitis. General assessment of cardiorespiratory function, blood pressure and perfusion is as important as examination of the abdomen.

Focal intestinal perforation is distinguished from NEC by pathology and clinical features. Focal intestinal perforation occurs earlier in life, characteristically in infants of low gestation who are receiving full intensive care, and is associated with blue discoloration of the abdomen (Pumberger et al. 2002).

Investigation

Immediate investigations include haemoglobin, white cell and platelet counts, coagulation studies, urea, electrolytes and albumin and blood gas analysis. The platelet count initially rises, but falls with disease progression and DIC. Blood and fluid losses into the abdomen are often larger than appreciated and abnormalities of perfusion, anaemia and electrolyte balance are common. Metabolic acidosis is usually a marker of shock. Carbon dioxide retention or hypoxia may represent respiratory failure due to apnoea or diaphragmatic splinting and indicates the need for ventilatory support.

Abdominal radiography is mandatory. The bowel appearance varies from a gasless abdomen (Fig. 29.26) to dilated loops of thick-walled gut with fluid levels. The pathognomonic radiographic appearance is pneumatosis intestinalis due to bubbles of gas in the gut wall (Fig. 29.27). In severe disease gas collects within the portal venous system (see below) (Rowe et al. 1994).

Radiological detection of perforation is not easy (Fig. 29.28). Free air may be seen in only two-thirds of infants in whom

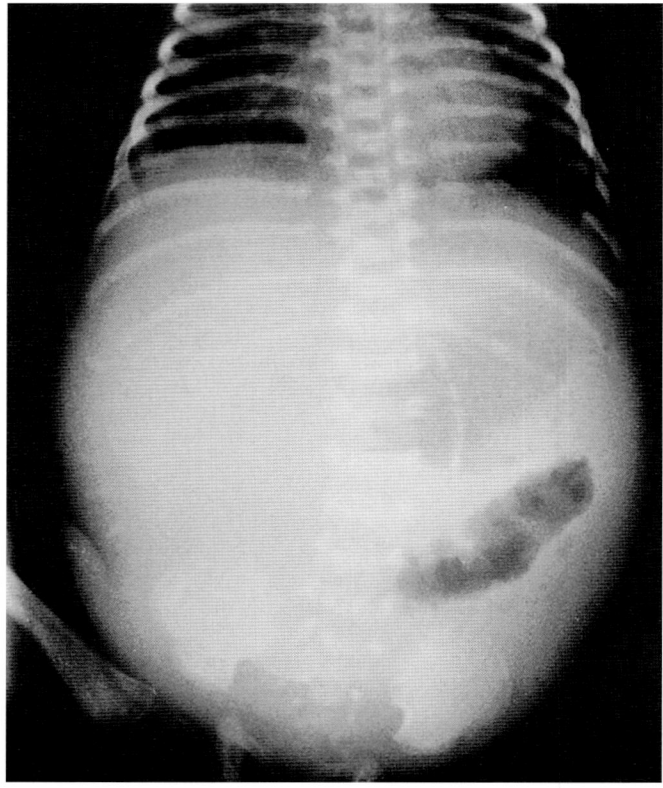

Fig. 29.26 Plain abdominal X-ray showing ascites in necrotising enterocolitis.

perforation is present. A lateral horizontal beam shoot-through X-ray may allow easier detection of anterior collection of gas (Fig. 29.29) but, on a supine film, free gas is best seen between the liver and the diaphragm. Free gas in a generally gasless abdomen without pneumatosis favours focal intestinal perforation (Pumberger et al. 2002).

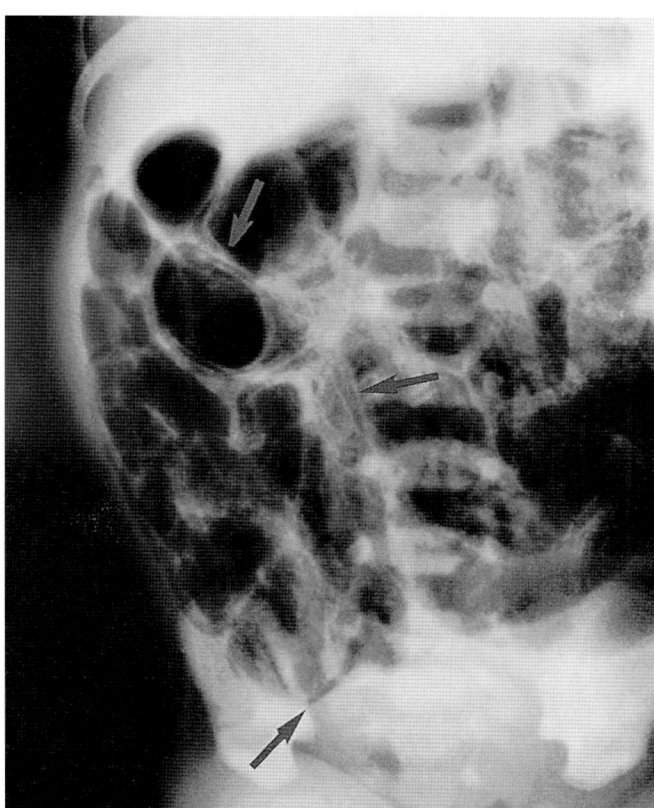

Fig. 29.27 Plain abdominal X-ray showing intraluminal gas (arrows) in necrotising enterocolitis.

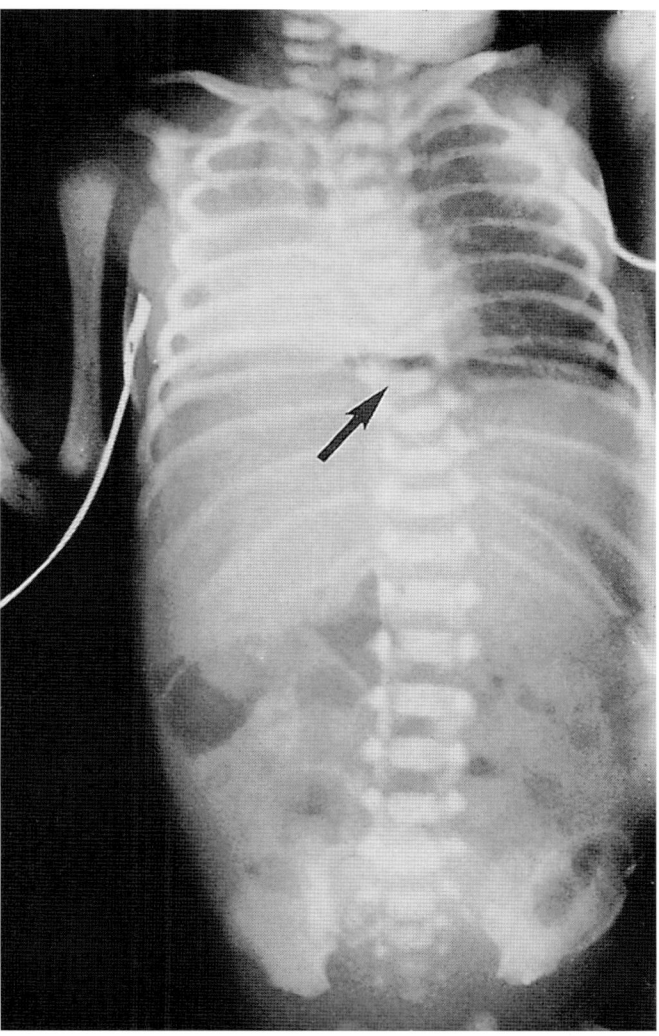

Fig. 29.28 Plain abdominal X-ray (anteroposterior supine) in the presence of a perforation: free gas is seen under the diaphragm (arrowed).

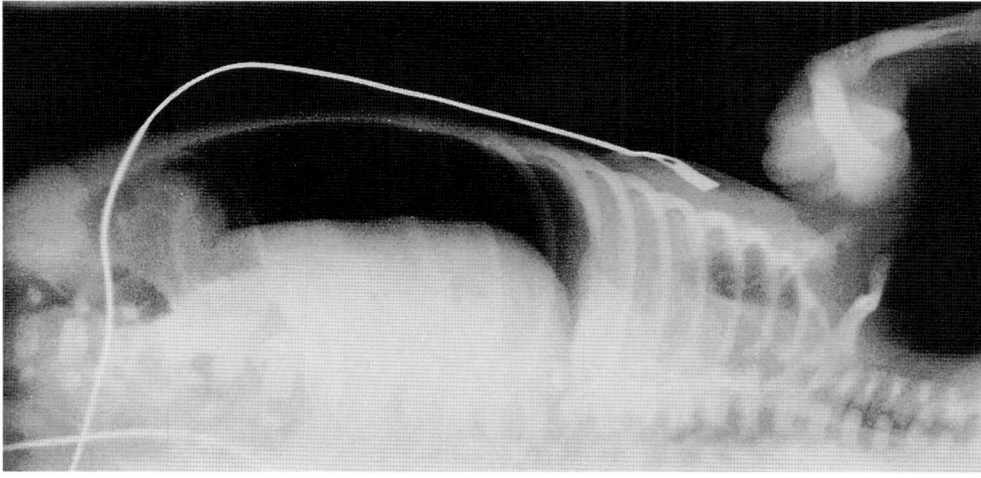

Fig. 29.29 Same infant as shown in Figure 29.28, radiographed lying on the left side with a shoot-through horizontal beam film.

Acute-phase proteins (C-reactive protein) are helpful in monitoring progress. Abdominal ultrasound may allow detection of masses or ascites. Contrast studies are avoided during the acute phase and should not be done outside a centre capable of providing immediate surgery.

Differential diagnosis

In most cases, recognition of NEC is not difficult. Other causes of gut ischaemia, including malrotation, volvulus and hernia, should be considered. Isolated rectal bleeding has a differential diagnosis, discussed above. Abdominal distension with regurgitation is common and, although NEC should be considered, it is reasonable to stop oral feeds for a few hours and observe the infant who has no other signs. 'NEC' may be the presenting feature of Hirschsprung disease or cystic fibrosis (Wood et al. 1995).

Treatment

The spectrum of clinical presentations makes it difficult and inappropriate to define a rigid regimen of management. Staging criteria are helpful in tailoring treatment (Bell et al. 1978; Walsh and Kliegman 1986) (Table 29.20).

Medical

The overall aim of treatment is to rest the gut, control infection, restore metabolic equilibrium and, with intensive or high-dependency care, maintain the infant in an optimal condition until the bowel heals. Suspension of enteral feeding means that parenteral nutrition should be provided. Surgery is indicated if intestinal perforation occurs, the infant's general condition deteriorates or intra-abdominal pathology persists beyond a few days.

The major components of medical management are:

- Cessation of enteral feeding.
- Nasogastric drainage with suction to minimise abdominal distension.
- Monitoring of temperature, pulse, respiratory rate, blood pressure, fluid balance.
- Plain abdominal radiography: if symptoms persist, radiographs should be repeated 6–12-hourly on the first day of NEC and while perforation remains likely.
- Peripheral venous access for antibiotics, blood and plasma.
- Blood cultures and septic screen; a lumbar puncture is not usually performed.
- Intravenous antibiotics: a triple-antibiotic regime is commonly used. Gram-negative cover: gentamicin or a third-generation cephalosporin (e.g. ceftazidime), although resistance to the latter is emerging. Gram-positive cover: amoxicillin or vancomycin. The broad-spectrum regimen should also include metronidazole. Second-generation beta-lactamase-resistant cephalosporins (e.g. cefuroxime) are not effective against Gram-negative organisms, notably *Enterobacter*. The local regimen may take account of the dominant neonatal intensive care unit flora.
- Volume replacement: fluid losses from the circulation into the gut or abdomen are easily underestimated. Immediate management of suspected NEC includes appropriate volume replacement and circulatory support. Monitoring must include peripheral perfusion, peripheral–core temperature gradient, urine output and plasma bicarbonate or base excess.
- Regular blood gas analysis and early recourse to assisted ventilation if there is evidence of shock, increasing metabolic acidosis, respiratory distress, respiratory failure or apnoeic episodes.
- Maintenance of normal urea, electrolytes, calcium and hydration by daily or twice-daily adjustments to rate and composition of intravenous fluids; prompt treatment of intercurrent problems such as hypoglycaemia, jaundice and DIC.
- Transfuse to maintain haemoglobin: the platelet count may fall and platelet transfusion will be necessary if the count is below 30×10^9/l or below 70×10^9/l before surgery.

Table 29.20 Modified Bell's staging for necrotising enterocolitis (Bell et al. 1978; Walsh and Kliegman 1986)

STAGE	CLINICAL FINDINGS	RADIOGRAPHIC FINDINGS	GASTROINTESTINAL FINDINGS
I: Suspected	Apnoea and bradycardia, temperature instability, lethargy	Normal or mild ileus	Mild abdominal distension, increased gastric residuals
IIA: Confirmed Features of stage I plus:	Apnoea and bradycardia, temperature instability, lethargy	Ileus pattern with one or more dilated loops, bowel wall oedema, focal pneumatosis	Bloody stools, prominent abdominal distension, absent bowel sounds, mild abdominal tenderness
IIB: Confirmed severe Features of stage IIA plus:	Thrombocytopenia and mild metabolic acidosis	Any of: widespread pneumatosis, ascites or portal venous gas	Abdominal wall oedema, palpable loops, tenderness, sometimes cellulitis
IIIA: Advanced Features of stage IIB plus:	Mixed acidosis, oliguria, hypotension, coagulopathy, disseminated intravascular coagulation	Prominent loops, worsening ascites, no free air	Signs of peritonitis: marked tenderness and distension. Abdominal wall oedema and induration
IIIB: Advanced plus perforation Features of stage IIIA plus:	Shock, deterioration in laboratory values and vital signs	Pneumoperitoneum	Perforated bowel

- Consider removal of umbilical cannulae – balance the risks: if an umbilical artery catheter is the only arterial access in an ill baby of less than 1000 g birthweight the balance may be in favour of keeping the catheter in situ.
- Insertion of a percutaneous central venous line for total parenteral nutrition (TPN) if possible.
- TPN (Ch. 17) is always necessary in NEC, for which enteral starvation for at least 7–10 days is needed. During the first 24–48 hours, if very ill, amino acid load is reduced and lipid infusion is avoided. If NEC is not confirmed, feeds may be recommenced after 48–72 h, and TPN may not be necessary.
- Analgesics should be used liberally: infants with NEC suffer pain and considerable stress. An opiate infusion (e.g. morphine or diamorphine) is recommended. Opiate-induced apnoea is not a problem in a neonatal unit where intermittent positive-pressure ventilation is available.
- Barrier nursing: scrupulous hand washing will prevent most cross-infection; true barrier nursing may be needed in an outbreak of NEC.

The majority of babies with NEC who are managed medically recover steadily. Stage I suspected or unconfirmed disease (Table 29.20) should be managed with 3 days of bowel rest, and if the baby rapidly improves he or she is unlikely to have NEC. For all confirmed cases, antibiotics, enteral starvation and TPN are usually prescribed for at least 7 days from the time of recovery from the initial severe illness. Perforation most often occurs in the first 48 hours but may become apparent at any time. By 7–14 days from diagnosis, most infants are free of signs of infection and have a soft abdomen, normal bowel sounds and a normal abdominal X-ray. Enteral feeding can then be restarted using 0.5–1.0 ml/h for the first 24 hours and thereafter increased cautiously. Expressed breast milk is the feed of choice; alternatively a preterm formula or donor expressed breast milk is used. Most infants who recover without surgery will tolerate one of these milks (see below for alternative feeds).

Surgical

In all, 20–50% of infants with NEC require surgery (Beeby and Jeffrey 1992; Spitz and Stringer 1993; Lucas and Morley 1998; Rees et al. 2010).

Indications

The cardinal indications for surgery in NEC are:

- failure to respond to medical management
- formation of a mass
- perforation.

The commonest indication for surgery is clinical deterioration with intestinal perforation, confirmed in 40–70% of infants who required surgery (Rowe et al. 1994; Horwitz et al. 1995; Rees et al. 2005). The commonest site of perforation is the terminal ileum, and multiple perforations are not unusual (Rowe et al. 1994; Horwitz et al. 1995). Perforation may occur without visible gas on the plain abdominal radiograph. Paracentesis showing at least 0.5 ml of brown-stained fluid, or bacteria on Gram stain, usually indicates perforation. Paracentesis is not widely used in the UK (Spitz and Stringer 1993).

Clinical deterioration despite medical treatment is more difficult to define. Abdominal signs, including a fixed dilated loop of intestine on serial radiographs, abdominal wall erythema or the development of an inflammatory mass, point to the need for surgery, as does general worsening in the infant's condition or a failure of intra-abdominal signs to resolve (Spitz and Stringer 1993).

Operation

At surgery, bowel necrosis is most commonly ileocaecal, and in around a third is limited to the colon, but it may occur at any point in the gut. Extensive gut necrosis may be inoperable and lethal (Rowe et al. 1994). The choice of operation depends upon the extent of gut necrosis, the extent of NEC in non-necrotic gut and the general condition of the infant. Among the numerous surgical procedures described, some main options exist (Rescorla 1995; Rees et al. 2005).

The commonest procedure is laparotomy, resection of necrotic bowel and creation of a proximal stoma and a distal mucous fistula (Horwitz et al. 1995; Rescorla 1995; Rees et al. 2005; Pierro et al. 2010). This necessitates a second procedure to restore gut continuity. Large fluid, electrolyte and nutrient losses may occur through a small bowel stoma, especially when milk is reintroduced. This has led to earlier timing of the second procedure, which is often performed within 2 months of the initial surgery. Postoperative complications include systemic, wound and intra-abdominal sepsis, which, perhaps surprisingly, are unusual (Horwitz et al. 1995). Stoma-related complications, such as dehiscence, are unusual and less likely with good nutritional status. Suspected stricture in the distal limb necessitates contrast study and may be resected (Schimpl et al. 1994).

Secondly, in the infant who is stable, with well-circumscribed disease, gut resection and primary anastomosis may be performed as one procedure. This is favoured in infants weighing over 1000 g (Rees et al. 2005). Problems with losses from the stoma are avoided and hospital stay may be reduced (Spitz and Stringer 1993). Primary anastomosis may reduce the likelihood of stricture.

'Clip and drop', referring to resection of necrotic bowel, while viable bowel is clipped and returned to the abdomen, pending further laparotomy in the following days, is used in some centres (Rees et al. 2005).

An alternative strategy is peritoneal drainage, at times performed on the neonatal intensive care unit under local anaesthesia (Pierro et al. 2010). One or two soft drains are inserted into the right lower quadrant, with broad-spectrum antibiotic cover and nasogastric aspiration. Initially used in babies who were too ill for surgery, some may avoid surgery altogether. In our practice, peritoneal drainage alone is usually reserved for small infants who are clinically unstable and unsuitable for laparotomy. After peritoneal drainage, laparotomy remains necessary in many (Pierro et al. 2010).

Finally, in the group with a poor prognosis (Spitz and Stringer 1993), disease may be so extensive that resection cannot be performed. Such extensive disease is usually lethal. A proximal jejunostomy can be used to defunction distal bowel. A 'second-look' laparotomy is performed if the baby survives, to reassess possible resection.

Postoperative management

Nutritional support and intensive care are usually needed for 2–3 weeks. Enteral feeds are reintroduced slowly using breast milk if available, as described above. If milk is not tolerated, a lactose-free formula containing hydrolysed protein and medium-chain triglycerides is used and, in some centres, this is the feed of choice after NEC. If rapid gut transit and diarrhoea persist, loperamide may be used. In the infant who is tolerating feeds but not gaining weight, salt and water depletion, malabsorption and intestinal, systemic or urinary tract infection should be considered. Calories and protein may be added to breast milk using a commercial breast milk fortifier. Formula may be supplemented with a powdered carbohydrate/fat mixture in 2–5% solution, but this may provoke or exacerbate diarrhoea. Advice from a paediatric dietician is essential.

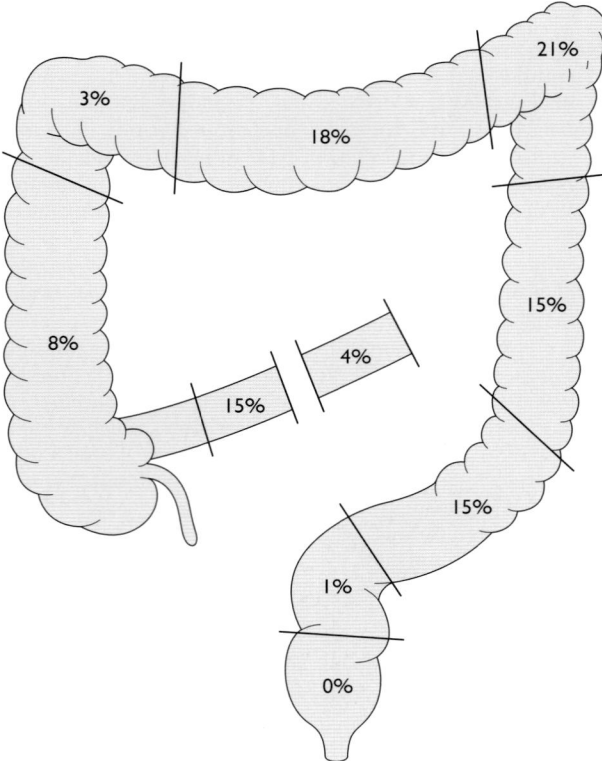

Fig. 29.30 Sites of intestinal stricture after necrotising enterocolitis. (*Redrawn from Janik et al. (1981).*)

Table 29.21 Late complications of necrotising enterocolitis

- Recurrence
- Intestinal stricture
- Enterocyst
- Short gut syndrome
- Enterocolic fistula
- Anastomotic leak
- Cholestasis
- Malabsorption
- Atresias and aganglionosis
- Salt and water depletion
- Polyposis
- Treatment complications

Late strictures due to submucosal thickening and fibrosis (Schimpl et al. 1994) may have become more common. In the baby who does not need surgery, strictures are less common and shorter (Lamireau et al. 1996). Most strictures manifest within 6 weeks and almost all do so within 4 months (Schimpl et al. 1994). Overall strictures occur in 10–40% and, although some narrowing seen on contrast studies may resolve spontaneously, most strictures need surgery. Most are colonic but strictures occur at the site of anastomosis and in the small bowel (Janik et al. 1981) (Fig. 29.30). Short bowel syndrome (SBS) may require long-term management, especially if the ileocaecal valve has been resected (see below).

Outcome

In 5–10%, NEC relapse occurs, usually within a month of initial presentation. Management is the same. It is not clear if management of the first attack can alter risk of recurrence. Late complications are important (Table 29.21).

Overall survival after NEC is 70–90% (Rowe et al. 1994; Horwitz et al. 1995). Mortality is higher in infants of less than 28 weeks' gestation despite similar severity of disease. In babies with a birthweight of less than 1000 g the survival rate is poor compared with larger infants (around 60% versus over 90%) (Chardot et al. 2003). Extensive disease, bacteraemia, DIC and persistent ascites are bad prognostic indicators (Kliegman and Fanaroff 1981; Rowe et al. 1994; Horwitz et al. 1995).

The nutrition, growth and gastrointestinal function of survivors depend upon the site and extent of disease and resection. In the absence of SBS (see below), major nutritional problems are unusual, although short-term problems with rapid gut transit, diarrhoea and malabsorption are seen as gut adaptation occurs (Liefaard et al.

1995). Specific nutritional deficiencies due to terminal ileal resection (particularly vitamin B_{12}) should not be forgotten.

Long-term neurodevelopmental follow-up is essential in view of the high rate of disability in survivors of severe NEC (Rees et al. 2007). Neurodevelopmental problems are more common after NEC (odds ratio 1.7 (1.3–2.2)) and in those needing surgery compared with those treated medically (odds ratio 2.3 (1.5–3.6)) (Rees et al. 2007). The link between NEC and periventricular leukomalacia may relate to common antenatal risk factors, or be the result of proinflammatory cytokine release or systemic illness and hypotension.

Prevention

Prevention in current practice includes:

- use of breast milk
- minimal enteral feeding (0.5 ml/h) for 7 days before increasing feeds
- slow feed advancement
- standardised feeding regimen
- probiotics.

Future progress in NEC lies in its prevention. Despite many suggested preventive strategies (Claud 2009), the central difficulty of studying a relatively infrequent, sporadic disease thwarts attempts at good, prospective, randomised studies.

In the term infant, avoidance of perinatal asphyxia might reduce NEC (Beeby and Jeffrey 1992; Clark and Miller 1996). In the infant with hypoxic–ischaemic encephalopathy, we avoid milk feeds during the acute encephalopathy and during cooling, starting low-volume feeds for at least 24 hours before full enteral feeding.

Maternal antenatal steroids reduce the risk of NEC by amelioration of preterm lung disease, or by a direct effect upon gut maturation and mucosal integrity (Claud 2009). Choice of antibiotic in preterm rupture of membranes is important, and co-amoxiclav should be avoided (Kenyon et al. 2001). The risk of NEC rises when antibiotics are continued for more than 5 days when cultures are negative (Cotton 2010). General measures including maintenance of good tissue perfusion, blood pressure and hydration and avoidance of hypotension, unnecessary H_2 receptor blockers, hypoxia and hypothermia are all likely to reduce NEC. In the preterm infant with hypotension resistant to volume expansion, inotropes improve gut perfusion (Hentschel et al. 1995). Umbilical artery catheters should be removed if there is evidence of thrombosis or reduced blood flow to buttocks or lower limbs. The role of blood transfusion is contentious. There is a temporal association with NEC after 4 weeks of age (Josephson et al. 2010) but the transfusion may be given in response to premonitory symptoms of NEC or relate to immaturity and generalised illness. In many centres, feeds are withheld a few hours around and during transfusion, although there is no strong evidence base for this practice (Agwu and Narchi 2005).

The timing, method and composition of enteral feeds in the face of immaturity of digestion, absorption, gut motility and barrier function have attracted most attention (Newell 2000). Breast milk should be given, and lactation supported whenever possible (Lucas and Cole 1990; Meinzen-Derr et al. 2009). Freezing breast milk for storage does not abolish benefit (Dvorak et al. 2003). Meta-analysis suggests that donor breast milk will reduce the risk of NEC fourfold compared with formula (McGuire and Anthony 2003). A substantial reduction in NEC may be achieved with the use of a structured feeding regimen (Patole and de Klerk 2005). Hyperosmolar feeds should be avoided, and care should be taken when adding electrolytes to milk.

Prolonged delay in enteral feeding for the prevention of NEC cannot be recommended but rapid, incautious introduction and increase of enteral feeds in the face of poor feed tolerance is likely to lead to NEC (McKeown et al. 1992; Berseth 1994). In the VLBW infant, most advise introduction of milk feeds at 20–25 ml/kg/day, increased by the same amount daily (Berseth et al. 2003). Administration of small amounts of milk (minimal enteral feeding) is widely used to promote gut development (McClure and Newell 2000; Bombell and McGuire 2009) and does not increase NEC risk and may reduce it (Berseth et al. 2003). Special care is needed with the introduction of milk in the infant with intrauterine growth restriction (Ewer et al. 1993; Dorling et al. 2005). In intrauterine growth restriction with abnormal fetal Doppler studies, early introduction of milk on day 2 is safe, and has the advantage of earlier feed tolerance (Leaf et al. 2010).

Control of infection is essential in the management of epidemic NEC and is good practice in all cases. Prophylactic use of systemic antibiotics is not advised. Administration of enteral aminoglycosides is not without risk, as absorption may occur, but may reduce the risk of NEC (Fast and Rosegger 1994). Manipulation of intestinal flora during gut colonisation towards the pattern seen in the breastfed infant, by administration of probiotics (bacteria) or prebiotics (oligosaccharides which favour selection of these bacteria), looks promising for NEC prevention. Meta-analysis of trials of a wide variety of prebiotic regimens, varying in organism, dose and timing, demonstrates a risk ratio for NEC in those given these live bacterial preparations of 0.35 (0.23–0.55), with a number needed to treat of 25 (17–34) to prevent a case of NEC (Deshpande et al. 2010). This evidence may indicate the need for a change in practice (Tarnow-Mordi et al. 2010), although clear guidance cannot be drawn from current evidence, and further trials are in progress (Soll 2010). Changes in gut flora during initial colonisation may have lasting effects, even into adult life, raising potential unforeseen consequences (Mshvildadze and Neu 2010).

Future possibilities include modification of cytokine activity and treatment with growth factors (Claud 2009).

Short bowel syndrome

SBS follows loss of a significant portion of the small intestine and comprises malabsorption, diarrhoea and growth failure due to loss of mucosal surface area and rapid gastrointestinal transit. Loss of bowel may follow pre- or postnatal damage to the gut (Liefaard et al. 1995, Stringer and Puntis 1995; Lao et al. 2010) (Table 29.22). NEC is the commonest cause of SBS and intestinal failure (Guarino and De Marco 2003), occurring at a time when, in fetal life, the

Table 29.22 Aetiology of short bowel

Prenatal
- Vascular accidents
- Intestinal atresia
- Abdominal wall defects
- Volvulus
- Meconium peritonitis

Postnatal
- Necrotising enterocolitis
- Volvulus
- Vascular thrombosis
- Abdominal trauma

small intestine is doubling in length. Among infants with NEC who require surgery and survive, 4–10% have SBS (Köglmeier et al. 2008).

Babies with less than 50% of their total bowel length, or less than 100 cm of small bowel, are at high risk of SBS (Chaet et al. 1994; Liefaard et al. 1995). Parenteral nutrition is usually needed when less than 40 cm of small intestine remains and is likely to be needed for longer if the ileocaecal valve is absent (Chaet et al. 1994).

The central tenet of management is nutritional support and maintenance of fluid and electrolyte balance, allowing gradual intestinal adaptation with bowel growth and mucosal hypertrophy (Chaet et al. 1994; Liefaard et al. 1995; Stringer and Puntis 1995; Vanderhoof et al. 2003) and permitting full enteral feeds with as little as 10 cm of small bowel (Stringer and Puntis 1995). Most babies will achieve 90% absorption of carbohydrate and fats by 3 months (Liefaard et al. 1995). Preservation of the ileum is important for adaptation, transit time and its unique ability to absorb vitamin B_{12} and bile acids.

Babies with SBS cannot survive without TPN. When TPN is needed long-term, home administration has allowed these children a good quality of life (Puntis 2001). Enteral feeding is essential for adaptation but is often difficult. Most infants tolerate a protein hydrolysate, with medium-chain triglycerides and glucose polymers but no lactose, and some require an amino acid formula. Increased caloric content may be needed, and some require modular feeds, allowing manipulation of individual nutrient components. Specific nutrients may be used as primary therapy (Stringer and Puntis 1995). The diet must contain adequate calcium, magnesium, iron, fat- and water-soluble vitamins and trace elements. Vitamin B_{12} supplements may be necessary after terminal ileal resection.

Possible pharmacotherapy includes oral decontamination regimens, antimotility drugs and hormonal therapies (Vanderhoof et al. 2003). Antimotility agents (loperamide) may be effective but should be used with care. The multidisciplinary team is key to successful management (Stringer and Puntis 1995; Puntis 2001). In intestinal failure, TPN dependence and associated complications, gut-lengthening surgery may be helpful. Procedures aim to slow intestinal transit time or increase absorptive surface area (Chaet et al. 1994; Stringer and Puntis 1995).

Small bowel transplantation is now available (Nayyar 2xnewrefs2). Outcome after transplant has improved, with mean survival over 50% at 5 years. Two-thirds require liver transplant for SBS-associated liver disease, and survival varies with primary pathology, between 44% for NEC and 75% for volvulus (Lao et al. 2010).

The prognosis for SBS is now vastly better than it was 20 years ago, with survival rates exceeding 90%, even in those with less than

40 cm of small bowel. Most children climb back into the normal weight range by their third year, albeit on the lower centiles (Liefaard et al. 1995).

Neonatal appendicitis

Appendicitis in the neonate is very rare, representing only 0.1–0.2% of childhood appendicitis (Jancelewicz et al. 2008). The commonest presentation is with perforation and diffuse peritonitis, with signs like those of NEC. Neonatal appendicitis may complicate NEC, Hirschsprung disease and cystic fibrosis and is more common in the preterm infant (Jancelewicz et al. 2008). Abnormal gas pattern on plain abdominal X-ray and red and white cells in the urine point to the diagnosis. Treatment is surgical, with intensive medical support and broad-spectrum antibiotic cover. Mortality is around 25%.

Intractable diarrhoea

Severe, protracted diarrhoea beginning soon after birth may be due to a congenital abnormality of gastrointestinal function. All are rare and investigation and management require the support of a specialist centre. Diarrhoea may be missed when watery stool is mistaken for urine in the nappy. Intestinal mucosal biopsy is indicated, and fluid and electrolyte balance and support of nutrition are the central objectives of treatment.

Microvillous inclusion disease (congenital microvillous atrophy)

This is an autosomal recessive disorder of the cytoskeleton of the apical region of the enterocyte in which there are atrophy and involution of microvilli of the small and large bowel (Canani et al. 2010). Massive diarrhoea is unresponsive to stopping feeds. To establish a diagnosis, mucosal biopsy is examined by electron microscopy. TPN is given but the poor prognosis has prompted use of small intestinal transplantation with good short-term survival (Bunn et al. 2000; Ruemmele et al. 2004).

Congenital electrolyte transport defects

Congenital chloride diarrhoea is autosomal recessive owing to a defect of the sodium-independent ($Cl^-HCO_3^-$) exchanger in the ileum and colon due to recognised mutations near the cystic fibrosis gene (Canani et al. 2010). Fetal diarrhoea produces polyhydramnios. Severe watery diarrhoea, abdominal distension, hypochloraemic alkalosis and rapid weight loss occur in the newborn period. Stool chloride is high. Congenital sodium diarrhoea, due to defective sodium/proton exchange, produces a similar picture (Booth 1985). Intravenous, and subsequently oral, fluid and mineral replacement is necessary.

Congenital lactase deficiency

Symptoms immediately follow introduction of milk feeds, with acidic stools which contain lactose. Diagnosis is made by withdrawal of lactose-containing feeds and the demonstration of absent lactase activity on a jejunal mucosal biopsy. It is very rare compared with secondary lactose intolerance (Heyman 2006).

Congenital glucose/galactose malabsorption

Watery acidic stools containing reducing substances, but possibly not lactose, are seen in the first days after birth. After rehydration, a fructose-based formula is given and the prognosis is good (Canani et al. 2010).

Autoimmune enteropathy

Intractable diarrhoea, characteristically with a family history of autoimmune disease, may be due to immune dysregulation with a variety of genetic abnormalities (Canani et al. 2010). Immunosuppressive or immunomodulatory therapy offers benefit (Montalto et al. 2009).

Gastro-oesophageal reflux

Clinical presentation

Gastro-oesophageal reflux disease (GORD) is difficult to define, diagnose and treat (Birch and Newell 2009; Vandenplas and Rudolph 2009). GORD may lead to vomiting, oesophagitis, recurrent apnoea, pulmonary aspiration, exacerbation of bronchopulmonary dysplasia, poor growth and longer stay in hospital. Most episodes of reflux occur during transient relaxation of the lower oesophageal sphincter (Omari et al. 2002). Reflux is more common in infancy than in childhood. The preterm infant is at high risk because of low resting lower oesophageal sphincter pressure and slow gastric emptying (Newell et al. 1993). Reflux is often seen after repair of oesophageal atresia. Feeds, the supine position, nursing care and chest physiotherapy increase reflux (Newell et al. 1989; Ewer et al. 1999).

GORD is a common diagnosis, made in over 20% of preterm infants (Dhillon and Ewer 2004). The clinical syndrome is difficult to define, and often the diagnosis is inferred from a positive response to a trial of therapy. Some infant behaviour patterns are associated with reflux, lending support to a score based upon clinical observations (Feranchak et al. 1994). Respiratory deterioration or recurrent apnoea without apparent precipitating cause, and resistant to usual therapy (e.g. caffeine), may respond to reflux therapy.

Investigations have poor predictive value. Contrast studies lack sensitivity but rule out anatomical abnormality (Dhillon and Ewer 2004). Prolonged oesophageal pH study, the gold standard in children, is limited by milk buffering of gastric acidity (Omari and Davidson 2003). Reference pH data vary according to prematurity and intensive care (Table 29.23) (Vandenplas and Sacre Smits 1987; Newell et al. 1989; Vandenplas et al. 1991; Ng and Quak 1998). Impedance monitoring and scintigraphy detect reflux that is not evident on pH study, but are largely confined to research (Dhillon and Ewer 2004; Lopez-Alonso et al. 2006; Birch and Newell 2009). The presence of acidic oropharyngeal secretions on litmus testing has a high positive predictive value for acid reflux (James and Ewer 1999).

Treatment

Best practice is difficult to define in the face of a limited evidence base for therapy (Birch and Newell 2009; Vandenplas and Rudolph 2009). We propose an inverse-pyramid, stepwise approach (Fig. 29.31). Prone or left lateral positioning, with cardiorespiratory monitoring, can be used while the infant is in hospital (Ewer et al. 1999; Omari et al. 2004). Clearly the prone position cannot be used

Table 29.23 Upper limits of reference range (median) for results of pH studies in infants without symptoms of gastro-oesophageal reflux

	NICU PRETERM INFANTS (Newell et al. 1989) (*n* = 35)	HEALTHY PRETERM INFANTS (Ng and Quak 1998) (*n* = 21)	INFANTS (Vandenplas et al. 1991) (*n* = 509)	CHILDREN 14–16 MONTHS (Vandenplas and Sacre Smits 1987) (*n* = 15)
Reflux index (%)	11 (3)	3 (1.1)	10 (4)	6.4 (2.7)
Episodes/24 h	29 (9.5)	30 (7.6)	70 (27)	46 (19)
Episodes >5 min/24 h	7 (3)	3 (1.1)	9 (3)	4.6 (2.2)
Longest episode (min)	41 (8)	16 (6.1)	41 (12)	22 (8.6)

NICU, neonatal intensive care unit.
The first study refers to preterm infants in neonatal intensive care units, the others to healthy infants. Almost all were receiving feeds.

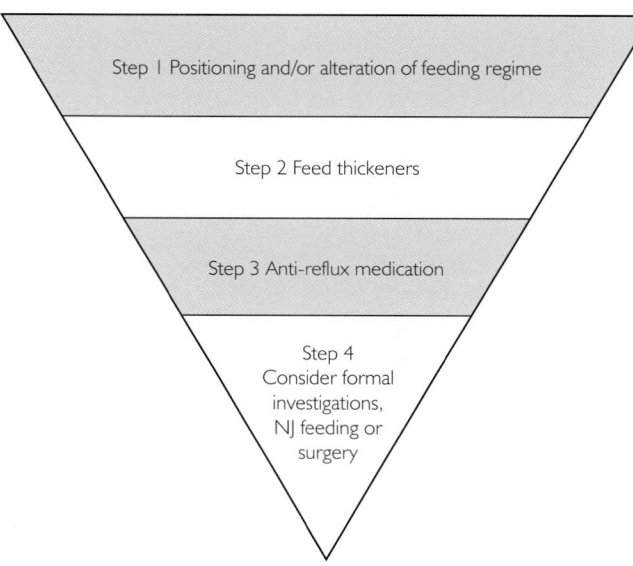

Fig. 29.31 The inverse pyramid of gastro-oesophageal reflux disease therapy. Most babies need only steps 1 or 2. NJ, nasojejunal.

Step 1 Positioning and/or alteration of feeding regime

Step 2 Feed thickeners

Step 3 Anti-reflux medication

Step 4 Consider formal investigations, NJ feeding or surgery

Table 29.24 Gastrointestinal manifestations of milk protein intolerance

– Vomiting
– Gastro-oesophageal reflux
– Diarrhoea
– Failure to thrive
– Colic
– Colitis
– Villous atrophy and malabsorption
– Eosinophilic gastroenteropathy
– Occult blood loss

Milk protein intolerance

Antigens provoking MPI include cow's milk whey proteins, β-lactoglobulin, α-lactalbumin and casein. Immunogenic proteins may be absorbed and secreted in breast milk, explaining cow's milk colitis in exclusively breastfed infants (Vandenplas et al. 2007). In the newborn, gut barrier function is poor (Table 29.15) and macromolecular absorption is high, although this does not fully account for allergic reactions. MPI may follow any gastrointestinal insult, such as NEC or surgery.

Over 90% of MPI presents in the first months of life, with an overall incidence of 2–5%, although over 50% with an atopic family history may develop MPI. Infants with MPI often react to other antigens.

Clinical features

The commonest gastrointestinal symptoms are vomiting and diarrhoea (Table 29.24) (Vandenplas et al. 2007). GORD is strongly linked with MPI. MPI is the commonest cause of colitis in the young infant, with rectal bleeding with loose stools containing mucus. MPI enteropathy may result in weight loss, abdominal distension and steatorrhoea with patchy subtotal villous atrophy and crypt hyperplasia. MPI may be accompanied by lactose intolerance. Non-gastrointestinal symptoms of MPI range from acute reactions, including urticaria, to chronic atopic disease. Anaphylaxis is rare in the neonate.

at home, with increased risk of sudden infant death syndrome. Feed thickening reduces regurgitation and is widely used. The prokinetic effects of erythromycin or domperidone suggest that they should reduce reflux, but evidence of efficacy is limited. Pain or irritability may suggest oesophagitis, and treatment with ranitidine or a proton pump inhibitor is often used. Surgical fundoplication is rarely necessary and is considered in recurrent aspiration, reflux-related life-threatening events or where severe reflux disease is unresponsive to medical therapy (Kiely 1990). In GORD resistant to therapy, transpyloric feeding may assist, and cow's milk protein intolerance (MPI) should be considered (Misra et al. 2007; Birch and Newell 2009; Vandenplas and Rudolph 2009).

Prognosis is good and in most infants reflux resolves with maturation of the antireflux barrier. Persistent reflux is more common in those with neurodevelopmental problems.

Diagnosis rests upon remission of symptoms on exclusion diet and relapse on challenge. Estimation of total IgE and specific antibodies (radioallergosorbent test) or skinprick testing may assist diagnosis and suggest prognosis (Vandenplas et al. 2007). A hypoallergenic, lactose-free, milk substitute containing extensively hydrolysed proteins or an amino acid-based formula is given. Infants with severe MPI, notably colitis, are more likely to require an amino acid formula. If breastfed, restriction of maternal diet, avoiding cow's milk and sometimes egg and soya, is recommended (Vandenplas et al. 2007). Soya milk is not recommended in MPI, and is not given before 6 months of age (Agostoni et al. 2006). Goat's milk is only suitable for goats.

Management demands close dietetic supervision. Challenge, to substantiate diagnosis and demonstrate resolution of MPI, can usually be performed under medical observation but out of hospital (Vandenplas et al. 2007). The vast majority of MPI resolves in the first 3 years.

Prevention

Early breastfeeding prevents atopic symptoms. Preventive strategies include exclusive breastfeeding and avoidance of solid foods for at least 4 months. In atopic families, hydrolysed formula prevents eczema (Berg et al. 2010). Immunomodulation may be important, using probiotic (*Lactobacillus*) (Kalliomaki et al. 2003) or prebiotic (Moro et al. 2006).

Pancreatic disease

Cystic fibrosis

Cystic fibrosis is an autosomal recessive condition affecting 1 : 3000 live births (Massie et al. 2010). The cystic fibrosis transmembrane conductance regulator (CFTR) regulates chloride and electrolyte transport across the cell membrane (Doull 2001; Welsh 2010). The commonest mutation is a single amino-acid substitution, ΔF508, which interferes with folding of CFTR so that it is held and degraded by the endoplasmic reticulum. Five classes of mutation are recognised and relate to prognosis and to potential therapy. In class I defects, where CFTR is not produced, for example, aminoglycosides inhibit the effect of a mutant stop codon so that full-length CFTR is made. Around 1000 mutations are known and result in a wide range of severity and clinical phenotype. The carrier rate of cystic fibrosis mutations is about 1 : 25.

Screening

Fetal diagnosis and family planning have reduced the incidence of cystic fibrosis by 17–30% (Massie et al. 2010). Neonatal screening uses the dried blood spot collected in the first week. Serum immune reactive trypsin is elevated in almost all infants with cystic fibrosis, but specificity is poor and so screening now includes DNA mutation analysis (Massie et al. 2010). Neonatal screening is now in place across Europe and North America. The detection of presymptomatic infants offers the chance to provide beneficial early management led by an expert multidisciplinary team from a cystic fibrosis centre, improving nutritional status and with anticipated long-term benefits (Borowitz et al. 2009; Robinson et al. 2009; Sermet-Gaudelus et al. 2010).

Clinical presentation

Most newborns with cystic fibrosis are asymptomatic and found on screening, but neonatal cystic fibrosis may present clinically (Table

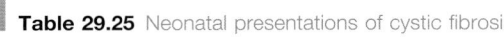

Table 29.25 Neonatal presentations of cystic fibrosis

- Antenatal mutation analysis
- Fetal hyperechogenic bowel
- Fetal gut dilatation
- Fetal intra-abdominal calcification
- Neonatal screening
- Meconium ileus
- Cholestasis
- Meconium peritonitis
- Respiratory infection
- Exocrine pancreatic insufficiency
- Failure to thrive

29.25). Fetal echogenic gut, noted on ultrasound, may mark cystic fibrosis, but it has a low predictive value (Stringer et al. 1996). A total of 10–15% of cystic fibrosis presents with meconium ileus resulting in intestinal obstruction within 48 hours of birth. It is associated with pre- or postnatal perforation, volvulus, chemical or bacterial peritonitis, intestinal atresia and microcolon. Conservative management with intravenous fluids, antibiotics and water-soluble, hyperosmolar contrast enema under fluoroscopic control should only be attempted in a specialised centre in collaboration with a paediatric surgeon. Neonatal mortality in meconium ileus is 10–20% but in survivors outcome is similar to that seen in other children with cystic fibrosis (Coutts et al. 1997).

Cystic fibrosis should not be forgotten as a cause of neonatal cholestasis. Liver function tests are abnormal but liver biopsy may not be diagnostic. Ursodeoxycholic acid is used and jaundice usually clears in infancy.

Sweat testing is possible in the neonatal period but is best attempted from 6 weeks postterm. A single sweat test is not diagnostic. Mutation analysis is usually diagnostic but there remain some unknown mutations.

Management

The support needed by the family whose baby has cystic fibrosis is considerable (Borowitz et al. 2009). The most important management step is referral to a specialised multidisciplinary team (Borowitz et al. 2009; Robinson et al. 2009; Sermet-Gaudelus et al. 2010). Confirmation of diagnosis, genetic counselling, nutritional supervision and monitoring of respiratory function are needed by all. Breastfeeding should be encouraged. Breast milk has lipolytic and anti-infective properties. Alternatively, a standard infant formula is used. Sodium supplements (2 mmol/kg/day) may be necessary. Energy supplements are provided if growth is suboptimal (Table 29.26). A lactose-free hydrolysed protein feed containing medium-chain triglycerides may be better tolerated after meconium ileus. Over 90% of European children with cystic fibrosis have pancreatic insufficiency with fat malabsorption by 12 months of age (Borowitz et al. 2009; Sermet-Gaudelus et al. 2010). Faecal elastase provides a convenient measure of pancreatic function and is reliable even in the preterm from 2 weeks of age. Enzyme replacement therapy is needed by all who are pancreatic-insufficient. Fat-soluble vitamin supplements are given.

Respiratory infection is treated aggressively. Chest physiotherapy to encourage clearance of secretions is commenced in the first months. Evidence does not support the use of prophylactic long-term antibiotics. Influenza immunisation is given and passive immunisation against respiratory syncytial virus is considered. Tobacco smoke exposure must be avoided.

Table 29.26 Nutritional management of cystic fibrosis (Borowitz et al. 2009; Sermet-Gaudelus et al. 2010)

Energy	
Routine	100–130 kcal/kg/day
Poor growth	150–200 kcal/kg/day
Milk	
Routine	Breast milk Standard infant formula
Poor growth	High-energy infant formula or supplement formula with glucose polymer or fat emulsion and glucose polymer or mixed fat and carbohydrate
Postoperative period, after meconium ileus or milk protein intolerance	Hydrolysed protein milk with medium-chain triglycerides
Pancreatic enzymes (acid-resistant microspheres)	
2000 IU lipase/100 ml milk	
Mix with milk or water and give immediately from a spoon before a feed	
Vitamins (daily dose)	
Vitamin A	1500 IU
Vitamin D	400 IU
Vitamin E	40–50 IU
Vitamin K	300 µg

Schwachman–Diamond syndrome

Pancreatic exocrine insufficiency is rare other than in cystic fibrosis. Pancreatic hypoplasia, isolated enzyme deficiencies and a number of rare syndromes (e.g. Johanson–Blizzard, Pearson's) may be associated with malabsorption.

Schwachman syndrome comprises pancreatic exocrine insufficiency, usually presenting in infancy, and variable or cyclical neutropenia, which may lead to clinical immunodeficiency. Short stature and metaphyseal dysplasia are characteristic. Pancreatic enzyme replacement is needed in infancy.

References

Agostoni, C., Axelsson, I., Goulet, O., et al., 2006. Soy protein infant formulae and follow-on formulae: a commentary by the ESPGHAN Committee on Nutrition. J Pediatr Gastroenterol Nutr 42, 352–361.

Agwu, J.C., Narchi, H., 2005. In a preterm infant, does blood transfusion increase the risk of necrotizing enterocolitis? Arch Dis Child 90, 102–103.

Bedu, A., Faure, C., Sibony, O., et al., 1994. Prenatal gastrointestinal bleeding caused by esophagitis and gastritis. J Pediatr 125, 465–467.

Beeby, P.J., Jeffrey, H., 1992. Risk factors for necrotising enterocolitis: the influence of gestational age. Arch Dis Child 67, 432–435.

Bell, M.J., Ternberg, J.L., Feigin, R.D., et al., 1978. Neonatal necrotizing enterocolitis: therapeutic decisions based upon clinical staging. Ann Surg 187, 1–7.

Berg, A., Krämer, U., Link, E., et al., 2010. Impact of early feeding on childhood eczema: development after nutritional intervention compared with the natural course – the GINIplus study up to the age of 6 years. Clin Exp Allergy 40, 627–636.

Berseth, C.L., 1994. Gut motility and the pathogenesis of necrotizing enterocolitis. Clin Perinatol 21, 263–270.

Berseth, C.L., Nordyke, C., 1993. Enteral nutrients promote postnatal maturation of intestinal motor activity in preterm infants. Am J Physiol 264, G1046–G1051.

Berseth, C.L., Bisquera, J.A., Paje, V.U., 2003. Prolonging small feeding volumes early in life decreases the incidence of necrotizing enterocolitis in very low birth weight infants. Pediatrics 111, 529–534.

Birch, J.L., Newell, S.J., 2009. Gastrooesophageal reflux disease in preterm infants: current management and diagnostic dilemmas. Arch Dis Child 94, F379–F383.

Bombell, S., McGuire, W., 2009. Early trophic feeding for very low birth weight infants. Cochrane Database Syst Rev (8), CD000504.

Book, L.S., Herbst, J.J., Atherton, S.O., et al., 1975. Necrotizing enterocolitis in low birth weight infants fed an elemental formula. J Pediatr 87, 602–605.

Booth, I.W., 1985. Defective jejunal brush border Na⁺/H⁺ exchange: a cause of congenital secretory diarrhoea. Lancet 1, 1066–1069.

Borowitz, D., Robinson, K.A., Rosenfeld, M., et al., 2009. Cystic fibrosis foundation evidence-based guidelines for management of infants with cystic fibrosis. J Pediatr 155, S73–S93.

Bunn, S.K., Beath, S.V., McKeirnan, P.J., et al., 2000. Treatment of microvillus inclusion disease by intestinal transplantation. J Pediatr Gastroenterol Nutr 31, 176–180.

Canani, R.B., Terrin, G., Cardillo, G., et al., 2010. Congenital diarrheal disorders: Improved understanding of gene defects is leading to advances in intestinal physiology and clinical management. J Pediatr Gastroenterol Nutr 50, 360–366.

Caplan, M.S., Hedlund, E., Adler, L., et al., 1994. Role of asphyxia and feeding in a neonatal rat model of necrotizing enterocolitis. Pediatr Pathol 14, 1017–1028.

Chaet, M.S., Farrell, M.K., Ziegler, M.M., et al., 1994. Intensive nutritional support and remedial surgical intervention for extreme short bowel syndrome. J Pediatr Gastroenterol Nutr 19, 295–298.

Chan, K.L., Saing, H., Yung, R.W.H., et al., 1994. A study of pre-antibiotic bacteriology in 125 patients with necrotizing enterocolitis. Acta Paediatr Suppl 396, 45–48.

Chardot, C., Rochet, J.S., Lezeau, H., et al., 2003. Surgical necrotizing enterocolitis: are intestinal lesions more severe in infants with low birth weight? J Pediatr Surg 38, 167–172.

Clark, D.A., 1977. Times of first void and first stool in 500 newborns. Pediatrics 60, 457–459.

Clark, D.A., Miller, M.J.S., 1996. What causes neonatal necrotising enterocolitis and how can it be prevented? In: Hansen, T.N., McIntosh, N. (Eds.), Current Topics in Neonatology 1. W B Saunders, London, pp. 160–176.

Claud, E.C., 2009. Neonatal necrotizing enterocolitis – inflammation and intestinal immaturity. Antiinflammatory Antiallergy Agents Med Chem 8, 248–259.

Communicable Disease Report, 1982. Neonatal necrotising enterocolitis surveillance. In: Communicable Disease Report 82/05. Communicable Disease Surveillance Centre, London.

Coppa, G.V., Zampini, L., Galeazzi, T., et al., 2006. Prebiotics in human milk: a review. Digest Liver Dis 38, S291–S294.

Cotton, C.M., 2010. Early, prolonged use of postnatal antibiotics increased the risk of necrotising enterocolitis. Arch Dis Child 95, 94.

Coutts, J.A., Docherty, J.G., Carachi, R., et al., 1997. Clinical course of patients with cystic fibrosis presenting with meconium ileus. Br J Surg 84, 555.

Davey, A.M., Wagner, C.L., Cox, C., et al., 1994. Feeding premature infants while low umbilical artery catheters are in place: a prospective, randomized trial. J Pediatr 124, 795–799.

De Boissieu, D., Dupont, C., Barbet, J.P., et al., 1994. Distinct features of upper gastrointestinal endoscopy in the newborn. J Pediatr Gastroenterol Nutr 18, 334–338.

De la Torre, L., Carrasco, D., Mora, M.A., et al., 2002. Vascular malformations of the colon in children. J Pediatr Surg 37, 1754–1757.

Deshpande, G., Rao, S., Patole, S., et al., 2010. Updated meta-analysis of probiotics for preventing necrotizing enterocolitis in preterm neonates. Pediatrics 125, 921–930.

Dhillon, A.S., Ewer, A.K., 2004. Diagnosis and management of gastroesophageal reflux in preterm infants in neonatal intensive care units. Acta Paediatr 93, 88–93.

Dorling, J., Kempley, S., Leaf, A., 2005. Feeding growth restricted preterm infants with abnormal antenatal Doppler results. Arch Dis Child 90, F359–F363.

Doull, I.J.M., 2001. Recent advances in cystic fibrosis. Arch Dis Child 85, 62–66.

Dvorak, B., Halpern, M.D., Holubec, H., et al., 2003. Maternal milk reduces severity of necrotizing enterocolitis and increases intestinal IL-10 in a neonatal rat model. Pediatr Res 53, 426–433.

Ewer, A.K., 2002. Role of platelet-activating factor in the pathophysiology of necrotizing enterocolitis. Acta Paediatr Suppl 91, 2–5.

Ewer, A.K., Yu, V.Y., 1996. Gastric emptying in pre-term infants the effect of breast milk fortifier. Acta Paediatr 85, 1112–1115.

Ewer, A.K., McHugo, J.M., Chapman, S., et al., 1993. Fetal echogenic gut: a marker of intrauterine gut ischaemia. Arch Dis Child 69, 510–513.

Ewer, A.K., Durbin, G.M., Morgan, M.E., et al., 1994. Gastric emptying in preterm infants. Arch Dis Child 71, F24–F27.

Ewer, A.K., James, M.E., Tobin, J.M., 1999. Prone and left lateral positioning reduce gastro-oesophageal reflux in preterm infants. Arch Dis Child Fetal Neonatal Ed 81, F201–F205.

Fast, C., Rosegger, H., 1994. Necrotizing enterocolitis prophylaxis: oral antibiotics and lyophilized enterobacteria vs oral immunoglobulins. Acta Paediatr (Suppl) 396, 86–90.

Feranchak, A., Orenstein, S., Cohn, J., 1994. Behaviours associated with onset of gastraoesophageal reflux episodes in infants. Clin Pediatr 33, 654–661.

Fitzgibbons, S.C., Ching, Y., Yu, D., et al., 2009. Mortality of necrotizing enterocolitis expressed by birth weight categories. J Pediatr Surg 44, 1072–1075.

Guarino, A., De Marco, G., 2003. Natural history of intestinal failure, investigated through a national network-based approach. J Pediatr Gastroenterol Nutr 37, 136–141.

Guillet, R., Stoll, B.J., Cotton, M., et al., 2006. Association of H_2-blocker therapy and higher incidence of necrotizing enterocolitis in very low birth weight infants. Pediatrics 117, e137–e142.

Hentschel, R., Hensel, D., Brune, T., et al., 1995. Impact of blood pressure and intestinal perfusion of dobutamine or dopamine in hypotensive preterm infants. Biol Neonate 68, 318–324.

Heyman, M.B., 2006. Lactose intolerance in infants, children, and adolescents. Pediatrics 118, 1279–1286.

Horwitz, J.R., Lally, K.P., Cheu, H.W., et al., 1995. Complications after surgical intervention in necrotizing enterocolitis: a multicenter review. J Pediatr Surg 30, 994–999.

James, M.E., Ewer, A.K., 1999. Acid oro-pharyngeal secretions can predict gastro-oesophageal reflux in preterm infants. Eur J Pediatr 158, 371–374.

Jancelewicz, T., Kim, G., Miniati, D., 2008. Neonatal appendicitis: a new look at an old zebra. J Pediatr Surg 43, E1–E5.

Janik, J.S., Ein, S.H., Mancer, K., 1981. Intestinal stricture after necrotizing enterocolitis. J Pediatr Surg 16, 438–443.

Jilling, T., Lu, J., Jackson, M., et al., 2004. Intestinal epithelial apoptosis initiates gross bowel necrosis in an experimental rat model of neonatal necrotizing enterocolitis. Pediatr Res 55, 622–629.

Jones, L.J., Craven, P.D., Attia, J., et al., 2011. Network meta-analysis of indomethacin versus ibuprofen versus placebo for PDA in preterm infants. Arch Dis Child 96, F45–F52.

Josephson, C.D., Wesolowski, A., Bao, G., et al., 2010. Do red cell transfusions increase the risk of necrotizing enterocolitis in premature infants? J Pediatr 157, 972–978.

Kalliomaki, M., Salminen, S., Poussa, T., et al., 2003. Probiotics and prevention of atopic disease: 4-year follow-up of a randomised placebo-controlled trial. Lancet 361, 1869–1871.

Kelly, E.J., Newell, S.J., 1994. Gastric ontogeny: clinical implications. Arch Dis Child 71, F136–F141.

Kempley, S.T., Bennett, S., Loftus, B.G., et al., 1993. Randomised trial of umbilical arterial position: clinical outcome. Acta Paediatr 83, 173–176.

Kennedy, K.A., Tyson, J.E., Chamnanvanakij, S., 2000. Rapid versus slow rate of advancement of feedings for promoting growth and preventing necrotizing enterocolitis in parenterally fed low-birth-weight infants. Cochrane Database Syst Rev (2), CD001241.

Kenyon, S.L., Taylor, D.J., Tarnow-Mordi, W., 2001. Broad-spectrum antibiotics for preterm, prelabour rupture of fetal membranes: the ORACLE I randomised trial. ORACLE Collaborative Group. Lancet 357, 979–988.

Kiely, E.M., 1990. Surgery for gastro-oesophageal reflux. Arch Dis Child 65, 1291–1292.

Kliegman, R.M., Fanaroff, A.A., 1981. Neonatal necrotizing enterocolitis: a nine year experience. I. Epidemiology and uncommon observations. Am J Dis Child 135, 603–607.

Kliegman, R.M., Walker, W.A., Yolken, R.H., 1993. Necrotizing enterocolitis: research agenda for a disease of unknown etiology and pathogenesis. Pediatr Res 34, 701–708.

Köglmeier, J., Day, C., Puntis, J.W.L., 2008. Clinical outcome in patients from a single region who were dependent on parenteral nutrition for 28 days or more. Arch Dis Child 93, 300–302.

Lamireau, T., Llanas, B., Chateil, J.F., et al., 1996. Frequence accrué et difficultés diagnostiques des stenose intestinales apres enterocolite ulceronecrosante. Arch Pediatr 3, 9–15.

Lao, O.B., Healey, P.J., Perkins, J.D., et al., 2010. Outcomes in children after intestinal transplant. Pediatrics 125, e550–e558.

Leaf, A., Dorling, J., Kempley, S., et al., 2010. Early or late enteral feeding for preterm growth-restricted infants? The abnormal Doppler enteral prescription trial. Arch Dis Child 95, A3.

Liefaard, G., Heineman, E., Molenaar, J.C., et al., 1995. Prospective evaluation of the absorptive capacity of the bowel after major and minor resections in the neonate. J Pediatr Surg 30, 388–391.

Llanos, A.R., Moss, M.E., Pinzon, M.E., et al., 2002. Epidemiology of neonatal necrotising enterocolitis: a population based study. Paediatr Perinatal Epidemiol 16, 342–349.

Lopez-Alonso, M., Moya, M.J., Cabo, J.A., et al., 2006. Twenty-four hour esophageal-impedance-pH monitoring in healthy preterm neonates: Rate and characteristics of acid, weakly acidic and weakly alkaline gastroesophageal reflux. Pediatrics 118, e299–308.

Lucas, A., Cole, T.J., 1990. Breast milk and neonatal necrotising enterocolitis. Lancet 336, 1519–1523.

Lucas, A., Morley, R., 1998. Necrotising Enterocolitis. British Paediatric Surveillance Unit, London.

Maki, M., Ruuska, T., Kuusela, A.-L., 1993. High prevalence of asymptomatic esophageal and gastric lesions in preterm infants in intensive care. Crit Care Med 21, 1863–1867.

Massie, J., Curnow, L., Gaffney, L., et al., 2010. Declining prevalence of cystic fibrosis since the introduction of newborn screening. Arch Dis Child 95, 531–533.

McClure, R.J., Newell, S.J., 1996. Effect of fortifying breast milk on gastric emptying. Arch Dis Child 74, F60–F62.

McClure, R.J., Newell, S.J., 1999. Randomised controlled trial of trophic feeding and gut motility. Arch Dis Child 80, F54–F58.

McClure, R.J., Newell, S.J., 2000. Randomised controlled trial of clinical outcome following trophic feeding. Arch Dis Child Fetal Neonatal Ed 82, F29–F33.

McGuire, W., Anthony, M.Y., 2003. Donor human milk versus formula for preventing necrotising enterocolitis in preterm infants: systematic review. Arch Dis Child Fetal Neonatal Ed 88, F11–F14.

McKeown, R.E., Marsh, T.D., Amarnath, U., et al., 1992. Role of delayed feeding and of feeding increments in necrotizing enterocolitis. J Pediatr 121, 764–770.

Meinzen-Derr, J., Poindexter, B., Wrage, L., et al., 2009. Role of human milk in extremely low birth weight infants' risk of necrotizing enterocolitis or death. J Perinatol 29, 57–62.

Misra, S., Macwan, K., Albert, V., 2007. Transpyloric feeding in gastroesophageal-reflux associated apnea ion premature infants. Acta Paediatr 96, 1426–1429.

Montalto, M., D'Onofrio, F., Santoro, L., et al., 2009. Autoimmune enteropathy in children and adults. Scand J Gastroenterol 44, 1029–1036.

Moro, G., Arslanoglu, S., Stahl, B., et al., 2006. A mixture of prebiotic oligosaccharides reduces the incidence of atopic dermatitis during the first six months of age. Arch Dis Child 91, 814–819.

Mshvildadze, M., Neu, J., 2010. The infant intestinal microbiome: Friend or foe? Early Hum Dev 86, S67–S71.

Newell, S.J., 1996. Gastrointestinal function and its ontogeny: how should we feed the preterm infant. In: Ryan, S. (Ed.), Seminars in Neonatology 1. W B Saunders, London, pp. 59–66.

Newell, S.J., 2000. Enteral feeding in the micropremie. Clin Perinatol 27, 221.

Newell, S.J., Booth, I.W., Morgan, M.E., et al., 1989. Gastro-oesophageal reflux in preterm infants. Arch Dis Child 64, 780–786.

Newell, S.J., Chapman, S., Booth, I.W., 1993. Ultrasonic assessment of gastric emptying in the preterm infant. Arch Dis Child 69, 32–36.

Ng, S.C., Quak, S.H., 1998. Gastroesophageal reflux in preterm infants: norms for extended distal esophageal pH monitoring. J Pediatr Gastroenterol Nutr 27, 411–414.

Omari, T.I., Davidson, G.P., 2003. Multipoint measurement of intragastric pH in healthy preterm infants. Arch Dis Child 88, F517–F520.

Omari, T.I., Barnett, C.P., Benninga, M.A., et al., 2002. Mechanisms of gastro-oesophageal reflux in preterm and term infants with reflux disease. Gut 51, 475–479.

Omari, T.I., Rommel, N., Staunton, E., et al., 2004. Paradoxical impact of body positioning on gastroesophageal reflux and gastric emptying in the premature neonate. J Pediatr 145, 194–200.

Ozek, E., Soll, R., Schimmel, M.S., 2010. Partial exchange transfusion to prevent neurodevelopmental disability in infants with polycythemia. Cochrane Database Syst Rev (20), CD005089.

Papaila, J.G., Wilmot, D., Grosfeld, J.L., et al., 1989. Increased incidence of delayed gastric emptying in children with gastroesophageal reflux. A prospective evaluation. Arch Surg 124, 933–936.

Patole, S.K., de Klerk, N., 2005. Impact of standardised feeding regimens on

incidence of neonatal necrotising enterocolitis: a systematic review and meta-analysis of observational studies. Arch Dis Child 90, 147–151.

Pierro, A., Eaton, S., Rees, C.M., et al., 2010. Is there a benefit of peritoneal drainage for necrotizing enterocolitis in newborn infants? J Pediatr Surg 45, 2117–2118.

Pritchard, J.A., 1966. Fetal swallowing and amniotic fluid volume. Obstet Gynaecol 28, 606–610.

Pumberger, W., Mayr, M., Kohlhauser, C., et al., 2002. Spontaneous localized intestinal perforation in very-low-birth-weight infants: a distinct clinical entity different from necrotizing enterocolitis. J Am Coll Surg 195, 796–803.

Puntis, J.W., 2001. Nutritional support at home and in the community. Arch Dis Child 84, 295–298.

Raval, N.C., Gonzalez, E., Bhat, A.M., et al., 1995. Umbilical venous catheters: evaluation of radiographs to determine position and associated complications of malpositioned umbilical venous catheters. Am J Perinatol 12, 201–204.

Rees, C.M., Hall, N.J., Eaton, S., et al., 2005. Surgical strategies for necrotising enterocolitis: a survey of practice in the United Kingdom. Arch Dis Child 90, F152–F155.

Rees, C.M., Pierro, A., Eaton, S., 2007. Neurodevelopmental outcomes of neonates with medically and surgically treated necrotizing enterocolitis. Arch Dis Child 92, F193–F198.

Rees, C.M., Simon Eaton, S., Agostino Pierro, A., 2010. National prospective surveillance study of necrotizing enterocolitis in neonatal intensive care units. J Pediatr Surg 45, 1391–1397.

Rescorla, F.J., 1995. Surgical management of pediatric necrotizing enterocolitis. Curr Opin Pediatr 7, 335–341.

Robinson, K.A., Saldanha, I.J., McKoy, N.A., 2009. Management of infants with cystic fibrosis: A summary of the evidence for the cystic fibrosis foundation working group on care of infants with cystic fibrosis. J Pediatr 155, S94–105.

Rotbart, H.A., Levin, M.J., 1983. How contagious is necrotizing enterocolitis? Pediatr Infect Dis J 2, 406–410.

Rouwet, E.V., Heineman, E., Buurman, W.A., et al., 2002. Intestinal permeability and carrier-mediated monosaccharide absorption in preterm neonates during the early postnatal period. Pediatr Res 51, 64–70.

Rowe, M.I., Reblock, K.K., Kurkchubasche, A.G., et al., 1994. Necrotizing enterocolitis in the extremely low birth weight infant. J Pediatr Surg 29, 987–990.

Ruemmele, F.M., Jan, D., Lacaille, F., et al., 2004. New perspectives for children with microvillous inclusion disease: early small bowel transplantation. Transplantation 77, 1024–1028.

Schimpl, G., Hollwarth, M.E., Fotter, R., et al., 1994. Late intestinal strictures following successful treatment of necrotizing enterocolitis. Acta Paediatr Suppl 396, 80–83.

Sermet-Gaudelus, I., Mayell, S.J., Southern, K.W., 2010. Guidelines on the early management of infants diagnosed with cystic fibrosis following newborn screening. J Cystic Fibrosis 9, 323–329.

Soll, R.F., 2010. Probiotics: are we ready for routine use? Pediatrics 125, 1071–1072.

Spitz, L., Stringer, M.D., 1993. Surgical management of neonatal necrotising enterocolitis. Arch Dis Child 69, 269–271.

Stringer, M.D., Puntis, J.W.L., 1995. Short bowel syndrome. Arch Dis Child 73, 170–173.

Stringer, M.D., Thornton, J.G., Mason, G.C., 1996. Hyperechoic bowel. Arch Dis Child 74, F1–F2.

Tarnow-Mordi, W.O., Wilkinson, D., Trivedi, A., et al., 2010. Probiotics reduce all-cause mortality and necrotizing enterocolitis: It is time to change practice. Pediatrics 125, 1068–1070.

Uauy, R.D., Fanaroff, A.A., Korones, S.B., et al., 1991. Necrotizing enterocolitis in very low birth weight infants: biodemographic and clinical correlates. National Institute of Child Health and Human Development Neonatal Research Network. J Pediatr 119, 630–638.

Vandenplas, Y., Rudolph, C.D., 2009. Pediatric gastroesophageal reflux clinical practice guidelines: Joint recommendations of the North American Society for Pediatric Gastroenterology, Hepatology, and Nutrition (NASPGHAN) and the European Society for Pediatric Gastroenterology, Hepatology, and Nutrition (ESPGHAN). J Pediatr Gastroenterol Nutr 49, 498–547.

Vandenplas, Y., Sacre Smits, L., 1987. Continuous 24-hour esophageal pH monitoring in 285 asymptomatic infants 0–15 months old. J Pediatr Gastroenterol Nutr 6, 220–224.

Vandenplas, Y., Goyvaerts, H., Helven, R., et al., 1991. Gastroesophageal reflux, as measured by 24-hour pH monitoring, in 509 healthy infants screened for risk of sudden infant death syndrome. Pediatrics 88, 834–840.

Vandenplas, Y., Brueton, M., Dupont, C., et al., 2007. Guidelines for the diagnosis and management of cow's milk protein allergy in infants. Arch Dis Child 92, 902–908.

Vanderhoof, J., Young, R., Thompson, J., 2003. New and emerging therapies for short bowel syndrome in children. Paediatr Drugs 5, 525–531.

Vinton, N.E., 1994. Gastrointestinal bleeding in infancy and childhood. Gastroenterol Clin North Am 23, 93–122.

Walsh, M.C., Kliegman, R.M., 1986. Necrotizing enterocolitis: treatment based on staging criteria. Pediatr Clin North Am 33, 179–201.

Weaver, L.T., Lucas, A., 1990. Maturation of large bowel function in relation to gestational and postnatal age, feed volumes and composition in the newborn. Pediatr Rev Commun 4, 250.

Welsh, M.J., 2010. Targeting the basic defect in cystic fibrosis. N Engl J Med 363, 2056–2057.

Wood, C.M., Spicer, R.D., Beddis, I.R., et al., 1995. Pancreatic exocrine failure in cystic fibrosis presenting as necrotising enterocolitis. J Pediatr Gastroenterol Nutr 20, 104–106.

Part 4: **Congenital defects and surgical problems**

Ian Sugarman   Mark D Stringer   Alistair G Smyth

Introduction

This chapter discusses the management of major surgical conditions affecting the neonatal alimentary tract. Most are congenital malformations and, as such, are frequently multiple. Conditions are discussed in sequence down the gut, rather than in order of importance or severity. Some preliminary general comments about neonatal gastrointestinal surgery are necessary.

The survival of babies with congenital malformations has improved progressively as a result of advances in neonatal care and the concentration of these infants within specialist paediatric surgical units. An integrated multidisciplinary approach is essential in the management of premature surgical neonates and in those with complex congenital malformations (British Association of Paediatric Surgeons/Royal College of Surgeons of England 1999).

Prenatal ultrasound diagnosis of major structural gastrointestinal anomalies presents parents and clinicians with the opportunity to terminate the pregnancy or to deliver the baby in a centre with ready access to paediatric surgical expertise; in rare instances, fetal intervention may be appropriate (Ch. 9). Prenatal diagnosis of gastrointestinal anomalies has had a major impact on the management of anterior abdominal wall defects in particular, not least because parents can be informed about management and prognosis. In other conditions, interpretation of ultrasound findings is less clear-cut. For example, hyperechogenic fetal bowel (bowel of similar or greater echogenicity than surrounding bone; Fig. 29.32) may indicate the presence of meconium ileus, cytomegalovirus infection or intestinal obstruction but it is a relatively soft marker of fetal pathology and most affected fetuses are normal after birth (Stringer et al. 1996). Similarly, intestinal dilatation is non-specific and may be seen in the fetus with midgut or hindgut atresia, meconium ileus, malrotation or Hirschsprung disease (Richards and Holmes 1995).

Many congenital gastrointestinal malformations present with symptoms and signs of intestinal obstruction in the newborn.

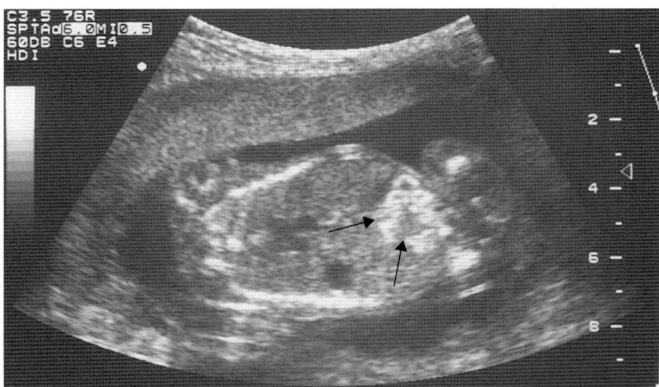

Fig. 29.32 Sonographic cross-section of the fetal abdomen at 18 weeks' gestation showing hyperechogenic fetal bowel as bright as bone (arrows).

Vomiting

This will be bile-stained if the obstruction is beyond the level of the ampulla of Vater. Bilious vomiting in the newborn should be attributed to intestinal obstruction until proven otherwise. In one prospective study of 63 consecutive neonates with bilious vomiting, a surgical cause was identified in 24 (38%): Hirschsprung disease in nine, small bowel atresia in five, intestinal malrotation in four, meconium ileus in three, meconium plug in one, colonic atresia in one and milk inspissation in one (Godbole and Stringer 2002). Most of these babies had abdominal signs and an abnormal abdominal radiograph. No surgical cause for bilious vomiting was found in 39 (62%) infants, whose symptoms resolved with conservative management. All neonates with bilious vomiting require careful review with a very low threshold for further investigation. Intestinal malrotation must be excluded. First-line investigations consist of a detailed clinical examination, a plain radiograph of the chest and abdomen, routine haematology and biochemistry, and blood and urine cultures. A more detailed septic screen may be indicated. Abdominal ultrasound and gastrointestinal contrast studies are often warranted and, in selected cases, a rectal biopsy may be necessary.

Abdominal distension

An algorithm for assessing a baby who develops marked abdominal distension soon after birth is shown in Figure 29.33. This must be interpreted in conjunction with the baby's gestational age and general condition.

Delay or failure to pass meconium

Over 95% of healthy term infants pass their first stool within 24 hours of birth (Sherry and Kramer 1955). Delayed passage of meconium after 48 hours in a term infant should always suggest the possibility of intestinal obstruction. However, such a delay is normal in premature infants (Weaver and Lucas 1993). In any baby who fails to pass meconium normally, the anus should be examined and its patency confirmed.

All babies with clinical features of intestinal obstruction should receive parenteral vitamin K. Bleeding is a rare manifestation of congenital gastrointestinal anomalies and more often indicates acquired disease. Upper gastrointestinal bleeding may be due to swallowed maternal blood, vitamin K deficiency bleeding or oesophagitis/gastritis. Peptic ulceration occurs occasionally and can be confirmed by endoscopy. Rectal bleeding in an otherwise well baby is most commonly due to an anal fissure or cow's milk protein intolerance. In a sick infant it may be from necrotising enterocolitis or malrotation with volvulus.

Mouth and nasopharynx

Cleft lip and palate

Cleft lip and palate is the commonest congenital anomaly in the craniofacial region, with an incidence in the UK of approximately 1:700 live births. Most clefts are diagnosed at birth but the diagnosis may be made by prenatal ultrasound scan. Cleft lip is twice as

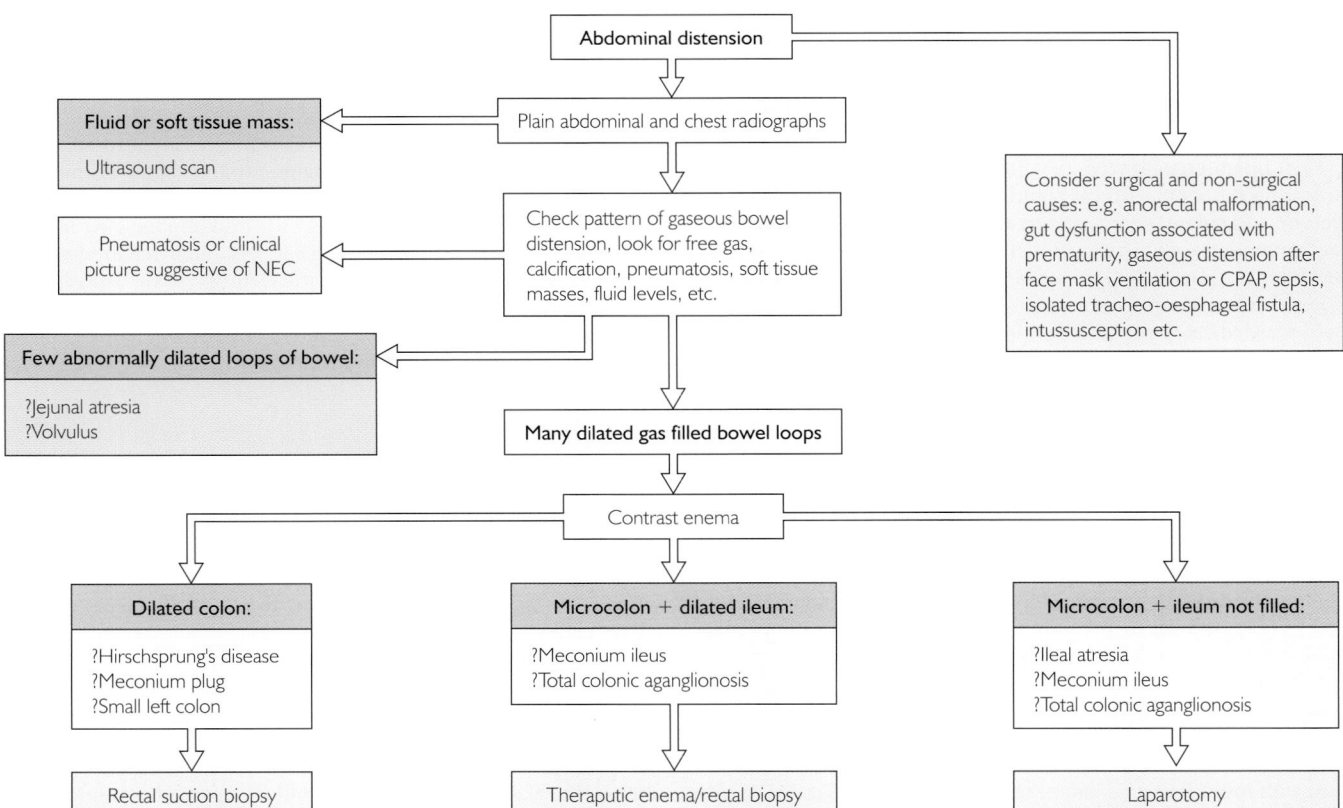

Fig. 29.33 An algorithm for investigating the neonate who develops abdominal distension soon after birth. This must be interpreted in conjunction with clinical and routine laboratory assessments. CPAP, continuous positive airway pressure; NEC, necrotising enterocolitis.

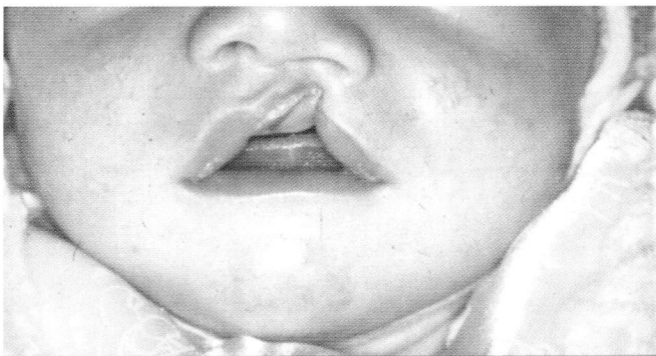

Fig. 29.34 Unilateral incomplete cleft lip.

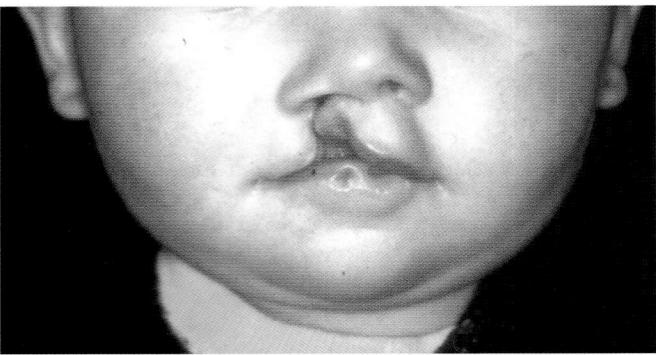

Fig. 29.35 Complete cleft lip and lower lip pits (Van der Woude syndrome).

common on the left side than on the right but the reason for this remains obscure. Cleft lip with or without cleft palate is more than twice as common in males, whereas cleft palate alone is twice as common in females. In most patients the orofacial cleft will be the only defect. However, approximately 15% of all patients with cleft lip and/or palate will have other associated abnormalities, which together may form part of a recognised syndrome. With regard to non-syndromic cleft lip and palate, a family history of the condition may be present or a history of maternal exposure to drugs such as phenytoin. All babies presenting with cleft lip and/or palate should have a full examination and a standard karyotype investigation.

Isolated cleft palate accounts for about 50% of all clefts, the remaining groups consisting of unilateral cleft lip and palate (20%), cleft lip (20%) and bilateral cleft lip and palate (10%). This complex deformity can affect many aspects of development, including speech, hearing, facial appearance, dental development and facial growth. Treatment requires a multidisciplinary approach from birth to maturity. Outcomes can be remarkably good when this is provided in a skilled and coordinated manner and remarkably bad when it is not (Shaw et al. 1996).

Cleft lip and palate services within the UK changed dramatically following the 1998 Clinical Standards Advisory Group report into cleft lip and palate services and treatment outcomes. This document recommended a reduction in cleft units within the UK from the previous 57 units to 8–15 specialist centres, allowing a concentration of expertise and resources. All patients should be cared for within a dedicated multidisciplinary cleft team with full access to the necessary specialist services.

Cleft lip

A cleft lip may result when fusion between the medial and lateral nasal processes with the maxillary process fails to occur. Cleft lip may occur in isolation or in conjunction with cleft palate. The lip cleft is usually to one side of the midline and may be incomplete (Fig. 29.34) or involve the full height of the lip (complete), extending into the floor of the nose. The cleft may be unilateral or bilateral and may extend on to the gum area (alveolus) of the upper jaw. Babies with isolated cleft lip usually manage to feed well from a soft bottle with teat and in many cases may also successfully breastfeed.

A rare midline cleft of the upper lip may occur as part of an orofacial–digital syndrome (type I). Cleft lip can also occur in conjunction with lower lip pits – Van der Woude syndrome (Fig. 29.35), an autosomal dominant condition with variable expressivity.

Outcomes from cleft lip treatment are often excellent and surgical repair is usually undertaken at around 3 months of age using a

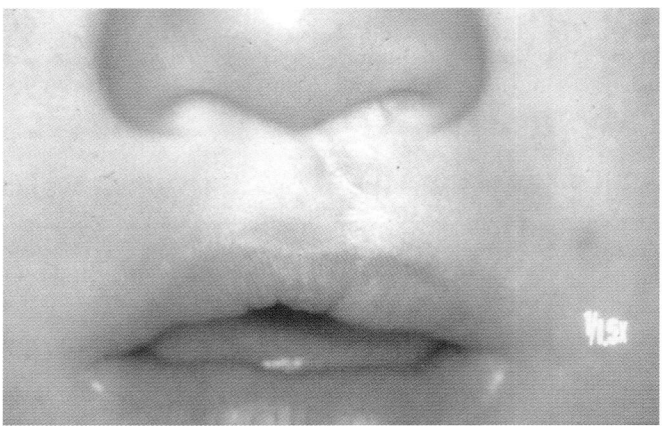

Fig. 29.36 Cleft lip and nose repair (same child as in Fig. 29.34).

modification of the Millard rotation–advancement method of repair. This includes a careful realignment and repair of the mid-facial and labial muscles. Primary nasal correction is carried out at the same time as lip repair (Fig. 29.36). In complete cleft lip and palate, the anterior palate (hard palate) is often repaired with a vomerine flap at the same time as the cleft lip repair. The alveolar bony cleft is usually not repaired at the same time as primary lip or palate surgery owing to maxillary growth impairment in the growing child, but delayed into later childhood.

Cleft palate

Palatal fusion begins around the 8th week of intrauterine life and occurs from the front of the palate to the back. Interference with palatal shelf fusion from extrinsic factors such as phenytoin or intrinsic factors such as genetic predisposition or obstructing tongue position may result in a cleft palate. Cleft palate may occur in isolation or in combination with cleft lip. Isolated cleft palate may involve the posterior palate alone (soft palate) or may extend further forward into the hard palate up to the incisive foramen just behind the front teeth (complete cleft palate). Cleft palate is a midline defect and may be incomplete or complete (Fig. 29.37).

Isolated cleft palate cannot be diagnosed antenatally and is noted after birth. Nasal regurgitation of milk is not pathognomonic of cleft palate and exclusion requires direct inspection of the full palate with a good light source with the tongue depressed. Digital palpation of the palate by itself is not sufficient, as incomplete clefts can

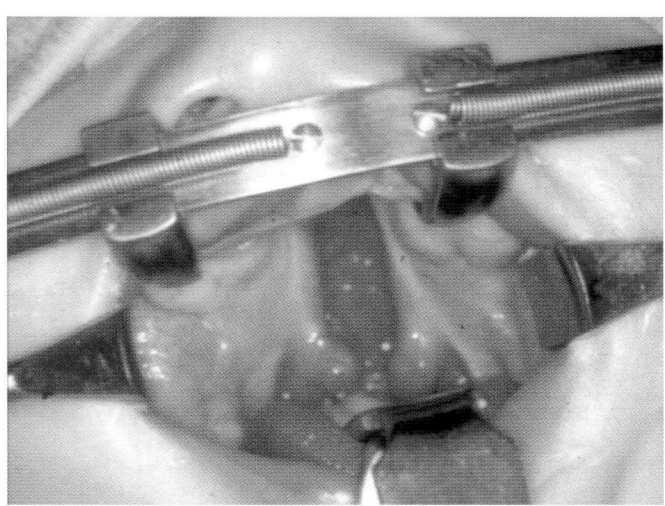

Fig. 29.37 Isolated cleft palate (seen at time of surgery).

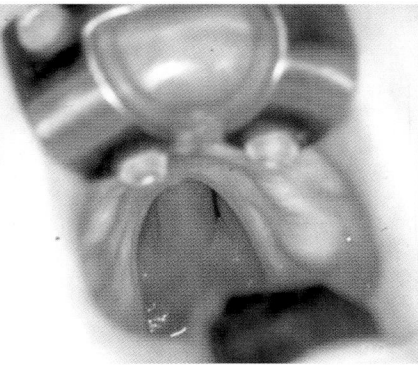

Fig. 29.39 Wide U-shaped cleft palate (Pierre Robin sequence).

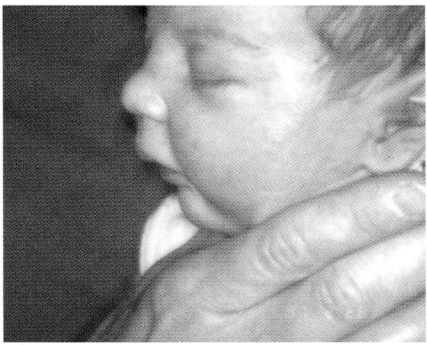

Fig. 29.38 Pierre Robin sequence (note micrognathia).

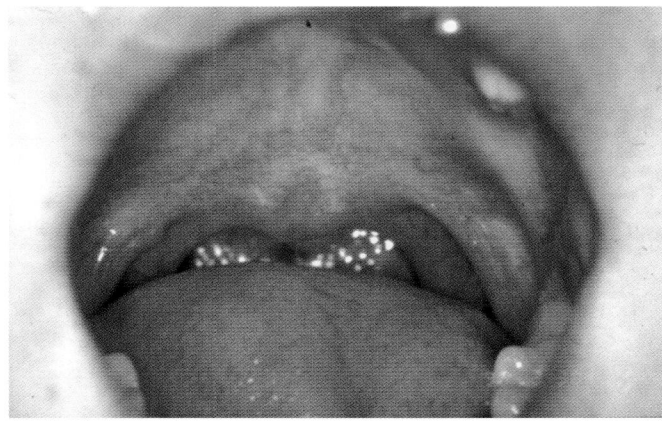

Fig. 29.40 Submucous cleft palate showing bifid uvula and midline groove/translucent line of soft palate.

be easily missed (Ch. 14). Babies with cleft palate have difficulty with suction and are unlikely to breastfeed properly. Assisted feeding (of formula or expressed breast milk) is often required using a soft bottle and teat. Midline clefts such as cleft palate are more likely to be associated with a chromosomal defect and therefore all babies born with cleft palate should have a fluorescent in situ hybridisation test for a chromosomal microdeletion on chromosome 22 (Catch-22, see Ch. 31) as well as a standard karyotype.

Pierre Robin sequence (Fig. 29.38) is the association of an often wide U-shaped cleft palate (Fig. 29.39) with a small mandible (micrognathia) and a posteriorly placed tongue. Upper airway obstruction is a common association, which may require intervention such as positioning the infant (side or prone) or insertion of a nasopharyngeal airway. Tracheostomy is rarely required. Pierre Robin-associated syndromes should be considered, such as Stickler syndrome and velo-cardio-facial syndrome (22q11 deletion).

Surgical repair of cleft palate is usually carried out at around 8–9 months of age using local tissues and includes repair of the soft palate muscles. When possible, cleft palate should be repaired before 18 months of age as later repairs are associated with reducing outcomes in speech quality. In Pierre Robin sequence cleft palate, the repair may be delayed to 1 year of age or older, depending on the degree of micrognathia and associated airway obstruction.

A subtype of cleft palate called a submucous cleft palate is often difficult to diagnose and typically may not present until the child

is 4 or more years of age, often with accompanying speech problems. Indicators of a submucous cleft palate may include a bifid uvula, midline translucent zone of the soft palate and a palpable notch at the back of the hard palate (Fig. 29.40).

Children with a history of cleft palate require screening for chronic otitis media with effusion, which may require insertion of grommets or provision of a hearing aid. Speech and language monitoring is required for the possible development of cleft-type characteristics and velopharyngeal incompetence during speech.

Alveolar bone grafts

Clefts that involve the gum area (alveolus) of the upper jaw may benefit from the insertion of a bone graft to allow tooth eruption, provide bone support for the teeth and upper jaw and close off any remaining fistula. Secondary bone grafting just before the eruption of the permanent canine tooth produces the best outcome and is usually carried out between 9 and 11 years of age (Fig. 29.41).

Other facial clefts

Other, more extensive facial clefts are rare. The pathogenesis of these facial clefts such as the lateral and oblique facial cleft remains uncertain. The soft-tissue clefts frequently involve the underlying facial bones and the orbit and a careful search is required for associated anomalies, including the central nervous system.

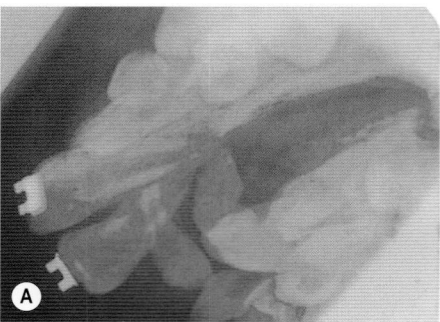 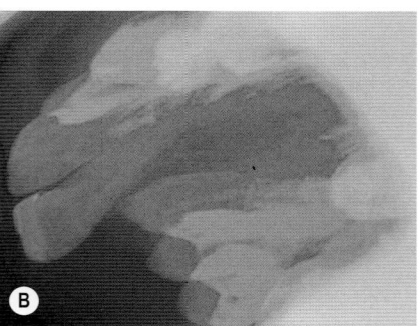

Fig. 29.41 Radiographs before (A) and 6 months after (B) alveolar bone graft operation.

Multidisciplinary management

Cleft lip and palate is a complex abnormality that demands coordinated care and treatment from a number of specialists and in the last 20 years there has been an increasing emphasis on the importance of the multidisciplinary team (Watson et al. 2001). The core team often consists of a cleft surgeon, orthodontist, speech and language therapist, paediatrician, clinical psychologist, clinical geneticist and specialist cleft nurses. While treatment interventions should be restricted to specific times to facilitate good outcomes and minimise the burden of care, follow-up by the cleft team is often required until growth has stopped (18–20 years of age). The Cleft Lip and Palate Association is an active parent/patient support group within the UK providing essential feeding equipment and information.

The provision of high-quality primary surgery reduces the need for future interventions and evidence is accumulating in support of high-volume operators achieving better outcomes (Williams et al. 1999). However, despite expert initial care, including surgery, some patients may require further operative procedures to improve speech (pharyngoplasty) or in early adult life to benefit facial appearance and function (rhinoplasty and orthognathic surgery).

Oesophagus and stomach

Oesophageal atresia

The commonest type of oesophageal atresia, accounting for 85% of all cases, consists of a dilated, blind-ended upper oesophageal pouch and a narrow, distal tracheo-oesophageal fistula (TOF; Fig. 29.42A). Nearly 10% of infants with oesophageal atresia do not have a fistula but have a long gap between the oesophageal segments (Fig. 29.42B). Rarely, there is a fistula between the upper oesophageal pouch and the trachea, with or without a distal fistula (Fig. 29.42D, E). An isolated TOF ('H' or 'N' fistula) is usually grouped with these anomalies, although there is no atresia (Fig. 29.42C). More detailed classifications of oesophageal atresia have been reported (Kluth 1976). The incidence of this spectrum of disorders is about 1:3500 births.

The trachea and oesophagus both develop from the primitive foregut but the pathogenesis of oesophageal atresia/TOF is uncertain. Some experimental studies have suggested that this malformation results from an abnormal separation of the primitive trachea and oesophagus while others have indicated that the fistula develops after these structures have separated. Oesophageal atresia is usually sporadic and rarely familial.

Maternal polyhydramnios and a small or absent fetal stomach bubble may suggest the possibility of oesophageal atresia prenatally but these sonographic findings are not specific (Stringer et al. 1995a). Occasionally, a dilated upper oesophageal pouch may provide further evidence. Additional malformations suggestive of trisomy 13 or 18 or the VACTERL association (vertebral defects, anal atresia, TOF, radial and renal dysplasia with cardiac and limb defects) may be detected by prenatal ultrasound.

Postnatally, the baby typically dribbles frothy saliva and has episodes of choking, coughing and cyanosis, often precipitated by attempts to feed. This is caused by overflow of secretions into the larynx and trachea. Attempted passage of a 10–12 Fr radiopaque nasogastric tube will reveal a hold-up about 10 cm from the lips (a smaller tube tends to curl up in the upper pouch). The diagnosis is confirmed by anteroposterior and lateral radiographs of the chest with the tube in situ (Figs 29.43 and 29.44). Air in the stomach indicates a TOF while a gasless abdomen usually signifies atresia without a fistula.

Associated congenital anomalies occur in 50% or more of infants (Chittmittrapap et al. 1989). Cardiovascular, genitourinary, skeletal and anorectal anomalies are found frequently. An echocardiogram, urinary tract ultrasound scan and radiographs of the chest, abdomen and spine will detect many of these additional malformations at an early stage. The VACTERL cluster has already been described. Duodenal atresia is the commonest associated gastrointestinal anomaly. Rarely, oesophageal atresia may be associated with the CHARGE association (coloboma, heart defects, choanal atresia (Ch. 31), retarded development and growth, genital hypoplasia and ear anomalies) (Kutiyanawala et al. 1992) or with midline defects such as cleft lip and palate and exomphalos.

Initial management is aimed at keeping the airway free of secretions and excluding additional major malformations. It is rarely necessary to operate immediately. The infant should be placed slightly head-up, with a 10 Fr double-lumen Replogle tube in the proximal pouch on continuous low-pressure suction. Routine neonatal care will include regulation of temperature, fluid balance and blood glucose. As soon as the baby is stable, he or she should be transferred to a neonatal surgical unit.

The vast majority of neonates with oesophageal atresia/TOF can be treated successfully by surgical division of the fistula between the trachea and oesophagus and primary anastomosis of the oesophagus. This was first successfully accomplished in 1941 (Haight and Towsley 1943). The operation is usually performed through a small right thoracotomy but minimally invasive repair using a thoracoscope is becoming more commonplace (Rothenberg 2002). A preliminary tracheoscopy is often carried out to search for an upper pouch fistula and to clarify the anatomy (Fig. 29.45). Postoperatively, after a straightforward operation, feeding is commenced enterally via a transanastomotic nasogastric tube or by mouth.

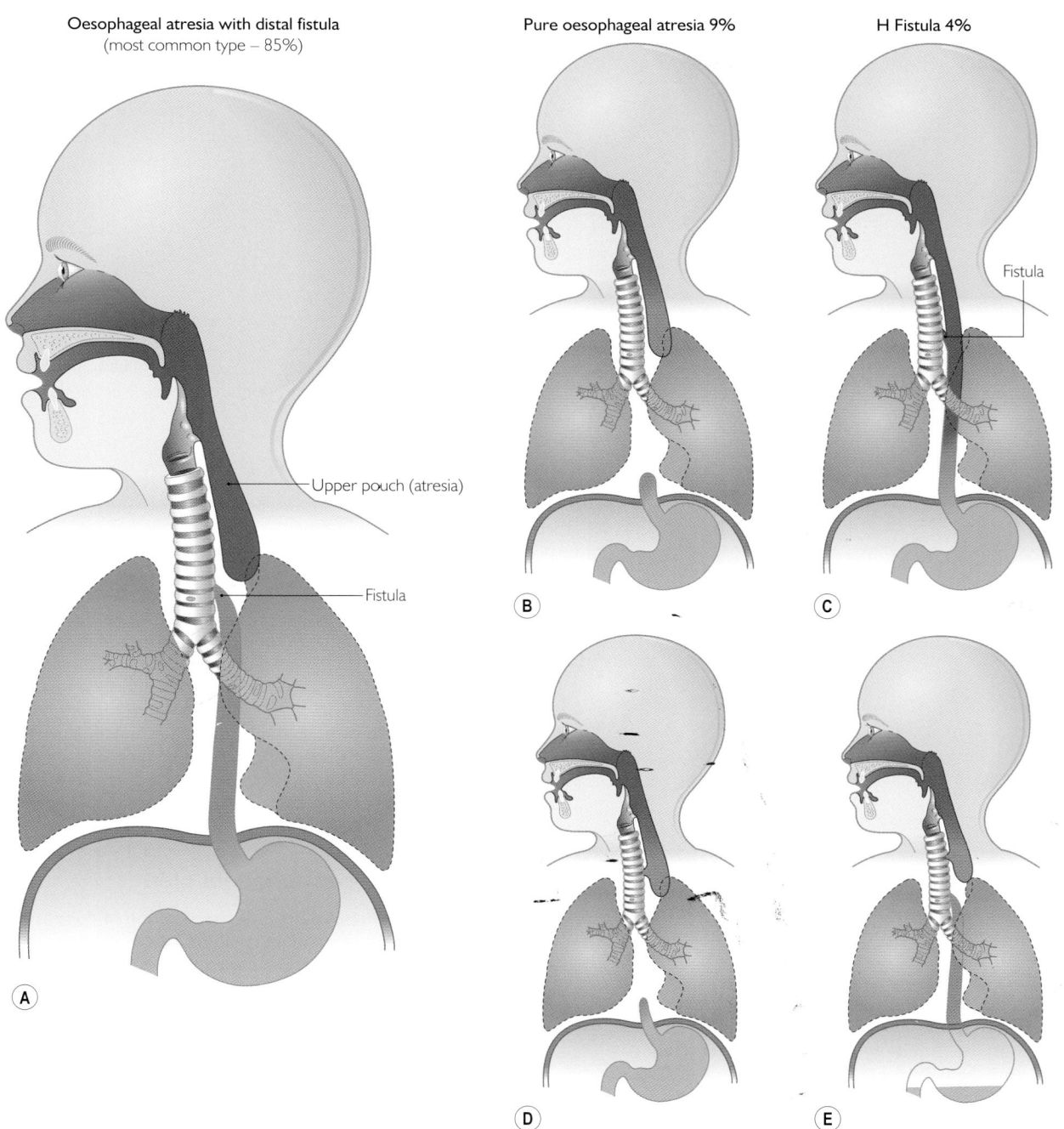

Oesophageal atresia with distal fistula
(most common type – 85%)

Upper pouch (atresia)

Fistula

(A)

Pure oesophageal atresia 9%

(B)

H Fistula 4%

Fistula

(C)

(D)

(E)

Fig. 29.42 Schematic representation of the spectrum of oesophageal atresia/tracheo-oesophageal fistula.

Two specific problems should be mentioned.

1. The baby with oesophageal atresia/TOF and severe respiratory distress (associated with prematurity or secondary to acid aspiration via the fistula) is in danger. The fistula provides a low-resistance pathway for inspiratory gases, thus preventing efficient ventilation. Gastric distension (and subsequently rupture) further compromises ventilation (Figs 29.46 and 29.47). Various temporising measures may be helpful, such as positioning the tip of the endotracheal tube below the fistula, using low-pressure ventilation or attempting balloon catheter

occlusion of the fistula, but the definitive treatment is emergency ligation of the fistula (Spitz 1996). Gastrostomy is hazardous because it provides an even easier pathway for the escape of respiratory gases.

2. The baby with long-gap oesophageal atresia may have oesophageal atresia without a fistula or a distal TOF but a wide gap between the oesophageal segments. In the former, surgery is typically delayed (delayed primary anastomosis). The upper and lower pouches are allowed to elongate and hypertrophy over a period of up to 3 months and can eventually be anastomosed. During this time the baby is fed

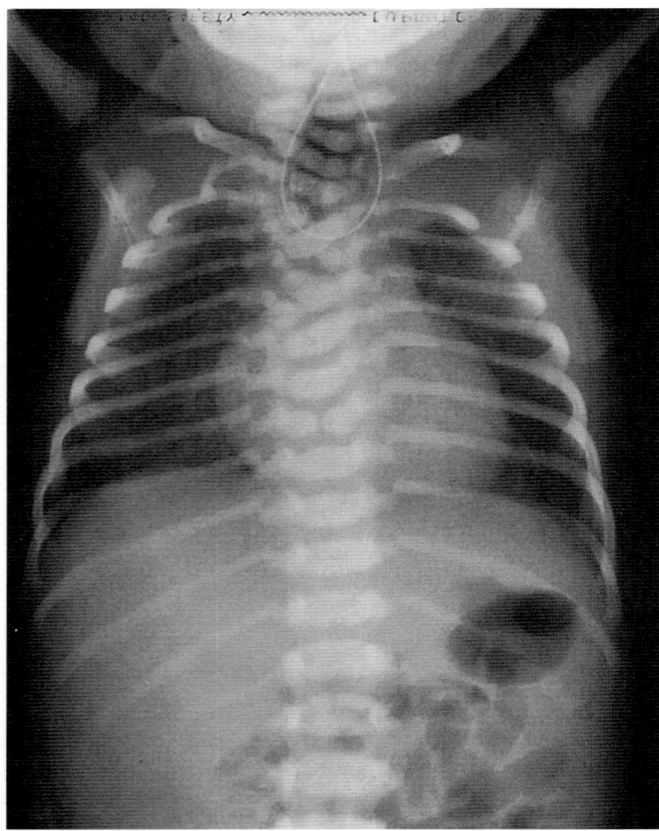

Fig. 29.43 Oesophageal atresia. Note the coiled feeding tube in the proximal pouch. Also note the vertebral and rib abnormalities. Distal gas confirms a tracheo-oesophageal fistula.

recurrent pneumonia, sometimes in the older child. In oesophageal atresia, the trachea is floppy and tends to collapse anteroposteriorly on expiration (tracheomalacia). Consequently, most children have a typical barking cough ('TOF cough'). In most, the tracheomalacia tends to improve during infancy but, in some cases, life-threatening cyanotic episodes develop, requiring treatment by aortopexy and/ or tracheopexy. All these complications can present with feeding difficulties and/or respiratory symptoms. Despite these problems, most children and adults enjoy a good quality of life after repair of oesophageal atresia/TOF (Chetcuti et al. 1988). In the UK, the Tracheo-Oesophageal Fistula Support (TOFS) group provides information for parents of affected children and a forum for sharing problems (www.tofs.org.uk) (Martin 1999).

The two most important factors determining survival are very low birthweight and major congenital cardiac defects (those causing cardiac failure or requiring surgery). Without either factor, predicted survival is greater than 95%. With one factor present it is 60% and with both it is only 20% (Spitz 1996).

Tracheo-oesophageal 'H' fistula

Congenital tracheo-oesophageal fistula without oesophageal atresia accounts for about 4% of all infants within the oesophageal atresia spectrum. It typically presents in the neonatal period with choking or cyanotic episodes associated with feeding. Some infants have marked gaseous abdominal distension from swallowed air. Right upper lobe pneumonia is common, especially when the fistula presents in older infants and children. In babies, a tube placed in the oesophagus with its external end under water may demonstrate bubbles of air. The fistula can be visualised by a prone tube oesophagogram: with the infant lying prone and a tube positioned in the distal oesophagus contrast is gradually injected as the tube is withdrawn (Fig. 29.49). The fistula can be confirmed by bronchoscopy. Treatment is to divide the fistula, which is best approached through a low cervical incision rather than a thoracotomy (Crabbe et al. 1996). Associated gastro-oesophageal reflux is common.

Laryngo-tracheo-oesophageal cleft

In this malformation, there is incomplete separation of the trachea and oesophagus. It can be associated with various other congenital anomalies, including oesophageal atresia and anorectal malformations. Clefts may be limited to the larynx and cricoid or involve the trachea. Recognising the disorder while intubating a baby with respiratory problems soon after birth is not easy. Difficulty in ventilating the infant may provide a clue. Any doubt about the anatomy of the posterior aspect of the larynx should prompt a detailed laryngoscopy, which will reveal whether it is cleft. Symptomatic or major clefts require surgical repair (Corbally 1993). Treatment of the condition is often difficult and the longer term problems of major clefts can be formidable.

Oesophageal perforation

Iatrogenic perforation of the upper oesophagus from the attempted passage of a nasogastric or endotracheal tube in a premature baby is rare (Krasna et al. 1987). It results in respiratory distress and feeding difficulties. A chest radiograph typically shows a right-sided pneumothorax or a pneumomediastinum (Fig. 29.50). A water-soluble contrast swallow helps to confirm the diagnosis, localise the perforation and direct treatment. Conservative management with chest tube drainage, antibiotics and parenteral nutrition is usually successful. Surgery is rarely required. Spontaneous rupture of the oesophagus in the neonate is extremely rare.

through a gastrostomy and the upper pouch is kept clear of secretions. This can be expediated by the Foker technique, which involves placing sutures on the upper and lower pouch and pulling them together by constant traction; this avoids the need for a gastrostomy (Foker et al. 2005). In wide-gap oesophageal atresia/TOF, the anastomosis is sometimes possible under tension. After the repair, disruptive forces at the anastomosis are minimised by electively paralysing and ventilating the baby for 5 days with the neck flexed. Alternatively, the proximal oesophagus can be lengthened by dividing its outer muscle (myotomy) or by tubularising a proximal flap. In some cases, the oesophagus has to be abandoned – the TOF is divided and a cervical oesophagostomy and gastrostomy are fashioned (Fig. 29.48). The baby is sham-fed and scheduled for oesophageal replacement (using the stomach or a segment of colon) when thriving.

Most infants can expect a good outcome after repair of oesophageal atresia/TOF but numerous complications may occur. An anastomotic leak is uncommon and typically manifests as a pneumothorax or sepsis; conservative management with chest drainage, antibiotics and nutritional support is usually sufficient. In contrast, an anastomotic stricture is common but is easily treated by oesophageal dilatation. Gastro-oesophageal reflux is also common and requires antireflux medication. Intractable symptoms or reflux associated with a recalcitrant anastomotic stricture may merit fundoplication. A recurrent TOF is rare and presents with

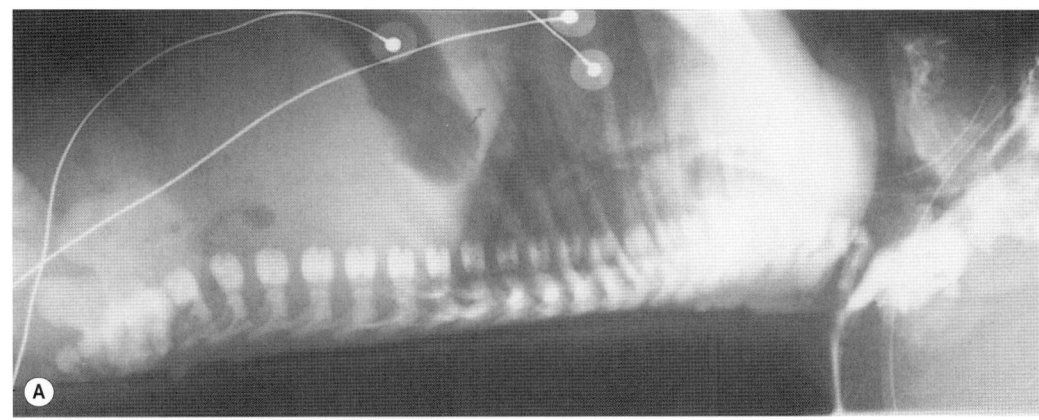

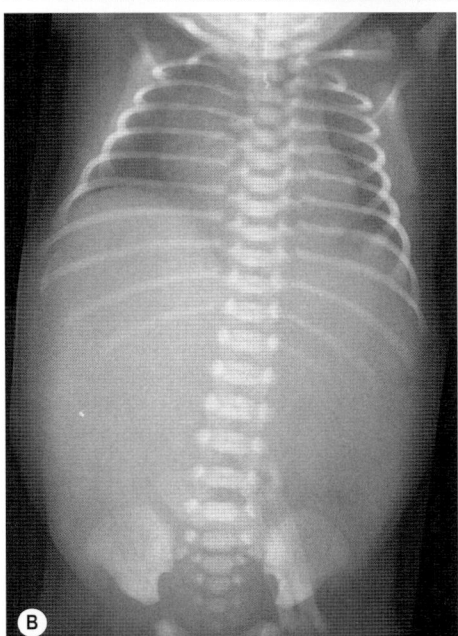

Fig. 29.44 (A) Lateral radiograph with a radiopaque tube in the proximal pouch confirming the diagnosis of oesophageal atresia. Gas in the stomach confirms a tracheo-oesophageal fistula. (B) Anteroposterior radiograph of oesophageal atresia with a tube in the upper pouch. A lack of gas in the abdomen usually indicates isolated oesophageal atresia with no distal tracheo-oesophageal fistula, as in this case.

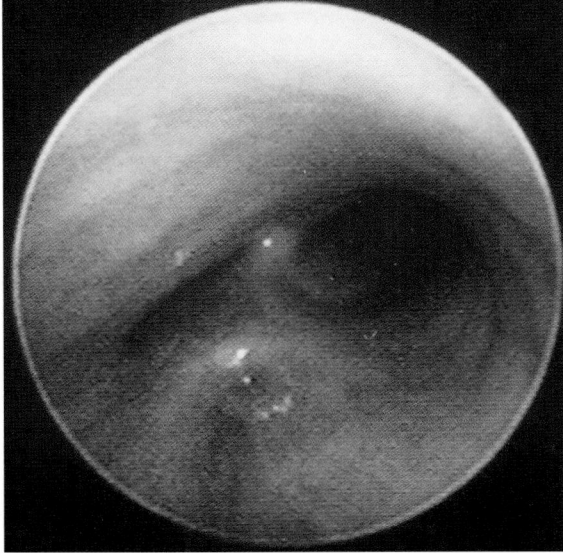

Fig. 29.45 Tracheoscopy in a baby with oesophageal atresia showing the site of a distal tracheo-oesophageal fistula just above the carina. The left main bronchus is partially collapsed from bronchomalacia.

Hypertrophic pyloric stenosis

In hypertrophic pyloric stenosis (HPS) the pylorus is increased in length and diameter as a result of hypertrophy and hyperplasia of the circular muscle layer. This causes projectile vomiting, typically between 2 and 8 weeks of age. The incidence of HPS in the UK is approximately 3:1000 live births but regional and temporal variations are well recognised. Boys are affected four times more often than girls. Occasionally, HPS is seen in a premature neonate (Tack et al. 1988) and it has even been described in the fetus. However, HPS is fundamentally an acquired condition. One ultrasound study of asymptomatic newborns failed to show any pyloric abnormality in those babies who subsequently developed HPS (Rollins et al. 1989). Its exact cause remains uncertain. Various neural and histo-chemical changes have been described in the pylorus in HPS but whether these are cause or effect is not clear. Infants born with oesophageal atresia are at increased risk, as are premature babies fed through a transpyloric tube (Evans 1982). A genetic predisposi-tion is apparent in some families.

Typically, the baby feeds hungrily and vomits toward the end of a feed. The vomit is non-bilious but may be blood-stained if there is an associated oesophagitis. Some affected infants are mildly

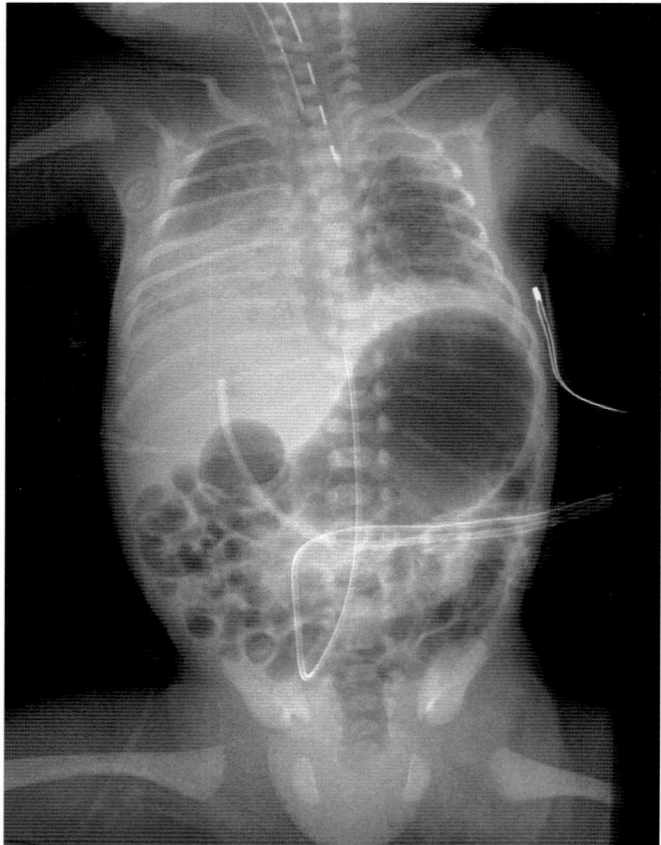 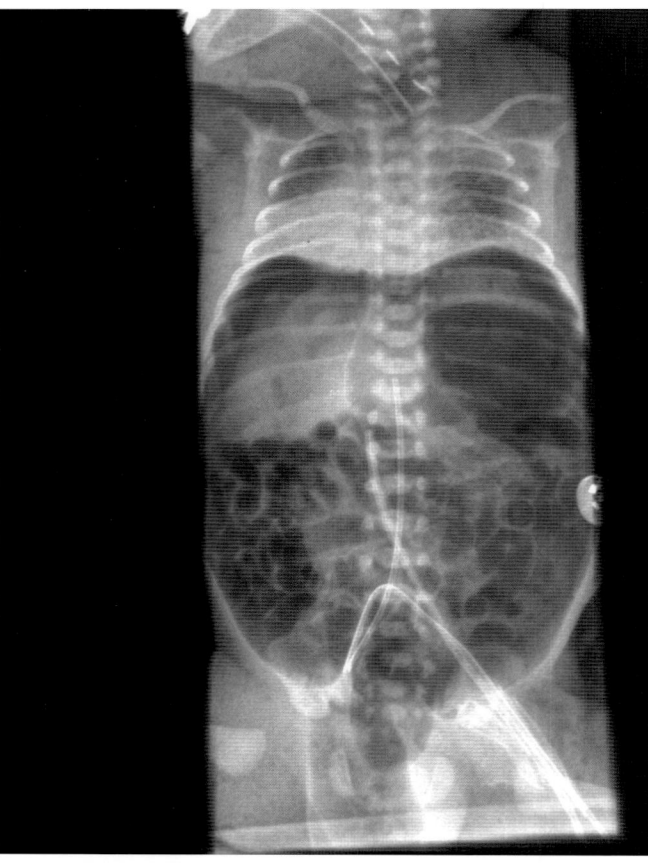

Fig. 29.46 Radiograph of a baby who is ventilated (endotracheal tube visible) and who has an oesophageal atresia (Replogle tube seen in the upper thorax) and also a tracheo-oesophageal fistula with a markedly dilated stomach.

Fig. 29.47 Radiograph of the same baby as in Fig. 29.46, taken 3 hours later, showing a gross pneumoperitoneum implying gastric rupture.

jaundiced because of an unconjugated hyperbilirubinaemia. Electrolyte abnormalities are common – characteristically, a hypochloraemic alkalosis (Touloukian and Higgins 1983). This disturbance may be severe and must be adequately corrected before surgery. Crystalloid solutions containing 0.45% saline and 5% dextrose with 20 mmol/l potassium chloride are useful. Blood glucose should be monitored.

The diagnosis of HPS is made by feeling the hypertrophied pyloric muscle (similar to an olive) while the baby's abdominal muscles are relaxed, such as during a test feed. Gastric peristalsis is often visible. If doubt remains, an ultrasound scan by an experienced sonographer is helpful (Blumhagen et al. 1988); the pyloric muscle is usually 3–4 mm thick and the pyloric length and diameter are increased (Fig. 29.51). Contrast studies are rarely necessary.

The treatment of HPS is by Ramstedt's pyloromyotomy (Fig. 29.52). This can be performed through a transverse upper abdominal incision, a circum-umbilical incision (Fig. 29.53) or laparoscopically. Feeding can be reintroduced within 24 hours of surgery. Minor, transient postoperative vomiting is common. Persistent vomiting is unusual and most often due to associated gastro-oesophageal reflux. Complications of pyloromyotomy, which include incomplete myotomy, duodenal perforation, haemorrhage, wound infection, wound dehiscence and incisional hernia, are rare (Zeidan et al. 1988). There are almost no significant long-term sequelae after a successful pyloromyotomy.

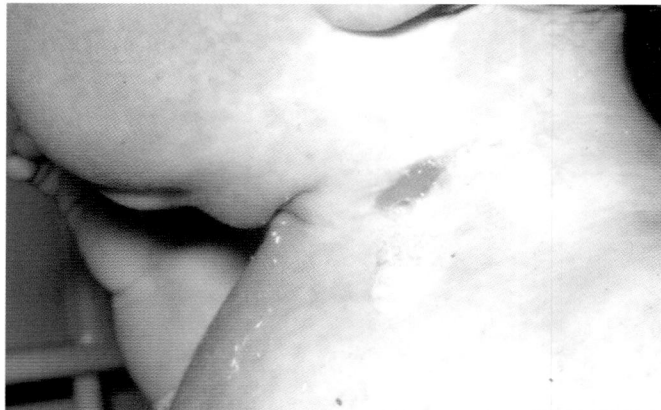

Fig. 29.48 Cervical oesophagostomy. This allows sham feeding.

Pyloric atresia

Pyloric atresia is rare and causes congenital gastric outlet obstruction. The stomach is distended and an abdominal radiograph shows a gasless abdomen beyond the pylorus (Fig. 29.54). Treatment is surgical. The condition is familial in some cases. Associations with

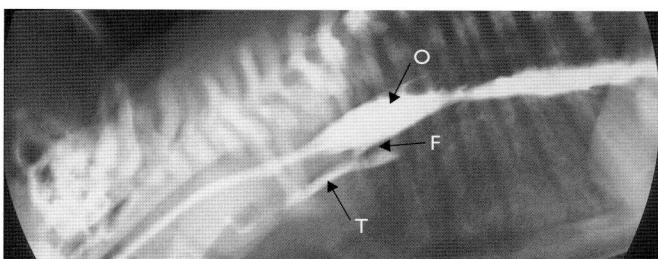

Fig. 29.49 An 'H' tracheo-oesophageal fistula outlined by contrast during a prone tube oesophagogram. A small amount of contrast has entered the trachea (T). O, oesophagus; F, fistula.

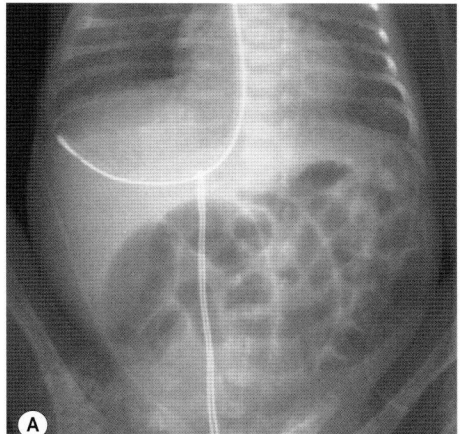

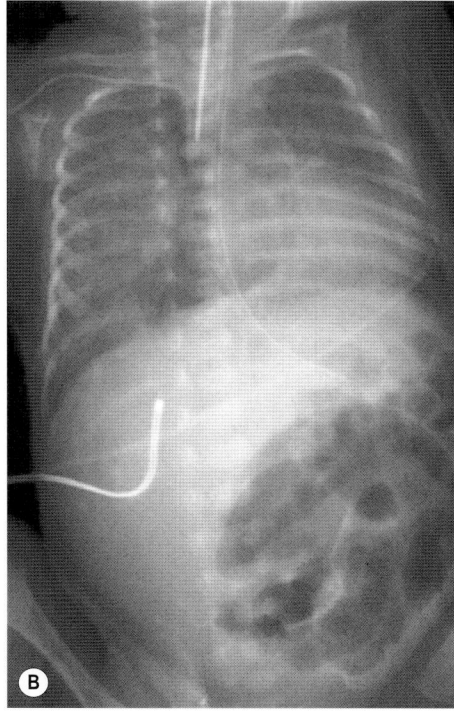

Fig. 29.50 (A) Abnormally positioned nasogastric tube in a premature baby following iatrogenic perforation of the upper oesophagus. (B) After the nasogastric tube was withdrawn and gently repassed into the stomach, a pneumomediastinum was evident. The baby recovered with conservative treatment.

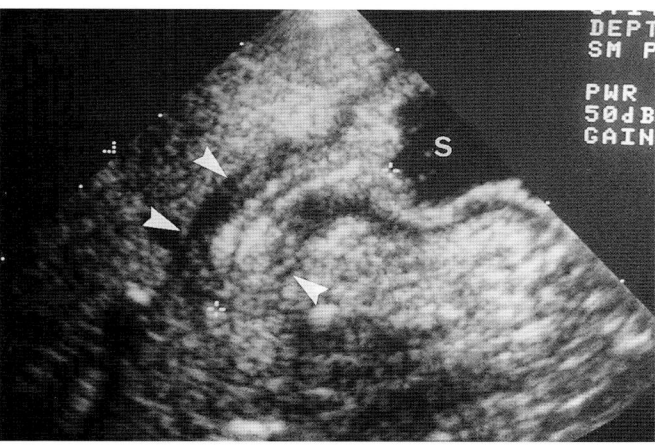

Fig. 29.51 Ultrasound appearance of hypertrophic pyloric stenosis. The arrowheads outline the hypertrophied pyloric muscle. S, stomach.

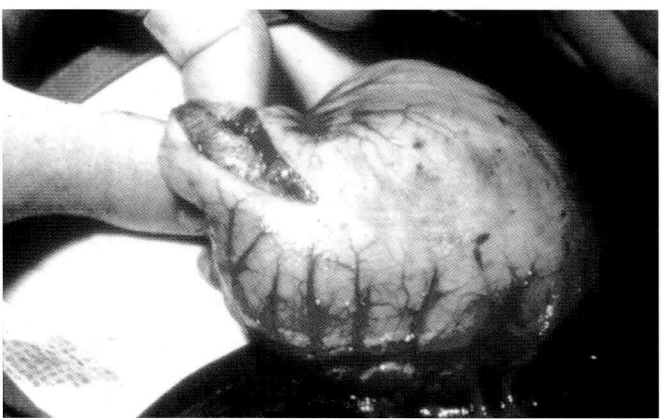

Fig. 29.52 Pyloromyotomy with mucosa projecting between the cut edges of the split hypertrophied muscle.

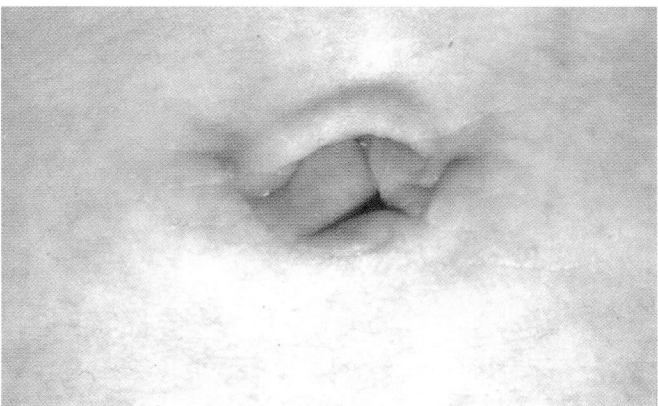

Fig. 29.53 Circum-umbilical wound a few weeks after surgery for hypertrophic pyloric stenosis.

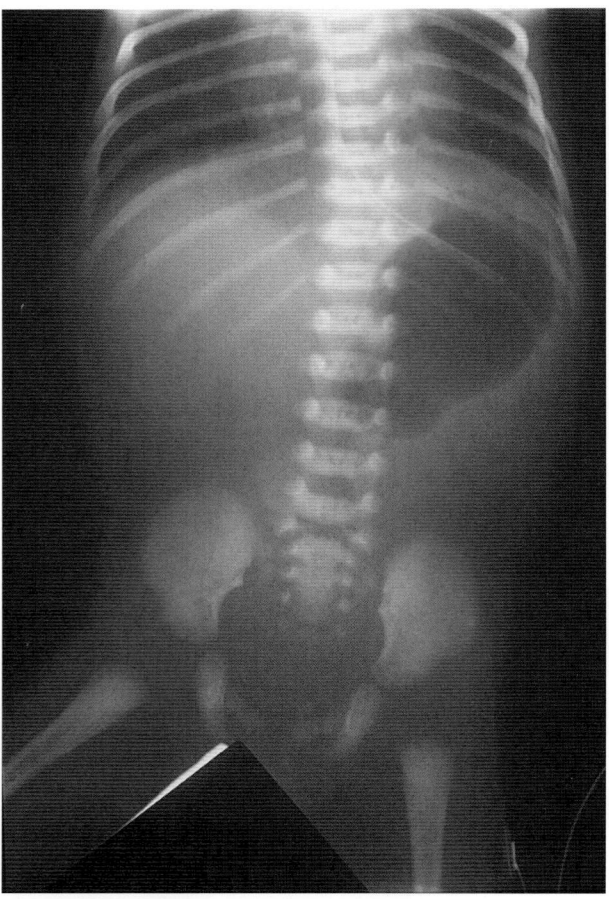

Fig. 29.54 Abdominal radiograph of a baby with pyloric atresia.

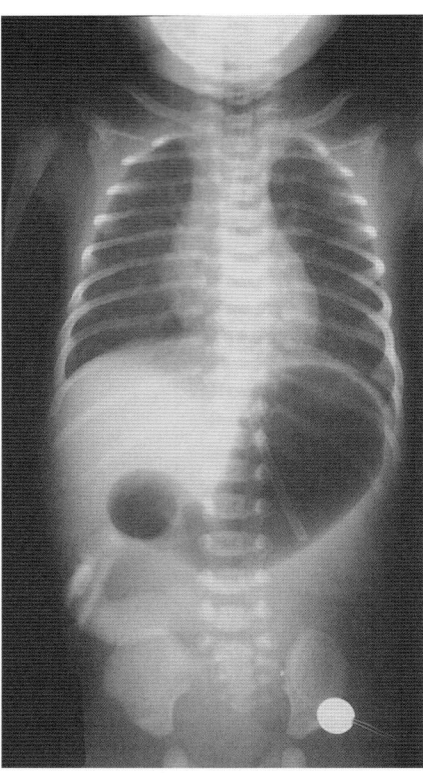

Fig. 29.55 Double bubble of duodenal atresia. Air has been injected through the nasogastric tube to highlight the anatomy.

epidermolysis bullosa and multiple intestinal atresias are well described (Okoye et al. 2000).

Gastric volvulus

Gastric volvulus is a rare, potentially life-threatening condition caused by abnormal rotation of the stomach about its axis resulting in a strangulating obstruction. Most instances of gastric volvulus in the newborn are associated with a diaphragmatic defect and/or deficient ligamentous attachments of the stomach (Stringer 2003). Vomiting, haematemesis and respiratory distress are the dominant symptoms. A distended stomach in an abnormal position on a plain abdominal or chest radiograph should raise the possibility of gastric volvulus. Contrast studies clarify the anatomy. If possible, the stomach should be decompressed by the gentle passage of a nasogastric tube. At surgery, the volvulus is reduced, the stomach is fixed and any associated diaphragmatic defect is repaired.

Duodenum and small bowel

Duodenal obstruction in the neonate may be intrinsic or extrinsic or occasionally combined.

Duodenal atresia and stenosis

Intrinsic obstruction may be secondary to duodenal atresia, where there is either a gap between the duodenal segments (often with interposed pancreas) or an intact duodenal membrane with continuity of the duodenal wall, or duodenal stenosis, typically with a perforated duodenal web. Intrinsic duodenal obstruction affects approximately 1:6000 live births. Additional anomalies may include intestinal malrotation and, in one-third of patients, Down syndrome. Whether the atresia is due to failure of recanalisation of the embryonic duodenum or to a later intrauterine event is not clear. The obstruction usually occurs in the region of the ampulla of Vater. Anomalies of the distal bile duct explain why, on rare occasions, an infant may have bile-stained vomiting and yet pass normal-coloured meconium (Astley 1969).

The frequent occurrence of polyhydramnios often results in duodenal atresia being detected by prenatal ultrasound (Gee and Abdulla 1978). The characteristic 'double bubble' may be seen only intermittently because of fetal vomiting. Prematurity is common.

Postnatally, duodenal atresia presents with bile-stained vomiting within hours of birth. In 20% of cases the obstruction is proximal to the common bile duct opening in the duodenum and the vomit is non-bilious. Duodenal stenosis causes partial obstruction and may not present during the neonatal period. Examination of the baby may show a distended stomach. A plain radiograph of the abdomen demonstrates the characteristic 'double bubble' sign of gas in the distended stomach and duodenum. This appearance is highlighted if the stomach is first aspirated via a nasogastric tube and 50 ml of air is instilled (Fig. 29.55). In most atresias there is no distal intestinal gas but occasionally a small amount of distal bowel gas may be seen if there is a Y-shaped termination of the common bile duct with limbs above and below the atresia. Significant amounts of distal gas with a distended stomach and duodenum should suggest the possibility of duodenal stenosis or intestinal malrotation and volvulus.

SINGLETON HOSPITAL
STAFF LIBRARY

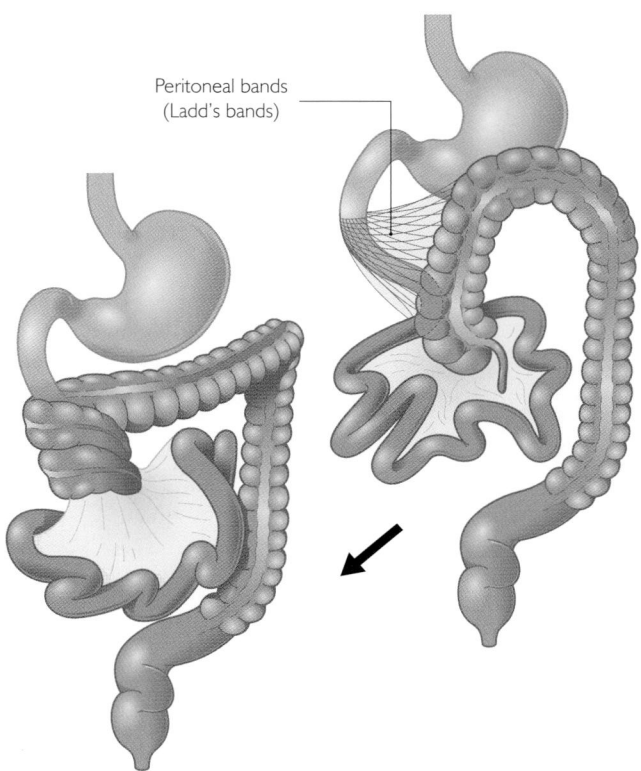

Fig. 29.56 Intestinal malrotation. The classical type of intestinal malrotation predisposes to midgut volvulus.

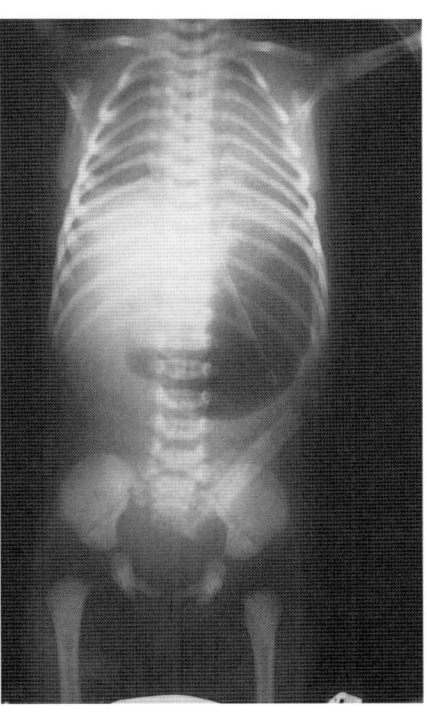

Fig. 29.57 Intestinal malrotation with neonatal midgut volvulus. The abdomen is virtually gasless beyond the distended stomach and duodenum.

Management consists of nasogastric decompression, correction of any metabolic alkalosis or electrolyte imbalance, and early surgery. An echocardiogram should be performed in babies with Down syndrome. At operation, the duodenum proximal to the site of atresia is anastomosed to the distal duodenum (duodeno-duodenostomy). Care must be taken not to damage the termination of the common bile duct. Because of the chronic nature of the obstruction, it may take a week or more before gastroduodenal function recovers sufficiently for the baby to tolerate full enteral feeding. Temporary parenteral nutrition is usually required. The outcome of intrinsic duodenal obstruction is related to associated anomalies, since the condition itself can be successfully corrected by surgery.

Intestinal malrotation

Unlike most cases of intrinsic duodenal obstruction, extrinsic obstruction due to intestinal malrotation with volvulus may be intermittent and incomplete and can present at any age. Boys are affected more often than girls. In classical intestinal malrotation, the midgut fails to complete its normal rotational development; the duodenojejunal flexure comes to lie on the right of the midline and the caecum is free-floating in the upper abdomen (Fig. 29.56). Consequently, the base of the small bowel mesentery, which extends between these two points, is a narrow pedicle. This predisposes to midgut volvulus around the superior mesenteric vessels, which can lead to fatal midgut strangulation. Most patients with midgut volvulus present during the first month of life with bilious vomiting. Intestinal strangulation manifests as abdominal distension and rectal bleeding progressing to hypovolaemic shock.

Because the obstruction may be intermittent and incomplete, the diagnosis may be delayed. While a plain abdominal radiograph may show an abnormal distribution of bowel gas, there is no single characteristic picture. The small bowel may be distributed more on the right and large bowel on the left of the abdomen. Alternatively, there may be a 'double bubble' of acute duodenal obstruction with a relatively gasless abdomen (Fig. 29.57). Any infant presenting with bile-stained vomiting should have an urgent upper gastro-intestinal contrast study if malrotation cannot be excluded (Figs 29.58 and 29.59). Colour Doppler imaging often demonstrates an abnormal relationship of the superior mesenteric artery and vein as a result of the malrotation (Pracros et al. 1992). A barium enema is less reliable in diagnosis but may confirm the abnormal position of the caecum.

Intestinal malrotation may be found in association with other congenital anomalies including congenital diaphragmatic hernia, abdominal wall defects, small bowel atresia, Hirschsprung disease, situs inversus, polysplenia and biliary atresia (Filston and Kirks 1981).

Surgery is mandatory for classical intestinal malrotation, even if the abnormality is diagnosed incidentally. This is because of the risk of midgut strangulation. Lesser degrees of intestinal malrotation rarely require surgery. The operation for classical intestinal malrotation is known as Ladd's procedure. It involves division of peritoneal bands extending from the caecum across the duodenum, broadening the base of the small bowel mesentery, placing the small bowel on the right of the abdomen and the colon on the left, and appendicectomy. Subsequent peritoneal adhesions stabilise the gut in a position of non-rotation, thereby reducing the likelihood of volvulus. In cases where there is a volvulus at the time of surgery, this must be promptly untwisted and as much viable bowel as possible preserved. A repeat laparotomy performed 24 hours later may be helpful if bowel viability is initially uncertain.

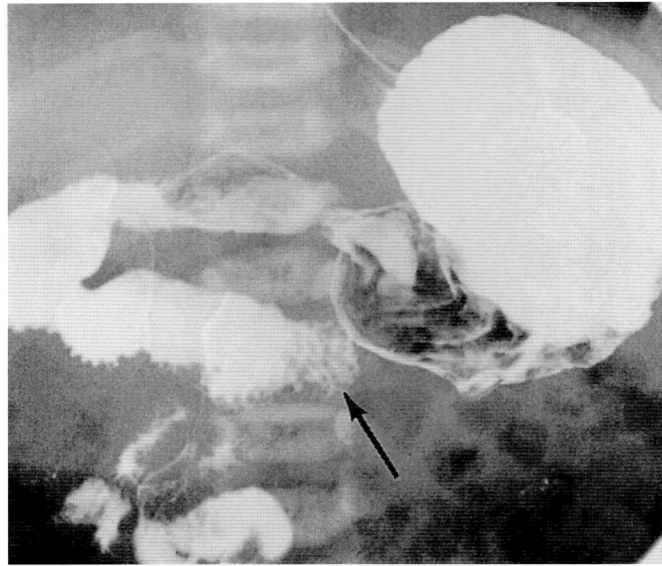

Fig. 29.58 Barium meal showing incomplete rotation of duodenum with the duodenojejunal flexure (arrow) in front of the vertebrae rather than to the left side of the abdomen.

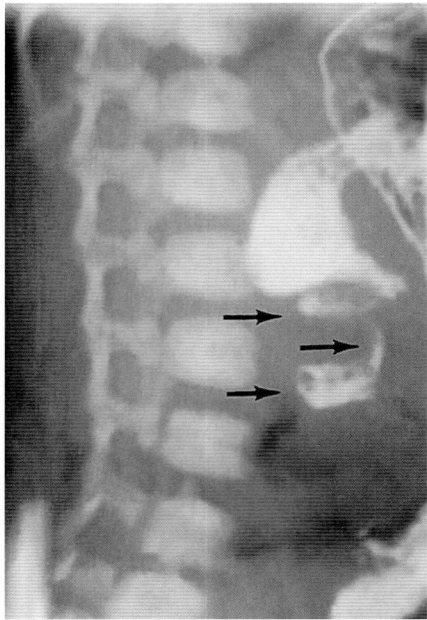

Fig. 29.59 Lateral radiograph showing barium passing down the duodenum and forming a corkscrew (arrows) configuration due to a midgut volvulus.

Jejunal and ileal atresia

Atresia of the jejunum or ileum is most often caused by a late gestational interruption to the blood supply of the fetal gut. This was shown experimentally by Louw (1959). This intrauterine mesenteric vascular accident may arise from intestinal volvulus (associated with midgut malrotation, cystic fibrosis (CF) or a duplication cyst), intussusception, the action of vasoconstrictor drugs such as cocaine or constriction of the mesentery in a tight abdominal wall defect.

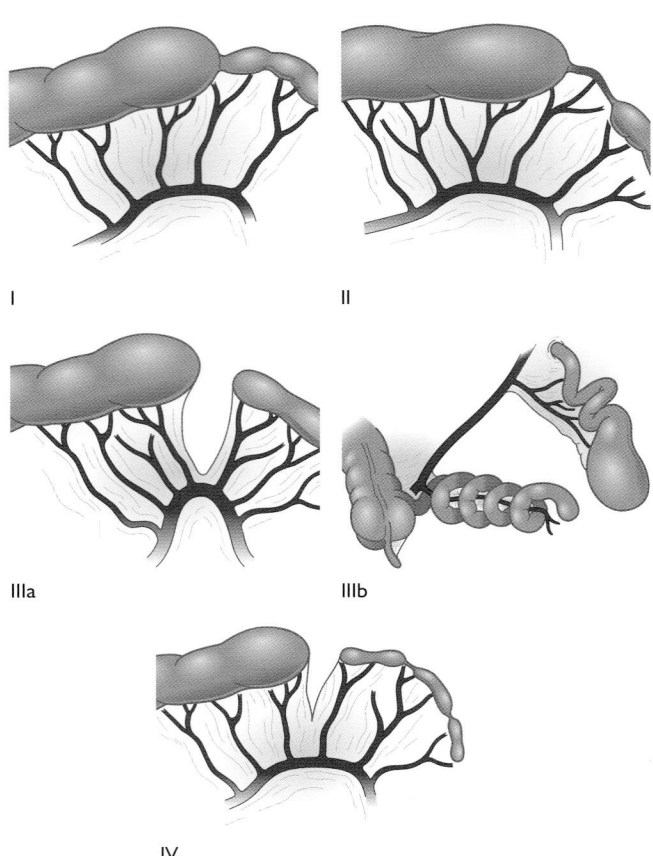

Fig. 29.60 Classification of intestinal atresia. Type I, membranous atresia with intact bowel wall and mesentery; type II, two atretic blind ends connected by a fibrous cord with an intact mesentery; type IIIa, two ends of atretic bowel separated by a V-shaped mesenteric defect; type IIIb, 'apple-peel' deformity; type IV, multiple atresias ('string of sausages'). *(Reproduced from Grosfeld et al. (1979) with permission.)*

A segment of small bowel is infarcted and reabsorbed, leaving a jejunal or ileal atresia. Multiple intestinal atresias are rare, may be familial and probably have a different pathogenesis (Noblett 1969; Puri and Fujimoto 1988).

Jejunoileal atresias can be classified into four types (Grosfeld et al. 1979) (Fig. 29.60). Type III is the commonest and is typically associated with a shorter bowel length. Type IIIb is known as an apple-peel deformity and consists of a proximal jejunal atresia, a wide mesenteric gap and a distal small bowel segment coiled around a marginal artery (Fig. 29.61). This classification is related more to the management and complications of intestinal atresia than to their presenting features.

Except for a lower mean birthweight, the baby with small bowel atresia often appears normal. There may be a history of maternal polyhydramnios or, rarely, dilated fetal bowel may have been detected by prenatal sonography (Richards and Holmes 1995). Vomiting begins within a day or two of birth – the higher the atresia, the earlier the vomiting. Bilious vomiting is a typical feature of jejunal atresia and abdominal distension is often prominent with ileal atresia. The baby fails to pass normal meconium. Inspection of the baby's abdomen may show distended bowel loops. A plain abdominal radiograph demonstrates the characteristic picture of intestinal obstruction with dilated loops of bowel and multiple fluid levels (Figs 29.62 and 29.63). The more distal the atresia, the

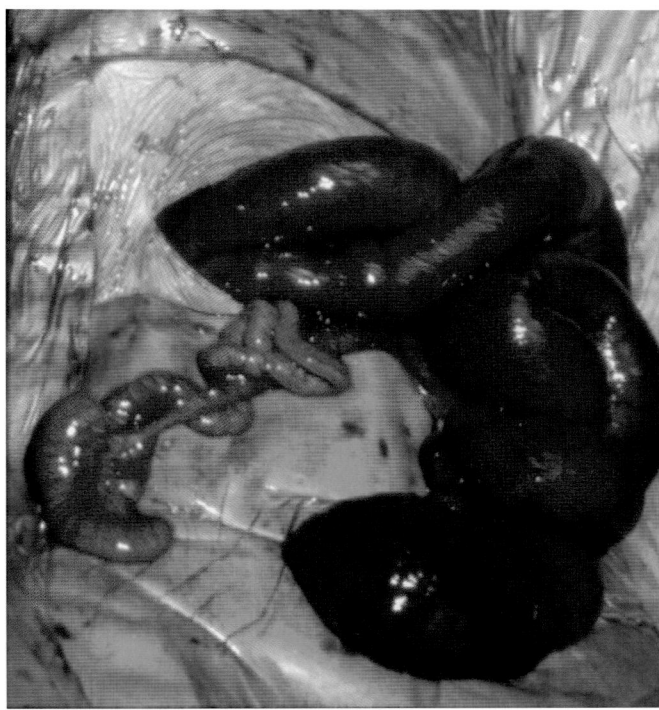

Fig. 29.61 Apple-peel atresia. The proximal bowel is dilated and congested.

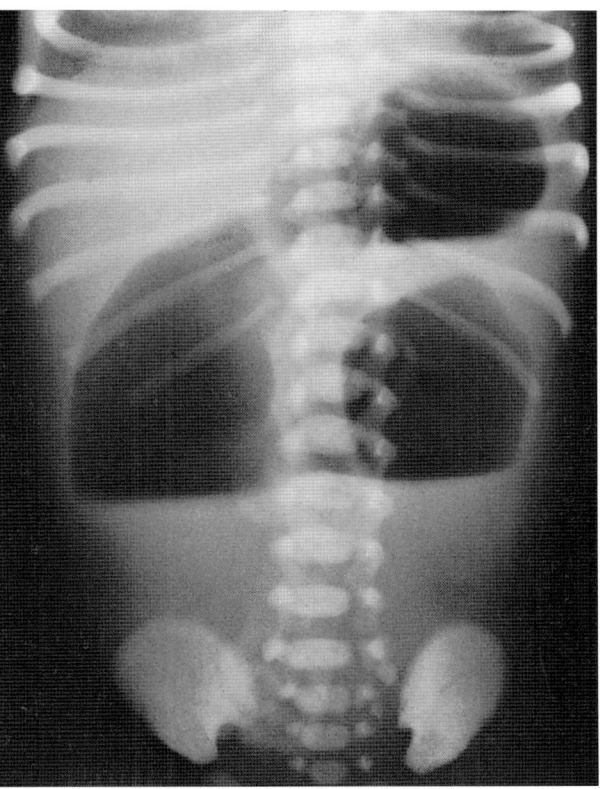

Fig. 29.62 Anteroposterior radiograph showing dilated bowel and fluid levels, indicating a proximal jejunal obstruction.

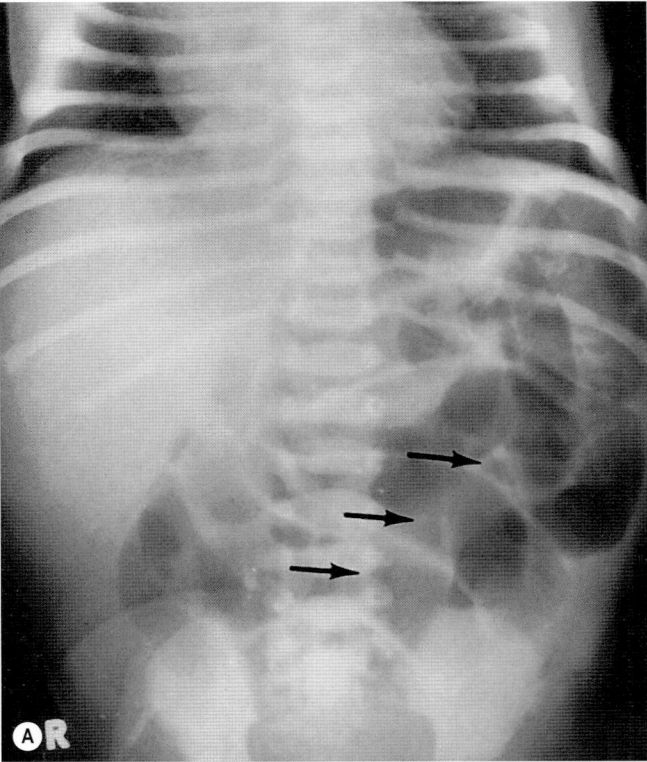

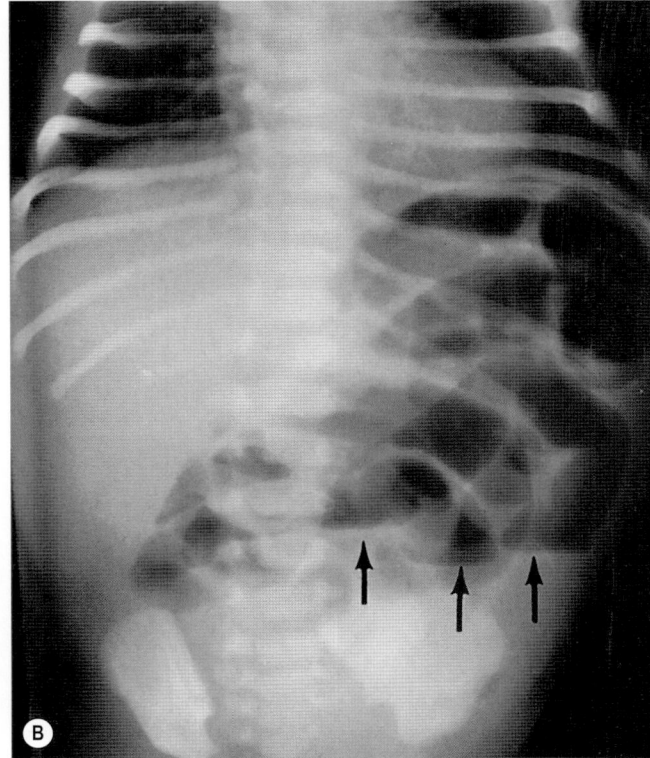

Fig. 29.63 (A) Supine radiograph showing ladder pattern of obstructed small bowel. (B) Erect film of the same baby showing dilated bowel with fluid levels indicating an ileal obstruction.

greater the number of distended bowel loops. Peritoneal calcification is a sign of intrauterine perforation. In a stable infant, a contrast enema may be required to clarify the cause of a distal bowel obstruction. Most infants with jejunoileal atresia have a microcolon.

After resuscitation, nasogastric decompression and any necessary urgent investigations, the baby should undergo surgery. At laparotomy the bowel distal to an obvious atresia must be examined carefully to exclude further atresias. Infants with type I and II atresias require resection of a short segment of dilated proximal bowel and an end-to-end anastomosis of the gut. Complications are infrequent and their long-term prognosis is good. Infants with type III defects require similar surgery but, because of the prenatal bowel loss, early postoperative digestive problems are common and parenteral nutrition is usually needed. Modified feeds may be necessary to optimise nutrition. An anastomotic leak or stenosis is rare but episodes of functional intestinal obstruction are common during the early postoperative period. Despite this, adaptation occurs rapidly and long-term parenteral feeding is seldom required. In babies with multiple intestinal atresias, several anastomoses may be needed to preserve the maximum length of bowel. A sweat test and DNA mutational analysis are undertaken to exclude CF in infants with jejunoileal atresia.

Infants with a short gut require long-term follow-up to monitor their growth and development, address any nutritional deficiencies and detect and treat potential complications such as gallstones and late anastomotic ulceration.

Meconium ileus

In this condition, obstruction of the small bowel lumen is caused by highly viscid meconium containing excess protein. CF is almost invariably the underlying cause, although exceptions do occur (Shigemoto et al. 1978). Approximately 10–15% of infants with CF present in this way.

Meconium ileus may be uncomplicated or complicated. In uncomplicated cases, there is small bowel obstruction, usually in the distal ileum. The proximal bowel is dilated and the distal small bowel is narrow and packed with grey-coloured meconium pellets. The unused colon is a narrow microcolon. Complicated meconium ileus is caused by a volvulus of meconium-laden bowel in the fetus. This may result in intestinal perforation, meconium peritonitis and meconium pseudocyst formation or an ileal atresia.

The neonate with meconium ileus usually has marked abdominal distension soon after birth, often accompanied by visible and palpable loops of bowel. There may be a palpable mobile abdominal mass.

The baby does not pass meconium, although small plugs or pellets of pale material may be passed. Vomiting becomes progressively worse and bile-stained.

There may be a family history of CF or prenatal genetic analysis may already have been performed. Hyperechogenic fetal bowel (see above) or meconium peritonitis may have been identified by prenatal sonography. Postnatally, CF mutation analysis and sweat testing will confirm the aetiology. There is no clear-cut genotype correlation with meconium ileus but an association with delta F508 and G542X mutations has been reported (Feingold and Guilloud-Bataille 1999).

A plain abdominal radiograph shows marked bowel distension. Fluid levels are uncommon because of the viscid meconium. A 'soap bubble' appearance, caused by the admixture of air and viscid meconium, may be noted (Fig. 29.64) but this is not pathognomonic for meconium ileus. In complicated cases intraperitoneal calcification or a cystic mass may be visible.

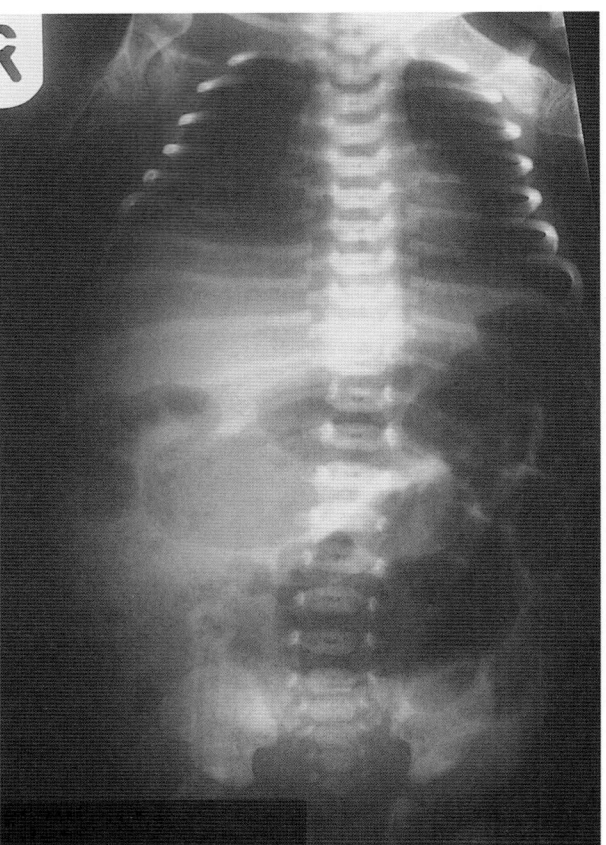

Fig. 29.64 Abdominal radiograph of a baby with meconium ileus. Note the lack of fluid levels and the 'soap bubble' appearance in the right lower quadrant.

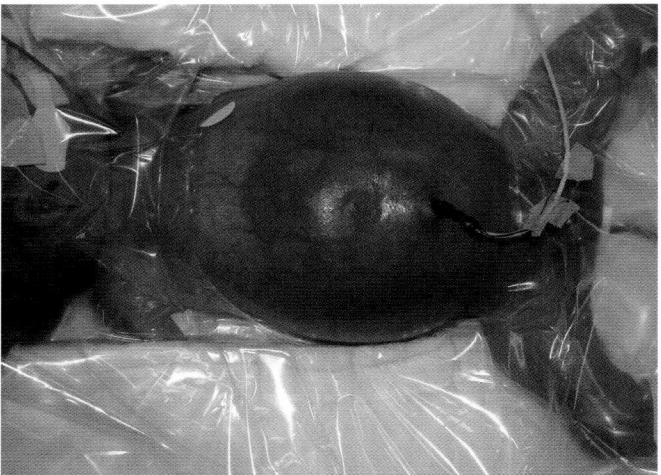

Fig. 29.65 A patient with complicated meconium ileus. Note the marked abdominal distension and discoloration of the anterior abdominal wall.

Neonates with complicated meconium ileus require surgery (Fig. 29.65). In uncomplicated cases, an isotonic contrast enema is diagnostic, showing an unused microcolon (Fig. 29.66) and inspissated meconium in the terminal ileum. Prophylactic antibiotics are advisable prior to giving the enema. Occasionally, this same appearance

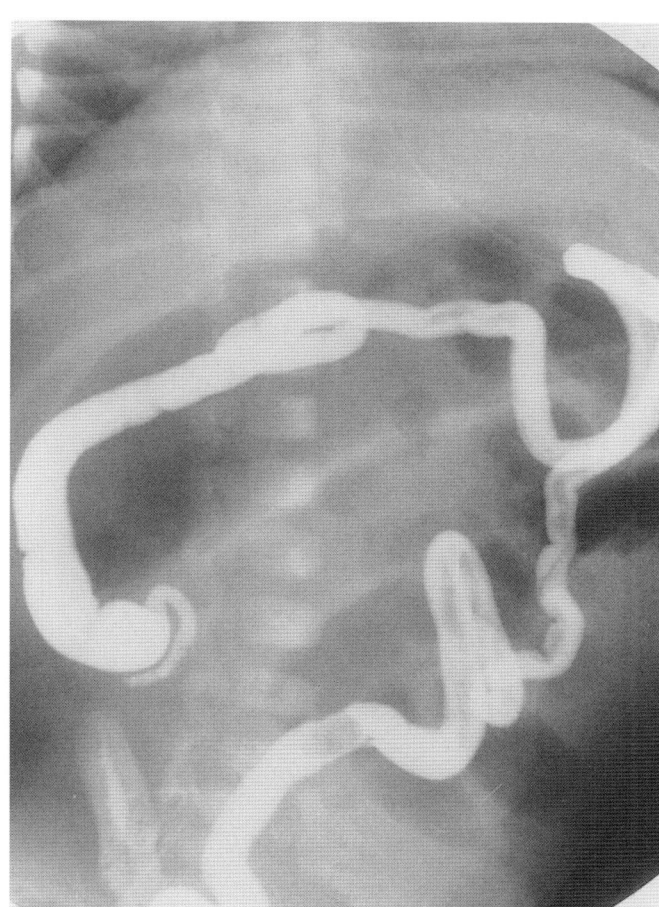

Fig. 29.66 Contrast enema showing a microcolon and dilated loops of proximal small bowel in meconium ileus.

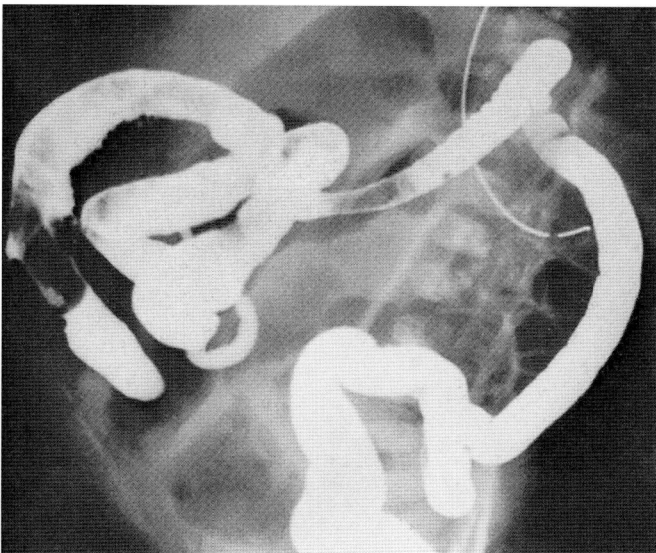

Fig. 29.67 Gastrografin enema filling the caecum and terminal ileum and outlining plugs of meconium in the distal ileum in a baby with meconium ileus.

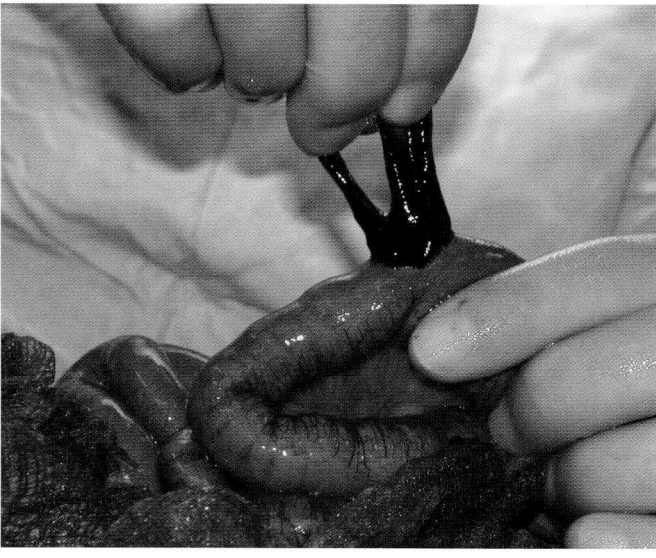

Fig. 29.68 Enterotomy in meconium ileus. The thick, tenacious meconium is milked out of the bowel lumen after irrigation.

is mimicked by total colonic aganglionosis. Passage of contrast into dilated proximal bowel confirms its patency. Once this is determined, a therapeutic enema can be used (Fig. 29.67). Hyperosmolar solutions, such as dilute Gastrografin, draw fluid into the lumen of the gut, making the meconium less tenacious and encouraging its evacuation (Noblett 1969). Additional intravenous fluids are required to compensate for this fluid loss. The enema may need to be repeated at daily intervals over the next few days before normal bowel movements are achieved (Boyd et al. 1988).

Non-operative management of uncomplicated meconium ileus is successful in about 50% of cases but it carries a risk of intestinal perforation. The presence of complicated meconium ileus precludes the use of a therapeutic enema and is an indication for surgery. Similarly, infants not responding to conservative management require operation. Various surgical procedures are used to treat meconium ileus, including intestinal resection and temporary stoma formation, resection and primary anastomosis and, in uncomplicated cases, enterotomy and irrigation of the bowel (Fig. 29.68).

Survival rates for infants with meconium ileus have improved progressively. Recent reports document survival rates of 90% for complicated meconium ileus and a higher figure for uncomplicated cases (Rescorla and Grosfeld 1993; Mushtaq et al. 1998). Advances in the overall management of CF have contributed to this success. Infants with CF who present with meconium ileus have a relatively good long-term prognosis (Coutts et al. 1997).

Alimentary tract duplications

Alimentary tract duplications are rare congenital malformations. Most are single, cystic lesions but some are tubular, running parallel to the gut. Typically, they are lined by alimentary tract mucosa and share a common smooth-muscle wall and blood supply with the adjacent gut. Some communicate directly with the lumen of the native alimentary tract. About 50% of duplications occur in the midgut and 35% in the foregut (Fig. 29.69) (Stringer et al. 1995b).

One-third of duplication cysts present in the neonate with symptoms of obstruction, bleeding or inflammation. Some only become apparent during investigation of more severe congenital anomalies

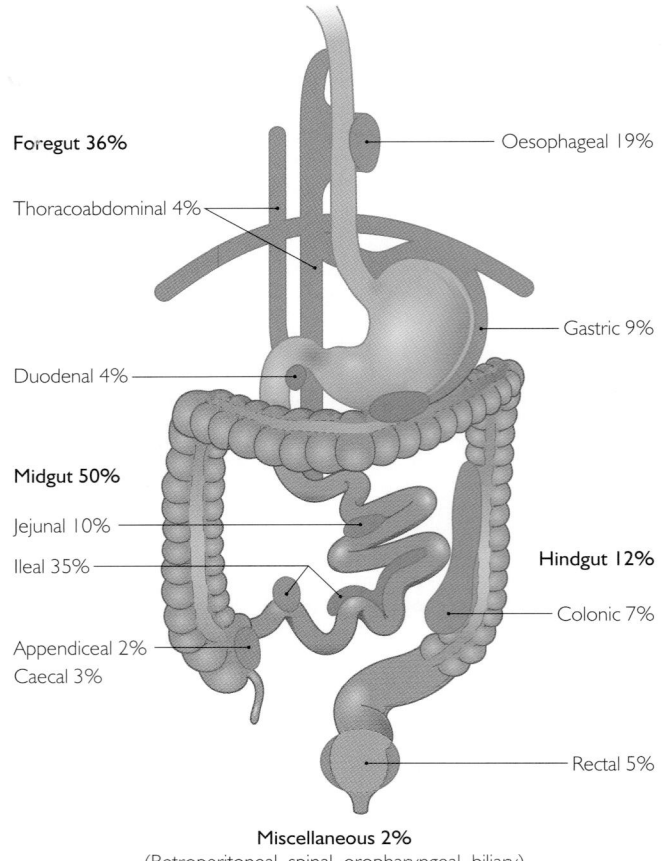

Foregut 36%

Oesophageal 19%

Thoracoabdominal 4%

Gastric 9%

Duodenal 4%

Midgut 50%

Jejunal 10%

Ileal 35%

Hindgut 12%

Colonic 7%

Appendiceal 2%
Caecal 3%

Rectal 5%

Miscellaneous 2%
(Retroperitoneal, spinal, oropharyngeal, biliary)

Fig. 29.69 Distribution of alimentary tract duplications. *(Reproduced from Stringer et al. (1995b).)*

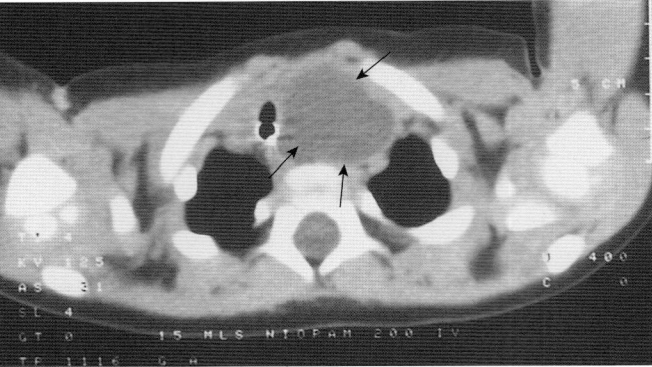

Fig. 29.70 Computed tomography scan of the thoracic inlet in an infant with a paraoesophageal duplication cyst (arrows) causing tracheal deviation and respiratory symptoms.

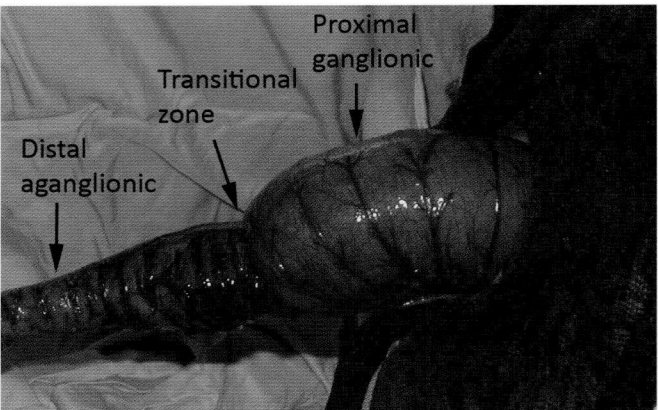

Proximal ganglionic

Transitional zone

Distal aganglionic

Fig. 29.71 Intraoperative picture of a baby with Hirschsprung disease showing the calibre change from aganglionic to ganglionic bowel.

such as anorectal malformations, oesophageal atresia or bladder/cloacal exstrophy. Additional congenital abnormalities are common. Examples include exstrophy or myelomeningocele with hindgut duplication, intestinal malrotation with midgut lesions, and oesophageal atresia with foregut duplication. Some duplications, particularly foregut lesions, are associated with vertebral anomalies and even intraspinal pathology. Heterotopic gastric mucosa is found in one-third of duplications and may cause ulceration and bleeding.

Paraoesophageal cysts may present with respiratory symptoms or be noticed first on a chest radiograph (Fig. 29.70). Thoracoabdominal duplications have the greatest potential for complications; they usually lie to the right of the oesophagus in the posterior mediastinum and may communicate distally, through the diaphragm, with the upper gastrointestinal tract. Intestinal duplications most often present with bowel obstruction (from local compression, volvulus or intussusception). An increasing proportion of duplication cysts are discovered during prenatal ultrasound scans.

Duplications are best managed by early complete excision to avoid complications, which include a small potential for malignant degeneration in adult life.

Other causes of neonatal small bowel obstruction

There are several other causes of intestinal obstruction in the newborn. Necrotising enterocolitis (pp. 708–717) and an incarcerated inguinal hernia (see below) are relatively common causes. Rarer conditions include neonatal acute appendicitis, segmental small bowel volvulus (not due to midgut malrotation, CF or duplication cyst), an adhesion band connected to a vitellointestinal remnant, distal small bowel obstruction from inspissated formula milk curds (Cook and Rickham 1969) and pseudo-obstruction from intestinal neuropathy or myopathy. Neonatal intussusception may mimic necrotising enterocolitis (Wang et al. 1998). An abdominal ultrasound scan and plain abdominal radiographs are often helpful in diagnosing these conditions.

Large bowel

Hirschsprung disease

In a neonate with delayed passage of meconium, increasing abdominal distension and bilious vomiting, Hirschsprung disease must be excluded (Stringer 1999).

Hirschsprung disease is characterised by a congenital absence of intramural ganglion cells in the rectum. This aganglionosis and the presence of hypertrophied nerve trunks lead to a tonic contraction of the involved segment of gut, which causes a functional intestinal obstruction (Fig. 29.71). The abnormalities of innervation extend into the proximal bowel to a variable degree.

Harald Hirschsprung, a Danish paediatrician, provided the first comprehensive account of the disease in 1887, although he wrongly believed that the proximal dilated colon was the cause of the condition (Hirschsprung 1887).

The aganglionosis is restricted to the rectum and sigmoid colon in 75% of patients (short-segment Hirschsprung disease), extends to the splenic flexure or transverse colon in 15% (long-segment Hirschsprung's disease) and along the entire colon and a variable length of terminal ileum in 8% (total colonic aganglionosis). Rarely, ganglion cells are absent as far proximally as the jejunum or duodenum.

Enteric ganglion cells are derived from vagal neural crest cells that migrate down the gut to the rectum in the embryo. Failure of this process is understood to be the cause of Hirschsprung disease. The incidence of the condition is about 1:5000 live births, with a male to female ratio of 4:1; this sex difference is less marked in longer segment disease.

Numerous conditions are associated with Hirschsprung disease. The most consistent association is with Down syndrome but various other chromosomal abnormalities and syndromes are recognised (Shaw et al. 1996). Cardiac, genitourinary, central nervous system and gastrointestinal abnormalities are each recorded in about 5% of patients. Links with congenital central hypoventilation (Croaker et al. 1998), Waardenburg syndrome (Moore and Johnson 1998), Mowat–Wilson syndrome (Mowat et al. 2003), multiple endocrine neoplasia and intestinal neuronal dysplasia are well described.

Advances in molecular genetics have confirmed that Hirschsprung disease is a genetic disorder (Kusafuka and Puri 1998). Most cases are sporadic but autosomal dominant, autosomal recessive and polygenic patterns of inheritance within families have been reported. Mutations in the *RET* proto-oncogene region of chromosome 10 are known to account for many cases. Other gene defects causing familial Hirschsprung disease have been mapped to the endothelin-B receptor gene on chromosome 13. The association of Hirschsprung disease with Down syndrome, chromosomal anomalies and genetically determined syndromes emphasises the genetic nature of the condition.

Hirschsprung disease typically presents during the neonatal period. Delayed passage of meconium is the cardinal clinical feature and is typically accompanied by progressive abdominal distension, reluctance to feed and vomiting, which is often bilious. Over 95% of healthy term infants pass their first stool within 24 hours of birth (Sherry and Kramer 1955). Delayed passage of meconium beyond 48 hours in a term infant should suggest the possibility of Hirschsprung disease. Delayed passage of meconium is normal in premature infants (Weaver and Lucas 1993) and this is therefore a less reliable feature of Hirschsprung disease in this group.

Rectal examination typically reveals a tightly contracted anorectum and withdrawal of the finger may be followed by an explosive discharge of stool and gas. In some cases, this induces a temporary remission but the baby continues to have problems with constipation. If the obstruction is not relieved the infant is at risk of intestinal perforation, enterocolitis and death.

Hirschsprung's enterocolitis is a serious and potentially fatal complication. It is characterised by marked abdominal distension, explosive diarrhoea, vomiting and fever. The clinical and radiological picture may be indistinguishable from necrotising enterocolitis. Obstruction, infection (e.g. *Clostridium difficile*) and impaired mucosal immunity are important predisposing factors. Bowel decompression by repeated rectal lavage with warm normal saline is the usual first-line treatment. Intravenous broad-spectrum antibiotics are given initially but ceased once washouts are established and the child is feeding normally.

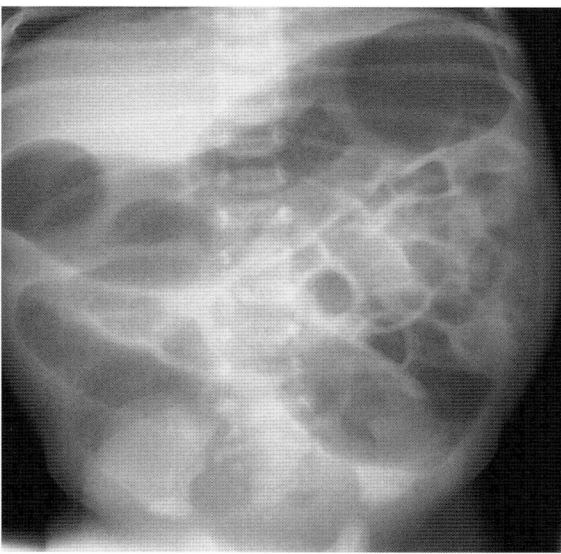

Fig. 29.72 Intestinal obstruction with an absence of gas in the rectum in a baby with Hirschsprung disease.

Histological examination of an adequate rectal biopsy by an experienced pathologist is the gold standard in the diagnosis of Hirschsprung disease. The main diagnostic tools are described below.

Radiology

Plain abdominal radiographs characteristically show multiple dilated loops of bowel with an absent rectal gas shadow (Fig. 29.72) but the latter is not specific for Hirschsprung disease. In infants with enterocolitis, thickening of the bowel wall, mucosal irregularity and/or a grossly dilated colon may be evident. A contrast enema performed by an experienced radiologist using an isotonic water-soluble contrast medium is often used to diagnose Hirschsprung disease but the results are not always reliable. Typically, contrast outlines a narrow distal segment of rectum and colon, a cone-shaped transition zone and a proximal dilated colon (Fig. 29.73). However, the cone is not necessarily the site of the transition zone between abnormal and healthy bowel.

Anorectal manometry

The resting pressure within the anal canal and lower rectum is raised and there is no anal relaxation in response to a distending stimulus in the rectum (absent rectoanal inhibitory reflex). Misleading results may occur and this technique is now used infrequently.

Rectal biopsy

A suction rectal biopsy is taken from above the anal canal (usually 2–4 cm from the anal verge) and must contain adequate amounts of submucosa, be appropriately oriented and sectioned, and be examined by an experienced histopathologist. Diagnosis rests on the absence of ganglion cells, the presence of thickened nerve trunks and a marked increase in acetylcholinesterase activity in the hypertrophied nerve bundles.

Initial treatment of Hirschsprung disease consists of decompressing the dilated proximal (ganglionic) bowel by rectal washouts using small volumes of warm saline (Fig. 29.74). Initially, this may

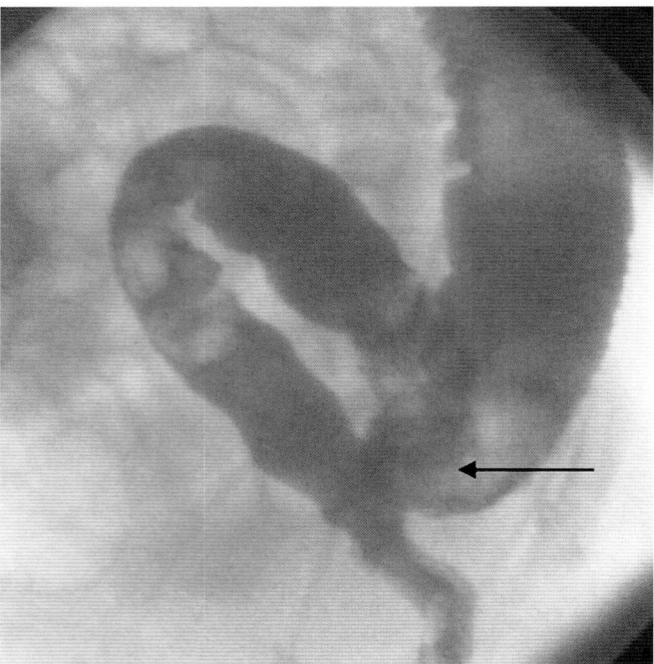

Fig. 29.73 Barium enema showing a 'transition zone' at the junction of the descending and colon (arrow). The actual transition zone was found to be proximal to this site.

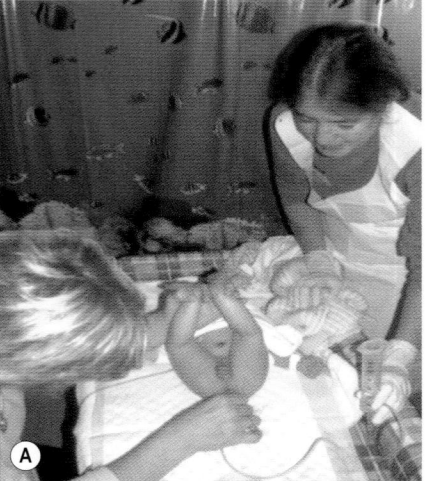

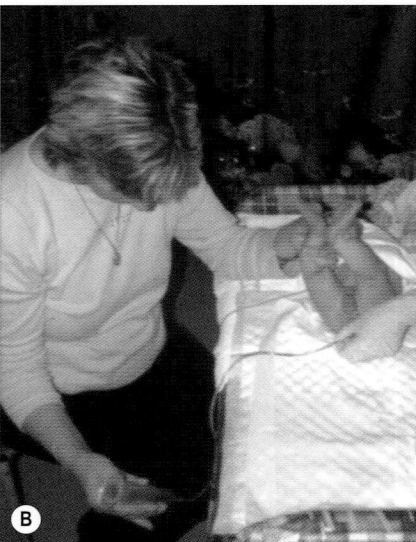

Fig. 29.74 Rectal washouts in Hirschsprung disease. The mother is being supervised by a specialist nurse.

be required twice daily but, with time, once a day is sufficient. If this fails to decompress the bowel then a stoma is necessary. The aim of definitive surgery for Hirschsprung disease is to resect the aganglionic bowel and to join healthy ganglionic proximal bowel to the anorectal stump.

Various techniques are described (e.g. Duhamel's, Soave's and Swenson's operations), and this implies that none is perfect. In the majority of infants, surgical correction is now performed as a single-stage procedure (primary pull-through) rather than the traditional approach of proximal stoma formation, definitive surgery and subsequent stoma closure. Recent developments include laparoscopically assisted procedures and transanal operations, which obviate the need for an abdominal incision in short-segment disease. Primary pull-through procedures are best avoided if the colon cannot be adequately decompressed by rectal washouts (and this includes most cases with total colonic aganglionosis), if enterocolitis cannot be rapidly controlled by medical treatment or if intestinal perforation has occurred.

Most patients can expect good long-term bowel function after definitive surgery for Hirschsprung disease. However, a significant proportion continue to have problems despite a technically adequate pull-through with fully ganglionic bowel. Potential long-term problems include enterocolitis, constipation and faecal incontinence. Long-term bowel function is influenced by early surgical complications, bowel training and the social background and intelligence of the child. In most series, about 75% of patients will achieve good bowel control as they reach adulthood (Engum and Grosfeld 1998). A UK support group for parents and families is called the Hirschsprung's and Motility Disorders Support Network (see Weblinks, below). Down syndrome has a major adverse impact on the acquisition of faecal continence in Hirschsprung disease.

The risk of disease in future offspring depends on the sex of the affected individual and the extent of the aganglionosis; increasingly, families of patients with Hirschsprung disease are routinely referred for genetic review (Badner et al. 1990).

Anorectal malformations

Anorectal malformations encompass a wide spectrum of congenital defects ranging from a minor malposition of the anus to complete agenesis of the anorectum. Classification of these anomalies is difficult but Pena (1995) has suggested a practical approach based on gender and differences in treatment and prognosis, although the Krickenbach classification is now being advocated (Holschneider et al. 2005). The common types of malformation are listed in Table 29.27 and shown in Figure 29.75.

In boys, an imperforate anus with the rectum terminating as a rectourethral fistula is the most frequent malformation. Next commonest is a low termination of the rectum and a perineal fistula. In girls, an anterior anus or perineal fistula or an imperforate anus with a rectovestibular fistula are the commonest lesions. Cloacal malformations account for about 10% of female defects.

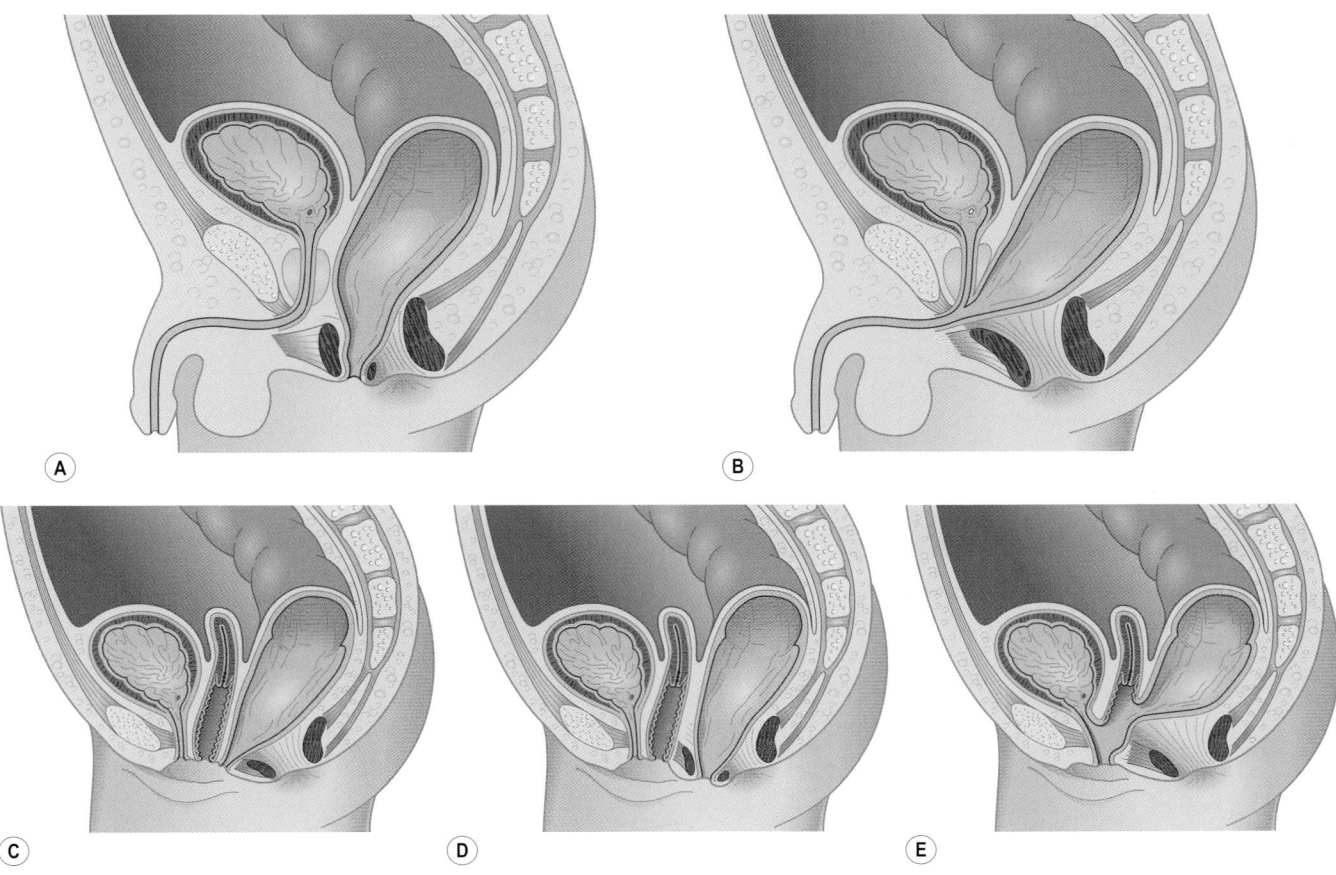

Fig. 29.75 Commoner varieties of anorectal malformations. (A) Perineal fistula in a boy; (B) rectourethral fistula in a boy; (C) rectovestibular fistula; (D) anterior stenotic anus in a girl; (E) cloacal anomaly.

Table 29.27 Types of anorectal malformation: Krickenbeck classification (Holschneider et al. 2005)

MAJOR CLINICAL GROUPS	RARE/REGIONAL VARIETIES
Perineal (cutaneous) fistula	Pouch colon
Rectourethral fistula: (a) prostatic or (b) bulbar	Rectal atresia or stenosis
Rectovesical	Rectovaginal
Vestibular	'H' fistula
Cloaca: (a) <3 cm or (b) >3 cm common channel	

The incidence of anorectal malformations is around 1:4000–5000 live births. The cause of these defects is unknown. Most are sporadic. Traditionally, anorectal malformations have been understood to arise as a result of abnormal partitioning of the embryonic cloaca by the caudal descent of the urorectal septum, but this view is almost certainly too simplistic (Kluth and Lambrecht 1997).

At least 40% of affected patients have additional congenital defects. This figure is higher in patients with high anorectal malformations (Rintala et al. 1991). Associated conditions include the following:

- Genitourinary: these are the commonest. Examples include absent, dysplastic, cross-fused or horseshoe kidneys, vesicoureteric reflux, hydronephrosis, hypospadias, bifid scrotum and cryptorchidism. Girls with cloacal anomalies may have vaginal and uterine malformations.
- Skeletal: lumbosacral vertebral anomalies are most common. Sacral defects are more frequent and more severe with high malformations. The absence of two or more sacral vertebrae is associated with a poor functional outcome (Rintala et al. 1991).
- Spinal cord: a range of spinal cord anomalies have been described since the advent of magnetic resonance imaging.
- Gastrointestinal: the best known association is with oesophageal atresia as part of the VACTERL complex (see above).
- Cardiovascular: various abnormalities may coexist.
- Syndromes: the commonest is the VACTERL association. Another example is the Currarino triad due to an autosomal dominant gene on chromosome 7, manifesting as partial sacral agenesis, anal stenosis and a presacral mass (e.g. meningocele or sacrococcygeal teratoma) (Currarino et al. 1981). Trisomy 21 is a recognised association in anorectal malformations and may involve a pure atresia rather than a fistula (Fig. 29.76).

Early diagnosis is important to avoid complications such as intestinal perforation and urinary tract infection. All infants should be

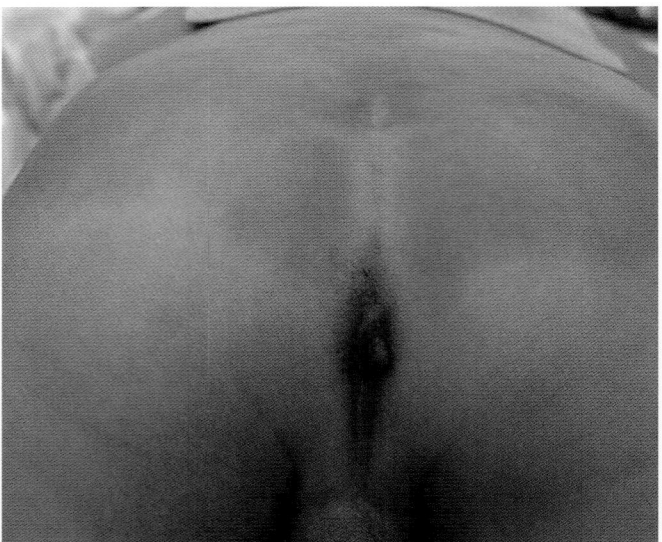

Fig. 29.76 A child with Down syndrome and a rectal atresia. An imperforate anus is visible, as is a large mongolian blue spot.

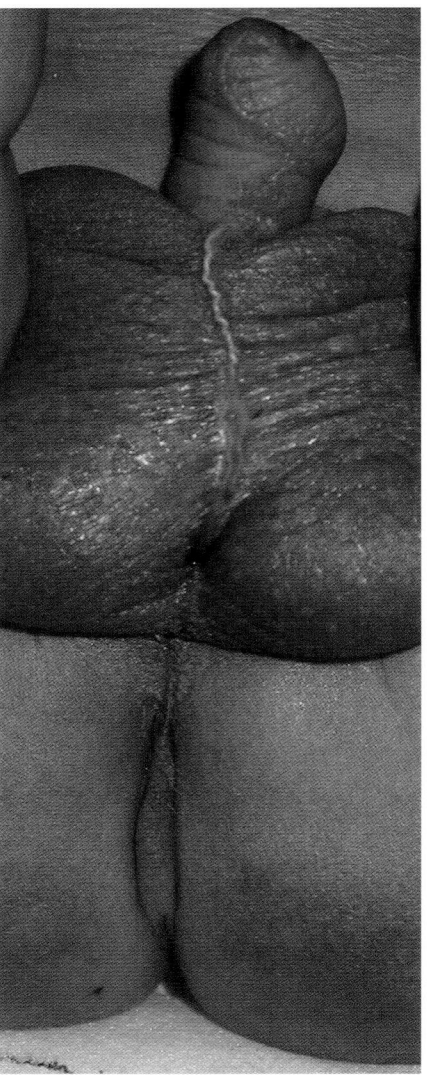

Fig. 29.77 Low anorectal anomaly. A perineal fistula with meconium seen at base of scrotum but also pearls of meconium seen tracking along the midline scrotal raphe on to the base of the penis.

examined thoroughly, including the spine and genitalia. In most cases, a detailed inspection of the perineum can distinguish low and high malformations.

In boys with low lesions, the anus is imperforate or appears abnormal. There is a single abnormal opening on the perineum or a track may be seen running along the midline raphe to the scrotum (Fig. 29.77). Boys with low lesions have a well-developed buttock cleft and anal dimple, good sphincter muscles and a normal sacrum. With higher lesions in boys, no perineal orifice is seen (Fig. 29.78) but meconium or bubbles may appear in the urine. In such cases, the pelvic and perineal muscles are less well developed and a sacral defect may be evident.

In normal girls, the anus is positioned midway between the posterior fourchette and the tip of the coccyx. A stenotic anterior anus (Fig. 29.79) is easily overlooked in the newborn and may not present until later, with severe constipation. In girls, it is important to count the number of perineal orifices. If only the vagina and urethra are visible, then the infant probably has a rectovestibular malformation in which the rectum opens immediately in front of the posterior fourchette (Fig. 29.80). Meconium is often passed through the fistula after birth. If there is only one perineal opening, then the baby has a cloacal malformation characterised by the confluence of rectum, vagina and urethra into a single common channel (Fig. 29.81). Neonatal hydrocolpos and urinary obstruction may complicate this anomaly.

If the clinical picture is unclear, a lateral prone radiograph at about 24 hours of age with the baby's pelvis elevated helps to distinguish high and low lesions. The anal dimple must be marked with a radiopaque marker (Fig. 29.82). The distance between the rectal termination and the anal skin can be measured. If this radiograph is performed too early, it may falsely suggest a high lesion because the gas has not yet reached the point of obstruction. The presence of air in the bladder is evidence of a rectourinary fistula.

Other useful investigations in a neonate with an anorectal malformation include lumbosacral and chest radiographs, a urinary tract ultrasound scan, echocardiography and, in selected cases, a karyotype.

Most low lesions can be successfully treated by an anoplasty soon after birth. Temporary use of an anal dilator is often needed.

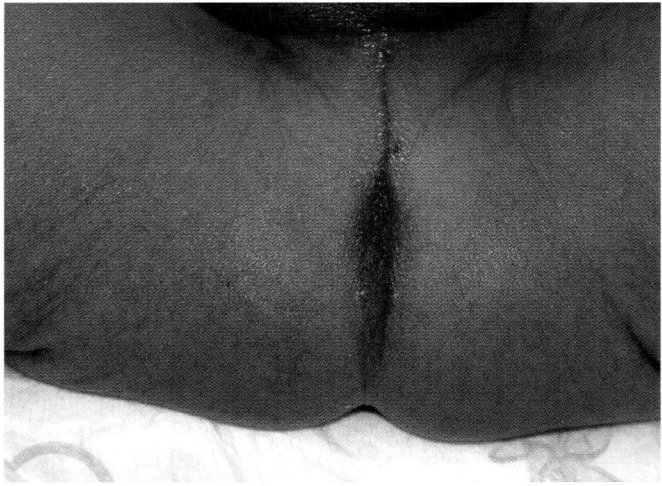

Fig. 29.78 Imperforate anus in a boy with a rectourethral fistula.

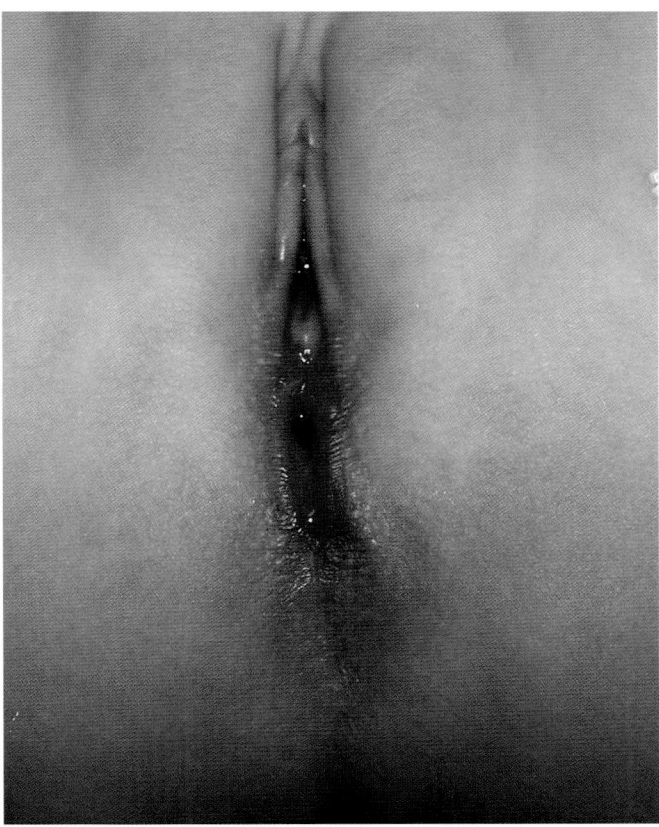

Fig. 29.79 An anterior stenotic anus in a girl. Note how narrow the perineal body is.

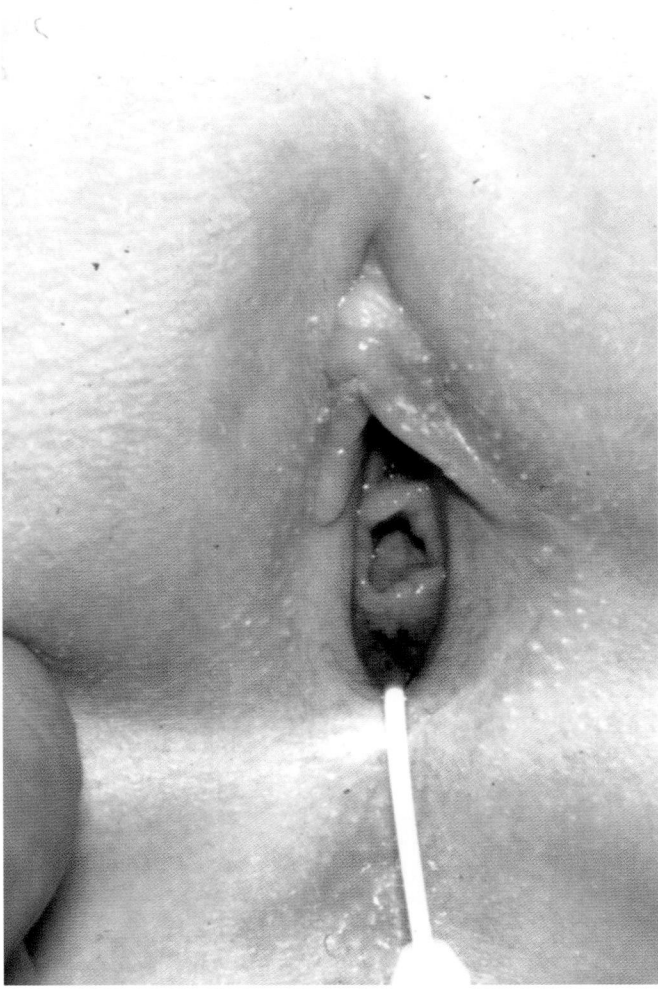

Fig. 29.80 A rectovestibular fistula demonstrated with a cannula in the fistula.

Constipation is a common problem but, provided this is managed aggressively, good bowel control can be achieved (Rintala et al. 1997). Higher malformations are usually treated by a diverting, proximal colostomy soon after birth and definitive repair of the malformation a few months later once the anatomy of the malformation has been defined and the infant is thriving. The posterior sagittal anorectoplasty is the current standard reconstructive operative procedure (Pena 1995); however, a laparoscopic approach to divide the fistula and then pull the bowel through a much smaller perineal incision is gaining popularity (El-Debeiky et al. 2009). Outcome in terms of constipation, soiling and faecal continence are affected by the type of anorectal malformation (many high lesions are associated with some faecal incontinence), the presence of a sacral defect and the method and timing of surgery. Many children require considerable help in achieving social continence and coping with psychosocial sequelae (Ludman 1998).

Colonic atresia

This is a rare form of atresia, accounting for only 5% of intestinal atresias. It may be associated with limb anomalies, abdominal wall defects, Hirschsprung disease or other atresias. Presentation is that of a low intestinal obstruction. The baby develops abdominal distension and progressive vomiting, and fails to pass meconium. An abdominal radiograph shows evidence of a distal bowel obstruction and a contrast enema demonstrates the level of the atresia. Staged surgery is often required, with initial relief of the obstruction by colostomy, followed later by large bowel anastomosis.

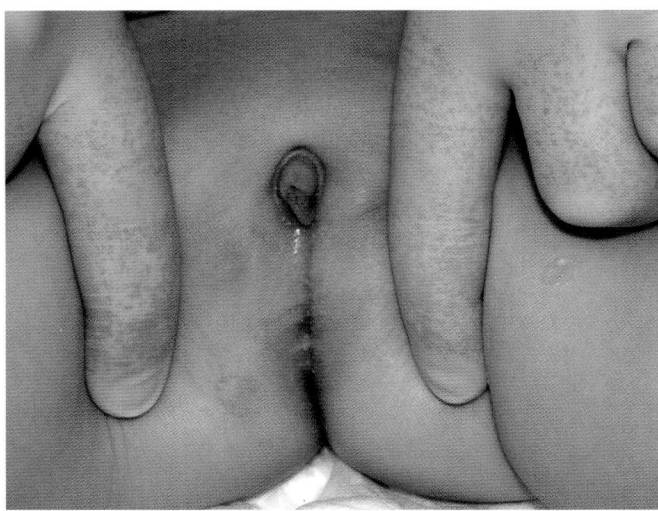

Fig. 29.81 A cloacal anomaly with a single perineal orifice only.

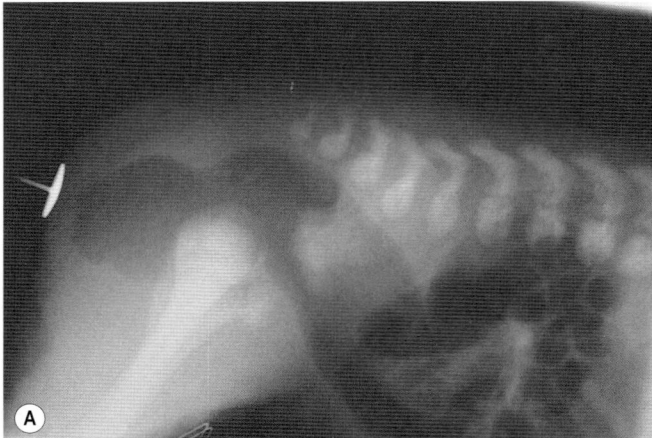

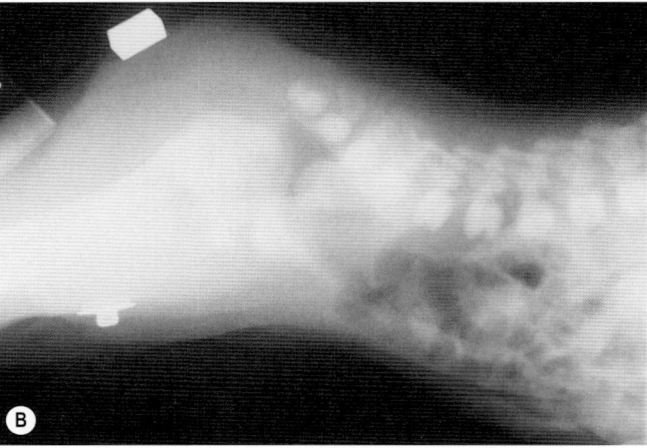

Fig. 29.82 Lateral prone radiograph with pelvic elevation at 24–36 hours of age in babies with (A) low and (B) high anorectal malformations. Note the distance between the rectal gas shadow and the anal marker in each case.

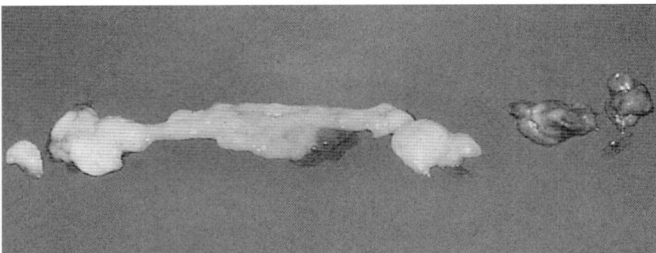

Fig. 29.83 Meconium plug.

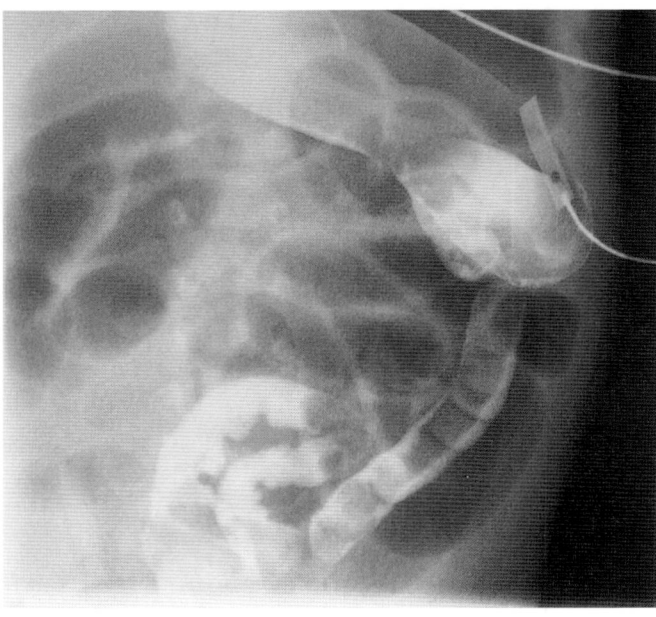

Fig. 29.84 Contrast enema in a baby with small left-colon syndrome.

Meconium plug obstruction

Meconium plug obstruction occurs most often in the low-birthweight baby who may also be compromised by other problems such as perinatal hypoxia, hypothermia and the effects of medication given to the mother in labour. It can be difficult to achieve a balance between subjecting the baby to potentially unnecessary investigations and overlooking genuine pathology. The main differential diagnosis is between meconium plug obstruction, Hirschsprung disease and CF, all of which can occur in low-birthweight infants. Contrast enema studies in this situation may be misinterpreted as showing evidence of Hirschsprung disease.

In preterm infants, expectant observation is usually the best approach. If abdominal distension is severe, gentle irrigation of the baby's rectum with warm saline usually relieves the obstruction and yields a pale plug of meconium (Fig. 29.83). Alternatively, warmed dilute Gastrografin may be instilled into the large bowel via a soft rectal catheter and a radiograph will demonstrate the meconium plug. This procedure often provokes passage of the plug and, once the infant has started passing motions, continuing difficulty is less marked. The infant with a meconium plug must be observed closely and followed up after discharge.

In full-term infants, delay in passage of meconium beyond 48 hours always merits investigation.

Megacystis–microcolon–intestinal hypoperistalsis syndrome

This rare entity, which is commoner in girls, is a form of visceral myopathy causing severe functional intestinal obstruction (Puri and Tsuji 1992). Intestinal and bladder motility are markedly impaired. Infants also have lax abdominal muscles and incomplete intestinal rotation. Most cases are reliant on long-term parenteral nutrition for survival.

Small left-colon syndrome

This term is used for a transient functional neonatal large bowel obstruction caused by a small-calibre left colon distal to the splenic flexure. It is associated with maternal insulin-dependent diabetes. The degree of obstruction is variable. A contrast enema is diagnostic and often therapeutic (Fig. 29.84). Hirschsprung disease must be excluded.

Stomas

An intestinal stoma may be temporarily required in the management of various neonatal surgical conditions, including necrotising enterocolitis, Hirschsprung disease, anorectal malformations,

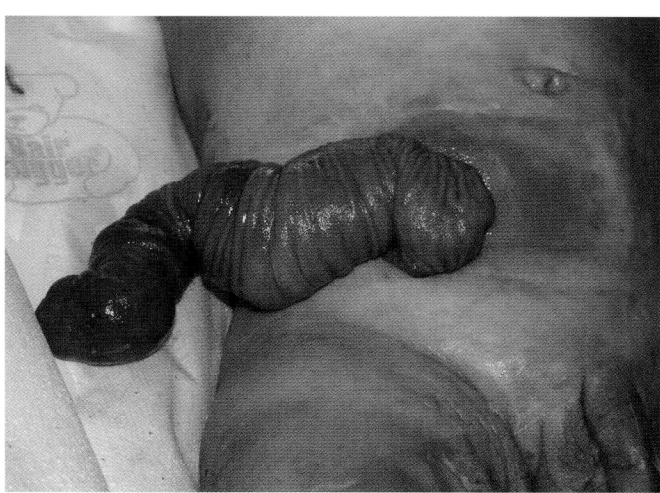

Fig. 29.85 Prolapse of an ileostomy.

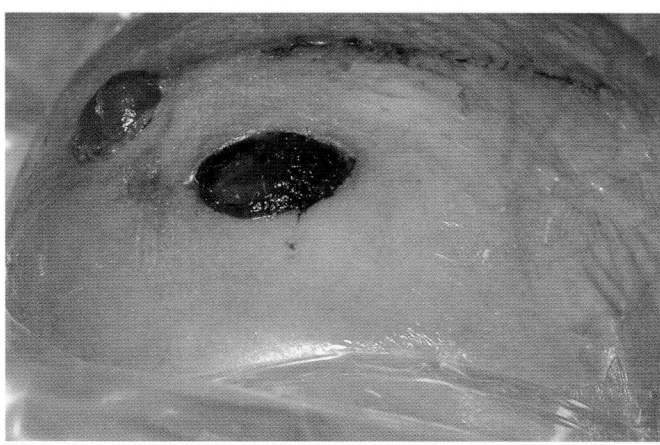

Fig. 29.86 A baby who had a split ileostomy and mucous fistula created for complicated necrotising enterocolitis. The ileostomy has become ischaemic.

intestinal atresia and complicated meconium ileus. Most are colostomies or ileostomies. Potential stoma complications include:

- mechanical, e.g. prolapse, stenosis, retraction – prolapse is more common with a loop stoma (Fig. 29.85)
- leakage and skin excoriation
- fluid and electrolyte losses – especially with small bowel stomas
- nutritional problems
- wound infection, candidiasis
- ischaemia (Fig. 29.86).

Expert surgical nursing care and appropriate stoma appliances are paramount.

Sodium deficiency occurs frequently with neonatal ileostomies or proximal colostomies. Plasma sodium levels are usually normal but urinary sodium concentrations are consistently less than 10 mmol/l, indicating a total body sodium deficit (Bower et al. 1988). A mild metabolic acidosis and growth failure ensue despite a good calorie intake. Before normal growth can be achieved, these babies must have their feeds supplemented with sodium chloride to restore normal urinary sodium excretion.

Anterior abdominal wall defects

Although gastroschisis was recognised as early as 1733 (Calder 1733), only in the last 50 years has it been clearly differentiated from exomphalos. A distinction between these two anterior abdominal wall defects is clinically important, but not all infants fall neatly into one or other category. The prevalence of gastroschisis is about 1 : 7000 total births (Curry et al. 2000) but there are significant regional variations within the UK and abroad (Stone et al. 1998; Di Tanna et al. 2002). Exomphalos is at least twice as common (Calzolari et al. 1995; Stone et al. 1998). Gastroschisis has become more prevalent in the past 25 years while the frequency of exomphalos has remained much the same. Both sexes are similarly affected. A UK parents support group can be found in the Weblinks section (see below):

- In simple terms, the anterior abdominal wall is formed by four separate embryological folds – cephalic, caudal and lateral – each of which has a splanchnic and somatic component. Failure of union of the cephalic fold results in exomphalos with a sternal/diaphragmatic defect or the pentalogy of Cantrell et al. (1958). Failure of the caudal fold to close results in exomphalos with bladder or cloacal exstrophy. Failure of the lateral folds to close results in exomphalos. The pathogenesis of gastroschisis is less clear. Suggested mechanisms include a local failure of differentiation of mesoderm forming the abdominal wall muscles, rupture of the membrane covering a hernia of the umbilical cord or a vascular insult interfering with the development of the somatopleure at the junction with the body stalk (Curry et al. 2000).
- Prenatal ultrasound is highly sensitive in the diagnosis of anterior abdominal wall defects. Most defects are detectable by 16–20 weeks' gestation and it is usually possible to differentiate between exomphalos and gastroschisis. This is important since exomphalos is frequently associated with chromosomal anomalies (e.g. trisomy 13, 18 and 21) and major congenital heart defects (Gilbert and Nicolaides 1987), indicating the need for fetal karyotyping and echocardiography. Although exomphalos is seen more often than gastroschisis in utero, this relationship is reversed at birth because of fetal deaths and terminations in the exomphalos group. For the same reasons, the observed incidence of additional congenital anomalies in neonates with exomphalos is less than expected. Gastroschisis is rarely associated with aneuploidy.

Exomphalos

This term encompasses a spectrum of abnormalities ranging from a small umbilical defect with gut prolapsing into the cord (a hernia into the cord; Fig. 29.87), through umbilical defects less than 5 cm wide (exomphalos minor; Fig. 29.88) to larger umbilical defects (exomphalos major or giant omphalocele; Fig. 29.89). Bowel and often liver are enclosed within the sac (unless it has ruptured). Since the developing bowel has failed to complete its normal return to the abdominal cavity from the umbilical cord, disorders of intestinal rotation may be found with all these umbilical defects, but classical midgut malrotation is uncommon:

- Urgent surgery is not indicated for the infant with an exomphalos and an intact amniotic sac. Echocardiography, karyotyping and, in selected cases, upper gastrointestinal contrast studies to assess gut rotation should be performed. Blood glucose must be monitored, particularly since

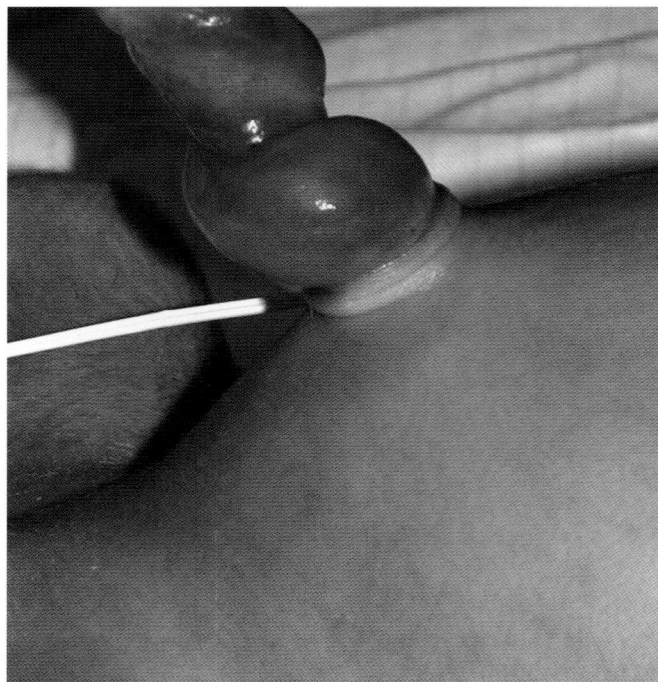

Fig. 29.87 A hernia into the cord containing the caecum and appendix. The infant had no other anomalies.

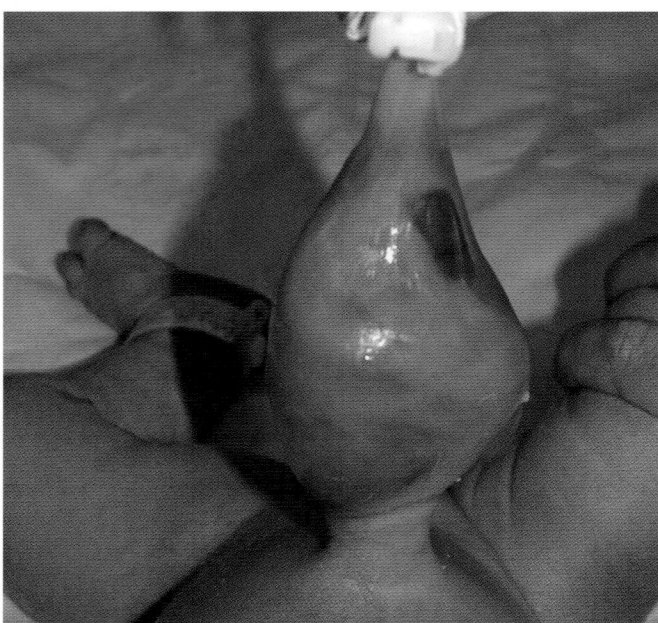

Fig. 29.88 An exomphalos minor.

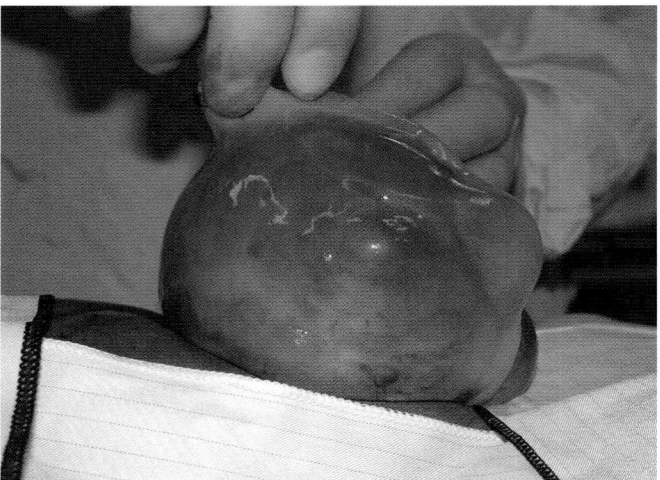

Fig. 29.89 Exomphalos major containing liver and bowel.

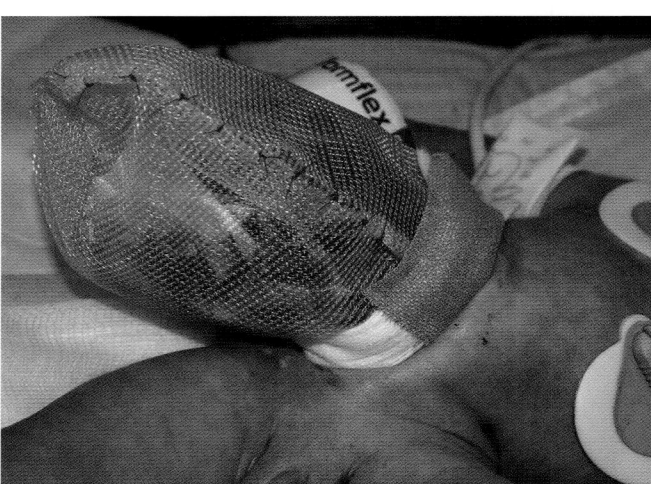

Fig. 29.90 Baby born with a ruptured exomphalos that required application of silo at birth.

Beckwith–Wiedemann syndrome (Ch. 31) may present with exomphalos. Other associations include intestinal atresia or stenosis.

- With a hernia into the cord or exomphalos minor, once the defect has been repaired the long-term outlook is good provided there is no associated syndrome or additional major congenital abnormality.

- In exomphalos major, reduction of the herniated bowel and liver into the abdominal cavity can be difficult. It may require the surgical application of sterile prosthetic material to the rim of the abdominal wall defect and gradual reduction of the contents of this silo over a period of 7–10 days (staged silo repair; Fig. 29.90). The fascia and skin are repaired as the final procedure. Temporary support with parenteral nutrition is often required. With this technique, potentially serious complications may occur. Consequently, a conservative approach is sometimes used. This involves treating the sac with desiccating antiseptic agents. Mercurochrome is potentially toxic (Fagan et al. 1977) and has been replaced by silver sulfadiazine ointment (Fig. 29.91) or povidone iodine spray. Thyroid function may be disturbed by prolonged use of the latter (Cosman et al. 1988). The sac gradually contracts, leaving a correctable abdominal wall defect.

- Outcome is largely dictated by the severity of associated malformations. In some infants, both the abdominal and thoracic cavities are poorly developed and pulmonary hypoplasia may pose additional problems. A ruptured exomphalos requires urgent surgery (Figs 29.90 and 29.92).

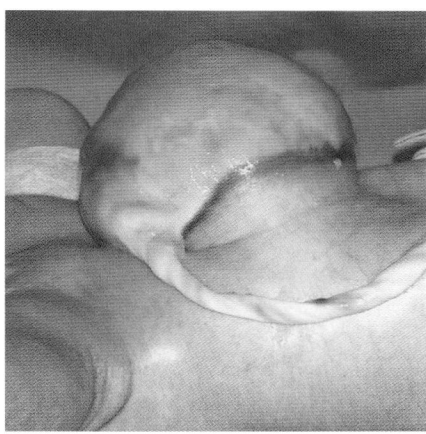

Fig. 29.91 Exomphalos major treated with flamazine. Note the epithelialisation of the sac at its edge.

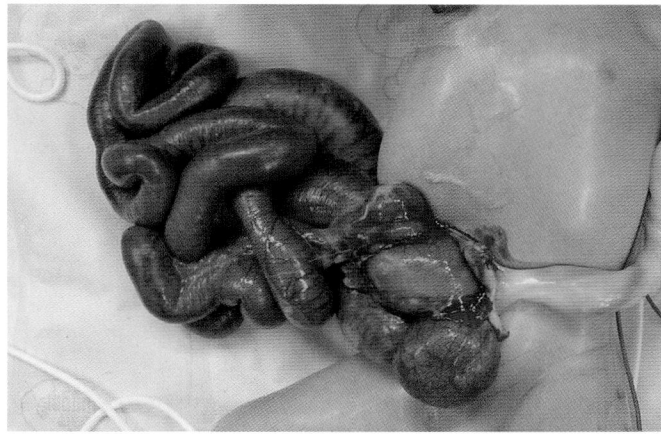

Fig. 29.93 Gastroschisis. The bowel is matted and has a fibrin peel. Note that the abdominal wall defect is just to the right of the umbilicus.

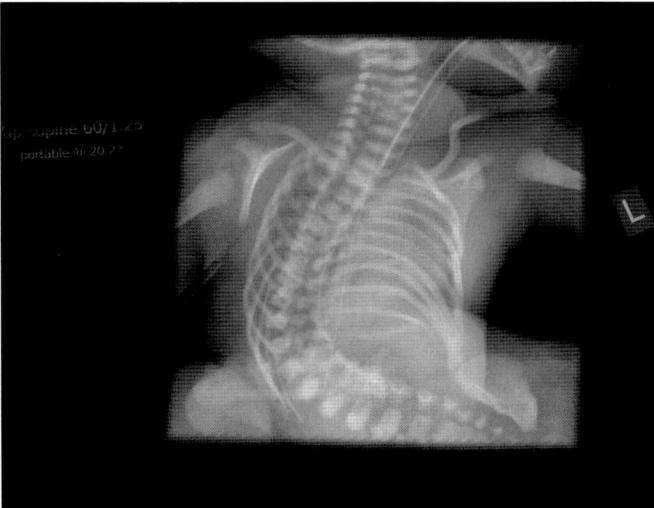

Fig. 29.92 Same baby as in Fig. 29.84. Radiograph confirmed a severe kyphoscoliosis with poorly developed thoracic and abdominal cavities.

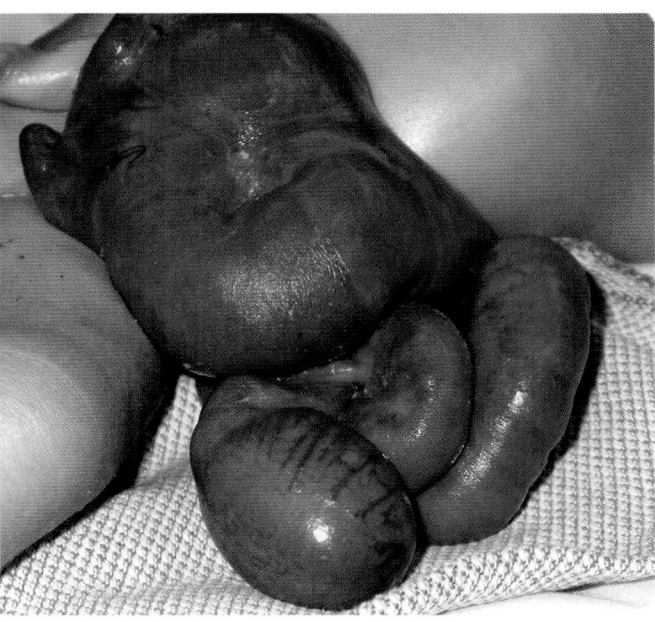

Fig. 29.94 Intestinal atresia associated with gastroschisis.

Gastroschisis

In gastroschisis, the bowel prolapses through a defect that is typically just to the right of the umbilicus (Fig. 29.93). Unlike exomphalos, there is no covering membrane. The extent of evisceration is variable but may include stomach, small bowel, colon, and ovary and fallopian tube or testis. Only rarely is the liver involved:

- Young maternal age (median 21 years) is consistently associated with the condition and other maternal risk factors have also been identified (Curry et al. 2000). Infants with gastroschisis are typically of low birthweight (median 2.3 kg) and do not usually have other life-threatening anomalies. Intestinal atresia is found in about 10% of cases (Fig. 29.94) and the bowel in gastroschisis is non-rotated. Rarely the gastroschisis defect narrows before birth, which leads to a potentially devastating outcome due to loss of the herniated bowel (Fig. 29.95).
- The postnatal appearance of the bowel varies from almost normal to a foreshortened, thickened mass covered in a dense fibrin 'peel'. The duration of exposure of the fetal gut to

amniotic fluid may determine this appearance but clinical and experimental evidence suggests that it is related more to vascular compression of the mesentery of the gut by the edges of the abdominal wall defect.

- Infants with gastroschisis lose fluid and heat readily from the exposed bowel. Immediately after delivery they require intravenous fluids, a nasogastric tube and measures to stabilise and insulate the bowel. Cellophane wrapping ('cling-film') allows the bowel to be inspected and prevents harmful traction on the mesentery (Fig. 29.96). In utero transfer to a centre with obstetric and paediatric surgical services is preferable to postnatal transfer since it facilitates prompt postnatal surgical treatment and enables mother and baby to be together.
- The management of gastroschisis has changed in many centres over the last few years. The standard treatment used to be (and still is for some surgeons) reduction under general anaesthesia, with repair of the defect (primary closure). This

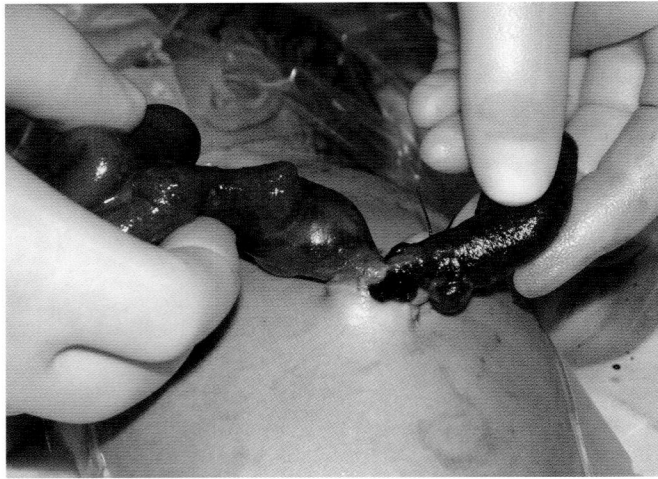

Fig. 29.95 A baby born with a closing gastroschisis. Note the small amount of bowel left, including one ischaemic loop.

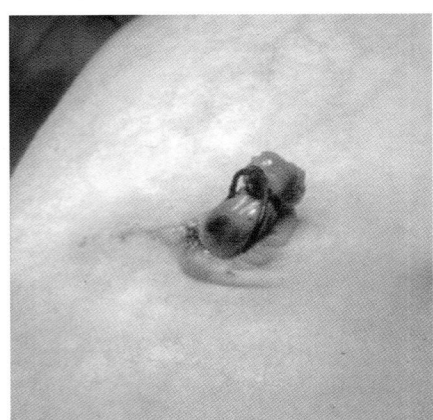

Fig. 29.97 Appearance of the umbilicus after primary repair of gastroschisis.

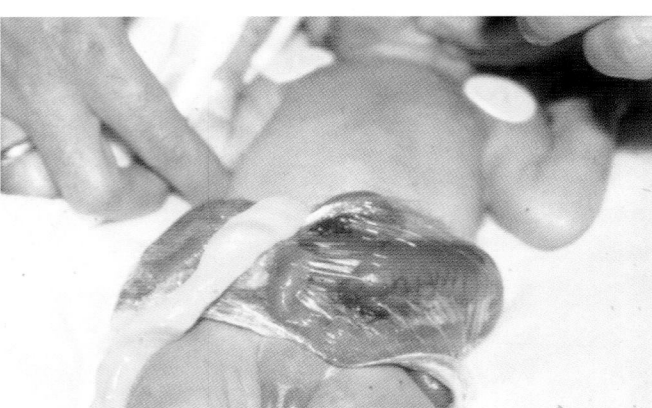

Fig. 29.96 The exposed gut can be temporarily insulated and stabilised with a 'cling-film' wrap.

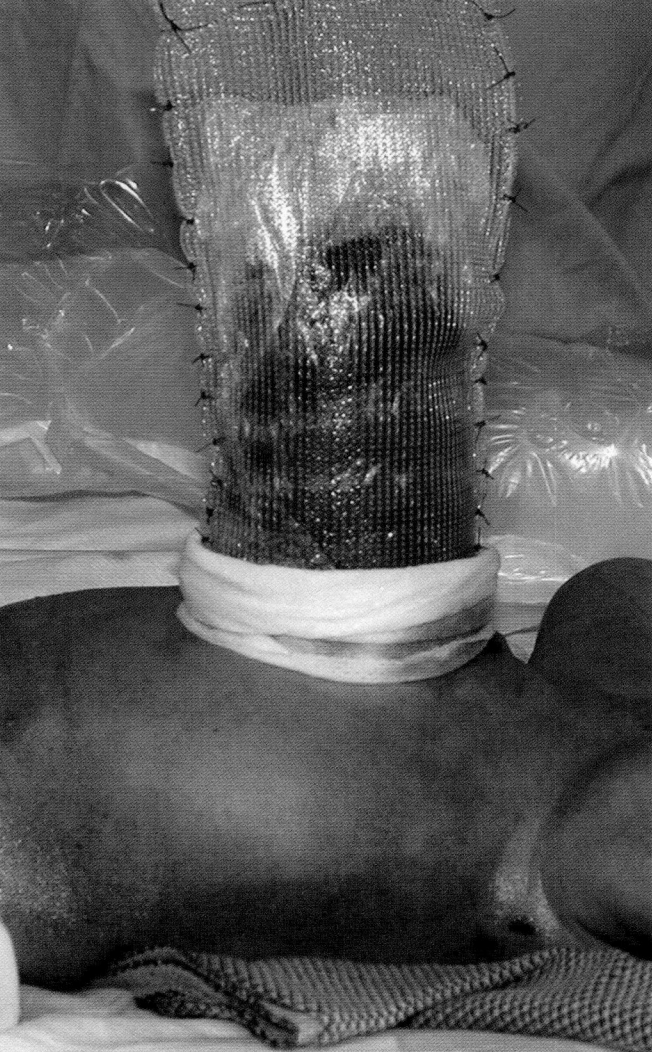

Fig. 29.98 Gastroschisis with a Prolene silo formed. This will be tucked daily to reduce the bowel into the abdominal cavity before the silo is removed.

usually leaves a good cosmetic appearance (Fig. 29.97). In cases where the abdominal cavity is not large enough to accommodate the viscera, a staged silo repair (see above) is necessary (Fig. 29.98). Recently, placing the bowel into a preformed silo (Fig. 29.99), with the baby awake on the neonatal unit, has become the alternative choice of treatment (Lansdale et al. 2009). This avoids the neonate requiring a general anaesthetic, prevents the bowel reduction being tight (which avoids the need for postoperative ventilation, with its associated complications) and the bowel contents can be reduced in a controlled manner over a few days. The silo is then removed and the abdomen closed on the unit without general anaesthesia. Occasionally, it is possible to reduce the gastroschisis fully with the baby awake.

- Although 90% or more of affected babies now survive, their postnatal course is often protracted. Full enteral feeding is usually not achieved for about 3 weeks after primary closure and during this period the infant requires total parenteral nutrition with its attendant risks and complications. Babies with gastroschisis often stay in hospital for several weeks. Those with atresias or severe short-gut syndrome may have a

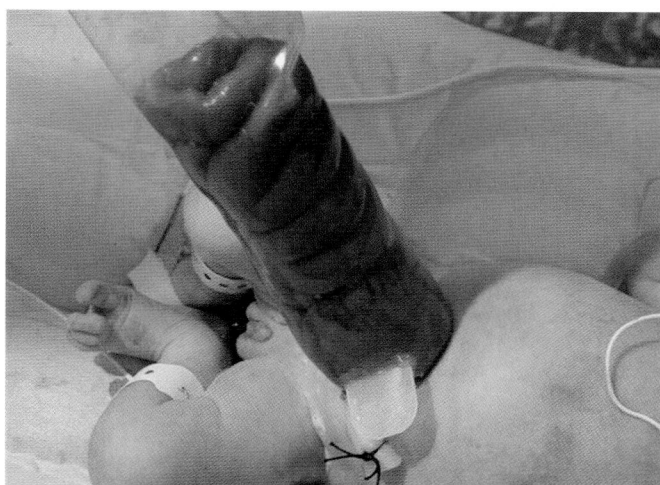

Fig. 29.99 Appearance of the bowel after being placed into a preformed silo (Medicina) whilst awake.

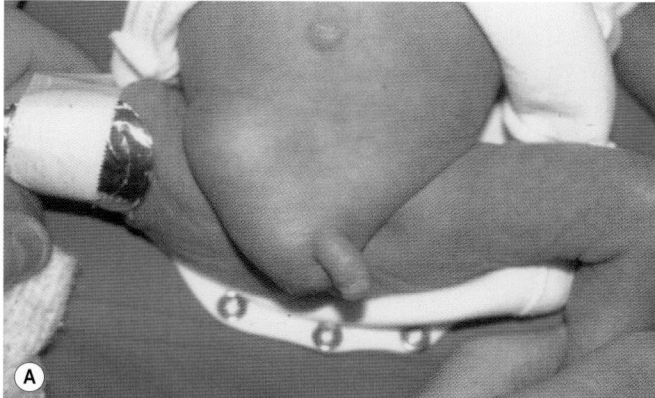

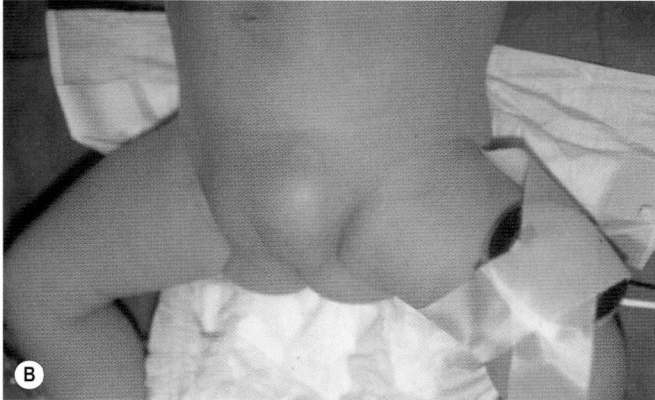

Fig. 29.101 Incarcerated inguinal hernias. (A) This boy's right inguinal hernia was reduced by taxis and subsequently repaired. (B) This baby girl had an ovary incarcerated in her irreducible inguinal hernia and required urgent surgery.

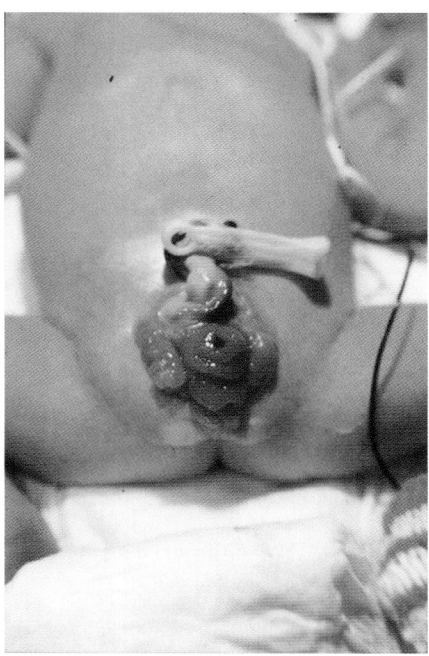

Fig. 29.100 Cloacal exstrophy. The gut is exposed between two hemibladders.

more complicated course. Necrotising enterocolitis is an additional potential complication.

Cloacal exstrophy

This is an uncommon condition that affects both the alimentary and urinary tracts. Typically, there is an exstrophic central segment of bowel (ileocaecal region) flanked by two hemibladders but many variations are described (Fig. 29.100). Gender assignment can be difficult and experienced multidisciplinary assessment is important. Major associated anomalies are common and reconstructive surgery is often complex (Lund and Hendren 2001).

Hernias

Inguinal

Although girls may develop an inguinal hernia, boys are affected much more frequently because of failure of closure of the processus vaginalis after testicular descent. The prevalence of inguinal hernia is greatest during infancy, when at least 1% of boys are affected. In boys, 60% of inguinal hernias occur on the right, 30% on the left and 10% are bilateral. Inguinal hernias in general and bilateral hernias in particular are much more common in premature babies, as are associated undescended testes:

* Inguinal hernias typically cause an intermittent swelling in the groin or scrotum when the baby cries or strains. If the hernia becomes obstructed (at the level of the external inguinal ring) it will manifest as a firm, tender lump in the groin or scrotum (Fig. 29.101). The baby may vomit and be irritable. Most incarcerated hernias in children can be successfully reduced by sustained gentle compression (taxis) after analgesia. Surgery is delayed for 24–48 hours to allow resolution of oedema. If reduction is impossible, emergency surgery is required because of the risk of strangulation of bowel (or ovary) and damage to the testis.
* The risk of incarceration/strangulation in an inguinal hernia is greatest in infancy and thus repair should generally be undertaken as soon as the infant is fit for surgery or prior to discharge from hospital in the case of a premature baby.

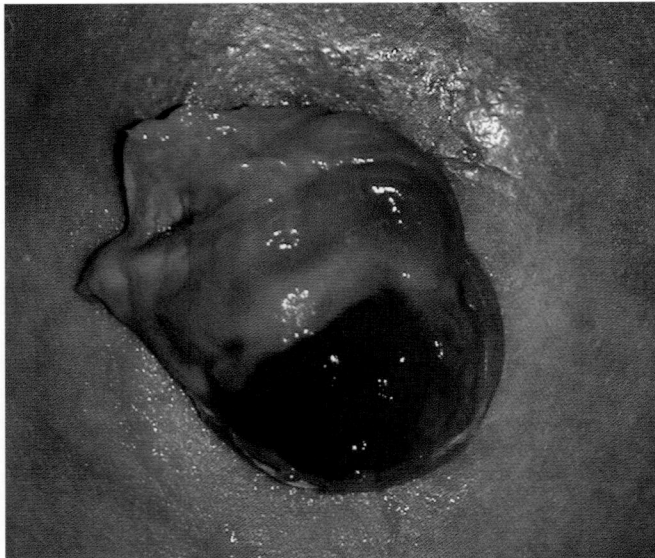

Fig. 29.102 A patent vitellointestinal duct causing an umbilical discharge. Excision of the duct was curative.

Postoperative apnoea is a potential hazard in infants less than 44 weeks' postconceptional age. Inguinal herniotomy is usually performed under general anaesthesia but regional anaesthetic techniques are valuable for some infants with respiratory problems (Peutrell and Hughes 1992). Most surgeons repair the hernia through an inguinal skin crease incision but laparoscopy has its advocates. Inguinal herniotomy is not a minor procedure in a neonate and demands anaesthetic and surgical expertise. Local complications are uncommon but may include recurrent hernia, interference with normal testicular descent and injury to the vas or vessels.

Umbilical

Incomplete regression of the vitelline duct may result in a patent vitellointestinal duct (Fig. 29.102) or a Meckel's diverticulum. An umbilical hernia is caused by incomplete closure of the umbilical ring. Most resolve spontaneously within a year or two and surgical repair is rarely necessary. Incarceration in an umbilical hernia is rare in western countries.

Acknowledgements

We are grateful to Mr Carl F Davis and Professor Dan G Young from the Royal Hospital for Sick Children in Glasgow, UK, for some of the illustrations taken from the previous editions of this chapter.

Weblinks

http://www.geeps.co.uk/: a website for parents of children with anterior abdominal wall defects.

http://www.hirschsprungs.info/: Hirschsprung's and Motility Disorders

Support Network: a website for parents of children with Hirschsprung disease and other motility disorders.

www.tofs.org.uk: a website for parents of children with tracheo-oesopheageal fistuls.

References

Astley, R., 1969. Duodenal atresia with gas below the obstruction. Br J Radiol 42, 351–353.

Badner, J.A., Sieber, W.K., Garver, K.L., et al., 1990. A genetic study of Hirschsprung's disease. Am J Hum Genet 46, 568–580.

Blumhagen, J.D., Maclin, L., Krauter, D., et al., 1988. Sonographic diagnosis of hypertrophic pyloric stenosis. American Journal of Roentgenology 150, 1367–1370.

Bower, T.R., Pringle, K.C., Soper, R.T., 1988. Sodium deficit causing decreased weight gain and metabolic acidosis in infants with ileostomy. J Pediatr Surg 23, 567–572.

Boyd, A., Carachi, R., Azmy, A., et al., 1988. Gastrografin enema in meconium ileus: the persistent approach. Pediatr Surg Int 3, 139–140.

British Association of Paediatric Surgeons/ Royal College of Surgeons of England, 1999. Surgical Services for the Newborn. British Association of Paediatric Surgeons and the Royal College of Surgeons of England, London.

Calder, J., 1733. Two examples of children with preternatural conformation of the guts. Medical Essays and Observations, Vol 1. T and W Ruddimans, Medical Society of Edinburgh, Edinburgh, p. 203.

Calzolari, E., Bianchi, F., Dolk, H., et al., 1995. Omphalocele and gastroschisis in Europe: a survey of 3 million births 1980–1990. EUROCAT Working Group. Am J Med Genet 58, 187–194.

Cantrell, J.R., Haller, Jr., J.A., Ravitch, M.M., 1958. A syndrome of congenital defects involving the abdominal wall, sternum, diaphragm, pericardium and heart. Surgery of Gynecology and Obstetrics 197, 602–614.

Chetcuti, P., Myers, N.A., Phelan, P.D., et al., 1988. Adults who survived repair of congenital oesophageal atresia and tracheo-oesophageal fistula. Br Med J 297, 344–346.

Chittmittrapap, S., Spitz, L., Kiely, E.M., et al., 1989. Oesophageal atresia and associated anomalies. Arch Dis Child 64, 364–368.

Clinical Standards Advisory Group, 1998. Cleft Lip and/or Palate. HMSO, London.

Cook, R.C.M., Rickham, P.P., 1969. Neonatal intestinal obstruction due to milk curds. J Pediatr Surg 4, 599–605.

Corbally, M.T., 1993. Laryngo-tracheo-oesophageal cleft. Arch Dis Child 532–533.

Cosman, B.C., Schullinger, J.N., Bell, J.J., et al., 1988. Hypothyroidism caused by topical povidone-iodine in a newborn with omphalocele. J Pediatr Surg 23, 356–358.

Coutts, J., Docherty, J.G., Carachi, R., et al., 1997. Clinical course of cystic fibrosis presenting with meconium ileus. Br J Surg 84, 555.

Crabbe, D.C.G., Kiely, E.M., Drake, D.P., et al., 1996. Management of the isolated congenital tracheo-oesophageal fistula. Eur J Pediatr Surg 6, 67–69.

Croaker, G.D.H., Shi, E., Simpson, E., et al., 1998. Congenital central hypoventilation syndrome and Hirschsprung's disease. Arch Dis Child 78, 316–322.

Currarino, G., Coln, D., Votteler, T., 1981. Triad of anorectal, sacral and presacral anomalies. American Journal of Roentgenology 137, 395–398.

Curry, J.I., McKinney, P., Thornton, J.G., et al., 2000. The aetiology of gastroschisis. Br J Obstet Gynaecol 107, 1339–1346.

Di Tanna, G.L., Rosano, A., Mastroiacovo, P., 2002. Prevalence of gastroschisis at birth: retrospective study. Br Med J 325, 1389–1390.

El-Debeiky, M.S., Safan, H.A., Shafei, I.A., et al., 2009. Long-term functional evaluation of fecal continence after laparoscopic-assisted pull-through for high anorectal malformations. Journal of laparoendoscopic & advanced surgical techniques 19 (Suppl 1), S51–S54.

Engum, S.A., Grosfeld, J.L., 1998. Hirschsprung's disease: Duhamel pull-through. In: Stringer, M.D., Oldham, K.T., Mouriquand, P.D.E., et al., (Eds.). Pediatric Surgery and Urology: Long Term Outcomes. W B Saunders, London, 329–339.

Evans, N.J., 1982. Pyloric stenosis in premature infants after transpyloric feeding. Lancet ii, 665.

Fagan, D.G., Pritchard, J.S., Clarkson, T.W., et al., 1977. Organ mercury levels in infants with omphaloceles treated with organic mercurial antiseptic. Arch Dis Child 52, 962–964.

Feingold, J., Guilloud-Bataille, M., 1999. Genetic comparisons of patients with cystic fibrosis with or without meconium ileus. Clinical Centers of the French CF Registry. Annals of Genetics 42, 147–150.

Filston, H.C., Kirks, D.R., 1981. Malrotation – the ubiquitous anomaly. J Pediatr Surg 16, 614–620.

Foker, J.E., Kendall, T.C., Catton, K., et al., 2005. A flexible approach to achieve a true primary repair for all infants with esophageal diversion. 14, 8–15.

Gee, H., Abdulla, U., 1978. Antenatal diagnosis of fetal duodenal atresia by ultrasonic scan. Br Med J ii, 1265.

Gilbert, W.M., Nicolaides, K.H., 1987. Fetal omphalocele: associated malformations and chromosomal defects. Obstet Gynecol 70, 633–635.

Godbole, P., Stringer, M.D., 2002. Bilious vomiting in the newborn: How often is it pathologic? J Pediatr Surg 37, 909–911.

Grosfeld, J.L., Ballantine, T.V.N., Shoemaker, R., 1979. Operative management of intestinal atresia and stenosis based on pathologic findings. J Pediatr Surg 14, 368–375.

Haight, C., Towsley, H.A., 1943. Congenital atresia of the esophagus with tracheo-esophageal fistula: extrapleural ligation of fistula and end-to-end anastomosis of esophageal segments. Surgery Gynecology and Obstetrics 76, 672–688.

Hirschsprung, H., 1887. Stuhltragheit Neugeborener in Folge von Dilatation und Hypertrophie des Colons. Jahrb Kinderheilk 27, 1–7.

Holschneider, A., Hutson, J., Pena, A., et al., 2005. Preliminary report on the International Conference for the Development of Standards for the Treatment of Anorectal Malformations. J Pediatr Surg 40, 1521–1526.

Kluth, D., 1976. Atlas of esophageal atresia. J Pediatr Surg 11, 901–919.

Kluth, D., Lambrecht, W., 1997. Current concepts in the embryology of anorectal malformations. Semin Pediatr Surg 6, 180–186.

Krasna, I.H., Rosenfeld, D., Benjamin, B.G., et al., 1987. Esophageal perforation in the neonate: an emerging problem in the newborn nursery. J Pediatr Surg 22, 784–790.

Kusafuka, T., Puri, P., 1998. Genetic aspects of Hirshsprung's disease. Semin Pediatr Surg 7, 148–155.

Kutiyanawala, M., Wyse, R.K.H., Brereton, R.J., et al., 1992. CHARGE and esophageal atresia. J Pediatr Surg 27, 1136–1141.

Lansdale, N., Hill, R., Gull, Z.S., et al., 2009. Staged reduction of gastroschisis using preformed silos: practicalities and problems. J Pediatr Surg 44, 2126–2129.

Louw, J.H., 1959. Congenital intestinal atresia and stenosis in the newborn. Observations of pathogenesis and treatment. Ann R Coll Surg Engl 25, 209–234.

Ludman, L., 1998. Anorectal malformations: psychological aspects. In: Stringer, M.D., Oldham, K.T., Mouriquand, P.D.E., et al., (Eds.), Pediatric Surgery and Urology: Long Term Outcomes. W B Saunders, Philadelphia, pp. 386–392.

Lund, D.P., Hendren, W.H., 2001. Cloacal exstrophy: a 25–year experience with 50 cases. J Pediatr Surg 36, 68–75.

Martin, V., 1999. The TOF Child. TOFS, Nottingham.

Moore, S.W., Johnson, A.G., 1998. Hirschsprung's disease: genetic and functional associations of Down's and Waardenburg syndromes. Semin Pediatr Surg 7, 156–161.

Mowat, D.R., Wilson, M.J., Goossens, M., 2003. Mowat–Wilson syndrome. J Med Genet 40, 305–310.

Mushtaq, I., Wright, V.M., Drake, D.P., et al., 1998. Meconium ileus secondary to cystic fibrosis. The East London experience, 1998. Pediatr Surg Int 13, 365–369.

Noblett, H., 1969. Treatment of uncomplicated meconium ileus by gastrografin enema: a preliminary report. J Pediatr Surg 4, 190–197.

Okoye, B.O., Parikh, D.H., Buick, R.G., et al., 2000. Pyloric atresia: five new cases, a new association and a review of the literature with guidelines. J Pediatr Surg 35, 1242–1245.

Pena, A., 1995. Anorectal malformations. Semin Pediatr Surg 4, 35–47.

Peutrell, J.M., Hughes, D.G., 1992. Epidural anaesthesia through caudal catheters for inguinal herniotomies in awake ex-premature babies. Anaesthesia 47, 128–131.

Pracros, J.P., Sann, L., Genin, G., et al., 1992. Ultrasound diagnosis of midgut volvulus: the 'whirlpool' sign. Pediatr Radiol 22, 18–20.

Puri, P., Fujimoto, T., 1988. New observations in the pathogenesis of multiple intestinal atresias. J Pediatr Surg 23, 221–225.

Puri, P., Tsuji, M., 1992. Megacystis-microcolon-intestinal hypoperistalsis syndrome (neonatal hollow visceral myopathy). Pediatr Surg Int 7, 18–23.

Rescorla, F.J., Grosfeld, J.L., 1993. Contemporary management of meconium ileus. World J Surg 17, 318–325.

Richards, C., Holmes, S.J., 1995. Intestinal dilatation in the fetus. Arch Dis Child 72, F135–F138.

Rintala, R., Lindahl, H., Louhimo, I., 1991. Anorectal malformations – results of treatment and long-term follow-up in 208 patients. Pediatr Surg Int 6, 36–41.

Rintala, R., Lindahl, H., Rasanen, M., 1997. Do children with repaired low anorectal malformations have normal bowel function? J Pediatr Surg 32, 823–826.

Rollins, M.D., Shields, M.D., Quinn, R.J.M., et al., 1989. Pyloric stenosis: congenital or acquired? Arch Dis Child 64, 138–140.

Rothenberg, S.S., 2002. Thoracoscopic repair of tracheoesophageal fistula in newborns. J Pediatr Surg 37, 869–872.

Shaw, W.C., Sandy, J.R., Williams, A.C., et al., 1996. Minimum standards for the management of cleft lip and palate: efforts to close the audit loop. Ann R Coll Surg Engl 78, 110–114.

Sherry, S.N., Kramer, I., 1955. The time of passage of first stool and first urine by the newborn infant. J Pediatr 46, 158–159.

Shigemoto, H., Endo, S., Isomoto, T., et al., 1978. Neonatal meconium obstruction in the ileum without mucoviscidosis. J Pediatr Surg 13, 475–479.

Spitz, L., 1996. Esophageal atresia: past, present, and future. J Pediatr Surg 31, 19–25.

Stone, D.H., Rimaz, S., Gilmour, W.H., 1998. Prevalence of congenital anterior abdominal wall defects in the United Kingdom: comparison of regional registers. Br Med J 317, 1118–1119.

Stringer, M.D., 1999. Hirschsprung's disease. In: Keighley, M.R.B., Williams, N.S. (Eds.), Surgery of the Anus, Rectum and Colon, second ed. W B Saunders, London, pp. 2635–2680.

Stringer, M.D., 2003. Gastric volvulus. In: Puri, P. (Ed.), Newborn Surgery, second ed. Arnold, London, pp. 399–404.

Stringer, M.D., McKenna, K.M., Goldstein, R.B., et al., 1995a. Prenatal diagnosis of esophageal atresia. J Pediatr Surg 30, 1258–1263.

Stringer, M.D., Spitz, L., Abel, R., et al., 1995b. Management of alimentary tract duplication in children. Br J Surg 82, 74–78.

Stringer, M.D., Thornton, J.G., Mason, G.C., 1996. Hyperechogenic fetal bowel. Arch Dis Child 74, F1–F2.

Tack, E.D., Perlman, J.M., Bower, R.J., et al., 1988. Pyloric stenosis in the sick premature infant. Clinical and radiological findings. American Journal of Disease in Childhood 142, 68–70.

Touloukian, R.J., Higgins, E., 1983. The spectrum of serum electrolytes in hypertrophic pyloric stenosis. J Pediatr Surg 18, 394–397.

Wang, N.L., Yeh, M.L., Chang, P.Y., et al., 1998. Prenatal and neonatal intussusception. Pediatr Surg Int 13, 232–236.

Watson, A.C.H., Sell, D.A., Grunwell, P. (Eds), 2001. Management of Cleft Lip and Palate. Wiley, Bognor Regis.

Weaver, L.T., Lucas, A., 1993. Development of bowel habit in preterm infants. Arch Dis Child 68, 317–320.

Williams, A.C., Sandy, J.R., Thomas, S., et al., 1999. Influence of surgeon's experience on speech outcome in cleft lip and palate. Lancet 354, 1697–1698.

Zeidan, B., Wyatt, J., Mackersie, A., et al., 1988. Recent results of treatment of infantile hypertrophic pyloric stenosis. Arch Dis Child 63, 1060–1064.

Haematology

30

Irene A G Roberts   Neil A Murray

CHAPTER CONTENTS

© 2012 Elsevier Ltd

Developmental haemopoiesis

Introduction

The process which ensures lifelong production of all haemopoietic cells is known as haemopoiesis. Sequential changes in the regulation of haemopoiesis during development help to explain the natural history of many neonatal haematological problems. Haemopoiesis in humans begins in the yolk sac in the third week of gestation (Huyhn et al. 1995). By 5 weeks' gestation, the main site of definitive haemopoiesis is found in the aorto-gonad-mesonephros region of the dorsal aorta. Haemopoiesis in the aorta is only transient and haemopoietic stem cells migrate from there a few weeks later to the liver, which remains the main site of blood cell production throughout fetal life (Huyhn et al. 1995; Marshall and Thrasher 2001). Even though signs of haemopoiesis are also found in the bone marrow from 11 weeks' gestation, this makes only a small contribution to overall haemopoiesis until after birth (Tavian et al. 1999). Thus, for preterm infants, the liver is the main haemopoietic organ at and shortly after birth; this is likely to be a contributory factor in a number of disorders, including the haematological abnormalities seen in neonates with Down syndrome (see later sections).

Erythropoiesis in the fetus and neonate

Erythropoiesis, production of red blood cells (RBCs), has a number of distinct characteristics in term and preterm neonates compared with older children which are relevant to our understanding of neonatal anaemias:

- *Rate of haemoglobin synthesis and RBC production*: the rates of haemoglobin synthesis and of RBC production fall dramatically after birth and remain low for the first 2 weeks of life, probably in response to the sudden increase in tissue oxygenation at birth (Oski 1993). The physiological rise in RBC production begins several weeks later and by 3 months of age a healthy infant, whatever the gestation at birth, should be able to produce up to 2 ml of packed RBCs per day (Oski 1993). Studies in preterm neonates suggest that over the first 2 months of life the maximal rate of RBC production is about 1 ml/day since preterm babies receiving erythropoietin are unable to maintain their haemoglobin if >1 ml of blood per day is venesected for diagnostic purposes but can do so when sampling losses are less than this (Ohls 2002).

- *Reduced RBC lifespan*: neonatal RBCs, particularly from preterm babies, have a reduced lifespan compared with adult red cells. Calculated RBC lifespans for preterm infants are 35–50 days compared with 60–70 days for term infants and 120 days for healthy adults (Pearson 1967). The main reason for this is the many differences in the membrane of neonatal versus adult RBCs, including increased resistance to osmotic lysis, increased mechanical fragility, increased total lipid content and an altered lipid profile, increased insulin-binding sites and reduced expression of blood group antigens such as A, B and I (Oski 1993).

- *Altered RBC metabolism*: there are numerous differences in the glycolytic and pentose phosphate pathways between neonatal and adult RBCs which lead to an increased susceptibility to oxidant-induced injury (Bracci et al. 1988).
  In addition, neonatal RBCs have reduced levels of NADH methaemoglobin reductase (about 60% of those in adult RBCs). This makes them more likely to develop methaemoglobinaemia as they are more susceptible to the toxic effects of chemicals (e.g. nitric oxide) which oxidise

haemoglobin iron more rapidly than the maximal rate of methaemoglobin reduction; methaemoglobin levels are correspondingly slightly higher in neonates than in adults (mean 0.43 g/dl in preterm neonates, 0.22 g/dl in term neonates and 0.11 g/dl in adults) (Oski 1993).

- *Changes in globin chain synthesis in the fetus and newborn*: the first globin chain produced is epsilon globin, followed almost immediately by α- and γ-globin chain production (Table 30.1). HbF ($\alpha_2\gamma_2$) is therefore produced from early in gestation (4–5 weeks) and is the predominant haemoglobin until after birth. Adult haemoglobin (HbA: $\alpha_2\beta_2$) remains at low levels (10–15%) until 30–32 weeks. After this, the rate of HbA production increases at the same time as HbF production falls, resulting in an average HbF level at term birth of 70–80%, HbA of 25–30%, small amounts of HbA$_2$ and sometimes a trace of Hb Barts (β_4) (Bard 1975). After birth, HbF falls, to ~2% at age 12 months with a corresponding increase in HbA. In term babies there is little change in HbF in the first 15 days after birth. In preterm babies who are not transfused, HbF may remain at the same level for the first 6 weeks of life before HbA production starts to increase. It is this delay in HbA production (i.e. the switch from the γ-globin of HbF to the β-globin of HbA) which can make the diagnosis of β-globin disorders difficult in the neonatal period. By contrast, the fact that α-globin chains are absolutely essential for the production of both HbF and HbA means that α-thalassaemia major causes severe anaemia from early in fetal life (Higgs 1993).
- *Erythropoietin production in the fetus and newborn*: erythropoietin is the principal cytokine regulating erythropoiesis in the fetus and newborn (Vora and Gruslin 1998; Halvorsen and Bechensteen 2002). Since erythropoietin does not cross the placenta, erythropoietin-mediated regulation of fetal erythropoiesis is predominantly under fetal control (Vora and Gruslin 1998). The liver is the main site of erythropoietin production in the fetus (Dame et al. 1998) and the only stimulus to erythropoietin production under physiological conditions is hypoxia with or without anaemia.

This explains the high erythropoietin levels in fetuses of mothers with diabetes or hypertension or those with intrauterine growth restriction (IUGR) or cyanotic congenital heart disease; erythropoietin is also increased in fetal anaemia of any cause, including haemolytic disease of the newborn (HDN) (Watts and Roberts 1999).

White cell production in the fetus and newborn

Neutrophils

There are few circulating neutrophils in first- and second-trimester blood ($0.1–0.2 \times 10^9$/l) (Campagnoli et al. 2000), after which the numbers gradually rise to reach over 2×10^9/l by term, with slightly lower numbers in preterm neonates (Table 30.2). The principal difference between neutrophil production in the newborn and the adult is the reduced neutrophil storage pool, particularly in preterm infants and most markedly in IUGR or exposure to maternal hypertension (Koenig and Christensen 1989; Ohls et al. 1995; Christensen et al. 2000). The neutrophil storage pool reflects the available reserve of neutrophils which the fetus or neonate can mobilise in response to infection. This may contribute to the frequency of bacterial infection in preterm infants. The neutrophil storage pool is defined as the numbers of segmented neutrophils, band neutrophils and metamyelocytes in the bone marrow and so is usually inferred (by the leukocyte response to bacterial sepsis) since bone marrow examination is rarely indicated in the newborn. Various cytokines stimulate neutrophil production in vitro and in vivo (e.g. granulocyte colony-stimulating factor (G-CSF) and granulocyte–macrophage colony-stimulating factor (GM-CSF)) (Ohls et al. 1995; Christensen et al. 2000).

Monocytes, eosinophils and lymphocytes

All types of leukocyte found in adult blood are also seen in the fetus and the newborn (Forestier et al. 1986): monocytes circulate from

---

Table 30.1 Composition of haemoglobins in the human embryo, fetus and neonate

HAEMOGLOBIN	GLOBIN CHAINS		GESTATION
	α-GLOBIN GENE CLUSTER	β-GLOBIN GENE CLUSTER*	
Embryonic			
Hb Gower-1	ζ_2	ε_2	From 3–4 weeks
Hb Gower-2	α_2	ε_2	
Hb Portland	ζ_2	γ_2	From 4 weeks
Fetal			
HbF	α_2	γ_2	From 4 weeks
Adult			
HbA	α_2	β_2	From 6–8 weeks
HbA$_2$	α_2	δ_2	From 30 weeks

*The α-globin gene cluster is situated on chromosome 16 and the β-globin gene cluster on chromosome 11. Note that fetuses and neonates with α-thalassaemia major, who are unable to synthesise α-globin chains, will have Hb Portland as well as Hb Barts (β_4) detectable by haemoglobin electrophoresis or high-performance liquid chromatography.

4–5 weeks' gestation and eosinophils from 14–16 weeks' gestation, increasing slowly to normal values at term (see Table 30.2). There are few studies of lymphopoiesis in the human fetus; both T lymphocytes and B lymphocytes are found in low numbers in fetal liver at 7 and 8 weeks' gestation, respectively (Hann 1991), and T lymphocytes are detectable in fetal blood, marrow and thymus during the second trimester (Pahal et al. 2000). By term, T lymphocytes form 40–45% of circulating mononuclear cells, with a CD4:CD8 ratio of around 5:1, slightly higher than in adult blood (3.1:1). B lymphocytes are found in fetal blood and bone marrow from 12 weeks' gestation and constitute 4–5% of circulating mononuclear cells by term (Hann 1991).

Table 30.2 Representative normal haematological values at birth and over the first 2 months of life in term babies*

	BIRTH	2 WEEKS	2 MONTHS
Hb (g/dl)	14.9–23.7	13.4–19.8	9.4–13
Haematocrit	0.47–75	0.41–0.65	0.28–0.42
MCV (fl)	100–125	88–110	77–98
Reticulocytes (×10⁹/l)	110–450	10–85	35–200
WBCs (×10⁹/l)	10–26	6–21	5–15
Neutrophils (×10⁹/l)	2.7–14.4	1.5–5.4	0.7–4.8
Monocytes (×10⁹/l)	0–1.9	0.1–1.7	0.4–1.2
Lymphocytes (×10⁹/l)	2.0–7.3	2.8–9.1	3.3–10.3
Eosinophils (×10⁹/l)	0–0.85	0–0.85	0.05–0.9
Basophils (×10⁹/l)	0–0.1	0–0.1	0.02–0.13
Nucleated RBCs (×10⁹/l)	<5	<0.1	<0.1
Platelets (×10⁹/l)	150–450	150–450	150–450

*These data are obtained from a number of sources and have been chosen to represent data most useful for interpreting the significance of haematological results.
Hb, haemoglobin; MCV, mean corpuscular volume; WBC, white blood cells; RBC, red blood cells.

Megakaryocytopoiesis and platelet production in the fetus and newborn

Platelets appear in the circulation at 5–6 weeks' gestation (Hann 1991). During the second trimester, the platelet count rises to normal adult values (175–250 × 10⁹/l) (Forestier et al. 1986). Thus, a platelet count of less than 150 × 10⁹/l is abnormal even in the most preterm neonate. The principal cytokine regulating platelet production in the fetus and newborn is thrombopoietin, as in adults (Watts et al. 1999). There are several differences between megakaryocytopoiesis and its regulation in the fetus and newborn compared with adults which may contribute to the frequent occurrence of thrombocytopenia in sick neonates. Fetal megakaryocytes are smaller and more immature (Hegyi et al. 1991; de Alarcon and Graeve 1996); the numbers of megakaryocyte progenitor cells, the precursor cells for maintaining megakaryocyte and platelet production, are reduced; and the ability to produce thrombopoietin is reduced, limiting the capacity to upregulate platelet production at times of increased demand, e.g. during thrombocytopenia in neonatal sepsis (Watts et al. 1999; Albert et al. 2000).

Neonatal anaemia and other red cell disorders

Introduction and definition

Anaemia is the commonest haematological abnormality in the newborn. In the majority of neonates, the causes are straightforward, since they reflect a combination of well-recognised physiological changes and iatrogenic blood letting. However, it is important to identify those neonates with pathological anaemia who require additional investigations and more tailored management. In the neonatal period, the most frequent diseases associated with anaemia are immune haemolysis and genetic red cell disorders. A logical approach and appropriate use of straightforward investigations, as outlined below, reveal the cause in most babies. Treatment options for neonatal anaemia are limited and are based mainly on sensible use of blood transfusion (see pp. 780–782) and prevention of anaemia.

Normal values for red blood cells and blood volume

Normal values at birth for haemoglobin, haematocrit and mean corpuscular volume (MCV) for term and preterm babies are shown in Table 30.2 and Table 30.3, respectively, and in Appendix 1.

Table 30.3 Representative normal haematological values at birth in preterm babies

	24–25 WEEKS	26–27 WEEKS	28–29 WEEKS	30–31 WEEKS
Hb (g/dl)	19.4 ± 1.5	19.0 ± 2.5	19.3 ± 1.8	19.1 ± 2.1
Haematocrit	0.63 ± 0.04	0.62 ± 0.08	0.60 ± 0.07	0.60 ± 0.08
MCV (fl)	135 ± 0.02	132 ± 14.4	131 ± 13.5	127 ± 12.7
Reticulocytes (×10⁹/l)	279 ± 23	454 ± 15	347 ± 12	278 ± 10
Platelets (×10⁹/l)	150–450	150–450	150–450	150–450

Hb, haemoglobin; MCV, mean corpuscular volume.
Adapted from Oski (1993).

In term babies, the haemoglobin, haematocrit and red cell indices fall slowly over the first few weeks, reaching a mean haemoglobin of 13–14 g/dl at 4 weeks of age and 9.5–11 g/dl at 7–9 weeks of age, with a lower limit of normal for the MCV and mean corpuscular haemoglobin (MCH) of 77 fl and 26 pg, respectively. For preterm infants, these changes may be difficult to interpret, because of their variable clinical course and transfusion requirements. However, studies of well preterm infants carried out in the 1970s show a more rapid and steeper fall in haemoglobin, reaching a mean of 6.5–9 g/dl at 4–8 weeks' postnatal age (Oski 1993). The reticulocyte count falls rapidly after birth as erythropoiesis is suppressed, and starts to increase in term babies at 7–8 weeks of age to reach 35–200 $\times 10^9$/l (1–1.8%) at 2 months of age, and in preterm babies at 6–8 weeks of age (Matoth et al. 1971; Brown et al. 1983; Oski 1993). Normal blood volume at birth varies with gestational age and the timing of clamping of the cord (Linderkamp et al. 1992). In term infants, the average blood volume is 80 ml/kg (range 50–100 ml/kg), and in preterm infants is higher at 106 ml/kg (range 85–143 ml/kg) (Sisson et al. 1959; Usher and Lind 1965). Term and preterm babies have adequate stores of iron, folic acid and vitamin B_{12} at birth. However, stores of both iron and folic acid are lower in preterm infants and are depleted more quickly, leading to deficiency after 2–4 months if the recommended daily intakes are not maintained (see Ch. 16, part 3). In general, even term neonates with a normal haemoglobin at birth will have depleted their iron stores by the time they have doubled their birthweight (Rao and Georgieff 2002).

There are no useful published normal ranges for the numbers of circulating nucleated red cells. Nevertheless, a useful 'rule of thumb' is that values of less than 5 nucleated RBCs per 100 white cells in a term baby and <20 nucleated RBCs per 100 white blood cells in a preterm baby can be considered normal for the first 1–2 days of life. The commonest causes of increased numbers of circulating nucleated RBCs are:

- haemolysis (common in rhesus haemolytic disease and α-thalassaemia major but uncommon in other types of haemolysis)
- haemorrhage (especially fetomaternal haemorrhage)
- chronic tissue hypoxia in utero (IUGR, maternal hypertension, maternal diabetes)
- perinatal asphyxia.

Definition of anaemia

Anaemia can be defined as a haemoglobin concentration below the normal range for a population of age- and sex-matched individuals. Normal values for term and preterm infants at birth are shown in Tables 30.2 and 30.3; from this it can be seen that, regardless of gestation, any neonate with a haemoglobin of <14 g/dl at birth in a properly taken blood sample should be considered anaemic. Not every neonate with a haemoglobin concentration at birth of <14 g/dl needs detailed further investigation, but thought should be given to the cause (Table 30.4) and appropriate investigations instituted. Where the reduced haemoglobin does not fit the clinical picture, the first step should be to repeat the sample, since in many cases the measured haemoglobin concentration is inaccurate because of the site of sampling (heelprick versus venous blood) or the way in which the sample was collected. The haemoglobin concentration in venous samples is lower than in heelprick samples collected simultaneously: in the first few hours of life this difference averages 2–4 g/dl and is greater at lower gestational ages (Thurlbeck and McIntosh 1987; Oski 1993). The difference between the venous and capillary haemoglobin falls with increasing gestational age, and also with increasing postnatal age, such that by the fifth day of life

Table 30.4 Causes of neonatal anaemia

Impaired red cell production
Diamond–Blackfan anaemia Congenital infection, e.g. cytomegalovirus, rubella Congenital dyserythropoietic anaemia Pearson syndrome Congenital leukaemia
Increased red cell destruction (haemolysis)
Alloimmune: haemolytic disease of the newborn (Rh, ABO, Kell, other) Autoimmune, e.g. maternal autoimmune haemolysis Red cell membrane disorders, e.g. hereditary spherocytosis Red cell enzyme deficiencies, e.g. pyruvate kinase deficiency Some haemoglobinopathies, e.g. α-thalassaemia major, HbH disease Infection, e.g. bacterial, syphilis, malaria, cytomegalovirus, *Toxoplasma*, herpes simplex Macro/microangiopathy, e.g. cavernous haemangioma, disseminated intravascular coagulation Galactosaemia
Blood loss
Occult haemorrhage before or around birth, e.g. twin-to-twin, fetomaternal, ruptured vasa praevia Internal haemorrhage, e.g. intracranial, subaponeurotic, intraperitoneal Iatrogenic: due to frequent blood sampling
Anaemia of prematurity
Impaired red cell production plus reduced red cell lifespan

there is almost no difference in haemoglobin concentration between a well-taken heelprick sample and a venous sample (Oski 1993).

The influence of cord clamping

The other major influence on haemoglobin concentration at birth is the timing of cord clamping and the position of the baby at the time of clamping. In term babies, the placental vessels contain around 100 ml of blood at birth. It has been estimated that 25% of the placental blood is transfused within the first 15 seconds and 50% (i.e. 50 ml in a term baby) by the end of the first minute (Linderkamp et al. 1992). The difference in haemoglobin concentration in the baby between early and late cord clamping is around 3 g/dl (Yao et al. 1969). Babies held below the level of the placenta continue to gain blood until the cord is clamped and have higher haemoglobin levels than those held above the level of the placenta, who may lose blood into the placenta until the cord is clamped (Yao et al. 1969).

Physiological impact of anaemia in the neonate

The clinical significance of anaemia in the newborn depends on whether or not the baby is able to maintain adequate tissue oxygenation. This does not depend solely upon the haemoglobin concentration since tissue oxygenation is also influenced by cardiopulmonary function and by the ability of the haemoglobin to unload the oxygen it is carrying. Fortunately, the oxygen-unloading capacity of blood increases progressively from birth, reflecting the position of the haemoglobin–oxygen dissociation curve.

In neonates, the two most important factors determining the position of the haemoglobin–oxygen dissociation curve are the concentrations of HbF and of 2,3-diphosphoglycerate (2,3-DPG) within the RBCs: high HbF and low 2,3-DPG both cause the curve to shift to the left, i.e. the affinity of haemoglobin for oxygen is increased, so less oxygen is released to the tissues. This is the situation just after birth in both term and preterm babies, as both have HbF concentrations above 50% at birth. The high oxygen affinity may be more of a problem for preterm babies since the HbF levels are >90% in babies of 24–28 weeks' gestation, although this may not be significant in practice since very preterm neonates are more likely to require transfusion over the first few weeks of life. Over the first few months of life, 2,3-DPG levels rise and HbF levels fall, so the haemoglobin–oxygen dissociation curve gradually shifts to the right, i.e. the oxygen affinity of haemoglobin falls and oxygen delivery to the tissues increases, to some extent ameliorating the effects of the falling haemoglobin over the first months of life.

Pathogenesis and causes of neonatal anaemia

Anaemia in the neonatal period has distinct physiological features compared with older children and a distinct pathogenesis. Interpretation of diagnostic investigations has to be made on a background of the developmental changes affecting the red cell membrane, red cell enzyme concentrations and the types and rate of haemoglobin production, which vary with gestational and postnatal age. Diagnostic tests are also often affected by whether the baby has been transfused. Furthermore, anaemia in the neonate may be due to pregnancy-related or pre-existing disorders in the mother, such as the presence of red cell alloantibodies or genetic disorders. It is therefore important to remember that in many cases evaluating the blood count and blood film of the parents is the quickest way of identifying the underlying diagnosis in the neonate.

The principal causes of neonatal anaemia are shown in Table 30.4. In general, anaemia can result from one or more of the following mechanisms:

- inappropriately reduced red cell production
- increased red cell destruction/reduced red cell lifespan
- blood loss
- a combination of these mechanisms (anaemia of prematurity).

Neonatal anaemia due to reduced red cell production

Anaemia due to reduced red cell production is not common in the neonatal period. Nevertheless, it is clinically important, because several of the disorders that present in this way are associated with severe, lifelong problems. The main diagnostic clues to reduced red cell production are the combination of a low reticulocyte count ($<20 \times 10^9$/l) together with a negative direct antiglobulin test (DAT; Coombs' test). The other useful diagnostic point is whether the disorder is confined to the red cell series (i.e. anaemia in the presence of a normal white cell and platelet count) or whether the blood count suggests that the white cells and/or platelets are also involved.

The most important causes are congenital infections (particularly due to parvovirus) and genetic disorders. Where failure of blood cell production is confined to the red cell series, as with

Diamond–Blackfan anaemia (DBA) and most episodes of parvovirus infection, the anaemia is said to be due to red cell aplasia. Reduced red cell production may also be part of a general failure of haemopoiesis and accompanied by leukopenia and/or thrombocytopenia, as seen in congenital infection due to cytomegalovirus (CMV), in congenital leukaemias (see p. 770 and Ch. 36) and in congenital bone marrow failure syndromes such as Pearson syndrome (see p. 761).

Anaemia and congenital infection

Infections which cause anaemia due to reduced red cell production include parvovirus B19, CMV, toxoplasmosis, congenital syphilis, rubella and herpes simplex (Brown and Abernathy 1998; Brown 2000). Identification of the causative organism is usually based on clinical suspicion prompted by well-recognised associated findings such as chorioretinitis, jaundice, pneumonitis, skin lesions, IUGR and hepatosplenomegaly, followed by specific diagnostic microbiological investigations. In infection due to CMV, toxoplasma or herpes simplex, the anaemia and reticulocytopenia are usually relatively mild (Brown and Abernathy 1998). In addition, the blood film often shows abnormal 'viral' lymphocytes, thrombocytopenia and/or neutropenia. Congenital parvovirus B19 can cause particular diagnostic difficulties and is discussed below (Brown 2000).

Parvovirus B19 and fetal/neonatal anaemia

Maternal infection with parvovirus B19 causes fetal anaemia which is severe enough to lead to intrauterine death in 9% of cases (Public Health Laboratory Service Working Party on Fifth Disease 1990; Miller et al. 1998; Brown 2000). A diagnosis of fetal parvovirus B19 should be considered in every 'unexplained' case of fetal hydrops (Table 30.5) since it has been estimated that parvovirus B19 is responsible for 15% of cases of non-immune hydrops (Yaegashi et al. 1994; Jordan 1996; Lallemand et al. 1999). In addition to anaemia, parvovirus infection causes marked reticulocytopenia (usually $<10 \times 10^9$/l) and thrombocytopenia may also occur. The diagnosis of parvovirus B19 infection is primarily based on maternal serology together with the demonstration of B19 DNA in the fetus/neonate by dot blot hybridisation or polymerase chain reaction (PCR) (Brown 2000; Heegaard and Brown 2002). Where results are negative on blood samples but clinical suspicion of parvovirus is high, PCR for B19 should also be carried out on bone marrow (Brown et al. 1983). Management depends on the severity

Table 30.5 Haematogical causes of hydrops fetalis (see Ch. 31 for other causes)

Reduced red cell production
Parvovirus B19
Diamond–Blackfan anaemia
Congenital dyserythropoietic anaemia
Congenital leukaemia

Increased red cell destruction (haemolysis)
Pyruvate kinase deficiency
α-thalassaemia major (or HbH hydrops)
Haemolytic disease of the newborn – rhesus, Kell, ABO (rare)

Blood loss
Twin-to-twin transfusion
Fetomaternal haemorrhage

of the anaemia – severe cases diagnosed in utero may be treated by intrauterine transfusion; for those that survive, the majority have no long-term sequelae. However, a small number of neonates with chronic red cell aplasia, with or without evidence of persistent B19 DNA by PCR, have been reported, and for such cases intravenous immunoglobulin (IVIG) should be given to try and eradicate persistent viral infection (Brown 2000; Fisch et al. 2000).

Failure of red cell production due to genetic disorders

Congenital or inherited disorders that usually or not infrequently present with neonatal anaemia due to reduced red cell production include DBA, congenital dyserythropoietic anaemia (CDA) and Pearson syndrome. The other inherited bone marrow failure syndromes, such as Fanconi's anaemia, rarely present at birth.

Diamond–Blackfan anaemia

The principal cause of congenital red cell aplasia is DBA (Fisch et al. 2000), which has an incidence of 5–7 cases per million live births. There is a clear family history in 20% of cases (both autosomal dominant and autosomal recessive inheritance are reported); the remaining 80% are sporadic. Affected children nearly always present in the first year of life; most diagnoses are made around 2–3 months of age, but 25% of cases present at birth and rare cases present as mid-trimester fetal anaemia and hydrops (Ball et al. 1996; Vlachos et al. 2008). The usual presentation is with anaemia in an otherwise healthy baby; 40% of infants have associated congenital anomalies, particularly craniofacial dysmorphism, IUGR, neck anomalies (Klippel–Feil syndrome) and thumb malformations (e.g. triphalangeal or bifid thumbs) (Ball et al. 1996; Vlachos et al. 2008) similar to those seen in Fanconi's anaemia. The important laboratory features are normochromic anaemia (which may be macrocytic), reticulocytopenia and absent erythroid precursors on the bone marrow aspirate. It is important to exclude parvovirus infection by appropriate serology and dot blot testing, and Fanconi's anaemia by diepoxybutane stress testing of peripheral blood lymphocytes (Giampietro et al. 1993). If these tests are negative, the only other differential diagnosis of red cell aplasia with absent red cell precursors is transient erythroblastopenia of childhood, which, in contrast to DBA, resolves within a couple of months. Although bone marrow examination is required to diagnose DBA, other useful tests include red cell adenosine deaminase levels, which are elevated in most affected patients and sometimes in parents (Vlachos et al. 2008) and genetic analysis for mutations in ribosomal protein genes, which are present in ~50% of families and can be investigated in specialised laboratories (Lipton and Ellis 2010). In the neonatal period, the treatment of DBA is red cell transfusion. Up to 75% of children with DBA respond to steroids and can often be weaned off transfusions, but this approach is not usually tried until after the first year of life (Vichinsky et al. 1988). DBA is a rather unpredictable disease: some cases resolve spontaneously; others wax and wane; but more than half of affected children have lifelong transfusion or steroid dependence and may be treated by bone marrow transplantation (Vlachos et al. 2008; Lipton and Ellis 2010).

Congenital dyserythropoietic anaemia

The CDAs are a rare group of disorders characterised by failure of red cell production due to ineffective erythropoiesis. Most cases are autosomal recessive and a history of parental consanguinity is not uncommon. In contrast to DBA, the bone marrow has vastly increased numbers of erythroid precursors but they are grossly abnormal and do not properly differentiate into mature RBCs. CDA usually presents during childhood. However, a number of neonates with CDA presenting at birth or during fetal life have been reported and in severe cases the presentation may be with hydrops fetalis (Remacha et al. 2002). Most affected babies are normally grown with no dysmorphic features, have a normocytic anaemia with normal white cells and platelets but a low reticulocyte count and transfusion-dependent anaemia. CDA type 1 is due to mutations in the codanin-1 gene (Dgany et al. 2002) and CDA type II, which is the most common type of CDA, has recently been shown to be due to mutations in the *SEC23B* gene (Schwarz et al. 2009). The prognosis of CDA is extremely variable. For transfusion-independent children with CDA, lifespan is usually normal and quality of life is good. For transfusion-dependent children, the treatment options are:

- splenectomy, which renders a small proportion of children transfusion-independent with a normal lifespan
- bone marrow transplantation, the only curative treatment, but one which carries a 10% risk of mortality or graft rejection
- lifelong red cell transfusion with iron chelation therapy, which carries a similar prognosis to children with β-thalassaemia major (i.e. median survival now >50 years with good treatment compliance).

Pearson syndrome

This rare disease is caused by mutations in mitochondrial DNA (Smith et al. 1995). It often presents in neonates who are small-for-gestational-age and thrive poorly in the first few weeks of life (Smith et al. 1995). The anaemia is normocytic and associated thrombocytopenia and neutropenia are common; abnormal leukocyte vacuolation may be seen in the peripheral blood and highly characteristic vacuolation of early erythoid cells on the marrow aspirate should prompt blood to be sent for mitochondrial DNA analysis to establish the diagnosis. The prognosis of Pearson syndrome is very poor: few children survive beyond the second year of life.

Anaemia due to increased red cell destruction (haemolytic anaemia)

After anaemia of prematurity and anaemia due to blood letting, haemolysis is the commonest cause of neonatal anaemia. Haemolysis should always be investigated even if the anaemia is mild and apparently trivial. This is because transient or mild haemolysis in the neonatal period may be the clue to an underlying problem with more serious manifestations later on in childhood (e.g. red cell enzymopathies) or to problems which might affect future siblings (e.g. alloimmune anaemia due to maternal red cell antibodies).

The principal clues which suggest a haemolytic anaemia are: increased numbers of reticulocytes and/or circulating nucleated RBCs, unconjugated hyperbilirubinaemia, a positive DAT (if immune) and characteristic changes in the morphology of the red cells on a blood film (e.g. hereditary spherocytosis). The main types of neonatal haemolytic anaemia are listed in Table 30.4 and a useful algorithm to guide investigations is shown in Figure 30.1. It is usually straightforward to distinguish the cause, although rarer causes require specialist investigations which should be discussed with a haematologist once the basic investigations are to hand. The first step should be a DAT, which will be positive only in the presence of immune haemolytic anaemia and not in non-immune haemolysis. The main cause of immune haemolytic anaemia is HDN (see below). The main causes of non-immune haemolysis in neonates are:

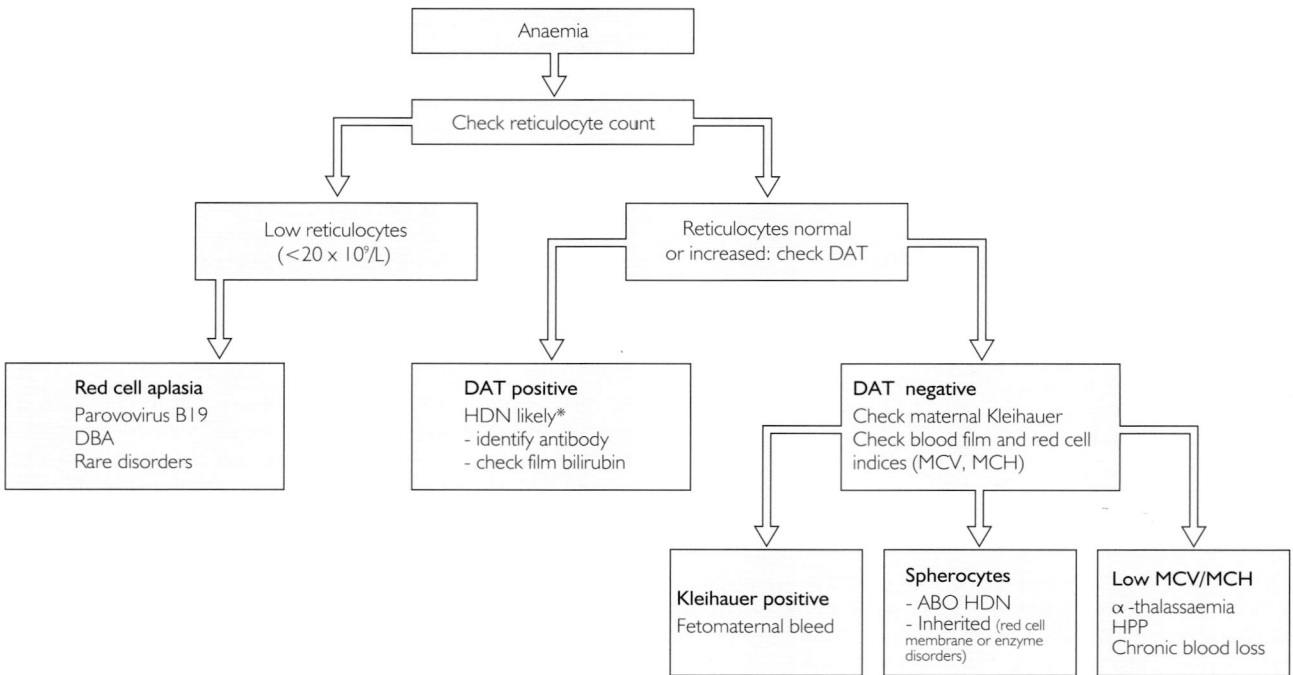

*Administration of prophylactic antenatal anti-D to Rhesus D-negative mothers may cause a weakly positive DAT in the baby at birth. Provided there is a clear history of antenatal prophylaxis and the FBC and blood film are normal, it is not necessary to arrange further investigation and follow up of such babies.

Fig. 30.1 A diagnostic algorithm for neonatal anaemia. The most useful screening tests for investigating unexplained neonatal anaemia are the reticulocyte count, the direct antiglobulin test and the mean cell volume (MCV) of the red blood cells. DAT, direct antiglobluin test (Coombs' test); DBA, Diamond–Blackfan anaemia; G6PD, glucose-6-phosphate dehydrogenase; HDN, haemolytic disease of the newborn; HS, hereditary spherocytosis; MCH, mean cell haemoglobin; HPP, hereditary pyropoikilocytosis; FBC, full blood count.

- red cell membrane disorders
- red cell enzymopathies
- haemoglobinopathies.

A number of congenital and primary infections can also cause haemolytic anaemia in the neonatal period, including CMV, toxoplasmosis, congenital syphilis, rubella, herpes simplex and, rarely, malaria.

Immune haemolytic anaemias, including haemolytic disease of the newborn

By far the most common cause of DAT-positive haemolysis is HDN due to transplacental passage of maternal IgG alloantibodies to red cell antigens. Although modern DAT reagents are very sensitive, a negative DAT is sometimes found in ABO HDN due to anti-A or anti-B (Herschel et al. 2002). Maternal autoimmune haemolytic anaemia very occasionally causes a positive DAT in the neonate; however, both haemolysis and anaemia in the baby are extremely rare.

The principal alloantibodies that cause significant anaemia due to HDN are those against rhesus antigens (anti-D, anti-c and anti-E), anti-Kell, anti-Kidd (J^k), anti-Duffy (F^y) and antibodies of the MNS blood group system, including anti-U. Anti-D remains the most frequent alloantibody to cause significant haemolytic anaemia, affecting 1 in 1200 pregnancies (Howard et al. 1998; Thompson 2002). Anti-Kell antibodies are less common but can cause severe

fetal and neonatal anaemia since they inhibit erythropoiesis as well as causing haemolysis (Vaughan et al. 1998). Most babies with HDN present with jaundice and/or anaemia and are born to women with known antibodies. In neonates with severe anaemia, there is often evidence of extramedullary haemopoiesis, including hepatosplenomegaly and occasionally skin lesions producing the clinical appearance of 'blueberry muffin baby' (Bowden et al. 1989; Waldron and de Alarcon 1999).

HDN due to ABO antibodies

ABO haemolytic disease occurs only in offspring of women of blood group O and is confined to the 1% of such women who have high-titre IgG antibodies. Haemolysis due to anti-A is more common (1 in 150 births) than anti-B. In contrast to anti-Rhesus antibodies, both anti-A and anti-B usually cause hyperbilirubinaemia without significant neonatal anaemia. This is mainly because there are relatively few group A or B antigen sites on neonatal red cells, allowing the antibody-coated cells to persist for longer in the circulation (Oski 1993). As a reflection of this, the blood film in ABO haemolytic disease characteristically shows very large numbers of spherocytes with little or no increase in nucleated red cells; this contrasts to rhesus HDN, where there are few spherocytes and vast numbers of circulating nucleated red cells. The DAT in ABO HDN may be negative. Management of ABO HDN usually just requires phototherapy; however, close monitoring is essential and exchange transfusion is occasionally required, particularly in cases of ABO HDN due to anti-B antibodies, which may cause severe anaemia as well as hyperbilirubinaemia (Waldron and de Alarcon 1999). Hydrops has occasionally been described.

Management of HDN

The antenatal diagnosis and management of pregnancies affected by red cell alloimmunisation require cooperation between obstetric, paediatric and haematology teams (Grant et al. 2000). All neonates at risk should have cord blood taken for measurement of haemoglobin, bilirubin and a DAT and should remain in hospital until hyperbilirubinaemia and/or anaemia have been properly managed. Phototherapy should be given from birth to all rhesus-alloimmunised infants with haemolysis, as the bilirubin can rise steeply after birth and this expectant approach will prevent the need for exchange transfusion in some infants. In HDN due to anti-Kell, anaemia is usually more prominent than jaundice and minimal phototherapy may be necessary despite severe anaemia (Grant et al. 2000). Systematic reviews have found that treatment of neonates with alloimmune haemolysis with IVIG does reduce the need for exchange transfusion (Alcock and Liley 2002; Gottstein and Cooke 2003). Current National Institute for Health and Clinical Excellence guidance (neonatal jaundice) is to use IVIG when the serum bilirubin continues to rise at more than 8.5 µmol/l/h in spite of phototherapy, although further research is recommended.

Exchange transfusion in HDN is required for:

- severe anaemia: haemoglobin <10 g/dl at birth (with the possible exception of anti-Kell, as mentioned above)
- severe or rapidly increasing hyperbilirubinaemia
- signs of bilirubin encephalopathy.

Details of the product to use for exchange transfusion are given on p. 782 and are summarised in the current British Committee for Standards in Haematology (BCSH) guidelines (2004).

'Late' anaemia presents at a few weeks of age in some babies with milder haemolytic disease who do not require exchange transfusion and in babies who have had earlier exchange transfusion. The blood film shows evidence of ongoing haemolysis and the anaemia is aggravated by the normal postnatal suppression of erythropoiesis. Such babies may require 'top-up' transfusion for symptomatic anaemia; conventional guidelines for neonatal transfusion can be followed (see Table 30.13) but irradiated blood must be used for infants previously receiving intrauterine transfusion, to prevent the risk of transfusion-associated graft-versus-host disease (TA-GVHD) (British Committee for Standards in Haematology, Transfusion Task Force 2004). Thus, all babies found to have a strongly positive DAT at birth and all treated by intrauterine transfusion must be followed up to monitor the rate of haemoglobin fall. It is important to note that administration of prophylactic antenatal anti-D to rhesus D-negative mothers quite commonly causes a weakly positive DAT in the baby at birth. Provided there is a clear history of antenatal prophylaxis and the Hb and the blood film are normal, it is not necessary to arrange further investigation and follow-up of such babies. It is worth noting that babies with ABO HDN rarely require 'top-up' transfusion unless severe anaemia in the first few days of life (Hb <10 g/dl) has been a feature. Where the haemoglobin is falling more rapidly than normal, particularly in babies with unconjugated hyperbilirubinaemia, monitoring must be continued until the jaundice resolves and the haemoglobin reaches a plateau. This may take 8 weeks and it may be helpful to ask the haematologist to review the blood films each time, to look for evidence of ongoing haemolysis. Folic acid (500 µg/kg/day) should be given to all babies with haemolytic anaemia until 3 months of age; folic acid is not necessary for babies with ABO HDN who are not anaemic. Erythropoietin has been used to prevent the need for 'top-up' transfusion

for late anaemia; both failures and successes of this approach have been reported and erythropoietin is unlikely to prevent the need for transfusion where ongoing haemolysis is brisk (Zuppa et al. 1999; Pessler and Hart 2002).

Neonatal haemolytic anaemia due to red cell membrane disorders

A number of red cell membrane disorders may present in the neonatal period. The three most common types of presentation are:

1. unexplained haemolysis with jaundice but usually only moderate anaemia (usually due to hereditary spherocytosis)
2. as an incidental finding on a routine blood film in the absence of unusual jaundice or anaemia (usually hereditary elliptocytosis)
3. severe, transfusion-dependent haemolytic anaemia with a characteristic very low MCV of 50–60 fl (usually due to hereditary pyropoikilocytosis (HPP)).

The main clues that a neonate has a red cell membrane disorder are a family history, otherwise unexplained haemolysis and an abnormal blood film. Red cell membrane disorders can nearly always be recognised by the characteristic shape of red cells on a blood film. However, the identification of the exact type of membrane abnormality is more complex and requires specialised investigations on both the neonate and the parents and close liaison with a haematologist. The osmotic fragility test has largely been replaced by the dye-binding test which is carried out on a small sample of peripheral blood but may need to be performed in a specialised centre (Tse and Lux 1999; King et al. 2008). It is important to carry out these definitive diagnostic investigations (red cell membrane studies) on pretransfusion blood samples to minimise diagnostic confusion due to transfused cells and to check the blood count and film of both parents if possible (Palek and Jarolim 1993).

A brief summary of the three main clinical disorders presenting in neonates is given below; for more detailed information, the reader is referred to comprehensive reviews (Tse and Lux 1999; Delaunay 2002; Bolton-Maggs et al. 2004).

Hereditary spherocytosis

This is the commonest red cell membrane defect. It occurs in 1 in 5000 live births to parents of northern European extraction, but is less frequently seen in other ethnic groups (Delaunay 2002). It is autosomal dominant, but around 25% of cases are sporadic due to new mutations. Hereditary spherocytosis is genetically heterogeneous – mutations in spectrin, ankyrin, protein 4.1 and protein 3 have all been reported (Delaunay 2002). The usual presentation of hereditary spherocytosis in the neonate is with unconjugated hyperbilirubinaemia. Most affected neonates are not anaemic, but a small proportion have anaemia severe enough to require transfusion. The blood film in hereditary spherocytosis shows moderate numbers of spherocytes; the appearance is identical to that of ABO haemolytic disease, but the two disorders are distinguishable by the negative DAT in hereditary spherocytosis. While some babies will require one or two transfusions during the first 1–2 months of life, very few remain transfusion-dependent after this time and it is important to stop transfusions to evaluate the nadir haemoglobin reached. All children with hereditary spherocytosis should also receive folic acid supplementation (from 500 µg/kg/day in the first 6 months of life and a total daily dose of 2.5 mg from 6 months until 10 years of life, increasing to 5 mg daily thereafter). Splenectomy almost invariably induces complete remission of haemolytic anaemia (and therefore the need for folic acid prophylaxis) but is only indicated for more severely affected children and virtually always deferred until after the age of 6 years.

Hereditary elliptocytosis

This is a more complex disorder. It is caused by different mutations in the genes for spectrin, ankyrin or protein 4.1 (Tse and Lux 1999; Delaunay 2002). In the common, autosomal dominant form of hereditary elliptocytosis, the heterozygotes have no clinical manifestations (i.e. no anaemia and no jaundice) apart from elliptocytes on the blood film. No treatment is required and folic acid prophylaxis is unnecessary, as folate deficiency is not a feature of this condition. Neonates who are homozygous or compound heterozygous for hereditary elliptocytosis mutations have severe haemolytic anaemia; the most common form is HPP.

Hereditary pyropoikilocytosis

Neonates with HPP have more than one mutation in a red cell membrane protein (they may be homozygous or compound heterozygotes) (Tse and Lux 1999; Delaunay 2002). HPP is uncommon but is important because it causes severe, transfusion-dependent haemolytic anaemia which does not improve with age. The diagnosis of HPP should easily be made by examining blood films from the baby (which shows lots of bizarre fragmented red cells and microspherocytes) and both parents (one or both often have red cell elliptocytosis); a useful diagnostic clue is the low MCV at birth (<60 fl). Red cell transfusion is usually necessary until the child is old enough to undergo splenectomy, to which there is an excellent response.

Neonatal haemolysis due to red cell enzymopathies

The principal red cell enzymopathies which present in the neonatal period are glucose-6-phosphate dehydrogenase (G6PD) deficiency and pyruvate kinase (PK) deficiency. They usually present with unconjugated hyperbilirubinaemia; clinically, they are indistinguishable from red cell membrane disorders, although anaemia is uncommon in neonates with G6PD deficiency. Unlike with the membrane disorders, there are often no diagnostic changes on the blood film.

Glucose-6-phosphate dehydrogenase deficiency

G6PD deficiency is seen in all ethnic groups but has a high prevalence in individuals from central Africa (20%) and the Mediterranean (10%). The G6PD gene is on the X chromosome and therefore most affected neonates are boys, although female carriers may sometimes be identified as a result of neonatal jaundice screens. In neonatal G6PD deficiency, jaundice usually presents within the first few days of life and is often severe; anaemia is extremely rare and the blood film is completely normal, thus the diagnosis must be made by assaying G6PD on a peripheral blood sample (Luzzatto 1993). It is not clear why some, but not all, G6PD-deficient neonates develop neonatal jaundice. In addition, the pathogenesis of the jaundice is also unclear, since most babies with G6PD deficiency have no evidence of haemolysis. The most important management issues in neonatal G6PD deficiency are close monitoring of the bilirubin, particularly where interactions with other risk factors for neonatal hyperbilirubinaemia are present, such as Gilbert syndrome or hereditary spherocytosis, since kernicterus has been reported in this setting (Kaplan 2001; Kaplan and Hammerman 2002), and counselling parents of affected babies about which medicines, chemicals and foods may precipitate haemolysis (Table 30.6). If exchange transfusion is required for severe hyperbilirubinaemia, conventional guidelines for exchange transfusion can be

Table 30.6 Drugs and chemicals associated with haemolysis in patients who are glucose-6-phosphate dehydrogenase (G6PD)-deficient

Antimalarials
Primaquine Pamaquine (Quinine)* (Chloroquine)*

Antibiotics
Nitrofurantoin Sulphones, e.g. dapsone Sulphonamides,† e.g. sulphamethoxazole (Septrin) Quinolones, e.g. nalidixic acid, ciprofloxacin (Chloramphenicol)‡

Analgesics
Aspirin (in high doses) Phenacetin

Chemicals
Naphthalene (mothballs) Divicine (fava beans – also known as broad beans) Methylene blue

*Acceptable in acute malaria.
†Some sulphonamides do not cause haemolysis in most G6PD-deficient patients, e.g. sulfadiazine.
‡To be avoided in some types of G6PD deficiency (can be taken by patients with the common, African A-form of G6PD deficiency).

followed (see Chs 29.2 and 44). Certain uncommon variants of G6PD deficiency are associated with chronic haemolysis, and for these children folic acid supplements should be given (Luzzatto 1993). However, for the vast majority of patients there is no chronic haemolysis and no anaemia and therefore folic acid supplements are not indicated.

Pyruvate kinase deficiency

PK deficiency is the second most common red cell enzymopathy in neonates. It is autosomal recessive and clinically heterogeneous, varying from anaemia severe enough to cause hydrops fetalis to a mild unconjugated hyperbilirubinaemia (Gilsanz et al. 1993; Zanella and Bianchi 2000). In severe cases, the jaundice has a rapid onset within 24 hours of birth and exchange transfusion may be required (Gilsanz et al. 1993). The diagnosis is made by measuring pretransfusion red cell PK activity; in mild cases, the PK activity may be relatively modestly reduced, making the diagnosis difficult, and it is often useful to assay levels in the parents for confirmation. The blood film is sometimes distinctive but more often shows non-specific changes of non-spherocytic haemolysis and therefore it is good practice to assay PK in all babies with unexplained haemolysis after the common causes have been excluded. Management in the neonatal period depends on the severity of the jaundice and anaemia; some, but not all, children are transfusion-dependent and folic acid supplements should be given to prevent deficiency due to chronic haemolysis.

Other red cell enzymopathies presenting in neonates

The other red cell enzymopathies are rare. The most important to be aware of in the neonatal period is triosephosphate isomerase deficiency, which is autosomal recessive (Schneider 2000). One-third of cases present with neonatal haemolytic anaemia and this may be the only presenting feature at this age; the devastating neurological features of this disorder only become apparent 6–12 months later (Schneider 2000). Persistent haemolysis should therefore always be investigated.

Neonatal haemolysis due to haemoglobinopathies

The haemoglobinopathies, with the exception of α-thalassaemia major, do not usually present in the neonatal period. Occasional non-thalassaemic, structural α-globin and γ-globin gene mutations, which are clinically completely silent in adults and children, cause transient haemolytic anaemia (and diagnostic confusion!) in the neonate (see below). Symptoms and signs of the major β-globin haemoglobinopathies (sickle-cell disease and β-thalassaemia major) are rare in neonates, although modern techniques (e.g. high-performance liquid chromatography (HPLC), isoelectric focusing) allow the diagnosis to be made on neonatal blood samples where family studies indicate that both parents are carriers (Davies et al. 2000). Many countries and regions with a high prevalence of haemoglobinopathies, including the UK, have neonatal screening programmes to facilitate early diagnosis, which is particularly important in sickle-cell disease in order to start penicillin prophylaxis as soon as possible (Vichinsky et al. 1988; Davies et al. 2000; Karnon et al. 2000).

Alpha-thalassaemia major

Alpha-thalassaemia major occurs when all four α-globin genes on chromosome 16 are deleted (Higgs 1993). It predominantly affects families of south-east Asian origin and presents with mid-trimester fetal anaemia or hydrops fetalis which is fatal within hours of delivery (occasional babies have lived a few days). The only long-term survivors of α-thalassaemia major are those who received intrauterine transfusions (Dame et al. 1999; Singer et al. 2000; Sohan et al. 2002). In recent years there have been several reports of normal growth and development where intrauterine transfusion is commenced during the second trimester (Dame et al. 1999; Sohan et al. 2002); however, there is a high incidence of hypospadias in boys and other survivors have limb defects and/or severe neurological problems (Dame et al. 1999; Singer et al. 2000). If intrauterine transfusions are delayed until the anaemia is severe, neonatal pulmonary hypoplasia is a cause of early mortality. The diagnosis of α-thalassaemia major should be suspected in any case of severe fetal anaemia presenting in the second trimester and any case of hydrops fetalis with severe anaemia in which the parents come from southeast Asia (it is also seen occasionally in families who originate from India, the Middle East or the Mediterranean). Checking the blood counts of the parents will immediately identify whether they are at risk of having a child with α-thalassaemia major – both parents will be carriers of a chromosome 16 in which both of the two α-globin genes are deleted and so they will have hypochromic, microcytic red cell indices (MCV usually <74 fl and MCH usually <24 pg). The diagnosis of α-thalassaemia major is confirmed by haemoglobin electrophoresis or HPLC (which shows only Hb Barts and Hb Portland; HbF and HbA are absent); the blood film shows hypochromic, microcytic red cells with vast numbers of circulating nucleated red cells. Neonatal management of α-thalassaemia major has no impact on survival unless the baby has received intrauterine transfusions; for these transfused neonates, management is the same as for β-thalassaemia, i.e. lifelong red cell transfusions or bone marrow transplantation after the age of 2 years (Chik et al. 1998; Sohan et al. 2002).

Alpha- and gamma-globin chain structural abnormalities

Most α- and γ-globin gene variants are clinically silent. Occasional α-globin gene variants may cause haemolytic anaemia in the newborn because when the abnormal α-globin associates with γ-globin the resultant haemoglobin is unstable whereas when the variant α-globin associates with β-globin the resultant haemoglobin is stable. An example of this is Hb Hasharon: $\alpha^{214Asp \rightarrow His}$-$\gamma_2$ is unstable; but as γ-globin chain production is physiologically switched off and β-globin chain production predominates, the $\alpha^{214Asp \rightarrow His}$-$\beta_2$ produced is stable and the haemolytic anaemia completely resolves (Oski 1993). A similar principle occurs in the γ-globin variant HbF-Poole, which causes neonatal haemolytic anaemia that resolves as the switch from γ- to β-globin occurs (Lee-Potter et al. 1975). These variants can be identified by haemoglobin HPLC and are worth considering when commoner causes of haemolysis have been excluded.

Beta-thalassaemias and sickle-cell disease

Although these disorders are asymptomatic in neonates, if they are identified as a result of neonatal screening programmes, specialist advice should be sought as soon as possible. Babies with sickle-cell disease (homozygous sickle-cell disease, SC disease or S-β-thalassaemia) should be started on prophylactic penicillin V (62.5 mg twice daily) and folic acid (500 μg/kg/day) (Vichinsky et al. 1988). Babies with β-thalassaemia major usually start to require transfusion around the age of 6 months but benefit from folic acid supplementation until regular transfusions begin (Olivieri 1999).

Anaemia due to blood loss

Blood loss causing neonatal anaemia may be very obvious, e.g. a large subgaleal haematoma or rupture of the cord, or be concealed and easy to miss unless specifically sought (e.g. fetomaternal bleeds). Conventionally, the causes of anaemia due to blood loss are classified according to the timing of the blood loss – during fetal life, at the time of delivery or postnatally (see Table 30.4). In neonates admitted to hospital the most common cause of anaemia is blood loss secondary to iatrogenic blood letting.

Blood loss prior to birth

Twin-to-twin transfusion

Twin-to-twin transfusion occurs in monochorionic twins with monochorial placentas (Ch. 23) (Wee and Fisk 2002). Bleeding may be acute, particularly during the second stage of labour, or chronic (Wee and Fisk 2002). Chronic twin-to-twin transfusion can cause a marked difference in birthweight between twins, although recent studies show that the majority of twin pairs have a discordance in haemoglobin of <5 g/dl (Wee and Fisk 2002). The diagnosis is now usually made in fetal life and antenatal treatment may be required (Chs 9 and 23). The donor twin is smaller and may be pale and lethargic or have overt cardiac failure; the recipient twin may be plethoric, with hyperviscosity and hyperbilirubinaemia and may rarely have a haemoglobin as high as 30 g/dl. Where the haemoglobin/haematocrit are very high, disseminated intravascular coagulation (DIC) can occur. Management of DIC is described on page 776, and that of polycythaemia on page 767.

Fetomaternal haemorrhage

This may occur spontaneously or secondary to trauma, such as road traffic accidents or falls. Most spontaneous fetomaternal bleeds occur in the third trimester or during labour. Fetomaternal bleeds may also be increased by invasive procedures such as fetal blood sampling and caesarean section. The degree of anaemia is variable and the clinical presentation depends on the amount and rate of blood loss. Most episodes involve very small quantities of blood (0.5 ml or less) but acute loss of >20% of the blood volume may cause intrauterine death, circulatory shock or hydrops (Giacoia 1997). Diagnostic clues are anaemia at birth in an otherwise well term baby with no or minimal jaundice. The most useful diagnostic tests are a DAT to exclude immune haemolysis, a reticulocyte count to exclude red cell aplasia, a Kleihauer test on maternal blood to quantify the number of HbF-containing fetal RBCs in the maternal circulation and a blood film (Howarth et al. 2002). Where the baby has bled acutely just prior to delivery, the blood film is normochromic/normocytic with large numbers of nucleated red cells. In this situation, the haemoglobin may be normal at delivery but fall rapidly as haemodilution occurs. Where there is chronic blood loss, the baby is often well but may present with cardiac failure; the blood film in this situation is hypochromic/microcytic, the nucleated red cells are less prominent and the Kleihauer result may be difficult to interpret. Another point of note is that, where there is ABO incompatibility between the mother and baby, the fetal cells may be rapidly destroyed within the maternal circulation – a high index of suspicion of fetomaternal haemorrhage as a cause of neonatal anaemia is needed because it is important to perform the Kleihauer test as soon as possible, to increase the chance of detection of fetal cells. In many cases, an acute fetomaternal bleed supervenes upon chronic fetomaternal blood loss. In this situation, severe anaemia (Hb <5 g/dl) has been shown to confer a poor prognosis, as most survivors have evidence of brain injury, although there are notable exceptions (Giacoia 1997).

Blood loss at or after delivery

Blood loss around the time of delivery is usually due to obstetric complications, including placenta praevia, placental abruption or incision of the placenta during caesarean section. Blood loss in this situation is from the maternal circulation, although the fetus can be subject to hypoxia as a result. Rarely, a vasa praevia is present, and is inevitably torn when the membranes rupture, leading to severe fetal blood loss. This can easily be missed because the volume of blood is relatively small in obstetric terms and it is not possible to distinguish fetal from maternal blood by eye. The incidence of vasa praevia is estimated to be around 1:2500 and the condition carries a high fetal mortality. The presence of a vasa praevia can be detected antenatally with a colour Doppler vaginal ultrasound but this is not routine practice; if a vasa praevia is found then the baby should be delivered by caesarean section before membrane rupture.

Haematological changes occur after massive internal bleeding in the baby, e.g. subaponeurotic or retroperitoneal bleeding, and may be particularly severe where there is damage to the liver. While most cases of internal bleeding are associated with traumatic delivery, it is important to search for any underlying bleeding diathesis in such babies, particularly haemophilia A or B and vitamin K deficiency. Inherited and acquired coagulation disorders that may present with bleeding at birth or during the neonatal period are discussed on pages 775–776.

Anaemia of prematurity

Pathogenesis

The haemoglobin falls after birth in all newborns, regardless of gestational age. This normal physiological fall in haemoglobin is greater in preterm than in term neonates and has been termed 'physiological anaemia of prematurity' since it does not appear to be associated with any abnormalities in the baby. The pathogenesis is not fully elucidated but contributory factors include the reduced red cell lifespan of fetal erythrocytes, the relatively low erythropoietin concentration and the rapid growth rate (Oski 1993). In practice, perhaps because of routine supplementation of preterm neonates with folic acid and iron, nutritional deficiency rarely plays a role (Fuller et al. 1992; Griffin et al. 1999; Rao and Georgieff 2002). On the other hand, for the majority of preterm infants in hospital, iatrogenic blood letting for diagnostic tests contributes to this physiological process. The clinical significance of anaemia of prematurity is mainly that the need for 'top-up' transfusion in preterm infants can be reduced if clinicians are aware of the normal nadir in erythropoiesis in neonates and the available measures to prevent the anaemia becoming severe.

Diagnosis

In a well term infant, the nadir in haemoglobin is as low as 9.4–11 g/dl and occurs at 8–12 weeks of age (see Table 30.2); for a preterm infant, the nadir in haemoglobin occurs earlier (4–8 weeks of age) and is lower (6.5–9 g/dl). The diagnosis is usually straightforward – a well preterm baby has a slowly falling haemoglobin with a completely unremarkable blood film showing normochromic/normocytic red cells, slightly low reticulocytes (20×10^9/l) and no nucleated red cells.

Management

There are three facets to the management of anaemia of prematurity. The first is to exclude other causes of anaemia using clinical features and a diagnostic algorithm (see p. 762, Fig. 30.1). Secondly, a decision whether or not to transfuse should be made (the indications and principles of neonatal transfusion are discussed in detail on pp. 782–785). Thirdly, with increasing recognition of potential transfusion hazards, amelioration of neonatal anaemia to reduce the need for transfusion has become extremely important.

The role of erythropoietin and haematinics

The severity of anaemia of prematurity and thereby the need for red cell transfusion can be reduced by a combination of the following approaches:

- limiting iatrogenic blood loss by appropriate use of blood tests (Lin et al. 2000)
- iron and folate supplementation for all preterm infants:
  - iron 3 mg/kg/day from 4–6 weeks of age (a pragmatic approach is to give 1 ml of sodium ironedetate (Sytron) once daily) or iron-fortified formula with 0.5–0.9 mg/dl iron (Griffin et al. 1999; Rao et al. 2002; Haiden et al. 2006)
  - folic acid 50 µg daily or 500 µg once weekly (Fuller et al. 1992)
- judicious use of erythropoietin (Vamvakas and Strauss 2001; Garcia et al. 2002).

The many controlled trials of erythropoietin for prevention of neonatal anaemia have been extensively reviewed (Ohls 2002), including two meta-analyses (Vamvakas and Strauss 2001; Garcia et al. 2002), and are only briefly summarised here. Recombinant erythropoietin is biologically effective in that it stimulates erythropoiesis in all preterm infants and there is no evidence of erythropoietin insensitivity. Erythropoietin is also able to reduce red cell transfusion requirements in preterm infants (Vamvakas and Strauss 2001;

Garcia et al. 2002; Maier et al. 2002; Meyer et al. 2003; Haiden et al. 2006). However, in most studies there is no evidence to support the clinical effectiveness of erythropoietin, i.e. that it reduces the number of transfusions to an extent which demonstrably reduces the hazards of transfusion. At best, the studies show that erythropoietin reduces the number of transfusions in relatively well infants with low transfusion requirements (Vamvakas and Strauss 2001; Garcia et al. 2002; Meyer et al. 2003; Haiden et al. 2006). One study has shown that the use of erythropoietin together with careful nutritional supplementaion and judicious use of laboratory tests to reduce iatrogenic blood loss can halve the transfusion requirements in a cohort of sick extremely-low-birthweight neonates (Haiden et al. 2006). However, most studies have shown that, even in high doses, the erythropoietin-mediated increase in red cell production is unable to increase sufficiently to cope with the need for frequent phlebotomy and multiple transfusions in sick preterm infants (Donalto et al. 2000; Ohls et al. 2001). Despite its marginal role in reducing transfusion requirements, erythropoietin may become more important again if worries over the safety of blood transfusion lead to reduced availability and parental acceptance of red cell transfusion. At present, the main therapeutic roles for erythropoietin in neonates are:

- in preventing anaemia in infants who have received intrauterine transfusions for alloantibody-mediated anaemia (Zuppa et al. 2009)
- in a non-emergency situation where red cell transfusions are against the parents' wishes and are not felt to be absolutely essential to save the life of the baby (e.g. preterm babies of Jehovah's witnesses) (Horan and Stutchfield 2001).

An effective dose of recombinant erythropoietin in this setting is 300 µg/kg as a single subcutaneous injection three times per week starting in the first week of life. Epoetin-β should be used in view of the potential risk of red cell aplasia described (in adults) with epoetin-α, the alternative form of recombinant erythropoietin (Casadevall et al. 2002). This is because the haemoglobin does not start to rise until about 10–14 days after erythropoietin has been commenced. In addition, iron supplements (Sytron, as above) should be started as soon as possible, to prevent the rapid development of iron deficiency in erythropoietin-treated infants (the dose may need to be increased up to a maximum of 9 mg/kg if iron deficiency develops on the standard dose of Sytron) (Bechensteen et al. 1993).

A simple diagnostic approach to neonatal anaemia

Red cell disorders associated with neonatal or fetal anaemia present in three main ways: with a low haemoglobin (anaemia), with jaundice due to haemolysis or with hydrops. Table 30.4 lists the most common causes of anaemia, and the most common haematological causes of jaundice and hydrops are shown in Table 30.7 and Table 30.5, respectively. A diagnostic algorithm to help identify the most likely cause of neonatal hyperbilirubinaemia and the investigations which are most useful is shown in Figure 30.2. This is based on simple observations and simple tests available in almost all haematology laboratories. When in doubt about the best investigations to use and the interpretation of the results, discussion with a haematologist at an early stage should be helpful.

Polycythaemia

For both term and preterm infants, polycythaemia can be defined as a central venous haematocrit of >0.65. At haematocrits in excess

Table 30.7 Haematological causes of neonatal jaundice

Immune
Haemolytic disease of the newborn
Maternal autoimmune haemolytic anaemia

Red cell membrane disorders
Hereditary spherocytosis
Homozygous hereditary elliptocytosis
Hereditary pyropoikilocytosis

Red cell enzymopathies
Glucose-6-phosphate dehydrogenase deficiency
Pyruvate kinase deficiency
Other: e.g. glucose phosphate isomerase deficiency

Haemoglobinopathies
α-thalassaemias (α-thalassaemia major; severe HbH disease)
γ-thalassaemias (e.g. Hb Hasharon)
Other: sickle-cell syndromes (occasionally)

Infection
Bacterial
Viral, e.g. cytomegalovirus, rubella, herpes simplex
Protozoal, e.g. *Toxoplasma*, malaria, syphilis

Table 30.8 Causes of neonatal polycythaemia

Intrauterine growth restriction
Maternal hypertension
Maternal diabetes
Chromosomal disorders: trisomy 21, 18 or 13
Twin-to-twin transfusion
Delayed clamping of the cord
Endocrine disorders: thyrotoxicosis, congenital adrenal hyperplasia

of 0.65, there is an exponential rise in blood viscosity (Werner 1995). However, even at haematocrits >0.70, only a minority of neonates exhibit clinical signs of hyperviscosity. The clinical manifestations include lethargy, hypotonia, hyperbilirubinaemia and hypoglycaemia (Watts and Roberts 1999). Polycythaemia may also be a contributory factor in neonatal seizures, stroke, renal vein thrombosis and necrotising enterocolitis (NEC) (Hakanson and Oh 1977). Causes of polycythaemia are shown in Table 30.8. Treatment of neonatal polycythaemia is controversial and is probably not necessary in infants with very minor symptoms (e.g. borderline hypoglycaemia or poor peripheral perfusion). However, most of the evidence supports active management of infants with a haematocrit >0.65 in association with symptoms or signs indicative of an adverse long-term outcome (e.g. refractory hypoglycaemia, neurological signs). For these infants, partial exchange transfusion using a crystalloid solution such as normal saline should be performed to reduce the haematocrit to 0.55 (Watts and Roberts 1999). There is no evidence to support the use of fresh frozen plasma (FFP) or albumin (Wong et al.1997) for this procedure, both of which carry the risk of transfusion-transmitted infection.

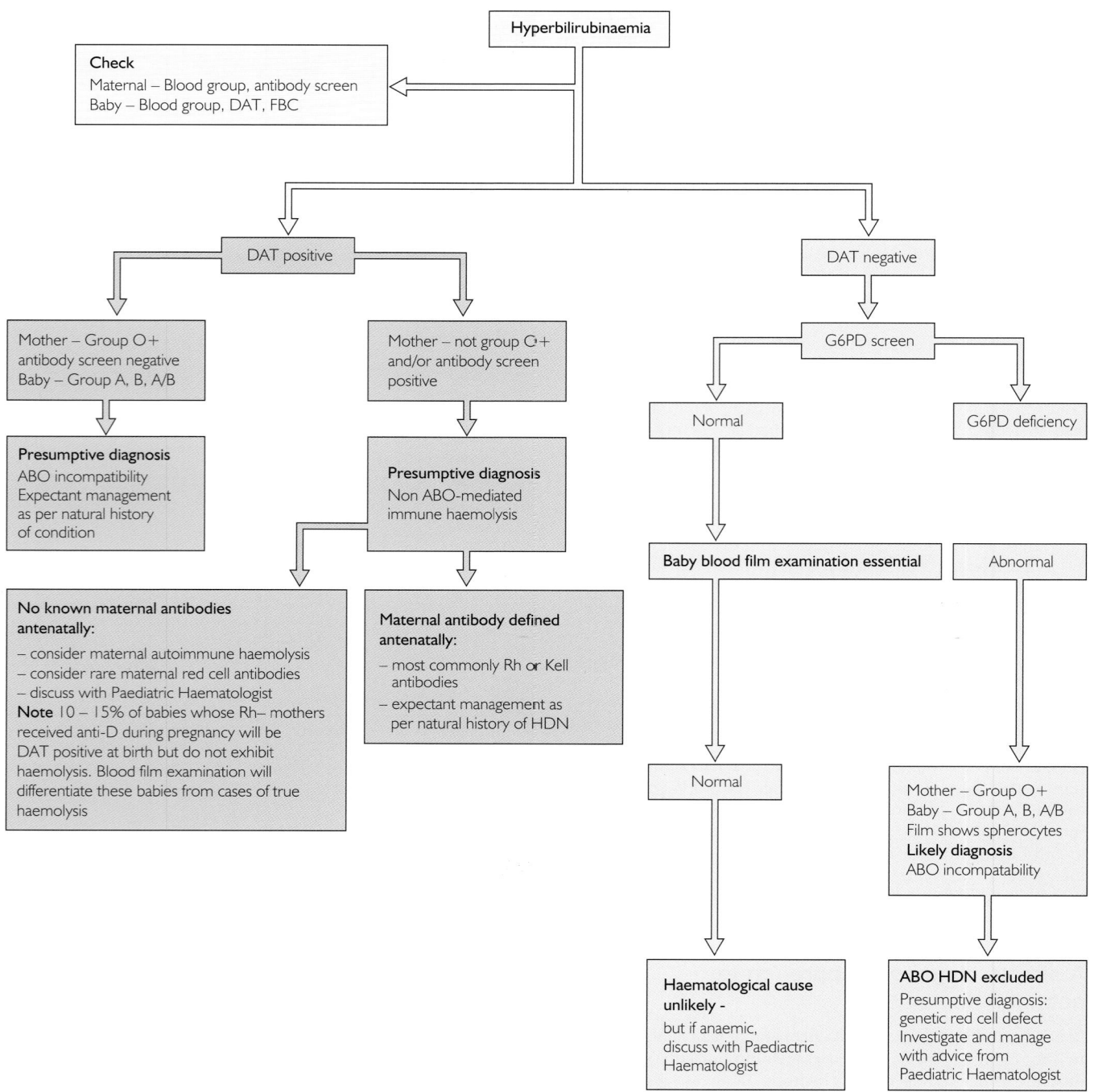

Fig. 30.2 A diagnostic algorithm for neonatal hyperbilirubinaemia. DAT, direct antiglobluin test (Coombs' test); FBC, full blood count; G6PD, glucose-6-phosphate dehydrogenase; HDN, haemolytic disease of the newborn.

White cell disorders

Introduction and normal values

Apart from alterations in the numbers of white blood cells in response to infection, disorders of white cells are not common in neonates. Nevertheless, some diagnostic dilemmas do present in the neonatal period, in particular the causes and investigation of neutropenia and

how to identify rare disorders such as congenital leukaemia (both described below). However, there is often a lot of very useful information that can be discovered just from looking carefully at the morphology of the white blood cells on a neonatal blood film. Not only can an early diagnosis of bacterial infection often be made in this way, but also there may be indicators of the type of bacterial infection, of NEC, of congenital viral infections, or even of rare genetic and metabolic disorders.

Normal values

Neutrophil and monocyte counts vary over the first few days of life even in healthy babies, increasing for the first 12 hours and then falling to a nadir at 4 days of age. Normal values for neutrophils at birth are also affected by other factors, including antenatal history, perinatal history and ethnic origin. The neutrophil count is higher in capillary samples and after vigorous crying; it is lower in neonates of African origin. All of the other types of white blood cell found in adult blood are also present in the newborn (see Table 30.2). Conversely, some cell types not found in healthy adults are seen in healthy preterm babies – these include blast cells, other early myeloid cells, nucleated red cells and even occasional megakaryocytes.

Neutropenia

Definition and causes of neonatal neutropenia

Transient neutropenia is fairly common in preterm neonates but is uncommon in term infants. The normal values for neutrophil counts vary both with gestational age and with postnatal age, particularly over the first few days of life. A pragmatic approach is to consider a neutrophil count at birth of $<2 \times 10^9/l$ as abnormal and worth monitoring and a neutrophil count during the first month of life of $<0.7 \times 10^9/l$ as significant enough to merit further investigation. The principal causes of neonatal neutropenia are shown in Table 30.9. The commonest cause in preterm neonates is neutropenia in association with IUGR and/or maternal hypertension (Koenig and Christensen 1989), while in term infants bacterial or

Table 30.9 Causes of neonatal neutropenia

Placental insufficiency
Maternal hypertension
Intrauterine growth restriction
Maternal diabetes
Infection
Acute, perinatal bacterial infection, e.g. group B streptococcus
Congenital infections, e.g. cytomegalovirus
Postnatal bacterial infections
Postnatal viral infections, e.g. cytomegalovirus
Necrotising enterocolitis
Immune
Alloimmune
Genetic
Trisomies: 21, 13 and 18
Severe congenital neutropenia (includes Kostmann syndrome)
Schwachman syndrome
Pearson syndrome
Reticular dysgenesis
Metabolic disorders, e.g. hyperglycinaemia, isovaleric, propionic and methylmalonic acidaemia
Marrow replacement
Congenital leukaemia

viral infection is the usual explanation. Other important causes of neutropenia, as they may be the cause of severe neonatal infection, are alloimmune neutropenia and congenital neutropenia due to failure of neutrophil production (e.g. Kostmann syndrome).

Neutropenia and infection

Any bacterial infection can cause acute neutropenia. Where this is short-lived (6–12 hours) it is a normal response, but neutropenia lasting >12 hours in the setting of acute bacterial infection may be a poor prognostic sign. Examination of the blood film is often helpful in differentiating neutropenia secondary to bacterial infection from viral infection or IUGR. The classical signs of acute bacterial infection are the presence of an increased percentage of band neutrophils and toxic granulation of immature and mature neutrophils, followed after 1–2 days by a mature neutrophilia and after 3–5 days by eosinophilia. By contrast, there is no increase in band cells or toxic granulation in viral infections; instead, atypical 'viral' lymphocytes are seen, particularly in congenital CMV infection, where they may persist for several months.

Neutropenia and intrauterine growth restriction

The commonest cause of neutropenia in preterm infants is IUGR and/or maternal hypertension or maternal diabetes. In these disorders, neutrophil production is reduced because of inadequate numbers of neutrophil progenitors; most affected neonates also have thrombocytopenia and increased erythropoiesis (polycythaemia and/or increased circulating nucleated red cells) (Watts and Roberts 1999). The exact pathogenesis is unknown but evidence suggests that the haematological abnormalities are secondary to fetal tissue hypoxia (Watts and Roberts 1999). The neutropenia resolves spontaneously, usually starting to recover 2–3 days after birth. However, both the duration and the severity of the neutropenia are directly related to the severity of the IUGR/maternal hypertension (Koenig and Christensen 1989; Watts and Roberts 1999). The main clinical significance of this form of neutropenia is firstly that recognition of its natural history prevents unnecessary treatment and investigations, and secondly that affected neonates do tend to have a 'blunted' neutrophil response to infection, i.e. the neutrophil response is both delayed and sometimes inadequate, which may lead to an increased frequency and duration of bacterial infections. There are no specific diagnostic tests for this form of neutropenia but clues that this is the explanation for the neutropenia are the clinical history, the concomitant presence of a platelet count $<150 \times 10^9/l$, an increased number of circulating nucleated RBCs (usually >20/100 white cells) and the severity (usually the neutrophil count is $>0.3 \times 10^9/l$). Neither of the recombinant haemopoietic growth factors available for therapeutic use in stimulating neutrophil production (G-CSF and GM-CSF) has been shown to be of clinical value in the treatment or prevention of IUGR-associated neutropenia (Carr et al. 2003).

Alloimmune neutropenia

Alloimmune neutropenia is the neutrophil equivalent of HDN and alloimmune thrombocytopenia. It occurs when fetal neutrophils express paternally derived neutrophil-specific antigens which are absent on maternal neutrophils and against which the mother produces IgG neutrophil alloantibodies (Maheshwari et al. 2002). The causative antibodies are usually anti-NA1 or anti-NA2 (Stroncek 2002). It is widely quoted that alloimmune neutropenia affects 3% of all deliveries (Maheshwari et al. 2002), although relatively few cases are reported and in our experience this is a very uncommon clinical problem. This suggests that, while the causative antibodies may be present in 3% of women, most neonatal cases are so mild that the signs do not merit medical attention. Therefore, from a practical perspective, the importance of neonatal alloimmune neutropenia is that it should be thought of as a possible cause of neutropenia in any neonate with a severe bacterial infection together with a neutropenia which persists for more than 3 days despite appropriate antibiotic treatment. Clinically significant neonatal alloimmune neutropenia presents in the first few days of life with fever and infections of the respiratory tract, urinary tract and skin, particularly due to *Staphylococcus aureus*. The diagnosis is made by demonstrating antineutrophil antibodies in the mother and baby which react against paternal, but not maternal, neutrophil antigens. The neutropenia is self-limiting, usually resolving within 1–2 months, and the mainstay of treatment is antibiotics. In severe cases, where there is clinical deterioration despite antibiotics, plasma exchange and/or G-CSF (10 μg/kg/day) may be useful.

Congenital and inherited neutropenias

All of the inherited and congenital neutrophil disorders are rare and are listed in Table 30.9. These should be sought where the neutropenia is prolonged, if there is a relevant family history or consanguinity, or if the baby has typical dysmorphic features (e.g. thumb/radial abnormalities in Fanconi's anaemia). The most likely of these to present in the neonatal period is severe congenital neutropenia (SCN), which used to be referred to as Kostmann syndrome; it is now recognised to be a heterogeneous group of conditions due to mutations in several different genes (Klein et al. 2007; Zeidler et al. 2009). SCN is defined as a condition in which neutrophil production is reduced due to an 'arrest' of differentiation at the myelocyte/promyelocyte stage. Infants with SCN usually present with severe infections within a few weeks of birth (Zeidler et al. 2009). Other clues to the diagnosis are that the neutropenia is marked (usually $<0.2 \times 10^9/l$) and there is often a marked compensatory monocytosis. SCN can be either autosomal recessive or autosomal dominant depending on the gene(s) which is/are mutated. The most common genetic cause is mutations of the elastase gene (*ELA2*) (Aprikyan et al. 2004), which is autosomal dominant; the original Kostmann syndrome is due to mutations in *HAX1*, which is autosomal recessive (Klein et al. 2007). The diagnosis is made on the basis of the severity of the neutropenia, the bone marrow appearances, the clinical history and the absence of antineutrophil antibodies. Where mutational analysis is available, this may prove useful for establishing the diagnosis and for prenatal diagnosis.

Congenital leukaemias and haematological abnormalities associated with Down syndrome

Congenital leukaemias

Congenital leukaemia is rare but the diagnosis is usually straightforward. The most common types are acute monoblastic leukaemia and acute megakaryoblastic leukaemia (Bresters et al. 2002). The usual presentation is with clinical signs of anaemia and skin lesions caused by focal infiltration by leukaemic cells. Rapid clinical deterioration due to severe anaemia and thrombocytopenia is common. Congenital leukaemia may also present as 'blueberry muffin' baby or hydrops fetalis (Bowden et al. 1989). Diagnostic clues to congenital leukaemia are the concomitant presence of severe and worsening anaemia and thrombocytopenia in a sick baby, usually with a very high white blood cell count. The diagnosis is established by examination of the blood film, which shows large numbers of primitive blast cells, and a bone marrow aspirate, bone marrow cytogenetics and immunophenotyping of the peripheral blood (or marrow) leukaemic cells. The prognosis is extremely poor; few are cured by chemotherapy, and bone marrow transplantation, which has been carried out successfully, may be the best option (Bajwa et al. 2001). Babies with Down syndrome may occasionally present with leukaemia but more often have a transient leukaemia known as transient myeloproliferative disorder or transient abnormal myelopoiesis (TAM) – see below (Roy et al. 2009).

Haematological abnormalities in neonates with Down syndrome and other trisomies

Haematological abnormalities are more common in neonates with chromosomal disorders, including Down syndrome, trisomy 13 and trisomy 18, all of which may be associated with pancytopenia. Most babies with Down syndrome have minor abnormalities (thrombocytopenia, neutrophilia or polycythaemia are the most common, but 5–10% have TAM).

TAM is frequently asymptomatic and is diagnosed when the blood count shows leukocytosis and the blood film is abnormal with increased numbers of circulating blast cells (Roy et al. 2009). Some babies develop signs of hepatic infiltration and abnormal liver function tests are frequently found. Mutations in GATA-1, a critical haemopoietic cell transcription factor, have recently been reported both in almost all neonates with TAM and in the megakaryoblastic leukaemia associated with Down syndrome (Wechsler et al. 2002; Hitzler et al. 2003; Roy et al. 2009). Usually, no treatment is indicated for TAM, which resolves by the age of 2–3 months in >70% of cases (Roy et al. 2009); occasionally neonates die from fulminant hepatic involvement and up to 30% will subsequently develop acute megakaryoblastic leukaemia within the first 5 years of life. For this reason, and because TAM is often asymptomatic, it is advisable to perform a full blood count and film on all neonates with Down syndrome (Roy et al. 2009).

Abnormal leukocytes in neonatal systemic disease

Careful examination of the blood film often provides clues to other underlying disorders in the newborn. As well as classical features of acute bacterial and viral infections, characteristic changes can be seen in fungal infection, where vacuolation of the neutrophils and monocytes may be prominent and fungi may be seen within the phagocytic cells. In NEC, neutrophil and monocyte vacuolation is almost always present and is usually a very early feature. A number of metabolic and storage disorders also produce changes in the appearance of leukocytes:

- leukocyte vacuolation in Pearson syndrome
- giant neutrophil granules in Chédiak–Higashi syndrome
- Alder Reilly leukocyte granules in Hunter syndrome, Hurler syndrome and Sanfilippo syndrome
- lymphocyte vacuolation in Wolman's disease, α-mannosidosis, sialidosis and Sanfilippo syndrome.

Haemostasis and thrombosis in the newborn

Introduction

Problems of disordered coagulation with or without obvious bleeding are relatively common in neonates, especially when they are sick. Thrombotic problems are also increasingly recognised in neonates, and the number of genetic and acquired causes of thrombophilia that can be identified in neonates and their families is rising. Therefore, in order to request and interpret the most useful laboratory tests, and to treat appropriately, it is important to have a basic understanding of normal haemostasis and how it differs in neonates compared with in older infants and children.

Haemostasis, the process of normal blood coagulation, takes place via a series of complex interactions involving both activators and inhibitors of coagulation (Hutton et al. 1999). In general, defects in the coagulation proteins (such as the vitamin K-dependent factors), in platelet number or function, or in the fibrinolytic pathway are associated with an increased risk of bleeding. In contrast, defects in the naturally occurring anticoagulants (such as protein C) or in the vessel wall (such as damage from vascular catheters) are associated with thrombosis. However, in many cases, both pro- and anticoagulant abnormalities can occur at the same time, as seen, for example, in DIC.

The process can be summarised as follows. In the first stage, tissue factor (TF) binds to the coagulation factor VIIa, and the TF–VIIa complex, by converting factor X to Xa, leads to the generation of small amounts of thrombin (Fig. 30.3A). In the second stage, amplification of the coagulation cascade occurs as the thrombin activates factor V and factor VIII, and the TF–VIIa activates factor IX, leading to rapid generation of more thrombin. Thrombin also activates factor XI, further amplifying its own generation (see Fig. 30.3B). Finally, thrombin converts fibrinogen to fibrin with subsequent cross-linking by factor XIII to stabilise the clot. The role of TF is of particular interest as it is produced not only by endothelial cells but also by monocytes (Mattsson et al. 2002). TF is increased by endotoxin and proinflammatory cytokines and so is likely to play an important role in the pathogenesis of sepsis-associated DIC (Osterud and Bjorklid 2001).

Platelets

The role of platelets in coagulation is also critical, as shown by the risk of severe bleeding in patients with thrombocytopenia. Endothelial damage leads to exposure not only of TF but also of collagen, which binds von Willebrand's factor (vWF) produced by the

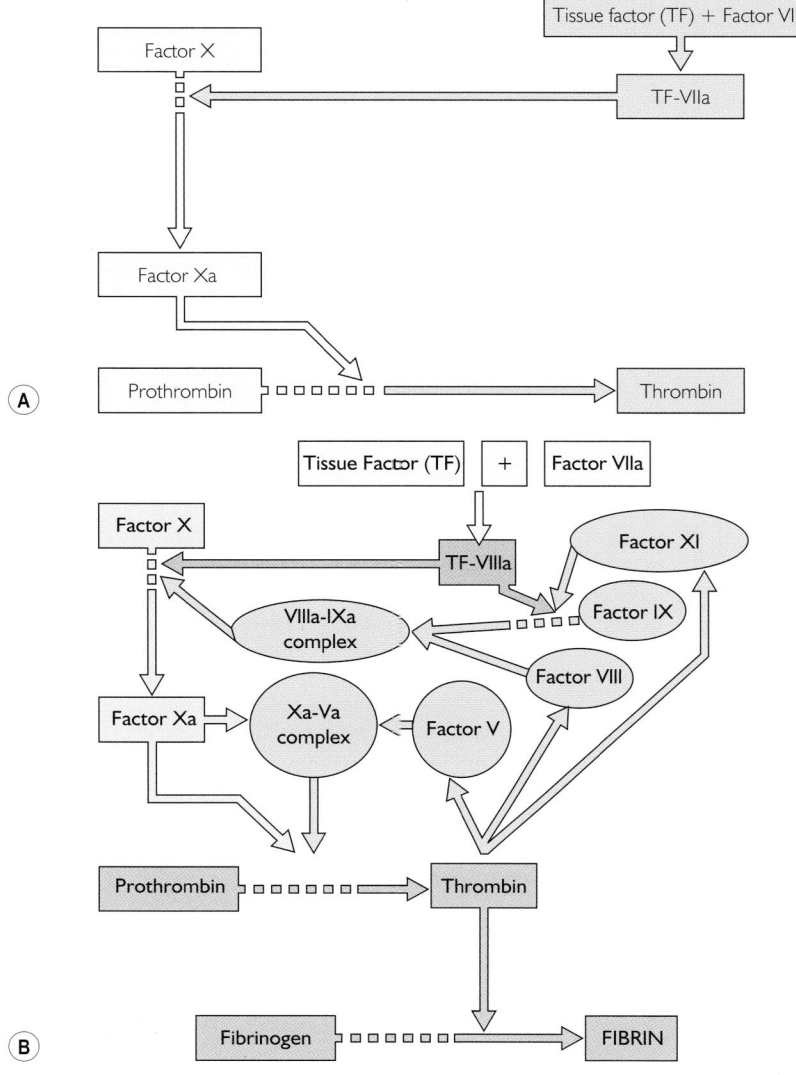

Fig. 30.3 A simplified scheme of the coagulation cascade. The first stage in the coagulation cascade is the binding of tissue factor (TF) to the coagulation factor VIIa. The TF–VIIa complex, by converting factor X to Xa, leads to the generation of small amounts of thrombin (A). In the second stage, amplification of the coagulation cascade then occurs as the thrombin activates factor V and factor VIII, and the TF–VIIa activates factor IX, leading to the rapid generation of more thrombin. Thrombin also activates factor XI, further amplifying its own generation (B). Finally, thrombin converts fibrinogen to fibrin with subsequent cross-linking by factor XIII to stabilise the clot.

endothelial cells. Platelets are first captured by the vWF via their glycoprotein 1b (Gp1b) receptors and are then 'tethered' by activation of their glycoprotein IIb/IIIa (GpIIb/IIIa) receptors, which bind to both vWF and fibrinogen. More and more platelets accumulate, followed by more vWF and fibrinogen, to form an occlusive platelet plug.

Regulation of the procoagulant process by endogenous anticoagulants and fibrinolysis

The procoagulant process is regulated by a large number of mechanisms. These include the natural anticoagulants (antithrombin; protein C/protein S/thrombomodulin), TF pathway inhibitor (TFPI) and the fibrinolytic pathway (Edstrom et al. 2000). The physiological importance of the natural anticoagulants is clear from the high risk of thrombosis in patients with deficiency of these factors. The main purpose of the natural anticoagulants is to limit the generation of thrombin and thereby prevent thrombosis. Antithrombin, heparin cofactor II and α_2-macroglobulin are direct inhibitors of thrombin. The protein C/protein S/thrombomodulin pathway is also activated by thrombin and does not function in the absence of thrombin. Current models (Fig. 30.4) indicate that activation of protein C requires binding of protein C to two receptors on the endothelial surface, thrombomodulin and the endothelial protein C receptor, which then act as a molecular switch to limit the procoagulant activity of thrombin (Kottke-Marchant and Comp 2002). Activated protein C then forms a complex with protein S and the protein C/S complex cleaves and inactivates factors Va and VIIIa, thus switching off thrombin generation. Consequently, vascular endothelium plays a key role in haemostasis not only by providing the principal initiator of coagulation (TF) but also by switching off the process via thrombomodulin.

A further mechanism preventing sustained activation of the procoagulant pathway is TFPI, which limits TF-induced initiation of coagulation. Finally, the risks of uncontrolled thrombosis due to activation of the procoagulant process are limited by the

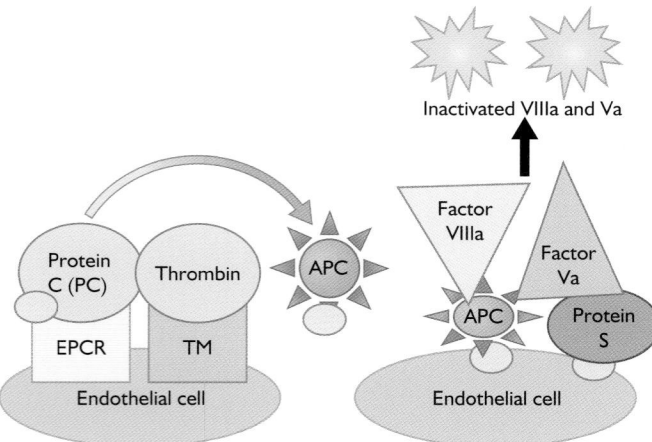

Fig. 30.4 Inactivation of activated factor VIII and factor V by the protein C/S pathway. The protein C/protein S/thrombomodulin pathway is activated by thrombin. The activation of protein C requires binding of protein C to two receptors on the endothelial surface, thrombomodulin (TM) and the endothelial protein C receptor (EPCR), which then act as a molecular switch to limit the procoagulant activity of thrombin. The activated protein C (APC) then forms a complex with protein S, and the protein C/S complex cleaves and inactivates factors Va and VIIIa, thus switching off thrombin generation.

fibrinolytic pathway. Fibrinolysis controls fibrin deposition at the site of injury via the activity of the serine protease plasmin and by thrombin-activated fibrinolysis inhibitor (TAFI) (Bouma et al. 2001). Like other aspects of the haemostatic system, this pathway is subject to feedback control to provide a balance between coagulation and fibrinolysis. For example, fibrin itself stimulates release of tissue plasminogen activator (t-PA) and urokinase-type plasminogen activator, which convert plasminogen into plasmin. Plasmin rapidly digests both fibrin and fibrinogen, leading to the production of fibrin degradation products. Plasmin is also able to digest fibrin cross-linked by factor XIII, leading to the generation of D-dimers.

Developmental haemostasis

Coagulation proteins are synthesised by the fetus from the fifth week of gestation onwards (Andrew 1997). Levels gradually rise during fetal life but, with some exceptions (see below), do not reach adult values until several months after birth, even in term babies. Thus, 'normal values' in the neonate vary not only with gestational but also with postnatal age (Appendix 2). Coagulation proteins do not cross the placenta, or do so in very small amounts, and therefore need to be independently synthesised by the fetus. However, fetal coagulation factor synthesis can be affected by maternal factors (e.g. warfarin, severe maternal vitamin K deficiency).

There are few data about the normal ranges of the coagulation factors at different gestational ages. In addition, the results can be difficult to interpret as there are differences between the levels measured in cord blood and the levels collected from fetal blood by fetoscopy at the same gestational age, perhaps because of activation of coagulation during birth (Andrew et al. 1987). The published data for coagulation factor levels in preterm neonates are for those born between 30 and 36 weeks' gestation (Appendix 2) (Andrew et al. 1988). Corresponding data are also available for term babies (Appendix 2) (Andrew et al. 1987). Data for babies at <30 weeks' gestation derive from fetoscopy samples and show that the levels of the vitamin K-dependent factors (II, VII, IX and X) and of factors XI and XII are all low (<40% of adult values) and remain so during the first month of life (Reverdiau-Moalic et al. 1996). By contrast, even in preterm babies (<30 weeks), levels of factor V, factor XIII and fibrinogen are normal at birth and levels of factor VIII and vWF are normal or increased.

Blood platelet counts at birth in term and preterm neonates are within the normal adult range (Roberts and Murray 2001). Many studies have found impaired function of neonatal platelets in vitro in term and preterm infants; the most consistent abnormalities are reduced aggregation in response to adrenaline (epinephrine), adenosine diphosphate and thrombin. Their significance in clinical practice is unclear since the bleeding time tested with adult and neonatal devices is normal in term and preterm infants (<135 seconds) (Stuart and Graeber 1998) and bleeding problems associated with abnormal platelet function are rare in neonates. There are also important gestational and postnatal age-related changes in the levels of the fibrinolytic and natural anticoagulant pathways.

Diagnostic approach to bleeding in neonates

Clinical presentation of bleeding disorders

The clinical presentation and likely cause(s) of bleeding in neonates depend on gestational age and whether the infant is sick or well. Particular patterns of bleeding may also suggest the underlying diagnosis, such as bleeding from the umbilical cord stump in factor XIII deficiency and bleeding after circumcision in haemophilia. The most common sites of bleeding in preterm neonates are oozing from venepuncture sites, pulmonary haemorrhage, gastrointestinal bleeding and intracranial haemorrhage. In term neonates, cephalo-haematomas are commonly seen following both normal and forceps deliveries. Subarachnoid (subgaleal) haemorrhages (Ch. 40.3) are increased following vacuum extraction (Wen et al. 2001) but in otherwise healthy neonates these bleeding manifestations are unlikely to be markers of disordered haemostasis. However, a neonate with a large subaponeurotic or subdural haemorrhage should be screened for coagulation defects (Davis 2000). Magnetic resonance imaging studies have shown that small peritentorial subdural collections are common after a normal delivery; in haemophilia it is probably the case that these continue to enlarge over the ensuing days, because the blood does not clot. Germinal matrix haemorrhage/intraventricular haemorrhage (GMH-IVH) in term babies is also rare and should point to a possible coagulation defect. GMH-IVH and thalamic haemorrhage in term babies is often secondary to venous thrombosis (Ch. 40.3) and a thrombophilia screen may be indicated. In any infant with abnormal bleeding, blood tests to identify the most likely cause should always be accompanied by a thorough clinical assessment, including sites of possible occult bleeding, and a careful history, including maternal/infant drugs (was vitamin K given?) and questions to elucidate a family history of bleeding disorders.

Screening tests for bleeding disorders

Nearly all significant bleeding disorders in neonates can be identified using simple screening tests, as summarised below. Notable exceptions are factor XIII deficiency (which requires a specific assay) and platelet function disorders (which require specialised tests and are usually performed after the neonatal period, because of the difficulties of sample size and data interpretation in neonates). Where an inherited defect is suspected or where bleeding and coagulation assay derangement are severe, it is extremely important to test both parents for coagulation abnormalities. There are several reasons for this: there is considerable interindividual variation in factor levels in neonates; there is also overlap between the deficiency states and the lower limit of normal, particularly in preterm neonates, when levels of many factors are physiologically low; and, finally, it is often difficult to obtain good-quality neonatal samples free from in vitro activation or contamination with heparin.

The most useful screening tests in neonates are:

- prothrombin time (PT) – this predominantly measures the activity of factors II, V, VII and X
- activated partial thromboplastin time (APTT) – this predominantly measures the activity of factors II, V, VIII, IX, X, XI and XII
- thrombin time (TT) – this tests for deficiency or dysfunction of fibrinogen
- quantitative fibrinogen assay
- platelet count.

The results of these tests along with the clinical history will guide subsequent investigation. A reptilase time (so named because snake venom is used in the test) can also be very helpful; it assesses the same components as a TT but is unaffected by heparin and so is useful when heparin contamination from an indwelling line is suspected. Bleeding times are generally unhelpful in neonates and have been abandoned in most centres. Instead, platelet function is usually assessed by platelet aggregometry using a limited range of agonists and by a newly developed machine which measures

platelet-dependent clot formation in whole blood (the platelet function analyser PFA-100) (Israels et al. 2001).

Interpretation of coagulation screen results

Interpretation can often be difficult, particularly in preterm babies and in those who are sick, because the cause is usually multifactorial. Broadly there are two ways to approach this: firstly, by considering the causes for an abnormality in each individual test (Table 30.10), and, secondly, by considering the pattern of results expected in the most common, clinically important conditions. These are discussed in more detail in the sections on inherited and acquired disorders (pp. 774–778).

Inherited coagulation disorders

While inherited coagulation disorders are rare, some of the most severe disorders may present in the neonatal period with life-threatening bleeding in otherwise healthy babies. The commonest are the X-linked disorders factor VIII deficiency (haemophilia A), which has a frequency of 1 in 5000 male births, and factor IX deficiency (haemophilia B), which occurs in 1 in 30 000 male births (Kulkarni and Lusher 2001). It is important to note that one-third of cases have no family history of haemophilia as they are due to new mutations. The other inherited coagulation disorders which may present with bleeding in the neonatal period are the severe

Table 30.10 Causes of abnormal coagulation tests in the newborn

Prolonged APTT alone	Inherited deficiency of factor VIII, factor IX, factor XI, factor XII
Heparin (therapeutic or heparin contamination*)
Prolonged PT alone	Inherited deficiency of factor VII
Vitamin K deficiency (haemorrhagic disease of the newborn)
Warfarin
Prolonged TT alone	Low fibrinogen
Artefact: contamination with heparin from line or sample bottle*
Prolonged APTT + PT	Inherited deficiency of factor II, factor V, factor X
Liver disease
Prolonged APTT, PT and TT	Inherited deficiency of fibrinogen
Disseminated intravascular coagulation
Severe liver disease
Normal APTT, PT	Factor XIII deficiency and TT
Platelet defect: thrombocytopenia or rare platelet function abnormality (e.g. Bernard Soulier syndrome)

APTT, activated partial thromboplastin time; PT, prothrombin time; TT, thrombin time.
*The effect of heparin contamination can be distinguished by checking the reptilase time on a coagulation sample; where a prolonged TT and/or a prolonged APTT is due to heparin contamination, the reptilase time will be normal, but where a prolonged TT or APTT is due to a true coagulation defect, the reptilase time will be abnormal.

forms of von Willebrand disease (vWD; type 3 and occasionally type 2b), factor XIII deficiency and deficiencies of factors II, V, VII, X and XI, which are all autosomal recessive and relatively rare.

Haemophilia A: factor VIII deficiency

Clinical presentation

Although the majority of cases of haemophilia A present in the second year of life, a recent review of the literature found that 3.5–4% of all boys with haemophilia born in countries with a good standard of healthcare suffer from intracranial haemorrhage in the neonatal period (Kulkarni and Lusher 1999; Looney et al. 2007). As discussed above, the problem is probably due to a slow expansion of a small subdural haemorrhage associated with delivery and it is sensible to warn parents about the signs of intracranial haemorrhage if their baby is known to have haemophilia. Other, slightly less common sites of bleeding typical of neonatal haemophilia are subgaleal collections, bleeding postcircumcision and bleeding from venous or arterial puncture sites (Kulkarni and Lusher 1999, 2001). Prolonged bleeding from the umbilical cord is less common and haemarthroses are rare. Haemorrhage into major organs such as the liver, spleen or lungs is also uncommon but has been reported in up to 5% of cases (Kulkarni and Lusher 2001).

Diagnosis

The diagnosis of haemophilia A in the neonatal period should be straightforward on either a cord blood or peripheral blood sample. The characteristic finding is a prolonged or very prolonged APTT together with a normal PT, TT, platelets and fibrinogen. The diagnosis is then established by measurement of factor VIII clotting activity, which is always reduced in haemophilia A (all other coagulation factors, including von Willebrand antigen, are normal). Clinically, the severity of the disease is classified according to the level of factor VIII activity: levels of <2% (i.e. <0.02 IU/ml) are classified as severe disease, 2–10% (0.02–0.1 IU/ml) as moderate disease, and >10% (>0.1 IU/ml) as mild haemophilia. Where there is a family history of haemophilia A, the diagnosis may be established prenatally by a variety of methods; most families choose early diagnosis by mutational analysis of the factor VIII gene on a chorionic villus biopsy in the first trimester (Kadir 1999).

Neonatal management

Acute management of the bleeding neonate with haemophilia requires intravenous administration of recombinant factor VIII. If absolutely necessary, FFP or cryoprecipitate (15–20 ml/kg) may be used for major haemorrhage if there is significant delay. The usual treatment dose of factor VIII in neonates is 50–100 units/kg intravenously twice daily (Kulkarni and Lusher 2001; British Committee for Standards in Haematology, Haemostasis and Thrombosis Task Force 2002). Since the half-life of factor VIII is shorter in children than in adults, more frequent dosing or a continuous factor VIII infusion may be required. The dose should be adjusted by monitoring plasma factor VIII activity to achieve factor VIII levels of 100% (1.0 IU/ml) (Kulkarni and Lusher 2001; British Committee for Standards in Haematology, Haemostasis and Thrombosis Task Force 2002). This is done by measuring plasma factor VIII activity and close liaison with a specialist haematologist. For neonates with intracranial bleeding, treatment with factor VIII should continue for at least 2 weeks. Note that venepuncture should be performed with great care in all haemophiliac neonates and arterial punctures should be avoided. In addition, lumbar punctures should be avoided unless essential for clinical management, and, if necessary, should be done by an experienced person in the presence of factor VIII cover. Fibrin glue may be useful in circumcision-associated bleeds.

Once the baby is ready for discharge it is vital to provide specialist family support and follow-up through a haemophilia centre. In the UK, all children are registered with such a centre and have access to clinical nurse specialists and haematologists with expertise in haemophilia. The UK Haemophilia Centres Doctors' Organization also publishes regularly updated guidelines on the recommended products for treatment of patients with hereditary coagulation disorders (United Kingdom Haemophilia Centre Doctors' Organization 2008). The Haemophilia Society provides very useful practical support and advice for families with affected children.

Prenatal management and delivery

For patients diagnosed prenatally, the best mode of delivery is controversial and accurate data about the risks are very limited. It is clear that significant haemorrhage may occur whatever the mode of delivery; in particular, there is no evidence that elective caesarean section eliminates the risk of bleeding (Kulkarni and Lusher 2001). Vaginal delivery is regarded as safe provided there are no difficulties anticipated (Looney et al. 2007); however, vacuum extraction should be avoided because several studies have shown a high rate of subgaleal bleeds and cephalohaematomas in this situation (Towner et al. 1999; Kulkarni and Lusher 2001). In known or suspected haemophiliac newborns, cord blood should always be taken for a coagulation screen and factor VIII level to confirm the diagnosis. Oral vitamin K should be given at birth because the intramuscular route should be avoided in view of the risk of haematoma formation. The role of prophylactic factor VIII administration to haemophiliac newborns following difficult delivery to reduce the risk of intracranial bleeding is controversial (Buchanan 1999; Kulkarni and Lusher 2001; Looney et al. 2007; United Kingdom Haemophilia Centre Doctors' Organization 2008). The risk of intracranial haemorrhage at around the time of birth in baby boys with haemophilia is ∼4%; at least half have significant sequelae (Ljung 2007). Any intervention that could reduce this morbidity deserves consideration. Magnetic resonance imaging studies in normal babies have shown that small peritentorial subdural haematomas are common (Looney et al. 2007). In a haemophilic baby boy, the collection is likely to continue to expand over several days because the blood will not clot, and hence parents should be warned to return to the hospital if they have any concerns (such as poor feeding, abnormal movements). The main disadvantage of prophylactic factor VIII is that it may increase the risk of inhibitor formation, leading to major problems with treatment later in childhood. Recent consensus advice from the European Paediatric Network for Haemophilia Management and the International Network of Pediatric Hemophilia recommended routine cranial ultrasound of all newborns born to known or suspected haemophilia carriers soon after delivery and administration of factor VIII only to those with signs of intracranial haemorrhage, while recognising that ultraound will not detect all types of intracranial haemorrhages, particularly small peritentorial bleeds (Ljung 2007).

Haemophilia B: factor IX deficiency

Haemophilia B is clinically indistinguishable from haemophilia A. From the diagnostic point of view, both diseases cause an isolated prolonged APTT, but the diagnosis of factor IX deficiency is made by demonstrating a low factor IX level. Occasional diagnostic confusion may arise with mild factor IX deficiency, as factor IX levels also fall in liver disease and vitamin K deficiency. Although this is usually straightforward to resolve since there will be concomitant reductions in the other vitamin K-dependent factors in this situation, it is important to recheck factor IX levels at 6 weeks and 6 months of age if in doubt.

Management of factor IX deficiency is similar to that of factor VIII deficiency. Treatment of bleeding is with recombinant factor IX concentrate. The usual dose is 100 units/kg intravenously once daily, and treatment should be monitored to achieve a factor IX level of 80–100% (1.0 IU/ml) (Kulkarni and Lusher 2001; British Committee for Standards in Haematology, Haemostasis and Thrombosis Task Force 2002). As for haemophilia A, treatment for intracranial haemorrhage should be continued for at least 2 weeks (Kulkarni and Lusher 2001). Similarly, lumbar punctures should be avoided where possible and venepunctures kept to a minimum. Recommendations for prenatal management are as for haemophilia A.

von Willebrand disease in neonates

vWD is caused by quantitative or qualitative defects in vWF. It is the commonest inherited bleeding disorder, affecting around 1% of the population (Castaman et al. 2003). There are several types of vWD, each of which has different clinical and genetic characteristics, but only two forms of the disease present in the neonatal period. Type 2b vWD is autosomal dominant and presents with thrombocytopenia; bleeding is uncommon. Type 3 vWD is the most severe form of the disease (Ikenboom 2001). It is autosomal recessive and has a clinical phenotype similar to haemophilia, as levels of both vWF and factor VIII are low. The diagnosis is made by measuring vWF and factor VIII, and determining the pattern of vWF multimers; clinical clues are the presence of a haemophiliac pattern of bleeding in girls or families without X-linked inheritance and a poor response to factor VIII concentrates. Type 3 vWD is currently treated with intermediate-purity factor VIII (Haemate-P is the most commonly used product) (British Committee for Standards in Haematology, Haemostasis and Thrombosis Task Force 2002).

Factor XIII deficiency

Factor XIII deficiency is a rare autosomal recessive disorder in which the routine diagnostic coagulation screen is normal. It usually presents clinically with delayed bleeding from the umbilical cord during the first 3 weeks of life (Anwar and Miloszewski 1999; Anwar et al. 2002). Intracranial haemorrhage has been reported in up to 30% of neonates with homozygous factor XIII deficiency (British Committee for Standards in Haematology, Haemostasis and Thrombosis Task Force 2002). The diagnosis is made by measuring clot solubility in 5 M urea solution as a screening test, followed by a specific factor XIII assay; molecular tests for the common mutations are also available (Smith 1990). The treatment of bleeding associated with factor XIII deficiency is factor XIII concentrate; cryoprecipitate (10 ml/kg) can be used prior to establishment of the diagnosis or where the specific concentrate is unavailable. Infants with homozygous factor XIII deficiency have a lifelong risk of intracranial haemorrhage, and current guidelines recommend monthly factor XIII to reduce this risk (United Kingdom Haemophilia Centre Doctors' Organization 2008).

Other inherited coagulation factor deficiencies

A number of rare coagulation deficiencies may present in neonates with bleeding or unexplained prolongation of coagulation tests. The majority are autosomal recessive and so a history of parental consanguinity is relatively common. Factor VII deficiency can produce a very severe bleeding disorder with a high incidence of intracranial haemorrhage. In some cases, factor VII has been shown to cross the placenta and in this way delay haemorrhage in severe factor VII deficiency until after birth. Recombinant factor VIIa is now available to treat this disorder but must be given at frequent intervals as it has a very short half-life (Chuansumrit et al. 2002). Factor XI deficiency is most frequent in Ashkenazi Jews and presents in a similar way to haemophilia. There are a number of rare congenital fibrinogen disorders, including dysfibrinogenaemias and hypo/afibrinogenaemia. They may present with umbilical stump bleeding but other sites of haemorrhage are extremely unusual in neonates. It is important to note that one of the commonest inherited causes of an isolated prolonged APTT in a healthy baby with no signs of bleeding is factor XII deficiency; despite what is often a markedly prolonged APTT, affected individuals have no clinically apparent bleeding disorder throughout life! Guidelines on the selection and use of therapeutic products to treat all hereditary bleeding disorders are produced by the UK Haemophilia Centre Doctors' Organisation and are regularly updated (United Kingdom Haemophilia Centre Doctors' Organization 2008).

Acquired disorders of coagulation

Vitamin K deficiency

Levels of the active forms of the vitamin K-dependent procoagulant factors (factors II, VII, IX and X), and of the natural anticoagulants protein C and protein S, are physiologically low at birth. There are many reasons for this. Vitamin K is essential for γ-carboxylation of these proteins, which converts them to their active form: placental transfer of vitamin K is insufficient to build up adequate stores in the neonate (Zipursky 1999); breast milk has a low vitamin K content; and bacterial vitamin K synthesis is lacking in the sterile neonatal gut. In neonates, vitamin K deficiency can lead to haemorrhagic disease of the newborn, now more commonly referred to as vitamin K-deficiency bleeding (VKDB) and comprehensively reviewed in two recent articles (van Winkel et al. 2008; Shearer 2009). It can be classified into early, classical and late disease according to the timing or presentation and the clinical features.

Early VKDB

This presents in the first 24 hours of life, usually with severe haemorrhage, including gastrointestinal bleeding and intracranial haemorrhage. It is caused by severe vitamin K deficiency in utero, usually as a result of maternal medication that interferes with vitamin K, e.g. anticonvulsants (phenobarbital, phenytoin), antituberculous therapy and oral anticoagulants. Guidelines for prevention of early VKDB are discussed below.

Classical VKDB

This presents at 2–7 days old in babies who have not received prophylactic vitamin K at birth. The risk is increased in breastfed babies and in those with poor oral intake. The incidence in babies not receiving vitamin K supplementation has been estimated at 0.25–1.7%, depending on the study population (Tripp et al. 1995), although studies have shown that it may now be less common even in communities without routine prophylaxis (Hey 2003). Numerous studies have shown that classical VKDB is prevented by a single intramuscular dose of vitamin K at birth (reviewed in Puckett and Offringa 2000; van Winkel et al. 2008; Shearer 2009). Routine prophylactic vitamin K has been the subject of much controversy, which is briefly summarised below.

Late VKDB

This occurs after the first week of life, most often between 2 and 8 weeks after birth, although presentation after 15 weeks of age has been reported (Sutor et al. 1999). The characteristic presentation is of sudden intracranial haemorrhage in an otherwise well, breastfed term baby, or in babies with liver disease (e.g. biliary atresia; Ch. 29.2) or malabsorptive states. Late VKDB in healthy breastfed babies can be prevented either by a single intramuscular dose of vitamin K or by repeated oral doses of vitamin K over the first 6 weeks of life. However, babies with chronic liver disease or malabsorption are likely to require prolonged vitamin K supplementation.

In all forms of VKDB, clotting studies show a prolonged PT with normal platelets and fibrinogen; in severe deficiency, the APTT may also be prolonged. In the presence of a typical clinical history, further diagnostic tests are usually unnecessary and correction of the PT following vitamin K administration provides additional confirmation. If doubt remains, factor assays of the vitamin K-dependent factors and of the inactive form of factor II (decarboxyprothrombin: PIVKA II) can be used to confirm the diagnosis (British Committee for Standards in Haematology, Haemostasis and Thrombosis Task Force 2002). Treatment of VKDB depends on the severity of the bleeding. In mild cases, vitamin K (1 mg), which should be given intravenously or subcutaneously (not intramuscularly because of the risk of haematoma), should suffice, as this increases the levels of active vitamin K-dependent coagulation factors within a few hours; where there is significant bleeding, FFP may be given, in addition to vitamin K (British Committee for Standards in Haematology, Haemostasis and Thrombosis Task Force 2002).

Vitamin K prophylaxis

Guidelines for the prevention of early VKDB (i.e. due to maternal medication that interferes with vitamin K) are to give a single intramuscular injection of vitamin K at birth together with antenatal administration of oral vitamin K to the mother during the last 4 weeks of pregnancy (British Committee for Standards in Haematology, Haemostasis and Thrombosis Task Force 2002). For classical and late VKDB, there are several options. This is because, although vitamin K supplementation undoubtedly prevents classical and late VKDB, controversy surrounds the route of administration since the publication of studies by Golding et al. (1992), which suggested a link between intramuscular vitamin K at birth and later childhood malignancies. These studies have been criticised on methodological grounds (Brousson and Klein 1996), and at least nine further studies have since investigated this link (reviewed in Zipursky 1999; Puckett and Offringa 2000; Roman et al. 2002; van Winkel et al. 2008; Shearer 2009). Although seven studies failed to confirm the link with malignancy, two produced equivocal results, and the controversy is unlikely to be resolved unequivocally in the short term. There is no link between oral vitamin K and malignancy.

The current situation is perhaps best summarised by the Cochrane review (Puckett and Offringa 2000), which concludes:

- Intramuscular vitamin K has been proven to prevent classical disease.
- Oral vitamin K has been proven to improve biochemical parameters of vitamin K deficiency in the first week of life.
- The efficacy of oral supplementation in preventing late disease is unproven. This probably reflects the unpredictable absorption and difficulties with compliance with repeated doses of oral vitamin K.

Both the American Academy of Paediatrics and the Royal College of Paediatrics and Child Health recommend vitamin K supplementation at birth. In healthy babies, the choice of administration route is increasingly being left to parents, who have to balance the remote risk of a borderline increase in leukaemia (odds ratio between 1.06 (confidence interval (CI) 0.89–1.25) and 1.16 (CI 0.97–1.39)) against the slightly higher risk of VKDB (2.7/100 000) in infants given various different oral vitamin K regimens. The best oral administration regimen has not yet been identified and is reviewed by Shearer (2009). It is clear that one or two oral doses is not sufficient and available data suggest that regimens employing a once-weekly or daily dose of vitamin K for the first 3 months of life are likely to be more effective (for example 2 mg at birth, followed by 1 mg weekly for 3 months, as used in Denmark, or 1 mg at birth followed by 25 μg daily for 3 months, as used in the Netherlands) (Shearer 2009).

Disseminated intravascular coagulation

The main precipitants of DIC in neonates are associated with severe hypoxia and/or acidosis and include peripartum haemorrhage, severe birth asphyxia, meconium aspiration and sepsis. The pathophysiology of DIC is complex and not fully understood. The process seems to be triggered by release of TF and cytokines from damaged endothelium and/or monocytes, which results in widespread activation of the coagulation cascade with subsequent consumption of clotting factors and a combination of thrombotic and haemorrhagic manifestations (Bick 2002). Clinically, DIC is seen in sick neonates and presents with generalised bleeding, including pulmonary haemorrhage and oozing from venepuncture sites. The usual pattern of coagulation abnormalities in DIC is prolongation of the PT, APTT and TT, together with low platelets and fibrinogen. D-dimers are increased but measurement is not necessary for diagnostic purposes and is often not done in neonates because of the need for an extra blood sample (results should also be interpreted with caution, as D-dimers are not specific and can be found in healthy neonates with no evidence of coagulopathy) (Karpatkin 1999). The most important aspect of management of DIC is treatment of the underlying cause. Blood product replacement is indicated for the treatment of clinical bleeding: FFP is a good source of procoagulant proteins as well as protein C, protein S and antithrombin; cryoprecipitate contains higher concentrations of factor VIII and fibrinogen and is useful when the fibrinogen levels are low (British Committee for Standards in Haematology, Haemostasis and Thrombosis Task Force 2002). There are no recent randomised trials that address optimum management of bleeding associated with neonatal DIC. However, a pragmatic approach is to aim to maintain the platelet count above 30×10^9/l and the fibrinogen >1 g/l. There is increasing experience of successfuly using recombinant factor VIIa for neonates with bleeding unresponsive, or poorly responsive, to coagulation factor replacement with FFP and/or cryoprecipitate (reviewed and comprehensively referenced by Puetz et al. (2009)). Although there are some reports of an increased frequency of thrombotic events in neonates receiving factor VIIa, there is no evidence that this was directly due to factor VIIa administration rather than the underlying poor condition of the baby. The factor VIIa regimens used vary hugely; overall the most common dose used was 100 μg/kg every 2 hours (Puetz et al. 2009).

Other acquired coagulation disorders

Other causes of acquired coagulopathy in neonates include liver disease, metabolic disorders (e.g. hyperammonemia), extracorporeal membrane oxygenation and the consumptive coagulopathy with thrombocytopenia secondary to giant haemangioendotheliomas (Kasabach–Merritt syndrome) (Hall 2001).

Table 30.11 Causes of neonatal thrombocytopenia

Early (<72 hours)	Placental insufficiency (PET, IUGR, diabetes)
	NAITP
	Birth asphyxia
	Perinatal infection (group B *Streptococcus*, *Escherichia coli*, *Listeria*)
	Congenital infection (CMV, toxoplasmosis, rubella, coxsackie virus)
	Maternal autoimmune (ITP, SLE)
	Severe Rh HDN
	Thrombosis (renal vein, aortic)
	Aneuploidy (trisomy – 21, 18, 13)
Late (>72 hours)	Late-onset sepsis and necrotising enterocolitis
	Congenital infection (CMV, toxoplasmosis, rubella)
	Maternal autoimmune (ITP, SLE)
	Congenital/inherited (TAR, Wiskott–Aldrich)

PET, pre-eclamptic toxaemia; IUGR, intrauterine growth restriction; NAITP, neonatal alloimmune thrombocytopenia; CMV, cytomegalovirus; ITP, idiopathic thrombocytopenic purpura; SLE, systemic lupus erythematosus; Rh, rhesus; HDN, haemolytic disease of the newborn; TAR, thrombocytopenia with absent radii.

Neonatal thrombocytopenia

Prevalence of neonatal thrombocytopenia

Thrombocytopenia (platelets $<150 \times 10^9/l$) is common in neonates. Several studies report a prevalence of thrombocytopenia of 1–5% of all newborns, around 10% of whom will have severe thrombocytopenia (platelets $<50 \times 10^9/l$). In neonatal intensive care units, thrombocytopenia develops in 22–35% of all admissions and in up to 50% of neonates who are preterm and sick (Roberts and Murray 2001).

Causes of neonatal thrombocytopenia

Conventional lists of the causes of thrombocytopenia include a large number of possible diagnoses, most of which are very rare. However, in routine clinical practice, it is more useful to be aware of the common causes and patterns of thrombocytopenia. Thrombocytopenia usually presents in one of two clinical patterns which reflect the most common causes: early thrombocytopenia (within 72 hours of birth) and late thrombocytopenia (after 72 hours of life). The principal causes of early and late thrombocytopenia are shown in Table 30.11.

Early thrombocytopenia

The most frequent causes of early thrombocytopenia in preterm infants are conditions resulting in fetal hypoxia. This thrombocytopenia is self-limiting, usually resolving within 10 days (Murray and Roberts 1996; Watts and Roberts 1999). It is seen in infants of mothers with pre-eclampsia, pregnancy-induced hypertension or diabetes; this form of thrombocytopenia is also seen in infants with IUGR (Murray and Roberts 1996; Watts and Roberts 1999). Thrombocytopenia is seen in virtually all such infants, although it is rarely severe (the platelet count usually remains above $50 \times 10^9/l$), except in neonates with severe IUGR. It is caused by reduced platelet production secondary to reduced megakaryocytopoiesis (this is

discussed in more detail below). The most important cause of severe early neonatal thrombocytopenia is neonatal alloimmune thrombocytopenia (NAITP), which is also discussed below.

Late thrombocytopenia

The most common and clinically important causes of late thrombocytopenia are sepsis and NEC, which together account for >80% of cases (Roberts and Murray 2001; Murray et al. 2002). This form of thrombocytopenia usually develops very rapidly over 1–2 days, is often very severe (platelets $<30 \times 10^9/l$) and takes 1–2 weeks to recover (Murray et al. 2002). Such babies frequently require platelet transfusion (Murray et al. 2002; Stanworth et al. 2009). The mechanism is likely to be a combination of increased platelet consumption, often but not always with evidence of DIC, and reduced platelet production.

Thrombocytopenia secondary to intrauterine growth restriction and maternal hypertension/diabetes

Neonates with IUGR have a number of distinctive haematological abnormalities which are present at birth, including neonatal thrombocytopenia, neutropenia, increased erythropoiesis (high numbers of circulating nucleated red cells with or without associated polycythaemia) and evidence on the blood film of hyposplenism (spherocytes, target cells and Howell–Jolly bodies) (Watts and Roberts 1999). The underlying cause of the haematological abnormalities appears to be chronic fetal hypoxia since the same pattern of abnormalities occurs in several types of placental insufficiency, both maternal disorders, such as pre-eclampsia, hypertension and diabetes mellitus, and fetal disorders, manifest as 'idiopathic' IUGR. Erythropoietin levels are increased in affected fetuses and neonates (Salvesen et al. 1993; Watts and Roberts 1999). In addition, the severity of the haematological abnormalities correlates both with serum erythropoietin levels and with the severity of the placental dysfunction (Salvesen et al. 1993). We and others have shown that megakaryocytopoiesis is severely impaired at birth in such neonates, as shown by a marked reduction in circulating megakaryocytes and their precursor and progenitor cells, and that this is likely to be the principal reason for the neonatal thrombocytopenia since there is no evidence of increased platelet destruction/consumption (Murray and Roberts 1996; Watts and Roberts 1999; Watts et al. 1999).

Immune neonatal thrombocytopenias

Neonatal alloimmune thrombocytopenia

This is the platelet equivalent of HDN and alloimmune neutropenia. NAITP affects around 1:1000 pregnancies (Bussel 2009). In addition to the summary below, there are several useful recent reviews to which the reader is referred for more detail about the diagnosis and treatment of this condition (Murphy and Bussel 2007; Roberts et al. 2008; Bussel 2009). NAITP is frequently severe and occurs in the first pregnancy in almost 50% of cases. Thrombocytopenia may present in the first few days of life or prenatally (as early as 20 weeks' gestation), in which case it is sometimes referred to as fetal alloimmune thrombocytopenia. The thrombocytopenia results from transplacental passage of maternal platelet-specific antibodies to human platelet antigens (HPAs), which the mother lacks but which the fetus inherits from the father. In 80% of cases these are anti-HPA-1a antibodies and in 10–15% anti-HPA-5b; the remaining cases are due to an increasing number of rare antibodies identified in specialised centres (Murphy and Bussel 2007; Bussel 2009). It is now clear that the ability of an HPA-1a-negative woman to form anti-HPA-1a is controlled by the HLA

DRB3*0101 allele such that HLA DRB3*0101-positive women are 140 times more likely to make anti-HPA-1a than those who are HLA DRB3*0101-negative (Murphy and Bussel 2007).

The main clinical problem in NAITP is intracranial haemorrhage; this occurs in 10% of cases, with long-term neurodevelopmental sequelae in 20% of survivors (Bussel and Kaplan 1998). Affected neonates may present with seizures or other signs of intracranial haemorrhage, with petechiae or bruising, or with an incidental thrombocytopenia. The platelet count is usually $<30 \times 10^9/l$. The diagnosis of NAITP is made by demonstrating platelet antigen incompatibility between mother and baby (in 80% of cases of NAITP, the mother is HPA-1a-negative and the baby is HPA-1a-positive). This can usually be done within 1–2 days either serologically or by PCR, and is carried out in reference transfusion laboratories (Murphy and Bussel 2007). In addition, most mothers have detectable anti-HPA antibodies. The recommended management for neonates with NAITP is to transfuse 'severely affected' babies with HPA-compatible platelets (usually available 'off the shelf' from transfusion centres) (Murphy and Bussel 2007); in an emergency random donor platelets may be used to raise the platelet count whilst HPA-compatible platelets are awaited. The definition of 'severely affected' varies in different studies but should be taken to include both asymptomatic neonates with severe thrombocytopenia (platelets $<30 \times 10^9/l$) and babies with evidence of haemorrhage despite less severe thrombocytopenia. If there is ongoing severe thrombocytopenia and/or haemorrhage despite HPA-compatible platelets, intravenous IgG (total dose 2 g/kg over 2–5 days) is often useful in ameliorating the thrombocytopenia until spontaneous recovery occurs 1–6 weeks after birth (Murphy and Bussel 2007). Prenatal management of NAITP has been controversial (see Ch. 9) (reviewed in Bussel and Kaplan 1998; Jolly et al. 2002; Murphy and Bussel 2007; Roberts et al. 2008). In recent years, the majority of centres recommend a non-invasive approach relying on maternal intravenous IgG therapy, reserving fetal transfusion with HPA-compatible platelets for selected pregnancies where the past maternal history predicts for a very high risk of fetal intracranial haemorrhage, especially where the father is known to be homozygous for the HPA against which maternal antibodies are directed (usually HPA-1a) (Jolly et al. 2002; Murphy and Bussel 2007; Roberts et al. 2008; Bussel 2009).

Neonatal autoimmune thrombocytopenia

This is secondary to transplacental passage of maternal platelet autoantibodies in maternal idiopathic thrombocytopenic purpura and, less often, systemic lupus erythematosus, which affects 1–5 in 10 000 pregnancies (Kelton 2002). Around 10% of infants of affected mothers develop thrombocytopenia. However, the thrombocytopenia is usually mild and intracranial haemorrhage occurs in <1% of at-risk babies. In affected babies with severe thrombocytopenia, treatment with intravenous IgG is usually effective (Gill and Kelton 2000).

Management of neonatal thrombocytopenia

Management of immune thrombocytopenias is described above. For other forms of neonatal thrombocytopenia, therapy depends upon the appropriate use of platelet transfusion. Evidence-based guidelines for neonatal platelet transfusion therapy are yet to be defined, although consensus guidelines are available (British Committee for Standards in Haematology, Transfusion Task Force; Roberts and Murray 2001; Roberts et al. 2008). Most recommend platelet transfusion for sick neonates where the platelet count is $<50 \times 10^9/l$; however, for stable, relatively well preterm and term

infants, platelet counts of $30–50 \times 10^9/l$ are not associated with an increased risk of haemorrhage (Murray et al. 2002; Stanworth et al. 2009); this approach conforms to the current UK guidelines (British Committee for Standards in Haematology, Haemostasis and Thrombosis Task Force 2002). The usual volume of platelets administered is 10–20 ml/kg, with no robust data yet available to show whether higher doses are either safer or more effective.

Neonatal thrombosis: physiology and developmental aspects

Physiological plasma concentrations of many of the inhibitors of coagulation are reduced in neonates. This, together with the frequent need for indwelling vascular catheters, is the main explanation for the increased risk of thrombosis in neonates (2.4 per 1000 hospital admissions) compared with in older infants and children. Of the direct inhibitors of thrombin, concentrations of antithrombin and heparin cofactor II are both decreased at birth while those of α_2-macroglobulin are increased and may partially compensate. In the protein C/S pathway, plasma concentrations of protein C are low at birth; total protein S levels are also low, but overall protein S activity is normal, as it exists mainly in its free active form owing to the virtual absence of its binding protein (C4b-BP) in neonates (Andrew 1997). Less is known about the third inhibitor pathway in neonates, TFPI, although neonates have slightly reduced TFPI levels in cord plasma compared with adult values. There are also several age-related differences in the neonatal fibrinolytic system. Levels of plasminogen at birth are only 50% of adult values; since even homozygous plasminogen deficiency is not associated with thrombosis, the main clinical significance of this is that there is a reduced ability to generate plasmin in response to fibrinolytic agents. In contrast, the plasma levels of t-PA and its inhibitor (plasminogen activator inhibitor-1) are high, the clinical significance of which is unclear (Andrew 1997).

Diagnostic approach to neonatal thrombosis: use of screening tests

The identification of an increasing number of risk factors for thrombosis in adults has led to increasing confusion about which of these factors are relevant to neonates and which neonates should be screened for congenital thrombophilia. Guidelines from the Haemostasis and Thrombosis Task Force of the BCSH (British Committee for Standards in Haematology, Haemostasis and Thrombosis Task Force 2002) state that congenital thrombophilia should be considered and screened for in the following situations:

- any child with clinically significant thrombosis, including spontaneous thrombotic events, unanticipated or extensive venous thrombosis, ischaemic skin lesions or purpura fulminans
- a positive family history of neonatal purpura fulminans.

In fact, the only inherited deficiencies for which there is a proven causative role in neonatal thrombosis are homozygous/double heterozygote deficiencies in protein C and protein S which cause purpura fulminans (see below). For other types of thrombosis, such as perinatal stroke, in which the cause is almost certainly multifactorial, the contribution to the thrombotic process made by less severe thrombophilic defects (e.g. factor V Leiden or a mutation in the promoter of the prothrombin gene, prothrombin[20210A]) is difficult to assess (reviewed by Grabowski et al. 2007; Mackay and Monagle 2008). While uncertainty remains, it is probably reasonable to carry out the tests listed below. An important proviso is that all the data from such investigations should, where possible, be entered into national and/or international registries of paediatric thrombosis so that the role of inherited abnormalities can be determined (Schmidt and Andrew 1995).

The screening tests that should be performed in all suspected cases of thrombophilia are:

- protein C activity
- protein S
- antithrombin
- factor V Leiden
- prothrombin[20210A].

These tests are all carried out on freshly collected anticoagulated blood samples (usually using the same type of sample bottle as employed for coagulation screen).

In addition, babies with thrombosis who are born to mothers with systemic lupus erythematosus and/or antiphospholipid syndrome should be tested for lupus anticoagulant, since antiphospholipid antibodies may cross the placenta and are a rare cause of neonatal thrombosis in such babies (Nowak-Gottl et al. 2001). Tests for factor V Leiden and prothrombin[20210A] are carried out on DNA extracted from white blood cells in the coagulation sample (see above). Associations between neonatal thrombosis and increased serum lipoprotein a and the methylene tetrahydrofolate reductase (MTHFR) genotype C677T have also been reported (Heller et al. 2000). However, the relevance of serum lipoprotein a and the MTHFR genotype to neonatal management remains unclear as there is no evidence that awareness of these laboratory abnormalities can be used to improve management (Grabowski et al. 2007; Mackay and Monagle 2008). Therefore they are not currently listed as recommended screening tests for neonatal thrombophilia by the BCSH (British Committee for Standards in Haematology, Haemostasis and Thrombosis Task Force 2002). On the other hand, where these tests are performed, it is logical to include such data, together with clinical details, in one of the national or international thrombosis registries, in order to understand their relevance in the future (Schmidt and Andrew 1995).

Inherited thrombotic disorders

Protein C deficiency

Babies who are homozygous or double heterozygotes for protein C deficiency have no normal protein C genes and as a result have undetectable or very low levels of plasma protein C. The condition is rare, occurring in 1 in 160 000 to 1 in 360 000 births (Marlar et al. 1989). Affected babies usually present within hours or days of birth with neonatal purpura fulminans in which there is DIC together with rapidly progressive, life-threatening, haemorrhagic necrosis due to dermal vessel thrombosis. Typically the lesions start as small ecchymoses, often in the extremities, buttocks or scalp and sometimes at sites of venepunctures. Neonates may also present with cerebral or renal vein thrombosis or with ophthalmic thrombosis, as suggested by vitreous and/or retinal haemorrhages and unreactive pupils.

The diagnosis of protein C deficiency is made by the characteristic clinical picture in conjunction with DIC and undetectable levels of protein C (<0.01 units/ml) in the patient, together with heterozygote levels in the parents (British Committee for Standards in Haematology, Haemostasis and Thrombosis Task Force 2002; Kottke-Marchant and Comp 2002). Molecular analysis can be used to confirm the diagnosis retrospectively and for prenatal diagnosis in future pregnancies (Millar et al. 2000). Patients who are heterozygous for protein C deficiency, and so have one normal protein C

gene, rarely present as neonates unless there are additional prothrombotic factors; these individuals have low protein C levels which may overlap with the lower limit of normal in the first few months of life, delaying diagnosis until after the age of 6 months and sometimes until later in childhood. The treatment of neonatal purpura fulminans due to protein C deficiency is protein C concentrate starting at a dose of 40 units/kg and aiming to maintain a plasma level of >0.25 units/ml, which may require frequent dosing in the initial stages when DIC is ongoing (British Committee for Standards in Haematology, Haemostasis and Thrombosis Task Force 2002; Monagle et al. 2008). FFP should be used until protein C concentrate is available, if any delay is likely. Heparin and antiplatelet agents are ineffective. In the long term, lifelong protein C replacement and/or anticoagulation are necessary (British Committee for Standards in Haematology, Haemostasis and Thrombosis Task Force 2002; Monagle et al. 2008).

Protein S deficiency

Homozygous or double heterozygosity for protein S deficiency is even rarer than protein C deficiency. It presents with features identical to those of protein C deficiency and the diagnosis is established by demonstrating undetectable levels of protein S (0.01 units/ml). Treatment is with FFP (10–20 ml/kg) to maintain a plasma protein S level of >0.25 units/ml (British Committee for Standards in Haematology, Haemostasis and Thrombosis Task Force 2002). As for protein C deficiency, lifelong replacement therapy and/or anticoagulation is necessary.

Antithrombin deficiency

Homozygous antithrombin deficiency is extremely rare and is only seen where the mutation involves the heparin-binding site. It usually presents later in childhood but neonatal thrombosis has been reported, including deep venous thrombosis and inferior vena caval thrombosis (Heller et al. 2000; Kuhle et al. 2001). Heterozygous antithrombin deficiency is more common (1 in 2000 to 1 in 5000 births); it usually presents in the second decade of life but neonatal presentation with venous and arterial thrombosis has been reported, including aortic thrombosis, myocardial infarction and cerebral dural sinus thrombosis. Neonatal purpura fulminans is not a feature. The diagnosis of both homozygous and heterozygous disease is made by measuring plasma antithrombin levels, although confirmation in heterozygotes may be delayed until 3–6 months of age because of the overlap with normal levels. The treatment of neonatal thrombosis due to antithrombin deficiency is replacement therapy with antithrombin concentrate together with heparin (British Committee for Standards in Haematology, Haemostasis and Thrombosis Task Force 2002).

Other inherited thrombotic disorders

The more recently discovered prothrombotic mutations such as factor V Leiden and the prothrombin 20210A promoter mutation (prothrombin[20210A]) (Heller et al. 2000; Nowak-Gottl et al. 2001) have not yet been reported to cause neonatal thrombotic problems in isolation. Even in adults, heterozygosity for factor V Leiden or prothrombin[20210A] only increases the thrombotic risk by fourfold and twofold, respectively. Thus, these prothrombotic genotypes may play a role in the presence of other acquired risk factors, but since the majority of individuals with these mutations do not suffer thrombotic events even during adulthood, there is so far no evidence that management of neonates found to be harbouring these mutations should be any different from that of neonates without the mutations (Mackay and Monagle 2008; Nowak-Gottl et al. 2008).

Acquired thrombotic problems

The most commonly identified risk factors for thrombosis are the presence of an intravascular catheter and shock in association with sepsis, hypoxaemia or hypovolaemia. The main sites, apart from catheters, of neonatal thrombosis are in the renal veins and, less commonly, in the aorta, aortic arch or cerebral vessels (Schmidt and Andrew 1995; Heller et al. 2000). Excellent guidelines for antithrombotic therapy in neonatal thrombosis are published regularly by the American College of Chest Physicians (Monagle et al. 2008).

Catheter-related thrombosis

This is the commonest cause of neonatal thrombosis; it is responsible for >80% of venous thrombosis and >90% of arterial thrombosis (Schmidt and Andrew 1995; British Committee for Standards in Haematology, Haemostasis and Thrombosis Task Force 2002). Symptomatic thrombosis occurs in 1% of neonates with indwelling vascular catheters, although postmortem studies suggest that asymptomatic thrombosis occurs in association with up to 20–30% of catheters. Arterial thrombosis can lead to peripheral gangrene or renal artery thrombosis with hypertension and heart failure (Ch. 44). Venous thrombosis can cause portal hypertension, varices and/or renal vein thrombosis with renal dysfunction (Ch. 44). The diagnosis of catheter-related thrombosis is usually made by Doppler ultrasound (Roy et al. 1997; Monagle et al. 2008) but this is notoriously unreliable, and may miss thrombosis in the aorta, right atrium or inferior vena cava, as well as in the upper limb. 'Linograms' (putting radiopaque dye into the line) may also miss extensive thrombosis. For this reason, contrast angiography has been identified as the 'gold standard' for confirmation of thrombotic vessel occlusion (Monagle et al. 2008).

The treatment of catheter-related thrombosis depends on the severity and extent of thrombosis. The first step is prompt removal of the umbilical venous catheter or umbilical arterial catheter where possible (Alkalay et al. 1993; Monagle et al. 2008). If, despite catheter removal, there is extension of thrombosis, anticoagulation with unfractionated heparin or low-molecular-weight heparin (LMWH) is recommended for 6–12 weeks (Table 30.12) (Monagle et al. 2008). Thrombolysis is not recommended unless there is major vessel occlusion causing critical organ or limb compromise; if thrombolysis is necessary, recombinant tissue plasminogen activator (tPA) is recommended (Monagle et al. 2008). However, thrombolytic therapy should be used judiciously in neonates because of the risk of life-threatening bleeding, including intracranial haemorrhage, and this risk may be higher in preterm infants (Lee-Potter et al. 1975; Leaker et al. 1996; Hartmann et al. 2001; Mercuri et al. 2001). The recommended dose for tPA is 0.1–0.6 mg/kg/h given over 6 hours, followed immediately by administration of heparin, omitting the loading dose (Monagle et al. 2008). It is often recommended to give FFP, as a source of plasminogen, immediately prior to tPA administration (Monagle et al. 2008). In any neonates treated with thrombolytic therapy, it is important to monitor the fibrinogen level (which should be maintained >1 g/l) as well as the APTT, PT and TT and the platelet count (which should be maintained >50 × 10^9/l). There is also no evidence that heparin prevents catheter-related thrombosis, although prophylactic low-dose heparin (heparin concentration 0.25–1 U/ml) has been shown to prolong umbilical artery catheter patency and is recommended (Monagle et al. 2008).

Non-catheter-related thrombosis

The commonest non-catheter-related thrombosis is renal vein thrombosis, which presents in the neonatal period in nearly 80% of cases and may even develop in utero. Renal vein thrombosis is usually unilateral (75% of cases) and presents with a flank mass, haematuria, proteinuria, thrombocytopenia and reduced function of the involved kidney (Heller et al. 2000). The most commonly identified risk factors which predispose to renal vein thrombosis are sepsis, maternal diabetes, polycythaemia, dehydration and prothrombotic mutations (therefore all such babies should have a thrombophilia screen performed). Management of renal vein thrombosis is controversial, as there are so few data. The most recent American College of Chest Physicians guidelines recommend, where there is unilateral renal vein thrombosis without renal impairment or inferior vena caval extension, either supportive care with monitoring for extension or therapeutic anticoagulation with unfractionated heparin or LMWH for 3 months; anticoagulation is suggested for all cases with inferior vena caval extension (Monagle et al. 2008). Thrombolysis with tPA followed by anticoagulation with unfractionated heparin or LMWH is indicated for more extensive thrombosis, where there is evidence of organ or limb dysfunction, e.g. bilateral renal vein thrombosis with renal failure (see Table 30.12 for suggested regimens) (Andrew and de Veber 1997; British Committee for Standards in Haematology, Haemostasis and Thrombosis Task Force 2002). It is essential to monitor LMWH therapy very carefully in neonates with renal impairment; in this situation unfractionated heparin may be preferable.

Neonatal stroke

Neonatal stroke occurs in about 1 in 4000 births (Ch. 40.3). An increased prevalence of thrombophilia in affected neonates, particularly factor V Leiden, is increasingly recognised and it is now considered that hypoxia–ischaemia is not the cause of neonatal stroke (Mercuri et al. 2001). However, it is important to note that all the evidence to date suggests that the aetiology of neonatal stroke is multifactorial and for the majority of thrombophilic mutations, including factor V Leiden, prothrombin[20210A] and the MTHFR genotype C677T, the presence of these genetic abnormalities alone has not been shown to be the direct cause of the stroke. For example, in the largest series reported, only 5 of the 24 children with neonatal stroke were factor V Leiden heterozygotes and in none of these children was there a family history of stroke (Mercuri et al. 2001). Genetic counselling requires great care and it is important that parents are informed both that the risk of stroke recurrence after neonatal stroke is very low (~2%) and that there is no evidence that stroke is more likely in siblings of a child with neonatal stroke when the only family risk factor identified on thrombophilic screening is factor V Leiden, prothrombin[20210A] or MTHFR C677T (Mackay and Monagle 2008). Thus, while it is likely that thrombophilia plays a role in neonatal stroke, additional risk factors may also be required and our current state of knowledge about the interactions between these factors does not suggest that siblings or future siblings should be screened for factor V Leiden, prothrombin[20210A] or MTHFR C677T.

Transfusion of blood and blood products in the newborn

Introduction

Although sick neonates are one of the most heavily transfused groups of patients in modern medicine, neonatal transfusion

Table 30.12 Heparin schedules for neonates

DRUG	ENOXAPARIN	
Low-molecular-weight heparin (LMWH)		
Dose	1.5 mg/kg/dose twice daily	
Monitoring	Measure anti-factor Xa level Therapeutic level is 0.5–1.0 U/ml anti-factor Xa Check anti-factor Xa 4–6 hours after first dose If in therapeutic range, check once weekly If dose adjusted (see below), recheck 4 hours after adjusted dose If <0.35 units/ml, increase by 25% If 0.35–0.49 units/ml, increase by 10% If 1.1–2 units/ml, decrease by 20–30% If >2 U/ml, withhold until anti-factor Xa is <0.5 U/ml; restart at 40% of original dose	
Unfractionated heparin		
	DOSE (U/kg/h)	**CHECK APTT OR FACTOR Xa LEVEL**
Loading dose	75	After 4 hours
Maintenance	28	Daily or 4 hours after dose change
Maintain anti-factor Xa level at 0.35–0.7 U/ml or adjust APTT as below:		
APTT <50 seconds	Increase by 20%	After 4 hours
APTT 50–59 seconds	Increase by 10%	After 4 hours
APTT 60–85 seconds	No change	24 hours
APTT 86–120 seconds	Decrease by 10%	After 4 hours
APTT >120 seconds	Stop for 1 hour then decrease by 15%	After 4 hours

Modified from Andrew and de Veber (1997).
APTT, activated partial thromboplastin time.

remains opinion based rather than evidence based and there is a wide diversity of opinion and practice between different clinicians and institutions (Calhoun et al. 2002; Bell 2008; Strauss 2008). As blood products convey a risk of transmitting potentially serious infections and are increasingly costly, it is clearly important to define evidence-based and/or standardised protocols for blood product use in neonatal medicine.

Red cell transfusion

Aims of red cell transfusion

The principal aims of red cell transfusion in the newborn are to ensure adequate tissue oxygenation, particularly during intensive care, and to treat significant symptomatic anaemia. Indeed, given that cardiopulmonary function during intensive care will be optimised, the only way to increase tissue oxygenation is red cell transfusion. Unfortunately there are relatively few data about using measures of tissue oxygenation to determine either the need for, or the effects of, red cell transfusion in neonates.

Near-infrared spectroscopy can be used to measure peripheral fractional oxygen extraction (FOE) and thereby estimate oxygen delivery to the tissues (Wardle et al. 2002). In a study of 74 neonates of birthweight <1500 g, half of the babies were transfused on the basis only of a high peripheral FOE (>0.47) (suggesting inadequate tissue oxygen delivery) while the remaining babies were transfused according to haemoglobin concentration. Neonates in the FOE group had lower median haemoglobin concentrations during the study, an increased time to first transfusion and no increase in major complications. Capillary whole-blood lactate concentration has also been used as an indicator of tissue oxygenation (in stable neonates, peripheral blood lactate decreases after red cell transfusions for 'symptomatic' anaemia) (Frey and Losa 2001). However, during intensive care, lactate levels are of little use in deciding the need for red cell transfusion, since capillary lactate levels are highly variable because they reflect tissue perfusion rather than haemoglobin-limited oxygen-unloading capacity to the tissues (Frey and Losa 2001). Overall, there is insufficient evidence that either FOE or lactate is a practical or superior substitute for haemoglobin/haematocrit as triggers for neonatal red cell transfusion.

Changing patterns of red cell transfusion in neonates

Numerous reports over the last 10–15 years show a trend towards increasingly restrictive use of red cell transfusions, even in the most preterm neonates (Hume 1997; Bell 2008; Strauss 2008; Von Kohorn and Ehrenkranz 2009). These changes have occurred without any significant increase in the need for respiratory support or oxygen therapy and without any increase in the incidence of IVH, NEC, sepsis or poor weight gain. These studies are well summarised in a number of reviews (Hume 1997; Franz and Pohlandt 2001; Bell 2008; Bishara and Ohls 2009). Despite two randomised clinical trials of restrictive versus liberal transfusion criteria (the Iowa trial and the Premature Infants in Need of Transfusion (PINT) trial: Kirpalani et al. 2006; Bell 2008), there is still too little evidence to show that a restrictive policy is superior to more liberal transfusion triggers. Both the Iowa and the PINT studies found that even restrictive transfusion guidelines did not reduce the number of donor exposures from red cell transfusion. In addition, the Iowa study, but not the PINT study, reported a higher frequency of major adverse outcomes, including the frequency of apnoeas, the frequency of major abnormalities on cranial ultrasound and the composite outcome or brain injury or death (Bell 2008).

Guidelines for transfusion of red cells in neonates

The BCSH provides comprehensive guidelines for transfusion of fetuses, neonates and older children and these are available through their website (British Committee for Standards in Haematology, Transfusion Task Force 2004). Their recommendations about the products and indications for red cell transfusion in neonates are briefly summarised here (for a full discussion of recommendations for blood components for use in the newborn, see British Committee for Standards in Haematology, Haemostasis and Thrombosis Task Force 2002).

Products for red cell transfusion in neonates

- Components for transfusion in utero or to children under 1 year of age must be prepared from donors who have given at least one donation within the previous 2 years which was negative for all mandatory microbiological markers.
- Dedicating aliquots from a single donation (multisatellite packs) to allow sequential transfusions from the same donor for neonates who are likely to be repeatedly transfused is considered good practice.
- All cellular components should be leukocyte-depleted at the point of manufacture (to reduce the risk of transmission of infectious agents); this has been mandatory for all cellular components in the UK since 2001.
- Components transfused in the first year of life should be CMV-seronegative.
- Irradiation of red cells prior to transfusion is necessary in several situations (for detail, see British Committee for Standards in Haematology, Transfusion Task Force 2004), including 'top-up' or exchange transfusion of neonates who have received an intrauterine transfusion, where a neonate has proven or suspected cellular immune deficiency and where the donated red cells are from a first- or second-degree relative.
- Blood group: samples from both the neonate and mother should be grouped to determine the ABO and rhesus group and screened for atypical red cell alloantibodies; small-volume 'top-up' transfusions can be given repeatedly over the first 4 months of life without further serological testing of the neonate provided that there are no atypical

red cell antibodies in the neonate's or mother's serum and the baby's DAT is negative (infants rarely produce atypical red cell antibodies unless they receive repeated large volume transfusions) (British Committee for Standards in Haematology, Transfusion Task Force 2004).

Volume of red cell transfusion in preterm neonates

The few studies available suggest that large volume (20 ml/kg) red cell transfusions not only lead to larger rises in haemoglobin and fewer overall transfusions than small volume transfusions (10 ml/kg), but are also well tolerated in the majority of preterm neonates (Paul et al. 2002).

Indications for red blood cell transfusion in preterm neonates

A number of groups have proposed RBC transfusion guidelines in preterm neonates, mostly in the setting of trials of erythropoietin to ameliorate neonatal anaemia (Maier et al. 1994; Bishara and Ohls 2009). These guidelines are based on combinations of ventilation requirements, oxygen requirements and haemoglobin/packed cell volume levels. However, as improvements in both antenatal and neonatal care have led to a reduced incidence and severity of acute lung disease, the recommendations of these guidelines are being increasingly superseded by a similar but more conservative approach (Table 30.13). What is clear, however, is that adherence to strict neonatal transfusion guidelines (in whatever form) reduces both the number of transfusions and donor exposure (Alagappan et al. 1998).

Whilst adverse transfusion reactions are rare in neonates, it should always be remembered that transfusion of all blood products is associated with finite risks and that serious adverse reactions do occasionally occur (Williamson et al. 2000).

Red blood cell T-antigen activation

The potential for transfusion-associated haemolysis in infants with T-activated RBCs has led to some centres screening infants and providing low-titre anti-T blood components. However, one study has shown that many 'T-activated' neonates are in fact expressing T-antigen variants (Th and Tx) and Tk antigen (Boralessa et al. 2002). This study also found no evidence of haemolysis in either T- or T-variant-activated neonates receiving standard blood components. The practice of providing low-titre anti-T blood components for neonates with sepsis or NEC cannot therefore be supported on current evidence.

Platelet transfusion

Studies of platelet transfusion to treat and prevent haemorrhage in neonates

Numerous studies suggest that neonatal thrombocytopenia is a risk factor for haemorrhage (particularly IVH), mortality and adverse neurodevelopmental outcome (reviewed in Roberts et al. 2008). However, whether these outcomes can be reduced by treating affected neonates with platelet transfusion is difficult to assess since there have been no neonatal trials which demonstrate reduced haemorrhage or improved outcome in neonates with non-immune-mediated thrombocytopenia treated with platelet transfusions. In the only randomised controlled trial in preterm neonates, Andrew et al. (1993) found no reduction in haemorrhage in neonates randomised to receive transfusions to maintain their platelet counts in the normal range ($>150 \times 10^9$/l) compared with control neonates

Table 30.13 Guidelines for red cell transfusion for preterm neonates

ASSISTED VENTILATION				CPAP		BREATHING SPONTANEOUSLY	
<28 days		>28 days		<28 days	>28 days	FiO$_2$ > 0.2 l	Well in air
FiO$_2$ > 0.3 l	FiO$_2$ < 0.3 l						
Hb < 12 g/dl or	Hb < 11 g/dl or	Hb < 10 g/dl or		Hb < 10 g/dl or	Hb < 8 g/dl or	Hb < 8 g/dl or	Hb < 7 g/dl or
PCV < 0.40	PCV < 0.35	PCV < 0.30		PCV < 0.30	PCV < 0.25	PCV < 0.25	PCV < 0.20

RBC transfusion may be considered at higher thresholds than the above for neonates with:
- hypovolaemia (unresponsive to crystalloid infusion)
- septic shock
- necrotising enterocolitis
- undergoing/recovering from major surgery.

CPAP, continuous positive airway pressure; Hb, haemoglobin; PCV, packed cell volume.

with moderate thrombocytopenia (platelets 50–150 × 10^9/l) who were not transfused.

Retrospective studies of neonatal platelet transfusion practice in the UK, USA and Mexico show not only that platelet transfusion remains a common procedure, occurring in 2–9.4% of all admissions, but that the majority of platelet transfusions are given prophylactically to non-bleeding neonates, suggesting that platelet transfusions are given to a large number of neonates who are unlikely to benefit (Sola et al. 2000; Garcia et al. 2001; Murray et al. 2002; Stanworth et al. 2009). Furthermore, these studies also show that thrombocytopenic neonates who receive platelets are up to 10 times more likely to die than neonates who do not receive platelet transfusion, although the high mortality was attributed to complications other than major haemorrhage. A recent prospective study also found that the majority of platelet transfusions were given to neonates with no bleeding or minor bleeding only and, importantly, showed that >90% of babies with severe thrombocytopenia (platelets <20 × 10^9/L) had no evidence of major haemorrhage (Stanworth et al. 2009).

Platelet transfusion guidelines

Until data from controlled trials become available, a number of countries have published consensus guidelines to help decide the indications for platelet transfusion in term and preterm neonates (Norfolk et al. 1998; British Committee for Standards in Haematology, Transfusion Task Force 2004). Our recent study (Stanworth et al. 2009) has led us to modify these guidelines to fit the clinical problems we face within our unit (summarised in Table 30.14) and take into account what is already known about the incidence and natural history of haemorrhage in the newborn. Most neonates who bleed (particularly those with GMH-IVH) do so in the first days of life. However, with the exception of perinatal asphyxia, the conditions precipitating the majority of episodes of severe thrombocytopenia (e.g. late-onset sepsis and NEC) usually develop after the first few days of life and are rarely accompanied by major haemorrhage. This suggests that prophylactic platelet transfusions are not required for such patients until the platelet count falls to between 20 and 30 × 10^9/l (see Table 30.14). However, we recommend a higher trigger level (<50 × 10^9/l) for platelet transfusion for patients with the greatest risk of haemorrhage, especially extremely-low-birthweight neonates (<1000 g) in the first week of life and neonates

with significant clinical instability, e.g. fluctuating ventilation requirements or blood pressure (see Table 30.14). Platelet transfusions in neonates with platelet counts greater than 50 × 10^9/l should be reserved for patients with active bleeding, since there is no evidence that higher platelet counts are of any benefit to non-bleeding neonates.

Platelet transfusion: the products to use

Platelets for transfusion to neonates should be both ABO- and RhD-compatible since the plasma in the transfused product will contain anti-A and/or anti-B depending on the blood group and this may be sufficient amounts to cause haemolysis (British Committee for Standards in Haematology, Haemostasis and Thrombosis Task Force 2002). All blood products in the UK are leukocyte-depleted and are therefore highly unlikely to transmit CMV; however, current guidelines recommend that platelets for transfusion to infants less than 12 months of age should be from CMV-seronegative donors (British Committee for Standards in Haematology, Transfusion Task Force 2004). There are no randomised studies evaluating the volume of platelets which should be administered; in our practice we have found that a transfusion volume of 20 ml/kg is well tolerated, even in very-low-birthweight babies, and produces both a higher increment in platelet count and a more sustained increase than a transfusion volume of 10 ml/kg.

Granulocytes

A number of small trials (summarised by Vamvakas and Pineda 1996) have suggested that granulocyte transfusion may convey benefit during neonatal sepsis. However, the practical difficulties of obtaining a sufficient dose of fresh granulocytes at the time of sepsis means that granulocyte transfusion has not entered routine practice in the UK for the treatment of neonatal sepsis.

Fresh frozen plasma and cryoprecipitate

Although FFP is widely used for a variety of indications in neonates, including prevention of IVH, volume replacement, as a source of 'opsonising factors' during sepsis and to 'support' haemostasis in neonates with thrombocytopenia, there is little or no evidence to

Table 30.14 Guidelines for platelet transfusion for neonates

PLATELET COUNT (×10⁹/l)	NON-BLEEDING NEONATE	BLEEDING NEONATE	NAITP (PROVEN OR SUSPECTED)
<30	Consider transfusion in all patients	Transfuse	Transfuse (with HPA-compatible platelets)
30–49	Do not transfuse if clinically stable Consider transfusion if: • <1000 g and <1 week of age • clinically unstable (e.g. fluctuating BP) • previous major bleeding • complication (e.g. GMH-IVH) • current minor bleeding (e.g. petechiae, puncture site oozing) • concurrent coagulopathy • requires surgery or exchange transfusion • platelet count falling and likely to fall below 30	Transfuse	Transfuse (with HPA-compatible platelets)
50–99	Do not transfuse	Transfuse	Transfuse (with HPA-compatible platelets if major bleeding present)
>99	Do not transfuse	Do not transfuse	Do not transfuse

NAITP, neonatal alloimmune thrombocytopenia; HPA, human platelet antigen; BP, blood pressure; GMH-IVH, germinal matrix haemorrhage/intraventricular haemorrhage.

support its use in any of these situations (Muntean 2002). The only indications for FFP in neonates recommended in the recent BCSH guidelines and supported by evidence are: DIC, vitamin K-dependent bleeding and inherited deficiencies of coagulation factors (British Committee for Standards in Haematology, Haemostasis and Thrombosis Task Force 2002; Muntean 2002). The large study conducted by the Northern Neonatal Network clearly shows that prophylactic FFP administered to preterm neonates at birth does not prevent IVH or improve outcome at 2 years of life (Northern Neonatal Nursing Initiative Trial Group 1996). Similarly, FFP is not superior to other colloid or crystalloid solutions as a volume replacement solution in standard neonatal practice (Niermeyer et al. 2000) and there is no evidence to support its use to 'correct' the results of abnormal coagulation screens (British Committee for Standards in Haematology, Haemostasis and Thrombosis Task Force 2002).

Fresh frozen plasma: the product to use

The current BCSH guidelines state that FFP for transfusion to neonates should be group AB (since this contains neither anti-A nor anti-B) or the same ABO blood group as the neonate. In the UK, Department of Health recommendations state that single-unit methylene blue-treated FFP (MB-FFP) should be used for neonates, as the 'standard' FFP carries a small risk of virus transmission (apart from CMV) and the residual levels of methylene blue have not been shown to be harmful in neonates (British Committee for Standards in Haematology, Transfusion Task Force 2004). The alternative to MB-FFP, solvent detergent FFP (SD-FFP), is made from pooled plasma of several hundred donations and, though shown to be generally safe in children in small studies, has been associated with transmission of parvovirus B19 (British Committee for Standards in Haematology, Transfusion Task Force 2004). The dose of FFP is 10–20 ml/kg, with the larger dose given if possible in order to limit donor exposure where repeated dosing is likely.

Cryoprecipitate

Cryoprecipitate contains a higher concentration of fibrinogen and factor VIII per unit volume than FFP. It is useful in treating DIC associated with hypofibrinogenaemia, inherited afibrinogenaemia or hypofibrinogenaemia and factor VIII deficiency (haemophilia A) if factor VIII concentrate is not immediately available.

Human albumin solution

The use of human albumin solution (HAS) has been reported to be associated with excess mortality in adults receiving intensive care. While data about the risks of HAS in neonates are not available, there are studies which clearly show that HAS is not superior to other colloid or crystalloid solutions for volume replacement in neonates (Wong et al. 1997). In addition, there is no evidence from randomised trials that HAS is of any benefit in hypoalbuminaemic neonates with clinically significant peripheral oedema (Greenough et al. 1993). Together these data suggest that there is no good indication for the use of HAS in standard neonatal practice.

Exchange transfusion

As severe rhesus HDN decreases in frequency, exchange transfusion is also becoming an increasingly rare procedure in neonatal medicine. Therefore, to ensure a high standard of practice, all neonatal units must adopt and maintain written practice guidelines for this procedure, as outlined in the BCSH guidelines (British Committee for Standards in Haematology, Transfusion Task Force 2004).

Indications for exchange transfusion

Established indications for exchange transfusion of neonates are severe anaemia, particularly in the presence of heart failure, and/or hyperbilirubinaemia (British Committee for Standards in Haematology, Haemostasis and Thrombosis Task Force 2002). Controversial indications for exchange transfusion, for which there is insufficient evidence, include metabolic disease, septicaemia and DIC (British Committee for Standards in Haematology, Haemostasis and Thrombosis Task Force 2002).

Principles of exchange transfusion and the product to transfuse

The current BCSH guidelines state that blood for exchange transfusion should be group O, RhD-identical with the neonate, Kell-negative and <5 days old (British Committee for Standards in Haematology, Transfusion Task Force 2004). They also state that the blood should be CMV-negative, although universal leukocyte depletion of red cells in the UK means that CMV-untested blood is likely to be of equivalent safety to CMV-negative blood even in the newborn. To prevent TA-GVHD, the blood should be irradiated if the baby has received intrauterine transfusion (British Committee for Standards in Haematology, Haemostasis and Thrombosis Task Force 2002); otherwise, irradiation of blood for exchange is recommended, but is not essential, and should only be requested where irradiation will not lead to a significant delay (the risks of severe hyperbilirubinaemia are greater than the remote risk of TA-GVHD) (British Committee for Standards in Haematology, Transfusion Task Force 2004).

There is no consensus about whether whole blood or plasma-reduced red cells should be used for exchange transfusion in neonates; however, the current BCSH guidelines state that plasma-reduced red cells with a haematocrit of 0.50–0.60 should be suitable for both hyperbilirubinaemia and severe anaemia and this product is available from the National Blood Service in the UK (British Committee for Standards in Haematology, Transfusion Task Force 2004). It is important to note that packed red cells as supplied for 'top-up' transfusion may have a haematocrit of up to 0.75, leading to an unacceptably high postexchange haematocrit, and, if used, will require dilution with colloid or saline. By contrast, whole blood, with a haematocrit of 0.35–0.45, may result in a postexchange haemoglobin of <12 g/dl in a severely anaemic baby and thus increase the need for subsequent 'top-up' transfusion (whole blood is no longer widely available) (British Committee for Standards in Haematology, Transfusion Task Force 2004). The pH of a unit of plasma-reduced red cells (and of whole blood) is around 7.0, which does not contribute to acidosis in the infant. Blood for exchange transfusion should be warmed to 37°C immediately prior to transfusion.

Dilutional exchange transfusion for polycythaemia

Dilutional exchange transfusion is undertaken to reduce whole-blood viscosity in neonates with polycythaemia. There is no evidence to support the use of FFP or albumin for this procedure (Wong et al. 1997), both of which carry the risk of transfusion-transmitted infection. In the assessment of such neonates it should always be remembered that umbilical venous catheterisation and dilutional exchange are not without complications. When considered clinically appropriate, a one-third whole-blood volume exchange (20–30 ml/kg) is usually performed.

Weblinks

www.bcshguidelines: transfusion guidelines.
www.diamondblackfan.org.uk: information for families with Diamond–Blackfan anaemia.
www.haemophilia.org.uk: information for families and professionals.
www.rcog.org.uk/vitamin-supplementation-in-pregnancy: vitamin K guidance.

www.sct.screening.nhs.uk: information about the UK national programme for neonatal screening for haemoglobinopathies (sickle-cell disease and thalassaemia).
www.sicklecellsociety.org: information for families with sickle-cell disease.

www.ukts.org: information for families with thalassaemia and their health professionals.
www.vasapraevia.co.uk: information for families and professionals.

References

Alagappan, A., Shattuck, K.E., Malloy, M.H., 1998. Impact of transfusion guidelines on neonatal transfusions. J Perinatol 18, 92–97.

Albert T.S.E., Meng, G., Simms, P., et al., 2000. Thrombopoietin in the thrombocytopenic term and preterm newborn. Pediatrics 105, 1286–1291.

Alcock, G.S., Liley, H., 2002. Immunoglobulin infusion for isoimmune haemolytic jaundice in neonates (Cochrane Review). Cochrane Database Syst Rev (3), CD003313.

Alkalay, A.L., Mazkereth, R., Santulli, T., et al., 1993. Central venous line thrombosis in premature infants: a case management and literature review. Am J Perinatol 10, 323–326.

Andrew, M., 1997. The relevance of developmental haemostasis to haemorrhagic disorders of newborns. Semin Perinatol 21, 70–85.

Andrew, M., de Veber, G., 1997. Paediatric Thromboembolism and Stroke Protocols. B C Decker, Hamilton, Ontario.

Andrew, M., Paes, B., Milner, R., et al., 1987. Development of the coagulation system in the full term infant. Blood 70, 165–172.

Andrew, M., Paes, B., Johnston, M., et al., 1988. Development of the human coagulation system in the healthy premature infant. Blood 72, 1651–1657.

Andrew, M., Vegh, P., Caco, V.C., et al., 1993. A randomized, controlled trial of platelet transfusions in thrombocytopenic premature infants. J Pediatr 123, 285–291.

Anwar, R., Miloszewski, K.J.A., 1999. Factor XIII deficiency. Br J Haematol 107, 468–484.

Anwar, R., Minford, A., Gallivan, L., et al., 2002. Delayed umbilical bleeding – a presenting feature for factor XIII deficiency: clinical features, genetics, and management. Pediatrics 109, E32143.

Aprikyan, A.A., Carlsson, G., Stein, S., et al., 2004. Neutrophil elastase mutations in severe congenital neutropenia patients of the original Kostmann family. Blood 103, 389.

Bajwa, R.P., Skinner, R., Windebank, K.P., et al., 2001. Chemotherapy and marrow transplantation for congenital leukaemia. Arch Dis Child Fetal Neonatal Ed 84, F47–F48.

Ball, S.E., McGuckin, C.P., Jenkins, G., et al., 1996. Diamond–Blackfan anaemia in the UK: analysis of 80 cases from a 20-year birth cohort. Br J Haematol 94, 645–653.

Bard, H., 1975. The postnatal decline in HbF synthesis in normal full-time infants. J Clin Invest 55, 395–398.

Bechensteen, A.G., Haga, P., Halvorsen, S., et al., 1993. Erythropoietin, protein, and iron supplementation and the prevention of the anaemia of prematurity. Arch Dis Child 69, 19–23.

Bell, E.F., 2008. When to transfuse preterm babies. Arch Dis Child 93, F469–F473.

Bick, R.L., 2002. Disseminated intravascular coagulation: a review of etiology, pathophysiology, diagnosis, and management: guidelines for care. Clin Appl Thromb Hemost 8, 1–31.

Bishara, N., Ohls, R.K., 2009. Current controversies in the management of the anemia of prematurity. Semin Perinatol 33, 29–34.

Bolton-Maggs, P.H., Stevens, R.F., Dodd, N.J., et al., 2004. Guidelines for the diagnosis and management of hereditary spherocytosis. Br J Haematol 126, 455–474.

Boralessa, H., Modi, N., Cockburn, H., et al., 2002. RBC T activation and hemolysis in a neonatal intensive care population: implications for transfusion practice. Transfusion 42, 1428–1434.

Bouma, B.N., Marx, P.F., Mosnier, L.O., et al., 2001. Thrombin-activatable fibrinolysis inhibitor (TAFI, plasma procarboxypeptidase B, procarboxypeptidase R, procarboxypeptidase U). Thromb Res 101, 329–354.

Bowden, J.B., Hebert, A.A., Rapini, R.P., 1989. Dermal hematopoiesis in neonates: report of five cases. J Am Acad Dermatol 20, 1104–1110.

Bracci, R., Martini, G., Buonocore, G., et al., 1988. Changes in erythrocyte properties during the first hours of life: electron spin resonance of reacting sulfhydryl groups. Pediatr Res 24, 391–395.

Bresters, D., Reus, A.C., Veerman, A.J., et al., 2002. Congenital leukaemia: the Dutch experience and review of the literature. Br J Haematol 117, 513–524.

British Committee for Standards in Haematology, Haemostasis and Thrombosis Task Force, 2002. The investigation and management of neonatal haemostasis and thrombosis. Br J Haematol 119, 295–309.

British Committee for Standards in Haematology, Transfusion Task Force, 2004. Transfusion guidelines for neonates and older children. Br J Haematol 124, 433–453.

Brousson, M.A., Klein, M.C., 1996. Controversies surrounding the administration of vitamin K to newborns: a review. CMAJ 154, 307–315.

Brown, K., 2000. Haematological consequences of parvovirus B19 infection. Baillieres Best Pract Res Clin Haematol 13, 245–259.

Brown, H.L., Abernathy, M.P., 1998. Cytomegalovirus infection. Semin Perinatol 22, 260–266.

Brown, M.S., Phibbs, R.H., Garcia, J.F., et al., 1983. Postnatal changes in erythropoietin levels in untransfused premature infants. J Pediatr 103, 612–617.

Buchanan, G.R., 1999. Factor concentrate prophylaxis for neonates with hemophilia. J Pediatr Hematol Oncol 21, 254–256.

Bussel, J.B., 2009. Diagnosis and management of the fetus and neonate with alloimmune thrombocytopenia. J Thromb Haemost 7 (Suppl 1), 253–257.

Bussel, J., Kaplan, C., 1998. The fetal and neonatal consequences of maternal alloimmune thrombocytopenia. Baillieres Clin Haematol 11, 391–408.

Calhoun, D.A., Christensen, R.D., Edstrom, C.S., et al., 2002. Consistent approaches to procedures and practices in neonatal hematology. Clin Perinatol 27, 733–753.

Campagnoli, C., Fisk, N., Overton, T., et al., 2000. Circulating hematopoietic progenitor cells in first trimester fetal blood. Blood 95, 1967–1972.

Carr, R., Modi, N., Doré, C., 2003. G-CSF and GM-CSF for treating or preventing neonatal infections. Cochrane Database Syst Rev (3), CD003066.

Casadevall, N., Nataf, J., Viron, B., et al., 2002. Pure red-cell aplasia and antierythropoietin antibodies in patients treated with recombinant erythropoietin. N Engl J Med 346, 469–475.

Castaman, G., Federici, A.B., Rodeghiero, F., et al., 2003. von Willebrand's disease in the year 2003: towards the complete identification of gene defects for correct diagnosis and treatment. Haematologica 88, 94–108.

Chik, K.W., Shing, M.M., Li, C.K., et al., 1998. Treatment of hemoglobin Bart's hydrops with bone marrow transplantation. J Pediatr 132, 1039–1042.

Christensen, R.D., Calhoun, D.A., Rimsza, L.M., 2000. A practical approach to evaluating and treating neutropenia in the neonatal intensive care unit. Clin Perinatol 27, 577–601.

Chuansumrit, A., Nuntnarumit, P., Okascharoen, C., et al., 2002. The use of recombinant activated factor VII to control bleeding in a preterm infant undergoing exploratory laparotomy. Pediatrics 110, 169–171.

Dame, C., Fahnenstich, H., Freitag, P., et al., 1998. Erythropoietin mRNA expression in human fetal and neonatal tissue. Blood 92, 3218–3225.

Dame, C., Albers, N., Hasan, C., et al., 1999. Homozygous alpha-thalassaemia and hypospadias – common aetiology or incidental association? Long-term survival of Hb Bart's hydrops syndrome leads to new aspects for counselling of alpha-thalassaemic traits. Eur J Pediatr 158, 217–220.

Davies, S.C., Cronin, E., Gill, M., et al., 2000. Screening for sickle cell disease and thalassaemia: a systematic review with supplementary research. Health Technol Assess 4, iii–v, 1–99.

Davis, D.J., 2000. Neonatal subgaleal hemorrhage: diagnosis and management. CMAJ 164, 1452–1453.

de Alarcon, P.A., Graeve, J.L., 1996. Analysis of megakaryocyte ploidy in fetal bone marrow biopsies using a new adaptation of the feulgen technique to measure DNA content and estimate megakaryocyte ploidy from biopsy specimens. Pediatr Res 39, 166–170.

Delaunay, J., 2002. Molecular basis of red cell membrane disorders. Acta Haematol 108, 210–218.

Dgany, O., Avidan, N., Delaunay, J., et al., 2002. Congenital dyserythropoietic anemia type I is caused by mutations in codanin-1. Am J Hum Genet 71, 1467–1474.

Donalto, H., Vain, N., Rendo, P., et al., 2000. Effect of early versus late administration of human recombinant erythropoietin on transfusion requirements in premature infants: results of a randomized, placebo-controlled, multicenter trial. Pediatrics 105, 1066–1072.

Edstrom, C.S., Calhoun, D.A., Christensen, R.D., 2000. Expression of tissue factor pathway inhibitor in human fetal and placental tissues. Early Hum Dev 59, 77–84.

Fisch, P., Handgretinger, R., Schaefer, H., 2000. Pure red cell aplasia. Br J Haematol 111, 1010–1022.

Forestier, F., Daffos, F., Galacteros, F., 1986. Hematological values of 163 normal fetuses between 18 and 30 weeks of gestation. Pediatr Res 20, 342–346.

Franz, A.R., Pohlandt, F., 2001. Red blood cell transfusions in very and extremely low birthweight infants under restrictive transfusion guidelines: is exogenous erythropoietin necessary? Arch Dis Child Fetal Neonatal Ed 84, F96–F100.

Frey, B., Losa, M., 2001. The value of capillary whole blood lactate for blood transfusion requirements in anaemia of prematurity. Intensive Care Med 27, 222–227.

Fuller, N.J., Bates, C.J., Cole, T.J., et al., 1992. Plasma folate levels in preterm infants, with and without a 1 mg daily folate supplement. Eur J Pediatr 151, 48–50.

Garcia, M.G., Duenas, E., Sola, M.C., et al., 2001. Epidemiologic and outcome studies of patients who received platelet transfusions in the neonatal intensive care unit. J Perinatol 21, 415–420.

Garcia, M.G., Hutson, A.D., Christensen, R.D., 2002. Effect of recombinant erythropoietin on 'late' transfusions in the neonatal intensive care unit: a meta analysis. J Perinatol 22, 108–111.

Giacoia, G.P., 1997. Severe fetomaternal hemorrhage: a review. Obstet Gynecol Surv 52, 372–380.

Giampietro, G.F., Adler-Brecher, B., Verlander, P.C., et al., 1993. The need for more accurate and timely diagnosis in Fanconi anemia: a report from the International Fanconi Anemia Registry. Pediatrics 91, 1116–1120.

Gill, K.K., Kelton, J.G., 2000. Management of idiopathic thrombocytopenic purpura in pregnancy. Semin Hematol 37, 275–289.

Gilsanz, F., Vega, M.A., Gomez-Castillo, E., et al., 1993. Fetal anaemia due to pyruvate kinase deficiency. Arch Dis Child 69, 523–524.

Golding, J., Greenwood, R., Birmingham, K., et al., 1992. Childhood cancer, intramuscular vitamin K, and pethidine given during labour. BMJ 305, 341–346.

Gottstein, R., Cooke, R.W.I., 2003. Systematic review of intravenous immunoglobulin in haemolytic disease of the newborn. Arch Dis Child Fetal Neonatal Ed 88, F6–F10.

Grabowski, E.F., Buonanno, F.S., Krishnamoorthy, K., 2007. Prothrombotic risk factors in the prevention and management of perinatal stroke. Semin Perinatol 31, 243–249.

Grant, S.R., Kilby, M.D., Meer, L., et al., 2000. The outcome of pregnancy in Kell alloimmunisation. Br J Obstet Gynaecol 107, 481–485.

Greenough, A., Emery, E., Hird, M.F., et al., 1993. Randomised controlled trial of albumin infusion in ill preterm infants. Eur J Pediatr 152, 157–159.

Griffin, I.J., Cooke, R.J., Reid, M.M., et al., 1999. Iron nutritional status in preterm infants fed formulas fortified by iron. Arch Dis Child Fetal Neonatal Ed 81, F45–F49.

Haiden, N., Klebermass, K., Cardona, F., et al., 2006. A randomized, controlled trial of the effects of adding vitamin B12 and folate to erythropoietin for the treatment of anemia of prematurity. Pediatrics 118, 180–188.

Hakanson, D.O., Oh, W., 1977. Necrotizing enterocolitis and hyperviscosity in the newborn infant. J Pediatr 90, 458–461.

Hall, G.W., 2001. Kasabach–Merritt syndrome: pathogenesis and management. Br J Haematol 112, 851–862.

Halvorsen, S., Bechensteen, A.G., 2002. Physiology of erythropoietin during mammalian development. Acta Paediatr Suppl 91, 17–26.

Hann, I.M., 1991. The normal blood picture in neonates. In: Hann, I.M., Gibson, B.E.S., Letsky, E.A. (Eds.), Fetal and Neonatal Haematology. Baillière Tindall, London.

Hartmann, J., Hussein, A., Trowitzscha, E., et al., 2001. Treatment of neonatal thrombus formation with recombinant tissue plasminogen activator: six years experience and review of the literature.

Arch Dis Child Fetal Neonatal Ed 85, F18–F22.

Heegaard, E.D., Brown, K.E., 2002. Human parvovirus B19. Clin Microbiol Rev 15, 485–505.

Hegyi, E., Nakazawa, M., Debili, N., et al., 1991. Developmental changes in human megakaryocyte ploidy. Exp Hematol 19, 87–94.

Heller, C., Schobess, R., Kurnik, K., et al., 2000. Abdominal venous thrombosis in neonates and infants: role of prothrombotic risk factors – a multicentre case-control study. For the Childhood Thrombophilia Study Group. Br J Haematol 111, 534–539.

Herschel, M., Karrison, T., Wen, M., et al., 2002. Isoimmunization is unlikely to be the cause of hemolysis in ABO-incompatible but direct antiglobulin test-negative neonates. Pediatrics 110, 127–130.

Hey, E., 2003. Vitamin K – what, why, and when. Arch Dis Child Fetal Neonatal Ed 88, F80–F83.

Higgs, D.R., 1993. Alpha-thalassaemia. Baillieres Clin Haematol 6, 117–150.

Hitzler, J.K., Cheung, J., Li, Y., Scherer, G.W., et al., 2003. GATA1 mutations in transient leukemia and acute megakaryoblastic leukemia of Down syndrome. Blood 101, 4301–4304.

Horan, M., Stutchfield, P.R., 2001. Severe congenital myotonic dystrophy and severe anaemia of prematurity in an infant of Jehovah's Witness parents. Dev Med Child Neurol 43, 346–349.

Howard, H., Martlew, V., McFadyen, I., et al., 1998. Consequences for fetus and neonate of maternal red cell alloimmunisation. Arch Dis Child Fetal Neonatal Ed 78, F62–F66.

Howarth, D.J., Robinson, F.M., Williams, M., et al., 2002. A modified Kleihauer technique for the quantitation of foetomaternal haemorrhage. Transfusion Med 12, 373–378.

Hume, H., 1997. Red blood cell transfusions for preterm infants: the role of evidence-based medicine. Semin Perinatol 21, 8–19.

Hutton, R.A., Laffan, M.A., Tuddenham, E.G.D., 1999. Normal haemostasis. In: Hoffbrand, A.V., Lewis, S.M., Tuddenham, E.G.D. (Eds.), Postgraduate Haematology, fourth ed. Butterworth-Heinemann, London, pp. 550–580.

Huyhn, A., Dommergues, M., Izac, B., et al., 1995. Characterization of hematopoietic progenitors from human yolk sacs and embryos. Blood 86, 4474–4485.

Ikenboom, J.C., 2001. Congenital von Willebrand disease type 3: clinical manifestations, pathophysiology and molecular biology. Baillieres Best Pract Res Clin Haematol 14, 365–379.

Israels, S.J., Cheang, T., McMillan-Ward, E.M., et al., 2001. Evaluation of primary

hemostasis in neonates with a new in vitro platelet function analyzer. J Pediatr 138, 116–119.

Jolly, M.C., Letsky, E.A., Fisk, N.M., 2002. The management of fetal alloimmune thrombocytopenia. Prenat Diagn 22, 96–98.

Jordan, J.A., 1996. Identification of human parvovirus B19 infection in non-immune hydrops fetalis. Am J Obstet Gynecol 174, 37–42.

Kadir, R.A., 1999. Women and inherited bleeding disorders: pregnancy. Semin Hematol 36, 28–35.

Kaplan, M., 2001. Genetic interactions in the pathogenesis of neonatal hyperbilirubinemia: Gilbert's syndrome and glucose-6-phosphate dehydrogenase deficiency. J Perinatol 21 (suppl. 1), S35–S39.

Kaplan, M., Hammerman, C., 2002. Glucose-6-phosphate dehydrogenase deficiency: a potential source of severe neonatal hyperbilirubinaemia and kernicterus. Semin Neonatol 7, 121–128.

Karnon, J., Zeuner, D., Ades, A.E., et al., 2000. The effects of neonatal screening for sickle cell disorders on lifetime treatment costs and early deaths avoided: a modelling approach. J Public Health Med 22, 500–511.

Karpatkin, M., 1999. Coagulation problems in the newborn. Semin Neonatol 4, 1–7.

Kelton, J.G., 2002. Idiopathic thrombocytopenic purpura complicating pregnancy. Blood Rev 16, 43–46.

King, M.J., Telfer, P., MacKinnon, H., et al., 2008. Using the eosin-5-maleimide binding test in the differential diagnosis of hereditary spherocytosis and hereditary pyropoikilocytosis. Cytometry B Clin Cytom 74, 244–250.

Kirpalani, H., Whyte, R.K., Andersen, C., et al., 2006. The Premature Infants in Need of Transfusion (PINT) study: a randomized, controlled trial of a restrictive (low) versus liberal (high) transfusion threshold for extremely low birth weight infants. J Pediatr 149, 301–307.

Klein, C., Grudzien, M., Appaswamy, G., et al., 2007. HAX1 deficiency causes autosomal recessive severe congenital neutropenia (Kostmann disease). Nat Genet 39, 86–92.

Koenig, J.M., Christensen, R.D., 1989. Incidence, neutrophil kinetics, and natural history of neonatal neutropenia associated with maternal hypertension. N Engl J Med 321, 557–562.

Kottke-Marchant, K., Comp, P., 2002. Laboratory issues in diagnosing abnormalities of protein C, thrombomodulin, and endothelial cell protein C receptor. Arch Pathol Lab Med 126, 1337–1348.

Kuhle, S., Lane, D.A., Jochmanns, K., et al., 2001. Homozygous antithrombin deficiency type II (99 Leu to Phe mutation) and childhood thromboembolism. Thromb Haemost 86, 1007–1011.

Kulkarni, R., Lusher, J.M., 1999. Intracranial and extracranial hemorrhages in newborns with hemophilia: a review of the literature. J Pediatr Hematol Oncol 21, 289–295.

Kulkarni, R., Lusher, J., 2001. Perinatal management of newborns with haemophilia. Br J Haematol 112, 264–274.

Lallemand, A.V., Doco-Fenzy, M., Gaillard, D.A., 1999. Investigation of nonimmune hydrops fetalis: multidisciplinary studies are necessary for diagnosis – review of 94 cases. Pediatr Dev Pathol 2, 432–439.

Leaker, M., Massicotte, M.P., Brooker, L.A., Andrew, M., 1996. Thrombolytic therapy in pediatric patients: a comprehensive review of the literature. Thromb Haemost 76, 132–134.

Lee-Potter, J.P., Deacon-Smith, R.A., Simpkiss, M.J., et al., 1975. A new cause of hemolytic anemia in the newborn. J Clin Pathol 28, 317–320.

Lin, J.C., Strauss, R.G., Kulhavy, J.C., et al., 2000. Phlebotomy overdraw in the neonatal intensive care nursery. Pediatrics 106, E19.

Linderkamp, O., Nelle, M., Kraus, M., Zilow, E.P., 1992. The effect of early and late cord clamping on blood viscosity and other hemorheological parameters in full-term infants. Acta Paediatr 81, 745–750.

Lipton, J.M., Ellis, S.R.. 2010. Diamond Blackfan anemia 2008–2009. Broadening the scope of ribosome biogenesis disorders. Curr Opin Pediatr 22, 12–19.

Ljung, R.C.R., 2007. Intracranial haemorrhage in haemophilia A and B. Br J Haematol 140, 378–384.

Looney, C.B., Smith, J.K., Merck, L.H., et al., 2007. Intracranial hemorrhage in asymptomatic neonates: prevalence on MR images and relationship to obstetric and neonatal risk factors. Radiology 242, 535–541.

Luzzatto, L., 1993. Glucose-6-phosphate dehydrogenase deficiency. In: Nathan, A., Oski, F.A. (Eds.), Hematology of Infancy and Childhood, fourth ed. WB Saunders, Philadelphia, pp. 674–695.

Mackay, M.T., Monagle, P., 2008. Perinatal and childhood stroke and thrombophilia. Pathology 40, 116–123.

Maheshwari, A., Christensen, R.D., Calhoun, D.A., 2002. Immune neutropenia in the neonate. Adv Pediatr 49, 317–339.

Maier, R.F., Obladen, M., Scigalla, P., et al., 1994. The effect of epoetin beta (recombinant human erythropoietin) on the need for transfusion in very-low-birth-weight infants. European Multicentre Erythropoietin Study Group. N Engl J Med 330, 1173–1178.

Maier, R.F., Obladen, M., Muller-Hansen, I., et al., 2002. Early treatment with erythropoietin beta ameliorates anemia and reduces transfusion requirements in infants with birth weights below 1000 g. J Pediatr 141, 8–15.

Marlar, R.A., Montgomery, R.R., Broekmans, A.W., 1989. Diagnosis and treatment of homozygous protein C deficiency. Report of the Working Party on Homozygous Protein C Deficiency. International Committee of Haemostasis and Thrombosis. J Pediatr 114, 528–534.

Marshall, C.J., Thrasher, A.J., 2001. The embryonic origins of human haematopoiesis. Br J Haematol 112, 838–850.

Matoth, Y., Zaizov, R., Varsano, I., 1971. Postnatal changes in some red cell parameters. Acta Paediatr Scand 60, 317–320.

Mattsson, E., Herwald, H., Bjorck, L., Egesten, A., 2002. Peptidoglycan from Staphylococcus aureus induces tissue factor expression and procoagulant activity in human monocytes. Infect Immun 70, 3033–3039.

Mercuri, E., Cowan, F., Gupte, G., et al., 2001. Prothrombotic disorders and abnormal neurodevelopmental outcome in infants with neonatal cerebral infarction. Pediatrics 107, 1400–1404.

Meyer, M.P., Sharma, E., Carsons, M., 2003. Recombinant erythropoietin and blood transfusion in selected preterm infants. Arch Dis Child Fetal Neonatal Ed 88, F41–F45.

Millar, D.S., Johansen, B., Berntorp, E., et al., 2000. Molecular genetic analysis of severe protein C deficiency. Hum Genet 106, 646–653.

Miller, E., Miller, C.K., Cohen, B.J., et al., 1998. Immediate and long-term outcome of human parvovirus B19 infection in pregnancy. Br J Obstet Gynaecol 105, 174–178.

Monagle, P., Chalmers, E., Chan, A., et al., 2008. Antithrombotic therapy in neonates and children. American College Of Chest Physicians Evidence-Based Clinical Practice Guidelines (8th Edition). Chest 133, 887S–968S.

Muntean, W., 2002. Fresh frozen plasma in the pediatric age group and in congenital coagulation factor deficiency. Thromb Res 107 (suppl. 1), S29.

Murphy, M.F., Bussel, J.B., 2007. Advances in the management of alloimmune thrombocytopenia. Br J Haematol 136, 366–378.

Murray, N.A., Roberts, I.A.G., 1996. Circulating megakaryocytes and their progenitors in neonatal thrombocytopenia. Pediatr Res 40, 1–8.

Murray, N.A., Howarth, L.J., Mcloy, M., et al., 2002. Platelet transfusion in the management of severe thrombocytopenia

in neonatal intensive care unit (NICU) patients. Transfusion Med 12, 35–41.

Niermeyer, S., Kattwinkel, J., Van Reempts, P., et al., 2000. International Guidelines for Neonatal Resuscitation: an excerpt from the Guidelines 2000. for Cardiopulmonary Resuscitation and Emergency Cardiovascular Care: International Consensus on Science. Contributors and Reviewers for the Neonatal Resuscitation Guidelines. Pediatrics 106, E29.

Norfolk, D., Ancliffe, P.J., Contreras, M., et al., 1998. Consensus Conference on Platelet Transfusion, Royal College of Physicians of Edinburgh, 27–28 November 1997. Synopsis of background papers. Br J Haematol 101, 609–617.

Northern Neonatal Nursing Initiative Trial Group, 1996. Randomised trial of prophylactic early fresh-frozen plasma or gelatin or glucose in preterm babies: outcome at 2 years. Lancet 348, 229–232.

Nowak-Gottl, U., Kosch, A., Schlegel, N., 2001. Thromboembolism in newborns, infants and children. Thromb Haemost 86, 464–474.

Nowak-Gottl, U., Albisetti, M., Bonduel, M., et al., 2008. Impact of inherited thrombophilia on venous thromboembolism in children: a systematic review and meta-analysis of observational studies. Circulation 118, 1372–1382.

Ohls, R.K., 2002. Erythropoietin in extremely low birthweight infants: blood in versus blood out. J Pediatr 141, 3–6.

Ohls, R.K., Li, Y., Abdel-Mageed, A., Buchanan Jr, G., et al., 1995. Neutrophil pool sizes and granulocyte colony-stimulating factor production in human mid-trimester fetuses. Pediatr Res 37, 806–811.

Ohls, R.K., Ehrenkrantz, R.A., Wright, L.L., et al., 2001. Effects of early erythropoietin on the transfusion requirements of preterm infants below 1250 grams birth weight: a multicenter, randomized, controlled trial. Pediatrics 108, 934–942.

Olivieri, N.F., 1999. The beta-thalassemias. N Engl J Med 341, 99–109.

Oski, F.A., 1993. The erythrocyte and its disorders. In: Nathan, A., Oski, F.A. (Eds.), Hematology of Infancy and Childhood. WB Saunders, Philadelphia, pp. 18–43.

Osterud, B., Bjorklid, E., 2001. The tissue factor pathway in disseminated intravascular coagulation. Semin Thromb Hemost 27, 605–617.

Pahal, G., Jauniaux, E., Kinnon, C., et al., 2000. Normal development of human fetal hematopoiesis between eight and seventeen weeks' gestation. Am J Obstet Gynecol 183, 1029–1034.

Palek, J., Jarolim, P., 1993. Clinical expression and laboratory detection of red blood cell membrane protein mutations. Semin Hematol 30, 249–283.

Paul, D.A., Leef, K.H., Locke, R.G., et al., 2002. Transfusion volume in infants with very low birth weight: a randomized trial of 10 versus 20 ml/kg. J Pediatr Hematol Oncol 24, 43–46.

Pearson, H.A., 1967. Life span of the fetal red blood cell. J Pediatr 70, 166–171.

Pessler, F., Hart, D., 2002. Hyporegenerative anemia associated with Rh hemolytic disease: treatment failure of recombinant erythropoietin. J Pediatr Hematol Oncol 24, 689–693.

Public Health Laboratory Service Working Party on Fifth Disease, 1990. Prospective study of human parvovirus (B19) infection in pregnancy. BMJ 300, 1166–1170.

Puckett, R.M., Offringa, M., 2000. Prophylactic vitamin K for vitamin K deficiency bleeding in neonates (Cochrane Review). Cochrane Database Syst Rev (4), CD002776.

Puetz, J., Darling, G., Brabec, P., et al., 2009. Thrombotic events in neonates receiving recombinant factor VIIa or fresh frozen plasma. Pediatr Blood Cancer 53, 1074–1078.

Rao, R., Georgieff, M.K., 2002. Perinatal aspects of iron metabolism. Acta Paediatr Suppl 91, 124–129.

Remacha, A.F., Badell, I., Pujol-Moix, N., et al., 2002. Hydrops fetalis-associated congenital dyserythropoietic anemia treated with intrauterine transfusions and bone marrow transplantation. Blood 100, 356–358.

Reverdiau-Moalic, P., Delahousse, B., Body, G., et al., 1996. Evolution of blood coagulation activators and inhibitors in the healthy human fetus. Blood 88, 900–906.

Roberts, I.A.G., Murray, N.A., 2001. Neonatal thrombocytopenia: new insights into pathogenesis and implications for clinical management. Curr Opin Pediatr 13, 16–21.

Roberts, I., Stanworth, S., Murray, N.A., 2008. Thrombocytopenia in the neonate. Blood Rev 22, 173–186.

Roman, E., Flear, N.T., Ansell, P., et al., 2002. Vitamin K and childhood cancer: analysis of individual patient data from six different case-control studies. Br J Cancer 86, 63–69.

Roy, M., Turner-Gomes, S., Gill, G., et al., 1997. Incidence and diagnosis of neonatal thrombosis associated with umbilical venous catheters. Thromb Haemost 78, PS2953.

Roy, A., Roberts, I., Norton, A., et al., 2009. Acute megakaryoblastic leukaemia (AMKL) and transient myeloproliferative disorder (TMD) in Down syndrome: a multi-step model of myeloid leukaemogenesis. Br J Haematol 147, 3–12.

Salvesen, D.R., Brudenell, J.M., Snijders, R.J., et al., 1993. Fetal plasma erythropoietin in pregnancies complicated by maternal diabetes mellitus. Am J Obstet Gynecol 168, 88–94.

Schmidt, B., Andrew, M., 1995. Neonatal thrombosis: report of a prospective Canadian and international registry. Pediatrics 96, 939–943.

Schneider, A.S., 2000. Triosephosphate isomerase deficiency: historical perspectives and molecular aspects. Baillieres Best Pract Res Clin Haematol 13, 119–140.

Schwarz, K., Iolascon, A., Verissimo, F., et al., 2009. Mutations affecting the secretory COPII coat component SEC23B cause congenital dyserythropoietic anemia type II. Nat Genet 41, 936–940.

Shearer, M.J., 2009. Vitamin K deficiency bleeding (VKDB) in early infancy. Blood Rev 23, 45–59.

Singer, S.T., Styles, L., Bojanowski, J., et al., 2000. Changing outcome of homozygous alpha-thalassemia: cautious optimism. J Pediatr Hematol Oncol 22, 539–542.

Sisson, T.R.C., Lund, C.J., Whalen, L.E., et al., 1959. The blood volume of infants. I. The full term infant in the first year of life. J Pediatr 55, 163–179.

Smith, P., 1990. Congenital coagulation protein deficiencies in the perinatal period. Semin Perinatol 14, 384–392.

Smith, O.P., Hann, I.M., Woodward, C.E., et al., 1995. Pearson's marrow/pancreas syndrome: haematological features associated with deletion and duplication of mitochondrial DNA. Br J Haematol 90, 469–472.

Sohan, K., Billington, M., Pamphilon, D., et al., 2002. Normal growth and development following in utero diagnosis and treatment of homozygous alpha-thalassaemia. Br J Obstet Gynaecol 109, 1308–1310.

Sola, M.C., Del Vecchio, A., Rimsza, L.M., 2000. Evaluation and treatment of thrombocytopenia in the neonatal intensive care unit. Clin Perinatol 27, 655–679.

Stanworth, S., Clarke, P., Watts, T., et al., 2009. Prospective observational study of outcomes in neonates with severe thrombocytopenia. Pediatrics 124, 826–834.

Strauss, R.G., 2008. How I transfuse red blood cells and platelets to infants with the anemia and thrombocytopenia of prematurity. Transfusion 48, 209–217.

Stroncek, D., 2002. Neutrophil alloantigens. Transfusion Med Rev 16, 67–75.

Stuart, M.J., Graeber, J.E., 1998. Normal hemostasis in the fetus and newborn: vessels and platelets. In: Polin, R.A., Fox, W.M. (Eds.), Fetal and Neonatal Physiology. WB Saunders, Philadelphia, pp. 1834–1848.

Sutor, A.H., von Kries, R., Cornelissen, E.A., et al., 1999. Vitamin K deficiency bleeding (VKDB) in infancy. ISTH Pediatric/ Perinatal Subcommittee. International Society on Thrombosis and Haemostasis. Thromb Haemost 81, 456–461.

Tavian, M., Hallais, M.F., Peault, B., 1999. Emergence of intraembryonic hematopoietic precursors in the pre-liver human embryo. Development 126, 793–803.

Thompson, J., 2002. Haemolytic disease of the newborn: the new NICE guidelines. J Fam Health Care 12, 133–136.

Thurlbeck, S.M., McIntosh, N., 1987. Preterm blood counts vary with sampling site. Arch Dis Child 62, 74–87.

Towner, D., Castro, M.A., Eby-Wilkens, E., et al., 1999. Effect of mode of delivery in nulliparous women on neonatal intracranial injury. N Engl J Med 341, 1709–1714.

Tripp, J.H., Cornelissen, M., Loughnan, P., et al., 1995. Suggested protocol for the reporting of prospective studies of vitamin K deficiency bleeding (previously called hemorrhagic disease of the newborn). In: Sutor, A.H., Hathaway, W.E. (Eds.), Vitamin K in Infancy. Stuttgart, Schattauer Verlag, pp. 395–401.

Tse, W.T., Lux, S.E., 1999. Red blood cell membrane disorders. Br J Haematol 104, 2–13.

United Kingdom Haemophilia Centre Doctors' Organization, 2008. Guideline approved by the British Committee for Standards in Haematology. Guidelines on the selection and use of therapeutic products to treart haemophilia and other hereditary bleeding disorders. Haemophilia 14, 671–684.

Usher, R., Lind, J., 1965. Blood volume of the newborn premature infant. Acta Paediatr Scand 54, 419.

Vamkakas, E.C., Pineda, A.A., 1996. Meta-analysis of clinical studies of the efficacy of granulocyte transfusions in the treatment of bacterial sepsis. J Clin Apher 11, 1–9.

Vamkakas, E.C., Strauss, R.G., 2001. Meta-analysis of controlled clinical trials studying the efficacy of rHuEPO in reducing blood transfusions in the anemia of prematurity. Transfusion 41, 406–415.

van Winkel, M., de Bruyne, R., van der Velde, S., et al., 2008. Vitamin K, an update for the paediatrician. Eur J Pediatr 168, 127–134.

Vaughan, J.I., Manning, M., Warwick, R.M., et al., 1998. Inhibition of erythroid progenitor cell growth by anti-Kell (K): a mechanism for fetal anemia in K-immunized pregnancies. N Engl J Med 338, 798–803.

Vichinsky, E., Hurst, D., Earles, A., et al., 1988. Newborn screening for sickle cell disease: effect on mortality. Pediatrics 81, 749–755.

Vlachos, A., Ball, S., Dahl, N., et al., 2008. Participants of Sixth Annual Daniella Maria Arturi International Consensus Conference. 2008. Diagnosing and treating Diamond Blackfan anaemia: results of an international clinical consensus conference. Br J Haematol 142, 859–876.

Von Kohorn, I., Ehrenkranz, R.A., 2009. Anemia in the preterm infant: erythropoietin versus erythrocyte transfusion – it's not that simple. Clin Perinatol 36, 111–123.

Vora, M., Gruslin, A., 1998. Erythropoietin in obstetrics. Obstet Gynecol Surv 53, 500–508.

Waldron, P., de Alarcon, P., 1999. ABO hemolytic disease of the newborn: a unique constellation of findings in siblings and review of protective mechanisms in the fetal-maternal system. Am J Perinatol 16, 391–398.

Wardle, S.P., Garr, R., Yoxall, C.W., et al., 2002. A pilot randomised controlled trial of peripheral fractional oxygen extraction to guide blood transfusions in preterm infants. Arch Dis Child Fetal Neonatal Ed 86, F22–F27.

Watts, T.L., Roberts, I.A.G., 1999. Haematological abnormalities in the growth-restricted infant. Semin Neonatol 4, 41–54.

Watts, T.L., Murray, N.A., Roberts, I.A.G., 1999. Thrombopoietin has a primary role in the regulation of platelet production in preterm babies. Pediatr Res 46, 28–32.

Wechsler, J., Greene, M., McDevitt, M.A., et al., 2002. Acquired mutations in GATA1 in the megakaryoblastic leukaemia of Down syndrome. Nat Genet 32, 148–152.

Wee, L.Y., Fisk, N.M., 2002. The twin-twin transfusion syndrome. Semin Neonatol 7, 187–202.

Wen, S.W., Liu, S., Kramer, M.S., et al., 2001. Comparison of maternal and infant outcomes between vacuum extraction and forceps deliveries. Am J Epidemiol 153, 103–107.

Werner, E.J., 1995. Neonatal polycythemia and hyperviscosity. Clin Perinatol 22, 693–710.

Williamson, L.M., 2000. Leucocyte depletion of the blood supply – how will patients benefit? Br J Haematol 110, 256–272.

Williamson, L., Cohen, H., Love, E., et al., 2000. The Serious Hazards of Transfusion (SHOT) initiative: the UK approach to haemovigilance. Vox Sang 78 (suppl. 2), 291–295.

Wong, W., Fok, T.F., Lee, C.H., et al., 1997. Randomised controlled trial: comparison of colloid or crystalloid for partial exchange transfusion for treatment of neonatal polycythaemia. Arch Dis Child Fetal Neonatal Ed 77, F115–F118.

Yaegashi, N., Okamura, K., Yajima, A., et al., 1994. The frequency of human parvovirus B19 infection in non-immune hydrops fetalis. J Perinat Med 22, 159–163.

Yao, A.C., Lin, J., Tiisala, R., et al., 1969. Placental transfusion in the premature infant with observation on clinical course and outcome. Acta Paediatr Scand 58, 561–566.

Zanella, A., Bianchi, P., 2000. Red cell pyruvate kinase deficiency: from genetics to clinical manifestations. Baillieres Best Pract Res Clin Haematol 13, 57–81.

Zeidler, C., Germeshausen, M., Klein, C., et al., 2009. Clinical implications of ELA2-, HAX1-, and G-CSF-receptor (CSF3R) mutations in severe congenital neutropenia. Br J Haematol 144, 459–467.

Zipursky, A., 1999. Prevention of vitamin K deficiency bleeding in newborns. Br J Haematol 104, 430–437.

Zuppa, A.A., Maragliano, G., Scapillati, M.E., et al., 1999. Recombinant erythropoietin in the prevention of late anaemia in intrauterine transfused neonates with Rh-haemolytic disease. Fetal Diagn Ther 14, 270–274.

SINGLETON HOSPITAL
STAFF LIBRARY

Malformation syndromes

31

Oana Caluseriu   William Reardon

CHAPTER CONTENTS

© 2012 Elsevier Ltd

Introduction

The demarcation between inborn errors of metabolism and genetic syndromes can be indistinct at a clinical level. Conditions of a primarily metabolic nature often manifest by multiple congenital anomalies, for example glutaric aciduria type II and Smith–Lemli–Opitz syndrome (Wilson et al. 1989; Kelley et al. 1996). Conversely, malformation syndromes can be underlined by changes in a metabolic enzyme, as recently demonstrated in the case of Miller syndrome (Ng et al. 2010). This indistinction between metabolic disease and malformation syndrome is understandable because of mutation in genes that are part of complex metabolic pathways.

It is estimated that about 5% of newborns have a serious congenital anomaly. Screening tests recognise 2–3% of these anomalies by invasive methods prenatally or at birth, and another 2% of newborns will have developmental or functional anomalies recognised during the first year of life (Kohut and Rusen 2002). A more refined presentation of the epidemiological basis of congenital malformation syndromes suggests that 6% of birth defects arise in the context of chromosomal abnormalities; 7.5% are considered monogenic in origin; 20% are multifactorial and 6–7% are caused by environmental factors, including teratogens, infections and maternal disease (Winter 1996a; Winter and Baraitser 2010). Although rare in absolute numbers, birth defects represent an important public heath problem. Some 20–30% of all infant deaths and 30–50% of deaths after the neonatal period are attributed to congenital anomalies (Mathews and Mac Dorman 2006). Birth defects account for 15–30% of pediatric hospitalisations and they incur proportionally higher healthcare costs than other hospitalisations (Yoon et al. 1997). For the main categories of birth defects the incidences are estimated at 0.43% for the nervous system and eye, 0.87% for the cardiovascular system, 0.77% for muscle and skeleton, 0.74% for the genitourinary tract and 0.11% for cleft lip and palate (CLP) defects (March of Dimes Perinatal Data Center 2000). The purpose of this chapter is to elucidate the diagnostic process in the newborn presenting with malformation.

Basic terms in dysmorphology

Malformations are the result of an intrinsic embryological process that fails to complete as specified by developmental genes. The process of development of a specific tissue or organ can be halted, delayed or misdirected, with the result that a structure is permanently abnormal. Malformations take place usually during the process of organogenesis in the first 2 months of embryonal life. Common examples would be congenital heart defects (CHDs), intestinal atresias and polydactylies.

- Example: Cleft lip with or without cleft palate (CL/P) is one of the most common congenital anomalies. It results from the failure of union of the frontonasal processes of the face with the lateral maxillary prominences at about 7 weeks' gestation. Isolated midline CP appears to be a different malformation process to that of CLP in the context of different syndromal associations. Up to 80% of affected patients are males and the defect shows a large variation in frequency based on ethnic origin. High rates are observed in babies from the southwestern USA and from the west coast of Canada. There is a 1/1000 incidence in Caucasians and 0.4/1000 in African Americans. A recent congenital anomalies review showed the overall prevalence of CL/P was 9.92 per 10 000. The prevalence of CL was 3.28 per 10 000 and that of CLP 6.64 per 10 000. About three-quarters of cases were isolated, 15.9% had malformations in other systems and 7.3% occurred as part of recognised

syndromes (Mastroiacovo et al. 2011). In common with many other malformations, CL/P arise as multifactorial conditions and the end point of the deviant developmental process can have a multitude of causes – chromosomal, monogenic, biochemical and environmental. CL can be identified in pregnancy by sonography at about 13 weeks of gestation and CP, although easily missed on ultrasound screening, may be seen at about 18 weeks' gestation. The finding of CL/P should prompt a careful examination for other anomalies, and this should be more detailed in the neonatal period. The challenge of correct diagnosis consists in discerning non-syndromal from syndromal conditions when the input of a geneticist can be pivotal.

In contrast to malformations, deformations are caused by extrinsic factors or mechanical forces that distort otherwise normal structures. They usually happen during the second trimester and are caused by intrauterine constraint, including oligohydramnios, maternal factors such as abnormalities of the uterus (bicornuate), small pelvic outlet or fetal factors such as twin pregnancy and abnormal presentation. Once the mechanical force is removed, most of the deformations will correct over the course of several months up to years using conservative (casts, braces, physiotherapy) or invasive (surgery) methods.

- Example: Arthrogryposis is a term used for a group of conditions characterised by usually non-progressive congenital joint contractures at multiple sites. In some situations there is only limb involvement, but in many instances there is a neuromuscular and/or central nervous system (CNS) involvement and only half of the children with arthrogryposis ever receive a specific diagnosis. What is common to various forms of arthrogryposis is reduced movement in utero. While some forms of arthrogryposis have an identified genetic defect, offering the possibility of confirmation of clinical diagnosis through molecular testing, the general evaluation of a newborn with joint contractures should bear in mind several possible forms of pathology. A problem of neurological origin is found in about 90% of patients (e.g. CNS anomaly). A muscular disorder such as a congenital myopathy or congenital myasthenia is found in 5–10% of cases, not counting the cases when the mother herself has a myopathic process (myasthenia gravis, myotonic dystrophy). While in some cases arthrogryposis is the effect of a deformation process as a result of constriction of the cavity by uterine fibroids or anomalies, maternal hyperthermia and maternal use of cocaine or exposure to misoprostol are rare but well-established alternative causes of this clinical presentation (Adam et al. 2003; Riel-Romero and Mattingly 2005).

When destruction of a previously normal tissue causes a structural defect, the result is called disruption. This can be produced not only as a result of mechanical forces, but also by phenomena such as haemorrhage, ischaemia, trauma and teratogens. An example would be the amniotic bands or amniotic disruption causing partial amputation of fetal limbs by constriction rings formed from strands of amniotic tissue. Examination of the placenta and membranes is usually diagnostic.

Both deformation and disruption are events that affect previously normally formed structures. As a consequence, there is no intrinsic factor acting, so no concern for mental handicap.

Dysplasias refer to abnormal cellular organisation within a specific tissue which results in structural changes that are persistent and can progress and worsen as the tissue grows and functions. In contrast with the other pathogenetic mechanisms, disruption can produce changes throughout the person's lifetime. There are many forms of dysplasia, examples of which might be storage disorders, skeletal dysostoses and ectodermal dysplasias.

- Example: Achondroplasia is the most common skeletal dysplasia, being present in 1/26 000 individuals. The disorder is transmitted as an autosomal-dominant trait with complete penetrance. Most cases are sporadic, and there is an association with advanced paternal age (Orioli et al. 1995). Although diagnosable in pregnancy by ultrasound because of micromelia and macrocephaly, many cases are likely to be missed, as foreshortening of bones is not evident until the third trimester. Molecular confirmation of diagnosis is available, there being a single common mutation identifiable in over 95% of cases. The physical characteristics which will alert the neonatologist to this likely diagnosis include proximal (rhizomelic) shortening of the arms and legs with redundant skin folds on limbs; the hands have a trident configuration and there is limitation of elbow extension (Fig. 31.1). These long-bone characteristics are accompanied by macrocephaly with frontal bossing and midface hypoplasia. Suggestive radiological findings include

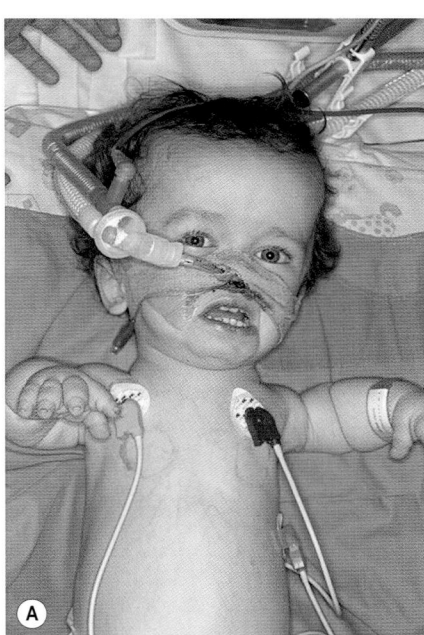

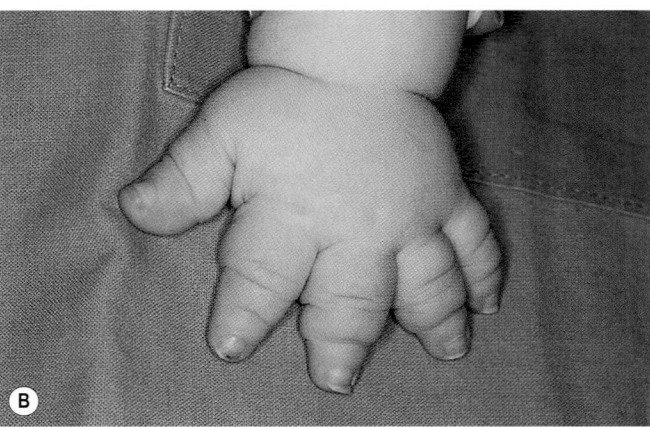

Fig. 31.1 (a) A baby with achondroplasia. Note the short upper limbs, particularly noteworthy in the humeri, and the relative narrowing of the chest. (b) The trident hand sign.

small skull base and foramen magnum, narrowing of the interpedicular distance in the lumbar spine and short vertebral bodies, square iliac wings, flat acetabula, narrowing of the sacrosciatic notch and the 'collar hoop' sign (Boulet et al. 2009). Of concern is the risk of premature sudden death arising from acute foraminal compression of the upper cervical cord or lower brainstem (Wynn et al. 2007). While there can be hypotonia in the neonatalperiod and delayed motor milestones initially, intelligence and life expectancy are normal.

Based on a clinical classification, birth defects can be classified as isolated defects, syndromes, associations and sequences.

Isolated defects

Most birth defects involve a single organ or region of the body. Common examples are CL/P, CHDs, club foot and neural tube defects (NTDs). Except for the involvement of some major genes that show a mendelian pattern of distribution in families, the majority of single defects show a multifactorial aetiology, indicating the involvement of both genetic and non-genetic factors. It is not unusual for different ethnic groups to show different frequencies of congenital anomalies (e.g. NTD incidence is lower in Japan than in Ireland).

- Example: NTDs represent a failure of closure of neural groove that is usually complete by 28 days' gestation (see Chs 8 and 9 for more information about the antenatal and postnatal diagnosis and prognosis of these conditions). In about 80% of cases this defect occurs in isolation. Such instances are considered multifactorial conditions with several non-genetic factors incriminated to date, including maternal diabetes, prepregnancy obesity and use of anticonvulsant medication, especially folic acid antagonists such as valproate (Mitchell 2005). Folic acid supplementation, an important public health intervention, has reduced the incidence of NTDs between 31% and 78% in countries such as Canada, the USA and Chile, but compliance remains a challenge. In addition, NTD prevalence varies with race and ethnicity. Recurrence risk can be variable (2–10%) and it is influenced by the number of cases identified in the pedigree (Eichholzer et al. 2006).

Syndrome

When a constellation of anomalies occurs repeatedly in the same combination, this pattern is called a syndrome. The fundamental point about a syndrome is that all the features may be explained by a common causative factor, whether that be a mutation in a single gene, the presence of additional chromosomal material or a teratogen. The clinical practice of dysmorphology teaches that a single underlying cause of birth defects can result in abnormalities in different organs, or in multiple structures at different times during the intrauterine period, a concept called pleiotropy. Another characteristic encountered in syndromal conditions is variable expressivity, which refers to different severity of a phenotype in individuals with the same genetic defect. Penetrance is a characteristic that refers to the probability that a gene will have a phenotypic expression at all. When an individual has a genetic mutation associated with a phenotype but fails to express it, the gene is said to show reduced penetrance.

- Example: A recognisable syndrome evident by the time of birth, with multiple dysmorphic features and birth defects, is Cornelia de Lange syndrome (Fig. 31.2). Newborns show marked growth retardation and often fail to thrive,

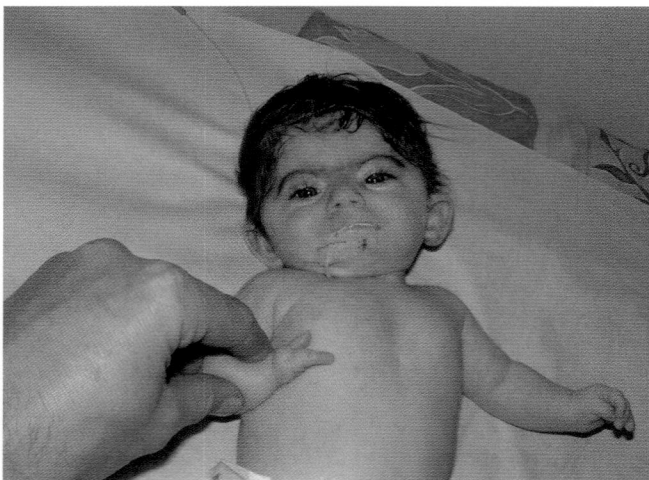

Fig. 31.2 Cornelia de Lange syndrome, showing the typical facial features and associated limb malformations. Note the nasogastric feeding tube.

manifesting with swallowing and feeding difficulties, and projectile vomiting. They initially present with hypertonicity and a low-pitched, weak cry. There is microbrachycephaly and the eyebrows are bushy with synophrys, long and curly eyelashes, a short nose with anteverted nostrils, and a long philtrum with thin upper lip. These infants are usually hirsute and may show cutis marmorata. Some 25% manifest severely malformed limbs with phocomelia or micromelia. Life-threatening complications relate to apnoea, aspiration, and complications related to bowel obstruction and cardiac defects.

Association

Some anomalies and physical features are seen happening together in a non-random fashion more often than would be expected by chance, but the link between these anomalies is not strong enough to justify a definition of a syndrome. This collection of features is called association. Variable expressivity can complicate the picture when deciding on classifying a combination of features a syndrome or an association. A good instance of an association is VACTERL, standing for vertebral anomalies (hemivertebrae, fused vertebrae, ± rib anomalies in upper, midthoracic and lumbar region), anal atresia (or fistulae, ± genital defects including hypospadias, bifid scrotum), cardiac anomalies (in 80% of cases, of various types), tracheo-oesophageal fistula, oesophageal atresia (80% have an associated tracheo-oesophageal fistula), renal anomalies (in 80% of cases including renal agenesis/dysplasia) and limb defects (restricted to the upper limbs, usually bilateral and preaxial). It is found in about 1.6/10 000 newborns, with most patients having three to four features. To secure a diagnosis of VACTERL there is need for at least one anomaly of the limbs, thorax and pelvis/lower abdomen (Hall 2010a).

Sequence

A sequence represents the clinical outcome of a chain of events that cause a pattern of multiple defects, all emanating from a single primary malformation. Robin sequence illustrates this concept very well. It is observed in 1/8500 births. The initiating defect is represented by the mandibular hypoplasia which determines that the

tongue be placed posteriorly and in the way of the closing palatal shelves that will remain open in a rounded U-shaped CP. Affected neonates should be monitored for the risk of airway obstruction and apnoea. Mortality rates up to 30% have been reported. The sequence of micrognathia, glossoptosis and cleft of the soft palate is accompanied by feeding difficulties requiring nasogastric tube feeding and is related in many cases to lower oesophageal sphincter hypertonia, failure of oesophageal sphincter relaxation at deglutition, and oesophageal dyskinesis (Baujat et al. 2001). Pierre Robin sequence is usually isolated, but can form part of a genetic syndrome (e.g. Stickler syndrome) (Reardon and Donnai 2007).

Clinical evaluation of a neonate with birth defects

The role of the geneticist is to diagnose a child with congenital anomalies and malformation syndromes by understanding the contribution of genetic and non-genetic factors to the aetiology of the child's condition.

The key elements of an ideal history and clinical examination are outlined as follows, recognising that the reality often falls short of the ideal.

Prenatal history

- Natural conception or pregnancy through assisted reproductive technologies
- Singleton or twin (may be diagnosed initially and lost after) gestation
- Maternal and paternal age at conception
- Parity
- Maternal health issues (pre-existent diseases, illnesses in pregnancy)
- Teratogenic exposures (medication, alcohol, tobacco, drugs)
- Periconceptional supplementation (folate, vitamins)
- Onset and quality of fetal movements, amniotic fluid volume
- Prenatal testing (nature of testing, when and where performed)
    - Non-invasive (first-trimester screen, maternal serum screen, ultrasound examination) versus invasive testing (chorionic villus sampling, amniocentesis, preimplantation genetic diagnosis) and results.

Perinatal history

- Duration of pregnancy
- Intrapartum course and duration
- Intrapartum drug and medication exposure
- Fetal presentation
- Mode of delivery
- Complications of delivery, need for resuscitation (methods used)
- Infant's condition at birth (growth parameters, Apgar score, physical examination)
- Examination of placenta
- Neonatal course.

Family history

- Three-generation family history with health information in all relatives (names, date of birth, date of diagnoses for affected individuals)

- Consanguinity
- Ethnic background
- Infertility
- Miscarriages, abortions, stillbirths, neonatal and childhood deaths
- Birth defects, birth marks
- Mental retardation (learning disabilities, schooling history), behavioural issues
- Disorders that 'run in the family'
- Prior genetic testing, screening
- Access to medical records (release of information forms), family photographs.

Clinical examination should address all systems in an organised manner, paying particular attention to major and minor malformations and to physical variations. In certain circumstances, such as a background family history suggestive of a similar condition, other family members should be examined. Medical photographs can be of particular value in the process of genetic evaluation of the family as part of reaching or confirming a diagnosis and documenting changes over time. A number of recent textbooks offer clear advice on the evaluation of dysmorphic features and growth parameters (Hall et al. 2007; Reardon 2008). Typically, the evaluation of the dysmorphic neonate might comprise:

- General examination:
  - Alertness, posture, positioning, colour, respiratory effort
- Growth parameters:
  - Assessment of proportionality and symmetry
  - Assessment of gestational age by physical parameter, including length, weight and head circumference expressed in percentiles or in standard deviations from the mean
  - Specific measurements to document subjective observations of physical features such as suspected hypertelorism (Hall et al. 2007)
- Detailed examination:
  - Head – observe shape, symmetry, sutures, fontanelles
  - Scalp – describe hair patterning, texture, colour, location of hair whorls, the presence of scalp aplasia
  - Facial features:
    - Forehead shape, bitemporal distance, supraorbital ridges, description of eyebrows
    - Eyes – pupils (reactivity to light, red reflexes), iris (colour, patterns, presence of colobomas), description of cornea, examination for cataracts, description of orbits (hyper- or hypotelorism, dystopia cantorum), palpebral fissure inclination (down-, upslanting or horizontal) and length, measurement of inner and outer canthal distance and interpupillary distance, description of eyelashes
    - Nose – appearance of nasal root, bridge and base, including columella and patency and shape of nares
    - Mouth – philtrum, appearance of upper (vermilion border) and lower lip, and intraoral examination, including soft and hard palate, uvula, alveolar ridges, teeth, tongue and frenulae
    - Mandible – shape and symmetry
    - Zygomatic area description
    - Ears – location, rotation, configuration and size, patency of ear canals and examination of tympanic membranes
  - Neck – posterior hairline, presence of sinus tracts, torticollis, redundant skin or webbing, apparent shortening
  - Chest – shape, symmetry, circumference, location of nipples, accessory nipples
  - Lungs – symmetry of breath sounds, note adventitious sounds

- Cardiovascular – colour, peripheral pulses, perfusion, heart sounds and murmurs, blood pressure
- Abdomen – shape, appearance of umbilicus, muscle tone, integrity of wall, enlarged organs or masses, presence of bowel sounds
- Genitalia – size, appearance, palpation of testes (in males), presence of ambiguity
- Anus – location and patency
- Skeletal system – proportions, appearance (presence of reduction or duplication of segments), length, range of motion (including hips) of limbs; symmetry of spine, presence of sinuses or hair tufts in intergluteal cleft, presence of clavicles, and scapular shape and position
- Hands and feet – shape, full length, finger length, description of nails and creases (palmar, phalangeal and flexion, plantar)
- Skin – pigmentation pattern (areas of increased or decreased pigmentation, correspondence with the lines of Blaschko), dimples, vascular or other lesions, or excessive peeling, lumps and bumps
- Neurological – tone, response, alertness, primitive and deep tendon reflexes, normal and abnormal movements.

Instant syndrome diagnosis by pattern recognition – gestalt

A gestalt diagnosis precludes the need for extensive investigation. Such an instance is represented by the case of Ellis–van Creveld syndrome, shown in Figure 31.3, where the postaxial polydactyly,

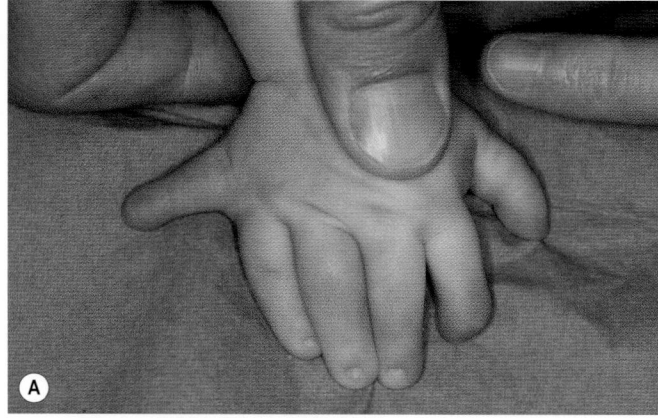

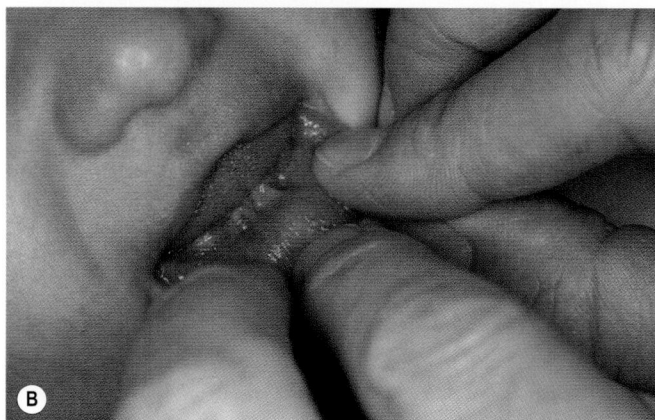

Fig. 31.3 (a, b) Ellis–van Creveld syndrome with typical postaxial polydactyly and small, deeply set nails. Note the multiple frenula.

deep-set small nails and natal teeth clearly signal the underlying condition and prompt the experienced dysmorphologist towards the cardiac evaluation which the diagnosis mandates (Carmi et al. 1992). Gestalt diagnosis is a powerful tool in the approach of the experienced dysmorphologist but can be misleading or downright harmful in the hands of the inexperienced. However, when deployed with accuracy and sensivity, the gestalt diagnosis can benefit patients, their families and neonatologists.

Investigating the malformed neonate in the absence of diagnosis

The range of investigations deployed by clinical geneticists is very broad, from histopathological examination, through biochemical analysis, to multiple different approaches to chromosome evaluation and the search for mutation at the single-gene level. Accordingly, the course of investigation pursued in any given case will vary. Sometimes very elaborate and wide-ranging investigation fails to clarify the diagnosis in a child whose clinical presentation strongly suggests a syndromal basis. From the many thousand different investigations open to the geneticist in respect of a specific case, the focus is on the series of investigations that maximise the likelihood of securing a definite diagnosis in any given case (Reardon and Donnai 2007).

A number of general investigations such as chest and abdominal X-rays and general chemistry are usually available by the time the geneticist sees the patient. Physical examination by the neonatologist often raises suspicions in the light of which more detailed investigations are undertaken, such as echocardiography in the event of a heart murmur being noted, or an abdominal ultrasound if hepatomegaly is identified.

Clinical photographs

Clinical photographs often act in conjunction with the physical examination when there is the need to document physical features and/or a facial gestalt. They can be used for different reasons:

1. A genetic condition said to 'run in the family' from information collected through family history and pictures of relatives can help in identifying a diagnosis in the index case (Fig. 31.4: Sheldon–Hall syndrome and arthrogryposis).
2. Photographs may be used to compare with similar phenotypes already published in the literature in order to reach a diagnosis.
3. Photographs may turn out to be useful at a later follow-up visit in a patient with an unknown diagnosis but nonetheless a likely syndromal presentation. In some conditions patients 'grow into their syndrome', meaning that facial gestalt may become more evident with time (Williams syndrome is a case in point).

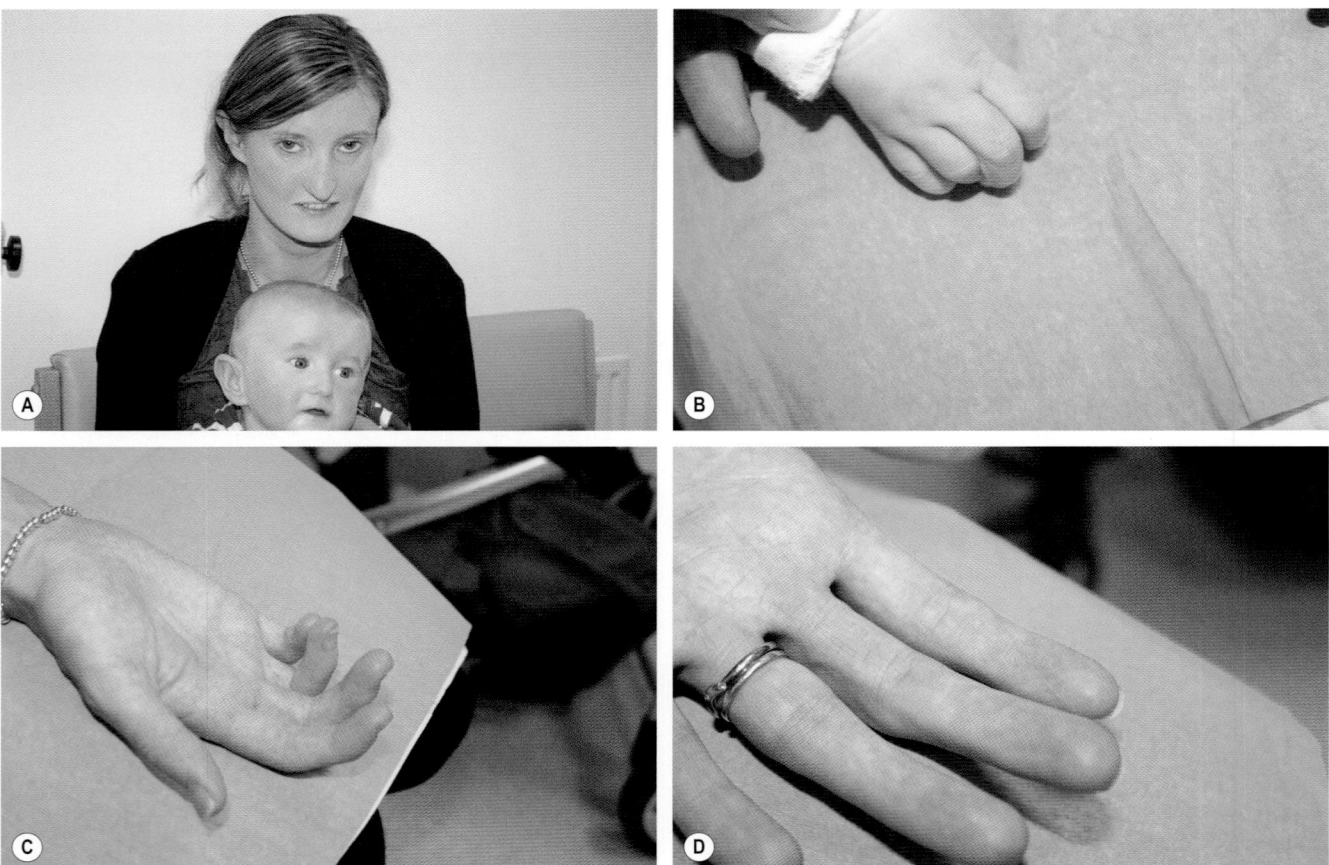

Fig. 31.4 This baby was referred with (a) immobile facies, (b) distal arthrogryposis and possible motor delay. However, maternal examination showed the same features with absence of the distal interphalangeal skin creases and distal arthrogryposis since infancy (c and d). The diagnosis is Sheldon–Hall syndrome, an autosomal-dominant cause of distal arthrogryposis associated with normal development.

Radiological images

The utility of X-rays in genetics, especially in regard to the skeletal system, cannot be overemphasised. A good example might be the finding of butterfly vertebrae in a neonate with cholestasis that should suggest a possible diagnosis of Alagille syndrome. In the event of neurological symptoms or the neonate with an abnormal head size (micro- or macrocephaly), or where there is an unusual contour of the skull, a head and brain magnetic resonance imaging will be the modality of choice (Battaglia and Carey 2003). For example, in the hypotonic neonate, the recognition of a 'molar tooth sign' suggests a diagnosis of Joubert syndrome (Fig. 31.5).

Chromosomal examination

Chromosomal examination has been part of the armamentarium of clinical geneticists for over 50 years. Many banding techniques have been developed over the years to permit the detection of aneuploidies and the identification of microscopically apparent structural aberrations, including deletions and translocations. Better techniques have improved the resolution of chromosome examination, offering the opportunity for better analysis and identification of microdeletions, microduplications or subtle translocations. At a resolution of more than 650 bands, alterations as small as 3–5 Mb can be detected using chromosome preparation on peripheral blood; for detection of subtle rearrangements in patients with either abnormal or normal standard karyotypes, molecular cytogenetics may be useful (e.g. fluorescence in situ hybridisation – FISH) (Shaffer 2005). A history of a 'normal' chromosome examination does not preclude a diagnosis of chromosomal disease, as improved techniques may identify previously unresolved/unresolvable and unidentified chromosomal disease.

Body asymmetry or streaks of pigmentation identified on the physical examination may be indicating an underlying diagnosis of a mosaic condition. A normal chromosome examination on blood may mislead the neonatologist as to the real diagnosis, and chromosome examination of another tissue may reveal the true cause of malformation. The condition of Pallister–Killian syndrome, caused by mosaicism of tetrasome 12p, exemplifies this. Presenting clinically with variable features comprising coarse facial features, temporal alopecia, diaphragmatic hernia, accessory nipples, poor feeding and hypotonia, the abnormal chromosome 12 is often absent on blood chromosomes, being lost in the rapid turnover of lymphocytes. However, skin biopsy and karyotype of the more slowly growing fibroblasts will generally reveal the true cause of the abnormal clinical profile by affording the identification of the abnormal chromosome 12 (Fig. 31.6 – clinical and cytogenetic). When ordering FISH, there is a need for a clear clinical hypothesis as to underlying diagnosis as this investigation is targeted to specific regions in the genome (e.g. FISH for 22q11.2 deletion syndrome, *ELN* on chromosome 7q11 for Williams syndrome). Chromosomal microarray is a new method for screening the chromosomes for abnormalities of dosage at a high-resolution scale and, offering a higher diagnostic yield (15–20%) than G-banding, it is suggested that it will become the first-tier cytogenetic diagnostic test for patients with multiple congenital anomalies (Miller et al. 2010). The results may be associated with significant counselling and diagnostic pitfalls and, at the time of writing, it is still a specialist tool of the experienced clinical geneticist and not suitable for more widespread use in clinical practice.

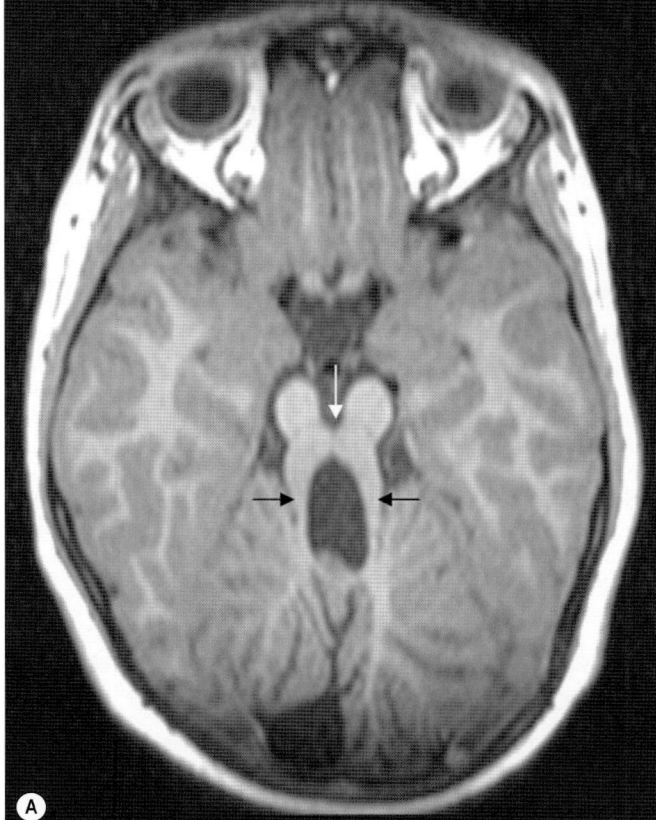

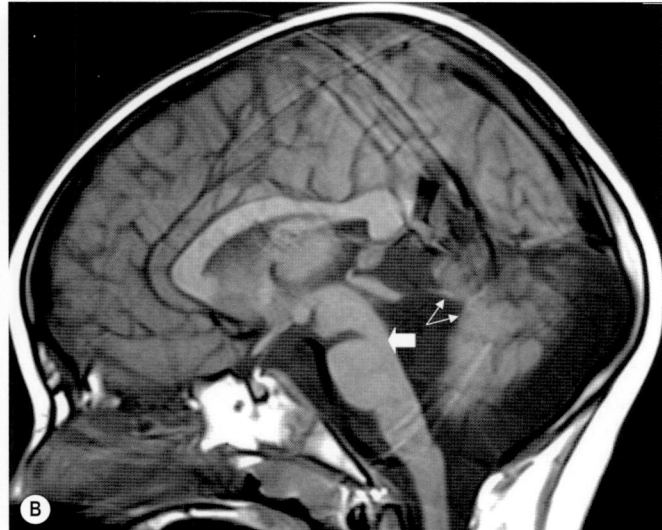

Fig. 31.5 (a) Axial T1-weighted image demonstrating the classical 'molar tooth' appearance of the midbrain caused by a narrow isthmus (white arrow) and large superior cerebellar peduncles (black arrows). (b) Sagittal T1-weighted image demonstrating a small dysplastic cerebellar vermis (white arrows) and small narrow isthmus (single solid white arrow). *(Courtesy of Dr Ethna Phelan.)*

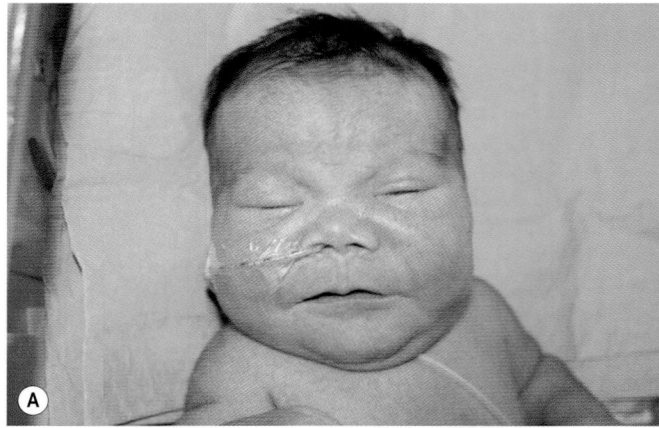

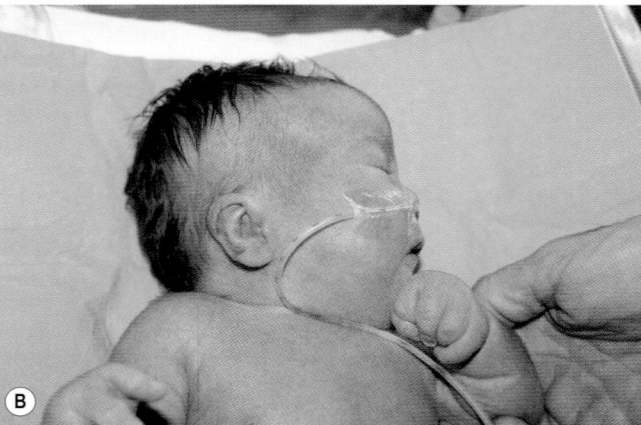

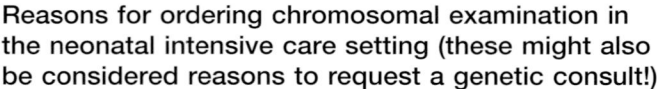

Fig. 31.6 (a, b) Newborn baby with Pallister–Killian syndrome. Note the coarse facial features and the paucity of temporal hair.

Reasons for ordering chromosomal examination in the neonatal intensive care setting (these might also be considered reasons to request a genetic consult!)

- Family history of a chromosomal anomaly in previous child
- Chromosomal rearrangement in one of the parents (e.g. balanced translocation)
- Problems of early growth and development in a previous child
- Stillbirth and neonatal death
- Infants with two or more major malformations
- Infants with a single major malformation or multiple minor malformations who are also small-for-dates
- Infants with a single major malformation who also have multiple minor anomalies.

Molecular genetics analysis

Molecular genetics analysis should always be based upon a strong diagnostic suspicion. The number of tests available in accredited laboratories around the globe continues to expand but the number of positive findings in respect of a specific analysis is often very low (<10%) which, in terms of the cost of these analyses, represents very poor value for money. Molecular testing done on a research basis in unaccredited laboratories may need further validation in a diagnostic laboratory in the event of wishing to use such data for predictive genetic purposes.

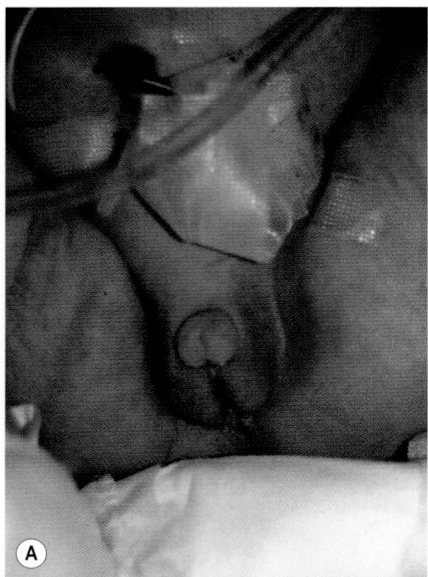

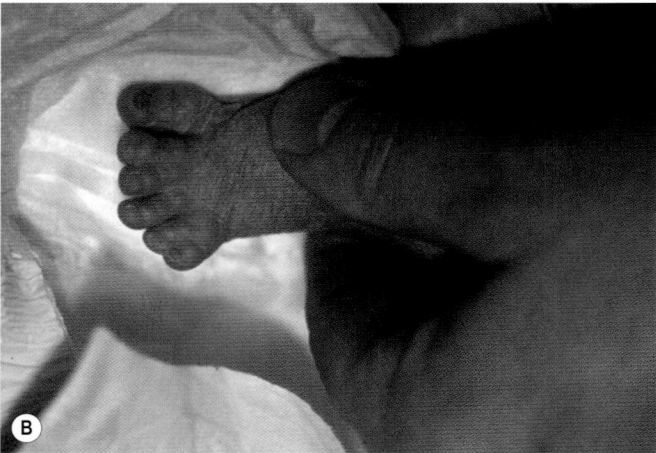

Fig. 31.7 (a, b) The combination of ambiguous genitalia, syndactyly and postaxial polydactyly in this neonate signals the diagnosis of Smith–Lemli–Opitz syndrome.

Metabolic testing

Metabolic testing needs to be done when specific signs of a metabolic disorder are raised during the neonatal clinical presentation. The metabolic genetics team will be the most appropriate to evaluate the need for specific tests (see Ch. 35, part 3). Pre- and postnatal growth deficiency, in a hypotonic neonate with microcephaly, ptosis, downslanting palpebral fissures, short nose, CP, a cardiac defect, hypospadias and/or cryptorchidism, Y-shaped 2–3 syndactyly and postaxial polydactyly, may clinically suggest Smith–Lemli–Opitz syndrome and be confirmed by the demonstration of abnormality of 7-dehydrocholesterol (Fig. 31.7).

Genetic counselling and support for families

The principal focus of the geneticist remains that of assisting the clinical team to reach a diagnosis in order to assist in prognosis and management, and to advise parents on recurrence risk. Frequently this requires the involvement of a multidisciplinary team who will need to continue to offer management to the child for several years.

Chromosomal anomalies/ microdeletion syndromes

Down syndrome

Down syndrome is by far the most common chromosomal disorder with prevalence highly dependent on maternal age. While about 1 in 1500 children are born with Down syndrome in mothers 20 years old, this incidence is about 1 in 100 in women 40 years of age. With the advent of prenatal diagnosis programmes for advanced maternal age the majority of children with Down syndrome are now born to younger women. About 78% of Down syndrome pregnancies end in spontaneous abortion. Babies are usually recognisable by their distinctive pattern of facial and extrafacial features. One of the first signs in a neonate with Down syndrome is hypotonia. Down syndrome babies can be microcephalic with a brachycephalic skull (short anteroposterior length), large fontanelles and midface hypoplasia that gives a flat appearance from the profile. The face is round in the neonate, and there are upslanted palpebral fissures and epicanthal folds. In children with light-coloured eyes, a pattern of peripheral spots on the irises can be observed (Brushfield spots: Fig. 31.8). The nose is short with a low nasal bridge and small nares and the mouth is small with downturned corners. Lips can be cracked, and the tongue can have a fissured aspect and a tendency to protrude that may give the impression of macroglossia. The ears are small, can have a cupped or squared shape and overfolded helices. It is not unusual for infants to have cutis marmorata and there can be an excess of folds in the nuchal area. The hands are short with a triangular shape of the middle phalanx on the fifth finger that gives a lateral curved aspect called clinodactyly. There can be a gap between the hallux and second toe, known as a sandal gap.

In addition to the distinctive physical features, children with Down syndrome frequently have congenital anomalies that may affect their chances of survival, especially CHDs. About half of Down syndrome neonates are found to have a heart defect, often requiring surgical repair. The most common heart defect is perimembranous ventricular septal defect (VSD), followed by patent ductus arteriosus and atrial septal defects (ASDs). Overall the incidence of congenital defects in Down syndrome children is increased twofold, including duodenal atresia and stenosis, and Hirschprung disease.

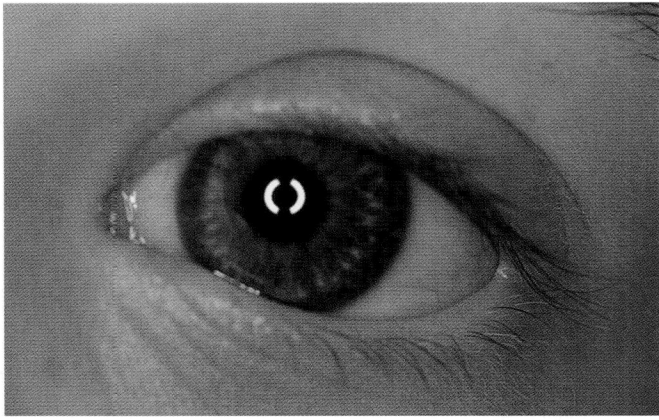

Fig. 31.8 Brushfield spots in the iris of a baby with Down syndrome.

In all, 95% of Down syndrome cases result from an extra full chromosome 21, known as trisomy 21. Most of the remaining 5% of cases arise from a robertsonian translocation (see Ch. 8, Fig 8.8 for definition) between chromosome 21 and another acrocentric chromosome, most commonly chromosome 14, in a parent, while a small number of cases represent mosaicism for trisomy 21. In the very rarely encountered situation where a robertsonian translocation involves the two chromosomes 21 in a parent, the recurrence risk approaches 100%. These cases involving parental chromosomal anomalies need specific counselling, best undertaken by specialists in a genetics clinic.

Turner syndrome

Turner syndrome is a rare sex chromosomal aneuploidy characterised by a complete or partial monosomy for one of the X chromosomes. It occurs in 1 in 5000 births, and in most cases is due to a 45,XO chromosomal complement that results from chromosomal nondisjunction and no maternal age effect has been noted. Over 95% of 45,XO conceptions are spontaneously aborted, mostly because of hydrops and nuchal cystic hygroma. Other characteristics include cardiac anomalies (20%), especially bicuspid aortic valve (30%) and coarctation of aorta (10%). In the surviving fetuses signs of congenital lymphoedema appear as residual puffiness over the dorsum of the fingers and toes with narrow, hyperconvex and/or deep-set nails. Small stature is also evident from birth and some subtle dysmorphic features may include low posterior hairline with the appearance of short neck with lateral webbing and loose skin. Facies may have a narrow maxilla (palate) with a relatively small mandible, inner canthal folds and prominent auricles. Newborns may have cubitus valgus, dislocated hips and broad chest with widely spaced nipples. About 60% of Turner syndrome patients can have renal anomalies, including horseshoe kidney, double or cleft renal pelvis, so an abdominal ultrasound as well as an echocardiogram is recommended in the neonatal period. A standard chromosomal examination will diagnose the condition. Girls with Turner syndrome are usually of normal intelligence; only about 10% have significant delays, need special education and require ongoing assistance in adult life.

Common microdeletion/duplication syndromes

Microdeletion/duplications are not usually visible by routine karyotype and may be the cause of several multiple congenital anomalies/mental retardation syndromes. Microdeletion/duplication means that an area of the chromosome (of several megabases) containing usually tens of genes is missing or duplicated respectively (contiguous gene syndrome). This large genetic imbalance explains the complexity of the phenotypes observed. While specific FISH analysis can be ordered to confirm a clinical diagnosis of such a microdeltion syndrome, syndromes caused by microdeletion/duplication may also be diagnosed using targeted microarray-based comparative genomic hybridisation (array-CGH) studies. Deletion and duplication are expected to occur with the same frequency, with the former expected to have more severe clinical consequences as the general rule, that trisomy is better tolerated than monosomy, may apply. Below are listed the most common microdeletion/duplication syndromes that can be diagnosed in the neonate or small infant and their chromosomal location:

- Sotos syndrome – 5q35
- Williams syndrome – 7q11.23
- Langer–Giedion syndrome – 8q24

- Wilms tumour–aniridia syndrome (Wilms, aniridia, genitourinary anomalies and mental retardation: WAGR) – 11p13
- Beckwith–Wiedemann syndrome (BWS) – 11p15
- Prader–Willi and Angelman syndrome – 15q11-13
- Smith–Magenis syndrome – 17p11.2
- Miller–Dieker syndrome – 17p13.3
- Velocardiofacial/22q11.2 deletion syndrome – 22q11.2.

Since velocardiofacial/22q11.2 deletion syndrome represents the most common microdeletion syndrome, a more detailed discussion is required. It is an extremely pleiomorphic condition, having been described by several different paediatric subspecialties in the absence of recognition that the different reports represented the same condition (Cayler et al. 1971; Scambler et al. 1992). A prevalence of 1 in 4000 births is based on a more severe phenotype and generally thought to be an underestimate (Shprintzen 2010). This condition encompasses DiGeorge sequence, characterised by a pattern of malformations as a result of developmental abnormalities in third and fourth branchial arches, emphasised by defects of thymus, parathyroids and great vessels (Kochilas et al. 2002). Hypoplasia (aplasia) of thymus with consequent deficit of cellular immunity is responsible for a predisposition to severe infections and the use of live vaccines should be avoided if this diagnosis is suspected or confirmed. Blood products should be irradiated to eliminate the risk of graft-versus-host disease. Hypoparathyroidism is responsible for hypocalcaemia that can produce easily treatable seizures in the neonatal period and thereafter.

Cardiovascular malformations derive from anomalies of the conotruncus and are found in 74% of affected individuals, representing the most important cause of death associated with this syndrome (Ryan et al. 1997). The most common heart defect is VSD followed closely by aortic arch defects and tetralogy of Fallot (Ryan et al. 1997). Most patients have palatal dysfunction, if not necessarily cleft, resulting in velopharyngeal insufficiency and a minority having overt CP (Ryan et al. 1997). Neonatal feeding problems, in particular nasal regurgitation of milk in term babies, is one of the most common clues to this syndrome, and should be an indication for genetic evaluation. Antenatal diagnosis is possible and indeed should be offered in the event of a conotruncal defect being identified – FISH for 22q11.2 is undertaken on amniocytes. The syndrome is inherited from one of the parents in about 7% of cases, in which event a history of learning disability and possible psychiatric disorder may be divined. The risk of learning difficulty reaches 70–90% in children with DiGeorge syndrome.

Single-gene disorders identifiable in the neonatal period

Single-gene disorder conditions indicate an aetiological origin attributable to mutations within a specific gene locus, which differentiates them from chromosomal aberrations where, by definition, a large amount of genetic material is involved. For didactic purposes, we will maintain the concept of single-gene disorders to introduce various examples of anomalies of genetic origin. Mendelian disorders usually refer to genetic diseases showing a mendelian pattern of inheritance of a trait (e.g. dominant, recessive), caused by a mutation in the nuclear DNA with pathogenic consequences. These disorders are listed in McKusick's reference Online Mendelian Inheritance in Man (OMIM) database, available on the internet through the National Library of Medicine (http://ncbi.nlm.nih.gov). As of March 2011, 21140 genetic conditions are listed, more than half of which have an established molecular basis.

Autosomal conditions relating to genes in chromosomes from 1 to 22 comprise 19845 disorders, and fewer than 1200 conditions relate to sex chromosomes (X and Y).

A particular mechanism of character transmission relevant to the neonatologist is imprinting. This phenomenon refers to the fact that some genes are expressed in a parent of origin manner.

Major anomalies are congenital malformations that have important functional consequences (e.g. CHD) and indicate that an important developmental process has been severely affected. Most of the time they may be identified during the prenatal period or at birth and medical intervention is needed to correct them. On the other hand, minor anomalies are unusual morphologic features of no medical importance, but can raise cosmetic concerns to the patient (e.g. preauricular tags). They are also indicators of some level of alteration of a normal morphogenetic process, and can be valuable 'handles' for a specific pattern of malformations. The significance of minor anomalies is to alert the clinician to the possibility of associated but undetected major malformations.

The face

The face offers many possible diagnostic clues to a clinical geneticist and it is often the recognition of an abnormal facial appearance by neonatologists that sets in train the chain of events leading to a diagnosis. As seen in the physical examination section, a large variety of facial features need to be observed by the trained eye in recognising normal and abnormal variants, and their interpretation in the context of the general clinical presentation. Facial structures develop from 4 weeks' gestational age and at about 8 weeks the embryonal face is recognisable. There are five primordial structures that contribute to face development, including paired maxillary and mandibulary prominences and a frontonasal prominence, and they derive from migration of the neural crest cells. A multitude of intrinsic genetic factors and local conditions contribute to the growth and development of these structures in a certain way that will culminate with a person's individual facial appearance (Winter 1996b).

A classical example of syndrome described in dysmorphology as having a recognisable gestalt is Rubinstein–Taybi syndrome (RTS) (Fig. 31.9). RTS is characterised by postnatal onset of growth deficiency and a well-described gestalt. Patients can have microcephaly with large anterior fontanelle, downslanting palpebral fissures, heavy eyebrows and long eyelashes and hypoplastic maxilla with narrow palate. There is a characteristic prominent or beaked nose with or without nasal septum extending below alae nasi and short columella (Allanson and Hennekam 1997). The classic hallmark of the condition is the broad great toes and thumbs, sometimes angled in a radial direction. Respiratory infections, constipation and feeding difficulties are frequent problems in infancy. The majority of cases are sporadic. Mutation of the CREBBP locus (>60%) is the main cause of the phenotype while mutation at a second locus, EP300, has been reported in a handful of cases in whom CREBBP analysis proved negative (Roelfsema et al. 2005).

Facial asymmetry

Facial asymmetry refers not to the usual slight differences observed in the majority of individuals between the two sides of the face or to the asymmetry that can often result during the process of birth. Facial asymmetry that is persistent and evident in time can be a reflection of an abnormal morphogenetic process of the skull as in craniosynostosis (described in craniosynostoses) or the direct result of lesser development of facial structures. The latter is best represented by a spectrum of defects known as oculoauriculovertebral

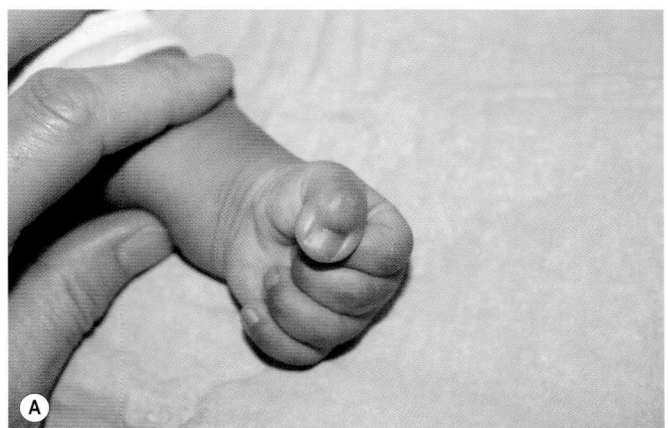

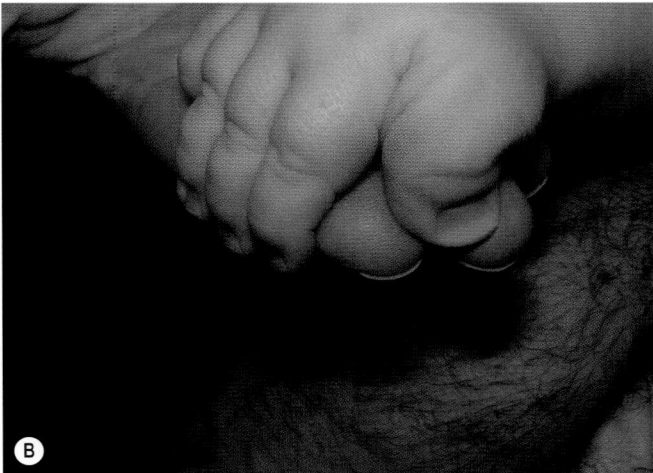

Fig. 31.9 The broad thumbs of Rubinstein–Taybi syndrome are shown in two patients. Note that the angulation of the thumb is not always present.

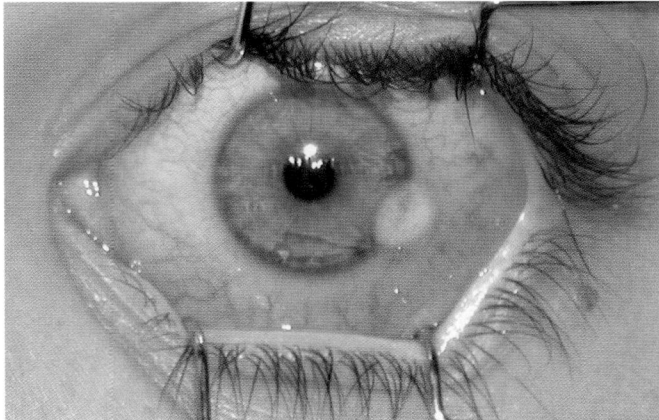

Fig. 31.10 A typical epibulbar dermoid is shown in a patient with Goldenhar syndrome.

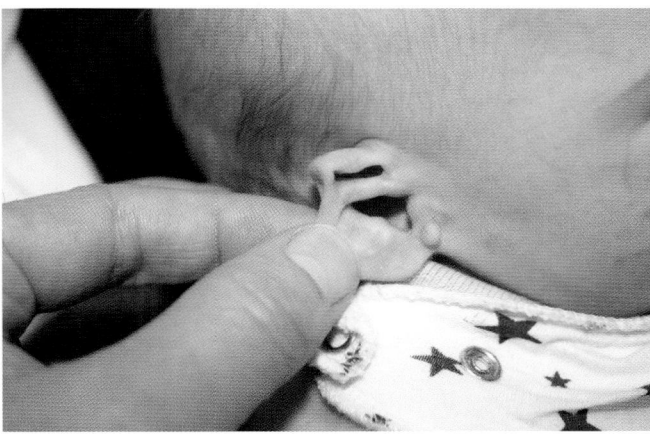

Fig. 31.11 A malformed ear in a patient with Goldenhar syndrome.

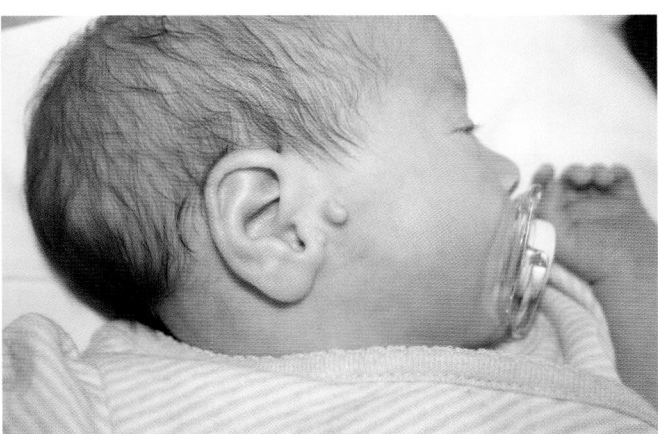

Fig. 31.12 A typical preauricular site of a skin appendage in a case of Goldenhar syndrome.

association. The defects described under this umbrella term are a result of abnormalities of the first and second branchial arches and present with a great variability of phenotypes, the most representative being Goldenhar syndrome (Fig. 31.10). In this condition, hemifacial microsomia reflecting maxillary and/or mandibulary hypoplasia is accompanied by uni- or bilateral epibulbar dermoids (benign solid tumours at the level of limbus, border between cornea and iris – Fig. 31.11) and vertebral anomalies (hypoplastic vertebrae, hemivertebrae). Preauricular or facial tags and/or pits are common, of different sizes and usually distributed along the skin overlying the mandibular ramus (Fig. 31.12). The ear on the affected side is typically small (microtia) with different degrees of malformation, which can extend to the middle ear and result in variable degrees of deafness. This is a relatively common presentation, the prevalence being 1/3000–5000 births and associated with a preponderance of male cases. Similar clinical features can be the presenting features of 22q11.2 deletion syndrome (Xu et al. 2008).

Hypotelorism

Hypotelorism or closely set eyes can be a subjective observation when looking at a face but objectively can be defined as smaller than normal interpupillary distance. Although sometimes seen as a harmless observation among the general population, to a geneticist the finding of hypotelorism prompts concern as to forebrain development and the possibility that such a face may represent a clinical presentation of the midline brain anomaly called holoprosencephaly (HPE) sequence (see below) (Fig. 31.13). If accompanied by syndactyly, especially of the fourth and fifth fingers, and third

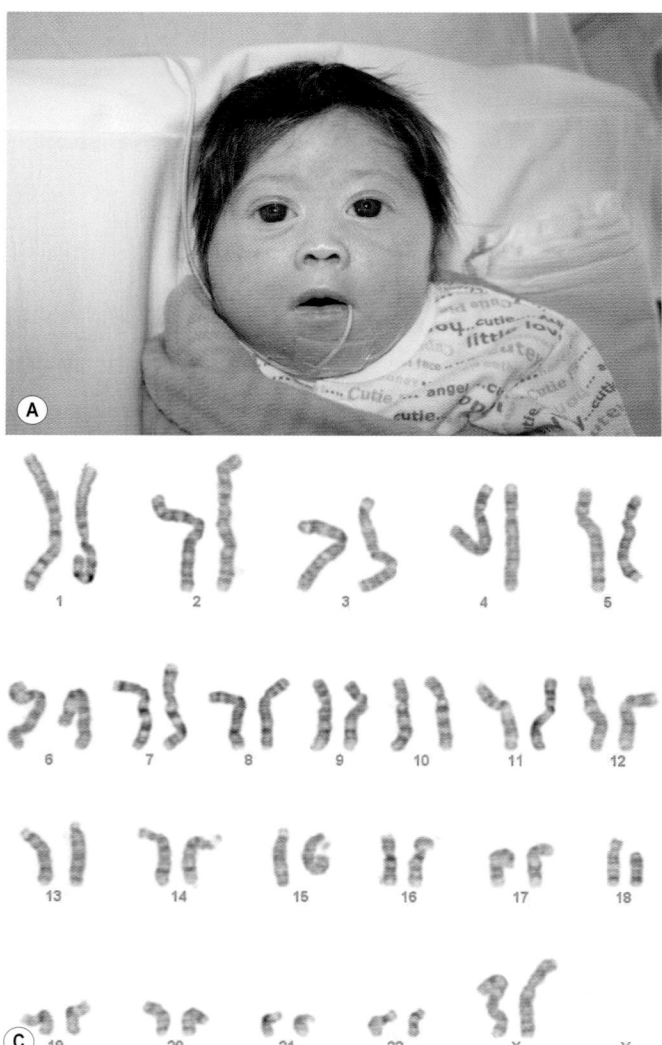

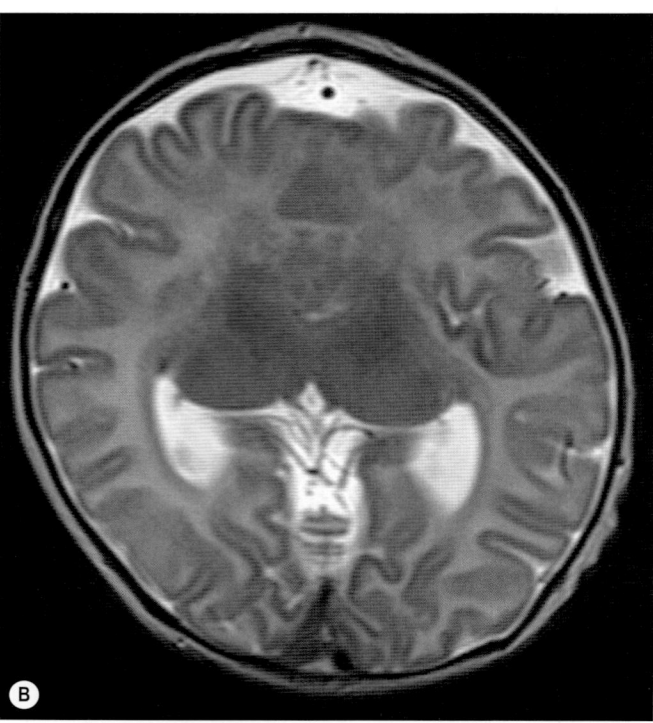

Fig. 31.13 (a) A newborn child with hypotelorism and poorly formed nasal columella. These clinical features signal the underlying holoprosencephaly seen in (b), where the failure of separation on the frontal lobes is seen. (c) Chromosome 18p deletion in this same child. One of the loci for holoprosencephaly, TGIF, is located at 18p11.3, whose deletion in this child has caused the holoprosencephaly.

and fourth toes, and small nose with hypoplastic alae nasi, hypotelorism may prompt the diagnosis of oculodentodigital syndrome (Fig. 31.14).

Hypertelorism

Hypertelorism or wide-set eyes refers objectively to an increased interpupillary distance. Hypertelorism is characteristic of Waardenburg syndrome type I, in which may also be observed iris heterochromia (different-coloured eyes or only speckled irises), white forelock and broad and high nasal bridge with hypoplastic alae nasi (Fig. 31.15). Deafness is the most serious characteristic of this syndrome that needs to be properly addressed.

Syndromal conditions

Most cases of CL/P are isolated, but up to 20% are part of a syndromal condition (Reardon and Donnai 2007). Chromosomal abnormalities are seen in approximately 10% of cases. Teratogens known to be associated with CL/P are alcohol, maternal diabetes and phenylketonuria. There are over 300 genetic syndromes in which CL/P have been described (Winter and Baraitser 2010). In the presence of a newborn with growth deficiency and

microcephaly, hypotonia, a prominent glabella and short upper lip, a chromosomal exam with specific request for FISH of 4p16.3 can confirm the diagnosis of Wolf–Hirschhorn syndrome or deletion 4p- syndrome (Fig. 31.16). These newborns have serious feeding difficulties that often require gastrostomy and are expected to have profound mental retardation. Very poor life expectancy is predicted in a newborn whose chromosomes show trisomy 13 who also have prenatal onset of growth deficiency, brain malformations including HPE or agenesis of corpus callosum, defects of the eye (microphthalmia, iris colobomas), polydactyly and scalp defects (Fig. 31.17).

The head

Macrocephaly

Macrocephaly refers to an abnormally large head inclusive of the scalp, cranial bone and intracranial contents. The measurement of head circumference, also known as occipital frontal circumference (OFC), encircles the largest diameter which includes the most prominent part of the glabella to the most prominent posterior area of the occiput. An OFC measurement of more than 2 SD above the mean is customary for the definition of macrocephaly.

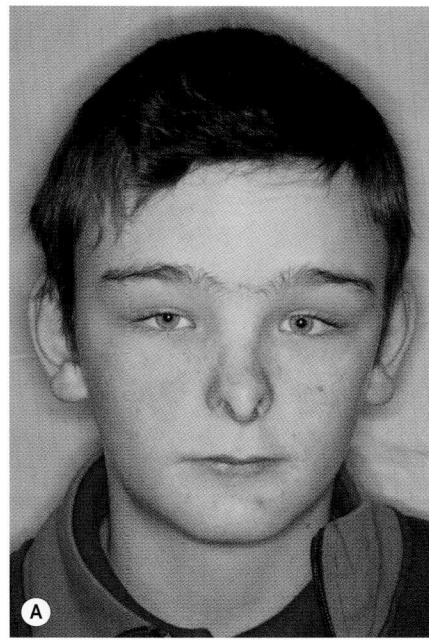

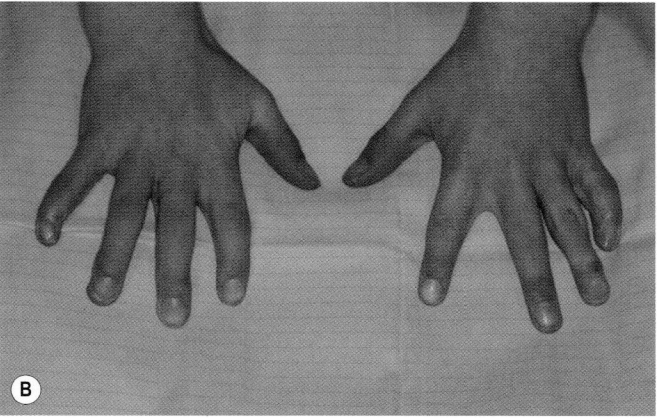

Fig. 31.14 (a–b) The face of an older child with oculodentodigital syndrome. Note the hypotelorism and the well-formed columella of the nose but hypoplasia of the alae nasi. Postsurgery the hands show the typical distribution of the syndactyly in this autosomal-dominant condition involving fingers 3–5.

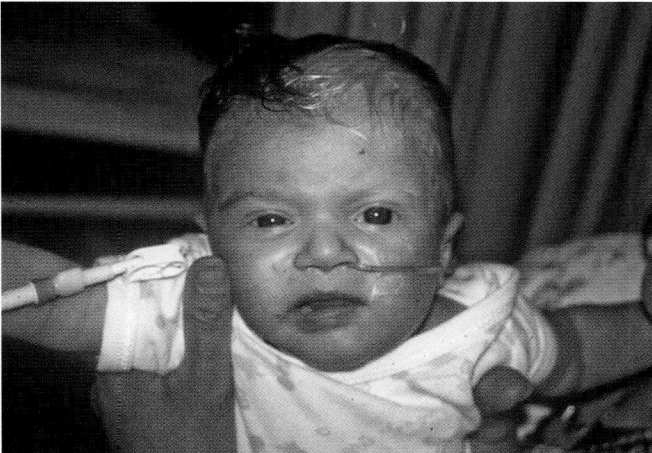

Fig. 31.15 The white forelock denoting underlying Waardenburg syndrome is well demonstrated in this newborn.

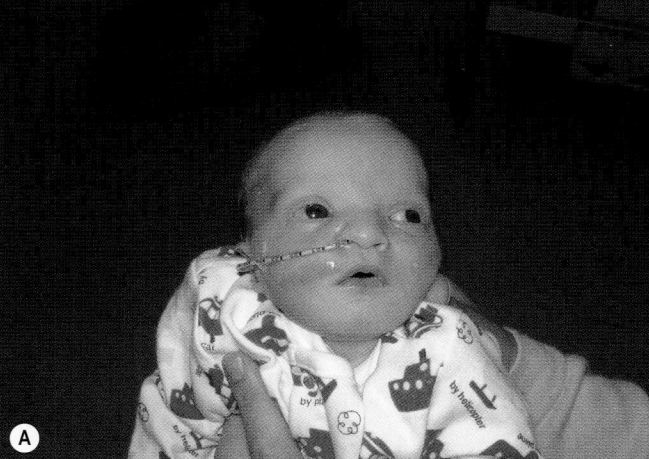

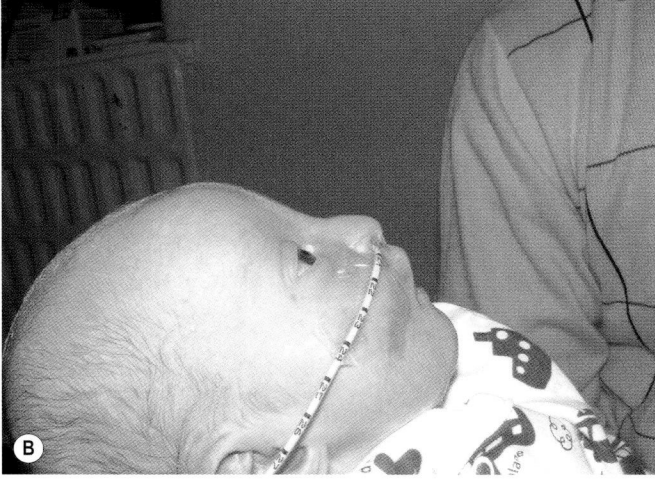

Macrocephaly may reflect a large variety of non-genetic (acquired) or genetic (non-syndromal and syndromal) causes. The genetic and acquired types of macrocephaly can be categorised based on associated physical, metabolic or brain imaging findings. Non-genetic macrocephalies are due to secondary effects of environment agents and these can include infections, hydrocephalus, subdural effusions, arachnoid cysts and neonatal intraventricular haemorrhage. Non-syndromic macrocephaly refers to conditions in which the enlarged brain is the predominant abnormality, not associated with other noteworthy major malformation or notable physical trait. An enlarged cranial vault may produce as a secondary effect minor craniofacial changes. These changes include a prominent or high forehead and a dolichocephalic (long skull) head shape. Increased width of the cranial base can occasionally cause mild hypertelorism and downslanting palpebral fissures. In contrast, the facial area may be relatively small, giving a triangular craniofacial appearance. Macrocephaly can be familial. Syndromic macrocephaly means that significant abnormalities (physical or behavioural) are associated

Fig. 31.16 The facial features of Wolf–Hirschorn syndrome, caused by deletion of chromosome 4p16.3, are instantly recognisable. Note the 'Greek helmet' appearance of the nose in profile.

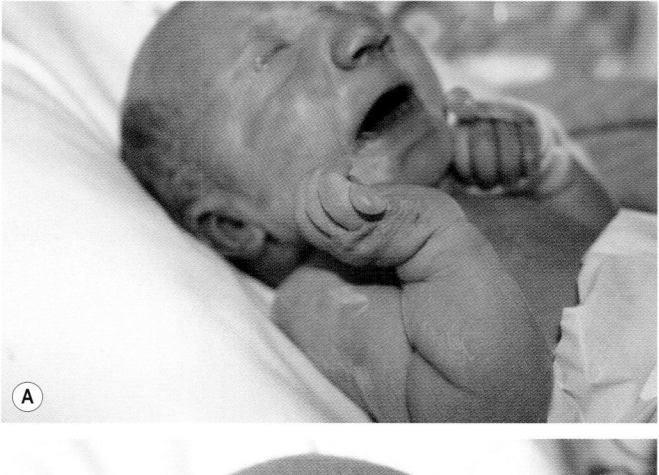

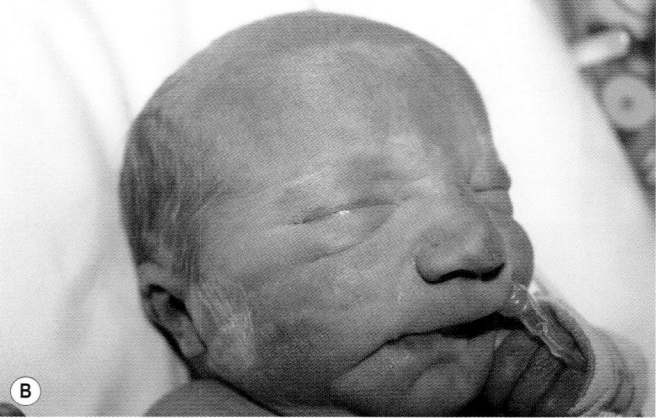

Fig. 31.17 (a, b) Note the postaxial polydactyly in this case of Patau syndrome. The face shows the uncommon anophthalmic presentation of Patau syndrome, the more common presentation being bilateral cleft lip. Patau syndrome is an important aspect of the differential diagnosis of the anophthalmic/microphthalmic neonate.

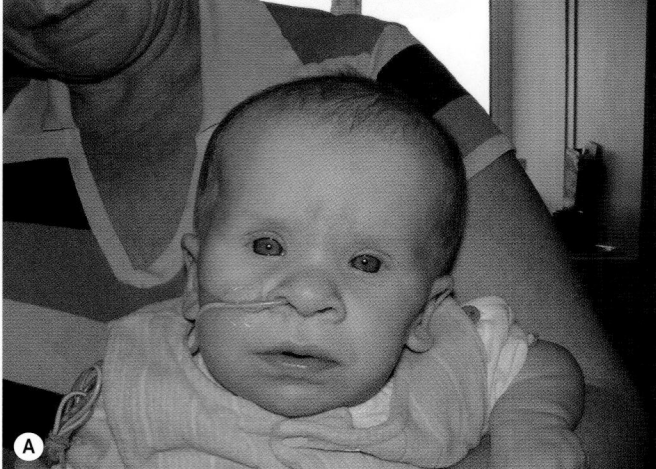

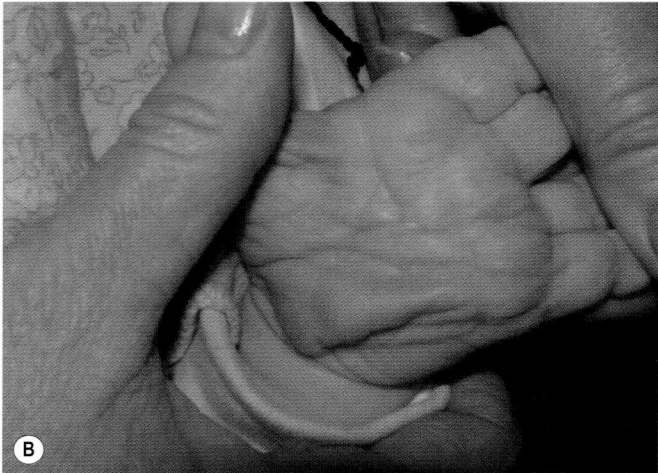

Fig. 31.18 (a, b) A patient with Costello syndrome. Note the coarse facial features and the excess skin of the hands. These patients need follow-up for tumour development and for cardiomyopathy.

with the generalised brain enlargement. The constellation of these abnormalities creates a recognisable pattern worthy of a syndromic designation. Syndromic macrocephalic conditions should be distinguished from other genetic syndromes in which macrocephaly is an occasional but not consistent, or clinically predominant, finding (Williams et al. 2008). An OMIM search for macrocephaly retrieved 258 genetic entries (OMIM, March 2011).

Among neurocardiofaciocutaneous syndromes, Costello syndrome has a distinctive facial appearance that may not be recognised in the newborn. Typically, the chin may be pointed and small and the ears are fleshy and may be cupped and posteriorly rotated. The hair can be sparse or normal or excessively curly. Full lips are characteristic (Allanson 2003) (Fig. 31.18). A cardiac anomaly can be detected in approximately two-thirds of individuals, including structural cardiovascular malformations, cardiac hypertrophy and rhythm disturbances, especially atrial tachycardia. They seem to be a risk factor for death, as was found in all patients of a series of 12 individuals diagnosed with Costello syndrome (Lin et al. 2002). Skin abnormalities are common and often discriminating. They include soft skin, deep palmar creases, premature ageing and wrinkling. The pregnancy may be characterised by polyhydramnios and swallowing difficulties, leading to failure to thrive, and the need for gavage feeding in the neonatal period is well described (Lin et al.

2010). Mutations in H-Ras gene can confirm the clinical diagnosis (Aoki et al. 2005).

When hydrocephalus is diagnosed prenatally in a male fetus a diagnosis to consider is aqueductal stenosis, an X-linked condition caused by mutations in LICAM gene (Finckh et al. 2000; De Angelis et al. 2002). The family history can be especially helpful in validating this suspected diagnosis if a history of male mental retardation and/or hydrocephalus is established. Macrocephaly also characterises Greig cephalopolysyndactyly, a diagnosis established clinically in macrocephalic patients by the associated limb anomalies. In more than three-quarters of cases, patients have postaxial polydactyly of the hands, but may also demonstrate broad thumbs, and variable degrees of syndactyly. By contrast, the feet in Greig syndrome present with preaxial polydactyly, broad halluces and syndactylies of toes 1–3. This syndrome is allelic to Pallister–Hall syndrome and both conditions are due to mutations involving the GLI3 locus on chromosome 7 (Debeer et al. 2003) (Fig. 31.19).

Microcephaly

Microcephaly is an important finding in a neonate and reflects impairment of the normal growth of the brain. Such an effect may

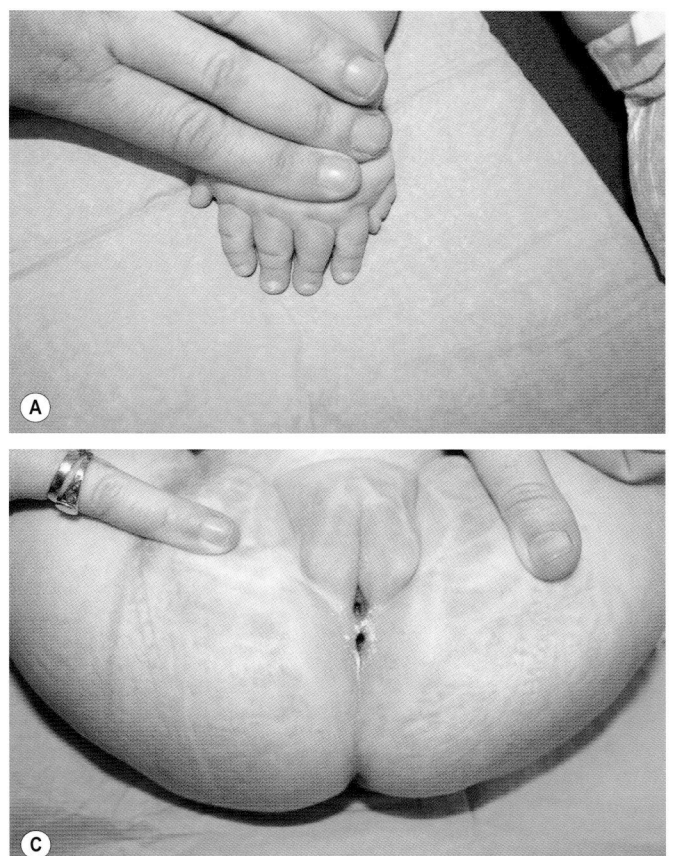
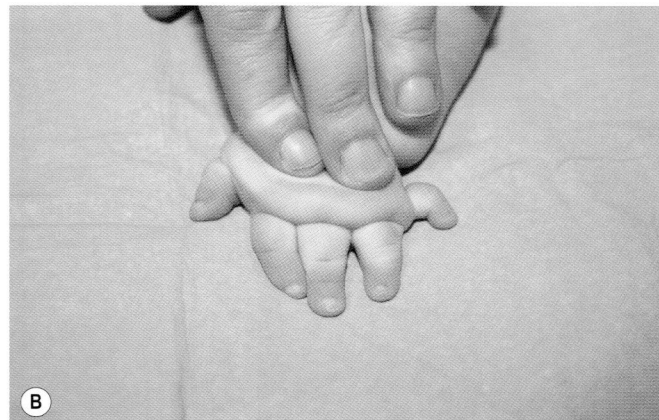

Fig. 31.19 (a, b) The various forms of polydactyly which can signal Pallister–Hall syndrome are shown in both hands from the same newborn. Note the right sided polydactyly in fig (a). (c) The anterior placement of the anus is another good pointer to this diagnosis.

be genetic or of other cause. By strict definition, microcephaly is diagnosed in any child with a head circumference 3 SD below the mean, when this head size is disproportionately small in relation to the rest of the body (Woods 2004). Regardless of aetiology, microcephaly may be congenital, also referred to as primary microcephaly, or of postnatal onset, known as secondary microcephaly. The finding of microcephaly in a newborn should start a comprehensive process of evaluation. Before embarking upon extensive investigations possible non-genetic causes for the microcephaly should be considered. Disruptive injuries, such as ischaemic and haemorrhagic stroke, intrauterine death of a monozygous twin, infectious causes (e.g. toxoplasmosis, other infections, rubella, cytomegalovirus and herpes simplex virus: TORCH), teratogens such as alcohol and maternal factors, including hypothyroidism, anaemia, malnutrition, folate deficiency and phenylketonuria, have all been established causes of acquired microcephaly. Much progress has been recorded in identifying loci causing inherited forms of microcephaly in recent years (Mochida 2009). Many of the microcephaly genes identified to date have been associated with specific phenotypes, facilitating targeted clinical testing. Chromosomal testing and related technologies such as FISH and comparative genomic hybridisation continue to have a role in particular situations and the finding of primitive chromatin condensation is an important clue to the rare autosomal-recessive form of microcephaly known as MCPH1 (Trimborn et al. 2004; Abuelo 2007).

Neuroimaging is useful in identifying structural malformations in the child with microcephaly (Ashwal et al. 2009). A search of the OMIM database revealed 738 conditions which involve microcephaly. Among the most common are trisomy 13, 18 and 21.

Likewise, microcephaly is a feature of several other conditions associated with a chromosomal basis, among the better known being cri-du-chat syndrome caused by terminal deletion of the short arm of chromosome 5. The name derives from the cat-like cry, the best clinical prompt to the diagnosis and its formal establishment by appropriate cytogenetic analysis.

Mild prenatal growth and microcephaly characterise Williams syndrome, which has an estimated prevalence of 1 in 10 000 births. Failure to thrive (80%), feeding problems (70%) and prolonged colic (70%) are common findings (Morris et al. 1988). The facial features of Williams syndrome are characteristic. Infants have a broad forehead, bitemporal narrowing, low nasal root, periorbital fullness, stellate/lacy iris pattern, strabismus, bulbous nasal tip, malar flattening, long philtrum, full lips, small jaw and prominent earlobes (Morris 2010). Since 1964, it has been known that Williams syndrome is associated with supravalvular aortic stenosis and this finding alone in a neonate should prompt a specific molecular cytogenetic testing for Williams syndrome (Garcia et al. 1964). Idiopathic hypercalcaemia of infancy has been documented in 15% of individuals with Williams syndrome and is usually present in the first 18 months of life (Kruse et al. 1992).

Wolf–Hirschhorn syndrome or 4p- deletion syndrome is another chromosomal condition which is typically associated with microcephaly (Fig. 31.20). Whereas microcephaly is an important feature of Seckel syndrome, the clinical picture is characterised by marked prenatal growth deficiency, the head circumference, length and birthweight all being greatly reduced, typically −5 to −10 SD. The face is characterised by a receding forehead, prominent nose, micrognathia, low-set, malformed ears and large eyes. Neuroimaging

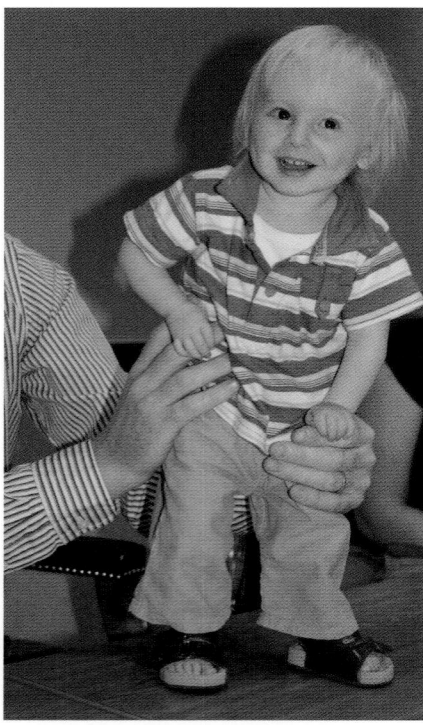

Fig. 31.20 Osteodysplastic primordial dwarfism, caused by mutation of the pericentrin gene, has caused a complete failure of growth in this boy, aged 2.5 years. His growth parameters at birth were already below the third centile for all measurements: birth weight at 38 weeks was 1.9 kg, while occipitofrontal circumference was 29.5 cm.

often shows cerebral gyral pattern simplification. This clinical presentation is genetically heterogeneous with some cases due to mutations in the gene encoding ataxia-teleangiectasia and Rad3-related protein (ATR) at 3q11.1 (O'Driscoll et al. 2003), while other cases are due to mutation of the pericentrin locus (Rauch et al. 2008).

Craniosynostosis

Craniosynostosis is a group of conditions caused by premature fusion of one or more cranial sutures. This arises in 1 per 2000 births. The function of the cranial suture is to allow adjustment for the growing brain. Fontanelles are formed at the junctional boundaries of the cranial sutures where, for a transitory period, larger areas of connective tissue occur without underlying bone. The fusion of sutures that accompanies normal development leads to closure of the posterior and anterior fontanelles by 3 and 20 months, respectively. Craniosynostosis results from premature ossification and fusion of the skull sutures and generally results in alteration of the shape of the cranial vault and/or premature closure of the fontanelles. Craniosynostosis may be classified as simple (involving one suture) or complex (involving two or more sutures); primary (caused by an intrinsic defect in the suture) or secondary (premature closure of normal sutures because of another medical condition such as deficient brain growth); isolated (occurring without other anomalies) or syndromic (accompanied by other dysmorphic features or developmental defects). The frequencies of the various sutures involved are sagittal 40–58%, coronal 20–29%, estimated one-third caused by single-gene mutations; metopic 4–10%, aetiology essentially unknown, though specific association with chromosome 11pdel and 9pdel lambdoid 2–4%, aetiology unknown (Kimonis et al. 2007).

The alteration in shape of the cranial vault varies with sutures fused, such that compensatory growth occurs in dimensions not restricted by sutures. Normally, the skull grows in planes perpendicular to the sutures, but premature fusion forces growth in a plane parallel to the closed suture. When associated anomalies or delays are present, the possibility of a syndrome should be considered. There are more than 180 syndromes which manifest craniosynostosis, and significant progress has been made in understanding their clinical and molecular aspects, in particular the contribution of mutation at the various fibroblast growth factor receptor (FGFR) loci (Wilkie 1997).

Clinical studies have found an unexpectedly high incidence of medical problems among children with non-syndromic craniosynostosis, such as increased intracranial pressure (Wilkie 1997), learning disabilities in sagittal craniosynostosis (Shipster et al. 2003) and strabismus and amblyopia in coronal craniosynostosis (Gupta et al. 2003).

Clinical evaluations should include indepth antenatal history and documentation of any teratogenic exposure because drugs such as fluconazole are associated with craniosynostosis (Aleck and Bartley 1997; Lopez-Rangel and Van Allen 2005). Because of the pleiotropic effects of various craniosynostosis syndromes, a comprehensive review of systems should be performed for other associated medical problems. The autosomal-dominant inheritance and variable expressivity of many disorders mandate that patients and available first-degree relatives should undergo detailed clinical examination. The initial diagnosis of craniosynostosis necessitates investigation for hydrocephalus and structural anomalies by appropriate neuroimaging. Three-dimensional computed tomography, allowing three-dimensional reconstructions of the bony anatomy of both endo- and ectocranial surfaces of the skull, has become the gold standard for diagnosing craniosynostosis. Plain radiographs of the axial skeleton and limbs such as syndactyly, carpal and tarsal fusions, and cervical spine abnormalities remain an integral part of the evaluation of the syndromic forms of craniosynostosis. Patients with craniosynostosis syndromes should be evaluated in craniofacial centres by a multidisciplinary team.

Saethre–Chotzen syndrome

In Saethre–Chotzen syndrome there may a disturbance of coronal, lambdoid and metopic sutures. Typically patients have brachycephaly with a high, flat forehead. The frontal hairline is low, often accompanied by maxillary hypoplasia with narrow palate. It is not unusual for these patients to have facial asymmetry with deviation of nasal septum, shallow orbits, hypertelorism and ptosis (Fig. 31.21). Limb examination may show partial cutaneous syndactyly, especially of second and third fingers or third and fourth toes. There can be short, angulated or flattened thumbs and broad great toes with valgus deformity (Reardon and Winter 1994). This is an autosomal-dominant condition and mutations in TWIST gene are responsible for the phenotype (Rose et al. 1997).

Apert syndrome

Apert syndrome is identifiable from other craniosynostosis syndromes by osseous and cutaneous syndactyly, most commonly with complete fusion of second, third and fourth fingers (Fig. 31.22). The anterior cranial fossa is very short with consequent shallow orbits and orbital hypertelorism. The middle third of the face is retruded and hypoplastic, resulting in relative mandibular prognathism. The nasal bridge is depressed, and hypertelorism, proptosis and downslanting palpebral fissures are observed, often resulting in sleep apnoea and related breathing difficulties. The palate is highly

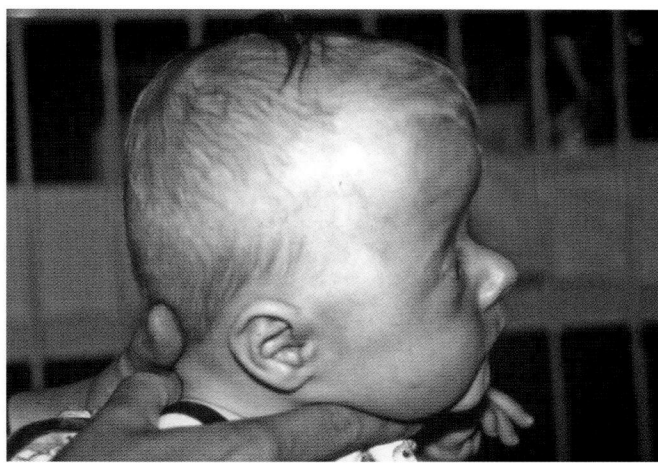

Fig. 31.21 The flat forehead and depressed midface are common features of Saethre–Chotzen syndrome. Also look out for partial syndactyly of the fingers.

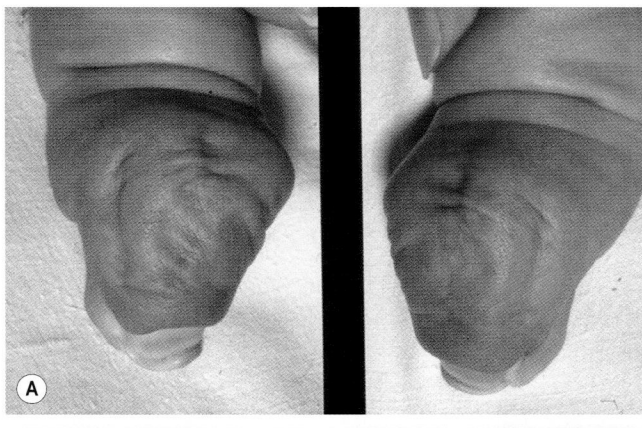

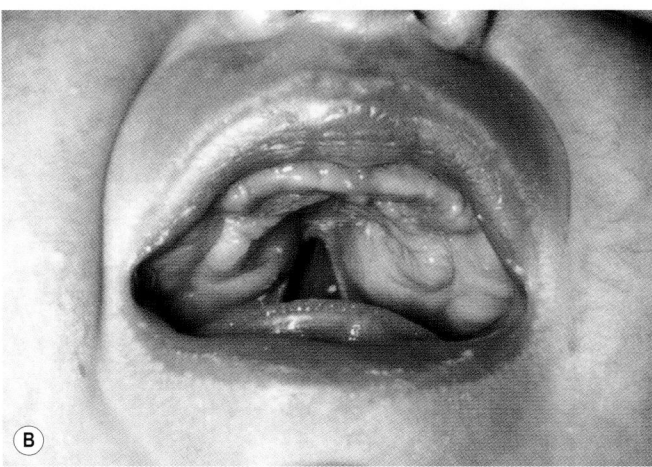

Fig. 31.22 (a, b) The mitten hand of Apert syndrome and the associated cleft palate seen in approximately 30% of cases is always worth checking for.

arched, and cleft of the soft palate is observed in 30% of cases (Slaney et al. 1996). The vast majority of cases are sporadic and have been associated with older paternal age. Most cases of Apert syndrome are caused by two specific mutations at the FGFR2 locus on chromosome 10q25 (Park et al. 1995).

Different mutations in the same gene cause Crouzon syndrome, in which a characteristic facial phenotype is observed without limb involvement. Ocular proptosis is the result of shallow orbits, and patients show hypertelorism, frontal bossing, parrot-beaked nose, short upper lip, hypoplastic maxilla and a relative mandibular prognathism (Carinci et al. 1994). Mutations of FGFR2 are responsible for Crouzon syndrome (Reardon et al. 1994).

Central nervous system

Neural tube defects

NTDs are mutifactorial anomalies which can happen in isolation, but can also be part of known genetic syndromes. About 20% of NTDs appear in the context of a chromosomal disorder such as triploidy or a single-gene condition. Always lethal, anencephaly is characterised by the absence of cranial vault with exposed neural tissue and is associated with spina bifida, facial and nasal clefts and omphalocele. It is first detectable at 11 weeks when the brain will have a 'floppy' outline since the skull is absent (Yang et al. 1992). Amniotic band disruption and environmental agents such as alcohol, antiepileptic medication with hepatic metabolism and rubella have been implicated as possible causes while rare families have been reported with an XL inheritance (Froster and Baird 1993). Anencephaly may be associated with rare malformation syndromes and the presentation of anencephaly with other malformations should be a prompt for a formal genetic assessment by a relevant specialist.

Encephaloceles

Encephaloceles are the result of a failure of neural tube closure in the cranial region. Polyhydramnios may be present and the head size is usually small despite ventriculomegaly. More than 30 genetic, sporadic, chromosomal and single-gene syndromes with encephalocele have been described; some are mentioned in other sections of this chapter, including trisomy 13, amniotic band disruption, Meckel–Gruber syndrome and Walker–Warburg syndrome. While encephaloceles in Meckel–Gruber syndromes are usually posterior, they tend to be anterior and multiple in limb–body wall complex. This lethal association seems to be the result of an early disruptive vascular defect characterised by thoraco- and abdominoschisis with occasional amputation-type limb defects (Van Allen et al. 1987).

Myelomeningocele

Myelomeningocele is the most common type of NTD characterised by protrusion of neural tissue and meninges through open vertebral arches with associated neurological deficits. They mostly occur in the lumbosacral area and are associated with hydrocephalus due to Arnold–Chiari malformation in 90% of cases (Biggio et al. 2001). If isolated the recurrence risk is low, but if part of a genetic syndrome, the recurrence risk is that of the underlying syndrome. This presupposes the assessment and evaluation that will lead to the syndrome identification. A meningomyelocele or encephalocele can be found in babies with renal agenesis and cryptophthalmos in whom the underlying diagnosis is Fraser syndrome. Renal and laryngeal defects are primarily responsible for the high mortality rate within the first year of life in this disorder (Van Haelst et al. 2007).

Holoprosencephaly

Holoprosencephaly (HPE) is a spectrum of disorders of early abnormalities of brain development resulting in a lack of separation of the cerebral hemispheres, including abnormalities of the optic and olfactory bulbs. It is quite rare in newborns (1/10 000) but a frequent abnormality in embryos (1/250). Developmental delay is present in virtually all individuals. The diagnosis may be suspected clinically by hypotelorism (Fig. 31.13) but is made by brain imaging. Although HPE has been associated with maternal diabetes (Barr et al. 1983), up to 50% of individuals with HPE have a chromosomal anomaly detectable by standard (e.g. trisomy 13) or molecular cytogenetics (e.g. FISH for 22q11.2). Another 25% of patients with HPE have recognisable syndromes and the remainder represent non-syndromal forms of HPE (Kauvar and Muenke 2010). To the latter category belong some rare families with autosomal-dominant and autosomal-recessive forms of HPE. The sonic hedgehog (SHH) located at 7q36 is one of the genes responsible for familial and sporadic cases of HPE.

If severe prenatal hydrocephalus is identified in the context of a pregnancy complicated by polyhydramnios and intrauterine growth deficiency, a diagnosis of hydrolethalus syndrome will likely be made, especially after the identification of further salient features at autopsy, including micrognathia and midline CL, with broad nose and microphthalmia, postaxial polydactyly of hands and preaxial polydactyly of feet, cardiac defects in about half of the patients, and multiple complex brain anomalies (Salonen and Herva 1990). A high rate of stillbirths characterises Fryns syndrome; this may be identified prenatally by cystic hygroma. It is likely that an autopsy will reveal a coarse face with CL/P, microretrognathia, diaphragmatic defects and anomalies of the genital tract (Ramsing et al. 2000).

Lissencephaly

Lissencephaly can be described as a smooth outer brain surface and refers to a paucity of gyral and sulcal development (Fig. 31.23). It encompasses a spectrum of gyral malformations ranging from complete agyria to regional pachygyria and includes subcortical band heterotopia. Lissencephaly has been traditionally classified in two distinct groups: classic (formerly lissencephaly type 1) and cobblestone complex (formerly lissencephaly type 2) based on both brain imaging and pathology (Jissendi-Tchofo et al. 2009). Lissencephaly type 1 is characterised by agyria and a thickened cortex and the genes responsible for this defect are LIS1 (17p13.3) and DCX (Xq22.3), with the former being situated in the microdeleted region involved in Miller–Dieker syndrome. Lissencephaly type 2 is characterised by a disorganised cortex, with migration of the cortical cells through defects in the pia. Some of the genes responsible for this group include severe congenital forms of muscular dystrophy like POMT1, involved in the pathogenesis of Walker–Warburg syndrome.

Miller–Dieker syndrome

Postnatal failure to thrive, severe feeding difficulties requiring gastrostomy and frequent complications of aspiration pneumonia are part of Miller–Dieker syndrome. Patients have a recognisable pattern of dysmorphic features, including microcephaly with bitemporal narrowing and high forehead with central furrowing when crying. As with any child who has a chromosomal microdeletion, there can be

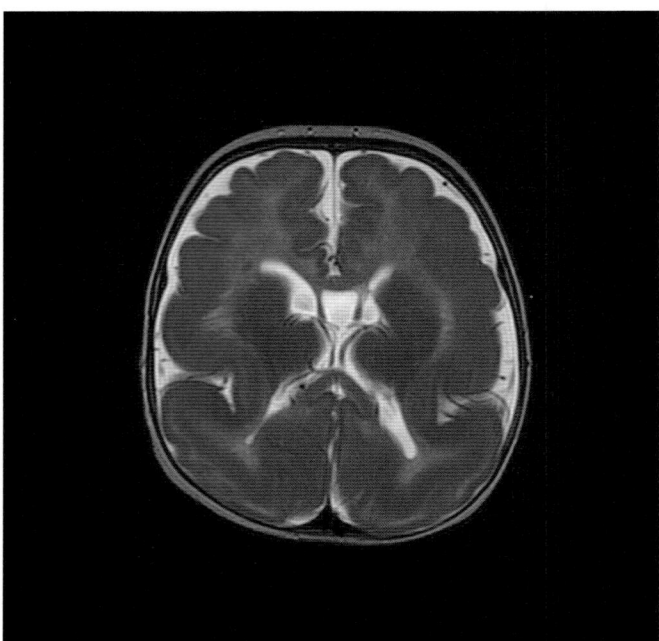

Fig. 31.23 Magnetic resonance imaging from a non-dysmorphic neonate whose feeding problems led to early investigation shows lissencephaly as the underlying condition.

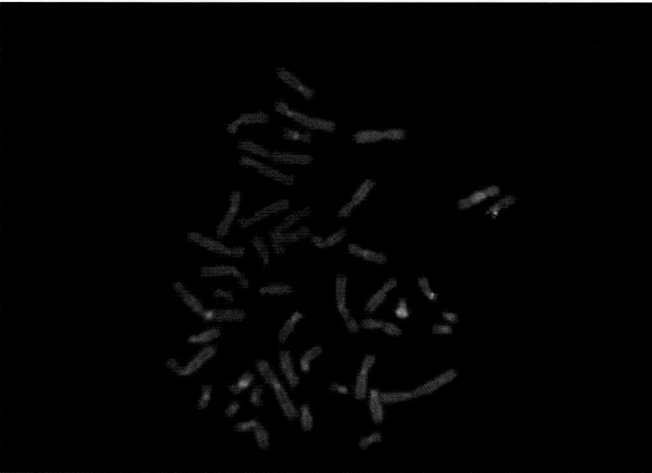

Fig. 31.24 Fluorescence in situ hybridisation showing the deletion of the LIS1 signal (red) on chromosome 17p in the sane patient as in Fig. 31.23.

an occasional congenital cardiac anomaly (especially tetralogy of Fallot), renal anomalies and, in addition to lissencephaly, absent or hypoplastic corpus callosum and large cavum septum pellucidum while brainstem and cerebellum appear grossly normal. FISH demonstrating a heterozygous deletion at 17p13.3 confirms the clinical diagnosis in most de novo cases (Fig. 31.24).

Walker–Warburg syndrome

An acronym is used alternatively to summarise associated defects in the autosomal-recessive condition also known as Walker–Warburg syndrome. HARD ± E stands for hydrocephalus, agyria, retinal dystrophy and sometimes encephalocele. Additionally there is hypoplasia of the cerebellum, ventriculomegaly and scattered areas of polymicrogyria. Besides retinal dysplasia, there are anterior-chamber malformations including cataract, corneal clouding and sometimes glaucoma. The majority of patients succumb within the first year of life to the severe brain anomalies. A minority who do survive longer are profoundly delayed. Mutational analysis of POMT1 locus is available on a clinical basis.

Cardiovascular system

Congenital heart defects

CHDs are present in nearly 1% of all newborns and continue to be a significant cause of death in infancy. Recent progress in disease gene discovery in patients with CHD prompts speculation that previous estimates of 2% for single-gene inheritance were too low (Gelb 2004). When confronted with a child with CHD, the geneticist's concerns are to decide if the situation represents an isolated defect, a possible familial form of CHD, CHD resulting from teratogenic exposures or maternal illness, a possible chromosomal basis or a syndromic condition. Several teratogenic factors have been implicated as causal in CHD, including alcohol, anticonvulsant medication, lithium, retinoic acid and intrauterine infections (e.g. rubella). Likewise a number of maternal illnesses are known to be associated with an increased prevalence of CHD in the fetus – notably diabetes (VSD, coarctation of aorta, truncus arteriosus), phenylketonuria (Fallot's tetralogy, coarctation of aorta) and systemic lupus erythematosus (complete heart block). Gross chromosomal anomalies account for 16% of children presenting with CHD (Sharland et al. 1991). A total of 40–50% of Down syndrome babies have CHDs, the most common being perimembranous VSD, followed by patent ductus arteriosus and ASD. Up to 90% of trisomy 18 patients have CHD (VSD, ASD).

Upwards of two-thirds of cases of 22q11.2 deletion syndrome manifest CHD, the most common lesions being VSD, Fallot's tetralogy, interrupted aortic arch and truncus arteriosus (CHD in 22q22.1). More than 200 features have been described in this genetic condition but the principal elements which challenge parents and carers relate to congenital heart disease, palatal anomalies (69%), hypotonia (about 70%) and transient neonatal hypocalcaemia, which occurs in 60% of cases and can lead to tetanic seizures. The facial features are not consistent (Botto et al. 2003). A deletion at 22q11.2 location can be identified in 95% of cases (Fernandez et al. 2005).

Pulmonary artery stenosis (20–50%), but also hypertrophic cardiomyopathy (20–30%), ASD, Fallot's tetralogy, aortic coarctation, mitral valve anomalies and atrioventricular canal are the most common CHDs found in Noonan syndrome. Cardinal clinical signs of this disorder comprise short stature, developmental delay, webbing of the neck and pectus excavatum and coagulation dysfunction. The most commonly described facial features consist of wide-set eyes with epicanthal folds, ptosis of eyelids, downslanting palpebral fissures, low nasal bridge and low-set and abnormal auricles (Fig. 31.25). Up to 20% of Noonan patients with cardiomyopathy die in the first 2 years of life. Approximately 90% of Noonan syndrome patients can be shown to have mutations in one of the four genes involved in the aetiology (PTPN11 50–60%, KRAS 5%, SOS1 10–15%, RAF1 3–8%) (Allanson 2007).

Gastrointestinal system

Gastroschisis

Gastroschisis is the intrauterine evisceration of the fetal intestine through a paraumbilical wall defect and affects 1 in 4000 births.

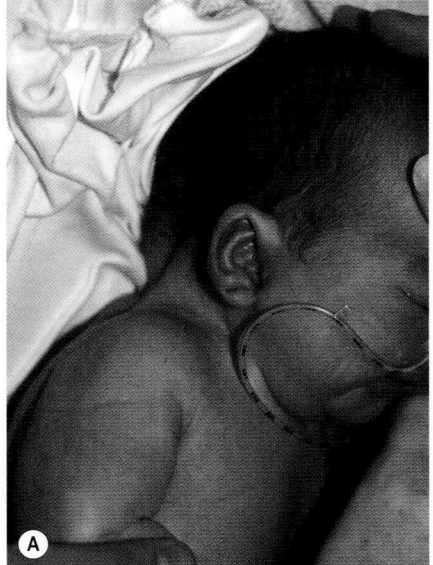

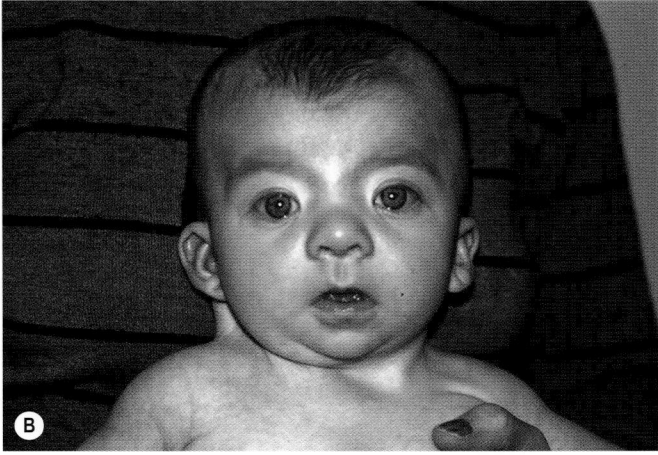

Fig. 31.25 Photograph in the neonatal period (a) and at 6 months of age (b) of a child with Noonan syndrome whose presentation was with polyhydramnios in utero. Note the nuchal redundancy.

Gastroschisis is usually detectable at around 13 weeks' gestational age as an isolated defect but prematurity and growth retardation are not unusual. Although this defect is sometimes associated with a widespread neuromuscular disorder, known as amyoplasia congenita, no specific genetic cause has been found for gastroschisis. However, epidemiological studies have demonstrated a significant increase in prevalence among births to young, nulliparous mothers (Mastroiacovo et al. 2007). The likelihood of a demonstrable chromosomal anomaly in a newborn with isolated gastroschisis is negligible (Hunter and Wand Stevensons 2008). Prompt surgical management has improved the rate of survival to 96% in developed countries (Nichol et al. 2008).

Omphalocele

Omphalocele (also termed exomphalos) represents herniated abdominal viscerae covered by a transparent sac of amnion attached to the umbilical ring. Like gastroschisis, this abnormality can be detected at about 11 weeks' gestational age if the liver is present in the mass. Polyhydramnios is often present. The prognosis depends on the presence or absence of associated malformations and the size of the defect. Mortality can be as high as 30%. Associated anomalies are found in about 60% and include CHDs, bladder exstrophy, NTDs, CL/P, imperforate anus and congenital diaphragmatic hernia (CDH) (Salihu et al. 2003). In contrast to gastroschisis, some 25% of cases have a chromosomal basis (trisomy 13, 18 and 21).

Omphalocele is one of the cardinal features of BWS, together with macrosomia, macroglossia, organomegaly and neonatal hypoglycaemia (see genetic conditions related to overgrowth, below).

Hirschsprung disease

Hirschsprung disease is a result of the complete absence of myenteric and submucosal plexuses in distal intestine development arising from the neural crest. Hirschsprung disease can be familial, syndromic or sporadic and occurs in 1 every 500 live births (Robertson et al. 1997). Symptoms usually begin at birth with delayed passage of meconium. Alternative presentations include neonatal intestinal obstruction or severe constipation in infants. In the majority of cases Hirschsprung disease occurs as a non-syndromal condition with a predominance of males, variable expressivity, incomplete penetrance and genetic heterogeneity (Badner et al. 1990). In about 12% of cases a chromosomal anomaly, such as trisomy 21, can be found while in 18% of cases Hirschsprung disease is part of a malformation syndrome.

Waardenburg syndrome type IV

An association between pigmentary anomalies, hearing loss and Hirschsprung disease is encountered in Waardenburg syndrome type IV. Mutations in the endothelin-B receptor gene (EDNRP), the gene for its ligand (EDN3) and the SOX10 gene can all result in a type 4 Waardenburg syndrome presentation (Ohtani et al. 2006; Bondurand et al. 2007; Barnett et al. 2009).

Mowat–Wilson syndrome

Hirschsprung disease can also arise in Mowat–Wilson syndrome, a sporadic entity characterised by microcephaly and distinctive facies. There is a low nasal bridge with a prominent tip, and the upper lip is full centrally and thin laterally (Fig. 31.26). The ears are

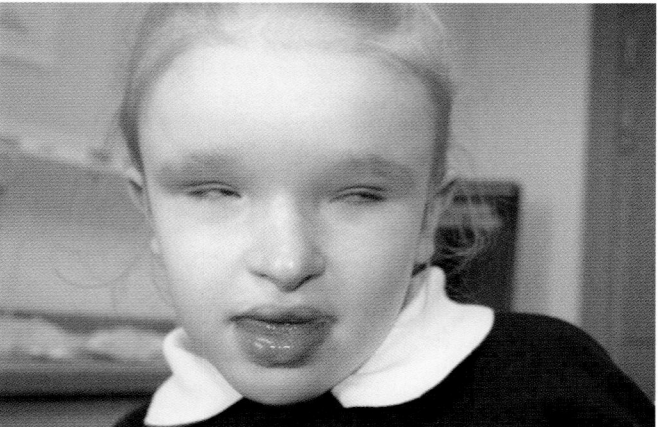

Fig. 31.26 Note the configuration of the upper lip in this child with Mowat–Wilson syndrome. The lip is full centrally but does not maintain the fullness across the full width of the upper lip, tapering to a narrower dimension laterally.

posteriorly rotated and large and have uplifted lobes. Almost half of the patients have cardiac anomalies and males can have hypospadias, cryptorchidism, hooding and webbed penis (Mowat et al. 1998). The condition results from a de novo or heterozygous mutation of the ZFHX1B gene (Zweier et al. 2002).

Congenital diaphragmatic hernia

Congenital diaphragmatic hernia (CDH) (Ch. 27, part 6) reflects a developmental defect in the formation of the diaphragm, in consequence of which some elements of the abdominal contents extend into the chest cavity. Left CDH can be detected as early as 12 weeks in some cases, with around 60% of cases being diagnosed antenatally by ultrasound (Garne et al. 2002). The two most important predictors for survival are the degree of pulmonary hypoplasia and the coexistence of associated anomalies. These include cardiac (20% of cases) as well as CNS (30% of cases) anomalies, but renal and vertebral anomalies have also been reported (Keijzer and Puri 2010). Most cases arise sporadically with a low recurrence risk (less than 2%). Rare kindreds have shown autosomal-dominant, X-linked and autosomal-recessive inheritance for isolated CDH, but CDH can be a component of several genetic syndromes (Enns et al. 1998). Trisomy 13 and 18 may both present with CDH. The same malformation may be the presenting feature of Cornelia de Lange syndrome (Fig. 31.2) and Pallister–Killian syndrome (Fig. 31.6).

Genitourinary system

The estimated incidence of clinically detectable ambiguous genitalia is about 2.2 per 10 000 births (Thyen et al. 2006). Given the controversy that has persisted for a long time in reference to disorders of sexual differentiation, a new nomenclature that removes gender differences and incorporates genetic aetiology and descriptive aetiology has been suggested (Hughes et al. 2006). Chromosomal sex is established at fertilisation and the differentiated gonads develop into either testes or ovaries. A child's phenotypic sex results from the differentiation of internal ducts and external genitalia under the influence of hormones and transcription factors. Any discordance during these complex processes results in ambiguous genitalia. Respectful multidisciplinary assessment is the recommended approach to sexually ambiguous presentations (Lambert et al. 2010). Genetic tests include a standard karyotype. If the clinical exam has revealed sufficient clues towards a specific diagnosis, direct sequencing of the causal gene is indicated. Examples of such situations that can be clarified by mutation analysis are androgen-insensitivity syndrome and congenital adrenal hyperplasia (CYP21). In the absence of a genetic cause following clinical, endocrine and radiological evaluation, array CGH should be undertaken to look for changes in the dosage of genetic material (deletions/duplications). Several genes are involved in testis determination and mutations in any of these genes may result in gonadal dysgenesis. Hence in 46,XY patients with masculinised genitalia, testing should be entertained for the loci SRY, DAX1, WT1 and SOX9.

Constitutional mutations in the WT1 gene can lead to different phenotypes. Denys–Drash syndrome is characterised by a triad of genitourinary anomalies, renal impairment and Wilms tumours, the latter being diagnosed in half of patients by 16 months of age (Pelletier et al. 1991). WAGR syndrome includes features such as Wilms tumour, aniridia, genitourinary anomalies and mental retardation. The mean age at diagnosis for Wilms tumour is 29 months. In this case the causative mechanism involves a deletion at 11p13 that includes WT1 gene. The external genitalia are usually normal in females with WAGR syndrome (Fischbach et al. 2005).

The most important diagnosis in 46,XX patients with masculinised genitalia is congenital adrenal hyperplasia. Congenital adrenal hyperplasia is estimated to occur in approximately 1 per 16 000 births. 21-hydroxylase (21-OHD) deficiency is the most common cause of congenital adrenal hyperplasia, a family of autosomal-recessive disorders involving impaired synthesis of cortisol from cholesterol by the adrenal cortex. In 21-OHD congenital adrenal hyperplasia, excessive adrenal androgen biosynthesis results in virilisation in all individuals and salt-wasting in some individuals. Newborns with salt-wasting 21-OHD congenital adrenal hyperplasia are at risk for life-threatening salt-wasting crises. Individuals with the non-classic form of 21-OHD congenital adrenal hyperplasia present postnatally with signs of hyperandrogenism; females with the non-classic form are not virilised at birth (Shaw 2010). More information on postnatal management can be found in Chapter 34 part 2.

Musculoskeletal system

Polydactyly describes one or more extra digits on hands or feet. The appearance can be very variable, from a complete extra digit to a minimal skin tag with intermediary forms of broad or bifid digits. Postaxial polydactyly occurs in 1 in 3000 live births of white infants, but it is 10 times more common in black populations. More than 100 malformation syndromes have been described with polydactyly, including many short-limbed skeletal dysplasias and chromosomal abnormalities such as trisomies 13, 18 and 21.

Short distal extremities, polydactyly, especially of fingers, and nail hypoplasia characterise Ellis–van Creveld syndrome. The babies are short and manifest hypoplastic distal phalanges. The thorax is short and narrow with poorly developed ribs. Clues leading to gestalt diagnosis include the presence of a natal tooth, multiple frenula of the upper lip and possible CHD, most commonly ASD (Fig. 31.3). This disorder has an autosomal-recessive pattern of inheritance and two genes located at 4p16 are responsible for the phenotype (Ruiz-Perez et al. 2003).

The observation of short limbs in a newborn indicating a disproportionate build should immediately alert the clinician to the possibility of a skeletal dysplasia. This group of genetic conditions, also known as osteochondrodysplasias, is a heterogeneous group of more than 350 disorders frequently associated with orthopaedic complications and varying degrees of dwarfism or short stature (Krakow and Rimoin 2010). Although individually rare, collectively the incidence of these disorders is in the range of 1 in 5000 (Orioli et al. 1986). Many of the prenatal-onset skeletal dysplasias are associated with lethality because of pulmonary insufficiency or concomitant visceral abnormalities.

What follows are a few examples of disorders that can be diagnosed early in life or prenatally. Resources such as the International Skeletal Dysplasias Registry (http://www.csmc.edu/skeletaldysplasia) and the European Skeletal Dysplasia Network (http://www.esdn.org) can be used for support with diagnosis.

In the group of disorders of poor bone mineralisation, osteogenesis imperfecta (OI) is a heterogeneous group of conditions characterised by excessive tendency to antenatal and/or postnatal fractures. Other clinical features include blue sclerae, adult-onset hearing loss and joint laxity. The severity is variable, from lethal in the perinatal period to a predisposition to occasional fractures. OI may be suspected in a fetus as early as 13–14 weeks' gestation for the severe form of OI II and at 16–20 weeks' gestation for OI III, the other forms usually being a diagnosis of later life (Sanders et al. 1994). Inheritance is generally autosomal-dominant but new mutations and recessive inheritance also appertain. When micromelia and undermineralisation of skeleton are found at 14–16 weeks'

gestation, the major differential diagnosis includes OI II, achondrogenesis IA, IB, and II, and the severe infantile form of hypophosphatasia. Aside from generalised undermineralisation, the perinatal lethal form of OI is indicated by the presence of wormian bones, platyspondyly, severely deformed, crumpled, bent, broad femurs and small beaded ribs. If the pregnancy is terminated on the basis of ultrasound findings, the specific diagnosis can be determined by detailed radiology, aided by biochemical study of cultured cells or analysis of DNA from the fetus. For OI, mutation analysis of COL1A1/COL1A2 will reveal a mutation in 98% of cases with the severe form of OI II.

Cleidocranial dysplasia is a skeletal dysplasia characterised by delayed closure of the cranial sutures, hypoplastic or aplastic clavicles and, in later life, multiple dental abnormalities. The most prominent clinical findings are abnormally large, wide-open fontanelles at birth which may remain patent into adult life, midface hypoplasia and abnormal dentition, including delayed eruption of secondary dentition, failure to shed the primary teeth, supernumerary teeth with dental crowding and malocclusion. Clavicular hypoplasia results in narrow, sloping shoulders that can be apposed at the midline and hand abnormalities such as brachydactyly, tapering fingers, and short, broad thumbs. Individuals with cleidocranial dysplasia are shorter than their unaffected siblings and are more likely to have orthopaedic problems, including pes planus, genu valgum and scoliosis. Three-dimensional fetal evaluation may suggest the diagnosis in utero by identifying signs such as large fontanelles, lack of nasal bones, clavicles without the typical S-form, as well as severe delay in calvarial ossification, especially in the midline (Hermann et al. 2009). The prenatal clinical suspicion can be confirmed immediately after birth by an experienced clinician. The diagnosis of cleidocranial dysplasia is based on clinical and radiographic findings that include imaging of the cranium, thorax, pelvis and hands. RUNX2 (CBFA1) is the only gene known to be associated with cleidocranial dysplasia. In all, 60–70% of cleidocranial dysplasia patients have mutations in this gene (Otto et al. 2002).

Campomelic dysplasia is a skeletal dysplasia characterised by distinctive facies, Pierre Robin sequence with CP, shortening and bowing of long bones and club feet. Other findings include laryngotracheomalacia with respiratory compromise and ambiguous genitalia or normal female external genitalia in most individuals with a 46,XY karyotype. Many affected infants die in the neonatal period; additional problems identified in long-term survivors include short stature, cervical spine instability with cord compression, progressive scoliosis and hearing impairment (Glimovsky et al. 2008). Mutations in SOX9 gene confirm the clinical diagnosis in 95% of cases (Meyer et al. 1997).

Skin

Skin defects

Aplasia cutis congenita commonly involves only the skin and is characterised by cutaneous ulcers that may look punched-out, stellate or elongated. At birth these lesions are usually covered by a glistening membrane which may then ulcerate (Fig. 31.27). The mortality associated with aplasia cutis congenita is related to the depth and size of the defect. With involvement of the dura, bone and scalp the mortality can approach 50%, with the risk of infection, meningitis, venous thrombosis and sagittal sinus haemorrhage (Bharti et al. 2011). The disorder is usually seen on the scalp, often as a solitary lesion without other anomalies (Irons and Olson 1980). If the aplasia patch is open the treatment is usually surgical using skin flaps; otherwise it can be conservative (Ribuffo et al.

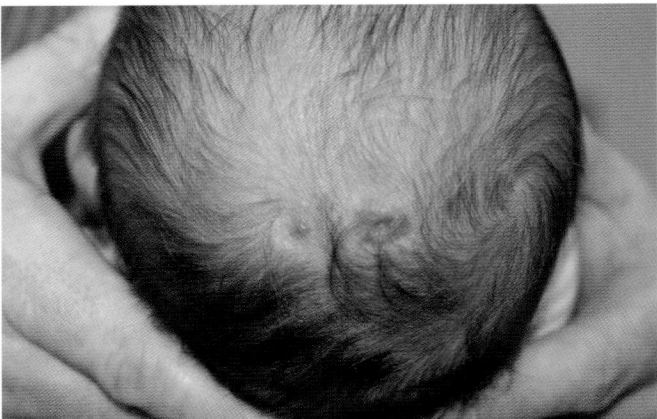

Fig. 31.27 Typical example of aplasia cutis congenita in a 3-day-old neonate.

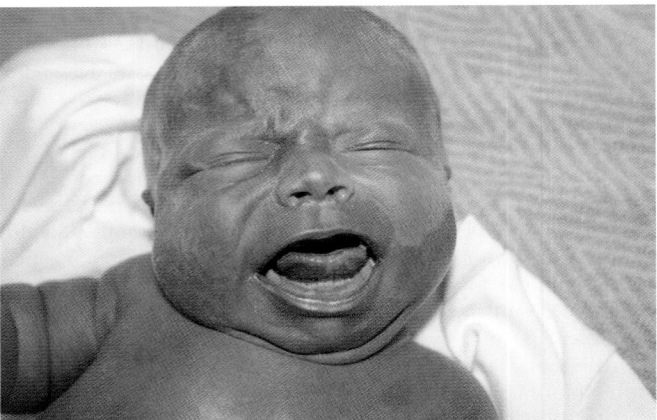

Fig. 31.28 Facial haemangioma in the distribution of the ophthalmic division of the fifth nerve signals the diagnosis of Sturge–Weber syndrome.

2003). Most cases are either autosomal-dominant familial or sporadic.

One specific syndrome associated with aplasia cutis is Adams–Oliver syndrome, an autosomal-dominant condition that manifests the combination of aplasia cutis and terminal transverse defects of limbs (Davis et al. 1993). The larger the scalp defect, the more likely it is to be associated with underlying defects of the bone. The terminal transverse defects can be very variable, including lower legs, feet, hands, fingers, toes or distal phalanges. In some cases there can be only short fingers or small toenails (Verdyck et al. 2003).

Cutis laxa is an acquired or inherited skin disorder characterised by wrinkled, inelastic skin. In the autosomal-dominant form skin and connective tissue symptoms are frequently apparent at birth or in early childhood. The presence of excessive skinfolds and loose, redundant skin leads to early diagnosis. Associated features include cardiac valve anomalies and hernias. It is important to ask about family members with a medical history of aortic dilatation or dissection. Patients with an X-linked cutis laxa syndrome have a distinct, unique presentation at birth. Besides generalised cutis laxa they have a thin face, long philtrum, hooked and beaked nose, brittle hair, high forehead and large fontanelle, giving a distinct facial appearance. Systemic involvement includes failure to thrive due to chronic diarrhoea, malabsorption, congenital hydronephrosis and urethral and bladder diverticula. Skeletal anomalies consist of large and late-closing fontanelle, narrow chest, pectus carinatum, coxa valga, short tubular bones, pelvic exostosis, kyphosis and platyspondyly. The specific sign of occipital horn exostoses of the skull is diagnostic for the disease. X-linked cutis laxa syndrome is allelic to Menkes disease and is caused by mutations in the copper transporter gene ATP7A (Morava et al. 2009).

Reduced skin elasticity identifiable in the neonatal period is the hallmark of restrictive dermopathy. This rare genetic disorder, mostly inherited in an autosomal-recessive manner, belongs to a large family of conditions called laminopathies. What all these condition have in common are mutations in one gene, Lamin A/C. Clinical and pathological findings are distinctive and allow for a specific diagnosis in most cases. Furthermore, polyhydramnios, decreased fetal movement, facial dysmorphisms and arthrogryposis are characteristic of restrictive dermopathy. Respiratory insufficiency leads to an early neonatal death. The typical characteristics are unusually tight and thick skin, joint contractures, wide sutures and characteristic facial features such as micrognathia, low-set ears, an amotile, open mouth or O mouth, a small pinched nose and

hypertelorism (Thill et al. 2008). The joint contractures present in the newborn are caused by the absent skin elasticity with consecutive intrauterine decreased fetal movement (also known as fetal akinesia deformation sequence) (Witters et al. 2002).

Vascular anomalies

Most malformations are present at birth and grow proportionally with the child. In the inherited forms, new lesions can appear, but they stay small. The aetiopathological genetic defects have been elucidated for some of these (e.g. Rendu–Osler–Weber syndrome, capillary malformation–arteriovenous malformation) (Brouillard and Vikkula 2007). A sporadic condition of unknown cause is Sturge–Weber sequence, the most common congenital vascular malformation, found in 0.3% of newborns, which is characterised by flat facial haemangiomata and sometimes meningeal haemangiomata with seizures (Fig. 31.28) (Jacobs and Walton 1976). Also called portwine capillary malformation, it is most commonly seen in a facial trigeminal distribution, at times involving the choroid of the eye. Lesions are usually bilateral, and particular care attends those that involve the ophthalmic branch as these cases are at risk of glaucoma. Glaucoma is common (60%) and is usually ipsilateral to the portwine stain (Sujansky and Conradi 1995). Approximately 83% of patients develop seizures of various severities between 2 and 7 months, grand mal and often asymmetric. Sometimes the leptomeninges can be involved without facial stigmata (Garzon et al. 2007). Ophthalmic consultation is essential in the newborn period to assess for glaucoma or buphthalmos caused by underlying choroidal angioma (Nowak 2007). With age, the portwine stain often darkens and can become nodular. However, there has been success at reducing the impact of the lesions using pulsed-dye laser treatments. Complete clearance of the lesion has been achieved in approximately 22% of cases, particularly those of smaller initial size. Results are best when started before age 7 years, and treatment is safe in the first few weeks of life (Ashinoff and Geronemus 1991).

Naevi

Melanocytic naevi are classically divided into those appearing at birth, or congenital melanocytic naevi (CMN), and those appearing after birth, or acquired naevi. Approximately 1% of newborns are born with small congenital naevi (Williams and Pennella 1994).

The estimated frequency of large CMN (LCMN) is 1 in 20 000 (Castilla et al. 1981). Large and giant naevi are always present at birth. Large CMN may be associated with symptomatic or asymptomatic (25%) systemic abnormalities. LCMN involving limbs have been associated with ipsilateral limb underdevelopment. It has been estimated that large naevi, defined as those that will exceed 20 cm in adulthood, carry a 5–15% lifetime risk of melanoma; between 50% and 60% of cutaneous melanomas arising in LCMN are diagnosed before the age of 5 (Kaplan 1974). LCMN may also be associated with the syndrome of neurocutaneous melanosis (NCM) – that is, melanocytic proliferation within the leptomeninges and brain parenchyma. NCM is particularly important to identify given that, when symptomatic, the prognosis is considerably worse than in with patients with LCMN alone (Eaves et al. 1995). Patients with symptomatic NCM frequently display neurological manifestations before the age of 2, namely signs and symptoms of increased intracranial pressure. Hydrocephalus was reported in 64% of cases. It is estimated that 40–62% of patients with NCM will develop leptomeningeal melanoma (Fox 1972).

A particular form of epidermal naevus with a sharp midline demarcation is seen in a genetic condition called CHILD syndrome, which is an acronym for congenital hemidysplasia with ichthyosiform erythroderma and limb defects. The naevus found in CHILD syndrome shows two different patterns of distribution. In more severe cases, there is a striking lateralisation diffusely affecting one side of the body with a strict midline demarcation. On the other hand, the lesions may follow Blaschko's lines. Another remarkable feature of CHILD naevus is its tendency to spontaneous involution and its hairlessness (Happle et al. 1980). Ipsilateral extracutaneous involvement may affect the bones, lung, kidney, heart and brain. The inflammatory lesions of CHILD naevus, which may wax and wane, are covered by large waxy, yellowish scales (Happle et al. 1995). Both patterns are often present and intermingled. The involved nails are dystrophic and often rather thick. A pathognomonic sign is the presence of strawberry-like lesions on the end phalanx of fingers or toes (Bittar and Happle 2004). Skeletal defects may range from a slightly shortened finger to the complete absence of a limb. Short stature and scoliosis are usually noted. During the first months of life, radiographs of the involved side may show epiphyseal stippling (chondrodysplasia punctata) of the long bones, ribs, scapula, vertebrae and pelvis, and sometimes even of the larynx and thyroid cartilage. Abnormally short limb bones may cause contractures. Clefting of hand or foot is frequently noted, and polydactyly has been reported. Associated cardiovascular defects are often fatal and can include the presence of one single ventricle or only one coronary ostium, mitral valve defect, septal defect, dilated right ventricle, coarctation of the aorta, subaortic stenosis and Fallot's tetralogy. Neurological anomalies include ipsilateral hypoplasia of the hemisphere or cranial nerves, electroencephalographic anomalies, mild intellectual impairment, hemiparesis, decreased sensation to touch and heat, and ipsilateral or bilateral sensorineural hearing loss (Happle 2010). This is an X-linked dominant genetic condition, lethal in males and caused by mutations in NSDHL gene, involved in cholesterol metabolism (Konig et al. 2000).

Genetic conditions related to growth deficiency

The evaluation of the small-for-gestational-age (SGA) newborn can be of particular challenge. A study that looked retrospectively at the aetiology of short stature in children showed that about half of the patients had either constitutional delay of growth or familial short stature, both conditions of isolated short stature. Nineteen per cent

of these patients had a cytogenetic abnormality, and about 3% have a recognisable multiple-malformation syndrome (Lam et al. 2002). A diagnosis of SGA requires detailed information regarding the onset of growth deficiency, exposure to teratogens, maternal height, nutritional status, presence of maternal disease during pregnancy or pre-existent conditions (e.g. high blood pressure), parity, presence of more than one fetus, presence or not of additional congenital anomalies, but also familial birth parameters and growth pattern, amniotic fluid volume and placental function (Ch. 10). Preliminary evaluation needs to exclude possible endocrinopathies, many of which can also have a genetic basis. Definitions of SGA vary and it is important to distinguish symmetrical from asymmetrical growth retardation. In babies with additional anomalies besides the short length, disproportion between the limbs and the trunk may signal a likely skeletal dysplasia, already discussed above. For the newborns with normal proportions, the identification of a specific syndrome by clinical means, confirmed, when available, by molecular testing, must be attempted. Adequate genetic tests of cytogenetic and/or molecular nature are important tools for the confirmation of the clinical suspicion, the former especially when no recognisable syndrome was identified in the clinical evaluation, and can include a karyotype or array studies (Seaver and Irons 2009). A few examples of syndromal intrauterine growth retardation (IUGR) conditions are presented below, and although of different genetic aetiology, they share some of the facial features and medical issues (Hall 2010b).

Body asymmetry in a term newborn with prenatal-onset short length and low birthweight always prompts consideration of a possible diagnosis of Russell–Silver syndrome. These babies have a triangular face shape and the head circumference may be in the normal range, thus seeming large relative to body length. Clinodactyly of the fifth finger is very common (69%) and half of the males can have hypospadias, inguinal hernia or cryptorchidism. Conduction heart defects or structural heart anomalies may be found. Newborns with Russell–Silver syndrome often have feeding problems and fail to thrive; half of the patients may present with hypoglycaemia, tachycardia and excessive sweating. About 12% are born with congenital hip dislocation and 20% have café-au-lait spots. There is an association with assisted reproduction (Wakeling et al. 2010). Three-quarters of patients clinically diagnosed with Russell–Silver syndrome have complex imprinting abnormalities involving chromosome 7 and 11 and most cases are sporadic (Bartholdi et al. 2009).

Taking the name from the initials of the authors who first described it, 3-M syndrome patients have a long cranium with frontal bossing and the head looks large relative to body size (Miller et al. 1975). Both length and weight are on the lower percentiles while head circumference is normal. The eyes are wide-set with full eyebrows, fleshy nasal tip, full lips, long philtrum and prominent ears, all in all having what was described as a 'gloomy' appearance (Le Merrer et al. 1991). A short, wide thorax and pectus excavatum are good clinical clues. Genetic heterogeneity seems to exist, but three-quarters of the clinically diagnosed 3-M patients have mutations in CUL7 gene in this autosomal-recessive syndrome (Huber et al. 2005).

On grounds of rarity, Mulibrey nanism is an autosomal-recessive condition whose name represents an abbreviation of the main features involving <u>mu</u>scle, <u>li</u>ver, <u>br</u>ain and <u>ey</u>e. Indeed, patients do have muscle wasting, making their hands and feet look prominent, and they also can be hypotonic. Constrictive pericarditis and heart failure may appear during infancy and underlie a large liver. The eye anomalies are multiple and include hypertelorism (64%), strabismus, hypoplasia of the choroid, coloboma and corneal dystrophy with yellow pigmentary deposits (Sorge et al. 2005).

Majewski osteodysplastic primordial dwarfism type 2 (MOPD2) is a rare syndrome diagnosed usually in term babies with extreme IUGR, where birth length, weight and head circumference, although proportionate, are normal for 28 weeks' gestational age. After birth, however, microcephaly becomes even more prominent (Fig. 31.20). There is a high forehead, the nasal bridge may be raised, the chin is small and the cheeks are full. Males can have criptorchidism and micropenis and occasionally hypospadias. Many complications are described progressively with age, including bone and endocrine changes. Affected individuals (about 25%) develop intracranial aneurysms, but it is not known if they are congenital or develop later (Bober et al. 2010). MOPD2 is an autosomal-recessive condition and the responsible gene, pericentrin, is involved in mitotic spindle activity (Rauch et al. 2008).

Genetic conditions related to overgrowth

Infant macrosomia or a fetus large for gestational age (LGA) is defined as a newborn with growth parameters of length and weight of more than 2 SD above the mean. The LGA infant can result from maternal effects of overweight, maternal diabetes or multiparity. As size is a reflection of increased extracellular fluid volume, an LGA baby can also be the result of a chorioangioma of the placenta, heart failure in utero or asphyxia. Somatic growth and placental growth are closely aligned; the total mass of the trophoblast limits fetal size (Stevenson et al. 1982). Overgrowth syndromes are genetic conditions characterised not only by excessive growth, but also by distinctive facial features, congenital anomalies, mental retardation and neoplasms, all of these aspects contributing to diagnosis (Cohen 1989).

The prototype of the overgrowth conditions is Beckwith–Wiedemann syndrome (BWS). BWS has a prevalence of 1/13 700 neonates, and is caused by imprinting defects in a cluster of genes located on chromosome 11. In about 85% of cases appropriate genetic analysis confirms the clinical diagnosis (Choufani et al. 2010). The clinical picture is variable and no two patients with BWS look the same, but they may have a combination of macrosomia, defects of the abdominal wall (from umbilical hernia to omphalocele), macroglossia, naevus flammeus, ear pits and creases, visceromegaly and propensity for developing embryonal tumours. Infants with BWS have an approximately 20% mortality rate, mainly caused by complications of prematurity. The risk of developing embryonal tumours is about 7.5% and this risk persists until about 8 years of age. The tumours which develop in patients with BWS are Wilms tumour, hepatoblastoma, neuroblastoma, adrenocortical carcinoma and rhabdomyosarcoma. Major and minor diagnostic criteria are well established (Cooper et al. 2005). Cardiomegaly sometimes appears in infancy but tends to resolve without treatment (Elliott and Maher 1994). It is important to identify and adequately treat hypoglycaemia both in the neonatal period and thereafter, in order to avoid easily treatable seizures and long-term consequences regarding developmental delay. There is an association between the observation of BWS in offspring and the use of assisted reproductive technology (Maher 2005).

Isolated hemihyperplasia can be seen in children with BWS and other overgrowth syndromes, but also as an entity on its own, posing a risk of 5.9% for embryonal tumour (Hoyme et al. 1998). Once a diagnosis of BWS or isolated hemihypertrophy is made, a tumour surveillance protocol is recommended for the first 7–8 years of life with regular measurements of plasma alpha-fetoprotein and abdominal ultrasound (Clericuzio and Martin 2009).

Sharing some similarities with BWS, the X-linked Simpson–Golabi–Behmel syndrome (SGBS) is also characterised by pre- and postnatal macrosomia and distinctive craniofacies features including macrocephaly, ocular hypertelorism and macroglossia. Mild to severe mental retardation is usual, in contrast to BWS. Other clinical clues that can help the diagnosis are supernumerary nipples, diastasis recti/umbilical hernia, congenital heart defects, renal defects, such as nephromegaly, multicystic kidneys, hydronephrosis, hydroureter and duplicated ureters. Polysplenia is well described, as is postaxial polydactyly. There is also an increased risk for tumours of about 10%; reported tumours include Wilms tumour, hepatoblastoma, adrenal neuroblastoma, gonadoblastoma and hepatocellular carcinoma (Neri et al. 1998). Up to 70% of SGBS patients have either a point mutation or a deletion in GPC3 gene located at Xq26 (Li et al. 2001).

References

Abuelo, D., 2007. Microcephaly syndromes. Semin Pediatr Neurol 14, 118–127.

Adam, M.P., Manning, M.A., Beck, A.E., et al., 2003. Methotrexate/misoprostol embryopathy: report of four cases resulting from failed medical abortion. Am J Med Genet 123A, 72–78.

Aleck, K.A., Bartley, D.L., 1997. Multiple malformation syndrome following fluconazole use in pregnancy: report of an additional patient. Am J Med Genet 72, 253–256.

Allanson, J., 2003. Costello syndrome: the face. Proc Greenwood Genet Ctr 22, 77.

Allanson, J.E., 2007. Noonan syndrome. Am J Med Genet 145C, 274–279.

Allanson, J.E., Hennekam, R.C.M., 1997. Rubinstein–Taybi syndrome: objective evaluation of craniofacial structure. Am J Med Genet 71, 414–419.

Aoki, Y., Niihori, T., Kawame, H., et al., 2005. Germline mutations in HRAS proto-oncogene cause Costello syndrome. Nat Genet 37, 1038–1040.

Ashinoff, R.A., Geronemus, R.G., 1991. Flashlamp-pumped pulsed tunable dye laser for port-wine stains in infancy: earlier versus later treatment. J Am Acad Dermatol 24, 467–472.

Ashwal, S., Michelson, D., Plawner, L., et al., 2009. Practice parameter: evaluation of the child with microcephaly (an evidence-based review). Neurology 73, 887–897.

Badner, J.A., Sieber, W.K., Garver, K.L., et al., 1990. A genetic study of Hirschprung disease. Am J Hum Genet 46, 568–580.

Barnett, C.P., Mendoza-Londono, R., Blaser, S., et al., 2009. Aplasia of cochlear nerves and olfactory bulbs in association with SOX10 mutation. Am J Med Genet 149A, 431–436.

Barr, Jr., M., Hanson, J.W., Currey, K., et al., 1983. Holoprosencephaly in infants of diabetic mothers. J Pediatr 102, 565–568.

Bartholdi, D., Krajewska-Walasek, M., Ounap, K., et al., 2009. Epigenetic mtations of the imprinted IGF-H19 domain in Silver-Russell syndrome (SRS): results from a large cohort of patients with SRS and SRS-like phenotypes. J Med Genet 46, 192–197.

Battaglia, A., Carey, J.C., 2003. Diagnostic evaluation of developmental delay/mental retardation: an overview. Am J Med Genet 117C, 3–14.

Baujat, G., Faure, C., Zaouche, A., et al., 2001. Oroesophageal motor disorders in Pierre Robin syndrome. J Pediatr Gastroenterol Nutr 32, 297–302.

Bharti, G., Groves, L., David, L.R., Sanger, C., Argenta, L.C., 2011. Aplasia cutis congenita: clinical management of a rare congenital anomaly. J Craniofac Surg Jan, 22 (1), 159–165.

Biggio, J.R., Owen, J., Weinstrom, K.D., 2001. Can prenatal findings predict ambulatory status in fetuses with open spina bifida? Am J Obstet Gynecol 185, 1016–1020.

Bittar, M., Happle, R., 2004. CHILD syndrome avant la lettre. J Am Acad Dermatol 50 (Suppl), S34–S37.

Bober, M.B., Khan, N., Kaplan, J., et al., 2010. Majewski osteodysplastic primordial dwarfism type II (MOPD II): expanding the vascular phenotype. Am J Med Genet 152A, 960–965.

Bondurand, N., Dastot-Le Moal, F., Stanchina, L., et al., 2007. Deletions at the SOX10 gene locus cause Waardenburg syndrome types 2 and 4. Am J Hum Genet 81, 1169–1185.

Botto, L.D., May, K., Fernhoff, P.M., et al., 2003. A population-based study of the 22q11.2 deletion: phenotype, incidence, and contribution to major birth defects in the population. Pediatrics 112, 101–107.

Boulet, S., Althuser, M., Nugues, F., et al., 2009. Prenatal diagnosis of achondroplasia: a new specific sign. Prenat Diagn 29, 697–702.

Brouillard, P., Vikkula, M., 2007. Genetic causes of vascular malformations. Hum Molec Genet 16, R140–R149.

Carinci, F., Avantaggiato, A., Curioni, C., 1994. Crouzon syndrome: cephalometric analysis and evaluation of pathogenesis. Cleft Palate Craniofac J 31, 201–209.

Carmi, R., Boughman, J.A., Ferencz, C., 1992. Endocardial cushion defect: further studies of 'isolated' versus 'syndromic' occurrence. Am J Med Genet 43, 569–575.

Castilla, E.E., Dutra, M.D.G., Oriolo-Parreiras, I.M., 1981. Epidemiology of congenital pigmented naevi. Br J Dermatol 104, 307–315.

Cayler, G.G., Blumenfeld, C.M., Anderson, R.L., 1971. Further studies of patients with the cardiofacial syndrome. Chest 60, 161–165.

Choufani, S., Shuman, C., Weksberg, R., 2010. Beckwith–Wiedemann syndrome. Am J Med Genet 154C, 343–354.

Clericuzio, C.L., Martin, R.A., 2009. Diagnostic criteria and tumor screening for individuals with isolated hemihyperplasia. Genet Med 11, 220–222.

Cohen, Jr., M.M., 1989. A comprehensive and critical assessment of overgrowth and overgrowth syndromes. In: Harris, H., Hirschhorn, K., (Eds.), Advances in Human Genetics, vol. 18. Plenum Press, New York, pp. 373–376.

Cooper, W.N., Luharia, A., Evans, G.A., et al., 2005. Molecular subtypes and phenotypic expression of Beckwith–Wiedemann syndrome. Eur J Hum Genet 13, 1025–1032.

Davis, P.M., Buss, P., Simpson, B.A., et al. 1993. Near fatal haemorrhage from the superior saggital sinus in Adams–Oliver syndrome. Arch Dis Child 68, 433.

De Angelis, E., Watkins, A., Schafer, M., et al., 2002. Disease-associated mutations in L1 CAM interfere with ligand interactions and cell-surface expression. Hum Mol Genet 11, 1–12.

Debeer, P., Peeters, H., Driess, S., et al., 2003. Variable phenotype in Grieg cephalopolysyndactyly syndrome: clinical and radiological findings in four independent families and three sporadic cases with identified GLI3 mutations. Am J Med Genet 120, 49–58.

Eaves, F.F., Brustein, F.D., Hudgins, R., et al., 1995. Primary temporal melanoma without diffuse leptomeningeal involvement: a variant of neurocutaneous melanosis. Plast Reconstr Surg 95, 133–135.

Eichholzer, M., Tonz, O., Zimmermann, R., 2006. Folic acid: a public health-challenge. Lancet 367, 1352–1361.

Elliott, M., Maher, E.R., 1994. Beckwith–Wiedemann syndrome. J Med Genet 31, 560–564.

Enns, G.M., Cox, V.A., Goldstein, R.B., et al., 1998. Congenital diaphragmatic defects and associated syndromes, malformations, and chromosome anomalies: a retrospective study of 60 patients and literature review. Am J Med Genet 79, 215–225.

Fernandez, L., Lapunzina, P., Arjona, D., et al., 2005. Comparative study of three diagnostic approaches (FISH, STRs and MLPA) in 30 patients with 22q11.2 deletion syndrome. Clin Genet 68, 373–378.

Finckh, U., Schroder, J., Ressler, B., et al., 2000. Spectrum and detection rate of L1CAM mutations in isolated and familial cases with clinically suspected L1-disease. Am J Med Genet 92, 40–46.

Fischbach, B.V., Trout, K.L., Lewis, J., et al., 2005. WAGR syndrome: a clinical review of 54 cases. Pediatrics 116, 984–988.

Fox, H., 1972. Neurocutaneous melanosis. In: Vinken, P.J., Bruyn, G.W., (Eds.), Handbook of Clinical Neurology, vol. 14. American Elsevier, New York, pp. 414–428.

Froster, U.G., Baird, P.A., 1993. Amniotic band sequence and limb defects: data from a population-based study. Am J Med Genet 46, 497–500.

Garcia, R.E., Friedman, W.F., Kaback, M.M., et al., 1964. Idiopathic hypercalcemia and supravalvular aortic stenosis. N Engl J Med 271, 117–120.

Garne, E., Haeusler, M., Barisic, I., et al., 2002. Congenital diaphragmatic hernia: evaluation of prenatal diagnosis in 20 European regions. Ultrasound Obstet Gynecol 19, 329–333.

Garzon, M.C., Huang, J.T., Enjolras, O., et al., 2007. Vascular malformations, part II. Associated syndromes. J Am Acad Dermatol 56, 541–564.

Gelb, B., 2004. Genetic basis of congenital heart disease. Curr Opin Cardiol 19, 110–115.

Glimovsky, M., Rosa, E., Tolbert, T., et al., 2008. Campomelic dysplasia: case report and review. J Perinatol 28, 71–73.

Gupta, P., Foster, J., Crowe, S., et al., 2003. Ophthalmologic findings in patients with nonsyndromeic plagyocephaly. J Craniofac Surg 14, 529–532.

Hall, B.D., 2010a. VATER association. In: Cassidy, S.B., Allanson, J.E., (Eds.), Management of Genetic Syndromes, third ed. Wiley-Liss, New Jersey, pp. 607–615.

Hall, J.G., 2010b. Review and hypothesis: syndromes with severe intrauterine growth restriction and very short stature – are they related to the epigenetic mechanism(s) of fetal survival involved in the developmental origins of adult health and disease? Am J Med Genet 152A, 512–527.

Hall, G.J., Allanson, J.E., Gripp, K.W., et al., 2007. Handbook of physical measurements. Oxford University Press, Oxford.

Happle, R., 2010. The group of epidermal nevus syndromes. Part I. Well defined phenotypes. J Am Acad Dermat 63, 1–22.

Happle, R., Koch, H., Lenz, W., 1980. The CHILD syndrome: congenital hemidysplasia with ichthyosiform erythroderma and limb defects. Eur J Pediatr 134, 27–33.

Happle, R., Mittag, H., Kuster, W., 1995. The CHILD nevus: a distinct skin disorder. Dermatology 191, 210–216.

Hermann, N.V., Hove, H.D., Jørgensen, C., et al., 2009. Prenatal 3D ultrasound diagnostics in cleidocranial dysplasia. Fetal Diagn Ther 25, 36–39.

Hoyme, H.E., Seaver, L.H., Jones, K.L., et al., 1998. Isolated hemihyperplasia (hemihypertrophy): report of a prospective multicenter study of the incidence of neoplasia and review. Am J Med Genet 79, 274–278.

Huber, C., Dias-Santagata, D., Gasser, A., et al., 2005. Identification of mutations in CUL7 in 3-M syndrome. Nat Genet 37, 1119–1124.

Hughes, I.A., Houk, C., Ahmed, S.F., Lee, P.A., et al., 2006. Consensus statement on management of intersex disorders. J Pediatr Urol 2, 148–162.

Hunter, A.G., Wand Stevensons, R.E., 2008. Gastroschisis: clinical presentation and associations. Am J Med Genet 148C, 219–230.

Irons, G.B., Olson, R.M., 1980. Aplasia cutis congenital. Plast Reconstr Surg 66, 199–203.

Jacobs, A.H., Walton, R.G., 1976. The incidence of birthmarks in the neonate. Pediatrics 58, 218–222.

Jissendi-Tchofo, P., Kara, S., Barkovich, A.J., 2009. Midbrain–hindbrain involvement in lissencephalies. Neurology 72, 410–418.

Kaplan, E.N., 1974. The risk of malignancy in large congenital nevi. Plast Reconstr Surg 53, 421–428.

Kauvar, E.F., Muenke, M., 2010. Holoprosencephaly: recommnedations for diagnosis and management. Curr Opin Pediatr. Dec; 25 (6): 687–695.

Keijzer, R., Puri, P., 2010. Congenital diaphragmatic hernia. Semin Pediatr Surg 19, 180–185.

Kelley, R.I., Roessler, E., Hennekam, R.C.M., et al., 1996. Holoprosencephaly in RSH/Smith–Lemli–Opitz syndrome: does abnormal cholesterol metabolism affect the function of sonic hedgehog? Am J Med Genet 66, 478–484.

Kimonis, V., Gold, J.A., Hoffman, T.L., et al., 2007. Genetics of craniosynostosis. Semin Pediatr Neurol 14, 150–161.

Kochilas, L., Merscher-Gomes, S., Lu, M.M., et al., 2002. The role of neural crest during cardiac development in a mouse model of DiGeorge syndrome. Dev Biol 251, 157–166.

Kohut, R., Rusen, I.D., 2002. Congenital Anomalies in Canada. Health Canada: A Perinatal Health Report 2002. Ministry of Public Health and Government Services Canada, Ottawa.

Konig, A., Happle, R., Bornholdt, D., et al., 2000. Mutations in the NSDHL gene, encoding a 3beta-hydroxysteroid dehydrogenase, cause CHILD syndrome. Am J Med Genet 90, 339–346.

Krakow, D., Rimoin, D.L., 2010. The skeletal dysplasias. Genet Med 12, 327–340.

Kruse, K., Pankau, R., Gosh, A., et al., 1992. Calcium metabolism in Williams Beuren syndrome. J Pediatr 121, 902–907.

Lam, W.F.F., Hau, W.L.K., Lam, T.S., 2002. Evaluation of referrals for genetic investigation of short stature in Hong Kong. Chin Med J 115, 607–611.

Lambert, S.M., Vilain, E.J.N., Kolon, T.F., 2010. A practical approach to ambiguous genitalia in the newborn period. Urol Clin North Am 37(2):195–205.

Le Merrer, M., Brauner, R., Maroteaux, P., 1991. Dwarfism with gloomy face: a new syndrome with features of 3-M syndrome. J Med Genet 28, 186–191.

Li, M., Shuman, C., Fei, Y.L., et al., 2001. GPC3 mutation analysis in a spectrum of patients with overgrowth expands the phenotype of Simpson–Golabi–Behmel syndrome. Am J Med Genet 102, 161–168.

Lin, A.E., Grossfeld, P.D., Hamilton, R., et al., 2002. Further delineation of cardiac anomalies in Costello syndrome. Am J Med Genet 111, 115–129.

Lin, A.E., Gripp, K.W., Kerr, B., 2010. Costello syndrome. In: Cassidy, S.B., Allanson, J.E., (Eds.), Management of Genetic Syndromes, third ed. Wiley-Liss, New Jersey, pp. 151–163.

Lopez-Rangel, E., Van Allen, M.I., 2005. Prenatal exposure to fluconazol: An identifiable dysmorphic phenotype. Birth Defects Res Clin Mol Teratol 73, 919–923.

Maher, E.R., 2005. Imprinting and assisted reproductive technology. Hum Mol Genet 14, Special No 1:R 133–138.

March Of Dimes Perinatal Data Center, 2000. http://www.marchofdimes.com/peristats/Peristats.aspx.

Mastroiacovo, P., Lisi, A., Castilla, E.E., et al., 2007. Gastroschisis and associated defects: an international study. Am J Med Genet Part 143A, 660–671.

Mastroiacovo, P., Working Group I.P., 2011. Prevalence at birth of cleft lip with or without cleft palate. Data from the International Perinatal Database of Typical Oral Clefts (IPDTOC). Cleft Palate Craniofac J 48(1), 66–81. Epub 2010 April 6.

Mathews, T.J., Mac Dorman, M.F., 2006. Infant Mortality Statistics from the 2003 Period Linked Birth/Infant Death Data Set. National Vital Statistics Reports: from the Centers for Disease Control and Prevention, national Center for Health Statistics, National Vital Statistics System 54(16), 1–29.

Meyer, J., Sudbeck, P., Held, M., et al., 1997. Mutational analysis of the SOX9 gene in campomelic dysplasia and autosomal sex reversal: lack of genotype/phenotype correlations. Hum Mol Genet 6, 91–98.

Miller, J.D., McKusick, V.A., Malvaux, P., et al., 1975. The 3-M syndrome: a heritable low birthweight dwarfism. Birth Defects Orig Artic Ser 11, 39–47.

Miller, D.T., Adam, M.P., Aradhya, S., et al., 2010. Consensus statement: chromosomal microarray is first-tier clinical diagnostic test for individuals with developmental disabilities or congenital anomalies. Am J Hum Genet 86, 749–764.

Mitchell, L.E., 2005. Epidemiology of neural tube defects. Am J Med Genet C Semin 135C, 88–94.

Mochida, G.H., 2009. Genetics and biology of microcephaly and lissencephaly. Semin Pediatr Neurol 16, 120–126.

Morava, E., Guillard, M., Lefeber, D.J., et al., 2009. Autosomal recessive cutis laxa syndrome revisited. Eur J Hum Genet 17, 1099–1110.

Morris, C.A., 2010. Williams syndrome. In: Cassidy, S.B., Allanson, J.E., (Eds.), Management of Genetic Syndromes, third ed. Wiley-Liss, Hoboken, New Jersey, pp. 655–665.

Morris, C.A., Dilts, C., Dempsey, S.A., et al., 1988. The natural history of Williams syndrome. Physical characteristics. J Pediatr 113, 318–326.

Mowat, D.R., Croaker, G.D., Cass, D.T., et al., 1998. Hirschprung disease, microcephaly, mental retardation and characteristic facial features: delineation of a new syndrome and identification of a locus of chromosome 2q22-q23. J Med Genet 35, 617–623.

Neri, G., Gurrieri, F., Zanni, G., et al., 1998. Clinical and molecular aspects of the Simpson–Golabi–Behmel syndrome. Am J Med Genet 79, 279–283.

Ng, S.B., Buckingham, K.J., Lee, C., et al., 2010. Exome sequencing identifies the cause of a medelian disorder. Nat Genet 42, 30–35.

Nichol, P., Byrne, J.L.B.B., Dodgion, C., et al., 2008. Clinical considerations in gastroschisis: incremental advance against a congenital anomaly with severe secondary effects. Am J Med Genet 148C, 231–240.

Nowak, C.B., 2007. The phakomatoses: dermatologic clues to neurologic anomalies. Semin Pedistr Neurol 14, 140–149.

O'Driscoll, M., Ruiz-Perez, V.L., Woods, C.G., et al., 2003. A splicing mutation affecting expression of ataxia-teleangiectasia and Rad3-related protein (ATR) results in Seckel syndrome. Nat Gen 33, 467–501.

Ohtani, S., Skinkai, Y., Horibe, A., et al., 2006. A deletion in the endothelin-B receptor gene is responsible for the Waardenburg syndrome-like phenotypes of WS4 mice. Exp Anim. 55, 491–495.

Orioli, I.M., Castilla, E.E., Barbosa-Neto, J.G., 1986. The birth prevalence rates for the skeletal dysplasias. J Med Genet 23, 328–332.

Orioli, I.M., Castilla, E.E., Scarano, G., et al., 1995. Effect of paternal age in achondroplasia, thanatophoric dysplasia, and osteogenesis imperfecta. Am J Med Gen 59, 209–217.

Otto, F., Kanegane, H., Mundlos, S., 2002. Mutations in the RUNX2 gene in patients with cleidocranial dysplasia. Hum Mutat 19, 209–216.

Park, W.J., Theda, C., Maestri, N.E., et al., 1995. Analysis of phenotypic features and FGFR2 mutations in Apert syndrome. Am J Hum Genet 57, 321–328.

Pelletier, J., Bruening, W., Kashtan, C.E., et al., 1991. Germline mutations in the Wilms tumor suppressor gene are associated with abnormal urogenital development in Denys–Drash syndrome. Cell 67, 437–447.

Ramsing, M., Gillessen-Kaesbach, G., Holzgreve, W., et al., 2000. Variability in the phenotypic expression of Fryns syndrome: a report of two sibships. Am J Med Genet 95, 415–424.

Rauch, A., Thiel, C.T., Schindler, D., et al., 2008. Mutations in the pericentrin (PCNT) gene cause primordial dwarfism. Science 319, 816–819.

Reardon, W., 2008. The bedside dysmorphologist. Classic clinical signs in human malformation syndromes and their diagnositic significance. Oxford University Press, Oxford.

Reardon, W., Donnai, D., 2007. Dysmorphology demystified. Arch Dis Child Fetal Neonatal Ed 92, F225–F229.

Reardon, W., Winter, R.M., 1994. Saethre–Chotzen syndrome. J Med Genet 31, 393–396.

Reardon, W., Winter, R.M., Rutland, P., et al., 1994. Mutations in the fibroblast growth factor receptor 2 gene cause Crouzon syndrome. Nat Genet 8, 98–103.

Ribuffo, D., Costantini, M., Gullo, P., et al., 2003. Aplasia cutis congenital of the scalp, the skull, and the dura. Scand J Plast Reconstr Surg Hand Surg 37, 176–180.

Riel-Romero, R.M.S., Mattingly, M., 2005. Developmental venous anomaly in association with neuromigrational anomalies. Pediatr Neurol 32, 53–55.

Robertson, K., Mason, I., Hall, S., 1997. Hirschprung's disease: genetic mutations in mice and men. Gut 41, 436–441.

Roelfsema, J.H., White, S.J., Ariyurek, Y., et al., 2005. Genetic heterogeneity in Rubinstein–Taybi syndrome: mutations in both the CBP and EP300 genes cause disease. Am J Hum Genet 76, 572–580.

Rose, C.S.P., Patel, P., Reardon, W., et al., 1997. The TWIST gene, although not disrupted in Saethre–Chotzen patients with apparently balanced translocations of 7p21, is mutated in familial and sporadic cases. Hum Mol Genet 6, 1369–1373.

Ruiz-Perez, V.L., Tompson, S.W.J., Blair, H.J., et al., 2003. Mutations in two nonhomologous genes in a head-to-head configuration cause Ellis–van Creveld syndrome. Am J Hum Genet 72, 728–732.

Ryan, A.K., Goodship, J.A., Wilson, D.I., et al., 1997. Spectrum of clinical features associated with interstitial chromosome 22q11 deletions: a European collaborative study. J Med Genet 34, 798–804.

Salihu, H.M., Perre-Louis, B.J., Druschel, C.M., et al., 2003. Omphalocele and gastroschisis in the State of New York, 1992–1999. Birth Defects Res A Clin Mol Teratol 67, 630–636.

Salonen, R., Herva, R., 1990. Hydrolethalus syndrome. J Med Genet 27, 756.

Sanders, R.C., Greyson-Fleg, R.T., Hogge, W.A., et al., 1994.Osteogenesis imperfecta and campomelic dysplasia: difficulties in prenatal diagnosis. J Ultrasound Med 13, 691–700.

Scambler, P.J., Kelly, D., Lindsay, E., et al., 1992. Velo-cardio-facial syndrome associated with chromosome 22 deletions encompassing the DiGeorge locus. Lancet 339, 1138–1139.

Seaver, L.H., Irons, M., 2009. ACMG practice guidelines: genetic evaluation of short stature. Genet Med 11, 465–470.

Shaffer. L., 2005. American College of Medical Genetics guidelines on cytogenetic evaluation of the individual with developmental delay or mental retardation. ACMG Practice Guidelines 7, 650–654.

Sharland, G.K., Allan, L.D., Chita, S.K., et al., 1991. Chromosomal anomalies in fetal congenital heart disease. Ultrasound Obstet Gynecol 1, 8–11.

Shaw, A.M., 2010. 21-hydroxylase deficiency congenital adrenal hyperplasia. Neonatal Netw 29, 191–196.

Shipster, C., Hearst, D., Sommerville, A., et al., 2003. Speech, language, and cognitive devepment in children with isolated sagittal synostosis. Dev Med Child Neurol 45, 34–43.

Shprintzen, R.J., 2010. Velo-cardio-facial syndrome. In: Cassidy, S.B., Allanson, J.E., (Eds.), Management of Genetic Syndromes, third ed. Wiley-Liss, Hoboken, New Jersey, pp. 615–633.

Slaney, S.F., Oldridge, M., Hurst, J.A., et al., 1996. Differential effects of FGFR2 mutations on syndactyly and cleft palate in Apert syndrome. Am J Hum Genet 58, 923–932.

Sorge, G., Greco, F., Mattina, T., et al., 2005. Mulibrey nanism. Clinical and molecular aspects. Ital J Pediatr 31, 340–344.

Stevenson, D.K., Hopper, A.O., Cohen, R.S., et al., 1982. Medical progress: macrosomia: causes and consequences. J Pediatr 100, 515–520.

Sujansky, E., Conradi, S., 1995. Outcome of Sturge–Weber syndrome in 52 adults. Am J Med Genet 57, 35–45.

Thill, M., Nguyen, T.D., Wehnert M., et al., 2008. Restrictive dermopathy: a rare laminopathy. Arch Gynecol Obstet 278, 201–208.

Thyen, U., Lanz, K., Holterus, P.M., et al., 2006. Epidemiology and initial management of ambiguous genitalia at birth in Germany. Horm Res 66, 195–203.

Trimborn, M., Bell, S.M., Felix, C., et al., 2004. Mutations in microcephalin cause aberrant regulation of chromosome condensation. Am J Hum Genet 75, 261–266.

Van Allen, M.E., et al., 1987. Limb–body-wall complex I: pathogenesis. Am J Med Genet 28, 529–548.

Van Haelst, M.M., Scambler, P.J., 2007. Fraser Syndrome Collaboration Group, Hennekam RCM. Fraser syndrome: a clinical study of 59 cases and evaluation of diagnostic criteria. Am J Med Genet 143A, 3194–3203.

Verdyck, P., Holder-Espinasse, M., Hul, W.V., et al., 2003. Clinical and molecular analysis of nine families with Adams–Oliver syndrome. Eur J Hum Genet 11, 457–463.

Wakeling, E.L., Amero, S.A., Alders, M., et al., 2010. Epigenotype-phenotype correlations in Silver–Russell syndrome. J Med Genet 47, 760–768.

Wilkie, A.O., 1997. Craniosynostosis: genes and mechanisms. Hum Mol Genet 6, 1647–1656.

Williams, M.L., Pennella, R., 1994. Melanoma, melanocytic nevi, and other melanoma risk factors in children. J Pediatr 124, 833–845.

Williams, C.A., Dagli, A., Battaglia, A., 2008. Genetic disorders associated with macrocephaly. Am J Med Genet 146A, 2023–2037.

Wilson, G.N., de Chadarevian, J.P., Kaplan, P., et al., 1989. Glutaric aciduria type II: review of the phenotype and report of an unusual glomerulopathy. Am J Med Genet 32, 395–401.

Winter, R.M., 1996a. Analysing human developmental abnormalities. Bioessay 18, 965–971.

Winter, R., 1996b. What's in a face? Nat Genet 12, 124–129.

Winter, R.M., Baraitser, M., 2010. Winter–Baraitser Dysmorphology Database. Medical Databases, London.

Witters, I., Moerman, P., Fryns, J.P., 2002. Fetal akinesia deformation sequence: a study of 30 consecutive in utero diagnoses. Am J Med Genet 113, 23–28.

Woods, C.G., 2004. Human microcephaly. Curr Opin Neurobiol 14, 112–117.

Wynn, J., King, T.M., Gambello, M.J., et al., 2007. Mortality in achondroplasia study: a 42-year follow up. Am J Med Gen 143A, 2502–2511.

Xu, J., Fan, Y.S., Siu, V.M., 2008. A child with features of Goldenhar syndrome and a novel 1.12 Mb deletion in 22q11.2 by cytogenetics and array CGH: is this a candidate region for the syndrome? Am J Med Genet 146A, 1886–1889.

Yang, Y.C., Wu, C.H., Chang, F.M., et al., 1992. Early prenatal diagnosis of acrania by transvaginal ultrasonography. J Clin Ultrasound 20, 343–345.

Yoon, P.W., Olney, R.S., Khoury, M.J., et al., 1997. Contribution of birth defects and genetic diseases to pediatric hospitalizations. Arch Pediatr Adoles Med 151, 1096–1103.

Zweier, C., Albrecht, B., Mitulla, B., et al., 2002. Mowat–Wilson syndrome with or without Hirschprung disease is a distinct, recognizable multiple congenital anomalies-mental retardation syndrome caused by mutations in the zinc finger homeo box 1B gene. Am J Med Genet 108, 177–181.

Neonatal dermatology

32

Maureen Rogers

© 2012 Elsevier Ltd

Box 32.1   Causes of cutis marmorata (livedo reticularis) in the neonate

Physiological cutis marmorata
Down syndrome
Trisomy 18
Homocystinuria
Cornelia de Lange syndrome
Neonatal lupus erythematosus
Congenital hypothyroidism
Cutis marmorata telangiectatica congenita
Macrocephaly–cutis marmorata syndrome

Introduction

There are important differences between the skin of the neonate, in particular the preterm neonate, and that of the child or adult, and an understanding of those differences is vital to the appropriate care of the baby.

Some skin disorders are very specific to the neonatal period. These are mostly benign and transient and their main importance is the fact that they can imitate more serious disorders. Cutaneous infections in the neonate are almost all potentially serious and may have atypical presentations; the first sign of certain systemic infections can be cutaneous. Some important systemic disorders present in the neonatal period with skin signs. Most naevi are present at birth and a number of skin tumours can be congenital or appear in the neonatal period. Finally, several important ongoing skin diseases may manifest in the first month of life. The recognition of these patterns of disease is important so that appropriate investigations and intervention can be instituted and so that the parents can be reassured or offered a realistic prognosis.

Structure and function of the neonatal skin

By 24 weeks' gestation, the anatomy of the skin is essentially similar to that of the older individual, but it is some years before functional maturity is achieved.

The epidermis of the baby is fragile (Lane 1987), especially in preterm neonates, with a susceptibility to fissuring and an increased risk of injury from adhesives, chemical burns from alcohol swabs and disinfectant solutions (Harpin and Rutter 1982) and thermal burns from transcutaneous oxygen monitors (Lane 1987).

Compared with that of the older child, there is an increased permeability of neonatal skin, especially in the preterm baby (Rutter 1987). This increases the risk of toxic effects of the application of agents such as iodine, hexachlorophene, gammabenzene hexachloride and phenol, and possibly some of the myriad over-the-counter preparations which are applied to the skin of babies. The absorption of topical steroid preparations is much increased, leading to potential side-effects, both local and systemic. This tendency to complications from the use of applied agents is exaggerated by the large surface area to bodyweight ratio of the baby.

Vasomotor instability is characteristic in the neonate and is responsible for certain essentially benign and physiological, but clinically striking, entities. A rubor or generalised redness is often present in the early hours of life. Peripheral acrocyanosis presents as a bilaterally symmetrical, intermittent, blue discoloration of the hands and feet, which usually disappears after the early weeks. Harlequin colour change is a vascular phenomenon probably caused by an immature autonomic regulatory mechanism (Selimoglu et al. 1995; Lucky 2008). When the neonate is lying on one side, the lower half of the body is red and the upper half is pale, with a clear midline separation. This colour change reverses on altering the baby's position. It is a very transient phenomenon and does not indicate any significant neural or vascular abnormality. Physiological cutis marmorata or livedo reticularis is a benign transient blue or purple cutaneous mottling, most marked when the baby is cool, lasting minutes to hours but reversing quickly on warming (Lucky 2008). The tendency to the condition lasts for weeks or months.

However, livedo is not always physiological (Box 32.1). A more persistent livedo may be seen in a number of syndromes, in congenital hypothyroidism and rarely in neonatal lupus. A very striking segmental livedo, associated with dilated veins and, sometimes, cutaneous atrophy, is a feature of cutis marmorata telangiectatica congenita, a rare vascular malformation.

Neonatal skin often manifests the same type of hyperpigmentation as is seen in pregnancy. This is believed to be due to the influence of maternal and placental hormones as part of the 'minipuberty' of the newborn. It affects particularly the external genitalia, and the linea alba is instead a linea nigra (Lucky 2008).

Lanugo is the fine silky hair found to cover neonates, especially preterm babies. It is most marked on the shoulders, back and cheeks. It is usually shed within 3 months. There is an extremely rare inherited disorder, congenital hypertrichosis lanuginosa, characterised by a very profuse and persistent, widespread covering of lanugo hair (Littler 1997). There are a number of causes of neonatal hypertrichosis featuring an excess of either vellus hair (normal childhood non-scalp hair) or terminal hair (adult or scalp-type hair). While this may occur alone, it is usually part of a syndrome with other diagnostic features. Certain drugs may cause a neonatal hypertrichosis. Some of these conditions are listed in Box 32.2.

Scalp hair may be sparse or abundant at birth. A well-defined patch of alopecia commonly develops in the occipital area. This is not, as commonly believed, due to rubbing the back of the head on the bedding surface. It is explained by understanding the fetal and neonatal hair cycles (Rogers 2008). By 20 weeks' gestation, there are well-developed hair follicles containing anagen (growing) hairs all over the scalp. Although the hair roots enter telogen (the

Box 32.2

Box 32.2   Causes of hypertrichosis in the neonate

Physiological lanugo hair
Congenital hypertrichosis lanuginosa
Primary isolated hypertrichosis
Hypertrichosis as part of various syndromes
 Hypertrichosis with gingival fibromatosis
 Congenital erythropoietic porphyria
 Familial porphyria cutanea tarda
 Cornelia de Lange syndrome
 Coffin–Siris syndrome
 Cantu syndrome
 Leprechaunism
 Seip–Berardinelli syndrome
 Rubenstein–Taybi syndrome
 Some mucopolysaccharidoses
Drug-induced hypertrichosis
 Diazoxide
 Fetal alcohol syndrome
 Maternal minoxidil

Box 32.3   Conditions which may present with pustules in the neonate

Toxic erythema of the newborn
Transient neonatal pustular dermatosis
Infantile acropustulosis
Eosinophilic pustulosis
Pustular miliaria
Neonatal cephalic pustulosis and neonatal acne
Varicella
Herpes simplex
Staphylococcal impetigo
Streptococcal impetigo
Candida
Scabies
Incontinentia pigmenti
Hyper-IgE syndrome
Myeloproliferative disorder in Down syndrome

Box 32.4   Conditions which may present with vesicles, blisters or erosions in the neonate

Sucking blisters
Herpes simplex
Varicella
Staphylococcal infections
 Impetigo
 Staphylococcal scalded-skin syndrome
Scabies
Aspergillus
Candida
Syphilis
Epidermolysis bullosa
Contact irritant dermatitis, chemical burn
Mastocytosis
Bullous ichthyosis
Incontinentia pigmenti
Neonatal pemphigus
Neonatal herpes gestationis
Congenital erosive and vesicular dermatosis
Zinc deficiency
Langerhans cell histiocytosis
Porphyrias
 Congenital erythropoietic porphyria
 Erythropoietic protoporphyria
 Transient porphyrinaemia in Rh incompatibility

Benign transient neonatal disorders presenting with sterile pustules

There are many benign conditions that may present in the neonatal period with sterile pustules (see Box 32.3), which can mimic serious infections (Nanda et al. 2002; Lucky 2008).

Toxic erythema of the newborn

This is a self-limiting, benign, idiopathic condition, which occurs in about two-thirds of all neonates (Lucky 2008) but almost never in premature babies. The onset is usually between 24 and 48 hours, but may occur at any time from birth to 14 days. The characteristic lesions are poorly demarcated erythematous macules, often surmounted by central pale papules, but occasionally pustules develop. The lesions may occur anywhere on the body surface apart from palms and soles, particularly on the face and trunk. When cases present at birth, lesions are more acrally distributed and are more often pustular. Smears taken from pustules and stained with Wright or Giemsa stain demonstrate numerous eosinophils and a peripheral blood eosinophilia is present. The disorder rarely lasts more than a few days.

Transient neonatal pustular dermatosis (transient neonatal pustular melanosis)

This condition presents at birth or in the first hours of life as lesions which quickly evolve from blisters to large flaccid pustules (Fig. 32.1) (Merlob et al. 1982; Lucky 2008). These lesions occur mainly on the trunk and buttocks, but may be widespread. Over the next 1–2 days, the pustules rupture, with the formation of a peripheral

resting stage, which lasts 10–12 weeks before the hairs inevitably fall) in a progressive manner from frontal to parietal areas at 26–28 weeks' gestation, those in the occipital area remain in anagen until birth, when they abruptly enter telogen. These hairs fall at 9–12 weeks of postnatal life. In some babies large numbers of hairs in the parietal area are still in telogen at birth and a more extensive postnatal alopecia occurs, with hair remaining only at the vertex.

Pustules, blisters and erosions in the neonate

There are a large number of conditions, some transient and benign and others serious, which present with pustules, blisters or erosions. Some of these are listed in Boxes 32.3 and 32.4.

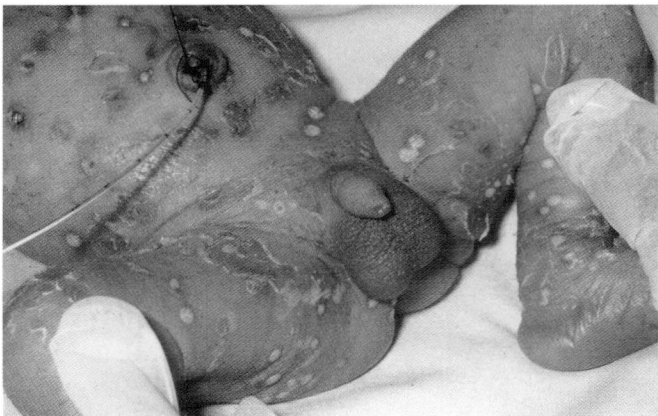

Fig. 32.1 Transient neonatal pustular dermatosis.

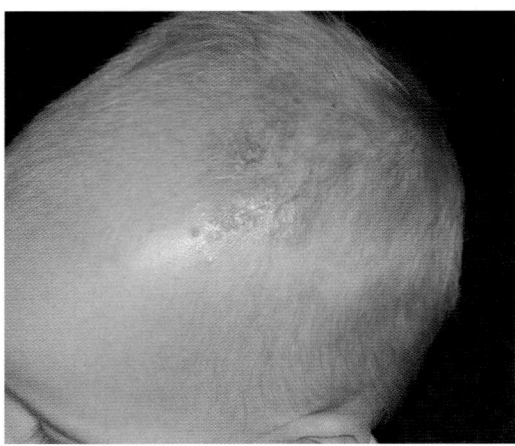

Fig. 32.3 Eosinophilic pustulosis.

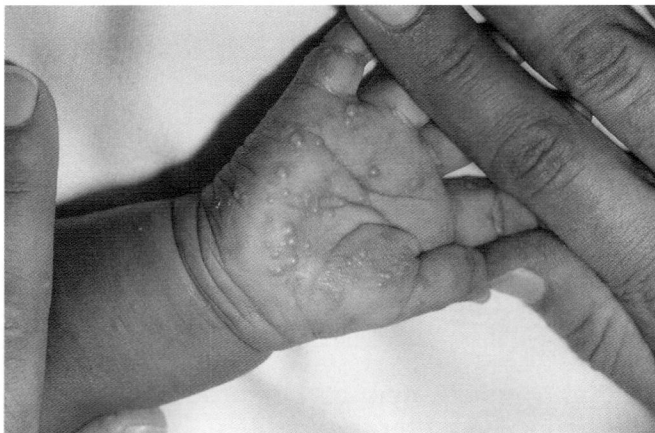

Fig. 32.2 Infantile acropustulosis.

collarette of scale, which separates after a further day or so to leave either normal skin or, in dark-skinned individuals, a temporary postinflammatory hyperpigmentation. Because the pigmentation depends on the skin colour, the term dermatosis is preferred to the earlier term melanosis. Occasionally, a few further crops of lesions appear. The pustules, which can closely simulate infective conditions, contain numerous neutrophils but are sterile on culture. The condition is entirely benign and does not require treatment; the prognosis is excellent.

Infantile acropustulosis

This is another benign idiopathic condition which commences in the neonatal period or early infancy (Mancini et al. 1998; Lucky 2008). Recurrent crops of extremely pruritic 2–4-mm vesicopustules develop on the hands and feet, especially on palmar and plantar surfaces (Fig. 32.2) (Jennings and Burrows 1983). Initially, each crop lasts 7–14 days and recurrences occur at 2–3-week intervals. With time, the duration of each attack becomes shorter and the time between attacks longer, until the condition resolves spontaneously after many months. Cultures of the pustules are sterile. A clinically identical condition occurs as a postscabetic reaction following successful treatment of severe neonatal or infantile scabies. When reports of infantile acropustulosis are studied, it becomes clear that almost all of the patients have been treated for scabies (Mancini et al. 1998) and the existence of the condition as a distinct entity

unrelated to scabies is in some doubt. The duration of the episode may be shortened with the use of strong topical steroids for a few days.

Eosinophilic pustulosis (eosinophilic pustular folliculitis)

This is a rare condition in which recurrent groups of sterile pustules, centred around hair follicles, develop on the scalp in the first few months of life (Ladrigan et al. 2008; Lucky 2008). Lesions begin as small, closely grouped red papules which quickly develop into pustules and then form crusted lesions which heal over several days (Fig. 32.3). Several groups may occur at one time on the scalp. The lesions are characteristically very itchy. Occasionally there are a few follicular lesions at other sites, and, in older infants, follicular and non-follicular lesions away from the scalp become more prominent. Cropping of lesions may continue for many months before there is eventual spontaneous resolution of the condition. Smears from the pustules show variable proportions of neutrophils and eosinophils and no evidence of infection on culture. There is often a peripheral blood eosinophilia present at the time of onset of new lesions. The use of fairly potent topical steroids may shorten the duration of each episode a little but has no effect on the overall course of the condition.

Miliaria

This is a sweat retention condition common in young babies and which is important to differentiate from milia (p. 827) (Lucky 2008). An obstruction, the nature of which is unknown, develops in the intraepidermal part of the sweat duct and sweat is trapped. The duct may rupture and sweat then leaks into the surrounding epidermis. Lesions begin as small red macules, soon surmounted by red papules (miliaria rubra) or pustules (pustular miliaria) (Fig. 32.4). Unlike miliaria in older individuals, the condition in infancy often occurs in the absence of fever or significant external occlusion of the skin. Lesions occur mainly on the face, scalp and upper trunk. There is often a mixture of red and pustular lesions, and the distribution and severity of the condition characteristically vary considerably from day to day or even within the same day. It is noted to be worse in areas of occlusion, such as where the face has been against the breast, and also at times of increased heat. It is important to stress to the parents that this is a benign phenomenon over which they have little control and which, if anything, will be worsened by the application of topical agents.

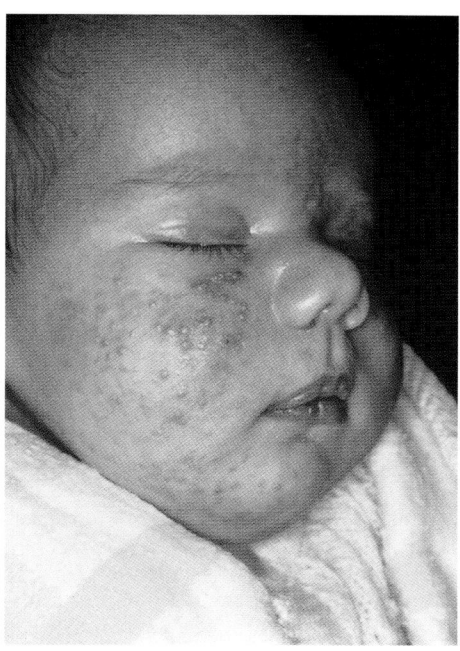

Fig. 32.4 Pustular miliaria.

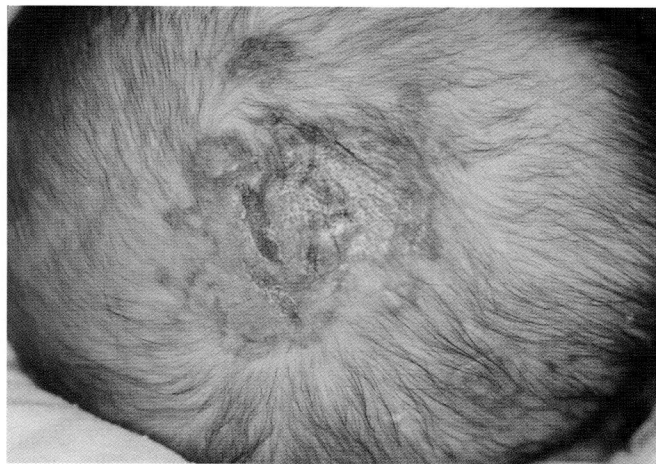

Fig. 32.5 Herpes simplex on the scalp.

Neonatal cephalic pustulosis and neonatal acne

Both of these terms are used to describe a condition presenting within the first 3–4 weeks of life with erythematous papules and pustules but no comedones, occurring primarily on the cheeks but scattered elsewhere on the face and extending to the scalp and resolving after several more weeks (Bergman and Eichenfield 2002; Lucky 2008). The condition is quite separate from infantile acne, which is predominantly comedonal, occurs almost entirely in boys and rarely presents before 3 months of age. There is an opinion that the term neonatal acne should be abandoned in favour of neonatal cephalic pustulosis (Lucky 2008). There is a suggestion that the lesions of cephalic pustulosis may be an inflammatory reaction to *Malassezia* species, but these are found as commensals on neonatal skin, so their pathogenic role is difficult to assess (Bergman and Eichenfield 2002). It is doubtful whether antifungal treatment significantly shortens the duration of this self-limiting condition. This condition is clinically very similar to pustular miliaria, and only biopsy, which clearly would be unjustified, could differentiate them in some cases.

Infective conditions presenting with pustules, blisters or erosions

A variety of infections can present in the neonatal period with pustules (see Box 32.3), blisters (see Box 32.4) or erosions. Some present predominantly with one or other type of lesion, but some infections can produce all types. Most of these conditions are described in more detail in Chapter 39, part 2 and only the cutaneous presentations are described here.

Varicella

Because the infection in the neonate is usually severe, there may be many lesions in the same stage of development. Hence, the condition may present as a widespread vesicular or pustular disorder with a wide differential diagnosis (Sauerbrei and Wutzler 2007a). It may not be recognised clinically as varicella until the characteristic crusts form several days later. Congenital varicella may present as erosions but often stellate scarring is already present at birth.

Herpes simplex

The skin lesions are grouped blisters, localised initially on the presenting part, usually the head, with the onset typically between the fourth and eighth days of life (Sauerbrei and Wutzler 2007b). They are often localised in the sites of application of scalp electrodes during delivery. Sometimes the lesions become pustular (Fig. 32.5), but they soon burst to form erosions, which may be deep and haemorrhagic. A characteristic pattern is individual lesions a few millimetres across coalescing to produce larger erosions with a geographical shape or scalloped border. On the thick skin of the palms or soles, the blisters or pustules may remain intact, producing a more confusing clinical picture. The diagnosis can be confirmed by electron microscopy (EM) of vesicle fluid. Treatment with intravenous aciclovir is urgent (Ch. 39).

Impetigo

This is usually a staphylococcal bullous impetigo, originating in an infected umbilical wound. The lesions first appear as intact vesicles, then become intact pustules, which eventually rupture to form fast-spreading erosions which, being very superficial, quickly dry out to form shiny crusts. Occasionally group A streptococcal infections present as pustules, but a non-specific omphalitis is more common. Systemic antibiotics are required.

Staphylococcal scalded-skin syndrome

The condition commences with a macular erythema, initially on the face and in the major flexures and then becoming generalised. The skin is exquisitely tender. After 2 days, flaccid bullae develop and the skin wrinkles and shears off (Fig. 32.6). The exfoliation is most marked in the groin, neck fold and around the mouth and may involve the entire body surface, but mucosae remain uninvolved. The child is usually febrile but, because of the superficial level of the split, fluid loss is rarely significant. The erosions crust and dry and heal with desquamation over 4–8 days leaving no sequelae. Cultures from affected skin and blister fluid are usually negative.

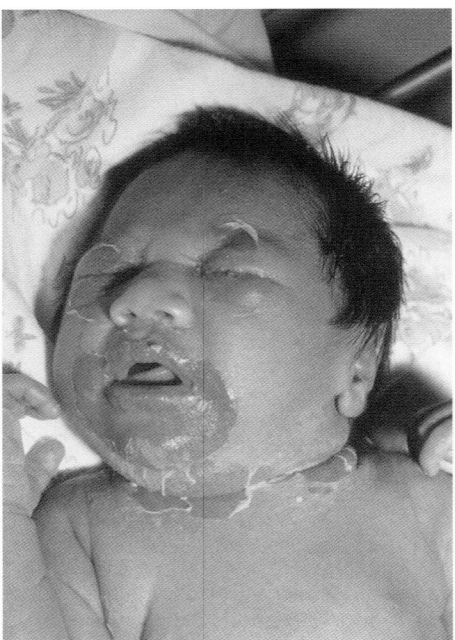

Fig. 32.6 Staphylococcal scalded-skin syndrome.

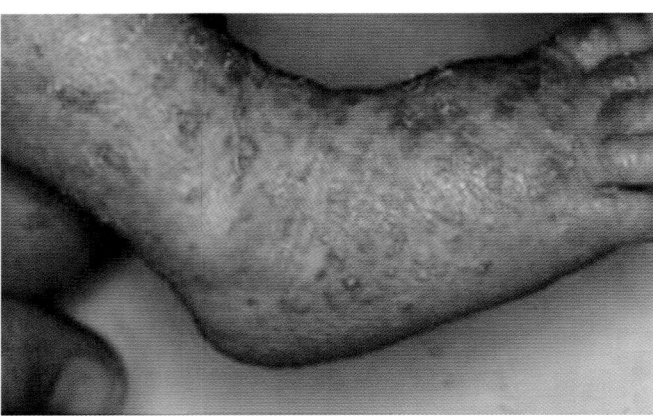

Fig. 32.7 Congenital candidiasis.

The usual source in a neonate is an infected umbilical stump. The condition responds quickly to intravenous antistaphylococcal antibiotics.

Candida

In congenital candidiasis, the infection is acquired in utero and presents in the first 2 days of life with a diffuse eruption of papules, papulovesicles and pustules, often on an erythematous base (Fig. 32.7) (Darmstadt et al. 2000). These usually settle in a few days with superficial desquamation.

In neonatal candidiasis, the infection is contracted during passage through an infected birth canal and there are several different presentations depending on the maturity and status of the neonate.

Localised neonatal candidiasis

This includes oral thrush and *Candida* napkin dermatitis (Carder 2008). The latter demonstrates a beefy-red erythema extending a variable distance from the groin folds, with a thick white accumulation deep in the fold. There are often satellite pustules which rupture to form a peripheral scale.

Invasive fungal dermatitis

This is a term used to describe primary cutaneous, erosive, crusted, sometimes necrotic lesions occurring in very-low-birthweight (VLBW) infants (Rowen et al. 1995). A similar condition can occur with other fungal infections, including *Aspergillus*.

Cutaneous lesions of systemic candidiasis

VLBW infants with systemic candidiasis can present with an extensive burn-like dermatitis followed by peeling (Carder 2008).

Scabies

Clinical manifestations of scabies have been reported as early as the second week of life (Quarterman and Lesher 1994). The lesions in neonatal scabies, which include papules, nodules, vesicles and pustules, tend to be very widespread, often with facial and scalp involvement, which is rare in older infants. Vesicles or pustules on the palms and soles are common features. Secondary eczematisation and infection may complicate the clinical picture. Permethrin 5% cream is regarded as safe at any age, except possibly in the VLBW infant. Nodules frequently persist, and even become more numerous, for some weeks, even after successful treatment. A common postscabetic phenomenon is recurrent episodes of pustules on the palms and soles, clinically identical to the condition designated infantile acropustulosis.

Syphilis

While macular or maculopapular eruptions are more frequently seen, neonates with congenital syphilis may present with vesicles, bullae and erosions (Chakraborty and Luck 2008). Blisters form on an erythematous base and rupture easily, leaving a macerated area, sometimes with a peripheral annular scale. Haemorrhagic bullae on the palms and soles are particularly suggestive of syphilis.

Dermatological conditions presenting with pustules, blisters or erosions
(see Boxes 32.3 and 32.4)

Epidermolysis bullosa

This is a group of diseases characterised by trauma-induced blistering of skin (Fig. 32.8) and mucosae (Marinkovich 1999; Fine et al. 2008). There are over 15 types now identified, separated on the basis of inheritance, clinical features and EM identification of the cleavage plane of the blister: within the epidermis, between the epidermis and dermis, or in the upper dermis. Blisters are clear or filled with serosanguineous material, depending on their level. They may rupture or spontaneously subside. Secondary bacterial infection is common. Milia are small retention cysts resulting from a split through pilosebaceous or sweat ducts; these eventually extrude. Permanent scarring is mainly a feature of the forms with a deeper level of split and varies from mild, with minor cosmetic significance, to severe, with gross deformity and functional disability. Sometimes epidermolysis bullosa presents with extensive areas of denuded skin, particularly on the legs, as well as blistering; some of these cases may be associated with pyloric atresia (Masunaga et al. 2004). A firm diagnosis and typing should always be established as soon as possible. The diagnostic techniques include EM, immunofluorescent microscopy using antibodies to antigens known

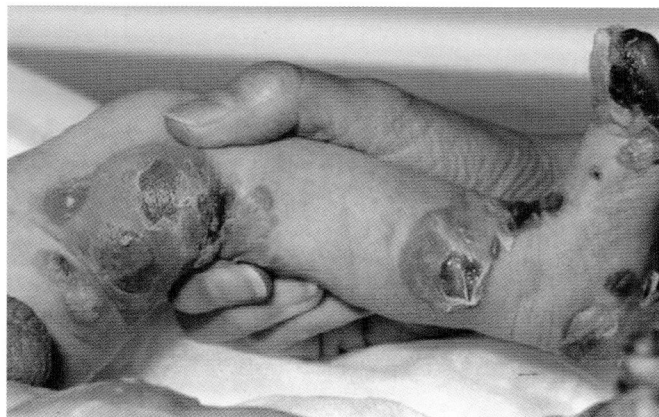

Fig. 32.8 Epidermolysis bullosa.

to be affected in EB and mutation analysis on DNA extracted from the blood of the patient and his or her family. This enables a prognosis to be given and a management plan to be established for the present and future.

In the severe forms with extensive neonatal blistering, the infant should initially be nursed naked in a humidified incubator, lying on non-adherent material, with barrier nursing to prevent infection. Blisters should be drained and antibacterial creams such as silver sulfadiazine applied to large erosions. Vaseline gauze or non-adherent plastic dressings should be used as required, covered by soft padding and secured with tubular cotton or by other means, but never taped to the skin with adhesive. A squeeze bottle or dropper should be used for feeding when there is severe oral ulceration. Nasogastric tubes should be avoided. Tourniquets, adhesive urine collection bags, identification bands and pacifiers should all be avoided. The parents should be encouraged to hold the baby, but the need for extreme gentleness in handling must be explained and demonstrated. Secondary bacterial infection is treated with topical or oral antibiotics. The severity of the pain and requirement for intensive treatment of this condition cause ethical dilemmas.

Mastocytosis

This is a condition in which the skin and sometimes other organs are infiltrated with benign mast cells. The cutaneous presentations vary from a single or a few isolated 1–5-cm lesions (mastocytoma), through multiple smaller often pigmented lesions (urticaria pigmentosa), to diffuse infiltration of the entire skin surface (diffuse cutaneous mastocytosis, bullous mastocytosis) (Briley 2008). Mast cells contain various mediators, of which the most important are histamine, prostaglandins and heparin, and the local and systemic effects of these account for many of the clinical features in this condition.

Urticaria pigmentosa is rarely present at birth but the other forms are usually congenital. Mastocytomas present as pink, pale-brown or yellowish nodules or plaques with a peau d'orange appearance on the surface. On rubbing, a red flush and oedema (urtication) are seen on the lesion and beyond it. Spontaneous or friction-induced blistering is common, as a result of local histamine release. Systemic spread of the histamine may lead to a generalised flushing. In diffuse cutaneous mastocytosis, there is a generalised thickening and oedema of the skin, usually with widespread haemorrhagic blistering (Fig. 32.9). Flushing, hypotension, shock, gastrointestinal haemorrhage, bronchospasm and diarrhoea may occur from the systemic effects of the mediators. There may be

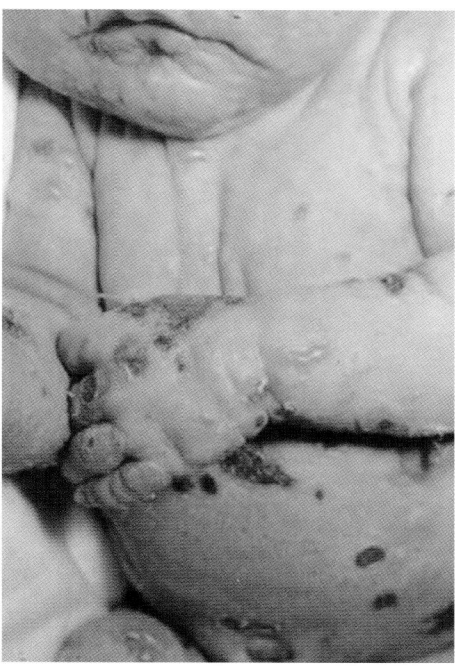

Fig. 32.9 Diffuse cutaneous mastocytosis.

hepatosplenomegaly and lymphadenopathy due to infiltration with mast cells. A number of drugs will cause degranulation of mast cells and release of mediators, and these should be avoided or used with caution; they include aspirin, opiates, tubocurarine, pilocarpine and iodine-containing radiographic agents.

All forms of mastocytosis improve with time, sometimes with complete resolution.

Bullous ichthyosis

This is an autosomal dominant condition, now known to be due to mutations in keratin genes (Ross et al. 2008). At birth the skin is diffusely erythematous with widespread erosions and maceration, and, sometimes, intact bullae (Fig. 32.10). In just a few days, the redness and blistering settle and the skin begins to thicken and become verrucous, taking on the appearance which will persist through life.

Incontinentia pigmenti

This is a multisystem disorder inherited as an X-linked dominant trait and usually lethal in males (Berlin et al. 2002). There are four cutaneous stages of the disease, vesiculopustular, verrucous, pigmented and hypopigmented, with stage 1 being present in the neonatal period. Abnormalities in other organ systems, especially neurological, ocular and skeletal, occur in about 70% of cases and seizures may occur in the neonatal period. It is therefore very important to recognise the stage 1 cutaneous lesions so that seizures may be anticipated or explained. These comprise linear groups of vesicles (Fig. 32.11), which quickly become pustular, situated mainly on the limbs and present at birth or appearing in the first days of life. They are accompanied by a peripheral blood eosinophilia and clear spontaneously over several weeks. The linear pattern is due to the fact that the lesions follow the lines of Blaschko, typical of mosaic disorders. Mosaicism in this X-linked condition occurs as a result of lyonisation.

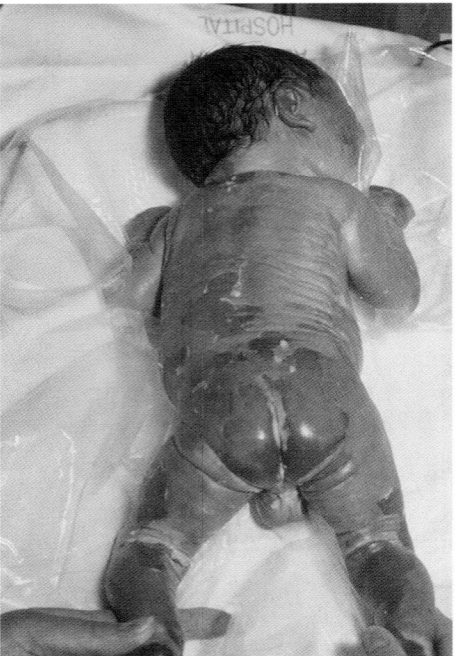

Fig. 32.10 Bullous ichthyosis.

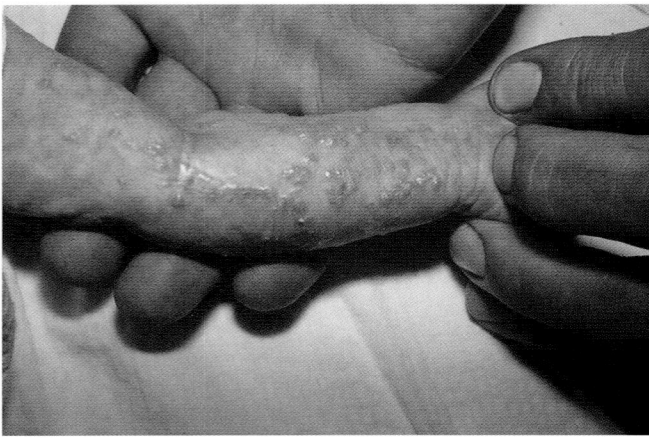

Fig. 32.11 Incontinentia pigmenti.

Neonatal pemphigus

Blisters may occur in the newborn as a result of transplacental passage of IgG antibodies from mothers who have pemphigus vulgaris or pemphigus foliaceus. The lesions are usually present at birth and vary from tense or flaccid bullae to large erosions. It is rare for new blisters to develop after the early days of life and the condition quickly resolves.

Neonatal herpes gestationis

Babies born to mothers with herpes gestationis in pregnancy (pemphigoid gestationis) may develop cutaneous disease as a result of transplacental passage of immunoglobulins formed against the maternal basement membrane zone (Al-Mutairi et al. 2004). The disorder may be evident at birth or within several hours, and red

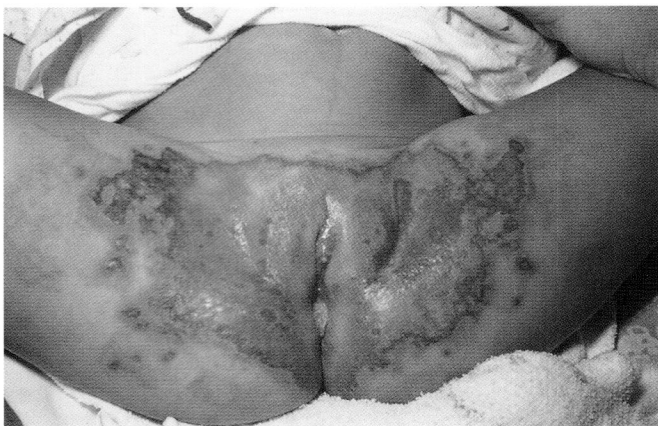

Fig. 32.12 Zinc-deficiency dermatosis.

macules or papules, often progressing to vesicles or bullae, can occur. Spontaneous resolution usually occurs by 1 month of age.

Congenital erosive and vesicular dermatosis

The aetiology of this rare disorder is unknown. It presents at birth with extensive blisters, erosions and crusts over most of the cutaneous surface (Goncalves et al. 2007). Lesions heal in several weeks with a strange supple and reticulated scarring. The babies are usually premature and may have underlying neurological defects, including developmental delay and seizures. The face, palms and soles are characteristically spared. Nails are absent or hypoplastic and patchy alopecia is seen on the scalp.

Disorders with systemic significance which can present with neonatal pustules, blisters or erosions

Zinc-deficiency dermatosis

This occasionally presents initially as a blistering rash. Acrodermatitis enteropathica is an autosomal recessive condition in which there is a defective absorption of zinc, possibly due to the absence of a specific carrier protein. The clinical features rarely appear in the early months of life. However, an identical condition occurs earlier in infants with nutritional zinc deficiency (Kiechl-Kohlendorfer et al. 2007). This may occur as a result of prematurity with low zinc stores, particularly in bottle-fed babies (as there is a lower bioavailability of zinc in bovine milk than in breast milk), or in babies born in any stage of maturity as a result of low maternal breast milk zinc (Kiechl-Kohlendorfer et al. 2007; Chue et al. 2008). The condition usually presents with a very well-marginated eczematous or psoriasiform rash occurring in a horseshoe shape on the chin and cheeks and in the napkin area (Fig. 32.12). It also often occurs around the eyes and nose and may involve fingers and toes. There is usually a very characteristic dark-coloured scale at the periphery. Sometimes it presents with bullae, particularly in the acral areas, but these soon become erosions and subsequently crust. The rash responds promptly to zinc supplementation. These children are very irritable and, if the condition goes untreated, may develop diarrhoea and alopecia and fail to thrive. Zinc deficiency also occurs in acquired immunodeficiency disease, cystic fibrosis and other causes of malabsorption, and in infants on parenteral nutrition solutions not containing adequate zinc. A clinically similar rash can occur with other metabolic conditions, including methylmaloni-cacidaemia and propionicacidaemia.

Langerhans cell histiocytosis

This can present at birth, or very soon after, as a widespread vesicular or bullous disorder (Herman et al. 1990), sometimes simulating staphylococcal scalded-skin syndrome. Usually some haemorrhagic changes point to the correct diagnosis. It may also present at birth as a small number of crusted nodules which often heal spontaneously after a few weeks. The most common presentation, however, is at several months of age, with a scaly and purpuric rash involving the major flexures, centrofacial area, scalp and ear canals. These children require a full assessment for systemic involvement, whether or not the lesions are apparently healing.

Hyper-IgE syndrome (Job syndrome)

This important immunodeficiency disorder (Ch. 39.1) may present in the neonatal period with inflammatory papules, vesicles and pustules, particularly on the face, scalp and upper trunk, but occasionally more widespread (Kamei and Honig 1988). The appearance may be very reminiscent of a pustular miliaria, but the condition is much more persistent and the pustules may be large and tense. As the lesions resolve, they develop a characteristic dark crust. Histologically, the lesions show an intense eosinophilic infiltrate; a peripheral blood eosinophilia is present and the IgE level starts to rise after the early weeks of life. The infant soon begins to develop troublesome infections, particularly with *Staphylococcus aureus* and *Candida*.

Myeloproliferative disorder in Down syndrome

Babies with Down syndrome are at increased risk of developing haematological abnormalities, including leukaemoid reaction, transient myeloproliferative disorder and congenital leukaemia. These entities may be accompanied by a very striking vesiculopustular disorder starting in the early days of life, most marked on the face but sometimes widespread (Wirges et al. 2006). It spontaneously resolves after a few weeks. The cells identified on skin smear or biopsy reflect those found in the peripheral blood.

Porphyrias

These are a group of disorders of haem synthesis leading to the accumulation of haem precursors which, when present in the skin, produce a photosensitivity. The porphyrias are designated hepatic or erythropoietic depending on the organ predominantly expressing the defect. They can be further separated by the assessment of plasma and red cell porphyrins and the pattern of porphyrin excretion in urine and faeces. Some of these may become symptomatic in the neonatal period.

Congenital erythropoietic porphyria presents soon after birth with severe photosensitivity, with bullae on areas exposed to sun or phototherapy machines and red urine. A later feature is red discoloration of the teeth and their fluorescence on Wood's light examination.

Erythropoietic protoporphyria usually presents later in childhood but occasionally erythema and blistering occur during phototherapy in the neonate. This has been reported also in the homozygous variants of coproporphyria and variegate porphyria.

A transient porphyrinaemia, of unclear aetiology, is described in haemolytic disease of the newborn (Mallon et al. 1995). This can produce marked erythema, purpura and blistering in areas exposed to phototherapy. There is a normalisation of the elevated plasma levels in a few weeks or months.

When photosensitivity occurs in the neonate, porphyrin levels in red cells, plasma, urine and faeces should be measured. The differential diagnosis of neonatal photosensitivity also includes neonatal lupus (see below), xeroderma pigmentosum (with early dark freckling) and drug-induced phototoxicity (e.g. furosemide, fluorescein dye).

Other transient neonatal conditions

Sebaceous hyperplasia

This is a common neonatal condition, probably representing the effect of maternal androgens on the neonatal glands (Lucky 2008). The hyperplastic sebaceous glands are seen as tiny yellow–white papules on the nose, especially at the tip. They disappear in several weeks.

Milia

These represent retention cysts of the pilosebaceous follicles (Lucky 2008). They occur in approximately 50% of neonates, manifesting as firm pearly-white 1–2-mm papules, particularly on the face. They usually disappear by 4 weeks of age. Persistent milia occur in certain syndromes, including Bazex syndrome, oral–facial–digital syndrome type I and Marie Unna hypotrichosis.

Sucking calluses or sucking pads

These develop on the lips as localised or extensive thickenings of the vermilion border. They may be present at birth, but more commonly occur postnatally, and are due to vigorous sucking (Lucky 2008).

Sucking blisters

These are present at birth and occur on the hands and forearms as a result of sucking in utero. The lesion is initially a tense fluid-filled blister, which ruptures to produce an erosion. Lesions in these areas may also appear as erosions of calluses.

Subcutaneous fat necrosis

This is a necrosis of subcutaneous fat in the newborn, probably induced by ischaemia. It occurs only in full-term infants. There is usually a history of a difficult labour and delivery, with complications such as prolonged labour, fetal distress and perinatal asphyxia. The lesions appear between the second and third weeks of life as tender, firm, skin-coloured or red–purple nodules or plaques occurring particularly on the buttocks, shoulders, upper back, proximal limbs and cheeks (Fig. 32.13). New nodules may develop over several weeks. They usually disappear spontaneously without complication in several months, leaving no trace. However, sometimes they become fluctuant, ulcerate or calcify. In patients with calcified lesions, troublesome hypercalcaemia may develop (Tran and Sheth 2003). Fluctuant lesions should be aspirated, secondary infection should be dealt with if it complicates ulcerated lesions and serum calcium levels should be monitored for some months.

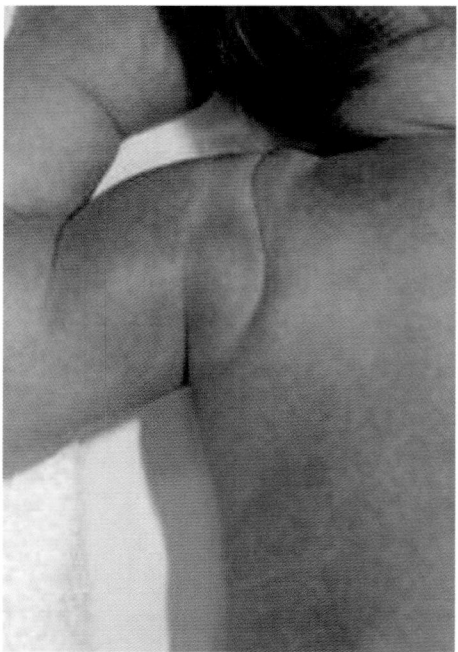

Fig. 32.13 Subcutaneous fat necrosis.

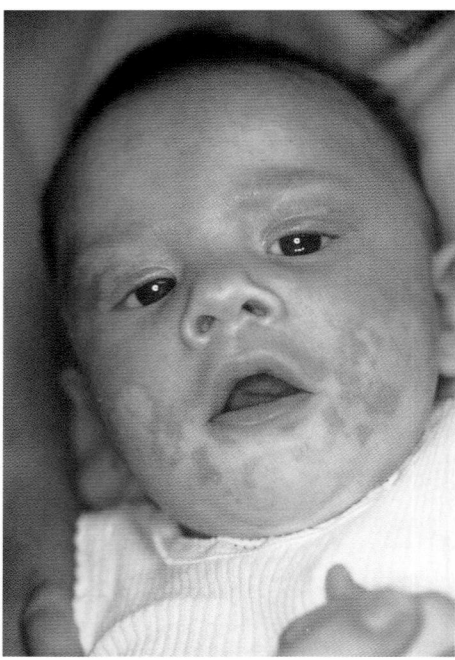

Fig. 32.14 Neonatal lupus erythematosus.

Neonatal lupus erythematosus

This occurs as a result of the passage of maternal SS-A or SS-B (anti-Ro, anti-La) antibodies through the placenta, when the mother suffers from clinical or subclinical lupus erythematosus or Sjögren syndrome (Buyon and Clancy 2003). The most important feature of neonatal lupus erythematosus is heart block, but there seems to be an inverse relationship between cutaneous and cardiac lesions. Other rare complications include autoimmune haemolytic anaemia, thrombocytopenia, hepatitis, pneumonitis and splenomegaly. Lesions appear soon after the first sun exposure. The most characteristic is a mauve erythema on the face with a clear lower border on the cheeks, extending up around the eyes into the hairline (Fig. 32.14). A similar erythema may occur on the arms. Occasionally lesions are annular, scaly or telangiectatic. The condition in the baby settles spontaneously in a few months, when the antibodies disappear. The finding of antibodies in either mother or child is adequate proof of the diagnosis and biopsy is unnecessary.

The red scaly baby

A number of important conditions can present with diffuse redness and variable scaliness (erythroderma) in the neonate or young baby (Box 32.5) (Pruszkowski et al. 2000). These babies can have major problems with temperature regulation and fluid balance and may fail to thrive.

Seborrhoeic dermatitis

There is a dull red erythema with a greasy yellow scale, involving particularly the scalp, centrofacial area and all the flexures but sometimes more widespread. The scale may be absent in the flexures and secondary candidiasis is common. It is usually asymptomatic and self-limiting after the early months of life. It responds to weak steroids and anticandidal agents.

Box 32.5	Conditions which may present with generalised erythema in the neonate

Seborrhoeic dermatitis
Atopic dermatitis
Psoriasis
Ichthyoses
    Collodion baby phenotype
    Netherton syndrome
    Harlequin ichthyosis
Immunodeficiency disorders
Congenital mastocytosis
Staphylococcal scalded-skin syndrome
Cystic fibrosis

Atopic dermatitis

Very rarely this condition presents in the neonatal period with a widespread red scaly and itchy rash. These patients are likely to go on to difficult long-term disease. Management involves emollients and careful use of weak topical steroids, sometimes with wet dressings.

Psoriasis

A dramatic form of psoriasis seen in babies is napkin (diaper) psoriasis with dissemination (Morris et al. 2001). A well-marginated, bright-red napkin rash develops initially and then small scaly patches spread beyond the margins. There is then an explosive spread of psoriatic lesions to the scalp and face and then all over the trunk (Fig. 32.15). This condition has become much less common with the popularity of superabsorbent disposable diapers. The baby remains well and the condition is usually self-limiting in

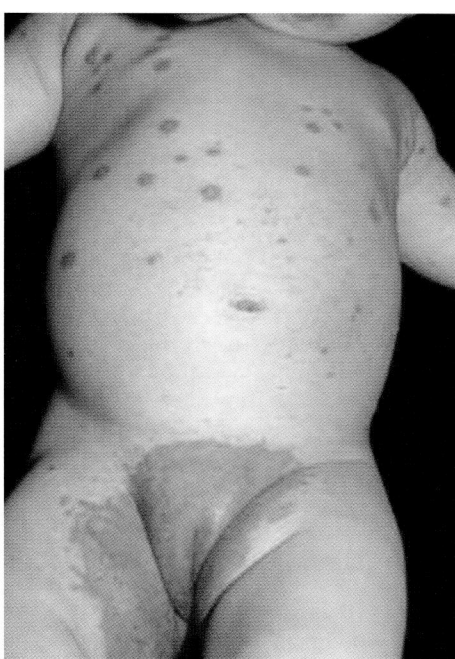

Fig. 32.15 Napkin psoriasis with dissemination.

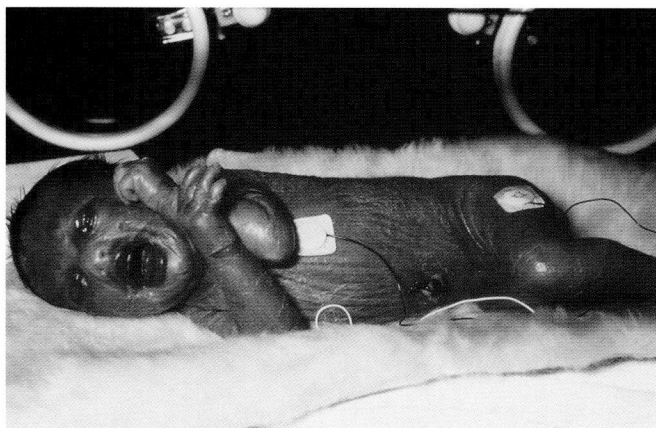

Fig. 32.16 Collodion baby.

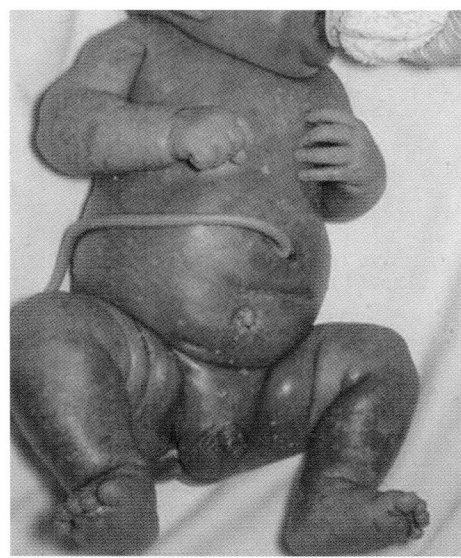

Fig. 32.17 Netherton syndrome.

a few weeks. Very rarely psoriasis may present in the neonatal period or even at birth as a generalised erythroderma, sometimes progressing to a pustular psoriasis. Infantile generalised pustular psoriasis may be associated with lytic bone lesions and the capillary leak syndrome (Pruzkowski et al. 2000).

Ichthyoses

Collodion baby phenotype

This is a descriptive term for the child who is encased at birth in a shiny tight membrane resembling collodion or plastic skin, producing ectropion and eclabium and fissuring (Fig. 32.16) (Buyse et al. 1993). The membrane peels off in days or weeks. This may be a presentation of various forms of ichthyosis, particularly congenital ichthyosiform erythroderma and lamellar ichthyosis, but also trichothiodystrophy, Gaucher disease, neutral lipid storage disease and Conradi–Hünermann syndrome. Rarely, the membrane peels off to leave normal skin; this condition is called lamellar exfoliation of the newborn. Collodion babies show temperature instability and excessive fluid loss. Corneal exposure may result if the eyes are not covered, and the eclabium may necessitate squeeze-bottle, tube or dropper feeding. As the fissures appear, secondary infection becomes a risk. The child should be nursed in high humidity. Emollients are best avoided in the early stages.

X-linked ichthyosis

This may present in the first month with pale shiny plates of scale, without redness, in a widespread distribution, lasting several days before exfoliating. It is only several months later that the typical dark scale of this condition appears.

Netherton syndrome

This is a genetic disorder, due to a *SPINK* gene mutation, which may present as a congenital erythroderma with generalised redness and scale (Fig. 32.17) (Chavanas et al. 2000). There is a severe failure to thrive and a significant risk of hypernatraemic dehydration. These babies usually have no hair at all at birth. When hair develops, it is fragile and appears short, broken and sparse and histologically shows trichorrhexis invaginata (bamboo hair).

Harlequin ichthyosis

It is only in recent years that survivors of this condition have been reported (Lawlor 1989; Rogers and Scarf 1989). In most patients, initial survival has been a result of retinoid therapy, but some patients have survived without specific therapy. These babies are at birth encased in a carapace of white hyperkeratotic skin, leading to severe distortion of facial features, ears, hands and feet. The skin soon splits, leaving bleeding fissures (Fig. 32.18), and then peels off, leaving red scaly skin beneath and a clinical picture similar to the severe end of the spectrum of congenital ichthyosiform erythroderma. Death in these infants occurs as a result of infection or respiratory failure due to prenatal collection in the lungs of exfoliated squamous material contaminating the amniotic fluid.

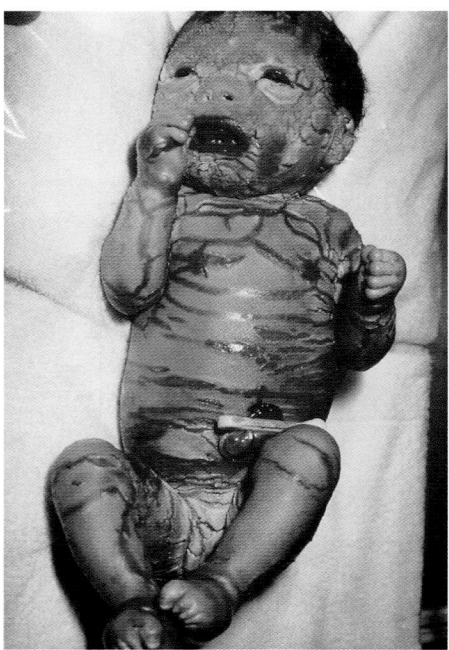

Fig. 32.18 Harlequin ichthyosis.

Immunodeficiencies

Patients with severe combined immunodeficiency, Omenn syndrome (T-cell deficiency, abnormal histiocytic cells and elevated IgE level; Ch. 39, part 1) and other immunodeficiencies may present with a widespread red scaly rash commencing in the neonatal period but not present at birth (Glover et al. 1988; Farrell et al. 1995; Ricci et al. 1997). In some cases this represents a congenital graft-versus-host reaction. These babies usually demonstrate a progressive alopecia, recurrent infections, diarrhoea and failure to thrive. What was described in the past as Leiner disease is now recognised as not a specific entity but a phenotype of non-congenital early-onset erythroderma, diarrhoea and failure to thrive. Some of the patients initially diagnosed as having Leiner disease have subsequently been recognised as having Netherton syndrome, while others have had a variety of immunodeficiencies. Skin biopsy and detailed study of immunological parameters is essential in any erythrodermic baby in whom another clear diagnosis has not been established. The terms Leiner disease and Leiner syndrome would be best abandoned.

Birthmarks, congenital tumours and other naevoid conditions

Pigmented birthmarks

Congenital melanocytic naevi

These occur at birth as raised verrucous or lobulated lesions of varying shades of brown to black, sometimes with blue or pink components, with an irregular margin and often growing long dark hairs. Giant-sized lesions may produce considerable redundancy of skin and often occur in a 'garment' distribution on the trunk and adjacent limbs. Malignancy in giant naevi can occur in childhood and the incidence over a lifetime is possibly of the order of 5%. In medium and small lesions, the risk is a lot lower and any development of malignancy is always postpubertal. Lesions

occurring over the spine, especially the upper part, may be associated with meningeal melanocytosis, which may be complicated by melanoma or obstructive hydrocephalus. Lesions over the lower spine may rarely be associated with spinal dysraphism and tethered cord. Large axial lesions or multiple scattered medium to large lesions may be associated with posterior cranial fossa malformations. All patients with these types of lesions should have imaging studies performed as soon as possible.

Naevoid pigmentary disorders

These are flat areas of hyperpigmented or hypopigmented skin which may be evident at birth. They occur in characteristic patterns – either segmental, or whirled and streaky following the lines of Blaschko (Nehal et al. 1996). Sometimes there is a combination of hypo- and hyperpigmented streaks. These distributions are now recognised as mosaic phenotypes, indicating that the individual comprises more than one population of cells as a result of a variety of mechanisms including chromosomal mosaicism, genomic mosaicism and chimerism. They may have smooth or irregular edges and occur anywhere on the trunk, limbs or face. They usually occur as isolated phenomena but, particularly when extensive, may be associated, as part of certain mosaic phenotypes, with neurological, skeletal and other abnormalities (Nehal et al. 1996).

Important in the differential diagnosis are the café-au-lait spots of neurofibromatosis and the hypopigmented macules of tuberous sclerosis, both of which may occasionally be present at birth but which tend to be smaller, do not follow mosaic patterns and increase in number with time.

Mongolian spots

These are flat, blue or slate-grey lesions with poorly defined margins. They may be single or multiple and occur particularly on the lumbosacral area, although the shoulders, upper back and occasionally other areas may be involved. They are found in over 80% of oriental and black infants and in up to 10% of white infants, particularly those of Mediterranean origin. They usually fade considerably by puberty, but may remain unaltered through life.

Naevus of Ota

This is a persistent patchy blue–grey discoloration of the skin of the face, particularly on the cheek, periorbital area and brow. It is usually unilateral and often there is a similar pigmentation of the sclera of the ipsilateral eye. It is most common in oriental individuals and is present at birth in over 50% of cases. Associated glaucoma (Lui and Ball 1991) and sensorineural deafness have been reported, and, very rarely, melanoma may occur in adult life.

Epidermal naevi

Epidermal naevi arise from the basal layer of the embryonic epidermis which gives rise to skin appendages as well as keratinocytes. These naevi have conventionally been classified according to the tissue of origin into keratinocytic, sebaceous and follicular types (Happle and Rogers 2002). They can involve any area of skin. They may be present at birth or appear in the first few years of life and may extend well beyond their original distribution. On the scalp and face they have a yellowish colour due to prominent sebaceous glands and present as a hairless, often linear plaque, usually flat in infancy and childhood and becoming verrucous at puberty. Sometimes they are more papillomatous. Lesions elsewhere are usually dark brown but occasionally are paler than the normal skin. They

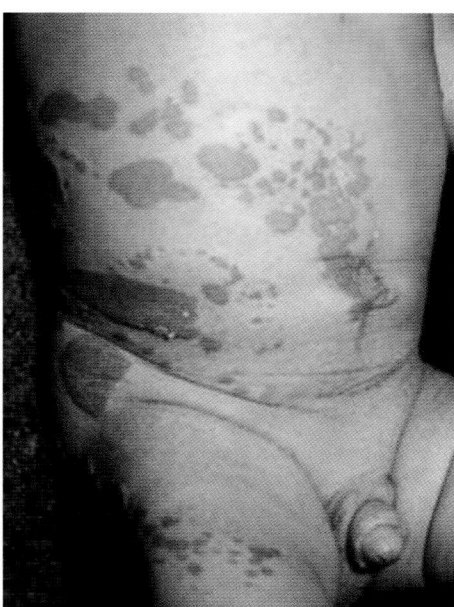

Fig. 32.19 Verrucous epidermal naevus.

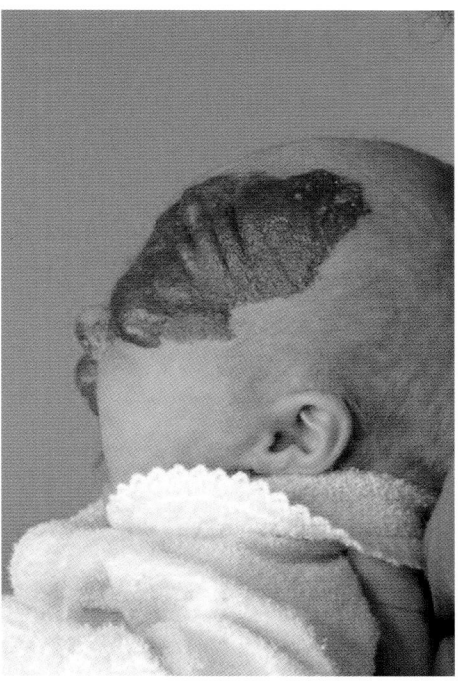

Fig. 32.20 Extensive segmental facial haemangioma.

occur as single or multiple warty plaques or lines (Fig. 32.19), often arranged in a linear or swirled pattern. It is now clear that the linear and swirled patterns taken by epidermal naevi follow the lines of Blaschko, and that all epidermal naevi can be explained on the basis of genetic mosaicism, with each type of naevus representing the cutaneous manifestation of a different mosaic phenotype. In most patients the naevus is the only detectable manifestation, but in some patients there are associated abnormalities in other organ systems, particularly skeletal, neurological and ocular. Skeletal abnormalities occur particularly with naevi of keratinocytic type on the limbs, and neurological and ocular abnormalities with naevi of sebaceous type on the head. These patients should have a careful physical examination, but imaging studies are generally not indicated in the absence of abnormal signs or symptoms.

Vascular birthmarks

These can be divided into haemangiomas, which are proliferative vascular tumours, and vascular malformations, which represent fixed collections of dilated abnormal vessels (Requena and Sangueza 1997; Bruckner and Frieden 2006).

Haemangiomas

Haemangiomas usually appear just after birth, undergo a fast growth phase, and then, over a long period, tend towards spontaneous resolution (Bruckner and Frieden 2006). It is now clear that haemangiomas, whether superficially or deeply located in the skin, have the same structure, being composed in the early stage of proliferating masses of endothelial cells with occasional lumina and later, as they resolve, of large endothelial lined spaces. The terms capillary, cavernous and capillary–cavernous are misleading and should be abandoned in favour of the simple term haemangioma.

Superficial haemangiomas are usually not present at birth but appear in the first weeks of life as an area of pallor followed by a telangiectatic patch. They then grow rapidly into a lobulated, well-demarcated, bright-red tumour (Fig. 32.20). Rapid growth

continues over the first 6 months; the growth rate then slows and further growth after 10 months is unusual, except in the case of extensive facial lesions which can continue to grow for over a year. After a stationary phase, signs of involution begin with the appearance of grey areas, which enlarge and coalesce. The lesions gradually fade and flatten, and, if uncomplicated, often resolve completely over several years. However residual telangiectasia may persist in the area and redundant tissue can remain in the place of large superficial lesions.

Deeper haemangiomas may occur alone or beneath a superficial lesion. They also usually appear after birth and undergo a growth phase. The overlying skin is normal or bluish in colour. As they resolve, deep haemangiomas soften and shrink, and complete disappearance occurs in almost all cases. Apparent deep haemangiomas which show no sign of resolution are now recognised as vascular malformations, usually of venous type, and are not haemangiomas at all.

Ulceration can occur during the rapid growth phase of superficial haemangiomas and can be associated with severe bleeding. If secondary infection is controlled, the ulcers usually heal in a few weeks, but some scarring is inevitable. Ulceration of lesions on eyelids, lips or ala nasae can lead to full-thickness tissue loss. Scarring following ulceration of lesions on or near the eyelids can result in a cicatricial ectropion, and alopecia may be permanent after scalp ulceration.

Haemangiomas may encroach on vital structures. A haemangioma closing the eye for as little as 4 weeks in infancy can produce amblyopia. However, even without occluding the pupil, an eyelid lesion, by pressing on the eye and producing astigmatism, can lead to failure of development of binocular vision and partial amblyopia. Large haemangiomas around the mouth may interfere with feeding and one blocking both nares can lead to respiratory difficulties while the child is being fed. A large deep haemangioma around the neck may displace the pharynx or trachea: also the upper respiratory tract may be directly involved with the haemangioma. The possibility of laryngeal involvement should be considered with an extensive lower face or neck haemangioma, particularly when there is accompanying intraoral involvement, and a lateral airways X-ray should be arranged. If there is stridor, urgent laryngoscopy is mandatory. Even when traumatised, uncomplicated haemangiomas rarely bleed significantly.

Lesions over the lower spine may be associated with spinal fusion abnormalities and a tethered spinal cord (Ch. 40.8); lesions involving the sacral area, with urogenital and rectal abnormalities; and large hemifacial lesions (Fig. 32.20), with Dandy–Walker and other posterior cranial fossa abnormalities, a vascular ring and other major vessel anomalies (Bruckner and Frieden 2006). Early imaging studies should be undertaken when haemangiomas are in these positions.

Simple observation and reassurance while awaiting natural resolution is the ideal approach for most haemangiomas. Showing serial photographs of resolved lesions is encouraging. Indications for active intervention are an alarming growth rate, threatening ulceration in areas where serious complications could ensue, interference with vital structures and severe bleeding. Oral corticosteroids will slow the growth of potentially dangerous or cosmetically serious lesions. They have no place once growth has ceased. A recent discovery is the frequent response of early haemangiomas to propranolol and controlled studies are being performed (Léauté-Labrèze et al. 2008). Vincristine is gaining favour as an additional or alternative agent in lesions which show inadequate response. Intralesional steroids may be used in very experienced hands to shrink periorbital haemangiomas that fail to respond to oral steroids. Cosmetic surgical procedures can improve the appearance when loose tissue remains. Laser therapy has a place for upper respiratory tract lesions and as an adjunct or alternative to surgery in some complicated lesions.

Diffuse infantile haemangiomatosis

This is a condition with multiple small haemangiomas in a widespread distribution (Bruckner and Frieden 2006). There is a benign form, with lesions limited to the skin; however, in the potentially serious systemic form, lesions may occur in many organs, particularly the liver, gastrointestinal tract, lungs and central nervous system, with or, rarely, without cutaneous lesions. These patients should be carefully assessed, with full blood count, chest X-ray and examination for cardiac failure due to arteriovenous shunts, and for bleeding from the gastrointestinal tract. Ultrasound should be performed to exclude hepatic involvement, and other organs should be further investigated as indicated. More sophisticated studies such as angiography and technetium-labelled red blood cell scans can delineate further the extent of internal involvement. With severe systemic involvement, high-dose corticosteroids are required along with management of cardiac failure and other complications.

Vascular malformations

Vascular malformations are structural abnormalities and, as such, are present at birth, grow in proportion to the patient's growth and have no tendency to resolution (Requena and Sangueza 1997). They can be further divided according to their vessel of origin into capillary, arterial, venous, lymphatic and mixed types. Ultrasound is the most useful non-invasive investigation and, along with history and clinical examination, can identify the elements of most vascular malformations and separate them from haemangiomas.

Capillary malformation

This has previously been called port-wine stain or naevus flammeus but the accurate descriptive term capillary malformation should be used. This is a vascular malformation composed of dilated mature capillaries. Lesions may be unilateral or, less often, bilateral and occur anywhere on the body, though most commonly on the face. They are deep pink in infancy, later becoming more purple. After puberty, they may become raised and nodular. Until recently, only cosmetic cover could be offered, but good results are now being achieved with the pulsed-dye laser and commencement of treatment in the early months of life gives the best results.

Sturge–Weber syndrome

This is the association of a facial capillary malformation and a vascular malformation of the ipsilateral meninges and cerebral cortex. The cutaneous lesion always involves the brow (Tallman 1991). The neurological manifestations of the syndrome include convulsions, hemiparesis and mental retardation. When the facial lesion involves both upper and lower eyelids congenital glaucoma may occur (Tallman 1991). Patients presenting with a capillary malformation in the appropriate distribution should have early neurological and ophthalmological consultation and continued close follow-up. A magnetic resonance imaging scan may demonstrate the intracranial malformations in the first few months of life.

Venous malformation

This appears as a bluish tumour, which empties with pressure when elevated, and fills when dependent.

Lymphatic malformation (lymphangioma, cystic hygroma)

Macrocystic deep lesions present as skin-coloured tumours, often with bruising (Fig. 32.21); superficial lesions present as groups of haemorrhagic vesicles or warty lesions (Davies and Rogers 2000).

Arteriovenous malformation

A localised arteriovenous malformation (AVM) presents as a skin-coloured lump which may demonstrate a bruit on auscultation. More often, an AVM is part of a complex mixed malformation.

Mixed malformations

All combinations of malformation can occur, with two, three or even four elements being present. The eponym Klippel–Trenaunay

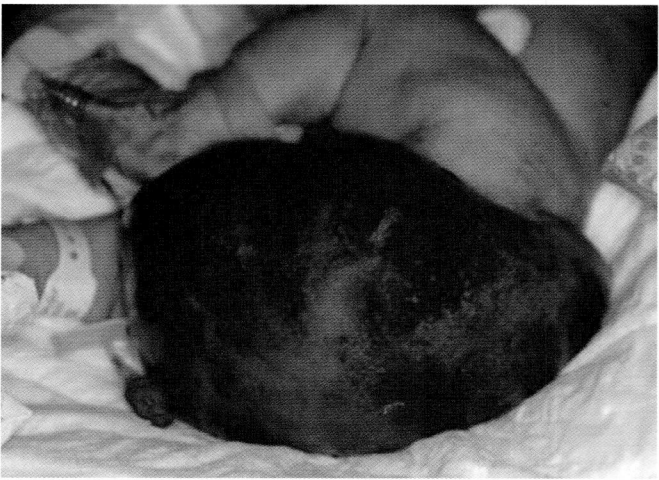

Fig. 32.21 Large lymphatic malformation with haemorrhage.

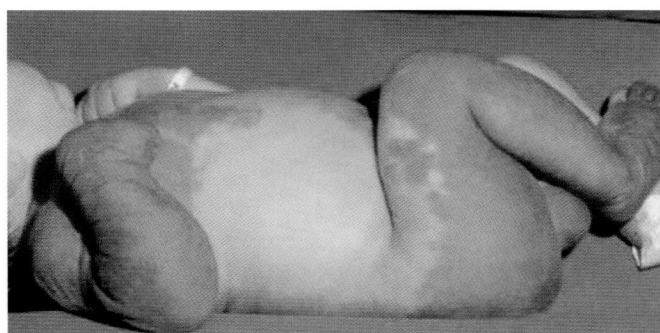

Fig. 32.22 Extensive capillary–venous malformation with limb hypertrophy (Klippel–Trenaunay syndrome)

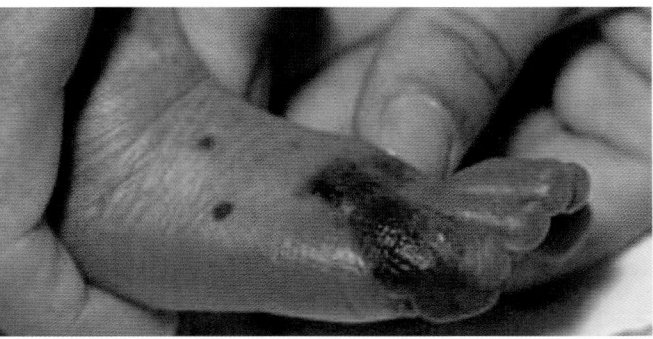

Fig. 32.23 Langerhans cell histiocytosis.

syndrome refers to a capillary malformation, venous malformation and sometimes lymphatic malformation associated with overgrowth of a limb, with soft-tissue hypertrophy and/or bony hypertrophy (Fig. 32.22), or, very rarely, hypotrophy. The eponym Parkes–Weber syndrome refers to a capillary malformation and AVM with limb hypertrophy. These mixed vascular malformations are best described by their component parts rather than using the eponyms.

Some congenital tumours

Vascular tumours

Rare vascular tumours that may be present at birth include tufted angioma, kaposiform haemangioendothelioma (KHE) and an entity presently designated congenital haemangioma (CH) (Rogers et al. 2002; Lyons et al. 2004). All of these have typical histological features and CH has a characteristic ultrasound appearance.

Tufted angioma is a rare vascular proliferation which may be congenital. It presents as a red to brown or violaceous plaque or nodule; some resolve, while others persist and spread. It is rarely associated with Kasabach–Merritt syndrome (KMS). KHE is a yellow, blue or red plaque-like lesion, usually present at birth and commonly associated with KMS (Lyons et al. 2004). Sometimes elements of both KHE and tufted angioma are found in the same lesion.

CH is a vascular tumour which bears some clinical resemblance to a common haemangioma of infancy but is quite distinct from it and has a characteristic ultrasound appearance (Rogers et al. 2002). It proliferates in utero and is fully developed at birth. It presents as a raised plaque or tumour, bluish or violaceous in colour, sometimes studded with telangiectases and often surrounded by a characteristic pale halo. Unlike standard haemangiomas, it does not demonstrate an accelerated postnatal growth phase. Instead, involution commences promptly and progresses rapidly, often leaving an area of atrophy. The majority regress totally by 12 months of age.

Kasabach–Merritt syndrome

This was initially believed to be a complication of large haemangiomas, but it is now clear that the associated lesions are not haemangiomas but represent other vascular tumours, including tufted angioma and KHE (see above). Thrombocytopenia is caused by entrapment of platelets within the lesion and is sometimes followed by disseminated intravascular coagulation. Initially there is bleeding into the lesion, which rapidly enlarges, and then widespread life-threatening haemorrhage may follow. When bleeding is confined to the tumour, the approach can be conservative. In severe cases, steroids and vincristine have been used to shrink the tumour, or removal can be considered if feasible. Management also involves resuscitation, transfusion and dealing with the disseminated intravascular coagulation.

Langerhans cell histiocytosis (Ch. 36)

This may occasionally present in the neonate with a single or small numbers of tumours. They are usually red nodules, often with an eroded or crusted surface (Fig. 32.23), and often resolve spontaneously.

Congenital leukaemia (Ch. 30)

This may present with multiple, skin-coloured or, more often, purpuric nodules, or, occasionally, a single nodule which histologically demonstrates a leukaemic infiltrate.

Sarcomas (Ch. 36)

Fibrosarcoma, rhabdomyosarcoma and undifferentiated sarcoma can all present as a deep red firm mass with a shiny surface and rapid growth.

Congenital neuroblastoma (Ch. 36)

Cutaneous metastases present at birth or soon after, as multiple bluish firm nodules, which may demonstrate persistent blanching on pressure.

Infantile myofibromatosis

In most cases, this presents at birth or soon after; the lesions may be solitary or multicentric, with possible involvement of bones and multiple internal organs (Stanford and Rogers 2000). Solitary lesions are usually large red tumours on the skin or involving mucosal surfaces (Fig. 32.24). In the multicentric form, cutaneous lesions present as small nodules or indented areas of skin due to surface tethering. Extensive imaging studies are required in these patients to detect internal involvement.

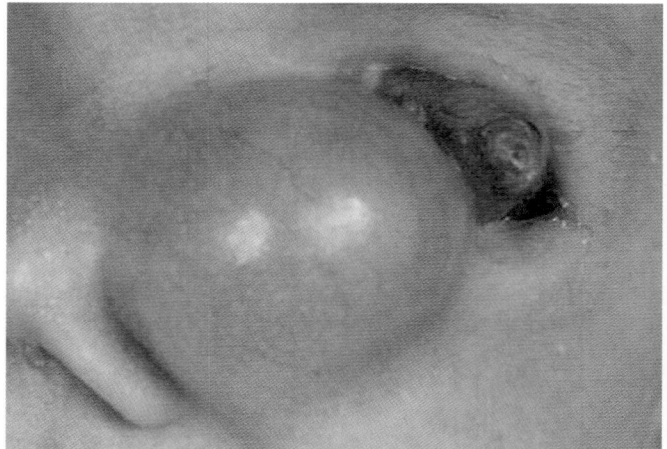

Fig. 32.24 Infantile myofibromatosis; large tumour in orbital area.

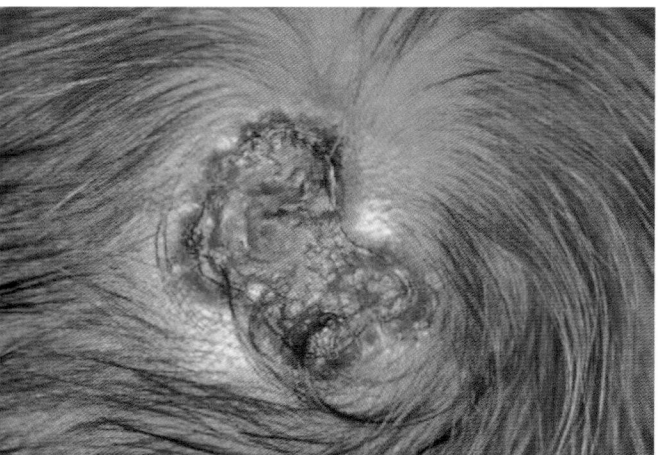

Fig. 32.25 Aplasia cutis presenting as a large stellate erosion.

Juvenile xanthogranuloma

These may be present at birth as yellow or red (the non-lipidised variant) nodules. They usually involve after many months. These patients are normolipaemic.

Dermoid cysts

These are congenital cysts occurring along embryonic fusion lines as asymptomatic, non-compressible nodules (Paller et al. 1991) with a typical ultrasound appearance. The commonest positions are over the anterior fontanelle, at the lateral end of the eyebrow and in the midline of the upper nose. Dermal sinuses are short tracks connecting the dermoid to the skin surface, where a punctum is seen. These occur particularly with nasal lesions. Dermoids have no malignant potential and cosmetic considerations are the main reason for their removal. However, as these lesions, with the exception of those in the eyebrow area, have a significant risk of underlying connections to the central nervous system, no surgery should ever be undertaken without imaging studies to identify whether such a connection exists so that an appropriate approach can be planned.

Encephalocele, meningocele and heterotopic brain tissue

See Chapter 40 part 8 for more detail. Local markers of these lesions include a capillary malformation and superimposed or surrounding hypertrichosis (Kos and Drolet 2008).

Aplasia cutis

Aplasia cutis (AC) is a congenital absence of skin, usually localised but sometimes occurring as multiple lesions in a widespread distribution. The commonest form is membranous AC, which presents as single or multiple round or oval lesions, with an intact but atrophic surface on the scalp or side of the face, sometimes with a surrounding hair collar, and probably representing incomplete closure of embryonic fusion lines (Drolet et al. 1995). Another form is as a large stellate erosion (Fig. 32.25) at or near the midline of the scalp, which crusts and finally, after some months, heals with a scar which is often hypertrophic. Imaging to detect an underlying skull defect is essential in all cases of scalp AC.

Scalp AC occurs in a number of syndromes, including trisomy 13, Johanson–Blizzard syndrome and Adams–Oliver syndrome.

Extensive truncal and limb AC may be associated with fetus papyraceus (Léauté-Labrèze et al. 1998).

Gluteal granulomas

These occur on top of a pre-existing napkin rash as impressive purplish nodules, histologically demonstrating a benign mixed inflammatory infiltrate. The nodules tend to be oval in shape, following the lines of the skin folds. The cause is unclear but they settle slowly with standard treatment with weak steroid and barrier preparations.

References

Al-Mutairi, N., Sharma, A.K., Zaki, A., et al., 2004. Maternal and neonatal pemphigoid gestationis. Clin Exp Dermatol 29, 202–204.

Bergman, J.N., Eichenfield, L.F., 2002. Neonatal acne and cephalic pustulosis: is malassezia the whole story? Arch Dermatol 138, 255–257.

Berlin, A.L., Paller, A.S., Chan, L.S., 2002. Incontinentia pigmenti: a review and update on the molecular basis of pathophysiology. J Am Acad Dermatol 47, 169–187.

Briley, L.D., 2008. Cutaneous mastocytosis: A review focusing on the pediatric population. Clin Pediatr 47, 757–761.

Bruckner, A.L., Frieden, I.J., 2006. Infantile hemangiomas. J Am Acad Dermatol 55, 671–682.

Buyon, J.P., Clancy, R.M., 2003. Neonatal lupus: review of proposed pathogenesis and clinical data from the US-based Research Registry for Neonatal Lupus. Autoimmunity 36, 41–50.

Buyse, L., Graves, C., Marks, R., et al., 1993. Collodion baby dehydration: the danger of high transepidermal water loss. Br J Dermatol 129, 86–88.

Carder, R., 2008. Fungal infections, infestations and parasitic infections in neonates. In: Eichenfield, L.F., Frieden, I.J., Esterly, N.B. (Eds.), Textbook of Neonatal Dermatology, second ed. WB Saunders, Philadelphia, PA, pp. 213–227.

Chakraborty, R., Luck, S., 2008. Syphilis is on the increase: the implications for child health. Arch Dis Child 93, 105–109.

Chavanas, S., Bodemer, C., Rochat, A., et al., 2000. Mutations in SPINK5, encoding a serine protease inhibitor, cause Netherton syndrome. Nat Genet 25, 141–142.

Chue, C.D., Rajpar, S.F., Bhat, J., 2008. An acrodermatitis enteropathica-like eruption secondary to acquired zinc deficiency in an exclusively breast-fed premature infant. Int J Dermatol 47, 372–373.

Darmstadt, G.L., Dinulos, J.G., Miller, Z., 2000. Congenital cutaneous candidiasis: Clinical presentation, pathogenesis, and management guidelines. Pediatrics 105, 438–444.

Davies, D., Rogers, M., 2000. Morphology of lymphatic malformations: a pictorial review. Aust J Dermatol 41, 1–7.

Drolet, B., Prendiville, J., Golden, J., et al., 1995. Membranous aplasia cutis with hair collars. Congenital absence of skin or neuroectodermal defect? Arch Dermatol 131, 1427–1429.

Farrell, A., Scerri, L., Stevens, A., et al., 1995. Acute graft-versus-host disease with unusual cutaneous intracellular vacuolation in an infant with severe combined immunodeficiency. Pediatr Dermatol 12, 311–313.

Fine, J.D., Eady, R.A., Bauer, E.A., et al., 2008. The classification of inherited epidermolysis bullosa (EB): Report of the Third International Consensus Meeting on Diagnosis and Classification of EB. J Am Acad Dermatol 58, 931–950.

Glover, M.T., Atherton, D.J., Levinsky, R.J., 1988. Syndrome of erythroderma, failure to thrive and diarrhea in infancy: a manifestation of immunodeficiency. Pediatrics 81, 66–72.

Goncalves, V., Pessoa, O., Lowy, G., 2007. Evaluation of a congenital erosive and vesicular dermatosis healing with reticulated supple scarring. Pediatr Dermatol 24, 384–386.

Happle, R., Rogers, M., 2002. Epidermal nevi. Adv Dermatol 18, 175–201.

Harpin, V.A., Rutter, N., 1982. Percutaneous alcohol absorption and skin necrosis in a premature infant. Arch Dis Child 57, 477–479.

Herman, L.E., Rothman, K.F., Harawi, S., et al., 1990. Congenital self-healing reticulohistiocytosis. A new entity in the differential diagnosis of neonatal papulovesicular eruptions. Arch Dermatol 126, 210–212.

Jennings, J.L., Burrows, W.M., 1983. Infantile acropustulosis. J Am Acad Dermatol 9, 733–738.

Kamei, R., Honig, P.J., 1988. Neonatal Job's syndrome featuring a vesicular eruption. Pediatr Dermatol 5, 75–82.

Kiechl-Kohlendorfer, U., Fink, F.M., Steichen-Gersdorf, E., 2007. Transient symptomatic zinc deficiency in a breast-fed preterm infant. Pediatr Dermatol 24, 536–540.

Kos, L., Drolet, B.A., 2008. Developmental abnormalities. In: Eichenfield, L.F., Frieden, I.J., Esterly, N.B. (Eds.), Textbook of Neonatal Dermatology, second ed. WB Saunders, Philadelphia, pp. 113–130.

Ladrigan, M.K., LeBoit, P.E., Frieden, I.F., 2008. Neonatal eosinophilic pustulosis in a 2-month old. Pediatr Dermatol 25, 52–55.

Lane, A.T., 1987. Development and care of the premature infant's skin. Pediatr Dermatol 4, 1–5.

Lawlor, F., 1989. Progress of a harlequin fetus to non-bullous ichthyosiform erythroderma. Pediatrics 82, 870–873.

Léauté-Labrèze, C., Depaire-Duclos, F., Sarlangue, J., et al., 1998. Congenital cutaneous defects as complications of surviving co-twins; aplasia cutis congenita and neonatal Volkmann ischemic contracture of the forearm. Arch Dermatol 134, 1121–1124.

Léauté-Labrèze, C., Dumas de la Roque, E., Hubiche, T., et al., 2008. Propranolol for severe hemangiomas of infancy. N Engl J Med 358, 2649–2651.

Littler, C.M., 1997. Laser hair removal in a patient with hypertrichosis lanuginosa congenita. Dermatol Surg 23, 705–707.

Lucky, A.W., 2008. Transient benign cutaneous lesions in the newborn. In: Eichenfield, L.F., Frieden, I.J., Esterly, N.B. (Eds.), Textbook of Neonatal Dermatology, second ed. WB Saunders, Philadelphia, pp. 85–97.

Lui, J.C., Ball, S.F., 1991. Nevus of Ota with glaucoma: report of three cases. Ann Ophthalmol 23, 286–289.

Lyons, L.L., North, P.E., Mac-Moune Lai, F., et al., 2004. Kaposiform hemangioendothelioma: a study of 33 cases emphasizing its pathologic, immunophenotypic, and biologic uniqueness from juvenile hemangioma. Am J Surg 28, 559–568.

Mallon, E., Wojnarowska, F., Hope, P., et al., 1995. Neonatal bullous eruption as a result of transient porphyrinemia in a premature infant with hemolytic disease of the newborn. J Am Acad Dermatol 33, 333–336.

Mancini, A.J., Frieden, I.J., Paller, A.S., 1998. Infantile acropustulosis revisited: history of scabies and response to topical corticosteroids. Pediatr Dermatol 15, 337–341.

Marinkovich, M., 1999. Update on inherited bullous dermatoses. Dermatol Clin 17, 473–485.

Masunaga, T., Ishiko, A., Takizawa, Y., et al., 2004. Pyloric atresia-junctional epidermolysis bullosa syndrome showing novel 594insC/Q425P mutations in integrin beta-4 gene (ITGB4). Exp Dermatol 13, 61–64.

Merlob, P., Metzker, A., Reisner, S.H., 1982. Transient neonatal pustular melanosis. AM J Dis Child 136, 521–522.

Morris, A., Rogers, M., Fischer, G., et al., 2001. Childhood psoriasis: a clinical review of 1262 cases. Pediatr Dermatol 18, 188–198.

Nanda, S., Reddy, B.S.N., Ramji, S., et al., 2002. Analytical study of pustular eruptions in neonates. Pediatr Dermatol 19, 210–215.

Nehal, K.S., PeBenito, R., Orlow, S.J., 1996. Analysis of 54 cases of hypopigmentation and hyperpigmentation along the lines of Blaschko. Arch Dermatol 132, 1167–1170.

Paller, A.S., Pensler, J., Tomita, T., 1991. Nasal midline masses in infants and children. Dermoids, encephaloceles, and nasal gliomas. Arch Dermatol 127, 362–366.

Pruszkowski, A., Bodemer, C., Fraitag, S., et al., 2000. Neonatal and infantile erythrodermas: A retrospective study of 51 patients. Arch Dermatol 136, 875–880.

Quarterman, M.J., Lesher, J.L., 1994. Neonatal scabies treated with permethrin 5% cream. Pediatr Dermatol 11, 264–266.

Requena, L., Sangueza, O.P., 1997. Cutaneous vascular anomalies. Part 1. Hamartomas, malformations and dilation of pre-existing vessels. J Am Acad Dermatol 37, 523–549.

Ricci, G., Patrizi, A., Specchia, F., 1997. Omenn syndrome. Pediatr Dermatol 14, 49–52.

Rogers, M., 2008. Hair disorders. In: Eichenfield, L.F., Frieden, I.J., Esterly, N.B. (Eds.), Textbook of Neonatal Dermatology, second ed. WB Saunders, Philadelphia, pp. 517–535.

Rogers, M., Scarf, C., 1989. Harlequin baby treated with etretinate. Pediatr Dermatol 6, 216–221.

Rogers, M., Lam, A., Fischer, G., 2002. Sonographic findings in a series of rapidly involuting congenital hemangiomas (RICH). Pediatr Dermatol 19, 5–11.

Ross, R., DiGiovanna, J.J., Capaldi, L., et al., 2008. Histopathologic characterization of epidermolytic hyperkeratosis: a systematic review of histology from the National Registry for Ichthyosis and Related Skin Disorders. J Am Acad Dermatol 59, 86–90.

Rowen, J.L., Atkins, J.T., Levy, M.L., et al., 1995. Invasive fungal dermatitis in the 1000-gram neonate. Pediatrics 95, 682–687.

Rutter, N., 1987. Percutaneous drug absorption in the newborn: hazards and uses. Clin Perinatol 14, 911–930.

Sauerbrei, A., Wutzler, P., 2007a. Herpes simplex and varicella-zoster virus infections during pregnancy: current concepts of prevention, diagnosis and therapy. Part 2. Varicella-zoster virus infections. Med Microbiol Immunol 196, 95–102.

Sauerbrei, A., Wutzler, P., 2007b. Herpes simplex and varicella-zoster virus infections during pregnancy: current concepts of prevention, diagnosis and therapy. Part 1. Herpes simplex virus infections. Med Microbiol Immunol 196, 89–94.

Selimoglu, M.A., Dilmen, U., Karakelleoglu, C., et al., 1995. Harlequin color change. Arch Pediatr Adolesc Med 149, 1171–1172.

Stanford, D., Rogers, M., 2000. Dermatological presentations of infantile myofibromatosis: a review of 27 cases. Aust J Dermatol 41, 156–161.

Tallman, B., 1991. Location of port-wine stain and the likelihood of ophthalmic and/or central nervous system complications. Pediatrics 87, 323–327.

Tran, J.T., Sheth, A.P., 2003. Complications of subcutaneous fat necrosis of the newborn: a case report and review of the literature. Pediatr Dermatol 20, 257–261.

Wirges, M.L., Stetson, M., Oliver, J.W., 2006. Pustular leukemoid reaction in a neonate with Down syndrome. J Am Acad Dermatol 52, S62–S64.

Ophthalmology

33

Brian Fleck

© 2012 Elsevier Ltd

When does a neonatologist need an ophthalmologist?

Neonatologists work closely with ophthalmologists in a number of areas. All neonatal units must have a retinopathy of prematurity (ROP) screening programme in place. All neonates must be screened for congenital cataract by examination of the red reflex. Congenital abnormalities of the eyes may be apparent at birth. The eyes may contain diagnostic clues to a number of dysmorphic syndromes and neonatal illnesses. At a slightly later age, neonatologists may encounter infants with reduced vision or abnormal eye movements.

Some common ophthalmic problems of neonates do not necessarily need the involvement of an ophthalmologist. Transient birth-induced eyelid bruising and subconjunctival haemorrhages may simply be observed. Retinal haemorrhages are seen in about 33% of infants following birth, and normally disappear within 1–2 weeks (Hughes et al. 2006). Neonatal conjunctivitis is common, and management is dependent on local microbiological investigation and treatment protocols. *Chlamydia* infection is prevalent in many countries (Rours et al. 2008; Yip et al. 2008), and should be treated with systemic antibiotics, because of the associated risk of pneumonia. Epiphora due to congenital delay of canalisation of the nasolacrimal duct is common in infants (MacEwen 2006). As the natural history is spontaneous resolution in the vast majority of cases (MacEwen 2006), no action is needed for typical cases with minor clinical signs.

Development of the eye

Premature infants show embryonic development features of the eyes. The eyelids are fused in infants born below about 26 weeks' gestation, and open spontaneously after about 5 days (Duerksen et al. 1994). The embryonic blood vessels that surround the lens of the eye – the tunica vasculosa lentis – involute at about 32 weeks' gestation. They inhibit visualisation of the posterior segment of the eye with an ophthalmoscope. They absorb laser energy during treatment of ROP, which may lead to the development of adhesions between the iris and the lens, or even to cataract (Salgado et al. 2010). The hyaloid artery may persist within the vitreous up to about 30 weeks' gestation, but involutes at about the same time as the tunica vasculosa lentis.

The fovea is immature at birth, and develops throughout infancy (Hendrickson 1992). Adult maturity is not achieved until age 5–6 years. Optic nerve myelination develops throughout infancy, and continues to mature during early childhood (Magoon and Robb 1981).

Development of vision

Visual functions develop rapidly during the first 8–12 weeks of life. Vernier visual acuity (Brown 1997; Calloway et al. 2001), visual acuity measured by 'sweep' visually evoked potentials (VEPs) (Weinacht et al. 1999; Lauritzen et al. 2004), stereoscopic vision (Calloway et al. 2001) and colour vision (Dobkins et al. 1997) may all be measured by 3 months of age. Visual acuity measured by VEP shows near-adult responses by age 8 months (Norcia and Tyler 1985). All visual functions continue to mature throughout childhood (Hargadon et al. 2010). Premature infants develop vision correct for their gestational age rather than postnatal age (Weinacht et al. 1999).

Amblyopia

Development of vision is highly dependent on visual experience. High levels of cortical plasticity are limited to the first weeks of life. If a patterned visual image is not experienced by 10–12 weeks, permanent 'visual deprivation' amblyopia will occur (Lloyd et al. 2007). Following surgery for congenital cataract, visual functions improve rapidly (Maurer et al. 1999). Eyelid abnormalities, such as severe congenital ptosis, corneal opacity or opacity of the vitreous, cause effects that are similar to congenital cataracts. Surgery for these conditions must therefore be performed urgently. Less severe forms of amblyopia develop at a later age. Strabismic amblyopia develops when input from a squinting eye is suppressed. Anisometropic amblyopia develops when the refractive focusing is significantly less normal in one eye. The treatment of amblyopia consists of treating the cause, and then temporarily reducing vision in the normal eye in order to allow competitive development of cortical connections using input from the amblyopic eye. Occlusion with an eye patch or blurring by cycloplegic eye drops may be used. Amblyopia treatment follows a dose–response curve, with a more rapid response in younger patients.

Eye conditions that require screening examinations

Retinopathy of prematurity

Premature birth may result in abnormal retinal blood vessel development, ROP, which may progress to blindness. Every neonatal unit requires an ROP screening service. Acute ROP develops approximately 6–12 weeks postnatally (gestational age approximately 32–38 weeks). The 'window' for treatment is narrow, 1–2 weeks in some cases, and failure to diagnose and treat ROP at the right time can lead to permanent, bilateral, complete blindness. ROP remains a leading cause of childhood blindness worldwide.

History and epidemiology

ROP was first described in 1942 (Terry 1942). An epidemic of blindness due to ROP occurred during the 1940s and early 1950s. In retrospect this was caused by the use of unrestricted oxygen. The results of a randomised controlled trial of restricted oxygen treatment published in 1956 (Kinsey 1956) led to a rapid reduction in the incidence of blindness due to ROP. Unfortunately, neurological morbidity (McDonald 1963) and mortality increased. A second 'epidemic' of ROP emerged during the 1970s because of improved survival of very-low-birthweight infants (Gibson et al. 1990). Currently, ROP is especially prevalent in 'middle-income' countries (Gilbert 2008). In these countries, neonatal care is sufficiently developed to allow the survival of premature infants, but the quality of perinatal and neonatal care is suboptimal. This results in a mixture of the effects of the first and second epidemics. It is estimated that at present at least 50 000 children are blind from ROP globally (Gilbert 2008). Blindness due to ROP also continues to occur in developed countries (Haines et al. 2005).

Retinal blood vessel development

The retinal blood vessels initially develop from cords of mesenchymal spindle-shaped cells that grow out from the optic disc, commencing at 15 weeks' gestation (Hughes et al. 2000). Further development of retinal blood vessels peripherally, and more deeply into the outer retina, is dependent on the process of angiogenesis.

Physiological hypoxia in tissues anterior to the developing blood vessels leads to hypoxia-inducible factor (HIF)-controlled production of vascular endothelial growth factor (VEGF) by glial cells (Stone et al. 1996). The nasal ora serrata (the anterior edge of the retina) is vascularised by about 34–36 weeks' gestation and the temporal ora serrata by 36–40 weeks' gestation.

International classification of ROP

Clinical ROP is described using an internationally agreed classification system (Anonymous 2005).

Retinal zones

ROP disease is primarily evident at the junction of vascularised and avascular retina. The position of the anterior edge of retinal vascularisation is defined in zones. Zone 1 retina is defined as a circle, centred on the centre of the optic disc, with a radius of twice the distance from the optic disc to the centre of the macula (Fig. 33.1). When parts of this zone remain avascular, the retinal vasculature is relatively immature. ROP in this zone progresses in an especially aggressive manner. Zone 2 retina is defined as the circle of retina,

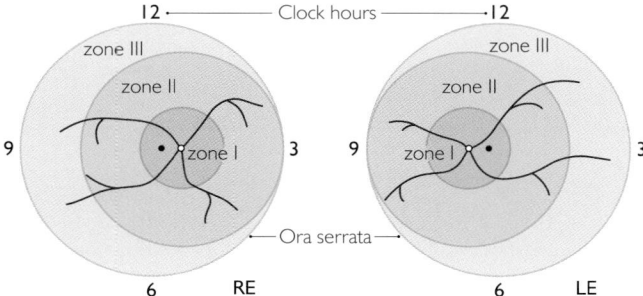

Fig. 33.1 Schematic representation of the retina of both eyes, showing the limits of each zone. The extent of disease may be described in clock hours as shown (the radius of zone 1 is twice the distance from the edge of the disc to the macula (shown as a red dot)). *(From Committee for the Classification of Retinopathy of Prematurity 1984 The international classification of retinopathy of prematurity. British Journal of Ophthalmology 68:690–697.)*

centred on the centre of the optic disc that lies anterior to zone 1, as far anteriorly as the nasal ora serrata. As the nasal ora serrata is closer to the optic disc than the temporal ora serrata, a peripheral crescent of retina lies anterior to zone 2 on the temporal side of the retina, and this is termed zone 3 retina. ROP confined to zone 3 carries a good prognosis.

Stages of ROP

The appearance of acute ROP disease at the junction of vascularised and avascular retina is described in stages. In stage 1 ROP a flat line delineates the junction of vascularised and avascular retina. Stage 2 ROP refers to the development of an elevated ridge of tissue (Fig. 33.2A). In stage 3 ROP, extraretinal angiogenesis is present – abnormal blood vessels grow out of the ROP ridge and the area immediately posterior to the ROP ridge into the vitreous. Stage 3 ROP represents a more severe form of ROP, with a potentially poor prognosis if not treated. The abnormal extraretinal blood vessels may proliferate further, and associated glial tissue may later contract. Contraction of the circular ring of glial tissue within the cavity of the eye causes the retina to be pulled out of position – traction retinal detachment. The presence of any area of traction retinal detachment is termed stage 4 ROP. The retina may become completely detached – stage 5 ROP. In general, stage 5 ROP causes complete, untreatable blindness.

Plus disease

More severe forms of ROP are associated with abnormalities of the posterior retinal blood vessels, and the iris blood vessels. This is termed plus disease (Fig. 33.2B). The posterior retinal blood vessels become dilated and tortuous, at least in part due to high levels of VEGF in the vitreous. The presence of plus disease is significant in the classification of ROP, as its presence is the main determinant of the need for interventional therapy (Early Treatment for Retinopathy of Prematurity Cooperative Group 2003).

Pathogenesis

Premature birth interrupts normal retinal blood vessel development. The physiological environment of the retina of a premature infant is very different from that found in utero. Oxygen therapy reduces the physiological hypoxia drive of normal retinal angiogenesis. Reduced HIF-controlled production of VEGF leads to reduced

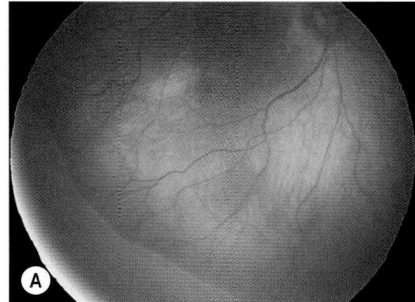 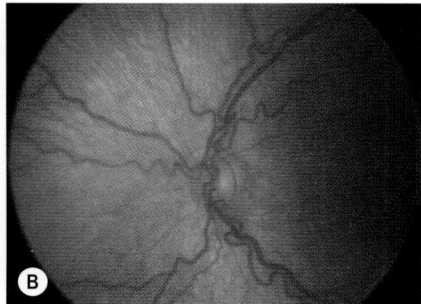 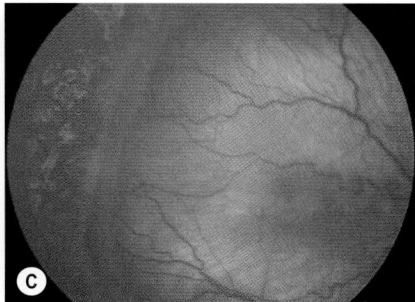

Fig. 33.2 (A) Stage 1 and 2 retinopathy of prematurity (ROP). White ridge (stage 2) at the advancing edge of the retinal vessels and lying at the junction of the vascularised and non-vascularised retina. Towards the left, the ridge is flatter, a line of stage 1 ROP. (B) Plus disease. Grossly engorged retinal venules and tortuous retinal arterioles – compare with (A). This baby had severe stage 3 ROP and this can be predicted from the plus disease alone without directly visualising the ROP lesion itself. (C) Stage 3 ROP and treatment. The retinal blood vessels are engorged and tortuous. Towards the left there is a raised neovascular lesion at the junction of the vascularised and non-vascularised retina. This is florid stage 3. Delta-like arborisation of vessels is seen running into the lesion, which is elevated above the retinal surface. This baby has been treated by laser – the pigmented laser lesions can be seen in the non-vascularised retina. The ROP lesion is not treated itself as the aim is to reduce vascular endothelial growth factor production in the non-vascularised retina. Images obtained by wide-field digital imaging.

endothelial cell proliferation and migration (McColm et al. 2004). In addition, reduced postnatal insulin-like growth factor 1 (IGF-1) appears to result in reduced retinal endothelial cell growth (Smith 2005). Reduced early retinal blood vessel development leads to inadequately vascularised retina at 6–10 weeks postnatally. The peripheral avascular retina continues to mature, but is avascular and becomes ischaemic. High levels of tissue VEGF are produced, and an abnormal angiogenesis response occurs (stage 3 ROP).

Risk factors for the development of ROP

Early gestation and low birthweight remain the strongest risk factors for the development of severe ROP (Dhaliwal et al. 2008). While infants of birth weight >1250 g born in developed countries are relatively unlikely to develop severe ROP (Dhaliwal et al. 2008), the birthweight-specific incidence of ROP varies between countries (Gilbert 2008).

Oxygen

The optimal level of oxygen therapy for premature infants remains unknown. While it is known that unrestricted oxygen greatly increases the risk of ROP (Kinsey 1956), optimal treatment levels have not been defined. In general, lower (Tin et al. 2001) and more stable (Cunningham et al. 1995) oxygen levels are thought to protect from ROP. However, the effects of lower levels of oxygen therapy on other tissues and organs may be detrimental (McDonald 1963). A number of collaborative international trials of oxygen therapy are currently in progress. Results from the SUPPORT trial indicate that, while lower oxygen levels are protective for ROP, they are associated with an increased risk of mortality (Anonymous 2010).

Nutrition and growth

Impaired early postnatal retinal blood vessel growth is important in the aetiology of ROP. Small-for-gestational-age infants are at higher risk of developing ROP (Dhaliwal et al. 2009b). Reduced postnatal growth velocity is an independent risk factor for the development of ROP (Hellstrom et al. 2009). Low levels of serum IGF-1 in the early postnatal period may predict the subsequent development of ROP (Hellstrom et al. 2003). Nutritional therapies that result in satisfactory early weight gain may prove to be important in the prevention of ROP (Hellstrom et al. 2003; Drenckpohl et al. 2008).

Blood transfusions and erythropoietin

Blood transfusions (Fortes Filho et al. 2009) and raised levels of erythropoietin (Suk et al. 2008) have been identified as risk factors for ROP. This may occur because of increased tissue delivery of oxygen. Alternatively, as with many risk factors identified for the development of ROP, ill infants may simply be at higher risk of developing ROP. Associations with necrotising enterocolitis, bronchopulmonary dysplasia and sepsis probably come within this category.

Screening

Screening guidelines have been developed in a number of countries. Guidelines developed in first-world countries are not applicable in less developed countries. The current UK guidelines are summarised in Table 33.1 (Wilkinson et al. 2009).

Eye drops are instilled 30 minutes prior to retinal examination. A combination of cyclopentolate 0.5% (an anticholinergic drug that relaxes the pupil sphincter) and phenylephrine 2.5% (an adrenergic

Table 33.1 Screening guidelines for retinopathy of prematurity (ROP)

Which infants should be screened?	
All infants born <32 weeks' gestation or <1500 g birthweight	
When should the first screening examination be performed?	
GESTATIONAL AGE AT BIRTH (WEEKS)	POSTNATAL AGE AT FIRST ROP EXAMINATION (WEEKS)
23	7
24	6
25	5
26	4
27	4
28	4
29	4
30	4
31	4

Adapted from Wilkinson et al. (2009).

agonist that stimulates the pupil dilator) is used in the UK, because of commercial availability. Reduced drug concentrations, available in some countries, are equally effective. Immediately before examination, local anaesthetic drops are instilled. An eyelid speculum is used to hold the eyelids open. Retinal examination is performed using a binocular indirect ophthalmoscope, or a digital camera system that comes into contact with the cornea (RetCam) (Dhaliwal et al. 2009a). This form of examination is painful (Dhaliwal et al. 2010) and some form of pain relief, such as sucrose (Boyle et al. 2006), is appropriate. Careful administration of ROP screening programmes is needed if infants are not to be lost to follow-up. This is especially the case when infants are transferred to other units, or discharged home prior to the completion of ROP screening.

Treatment

The severity of disease that requires intervention has been defined by the Early Treatment of ROP study (Early Treatment for Retinopathy of Prematurity Cooperative Group 2003). ROP in zone 1 retina that has reached stage 3, or is accompanied by plus disease, should be treated. ROP in zone 2 that has reached stage 2 or 3, and is accompanied by plus disease, should be treated. Thus, the presence or absence of plus disease is critical to treatment decisions. Once a treatment decision has been made, treatment should be performed within 48–72 hours. Treatment currently consists of laser ablation of peripheral avascular, ischaemic retina (Fig. 33.2C). A general anaesthetic, topical anaesthetic with sedation or a combination of opiate analgesia, muscle relaxant and ventilation may be used. Laser is delivered to the retina anterior to the ROP ridge. This retina is ischaemic, and ablation leads to reduced VEGF production, with resolution of ROP. The treatment should be performed carefully in order to ablate all ischaemic retina and reduce the likelihood of the

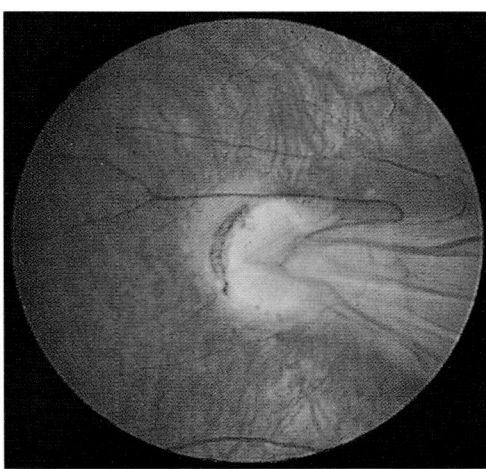

Fig. 33.3 Cicatricial retinopathy of prematurity with dragging of the retinal vessels towards the retinal periphery.

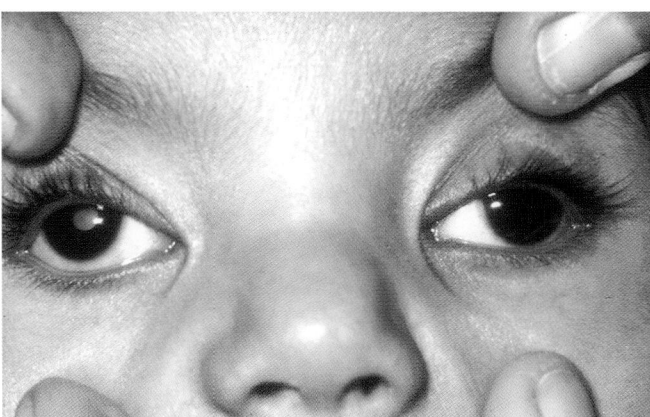

Fig. 33.4 Appearances of a cataract due to congenital rubella.

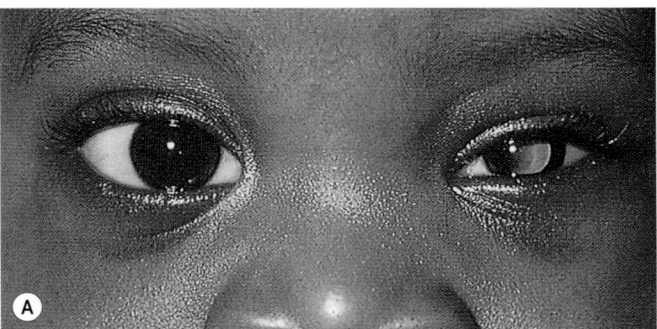

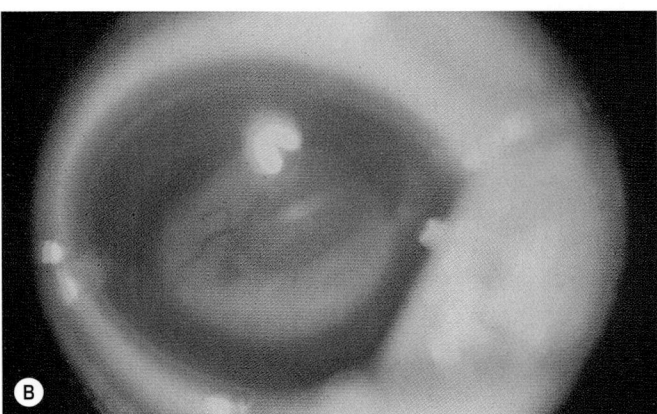

Fig. 33.5 (A) Infant with leukocoria of the left eye. (B) Infant with leukocoria due to a total retinal detachment.

need for retreatment later. Potential complications include intraocular bleeding, iritis and cataract development. Steroid eye drops and pupil-dilating eye drops should be given for 1 week after laser treatment to prevent iritis and the subsequent development of adhesions between the lens and iris. Treatment is usually successful, leading to arrest and reversal of acute ROP changes. However, in a small proportion of cases, especially those with aggressive posterior disease, laser treatment may fail. Vitreoretinal surgery may then become necessary in order to preserve vision.

An alternative approach to treatment is the use of anti-VEGF monoclonal antibodies, injected into the vitreous. Trials are underway, and the initial results indicate that this form of therapy is a satisfactory alternative to laser ablation (Mintz-Hittner and Best 2009).

Outcome of treatment

Treatment for acute ROP generally results in normal or near-normal anatomy of the macula and posterior retina. However, treatment fails in a small proportion of cases. Retinal detachment ensues, and prompt vitreoretinal surgery may then be needed to preserve vision. Severe visual impairment continues to occur in some infants.

Less severe forms of visual abnormality occur in many ex-premature children, irrespective of whether acute ROP occurred in the neonatal period (Holmstrom and Larsson 2008). Ocular causes of reduced vision include forms of retinal scarring (Fig. 33.3), refractive errors, strabismus and amblyopia. Neurological causes of visual impairment are common, and are frequently under-recognised. Mild forms of cerebral visual impairment (CVI) are relatively common, especially when periventricular leukomalacia is present.

Congenital cataract

The incidence of congenital cataract in the UK is approximately 2.5 per 10 000 live births per year (Rahi and Dezateux 2001). Surgery is required for most cases, and must be done within 6–8 weeks of birth in order to avoid irreversible visual loss due to amblyopia. Neonatal screening of all infants is necessary (Fry and Wilson 2005). The 'red reflex' is examined, using a direct ophthalmoscope. When a clear red reflex appearance is not obtained, prompt referral to an ophthalmologist is required (Fig. 33.4).

How to examine the red reflex

The examination should ideally be done in a dark or dimly lit room. The infant should be awake. The examiner should be about 30 cm from the infant's face. Each of the infant's eyes is observed through a direct ophthalmoscope. When light is directed into the pupil, a red reflection (from the choroidal circulation) is visible. If the reflex is dark, a cataract may be present. Darkly pigmented eyes can produce less clear red reflex appearances than lightly pigmented eyes. An abnormally white reflex can indicate the presence of cataract, but can also indicate the presence of retinoblastoma, or other pathology (Fig. 33.5 and Box 33.1).

Box 33.1 Differential diagnosis of white pupil (leukocoria) in infants

Retinoblastoma
Congenital cataract
Persistent hyperplastic primary vitreous
Coats' disease
Chorioretinal colobomas

Table 33.2 Associations of bilateral congenital cataracts*

	PERCENTAGE OF CASES
Idiopathic	38
Hereditary, with no systemic disorder	37
Autosomal dominant isolated congenital cataract	(25)
Hereditary, with systemic disorder	19
Down syndrome	(7)
Autosomal recessive systemic syndromes	(11)
Not hereditary, associated with a systemic disorder	6
Prenatal infection	(1)

*Numbers in brackets are percentage subsets of the categories given in the blue boxes.
Adapted from Rahi and Dezateux (2001).

Causes of congenital cataracts

Two-thirds of cases are bilateral (Rahi and Dezateux 2000). Unilateral cases are more frequently associated with additional ocular abnormalities, and are less likely to be associated with hereditary or systemic diseases (Rahi and Dezateux 2000). Common associations of bilateral congenital cataracts are shown in Table 33.2. Prenatal infections, due to rubella or toxoplasmosis, are now rare causes of congenital cataracts. All infants diagnosed as having congenital cataracts should be assessed for related systemic disease.

Ophthalmic management of congenital cataracts

A complete ocular examination should be performed, in order to detect associated ocular abnormalities. When the fundus cannot be visualised, ultrasound examination of the posterior segment of the eye should be done. Occasionally, congenital cataracts are not sufficiently opaque to reduce vision significantly. A clinical decision must be made as to whether surgical treatment is required.

Surgery should be done promptly, in order to avoid irreversible amblyopia. In general, surgery is now avoided during the first 4 weeks of life, because of increased anaesthetic risk, and an increased risk of the later development of glaucoma (Vishwanath et al. 2004; Khan and Al Dahmesh 2009). The optimal timing of surgery is 4–6 weeks postnatally. Generally, the two eyes are not operated on at the same time, because of risks of operative infection.

Cataract surgery results in loss of the normal focusing power of the lens of the eye. This may be replaced by: insertion of a prosthetic plastic lens implant; use of specialised contact lenses; or use of high-powered spectacles (Solebo et al. 2009). Long-term follow-up is required. The majority of children in developed countries have a good visual outcome following treatment of congenital cataract, and lead a normal life.

Prenatal infections and the eyes

Ophthalmologists may be asked to examine the eyes of infants with suspected prenatally acquired infection. The acronym TORCH is useful – toxoplasmosis, rubella, cytomegalovirus, herpes simplex infection. Prenatal toxoplasmosis infection frequently causes patches of retinal inflammation, especially at the macula (Mets et al. 1996). When bilateral, visual impairment may result. Prenatal rubella infection causes cataracts and a pigmentary retinopathy. In the longer term, glaucoma may develop (Givens et al. 1993). Prenatal cytomegalovirus infection typically results in retinitis at the macula (Wren et al. 2004). Herpes simplex infection of the cornea may be acquired during birth. In addition, occasional cases of herpes simplex retinitis have been reported (Malik et al. 2008). In summary, infants with suspected prenatal infection should be examined for corneal disease, cataract and retinal inflammation.

Teratogens and the eyes

Prenatal exposure to significant amounts of alcohol, opiates, 'street drugs' and some prescribed medicines may lead to ocular abnormalities. Shortened palpebral fissure length is a diagnostic feature of fetal alcohol syndrome (Ribeiro et al. 2007) and optic nerve hypoplasia occurs in up to 25% of cases (Garcia et al. 2006; Ribeiro et al. 2007). Nystagmus, strabismus and optic nerve hypoplasia are associated with prenatal exposure to methadone (Mulvihill et al. 2007). Isotretinoin (Roaccutane), used to treat acne vulgaris, is a potent teratogen. A wide range of effects may occur, including eye movement abnormalities (Morrison et al. 2005).

Endogenous endophthalmitis in infants

Systemic sepsis can lead to intraocular infection (endophthalmitis). A range of bacteria have been reported to cause endogenous endophthalmitis. *Pseudomonas* infections appear to be particularly virulent. In contrast, systemic *Candida* infections in neonates, when treated effectively, only rarely result in endophthalmitis (Fisher et al. 2005). It is questionable as to whether regular retinal examinations of neonates with bacteraemia or *Candida* infection are helpful. However, if signs of eye inflammation develop in a neonate with sepsis, prompt ophthalmic examination should be requested.

Diagnostic clues seen in the eyes of dysmorphic or ill infants

Ocular abnormalities may be present in a wide range of dysmorphic syndromes and metabolic disorders. Ophthalmic examination may therefore provide diagnostic information. A list of more common associations is given in Table 33.3.

Congenital abnormalities of the eyes: unusual appearances seen by the neonatologist

A number of abnormalities of the eyelids, orbits, ocular surface and anterior segment of the eyes may be evident on neonatal examination. Referral to an ophthalmologist for diagnosis and management will be appropriate in most cases. Urgent action is needed if eyelid closure is inadequate to protect the ocular surface, for example in the presence of large eyelid colobomas (failure of development of part of the eyelid) or facial palsy. A list of the more common abnormalities is given in Table 33.4.

The infant with poor vision

Visual behaviour, initially fixation to a face, is evident soon after birth in most infants. Concern that vision development is abnormal should arise when an infant shows no evidence of visual fixation by age 2–3 months. When nystagmus accompanies poor visual behaviour, the abnormality is likely to be ocular, optic nerve, optic chiasm or optic tract. CVI involving the occipital lobes, or more global involvement of the visual association areas, is less frequently associated with nystagmus. Infants with poor vision should be referred promptly to an ophthalmologist.

Causes of reduced vision in infants and that are evident on ophthalmic examination

Ophthalmic examination may detect the cause of reduced vision in some infants. The following are the common abnormalities that may be detected:

- corneal opacity
- congenital cataract
- vitreous opacity (e.g. vitreous haemorrhage)
- retinal detachment (e.g. following ROP; Norrie's disease)
- optic nerve hypoplasia (e.g. septo-optic dysplasia)
- chorioretinal coloboma.

Causes of reduced vision in infants with normal ocular appearances

Ophthalmic examination may be normal in some infants with reduced vision. The more common abnormalities that cause reduced vision with normal ocular appearances include:

- delayed visual maturation (DVM)
- CVI
- retinal dystrophy (Leber's congenital amaurosis).

Disorders of the eyes and related tissues

Eyelid abnormalities

Capillary haemangioma

Capillary haemangiomas may involve the eyelids, and may interfere with visual development by causing distorted focusing due to pressure effects on the eye or by occluding the pupil. Prompt referral to an ophthalmologist is appropriate. The lesions often enlarge in size during the first few months of life, before starting to involute slowly. Interestingly, capillary haemangiomas share antigens with placenta (Mulliken et al. 2007). The lesions often respond to oral propranolol (Siegfried et al. 2008).

Table 33.3 Diagnostic clues seen in the eyes of dysmorphic or ill infants

SYNDROME/DISEASE	OCULAR FEATURES
Down syndrome	Congenital cataract; refractive errors
Tuberous sclerosis	Retinal astrocytomas
Mucopolysaccharidoses	Corneal clouding; retinal 'cherry-red' spot
Stickler syndrome with cleft lip/palate	Myopia; abnormal vitreous structure
Aicardi syndrome	Optic disc anomalies; lacunar defects of retina and choroid

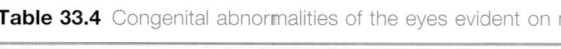

Table 33.4 Congenital abnormalities of the eyes evident on neonatal examination

STRUCTURE	ABNORMALITY	ASSOCIATIONS
Whole eye	Microphthalmia, anophthalmia, coloboma	
Eyelids	Coloboma	
	Ptosis	Third-nerve palsy
		Horner syndrome
	Facial palsy	Moebius syndrome (associated bilateral sixth cranial nerve palsy)
Tear sac	Dacrocele	Intranasal cyst
Cornea	Opacity	Peter's anomaly
		Congenital dystrophy
		Congenital glaucoma
Iris	Coloboma	
	Aniridia	
	Reduced iris pigmentation	Oculocutaneous and ocular albinism

Ptosis

Ptosis in neonates may be caused by birth-related bruising, developmental dystrophy of the levator muscle, third cranial nerve palsy or as part of a congenital eyelid development abnormality such as blepharophimosis. Congenital Horner syndrome can be associated with neuroblastoma. If ptosis occludes the pupil, prompt surgery is required, to allow visual development.

The whole eye: microphthalmia, anophthalmia and coloboma

Microphthalmia, anophthalmia and ocular coloboma co-segregate in families and may be grouped together. Ocular coloboma and some cases of microphthalmia are due to developmental optic fissure closure defects. The incidence is approximately 2 per 10 000 live births (Morrison et al. 2002). The abnormality may be subtle, or profound. Cases should be referred to an ophthalmologist. In addition to maximising visual function using glasses, management with tissue expanders may be needed in order to optimise orbit and eyelid growth (Gossman et al. 1999).

Watering eyes: lacrimal problems

Approximately 20% of infants have symptomatic epiphora (watering eye) due to delayed canalisation of the nasolacrimal duct mucosa (MacEwen 2006). The majority of cases resolve spontaneously. Intermittent stickiness of the eyes may occur, but tissue inflammation is rare and antibiotic treatment is generally not required. Massage over the tear sac shortens the time to resolution of epiphora. Probing of the nasolacrimal duct may be postponed until the age of 18 months in most cases (Young et al. 1996).

Swelling of the lacrimal sac may occur in the neonatal period – congenital dacryocele. An intranasal cyst may be present in association with a dacryocele, and can cause breathing difficulties. Infection may develop – dacrocystitis – and treatment with antibiotics is then required. While spontaneous resolution may occur, surgical probing of the nasolacrimal duct is required in most cases (Wong and Vanderveen 2008).

Congenital glaucoma

Congenital glaucoma is a rare condition (Aponte et al. 2010) that presents with watering, photophobia and enlargement and oedema of the corneas (Fig. 33.6). The disease may be evident at birth, or develop during infancy. The most commonly identified causative mutation is in the *CYP1B1* gene (Fuse et al. 2010), and while the disease is autosomal recessive, it is more common in males. Cases of suspected congenital glaucoma should be referred urgently to an ophthalmologist. The diagnosis is based on measurement of intraocular pressures, examination of the corneas and assessment of the optic discs. The treatment is usually surgical. Glaucoma eye drop treatment may be used for limited periods. Brimonidine should be avoided, because of the risk of collapse in infants (Lai Becker et al. 2009).

Congenital abnormalities of the iris and choroid

Albinism

Oculocutaneous albinism (OCA) is a relatively common autosomal recessive disease of tyrosine metabolism. Most commonly, tyrosinase function is defective – OCA type 1. Gene therapy animal

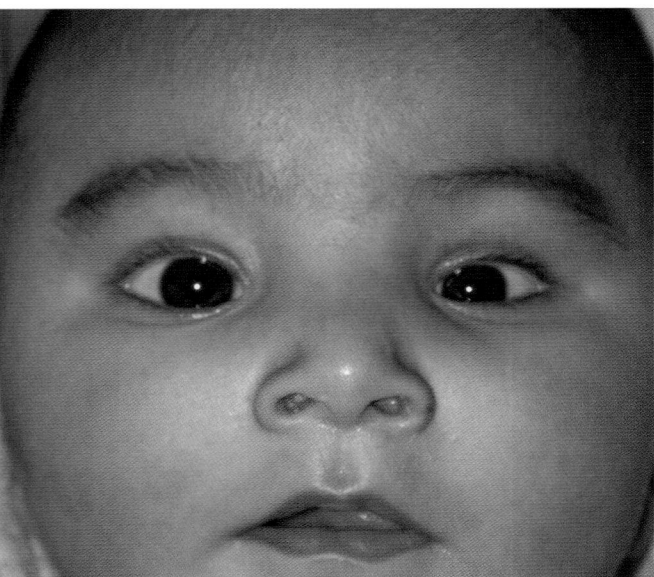

Fig. 33.6 Congenital glaucoma of the right eye.

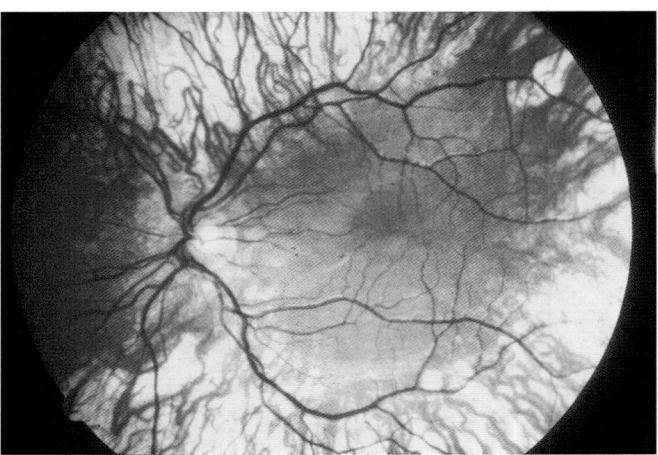

Fig. 33.7 The fundus in albinism.

model studies of therapy for OCA1 show promising results (Gargiulo et al. 2009).

When associated with a bleeding disorder, Hermansky–Pudlak syndrome should be suspected (Sandrock et al. 2010). When associated with immune deficiency, Chédiak–Higashi syndrome should be suspected (Manoli et al. 2010). Rare X-linked forms of albinism show ocular features of albinism, with normal skin – 'ocular albinism'.

The ocular features of OCA show a spectrum of severity and include: nystagmus, DVM, iris transillumination, photophobia, reduced fundus pigmentation (Fig. 33.7), foveal hypoplasia and optic chiasm decussation abnormalities. Normally, 50% of fibres cross at the chiasm, and 50% remain uncrossed. In albinism, almost all fibres decussate. This results in a typical, asymmetrical VEP response pattern (dem Hagen et al. 2008).

Ophthalmic treatment is at present limited to the treatment of associated refractive errors, strabismus and amblyopia. Tinted lenses may be used to reduce symptoms of photophobia.

Aniridia

While absence or near absence of iris tissue is the most striking phenotype abnormality of aniridia, multiple ocular abnormalities are usually present in this condition. Aniridia is an autosomal dominant condition, caused by mutations in the *PAX6* homeobox gene (chromosome 11p13 in humans) (Kokotas and Petersen 2010). Systemic abnormalities, including nephroblastoma, genitourinary malformations and developmental delay, may be present in sporadic cases that have a large underlying gene deletion (Xu et al. 2008). Ocular features include nystagmus, corneal epithelium stem cell abnormalities, cataract, glaucoma and foveal hypoplasia.

Congenital abnormalities of the vitreous and retina

Chorioretinal coloboma

Colobomas of the retina and choroid may be found in infants who have iris colobomas or microphthalmia. The area of bare sclera present in a coloboma may cause a white pupil reflex, and the condition therefore forms part of the differential diagnosis of leukocoria. When the optic disc and central part of the retina (macula) are involved, a variable degree of visual impairment will occur. Associated amblyopia and refractive errors should be treated. Retinal detachment may occur (Morrison and Fleck 1999).

Persistent hyperplastic primary vitreous

Failure of regression of fetal hyaloid vessels in the vitreous may result in the development of a fibrovascular membrane immediately behind the lens of the eye. This results in a white pupil reflex. The condition is usually unilateral, and the affected eye is relatively small. An abnormality of the Norrie's disease protein (*NDP*) gene is found in some cases (Pendergast et al. 1998).

Vitreous haemorrhage

Vitreous haemorrhage is occasionally seen in neonates, secondary to retinal haemorrhages that occur at birth. Vitrectomy surgery may be considered in some cases.

Retinal detachment

Retinal detachment may be found in neonates, as a sequel to ROP or as part of Norrie's disease. Once again, vitreoretinal surgery may be considered.

Leber's congenital amaurosis

The term Leber's congenital amaurosis (LCA) is used to describe a group of hereditary retinal dystrophies that present in infancy. Typically, the infant fails to develop normal visual behaviour, and nystagmus develops at about age 3 months. The fundus appears normal. Refractive error, such as a high degree of hypermetropia, may be present. The electroretinogram (ERG) shows a severely attenuated or no response. Inheritance is usually autosomal recessive. Promising gene therapy trials are underway for the RPE 65 retinal dystrophy (Maguire et al. 2009).

Norrie's disease

Bilateral congenital retinal detachment, deafness and intellectual impairment are the dominant features of Norrie's disease. The condition is X-linked recessive and occurs in males. Mutations of the *NDP* gene cause a spectrum of neonatal retinal diseases (Black and Redmond 1994).

Optic nerve hypoplasia

Optic nerve hypoplasia is a relatively common cause of visual impairment in infants (Khan et al. 2007). There is a wide spectrum of severity. Most cases may be diagnosed by ophthalmoscopic appearance of the optic discs, although caution should be exercised as the optic disc appearances in neonates are rather variable. Neuroimaging may demonstrate small optic nerves. The abnormality may be isolated, associated with septo-optic dysplasia, or associated with more widespread developmental abnormalities of the brain.

Delayed visual maturation

DVM is a retrospective diagnosis – an infant is initially visually unresponsive, but vision later improves. DVM is the commonest cause of reduced vision in early infancy. The infant is initially 'blind', with no response to a smile, or a moving visual stimulus. Infants with type 1 DVM are otherwise normal, do not have nystagmus, have normal ERG and VEP responses and go on to develop normal vision. Typically, they show dramatic improvement of vision at age 3–5 months (Tresidder et al. 1990).

Type 2 DVM is associated with severe neurodevelopmental abnormalities. Improvement is slow, and incomplete. Type 3 DVM is associated with albinism, and nystagmus is a prominent feature. Improvement of vision takes place at 3–5 months, as for type 1 DVM. Type 4 DVM is associated with severe, bilateral structural abnormalities of the eyes, such as colobomas, and is also associated with nystagmus. As with type 2 DVM, improvement of vision is slow, and incomplete.

Cerebral visual impairment

Brain disease is the most common cause of visual impairment in children (CVI) (Bunce and Wormald 2008). Perinatal insults such as hypoxic–ischaemic encephalopathy, and, in premature neonates, periventricular haemorrhage, make up a significant proportion of CVI cases.

A wide variety of types of visual impairment may occur, based on the areas of the visual pathways, primary visual cortex and visual association areas damaged. Damage to the anterior visual pathways, optic radiations and primary visual cortex leads to reduced visual acuity and a variety of visual field defects.

Damage to visual association areas typically causes more subtle visual impairments, which may only become apparent in later childhood. Awareness of these types of visual impairment will facilitate appropriate counselling of parents, and appropriate follow-up arrangements. Two main groups (streams) of association pathways and areas, the ventral and dorsal streams, have been identified (Dutton and Jacobson 2001). The ventral stream runs from the primary visual cortex to the fusiform gyri of the inferior temporal lobes. Damage to these areas leads to difficulty recognising faces and objects, and difficulty orienting within a familiar environment. These areas of cortex may be thought of as containing a 'library' of learned images.

The dorsal stream runs from the primary visual cortex to the posterior parietal lobes, and related association pathways. Damage to these areas leads to poor visually guided movement, poor visual attention and poor orientation in space.

Some typical clusters of symptoms exist, based on the aetiology and timing of the insult. Premature infants who sustain damage to the periventricular white matter following periventricular haemorrhage in the early neonatal period may develop a constellation of visual symptoms, and diplegia. Reduced visual acuity, inferior visual field defects, an inability to process complex visual scenes ('crowding'), nystagmus and cupped optic discs occur (Jacobson and Dutton 2000).

A more global form of CVI occurs following hypoxic–ischaemic encephalopathy. Optic atrophy when present carries a worse visual prognosis. Visual impairments are common in children with cerebral palsy, and are often underrecognised (Ghasia et al. 2008).

The infant with unusual eye movements

Abnormal alignment of the eyes in neonates

Inturning strabismus (esodeviation) of one or both eyes may occur as a result of sixth cranial nerve palsy due to birth trauma (Galbraith 1994). Typically this resolves spontaneously over a period of weeks. In Moebius syndrome, weakness of sixth and seventh nerve function due to hypoplasia of brainstem nuclei results in esodeviation and reduced eyelid closure. Some cases of Duane syndrome, where 'miswiring' of the nerve supply to the medial and lateral rectus muscles occurs, also have reduced sixth-nerve function. Relatively early strabismus surgery may be appropriate for some of these conditions, and early referral to an ophthalmologist is appropriate.

Infantile esotropia is a relatively common type of strabismus in infants. However, it is rarely seen at birth, and usually becomes apparent at age 2–4 months. The eyes deviate inwards, and may appear to show reduced sixth-nerve function. However, if one eye is covered, the uncovered eye may be shown to have a full range of movement while following an object. In addition to esotropia, manifest latent nystagmus may be present. This form of nystagmus has greater amplitude when one eye is occluded, and the fast phase of the nystagmus 'beat' is towards the fixing eye. Infantile esotropia is more common in infants with neurological impairment. Early surgery is usually appropriate (Gerth et al. 2008), and the infant should be referred to an ophthalmologist.

Outturning (exodeviation) and vertical forms of strabismus are rare in infants, and should be referred, as underlying neurological disease may be present. A variety of patterns occur – for instance, congenital third-nerve palsy is generally incomplete, with variable ptosis and reduced eye movement.

Brief episodes of esodeviation frequently occur in neonates and young infants while feeding or viewing near objects. This is a normal developmental stage. All other cases of strabismus should be referred to an ophthalmologist. Not only is early surgical treatment appropriate in some cases, but strabismus may be the presenting feature of a more significant underlying ocular disease, such as retinoblastoma, or of neurological disease.

Nystagmus

Nystagmus may occur as a primary disorder or secondary to sensory visual impairment or to neurological disease. While some typical patterns of nystagmus may be identified, all cases should be carefully evaluated by an ophthalmologist and a neurologist. Evoked potential studies of the retina and optic nerve (ERG and VEPs) are usually indicated. Neuroimaging is appropriate in many cases.

Idiopathic infantile nystagmus develops during the first 2–3 months of life, and is a diagnosis of exclusion. In most cases a horizontal nystagmus, present in all directions of gaze, is seen. Ocular and brain structure and function are otherwise normal. Cases may be familial.

Nystagmus may occur as a result of reduced visual function of the eyes or anterior visual pathways, and in association with periventricular leukomalacia. Ocular examination may be abnormal, but, even when normal, electrophysiology investigation of retinal and optic nerve function is appropriate.

Acquired nystagmus in later infancy, and vertical forms of nystagmus, are especially likely to be related to underlying neurological disease. Prompt assessment by a neurologist, and neuroimaging, should be arranged.

Spasmus nutans is a syndrome of nystagmus, head nodding and torticollis with onset from age 4 months to 18 months. The diagnosis may only be made in retrospect, after spontaneous resolution of the condition has occurred, usually after 1–2 years. As the abnormal signs may be related to underlying neurological disease, assessment by a neurologist and neuroimaging are required.

Ocular motor apraxia

Horizontal saccadic eye movements are absent in this condition, which may be mistaken for severe visual impairment. The ERG may also show reduced amplitude, further increasing the possibility of incorrect diagnosis. From about the age of 6 months compensatory jerking head thrusts are used to alter the position of gaze. The condition remains unchanged thereafter, and is not associated with significant visual impairment. Underlying neurological abnormalities may be present in some cases (Harris et al. 1996), and neurological investigation and neuroimaging should be considered.

Other patterns of eye movement disorder

'Sunsetting' of the eyes may occur when the third ventricle is enlarged due to intraventricular haemorrhage in a premature neonate, or infantile hydrocephalus (Chattha and Delong 1975; O'Keefe et al. 2001). Pressure on the vertical gaze centre causes downward deviation of the eyes, and associated upper eyelid retraction. Transient ocular flutter movements – opsoclonus – may occur in association with encephalitis, and as a feature of neuroblastoma.

References

Anonymous, 2005. The International Classification of Retinopathy of Prematurity revisited. Arch Ophthalmol 123, 991–999.

Anonymous, 2010. Target ranges of oxygen saturation in extremely preterm infants. N Engl J Med 362, 1959–1969.

Aponte, E.P., Diehl, N., Mohney, B.G., 2010. Incidence and clinical characteristics of childhood glaucoma: a population-based study. Arch Ophthalmol 128, 478–482.

Black, G., Redmond, R.M., 1994. The molecular biology of Norrie's disease. Eye (Lond) 8, 491–496.

Boyle, E.M., Freer, Y., Khan-Orakzai, Z., et al., 2006. Sucrose and non-nutritive sucking for the relief of pain in screening for retinopathy of prematurity: a randomised controlled trial. Arch Dis Child Fetal Neonatal Ed 91, F166–F168.

Brown, A.M., 1997. Vernier acuity in human infants: rapid emergence shown in a longitudinal study. Optom Vis Sci 74, 732–740.

Bunce, C., Wormald, R., 2008. Causes of blind certifications in England and Wales: April 1999–March 2000. Eye (Lond) 22, 905–911.

Calloway, S.L., Lloyd, I.C., Henson, D.B., 2001. A clinical evaluation of random dot stereoacuity cards in infants. Eye (Lond) 15, 629–634.

Chattha, A.S., Delong, G.R., 1975. Sylvian aqueduct syndrome as a sign of acute obstructive hydrocephalus in children. J Neurol Neurosurg Psychiatry 38, 288–296.

Committee for the Classification of Retinopathy of Prematurity, 1984. The international classification of retinopathy of prematurity. Br J Ophthalmol 68, 690–697.

Cunningham, S., Fleck, B.W., Elton, R.A., et al., 1995. Transcutaneous oxygen levels in retinopathy of prematurity. Lancet 346, 1464–1465.

dem Hagen, E.A., Hoffmann, M.B., Morland, A.B., 2008. Identifying human albinism: a comparison of VEP and fMRI. Invest Ophthalmol Vis Sci 49, 238–249.

Dhaliwal, C., Fleck, B., Wright, E., et al., 2008. Incidence of retinopathy of prematurity in Lothian, Scotland, from 1990 to 2004. Arch Dis Child Fetal Neonatal Ed 93, F422–F426.

Dhaliwal, C., Wright, E., Graham, C., et al., 2009a. Wide-field digital retinal imaging versus binocular indirect ophthalmoscopy for retinopathy of prematurity screening: a two-observer prospective, randomised comparison. Br J Ophthalmol 93, 355–359.

Dhaliwal, C.A., Fleck, B.W., Wright, E., et al., 2009b. Retinopathy of prematurity in small-for-gestational age infants compared with those of appropriate size for gestational age. Arch Dis Child Fetal Neonatal Ed 94, F193–F195.

Dhaliwal, C.A., Wright, E., McIntosh, N., et al., 2010. Pain in neonates during screening for retinopathy of prematurity using binocular indirect ophthalmoscopy and wide-field digital retinal imaging: a randomised comparison. Arch Dis Child Fetal Neonatal Ed 95, F146–F148.

Dobkins, K.R., Lia, B., Teller, D.Y., 1997. Infant color vision: temporal contrast sensitivity functions for chromatic (red/green) stimuli in 3-month-olds. Vision Res 37, 2699–2716.

Drenckpohl, D., McConnell, C., Gaffney, S., et al., 2008. Randomized trial of very low birth weight infants receiving higher rates of infusion of intravenous fat emulsions during the first week of life. Pediatrics 122, 743–751.

Duerksen, K., Barlow, W.E., Stasior, O.G., 1994. Fused eyelids in premature infants. Ophthalm Plast Reconstr Surg 10, 234–240.

Dutton, G.N., Jacobson, L.K., 2001. Cerebral visual impairment in children. Semin Neonatol 6, 477–485.

Early Treatment for Retinopathy of Prematurity Cooperative Group, 2003. Revised indications for the treatment of retinopathy of prematurity: results of the early treatment for retinopathy of prematurity randomized trial. Arch Ophthalmol 121, 1684–1694.

Fisher, R.G., Gary, Karlowicz, M.G., Lall-Trail, J., 2005. Very low prevalence of endophthalmitis in very low birthweight infants who survive candidemia. J Perinatol 25, 408–411.

Fortes Filho, J.B., Eckert, G.U., Procianoy, L., et al., 2009. Incidence and risk factors for retinopathy of prematurity in very low and in extremely low birth weight infants in a unit-based approach in southern Brazil. Eye (Lond) 23, 25–30.

Fry, M., Wilson, G.A., 2005. Scope for improving congenital cataract blindness prevention by screening of infants (red reflex screening) in a New Zealand setting. J Paediatr Child Health 41, 344–346.

Fuse, N., Miyazawa, A., Takahashi, K., et al., 2010. Mutation spectrum of the CYP1B1 gene for congenital glaucoma in the Japanese population. Jpn J Ophthalmol 54, 1–6.

Galbraith, R.S., 1994. Incidence of neonatal sixth nerve palsy in relation to mode of delivery. Am J Obstet Gynecol 170, 1158–1159.

Garcia, M.L., Ty, E.B., Taban, M., et al., 2006. Systemic and ocular findings in 100 patients with optic nerve hypoplasia. J Child Neurol 21, 949–956.

Gargiulo, A., Bonetti, C., Montefusco, S., et al., 2009. AAV-mediated tyrosinase gene transfer restores melanogenesis and retinal function in a model of oculo-cutaneous albinism type I (OCA1). Mol Ther 17, 1347–1354.

Gerth, C., Mirabella, G., Li, X., et al., 2008. Timing of surgery for infantile esotropia in humans: effects on cortical motion visual evoked responses. Invest Ophthalmol Vis Sci 49, 3432–3437.

Ghasia, F., Brunstrom, J., Gordon, M., et al., 2008. Frequency and severity of visual sensory and motor deficits in children with cerebral palsy: gross motor function classification scale. Invest Ophthalmol Vis Sci 49, 572–580.

Gibson, D.L., Sheps, S.B., Uh, S.H., et al., 1990. Retinopathy of prematurity-induced blindness: birth weight-specific survival and the new epidemic. Pediatrics 86, 405–412.

Gilbert, C., 2008. Retinopathy of prematurity: a global perspective of the epidemics, population of babies at risk and implications for control. Early Hum Dev 84, 77–82.

Givens, K.T., Lee, D.A., Jones, T., et al., 1993. Congenital rubella syndrome: ophthalmic manifestations and associated systemic disorders. Br J Ophthalmol 77, 358–363.

Gossman, M.D., Mohay, J., Roberts, D.M., 1999. Expansion of the human microphthalmic orbit. Ophthalmology 106, 2005–2009.

Haines, L., Fielder, A.R., Baker, H., et al., 2005. UK population based study of severe retinopathy of prematurity: screening, treatment, and outcome. Arch

Dis Child Fetal Neonatal Ed 90, F240–F244.

Hargadon, D.D., Wood, J., Twelker, J.D., et al., 2010. Recognition acuity, grating acuity, contrast sensitivity, and visual fields in 6-year-old children. Arch Ophthalmol 128, 70–74.

Harris, C.M., Shawkat, F., Russell-Eggitt, I., et al., 1996. Intermittent horizontal saccade failure ('ocular motor apraxia') in children. Br J Ophthalmol 80, 151–158.

Hellstrom, A., Engstrom, E., Hard, A.L., et al., 2003. Postnatal serum insulin-like growth factor I deficiency is associated with retinopathy of prematurity and other complications of premature birth. Pediatrics 112, 1016–1020.

Hellstrom, A., Hard, A.L., Engstrom, E., et al., 2009. Early weight gain predicts retinopathy in preterm infants: new, simple, efficient approach to screening. Pediatrics 123, e638–e645.

Hendrickson, A., 1992. A morphological comparison of foveal development in man and monkey. Eye (Lond) 6, 136–144.

Holmstrom, G., Larsson, E., 2008. Long-term follow-up of visual functions in prematurely born children – a prospective population-based study up to 10 years of age. J AAPOS 12, 157–162.

Hughes, S., Yang, H., Chan-Ling, T., 2000. Vascularization of the human fetal retina: roles of vasculogenesis and angiogenesis. Invest Ophthalmol Vis Sci 41, 1217–1228.

Hughes, L.A., May, K., Talbot, J.F., et al., 2006. Incidence, distribution, and duration of birth-related retinal hemorrhages: a prospective study. J AAPOS 10, 102–106.

Jacobson, L.K., Dutton, G.N., 2000. Periventricular leukomalacia: an important cause of visual and ocular motility dysfunction in children. Surv Ophthalmol 45, 1–13.

Khan, A.O., Al Dahmesh, S., 2009. Age at the time of cataract surgery and relative risk for aphakic glaucoma in nontraumatic infantile cataract. J AAPOS 13, 166–169.

Khan, R.I., O'Keefe, M., Kenny, D., et al., 2007. Changing pattern of childhood blindness. Ir Med J 100, 458–461.

Kinsey, V.E., 1956. Retrolental fibroplasia; cooperative study of retrolental fibroplasia and the use of oxygen. AMA Arch Ophthalmol 56, 481–543.

Kokotas, H., Petersen, M.B., 2010. Clinical and molecular aspects of aniridia. Clin Genet 77, 409–420.

Lai Becker, M., Huntington, N., Woolf, A.D., 2009. Brimonidine tartrate poisoning in children: frequency, trends, and use of naloxone as an antidote. Pediatrics 123, e305–e311.

Lauritzen, L., Jorgensen, M.H., Michaelsen, K.F., 2004. Test–retest reliability of swept visual evoked potential measurements of infant visual acuity and contrast sensitivity. Pediatr Res 55, 701–708.

Lloyd, I.C., Ashworth, J., Biswas, S., et al., 2007. Advances in the management of congenital and infantile cataract. Eye (Lond) 21, 1301–1309.

MacEwen, C.J., 2006. Congenital nasolacrimal duct obstruction. Compr Ophthalmol Update 7, 79–87.

Magoon, E.H., Robb, R.M., 1981. Development of myelin in human optic nerve and tract. A light and electron microscopic study. Arch Ophthalmol 99, 655–659.

Maguire, A.M., High, K.A., Auricchio, A., et al., 2009. Age-dependent effects of RPE65 gene therapy for Leber's congenital amaurosis: a phase 1 dose-escalation trial. Lancet 374, 1597–1605.

Malik, A.N., Hildebrand, G.D., Sekhri, R., et al., 2008. Bilateral macular scars following intrauterine herpes simplex virus type 2 infection. J AAPOS 12, 305–306.

Manoli, I., Golas, G., Westbroek, W., et al., 2010. Chédiak–Higashi syndrome with early developmental delay resulting from paternal heterodisomy of chromosome 1. Am J Med Genet A 152A, 1474–1483.

Maurer, D., Lewis, T.L., Brent, H.P., et al., 1999. Rapid improvement in the acuity of infants after visual input. Science 286, 108–110.

McColm, J.R., Cunningham, S., Wade, J., et al., 2004. Hypoxic oxygen fluctuations produce less severe retinopathy than hyperoxic fluctuations in a rat model of retinopathy of prematurity. Pediatr Res 55, 107–113.

McDonald, A.D., 1963. Cerebral palsy in children of very low birth weight. Arch Dis Child 38, 579–588.

Mets, M.B., Holfels, E., Boyer, K.M., et al., 1996. Eye manifestations of congenital toxoplasmosis. Am J Ophthalmol 122, 309–324.

Mintz-Hittner, H.A., Best, L.M., 2009. Antivascular endothelial growth factor for retinopathy of prematurity. Curr Opin Pediatr 21, 182–187.

Morrison, D.A., Fleck, B., 1999. Prevalence of retinal detachments in children with chorioretinal colobomas. Ophthalmology 106, 645–646.

Morrison, D., FitzPatrick, D., Hanson, I., et al., 2002. National study of microphthalmia, anophthalmia, and coloboma (MAC) in Scotland: investigation of genetic aetiology. J Med Genet 39, 16–22.

Morrison, D.G., Elsas, F.J., Descartes, M., 2005. Congenital oculomotor nerve synkinesis associated with fetal retinoid syndrome. J AAPOS 9, 166–168.

Mulliken, J.B., Bischoff, J., Kozakewich, H.P., 2007. Multifocal rapidly involuting congenital hemangioma: a link to chorangioma. Am J Med Genet A 143A, 3038–3046.

Mulvihill, A.O., Cackett, P.D., George, N.D., et al., 2007. Nystagmus secondary to drug exposure in utero. Br J Ophthalmol 91, 613–615.

Norcia, A.M., Tyler, C.W., 1985. Spatial frequency sweep VEP: visual acuity during the first year of life. Vision Res 25, 1399–1408.

O'Keefe, M., Kafil-Hussain, N., Flitcroft, I., et al., 2001. Ocular significance of intraventricular haemorrhage in premature infants. Br J Ophthalmol 853, 357–359.

Pendergast, S.D., Trese, M.T., Liu, X., et al., 1998. Study of the Norrie disease gene in 2 patients with bilateral persistent hyperplastic primary vitreous. Arch Ophthalmol 116, 381–382.

Rahi, J.S., Dezateux, C., 2000. Congenital and infantile cataract in the United Kingdom: underlying or associated factors. British Congenital Cataract Interest Group. Invest Ophthalmol Vis Sci 41 (8), 2108–2114.

Rahi, J.S., Dezateux, C., 2001. Measuring and interpreting the incidence of congenital ocular anomalies: lessons from a national study of congenital cataract in the UK. Invest Ophthalmol Vis Sci 42, 1444–1448.

Ribeiro, I.M., Vale, P.J., Tenedorio, P.A., et al., 2007. Ocular manifestations in fetal alcohol syndrome. Eur J Ophthalmol 17, 104–109.

Rours, I.G., Hammerschlag, M.R., Ott, A., et al., 2008. Chlamydia trachomatis as a cause of neonatal conjunctivitis in Dutch infants. Pediatrics 121, e321–e326.

Salgado, C.M., Celik, Y., Vanderveen, D.K., 2010. Anterior segment complications after diode laser photocoagulation for prethreshold retinopathy of prematurity. Am J Ophthalmol 150, 6–9.

Sandrock, K., Bartsch, I., Rombach, N., et al., 2010. Compound heterozygous mutations in 2 siblings with Hermansky–Pudlak syndrome type 1 (HPS1). Klin Padiatr 222, 168–174.

Siegfried, E.C., Keenan, W.J., Al Jureidini, S., 2008. More on propranolol for hemangiomas of infancy. N Engl J Med 359, 2846–2847.

Smith, L.E., 2005. IGF-1 and retinopathy of prematurity in the preterm infant. Biol Neonate 88, 237–244.

Solebo, A.L., Russell-Eggitt, I., Nischal, K.K., et al., 2009. Cataract surgery and primary intraocular lens implantation in children < or = 2 years old in the UK and Ireland: finding of national surveys. Br J Ophthalmol 93, 1495–1498.

Stone, J., Chan-Ling, T., Pe'er, J., et al., 1996. Roles of vascular endothelial growth factor and astrocyte degeneration in the genesis of retinopathy of prematurity. Invest Ophthalmol Vis Sci 37, 290–299.

Suk, K.K., Dunbar, J.A., Liu, A., et al., 2008. Human recombinant erythropoietin and the incidence of retinopathy of prematurity: a multiple regression model. J AAPOS 12, 233–238.

Terry, T.L., 1942. Fibroblastic overgrowth of persistent tunica vasculosa lentis in infants born prematurely. II. Report of cases – clinical aspects. Trans Am Ophthalmol Soc 40, 262–284.

Tin, W., Milligan, D.W., Pennefather, P., et al., 2001. Pulse oximetry, severe retinopathy, and outcome at one year in babies of less than 28 weeks gestation. Arch Dis Child Fetal Neonatal Ed 84, F106–F110.

Tresidder, J., Fielder, A.R., Nicholson, J., 1990. Delayed visual maturation: ophthalmic and neurodevelopmental aspects. Dev Med Child Neurol 32, 872–881.

Vishwanath, M., Cheong-Leen, R., Taylor, D., et al., 2004. Is early surgery for congenital cataract a risk factor for glaucoma? Br J Ophthalmol 88, 905–910.

Weinacht, S., Kind, C., Monting, J.S., et al., 1999. Visual development in preterm and full-term infants: a prospective masked study. Invest Ophthalmol Vis Sci 40, 346–353.

Wilkinson, A.R., Haines, L., Head, K., et al., 2009. UK retinopathy of prematurity guideline. Eye (Lond) 23, 2137–2139.

Wong, R.K., Vanderveen, D.K., 2008. Presentation and management of congenital dacryocystocele. Pediatrics 122, e1108–e1112.

Wren, S.M., Fielder, A.R., Bethell, D., et al., 2004. Cytomegalovirus retinitis in infancy. Eye (Lond) 18, 389–392.

Xu, S., Han, J.C., Morales, A., et al., 2008. Characterization of 11p14-p12 deletion in WAGR syndrome by array CGH for identifying genes contributing to mental retardation and autism. Cytogenet Genome Res 122, 181–187.

Yip, P.P., Chan, W.H., Yip, K.T., et al., 2008. The use of polymerase chain reaction assay versus conventional methods in detecting neonatal chlamydial conjunctivitis. J Pediatr Ophthalmol Strabismus 45, 234–239.

Young, J.D., MacEwen, C.J., Ogston, S.A., 1996. Congenital nasolacrimal duct obstruction in the second year of life: a multicentre trial of management. Eye (Lond) 10, 485–491.

Metabolic and endocrine disorders

Jane Hawdon   Tim Cheetham   Daniel J Schenk
James E Wraith   Simon A Jones   Nick Bishop

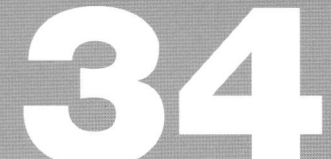

CHAPTER CONTENTS

© 2012 Elsevier Ltd

Part 1: **Disorders of metabolic homeostasis in the neonate**

Jane Hawdon

Introduction

Neonatal hypoglycaemia has been recognised for a century (Cobliner 1911; Sedgwick and Ziegler 1920; Spence 1921), although over these years there have been wide swings of opinion regarding the definition of the condition, its clinical significance and its optimal management. For example, in the era when routine postnatal management involved the withholding of feeds from healthy infants for up to 24 hours, and even longer in sick or small babies, many were found to have low blood glucose concentrations, and this became accepted as a normal finding (Cornblath and Schwartz 1976). Healthy term babies have a number of protective mechanisms to prevent the postnatal physiological fall in blood glucose causing harm and these mechanisms are discussed below. However, some babies have impaired protective responses and display clinical signs of hypoglycaemia. The risk of reduced glucose availability to the brain in such circumstances is acknowledged (Cornblath and Reisner 1965; Neligan 1965).

Neligan (1965) wrote: 'Certainly the risk of such complications forms a cogent incentive to all concerned to make the diagnosis as early as possible in every case'.

More recently, practice swung towards the treatment of large numbers of infants, often unnecessarily, with intravenous glucose, resulting in separation from their mothers and jeopardising breast-feeding. It is important to identify those infants most at risk of adverse effects of hypoglycaemia and determine the most effective and least invasive regimens for prevention of hypoglycaemic brain injury (Cornblath et al. 2000). To date, no controlled study has addressed either of these issues.

Hyperglycaemia was also recognised as a neonatal complication over a century ago (Kitselle 1852) and until recent times was a rare phenomenon. However, it is now commonly seen in the increasing numbers of extremely low-birthweight infants who are cared for in our neonatal units. Despite this history and current frequency, uncertainty as to its clinical significance and optimal management remains.

To manage these disorders of blood glucose homeostasis it is essential to understand the metabolism of the fetus and neonate and the changes that occur at birth in the healthy infant. This chapter will summarise the current knowledge of the disorders of blood glucose homeostasis, and aims to provide a practical and pragmatic approach to the management of babies with hypoglycaemia and hyperglycaemia.

Glucose homeostasis in the healthy fetus and neonate

Fetal metabolism

During pregnancy the human fetus receives from its mother, via the placental circulation, a supply of substrates necessary for growth, for the deposition of fuel stores which are essential after birth (see below) and for energy to meet the basal metabolic rate and requirements for growth. Glucose is transported across the placenta by facilitated diffusion, but during maternal starvation or placental insufficiency the fetus is capable of endogenous glucose production (Hay and Sparks 1985). Glucose metabolism accounts for 65% of fetal energy production, with lactate probably accounting for most of the remainder (Hay and Sparks 1985). Glucose is not the only fuel utilised by the fetal brain. Studies of perfused human fetal brain have demonstrated that uptake of ketone bodies, the products of β oxidation of fatty acids, is greater than that of glucose and it is likely that the fate of ketone bodies is both incorporation into brain lipids and for use as a cerebral energy source (Adam et al. 1975). Lactate may also be metabolised.

The fetus is usually capable of regulating its circulating glucose concentration independently of maternal glucose level and placental transfer. This capacity is seen in some cases of placental insufficiency when fetal gluconeogenesis is activated at the expense of growth and storage, and in the fetus of the mother with suboptimal control of diabetes (Ch. 22) when the fetal response to the high placental transfer of glucose is increased secretion of insulin, in turn resulting in greater than normal fetal growth and storage. However, the healthy fetus differs from adults in that there is a blunted insulin response to high glucose concentrations, and that insulin secretion is more sensitive to amino acids than glucose (Obershain et al. 1970). It appears that insulin has a greater role in fetal growth than in fetal metabolic control. Similarly, the fetus is less sensitive than the neonate to the glucose-mobilising actions of glucagon, although sensitivity increases with gestational age (Sperling et al. 1976, 1984).

Under extreme circumstances fetal blood glucose control fails; for example, in cases of severe and prolonged placental insufficiency (Soothill et al. 1987). It must be questioned whether it is possible that such profound and prolonged fetal hypoglycaemia has adverse effects on the developing brain and may explain some of the disability following severe intrauterine growth restriction (IUGR), even when there have been no postnatal complications.

Metabolic changes at birth

When the continuous flow of nutrients from the placenta is abruptly discontinued, immediate postnatal metabolic changes preserve fuel supplies for vital organ function. Oxygen supply temporarily fails during delivery and anaerobic metabolism must occur: this requires higher substrate availability than aerobic metabolism. In addition, the newborn infant must adapt to the fast-feed cycle and to the change in major energy source, from glucose transfer across the placenta to using fat from adipose tissue stores and milk feeds. After birth, plasma insulin levels fall and there are rapid surges of catecholamine and pancreatic glucagon release (Sperling et al. 1976; Hägnevik et al. 1984). These endocrine changes switch on the essential enzymes for glycogenolysis (the release of glucose stored as glycogen in liver, cardiac muscle and brain), for gluconeogenesis (glucose production from 3-carbon precursor molecules by the liver), lipolysis (release of fatty acids from adipose tissue stores) and ketogenesis (the β oxidation of fatty acids by the liver). Although glucose is the major metabolic fuel for most organs in the immediate postnatal period, there is evidence that lactate may be the preferred cerebral fuel over glucose and ketone bodies at this time (Medina et al. 1990).

Neonatal metabolism

The metabolic switch at birth is repeated on a smaller scale during the milk-fed infant's fast-feed cycles. Immediately after a feed there is availability of metabolic fuels, namely fatty acids and, to a lesser extent, sugars from milk. Some tissues, for example the kidney, are obligate glucose users, but others burn fatty fuels and the overall respiratory quotient falls after birth, reflecting the fact that fat oxidation accounts for about 75% of oxygen consumption. Of the organs that utilise alternative fuels to glucose, the brain is the most important in that it takes up and oxidises ketone bodies at higher rates than seen in adults, and the neonatal brain uses ketone bodies more efficiently than glucose (Edmond et al. 1985).

Any excess glucose available after a feed is stored as glycogen in the liver or converted to fat for deposition in adipose tissue, along with fatty acids absorbed after milk feeds.

Some time after each feed, the blood glucose level starts to fall and glycogenolysis and gluconeogenesis are again activated to ensure energy availability for organs which are obligate users (Fig. 34.1). Glycogenolysis is an exhaustible source of glucose whose capacity varies according to fetal growth and maturity (Shelley and Neligan 1966) and around 2 hours after birth gluconeogenesis must become the major glucose-providing process. Stable isotope turnover studies have shown that neonatal glucose production rates are 4–6 mg/kg/min (Bougneres 1987). Between feeds, lipolysis and ketogenesis provide alternative fuels to glucose for organs such as the brain, which are not obligate glucose utilisers (Hawdon and Ward Platt 1992). The process of ketogenesis also provides energy and cofactors which are utilised in gluconeogenesis, again highlighting the importance of fatty fuels.

The control of neonatal metabolism is dependent first on the synthesis of key enzymes, such as hepatic phosphorylase for glycogenolysis, phosphoenolpyruvate carboxykinase for gluconeogenesis and carnitine acyltransferases for ketogenesis, and, secondly, on the induction of enzyme activity by hormonal changes. Glucagon is the major neonatal glucoregulatory hormone (Sperling et al. 1976). Its concentration increases when blood glucose levels fall, and it induces activity of the enzymes of glycogenolysis, gluconeogenesis and ketogenesis in the liver. The glucoregulatory role of insulin in the neonate is less clear and may well differ from that in the adult. In most neonates, insulin does not appear to have a major influence on normal blood glucose homeostasis, but in some extreme cases (see below) high insulin concentrations may result in hypoglycaemia. Finally, it is unlikely that other hormones, such as the catecholamines, cortisol, thyroid hormones and growth hormone, are important regulators in the fast-feed cycle of the healthy neonate, but rare cases of hypopituitarism or cortisol deficiency (see below) may present with neonatal hypoglycaemia, which suggests that minimum basal levels are needed to maintain normoglycaemia.

Finally, the change from fetal to neonatal metabolism must take into account the important role of gastrointestinal adaptation. The introduction of enteral feeding has been shown to trigger the

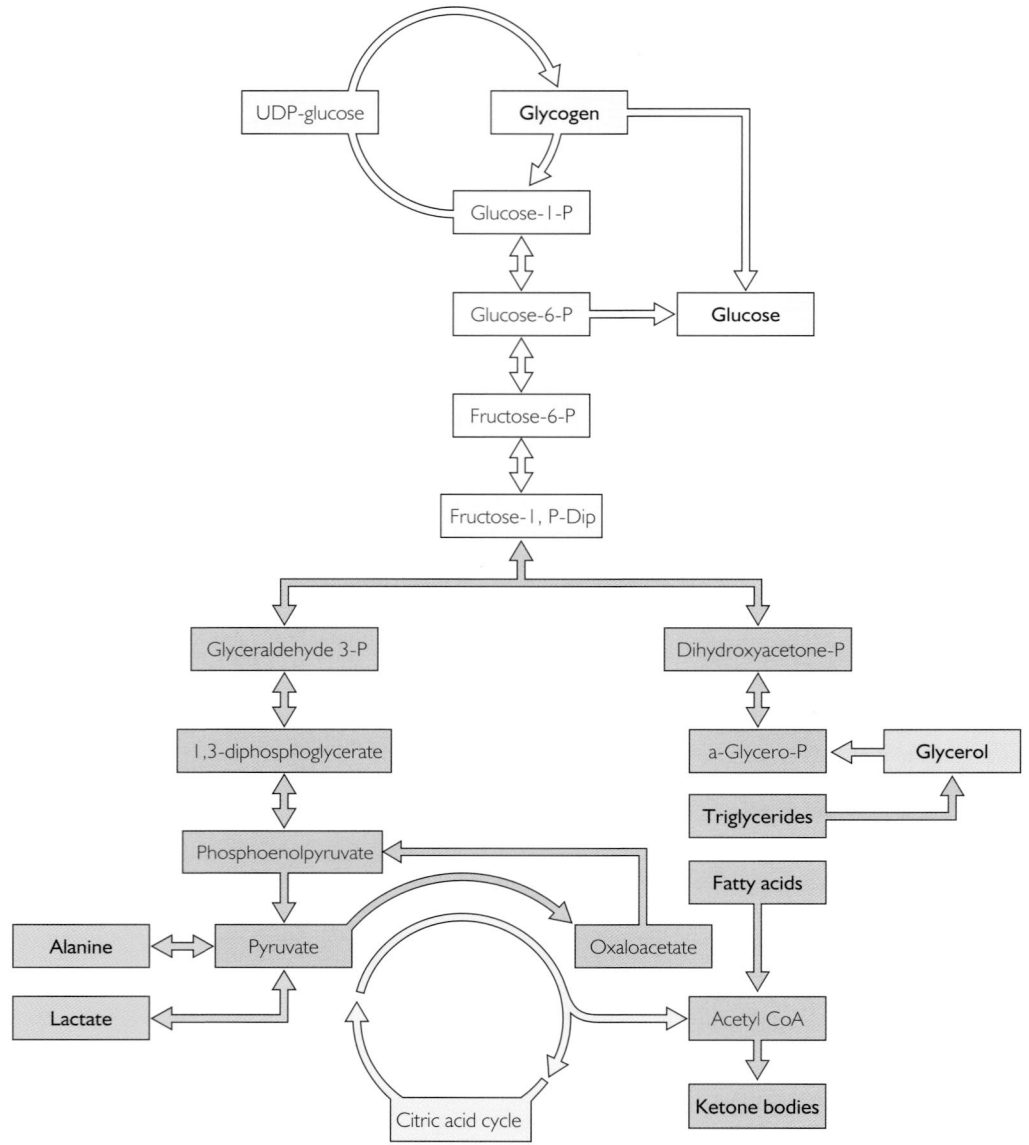

Fig. 34.1 Metabolic pathways involved in gluconeogenesis (pathways below glucose-6-P) and in glycogen synthesis (above glucose-6-P) and glycogenolysis. Galactose enters the pathways above glucose-6-P.

secretion of gastrointestinal regulatory peptides and hormones, which in turn induce the features of gut adaptation, namely gut growth, mucosal differentiation, induction of motor activity and the development of digestion and absorption (Lucas et al. 1981; Aynsley-Green 1988).

Differences between neonatal and adult metabolism

The differences between neonatal and adult metabolism are most likely to be evolutionary protective responses. Milk-fed neonates during their normal fast-feed cycle produce and utilise ketone bodies to the extent seen in adults only after a prolonged fast. Other fuels such as lactate may also be used in addition to glucose and

ketone bodies. Insulin plays a lesser role in neonatal glucoregulation than in the adult, in that its release in response to glucose is blunted and delayed when compared with the adult, and that there may be end-organ insensitivities to its action (Johnston et al. 1991). In fact, healthy neonates have insulin–glucose relationships that differ markedly from those of older subjects (Hawdon et al. 1993a, 1995). Therefore, when investigating a neonate for possible impaired neonatal glucoregulation it is essential to have reference data from healthy infants, rather than comparing the neonatal concentrations and interrelationships of fuels and hormones with those of adults. Also, it is impossible to consider glucose alone – the availability of alternative fuels must be established. Therefore, hypoglycaemia cannot strictly be applied as a pathological diagnostic term and it is preferable to consider a diagnosis of impaired metabolic adpatation.

Hypoglycaemia

Clinical significance

The continuing controversy regarding the clinical significance of neonatal hypoglycaemia arises from a failure to consider the changes of metabolic adaptation in their totality (Cornblath et al. 2000). Blood glucose levels fall immediately after birth but rise after a few hours either spontaneously or in response to feeding in healthy full-term babies (Srinivasan et al. 1986; Hawdon et al. 1992). In many babies, blood glucose levels then remain below what would be the normal range for an adult. This physiological pattern in the healthy baby with no risk factors for impaired metabolic adaptation and no clinical signs cannot be considered to be of clinical significance.

A factor not commonly recognised is that babies vary in their ability to mount protective metabolic responses when blood glucose levels are low. Indeed, there is evidence that glucose utilisation by the neonatal brain is less than in subsequent months, because of utilisation of alternative fuels (Kinnala et al. 1996; Kapoor et al. 2009). Low blood glucose concentrations (less than 2.6 mmol/l) are commonly found during the first postnatal days in healthy appropriate-for-gestational-age (AGA) and small-for-gestational age term neonates, particularly those who are breastfed. However, these infants have high ketone body levels when blood glucose concentrations are low, and it is likely that this protects them from neurological sequelae (Thurston et al. 1986; Hawdon et al. 1992; De Boissieu et al. 1995; de Rooy and Hawdon 2002; Hay et al. 2009).

Therefore, it is not always appropriate to consider low blood glucose levels to represent a pathological process. However, in some circumstances, such as following preterm delivery, IUGR, perinatal hypoxia–ischaemia or suboptimal control of diabetes in pregnancy, there may be impaired ketone body production and in these babies circulating blood glucose concentrations acquire greater clinical significance and hypoglycaemia, if present, must be diagnosed and treated effectively (Hawdon and Ward Platt 1992; Hawdon et al. 1992, 1993a; Cornblath et al. 2000).

No study has yet satisfactorily addressed the duration of absent or reduced availability of metabolic fuels which is harmful to the human neonate. Studies in neonatal rats have demonstrated that prolonged insulin-induced hypoglycaemia, but not starvation-induced hypoglycaemia and not short-period hypoglycaemia, resulted in neurodegenerative changes (Zhou et al. 2008). A study of rhesus monkeys has shown that a duration of insulin-induced neonatal hypoglycaemia (blood glucose <1.5 mmol/l) of 6.5 hours had no demonstrable long-term effects, whereas 10 hours of hypoglycaemia was associated with 'motivational and adaptability problems' but no motor or cognitive deficit on testing at 8 months of age (Schrier et al. 1990).

In the light of the paucity of human neonatal data and the variability between babies with regard to exacerbating factors and protective mechanisms, it is impossible to state the duration of hypoglycaemia that is harmful to human neonates. It is very unlikely that brief self-limiting episodes are of neurological significance if not accompanied by clinical signs or coexisting clinical complications, but for some babies protective metabolic responses will fail after a period of hypoglycaemia (measured in hours rather than minutes) resulting first in abnormal neurological signs and then, in the untreated baby, brain injury (Cornblath et al. 2000).

Acute neurophysiological changes at low blood glucose levels have been demonstrated in human neonates and the newborn of other species (Vannucci et al. 1981; Koh et al. 1988a). However, the long-term significance of these acute changes is not clear. There is no doubt that a number of infants have fits or a reduced level of consciousness when blood glucose levels are low and protective metabolic responses fail or are exhausted, and adverse long-term outcomes have been reported when neurological signs have been present (Boluyt et al. 2006; Rozance and Hay 2006). In extreme cases, profound hypoglycaemia, usually the result of serious inborn errors of metabolism, may even result in 'cot death' or apparent life-threatening events. A multitude of clinical signs have often been associated with hypoglycaemia, namely tremor, irritability, 'jitteriness', apnoea, hypotonia, abnormal cry, tachypnoea, pallor and feeding difficulties. However, these are as likely to be the result of coexisting clinical complications, such as perinatal hypoxia–ischaemia, or the cause of hypoglycaemia (e.g. poor feeding) as the specific effects of hypoglycaemia.

No study has clearly demonstrated the independent contribution of hypoglycaemia (with or without clinical signs) to neurodevelopmental outcome because all studies to date are of neonates who had other adverse clinical factors (Cowett 1999; Cornblath et al. 2000; Boluyt et al. 2006; Rozance and Hay 2006). There is also a paucity of information regarding the histopathological and neuroradiological changes associated with neonatal hypoglycaemia, and the reports of past studies are conflicting. However, there is evidence from case reports that profound and prolonged hypoglycaemia is associated with both transient and permanent structural changes in the brain (Anderson et al. 1967; Banker 1967; Griffiths and Lawrence 1974; Auer and Siesjo 1993; Barkovich et al. 1998; Murakami et al. 1999; Kinnala et al. 2000; Filan et al. 2006; Burns et al. 2008). Grey-matter damage is most commonly reported, with the parieto-occipital regions being most affected.

Impaired metabolic adaptation is likely to be most common following or coincident with other insults, such as hypoxia–ischaemia. Although concurrent hypoglycaemia and hypoxia–ischaemia are more damaging than either insult alone, there is no evidence that hypoglycaemia following cessation of a hypoxic–ischaemic insult worsens hypoxic–ischaemic injury (Vannucci and Vannucci 2001). For infants with multisystem problems (for example, after preterm delivery or perinatal hypoxia–ischaemia) all potential causes of neurological dysfunction should be prevented and treated as far as possible, and in practice the prevention of hypoglycaemia is often the easiest of clinical issues.

Unfortunately, even in cases where clinical significance is tenuous, hypoglycaemia has acquired legal and costly significance (Cornblath et al. 2000). This can be avoided on many occasions by following local guidelines and paying close attention to documentation, especially of normal findings (Williams 2005; Hawdon 2007).

Finally, the impact of hypoglycaemia and its treatment on the mother and baby must be considered. The early neonatal period is an emotionally sensitive time, and the diagnosis of hypoglycaemia may create or add to anxiety for the parents. Treatment of the infant with intravenous glucose involves separation of the baby and mother, and may be perceived as invasive or painful. The implications for the establishment of breastfeeding must also not be forgotten, especially as there is evidence that separation disrupts breastfeeding and in turn breastfeeding and avoidance of formula supplementation augment ketogenesis (Elander and Lindberg 1984; Hawdon 1993; de Rooy and Hawdon 2002). Therefore, emphasis should be on the early prevention of hypoglycaemia and strategies of management that do not involve the separation of mother and baby (National Childbirth Trust 1997; Haninger and Farley 2001).

Definition

Much controversy and confusion has surrounded the definition of hypoglycaemia. Some authors (Koh et al. 1988b; Cornblath et al.

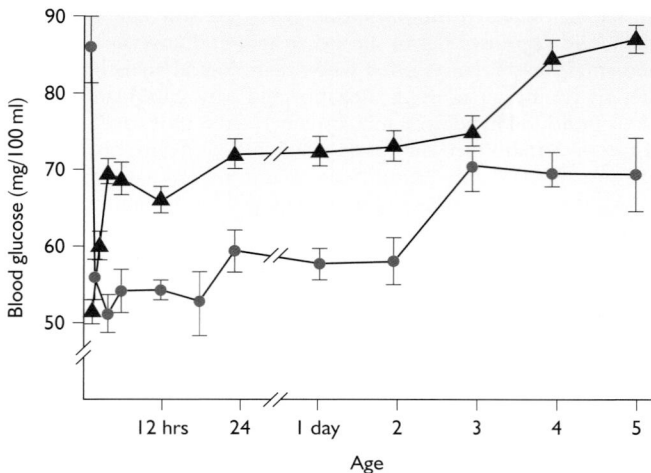

Fig. 34.2 Blood glucose levels (mean ± SE) in full-term infants, showing the changing pattern of development during the first postnatal days in 1965 compared with 1986 (circles, Cornblath and Reisner (1965); triangles, Srinivasan et al. (1986)). To convert mg/100 ml into mmol/l, divide by 18.

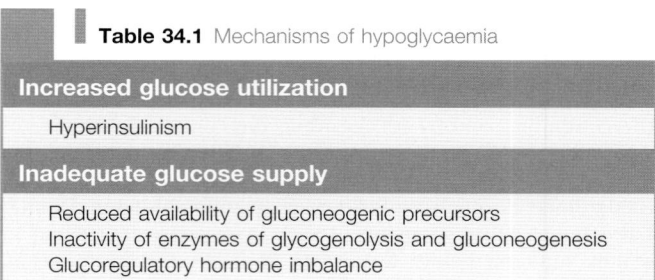

Table 34.1 Mechanisms of hypoglycaemia

Increased glucose utilization
Hyperinsulinism
Inadequate glucose supply
Reduced availability of gluconeogenic precursors
Inactivity of enzymes of glycogenolysis and gluconeogenesis
Glucoregulatory hormone imbalance

2000; Hay et al. 2009) demonstrated that the definition varied widely not only among standard paediatric textbooks but also among neonatologists, with values given ranging from below 1 mmol/l to below 4 mmol/l. Cornblath et al. (2000) wrote: 'The definition of clinically significant hypoglycaemia remains one of the most confused and contentious issues in contemporary neonatology.'

Previous widely used definitions were based on cross-sectional samples from newborn babies, with the assumption that the lowest blood glucose levels were abnormal. However, these definitions were proposed at a time when, unlike the present, infants were starved for considerable periods after birth, and small and preterm infants received less milk than healthy term infants. Therefore, it is not surprising that many infants on the first postnatal day had very low blood glucose levels. The current practice of early feeding of infants has been associated with a more rapid increase in blood glucose concentration after the immediate postnatal fall (Fig. 34.2) (Srinivasan et al. 1986; Aynsley-Green 1988). Fortunately, the long-standing belief that the brains of preterm infants were more able to withstand low blood glucose levels than those of term infants is now less widely accepted (Koh et al. 1988b).

Later, this statistical definition of hypoglycaemia was challenged and a 'functional' definition was proposed, which is 'at what level of blood glucose is the body's function, particularly that of the brain, compromised?' In reality, this threshold level will vary between babies, and is only of significance when protective metabolic responses are impaired and there are no alternative fuels to glucose. It is not possible to describe a functional definition of hypoglycaemia in terms of the blood glucose level at which symptoms occur because, unlike adults and older children, babies cannot complain of symptoms and by the time blood glucose levels have fallen so low that clinical signs of cerebral dysfunction have been allowed to persist, there is a risk that brain injury may have been sustained. There is no doubt that any low blood glucose concentration of any duration which causes clinical signs, such as fits or coma, is too low, regardless of its numerical value, and must be treated. In fact, the rapid clinical resolution of the signs after the intravenous administration of glucose confirms the diagnosis of acute cerebral dysfunction secondary to hypoglycaemia.

Only two studies have attempted to define the 'safe level' for blood glucose concentrations in neonates without apparent clinical signs (Koh et al. 1988a; Lucas et al. 1988). In a neurodevelopmental follow-up study of very-low-birthweight preterm infants, Lucas et al. (1988) found that neonatal blood glucose concentrations below 2.6 mmol/l on at least 3 days were associated with a poor neurodevelopmental outcome. The neurophysiological study of Koh et al. (1988a) demonstrated that, in a group of subjects which included five neonates of varying birthweights and gestations, no baby with a blood glucose level above 2.6 mmol/l had abnormal sensory-evoked brainstem potentials. No differences were found in the blood glucose threshold for abnormal sensory-evoked potentials between subjects who had signs of hypoglycaemia and those who did not. Both studies concluded with the suggestion that blood glucose levels less than 2.6 mmol/l are associated with abnormal acute and prolonged neurological function, and that levels above this could be considered safe. However, these conclusions are not entirely supported by data from the studies and cannot be extrapolated to other groups of neonates (Cornblath et al. 2000).

An evidence-based definition of hypoglycaemia should include the blood glucose concentration considered to be the minimum safe level, the duration beyond which the low blood glucose level is considered to be harmful, the presence of clinical signs, the group of infants studied, the consideration of alternative fuel availability, the conditions of sampling and the assay methods. Most of these criteria have never been adequately addressed by previous studies or publications (Boluyt et al. 2006; Rozance and Hay 2006; Hay et al. 2009). This paucity of data has resulted in a pragmatic approach proposed by a group of clinicians based on thresholds for intervention rather than attempting to define hypoglycaemia as a single numerical term (Cornblath et al. 2000). This group proposed that, regardless of the blood glucose concentration, neurological signs in association with low blood glucose levels should prompt investigations to establish a firm diagnosis of hypoglycaemia and its underlying cause, and the institution of urgent treatment. For infants without clinical signs but at risk of neurological sequelae by virtue of their impaired ability to mobilise ketone bodies at low blood glucose levels (Table 34.1), intervention to raise blood glucose should be considered if two consecutive blood glucose levels are below 2 mmol/l (measured using accurate device) or a single blood glucose level is below 1 mmol/l.

Diagnosis

The accurate measurement of blood glucose levels is essential in the diagnosis of hypoglycaemia. It is well known that glucose reagent strips, commonly used in neonatal and maternity units, are insufficiently reliable for the diagnosis (Medical Devices Agency 1996; Cornblath et al. 2000; Hay et al. 2009). Therefore, if these strips are used for neonatal screening all low values should be confirmed by accurate measurement. These samples should be assayed promptly

Table 34.2 Infants who are at risk for the neurological sequelae of neonatal hypoglycaemia

AT-RISK GROUP	MECHANISMS	MANAGEMENT
Preterm (≤36 weeks)	Low substrate stores Immature hormone and enzyme responses Fluid/energy restriction Feeding difficulties Poor temperature control	Early, frequent, adequate feeds Intravenous glucose if necessary Thermoprotection
Intrauterine growth restriction (birthweight ≤2nd centile or clinically wasted)	Low substrate stores Immature hormone and enzyme responses Feeding difficulties Poor temperature control	Early, frequent, adequate feeds Intravenous glucose if necessary
Infant of diabetic mother (poor antenatal control) Beckwith–Wiedemann syndrome Rhesus haemolytic disease	Hyperinsulinism	Early, frequent, adequate feeds Intravenous glucose if necessary Early, frequent, adequate feeds
Congenital hyperinsulinaemic hypoglycaemia Islet cell adenoma	Hyperinsulinism	Intravenous glucose, often >8 mg/kg/min Diazoxide Somatostatin Surgery (if necessary)
Moderate to severe perinatal hypoxia–ischaemia	Low substrate stores 'Exhausted' stress response Enzyme dysfunction Hyperinsulinism Fluid/energy restriction Feeding difficulties	Adequate energy provision
Maternal beta-blocker medication	Suppressed catecholamine release	Early, frequent, adequate feeds
Septicaemia	'Exhausted' stress response Enzyme dysfunction Fluid/energy restriction Feeding difficulties	Adequate energy provision
Pituitary/adrenal insufficiency	Impaired cortisol response	Early, frequent, adequate feeds Intravenous glucose (if necessary)
Inborn errors of metabolism	Defects of enzymes of glycogen production, glycogenolysis, gluconeogenesis, fatty acid oxidation	Investigate Adequate energy provision

as blood glucose levels diminish with time, even in fluoridated tubes (Joosten et al. 1991). Accurate determination may be conveniently performed using a blood glucose analyser sited in a neonatal unit laboratory. Usually whole blood samples are taken. Plasma glucose sample results are 13–18% higher than in whole blood. In terms of safety, accurate blood glucose measurements in whole blood samples will not underestimate the severity of hypoglycaemia, except in polycythaemia.

Interesting new techniques of glucose monitoring by subcutaneous microdialysis may in time reduce the need for venepuncture and heelpricks (Baumeister et al. 2001). However, the clinical significance and validity of glucose measurements using these techniques are not fully evaluated.

In addition to diagnosing hypoglycaemia, the underlying cause must be determined. This is usually self-evident from the obstetric history or clinical examination, but if this is not the case and the hypoglycaemia is profound or persistent despite treatment, further

investigations must be performed to identify rare but serious inborn errors of metabolism or hormone deficiencies (Table 34.2). As these tests are most informative when carried out at the time of hypoglycaemia, it is important to take the necessary blood and urine samples during such episodes and process and store them if necessary out of laboratory working hours. Each unit should devise an appropriate protocol for this in liaison with local and regional specialised laboratories.

Prevalence of neonatal hypoglycaemia

Because clinical practices have changed to such an extent since the risks of hypoglycaemia were first identified, and because of the controversy surrounding definition, it is difficult to ascertain the prevalence of hypoglycaemia in at-risk groups. For example, using the definition proposed by Cornblath and Schwartz (1976), prevalences ranged from 5% to 7.9% in term infants and from 3.2% to

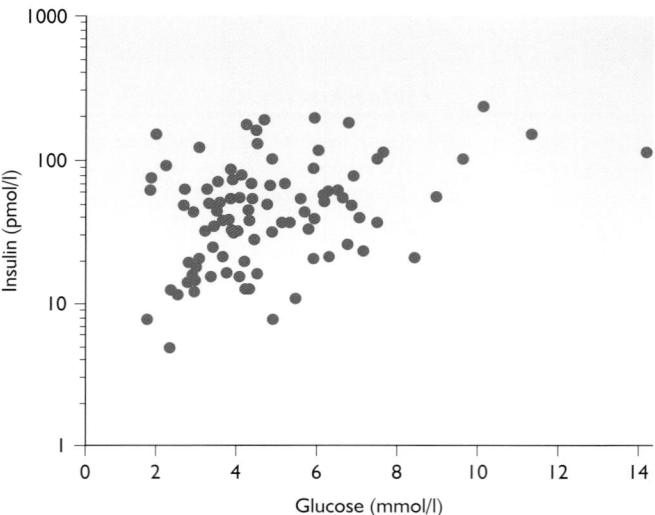

Fig. 34.3 Insulin–glucose relationship in preterm neonates; insulin concentrations measured using a highly specific immunoradiometric assay. *(Reproduced from Hawdon et al. (1995).)*

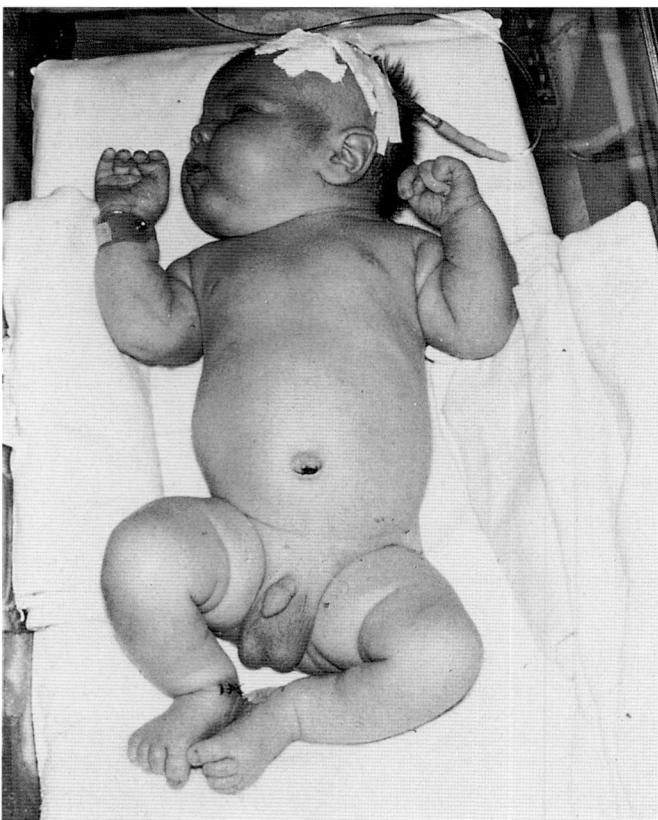

Fig. 34.4 Newborn infant with hyperinsulinism showing increased adiposity and resemblance to an infant of a diabetic mother.

15% in preterm infants (Fluge 1974; Cornblath and Schwartz 1976; Heck and Erenberg 1987; Hawdon et al. 1992). Using the suggested 'safe' level for blood glucose concentrations (2.6 mmol/l) proposed by Lucas et al. (1988), this group reported a prevalence of 67%, whereas a more recent study of clinically stable, AGA, term and preterm neonates reported prevalences of 10% and 4%, respectively (Hawdon et al. 1992).

Mechanisms and at-risk groups

Hypoglycaemia may be secondary to increased utilisation of glucose, to inadequate endogenous or exogenous supply of glucose, or to a combination of the two (Table 34.1).

Increased glucose utilisation

The most common cause of excessive utilisation of glucose is neonatal hyperinsulinism. Hyperinsulinism should be confirmed by the use of a highly specific insulin assay for plasma insulin concentrations and its interpretation with reference to normal neonatal insulin–glucose relationships (Hawdon et al. 1993a, 1995) (Fig. 34.3). Clinical features are that glucose requirements to maintain normoglycaemia are high, in excess of 8 mg/kg/min, as compared with 4–6 mg/kg/min usually required by neonates, and the infant may be macrosomic if hyperinsulinism was of fetal origin (Fig. 34.4). Investigation of suspected hyperinsulinism will demonstrate low fatty acid and ketone body concentrations during hypoglycaemia, but this feature is not specific to hyperinsulinism as some infants who are not hyperinsulinaemic, such as some who are preterm or have IUGR, also fail to mount lipolytic and ketogenic responses.

Self-limiting hyperinsulinism

Hyperinsulinism may be a temporary phenomenon when the fetus has been rendered hyperglycaemic by poorly controlled maternal diabetes (see Ch. 22), antenatal administration of thiazide diuretics or the administration of glucose to the mothers in labour, and in infants shortly after abrupt discontinuation of intravenous glucose

infusions, after bolus doses of glucose or if glucose has been infused through an umbilical arterial catheter whose tip is close to the coeliac axis (Senior et al. 1976; Lucas et al. 1980). Rhesus haemolytic disease and perinatal asphyxia have also been associated with transient fetal and neonatal hyperinsulinism, although the aetiological link is not known (Molsted-Pedersen et al. 1973; Collins and Leonard 1984; Hawdon and Ward Platt 1992). It has been suggested that hyperinsulinism contributes to hypoglycaemia after intrauterine growth retardation, but normal insulin–glucose relationships (using neonatal reference data) have been demonstrated in IUGR neonates (Chaivorarat and Dweck 1976; Collins et al. 1990; Hawdon et al. 1993a, b, c).

Iatrogenic or factitious hyperinsulinism

Hyperinsulinism may result from erroneous or malicious administration of insulin. Although rare, these conditions should be suspected if hypoglycaemia is unexpected, profound or resistant to treatment.

Beckwith–Wiedemann syndrome

This condition, described independently by Beckwith (1963) and Wiedemann (1964), is characterised by exomphalos, macroglossia, visceromegaly, earlobe abnormalities and an increased later incidence of malignancies. Hyperinsulinism is a common but not invariable feature causing high glucose requirements in the early neonatal period; it usually resolves some time after birth. It is likely that the previously reported long-term developmental difficulties were related to undiagnosed and untreated hypoglycaemia, and it is anticipated that awareness of the condition and prevention of hypoglycaemia should result in improved outcome.

Congenital hyperinsulinaemic hypoglycaemia

Although a rare condition, this is the most common cause of recurrent and persistent hypoglycaemia in infancy and childhood (Kapoor et al. 2009). It is usually associated with macrosomia and always with extreme hyperinsulinism and high glucose requirements. The condition may be self-limiting in the neonatal period but more often extends beyond this time. As there is no protective ketone body response to hypoglycaemia, there are usually neurological signs and the risk of brain injury is high. Therefore, urgent treatment is required (see below). Many descriptive terms, such as 'nesidioblastosis', 'islet-cell dysregulation syndrome' or 'persistent hyperinsulinaemic hypoglycaemia of infancy', have been applied to the condition over the years. Currently, histological classification is into diffuse and focal forms (Kapoor et al. 2009).

The condition is more often familial than sporadic. Several underlying pathologies have been demonstrated (Kapoor et al. 2009). In severe cases of hyperinsulinaemic hypoglycaemia there are mutations in the genes encoding for subunits of the K^+ATP channel and the involvement of the pancreas is diffuse. The functional loss of this channel results in dysregulation of calcium fluxes and thus unregulated insulin release. Other forms of hypersinsulinism, which tend to be milder or present later, are linked to defects in genes coding for glutamate dehydrogenase and glucokinase, with activation of these genes in turn affecting the function of the beta cell. The former is the second most common form of congenital hyperinsulinaemic hypoglycaemia and is associated with hyperammonaemia, so ammonia levels should always be measured when hyperinsulinaemia is suspected (De Lonlay et al. 2002). Other mutations are those coding for hepatocyte nuclear factor-4 α protein and HADH (a mitochondrial enzyme of fatty acid metabolism) (Clayton et al. 2001).

Rarely, an isolated islet-cell adenoma may present with neonatal hyperinsulinaemic hypoglycaemia.

Recognition of hyperinsulinism and early prevention and treatment of hypoglycaemia, with referral to a specialist centre, are essential to reduce the incidence of permanent neurological damage, which has been widely reported (Jacobs et al. 1986; Meissner et al. 1997; Menni et al. 2001; Kapoor et al. 2009).

'Leucine-sensitive hypoglycaemia'

This was previously described as a distinct entity, but it is more likely that hypoglycaemia in response to leucine administration represents underlying hyperinsulinism sensitive to protein and should be investigated and treated as such (Kapoor et al. 2009).

Insufficient supply of glucose

Hypoglycaemia is most often the result of reduced delivery of glucose into the blood. In the enterally fed infant all the circulating glucose is provided either by the absorption and conversion of sugars or by glycogenolysis and gluconeogenesis, and in some babies there may be a contribution from intravenous glucose infusion. Thus, if the infant fails to switch on glycogenolysis or gluconeogenesis in response to falling blood glucose levels, or clinicians prescribe insufficient intravenous glucose, hypoglycaemia may occur. This will be most significant when production of alternative fuels to glucose is also impaired. Three possible mechanisms may cause the failure of glucose production: (1) reduced availability of gluconeogenic precursors; (2) reduced activity of enzymes of glycogenolysis and gluconeogenesis; or (3) impaired counterregulatory hormone response.

Reduced availability of gluconeogenic precursors

Glycogenolysis and gluconeogenesis may be limited by availability of glycogen, gluconeogenic precursors or the energy provided by fatty acid oxidation. This may occur after preterm delivery, IUGR, maternal alcohol abuse or perinatal hypoxia–ischaemia, or as a consequence of inadequate substrate intake after birth (Shelley and Basset 1975; Ogata 1986; Singh et al. 1988).

Reduced activity of enzymes of glycogenolysis and gluconeogenesis

There may be failure of synthesis and activation of the key enzymes described above, and enzymes of lipolysis and ketogenesis will also be affected. This may be the result of a specific inherited metabolic disorder, in which case hypoglycaemia is usually severe, and recurrent or persistent, or there may be generalised immaturity of enzymes, as in preterm infants. The infant is resistant to the effects of the postnatal surges of counterregulatory hormones. Finally, enzyme activity may be suppressed by acquired conditions, such as perinatal bacterial infection or impaired liver function. Defective gluconeogenesis may also be the cause of hypoglycaemia complicating cases of congenital heart disease and cold injury (Mann and Elliot 1957; Haymond et al. 1979).

Impaired counterregulatory hormone response

This will result in failure to activate enzymes of glycogenolysis, gluconeogenesis, lipolysis and ketogenesis. Hyperinsulinism has a dual mechanism in that glucose utilisation is increased (see above) but also counterregulatory hormone release is inhibited. Failure of release of counterregulatory hormones may play a role in hypoglycaemia in preterm and IUGR babies, and after maternal medication with beta-blockers in pregnancy (Ogata 1986; Munshi et al. 1992). Finally, there may be rare permanent disorders which result in insufficiency of counterregulatory hormones, for example low growth hormone and cortisol levels in septo-optic dysplasia and congenital hypopituitarism, and low glucocorticoid levels in adrenocortical deficiencies (Lovinger et al. 1975; Gemelli et al. 1979; Costello and Gluckman 1988).

Mechanisms of hypoglycaemia vary among groups of infants, and for some there may be more than one aetiological mechanism (Table 34.2). This is most applicable to neonates who have been subject to IUGR, which for many reasons may result in failure of glycogenolysis and gluconeogenesis after birth. Animal and clinical studies have demonstrated that IUGR may reduce the availability of alternative fuels for cerebral metabolism (Dahlquist 1976; Hawdon and Ward Platt 1993). However, another clinical study has shown that healthy breastfed IUGR babies can mount a ketogenic response, and that excessive formula milk supplementation may be the cause of the suppressed response (de Rooy and Hawdon 2002). It is important to note that not all IUGR infants will be 'small for gestational age' (see Ch. 10), and clinical examination is important for the identification of the 'wasted' neonate with disproportionate birthweight and head circumference centiles. Conversely, not all small-for-gestational-age infants will have been subject to placental insufficiency – they may be constitutionally small and will not experience impaired postnatal metabolic adaptation. In summary, the early identification of at-risk neonates and the understanding of underlying mechanisms of hypoglycaemia are important for the diagnosis and treatment of the disorder.

Prevention and management of neonatal hypoglycaemia (Table 34.3)

Normal babies

As described above, healthy full-term AGA neonates often have low blood glucose concentrations in the first postnatal days, but are protected by the presence of ketone bodies and lactate as alternative fuels. Thus, it is now recognised in Europe and North America that, for this group, it is not appropriate to carry out routine blood glucose monitoring, to label low blood glucose as a pathological entity or to initiate treatment which is invasive or which may interfere with the establishment of breastfeeding (National Childbirth Trust 1997; Cornblath et al. 2000; Eidelman 2001; Haninger and Farley 2001). Because of the healthy infant's ability to counterregulate, problems with establishment of successful breastfeeding are equally likely to present with excessive weight loss (in excess of 10% birthweight), dehydration and jaundice as with clinically significant hypoglycaemia. Therefore, breastfeeding advice and intervention should not be based on blood glucose levels, but on full assessment of the baby – proceeding to blood glucose measurement if there are clinical concerns. Midwives and doctors must be alert to the possibility that other conditions, such as infection or, more rarely, inborn errors of metabolism, may present with the neurological signs and hypoglycaemia and specific investigations should be performed (Table 34.4).

At-risk babies (Table 34.2)

For practical purposes, the following discussion focuses only on the infants who are at risk of the impaired metabolic adapatation and the neurological sequelae of hypoglycaemia (Table 34.2). Early prevention of hypoglycaemia is optimal for these infants, so the first step in management must be to identify them. Although this is easy in some cases (such as the preterm baby), for others clinical observations are important (for example, to identify the wasted appearance of the growth-restricted neonate who may not necessarily have a low birthweight).

At-risk infants should have regular pre-feed blood glucose monitoring (at least 4–6-hourly initially). In addition, it is imperative that any infant with neurological signs, even if not in an at-risk group, should have urgent, accurate blood glucose measurement. The monitoring schedule for at-risk infants will vary according to local protocols, but we suggest that monitoring should be commenced before the second feed and that pre-feed monitoring be continued until the infant has had at least two satisfactory measurements. Monitoring should be recommenced if the infant's clinical condition worsens or energy intake decreases. If monitoring is by reagent strip, low levels must be confirmed by accurate measurement (see above).

The importance of early milk feeding has been appreciated for many years (Smallpiece and Davies 1964). Both breast and formula milks provide important gluconeogenic precursors and fatty acids for β oxidation. As they contain sources of energy other than carbohydrate they have a higher joule/ml content than 10% dextrose. In addition, enteral milk feeding stimulates the secretion of gut hormones, which may facilitate postnatal metabolic adaptation (Lucas et al. 1981). Therefore, all infants who are expected to tolerate enteral feeds should be fed with milk as soon as possible after birth, and at frequent intervals thereafter. Babies who are capable of sucking should be offered the breast at each feed (if this is the mother's wish). If it is likely that babies will need complementary or supplementary feeds, maternal breast milk expression should be encouraged. The need for formula supplementation will vary between babies, will diminish with the successful establishment of breastfeeding, and will be guided by the availability of expressed breast milk, regular pre-feed blood glucose monitoring, the clinical condition of the baby and assessment of breastfeeding. In the breastfed baby, formula intake should be kept to the minimum necessary, so as to enhance breastfeeding and avoid suppression of normal metabolic adaptation (de Rooy and Hawdon 2002).

In the at-risk baby who is establishing oral feeds there is a potential nadir at which body stores are steadily reducing but milk feeds have not yet started to replenish these stores. Even if the baby is feeding well, this may not occur until at least 48 hours. For this reason, vulnerable babies should not be transferred to the community at less than 48 hours, and only when experienced staff are satisfied that feeding is effective.

When full enteral feeding is not anticipated, for example in the very preterm or sick infant, an intravenous glucose infusion should be commenced as soon as possible after birth. Usually 10% dextrose at 3 ml/kg/h (5 mg glucose/kg/min) is sufficient to prevent hypoglycaemia, but in some cases (such as hyperinsulinism) more is required. If the amount of glucose administered is limited by fluid restriction, more concentrated dextrose solutions may be required and central venous lines should be used, because these solutions are sclerotic to peripheral veins and cause tissue damage if they leak.

If low blood glucose levels persist or are associated with clinical signs in the milk-fed infant despite the above measures, it may be possible to increase further the volumes and/or frequencies of feeds. If this is not possible, or if the hypoglycaemia is resistant to this strategy, intravenous glucose will be required. If the infant is tolerating milk feeds these should be neither stopped nor reduced. The initial rate of 10% glucose infusion should be 3 ml/kg/h (5 mg/kg/min; Table 34.5), but adjusted according to frequent accurate blood glucose measurements. If the need for fluid restriction limits the amount of glucose that may be given, more concentrated solutions may need to be infused (Table 34.5). If hypoglycaemia persists despite intravenous glucose, it is important to check the infusion site and the infusion apparatus to confirm glucose delivery. Leaking drips should be promptly resited. Boluses of concentrated glucose solution should be avoided because of the risk of rebound hypoglycaemia and cerebral oedema (Shah et al. 1992); if boluses are required (for example, if there are neurological signs of hypoglycaemia), they should be of 10% dextrose (3–5 ml/kg), given slowly, and always followed by an infusion. All reductions in infusion rate should be gradual. In cases of hyperinsulinism, intramuscular glucagon will have a temporary glycaemic effect if there is delay in siting an intravenous infusion (see below).

Specific treatments

Hyperinsulinism

It should be stressed again that, when hyperinsulinism is not self-limiting and requires or is resistant to very high glucose infusion rates, referral to a specialist centre must be made (Aynsley-Green et al. 2000). The treatments outlined below should only be administered in non-specialist units on the advice of a specialist centre and as a holding measure pending transfer. The risk of precipitating heart failure, especially if there is a coexisting hypertrophic cardiomyopathy, must be considered.

Glucose delivery should be prescribed to maintain blood glucose levels above 3 mmol/l and early siting of an umbilical venous catheter or venous central line is essential to allow adequate delivery rates. If hypoglycaemia is still resistant to high glucose delivery rates,

Table 34.3

| **1. Identify at-risk infants (see Table 34.2)** |
| **2. Early energy provision (within 1 hour of birth)** |

If enteral feeding planned:	If enteral feeding contraindicated
Breastfeed if mother's wish Encourage kangaroo care and unlimited access to breast Support mother to express breast milk and give colostrum If not breastfed, formula feed of 12 ml/kg Minimum interval between feeds of 3–4 hours	IV 10% glucose infusion of at least 3 ml/kg/h

3. Blood glucose monitoring

Pre-feed measurement
Before second feed, then frequency according to progress (at least 4–6-hourly in first 48 hours)
Accurate method or confirm reagent stick measurements <3.0 mmol/l with accurate method
Discontinue when two readings at least 2.0 mmol/l (3.0 mmol/l for hyperinsulinism)
Recommence if energy intake falls, e.g. vomiting or condition of baby changes
Measure blood glucose in any baby with abnormal clinical signs

4. Maintain energy provision

Increase feed interval if blood glucose ≥2.0 mmol/l (3.0 mmol/l for hyperinsulinism)

Mother plans to breastfeed:	Mother plans to bottle-feed:

Encourage kangaroo care and unlimited access to breast
Offer breast before formula feeds
Support mother to express breast milk
Expressed breast milk/formula supplements by gavage, cup or bottle
    Volume and frequency as indicated by blood glucose monitoring and clinical condition
    Discontinue when blood glucose ≥2.0 mmol/l (3.0 mmol/l for hyperinsulinism)
Continue milk feeds if tolerated even if IV therapy is commenced
	Start at 100 ml/kg/day
	Demand feed when blood glucose ≥2.0mmol/l
	    (3.0 mmol/l for hyperinsulinism)

IV therapy:

Make gradual reductions, e.g. by 1–2 ml/h if blood glucose ≥2.0 mmol/l (3.0 mmol/l for hyperinsulinism)
Resite drips promptly

5. If blood glucose <2.0 mmol/l on at least two occasions but no clinical signs

If enterally fed:	If IV glucose already running:
Increase feed volume and frequency Commence IV glucose if blood glucose remains <2.0 mmol/l despite above If blood glucose persistently low, investigate for underlying cause	Increase infusion rate or concentration

6. If blood glucose <1.0 mmol/l and/or major clinical signs, e.g. fits/coma

Take sample for accurate blood glucose but do not wait for result
If possible, take diagnostic hormone and metabolite samples
IV 10% glucose bolus of 3 ml/kg, repeated if signs do not resolve
Followed immediately by IV glucose infusion of at least 3 ml/kg/h; adjust according to signs and blood glucose
If problems siting IV and diagnosis is hyperinsulinism, give glucagon IM/IV 100 μg/kg
Investigate for underlying cause, e.g. infection
Collect and freeze next urine sample
Hourly blood glucose measurements until ≥2.0 mmol/l

7. If hypoglycaemia is severe or persistent

Investigate as in Table 34.4

8. Summary

Milk feeds: to maximum volume tolerated
IV glucose: minimum necessary to maintain blood glucose ≥2.0 mmol/l (3.0 mmol/l for hyperinsulinism)

IV, intravenous; IM, intramuscular.

Table 34.4 Samples for the investigation of severe or persistent hypoglycaemia (NB. each condition is a rare cause of neonatal hypoglycaemia)

SAMPLE	ASSAY	DIAGNOSIS
Blood	Glucose*	Confirm diagnosis
Blood	pH*	Lactic acidosis in: glucose-6-phosphatase deficiency, fructose-1,6-diphosphatase deficiency, pyruvate carboxylase deficiency, phosphoenolpyruvate carboxykinase deficiency
	Lactate*	Acidosis in disorders of amino acid metabolism
Blood	Intermediary metabolites	Disorders of gluconeogenesis
Blood	Ketone bodies	Disorders of fatty acid β oxidation (NB. low ketone body levels in preterm, intrauterine growth restriction and hyperinsulinaemic infants)
Plasma	Ammonia	Disorders of amino acid metabolism Hyperinsulinism
Plasma	Fatty acids	Disorders of fatty acid β oxidation
Plasma	Insulin†	Hyperinsulinism
Plasma	Glucagon Catecholamines Corticosteroids Growth hormone	Isolated hormone deficiency or in association with others, e.g. septo-optic dysplasia
Plasma/urine	Amino acid profile	Disorders of amino acid metabolism
Urine	Organic acids	Disorders of fatty acid β oxidation
Fibroblasts/leukocytes	Enzyme activities	Selected inborn errors of metabolism

*Analysers available for use in neonatal unit laboratory.
†Use specific assay and neonatal reference data (Hay and Sparks 1985; Hawdon et al. 1995).

Table 34.5 Chart for conversion of rate of glucose infusion from ml/kg/24 h to mg/kg/min depending on strength of dextrose solution

RATE OF INFUSION		STRENGTH DEXTROSE SOLUTION (mg/kg/min)			
ml/kg/24 h	ml/kg/h	4%	10%	15%	20%
60	2.5	1.7	4.2	6.2	8.4
72	3.0	2.0	5.0	7.5	10.0
80	3.3	2.2	5.6	8.3	11.2
100	4.2	2.8	6.9	10.4	13.8
120	5.0	3.3	8.3	12.5	16.6
150	6.3	4.2	10.4	15.6	20.8
180	7.5	5.0	12.5	18.7	25.0
200	8.3	5.6	13.9	20.8	27.8

it is possible to administer diazoxide (10–20 mg/kg/day), which suppresses pancreatic insulin release. The effect is optimal if a daily dose of chlorthiazide (7–10 mg/kg) is given to potentiate the hyperglycaemic effect and prevent the fluid-retentive effect of diazoxide. In cases of persistent hyperinsulinism response to diazoxide is variable, patients with mutations in the genes coding for HI-GK and HI-GLUD tend to show the best response.

Work defining the molecular basis of hyperinsulinism has demonstrated that some cases respond to the calcium channel blocker nifedipine (Bas et al. 1999; Kapoor et al. 2009).

Somatostatin analogue (octreotide, Sandostatin, Sandoz Pharmaceuticals) administered intravenously or subcutaneously at a dose of 10 μg/kg/day also suppresses insulin release (Aynsley-Green et al. 2000). However, tolerance may develop and there is concern about possible effects on the secretion of other hormones, and for this latter reason glucagon is administered simultaneously at a dose of 1 μg/kg/h (Hawdon et al. 1990).

Glucagon (200 μg/kg bolus intravenously or intramuscularly or infusion 5–10 μg/kg/h) has a temporary glycaemic effect via its glycogenolytic action and given alone may be a useful holding measure, for example when resiting glucose infusions. However, its prolonged use is limited because glucagon further stimulates insulin release.

Some cases of neonatal hyperinsulinism, especially those caused by recessive mutations of the genes encoding the SUR1 and Kir6.2 proteins, are unresponsive to medical treatment and near-total pancreatectomy is required. Referral should be made to specialist surgical centres. In specialist centres, rapid genetic testing allows clinicians to identify those who are likely to have focal disease and then ^{18}F-L-DOPA positron emission tomography imaging is indicated for the preoperative identification and precise anatomical location of focal lesions (De Lonlay et al. 1997, 1999; Kapoor et al. 2009). This is followed by laparoscopic or open surgery for targeted focal pancreatectomy.

Intrauterine growth restriction

Glucagon has a potential role when hypoglycaemia is secondary to IUGR. It appears that its mechanism of action when given in pharmacological doses (30–200 µg/kg) is to mimic the postnatal glucagon surge and the 'switching on' of the enzymes of gluconeogenesis (Hawdon et al. 1993c). Thus it is a useful adjunct to intravenous glucose therapy.

Adrenocortical insufficiency

Although parenteral hydrocortisone has been used for many years for the treatment of hypoglycaemia of various aetiologies, its place is solely as a replacement therapy for cortisol deficiency.

Inborn errors of metabolism

The management of the rare inborn errors of metabolism varies according to diagnosis and is beyond the scope of this chapter. In general, the aim is to provide adequate calories to prevent hypoglycaemia and catabolism.

Summary

The prevention and management of hypoglycaemia in babies at risk of impaired metabolic adaptation depend upon the administration of sufficient energy via either enteral or parenteral routes. In fact, many cases of hypoglycaemia are iatrogenic as a result of a failure to ensure adequate intake for at-risk babies, or to prescribe sufficient glucose to fluid-restricted babies. Correcting these deficiencies is usually sufficient and only rarely are additional treatments required.

Neonatal hypoglycaemia is a common but usually preventable condition. Prompt recognition of risk factors and prevention and management are important to reduce the risk of neurological sequelae.

Hyperglycaemia

Neonatal hyperglycaemia has been recognised for over a century (Kitselle 1852) and during this time it has become apparent that it represents several distinct clinical entities. As with hypoglycaemia, much uncertainty exists regarding definition, clinical significance and treatment.

Neonatal diabetes mellitus

Diabetes mellitus has been described as first presenting in the neonatal period (and onset may be after discharge from the neonatal unit or maternity ward). It was the subject of a British Paediatric Surveillance Unit study and there are now exciting data regarding the genetics of the condition (Temple et al. 1996; Shield 2000; Barbetti 2007; Aguilar-Bryan and Bryan 2008). The condition is rare (1 : 500 000) (Shield et al. 1996). Early reports suggested that the condition was usually transient, characteristically occurring in small-for-gestational-age infants in the first 6 postnatal weeks and presenting with very high blood glucose levels, low plasma insulin concentrations, dehydration, fever and failure to thrive despite adequate feeding (Hutchinson et al. 1962; Pagliara et al. 1973; Hoffman et al. 1980). The mean duration of insulin therapy, if required, was 69 days for the transient form, and it was thought that very few infants developed permanent diabetes in later life (Cornblath and Schwartz 1976). However, more recent reviews of reported cases of neonatal diabetes mellitus have confirmed its occurrence in predominantly small-for-gestational-age infants.

They demonstrated that 46% developed permanent diabetes in the neonatal period, 23% developed permanent diabetes in childhood or adolescence and in 31% diabetes resolved in the neonatal period. Ten cases had coexisting clinical conditions and six families had more than one affected individual (including two pairs of twins) (Von Muhlendahl and Herkenhoff 1995; Shield et al. 1996).

Self-limiting neonatal hyperglycaemia

Neonatal hyperglycaemia is most often a transient disorder which resolves spontaneously and has few features in common with classic diabetes mellitus. The prevalence of transient hyperglycaemia appears to be increasing in parallel with the increased survival of extremely low-birthweight infants and the early use of parenteral nutrition solutions and corticosteroid therapy in these babies (Lindblad et al. 1977). Iatrogenic or factitious hyperglycaemia must also be considered. The following sections refer to the most common condition, transient hyperglycaemia in small or sick infants.

Clinical significance

It is of the utmost importance to remember that neonatal hyperglycaemia may be a sign of a serious underlying disorder, such as infection. However, despite reports of associations between hyperglycaemia and adverse outcomes in exteremely low-birthweight babies, it is still not known whether the high glucose concentrations themselves place the infant at further risk or whether the high blood glucose levels simply reflect the fragile and unstable condition of the babies most at risk of adverse outcome (Hays et al. 2006). Unlike adults with insulin deficiency, hyperglycaemic neonates do not develop ketosis or metabolic acidosis (Gentz and Cornblath 1969). There is a risk that glycosuria and osmotic diuresis may cause fluid and electrolyte imbalance with dehydration. These disturbances are more likely to be comorbidities rather than the result of hyperglycaemia as studies of large numbers of infants have reported that osmotic diuresis is not an invariable consequence of neonatal hyperglycaemia (Pollack et al. 1978; Cowett and Schwartz 1979; Coulthard and Hey 1999; Hey 2005). There is also concern that changes in blood osmolality and fluid shifts may result in cerebral damage. However, cerebral pathology and adverse neurodevelopmental outcome have never been demonstrated to occur as the direct result of hyperglycaemia, and it is thought that blood glucose levels above 20 mmol/l are required to exert significant osmolar effects (Dweck and Cassady 1974; Miranda and Dweck 1977; Arant and Gorsh 1978).

As described above, neonatal hyperglycaemia is clinically significant in that it may herald a serious underlying disorder. Once such disorders have been ruled out and treated, there is no evidence that self-limiting hyperglycaemia secondary to immaturity of glucoregulation or excessive glucose intakes and not associated with osmotic diuresis has adverse effects at blood glucose levels below 20 mmol/l.

Definition and diagnosis

There is no established definition of neonatal hyperglycaemia, but blood glucose levels above 7 mmol/l are usually considered to be above the normal range and the majority of units recently surveyed define hyperglycaemia as a blood glucose level above 10 mmol/l (Alsweiler et al. 2007). However, the upper 'safe' limit of blood glucose concentration in the neonate is likely to be above this level. As with hypoglycaemia, there is great variation in terms of the diagnosis and management of hyperglycaemia (Alsweiler et al. 2007).

Glucose reagent strips are more useful in the diagnosis of hyperglycaemia than for hypoglycaemia because the strips are more reliable at high blood glucose levels, and inaccuracies of 0.5–1.0 mmol/l are of less clinical relevance in the context of hyperglycaemia. It may also be useful to monitor urine for glycosuria, but it should be remembered that neonates, particularly those who are preterm, have a low renal threshold for glucose and fractional excretion of glucose varies widely, so that glycosuria may be present even in normoglycaemia and is independent of circulating blood glucose concentration (Wilkins 1992; Hey 2005).

Prevalence

Without a clear definition of hyperglycaemia it is difficult to comment on its frequency. Studies of prevalence vary according to their subjects, with hyperglycaemia found most frequently in very low-birthweight and preterm infants (Chaivorarat and Dweck 1976; Zarif et al. 1976). Small-for-gestational-age infants who are preterm are more at risk for developing hyperglycaemia than hypoglycaemia when receiving standard intravenous infusions (Chance and Bower 1966). Reported prevalences vary from 29% to 86% in very low-birthweight neonates (Dweck and Cassady 1974; Louik et al. 1985).

Mechanisms and at-risk groups

The mechanisms underlying neonatal hyperglycaemia vary and, as with hypoglycaemia, are best understood with reference to the expected metabolic changes at birth. In contrast to hypoglycaemia resulting from a low glucose production rate or a high glucose uptake rate, hyperglycaemia may be the result of a high glucose production or infusion rate or a low glucose uptake rate.

Neonatal hyperglycaemia is usually secondary to a high glucose appearance rate, that is, failure of the baby to suppress endogenous glucose production even if glucose infusion rate is high (Miranda and Dweck 1977; Louik et al. 1985; Hawdon et al. 1993b). To maintain control, the infant must be able to adapt to the exogenous administration of glucose by suppressing glucose production by the liver. The ability to glucoregulate in this way has been demonstrated in normoglycaemic neonates (Lafeber et al. 1990). However, there is evidence from clinical and animal studies that some neonates do not suppress glucose production in response to glucose infusion and/or increased blood glucose levels (Cowett et al. 1988; Hawdon et al. 1993b; Van Goudoever et al. 1993).

The inability to suppress gluconeogenesis may in turn be the result of disordered glucoregulatory hormone control. Although the glucoregulatory role of insulin in the neonate is unclear and may vary between infants, it has been suggested that hyperglycaemia results from decreased insulin secretion in immature subjects (Milner et al. 1971; Zarif et al. 1976). This is analogous to the adult insulin-dependent diabetic. Animal studies have also shown that, after chronic hyperglycaemia, the fetal pancreas cannot mount an insulin response to a further glucose surge (Carver et al. 1995). This may be analogous to the condition in preterm babies receiving constant high-rate glucose infusions, whose pancreatic response to hyperglycaemia may be 'exhausted'.

Alternatively, circulating insulin concentrations may be appropriate for the blood glucose concentration, but hyperglycaemia may result from end-organ insensitivity to insulin. This is analogous to type 2 diabetes, which is characterised by insulin resistance.

Neonatal insulin resistance has been demonstrated by the persistence of hyperglycaemia in the presence of raised insulin concentrations, by the poor hypoglycaemic response to large exogenous doses of insulin and by the high insulin concentrations needed to suppress gluconeogenesis (Le Dune 1971; Pollack et al. 1978; Susa et al. 1979; Issad et al. 1990). Insulin resistance may be secondary to immaturity or downregulation of peripheral receptors, to the effect of high fatty acid levels resulting from infusion of fat emulsion or to the peripheral actions of counterregulatory hormones (Yunis et al. 1989).

Clinical data demonstrate that some hyperglycaemic preterm infants have inappropriately low plasma insulin concentrations and high plasma catecholamine levels, whereas others have apparently appropriate insulin concentrations and may have insulin resistance (Fig. 34.5) (Hawdon et al. unpublished data). The former group were those who had other clinical complications such as infection, and the latter were either very preterm or preterm and small for gestational age.

The excess secretion of counterregulatory hormones, which themselves stimulate glycogenolysis and gluconeogenesis, may in addition block the secretion of insulin and inhibit its peripheral action, thereby contributing to insulin resistance (Collins et al. 1991). This is the mechanism of hyperglycaemia secondary to exogenous corticosteroids, sometimes administered in large doses to neonates with lung disease (The Vermont Oxford Network Steroid Study Group 2001). It has even been suggested that antenatal corticosteroid administration contributes to the failure to suppress postnatal gluconeogenesis (Van Goudoever et al. 1993). Aminophylline, used for the prevention of apnoea of prematurity, mimics the action of catecholamines and induces glycogenolysis (Wilkinson et al. 1984). To date, growth hormone has not been implicated in the aetiology of neonatal hyperglycaemia (Zarif et al. 1976).

These hormonal disturbances may be the consequence of underlying clinical stresses such as infection, respiratory distress, pain or surgery (Stubbe and Wolf 1971; Bryan et al. 1973; Zarif et al. 1976; Lilien et al. 1979; Anand et al. 1985a, b; Louik et al. 1985). Studies by Anand et al. (1985a, b, 1987, 1988; Anand and Hickey 1987; Anand and Aynsley-Green 1988) demonstrated that, with minimal anaesthesia for major surgical procedures in term and preterm neonates, high glucagon and catecholamine levels and inhibition of insulin secretion led to a number of metabolic abnormalities,

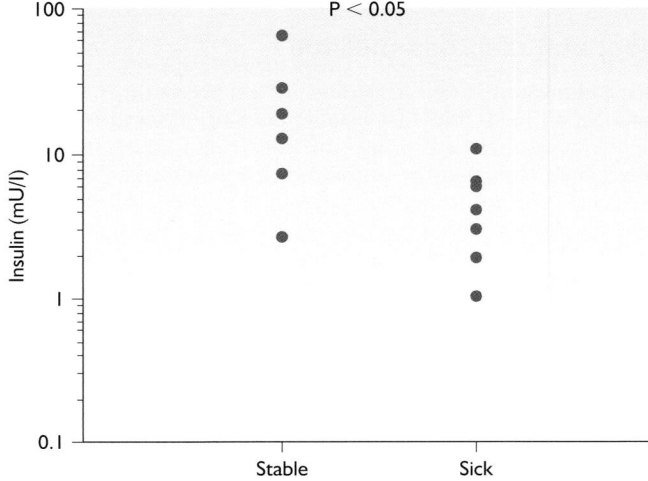

Fig. 34.5 Plasma insulin concentrations in preterm infants who were clinically stable or who had clinical complications such as infection or necrotising enterocolitis (sick infants).

including hyperglycaemia and hyperlactataemia. This response was in proportion to the severity of surgical stress and could be prevented by the addition of opioid analgesia or halothane to anaesthetic regimens. In some conditions associated with severe clinical stress, such as perinatal asphyxia, hyperglycaemia may occur as the result of high counterregulatory hormone concentrations but hypoglycaemia is more often seen, probably because the latter represents the situation found after the stress response is exhausted.

Despite the frequency with which hyperglycaemia is now observed, the aetiology and optimal management of this metabolic disorder have not been established. Clinical, animal and laboratory studies suggest that glucose production is not suppressed in the face of hyperglycaemia, but there are conflicting data regarding the role of defective glucoregulatory hormone responses.

Prevention and management (Fig. 34.6)

As neonatal hyperglycaemia is usually self-limiting and not associated with adverse sequelae, many clinicians choose not to treat raised blood glucose concentrations aggressively. However, the first step in management, especially in a baby who has previously been normoglycaemic, must be to seek and treat serious underlying disorders. The second step is to prevent the occurrence of high blood glucose concentrations secondary to high glucose infusion rates by instituting careful management of intravenous fluid prescriptions. Clinicians often increase fluid infusion rates to counter renal and extrarenal losses in the immature neonate. The condition is usually self-limiting and may be prevented by the more gradual increase in glucose intake in those at risk. For example, 200 ml/kg/day of 10% dextrose provides 14 mg/kg/min glucose, which is well in excess of the neonate's requirements. Thus it is not surprising that hyperglycaemia occurs and the extra glucose given is 'wasted'. Therefore, glucose infusion rates should be calculated and, if they are found to be excessive (for example, above 4–6 mg/kg/min), more dilute solutions should be used.

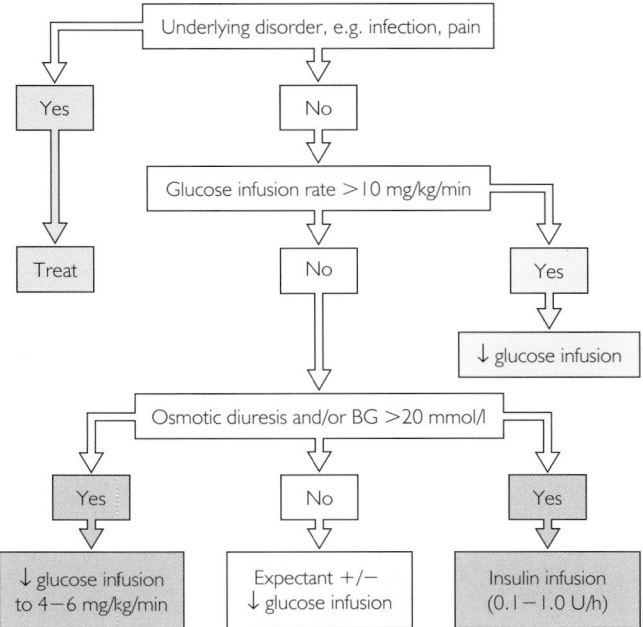

Fig. 34.6 Steps in the management of neonatal hyperglycaemia. BG, blood glucose.

Hyperglycaemia may still occur in some neonates who are clinically stable and who are not receiving excessive glucose intakes. These infants are usually of extremely low birthweight and less than 1 week old. Often they have received early parenteral nutrition and thus fairly high rates of glucose infusion in combination with amino acids. At the same time they may have high counterregulatory hormone levels, rendering them 'catabolic' with or without peripheral insulin resistance, so that they cannot utilise the infused substrates. The condition is usually self-limiting and may be prevented by the more gradual increase in glucose intake in those at risk.

There are three strategies for management of hyperglycaemia when it occurs in these circumstances.

First, moderate hyperglycaemia may be 'tolerated' if it does not appear to be causing osmotic diuresis. In most instances the condition resolves within a few days even if no action is taken.

Second, the rate of glucose infusion may be carefully reduced to the rate at which blood glucose levels become normal, and then gradually increased as tolerated. This carries the possible disadvantage of reducing the infant's energy intake, but it is likely that immature infants are unable to utilise effectively all the glucose offered, especially if at a rate in excess of 5 mg/kg/min (Van Goudoever et al. 1993).

Third, insulin may be administered in order to lower the blood glucose concentration without reducing the glucose infusion rate. If insulin is to be used, there needs to be priming of infusion tubing as insulin is adsorbed to plastic to a variable extent. Controlled studies of insulin administration to adult intensive care patients on intravenous nutrition have demonstrated that, although there is a short-term improvement in nitrogen balance, there is no advantage in terms of either weight gain or body composition, and that a number of patients become hypoglycaemic (Ross et al. 1991). Although there are a number of reports of this practice in the neonatal literature, there is no consistency regarding the clinical situations in which insulin has been given, only short-term outcome measures have been reported and there are few prospective controlled trials (Vaucher et al. 1982; Ostertag et al. 1986; Binder et al. 1989; Collins et al. 1991; Beardsall et al. 2008). All of these studies reported hypoglycaemia in some infants even after the discontinuation of insulin infusion. Therefore, insulin should not be prescribed without availability of prompt and accurate blood glucose testing. Recent systematic reviews have not supported the strategy of routinely infusing insulin to achieve a specific glucose delivery rate or prevent neonatal hyperglycaemia, and recommend reserving the use of exogenous insulin for infants with severe hyperglycaemia (above 14–16 mmol/l) because the safety of the practice has not yet been determined (Raney et al. 2008; Sinclair et al. 2009).

There is marked variation between and within studies regarding the doses of insulin required, and some authors have raised the possibility of the development of tolerance in some babies, so that hyperglycaemia recurs despite large increases in insulin dosage (Ostertag et al. 1986; Binder et al. 1989; Collins et al. 1991). Considering the clinical observation that without insulin treatment neonatal hyperglycaemia is usually a transient and self-limiting condition, it may be that insulin administration in some way hinders spontaneous recovery.

Epidemiological studies have suggested that intrauterine nutritional and endocrine status may influence adult metabolism and susceptibility to disease (Barker 1992). The long-term clinical significance of early high energy intakes in association with large doses of exogenous insulin in the preterm neonate, and of possible up- or downregulation of insulin receptors, has not yet been considered.

Finally, the introduction of enteral feeding with small volumes of milk as soon as the infant's gastrointestinal tract will tolerate this may hasten the control of blood glucose homeostasis by inducing surges of gut hormones which promote insulin secretion (the entero-insular axis) (Aynsley-Green 1988).

Accidental hyperglycaemia should be prevented by strict attention to stocked glucose solutions, pharmacy total parenteral nutrition production quality control and glucose infusion devices.

The pathogenesis of neonatal hyperglycaemia and the mechanism of action of exogenous insulin administration are not clearly understood. Therefore, the increasing practice of prescribing insulin to neonates without understanding its mode of action is of concern. It is not known whether insulin administration promotes linear growth in neonates, or merely converts glucose into fat. Further prospective randomised controlled trials of insulin therapy in preterm neonates who become glucose-intolerant would assess the impact of insulin therapy on glucose tolerance, metabolism and growth in the short and long term. It is currently impossible to judge whether insulin therapy does confer clinical advantage over expectant management of a condition which is usually self-limiting.

Summary

An approach to the controversy surrounding the definition, diagnosis and management of babies with neonatal hypoglycaemia has been presented. The present pragmatic approach, based on the available evidence and clinical experience, is unlikely to be established on a more secure scientific basis in the near future. The following summarises the key questions that still need to be addressed.

First, the long-term effects of moderate hypoglycaemia must be established. For example, we do not know whether the preterm infant's brain is more or less vulnerable to hypoglycaemia than that of the term infant, what duration of hypoglycaemia results in permanent disability and whether the effects of hypoglycaemia are exacerbated by concurrent complications such as hyperbilirubinaemia. We do not know whether the differences that have been demonstrated between preterm and term infants in metabolic adaptation persist beyond the first postnatal week, and whether there are implications for the preterm infant in terms of persistent impairment of metabolic responses.

Second, more information must be gathered relating to other factors regulating glucose availability to the brain, namely cerebral blood flow, the ontogeny of glucose transporter proteins and the role of the astrocyte in neuronal metabolic support.

Finally, as we realise the inadequacy of glucose reagent sticks for the diagnosis and monitoring of hypoglycaemia, improved accurate near-patient systems should be developed for the measurement of blood glucose concentrations and the ability to measure blood ketone body concentrations in these circumstances would markedly enhance management.

In 1954, McQuarrie urged the physician caring for children to be constantly aware of the risk of hypoglycaemia. This exhortation is still relevant in the 21st century, but much still needs to be learned and there are many challenging areas of research for the clinical investigator.

Acknowledgement

The author wishes to thank Dr K Hussain for contributing to the section on hyperinsulinism.

References

Adam, P.A.J., Raiha, N., Rahiala, E.C., et al., 1975. Oxidation of glucose and D-beta-hydroxybutyrate by the early human fetal brain. Acta Paediatr Scand 64, 17–24.

Aguilar-Bryan, L., Bryan, J., 2008. Neonatal diabetes mellitus. Endocrinol Rev 29, 265–291.

Alsweiler, J.M., Kuschel, C.A., Bloomfield, F.H., 2007. Survey of the management of neonatal hyperglycaemia in Australasia. J Paediatr Child Health 43, 632–635.

Anand, K.J.S., Aynsley-Green, A., 1988. Measuring the severity of surgical stress in newborn infants. J Pediatr Surg 23, 297–305.

Anand, K.J.S., Hickey, P.R., 1987. Pain and its effects on the human neonate and fetus. NEJM 317, 1321–1329.

Anand, K.J.S., Brown, M.J., Causon, R.C., et al., 1985a. Can the human neonate mount an endocrine and metabolic response to surgery? J Pediatr Surg 20, 41–48.

Anand, K.J.S., Sippell, W.G., Aynsley-Green, A., 1985b. Metabolic and endocrine effects of surgical ligation of patent ductus arteriosus in the human neonate: are there implications for further improvement

of postoperative outcome? In: Falkner, R., Kretchner, N., Rossi, E. (Eds.), Modern Problems in Paediatrics. Karger, Basel, pp. 145–157.

Anand, K.J.S., Sippel, W.G., Aynsley-Green, A., 1987. Randomised trial of fentanyl anaesthesia in preterm neonates undergoing surgery. Effects on the stress response. Lancet i, 243–248.

Anand, K.J.S., Sipell, W.G., Schofield, N., et al., 1988. Does halothane anaesthesia decrease the metabolic and endocrine stress response of newborn infants undergoing surgery? Br Med J 296, 668–672.

Anderson, J.M., Milner, R.D.G., Strich, S.J., 1967. Effects of neonatal hypoglycaemia on the nervous system: a pathological study. J Neurol Neurosurg Psychiatry 30, 295–310.

Arant, B.S., Gorsh, W.M., 1978. Effects of acute hyperglycemia on the central nervous system of neonatal puppies. Pediatr Res 12, 549.

Auer, R.N., Siesjo, B.K., 1993. Hypoglycaemia: brain neurochemistry and neuropathology. Baillières Clinical Endocrinology and Metabolism 7, 611–625.

Aynsley-Green, A., 1988. Metabolic and endocrine interrelationships in the human fetus and neonate: an overview of the control of the adaptation to postnatal nutrition. In: Lindblad, B.A. (Ed.), Perinatal Nutrition. Academic Press, New York, pp. 162–191.

Aynsley-Green, A., Hussain, K., Hall, J., et al., 2000. Prcatical management of hyperinsulinism in ingancy. Arch Dis Child 82, F98–F107.

Banker, B.Q., 1967. The neuropathological effects of anoxia and hypoglycaemia in the newborn. Dev Med Child Neurol 9, 544–550.

Barbetti, F., 2007. Diagnosis of neonatal and infancy-onset diabetes. Endocrinol Dev 11, 83–93.

Barker, D.J.P., 1992. Fetal and Infant Origins of Adult Disease. BMJ Publishing, London.

Barkovich, A.J., Ali, F.A., Rowley, H.A., et al., 1998. Imaging patterns of neonatal hypohglycaemia. Am J Neuroradiol 19, 523–528.

Bas, F., Darendeliler, F., Demirkol, D., et al., 1999. Succesful therapy with calcium channel blocker (nifedipine) in persistent neonatal hyperinsulinaemic hypoglycaemia of infancy. J Pediatr Endocrinol Metab 12, 873–878.

Baumeister, F.A., Rolinski, B., Busch, R., et al., 2001. Glucose monitoring with long-term subcutaneous microdialysis in neonates. Pediatrics 108, 1187–1192.

Beardsall, K., Vanhaesebrouck, S., Ogilvy-Stuart, A., et al., 2008. Early insulin therapy in very-low-birth-weight infants. N Engl J Med 359, 1873–1884.

Beckwith, J.B., 1963. Extreme cytomegaly of the adrenal fetal cortex, omphalocele, hyperplasia of kidneys and pancreas and Leydig cell hyperplasia. Another syndrome? Proceedings of the Western Society for Pediatric Research, November 1963, Los Angeles.

Binder, N.D., Raschko, R.K., Benda, G.I., et al., 1989. Insulin infusion with parenteral nutrition in extremely low birthweight infants with hyperglycemia. J Pediatr 114, 273–280.

Boluyt, N., van Kempen, A., Offringa, M., 2006. Neurodevelopment after neonatal hypoglycaemia: A systematic review and design of optimal future study. Pediatrics 117, 2231–2243.

Bougneres, P.F., 1987. Stable isotope tracers and the determination of fuel fluxes in newborn infants. Biol Neonate 52 (Suppl. 1), 87–96.

Bryan, M.H., Wei, P., Hamilton, J.R., et al., 1973. Supplemental intravenous alimentation in low birthweight infants. J Pediatr 82, 940–944.

Burns, C.M., Rutherford, M.A., Boardman, J.P., et al., 2008. Patterns of cerebral injury and neurodevelopmental outcomes after symptomatic neonatal hypoglycaemia. Pediatrics 122, 65–74.

Carver, T.D., Anderson, S.M., Aldoretta, P.A., et al., 1995. Glucose suppression of insulin secretion in chronically hyperglycemic fetal sheep. Pediatr Res 38, 754–762.

Chaivorarat, O., Dweck, H.S., 1976. Effect of prolonged continuous glucose infusion in preterm neonates. Pediatr Res 10, 406.

Chance, G.W., Bower, B.D., 1966. Hypoglycaemia and temporary hyperglycaemia in infants of low birth weight for maturity. Arch Dis Child 41, 279–285.

Clayton, P.T., Eaton, S., Aynsley-Gree, A., et al., 2001. Hyperinsulinism in short-chain L-3-hydroxyacyl-CoA dehydrogenase deficiency reveals the importance of beta-oxidation in insulin secretion. J Clin Invest 108, 457–465.

Cobliner, S., 1911. Blutzuckeruntersuchungen bei Säuglingen. Zeitschrift für Kinderheilkunde 1, 207–216.

Collins, J.E., Leonard, J.V., 1984. Hyperinsulinism in asphyxiated and small for dates infants with hypoglycaemia. Lancet ii, 311–313.

Collins, J.E., Leonard, J.V., Teale, D., et al., 1990. Hyperinsulinaemic hypoglycaemia in small for dates babies. Arch Dis Child 65, 1118–1120.

Collins, Jr., J.W., Hoppe, M., Brown, K., et al., 1991. A controlled trial of insulin infusion and parenteral nutrition in extremely low birthweight infants with glucose intolerance. J Pediatr 118, 921–927.

Cornblath, M., Reisner, S.H., 1965. Blood glucose in the neonate, clinical significance. NEJM 272, 378–381.

Cornblath, M., Schwartz, R., 1976. Disorders of Carbohydrate Metabolism in Infancy, second ed. W B Saunders, Philadelphia.

Cornblath, M., Hawdon, J.M., Williams, A.F., et al., 2000. Controversies regarding definition of neonatal hypoglycemia: suggested operational thresholds. Pediatrics 105, 1141–1145.

Costello, J.M., Gluckman, P.D., 1988. Neonatal hypopituitarism: a neurological perspective. Dev Med Child Neurol 30, 190–199.

Coulthard, M.G., Hey, E.N., 1999. Renal processing of glucose in well and sick neonates. Arch Dis Child 81, F92–F98.

Cowett, R.M., 1999. Neonatal hypoglycaemia: A little goes a long way. J Pediatr 134, 389–391.

Cowett, R.M., Schwartz, R., 1979. The role of hepatic control of glucose homeostasis in the aetiology of neonatal hypo and hyperglycemia. Semin Perinatol 3, 327.

Cowett, R.M., Andersen, G.E., Maguire, C.A., et al., 1988. Ontogeny of glucose homeostasis in low birth weight infants. J Pediatr 112, 462–465.

Dahlquist, G., 1976. Cerebral utilization of glucose, ketone bodies and oxygen in starving infant rats and the effect of intrauterine growth retardation. Acta Paediatr Scand 98, 237–247.

De Boissieu, D., Rocchiccioli, F., Kalach, N., et al., 1995. Ketone body turnover in term and in premature newborns in the first two weeks after birth. Biol Neonate 67, 84–93.

De Lonlay, P., Fournet, J.C., Rahier, J., et al., 1997. Somatic deletion of the imprinted 11p15 region in sporadic persistent hyperinsuliaemic hypoglycaemia of infancy is specific of focal adenomatous hyperplasia and endorses partial pnacreatectomy. J Clin Invest 100, 802–807.

De Lonlay-Debeny, P., Poggi-Travert, F., Fournet, J.C., et al., 1999. Clinical features of 52 infants with hyperinsulinism. NEJM 340, 1169–1175.

De Lonlay, P., Fournet, J.C., Touati, G., et al., 2002. Heterogeneity of persistent hyperinsulinaemic hypoglycaemia. A series of 175 cases. Eur J Pediatr 161, 37–48.

de Rooy, L.J., Hawdon, J.M., 2002. Nutritional factors that affect the postnatal metabolic adaptation of full-term small- and large-for-gestational-age infants. Pediatrics 109 (3), E42.

Dweck, H.S., Cassady, G., 1974. Glucose tolerance in infants of very low birthweight. I. Incidence of hyperglycemia in infants of birthweights 1100 grams or less. Pediatrics 53, 189–195.

Edmond, J., Auestad, N., Robbins, R.A., et al., 1985. Ketone body metabolism in the neonate: development and effect of diet. Federal Proceedings 44, 2359–2364.

Eidelman, A.I., 2001. Hypoglycemia and the breastfed neonate. Pediatr Clin North Am 48, 377–387.

Elander, G., Lindberg, T., 1984. Short mother–infant separation during first week of life influences the duration of breast feeding. Acta Paediatr Scand 73, 237–240.

Filan, P.M., Inder, T.E., Cameron, F.J., et al., 2006. Neonatal hypoglycaemia and occipital cerebral injury. J Pediatr 148, 552–555.

Fluge, G., 1974. Clinical aspects of neonatal hypoglycaemia. Acta Paediatr Scand 63, 826–832.

Gemell, M., De Luca, F., Barberio, G., 1979. Hypoglycaemia and congenital adrenal hyperplasia. Acta Paediatr Scand 68, 285–286.

Gentz, J.C.H., Cornblath, M., 1969. Transient diabetes of the newborn. Adv Pediatr 16, 345–363.

Griffiths, A.D., Lawrence, K.M., 1974. The effects of hypoxia and hypoglycaemia on the brain of the newborn human infant. Dev Med Child Neurol 16, 308–319.

Hägnevik, K., Faxelius, G., Irestedt, L., et al., 1984. Catecholamine surge and metabolic adaptation in the newborn after vaginal delivery and caesarean section. Acta Paediatr Scand 73, 602–609.

Haninger, N.C., Farley, C.L., 2001. Screening for hypoglycemia in healthy term neonates: effects on breastfeeding. J Midwifery Womens Health 46, 292–301.

Hawdon, J.M., 1993. Neonatal hypoglycaemia: the consequences of admission to the special care nursery. Maternal and Child Health Feb, 48–51.

Hawdon, J.M., 2007. The medico-legal implications of hypoglycaemia in the newborn. Clinical Risk 13, 135–137.

Hawdon, J.M., Ward Platt, M.P., 1992. Metabolic and hormonal interrelationships in perinatal asphyxia. Biol Neonate 62, 300.

Hawdon, J.M., Ward Platt, M.P., 1993. Metabolic adaptation in small for gestational age infants. Arch Dis Child 68, 262–268.

Hawdon, J.M., Ward Platt, M.P., Lamb, W.H., et al., 1990. Tolerance to sandostatin in neonatal hyperinsulinaemic hypoglycaemia. Arch Dis Child 65, 341–343.

Hawdon, J.M., Ward Platt, M.P., Aynsley-Green, A., 1992. Patterns of metabolic adaptation for preterm and term infants in the first neonatal week. Arch Dis Child 67, 357–365.

Hawdon, J.M., Aynsley-Green, A., Alberti, K.G.M.M., et al., 1993a. The role of pancreatic insulin secretion in neonatal glucoregulation. I Healthy term and preterm infants. Arch Dis Child 68, 274–279.

Hawdon, J.M., Aynsley-Green, A., Bartlett, K., et al., 1993b. The role of pancreatic insulin secretion in neonatal glucoregulation. II Infants with disordered blood glucose homeostasis. Arch Dis Child 68, 280–285.

Hawdon, J.M., Aynsley-Green, A., Ward Platt, M.P., 1993c. Neonatal blood glucose concentrations: Metabolic effects of intravenous glucagon and intragastric medium chain triglyceride. Arch Dis Child 68, 255–261.

Hawdon, J.M., Hubbard, M., Hales, C.N., et al., 1995. Use of a specific immunoradiometric assay to determine preterm neonatal insulin–glucose relations. Arch Dis Child 73, F166–F169.

Hay, Jr., W.W., Sparks, J.W., 1985. Placental, fetal and neonatal carbohydrate metabolism. Clin Obstet Gynecol 28, 473–485.

Hay, Jr., W.W., Raju, T.N., Higgins, R.D., et al., 2009. Knowledge gaps and research needs for understanding and tretaing neonatal hypoglycaemia: workshop report from Eunice Kennedy Shriver National Institute of Child Health and Human Development. J Pediatr 155, 612–617.

Haymond, M.W., Strauss, A.W., Arnold, K.J., et al., 1979. Glucose homeostasis in children with severe cyanotic congenital heart disease. J Pediatr 95, 220–227.

Hays, S.P., Smith, E.O., Sunehag, A.L., 2006. Hyperglycaemia is a risk factor for early death and morbidity in extremely low birth-weight infants. Pediatrics 118, 1811–1818.

Heck, L.J., Erenberg, A., 1987. Serum glucose levels in term neonates during the first 48 hours of life. J Paediatr 110, 119–122.

Hey, E., 2005. Hyperglycaemia and the very preterm baby. Semin Fetal Neonatal Med 10, 3677–3387.

Hoffman, W.H., Knoury, C., Byrd, H.A., 1980. Prevalence of permanent congenital diabetes mellitus. Diabetologia 19, 487–488.

Hutchinson, J.H., Keay, A.J., Kerr, M.N., 1962. Congenital temporary diabetes mellitus. Br Med J ii, 436–440.

Issad, T., Pastor-Anglada, M., Coupe, C., et al., 1990. Glucose metabolism and insulin sensitivity during suckling period in rats. In: Cuezva, J.M., Paseaud-Leone, A.M., Patel, M.S. (Eds.), Endocrine

Development of the Fetus and Neonate. Plenum Press, New York, pp. 61–66.

Jacobs, D.G., Haka-Ikse, K., Wesson, D.E., et al., 1986. Growth and development in patients operated on for islet cell dysplasia. J Pediatr Surg 21, 1184–1189.

Johnston, V., Frazzini, V., Davidheiser, S., et al., 1991. Insulin receptor number and binding affinity in newborn dogs. Pediatr Res 29, 611–614.

Joosten, K.J., Schellehens, A.P., Waellens, J.J., et al., 1991. Erroneous diagnosis 'neonatal hypoglycaemia' due to incorrect preservation of blood samples. Nederlands Tijdschrift Geneeskunde 135, 1691–1694.

Kapoor, R.R., James, C., Hussain, K., 2009. Advances in the diagnosis and management of hyperinsulinaemic hypoglycaemia. Nat Clin Pract Endocrinol Metab 5, 101–112.

Kinnala, A., Suhonen-Polvi, H., Aarimaa, T., et al., 1996. Cerebral metabolic rate for glucose during the first six months of life: an FDG positron emission tomography study. Arch Dis Child 74, F153–F157.

Kinnala, A., Korvenranta, H., Parkkola, R., 2000. Newer techniques to study neonatal hypoglycemia. Semin Perinatol 24, 116–119.

Kitselle, J.F., 1852, Kinderh Leipsic XVIII 313.

Koh, T.H.H.G., Eyre, J.A., Aynsley-Green, A., 1988a. Neural dysfunction during hypoglycaemia. Arch Dis Child 63, 1353–1358.

Koh, T.H.H.G., Eyre, J.A., Aynsley-Green, A., 1988b. Neonatal hypoglycaemia – the controversy regarding definition. Arch Dis Child 63, 1386–1389.

Lafeber, H.N., Sulkers, E.J., Chapman, T.E., et al., 1990. Glucose production and oxidation in preterm infants during total parenteral nutrition. Pediatr Res 28, 153–157.

Le Dune, M.A., 1971. Insulin studies in temporary neonatal hyperglycaemia. Arch Dis Child 46, 392–394.

Lilien, L.D., Rosenfield, R.C., Pildes, R.S., 1979. Hyperglycemia in small stressed neonates. J Pediatr 94, 454–459.

Lindblad, B.S., Settegren, G., Feychting, H., 1977. Total parenteral nutrition in infants. Blood levels of glucose, lactate, pyruvate, free fatty acids, glycerol, D? hydroxybutyrate, triglycerides, free amino acids and insulin. Acta Paediatr Scand 66, 409–419.

Louik, C., Mitchell, A.A., Epstein, M.F., et al., 1985. Risk factors for neonatal hyperglycemia associated with 10% dextrose infusion. Am J Dis Child 139, 783–786.

Lovinger, R.D., Kaplan, S.L., Grumback, M.M., 1975. Congenital hypopituitarism associated with neonatal hypoglycemia and microphallus. J Pediatr 87, 1171–1181.

Lucas, A., Adrian, T.E., Aynsley-Green, A., et al., 1980. Iatrogenic hyperinsulinism at birth. Lancet i, 144–145.

Lucas, A., Aynsley-Green, A., Bloom, S.R., 1981. Gut hormones and the first meals. Clin Sci 60, 349–353.

Lucas, A., Morley, R., Cole, T.F., 1988. Adverse neurodevelopmental outcome of moderate neonatal hypoglycaemia. Br Med J 297, 1304–1308.

Mann, T.P., Elliot, R.I.K., 1957. Neonatal cold injury due to accidental exposure to cold. Lancet i, 229–231.

McQuarrie, I., 1954. Idiopathic spontaneously occurring hypoglycemia in infants. Am J Dis Child 87, 399–428.

Medical Devices Agency, 1996. Extra-laboratory use of blood glucose meters and test strips: contraindications, training and advice to the users. Safety Notice MDA SN 9616.

Medina, J.M., Fernandez, E., Bolaros, J.P., et al., 1990. Fuel supply to the brain during the early postnatal period. In: Cueza, J.M., Pasaud-Leone, A.M., Patel, M.S. (Eds.), Endocrine Development of the Fetus and Neonate. Plenum Press, New York, pp. 175–194.

Meissner, T., Brune, W., Mayatepak, E., 1997. Persistent hyperinsulinaemic hypoglycaemia of infancy: Therapy, clinical outcome and mutational analysis. Eur J Pediatr 156, 754–757.

Menni, F., de Lonlay, P., Sevin, C., et al., 2001. Neurologic outcomes of 90 neonates and infants with persistent hyperinsulinaemic hypoglycemia. Pediatrics 107, 476–479.

Milner, R.D.G., Ferguson, A.W., Naidu, S.H., 1971. Aetiology of transient neonatal diabetes. Arch Dis Child 46, 724–726.

Miranda, L., Dweck, H.S., 1977. Perinatal glucose homeostasis: the unique character of hyperglycemia and hypoglycemia in infants of very low birthweight. Clin Perinatol 4, 351–365.

Molsted-Pedersen, L., Trautner, H., Jorgensen, K.R., 1973. Plasma insulin and K values during intravenous glucose tolerance test in newborn infants with erythroblastosis fetalis. Acta Paediatr Scand 62, 11–16.

Munshi, U.K., Deorari, A.K., Paul, V.K., et al., 1992. Effects of maternal labetalol on the newborn infant. Indian Pediatr 29, 1507–1512.

Murakami, Y., Yamashita, Y., Matsuishi, T., et al., 1999. Cranial MRI of neurologically impaired children suffering from neonatal hypoglycaemia. Pediatr Radiol 29, 23–27.

National Childbirth Trust, 1997. Hypoglycaemia of the newborn. Mod Midwife 7, 31–33.

Neligan, G., 1965. Idiopathic hypoglycaemia in the newborn. In: Gairdner, D. (Ed.), Recent Advances in Paediatrics III. Churchill, London.

Obershain, S.S., Adam, P.A.J., King, K.C., et al., 1970. Human fetal response to sustained maternal hyperglycemia. NEJM 283, 566–572.

Ogata, E.S., 1986. Carbohydrate metabolism in the fetus and neonate and altered neonatal glucoregulation. Pediatr Clin North Am 33, 25–45.

Ostertag, S.G., Jovanovic, L., Lewis, B., et al., 1986. Insulin pump therapy in the very low birthweight infant. Pediatrics 78, 625–630.

Pagliara, A.S., Karl, I.E., Kipnis, D.B., 1973. Transient neonatal diabetes: delayed maturation of the pancreatic beta cell. J Pediatr 82, 97–101.

Pollack, A., Cowett, R.M., Schwartz, R., et al., 1978. Glucose disposal in low birthweight infants during steady state hyperglycemia: effects of exogenous insulin administration. Pediatrics 61, 546–549.

Raney, M., Donze, A., Smith, J.R., 2008. Insulin infusion for the treatment of hyperglycaemia in low birth weight infants: eaxmining the evidence. Neonatal Netw 27, 127–140.

Ross, R.J.M., Miell, J.P., Buchanan, C.R., 1991. Avoiding autocannibalism. Br Med J 303, 1147–1148.

Rozance, P.J., Hay, W.W., 2006. Hypoglycaemia in newborn infants: Features assoicated with adverse outcomes. Biol Neonate 90, 74–86.

Schrier, A.M., Wilhelm, P.B., Church, R.M., et al., 1990. Neonatal hypoglycaemia in the Rhesus monkey: effect on development and behaviour. Infant Behaviour and Development 13, 189–297.

Sedgwick, J.P., Ziegler, M.R., 1920. The nitrogenous and sugar content of the blood of the newborn. Am J Dis Child 19, 429–432.

Senior, B., Slone, D., Shapiro, S., 1976. Benzothiazides and neonatal hypoglycaemia. Lancet ii, 377.

Shah, A., Stanhope, R., Matthew, D., 1992. Hazards of pharmacological tests of growth hormone secretion in childhood. Br Med J 304, 173–174.

Shelley, H.J., Basset, J.M., 1975. Control of carbohydrate metabolism in the fetus and newborn. Br Med Bull 31, 37–43.

Shelley, H.J., Neligan, G.S., 1966. Neonatal hypoglycaemia. Br Med Bull 22, 34–39.

Shield, J.P., 2000. Neonatal diabetes: new insights into aetiology and implications. Horm Res. 53 (Suppl. 1), 7–11.

Shield, J.P.H., Gardner, R.J., Wadsworth, E.J.K., et al., 1996. Transient neonatal diabetes: a study of its aetiopathology and genetic basis. Arch Dis Child 76, F39–F42.

Sinclair, J.C., Bottino, M., Cowett, R.M., 2009. Interventions for prevention of neonatal hyperglycaemia in very low birth weight infants. Cochrane Database Syst Rev (3), CD007615.

Singh, S.P., Pullen, G.L., Snyder, A.K., 1988. Effects of ethanol on fetal fuels and brain growth in rats. J Lab Clin Med 112, 704–710.

Smallpiece, V., Davies, P.A., 1964. Immediate feeding of premature infants with undiluted breast milk. Lancet ii, 1349–1356.

Soothill, P.W., Nicolaides, K.H., Campbell, S., 1987. Prenatal asphyxia, hyperlacticaemia, hypoglycaemia and erythroblastosis in growth retarded fetuses. Br Med J 294, 1051–1053.

Spence, J.C., 1921. Some observations on sugar tolerance, with special reference to variations found at different ages. Q J Med 14, 314–326.

Sperling, M.A., Grajwer, L.A., Leake, R., et al., 1976. Role of glucagon in perinatal glucose homeostasis. Metabolism 25 (Suppl. 1), 1385–1386.

Sperling, M.A., Ganguli, S., Leslie, N., et al., 1984. Fetal–perinatal catecholamine secretion: role in perinatal glucose homeostasis. Am J Physiol 247, E69–E74.

Srinivasan, G., Pildes, R.S., Cattamanchi, G., et al., 1986. Plasma glucose values in normal neonates: a new look. Journal of Pediatrics Surgery 21, 114–117.

Stubbe, P., Wolf, H., 1971. The effect of stress on growth hormone, glucose and glycerol levels in newborn infants. Hormone Metabolism Research 3, 175–179.

Susa, J.B., Cowett, R.M., Oh, W., 1979. Suppression of gluconeogenesis and endogenous glucose production by exogenous insulin administration in the newborn lamb. Pediatr Res 13, 594–599.

Temple, I.K., Gardner, R.J., Robinson, D.O., et al., 1996. Further evidence for an imprinted gene for neonatal diabetes localised to chromosome 6q22-q23. Hum Mol Genet 5, 1117–1121.

The Vermont Oxford Network Steroid Study Group, 2001. Early postnatal dexamethasone therapy for the prevention of chronic lung disease. Pediatrics 108, 741–748.

Thurston, J.H., Hawhart, R.E., Schiro, J.A., 1986. β-hydroxybutyrate reverses insulin-induced hypoglycaemic coma in suckling–weanling mice despite low blood and brain glucose levels. Metabolism and Brain Research 1, 63–82.

Van Goudoever, J.B., Sulkers, E.J., Chapman, T.E., 1993. Glucose kinetics and glucoregulatory hormone levels in ventilated preterm infants on the first day of life. Pediatr Res 33, 583–589.

Vannucci, R.C., Vannucci, S.J., 2001. Hypoglycemic brain injury. Semin Perinatol 6, 147–155.

Vannucci, R.C., Nardis, E.E., Vannucci, J.S., et al., 1981. Cerebral carbohydrate and energy metabolism during hypoglycemia in newborn dogs. Am J Physiol 240, R192–R199.

Vaucher, Y.E., Watson, P.D., Morrow, G., 1982. Continuous insulin infusion in hyperglycemic, very low birthweight infants. J Pediatr Gastroenterol Nutr 1, 211–217.

Von Muhlendahl, K.E., Herkenhoff, H., 1995. Long term outcome of neonatal diabetes. NEJM 333, 704–708.

Wiedemann, H.R., 1964. Complexe malformatif familial avec hernie umbilicale et macroglossie. Un 'syndrome nouveau'? Journal de Génétique Humaine 13, 223–232.

Wilkins, B.H., 1992. Renal function in sick very low birthweight infants: 4: Glucose excretion. Arch Dis Child 67, 1162–1165.

Wilkinson, A.R., Fok, T.-F., Au-Yeung, H., 1984. High incidence of clinical problems in the newborn possibly attributable to theophylline therapy (abstract). Pediatr Res 18, 89.

Williams, A.F., 2005. Neonatal hypoglycaemia: Clinical and legal aspects. Semin Fetal Neonatal Med 10, 363–368.

Yunis, K.A., Oh, W., Kalhan, S., et al., 1989. Mechanisms of glucose perturbation following intravenous fat infusion in the low birthweight infant. Pediatr Res 25, 299A.

Zarif, M., Pildes, R.S., Vidyasagar, D., 1976. Insulin and growth hormone responses in neonatal hyperglycemia. Diabetes 25, 428–433.

Zhou, D., Qian, J., Liu, C.X., et al., 2008, Repetitive and profound insulin-induced hypoglycaemia results in brain damage in newborn rats: an approach to establish an animal model of brain injury induced by neonatal hypoglycaemia. Eur J Pediatr 167, 1169–1174.

Tim Cheetham   Daniel J Schenk

Endocrine disorders in the newborn may be serious and potentially life-threatening, but are nearly always treatable. It is therefore particularly important that they are identified as soon as possible.

Advances in the field of molecular biology have now clarified the cellular basis of many endocrine disorders but this chapter will focus on the presentation, differential diagnosis and management of these conditions. For fuller discussions of the clinical and molecular aspects of endocrine disease the reader is referred to works on paediatric or general endocrinology, such as Sperling (2008), Brook et al. (2010), Kronenburg et al. (2008) or Ogilvy-Stuart and Midgley (2006).

Hypothalamus and anterior pituitary

Normal function

The hypothalamus and anterior pituitary form a neuroendocrine unit that mediates between the central nervous system (CNS) and peripheral tissues. The hypothalamic nerve fibres release humoral substances into the capillaries of the primary plexus in the median eminence, to be carried by the portal vessels to excite or inhibit the secretion of the cells of the anterior pituitary. The principal hypothalamic-releasing hormones are corticotrophin-releasing hormone (CRH), thyrotrophin-releasing hormone (TRH), gonadotrophin-releasing hormone (GnRH) and growth hormone-releasing hormone (GHRH), with two inhibitory hormones, somatostatin and dopamine. These factors regulate the secretion of the pituitary trophic hormones adrenocorticotrophic hormone (ACTH), thyroid-stimulating hormone (TSH), follicle-stimulating hormone (FSH), luteinising hormone (LH), growth hormone (GH) and prolactin into the circulation. They, in turn, stimulate the production of cortisol, thyroxine (T_4), sex steroids and insulin-like growth factor-I (IGF-I), which will then feed back and modulate hypothalamic and pituitary hormone release. Many other neurotransmitters and neuropeptides are involved in the regulation of pituitary hormone release and there is considerable interaction between the various axes; GH production is, for example, modulated by T_4, cortisol and sex steroids as well as by IGF-I.

Hypothalamic and anterior pituitary disease

Children with congenital pituitary hormone deficiency (PHD) have quantitative and qualitative abnormalities of the production of one or more pituitary hormones and represent a spectrum of hormonal and associated midline abnormalities. At one end of the spectrum is the child with isolated GH deficiency and a structurally normal brain. At the other end of the spectrum is the patient with septo-optic dysplasia (SOD) and associated combined PHD (CPHD) (Parks et al. 1999; Dattani and Robinsonn 2000). Many children with 'hypopituitarism' have an abnormal hypothalamus which cannot manufacture and release the relevant hypothalamic hormones appropriately. The incidence of isolated GH deficiency is approximately 1 in 4000–10 000 (Millar et al. 2003; Kelberman et al. 2009) and that of SOD around 1 in 10 000 (Patel et al. 2006). Inheritance of CPHD may be recessive, dominant or X-linked and chromosomal defects such as 18p – may be associated with PHD (Artman et al. 1992).

There is an association between PHD and midline CNS malformations as well as midline malformations elsewhere in the body such as cleft lip or cleft palate (Rudman et al. 1978; Traggiai and Stanhope 2002) or a single central incisor (Dattani 2004). More than 90% of those with CPHD have midline CNS abnormalities on magnetic resonance imaging (MRI). These include an abnormal pituitary gland and/or hypothalamus as well as the absent septum pellucidum and optic nerve hypoplasia characteristic of SOD (Barkovich et al. 1989; Triulzi et al. 1994; Hamilton et al. 1998). The fact that SOD is more common in areas of high unemployment and high teenage pregnancy has led to suggestions that environmental factors may play a role in disease development (Patel et al. 2006). A normal MR in infancy and the MR from a patient with combined PHD is shown in Figure 34.7.

Holoprosencephaly is a midline brain malformation where the forebrain fails to develop into separate hemispheres correctly. Holoprosencephaly is associated with aplasia of the olfactory bulbs and craniofacial abnormalities and patients may also have anterior and posterior PHD. Patients may have an underlying chromosomal abnormality (Bullen et al. 2001) and a number of single-gene defects have been identified in these babies (Nanni et al. 1999; Wallis and Muenke 2000). The prevalence appears to be higher in young mothers (Olsen et al. 1997) and in mothers with diabetes (Barr et al. 1983). MR images may show an abnormal pituitary gland as well as the characteristic forebrain abnormalities seen in this disorder.

Hypopituitarism has been linked to traumatic delivery in the past and there is a high incidence of breech and forceps delivery in some series (Craft et al. 1980). Rona and Tanner (1977) calculated that a male firstborn delivered by breech has an 11-fold increased risk of GH deficiency. Most children with hypopituitarism still present in the cephalic position and altered movement in utero secondary to the underlying defect in brain development may be the common link between hypopituitarism and breech delivery (De Zegher et al. 1995b; Pinto et al. 1999).

Molecular basis

The molecular background to some cases of PHD has been established. Isolated deficiencies of GH (Vulsma et al. 1989; Procter et al. 1998), TSH (Doeker et al. 1998), ACTH (Krude et al. 1998; Vallette-Kasic et al. 2004) or gonadotrophins (Weiss et al. 1992; Layman et al. 1997, 2002; Phillip et al. 1998; Weiss and Refetoff 1999) may reflect mutations of the respective genes. Mutations of the *GH-1* gene can result in recessive and dominantly inherited isolated GH deficiency (Phillips et al. 1981; Igarashi et al. 1993; Binder and Ranke 1995; Cogan et al. 1995) and defects of the GHRH receptor can also result in isolated GH deficiency (Wajnrajch et al. 1996). Severe isolated ACTH deficiency presenting in the neonatal period may be due to mutations in *TBX19* (*TPIT*) (Vallette-Kasic et al. 2004).

A defect in one of the genes involved in the development of the pituitary may result in a more severe endocrinopathy with deficiencies of more than one hypothalamic and/or pituitary hormone. Defects of the gene *POU1F1* (*Pit-1*) are typically associated with a deficiency of GH, TSH and prolactin (Pfaffle et al. 1992; Radovick et al. 1992; Tatsumi et al. 1992; De Zegher et al. 1995b) whilst the gene *PROP1*, active at an earlier stage of pituitary gland development, is associated with deficiency of GH, TSH, prolactin, gonadotrophins (Wu et al. 1998; Deladoey et al. 1999) and sometimes

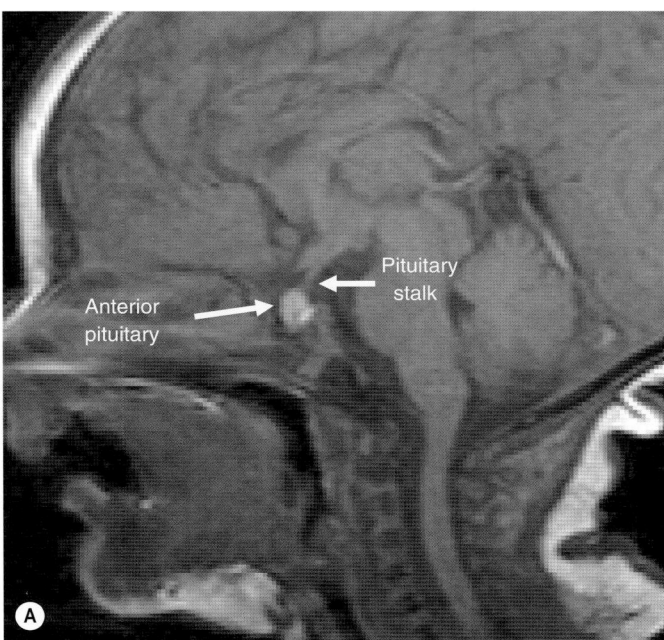
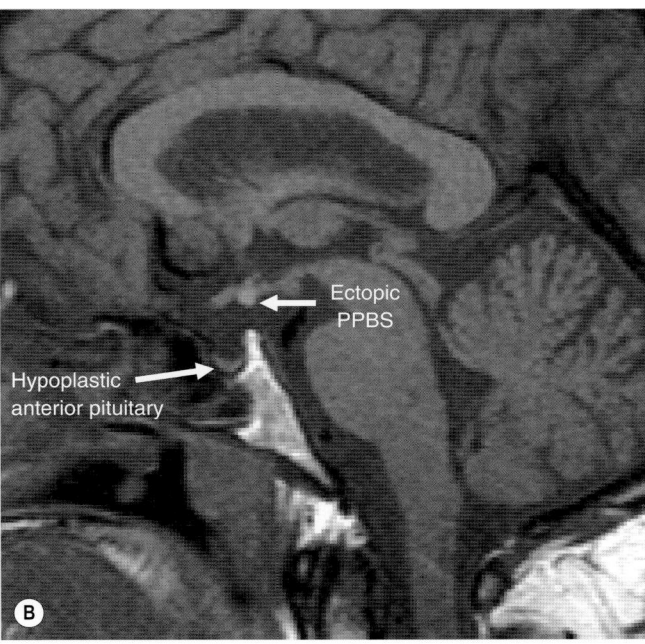

Fig. 34.7 (A) Magnetic resonance (MR) scan of infant brain (1 month old). The anterior pituitary has a relatively bright appearance in early life on T_1-weighted images. (B) MR scan of baby with pituitary hormone deficiency.

Table 34.6 Principal human mutations causing abnormal hypothalamopituitary development and function

GENE	PHENOTYPE	INHERITANCE
POU1F1	CPHD: GH, TSH, prolactin deficiencies; usually severe; small or normal AP	Recessive, dominant
PROP1	CPHD: GH, TSH, LH, FSH, prolactin deficiencies; evolving ACTH deficiency; small, normal or enlarged AP	Recessive
HESX1	IGHD, CPHD, septo-optic dysplasia; APH, EPP, absent infundibulum, ACC	Recessive, dominant
LHX3	CPHD (GH, TSH, LH, FSH, prolactin deficiencies), short neck, limited rotation; small, normal or enlarged AP, short cervical spine	Recessive
LHX4	CPHD (GH, TSH, ACTH deficiencies); small AP, EPP, cerebellar abnormalities	Dominant
SOX3	IGHD and mental retardation, panhypopituitarism; APH, infundibular hypoplasia, EPP	X linked
SOX2	Hypogonadotrophic hypogonadism; APH, bilateral anophthalmia/microphthalmia, abnormal corpus callosum, learning difficulties, oesophageal atresia, sensorineural hearing loss	De novo

CPHD, combined pituitary hormone deficiency; GH, growth hormone; TSH, thyroid-stimulating hormone; LH, luteinising hormone; FSH, follicle-stimulating hormone; APH, anterior pituitary hypoplasia; ACTH, adrenocorticotrophic hormone; EPP, ectopic posterior pituitary; IGHD, isolated growth hormone deficiency; ACC, agenesis of corpus callosum.

ACTH deficiency as well (Van Esch et al. 2000; Vallette-Kasic et al. 2001) (Table 34.6). HESX1 has a fundamental role in CNS development and homozygous and heterozygous mutations of HESX1 are a recognised cause of SOD. Heterozygous defects can also cause isolated GHD (Dattani et al. 1998; Thomas et al. 2001; Tajima et al. 2003). Defects of SOX3 may result in PHD in association with mental retardation whilst defects in LHX4 may result in PHD in association with abnormalities of the cerebellar tonsils.

Clinical features (Table 34.7)

Clinical recognition of hypopituitarism in the newborn can be difficult. GH deficiency leads to relatively subtle changes in body form

and whilst some authors report a reduction in length of about 1 SD with a normal birthweight (Gluckman et al. 1992) other studies indicate that birth length is largely unaffected (Pena-Almazan et al. 2001; Mehta et al. 2005). GH-deficient children grow slowly in infancy and may be more than 2 SD below the mean for length by the end of the first year of life (Mehta et al. 2005). Micropenis can be a feature of GH deficiency but is more typically associated with gonadotrophin deficiency (Salisbury et al. 1984). GH promotes longitudinal growth but also has lipolytic and ketogenic activity. Ketones are an important fuel in the newborn period and babies with isolated GH deficiency are therefore more susceptible to hypoglycaemia. Hypoglycaemia is typically more profound in the infant with adrenocortical insufficiency and a deficiency of one or

Table 34.7 Clinical and biochemical assessment of the infant with suspected hypopituitarism

Clinical features

Micropenis
Hypoglycaemia – may present as episodes of colour change and/ or fits
Prolonged jaundice – typically conjugated hyperbilirubinaemia
Associated defects, e.g. cleft palate

Investigations

Baseline investigations

Electrolytes – hyponatraemia may reflect cortisol deficiency
Random growth hormone – produced continuously in the first days of life, unmeasurable levels suspicious
Thyroid function (thyroid-stimulating hormone may, paradoxically, be mildly elevated)
Prolactin – usually high in the newborn period
Luteinising hormone/follicle-stimulating hormone – unrecordable levels, particularly at 2–3 months of age, suggest gonadotrophin deficiency

Biochemistry at the time of hypoglycaemia

Cortisol (values greater than 500 nmol/l make adrenocorticotrophic hormone deficiency unlikely)
Growth hormone

Other

Dynamic testing (may not always be feasible)
Glucagon (to assess pituitary growth hormone and adrenocorticotrophic hormone/cortisol production)
Thyroid-releasing hormone testing (of questionable value)
Other dynamic tests to assess the hypothalamopituitary axis
Synacthen

both of these hormones should be considered in the hypoglycaemic baby. Prolonged neonatal jaundice with a conjugated hyperbilirubinaemia is a further well-recognised feature of congenital hypopituitarism (Herman et al. 1975) and is closely linked to cortisol deficiency. All neonates with suspected PHD should have an opthalmological assessment because of the possiblility of underlying SOD.

Further investigations (Table 34.7)

Diagnosing PHD typically involves piecing together a range of clinical and biochemical parameters. The neonate with microphallus, hypoglycaemia and a low free T_4 (fT_4) is at high risk of having CPHD. The diagnosis is even more likely if the infant has a conjugated hyperbilirubinaemia and small optic discs on opthalmological examination. Random measurements of pituitary hormones (particularly TSH and fT_4) can be helpful but hypoglycaemia may not be an effective stimulus for GH and cortisol production (babies who prove to be GH- and ACTH-'sufficient' may have low levels at the time of hypoglycaemia). Hence stimulation tests may be required as part of the diagnostic work-up. Biochemical testing can be extremely helpful but requires careful planning and is potentially misleading because, like all tests, there are false positives and negatives. GH levels are often elevated in the first days of life and a low random GH concentration raises the possiblity of hypothalamo-pituitary disease.

It is important to remember the TSH surge and associated increase in thyroid hormone levels that occur in healthy babies around the time of delivery when interpreting thyroid function tests (Fig. 34.8). Laboratories may not have appropriate age-related data for babies in the first days of life and so a 'normal' adult fT_4 may be abnormally low at this time of life. TSH levels can, paradoxically, be mildly elevated in secondary hypothyroidism and there may be an exaggerated response to TRH (Gruneiro de Papendieck et al. 1982). The increase in TSH levels and exaggerated response in hypothalamic hypothyroidism may reflect the presence of detectable but bioinactive TSH (Persani et al. 2000) or alternatively the abnormal production of TSH in the absence of hypothalamic hormones such as somatostatin. Although the TRH test has its advocates (Van Tijn et al. 2008), many feel that the diagnosis of secondary hypothyroidism can be made with a single or serial measurements of TSH and thyroid hormone (Mehta et al. 2003).

Cortisol deficiency secondary to ACTH deficiency can be associated with hyponatraemia because cortisol inhibits arginine vasopressin (AVP) production and is required to excrete a water load. Potassium levels are not typically raised because mineralocorticoid production is primarily regulated by the renin–angiotensin system and not ACTH. The Synacthen test is still an appropriate test with which to investigate possible secondary hypoadrenalism (ACTH deficiency) prior to commencing hydrocortisone in the infant with hypoglycaemia and suspected hypopituitarism. The CRH test has theoretical advantages but both tests are hampered by concerns about sensitivity and specificity, a lack of reliable normative data as well as the more complex and, in the case of the CRH test, more limited availability of the ACTH assay. GnRH administration with assessment of LH and FSH levels may be helpful (Segal et al. 2009) but the assessment of other axes is more important if there is a limited amount of blood available. It should be remembered that drugs such as dopamine may interfere with endocrine investigations (De Zegher et al. 1993).

It can be difficult to balance the desire to obtain comprehensive biochemical data with the need to treat the sick, hypoglycaemic neonate. If the clinical picture strongly suggests hypopituitarism then it is wise to treat and then reassess the neonate biochemically at a later stage. Hormone deficiencies can evolve with time (see above) and a neonate who is ACTH-'sufficient' can become ACTH- and hence cortisol-'insufficient' in later childhood.

MRI can provide extremely helpful information about pituitary/hypothalamic anatomy as well as information about other CNS developmental abnormalities such as optic nerve hypoplasia or migrational abnormalities such as schizencephaly, which are more common in babies with CPHD (Fig. 34.7).

Treatment

Hypopituitarism is treated by replacing the missing pituitary hormone (GH) or the product of its target organs (T_4 or hydrocortisone). Although the cortisol production rate in the newborn is 6.6–8.8 mg/m^2/24 h (Metzger et al. 1993), the absorption and bioavailability of hydrocortisone can vary (Charmandari et al. 2001). Adrenal replacement (secondary to ACTH deficiency) should be with hydrocortisone in a dose around 8–10 mg/m^2/24 h (in three or four divided doses). There are concerns about the bioavailability of some hydrocortisone suspensions and these need to be borne in mind (Merke et al. 2001). For thyroid replacement, T_4 in a single dose of approximately 8–10 µg/kg/24 h in the newborn is suitable initially. The objective is to obtain T_4 levels in the upper part of the normal range and the dose should be adjusted accordingly. TSH levels will be low in secondary hypothyroidism once therapy has commenced and cannot be used to guide replacement. GH replacement may be needed to control the hypoglycaemia of hypopituitarism if this proves intractable and therapy may also be warranted from an early stage if growth is to be optimised.

Resistance to the actions of anterior pituitary hormones

Endocrine disorders in which hormone action is impaired or absent owing to abnormalities of the receptor or abnormal postreceptor events are well recognised. The phenotypic features of these rare conditions may suggest hypopituitarism, but the levels of pituitary hormones are usually normal or elevated. The best-described example is insensitivity to GH (Laron syndrome), which can present with hypoglycaemia and micropenis in the newborn period (Godowski et al. 1989; Savage et al. 2010).

Abnormalitites of the TSH receptor leading to hypothyroidism (see below), the ACTH receptor leading to glucocorticoid deficiency and the LH receptor leading to genital ambiguity are considered in more detail in the appropriate sections below (Kremer et al. 1995; Sunthornthepvarakul et al. 1995; Weber et al. 1995).

Posterior pituitary (Robertson 2001)

Normal function

AVP, a nonapeptide, is the major determinant of renal solute-free water excretion. AVP acts to conserve body water by altering the permeability of the distal convoluted and renal collecting tubules, thereby increasing urine osmolality. AVP is produced by secretory neurons residing in the supraoptic nuclei and paraventricular nuclei from the end of the first trimester. The neurons project along the supraoptic–hypophyseal tract and terminate in the posterior pituitary. The generation and release of mature peptide from the axon terminal is the consequence of the processing and cleavage of a large precursor molecule, preproAVP, encoded by the AVP-neurophysin II gene. Cleavage of the signal peptide occurs as preproAVP translocates into the endoplasmic reticulum. Dimerisation occurs as the molecules pass into the neurosecretory granules from the Golgi apparatus. Further oligomerisation and processing occur as the neurosecretory granules move along towards the axon terminal, with cleaved neurophysin II and copeptin binding to AVP. Exocytosis and release of the mature AVP–neurophysin complex from the nerve endings in the posterior pituitary follow neurotransmitter-induced depolarisation. The AVP–neurophysin complex then dissociates to release free hormone. Secretion is primarily controlled by the osmoreceptors of the hypothalamus, although non-osmotic stimuli, notably blood volume and blood pressure, also influence vasopressin release via the stretch receptors of the left atrium and the baroreceptors in the carotid sinus. Mature AVP has a circulating half-life of 5–15 minutes.

Cranial diabetes insipidus (Cheetham and Bayliss 2002)

In the absence of vasopressin, urine volume and tonicity are changed only minimally in the distal tubule and collecting ducts. Urine volume can reach nearly 10% of the glomerular filtrate, with an osmolality of 100 mmol/kgH$_2$O or less. The infant with AVP deficiency (cranial diabetes insipidus or CDI) will therefore tend to pass inappropriately large amounts of dilute urine for a given plasma osmolality.

The causes of diabetes insipidus in the newborn are shown in Table 34.8 and include congenital brain malformations such as

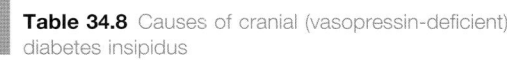

Table 34.8 Causes of cranial (vasopressin-deficient) diabetes insipidus

Primary
Genetic
Autosomal dominant (vasopressin – neurophysin gene) Autosomal recessive (vasopressin – neurophysin gene) Autosomal recessive – Wolfram (DIDMOAD) syndrome
With congenital malformations (which may also have a genetic, single-gene basis)
Hypopituitarism Septo-optic dysplasia Holoprosencephaly Midline defects
Secondary
Trauma – neurosurgery or following head injury Tumours – craniopharyngioma, optic glioma Infection/inflammation Vascular, including haemorrhage or malformations Hypoxic–ischaemic encephalopathy Langerhans cell hystiocytosis
DIDMOAD, diabetes insipidus, diabetes mellitus, optic atrophy and deafness.

SOD and holoprosencephaly (Traggiai and Stanhope 2002). Trauma can cause diabetes insipidus, although the site of injury will determine whether or not this is permanent. Damage to the supraoptic nucleus or high stalk section causes permanent CDI, with more distal lesions usually causing transient dysfunction.

Clinically the condition is characterised by excessive fluid output and intake. Diagnosis is difficult in the newborn because a high urine output is easily overlooked and persistent crying and weight loss can easily be attributed to a cause other than water loss. Infants may therefore present late, with non-specific symptoms such as anorexia, vomiting, poor weight gain, constipation or delayed development. Failure to thrive can occur (Nijenhuis et al. 2001) but is less pronounced than in children with nephrogenic diabetes insipidus, because the urine tends to be less dilute. The low osmolar load associated with breastfeeding may help to maintain a normal serum osmolality and reduce symptoms.

The diagnosis is confirmed by a failure to concentrate the urine in spite of plasma hypertonicity, with reversal by administration of the vasopressin analogue desmopressin (DDAVP). Polyuria due to hypercalcaemia or potassium deficiency must be excluded, and allowance made for the lesser concentrating power of the neonatal kidney. Circulating vasopressin concentrations can be measured, although a relatively large amount of plasma is required. The principal differential diagnosis is nephrogenic diabetes insipidus, where there is resistance to the effects of circulating AVP

Treatment

Treatment is usually with the vasopressin analogue DDAVP. This compound is more potent than the native molecule and has a longer half-life (Ng et al. 2002). It is important to be aware of the danger of water overload, which will develop if urine is inappropriately concentrated for a given fluid intake. Babies have been treated with DDAVP administered nasally but the likelihood of water intoxication is markedly reduced with oral therapy and this is the preferred route of administration (Stick and Betts 1987; Cheetham and Bayliss 2002). Capillary or serum sodium osmolality should be checked regularly, particularly in the initial phase as the dose is being adjusted. It is safer in both the short and the long term for an infant with diabetes insipidus (and an intact sense of thirst) to be allowed to compensate for a relatively low dose of DDAVP by feeding or drinking more and babies should be offered water on occasions as well as milk. Parents should be actively involved in management from an early stage and encouraged to gauge fluid input and output.

A suitable starting dose of oral DDAVP is around 1–4 µg daily, increased to twice a day once the impact of the first dose has been established. The dose can be administered orally using the desmopressin injection solution (4 µg/ml), although some people have used an aliquot of a DDAVP tablet dispersed in water. If the baby is sleeping longer overnight then the logical time to administer a single daily dose or the larger dose of a twice-daily regimen is in the evening. We do not recommend the nasal route of administration but if there is no alternative then the standard solution (100 µg/ml) can be diluted with 0.9% NaCl solution to create a more manageable volume (for example, 10 µg/ml – discuss with the hospital pharmacy). This can then be instilled into the nose using a 1-ml syringe. A suitable starting dose in the newborn is 0.1–1.0 µg once or twice daily. Initially it is wise to administer the second dose only when the impact of the first has been established.

Low-dose subcutaneous DDAVP has been advocated as a safe means of managing CDI in infancy (Blanco et al. 2006). A low dose (usually 0.01 µg, s.c.) used once a day can be initiated and then increased to maintain a normal serum sodium. DDAVP (4 µg/ml) can be diluted 1:10 in a syringe with the required dose ranging from 0.02 to 0.08 µg DDAVP s.c. twice daily.

Finally, 5 mg/kg of chlorothiazide administered twice a day has also been used to treat CDI on the basis that, as with nephrogenic diabetes insipidus, the associated increase in urine osmolality will compensate for vasopressin deficiency (Rivkees et al. 2007).

Excess vasopressin secretion (syndrome of inappropriate antidiuretic hormone secretion)

This is described in Chapter 18.

The hormonal regulation of appetite and feeding behaviour

An increasing number of hormones and receptors are known to be involved in the regulation of feeding behaviour and growth. The hormone leptin is produced by the *ob* gene in the adipocyte and circulating levels provide the hypothalamus with information about nutritional status. This in turn will influence feeding behaviour, as vividly illustrated by rare examples of leptin deficiency or resistance (Farooqi et al. 1999; Montague et al. 1997). Leptin levels are a reflection of fat mass and cord leptin levels are positively related to birthweight (Sivan et al. 1997; Christou et al. 2001). Feeding behaviour will influence growth, and leptin status has been shown to be related to weight gain in the first months of life (Ong et al. 1999).

As many as 5% of children with severe early-onset obesity may have defects of the MC4 receptor (Farooqi et al. 2000, 2003) and patients with rare abnormalities of the *POMC* gene can present with ACTH deficiency and demonstrate obesity with associated rapid growth in early life (Krude et al. 1998).

Other components of the appetite-regulatory pathway are steadily being elucidated and the gut peptide PYY has been shown to

inhibit food intake (Batterham et al. 2002) whilst ghrelin (Broglio et al. 2003), a GH secretogogue produced by a number of tissues including the gastrointestinal tract and the hypothalamus, promotes feeding. Reduced insulin levels between feeds are associated with a rise in ghrelin release and GH production. Hence there is a complex interplay between feeding, fasting, hormone production and the regulation of intermediate metabolism and fuel supply in the newborn period (Chanoine et al. 2002; Iniguez et al. 2002; Haqq et al. 2003).

Thyroid

Disorders of thyroid gland development and/or function are relatively common, affecting approximately one newborn infant in 3000. Recent advances in this field reflect the development of more refined biochemical assays, the elucidation of genes involved in thyroid gland development and hormone synthesis, as well as information gained from screening programmes for congenital hypothyroidism (CHT).

Normal function

Thyroid function in utero

TSH, modulated by TRH, stimulates the synthesis and release of T_4 and triiodothyronine (T_3) from the thyroid into the plasma, where they circulate, strongly bound to proteins. Maternal T_4, but not TSH or T_3, can cross the placenta in physiologically significant amounts and this explains the relatively normal phenotype in infants with CHT at birth with levels that are one-third to one-half normal values in babies unable to manufacture thyroid hormone (Vulsma et al. 1989). The importance of maternal T_4 delivery to the fetus in early gestation, whilst the fetal thyroid axis is developing, is supported by studies of neurodevelopment in infants of mothers with relatively low T_4 levels (Gruneiro de Papendieck et al. 1982; Haddow et al. 1999). The significance of T_4 transfer in the latter stages of pregnancy is illustrated by the life-threatening illness seen in hypothyroid infants of hypothyroid mothers (De Zegher et al. 1995a; Yasuda et al. 1999).

The greater part of circulating T_3 is derived from peripheral monodeiodination of the outer ring of T_4, which therefore acts as a reservoir or prohormone for the more active T_3. An alternative monodeiodination affects the inner ring of T_4 and produces inactive reverse T_3 (rT_3). This mechanism permits a balance between production of the most and least active thyroid hormones. There are three deiodinases – type I (D1), which has inner and outer deiodination activity; type II deiodinase (D2), which catalyses outer-ring deiodination; and type III deiodinase (D3), which catalyses inner-ring deiodination.

Fetal thyroid hormone metabolism is characterised by a predominance of D3 activity outside the CNS in tissues such as the liver, kidney and placenta. This converts maternal and endogenous T_4 preferentially to rT_3 and presumably helps to reduce tissue thermogenesis and enhance tissue anabolism. T_4 (rather than T_3) is required by the developing brain, and the appropriate deiodinases (particularly D2) are expressed in a temporal and spatial manner in different brain regions. Sulphotransferase enzymes also have an important role in thyroid hormone metabolism. T_4 sulphation blocks outer-ring deiodination to T_3 whilst promoting inner-ring conversion to inactive rT_3. The activity of sulphotransferase enzymes in tissues like the liver will also, therefore, play a key role in determining thyroid hormone availability (Fisher 2002). A key determinant of thyroid hormone transport into cells has been identified with defects of this

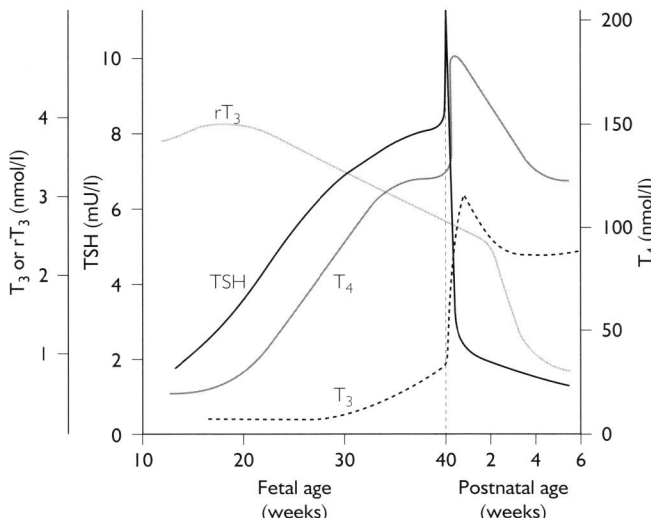

Fig. 34.8 The trend in fetal and neonatal plasma thyroid-stimulating hormone (TSH), thyroxine (T₄), triiodothyronine (T3) and reverse T3 (rT3) levels. *(Adapted from Fisher 1999.)*

protein resulting in a phenotype that includes profound neuro-developmental delay (Friesma et al. 2004).

Thyroid function in the neonatal period

After birth there is an acute discharge of TSH which reaches a peak at 30 minutes, before falling towards basal levels within the first 3 days. There is an associated release of thyroid hormones and enhanced peripheral conversion of T_4 (closely linked to D2 activity), which results in a pronounced increase in T_3 in the first hours of life. There is a further increase in total T_3 and free T_3 levels for about 36 hours around the time of the postnatal peak in T_4 (Fig. 34.8) and fT_4 levels remain relatively high for the first weeks of life (Fisher et al. 2000). In preterm infants the levels of T_3 remain higher than the cord values of babies of equivalent gestational age for several weeks (Williams et al. 2004). Preterm infants (down to 30 weeks) show similar but lesser changes in TSH and thyroid hormone concentrations, although the most preterm babies (23–27 weeks) have relatively low T_4 values (Williams et al. 2004). By 1–2 months of age, thyroid hormone levels are comparable to those in term infants. In the case of infants under 30 weeks' gestation, the postnatal surge does not occur (Biswas et al. 2002) and T_4 levels frequently fall to a nadir around 1–2 weeks of age, which is more pronounced with increasing prematurity (Mercado et al. 1988; Van Wassenaer et al. 1997). T_4 levels remain below those of full-term infants through the first few weeks of life (Frank et al. 1996) and climb gradually to normal postnatal levels.

Congenital hypothyroidism

This is a heterogeneous group of patients, some of whom will have functioning thyroid tissue and some of whom will not. In those with functioning tissue, the gland may be normally sited and of normal size, hypoplastic or ectopic. Despite significant developments in our understanding of the aetiology of CHT, the cause is still unknown in most patients. Malformations besides defects of thyroid gland development and function are more common in infants with CHT (Olivieri et al. 2002). It is helpful to divide patients into those with thyroid dysgenesis and those with an abnormality of one of the enzymes or factors involved in thyroid hormone synthesis (dyshormonogenesis).

Thyroid dysgenesis

Embyrological defects resulting in thyroid dysgenesis are the most common cause of CHT, and range from thyroid agenesis (no gland present) to an ectopic and/or hypoplastic gland. Some thyroid tissue is demonstrable in approximately two-thirds of affected infants, and there is a spectrum of biochemical severity. The frequency is around 1 in 3000–4000 and is twice as common in females as in males, with only minor racial and seasonal differences in incidence described. As genetic factors involved in thyroid development and thyroid-specific gene expression have been described, so abnormalities of these same genes have been identified in a small number of patients with thyroid dysgenesis. Mutations in the TSH receptor (TSHR) (Sunthornthepvarakul et al. 1995; Biebermann et al. 1997) and transcription factors such as TTF1 (NKX2-1), TTF2 and Pax-8 have been published, but a strict mendelian inheritance pattern is relatively uncommon (Krude et al. 2002; Perry et al. 2002b) and the aetiology of thyroid dysgenesis in most patients is unknown (Castanet et al. 2010).

Thyroid hormone replacement abolishes the physical manifestations of hypothyroidism but intellectual and neurological prognosis is compromised in those babies at the more severe end of the spectrum unless treatment is started within the first few weeks of life (Alm et al. 1984).

Dyshormonogenesis (Fig. 34.9)

Recessively inherited biochemical defects of iodothyronine synthesis are the second most common cause of permanent CHT, with a frequency in Europe and North America of approximately 1 in 30 000–50 000, accounting for some 10–15% of patients identified by screening. The sex incidence is equal. A goitre may be present at birth but, unless large, may be difficult to detect and may not develop until later in life. The degree of hypothyroidism is variable with some patients clinically and even biochemically euthyroid. Dyshormonogenesis can be a cause of transient hypothyroidism when the extra demands in early life cannot be met. Thyroid ultrasonography usually shows normal thyroid anatomy and site (a eutopic gland). In many dyshormonogeneses there is excessive discharge of iodide from the thyroid gland after administration of perchlorate (the perchlorate discharge test), due to an abnormality of iodide organification into thyroglobulin. Recognised abnormalities of thyroid hormone synthesis include defects in iodide transport across the basolateral membrane (sodium iodide symporter) (Fujiwara et al. 1997; Pohlenz et al. 1998) and then into the colloid lumen (Everett et al. 1997; Coyle et al. 1998). Other causes include abnormalities of the thyroglobulin gene (Ieiri et al. 1991), thyroid peroxidase (Bakker et al. 2000; Ambrugger et al. 2001) and THOX (Moreno et al. 2002), which is involved in the generation of H_2O_2 required by thyroid peroxidase to oxidise iodide. Delineation of the precise biochemical defect in these disorders does not alter the need for T_4 replacement, but can help when counselling families about the likelihood of recurrence.

Neonatal screening for congenital hypothyroidism (Fisher 1999; Rose et al. 2006; LaFranchi 2010)

The development of radioimmunoassays for measurement of T_4 and TSH in very small samples of serum or whole blood spotted on to filter paper resulted in the rapid adoption of screening in many countries. Most programmes used a single blood sample taken between the fifth and 10th days of life, by which time relative stability has returned to the thyroid axis after the abrupt postnatal

Table 34.9 The advantages and disadvantages of the different approaches to identifying babies with congenital hypothyroidism

DISORDER	INCIDENCE IN NEWBORNS	PRIMARY TSH	PRIMARY T$_4$, FOLLOW-UP TSH	COMBINED T$_4$ AND TSH
Primary CHT	~1 in 2500–4000	Good	Good	Very good
Hypopituitary hypothyroidism (most will have combined pituitary hormone deficiency)	~1:16000	No	Some	Some
Transient hypothyroidism and hyperthyrotropinaemia	~1 in 30000	Yes, but may require second specimen in preterms	Some	Yes
Recall rate		0.3–1% (cut-off-dependent)	1–2%	~2%

TSH, thyroid-stimulating hormone; T$_4$, thyroxine; CHT, congenital hypothyroidism.

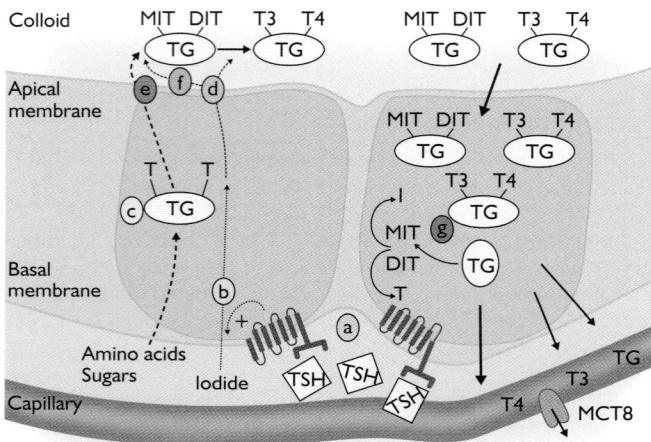

Fig. 34.9 Dyshormonogenesis. Thyroid hormone production and disorders of thyroid hormone synthesis (dyshormonogeneses). Thyroid hormone production: amino acids and glucose are used to produce thyroglobulin to which tyrosine residues are attached. Iodine is incorporated into these residues at the apical membrane to produce iodotyrosines. These are stored as extracellular colloid. Thyroid hormone secretion: colloid droplets are invaginated to release thyroglobulin and the iodotyrosines, including thyroxine (T$_4$) and triiodothyronine (T$_3$), which are released into the circulation. The other iodotyrosinases (DIT and MIT) are deiodinated and the iodine reused. Dyshormongeneses: a, thyroid-stimulating hormone (TSH) receptor defects; b, abnormalities of iodide uptake (sodium iodide symporter); c, defects of thyroglobulin synthesis; d, abnormalities of iodine transport at the apical membrane (pendrin); e, abnormalities of the enzyme system incorporating iodine into tyrosine (thyroid peroxidase); f, abnormalities of the enzyme system involved in H$_2$O$_2$ generation (Thox); g, abnormalities of the deioidinase system.

perturbation. T$_4$ screening alone proved inadequate because of the overlap between normal and hypothyroid values. The alternatives were to add a TSH assay in all cases or for the lower range of T$_4$ values, or to use TSH as the primary test and accept that the rare cases of secondary hypothyroidism (hypopituitary hypothyroidism) may be missed. Many European countries have adopted the primary TSH approach whilst a combined approach with the simultaneous measurement of both TSH and T$_4$ is used in some parts of the USA (Asakura et al. 2002). A comparison of the three principal strategies is shown in Table 34.9.

The returns from screening proved even greater than had been expected: in both the USA and Europe, the frequency of CHT was approximately 1 in 3500, almost double that suggested by retrospective surveys (Fisher et al. 1979). The early manifestations of CHT are non-specific and development of the typical features usually occurs slowly (Table 34.10). Even in the most medically advanced countries, no more than half the affected infants could be diagnosed clinically by the age of 3 months (Alm et al. 1978). With screening, treatment could be started by 4 weeks and ideally by 2 weeks of age (Toublanc 1999; Working Group on Neonatal Screening of the European Society for Paediatric Endocrinology 1999).

One of the key issues in countries using bloodspot TSH as a screening tool centres on the question of the TSH screening cut-off. TSH assays have become more refined and there has been a temptation to use an increasingly lower cut-off value. Reducing the screening cut-off and collecting samples relatively early (within the first 2 days of life) will increase sensitivity but reduce specificity. Whilst it is possible that true CHT is becoming more common (Hertzberg et al. 2010), reports of a rising incidence will, in some instances, reflect changes in screening practice. A lower TSH cut-off and repeat testing will detect subtle fluctuations in TSH or T$_4$ that may occur in the absence of classical thyroid dysgenesis or dyshormonogenesis (see the sections on a delayed TSH rise, transient hypothyroidism and hyperthyrotropinaemia below). The incidence of CHT in countries using the combined TSH/T$_4$ approach is around 1 in 2500. Dropping the TSH screening cut-off in a region of Italy using a primary TSH strategy resulted in the incidence rising from around 1 in 2600 to around 1 in 1400 (Corbetta et al. 2009). Not surprisingly, the proportion of babies with established defects of thyroid gland development tends to fall as the reported incidence of CHT increases. Only longer term surveillance will establish which infants have permanent CHT. A key question is the extent to which babies with the more subtle biochemical abnormalities benefit from intervention with T$_4$.

Diagnosis

The diagnosis of CHT is confirmed by finding low serum thyroid hormone concentrations (fT$_4$) and a high TSH. The fT$_3$ level is variable and is preserved in the normal range for longer. It remains

Table 34.10 Clinical features of congenital hypothyroidism

At birth
Postmaturity, large size
Large posterior fontanelle
Umbilical hernia
Goitre
Macroglossia

Early signs
Placid, sleepy
Poor feeding
Constipation, abdominal distension
Respiratory problems
Peripheral cyanosis
Oedema
Prolonged jaundice
Subtle dysmorphism

Later signs
Large tongue
Hoarse cry
Dry skin, hair
Slow responses
Delayed development
Growth failure

essential to exclude hypothyroidism in any infant in whom there is clinical suspicion, because, first, errors inevitably occur in all screening programmes; second, mild hypothyroidism may escape detection by all screening methods (see below); and third, there may be a late rise in TSH levels. The major clinical features of CHT are summarised in Table 34.10. Infants with low T_4 values are more likely to have clinical signs such as feeding difficulties, lethargy, prolonged jaundice, umbilical hernia and macroglossia (Grant et al. 1992). Such infants are more likely to have an aplastic rather than a hypoplastic or ectopic gland. A gestation over 40 weeks, induction of labour and a birthweight above 3500 g are all more common among infants with hypothyroidism.

Further investigation

The laboratory tests of thyroid function primarily determine whether an infant requires T_4 treatment. Isotope scanning (technetium or ^{123}I) can be undertaken before or within a few days of starting T_4 replacement treatment, ideally when the TSH levels are still high (Clerc et al. 2008). Thyroid ultrasonography is also performed in some centres (Perry et al. 2002a, 2006) and, whilst it is a highly operator-dependent technique, it can provide information about gland morphology and hence more detail than isotope scanning alone. An ultrasound can be conducted on the neonatal unit and may be of particular value in the infant exposed to iodine-containing compounds whose isotope scan may be hard to interpret.

In thyroid dysgenesis, an isotope scan or ultrasound will reveal an absent, small or ectopic gland. This condition has a low risk of recurrence in further children (Castanet et al. 2010). The infant with thyroid aplasia or ectopia will need treatment for life and is unlikely to benefit from a trial off therapy in later childhood. If the gland is anatomically normal and the isotope uptake is high, then hypothyroidism is probably due to a dyshormonogenesis and may be

inherited in an autosomal recessive (AR) manner. Absent isotope uptake in a normally sited gland on ultrasonography also suggests a dyshormonogenesis with abnormal iodine trapping.

Advocates of investigations in CHT highlight the fact that this information can be used to refine the T_4 dose (Mathai et al. 2008) and can provide information about recurrence risk and prognosis. On the other hand investigations can be operator-dependent, difficult to interpret and may involve intravenous access and ionising radiation. Some clinicians still prefer to rely on the biochemistry (TSH and thyroid hormone levels) alone. A plain radiograph of the knee to assess epiphyseal maturity was frequently performed in the past. This may reflect the degree of fetal hypothyroidism but is of limited clinical value.

A TRH stimulation test is rarely indicated, but has been used in babies with mild thyroid dysfunction. An exaggerated and prolonged TSH response is observed if TSH levels are mildly elevated because of a compromised thyroid gland (Rapaport et al. 1993). TRH testing has been advocated as a way of teasing out central hypothyroidism in babies found to have low T_4 levels on screening (Van Tijn et al. 2008).

Treatment

T_4 is used for replacement and there is no advantage in giving T_3 (see above). It is a matter of some urgency to start treatment, and when the diagnosis is reasonably certain it may be preferable to collect further specimens and start treatment without waiting for the results.

The aim of therapy is to normalise T_4 and TSH concentrations quickly, and an appropriate starting dose of T_4 in the newborn with low T_4 levels is 10–12 µg/kg/24 h given as a single daily dose (Bongers-Schokking et al. 2000; Salerno et al. 2002; Corbetta et al. 2009). Full-term infants of normal birthweight should be commenced on 37.5–50 µg daily. This will usually bring the TSH into the normal range quickly and the dose of T_4 may then need to be reduced. Babies with significant endogenous thyroid hormone production may normalise TSH values on a smaller dose. The smallest tablet available contains 25 µg T_4 but as the hormone has a long half-life (in excess of a week) the dose can be adjusted in smaller increments by (for example) giving a higher or lower dose on alternate days as well as by dividing them. T_4 solutions are available, although there have been concerns about the stability of some of these preparations and parents need to be aware that they may come in different strengths.

Relatively high fT_4 levels may be seen after treatment is commenced but this picture does not necessarily indicate overtreatment if TSH levels are normal or raised. The dose of T_4 will fall with time when calculated according to weight and a suppressed TSH indicates overtreatment. The heterogeneity of CHT has been highlighted earlier and babies with only mild or moderately elevated baseline TSH levels may require smaller doses of T_4 than babies with agenesis, in whom the baseline TSH is typically very high (Hanukoglu et al. 2001). Replacement is usually satisfactory if the serum total T_4 and fT_4 are in the upper part of the quoted laboratory normal range for age, but suboptimal compliance needs to be excluded if TSH values remain elevated despite a substantial T_4 dose.

There is evidence to suggest that higher initial starting doses of T_4 may have a beneficial impact on neurodevelopment (Dubuis et al. 1996; Bongers-Schokking et al. 2000; Salerno et al. 2002), although there has been concern that this might be at the expense of an increase in behavioural problems (Rovet and Ehrlich 1995; Hindmarsh 2002). Severe overdosage may also cause accelerated growth and even craniosynostosis, but the danger of impaired neurological development from underdosage is probably greater.

Higher doses of T_4 treatment in early life as well as a milder baseline biochemical picture have been associated with increased stature in mid-childhood and at final height (Grant 1994; Dickerman and De Vries 1997; Heyerdahl et al. 1997), although this has not been a consistent observation (Salerno et al. 2001).

Follow-up and prognosis

Growth, clinical progress and thyroid function should be checked after 2 and then 4 weeks on treatment, and then at 1–2-monthly intervals in the first 6 months and then every 3–4 months up to 3 years of age. Definitive reassessment of thyroid status can be undertaken after the age of 2 years, when brief cessation of treatment will have no adverse effects. Most children with a permanent defect of thyroid hormone generation will develop abnormal biochemistry without any adverse symptoms if T_4 is stopped for 2–4 weeks at this stage. In addition to a biochemical assessment of thyroid function, the opportunity can be taken to obtain or repeat an isotope thyroid scan. If the T_4 dose has been increased during the first 2 years of life because of an elevated TSH then this may not be necessary.

CHT is associated with impaired motor development, a reduced intelligence quotient (IQ) and impaired hearing and language problems (Alm et al. 1984; Derksen-lubsen Verkerk 1996; Rovet et al. 1996). These features are related to the severity of hypothyroidism at birth (Rovet 1999). In one study, total T_4 levels below 42 nmol/l in the neonatal period were associated with a 10-point deficit in IQ at school entry (Tillotson et al. 1994). Individuals with T_4 values above 42 nmol/l were no different from controls, suggesting a 'threshold' effect. Thus it seems that the degree of pre- and perinatal hypothyroidism has implications for CNS function in the long term. A formal hearing assessment is recommended in the hypothyroid infant because of the 10-fold increase in hearing loss in these babies (Van Wassenaer et al. 1993).

Neonatal screening and the preterm infant: the delayed TSH rise

A well-recognised phenomenon is that of the infant in whom the initial neonatal screening TSH is normal but who then develops an elevated TSH in the context of low thyroid hormone levels in the subsequent few weeks. Many such cases are infants born preterm or of low birthweight. Mandel and colleagues (2000) referred to this as 'atypical hypothyroidism' and this pattern is the principal reason why some countries opt for a second bloodspot screen in all babies or in those born preterm. It is likely that many of the preterm infants will have transient abnormalities of thyroid function related to illness, exposure to drugs such as dopamine, a negative iodine balance or exposure to topical iodine-containing compounds. Many paediatricians feel that abnormalities of thyroid gland development per se are not more common in preterm infants but that some preterm infants with CHT, in contrast to term infants, may not generate increased levels of TSH because of 'immaturity' of the hypothalamopituitary–thyroid axis. Lowering the initial TSH screening threshold may identify 'at-risk' infants and reduce the need for a second dried bloodspot sample (Korada et al. 2008).

Other abnormalities of thyroid function in the neonatal period

Transient hypothyroidism and hyperthyrotropinaemia (subclinical hypothyroidism)

In this heterogeneous group of disorders, the TSH is raised and thyroid hormone concentrations are within the age-related

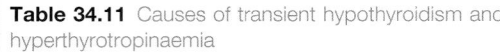

Table 34.11 Causes of transient hypothyroidism and hyperthyrotropinaemia

Congenital hypothyroidism at the milder end of the spectrum (e.g. dysgenesis associated with a hemithyroid)
Maternal antibodies
Exposure to iodine-containing compounds
Exposure to antithyroid drugs in utero
Iodine deficiency
Down syndrome
In association with prematurity
Pseudohypoparathyroidism

reference range (hyperthyrotropinaemia) or temporarily low (hypothyroidism). Babies may have had a mild abnormality of thyroid function detected by the screening programme or may have had thyroid function checked for other reasons. Although thyroid function may normalise within the first few months of life, some of these infants may have a permanent, albeit subtle, abnormality of thyroid function (Daliva et al. 2000; Calaciura et al. 2002). There are well-established causes of transient thyroid dysfunction but some of these children will lie at the mild end of the CHT phenotypic spectrum. The overlap with CHT is illustrated by the transient hyperthyrotropinaemia that can occur in infants with an underlying dyshormonogenesis (Moreno et al. 2002). These babies are presumably unable to meet the demand for T_4 in the early neonatal period. Some babies with hyperthyrotropinaemia will have abnormal thyroid gland morphology (Calaciura et al. 2002).

A list of causes of hyperthyrotropinaemia/transient hypothyroidism is given in Table 34.11. Noteworthy causes of transient hypothyroidism include intrauterine exposure to antithyroid drugs (Cheron et al. 1981), iodine deficiency (Köhler et al. 1996; Ares et al. 1997) and exposure to topical iodinated antiseptic agents. The last are readily absorbed and should be avoided or carefully removed following initial application (Smerdely et al. 1989; Brown et al. 1997; Linder et al. 1997). Transient hypothyroidism may also be due to the transplacental passage of thyrotropin receptor-blocking antibodies in approximately 2% of cases of CHT (Brown et al. 1996) and it is wise to check a mother's thyroid status in these circumstances. Causes of permanent hyperthyrotropinaemia include abnormalities of thyroid gland development (Zung et al. 2010) and abnormalities of the TSH receptor (Alberti et al. 2002). Abnormal thyroid imaging is, not surprisingly, more common in babies with permanent hyperthyrotropinaemia (Zung et al. 2010). Transient hypothyroidism and hyperthyrotropinaemia appear to be more common in the preterm infant with some infants demonstrating the delayed TSH rise described above. Hence iodine deficiency or exposure to excess iodine could result in a 'delayed' TSH rise as well as transient hypothyroidism and hyperthyrotropinaemia.

Intervention is important in those patients with low thyroid hormone levels and some clinicians may treat relatively subtle increases in TSH that persist on the basis that this is a marker of thyroid hormone insufficiency within the developing CNS (Fisher 1999; Rapaport 2000). Intervention is of unproven benefit but likely to be safe provided the infant is monitored appropriately and TSH suppression avoided.

Transient hypothyroxinaemia (Rapaport et al. 2001)

All premature infants have some degree of hypothyroxinaemia because cord serum T_4 values increase with gestational age. Low T_4 levels in the preterm infant reflect the loss of the normal maternal

T_4 supply, immaturity of the hypothalamopituitary–thyroid axis, as well as other factors such as the ongoing fetal tendency to convert thyroid hormone to inactive rT_3. Low thyroid hormone values persist in the first 1–2 weeks in association with low fT_4 and normal TSH levels. This biochemical picture tends to be more profound in the most preterm babies (Van Wassenaer et al. 1997). This was thought to be of little consequence, but more recent evidence indicates that there is a relationship between T_4 concentrations in preterm and low-birthweight (LBW) infants and subsequent neurodevelopmental outcome (Meijer et al. 1992; Den Ouden et al. 1996; Reuss et al. 1996; Leviton et al. 1999).

The impact of thyroid hormone administration on the short- and longer-term outcome following preterm delivery has yet to be established. Improvements in survival have been reported in some studies (Schonberger et al. 1981) but not others (Chowdhry et al. 1984) and early neurodevelopmental outcome does not appear to be affected by treatment. A subgroup analysis in the study by Van Wassenaer et al. (1997) suggested a potential benefit of T_4 treatment (8 µg/kg/day) on the Bayley Mental Development Index in babies of 25–26 weeks' gestation. However, evidence from the same and other studies has suggested that increasing T_4 delivery in babies born at 27–29 weeks may have an adverse effect on neurodevelopment. A more recent report from the same group, as the children reach school age, has confirmed the improved IQ with a reduction in behavioural problems in those receiving T_4 at less than 27 weeks, and lower IQ with more developmental problems in those receiving T_4 at 29 weeks (Briet et al. 2001). The effects of T_4 administration may therefore depend on the gestation and age of the infant treated, with protective mechanisms ensuring an adequate supply of T_3 in all but the most preterm. At this time, the routine supplementation of babies of any gestation in whom TSH levels are normal is not recommended, but we do recommend following the thyroid hormone levels until they normalise.

It is important to remember that preterm infants with hypothyroxinaemia may have a permanent abnormality of thyroid function which will only become apparent with longer term follow-up (Hunter et al. 1998).

Secondary (hypopituitary) hypothyroidism

Secondary hypothyroidism (TSH deficiency) should be suspected if fT_4 and T_3 levels are low in the presence of a low, normal or paradoxically mildly elevated TSH. The differential diagnosis of this biochemical picture includes euthyroid illness and prematurity (see below). Isolated TSH deficiency is very rare and most infants with secondary hypothyroidism will have other PHDs with associated clinical and biochemical features. Screening programmes using the combination of TSH and T_4 suggest that the incidence of secondary hypothyroidism is around 1 in 16 000. The TSH response to TRH in patients with secondary hypothyroidism may be normal, poor or even exaggerated (Gruneiro de Papendieck et al. 1982).

The 'low T_3 syndrome' (non-thyroidal illness)

This term is used to describe thyroid function tests characterised by low serum T_3 concentrations, normal or raised rT_3, variable T_4 and normal TSH. Fetal T_3 levels are low throughout gestation because of enhanced conversion of T_4 to rT_3, and this picture is frequently observed in preterm infants. As in older patients, T_3 levels may be further reduced by intercurrent illness and by poor nutrition in infants of all gestational ages. Low T_3 levels, like T_4, have been linked to a reduction in IQ in later life (Lucas et al. 1996). T_4 administration to infants of less than 30 weeks' gestation does not increase T_3 levels (Van Wassenaer et al. 1993).

Peripheral abnormalities of thyroid hormone binding, transport or action

Abnormalities of binding proteins: thyroxine-binding globulin deficiency and familial dysalbuminaemic hyperthyroxinaemia

The major carrier protein of the thyroid hormones is thyroxine-binding globulin (TBG). Deficiency of TBG is usually inherited as an X-linked dominant trait and has an incidence in male infants of 1 : 2400 with an overall frequency around 1:4000–4300 in North America (Mandel et al. 1993; Hunter et al. 1998). Affected patients are euthyroid. Total T_4 and T_3 levels are low, but the free fractions are normal and the resting and stimulated TSH values are also normal. TBG measurement is needed for a definitive diagnosis.

Familial dysalbuminaemic hyperthyroxinaemia is a relatively common disorder, affecting 1 in 100 people. It is characterised by increased T_4 levels in clinically euthyroid individuals because of an abnormal albumin molecule that has an increased affinity for thyroid hormone. The abnormal albumin molecule will also interfere with some thyroid hormone assays, leading to spurious and potentially confusing results (Pohlenz et al. 2001). This condition underlines the importance of measuring TSH concentrations in infants with raised thyroid hormone concentrations.

Abnormal thyroid hormone transport into the cell

Thyroid hormone transport across the cell membrane is an active process that involves the membrane protein monocarboxylase transporter 8 (MCT8). MCT8 action is crucial if thyroid hormone is to enter the cell and then exert its biological effects by binding to nuclear thyroid receptors. Mutations in MCT8, located on the X chromosome, result in severe psychomotor retardation with a biochemical picture that classically involves elevated T_3 levels and a normal or mildly elevated TSH. Hemizygous males with MCT8 mutations are severely affected whilst heterozygous females with one abnormal and one normal allele have a normal phenotype in the presence of a milder biochemical abnormality (Friesma et al. 2004).

Thyroid hormone resistance
(Refetoff and Weiss 1997; Weiss and Refetoff 1999)

Resistance to thyroid hormone is caused by mutations in the thyroid hormone receptor (TR beta) gene. The clinical presentation of resistance to thyroid hormone is highly variable and the majority of individuals are completely asymptomatic. Occasionally neonates will be found to have this disorder because of a goitre or because of a raised TSH. A minority may have symptoms suggestive of hypothyroidism such as growth retardation and impaired cognitive ability, whilst others have signs of thyroid hormone excess such as tachycardia or hyperactivity (Blair et al. 2002). The typical picture is of a healthy, clinically euthyroid infant with a raised TSH and raised fT_4 and fT_3. The disorder is usually inherited in an autosomal dominant (AD) manner and so a parent may have similar biochemistry.

Hyperthyroidism

Neonatal thyrotoxicosis

Neonatal thyrotoxicosis is a rare but potentially serious condition, usually caused by the transplacental passage of TSH receptor-stimulating antibodies from the serum of a mother with active, inactive or treated Graves disease (Teng et al. 1980). It may also occur when the mother has autoimmune thyroid disease other than Graves (Hoffman et al. 1982). The disease is usually transient, resolving within the timespan of the circulating antibodies. Neonatal hyperthyroidism is underrecognised but it can often be predicted and treated prenatally.

TSH receptor-stimulating antibodies may be demonstrated in the majority of patients with Graves disease and they cross the placenta freely. Thyrotoxicosis in the fetus may lead to preterm labour, LBW, stillbirth and neonatal death. Approximately 1% of babies of mothers with Graves disease become overtly thyrotoxic, although the absolute risk is related to the concentration of TSH receptor-stimulating antibodies in the maternal serum (Munro et al. 1978; Zakarija et al. 1986; Skuza et al. 1996) and some babies will be biochemically toxic but asymptomatic. Thyroid dysfunction has been detected in as many as 16.5% of babies born to women with Graves disease (Mitsuda et al. 1992). TSH receptor-blocking antibodies may be present as well, and the clinical and biochemical picture will reflect a range of factors, including the impact of altered maternal and fetal thyroid hormone levels on fetal hypothalamo-pituitary function as well as the nature and concentration of prevailing antibody concentrations. Exposure to antithyroid drug treatment in utero will also influence the neonatal picture. Hence, an infant who is initially hyperthyroid can subsequently become hypothyroid (requiring T_4 replacement) and an initially hypothyroid infant can become hyperthyroid (Cheron et al. 1981; Hashimoto et al. 1995; Matsuura et al. 1997).

Although neonatal thyrotoxicosis is usually due to the transplacental passage of TSH receptor-stimulating antibodies, activating mutations of the TSH receptor can also give rise to a similar picture. This form of hyperthyroidism is typically inherited in an AD fashion (a parent may have a history of thyroidectomy) and will not resolve spontaneously. Treatment is with total thyroidectomy (Duprez et al. 1994; Kopp et al. 1995).

Clinical features (Table 34.12)

The signs of thyrotoxicosis in the fetus include tachycardia and intrauterine growth retardation. Infants with perinatal thyrotoxicosis may show signs of hyperthyroidism immediately after birth, but

Table 34.12 Clinical features of neonatal hyperthyroidism

Thyroid	Goitre
Central nervous system	Irritability, restlessness, jitteriness, microcephaly
Eyes	Stare, lid retraction, periorbital oedema, exophthalmos
Cardiovascular system	Tachycardia, cardiac failure, arrhythmia, hypertension
Gastrointestinal tract	Excessive appetite, weight loss, failure to thrive, diarrhoea, hepatosplenomegaly
Other	Sweating, flushing, acrocyanosis, lymphadenopathy, thymic enlargement, thrombocytopenia, bruising, petechiae, hyperviscosity, advanced skeletal maturation, craniosynostosis, microcephaly

symptoms may be delayed as long as 4–7 weeks (Zakarija and McKenzie 1983; Skuza et al. 1996). This may be due to the effect of maternal antithyroid drugs or to the relative effects of both blocking and stimulating antibodies. Infants may have a palpable goitre, and although eye signs, especially proptosis and lid retraction, can be present at birth, they are often mild or absent throughout the course of the disease. Rarely, a mother with euthyroid ophthalmic Graves disease may produce an infant with eye involvement but no evidence of thyrotoxicosis. Signs of CNS stimulation, such as irritability, restlessness and jitteriness, usually predominate and there is tachycardia and occasionally arrhythmia, which may progress rapidly to severe and intractable heart failure. Other signs of hypermetabolism include an excessive appetite with weight loss or inadequate weight gain, diarrhoea, sweating and flushing. Less predictable clinical features include hepatosplenomegaly, jaundice and accelerated bone maturation, which can cause premature closure of the skull sutures. Mortality rates of 16–25% have been reported and the long-term outcome is uncertain (Skuza et al. 1996).

Management (Fig. 34.10)

Hyperthyroid pregnant women should be treated with the antithyroid thiourea derivatives carbimazole or propylthiouracil (Roti et al. 1996). The use of radioactive iodine is absolutely contraindicated during pregnancy (Carabinas and Tolis 1998) and surgery may precipitate preterm delivery. The antithyroid drugs cross the placenta, and the lowest dose that controls the hyperthyroidism should be used. Propylthiouracil is excreted into breast milk in lower concentrations than carbimazole and hence may be preferable. The 'block and replace' regimen, using higher doses of antithyroid drugs in combination with replacement T_4, should be avoided. If maternal antithyroid treatment causes goitre formation and bradycardia in the fetus, it is possible to give T_4 by intra-amniotic injection. There may be biochemical evidence of transient hypothyroidism in clinically euthyroid babies of mothers treated with antithyroid drugs (Cheron et al. 1981). If fetal tachycardia suggests hyperthyroidism, treatment should be adjusted to maintain the fetal heart rate below 160 beats/min and careful assessment of fetal growth is necessary. Cordocentesis may be used to confirm the diagnosis.

Severe hyperthyroidism carries a high mortality in the newborn. The key to successful management is, first, anticipation and prevention, then control of thyroid status until the disease runs its self-limited course. If the fetus was hyperthyroid and the mother received a thionamide during pregnancy, then the wisest course will usually be to continue the thionamide medicine (CBZ is preferred in children: Rivkees and Mattison 2009) in a suitable neonatal dosage, which is carbimazole 0.5–1.5 mg/kg/24 h in divided doses every 8 hours. Regular assessment of thyroid function is necessary. Babies who are clinically euthyroid but subsequently show signs of hyperthyroidism will also need to be treated. Neonatal thyrotoxicosis usually remits after 2–5 months and so antithyroid medication can be withdrawn around this time.

Administration of a generous dose of antithyroid drug and simultaneous replacement with T_4 ('block and replace') has been used in thyrotoxic infants but the relatively short duration of the hyperthyroid phase makes this approach impractical in most babies. If a baby is thought to be at particular risk of hyperthyroidism, if a sibling was symptomatic or if there is a high titre of maternal antibodies, then close clinical and biochemical surveillance should be continued for the first weeks of life. Treatment with an antithyroid preparation should be started promptly if necessary.

If acute thyrotoxicosis does occur, then in addition to a thionamide, propranolol 2.0 mg/kg/24 h in divided doses by mouth

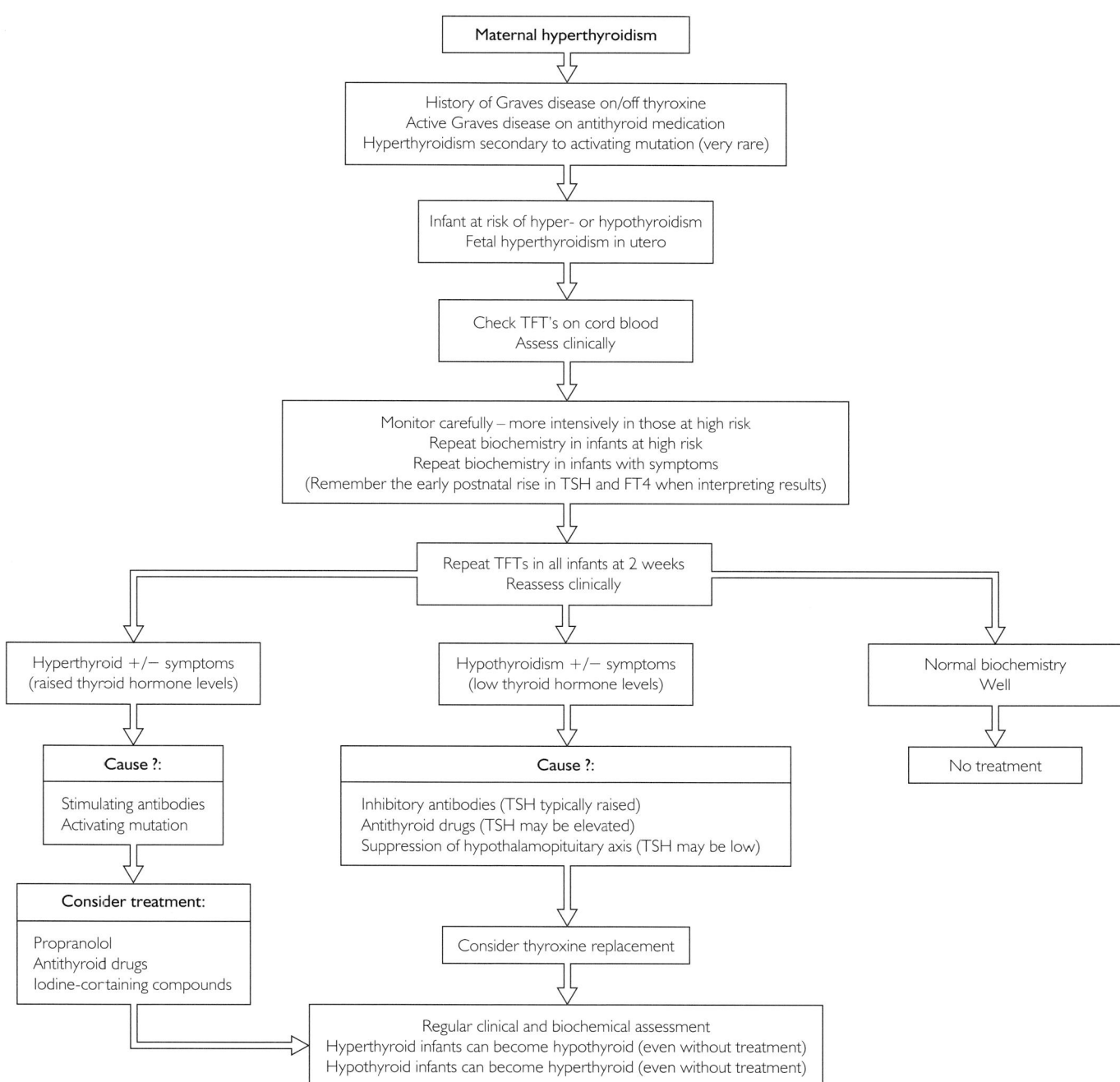

Fig. 34.10 Maternal hyperthyroidism – an approach to the assessment and management of children who are therefore at risk of neonatal hyper- or hypothyroidism. TFT, thyroid function tests; TSH, thyroid stimulating hormone; FT₄, free thyroxine.

6–8-hourly can be used to control the peripheral stimulatory effects of thyroid hormones and/or potassium iodide, as aqueous iodine solution (5% potassium iodide, 130 mg/ml) 0.05–0.1 ml 8-hourly can be administered to prevent synthesis and release of thyroid hormones from the gland. Radiographic iodine-containing agents such as sodium ipodate (0.5 mg every 3 days) have also been used in the treatment of neonatal Graves disease (Karpman et al. 1987). Severely ill babies can be treated with sedatives as well as a glucocorticoid such as prednisolone (2 mg/kg/day) which suppresses T_4 to T_3 conversion.

Occasionally an infant born to a mother with Graves disease will be found to have a hypothyroid picture with low thyroid hormone levels and a raised or suppressed TSH. In some instances, a low TSH and low T_4 reflect suppression of the hypothalamopituitary–thyroid axis by the transplacental passage of thyroid hormone from a hyperthyroid mother, and these babies will need T_4 replacement whilst the axis recovers (Mitsuda et al. 1992; Matsuura et al. 1997; Lee et al. 2002). The transplacental passage of blocking antibodies and exposure to antithyroid drug may account for low thyroid hormone levels.

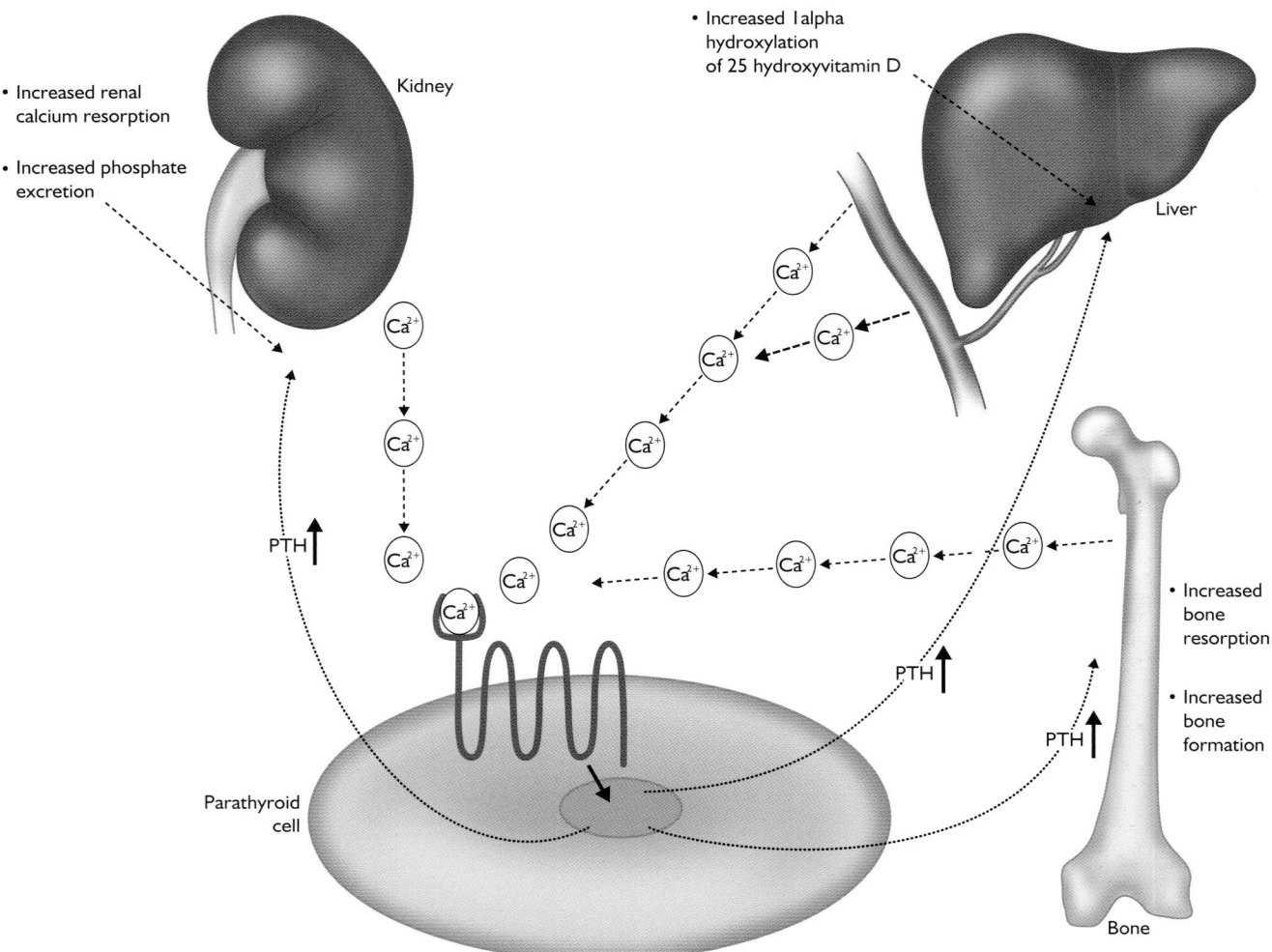

• Increased renal
calcium resorption

• Increased phosphate
excretion

Kidney

• Increased 1 alpha
hydroxylation
of 25 hydroxyvitamin D

Liver

PTH ↑

Ca²⁺

Ca²⁺

Ca²⁺

Ca²⁺

Ca²⁺

Ca²⁺

Ca²⁺

Ca²⁺

Ca²⁺

Ca²⁺

Ca²⁺

Ca²⁺

Ca²⁺

Ca²⁺

Ca²⁺

PTH ↑

• Increased
bone
resorption

• Increased
bone
formation

PTH ↑

Parathyroid
cell

Bone

Fig. 34.11 Calcium. The role of the calcium-sensing receptor and parathyroid hormone (PTH) production in calcium homeostasis. Calcium is detected by the calcium-sensing receptor on the surface of the parathyroid chief cell. Low calcium concentrations result in a rise in PTH release. The effects of PTH include enhanced calcium resorption by the kidney, increased 1α-hydroxylation of 25 hydroxyvitamin D by the liver and increased bone resorption.

Disorders of calcium metabolism

Normal physiology

Calcium is the most plentiful mineral in the body and has a central role in many physiological processes including haemostasis, hormone secretion and action, enzyme activation and inhibition, transmission across cellular membranes and muscle contraction. Calcium is also key to the formation of mineralised connective tissue that provides the skeleton with its structural integrity.

Of the total body stores of calcium, approximately 99% is found in bone and can be considered metabolically inactive as it is mobilised from this pool only slowly. Of the remaining 1%, around half (0.5% of the body total) is the 'biologically active' ionised form. A further 40% is bound to circulating proteins albumin (80%) and globulin (20%), although the exact proportion varies with the serum concentration of albumin and pH. The remainder exists as diffusible non-ionised calcium present in complexes with phosphate and citrate (Hsu and Levine 2004). Because hydrogen ions compete with calcium for protein-binding sites, an increase in acidity will result in a release of calcium from albumin and increase

the ionised fraction of total body calcium. An alkalosis will result in the opposite effect.

The maintenance of serum calcium levels in the physiological range is a complex process that primarily reflects the function of, and interaction between, parathyroid hormone (PTH), vitamin D and the calcium-sensing receptor (CaSR) (Fig. 34.11).

The calcium-sensing receptor

The extracellular CaSR is one of a group of G protein-coupled cell surface receptors. The CaSR modulates the production and secretion of PTH by the chief cells in the parathyroid gland (Tfelt-Hansen and Brown 2005). The CaSR has been termed the 'calciostat' (Egbuna and Brown 2008) because of its fundamental role in maintaining the narrow normal range (Don-Wauchope et al. 2009) of ionised calcium in blood. Rising calcium levels inhibit chief cell activity whilst falling levels of serum calcium will result in a rise in CaSR-induced cellular function. The CaSR is also known to be expressed in other tissues involved in calcium homeostasis, such as bone, gut and kidneys.

Gene defects that result in impaired or enhanced receptor activity can alter the 'set-point' and lead to hypo- or hypercalcaemia. For instance, AD familial benign hypocalciuric hypercalcaemia (impaired receptor function) and hypercalciuric hypocalcaemia (enhanced receptor function) may present in the neonatal period. These rare but important causes of neonatal hyper- and hypocalcaemia are described in more detail below.

Parathyroid hormone

PTH, a polypeptide with 84 amino acid residues, is secreted by the four (occasionally up to seven) parathyroid glands that usually lie behind the thyroid gland. The 34 amino-terminal residue has full biological activity and the function of the remainder of the polypeptide is unknown. Reduced calcium binding on the extracellular side of the CaSR results in an increase in PTH release via exocytosis from the chief cell of the parathyroid gland (Coburn et al. 1999). An increase in circulating phosphate will have a similar effect as it will complex with free ionised calcium to form calcium phosphate which is not detected by the CaSR. Low magnesium levels inhibit PTH secretion and so serum levels of this mineral should be measured whenever hypocalcaemia is being investigated.

When PTH is released, it is rapidly degraded into a number of fragments, the more active of which include the amino-terminal sequence. The half-life of PTH is a few minutes but some inactive fragments remain in the circulation longer.

PTH has three key actions:

1. osteoclast stimulation with an associated release of calcium from bone
2. to promote renal phosphate excretion (and sodium, potassium and bicarbonate) and decrease renal tubular calcium reabsorption (and magnesium and hydrogen ions)
3. the stimulation of 1-α hydroxylase enzyme activity in the proximal renal tubule, thereby increasing the formation of 1,25-dihydroxyvitamin D. This will, in turn, promote intestinal calcium absorption.

The first two actions will regulate calcium levels acutely whilst the third has a more delayed onset of action.

Vitamin D

The two naturally occurring forms of vitamin D are ergocalciferol (D_2), which is derived from ingested vegetables, and cholecalciferol (D_3), which is formed from 7-dehydrocholesterol by the effects of ultraviolet light on the skin. Vitamin D_3 is also absorbed from animal sources in the diet by the upper part of the small intestine. The formed cholecalciferol and absorbed ergo-/cholecalciferol are hydroxylated, primarily by the liver, to 25-hydroxyvitamin D, which is the major circulating vitamin D metabolite. This undergoes 1-hydroxylation in the kidney to 1,25-dihydroxyvitamin D, the metabolically active form, or to the less active 1,24,25-trihydroxyvitamin D or 24,25-dihydroxyvitamin D. 1-hydroxylation is stimulated and 24-hydroxylation inhibited by hypocalcaemia, hypophosphataemia and PTH. Only 1–3% of circulating vitamin D is free, with most bound to vitamin D-binding protein, an α_2-globulin.

The major effect of vitamin D is to increase serum levels of calcium and phosphate by facilitating their absorption from the gut. Vitamin D also enhances the mobilisation of calcium and phosphate from bone when dietary calcium is inadequate and promotes bone mineralisation by maintaining adequate concentrations of calcium and phosphate in the vicinity of unmineralised osteoid.

Fetal 1,25-dihydroxyvitamin D is probably the major stimulus for the placental transfer of calcium.

Other peptide hormones with a more peripheral role in calcium homeostasis

PTH-related peptide (PTHrP)

The circulating levels of PTHrP are low but it is found in breast milk and may have a role in calcium homeostasis in the fetus (Kovacs et al. 2001). PTHrP has an important paracrine role in chondrocyte proliferation and maturation whilst the production of PTHrP by tumour cells is responsible for some cases of tumour-related hypercalcaemia.

Calcitonin

This 32-amino-acid peptide hormone is secreted by the parafollicular C cells of the thyroid in response to hypercalcaemia. It lowers serum calcium by inhibiting bone resorption, increasing urinary calcium and phosphate loss, and probably by decreasing intestinal calcium absorption. Although it can produce hypocalcaemia in humans, neither removal of the thyroid gland nor massive hypersecretion in medullary thyroid carcinoma affects the serum calcium. Hence its physiological significance in humans is unclear, although it may have a role in promoting fetal skeletal mineralisation.

Perinatal calcium metabolism (Hsu et al. 2004)

A baby accumulates 30 g of calcium by term, with 80% of this process occurring during the third trimester (Bowyer et al. 2009). Active transport of calcium and phosphate to the fetus across the placenta is driven by a magnesium adenosine triphosphate-dependent pump which maintains a 1:1.4 mother/fetus gradient, thereby ensuring that the fetus is relatively hypercalcaemic compared with mother (Kovacs and Kronenberg 1997; Bass and Chan 2006). This active transport is regulated by CaSRs present in the placenta. The fetus is not affected directly by maternal PTH, 1,25-dihydroxyvitamin D or calcitonin levels as these hormones do not cross the placenta. However, maternal 25-hydroxyvitamin D does cross the placenta, where it may then promote fetal bone mineralisation by stimulating bone osteoblast activity (Bass and Chan 2006).

Serum total and ionised calcium concentrations are high in cord blood but fall quickly in the first few hours of life as the maternal supply is interrupted. The greatest fall is in ionised calcium, with three-quarters of the total reduction in serum calcium occurring in this fraction (Loughead et al. 1988). A degree of PTH resistance may also be present, although the levels of this hormone are not usually low (Romagnoli et al. 1987). A low milk intake, or blood transfusions that can cause non-ionisable salt formation, may exacerbate hypocalcaemia still further. The nadir in ionised calcium levels occurs around days 2–4 of life, with the low levels stimulating PTH release and a return to adult levels by 2 weeks of age (Mayne and Kovar 1991).

Hypocalcaemia (Singh et al. 2003)

The clinical features of hypocalcaemia in infants include irritability, tremors, twitching and seizures. In contrast, others may be lethargic, feed poorly or vomit. The Chvostek (Hopkins 1964) and Trousseau signs can be unreliable in the newborn examination but the QT interval of the ECG is increased (Giacoia and Wagner 1978).

Table 34.13 Causes of hypocalcaemia

Neonatal hypocalcaemia
   Early (preterm, asphyxiated, infants of diabetic mothers)
   Late (inappropriate feeds)
Hypoparathyroidism
   Microdeletions of chromosome 22q11 and 10p (including
     DiGeorge syndrome)
   X-linked
   Autosomal dominant, including HDR syndrome
   Autosomal recessive
Mitochondrial DNA mutations
Secondary to hypomagnesaemia
Maternal hypercalcaemia
Calcium-sensing receptor defects (activating – hypercalciuric
   hypocalcaemia)
Vitamin D deficiency
Vitamin D-dependent rickets (types I and II)
Pseudohypoparathyroidism (seldom presents in the newborn)
Alkalosis, bicarbonate therapy, citrate in blood transfusion
Renal failure
Malabsorption
Hypoalbuminaemia

HDR, hypoparathyroidism, deafness and renal dysplasia.

Causes

The causes of hypocalcaemia are shown in Table 34.13.

Treatment

Severe symptoms of hypocalcaemia, such as seizures, may be treated with 10% calcium gluconate 0.5–2 ml/kg (0.11–0.46 mmol/kg) by slow i.v. injection over 5–10 minutes. If necessary, this may be followed by continuous infusion of diluted 10% calcium gluconate, 2.5 ml/kg/24 h, with careful monitoring of cardiac rate and rhythm and serum calcium concentration. Calcium solutions are irritant to veins and should ideally be administered via a central venous catheter. Oral calcium supplements (0.25 mmmol/kg qds adjusted according to response) and vitamin D or a vitamin D analogue may be needed for long-term management.

Early hypocalcaemia

Symptomatic hypocalcaemia during the first 3 days of life occurs more commonly in preterm babies, infants of mothers with pre-eclampsia or diabetes and those who suffer birth asphyxia, sepsis or other perinatal stress. To some extent this can be viewed as an exaggeration of the normal postnatal fall in calcium levels. In the preterm infant this reflects a somewhat delayed PTH response to low calcium levels which is compounded by a relative renal resistance to the phosphaturic actions of of PTH. Many infants with early neonatal hypocalcaemia, especially those with diabetic mothers, also have low serum magnesium levels, which, like the hypocalcaemia, usually improve spontaneously.

Late hypocalcaemia due to inappropriate feeds

This clinical picture is now much less common than it was when unmodified cow's milk formulas were widely used. It usually presented with seizures in apparently normal term infants on the fifth to 10th days of life. Classically this was due to the high phosphate and relatively low calcium content of cow's milk. Increased absorption of phosphate caused hyperphosphataemia, which in turn depressed the serum calcium.

Hypoparathyroidism (Shoback 2008)

Hypoparathyroidism is a rare cause of hypocalcaemia in the newborn period. It usually presents after 5 days of age with overt signs of hypocalcaemia. Other biochemical findings include hyperphosphataemia, hypomagnesaemia and a normal or low alkaline phosphatase. The diagnosis is confirmed by the finding of low or absent immunoreactive PTH levels at the time of hypocalcaemia.

The condition may be familial, with X-linked recessive, AD and AR inheritance patterns described, and the underlying cause typically reflects an abnormality of gland development, abnormalities of the PTH molecule itself or abnormalities in other aspects of cellular function. Hypoparathyroidism may be an isolated disorder or it may occur in association with other abnormalities.

Isolated hypoparathyroidism

Defects in the the preproPTH gene can give rise to AD and AR isolated hypoparathyroidism (Arnold 1990; Parkinson and Thakker 1992). The transcription factors GCMB and SOX-3 are involved in parathyroid gland development and mutations can give rise to AR and X-linked recessive hypoparathyroidism, both of which can present in the neonatal period.

DiGeorge syndrome

The most well-known syndrome associated with hypoparathyroidism is the DiGeorge syndrome, which overlaps with the velo-cardiofacial syndrome (Ch. 32). In this spectrum of phenotypes hypoparathyroidism, thymic aplasia, congenital abnormalities of the heart and great vessels, and other dysmorphic features result from deletions within chromosome 22q11. The deletions involve a variable length of chromosome 22 but when hypoparathyroidsm is present there is typically an abnormality of the *TBX1* gene. A small number of cases of DiGeorge syndrome have defects in other chromosomes, notably 10p13 (Daw et al. 1996). The presence of hypocalcaemia with congenital abnormalities should prompt detailed genetic analysis, although it should be remembered that calcium levels may return to normal spontaneously.

Other causes of neonatal hypoparathyroidism

Causes of hypoparathyroidism also include the HDR syndrome (hypoparathyroidism, deafness and renal dysplasia) due to defects in the *GATA3* gene at 10p15 (Van Esch et al. 2000). This is an AD disorder which can present with hypocalcaemia in early life, although the diagnosis of hypoparathyroidism may be delayed by many years. Other rare causes of hypoparathyroidism include the Kenny–Caffey syndrome (short stature, osteosclerosis and ocular abnormalities) and Sanjad–Sakati syndrome (short stature, ocular abnormalities and learning difficulties). Mitochondrial disease such as Kearns–Sayre syndrome and MELAS (mitochondrial encephalomyopathy, lactic acidosis and stroke-like episodes) can also be associated with hypoparathyroidism.

Management of hypoparathyroidism

The potent water-soluble analogues of vitamin D should be used to treat hypoparathyroidism. A suitable dose in the newborn is alpha-calcidol (1α-hydroxycholecalciferol) or calcitriol (1,25-dihydroxycholecalciferol) 0.03–0.08 μg/kg/24 h up to a maximum of 1–2 μg. The maintenance dose needed varies not only between patients but also in the same patient at different times;

frequent measurement of the serum calcium is therefore necessary, with dose adjustments to keep the level within the normal range. Supplementary oral calcium is not essential but may help to stabilise the serum calcium. It should be remembered that a suboptimal vitamin D status is common in early life and so a vitamin D supplement may be required as well (see below).

Other causes of hypocalcaemia

Hypomagnesaemia

Hypomagnesaemia may cause clinically significant hypocalcaemia both by inhibiting the secretion of PTH and by reducing PTH responsiveness (Visudhiphan 2005). As many as 80% of infants with hypocalcaemic fits may be relatively hypomagnesaemic as well, and the hypocalcaemia may prove to be difficult to correct until the hypomagnesaemia has been addressed. This is most easily done by giving intramuscular (i.m.) or intravenous (i.v.; over at least 10 minutes) magnesium sulphate 0.4 mmol/kg Mg^{2+} (100 mg/kg magnesium sulphate) every 8–12 hours. The serum magnesium should therefore be measured in all infants with persistent hypocalcaemia.

There are other, rare, primary abnormalities of intestinal magnesium absorption (AR familial hypomagnesaemia with hypocalcaemia) and renal magnesium handling (primary hypomagnesaemia) which need to be considered in the hypomagnesaemic, hypocalcaemic patient. Hypomagnesaemia may be a feature of Gitelman syndrome and Bartter syndrome.

Maternal hypercalcaemia

In the presence of maternal hypercalcaemia, the fetus is exposed to chronic hypercalcaemia from excessive transplacental passage of calcium and subsequent parathyroid suppression after birth. Whilst this generally resolves spontaneously, maternal calcium levels should be checked whenever there is unexplained hypocalcaemia in the newborn (Thomas and Bennett 1995).

Hypercalciuric hypocalcaemia

Hypocalcaemia with hypercalciuria due to activating mutations of the CaSR may present in childhood with seizures. This rare condition should be suspected when hypocalcaemia is associated with hypercalciuria and PTH levels that are within the normal range, in contrast to infants with hypoparathyroidism (Pearce et al. 1996). It is important to be aware of this condition because vitamin D administration may lead to nephrocalcinosis. No active treatment is needed.

Vitamin D deficiency

Maternal and hence infant vitamin D status is a key determinant of bone mineralisation in the newborn (Viljakainen et al. 2010). Vitamin D deficiency can present as neonatal seizures before any change in skeletal phenotype has become apparent. The vitamin D status of an infant will reflect the mother's diet and her exposure to sunlight, as well as postnatal factors such as the type of feed. Maternal vitamin D deficiency, although particularly common in racial groups with pigmented skin, is found in up to a third of all mothers at the time of delivery even in industrialised nations (Merewood et al. 2010). Less common but important manifestations of vitamin D deficiency include dilated cardiomyopathy (Maiya et al. 2008).

Most commercial milk preparations contain enough vitamin D to prevent rickets, but supplementation is still advisable (Shaw and Pal 2002; Taylor et al. 2010). Current recommendations are that all breastfed infants receive 280–400 IU of vitamin D daily from the age of 6 months if consuming <500 ml/day of infant formula, and that 'at-risk' groups should start supplements before 6 months. Babies with vitamin D deficiency should be treated with vitamin D (ergo- or cholecalciferol) in a dose of 3000 IU for 2–3 months, with supplements thereafter.

Vitamin D-dependent rickets (VDDR)

VDDR type I is due to defective renal hydroxylation of vitamin D (Kitanaka et al. 1998) whereas in VDDR type II there is cellular resistance to hormone action, which is usually due to mutations in the steroid-binding domain or the DNA-binding domain of the vitamin D receptor (Hughes et al. 1988). Both of these disorders can present with rickets in infancy. Levels of 1,25-dihydroxyvitamin D are reduced in type I VDDR but elevated in type II. The terminology is confusing because VDDR type II will not respond to physiological levels of vitamin D but might to very high doses. VDDR type I is treated with hydroxylated vitamin D metabolites – calcitriol or 1α-calcidol.

Pseudohypoparathyroidism

The term 'pseudohypoparathyroidism' is used to describe several related disorders characterised by peripheral unresponsiveness to the action of PTH because of a receptor or postreceptor defect. This is an uncommon cause of hypocalcaemia in infancy which can, for similar reasons, result in TSH resistance and neonatal hyperthyrotropinaemia (see above). The characteristic biochemical findings are hypocalcaemia with hyperphosphataemia, raised levels of PTH and an absent or impaired response to exogenous PTH. These conditions are usually inherited as an AD trait with variable penetrance. Treatment of hypocalcaemia in this disorder requires calcium supplements and a vitamin D analogue (see below).

Miscellaneous causes of neonatal hypocalcaemia

Hypocalcaemia may occur in alkalosis, with citrate administration in blood transfusion, and in hypoalbuminaemic states. It may also arise in infants with renal failure who have hyperphosphataemia.

Hypercalcaemia (Rodd and Goodyer 1999)

Hypercalcaemia is an uncommon problem in infancy and can be defined as a serum calcium above 2.75 mmol/l. The causes of hypercalcaemia are shown in Table 34.14 and are described in more detail below, but conceptually can be thought of as reflecting vitamin D or calcium excess, disease associated with reduced bone formation (hypophosphatasia) or increased bone resorption (e.g. some tumours). Occasionally a raised serum calcium can reflect an abnormality of the CaSR (hypocalciuric hypercalcaemia) (Zajickova et al. 2007) with an associated altered 'set-point', and it may also be a manifestation of Williams syndrome. Primary hyperparathyroidism (as opposed to neonatal severe hyperparathyroidism resulting from a CaSR defect) does not occur in infancy. Clinical manifestations of hypercalcaemia include hypotonia, weakness and irritability, poor feeding, weight loss, constipation, vomiting, polydipsia and polyuria. Hypercalciuria can give rise to nephrocalcinosis.

Treatment

Whilst the primary cause must be corrected if possible, the key component of short-term treatment of neonatal hypercalcaemia is a reduction in dietary calcium intake using low-calcium feed. Generous hydration and furosemide diuresis promote urinary calcium loss if a more acute reduction is needed. Glucocorticoids (e.g. hydrocortisone 1 mg/kg 6-hourly) reduce intestinal calcium

Table 34.14 Causes of hypercalcaemia

Excess vitamin D
Idiopathic infantile hypercalcaemia
Williams syndrome
Phosphate depletion in low-birthweight infants
Calcium-sensing receptor defects (inactivating)
   Benign familial hypercalcaemia with hypocalciuria
   Neonatal severe hyperparathyroidism
Maternal hypoparathyroidism
Subcutaneous fat necrosis
Hypophosphatasia
Malignancy
Vitamin A intoxication
Activating parathyroid hormone receptor mutations (Jensen
   syndrome)

absorption but the effect is slow and they should not be used if neoplasia is suspected. Calcitonin (10 U/kg i.v.) may be useful and has its maximum effect in 1 hour; infusions may be repeated 4-hourly. The hormone is antigenic and so the synthetic derivative salcatonin should be used in the longer term. Experience with the bisphosphonates is increasing (Fox et al. 2007) and pamidronate in a dose of 0.5–1.0 mg/kg as an i.v. infusion may be worth considering in particularly difficult cases (Waller et al. 2004). Long-term safety data following administration in infancy are not yet available.

Causes of hypercalcaemia (Table 34.14)

Hypercalcaemia in association with excess vitamin D

Infantile hypercalcaemia was relatively common in the UK when foods were liberally supplemented with vitamin D. It generally presented with signs of hypercalcaemia in the early months of life, but was generally mild and self-limiting (Lightwood syndrome). The incidence fell when the use of vitamin D supplements was reduced. It is thought to have affected infants with a particular sensitivity to vitamin D in whom the cumulative daily vitamin D dose could reach 2000–4000 IU or more. Hypercalcaemia due to excessive vitamin D intake has been reported in association with prolonged administration of preterm formula (Nako et al. 1993).

Williams syndrome (Ch. 31)

Williams syndrome is a contiguous gene deletion disorder caused by hemizygous loss of 1.5–1.8 Mb on chromosome 7q11.23 (see Ch. 32 for details of the phenotype). Hypercalcaemia is present in around 15% and tends to resolve spontaneously, but the other features persist. The condition is usually sporadic, although familial AD inheritance has also been observed. In the hypercalcaemic phase, treatment is with a low-calcium milk/diet and then a cautious reintroduction of calcium once the biochemistry has been normalised. Controlling serum calcium does not affect the progression of the other features of the disease.

Hypercalcaemia due to phosphate depletion

Severe hypercalcaemia may occur in LBW preterm infants with hypophosphataemia due to a low phosphate intake from breast milk or parenteral feeding. The hypercalcaemia responds to phosphate repletion (Miller et al. 1984).

Benign familial hypocalciuric hypercalcaemia and neonatal severe hyperparathyroidism

These disorders are associated with mutations in the extracellular calcium ion-sensing receptor which lead to loss of function. The 'set-point' at which PTH is released is therefore altered. Benign familial hypercalcaemia is inherited as an AD trait (one abnormal allele), whereas the severe neonatal form is associated with both heterozygous and homozyous mutations of the CaSR gene (Pidasheva et al. 2004). Factors influencing the phenotype in this disorder include the number of mutant genes as well as the extent to which the calcium receptor is compromised. The phenotype may also be influenced by the pattern of inheritance: if the infant inherits the mutant allele from the father, then PTH production will be more exaggerated, because of the discrepancy between the maternal and fetal CaSR 'set-point' in utero. The neonatal form can lead to hypotonia, respiratory distress and failure to thrive, in association with hypercalcaemia and elevated PTH levels. There is skeletal undermineralisation, with rib fractures and subperiosteal erosions. The treatment of severe cases, usually homozygous for receptor mutations, may entail urgent parathyroidectomy, but some neonatal cases appear to run a milder, self-limiting course (Wilkinson and James 1993). Some of these cases will be heterozygote infants with the abnormal allele inherited from the father. Earlier reports of primary hyperparathyroidism in neonatal life probably included children with calcium receptor abnormalities. Bisphosphonates may help to protect the skeleton from the harmful effects of hyperparathyroidism prior to surgical intervention (Waller et al. 2004).

Hyperparathyroidism secondary to maternal hypoparathyroidism

Secondary hyperparathyroidism may be due to untreated maternal hypoparathyroidism, which causes fetal hypocalcaemia and parathyroid hyperplasia; this condition is self-limiting but the hypercalcaemia may need treatment with hydration and calcitonin.

Subcutaneous fat necrosis

Hypercalcaemia may occur in association with extensive neonatal subcutaneous fat necrosis, which is seen especially after traumatic delivery of large infants, or cold injury. This may be due to unregulated production of 1,25-dihydroxyvitamin D by the affected adipose tissue (Kruse et al. 1993).

Hypophosphatasia (Whyte 1994)

Hypophophatasia is an AR disorder due to defects in the gene for tissue non-specific (bone/liver/kidney) alkaline phosphatase.

The perinatal form is characterised by extreme skeletal hypomineralisation and babies often die in utero or in early postnatal life. The infantile form is defined by a presentation before the age of 6 months. Clinical features include poor feeding, hypotonia, craniotabes, blue sclerae and a rachitic deformity of the limbs. Hypercalcaemia and hypercalciuria reflect poor skeletal growth and mineralisation. The infantile form of the disease is fatal in approximately 50% of patients and, whilst treatment options are limited, trials of recombinant alkaline phosphatase are showing promising results.

Idiopathic infantile hypercalcaemia (Langman 1999)

Idiopathic infantile hypercalcaemia remains a poorly defined entity that is diagnosed once other causes have been excluded. Infants can present with the symptoms and signs of hypercalcaemia, including polyuria and polydipsia, and some have features in common with Williams syndrome, such as facial dysmorphism and cardiac defects (Martin et al. 1984). There is recent evidence to suggest that the hypercalcaemia is linked to abnormal vitamin D metabolism as well as abnormal PTHrP production. The hypercalcaemia can be more difficult to treat than in Williams syndrome and may persist for longer.

Miscellaneous causes of hypercalcaemia

Vitamin A excess, adrenal failure, drugs such as thiazide diuretics, muscle disease with associated inactivity and malignancy are rare causes of hypercalcaemia in early life. Constitutively activating PTH receptor mutations result in Jansen syndrome and a phenotype that includes hypercalcaemia and short-limbed dwarfism (Schipani et al. 1996).

Adrenal

Normal development and function

The adrenal gland lies adjacent to the upper pole of the kidney and has two embryologically and functionally distinct components. The medulla is formed from neural crest cells which enter the gland at about the seventh week of gestation and secrete catecholamines. Clinically significant abnormalities of medullary function are not recognised in the newborn. The cortex is derived from mesodermal cells near the cephalic part of the mesonephros. It shares common primordial cells with the gonads, which also secrete steroids and may express similar enzyme deficiencies. The fetal adrenal is 20–30 times larger than the adult gland relative to body weight (twice as large in absolute terms), which reflects its contribution to oestrogen production in utero. At birth both glands together weigh 7–9 g. They are largely composed of the histologically distinct fetal cortex, which constitutes 80% of the gland at birth and which then involutes rapidly, reducing to half its size by 2 weeks and disappearing by 6 months.

The enzyme activities of the fetal adrenal and the placenta are complementary; thus the placenta lacks the enzymatic activity necessary to generate androgens from the precursors, pregnenolone and progesterone (17α-hydroxylase and 17,20-desmolase; Fig. 34.12), whereas the fetal adrenal lacks the enzymatic activity to produce oestrogen from androgens, until the later stages of gestation. The adrenal androgens (primarily dehydroepiandrosterone and its sulphate) are converted to oestrogen by the placenta, which expresses the necessary sulphatase and aromatase enzyme activity. Hence the fetal adrenal provides the precursors necessary for placental oestrogen production, and steroid production by the fetoplacental unit as a whole promotes maturation of organs such as the lungs (Ng 2000). A deficiency of placental aromatase leads to virilisation of both the mother and female infants during pregnancy (Shozu et al. 1991; Belgorosky et al. 2009).

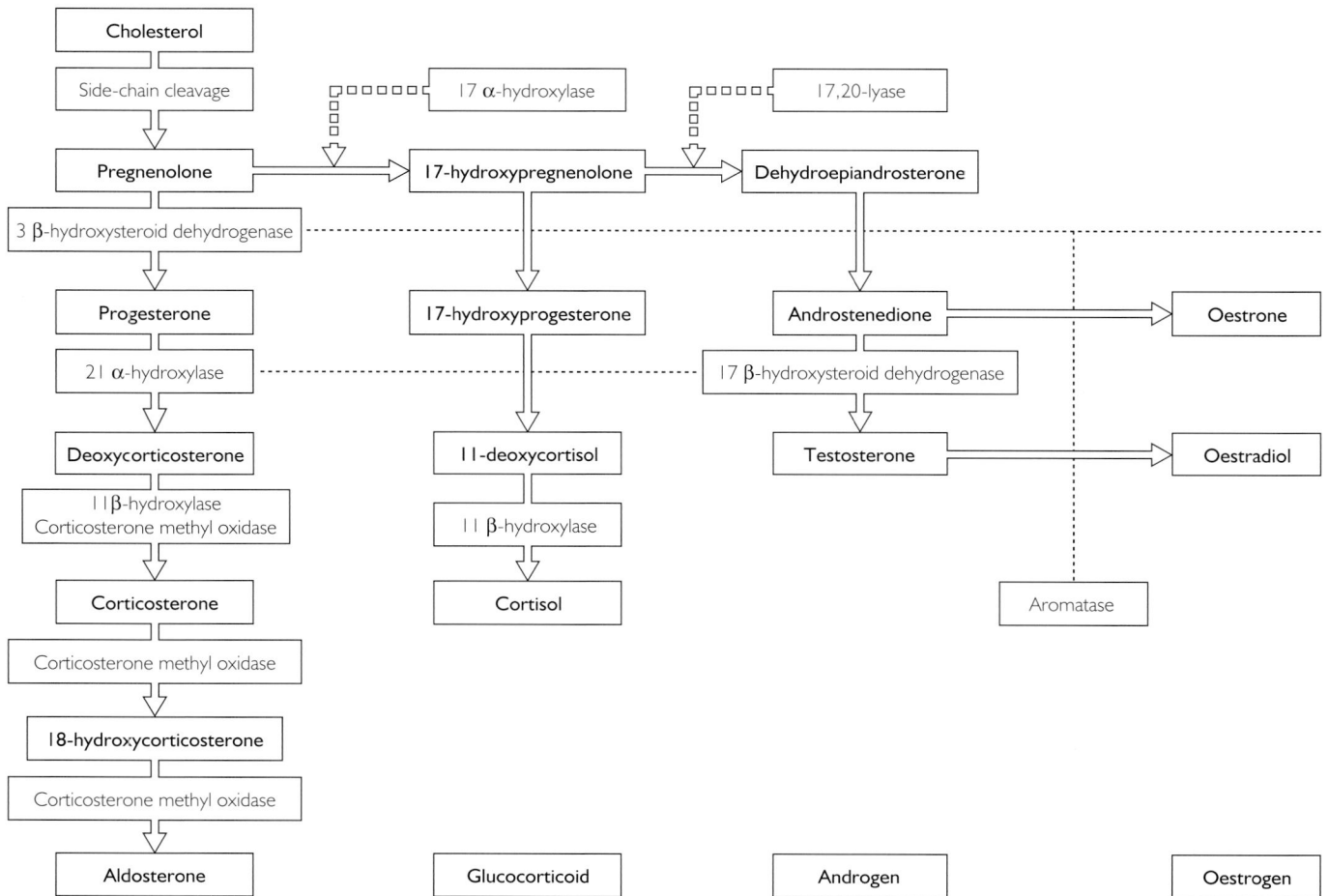

Fig. 34.12 Steroidogenic pathway: adrenal steroid biosynthesis. Steroids and steroid precursors are in bold.

The adrenal cortex secretes three major groups of steroid hormones: glucocorticoids, mineralocorticoids and androgens, all of which are derived from cholesterol. The gland has three histologically distinct zones. The outer zone, the zona glomerulosa, contains the enzymes for aldosterone biosynthesis but little 17α-hydroxylase, so it produces little cortisol or androgen. Aldosterone release is primarily controlled by the renin–angiotensin system and by the plasma concentrations of sodium and potassium, with ACTH playing a minor role. The two inner zones, fasciculata and reticularis, secrete cortisol and androgens, respectively, but no aldosterone. ACTH is the primary regulator of cortisol synthesis and also has a role in the regulation of androgen production.

Whilst umbilical cord cortisol concentrations are positively related to gestation (Kari et al. 1996), cortisol concentrations subsequently fall with increasing postnatal and postconceptional age (Midgley et al. 2001). Cortisol levels reach a nadir in the first weeks of life in well term and preterm infants, although the pattern will be influenced by general well-being (Scott and Watterberg 1995). Cortisol levels tend to be lower in the very sick, preterm infant, although the more mature preterm infant (greater than 30 weeks' gestation) may be able to mount a more appropriate stress response (Grofer et al. 2010). Hence, the postnatal trend in cortisol concentrations is linked to gestational age and postnatal age as well as other factors, such as intrauterine growth and the presence of intercurrent illness. The apparent inability of the more preterm infant to mount an appropriate stress response, which can be associated with clinically significant hypotension, may be linked to enzymatic immaturity of the adrenal gland and with an associated inability to manufacture cortisol directly from cholesterol (Hingre et al. 1994).

The ability of the adrenal gland to respond more appropriately to ACTH production has developed by 2 weeks of age (Ng 2000). The normal circadian pattern of cortisol release is usually established by 3 months of age, but has been identified as early as 2 weeks postdelivery (Santiago et al. 1996). The assessment of steroid concentrations is complicated by the limitations of immunoassays, including crossreactivity, and accurate determination of steroids is increasingly being undertaken using high-performance liquid chromatography/tandem mass spectrometry.

Inherited disorders of steroidogenesis: the congenital adrenal hyperplasias

Congenital adrenal hyperplasia (CAH) is a generic term used to describe a series of AR disorders that prevent normal adrenal steroidogenesis. Chronic ACTH stimulation and impaired cortisol synthesis result in a histological appearance characterised by hyperplastic adrenal tissue. The phenotype of an affected infant is the result of steroid hormone deficiency coupled with the effects of excess steroidogenic precursors. CAH is one of the leading causes of ambiguous genitalia. More than 95% of cases of CAH are due to 21α-hydroxylase deficiency, with the remaining 5% due to deficiencies in one of the other steroidogenic enzymes. Some of the steroidogenic steps are common to the adrenal gland and gonad and so impaired glucocorticoid and mineralocorticoid production can be associated with reduced gonadal sex steroid production.

Pathogenesis

A simplified schematic representation of adrenal steroid biosynthesis is shown in Figure 34.12, and, with this background, some of the consequences of a given enzyme defect can be elucidated. These are summarised in Table 34.15.

21α-hydroxylase deficiency

This condition classically presents as salt-losing, simple virilising or non-classical forms. There is a close link between residual enzyme activity and phenotype: the more severe gene defects result in the salt-losing form, whilst patients with significant residual enzyme activity will have the milder, non-classical or late-onset form. Boys are underrepresented in most series and some have presumably succumbed to adrenal insufficiency before the diagnosis was made in early life or have signs of androgen production in later life that are considered normal. The overall prevalence in the UK and Europe is approximately 1 in 18,000, whilst this rate (Pang et al. 1982), whilst this rate is known to increase dramatically in certain ethnic and population groups, such as Yupik Eskimos where the rate is 1 in 282 (Pang et al. 1982). The majority of affected individuals

Table 34.15 Major clinical and biochemical features of enzymatic blocks in adrenocortical steroid biosynthesis

ENZYME DEFECT	CLINICAL FEATURES		
	Male	Female	Salt status
21α-Hydroxylase			
Simple virilising	N	Virilised	N
Salt-losing	N	Virilised	Loss
11β-Hydroxylase	N	Virilised	Retention (salt loss may occur in early life)
3β-Hydroxysteroid	Undervirilisation	N or mild virilisation	N or loss
17α-Hydroxylase	Undervirilisation Undervirilisation	N	Retention with hypertension
Lipoid CAH (StAR and side-chain cleavage defects)	Undervirilisation	N	Severe loss
P450-Oxidoreductase	Undervirilisation	Virilised	N
Corticosterone methyloxidase	N	N	Loss

CAH, congenital adrenal hyperplasia; StAR, steroidogenic regulatory protein.

presenting in early life have salt loss, but some produce enough mineralocorticoid to maintain sodium homeostasis; these children generate sufficient aldosterone while on appropriate glucocorticoid replacement, despite impaired enzyme activity. The genetics of 21α-hydroxylase deficiency have been extensively studied. There are two 21α-hydroxylase genes, one of which is inactive (*CYP21A*) and one active (*CYP21B*). They are both located on chromosome 6, interspersed between the genes encoding the C4 component of complement and in close proximity to the human leukocyte antigen (HLA) complex (Krone and Arlt 2009). Most affected individuals will be compound heterozygotes for a relatively small number of gene defects: the *CYP21B* locus (normally the active gene sequence) is affected by a gene conversion whereby part or all of this gene is converted to the inactive gene sequence of *CYP21A*. Most patients with salt loss have gene deletions or conversions that severely impair enzyme activity, whilst patients with the non-classical form will have two abnormal alleles but there will be enough residual enzyme activity to maintain health and a normal phenotype in the newborn period.

Clinical presentation

The clinical features reflect the combination of impaired cortisol/aldosterone production and androgen excess. Reduced cortisol generation leads to enhanced ACTH production with hyperplasia of the adrenal cortex and excess androgen release as the gland attempts to overcome the steroidogenic block. In the simple virilising form the steroidogenic defect is not as profound as in the salt-wasting form and residual enzyme activity can generate sufficient cortisol and aldosterone to survive but not enough to prevent excess androgen release. In male babies there may be some increase in pigmentation, especially of the scrotum, but there is no anatomical abnormality. If the infant with simple virilising CAH is not treated, then continued postnatal overproduction of androgen causes further virilisation and rapid growth.

In females the prenatal androgen overproduction will virilise the external genitalia. In the least affected infants there may be only slight clitoral enlargement, whilst in the more severely virilised

cases there is fusion of the labioscrotal folds and the clitoris becomes almost as large as a normal neonatal penis. These female babies can resemble a cryptorchid male and may be misdiagnosed as such. A moderately severely virilised female with CAH is shown in Figure 34.13 and the spectrum through from normal female to an apparently normal male is shown in Figure 34.14.

In salt-losing CAH, inadequate production of aldosterone leads to renal salt loss. Affected neonates can become seriously unwell because of sodium depletion, with typical presentation in the second week of life. The early signs are vomiting, anorexia and, sometimes, diarrhoea, which, if untreated, may develop into full addisonian crisis. Further investigations reveal hyponatraemia, hyperkalaemia and acidosis and this picture should raise the possibility of CAH if it has not been suspected previously. Conditions that may be confused with salt-wasting CAH include renal tract malformations, urinary tract infection and pyloric stenosis. Cortisol deficiency can also result in hypoglycaemia.

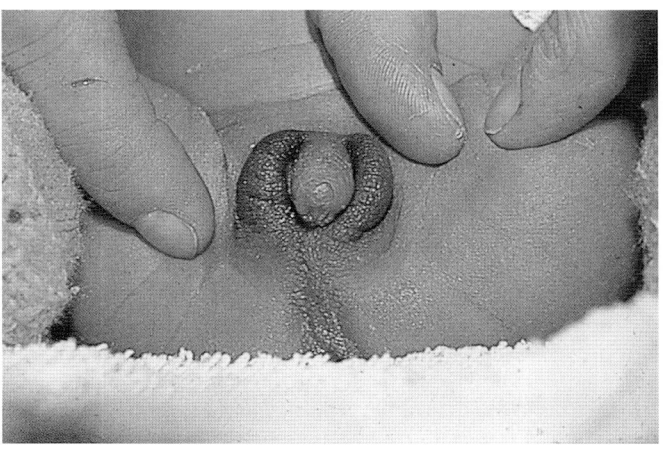

Fig. 34.13 Ambiguous genitalia. Genitalia of a female infant with 21α-hydroxylase deficiency.

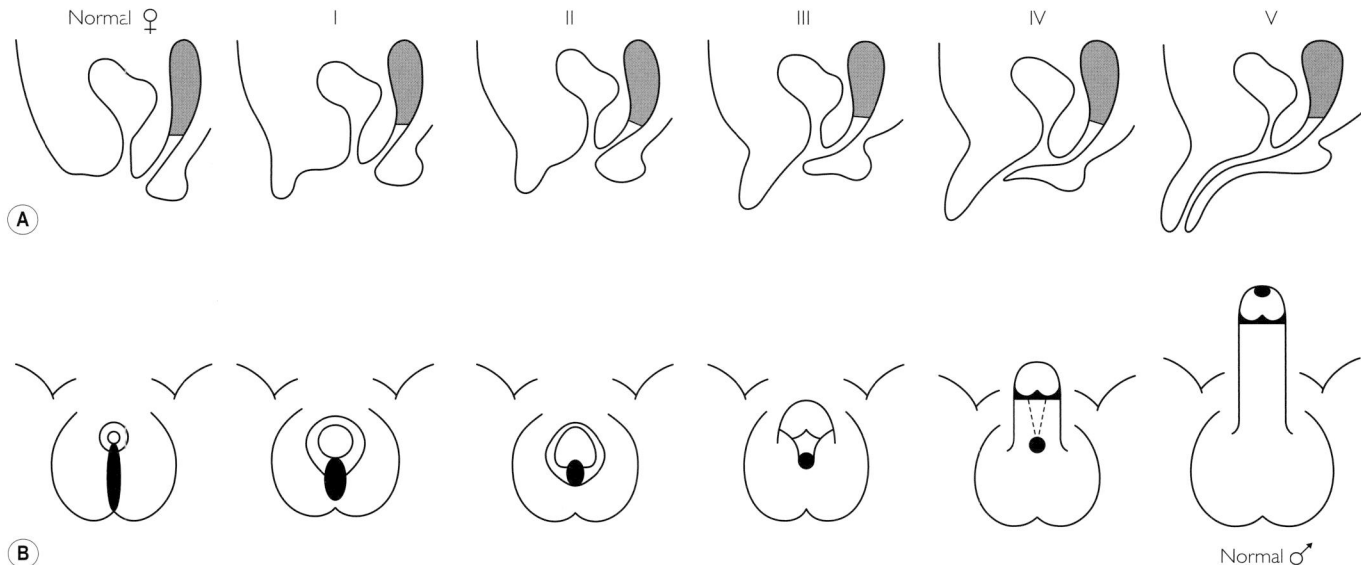

Fig. 34.14 Prader staging. Virilisation of the external genitalia based on the staging system of Prader and adapted from Miller (2001). A spectrum from normal female through to normal male is shown. Virilisation of a normal female (as in congenital adrenal hyperplasia) will result in any stage from I to V, and undervirilisation of a male (XY karyotype) will result in any appearance from IV through to normal female (as in partial or complete androgen insensitivity syndrome – see section 0895).

Diagnosis

A baby presenting with a biochemical picture suggestive of a salt-wasting crisis requires resuscitation and an urgent renal and pelvic ultrasound. This can help to exclude renal malformations, and the identification of enlarged echogenic adrenals is a helpful pointer towards CAH at a time when 17-hydroxyprogesterone (17-OHP) levels are awaited. When the genitalia are ambiguous, establishing the genetic sex of the infant by examination of the karyotype is a priority. In 21α-hydroxylase deficiency, there is gross elevation of plasma 17-OHP concentrations. Levels are relatively high in healthy infants in the first hours of life and seriously ill preterm infants may also show moderate elevation of plasma 17-OHP in the absence of adrenal hyperplasia (Ng 2000; Murphy et al. 1983). However, by 24 hours of age, the elevated plasma 17-OHP is usually diagnostic of CAH. Babies with congenital adrenal hypoplasia (see later) can present with a similar electrolyte imbalance but 17-OHP levels will not be raised. The plasma ACTH level is raised in many states of cortisol deficiency, so this is a non-specific test. 11β-hydroxylase deficiency can be misdiagnosed as 21α-hydroxylase deficiency and so it is wise to collect a sample of urine at presentation for urinary steroid profile analysis by gas chromatography mass spectrometry. If this is collected before or in the very early stages of treatment, then the precise enzyme defect can be established defect can be established. It is possible to measure plasma 11-deoxycortisol (raised in 11β-hydroxylase deficiency) as well as 17-OHP, but poor assay specificity can lead to confusion. A case has been made for confirming the diagnosis of 21α-hydroxylase deficiency at the molecular level, partly because it can help to define the severity of 21α-hydroxylase deficiency (Nordenstrom et al. 1999).

Prenatal diagnosis and treatment

The prenatal administration of glucocorticoids to the mother of a female fetus with 21α-hydroxylase deficiency can reduce the degree of fetal virilisation and hence the need for postnatal surgery (Forest 1998; New 2001). Girls with CAH have a more 'masculine' pattern of play than is usual (Nordenstrom et al. 2002) and so there may be behavioural implications of reducing androgen exposure in utero. The role and in particular the risk/benefit ratio of this intervention are still unclear, with particular concerns about the impact of high doses of glucocorticoid on growth and CNS function.

Before the pregnancy, the potential benefits and risks of prenatal treatment must therefore be explained to the parents. There may be less inclination to intervene if a child was only mildly virilised but the phenotype can vary within families and so it is not possible to state that subsequent children will not be more severely affected (Chemaitilly et al. 2005).

In a pregnancy at risk, the mother can be given dexamethasone in a dose of 20 μg/kg/day in two or three divided doses as soon as the pregnancy is confirmed. Dexamethasone crosses the placenta and suppresses fetal ACTH secretion, and so the excess androgen production is curtailed. The treatment needs to be started as early as possible, and certainly before 8 weeks' gestation. It is then necessary to establish the sex of the fetus and whether or not it is affected. As the treatment is needed only for female fetuses with homozygous or compound heterozygous 21α-hydroxylase deficiency, glucocorticoid can be stopped in the seven out of eight pregnancies where the fetus is either male or an unaffected female.

The prenatal diagnosis of 21α-hydroxylase deficiency was originally made by finding raised 17-OHP levels in amniotic fluid. More recently, the likelihood of a pregnancy being affected has been established by HLA typing of the parents, index case and fetus, or by linkage analysis using markers in the region of the 21α-hydroxylase gene (Nimkarn and New 2010). These techniques depend on the proximity of the locus for the 21α-hydroxylase gene to the HLA antigens on chromosome 6 or other adjacent genes. Specific DNA probes or allele-specific polymerase chain reaction can also be used to screen tissue obtained by chorionic villus sampling at 10–12 weeks for mutations previously identified in family members. Recently it has become possible to establish the sex of the fetus at an even earlier stage by identifying fetal cells in the maternal circulation. In the case of a male fetus dexamethasone can then be stopped.

Treatment of the mother with a potent steroid throughout pregnancy clearly carries some risk, and excessive weight gain, glucose intolerance, a rise in blood pressure, gastrointestinal upset and cushingoid features have been recorded. No clear adverse effects on the fetus have been observed to date; however, long-term follow-up studies have demonstrated negative effects on verbal working memory in childhood (Lajic et al. 2008).

Population screening

Measurement of 17-OHP in dried capillary blood samples (like those collected for screening for phenylketonuria and hypothyroidism) is possible and screening has been implemented in many parts of the developed world, including the USA and some western European countries (Honour and Torresani 2001; Riepe and Sippell 2007). Screening programmes have been shown to operate effectively despite the need for a rapid turnaround (Pitt 2010). There are no plans to include CAH in the UK national neonatal screening programme at present.

Treatment (Joint LWPES/ESPE CAH Working Group 2002)

This entails replacing glucocorticoid and, if necessary, mineralocorticoid. The majority of affected girls will also require surgical correction of the virilisation.

A baby presenting in Addisonian crisis should be treated as detailed below. Thereafter the need to suppress ACTH, and hence androgen levels, means that a dose of hydrocortisone of 10–14 mg/m^2/24 h administered as a thrice-daily regimen is appropriate in most infants. This should be trebled to cover significant acute illness and must be given parenterally if oral therapy cannot be tolerated. Pre-prepared liquid preparations may be unpredictable (Merke et al. 2001) but the smallest available tablet contains 2.5 mg hydrocortisone. Fludrocortisone can be given in an initial dose of 100–200 μg twice daily and then adjusted according to sodium levels, blood pressure and renin levels; divisible 100-μg tablets are available. Salt supplements should also be provided to the salt-wasting infant and can be added to the milk. A daily dose of 2–8 mmol/kg/day of additional sodium chloride will ensure adequate intake until the diet contains more salt and until the infant's renal function becomes more refined (Fig. 34.15).

The long-term management consists of, firstly, giving enough glucocorticoid to maintain suppression of the excess androgen production but not enough to cause iatrogenic Cushing syndrome and growth retardation, and, secondly, giving enough mineralocorticoid to ensure normal salt balance without excessive salt retention and hypertension. Although treatment in infancy requires close observation with careful measurement of growth, blood pressure, electrolytes, renin activity and plasma steroid measurement, the skeleton is relatively resistant to the growth-promoting effects of sex steroids at this stage of life. The glucocorticoid dose will rise in infancy as the child grows, but the fludrocortisone dose will fall as the infant kidney becomes more sensitive to mineralocorticoid (Miller 2001). A profile of plasma 17-OHP (which can be estimated on fingerprick samples) probably gives the best simple estimate of biochemical

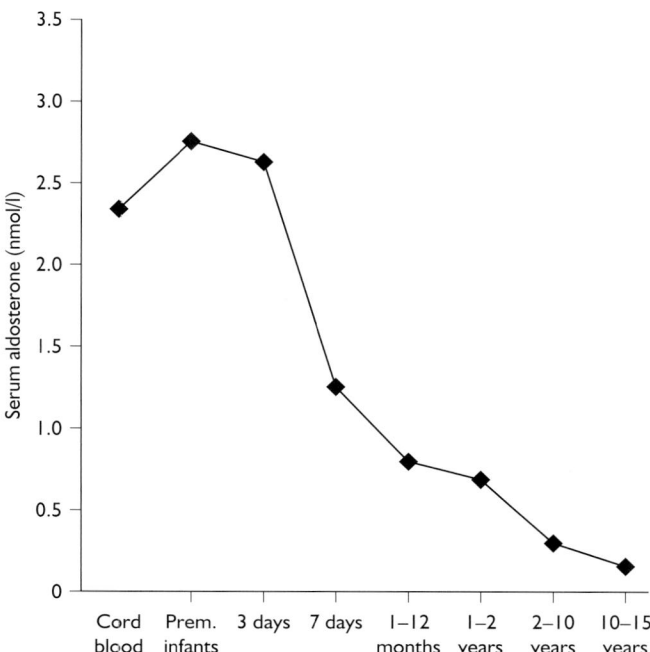

Fig. 34.15 Aldosterone levels as a function of age. This helps to explain why the neonate is more susceptible to salt-wasting than are older children and why such a relatively large dose of aldosterone is required. (*Adapted from Miller (2001).*)

control. Levels should be relatively low but not suppressed and later in infancy there should be evidence of diurnal variation. The sodium dose can usually remain unchanged beyond the neonatal period and the supplements stopped before the child's first birthday.

The management of 21α-hydroxylase deficiency in childhood and adolescence is not straightforward because of frequent difficulties achieving a balance between the need to suppress androgens on one hand and avoiding glucocorticoid toxicity on the other. Medical treatment with additional agents that block sex steroid effects may enable a more physiological replacement dose of glucocorticoid to be used (Merke et al. 2000). The nature and timing of surgery in virilised girls remain controversial and early assessment by a multi-disciplinary team that includes an experienced paediatric urologist is important. One possible approach to the surgical management of the profoundly virilised girl with CAH is to perform a clitoral reduction or recession in early life, with reassessment and possible vaginoplasty in the teenage years, when tissues have grown and matured. The family and health professionals may also feel that it is appropriate to defer any decision regarding surgical management until a later date. A single-stage procedure in early life which involves both clitoral reduction and vaginoplasty has seemed an attractive option in the past but there are concerns about long-term outcome, including susceptibility to scarring and vaginal stenosis. Increased steroid cover is, of course, needed for surgery.

11β-hydroxylase deficiency

This is the second most common cause of CAH, but accounts for less than 5% of cases in the UK. There is a relatively high incidence in the Middle East. Affected females are virilised but males have a normal phenotype at birth. Plasma 11-deoxycortisol, deoxy-corticosterone (DOC) and their metabolites are increased and there

is also an increase in 17-OHP. The increased intermediate compounds in the aldosterone pathway (notably DOC) can cause hypertension in later life but there may be salt-wasting in infancy because of a relative mineralocorticoid resistance at this stage. It is important to be aware of the potential for confusing 11β-hydroxylase deficiency with 21α-hydroxylase deficiency because assays for 11-deoxycortisol may have suboptimal specificity. The antenatal treatment of affected pregnancies with dexamethasone in an attempt to reduce virilisation has been successful in some cases (Cerame et al. 1999).

3β-hydroxysteroid dehydrogenase deficiency

In this condition, the variable degree of impaired enzyme activity can cause considerable phenotypic heterogeneity, including varying degrees of adrenal insufficiency. There are two 3β-hydroxysteroid dehydrogenase isoenzymes and it is type 2 (expressed in gonads and adrenals) rather than type 1 (expressed in placenta, prostate and skin) that is abnormal. Affected males may have perineal hypospadias. Females are either normal in appearance or are virilised, probably because of increased ACTH-stimulated production of the weak androgen dehydroepiandrosterone, which can be converted to more potent androgens. Some, but not all, affected children develop salt-wasting or signs of glucocorticoid deficiency.

17α-hydroxylase deficiency and 17,20-desmolase deficiency

A single protein is responsible for these two separate enzyme activities. When this is deficient, there are varying degrees of cortisol deficiency with excessive mineralocorticoid production, driven primarily by ACTH feedback, sometimes causing hypertension and hypokalaemic alkalosis in infancy. The glucocorticoid activity of the excess mineralocorticoid may in part compensate for a lack of cortisol. In later life, affected females develop minimal secondary sexual characteristics and are amenorrhoeic. Males show absent or inadequate virilisation. This defect should be considered in the differential diagnosis of undervirilised males and primary hypogonadism in females.

Congenital lipoid adrenal hyperplasia

Congenital lipoid adrenal hyperplasia (lipoid CAH) is usually due to mutations in the steroidogenic regulatory protein (StAR) which promotes cholesterol transport into the mitochondria. Impaired StAR activity leads to deficient synthesis of all steroid products, including aldosterone, cortisol and androgen. The synthesis of adrenal and gonadal steroids is impaired and so there is typically salt loss and hypoglycaemia in infancy and the genitalia will be female in appearance in the XY individual. At postmortem the adrenals are enlarged and full of accumulated cholesterol. Survival is possible with prompt recognition and appropriate treatment. The phenotypic heterogeneity described in this disorder probably reflects reduced but significant steroidogenesis occurring in the absence of StAR as well as residual enzyme activity. Cholesterol may then accumulate and damage cellular function with a further reduction in steroid production. Congenital lipoid adrenal hyperplasia can also present as isolated glucocorticoid deficiency.

P450 oxidoreductase deficiency (POR)

This disorder reflects an abnormality in a flavoprotein that is involved in electron transfer from NADPH to P450 microsomal enzymes, including 21 hydroxylase, 17α-hydroxylase and aromatase.

Patients with biochemical abnormalities in keeping with CAH and apparent combined P450C17 and P450C21 deficiency (impaired activity of 17α-hydroxylase and 21-hydroxylase) have been found to harbour mutations in POR. Female infants can have genital ambiguity due to androgen excess whilst males have hypopadias and micropenis. Some patients also have features of a condition called Antley–Bixler syndrome, which is characterised by dysmorphic features and skeletal abnormalities, including craniosynostosis, midfacial hypoplasia, choanal atresia, dysplastic ears and femoral bowing. The disorder is associated with characteristic abnormalities on urinary steroid profile and medical treatment may involve cortisol replacement and androgen supplementation in males (Arlt et al. 2004).

Corticosterone methyloxidase deficiency

This enzyme is responsible for the distal steps in aldosterone synthesis in the zona glomerulosa. It is very similar in sequence and structure to 11β-hydroxylase and is able to convert DOC to corticosterone in the zona glomerulosa (like 11β-hydroxylase), as well as corticosterone to aldosterone via 18-hydroxycorticosterone (Fig. 34.15). Enzyme defects lead to salt-wasting in early life and investigation demonstrates high plasma renin activity with low aldosterone levels. 17-OHP levels are not grossly elevated as they are in 21-hydroxylase deficiency and cortisol production is not impaired. These patients will respond to treatment with fludrocortisone, although ongoing production of DOC by 11β-hydroxylase helps to explain why these patients may be able to manage off therapy in later life when the kidney becomes more sensitive to mineralocorticoid. Corticosterone methyloxidase (CMO) deficiency can be divided into CMOI and CMOII, depending upon the impact of mutations on enzyme function. CMOI deficiency results from a loss of 18-hydroxylase and methyloxidase activity, whilst CMOII deficiency is the consequence of a selective deficiency in the ability of the enzyme to convert 18-hydroxycorticosterone to aldosterone (18-methyloxidase activity).

Other causes of adrenocortical insufficiency

There are a number of other disorders that can result in adrenal insufficiency in the newborn in addition to the CAHs. A classification of the causes of adrenocortical insufficiency is shown in Table 34.16.

Smith–Lemli–Opitz syndrome

Although not stricly one of the adrenal hyperplasias, there are similarities between Smith–Lemli–Opitz syndrome and other early abnormalities of steroidogenesis. The reduction in 7-dehydrocholesterol reductase activity results in decreased generation of cholesterol from 7-dehydrocholesterol. This impairs steroidogenesis and can lead to adrenal insufficiency as well as undervirilisation in genetic males (Porter 2008). It is an AR disorder with varying phenotypic features, including failure to thrive, syndactyly of the second and third toes, behavioural problems and learning difficulties. Smith–Lemli–Opitz syndrome is caused by defective cholesterol formation from dehydrocholesterol. Patients have a characteristic facies (microcephaly, cleft palate, anteverted nares) and may also have cardiac and CNS malformations. The impaired enzyme activity (3β-hydroxysteroid delta 7 reductase) results in an increase in cholesterol precursors (notably 7-dehydrocholesterol) and gonadal and occasionally adrenal steroidogenesis may be compromised. The external genitalia in XY infants with Smith–Lemli–Opitz syndrome can vary from normal

Table 34.16 Causes of adrenocortical insufficiency

Primary
Congenital adrenal hyperplasia
Deficiency of glucocorticoid and mineralocorticoid
21α-hydroxylase deficiency, salt-losing 11β-hydroxylase deficiency (in early life) 3β-hydroxysteroid dehydrogenase deficiency 17α-hydroxylase deficiency and 17,20-desmolase deficiency Lipoid congenital adrenal hyperplasia (steroidogenic acute regulatory protein and side-chain cleavage defects) P450 oxidoreductase (POR) deficiency
Deficiency of glucocorticoid
21α-hydroxylase deficiency, non-salt-losing
11β-hydroxylase deficiency 17α-hydroxylase deficiency
Deficiency of mineralocorticoid
Corticosterone methyl oxidase deficiency I Corticosterone methyl oxidase deficiency II
Early abnormalities of steroidogenesis
Smith–Lemli–Opitz (7-dehydrocholesterol reductase deficiency) Lysosomal acid lipase deficiency (Wolman syndrome)
Congenital adrenal hypoplasia
X-linked (abnormalities of DAX-I/NROB1) Autosomal recessive
Adrenal hypoplasia in association with SF-1 mutations
Adrenoleukodystrophy
Adrenal necrosis or haemorrhage
Acute infection (Waterhouse–Friderichsen syndrome)
Familial glucocorticoid deficiency (FGD)
FGD type 1 (ACTHR) FGD type 2 (MRAP)
Triple-A syndrome (AAAS)
Iatrogenic, post-glucocorticoid therapy
Secondary
Hypopituitarism Withdrawal from glucocorticoid therapy Maternal Cushing's

male to normal female depending on the extent to which testosterone synthesis is affected. Prenatal diagnosis is possible, and parents of an affected child should be offered genetic counselling.

Wolman disease

In this disorder there is a failure to mobilise cholesterol from lipid droplets because of an abnormality of lysosomal acid lipase. Adrenal insufficiency is a consequence of the inadequate supply of cholesterol to facilitate normal steroidogenesis. The severe infantile-onset

Wolman disease and the milder late-onset cholesteryl ester storage disease are caused by mutations in different parts of the lysosomal acid lipase gene (Anderson et al. 1994).

Congenital adrenal hypoplasia

Primary adrenocortical insufficiency due to congenital hypoplasia or atrophy of the glands has been estimated to have a frequency of 1 in 12 500 births. The X-linked recessive form is due to mutations of the gene encoding a nuclear hormone receptor, *NROB-1* or *DAX-1* (Ferraz-de-Souza and Achermann 2008), which resides in the region Xp21. *NROB-1* is expressed in the adrenal and testis, and also has a role in the normal production of gonadotrophins by the hypothalamopituitary axis. Hence, this form of adrenal hypoplasia is also associated with primary and secondary gonadal failure, although gonadotrophin and gonadal function may appear normal in early life.

Congenital adrenal hypoplasia is a well-recognised cause of an addisonian crisis in the neonatal period and later childhood. Poor feeding, vomiting, poor weight gain and dehydration, apnoeas, fits and shock may all be manifestations of glucocorticoid and mineralocorticoid deficiency. The biochemical findings include hypoglycaemia, hyponatraemia, hyperkalaemia and a metabolic acidosis. Hyperpigmentation is rare until the third week of life, and cortisol deficiency may also present as prolonged jaundice.

The clinical and biochemical picture in the neonatal period is very similar to CAH but 17-OHP levels are not raised in congenital adrenal hypoplasia (see below). ACTH and renin levels are raised but cortisol and aldosterone are reduced. Adrenal stimulation tests are not usually necessary but tetracosactrin stimulation shows an absent or greatly reduced cortisol response.

The diagnosis may be suspected antenatally if maternal oestriol values are very low, but adrenal hypoplasia cannot be differentiated on this basis from the more common – and also X-linked – placental sulphatase deficiency. It is important to remember that there is not always a close correlation between genotype and phenotype and so brothers with the same genetic defect can present at different ages.

Congenital adrenal hypoplasia has been described in association with small-for-gestational age (SGA), metaphyseal dysplasia and genital anomalies. The inheritance is believed to be AR and the term IMAGe association has been coined (Lienhardt et al. 2002).

Steroidogenic factor-1 (see below)

Steroidogenic factor-1 (SF-1) is a nuclear receptor which has a crucial role in the development of steroidogenic tissue. Defects of SF-1 can therefore lead to adrenal failure and abnormal gonadal development (Lin et al. 2006).

Adrenal haemorrhage

The large hyperaemic fetal gland is vulnerable to vascular damage. The reported incidence of neonatal adrenal haemorrhage ranges from 1.7 per 1000 found on postmortem examination (DeSa and Nicholls 1972) to around 30 per 1000 on abdominal ultrasound scanning (Velaphi and Perlman 2001). Predisposing factors include large fetal size, hypoxic episodes, thrombocytopenia, coagulation defects, disseminated thromboembolic disease and sepsis (Black and Williams 1973). The bleeding may be sufficient to form a palpable mass, which can be mistaken for a tumour, especially if unilateral, or may rupture into the peritoneum and cause intestinal obstruction or a scrotal haematoma. There may also be signs of acute blood loss or, at a later stage, anaemia and jaundice (Velaphi

and Perlman 2001). If both glands are infarcted, the baby may present acutely with an addisonian crisis (see below).

The diagnosis can be difficult to make unless there is scrotal/perineal bruising or a mass is palpable, but abdominal ultrasound is useful to confirm suspected haemorrhage (Velaphi and Perlman 2001). Adrenal calcification has been observed as early as the fifth day, but usually occurs much later. The presentation of adrenal insufficiency may be delayed but the regenerative capacity of the adrenal is great, and most adrenal haemorrhage is not associated with significantly impaired function (Black and Williams 1973).

Adrenoleukodystrophy

See Chapter 40, part 6.

Familial glucocorticoid deficiency

There are a number of causes of familial glucocorticoid deficiency (FGD), characterised by high circulating ACTH levels. FGD presents with signs of cortisol deficiency in infancy, or later in childhood, when hyperpigmentation may provide a diagnostic clue (Clark et al. 2009). It may reflect abnormalities of the ACTH receptor (FGD type 1) or of the melanocortin 2 receptor accessory protein, MRAP (FGD type 2). MRAP seems to be involved in transporting the ACTH receptor from the endoplasmic reticulum to the cell membrane. The triple-A syndrome describes the association of glucocorticoid deficiency with achalasia of the cardia and deficient tear production. It is caused by mutations of the AAAS gene on chromosome 12. Congenital lipoid adrenal hyperplasia can also present as isolated glucocorticoid deficiency.

Adrenal (Addisonian) crisis

An adrenal crisis may supervene in all forms of adrenal insufficiency pre- or postdiagnosis. It may develop insidiously, be precipitated by acute illness or surgery and hypoglycaemia can occur independently of salt and water loss. Features include poor feeding, poor weight gain, vomiting, diarrhoea and latterly vascular collapse, prostration and coma. Hypoglycaemia, hyponatraemia, hyperkalaemia and metabolic acidosis may all be present.

Treatment consists of i.v. fluid, glucose and electrolyte replacement, steroid replacement, and treatment of any underlying disease. A bolus of i.v. glucose (0.5–1.0 g/kg over several minutes) and a rapid infusion of normal saline (20 ml/kg initially) may be needed. If the response is satisfactory, rehydration can be continued with i.v. normal saline and added glucose. Intravenous hydrocortisone 10 mg should be given immediately in the neonate, then 100–200 mg/m²/day as 4-hourly bolus therapy or by continuous infusion. When the baby's condition is stable, the dose can be reduced. Hydrocortisone may also be administered i.m. if venous access is difficult. The mineralocorticoid effect of hydrocortisone is adequate at these doses.

Glucocorticoids and adrenal function in the neonate

There are a number of situations where the fetus or neonate may be exposed to or treated with exogenous glucocorticoid.

Maternal steroid administration and fetal adrenal function (Roberts and Dalziel 2010)

Antenatal betamethasone is of proven benefit when given to mothers who are likely to deliver preterm in order to accelerate fetal lung maturation. Transient biochemical changes in adrenal function have been identified in these infants, including reduced baseline cortisol levels, but these are of little clinical importance (Schäffer et al. 2009). Adrenocortical insufficiency in the newborn may occasionally arise if the mother received glucocorticoid therapy during pregnancy or following maternal Cushing syndrome.

Ventilator dependency and glucocorticoid administration (Halliday et al. 2009, 2010)

Ventilator-dependent neonates are still treated with exogenous glucocorticoids, now usually hydrocortisone, in order to assist weaning, although use has declined considerably over the last decade.

Large doses of dexamethasone (500 µg/kg/day) suppress the hypothalamopituitary–adrenal (HPA) axis but smaller doses, as well as inhaled steroids, can also affect HPA function. If an infant has received glucocorticoid for more than 1 week, it is wise to reduce the dose gradually and/or change to an alternate-day regimen prior to stopping treatment, bearing in mind that 50 µg of dexamethasone will probably suppress the adrenal gland completely (Hindmarsh and Brook 1985). It should also be remembered that an infant who has recently stopped glucocorticoid treatment may require steroid cover in association with subsequent illness or surgery. Children on pharmacological doses of steroids (an equivalent dose of prednisolone 2 mg/kg/day for >1 week, or 1 mg/kg/day for >1 month) or other immunosuppressive therapy should not be given live vaccines until 3 months after ceasing therapy.

Hypotension, respiratory function and relative adrenal insufficiency

Sick preterm infants may have inappropriately low baseline and stimulated cortisol levels. This relative adrenal insufficiency may be linked to immaturity of the steroidogenic pathway and has been associated with haemodynamic instability (Ng et al. 2004; Noori and Seri 2005; Quintos and Boney 2010). There may be a role for a short course of hydrocortisone in the sick hypotensive infant (e.g. 0.25–2.5 mg/kg every 6 hours), although this is an area of neonatal practice that requires further study.

Biochemical assessment of adrenal function in the neonate

The assessment of HPA integrity is not straightforward. Differences in cortisol assay performance and the absence of appropriate reference data remain significant confounding factors when assessing adrenal function in babies (see below).

The cortisol response to i.v. Synacthen administration is used by many units to assess the HPA axis. In many primary adrenal pathologies cortisol production is compromised. If secondary hypoadrenalism is suspected then the test is conducted on the basis that an understimulated adrenal will be hypoplastic and will produce less cortisol. Sensitivity and specificity issues explain the large number of Synacthen protocols described in the literature. Higher Synacthen doses represent a pharmacological rather than a physiological stimulus and it is well known that a normal response does not exclude a degree of adrenal suppression ('false negatives').

As a general rule, a baseline or 20–30-minute post-Synacthen cortisol response (any dose of Synacthen) that is greater than 560 nmol/l makes adrenal insufficiency (primary or secondary) very unlikely. However, it needs to be recognised that some healthy infants will have a response that is below this threshold. Random plasma cortisol concentrations may be difficult to interpret, but adrenal suppression or insufficiency should be suspected if baseline cortisol values are below 140 nmol/l in stressed preterm infants or when the response to Synacthen stimulation is below 360 nmol/l in preterm infants.

Data from children and adolescents that can be applied with caution to the infant population indicate that hypoadrenalism is also unlikely if the cortisol peak at 20 or 30 minutes is 500 nmol/l and/or the increment is 200 nmol/l following Synacthen administration using a 'low' dose of 0.5 µg/1.73 m² (Agwu et al. 1999). The 'usual' dose is 36 µg/kg.

Concern about the performance of the Synacthen test has generated interest in other approaches to the assessment of HPA axis integrity. The ACTH response (typically measured at 20–30 minutes) and cortisol response (typically measured at 60 minutes) to CRH is a more logical approach to the assessment of the adrenal axis because it is examining pituitary function directly, although there are still issues about the optimum CRH dose (Bolt et al. 2002). A cortisol response that is below 360 nmol/l at 60 minutes post CRH administration (CRH 1.0 µg/kg) suggests adrenal insufficiency.

Adrenal hyperfunction

There are very few causes of adrenal hyperfunction in early life apart from CAH. Infants with adrenal hyperfunction usually have abnormal cell signalling (McCune–Albright syndrome) or an underlying neoplasia.

McCune–Albright syndrome is a well-recognised cause of endocrine gland hyperfunction in childhood. It results from activating mutations of the G protein component adjacent to the cell surface receptor. Hyperfunction of the gonadotrophin receptor–G protein complex explains the precocious puberty in this disorder (characterised by the triad of precocious puberty, café-au-lait lesions and polyostotic fibrous dysplasia), but activation of the ACTH receptor can also lead to glucocorticoid excess and Cushing syndrome.

Adrenal tumours have been reported in early life and when they occur the possibility of an underlying tumour predisposition syndrome such as Li–Fraumeni syndrome must be considered. The clinical picture will reflect the adrenal steroid produced in excess, with glucocorticoid leading to signs of Cushing syndrome and androgens resulting in virilisation (Sandrini et al. 1997).

Disorders of sex development

Disorders of sex development (DSD) can be defined as congenital conditions in which the development of chromosomal, gonadal or anatomical sex is atypical (Diamond and Sigmundson 1997).

Normal sexual differentiation

The physical basis of a person's sex reflects many factors, including genotype, type of gonad present, the nature of the internal and external sexual organs and the development of secondary sexual characteristics. In DSD there is atypical development of one or more of these factors.

The primary event in sexual determination is the fertilisation of an ovum by either an X- or a Y-bearing spermatozoon. Normally this initiates a cascade of events which culminates in female or male development. A 46,XX genotype results in the undifferentiated bipotential gonads developing into ovaries by the 12th week of fetal life. Subsequent female development is associated with persistence and development of the müllerian ducts, which form the fallopian tubes, uterus and upper vagina, and the external genitalia will take a female form. The classic studies of Jost (1953) demonstrated that this process occurred in a castrated fetus irrespective of the genetic sex. However, this is a rapidly expanding field and it is clear that genetic factors contribute to the process of both ovarian as well as testicular development (see below). In the individual with a normal 46,XY genotype, the sex-determining region of the Y chromosome (*SRY*) is the first of a series of genes involved in testicular determination (Koopman et al. 1991). *SRY* is a sequence of 14 kilobases adjacent to the pseudoautosomal region on the short arm of the Y chromosome at Yp11.3 that encodes a DNA-binding regulatory protein. The presence of testicular tissue therefore indicates the presence of a Y chromosome except in rare instances such as XX males in whom *SRY* may reside somewhere in the genome. In the presence of *SRY* and other downstream genes the indifferent gonads transform into testes by the fifth to sixth week of intrauterine life and then play an active role in further development by secreting testosterone and antimüllerian hormone (AMH). Abnormalities of the same genes can result in abnormal gonadal development with associated genital malformations in XY individuals (see below).

Testosterone is secreted from the Leydig cells, initially under the stimulus of placental chorionic gonadotrophin, which is why gonadotrophin deficiency results in micropenis and/or cryptorchidism rather than true ambiguity. Testosterone acts locally to stimulate development of the wolffian ducts into epididymis, vas deferens and seminal vesicles. It also reaches androgen-sensitive peripheral cells via the circulation, where it binds to the androgen receptor in the cell cytoplasm and nucleus. Testosterone is also converted to the potent androgen dihydrotestosterone (DHT) in peripheral tissues by the enzyme 5α-reductase. In the fetus, testosterone and DHT induce virilisation of the urogenital sinus and the external genitalia. This process is complete by 13 weeks of embryonic life. The normal pattern of human chorionic gonadotrophin (hCG), gonadotrophin and androgen release in the male fetus is shown in Figure 34.16.

The fetal testes also produce AMH, a high-molecular-weight glycoprotein secreted by the Sertoli cells, which causes regression of the müllerian ducts.

Disorders of sex development

Patterns of abnormal sex development

In the neonatal period the most common presentation of DSD is genital ambiguity. The prevalence of genital anomalies per se may be as high as 1 in 300 births (Ahmed et al. 2004), but complex anomalies with true ambiguity are much less common, at 1 in 5000 births (Thyen et al. 2006). The abnormalities can vary from a minor degree of labial fusion in the female or hypospadias in the male to profound virilisation in a genetic female or what appear to be female external genitalia in a genetic male (Fig. 34.17). A scoring system for genital anomalies in cases of undermasculinisation has been described (Ahmed et al. 2000b).

The terminology used to describe particular types of DSD has changed on a number of occasions over the last 20 years. A consensus statement on the management of intersex disorders is a valuable resource when considering this topic and a DSD classification used in this document is as follows (Hughes et al. 2006):

- sex chromosome DSD, for example 45,X Turner syndrome or 45,X/46,XY mixed gonadal dysgenesis
- 46,XY DSD: the karyotype is XY but the gonad has failed to develop, there are abnormalities of androgen synthesis or action or there are abnormalities such as severe hypospadias of unknown cause

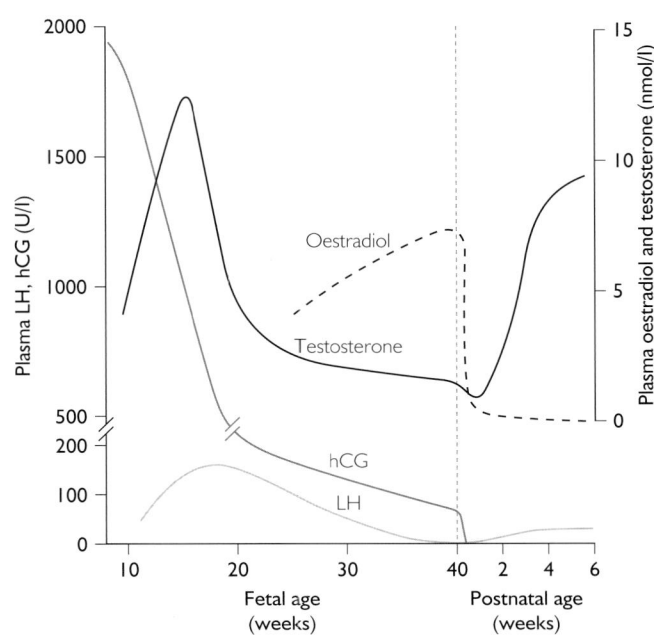

Fig. 34.16 Trend in fetal and neonatal human chorionic gonadotrophin (hCG), luteinising hormone (LH), testosterone and oestradiol concentrations in the male. *(Adapted from Fisher.)*

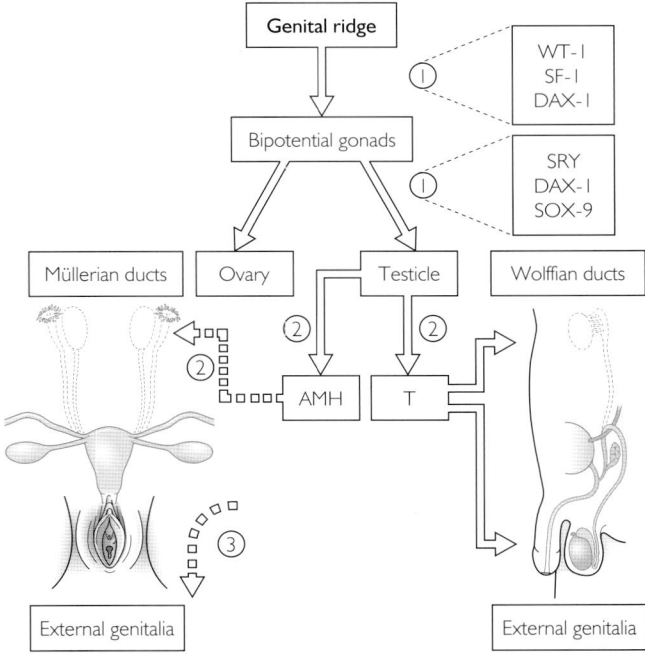

Fig. 34.17 Abnormal sexual development. 1, Disorders of urogenital and gonadal development. 2, Undervirilised males: XY individuals with abnormalities of steroidogenesis/antimüllerian hormone (AMH) production or who are unable to respond to androgen or AMH in the normal way. 3, Virilised females: XX individuals exposed to excess androgen (see text for further details).

- 46,XX DSD: the karyotype is 46,XX but the gonad has not developed in the usual manner, there has been exposure to excess androgen or there are abnormalities such as abnormal vaginal/müllerian structure development.

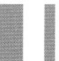

Table 34.17 Disorders of urogenital and gonadal development

Genes involved in development of the bipotential gonad
WT-1 SF-1
Genes involved in development of the testis
SRY Sox-9
Genes involved in development of the ovary
FOXL2
Other causes of abnormal gonadal development
True hermaphroditism XX males Klinefelter Mixed gonadal dysgenesis Turner syndrome Pure gonadal dysgenesis Anorchia

Table 34.18 Incomplete virilisation in a baby with an XY karyotype including disorders of androgen production or action

Testosterone deficiency
Androgen insensitivity
Partial Complete
Antimüllerian hormone resistance and deficiency
Idiopathic
Including the association with intrauterine growth retardation and dysmorphic syndromes

Table 34.19 Patients with an XX karyotype who have been exposed to excess androgen

Virilising congenital adrenal hyperplasia

Deficiency of:
   21α-hydroxylase
   11β-hydroxylase
   3β-hydroxysteroid dehydrogenase

Aromatase deficiency
Maternal androgen excess
Endogenous Exogenous

The foundation for the above classification is the underlying karyotype but gives little insight into the clinical phenotype. For the purposes of this chapter we have divided the causes of intersex disorders into the following broad areas (Fig. 34.17):

- Disorders of urogenital (gonadal) ridge development and gonadal (ovarian and testicular) determination. These abnormalities frequently reflect an abnormal karyotype or a single-gene defect affecting gonadal development (Table 34.17).
- Disorders of androgen production or action. These are individuals with an XY karyotype but with abnormalities of steroidogenesis/AMH production or who are unable to respond to androgen or AMH in the normal way. These patients have 46,XY DSD in the above classification (Table 34.18).
- Patients with an XX karyotype who have been exposed to excess androgen (Table 34.19).

The sexual organs may also be affected in a wide variety of dysmorphic syndromes which are not currently known to be related to specific disorders of sexual development.

Disorders of urogenital and gonadal development (Fig. 34.17 and Table 34.17) (Sarafoglou and Ostrer 2000; Ahmed and Hughes 2002)

These disorders may be the consequence of a single-gene defect affecting urogenital and/or gonadal development or may arise because of chromosomal mosaicism. There is the potential for both müllerian and wolffian duct development in one individual and variable potential for germ cell development and gonadal endocrine function as well as neoplasia. The renal tract may also be abnormal. Diagnosis in the newborn period usually depends on recognising an abnormality of the external genitalia, which is frequently present.

Studies in mice have highlighted many genes which appear to be important in gonadal development but in this section we will focus on factors that, when mutated, give rise to abnormalities in humans.

Genes involved in the formation of the bipotential urogenital (gonadal) ridge

A number of genes operating 'upstream' from *SRY* are important in the development of the bipotential urogenital (gonadal) ridge. These include *SF-1* and *WT-1*. Both of these genes are expressed during formation of the bipotential gonadal ridge as well as during the process of gonadal differentiation. Some of these genes have a role that extends beyond that of gonadal development and as such the DSD may form part of a 'syndrome'.

WT-1

The WAGR (Wilms tumour, aniridia, genitourinary anomalies and mental retardation), Denys–Drash and Frasier syndromes result from abnormalities of the gene *WT-1* located at 11p13. The nature of the underlying defect in the *WT-1* gene determines phenotype. The Denys–Drash syndrome is characterised by childhood renal cancer, glomerular nephropathy and abnormal gonadal and genital development. Gonadal abnomalities are also found in XX individuals (Little and Wells 1997).

Steroidogenic factor-1 (NR5A1)

SF-1 or *NR51A* (nuclear receptor subfamily 5, group A, member 1) is a nuclear receptor which has a crucial role in the development of steroidogenic tissue. Mutations of *SF-1* in humans can be associated with failure of both adrenal and gonadal development (Achermann et al. 1999). Infants may present with adrenal failure, and XY individuals at the severe end of the phenotypic spectrum can have a female phenotype with persistent müllerian structures. The effects of *SF-1* are complex and sensitive to a gene dosage effect as well as gene activity. Hence phenotypes will include severe penoscrotal hypospadias in the presence of normal adrenal function (Köhler et al. 2009).

Genes involved in normal testicular development

SRY

SRY encodes a protein that is highly conserved amongst mammalian species. SRY appears to bend DNA, thereby allowing other proteins access to genes along the DNA sequence. Defects in the *SRY* gene can be identified in some patients with XY sex reversal, streak gonads and müllerian structures (Hawkins et al. 1992). However, most patients with this phenotype have a normal *SRY* gene, suggesting that many other genetic factors are involved in testicular development. This view has been reinforced by the report of an *SRY* gene mutation associated with XY sex reversal in one family member but not her father (Jordan et al. 2002).

SOX9

SOX proteins (SRY-type HMG box) are important in many aspects of human development and *SOX9* has an important role in testis determination, acting downstream from *SRY*. Heterozygous loss-of-function mutations of *SOX9* are associated with campomelic dysplasia, which is a skeletal abnormality associated with male-to-female sex reversal (Savage et al. 2001). The skeletal features include micrognathia, cleft palate, 11 pairs of ribs and bowing of the long bones, and most individuals die from respiratory failure in early life. A total of 75% of XY fetuses have abnormal gonadal development with female or ambiguous genitalia.

Factors involved in normal ovarian development

Absence of *SRY* in 46,XY individuals results in female internal and external genitalia but ovaries do not develop normally in these circumstances, which underlines the fact that this process is not passive. This process is, nevertheless, poorly understood, although genes such as *Wnt-4* may be important.

Other causes of abnormal gonadal development

True hermaphroditism

This diagnosis rests on the histological demonstration of ovarian and testicular tissue in a single individual, either in separate gonads or, more commonly, in ovotestes. There is nearly always some genital ambiguity and the internal sexual organs are variable. Most patients have an XX karyotype, although molecular analysis has identified Y sequences in some of these patients (Queipo et al. 2002). Pedigrees with XX true hermaphrodites and XX males have been described, which suggests varying penetrance of a mutated gene involved in sexual differentiation (Ramos et al. 1996). Many affected children have been raised as males, but female gender assignment can be considered as well because there is good potential for sexual function and even fertility with a high risk of tumour formation in dysgenetic testicular tissue (Hadjiathanasiou et al. 1994).

46,XX testicular DSD (XX males)

Individuals with this rare condition (1 in 20 000) have testes despite an XX karyotype. The genitalia are usually male, although there may be ambiguity, which can lead to presentation in infancy. Y-specific

DNA sequences, sometimes including the *SRY* gene, can be identified in 80–90% of cases (Weil et al. 1994) and duplication of SOX9 has also been shown to result in this phenotype.

Klinefelter syndrome

This relatively common condition (around 1–2 per 1000 live male births) is associated with a 47,XXY karyotype. Many patients remain undiagnosed (Bojesen et al. 2003), but when the diagnosis is made it is typically because the karyotype is checked antenatally or because of concerns about learning difficulties, a small phallus or small testes (Schwartz and Root 1991). The diagnosis is sometimes made when a couple are investigated for infertility.

Mixed gonadal dysgenesis

Children with this condition have genetic mosaicism, including cell lines with and without Y-chromosome material. The phenotype is extremely varied, ranging from apparently normal male to apparently normal female, but is typified by a child with a dysgenetic testis and wolffian structures on one side of the body and a streak gonad with müllerian structures on the other. The karyotype in peripheral blood is frequently 45,X/46,XY (Telvi et al. 1999). Stigmata of Turner syndrome may be present. There is a significant risk of gonadoblastoma, and laparoscopy with removal of dysgenetic tissue or orchidopexy to facilitate the assessment of gonadal health may be appropriate. Studies on prenatal diagnosis have shed new light on the condition, with 80% of 45,X/46,XY cases detected having an apparently male phenotype (Hsu 1989).

Turner syndrome

A clinical diagnosis may be made in the newborn period because of the characteristic lymphoedema of the hands and feet, or suspected because of the presence of other associated abnormalities such as aortic coarctation. This permits early counselling and detection of problems such as growth failure and primary gonadal failure.

XY female pure gonadal dysgenesis

Affected infants are phenotypic females with normal external genitalia and bilateral streak or absent gonads. This condition usually presents in adolescence with primary amenorrhoea, rather than in the neonatal period.

Bilateral anorchia

The aetiology of most cases of bilateral anorchia is unclear. It has been suggested that testicular torsion in utero or in the perinatal period may be responsible for some cases (Smith et al. 1991), although familial cases suggest a genetic aetiology in some families and a defect in SF-1 in a boy with testicular regression and micropenis has been identified (Philibert et al. 2007). The incidence is estimated to be around 0.5–1 in 20 000 males (Zenaty et al. 2006). The impact of bilateral anorchia on phenotype depends on the stage of development at which it occurs but the presence of micropenis in 50% suggests that in these children the insult occurred in midgestation.

Disorders of androgen production or action: incomplete virilisation in a baby with an XY karyotype (Fig. 34.17 and Table 34.18) (Ahmed and Hughes 2002)

These disorders arise when a genetic male with well-differentiated testes fails to virilise normally because of an inability to manufacture androgen normally or a failure to respond to androgen appropriately. The phenotype can vary from that of a normal female through all degrees of ambiguity to normal male external genitalia.

Testosterone or dihydrotestosterone deficiency

The biosynthesis of testosterone can be affected at one of various stages, resulting in suboptimal testosterone production and fetal and usually postnatal undervirilisation. Steroid synthesis in the adrenal cortex as well as in the testis can be affected if the enzyme block occurs at a relatively early stage of steroidogenesis. These defects can produce severe undervirilisation, and associated cortisol/aldosterone deficiency can produce an adrenal crisis with hyponatraemia and hypoglycaemia.

Luteinising hormone receptor defects

Impaired androgen production by the testis may be due to end-organ insensitivity arising from molecular defects in the LH receptor. The gonad is unable to respond normally to hCG in early pregnancy and then to LH in later gestation. Affected individuals may be described as having Leydig cell hypoplasia because of the associated histological findings.

Smith–Lemli–Opitz syndrome (see above)

Patients with Smith–Lemli–Opitz syndrome are unable to manufacture cholesterol from dehydrocholesterol and so adrenal and gonadal steroidogenesis is compromised. The external genitalia in XY infants with Smith–Lemli–Opitz syndrome can vary from normal male to normal female depending on the extent to which testosterone synthesis is affected (Kelley and Hennekam 2000).

Congenital adrenal hyperplasia

Some of the CAHs can be associated with impaired androgen production. These disorders are described in more detail under the adrenal section of this chapter (see above), but include congenital lipoid adrenal hyperplasia, 3β-hydroxysteroid dehydrogenase deficiency, 17α-hydroxylase deficiency/17,20-desmolase deficiency and POR deficiency.

17β-hydroxysteroid dehydrogenase deficiency

This enzyme is responsible for the last step in testosterone production (Geissler et al. 1994). At birth, affected males are poorly virilised and infants can present with herniae and palpable gonads (Gregory et al. 1993). Many XY babies have been reared as females, although virilisation can occur at puberty if the gonads are in situ (Tullio-Pelet et al. 2000). Females with an XX karyotype are unaffected.

5α-reductase deficiency

Genetic males with 5α-reductase deficiency have external genitalia that are largely female in appearance. The defect was described in families living in an isolated community in the Dominican Republic, where affected individuals were raised as females but at puberty there was virilisation of the genitalia and body habitus and the development of male psychosexual orientation; most then converted to the male role (Imperato-McGinley et al. 1979). Clinically, there is normal fetal development of wolffian structures, which are testosterone-dependent, but poor development of the external genitalia, which require DHT. Biochemically, the key finding is a high testosterone/DHT ratio in serum and analogous changes on urinary steroid analysis (Pearce et al. 2010). Male gender assignment is

appropriate and topical DHT cream can be used to induce phallic enlargement.

Androgen insensitivity (Ahmed et al. 2000a)

Partial androgen insensitivity

In this X-linked recessive condition, the genital abnormality arising from the insensitivity to androgen varies widely, ranging from a near-normal female appearance to normal male virilisation with azoospermia. This is an important cause of perineal hypospadias (Batch et al. 1993). Many affected children have inherited defects of the androgen receptor (which maps to the long arm of the X chromosome). The genetics of this disorder have been studied in detail.

Complete androgen insensitivity

Complete androgen insensitivity, also inherited as an X-linked recessive condition, is seldom diagnosed in the neonatal period unless there is a positive family history or gonads are palpable in the groin. Affected infants are otherwise indistinguishable from normal females. Müllerian regression occurs normally under the influence of AMH but the wolffian ducts fail to differentiate because of end-organ insensitivity to androgen. The normal postnatal surge in LH and testosterone (Forest et al. 1973) is absent in complete androgen insensitivity syndrome, presumably because the hypothalamus and pituitary are unable to respond to androgen (Bouvattier et al. 2002). Breast development occurs at puberty because of oestrogen generation from androgen.

AMH resistance and deficiency

In the persistent müllerian duct syndrome, the uterus and fallopian tubes fail to regress during development. Affected infants usually present when undergoing surgery for cryptorchidism or inguinal hernia repair, when the müllerian structures are identified. A number of mutations of the AMH gene, leading to AMH deficiency, or of the type II AMH receptor, resulting in AMH resistance, have been described in these patients (Belville et al. 1999).

Patients with an XX karyotype who have been exposed to excess androgen
(Fig. 34.17 and Table 34.19)

These conditions are characterised by a normal female karyotype, normal ovaries, and normal female internal genitalia but virilised external genitalia. Exposure of a female fetus to excess androgen can occur in a number of ways, although the commonest cause of this picture by far is CAH due to 21α-hydroxylase deficiency. The remaining causes, shown in Table 34.19, are very rare.

Congenital adrenal hyperplasia

The three virilising forms of CAH, 21-hydroxylase, 11β hydroxylase and 3β HSD, are described in the adrenal section of this chapter (see above).

Aromatase deficiency (Pohlenz et al. 1998)

Normal conversion of fetal and maternal androgens to oestrogen by placental aromatase enzyme activity was thought to be essential for survival of the conceptus, but there are now reports of aromatase gene mutations leading to impaired placental enzyme activity and subsequent maternal and fetal virilisation (Conte et al. 1994). It therefore appears that a pregnancy can be viable despite a marked reduction in oestrogen production.

Excess maternal androgens

Fetal virilisation may rarely occur in response to excess maternal androgen production from an adrenal or ovarian tumour. The degree of virilisation will depend on the timing and degree of androgen overproduction.

Small for gestational age and gonadal function

An association between small size at birth and hypospadias has been recognised for some time (Calzolari et al. 1986; Fredell et al. 2002) and a link between SGA and altered gonadal (and adrenal) function in later life has now also been identified. Prenatal growth restriction is associated with a reduction in uterine and ovarian size (Ibanez et al. 2000) and an increase in FSH production in males and females, with oligo-ovulation and anovulation at adolescence (Ibanez et al. 2002a, 2002b).

The clinical approach to problems of intersex
(Meyer-Bahlburg 1999; American Academy of Pediatrics Committee on Genetics 2000)

There is inevitable distress when parental questions about infant sex and well-being cannot be answered immediately. The initial discussions should emphasise that:

- A range of laboratory staff and health professionals will need to be involved in establishing the correct diagnosis and planning treatment.
- This process may take a matter of a few days but can take longer than this and the emphasis will be on making the right decision about gender assignment; it is important to avoid hasty decisions that subsequently turn out to be ill advised.
- The prognosis for life and health and also for sexual function is good, but that for fertility must be guarded.

An early anxiety of the parents will be what to tell friends and relatives. It may be possible to delay announcing the birth, or, alternatively, to announce only that the baby has a problem requiring treatment and that the parents would prefer not to discuss progress for a few days. The birth should not be registered until the sex of rearing is decided. Choice of a name suitable for either sex is probably unwise at this early stage.

Successful integration in either sexual role depends upon the social and cultural setting as well the genetic status, the internal sexual organs and the configuration and function of the external genitalia. It is impossible, even with the most expert modern reconstructive surgery, to create a normal-sized, functioning penis from inadequate tissue, although a profound increase in phallic size can be seen in, for example, XY patients with 5α-reductase deficiency exposed to DHT. Conversely, the impact of androgen exposure on the infant brain and the well-recognised instances of female-assigned XY patients subsequently requesting gender change must be considered. The prospects for fertility must also be borne in mind and there may be strong ethnic, social or religious pressures influencing the family's choice. Psychological adjustment to the sex of rearing does not usually cause problems as long as this is chosen early and accepted by those handling the child (Meyer-Bahlburg 1999). Experience with 5α-reductase deficiency and other conditions has shown that greater flexibility in sexual role is possible than

was previously believed. Many physicians feel that the sex of rearing should be selected as early in infancy as possible and there is frequently a desire on the part of physician and parents to complete any genital surgery necessary to produce cosmetically acceptable external genitalia as early as is practicable. However, this is a contentious topic that is complicated by a dearth of long-term data and a desire to involve the patient in the decision-making process (Diamond and Sigmundson 1997; Creighton et al. 2001).

Initial assessment

The history should include details about the pregnancy. Was there any maternal virilisation in pregnancy that might suggest a problem, such as aromatase deficiency or a maternal androgen-secreting tumour? If the parents are consanguineous then an AR cause of clinical picture is more likely.

The examination should include an overall assessment of the infant looking to see if there is evidence of dehydration (salt-wasting CAH) and looking for dysmorphic features (e.g. Smith–Lemli–Opitz). The degree of virilisation should be determined and this will include an assessment of phallus dimensions, position of urethral opening and the extent of labioscrotal fold fusion. The genitalia can be described using the Prader staging system (Fig. 34.14), although the calibre of the corpora and not merely the amount of shaft and preputial skin should be assessed. Attention should be paid to the presence/absence and location of the gonads:

- Severe hypospadias with bilateral descended gonads is likely to be a case of 46,XY DSD. A definitive hormonal or endocrine cause will not be found in many of these children.
- A neonate with any degree of virilisation and without palpable gonads may have 46,XX DSD due to CAH and the measurement of 17-OHP levels is a particularly crucial investigation in such circumstances.
- Genital ambiguity with asymmetry and unilateral gonadal descent increases the likelihood of gonadal dysgenesis (Kaefer et al. 1999).

Most patients with ambiguous genitalia should be discussed with, or transferred to, the local tertiary centre at an early stage because of the need for multidisciplinary input from individuals who manage these complex cases regularly. Urgent investigations in the neonate with ambiguous genitalia include a karyotype and pelvic and renal imaging. 17-OHP should also be measured (beyond 36 hours of age) and serum stored so that LH, FSH and androgens can be measured. It may also be appropriate to image the internal genitalia more precisely by endoscopy or laparoscopy. Babies with genital ambiguity may have adrenal insufficiency and so electrolytes and glucose will need to be monitored in the neonatal period until a diagnosis has been reached or adrenal insufficiency excluded.

Subsequent assessment

Patients can usually be assigned to one of the three main categories of abnormal sexual development when the karyotype and imaging results are available. The more common scenarios are described first.

Genital ambiguity in a baby with a 46,XX karyotype and probable müllerian structures on pelvic imaging: probable virilisation of a genetic female

This is one of the more common scenarios and often reflects CAH, the commonest cause of which is 21-hydroxylase. Gonads will not be palpable in the groin. Salt-losing CAH will be manifest by a rising potassium and falling sodium, although this will not be apparent until the baby is several days old. 17-OHP levels will typically be markedly elevated in 21-hydroxylase (ideally measure beyond 36 hours to avoid false positives) and the child will need glucocorticoid and mineralocorticoid replacement. A urinary steroid profile for analysis by mass spectrometry will be taken before, or in the early stages of, therapy and can identify many steroidogenic defects. More uncommon causes of androgen exposure in utero include placental aromatase deficiency and a maternal androgen-producing tumour. Girls with these defects have normal female internal genitalia, are potentially fertile and most will have a female gender identity. Most physicians feel that, whatever the degree of virilisation, individuals in this category should be reared as females.

Karyotype XY in the presence of severe hypospadias or microphallus with or without descended gonads and no evidence of müllerian structures on pelvic ultrasonography: possible disorder of androgen production or action

The cause of this clinical picture frequently remains unknown although there is a well-described association with SGA. It is important to look for dysmorphic features that may help to establish a diagnosis (e.g. Smith–Lemli–Opitz syndrome). If a definitive 'endocrine' diagnosis is reached then this will usually reflect insufficient androgen generation or impaired androgen action:

- testosterone biosynthetic or metabolism defect, e.g. 17β-hydroxysteroid dehydrogenase deficiency
- partial androgen insensitivity syndrome.

Important investigations include measurement of:

- testosterone/DHT (abnormal ratio in 5α-reductase deficiency)
- androstenedione (raised relative to testosterone in 17β-hydroxysteroid dehydrogenase deficiency)
- urinary steroid profile (to exclude disorders such as 3β-hydroxysteroid dehydrogenase deficiency).

hCG stimulation with measurement of androstenedione, testosterone and DHT response may also be helpful. Serum should be stored for the subsequent measurement of factors such as AMH, which is a potentially useful marker of Sertoli cell function (Rey et al. 1999). Levels tend to be low in patients with abnormal gonadal development, normal in conditions associated with impaired testosterone secretion and high in androgen insensitivity syndrome. Techniques to delineate the internal anatomy include cystoscopy or laparoscopy.

If surgery is required, a genital skin biopsy should be taken for androgen-binding studies and it may also be appropriate to discuss androgen receptor sequencing if the clinical and biochemical picture points towards this diagnosis (Ahmed et al. 2000b). The choice of sex of rearing will depend to some extent on the external genitalia but assigning sex according to the appearance of the external genitalia alone and without a definitive diagnosis is unwise. A substantial phallus in association with an XY karyotype, and significant circulating androgen concentrations with associated CNS exposure, should normally result in male sex of rearing. Children with 5α-reductase deficiency can have apparently normal female external genitalia but typically have a male gender identity. The phallic response to DHT cream in these children can be striking. If there is remaining doubt, a course of depot testosterone, 25 mg i.m. monthly for 3 months, can be given. Good phallic growth confirms the potential for virilisation at puberty.

Gonadal dysgenesis/abnormal gonadal differentiation

Scenario 1: müllerian structures in an individual with an XY karyotype and no identifiable or abnormal streak gonadal tissue

If there is no or minimal evidence of virilisation then these patients are likely to have an underlying abnormality of gonadal formation. Sex of rearing should be female because the CNS has not usually been exposed to androgen. Many of these individuals present in the teenage years as girls with pubertal delay rather than in the neonatal period. A laparotomy to assess the pelvic structures and, potentially, to remove dysgenetic gonadal tissue which is at high risk of tumour formation is important.

Scenario 2: genital ambiguity in an individual with an abnormal karyotype, e.g. XO/XY or XX/XY

In the disorders of gonadal development there is considerable diversity and discordance between the genetic and anatomical findings. Patients with a mosaic karyotype are at risk of abnormal gonadal differentiation with a highly variable phenotype that can lie on the spectrum that runs from an undervirilised 'male' with bilateral dysgenetic gonads, through mixed gonadal dysgenesis (see above) to an individual with features of Turner syndrome. There is frequently structure asymmetry and imaging, including a renal/pelvic ultrasound and MRI, as well as laparoscopy and gonadal biopsy may be necessary in order to obtain a comprehensive understanding of the underlying picture.

References

Achermann, J.C., Ito, M., Hindmarsh, P.C., et al., 1999. A mutation in the gene encoding steroidogenic factor-1 causes XY sex reversal and adrenal failure in humans. Nat Genet 22, 125–126.

Agwu, J.C., Spoudeas, H., Hindmarsh, P.C., et al., 1999. Tests of adrenal insufficiency. Arch Dis Child 80, 330–333.

Ahmed, S.F., Hughes, I.A., 2002. The genetics of male undermasculinization. Clin Endocrinol 56, 1–18.

Ahmed, S.F., Cheng, A., Dovey, L., et al., 2000a. Phenotypic features, androgen receptor binding, and mutational analysis in 278 clinical cases reported as androgen

insensitivity syndrome. J Clin Endocrinol Metab 85, 658–665.

Ahmed, S.F., Khwaja, O., Hughes, I.A., 2000b. The role of a clinical score in the assessment of ambiguous genitalia. Br J Urol Int 85, 120–124.

Ahmed, S.F., Dobbie, R., Finlayson, A.R., et al., 2004. Prevalence of hypospadias and other genital anomalies among singleton births, 1988–1997, in Scotland. Arch Dis Child Fetal Neonatal Ed 89, F149–F151.

Alberti, L., Proverbio, M.C., Costagliola, S., et al., 2002. Germline mutations of TSH receptor gene as cause of nonautoimmune

subclinical hypothyroidism. J Clin Endocrinol Metab 87, 2549–2555.

Alm, J., Larsson, A., Zetterstrom, I.R., 1978. Congenital hypothyroidism in Sweden. Incidence and age at diagnosis. Acta Paediatr Scand 67, 1–3.

Alm, J., Hagenfeldt, L., Larsson, A., et al., 1984. Incidence of congenital hypothyroidism: retrospective study of neonatal laboratory screening versus clinical symptoms as indicators leading to diagnosis. Br Med J 289, 1171–1175.

Ambrugger, P., Stoeva, I., Biebermann, H., et al., 2001. Novel mutations of the thyroid peroxidase gene in patients with permanent congenital hypothyroidism. Eur J Endocrinol 145, 19–24.

American Academy of Pediatrics Committee on Genetics, 2000. Evaluation of the newborn with developmental anomalies of the external genitalia. Pediatrics 106, 138–142.

Anderson, R.A., Byrum, R.S., Coates, P.M., et al., 1994. Mutations at the lysosomal acid cholesteryl ester hydrolase gene locus in Wolman disease. Proc Natl Acad Sci U S A 91, 2718–2722.

Ares, S., Escobar-Morreale, H.F., Quero, J., et al., 1997. Neonatal hypothyroxinemia: effects of iodine intake and premature birth. J Clin Endocrinol Metab 82, 1704–1712.

Arlt, W., Walker, E.A., Draper, N., et al., 2004. Congenital adrenal hyperplasia caused by mutant P450 oxidoreductase and human androgen synthesis: analytical study. Lancet 363, 2128–2135.

Arnold, A., 1990. Mutation of the signal peptide-encoding region of the preproparathyroid hormone gene in familial isolated hypoparathyroidism. J Clin Invest 86, 1084–1087.

Artman, H.G., Morris, C.A., Stock, A.D., 1992. 18p- syndrome and hypopituitarism. J Med Genet 29, 671–672.

Asakura, Y., Tachibana, K., Adachi, M., et al., 2002. Hypothalamo-pituitary hypothyroidism detected by neonatal screening for congenital hypothyroidism using measurement of thyroid-stimulating hormone and thyroxine. Acta Paediatr 91, 172–177.

Bakker, B., Bikker, H., Vulsma, T., et al., 2000. Two decades of screening for congenital hypothyroidism in The Netherlands: TPO gene mutations in total iodide organification defects (an update). J Clin Endocrinol Metab 85, 3708–3712.

Barkovich, A.J., Fram, E.K., Norman, D., 1989. Septo-optic dysplasia: MR imaging. Radiology 171, 189–192.

Barr, Jr., M., Hanson, J.E., Currey, K., et al., 1983. Holoprosencephaly in infants of diabetic mothers. J Pediatr 102, 565–568.

Bass, J.K., Chan G.M., 2006. Calcium nutrition and metabolism during infancy. Nutrition 22, 1057–1066.

Batch, J.A., Evans, B.A.J., Hughes, I.A., et al., 1993. Mutations of the androgen receptor gene identified in perineal hypospadias. J Med Genet 30, 198–201.

Batterham, R.L., Cowley, M.A., Small, C.J., et al., 2002. Gut hormone PYY(3–36) physiologically inhibits food intake. Nature 418, 650–654.

Belgorosky, A., Guercio, G., Pepe, C., et al., 2009. Genetic and clinical spectrum of aromatase deficiency in infancy, childhood and adolescence. Hormone Res 72, 321–330.

Belville, C., Josso, N., Picard, J.Y., 1999. Persistence of Mullerian derivatives in males. Am J Med Genet 89, 218–223.

Biebermann, H., Schoneberg, T., Krude, H., et al., 1997. Mutations of the human thyrotropin receptor gene causing thyroid hypoplasia and persistent congenital hypothyroidism. J Clin Endocrinol Metab 82, 3471–3480.

Binder, G., Ranke, M.B., 1995. Screening for growth hormone (GH) gene splice-site mutations in sporadic cases with severe isolated GH deficiency using ectopic transcript analysis. J Clin Endocrinol Metab 80, 1247–1252.

Biswas, S., Buffery, J., Enoch, H., et al., 2002. A longitudinal assessment of thyroid hormone concentrations in preterm infants younger than 30 weeks' gestation during the first 2 weeks of life and their relationship to outcome. Pediatrics 109, 222–227.

Black, J., Williams, D.I., 1973. Natural history of adrenal haemorrhage in the newborn. Arch Dis Child 48, 183–190.

Blair, J.C., Mohan, U., Larcher, V.F., et al., 2002. Neonatal thyrotoxicosis and maternal infertility in thyroid hormone resistance due to a mutation in the TRbeta gene (M313T). Clin Endocrinol 57, 405–409.

Blanco, E.J., Lane, A.H., Aijaz, N., 2006. Use of subcutaneous DDAVP in infants with central diabetes insipidus. J Pediatr Endocrinol Metab 19, 919–925.

Bojesen, A., Juul, S., Gravholt, C.H., 2003. Prenatal and postnatal prevalence of Klinefelter syndrome: a national registry study. J Clin Endocrinol Metab 88, 622–626.

Bolt, R.J., van Weissenbruch, M.M., Cranendonk, A., et al., 2002. The corticotrophin-releasing hormone test in preterm infants. Clin Endocrinol 56, 207–213.

Bongers-Schokking, J.J., Koot, H.M., Wiersma, D., et al., 2000. Influence of timing and dose of thyroid hormone replacement on development in infants with congenital hypothyroidism. J Pediatr 136, 292–297.

Bouvattier, C., Carel, J.C., Lecointre, C., et al., 2002. Postnatal changes of T, LH, and FSH in 46,XY infants with mutations in the AR gene. J Clin Endocrinol Metab 87, 29–32.

Bowyer, L., Catling-Paull, C., Diamond, T., et al., 2009. Vitamin D, PTH and calcium levels in pregnant women and their neonates. Clin Endocrinol 70, 372–377.

Briet, J.M., van Wassenaer, A.G., Dekker, F.W., et al., 2001. Neonatal thyroxine supplementation in very preterm children: developmental outcome evaluated at early school age. Pediatrics 107, 712–718.

Broglio, F., Gottero, C., Arvat, E., et al., 2003. Endocrine and non-endocrine actions of ghrelin. Hormone Res 59, 109–117.

Brook, C.D.G., Clayton, P.E., Brown, R.S. (Eds.), 2010. Clinical Pediatric Endocrinology, sixth ed. Blackwell Science, Oxford.

Brown, R.S., Bellisario, R.L., Botero, D., et al., 1996. Incidence of transient congenital hypothyroidism due to maternal thyrotropin receptor-blocking antibodies in over one million babies. J Clin Endocrinol Metab 81, 1147–1151.

Brown, R.S., Bloomfield, S., Bednarek, F.J., et al., 1997. Routine skin cleansing with povidone-iodine is not a common cause of transient neonatal hypothyroidism in North America: a prospective controlled study. Thyroid 7, 395–400.

Bullen, P.J., Rankin, J.M., Robson, S.C., 2001. Investigation of the epidemiology and prenatal diagnosis of holoprosencephaly in the North of England. Am J Obstet Gynecol 184, 1256–1262.

Calaciura, F., Motta, R.M., Miscio, G., et al., 2002. Subclinical hypothyroidism in early childhood: a frequent outcome of transient neonatal hyperthyrotropinemia. J Clin Endocrinol Metab 87, 3209–3214.

Calzolari, E., Contiero, M.R., Roncarati, E., et al., 1986. Aetiological factors in hypospadias. J Med Genet 23, 333.

Carabinas, C.D., Tolis, G.J., 1998. Thyroid disorders and pregnancy. J Obstet Gynaecol 18, 509–515.

Castanet, M., Marinovic, D., Polak, M., et al., 2010. Epidemiology of thyroid dysgenesis: the familial component. Hormone Res Paediatr 73, 231–237.

Cerame, B.I., Newfield, R.S., Pascoe, L., et al., 1999. Prenatal diagnosis and treatment of 11beta-hydroxylase deficiency congenital adrenal hyperplasia resulting in normal female genitalia. J Clin Endocrinol Metab 84, 3129–3134.

Chanoine, J.P., Yeung, L.P., Wong, A.C., et al., 2002. Immunoreactive ghrelin in human cord blood: relation to anthropometry, leptin, and growth hormone. J Pediatr Gastroenterol Nutr 35, 282–286.

Charmandari, E., Johnston, A., Brook, C.G., et al., 2001. Bioavailability of oral hydrocortisone in patients with congenital adrenal hyperplasia due to 21-hydroxylase deficiency. J Endocrinol 169, 65–70.

Cheetham, T.D., Bayliss, P.B., 2002. Diabetes insipidus in children. Pathophysiology, diagnosis and management. Pediatr Drugs 4, 785–796.

Chemaitilly, W., Betensky, B.P., Marshall, I., et al., 2005. The natural history and genotype-phenotype nonconcordance of HLA identical siblings with the same mutations of the 21-hydroxylase gene. J Pediatr Endocrinol Metab 18, 143–153.

Cheron, R.G., Kaplan, M.M., Larsen, P.R., et al., 1981. Neonatal thyroid function after propylthiouracil therapy for maternal Graves' disease. N Engl J Med 304, 525–528.

Chowdhry, P., Scanlon, J.W., Auerbach, R., et al., 1984. Results of controlled double blind study of thyroid replacement in very low birth weight premature infants with hypothyroxinaemia. Pediatrics 73, 301–305.

Christou, H., Connors, J.M., Ziotopoulou, M., et al., 2001. Cord blood leptin and insulin-like growth factor levels are independent predictors of fetal growth. J Clin Endocrinol Metab 86, 935–938.

Clark, A.J., Chan, L.F., Chung, T.T., et al., 2009. The genetics of familial glucocorticoid deficiency. Best Pract Res Clin Endocrinol Metab 23, 159–165.

Clerc, J., Monpeyssen, H., Chevalier, A., et al., 2008. Scintigraphic imaging of paediatric thyroid dysfunction. Hormone Res 70, 1–13.

Coburn, J.W., Elangovan, L., Goodman, W.G., et al., 1999. Calcium-sensing receptor and calcimimetic agents. Kidney Int. 73, S52–S58.

Cogan, J.D., Ramel, B., Lehto, M., et al., 1995. A recurring dominant negative mutation causes autosomal dominant growth hormone deficiency – a clinical research center study. J Clin Endocrinol Metab 80, 3591–3595.

Conte, F.A., Grumbach, M.M., Ito, Y., et al., 1994. A syndrome of female pseudohermaphrodism, hypergonadotropic hypogonadism, and multicystic ovaries associated with missense mutations in the gene encoding aromatase (P450arom). J Clin Endocrinol Metab 78, 1287–1292.

Corbetta, C., Weber, G., Cortinovis, F., et al., 2009. A 7-year experience with low blood TSH cutoff levels for neonatal screening reveals an unsuspected frequency of congenital hypothyroidism (CH). Clin Endocrinol 71, 739–745.

Coyle, B., Reardon, W., Herbrick, J.A., et al., 1998. Molecular analysis of the PDS gene in Pendred syndrome. Hum Mol Genet 7, 1105–1112.

Craft, W.H., Underwood, L.E., Van Wyk, J.J., 1980. High incidence of perinatal insult in children with idiopathic hypopituitarism. J Pediatr 96, 397–402.

Creighton, S.M., Minto, C.L., Steele, S.J., 2001. Objective cosmetic and anatomical outcomes at adolescence of feminising surgery for ambiguous genitalia done in childhood. Lancet 358, 124–125.

Daliva, A.L., Linder, B., DiMartino-Nardi, J., et al., 2000. Three-year follow-up of borderline congenital hypothyroidism. J Pediatr 136, 53–56.

Dattani, M.T., 2004. Novel insights into the aetiology and pathogenesis of hypopituitarism. Hormone Res 62 (S3), 1–13.

Dattani, M.T., Robinson, I.C., 2000. The molecular basis for developmental disorders of the pituitary gland in man. Clin Genet 57, 337–346.

Dattani, M.T., Martinez-Barbera, J.P., Thomas, P.Q., et al., 1998. Mutations in the homeobox gene HESX1/Hesx1 associated with septo-optic dysplasia in human and mouse. Nat Genet 19, 125–133.

Daw, S.C.M., Taylor, C., Kraman, M., 1996. A common region of 10p deleted in DiGeorge and velocardiofacial syndromes. Nat Genet 13, 458–461.

Deladoey, J., Fluck, C., Buyukgebiz, A., et al., 1999. 'Hot spot' in the PROP1 gene responsible for combined pituitary hormone deficiency. J Clin Endocrinol Metab 84, 1645–1650.

De Zegher, F., Van den Berghe, G., Devlieger, H., et al., 1993. Dopamine inhibits growth hormone and prolactin secretion in the human newborn. Pediatr Res 34, 642–645.

De Zegher, F., Kaplan, S.L., Grumbach, M.M., et al., 1995a. The foetal pituitary, postmaturity and breech presentation. Acta Paediatr 83, 1100–1102.

De Zegher, F., Pernasetti, F., Vanhole, C., et al., 1995b. The prenatal role of thyroid hormone evidenced by fetomaternal Pit-1 deficiency. J Clin Endocrinol Metab 80, 3127–3130.

Den Ouden, A.L., Kok, J.H., Verkerk, P.H., et al., 1996. The relation between neonatal thyroxine levels and neurodevelopmental outcome at age 5 and 9 years in a national cohort of very preterm and/or very low birth weight infants. Pediatr Res 39, 142–145.

Derksen-lubsen Verkerk, P.H., 1996. Neuropsychologic development in early treated congenital hypothyroidism: analysis of literature data. Pediatr Res 39, 561–566.

DeSa, D.J., Nicholls, S., 1972. Hemorrhagic necrosis of the adrenal gland in perinatal infants: a clinic-pathological study. J Pathol 106, 133–149.

Diamond, M., Sigmundson, H.K., 1997. Management of intersexuality. Guidelines for dealing with persons with ambiguous genitalia. Arch Pediatr Adolesc Med 151, 1046–1050.

Dickerman, Z., de Vries, L., 1997. Prepubertal and pubertal growth, timing and duration of puberty and attained adult height in patients with congenital hypothyroidism (CH) detected by the neonatal screening programme for CH – a longitudinal study. Clin Endocrinol 47, 649–654.

Doeker, B.M., Pfaffle, R.W., Pohlenz, J., et al., 1998. Congenital central hypothyroidism due to a homozygous mutation in the thyrotropin beta-subunit gene follows an autosomal recessive inheritance. J Clin Endocrinol Metab 83, 1762–1765.

Don-Wauchope, A.C., Wang, L., Grey, V., 2009. Pediatric critical values: Laboratory–pediatrician discourse. Clin Biochem 42, 1658–1661.

Dubuis, J.-M., Glorieux, J., Richer, F., et al., 1996. Outcome of severe congenital hypothyroidism: closing the developmental gap with early high dose levothyroxine treatment. J Clin Endocrinol Metab 81, 222–227.

Duprez, L., Parma, J., Van Sande, J., et al., 1994. Germline mutations in the thyrotropin receptor gene cause non-autoimmune autosomal dominant hyperthyroidism. Nat Genet 7, 396–401.

Egbuna, O.I., Brown, E.M., 2008. Hypercalcaemic and Hypocalcaemic conditions due to Calcium-sensing receptor mutations. Best Pract Res Clin Rheumatol 22, 129–148.

Everett, L.A., Glaser, B., Beck, J.C., et al., 1997. Pendred syndrome is caused by mutations in a putative sulphate transporter gene (PDS). Nat Genet 17, 411–422.

Farooqi, I.S., Jebb, S.A., Langmack, G., et al., 1999. Effects of recombinant leptin therapy in a child with congenital leptin deficiency. N Engl J Med 341, 879–884.

Farooqi, I.S., Yeo, G.S., Keogh, J.M., et al., 2000. Dominant and recessive inheritance of morbid obesity associated with melanocortin 4 receptor deficiency. J Clin Invest 106, 271–279.

Farooqi, I.S., Keogh, J.M., Yeo, G.S., et al., 2003. Clinical spectrum of obesity and mutations in the melanocortin 4 receptor gene. N Engl J Med 348, 1085–1095.

Ferraz-de-Souza, B., Achermann, J.C., 2008. Disorders of adrenal development. Endocr Dev.13, 19–32.

Fisher, D.A., 1999. Hypothyroxinemia in premature infants: is thyroxine treatment necessary? Thyroid 9, 715–720.

Fisher, D.A., 2002. Disorders of the thyroid in the newborn and infant. In: Sperling, M., (Ed.), Pediatric Endocrinology. W B Saunders, Philadelphia, pp. 161–185.

Fisher, D.A., Dussault, J.H., Foley, Jr., T.P., et al., 1979. Screening for congenital hypothyroidism: results of screening one million North American infants. J Pediatr 94, 700–705.

Fisher, D.A., Nelson, J.C., Carlton, E.I., et al., 2000. Maturation of human hypothalamic-pituitary-thyroid function and control. Thyroid 10, 229–234.

Forest, M., 1998. Prenatal diagnosis, treatment, and outcome in infants with congenital adrenal hyperplasia. Curr Opin Endocrinol Diabetes. 4, 209–217.

Forest, M.G., Cathiard, A.M., Bertrand, J.A., 1973. Total and unbound testosterone levels in the newborn and in normal and hypogonadal children: use of a sensitive radioimmunoassay for testosterone. J Clin Endocrinol Metab 36, 1132–1142.

Fox, L., Sadowsky, J., Pringle, K.P., et al., 2007. Neonatal hyperparathyroidism and pamidronate therapy in an extremely premature infant. Pediatrics 120, 1350–1354.

Frank, J.E., Faix, J.E., Hermos, R.J., et al., 1996. Thyroid function in very low birth weight infants: effects on neonatal hypothyroidism screening. J Pediatr 128, 548–554.

Fredell, L., Kockum, I., Hansson, E., et al., 2002. Heredity of hypospadias and the significance of low birth weight. J Urol 167, 1423–1427.

Friesma, E.C., Grueters, A., Biebermann, H., et al., 2004. Association between mutations in a thyroid hormone transporter and severe X-linked psychomotor retardation. Lancet 364, 1435–1437.

Fujiwara, H., Tatsumi, K., Miki, K., et al., 1997. Congenital hypothyroidism caused by a mutation in the Na$^+$/L$^-$ symporter. Nat Genet 16, 124–125.

Geissler, W.M., Davis, D.L., Wu, L., et al., 1994. Male pseudohermaphroditism caused by mutations of testicular 17 beta-hydroxysteroid dehydrogenase 3. Nat Genet 7, 34–39.

Giacoia, G.P., Wagner, H.R., 1978. Q-oTc Interval and blood calcium levels in newborn infants. Pediatrics 61, 877–882.

Gluckman, P.D., Gunn, A.J., Wray, A., et al., 1992. Congenital idiopathic growth hormone deficiency is associated with prenatal and early postnatal growth failure. J Pediatr 121, 920–923.

Godowski, P.J., Leung, D.W., Meacham, L.R., et al., 1989. Characterization of the human growth hormone receptor gene and demonstration of a partial gene deletion in two patients with Laron-type dwarfism. Proc Natl Acad Sci U S A 86, 8083–8087.

Grant, D.B., 1994. Growth in early treated congenital hypothyroidism. Arch Dis Child 70, 464–468.

Grant, D.B., Smith, I., Fuggle, P.W., et al., 1992. Congenital hypothyroidism detected by neonatal screening: relationship between biochemical severity and early clinical features. Arch Dis Child 67, 87–90.

Gregory, J.W., Aynsley-Green, A., Evans, B.A., et al., 1993. Deficiency of 17-ketoreductase presenting before puberty. Hormone Res 40, 145–148.

Grofer, B., Bodekere, R.H., Gortner, L., et al., 2010. Maturation of adrenal function determined by urinary glucocorticoid steroid excretion rates in preterm infants of more than 30 weeks of gestational age. Neonatology 98, 200–220.

Gruneiro de Papendieck, L., Iorcansky, S., Rivarola, M.A., et al., 1982. Patterns of TSH response to TRH in children with hypopituitarism. J Pediatr 100, 387–392.

Haddow, J.E., Palomaki, G.E., Allan, W.C., et al., 1999. Maternal thyroid deficiency during pregnancy and subsequent neuropsychological development of the child. N Engl J Med 341, 549–555.

Hadjiathanasiou, C.G., Brauner, R., Lortat-Jacob, S., et al., 1994. True hermaphroditism: genetic variants and clinical management. J Pediatr 125, 738–744.

Halliday, H.L., Ehrenkranz, R.A., 2010. Early (<8 days) postnatal corticosteroids for preventing chronic lung disease in preterm infants. Cochrane Database Syst Rev CD001146.

Halliday, H.L., Ehrenkranz, R.A., Doyle, L., 2009. Late (>7 days) postnatal corticosteroids for chronic lung disease in preterm infant. Cochrane Database Syst Rev CD00114.

Hamilton, J., Blaser, S., Daneman, D., 1998. MR imaging in idiopathic growth hormone deficiency. AJNR. Am J Neuroradiol 19, 1609–1615.

Hanukoglu, A., Perlman, K., Shamis, I., et al., 2001. Relationship of etiology to treatment in congenital hypothyroidism. J Clin Endocrinol Metab 86, 186–191.

Haqq, A.M., Farooqi, I.S., O'Rahilly, S., et al., 2003. Serum ghrelin levels are inversely correlated with body mass index, age, and insulin concentrations in normal children and are markedly increased in Prader–Willi syndrome. J Clin Endocrinol Metab 88, 174–178.

Hashimoto, H., Maruyama, H., Koshida, R., et al., 1995. Central hypothyroidism resulting from pituitary suppression and peripheral thyrotoxicosis in a premature infant born to a mother with Graves' disease. J Pediatr 127, 809–811.

Hawkins, J.R., Taylor, A., Goodfellow, P.N., et al., 1992. Evidence for increased prevalence of SRY mutations in XY females with complete rather than partial gonadal dysgenesis. Am J Hum Genet 51, 979–984.

Herman, S.P., Baggenstoss, A.M., Cloutier, M.D., 1975. Liver dysfunction and istologic abnormalities in neonatal hypopituitarism. J Pediatr 87, 892–895.

Hertzberg, V., Mei, J., Therrell, B.L., 2010. Effect of laboratory practices on the incidence rate of congenital hypothyroidism. Pediatrics 125 (S2), S48–S53.

Heyerdahl, S., Ilicki, A., Karlberg, J., et al., 1997. Linear growth in early treated children with congenital hypothyroidism. Acta Paediatr 86, 479–483.

Hindmarsh, P.C., 2002. Optimisation of thyroxine dose in congenital hypothyroidism. Arch Dis Child 86, 73–75.

Hindmarsh, P.C., Brook, C.G.D., 1985. Single dose dexamethasone suppression test in children: dose relationship to body size. Clin Endocrinol 23, 67–70.

Hingre, R.V., Gross, S.J., Hingre, K.S., et al., 1994. Adrenal steroidogenesis in very low birth weight preterm infants. J Clin Endocrinol Metab 78, 266–270.

Hoffman, W.H., Sahasrananan, P., Ferandos, S.S., et al., 1982. Transient thyrotoxicosis in an infant delivered to a longacting thyroid stimulator (LATS) and LATS protector negative, thyroid stimulating antibody positive woman with Hashimoto's thyroiditis. J Clin Endocrinol Metab 54, 354–356.

Honour, J.W., Torresani, T., 2001. Evaluation of neonatal screening for adrenal hyperplasia. Hormone Res 55, 206–211.

Hopkins, I.J., 1964. Chvostek's sign and facial reflexes in normal newborn infants. Dev Med Child Neurol 6, 389–392.

Hsu, L.Y.F., 1989. Prenatal diagnosis of 45X/46XY mosaicism – a review and update. Prenatal Diagn 9, 31–48.

Hsu, S.C. Levine, M.A., 2004. Perinatal Calcium metabolism: physiology and pathophysiology. Semin Neonatol 23–36.

Hughes, M.R., Malloy, P.J., Kieback, D.G., 1988. Point mutations in the human vitamin D receptor gene associated with hypocalcemic rickets. Science 242, 1702–1705.

Hughes, I.A., Houk, C., Ahmed, S.F., et al., 2006. Consensus statement on management of intersex disorders. Arch Dis Child 91, 554–563.

Hunter, M.K., Mandel, S.H., Sesser, D.E., et al., 1998. Follow-up of newborns with low thyroxine and nonelevated thyroid-stimulating hormone-screening concentrations: results of the 20-year experience in the Northwest Regional Newborn Screening Program. J Pediatr 132, 70–74.

Ibanez, L., Potau, N., Enriquez, G., et al., 2000. Reduced uterine and ovarian size in adolescent girls born small for gestational age. Pediatr Res 47, 575–577.

Ibanez, L., Potau, N., Ferrer, A., et al., 2002a. Reduced ovulation rate in adolescent girls born small for gestranional age. J Clin Endocrinol Metab 87, 3391–3393.

Ibanez, L., Valls, C., Cols, M., et al., 2002b. Hypersecretion of FSH in infant boys and girls born small for gestational age. J Clin Endocrinol Metab 87, 1986–1988.

Ieiri, T., Cochaux, P., Targovnik, H.M., et al., 1991. A 3' splice site mutation in the thyroglobulin gene responsible for congenital goiter with hypothyroidism. J Clin Invest 88, 1901–1905.

Igarashi, Y., Ogawa, M., Kamijo, T., et al., 1993. A new mutation causing inherited growth hormone deficiency: a compound heterozygote of a 6.7 kb deletion and a two base deletion in the third exon of the GH-1 gene. Hum Mol Genet 2, 1073–1074.

Imperato-McGinley, J., Peterson, R.E., Gautier, T., et al., 1979. Androgens and the evolution of male-gender identity among pseudohermaphrodites with 5α-reductase deficiency. N Engl J Med 300, 1233–1237.

Iniguez, G., Ong, K., Pena, V., et al., 2002. Fasting and post-glucose ghrelin levels in SGA infants: relationships with size and weight gain at one year of age. J Clin Endocrinol Metab 87, 5830–5833.

Joint LWPES/ESPE CAH Working Group, 2002. Consensus statement on 21-hydroxylase deficiency from the Lawson Wilkins Pediatric Endocrine Society and the European Society for Paediatric Endocrinology. J Clin Endocrinol Metab 87, 4048–4053.

Jordan, B.K., Jain, M., Natarajan, S., et al., 2002. Familial mutation in the testis-determining gene SRY shared by an XY female and her normal father. J Clin Endocrinol Metab 87, 3428–3432.

Jost, A., 1953. Problems of fetal endocrinology: the gonadal and hypophyseal hormones. Rec Progr Hormone Res 8, 379–413.

Kaefer, M., Diamond, D., Hendren, W.H., et al., 1999. The incidence of intersexuality in children with cryptorchidism and hypospadias: stratification based on gonadal palpability and meatal position. J Urol 162, 1003–1006.

Kari, M.A., Raivio, K.O., Stenman, U.H., et al., 1996. Serum cortisol, dehydroepiandrosterone sulfate, and steroid-binding globulins in preterm neonates: effect of gestational age and dexamethasone therapy. Pediatr Res 40, 319–324.

Karpman, B.A., Rapoport, B., Filetti, S., et al., 1987. Treatment of neonatal hyperthyroidism due to Graves disease with sodium ipodate. J Clin Endocrinol Metab 64, 119–123.

Kelberman, D., Rizzoti, K., Lovell-Badge, R., et al., 2009. Genetic regulation of pituitary gland development in human and mouse. Endocr Rev 30, 790–829.

Kelley, R.I., Hennekam, R.C., 2000. The Smith–Lemli–Opitz syndrome. J Med Genet 37, 321–335.

Kitanaka, S., Takeyama, K., Murayama, A., 1998. Inactivating mutations in the 25-hydroxyvitamin D3 1alpha-hydroxylase gene in patients with pseudovitamin D-deficiency rickets. N Engl J Med 338, 653–661.

Köhler, B., Schnabel, D., Biebermann, H., et al., 1996. Transient congenital hypothyroidism and hyperthyrotropinemia: normal thyroid function and physical development at the ages of 6–14 years. J Clin Endocrinol Metab 81, 1563–1567.

Köhler, B., Lin, L., Mazen, I., et al., 2009. The spectrum of phenotypes associated with mutations in steroidogenic factor 1 (SF-1,

NR5A1, Ad4BP) includes severe penoscrotal hypospadias in 46,XY males without adrenal insufficiency. Eur J Endocrinol 161, 237–242.

Koopman, P., Gubbay, J., Vivian, N., et al., 1991. Male development of chromosomally female mice transgenic for Sry. Nature 351, 117–121.

Kopp, P., van Sande, J., Parma, J., et al., 1995. Brief report: Congenital hyperthyroidism caused by a mutation in the thyrotropin-receptor gene. N Engl J Med 332, 183–185.

Korada, M., Pearce, M.S., WardPlatt, M.P., et al., 2008. Repeat testing for congenital hypothyroidism in preterm infants is unnecessary with an appropriate thyroid stimulating hormone threshold. Arch Dis Child Fetal Neonatal Ed 93, F286–F288.

Kovacs, C.S. Kronenberg, H.M., 1997. Maternal-fetal calcium and bone metabolism during pregnacy, puerperium and lactation. Endocr Rev 18, 832–872.

Kovacs, C., Chafe, L., Fudge, N., et al., 2001. PTH regulates fetal blood calcium and skeletal mineralization independently of PTHrP. Endocrinology 142, 4983–4993.

Kremer, H., Kraaij, R., Toledo, S.P.A., et al., 1995. Male pseudohermaphroditism due to a homozygous missense mutation of the luteinizing hormone receptor gene. Nat Genet 9, 160–164.

Krone, N., Arlt, W., 2009. Genetics of congenital adrenal hyperplasia. Best Pract Res Clin Endocrinol Metab 23, 181–192.

Kronenburg, H.M., Melmed, S., Polonsky, K.S., Larsen, P.R. (Eds.), 2008. Williams Textbook of Endocrinology, 11th ed. W B Saunders, Philadelphia.

Krude, H., Biebermann, H., Luck, W., et al., 1998. Severe early-onset obesity, adrenal insufficiency and red hair pigmentation caused by POMC mutations in humans. Nat Genet 19, 155–157.

Krude, H., Schutz, B., Biebermann, H., et al., 2002. Choreoathetosis, hypothyroidism, and pulmonary alterations due to human NKX2-1 haploinsufficiency. J Clin Invest 109, 475–480.

Kruse, K., Irle, U., Uhlig, R., 1993. Elevated 1,25-dihydroxyvitamin D serum concentrations in infants with subcutaneous fat necrosis. J Pediatr 122, 460–463.

LaFranchi, S.H., 2010. Newborn screening stratergies for congenital hypothyroidism: an update. J Inherit Metab Dis 2010; 33 (Suppl. 2), S225–S233.

Lajic, S., Nordenström, A., Hirvikoski, T., 2008. Long-term outcome of prenatal treatment of congenital adrenal hyperplasia. Endocr Dev 13, 82–89.

Langman, C.B., 1999. Hypercalcemic syndromes in infants and children. In: Favus, M.J. (Ed.), Primer on the Metabolic Bone Diseases and Disorders of Mineral

Metabolism. Lippincott Williams & Wilkins, Philadelphia, pp 219–223.

Layman, L.C., Lee, E.J., Peak, D.B., et al., 1997. Delayed puberty and hypogonadism caused by mutations in the follicle-stimulating hormone beta-subunit gene. N Engl J Med 337, 607–611.

Layman, L.C., Porto, A.L., Xie, J., et al., 2002. FSH beta gene mutations in a female with partial breast development and a male sibling with normal puberty and azoospermia. J Clin Endocrinol Metab 87, 3702–3707.

Lee, Y.S., Loke, K.Y., Ng, S.C., et al., 2002. Maternal thyrotoxicosis causing central hypothyroidism in infants. J Paediatr Child Health 38, 206–208.

Leviton, A., Paneth, N., Reuss, M.L., et al., 1999. Hypothyroxinemia of prematurity and the risk of cerebral white matter damage. J Pediatr 134, 706–711.

Lienhardt, A., Mas, J.C., Kalifa, G., et al., 2002. IMAGe association: additional clinical features and evidence for recessive autosomal inheritance. Hormone Res 57 (S2), 71–78.

Lin, L., Gu, W.X., Ozisik, G., et al., 2006. Analysis of DAX1 (NR0B1) and steroidogenic factor-1 (NR5A1) in children and adults with primary adrenal failure: ten years' experience. J Clin Endocrinol Metab 91, 3048–3055.

Linder, N., Davidovitch, N., Reichman, B., et al., 1997. Topical iodine-containing antiseptics and subclinical hypothyroidism in preterm infants. J Pediatr 131, 434–439.

Little, M., Wells, C., 1997. A clinical overview of WT1 gene mutations. Hum Mutat 9, 209–225.

Loughead, J.L., Mimouni, F., Tsang, R.C., 1988. Serum ionized calcium concentrations in normal neonates. Am J Dis Child 142, 516–518.

Lucas, A., Morley, R., Fewtrell, M.S., 1996. Low triiodothyronine concentration in preterm infants and subsequent intelligence quotient (IQ) at 8 year follow up. Br Med J 312, 1132–1133.

Maiya, S., Sullivan, I., Allgrove, J., et al., 2008. Hypocalcaemia and vitamin D deficiency: an important, but preventable, cause of life-threatening infant heart failure. Heart 94, 581–584.

Mandel, S., Hanna, C., Boston, B., et al., 1993. Thyroxine-binding globulin deficiency detected by newborn screening. J Pediatr 122, 227–230.

Mandel, S.J., Hermos, R.J., Larson, C.A., et al., 2000. Atypical hypothyroidism and the very low birthweight infant. Thyroid 10, 693–695.

Martin, N.D., Snodgrass, G.J., Cohen, R.D., 1984. Idiopathic infantile hypercalcaemia – a continuing enigma. Arch Dis Child 59, 605–613.

Mathai, S., Cutfield, W.S., Gunn, A.J., et al., 2008. A novel therapeutic paradigm to treat congenital hypothyroidism. Clin Endocrinol 69, 142–147.

Matsuura, N., Harada, S., Ohyama, Y., et al., 1997. The mechanisms of transient hypothyroxinemia in infants born to mothers with Graves' disease. Pediatr Res 42, 214–218.

Mayne, P.D., Kovar, I.Z., 1991. Calcium and phosphate metabolism in the premature infant. Ann Clin Biochem 28, 131–142.

Mehta, A., Hindmarsh, P.C., Stanhope, R.G., et al., 2003. Is the thyrotropin-releasing hormone test necessary in the diagnosis of central hypothyroidism in children. J Clin Endocrinol Metab 88, 5696–5703.

Mehta, A., Hindmarsh, P.C., Stanhope, R.G., et al., 2005. The role of growth hormone in determining birth size and early postnatal growth, using congenital growth hormone deficiency (GHD) as a model. Clin Endocrinol 63, 223–231.

Meijer, W.J., Verloove-Vanhorick, S.P., Brand, R., et al., 1992. Transient hypothyroxinaemia associated with developmental delay in very preterm infants. Arch Dis Child 67, 944–947.

Mercado, M., Yu, V.Y., Francis, I., et al., 1988. Thyroid function in very preterm infants. Early Hum Dev 16, 131–141.

Merewood, A., Mehta, S., Grossman, X., 2010. Widespread vitamin D deficiency in urban Massachusetts newborns and their mothers. Pediatrics 125, 640–647.

Merke, D.P., Keil, M.F., Jones, J.V., et al., 2000. Flutamide, testolactone, and reduced hydrocortisone dose maintain normal growth velocity and bone maturation despite elevated androgen levels in children with congenital adrenal hyperplasia. J Clin Endocrinol Metab 85, 1114–1120.

Merke, D.P., Cho, D., Calis, K.A., et al., 2001. Hydrocortisone suspension and hydrocortisone tablets are not bioequivalent in the treatment of children with congenital adrenal hyperplasia. J Clin Endocrinol Metab 86, 441–445.

Metzger, D.L., Wright, N.M., Veldhuis, J.D., et al., 1993. Characterization of pulsatile secretion and clearance of plasma cortisol in premature and term neonates using deconvolution analysis. J Clin Endocrinol Metab 77, 458–463.

Meyer-Bahlburg, H.F., 1999. Gender assignment and reassignment in 46,XY pseudohermaphroditism and related conditions. J Clin Endocrinol Metab 84, 3455–3458.

Midgley, P.C., Holownia, P., Smith, J., et al., 2001. Plasma cortisol, cortisone and urinary glucocorticoid metabolites in preterm infants. Biol Neonate 79, 79–86.

Millar, D.S., Lewis, M.D., Horan, M., et al., 2003. Novel mutations of the growth hormone 1 (GH1) gene disclosed by modulation of the clinical selection criteria for individuals with short stature. Hum Mutat 21, 424–440.

Miller, W., 2001. The adrenal cortex and its disorders. In: Brook, C.D.G., Hindmarsh, P.C. (Eds.), Clinical Pediatric Endocrinology. Blackwell Science, Oxford, pp 321–337.

Miller, R.R., Menke, J.A., Menster, M.I., 1984. Hypercalcaemia associated with phosphate depletion in the neonate. J Pediatr 105, 814–817.

Mitsuda, N., Tamaki, H., Amino, N., et al., 1992. Risk factors for developmental disorders in infants born to women with Graves disease. Obstet Gynecol 80, 359–364.

Montague, C.T., Farooqi, I.S., Whitehead, J.P., et al., 1997. Congenital leptin deficiency is associated with severe early-onset obesity in humans. Nature 387, 903–908.

Moreno, J.C., Bikker, H., Kempers, M.J., et al., 2002. Inactivating mutations in the gene for thyroid oxidase 2 (THOX2) and congenital hypothyroidism. N Engl J Med 347, 95–102.

Munro, D.S., Dirmikis, S.M., Humphries, H., et al., 1978. The role of thyroid stimulating antibodies of Graves' disease in neonatal thyrotoxicosis. Br J Obstet Gynaecol 85, 837–843.

Murphy, J.F., Joyce, B.G., Dyas, J., et al., 1983. Plasma 17-hydroxyprogesterone concentration in ill newborn infants. Arch Dis Child 58, 532–534.

Nako, Y., Fukushima, N., Tomomasa, T., et al., 1993. Hypervitaminosis D after prolonged feeding with a premature formula. Pediatrics 92, 862–864.

Nanni, L., Ming, J.E., Bocian, M., et al., 1999. The mutational spectrum of the Sonic hedgehog gene in holoprosencephaly: SHH mutations cause a significant proportion of autosomal dominant holoprosencephaly. Hum Mol Genet 8, 2479–2488.

New, M., 2001. Extensive personal experience: prenatal diagnosis for congenital adrenal hyperplasia in 532 pregnancies. J Clin Endocrinol Metab 86, 5651–5657.

Ng, P.C., 2000. The fetal and neonatal hypothalamic–pituitary–adrenal axis. Arch Dis Child Fetal Neonatal Ed 82, F250–F254.

Ng, P.C., Lam, C.W., Lee, C.H., et al., 2002. Reference ranges and factors affecting the human corticotropin-releasing hormone test in preterm, very low birth weight infants. J Clin Endocrinol Metab 87, 4621–4628.

Ng, P.C., Lee, C.H., Lam, C.W., et al., 2004. Transient adrenocortical insufficiency of prematurity and systemic hypotension in very low birthweight infants. Arch Dis Child Fetal Neonatal Ed 89, F119–F126.

Nijenhuis, M., van den Akker, E.L.T., Zalm, R., et al., 2001. Familial neurohypophysial diabetes insipidus in a large Dutch kindred: effect of the onset of diabetes on growth in children and cell biological defects of the mutant vasopressin prohormone. J Clin Endocrinol Metab 86, 3410–3420.

Nimkarn, S. New M.I., 2010. Congenital adrenal hyperplasia due to 21-hydroxylase deficiency: A paradigm for prenatal diagnosis and treatment. Ann N Y Acad Sci 1192, 5–11.

Noori, S., Seri, I., 2005. Pathophysiology of newborn hypotension outside the transitional period. Early Hum Dev 81, 399–404.

Nordenstrom, A., Thilen, A., Hagenfeldt, L., et al., 1999. Genotyping is a valuable diagnostic complement to neonatal screening for congenital adrenal hyperplasia due to steroid 21-hydroxylase deficiency. J Clin Endocrinol Metab 84, 1505–1509.

Nordenstrom, A., Servin, A., Bohlin, G., et al., 2002. Sex-typed toy play behaviour correlates with the degree of prenatal androgen exposure assessed by CYP21 genotype in girls with congenital adrenal hyperplasia. J Clin Endocrinol Metab 87, 5119–5124.

Ogilvy-Stuart, A., Midgley, P., 2006. Practical Neonatal Endocrinology. Cambridge University Press, Cambridge.

Olivieri, A., Stazi, M.A., Mastroiacovo, P., et al., 2002. The Study Group for Congenital Hypothyroidism. A population-based study on the frequency of additional congenital malformations in infants with congenital hypothyroidism: data from the Italian Registry for Congenital Hypothyroidism (1991–1998). J Clin Endocrinol Metab 87, 557–562.

Olsen, C.L., Hughes, J.P., Youngblood, L.G., et al., 1997. Epidemiology of holoprosencephaly and phenotypic characteristics of affected children: New York State, 1984–1989. Am J Med Genet 73, 217–226.

Ong, K.K., Ahmed, M.L., Sherriff, A., et al., 1999. Cord blood leptin is associated with size at birth and predicts infancy weight gain in humans. ALSPAC Study Team. Avon Longitudinal Study of Pregnancy and Childhood. J Clin Endocrinol Metab 84, 1145–1148.

Pang, S., Murphey, W., Levine, L.S., 1982. A pilot newborn screening for congenital adrenal hyperplasia in Alaska. J Clin Endocrinol Metab 55, 413–420.

Parkinson, D., Thakker, R., 1992. A donor splice mutation in the parathyroid hormone gene is associated with autosomal recessive hypoparathyroidism. Nat Genet 1, 149–152.

Parks, J.S., Brown, M.R., Hurley, D.L., et al., 1999. Heritable disorders of pituitary development. J Clin Endocrinol Metab 84, 4362–4370.

Patel, L., McNally, R.J., Harrison, E., et al., 2006. Geographical distribution of optic nerve hypoplasia and septo-optic dysplasia in Northwest England. J Pediatrics.148, 85–88.

Pearce, S.H.S., Williamson, C., Kifor, O., et al., 1996. A familial syndrome of hypocalcemia with hypercalciuria due to mutations in the calcium-sensing receptor. N Engl J Med 335, 1115–1122.

Pearce, S., Tim, D., Cheetham, T., 2010. Diagnosis and management of vitamin D deficiency. Br Med J 340, b5664.

Pena-Almazan, S., Buchlis, J., Miller, S., et al., 2001. Linear growth characteristics of congenitally GH-deficient infants from birth to one year of age. J Clin Endocrinol Metab 86, 5691–5694.

Perry, R.J., Hollman, A.S., Wood, A.M., et al., 2002a. Ultrasound of the thyroid gland in the newborn: normative data. Arch Dis Child Fetal Neonatal Ed 87, F209–F211.

Perry, R., Heinrichs, C., Bourdoux, P., et al., 2002b. Discordance of monozygotic twins for thyroid dysgenesis: implications for screening and for molecular pathophysiology. J Clin Endocrinol Metab 87, 4072–4077.

Perry, R.J., Maroo, S., MacLennan, A.C., et al., 2006. Combined ultrasound and isotope scanning is more informative in the diagnosis of congenital hypothyroidism than single scanning. Arch Dis Child 91, 972–976.

Persani, L., Ferretti, E., Borgato, S., et al., 2000. Circulating thyrotropin bioactivity in sporadic central hypothyroidism. J Clin Endocrinol Metab 85, 3631–3635.

Pfaffle, R.W., Di Mattia, G.E., Parks, J.S., et al., 1992. Mutation of the POU-specific domain of Pit-1 and hypopituitarism without pituitary hypoplasia. Science 257, 1118–1121.

Philibert, P., Zenaty, D., Lin, L., et al., 2007. Mutational analysis of steroidogenic factor 1 (NR5a1) in 24 boys with bilateral anorchia: a French collaborative study. Hum Reprod 22, 325–3261.

Phillip, M., Arbelle, J.E., Segev, Y., et al., 1998. Male hypogonadism due to a mutation in the gene for the beta-subunit of follicle-stimulating hormone. N Engl J Med 338, 1729–1732.

Phillips, III, J.A., Hjelle, B., Seeburg, P.H., et al., 1981. Molecular basis for familial isolated growth hormone deficiency. Proc Natl Acad Sci U S A 78, 6372–6375.

Pidasheva, S., D'Souza-Li, L., Canaff, L., et al., 2004. CASRdb: calcium-sensing receptor locus-specific database for mutations causing familial (benign) hypocalciuric hypercalcemia,neonatal severe hyperparathyroidism and autosomal dominant hypocalcemia. Hum Mutat 24, 107–111.

Pinto, G., Netchine, I., Sobrier, M.L., et al., 1999. Pituitary stalk interruption syndrome: a clinical-biological-genetic assessment of its pathogenesis. J Clin Endocrinol Metab 82, 3450–3454.

Pitt, J.J., 2010. Newborn screening. Clin Biochem Rev 31, 57–68.

Pohlenz, J., Rosenthal, I.M., Weiss, R.E., et al., 1998. Congenital hypothyroidism due to mutations in the sodium/iodide symporter. Identification of a nonsense mutation producing a downstream cryptic 3' splice site. J Clin Invest 101, 1028–1035.

Pohlenz, J., Sadow, P.M., Koffler, T., et al., 2001. Congenital hypothyroidism in a child with unsuspected familial dysalbuminemic hyperthyroxinemia caused by a mutation (R218H) in the human albumin gene. J Pediatr 139, 887–891.

Porter, F.D., 2008. Smith–Lemli–Opitz syndrome: pathogenesis, diagnosis and management. Eur J Hum Genet 16, 535–541.

Procter, A.M., Phillips, 3rd, J.A., Cooper, D.N., 1998. The molecular genetics of growth hormone deficiency. Hum Genet 103, 255–272.

Queipo, G., Zenteno, J.C., Pena, R., et al., 2002. Molecular analysis in true hermaphroditism: demonstration of low-level hidden mosaicism for Y-derived sequences in 46,XX cases. Hum Genet 111, 278–283.

Quintos, J.B., Boney, C.M., 2010. Transient adrenal insufficiency in the premature newborn. Curr Opin Endocrinol Diabetes Obesity 17, 8–12.

Radovick, S., Nations, M., Du, Y., et al., 1992. A mutation in the POU-homeodomain of Pit-1 responsible for combined pituitary hormone deficiency. Science 7, 1115–1118.

Ramos, E.S., Moreira-Filho, C.A., Vicente, Y.A., et al., 1996. SRY-negative true hermaphrodites and an XX male in two generations of the same family. Hum Genet 97, 596–598.

Rapaport, R., 2000. Congenital hypothyroidism: expanding the spectrum. J Pediatr 136, 10–12.

Rapaport, R., Sills, I., Patel, U., et al., 1993. Thyrotropin-releasing hormone stimulation tests in infants. J Clin Endocrinol Metab 77, 889–894.

Rapaport, R., Rose, S.R., Freemark, M., 2001. Hypothyroxinemia in the preterm infant: the benefits and risks of thyroxine treatment. J Pediatr 139, 182–188.

Refetoff, S., Weiss, R.E., 1997. Resistance to thyroid hormone. In: Thakker, T.V. (Ed.), Molecular Genetics of Endocrine Disorders. Chapman & Hill, London, pp 85–122.

Reuss, M.L., Paneth, N., Pinto-Martin, J.A., et al., 1996. The relation of transient hypothyroxinemia in preterm infants to neurologic development at two years of age. N Engl J Med 334, 821–827.

Rey, R.A., Belville, C., Nihoul-Fekete, C., et al., 1999. Evaluation of gonadal function in 107 intersex patients by means of serum antimullerian hormone measurement. J Clin Endocrinol Metab 84, 627–631.

Riepe, F.G., Sippell, W.G., 2007. Recent advances in diagnosis, treatment, and outcome of congenital adrenal hyperplasia due to 21-hydroxylase deficiency. Rev Endocrinol Metab Disord 8, 349–363.

Rivkees, S.A., Mattison, D.R., 2009. Propylthiouracil (PTU) hepatotoxicity in children and recommendations for discontinuation of use. Intl J Pediatr Endocrinol 132041.

Rivkees, S.A., Dunbar, N., Wilson, T.A., 2007. The management of central diabetes insipidus in infancy: desmopressin, low renal solute load formula, thiazide diuretics. J Pediatr Endocrinol Metab. 20, 459–469.

Roberts, D., Dalziel, S., 2010. Antenatal corticosteroids for accelerating fetal lung maturation for women at risk of preterm birth. Cochrane Database Syst Rev (3):CD00445.

Robertson, G.L., 2001. Disorders of water balance. In: Brook, C.G.D., Hindmarsh, P.C. (Eds.), Clinical Pediatric Endocrinology. Blackwell Scientific, Oxford, pp 193–221.

Rodd, C., Goodyer, P., 1999. Hypercalcemia of the newborn: etiology, evaluation, and management. Pediatr Nephrol 13, 542–547.

Romagnoli, C., Zecca, E., Tortorolo, G., et al., 1987. Plasma thyrocalcitonin and parathyroid hormone concentrations in early neonatal hypocalcaemia. Arch Dis Child 62, 580–584.

Rona, R.J., Tanner, J.M., 1977. Aetiology of idiopathic growth hormone deficiency in England and Wales. Arch Dis Child 52, 197–208.

Rose, S.R., 2006. Newborn screening for congenital hypothyroidism: recommended guidelines. Pediatrics 117, 2290–2303.

Roti, E., Minelli, R., Salvi, M., 1996. Management of hyperthyoidism and hypothyroidism in the pregnant woman. J Clin Endocrinol Metab 781, 1679–1682.

Rovet, J.F., 1999. Congenital hypothyroidism: long-term outcome. Thyroid 9, 741–748.

Rovet, J.F., Ehrlich, R.M., 1995. Long-term effects of L-thyroxine therapy for congenital hypothyroidism. J Pediatr 126, 380–386.

Rovet, J., Walker, W., Bliss, B., et al., 1996. Long-term sequelae of hearing impairment in congenital hypothyroidism. J Pediatr 128, 776–783.

Rudman, D., Davis, T., Priest, J.H., et al., 1978. Prevalence of growth hormone deficiency in children with cleft lip and palate. J Pediatr 93, 378–382.

Salerno, M., Micillo, M., Di Maio, S., et al., 2001. Longitudinal growth, sexual maturation and final height in patients with congenital hypothyroidism detected by neonatal screening. Eur J Endocrinol 145, 377–383.

Salerno, M., Militerni, R., Bravaccio, C., et al., 2002. Effect of different starting doses of levothyroxine on growth and intellectual outcome at four years of age in congenital hypothyroidism. Thyroid 12, 45–52.

Salisbury, D.M., Leonard, J.V., Dezateux, C.A., et al., 1984. Micropenis: an important early sign of congenital hypopituitarism. Br Med J 288, 621–622.

Sandrini, R., Ribeiro, R.C., DeLacerda, L., 1997. Childhood adrenocortical tumors. J Clin Endocrinol Metab 82, 2027–2031.

Santiago, L.B., Jorge, S.M., Moreira, A.C., 1996. Longitudinal evaluation of the development of salivary cortisol circadian rhythm in infancy. Clin Endocrinol 44, 157–161.

Sarafoglou, K., Ostrer, H., 2000. Clinical review 111: familial sex reversal: a review. J Clin Endocrinol Metab 85, 483–493.

Savage, M.O., Burren, C.P., Blair, J.C., et al., 2001. Growth hormone insensitivity: pathophysiology, diagnosis, clinical variation and future perspectives. Hormone Res 55 (Suppl. 2), 32–35.

Savage, M.O., Cohen, L., Cohen, A.J., et al., 2010. Pathophysiology, assessment and management of the child with growth hormone resistance. Pediatr Endocrinol Rev 7, 347–356.

Schäffer, L., Luzi, F., Burkhardt, T., et al., 2009. Antenatal Betamethasone administration alters stress physiology in healthy neonates. Obstet Gynecol 113, 1082–1088.

Schipani, E., Langman, C.B., Parfitt, A.M., et al., 1996. Constitutively activated receptors for parathyroid hormone and parathyroid hormone-related peptide in Jansen's metaphyseal chondrodysplasia. N Engl J Med 335, 708–714.

Schonberger, W., Grimm, W., Emmrich, P., et al., 1981. Reduction of mortality rate in premature infants by substitution of thyroid hormones. Eur J Pediatr 135, 245–253.

Schwartz, I.D., Root, A.W., 1991. The Klinefelter syndrome of testicular dysgenesis. Endocrinol Metab Clin North Am 20, 153–163.

Scott, S.M., Watterberg, K.L., 1995. Effect of gestational age, postnatal age, and illness on plasma cortisol concentrations in premature infants. Pediatr Res 37, 112–116.

Segal, T., Mehta, A., Anazodo, A., et al., 2009. Role of gonadotrophin-releasing hormone and human chorionic gonadotrophic stimulation tests in differentiating patients with hypogonadotropic hypogonadism and those with constitutional delay of growth and puberty. J Clin Endocrinol Metab 94, 780–785.

Shaw, N.J., Pal, B.R., 2002. Vitamin D deficiency in UK Asian families: activating a new concern. Arch Dis Child 86, 147–149.

Shoback, D., 2008. Clinical practice: hypoparathyroidism. N Engl J Med 359, 391–403.

Shozu, M., Akasofu, K., Harada, T., et al., 1991. A new cause of female pseudohermaphroditism: placental aromatase deficiency. J Clin Endocrinol Metab 72, 560–566.

Singh, J., Pearce, S., Moghal, N., Cheetham, T.D., 2003. The investigation of hypocalcaemia and rickets. Arch Dis Child 88, 403–407.

Sivan, E., Lin, W.M., Homko, C.J., et al., 1997. Leptin is present in human cord blood. Diabetes 46, 917–919.

Skuza, K.A., Sills, I.N., Stene, M., et al., 1996. Prediction of neonatal hyperthyroidism in infants born to mothers with Graves disease. J Pediatr 128, 264–267.

Smerdely, P., Lim, A., Boyages, S.C., et al., 1989. Topical iodine-containing antiseptics and neonatal hypothyroidism in very-low-birthweight infants. Lancet ii, 661–664.

Smith, N.M., Byard, R.W., Bourne, A.J., 1991. Testicular regression syndrome – a pathological study of 77 cases. Histopathology 19, 269–272.

Sperling, M. (Ed.), 2008. Pediatric Endocrinology, third ed. W B Saunders, Philadelphia.

Stick, S.M., Betts, P.R., 1987. Oral desmopression in neonatal diabetes insipidus. Arch Dis Child 62, 1177–1178.

Sunthornthepvarakul, T., Gottschalk, M.E., Hayashi, Y., et al., 1995. Resistance to thyrotropin caused by mutations in the thyrotropin-receptor gene. N Engl J Med 332, 155–160.

Tajima, T., Hattorri, T., Nakajima, T., et al., 2003. Sporadic heterozygous frameshift mutation of HESX1 causing pituitary and optic nerve hypoplasia and combined pituitary hormone deficiency in a Japanese patient. J Clin Endocrinol Metab 88, 45–50.

Tatsumi, K.-I., Miyai, K., Notomi, T., et al., 1992. Cretinism with combined hormone deficiency caused by a mutation in the PIT1 gene. Nat Genet 1, 56–58.

Taylor, J.A., Geyer, L., Feldman, K., 2010. Use of supplemental vitamin D among infants breastfed for prolonged periods. Pediatrics 125, 105–111.

Telvi, L., Lebbar, A., Del Pino, O., et al., 1999. 45,X/46,XY mosaicism: report of 27 cases. Pediatrics 104, 304–308.

Teng, C.S., Tong, T.C., Hutchinson, J.H., et al., 1980. Thyroid stimulating immunoglobulins in neonatal Graves' disease. Arch Dis Child 55, 894–895.

Tfelt-Hansen, J., Brown, E.M., 2005. The calcium-sensing receptor in normal physiology and pathophysiology: a review. Crit Rev Clin Lab Sci 42, 35–70.

Thomas, B.R., Bennett, J.D., 1995. Symptomatic hypocalcemia and hypoparathyroidism in two infants of mothers with hyperparathyroidism and familial benign hypercalcemia. J Perinatol 15, 23–26.

Thomas, P.Q., Dattani, M.T., Brickman, J.M., et al., 2001. Heterozygous HESX1 mutations associated with isolated congenital pituitary hypoplasia and septo-optic dysplasia. Hum Mol Genet 10, 39–45.

Thyen, U., Lanz, K., Holterhus, P.-M., et al., 2006. Epidemiology and initial management of ambiguous genitalia at birth in Germany. Hormone Res 66, 204–205.

Tillotson, S.L., Fuggle, P.W., Smith, I., et al., 1994. Relation between biochemical severity and intelligence in early treated congenital hypothyroidism: a threshold effect. Br Med J 309, 440–445.

Toublanc, J.E., 1999. Guidelines for neonatal screening programs for congenital hypothyroidism. Working Group for Neonatal Screening in Paediatric Endocrinology of the European Society for Paediatric Endocrinology. Acta Paediatr Supplement 88, 13–14.

Traggiai, C., Stanhope, R., 2002. Endocrinopathies associated with midline cerebral and cranial malformations. J Pediatr 140, 252–255.

Triulzi, F., Scotti, G., di Natale, B., et al., 1994. Evidence of congenital midline brain anomaly in pituitary dwarfs: a magnetic resonance imaging study in 101 patients. Pediatrics 93, 409–416.

Tullio-Pelet, A., Salomon, R., Hadj-Rabia, S., et al., 2000. Mutant WD-repeat protein in triple-A syndrome. Nat Genet 26, 332–335.

Vallette-Kasic, S., Barlier, A., Teinturier, C., et al., 2001. PROP 1 gene screening in patients with multiple pituitary hormone deficiency reveals two sites of hypermutability and a high incidence of corticotroph deficiency. J Clin Endocrinol Metab 86, 4529–4535.

Vallette-Kasic, S., Pulichino, A.M., Gueydan, M., et al., 2004. A neonatal form of isolated ACTH deficiency frequently associated with Tpit gene mutations Endocr Res 30, 943–944.

Van Esch, H., Groenen, P., Nesbit, M., 2000. GATA3 haplo-insufficiency causes human HDR syndrome. Nature 406, 419–422.

Van Tijn, D.A., de Vijlder, J.J., Vulsma, T., 2008. Role of the thyrotropin-releasing hormone stimulation test in diagnosis of congenital central hypothyroidism in infants. J Clin Endocrinol Metab 93, 410–419.

Van Wassenaer, A.G., Kok, J.H., Endert, E., et al., 1993. Thyroxine administration to infants of less than 30 weeks' gestational age does not increase plasma triiodothyronine concentrations. Acta Endocrinol (Copenhagen) 129, 139–146.

Van Wassenaer, A.G., Kok, J.H., de Vijlder, J.J.M., et al., 1997. Effects of thyroxine supplementation on neurologic development in infants born at less than 30 weeks' gestation. N Engl J Med 336, 21–26.

Velaphi, S.C., Perlman, J.M., 2001. Neonatal adrenal hemorrhage: clinical and abdominal sonographic findings. Clin Pediatr 40, 545–548.

Viljakainen, H.J., Saarnio, E., Hytinantti, T., et al., 2010. Maternal vitamin D status determines bone variables in the newborn. J Clin Endocrinol Metab 95, 1749–1757.

Visudhiphan, P., 2005. Neonatal seizures and familial hypomagnesemia with secondary hypocalcemia. Pediatr Neurol 33, 202–205.

Vulsma, T., Gons, M.H., de Vijlder, J.J., 1989. Maternal-fetal transfer of thyroxine in congenital hypothyroidism due to a total organification defect or thyroid agenesis. N Engl J Med 321, 13–16.

Wajnrajch, M.P., Gertner, J.M., Harbison, M.D., et al., 1996. Nonsense mutation in the human growth hormone-releasing hormone receptor causes growth failure analogous to the little (lit) mouse. Nat Genet 12, 88–90.

Waller, S., Kurzawinski, T., Spitz, L., et al., 2004. Neonatal severe hyperparathyroidism: genotype/phenotype correlation and the use of pamidronate as

rescue therapy. Eur J Pediatr 163, 589–594.

Wallis, D., Muenke, M., 2000. Mutations in holoprosencephaly. Hum Mutat 16, 99–108.

Weber, A., Toppari, J., Harvey, R.D., et al., 1995. Adrenocorticotropin receptor gene mutations in familial glucocorticoid deficiency: relationships with clinical features in four families. J Clin Endocrinol Metab 80, 65–71.

Weil, D., Wang, I., Dietrich, A., et al., 1994. Highly homologous loci on the X and Y chromosomes are hot-spots for ectopic recombinations leading to XX maleness. Nat Genet 7, 414–419.

Weiss, R.E., Refetoff, S., 1999. Treatment of resistance to thyroid hormone – primum non nocere. J Clin Endocrinol Metab 84, 401–404.

Weiss, J., Axelrod, L., Whitcomb, R.W., et al., 1992. Hypogonadism caused by a single amino acid substitution in the beta subunit of luteinizing hormone. N Engl J Med 326, 179–183.

Whyte, M.P., 1994. Hypophosphatasia and the role of alkaline phosphatase in skeletal mineralization. Endocr Rev 15, 439–461.

Wilkins, L.M., 1960. Masculinisation of the female fetus due to the use of orally given progestagens. JAMA 172, 1028–1032.

Wilkinson, H., James, J., 1993. Self limiting neonatal primary hyperparathyroidism associated with familial hypocalciuric hypercalcaemia. Arch Dis Child 69, 319–321.

Williams, F.L., Simpson, J., Delahunty C., et al., 2004. Developmental trends in cord and postpartum serum thyroid hormones in preterm infants. J Clin Endocrinol Metab 89, 5314–5320.

Working Group on Neonatal Screening of the European Society for Paediatric Endocrinology, 1999. Revised guidelines for neonatal screening programmes for primary congenital hypothyroidism. Hormone Res 52, 49–52.

Wu, W., Cogan, J.D., Pfaffle, R.W., et al., 1998. Mutations in PROP1 cause familial combined pituitary hormone deficiency. Nat Genet 18, 147–149.

Yasuda, T., Ohnishi, H., Wataki, K., et al., 1999. Outcome of a baby born from a mother with acquired juvenile hypothyroidism having undetectable thyroid hormone concentrations. J Clin Endocrinol Metab 84, 2630–2632.

Zajickova, K., Vrbikova, J., Canaff, L., et al., 2007. Identification and functional characterization of a novel mutation in the calcium-sensing receptor gene in familial hypocalciuric hypercalemia: modulation of clinical severity by vitamin D status. J Clin Endocrinol Metab 92, 2616–2623.

Zakarija, M., McKenzie, J.M., 1983. Immunoglobulin G inhibitor of thyroid-stimulating antibody is a cause of delay in the onset of neonatal Graves' disease. J Clin Invest 72, 1352–1356.

Zakarija, M., McKenzie, J.M., Hoffman, W.H., 1986. Prediction and therapy of intrauterine and late onset neonatal hyperthyroidism. J Clin Endocrinol Metab 62, 368–371.

Zenaty, D., Dijoud, F., Morel, Y., et al., 2006. Bilateral anorchia in infancy: occurence of micropenis and the effect of testosterone treatment. J Pediatr 149, 687–691.

Zung, A., Tenenbaum-Rakover, Y., Barkan, S., et al., 2010. Neonatal hyperthyrotropinemia: population characteristics, diagnosis, management and outcome after cessation of therapy. Clin Endocrinol 72, 264–271.

Part 3: Inborn errors of metabolism in the neonate

Simon A Jones   James E Wraith

Introduction

All paediatricians have been presented with a desperately sick neonate for whom no diagnosis is readily available. It is in this group of patients that an inborn error of metabolism (IEM) is near the top of the differential diagnostic list. It is important to keep IEMs in mind as a possible cause of symptoms in the neonatal period, and to accept that it is worth investigating 10 babies to diagnose one. Most neonatologists find it easy to maintain this attitude towards bacterial infection, but more difficult to sustain the same approach to IEMs. It is important that a diagnosis of an IEM is established promptly, not only because many disorders are now

amenable to effective treatment, but also because of the genetic implications for the families concerned. Even in disorders for which there is as yet no effective treatment, prenatal diagnosis in subsequent pregnancies may allow parents to choose termination of an affected fetus or seek preimplantation diagnosis in the few conditions for which this is currently possible.

In most cases, an IEM will be diagnosed during the newborn period because of severe clinical signs (Table 34.20), and the bulk of this chapter will concentrate upon the recognition of IEMs in babies who become ill without any prior warning. In some families, the neonatologist or preferably the obstetrician will be alerted to the risk of a particular IEM which has been present in a previous

Table 34.20 Clues to the presence of an inborn error of metabolism

Antenatal
Consanguinity
Previous neonatal death
Recurrent non-immune hydrops fetalis
Siblings with known inborn error of metabolism
Maternal HELLP syndrome or AFLP

Clinical
Unexplained clinical deterioration in an infant who was well at birth
Persistent vomiting with no anatomical cause
Persistent hiccups
Major organ failure, e.g. heart or liver
Cardiomyopathy
Dysmorphism or multiple congenital anomalies
Unusual odours
Cataracts
Encephalopathy/coma and/or seizures

Biochemical
Unexplained metabolic acidaemia
Ketosis
Unexpected hypoglycaemia
Hyperammonaemia

Haematological
Neutropenia and thrombocytopenia

Postmortem
Fatty liver and/or heart

HELLP, haemolysis, elevated liver enzymes, low platelets; AFLP, acute fatty liver of pregnancy.

Table 34.21 Investigations for diagnosis of an inborn error of metabolism

First-line investigations (available in all units providing neonatal care)
Full blood count
Urea and electrolytes
Blood gas and acid–base analysis
Blood ammonia blood lactate
Urine-reducing substances add row, blood lactate
Urine ketones (dipstick)

Second-line investigation (available in each region)
Urine amino acids
Urine organic acids
Plasma amino acids
Blood and cerebrospinal fluid lactate and/or pyruvate
Plasma carnitine and acylcarnitine analysis
Urine orotic acid
Beutler test (for galactosaemia)

Specialised investigations (available on a supraregional basis)
Specific enzyme assays on blood or skin fibroblasts, e.g. lysosomal enzyme studies
DNA mutation analysis
Special metabolite studies, e.g. very long-chain fatty acids, bile acid analysis

sibling (or other family members in the case of X-linked disorders). In other families, less specific but equally important clues may exist, such as previous unexplained neonatal deaths, particularly if there is a history of parental consanguinity. It is important always to take a careful family history and examine the obstetric notes carefully.

The importance of being forewarned about the possibility of an IEM cannot be overemphasised. Most disorders are much easier to treat before the onset of symptoms, and the prognosis for a good neurological outcome is often directly related to the age at which effective treatment commences. This is particularly true for disorders associated with neonatal encephalopathy, such as maple syrup urine disease, organic acidaemias or urea cycle defects. Remember: the outcome is directly related to the speed of diagnosis in treatable IEMs.

IEMs can present in other ways, for instance as a result of mass screening of newborn babies, giving the clinician the opportunity of starting treatment before damage is done. In the UK this is currently offered for medium-chain acyl coenzyme A (CoA) dehydrogenase deficiency and phenylketonuria; in North America and continental Europe many other disorders of intermediary metabolism are screened for by an expanded programme utilising tandem mass spectrometry.

A pilot study in England which commenced in 2012 will examine screening for maple syrup urine disease, homocystinuria, glutaric acidaemia type 1, isovaleric acidaemia and long chain fatty acid acidaemia.

Although the primary concern of this chapter is with those IEMs that cause signs in the newborn period, it is important to recognise that a number of disorders which normally present in older infants are capable of producing profound abnormalities in the neonate. The neonatologist needs to be alert to the possibility of encountering these conditions for the first time, or even of encountering a new IEM not previously described.

Finally, it is important to remember that infants with IEMs can be severely dysmorphic, and investigation of this latter group of patients can never be considered complete until one has considered the possibility of an IEM in the infant, or indeed in the mother.

Details of the long-term management of individual IEMs and the laboratory methods used for detection and follow-up are beyond the scope of this chapter. This information is available in the major reference work on IEMs which is now available online (Valle 2010).

The organisation of clinical and laboratory services

A large number of IEMs present in the newborn period. A wide range of techniques are required for diagnosis, and the level of clinical and biochemical experience required for their effective treatment is substantial. Ideally, clinical and laboratory services for IEMs should be integrated, as prompt clinical interpretation of abnormal results is required if treatment is to proceed smoothly. Neonatologists must initiate appropriate investigations (Table 34.21), but they must also recognise that rapid and correct diagnosis and treatment of these conditions is a highly specialised skill. A high index of suspicion of an IEM is a reason for referral to a paediatrician expert in the management of metabolic diseases, and not just a reason for sending blood and urine samples to a laboratory.

Some of the investigations performed in the laboratory are relatively simple and can be applied to every patient in whom there is the slightest suspicion of an IEM. Other tests are complex and should only be used in carefully defined situations. Errors or delays in the use of the right tests or the best forms of therapy can prove damaging – even fatal – to the affected neonate, especially those with a disorder of intermediary metabolism such as an organic acid defect or a urea cycle disorder. Close collaboration between clinician and laboratory is essential. Each health region within the UK should have the facilities to screen for the more common IEMs, as well as a clinician specialising in the clinical management of affected patients. Laboratory services for subacute and chronic disorders can be centralised for much larger populations and areas, giving rise to national reference laboratories for these groups of IEMs.

Before sending samples always:

- phone the laboratory to indicate urgency
- give all details of drugs, diet and previous blood transfusions
- arrange suitable transport for samples
- discuss which tests are indicated with the metabolic consultant.

Pathogenesis of inborn errors of metabolism

The majority of disorders are autosomal recessive but a few are X-linked recessive, e.g. ornithine carbamoyltransferase (OCT) deficiency. Deficiency of the E1 α-subunit of pyruvate dehydrogenase is X-linked dominant, with almost all cases, both male and female, due to new mutations (Brown et al. 1989). In the X-linked recessive disorders, one occasionally sees partial manifestation in heterozygous females, e.g. OCT deficiency. The defective genotype is present from conception and in most cases the enzyme controlled by the gene in question is active during fetal life. Nonetheless, most IEMs have no effect on the health and development of the fetus, because placental perfusion can correct the disturbance in systemic metabolite levels caused by the enzyme defect. Consequently, most babies with IEMs are of normal birthweight and are in good general condition at birth.

This statement applies to those IEMs in which systemic accumulation of a toxic metabolite (or deficiency of an essential metabolite) damages cells of organs such as the brain. Hyperammonaemia can be taken as a classic example of this. Defective conversion of ammonia to urea in the liver leads to elevated levels of circulating ammonia and intoxicating effects on the brain. A readily dialysed compound such as ammonia is removed effectively by the placenta before birth, and accumulation commences only after delivery.

There are some exceptions to this concept of 'placental protection'. Defects in cellular energy production (e.g. mitochondrial disorders) may have severe effects prenatally, including defects in embryonic development presenting as physical malformations at birth, or destructive processes later in fetal life (e.g. patchy brain destruction). In lysosomal storage disorders, intracellular accumulation of the substrate of the defective enzyme can be demonstrated early in fetal life, even though the serious symptoms may not develop until some years after birth.

In some IEMs the primary defect is in cerebral metabolism (e.g. glycine encephalopathy) and the abnormalities observed in blood and urine merely represent overflow from the brain. Placental perfusion may have a small effect on this disease in utero, but not enough to prevent affected infants from being born with hypotonia, lethargy, seizures and often established structural brain damage.

Finally, symptoms of some IEMs develop after birth because the substrate of the defective enzyme becomes available in large amounts only after the baby begins to feed, as in galactosaemia and hereditary fructose intolerance.

Clinical presentation of inborn errors of metabolism

The affected child is likely to be normal at birth. The signs and symptoms produced by IEMs are non-specific and most are shared by many other more common neonatal disorders, especially serious generalised infections. The high frequency of bacterial infections in the newborn period makes it easy to forget the possibility of an IEM. To complicate the matter further, septicaemia is a frequent secondary event in some IEMs, e.g. galactosaemia.

A metabolic cause is particularly likely in babies who develop symptoms one or several days after birth, having been entirely normal for an initial period. Dramatic improvements during a period of intravenous fluid administration, followed by relapse when put back on milk feeding, is another strongly suggestive feature.

Although the range of possible symptoms is wide indeed, there are two particularly frequent patterns of illness. The first begins with vomiting, acidosis and circulatory disturbance, followed by depressed consciousness and convulsions, and is particularly suggestive of one of the organic acidaemias. The second is dominated by neurological features, with lethargy, refusal to feed, drowsiness, unconsciousness and apnoea. Hypotonia may be a prominent feature. Primary defects of the urea cycle and glycine encephalopathy present in this way.

There are a few more specific symptoms of IEMs. Abnormal body odour is noted in some organic acidaemias, e.g. the smell of maple syrup in maple syrup urine disease, and of sweaty feet in isovaleric acidaemia or glutaric aciduria type II. Most babies who have an unusual or powerful odour do not have an IEM, but there are exceptions.

Jaundice and a haemorrhagic tendency occur in those diseases that damage the liver (galactosaemia and acute hereditary tyrosinaemia), but may also be seen as a late sign in other IEMs, such as urea cycle defects. The presence of cataracts in an infant with liver disease should lead to urgent investigation to exclude galactosaemia.

Although convulsions may occur in many different IEMs, the pattern of convulsions in pyridoxine (vitamin B_6) dependency is particularly characteristic and the onset is usually early (Mills et al. 2006). This classic pattern does not occur in every instance, and patients have been described whose convulsions began later than the first 24 hours or were of a minor type, and some in whom there were considerable periods of freedom from convulsion without specific administration of pyridoxine (Bankier et al. 1983; Goutieres and Aicardi 1985). Formal exclusion of this condition is desirable in all babies with persistent convulsions, regardless of the pattern of onset and progression and regardless of the existence of other apparent aetiological factors (e.g. birth asphyxia). This is now possible by measuring aminoadipic semialdehyde levels or mutation analysis as the genetic defect has been characterised (Mills et al. 2006). Pyridoxal phosphate is the active form of pyridoxine and a defect in this reaction is now described (Mills et al. 2005); these infants present in a similar way but do not respond to pyridoxine and must be treated with pyridoxal phosphate.

Hypoglycaemia is a common finding in the newborn period and is only occasionally due to an IEM. Fat oxidation defects (e.g. medium-chain acyl CoA dehydrogenase deficiency or MCADD) usually present later in the first year with hypoglycaemia in the context of an intercurrent illness but can indeed present in the first few days of life, usually in the underfed infant, and can be fatal. To have the best chance of making a diagnosis in a hypoglycaemic infant, collect the samples whilst the sugar is low.

Some patients with IEMs present with prominent cardiac disease. Cardiac failure, particularly with an accompanying cardiomyopathy and hypotonia, is suggestive of a mitochondrial respiratory chain disorder, or glycogen storage disease (GSD) type II (Pompe disease) or a defect in long-chain fatty acid oxidation. The multisystem congenital disorders of glycosylation (e.g. congenital disorder of glycosylation type I (CDG)) may also present soon after birth with pericardial effusion. In addition, affected patients fail to thrive and have a variable dysmorphic appearance, which often includes abnormal fat distribution ('fat pads'), large ears and inverted nipples (Leonard et al. 2001a).

Dysmorphic features can also be produced by other metabolic disturbances in the embryo. The resulting infants have physical malformations at birth, including abnormal facies and cardiac, cerebral, renal and skeletal defects. The conditions responsible include those that affect mitochondrial energy production directly (glutaric aciduria type II, pyruvate dehydrogenase deficiency) or indirectly (3-hydroxy isobutyryl CoA deoxylase deficiency). Multiple morphogenic and congenital anomalies are also a feature of the inherited disorders of cholesterol biosynthesis (Waterham 2002). Always remember IEMs as a possible cause of multiple congenital anomalies.

Hypothermia may be environmental or suggest hypothyroidism or, less often, Menkes disease. The majority of infants with this X-linked recessive disorder have temperature instability which can be noted in the newborn period, although most are not diagnosed until other features of the disease appear in later infancy.

Microcephaly, hydranencephaly and porencephaly with severe neurological deficits are other important presenting features seen in some peroxisomal defects and in pyruvate dehydrogenase deficiency. Rapidly progressive cerebral degeneration starting in the newborn period is seen in both molybdenum cofactor deficiency and isolated sulphite oxidase deficiency. Severe peripheral arteriospasm with marked pallor may occur in primary lactic acidosis. This causes a particularly difficult differential because poor perfusion may cause secondary lactic acidosis.

Finally, one group of disorders in the fetus has the potential to produce severe illness in the mother during pregnancy. Fetal long-chain L-3-hydroxyacyl-coenzyme A dehydrogenase deficiency is associated with several pregnancy-specific disorders, including pre-eclampsia, HELLP syndrome (haemolysis, elevated liver enzymes, low platelets), hyperemesis gravidarum, acute fatty liver of pregnancy and maternal floor infarct of the placenta (Rakheja et al. 2002). A floor infarct is a lesion in which fibrin is deposited in the placenta, leading to necrosis of villi.

A summary of some of the commoner presentations is given in Table 34.22. It should be recognised that this is not an exhaustive list and that some symptoms, such as poor feeding, lethargy and failure to thrive, are almost universal in infants with IEMs. Those who find algorithms useful are guided to Leonard and Morris (2006).

Investigation of a baby who may have an inborn error of metabolism

General approach

The approach to diagnosis varies with the severity and nature of the symptoms. In some babies, one can make a good guess at the diagnosis clinically and choose the test or tests most likely to give the answer – for example, a baby hypotonic at birth who becomes more depressed within the first 24 hours and who develops seizures with a burst suppression pattern on electroencephalogram (EEG) is likely to have glycine encephalopathy. However, it is more usual to need to perform a group of tests to reach a diagnosis, as many different IEMs may cause similar symptoms.

It is important to discuss investigations with the laboratory and also to give some indication of urgency. Many non-urgent samples for amino acid and organic acid analysis are received by metabolic laboratories, and it is often difficult from the clinical information (if any is provided!) on the sample cards to obtain any idea of the urgency of the situation. In addition, appropriate transportation to the laboratory must be arranged if an urgent analysis is requested. Full details of drugs and feeding history should be provided so that proper interpretation of results can be made. If an infant has received a blood transfusion prior to metabolic screening, this should be made known to the laboratory, as this will interfere with the commonly used screening test to exclude galactosaemia.

Some general tests are easily performed and should be used in all infants in whom there is even a slight possibility of an IEM (see Table 34.22). These will include routine tests of electrolyte analysis, bilirubin, acid–base balance, blood glucose and calcium, as well as haematological assessment. Plasma ammonia should be measured in all infants with neurological depression. A simple bedside test for ketones can be useful, as a heavy ketonuria in a neonate with unexplained illness, especially if associated with metabolic acidosis, should be followed by urgent organic acid analysis. Urine testing for reducing substances should not be relied upon to make or refute a diagnosis of possible galactosaemia. Infants presenting with vomiting and acute liver disease, often with a secondary coagulopathy, must be screened urgently for galactosaemia using a specific screening test on blood. In patients with acidosis, calculation of the anion gap – the sum of the serum concentrations of sodium and potassium minus the sum of the serum concentrations of chloride and bicarbonate – can be helpful. Patients with an increased anion gap, and especially those with a value greater than 25 mmol/l (normal range 12–16 mmol/l), are likely to have a specific organic acidaemia. Patients with a normal anion gap and acidosis are most likely to have renal tubular acidosis or intestinal bicarbonate loss (Gabow et al. 1980). Never ignore a raised anion gap: if it is associated with ketosis, an organic acidaemia is likely (Jones and Walter 2007).

Specific tests: 'the metabolic screen'

Occasionally, experts are asked to give advice after a baby's death, and although it is possible to perform some investigations postmortem, early suspicion and collection of the appropriate tissues and samples from a living child permit a more comprehensive screen for metabolic disease.

Although techniques will vary, most metabolic laboratories will require a sample of blood (1–2 ml in a heparinised tube) and urine (5–10 ml in a sterile container with no preservatives) for a metabolic screen. It is now essential that these basic samples are supplemented by a sample of blood (3–5 ml in an ethylene diaminetetraacetic acid bottle) for subsequent DNA extraction and storage. In addition, a capillary blood sample on filter paper should be collected for acylcarnitine analysis by tandem mass spectrometry. This powerful technique is the easiest and quickest way of diagnosing most fat oxidation disorders. The technique can also be used to diagnose amino acid disorders and some organic acidaemias (Jones and Bennett 2002).

In the laboratory, amino acid concentrations can be accurately determined in blood and urine with high-performance liquid

Table 34.22 Signs and symptoms suggestive of an inborn error of metabolism

SIGN OR SYMPTOM	DISORDER	TEST(S)
Hydrops fetalis	Lysosomal storage disease	Urine MPS, WCEs
Coma/encephalopathy	Organic acidaemias	UOAs, acylcarnitines
	Maple syrup urine disease	UAAs/PPAs
	Urea cycle disorders	NH_4, orotic acid, UAAs/PAAs
	Non-ketotic hyperglycinaemia	CSF/P glycine ratio
	Mitochondrial disease	P/CSF lactate
Coma + hypoglycaemia	GSD 1	Enzyme assay
	Organic acidaemias	UOAs, acylcarnitines
	Fructose 1,6-bisphosphatase	Enzyme assay
	Fat oxidation defects	UOAs, acylcarnitines
	Hyperinsulinism	Insulin, c-peptide
	Other endocrine causes	GH, cortisol
Odours	Maple syrup urine disease	UAAs/PAAs
	Isovaleric acidaemia	UOAs
	Glutaric aciduria type II	UOAs
Cataracts	Galactosaemia	Beutler test
Seizures	Pyridoxine dependency	Pyridoxine intravenously
	Non-ketotic hyperglycinaemia	CSF/P glycine ratio
Liver disease	Galactosaemia	Beutler test
	Tyrosinaemia	UOAs, PAAs/UAAs
	α_1-antitrypsin deficiency	α_1-AT level
	Niemann–Pick type C	Filipin staining of cultured fibroblasts or DNA
	Fat oxidation defects	UOAs, acylcarnitines
	Mitochondrial disease	P/CSF lactate
Severe diarrhoea	Congenital chloride diarrhoea	Blood and stool chloride
	Glucose/galactose malabsorption	Faecal sugars
	CDG syndrome	Plasma transferrins
Cardiomyopathy	Fat oxidation defects	UOAs
	Primary carnitine deficiency	Acylcarnitine
	Mitochondrial disease	P/CSF lactate
Severe hypotonia	Zellweger syndrome	VLCFAs, DHAP-AT
	Mitochondrial disease	P/CSF lactate
Dysmorphism	Peroxisomal disorders	VLCFAs, DHAP-AT
	Glutaric acidura II	UOAs
	PDH deficiency	P/CSF lactate
	CDG syndrome	Plasma transferrins
	Smith–Lemli–Opitz	Plasma 7-dehydrocholesterol and fasting cholesterol

MPS, mucopolysaccharides; WCEs, white cell enzymes; UOAs, urine organic acids; UAAs, urine amino acids; PAAs, plasma amino acids; CSF, cerebrospinal fluid; P/CSF, plasma/CSF ratio; GSD, glycogen storage disease; GH, growth hormone; α_1-AT, α_1-antitrypsin; CDG, congenital disorder of glycosylation; VLCFAs, very-long-chain fatty acids; DHAP-AT, dihydroacetone phosphate acyl-transferase; PDH, pyruvate dehydrogenase.

chromatography. Gas–liquid chromatography with mass spectrometry should be used for urinary organic acid analysis. In infants who are hyperammonaemic, amino acid analysis should be performed, and the urinary orotic acid level measured urgently. Fat oxidation defects as well as other organic and amino acid disorders can be detected rapidly by assessment of the free carnitine level and acylcarnitine profile of a blood spot on a newborn screening card. Occasionally, more specialised investigations will be required, e.g. amino and organic acid analysis of cerebrospinal fluid (CSF). If this is the case, it is best to discuss the clinical problem with the laboratory to ensure that the appropriate samples are collected.

Babies with lactic acidosis present a difficult problem. It is often impossible to distinguish those with a primary defect in pyruvate metabolism from those with lactic acidosis secondary to hypoxia, cardiac disease, infection or convulsions. It is necessary to treat possible underlying causes aggressively while attempting to separate the two groups. Venous obstruction by tourniquet, crying or breath-holding may raise venous lactate and pyruvate levels as much as two- or threefold. Arterial samples are generally required, preferably from an arterial line that has been in place for some time. A persistent elevation of blood lactate greater than 2 mmol/l in a baby who was not asphyxiated and who was not hypoxic or suffering from other organ failure at the time of collection should lead to further mitochondrial investigations, especially if the clinical presentation is suggestive, e.g. prominent neuromuscular symptoms. This can clearly be even more difficult in infants with cardiomyopathy, who may have a primary or secondary lactic acidosis.

In those patients with secondary lactic acidosis, the plasma lactate will usually fall (although this may take 2–3 days) as the underlying disorder improves, but babies with a primary defect in pyruvate metabolism presenting in the newborn period are generally unresponsive to treatment. Often the child dies before a clear distinction can be made, and one has to rely upon formal assay of the enzymes known to cause lactic acidosis. This is an unsatisfactory approach, as some patients with strong evidence of a primary defect have no biochemical abnormality detectable on enzyme testing. Lactic acidosis is a heterogeneous group of disorders, and it is likely that many defects have not been fully defined or are tissue-specific, e.g. limited to muscle or the central nervous system (CNS). Those defects that are identified often have abnormalities of the respiratory chain (performed in muscle) or of the pyruvate dehydrogenase complex (assayed in fibroblasts).

In many cases these investigations will provide a definitive diagnosis or a high suspicion of a known IEM, and appropriate treatment can be commenced. The complete characterisation of the particular condition often involves more specific studies, such as enzyme assays, studies of in vitro cofactor requirements and DNA mutation analysis. Much of the biochemical work-up can often be performed on cultured skin fibroblasts.

Management while awaiting results

The severity of symptoms dictates the management. Mild symptoms may occasion no change in management while awaiting results. It may be prudent to cease milk-containing feeds if symptoms are more than mild, as protein catabolism (endogenous as well as exogenous) is generally the source of the toxic metabolites. Glucose can be given orally or intravenously, but care must be taken to avoid inducing intestinal sugar intolerance by too large an oral glucose load.

In more severe cases, intravenous fluids will certainly be needed, and bicarbonate may be necessary to correct acidosis. Other additives should be dictated by laboratory results, the aim being to achieve glucose and electrolyte homeostasis. Dextrose 10% (with appropriate additives) should generally be used to try and inhibit catabolism, except when a primary lactic acidosis is possible, as some forms will be aggravated by a carbohydrate load.

If the patient is extremely ill, or is deteriorating rapidly (e.g. hyperammonaemia or profound acidosis), then aggressive therapy may be warranted even before a diagnosis has been made.

Management of babies with severe acute inborn errors of metabolism

There can be no doubt that the greatest impact on the prognosis for infants with severe acute IEMs has been the improvement in neonatal intensive care that has occurred over the last 20 years or so. In particular, improvements in mechanical ventilation techniques, the use of central access and the ability to dialyse small infants have been critical, but if treatment is to be successful, great emphasis must be placed on precision and attention to detail.

Appropriate intravenous fluids must be given, but care must be taken to avoid overhydration in the presence of impaired renal function.

Acid–base imbalance must be corrected promptly and adequately. This may require large doses of sodium bicarbonate (e.g. 20–30 mmol/kg/day) in some of the organic acidaemias, and this may lead to hypernatraemia of a degree sufficient to necessitate dialysis or haemofiltration, especially in the presence of impaired renal function. Correction of acidosis may unmask hypokalaemia, which must be corrected quickly. It is always important to check the electrolyte levels frequently (e.g. 6-hourly) during correction of acidosis and liaise closely with the metabolic team who will be involved in the acute management of these patients.

Good tissue perfusion is essential if secondary lactic acidosis is to be avoided. Oxygen therapy may be needed as well as blood transfusion to correct anaemia (which may occur as an iatrogenic problem). The most common reason for poor tissue oxygenation is hypoventilation due to cerebral depression, and most babies with severe IEMs will require mechanical ventilation. Direct toxic effects of accumulating metabolites (e.g. ammonia) upon the brain may cause cerebral oedema, and this can be easily aggravated by hypercapnia due to inadequate ventilation. Ventilatory support should therefore be used early in order to treat carbon dioxide retention long before measurable hypoxia develops, and should be continued until the baby is breathing vigorously; mechanical ventilation will also reduce the infant's metabolic demand which can be helpful in management. If an IEM causes coma (as in hyperammonaemia) one usually has to wait at least 48 hours after metabolic correction before clinical recovery occurs to a degree sufficient to cease ventilator support. Hypoglycaemia or hypocalcaemia may require correction initially or during the recovery phase.

Nutrition in the acute phase requires careful attention, as most IEMs are aggravated by tissue catabolism, which is difficult to reverse during the first 24 hours of severe illness. Intravenous glucose (with appropriate electrolyte additives) should be used initially and, when acid–base balance has been restored and tissue perfusion and oxygenation improved, one should attempt to encourage the development of an anabolic state. This may mean infusing 20% dextrose via a central venous catheter, the amount given being increased until a mild hyperglycaemia is induced (e.g. blood glucose 7–12 mmol/l). Small doses of insulin (e.g. 0.05 U/kg/h as an infusion) may be used to help initiate anabolism, but this must be used with caution as some infants are exquisitely sensitive and become hypoglycaemic rapidly. If tolerated, intravenous lipid emulsions can be used as a source of calories, and, in some units, growth hormone is also being used as an anabolic agent (Marsden et al. 1994). Total parenteral nutrition (TPN) will be needed in those patients who are so unwell that enteral feeding seems unlikely to be achieved quickly. Initially, protein should be added in an amount sufficient to meet minimal daily requirements, and then carefully titrated according to the results of biochemical monitoring (Ogier de Baulny 2002). Intravenous L-carnitine (100 mg/kg/day) may be given to compensate for urinary losses, and, for some disorders, more specific therapies may be indicated (Chakrapani and Wraith 2002; Walter 2002). Oxygenation, good tissue perfusion, the correction of acidosis and the promotion of anabolism are the cornerstones of supportive therapy.

Once the infant's catabolic state has been stabilised – often apparent as an increase in the amount of glucose tolerated, and accompanied by a diuresis (as well as improvement in general condition) – one should introduce oral protein into the diet fairly quickly. This should start at 0.5 g protein per kilogram bodyweight for the first 24 hours; this can then be increased (if tolerated) by 0.25–0.5 g/kg/day on successive days up to 1.5–2.5 g/kg/day (depending on the underlying IEM). In addition, one should supply 120 kcal/kg, and this combination of protein and energy should be sufficient to promote and sustain anabolism. In some infants, especially those with urea cycle defects, protein may need to be maintained at slightly lower levels (1.2 g/kg/day), but, in all cases, sufficient must be given to allow the infant to grow and gain weight. Usually the infant has recovered sufficiently to tolerate the protein as a formula given by nasogastric tube, but, if not, parenteral feeding regimens can also be used.

Haemodialysis and haemofiltration have largely replaced peritoneal dialysis and are important in the management of these patients. Exchange transfusion is not a useful adjunct to therapy, except in exceptional circumstances when access to dialysis is not immediately available. Often one will have to start one or other of these treatments while awaiting biochemical results, especially if the baby has a history strongly suggestive of an IEM and is unconscious or deteriorating rapidly despite supportive treatment. Peritoneal dialysis can be effective in infants with organic acid defects or hyperammonaemia due to a urea cycle defect, and it can be used with safety in infants in whom vascular access proves difficult, although haemodialysis or haemofiltration remain the methods of choice as clearance of toxic metabolites is faster. Dialysis or haemofiltration will generally be required for 2–4 days, and one should continue with therapy until the baby is established on enough protein and calories to maintain anabolism.

A number of metabolic disorders are known to have vitamin-responsive forms, and it has become traditional to administer a combination of vitamins in pharmacological dosages to sick infants while awaiting results. It is difficult to justify this blind approach to therapy, as the ready availability of metabolic investigations in most regions should allow for diagnosis to proceed rapidly. This can be followed by the use of the appropriate vitamin cofactor (in a dose approximately 100 times the daily requirement) once diagnosis has been confirmed. 'Blunderbuss' vitamin therapy is never indicated.

Long-term management after the acute phase has passed

The first problem is to achieve a form of treatment which can be continued in the long term and which is compatible with normal growth and development. This can be difficult when the mainstay of treatment is protein restriction, as the amount of protein tolerated may be insufficient for growth.

The next step is to obtain some information about the margin of latitude available in the treatment of a particular patient. A patient who tolerates little protein (e.g. 1.5 g/kg/day) will demonstrate metabolic imbalance rapidly during the course of intercurrent infections, and will be at great risk if the parents or local paediatricians are not familiar with the child's illness. An emergency regimen, giving clear, written instructions on how to deal with infections, particularly those associated with anorexia, diarrhoea or vomiting, should be discussed with the parents before the baby is discharged from hospital. A copy should also be made available for the general practitioner and referring paediatrician. We instruct the parents to be cautious and to bring the child early to hospital for assessment, particularly during the first two or three episodes of intercurrent illness. This allows the metabolic team as well as the parents to get some idea of how the individual child responds to different stresses. With experience, the parents become experts in judging how to respond to these intercurrent episodes. One must guard against undue complacency on the part of parents or of doctors in hospital emergency departments as well as doctors in the community, who are not experienced with these conditions.

Management when no diagnosis can be made

As all metabolic disorders have genetic implications for the family, every effort must be made to keep the infant alive so that investigations can be completed. Even if the initial metabolic screen is normal, biochemical correction by dialysis or haemofiltration is still indicated in infants with hyperammonaemia, as severe transient hyperammonaemia is well recognised. These infants, often premature, may have high plasma ammonia levels, but with aggressive treatment can have a good prognosis without long-term metabolic disturbance.

Further management when death is inevitable

If a baby cannot be kept alive, it is still important to think carefully about the possibility of an underlying metabolic disorder. An autopsy can be extremely valuable, and this must be performed quickly if metabolic studies are to be interpretable (Perry 1981). In this situation it is always best to discuss the infant's poor prognosis fully and frankly with the parents and obtain written permission for the autopsy or biopsies before the infant's demise. In the absence of a full autopsy it may be permissible for tissue samples (usually liver or muscle) to be taken either just before or just after death; these should be snap-frozen in liquid nitrogen. Parallel samples should be taken for histology and histochemistry, and it is best to work in close liaison with the pathologist and metabolic specialist to ensure that the correct specimens are collected. It is important not to forget the appropriate viral and bacterial cultures.

Special management when an inborn error of metabolism can be anticipated

Sometimes one knows in advance that a baby may be born with a particular IEM. This may be true when a sibling has the condition, or when the mother is a proven or suspected carrier of the gene for an X-linked IEM. The optimal treatment can be planned in advance and one can decide whether to treat the baby as affected from the time of delivery (or before), or to investigate promptly and treat only after a diagnosis has been established. The choice will vary from one disease to another.

In other circumstances, the birth of a child who may have an IEM is anticipated without any precise information about what IEM may be present, e.g. when one or two children in a family have died in circumstances that suggest an IEM but without adequate investigation or without achieving a diagnosis. In families like this, consideration should be given to transfer to the metabolic unit soon after delivery (Danks 1974). All the investigations listed above should be done immediately, and repeated after the infant has started protein-containing feeds if the initial set is negative.

By using this approach it is hoped to achieve a diagnosis before symptoms develop, and to initiate appropriate therapy. If symptoms develop without any diagnostic biochemical findings, the prognosis is poor.

Detection of inborn errors of metabolism by mass screening

Screening for hypothyroidism is considered on page 875. Phenylketonuria (PKU) and MCADD are the only IEMs which have received universal acceptance for mass newborn screening in the UK and this has been a source of frustration to metabolic paediatricians. It is worth reflecting on the characteristics of PKU, as it illustrates an almost ideal situation for mass screening and is serving as the yardstick against which other mass screening programmes for other IEMs in the newborn period are being measured.

Babies with PKU are born in good health, protected by the intrauterine environment. They begin to be affected by their metabolic disorder after birth, but these effects are gradual and probably take several weeks before leading to severe, irreversible change. The outcome of treatment is excellent if it is initiated within the first 2–3 weeks of life, but is not good if treatment is delayed until symptoms are apparent. In addition, this condition is reliably diagnosed by tandem mass spectrometry, a technique well adapted for mass screening for a range of disorders. Finally, PKU occurs with a frequency (1 in 10 000 in the UK) sufficient to justify detection by screening.

Tests suitable for mass screening have been developed for a large number of IEMs but none of these has achieved universal acceptance within the UK (Bamforth 1994). Presymptomatic identification of the conditions that cause acute illness in the newborn period would be an advantage and for many conditions this can now be achieved with introduction of tandem mass spectrometry techniques (Sweetman 1996). The sample used for PKU screening is collected between the fifth and seventh days of life. This is too late for conditions that cause severe symptoms within the first day or so of life. Tandem mass spectrometry is a sensitive technique and samples may be collected much earlier (at 48–72 hours), allowing for the diagnosis of many disorders before initial decompensation. If an earlier sample were collected (before discharge from the maternity hospital), it would be a challenge to organise a system that could handle the large number of samples concerned and get results back within the 24-hour period that might be available before decompensation in some disorders. Despite this many parts of the world have started expanded screening programmes using tandem mass spectrometry to detect disorders of intermediary metabolism. Umbilical cord blood is probably unsuitable for the vast majority of disorders, as metabolite levels are too close to normal in the cord blood to be diagnostic in most diseases, although this approach may work for some disorders of intermediary metabolism and requires further study.

False-negative results for PKU may occur if samples are taken too early or if the infant has not been established on a good protein intake (Starfield and Holtzman 1975), and this would be a concern if an earlier age of screening was introduced. Premature or sick babies may be receiving intravenous fluids at the time of the test. A false-positive result may be obtained from a sick neonate on TPN. The elevation of phenylalanine will be accompanied by increases in the level of other amino acids, and in practice is not a diagnostic problem. Details of feeds should be recorded on the screening card and a further test performed when the infant has been established on a normal protein intake for 48–72 hours.

The PKU screening test identifies all babies with elevated levels of blood phenylalanine, but not all will have 'classic' PKU. Some will have mild hyperphenylalaninaemia (blood phenylalanine >400 µmol/l) and will not require dietary therapy, but all should be seen in the metabolic unit for assessment. Infants with defects in the synthesis or recycling of the tetrahydrobiopterin cofactor for phenylalanine hydroxylase activity (Fig. 34.18) need to be distinguished from those with 'classic' PKU, as the low-phenylalanine diet has to be supplemented with neurotransmitter therapy in these patients. Specific enzyme assays for cofactor defects, combined with urine pterin analysis, are necessary in all patients found to have raised phenylalanine on neonatal screening. It is important to remember that blood phenylalanine may only be marginally elevated in infants with cofactor disorders.

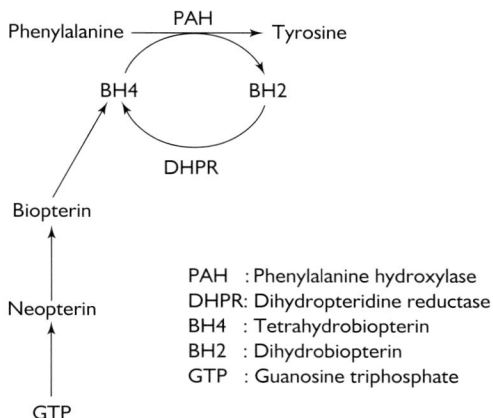

Fig. 34.18 Metabolic pathways for hyperphenylalaninaemia, which, in the classic form, is due to lack of phenylalanine hydroxylase. Rarer variants are due to defects in the tetrahydrobiopterin cofactor system.

Each metabolic unit will have its own approach to the management of PKU. We recommend dietary treatment for all infants with a blood phenylalanine >400 µmol/l. The treatment of PKU (like other metabolic disorders) should be carried out only by those with substantial experience, and details of management are beyond the scope of this chapter. In principle, most of the infant's amino acid requirements are provided in synthetic form, and natural proteins are used in portions sufficient to supply the phenylalanine required for growth, leaving no excess to be broken down to tyrosine.

MCADD has been screened for in all UK screening laboratories since 2008, after a national study. This is the commonest defect in fat oxidation in the UK (1:6000–10 000) and presents in the first 3 years of life with hypoketotic hypoglycaemia, usually in the context of an intercurrent illness. Up to 25% of those presenting clinically die at first presentation (Fernandes et al. 2006) and others suffer neurological damage. Diagnosis is usually straightforward with a typical pattern on urine organic acids; however the elevated octanoylcarnitine on tandem mass spectrometry acylcarnitine scan makes newborn screening straightforward for this condition. Treatment of MCADD is less onerous than that of PKU and simply involves adequate provision of carbohydrate during intercurrent infections. A glucose polymer is drunk regularly through the period of illness, providing adequate calories and preventing major fat breakdown by stimulating endogenous insulin production. If the child refuses or vomits the glucose drink then intravenous glucose should be provided until the illness resolves. Outcome of treated cases is excellent if diagnosed at screening and the treatment plan is followed (Leonard and Dezateux 2009). A small number of MCADD cases present in the first few days of life (Wilcken et al. 1993), often in those breastfed infants who have failed to establish adequate intake. Newborn screening cannot prevent these fatalities, but provision of adequate feeds for at least those babies known to be at higher risk for MCADD is important.

Screening for other IEMs now varies tremendously throughout the world. Many centres, including a number in Australasia, Japan, USA and Europe (not the UK), have introduced comprehensive metabolic screening programmes based on tandem mass spectrometry. The simultaneous detection of more than 30 disorders affecting either fatty acid or amino acid metabolism is now possible. Concerns remain about this approach in the UK, since many individuals may be detected who would have otherwise remained asymptomatic, as the natural history of a number of the conditions detected is not yet fully established (Leonard and Dezateux 2002). As mentioned above, a pilot study of several more defects in intermediary metabolism will commence in 2012, in some areas of England.

Consideration of specific inborn errors of metabolism

Amino acid disorders (Fig. 34.19)

Maple syrup urine disease

This rare disorder usually presents towards the end of the first week of life, with vomiting and an encephalopathy characterised by drowsiness, seizures and dystonia. A maple syrup odour is often detectable and affected infants have severe ketosis and are often hypoglycaemic. They can also have apnoea and mild hyperammonaemia.

Elevated levels of the branched-chain amino acids (leucine, isoleucine and valine) in blood and urine and of the corresponding 2-ketoacids in urine are characteristic. Deficiency of the branched-chain 2-ketoacid dehydrogenase complex can be demonstrated in cultured skin fibroblasts. The prognosis is directly related to the age at diagnosis (Kaplan et al. 1991) and reports suggest a

good outcome is possible with careful nutritional treatment (Morton et al. 2002). Rarely, the disorder occurs as a thiamine-responsive variant.

Acute hereditary tyrosinaemia (tyrosinaemia type I)

The acute neonatal form of this disorder presents with progressive synthetic liver failure (occasionally, acute hepatic necrosis) and renal tubular dysfunction. A diffuse hyperplasia of the pancreatic islet cells is seen in florid cases, and the subsequent hypoglycaemia can be resistant to treatment. Plasma tyrosine and methionine levels are raised, phosphate and potassium levels are low, and there is usually a gross generalised aminoaciduria, glycosuria and phosphaturia. The diagnosis is established by demonstrating increased urinary succinylacetone excretion on urinary organic acid analysis. The enzyme fumarylacetoacetase is deficient when assayed in lymphocytes or fibroblasts.

The prognosis for affected infants has been revolutionised by the introduction of treatment with 2-(2-nitro-4-trifluoromethylbenzoyl)-1,3-cyclohexanedione (NTBC) (Lindstedt et al. 1992). This chemical prevents the formation of succinylacetone at the expense of raising tyrosine levels. Treatment therefore must include a low-tyrosine diet as well as NTBC therapy.

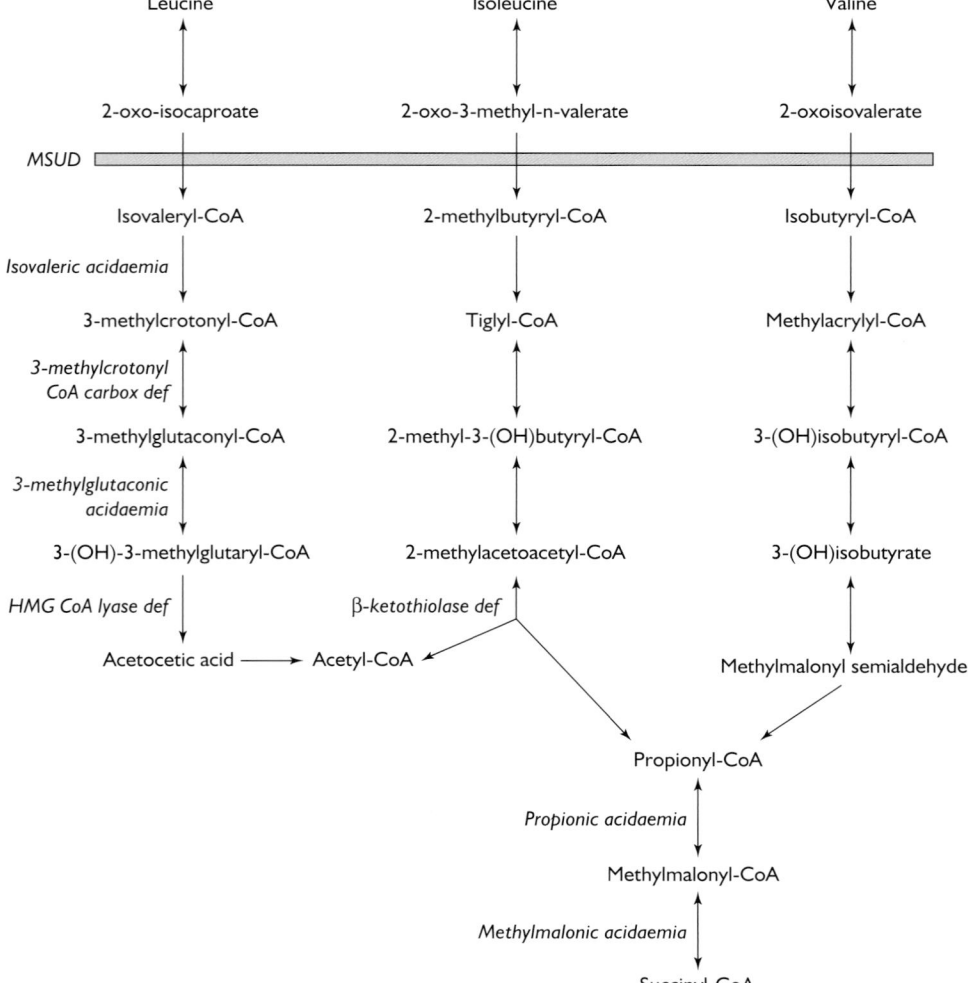

Fig. 34.19 Metabolic pathways in several important inborn errors of metabolism presenting in the neonatal period. The disorders (italics) are placed next to the metabolic step for which the enzyme (see text) is lacking.

Although there is a panethnic incidence, the disorder is particularly common in a French-Canadian isolate in Quebec, as well as in certain areas of Scandinavia.

Non-ketotic hyperglycinaemia (glycine encephalopathy)

This usually presents in the neonatal period, with drowsiness and lethargy, hypotonia and hypoventilation. Seizures are prominent and are often myoclonic in nature. The EEG often shows a burst suppression pattern. Hiccupping and opisthotonus are common features. These may be present at birth and some mothers have reported reduced fetal movements in utero. In these latter cases, intracranial anomalies have been reported, and the disorder is one cause of agenesis of the corpus callosum.

Plasma glycine levels are variable in affected patients, and can be normal. Large amounts of glycine are usually excreted in the urine, but the glycine elevation is much more marked in the CSF, reflecting the primary disturbance of neuronal glycine metabolism. Organic acids are not increased in the urine as they are in the various forms of ketotic hyperglycinaemia. Diagnosis is usually possible by demonstration of an abnormal CSF/plasma glycine ratio (>0.06).

The effects of the disease are caused by the excitatory effects of glycine at the cortical *N*-methyl-D-aspartic acid (NMDA) receptor. Treatment that modifies the systemic levels of glycine (sodium benzoate) has little effect on the disease, and specific inhibitors of glycine at the NMDA receptor, such as dextromethorphan, may lead to an improvement in seizure control and hypotonia but do not usually affect the prognosis, which is gloomy: little developmental progress is ever achieved in these children.

The basic defect is in the multicomplex glycine cleavage enzyme, and diagnosis can be confirmed by liver biopsy and enzyme analysis or mutation studies (Hayasaka et al. 1987).

Urea cycle disorders (Table 34.23)

The predominant clinical features of all of these conditions are similar and are a result of the accumulation of ammonia and glutamine. Presentation in the neonatal period is usually with episodes of vomiting and drowsiness, proceeding to unconsciousness and seizures. The absence of acidosis is an important point.

Once hyperammonaemia (levels above 200 μmol/l are usually due to an IEM) has been established by measurement of the blood ammonia level, the diagnosis of a primary urea cycle defect can usually be made after measuring plasma and urine amino acids and by screening the urine for organic acids and orotic acid. Hyperammonaemia secondary to an organic acidaemia will be excluded by a normal urinary organic acid profile and the absence of ketosis and metabolic acidosis.

In carbamoyl phosphate synthetase (CPS) deficiency and OCT deficiency, plasma ammonia levels are grossly elevated (2000–3000 μmol/l), but plasma amino acid levels are usually normal apart from elevation of glutamine and perhaps a low citrulline level. The two conditions can be differentiated by measuring urinary orotic acid, which is grossly elevated in OCT deficiency but not in CPS deficiency. Citrullinaemia, argininosuccinic aciduria and arginase deficiency all show characteristic elevations of the respective amino acids in plasma and urine.

Definitive diagnosis is obtained by measuring the individual enzymes in a liver biopsy (all defects), cultured skin fibroblasts (citrullinaemia, argininosuccinic aciduria and arginase deficiency) or by mutation analysis.

Treatment of urea cycle disorders includes arginine (which becomes an essential amino acid in all but arginase deficiency) supplementation (200–600 mg/kg/day arginine) and the use of alternative pathways to excrete nitrogen waste. Amino acid nitrogen may be excreted as hippuric acid if sodium benzoate (250–500 mg/kg/day) is administered, or as phenylglutamine after sodium phenylbutyrate (250–500 mg/kg/day) administration. These methods have made a great difference to the outcome of this group of patients (Batshaw et al. 1982, 1984). Essential amino acid supplements can also be used to provide some of the nitrogen requirement in the introduction of a low-protein diet, which is the mainstay of long-term management. Acute severe hyperammonaemia in the neonatal period may well require haemofiltration to control the levels, as discussed earlier.

It is important to remember that OCT deficiency is one of the X-linked IEMs. Female heterozygotes can be symptomatic in the newborn period and are often protein-intolerant later in life. In this disorder, the neurological outcome is directly related to the plasma ammonia at diagnosis (Nicolaides et al. 2002). The OCT gene has been identified and many mutations characterised (Tuchman et al. 2002). Direct mutation analysis has replaced liver biopsy and enzyme analysis in the diagnosis of OCT deficiency. The role of liver and hepatocyte transfer is unclear but probably increasing (Puppi et al. 2008).

Transient neonatal hyperammonaemia

Plasma ammonia levels of over 1500 μmol/l have been described in a small number of comatose newborn infants who have recovered completely after aggressive treatment, with no biochemical evidence of a specific enzyme defect in the urea cycle. These babies have subsequently tolerated a normal protein intake without any symptoms. The biochemical basis of the condition is unknown, but immaturity of enzyme systems or venous malformations has been postulated.

Table 34.23 Urea cycle disorders

	CPS	OTC	ASAS	ASAL	ARG
Incidence	1:100000	1:100000	1:100000	1:100000	1:100000
Inheritance	AR	XLR	AR	AR	AR
Enzyme deficiency	CPS	OTC	ASAS	ASAL	ARG
Mutations	2p	Xp21.1	9q34	7cen-p21	6q23
Prenatal	Fetal liver or DNA	Fetal liver or DNA	Enz-CVB	Enz-CVB	Fetal blood or DNA

CPS, carbamyl phosphate synthetase; OTC, ornithine transcarbamylase; ASAS, argininosuccinic acid synthetase (citrullinaemia); ASAL, argininosuccinic acid lyase (argininosuccinic aciduria); ARG, arginase (argininaemia); AR, autosomal recessive; XLR, X-linked recessive; Enz-CVB, enzyme assay on chorion villus biopsy.

Organic acid disorders (Fig. 34.19)

Propionic acidaemia

In its acute form, this disorder presents early in the newborn period, with severe metabolic acidosis, poor feeding, vomiting and drowsiness which rapidly proceeds to coma. Hyperammonaemia and hypoglycaemia are often present. The blood ammonia may be elevated to levels similar to those seen in primary urea cycle defects. Treatment of the high ammonia in this condition is similar to that in urea cycle disorders, with the addition of carnitine (100 mg/kg/day) and possibly carglumic acid for high ammonia levels (Jones et al. 2008).

In less severe forms, the features are poor feeding, failure to thrive and recurrent vomiting. Ketoacidosis and hyperglycinaemia are the main biochemical features, and some patients have bone marrow suppression during decompensation.

The urine contains large amounts of a wide variety of organic acids, including 3-hydroxypropionate, methylcitrate and tiglylglycine, as well as some unusual ketone bodies. Diagnosis is suggested by a characteristic pattern of acylcarnitine metabolites on tandem mass spectrometry of a blood spot and confirmed by assay of propionyl-CoA carboxylase in cultured skin fibroblasts.

Long-term treatment relies upon protein restriction, alkali therapy, sodium benzoate (in some patients) and carnitine replacement. Because of the poor prognosis for neurological outcome in most patients on conventional therapy, liver transplantation may offer a better long-term prognosis, although this is by no means certain (Leonard et al. 2001b).

Methylmalonic acidaemia

The clinical features of this disorder are similar to those of propionic acidaemia. However, it can be distinguished by the pattern of acylcarnitine metabolites, excretion of methylmalonic acid in the urine and by specific enzyme assay. Methylmalonic acidaemia can be subdivided into a number of different categories, depending on whether the defect is in the methylmalonyl-CoA mutase enzyme or in one of the steps in the formation of its cofactor adenosylcobalamin. They all present with vomiting, acidosis and neurological symptoms and they can be differentiated only by careful enzyme studies in cultured cells to distinguish defects of different steps in adenosylcobalamin synthesis as well as responsiveness to vitamin B_{12} therapy (Fowler et al. 2008). The degree of response to vitamin B_{12} varies depending on the step in cofactor synthesis that is affected.

Hyperammonaemia can occur in any of the more severe forms of methylmalonic acidaemia, as in propionic acidaemia, although it is usually not so severe. The other treatment modalities used in propionic acidaemia apply here also. Methylmalonic acidaemia plus homocystinuria may be seen in defects in the early steps of cobalamin cofactor biosynthesis. Long-term therapy is relatively simple and effective in the vitamin B_{12}-responsive cases, but difficult in the remainder, in whom stringent protein restriction is required. Intercurrent infective illnesses frequently cause exacerbations of acidosis requiring intravenous therapy. Long-term complications such as progressive renal damage and acute infarction of the basal ganglia may occur, rendering the long-term prognosis poor. The role of liver and/or renal transplantation remains unclear.

Isovaleric acidaemia

This disorder, caused by a deficiency of the enzyme isovaleryl-CoA dehydrogenase, may present in the newborn period with vomiting and severe ketoacidosis. Affected infants are often neutropenic and thrombocytopenic during the acute episode, and the urine has a characteristic 'sweaty feet' odour owing to the excretion of isovaleric acid. Treatment with protein restriction, carnitine and glycine supplementation generally results in relatively normal development in those infants who survive the newborn period unscathed.

Defects in carbohydrate metabolism

Galactosaemia

Infants with 'classical' galactosaemia due to deficiency of the enzyme galactose-1-phosphate uridyl transferase present towards the end of the first week of life with vomiting, failure to thrive and jaundice. Neurological symptoms are common and 30–40% develop a superadded septicaemia, usually due to *Escherichia coli* infection, which often starts as a urinary tract infection. This may be diagnosed and treated without recognising the underlying metabolic disease, especially as milk feeds are stopped during the treatment of this acute illness. Recurrence of symptoms when milk is reintroduced may alert the neonatologist to the principal diagnosis. Hepatomegaly is always present and the clinical course is dominated by the progressive liver damage. Cataracts may appear even in the first week, and there may be a proximal tubulopathy.

The diagnosis may be suspected by the urinary excretion of galactose and is readily confirmed by measurement of erythrocyte galactose-1-phosphate uridyl transferase. If the infant has had a prior blood transfusion, enzyme analysis is unreliable and diagnosis can be achieved by measuring galactose-1-phosphate levels in blood.

Long-term treatment is with a milk-free diet. Cataracts regress and the liver heals, but the intellectual outcome remains poor, with most affected adults having IQ scores of 60–80. There is often a specific speech delay, and a cerebellar syndrome with ataxia becomes prominent in some affected adults. Ovarian failure occurs in at least 80% of affected female patients and is not related to delays in postnatal treatment. This may be related to abnormal glycosylation of female hormones.

Fructose-1,6-bisphosphatase deficiency

This disorder may present in the newborn period with severe lactic acidosis. Affected infants hyperventilate, are often hypoglycaemic and can deteriorate rapidly with apnoea and death. Hepatomegaly is often present acutely and urine organic analysis can show glycerol excretion. Later episodes in survivors are often triggered by intercurrent fasting or infections. Gluconeogenesis is severely impaired and hypoglycaemia is prominent, with the accumulation of gluconeogenic precursors such as lactate, amino acids and ketones. Unlike hereditary fructose intolerance, patients do not vomit after ingesting fructose and an aversion to sweets does not develop. The diagnosis can be established on white blood cell enzyme assay and mutation analysis. Affected children usually respond to intravenous glucose during acute crises.

Glycogen storage disease type I

All variants of GSD type I (e.g. GSD Ia and Ib) can present in the newborn period with profound hypoglycaemia. In addition there is lactic acidosis, hyperuricaemia and hyperlipidaemia. Hepatomegaly is usually obvious, but the soft liver in GSD I may be difficult to define by palpation. The diagnosis is usually obvious clinically and mutation analysis has replaced liver biopsy as the confirmatory test. Treatment is aimed at maintaining normoglycaemia with frequent daytime feeds and continuous nocturnal intragastric infusion of glucose. Patients with type Ib disease also suffer from chronic neutropenia and functional deficiencies of neutrophils and monocytes, which requires therapy with granulocyte colony-stimulating factor to restore myeloid function (Rake et al. 2002).

Primary disorders of pyruvate metabolism

All the primary disorders of pyruvate metabolism are associated with lactic acidosis and all have similar clinical features, with profound peripheral circulatory disturbance and severe neurological abnormalities. Pyruvate dehydrogenase deficiency deserves special mention.

Pyruvate dehydrogenase deficiency

Pyruvate dehydrogenase, a multienzyme complex, is a major metabolic control point in the aerobic oxidation of carbohydrates and some gluconeogenic amino acids. The action of pyruvate dehydrogenase is controlled by a specific kinase (inactivation) and phosphorylase (activation), which are tightly regulated in response to metabolite concentrations within the mitochondrion. The enzyme complex itself comprises three main enzymes: E1 or pyruvate decarboxylase (with α and β subunits), E2 or lipoyl transacetylase, and E3, a dihydrolipoyl-dehydrogenase. Defects in all three main components have been described, and early presentation is generally with severe acidosis or with profound neurological deficit in a baby with minimal or no acidosis (often with structural brain lesions, 'cerebral lactic acidosis'). Milder cases may present later, with intermittent ataxia or acidosis. Deficiency of the E1 α-subunit (the subunit which is subject to most of the acute metabolic controls over enzyme activity) is the most frequent defect. The gene for this subunit is on the short arm of the X chromosome. Both hemizygous males and heterozygous females are affected, most being the result of de novo mutations. The patients with the 'cerebral' form are more often females with severe enzyme lesions which destroy patches of the brain in which the mutant gene is active. Males predominate among those with early severe acidosis, and usually have an incomplete enzyme deficiency.

Patients with E3 deficiency may excrete large amounts of 2-ketoglutarate and branched-chain 2-ketoacids in addition to lactate, as this component appears to be common to all 2-ketoacid dehydrogenase complexes.

Patients with these defects deteriorate when given a high glucose intake, and prompt recognition is therefore important. It is difficult to give the high-lipid, high-protein, low-carbohydrate regimens that in theory would be best for these patients. Occasional patients have been described who respond to large doses of thiamine, but there is no way of differentiating these patients clinically or biochemically from those with unresponsive forms (Wick et al. 1977). Lactic acidosis presents a complex set of problems. The first difficulty arises in diagnosis in an acutely ill newborn infant. Primary lactic acidosis can cause the effects (vasoconstriction, convulsions, severe acidosis) that can cause secondary lactic acidosis when present for other reasons. The matter is further complicated by the existence of some disorders leading to lactic acidosis which require treatment with carbohydrate supplementation (e.g. fructose 1,6-bisphosphatase deficiency and some other gluconeogenic defects), and others which are made worse by this regimen (e.g. pyruvate dehydrogenase deficiency and some other mitochondrial disorders). The presence of structural CNS defects makes the latter group more likely, but often one has to gamble. As the gluconeogenic defects generally have the better prognosis, it is usually preferable to err on the side of carbohydrate supplementation in practice, especially as the profound hypoglycaemia which can occur in these disorders can cause severe brain damage.

In all forms of severe lactic acidosis, muscle paralysis and ventilatory support have a specific role in reducing muscle lactate production and, as with other IEMs that can affect the brain, ventilatory support should be considered early, especially in infants with significant (pH < 7.1) or persistent metabolic acidosis.

Some patients who survive the newborn period with pyruvate dehydrogenase deficiency seem to respond to the ketogenic diet and this should be attempted in older patients if possible (Barnerias et al. 2009).

Fatty acid oxidation defects

A number of defects in fatty acid oxidation have been identified. Some prevent uptake of fatty acids into the mitochondria and others affect specific steps in the β-oxidation within the mitochondria. These enzymes have specificity based on the length of the fatty acid carbon chain. All can present in the newborn period and can commonly present with life-threatening or fatal illness. MCADD is the most frequently recognised, as discussed in the section on detection of IEMs by mass screening, above. Our ability to diagnose disorders of fat oxidation has been considerably enhanced by the introduction of acylcarnitine analysis by tandem mass spectrometry.

One other serious presentation of this group of disorders is with hypertrophic cardiomyopathy, which can cause heart failure or cardiorespiratory arrest in the newborn period. This occurs in multiple acyl-CoA dehydrogenase deficiency (glutaric aciduria type II), long-chain fatty acyl-CoA dehydrogenase deficiency, 3-hydroxyacyl-CoA dehydrogenase deficiency and the primary disorders of carnitine metabolism (Servidei et al. 1994). As mentioned earlier, these disorders, when present in the fetus, can be associated with severe maternal disease during pregnancy.

Diagnosis of defects in fatty acid metabolism relies on a combination of biochemical abnormalities, which may include evidence of liver disease (raised transaminases, hyperammonaemia) and muscle disease (raised creatine phosphokinase). A characteristic pattern of blood acylcarnitine metabolites and abnormal urinary organic acid profiles is usually enough to clinch the diagnosis. Specific enzyme assays on cultured skin fibroblasts are a difficult and specialised investigation and are not readily available. Decreased rates of catabolism of radiolabelled fatty acid substrates can be used to demonstrate a defect somewhere in the β-oxidation pathway, and can be helpful when interpreted with the clinical presentation and supporting biochemical abnormalities. Mutation analysis is also available for all the known defects.

Treatment of these defects varies with the condition but tends to rely on suppression of fat oxidation by provision of large quantities of glucose. In isolated long-chain defects medium-chain triglyceride-based feeds can be helpful (Spiekerkoetter et al. 2009).

Disorders of subcellular organelles

Mitochondrial disease

Mitochondria are unique among cytoplasmic organelles as they contain their own genetic material. The mitochondrial genome is a circular DNA molecule of approximately 16 500 basepairs which encodes some (but not all) of the polypeptides of the respiratory transport chain and some other components of mitochondrial transcription and translation (22 transfer RNAs and two ribosomal RNAs). There are multiple copies of mitochondrial DNA (mtDNA) in each mitochondrion and many mitochondria in each cell, so that each cell contains several thousand mtDNA molecules. The phenotype and rate of progression of mitochondrial disorders appear to be determined by the proportion and segregation of abnormal mtDNA molecules at cell division, combined with a 'threshold effect' in various tissues, depending on energy requirements and functional reserve. Brain and muscle appear to be most sensitive to mitochondrial dysfunction.

The other major characteristic of mtDNA is that it is transmitted between generations only by the mother, probably because at fertilisation only the head of the sperm enters the egg and the mitochondria in the rest of the sperm are lost. Maternal inheritance patterns are seen in those disorders where there is a primary mtDNA mutation responsible for the disease.

It should be noted that not all mitochondrial disease is due to defects in mitochondrial DNA and the others are often inherited in an autosomal recessive manner.

Clinical features are extremely variable and the diagnosis should be suspected in infants where there is multiple organ involvement. Lactic acidosis is common but not a requirement for the diagnosis and there may be abnormalities on routine haematological and biochemical analyses, depending on the main target organs affected. Raised lactate in the CSF is more specific than in the plasma. Specific biochemical investigation will include assay of respiratory chain activity on muscle biopsy material. Histological changes in muscle tissue can be important; however it is usually the pattern of organ involvement ± lactic acidosis that suggests the diagnosis. The organs most typically involved are the brain (including Leigh disease), liver, kidney (tubulopathy), skeletal muscles and heart (cardiomyopathy). The clinical presentation of these disorders in childhood has been reviewed (Borchert et al. 2002; Di Donato 2009). The overlap in clinical phenotype and radiological features between a baby with mitochondrial disease and hypoxic-ischaemic injury can be problematic.

In a number of mitochondrial disorders, underlying or associated genetic changes have been defined in mtDNA. These include large structural rearrangements (deletions and duplications) and point mutations. When present, these are a highly specific and sensitive addition to the biochemical investigations. It should be noted however that most mitochondrial disorders presenting in the newborn period have a genetic defect in nuclear genes affecting mitochondrial function.

Peroxisomal disorders

These disorders present in the neonatal period and are all disorders of peroxisomal biogenesis or peroxisomal protein transportation. Not all defects have been fully categorised and there are a number of different complementation groups described. Single peroxisomal enzyme defects have been described and some can present neonatally (Baumgartner and Saudubray 2002).

There are over 20 different peroxisomal disorders, caused by an impairment of one or more peroxisomal functions. The more profound and complex disorders of peroxisomal biogenesis or of multiple peroxisomal enzyme deficiency present in the newborn period with severe neurological abnormalities plus various other features, including abnormal facies and body build, cataracts, punctate epiphyseal calcification, liver fibrosis, renal cysts and adrenal or hepatic failure. Increased levels of very-long-chain fatty acids (Ch. 26.1) in plasma and decreased plasmalogens are useful biochemical markers. The absence of peroxisomes on liver histology is typical of Zellweger syndrome. There is no effective treatment, but prenatal diagnosis is possible.

Lysosomal disorders

The lysosomal disorders are conditions in which a defective lysosomal enzyme leads to the accumulation of specific substrates within the cell which eventually interfere with normal cellular function. The disorders are progressive and usually present in childhood or later, but some can produce dramatic neonatal presentation, usually in such cases with hydrops fetalis as a prominent feature.

Diagnosis is established by enzyme assay on white blood cells or cultured skin fibroblasts. The neonatal presentation of these disorders has been reviewed (Wraith 2002) the exception to this rule is Mucolipidosis II (I cell disease) which can present with coarse features, gingivial hypertrophy and severe dysostosis in the neonatal period, even including neonatal fractures.

Miscellaneous disorders

Congenital disorders of glycosylation

This newly described group of metabolic disorders is characterised by a deficiency in the carbohydrate moiety of secretory glycoproteins, including a characteristic change in transferrin, which can be used as a diagnostic test (transferrin isoelectric focusing). A number of variants have been described, including a type that can produce severe neonatal disease (Leonard et al. 2001a; Jaeken 2011).

During the first 24 hours of life, many infants with CDG feed poorly and are often floppy and hypothermic; hyperinsulinaemic hypoglycaemia can also occur (Freeze 2007). Birthweight is usually normal, but a variable dysmorphism is often present, including abnormalities of the skin (*peau d'orange*) or subcutaneous tissue (fat pads). A number of serious complications can develop, including pericardial effusion and liver dysfunction. Failure to thrive and psychomotor delay are usual.

Menkes disease

Most babies with this X-linked recessive disease have difficulty in maintaining body temperature in the neonatal period, but few are diagnosed at this stage. Most are diagnosed at 2–4 months because of poor development, seizures and abnormal 'steely' hair. Low plasma levels of copper confirm the diagnosis.

The basic defect is in copper transport across the intestinal mucosa and in body cells. Daily parenteral copper therapy improves copper levels, but has little effect on development unless commenced early in life. Treatment after symptomatic diagnosis can only prolong existence with severe brain damage.

Inherited disorders of cholesterol biosynthesis

Cholesterol plays a crucial role in fetal development, and a number of inherited disorders of cholesterol biosynthesis show that low cholesterol levels may have severe consequences for human development. At least seven different defects linked to the cholesterol biosynthetic pathway have been described, the most common of which is the Smith–Lemli–Opitz syndrome (Waterham 2002).

Smith–Lemli–Opitz syndrome had been recognised as a 'dysmorphic syndrome' for many years prior to the identification of the defect in cholesterol metabolism responsible for the clinical phenotype. Affected patients have characteristic craniofacial features, cleft palate, hypospadias, postaxial polydactyly and toe syndactyly. A number of biochemical abnormalities were known to be associated with the syndrome, including a low plasma cholesterol level. Further investigation led to the finding of grossly elevated 7-dehydrocholesterol levels in the plasma of affected children, and this is now the basis of the biochemical confirmation of this disorder. This compound is the immediate precursor in the cholesterol biosynthetic pathway. A deficiency of the enzyme 3β-hydroxysterol Δ7-reductase has been shown to be the primary genetic lesion in affected infants. Treatment with statins and a high-cholesterol diet has been attempted in a number of patients, but it is too early to say whether this will be of major clinical benefit (Jira et al. 2000).

Weblinks

www.bimdg.org.uk: British Inherited Metabolic Disease Group. Useful information, including emergency management protocols.

http://www.ommbid.com/: online metabolic disease and molecular basis of inherited disease. Subscription required to access full content.

References

Bamforth, F.J., 1994. Laboratory screening for genetic disorders and birth defects. Clin Biochem 27, 333–342.

Bankier, A., Turner, M., Hopkins, I.J., 1983. Pyridoxine-dependent seizures – a wider clinical spectrum. Arch Dis Child 58, 415–418.

Barnerias, C., Saudubray, J.M., Touati, G., et al., 2009. Pyruvate dehydrogenase complex deficiency: four neurological phenotypes with differing pathogenesis. Dev Med Child Neurol, 52, e1–e9.

Batshaw, M.L. Brusilow, S., Waber, L., et al., 1982. Treatment of inborn errors of urea synthesis. Activation of alternative pathways of waste nitrogen synthesis and excretion. NEJM 306, 1387–1392.

Batshaw, M.L., Brusilow, S.W., Danney, M., et al., 1984. Treatment of episodic hyperammonemia in children with inborn errors of urea synthesis. NEJM 310, 1630–1634.

Baumgartner, M.R., Saudubray, J.M., 2002. Peroxisomal disorders. Semin Neonatol 7, 85–94.

Borchert, A., Wolf, N.I., Wilichowski, E., 2002. Current concepts of mitochondrial disorders in childhood. Semin Pediatr Neurol 9, 151–159.

Brown, R.M., Dahl, H.H., Brown, G.K., 1989. X-chromosome localization of the functional gene for the E1α subunit of the human pyruvate dehydrogenase complex. Genomics 4, 174–181.

Chakrapani, A., Wraith, J.E., 2002. Principles of management of the more common metabolic disorders. Current Paediatrics 12, 117–124.

Danks, D.M., 1974. Management of newborn babies in whom serious metabolic disease is anticipated. Arch Dis Child 49, 576–578.

Di Donato, S., 2009. Multisystem manifestations of mitochondrial disorders. J Neurol 256, 693–710.

Fernandes, J., Saudubray, J.-M., Van Den Berghe, G., et al., (Eds.), 2006. Inborn Metabolic Diseases: Diagnosis and Treatment, fourth ed. Springer, Berlin.

Fowler, B., Leonard, J.V., Baumgartner, M.R., 2008. Causes of and diagnostic approach to methylmalonic acidurias. J Inherit Metab Dis 31, 350–360.

Freeze, H.H., 2007. Congenital disorders of glycosylation: CDG-I, CDG-II, and beyond. Curr Mol Med 7, 389–396.

Gabow, P.A., Kaeburg, W.D., Fennessey, P.V., et al., 1980. Diagnostic importance of an increased anion gap. NEJM 330, 854–858.

Goutieres, F., Aicardi, J., 1985. Atypical presentation of pyridoxine-dependent seizures: a treatable cause of intractable epilepsy in infants. Neurology 17, 117–120.

Hayasaka, K., Tada, K., Fueki, N., et al., 1987. Non-ketotic hyperglycinaemia: analysis of glycine cleavage system in typical and atypical cases. J Pediatr 110, 873–877.

Jaeken, J., 2011. J Inherit Metab Dis 34 (4), 853–858. Epub 2011 Mar 8. Review.

Jira, P.E., Wevers, R.A.J., de Jong, J., et al., 2000. Simvastatin:a new therapeutic approach for Smith–Lemli–Opitz syndrome. J. Lipid Res. 41, 1339–1346.

Jones, P., Bennett, M., 2002. The changing face of newborn screening: diagnosis of inborn errors of metabolism by tandem mass spectrometry. Clin Chim Acta 324, 121–128.

Jones, A. Walter J.H., 2007. Diagnosis and treatment of severe metabolic acidosis. Paediatr Child Health 17, 260–265.

Jones, S., Reed, C.A., Vijay, S., et al., N-carbamylglutamate for neonatal hyperammonaemia in propionic acidaemia [published online ahead of print February 21, 2008]. J Inherit Metab Dis.

Kaplan, P., Mazur, A., Field, M., et al., 1991. Intellectual outcome in children with maple syrup urine disease. J Pediatr 119, 46–50.

Leonard, J.V., Dezateux, C., 2002. Screening for inherited metabolic disease in newborn infants using tandem mass spectrometry. Br Med J 324, 4–5.

Leonard, J.V., Dezateux, C., 2009. Newborn screening for medium chain acyl CoA dehydrogenase deficiency. Arch Dis Child 94, 235–238.

Leonard, J.V., Morris, A.A., 2006. Diagnosis and early management of inborn errors of metabolism presenting around the time of birth. Acta Paediatr 95, 6–14.

Leonard, J., Grunewald, S., Clayton, P., 2001a. Diversity of congenital disorders of glycosylation. Lancet 357, 1382–1383.

Leonard, J.V., Walter, J.H., McKiernan, P.J., 2001b. The management of organic acidaemias: the role of transplantation. J Inherit Metab Dis 24, 309–311.

Lindstedt, S., Holme, E., Lock, E.A., et al., 1992. Treatment of hereditary tyrosinaemia type I by inhibition of 4-hydroxyphenylpyruvate dioxygenase. Lancet 340, 813–817.

Marsden, D., Barshop, B.A., Capistrano-Estrada, S., et al., 1994. Anabolic effect of human growth hormone: management

of inherited disorders of catabolic pathways. Biochemical Medicine, Metabolism and Biology 52, 145–154.

Mills, P.B., Surtees, R.A., Champion, M.P., et al., 2005. Neonatal epileptic encephalopathy caused by mutations in the PNPO gene encoding pyridox(am)ine 5′-phosphate oxidase. Hum Mol Genet 14, 1077–1086.

Mills, P.B., Struys, E., Jakobs, C., et al., 2006. Mutations in antiquitin in individuals with pyridoxine-dependent seizures. Nat Med 12, 307–309.

Morton, D.H., Strauss, K.A., Robinson, D.L., et al., 2002. Diagnosis and treatment of maple syrup urine disease. Pediatrics 109, 999–1008.

Nicolaides, P., Liebsch, D., Dale, N., et al., 2002. Neurological outcome of patients with ornithine carbamyltransferase deficiency. Arch Dis Child 86, 54–56.

Ogier de Baulny, H., 2002. Management and emergency treatments of neonates with a suspicion of inborn errors of metabolism. Semin Neonatol 7, 17–26.

Perry, T.L., 1981. Autopsy investigation of disorders of amino acid metabolism. In: Barson, A.J. (Ed.), Laboratory Investigation of Fetal Disease. Wright, Bristol, pp. 429–451.

Puppi, J., Tan, N., Mitry, R.R., et al., 2008. Hepatocyte Transplantation Followed by Auxiliary Liver Transplantation—a Novel Treatment for Ornithine Transcarbamylase Deficiency. Am J Transplant 8, 452–457.

Rake, J.P., Visser, G., Labrune, P., et al., 2002. Guidelines for management of glycogen storage disease type I – European Study on Glycogen Storage Disease Type I (ESGSD I). Eur J Pediatr. 161 (Suppl. 1), S112-S119.

Rakheja, D., Bennett, M.J., Rogers, B.B., 2002. Long chain L-3-hydroxyacyl-coenzyme A dehydrogenase deficiency: a molecular and biochemical review. Lab Invest 82, 815–824.

Servidei, S., Bertini, E., DiMauro, S., 1994. Hereditary metabolic cardiomyopathies. Adv Pediatr 41, 1–32.

Spiekerkoetter, U., Lindner, M., Santer, R., et al., 2009. Treatment recommendations in long-chain fatty acid oxidation defects: consensus from a workshop. J Inherit Metab Dis. 32, 498–505.

Starfield, B., Holtzman, N.A., 1975. A comparison of screening for phenylketonuria in the United States, United Kingdom and Ireland. NEJM 293, 118–121.

Sweetman, L., 1996. Newborn screening by tandem mass spectrometry (MS-MS). Clin Chem 42, 345–346.

Tuchman, M., Jaleel, N., Morizono, H., et al., 2002. Mutations and polymorphisms in the human ornithine transcarbamylase gene. Hum Mutat 19, 93–107.

Valle, D. (Ed.), 2010. The Online Metabolic and Molecular Bases of Inherited Disease. Available online at: http://www.ommbid.com/.

Walter, J.H., 2002. Investigation and initial management of suspected metabolic disease. Current Paediatrics 12, 110–116.

Waterham, H.R., 2002. Inherited disorders of cholesterol biosynthesis. Clin Genet 61, 393–403.

Wick, H., Schweizer, K., Baumgartner, R., 1977. Thiamine dependency in a patient with congenital lactic acidaemia due to pyruvate dehydrogenase deficiency. Agents Actions 7, 405–410.

Wilcken, B., Carpenter, K.H., Hammond, J., 1993. Neonatal symptoms in medium chain acyl coenzyme A dehydrogenase deficiency. Arch Dis Child 69, 292–294.

Wraith, J.E., 2002. Lysosomal disorders. Semin Neonatol 7, 75–83.

Part 4: Metabolic bone disease

Nick Bishop

Background

The majority of neonatal metabolic bone disease is seen in infants born prematurely, and is due largely to substrate deficiency. Additional adverse effects on the skeleton may result from administration of steroids (suppression of bone turnover), diuretics and immobilisation. Diagnostic criteria vary considerably between centres, leading to estimates of incidence that range from 32% to 92% (Callenbach et al. 1981; Hillman et al. 1985; Lyon et al. 1987).

Diagnosing metabolic bone disease in preterm infants

Bone disease in preterm infants is characterised in the short term by a sequence of events which begins with biochemical evidence of disturbed mineral metabolism (Sagy et al. 1980; Senterre and Salle 1982; Atkinson et al. 1983; Gross 1983; Lyon et al. 1984; Carey et al. 1985; Carey and Hopfer 1987; Lucas et al. 1989), continues with reduced bone mineralisation (Steichen et al. 1980, 1988; James et al. 1986; Chan et al. 1988; Greer and McCormick 1988; Venkataraman and Blick 1988) and results in abnormal bone remodelling (Eek and Gabrielson 1957) and reduced linear growth velocity (Lucas et al. 1989). In extreme forms, fractures of ribs and the distal ends of long bones (Koo et al. 1988) and craniotabes have been reported (Eek and Gabrielson 1957; Lyon et al. 1987). The progression of radiological changes is most clearly recorded in the literature prior to the introduction of formula and breast milk supplementation, in particular in the work of Eek and Gabrielson (1957).

In the longer term, height may be reduced (Lucas et al. 1989). There is a trend towards earlier presentation with fracture (excluding non-accidental injury cases) (Dahlenburg et al. 1989) and bone mineral accretion (Bishop et al. 1996); bone turnover and height in later childhood may also be influenced (Fewtrell et al. 1999, 2000a, b).

Aetiology

Disturbed mineral metabolism in the neonatal period

Calcium and phosphate

Whole blood ionised calcium falls within 18–24 hours of delivery. This is a physiological rather than pathological event, reflecting continued calcium accretion into bone in the face of reduced exogenous calcium input, and a postnatal surge in calcitonin production of unknown aetiology (Romagnoli et al. 1987). In term infants, symptomatic neonatal hypocalcaemia may reflect maternal vitamin D insufficiency (Delvin et al. 1986; Venkataraman et al. 1987). The initial manifestation of disturbed mineral metabolism in the premature infant is hypophosphataemia (Sagy et al. 1980; Carey et al. 1985). Plasma phosphate falls below 1.0 mmol/l between 7 and 14 days of age and is then accompanied by hypophosphaturia, with tubular reabsorption of phosphorus, typically <90% (Senterre and Salle 1982; Atkinson et al. 1983). Where persistent phosphate wasting is observed, investigations for renal tubular problems should be undertaken.

In phosphate-depleted infants, both hypercalcaemia (plasma calcium >2.7 mmol/l) and hypercalciuria are frequently observed (Lyon et al. 1984; Carey and Hopfer 1987). These changes may also occur secondary to immobilisation.

Phosphate depletion can be monitored by serial urinary calcium:phosphate ratios (Senterre 1991). This test can be performed on a spot sample (ideally immediately pre-feed) and should be <1 by age 3 weeks if the infant is phosphate-replete (calcium and phosphate both measured in mmol/l).

Lucas et al. (1989), in a prospective study of 857 preterm infants fed different diets, could not demonstrate a relationship between initial or later linear growth and plasma phosphate, after adjusting for the effects of diet and plasma alkaline phosphatase activity. Ryan and colleagues (1993) found a weak negative correlation of serum phosphate concentrations with forearm bone mineral content.

Bone turnover

There are now available a range of assays for assessing bone turnover (Tables 34.24 and 34.25). It is important to remember that the values obtained reflect the summation of both bone modelling – bone formation from the calcified cartilage of the growth plate and the combined effects of periosteal apposition and endosteal resorption – and remodelling activity which results from the resorption of discrete packets of bone and new bone formation at the same site.

In general, the studies show a period of increased bone turnover in the initial weeks after birth, followed by a period of stability and then a subsequent decline (Crofton et al. 1999). Crofton et al. (2000) also looked at the effects of steroids: dexamethasone suppressed bone activity (both formation and resorption) in a dose-dependent manner, in keeping with results at later ages. Only plasma (tissue non-specific) alkaline phosphatase is routinely

Table 34.24 Bone turnover markers

FORMATION	MEASURES	RESORPTION	MEASURES
Alkaline phosphatase (ALP)	New bone formation and/or rate of mineralisation	Cross-linked N-telopeptide of type I collagen (NTx)	Rate of bone type I collagen breakdown
N-terminal propeptide of type I collagen (PINP)	Rate of type I collagen incorporation into matrix	Cross-linked C-telopeptide of type I collagen (CTx)	Rate of bone type I collagen breakdown
C-terminal propeptide of type I collagen (PICP)	Rate of type I collagen incorporation into matrix	TRAP-5b	Number of osteoclasts
Osteocalcin	New bone formation	Type I collagen C-terminal telopeptide (ICTP)	Rate of type I collagen breakdown
		Pyridinoline	Rate of type I collagen breakdown (non-specific)
		Deoxypyridinoline	Rate of type I collagen breakdown
		Hydroxyproline	Rate of type I collagen breakdown (non-specific)

Table 34.25 Summary of change in markers over time in infants born prematurely

	0–4 WEEKS	4–10 WEEKS: 'POOR' DIET	4–10 WEEKS: 'GOOD' DIET	>10 WEEKS
Formation	↑↓	↑	→/↑ then ↓	↓
Resorption	↑↓	No data	→/↑ then ↓	↓

measured in neonatal units. It has been reported often in the context of bone health in infants born prematurely.

Plasma alkaline phosphatase activity typically rises over the first 3 weeks of postnatal life to levels two- to threefold greater than the maximum of the adult normal range. Activity increases further (from age 5–6 weeks) in infants who receive diets low in mineral substrate compared with those who receive diets with increased mineral content (Gross 1983; Lucas et al. 1989). In the short term, plasma alkaline phosphatase activity greater than five times the maximum of the adult normal range is associated with progressive slowing of linear growth velocity (Lucas et al. 1989). In the longer term (18 months and 9–12 years), such levels are associated with reduced height (Fewtrell et al. 2000b).

Vitamin D and its metabolites

Where routine supplementation of cow's milk and cereals is practised, cord blood levels of 25-hydroxyvitamin D_3 are typically >20 nmol/l, indicating vitamin D sufficiency. In the UK, spreading margarines and breakfast cereals are supplemented; dairy products are not. Maternal supplementation with vitamin D results in higher cord blood levels of 25-hydroxyvitamin D, but not 1,25-dihydroxyvitamin D (Delvin et al. 1986). Where maternal vitamin D intake during pregnancy has been poor, or where there is pre-existing maternal vitamin D deficiency, neonatal vitamin D stores may be low, and supplemental vitamin D of more than the normal 400 IU/day may be required. South Asian children living in the UK are at particular risk of vitamin D insufficiency (Lawson and Thomas 1999; Mughal et al. 1999). Insufficiency tends to be familial, and parents and other siblings should be tested (plasma 25-hydroxyvitamin D, parathyroid hormone) if a neonate presents with features of insufficiency. Formula feeding may not provide sufficient vitamin D to prevent hypocalcaemic fits if infants are severely deficient at birth (Callaghan et al. 2006).

A number of studies have identified low/borderline plasma 25-hydroxyvitamin D and elevated 1,25-dihydroxyvitamin D levels in plasma of preterm infants fed unsupplemented human milk (Greer et al. 1982; Salle et al. 1988), suggesting an increased requirement for vitamin D during rapid bone turnover in phosphate-depleted infants. Many studies indicate that vitamin D supplementation does improve calcium absorption and retention, although the magnitude of this improvement is variable, possibly reflecting mineral as well as vitamin D status. There are no data indicating improved long-term outcome for infants receiving higher doses of vitamin D (>1000 IU/day). There is no good evidence suggesting frank vitamin D deficiency in the majority of preterm infants.

Reduced or static bone mineral accretion

Bone is composed of two elements, matrix and mineral. The commonly used methods of measuring bone mass utilise the attenuation of one or more X-ray beams. The values obtained reflect both total amount of bone material and the degree of its mineralisation.

Most of the published literature up to the early 1990s reported data obtained using single-photon absorptiometry (SPA) measuring principally cortical bone at an appendicular site such as the distal forearm. Dual-energy X-ray absorptiometry (DXA) measures total and regional body bone mineral and can also estimate total body lean and fat mass (Lapillonne and Salle 1999). SPA is now rarely used. Both SPA and DXA are 'areal' techniques that reduce a three-dimensional quantity to two dimensions (volume becomes area). Both therefore measure bone mass rather than bone density. The effects of body (and bone) size must be considered, since an areal technique gives a greater value for the same true volumetric density in larger bones. Neither technique gives any indication of cortical thickness (relevant when considering fracture risk, particularly post-discharge). Current computed tomography-based techniques are insufficiently precise to use in infants.

The estimation of bone mineral content (BMC) in both term and premature infants has been reported from many centres but remains largely a research technique. The studies undertaken of mineralised bone mass accretion, irrespective of the technique used, have shown lower values than those expected had the infant remained in utero (James et al. 1986; Chan et al. 1988; Greer and McCormick 1988; Steichen et al. 1988; Venkataraman and Blick 1988). In general terms, healthy preterm infants who receive cow's milk-based diets supplemented with large amounts of calcium and phosphorus show improved mineral accretion that approaches the in utero accretion rate (James et al. 1986; Chan et al. 1988; Greer and McCormick 1988; Steichen et al. 1988; Venkataraman and Blick 1988; Wauben et al. 1998; Lapillonne et al. 2004). However, many studies do not relate BMC to body size; it remains unclear whether low BMC reflects the infant's smaller body and bone size, or true undermineralisation. Growth-retarded infants may have low BMC compared with appropriate-for-gestational-age (AGA) infants, although the differences frequently disappear when BMC is related to body size rather than gestation (Minton et al. 1983). There have been no reports of reduced mineral accretion during the period of initial hospitalisation being predictive of later outcomes such as growth, fracture risk, later mineral accretion or skeletal homeostasis. Continuing mineral supplementation postdischarge can enhance bone mass at 6–9 months (Bishop et al. 1993; Lapillonne et al. 2004).

Radiological changes

Radiological abnormalities are occasionally seen at birth in very growth-retarded infants, often in association with severe maternal malnutrition, including coeliac disease (Krishnamachari and Iyengar 1975). Early osteopenia can also follow chronic maternal magnesium administration (for preterm labour) (Kaplan et al. 2006). The majority of infants developing radiological abnormalities (Fig. 34.20) (rachitic changes, cortical thinning, periosteal elevation, fractures) either weigh <1000 g at birth or receive diets grossly deficient in mineral substrate (<1 mmol/kg/day calcium and phosphate).

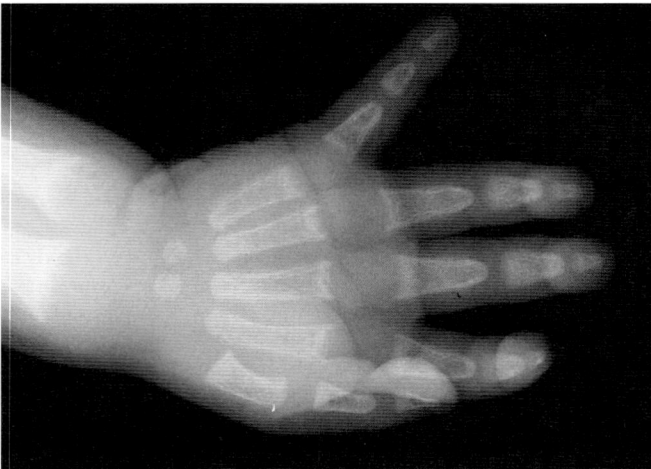

Fig. 34.20 X-ray of an ex-preterm infant showing rachitic changes.

Koo et al. (1982), described a scoring system based on single-view radiographs of the wrist or ankle at postnatal ages 5 and 10 weeks. Lyon and colleagues (1987) found that over 70% of infants weighing less than 1000 g had evidence of abnormal remodelling using this system. In older reports, metaphyseal cupping, splaying and fraying, and craniotabes were observed in half of all infants born before 33 weeks' gestation. Fractures of the ribs and long bones were also widely reported (Von Sydow 1946; Eek and Gabrielson 1957; Tulloch 1974) along with periosteal double contours, presumably reflecting the periosteal deposition of unmineralised osteoid. A review of 262 cases of unexplained fractures in infancy referred for the exclusion of osteogenesis imperfecta (OI) to a centre in Seattle identified a higher than expected proportion of infants born prematurely amongst the referral population (Marlowe et al. 2002).

Fractures

Fractures are more common in infants who have had necrotising enterocolitis; take more than 30 days to establish full enteral nutrition; have conjugated hyperbilirubinaemia; have chronic pulmonary disease; receive chronic furosemide; or receive physiotherapy (Amir et al. 1988; Koo et al. 1988; Dabezies and Warren 1997). The numbers of fractures reported can be up to 15; between a third and half of all fractures are rib fractures. Timing is typically around 10–11 weeks' chronological age (Bishop et al. 2007). These associations probably reflect the combined effects of reduced mineral intake and immobility, with the added loss of calcium from furosemide therapy. Bending forces exerted during procedures (Habert and Haller 2000) cause some fractures, as do forces exerted during physiotherapy that the thinned cortices cannot resist (Dabezies and Warren 1997). The excess of rib fractures may reflect a preponderance of chest X-rays in infants with chronic lung disease. The association with hyperbilirubinaemia is unexplained.

Long-term outcome

There is evidence to suggest that premature infants who have raised alkaline phosphatase during their initial period of hospitalisation have reduced stature at age 18–20 years (Fewtrell et al. 2009b). In addition, use of parenteral nutrition solutions containing aluminium (a common contaminant of mineral additive solutions added from glass ampoules) was associated with reduced femoral neck bone density at age 20 years (Fewtrell et al. 2009a).

Effects of drugs and immobilisation

Steroids reduce bone turnover (see above) and reduce linear growth. Oral steroid is associated with slowing of growth, reduced calcium absorption and increased renal losses of calcium and phosphate that recover after steroid cessation (Gibson et al. 1993; Shrivastava et al. 2000). Longer term skeletal effects of steroids have been difficult to evaluate because of multiple confounders. Furosemide may cause hypercalciuria and nephrocalcinosis (Hein et al. 2004) but without a clear effect on growth or mineral homeostasis. Steroids and furosemide together have been reported to cause nephrocalcinosis; immobilisation in infants receiving such treatment is likely to exacerbate this problem (Ezzedeen et al. 1988).

Immobilisation leads to disuse osteoporosis in older children and adults. Moyer-Mileur et al. (1995, 2000) showed a substantial gain in forearm BMC in infants undergoing up to 10 minutes of passive exercise per day over a 4-week period compared with matched controls.

Treatment: prevention is better than cure

The objectives of treatment are:

- prevention of abnormal bone-remodelling activity during the period of hospitalisation
- optimisation of growth potential, including effects on bone size and mass.

The principal aetiological factor remains inadequate mineral supply and therapeutic strategies are suggested with this in mind.

Organic phosphate solutions such as sodium glycerophosphate and glucose-1-phosphate are available. These will not co-precipitate with inorganic calcium solutions. They could provide adequate mineral substrate even before intravenous feeding is started.

All enterally fed preterm babies should receive 2 mmol/kg/day phosphate. Phosphate retention is of the order of 90–95%. For the baby receiving human milk, with a typical phosphate content of 0.5 mmol/100 ml, this equates to a total daily supplement when on full feeds of 1 mmol/kg/day phosphate.

For infants receiving preterm formula, no further supplements should be necessary. Term formula is not an acceptable diet for preterm infants (Lucas et al. 1990). In practical terms it seems reasonable to start oral phosphate supplements when oral intake is >2 ml/h.

Once phosphate supplementation is adequate, a relative deficiency of calcium may become evident (Senterre 1991). Such a deficiency is evidenced by radiological osteopenia and high plasma alkaline phosphatase activity in the face of normal plasma phosphate ($\geq$1.8 mmol/l). Calcium supplementation is then warranted.

If both calcium and phosphate are being added to human milk, the phosphate should be added first and allowed to stand for at least 5 minutes, and then the calcium added subsequently; co-precipitation is kept to a minimum by this method.

There is no place for the use of active metabolites of vitamin D, other than the treatment of rare inherited disorders (see below).

All infants should receive 400 IU/day vitamin D. It is not at all clear that supplements beyond this amount are associated with improved long-term outcome, but growth is certainly slower in unsupplemented term infants. Some authors believe that 1000 IU/day vitamin D is needed for the more immature infants and there is no indication from the literature that this is an excessive or unsafe dose.

Passive physical exercise substantially improves weight gain and bone mineral accretion in preterm infants and should be considered a routine part of care in the prevention of immobilisation-induced bone loss, whilst bearing in mind the issue of bone fragility.

Monitoring and adjusting treatment in affected infants

Most infants will have a weekly biochemical profile during their period in the neonatal intensive care unit. Senterre and Salle (1988) suggested the use of a random calcium:phosphate urine sample at age 3 weeks to identify infants who were becoming phosphate-depleted. Expressing both measurements as mmol, the ratio should be less than 1 in phosphate-replete infants. Later (from age 4 weeks onwards), persistently elevated serum alkaline phosphatase activity (more than three times the upper limit of the adult normal range) should lead the clinician to suspect metabolic bone disease. In each case, the remedy is the same – consider first the intake of mineral substrates and adjust the intake accordingly. Immobility leading to hypercalcaemia and hypercalciuria should be addressed with gentle passive physiotherapy.

There is no evidence that the use of vitamin D in high doses or by the intramuscular route is an effective intervention in any of these situations. Active metabolites are only indicated in highly specialised circumstances (see below); their use in metabolic bone disease of prematurity may lead to hypercalcaemia and nephrocalcinosis.

Inherited metabolic bone disease

Rachitic disorders

The three principal inherited types of rickets – X-linked hypophosphataemic rickets (*PHEX* gene defects), pseudo-vitamin D deficiency rickets (PDDR; 25-hydroxyvitamin D 1-α hydroxylase gene defects), or hereditary vitamin D receptor deficiency rickets (HVDRR; vitamin D receptor defects) – rarely present in the neonatal period, but clinical suspicion may indicate investigation where there is a relevant family history. Treatment in the neonatal period is indicated for the last two defects; replacement of 1,25 dihydroxyvitamin D with calcitriol or 1-α calcidol for PDDR; and high-dose calcium (initially intravenously) ± calcitriol for HVDRR (al-Aqeel et al. 1993).

Hypophosphatasia

Hypophosphatasia is the congenital absence of bone/liver/kidney-specific alkaline phosphatase in all tissues and serum (Whyte 1994). Cases presenting early (infantile form) are characterised by severely defective osteogenesis with rachitic changes, low/absent circulating alkaline phosphatase, with elevated urinary excretion of inorganic pyrophosphate and phosphoethanolamine. Studies of a recombinant bone-targeted alkaline phosphatase have been successful in TNSALP –/– mice (Millan et al. 2008); studies in infants show substantial resolution of bone disease with 12–18 months treatment (Whyte et al. 2012).

Disorders of osteogenesis

A problem with osteogenesis may be suggested antenatally by ultrasound demonstration of shortened limbs.

Osteogenesis imperfecta

The diagnosis of OI remains difficult because of the extreme variability in phenotype (Sillence et al. 1979), the lack of a definitive biochemical test and the heterogeneity of the genetic alterations – more than 800 separate mutations in the type I collagen genes have been described to date (Marini et al. 2007). Genetic studies looking for the individual mutations typical in types III and IV can now be undertaken on genomic DNA (i.e. on 5 ml of blood) using exon-spanning primers on high-throughput DNA-sequencing instruments with 99.9% ascertainment, but the procedure remains labour-intensive and costly. In those with a clear family history (frequent fractures and/or dislocations, hearing loss, hernias, fragile teeth, early-onset osteoporosis), 90% will have a mutation in the type I collagen genes (Sykes et al. 1990).

Fractures at birth may occur in any type of OI, but are more often seen in children with types II, III and IV.

OI type I (characterised by a 50% deficit in type I collagen production, autosomal dominant inheritance) rarely causes problems in the neonatal period. Types II–IV result from mutations in the collagen gene that affect the protein's ability to form the normal triple helices.

Type II is uniformly lethal. It is important to make the diagnosis, however, since parental germline mutations effectively create an autosomal dominant inheritance, engendering a significant risk (empirically approximately 7%) of a second affected child (Cole 1994).

Multiple early fractures leading to limb shortening are characteristic of OI III; affected infants typically have blue sclerae. In contrast to infants with OI II, there are few rib fractures and thus no thoracic dysplasia. Differentiating types III and IV is really only possible postneonatally, although children with OI IV may have white rather than blue sclerae. Lax skin and ligaments may be seen in all types of OI.

Postneonatally, the principal differential diagnosis is non-accidental injury; in such cases, the importance of family history and clinical examination is evident. Recently, five more forms of relatively severe OI have been described: three of these are due to mutations in the protein complex that performs 3-prolyl hydroxylation and are recessively inherited (Cabral et al. 2007; Baldridge et al. 2008; Marini et al. 2010; van Dijk et al. 2009; Willaert et al. 2009). Genetic testing is available for all three. The other two types present initially outside the neonatal period (Glorieux et al. 2000, 2002).

Treatment of severely affected infants with OI should be undertaken in a specialist centre that has a dedicated multidisciplinary team. Pamidronate given intravenously has been used to treat infants as young as 2 weeks old with type III OI (Plotkin et al. 2000; Senthilnathan et al. 2008). The available data suggest that such treatment, in combination with occupational and physiotherapy, improves bone mass, reduces fracture rates, reduces bone pain and enables the reconstruction of previously crush-fractured vertebrae. There is, as yet, no information on the long-term outcome of treated infants, and the ideal dose and preferred drug are still the subject of research endeavours.

Thanatophoric dwarfism

Both type I (cloverleaf skull, curved femora, marked platyspondyly) and type II (cloverleaf skull, short, straight long bones, mild platyspondyly) thanatophoric dwarfism result from mutations in fibroblast growth factor receptor 3 gene (Tavormina et al. 1995). Mutations in other parts of the same gene are responsible for achondroplasia and hypochondroplasia.

Osteopetrosis

A large number of mutations in different genes involved in cellular processes such as ion transport and energy production within osteoclasts have been found (Frattini et al. 2000; Chalhoub et al. 2003; Teitelbaum and Ross 2003). Rarely, osteopetrosis may arise as a result of the absence of osteoclasts due to lack of key factors in osteoclastogenesis (Sobacchi et al. 2007; Villa et al. 2009). The clinical features of 'marble bones' and immunodeficiency in the autosomal recessive form arise from defective osteoclastic (bone-resorbing) activity and reduced leukocyte superoxide production.

Pancytopenia is common, and retinal degeneration reported from age 2 months (Gerritsen et al. 1994). Treatment with interferon gamma-1b may be effective initially (Key et al. 1995) but later bone marrow or stem cell transplantation is still likely to be needed and management in a specialist centre is recommended.

References

Al-Aqeel, A., Ozand, P., Sobki, S., et al., 1993. The combined use of intravenous and oral calcium for the treatment of vitamin D dependent rickets type II (VDDRII). Clin Endocrinol (Oxf) 39, 229–237.

Amir, J., Katz, K., Grunebaum, M., et al., 1988. Fractures in premature infants. J Pediatr Orthop 8, 41–44.

Atkinson, S.A., Radde, I.C., Anderson, G.H., 1983. Macromineral balances in premature infants fed their own mothers' milk or formula. J Pediatr 102, 99–106.

Baldridge, D., Schwarze, U., Morello, R., et al., 2008. CRTAP and LEPRE1 mutations in recessive osteogenesis imperfecta. Hum Mutat 29, 1435–1442.

Bishop, N.J., King, F.J., Lucas, A., 1993. Increased bone mineral content of preterm infants fed with a nutrient enriched formula after discharge from hospital. Arch Dis Child 68, 573–578.

Bishop, N.J., Dahlenburg, S.L., Fewtrell, M.S., et al., 1996. Early diet of preterm infants and bone mineralization at age five years. Acta Paediatr 85, 230–234.

Bishop, N., Sprigg, A., Dalton, A., 2007. Unexplained fractures in infancy: looking for fragile bones. Arch Dis Child 92, 251–256.

Cabral, W.A., Chang, W., Barnes, A.M., et al., 2007. Prolyl 3-hydroxylase 1 deficiency causes a recessive metabolic bone disorder resembling lethal/severe osteogenesis imperfecta. Nat Genet 39, 359–365.

Callaghan, A.L., Moy, R.J., Booth, I.W., et al., 2006. Incidence of symptomatic vitamin D deficiency. Arch Dis Child 91, 606–607.

Callenbach, J.C., Sheehan, M.B., Abramson, S.J., et al., 1981. Etiologic factors in rickets of very-low-birth-weight infants. J Pediatr 98, 800–805.

Carey, D.E., Hopfer, S.M., 1987. Hypophosphatemic rickets with hypercalciuria and microglobulinuria. J Pediatr 111, 860–863.

Carey, D.E., Goetz, C.A., Horak, E., et al., 1985. Phosphorus wasting during phosphorus supplementation of human milk feedings in preterm infants. J Pediatr 107, 790–794.

Chalhoub, N., Benachenhou, N., Rajapurohitam, V., et al., 2003. Grey-lethal mutation induces severe malignant autosomal recessive osteopetrosis in mouse and human. Nat Med 9, 399–406.

Chan, G.M., Mileur, L., Hansen, J.W., 1988. Calcium and phosphorus requirements in bone mineralization of preterm infants. J Pediatr 113, 225–229.

Cole, G.C., 1994. Osteogenesis imperfecta as a consequence of naturally occurring and induced mutations of type I collagen. Bone and Mineral Research 8, 167–204.

Crofton, P.M., Shrivastava, A., Wade, J.C., et al., 1999. Bone and collagen markers in preterm infants: relationship with growth and bone mineral content over the first 10 weeks of life. Pediatr Res 46, 581–587.

Crofton, P.M., Shrivastava, A., Wade, J.C., et al., 2000. Effects of dexamethasone treatment on bone and collagen turnover in preterm infants with chronic lung disease. Pediatr Res 48, 155–162.

Dabezies, E.J., Warren, P.D., 1997. Fractures in very low birth weight infants with rickets. Clin Orthop 233–239.

Dahlenburg, S.L., Bishop, N.J., Lucas, A., 1989. Are preterm infants at risk for subsequent fractures? Arch Dis Child 64, 1384–1385.

Delvin, E.E., Salle, B.L., Glorieux, F.H., et al., 1986. Vitamin D supplementation during pregnancy: effect on neonatal calcium homeostasis. J Pediatr 109, 328–334.

Eek, S., Gabrielson, L.H., 1957. Prematurity and rickets. Pediatrics 20, 63–77.

Ezzedeen, F., Adelman, R.D., Ahlfors, C.E., 1988. Renal calcification in preterm infants: pathophysiology and long-term sequelae. J Pediatr 113, 532–539.

Fewtrell, M.S., Prentice, A., Jones, S.C., et al., 1999. Bone mineralization and turnover in preterm infants at 8–12 years of age: the effect of early diet. J Bone Miner Res 14, 810–820.

Fewtrell, M.S., Prentice, A., Cole, T.J., et al., 2000a. Effects of growth during infancy and childhood on bone mineralization and turnover in preterm children aged 8–12 years. Acta Paediatr 89, 148–153.

Fewtrell, M.S., Cole, T.J., Bishop, N.J., et al., 2000b. Neonatal factors predicting childhood height in preterm infants: evidence for a persisting effect of early metabolic bone disease? J Pediatr 137, 668–673.

Fewtrell, M.S., Bishop, N.J., Edmonds, C.J., et al., 2009a. Aluminum exposure from parenteral nutrition in preterm infants: bone health at 15-year follow-up. Pediatrics 124, 1372–1379.

Fewtrell, M.S., Williams, J.E., Singhal, A., et al., 2009b. Early diet and peak bone mass: 20 year follow-up of a randomized trial of early diet in infants born preterm. Bone 45, 142–149.

Frattini, A., Orchard, P.J., Sobacchi, C., et al., 2000. Defects in TCIRG1 subunit of the vacuolar proton pump are responsible for a subset of human autosomal recessive osteopetrosis. Nat Genet 25, 343–346.

Gerritsen, E.J., Vossen, J.M., Van Loo, I.H., et al., 1994. Autosomal recessive osteopetrosis: variability of findings at diagnosis and during the natural course. Pediatrics 93, 247–253.

Gibson, A.T., Pearse, R.G., Wales, J.K., 1993. Growth retardation after dexamethasone administration: assessment by knemometry. Arch Dis Child 69, 505–509.

Glorieux, F.H., Rauch, F., Plotkin, H., et al., 2000. Type V osteogenesis imperfecta: a new form of brittle bone disease. J Bone Miner Res 15, 1650–1658.

Glorieux, F.H., Ward, L.M., Rauch, F., et al., 2002. Osteogenesis imperfecta type VI: a form of brittle bone disease with a mineralization defect. J Bone Miner Res 17, 30–38.

Greer, F.R., Mccormick, A., 1988. Improved bone mineralization and growth in premature infants fed fortified own mother's milk. J Pediatr 112, 961–969.

Greer, F.R., Searcy, J.E., Levin, R.S., et al., 1982. Bone mineral content and serum 25-hydroxyvitamin D concentrations in breast-fed infants with and without supplemental vitamin D: one-year follow-up. J Pediatr 100, 919–922.

Gross, S.J., 1983. Growth and biochemical response of preterm infants fed human milk or modified infant formula. N Engl J Med 308, 237–241.

Habert, J., Haller, J.O., 2000. Iatrogenic vertebral body compression fracture in a premature infant caused by extreme flexion during positioning for a lumbar puncture. Pediatr Radiol 30, 410–411.

Hein, G., Richter, D., Manz, F., et al., 2004. Development of nephrocalcinosis in very low birth weight infants. Pediatr Nephrol 19, 616–620.

Hillman, L.S., Hoff, N., Salmons, S., et al., 1985. Mineral homeostasis in very premature infants: serial evaluation of serum 25-hydroxyvitamin D, serum minerals, and bone mineralization. J Pediatr 106, 970–980.

James, J.R., Congdon, P.J., Truscott, J., et al., 1986. Osteopenia of prematurity. Arch Dis Child 61, 871–876.

Kaplan, W., Haymond, M.W., Mckay, S., et al., 2006. Osteopenic effects of MgSO4 in multiple pregnancies. J Pediatr Endocrinol Metab 19, 1225–1230.

Key, L.L., Jr., Rodriguiz, R.M., Willi, S.M., et al., 1995. Long-term treatment of osteopetrosis with recombinant human interferon gamma. N Engl J Med 332, 1594–1599.

Koo, W.W., Gupta, J.M., Nayanar, V.V., et al., 1982. Skeletal changes in preterm infants. Arch Dis Child 57, 447–452.

Koo, W.W., Sherman, R., Succop, P., et al., 1988. Sequential bone mineral content in small preterm infants with and without fractures and rickets. J Bone Miner Res 3, 193–197.

Krishnamachari, K.A., Iyengar, L., 1975. Effect of maternal malnutrition on the bone density of the neonates. Am J Clin Nutr 28, 482–486.

Lapillonne, A., Salle, B.L., 1999. Methods for measuring body composition in newborns–a comparative analysis. J Pediatr Endocrinol Metab 12, 125–137.

Lapillonne, A., Salle, B.L., Glorieux, F.H., et al., 2004. Bone mineralization and growth are enhanced in preterm infants fed an isocaloric, nutrient-enriched preterm formula through term. Am J Clin Nutr 80, 1595–1603.

Lawson, M., Thomas, M., 1999. Vitamin D concentrations in Asian children aged 2 years living in England: population survey. Br Med J 318, 28.

Lucas, A., Brooke, O.G., Baker, B.A., et al., 1989. High alkaline phosphatase activity and growth in preterm neonates. Arch Dis Child 64, 902–909.

Lucas, A., Morley, R., Cole, T.J., et al., 1990. Early diet in preterm babies and developmental status at 18 months. Lancet 335, 1477–1481.

Lyon, A.J., Mcintosh, N., Wheeler, K., et al., 1984. Hypercalcaemia in extremely low birthweight infants. Arch Dis Child 59, 1141–1144.

Lyon, A.J., Mcintosh, N., Wheeler, K., et al., 1987. Radiological rickets in extremely low birthweight infants. Pediatr Radiol 17, 56–58.

Marini, J.C., Forlino, A., Cabral, W.A., et al., 2007. Consortium for osteogenesis imperfecta mutations in the helical domain of type I collagen: regions rich in lethal mutations align with collagen binding sites for integrins and proteoglycans. Hum Mutat 28, 209–221.

Marini, J.C., Cabral, W.A., Barnes, A.M., 2010. Null mutations in LEPRE1 and CRTAP cause severe recessive osteogenesis imperfecta. Cell Tissue Res 339, 59–70.

Marlowe, A., Pepin, M.G., Byers, P.H., 2002. Testing for osteogenesis imperfecta in cases of suspected non-accidental injury. J Med Genet 39, 382–386.

Millan, J.L., Narisawa, S., Lemire, I., et al., 2008. Enzyme replacement therapy for murine hypophosphatasia. J Bone Miner Res 23, 777–787.

Minton, S.D., Steichen, J.J., Tsang, R.C., 1983. Decreased bone mineral content in small-for-gestational-age infants compared with appropriate-for-gestational-age infants: normal serum 25-hydroxyvitamin D and decreasing parathyroid hormone. Pediatrics 71, 383–388.

Moyer-Mileur, L., Luetkemeier, M., Boomer, L., et al., 1995. Effect of physical activity on bone mineralization in premature infants. J Pediatr 127, 620–625.

Moyer-Mileur, L.J., Brunstetter, V., Mcnaught, T.P., et al., 2000. Daily physical activity program increases bone mineralization and growth in preterm very low birth weight infants. Pediatrics 106, 1088–1092.

Mughal, M.Z., Salama, H., Greenaway, T., et al., 1999. Lesson of the week: florid rickets associated with prolonged breast feeding without vitamin D supplementation. Br Med J 318, 39–40.

Plotkin, H., Rauch, F., Bishop, N.J., et al., 2000. Pamidronate treatment of severe osteogenesis imperfecta in children under 3 years of age. J Clin Endocrinol Metab 85, 1846–1850.

Romagnoli, C., Zecca, E., Tortorolo, G., et al., 1987. Plasma thyrocalcitonin and parathyroid hormone concentrations in early neonatal hypocalcaemia. Arch Dis Child 62, 580–584.

Ryan, S.W., Truscott, J., Simpson, M., et al., 1993. Phosphate, alkaline phosphatase and bone mineralization in preterm neonates. Acta Paediatr 82, 518–521.

Sagy, M., Birenbaum, E., Balin, A., et al., 1980. Phosphate-depletion syndrome in a premature infant fed human milk. J Pediatr 96, 683–685.

Salle, B.L., Glorieux, F.H., Delvin, E.E., 1988. Perinatal vitamin D metabolism. Biol Neonate 54, 181–187.

Senterre, J., 1991. Osteopenia versus rickets in premature infants. Rickets 145–154.

Senterre, J., Salle, B., 1982. Calcium and phosphorus economy of the preterm infant and its interaction with vitamin D and its metabolites. Acta Paediatr Scand Suppl 296, 85–92.

Senterre, J., Salle, B., 1988. Renal aspects of calcium and phosphorus metabolism in preterm infants. Biol Neonate 53, 220–229.

Senthilnathan, S., Walker, E., Bishop, N.J., 2008. Two doses of pamidronate in infants with osteogenesis imperfecta. Arch Dis Child 93, 398–400.

Shrivastava, A., Lyon, A., Mcintosh, N., 2000. The effect of dexamethasone on growth, mineral balance and bone mineralisation in preterm infants with chronic lung disease. Eur J Pediatr 159, 380–384.

Sillence, D.O., Senn, A., Danks, D.M., 1979. Genetic heterogeneity in osteogenesis imperfecta. J Med Genet 16, 101–116.

Sobacchi, C., Frattini, A., Guerrini, M.M., et al., 2007. Osteoclast-poor human osteopetrosis due to mutations in the gene encoding RANKL. Nat Genet 39, 960–962.

Steichen, J.J., Gratton, T.L., Tsang, R.C., 1980. Osteopenia of prematurity: the cause and possible treatment. J Pediatr 96, 528–534.

Steichen, J.J., Asch, P.A., Tsang, R.C., 1988. Bone mineral content measurement in small infants by single-photon absorptiometry: current methodologic issues. J Pediatr 113, 181–187.

Sykes, B., Ogilvie, D., Wordsworth, P., et al., 1990. Consistent linkage of dominantly inherited osteogenesis imperfecta to the type I collagen loci: COL1A1 and COL1A2. Am J Hum Genet 46, 293–307.

Tavormina, P.L., Shiang, R., Thompson, L.M., et al., 1995. Thanatophoric dysplasia (types I and II) caused by distinct mutations in fibroblast growth factor receptor 3. Nat Genet 9, 321–328.

Teitelbaum, S.L., Ross, F.P., 2003. Genetic regulation of osteoclast development and function. Nat Rev Genet 4, 638–649.

Tulloch, A.L., 1974. Rickets in the premature. Med J Aust 1, 137–140.

Van Dijk, F.S., Nesbitt, I.M., Zwikstra, E.H., et al., 2009. PPIB mutations cause severe osteogenesis imperfecta. Am J Hum Genet 85, 521–527.

Venkataraman, P.S., Tsang, R.C., Chen, I.W., Sperling, M.A., 1987. Pathogenesis of early neonatal hypocalcemia: studies of serum calcitonin, gastrin, and plasma glucagon. J Pediatr 110, 599–603.

Venkataraman, P.S., Blick, K.E., 1988. Effect of mineral supplementation of human milk on bone mineral content and trace element metabolism. J Pediatr 113, 220–224.

Villa, A., Guerrini, M.M., Cassani, B., et al., 2009. Infantile malignant, autosomal recessive osteopetrosis: the rich and the poor. Calcif Tissue Int 84, 1–12.

Von Sydow, G., 1946. A study of the development of rickets in premature infants. Acta Paediatr 22.

Wauben, I.P., Atkinson, S.A., Grad, T.L., et al., 1998. Moderate nutrient supplementation of mother's milk for preterm infants supports adequate bone mass and short-term growth: a randomized, controlled trial. Am J Clin Nutr 67, 465–472.

Whyte, M.P., 1994. Hypophosphatasia and the role of alkaline phosphatase in skeletal mineralization. Endocr Rev 15, 439–461.

Whyte, M.P., Greenberg, C.R., Salman, N.J., et al., 2012. Enzyme-replacement therapy in life-threatening hypophosphatasia. N Engl J Med 366, 904–913.

Willaert, A., Malfait, F., Symoens, S., et al., 2009. Recessive osteogenesis imperfecta caused by LEPRE1 mutations: clinical documentation and identification of the splice form responsible for prolyl 3-hydroxylation. J Med Genet 46, 233–241.

Disorders of the kidney and urinary tract

35

Neena Modi   Naima Smeulders   Duncan T Wilcox

Part 1: Renal function and renal disease in the newborn

Neena Modi

Morphological development of the kidney

The kidney develops from the caudal segment of the nephrogenic ridge, the metanephros, a population of mesodermal cells that condense around the tip of the ureteric bud from about 5 weeks' gestation. Nephron formation is induced as the ureteric bud branches and rebranches, forming first the major, then the minor calices, and finally the arborising system of collecting ducts. Nephrogenesis proceeds centrifugally with the juxtamedullary nephrons that lie deepest in the cortex developing first, and those in the superficial (subcapsular) cortex last. Urine production begins

© 2012 Elsevier Ltd

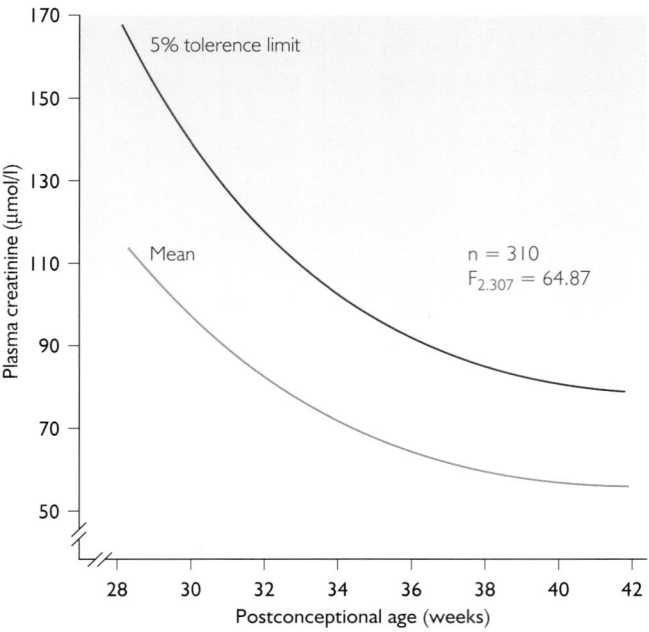

Fig. 35.1. Normal ranges for plasma creatinine by postconceptional age. *(Adapted from Trompeter et al. (1983).)*

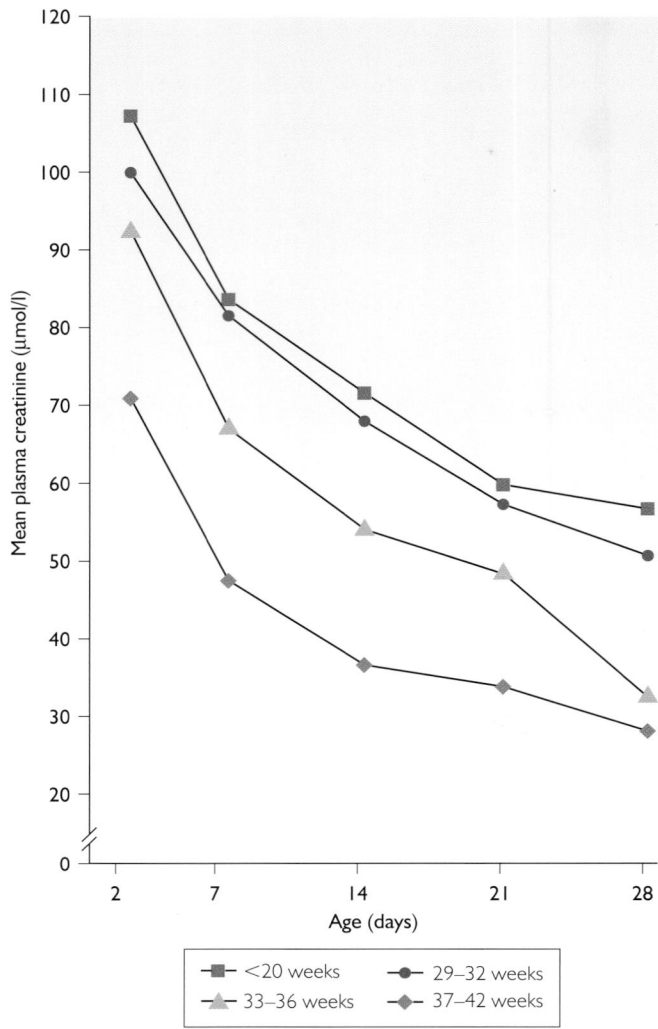

Fig. 35.2 Relationship between plasma creatinine and postnatal age in different gestational age groups. *(Adapted from Rudd et al. (1983).)*

at 8–10 weeks' gestation. The total complement of around 1 million nephrons is complete by 36 weeks. Nephrons that die are not replaced and subsequent increase in renal mass is due to tubular growth.

Assessing renal function

Glomerular filtration rate

Although widely described as 'low' in the newborn, glomerular filtration rate (GFR) is adequate for need. Formal measurement is not usually made and the serum or plasma creatinine (Pcr) is used as a proxy. Creatinine is derived from the turnover of phosphocreatine in muscle and excreted in the urine. The Pcr at birth reflects the maternal concentration. Subsequently this changes at a rate based on the balance between creatinine production rate, dependent on muscle mass (Modi and Hutton 1990), and clearance, dependent on GFR, that varies with postconceptional age (Fig. 35.1). The wide range in Pcr against postnatal age is due predominantly to the large variation that exists in weight for postconceptional age.

Pcr initially falls rapidly as the maternally derived load is excreted, then more gradually (Rudd et al. 1983). In term newborns, the Pcr at birth is typically 70–90 µmol/l (about 1 mg/dl), falling to about 30 µmol/l (0.3 mg/dl), with a range of 15–40 µmol/l (0.17–0.45 mg/dl), by 1 week of age and remaining at this level for the rest of the first month. A single measure of Pcr provides no more than a crude estimate of renal function. Observing the change over days is of more help. In the neonate, a sustained rise in Pcr, or a failure to fall, is often indicative of reduced GFR (Fig. 35.2). Blood urea is not recommended for assessment of renal function as it is influenced by numerous non-renal factors such as an elevated level from sequestered blood in the gastrointestinal tract.

Tubular function

Amino acids

In term neonates mild aminoaciduria is present, particularly affecting glycine, imino acids (proline and hydroxyproline), dibasic amino acids and taurine. Fractional reabsorption of other amino acids is relatively complete (Brodehl and Gellissen 1968).

Glucose

Mean urinary glucose concentration in the term newborn is slightly higher than in older children and adults (mean values 0.83 mmol/l (15 mg/dl) versus 0.33 mmol/l (6 mg/dl)) (Arant 1973). More marked glycosuria in a term infant cannot be attributed to physiological immaturity and should be investigated. Even moderate hyperglycaemia in the presence of a low threshold leads to substantial glycosuria and osmotic diuresis. It is essential that blood glucose is closely monitored in infants receiving intravenous fluids and parenteral nutrition.

Phosphate

Normal plasma phosphate concentration is higher in the fetus and healthy newborn infant than in older subjects. This is associated with a renal tubular phosphate threshold (plasma phosphate concentration above which phosphate appears in the urine) that is higher than that in adults (Kaskel et al. 1988), reflecting the need for phosphate retention in the rapidly growing infant, mainly to support skeletal growth. Since human milk contains little or no excess phosphate over the dietary needs of the infant, urinary phosphate excretion is normally low. Preterm infants are vulnerable to metabolic bone disease secondary to phosphate deficiency. Phosphaturia in the presence of normal or low plasma phosphate concentrations should be investigated.

Sodium

Healthy term infants are able to produce virtually sodium-free urine but the capacity to excrete a sodium load is less well developed than in older individuals (Aperia et al. 1975). The preterm newborn's ability to conserve and excrete sodium is compromised, and hence these babies are vulnerable to both sodium depletion and overload. In adults, approximately 80–90% of filtered sodium is reabsorbed in the proximal tubule (Fig. 35.3) (Cumming and Swainson 1995) and in the thick ascending limb of the loop of Henle. Unabsorbed sodium passes into the distal tubule and collecting duct where absorption occurs in exchange for potassium and hydrogen. Distal tubular sodium reabsorption is regulated by the renin–angiotensin–aldosterone system (RAAS). In neonates, a smaller proportion of filtered sodium is absorbed in the proximal tubule and a correspondingly larger proportion delivered distally. The sodium retention that characterises growth is due to the influence of very high RAAS activity (Spitzer 1982). The preterm neonate has a reduced capacity to retain sodium owing to impaired reabsorption at the proximal tubule, resulting in a higher distal sodium delivery, and to limited aldosterone responsiveness at the distal tubule (Sulyok et al. 1979b). Intestinal absorption, though also limited (Al-Dahhan et al. 1983b), is an important route for sodium conservation, with stool sodium loss generally less than 10% of intake.

The limited capacity to excrete a sodium load is not due to a low GFR, because filtration in even the most immature neonate greatly exceeds the amount that is ultimately retained, but because acute sodium loading results in only a blunted fall in RAAS activity and a limited natriuretic response (Drukker et al. 1980). Homeostasis is dependent on the regulation of tubular reabsorption, a process that in turn is dependent upon the stage of developmental maturation.

Tubular epithelial cells are bound by an apical membrane that faces the tubular lumen, and a basolateral membrane that lines the lateral and basal intercellular space and faces the peritubular capillaries. The lipid bilayer of the cell membrane is poorly permeable and solutes cross the membrane via transporters. These are specialised proteins inserted into the cell membrane. Their regulation is complex and involves hormones, intracellular signalling systems, protein phosphorylation, and endo- and exocytosis, each of which undergoes developmental regulation. Na^+/K^+-ATPase is the enzyme responsible for active sodium transport in all eukaryotic cells. There are many forms of Na^+/K^+-ATPase, each encoded by specific groups of Na^+/K^+-ATPase genes. In renal tubular cells, Na^+/K^+-ATPase, present on the basolateral membrane, creates an electrochemical gradient which is the energy source for the co-transport, involving specific transporter proteins, of Na^+ and glucose, and Na^+ and amino acids, and the countertransport of Na^+ and H^+ across the luminal membrane (Jorgensen 1986). The long-term regulation of

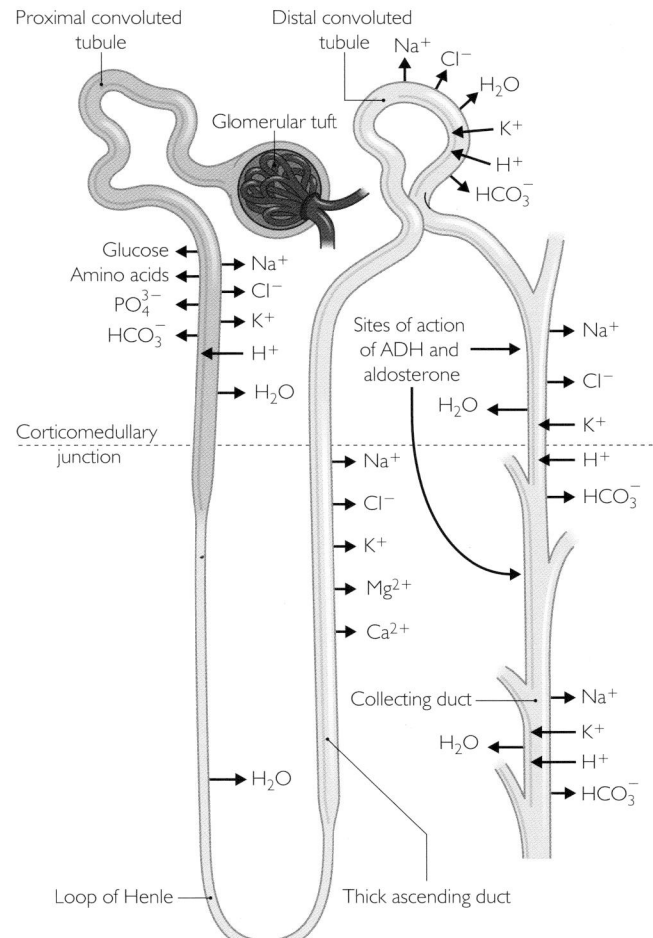

Fig. 35.3 Excretion of water and electrolytes. Water is reabsorbed in the proximal tubule together with glucose, amino acids, phosphate, sodium and bicarbonate, and from the distal nephron under the influence of arginine vasopressin and the hypertonic medulla. In the distal tubule, sodium is reabsorbed under the influence of aldosterone with associated excretion of potassium and hydrogen ions. ADH, antidiuretic hormone. *(Adapted from Cumming and Swainson (1995).)*

sodium balance is brought about by changes in the abundance of sodium transporters. During ontogenesis, there are tissue-specific patterns of increase in activity accompanied by an increase in Na^+/K^+-ATPase mRNA (Orlowski and Lingrel 1988). Antenatal glucocorticoid treatment increases the abundance of Na^+/K^+-ATPase in both lungs and kidney and enhances the maturation of renal tubular transport.

The postnatal enhancement in sodium conservation is brought about by the increasing responsiveness of the distal tubule to aldosterone (Sulyok et al. 1979a; Al-Dahhan et al. 1983a) and by an increase in the abundance of Na^+/K^+-ATPase and transporter proteins (Haycock and Aperia 1991; Herin and Aperia 1994). The ability to excrete a sodium load also matures during development. An increase or decrease in activity of renal Na^+/K^+-ATPase is the final common pathway for the short-term regulation of natriuresis (Aperia et al. 1994). Downregulatory factors that cause natriuresis include atrial natriuretic peptide (ANP), dopamine and diuretics. Noradrenaline is an upregulatory factor, which results in sodium retention. The peptide regulatory factors bind to cell membrane receptors and exert their effects via a cascade of intracellular messengers. Developmental maturation of these intracellular signalling systems fine-tunes the regulation of sodium balance (Kinoshita et al. 1989; Sposi et al. 1989; Fukuda et al. 1991; Ekblad et al. 1992; Midgley et al. 1992). Clinical observations offer some substantiation of these in vitro studies. ANP stimulates membrane-bound guanylate cyclase, which leads to an increase in the intracellular second messenger, cyclic guanosine monophosphate (cGMP), generated from endogenous guanosine triphosphate. cGMP interacts with specific protein kinases which in turn catalyse the phosphorylation of several protein substrates and this finally leads to a biological effect such as inhibition of sodium reabsorption. In a study of preterm babies (Midgley et al. 1992) the ratio of urinary cGMP to ANP was found to increase exponentially in the first 3 days after birth and then to reach a plateau. The ratio of sodium excretion to cGMP continued to increase over the 10 days of the study. This suggests a postnatal maturation in the ANP/cGMP/sodium excretion cascade and thus an increasing postnatal ability to excrete sodium.

Potassium

Potassium is the principal intracellular cation. Total body potassium is approximately 46 mmol/kg, a value that is similar in babies and adults. Unrecognised negative potassium balance may be relatively common in neonates receiving intensive care as it is easy to mask a falling serum potassium concentration if blood samples are slightly haemolysed. Preterm neonates should receive a potassium intake of 2 mmol/kg/day, commencing within 48 hours of birth if urine output is satisfactory and there are no concerns about renal function. Most gastrointestinal disorders are also associated with sodium loss and the resulting increase in circulating aldosterone exacerbates potassium loss. Hypokalaemia is usually accompanied by a metabolic alkalosis. Causes of potassium depletion are listed in Table 35.1.

The serum potassium may be spuriously elevated if there has been difficulty in obtaining the blood sample or a delay in processing it, as potassium is released from damaged cells. True hyperkalaemia occurs in the context of extensive tissue damage, shock and ischaemia, and in renal failure. The management of hyperkalaemia is discussed below.

Renal water handling: urine flow rate

As nutrition can be provided to babies only in liquid form, a high fluid intake is necessary and a high urine flow rate must be sustained to maintain water balance. This is achieved by a much greater fractional excretion of glomerular filtrate (Fe_{H2O}). In newborn babies, lower hydrostatic and osmotic forces across the peritubular space result in decreased proximal tubular reabsorption of filtered water and a greater proportion of water is delivered distally in comparison with in older subjects. Water reabsorption in the distal nephron is regulated by the antidiuretic hormone (ADH), arginine vasopressin (AVP). The ADH-dependent increase in water permeability is brought about by the insertion of water channels, the aquaporins (AQP), from an intracellular vesicular reservoir into the apical membranes of cells of the collecting ducts (Deen and Knoers 1998), allowing the movement of water across the tubular membrane in response to the high concentration of the medullary interstitium. Not all AQP isoforms are expressed in the human kidney and there are differences in expression during development, but fetal animals and preterm babies are sensitive to ADH (Ervin 1988). The regulation of collecting-duct water permeability by vasopressin is mediated by *AQP2* expression.

The capacity to concentrate urine develops progressively during postnatal life. The adult kidney can concentrate urine to 1200–1400 mOsmol/kg water. Infants are normally in a state of marked anabolism and have a lower urea production rate than adults, hence maximum osmolality is of the order of 600–800 mOsmol/kg. This difference is due to a shorter loop of Henle, reduced tonicity of the medullary interstitium as urea concentrations are low because of the highly anabolic state of the rapidly growing infant, and reduced expression of *AQP2*. A higher urine concentration, however, can be produced under conditions of severe dehydration stress, in response to antenatal glucocorticoid therapy (Yasui et al. 1996) and if the urea production rate is increased by high protein feeding. Very immature babies in the first days after birth may have more limited concentrating ability and hence become dehydrated while continuing to pass urine of low osmolality.

The capacity of the healthy term and preterm neonate to dilute urine matches that of adults (minimum urine osmolality 50 mOsmol/kg H_2O) (Ziegler and Ryu 1976; Coulthard and Hey 1985), hence diluting ability is unlikely to limit water excretion. Coulthard and Hey (1985) showed that healthy preterm babies are able to adjust water excretion appropriately from the second day after birth, when their daily intakes were varied between 95 and 200 ml/kg, with sodium intake remaining constant. The Fe_{H2O} increased from a mean of 7.4% to 13.1% of the filtered volume with the higher intake. A similarly high Fe_{H2O} in adults would result in a daily urine volume of over 20 litres. Of note is that there was no concomitant increase in the loss of sodium in the urine, an observation that refutes the widely held view that babies are unable to sustain a high urine flow without an inevitable increase in the loss of sodium.

Given a diluting and concentrating capacity that extends from 50 to 600 mOsmol/kg and a daily renal solute load of approximately 10–15 mOsmol/kg (Ziegler and Ryu 1976), the maximum and minimum urine flow rates that can be achieved are 300 ml/kg/24 h (12 ml/kg/h) (Leake et al. 1976) and 25 ml/kg/24 h (1 ml/kg/h) respectively. The latter value, which represents the minimum urine flow rate beyond which solute retention would result, is the

Table 35.1 Causes of potassium depletion

Inadequate intake
Gastrointestinal loss
Unreplaced nasogastric aspirates
Vomiting
Pyloric stenosis
Ileostomy loss
Diarrhoea
Renal loss
With metabolic alkalosis
Excessive base administration
Furosemide and other loop diuretics
Congenital chloride diarrhoea
Hyperaldosteronism
Bartter syndrome
Cushing syndrome
With metabolic acidosis
Renal tubular acidosis
Diuresis during recovery from acute renal failure

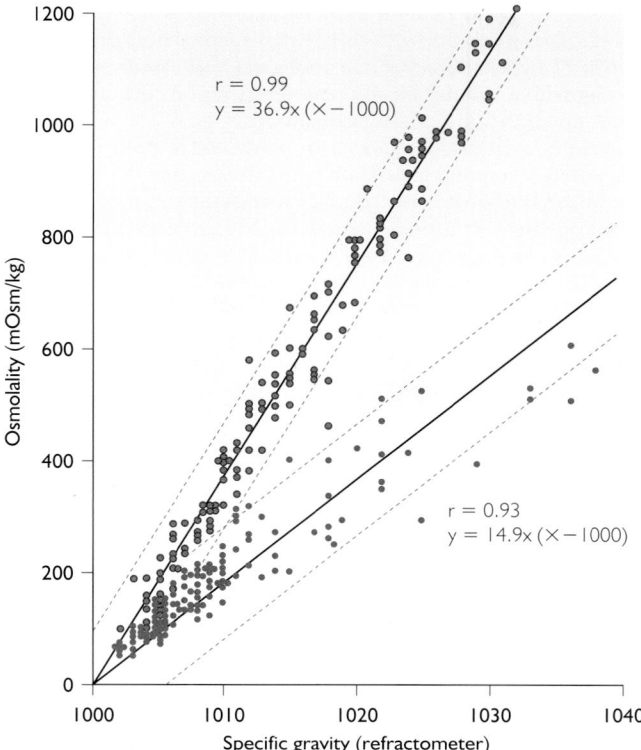

Osmolality (mOsm/kg) vs Specific gravity (refractometer)

r = 0.99
y = 36.9x (X − 1000)

r = 0.93
y = 14.9x (X − 1000)

Fig. 35.4 Relationship between specific gravity and urinary osmolality in newborn infants (•) and older children (•). Dotted lines show 95% prediction limits for individual observations. *(Adapted from Benitez et al. (1986).)*

justification for the use of this figure as a clinical indication of renal failure. Healthy infants, demand-fed on their mother's milk, usually produce urine approximately isotonic to plasma at a rate of about 3 ml/kg/h. A urine osmolality that lies between 200 and 400 mOsmol/kg usually suggests that fluid intake is satisfactory.

Specific gravity is often measured in place of osmolality as it can easily be performed on the ward. The presence of glucose or protein (both often found in samples from sick preterm babies) will, however, falsely elevate the specific gravity. In addition, the relationship between specific gravity, as measured with a refractometer, and osmolality differs between the newborn and older children, so that, in the newborn, an osmolality of 400 mOsmol/kg is indicative of a specific gravity anywhere between 1020 and 1030 (Fig. 35.4) (Benitez et al. 1986). Reagent strip test measurement of urinary specific gravity is unsatisfactory (Gouyon and Houchan 1993).

As neonates do not empty their bladders completely on voiding and as 7% fail to void during the first 24 hours after birth, external urine collections of short duration may be inaccurate. Urine can be collected using adhesive urine bags, taking care to protect the skin. Collection into preweighed nappies or cotton wool balls is widely practised, but can be misleading, as evaporation, leading to volume loss and increased osmolality, may be appreciable. Catheterisation is practicable even in the tiniest of babies.

Other urinary indices

Dipstick urinalysis may be used as a screening test for proteinuria, haematuria and glycosuria. Bilirubin causes dark-yellow to brown discoloration and suggests a conjugated hyperbilirubinaemia. Dark brown or red urine usually suggests haematuria, but may be caused by bile pigments, haemoglobin, rifampicin, porphyrins or urates. Haematuria may occur in renal venous and arterial thrombosis, cortical and tubular necrosis, neoplasia, obstructive uropathy, coagulopathy, nephritis and infection. Haemoglobinuria results from intravascular haemolysis and should raise suspicion of transfusion of incompatible blood, T-antigen activation or clostridial infection. Urine microscopy is necessary to detect red blood cells, leukocytes and casts. Red blood cell casts imply renal parenchymal pathology. A clean catch, catheter or suprapubic aspirate of urine should contain fewer than 5 white blood cells per cm^3 (Littlewood 1971). Leukocyturia is most often caused by infection but pyrexia or any inflammatory process may also be responsible. Newborns normally excrete small amounts of protein (De Luna and Hallet 1967).

Acid–base balance

The normal pH range of extracellular fluid is 7.35–7.45, corresponding to an H^+ concentration of 35–45 mmol/l. The regulation of acid–base balance involves, in order of speed of response, body buffers, respiratory function and renal function. In the proximal tubular cells, carbon dioxide, derived from cellular metabolism or diffusion from the tubular lumen, combines with water to form carbonic acid. This dissociates to H^+ and HCO_3^-. The H^+ is actively pumped into the tubular lumen and combines with filtered bicarbonate to form carbonic acid, which dissociates to water and CO_2. The CO_2 then diffuses back into the tubular cell to repeat the cycle. The net effect is that, for each hydrogen ion excreted, one bicarbonate ion is retained, so that bicarbonate reserves are continuously regenerated:

$$CO_2 + H_2O \leftrightarrow H_2CO_3 \leftrightarrow H^+ + HCO_3^-$$

In mature subjects, bicarbonate is regenerated by this process to maintain a plasma concentration of about 25 mmol/l, but preterm babies have a lower threshold (Brewer 1992). The capacity to excrete an acid load depends on the presence of urinary buffers. Hydrogen ions are excreted all along the nephron and combine with base buffers, chiefly phosphate, sulphate and ammonia, in the tubular fluid, when bicarbonate reabsorption is complete. In health, renal excretion is the only route for acid loss. Acid gain may arise from respiratory or metabolic disorders. Newborn infants can acidify urine to the same extent as healthy adults (Edelmann et al. 1967).

Acidosis

Acidosis may be respiratory, metabolic or mixed. In respiratory failure, carbon dioxide retention shifts the equation above to the right, with an increase in carbonic acid. Renal compensation is accomplished over a period of several days, by an increase in hydrogen ion excretion and bicarbonate regeneration. Blood gas analysis will reveal a compensated respiratory acidosis, with a high PCO_2, raised bicarbonate and a normal pH (Fig. 35.5). In an otherwise normal subject, a fall in pH will stimulate hyperventilation, shift the carbonic acid equation to the left and increase CO_2 elimination. The features of a compensated metabolic acidosis are a low bicarbonate, low PCO_2 and normal pH. Infants with both respiratory disease and a metabolic acidosis will show a mixed picture, with a high PCO_2, low bicarbonate and low pH. Renal tubular acidosis (RTA) is discussed below. In a ventilated infant acute respiratory acidosis is managed by increasing the tidal volume or respiratory rate to lower the PCO_2. Once compensatory changes have taken place, lowering the PCO_2 will lead to a respiratory alkalosis, hence the importance of recognising if compensation has taken place and,

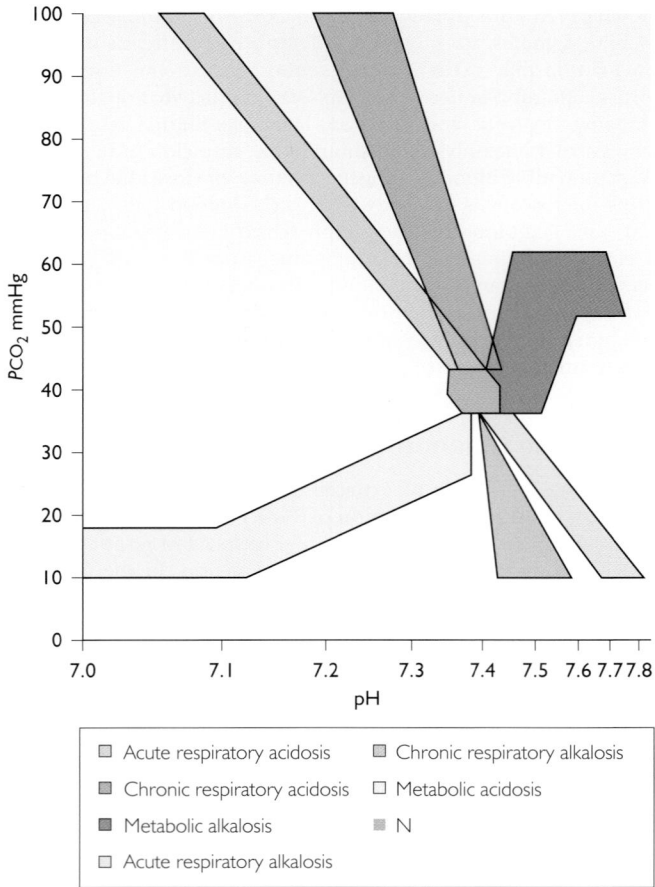

an extracellular anion and the normal serum level is 90–110 mmol/l. Partly replacing chloride with acetate in parenteral nutrition reduces the risk of hyperchloraemic metabolic acidosis. Medications that affect proximal tubular bicarbonate regeneration include the carbonic anhydrase inhibitor acetazolamide.

Metabolic acidosis arising as a consequence of poor peripheral perfusion will respond to a saline bolus. Treatment with base, such as sodium bicarbonate or tris(hydroxymethyl)aminomethane, may be appropriate. The formula widely used to calculate the quantity to achieve complete correction is mmol/l base=0.3×bodyweight (kg)×SBE (mmol/l), with 'half-correction' obtained by dividing this by two. This assumes that the extracellular fluid volume (ECFV) is 20% of bodyweight and, as administered base equilibrates to some extent with the intracellular compartment, this factor is increased to 0.3. The inherent imprecision in this approach should be appreciated; ECFV is considerably higher in the neonate, and the volume of distribution and rate of acid accumulation cannot be estimated with any degree of certainty.

Alkalosis

Respiratory alkalosis results from hyperventilation and the PCO_2 will be low. The commonest cause in the neonatal unit is iatrogenic and occurs during assisted ventilation, particularly high-frequency oscillatory ventilation. This is dangerous and is further discussed in Chapter 27 part 2.

Metabolic alkalosis is caused by gain of base, as in the injudicious use of sodium bicarbonate or from loss of acid. A common cause is loss of gastric acid and chloride in high intestinal obstruction, vomiting or failure to replace gastric aspirates. In the distal tubule and collecting duct, sodium is reabsorbed in exchange for either potassium or hydrogen ions, under the influence of aldosterone. If intracellular H$^+$ is low, potassium is preferentially lost and vice versa, explaining the association between alkalosis and hypokalaemia. Hypokalaemia is both a cause and a consequence of metabolic alkalosis. Chronic diuretic therapy results in metabolic alkalosis through multiple mechanisms. Causes of metabolic alkalosis are shown in Table 35.2.

Acute renal failure

Acute renal failure (ARF) is the syndrome that results from an abrupt reduction in GFR. The spectrum of renal injury extends from mild tubular dysfunction to acute tubular necrosis or cortical necrosis. There may be full recovery from acute renal failure, or injury may be irreversible and fatal, or partial, leading to renal impairment many years later.

Formerly most often seen in the context of severe respiratory disease, perinatal asphyxia, sepsis and necrotising enterocolitis have emerged as the most common predisposing causes in neonatal intensive care. Renal injury may arise as a result of reduced renal perfusion, ischaemic injury, myoglobinuria following rhabdomyolysis or haemoglobinuria due to intravascular haemolysis. Antenatal exposure to angiotensin-converting enzyme inhibitors and angiotensin receptor blockers may present as renal impairment in the newborn and should be suspected if there is accompanying undermineralisation of the calvarium (Mehta and Modi 1989).

There is no agreed definition for ARF in the newborn, nor is this unreasonable as this is not a steady-state period. A practical approach is to consider the possibility of renal impairment if the expected postnatal decline in PCr does not occur (Fig. 35.2) or if it remains persistently above 1.5 mg/dl (about 130 μmol/l) (Stapleton et al. 1987).

in this case, targeting ventilation management upon achieving a normal pH, and not a normal PCO_2. Metabolic acidosis is due to an increase in acid or a decrease in base. The best measure of metabolic acidosis is the standard base excess (SBE) as this is independent of PCO_2.

In cases of unexplained metabolic acidosis at any age, measure the anion gap (AG), the difference between the sodium concentration (sometimes summated with potassium) and the sum of the chloride and bicarbonate:

$$AG = Na^+ - (Cl^- + HCO_3^-)$$

The normal value is 8–16 mmol/l or, if sodium and potassium concentrations are summated, about 4 mmol/l higher. The normal gap is due to unmeasured anions, mainly albumin, phosphate and small amounts of organic anions, including lactate. A raised anion gap is due to an increase in either one of the 'normal' unmeasured anions (e.g. lactate) or another organic anion normally present in no more than trace amounts (e.g. ketoacids, complex organic anions in various inborn errors of metabolism). In patients with a normal anion gap metabolic acidosis the fall in HCO_3^- is compensated for by an increase in Cl$^-$.

A common cause of metabolic acidosis in neonatal intensive care is tissue hypoxia. Metabolic acidosis also occurs in renal failure, from amino acid intolerance during parenteral nutrition, and in inborn errors of metabolism. Hyperchloraemia may occur with some parenteral nutrition formulations. Chloride is predominantly

Table 35.2 Causes of metabolic alkalosis

Gastric loss	Vomiting
	Pyloric stenosis and other high intestinal obstruction
	Unreplaced gastric aspirates
Stool loss	Diarrhoea
Bartter syndrome	Hypokalaemic metabolic alkalosis; may present with polyhydramnios, polyuria and dehydration
Diuretic therapy	Secondary hyperaldosteronism due to volume depletion, chloride depletion, potassium depletion
Hypokalaemia	
Refeeding syndrome	Associated with restoration of homeostasis, intracellular water and electrolyte shift, and hypokalaemia
Adrenal hypersecretion	Primary and secondary hyperaldosteronism
Excessive bicarbonate administration	

Table 35.3 Urinary biochemical indices in prerenal failure and acute tubular necrosis in term babies

TEST	PRERENAL FAILURE	ACUTE TUBULAR NECROSIS
Urine urea	High	Low
Urine creatinine	High	Low
Urine osmolality	High (>500 mOsmol/kg)	Low (>300 mOsmol/kg)
Specific gravity	High (>1.025)	Low (>1010)
Urine sodium	Low (<10 mmol/l)	High (>20 mmol/l)
U:P urea	High (>10)	Low
U:P creatinine	High (>40)	Low
U:P osmolality	High (>2)	Low (>1)
FE_{Na}	Low (<1%)	High (>3%)
RFI	Low (<1)	High (>4)

FE_{Na}, fractional sodium excretion; RFI, renal failure index. See text for calculation and interpretation in extremely preterm babies.

Presentation, investigation and management

Anticipate problems. Careful monitoring of urine output should commence on admission to neonatal intensive care. Delayed recognition of oligoanuria will increase the risk of prerenal impairment progressing to intrinsic renal failure. In term asphyxiated babies restrict initial fluid intake to 30–40 ml/kg/day until the situation is clear. This will not result in dehydration as it is considerably more than their transepidermal insensible loss, which is around 12 ml/kg/day. Hypoglycaemia may be a problem at low infusion volumes, and hypertonic glucose, infused centrally, may be necessary. Intravenous sodium should be avoided.

Though non-oliguric ARF is probably more frequent than oliguric ARF and represents the mild end of the spectrum of renal injury (Chevalier et al. 1984), it is infrequently diagnosed. Oligoanuria is the commonest presenting sign and may indicate impaired renal perfusion (prerenal failure), established renal failure with damage to the renal parenchyma or urinary obstruction. If the urine flow rate falls below 1 ml/kg/h, immediate investigation is required. Consider the clinical context and whether the problem is likely to be prerenal, renal or postrenal. Ultrasound examination of the renal tract will identify congenital abnormalities, obstructive lesions such as posterior urethral values, postoperative urinary retention and the large, swollen kidneys of renal venous thrombosis.

Radionuclide imaging studies are of little initial value in distinguishing between causes of ARF in the newborn. Clinical examination should include assessment of perfusion (capillary refill time, toe–core temperature gap, blood pressure, metabolic acidosis), presence of renal masses and bladder palpation. Renal underperfusion leads to the production of urine of 'poor quality' (high osmolality, high urea and creatinine and low sodium concentration) (Table 35.3). Some authors suggest that the best indicator to distinguish prerenal from established renal failure in the oliguric neonate is the fractional excretion of sodium (FeNa). This is calculated from the sodium and creatinine concentrations of plasma (P) and a spot urine (U) sample:

$$Fe_{Na} \% = (U/P)\,sodium \times (P/U)\,creatinine \times 100$$

If tubular function is intact and sodium reabsorption continues, the infant is in oliguric prerenal failure and the Fe_{Na} will be less than 3% (6% in very preterm babies) (Mathew et al. 1980). Unfortunately, the Fe_{Na} and other indices such as the renal failure index (U sodium × P/U creatinine) have poor sensitivity and specificity (Modi 1989). The urinary sodium concentration cannot be interpreted clearly if furosemide has already been used, nor is it acceptable to delay further action until urinary sodium and creatinine estimations have been obtained.

A suspicion of prerenal failure demands urgent attention to restoration of renal perfusion. A high Fe_{Na} suggests established renal failure and the equally urgent need for restriction of fluid intake. If prerenal impairment is suspected administer a fluid challenge of 10–20 ml/kg 0.9% saline followed by a single dose of furosemide. A dose of 1–2 mg/kg is often used but a single dose of 4 mg/kg is probably more appropriate in babies less than 31 weeks' postconceptional age as furosemide secretory clearance is low, resulting in reliance on glomerular filtration for delivery to the main site of action within the lumen of the loop of Henle, and a high plasma level is necessary when GFR is reduced (Modi and Coulthard 1999). As the half-life of furosemide exceeds 24 hours in healthy preterm infants, repeated doses and dose scheduling more frequently than every 24 hours will lead to accumulation and increased risk of ototoxicity, interstitial nephritis and possibly persistence of ductal patency through stimulation of prostaglandin release. If a volume challenge does not produce a prompt diuresis, further management is that of established renal failure.

Management of acute renal failure

General principles

The goal of management is to maintain the baby in stable fluid and electrolyte balance, avoid catabolism and support growth while awaiting recovery. Calculate the maintenance fluid requirement as the sum of measured urine and gastrointestinal losses and estimated insensible water loss. Correct hypovolaemia with isotonic fluid. Weigh the baby daily. Monitor acid–base balance, serum creatinine and electrolytes. An adequate energy intake is necessary to minimise catabolism, which potentiates hyperkalaemia, hyperphosphataemia and acidosis, but may be limited by the need for fluid restriction. Enteral nutrition is preferred if the patient's condition allows, but parenteral nutrition may be necessary. Dietary sodium should not exceed 1 mmol/kg/day. It may be preferable to give this as bicarbonate if metabolic acidosis is present. Hyperphosphataemia is managed by the addition of oral calcium carbonate to feeds. This binds phosphate, rendering it insoluble, thereby reducing intestinal absorption. Aluminium hydroxide should not be used as a phosphate binder in neonates, because of the risk of neurotoxicity. Hyperphosphataemia is usually accompanied by hypocalcaemia but additional calcium should not be given until the plasma phosphate has been reduced to normal, or ectopic calcification may occur. The management of hypertension is discussed in Chapter 28.

Unproven therapies include furosemide by infusion (0.1 mg/kg/h) (discussed above) and low-dose dopamine (2–5 µg/kg/min). In addition to cardiovascular effects which influence renal function, dopamine has direct renal actions, inhibiting renal Na^+/K^+-ATPase and Na^+H^+ exchanger activity and attenuating the actions of aldosterone and AVP (Seri et al. 1993). The cellular signalling system that transduces the signal from activated dopamine receptors to inhibit renal Na^+/K^+-ATPase undergoes developmental regulation (Fukuda et al. 1991). In healthy volunteers, low-dose dopamine increases renal blood flow and induces natriuresis and diuresis. The hope has been that, by increasing renal blood flow, low-dose dopamine might help preserve renal cellular oxygenation, GFR and urine output in renal ischaemia. Seri et al. (1993) showed that dopamine at a dose of 2 µg/kg/min induced maximal diuresis and natriuresis in sick preterm neonates if systemic blood pressure was within the normal range. An increase to 4 µg/kg/min resulted in a further increase in blood pressure, but no change in urine output and sodium excretion. Dopamine is also a proximal tubular diuretic, increasing the presentation and reabsorption of chloride by the ascending limb of the loop of Henle, an effect that may increase medullary oxygen consumption and exacerbate medullary ischaemia. In critically ill adult patients, low-dose dopamine does not protect against renal dysfunction (Bellomo et al. 2000). As dopamine raises blood pressure through its vasoconstrictor actions, renal perfusion may in fact be impaired at higher doses. To date, there is insufficient evidence to support the use of low-dose dopamine to improve urine output in very immature infants and, given the side-effects that include renal, pulmonary and mesenteric vasoconstriction, and impaired growth hormone, thyroid and prolactin secretion, use for this indication is not recommended.

Low-dose theophylline, a xanthine derivative and adenosine antagonist, has been used in the hope of blunting the efferent arteriolar adenosine-mediated vasodilatation induced by hypoxia. Placebo-controlled trials of a single 8 mg/kg dose of theophylline given after delivery in term asphyxiated newborns significantly improved renal function (Jenik et al. 2000; Bakr 2005; Bhat et al. 2006).

Table 35.4 Emergency management of hyperkalaemia

Intravenous salbutamol (4 µg/kg over 5 minutes) or nebulised salbutamol (2.5–5 mg); repeated as necessary

Intravenous glucose and insulin infusion (12 units soluble insulin in 100 ml 25% glucose; 5 ml/kg given over 30 minutes); has an additive effect with salbutamol; monitor blood glucose closely during and after treatment

Intravenous sodium bicarbonate 1 mmol/kg (2 ml/kg 4.2%); effective even if infant is not acidotic

10% calcium gluconate (0.1 ml/kg) by intravenous injection over 10 minutes; repeated as necessary to maintain normocalcaemia (caution: do not administer in same line as bicarbonate; risk of precipitation)

Hyperkalaemia

Severe hyperkalaemia is a medical emergency since it may cause potentially lethal ventricular fibrillation. Electrocardiogram changes, initially peaked T waves, followed by prolongation of the PR interval, flattening of the P waves, and widening of QRS complexes, are not usually seen in extremely preterm babies until the serum potassium exceeds 8 mmol/l. Short-term measures to shift potassium from the extracellular to the intracellular compartment and protect against cardiotoxic effects while preparing for dialysis are shown in Table 35.4. Oral/rectal cation exchange resins, such as calcium polystyrene sulphate (Resonium), are effective in permanent removal of potassium but use may be complicated by bowel obstruction. Although exchange resins can be given rectally and then removed by gentle saline lavage, dialysis is preferable (Table 35.4).

Dialysis

Dialysis is the removal of small solutes across a semipermeable membrane by diffusion across a concentration gradient. The membrane may be the peritoneum, separating blood in the splanchnic capillaries from dialysis fluid within the peritoneal cavity, or may be synthetic, as in haemodialysis, with blood and dialysis fluid pumped on opposite sides of the membrane. This process differs from ultrafiltration, in which there is convective removal of plasma water and small solutes as a result of a pressure gradient across a highly permeable membrane. Treatments can consist of pure dialysis, pure filtration or both. Peritoneal and haemodialysis are possible in infants weighing <1 kg. The main indications for dialysis are inability to meet the baby's nutritional needs because of limitation in the amount of fluid or sodium that can be given, intractable metabolic acidosis, volume overload, hyperkalaemia and hyperphosphataemia/hypocalcaemia.

Peritoneal dialysis

Peritoneal dialysis (PD) is the modality of choice in most neonates, the advantage being relative ease of access and technical simplicity in comparison with haemodialysis. The preferred means of access to the peritoneal cavity is with a Silastic Tenckhoff catheter inserted using a sterile technique by an experienced surgeon. Catheters can be inserted over a guidewire using the Seldinger technique, but these have a shorter functional life and are more prone to blockage, leakage and infection than those placed surgically. In very small infants, in whom insertion is not feasible, PD can be carried out using an angiography catheter, intravenous cannula or thoracic drain.

Commercial 1.36%, 2.27% and 3.86% glucose solutions are available for neonatal PD (osmolality 347, 398 and 486 mOsmol/kg). As these contain lactate, bicarbonate buffered solution should be used in the neonate with lactic acidosis. Calcium-free solutions are also available. Hypertonic glucose dialysate can cause hyperglycaemia and hypovolaemia, and it is usual to use the 1.36% solution in preterm neonates, introducing higher concentrations with caution and only if considered essential. A fill volume, warmed to body temperature, of 10–20 ml/kg is used initially, increasing to 30 ml/kg if tolerated. The dialysate is run into the abdomen by gravity. An automatic cycler may be used but for small cycle volumes dialysis must be performed manually, usually using modified intravenous giving sets with suitably sized burettes.

A relative, though not absolute, contraindication to PD is major abdominal surgery. Common complications include peritonitis, catheter site infection, catheter blockage or occlusion by omentum. To reduce the risk of blockage, some surgeons perform an omentectomy when inserting a catheter. Substantial fluid and electrolyte imbalances can occur during PD. Hypokalaemia or hypophosphataemia is managed by adding 3–5 mmol/l KCl or 2–3 mmol/l KPO_4 to the dialysate.

Haemofiltration and haemodialysis

If PD fails or is contraindicated haemofiltration and/or haemodialysis provide alternative options. It is preferable to perform these techniques continuously in order to avoid swings in intravascular volume and biochemistry, but intermittent haemodialysis has been used successfully in neonates (Sadowski et al. 1994). The advantage of haemofiltration with or without dialysis is that fluid removal is rapid; the disadvantages are the need for heparinisation, blood priming of the circuit in the smallest babies, and the potential for severe fluid and electrolyte imbalance because of the large volume of fluid removed and subsequently replaced.

The simplest technique is continuous arteriovenous haemofiltration (CAVH), in which an artery and a vein are cannulated and blood is driven across a filter by the patient's systemic blood pressure (Lieberman et al. 1985). Arterial access is via the umbilical or femoral vessels and venous access via the umbilical, femoral or jugular veins. A systemic blood pressure of at least 40 mmHg is required to maintain adequate flow across the filter. If necessary a volumetric infusion pump can be inserted into the circuit to improve this (Heney et al. 1989). The ultrafiltration pressure can be increased by increasing the vertical height between the filter and the collection vessel and further adjusted by applying gentle suction with a pump across the filter. The pump also prevents excessive ultrafiltration. Using this system, ultrafiltration rates of up to 5 ml/kg/h have been achieved (Bauer and Stewart 1988). Replacement fluid and parenteral nutrition can be infused into the venous port of the circuit. CAVH may not be possible in patients who have refractory hypotension or poor cardiac function. Most infants will tolerate a maximum extracorporeal volume of 10% of their blood volume.

An alternative technique is continuous venovenous haemofiltration, in which access is obtained either via two venous lines or via a single double-lumen venous line, and a pump is used to control blood flow through the circuit.

Haemofiltration removes solute by convection but not diffusion. If this is inadequate, for example if the infant is catabolic with a raised urea generation rate, diffusive clearance can be added by running dialysis fluid through the ultrafiltrate compartment of the filter in the opposite direction to blood flow (Assadi 1988; Bishof et al. 1990). Figure 35.6 illustrates the principles of haemofiltration and haemodiafiltration.

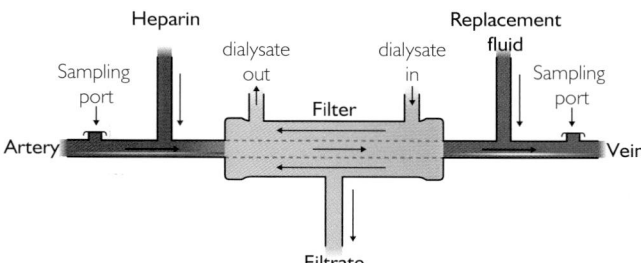

Fig. 35.6 Schematic representation of arteriovenous haemofiltration and haemodiafiltration (see text for details).

Outcome

The extent and time course of renal functional recovery are very variable and depend upon the underlying aetiology and associated morbidities. Return of function may include a diuretic phase necessitating a change from sodium and water restriction to equally careful replacement of a large volume of dilute urine and large sodium losses. Mortality is highest when ARF occurs in a setting of multiorgan failure. Survivors are at risk of increased late mortality and renal sequelae, indicating the need for long-term follow-up.

Chronic renal failure

Causes

Bilateral renal agenesis and bilateral multicystic renal dysplasia are incompatible with survival. The severe oligohydramnios caused by absence of fetal urine production leads to the Potter sequence and lethal pulmonary hypoplasia. Renal dysplasia, usually associated with gross bilateral vesicoureteric reflux (VUR) or obstructive uropathy, is the commonest cause of 'true' congenital chronic renal failure (CRF). It is about twice as common in boys as girls because of the male predominance in posterior urethral valves and severe VUR. Acquired causes include bilateral renal arterial or venous thrombosis and severe acute tubular necrosis progressing to renal cortical necrosis. It is unusual for congenital renal dysplasia to be severe enough to require dialysis in the newborn period. The recessive form of polycystic kidney disease (see below), a rare disease, may occasionally cause renal failure in the neonatal period.

Clinical features

Cord blood biochemistry reflects maternal, not fetal, renal function. The presentation of CRF may be subtle with failure to thrive, or serendipitous through detection of an elevated serum creatinine, and may be missed for several weeks. Many babies with renal dysplasia have obligate high urinary sodium excretion, and are prone to become salt-depleted if adequate replacement is not provided. Arterial hypertension may be present, but usually not in those with significant urinary salt loss. There are numerous rare inherited syndromes with renal involvement that may lead to CRF, but it is exceptional for them to present in the neonatal period and they will not be discussed further here.

Management

The principal problem in babies with CRF is achieving an adequate energy intake. Uraemia causes anorexia, nausea and vomiting, requiring total or partial nasogastric tube feeding. The ideal feed is breast milk with added energy supplements or a low-phosphate artificial formula. The target energy intake is 150–180 kcal/kg/day, more than required by healthy infants. A common stratagem is to administer intermittent feeds by day with continuous intragastric infusion by night. Sodium bicarbonate is added to the feed in an amount sufficient to maintain the plasma bicarbonate at 22–24 mmol/l. If there is any tendency to hyponatraemia, or if weight gain is poor despite adequate energy intake, sodium chloride should also be added in a dose that maintains normal plasma sodium concentrations without inducing fluid overload or hypertension. Calcium carbonate is often necessary to maintain the plasma phosphate in the normal range. When serum phosphate is adequately controlled, calcidiol or calcitriol should be added if the plasma calcium concentration is low. This is a difficult and demanding regimen and requires skilled and sympathetic coaching of the parents by a team of experienced nurses, dieticians and nephrologists (Rigden et al. 1987).

Polycystic kidney disease

Autosomal dominant polycystic kidney disease (ADPKD) is a fairly common condition (incidence about 1 in 500–600) that seldom causes clinical problems in the newborn period. Hyperechoic kidneys may be detectable in utero or in the neonatal period (Fick et al. 1993). Cysts are identifiable in 60% of those affected by the age of 5 years (Kaplan et al. 1977; Michaud et al. 1994). Affected children have large kidneys and a tendency to higher blood pressure, although few progress to overt hypertension. Of the two known loci for ADPKD, PKD-1 is more likely to present early than PKD-2. With very rare exceptions, GFR does not begin to decline measurably during infancy and childhood.

Autosomal recessive polycystic kidney disease (ARPKD) is rare (1 in 10 000–40 000 births) and very variable in expression. When arising from a known mutation such as in a gene at 6p21, which codes for a protein recently identified and named fibrocystin (Zerres et al. 2003), antenatal diagnosis is a possibility, but not all cases have this mutation. The most severely affected cases have a version of Potter syndrome and die of pulmonary insufficiency. Many cases are now detected antenatally by ultrasonography. Neonatal survivors are destined to develop end-stage renal failure, in infancy, childhood, adolescence or early adult life. Congenital periportal hepatic fibrosis is a consistent associated finding. End-stage renal failure developing in infancy should be managed like other causes, with two provisos. Firstly it may be necessary to remove both kidneys to make PD a practical proposition. Secondly hypertension is a frequent feature of ARPKD. The combination of hypertension and renal salt loss is unusual and can be particularly difficult to manage.

Congenital nephrotic syndrome

The nephrotic syndrome is rare in the neonatal period. Acquired causes include congenital infection due to syphilis, toxoplasmosis, rubella, cytomegalovirus, human immunodeficiency virus and malaria. Congenital nephrotic syndrome of the Finnish type is the least rare cause. This is an autosomal recessive condition due to mutations in a gene, NPHS1, at 19q13.1 that codes for nephrin, a protein that is an essential part of the glomerular ultrafilter, preventing leakage of albumin from the glomerular capillaries into Bowman's space (Mannikko et al. 1995; Khoshnoodi and Tryggvason 2001). The name derives from the fact that the gene frequency is uniquely high in Finns, leading to an incidence of the disease of

1 : 8200 live births. Though much less common, the condition has been described in most ethnic groups. Heavy albuminuria is invariably present from early gestation, as shown by the consistent finding of very high amniotic fluid α-fetoprotein levels before 16–20 weeks' gestation.

Most affected babies are born preterm, typically at about 36 weeks. The placenta is large, the mean ratio of placental to infant weight being 0.43 (average normal 0.18). Clinically evident oedema and abdominal distension are present in 25% of cases at birth and in 90% within the first week. Typical facies include wide sutures and fontanelle, a small nose, wide-set eyes and low-set ears, although these may not be apparent at birth (Huttunen 1976). Without replacement therapy, the serum albumin concentration remains below 10 g/l.

Conservative treatment is difficult and involves frequent infusion of albumin, use of angiotensin-converting enzyme inhibitors and non-steroidal anti-inflammatory drugs aiming to reduce proteinuria by altering glomerular filtration dynamics, and, occasionally, elective unilateral nephrectomy (Coulthard 1989). Growth and nutrition can often be improved, though not restored to normal. The definitive treatment is bilateral nephrectomy and renal transplantation. The interposition of a period of several months on dialysis between nephrectomy and transplantation, to optimise nutrition and growth and to normalise the plasma albumin concentration and secondary metabolic abnormalities such as hyperlipidaemia, may be necessary. Newborns with congenital nephrotic syndrome should be transferred at diagnosis to a regional paediatric nephrology unit with full dialysis and transplant facilities as well as an appropriate level of neonatal care.

Tubulopathies
Bartter syndrome(s)

Bartter syndrome is caused by mutations in one of three membrane transporters in the thick segment of the ascending limb of the loop of Henle. This results in failure of reabsorption of sodium, potassium and chloride (Simon et al. 1996a, b, 1997), consequential increased salt delivery to the distal nephron, and the salt loss, volume depletion, hyperaldosteronism, hypokalaemia and metabolic alkalosis typical of the disease. Polyuria may be of sufficient degree to cause polyhydramnios (Proesmans 1997). Neonatal presentation is with failure to thrive, dehydration and polyuria. The features of Bartter syndrome are mimicked by the loop diuretics, an important point in differential diagnosis. Similar biochemical findings can occur as a result of non-renal electrolyte losses in cystic fibrosis (transcutaneous) and congenital chloride-losing diarrhoea (intestinal). The crucial diagnostic investigation is the urinary chloride concentration, which is high in Bartter syndrome but low (virtually chloride-free urine) if the losses are non-renal. The diagnosis can be confirmed by DNA analysis. Treatment consists of potassium supplementation in all cases, salt supplementation in some and the use of indometacin in a dose of up to 3 mg/kg/day in divided doses. The closely related syndrome of Gitelman is a much milder disease and seldom, if ever, presents in the neonatal period.

Nephrogenic diabetes insipidus

Nephrogenic diabetes insipidus is due to renal resistance to ADH. The commonest inherited variety is X-linked recessive, due to mutations in the tubular ADH receptor (V_2 receptor) (Knoers et al. 1994). A less common form is inherited as an autosomal recessive mutation of the *AQP2* gene (van Lieburg et al. 1994). The two forms are clinically identical and it is important not to exclude the diagnosis merely because the baby is female.

As ADH has a limited role in fetal life and breast milk is relatively low in solute, the clinical features of polyuria, hypernatraemic dehydration and failure to thrive do not usually occur in the immediate neonatal period. However the condition should be considered in any baby with recurrent hypernatraemic dehydration. A formal water deprivation test is unnecessary in the newborn and may be dangerous. If the plasma osmolality is above 300 mOsmol/kg H$_2$O and the sodium above 150 mmol/l, the urine should be maximally concentrated for age (see above). If it is not, and certainly if the urine is hypotonic to plasma, the diagnosis should be provisionally assumed and water supplementation given to maintain normonatraemia.

Renal tubular acidosis

Distal RTA results from impaired hydrogen ion secretion in the distal tubule. The urine pH is high (>5.5) and plasma HCO$_3$ is usually <15 mmol/l. Hypokalaemia, hypercalciuria and decreased citrate excretion are often present. Hypercalciuria is the primary abnormality in some familial cases with calcium-induced tubular damage. Nephrocalcinosis and nephrolithiasis are possible complications. Distal RTA is rare. Familial cases usually present in childhood and are most often autosomal dominant.

Proximal RTA is also rare. It is caused by impaired HCO$_3$ reabsorption in the proximal tubule. It occurs in infants with the renal Fanconi syndrome, of which the commonest cause in British children is cystinosis, but it is relatively unusual for it to be apparent in the neonatal period. The presence of other features of the Fanconi syndrome (glycosuria, generalised aminoaciduria, phosphaturia) should lead to suspicion. Treatment goals involve correction of acidosis and hypokalaemia, avoidance of osteopenia and maintenance of growth velocity.

A generalised RTA occurs in aldosterone deficiency or unresponsiveness of the distal tubule to aldosterone. As aldosterone induces Na resorption in exchange for K and H, there is reduced K excretion, causing hyperkalaemia, and reduced acid excretion. The urine pH is usually appropriate for serum pH and plasma HCO$_3$ is usually >17 mmol/l. This form of RTA may also occur in congenital adrenal hyperplasia, particularly 21-hydroxylase deficiency.

The renal sequelae of preterm birth

Several groups around the world have described higher blood pressure in young adults born preterm (Johansson et al. 2005; Keijzer-Veen et al. 2005). The pathophysiological basis is unclear and may reflect aberrant renal and/or vascular development. A reduction in nephron number is well described in intrauterine growth restriction (Hinchcliffe et al. 1992) and is a plausible consequence of the compromised third-trimester development of the extremely preterm infant. Nephron deficit is postulated to lead to compensatory hyperfiltration, glomerulosclerosis, deteriorating renal function and ultimately hypertension. Preterm cohort studies have not to date shown consistent alterations in renal function but, as these subjects are still in young adulthood, further assessments must be awaited.

References

Al-Dahhan, J., Haycock, G.B., Chantler, C., et al., 1983a. Sodium homeostasis in term and preterm neonates. I. Renal aspects. Arch Dis Child 58, 335–342.

Al-Dahhan, J., Haycock, G.B., Chantler, C., et al., 1983b. Sodium homeostasis in term and preterm neonates. II. Gastrointestinal aspects. Arch Dis Child 58, 343–345.

Aperia, A., Broberger, O., Thodenius, K., et al., 1975. Development of renal control of salt and fluid homeostasis during the first year of life. Acta Paediatr Scand Suppl 64, 393–398.

Aperia, A., Holtback, U., Syren, M.L., et al., 1994. Activation/deactivation of renal Na+,K(+)-ATPase: a final common pathway for regulation of natriuresis. FASEB J 8, 436–439.

Arant, B.S.J., 1973. Developmental patterns of renal functional maturation compared in the human neonate. J Pediatr 92, 705–712.

Assadi, F.K., 1988. Treatment of acute renal failure in an infant by continuous arteriovenous hemodialysis. Pediatr Nephrol 2, 320–322.

Bakr, A.F., 2005. Prophylactic theophylline to prevent renal dysfunction in newborns exposed to perinatal asphyxia – a study in a developing country. Pediatr Nephrol 20, 1249–1252.

Bauer, M., Stewart, S., 1988. Renal failure following cardiac surgery in a 2.8 kg infant managed with continuous arteriovenous hemofiltration. Ann Thorac Surg 45, 225–226.

Bellomo, R., Chapman, M., Finfer, S., et al., 2000. Low-dose dopamine in patients with early renal dysfunction: a placebo-controlled randomised trial. Australian and New Zealand Intensive Care Society (ANZICS) Clinical Trials Group. Lancet 356, 2139–2143.

Benitez, O.A., Benitez, M., Stijnen, T., et al., 1986. Inaccuracy in neonatal measurement of urine concentration with a refractometer. J Pediatr 108, 613–616.

Bhat, M.A., Shah, Z.A., Makhdoomi, M.S., et al., 2006. Theophylline for renal function in term neonates with perinatal asphyxia: a randomized, placebo-controlled trial. J Pediatr 149, 180–184.

Bishof, N.A., Welch, T.R., Strife, F., et al., 1990. Continuous hemodiafiltration in children. Pediatrics 85, 819–823.

Brewer, E.D., 1992. Urinary acidification. In: Polin, R.A., Fox, W.W. (Eds.), Fetal and Neonatal Physiology. W.B. Saunders, Philadelphia.

Brodehl, J., Gellissen, K., 1968. Endogenous renal transport of free amino acids in infancy and childhood. Pediatrics 42, 395–404.

Chevalier, R.L., Campbell, F., Brenbridge, A.N., 1984. Prognostic factors in neonatal acute renal failure. Pediatrics 74, 265–272.

Coulthard, M.G., 1989. Management of Finnish congenital nephrotic syndrome by unilateral nephrectomy. Pediatr Nephrol 3, 451–453.

Coulthard, M.G., Hey, E.N., 1985. Effect of varying water intake on renal function in healthy preterm babies. Arch Dis Child 60, 614–620.

Cumming, A.D., Swainson, C.P., 1995. Disturbances in water, electrolyte and acid–base balance. In: Edwards, C.R.W., Bouchier, I.A.D., Haslett, C., et al. (Eds), Davidson's Principles and Practice of Medicine. Churchill Livingstone, Edinburgh.

Deen, P.M., Knoers, N.V., 1998. Vasopressin type-2 receptor and aquaporin-2 water channel mutants in nephrogenic diabetes insipidus. Am J Med Sci 316, 300–309.

De Luna, M.B., Hallet, W.H., 1967. Urinary protein excretion in healthy infants, children and adults. Proc Am Soc Nephrol 16, 16.

Drukker, A., Goldsmith, D.I., Spitzer, A., et al., 1980. The renin angiotensin system in newborn dogs: developmental patterns and response to acute saline loading. Pediatr Res 14, 304–307.

Edelmann, C.M.J., Boichis, H., Soriano, J.R., et al., 1967. The renal response of children to acute ammonium chloride acidosis. Pediatr Res 1, 452–460.

Ekblad, H., Aperia, A., Larsson, S.H., 1992. Intracellular pH regulation in cultured renal proximal tubule cells in different stages of maturation. Am J Physiol 263, F716–F721.

Ervin, M.G., 1988. Perinatal fluid and electrolyte regulation: role of arginine vasopressin. Semin Perinatol 12, 134–142.

Fick, G.M., Johnson, A.M., Strain, J.D., 1993. Characteristics of very early onset autosomal dominant polycystic kidney disease. J Am Soc Nephrol 3, 1863–1870.

Fukuda, Y., Bertorello, A., Aperia, A., 1991. Ontogeny of the regulation of Na+,K(+)-ATPase activity in the renal proximal tubule cell. Pediatr Res 30, 131–134.

Golberger, E., 1986. A Primer of Water, Electrolyte and Acid–Base Disorders, seventh ed. Lea & Febiger, Philadelphia, p. 55.

Gouyon, J.B., Houchan, N., 1993. Assessment of urine specific gravity by reagent strip test in newborn infants. Pediatr Nephrol 7, 77–78.

Haycock, G.B., Aperia, A., 1991. Salt and the newborn kidney. Pediatr Nephrol 5, 65–70.

Heney, D., Brocklebank, J.T., Wilson, N., 1989. Continuous arteriovenous haemofiltration in the newlyborn with acute renal failure and congenital heart disease. Nephrol Dial Transplant 4, 870–876.

Herin, P., Aperia, A., 1994. Neonatal kidney, fluids, and electrolytes. Curr Opin Pediatr 6, 154–157.

Hinchcliffe, S.A., Lynch, M.R.J., Sargent, P.H., et al., 1992. The effect of intrauterine growth retardation on the development of renal nephrons. Br J Obstet Gynaecol 99, 296–301.

Huttunen, N.P., 1976. Congenital nephrotic syndrome of Finnish type. Study of 75 patients. Arch Dis Child 51, 344–348

Jenik, A.G., Ceriani Cernadas, J.M., Gorenstein, A., et al., 2000. A randomized, double-blind, placebo-controlled trial of the effects of prophylactic theophylline on renal function in term neonates with perinatal asphyxia. Pediatrics 105, E45.

Johansson, S., Iliadou, A., Bergvall, N., et al., 2005. Risk of high blood pressure among young men increases with the degree of immaturity at birth. Circulation 112, 3430–3436.

Jorgensen, P.L., 1986. Structure, function and regulation of Na,K-ATPase in the kidney. Kidney Int 29, 10–20.

Kaplan, B.S., Rabin, I., Nogrady, M.B., et al., 1977. Autosomal dominant polycystic

renal disease in children. J Pediatr 90, 782–783.

Kaskel, F.J., Kumar, A.M., Feld, L.G., et al., 1988. Renal reabsorption of phosphate during development: tubular events. Pediatr Nephrol 2, 129–134.

Keijzer-Veen, M.G., Finken, M.J., Nauta, J., et al., 2005. Is blood pressure increased 19 years after intrauterine growth restriction and preterm birth? A prospective follow-up study in The Netherlands. Pediatrics 116, 725–731.

Khoshnoodi, J., Tryggvason, K., 2001. Congenital nephrotic syndromes. Curr Opin Genet Dev 11, 322–327.

Kinoshita, S., Jose, P.A., Felder, R.A., 1989. Ontogeny of the dopamine 1 receptor in rat renal proximal convoluted tubule. Pediatr Res 25, 68A.

Knoers, N.V., Van Den Ouweland, A.M., Verdijk, M., et al., 1994. Inheritance of mutations in the V2 receptor gene in 13 families with nephrogenic diabetes insipidus. Kidney Int 46, 170–176.

Leake, R.D., Zakauddin, S., Trygstad, C.W., et al., 1976. The effect of large volume intravenous fluid infusion on neonatal renal function. J Pediatr 89, 968–972.

Lieberman, K.V., Nardi, L., Bosch, J.P., 1985. Treatment of acute renal failure in an infant using continuous arteriovenous hemofiltration. J Pediatr 106, 646–649.

Littlewood, J.M., 1971. White cells and bacteria in voided urine of healthy newborns. Arch Dis Child 46, 167–172.

Mannikko, M., Kestaila, M., Holmberg, C., 1995. Fine mapping and haplotype analysis of the locus for congenital nephrotic syndrome on chromosome 19q13.1. Am J Hum Genet 57, 1377–1383.

Mathew, O.P., Jones, A.S., James, E., et al., 1980. Neonatal renal failure: usefulness of diagnostic indices. Pediatrics 65, 57–60.

Mehta, N., Modi, N., 1989. ACE inhibitors in pregnancy. Lancet ii 96.

Michaud, J., Russo, P., Grignon, A., 1994. Autosomal dominant polycystic kidney disease in the fetus. Am J Med Genet 51, 240–246.

Midgley, J., Modi, N., Littleton, P., et al., 1992. Atrial natriuretic peptide, cyclic guanosine monophosphate and sodium excretion during postnatal adaptation in male infants below 34 weeks gestation with severe respiratory distress syndrome. Early Hum Dev 28, 145–154.

Modi, N., 1989. Treatment of renal failure in neonates. Arch Dis Child 64, 630–631.

Modi, N., Coulthard, M., 1999. Renal function. In: Levitt, G., Harvey, D., Cooke, R.W.I. (Eds.), Practical Perinatal Care – the Baby Under 1000 g. Butterworth Heinemann, Oxford.

Modi, N., Hutton, J.L., 1990. Urinary creatinine excretion and estimation of muscle mass in infants of 25–34 weeks

gestation. Acta Paediatr Scand 79, 1156–1162.

Orlowski, J., Lingrel, J.B., 1988. Tissue-specific and developmental regulation of rat Na,K-ATPase catalytic alpha isoform and beta subunit mRNAs. J Biol Chem 263, 10436–10442.

Proesmans, W., 1997. Bartter syndrome and its neonatal variant. European J Pediatr 156, 669–679.

Rigden, S.P., Start, K.M., Rees, L., 1987. Nutritional management of infants and toddlers with chronic renal failure. Nutrition Health 5, 163–174.

Rudd, P.T., Hughes, E.A., Placzek, M.M., et al., 1983. Reference ranges for plasma creatinine during the first month of life. Arch Dis Child 58, 212–215.

Sadowski, R.H., Harmon, W.E., Jabs, K., 1994. Acute hemodialysis of infants weighing less than five kilograms. Kidney Int 45, 903–906.

Seri, I., Rudas, G., Bors, Z., et al., 1993. Effects of low-dose dopamine infusion on cardiovascular and renal functions, cerebral blood flow, and plasma catecholamine levels in sick preterm neonates. Pediatr Res 34, 742–749.

Simon, D.B., Karet, F.E., Hamdan, J.M., et al., 1996a. Bartter's syndrome, hypokalemic alkalosis with hypercalciuria, is caused by mutations in the Na-K-2Cl transporter $NKCC_2$. Nature Genet 13, 183–188.

Simon, D.B., Karet, F.E., Rodriguez-Soriano, J., 1996b. Genetic heterogeneity of Bartter's syndrome revealed by mutations in the K^+ channel, ROMK. Nature Genet 14, 152–156.

Simon, D.B., Bindra, R.S., Mansfield, T.A., 1997. Mutations in the chloride channel gene, CLCNKB, cause Bartter's syndrome type III. Nature Genet 17, 171–178.

Spitzer, A., 1982. The role of the kidney in sodium homeostasis during maturation. Kidney Int 21, 539–545.

Sposi, N.M., Bottero, L., Cossu, G., et al., 1989. Expression of protein kinase C genes during ontogenic development of the central nervous system. Mol Cell Biol 9, 2284–2288.

Stapleton, F.B., Jones, D.P., Green, R.S., 1987. Acute renal failure in neonates: incidence, etiology and outcome. Pediatr Nephrol 1, 314–320.

Sulyok, E., Nemeth, M., Tenyi, I., et al., 1979a. Postnatal development of rennin–angiotensin–aldosterone system, RAAS, in relation to electrolyte balance in premature infants. Pediatr Res 13, 817–820.

Sulyok, E., Varga, F., Gyory, E., et al., 1979b. Postnatal development of renal sodium handling in premature infants. J Pediatr 95, 787–792.

Trompeter, R.S., Al-Dahhan, J., Haycock, G.B., et al., 1983. Normal values for plasma creatinine concentration related to maturity in normal term and preterm infants. Int J Pediatr Nephrol 4, 145–148.

Van Lieburg, A.F., Verdijk, M.A., Knoers, V.V., 1994. Patients with autosomal nephrogenic diabetes insipidus homozygous for mutations in the aquaporin 2 water-channel gene. Am J Hum Genet 55, 648–652.

Yasui, M., Marples, D., Belusa, R., et al., 1996. Development of urinary concentrating capacity: role of aquaporin-2. Am J Physiol 271, F461–F468.

Zerres, K., Rudnik-Schoneborn, S., Senderek, J., et al., 2003. Autosomal recessive polycystic kidney disease (ARPKD). J Nephrol 16, 453–458.

Ziegler, E.E., Ryu, J.E., 1976. Renal solute load and diet in growing premature infants. J Pediatr 89, 609–611.

Part 2: **Urology**

Naima Smeulders   Duncan T Wilcox

Urinary tract anomalies

Urinary tract abnormalities are increasingly detected by antenatal ultrasound, with 1:800 pregnancies having an antenatally diagnosed uropathy (Smith et al. 1987; Scott and Renwick 1988; Arthur et al. 1989). Those not detected prenatally may present symptomatically during childhood, often with a urinary tract infection (UTI). Antenatally diagnosed dilatation of the urinary tract can result from either impairment of urine flow or retrograde reflux of urine. Urine flow impairment can occur at any level in the urinary tract, and may affect one or both sides. Dilatation of the renal pelvis and calyces is the first anatomical response to impairment of urine flow and may lead to histological damage of the renal parenchyma and changes in renal function. Histological damage is related to the degree and level of urine flow impairment and its duration. Renal atrophy, as seen in patients with multicystic dysplastic kidney, is the ultimate response to impairment of urine flow related to the onset of apoptosis (Gobe and Axelsen 1987). When urine flow impairment is present early in pregnancy, the renal parenchyma develops dysplasia (Glick et al. 1983), and in severe cases there is a reduction of the ipsilateral glomerular filtration rate (GFR) and an increase in the contralateral GFR. Where outflow of urine from both kidneys is significantly impaired, this will result in fetal oliguria or anuria. While fetal urine is not a major contributor to amniotic fluid volume in the first trimester, oliguria or anuria thereafter leads to oligo- or anhydramnios (Mure and Mouriquand 2008). When urine flow impairment becomes significant later in gestation or is partial, it generates dilatation of the excretory system (Beck 1971; Harrison et al. 1982) without affecting the parenchymal structure.

Evaluation of a neonate with antenatally detected uropathy

When an antenatal uropathy is discovered, it is imperative to confirm the diagnosis postnatally. Knowledge of the prenatal evaluations during the progression of pregnancy forms the starting point of the assessment of the newborn (Becker 2009). The degree of unilateral or bilateral 'hydronephrosis' (pyelectasis) (defined as fetal renal pelvic diameter ≥5 mm in the second trimester and ≥7 mm in the third trimester), ureteric dilatation, renal size and parenchymal appearance, visualisation and size of the fetal bladder as well as the amniotic fluid volume in relation to gestational age are the key facts to obtain from antenatal ultrasound (Mure and Mouriquand 2008).

A thorough physical examination of the neonate is required. This may reveal a palpable abdominal mass in neonates with a pelviureteric junction (PUJ) anomaly, multicystic dysplastic kidney,

autosomal recessive polycystic kidney disease and in congenital bladder outflow obstruction, such as posterior urethral valves (PUVs) and urethral atresia (Becker 2009). Urinary tract abnormalities can occur secondary to other congenital anomalies, for example neural tube defects, and feature in many chromosomal anomalies and syndromes (Desphande and Hennekam 2008). For instance, deficient abdominal wall musculature with bilateral cryptorchism raises the possibility of prune-belly syndrome, whereas anorectal or oesophageal atresia may point to the VACTERL association (vertebral anomalies, anal atresia, cardiovascular anomalies, tracheo-oesophageal fistula, oesophageal atresia, renal and/or radial anomalies, limb defects). Secondary effects of oligohydramnios – due to oliguria or anuria in the second half of pregnancy – may be present, culminating in the Potter sequence or talipes (Ch. 37) (Becker 2009). Whilst the appearance of the open bladder in the anterior abdominal wall in vesical exstrophy is striking, other uropathies may have no obvious manifestations on physical examination. A postnatal ultrasound is therefore necessary.

Postnatal ultrasound should be done after day 2 or 3 of life (Dhillon 1995) because ultrasonography earlier than this can lead to a false-negative result (Aksu et al. 2005), owing to the relative oliguria of the newborn period (De Bruyn and Marks 2008). If no abnormality is detected, a repeat ultrasound scan is advisable at 6 weeks of age (Lee et al. 2006; Becker 2009). The ultrasound evaluation must comprise images of the bladder including the bladder wall thickness and the presence of dilated distal ureters or ureteroceles, prone views of the kidneys for accurate measurement of the renal length and the renal pelvic diameter in the anterior–posterior plane, as well as an assessment of calyceal dilation and the renal parenchyma (De Bruyn and Marks 2008). Figure 35.7A summarises the initial steps in the investigation of the neonate with antenatal hydronephrosis.

Neonates who have potentially life-threatening urinary tract anomalies require urgent investigation before discharge. An early postnatal ultrasound is essential for all fetuses with an abnormal bladder, a history of oligo- or anhydramnios, bilateral hydronephrosis >20 mm or hydronephrosis >20 mm in a solitary kidney, and bilateral echogenic kidneys (Fig. 35.7A). Many of these neonates require referral to a paediatric urologist. Early ultrasound, ideally between day 3 and 7 of life, is also recommended where details of the prenatal history are incomplete or a reliable late third-trimester scan is missing. Ultrasound assessment of the neonate with antenatal unilateral or bilateral hydronephrosis >15 mm, with or without ureteric dilatation, duplex kidneys with a ureterocele or a large multicystic dysplastic kidney is advised in the first 7–10 days of life. These babies require antibiotic prophylaxis.

For the remainder (antenatal hydronephrosis >7 mm in the second trimester and/or >10 mm in the third trimester, but less

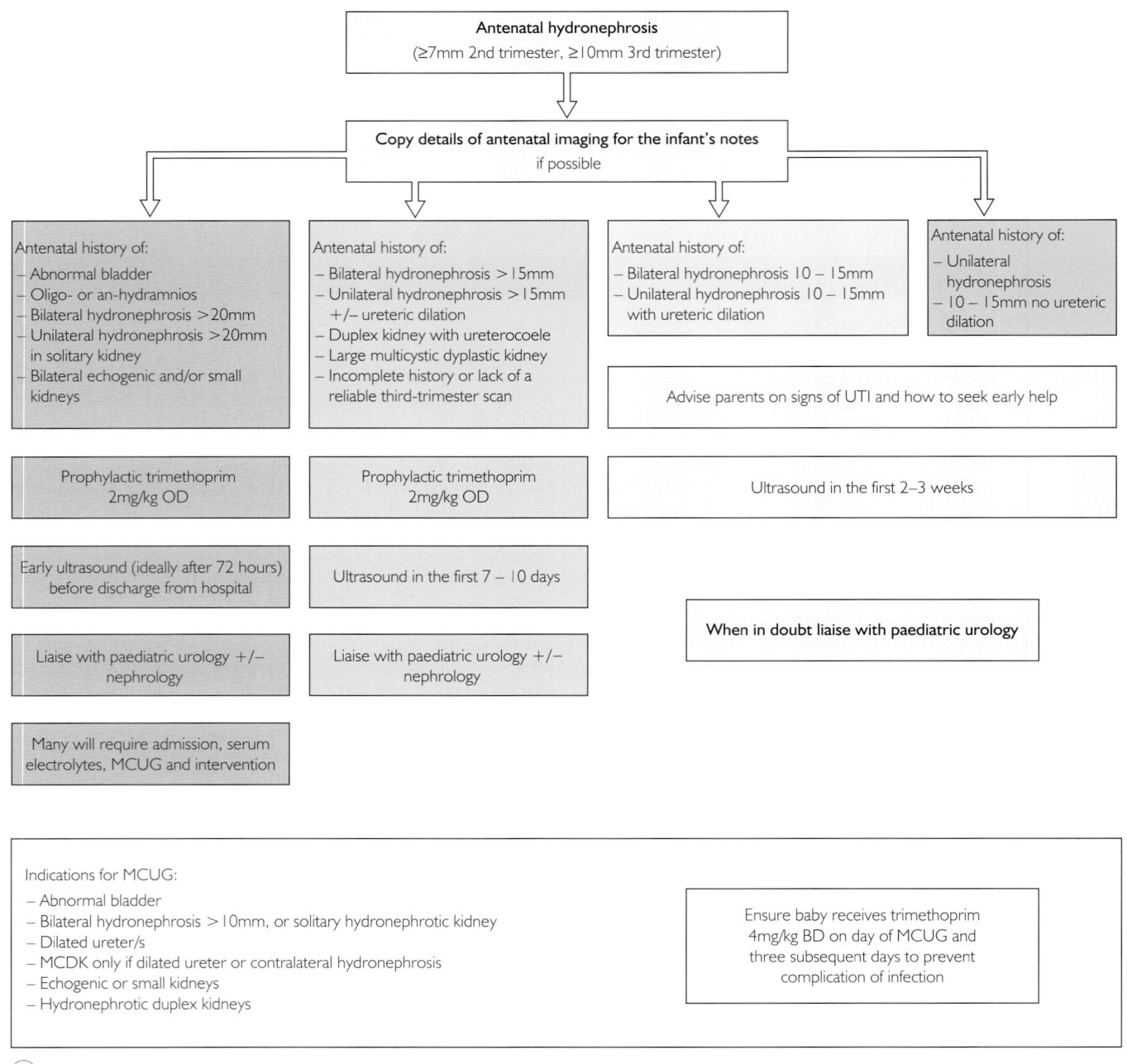

Antenatal hydronephrosis
(≥7mm 2nd trimester, ≥10mm 3rd trimester)

Copy details of antenatal imaging for the infant's notes
if possible

Antenatal history of:
– Abnormal bladder
– Oligo- or an-hydramnios
– Bilateral hydronephrosis >20mm
– Unilateral hydronephrosis >20mm in solitary kidney
– Bilateral echogenic and/or small kidneys

Antenatal history of:
– Bilateral hydronephrosis >15mm
– Unilateral hydronephrosis >15mm +/− ureteric dilation
– Duplex kidney with ureterocoele
– Large multicystic dyplastic kidney
– Incomplete history or lack of a reliable third-trimester scan

Antenatal history of:
– Bilateral hydronephrosis 10 – 15mm
– Unilateral hydronephrosis 10 – 15mm with ureteric dilation

Antenatal history of:
– Unilateral hydronephrosis
– 10 – 15mm no ureteric dilation

Advise parents on signs of UTI and how to seek early help

Prophylactic trimethoprim 2mg/kg OD

Prophylactic trimethoprim 2mg/kg OD

Ultrasound in the first 2–3 weeks

Early ultrasound (ideally after 72 hours) before discharge from hospital

Ultrasound in the first 7 – 10 days

Liaise with paediatric urology +/− nephrology

Liaise with paediatric urology +/− nephrology

When in doubt liaise with paediatric urology

Many will require admission, serum electrolytes, MCUG and intervention

Indications for MCUG:
– Abnormal bladder
– Bilateral hydronephrosis >10mm, or solitary hydronephrotic kidney
– Dilated ureter/s
– MCDK only if dilated ureter or contralateral hydronephrosis
– Echogenic or small kidneys
– Hydronephrotic duplex kidneys

Ensure baby receives trimethoprim 4mg/kg BD on day of MCUG and three subsequent days to prevent complication of infection

(A)

Fig. 35.7 (A) Flow chart detailing the initial steps in the investigation of the neonate with antenatally diagnosed hydronephrosis. UTI, urinary tract infection; MCUG, micturating cystourethrogram; MCDK, multicystic dysplastic kidney.

than 15 mm) an ultrasound can be performed in the first 2–3 weeks of life, and antibiotic prophylaxis is no longer recommended (see below and Fig. 35.7A). Parents should be given information about the signs of UTI and advised to seek help early if their baby develops such signs.

If the postnatal ultrasound scan shows unilateral renal pelvic dilatation, no further investigations need to be done until 4–6 weeks of age. Isotope renography (p. 943) can then be performed at 4–12 weeks, when the kidneys have matured sufficiently for this to be reliable. As a guide, we advocate a MAG3 study at 4 weeks for hydronephrosis >30 mm, at 4–6 weeks for hydronephrosis >20 mm

and at 3 months for hydronephrosis of 15–20 mm and 10–15 mm with calyceal dilatation. Bilateral dilatation requires an early micturating cystourethrogram (MCUG) to exclude bladder outlet obstruction.

The role of the MCUG in neonates with unilateral dilatation is less well established, and there is still controversy (Lee et al. 2006). Initially it was felt that all babies with pelvic dilatation of any degree required a MCUG in order to exclude reflux, which is present in approximately 15–20% (Tibballs and De Bruyn 1996). More recent studies have questioned the clinical significance of this reflux. We, like many other centres (Yerkes et al. 1997), advocate performing

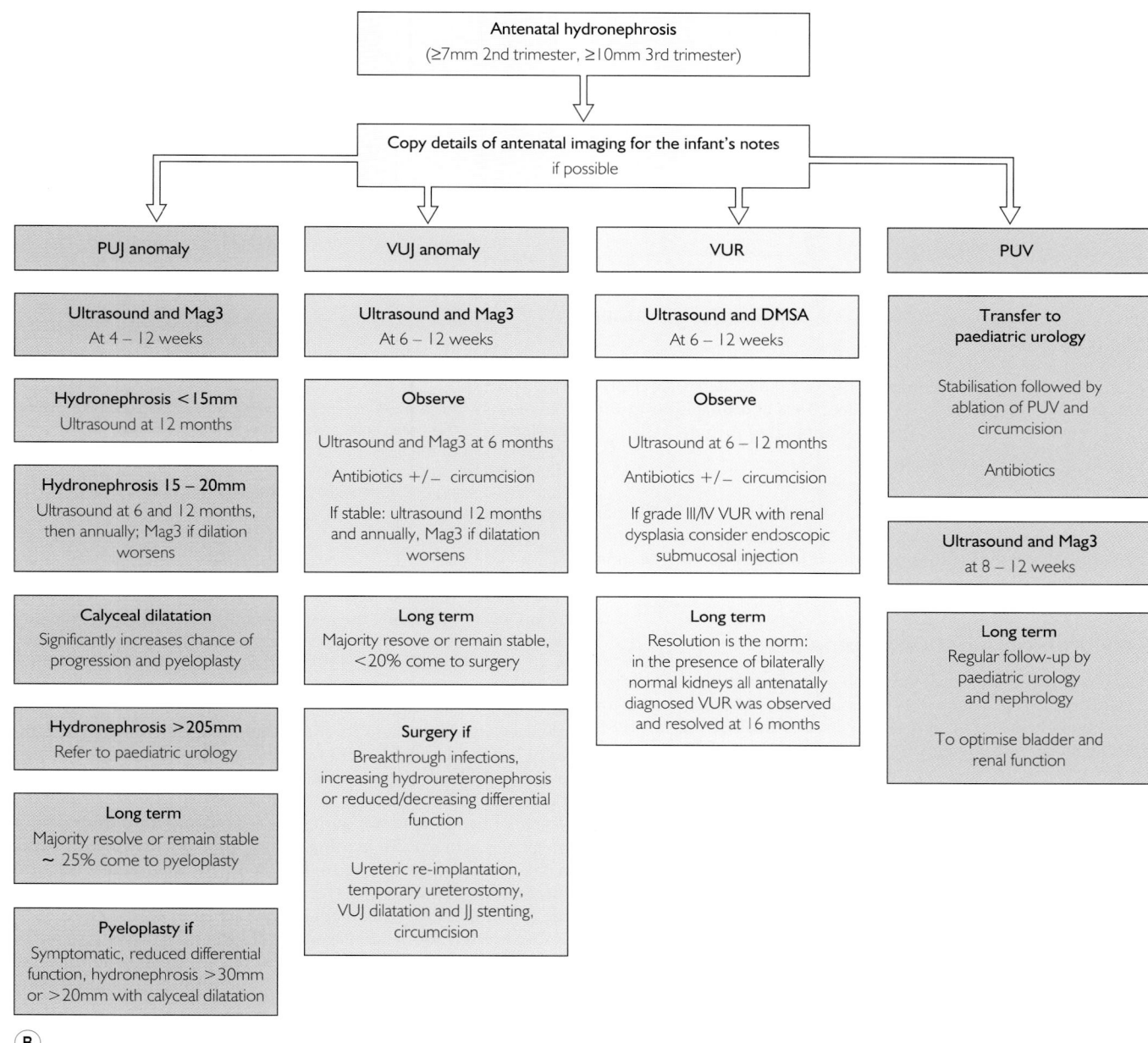

Fig. 35.7 (B) Flow chart detailing the subsequent postnatal investigation pathways of a child born with antenatally diagnosed dilatation. PUJ, pyeloureteric junction; VUJ, vesicoureteric junction; VUR, vesicoureteric reflux; PUV, posterior urethral valve; DMSA, dimercaptosuccinic acid; Mag 3, mercaptotriglycylglycine dynamic renography.

MCUG only in patients with bilateral or unilateral hydronephrosis >10 mm in a solitary kidney, with a dilated ureter or where there is a suspicion of an abnormal bladder. An MCUG is not necessary when there is unilateral hydronephrosis and a normal contralateral kidney. Others, however, still recommend that an MCUG is done in all cases where significant hydronephrosis persists postnatally (Becker 2009; Estrada et al. 2009). Babies should receive treatment dose antibiotics (trimethoprim 4 mg/kg BD) on the day of the MCUG and on the subsequent 3 days, to prevent the complication of infection.

The use of prophylactic antibiotics is also debated (Lee et al. 2006; Song et al. 2007; Roth et al. 2009). While some units advocate their use in all neonates undergoing investigation for antenatal hydronephrosis (Song et al. 2007; Estrada et al. 2009), others advise that instead of routine prophylaxis families should be educated on the signs and symptoms of UTI to enable prompt diagnosis and treatment if infection occurs (Becker 2009). We advocate prophylactic trimethoprim at 2 mg/kg nocte initially for all neonates who fulfil the criteria for MCUG, and subsequently for those who are found to have vesicoureteric reflux (VUR), in the absence of VUR

Box 35.1 Common causes of antenatally diagnosed uropathy

Pelviureteric junction anomaly
Vesicoureteric reflux
Vesicoureteric junction anomaly
Multicystic dysplastic kidney
Duplex kidney
Posterior urethral valves

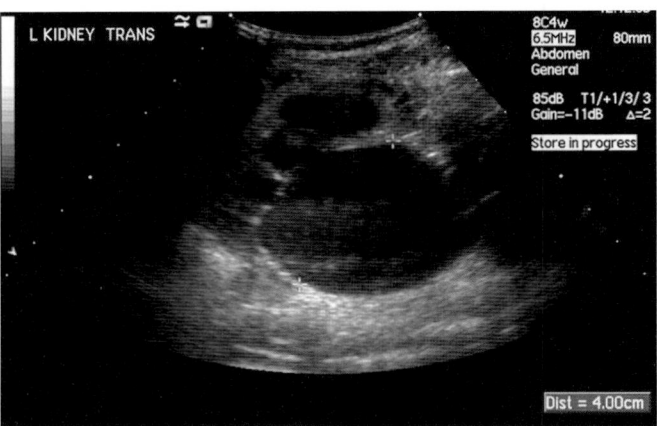

Fig. 35.8 Ultrasound scan showing a pyeloureteric junction anomaly. The markers indicate the anterior–posterior (AP) diameter of the dilated renal pelvis in the transverse plane at the level of the renal hilum. Measurement of the renal pelvic diameter at this point allows standardisation and comparison of the severity of hydronephrosis. Note the layering of debris within the renal pelvis as well as the calyceal dilatation.

but presence of ureteric dilatation >10 mm, and for those with hydronephrosis >20 mm.

Following the initial newborn and 6–12-week investigations, a diagnosis can be made in the majority of infants. Renal parenchymal anomalies occur in approximately 13% and dilatation in the remainder (Thomas 1998). The renal anomalies include:

- multicystic dysplastic kidney
- unilateral and bilateral renal agenesis.

The common causes of dilatation are listed in Box 35.1 (Thomas 1998). The routine postnatal management of these patients with dilatation due to these causes is outlined in Figure 35.7B. The individual diagnoses are discussed below.

Pelviureteric junction anomalies

PUJ anomalies are the most common antenatally diagnosed uropathy (Turnock and Shawis 1984; Thomas et al. 1995), accounting for approximately half of all antenatal hydronephrosis (Dhillon 1998). The diagnosis of unilateral or bilateral PUJ anomaly can be suspected antenatally when an ultrasound scan of the fetus shows a dilated renal pelvis without ureteric dilatation. The likelihood of significant postnatal pathology correlates to the severity of antenatal hydronephrosis (Lee et al. 2006).

Although many PUJ anomalies are diagnosed prenatally, some may present as problems in infancy and childhood. Abdominal mass was one of the principal symptoms of PUJ anomaly in babies before the ultrasound era (Flashner and Lower 1992). Loin or renal-angle pain reflects intermittent distension of the renal pelvis. Haematuria, hypertension and UTIs are rare problems of PUJ anomalies.

Associated urological anomalies include ureteric hypoplasia (Allen and Husmann 1989), VUR (Hollowell et al. 1989; Paltiel Lebowitz 1989), partial or complete ureteric duplication (Mesrobian 1986; Joseph et al. 1989) and horseshoe kidney. PUJ anomalies also can be associated with anorectal anomalies, congenital heart disease and VATER syndrome (Ch. 31) (Flashner et al. 1993).

Congenital PUJ anomalies are typically characterised histologically by abnormal fibromuscular and neural arrangements at the PUJ (Kajbafzadeh et al. 2006), interfering with the normal peristalsis of urine at this point. Alternatively or additionally, extrinsic compression of the PUJ, which may be intermittent, can result from, for instance, aberrant vessels crossing to the lower pole of the kidney (Mure and Mouriquand 2008). Intraluminal obstruction is rare.

With the introduction of antenatal ultrasound to routine obstetric care in the 1980s, many more children with isolated hydronephrosis were detected than had previously come to surgery for a symptomatic PUJ anomaly (Mallik and Watson 2008). Since then, numerous clinical studies have sought to elucidate the natural history of antenatally diagnosed upper tract dilatation (Ransley

et al. 1990; Madden et al. 1991; Blyth et al. 1993; Koff and Campbell 1994). While the majority of patients improve spontaneously, some proceed to progressive loss of renal function (Ransley et al. 1990; Madden et al. 1991; Koff and Campbell 1994; Dhillon 1998). The management of PUJ anomaly is thus a balance between preventing renal deterioration on the one hand, and avoiding unnecessary surgery and its complications on the other. The difficulty lies in identifying who benefits from an operation. This can only be decided after a period of regular assessment (Koff and Campbell 1994; Ulman et al. 2000; Onen et al. 2002), with the degree of hydronephrosis during the second and third trimesters of pregnancy acting as the starting point. Approximately 25% of antenatal hydronephrosis due to PUJ anomaly will require surgical intervention (Dhillon 1998), usually within the first few years of life (Dhillon 1998; Ulman et al. 2000; Onen et al. 2002).

Close observational management of PUJ anomalies is justified in most patients during the first year(s) of life. Three conditions are required before it can be considered appropriate to follow a baby with unilateral PUJ anomaly conservatively:

- The baby must be asymptomatic.
- The degree of pelvic dilatation, measured with repeated ultrasound, should be stable or decreasing.
- The relative function of the affected kidney (measured with radioisotope studies) should be either stable or improving.

This conservative approach, initially proposed by Ransley et al. (1990), is now adopted by many centres and requires 3-monthly ultrasound scans during the first year of life. The anterior–posterior diameter of the renal pelvis in the transverse plane should be measured with ultrasound, as this is a good predictor of significant UTI (Fig. 35.8) (Dhillon 2002). In addition, nuclear renography should be performed at 6–12 weeks and again at 1 year (Fig. 35.9). Many centres recommend prophylactic antibiotic cover (Song et al. 2007), although no studies have to date proved that it prevents UTI.

Surgical treatment of a PUJ anomaly is advocated by most urologists when the following conditions exist:

- a symptomatic PUJ anomaly
- declining function in the dilated kidney (Onen et al. 2002; Koff and Campbell 1994; Dhillon 1998; Ulman et al. 2000)

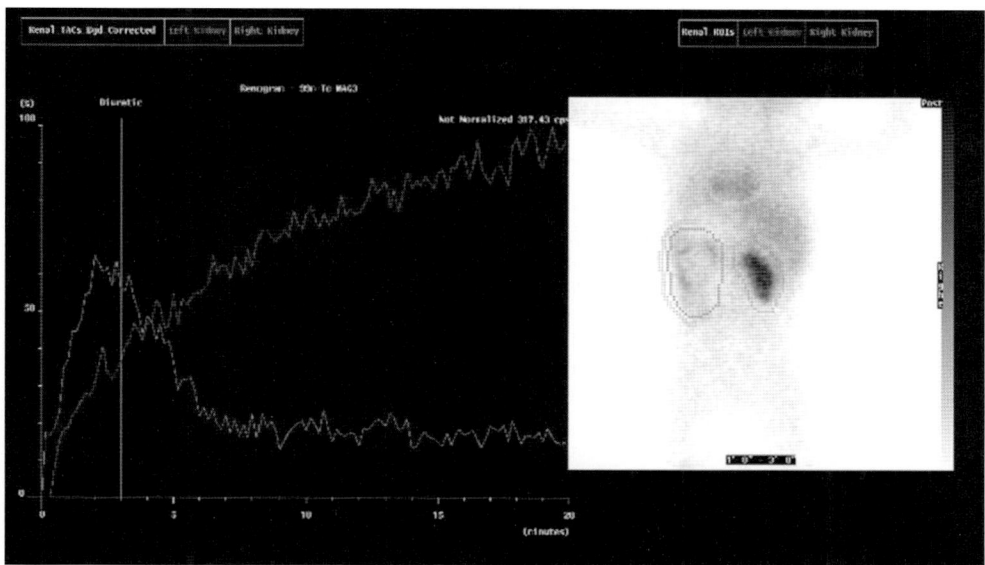

Fig. 35.9 MAG3 renogram showing a left unilateral pyeloureteric junction anomaly. Tc99m-labelled MAG3 followed by furosemide is injected. The uptake image (left-hand image) demonstrates a left kidney stretched around a grossly dilated collecting system. The right kidney (green line) handles the tracer normally. The left kidney (red line) shows delayed transit of the tracer through the parenchyma into the renal pelvis with poor drainage from the renal pelvis even after a change in posture and micturition (image not shown). The right kidney contributes 66% and the left 34% to overall renal function.

- an increasing pelvic dilatation (Onen et al. 2002; Koff and Campbell 1994; Dhillon 1998; Ulman et al. 2000)
- moderate pelvic dilatation (>20 mm) with dilatation of the calyces
- bilateral moderate to severe dilatation of the pelvis (Dhillon 1998).

These indications are not accepted by all: some operate on all infants during the first year of life, arguing that the outcome of pyeloplasty is usually excellent in terms of drainage and preserved renal function (Hanna 1991). Conversely, others will follow a conservative approach even with severe pelvic dilatation (Onen et al. 2002; Koff and Campbell 1994; Ulman et al. 2000). When surgery is performed, the most common operation is a pyeloplasty.

Temporary diversion of the pelvic urine via a percutaneous nephrostomy for 3–4 weeks may be considered to assess whether renal function may be partially recovered in a poorly functioning, severely dilated kidney (Ransley et al. 1990). However, kidneys with very poor relative function (<10%) fail to recover (Ransley et al. 1990). Nephrectomy is therefore recommended for infants with severe pelvic dilatation and very poor relative function (<10%) in the presence of a normal contralateral kidney (Dhillon 1998).

Vesicoureteric junction anomaly (megaureter)

Many classifications of megaureter have been reported (Kass 1992) but practically there are only two: megaureter with or without reflux. However, distal anatomical obstruction of the ureter and VUR may occur together. Investigations include ultrasound scan of the urinary tract (Fig. 35.10) and an MCUG. Functional studies (diuresis renography) are useful to assess the differential function. Coexisting anomalies occur in 16% and include PUJ anomaly, multicystic dysplastic kidney, pelvic kidney and renal agenesis (Rickwood et al. 1992). It is sometimes difficult to distinguish a PUJ from a vesicoureteric junction (VUJ) anomaly, and a contrast antegrade pyelogram may be the only way to differentiate the two conditions.

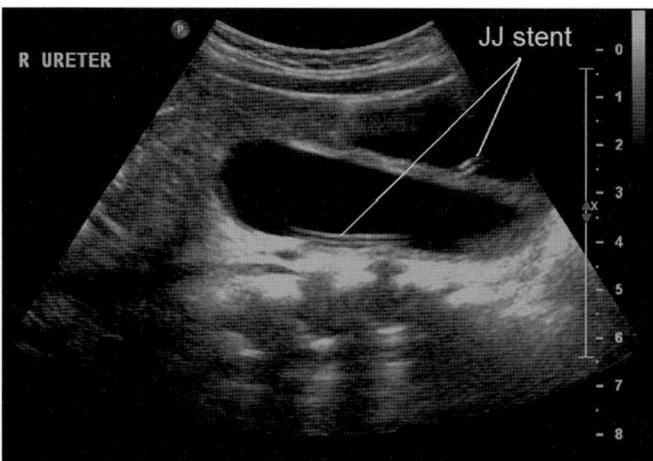

Fig. 35.10 Ultrasound scan showing an obstructed megaureter which has been stented. The 'tramline' of the JJ stent can be seen in both the bladder and the distal right ureter behind.

Spontaneous improvement of ureteric dilatation is a frequent event in megaureters related to a faulty VUJ (McLellan et al. 2002). Conservative management of megaureters is recommended when renal function and dilatation of the upper tract remain stable (or improve), and when the child remains asymptomatic (Rickwood et al. 1992; Shukla et al. 2005). Antibiotic prophylaxis is recommended (Song et al. 2007), especially in refluxing megaureters. Some also advise circumcision to reduce the risk of infection (Mure and Mouriquand 2008). Regular isotope assessments are required to follow these children.

When the conservative approach fails, i.e. when infections recur in spite of adequate antibiotic prophylactic cover, or when renal function decreases on repeated isotope studies or when dilatation of the urinary tract increases, ureteric reimplantation is usually recommended, except where renal function is poor (<10%), when nephroureterectomy is indicated. The aim of the operation is to excise the distal obstructive segment of the ureter and reimplant the ureter with an antireflux mechanism. The temporary placement of a double-J stent across the VUJ may be of value in infants to avoid extensive dissection in a small bladder (Castagnetti et al. 2006; Farrugia et al. 2009). Stent-related complications are common. However, in a significant proportion, primarily in those with preserved renal function, good drainage was observed after a period of double-J stenting, thereby eluding ureteric reimplantation (Castagnetti et al. 2006; Farrugia et al. 2009).

Ureteroceles

Ureteroceles are a cystic dilatation of the distal portion of the ureter. They occur in approximately 1:500 people (Uson et al. 1961). Ureteroceles occur more frequently in girls and in the Caucasian population (Whitten and Wilcox 2001). In children they are almost always associated with the upper moiety of a duplex kidney, although rarely they can occur in a simplex system (Whitten and Wilcox 2001). Ureteroceles have been classified in many ways, but a simple classification is to divide them into those arising from a single or duplex kidney, and then further into intravesical and extravesical types.

Postnatally these babies need to be placed on prophylactic antibiotics and investigated with an ultrasound scan (Fig. 35.11); in addition, functional studies are required to assess the relative function in the upper and lower poles of a duplex kidney. As reflux occurs in approximately 30% into the lower moiety and 20% into the contralateral kidney, many centres recommend an MCUG (Castagnetti et al. 2004). Bladder outflow obstruction can result from prolapse of a ureterocele into the urethra. Dysplasia and obstructive nephropathy are commonly seen in the renal moiety drained by the ureterocele.

There is considerable controversy over the management of ureteroceles, which varies from simple endoscopic puncture of the ureterocele to upper-pole heminephrectomy and bladder reconstruction (Mure and Mouriquand 2008). Increasingly a more conservative approach is being adopted. In patients who present in the neonatal period, the appropriate first procedure is endoscopic puncture: this was the only procedure required in 73% of babies, and resulted in drainage and preservation of the upper pole in over 90% (Blyth

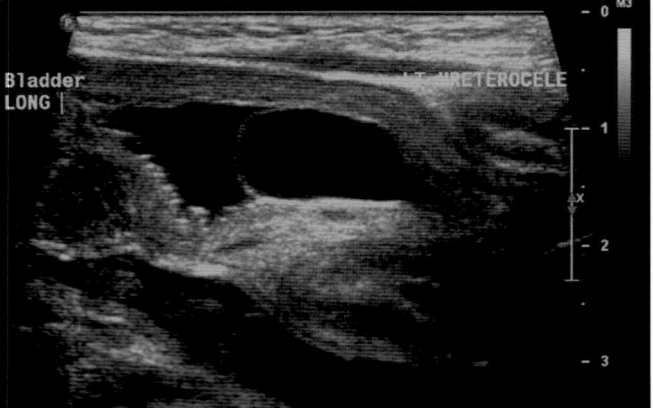

Fig. 35.11 Ultrasound scan of a thick-walled bladder with a left-sided ureterocele (thin-walled cystic structure) prolapsing into the urethra, causing bladder outflow obstruction.

et al. 1993). In this and other studies, ureteric reflux was created in 20–40% of patients, and further surgery, including upper-pole heminephrectomy plus or minus bladder reconstruction, was required in 20–80% (Blyth et al. 1993; Di Benedetto et al. 1995).

Posterior urethral valves

A PUV is a congenital membrane obstructing or partially obstructing the posterior urethra. It is the most common cause of lower urinary obstruction in males, but has extremely rarely been described in females (Bakker 1958). The incidence is between 1:4000 and 1:25000 (Atwell 1983; Kaplan and Scherz 1992).

PUV should be suspected in a fetus with a thick-walled bladder and bilateral dilatation of the upper urinary tract, whether or not associated with renal dysplasia and oligohydramnios. Oligohydramnios is usually noticed during the second part of pregnancy, when most of the amniotic fluid is fetal urine. Despite modern ultrasonic equipment, only 16–55% of patients with PUV are detected before 24 weeks' gestation (Dinneen et al. 1993).

In the newborn, there can be symptoms of severe metabolic disorders related to renal failure, respiratory problems (spontaneous pneumothorax or pneumomediastinum) and UTI (Sheldon 1995). Palpation of the kidney(s) and the bladder is usually easy. In infants and young children, urinary symptoms are more common (dysuria, haematuria, UTI, septicaemia), sometimes accompanied by rectal prolapse. Renal failure may be present. In the older child, urinary incontinence, urgency and dysuria are also sometimes seen. The quality of the urinary stream is misleading: voiding pressures in boys with PUV are as high as in normal male infants (Taskinen et al. 2009).

Ultrasound scan of the urinary tract is the first-line investigation. This shows the dilatation of the upper urinary tract, and, sometimes, abnormal echogenicity of the renal parenchyma is seen. There is usually a thick bladder wall and a dilated posterior urethra. MCUG is still the gold-standard investigation to detect PUV (Fig. 35.12), although compared with cystourethroscopy its sensitivity is only 80–90% (De Kort et al. 2004; Schober et al. 2004; De Jong et al. 2008). As the insertion of a transurethral catheter can damage the anatomy of the valve, some paediatric urologists prefer to perform the MCUG via a suprapubic catheter. Others have found the presence of a urethral catheter even during the voiding phase of the test not to hinder the detection of PUV fluoroscopically (Ditchfield et al. 1994). Serum creatinine, followed by a formal assessment of the GFR in due course, and isotope studies are essential to assess the renal consequences of PUV (Groshar et al. 1988; van der Vis-Melsen et al. 1989).

Antenatal treatment is rarely indicated but may be justified when the liquor volume is reducing in a fetus with bilateral dilatation of the upper urinary tract (Hendron et al. 2000). Insertion of a double-J stent between the fetal bladder (or the dilated kidneys) and the amniotic cavity, under ultrasound guidance, allows decompression of the urinary tract, possible preservation of development of the fetal kidney and maturation of the fetal lungs by restoration of an adequate volume of amniotic fluid. These antenatal diversions are usually done quite late in pregnancy and the benefit of such interventions in children with PUV has not been demonstrated (Hendron et al. 2000). A multicentre trial across the UK and Europe (Pluto Collaborative Study Group 2007) is currently studying the outcome of vesicoamniotic shunting in a randomised controlled manner.

After birth, three main principles of treatment are to resuscitate the child, adequately drain the bladder and destroy the valves. Resuscitation implies hydration, electrolyte replacement and antibiotics. Urine drainage can usually be achieved by inserting either

Staff Library
Singleton Hospital
Tel: 01792 285678 Ext. 5281

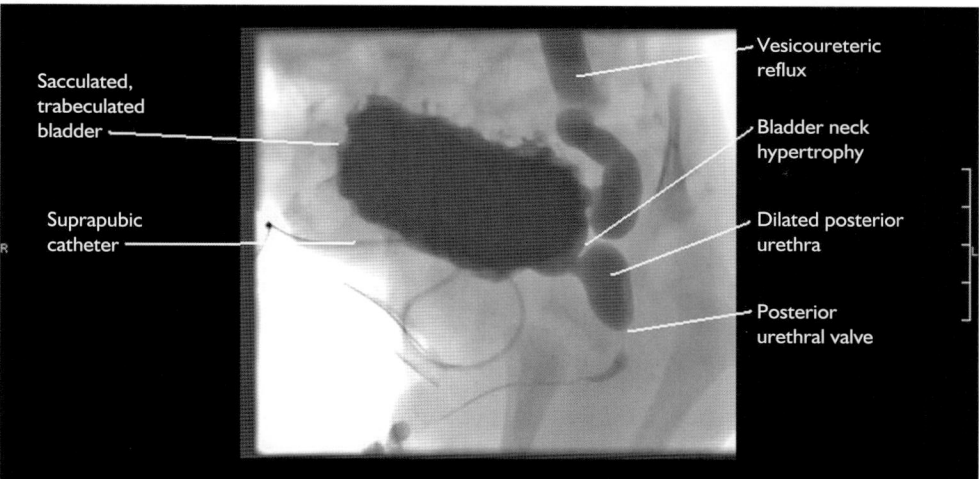

Fig. 35.12 Micturating cystogram showing a posterior urethral valve. The bladder was filled with contrast via the suprapubic catheter. Note the irregular outline of the trabeculated and sacculated bladder and the vesicoureteric reflux into a dilated ureter. The hypertrophied bladder neck produces an indentation between the bladder and the dilated posterior urethra below. The posterior urethral valve is situated at the inferior aspect of the dilated posterior urethra. Contrast flows through the valve so slowly that it fails to fill the distal urethra beyond it.

a transurethral or a suprapubic catheter. Occasionally, a surgical vesicostomy is required to drain the bladder. If the baby is severely ill and infected, drainage of the upper tract may be the best option (ureterostomy or percutaneous nephrostomy). Destruction of the valve is performed when resuscitation is achieved, usually within a week of birth. Surgical incision of the valve is performed endoscopically.

Renal failure is a common complication of PUV and is seen in 40–50% of cases at the time of diagnosis. The type of primary surgical treatment does not seem to influence the progression of renal failure, which occurs in almost 50% of children with PUV (Reinberg et al. 1992). Four factors have been identified as being associated with poor long-term outcome: presentation before the age of 1 year, bilateral VUR, proteinuria, and daytime incontinence at the age of 5 years (Parkhouse et al. 1988). Until recently, antenatal diagnosis appeared to carry a worse prognosis (Reinberg et al. 1992). However, a long-term outcome study from Leeds observed better renal function in the second decade of life for antenatally detected PUV than for those presenting clinically later in life (Kousidis et al. 2008). While mortality or end-stage renal failure in the first decade of life seems predetermined by renal dysplasia and the severity of in utero obstruction, retention of renal function thereafter appears improved by early diagnosis and nephrourological care.

Incontinence is reported to occur in between 14% and 38% (Johnson and Kulatilake 1971; Cass and Stephens 1974) of boys after treatment of PUV. The association of poor renal outcome with urinary incontinence suggests that continuing bladder dysfunction plays a major role in secondary renal damage in these boys with PUV. Indeed, today the need for careful management of the bladder in boys with PUV is well recognised (Desai 2007).

Prune-belly syndrome

Prune-belly syndrome is an extremely rare condition in which the male infant has three characteristic features: bilateral undescended testes, absence of the muscle of the anterior abdominal wall, and anomalies of the urinary tract. Renal dysplasia is common. Other associated anomalies include cardiac (atrial or ventricular septal defect, tetralogy of Fallot), pulmonary (hypoplasia),

gastrointestinal (malrotation volvulus, gastroschisis, exomphalos, Hirschsprung's, anorectal anomaly) and orthopaedic abnormalities (Becker 2009). In view of the wide range of severity, from in utero demise to near-normal life expectancy, management needs to be individualised (Keating and Rich 2005).

Vesicoureteric reflux

VUR occurs when urine flows retrogradely from the bladder into the ureters. Previously, reflux was diagnosed in patients being investigated for UTIs; however, with improvements in antenatal scanning, pelvicalyceal dilatation can be identified during pregnancy, which subsequently is diagnosed as reflux and accounts for approximately 25% of all antenatally diagnosed dilatation (Arthur et al. 1989). Over 90% of those with antenatally diagnosed reflux are boys; this is in contrast to those with postnatally diagnosed reflux, who are mainly girls, and may be explained by the increased voiding pressure required in male fetuses (Anderson and Rickwood 1991). Spontaneous improvement of VUR is the norm, with persistent VUR more likely with greater severity, bilaterality and older age at presentation (Dave and Khoury 2007). With the advent of detailed antenatal anomaly scanning, many offspring (50% risk of VUR if mother has VUR) and siblings (34% of siblings have VUR) with significant VUR are identified on prenatal scanning and can be investigated postnatally as indicated by their prenatal history. When reflux has been identified (Fig. 35.13), it is important to proceed to a dimercaptosuccinic acid (DMSA) isotope scan so that split renal function and the presence of renal scarring can be assessed. Before the advent of antenatal scanning all renal damage (scars) seen in patients with VUR was thought to be secondary to postnatal infection. Subsequently, early preinfection studies on neonates detected renal scars in approximately 60% of kidneys with reflux (Anderson and Rickwood 1991). In these kidneys the scarring was global, compared with the segmental scarring seen following infection (Yeung et al. 1997). Mackie and Stephens (1975) postulated that an abnormal development of the ureteric bud would lead to anomalous development of the kidney, resulting in renal dysplasia. Indeed, VUR is now recognised as part of a more generalised urinary tract abnormality, including renal dysplasia and hypoplasia, bladder

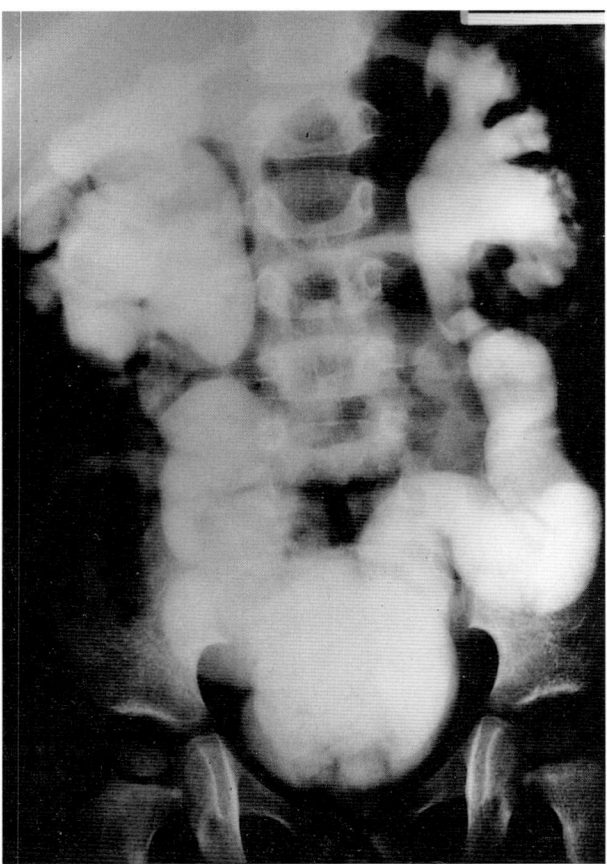

Fig. 35.13 Micturating cystogram showing bilateral vesicoureteric reflux. There is gross bilateral dilatation of the ureters and marked clubbing of the calyces and renal pelvis.

dysfunction and a possible predisposition to UTIs (Dave and Khoury 2007).

The goal of treatment is the prevention of renal injury, leading to hypertension and renal failure. The management of VUR is once again intensely debated. Previously, randomised controlled studies centred on surgical versus medical management (Dave and Khoury 2007). Surgical correction of VUR was found to offer no advantage on renal outcome over antibiotic prophylaxis. Today, antibiotic prophylaxis is the focus of randomised controlled trials. The incidence of UTI and renal scarring has been observed to be the same in infants with grade II–IV VUR with or without prophylactic antibiotics (Pennesi et al. 2008). This is leading many to advise prompt treatment of infection when this occurs rather than continuous antibiotic prophylaxis (Pennesi et al. 2008; Becker 2009). In addition, adequate and regular bladder and bowel emptying must be achieved (Capozza et al. 2004). Some centres suggest that circumcision can reduce the number of UTIs, but this has not been proved by a controlled trial despite being supported by considerable anecdotal evidence (Wiswell et al. 1985). Only when these methods fail to prevent recurrent UTIs, or where there is a significant decrease in renal function associated with scarring, is reimplantation of the ureter required to correct the reflux surgically. Endoscopic submucosal injection of a bulking agent at the VUJ is increasingly advocated as an alternative treatment modality to open surgery, and to antibiotic prophylaxis (Capozza et al. 2004). Indeed, a success rate of 70–90% – depending on the grade of reflux – combined with a low risk of transient ureteric obstruction (less than 0.5%), makes endoscopic submucosal injection an ideal first-line intervention for VUR.

Abnormal formation, migration and fusion of the kidney

The absence of a kidney on ultrasound can be due to a congenital deficiency (unilateral or bilateral), involution of a multicystic dysplastic kidney or, alternatively, it could represent an ectopically placed kidney which has yet to be identified.

Renal agenesis

Renal agenesis can be unilateral or bilateral and probably results from a failure of the ureteral bud to induce development in the kidney. This may be due to a defect either in the ureteral bud or in the developing kidney (Mesrobian and Sulik 1992). The incidence of unilateral agenesis is between 1:1000 and 1:1500 (Ritchey 1992). An ectopic kidney needs to be excluded by performing a renal isotope scan (DMSA) that visualises all functioning renal tissue. Associated urogenital anomalies are common. The ipsilateral ureter is absent or partially atretic in all cases. The contralateral kidney is either malrotated or ectopic in 15% of cases, and has associated VUR in 37% (Song et al. 1995).

The incidence of bilateral renal agenesis (Potter syndrome) is 1:4000 births. Bilateral renal agenesis is more common in males and within the same family, suggesting a genetic component (Rizza and Downing 1971). Diagnosis is usually made antenatally by ultrasonography, which reveals oligohydramnios and absence of the kidneys. The ureters are usually absent or partially developed. Testicular absence has been found in approximately 10% of cases, but the vas deferens is often present, suggesting that renal agenesis is not due to a failure of the wolffian duct to develop (Ashley and Mostofi 1960). Potter syndrome is, of course, fatal. The main differential diagnosis is bilateral involuted multicystic dysplastic kidneys.

Multicystic dysplastic kidney

Multicystic dysplastic kidney is increasingly being diagnosed during pregnancy, affecting approximately 1 in 4000 live births (Hains et al. 2009). It is more commonly unilateral, although bilateral cases have been reported. Postnatally, the diagnosis is confirmed with an ultrasound showing multiple cysts that have completely replaced the kidney (Fig. 35.14). Nuclear renograms show that the multicystic dysplastic kidney is non-functioning. Anomalies in the contralateral kidney are seen in 25% of patients: these include PUJ anomalies and VUR.

The management of these patients has gradually changed to a non-operative approach. Serial ultrasounds show that these kidneys involute: approximately one-third by 2 years of age, half by 5 years and two-thirds by 10 years of age (Aslam et al. 2006). However, if the kidney fails to decrease in size nephrectomy is offered. Hypertension and malignant change associated with multicystic dysplastic kidneys have been reported, although their incidence is roughly similar to that in the normal population (Hains et al. 2009).

Ectopic kidneys

Ectopic kidneys are caused by an abnormality in renal ascent and/or renal fusion. If an ectopic kidney is suspected, an ultrasound and DMSA scan should be performed for diagnostic reasons. Ectopic

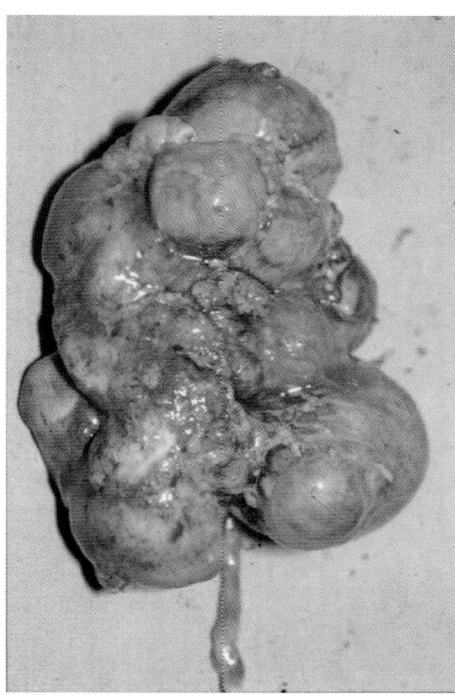

Fig. 35.14 Pathology specimen showing a multicystic dysplastic kidney. Note the pearly appearance of the partly atretic ureter.

kidneys can be divided into simple, horseshoe, and crossed renal ectopia.

Simple ectopic kidney

The most common location for a simple ectopic kidney is pelvic; this occurs in 60% of cases. It is usually unilateral, with a slight predilection for the left side, but is found bilaterally in 10% of cases (Ritchey 1992). In addition to its abnormal location, a pelvic kidney is frequently small and irregular in shape. The remaining ectopic kidneys lie between the pelvis and the normal position. Very rarely, the kidney can be found within the thorax.

Ectopic kidneys are associated with genital and contralateral urinary abnormalities, such as absence of the vagina (Hendren and Donahoe 1986), retrocaval ureter, bicornuate uterus, supernumerary kidney (Flyer et al. 1994) and contralateral ectopic ureter (Borer et al. 1993).

Horseshoe kidney

The incidence of horseshoe kidney varies between 1:400 and 1:1800 (Campbell 1970), and is more common in males. In 95% of cases, the lower poles of the two kidneys are joined by a bridge of renal tissue, which can be normal, dysplastic or fibrous (Fig. 35.15). In about 40% of cases, the isthmus lies at the level of L4, just beneath the origin of the inferior mesenteric artery. In 20% the isthmus is in the pelvis; in the rest it lies at the level of the lower poles of normally placed kidneys (Hendren and Donahoe 1986). A small number of horseshoe kidneys have fusion at their upper poles. The ureters arch anteriorly to pass over the isthmus (Boullier et al. 1992), which may explain the relatively high incidence of pyeloureteric anomalies (20%) associated with horseshoe kidneys. Associated abnormalities are common: these can involve the central nervous system, gastrointestinal tract, and the skeletal and cardiovascular systems.

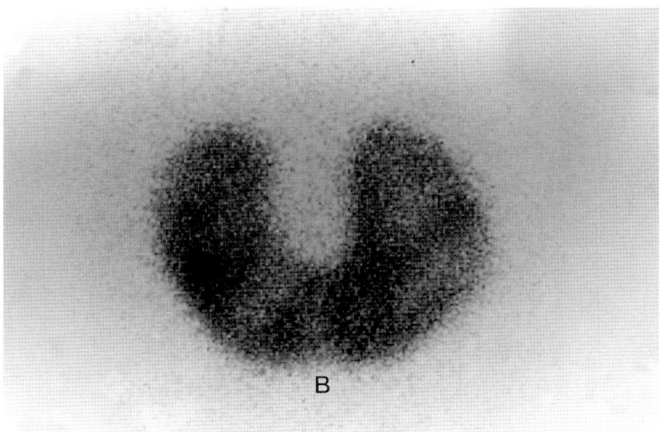

Fig. 35.15 MAG3 renogram showing a horseshoe kidney; the bridge of renal tissue connecting the right and left kidneys can be seen (B).

Crossed renal ectopia

Crossed renal ectopia can occur either with renal fusion (80%) or without fusion. It is slightly more common in boys and the left kidney usually crosses to the right side, where the upper pole of the crossed kidney fuses with the lower pole of the uncrossed kidney. As with all renal ectopia, treatment is only required for clinically significant consequences, which are fortunately rare, such as VUR or PUJ obstruction (Fig. 35.16).

Genitourinary tract anomalies

Hypospadias

Hypospadias occurs in 1 in 300 male births. This congenital abnormality consists of three features: an abnormally placed urethral meatus, which can be found anywhere from the glans to the perineum junction; chordee of the penis, which forces the penis to point towards the scrotum when erect; and a foreskin which, instead of being wrapped around the penis, is present only on the dorsal side (Fig. 35.17) (Mouriquand and Mollard 1995). The underlying pathology is not fully understood, but it is probably caused by an incomplete virilisation of the penis. The important consideration when examining a child with hypospadias is to be certain that this is not a virilised female or an XY/XO mosaic. This can be assessed by palpation of the testes: if there are two, the karyotype is XY; however, if one or both testes are undescended, then intersex problems must be excluded (see Ch. 34 part 2) (Rajfer and Walsh 1976). In the majority, the hypospadias is an isolated problem that necessitates appropriate referral and requires surgical reconstruction between 1 and 2 years of age.

Undescended testicle

Testicular descent typically occurs from the fifth to the seventh months of gestation. In term boys, both testicles are therefore usually descended at birth. The incidence of undescended testicles at term is 1:50 to 1:100. Premature boys have an increased risk of undescended testicles (Chilvers et al. 1986). Postnatally, descent can still occur spontaneously but is rare after the first few months of life. The left testicle descends first; a right undescended testis is therefore more common. Undescended testicles can be of two types: true undescended testicles, which lie along the original line of

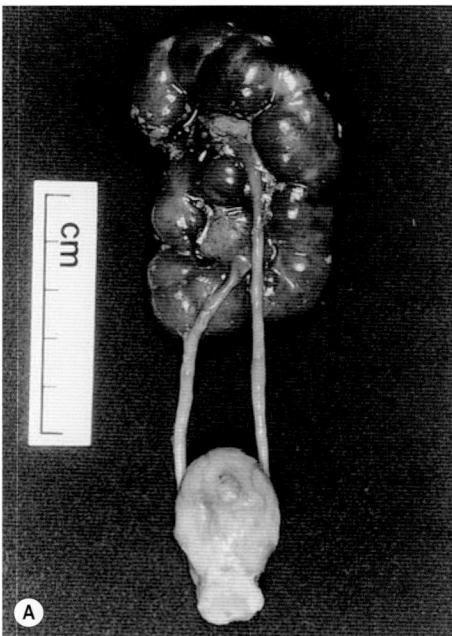
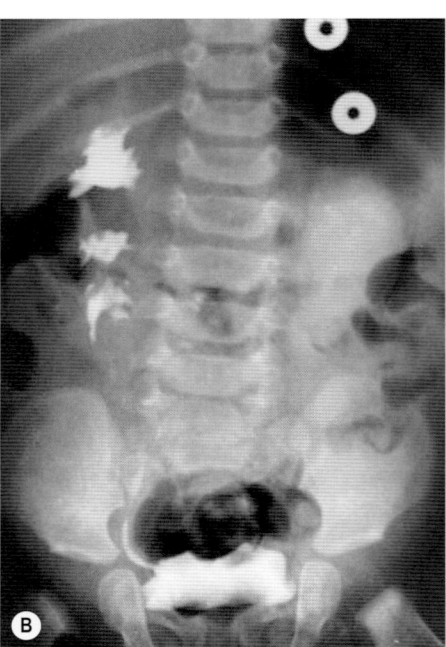

Fig. 35.16 (a) Postmortem specimen showing a crossed fused ectopia. (b) Intravenous urogram showing a crossed fused ectopia, with both collecting systems visualised on the right side.

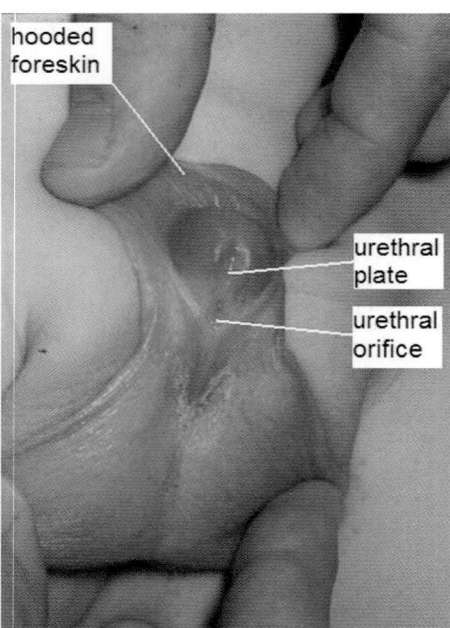

Fig. 35.17 Boy with hypospadias. This shows the urethral plate with the urethral opening on the ventral aspect of the penis and the hooded foreskin all behind the penis.

descent but which have not reached the scrotum, and ectopic testes, which have deviated from the normal line of descent. Approximately 20% of undescended testes are impalpable, mostly due to an intra-abdominal location of the testis, the vanishing testis syndrome or a testis sited in the inguinal canal that was missed on palpation.

A retractile testis, pulled into the inguinal canal by the cremasteric reflex, is often incorrectly diagnosed as an undescended testis. A retractile testis can be milked into the scrotum. These testes are normal and do not require further treatment, as they will become permanently situated in the scrotum with puberty, secondary to the androgen effect on the cremaster.

There is a strong association between undescended testicle and a hernial sac (see Ch. 29 part 4 for surgical management of inguinal hernia). If a hernia occurs, it is necessary both to repair the hernia and to perform an orchidopexy soon, in order to prevent an incarcerated hernia. In most cases of undescended testicle, a definitive operation to bring the testicle down into the scrotum is performed around 1 year of age.

The benefits of orchidopexy include the following:

- cosmetic and psychological benefits of having two testes in the scrotum
- the undescended testis has an increased risk of malignancy – placement in the scrotum enables easy palpation
- it places the testis in a lower temperature environment, which may improve the long-term chances of fertility. Recent evidence suggests benefit to germ and Leydig cell numbers (Tasian et al. 2004) and sperm count and motility from early orchidopexy (Canavese et al. 2009)
- a malpositioned testis is more susceptible to damage from trauma.

Hydroceles

Congenital hydrocele results from an incomplete obliteration of the patent processus vaginalis. Normally, the processus vaginalis, which accompanies the descending testicle into the scrotum, has been obliterated by the seventh month of pregnancy. If the processus remains patent around the testicle and there is a small lumen connecting it to the peritoneal cavity, fluid can enter and stay in the processus vaginalis, forming a hydrocele. The only difference between a hydrocele and hernia, therefore, in anatomical terms, is that in a hernia the lumen allows the bowel to enter the processus.

Hydroceles usually present with a scrotal swelling. The features which differentiate hydrocele from hernia are that hydroceles transilluminate, and that it is possible to 'get above' a hydrocele, whereas a hernia extends into the peritoneal cavity. It is vital that a hernia is excluded in the diagnosis, as the two conditions have very different treatments. Most hydroceles can be left alone, as the vast majority spontaneously resolve by 3 years of age. Surgical ligation of the processus vaginalis should be carried out if the hydrocele remains, becomes symptomatic (rare), or cannot be differentiated from a hernia.

Neonatal testicular torsion

Neonatal or intrauterine torsion of the testicle usually presents as a swollen testicle. The scrotum is often red and oedematous, and may be tender on examination. Often a black testicle can be identified within the scrotum. Occasionally the initial event is not identified and the torted testicle is only noticed when a fibrotic atrophied testicle is seen during exploration for an undescended testicle. The established treatment is early surgical exploration and fixation of the contralateral testis. However, if the scrotum has been red and oedematous from birth, the testicle is always necrotic and it is now common practice to treat the boy with analgesia and antibiotics alone. Controversy exists about whether to fix the contralateral testis, but because asynchronous torsion has been described we believe it is prudent to perform surgical fixation of the contralateral testis before discharge. If at the time of presentation both testicles appear torted, then surgical exploration is recommended (Driver and Losty 1998).

Tight foreskin

At birth the prepuce and the glans of the penis are firmly adherent, gradually separating over the first 4 years. During this time, retraction of the foreskin is not possible – so-called physiological phimosis. It is unusual to require circumcision during the neonatal period. The indications for circumcision are:

- religious reasons
- a fibrous scarred foreskin
- babies under a year with severe underlying uropathies who continue to present with recurrent UTIs despite prophylaxis.

All other indications are considerably less definite. Pathological tightness of the foreskin (pathological phimosis) does occur but is rare before 5 years of age, and even then can usually be successfully treated with gentle parental retraction of the foreskin and local steroid cream (after the age of 4 years). Many factors have been put forward in defence of circumcision, including a decreased incidence of penile and cervical cancer and a reduction in the incidence of UTIs (Wiswell et al. 1985) and female-to-male human immunodeficiency virus (HIV) transmission. The one definite contraindication for circumcision is in boys with other penile anomalies, where the prepuce may be required to reconstruct the urethra; for religious reasons, parents can be reassured that once the hypospadias repair has been performed their child will be circumcised.

Epispadias and bladder exstrophy

Epispadias, bladder exstrophy and cloacal exstrophy represent a spectrum of congenital malformations in which there is an abnormal development of the cloacal membrane and consequently incomplete midline fusion of the cloacal structures.

Epispadias is the mildest form: it is rare, with an incidence of 1 in 100 000, and can occur in both sexes, although it is more common

in boys. In epispadias, the bladder is covered and the urethra opens onto the dorsal surface of the penis; in addition, the penis is often short and wide, with marked dorsal chordee. In girls the urethra is patulous and the clitoris has not fused in the midline. Treatment consists of reconstructing the genitalia; however, as the bladder neck and sphincter are often involved, further treatment to ensure urinary continence is often required.

Bladder exstrophy occurs in 1 in 50 000 live births. In this anomaly, the bladder opens onto the abdominal wall; there is marked separation of the pubic bones and epispadias of the genitalia (Fig. 35.18). Like epispadias, this is more common in boys. Treatment requires closure of the bladder and pubic ring within the first few days of life, then a staged approach to correct the epispadias

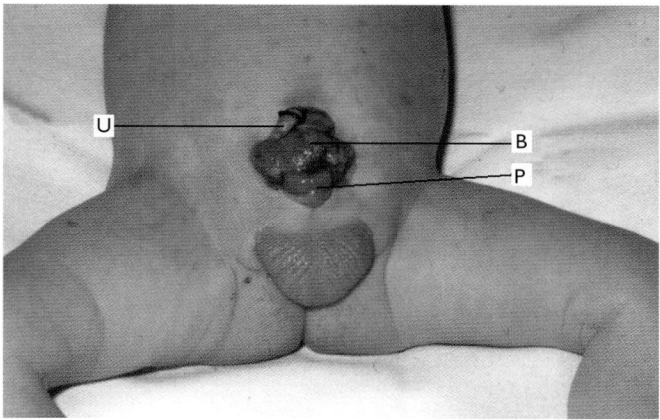

Fig. 35.18 A child with bladder exstrophy. The umbilicus is at the top of the photograph (U); below this is the bladder plate (B) with an open bladder neck and an epispadic penis (P).

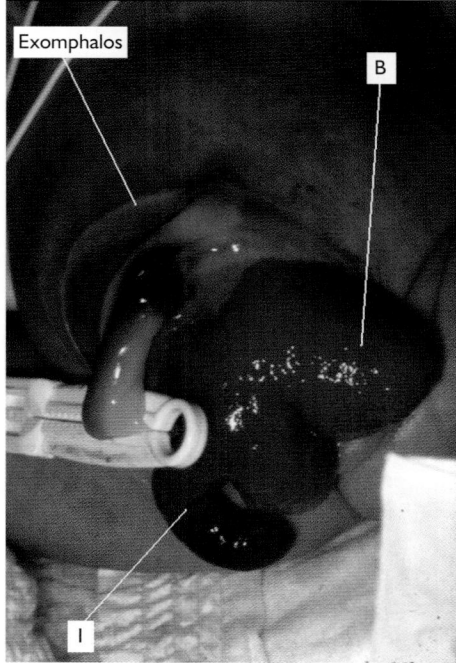

Fig. 35.19 Child with cloacal exstrophy. Prolapsed ileum (I) is seen coming from the exstrophied caecum; on the left side is an exstrophied hemibladder (B).

and reconstruct the bladder neck. These patients will require life-long follow-up, but despite the many problems the majority are socially continent and sexually active.

Cloacal exstrophy is the most severe and fortunately the rarest form of the exstrophy complex. It has an incidence of 1 in 250 000 and, unlike bladder exstrophy, is more common in girls (Diamond 1990). In cloacal exstrophy, the bowel, usually at the ileocaecal valve, opens in the midline with two hemibladders lateral to it (Fig. 35.19). There is also epispadias of the genitalia and pubic bone separation (Hurwitz et al. 1988). Until 1960 this was uniformly fatal, but since 1980 the survival rate has been over 90% (Hurwitz et al. 1988).

References

Aksu, N., Yavascan, O., Kangin, M., et al., 2005. Postnatal management of infants with antenatally detected hydronephrosis. Pediatr Nephrol 20, 1253–1259.

Allen, T.D., Husmann, D.A., 1989. Ureteropelvic junction obstruction associated with ureteral hypoplasia. J Urol 142, 353–355.

Anderson, P.A., Rickwood, A.M.K., 1991. Features of primary vesicoureteric reflux detected by prenatal sonography. Br J Urol 67, 267–271.

Arthur, R.J., Irving, H.C., Thomas, D.F.M., 1989. Bilateral fetal uropathy; what is the outlook? BMJ 298, 1419–1420.

Ashley, D.J.B., Mostofi, F.K., 1960. Renal agenesis and dysgenesis. J Urol 83, 211–230.

Aslam, M., Watson, A.R., on behalf of the Trent, Anglia MCDK study group, 2006. Unilateral multicystic dysplastic kidney; long term outcomes. Arch Dis Child 91, 820–823.

Atwell, J.D., 1983. Posterior urethral valves in the British Isles: a multicenter BAPS review. J Pediatr Surg 18, 70–74.

Bakker, N.J., 1958. Valves in the female urethra. Urol Int 6, 187–190.

Beck, A.D., 1971. The effect of intra-uterine urinary obstruction upon the development of the fetal kidney. J Urol 105, 784–789.

Becker, A.M., 2009. Postnatal evaluation of infants with an abnormal antenatal renal sonogram. Curr Opin Pediatr 21, 207–213.

Blyth, B., Snyder, H.M., Duckett, J.W., 1993. Antenatal diagnosis and subsequent management of hydronephrosis. J Urol 149, 693–698.

Borer, J.G., Corgan, F.J., Krantz, R., et al., 1993. Unilateral single vaginal ectopic ureter with ipsilateral hypoplastic pelvic kidney and bicornuate uterus. J Urol 149, 1124–1127.

Boullier, J., Chehval, M.J., Purcell, M.H., 1992. Removal of a multicystic half of a horseshoe kidney: significance of preoperative evaluation in identifying abnormal surgical anatomy. J Pediatr Surg 27, 1244–1246.

Campbell, M.F., 1970. Anomalies of the kidney. In: Campbell, M.F., Harrison, J.H. (Eds.), Urology, third ed, vol. 2. W.B. Saunders, Philadelphia, p. 1416.

Canavese, F., Mussa, A., Manenti, M., et al., 2009. Sperm count of young men surgically treated for cryptorchidism in the first and second year of life: fertility is better in children treated at a younger age. Eur J Pediatr Surg 19, 388–391.

Capozza, N., Lais, A., Nappo, S., et al., 2004. The role of endoscopic treatment of vesicoureteral reflux: a 17-year experience. J Urol 172, 1626–1628.

Cass, A.S., Stephens, F.D., 1974. Posterior urethral valves: diagnosis and management. J Urol 112, 519–525.

Castagnetti, M., Cimador, M., Sergio, M., et al., 2004. Transurethral incision of duplex system ureteroceles in neonates: does it increase the need for secondary surgery in intravesical and ectopic cases? BJU Int 93, 1313–1317.

Castagnetti, M., Cimador, M., Sergio, M., et al., 2006. Double-J stent insertion across vesicoureteral junction – is it a valuable initial approach in neonates and infants with severe primary nonrefluxing megaureter? Urology 68, 870–875.

Chilvers, C., Dudley, N.E., Gough, M.H., et al., 1986. Undescended testis: the effect of treatment on subsequent risk of subfertility and malignancy. J Pediatr Surg 21, 691–696.

Dave, S., Khoury, A.E., 2007. The current evidence based medical management of vesicoureteral reflux: the Sickids protocol. Indian J Urol 23, 403–413.

De Bruyn, R., Marks, S.D., 2008. Postnatal investigation of fetal renal disease. Semin Fetal Neonatal Med 13, 133–141.

De Jong, T.P.V.M., Radmayr, C., Dik, P., et al., 2008. For the Pediatric Urology Club Meeting, Stans, Austria, January 2007: Posterior urethral valves: search for a diagnostic reference standard. Urology 72, 1022–1025.

De Kort, L.M.O., Uiterwal, C.S.P.M., Beek, E.J.A., et al., 2004. Reliability of voiding cystourethrography to detect urethral obstruction in boys. Urology 63, 967–971.

Desai, D.Y., 2007. A review of urodynamic evaluation in children and its role in the management of boys with posterior urethral valves. Indian J Urol 23, 435–442.

Desphande, C., Hennekam, R.C.M., 2008. Genetic syndromes and prenatally detected renal anomalies. Semin Fetal Neonatal Med 13, 171–180.

Dhillon, H.K., 1995. Imaging and follow up of neonatal hydronephrosis. Curr Opin Urol 5, 75–78.

Dhillon, H.K., 1998. Prenatally diagnosed hydronephrosis: the Great Ormond Street experience. Br J Urol 81 (suppl. 2), 39–44.

Dhillon, H.K., 2002. Prenatally diagnosed hydronephrosis: selective postnatal intervention. Dial Pediatr Urol 25, 5–7.

Diamond, D.A., 1990. Cloacal exstrophy: associated anomalies. Dial Pediatr Urol 13, 6–8.

Di Benedetto, V., Meyrat, B.J., Sorrentino, G., et al., 1995. Management of duplex ureteroceles detected by prenatal ultrasound. Pediatr Surg Int 10, 485–487.

Dinneen, M.D., Dhillon, H.K., Word, H.C., et al., 1993. Antenatal diagnosis of PUV. Br J Urol 72, 364–369.

Ditchfield, M.R., Grattan-Smith, J.D., De Campo, J.F., et al., 1994. Voiding cystourethroscopy in boys: does the presence of the catheter obscure the diagnosis of posterior urethral valves? AJR Am J Roentgenol 164, 233–1235.

Driver, C.D., Losty, P.D., 1998. Neonatal testicular torsion. Br J Urol 82, 855–858.

Estrada, C.R., Peters, C.A., Retik, A.B., et al., 2009. Vesicoureteral reflux and urinary tract infection in children with a history of prenatal hydronephrosis – should voiding cystourethrography be performed in all cases of persistent grade II hydronephrosis? J Urol 181, 801–806.

Farrugia, M.K., Steinbrecher, H.A., Malone, P.S., 2009. The outcome of double-J stents in the management of primary obstructive megaureters presenting before one year of age. Available online at: http://aap.confex.com/aap/2009/webprogram/Paper5484.html.

Flashner, S.C., Lower, R.K., 1992. Ureteropelvic junction. In: Kelalis, P.P., King, L.R., Belman, A.B. (Eds.), Clinical Pediatric Urology, third ed. W.B. Saunders, Philadelphia, pp. 693–725.

Flashner, S.C., Mesrobian, H.G.J., Flatt, J.A., et al., 1993. Nonobstructive dilatation of upper urinary tract may later convert to obstruction. Urology 42, 569–573.

Flyer, M.A., Haller, J.O., Feld, M., et al., 1994. Ectopic supernumerary kidney: another cause of a pelvic mass. Abdom Imag 19, 374–375.

Glick, P.L., Harrison, M.R., Noall, R.A., et al., 1983. Correction of congenital hydronephrosis in utero. III. Early mid-trimester ureteral obstruction produces renal dysplasia. J Pediatr Surg 18, 681–687.

Gobe, G.C., Axelsen, R.A., 1987. Genesis of renal tubular atrophy in experimental hydronephrosis in the rat. Role of apoptosis. Lab Invest 56, 273–281.

Groshar, D., Embdon, O.M., Sazbon, A., et al., 1988. Radionuclide assessment of bladder outlet obstruction: a noninvasive (1-step) method for measurement of voiding time, urinary flow rates and residual urine. J Urol 139, 266–269.

Hains, D.S., Bates, C.M., Ingraham, S., et al., 2009. Management and etiology of the unilateral multicystic dysplastic kidney: a review. Pediatr Nephrol 24, 233–241.

Hanna, M.K., 1991. Neonatal UPJ obstruction. Current controversies: The case for early operation. Dialogues in Pediatric Urology 14, 2–4.

Harrison, M.R., Nakayama, D.K., Noall, R., et al., 1982. Correction of congenital hydronephrosis in utero; decompression reverses the effects of obstruction on the fetal lung and urinary tract. J Pediatr Surg 17, 965–974.

Hendren, W.H., Donahoe, P.K., 1986. Renal fusions and ectopia. In: Welch, K.J., Randolph, J.G., Ravitch, M.M., et al. (Eds.), Pediatric Surgery, fourth ed. Year Book Medical Publishers, Chicago, pp. 1134–1145.

Hendron, C.D., Ferrer, F.A., Freedman, A., et al., 2000. Consensus on the prenatal management of antenatally detected urological abnormalities. J Urol 164, 1052–1056.

Hollowell, J.G., Altman, H.G., Snyder, H.M., et al., 1989. Coexisting ureteropelvic junction obstruction and vesicoureteral reflux: diagnostic and therapeutic implications. J Urol 142, 490–493.

Hurwitz, R.S., Mansoni, G.A.M., Ransley, P.G., et al., 1988. Cloacal exstrophy: a report of 34 cases. J Urol 138, 1065–1068.

Johnson, J.H., Kulatilake, A.E., 1971. The sequelae of posterior urethral valves. Br J Urol 43, 743–748.

Joseph, D.B., Bauer, S.B., Colodny, A.H., et al., 1989. Lower pole ureteropelvic junction obstruction and incomplete renal duplication. J Urol 141, 896–899.

Kajbafzadeh, A.M., Payabvash, S., Hassanzadeh, S., et al., 2006. Smooth muscle cell apoptosis and defective neural development in congenital ureteropelvic junction obstruction. J Urol 176, 718–723.

Kaplan, G.W., Scherz, H.L., 1992. Infravesical Obstruction in Clinical Pediatric Urology, third ed. W.B. Saunders, Philadelphia, pp. 821–864.

Kass, E.J., 1992. Megaureter. In: Kelalis, P.P., King, L.R., Belman, A.B., (Eds.), Clinical Pediatric Urology. W.B. Saunders, Philadelphia, p. 782.

Keating, M.A., Rich, M.A., 2005. Prune-belly syndrome. In: Ashcraft, K.W., Holcomb III G.W., Murphy, J.P. (Eds.), Pediatric Surgery, fourth ed. W.B. Saunders, Philadelphia, pp. 831–850.

Koff, S.A., Campbell, K.D., 1994. The nonoperative management of unilateral neonatal hydronephrosis: natural history of poorly functioning kidneys. J Urol 152, 593–595.

Kousidis, G., Thomas, D.F.M., Morgan, H., et al., 2008. The long-term outcome of prenatally detected posterior urethral valves: a 10 to 23-year follow-up study. BJU Int 102, 1020–1024.

Lee, R.S., Cendron, M., Kinnamon, D.D., et al., 2006. Antenatal hydronephrosis as a predictor of postnatal outcome: a meta-analysis. Pediatr Nephrol 22, 1727–1734.

Mackie, G.G., Stephens, F.D., 1975. Duplex kidneys: a correlation of renal dysplasia with position of the ureteral orifice. J Urol 114, 274–280.

Madden, N.P., Thomas, D.F.M., Gordon, A.C., et al., 1991. Antenatally detected pelviureteric junction obstruction. Is non-operation safe? Br J Urol 68, 305–310.

Mallik, M., Watson, A.R., 2008. Antenatally detected urinary tract anomalies: more detection but less action. Pediatr Nephrol 23, 897–904.

McLellan, D.L., Retik, A.B., Bauer, S.B., et al., 2002. Rate and predictors of spontaneous resolution of prenatally diagnosed primary non-refluxing megaureter. J Urol 168, 2177–2180.

Mesrobian, H.G.J., 1986. Ureteropelvic junction obstruction of the upper pole moiety in complete ureteral duplication. J Urol 136, 452–453.

Mesrobian, H.G.J., Sulik, K.K., 1992. Characterization of the upper urinary tract anatomy in the Danforth spontaneous murine mutation. J Urol 148, 752–755.

Mouriquand, P.D.E., Mollard, P., 1995. Hypospadias repair: the paediatric urologist's point of view. Eur Urol Update Series 4, 106–111.

Mure, P.-Y., Mouriquand, P.D.E., 2008. Upper urinary tract dilatation: Prenatal diagnosis, management and outcome. Fetal Neonatal Med 13, 152–163.

Onen, A., Jayanthi, V.R., Koff, S.A., 2002. Long-term followup of prenatally detected severe bilateral newborn hydronephrosis initially amanged nonoperatively. J Urol 168, 1118–1120.

Paltiel, H.J., Lebowitz, R.L., 1989. Neonatal hydronephrosis due to primary vesico-ureteric reflux: trends in diagnosis and treatment. Radiology 170, 787–789.

Parkhouse, H.F., Barratt, T.M., Dillon, M.J., et al., 1988. Long-term outcome of boys with posterior urethral valves. Br J Urol 62, 59–62.

Pennesi, M., Travan, L., Peratoner, L., et al., 2008. Is antibiotic prophylaxis in children with vesicoureteral reflux effective in preventing pyelonephritis and renal scars? A randomized, controlled trial. Pediatrics 121, e1489–e1494.

Pluto Collaborative Study Group, 2007. PLUTO trial protocol: percutaneous shunting for lower urinary tract obstruction randomised controlled trial. Br J Obstet Gynaecol 114, 904–905.

Rajfer, J., Walsh, P.C., 1976. The incidence of intersexuality in patients with hypospadias and cryptorchidism. J Urol 116, 769–770.

Ransley, P.G., Dhillon, H.K., Gordon, I., et al., 1990. The postnatal management of hydronephrosis diagnosed by prenatal ultrasound. J Urol 144, 584–587.

Reinberg, Y., De Castano, I., Gonzales, R., 1992. Prognosis for patients with prenatally diagnosed posterior urethral valves. J Urol 148, 125–126.

Rickwood, A.M.K., Jee, L.D., Williams, M.P.L., et al., 1992. Natural history of obstructed and pseudo-obstructed megaureters detected by prenatal ultrasonography. Br J Urol 70, 322–325.

Ritchey, M., 1992. Anomalies of the kidney. In: Kelalis, P.P., King, L.R., Belman, A.B. (Eds.), Clinical Pediatric Urology, third ed. W.B. Saunders, Philadelphia, pp. 500–529.

Rizza, J.M., Downing, S.E., 1971. Bilateral renal agenesis in two female siblings. Am J Dis Child 121, 60–63.

Roth, C.C., Hubanks, J.M., Bright, B.C., et al., 2009. Occurrence of urinary tract infection in chidren with significant urinary tract obstruction. Urology 73, 74–78.

Schober, J.M., Dulabon, L.M., Woodhouse, C.R., 2004. Outcome of valve ablation in late-presenting posterior urethral valves. BJU Int 94, 616–619.

Scott, J.E.S., Renwick, M., 1988. Antenatal diagnosis of congenital abnormalities in the urinary tract. Results from the northern region fetal abnormality survey. Br J Urol 62, 295–300.

Sheldon, C.A., 1995. Male external genitalia. In: Rowe, M.I., O'Neill, J.A., Grosfeld, J.L., et al. (Eds.), Essentials of Pediatric Surgery. Mosby, St Louis, pp. 775–776.

Shukla, A.R., Cooper, J., Patel, R.P., et al., 2005. Prenatally detected primary megaureter; a role for extended followup. J Urol 173, 1353–1356.

Smith, D., Egginton, J.A., Brookfield, D.S.K., 1987. Detection of abnormality of fetal urinary tract as a predictor of urinary tract disease. BMJ 294, 27–28.

Song, J.T., Ritchey, M.L., Zerin, M., et al., 1995. Incidence of vesicoureteral reflux in children with renal agenesis. J Urol 153, 1249–1251.

Song, S.H., Lee, S.B., Park, Y.S., et al., 2007. Is antibiotic prophylaxis necessary in infants with obstructive hydronephrosis? J Urol 177, 1098–1101.

Tasian, G.E., Hittelman, A.B., Kim, G.E., et al., 2004. Age at orchidopexy and testis palpability predict germ and Leydig cell loss: clinical predictors of adverse histological features of cryptorchidism. J Urol 182, 704–709.

Taskinen, S., Heikkila, J., Rintala, R., 2009. Posterior urethral valves: primary voiding pressures and kidney function in infants. J Urol 182, 699–702.

Thomas, D.F., 1998. Prenatally detected uropathy: epidemiological considerations. Br J Urol 81 (suppl. 2), 8–12.

Thomas, D.F., Irving, H.C., Arthur, R.J., 1995. Prenatal diagnosis: how useful is it? Br J Urol 57, 784–787.

Tibballs, J.M., De Bruyn, R., 1996. Primary vesicoureteric reflux – how useful is postnatal ultrasound? Arch Dis Child 75, 444–447.

Turnock, R.R., Shawis, R., 1984. Management of fetal urinary tract anomalies detected by prenatal ultrasonography. Arch Dis Child 59, 962–965.

Ulman, I., Jayanthi, V.R., Koff, S.A., 2000. The long-term followup of newborns with severe unilateral hydronephrosis initially treated non-operatively. J Urol 164, 1101–1105.

Uson, A.C., Lattimer, J.K., Melicow, M.M., 1961. Ureteroceles in infants and children: a report based on 44 cases. Pediatrics 27, 971.

van der Vis-Melsen, M.J.E., Baert, R.J.M., Rajnherc, J.R., et al., 1989. Scintigraphic assessment of lower urinary tract function in children with and without outflow tract obstruction. Br J Urol 64, 263–269.

Whitten S.M., Wilcox D.T., 2001. Duplex systems. Prenatal Diagn 21, 952–957.

Wiswell T.E., Smith F.R., Bass J.W., 1985. Decreased incidence of urinary tract infections in circumcised male patients. Pediatrics 75, 901–903.

Yerkes E.B., Adams M.C., Pope 4th J.C., et al., 1999. Does every patient with prenatal hydronephrosis need voiding cystourethrography? J Urol 162, 1218–1220.

Yeung C.K., Godley M.L., Dhillon H.K., et al., 1997. The characteristics of primary vesico-ureteric reflux in male and female infants with pre-natal hydronephrosis. Br J Urol 80, 319–327.

Neonatal malignancy

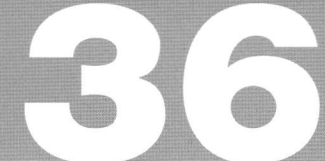

Roger D Palmer   Denise M Williams

Introduction

Neonatal cancer is rare, a surprising fact in view of the rapid cell division and growth occurring throughout fetal life. Our understanding of the factors affecting cell growth and the genetic events responsible for the development or progression of malignant disease continues to increase at a rapid rate. Genes controlling cell growth are termed proto-oncogenes. Research efforts have led to the identification of two major classes of genes associated with malignancy. Oncogenes are mutated proto-oncogenes and give rise to excessive cell growth and proliferation, whilst tumour-suppressor genes act in normal cells to suppress proliferation, but, if inactivated, remove the normal constraint to growth, and target cells are allowed to proliferate in an uncontrolled way (Friend et al. 1988).

Knudson's 'two-hit' theory of carcinogenesis has been verified by this knowledge of the genetic factors that control cell growth (Knudson 1985). The 'hits' could be a wide variety of agents – viral, chemical or radiation – and cause mutation of a proto-oncogene or inactivation or loss of a tumour-suppressor gene. This first 'hit' would allow all cells in the body, including the germ cells, to carry the defect, which could then be passed on to the next generation. The second 'hit' would be in the somatic cells of a target organ. The

© 2012 Elsevier Ltd

proto-oncogene would become an oncogene, or the loss of a homologous tumour-suppressor gene would allow uncontrolled cellular growth. The time during which the second 'hit' could occur is probably confined to the period when the cells of the target organ are undergoing mitotic activity, but ceases when they are fully mature. For example, retinoblasts differentiate to become photoreceptor cells by the age of 3 years, and this may explain why retinoblastoma is unusual in older children or adults.

Oncogenes exert their effect on cells through a variety of mechanisms. These include control of cellular growth factors or their receptors, or by modifying the signals sent from growth receptors to the nucleus of the cell. This may result in an effect on DNA repair, apoptosis or the cells' ability to metabolise toxins.

Neonatal malignancy presents many therapeutic challenges. Chemotherapy is poorly tolerated in young infants, and myelosuppression and life-threatening complications of therapy are common (Weitzman and Grant 1997). This may be because of altered pharmacokinetics in the neonatal age group (Weitzman and Grant 1997). The long-term effects of chemotherapy, surgery and radiation in terms of growth, development and second tumours (Weitzman and Grant 1997) have been recognised for many years, and both short-term and long-term effects of treatment should be taken into account when planning therapy. Improvements in surgery, anaesthesia and supportive care, including avoidance of therapeutic complications such as tumour lysis syndrome with new agents like raspuricase, have all contributed to better survival (McNutt et al. 2006). Increasingly, cancer research is attempting to exploit the underlying genetic mutations for therapeutic purposes. This, in the future, may provide more specific tumour-targeted therapies, increasing cure rates with a reduction in toxicity.

The routine use of antenatal ultrasound, and the improved quality of the images, has led to an increase in the diagnosis of congenital tumours, particularly teratomas and neuroblastomas, and an increase in the understanding of their natural history (Sbragia et al. 2001). It allows close monitoring of affected pregnancies and management planning with appropriate multidisciplinary team involvement (Sebire and Jauniaux 2009).

Incidence and survival

Neonatal malignancy is disproportionately represented within childhood, where the incidence of cancer is 11–15 per 100 000 population less than 15 years of age (Table 36.1). Defining neonatal malignancy as malignant and central nervous system (CNS) tumours diagnosed in the first 6 weeks of life, the UK National Registry of Childhood Tumours (NRCT) incidence between 1981 and 2000, from 394 cancer registrations, was 2.74 per 100 000 live births, with 45.4% of these tumours presenting in the first week of life, 14.8% in the second and approximately 10% per week thereafter. This is similar to reports from other cancer registries (Table 36.1B). Suspected risk factors for the development of childhood cancer include certain congenital abnormalities (Agha et al. 2005) (Table 36.2), in utero exposure to certain drugs (e.g. diethylstilbestrol), vaginal adenocarcinoma and irradiation (all cancer types). There remains no convincing evidence that intramuscular vitamin K given at birth is associated with an increased risk of childhood leukaemia (Roman et al. 2002). However, childhood leukaemia might be initiated in utero and more than one study has suggested that high birthweight is associated with this risk (Caughey and Michels 2009).

Survival is dependent upon tumour type and site, and condition of the infant at diagnosis. Survival statistics, although improving (Table 36.1), are inherently unreliable owing to the rarity of neonatal malignancy and advances in treatment over the decades. The NRCT reports a 1- and 5-year survival of 57% and 52%, respectively, for neonatal malignancy diagnosed between 1981 and 2000. This remains lower than for malignancy during childhood as a whole.

Neuroblastoma

Neuroblastoma is the commonest neonatal malignancy, accounting for 30–50% of all tumours in the newborn period. Approximately 30% of cases are diagnosed on the first day of life and a further 20% within the first week (Isaacs 2007b). Neuroblastomas originate from neural crest cells, which give rise to the adrenal medulla and the sympathetic ganglia, but are also found in nearly all organs, including skin. Spontaneous differentiation and apoptosis may explain the 50-fold increase in frequency of small foci of neuroblastoma cells found at perinatal autopsies compared with documented cases of neuroblastoma.

Tumour genetics may be important in predicting rates of tumour progression and response to treatment and are important to determine at the time of diagnosis. Deletion of the short arm of chromosome 1, probably resulting in the loss of a tumour-suppressor gene, is associated with a poor prognosis (Brodeur et al. 1997). Hyperdiploid tumours occur more commonly in infants and are associated with a good response to chemotherapy, while a diploid DNA index is associated with advanced and aggressive disease. Amplification of *MYCN*, the *c-myc*-related oncogene, found on chromosome 2, is an adverse prognostic biological marker associated with rapid disease progression and a poor outcome (Brodeur et al. 1997).

Clinical features

A neuroblastoma arises anywhere in the neural crest tissues. Around 45% arise within the adrenal medulla, presenting as an abdominal mass (Fig. 36.1), while those arising in the posterior mediastinum may present with respiratory difficulties, swallowing problems or a unilateral Horner syndrome. Approximately 60% of infants will have metastatic disease at presentation, common sites being bone, bone marrow and skin. The so-called blueberry muffin skin deposits (Fig. 36.2) are indistinguishable clinically from those seen in congenital leukaemia. Spinal cord compression due to intraspinal extension of tumour may give rise to paraplegia or neurological signs.

Hypertension secondary to circulating catecholamines is not uncommon. Rarely, neonatal neuroblastoma may metastasise to the placenta and lead to placental insufficiency or hydrops fetalis. Maternal pre-eclampsia secondary to catecholamine release has been reported (Voute et al. 1970).

The use of antenatal ultrasound has led to an increase in prenatal diagnosis (Sbragia et al. 2001).

Staging

The international staging system for neuroblastoma (INSS) (Lukens 1999) is based on the clinical and radiological features and the operability of the tumour. The clinical stage at diagnosis is a good predictor of overall survival, and, together with knowledge of biological factors, dictates treatment.

Stage 4s disease

Stage 4s denotes an infant with a localised primary lesion and dissemination restricted to skin, bone marrow and liver but excluding bone. Spontaneous regression usually occurs (Pritchard and

Table 36.1 UK registration data and previously published series of neonatal tumours

Table 36.1A Single-centre experience

INSTITUTION	TORONTO, CANADA (Campbell et al. 1987)	PHILADELPHIA, USA (Gale et al. 1982)	LOS ANGELES, USA (Isaacs 1985)	TEXAS, USA (Xue et al. 1995)	GLASGOW, UK (Davis et al. 1988)	DURHAM, USA (Halperin 2000)	MEMPHIS, USA (Crom et al. 1989)
Years	1922–1982	1952–1978	1958–1982	1941–1981	1955–1986	1930–1998	1962–1988
Percentage of all paediatric cancers	2%	2.6%	2.6%			2%	3.2%
Male:female ratio	1.7:1	1:1.1			1:1.4	1:2.3	1:1
Survival	42%	2-year 45%	37%	78% (solid tumours only)	Approx. 50%[†] (solid only)[‡]	Approx. 60%[§]	68%
Tumour numbers	102	22	49 (61*)	45	16 (35)	15 (8)	34
Neuroblastoma	48	11	14	6	7	5	19
Retinoblastoma	17		2	3	3	4	3
Sarcoma	12	3	8 (16)	15	4 (4)	1	
Central nervous system	9		5	5		4	
Leukaemia	8	3	11	13			6
Wilms' tumour	4	1	3 (3 mesoblastic nephroma)	1	(9 mesoblastic nephroma)		2
Liver tumours	1 hepatoblastoma		1 hepatoblastoma (3 hamartoma)		(2 haemangioma, 1 hamartoma)		
MGCTs (teratoma)	1	3	1 (39 other teratomas)		1 (18 SCT, 1 orbital teratoma)	1 retroperitoneal (6 other teratomas)	1 SCT 1 oropharyngeal
Others	1 schwannoma, 1 YST testis	1 parotid carcinoma	2 carcinoma, 2 LCH	2 melanoma	1 squamous cell carcinoma	(1 glossal glial choristoma, 1 haemangioma with Kasabach–Merritt)	2 melanoma

MGCT, malignant germ cell tumour; YST, yolk sac tumour; LCH, Langerhans' cell histiocytosis; SCT, sacrococcygeal teratoma.
( ) Number and type of benign neoplasms also reported.
* Haemangiomas (five hepatic haemangiomas reported) and lymphangiomas excluded.
[†] One patient unaccounted for (malignant SCT).
[‡] Central nervous system tumours and leukaemias excluded.
[§] One patient unaccounted for (rhabdomyosarcoma)

Table 36.1 Continued
Table 36.1B Cancer registry experience

CANCER REGISTRY	DENMARK (Borch et al. 1992)	WEST MIDLANDS, UK (Parkes et al. 1994)	THIRD NATIONAL CANCER SURVEY, USA (Bader and Miller 1979)	NATIONAL REGISTRY OF CHILDHOOD TUMOURS, UK*
Years	1943–1985	1960–1989	1969–1971	1981–2000
Incidence per 100 000				
Live births	2.38 (up to 28 days old)	7.2 (up to 3 months old)	3.65 (up to 28 days old)	2.74 (up to 6 weeks old)
Male : female ratio	1 : 1.4	1 : 1.1	Not reported	1 : 1
Survival	5-year 25%	1-year 55%†, 5-year 47%†	Not reported	1-year 57%, 5-year 51%
Tumour numbers	76	98 (72)	39	394 (213†)
Neuroblastoma	20	31	21	113
Retinoblastoma	2	14		37
Sarcoma	14	6 (11)	4	38
Central nervous system	8	14	1	61
Leukaemia	12	21	5	74
Wilms' tumour	4	1 (7 mesoblastic nephroma)	5 including mesoblastic nephromas	7
Liver tumours		2 hepatoblastoma, 1 rhabdoid tumour (5 unspecified)		9 hepatoblastoma
MGCTs (teratoma)	4 (2 other teratomas), all retroperitoneal	(49 mature teratoma – 4 malignant recurrences)		40 MGCT, of which 2 gonadal
Others	8 unspecified	3 HLH, 3 LCH, 1 malignant thymoma, 1 malignant stromal cell tumour of testes	1 carcinoma, 1 lymphoma, 1 unspecified	5 extrarenal rhabdoid tumours, 4 peripheral PNET, 3 melanoma, 1 malignant histiocytosis, 1 pancreatoblastoma, 1 unspecified

MGCT, malignant germ cell tumour; LCH, Langerhans' cell histiocytosis; HLH, haemophagocytic lymphohistiocytosis; PNET, primitive neuroectodermal tumour.
( ) Number and type of benign neoplasms also reported.
* With thanks to Mr C Stiller, Childhood Cancer Research Group, University of Oxford, for providing data from the National Registry of Childhood Tumours.
†Includes benign tumours.
‡Further 213 non-malignant tumours reported (not population-based): 2 myelodysplasia/myeloproliferative disease, 26 mesoblastic nephroma, 12 LCH, 8 HLH, 10 fibromatosis, 9 haemangiopericytoma, 14 other non-malignant soft-tissue sarcoma, 5 neurofibromatosis, 120 (benign) teratomas, 7 unspecified.

Table 36.2 Tumours associated with specific malformations, syndromes and chromosomal abnormalities

INHERITED SYNDROME	CHILDHOOD CANCER
Hamartoses	
Tuberous sclerosis	Giant cell astrocytoma
Neurofibromatosis	Gliomas
Basal cell naevus (Gorlin) syndrome	Medulloblastoma, basal cell carcinoma
Turcot syndrome	Medulloblastoma
Multiple mucosal neuroma syndrome	Medullary thyroid carcinoma, phaeochromocytoma
Neurocutaneous melanosis sequence	Melanoma
Aicardia syndrome	Germ cell tumour, hepatoblastoma
Metabolic disorders	
Glycogenosis type I, hereditary tyrosinaemia and α_1-antitrypsin deficiency	Hepatocellular carcinoma
Chromosome breakage and repair defects	
Bloom syndrome	Leukaemia, Wilms' tumour and gastrointestinal tumours
Ataxia telangiectasia	Leukaemia, lymphoma
Fanconi's anaemia	Leukaemia, hepatoma, hepatoblastoma
Xeroderma pigmentosum	Skin cancers, melanoma
Werner syndrome	Sarcomas, meningioma
Immune deficiency disorders	
Wiscott–Aldrich syndrome	Leukaemia, lymphoma (often in the central nervous system)
X-linked lymphoproliferative disease (Duncan disease)	B-cell lymphoma
Severe combined immunodeficiency	Leukaemia, lymphoma
Bruton's agammaglobulinaemia	Leukaemia, lymphoma
Xeroderma pigmentosa	Non-melanomatous skin carcinomas
Chromosomal anomaly	
Down syndrome (trisomy 21)	Acute leukaemias
Turner syndrome (45XO)	Neurogenic tumours, germ cell tumours
13q syndrome	Retinoblastoma
11p syndrome	Wilms' tumour (nephroblastoma)
Monosomy 7	Preleukaemia and non-lymphoblastic leukaemia
XY gonadal dysgenesis, aniridia–Wilms' tumour association	Gonadoblastoma
Edwards syndrome (trisomy 18)	Wilms' tumour (nephroblastoma)
Klinefelter syndrome (XXY)	Leukaemia, teratoma, breast carcinoma
Congenital anomaly	
Hemihypertrophy and Beckwith–Wiedemann syndrome	Wilms' tumour, adrenal cortical carcinoma and hepatoblastoma
Sporadic aniridia, Denys–Drash syndrome, Fraser syndrome and Perlman syndrome, Sotos syndrome	Wilms' tumour (nephroblastoma)
Simpson–Golabi–Behmel syndrome	Germ cell tumour, Wilms' tumour

Table 36.2 Continued

INHERITED SYNDROME	CHILDHOOD CANCER
Poland anomaly	Leukaemia
Hirschsprung disease	Neuroblastoma
Pyloric stenosis	Germ cell tumour
Other	
Monozygotic twins	Sacrococcygeal teratoma
Very low birthweight (<1 kg)	Hepatoblastoma
After Berry (1987).	

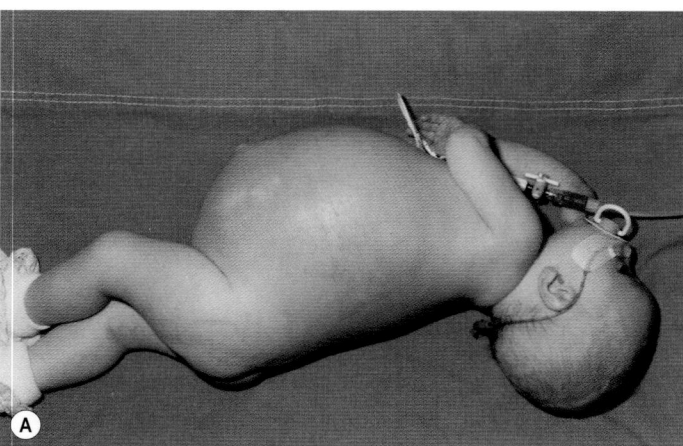 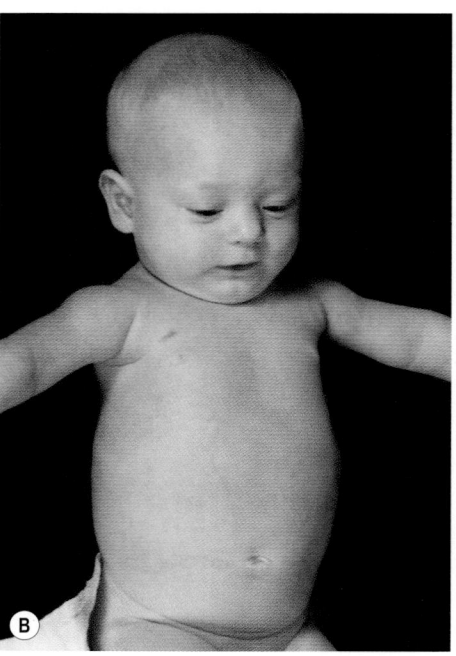

Fig. 36.1 (A) Enlarged abdomen in stage 4s neuroblastoma (left adrenal gland), presenting in the neonatal period with poor feeding, hepatomegaly and coagulopathy. (B) Same patient 5 months later, following a single course of low-dose OJEC chemotherapy (vincristine, cyclophosphamide, etoposide and carboplatin).

Hickman 1994), although close observation is necessary, as a grossly enlarging liver may result in respiratory compromise, hepatic dysfunction and coagulopathy, renal dysfunction or failure to thrive, any of which may be an indication for chemotherapy.

Diagnosis

A tissue diagnosis, although often confirming the diagnosis in a baby with a typical presentation and elevated catecholamines, vanil-lylmandelic acid and homovanillic acid (Lukens 1999) is important to provide additional biological and prognostic information. The presence of *MYCN* amplification will influence treatment. Staging involves a bone scan and bone marrow examination. Use of ^{131}I-labelled meta-iodobenzyl guanidine (MIBG), taken up by

neurosecretory granules, will give a positive scan in about 90% of patients.

Treatment

Total surgical excision is usually curative in stages 1 and 2, and chemotherapy is not indicated. However, a recent report also suggests that small, localised tumours can be watched as many undergo spontaneous regression (Hero et al. 2008). A number of chemotherapeutic agents are active for higher stage disease and, as numbers are small, in the UK such babies are treated as part of a European collaborative study. Spinal cord compression requires urgent treatment with dexamethasone and chemotherapy. Surgery may have a role in removing residual disease, although there is increasing

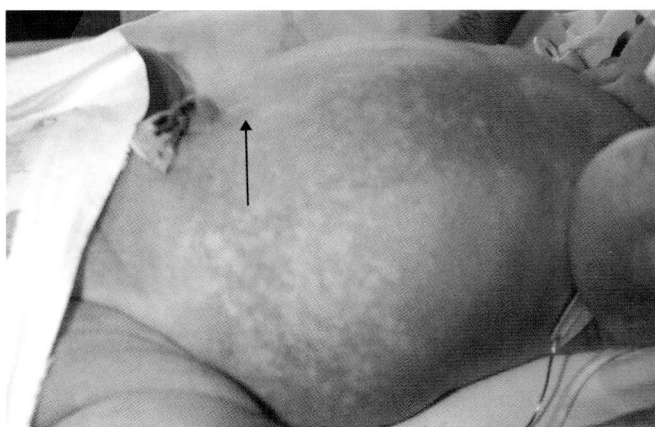

Fig. 36.2 Stage 4s neuroblastoma presenting on the first day of life with abdominal distension and marked hepatomegaly. 'Blueberry muffin' skin deposit adjacent to the umbilicus and intense cutaneous vasomotor reaction in response to handling.

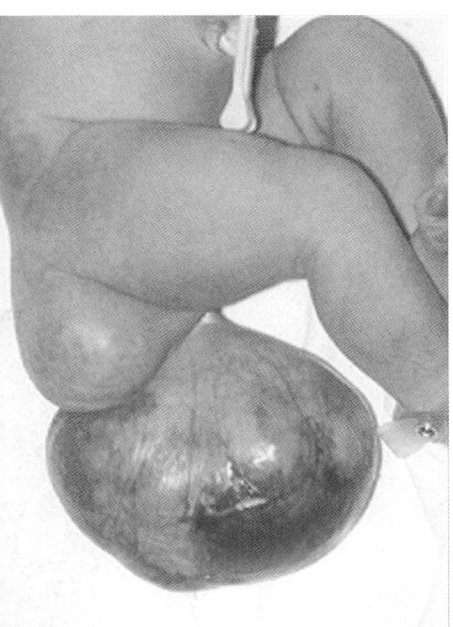

Fig. 36.3 Sacrococcygeal teratoma. *(Courtesy of Dr J. Berry.)*

evidence that complete resection is not necessary in those patients without poor-risk biological factors (Kaneko et al. 1998).

Prognosis

At all stages, infants with neuroblastoma have a much better prognosis than older children. The overall survival in infants with no adverse biological factors, even in the presence of metastatic disease, is >90% (De Bernardi et al. 2009). Deaths in those with stage 4s disease may rarely occur as a result of hepatic dysfunction or respiratory compromise. As in older children, the presence of adverse biological factors, particularly *MYCN* amplification, significantly affects the prognosis with a 2-year overall survival of around 30% (Canete et al. 2009).

Screening

Approximately 90% of infants with neuroblastoma have raised urinary catecholamines and these can be measured quantitatively to screen for disease. Screening programmes for children under 1 year of age were introduced in Japan in 1985. However, a number of studies have now shown that infant screening is associated with a twofold increase in the documented incidence of neuroblastoma but no decrease in the incidence of advanced-stage disease in older children (Woods et al. 1996) and no improvement in overall survival. Of interest is the increased number of early-stage patients diagnosed clinically during and after the screening programmes. This might have been due to the publicity surrounding the screening and increased awareness on the part of clinicians. This effect seemed to disappear within a few years of the termination of the screening programme (Barrette et al. 2007).

Teratoma and other germ cell tumours

Teratomas (the word is derived from the Greek *teras-atos*, meaning monster, and *-oma*, denoting tumour) are tumours derived from the three embryonic germ cell layers – ectoderm, mesoderm and endoderm. They are predominantly benign and arise in the gonads or in midline extragonadal sites. In the neonate, the commonest site is the sacrococcygeal region, occurring in 1 : 35 000–45 000 live births

(the commonest tumour of the newborn) with a 3 : 1 female to male preponderance (Rescorla et al. 1998). Tumours in this region may be postsacral (external), presacral (internal) or dumbbell-shaped (external and internal portions). Sacrococcygeal teratomas (SCTs) are mature in 65–70% of cases, immature in 5–15% (both benign) and classified as mixed malignant germ cell tumours (GCTs) in 15–30% of cases. The risk of malignancy, invariably yolk sac tumour, is greater in males and in cases with delayed surgery, and increases with the proportion of internal (presacral) tumour. Of neonatal teratomas, 45% arise in the sacral area, 20% in the ovary, 20% in the testis, 10% intracranially, with the cervical region and the mediastinum accounting for 5%.

Clinical features

The most common presentation in the newborn is that of an SCT, with a readily recognisable tumour lying between the buttocks. The tumour varies in size, from one that appears as a slight elevation or discoloration over the coccyx to one which equals the size of the baby and may cause hydrops fetalis or obstruction of labour. Diagnosis by antenatal ultrasound allows elective caesarean section, which must be weighed up against the risk from prematurity, although the baby may still succumb if the tumour is in a site causing vital organ obstruction or heart failure. With the huge postsacral SCTs (Fig. 36.3) there is usually very little presacral extension. However, presacral tumours may not be as rare in this age group as supposed and only become apparent in the older child, by which time they have a greater chance of being malignant.

Investigations

A lateral X-ray of the abdomen may show anterior displacement of the rectum and possible calcification within the tumour. A chest X-ray including a lateral view is important to rule out pulmonary metastases. Computed tomography (CT) scan of the abdomen and pelvis with bowel contrast may determine whether primary surgery is feasible. Serum tumour markers, alpha-fetoprotein (AFP) and human chorionic gonadatrophin (hCG) should be measured. High AFP levels are found in the normal newborn (mean 50 000 kU/l), and these gradually fall to adult levels (less than 10 kU/l) over the first year of life (Blair et al. 1987). This protein is produced by cells derived embryologically from either fetal yolk sac or liver, and the level is grossly elevated, often to several million kU/l, in teratomas containing malignant yolk sac tumour tissue. High AFP readings, as found in the normal newborn, should fall sequentially at an expected rate based on the half-life of AFP (5–7 days) in the absence of a malignant yolk sac tumour and fall at a similar rate after surgery. Failure to fall at the expected rate after surgery, or a subsequent rise, would indicate residual malignant yolk sac elements or the development of metastases.

Choriocarcinomas are occasionally seen and may secrete hCG. In infancy, they probably result from migration of maternal or placental tissue, and are perhaps better termed 'gestational trophoblastic tumours', being less aggressive than the highly malignant pure choriocarcinoma of adolescence and adulthood. Testicular yolk sac tumours may also present in this period.

Treatment

The treatment of benign SCTs is surgical removal. Removal of the entire coccyx en bloc is essential. Failure to do this will result in a local recurrence, approaching 40%. Approximately 10% of neonatally detected SCTs recur as malignant GCTs up to 3 years of age (Palmer et al. 2003). Follow-up of neonates with tumour markers for this period is therefore essential. Malignant recurrence usually requires chemotherapy, although the key prognostic intervention is the completeness of subsequent surgical resection. Surgery alone with long-term monitoring may be sufficient for small local relapses.

Where malignancy is suspected at the initial presentation (usually late diagnosis with raised AFP, bulky infiltrating lesion on imaging or metastases identified), preoperative chemotherapy is preferable and significantly increases the chance of complete resection and long-term survival (Gobel et al. 2001).

Functional impairment after surgery, particularly for large tumours and those with intrapelvic extension, may be commoner than previously thought. Follow-up to detect bladder or bowel dysfunction or lower limb weakness is mandatory (Rescorla et al. 1998).

Other malignant GCTs are generally treated with chemotherapy until the tumour markers have returned to normal, although surgery may be required to remove residual disease. The exception is stage 1 gonadal tumours, where surgical excision alone suffices. With modern chemotherapy using platinum-based drug regimens, the few neonates with malignant GCTs have an excellent chance of cure.

Acute leukaemia

Congenital and neonatal leukaemia represents 1% of all childhood leukaemia (Bresters et al. 2002) but is the second most common neonatal malignancy, exceeded only by neuroblastoma. Acute leukaemia in the neonatal period is equally distributed between acute lymphoblastic (ALL) and acute myeloid (AML) subtypes, unlike older children, where ALL accounts for about 80% of cases of leukaemia.

Clinical features

Babies may present with a range of clinical symptoms. Hepatosplenomegaly is common, together with symptoms of anaemia and thrombocytopenia such as bruising, pallor and poor feeding. CNS involvement is common and may present as a bulging fontanelle or neurological signs. A high white cell count with hyperviscosity may be responsible for respiratory, cardiac or neurological compromise. Skin infiltration, seen in about 20% of cases (Frangoul and Patterson 1998), presents as firm mobile nodules ranging in colour from blue to brown which typically wax and wane. Congenital leukaemia is a rare cause of hydrops fetalis and stillbirth.

Diagnosis

As congenital and infant leukaemia frequently present with a high white count, diagnosis may be possible by morphology and the appropriate immunohistochemistry of the peripheral blood. If non-diagnostic, a bone marrow aspirate is necessary. Biopsy of the skin nodules will show immature blast cells.

Up to 75% of cases of neonatal leukaemia have chromosome rearrangements involving the mixed lineage leukaemia (MLL) gene, usually arising from the translocation t(4;11)(q21;q23) (Greaves 1996). Other translocations found in infant leukaemia include t(1;11), t(11;19) in ALL and t(9;11), t(8;21) in AML (Greaves 1996). Recent studies of twins with concordant leukaemia suggest that acute leukaemia in childhood may have a prenatal origin. This has been further supported by the finding of chromosomal fusion sequences in archived Guthrie blood spots matched to children who later developed leukaemia (Wiemels et al. 2002).

Treatment/prognosis

Acute lymphoblastic leukaemia

The current treatment protocol is an intensive hybrid therapy consisting of both ALL and AML elements. The first such study, Interfant-99, reported a 47% event-free survival (EFS) at 4 years (Pieters et al. 2007). Analysis of prognostic factors showed that rearrangements in the MLL gene, a high white blood cell count, age younger than 6 months, and a poor response to the prednisone prephase were independently associated with inferior outcomes, as part of an international collaboration (Pieters et al. 2007). Congenital ALL (i.e. those diagnosed in the first month of life) is very rare and only 30 such infants were registered on the Interfant-99 study. Their disease was characterised by a higher white cell count, a higher incidence of MLL rearrangements and a higher relapse rate than in the older infants, with a 2-year EFS of only 20% (van der Linden et al. 2009). Several studies in children and adults with ALL have shown that minimal residual disease status is a strong prognostic factor. The same is true for infant disease and allows stratification according to risk (Van der Velden et al. 2009).

Acute myeloid leukaemia

Despite the many poor prognostic factors found in neonatal AML, such as high presenting white count and extramedullary disease (CNS and skin involvement), the outcome after intensive chemotherapy is similar to that of older children with AML, with 60–65% overall survival (Chessells et al. 2002).

Transient myeloproliferative disorder and Down syndrome

A number of neonates with Down syndrome will have a transient leukaemia or myeloproliferative disorder associated with a high incidence of spontaneous remission. Infants with this condition may be relatively asymptomatic or may have fulminant hepatic and multiorgan failure resulting in death in utero or infancy. Circulating blasts are myeloid and may range from a count of 5 to 384 000 (Homans et al. 1993). Somatic mutations in the haemopoietic transcription factor gene *GATA1*, located on the X chromosome and encoding a transcription factor essential for normal erythroid and megakaryocytic differentiation, have been found in almost all cases of Down-associated transient leukaemia (Massey 2005; Pine et al. 2007). Leukopheresis and/or exchange transfusion may be necessary to treat signs or symptoms of hyperviscosity, or organ failure. Chemotherapy is rarely needed, although low-dose cytarabine has been used to treat leukocytosis refractory to leukopheresis (Tchernia et al. 1996). It is estimated that approximately 30% of Down syndrome infants with transient myeloproliferative disorder will go on to develop acute leukaemia, most commonly acute megakaryocytic leukaemia (AMKL) during the first 4 years of life: the incidence is 500 times higher in Down syndrome than in normal children. *GATA1* mutations are also found in those children with Down syndrome who develop AMKL, but not in non-Down syndrome-related AMKL (Pine et al. 2007).

Renal tumours

Mesoblastic nephroma accounts for approximately 80% of solid renal masses in the neonate and for around 4% of early-infancy tumours. Although considered benign, they may rarely metastasise. They are composed of immature stromal cells that infiltrate the kidney parenchyma, synonymous with leiomyomatous hamartoma. Wilms' tumour and rhabdoid tumour are malignant renal neoplasms, and, although both are treated similarly, the latter has a considerably worse outcome (Isaacs 2008).

Wilms' tumour, or nephroblastoma, is rare in the neonatal period, accounting for 1% of all Wilms' tumours, with an incidence of 0.49 per million live births. This represents 1.8% of tumours diagnosed in the first 6 weeks of life (NRCT data). Various congenital abnormalities are associated with an increased risk of developing Wilms' tumour, many involving chromosome 11p, where the tumour-suppressor gene *WT1* (11p13) is found (Bove 1999). Loss of *WT1* is seen in WAGR syndrome (Wilms' tumour, aniridia, genitourinary tract abnormalities and mental retardation), Denys–Drash syndrome (congenital nephrotic syndrome and ambiguous genitalia) and the related Fraser syndrome, along with 10–15% of sporadic Wilms' tumours. The *WT2* gene (11p15) is affected in Beckwith–Wiedemann syndrome (Bove 1999). Additionally, 40% of all Wilms' tumours show loss of heterozygosity for alleles on chromosome 11 (Bove 1999). Other associated clinical conditions where 11p is not implicated include Edwards syndrome (trisomy 18), Sotos syndrome (5q35) and Bloom syndrome (15q26).

Clinical features

Most neonatal Wilms' tumours are discovered on clinical examination at a median age of 2 days, although more recently there has been an increase in antenatally detected masses (Leclair et al. 2005). Haematuria, unexplained anaemia and hypertension may be presenting features. Mesoblastic nephroma is typically diagnosed in the first week of life; it is uncommon beyond 3 months, and sometimes is associated with hypercalcaemia. The resulting polyuria is potentially a cause of polyhydramnios, occasionally seen with the condition (Fung et al. 1995).

Hydrocephalus, due to cerebral deposits of renal rhabdoid tumour, has also been reported (Bonnin et al. 1984).

Investigations

Abdominal CT with intravenous contrast will delineate the primary tumour. Chest X-ray is required as a minimum to identify metastases. Hypercalcaemia responds to nephrectomy, but hypertension needs careful evaluation as it is associated with a high intraoperative morbidity (Howell et al. 1982).

Treatment

Mesoblastic nephroma is treated by nephrectomy alone. Chemotherapy is only considered with incomplete excision or tumour rupture of the atypical/cellular histological type rather than the classical, leiomyomatous form.

For unilateral Wilms' tumours, current practice is surgery and postoperative chemotherapy according to surgical staging. Following biopsy, bilateral tumours receive chemotherapy first, in the hope that renal-sparing surgery may be possible later. Radiotherapy is avoided because of long-term sequelae.

Prognosis

The prognosis for mesoblastic nephroma is excellent (95% overall survival). Patients with a cellular mesoblastic nephroma, patients aged 3 months or older, and those with stage 3 disease had lower EFS (Furtwaengler et al. 2006). Wilms' tumours are invariably of favourable histology and predominantly stage 1. Their survival is excellent – 86% (van den Heuvel-Eibrink et al. 2008).

Rhabdoid tumours are usually fatal, irrespective of treatment (Ritchey et al. 1995).

Screening

Routine radiological screening for at-risk groups has been debated for many years and some would advocate that it is of dubious benefit where simple clinical examination may suffice (Craft et al. 1995). There is increasing support internationally for routine ultrasound for those with at least a 5% risk, 3-monthly and continuing until 7 years of age (Bove 1999). This generally includes those with Beckwith–Wiedemann syndrome (4–10% risk), *WT1*-associated syndromes, familial Wilms' or offspring of a parent previously treated for bilateral disease (if unilateral, risk 5%). Certain hemihypertrophy associations are likely to become included as more becomes known about the natural history.

Brain tumours

Although the most common solid malignancy in childhood, CNS malignancies are rare in the neonatal period, accounting for only 0.5–1.5% of all childhood CNS neoplasms (Wakai et al. 1984). Between 1981 and 2000, 15.5% of NRCT registrations in the first 6 weeks of life were CNS tumours, an incidence of 4.24 per million live births.

Neonatal brain tumours are predominantly supratentorial, and teratomas account for a third to a half of all cases. Teratomas frequently occur in the pineal or suprasellar region and may contain calcium visible on CT scan. Typically they are very large, rapidly growing and often histologically mature. Because of their size, they are rarely totally excised and there is a high operative mortality (Isaacs 2002a, b).

Glial tumours such as astrocytomas account for 20–30% of neonatal tumours, with primitive neuroectodermal tumours (PNETs or medulloblastoma if infratentorial) the next most common. Choroid plexus papillomas are infrequent but overrepresented in this age group, whilst others, such as craniopharyngiomas, ependymomas and meningiomas, are rarely seen (Isaacs 2002a, b).

Clinical features

The majority will present with macrocephaly, which may be diagnosed antenatally, or present with obstructed labour. Otherwise, a rapidly enlarging head circumference may become evident in the first week, frequently associated with hydrocephalus. Vomiting, listlessness, poor weight gain, neurological signs and seizures may occur but are less common, owing to the ability of the skull to expand (Wakai et al. 1984; Isaacs 2002a, b).

Investigations

Neonatal brain tumours are often large, heterogeneous and rapidly growing. CT or magnetic resonance imaging (MRI) will delineate the tumour (Fig. 36.4), and determine operability and the presence of metastases. Extracranial metastases are seen in some cases of PNET (Isaacs 2002a, b).

Low-grade gliomas, particularly of the optic tract, may be predictive of type 1 neurofibromatosis, whilst subependymal giant cell astrocytomas are unique to tuberous sclerosis and are usually seen outside the neonatal period (see Table 36.2).

Treatment

Complete surgical resection is the treatment of choice for most tumours, although operability is dependent upon the site and size of the primary. Chemotherapy may be used as part of an aggressive treatment approach for PNET and ependymomas, although it is unclear whether this confers any survival advantage in neonates owing to the small numbers reported to date. However, in infants below 36 months of age, surgery followed by intensive chemotherapy, thereby delaying or avoiding radiotherapy, resulted in equivalent survival to historical studies universally including

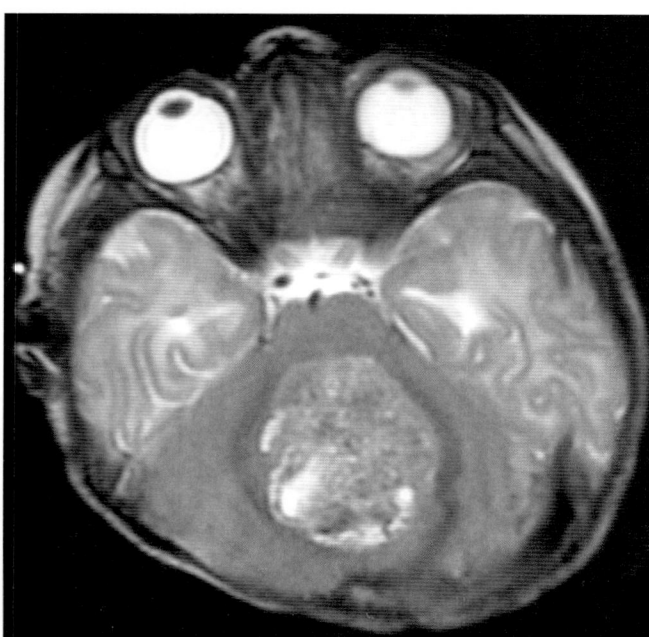

Fig. 36.4 Posterior fossa brain tumour.

radiotherapy (Geyer et al. 2005). Radiotherapy is avoided owing to the high incidence of cognitive, endocrine and neuropsychological sequelae, and together with high-grade malignant lesions and/or tumour progression is associated with poor functional outcomes (Gerber et al. 2008).

Prognosis

A literature review of 250 published neonatal cases determined an overall 5-year survival of 28% (Isaacs 2002a, b) and this is similar to larger series studying neonates and infants (Geyer et al. 2005). Teratomas and PNETs generally had a very poor outcome, whilst survival was significantly better for astrocytomas and choroid plexus papillomas.

Retinoblastoma

Retinoblastoma is the commonest intraocular tumour in children and accounts for 3% of all childhood tumours. It produces progressive destruction of the retina, and occupies the globe, before spreading to the orbit and brain. Familial (i.e. indicative of an inherited germline mutation) in up to 70% of cases and with a female preponderance of 1.5:1 (Abramson et al. 2002), the incidence in the neonatal period will depend on the local screening policy regarding those with a family history. The NRCT has recorded 37 cases of retinoblastoma over a 20-year period (1981–2000), accounting for 9% of malignancies in the first 6 weeks of life, with an incidence of 2.57 per million live births. A review of all neonatal retinoblastomas seen in New York (Abramson et al. 2002) identified 46 cases diagnosed in the first 30 days of life (2.5% of all retinoblastomas), of which 56% were unilateral. Of these unilateral cases, 85% subsequently developed a tumour in the contralateral eye during follow-up (i.e. 91% had bilateral disease at some point).

The retinoblastoma gene was identified on chromosome 13q14, and is either partially or totally deleted in retinoblastoma (Friend et al. 1986). As more becomes known about the retinoblastoma gene (*Rb1*) and there is further progress in molecular and cytogenetic techniques, it may be possible to predict the occurrence of these tumours by fetal chromosome analysis, especially in familial cases.

Clinical features

Those tumours not detected by elective screening are most likely to present with leukocoria (Fig. 36.5), heterochromia of the iris and strabismus.

Investigations

Staging by the Reese–Ellsworth classification (Abramson et al. 2002), or the International Intraocular Retinoblastoma Classification, is based on the size, number, distribution and local dissemination of the tumours (Gallie et al. 2009). Assessment of tumours is by ophthalmoscopic examination under anaesthetic, together with CT scanning or MRI, which also have the benefit of identifying any extraocular spread.

Treatment

Treatment is dependent upon tumour extent and there has been a move towards eye-sparing therapy. The choice of therapy depends upon the location as well as the size of the tumour, and may include

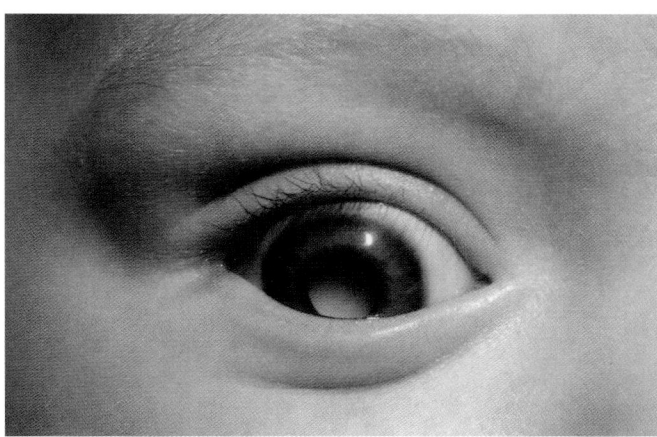

Fig. 36.5 Leukocoria.

cryotherapy, laser or plaque therapy, or cyclical chemotherapy. In the New York series (Abramson et al. 2002), 79% of diseased eyes were salvaged. Reese–Ellsworth group 5 tumours typically require early enucleation. If bilateral, conservative management is usually attempted first in order to preserve the less severely affected eye, although primary enucleation of the most severely affected eye may be required to reduce the likelihood of extraocular spread. External-beam radiotherapy is avoided where possible because of the physical effects and a marked increase in secondary tumour risk.

Prognosis

For unilateral neonatal retinoblastoma there is an 85% chance of retinoblastoma development in the contralateral eye (Abramson et al. 2002), hence regular ophthalmic follow-up is required. The prognosis is dependent upon the treatment modality employed, but generally 5-year survival exceeds 90%. However, the outcome in cases of metastatic disease is exceedingly poor.

Pineoblastoma is the second tumour most frequently seen in familial (bilateral) retinoblastoma. There is an increased risk of such tumours in the first 4 years of life, and because of retinal differentiation seen on histology these have been termed 'trilateral retinoblastomas'. They are thought to be multicentric primaries rather than metastatic deposits and are usually fatal.

There is also an increased chance of developing another second tumour, most frequently an osteosarcoma, the locus for which is closely linked to that of the retinoblastoma gene. This usually follows local irradiation, with a cumulative risk of 1–2% per year for a secondary non-ocular malignancy (Abramson et al. 2002), although there is also concern surrounding the contribution of repeated CT scans. Secondary malignancies are predominantly of high grade and carry a poor prognosis.

Risk to offspring

Following identification of retinoblastoma with a germline *Rb1* mutation, screening the family for this mutation is recommended (Gallie et al. 2009). Germline mutations in familial disease are inherited in an autosomal dominant fashion with 90% penetrance. Hence, there is a 50% risk of carriage and a 45% risk of disease, and, even if retinoblastoma does not develop, the future risk of developing other tumours and of passing the gene to subsequent offspring remains. Where neither parent is affected, the sibling risk for retinoblastoma is 1% in unilateral disease and 6% in bilateral

or multifocal disease. This risk falls with every subsequent unaffected child (Margo et al. 1998).

Sarcomas

Soft-tissue tumors account for approximately 25% of neonatal tumors and are benign in more than two-thirds of cases (Minard-Colin et al. 2009). Malignant soft-tissue tumours account for 11% of neonatal tumours, but only 2% of childhood sarcomas are diagnosed in the newborn period.

Infantile fibrosarcoma is one of the commonest soft-tissue sarcomas. Although histologically similar to fibrosarcoma in adults, the biology is often not malignant and classification as a true sarcoma is questionable. It presents as a soft-tissue mass, most commonly in the head, neck or extremities. Cytogenetic abnormalities have been described (Alaggio et al. 2008). The treatment of choice is surgical excision, although local recurrences have been reported. Metastases are rare. Because of the overall benign nature of the condition, the role of chemotherapy is limited to those where surgical resection would be disfiguring. The most commonly used agents are vincristine, actinomycin D and cyclophosphamide (Russell et al. 2009).

Rhabdomyosarcomas rarely present at birth. Of the 3217 patients entered on the Intergroup Rhabdomyosarcoma Study, 14 were less than 30 days of age (Lobe et al. 1994). Similar figures have been reported for the International Society of Paediatric Oncology malignant mesenchymal studies where, of 102 registered infants less than 1 year of age, 24 were less than 3 months and 16 less than 1 month (Orbach et al. 2005). The most common primary sites are the genitourinary system, extremities or head and neck. Rhabdomyosarcoma has been classified histologically as alveolar, embryonal or botyroid. The last two are the most common types in the neonatal period. Chromosomal abnormalities are commonly found and may be helpful both in diagnosis and in the understanding of tumorigenesis (Barr 1997).

Treatment consists of chemotherapy and surgery. Radiotherapy is generally avoided because of the effects on growth and function. Prognosis depends on the presence of metastases and, to a lesser extent, on the site of disease. Approximately 20–25% of patients with metastatic disease are expected to be long-term survivors, as compared with 82% of those with localised disease. Infants with the alveolar histological subtype have a poorer overall survival (37% at 5 years) than those with non-alveolar rhabdomyosarcoma (82% at 5 years) (Orbach et al. 2005).

Rare neonatal sarcomas include Ewing's tumour, extraosseous Ewing's tumours, liposarcomas and leiomyosarcomas (van den Berg et al. 2008; Minard-Colin et al. 2009).

Liver tumours

The only primary liver malignancy seen in the neonatal period is hepatoblastoma, which may be associated with hemihypertrophy or Beckwith–Wiedemann syndrome (see Table 36.2) or very low birthweight (<1000 g) (Spector et al. 2008). The differential diagnosis of liver masses includes secondary deposits from neuroblastoma or choriocarcinoma, along with benign lesions such as haemangiomas, hamartomas, adenomas and cysts (Isaacs 2007a). Haemangioma and hepatoblastoma are the commonest lesions, often difficult to distinguish by imaging (angiogram or MRI), or by tumour markers due to the normally high AFP seen at birth (Blair et al. 1987) and may require biopsy for diagnosis. Around 40 cases of neonatal hepatoblastoma have been reported in the literature, although few have received standard infant treatment (chemotherapy followed by surgery) and consequently the reported mortality rate is high (Ammann et al. 1999). Metastases are usually pulmonary in the older child, although this is rarely seen in the neonate, where 10–15% have metastases, but usually at non-pulmonary sites. This is thought to be due to the fetal circulation bypassing the pulmonary vasculature. Bone scan and MRI of the brain are required for staging.

Histiocytosis

The histiocytoses are a group of poorly understood conditions resulting from abnormal proliferation of histiocyte/mononuclear cells (including antigen-presenting cells). Predominantly benign conditions, they are frequently overseen by paediatric oncologists, as they may require intervention with chemotherapy or, rarely, irradiation, despite a strong immunological basis to the disease, with cytotoxic T-cell deficiency and excessive interleukin and prostaglandin E_2 production.

Langerhans' cell histiocytosis (LCH) is a clonal proliferation of Langerhans' cells distinguished by the presence of Birbeck granules on electron microscopy, and is usually benign. It may present in the neonate with single-system (SS) or, more typically, multisystem (MS) disease. Skin lesions are extremely common in neonatal LCH irrespective of type (Minkov et al. 2005), although solitary painful swelling or incidental discoveries on X-ray may also be a presenting feature (for either SS or MS-LCH), as well as the possibility of failure to thrive, hepatospenomegaly, lymphadenopathy and/or dyspnoea in MS-LCH (Isaacs 2006) Diagnosis is confirmed on biopsy. Many SS-LCH lesions spontaneously involute, although local treatments may become necessary, including topical corticosteroids for skin lesions, surgical excision, intralesional or systemic steroids (with or without vinblastine) for persistent or progressive disease (Minkov et al. 2005). Generally the prognosis is excellent, although in a minority the disease can recur.

The term Hashimoto–Pritzker disease is still sometimes used to describe the congenital self-healing reticulohistiocytosis and purely cutaneous form of LCH. Red–purple nodules, similar to healing chickenpox lesions, occur predominantly on the scalp, spontaneously regressing over a few weeks or months.

MS-LCH is considerably less likely to resolve spontaneously, and the presence of 'risk organ' involvement (liver, spleen, haemopoietic system, lungs), which is more common in neonatal presentations, necessitates treatment with chemotherapy to avert organ dysfunction. Response to chemotherapy is variable with a 5-year survival of 57%, which is significantly lower than for infants below 1 year of age and for children more generally is probably attributable to risk organ involvement (Minkov et al. 2005).

Haemophagocytic lymphohistiocytosis (HLH) is rarely seen in the neonatal period. This is usually the familial form and there may be a family history (autosomal recessive) or consanguinity. HLH is a non-clonal proliferation of histiocytes without Birbeck granules. This manifests with fever, splenomegaly, pancytopenia, hypofibrinogenaemia and hypertriglyceridaemia. Haemophagocytosis is seen in lymph node biopsy or bone marrow, and, untreated, is rapidly fatal. Treatment involves chemotherapy and allogeneic bone marrow transplantation, with a 3-year EFS of 44% (Baker et al. 1997). Secondary HLH is a consequence of infection or malignancy, for which supportive therapy and chemotherapy alone are preferred.

Juvenile xanthogranuloma is a very rare form of dendritic cell histiocytosis that may present with neonatal skin rashes and/or organ involvement in a similar way to LCH.

Other rare tumours

Many other rare malignancies may also occur in the neonatal period and appear as isolated cases within incidence series (Gale et al. 1982; Isaacs 1985; Campbell et al. 1987; Davis et al. 1988).

Melanoma is the most frequent, and may arise in large congenital pigmented naevi or following transplacental spread. These lesions can regress spontaneously. Treatment is surgery and, rarely, chemotherapy, with less than 60% surviving 18 months (Richardson et al. 2002).

Throughout this chapter, histologically benign tumours have been included, as they are important in the differential diagnosis of malignant tumours (e.g. mature teratomas, mesoblastic nephroma) or may be fatal, often because of the site of disease (e.g. CNS tumours, hepatic haemangiomas).

Haemangiomas may occur at any site and may be associated with high-output cardiac failure or thrombocytopenia, the Kasabach – Merritt syndrome. They may respond to α-interferon, although spastic diplegia has been reported as a consequence of treatment (Barlow et al. 1998).

Cystic hygromas (congenital lymphatic malformation) are most frequently seen in the posterior neck, often associated with Turner syndrome or the trisomies. Surgery is preferred, although inoperable or recurrent malformations may respond to intralesional bleomycin or OK-432 (Howarth et al. 2005).

Other benign lesions include rhabdomyomas (seen in tuberous sclerosis), myofibromatoses, lipomas, ovarian cysts and epidermal or dermal cysts. Many are excised, although some spontaneously regress or require no intervention.

References

Abramson, D.H., Du, T.T., Beaverson, K.L., 2002. (Neonatal) retinoblastoma in the first month of life. Arch Ophthalmol 120, 738–742.

Agha, M.M., Williams, J.I., Marrett, L., et al., 2005. Congenital abnormalities and childhood cancer. Cancer 103, 1939–1948.

Alaggio, R., Barisani, D., Ninfo, V., et al., 2008. Morphologic overlap between infantile myofibromatosis and infantile fibrosarcoma: a pitfall in diagnosis. Pediatr Dev Pathol 11, 355–362.

Ammann, R.A., Plaschkes, J., Leibundgut, K., 1999. Congenital hepatoblastoma: a distinct entity? Med Pediatr Oncol 32, 466–468.

Bader, J.L., Miller, R.W., 1979. US cancer incidence and mortality in the first year of life. Am J Dis Child 133, 157–159.

Baker, K.S., DeLaat, C.A., Steinbuch, M., et al., 1997. Successful correction of hemophagocytic lymphohistiocytosis with related or unrelated bone marrow transplantation. Blood 89, 3857–3863.

Barlow, C.F., Priebe, C.J., Mulliken, J.B., et al., 1998. Spastic diplegia as a complication of interferon Alfa-2a treatment of hemangiomas of infancy. J Pediatr 132, 527–530.

Barr, F.G., 1997. Molecular genetics and pathogenesis of rhabdomyosarcoma. J Pediatr Hematol Oncol 19, 483–491.

Barrette, S., Bernstein, M.L., Robison, L.L., et al., 2007. Incidence of neuroblastoma after a screening program. J Clin Oncol 25, 4929–4932.

Berry, P.J., 1987. Fetal and Neonatal Pathology. Springer-Verlag, London.

Blair, J.I., Carachi, R., Gupta, R., et al., 1987. Plasma alpha fetoprotein reference ranges in infancy: effect of prematurity. Arch Dis Child 62, 362–369.

Bonnin, J.M., Rubinstein, L.J., Palmer, N.F., et al., 1984. The association of embryonal tumors originating in the kidney and in the brain. A report of seven cases. Cancer 54, 2137–2146.

Borch, K., Jacobsen, T., Olsen, J.H., et al., 1992. Neonatal cancer in Denmark 1943–1985. Pediatr Hematol Oncol 9, 209–216.

Bove, K.E., 1999. Wilms' tumor and related abnormalities in the fetus and newborn. Semin Perinatol 23, 310–318.

Bresters, D., Reus, A.C., Veerman, A.J., et al., 2002. Congenital leukaemia: the Dutch experience and review of the literature. Br J Haematol 117, 513–524.

Brodeur, G.M., Maris, J.M., Yamashiro, D.J., et al., 1997. Biology and genetics of human neuroblastomas. J Pediatr Hematol Oncol 19, 93–101.

Campbell, A.N., Chan, H.S., O'Brien, A., et al., 1987. Malignant tumours in the neonate. Arch Dis Child 62, 19–23.

Canete, A., Gerrard, M., Rubie, H., et al., 2009. Poor survival for infants with MYCN-amplified metastatic neuroblastoma despite intensified treatment: the International Society of Paediatric Oncology European Neuroblastoma Experience. J Clin Oncol 27, 1014–1019.

Caughey, R.W., Michels, K.B., 2009. Birth weight and childhood leukemia: a meta-analysis and review of the current evidence. Int J Cancer 124, 2658–2670.

Chessells, J.M., Harrison, C.J., Kempski, H., et al., 2002. Clinical features, cytogenetics and outcome in acute lymphoblastic and myeloid leukaemia of infancy: report from the MRC Childhood Leukaemia working party. Leukemia 16, 776–784.

Craft, A.W., Parker, L., Stiller, C., et al., 1995. Screening for Wilms' tumour in patients with aniridia, Beckwith syndrome, or hemihypertrophy. Med Pediatr Oncol 24, 231–234.

Crom, D.B., Wilimas, J.A., Green, A.A., et al., 1989. Malignancy in the neonate. Med Pediatr Oncol 17, 101–104.

Davis, C.F., Carachi, R., Young, D.G., 1988. Neonatal tumours: Glasgow 1955–86. Arch Dis Child 63, 1075–1078.

De Bernardi, B., Gerrard, M., Boni, L., et al., 2009. Excellent outcome with reduced treatment for infants with disseminated neuroblastoma without MYCN gene amplification. J Clin Oncol 27, 1034–1040.

Frangoul, H.A., Patterson, K., 1998. Complications of acute leukemia. Case one: congenital acute myelogenous leukemia with cutaneous involvement. J Clin Oncol 16, 3199–3200.

Friend, S.H., Bernards, R., Rogelj, S., et al., 1986. A human DNA segment with properties of the gene that predisposes to retinoblastoma and osteosarcoma. Nature 323, 643–646.

Friend, S.H., Dryja, T.P., Weinberg, R.A., 1988. Oncogenes and tumor-suppressing genes. N Engl J Med 318, 618–622.

Fung, T.Y., Fung, Y.M., Ng, P.C., et al., 1995. Polyhydramnios and hypercalcemia associated with congenital mesoblastic nephroma: case report and a new appraisal. Obstet Gynecol 85, 815–817.

Furtwaengler, R., Reinhard, H., Leuschner, I., et al., 2006. Mesoblastic nephroma – a report from the Gesellschaft für Pädiatrische Onkologie und Hämatologie (GPOH). Cancer 106, 2275–2283.

Gale, G.B., D'Angio, G.J., Uri, A., et al., 1982. Cancer in neonates: the experience at the Children's Hospital of Philadelphia. Pediatrics 70, 409–413.

Gallie, B.L., Gronsdahl, P., Dimaras, H., et al., 2009. National Retinoblastoma Strategy Canadian Guidelines for Care: Stratégie thérapeutique du retinoblastome guide clinique canadien. Can J Ophthalmol 44 (Suppl 2), S1–88.

Gerber, N.U., Zehnder, D., Zuzak, T.J., et al., 2008. Outcome in children with brain tumours diagnosed in the first year of life: long-term complications and quality of life. Arch Dis Child 93, 582–589.

Geyer, J.R., Sposto, R., Jennings, M., et al., 2005. Multiagent chemotherapy and deferred radiotherapy in infants with malignant brain tumors: a report from the Children's Cancer Group. J Clin Oncol 23, 7621–7631.

Gobel, U., Schneider, D.T., Calaminus, G., et al., 2001. Multimodal treatment of malignant sacrococcygeal germ cell tumors: a prospective analysis of 66 patients of the German cooperative protocols MAKEI 83/86 and 89. J Clin Oncol 19, 1943–1950.

Greaves, M.F., 1996. Infant leukaemia biology, aetiology and treatment. Leukemia 10, 372–377.

Halperin, E.C., 2000. Neonatal neoplasms. Int J Radiat Oncol Biol Phys 47, 171–178.

Hero, B., Simon, T., Spitz, R., et al., 2008. Localized infant neuroblastomas often show spontaneous regression: results of the prospective trials NB95-S and NB97. J Clin Oncol 26, 1504–1510.

Homans, A.C., Verissimo, A.M., Vlacha, V., 1993. Transient abnormal myelopoiesis of infancy associated with trisomy 21. Am J Pediatr Hematol Oncol 15, 392–399.

Howarth, E.S., Draper, E.S., Budd, J.L., et al., 2005. Population-based study of the outcome following the prenatal diagnosis of cystic hygroma. Prenat Diagn 25, 286–291.

Howell, C.G., Othersen, H.B., Kiviat, N.E., et al., 1982. Therapy and outcome in 51 children with mesoblastic nephroma: a report of the National Wilms' Tumor Study. J Pediatr Surg 17, 826–831.

Isaacs Jr, H., 1985. Perinatal (congenital and neonatal) neoplasms: a report of 110 cases. Pediatr Pathol 3, 165–216.

Isaacs, H., 2002a. I. Perinatal brain tumors: a review of 250 cases. Pediatr Neurol 27, 249–261.

Isaacs Jr, H., 2002b. II. Perinatal brain tumors: a review of 250 cases. Pediatr Neurol 27, 333–342.

Isaacs Jr, H., 2006. Fetal and neonatal histiocytoses. Pediatr Blood Cancer 47, 123–129.

Isaacs Jr, H., 2007a. Fetal and neonatal hepatic tumors. J Pediatr Surg 42, 1797–1803.

Isaacs Jr, H., 2007b. Fetal and neonatal neuroblastoma: retrospective review of 271 cases. Fetal Pediatr Pathol 26, 177–184.

Isaacs Jr, H., 2008. Fetal and neonatal renal tumors. J Pediatr Surg 43, 1587–1595.

Kaneko, M., Iwakawa, M., Ikebukuro, K., et al., 1998. Complete resection is not required in patients with neuroblastoma under 1 year of age. J Pediatr Surg 33, 1690–1694.

Knudson Jr, A.G., 1985. Hereditary cancer, oncogenes, and antioncogenes. Cancer Res 45, 1437–1443.

Leclair, M.D., El-Ghoneimi, A., Audry, G., et al., 2005. The outcome of prenatally diagnosed renal tumors. J Urol 173, 186–189.

Lobe, T.E., Wiener, E.S., Hays, D.M., et al., 1994. Neonatal rhabdomyosarcoma: the IRS experience. J Pediatr Surg 29, 1167–1170.

Lukens, J.N., 1999. Neuroblastoma in the neonate. Semin Perinatol 23, 263–273.

Margo, C.E., Harman, L.E., Mulla, Z.D., 1998. Retinoblastoma. Cancer Control 5, 310–316.

Massey, G.V., 2005. Transient leukemia in newborns with Down syndrome. Pediatr Blood Cancer 44, 29–32.

McNutt, D.M., Holdsworth, M.T., Wong, C., et al., 2006. Rasburicase for the management of tumor lysis syndrome in neonates. Ann Pharmacother 40, 1445–1450.

Minard-Colin, V., Orbach, D., Martelli, H., et al., 2009. [Soft tissue tumors in neonates.] Arch Pediatr 16, 1039–1048.

Minkov, M., Prosch, H., Steiner, M., et al., 2005. Langerhans cell histiocytosis in neonates. Pediatr Blood Cancer 45, 802–807.

Orbach, D., Rey, A., Oberlin, O., et al., 2005. Soft tissue sarcoma or malignant mesenchymal tumors in the first year of life: experience of the International Society of Pediatric Oncology (SIOP)

Malignant Mesenchymal Tumor Committee. J Clin Oncol 23, 4363–4371.

Palmer, R.D., Nicholson, J.C., Hale, J.P., 2003. Management of germ cell tumours in childhood. Curr Paediatr 13, 213–220.

Parkes, S.E., Muir, K.R., Southern, L., et al., 1994. Neonatal tumours: a thirty-year population-based study. Med Pediatr Oncol 22, 309–317.

Pieters, R., Schrappe, M., De Lorenzo, P., et al., 2007. A treatment protocol for infants younger than 1 year with acute lymphoblastic leukaemia (Interfant-99): an observational study and a multicentre randomised trial. Lancet 370, 240–250.

Pine, S.R., Guo, Q., Yin, C., et al., 2007. Incidence and clinical implications of GATA1 mutations in newborns with Down syndrome. Blood 110, 2128–2131.

Pritchard, J., Hickman, J.A., 1994. Why does stage 4s neuroblastoma regress spontaneously? Lancet 344, 869–870.

Rescorla, F.J., Sawin, R.S., Coran, A.G., et al., 1998. Long-term outcome for infants and children with sacrococcygeal teratoma: a report from the Childrens Cancer Group. J Pediatr Surg 33, 171–176.

Richardson, S.K., Tannous, Z.S., Mihm Jr, M.C., 2002. Congenital and infantile melanoma: review of the literature and report of an uncommon variant, pigment-synthesizing melanoma. J Am Acad Dermatol 47, 77–90.

Ritchey, M.L., Azizkhan, R.G., Beckwith, J.B., et al., 1995. Neonatal Wilms tumor. J Pediatr Surg 30, 856–859.

Roman, E., Fear, N.T., Ansell, P., et al., 2002. Vitamin K and childhood cancer: analysis of individual patient data from six case-control studies. Br J Cancer 86, 63–69.

Russell, H., Hicks, M.J., Bertuch, A.A., et al., 2009. Infantile fibrosarcoma: clinical and histologic responses to cytotoxic chemotherapy. Pediatr Blood Cancer 53, 23–27.

Sbragia, L., Paek, B.W., Feldstein, V.A., et al., 2001. Outcome of prenatally diagnosed solid fetal tumors. J Pediatr Surg 36, 1244–1247.

Sebire, N.J., Jauniaux, E., 2009. Fetal and placental malignancies: prenatal diagnosis and management. Ultrasound Obstet Gynecol 33, 235–244.

Spector, L.G., Johnson, K.J., Soler, J.T., et al., 2008. Perinatal risk factors for hepatoblastoma. Br J Cancer 98, 1570–1573.

Tchernia, G., Lejeune, F., Boccara, J.F., et al., 1996. Erythroblastic and/or megakaryoblastic leukemia in Down syndrome: treatment with low-dose arabinosyl cytosine. J Pediatr Hematol Oncol 18, 59–62.

van den Berg, H., Dirksen, U., Ranft, A., et al., 2008. Ewing tumors in infants. Pediatr Blood Cancer 50, 761–764.

van den Heuvel-Eibrink, M.M., Grundy, P., Graf, N., et al., 2008. Characteristics and survival of 750 children diagnosed with a renal tumor in the first seven months of life: A collaborative study by the SIOP/GPOH/SFOP, NWTSG, and UKCCSG Wilms tumor study groups. Pediatr Blood Cancer 50, 1130–1134.

van der Linden, M.H., Valsecchi, M.G., De Lorenzo, P., et al., 2009. Outcome of congenital acute lymphoblastic leukemia treated on the Interfant-99 protocol. Blood 114, 3764–3768.

Van der Velden, V.H., Corral, L., Valsecchi, M.G., et al., 2009. Prognostic significance of minimal residual disease in infants with acute lymphoblastic leukemia treated within the Interfant-99 protocol. Leukemia 23, 1073–1079.

Voute Jr, P.A., Wadman, S.K., van Putten, W.J., 1970. Congenital neuroblastoma. Symptoms in the mother during pregnancy. Clin Pediatr (Phila) 9, 206–207.

Wakai, S., Arai, T., Nagai, M., 1984. Congenital brain tumors. Surg Neurol 21, 597–609.

Weitzman, S., Grant, R., 1997. Neonatal oncology: diagnostic and therapeutic dilemmas. Semin Perinatol 21, 102–111.

Wiemels, J.L., Xiao, Z., Buffler, P.A., et al., 2002. In utero origin of t(8;21) AML1-ETO translocations in childhood acute myeloid leukemia. Blood 99, 3801–3805.

Woods, W.G., Tuchman, M., Robison, L.L., et al., 1996. A population-based study of the usefulness of screening for neuroblastoma. Lancet 348, 1682–1687.

Xue, H., Horwitz, J.R., Smith, M.B., et al., 1995. Malignant solid tumors in neonates: a 40-year review. J Pediatr Surg 30, 543–545.

Orthopaedic problems
in the neonate

Christopher J Dare   N M P Clarke

37

© 2012 Elsevier Ltd

Introduction

With the advent of high-resolution ultrasound scanning (USS), orthopaedic problems are being increasingly detected during routine antenatal screening – for example, talipes equinovarus, limb deficiency and complex syndactyly. This is creating a need for neonatologists and those in fetal medicine to have a better knowledge of orthopaedic problems relevant to the newborn infant. Early diagnosis should facilitate appropriate referral and counselling, which should lead to an improvement in parent satisfaction and outcome for the child.

A whole range of factors can have an impact on the developing fetus, resulting in orthopaedic problems in the neonate. Some of these are well understood, such as genetic influences in achondroplasia and drug-related problems such as thalidomide; others are less well understood, such as congenital talipes equinovarus (CTEV) and developmental dysplasia of the hip (DDH). In this chapter we aim to give the reader some understanding and a working knowledge of the common and rarer orthopaedic problems affecting the neonate.

Lower limb abnormalities

Developmental dysplasia of the hip

Terminology

The nomenclature of this condition has been open to debate recently, as it encompasses a whole range of conditions other than frank dislocation of the hip. These include congenital subluxation of the hip, developmental dysplasia and dislocatable hip. It is now accepted that hips are rarely truly dislocated at birth but are merely unstable and go on to develop problems at a later stage. Therefore, the condition formerly known as congenital dislocation of the hip is more correctly referred to as developmental dysplasia of the hip or DDH (Klisic 1989). DDH is the term used throughout this book.

Hips that are truly dislocated at birth are rare, and the cause usually involves teratological factors. The aetiology is thus entirely different to DDH, and is usually secondary to neuromuscular conditions such as arthrogryposis multiplex congenita (AMC) and spina bifida.

Incidence of developmental dysplasia of the hip

The incidence of DDH is approximately 1–2 per 1000 live births. The incidence of unstable hips at birth ranges from 5 to 20 per 1000 live births, but the majority (60%) of these go on spontaneously to stabilise (Barlow 1962). The difference in incidence is thought to be due to transplacental passage of maternal relaxin causing temporary ligamentous instability in the early neonatal period, as well as to differences in diagnostic method and timing of evaluation. There are geographical variations thought to be genetic in northern Italians and environmental in North American Indians (Haynes 2001).

Risk factors

For 60% of neonates with DDH, no known risk factor(s) can be identified (Standing Medical Advisory Committee, Standing Nursing and Midwifery Advisory Committee Working Parties for the Secretary of State for Social Services and Wales 1986). In 20% of cases, the condition is bilateral. There are, however, well-documented risk factors for DDH, such as positive family history, female sex, first-born children, oligohydramnios, macrosomia and breech presentation. When there is a positive family history, there is a 6% risk for one affected child, a 12% risk with one affected parent and a 36% risk with one affected child and one affected parent. In monozygotic twins there is 43% concordance, with 3% concordance in dizygotic twins. Girls are affected more than boys at a ratio of 5:1. There is an increased incidence in first-born Caucasian children (Haynes 2001). Oligohydramnios and macrosomia increase the risk owing to the simple mechanics of a crowded intrauterine environment. The left hip is more often affected than the right, which is attributed to the right shoulder more often being anterior in breech presentation. With the right shoulder anterior, the left hip is compressed against the maternal sacral promontory, a position favouring dislocation. Breech presentation increases the risk, particularly in breech with extended knees, which increases the incidence by a factor of 10 (Broughton 1997). Extrauterine factors that increase the risk of DDH include swaddling clothes and the now historic use of cradle boards to hold the hips in the extended position.

DDH is also associated with other congenital anomalies, including torticollis, metatarsus adductus, CTEV, congenital vertical talus (CVT) and calcaneovalgus (see below) (Broughton 1997).

Screening

Since 1966, as part of routine postnatal screening, the hips of newborn children are clinically examined by employing the Ortolani and Barlow tests (Ortolani 1937; Barlow 1962) (pp. 257–258). Both these tests are subject to inter- and intraobserver variability and hence their sensitivity varies with the experience of the examiner. In some reported studies, as many as 50% of established cases of clinical hip abnormality are missed by clinical examination alone. They remain, however, the standard screening test for DDH in the newborn infant in the UK (Bialik et al. 1999).

Prior to the advent of routine screening, the number of cases of DDH matched the number requiring surgery (1–2/1000). However, since the introduction of routine clinical screening, the number of identified cases of DDH has increased significantly (5–20/1000) along with the number undergoing abduction splinting (3–4/1000). Alongside this increase has been a significant decrease in the number undergoing surgery for DDH (0.2–0.7/1000). However, since the introduction of clinical screening, the number of late-presenting cases of DDH has changed very little and may have increased slightly. This may be because primary clinical examination fails to identify hip displacement or that no clinical abnormality was present or detectable at that stage. This questions the validity of clinical examination alone as a screening tool and it is now accepted that the clinical tests are not 100% specific or sensitive.

Clinical examination and findings

Ortolani's test is performed by flexing and abducting the hips. A dislocated hip will 'clunk' back into the normal acetabular position as the hip is abducted. The Barlow test, however, is a provocative test, which aims to displace a dysplastic hip from its normal acetabular position. This test is performed by adducting and flexing the hip to 90°, and applying downward force through the femur in a posterolateral direction while the pelvis is stabilised. A positive test is indicated by the hip displacing posteriorly when this force is applied. With older children, these tests become less appropriate, because secondary signs develop (restriction of abduction, shortening and thigh crease asymmetry). Finally, a child with undiagnosed unilateral DDH will often be noted to have asymmetric limb lengths and will walk with a limp.

Investigations

The femoral head in the newborn is an entirely cartilaginous structure and only begins to ossify between 4 and 7 months of age. Radiological assessment of the hip in the first few months of life is difficult, and, in most centres, ultrasound is employed.

USS has proved to be a very cost-effective, non-invasive, non-irradiating way of assessing hip stability (Fig. 37.1). Ultrasound visualises the cartilaginous and soft-tissue structures around the hip (Fig. 37.2) and is now the first-line investigation for DDH in neonates with clinical suspicion or when there are risk factors (Clarke et al. 1985; Boeree and Clarke 1994).

In some centres in the UK, both static and dynamic ultrasonography are now routinely used in the initial assessment and for the assessment of treatment of DDH (Taylor and Clarke 1997).

There currently exist no national set guidelines on the initial diagnosis and management of DDH. Some children will be splinted on clinical suspicion alone, while others will also undergo USS in addition to clinical assessment. The UK Hip Trial recommends the use of ultrasound assessment of clinically unstable hips but advocates caution with clinically stable hips in at-risk children (Elbourne et al. 2002). This stance is taken because of the risk of exposing babies to unnecessary abduction splinting when the natural history of ultrasound-diagnosed hip dysplasia is not clearly understood.

Referral and treatment

Following detection of the at-risk neonate by either clinical assessment or risk factor identification, the baby is referred on for further assessment by ultrasonography. The authors use treatment algorithms for subsequent management (Figs 37.3 and 37.4) (Taylor

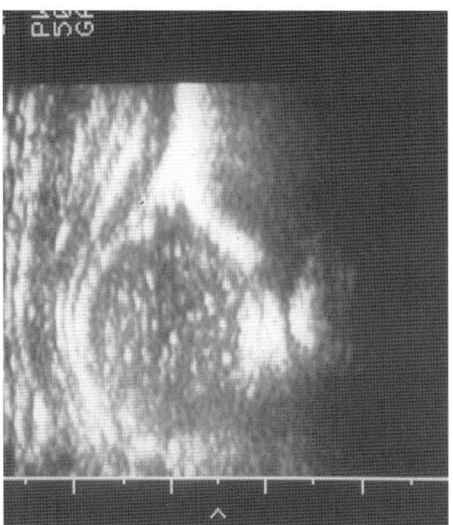

(A)

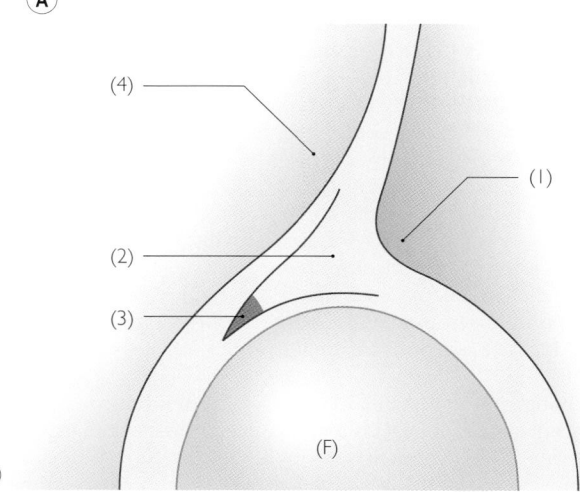

(B)

Fig. 37.2 (A) Ultrasound scan image of a normal neonatal hip. (B) The acetabular rim area of the right hip: 1, osseous rim; 2, cartilaginous rim; 3, fibrocartilaginous limbus; 4, joint capsule; F, femoral head. *(Reproduced from Graf (1984).)*

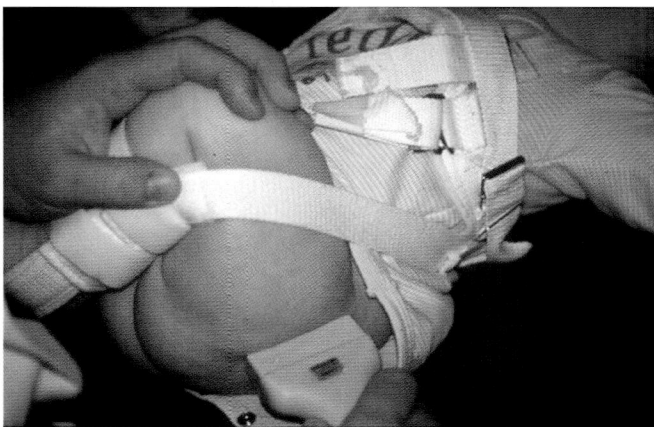

Fig. 37.1 Dynamic ultrasound of a left hip of a child in a Pavlik harness.

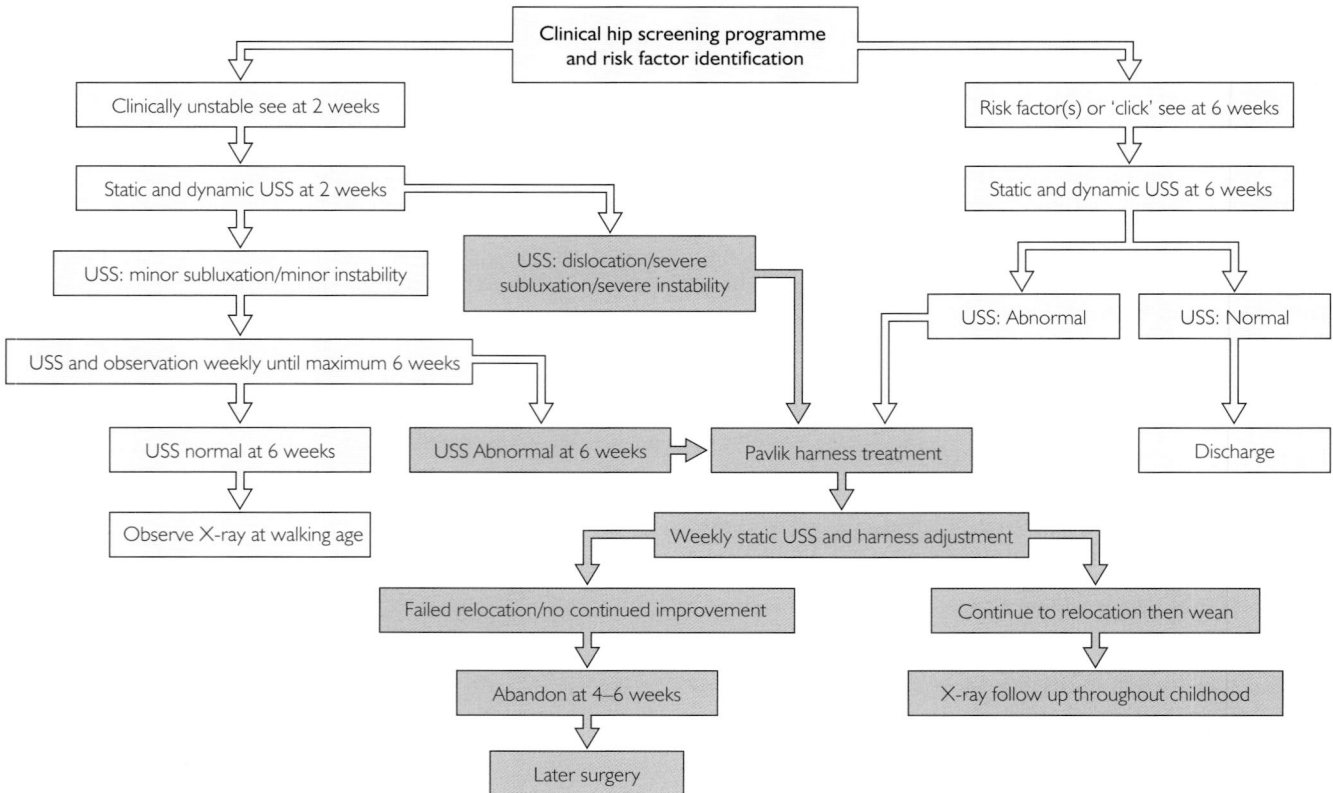

Fig. 37.3 Treatment algorithm for developmental dysplasia of the hip in the newborn. USS, ultrasound scanning.

and Clarke 1997). Those neonates with clinically unstable hips are referred and seen urgently within 2 weeks, and those with identified risk factors or 'clicky' hips are seen at 6 weeks.

There has been much debate about the role of ultrasound in the screening process, as some believe that ultrasonographic screening is too sensitive and therefore overdiagnoses DDH. As a result, a small percentage of babies are exposed to the risks of unnecessary splinting. As more information is gathered on the natural history of subtle ultrasound abnormalities of the neonatal hip, and abduction splintage is delayed in these cases until persistent ultrasonographic abnormalities are present at 6 weeks, this overdiagnosis of significant DDH is likely to decrease in the future.

Once assessed by ultrasound, subsequent management is dictated by the degree or otherwise of hip instability, with the mainstay of treatment being the abduction harness (Fig. 37.5).

The Pavlik harness is the commonest abduction device which encourages dynamic hip relocation (Pavlik 1992; Cashman et al. 2002). Other abduction devices do exist, such as the Von Rosen and Denis Browne splints, which are rigid in structure. Failure to respond to treatment or delay in presentation results in a more invasive surgical treatment which includes arthrography (Fig. 37.6).

Although it is now standard practice to apply abduction splintage when a diagnosis of DDH is made, concerns have been raised about how sound this treatment strategy is. Despite abduction splinting commencing before 8 weeks of age, a small percentage of babies will still have radiological evidence of hip dysplasia and 12% will have undergone surgery by the age of 2 years. It is clear that some babies will develop dysplasia despite splinting and these babies will be exposed to the risks of abduction splinting. Because the

unaffected hip in unilateral DDH is also splinted, there is a small risk of iatrogenic complications. These include avascular necrosis (1–4% of cases), pressure sores, epiphysitis, femoral nerve palsy, inferior dislocation of the hip and medial instability of the knee joint. These risks are inevitable when treating an affected hip but may be unacceptable if they affect the 'normal' hip. Therefore, much of the current research on the management of DDH is focused on identifying those 'clicky' hips that will resolve spontaneously and those that will definitely require some form of intervention.

The efficacy of abduction splinting has been shown in prospective longitudinal trials but this method of treatment has not yet been subject to a randomised trial. It is now apparent that this will be necessary to develop treatment strategies for hips which are clinically stable but demonstrate borderline abnormalities on ultrasound.

As has been previously stated, the current clinical screening tests are not the most reliable, and much debate has been generated about the inclusion of routine USS to identify those hips that require treatment and those that do not. This is an important issue, as there may be significant adverse long-term sequelae if DDH is not diagnosed and treated. Therefore, a dichotomy exists between overdiagnosing and overtreating DDH that may settle spontaneously, exposing the baby to unnecessary risk, and underdiagnosing DDH, which may result in degenerative changes of the hip in early adult life.

This begs the question of whether there is a need for a national screening programme inclusive of ultrasound assessment, for all children, to identify all cases of DDH in the absence of clinical instability. However, until the use of abduction harnesses has been properly evaluated and further expertise in neonatal hip

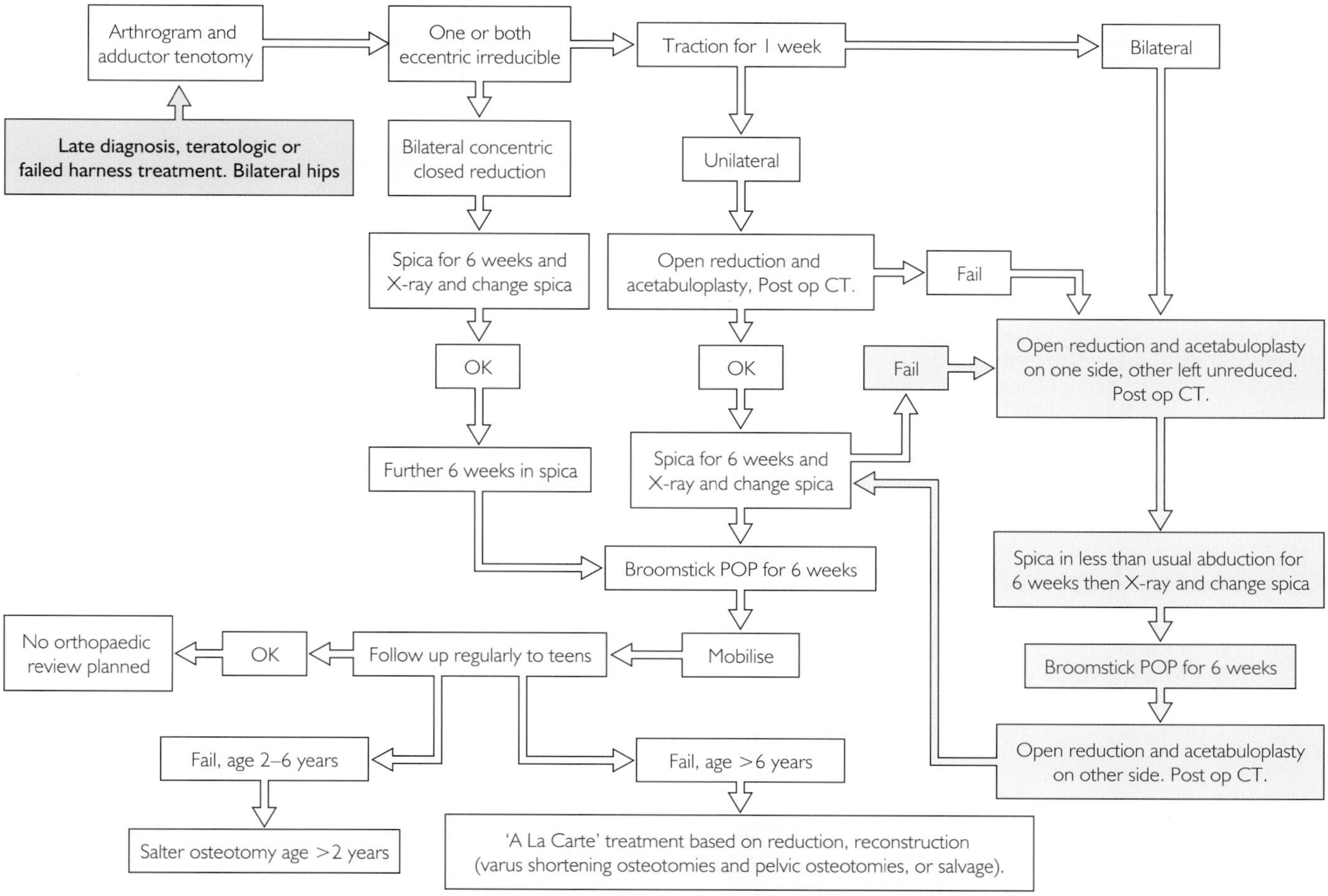

```
                                                       ┌──────────────────┐
┌──────────────────┐      ┌──────────────────┐         │ Traction for 1   │────────────────────────────► ┌──────────────┐
│ Arthrogram and   │─────►│ One or both      │────────►│ week             │                              │ Bilateral    │
│ adductor tenotomy│      │ eccentric irreducible│     └──────────────────┘                              └──────────────┘
└──────────────────┘      └──────────────────┘                  │                                                │
         ▲                         │                             ▼                                                │
┌──────────────────────────┐       ▼                   ┌──────────────────┐                                       │
│ Late diagnosis, teratologic or │ ┌──────────────────┐│ Unilateral       │                                       │
│ failed harness treatment. Bilateral hips │ │ Bilateral concentric ││                  │                         │
└──────────────────────────┘       │ closed reduction  │└──────────────────┘                                     │
                            └──────────────────┘         │                                                        │
                                    │                    ▼                                                        │
                                    ▼          ┌──────────────────────┐   ┌──────┐                                ▼
                          ┌──────────────────┐ │ Open reduction and   │──►│ Fail │    ┌────────────────────────────────────┐
                          │ Spica for 6 weeks and│ │ acetabuloplasty, Post op CT.│ └──────┘   │ Open reduction and acetabuloplasty │
                          │ X-ray and change spica│└──────────────────────┘             │ on one side, other left unreduced. │
                          └──────────────────┘         │              ┌──────┐          │ Post op CT.                        │
                                    │                   ▼              │ Fail │──►       └────────────────────────────────────┘
                                    ▼          ┌──────────────┐        └──────┘                        │
                              ┌──────────┐     │ OK           │                                         │
                              │ OK       │     └──────────────┘                                         ▼
                              └──────────┘           │                            ┌────────────────────────────────────┐
                                    │                ▼                            │ Spica in less than usual abduction for │
                                    ▼          ┌──────────────────┐               │ 6 weeks then X-ray and change spica    │
                          ┌──────────────────┐ │ Spica for 6 weeks and│           └────────────────────────────────────┘
                          │ Further 6 weeks in spica│ │ X-ray and change spica│                        │
                          └──────────────────┘ └──────────────────┘                                    ▼
                                    │                │                            ┌────────────────────────────────────┐
                                    └───────►┌──────────────────────┐             │ Broomstick POP for 6 weeks         │
                                             │ Broomstick POP for 6 weeks│        └────────────────────────────────────┘
                                             └──────────────────────┘                          │
                                                      │                                         ▼
┌──────────────┐  ┌──────┐ ┌──────────────────────┐ ┌──────────┐        ┌────────────────────────────────────┐
│ No orthopaedic │◄─│ OK   │◄│ Follow up regularly to teens │◄│ Mobilise │  │ Open reduction and acetabuloplasty │
│ review planned │ └──────┘ └──────────────────────┘ └──────────┘        │ on other side. Post op CT.         │
└──────────────┘                  │            │                        └────────────────────────────────────┘
                    ┌──────────────────┐   ┌──────────────────┐
                    │ Fail, age 2–6 years│◄─│ Fail, age >6 years │
                    └──────────────────┘   └──────────────────┘
                             │                     │
                             ▼                     ▼
               ┌──────────────────────┐ ┌────────────────────────────────────────────┐
               │ Salter osteotomy age >2 years│ │ 'A La Carte' treatment based on reduction, reconstruction │
               └──────────────────────┘ │ (varus shortening osteotomies and pelvic osteotomies, or salvage). │
                                         └────────────────────────────────────────────┘
```

Fig. 37.4 Treatment algorithm for developmental dysplasia of the hip in children with delayed presentation or failed Pavlik treatment. CT, computed tomography; POP, plaster of Paris.

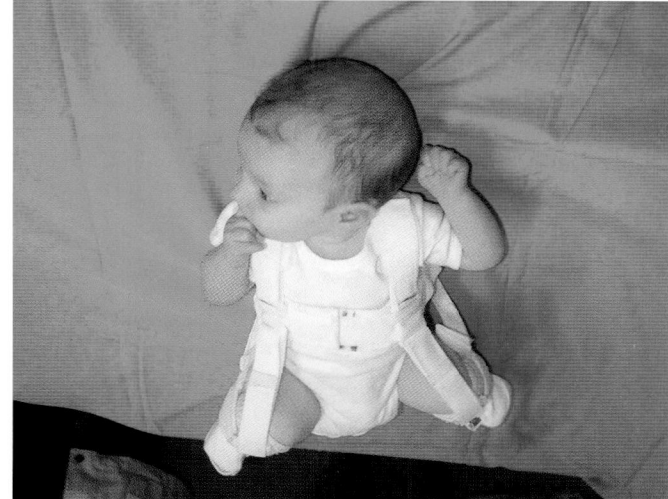

Fig. 37.5 Child in a Pavlik harness.

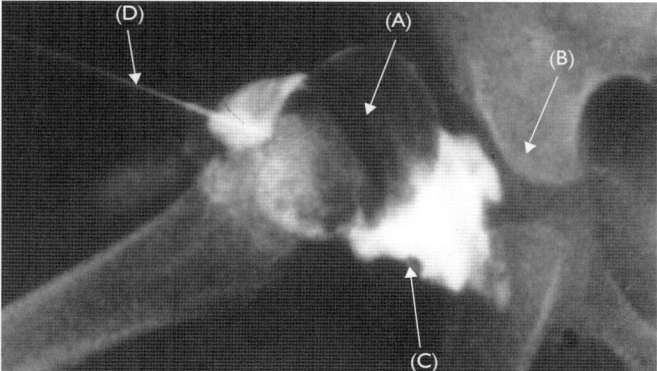

Fig. 37.6 Arthrogram of a dislocated right hip: (A) femoral head (dislocated); (B) dysplastic acetabulum; (C) medial pooling of contrast; (D) spinal needle to introduce contrast.

ultrasonography is developed nationally, this would be premature. A national screening programme incorporating USS, as seen in Germany and Norway, is unlikely to be instigated in the UK in the foreseeable future because of financial and personnel resource problems.

Congenital dislocation of the knee

Incidence

The incidence of congenital dislocation of the knee (CDK) is approximately 1 per 100 000 live births, which is about 100 times less than that of DDH, making it exceedingly rare. It is commonly associated with other congenital anomalies – DDH in 45% of cases and CTEV in 35% of cases – as well as torticollis and congenital dislocation of the elbow. It is a more frequent finding in children with AMC and myelodysplasia and those with Larsen syndrome (a condition of ligamentous laxity). It is bilateral in approximately a third of cases and has a predilection for females at a ratio of 2 : 1 (Neibauer and King 1960; Stern 1968; Curtis and Fisher 1969; Nogi and MacEwen 1982; Austwick and Dandy 1983).

Aetiology

The underlying cause for CDK is poorly understood but several factors have been postulated. In an otherwise normal breech child, oligohydramnios has been proposed as a mechanical cause, with crowding in utero holding the legs in an extended position with the feet locked under the mandible or axillae. Other suggestions include congenital abnormalities of the quadriceps (fibrous contracture) and absent cruciate ligaments, although these may be secondary findings as a result of the dislocation.

It has also been described in children with Down syndrome and in children with other chromosomal defects.

Clinical findings and presentation

The abnormality is usually obvious at birth, with the knee(s) hyper-extended (recurvatum) (Fig. 37.7A). In severe forms, the tibia may be in contact with the chest, with the feet tucked under the axilla or mandible (Stern 1968). X-ray evaluation (Fig. 37.7B) will reveal complete dislocation in the severe form, with the proximal tibia

anterior and lateral to the distal femur. Clinically, the patella may be subluxed laterally and the femoral condyles are prominent posteriorly. In the first few hours after birth the knee is usually flexible but any delay in treatment can result in a fixed deformity.

Referral and treatment

CDK is an orthopaedic emergency and immediate orthopaedic referral is essential. The optimal treatment for CDK remains controversial, with some advocating early surgical intervention and others conservative treatment (Austwick and Dandy 1983). Success of conservative treatment is dependent on early referral within the first 24 hours following delivery. The exception to this is when CDK is found in association with Larsen syndrome and arthrogryposis. A variety of conservative treatments are available, including serial casting, Pavlik harness, skin traction and skeletal traction.

If it is possible, gentle traction and direct reduction should be attempted in the first 24 hours, followed by splinting or casting with the knee in 90° of flexion. If this is not possible, then passive stretching of the quadriceps and the anterior knee capsule, combined with splinting or serial casting of the knee in an increasingly flexed position, is an alternative method.

It has been suggested that the pathoanatomy of CDK resembles that of DDH in that failure to reduce the joint early results in soft-tissue contracture with a resultant fixed deformity, which requires surgical correction (Stern 1968; Curtis and Fisher 1969; Nogi and MacEwen 1982).

Prognosis

When CDK is treated in the early stages, i.e. the first day of life, then conservative measures are most likely to produce a good functional range of movement of the knee with no further intervention required. In those cases of CDK associated with other musculoskeletal abnormalities, the prognosis remains good but conservative treatment tends to be more protracted. In older children with moderate to severe subluxation or with dislocation, surgical intervention is invariably required.

Congenital talipes equinovarus

This is a structural abnormality affecting the feet of children. It may be unilateral or bilateral, with the feet held in an adducted, supinated, plantar-flexed position (Fig. 37.8). This position is achieved by a combination of adduction and supination of the forefoot with

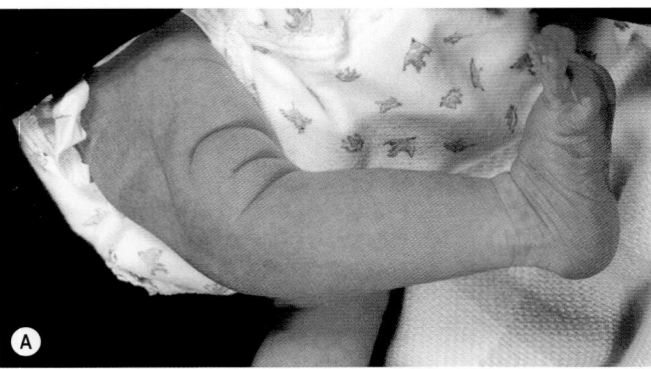
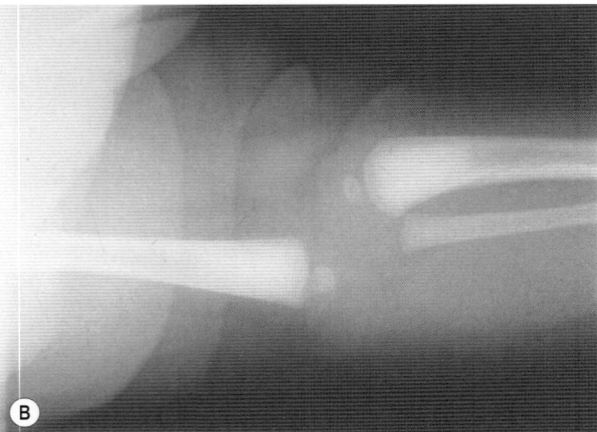

Fig. 37.7 (A) Clinical appearance of a right congenitally dislocated knee. (B) X-ray demonstrating the radiological appearance of a right congenitally dislocated knee.

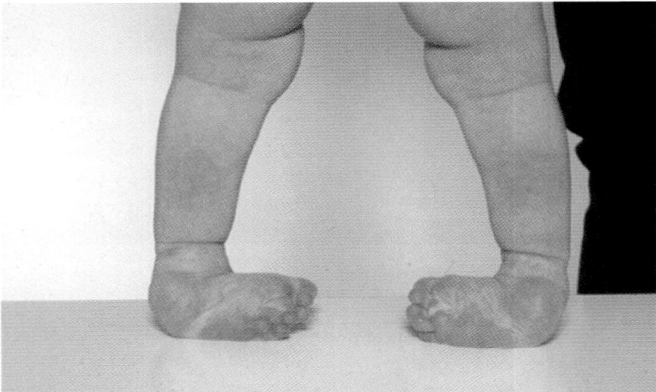

Fig. 37.8 Typical appearance of bilateral congenital talipes equinovarus.

a varus deformity of the heel and with the whole foot held in equinus at the ankle. The abnormal position is reflected in the bony architecture of the foot. The lateral malleolus is positioned postero-laterally and the head of the talus points anterolaterally (instead of anteromedially); the navicular is subluxed medially around the head of the talus and may even be in contact with the medial malleolus. With the talus lying obliquely in relation to the calcaneum, excess pressure on the anteromedial part of the calcaneum forces it into varus and equinus to compensate for the abnormally positioned talus (Carroll et al. 1978).

Incidence

In the UK, the incidence of CTEV is approximately 1 per 1000 live births, but geographical variations exist worldwide, with an incidence of 0.57 per 1000 for Orientals and 6.81 per 1000 in Polynesians. There is a sex difference, with a male preponderance of 2–3:1, and the condition is bilateral in 50% of cases (Barlow and Clarke 1994).

Aetiology

The aetiology of CTEV is poorly understood but a variety of hypotheses have been put forward, including external compression in utero, abnormal tendon and ligament attachments, neuromuscular dysfunction and germ plasm defect (Carroll et al. 1978; Tachdjian 1990).

External compression in utero is thought to account for postural talipes, a variety of talipes deformity which is fully correctable at birth and resolves spontaneously with stretching. Abnormalities in the ligaments and tendons of CTEV feet have been well documented. Neurological dysfunction with abnormalities in muscle innervation and muscle imbalance and delayed muscle maturation have also been proposed as aetiological factors. However, the most widely accepted hypothesis is the germ plasm defect theory, which suggests that the primary defect is in the development of the bones of the tarsus (principally the talus), and the other abnormalities are adaptive to this underlying defect (Carroll et al. 1978; Tachdjian 1990; Barlow and Clarke 1994; Broughton 1997).

Clinical features and classification

The affected feet are held adducted, supinated and plantar-flexed (equinus) and classically have been graded as benign, moderate, severe and very severe. This classification is subjective and open to inter- and intraobserver errors. A variety of more objective grading systems do exist but the most widely adopted is the Dimeglio classification (Dimeglio et al. 1995).

Dimeglio grading system for CTEV

Dimeglio devised a scoring system based on the morphological characteristics and the stiffness of the foot, in an attempt to standardise the grading of CTEV and hence prognostic outlook and response to treatment. A score is attributed for morphological features, i.e. deep plantar crease and a deep heel crease. A second score is attributed for the suppleness of the foot. The sum of the scores attributes a Dimeglio grade to the feet. This is a complex and comprehensive system for producing a reproducible assessment of club feet, and should be employed at the first orthopaedic appointment. A simpler, easier, but less exact assessment, also described by Dimeglio, can be employed at the bedside to give a rough assessment of Dimeglio grade and hence prognosis.

A foot that is held in the classic position but is 90% correctable (20% of all club feet), and appears very similar to positional talipes,

is said to be soft–soft (Dimeglio grade I). A foot that is reducible but partly resistant is said to be soft–stiff (Dimeglio grade II, 33% of all club feet). A foot that is resistant but partly reducible is said to be stiff–soft (Dimeglio grade III, 35% of all club feet). Feet that are almost irreducible are said to be stiff–stiff (Dimeglio grade IV, 12% of all club feet).

Radiological assessment of the feet plays no part in initial management of the feet in the neonate, as most of the bony structures of the foot remain cartilaginous anlages, making radiological assessment inaccurate. It is of more benefit in the older child, when ossification of the bony elements of the foot has occurred.

Referral and treatment

Antenatal diagnosis of CTEV is becoming increasingly common with the advent of high-resolution ultrasound, allowing time for appropriate antepartum counselling.

Early referral is important postnatally, even in the premature infant, as treatment should begin as soon as is practicable.

In the first instance, even before or simultaneously with orthopaedic referral, physiotherapy is required. Stretching exercises should be taught to the parent(s) and commenced as soon as possible, in order to stretch the tight ligaments and capsules at a time when they are likely to be most lax. Forceful correction of the deformity should, however, be avoided, as this may lead to harm.

Following orthopaedic assessment and grading, treatment will be either conservative or interventional. Conservative treatment is applied to Dimeglio grade I feet and consists of stretching exercises and regular orthopaedic review to assess progress and resolution.

Conservative treatment, proposed by Ponseti and Smoley (1963), consists of application of serial above-knee plaster casts changed on a weekly basis for 5 weeks, gradually correcting the adductus and supination deformity by reducing the forefoot around the talus (Fig. 37.9). On the sixth week, a tendo-Achilles tenotomy is undertaken to correct the equinus deformity and the plaster is applied for a further 4 weeks (Fig. 37.10). At the end of this period, the casts are removed and the child placed in a splint – so-called boots on a bar (Fig. 37.11) – to maintain the correction until walking age.

Early relapse or failure to respond to treatment requires further intervention, as outlined in the treatment algorithm for CTEV (Fig. 37.12) (Uglow and Clarke 2000a, b).

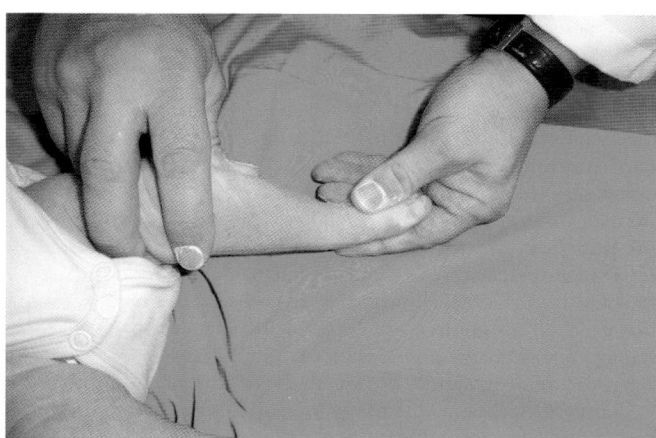

Fig. 37.9 Child undergoing the Ponseti regimen for congenital talipes equinovarus, demonstrating the maximum amount of correction of the foot prior to application of the plaster cast.

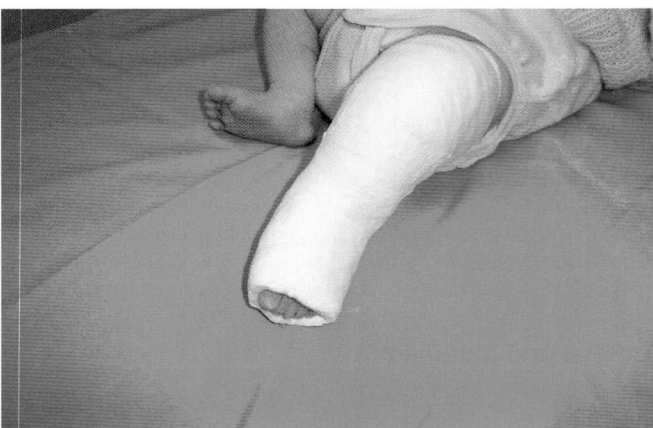

Fig. 37.10 The same foot as in Fig. 37.9, showing the cast in situ, demonstrating how the forefoot adductus, supination and equinus are held in a corrective position along with correction of the internal tibial torsion.

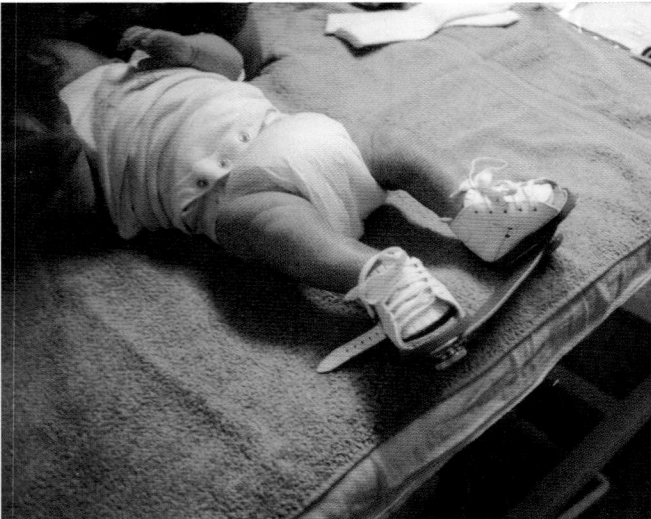

Fig. 37.11 Boots on a bar, showing how the corrective position is maintained when the child is out of plaster following tendo-Achilles tenotomy.

Prognosis

The prognosis for CTEV is difficult to quantify at present. On the whole, the long-term outlook is very good for all grades of feet, with only a very small number going on to require salvage surgery. But measures of outcome clearly differ between clinicians and parents. The principal aim of orthopaedic surgeons is to produce a functional pain-free foot, with cosmesis not being a clinical indication for intervention. With Dimeglio grade II–IV feet, in most cases the foot is never morphologically 'normal'. Parents, however, focus on the appearance of the child and look at appearance posttreatment as a measure of outcome. Parents need to be made aware that the condition affects the whole of the lower limb as a unit and a small foot and calf are normal features, particularly with Dimeglio grade IV feet. There may be significant variation in shoe size between affected and unaffected feet. A degree of forefoot adductus and dynamic supination may need to be accepted providing the foot is functional and pain free, as to correct minor variations would involve major surgery for little gain.

Metatarsus adductus

This is a relatively common condition in the neonate, and parents should be reassured that it is usually self-correcting in 85% of cases.

It is important to note that approximately 5–10% of neonates with metatarsus adductus will have an associated DDH, and careful screening of the hips is therefore required.

The typical appearance is of a kidney-bean shape to the sole of the foot, with a curve on the lateral side beginning at the base of the fifth metatarsal and with the toes pointing inwards (Fig. 37.13). It is usually bilateral but not symmetrical and may have an associated internal tibial torsion. The abnormality is usually flexible and the forefoot can be corrected to the neutral position.

It is thought to occur in simple cases because of intrauterine moulding and can be compounded postnatally by neonates sleeping in the prone position, a sleeping position no longer advocated by paediatricians.

If there is still a significant problem at 12 months, serial casting or soft-tissue release may be indicated (Ghali et al. 1984; Berg 1986).

In all but a very few children the deformity will be corrected by conservative measures alone.

Calcaneovalgus

This benign condition is not an infrequent neonatal finding. The ankle is unusually lax and the foot is noted to be excessively dorsiflexed – so much so, the forefoot touches the tibia (Fig. 37.14). The foot is also in valgus (away from the midline) and may even rest on the lateral side of the lower limb.

This condition is frequently associated with hip dysplasia, meaning that examination of the hips is required. We recommend USS of the hips in all babies with calcaneovalgus feet.

It is thought that the aetiology of this condition is related to intrauterine moulding and hence it is a more frequent finding in oligohydramnios. Calcaneovalgus is also more common in first-born children.

Treatment is by passive stretching of the foot in the direction of neutrality. A paediatric physiotherapist should be involved early to educate the parent(s) and give instruction on stretching exercises. Occasionally the deformity is more rigid and serial casting may need to be employed gradually to correct the deformity.

The majority of cases resolve completely with these simple conservative measures.

Congenital vertical talus ('rocker-bottom' foot, congenital pes planus, congenital convex pes valgus)

This is a rare condition in the neonate and is characterised by a dysmorphic foot (Fig. 37.15A). The forefoot is dorsiflexed and abducted and the heel is in valgus and equinus. When viewed laterally, the plantar surface of the foot is curved, with the apex at the midtarsal joint. In contrast to calcaneovalgus, which may have a similar appearance, the deformity is fixed and non-flexible. If doubt exists about the diagnosis, X-rays are usually diagnostic (Fig. 37.15B). In 85% of cases there is an associated congenital anomaly such as AMC, myelomeningocoele, myelodysplasia, diastematomyelia, sacral agenesis, DDH, or Turner or Edward syndrome (Tachdjian 1990; Broughton 1997).

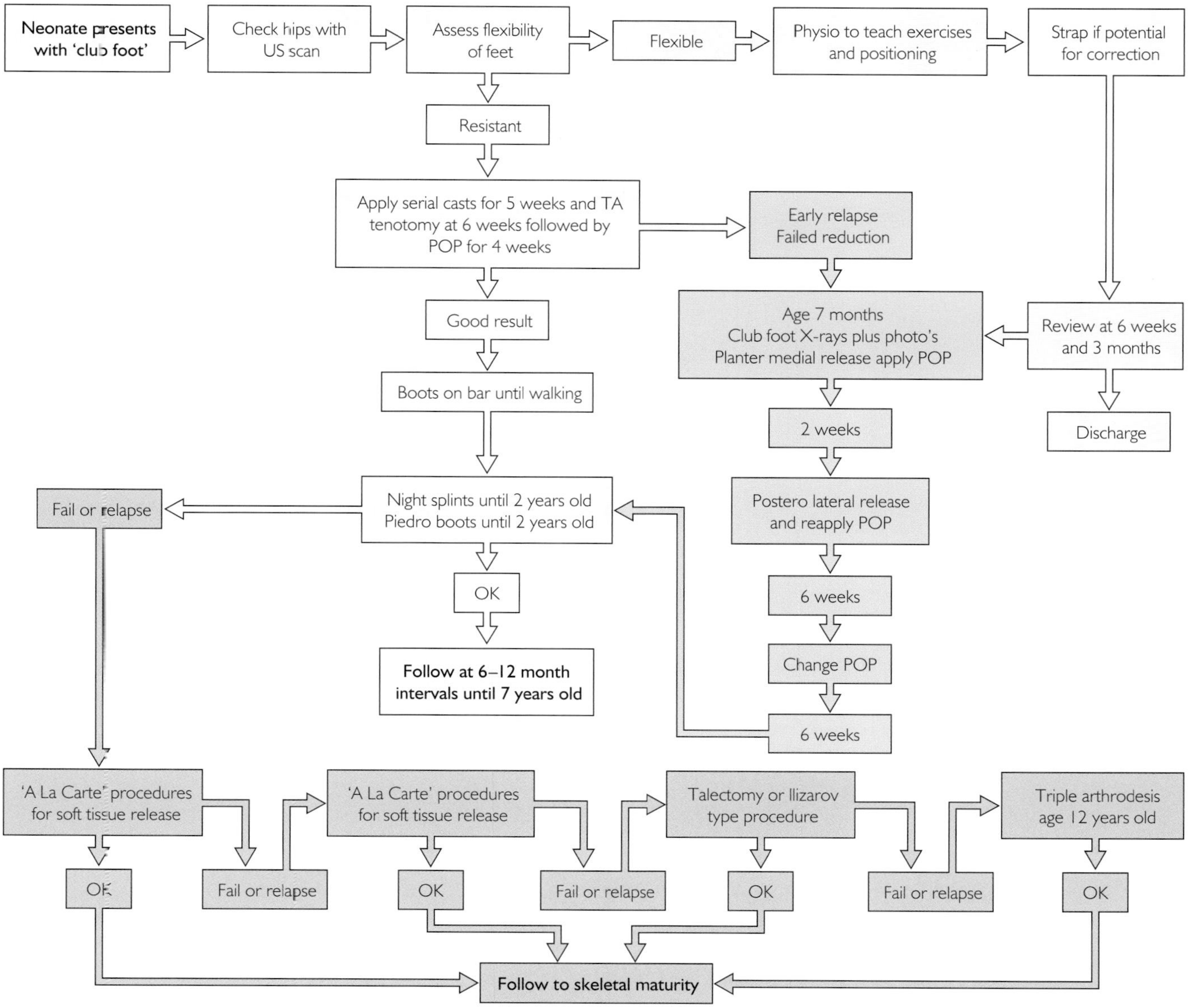

Neonate presents with 'club foot' → Check hips with US scan → Assess flexibility of feet → Flexible → Physio to teach exercises and positioning → Strap if potential for correction

Resistant

Apply serial casts for 5 weeks and TA tenotomy at 6 weeks followed by POP for 4 weeks → Early relapse Failed reduction

Good result

Boots on bar until walking

Age 7 months Club foot X-rays plus photo's Planter medial release apply POP ← Review at 6 weeks and 3 months

2 weeks

Discharge

Fail or relapse ← Night splints until 2 years old Piedro boots until 2 years old

Postero lateral release and reapply POP

OK

6 weeks

Follow at 6–12 month intervals until 7 years old

Change POP

6 weeks

'A La Carte' procedures for soft tissue release | 'A La Carte' procedures for soft tissue release | Talectomy or Ilizarov type procedure | Triple arthrodesis age 12 years old

OK | Fail or relapse | OK | Fail or relapse | OK | Fail or relapse | OK

Follow to skeletal maturity

Fig. 37.12 Treatment algorithm for congenital talipes equinovarus. US, ultrasound; TA, tendo-Achilles; POP, plaster of Paris.

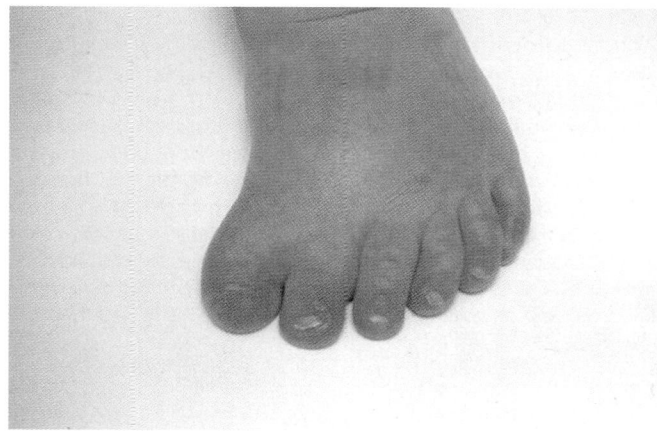

Fig. 37.13 Complex metatarsus adductus, demonstrating the curve of the lateral side of the foot beginning at the base of the fifth metatarsal (in this case associated with duplication of the hallux).

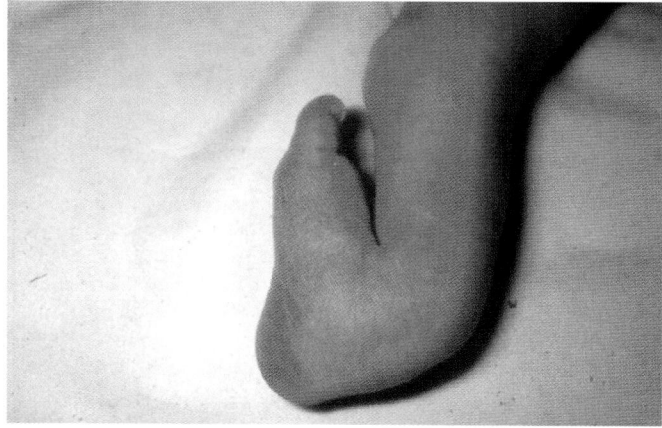

Fig. 37.14 Calcaneovalgus and tibial kyphoscoliosis in the same leg. The bow of the leg is directed posteromedially and the foot is in contact with the shin.

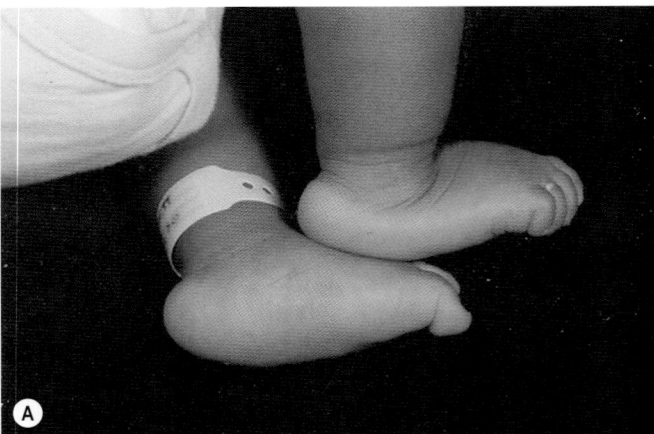

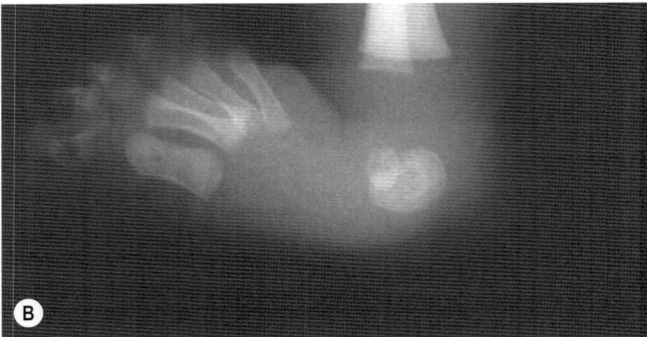

Fig. 37.15 (A) Clinical appearance of congenital vertical talus (CVT). (B) X-ray demonstrating the radiological appearance of CVT. The soft-tissue shadow clearly shows the rocker-bottom appearance of the sole of the foot.

Pathoanatomy

The talus is in a vertical position. There is lateral displacement of the calcaneum and hypoplasia of the sustentaculum tali, which results in subluxation of the talus medial to the calcaneum, making it palpable on the plantar surface of the foot. The talonavicular joint is dislocated, with the navicular lying on the dorsum and neck of the talus. The calcaneus is in an equinus position due to contracture of the tendo-Achilles. The tibialis anterior, extensor hallucis longus and extensor digitorum tendons are shortened, as are the peroneal tendons, which are often subluxed anterior to the medial malleolus, causing the characteristic abduction and dorsiflexion.

Management

Early intervention is advocated, as late surgical correction has a poor outcome.

Initially treatment is conservative, with serial casting, which may be of benefit in stretching the soft tissues and aiding later surgical reduction. The optimum time for surgical intervention is at about 12 weeks. This involves lengthening the shortened tendons and open reduction of the navicular and talus, which are held in place with temporary wires and a well-moulded plaster. At 3 weeks postoperatively, the wires are removed and the plaster changed. A further 12 weeks are required in plaster, and the plaster is then replaced with an ankle–foot orthosis until the child is walking.

Lower limb deficiencies

In the developing fetus, the limb buds appear at the beginning of the fifth week. Specialised cells at the tip of the limb bud (apical ectodermal ridge) are instrumental in the normal development of the limbs, which develop in a longitudinal direction from proximal to distal. Any disruption in the intimate relationship between the apical ectodermal ridge and the underlying mesenchyme may result in a congenital limb deformity (Achterman and Kalamchi 1979; Kalamchi and Dawe 1985; Sadler 1990).

These deformities can be classified according to the part of the limb affected. Arrest of longitudinal growth results in a transverse defect. Failure of development of the medial (postaxial) or lateral (preaxial) elements of the limb results in a longitudinal defect. Deficiencies of the central portion of the limb result in a central deficiency.

As with upper limb deficiencies, the deformity may be either transverse or longitudinal. Transverse abnormalities are usually obvious, with congenital absence of a whole or part of a limb.

Longitudinal deficiencies of the lower limb present with a shortened or abnormal-looking limb. Conditions that may be seen include hypolastic conditions of the femur, with shortening of the proximal limb and normally formed elements distally. Other conditions present with hypoplasia or absence of the fibula or tibia, with a variety of clinical deformities of the lower leg, knee and ankle joint.

Congenital femoral deficiencies

Abnormalities of the femur have been variously classified. Gillespie and Torode (1983) classified proximal deficiencies of the femur into group 1 (congenital short femur) and group 2 (true proximal focal femoral deficiencies).

Group 1

Group 1 conditions are truly hypoplastic and result in a leg-length discrepancy. The defect is obvious at birth, with asymmetric leg lengths and the foot on the affected side being at the mid-tibial level of the contralateral limb. The hip develops normally and there is a valgus deformity of the knee on the affected side. The femur is between 40% and 60% shorter than the normal femur. In the milder forms of congenital short femur, limb lengthening is a realistic treatment option at a later stage.

Group 2

Group 2 deficiencies have been further classified by Aitken (1969) based on the radiological findings (Fig. 37.16). There are four categories in the classification, ranging from A to D, with A being the most mild and D the most severe deformity. Once again, the deformity is obvious at birth, but differs from hypoplastic femur in that the proximal leg is very much shorter, with the foot being at the level of the contralateral knee (Fig. 37.17). There is also a fixed flexion deformity of the hip and knee which fails to improve with growth. In group 2 children, surgery is aimed at modification of the limb to fit a suitably functional and cosmetically acceptable prosthesis, as limb lengthening is not possible.

Congenital deficiencies of the tibia (tibial hemimelia)

This is a rare condition, with an incidence of 1 : 1 000 000 livebirths. It has been classified by Kalamchi and Dawe (1985) (Fig. 37.18) into types I–III, with type I being the most severe. The classification

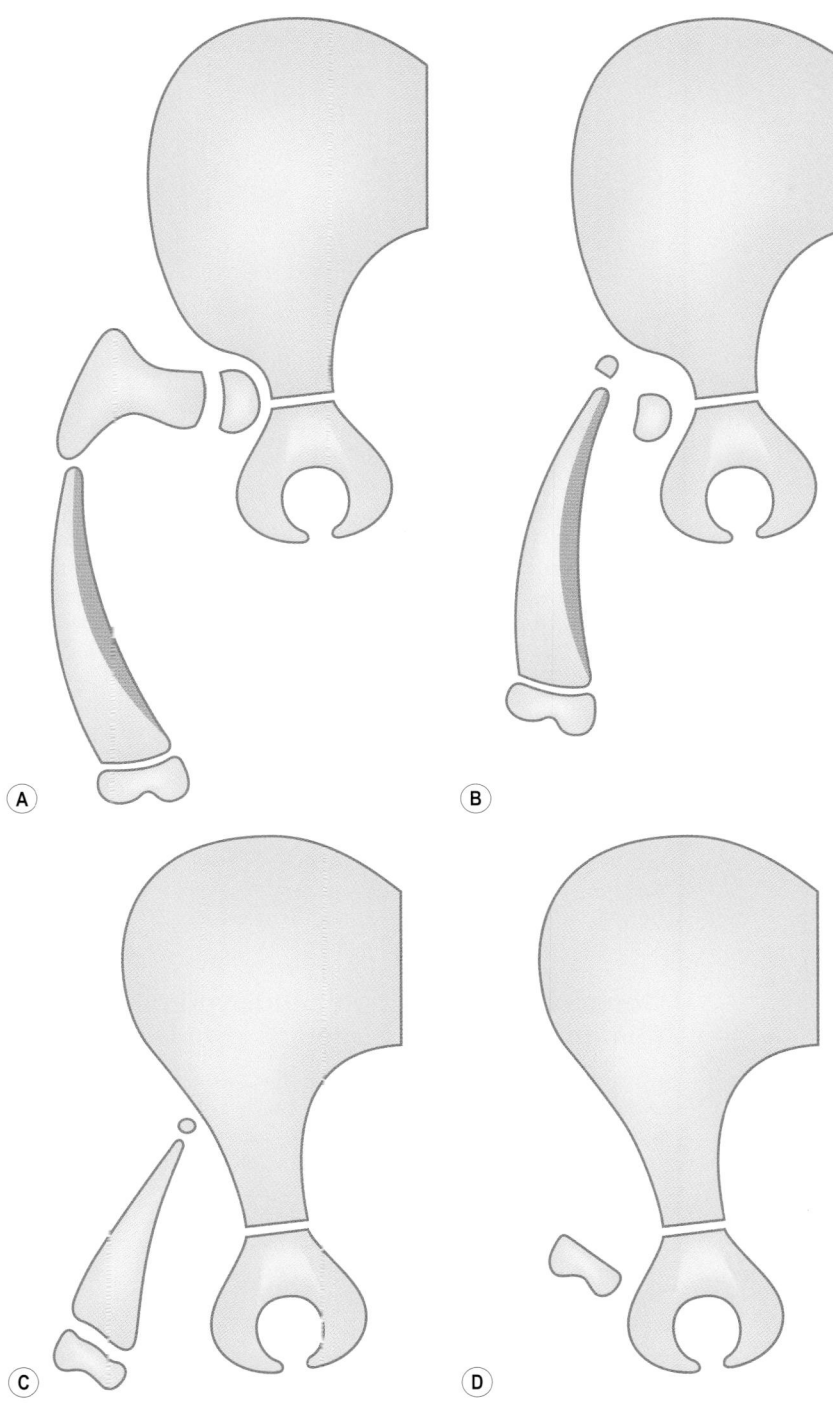

Fig. 37.16 Aitken (1969) classification of proximal femoral focal deficiency. (A) Type A, short femur with coxa vara and lateral bowing with thickening of the medial cortex. Adequate acetabulum with femoral head. (B) Type B, mildly dysplastic acetabulum with delayed ossification of the femoral head. Displacement of the proximal femur superiorly with a bony tuft connected to the femoral shaft by defective cartilage which will fail to ossify. (C) Type C, very dysplastic acetabulum and femoral head. No synchronous movement between the femoral shaft and head, with the proximal femoral shaft articulating with the iliac wing. (D) Type D, most severe deformity, with absent femoral head and acetabulum, and very short femoral shaft with no tufting. As is represented here, the femoral shaft may be represented by the femoral condyles only.

is based on the radiological findings. In type I deformity there is complete absence of the tibia, which results in marked inversion and adduction of the foot, with or without absence of the medial rays. There is a fixed flexion contracture of the knee, with weak or absent quadriceps function. In type II, the distal tibia is absent, with the knee joint reasonably well preserved and a mild fixed flexion deformity. In the mildest form (type III), the distal tibia is dysplastic, with the foot in varus and a prominent lateral malleolus.

Management is aimed at producing a functional lower limb. In the milder forms, surgery is aimed at stabilisation of the ankle joint

and correcting the leg-length discrepancy. In the more severe forms, surgery is aimed at fitting a prosthesis.

Congenital deficiency of the fibula (fibular hemimelia)

Congenital deficiency of the fibula is a rare condition in which there is partial or complete absence of the fibula. It is seldom found in isolation but is frequently associated with anomalies of the foot, tibia and femur. The condition has been classified by Achterman

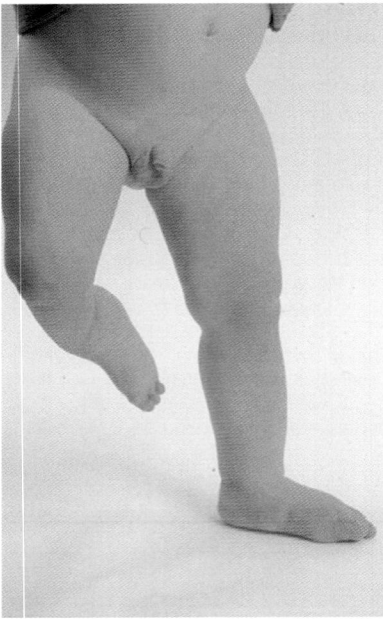

Fig. 37.17 Proximal femoral focal deficiency of the right leg in a boy, with the foot of the affected leg at the level of the knee of the unaffected contralateral leg.

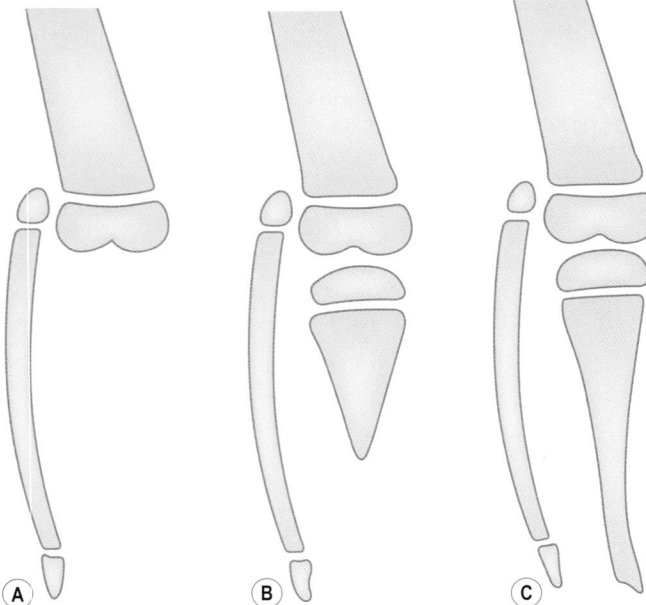

Fig. 37.18 Kalamchi and Dawe (1985) classification of congenital deficiencies of the tibia. (A) Type I, complete absence of the tibia; (B) type II, the distal tibia is absent, with presence of the proximal tibia to varying degrees; (C) type III, dysplasia of the distal tibia with diastasis of the distal tibiofibular joint.

and Kalamchi (1979) and Coventry and Johnson (1952), the former classification being based on the radiological findings and the latter on the progressive severity of the deformity and the prognosis. In the most severe form (type III), there is complete absence of the fibula. This is frequently bilateral and associated with other limb deficiencies. The functional and cosmetic outlook is poor and treatment is usually by amputation and fitting of a prosthesis. In type II, the deficiency is unilateral, with complete absence of the

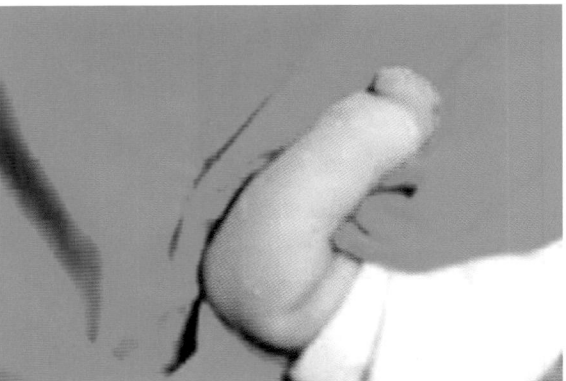

Fig. 37.19 Transverse deficiency of the upper limb secondary to congenital constriction band syndrome.

fibula, marked hypoplasia of the entire lower limb and foot abnormalities. As with type I, the outlook is poor and management is usually with amputation. In the mildest form (type I), there is shortening or partial absence of the fibula, the foot is usually normal, with minimal leg-length inequality, and is associated with a good prognosis. With all types, there may be absence of the lateral rays of the foot.

As with any other skeletal anomaly, careful assessment of the neonate for other abnormalities should be undertaken along with referral to an orthopaedic surgeon with a specialist interest in paediatrics.

There is a whole spectrum of treatments available for congenital limb abnormalities, ranging from reconstruction to amputation. Those involved include orthopaedic and plastic surgeons, physiotherapists, occupational therapists and orthotists. The principle underlying any treatment is primarily to preserve or restore function, with cosmesis being a secondary issue.

Congenital constriction band syndrome (Simonart's bands, Streeter's dysplasia)

Congenital constriction band syndrome has a gamut of clinical presentations, ranging from simple bands around digits to limb amputation (Fig. 37.19). The aetiology is poorly understood and several theories have been proposed. The most popular aetiological theory is that a sequence of events occurs in utero: initially, early amniotic rupture, followed by temporary oligohydramnios, with resultant intrauterine compression and subsequent constriction of the fetal appendages by cords of torn amnion (Patterson 1961; Torpin and Faulkner 1966; Foulkes and Reinker 1994).

The typical presentation of congenital constriction band syndrome is that of limb reduction, constriction bands or syndactyly (especially acrosyndactyly). Other presentations include pseudoarthrosis, impending gangrene, peripheral nerve palsy and skin tube pedicles. Amniotic bands can also produce fetal death via a number of mechanisms.

Treatment is aimed at optimising early function and cosmesis, and should involve orthopaedic and plastic surgeons as well as physiotherapists.

Tibial kyphosis (posteromedial bowing of the tibia)

This is a dramatic-looking deformity of the lower limb (Fig. 37.14). Clinically, the foot is in extreme dorsiflexion and valgus, with the forefoot touching the anterolateral aspect of the shin (as seen in

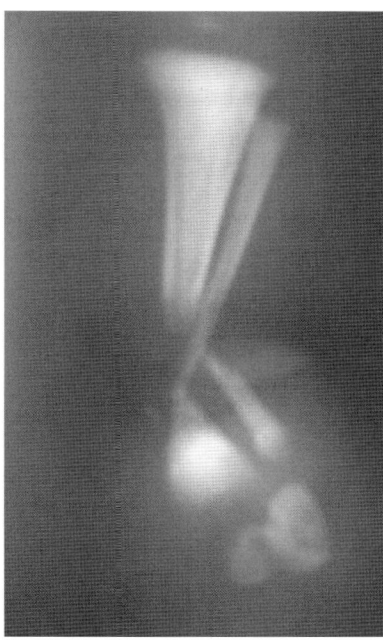

Fig. 37.20 Radiological appearance of congenital pseudoarthrosis of the tibia.

calcaneovalgus). In association with this is a posteromedial bow of the tibia, most marked distally. There is shortening of the lower leg on the affected side, with wasting of the muscles.

Fortunately, the condition is relatively benign, with rapid improvement in the foot position and the tibial bow in the first year of life.

Initial treatment consists of stretching exercises, as taught by a physiotherapist, which should begin as soon after birth as possible. For a marked deformity, serial casts may be applied. Residual deformity after the age of 3 years may require surgical intervention to correct the bow and leg-length discrepancy.

Congenital pseudoarthrosis of the tibia

This is a complex anomaly of the lower leg, of unknown aetiology, whose treatment and management are difficult and protracted. It is associated with neurofibromatosis type 1 in more than half of cases and has an incidence of approximately 1 : 200 000 livebirths. Other stigmata of neurofibromatosis may be present.

Rarely is there a fracture present at birth, but pathological fracture and pseudoarthrosis readily occur at some stage thereafter.

The deformity may be very slight or there may be mild or marked anterolateral bowing of the tibia. The condition is diagnosed by X-ray (Fig. 37.20) and attempts have been made to classify the condition radiologically. Initial treatment consists of protecting the tibia, which is at risk of fracture, until definitive treatment can be undertaken. There should be early involvement of an orthopaedic surgeon.

Upper limb abnormalities

Other anomalies of the hand

Syndactyly (congenital webbing of the hand, Fig. 37.21) occurs because of failure of apoptosis of the web spaces of the hand plate in utero. This is the most common congenital anomaly in the hand.

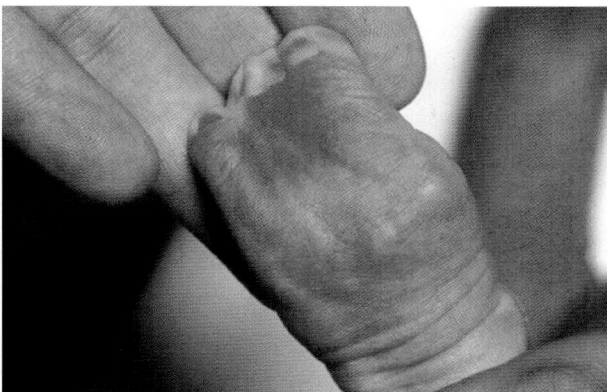

Fig. 37.21 Complex syndactyly in a neonate, showing fusion of all the web spaces in the right hand and bony union of the middle and ring fingers.

The incidence is 1 : 2250 live births and the condition is bilateral and symmetrical in 50% of cases. Boys are affected more than girls at a ratio of 2 : 1. Simple syndactyly involves simple skin bridges between the fingers, whereas complex syndactyly involves skin and bone. In acrosyndactyly, only the tips of the fingers are fused.

Varying degrees of complex syndactyly are seen in Apert syndrome. Polydactyly and oligodactyly refer to excess or insufficient digits, respectively. Macrodactyly refers to overgrowth of a digit.

Trigger thumb is a common deformity, presenting with flexion of the interphalangeal joint of the thumb. Examination reveals a thickening of the flexor pollicis longus tendon. In 25% of cases the deformity is present at birth, with bilateral involvement in 50%. Left untreated, 30% will resolve spontaneously by 1 year.

Thumb-in-palm deformity (congenital clasped thumb) – characterised by marked flexion at the metocarpophalangeal joint with adduction of the thumb – is a rare anomaly which is familial. It affects males more than females at a ratio of 2 : 1 and is almost always bilateral. The deformity is caused by muscle imbalance in the thumb and may be seen in cerebral palsy and arthrogryposis but frequently has no other associated congenital anomalies. Treatment ranges from physiotherapy and splinting to tendon transfers, depending on the type and severity of the deformity.

Upper limb deficiencies
Transverse failure

Arrest of longitudinal growth of the arm can affect any part of the limb from the shoulder distally, with the most common being the proximal third of the forearm (Fig. 37.22A).

Longitudinal failure

Preaxial deficiencies present with hypoplasia or partial or complete absence of the radius and thumb, the 'radial club hand', with marked deviation of the hand radially. The incidence is approximately 1 : 100 000 livebirths, with 50% being bilateral. In unilateral cases, the right arm is involved twice as often as the left. Males are affected more than females at a ratio of 1.5 : 1. Half the cases are found in association with congenital syndromes, including thrombocytopenia–absent radius syndrome (Fig. 37.22B), Fanconi syndrome, Holt–Oram syndrome and Vater syndrome (Tachdjian 1990; Broughton 1997).

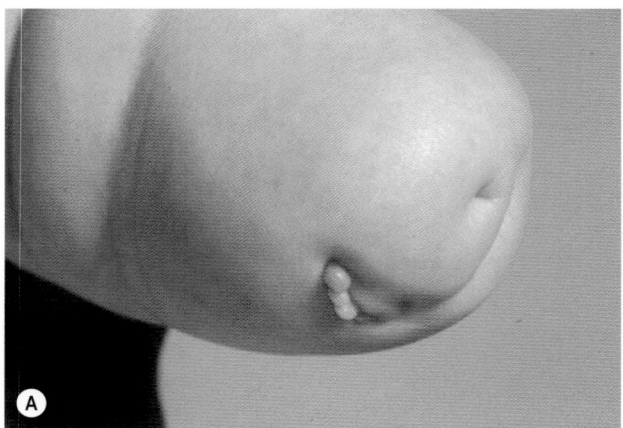

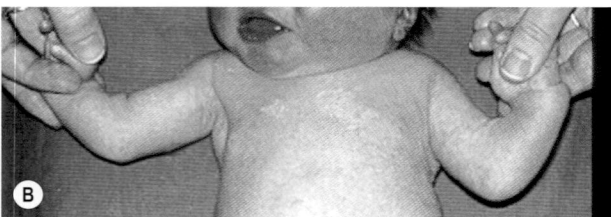

Fig. 37.22 (A) Transverse upper limb deficiency, showing absence of the arm just below the elbow. (B) Neonate with the thrombocytopenia–absent radius syndrome.

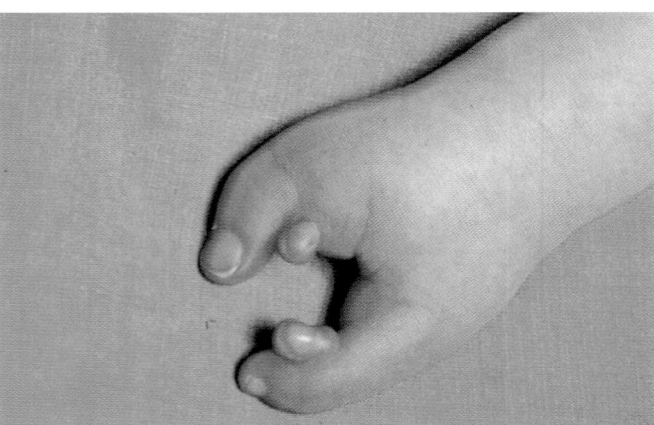

Fig. 37.23 Central longitudinal deficiency of the upper limb resulting in a 'lobster claw' hand.

Treatment is aimed at producing a functional hand. Initial treatment is passive stretching and splinting in the early phases. There are then a variety of surgical procedures aimed at centralising the carpus on the ulna and maintaining muscle balance in the forearm and creating a thumb. Functional outcome is usually good and in only a very few cases is a salvage wrist fusion required.

Postaxial longitudinal deficiencies of the arm present as absence of the ulna and a varying number of digits from the ulnar half of the hand. This condition is referred to as 'ulnar club hand'. It is one of the rarest upper limb anomalies and is associated with other skeletal anomalies rather than visceral defects.

Central longitudinal deficiency presents with absence of the second, third and fourth rays of the hand, with or without associated absence of the carpals. This results in a cleft or 'lobster claw' hand (Fig. 37.23). It accounts for approximately 2% of congenital hand anomalies. There is a male preponderance, with the condition usually being bilateral. In 50% of cases, cleft feet are also present. Associated anomalies include cleft lip and palate, cataracts, deafness, absence of nails, heart defects and imperforate anus.

Abnormalities of the spine and axial skeleton

Congenital spinal abnormalities (kyphosis and scoliosis)

During early embryonic life, at around the fourth week of gestation, the polymorphous mesenchyme of the segmented ventromedial somite, the sclerotome, surrounds the neural tube and notochord in development of the vertebral column. During further development, the cranial and caudal parts of the sclerotome proliferate and condense, ultimately uniting to form the precartilaginous vertebral body.

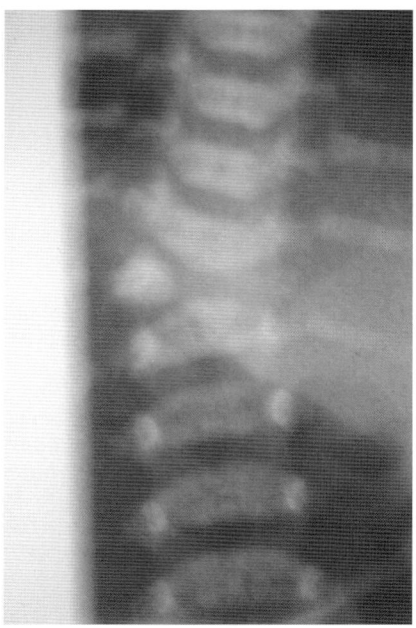

Fig. 37.24 X-ray showing a hemivertebra on the right in the thoracic region with an associated scoliosis.

The formation and subsequent rearrangement of the segmental sclerotomes into the definitive vertebrae is a complex process. It is not uncommon for adjacent vertebrae to fuse symmetrically or asymmetrically or for half the vertebrae to be missing (hemivertebra) (Fig. 37.24), or for the vertebrae to be wedged, resulting in congenital spinal anomalies (Sadler 1990). With abnormalities of the spine, the overlying skin may contain angiomas, naevi and patches of hair, dimples or a pad of fat (p. 1204).

Osteopathic (congenital) scoliosis

Scoliosis refers to a lateral deviation of the spine. The most common cause of congenital scoliosis is failure of one side of a vertebra or adjacent vertebrae to segment, resulting in a unilateral unsegmented bar (an unbalanced anomaly). These are most commonly seen in the thoracic area. There is restricted growth of the unsegmented portion of the vertebra, with normal growth of the contralateral side, resulting in a curvature of the spine towards the bar. When there is one hemivertebra or two hemivertebrae on the same side, the curve will be severe. This deformity is progressive and carries the worst prognosis. Hemivertebrae present on opposite sides of the vertebral column, however, balance each other (balanced anomaly) and result in a relatively mild deformity.

Congenital scoliosis may be apparent at birth but may not manifest until later years. It is associated with a variety of congenital defects involving the spinal cord (diastematomyelia), cardiac system, renal system, gastrointestinal system (e.g. tracheo-oesophageal fistula) and limbs (e.g. congenital absence of the radius and hypoplasia of the thumb) (MacEwen and Hardy 1972; Hensinger and Jones 1981). Careful and thorough clinical assessment is therefore required for any neonate presenting with a scoliosis.

Referral to an orthopaedic surgeon specialising in paediatric spines should be made. Surgical intervention is required for curves greater than 50° and for those children with a progressive curve that is likely to reach more than 50°. Initial treatment may consist of bracing, which does little to influence progression of the condition but may help in delaying surgery until the child is of a more appropriate age. Surgery is only undertaken following further assessment of the spinal cord with magnetic resonance imaging (MRI) to exclude a spinal cord abnormality. The surgical options consist of spinal fusion, correction with rods, hemivertebrae excision or osteotomy, depending on the age of the child and whether the deformity is fixed or flexible (Harrington 1960; Winter 1981). Corrective surgery usually results in permanent correction.

Congenital kyphosis

Kyphosis refers to an excessive outward curvature of the spine, causing forward bend of the back.

Congenital kyphosis is more often progressive than scoliosis, leading to a severe deformity in early life. It is categorised as type I or II. In type I, there is failure of formation of the vertebrae; in type II, there is failure of segmentation of the vertebrae. Kyphosis may result from a combination of the two.

The common site for kyphosis is at the thoracolumbar junction between T10 and L2. Type I is the most common form and has a poorer prognosis than type II. Absence or hypoplasia of the anterior part of the vertebra results in progressive kyphosis and posterior displacement of the posterior hemivertebra, with a risk of cord compression.

Type II is characterised by an anterior unsegmented bar. As the posterior vertebrae grow, so there is progressive kyphosis.

Treatment is either surgical or conservative and is dictated by the type of kyphosis, the severity of the deformity and the age of the patient. If the curvature is greater than 50°, bracing with a Milwaukee brace is indicated. If the curvature is greater than 75°, corrective surgery is indicated. For less severe curves with no documented evidence of progression, careful follow-up is required.

The mainstay of treatment is spinal fusion, and, for severe fixed deformities, osteotomies and correction with rods (Winter et al. 1973; Winter 1981).

Klippel–Feil syndrome (congenital synostosis of the cervical vertebrae, brevicollis, congenital short neck)

Klippel–Feil syndrome is a condition characterised by failure of vertebral segmentation in the neck, resulting in fusion of two (congenital block vertebrae) or more vertebrae, and may involve the

whole neck. Other associated physical features, classically described but not always present, include a low posterior hairline and restricted head and neck movements.

This syndrome is associated with other congenital anomalies, the most common being a scoliosis. Other congenital anomalies include deafness, congenital heart disease and urological anomalies, particularly unilateral renal agenesis (Hensinger et al. 1974). Any neonate with congenital cervical spine abnormalities should undergo USS of the renal tract.

The condition itself is relatively asymptomatic, except in a partial fusion there is a risk of non-traumatic spontaneous dislocation. Treatment is conservative with passive stretching exercises to obtain maximum range of movement, which should begin immediately after birth, initially under the guidance of a physiotherapist.

Spina bifida (dysraphism) (see Ch. 40.8)

Spina bifida is a condition of the vertebral column with or without defects in the neural tube and has a spectrum ranging from a benign incidental finding to one causing significant disability.

During development of the vertebral column in utero, there is failure of the vertebral arch or arches to develop posteriorly and the lamina and spinous processes are absent at either one or multiple vertebral levels. In association with this, there may be a defect in the neural tube ranging from failure of separation of the skin from the neural tissue to complete exposure of the neural tissue to the surface.

Incidence

The incidence of spina bifida affecting the neural tube is approximately 2–4 per 1000 live births in the UK, and less than 1 per 1000 in the USA and Australia. There is a very slight sex difference, with girls more affected than boys, and a suggested polygenic mode of inheritance. There is a 10-fold increase in incidence with an affected sibling.

Aetiology

Environmental factors have been implicated, including folate and selenium deficiency, poor maternal nutrition, a high maternal alcohol intake and maternal diabetes. Teratogens such as valproate have also been implicated. As yet, no single factor has been identified and therefore the aetiology is likely to be multifactorial.

The use of folic acid supplements preconceptually and during the first trimester of pregnancy is now advocated.

Screening

In the UK, antenatal ultrasound has replaced serum alpha-fetoprotein as the screening method of choice (Ch. 9).

Clinical presentation

Spina bifida occulta is one of the most common congenital anomalies, with approximately 25% of children showing some minor defect of the vertebral arches on X-ray. It may not manifest itself in the neonate but may be a serendipitous finding at a later stage. The skin overlying the defect is usually normal, but there may be failure of separation of the skin from the underlying neural tissue and it may contain pigmentation, dimples, pits, lipomas or hairy patches. The presence of these clinical findings should alert the examiner to the possibility of spina bifida, particularly if in association with neurological defects, which are rare in spina bifida occulta.

The remaining forms of spina bifida are collectively known as spina bifida cystica. The most benign form is a meningocele, which is a cystic swelling overlying the bony defect with normal skin covering. The swelling is a bulge of cerebrospinal fluid-filled meninges protruding through the underlying bony defect with the spinal cord remaining contained between the neural arches. This condition represents 5% of the spina bifidas and is rarely associated with neuromuscular deficiencies. In contrast, a myelomeningocele, which is similar to a meningocele except the spinal cord is contained in the fundus of the sac (closed myelomeningocele), is always associated with neuromuscular deficiencies. The most severe defect is a myelocele (open myelomeningocele), in which the primitive unfolded neural tube forms the roof of the cystic swelling and may be open to the air.

Associated lower limb deformities such as teratological DDH, CTEV, claw toes and recurvatum are common with the myelomeningoceles. In a third of neonates with myelomeningocele there is complete lower motor neuron paralysis with loss of sensation and sphincter control below the affected level. In one-third there is a complete segmental lesion with preservation of a distal spinal segment, which results in a mixed neurological picture with intact reflexes and spastic muscle groups. In the final third the lesion is incomplete and there is some movement and sensation below the affected level.

Management

Management of spina bifida requires a multidisciplinary approach. The team is usually headed by a paediatrician, who coordinates the care. Others who input care include orthopaedic and neurosurgeons, urologists, physiotherapists and occupational therapists, and orthotists.

Congenital high scapula (Sprengel's deformity)

The scapula develops as a cervical appendage in the fifth week of gestation. It descends to the level of the posterior thorax by the end of the third month of gestation. Sprengel's deformity, described in 1863 (Eulenberg 1863), occurs because of failure of separation and descent of the scapula at about 12 weeks' gestation. As a result, the scapula remains small and abnormally high and may remain tethered to the cervical spine by a tough fibrous band or by a cartilaginous or bony bar (the omovertebral bar).

The condition usually occurs sporadically but can be transmitted as an autosomal dominant trait. It is more common in female offspring, with the left shoulder being more affected than the right, and is occasionally bilateral.

It is frequently associated with other congenital abnormalities such as torticollis, scoliosis, kyphosis, diastematomyelia and Klippel–Feil syndrome.

Clinical presentation

The deformity is usually noticed at birth, with asymmetry of the shoulders. The elevation of the scapula is variable, depending on the severity of the condition. The clavicle is abnormally positioned and the pectoral girdle is hypoplastic due to wasting of the muscles. Abduction of the shoulder is limited owing to decreased scapulothoracic motion. With a bilateral deformity, there may be a low hairline and webbing of the neck.

Management

Management depends on the severity of the deformity and the degree of disability encountered. Mild cases are usually observed with no need for surgical intervention. Surgery is considered for

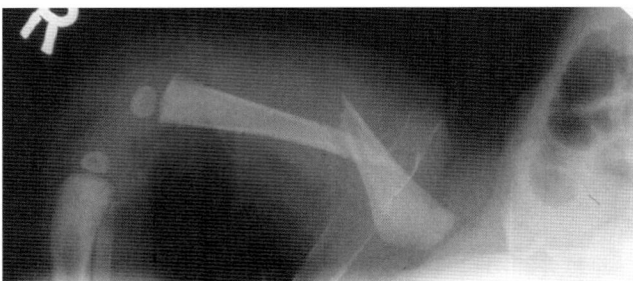

Fig. 37.25 X-ray demonstrating a birth fracture of the right femoral shaft.

cosmetic reasons and if the deformity is very fixed. Conjecture exists over the timing of surgery, some advocating early intervention in the first year and others before the age of 6.

Fractures in the newborn

Childbirth complicated by the necessity for rapid delivery, breech presentation or macrosomia may result in a birth fracture (Madsen 1955). The sites of fractures in descending order of frequency are: clavicle, humeral shaft, femoral shaft (Fig. 37.25), epiphyseal separation at the upper and lower humerus, and, finally, separation of the upper and lower femoral epiphyses. Distal fractures below the elbow and the knee are rare (Madsen 1955; Tachdjian 1990; Broughton 1997).

Long bone fractures are usually obvious and detected immediately by the obstetrician, as the bone can be heard and felt to break. There is usually associated pseudoparalysis of the affected limb. Long bone fractures are more likely when there is osteopenia, sometimes due to lack of fetal movements because of myopathy.

Clavicular fractures may go unnoticed, with the majority being relatively asymptomatic. All are unilateral, with most involving the anterior shoulder. The diagnosis may not come to light until callus formation creates the telltale lump seen in clavicular fractures. If suspected after birth, crepitus, tenderness and swelling are present on palpation of the clavicle and the diagnosis is confirmed by X-ray. There may be an associated brachial plexus injury. Treatment is conservative.

Long bone fractures of the humerus and femur are usually midshaft. Humeral shaft fractures may be associated with a radial nerve palsy. Such palsies are usually temporary and most have resolved by 6 weeks. Treatment is by immobilisation of the affected limb, with healing taking 2–3 weeks. Any residual angular deformity will invariably remodel with growth of the infant.

Physeal injuries are more difficult to diagnose and may go unnoticed if clinical suspicion is not present. However, if a birth is particularly difficult and there has been excess traction on a limb followed by swelling and immobility of the limb, then physeal injury should be considered. Immobility due to long bone fracture can easily be excluded by plain X-ray. Radiological findings in physeal injuries are initially difficult to interpret and a history of the clinical concern should be discussed with a paediatric musculoskeletal radiologist to aid interpretation. X-rays at a later stage of the injury reveal a florid periosteal reaction and callus formation.

If diagnosed early, treatment occasionally consists of manipulation, depending on the type of injury, and all early-diagnosed injuries should undergo a period of immobilisation of the affected limb for comfort. If diagnosis is delayed and healing has occurred, no treatment is necessary.

Multiple birth fractures are seen in AMC and osteogenesis imperfecta (Ch. 34.4).

Vascular conditions associated with orthopaedic problems in the newborn

Neonatal gangrene and amputation

Ischaemic gangrene of the extremity in the neonate has been recognised since 1828. It is a relatively uncommon condition, but failure to recognise the problem early can result in catastrophic sequelae, with loss of digits or limbs. It is important to make the distinction between ischaemic necrosis and necrotising fasciitis, a completely different entity requiring different treatment.

There are four main causes of gangrene of the extremity in the neonate: following a complicated delivery, secondary to invasive monitoring, extravasation of intravenous fluids, and secondary to sepsis.

Any delivery complicated by a long second stage of labour with an abnormal fetal position resulting in compression of a limb for prolonged periods may result in thrombosis of the limb. There is an increased incidence in diabetic mothers because of macrosomia of the infant and increased blood viscosity. Twin delivery with twin-to-twin transfusion results in polycythaemia and hypercoagulability in one of the infants, increasing the risk of thrombosis of an extremity (Fig. 37.26) (Letts et al. 1997).

Peripheral arterial cannulation in the neonatal intensive care setting may compromise the circulation to the distal limb (Ch. 44). Cannulation of the femoral artery has been linked with ischaemia of the leg, as this site is an end artery. Also, failure to perform Allen's test prior to radial artery cannulation can compromise the circulation to the hand. Care also needs to be taken with repeated arterial

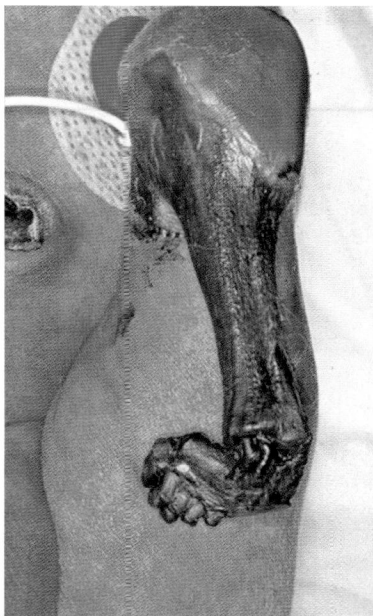

Fig. 37.26 Neonatal gangrene of the lower leg secondary to polycythaemia following twin-to-twin transfusion in utero.

blood sampling. With any insult of the peripheral arteries there is not only local trauma to the vessel but also possibly an associated intense vasospasm of the vessel proximally, with a risk of extensive gangrene.

Cannulation of the umbilical artery has been associated with aortic thrombosis and aortic branch occlusion, as well as digital thrombosis.

One of the most common procedures undertaken in the sick neonate is peripheral venous cannulation. Frequently, the cannula either erodes through the vessel wall or thromboses, with a risk of extravasation of fluid into the surrounding tissues. If the fluid being infused is hypertonic or irritant, such as total parenteral nutrition or calcium salts, there is blistering of the skin with local tissue necrosis (Ch. 44). Therefore, extreme vigilance is required when infusing such solutions through a peripheral cannula, and infusion pumps that alarm when the line is occluded are mandatory, as is regular observation of the infusion site.

Severe infections that cause disseminated intravascular coagulation can cause digital gangrene and skin necrosis.

It is important to look for peripheral ischaemia in at-risk neonates. Early clinical signs may be difficult to detect, but asymmetrically cool peripheries and absent pulses with skin mottling should alert the examiner. If there is a high index of clinical suspicion, there should be an aggressive search for the occlusion with Doppler ultrasound and angiography. If an occlusion is found, then either thrombolysis (pp. 780–781) or thrombectomy should be considered and undertaken.

Despite best measures, it may not be possible to salvage a limb and the need for amputation arises. In the neonate, there is no urgency to amputate, as the early level of gangrene may be significantly lower than the final level. It is therefore important to wait for unequivocal demarcation of the gangrene prior to amputation.

Nerve and muscle conditions associated with orthopaedic problems in the newborn

Brachial plexus palsy

Damage to the brachial plexus during childbirth has long been recognised, first being reported in 1764.

Incidence

The reported incidence ranges from 0.4 to 2.5 cases per 1000 live births. There has been no reduction in incidence over the last few decades but much progress has been made in recovery rates. Recovery is dependent on the level and extent of the injury, which can range from a neuropraxic injury to complete neurotmesis.

Historically, recovery rates were bleak, with only 13–18% regaining full function. Today, rates of full recovery are in excess of 70–90% for upper plexus palsies (Adler and Patterson 1967).

Risk factors

Brachial plexus injury is associated with gestational diabetes, grand multiparity, instrumental deliveries, shoulder dystocia, fetal macrosomia, prematurity and postmaturity, breech delivery and oxytocin use. More recent findings have associated obstetric brachial plexus palsy (OBPP) with the passage of meconium during delivery and neonatal hyperbilirubinaemia (Aston 1977; Hardy 1981; Jackson et al. 1988).

Aetiology

The cause of many cases of upper OBPP (Erb's palsy), which involves the C5 and C6 nerve roots, is widening of the head–shoulder angle at delivery, and this is by far the most common brachial plexus injury. Klumpke's palsy, which involves the lower brachial plexus roots, C8 and T1, is a much less common finding, with an incidence of 0.6/1000 live births. The reduced incidence of lower OBPP is thought to be attributable to the decline in vaginal breech deliveries. These deliveries are associated with forced hyper-abduction of the upper limb, with risk to the lower brachial plexus (Jennett et al. 2002).

Complete plexus palsies are more common than lower plexus palsies. The long-term outcome of complete brachial plexus palsy is very poor, with 66% having permanent dysfunction (Jennett et al. 2002).

Clinical presentation

The signs at birth are obvious. With an upper plexus palsy, the abductors and external rotators of the shoulder and the supinators are paralysed. Therefore, the arm is held to the side internally rotated and pronated and there may also be loss of finger extension, the classic 'waiter's tip' sign (Fig. 37.27). In an adult, one would expect to find sensory loss over the deltoid; however, tests of sensation are unreliable in a baby. Lower plexus palsies result in clawing and wasting of the muscles of the hand. Complete plexus palsies result in a flail arm. The arm is pale with no motor function and there may be vasomotor impairment with a Horner syndrome (meiosis, anhydrosis, ptosis and enopthalmos) on the affected side. Motor function of the arms can be tested in the neonate using the Moro reflex (p. 1073).

Referral and treatment

All babies with a suspected OBPP should be referred for an orthopaedic opinion. Occasionally, a birth fracture of the clavicle or the proximal humerus compounds the paralysis of the affected limb.

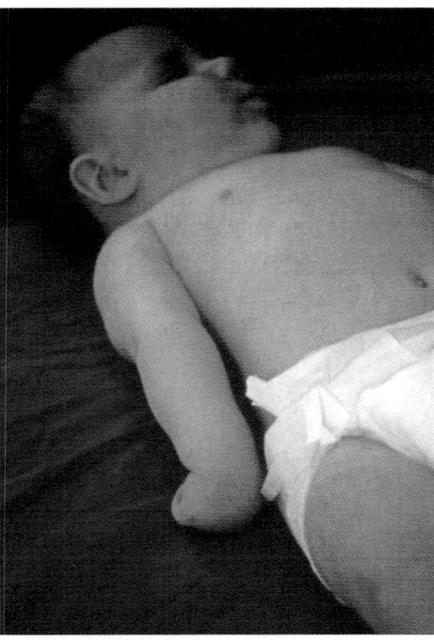

Fig. 37.27 The classic 'waiter's tip' posture of Erb's palsy following brachial plexus injury at birth.

Prognosis

As most palsies are in the upper plexus with an excellent prognosis, the mainstay of treatment is to prevent stiffness and contractures, and early involvement of the paediatric physiotherapist is essential. The same applies for lower and complete plexus palsies, which have a higher risk of permanency. Regular orthopaedic review to monitor progress is essential. Absence of any motor function of the biceps at 3 months is an indication for further investigation with electro-physiological studies and possible surgical repair or grafting of the plexus.

Arthrogryposis multiplex congenita

Arthrogryposis is a generic term referring to a congenital, non-progressive fibrous ankylosis of joints resulting in reduced range of movement. It covers a heterogeneous group of syndromes, the most common being AMC.

AMC is an uncommon problem characterised by multiple joint contractures and absence of skin creases around joints, with occasional webbing on the flexor surface of immobile joints. It occurs sporadically with no known hereditary pattern.

Distal arthrogryposis causing clenched fists and foot deformities, however, is an autosomal dominant condition (Wynne-Davies 1978).

Affected neonates with classic AMC have normal chromosomes and will generally develop normal intelligence.

Aetiology

As yet, no known cause for AMC has been found. Several aetiological theories have been postulated, including intrauterine infection (a similar condition is found in sheep, cows and horses secondary to Akabane virus), teratogens, environmental agents or a metabolic cause.

AMC may be either neurogenic or myopathic. In the neurogenic form, there is depletion of motor neurons in the anterior horns of the spinal cord. In the myopathic form, there is depletion of muscle spindle fibres, although this may be secondary to neuropathic AMC.

It may be mimicked by other conditions which restrict fetal movements, resulting in contracture deformities such as spina bifida, sacral agenesis and cerebral palsy.

Clinical presentation

The neonate presents with multiple rigid deformities which are usually bilateral and symmetrical. A characteristic posture is adopted in that the upper limb is adducted and internally rotated with the elbows extended and the wrists and fingers flexed (Fig. 37.28A). The legs are held in a diamond shape, flexed and externally rotated at the hip with the knees partially flexed, with the feet invariably in the equinovarus position (Fig. 37.28B). There is marked muscle wasting proximal and distal to the joint contracture, with featureless skin and occasional webbing. In 92% of cases of AMC, all four limbs are affected; in 7%, lower limb only; and in 1%, upper limb only (Broughton 1997). The condition is commonly associated with CVT, CTEV and DDH of the teratological variety.

Management

The deformities are at their worst at birth and, as the condition is non-progressive, are unlikely to advance with appropriate treatment. It is important that the baby is referred to an orthopaedic surgeon familiar with managing this condition.

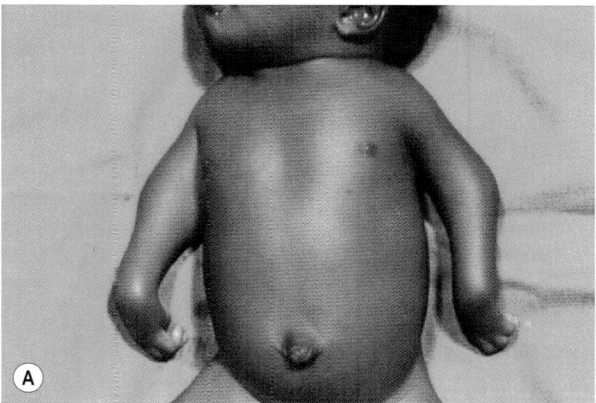

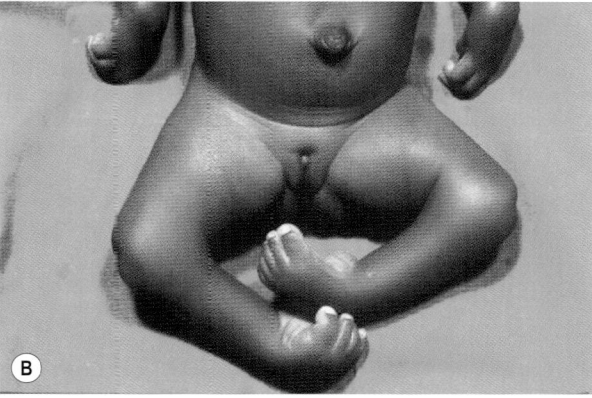

Fig. 37.28 (A) Clinical picture of the upper limbs in a baby with arthrogryposis. (B) The 'diamond' posture of the lower limbs in arthrogryposis.

The mainstay of treatment in the initial phase is gentle stretching and splinting to correct the deformities and this requires the input of specialist paediatric physiotherapists and occupational therapists. Care must be taken to avoid undue force when stretching, as the bones are thin and fracture easily. The therapists are closely involved with the family and provide invaluable support and advice, initially in the hospital setting and ultimately in the community (Williams 1978; Palmer et al. 1985).

Invariably, affected children require some kind of surgical intervention in the form of soft-tissue release or tendon transfers, as well as management of DDH, CTEV or CVT if present.

On the whole, the outlook is good for genetically normal children with AMC, with 85% walking independently and having good wrist and hand function (Drennan 1990).

Congenital muscular torticollis

The name torticollis is derived from Latin, *tortus* meaning twisted and *cullum* meaning neck. It presents with an abnormal head posture caused by shortening of one of the sternocleidomastoid (SCM) muscles in the neck. There is no information on incidence; it affects the right-hand side in 70% of cases and in 29% of cases is associated with DDH. This contracture prevents normal rotation of the head, pulling the chin away from the affected side when observed from the front and the ear towards the shoulder of the affected side when viewed from behind – the 'cock robin' posture (Fig. 37.29A).

The aetiology of congenital muscular torticollis (CMT) is poorly understood, but the condition is seen more commonly in traumatic births, leading to the suggestion that it is due to direct damage to the muscle resulting in a fibrous contracture following haematoma formation. CMT is seen in association with DDH and CTEV. Occasionally, the swelling of the muscle can be palpated in the affected SCM and is referred to as a 'tumour'. In other mature cases there is simply clinical thickening and tightness of the muscle and in some there is a torticollis posture with an absence of tightness or thickening of the SCM muscle.

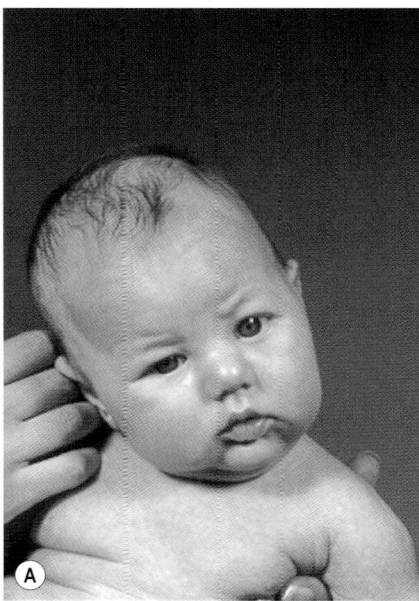

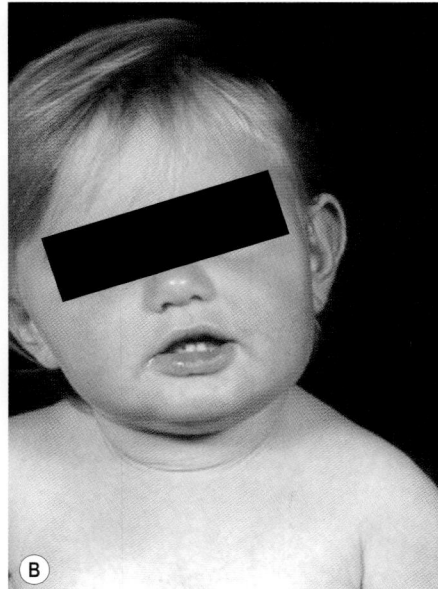

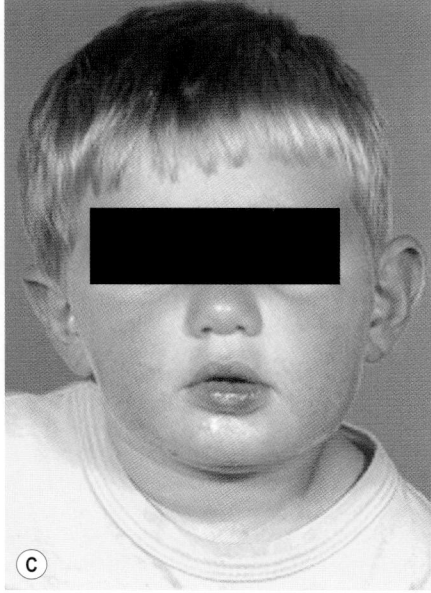

Fig. 37.29 (A) Congenital torticollis at birth. (B) The same child at the age of 1 year. (C) The same child at the age of 2 years.

Treatment initially is conservative with physiotherapy to increase range of movement. In most cases, the mass or thickening gradually disappears over the first year of life, and manual stretching is effective in 95% of cases referred before 1 year of age (Cheng et al. 2001).

Persistence of torticollis after 1 year (Fig. 37.29B) requires further investigation and possible treatment. Occasionally, abnormal head posture may be due to an ocular or cerebral cause: in the absence of an obvious SCM tumour or tightening, ocular pathology should be excluded by ophthalomogical examination and cerebral pathology by MRI of the posterior fossae (Williams et al. 1996).

Ultrasound assessment of the SCM muscle has been used to assess prognosis and need for surgical intervention. Ultrasound involvement of the distal third usually responds to conservative treatment, whereas involvement of the middle and distal thirds requires surgery in 6% of cases, and with whole muscle involvement, 35% of patients require surgery (Lin and Chou 1997). Failure to treat resistant CMT may result in facial moulding and asymmetry (plagiocephaly), and subsequent treatment is surgical, with release of the SCM muscle.

Infectious disease associated with orthopaedic problems in the newborn

Septic arthritis

Septic arthritis is an orthopaedic emergency and early involvement of an orthopaedic surgeon is mandatory (Nade 1983a). If there is any clinical suspicion of septic arthritis, an orthopaedic opinion should be sought urgently. It cannot be overemphasised that neonates may manifest very few systemic symptoms, making early diagnosis difficult, but if not considered in the differential of a child failing to thrive, the opportunity of early diagnosis and treatment will be missed.

Infection of a joint originates from three main sources: (1) haematogenous, in which the synovium of the joint is inoculated from a distant source, i.e. the umbilicus; (2) direct extension from an adjacent osteomyelitis; and (3) direct inoculation from joint aspiration or arthrotomy. It must be remembered that taking blood from the femoral vein may lead to inadvertent joint puncture.

In order of frequency, the joints most often affected in the neonate are hip, knee and elbow, although any joint can be affected. The most common infecting organism is *Staphylococcus aureus* (60–80%), followed by *Streptococcus* and *Haemophilus* species. Unfortunately, only 50% of hip aspirates yield a positive culture.

As previously stated, clinical features may be slight and the characteristic high fever, systemic upset and immobility of the affected limb (pseudoparalysis) as seen in a child may be absent in the neonate. Failure to thrive may be the first clinical clue and careful clinical examination of the infant should be undertaken. Attention should be paid to any swelling, redness or tenderness of a joint, pain and stiffness on movement of a joint, pseudoparalysis, and observation of the position of the limbs. In septic arthritis of the hip, the limb is held in the position of most comfort, notably 40–60° of flexion, 10–20° of abduction and 10–15° of external rotation.

Markers of infection should be measured, including white cell count, C-reactive protein and a falling platelet count. These investigations are useful if the markers are raised, as they help to support the diagnosis. However, in the neonate these may be misleadingly normal, and, if clinically suspected, further investigation is warranted.

Urgent ultrasound examination of the joint should be undertaken. This may simply identify a joint effusion, but the presence of echogenic debris may be more suggestive of infection. Bone scanning may be undertaken if the diagnosis is uncertain and may demonstrate increased activity around the joint. Plain X-rays in septic arthritis of the hip may be helpful, demonstrating lateral displacement of the hip or dislocation, but may also be entirely normal.

Delay in diagnosis and treatment results in joint destruction with secondary osteoarthritis or ankylosis, growth plate arrest, dislocation and avascular necrosis.

Management

If there is clinical suspicion, the neonate should be prepared for surgery while investigations are taking place. Septic joints should be washed out and specimens sent for culture and sensitivity, and parenteral antibiotics commenced. The affected joint should be immobilised. Response to treatment can be monitored by the general well-being of the infant and, if raised initially, the restoration to normal values of inflammatory markers. Antibiotics must be continued for a minimum of 6 weeks, after which time splintage can be removed and clinical assessment of the joint made. After careful consideration, and only if the baby is doing well, it may be possible to convert parenteral antibiotics to enteral.

Osteomyelitis

Neonatal osteomyelitis (Fig. 37.30) presents with swelling of the limb and septicaemia (Mollan and Piggot 1977; Nade 1983b). Most commonly the infection is haematogenous in origin. The metaphyseal blood supply is sluggish, rendering this region of the bone susceptible to seeding of infection. In the neonate, the umbilicus is implicated as the portal for infection, particularly in the sick neonate who has undergone umbilical artery cannulation. In 70% of cases the adjacent joint becomes involved, because invariably the infected metaphysis is intracapsular.

Infecting organisms include group B beta-haemolytic streptococcus, *Streptococcus* species, *Staphylococcus aureus* and *Escherichia coli*.

In the newborn, there is often very little systemic response and, as with many childhood illnesses, there may simply be a failure to thrive. The most obvious clinical finding is absence of movement in the affected limb, 'pseudoparalysis'; other clues include

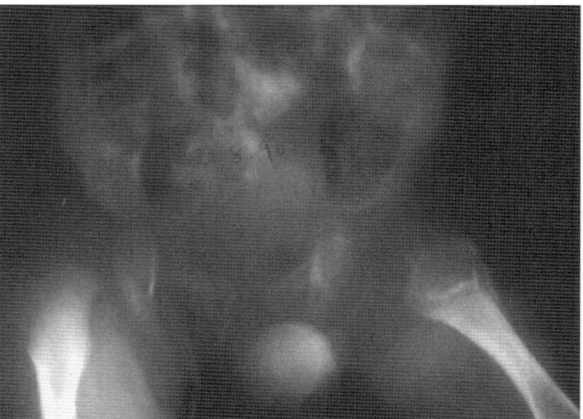

Fig. 37.30 Neonatal osteomyelitis of the left hip, showing lucency around the proximal femur and lifting of the periosteum.

instant crying when the affected limb is palpated or moved. There may also be local swelling and heat. There is spasm of the surrounding muscles that manifests as stiffness when the limb is moved.

Frequently, the signs of osteomyelitis are soft, and, if it is clinically suspected, a bone scan should be organised. This may be helpful in determining all sites involved, as these may be multiple in the neonate. The scan may highlight a hot spot at the site of hyperaemia or a cold spot if bone infarction has occurred. A negative scan in the presence of high clinical suspicion should be followed by a gallium study, which is more sensitive in this age group.

Failure to make the diagnosis results in late sequelae of growth plate arrest, chondrolysis of the joint, early degenerative changes and avascular necrosis.

The mainstay of treatment is parenteral antibiotic therapy, ideally started after specimens and cultures have been obtained. However, commencement of treatment should not be delayed. Antibiotic choice depends on local policy and advice should be sought from the microbiology department. As a guide, cefotaxime is a reasonable first-choice antibiotic, which should be continued until specific sensitivities are known. The affected limb should be splinted for comfort.

References

Achterman, C., Kalamchi, A., 1979. Congenital absence of the fibula. J Bone Joint Surg 61-B, 133–137.

Adler, J.B., Patterson, R.L., 1967. Erb's palsy: long term results of treatment in 88 cases. J Bone Joint Surg 49-A, 1052–1064.

Aitken, G.T., 1969. Proximal focal femoral deficiency – definition, classification, and management. In: Aitken, G.T. (Ed.), Proximal Focal Femoral Deficiency: A Congenital Anomaly. Washington, DC, National Academy of Sciences, pp. 1.

Aston Jr, J.W., 1977. Brachial plexus birth palsy. Orthopedics 2, 594–601.

Austwick, D.H., Dandy, D.J., 1983. Early operation for congenital subluxation of the knee. J Pediatr Orthop 3, 85–87.

Barlow, T.G., 1962. Early diagnosis and treatment of congenital dislocation of the hip. J Bone Joint Surg 44-B, 292–301.

Barlow, I.W., Clarke, N.M.P., 1994. Congenital talipes equinovarus. Surgery 12, 211–215.

Berg, E.E., 1986. A reappraisal of metatarsus adductus and skewfoot. J Bone Joint Surg 68-A, 1185–1196.

Bialik, V., Bialik, G.M., Blazer, M., et al., 1999. Developmental dysplasia of the hip: a new approach to incidence. Pediatrics 103, 93–99.

Boeree, N.R., Clarke, N.M.P., 1994. Ultrasound imaging and secondary screening for congenital dislocation of the hip. J Bone Joint Surg 76-B, 525–533.

Broughton, N.S., 1997. A Textbook of Paediatric Orthopaedics. WB Saunders, Philadelphia.

Carroll, N.C. McMurty. R., Leete, S.F., 1978. The pathoanatomy of congenital clubfoot. Orthop Clin North Am 9, 225–231.

Cashman, J.F., Round, J., Taylor, G., et al., 2002. The natural history of developmental dysplasia of the hip after early supervised treatment with a Pavlik harness. A prospective longitudinal follow up. J Bone Joint Surg 84-B, 418–425.

Cheng, J.C.Y. Wong, M.W.N., Tang, S.P., et al, 2001. Clinical determinants of the outcome of manual stretching in the treatment of congenital muscular torticollis in infants. A prospective study of 821 cases. J Bone Joint Surg 83-A, 679–687.

Clarke, N.M.P., Harcke, H.T., McHugh, P., et al., 1985. Real-time ultrasound in the diagnosis of congenital dislocation and dysplasia of the hip. J Bone Joint Surg 67-B, 406–412.

Coventry, M.B., Johnson, E.W.J., 1952. Congenital absence of the fibula. J Bone Joint Surg 34-A, 941–945.

Curtis, B.H., Fisher, R.L., 1969. Congenital hyperextension with anterior subluxation of the knee. J Bone Joint Surg 51-A, 255–269.

Dimeglio, A., Bensahel, H., Souchet, P., et al., 1995. Classification of clubfoot. J Pediatr Orthop 4-B, 129–136.

Drennan, J.C., 1990. Neuromuscular disorders. In: Morrissy, R.T. (Ed.), Lovell and Winter's Pediatric Orthopaedics, third ed. JB Lippincott, Philadelphia, pp. 381–463.

Elbourne, D., Dezateux, C., Arthur, R., et al., 2002. Ultrasonography in the diagnosis and management of developmental hip dysplasia (UK Hip Trial): clinical and economic results of a multicentre randomised controlled trial. Lancet 360, 2009–2017.

Eulenberg, M., 1863. Beitrag zur Dislocation der Scapula. Amtliche Berichte über die Versammlungen deutscher Naturforscher und Aerzte fur die Jahre 37, 291.

Foulkes, G.D., Reinker, K., 1994. Congenital constriction band syndrome: a 70 year experience. J Pediatr Orthop 14, 242–248.

Ghali, N.N., Abberton, M.J., Silk, F.F., 1984. The management of metatarsus adductus et supinatus. J Bone Joint Surg 66-B, 376–380.

Gillespie, R., Torode, I.P., 1983. Classification and management of congenital abnormalities of the femur. J Bone Joint Surg 65-B, 557–568.

Graf, R., 1984. New possibilities of the diagnosis of congenital hip joint dislocation by ultrasonography. J Pediatr Orthop 3, 354–359.

Hardy, A.E., 1981. Birth injuries of the brachial plexus: incidence and prognosis. J Bone Joint Surg 63-B, 98–101.

Harrington, P.R., 1960. Surgical instrumentation for management of scoliosis. J Bone Joint Surg 42-A, 1448.

Haynes, R.J., 2001. Developmental dysplasia of the hip: etiology, pathogenesis, and examination and physical findings in the newborn. AAOS Instruct Course Lect 50, 535–540.

Hensinger, R.N., Jones, E.T., 1981. Neonatal Orthopaedics. Grune and Stratton, New York.

Hensinger, R.N., Lang, J.R., MacEwen, G.D., 1974. The Klippel–Feil syndrome: a constellation of related anomalies. J Bone Joint Surg 56-A, 1246–1253.

Jackson, S.T., Hoffer, M.M., Parrish, N., 1988. Brachial plexus palsy in the newborn. J Bone Joint Surg 70-A, 1217–1220.

Jennett, R.J., Tarby, T.J., Krauss, R.L., 2002. Erb's palsy contrasted with Klumpke's and total palsy: different mechanisms are involved. Am J Obstet Gynecol 186, 1216–1220.

Kalamchi, A., Dawe, R.V., 1985. Congenital deficiency of the tibia. J Bone Joint Surg 67-B, 581–584.

Klisic, P.G., 1989. Congenital dislocation of the hip – a misleading term. J Bone Joint Surg 71-B, 136.

Letts, M., Blastorah, B., Al-Azzam, S., 1997. Neonatal gangrene of the extremities. J Pediatr Orthop 17, 397–401.

Lin, J.N., Chou, M.L., 1997. Ultrasonographic study of the sternocleidomastoid muscle in the management of congenital muscular torticollis. J Pediatr Surg 32, 1648–1651.

MacEwen, G.D., Hardy, J.H., 1972. Evaluation of kidney anomalies in congenital scoliosis. J Bone Joint Surg 54-A, 1451–1454.

Madsen, E.T., 1955. Fractures of extremities in the newborn. Acta Obstet Gynaecol Scand 34, 41–75.

Mollan, R.A.B., Piggot, J., 1977. Acute osteomyelitis in children. J Bone Joint Surg 59-B, 2–7.

Nade, S., 1983a. Acute septic arthritis in infancy and childhood. J Bone Joint Surg 65-B, 234–241.

Nade, S., 1983b. Acute haematogenous osteomyelitis in infancy and childhood. J Bone Joint Surg 65-B, 109–119.

Neibauer, J.J., King, D.E., 1960. Congenital dislocation of the knee. J Bone Joint Surg 42-A, 207–225.

Nogi, J., MacEwen, G.D., 1982. Congenital dislocation of the knee. J Pediatr Orthop 2, 509–513.

Ortolani, M., 1937. Un sengo poco noto e sua importanza per la diagnosi precoce di prelussazione congenital dell'anca. Pediatrica (Napoli) 45, 129–136.

Palmer, P.M., MacEwen, G.D., Bowen, J.R., et al., 1985. Passive motion therapy for infants with arthrogryposis multiplex congenita. Clin Orthop Rel Res 195, 53–59.

Patterson, T.J.S., 1961. Congenital ring constrictions. Br J Plast Surg 14, 1–31.

Pavlik, A., 1992 .The functional method of treatment using a harness with stirrups as the primary method of conservative therapy for infants with congenital dislocation of the hip. 1957. Clin Orthop Rel Res 281, 4–10.

Ponseti, I.V., Smoley, E.N., 1963. Congenital clubfoot: the results of treatment. J Bone Joint Surg 45-A, 261–275.

Sadler, T.W., 1990. Langman's Medical Embryology, sixth ed. Williams and Wilkins, Baltimore.

Standing Medical Advisory Committee, Standing Nursing and Midwifery Advisory Committee Working Parties for the Secretary of State for Social Services and Wales, 1986. Screening for the detection of congenital dislocation of the hip. Arch Dis Child 61, 921–926.

Stern, M.B., 1968. Congenital dislocation of the knee. Clin Orthop Rel Res 61, 261–268.

Tachdjian, M.O., 1990. Pediatric Orthopaedics, second ed. WB Saunders, Philadelphia.

Taylor, G.R., Clarke, N.M.P., 1997. Monitoring the treatment of developmental dysplasia of the hip with the Pavlik harness. The role of ultrasound. J Bone Joint Surg 79-B, 719–723.

Torpin, R., Faulkner, A., 1966. Intrauterine amputation with the missing member found in the fetal membranes. JAMA 198, 185–187.

Uglow, M.G., Clarke, N.M.P., 2000a. Relapse in staged surgery for congenital talipes equinovarus. J Bone Joint Surg 82-B, 739–743.

Uglow, M.G., Clarke, N.M.P., 2000b. The functional outcome of staged surgery for the correction of talipes equinovarus. J Pediatr Orthop 20, 517–523.

Williams, P., 1978. The management of arthrogryposis. Orthop Clin North Am 9, 67–88.

Williams, C.R.P., O'Flynn, E., Clarke, N.M.P., et al., 1996. Torticollis secondary to ocular pathology. J Bone Joint Surg 78-B, 620–624.

Winter, R.B., 1981. Convex anterior and posterior hemiarthrodesis and hemiepiphysiodesis in young children with progressive congenital scoliosis. J Pediatr Orthop 1, 361–366.

Winter, R.B., Moe, J.H., Wang, J.F., 1973. Congenital kyphosis. Its natural history and treatment as observed in a study of 130 patients. J Bone Joint Surg 55-A, 223–256.

Wynne-Davies, R., 1978. Heritable disorders in orthopedics. Orthop Clin North Am 9, 1–14.

Neonatal gynaecology

38

D Keith Edmonds

CHAPTER CONTENTS

Gynaecological problems in neonatal life are unusual and rare. Many conditions that are thought to be pathological are commonly physiological or anatomical variants, but these variants cause considerable anxiety amongst parents. Knowledge of the physiology and anatomy of the development of the genital tract during fetal life is therefore important, so that an explanation of these variations can be offered to parents in a reassuring manner.

The physiology of the fetal hypothalamopituitary axis

The early fetal brain undergoes rapid development, and, by 5 weeks of gestation, gonadotrophin-releasing hormone (GnRH) can be detected in whole-brain extract (Winters et al. 1974). GnRH can be localised to the hypothalamus by 8–13 weeks' gestation (Kaplan et al. 1976; Aubert et al. 1977), and the hypothalamic GnRH content of female fetuses reaches a maximum at between 22 and 25 weeks' gestation and thereafter declines (Siler-Khodr and Khodr 1978). This is almost certainly in response to negative feedback of circulating oestradiol.

Luteinising hormone (LH) and follicle-stimulating hormone (FSH) can be identified within the pituitary gland by 9–11 weeks'

gestation (Hagen and McNeilly 1977; Currie et al. 1981) and the portal circulation linking the hypothalamus with the pituitary is known to be intact by 12 weeks' gestation (Thliveris and Currie 1980). In response to GnRH release, FSH and LH reach their maximum between 16 and 24 weeks (Takagi et al. 1977). Subsequently, FSH levels decline, almost certainly owing to active secretion of inhibin from the granulosa cells in the ovary. During the latter part of fetal life, gonadotrophin levels are reduced and remain at low levels until birth (Takagi et al. 1977). Both inhibin and circulating oestradiol exhibit this negative-feedback mechanism.

Following birth, the contribution of placental oestradiol to the fetal circulation is withdrawn, the fetal hypothalamopituitary axis becomes activated and both GnRH and gonadotrophin levels rise immediately (Winter et al. 1975). FSH levels and LH levels remain elevated for several months after birth, but subsequent central suppression of GnRH leads to decline in gonadotrophin levels by around 6 months of age. The central suppression of the pulse generator in the arcuate nucleus of the hypothalamus may be brought about by several modulators, including noradrenaline (norepinephrine), dopamine, central opiates, neuropeptide Y, glutamate or aspartate (Lee 1988; Gore et al. 1993; Prasad et al. 1993; Brann 1995). The cell receptors on the GnRH-secreting neurons are controlled by a gene encoding for transforming growth factor-alpha (Ma et al. 1994), and this gene may well itself be controlled by the secretion of leptin (MacDougald et al. 1995), a hormone produced by adipose tissue; decreasing the body mass index towards later infancy and increasing body mass at puberty may be intimately involved in the activation of the gene.

Thus, throughout fetal and early neonatal life, the hypothalamopituitary ovarian uterine axis is fully developed and active, and capable of responding to all of the appropriate integrated mechanisms. It is only the genetic downregulation of central receptors that suppresses activity after birth.

Neonatal breast development

Breast development occurs during fetal life and is well described as proceeding in female infants for several months after birth (Fig. 38.1). It is occasionally associated with secretions similar to lactation. Two studies suggest that, after birth, circulating levels of oestriol, which would be maternally derived, decline rapidly, and yet breast development continues for several months after birth

© 2012 Elsevier Ltd

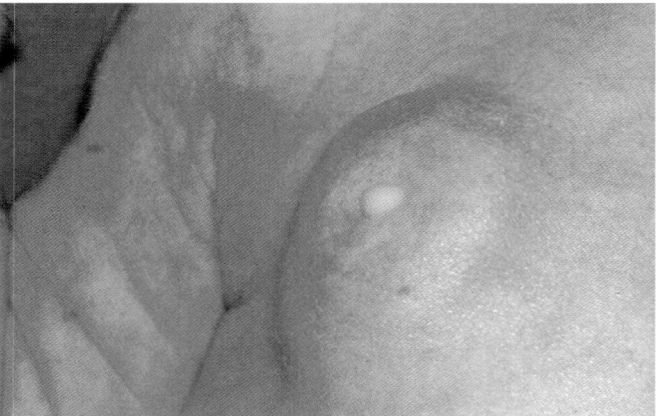

Fig. 38.1 Neonatal gynaecomastia.

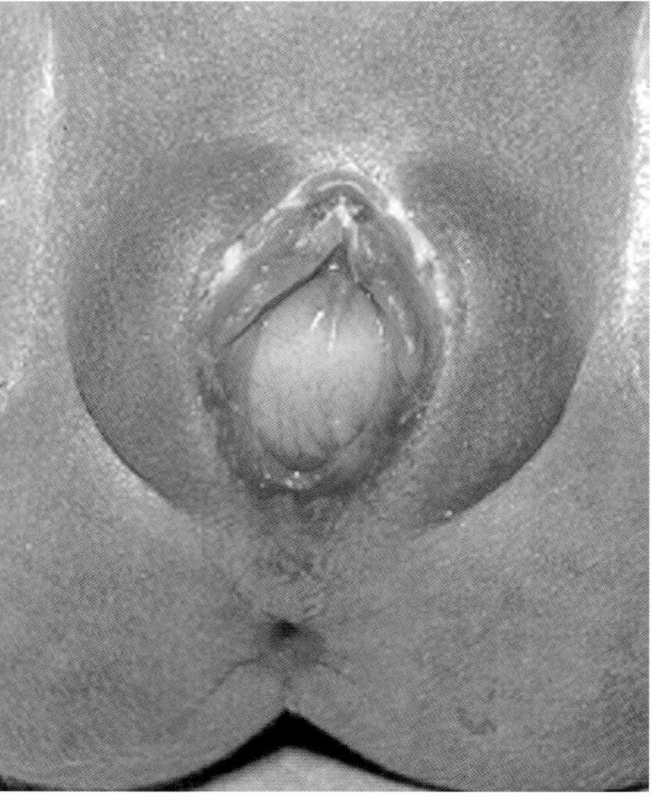

Fig. 38.2 Bulging membrane at the introitus in a case of transverse vaginal septum presenting in a newborn.

(McKiernan and Hull 1981; Anbazhagan et al. 1991). Elevated levels of oestradiol and prolactin in the neonate are directly related to breast size, the relationship being particularly strong with pro-lactin. Therefore it would seem that the infant's own gonadal secretions are responsible for the control of the breast. Histological studies further support this theory (McKiernan et al. 1988). Breast development in early neonatal life thus is a normal physiological process and ceases at 3–6 months of age; the breast bud may thereafter regress.

A recent study (Zung et al. 2008) suggests that breast regression is delayed in infants who are fed soy-based infant formulas. It is suggested that phyto-oestrogens in soy-based milk preserve breast tissue in the neonate until cessation of this type of formula feed and thereafter breast tissue regresses.

Supernumerary nipples are a common finding; they extend along the nipple line on either side of the chest wall, down the abdomen and may occur in the labia. Bilateral ectopic breast tissue has been described in the vulva (Levin and Diener 1968).

Vulval problems

Labial cysts in the newborn are rare, and occur in about 6 per 1000 female infants. These congenital cysts require no treatment whatsoever, and conservative management leads to complete resolution within 2–3 months of life. No surgical approach should be taken in these circumstances (Merlob et al. 1978).

Inguinal hernia in infants is very common and is encountered in approximately 1–3% of full-term newborns and 3–5% of premature babies (Dassonville et al. 1985). Surgical management of this involves closure of the hernia (Ch. 29, part 4). It is important to be aware that, in female infants, a differential diagnosis of an irreducible inguinal mass must include the presence of either a prolapsed ovary or the uterus and ovary, and, in female infants with ambiguous genitalia, the inguinal mass may be a testis. It is unusual for these to be seen immediately after birth, but they may become obvious in the ensuing months. Ultrasound of these masses can be extremely useful and may help to differentiate the presence of ovarian tissue in the hernia sac and also aid in differentiating the presence of an ovary or a testis. It is important that, when these masses are detected, early treatment is offered, as correction of this anatomical defect will reduce the risk of torsion and infarction and subsequent loss of the gonad. This is particularly important when the herniation is an ovary, which requires conservation.

Abnormalities of the hymen

The hymen at birth is usually annular or fimbriated and commonly associated with external ridges. Hymenal tags are extremely common at birth (Mor et al. 1983), and are often misdiagnosed as 'prolapse'. The hymen changes its characteristics during the first 3 years of life and becomes crescentic by age 3 years in the vast majority, with the external ridges disappearing (Berenson 1995). Problems in neonatal life that are associated with peripheral oedema often lead to oedema of the hymen, which may protrude beyond the vulval entrance and again be mistaken for a prolapse.

Failure of the hymen to perforate during embryological life may lead to retention of vaginal secretions which cannot escape and the vagina distends proximal to the hymen. Although these membranes are often referred to as imperforate hymen, it is likely that this is not strictly correct and that these membranes are transverse vaginal septa, resulting from failure of fusion of the urogenital sinus and the downgrowth of the vaginal plate from the müllerian structures. When a large quantity of fluid collects, there may be difficulty in emptying the bladder, as the distended vagina fills the pelvis, and the child may be very fretful and clearly in discomfort. The physical signs are of a lower abdominal cystic swelling and a bulging membrane at the introitus (Fig. 38.2). Diagnosis is extremely important, as misdiagnoses abound in which laparotomy has been performed, and even hysterectomy, and this is absolutely unnecessary. The most common misdiagnoses are to believe that this is either a swelling which is an ovarian cyst or, occasionally, a full bladder with urethral prolapse. Ultrasound imaging may diagnose a hydrocolpos both antenatally and after delivery, and the condition has been described as early as 25 weeks' gestation (Winderl and Silverman 1995). With ultrasound, it is simple to demonstrate the uterus sitting above a distended vagina, when the diagnosis of hydrocolpos can be made. Treatment is straightforward in most cases: the intact membrane is incised and the retained fluid released. Redundant portions of the membrane may be excised and the procedure completed. If the obstruction is more extensive owing to a wide transverse septum, great care is needed to avoid damage to the bladder and rectum, but an end-to-end anastomosis can be achieved to result in a normal vagina. These cases of hydrocolpos are probably exceptional, as most cases of transverse vaginal septum are not diagnosed until puberty (Edmonds 1988).

Vaginal bleeding problems

Bleeding from the genital tract in the newborn period is well described. A study from Huber in 1976 showed that vaginal bleeding occurs in 25% of newborn girls, although it is only macroscopically visible in 3.3%. Vaginal bleeding in the first week of life is extremely common due to the influence of maternal oestriol and therefore should cause no alarm. However, persistent vaginal bleeding, particularly beyond the first year of life, demands further investigation. The development of rhabdomyosarcoma, whilst extraordinarily rare in immediate neonatal life, may present as bleeding at 2–3 months of age. Most of the genital lesions associated with rhabdomyosarcoma of the perineum, vulva and vagina occur in early childhood.

Uterine prolapse

Prolapse in the neonatal period is extremely rare, but may present with the cervix protruding through the vagina. A number of cases have been described and, although the aetiology of the problem remains obscure, some cases are associated with neurological abnormalities, e.g. spina bifida. Treatment is conservative and involves digital replacement of the prolapse into the vagina. This may have to be repeated on a number of occasions, but eventually, by 3 months of age at the latest, all of these prolapses have resolved. Occasionally, pessaries may be required if the prolapse remains persistent, although these are very difficult to design for infants (Johnson et al. 1984). Surgical management using a ventrosuspension has been performed in an infant with a persisting problem (Banieghbal and Fonseca 1998). No data exist to suggest whether or not these female infants will develop prolapse problems in a later stage of their lives, but it is likely that this will be the case, as the occurrence of prolapse in these circumstances may be associated with poor collagen development in the supporting tissue of the genital tract

Urethral prolapse

Urethral prolapse in the neonatal period is extremely rare, but may present with vaginal bleeding. If the urethral mucosa prolapses through the meatus it may form a sensitive vulval mass that bleeds to touch. This urethral mucosal prolapse in the neonatal period is extremely rare and usually presents with bleeding. The passage of urine may be unimpaired when the lesion is small, and in these circumstances the use of oestrogen cream may be beneficial. However, occasionally, urinary retention may be present, or the prolapse may recur following repeated oestrogen treatments and recurrence may require surgical excision if the lesion is large. This tends to be only rarely necessary and is usually only employed when urinary retention is present.

Paraurethral cysts

This rare condition has been described in the neonatal period and the cyst may obscure the urethra. These cysts tend to resolve spontaneously and only rarely require surgical intervention (Fujimoto et al. 2009).

Ovarian cysts

Ultrasound of the fetus during pregnancy is now sophisticated enough to diagnose ovarian cysts in mid-pregnancy, and these may be detected as early as 16–18 weeks' gestation. The vast majority of these cysts are functional, benign follicular cysts and do not interfere with the course of pregnancy or birth. If these cysts are less than 5 cm in diameter as diagnosed during the postnatal period, then they may be managed conservatively with serial ultrasound and the vast majority will resolve spontaneously (Brandt et al. 1991). This may take as long as 6 months to a year and this relates to stimulation of the ovary by elevated FSH levels which persist during this time. Cysts that are larger than 5 cm in diameter (Fig. 38.3) that do not contain any solid elements should be managed conservatively

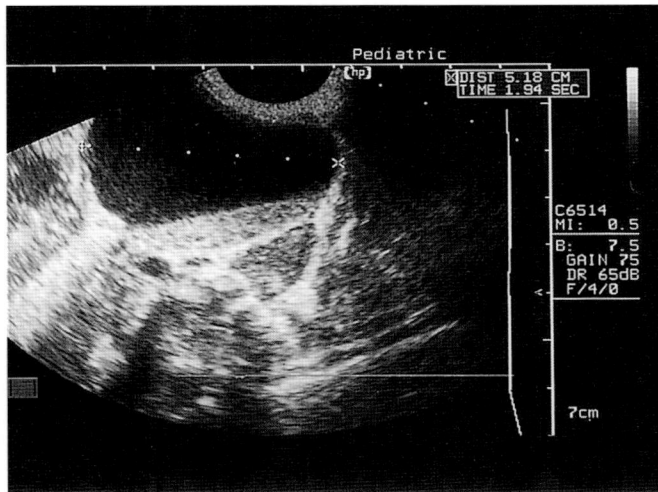

Fig. 38.3 Pelvic ultrasound scan showing an ovarian cyst 5 cm in diameter in a newborn girl.

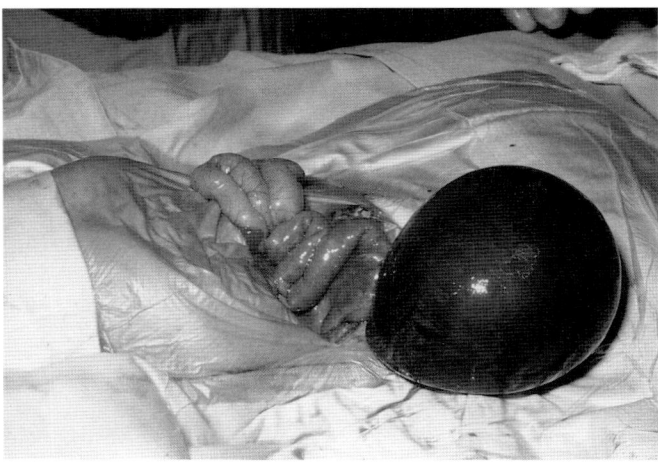

Fig. 38.4 Torted ovarian cyst at laparotomy in a young girl.

unless there are complications. These include torsion or haemorrhage and in these circumstances may require either cystectomy or aspiration of the cyst. Parents should be advised about the risk of torsion and any symptoms of acute pain should be acted upon. If this is performed, cytology should always be carried out for confirmation of a benign lesion. All cysts of 4 cm or more have the risk of torsion, and therefore care must be taken in their management

and also in the advice that is given to parents. All larger cysts and complex cysts require more careful assessment and may require a surgical approach (Fig. 38.4) to ensure that the cyst is benign. This may be carried out laparoscopically or via laparotomy (Esposito et al. 1998). Antenatal torsion of a cyst has been described in a pregnancy that resulted in premature birth, although the clinical course of the neonate was uneventful.

References

Anbazhagan, R., Bartek, J., Monaghan, P., et al., 1991. Growth and development of the human infant breast. Am J Anat 192, 407–417.

Aubert, M.L., Grumbach, M.M., Kaplan, S.L., 1977. The autogenesis of human fetal hormones. IV. Somatostatin, luteinizing hormone releasing factor, and thyrotropin releasing factor in hypothalamus and cerebral cortex of human fetuses 10–22 weeks of age. J Clin Endocrinol Metab 44, 1130–1141.

Banieghbal, B., Fonseca, J., 1998. Surgical management of uterine prolapse in an infant. Eur J Pediatr Surg 8, 119–120.

Berenson, A.B., 1995. A longitudinal study of hymenal morphology in the first 3 years of life. Pediatrics 95, 490–496.

Brandt, M.L., Luks, F.I., Filiatrault, D., et al., 1991. Surgical indications in antenatally diagnosed ovarian cysts. J Pediatr Surg 26, 276–281.

Brann, D.W., 1995. Glutamate: a major excitatory transmitter in neuroendocrine regulation. Neuroendocrinology 61, 213–225.

Currie, R.W., Faiman, C., Thliveris, J.A., 1981. An immunocytochemical and routine electron microscopic study of LH and FSH cells in the human fetal pituitary. Am J Anat 161, 281–297.

Dassonville, M., Verstreken, L., De Laet, M.H., 1985. [Inguinal hernia in infants and children.] Acta Chir Belg 85, 341–347.

Edmonds, D.K., 1988. Practical Paediatric and Adolescent Gynaecology. Butterworths, London, pp. 86–95.

Esposito, C., Garipoli, V., Di Matteo, G., et al., 1998. Laparoscopic management of ovarian cysts in newborns. Surg Endosc 12, 1152–1154.

Fujimoto, T., Suwa, T., Ishii, N., et al., 2009. Paraurethral cyst in female newborn: is surgery always advocated? J Pediatr Surg 42, 400–403.

Gore, A.C., Mitsushima, D., Terasawa, E., 1993. A possible role of neuropeptide Y in the control of the onset of puberty in female rhesus monkeys. Neuroendocrinology 58, 23–34.

Hagen, C., McNeilly, A.S., 1977. The gonadotrophins and their subunits in foetal pituitary glands and circulation. J Steroid Biochem 8, 537–544.

Huber, A., 1976. [The frequency of physiologic vaginal bleeding of newborn infants.] Zentralbl Gynakol 98, 1017–1020.

Johnson, A., Unger, S.W., Rodgers, B.M., 1984. Uterine prolapse in the neonate. J Pediatr Surg 19, 210–211.

Kaplan, S.L., Grumbach, M.M., Aubert, M.L., 1976. The ontogenesis of pituitary hormones and hypothalamic factors in the human fetus: maturation of central nervous system regulation of anterior pituitary function. Recent Progr Horm Res 32, 161–243.

Lee, P.A., 1988. The neuroendocrinology of puberty. Semin Reprod Med 6, 13–20.

Levin, N., Diener, R.L., 1968. Bilateral ectopic breast of the vulva. Report of a case. Obstet Gynecol 32, 274–276.

Ma, Y.J., Costa, M.E., Ojeda, S.R., 1994. Developmental expression of the genes encoding transforming growth factor alpha and its receptor in the hypothalamus of female rhesus macaques. Neuroendocrinology 60, 346–359.

MacDougald, O.A., Hwang, C.S., Fan, H., et al., 1995. Regulated expression of the obese gene product (leptin) in white adipose tissue and 3T3-L1 adipocytes. Proc Natl Acad Sci USA 92, 9034–9037.

McKiernan, J.F., Hull, D., 1981. Prolactin, maternal oestrogens, and breast development in the newborn. Arch Dis Child 56, 770–774.

McKiernan, J., Coyne, J., Cahalane, S., 1988. Histology of breast development in early life. Arch Dis Child 63, 136–139.

Merlob, P., Bahari, C., Liban, E., et al., 1978. Cysts of the female external genitalia in the newborn infant. Am J Obstet Gynecol 132, 607–610.

Mor, N., Merlob, P., Reisner, S.H., 1983. Tags and bands of the female external genitalia in the newborn infant. Clin Pediatr 22, 122–124.

Prasad, B.M., Conover, C.D., Sarkar, D.K., et al., 1993. Feed restriction in prepubertal lambs: effect on puberty onset and on in vivo release of luteinizing-hormone-releasing hormone, neuropeptide Y and beta-endorphin from the posterior-lateral median eminence. Neuroendocrinology 57, 1171–1181.

Siler-Khodr, T.M., Khodr, G.S., 1978. Studies in human fetal endocrinology. I. Luteinizing hormone-releasing factor content of the hypothalamus. Am J Obstet Gynecol 130, 795–800.

Takagi, S., Yoshida, T., Tsubata, K., et al., 1977. Sex differences in fetal gonadotropins and androgens. J Steroid Biochem 8, 609–620.

Thliveris, J.A., Currie, R.W., 1980. Observations on the hypothalamo-hypophyseal portal vasculature in the developing human fetus. Am J Anat 157, 441–444.

Winderl, L.M., Silverman, R.K., 1995. Prenatal diagnosis of congenital imperforate hymen. Obstet Gynecol 85, 857–860.

Winter, J.S., Faiman, C., Hobson, W.C., et al., 1975. Pituitary–gonadal relations in infancy. I. Patterns of serum gonadotropin concentrations from birth to four years of age in man and chimpanzee. J Clin Endocrinol Metab 40, 545–551.

Winters, A.J., Eskay, R.L., Porter, J.C., 1974. Concentration and distribution of TRH and LRH in the human fetal brain. J Clin Endocrinol Metab 39, 960–963.

Zung, A., Glaser, T., Kerem, T., et al., 2008. Breast development in first 2 years of life: an association with soy-based infant formulas. J Pediatr Gastroenterol Nutr 46, 191–195.

Neonatal infection

Andrew J Cant   Andrew R Gennery
Alison Bedford Russell   David Isaacs

CHAPTER CONTENTS

© 2012 Elsevier Ltd

Part 1: **Immunodeficiency**

Andrew J Cant   Andrew R Gennery

Introduction

The immune system distinguishes 'self' from 'non-self', destroying microorganisms but leaving other proteins intact. Immunological abnormalities result in an increased susceptibility to infection, as well as allergy and autoimmunity. The term baby's immune system will generally respond appropriately, but failure may occur because of naïvety to an antigen or lack of fine-tuning (e.g. the antibody response to polysaccharide antigen). The preterm infant is immature in several respects, and is often subject to breaches of protective barriers by intravenous catheters and endotracheal tubes.

The immune system

Every effort should be made to exclude pathogens, particularly from the neonatal intensive care unit environment. The importance of hand-washing and high standards of hygiene cannot be overemphasised. The baby's epithelial surfaces and mucous membranes

Table 39.1 Differences between innate and adaptive immunity

	INNATE IMMUNITY	ACQUIRED (ADAPTIVE) IMMUNITY

Cellular elements	Cellular:
	  Phagocytes Neutrophils
	          Basophils
	          Eosinophils
	          Macrophages
	Natural killer cells
		T lymphocytes
		CD4+ helper T cells T_H1 cells T_H2 cells
		CD8+ cytotoxic T cells
		CD19+ B lymphocytes
		Plasma cells – secrete immunoglobulin

Humoral elements	Chemical:
	  Complement
	  Mannose-binding lectin
	  C-reactive protein
	Cytokines
		Immunoglobulin (Ig)3
		          IgM
		          IgA
		          IgG
		          IgE
		Cytokines

Response to infection	Rapid: 0–4 hours	Delayed. Slow at first encounter (>96 hours)
Receptor characteristics	Germline encoded Expressed by all cells of a particular type Broad specificity	Encoded in multiple gene segments requiring gene rearrangement Clonal distribution Antigen specificity
Memory	Common to species, static	Specific to individual Updatable

provide the initial defence, augmented by cilia and respiratory tract mucus secretions, stomach acids and other mucous membrane secretions. Commensal intestinal and skin flora produce locally acting antibiotics. These barriers are particularly important in neonates, whose immunological immaturity predisposes them to infections.

Specific and non-specific mechanisms of immunity

Pathogens that breach the barrier defences first encounter non-specific and then specific components of the immune system. These are interdependent; many specific immune mechanisms use non-specific elements to exert their effects, and factors produced by the specific immune response can greatly potentiate non-specific functions.

Phagocytes such as neutrophils or monocytes, as well as the complement system, deliver highly effective non-antigen-specific immune responses using a limited number of pattern recognition receptors specific for conserved microbial structures, including Toll-like receptors and nucleotide-binding olgomerisation domain (NOD)-like receptors.

The specific immune system responds to antigens by proliferation of antigen-specific T and B lymphocytes following antigen presentation to their receptor by cells of the non-specific (innate) system. These responses are then committed to 'immunological memory', resulting in more rapid and enhanced responses upon subsequent antigen exposure. The differences between the innate and adaptive immune systems are summarised in Table 39.1.

Non-specific immune mechanisms

Humoral

Complement is the major humoral component of the innate response. When the central component, C3b, which can be activated by at least three pathways, is bound to an antigen, it interacts

powerfully with C3b receptors on neutrophils and monocytes, enhancing phagocytosis. C3b also initiates a cascade activating further components such as C5–C9, which lyse cell membranes, a mechanism particularly important in the handling of systemic neisserial infections.

Mannan-binding lectin, which binds to mannose on the surface of microorganisms, activates the classical complement pathway; this is important in the early stages of infection before antibody production, particularly in young children whose antibody-producing ability is immature.

Alpha- and beta-interferon (IFN-α, IFN-β) proteins are produced by virally infected cells. They render other cells immune to virus infection by producing an antiviral state. They also increase natural killer (NK) cell activity and increase human leukocyte antigen (HLA) class I antigen expression on cells. Gamma-interferon (IFN-γ), though having some antiviral effect, upregulates immune responses by enhancing intracellular killing of microorganisms such as mycobacteria.

Many bacteria require iron for growth, and decreasing iron availability is one mechanism of defence used by the host. An avid iron-binding protein, lactoferrin, present in human milk, reduces the growth of *Escherichia coli*. The removal of serum iron, which occurs during infections, increases the bacteriostatic effect of serum.

Lysozyme is found in neutrophil lysosomes and body secretions, including tears, saliva, and at increased concentrations on newborn skin, and has antibacterial properties.

Cellular

Phagocytic cells such as neutrophils and monocyte/macrophages migrate to the site of infection attracted by products of the acute inflammatory response (chemotaxis), including cleaved complement fragments. Adherence to the bacterium and ingestion (phagocytosis) follow, aided by immunoglobulin G (IgG) and complement (C3b), which stick to bacteria and phagocyte cell surface receptors Fcg and CR1/3, respectively (opsonisation). Following phagocytosis, lysosomes fuse with the bacterium-containing phago-some and release lysosomal enzymes (e.g. myeloperoxidase) and free oxygen radicals, which kill and digest microorganisms. Neutrophil numbers and function are enhanced by the inflammatory response.

Monocytes and macrophages kill extracellular bacteria more slowly and less efficiently than neutrophils but are important in defences against intracellular microorganisms, such as *Mycobacterium tuberculosis* and *Listeria monocytogenes*, because their activity is greatly enhanced by cytokines, particularly IFN-γ, produced by T lymphocytes.

NK cells are part of the non-T, non-B-cell lymphoid population and recognise and kill tumour and virus-infected cells.

Specific immune mechanisms

Specific responses are generated by T and B lymphocytes, whose receptors are antigen-specific. Binding of antigen to receptor initiates antibody production or the generation of specific cytotoxic T lymphocytes (Fig. 39.1).

Antigen-presenting cells (APC) present antigens to T lymphocytes, degrade them to small peptide fragments and then express them on

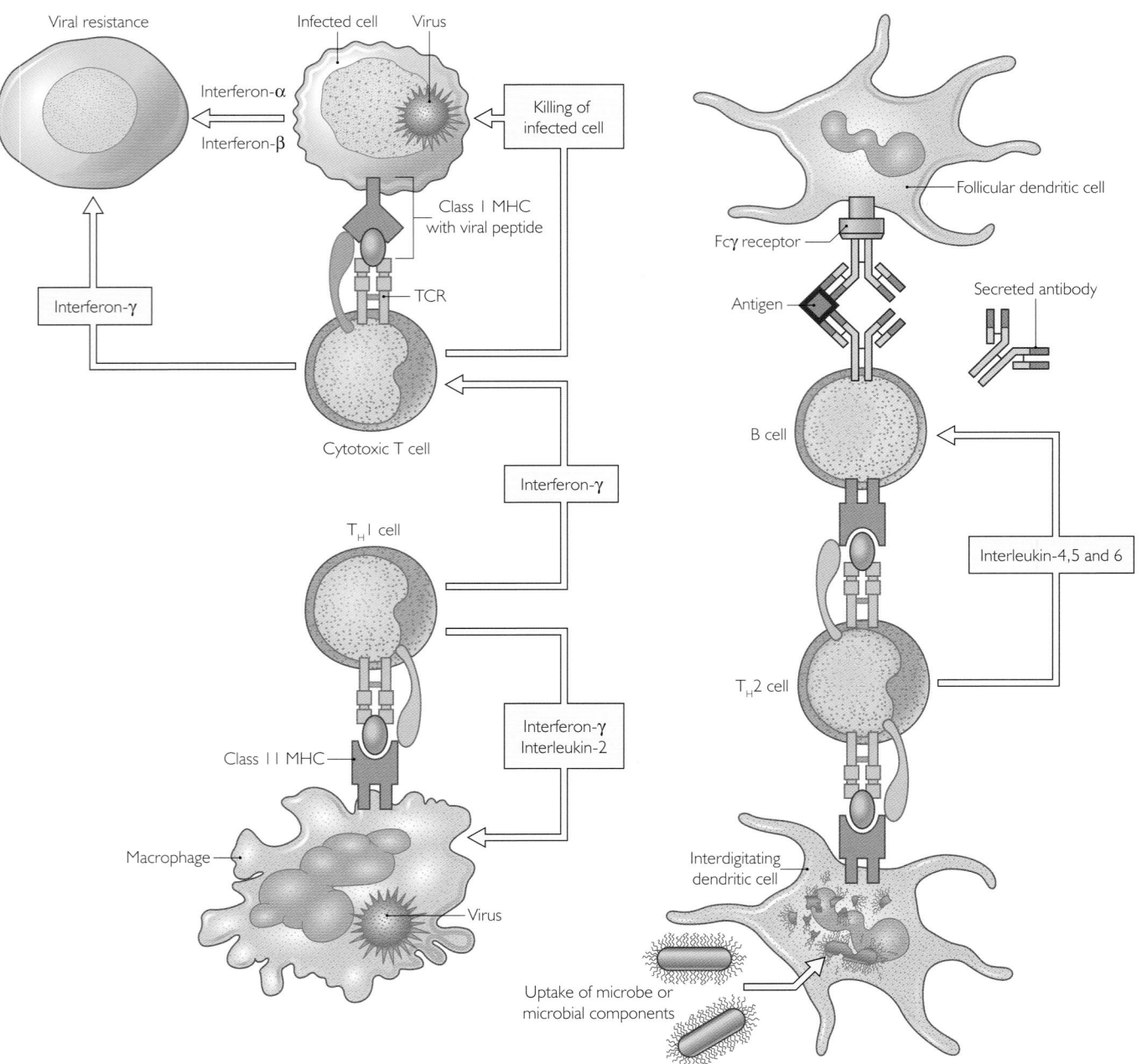

Fig. 39.1 Lymphocyte responses. T-lymphocyte receptors (TCR) recognise specific processed antigen presented in association with major histocompatibility (MHC) molecules by antigen-presenting cells. Cytotoxic (CD8+) T cells kill infected cells and prevent viral replication (left). Helper T cells (CD4+) either activate cytotoxic T cells and macrophages to kill intracellular organisms (T_H1) or secrete cytokines to help B cells secrete antibody (T_H2) (right). *(Adapted with permission from Delves and Roitt 2000; copyright © 2004 Massachusetts Medical Society. All rights reserved.)*

the cell surface in association with the major histocompatibility complex (MHC) molecules. The T-lymphocyte receptor (T-cell receptor, TCR) recognises the peptide in association with a self MHC molecule. CD4+ helper T lymphocytes respond to antigen bound within the groove of class II MHC molecules (HLA-DR) whilst CD8+ cytotoxic T lymphocytes respond to antigen bound within the groove of class I (HLA-AB) molecules. There are two arms of the specific immune system – antibody-mediated and cell-mediated.

Antibodies

These are produced by B lymphocytes and their derivatives, plasma cells, in response to specific antigens such as microbial or vaccine peptide.

The immunoglobulin class (isotype) is determined by the heavy chain. During B-lymphocyte development, genes coding for the variable and constant parts of the immunoglobulin chain are rearranged. One each of the variable (V), diversity (D) and joining (J) heavy-chain genes are rearranged to lie adjacent to the relevant heavy-chain constant-region gene, so that transcription produces a single protein with a constant and a variable portion (Fig. 39.2). Approximately 10^{16} different specific B-lymphocyte receptors (with a similar number of TCR) are generated. Further rearrangement to bring a particular variable gene combination to lie adjacent to a different heavy-chain constant-region gene allows the B lymphocyte to switch to another antibody isotype with the same antigen

specificity. The m chain is always produced first; class switching to other isotypes occurs later. Specific antibody diversity is created by the large number of possible combinations of variable-region genes that can be selected and is increased further by a very high mutation rate in V genes. A similar but slightly less complex process takes place with light chains, of which there are two types, kappa and lambda.

IgM is the first antibody class produced in primary immune responses. For most antigens, there is a subsequent switching to other classes. Its large pentameric structure confines it to the intravascular space, where it fixes complement.

IgG is the main class of antibody produced in secondary immune responses. Functions include opsonisation, complement fixation leading to C3 opsonisation and complement-mediated lysis, neutralisation of toxins or viruses, and participation in antibody-dependent cellular cytotoxicity. Though there is considerable overlap, the four subclasses of IgG tend to have different functions. Responses to protein antigens are mainly in the IgG_1 and IgG_3 subclasses. IgG_2 binds polysaccharide, such as group B streptococcal surface antigen. The role of IgG_4 is, as yet, unclear.

IgA is the main antibody in secretions, where it forms a dimeric molecule. In addition to protecting mucous membranes and the gastrointestinal tract from infection, IgA may have a role in limiting food antigen uptake from the gut. Serum IgA is mainly in monomeric form, though dimeric and trimeric forms are also found. It is secreted in breast milk.

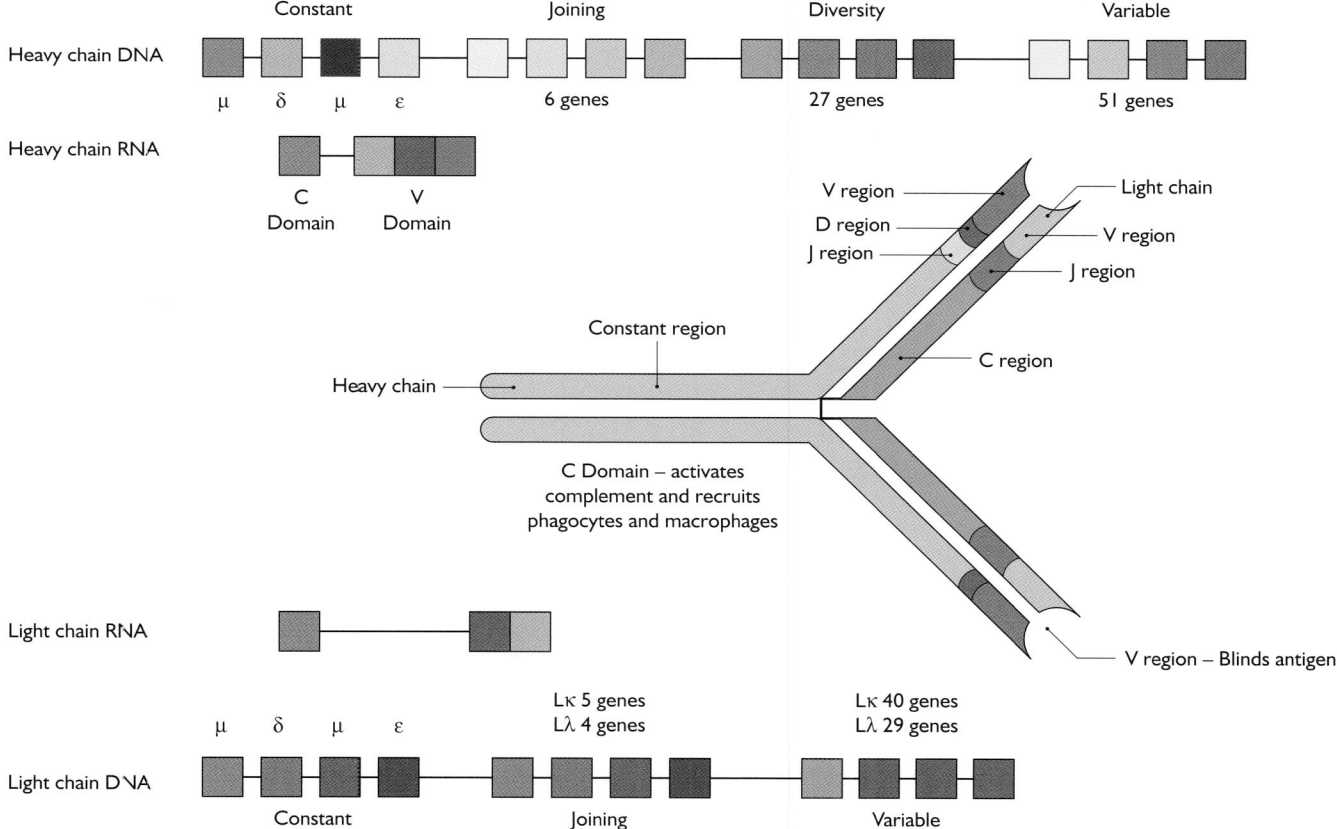

Fig. 39.2 Immunoglobulin heavy- and light-chain gene rearrangements. Discrete segments of the V, D and J heavy-chain genes are rearranged to lie adjacent to the relevant heavy-chain constant-region gene. Light-chain gene rearrangements using V and J segments from either kappa or lambda light chains complete the process. Transcription produces a single protein with a constant and a variable portion. *(Adapted with permission from Gennery and Cant 2001.)*

Mast cells and basophils have receptors for the Fc part of IgE. Antigen binding causes degranulation of the cells, triggering an immediate hypersensitivity response.

The final stages of B-lymphocyte differentiation require stimulation with the appropriate antigen, leading to maturation into plasma cells. The full process requires the cooperation of antigen-specific T helper (CD4+) lymphocytes. Isotype switching from IgM production to the other antibody classes is critically dependent on T/B-lymphocyte interaction via the B-lymphocyte CD40 antigen and the CD40 ligand expressed on activated T lymphocytes (CD40L, CD154).

Cell-mediated immunity

T (thymus-derived) lymphocytes kill intracellular microbes and regulate immune responses by secreting cytokines and growth factors.

T lymphocytes develop from bone marrow stem cells, but mature in the thymus, where their receptor genes (TCR) are rearranged to generate the diversity of lymphocyte receptors needed to counter every potential antigen. Self-reactive T lymphocytes are deleted and only those recognising antigen in association with self MHC are preserved and exit the thymus. Regulatory CD4+ T lymphocytes (T_{REG}) help maintain peripheral tolerance to self antigens.

The TCR is similar to the immunoglobulin molecule, with constant and variable parts and the generation of diverse specificity achieved in a similar way. Recombinase activating genes 1 and 2 (*RAG1, 2*) are critical for TCR gene rearrangement. During thymic maturation, T lymphocytes also acquire important functional surface molecules. CD3 is closely associated with the TCR. The CD4+ T-helper lymphocyte is the primary effector cell. Once switched on by antigen presentation via the MHC II molecule, these cells develop either by the T_H1 route, with production of the cytokines interleukin-2 (IL-2) and IFN-γ, stimulating macrophage function, cell-mediated immunity and B-lymphocyte class switching to IgG_2 production, or to T_H2 cells, which produce predominantly IL-4 and IL-10, which promote antibody responses and class switching, particularly towards IgG_1, IgG_4 and IgE. Allergic responses and those against parasites are of T_H2 type. Antigen responses may follow a T_H1 or T_H2 route, depending on a complex set of circumstances. CD8+ cytotoxic lymphocytes are activated by antigen presentation via the MHC I molecule, and directly kill virally infected cells.

The development of the immune system

Prenatal development

T- and B-lymphocyte development commences early in human embryogenesis (Holt 2000). Cells capable of responding in mixed lymphocyte culture, or to mitogens, and recognisable NK cells are present in fetal liver from 6 weeks. T- and B-lymphocyte precursors are identifiable from 7–8 weeks. Thymic stroma starts to form from the sixth week; T-lymphocyte precursors and stem cells colonise the rudimentary thymus from the ninth week. By the second trimester, circulating lymphocytes with mature T-lymphocyte surface markers, including CD3+, CD4+ and CD8+, are present in fetal blood. Surface B-lymphocyte markers, including surface immunoglobulin, are also expressed at this stage. However, lymphocyte response to antigens, especially by making immunoglobulin, is limited until birth.

Absence of these lymphocyte markers can be used for the antenatal diagnosis of severe combined immunodeficiency (SCID) by fetal blood sampling.

The non-specific elements of immunity also develop early. Neutrophil precursors can be identified in the yolk sac; mature neutrophils appear in the circulation in the second trimester, but numbers are low until the onset of labour. Complement components are present by 6 weeks of gestation.

The immune system in the newborn

The primary mechanism for distinguishing harmful from benign antigens depends on the activation status of APCs, especially dendritic cells, also known as 'professional' APCs. Lymphocyte responses can be activated by costimulatory molecules in the presence of 'alarm signals' from the environment, e.g. proinflammatory cytokines when tissues are under stress, or when pathogenic microbial products are present; and rendered tolerant in the absence of such costimulatory signals. Hence, mature virgin neonatal cells can be immunised, tolerised, or switched to T_H1 or T_H2 responses according to the dose of antigen (Sarzotti et al. 1996), the type of antigen in the environment (Forsthuber et al. 1996) or the type of APC (Ridge et al. 1996).

Neonatal T lymphocytes, therefore, can behave like adult T lymphocytes (Ridge et al. 1996) and are similarly capable of activation if appropriately stimulated by APCs. The immune system is dependent on evolutionarily conserved pathogen pattern recognition receptors on cells of the innate immune system; these allow recognition of certain pathogen-associated molecular patterns not found in the host, e.g. human Toll-like receptors. These pattern recognition molecules induce activation in cells of the innate immune system such as dendritic cells. However, the immune systems of both full-term and preterm infants exhibit a physiological immunodeficiency (Marshall-Clarke et al. 2000), though it is more marked in the premature, and particularly in the sick or stressed infant. This accounts for the newborn's increased susceptibility to infection, whether overwhelming group B streptococcal sepsis or disseminated herpes simplex infection. Placentally transferred IgG partially offsets the deficiency, but transfer of immunoglobulin occurs late in gestation, and so preterm infants have significantly reduced levels; those at the limit of viability (23–24 weeks) have extremely low levels. The protective effect of maternal immunoglobulin depends on the mother having the appropriate antigen-specific IgG antibody, and in group B streptococcal sepsis, lack of specific maternal antibody is a major risk factor. The newborn infant shows particularly poor antibody responses to polysaccharide antigens, does not switch from making IgM to IgA and IgG so readily and does not produce tightly sticking antibody.

Neonatal T lymphocytes differ in other ways. There is a high CD4:CD8 ratio, and there is usually less than 10% of the memory isoform and predominant expression of the naïve isoform. These proportions gradually reverse during childhood. Exposure to intrauterine infection often provokes a more 'mature' picture.

Naïve T lymphocytes are harder to stimulate, accounting for poorer responses in neonates. Furthermore, the overall balance of neonatal T-lymphocyte responsiveness is tilted towards a T_H2 rather than a T_H1 response. This may contribute to the susceptibility to intracellular bacterial pathogens, such as *Listeria monocytogenes* or *Salmonella* species, since defences to these pathogens rely on a T_H1 pattern response.

Non-specific immune mechanisms are also immature at birth. Neutrophil bone marrow reserves are easily exhausted, leading to neutropenia; chemotaxis and cell deformability are also reduced (Hill et al. 1999), whilst neutrophil numbers and function tend to deteriorate in the presence of infection. At term, complement levels and function are at approximately two-thirds of the adult value, and often below one-half in preterm babies, although it is not clear whether these findings significantly predispose to neonatal sepsis.

Whilst low immunoglobulin and complement levels are directly proportional to gestational age, depressed T-lymphocyte function may occur in infants who have suffered severe intrauterine growth restriction. Intrauterine growth restriction has been demonstrated up to 5 years of age, though the clinical significance of such findings is unclear. The placental transfer of immunoglobulin in situations of severe intrauterine growth restriction is probably also compromised, though not all studies have confirmed this (Shapiro et al. 1989).

Postnatal development

Following birth, exposure to a wide variety of antigenic stimuli triggers immunological maturation, regardless of gestational age. Initially IgM is mostly produced, but gradually IgG responses develop, and by 2 months of age, infants are able to produce good IgG antibody responses to protein vaccines, such as tetanus toxoid. During this period, maternal IgG levels fall due to catabolism, and a physiological nadir in IgG level occurs at 3–6 months of age, before the infant's production picks up (Fig. 39.3). Thereafter, isotype levels rise at different rates; adult levels of IgM are achieved by 4–5 years, IgG by 7–8 years, whilst serum IgA levels and secretory IgA (SIgA) rise only very slowly, not achieving adult values until the teenage years. Most antipolysaccharide IgG antibody in adults is found in the G2 subclass, and whilst young children make G1 polysaccharide responses, this immaturity probably explains infants' susceptibility to polysaccharide-encapsulated organisms such as pneumococcus and the lack of responsiveness of children under the age of 18–24 months to pure polysaccharide vaccines, such as pneumococcal vaccine (Klouwenberg and Bont 2008). Conjugation of the polysaccharide to a protein or peptide facilitates early responsiveness to

both components, as demonstrated by the high efficacy of Hib conjugate vaccine and the pneumococcal conjugate vaccines, although prematurity can blunt the antibody responses when certain vaccine combinations are used (Berrington et al. 2007; Moss et al. 2010).

T-lymphocyte immunity matures rapidly in the early weeks of life following antigen exposure. T-lymphocyte expression of CD40 ligand improves, as does cytokine production, with the T_H1/T_H2 balance shifting towards T_H1. However, maturation and development of the cell-mediated immune system continue through early childhood. Subtle immaturities in cell-mediated immunity probably account for the increased susceptibility of young children to tuberculosis and of young infants to invasive salmonellosis and listeriosis.

The maternofetal immunological relationship

The close physiological contact at the placental interface of the fetus and mother has important effects on immunological development and disease. During pregnancy, the mother and her incompatible fetus are relatively immunologically hyporesponsive, preventing rejection of the fetus and allowing pregnancy to be maintained. The changes involve polarisation of T-helper lymphocytes towards T_H2 and regulatory (T_{reg}) responses in both mother and fetus. In humans, during the third trimester, fetal T cells are able to mount antigen-specific responses to environmental and food-derived antigens. Antigen-specific T lymphocytes are detectable in cord blood almost universally, indicating that in utero sensitisation occurs. If the pre-existing T_H2 dominance is not counterregulated effectively, an allergic phenotype may well develop. The neonate possesses all the elements to develop a robust immune system, but most are downregulated. During the initial period of immune maturation, the neonate is at risk of infection, and relies on the mother for 'immune protection' via transplacental transfer of immunoglobulins, and by immune protective agents in breast milk. The fact that the innate immune system of a newborn baby is able to mount a robust, and occasionally exaggerated, proinflammatory response under certain conditions (Karlsson et al. 2002) is testimony to the fact that all of the elements for the development of a robust immune system are present, but most elements are downregulated at birth.

Maternal IgG is actively transferred across the placenta to the fetus from about 12 weeks' gestation, and by term, cord blood IgG levels are higher than those in maternal blood. IgG_1 and IgG_3 are principally transferred but little IgG_2 is transferred, compounding the poor neonatal response to encapsulated bacteria such as the group B streptococcus.

Placentally transferred maternal IgG occasionally causes fetal or neonatal disease. Most maternal antifetal immunoglobulins bind to fetal antigen expressed at the centre of the placental villus, and thus never cross to the fetus. However, some antigens expressed on highly differentiated fetal cells are not expressed at the placental villus, and so antibody can cross and cause disease such as Rhesus disease, neonatal thyrotoxicosis and myasthenia gravis. Neonatal haemochromatosis is a rare and often fatal disease which can be ameliorated by giving high-dose immunoglobulin to the mother during pregnancy, and hence may have an autoimmune basis (Whitington and Hibbard 2004). Maternal anti-Ro antibodies, found in systemic lupus erythematosus (SLE), can cause a transient neonatal SLE, but also damage the fetal cardiac conduction pathway, leading to permanent neonatal heart block which may require cardiac pacing. Maternal hypogammaglobulinaemia may be manifest in the newborn infant, as there will have been no placental

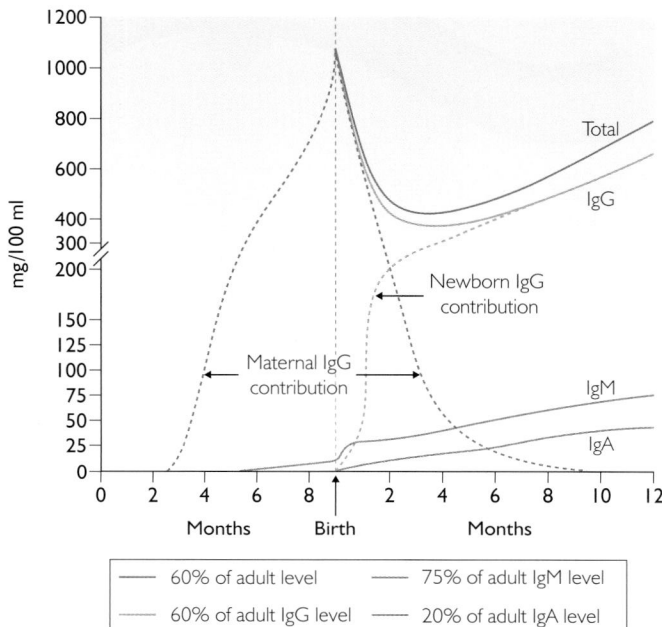

Fig. 39.3 Immunoglobulin (Ig) levels in fetal life and the first year of postnatal life *(Adapted with permission from Stiehm et al. 2004.)*

transfer of IgG. Maternal medication can also cross the placental barrier, and maternally acquired immunosuppressive medication such as ciclosporin or azathioprine can lead to transient neonatal lymphopenia and hypogammaglobulinaemia. Viruses such as cytomegalovirus (CMV) can also cross the placenta and are not effectively excluded by fetal cell-mediated immunity, allowing progressive infection or persistent viral excretion.

Immune development and the neonatal gut
(written with Alison Bedford Russell)

The newborn gut is critical to the development of normal immune defence mechanisms in the infant, through the interaction of colonising organisms, nutrients and gut-associated lymphoid tissue, and nutrition and immune function are closely interlinked. Understanding the importance of early exposure to maternal breast milk and the benefits of prophylactic use of pre- and probiotics and lactoferrin in reducing neonatal sepsis and necrotising enterocolitis (NEC) rates, require knowledge of gut immune mechanisms.

In utero, the fetal gut is active and the fetus starts to swallow up to 200–250 ml/kg/day of amniotic fluid, containing carbohydrates, proteins, peptides, lipids and trophic growth factors (Hirai et al. 2002) at around 8 weeks (Brace and Wolf 1989), contributing to gut development (Mulvihill et al. 1986; Jauniaux et al. 1999; Hirai et al. 2002). Normally, in the immediate peripartum period, the gut becomes colonised with maternal skin and gut bacteria, inducing the development of a competent and functional immune system. This exposure to maternal bacteria and concurrent provision of immunological factors in breast milk are key events which promote gut-associated and systemic immunity, and also nutritional and functional gut maturation (Calder et al. 2006).

The gut of the human adult contains 10 times as many bacterial cells as there are human cells in the body (10^{14} in the gut versus 10^{13} human cells) and more than 400 different species of bacteria, mostly commensals (Backhed et al. 2005). In addition to microbial antigens, the gut is exposed to a large number of complex dietary antigens. It is important that each individual develops tolerance of commensal faecal flora and dietary antigens, whilst able to react vigorously to intestinal pathogens (Backhed et al. 2005; Turner 2009). Such balance of immunological response is facilitated through the interaction of innate and adaptive immune systems (Duerkop et al. 2009).

Toll-like receptors and NOD proteins on dendritic cells and M cells sense luminal and mucosally adherent bacteria (Murch 2001), in organised lymphoid tissue of Peyer's patches or mesenteric lymph nodes, or away from organised lymphoid tissue, as dendritic cells can interdigitate between enterocytes and extend processes into the lumen (Macpherson and Uhr 2004). The local cytokine environment is critical in shaping dendritic cell–lymphocyte interactions (Coombes and Powrie 2008). B lymphocytes switch from IgM production to other immunoglobulin isotypes, dependent on the local cytokine environment and cell–cell contact with T lymphocytes (Brandtzaeg and Johansen 2005; Spencer et al. 2009). Generally, IgA responses protect against inflammation, whereas IgG is proinflammatory and promotes bacterial opsonisation. IgE responses may promote inflammation by disrupting epithelial barrier and neural function. Three major groups of CD4+ T helper lymphocytes can drive different forms of intestinal inflammation – T_H1, T_H2 and T_H17 cells. T_H17 cells are generated in response to transforming growth factor-β (TGF-β), IL-23 and IL-6 (Brandtzaeg and Johansen 2005) and produce IL-17 (Neurath et al. 2002; van Wijk and Cheroutre 2009). T_{REG} populations, produced in response

to TGF-β or IL-10 (Neurath et al. 2002; Coombes and Powrie 2008; Wershil and Furuta 2008; van Wijk and Cheroutre 2009), include T_H3 cells, which produce TGF-β – a key cytokine for mucosal IgA responses. If pathogens induce inflammatory local cytokine production at the time of initial priming, sensitisation, rather than tolerance, may develop.

There are two ways in which this flora-driven immune programming may be disrupted: either by alterations in the colonising flora in early life, or by reduced host immune reactivity. The basis of the 'hygiene' hypothesis relating to allergic, autoimmune and inflammatory diseases is now thought to relate to failed induction of regulatory immune responses in abnormal early-life infectious exposure, rather than the straightforward deviation of T_H1/T_H2 balance previously postulated. First infectious exposures of the nascent immune system shortly after birth may be of much greater importance to immune development than later exposures, and disordered immune programming may result in immune dysregulation with lifelong effects.

The bacteria which arrive in the newborn gut first, usually coliforms and other maternal gut bacteria, establish a permanent niche by interacting with gut-associated lymphoid tissue, and are at a competitive advantage to those arriving late. The normally born infant will be exposed to normal maternal gut flora, which induces normal gut and immune maturation (Hanson et al. 2003). Colonisation of the newborn is supported and 'made safe' by the baby receiving its own mother's breast milk as soon as possible after delivery. The mother's breast milk contains maternal flora-specific SIgA, which prevents invasion of gut mucosa by potentially pathogenic species, as well as lactobacilli and bifidobacteria (known as probiotic species), and complex carbohydrates which have prebiotic activity (Fig. 39.4). A baby born by caesarean section will have very different colonising gut bacteria than one born by normal vaginal

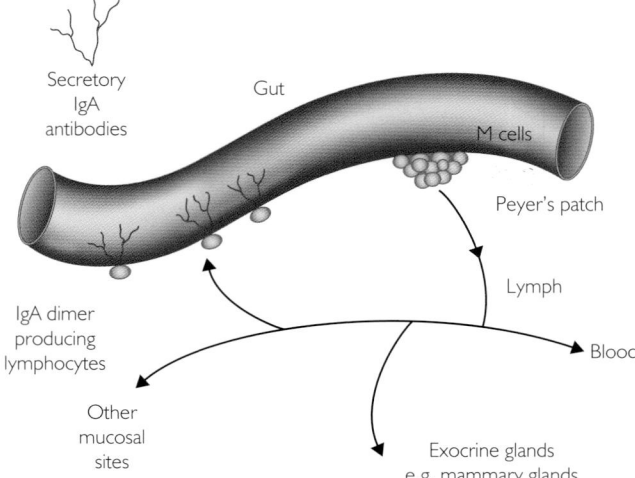

Fig. 39.4 The role of breastfeeding in the prevention of neonatal infection. In maternal gut, food and microbial antigens are taken up into the maternal gut-associated lymphoid tissue including Peyer's patches. B lymphocytes produce secretory antigen-specific immunoglobulin A (IgA) dimers with adjoining J chains. These lymphocytes migrate to various mucous membranes and exocrine sites, including the mammary glands, hence forming the 'enteromammaric link'. Here the cells produce the IgA dimer J chains, which become complete SIgA antibodies when transported through the mammary gland epithelium. Thus a mother's breast milk contains specific antibodies against all the elements of her intestinal flora. *(Reproduced from Hanson and Korotkova, 2003; Semin Neonatol, 2002; 275–281).*

delivery, face to anus (Grönlund et al. 1999). Peripartum antibiotics inevitably alter the composition of gut flora, with possible later consequences for the child's immune health (Bedford Russell and Murch 2005), and antibiotic therapy is associated with abnormal faecal flora profiles in preterm babies within a neonatal unit (Gewolb et al. 1999).

Colostrum contains a rich supply of maternal faecal flora-specific SIgA. The major breast milk protein, lactoferrin, has microbicidal, immunostimulatory and anti-inflammatory activities as a result of blocking production of Il-6, Il-8, Il-1β and TNF-α. In addition, breast milk contains immunoregulatory cytokines such as TGF-β, and lymphocytes expressing gut homing markers (Field 2005). Other protective factors in breast milk include lysozyme, neutrophils and macrophages. Importantly, bacteria, particularly bifidobacteria, are also transported via breast milk and have an important role in modifying the microbiota of the neonatal gastrointestinal tract, which in turn influence mucosal immunological maturation (M'Rabat, et al. 2008). The naïve gut thereby becomes colonised with more normal bacteria, with responses modulated by transferred maternal antibody and immune cells, which further assist with inducing normal gut and immune development (Hooper and Macpherson 2010).

However, breast milk may also be a vehicle through which CMV can be transmitted, which may be of particular concern in preterm or immunodeficient infants (Vochem et al. 1998).

Immunodeficiency disorders: general principles

Classification and genetics

Immunodeficiency may be due to primary or secondary defects. The World Health Organization working party on immunodeficiency has classified the primary disorders (Notarangelo et al. 2009) (Table 39.2). The incidence of any significant immune deficiency disorder (excluding selective IgA deficiency) is 1 in 10 000.

In many of the primary disorders, the molecular basis is understood (Fischer 2007). These discoveries have enhanced understanding of the immune response and led to more focused treatment of primary immune deficiencies. Precise genetic diagnosis has also aided antenatal diagnosis.

Diagnosis and investigation of immunodeficiency

A careful history and examination should precede any laboratory tests for immunodeficiency, as this will help indicate which children should be investigated further and determine the nature and extent of investigations (Table 39.3).

Table 39.2 Primary immunodeficiencies

IMMUNODEFICIENCY	CELLS AFFECTED	GENE DEFECT	INHERITANCE	NEONATAL PRESENTATION
Cell-mediated				
SCID				
T⁻B⁺NK⁻	T, NK	CgC	XL	Yes
T⁻B⁺NK⁻	T, NK	JAK3	AR	Yes
T⁻B⁺NK⁺	T	IL7Ra	AR	Yes
T⁻B⁻NK⁺	T, B	RAG 1,2	AR	Yes
T⁻B⁻NK⁺	T, B	Radiosensitive SCID (artemis, DNA PKcs)	AR	Yes
T⁺B⁻NK⁺		T-B-SCID with MFE or Omenn syndrome	AR	Yes
Reticular cysgenesis	T, B+/−, NK, neutrophils	AK2 (deafness)	AR	Yes
ADA deficiency	T, B, NK	Adenosine deaminase	AR	Yes
PNP deficiency	T, B, NK	Purine nucleoside phosphorylase	AR	No
CID				
MHC II deficiency	Low T (CD4)	Defective MHC II expression	AR	No
MHC I deficiency	Low T (CD8)	Defective MHC I expression	AR	No
CD40L deficiency (XL hyper-IgM)	T	Defective CD40L	XL	No
Wiskott–Aldrich syndrome	T, B, platelet	WAS	XL	Yes
ZAP 70 kinase deficiency	T (low CD8)	ZAP 70 kinase	AR	No

Table 39.2 Continued

IMMUNODEFICIENCY	CELLS AFFECTED	GENE DEFECT	INHERITANCE	NEONATAL PRESENTATION
XL lymphoproliferative disease	T, B	SAP	XL	No
DiGeorge syndrome	T, B	22q11 deletion	Sporadic, occasional AD	Yes
Cartilage hair hypoplasia	T, B	RMRP gene	AR	Yes
Ataxia telangiectasia	T, B	ATM gene	AR	No
Nijmegen breakage syndrome	T, B	NBS1 gene	AR	Yes
Antibody deficiency				
XL agammaglobulinaemia	Absent B	Btk	XL	No
XL hyper-IgM (see CD40L deficiency)				
AR hyper-IgM syndrome	B	AID, CD40	AR	No
AR agammaglobulinaemia	Absent B	m chain	AR	No
Transient hypogammaglobulinaemia of infancy		Unknown	Unknown	No
Phagocyte defects				
XL chronic granulomatous disease	Neutrophils	Killing gp91phox	XL	Yes
AR chronic granulomatous disease	Neutrophil killing	Killing gp22phox, gp47phox, gp67phox, p40phox Killing gp67phox	AR	Unusual
LAD I	Neutrophil adherence	CD18	AR	Yes
Chédiak–Higashi	Chemotaxis		AR	Yes
Griscelli	Chemotaxis		AR	Yes
Congenital neutropenia	Absent neutrophils	ELA2, HAX1 WAS	AR XL	Yes
(Kostmann's syndrome)			Sporadic	
Shwachman syndrome	Chemotaxis	SBDS	AR	Yes
Hyper-IgE syndrome	Macrophages, neutrophils, lymphocytes	STAT3, TYK2	AD, AR	Yes
Mycobactericidal defect	Macrophages, T	IFN-γ receptor 1, 2 IL-12 receptor IL-12	AR	Yes
Complement deficiencies				
C1–9		C1–9 gene defects	AR	No
Properdin		Properdin gene	XL	No
Factor H, I		Factor H, I gene	AR	No

SCID, severe combined immunodeficiency; NK, natural killer; XL, X-linked; AD, autosomal dominant; AR, autosomal recessive; MFE; ADA, adenosine deaminase; PNP, purine nucleoside phosphorylase; CID, combined immunodeficiency; MHC, major histocompatibility complex; WAS, Wiskott–Aldrich syndrome; ZAP; SAP; AID; LAD I; IFN-γ, interferon-γ; IL, interleukin.
(Adapted from Notarangelo et al. 2009.)

Table 39.3 Neonatal immunodeficiency – diagnostic clues

History

Parental consanguinity
Family history of immunodeficiency
History of early infectious deaths
Autoimmune disease in the mother (e.g. systemic lupus erythematosus)
Immunosuppressive drug therapy in the mother (e.g. azathioprine)
Infection during pregnancy (e.g. cytomegalovirus)
Extreme intrauterine growth retardation with maternal hypertension
Risk factors for human immunodeficiency virus
Persistent diarrhoea
Recurrent/chronic superficial candidiasis
Recurrent bacterial infections
Infection with unusual or opportunistic organism
Failure to thrive

Examination

Skin rash, eczema, pustulosis
Hepatosplenomegaly
Absence of lymphoid tissue
Axillary or inguinal lymphadenopathy
Cardiac disease, especially truncus, Fallot, with reduced thymic shadow on X-ray
Oculocutaneous albinism
Unusual facies and cleft palate
Delayed separation of the umbilical cord
Sparse light hair and short length

Investigations

Lymphopenia ($<2.7 \times 10^9$/l)
Neutropenia
Abnormal blood film – leukocyte granules or Howell–Jolly bodies
Low immunoglobulins
Autoantibodies (may be maternal)
Thrombocytopenia with small platelets
Lack of thymic shadow on X-ray
Adenosine deaminase skeletal abnormalities (cupping deformities of the ends of the ribs, abnormal transverse vertebral processes, scapulae)

History

Pregnancy and birth history may suggest possible congenital infection, intrauterine growth retardation or prematurity, all of which are associated with immune defects. Delayed separation of the umbilical cord, in the absence of local infection, may suggest a neutrophil defect. Risk factors for human immunodeficiency virus (HIV) in the parents should be sought. A family history may reveal other children with unusual or fatal infectious complications, suggesting an autosomal-recessive (AR) or X-linked pattern of inheritance. A history of consanguinity is important. In some disorders, such as IgA deficiency, there may be a family history of collagen vascular or other immunopathological disease. Older relatives who are carriers of, or who are affected by, milder variants of primary immune defects may have autoimmune manifestations (e.g. mouth ulcers and SLE variant in chronic granulomatous disease (CGD)) or have a history of malignant disease (lymphoma in X-linked lymphoproliferative disease).

Examination

Examination should be directed towards potential sites of infection, including the throat, ears and mouth, and nappy area for candidiasis (Table 39.3). The presence or absence of lymphoid tissue should be noted. In more severe immunodeficiency states such as SCID and X-linked agammaglobulinaemia, there is a lack of tonsils and lymphoid tissues, although visualising tonsillar tissue in neonates and small infants can be very difficult. Some diseases may have specific physical signs, such as oculocutaneous albinism in Chédiak–Higashi syndrome, typical facies and/or cleft palate in DiGeorge syndrome, and disproportionate short stature in some forms of combined immune deficiency, such as cartilage hair hypoplasia. Microcephaly with developmental delay may be seen in some DNA repair disorders associated with immunodeficiency (Slatter and Gennery 2010). Neonatal pustulosis may be seen in the hyper-IgE syndrome due to STAT3 deficiency, or in chronic granulomatous disease (CGD).

Radiological evaluation

Radiological evaluation, directed by findings from history and examination, may be useful. Bony abnormalities may be seen in adenosine deaminase (ADA) deficiency (Cederbaum et al. 1976), in Shwachman–Diamond syndrome, or in other dysplasias associated with immune defects. Absence of a thymus on anteroposterior and lateral chest radiographs is consistent with a combined immune defect in infants and young children, but thymic atrophy may also occur in response to stress (e.g. infection), and this finding is not diagnostic.

Laboratory investigation

The following should trigger investigation:

- family history consistent with immune deficiency
- single infection with an unusual/opportunistic organism (e.g. *Pneumocystis jiroveci*)
- single infection which is atypically severe or has an atypical course
- more than one episode of serious bacterial infection (Table 39.3).

Haematology

A full blood count and blood film examination will readily detect neutropenia. Bone marrow aspiration will distinguish between failure of production and increased peripheral destruction, and exclude a myelodysplastic or malignant process. Neutrophilia in the absence of overt infection may suggest a neutrophil adhesion defect or functional problem (e.g. CGD). Lymphopenia, using appropriate age-related ranges, is highly suggestive of a combined immune deficiency of primary or secondary aetiology (Hague et al. 1994), but a normal lymphocyte count does not exclude SCID. A manual differential will differentiate nucleated red cells in infants and abnormal leukocyte morphology in sick children. Abnormal leukocyte granules are characteristic of Chédiak–Higashi syndrome. Platelet volume is universally low in Wiskott–Aldrich syndrome (WAS). Eosinophilia may be marked in Omenn syndrome, immunodysregulation polyendocrinopathy enteropathy X-linked (IPEX) syndrome and hyper-IgE syndrome.

Tests of innate immunity

Complement function should be assayed by testing the ability of patient serum to lyse sensitised red blood cells, thus testing the whole pathway. Deficiency in any one component will result in a failure of lysis. Samples must be separated and frozen within 2 hours of venesection. If repeat testing shows a persistent abnormality, evaluation of individual complement components should be performed. Mannan-binding lectin deficiency is detected by analysing the genotype; complete deficiency may be associated with severe infection.

Neutrophil function tests are technically difficult, as neutrophils activate and then quickly die after venesection. The nitroblue tetrazolium (NBT) test is a rapid and sensitive test for CGD, but false normal results can be seen when the test is performed infrequently; it is now being superseded by the more reliable flow cytometric evaluation of the neutrophil oxidative burst.

Adaptive immune system

Test of humoral immunity

Immunoglobulins

IgG is the predominant circulating immunoglobulin, and in the neonate, most is maternal in origin. Smaller amounts of IgA, IgM, IgD and IgE are found in serum. Results must be compared with age-specific normal ranges (Appendix 6), as production of all five classes of immunoglobulin is low at birth and gradually matures over the first 5 years of life. Immunoglobulin can be lost via the gut or urinary tract. Low levels of immunoglobulin can only be attributed to a production defect if gut or renal losses have been excluded and the serum albumin is within the normal range. Measurement of IgE is indicated if hyper-IgE (Job's) syndrome, IPEX syndrome or Omenn syndrome is included in the differential diagnosis; however, in hyper-IgE syndrome the level may be normal in the neonatal period.

Measures of in vivo antibody responses

Functional antibody is more important than the amount of circulating antibody. Functional tests of IgG production rely on measuring antibody titres to antigens to which the child is known to have been exposed either naturally or by vaccination. Responses to protein antigens such as tetanus and the conjugated Hib vaccine are widely available.

Cell-mediated immunity

Cell-mediated defects are likely to result in poor antibody responses, as these depend on T-lymphocyte help in making an antibody response with memory.

Quantification of cell numbers

Lymphocytes can be enumerated using flow cytometry, characterised by their cell surface markers and expressed either as a percentage of the lymphocyte pool or as an absolute number. Proportions of different lymphocytes and absolute numbers vary with age, and age-related normal ranges should be consulted (Berrington et al. 2005).

In vitro lymphocyte proliferation assays

Culturing lymphocytes for a defined time period with an appropriate non-specific stimulus and using the incorporation of tritiated thymidine or a non-radioactive marker such as bromodeoxyuridine into the DNA of dividing cells acts as a surrogate measure of cell proliferation. An alternative method utilises the stable incorporation of the intracellular fluorescent dye 5-carboxyfluorescein diacetate succinimidyl ester (CFSE) into cells to quantify cell division, because of the sequential decrease in fluorescent labelling in daughter cells. CFSE labelling enables a specific lymphocyte sub-population proliferation to be analysed.

Definition of molecular defects

The genetic basis of an increasing number of immune deficiencies is well defined. Usually, a gene defect coding for the protein results in no protein expression, expression of low amounts or expression of abnormally sized protein, and can be detected by Western blotting and flow cytometry (Gilmour et al. 2001). In the presence of an appropriate history or abnormal protein expression, genetic analysis may be undertaken.

Carrier testing

When a primary immunodeficiency is diagnosed, families should be offered genetic counselling. Parents can be tested for carrier status by mutation analysis if the mutation has been defined. Carrier status can also be determined by other tests such as the NBT, in which intermediate numbers of neutrophils will reduce NBT in mothers who carry the mutation.

Antenatal diagnosis

Appropriate counselling by an individual conversant with the outcome of immune deficiencies in the modern era should be undertaken before antenatal diagnosis is offered. Testing confers a small risk of miscarriage, and so screening should be offered only to mothers in whom the result would materially influence the outcome of the pregnancy, although antenatal tissue typing can be performed, and potential donors identified if the disease is treatable by haematopoietic stem cell transplantation.

Neonatal screening

Outcome of stem cell transplantation is much better for patients with SCID transplanted in the neonatal period when infection-free, than for older infants (Kane et al. 2001). Screening programmes measuring molecular markers of T-lymphocyte production, absent in SCID, have been successfully developed from the Newborn Bloodspot Screening Program in the USA (Baker et al. 2009).

Specific primary immunodeficiencies

The complete spectrum of primary immunodeficiency is beyond the scope of this chapter, which will focus on those disorders that present very early in life. More comprehensive texts are recommended for those requiring more information (Stiehm et al. 2004; Ochs et al. 2007).

Disorders of cell-mediated immunity: severe combined immunodeficiencies

Failure to develop normal T and B lymphocytes is usually due to a specific gene defect affecting early lymphocyte development or subsequent signalling pathways, but as T lymphocytes are critical for the maturation and function of B lymphocytes, the more severe T-lymphocyte deficiencies are often accompanied by defective antibody responses and also result in combined deficiency. Combined immunodeficiency results from a large number of disorders with X-linked or AR inheritance, most of which are now molecularly

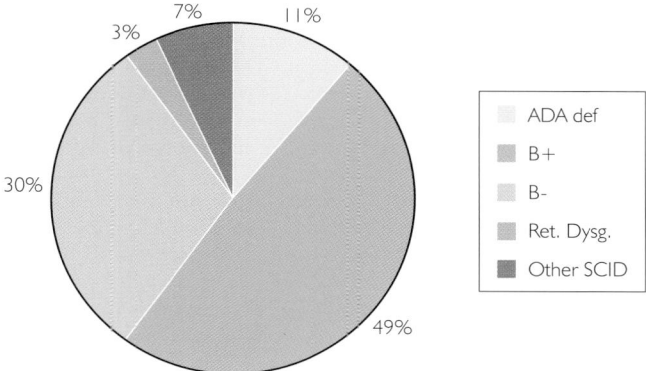

7% 11%

3%

30%

49%

- ADA def
- B+
- B-
- Ret. Dysg.
- Other SCID

Fig. 39.5 Felative frequencies of the various types of severe combined immunodeficiency (SCID) among 699 European patients. ADA, adenosine deaminase; Ret. Dysg., reticular dysgenesis. (*Adapted from* Gennery *et al.* 2010.)

defined (Table 39.2). The most severe phenotype is SCID (Fig. 39.5) associated with a profound T lymphopenia and panhypogamma-globulinaemia, with early death from infection. Whilst the usual clinical features of this group of diseases are well characterised, atypical presentations and 'leaky' forms with an attenuated phenotype are increasingly recognised. Circulating T-lymphocyte numbers are usually low or absent but may be normal. In the classic SCID presentation, lymphocyte responses to mitogen are absent. Patients usually have a limited diversity of T-lymphocyte receptor and immunoglobulin gene rearrangements. Identifying the molecular defect in specific patients with combined immunodeficiency or SCID is important for prognosis, treatment and genetic counselling.

General features of severe combined immunodeficiency

Affected infants appear well at birth but within the first few months of life fail to clear infection and present with persistent respiratory tract or gut infection, failure to thrive and, sometimes, apparent food intolerance (Fischer 2000). Persistent respiratory tract infection with respiratory syncytial virus or parainfluenza viruses is common, with failure to clear virus accompanying persistent bronchiolitic-like signs. An insidiously progressive persistent respiratory infection with radiological evidence of interstitial pneumonitis should raise the suspicion of *Pneumocystis jiroveci* infection, often a co-pathogen with respiratory viruses (Berrington et al. 2000). Other presentations include prolonged otitis media and invasive bacterial infections, particularly staphylococcal or *Pseudomonas* septicaemia and pneumonia, which may respond poorly to appropriate treatment. Severe invasive fungal infection is rare, but often fatal. Extensive persistent superficial candidiasis is more common. Occasionally infants present with disseminated bacille Calmette–Guérin (BCG).

Congenital graft-versus-host disease (GvHD) occurs because many infants with SCID are unable to reject foreign lymphocytes, acquired either from the mother in utero (Muller et al. 2001) or from a non-irradiated blood transfusion. When the disease is clinically apparent, there is typically a mild reticular skin rash, sometimes with abnormal liver function tests. GvHD following transfusion with non-irradiated blood or white cell or platelet concentrates is generally more severe and can be fatal. In these cases, the skin rash is severe and lymphadenopathy and

hepatosplenomegaly may be present. The clinical picture may be indistinguishable from Omenn syndrome, but identification of maternal cells by karyotype or DNA fingerprinting will distinguish maternofetal GvHD from Omenn syndrome.

Examination usually reveals a wasted child who has dropped through the growth centiles, with evidence of candidiasis and other infections. Skin rashes may indicate infection or GvHD. There is no clinically detectable lymphoid tissue. There may be hepatomegaly.

Investigation usually shows severe lymphopenia from birth. It should be remembered that in infancy a normal lymphocyte count is $>2.7 \times 10^9/l$ (unlike adults, where it is $>1.0 \times 10^9/l$). Lymphocytic phenotyping shows severely depleted T-lymphocyte numbers; B lymphocytes and NK cells may be present or absent, depending on the type of SCID. Occasional variants show unusual patterns of immature T-lymphocyte markers; in such cases, maternal engraftment should be excluded. Mitogen responses are usually absent. Immunoglobulin estimations show low levels of IgG, IgA and IgM but residual maternal IgG may give a falsely reassuring result and it can be difficult distinguishing IgA and IgM levels in SCID from the low levels seen in normal infants. Isohaemagglutinins are a useful measure of in vitro IgM production, and absence is significant. If SCID is suspected, lymphocyte phenotyping is more reliable than immunoglobulin estimation. Chest radiographs show an absent thymus and, if infection is present, hyperinflation and/or interstitial pneumonia.

In children who die, postmortem examination reveals severely depleted lymphoid tissue, with nodes and thymus showing no lymphoid follicles and absent Hassall's corpuscles in the thymus. Without treatment, patients die from infection by about 12 months of age. Currently, the only curative treatment is haematopoietic stem cell transplantation (HSCT), although clinical gene therapy trials for common gamma chain and ADA deficiency are in progress. Supportive interim treatments include antibiotic prophylaxis with co-trimoxazole as anti-*Pneumocystis* treatment, antifungal prophylaxis and immunoglobulin replacement. Live vaccines, including BCG, must be avoided. The diagnosis of SCID is a paediatric emergency, and suspected cases should be urgently referred to a designated treatment centre for assessment and treatment.

Newborns suspected of having a severe immunodeficiency disorder should be protected using isolation techniques, including limitation of the numbers of persons involved with care; individuals with respiratory or gastrointestinal symptoms of infection should avoid contact. If the mother is CMV-negative, breastfeeding should be encouraged; otherwise it should be discontinued to prevent neonatal CMV infection being transmitted through the milk. Wherever the child is managed, the importance of strict hand-washing procedures cannot be overemphasised. Blood products should be CMV-negative and irradiated to avoid the risk of transfusion GvHD.

Types of severe combined and combined immunodeficiencies

Severe combined immunodeficiency

SCID can be classified according to the presence or absence of T, B and NK lymphocytes, each phenotype being due to a number of distinct molecular defects, so enabling classification by mechanism (Table 39.2). The genetic basis of a few disorders remains to be elucidated. Other rare phenotypes may be due to atypical presentation of known molecular defects.

Omenn syndrome

Omenn syndrome is characterised by a generalised erythematous rash, together with scaling and erythroderma, lymphadenopathy,

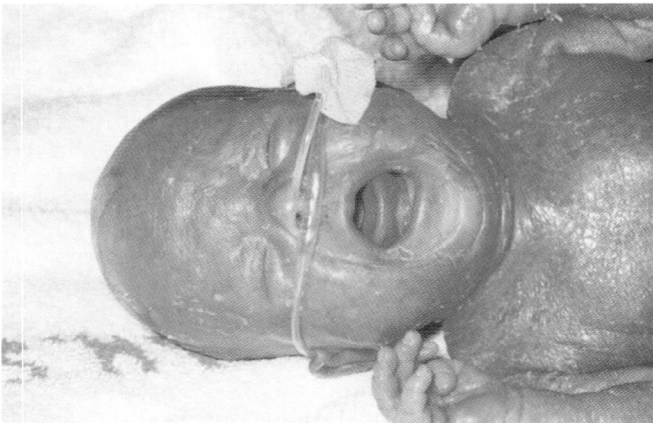

Fig. 39.6 Omenn syndrome. A newborn infant showing the typical features of Omenn syndrome, including generalised scaly erythroderma, alopecia, lymphadenopathy and hepatosplenomegaly. *(Courtesy of the Audiovisual Department, University of Newcastle.)*

hepatosplenomegaly, increased serum IgE levels with a marked eosinophilia and the usual clinical features of SCID (Fig. 39.6) (Notarangelo et al. 1999). The syndrome is a 'leaky' form of SCID in that small numbers of very abnormal T lymphocytes 'leak' past the block in T-lymphocyte development. The underlying defect in many cases is a mutation in the RAG genes, although other gene mutations have been associated with the phenotype (Villa et al. 2008). HSCT is the only curative treatment.

Netherton syndrome

This triad of generalised infantile erythroderma, diarrhoea and failure to thrive may be associated with a variable immunodeficiency, including mild lymphopenia. The clinical features are similar to those seen in Omenn syndrome and in SCID and maternofetal engraftment. Distinguishing these entities is important, as the other conditions are treated by HSCT, whereas Netherton syndrome is not (Renner et al. 2009). Mutations in the serine protease inhibitor Kazal-type 5 (SPINK5) gene, are reported in most patients. Hair shaft abnormalities with trichorrhexis invaginata (bamboo hairs) are diagnostic.

Reticular dysgenesis

This rare AR-inherited form of SCID, due to a defect in mitochondrial adenylate kinase 2, is characterised by defective lymphoid and myeloid differentiation (Pannicke et al. 2009). Neural deafness is an associated feature.

Adenosine deaminase deficiency

This disorder, due to a single gene defect, results in absence of the purine salvage pathway enzyme ADA, leading to accumulation of the toxic DNA breakdown products. Neurodevelopmental problems may also occur in some patients (Rogers et al. 2001). Treatment is by HSCT or by use of replacement polyethelene glycol-coupled ADA. Gene therapy trials are in progress for this form of SCID (Gaspar et al. 2006).

Major histocompatibility complex class II deficiency

MHC class II antigens (HLA DR, DP, DQ) are expressed on a limited repertoire of cells and present antigen to CD4+ T lymphocytes, which, with the help of an appropriate second signal, leads to the activation of T-helper lymphocytes specific for that antigen and an effective immune response. Expression of MHC II in the thymus is also essential for positive selection of CD4+ T lymphocytes. Since HLA antigens are of vital importance for lymphocyte development and function, lack of MHC II expression results in a profound susceptibility to viral, bacterial, fungal and protozoal infections (Klein et al. 1993).

Autosomal-recessive MHC II deficiency is rare and can result from mutations in several different genes which code for a complex of regulatory factors controlling transcription of MHC II genes.

The clinical picture resembles SCID. The diagnosis can be confirmed flow cytometrically by showing absent or significantly reduced levels of class II molecules on B lymphocytes and monocytes. Definitive treatment is HSCT, although this has had limited success in comparison with that achieved in other types of SCID (Renella et al. 2006).

Combined immunodeficiency forming part of other syndromes

DiGeorge anomaly

This condition results from abnormal cephalic neural crest cell migration into the third and fourth pharyngeal arches in early embryological development. A microdeletion at chromosome 22q11.2 is present in 90% of cases, while the remainder are associated with other chromosomal anomalies, particularly 10p–. Whilst classically recognised by the triad of congenital heart defects, immunodeficiency secondary to thymic hypoplasia and hypocalcaemia secondary to parathyroid gland hypoplasia, an expanded phenotype is increasingly recognised. Conotruncal heart defects are most often associated with the syndrome, but other defects include tetralogy of Fallot, septal defects, pulmonary atresia and aberrant subclavian vessels.

Severe T-lymphocyte immunodeficiency presenting with a SCID phenotype of profound lymphopenia and poor lymphocyte proliferation is rare and accounts for <1.5% of cases. A similar clinical picture has been described in some patients with CHARGE syndrome (coloboma of the eye, heart defects, atresia of the choanae, retardation of growth and/or development, genital and/or urinary abnormalities and ear abnormalities and deafness) (Gennery et al. 2008).

All children suspected of having DiGeorge syndrome (with or without 22q11.2 deletion) should have an immunological evaluation including lymphocyte subset analysis, T-lymphocyte proliferative responses, immunoglobulin levels and specific antibody responses to vaccination antigens.

Blood products should be irradiated if T-lymphocyte mitogen responses are poor. Patients with severe immune deficiency have been successfully treated with HSCT: thymic transplantation may be a preferred option for some patients, although it is available in only a few centres worldwide (Janda et al. 2010). In the partial phenotype with normal T-lymphocyte function, the usual infant vaccination schedule can be followed. It is safe to give live vaccines such as measles, mumps, rubella vaccine or varicella-zoster vaccine as long as the CD4 count exceeds 400 cells/ml, and there are normal T-lymphocyte mitogen responses. Demonstration of good antibody responses to tetanus and *Haemophilus influenzae* type B vaccination give further reassurance that live vaccines can be safely administered (Driscoll and Sullivan 1999). Prophylactic antibiotics and, occasionally, intravenous immunoglobulin (IVIG) can be helpful, particularly for young children with recurrent infection due to humoral deficiency.

Wiskott–Aldrich syndrome

Immunodeficiency, thrombocytopenia, eczema and an increased risk of autoimmune disorders and malignancy characterise this X-linked recessive condition. Mutations in the same gene are found in patients with X-linked thrombocytopenia and X-linked neutropenia.

Clinical features can be surprisingly mild, especially in the newborn. Thrombocytopenia with a low mean platelet volume (<5 fl) is always present and should raise suspicion of the diagnosis even if bruising and bleeding are minimal.

Acute bleeding episodes may require platelet transfusions (irradiated to prevent GvHD). IVIG, with or without prophylactic antibiotics, reduces infections, and splenectomy may suppress autoimmune phenomena. Without HSCT, the prognosis is variable, but median survival is between 3 and 15 years. The presence or absence of WAS protein correlates with outcome, with patients who have no expressed protein having a worse outcome than those with expressed protein (Imai et al. 2004). The efficacy of HSCT for patients with WAS is long established, with good outcomes following related and unrelated donor HSCT (Pai et al. 2006).

X-linked hyper-IgM syndrome (CD40 ligand deficiency)

X-linked hyper-IgM syndrome is a combined immunodeficiency caused by a T-lymphocyte defect and not an isolated antibody deficiency, as was previously thought. The defect is in the gene encoding for the CD40 ligand (CD154) expressed on T lymphocytes which activate B lymphocytes and monocyte/macrophage-derived cells. Without CD40L binding, B lymphocytes cannot switch from producing IgM to producing IgA IgG and IgE. Pulmonary macrophages are not activated, resulting in *Pneumocytis jiroveci* pneumonia, and ineffective Kupffer cell function allows repeated infection with *Cryptosporidium parvum* and similar organisms, leading to sclerosing cholangitis, pancreatitis and malignancy. Absent IgA and IgG results in sinopulmonary and invasive bacterial infection. Neutropenia with oral ulceration is common and this, together with low or absent IgA and IgG, and normal or raised IgM, should suggest the diagnosis (Notarangelo and Hayward 2000).

Patients should receive co-trimoxazole, as *Pneumocystis carinii* pneumonia (PCP) prophylaxis, and immunoglobulin replacement therapy. With adequate replacement, the rising IgM levels may normalise. The neutropenia sometimes responds to granulocyte colony-stimulating factor (G-CSF) and IVIG. All drinking water should be boiled. Azithromycin prophylaxis may lessen the risks of *Cryptosporidium parvum*. HSCT should be considered for this condition (Gennery et al. 2004). A much rarer, but similar, AR disease, CD40 deficiency, presents with similar features; treatment is the same as for CD40 ligand deficiency (Ferrari et al. 2001).

Immunodeficiency and short-limbed dwarfism

Cartilage hair hypoplasia is the best described form, inherited in an AR manner and associated with mutations in the RMRP gene, which encodes endoribonuclease Rnase mitochondrial RNA processing (MRP). Severe short-limbed short stature (211.8–22.1 sd) with X-ray appearances of metaphyseal and spondyloepiphyseal dysplasia are always present, accompanied by sparse light hair in most patients. Severe anaemia and Hirschsprung disease are uncommon but well-recognised associations, as are malignancies, notably lymphoma and skin carcinoma. The immunodeficiency is surprisingly variable; most have T lymphopenia and impaired in vitro mitogen proliferative responses, but only half suffer recurrent infection. However, some have IgA and/or IgG subclass deficiencies, with frequent ear infections. Patients are excessively vulnerable to viral infections, particularly varicella-zoster virus, Epstein–Barr virus and other human herpesvirus infections, and the risk of infective death is 300 times greater than normal. Rare patients can present with a SCID immunophenotype, but no limb dysplasia (Kavadas et al. 2008). Severely affected patients should be assessed for bone marrow transplantation (BMT), which has been successful in correcting the immunodeficiency (Bordon et al. 2010).

Abnormalities of T- and B-lymphocyte function are seen in a number of other osteochondrodysplasias, including Shwachman syndrome, in which there are neutropenia and pancreatic insufficiency and Schimke immuno-osseous dysplasia, which features radiographic changes of spondyloepiphyseal dysplasia, nephrotic syndrome and cellular immunodeficiency.

DNA repair defects and immunodeficiency

The immune system uses cellular DNA repair mechanisms to generate the diversity of specific immune responses by rearrangement of the variable (V), diversity19 (D) and joining (J) gene segments that code for T- or B-lymphocyte receptor genes (VDJ recombination). Inability to repair DNA damage causes cellular apoptosis or malignant proliferation, and so individuals with defective DNA repair mechanisms have a predisposition to neurodegeneration, developmental anomalies and cancer, as well as defective immunity (Slatter and Gennery 2010).

Single-gene defects cause a number of distinct clinical entities, of which ataxia telangiectasia is the best known, although the features are not apparent in the neonatal period. Nijmegen breakage syndrome, an AR disorder, is characterised by microcephaly, mental retardation, bird-like facies, immunodeficiency, clinical radiation sensitivity and chromosomal instability. It should be considered when investigating an infant with features of bird-headed dwarfism. Fanconi's anaemia presents with progressive bone marrow failure leading to pancytopenia. There may also be skeletal malformations, and immunodeficiency can occur.

Immunoregulation disorders

Increasingly, patients with complex autoimmune manifestations are being recognised, often with coexistent infectious problems. Patients with classical primary immunodeficiency such as WAS or DiGeorge syndrome present with autoimmune manifestations, and it is logical to consider genetic disorders of immune regulation as primary immunodeficiencies in the broadest sense.

Defects of lymphocyte apoptosis

Autoimmune lymphoproliferative syndrome

Apoptosis (programmed cell death) regulates immune responses once an infection has been countered, to delete many antigen-specific lymphocytes that clonally expanded to deal with the infection. Apoptosis defects lead to marked autoimmune and lymphoproliferative features which characterise autoimmune lymphoproliferative syndrome (ALPS) (Bleesing et al. 2000).

Chronic mucocutaneous candidiasis

Chronic mucocutaneous candidiasis (CMC) describes a heterogeneous group of primary or secondary disorders characterised by chronic infection of skin, nails and mucous membranes by organisms of the genus *Candida*, most commonly *Candida albicans*. The precise molecular defect is not known for most forms of primary CMC, although defects in cytokine signalling are apparent in some patients (Ferwerda et al. 2009; Glocker et al. 2009). Recurrent and persistent *Candida* of the mouth, napkin area, skins and nails is the hallmark of this condition, but the severity varies considerably and invasive disease almost never occurs. Failure of usually effective antifungal drugs to clear *Candida* distinguishes primary CMC from other conditions that predispose to *Candida*, such as secondary immunodeficiency, steroid treatment or systemic antibiotics. Candidiasis is usually first noticed early in infancy and in severe cases gross oesophageal involvement causes dysphagia, gastro-oesophageal reflux and failure to thrive, whilst skin lesions may be extremely disfiguring and distressing. Cases may be familial or sporadic with recessive or dominant patterns of inheritance.

Treatment with azole antifungals, such as fluconazole, can be very effective, even in severe cases, but may not completely eradicate infection, and infection often recurs on stopping treatment.

IPEX syndrome

Immunodysregulation polyendocrinopathy enteropathy X-linked (IPEX) syndrome is characterised by early-onset type 1 insulin-dependent diabetes mellitus, infantile ichthyosiform dermatitis, protracted diarrhoea and severe total parenteral nutrition-dependent enteropathy and thyroiditis. Mutations in the FOXP3 gene have been described in affected patients (Gambineri et al. 2008).

Other immunodeficiencies

A number of syndromes that include primary immunodeficiency as part of the phenotype have been described. Although most lack clear definition, the syndrome is well described in some, and the underlying molecular defect has been elucidated in some.

Hoyeraal–Hreidarsson syndrome

This X-linked disorder is characterised by microcephaly, cerebellar hypoplasia, aplastic anaemia and growth retardation. A progressive combined immunodeficiency, with hypogammaglobulinaemia and lymphopenia, is a well-recognised association.

ICF syndrome

Immunodeficiency, centromeric instability and facial anomalies (ICF) syndrome is an AR disorder characterised by structural chromosomal abnormalities in chromosomes 1, 9 and 16 in lymphocytes, easily seen on chromosome analysis. Other cells do not show these changes. Affected children develop severe recurrent infections and have immunoglobulin deficiency, often with agammaglobulinaemia but with normal numbers of T and B lymphocytes (Hagleitner et al. 2008). T-lymphocyte immunity is not normal and affected children can present with *Pneumocystis carinii* infection in infancy; severe viral warts and cutaneous fungal infection also occur. HSCT may be curative for selected patients.

Defects of antibody production

Isolated antibody deficiency does not usually present in the neonatal period because the presence of transplacentally acquired immunoglobulin obscures the affected child's inability to make antibody.

Neonates can present with severe or recurrent bacterial infection and may be found to have hypogammaglobulinaemia because of:

- failure of transfer of immunoglobulin due to prematurity
- failure of transfer of immunoglobulin due to unrecognised maternal hypogammaglobulinaemia
- immunoglobulin loss from the thoracic duct in chylothorax
- immunoglobulin loss from gut in lymphangiectasia.

Table 39.2 describes the main causes of primary hypogammaglobulinaemia; these can often be screened for in the neonatal period when there is a positive family history.

Disorders of phagocytic cells

Chronic granulomatous disease

Chronic granulomatous disease (CGD) results from inherited defects of the phagocyte nicotinamide adenine dinucleotide phosphate (NADPH) oxidase enzyme complex, which generates free oxygen species needed to kill microorganisms ingested into phagosomes. The X-linked form is more common than the AR form.

The disease has protean clinical manifestations, but the hallmark is acute, and potentially fatal, bacterial or fungal infection (Jones et al. 2008). In the neonatal period, a non-specific generalised pustulosis can be seen, and the most common manifestation, acute suppurative lymphadenitis in the neck, axilla or groin, can sometimes be seen very early in life. Other frequent pyogenic infections include liver abscesses, osteomyelitis, arthritis, pneumonia, skin sepsis and perianal abscesses. Pathogens such as *Staphylococcus aureus*, *Burkholderia cepacia*, *Aspergillus* species and *Serratia marcescens*, are common. Infections with catalase-negative organisms, such as *Streptococcus pneumoniae*, are rare. Fungal infection often manifests as pneumonia, but disseminated infection is frequently seen, with osteomyelitis and hepatic involvement. Once established, fungal infection is hard to treat and frequently fatal.

Diagnosis is suggested by failure of reduction of NBT or dihydrorhodamine by neutrophils. Prophylactic antibiotics, particularly co-trimoxazole, which is concentrated in neutrophils, can significantly reduce morbidity and mortality from bacterial infections. Oral antifungal prophylaxis with an agent such as itraconazole probably reduces the incidence of fatal fungal disease.

Infections or unexplained fevers should be treated aggressively. IFN-γ is a useful adjunctive treatment in severe bacterial or fungal infections. White cell infusions may also be used as adjunctive therapy in severe infection. Despite these therapeutic advances, considerable morbidity and mortality still occur, and HSCT should be considered (Seger et al. 2002).

Other neutrophil disorders

Neutropenia

Neutropenia may result from reduced production in the bone marrow or from increased peripheral destruction, distinguished by the findings on bone marrow examination. It most frequently follows decreased production induced by disease processes or drug treatments, as well as sepsis in preterm or stressed neonates. Increased consumption may occur in autoimmune states, including neonatal alloimmune neutropenia and those associated with immune deficiency. The degree of neutropenia will influence the clinical picture: neutrophil counts of less than $0.5 \times 10^9/l$ carry a major risk of infection, whilst counts below $0.2 \times 10^9/l$ are associated with a significant risk of life-threatening sepsis.

Severe congenital neutropenia (Kostmann's syndrome)

This AR disease was originally described by Kostmann (1956). Onset is within the first year of life with recurrent and life-threatening infections. Symptoms include cellulitis, perirectal abscesses, peritonitis, stomatitis and meningitis. Bone marrow examination shows an arrest at the promyelocyte to myelocyte maturation stage. Kostmann's syndrome is due to mutations in Hax1, but defects in other genes can lead to a similar clinical picture (Pessach et al. 2009).

Shwachman–Diamond syndrome

This rare AR disorder is characterised by exocrine pancreatic insufficiency, skeletal abnormalities, bone marrow dysfunction and recurrent infections. Neutropenia occurs in all patients, whilst 10–25% of patients also have pancytopenia. There is an increased incidence of malignancy.

Treatment of neutropenia with G-CSF results in increased counts and fewer infections in almost all patients with neutropenia not secondary to peripheral destruction. Concerns about the induction of leukaemias with prolonged use have not been realised, although pretreatment and annual bone marrow aspirates are recommended. BMT may be indicated in selected cases.

Haemophagocytic lymphohistiocytosis

Congenital neutropenia or neutrophil dysfunction, with or without associated hypopigmentation, is a feature of diseases with defects in proteins that control lysosomal secretion in melanocytes and immune cells. An important presentation of these diseases is haemophagocytic lymphohistiocytosis (HLH), a fatal inflammatory disease characterised by high swinging fevers, hepatosplenomegaly, jaundice and erythematous rash, respiratory distress and pancytopenia, consequent to hypercytokinaemia and organ infiltration by CD8+ lymphocytes and macrophages. Patients appear septic but blood cultures are usually sterile. Laboratory findings include an acute-phase response, elevated ferritin and elevated fasting triglycerides. Examination of bone marrow, cerebrospinal fluid, pleural effusions or ascitic fluid may demonstrate haemophagocytosis. Haemophagocytosis may occur secondary to a number of infections, in particular viral infections, and careful exclusion of infections by serology/polymerase chain reaction should be undertaken. Haemophagocytosis is seen in a number of immunodeficient states, including Chédiak–Higashi syndrome, Griscelli syndrome and X-linked lymphoproliferative disease (XLP) (Table 39.2). Chédiak–Higashi syndrome is a rare AR disease with partial oculocutaneous albinism, recurrent bacterial infections and a high risk of developing HLH, which is usually fatal. Variable neurological manifestations are also recognised. Characteristic giant lysosomal granules are seen in the cytoplasm of all cells containing these organelles, and are easily detected on a peripheral blood film. Individuals with Griscelli syndrome resemble those with Chédiak–Higashi syndrome in that they have variable hypopigmentation of the skin and hair and recurrent pyogenic infections associated with absent delayed-type cutaneous hypersensitivity and impaired NK cell function. Hypogammaglobulinaemia can be seen as a secondary phenomenon. In contrast to Chédiak–Higashi syndrome, large lysosomal granules are not seen, and examination of the hair by electron microscopy shows large clumps of pigment, with the accumulation of mature melanosomes in melanocytes. Neurological abnormalities are absent in these patients. They are also at high risk of developing macrophage activation syndrome unless treated by BMT.

Leukocyte adhesion deficiency

Inherited defects in leukocyte cell surface molecules can prevent their egress into infected tissue, resulting in a characteristic clinical presentation. In leukocyte adhesion deficiency type I, deficiency of the 95-kD β chain (CD18), common to the β2 integrin family of cell surface adhesive molecules, leads to a profound immunodeficiency affecting the function of neutrophils, monocytes and certain lymphocytes, including T and NK cytotoxic cells (Crowley et al. 1980). Inheritance is AR. Chemotaxis, adherence and phagocytosis are markedly depressed. The phenotype varies according to the severity of the mutation. Leukocytes are attracted to areas of infection and become fixed to the vessel walls at sites of inflammation in the usual way but cannot pass out into the tissues, causing infarction of small vessels and rapidly expanding necrotic lesions without pus.

Individuals with the most severe phenotype (<1% expression) present in the first weeks of life with delayed umbilical cord separation (the cord fails to shrink down and may not separate until 3–4 weeks of age) and rapidly progressive erosive perianal ulcers. Delayed umbilical cord separation does not occur in patients with some expression of the molecule (usually in the range 2–10% of normal expression). In all forms there is excessive susceptibility to bacterial and fungal infections. Gingivitis and periodontitis are common, and more deep-seated infections of bone, respiratory tract and gastrointestinal tract are often seen. Non-infective inflammatory lesions, particularly affecting the skin and resembling pyoderma gangrenosum, can occur in the partial forms of the deficiency and are often responsive to steroids.

There is almost always a neutrophilia (because of failure of the cells to migrate out of the circulation) and a profound neutrophil chemotactic defect. Diagnosis is confirmed by demonstrating the absence of the cell surface markers recognised by anti-CD11/CD18 monoclonal antibodies.

In the severe form, early death from infection occurs unless a successful BMT can be performed. In the partial forms, supportive and expectant management is pursued in the first instance, but BMT may become necessary.

Hyper-IgE syndromes

These complex disorders are characterised by extreme elevation of the serum IgE level (usually in the range 2000–40 000 U/l), chronic dermatitis and repeated lung and skin infections (Freeman and Holland 2009). Patients present in infancy with eczema, but in the neonatal period a vesicular rash may be present in the first few days of life. *Staphylococcus aureus*, the predominant pathogen, can cause pneumatoceles and chronic lung damage. Recurrent candidiasis may be a feature. Treatment is long-term antistaphylococcal antibiotic prophylaxis, usually with flucloxacillin. Three genes have been identified, leading to the clinical picture. Defects in STAT3 give rise to the classical autosomal-dominant clinical picture, whereas AR defects in TYK2 and DOCK8 are associated with severe molluscum contagiosum and herpesvirus infection.

Anhydrotic ectodermal dysplasia, incontinentia pigmenti and defects in the NEMO gene

Until recently, incontinentia pigmenti and X-linked anhydrotic ectodermal dysplasia were thought to be unrelated disorders. Incontinentia pigmenti is a rare X-linked dominant condition characterised by developmental abnormalities of the skin, hair, teeth and central nervous system. Affected female infants present with a characteristic rash, occurring in four phases of erythema and vesicles, hyperkeratosis, hyperpigmentation and finally pallor and atrophy. Previously thought lethal in male fetuses carrying the affected X chromosome, rare male infants with a progressive combined immunodeficiency have been described. Patients with X-linked anhydrotic ectodermal dysplasia present with sparse scalp hair, conical teeth and absent sweat glands. Some suffer from recurrent sinopulmonary infection, often with encapsulated organisms, and have poor antibody responses to polysaccharide antigens, or frank hypogammaglobulinaemia. Hypofunctional mutations in the NEMO gene encoding a protein required to activate the transcription factor NF-κB have been described in male patients with both incontinentia pigmenti and X-linked anhydrotic ectodermal dysplasia, suggesting that these conditions represent variants of the same disorder (Doffinger et al. 2001). Other proteins in the same signalling pathway can cause a similar clinical picture, although inheritance is AR.

Congenital asplenia

Asplenia is seen when congenital cardiac defects are associated with right isomerism, and the presence of Howell–Jolly and Heinz bodies on a blood film should raise suspicion, asplenia being confirmed by abdominal ultrasound. Asplenic infants are at lifelong risk from invasive infection by organisms with polysaccharide coats, such as group B streptococcus and pneumococcus. Treatment is with lifelong prophylactic antibiotics. Penicillin is the antibiotic of choice, although in children less than 5 years of age we advocate using co-trimoxazole in order to prevent infection with the greater range of pathogens, including *Haemophilus influenzae* and Gram-negative organisms, to which younger children with asplenia are susceptible. Vaccination with conjugate pneumococcal and quadravalent meningococcal vaccines is recommended before 2 years of age, and thereafter with polysaccharide pneumococcal and meningococcal vaccines.

Treatment of immunodeficiency

Vaccination of the child with a potentially impaired immune response

Immunocompromised children are more in need of the protection vaccination can offer because of their greater risk from infection, and yet are less likely to be vaccinated because of concerns about the underlying immunodeficiency. Children with primary immunodeficiency should be immunised. Live vaccines should be avoided in those with T-lymphocyte-mediated immunodeficiency; all other forms of immunodeficiency can safely have live vaccine administered, except BCG in patients with CGD. Preterm infants should be vaccinated routinely, following the national immunisation programme. Children on pharmacological doses of steroids (an equivalent dose of prednisolone 2 mg/kg/day for >1 week, or 1 mg/kg/day for >1 month) or other immunosuppressive therapy should not be given live vaccines until 3 months after ceasing therapy (Skinner et al. 2002). At-risk infants should receive passive immunisation with appropriate antigen-specific immunoglobulin.

Supportive care

Children with immunodeficiency disorders often require the full spectrum of paediatric care. Particular attention needs to be paid to nutritional status and the management of dietary intolerances secondary to the gastrointestinal problems which frequently occur.

Advice from paediatric gastroenterologists and respiratory paediatricians should be sought early, to minimise the impact of the disease on gut and lungs and to maximise supportive therapy. Supporting the emotional needs of the family is also very important. Prevention and treatment of infections are mainstays of supportive care.

Specific measures for prevention of infections

Co-trimoxazole as prophylaxis against *Pneumocystis jiroveci* should be given for defects involving cell-mediated immunity mechanisms. For PCP prophylaxis only, co-trimoxazole need only be given on 2 or 3 days a week. If this is not tolerated, alternatives include dapsone and atovaquone. Co-trimoxazole probably also reduces the incidence of pyogenic infections in these patients and those with phagocytic or humoral immune deficiencies, and for this purpose it is usually given daily (dose 30 mg/kg/day in one or two doses). In circumstances of poor nutrition, increased bone marrow turnover and in all cases after BMT, weekly folinic acid supplements are given to lessen the risk of bone marrow depression without compromising the antimicrobial efficacy. Antifungal prophylaxis should be used in combined immunodeficiencies or phagocytic cell defects. In CGD and other conditions where the risk of *Aspergillus* infection is high, itraconazole is preferred. Otherwise, fluconazole or non-absorbed agents such as nystatin are used. Antiviral prophylaxis with aciclovir is used in patients with cell-mediated immunodeficiency and previous herpes simplex infection. It is also used in the context of BMT to prevent herpes simplex and CMV reactivation.

Treatment of infections

A policy of vigorous and early antimicrobial treatment of infections should be observed. Unusual agents may cause infection, and broader-spectrum antimicrobial cover may therefore be needed. In neutrophil disorders, it is particularly important to cover *Pseudomonas* and other Gram-negative bacilli. Early treatment of an infection may be life-saving, but its initiation should not detract from full attempts at identification of the causative agent. Invasive diagnostic procedures, such as bronchoalveolar lavage or, if this fails to produce a diagnosis, open-lung biopsy, can be fully justified on the basis that they will facilitate precise and optimal therapy. The mainstay of treatment for systemic fungal infection remains amphotericin B, mostly used in its liposomal form to reduce toxicity and enable larger doses to be given. Promising new agents for treating invasive aspergillosis include voriconazole and caspofungin.

Antivirals such as the broad-spectrum agent ribavirin and the anti-CMV agents ganciclovir and foscarnet are particularly useful in the immunocompromised infant. Cidofovir is useful against resistant CMV, adenovirus and severe molluscum contagiosum.

Replacement immunoglobulin

Immunoglobulin is a blood product, and so its use is associated with all the risks of giving such products, such as hypersensitivity reactions (including anaphylaxis) during administration. Although modern manufacturing processes include steps which screen for and inactivate viruses such as hepatitis B and C, and HIV, transmission of infectious agents remains theoretically possible. Particular current concerns revolve around the issue of transmission of prion disease, although the risk of this is probably very small. Such factors mean that immunoglobulin treatment should be initiated only after due consideration of the risks and benefits, and in line with published national guidelines (Provan et al. 2008). Before administration, liver function tests should be measured, and a sample of serum taken for long-term storage in case of future infective complications which may be attributable to the immunoglobulin. Many studies have examined the role of immunoglobulin in either the prophylaxis or treatment of infection in preterm or low-birthweight (LBW) infants. Taken overall, whilst IVIG prophylaxis gives a small (4–5%) reduction in the incidence of sepsis or serious infection, there is no difference in mortality, and only a trend towards shorter hospital stay. This has to be balanced against cost, risk of side-effects (including potential transmission of infection) and recurrent venous access. There is no justification for the routine use of IVIG as prophylaxis against Gram-negative infection in preterm or LBW infants (Ohlsson and Lacy 2004).

IVIG has also been advocated as an adjunctive treatment to antibiotics in sepsis or suspected sepsis. A recent meta-analysis showed a borderline statistically significant reduction in mortality in cases of suspected sepsis given immunoglobulin, although the difference was more significant in cases that were proven sepsis (Ohlsson and Lacy 2010). Immunoglobulin treatment for this indication is not recommended in the current national guidelines, and should only be administered in the context of a clinical trial. Pathogen-specific immunoglobulin such as palivizumab may have a role in preventing respiratory syncytial virus-associated pneumonitis in at-risk infants, particularly those with impaired T-lymphocyte immunity.

Granulocyte colony-stimulating factor

Septic sick or preterm neonates become neutropenic because neutrophil stores are rapidly depleted, and granulopoiesis is depressed. G-CSF mobilises preformed neutrophils from the marrow into the circulation, and enhances neutrophil precursor proliferation. Several studies have examined the effect of administering G-CSF to septic infants. Other studies have addressed the issue of using G-CSF as prophylaxis by prospectively stimulating neutrophil production.

There is no evidence to support these treatment modalities (Carr et al. 2003). G-CSF has a role in treating infants with congenital neutropenia.

Blood product support

All blood products except IVIG and fresh frozen plasma contain viable leukocytes, and so before being given to patients with combined immunodeficiency or to those receiving intense immunosuppression should be irradiated with 25–50 Gy to prevent possible GvHD (Treleaven et al. 2010). In those with no evidence of previous exposure to CMV, blood products should be obtained from CMV antibody-negative donors. White cell infusions can benefit patients with CGD and other neutrophil disorders with invasive infections who respond poorly to antibiotic treatment, particularly if the leukocytes are harvested from G-CSF-primed donors.

Haematopoietic stem cell transplantation

Most primary T-lymphocyte and phagocyte immunodeficiency disorders can be corrected by HSCT, using stem cells from marrow, mobilised peripheral blood stem cells or those harvested from umbilical cord blood (Gennery et al. 2010). Best results are obtained using HLA-matched sibling donors, but these are available for only about 20% of patients. Since the early 1980s, techniques have been developed to allow HLA-mismatched parent-to-child (haploidentical) grafts, by removing mature T lymphocytes that would otherwise cause fatal GvHD. Broadly matched volunteer-unrelated donor transplants are being increasingly used, particularly for non-SCID immunodeficiencies, and peripheral blood or umbilical cord stem cells are increasingly used instead of bone marrow. Gene therapy has been used for selective specific disorders, and clinical trials are ongoing (Qasim et al. 2009).

References

Backhed, F., Ley, R.E., Sonnenburg, J L., et al., 2005. Host–bacterial mutualism in the human intestine. Science 307, 1915–1920.

Baker, M.W., Grossman, W.J., Laessig, R.H., et al., 2009. Development of a routine newborn screening protocol for severe combined immunodeficiency. J Allergy Clin Immunol 124, 522–527.

Bedford Russell, A.R., Murch, S.H., 2006. Could peripartum antibiotics have delayed health consequences for the infant? Br J Obstet Gynaecol 113, 758–765.

Brace, R.A., Wolf, E.J., 1989. Normal amniotic fluid volume changes throughout pregnancy. Am J Obstet Gynecol 161, 382–388.

Brandtzaeg, P., Johansen, F.-E., 2005 Mucosal B cells: phenotypic characteristics, transcriptional regulation, and homing properties. Immunol Rev 206, 32–63.

Berrington, J.E., Flood, T.J., Abinun, M., et al., 2000. Unsuspected *Pneumocystis carinii* pneumonia at presentation of severe primary immunodeficiency. Arch Dis Child 82, 144–147.

Berrington, J.E., Barge, D., Fenton, A.C., et al., 2005. Lymphocyte subsets in term and significantly preterm UK infants in the first year of life analysed by single

platform flow cytometry. Clin Exp Immunol 140, 289–292.

Berrington, J.E., Fenton, A.C., Cant, A.J., et al., 2007.

Bleesing, J.H.J., Straus, S.E., Fleisher, T.A., 2000. Autoimmune lymphoproliferative syndrome: a human disorder of abnormal lymphocyte survival. Pediatr Clin North Am 47, 1291–1310.

Bordon, V., Gennery, A.R., Slatter, M.A., et al., 2010. Clinical and immunological outcome of patients with cartilage hair hypoplasia after hematopoietic stem cell transplantation. Blood 116, 27–35. Epub 2010 Apr 7.

Calder, P.C., Krauss-Etschmann, S., de Jong, E.C., et al., 2006. Early nutrition and immunity – progress and perspectives. Br J Nutr 96, 774–790.

Carr, R., Modi, N., Doré, C., 2003. G-CSF and GM-CSF for treating or preventing neonatal infections. Cochrane Database Syst Rev (3), CD003066.

Coombes, J.L., Powrie, F., 2008. Dendritic cells in intestinal immune regulation. Nat Rev Immunol 8, 435–446.

Crowley, C.A., Curnutte, J.T., Rosin, R.E., et al., 1980. An inherited abnormality of neutrophil adhesion: its genetic

transmission and its association with a missing protein. N Engl J Med 302, 1163–1168.

Delves, P.J., Roitt, I.M., 2000. The immune system: second of two parts. N Engl J Med 343, 108–117.

Doffinger, R., Smahi, A., Bessia, C., et al., 2001. X-linked anhidrotic ectodermal dysplasia with immunodeficiency is caused by impaired NF-kB signalling. Nature Genet 27, 277–285.

Driscoll, D.A., Sullivan, K.E., 1999. DiGeorge syndrome: a chromosome 22q11.2 deletion syndrome. In: Ochs, H.D., Smith, C.I.E., Puck, J.M. (Eds.), Primary Immunodeficiency Diseases: A molecular and genetic approach. Oxford University Press, New York, pp. 198–207.

Duerkop, B.A., Vaishnava, S., Hooper, L.V., 2009. Immune responses to the microbiota at the intestinal mucosal surface. Immunity 31, 368–376.

Ferrari, S., Giliani, S., Insalaco, A., et al., 2001. Mutations of CD40 gene cause an autosomal recessive form of immunodeficiency with hyper IgM. Proc Natl Acad Sci 98, 12614–12619.

Ferwerda, B., Ferwerda, G., Plantinga, T.S., et al., 2009. Human dectin-1 deficiency and mucocutaneous fungal infections. N Engl J Med 361, 1760–1767.

Field, C.J., 2005. The immunological components of human milk and their effect on immune development in infants. J Nutr 135, 1–4.

Fischer, A., 2000. Severe combined immunodeficiencies (SCID). Clin Exp Immunol 122, 143–149.

Fischer, A., 2007. Human primary immunodeficiency diseases. Immunity 27, 835–845.

Forsthuber, T., Yip, H.C., Lehmann, P.V., 1996. Induction of TH1 and TH2 immunity in neonatal mice. Science 271, 1728–1730.

Freeman, A.F., Holland, S.M., 2009. Clinical manifestations, etiology, and pathogenesis of the hyper-IgE syndromes. Pediatr Res 65, 32R–37R.

Gambineri, E., Perroni, L., Passerini, L., et al., 2008. Clinical and molecular profile of a new series of patients with immune dysregulation, polyendocrinopathy, enteropathy, X-linked syndrome: inconsistent correlation between forkhead box protein 3 expression and disease severity. J Allergy Clin Immunol 122, 1105–1112.e1.

Gaspar, H.B., Bjorkegren, E., Parsley, K., et al., 2006. Successful reconstitution of immunity in ADA-SCID by stem cell gene therapy following cessation of PEG-ADA and use of mild preconditioning. Mol Ther 14, 505–513.

Gennery, A.R., Cant, A.J., 2001. Applied physiology: immune competence. Curr Paediatr 11, 458–464.

Gennery, A.R., Khawaja, K., Veys, P., et al., 2004. Treatment of CD40 ligand deficiency by hematopoietic stem cell transplantation: a survey of the European experience, 1993–2002. Blood 103, 1152–1157.

Gennery, A.R., Slatter, M.A., Rice, J., et al., 2008. Mutations in CHD7 in patients with CHARGE syndrome cause T-B + natural killer cell + severe combined immune deficiency and may cause Omenn-like syndrome. Clin Exp Immunol 153, 75–80.

Gennery, A.R., Slatter, M.A., Grandin, L., et al., 2010. Transplantation of hematopoietic stem cells and long-term survival for primary immunodeficiencies in Europe: entering a new century, do we do better? J Allergy Clin Immunol 126, 602–610.

Gewolb, I.H., Schwalbe, R.S., Taciak, V.L., et al., 1999. Stool microflora in extremely low birthweight infants. Arch Dis Child Fetal Neonatal Ed 80, F167–F173.

Gilmour, K.C., Cranston, T., Loughlin, S., et al., 2001. Rapid protein-based assays for the diagnosis of T-B 1 severe combined immunodeficiency. Br J Haematol 112, 671–676.

Glocker, E.O., Hennigs, A., Nabavi, M., et al., 2009. A homozygous CARD9 mutation in a family with susceptibility to fungal infections. N Engl J Med 29, 1727–1735.

Grönlund, M.M., Salminen, S., Mykkänen, H., et al., 1999. Development of intestinal bacterial enzymes in infants–relationship to mode of delivery and type of feeding. APMIS 107, 655–660.

Hagleitner, M.M., Lankester, A., Maraschio, P., et al., 2008. Clinical spectrum of immunodeficiency, centromeric instability and facial dysmorphism (ICF syndrome). J Med Genet 45, 93–99.

Hague, R.A., Rassam, S., Morgan, G., et al., 1994. Early diagnosis of severe combined immune deficiency syndrome. Arch Dis Child 70, 260–263.

Hanson, L.A., Korotkova, M., Telemo, E., 2003. Breast-feeding, infant formulas, and the immune system. Ann Allergy Asthma Immunol 90 (Suppl 3), 59–63.

Hill, H.R., Joyner, J.L., Augustine, N.H., 1999. The pathophysiology of neonatal neutrophil dysfunction. Pediatr Res 45, 761.

Hirai, C., Ichiba, H., Saito, M., et al., 2002. Trophic effect of multiple growth factors in amniotic fluid or human milk on cultured human fetal small intestinal cells. J Pediatr Gastroenterol Nutr 34, 524–528.

Holt, P.G., 2000. The development of the immune system during pregnancy and early life. Allergy 55, 688–697.

Hooper, L.V., Macpherson, A.J., 2010. Immune adaptations that maintain homeostasis with the intestinal microbiota. Nat Rev Immunol 10, 159–169.

Imai, K., Morio, T., Zhu, Y., et al., 2004. Clinical course of patients with WASP gene mutations. Blood 103, 456–464.

Janda, A., Sedlacek, P., Hönig, M., et al., 2010. Multicenter survey on the outcome of transplantation of hematopoietic cells in patients with the complete form of DiGeorge anomaly. Blood 116, 2229–2236.

Jauniaux, E., Gulbis, B., Gerloo, E., 1999. Free amino acids in human fetal liver and fluids at 12–17 weeks of gestation. Hum Reprod 14, 1638–1641.

Jones, L.B.K.R., McGrogan, P., Flood, T.J., et al., 2008. Chronic granulomatous disease in the UK and Ireland – a comprehensive national patient based registry. Clin Exp Immunol 152, 211–218.

Kane, L.C., Gennery, A.R., Crooks, B.N.A., et al., 2001. Neonatal bone marrow transplantation for severe combined immunodeficiency. Arch Dis Child Fetal Neonatal Ed 85, F110–F113.

Karlsson, H., Hessle, C., Rudin, A., 2002. Innate immune responses of human neonatal cells to bacteria from the normal gastrointestinal flora. Infect Immun 70, 6688–6696.

Kavadas, F.D., Giliani, S., Gu, Y., et al., 2008. Variability of clinical and laboratory

features among patients with ribonuclease mitochondrial RNA processing endoribonuclease gene mutations. J Allergy Clin Immunol 122, 1178–1184.

Klein, C., Lisowska-Grospierre, B., LeDeist, F., et al., 1993. Major histocompatibility complex class II deficiency: clinical manifestations, immunologic features, and outcome. J Pediatr 123, 921–928.

Klouwenberg, P.K., Bont, L., 2008. Neonatal and infantile responses to encapsulated bacteria and conjugate vaccines. Clin Dev Immunol 2008:628963. Review.

Kostmann, R., 1956. Infantile genetic agranulocytosis. A review with presentation of ten new cases. Acta Paediatr Scand 64, 362–366.

Macpherson, A.J., Uhr, T., 2004. Induction of protective IgA by intestinal dendritic cells carrying commensal bacteria. Science 303, 1662–1665.

Marshall-Clarke, S., Reen, D., Tasker, L., et al., 2000. Neonatal immunity: how well has it grown up? Immunol Today 21, 35–41.

Moss, S.J., Fenton, A.C., Toomey, J., et al., 2010. Immunogenicity of a heptavalent conjugate pneumococcal vaccine administered concurrently with a combination diphtheria, tetanus, five-component acellular pertussis, inactivated polio, and Haemophilus influenzae type B vaccine and a meningococcal group C conjugate vaccine at 2, 3, and 4 months of age. Clin Vaccine Immunol 17, 311–336.

M'Rabat, L., Vos, A.P., Boehm, G., et al., 2008. Breast feeding and its role in early development of the immune system in infants: consequences for health in later life. J Nutr 138, 1782S–1790S.

Muller, S.M., Ege, M., Pottharst, A., et al., 2001. Transplacentally acquired maternal T lymphocytes in severe combined immunodeficiency: a study of 121 patients. Blood 98, 1847–1851.

Mulvihill, S.J., Stone, M.M., Fonkalsrud, E.W., et al., 1986. Trophic effect of amniotic fluid on fetal gastrointestinal development. J Surg Res 40, 291–296.

Murch, S.H., 2001. Toll of allergy reduced by probiotics. Lancet 357, 1057–1059.

Neurath, M.F., Finotto, S., Glimcher, L.H., 2002. The role of Th1/Th2 polarization in mucosal immunity. Nat Med 8, 567–573.

Notarangelo, L.D., Hayward, A.R., 2000. X-linked immunodeficiency with hyper-IgM (XHIM). Clin Exp Immunol 120, 399–405.

Notarangelo, L.D., Villa, A., Schwarz, K., 1999. RAG and RAG defects. Curr Opin Immunol 11, 435–442.

Notarangelo, L.D., Fischer, A., Geha, R.S., et al., 2009. Primary immunodeficiencies: 2009 update. J Allergy Clin Immunol 124, 1161–1178.

Ochs, H.D., Smith, C.I.E., Puck, J.M. (Eds.), 2007. Primary Immunodeficiency Diseases: A Molecular and Genetic

Approach, second ed. Oxford University Press, New York.

Ohlsson, A., Lacy, J.B., 2004. Intravenous immunoglobulin for preventing infection in preterm and/or low-birth-weight infants. Cochrane Database Syst Rev (1), CD000361.

Ohlsson, A., Lacy, J.B., 2010. Intravenous immunoglobulin for suspected or subsequently proven infection in neonates. Cochrane Database Syst Rev (3), CD001239.

Pai, S.Y., DeMartiis, D., Forino, C., et al., 2006. Stem cell transplantation for the Wiskott–Aldrich syndrome: a single-center experience confirms efficacy of matched unrelated donor transplantation. Bone Marrow Transplant 38, 671–679.

Pannicke, U., Hönig, M., Hess, I., et al., 2009. Reticular dysgenesis (aleukocytosis) is caused by mutations in the gene encoding mitochondrial adenylate kinase 2. Nat Genet 41, 101–105.

Pessach, I., Walter, J., Notarangelo, L.D., 2009. Recent advances in primary immunodeficiencies: identification of novel genetic defects and unanticipated phenotypes. Pediatr Res 65, 3R–12R.

Provan, D., Nokes, T.J.C., Agrawal, S., et al., 2008. Clinical Guidelines for Immunoglobulin Use. Department of Health, London.

Qasim, W., Gaspar, H.B., Thrasher, A.J., 2009. Progress and prospects: gene therapy for inherited immunodeficiencies. Gene Ther 16, 1285–1291.

Renner, E.D., Hartl, D., Rylaarsdam, S., et al., 2009. Comèl–Netherton syndrome defined as primary immunodeficiency. J Allergy Clin Immunol 124, 536–543.

Renella, R., Picard, C., Neven, B., et al., 2006. Human leucocyte antigen-identical haematopoietic stem cell transplantation in major histocompatiblity complex class II immunodeficiency: reduced survival correlates with an increased incidence of acute graft-versus-host disease and pre-existing viral infections. Br J Haematol 134, 510–516.

Ridge, J.P., Fuchs, E.J., Matzinger, P., 1996. Neonatal tolerance revisited: turning on newborn T cells with dendritic cells. Science 271, 1723–1726.

Rogers, M., Lwin, R., Fairbanks, L., et al., 2001. Cognitive and behavioural abnormalities in adenosine deaminase deficient severe combined deficiency. J Pediatr 139, 44–50.

Sarzotti, M., Robbins, D.S., Hoffman, P.M., 1996. Induction of protective CTL responses in newborn mice by a murine retrovirus. Science 271, 1726–1728.

Seger, R.A., Gungor, T., Belohradsky, B.H., et al., 2002. Treatment of chronic granulomatous disease with myeloablative conditioning and an unmodified hematopoietic allograft: a survey of the European experience 1985–2000. Blood 100, 4344–4350.

Shapiro, R., Beatty, D.W., Woods, D.L., et al., 1989. Serum complement and immunoglobulin values in small for gestational age infants. J Pediatr 99, 139–142.

Skinner, R., Cant, A., Davies, G., et al., 2002. Immunisation of the immunocompromised child. Best Practice Statement. Royal College of Paediatrics and Child Health, London.

Slatter, M.A., Gennery, A.R., 2010. Primary immunodeficiencies associated with DNA-repair disorders. Expert Rev Mol Med 12, e9.

Spencer, J., Barone, F., Dunn-Walters, D., 2009. Generation of immunoglobulin diversity in human gut-associated lymphoid tissue. Semin Immunol 21, 139–146.

Stiehm, R.E., Ochs, H.D., Winkelstein, J.A. (Eds.), 2004. Immunological Disorders in Infants and Children, fifth ed. Elsevier Saunders, Philadelphia.

Treleaven, J., Gennery, A., Marsh, J., et al., 2010. Guidelines on the use of irradiated blood components. Available online at: www.bcshguidelines.com.

Turner, J.R., 2009. Intestinal mucosal barrier function in health and disease. Nat Rev Immunol 9, 799–809.

van Wijk, F., Cheroutre, H., 2009. Intestinal T cells: facing the mucosal immune dilemma with synergy and diversity. Semin Immunol 21, 130–138.

Villa, A., Notarangelo, L.D., Roifman, C.M., 2008. Omenn syndrome: inflammation in leaky severe combined immunodeficiency. J Allergy Clin Immunol 122, 1082–1086.

Vochem, M., Hamprecht, K., Jahn, G., et al., 1998. Transmission of cytomegalovirus to preterm infants through breast milk. Pediatr Infect Dis J 17, 53–58.

Wershil, B.K., Furuta, G.T., 2008. 4. Gastrointestinal mucosal immunity. J Allergy Clin Immunol 121, S380–S383.

Whitington, P.F., Hibbard, J.U., 2004. High-dose immunoglobulin during pregnancy for recurrent neonatal haemochromatosis. Lancet 364, 1690–1698.

Part 2: **Infection in the newborn**

Alison Bedford Russell   David Isaacs

In spite of significant advances in neonatal intensive care and the development of broad-spectrum antibiotics, sepsis remains a leading cause of morbidity and mortality in the newborn, especially those born prematurely (Hemming et al. 1976; Stoll et al. 1996a, b, 2002a, b) and with low birthweight (Isaacs and Moxon 1991; Fanaroff et al. 1998; Heath et al. 2004).

The incidence of sepsis is inversely proportional to birthweight. In very-low-birthweight (VLBW) infants, infection is associated with significant risk of death and morbidity, including prolonged ventilation and hospital stay, and increased risk of chronic lung disease (CLD) (Thompson et al. 1992; Fanaroff et al. 1998; Marshall et al. 1999), interventricular haemorrhage and death (Stoll et al. 1996a, b). Perinatal infection has also become recognised as an important aetiological factor in the pathogenesis of cerebral cortical lesions (Dammann and Leviton 1997) and subsequent neurodevelopmental delay in both preterm (Murphy et al. 1995; Stoll et al. 2004) and term infants (Grether and Nelson 1997; Inder and Volpe 2000; Jacobsson and Hagberg 2004). Chemical mediators of this damage include proinflammatory cytokines, e.g. tumour necrosis factor-α

(TNF-α) and interleukin-6 (IL-6), as well as free radicals generated by activation of the neutrophil respiratory burst (Buonocore et al. 1994). Infection has been shown to induce damaging activation of glial cells, with infiltration of macrophages, leading ultimately to neuronal apoptosis (Pang et al. 2005). High concentrations of proinflammatory cytokines are associated with an increased risk of cardiovascular compromise, septic shock and death (Girardin et al. 1990; Roman et al. 1993). Proinflammatory cytokines also have effects on the developing brain during sepsis episodes, and are strongly associated with the development of brain lesions, even in the absence of meningitis (Inder and Volpe 2000; Jacobsson and Hagberg 2004).

The origins of nosocomial infection related to feeding practices

The gut of a baby admitted to a neonatal unit becomes colonised with abnormal bacteria as a result of obstetric practices, exposure to the neonatal unit bacterial flora and antibiotic administration. Recent evidence points to the huge importance of specific components of the gut flora in programming both intestinal function and immunological responses (both mucosal and systemic) in the host (Hooper et al. 2001; Hooper 2004; Backhed et al. 2005; Murch 2011). Thus abnormalities of initial colonisation patterns induced by preterm delivery, caesarean section and antibiotic administration may have potential delayed effects upon the infant, although so far there has been little focused study of this (Bedford Russell and Murch 2006).

Faecal flora in preterm babies is dominated by coagulase-negative staphylococci (CoNS) (Gewolb et al. 1999), which are the most common organisms causing late-onset sepsis (LOS) (Eastick et al. 1996; Stoll et al. 2002a, b; Vergnano et al. 2011), and enteric Gram-negative bacilli (Eriksson et al. 1982, 1986). It is likely that bacteria from the gut translocate across immature gut mucosa (Van Camp et al. 1994; Pierro et al. 1996) as the gut mucosa presents a poor barrier to infection, particularly in a non-fed newborn baby. Translocating bacteria may colonise indwelling devices such as catheters and give rise to systemic infection (Pierro et al. 1996).

The amniotic fluid-induced growth and development of the fetal gut are interrupted by preterm birth. Unit practices, such as delaying the introduction of maternal breast milk, may reduce the ability to undergo postnatal adaptation, and compromise normal immune development. Timing of introduction of colostrum is likely to be a key factor in postnatal intestinal development. Animal studies have demonstrated that delaying the introduction of milk feeds for even 2–3 days is associated with significant gut atrophy (Hughes and Dowling 1980; Sangild et al. 2002; Oste et al. 2005, 2010a and b) and necrotising enterocolitis (NEC) (Petersen et al. 2003). Formula feeding is associated with an increased risk of gut atrophy, reduced gut function and NEC-like lesions (Bjornvad et al. 2005; Oste et al. 2010b).

Because abnormal gut colonisation patterns may have very broad effects on immune development (Bedford Russell and Murch 2006; Murch 2011) and postnatal gut adaptation, delaying the introduction of human milk feeds may also contribute to an increased risk of infection. The introduction of any milk feed may be delayed for up to a week or more as a result of concerns regarding medical stability and the risk of necrotising enterocolitis (NEC) in particular 'high-risk' groups such as those with intrauterine growth retardation (IUGR). However this practice in babies has not been validated (La Gamma et al. 1985; Brown et al. 1987; Leaf et al. 2009), except for babies receiving formula feeds; the giving of human breast milk has not been associated with increased risk of NEC (Lucas and Cole 1990; McGuire and Anthony 2003). Indeed, breast milk has only ever been shown to protect babies from NEC (McGuire and Anthony 2003; Meinzen-Derr et al. 2009). Breast milk has also been shown to protect babies from late-onset infection (Hanson and Korotkova 2002; Hanson et al. 2003; Rønnestad et al. 2005; Meinzen-Derr et al. 2009).

Conversely, the introduction of even very small quantities of oral nutrients prevents intestinal mucosal atrophy and bowel villi flattening (Dworkin et al. 1976; Feldman et al. 1976). This effect is most marked following exposure to colostrum (Sangild et al. 2002; Bjornvad et al. 2005; Oste et al. 2005, 2010a and b). In vitro studies have demonstrated increased intestinal mass and deoxyribonucleic acid synthesis rates as a result of gut exposure to human breast milk (Klagsbrun 1978). Epidemiological studies indicate that the risk of infection is greatly increased for every day a baby is not enterally fed (Stoll et al. 2002a; Flidel-Rimon et al. 2004; Rønnestad et al. 2005; Meinzen-Derr et al. 2009). Conversely the earlier enteral feeds are commenced, and the sooner a baby is receiving full enteral feeds, the less likely that baby is to develop nosocomial (late-onset) infection

and NEC (Rønnestad et al. 2005; Meinzen-Derr et al. 2009). In one study of babies <1000 g, early breast milk feeding (initiated in 98% of babies within 3 days of life) was the most significant factor in reducing the risk of nosocomial sepsis, without increasing the risk of NEC (Rønnestad et al. 2005). Indeed, the incidence of all NEC was low, at a rate of 4% (published ranges 5.6–7.2%: Fanaroff et al. 2003; Fitzgibbons et al. 2009). The effect of early feeding is independent of the increased risk of infection with indwelling catheters (long lines, umbilical venous and arterial lines), and total parenteral nutrition (TPN) (Stoll et al. 2002; Rønnestad et al. 2005). However the nutritional needs of a baby have to be balanced against risk of infection, so that almost all babies <1 kg are likely to require at least a short period of TPN to 'feed the brain', and this is most safely delivered by a central venous catheter.

Introducing even 0.5 ml/kg of trophic maternal breast milk (and only breast milk) in the first hours of life at infrequent intervals of up to daily, in very immature babies, will facilitate the colonisation of the naïve gut with normal bacteria (lactobacilli and bifidobacteria). Although many of the potential benefits of trophic feedings still require confirmation by good clinical studies, clinical benefits may include improved milk tolerance, greater postnatal growth, reduced systemic sepsis, reduced NEC risks and shorter hospital stay (Bombell and McGuire 2009). There is currently no evidence of any adverse effects following trophic feeding with human breast milk (Bombell and McGuire 2009).

Recent findings emphasise the role of the normal flora in conditions such as NEC, and have shown benefit from use of probiotic organisms (Bin-Nun et al. 2005; Stenger et al. 2011). The links between trophic feeding, breast milk, the gut flora and the mucosal immune system are complex but highly important.

Neonatal skin and infection

Neonatal skin has innate immune functions, and provides a physical barrier, albeit fragile, as well as serving as a repository of antimicrobial proteins. In utero, the human fetus is encased in vernix caseosa and bathed in amniotic fluid, both of which are highly enriched with host defence proteins (HDPs) such as lysozyme and lactoferrin (Marchini et al. 2002; Akinbi et al. 2004; Walker et al. 2008). The latter permit a homeostatic balance between the presence of normal commensal bacteria and deterrence of pathogenic organisms (Gallo et al. 2002; Bowdish et al. 2005). In the immediate postnatal period an acid mantle covering the skin surface is rapidly established, and may enhance host defence mechanisms against pathogenic bacterial colonisation and infection (Dorschner et al. 2003). There has been much debate about the potential harmful effects versus the presumed benefits of bathing newborns (Gfatter et al. 1997; Quinn et al. 2005; Trotter 2006; Blume-Peytavi et al. 2009). Bathing may remove HDPs in vernix as well as reduce pathogen load (Medves and O'Brien 2001; Akinbi et al. 2004). The World Health Organization (WHO) recommends that newborns should not be bathed for at least 6 hours after birth to prevent deleterious effects of hypothermia (Bergstrom et al. 2005). Term newborn skin is replete with HDPs, which may not be significantly affected by a single bath (Walker et al. 2008), but may be affected by frequent bathing with soap. Skin colonisation on the neonatal intensive care unit (NICU) is mainly by CoNS, which can be isolated from over 90% of all positive cultures (Keyworth et al. 1992).

A clearer understanding of the role of HDPs in the cutaneous innate immune system, and of the impact of neonatal skin adaptation and skin care practices, such as bathing and the use of soap, will be important in the quest to reduce newborn infections. The benefits of frequent bathing with soap need to be properly evaluated in order to avoid potential harm.

Incidence of infection and causative organisms

Neonatal infection surveillance networks

When a neonate has suspected sepsis, antibiotic therapy is empirical, and should be commenced without delay, before knowing the exact nature of the infecting organism and its antimicrobial susceptibility. Since the aim of empirical therapy is to target the most likely infecting organism(s), it is crucial for neonatal units to survey the profile of causative organisms and their susceptibilities, in order to direct antimicrobial treatments effectively. Microbial pathogens, their antimicrobial sensitivities and patterns change over time (Isaacs et al. 1995, 2004; Isaacs and Royle 1999; Stoll et al. 2002b, May et al. 2005) and between countries (Zaidi et al. 2005; Geffers et al. 2008).

Neonatal infection surveillance networks have been established in a number of countries, including the Australasian Study Group for Neonatal Infections (ASGNI) (Daley and Isaacs 2004), the Israeli National VLBW Infant Database (Makhoul et al. 2005), the Canadian Neonatal Network (http://www.canadianneonatalnetwork.org), the US National Institute of Child Health and Human Development Neonatal Research Network (http://www.nichd.nih.gov), the Vermont Oxford Network (http://www.vtoxford.org/home.aspx) and the German Krankenhaus-Infektions-Surveillance-Systäm (Gastmeier et al. 2004). Apart from the ASGNI and Canadian groups, these neonatal infection networks focus on infection rates in VLBW babies.

In the UK, a Neonatal Infection Surveillance Network (NeonIN) was established in 2004 to collect clinical and microbiological data on episodes of neonatal infection longitudinally. The incidence, pathogens and antibiotic resistance profiles of infections captured in NeonIN in the 3 years between January 2006 and December 2008 have recently been reported (Vergnano et al. 2011).

Additionally the Health Protection Agency has a voluntary surveillance scheme in England and Wales, whereby bacteraemias but not clinical data are reported. The British Paediatric Surveillance Unit has also continued to conduct studies of the epidemiology of infections over defined time periods, such as herpes simplex virus (HSV) (Tookey and Peckham 1996), group B streptococcus (GBS) (Heath et al. 2004), meticillin-resistant *Staphylococcus aureus* (MRSA) (Johnson et al. 2010), fungal infections in VLBW babies (Clerihew et al. 2007) and neonatal meningitis (Holt et al. 2001), which have provided invaluable data. Surveillance of human immunodeficiency virus (HIV) infections in children is ongoing, and current specific studies include surveillance of congenital syphilis and congenital rubella.

A variety of data are collected on culture-proven sepsis, as well as presumed and possible sepsis (Gastmeier et al. 2004). Definitions of sepsis vary between surveillance networks but all consist of a combination of clinical and laboratory parameters (May et al. 2005). These networks have been able to monitor changes in pathogens (May et al. 2005) and their antibiotic resistance over time (Daley and Isaacs 2004; Stoll et al. 2005), so can be used to inform antibiotic policy. They provide data for comparisons between different countries, and have been used to document changes in clinical practice and their effects (Lee et al. 2000; Stoll et al. 2002b), and provide a system to identify what constitutes effective practice, and thus improve quality of care (Horbar et al. 2001). Surveillance systems can also be used to provide data for the planning of interventional studies, as well as systems for data capture, following interventions (Edwards et al. 2004; Vergnano et al. 2011).

Incidence of infection

The UK NeonIN data demonstrate that, with the inclusion of CoNS, the incidence of all neonatal infection is 0.8% of live births and 7.1% of neonatal admissions. The incidence of culture-confirmed neonatal sepsis in the USA is in the region of 0.7% (Philip 1994). One study in Australia reported an incidence of 0.22% for early-onset sepsis (EOS) and 0.44% for late-onset sepsis (LOS), with mortality rates 15% and 9% respectively (Isaacs et al. 1995). In resource-poor countries, neonatal sepsis rates are as high as 5–10%, with case-fatality rates of between 23% and 52%. Septicaemia accounts for between 11% and 30% of all neonatal deaths (Boo and Chor 1994).

Classification of neonatal infections

Neonatal infection is broadly classified into early- or late-onset neonatal sepsis.

Early-onset sepsis (EOS) is variably defined as sepsis (e.g. bacteraemia and meningitis) within 48–72 hours of birth (some define it as <7 days) and usually presents as a fulminating septicaemic illness, often complicated by pneumonia. The main routes of infection are vertical transmission from the mother via transplacental or ascending vaginal routes, and postnatally from the environment. Other terms used for this pattern of infection are 'vertically transmitted' (meaning from mother to infant) and 'perinatally acquired'. The pattern of presentation is similar with most of the causative bacteria.

Late-onset sepsis

Late-onset infection in neonates is defined as infection becoming clinically evident more than 48–72 hours after birth, and is usually the result of nosocomially acquired organisms, hence the term 'healthcare-acquired infection'.

Early-onset sepsis

The risk of sepsis and mortality increases with decreasing gestational age and birthweight and is highest in babies <1000 g. The reported incidence of EOS in VLBW infants ranges from 1.5% (Stoll et al. 2002b) to 2.7% (López Sastre 2000), with high case-fatality rates of 26–36% (Stoll et al. 1996a).

The overall incidence of EOS in the UK is 0.9/1000 of all live births and 0.9% of all neonatal admissions. GBS and *Escherichia coli* are the most common causative organisms, if CoNS are excluded, and account for 58% and 18% of bacteraemias respectively in the UK (Muller-Pebody et al. 2011; Vergnano et al. 2011).

In the USA, widespread universal screening for maternal GBS colonisation was introduced in the mid-1990s, and intrapartum antibiotic prophylaxis (IAP) was adopted as routine practice. Since then, there has been a significant decline in GBS-EOS (Centers for Disease Control 2002; Stoll et al. 2005), and an accompanying change in the distribution of pathogens, from predominantly Gram-positive organisms to Gram-negative Enterobacteriaceae, particularly *E. coli* (McDuffie et al. 1993; Nambiar and Singh 2002; Gilbert 2004; Stoll et al. 2005). In the USA, there has also been an increase in frequency of multiply resistant *E. coli* isolates in VLBW infants (Stoll et al. 2002b). The reason for this shift in causative organisms, although tentatively linked to IAP use in VLBW babies (Stoll et al. 2002b), is uncertain since many factors affect the maternal vaginal flora (including intrapartum antibiotic treatment, both in the community and in hospital, ethnic group, underlying medical condition and age). In Australia, the introduction of IAP for GBS

Table 39.4 Pathogens causing early-onset sepsis: a comparison between US National Institute of Child Health and Human Development (NICHD) data and UK Neonatal Infection Surveillance Network (NeonIN) data

	USA: NICHD 2002–2003 Incidence/1000 VLBW	UK: NeonIN 2007–2008 Incidence/1000 VLBW	P
All infections	17	22	
Gram-positive	8	17	0.002
Group B streptococcus	2	11	0.06
Listeria	0.3	5	
CoNS	2	8	0.005
Other	3	3	
Gram-negative	9	4	0.002
Escherichia coli	7	3	0.02
Other	2	0.4	
Fungal			
Candida albicans	0.3	0.4	

VLBW, very low birthweight; CoNS, coagulase-negative staphylococci.

prophylaxis has not been accompanied by the same increase in resistant Gram-negative infections (Daley and Isaacs 2004). Recent studies in the UK report national incidence rates of GBS infection in infants similar to those seen in the USA following the introduction of universal screening and IAP (Heath et al. 2004). Hence in the UK the National Screening Committee has not recommended the introduction of a UK GBS screening programme. Pathogens associated with EOS are summarised in Table 39.4.

Group B streptococcus

GBS is an important cause of serious infection in neonates, infants and immunocompromised or pregnant adults. The overall incidence of GBS infection in the UK is 0.72/1000 live births, though there are regional variations, with the highest incidence being in Northern Ireland and the lowest in Scotland (Heath et al. 2004). GBS is a commensal of the gastrointestinal tract and vagina, and colonises some 10–30% of pregnant women in the UK. There are numerous identifiable serotypes of GBS, based on capsular polysaccharide antigens: Ia, Ib, II, III, IV, V, VI, VII and VIII. All are implicated in early-onset disease, with national variations in prevalence. In the UK, enhanced surveillance has demonstrated that GBS serotypes III, Ia and V are the most commonly identified isolates causing early-onset infection (Weisner et al. 2004). Simultaneous infection with two distinct serotypes has been described (Fernandez et al. 1999). In addition to the polysaccharide antigens there are surface-exposed protein antigens which may also contribute to the pathogenicity of particular strains (Chun et al. 1991).

It is well established that GBS can cross intact fetal membranes. While prolonged rupture of fetal membranes (>18 hours) is a feature in 44% of newborns with invasive GBS infection, for 56% of affected babies, membrane rupture occurred less than 18 hours before birth (Heath et al. 2004). Although GBS infection is uncommon, mortality and morbidity are high, especially for preterm babies (Heath et al. 2004). This may partly be a consequence of the acute inflammatory response to GBS. GBS is able to invade

pulmonary endothelial cells, leading to release of eicosanoids such as prostacyclin and prostaglandin E2 (Gibson et al. 1995). In animal models, GBS causes a dose-dependent increase in pulmonary arterial pressure and pulmonary and systemic vascular resistance, and decreases cardiac output and heart rate. The quantitative response of the pulmonary vascular resistance is GBS strain-dependent in animal models, with serotype Ib having a greater effect than serotype III (Covert and Schreiber 1993). Postmortem examination demonstrates that many infants develop alveolar hyaline membranes, as well as pneumonia (Ablow et al. 1976). In the preterm infant, this is likely to represent coexistent surfactant-deficient hyaline membrane disease of prematurity (Jacob et al. 1980), but in term babies the hyaline membranes are a non-specific change associated with GBS infection (Rojas and Stahlman 1984), and may reflect a secondary surfactant insufficiency.

Most incidence figures are based on 'culture-proven' GBS whereby GBS is grown in blood or cerebrospinal fluid (CSF). Various factors may decrease the yield of blood and CSF cultures in the presence of true infection. Blood cultures are often negative in pneumonia (Webber et al. 1990). Other possible explanations include prior use of antibiotics (e.g. when given to the mother as IAP) (Kenyon et al. 2001), inadequate blood volumes obtained (Isaacman et al. 1996) or low-level bacteraemia. In the case of GBS, 'probable' infection has been defined as an episode of clinical sepsis likely to have been caused by GBS, and indicated by GBS surface colonisation together with clinical features of sepsis but with negative blood cultures. Prospectively collected data in a UK tertiary neonatal unit from all neonates requiring a sepsis screen in the first 72 hours of life demonstrated a combined rate of definite and probable GBS infection of 3.6/1000 live births (Luck et al. 2003). This suggests a much greater disease burden in the UK than the incidence based on culture-proven sepsis.

Prior to the introduction of a national GBS-screening programme and IAP, the reported prevalence of early-onset GBS sepsis in the USA was 1.8 per 1000 live births (Boyer 1995); in Canada, 1.75 per 1000 (Cimolai and Roscoe 1995); in Australia, 1.3 per 1000 (Isaacs et al. 1995); and in Spain, 1.2 per 1000 (Hervas et al. 1993). The prevalence in Finland is around 0.76 per 1000 (Kalliola et al. 1999).

Risk factors for early-onset GBS infection can be identified in up to 60% of cases and include preterm delivery (<37 weeks), prolonged rupture of membranes (PROM ≥ 18 hours) or known genital carriage of GBS during pregnancy (Heath et al. 2004), although GBS can cross intact membranes. Infection is the most common identifiable reason for spontaneous vaginal preterm delivery, so preterm delivery alone represents a risk factor for infection. The overall mortality is approximately 10% but is significantly higher among infants born prematurely (Heath et al. 2004). Up to 7% of survivors of GBS infection may suffer some disability; the risk is obviously higher if there is meningitis. Opportunities to prevent GBS infection using a risk factor based approach to GBS-prevention are often missed (Vergnano et al. 2011).

The mode of presentation and frequency of infection differ according to age at onset: GBS most commonly causes early-onset disease, defined as being <7 days (0.47/1000), manifesting as sepsis or pneumonia. Late-onset GBS disease can occur from 7 days to 3 months of life and is less common (0.25/1000); the more frequent presentation is with meningitis and sepsis. Late-onset GBS infection may result from invasion of colonising organisms acquired at birth or nosocomially or possibly from breast milk (Olver et al. 2000; Dinger et al. 2002).

GBS colonisation

GBS resides in the lower gut and vagina in 12–23% of mothers (Gibbs et al. 1994; Jeffery and McIntosh 1994; Stoll and Schuchat 1998). Such women are described as being 'carriers' of GBS or 'colonised' with GBS. GBS is passed from one person to another by skin-to-skin contact and can be exchanged between mother and father through sexual contact. However, there are no known harmful effects of carriage itself and, since the GBS bacteria do not cause genital symptoms or discomfort, GBS is not a sexually transmitted disease. Neither is GBS carriage a sign of ill health or poor hygiene. The likelihood of GBS isolation increases if samples are obtained from the lower vagina and rectum (Badri et al. 1977) and placed in selective broth, and decreases if the sample is limited to a high vaginal swab.

Babies are far more frequently 'colonised' than 'infected' with GBS. If a term baby is well, has a normal examination (specifically a normal respiratory rate and heart rate) and no other risk factors for infection, the baby is most likely simply to be colonised with GBS. The National Institute for Health and Clinical Excellence (NICE) intrapartum care guideline recommends monitoring of general well-being, temperature, perfusion, respiration rate, pulse and heart rate for a minimum of 12 hours in babies whose mothers had PROM at term (NICE 2007) for management of babies at risk for GBS infection (see Fig. 21.1 in Ch. 21 for a suggested observation chart). A preterm baby, especially one delivered after spontaneous onset of labour, warrants an infection screen and treatment with antibiotics, including penicillin, until cultures are known to be negative. This is because infection is the most common identifiable reason for spontaneous preterm delivery, as stated above.

Presentation of GBS infection

Nearly 90% of neonates with early-onset GBS have signs of infection within 12 hours of delivery (Escobar et al. 2000; Lin and Troendle 2006). Early stages of infection may be very subtle. A baby may simply not be feeding well or be excessively sleepy. Tachypnoea, apnoea or other respiratory distress are the most common presenting signs (Boyle et al. 1978; Luck et al. 2003). GBS sepsis may alternatively present with respiratory failure, cyanosis and shock, and the baby's condition at delivery may be clinically indistinguishable from perinatal hypoxic ischaemia. GBS infection should always be suspected in a baby who has more severe respiratory distress syndrome (RDS) than would have been anticipated, as RDS and GBS pneumonia are radiologically indistinct. In severe cases, persistent pulmonary hypertension of the newborn, hypotension, metabolic acidaemia, tachycardia and poor peripheral perfusion may develop and are poor prognostic features.

If infection is suspected in a baby, the baby should be promptly investigated (including a chest radiograph (CXR)), and treated with antibiotics. C-reactive protein (CRP) measurements may be normal in the early stages of infection (Luck et al. 2003) as it takes at least 12 hours for a CRP level to become raised (Black et al. 2004). A normal CRP does not exclude GBS infection, but may rise after 12–24 hours in infection. A raised CRP may be due to infection or other causes of inflammation. Some use the CRP to monitor the response to therapy, but there is no evidence that this is superior to clinical response.

Benzylpenicillin is the antibiotic of choice for GBS. Any organisms present in blood usually require a minimum of 48 hours to culture. During this time babies are treated with antibiotics until the results of the cultures are known. It is not uncommon for a baby to have signs of infection but for the tests on blood, swabs or CSF to be negative. Pneumonia is the most common focal infection caused by GBS, and, as already stated, can mimic RDS radiologically, with bilateral ground-glass shadowing and air bronchograms (Fig. 39.7). Signs of pneumonia may be minimal and only manifest on a radiograph and with clinical signs and raised inflammatory markers (raised CRP, alterations in absolute neutrophil count (ANC) and low platelet count). It is common practice to treat such babies with antibiotics for many days because of the difficulty in being certain about whether or not bacteria are causing their illness (Stoll et al. 1996a). As a result not only do many infants receive antibiotics that are ultimately not required, but they may also receive them for a long time. In the prospective study referred to

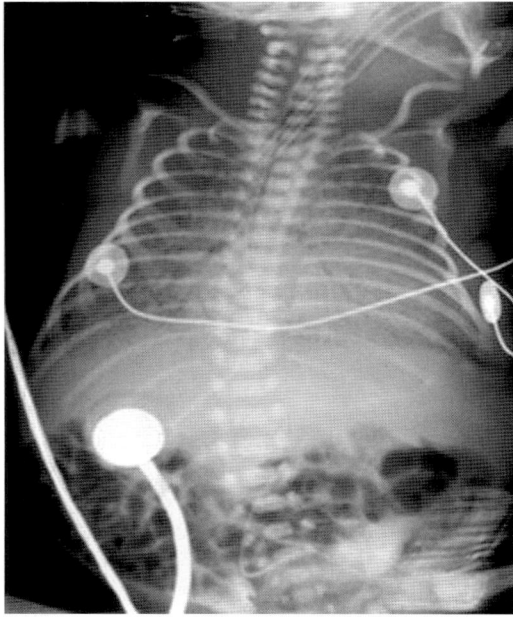

Fig. 39.7 Chest radiograph of baby with culture-proven group B streptococcus and more severe respiratory distress syndrome then was anticipated.

above (Luck et al. 2003), <5% of infants treated for infection had either culture-proven or culture-negative clinical sepsis; thus >95% of babies receiving antibiotics did not need them. Excessive antibiotic use may alter antibiotic susceptibilities as well as the types of colonising microbial flora, especially in the gut. Possible consequences include the emergence of antibiotic resistance in common bacterial pathogens, such as *E. coli* (Stoll et al. 2002b; Moore et al. 2003; Alarcon et al. 2004), the emergence of new pathogens, such as *Enterobacter* sp. (Van Houten et al. 2001), and an increased risk of atopy and asthma in childhood (McKeever et al. 2002; Benn et al. 2002; Bedford Russell and Murch 2006).

Recurrent GBS infection

Reccurrent GBS sepsis occurs in <1% of infants. In a series of nine cases (Green et al. 1994), the mean age at second infection was 42 days; six cases had septicaemia without a focus of infection and three had meningitis. The organism causing the first and subsequent infection was shown to be the same in more than half of the cases. Whether these cases represent a relapse of the initial infection or a reinfection is unclear. Rifampicin has been used, with limited success, to eradicate carriage in some children with recurrent GBS infection.

Detection of GBS with PCR

There are a number of studies in progress to evaluate polymerase chain reaction (PCR) as a diagnostic tool in the detection of GBS and *E. coli* in neonates undergoing sepsis screens in the first 72 hours of life. PCR can be used to detect specific bacterial proteins in body fluids and swabs. Such methods do not depend on having to culture bacteria. In animals PCR has been shown to result in a significantly more rapid detection rate of organisms than conventional culture methods (Heininger et al. 1999; Straka et al. 2004; Natarajan et al. 2006).

In future, PCR may be able to detect bacteraemia in cases of clinical sepsis with a greater sensitivity and frequency than is currently detected by conventional blood cultures. Furthermore for infants with GBS or *E. coli* bacteraemia, diagnosis will be made in hours rather than days.

Improvements in diagnostic techniques may thus better inform antibiotic management of the newborn (Natarajan et al. 2006). Negative results should enable clinicians to have confidence in prescribing antibiotics for short periods of time, or not at all.

Prevention of GBS

In the absence of a vaccine, the most effective strategy for prevention of GBS disease is to give antibiotic prophylaxis to mothers during labour. In the USA, where GBS was very much more common than in the UK, all mothers have a vaginal swab to look for GBS at 35–37 weeks' gestation. GBS swab-positive mothers are treated with a penicillin (usually ampicillin) during labour. This has resulted in a significant reduction in babies with invasive GBS disease. In the UK, approximately 625 women with one or more risk factors (intrapartum fever, PROM >18 hours, prematurity <37 weeks, previous infant with GBS) need to be treated to prevent one case of disease, and 5882 women need to be treated to prevent one death (Hughes et al, 2003). There is increasing concern that unnecessary use of antibiotics is associated with an increase in infections with resistant bacteria (Stoll et al. 2002b). IAP may therefore be useful in the short term, but in the long term may facilitate the development of resistant Gram-negative organisms, which result in as much, if not greater, harm. Routine screening and antibiotic prophylaxis are not currently recommended in the UK (NICE 2007; Royal College of Obstetricians and Gynaecologists 2003). Studies of GBS vaccines which may prevent GBS infection in the future are promising, but vaccine development is in the early phases, and at present there is no GBS vaccine available (Heath and Feldman 2005).

Listeria

Listeria monocytogenes is a short Gram-positive intra- and extracellular rod. The most important reservoir for transmission to humans is probably food, especially dairy products, contaminated by infected farm animals (Fleming et al. 1985, Gellin and Broome 1989). Neonatal infection in the UK is now uncommon (Table 39.4). Women infected with HIV are considerably more susceptible to *L. monocytogenes* than are the general population (Ewert et al. 1995). Three main types of fetal and neonatal infection are found: (1) transplacental infection; (2) early-onset infection acquired intrapartum; and (3) late-onset infection, usually meningitis, probably due to nosocomial infection.

Transplacental infection

L. monocytogenes causes a non-specific influenzal or gastroenteritic illness in the pregnant woman, during which the organism may infect the fetus, either by haematogenous spread across the placenta or via infection of the amniotic fluid. First- or second-trimester infection may cause fetal death or miscarriage, and recurrent abortion due to *Listeria* has been recorded in humans (Gray 1960). Later in pregnancy, infection may precipitate preterm labour (Gellin and Broome 1989), with spontaneous PROM, and fetal distress. Meconium staining of the liquor is not specific to *Listeria* infection (Romero et al. 1991). Liveborn babies are often extremely ill at birth. They may have severe pneumonia, and hepatosplenomegaly and meningitis may already be present. Blood and stool cultures are invariably positive. Characteristically, small (2–3 mm) pinkish-grey cutaneous granulomas are present and, at autopsy, similar small granulomatous lesions are widespread in the lung, liver, central nervous system (CNS) and many other tissues and organs.

Early-onset infection, acquired intrapartum

Most cases of neonatal listeriosis are sporadic, but epidemics have been described. The mother of a case is likely to be carrying the organism in her stool and presents an infection risk in a maternity hospital. She and her baby should be isolated. At least two-thirds of infants who acquire *Listeria* infection intrapartum are preterm, and almost all become ill within 24 hours of birth (MacGowan et al. 1991). Most have disseminated infection, with pneumonia, meningitis, thrombocytopenia, anaemia and sometimes conjunctivitis. Small cutaneous granulomas may be found in some babies.

Late-onset infection, usually meningitis, probably due to nosocomial infection

Nosocomial spread of *Listeria* is well documented, and asymptomatic mothers of affected babies should be isolated, as discussed above (Farber et al. 1991; MacGowan et al. 1991). Late-onset *Listeria* infection is usually in the form of meningitis with or without concomitant septicaemia or colitis. The median age of onset is about 2 weeks. Associated brain abscess has been described (Banerjee and Noya 1999).

Investigation

The routine investigations of EOS and meningitis reveal the diagnosis. However, *Listeria* can pose problems for the microbiologist, as its uptake of the Gram stain can be variable and it may be slow-growing.

Therapy

The most effective antibiotic therapy is ampicillin plus gentamicin, although *Listeria* is sensitive to benzylpenicillin. *Listeria* is resistant to all third-generation cephalosporins.

Outcome

The mortality for neonatal listeriosis ranges between 5% and 15% (Frederiksen and Samuelsson 1992; Jones et al. 1994).

Late-onset sepsis

The majority of LOS occurs in premature (<37 weeks' gestation) and low-birthweight (<2500 g) babies, the risk being greater for the smallest and most immature babies (Stoll et al. 1996b, 2002a; Fanaroff et al. 1998; Brodie et al. 2000; López Sastre et al. 2002; Makhoul et al. 2002; Rønnestad et al. 2005; Geffers et al. 2008; Vergnano et al. 2011).

The incidence of LOS among VLBW infants ranges between 16% and 30% (Brodie et al. 2000; López Sastre et al. 2002; Makhoul et al. 2002; Stoll et al. 2002a; Vergnano et al. 2011) and approaches 50% in infants with a birthweight <1000 g (Makhoul et al. 2002; Vergnano et al. 2011). Mortality rates vary between 17% and 21% (Fanaroff et al. 1998; Stoll et al. 2002a). The incidence of LOS in the UK is 0.7% of live births and 6.1% of neonatal unit admissions.

Organisms

The most common organisms causing late sepsis in industrialised countries are CoNS, which comprise 45–55% of isolates (Freeman et al. 1987; Stoll et al. 1996b; Rønnestad et al. 1998; Vergnano et al. 2011) (Table 39.5). CoNS predominate amongst gut flora of babies in neonatal units (Eastick et al. 1996; Gewolb et al. 1999) and may translocate across gut mucosa (Pierro et al. 1996) or invade via skin surfaces or indwelling catheters. CoNS can cause sepsis but are also frequent contaminants of blood and CSF cultures. Epidemiological studies vary in their definition of true CoNS infection and contaminants (Hyde et al. 2002; Stoll et al. 2005). In one study, more than half of late-onset CoNS-positive neonatal bacteraemias were considered to be true infections (Huang et al. 2003). Rapid time (≤36 hours) to blood culture positivity is a surrogate for organism load and has been used as a marker of true infection (Kumar et al. 2001). CoNS rarely cause fulminant infection or death, and empiric antibiotic regimens that include vancomycin to cover CoNS are no more effective than those that use a semisynthetic penicillin such as flucloxacillin (Isaacs 2003). That said, in the largest study of outcomes in extremely low-birthweight (ELBW) infants, CoNS were the predominant isolates, and all adverse neurodevelopmental outcomes, except hearing impairment, were higher among infected children regardless of type of pathogen (Stoll et al. 2004). This may be because the babies with Gram-negative bacillary infection were more likely to have died.

Selection pressure due to intensive use of antimicrobials in neonatal units has led to changes in antimicrobial susceptibility patterns of organisms associated with LOS. Changes in the epidemiology of nosocomial infections and outbreaks of MRSA (Boyce et al. 2005), ampicillin-resistant *E. coli*, vancomycin-resistant enterococci and multiresistant Gram-negative bacilli are increasingly being reported from neonatal units. This is a major concern, especially since resistant Gram-negative bacteria make the choice of empirical therapy more difficult, and result in a poorer prognosis for the patient treated with antibiotics to which the organisms are resistant (Kang et al. 2005).

Other isolates causing LOS include Enterobacteriaceae (9–21%) and *Staphylococcus aureus* (13–18%, 11% of which were MRSA),

Table 39.5 Organisms causing late-onset sepsis: comparison between Neonatal Infection Surveillance Network (NeonIn), Krankenhaus-Infektions-Surveillance-Systäm (NeoKISS) and National Institute of Child Health and Human Development (NICHD) surveillance data

	USA: NICHD 1998–2000 n = 1313 Incidence/1000 VLBW	UK: NeoNIN 2007–2008 n = 524 Incidence/1000 VLBW	Germany NeoKISS 2000–2005 n = 1844 Incidence/1000 VLBW
All infections	21	24	21
Gram-positive	15	18	
CoNS	10	13	6.6
Staphylococcus aureus	1.6	1.9	1.2
Enterococcus	0.7	2.0	0.5
Gram-negative	3.7	4.4	
Escherichia coli	1.0	1.6	0.6
Enterobacteriacae	1.8	1.9	
Pseudomonas	0.6		4.0
Candida spp.	2.6	0.8	0.4

P-values represent significant differences between NICHD and NeonIn data. Enterobacteriaceae include *Klebsiella*, *Enterobacter* and *Serratia* (NICHD 45%, 30% and 25% of isolates respectively); *Klebsiella*, *Enterobacter* and *Serratia* (NeonIN 53%, 37% and 9% of isolates), and equal numbers of *Enterobacter* and *Klebsiella* (NeoKISS).
n = number of infection episodes for which data are available.
VLBW, very low birthweight; CoNS, coagulase-negative staphylococci.

Table 39.6 Commonly known Enterobacteriaceae associated with opportunistic infection

Escherichia coli
Klebsiella
Enterobacter
Serratia
Proteus
Morganella
Citrobacter

E. coli (Health Protection Agency, HPA), GBS (HPA) and fungi 9% (72% *C. albicans*).

Systemic fungal infection has become a major problem for ELBW infants <1000 g, with published infection rates varying widely between countries at 1.5–20%.

Enterobacteriaceae

The family Enterobacteriaceae includes many genera and species (Table 39.6). Members are Gram-negative, facultatively anaerobic bacilli, which may appear as coccobacilli on Gram stain. The virulence of these species is controlled by a number of factors, including the ability to adhere, colonise, invade tissues and produce various toxins. Different antigens can be used to differentiate different serologic groups. The capsular antigen K1, present in certain strains of *E. coli*, has been the most documented virulence factor associated with *E. coli* meningitis and sepsis. These strains are distinct from those associated with diarrhoeal disease. Some Enterobacteriaceae harbour plasmids providing antimicrobial resistance genes. An increasing number of *E. coli* and *Klebsiella* strains produce plasmid-mediated extended-spectrum β-lactamases, which can inactivate cephalosporins, penicillins and aztreonam. Family members are ubiquitous in nature but almost all share the gastrointestinal tract as a common niche, and, apart from *Yersinia*, *Shigella* and *Salmonella*, can be normal resident flora if confined to their natural environment. *E. coli* is so commonly isolated from colonic flora that it is used as a primary marker of faecal contamination in water purification. Although Enterobacteriaceae can cause opportunistic infection, they are often harmless commensals. Members are broadly divided into opportunistic and primary pathogens. Opportunistic pathogens are often part of the normal faecal flora. They may produce serious extraintestinal opportunistic infections, however; for example *E. coli* is a member of the normal bowel flora but can cause urinary tract infections (UTIs), septicaemia and meningitis. Primary pathogens include *Salmonella*, *Shigella* and *Yersinia*, and are not part of normal gut flora. They are true pathogens and will cause infections if ingested.

Gram-negative bacteraemia and antimicrobial non-susceptible Enterobacteriaceae

The Centers for Disease Control National Nosocomial Infection Surveillance System has reported a substantial increase in third-generation cephalosporin-resistant enteric Gram-negative bacilli causing nosocomial infections in intensive care units (Fridkin et al. 2001, 2002; Sohn et al. 2001). Gram-negative bacteraemia in children has also been positively associated with the use of antibiotics in addition to cephalosporins, including aminoglycosides and vancomycin, but also correlates with surgical interventions, central venous catheters, parenteral nutrition, antacids and dexamethasone. The strongest association in one study was with the use of

vancomycin (van Houten et al. 2001), hence the recommendation that vancomycin should not be used for empirical treatment on the basis of suspicion of bacteraemia.

ELBW babies, <1000 g, who are colonised with antimicrobial non-susceptible Enterobacteriaceae (ANE) and those who receive prolonged exposure to antimicrobial agents are at increased risk of ANE infections (Singh et al. 2002). Such ANE include *E. coli*, *Enterobacter* spp., *Citrobacter* spp., *Klebsiella* spp. and *Serratia* spp. They are defined as being 'members of the Enterobacteriaceae family exhibiting non-susceptibility to ceftazidime or with evidence of extended spectrum beta-lactamase production'. Multiply resistant Enterobacteriaceae strains (MRE, defined as 'strains resistant to three or more classes of antibiotic'), have been found at high frequency in NICU infants, and persist in a significant proportion of infants for at least 6 months, even after discharge from hospital (Millar et al. 2008). Such high prevalence of colonisation increases the probability of MRE infection in vulnerable infants and outbreaks are increasingly described within NICUs (Musoke and Revathi 2000; Bromiker et al. 2001; Kartali et al. 2002; Dent and Toltzis 2003; Nambiar et al. 2003; Sherer et al. 2005).

Colonisation with MRE strains has been detected as early as on the first day of hospitalisation (Almuneef et al. 2001), and may follow transmission from other NICU patients, or may evolve endogenously from selective pressures exerted by antimicrobial therapy.

In the UK, the majority of pathogens, other than CoNS, causing EOS (>94%) are susceptible to commonly used empiric first-line antibiotic regimens of penicillin/gentamicin or amoxicillin, amoxicillin combined with cefotaxime or cefotaxime monotherapy (Health Protection Agency 2007; Vergnano et al. 2011). More than 95% of organisms causing LOS are susceptible to gentamicin with either flucloxacillin (Health Protection Agency 2007; NeonIN), or amoxicillin and amoxicillin with cefotaxime, but only 79% are susceptible to cefotaxime monotherapy (Health Protection Agency 2007). This supports the use of narrow-spectrum antimicrobials in the form of penicillin/gentamicin as 'first-line' therapy for EOS and flucloxacillin/gentamicin for LOS, with use of vancomycin restricted to situations where there is a serious risk of CoNS infection.

Suboptimal empiric antibiotic therapy potentially leads to worse outcomes (Kang et al. 2005; Zaoutis et al. 2005), but must be balanced against the hazards of routine use of broad-spectrum antibiotics for empiric therapy, since administration of these correlates with the development of resistant organisms (de Man et al. 2000; Fridkin et al. 2001, 2002).

Enterococci

Previously classified as group D streptococci, enterococci are Gram-positive cocci that are natural inhabitants of the human intestinal tract. They have a survival advantage over other organisms in that they can grow in extreme conditions and are resistant to multiple antimicrobial agents. Enterococci are associated with nosocomial infection, most commonly bacteraemia and UTI. Prolonged hospitalisation, immunocompromise and prior surgical procedures are risk factors. Because of intrinsic or acquired resistance to several antimicrobial agents, including aminoglycosides, beta-lactams and glycopeptides, e.g. vancomycin and teicoplanin, differentiation of enterococci from other streptococci and susceptibility testing are important.

Fungal infection

Systemic candidiasis is a leading cause of death and morbidity, specifically poor neurodevelopmental outcome, in ELBW infants

(Benjamin et al. 2010). The incidence of *Candida* infection in ELBW babies in a recent surveillance study of 13 USA centres varied between 2% and 28% (Benjamin et al. 2010), with an overall incidence across 19 units of 9%. Recent UK data estimated the annual incidence of invasive disease to be 1.0% (0.8–1.2%) amongst VLBW infants and 2.1% (1.65–2.57%) in ELBW infants (Clerihew et al. 2007). The vast majority of cases are of late onset (>72 hours after birth). Mortality rates range from 25% to 40%, which is higher than those for bacterial infection. Risk factors include birthweight <1500 g, TPN, presence of indwelling catheters, not receiving enteral feeds, mechanical ventilation, exposure to broad-spectrum antibiotics, especially third-generation cephalosporins, and exposure to antenatal antibiotics (Benjamin et al. 2010), H_2 receptor antagonists, abdominal surgery and peritoneal dialysis (Clerihew et al. 2007).

Signs and symptoms may be very non-specific and include: temperature instability; respiratory distress; lethargy, apnoeas with or without bradycardia; abdominal distension, bilious aspirates and blood in stools mimicking NEC, but without pneumatosis coli; and glucose intolerance.

Clinical presentation, investigation and management of neonatal sepsis

Clinical presentation and assessment of the infant

Early recognition, diagnosis and treatment of serious infection in the neonate are essential because of the risk of permanent morbidity or mortality. Progression from mild symptoms to death can occur in less than 24 hours. Clinical signs may be subtle in the early stages of bacteraemia, but this is when treatment must be started if there is to be intact survival. This leads to a tendency to overinvestigate and overtreat. Over 95% of infants screened and treated for early-onset infection had no evidence of infection in one study (Luck et al. 2003). However, the consequences of procrastination when infection is the cause of signs and symptoms can be fatal.

History

It is important to ask specific questions about maternal, perinatal and neonatal events. Apparently trivial episodes of pyrexia or skin rash may be significant, as well as contact with known cases of infectious disease; whether a mother was unwell or febrile; had a tender uterus or a vaginal discharge; the exact time of membrane rupture; potentially infectious lesions on her cervix or vulva; presence of a cervical suture; fetal tachycardia; raised maternal CRP or white cell count. The smaller and more preterm a baby, the higher the risk of infection and mortality (Heath et al. 2004).

If the mother has overt intrapartum infection, 15.2% of preterm babies and 4.1% of term babies will develop infection. Maternal UTI is an important risk factor for neonatal sepsis.

Factors predisposing to nosocomial infection include a history of possible contact with an infected person or environment, not receiving enteral feeds (Stoll et al. 2002a; Rønnestad et al. 2005), indwelling catheters or receiving TPN (Stoll et al. 2002a; Shinwell et al. 2004). Babies who have had gut surgery or gut-related problems also have a significant risk of nosocomial sepsis. Infection is more likely to occur in a baby in intensive care, and infection will prolong hospital stay and morbidity (Thompson et al. 1992; Stoll et al. 1996b; Fanaroff et al. 1998; Marshall et al. 1999).

Signs of neonatal sepsis

In the early stages, signs may be subtle and, although difficult to define, a mother or nurse may report that a baby is simply 'not right'. Isolated tachypnoea (respiratory rate sustained above 60 breaths/min and slight recession) and feeding difficulties (not feeding or poor suck) are the most frequent early signs of infection.

Temperature

After excluding the effect of pyrexia in the first 1–2 hours following birth in a baby of a pyrexial mother, which may be associated with epidural anaesthetic and an abnormal environmental temperature, temperature below 36°C or above 37.8°C, sustained for more than an hour, must be regarded as probably due to infection until proved otherwise. An unremitting fever is likely to be viral in origin.

Irritability

Infection may cause pain and may make the baby restless or whimper.

Skin

Petechiae may be present, or there may be septic spots, paronychia or omphalitis. Poor cutaneous circulation is indicated by mottling and delayed capillary filling (>3 seconds).

Jaundice

Unexplained jaundice may result from the effect of increased haemolysis.

Cardiovascular

Tachycardia of 160 beats/min may be a sign of sepsis and may be more marked in cases of myocarditis or endocarditis.

Gastrointestinal

The baby may vomit, have mild diarrhoea, or may develop an ileus with associated abdominal distension. The differential diagnosis includes NEC and structural malformations of the gastrointestinal tract.

Respiratory

Apnoea, cyanosis, grunting and dyspnoea are all signs of respiratory distress. Pneumonia is a possibility, but many other diagnoses are also possible, including generalised sepsis, meningitis and cardiac disease. Persistent moaning respiration is an ominous early sign.

For ventilated babies, an increase in ventilation requirements often accompanies generalised sepsis as well as pneumonia.

Central nervous system

A high-pitched cry, neck retraction, bulging fontanelle and convulsions are late features of neonatal meningitis.

Haemorrhagic diathesis

Disseminated intravascular coagulation (DIC) with petechiae and bleeding from puncture sites, the gut or the renal tract is a late sign of sepsis. Thrombocytopenia without evidence of DIC is a more common feature of infection and NEC.

Sclerema

This is often associated with Gram-negative infection but may be a non-specific feature of any serious neonatal illness (Box 39.1).

Box 39.1 Physical examination

It is important to examine the completely naked baby in a warm environment, as subtle signs will otherwise be missed. Inspect for the following:

- Tone – is the baby floppy?
- Irritability and responsiveness
- Signs of dehydration
- Colour and lesions of the skin, e.g. erythematous umbilicus or subcutaneous tissues, mottling (with cutis marmorata)
- Fontanelle tension, spinal column and skull for pits or other skin defects, which might be the entry site for meningeal infections
- Signs of respiratory distress, such as tachypnoea or grunting, recession, abnormal breath sounds
- Heart rate and pulses, and note pulse volume. Murmurs or a triple rhythm may suggest congenital cardiac disease or myocarditis or endocarditis
- Abdomen for distension, rigidity, masses and bowel sounds
- Hepatosplenomegaly, which may accompany generalised septicaemia as well as hepatitis
- Kidney enlargement
- Limbs for signs of osteomyelitis and septic arthritis

Investigation of neonatal sepsis

Any baby with a history and examination suggestive of infection should be promptly evaluated, investigated and treated if there is any suspicion that infection could be present. Although antibiotics are administered to a considerable number of non-infected infants (Luck et al. 2003), a bacteraemic baby with early features of sepsis may deteriorate rapidly if not treated. New diagnostic methods, including PCR, continue to be evaluated but none so far has been of sufficient worth to replace conventional blood culture and clinical acumen. A number of additional investigations may provide information to support or refute a diagnosis of sepsis.

Microbiological investigation

Blood culture remains the 'gold standard' for diagnosing infection, though it has limitations (Buttery 2002). The majority of significant blood cultures are positive by 48 hours (Kumar et al. 2001).

Collecting blood for culture

Blood for culture should be drawn from a freshly punctured blood vessel using strict aseptic technique and a closed system. The greater the volume of blood, the higher the yield of organisms, but 0.5 ml of blood is usually sufficient for a successful culture (Buttery 2002). Taking two cultures from separate sites reduces false-positive diagnoses of infection.

Antibiotic therapy should be stopped after 36–48 hours if cultures are negative and there are no further signs of infection. Alternatively, when there is a suspicion that clinical progress is suboptimal, consideration should always be given to an empiric change of antibiotic therapy to include a broader spectrum of pathogens. Such analyses should be validated in other data sets but have the potential to improve neonatal outcome by ensuring appropriate antibiotics are used as early as possible. Once a bacterium is identified, the antibiotic regimen should be targeted appropriately.

Surface swabs, tracheal secretions, endotracheal tube tip culture and gastric aspirates

Routine swabbing of sites such as the umbilicus, groin, ear, nose, throat, pharynx and rectum are informative about colonisation, but numerous studies have shown that the results of surface cultures are of limited value in diagnosis (Dobson et al. 1992; Puri et al. 1995). Colonisation of babies, for example of endotracheal secretions or of skin and mucosal surfaces, without clinical signs of infection does not warrant antibiotic treatment (Webber et al. 1990). The same applies to gastric aspirates and maternal vaginal swabs which are indicative of colonisation but not invasive infection. The latter may be helpful in a baby who is symptomatic of infection if positive for GBS.

Urine

A UTI is defined by there being a pure growth of at least 10^8 organisms per litre of urine (10^5/ml) in a specimen of urine. In order to avoid the problems of contamination of urine specimens, suprapubic aspiration of urine or fresh catheter urine specimens should be obtained in the initial assessment of the sick baby who is thought to be septicaemic, though this may be impracticable. A clean-catch sample may be helpful if the genitalia have been adequately cleaned. The only value of 'bag urines' is that if they are clear they exclude UTI. Positive bag urines, even when the genitalia have been adequately cleaned, should always be viewed with suspicion, even in the presence of white cells, as babies may have sterile pyuria.

Vascular lines and thoracocentesis tubes

The tips of umbilical cannulae, central lines and thoracocentesis tubes are usually sent for culture, though they have a limited role for diagnosing infection as they are indicative of colonisation, including of the skin through which they are withdrawn.

Lumbar puncture

A lumbar puncture should be performed as part of the sepsis screen in most ill babies before antibiotics are started. Exemptions include babies with acute RDS (Hendricks Munoz and Shapiro 1990), pulmonary infection complicating long-term intermittent positive-pressure ventilation (IPPV), babies with overt localised infection, such as NEC or pneumonia, and babies who would not be able to tolerate the procedure (Halliday 1989). A low platelet count is a contraindication to lumbar puncture; if the investigation is essential a platelet transfusion should be given first. Asymptomatic term babies undergoing investigation because of risk factors for sepsis do not require a lumbar puncture, nor is jaundice requiring treatment in a well baby an indication for lumbar puncture (Johnson et al. 1997; Hristeva et al. 2003). Meningitis is more frequently a feature of LOS than EOS (Schwersenski et al. 1991; Heath et al. 2003).

Lumbar puncture must be performed with strict sterile precautions, avoiding excessive flexion of the trunk, which may otherwise cause respiratory embarrassment or apnoea. It is safer to intubate and ventilate a very unstable baby before proceeding.

CSF analysis

High white blood cell counts in CSF have sometimes been reported in babies without meningitis, but a polymorphonuclear count higher than $20/mm^3$ should be regarded with suspicion (Ahmed et al. 1996), and counts above $30/mm^3$ are strongly indicative of meningitis (Appendix 8). For blood-stained CSF the ratio of red cells to white cells should be 500:1 in uninfected CSF.

The upper normal limit of CSF protein is 1.5–2.0 g/l in the term baby (Appendix 8). Preterm babies may have higher CSF protein concentrations but rarely greater than 3.0 g/l. Protein levels are usually raised in meningitis. CSF glucose levels should be compared to a simultaneous measurement of blood glucose, and should be at least 50% of the blood glucose level. A low level, less than 30% of the blood glucose, suggests bacterial meningitis.

The CSF should be Gram-stained, examined under a microscope, and cultured for bacteria. Other tests which may be indicated include PCR tests for GBS, herpesvirus and enteroviruses.

Radiology

All babies with suspected sepsis should have a CXR. An abdominal radiograph may also be helpful in the differentiation between septic ileus and NEC. Radiographs may not detect bone or joint infection in the early stages.

Haematological investigation

Total white cell count

This is the least useful index, because the normal range is so wide (Appendix 1), varies with gestation and postnatal age, can be confused by machines including nucleated red blood cells in the count, and can be 30–40% lower in blood obtained from a central catheter than in a capillary sample. Furthermore, the white blood cell count is raised in many non-infective conditions such as periventricular haemorrhage, convulsions and hypoxic–ischaemic encephalopathy (HIE).

Neutrophil count

Normal ranges for neonatal ANC are different from those of infants and children, and there are a variety of published ranges. The most widely used reference ranges for normal neonatal neutrophil counts are derived from those published by Manroe et al. (1979). These data are limited by the small numbers of babies of lower gestational age, with very few of 26 weeks' gestation or lower. Revised Manroe reference ranges have been published by Schelonka et al. (1994) and Mouzinho et al. (1994). Although both neutropenia and neutrophilia ($<5 \times 10^9$/l or $>20 \times 10^9$/l respectively) have useful predictive power (Metsvaht et al. 2009), in neither case is the specificity or sensitivity greater than about 80%.

The ANC in babies born small for gestational age are lower than those born at weights appropriate for gestational age and may take up to 2 weeks of age to normalise (McIntosh et al. 1988).

Similarly, infants born to mothers with pregnancy-induced hypertension (PIH) are more frequently neutropenic and may be at higher risk of infection (Brazy et al. 1982; Koenig and Christensen 1989; Cadnapaphornchai and Faix 1992). The mechanism for this is thought to be related to there being a circulating inhibitor of granulocyte (G)-CSF in mothers with PIH (Koenig and Christensen 1989, 1991) Such infants are also more likely to be thrombocytopenic (Brazy et al. 1982).

Immature circulating neutrophils, known as band forms, are seen in the peripheral blood in response to infection. In the most severely affected infants band cell production becomes limited as the marrow becomes exhausted. There is a high mortality rate in neonates who fail to mount a neutrophil response to infection (Gregory and Hey 1972; Rodwell et al. 1988, 1993).

The I/T ratio may be useful in diagnosing and monitoring infection (Metsvaht et al. 2009). The maximum normal value is 0.16 during the first 24 hours, 0.14 by 48 hours and 0.13 by 60 hours, where it remains until 5 days of age. Thereafter, the maximum

normal I/T ratio is 0.12 until the end of the first month. Several studies have found that an I/T ratio of ≥0.2 is a useful marker of infection (Metsvaht et al. 2009). Another feature suggesting infection is the presence of toxic granulation in the neutrophils. Manroe et al. (1979) found this in only 11% of normal infants, compared with 63% of infants with confirmed sepsis.

Lymphocyte count

Babies who have lymphocyte counts persistently below 2.8×10^9/l should be investigated for severe combined immunodeficiency (Hague et al. 1994).

Platelet count

In 50% of babies with bacterial infection, the platelet count will fall below 100×10^9/l.

Thrombocytopenia is a common feature of NEC and infection but may also be a feature of non-infective conditions such as HIE. Thrombocytopenia as well as neutropenia is a feature of IUGR and PIH (Brazy et al. 1982; Koenig and Christensen 1989, 1991; Cadnapaphornchai and Faix 1992). Viral infections, both congenital (e.g. rubella, cytomegalovirus (CMV) and herpes) and acquired (e.g. enterovirus, CMV, herpes), may cause a profound thrombocytopenia. Conversely, thrombocytosis can be a manifestation of chronic inflammation, particularly within the gut.

Abnormal liver function tests, jaundice or a bleeding tendency are further indications of viral infection, though they can also be features of bacterial infection.

Acute-phase proteins

C-reactive protein

CRP levels rise after inflammatory mediators such as IL-6 stimulate synthesis in the liver (Black et al. 2004). It is not uncommon for babies with positive blood cultures to have negligible CRP levels at birth but the CRP rises some 12 hours or more later. CRP may also rise in response to apparently non-infective inflammation such as with HIE (Inder and Volpe 2000; Shalak and Perlman 2002; Silveira and Procianoy 2003; Jacobsson and Hagberg 2004), which is consistent with data demonstrating elevation in IL-6 concentrations in babies with HIE (Silveira and Procianoy 2003).

Intrauterine infection and inflammation giving rise to a fetal inflammatory response, and resulting in elevated IL6 in fetal plasma (and thus elevation of CRP), have been related to white-matter injury and cerebral palsy (Inder and Volpe 2000; Jacobsson and Hagberg 2004). While there may be rises in CRP as a result of HIE, autopsy findings suggest congenital infection may mimic perinatal asphyxia, but are missed diagnostically, in the absence of placental histology and autopsy (Elder et al. 2005).

Severe hypoxic respiratory failure has been associated with raised blood concentrations of CRP, IL-6 and IL-8 and a greater incidence of histological chorioamnionitis and funisitis (Woldensbet et al. 2008), which suggests that inflammation, whether infective or non-infective, contributes to the severity of hypoxic respiratory failure.

Meconium-stained liquor is by no means specific for infection (Maymon et al. 1998), yet may be associated with inflammation and hence a CRP response. Some babies never mount a CRP response. This may be related to genetic polymorphisms in the immune response (Lorenz et al. 2002; Burgner and Levin 2003; Hedberg et al. 2004).

Serial measurements of CRP may be useful in monitoring the progress of infection or other inflammatory conditions such as NEC, and may help to guide treatment. Persistently elevated CRP during antibiotic therapy for presumed bacterial infection suggests ongoing infection or inflammation.

Serum procalcitonin

Procalcitonin is the prehormone of calcitonin, which is normally secreted by thyroid C cells, and rises within 3–6 hours of exposure to infection. Elevated serum concentrations of procalcitonin appear to be more sensitive and specific in the differentiation between neonatal infection and inflammation than CRP (Simon et al. 2004) and may also differentiate between bacterial and viral infection (Gendrel and Bohuon 2000). Procalcitonin measurements are undertaken by some laboratories as routine clinical tests.

Cytokines

TNF-α and IL-6

Elevations of plasma TNF-α and IL-6 concentrations in plasma may provide an early indication of sepsis, but levels may also be raised as a result of non-infective inflammation. Plasma IL-6 but not TNF-α has been shown to increase in term newborns with HIE, and both CSF (TNF-α) and CSF (IL-6) are significantly higher in babies with HIE compared with sepsis and controls (Silveira and Procianoy 2003). Because of difficulties in excluding any contributing infection without autopsy (Elder et al. 2005), the exact mechanism of rises in proinflammatory cytokines in non-infective inflammatory conditions is unclear. IL-6 may be a better marker of EOS than CRP; however, these cytokine assays have largely been used in research (Mehr and Doyle 2000) and have not been introduced into routine clinical practice.

IL-8 is also an early indicator of sepsis, being involved in neutrophil release from bone marrow, and neutrophil activation.

Serum granulocyte colony-stimulating factor

Neonates are able to produce endogenous, immunoreactive G-CSF which is measurable in the plasma, and levels are inversely related to ANCs, but the relationship is variable. As with many other measurable cytokines and growth factors, plasma G-CSF is variably raised at birth. Plasma G-CSF rises in response to infection and inflammation, but responses are no more sensitive or specific then CRP measurements, and thus should not be relied upon as a marker of infection or inflammation (Bedford Russell 2009).

Mannose-binding lectin

Mannose-binding lectin (MBL) is a protein of the innate immune system which activates complement after binding to repeating mannose units present on a number of different pathogens. Binding results in opsonisation and individuals with low MBL levels are associated with a decreased ability to opsonise bacteria and hence an increased susceptibility to infection. MBL2 gene polymorphisms are present on approximately one third of white people, and thus deficiency of MBL presents a potential risk factor for infection. In a recent review of MBL studies, newborns with low MBL levels had a greater risk of culture-positive sepsis then those with normal MBL levels, but the results for MBL2 genotype and infection were contradictory (Israels et al. 2010).

Immunological tests

Antigen detection tests

Rapid screening for GBS using latex particle agglutination is widely used, for detecting both maternal and neonatal colonisation (Green et al. 1993). The main value of the test may be in providing reassurance of the absence of GBS.

Box 39.2 Additional investigations if fungal infection is suspected or diagnosed

- End-organ evaluation to include (Benjamin et al. 2010):
  - Abdominal ultrasound (including renal ultrasound)
  - Cerebral ultrasound
  - Lumbar puncture
  - Fundoscopy
  - Echocardiogram
- Blood cultures at 24–48-hourly intervals to ensure clearance
- Suprapubic or catheter specimen of urine

Antibody detection tests

These are of more value in viral infections, when a fourfold or greater rise in antibody titre in samples drawn 2 weeks apart is diagnostic. If there is suspicion of congenital infection, organism-specific immunoglobulin M (IgM) should be sought.

Genetic techniques

It is now possible to amplify highly conserved DNA sequences from a variety of Gram-positive and Gram-negative organisms, as well as many viruses, using PCR, while avoiding the simultaneous amplification of associated human DNA. This method has the potential to be automated and to provide rapid diagnosis of bacteraemia.

In a meta-analysis of various intrapartum group B streptococcus colonisation tests, the most accurate was the real-time PCR test, although it took 10 minutes longer to perform PCR as compared to the Optical immunoassay (OIA) test (40 versus 30 minutes) (Honest et al. 2006) (Box 39.2).

Treatment of neonatal sepsis

Prompt treatment of neonatal infection with appropriate antibiotics can be life-saving; however, the availability of effective antibiotics may become limited by the development of resistant organisms.

Antibiotic therapy should be with narrow-spectrum antibiotics wherever possible and only used when significant infection is likely. Broad-spectrum antibiotics should be held in reserve (Webber et al. 1990). Colonisation of babies, for example of endotracheal secretions or of skin and mucosal surfaces, without clinical signs of infection does not warrant antibiotic treatment (Webber et al. 1990; Isaacs 2000).

There are no definitive randomised controlled trials of the best antibiotic regimens for the newborn. Each antibiotic has benefits and side-effects which should be evaluated every time antibiotics are prescribed. Best-practice recommendations based on currently available data are summarised in Table 39.7.

Antibiotic choices for early-onset infection

The empiric combination of benzylpenicillin with an aminoglycoside such as gentamicin provides excellent coverage for UK EOS pathogens while maintaining a relatively narrow spectrum. A cephalosporin-based combination does not provide significantly better coverage of likely bacteria yet is clearly associated with a broader spectrum and therefore is of greater potential harm (Bryan et al. 1985). Both combinations, however, neglect *Staphylococcus aureus*. Clinical correlates of *S. aureus* infection should be sought in future studies to enable empiric use of flucloxacillin where this pathogen is more likely. Additionally, when there is a suspicion that

Table 39.7 Summary of suggested antibiotic regimens

EARLY OR LATE INFECTION	CHOICE OF ANTIBIOTIC
Early	**First-line**
<48 hours–1 week	Benzylpenicillin with gentamicin Consider amoxicillin if *Listeria* suspected Consider flucloxacillin if *Staphylococcus aureus* suspected
Late	**First-line**
>48 hours–1 week	Flucloxacillin with gentamicin
	Second-line
	Vancomycin and gentamicin (with caution) Alternatives to gentamicin to extend Gram-negative cover: piperacillin/tazobactam (Tazocin)
	Third-line
	Meropenem, ciprofloxacin
Meningitis	Cefotaxime with amoxicillin or benzylpenicillin ± gentamicin
	Second-line
	Meropenem

clinical progress is suboptimal, consideration should always be given to an empiric change of antibiotic therapy to include a broader spectrum of pathogens. A recent MLR analysis revealed that EOS empiric treatment failure could be predicted at 24 hours using the following variables: need for vasoactive treatment (OR 2.83 (1.21–666)); white blood cell count <5000 or >20 000 per mm³ on day 1 (2.51 (1.09–5.81)); I/T ratio >0.2 on day 1 (2.79 (1.10–7.11)) and platelet count on day 1 (per 10 000 mm³ increase) 0.92 (0.86–0.98) (Metsvaht et al. 2009). Such analyses should be validated in other data sets but have the potential to improve neonatal outcome by ensuring appropriate antibiotics are used as early as possible.

Once a bacterium is identified, the antibiotic regimen should be targeted appropriately. In the case of suspected *Listeria monocytogenes*, for example, ampicillin or amoxicillin is usually given in place of benzylpenicillin.

Disadvantages of aminoglycosides

Although gentamicin is an excellent narrow-spectrum antibiotic to which most Gram-negative infections in the UK (the second commonest cause of early-onset infection) are sensitive (Vergnano et al. 2011), the disadvantage of using an aminoglycoside is the need to monitor levels and the dosing errors which may occur (National Patient Safety Agency 2010). There is also anxiety regarding gentamicin-induced ototoxicity and sensorineural hearing loss (SNHL). There are two mechanisms for gentamicin-associated toxicity: the result of sustained high trough gentamicin concentrations, and genetically determined ototoxicity. The link with high trough gentamicin levels is based on published case series from times when

extended-interval gentamicin dosing regimens were not in common use. As the bactericidal activity of gentamicin depends on the peak gentamicin concentration, and gentamicin continues to have a bactericidal effect even after this peak has been obtained (the so-called postantibiotic effect), extended interval dosing regimens have been developed. Such regimens result in high peak levels but safer trough concentrations (Rao et al. 2006). Gentamicin continues to be a significant source of medication errors (National Patient Safety Agency 2010), and the large number of recommendations on doses and monitoring that exist in the literature and in local guidelines may well explain this. There is an urgent need for a standardised approach to gentamicin dosing and monitoring.

The genetic link between gentamicin and SNHL is also of concern, following the finding that approximately 1:500 of the population carry the mitochondrial DNA mutation m.1555A→G. Carriers of this mutation have permanent and profound hearing loss after receiving aminoglycosides even when drug levels are within the therapeutic range (Bitner-Glindzicz et al. 2009; Vandebona et al. 2009). For this reason, elective genetic testing is increasingly being considered prior to gentamicin administration, although this has not been evaluated in routine practice, and would be very difficult to implement in neonatal practice, which requires short decision to administration times. Further studies are required to evaluate the risk of genetically determined SNHL with neonatal gentamicin use, the practicalities of screening for such mutations and the best alternative antibiotics when gentamicin is contraindicated. There may be a role for ciprofloxacin in this situation. An ongoing European study will provide much needed data in this area (TINN 2010).

Antibiotic choices for late-onset infection

CoNS are the most frequent bacteria isolated from blood cultures in the context of late-onset infections. Vancomycin and teicoplanin are the antibiotics of choice for CoNS infections but their excessive use has been associated with the development of vancomycin-resistant enterococcal infections and of Gram-negative infections (van Houten et al. 2001; Singh et al. 2002). Targeting empiric use of these agents only to those babies with the highest risk of complicated CoNS infections would greatly minimise their exposure in the neonatal unit. Their use as first-line antibiotics for nosocomial infection should be avoided (Kumar et al. 2001; Muller-Pebody et al. 2011; Vergnano et al. 2011).

The majority of the other leading causes of LOS can be appropriately treated by a relatively narrow combination such as flucloxacillin and gentamicin. This includes meticillin-sensitive *S. aureus*, the second most common cause of late-onset bacteraemia and an organism capable of causing overwhelming infection if not treated early (Isaacs et al. 2004). It also includes most of the Gram-negative bacteria, some of which, such as *Pseudomonas*, have a significant mortality. In contrast, while the overall coverage is similar to that of flucloxacillin and gentamicin, a cephalosporin alone or in combination with ampicillin may not adequately cover a number of the Enterobacteriaceae (Muller-Pebody et al. 2011; Vergnano et al. 2011). As with EOS, in situations where clinical improvement is not evident or deterioration is occurring, an empiric change from flucloxacillin to vancomycin or teicoplanin should be considered, together with another antibiotic with broader activity against Gram-negative bacteria: piperacillin/tazobactam (Tazocin) is one such example. The use of piperacillin/tazobactam rather than ceftazidime has been associated with a reduction in neonatal *Klebsiella* infections (Flidel-Rimon et al. 2004). A combination of vancomycin and gentamicin provides good Gram-negative and Gram-positive cover but potentially has additive toxicity; this combination should therefore be used with caution.

The bactericidal activity of vancomycin is related to its trough concentration. It is vital therefore that the concentration of vancomycin is maintained well above the minimal inhibitory concentration (MIC) of the organism (e.g. at least 3–4 times) at all times during treatment. This is the rationale for developing vancomycin dosing regimens whereby a continuous infusion of vancomycin is given. As many organisms including CoNS have become more resistant over time (Tenover et al. 2001), this level is now set at 10–15 µg/ml rather then 5–10 µg/ml. There is a need for more contemporary data on the vancomycin MICs of relevant pathogens as well as on the best dosing schedules (i.e. doses and intermittent versus continuous infusion), especially for very premature babies.

Stopping therapy

Antibiotic therapy should be stopped after 36–48 hours if cultures are negative and there are no further signs of infection. It is very unlikely that a culture that becomes positive after more than 48 hours in an asymptomatic baby is of clinical significance (Kumar et al. 2001). Furthermore a 3-day period of incubation is sufficient to detect all clinically relevant infections using the BacT/Alert microbial detection system (Kumar et al. 2001). Conversely, once a relevant isolate been obtained, treatment should be adapted appropriately to ensure that an effective antibiotic with the narrowest spectrum possible is being used (Isaacs 2000; van Houten et al. 2001; Fernando et al. 2008).

Monitoring response to therapy

Antibiotic therapy alone may not clear infection. If the baby remains unwell, or in the presence of other laboratory indicators, including persisting thrombocytopenia and/or neutropenia, raised CRP, procalcitonin or plasma lactate, and always if there is persistence of positive blood cultures, further sets of blood cultures should be taken. As discussed earlier, more work is needed on timely clinical markers that indicate an inadequate response to treatment. Reasons for persistent positive blood cultures include: inadequate antibiotic levels or regimens; resistant organisms, colonisation of indwelling 'foreign bodies', for example long line, umbilical arterial or venous lines; focal infection, for example necrosis of the gut, especially during 'conservative' management of NEC, abscess formation, osteomyelitis or endocarditis. Evaluation by paediatric surgeons, paediatric orthopaedic surgeons and cardiologists, as appropriate, should be sought for such cases.

Apart from repeating blood cultures, further investigations for consideration should include lumbar puncture and suprapubic urine aspirate, checking antibiotic levels, ultrasound of potential foci of infection, skeletal radiographs and echocardiogram. Consideration should also be given to therapeutic options such as optimising antibiotic doses, changing antibiotic regimens or removing indwelling catheters.

Length of treatment

This will depend on a number of variables such as the type of organism, antibiotic levels that have been achieved, the presence of indwelling catheters and clinical response. There is little published evidence to suggest the optimal length of a course of antibiotics for culture-proven infection in neonates (Cotten 2009). Prolonged duration of initial empirical antibiotic treatment (defined as >5 days) is associated with increased rates of NEC and death in ELBW infants, with each empirical treatment day being associated with

increased OR for these outcomes (Cotten et al. 2009). Although there are methodological limitations to this study, the findings are consistent with the recommendation that, while antibiotic therapy should be commenced promptly for suspected infection, treatment should be stopped as soon as sepsis has been excluded.

As a general rule, if antibiotics are started because of the possibility of infection, but there is no subsequent clinical evidence of infection, and cultures are all negative at 36–48 hours, antibiotics should be stopped (Kumar et al. 2001; Cotten et al. 2009). This should be the norm and depends on having robust communication systems with the microbiology department. If antibiotics are started on suspicion of infection, but cultures are negative (perhaps as a result of prior antibiotics), yet the clinical impression at the start of treatment was that sepsis was likely, then a longer course may be warranted – usually 5 days. It is in this category of patients that most uncertainty lies, and where non-culture methods of pathogen detection, as well as reliable markers of host inflammation, offer most potential benefit. Likewise, if there is pneumonia on a CXR, but blood cultures are negative, a 5-day course may be appropriate. If there are positive blood cultures but negative CSF cultures, treatment should be for a minimum of 10 days. Treatment should be for at least 14 days for *S. aureus*, because of its propensity to seed other tissues, but this decision should be taken in partnership with microbiology or infectious diseases colleagues, if possible. For a baby with positive CSF cultures or a clinical diagnosis of meningitis, treatment may be required for at least 21 days, depending on the infecting organism (Heath et al. 2003).

Osteomyelitis, endocarditis and deep abscesses which are not surgically drained may require several weeks of antibiotic therapy. The length of treatment course may require extension in those with slow clinical and microbiological resolution, and requires specialist input.

Potential hazards of antibiotics

Antibiotics are increasingly prescribed in the peripartum period, for both maternal and fetal indications. Their effective use undoubtedly reduces the incidence of specific invasive infections in the newborn, such as GBS infection, but a number of potential adverse consequences must also be recognised.

One concern has recently been highlighted by the findings from the 7-year follow-up of the ORACLE trial. In this study women with spontaneous preterm labour with intact membranes and no overt infection were randomised to receive either erythromycin or co-amoxiclav, or both, or neither in a factorial design. The study found increased numbers of children with any functional impairment, OR 1.18 (95% confidence interval (CI) 1.02–1.37) with the prescription of erythromycin (either with or without co-amoxiclav) and an increased risk of cerebral palsy with the prescription of either or any erythromycin, OR 1.93 (95% CI 1.21–3.09), or any co-amoxiclav, OR 1.69 (95% CI 1.07–2.67) (Kenyon et al. 2008). These results demonstrate that the widespread use of antibiotics in late pregnancy may be associated with unexpected long-term consequences in the baby, and confirms that antibiotic use is not risk-free (Bedford Russell and Steer 2008).

All antibiotics, particularly broad-spectrum antibiotics, alter the natural microflora of the patient, particularly in the gastrointestinal tract. This may result in an increase in antibiotic resistance among normal commensal organisms or the emergence of other pathogens. One pathogen may simply be replaced by another pathogen, which itself may be more hazardous, and the total burden of neonatal infection may be unchanged (Stoll et al. 2002b). Widespread use of broad-spectrum antibiotics within a maternity unit will also increase local persistence of resistant organisms, and favour opportunistic transmission within the unit (van Houten et al. 2001; Singh et al. 2002). Such organisms can then persist within hospitals and even in the community (Millar et al. 2008).

A further possible hazard of peripartum antibiotics relates to the potential link with immune dysregulation in later childhood. The developed world has witnessed a substantial increase in the incidence of allergic and autoimmune disease in young children over the past three decades. The suggestion is that immune development becomes abnormal because the naïve immune system is exposed to abnormal bacterial challenge, as a result of obstetric practices and inappropriate antibiotic use (Bedford Russell and Murch 2006).

Longitudinal studies are needed to investigate the potential link between peripartum antibiotic use and immunological health problems in later life. In the meantime all those involved with caring for the newborn should be aware of these issues; many parents already are, particularly if they already have children with allergies.

Suggested action plan

The future for development of new antibiotics is extremely limited. There are very few new antibiotics under development with activity against Gram-negative bacteria. Evidence from around the world demonstrates that neonatal units are a high-risk area for the selection and transmission of multiresistant organisms. The risk is that recurrent outbreaks of multiresistant organisms become very difficult to treat and could cause significant disruption to movement of babies between hospitals in neonatal networks (with serious potential clinical and financial consequences). The balance is switching towards recognition of the need to conserve antibiotics as a finite resource (So et al. 2010). Conservation of antibiotics in hospitals can be performed using some form of Antibiotic Stewardship Program (Lesprit and Brun-Buisson 2008; Sharland 2007). The implementation of such a programme has been shown to reduce vancomycin utilisation and vancomycin-prescribing errors with concomitant improvements in quality of care and safety of hospitalised children (Di Pentima and Chan 2010). The optimal programme for neonatal units still needs to be developed, but first steps that can be taken now include:

1. Establish systematic regular infection surveillance of bloodstream infections, either at a local level, for example by performing an annual audit in collaboration with the local microbiology department, and/or through a network such as NeoNIN (neonin@sgul.ac.uk).
2. Strengthen links between local microbiology and infection control teams and local pharmacists. Have regular (e.g. weekly) reviews of infections and antibiotic use. This could be formalised into a weekly neonatal 'infection round', though the evidence base for this has yet to be established.
3. Use a narrow-spectrum empiric antibiotic policy and audit compliance with this.
4. Reinforce to all staff that the routine policy is for empiric antibiotics to be stopped when blood cultures are negative and audit compliance with this.
5. Ensure that continuation of antibiotics after negative blood cultures requires a new prescription to be written.
6. Ensure that the duration of antibiotics to treat an infection episode (whether culture-positive or -negative) is prespecified and only prolonged with the writing of a new prescription.
7. Ensure that the narrowest-spectrum antibiotics possible are used for treatment of proven infections and audit this.
8. Identify a panel of consultant decision-only antibiotics, such as third-generation cephalosporins, vancomycin and

meropenem. Audit compliance with this and review individual cases where such antibiotics were prescribed.

Putting these measures in place now, while we develop the evidence base for optimal antibiotic prescribing, is the best way of ensuring that neonatal networks can be maintained in the future and that neonatal infections remain treatable.

Treatment of fungal infection

Liposomal amphotericin, which is a fungicidal agent, is the first-choice treatment, as side-effects with non-liposomal amphotericin can be avoided and doses maximised. A low dose is usually commenced (e.g. 1–2 mg/kg) and the dose is increased as tolerated to a maximum of 6 mg/kg. Higher doses can be used but require close monitoring and collaboration with infectious disease or microbiology specialists. Fluconazole, which is a fungistatic agent, may be used if the *Candida* species is fluconazole-sensitive, the baby is well, and all anti-inflammatory markers have settled. This is well absorbed orally so can be given in order to complete a long course of antifungal treatment, especially when intravenous access is compromised. Any indwelling catheters should be removed (Karlowicz et al. 2000). A fungal infection will not clear unless 'foreign bodies' are removed, unlike infection with CoNS, which can respond to antibiotic treatment in the presence of indwelling catheters in some instances.

Fungal prophylaxis

The Infectious Diseases Society of America has suggested that *Candida* prophylaxis should be considered at high incidence for infection centres (Pappas et al. 2009). However, widespread use of antifungal therapy may lead to antifungal resistance which presents an even greater public health threat. In the UK (as opposed to the USA), the incidence of fungal infection does not justify routine use of prophylactic fluconazole even in babies of birthweight <1000 g (Clerihew et al. 2007), although in certain high-risk babies prophylaxis may be appropriate as detailed below. The situation is different in the USA where the incidence of *Candida* infection is much higher than in the UK (Clerihew et al. 2006). Oral nystatin prophylaxis has been associated with a significantly reduced incidence of fungal invasive disease, compared to no prophylaxis (Howell et al. 2009). Prophylaxis with either nystatin or fluconazole may be considered in individual babies at high risk of sepsis, e.g. those preterm babies <1500 g who have not received enteral nutrition, who have had gut surgery or received broad-spectrum antibiotics for an extended period of time. Although no study has yet reported increasing resistance to fluconazole as a result of prophylaxis, routine prophylaxis risks selecting for resistant species, and should therefore be used with caution (Benjamin et al. 2010). Wide variations in the incidence of *Candida* infection between units suggests that components of clinical care may be modified in order to reduce the risk of *Candida* infection. Such factors include avoiding the use of broad-spectrum antibiotics, especially cephalosporins, reducing use of central catheters and TPN and modifying antenatal antibiotic exposure (Benjamin et al. 2010). These factors are likely to be more critical than antifungal prophylaxis in preventing *Candida* infection.

Treatment of 'very sick septic neonates'

In addition to prompt antibiotic therapy, babies with infection may require intensive care support, including ventilation, which should be considered early. Inotropes may be needed to support circulation, in addition to blood products. Sepsis is often associated with renal impairment so urine output should be monitored routinely and urine tested for blood and protein in addition to monitoring the serum urea, electrolytes and creatinine. The gut will almost certainly stop working in sepsis, therefore enteral feeding may need to be stopped; indeed, sepsis may present with a paralytic ileus, clinically indistinguishable from NEC. Liver dysfunction is common in sepsis with raised aspartate transaminase and conjugated hyperbilirubinaemia, particularly if a baby is receiving TPN. The coagulation profile should be checked and additional doses of vitamin K should be considered if coagulation is found to be abnormal. Glucose instability is a well-recognised sign of neonatal sepsis, so that institution of insulin therapy should always be accompanied by investigation of why it is necessary. Metabolic acidosis may also require active management, including investigation of plasma lactate and chloride values, to assist diagnosis.

Additional (adjuvant) treatments for infection

Antibiotic therapy alone may be insufficient to treat infection in an immune-compromised host, and long-term or recurrent use of antibiotics facilitates antibiotic resistance, as described above (Levy 1998; Van Houten et al. 2001; Singh et al. 2002), as well as having potential longer-term consequences on immunological health in childhood (Bedford Russell and Murch 2006). Efforts have therefore been directed at ways of enhancing neonatal host defence mechanisms. Such therapies have included immunoglobulins, haemopoietic growth factors (rhG-CSF and rhGM-CSF), pre- and probiotics and pentoxifilline. Because of inadequate sample sizes of randomised controlled trials, few immunological interventions to treat or prevent neonatal sepsis have been reliably evaluated. In the future, international collaboration will be essential in achieving timely, adequate samples reliably to assess effects on mortality or morbidity. Promising or possible therapeutic interventions in severe or Gram-negative sepsis include exchange transfusions, pentoxifylline and IgM-enriched intravenous immunoglobulin (IVIG). Promising or possible prophylactic interventions include lactoferrin, with or without a probiotic; selenium; early curtailment of antibiotics after sterile cultures; breast milk; and earlier initiation of colostrum in high-risk preterm infants (Tarnow-Mordi et al. 2010a). Prophylactic oral probiotics are discussed further below.

Intravenous immunoglobulin therapy

There have been many studies investigating the potential benefits of giving immunoglobulins to babies prophylactically, as well as at the time of infection. So far no study has demonstrated conclusively that pooled IVIG is of any benefit in the prophylaxis or treatment of neonatal sepsis, though there is a suggestion of benefit from using immunoglobulins in the treatment of infection (Ohlsson and Lacy 2006). For this reason, the International Neonatal Immunotherapy Study (2008) investigated the potential benefit of giving pooled IVIG to neonates with infection, and concluded that IVIG have neither short-term nor long-term benefits in the adjuvant treatment of neonatal sepsis.

One factor that may have contributed to lack of efficacy in prophylaxis studies was the enrolment of many higher-birthweight infants who had a low risk of developing sepsis. Another factor may have been the variability of CoNS-specific activity of pooled IVIG, with opsonic activity being low for such isolates (Fanaroff et al. 1994; Fischer et al. 1994; Weisman et al. 1996). Despite the use of

thousands of donors for each lot of standard immune globulin G, substantial batch-to-batch variation has been noted in the antibody profile (Fanaroff et al. 1994; Weisman and Cruess 1994; Weisman et al. 1996). Based on this experience, it is unlikely that any preventive strategy for neonatal sepsis will demonstrate efficacy unless it is studied in the population at highest risk, i.e. those infants weighing less than 1500 g at birth, and with an immunoglobulin preparation that has known antistaphylococcal activity.

In a study of an intravenous immune globulin derived from donors with high titres of antibody to surface adhesins of *Staphylococcus epidermidis* and *S. aureus* (INH-A21), immunoglobulin infusion was well tolerated but there was no reduction in the incidence of these infections (De Jonge et al. 2007).

An antistaphylococcus-specific chimeric monoclonal antibody (BSYX-A110, also known as pagibaximab) has been developed by recombinant DNA technology (Weisman et al. 2009) for the prevention of staphylococcal infections in VLBW babies. This antibody is directed against lipoteichoic acid, which is a highly conserved cell wall macromolecule in all strains of staphylococci; it is necessary for staphylococcal survival and important for cell division (Ginsberg 2002). Lipoteichoic acid inhibits phagocytosis of bacteria and induces proinflammatory cytokine expression, resulting in sepsis syndrome with concomitant multiorgan failure (Ginsberg 2002). Pagibaximab inhibits these actions, thus promoting bacterial phagocytosis and downmodulating proinflammatory cytokine expression. In clinical studies to date, pagibaximab has been well tolerated by VLBW infants with no evidence of immunological reaction to the antibody (Weisman et al. 2009). Studies are currently under way to investigate the potential efficacy of pagibaximab in the prevention of staphylococcal sepsis in VLBW infants.

Potential therapeutic use of recombinant human G-CSF and GM-CSF (rhG-CSF and rhGM-CSF) in neonates

Neonatal sepsis may result in depletion of the bone marrow-proliferative pool, resulting in neutropenia, often with fatal consequences (Christensen and Rothstein 1980). In some infants neutropenia is a particularly frequent finding, for example babies born to mothers with PIH, exposing them to an increased risk of sepsis (Koenig and Christensen 1989, 1991).

Treatment of neonates, as well as adults, with rhG-CSF is known to produce a measurable rise in ANC, with a peak response between 12 hours and 10 days (de Haas et al. 1994; Gillan et al. 1994; Kocherlakota and La Gamma 1997, 1998), depending upon duration of treatment. No single study has demonstrated an improved clinical outcome for neonates treated with rhG-CSF, but few have concentrated on recruiting those neonates at highest risk of sepsis and its complications, namely the smallest and most immature, and those with any degree of neutropenia.

In case-control studies rhG-CSF has been shown to have a potential benefit for babies with NEC (Kocherlakota and La Gamma 1997). This has been related to the potential for rhG-CSF to downregulate inflammation (Hartung et al. 1995; Gorgen et al. 1999), yet improve the quantitative and qualitative neutrophil response.

RhG-CSF therapy may have a role in neonates who are both neutropenic and septic, especially those of lower birthweights, <2 kg (Bedford Russell et al. 2000; Bernstein et al. 2001). The authors of the Cochrane review of rhG-CSF and rhGM-CSF for treating or preventing neonatal infections concluded that there is no evidence to support the introduction of either rhG-CSF or rhGM-CSF for the treatment or prophylaxis of infection (Carr et al. 2006). This may be overstating the lack of evidence for the use of rhG-CSF from large randomised controlled studies in babies who have both sepsis and/or NEC, and who are neutropenic.

There are no published studies of the prophylactic administration of rhG-CSF in human neonates, although animal models suggest that both rhG-CSF and rhGM-CSF are more effective when administered before bacterial inoculation (Cairo et al. 1992). In the PRO-GRAMS trial, Carr et al. (2009) assessed whether or not rhGM-CSF administered as prophylaxis to small-for-gestational-age, preterm neonates who are at high risk of neutropenia would reduce sepsis, mortality and morbidity. The PROGRAMS trial demonstrated that, while early postnatal rhGM-CSF corrects neutropenia, sepsis rates, survival and short-term outcomes are not improved (Carr et al. 2009). This trial illustrates the great importance of studies which are large enough to be sufficiently powered to yield statistically meaningful results: having observed a potential benefit for prophylactic rhGM-CSF in a small pilot study (Carr et al. 1999), there was no benefit in a large randomised controlled study (Carr et al. 2009).

Following chronic administration of rhG-CSF to patients with congenital neutropenia a malignant myeloid disorder develops in approximately 10–20% (Dale et al. 2003, 2006; Kaushansky 2006; Rosenberg et al. 2006).

RhG-CSF therapy is unlikely to benefit more than a few infants, as there are relatively few who become both septic and neutropenic. Immune host defence requires a complex interaction and partnership, between innate and immune systems, and simply altering one element may be insufficient to make a difference to the other elements.

A risk:benefit evaluation has to be applied to each individual's case, in the evaluation of whether or not rhG-CSF could benefit outcome. While there may be a benefit in a small population of neutropenic, septic babies, the long-term risk of malignant transformation, though small in this population, remains a matter of debate, and must be considered in any evaluation.

Evidence to date does not support the routine use of rhG-CSF or rhGM-CSF for either prophylaxis or treatment of newborn sepsis, but use in preterm, neutropenic and septic babies <1500 g may be of benefit and should be considered in extreme situations after consultation with parents.

Granulocyte infusions

Granulocyte infusions have been used successfully in small studies of neutropenic and non-neutropenic sepsis (Cairo et al. 1992). No adverse side-effects had been reported but human leukocyte antigen and blood group sensitisation (Bedford Russell et al. 1993), viral and prion transmission and graft-versus-host disease remain theoretical risks. The practicalities of preparing fresh neutrophil concentrates and the resources required to do so have further limited use. As leucophoresis has become a much easier procedure, there has been speculation that the time is perhaps right for further large randomised trials of granulocyte transfusions in neonatal sepsis (Shan 2009).

Prebiotics and probiotics

More recently, and in recognition of the importance of the gut flora in immune development, there have been trials of prebiotics and probiotics in neonates. These are often termed 'good bacteria' and include lactobacilli and bifidobacteria found in breast milk. A probiotic is defined as 'a live microbial food supplement that beneficially affects the host by alteration of its intestinal microbial balance'. A prebiotic is defined as 'a non-digestible food ingredient that beneficially affects the host by stimulating the growth or activity of one or more bacterial species already present in the gut'. The benefits of these are thought to derive from normalising gut flora. Animal studies support the probability that probiotics act by normalising gut flora, and thereby upregulate mucosal barrier proteins and nutritional functions, as well as stimulate development of normal immune responses, but the responses are probiotic-specific (Hooper et al. 2001; Murch 2011; Hooper 2004).

Different probiotics have different actions, as already described, and have been shown to reduce the development of allergy duration of diarrhoea in older children. Although some milk-marketing companies now supply infant milks and breast milk fortifiers with added prebiotics or probiotics, these additives have not been subjected to rigorous scientific evaluation and the benefits are unclear (Schanler 2006). A systematic review of probiotics for prevention of NEC in VLBW preterm infants suggested that probiotics may reduce NEC risk (Deshpande et al. 2007). Risk of sepsis was not reduced by probiotics in this systematic review, although in a single-centre study of a combination of two species, given with breast milk only in both control and treatment groups, *Lactobacillus acidophilus* and *Bifidobacterium infantis*, sepsis rates were reduced (Lin et al. 2005). Probiotics appear to be safe and effective in reducing all-cause mortality and NEC in preterm infants by over half, but overall do not reduce sepsis (Tarnow-Mordi et al. 2010b). Optimal probiotic regimens and doses remain under investigation in ongoing studies in Australia and the UK. The ideal choice of probiotic is unclear. In the meantime, probiotics should not be used routinely until the results of these further studies can better inform practice.

Prevention of infection – infection control

Every baby should always be cared for with the strictest attention to protecting him or her from cross-infection. Staff and visitors should remove coats and leave bags outside the nurseries. Arms should be naked from elbows down and freshly cleaned, either with alcohol or soap and water, before touching any baby or equipment for that baby. Bacteria live on all jewellery, particularly stones, so these should not be worn at work. Hair and clothing should not be allowed to dangle on to a baby, and theatre scrubs should not be worn outside the unit or theatre. Gloves should be worn for any procedures involving bodily secretions, and discarded as soon as the procedure is completed. Hands should have alcohol applied or should be rewashed on exiting and entering a nursery from a different area, such as the nurse's station or staff room. A baby should have his or her own stethoscope, scissors, laryngoscope and any other small items of equipment. Nothing should be shared. Where equipment has to be shared, such as ultrasound machine heads and cold lights, these must always be carefully cleaned between babies.

Cohorting of babies may be necessary when a baby has a particularly resistant bacteria, such as MRSA, or an easily transmissible infection, such as respiratory syncytial virus (RSV). Organisms are readily transferred on objects around a baby as well as between babies themselves. Strict attention to infection control can be achieved by placing tape on the floor around a cot to create virtual 'baby space'. No one should be allowed across the tape to gain access to any part of the baby and baby's equipment, including to observe baby or drug charts, or to adjust monitor or ventilator buttons, unless they wash their hands, put on gloves (and gowns if touching the baby) and 'decontaminate' themselves afterwards. Each baby cot should have separate pens as well as stethoscopes, scissors and other such equipment. The notes should stay outside the baby domain and not be touched by any individual on the inside of the 'baby space'. This may seem obsessive, but it is only with such attention to detail that cross-infection can be averted.

Neonates who have been home are often not allowed to be readmitted to a neonatal unit because of 'infection control'. This is a somewhat illogical policy: babies are more likely to acquire abnormal bacteria as inpatients. RSV infection may have been acquired in the community, particularly during the winter months, and admission to the neonatal unit would be a contraindication if suspected. With proper attention to infection control and use of cohorting until the results of screening cultures are known, babies can be readmitted to a neonatal unit if that is the most appropriate place for their needs to be met.

Within neonatal units, high cot occupancy rates and high numbers of babies cared for by one nurse contribute to a greater mortality (Tucker and UK Neonatal Staffing Study 2002). The effect of overcrowding on positive blood culture rates is less easy to discern, because bigger and busier units are likely to look after sicker babies and take more blood cultures, but the perceived wisdom is that overcrowding and high-volume workload lead to greater risk of infection. Nosocomial bacteraemia rates are high in NICUs with high consultant provision and the suggestion is that increased use of invasive procedures, poor compliance with hand-washing by doctors and reduced compliance with all infection control measures within busy intensive care settings are associated with a higher risk of true nosocomial infection.

Care bundles in the reduction of nosocomial infection

Variations in nosocomial infection rates between neonatal units have been observed by the Canadian NICU network, National Nosocomial Infection Surveillance System and the Vermont Oxford Network, suggesting that the site of care influences acquired infection rates (Lee et al. 2000; Bloom et al. 2003; Benjamin et al. 2010). 'Best demonstrated process' has been developed as a method for quality improvements in reducing nosocomial infection with neonatal units (Bloom et al. 2003), but does require collaboration (Horbar et al. 2001). How interventions are implemented is as important as what changes in practices are chosen. Such best practices which have been individually proven to reduce infection risk have been grouped together as 'care bundles', in anticipation of better outcomes than if the practices were implemented individually (Marwick and Davey 2009). The implementation of care bundles within neonatal units has been gaining momentum (Lachman 2009). Significant improvements in practice development can be facilitated by the implementation of random safety audits (Lee et al. 2009).

Focal bacterial infections in the newborn

Meningitis

The incidence of bacterial meningitis in the newborn ranges from 0.21/1000 (Heath et al. 2003) to 1/1000 livebirths. The current prevalence in England and Wales has remained stable since 1985, and is reported as 0.39 cases per 1000 births, of which 0.21 cases were bacterial in origin (De Louvois et al. 1991; Holt et al. 2001). In the developing world it is more like 2 per 1000 (Airede 1993). Meningitis formerly complicated 10% of cases of LOS, but the incidence is probably lower now (Isaacs et al. 1996). The risk

increases with decreasing gestational age, and, as a group, preterm infants carry two or three times the risk of term infants, and account for an even greater majority of the late-onset cases.

Organisms

The most common pathogens causing neonatal bacterial meningitis are GBS and *E. coli*. In a Canadian study, GBS were responsible for 50% of cases, 25% of *E. coli*, 8% of other Gram-negative rods and *Listeria monocytogenes* for 6% of cases, with 3% being non-typable *Haemophilus influenzae* (Doctor et al. 2001).

In a comparison of two studies of neonatal meningitis conducted in England and Wales between 1985–87 and 1996–97, it is apparent that the bacteria responsible for meningitis changed very little up until 1997.

Other studies have noted an increase in disease caused by *Enterobacter* spp. and *Serratia marcescens*: the majority of these Gram-negative organisms were isolated from premature infants with late-onset meningitis (Campbell et al. 1992; Hervas et al. 2001). Gram-negative enteric organisms appear to account for the majority of early-onset meningitis and *Streptococcus pneumoniae* for late-onset meningitis in developing countries.

Clinical features

Early signs of neonatal meningitis may be minimal and are often non-specific and unreliable (Wiswell et al. 1995, Visser and Hall 1980), hence the recommendation to perform a lumbar puncture in the evaluation of all neonates with suspected or proven sepsis or meningitis (Heath et al. 2003). This is not the case for asymptomatic babies at risk of early-onset infection because of maternal risk factors, where the yield of positive lumbar puncture has been shown to be low (Schwersenski et al. 1991). Advanced signs include a bulging fontanelle, a high-pitched cry, altered consciousness or seizures.

During clinical examination, the head circumference should be measured and the skull and axial skeleton scrutinised for skin defects or pits that might have provided a portal of entry for infection.

Pathology

Inflammation, oedema and arachnoiditis are widespread in most cases of neonatal meningitis, as are vasculitis and superficial cortical thrombophlebitis, which cause superficial ischaemic damage to the brain. Ventriculitis occurs in 70–90% of cases of neonatal meningitis, but is less common with GBS than with Gram-negative organisms. Severe encephalopathic changes often occur, probably as a result of direct penetration of the infection into the brain, and may result in widespread cerebral atrophy. The choroid plexus may be damaged, permanently compromising CSF production, and exudate may obstruct intraventricular foramina and arachnoid granulations, leading to hydrocephalus in around one-third of cases.

Abscess formation is commonly seen with meningitis caused by *Citrobacter* and *Proteus* species, and occasionally with other coliforms. Abscess formation begins with a suppurative ventriculitis and progresses to periventricular abscess formation.

Investigation

CSF analysis

The criteria for diagnosing meningitis are given in Appendix 8. In most cases, bacteria can be identified when the CSF is stained by the Gram staining; if no bacteria are seen, the possibility of a viral pathogen such as HSV should be considered. If the CSF cytology suggests meningitis but no organisms are seen, treatment with aciclovir should be started pending the results of further tests. Occasionally, in the early stages of fulminating infection, organisms may be seen without a significant pleocytosis. Lumbar puncture may safely be deferred if the baby is too ill to tolerate handling.

The need for repeat lumbar punctures is debatable but is definitely worth considering in babies who have not responded to treatment after 48 hours of therapy. Failure of the lumbar CSF to improve is an indication for further investigation by ultrasound or magnetic resonance imaging (MRI) scan. A lumbar puncture following cessation of treatment in a clinically well baby is unnecessary (Heath et al. 2003). In a baby with ventriculomegaly and symptoms suggestive of meningitis, a ventricular tap may be warranted for the investigation of meningitis.

Blood culture

Blood culture is commonly positive, but may be negative in 15% of cases (Visser and Hall 1980; Wiswell et al. 1995).

Neuroimaging

Cerebral ultrasonography should be performed for complications including evidence of ventriculitis or any structural changes as a result of meningitis. Ultrasound should be performed early to establish a baseline and after 7–10 days at minimum. The presence of parenchymal changes or ventriculomegaly places babies in a group at high risk of sequelae. MRI may give greater definition of meningitis-induced cerebral damage.

If there are abnormal movements an electroencephalogram should be performed, and continuous EEG monitoring in the acute phase is worth considering if available – the background EEG can give useful information about prognosis (see below) and subclinical seizures may be identified.

Head circumference should be measured routinely and may be helpful in monitoring the increasing cranial volume that occurs with cerebral oedema, hydrocephalus or subdural effusion (although the latter is rare in neonatal meningitis).

Treatment

Appropriate empirical regimens are summarised in Table 39.7.

Initial antibiotic choice is empirical, based on age of onset, most likely pathogens (GBS and *Escherichia coli*), and likely antibiotic sensitivities and the most common choice would be as in Table 39.7. In an individual neonatal unit, empirical therapy should consider unit pathogens and susceptibility if known, for example if there is a known outbreak of *Serratia*, meropenem should be considered as empirical therapy. If the initial Gram stain is negative or heavily blood-stained but meningitis is a distinct possibility, herpes simplex is a rare but devastating cause of meningoencephalitis so aciclovir should be commenced promptly. While aminoglycosides have relatively good CSF penetration, the CSF concentration achieved may only be minimally above the minimal bactericidal concentration for Gram-negative organisms. Aminoglycoside toxicity limits using high doses to achieve satisfactory concentrations. Although CSF penetration by third-generation cephalosporins may only be modest, the CSF concentrations achieved are much higher than the minimal bactericidal concentrations of the organisms and not limited by toxicity (Lutsar et al. 1998). Cefotaxime is therefore suggested as the choice for suspected Gram-negative meningitis in combination with an aminoglycoside until sensitivities are known. Once-daily ceftriaxone may also be used but there is less experience

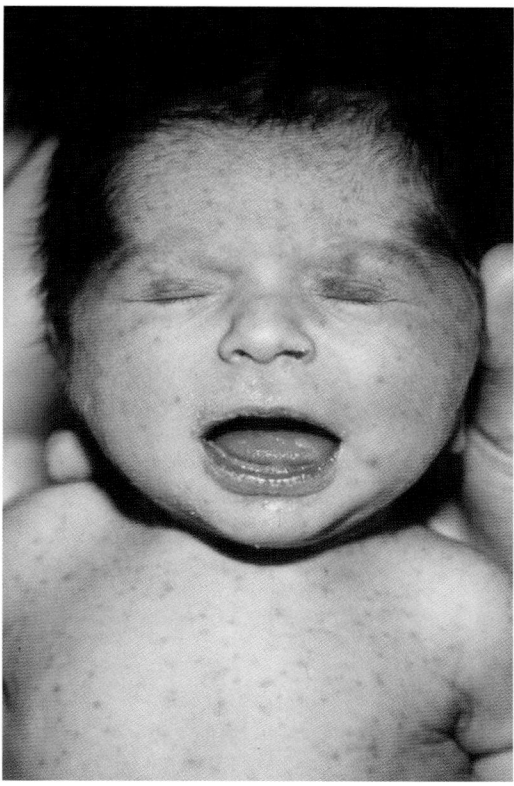

Fig. 39.8 Baby with typical rash due to *Listeria* infection.

with this antibiotic in neonates, it displaces bilirubin from binding to plasma proteins and has been reported to be associated with cholestasis and gallbladder hydrops. Benzylpenicillin is the choice for confirmed GBS meningitis in doses of up to 270 mg/kg/day divided 8-hourly if <7 days of age and 6-hourly if >7 days (Heath et al. 2003).

Listeria meningitis is best treated with amoxicillin. *Streptococcus pneumoniae* is usually susceptible to benzylpenicillin but as resistance does occur it is recommended to commence empirical therapy with a penicillin in combination with a cephalosporin. CoNS meningitis is rare but may complicate bacteraemia in a VLBW baby, in the presence of a ventriculoperitoneal shunt or following ventricular tap (Fig. 39.8).

There is no established place for dexamethasone in the adjuvant treatment of neonatal meningitis (Daoud et al. 1999), and so far no other therapies, including immunoglobulins, growth factors and pentoxyfilline, have demonstrated benefit.

Duration of therapy

There are no randomised controlled trials to inform clinicians about optimal duration of treatment. The perceived wisdom is that antibiotic therapy should be continued for 2–3 weeks following sterilisation of CSF with adequate antibiotic concentrations. This equates to a minimum of 2–3 weeks for GBS and *Listeria* meningitis and 3 weeks for Gram-negative meningitis.

Intraventricular antibiotic therapy

Ventriculitis is common in neonatal meningitis, especially when caused by Gram-negative bacilli. Before the introduction of the third-generation cephalosporins, ventriculitis with persistently positive CSF cultures was relatively common. This was probably related to the poor CSF penetration of aminoglycoside antibiotics described above. Intraventricular gentamicin therapy has been associated with an increased mortality and is not recommended unless there is significant ventriculomegaly (see below) (McCracken et al. 1980).

Neurological complications

Cerebral abscess

This mainly occurs when meningitis is caused by *Citrobacter* or *Proteus* species, but may occasionally complicate meningitis caused by many other organisms, including *E. coli*, *Staphylococcus aureus*, *Mycoplasma hominis* and GBS (Fischer et al. 1981). Abscesses may present with signs of increased intracranial pressure in a baby who is responding poorly to treatment, but in some cases produce no obvious change in the clinical state. Ultrasound or MRI can be used to establish the diagnosis, and neurosurgical advice should be sought regarding management. Multiple or small abscesses can be treated with high-dose intravenous antibiotics. If only one or two abscess cavities are present, or if abscesses fail to resolve with antibiotics, the cavities generally require aspiration and instillation of an appropriate antibiotic. Systemic antibiotic therapy should be maintained for at least 4 weeks.

Hydrocephalus

This may occur during the second week of the illness while the infant still has ventriculitis, or may present with increased head growth and CNS signs at almost any stage after bacteriological cure of the meningitis. If infection is still present, an intraventricular reservoir should be inserted and intraventricular and systemic antibiotics continued. External ventricular drainage is an alternative. In most cases, a permanent CSF shunt will be required after the infection is controlled.

Deafness

Bacterial meningitis is the single most important cause of acquired SNHL in childhood, and neonates are especially vulnerable (Fortnum and Davis 1997). All survivors of neonatal meningitis should routinely undergo audiological screening soon after recovery, and audiological follow-up.

Prognosis following meningitis

In England and Wales, the mortality rate from culture-proven neonatal meningitis has declined over the last two decades from 25% to around 10% (Holt et al. 2001; Heath et al. 2003). However, the frequency of long-term consequences remains unchanged and is generally greater in neonates than older infants and children with meningitis (De Louvois et al. 1991; Bedford et al. 2001). As with many other infections, mortality is higher in preterm infants, with a reported mortality in *E. coli* meningitis of 66% in babies of 31 weeks' gestation, 30% at 32–34 weeks' and 19% in babies >35 weeks' gestation (Mulder and Zanen 1984).

In most series, adverse neurological sequelae occur in 30–50% of survivors. All forms of cerebral palsy, global developmental delay, epilepsy, SNHL and cortical blindness may occur singly or in combination. The neurodevelopmental outcome at 5 years of age of cases from the 1985–87 national neonatal meningitis cohort demonstrated an approximately 50% disability rate following both *E. coli* and GBS meningitis, but a much poorer outcome with other Gram-negative organisms (Bedford et al. 2001). Previous reports had suggested mortality rates from Gram-negative meningitis were greater than that seen with meningitis caused by Gram-positive organisms. Similarly, approximately 50% of VLBW babies had poor neurodevelopmental outcome at 20 months' corrected age (Doctor et al. 2001). Although mortality has declined, morbidity has not altered significantly from the 1970s to the 1990s (Edwards et al. 1985; Unahand et al. 1993; Klinger et al. 2000).

Predictors of adverse outcome, including mortality and moderate or severe disability, at 12 hours following admission include: presence of seizures or coma, use of inotropes and leukopenia <5 × 10^9/l (Klinger et al. 2000).

In a retrospective study babies with a normal or mildly abnormal EEG background had a normal outcome, whereas babies with an abnormal EEG were more likely to die or have an adverse neurological outcome (Chequer et al. 1992).

Pneumonia

Neonatal pneumonia may be an isolated focal infection but may also be part of generalised sepsis. Colonisation of endotracheal secretions without clinical signs of infection does not warrant antibiotic treatment (Webber et al. 1990; Isaacs 2000).

Early-onset pneumonia

The reported incidence of early-onset pneumonia is 1.79 per 1000 live births (Webber et al. 1990). GBS accounts for 70% of cases, but *Haemophilus influenzae* (Rusin et al. 1991; Kinney et al. 1993), *Streptococcus pneumoniae* (Jacobs et al. 1990; Gomez et al. 1999), *L. monocytogenes* (Hirschl et al. 1994) and Gram-negative enteric bacilli contribute. Rarely, yeasts may be involved (Ng et al. 1994). The same predisposing factors operate as for early-onset septicaemia and bronchoalveolar lavage fluid from ventilated babies, born following prolonged rupture of the membranes, contains increased numbers of white blood cells and a high concentration of IL-6 (Grigg et al. 1992). Numerous viruses may also cause early-onset pneumonia, for example adenovirus (Piedra et al. 1992; Chiou et al. 1994) and CMV (Schwebke et al. 1995).

It has been hypothesised that intrapartum penicillin prophylaxis might cause respiratory distress in infants who were colonised with GBS but were not considered to have early-onset GBS disease on the basis of negative blood cultures (Lin and Troendle 2006). They identified an incidence of approximately 2.5 cases of pneumonia per 1000 births in the general population studied, compared with a rate of proven early-onset GBS disease of 1.2 per 1000 births. This may, however, be a feature of partially treated early-onset GBS disease, with IAP rendering them blood culture-negative. In support of this, 93% developed their symptoms within 24 hours of birth (similar timing to those with culture-proven GBS infection) and 85% had a sepsis evaluation performed. This study raises the possibility that IAP may be less effective in preventing GBS disease than has been assumed (Stenson et al. 2007).

Clinical features

Tachypnoea, apnoea and other respiratory distress are the most common presenting signs. Clinical signs of pneumonia are not always predictive of pneumonia, even in older children, and a radiograph may be the only way to detect pneumonia. Appearances of GBS pneumonia may mimic hyaline membrane disease. This is because in a sick baby pneumonia can 'switch off' the type II cells that produce surfactant and so give rise to a secondary surfactant insufficiency. Infection should always be suspected in a newborn baby with disproportionately severe RDS, especially if accompanied by a metabolic acidosis and hypotension. As already noted, severe hypoxic respiratory failure, requiring inhaled nitric oxide and high-frequency ventilation, has been associated with raised blood concentrations of CRP, IL-6 and IL-8 and a greater incidence of histological chorioamnionitis and funisitis (Woldensbet et al. 2008), which suggests that inflammation, whether infective or non-infective, contributes to the severity of hypoxic respiratory failure.

Investigation

Blood culture may or may not be positive and organisms isolated from endotracheal secretions may be typical colonising organisms, such as CoNS, and not necessarily the cause of pneumonia (Webber et al. 1990, Isaacs 2000). If intubation is necessary, tracheal secretions should be obtained for microscopy and culture. While positive cultures from respiratory secretions do not prove pneumonia, it may be important to know what is grown in rationalising the choice of antibiotics.

To make the diagnosis of pneumonia there should be convincing CXR appearances, evidence of an inflammatory process, such as a rise in the CRP, an abnormal white blood cell count, or thrombocytopenia, and/or a positive blood culture.

Differential diagnosis

The principal differential diagnosis in the preterm infant is RDS, and, as pneumonia can damage surfactant production and function, the two conditions may coexist (Lee et al. 1991). Other causes of respiratory distress include transient tachypnoea of the newborn with retained lung fluid, pneumothorax, congenital structural abnormalities such as diaphragmatic hernia, oesophageal atresia with tracheo-oesophageal fistula, and cystic malformation of the lung; cardiac abnormalities and metabolic abnormalities resulting in metabolic acidosis.

Treatment

Respiratory distress should be considered as being secondary to infection until proven otherwise and treated with antibiotics until results of cultures are known. Antibiotic regimens are as shown in Table 39.7.

Outcome

Early-onset pneumonia in otherwise normal term babies carries a low mortality rate, but among preterm babies the mortality rate approaches 50%, especially when the CXR shows widespread atelectasis (Webber et al. 1990). In infants with staphylococcal or coliform pneumonia, pneumatocoeles may develop, as, rarely, may lung abscess and empyema. Abscesses and pneumatocoeles should be treated conservatively in the first place, using long-term intravenous antibiotics for the abscess. Empyema requires insertion of a thoracentesis tube for closed chest drainage, and intravenous antibiotics for several weeks.

Late-onset pneumonia

Pneumonia developing more than 48 hours after birth is commonest among preterm babies who are receiving IPPV. The reported incidence of pneumonia in intubated babies varies from 10% (Webber et al. 1990) to 35% (Halliday et al. 1984).

Organisms and pathogenesis

The organisms implicated in late-onset pneumonia are similar to those already described as causing late-onset septicaemia, except that Gram-negative bacilli are potentially more prevalent as causes of pneumonia than CoNS. In long-stay patients with CLD, unusual organisms, including fungi, Mycoplasma and Chlamydia, as well as viruses such as RSV and CMV, must be considered (Campbell

1996). Other unusual causes of nosocomial neonatal pneumonia are reported, for example *Legionella pneumophila* (Holmberg et al. 1993; Luck et al. 1994), *Serratia marcescens* (Khan et al. 1997), coronavirus (Sizun et al. 1995) and rhinovirus (Chidekel et al. 1997). Pneumonia in ventilated babies can occur secondary to septicaemia or secondary to colonisation of the endotracheal tube. Blood cultures are often negative in late-onset pneumonia.

Clinical features

In an infant with primary lung disease already on IPPV, infection presents with deteriorating lung function plus non-specific signs of infection. An increase in endotracheal tube aspirate suggests infection, but can be confused with the bronchorrhoea seen in CLD. Localised and generalised crepitations may be heard.

Investigation

Investigations include CXR, blood cultures, full blood count, CRP and culture of respiratory secretions as appropriate. In older babies, viral cultures and immunofluorescence studies for *Chlamydia* and RSV are indicated.

Treatment

Empirical antibiotic choice is as in Table 39.7. Alterations to the regimen should be dictated by a knowledge of colonising organisms and their sensitivities.

Pneumonia in the baby with chronic lung disease

In babies with long-term respiratory disease, pneumonia should always be considered if the lung disease deteriorates. In addition to the usual pathogens, respiratory viral infections are characteristic of that age group (Piedra et al. 1992). Viral respiratory infections in babies with CLD lead to a worsening of chronic respiratory morbidity, with signs of increased airway resistance, compared with those who avoid viral infection (Yuksel and Greenough 1994).

Specific neonatal lung infections

Ureaplasma urealyticum

Ureaplasma urealyticum is a common vaginal commensal. It may be implicated in some cases of chorioamnionitis and premature delivery (Dyke et al. 1993), along with *Mycoplasma hominis* (Valencia et al. 1993). There is speculation that these organisms may cause acute neonatal pneumonia and have a role in the pathogenesis of CLD, although the literature is variable (Cassell et al. 1993; Ollikainen et al. 1993; Da Silva et al. 1997; Maxwell et al. 2009; Viscardi and Hasday 2009). Ureaplasmas require a special culture medium and may take several weeks to grow, although there have been recent improvements in detection methods. Erythromycin is the antibiotic of choice for both *Ureaplasma* and *Mycoplasma* infections in the newborn (Waites et al. 1993).

Respiratory syncytial virus

RSV infections are comparatively rare on the neonatal unit, but small epidemics occur from time to time and the effects on individual babies can be devastating, especially among those with severe CLD. Such babies may rapidly develop almost complete airway obstruction and become impossible to ventilate. Recurrent bradycardia is a common presenting feature, and the clinical course is occasionally complicated by atrial tachycardia (Donnerstein et al.

1994). RSV infection must always be considered when a baby with CLD experiences a deterioration in lung function, even if the typical physical signs of a bronchiolitis are absent. RSV is easily diagnosed by immunofluorescence on respiratory secretions. Stringent measures to limit cross-infection are required if a case of RSV infection occurs on a NICU (Madge et al. 1992). Extracorporeal membrane oxygenation should be considered early in deteriorating cases (Greenough 2009). Babies with CLD also remain very vulnerable to RSV infection for many months after discharge from the NICU and hospital readmission is common (Paramore et al. 2010). There is evidence for the effectiveness of prophylaxis using palivizumab (a humanised RSV monoclonal antibody). Recommendations have recently been revised in the UK, but there is universal agreement that palivizumab should be offered to babies at home in oxygen during the RSV season (Sharland and Bedford Russell 2001) (Ch. 27, part 3).

Other respiratory viruses

VLBW babies who remain on the NICU for many months may contract the usual viral respiratory infections of early childhood from their visitors and from nursing and medical staff. Symptoms are usually of a mild upper respiratory tract infection (URTI) accompanied by a low-grade pyrexia. More severe viral pneumonia, other than that caused by RSV, may also occur at any time in the neonatal period, and adenoviruses and coronaviruses are often responsible (Piedra et al. 1992; Sizun et al. 1995).

Pertussis

Severe pertussis can occur in the late neonatal period, presenting with paroxysmal cough, vomiting, apnoea and choking spells. Whooping is rare. Prolonged ventilatory support is often required (Hampl and Olson 1995). Diagnosis is by culture of nasopharyngeal swabs or, in the case of babies who have started antibiotic therapy, by PCR (Edelman et al. 1996). Treatment is with erythromycin and sedation. There is one report of fatal pertussis in an infant who contracted the infection from his unimmunised mother (Beiter et al. 1993).

Chlamydia

Chlamydia trachomatis and C. pneumoniae can cause severe early-onset disease similar to that seen with GBS. Even birth by caesarean section with intact membranes does not preclude the possibility of vertical transmission, and the organism can cross the intact membranes, causing fetal pneumonic stillbirth (Bell et al. 1994). Chlamydial infection during pregnancy should be treated with either ampicillin or erythromycin in order to prevent perinatal transmission (Samson and MacDonald 1995). Chlamydial pneumonia in term infants is characteristically a disease in those over 4 weeks of age, but it can occur in the first week of life. The diagnosis is made by culture or immunofluorescence techniques in the presence of a suggestive clinical picture, which includes an afebrile pneumonia with tachypnoea and rales, diffuse CXR changes, an eosinophilia and previous neonatal conjunctivitis. Like other neonatal lung diseases, chlamydial pneumonia can cause long-term pulmonary damage. Treatment is with erythromycin.

Lung abscess

This is a rare occurrence in the newborn, presenting usually with dyspnoea and an area of opacification on CXR. It usually follows previous pneumonia and is usually caused by Gram-negative organisms, but can be caused by *Staphylococcus aureus*. It should be treated initially with broad-spectrum antibiotics. If the lesion does not resolve, bronchoscopy or surgery may be indicated.

Cardiac infection

Endocarditis

Endocarditis is being recognised with increasing frequency in VLBW babies with structurally normal hearts. Virtually all of these babies have had central lines lying in the right atrium or right ventricle. The organisms responsible for most cases are CoNS, and it is notable that breastfeeding is associated with shorter disease duration (Linder et al. 2011). Enterococci, *S. aureus* and *Candida* species are other well-recognised causal agents (Rastogi et al. 1993; Mecrow and Ladusans 1994). Endocarditis in this group of infants usually presents with no more than persistent signs of sepsis and positive blood cultures despite appropriate antibiotic therapy, although in a few cases there are changing murmurs, heart failure, persisting haematuria or thrombocytopenia. A baby who presents with any of these features and who has, or has recently had, an intracardiac central line should have an echocardiogram performed. The demonstration of intracardiac vegetations, which are present in most patients, confirms the diagnosis.

Treatment and outcome

Remove the central line and check that the appropriate antibiotics are being given for the organism grown from the blood, at the correct dose and dose interval. If the signs of sepsis remit within a few days, and blood cultures become negative, antibiotic therapy should be continued for 10–14 days (Raad and Sabbagh 1992). The prognosis for catheter-related endocarditis due to CoNS is better than might be thought, with recovery rates of more than 60% reported from small series (Rastogi et al. 1993; Mecrow and Ladusans 1994; Linder et al. 2011). Endocarditis due to *Candida albicans* carries a poor prognosis. Rarely, vegetations persist or severe valve damage occurs, and then surgery may be indicated.

Pericarditis

This is extremely rare, and usually develops as a complication of pre-existing sepsis or an abscess near the mediastinum. Implicated organisms include *S. aureus*, *E. coli*, *H. influenzae*, *Klebsiella* species, *Pseudomonas* species and *Candida* species (Feldman 1979). The CXR shows an increase in the size of the cardiac silhouette, but signs of tamponade are unusual. ECG changes are present, and the diagnosis can be confirmed by echocardiography and pericardial tap. The treatment is surgical drainage and long-term antibiotics.

Myocarditis

Myocarditis is classically caused by enterovirus infection, with coxsackieviruses being the predominant causative agents. It is a rare but severe disease with death or cardiac sequelae including chronic heart failure and aneurysm formation in the majority. Fewer than 25% make a full recovery (Freund et al. 2010). The myocardium is damaged primarily by direct lysis of infected myocytes with apoptotic degeneration of infected myocytes. Presenting clinical signs include fever, lethargy, poor feeding, respiratory distress, irritability and poor peripheral perfusion, and may be associated with hepatitis. Diagnosis is usually made by enterovirus PCR.

There is no specific antiviral treatment, though pleconaril has been used sporadically. Early treatment with IVIG has also been used with limited success. Mortality thus remains high in spite of high-quality intensive care.

Bone and joint infection

Septic arthritis and osteomyelitis are rare in the newborn, although incidence rates up to 9.6 cases per 1000 NICU admissions have been reported (Isaacs et al. 1996). Osteomyelitis and septic arthritis are mainly caused by *S. aureus* (Ish Horowicz et al. 1992), but GBS is important (Yagupsky et al. 1991) and several other organisms may be involved, including *H. influenzae, U. urealyticum, Candida* species, *Neisseria gonorrhoeae, N. meningitides* and *Streptococcus pneumoniae* (Wong and Ng 1991; Weisse et al. 1993; Eisenstein and Gesundheit 1998; Babl et al. 2000; Cigni et al. 2004; Pinna et al. 2006). Osteomyelitis and septic arthritis often coexist, and are often indistinguishable clinically. There are two reasons for this. The infected metaphysis of the bone often lies within the capsule of the joint, and when the thin metaphyseal cortex collapses, infection enters the joint. In addition, blood vessels frequently pass through the thin epiphyseal plate of neonatal long bones, transmitting metaphyseal infection to the joint capsule.

Osteomyelitis/septic arthritis takes two forms. One is seen in acutely ill babies with complex problems, and often with indwelling cannulae, in whom multiple bone involvement may occur (Ish Horowicz et al. 1992). The other form is a more subtle presentation and usually only one site is affected. GBS is quite often responsible for this latter form. The sites most commonly affected are the pelvis, hip, knee and humerus, but any site may be involved. Skull osteomyelitis may occur following infection of a cephalhaematoma or a scalp puncture for fetal pH monitoring. Vertebral disease occasionally develops, and calcaneal disease may follow heel puncture. Isolated arthritis is rarely reported, but the organisms isolated are similar to those reported for osteomyelitis, except for the preponderance of coliform arthritis of the hip when this complicates femoral venepuncture (Ho et al. 1989).

Clinical features

These disorders usually present in one of three ways:

1. with pseudoparalysis of the affected limb due to pain – the affected area may be warm and swollen
2. following investigation of the baby with non-specific signs of sepsis
3. incidentally on X-ray in a baby with multisystem disease.

Investigation and diagnosis

The affected bone or joint must be X-rayed as a baseline, although no changes are usually seen for 10–14 days, when bone rarefaction, lytic lesions, periosteal elevation and periosteal new bone formation are seen. Isotope scans are also useful in identifying 'hot spots' in joints or bones. MRI can be very valuable, especially to look at the spine and pelvis (Mazur et al. 1995). Aspiration of the affected joint or bone should usually be attempted, not only to achieve prompt bacteriological diagnosis by Gram stain and culture, but also because decompression is an important part of therapy.

Treatment

Vancomycin and a third-generation cephalosporin is a reasonable starting point until the results of blood cultures are available, but this should be discussed with the local microbiologist. Antibiotics should be given intravenously for at least 4–6 weeks. When pus is obtained at aspiration, orthopaedic advice should always be sought about surgical drainage of the bone or joint.

Prognosis

Mortality relates almost entirely to multisytem disease, but there is a high morbidity rate. Following staphylococcal and Gram-negative infections, permanent damage to the epiphyseal plate or the metaphysis is common. This may cause permanent arthritis, long-term growth problems or deformity, particularly in those with an acute onset or multiple sites of involvement, in whom up to 50% may have significant long-term orthopaedic problems (Peters et al. 1992). Long-term clinical and radiological follow-up is essential, especially as impaired growth may not become evident for several years (Peters et al. 1992). The prognosis for complete recovery from GBS infections is somewhat better.

Gastroenteritis

Neonatal gastroenteritis in the UK is commonly sporadic and usually mild. Infection may be acquired from the mother during birth, or subsequently by cross-infection, or from contaminated feeds. Many nursery outbreaks are initiated by an asymptomatic infant who sheds the virus or bacterium. For some viral pathogens, such as rotavirus, nursery outbreaks often coincide with seasonal peaks of the disease in the community (Steele and Sears 1996). Breastfeeding is strongly protective in both developing and developed world populations (Plenge-Bönig et al. 2010).

Organisms

Most neonatal gastroenteritis is due to rotavirus which may also be endemic in some nurseries without obvious symptoms, especially in preterm infants (Sharma et al. 2002). Astrovirus infection, although less common, is more likely to cause systemic infection or NEC (Bagci et al. 2010). *E. coli, Salmonella* species and *Shigella* species all may cause neonatal gastroenteritis (Umasankar et al. 1996). Neonatal *Campylobacter* gastroenteritis has been described, often contracted from the baby's mother, as have infections with adenovirus, echovirus, coxsackievirus and astrovirus.

Symptoms and signs

Diarrhoea, rather than vomiting, is usually the predominant feature in neonatal gastroenteritis, and copious watery stools may be passed. Bloody stools are rare, except in infection with *Salmonella, Shigella* or *Campylobacter* species. Signs of dehydration soon appear and shock may develop, especially in preterm babies, who may rapidly lose more than 10% of their bodyweight. The infant is often pale and listless, with a distended abdomen and a metabolic acidosis.

Differential diagnosis and investigation

Healthy breastfed babies may pass up to 10 loose yellow stools per day, but are thriving and otherwise completely asymptomatic. Frequent loose green stools are often seen in infants receiving phototherapy and do not require further investigation. Severe diarrhoea can occasionally be caused by the inherited abnormalities of sugar absorption, congenital chloride diarrhoea or cystic fibrosis. If these conditions are excluded, copious diarrhoea is almost always due to gastroenteritis. Stool culture is essential and, if appropriate, stools should also be examined by electron microscopy for virus particles.

Treatment

If the symptoms are mild and dehydration minimal, breastfeeding should continue. It may even be worth persisting with formula feeding if this is the chosen method of feeding, giving small frequent feeds. If the major problem is vomiting, this can usually be controlled with a glucose–electrolyte solution. In more severe cases, oral feeds should be stopped for 48 hours and intravenous fluids started. Infusions of sodium bicarbonate may need to be given to acidaemic preterm babies. After 48 hours, oral glucose–electrolyte solutions are usually well tolerated, and the baby can promptly restart milk feeds in the next 24–48 hours. There is no need to regrade the feeds from quarter to half to full strength. If diarrhoea returns, milk protein intolerance should be considered, which may downregulate lactase production temporarily, resulting in stool positive for reducing substances. If present, the baby may respond to an appropriate semihydrolysed milk such as Pregestimil.

Antibiotics should not be given routinely. However, if an epidemic of bacterial gastroenteritis develops, oral non-absorbable antibiotics such as neomycin or colomycin may be indicated (Umasankar et al. 1996). If *Salmonella* species, *Shigella* species or *Campylobacter* are grown, and particularly if the infant has systemic symptoms or is premature, parenteral antibiotics should be given using co-trimoxazole or a third-generation cephalosporin for *Salmonella*, ampicillin or co-trimoxazole for *Shigella*, and erythromycin or gentamicin for *Campylobacter*. Antidiarrhoeal agents should not be used in the neonatal period.

Isolation

Term babies who develop mild symptoms on a postnatal ward can be isolated with their mothers. Sporadic cases on a neonatal unit should be isolated within the unit or, if appropriate facilities exist, transferred to the paediatric infectious disease unit. The management of epidemics is outlined above.

Urinary tract infection

The true incidence of UTI in the newborn is difficult to establish because the methods of urine collection employed in epidemiological surveys are all likely to lead to overdiagnosis, because of contamination. In term infants, the reported incidence is in the range 0.1–3%; among LBW infants, it is at least three times as high and possibly as much as 10 times as high (Edelman et al. 1973; Wettergren et al. 1985). If the higher quoted figures are true, most neonatal UTIs remain undiagnosed. There is a two- to three-fold higher incidence in males at any gestation. Infants of cocaine users seem to be unusually susceptible to UTI (Gottbrath Flaherty et al. 1995). UTI in the newborn is believed to occur mainly as a result of bloodstream spread of organisms to the kidney during septicaemia, although no doubt the reverse situation can also apply. Breastfeeding offers a significant degree of protection (Levy et al. 2009).

Organisms

The commonest pathogen by far is *E. coli*. Important bacterial virulence factors include fimbriae, toxins, flagellae and proteins that evade host immune responses (Nielubowicz and Mobley 2010). Host factors, including Toll-like receptors and chemokine receptors are also important determinants of susceptibility to infection (Ragnarsdóttir et al. 2008), although these have yet to be characterised in preterm infants with UTI. In addition, many Gram-negative enteric bacteria and some Gram-positive cocci, including CoNS, *Staphylococcus aureus* and enterococci, can cause neonatal UTI. *C. albicans* accounts for some 40% of UTIs in a neonatal unit setting (Phillips and Karlowicz 1997). Candiduria was associated with

a significant risk of disseminated disease and a high mortality rate (30%) in a large Canadian multicentre study (Robinson et al. 2009).

Symptoms and signs

Neonatal UTI may present acutely with all the signs of septicaemia or insidiously with poor feeding, listlessness, poor weight gain and low-grade fever. Some infections only come to light if urinalysis is done as part of the routine investigation of a baby with, say, persisting jaundice, unexplained anaemia or poor weight gain. On examination, signs particularly relevant to the diagnosis of UTI include distress during renal palpation, renal enlargement due to hydronephrosis or some other congenital abnormality, and an enlarged bladder, suggesting outflow tract obstruction. The external genitalia must be examined to exclude stenoses or fistulae, and the blood pressure should be checked.

Investigation

If the UTI is part of a septicaemic illness, as it is in around a quarter of cases (Phillips and Karlowicz 1997), there will commonly be a positive blood culture in addition to a positive urine culture. The technique of urine collection and the diagnostic criteria for UTI are given on, and should be adhered to. All babies with a proven UTI must have their serum biochemistry checked.

Further investigation is essential, as between 35% and 50% of infants will have an underlying abnormality, which in about two-thirds will be vesicoureteric reflux. A renal ultrasound scan will demonstrate the presence, position and size of the kidneys, the size and thickness of the bladder, and dilatation of the collecting systems. Ultrasound may also show echogenic fungal material in the renal pelvis or ureter in around a third of cases of proven UTI due to *C. albicans*. Ultrasound alone, however, cannot be relied upon to show scars or exclude vesicoureteric reflux, and all children under the age of 1 year being investigated following proven UTI should have a micturating cystourethrogram (MCUG) and a dimercaptosuccinic acid (DMSA) scan in addition to ultrasound. The MCUG will exclude bladder neck obstruction and urethral valves, but its most important role is to exclude vesicoureteric reflux. The DMSA scan can show scarring, which is probably commoner after renal infection than was once thought to be the case. The intravenous urogram has fallen out of fashion but may be necessary on occasion to delineate an abnormality fully and plan further treatment.

Treatment

If the baby presents with a systemic illness, the usual antibiotic combinations for either EOS or LOS should be used, and the treatment refined when the results of cultures are available. If UTI is confirmed, antibiotics should be continued for 10–14 days. Resolution of infection should be confirmed with further urine cultures. Once the infection has been treated, prophylaxis with low-dose trimethoprim, given in a single dose at night, should continue until radiological investigations have excluded underlying abnormalities. If the investigations are normal, prophylaxis can be discontinued, but the infant should be followed with urinalyses every 3 months for at least a year. If there is evidence of reflux, antibiotic prophylaxis should be continued. There is significant variability in treatment of candiduria in infants, although most centres use fluconazole and amphotericin B (either deoxycholate or lipid-based) in combination or sequentially (Robinson et al. 2009).

Superficial infections

Umbilical cord infections

Despite good cord care, minor umbilical infection still occurs in 2% of preterm and 0.5% of term neonates. Although *S. aureus* is still the most important pathogen, Gram-negative enteric bacilli, especially *E. coli* and *Klebsiella* species, are relatively common. In most cases the clinical features are limited to periumbilical erythema, often with a small amount of discharge, but in other cases there is a spreading cellulitis of the abdominal wall, or even fasciitis (Fraser et al. 2006). In the developing world, neonatal tetanus occurs mainly as a result of contamination of the umbilical cord stump by *Clostridium tetani*.

Investigation and treatment

Swabs of the umbilicus should be taken, and a blood culture unless the baby is completely well. Local treatment should usually suffice, but if there is evidence of invasion of the surrounding tissues or of systemic upset, empiric treatment against *S. aureus* with flucloxacillin should be given intravenously or orally depending on the condition of the baby.

Skin infections

Staphylococcal

The commonest presentation is with a few flaccid intraepidermal bullae which are filled with a yellowish opalescent fluid, but occasionally larger bullae may be present, in which case the condition merges into bullous impetigo. Paronychia may also occur. It is important not to misdiagnose (and hence treat) the benign condition of neonatal pustular melanosis. The infant is usually well, with little or no local inflammation and no regional lymphadenitis. After taking swabs from the lesions, treatment should be with oral flucloxacillin. If there is any suggestion of a systemic illness, staphylococcal septicaemia should be suspected, appropriate investigations carried out and parenteral antibiotics started.

Conjunctivitis

Up-to-date and useful epidemiological information on neonatal conjunctivitis has been hard to come by. A recent study from Israel identified CoNS as the most common early pathogen, with a shift from Gram-negative to Gram-positive, often resistant, microorganisms during the infants' stay (Borer et al. 2010).

Organisms

Infective conjunctivitis can be caused by a wide variety of pathogens and the pattern varies considerably between reported series. In the UK, the top five would normally include *Staphylococcus aureus*, *C. trachomatis*, *H. influenzae*, *Streptococcus pneumoniae* and *S. viridans*. *N. gonorrhoeae* is rare in the UK at the present time. In all ill children with conjunctival discharge, in addition to the organisms mentioned, always consider HSV, *L. monocytogenes* and *N. meningitidis*.

General considerations

Conjunctivitis can develop at any stage in the neonatal period. Late-onset and recurrent conjunctivitis is much more common if there is a blocked lacrimal duct with epiphora. The spectrum of severity ranges from mild crusting on the eyelids, through purulent discharge, conjunctival injection and eyelid oedema, to invasion of the eye and retro-orbital structures.

In infants with mild conjunctivitis, no treatment other than regular cleaning/bathing of the lids with a sterile saline swab 4–6-hourly for 2–3 days is required. However, if cultures are positive, discharge persists for more than 48 hours or there is conjunctival or lid oedema, topical antibiotics should be started. Chloramphenicol, neomycin or gentamicin eye drops are common choices, administered 6-hourly. Because an important part of the therapy is irrigation, drops are preferable to ointment. Both eyes should be treated, even though infection is only apparent in one. In infants with epiphora, after instilling the antibiotics the lacrimal duct should be gently massaged towards the eye in an attempt to unblock it. Rarely, probing the lacrimal duct under anaesthesia may be necessary later in infancy.

Gonococcal ophthalmia

This usually presents within 24 hours of delivery with a profuse, bilateral, purulent conjunctival discharge, but can present less dramatically at any time in the first month. Significant systemic upset is unusual, but because of the speed with which the infection can damage the cornea it is important that the diagnosis is made and treatment started immediately. A swab must be sent to the laboratory promptly for Gram stain and culture in an enriched medium. If Gram-negative intracellular diplococci are seen on microscopy, treatment must be started immediately, pending culture. Traditionally, treatment has been with systemic penicillin and penicillin eye drops and this is an effective regimen. Currently recommended treatment is with a single dose of ceftriaxone, 25–50 mg/kg intravenously or intramuscularly to a maximum dose of 125 mg. However, there has been an increasing incidence of resistant strains, and thus local resistance patterns should be taken into account in determining treatment regimens (Woods 2005). The infected baby must be isolated together with the mother from all other babies, and the mother and her contacts should be treated.

Chlamydial ophthalmia

This is now among the commonest causes of neonatal conjunctivitis, and some babies infected as neonates will develop chlamydial pneumonia later in infancy, which is often severe enough to require hospital admission. In western Europe, chlamydial pneumonia is now less common than previously, but within the developing world a high proportion of all pneumonia in early infancy may be due to this organism. Amongst mothers infected with *Chlamydia*, around 25–50% of infants will develop infection.

Chlamydial conjunctivitis usually presents between 5 and 12 days postnatal age (Darville 2005). It may be unilateral initially, but often becomes bilateral. Rarely it can cause adhesions between the bulbar and tarsal conjunctiva, with some persisting pannus, but it almost never causes permanent visual impairment. Conventional cultures are negative and treatment with standard topical antibiotics is rarely successful: in many cases *Chlamydia* is first suspected for these very reasons. Several tests are available for the identification of *Chlamydia* from eye swabs, including enzyme immunoassay, immunofluorescence techniques and PCR (Darville 2005). Chlamydial eye infection is usually treated with oral erythromycin for 2 weeks, which may be effective without the need for additional topical treatment (Zar 2005). Azithromycin and clarithromycin may also be effective, although these are less well studied.

Attempts have been made to prevent both the neonatal conjunctivitis and pneumonia in infancy by some form of early neonatal prophylaxis. Silver nitrate eye drops and tetracycline or erythromycin eye ointment applied at delivery have all been used, with varying degrees of success. A 2.5% ophthalmic solution of povidone-iodine is a more effective form of prophylaxis than either silver nitrate or erythromycin, and does not have the potential for promoting antibiotic ressistance (Zar 2005). If maternal infection is detected antenatally, treatment with erythromycin for 1 week may reduce the risk of neonatal infection.

Pseudomonal ophthalmia

Although a relatively rare cause of neonatal ophthalmia, *Pseudomonas aeruginosa* has a remarkable ability to invade ocular tissue and to cause severe damage (Boyle et al. 2001). Most cases occur in preterm infants, usually as a result of cross-infection from an environmental source. Many of these infants develop septicaemia as well as ophthalmia. If pseudomonal ophthalmia is suspected, or if the organism is grown from an eye swab, parenteral therapy with a suitable antibiotic combination, such as gentamicin and ceftazidime, should be begun at once, in addition to locally applied gentamicin drops or ointment. Urgent ophthalmological opinion is required if invasive disease is suspected.

Dacrocystitis

This presents within the first week as a reddish-purple swelling over the course of the lacrimal duct and sac on the medial and inferior margin of the eye. Local pressure often results in a squirt of purulent material from the lacrimal punctum. The usual cause is *Staphylococcus aureus*, but anaerobes may sometimes be involved. Treatment is with systemic and topical antibiotics, usually in drops rather than ointment. Sequelae are rare.

Otitis media

This diagnosis is often ignored in the neonatal period, probably because of the great difficulty in visualising the oblique, downward-facing immobile tympanic membrane through the hairy, narrow neonatal external auditory meatus. However, otitis media has been reported to occur in two-thirds of infants ventilated through a nasotracheal tube, which compromises normal function at the lower end of the eustachian tube, and infection may still be present at autopsy. However, in those who survive, the infection resolves. Otitis media is virtually universal in infants with cleft palate, in whom there is reflux of milk and secretions into the eustachian tube. Finally, otitis media may occur in a previously healthy baby and in long-stay patients on a NICU who develop signs of an URTI.

Among the inmates of a NICU, the organisms responsible are often *E. coli* and *S. aureus*, but *H. influenzae* and *Streptococcus pneumoniae* may be grown from previously asymptomatic babies who present later in the neonatal period. In many cases, fluid obtained by tympanocentesis is sterile.

Treatment of otitis media in the ill LBW baby on IPPV should be with the usual broad-spectrum antibiotic combination. In older infants with URTI and/or cleft palate, oral treatment with an antibiotic active against *S. pneumoniae* and *H. influenzae*, such as amoxicillin or trimethoprim, is usually adequate.

Other neonatal bacterial infections

Localised abscesses

These may develop anywhere, but are most common at the site of heelpricks, intravenous infusions, or where the skin has been abraded by electrode adhesive or some other piece of monitoring equipment. There is localised swelling, redness and tenderness. The infection may spread to more important local tissues, such as bone, causing osteomyelitis, or, rarely, septicaemia may develop. If a fluctuant area develops, incision or aspiration under local anaesthesia, using a wide-bore needle, is helpful. Broad-spectrum antibiotic cover should be given intravenously, but if the baby is well this can be changed to an appropriate oral antibiotic once the culture and sensitivities are available. Treatment should usually be given for 7–10 days.

Breast abscess

Breast enlargement and redness in babies of either sex are not unusual and represent a transient hormonal stimulus, rather than infection. However, if tenderness and erythema are present with fluctuation, pyrexia or a purulent discharge from the nipple (not to be confused with neonatal breast milk/lactorrhoea, then treatment with systemic antibiotics should be given.

Liver abscess

Postmortem examinations indicate that multiple microabscesses in the liver may occur in both preterm and term babies as a complication of generalised sepsis, vascular cannulae or abdominal surgery. In life there are few clues to their presence, although they may be associated with hepatomegaly and abnormal liver enzymes. Solitary liver abscesses have occasionally been reported in the newborn, mostly in preterm infants who have had umbilical vein catheterisation (Tan et al. 2005). Early recognition may allow good outcome, and persistence of positive blood cultures despite treatment in an infant with sepsis should prompt abdominal ultrasound examination. True bacterial hepatitis is very rare, but is a well-documented feature of congenital listeriosis. *C. albicans* can cause multiple liver abscesses in babies with immunodeficiency states.

Therapy for multiple microabscesses is that for septicaemia. Solitary abscesses may require drainage in addition, either percutaneously under ultrasound guidance or by open operation.

Sialadenitis

The parotid or submandibular glands may become infected, with the latter more often involved in premature babies. Presentation is with a red indurated area over the gland, with pus draining from either Stensen's or Wharton's duct. *Staphylococcus aureus* is the commonest pathogen, but *E. coli* and *P. aeruginosa* may also be implicated. Rarely this can be the presenting feature of late-onset GBS infection (Walter et al. 2009). Suppurative parotitis caused by anaerobic organisms has also been reported. Treatment is with intravenous antibiotics, which should always include flucloxacillin.

Necrotising fasciitis

Bacterial infection of the subcutaneous tissues and fascia is a rare but potentially very serious condition in the newborn. The organisms most commonly implicated are streptococci of groups B, A and D, staphylococci, Gram-negative enterobacteria and various anaerobes. Necrotising fasciitis can arise at any site, but the commonest is the abdominal wall, secondary to omphalitis (Fraser et al. 2006). There is commonly marked tissue oedema and inflammation, which spreads rapidly. There are signs of systemic toxicity but blood cultures are positive in only about half the cases. The keys to a successful outcome are a high level of clinical suspicion, appropriate antibiotics, and prompt and aggressive surgical intervention.

Mycoplasma and *Ureaplasma* infections

If present in the mother's birth canal, these organisms may colonise as many as 50% of babies. They may play a role in triggering preterm labour and may potentially cause disease in the infant, although variation in host defences may account for the wide differences in response between individuals (Larsen and Hwang 2010).

The probable role of *U. urealyticum* in neonatal pneumonia and CLD has been discussed. The evidence that *U. urealyticum* in particular is an important pathogen in preterm infants is accumulating (Viscardi 2010). The most effective antibiotic against both mycoplasmas and ureaplasmas is erythromycin, and this should be given intravenously.

Tuberculosis

Tuberculosis (TB) is prevalent in almost all tropical developing countries and constitutes a special risk during pregnancy and lactation to mothers and babies (Figueroa-Damian and Arredondo-Garcia 2001). In the UK, perinatal TB is extremely rare, although may increase because of migration. Transplacental haematogenous infection usually occurs when the pregnant woman has clinical TB or a recent primary infection. In disseminated maternal infection, miliary lesions may be present in the placenta. There is an absence of cellular response in the baby, and the primary focus and lymph nodes are caseous, with abundant tubercle bacilli. The peripheries of the lesions contain few lymphocytes and no giant cells. Coinfection with HIV is well recognised.

Criteria for the diagnosis of congenital TB were first laid down by Beitzke in 1935. There must be proof that the lesion is tuberculous. A primary complex in the liver is almost certainly of intrauterine origin. If the liver primary complex is absent, the infection should be obvious in the fetus or in the neonate at birth or during the first week. Neonatal TB is the result of either intrauterine infection or inhalation of tubercle bacilli during or soon after birth, through intimate contact with an adult with active pulmonary TB.

Clinical picture

The onset of symptoms is usually in the first month of life. The primary focus is often in the liver, and congenitally infected infants may present with hepatomegaly and jaundice caused by obstruction of bile drainage by enlarged lymph nodes at the porta hepatis. Sometimes a primary complex is found in the lung as a result of dissemination through the ductus venosus, probably from the amniotic fluid or the maternal genital tract (Gogus et al. 1993). The infant may then present with pneumonia, anaemia and hepatosplenomegaly, with radiological evidence of widespread pulmonary infection with mediastinal and hilar lymphadenopathy, but usually no liver lesion. Gastric aspirate microscopy for acid-fast bacilli and culture for mycobacteria are the best diagnostic tests. The infected neonate is not sensitive to tuberculin. Occasionally, localised infection is reported, such as otitis or cutaneous involvement, and occasionally the presentation is with an acute sepsis syndrome (Mazade et al. 2001).

Management

The prognosis is best when infected mothers have been detected by antenatal screening and antituberculous treatment instituted during pregnancy (Mnyani and McIntyre 2011). The management of an infant of a mother with active TB infection poses special problems.

> **Box 39.3** The following policy is advocated for asymptomatic infants of mothers with sputum-positive tuberculosis (TB)
>
> - Test mother for human immunodeficiency virus
> - Treat the mother for TB
> - Maintain breastfeeding (except where this is precluded by the gravity of the maternal illness)
> - Exclude congenital TB with chest X-ray and lumbar puncture
> - If no congenital TB, give the infant prophylactic isoniazid 10 mg/kg once daily for 3–4 months
> - Consider immunising the infant with isoniazid-resistant bacille Calmette-Guérin (BCG), if available, or BCG vaccine if not
> - At 3–4 months of age, perform tuberculin skin test (TST) on infant: if TST negative and infant well, stop isoniazid
> - If TST positive at 3 months, re-evaluate infant for TB

Isolation of the baby from the infected mother is usually not feasible and is in any case undesirable, because it would signal the end of breastfeeding and expose the infant to all the hazards of artificial feeding. Breastfeeding is deemed safe for the infant of a mother taking antituberculous drugs (Box 39.3).

Neonatal TB infection is rare and treatment is empiric. One recommended regimen is isoniazid (10 mg/kg/day) plus rifampicin (15 mg/kg/day) and pyrazinamide (25 mg/kg/day) for 2 months, followed by 4 months of isoniazid and rifampicin. If isoniazid resistance is suspected, usually on the basis of the likely geographical source of the infection, at least one additional drug should be used until sensitivities are known. Ethambutol (20 mg/kg/day) is one possibility. Steroids have no place in treatment because of the lack of a host reaction. Isoniazid prophylaxis is recommended for skin test-negative neonatal contacts.

Neonatal tetanus

Tetanus is an important cause of neonatal death (up to 60 per 1000 livebirths) worldwide because of local conditions and customs, rather than climate. Neonatal tetanus still accounts for between 25% and 65% of all neonatal deaths in some countries. In rural India, the walls of the village houses are made of a mixture of earth and cow dung, and the ash of cow dung fires is used to dress the umbilical stump. Neonatal tetanus is known as the '8-day disease' in the Punjab, because so many babies die of tetanus on the eighth day of life. Infection of the umbilical stump caused by septic management of the cord and harmful cultural practices are the main reasons for the high frequency of neonatal tetanus in rural communities in the tropics.

The organism

Clostridium tetani is a Gram-positive rod and a strict anaerobe. It is present in animal faeces, though usually absent from human faeces. Spores of *C. tetani* are highly resistant to heat, chemicals and antibiotics, but can be destroyed if autoclaved. They can survive for many years in dry dust or earth. During germination and growth in anaerobic conditions, the organism produces two toxins, tetanospasmin and tetanolysin. Tetanospasmin is a potent exotoxin with high affinity for nervous tissue. It is produced by the vegetative form of *C. tetani* in conditions of reduced oxygen. Within the CNS, the toxin is bound to gangliosides, where it suppresses inhibitory influences on motor neurons and interneurons, directly enhancing excitatory synaptic action. Its action is similar to that of strychnine, inducing hypertonicity, spasms and seizures. The toxin also produces overactivity of the sympathetic nervous system, resulting in tachycardia, arrhythmias, labile hypertension, peripheral vasoconstriction, sweating, hypercarbia and increased urinary excretion of catecholamines. The site of absorption of tetanus toxin is at the peripheral motor and autonomic nerve endings. Toxin ascends the nerve fibres and crosses the synaptic cleft into the presynaptic endings of adjacent inhibitory spinal interneurons, where it is bound. Antitoxin inhibits tetanospasmin only before it is fixed on to the presynaptic terminal.

Clinical features

The incubation period of neonatal tetanus varies from 3 to 14 days or more, the severity of the disease being greater with a shorter incubation period (Saltigeral Simental et al. 1993). Both muscle rigidity and spasms are typical of tetanus.

Trismus, caused by spasm of the masseter muscles, a few days after birth is the presenting symptom in more than half of patients with neonatal tetanus. This is followed by stiffness of the neck muscles and difficulty in swallowing. The infant is irritable, restless and unable to feed. Spasm of the facial muscles produces risus sardonicus. Tonic contractions of the lumbar and abdominal musculature occur next, and result in opisthotonus. This is accompanied by flexion and adduction of the arms and clenching of the fists. Spasms which initially last a few seconds become more prolonged, and may persist for minutes as the disease progresses. The baby is conscious and crying because of intense pain from muscle spasms that become more powerful. Fever is a feature, probably because of overactivity of the muscles. Spasms of laryngeal and respiratory muscles may lead to obstruction, asphyxia and cyanosis. The natural history of tetanus is one of increasing severity during the first 7 days, followed by a plateau in the second week and gradual abatement over the next 2–6 weeks. Tetanus is often fatal in the neonate, with mortality as high as 50–90% (Kurtoglu et al. 1998). Bronchopneumonia, aspiration pneumonia and atelectasis are common complications. When assisted ventilation and intensive care are available, the death rate can be substantially reduced (Saltigeral Simental et al. 1993).

Management

There is currently no agreed standard regimen of management of neonatal tetanus and care is supportive, with respiratory support where it is available. The aims of treatment are to neutralise existing toxin before it enters the nervous system, to reduce further production of toxin, to control the neuromuscular and autonomic features, and to sustain the patient until the effects of toxin resolve.

General management includes skilful nursing care to prevent aspiration pneumonia and atelectasis, and the reduction to a minimum of stimuli that can precipitate a convulsion.

Penicillin 60 mg (100 000 units)/kg/day is given for 5 days to eliminate *C. tetani*. Concomitant infections should be treated with appropriate broad-spectrum antibiotics.

Specific therapy is in the form of antitetanus human immunoglobulin, which neutralises unbound circulating toxin and has no effect on toxin fixed in nerve cells. Although the CNS is often affected by toxin before symptoms appear, patients given antitoxin usually fare better than those not given antitoxin. A single dose of 3000–5000 units given by intramuscular injection is recommended. Equine antitetanus serum (ATS) remains the most widely used tetanus antitoxin. It should be used as early as possible in the course of the disease, as either a single intramuscular injection of 5000

units or 750–1500 units daily for three doses. Massive doses of ATS have no significant advantage over smaller doses. There may be benefit in giving 1500 units of ATS intrathecally early in the disease. There is a significantly lower death rate in babies given intrathecal therapy (45%) compared with controls given intramuscular ATS (82%). Infants who receive intrathecal ATS also have fewer complications than controls. There is no convincing evidence that periumbilical infiltration of ATS has a significant effect on the outcome of neonatal tetanus.

Paraldehyde for immediate control of spasms, followed by phenobarbital and chlorpromazine or diazepam for continued sedation, is effective in the control of spasms. Combination therapy using phenobarbital, chlorpromazine and diazepam may help reduce mortality (Kurtoglu et al. 1998). The mortality from neonatal tetanus has been strikingly reduced by the use of muscle relaxants and IPPV, and this approach should be used wherever the facilities to apply it exist.

Prevention

Tetanus in the newborn can be prevented by aseptic management of the umbilical cord at birth. The persistence of neonatal tetanus in many developing countries reflects the lack of rudimentary obstetric services for large sections of the population. Education of traditional birth attendants in hygienic handling of the umbilical cord at birth has resulted in a sharp decline in the prevalence of neonatal tetanus.

Active immunisation of pregnant women with tetanus toxoid reduces the risk of the disease by almost 90% (Gupta and Keyl 1998). Two doses of tetanus toxoid, 0.5 ml each, separated by 2 months, affords excellent immunity, but even one dose is effective. Passive immunisation of neonates in high-risk circumstances with 750 units of ATS will provide protection.

Leprosy

Babies of mothers with leprosy

Babies of mothers with leprosy are of lower than average birthweight, with IUGR being observed as early as the 16th week of pregnancy. IgA antibodies to *Mycoplasma leprae* have been found in 30% of cord sera of babies of mothers with active lepromatous leprosy. Specific IgA and IgM anti-*M. leprae* antibody production occurs during the first 6 months of life of these babies infected in utero. The prevalence of leprosy in children under 2 years of age whose mothers have active lepromatous leprosy is 5%. Diagnosis in these children has been made with positive skin tests to *M. leprae*, together with a marked increase in serum IgA and IgM anti-*M. leprae* antibody activity.

Management

The pregnant mother should receive multidrug therapy of dapsone 2 mg/kg daily, clofazimine 1 mg/kg daily and rifampicin 10 mg/kg monthly. Folate supplements should be given. Clofazimine will turn her milk pink but women with leprosy should be encouraged to breastfeed their babies while they are receiving effective treatment. Heavy breast milk infection only occurs in advanced leprosy involving the nipple and milk ducts.

Newborn babies of mothers who were not treated during pregnancy should be treated with clofazimine 1 mg/kg daily, which may also be given to babies of treated women if indicated. Unlike dapsone, clofazimine will not induce haemolysis in children with glucose-6-phosphate dehydrogenase (G6PD) deficiency.

Congenital syphilis

Congenital syphilis remains an important worldwide problem, with 750 000–1.5 million cases estimated annually, most in resource-poor countries (Krüger and Malleyeck 2010). All women who have positive treponemal serology in pregnancy should be treated according to British Association for Sexual Health and HIV national guidelines for the management of syphilis (http://www.bashh.org/guidelines). All women with positive syphilis serology should also be offered screening for hepatitis B and C, HIV and other sexually transmitted infections.

After birth, all babies born to women with positive syphilis serology should be examined and have their blood sent for syphilis serology. Babies should be managed as 'possible' or 'unlikely' congenital syphilis depending on antenatally assessed risk category, including maternal treatment and the mother's serological response examination findings and the infant's postnatal serology results.

All women without documented antenatal syphilis serology should be offered a test immediately after birth. Women who acquire syphilis after a negative booking test in pregnancy are at very high risk of delivering a baby with congenital syphilis. The possibility of congenital syphilis should be considered in all babies with signs or symptoms regardless of maternal booking serology results, but especially if no antenatal maternal serology results are available.

The classic sequence of events in untreated syphilis in a woman of childbearing age is one or more miscarriages followed by stillbirth or the livebirth of an affected infant. Fetal infection occurs in 40–50% of women with primary syphilis. Reactive syphilis serology is a significant risk factor for perinatal mortality in developing countries, where the prevalence of seropositivity among pregnant women may be as high as 10%.

Clinical manifestations of congenital syphilis

The commonest early abnormality in babies with congenital syphilis is hepatitis, so syphilis serology should be requested on any baby with unexplained abnormal liver function tests.

Early-onset congenital syphilis may present with general constitutional disturbance such as anaemia, oedema, jaundice, failure to thrive and pyrexia, in the absence of the more typical mucocutaneous lesions and other local signs of the disease. Conversely, the infant may initially show quite florid mucocutaneous lesions in the absence of significant constitutional disturbance (Bennett et al. 1997). Hepatomegaly is usual and splenomegaly and lymphadenopathy are common. A characteristic early sign is rhinitis, and ulceration of the nasal mucosa produces a profuse mucopurulent discharge which may be blood-stained and frequently causes excoriation around the nose and on the upper lip. Destruction of the nasal cartilage and bone will in time produce the flattened nasal bridge and 'saddle nose' of congenital syphilis.

Skin eruptions vary in character and distribution. Usually the rash is maculopapular, but circinate lesions occur and are among the most characteristic eruptions. Involvement of the skin of the palms and the soles provides one of the typical localising features of the rash of congenital syphilis. Lesions at the mucocutaneous junctions of the mouth, nose, anus and vulva are common and produce moist fissuring and bleeding. Healing of deep fissures around the mouth leads to radiating scars called rhagades, one of the typical stigmata of congenital syphilis. Flat raised plaques with moist surfaces, called condylomata, may occur around the anus and female genitalia. Osteochondritis is a frequent and typical manifestation of the disease and may present as dactylitis, fracture or pseudoparalysis. Pulmonary abscesses may occur (Bell and Taxy 2002).

Signs of meningitis may occur with congenital syphilis, as may evidence of hydrocephalus. The classic changes in the CSF are a moderate increase in cells, mainly lymphocytes, an increased protein, normal sugar levels and positive serological tests for syphilis.

Investigation and diagnosis

If there are any symptoms on examination, obtain liver function tests, full blood count and long-bone X-rays (see below). HIV, hepatitis B and C status should be checked as women can catch these infections whilst pregnant. A negative test at booking is not a guarantee of negativity at delivery.

Direct identification of treponemes

Treponemes are identified by darkfield microscopy from lesions of placenta, cord, fluid from any skin lesions or nasal discharge, CSF or skin. There is a high false-negative rate.

PCR is not yet routinely available.

Culture is not relevant – the organism does not grow in any culture medium.

Serology

Non-treponemal tests

These include the Venereal Disease Research Laboratory (VDRL) test. A fourfold decrease in titre suggests effective treatment. A fourfold increase after treatment suggests relapse or reinfection.

False-negative results occur in infants with acquisition of congenital syphilis in late pregnancy and in individuals with extremely high antibody titres prior to dilution (prozone phenomenon).

There are false-positive results in Epstein–Barr virus, varicella-zoster virus, hepatitis, measles, TB, subacute bacterial endocarditis, malaria, lymphoma, connective tissue disease, pregnancy, intravenous drug use and Wharton jelly contamination of cord blood samples. The VDRL titre correlates with disease activity.

Treponemal tests

- Screening enzyme-linked immunosorbent assay (ELISA: IgG and IgM combined)
- Fluorescent treponemal antibody absorption (FTA-Abs)
- *T. pallidum* particle agglutination (TPPA) test.

These tests may also be positive in other spirochaetal disease, for example yaws, pinta, leptospirosis, and Lyme disease. The patient will remain positive for life but titres correlate poorly with disease activity.

Transplacental antibody transmission occurs. In the infant transplacental non-treponemal antibodies wane in 4–6 months, whereas treponemal antibodies persist for longer than 1 year.

Serological screening should be performed on all infants born to infected mothers, especially those in the following groups:

- Inadequate maternal treatment or titres unknown
- Treatment with a non-penicillin regimen
- Maternal syphilis TPPA titre > 1 in 18 or failure of treatment to produce a fourfold reduction in VDRL titre
- Maternal syphilis treatment less than 1 month prior to delivery
- Infant symptomatic or antibody titre four times greater than that of mother at birth.

Quantitative non-treponemal and treponemal serology on serum (paired maternal and infant samples) is not routinely carried out but may be helpful. If maternal/infant paired serology is deemed

Table 39.8 Interpretation of serological tests for syphilis

NON-TREPONEMAL TESTS MOTHER	TREPONEMAL TESTS MOTHER	INTERPRETATION
−	−	No syphilis. However, very early syphilis in the mother and infant, or prozone effect is possible
+	−	No syphilis or false-positive mother. Passive transfer to infant may occur
+	+	Maternal syphilis with possibility of infant infection, or mother treated for syphilis during pregnancy or mother with latent syphilis and possibility of infant infection
−	+	Mother successfully treated for syphilis before or early in pregnancy, or mother with false-positive serology, e.g. yaws, pinta, Lyme

essential, current maternal serum should accompany that from the infant. These investigations should always be discussed with the microbiology team first (Table 39.8).

Table 39.8 is a guide and not the definitive interpretation of serological tests for syphilis. Maternal history is the most important aspect of the interpretation of test results. Factors which should be included are the timing of maternal infection, the nature and timing of maternal treatment, quantitative maternal and infant titres, and serial determination of test titres in both mother and infant.

Indications for CSF examination in the infant at risk of congenital syphilis

- Examination features suggestive of congenital syphilis
- Infant antitreponemal titre more than four times greater than maternal maternal titres
- Positive darkfield microscopy from lesion.

CSF investigations require at least 0.5 ml CSF; request cell count, protein, glucose, VDRL and TPPA titres with paired serum titres.

CSF is considered positive if there are increased white blood cells and protein and reactive TPPA and VDRL titres. (A negative VDRL does not exclude neurosyphilis.)

FTA has increased sensitivity but less specificity and is performed if the VDRL or TPPA is positive.

Radiology

The radiological signs of congenital syphilis may not be very evident in the immediate neonatal period, but become more obvious during the early months of life. They may show spontaneous regression after the sixth month. If present, radiological changes are usually multiple and widespread, and most easily evident around the wrists, elbows and knees. Osteochondritis is manifest by widening and alteration in the density of the epiphyseal line and by irregular destructive lesions in the epiphyseal end of the metaphyses. Periostitis can be widespread in the bones of the limbs and may also involve the skull.

Treatment

Penicillin is the drug of choice in treatment, preferably aqueous penicillin G (benzylpenicillin) 50000 units/kg (i.e. 30 mg/kg) intravenously, twice daily for 10 days. In circumstances where follow-up is unlikely or doubtful, and meningeal involvement has been excluded, long-acting benzathine penicillin 100000 units/kg may be given in a single intramuscular dose, although published evidence on the efficacy of this approach is lacking.

All pregnant women with positive syphilis serology must be referred to a genitourinary medicine clinic, and booked to see an obstetric consultant with specific expertise in caring for mothers with syphilis infection. All babies should be followed up by a neonatologist with specific expertise in infection or a paediatric infectious diseases consultant.

Perinatal viral infections

Several viral agents can cause serious neonatal illness with high mortality and morbidity rates. Most of these infections are acquired by vertical transmission, but some are the result of cross-infection postnatally.

HIV infection and AIDS

In 2010, an estimated 390,000 children were newly infected with HIV, the majority through mother-to-child transmission (MTCT) during pregnancy, delivery and/or breastfeeding (WHO 2011). The vast majority of these infections occur in sub-Saharan Africa owing to limited access to effective interventions for testing pregnant women, treating HIV-infected mothers and preventing MTCT. Without these interventions, MTCT rates ranges from 5% to 20% (WHO 2006). Recent UK guidelines for the management of paediatric HIV infection (the CHIVA guidelines) have been published (http://www.chiva.org.uk/health/guidelines/standards).

Risk factors for transmission

The risk of MTCT relates to the duration of ruptured membranes: membrane rupture for more than 4 hours before delivery is associated with an increased rate of MTCT. Risk of transmission is also related to the amount of virus to which the infant is exposed in utero, in cervicovaginal fluid during delivery, and through breast milk. Thus, the use of antiretroviral drugs can reduce MTCT by decreasing maternal viral load in these compartments, as well as providing antepartum and intrapartum prophylaxis for the infant. Another key component of prevention of MTCT is the administration of postpartum antiretroviral prophylaxis to the infant. The risk of transmission is heightened if the mother is severely immunodeficient, as evidenced by a low CD4 lymphocyte count and the presence of immune complex-dissociated p24 antigenaemia, which may in turn be reflections of a high maternal viral load. Preterm birth is associated with a higher transmission rate, and in a European Collaborative Study (1991), babies of less than 34 weeks' gestation were three times more likely to be infected than mature babies. How much of this effect is directly due to HIV status and how much to confounding factors, such as intravenous drug abuse, is unclear. Breastfeeding is an established mechanism for vertical transmission of HIV, but recent advances in maternal and infant prophylaxis may reduce the rates of MTCT in resource-poor countries where breastfeeding is of critical overall benefit to the infant (Mepham et al. 2011).

The number of new infections from MTCT has declined since prevention of MTCT services have expanded. However, limitations in resources and access to comprehensive HIV care services (testing and counselling, pre-, intra- and postnatal care, HIV care and treatment) continue to restrict the full implementation of successful prevention of MTCT programmes.

Recognising the rapidly emerging scientific understanding of HIV treatment and care, and the dynamics of scale-up efforts in resource-constrained settings, the WHO guidelines and recommendations are updated routinely every few years and are based on systematic reviews of the peer-reviewed literature.

In the UK in 1993, the vertical transmission rate was almost 20%, but this had fallen to just over 2% by 2004, by which time antiretroviral treatment was used in 97% of affected pregnancies.

Prevention of vertical transmission

The WHO recommends a four-component approach to the prevention of MTCT, including: (1) primary prevention of HIV infection in women; (2) prevention of unintended pregnancies; (3) prevention of MTCT in HIV-infected pregnant women; and (4) treatment and support of HIV-infected mothers and their families. Implementation of all four components is required in order to maximise program effectiveness and achieve the overall goal of improving maternal and child health in the context of the HIV pandemic.

The WHO publishes guidelines on the use of antiretroviral therapy (ART) in adults, including pregnant women (WHO 2006). In 2006, the WHO published guidelines on the use of antiretroviral drugs for the prevention of MTCT in HIV-infected pregnant women with the aim of reducing the proportion of infants infected with HIV by 50% by 2010. These guidelines issued recommendations based on an HIV-infected pregnant woman's need for ART for her own health as well as recommendations for prophylaxis to prevent HIV transmission to the fetus. The UK babies are managed by networks of professionals overseen by the Children's HIV association (CHIVA since 2002). CHIVA has a centralized website that provides information guidance and online support for professionals, parents and young people with HIV.

The British HIV Association has recently published detailed guidelines for managing HIV infection in pregnancy and preventing MTCT (de Ruiter et al. 2008). Management of the baby depends on the circumstances (PENTA 2009).

Diagnosis

For HIV in children aged less than 18 months, HIV infection should be diagnosed by a positive RNA or DNA PCR, and by positive serology in older children. A repeat test should always be performed to confirm the diagnosis. Maternal IgG to HIV crosses the placenta, resulting in all babies born to HIV-positive women being initially seropositive. Most non-infected children become seronegative by about 9 months of age, although some may remain so for up to twice as long. A small number of at-risk but seronegative infants have evidence of infection on clinical or virological grounds (Borkowsky et al. 1987). Because of the prolonged persistence of maternal antibody, an infant can only be declared free from HIV if

there are no stigmata of disease and the baby is free of antigen and antibody after 18 months of age.

PCR tests should be performed on day 1 (but not from cord blood, because of the risk of contamination by maternal blood) and at 1 and 3 months. If all of these tests are negative and the baby is not being breastfed, the baby can be declared free of infection with a high level of confidence, although not with absolute certainty.

Cross-infection

HIV is not a highly contagious disease, unless there is direct contact with the patient's body fluids. The number of hospital staff infected by contact with HIV-positive patients worldwide is in the region of 100 cases, and the estimated risk of acquiring infection from a single cutaneous exposure is 0.3% (95% CI 0.18–0.46%). Mothers who decline testing are more likely to be HIV-positive.

Breastfeeding and breast milk banking

The advice from both the American Academy of Pediatrics and the Department of Health is that HIV-positive mothers should not breastfeed. In resource-poor countries, the risk of HIV-acquistition from breastfeeding remains, as the decrease in mortality may outweigh the risk of acquiring HIV. A study in South Africa found that exclusive breastfeeding up to 6 months posed no additional risk over non-breastfeeding, whereas mixed breast/formula feeding posed a substantially increased risk of transmission (Coutsoudis et al. 2001). Beyond about 6 months of age, this risk/benefit balance of breastfeeding may reverse, possibly related to enteropathy and micronutrient deficiency following introduction of solids, and there is a significant late-postnatal rate of acquisition of HIV by babies of infected mothers of around 4% (Nduati et al. 1995).

Immunisation

Infants of HIV-positive mothers should be immunised at the normal times with diphtheria, pertussis and tetanus (DPT) vaccine using the Salk killed-polio vaccine. Measles, mumps and rubella (MMR) should also be given, as the severity of these illnesses, especially measles, is increased in infants with acquired immunodeficiency syndrome (AIDS). For measles immunisation to be maximally effective in HIV-infected children it should be given between 6 and 12 months of age.

Bacille Calmette-Guérin (BCG) should be withheld until results of testing are known, to avoid disseminated infection if immunodeficiency has developed. Hepatitis B vaccination is relatively unsuccessful in babies who subsequently progress to AIDS, and failure to seroconvert may be a marker for a poor prognosis. Infected infants may make suboptimal responses to other immunisations. By contrast, uninfected infants of HIV-positive South African mothers had lower specific antibody responses at birth compared to uninfected infants, but made robust responses to normal immunisation (Jones et al. 2011).

Prognosis

A few babies with undoubted HIV infection seem to recover completely and become seronegative (Bryson et al. 1995; Newell et al. 1996). For the rest, the prognosis is poor. In a large outcome study involving 2148 perinatally HIV-infected children, there was a 50% chance of developing AIDS, and a 25% chance of dying, by 5 years of age. The mean time from birth to developing AIDS was 4.8 years and the mean survival time was 9.4 years (Barnhart et al. 1996).

Early introduction of highly active ART (HAART) improves outcome, as demonstrated recently in Ukraine, the country with the highest prevalence in Europe (Mahdavi et al. 2010). The prognosis is worse in those born with hepatosplenomegaly or adenopathy, in those with a low proportion of CD4+ cells at birth, and in those who are culture- or PCR-positive (Smith et al. 2000). HIV-infected infants also exhibit impaired physical growth and development relative to controls. Respiratory infection and cor pulmonale are common findings, even in the first year of life. Early treatment, especially of *Pneumocystis carinii* pneumonia, may improve the outlook. In general, those who present early or are born prematurely do less well. Coinfection with CMV is associated with a more rapid disease progression (Kovacs et al. 1999).

Congenital HTLV I/II infection

These viruses, the cause of T-cell lymphoma and adult T-cell leukaemia, are carried by a large number of women from Japan and the Caribbean. In the UK, up to 5% of women in London of African-Caribbean descent are antibody-positive.

Although congenital infection with this virus is thought not to occur, some 40% of babies of infected women become infected, probably by breast milk (Nyambi et al. 1996). Seropositive women should therefore be counselled not to breastfeed their babies, with the intention of significantly reducing the incidence of lymphatic malignancy in their babies 50 years later.

Human papillomavirus

Perinatal transmission of human papillomavirus and the persistence of viral DNA in infants are well described, occurring in up to a quarter of exposed infants (Rombaldi et al. 2009). Infected infants may present with minor hyperplastic growths of the oral mucosa or, rarely, with laryngeal papillomatosis. The human papillomavirus is associated with anogenital carcinoma in adults, although the potential seriousness of perinatal transmission has yet to be established. The widespread introduction of human papillomavirus vaccination to teenage girls is likely to reduce the incidence of transmission to infants.

Herpesviruses

Herpes simplex virus

HSV is a large virus containing double-stranded DNA, which exists in two antigenically distinct forms: (1) HSV-1, the cause of oral or ophthalmic herpes, and sometimes encephalitis; and (2) HSV-2, the most common cause of genital herpes. Both HSV-1 and HSV-2 may cause neonatal infection, particularly in preterm infants, with an incidence in the UK around 1 per 50000 births (Tookey and Peckham 1996), but much higher in North America. Neonatal herpes is often fatal and neurological handicap is common in survivors.

Modes of transmission

Transplacental infection

Transplacental transmission of HSV is rare and usually associated with primary maternal infection with HSV-2. The congenitally infected baby is usually profoundly damaged with microcephaly or hydranencephaly, chorioretinitis and skin lesions, but occasionally may just have mild eye involvement. No treatment is available for these babies.

Vertical transmission

Neonatal HSV occurs as a result of maternal genital herpes in about 85% of cases, although most of the mothers are either asymptomatic at the time of birth or have no history of genital herpes. Rarely, the virus may reach the fetus in utero following prolonged rupture of the membranes, in which case the baby may be born with skin and eye lesions. This form of infection is rare and carries a relatively good prognosis with effective antiviral treatment (Whitley 1993). Usually, infection is acquired during passage down the birth canal. If the mother has an active primary infection at the time of vaginal delivery, the risk of neonatal infection is about 50% (Brown et al. 1987), but if the mother has a secondary recurrence of genital herpes the risk is only around 3% (Brown et al. 1991).

Nosocomial infection

HSV can be acquired from other neonatal cases, or from lesions in staff or family. The incidence of type 1 neonatal HSV is roughly double that of type 1 genital herpetic infections, suggesting that non-genital sources of neonatal infection may be more common than previously thought.

Clinical features

Neonatal HSV infection occurs in three forms, which may overlap: (1) superficial infection; (2) CNS disease; and (3) disseminated disease.

Superficial infection

Localised to skin, mouth and eyes, superficial infection ordinarily occurs during the second week of life and is usually associeted with recurrent maternal infection. The baby may develop a vesicular skin rash, keratoconjunctivitis or, rarely, intraoral vesicles. Although babies presenting with superficial infection generally do not develop disseminated disease, up to 30% may show subsequent neurodevelopmental abnormalities (Whitley 1993).

CNS disease

About one-third of babies with HSV infection present with isolated meningoencephalitis and symptoms similar to those seen in neonatal bacterial meningitis. The usual age of onset is around 10–14 days. Many subsequently develop cutaneous or ocular herpes. This form of the disease may result either from haematogenous spread or from retrograde axonal transmission of the virus to the CNS.

Disseminated disease

This most severe form of neonatal herpes presents during the first week of life, and is probably a viraemia with secondary seeding of the CNS. About half of the cases will have only system disease and/or pneumonia, but the rest will have coexisting meningoencephalitis. Twenty per cent have no cutaneous manifestations, making diagnosis difficult. Infants with disseminated disease present like any critically ill septic baby. They have respiratory distress as a result of pneumonitis, and usually require IPPV. They are often hypotensive, peripherally vasoconstricted, and have renal failure. Severe hepatitis or liver failure may occur with or without hepatosplenomegaly (Verma et al. 2006), and DIC, causing petechiae and generalised bleeding, is common. Hypotonia, seizures and coma are common whether or not meningoencephalitis is present. Pneumonia and pleural effusions may occur. Hydrops due to intrauterine HSV has been reported (Anderson and Abzug 1999).

Diagnosis

Vesicular cutaneous, ocular or oral lesions strongly suggest herpes. Other vesicular lesions, such as staphylococcal skin infection or varicella, are usually easily differentiated by the history and their clinical appearance.

The most rapid and useful diagnostic test is PCR for viral DNA on both serum and CSF. Negative results in a baby with clinically suspected HSV infection should not stop appropriate treatment being provided. Viral culture should also be undertaken on vesicle fluid, conjunctival scrapings, nasopharyngeal swab and, where obtained, CSF. The virus may also grow from blood. Serology is much less useful because of the difficulty in distinguishing between passively acquired maternal antibody and endogenously produced antibody.

In the absence of a maternal history of genital disease or of suspicious lesions, disseminated HSV infection will only be diagnosed if viral cultures are performed in investigation of septic babies from whom no bacterial pathogen is identified. Neonatal viral meningitis is usually a mild illness, so that if the CSF findings suggest it but the baby is seriously ill, herpes is the most likely diagnosis. In some cases of herpetic meningoencephalitis, however, the CSF may show findings similar to bacterial meningitis (Isaacs and Moxon 1991). If herpes is suspected, an EEG should be performed, as it may show characteristic temporoparietal high-voltage low-frequency activity. A CT scan should be performed to look for the characteristic necrosis and haemorrhage in the temporal lobes. These may only appear late in the disease, although MRI changes may occur earlier. Visceral calcification has been reported with disseminated disease.

If there is even a suspicion that systemic illness in a baby is due to herpes, treatment should be begun (see below) until a definite diagnosis is established. Nevertheless, some fulminating cases only come to light at postmortem.

Treatment

Aciclovir is the current drug of choice, given intravenously, 8-hourly, in a total daily dose of 30 mg/kg for at least 14 days. Topical aciclovir should be applied to eye and skin lesions. Consideration should be given to prolonging therapy in babies with a positive PCR test for HSV DNA at the end of a normal course of treatment.

Prognosis

The mortality rate for disseminated disease is now between 35% and 60%, and for disease isolated to the CNS between 10% and 15%. HSV-2 carries a much higher mortality rate than HSV-1. In terms of morbidity, the picture remains poor, with major adverse sequelae in some 85% of survivors of disseminated disease and in 50–75% of survivors of meningoencephalitis (Isaacs and Moxon 1991). HSV-2 infection has a worse prognosis than HSV-1: in one study, only 25% of babies with HSV-2 infection were normal on follow-up compared to 100% of those with HSV-1 (Corey et al. 1988). An abnormal EEG in the neonatal period is a poor prognostic sign (Thompson and Whitley 2011).

Recurrent infection

Despite apparent complete resolution of the initial infection, there is a high incidence of late recurrence due to poor immunological response to the virus. The virus, however, remains sensitive to further courses of antiviral drugs. There is no good evidence supporting prophylactic antiviral therapy.

Prevention

The risk of transplacental infection is low and the risk of neonatal infection is extremely small in babies born to asymptomatic HSV excretors (Brown et al. 1991). However, most cases of neonatal herpes occur in babies whose mothers have no history of genital herpes or evidence of intrapartum infection. Thus there is no good evidence favouring routine screening for HSV during pregnancy or elective caesarean section in asymptomatic women with a history of herpes. By contrast, the risk of neonatal infection after vaginal delivery when the mother has overt primary genital herpes is around 50%, but falls to below 20% if delivery is by caesarean section within 24 hours of membrane rupture.

Postnatally, the baby of the mother with covert genital herpes requires no treatment. Following vaginal delivery in the presence of overt genital herpes, the baby should stay with the mother and be treated with intravenous aciclovir. If the mother has orolabial or cutaneous herpes, the baby should stay with her but her lesions should be covered, treated with topical aciclovir, and her hand-washing technique should be meticulous. Other family members or staff with open herpes should stay away.

Varicella-zoster virus

This member of the herpesvirus family causes varicella (chickenpox) as an acute primary infection, but when reactivated from its dormant site in the dorsal root ganglia it causes the cutaneous eruption known as zoster (shingles). Primary infection can occur in the fetus and newborn, sometimes with devastating effect. Reactivation of the virus to cause zoster is rare in the newborn period. Primary varicella-zoster infections can be classified as congenital, perinatal or postnatal.

Perinatally acquired varicella

If a mother develops varicella during the 3 weeks prior to delivery, there is a 25% chance of her baby developing the illness. The usual interval between the onset of the rash in the mother and the infant is 9–15 days, so the timing of birth in relation to maternal infection is critical to outcome. Babies born 5 or more days after the mother develops the rash receive transplacental immunity, and have an excellent prognosis. Babies born less than 5 days after the mother develops the rash develop the disease some 5–10 days after delivery and have high mortality. Varicella acquired later in the neonatal period is usually, though not always, a benign disease. The disease in the newborn can range from a few vesicles in a relatively well baby to severe disseminated infection complicated by pneumonitis and with high mortality.

Treatment

Babies born to mothers who develop varicella between 7 days antenatally and 7 days postnatally should receive a dose of zoster immune globulin (ZIG), 100 mg, as soon after delivery or onset of maternal symptoms as possible. This reduces the severity of the disease in the baby but will usually not prevent it (Miller et al. 1989). If vesicles develop despite use of ZIG, aciclovir should be considered, as there have been reports of death in ZIG-treated infants (Holland et al. 1986). Babies born to mothers with perinatal varicella should be isolated from other babies from birth. If a baby is exposed to varicella postnatally, the decision about treatment depends on the infant's varicella-zoster virus serology. If the baby has varicella-zoster virus antibody, there is no need to give ZIG, unless the baby is more than 2 months old and still in a NICU.

Enteroviruses

These are small spherical viruses containing a single strand of RNA (Sawyer 1999). There are traditionally three main subgroups, polioviruses, echoviruses and coxsackieviruses, but newly classified enteroviruses may also cause disease in infants (Tebruegge and Curtis 2009).

Most neonatal enterovirus infections are mild and occur after the first week, often coinciding with epidemics in the community. Although poliovirus infections are rare, both echoviruses and coxsackieviruses regularly cause serious neonatal infection. Enterovirus infection in the newborn can be acquired by both vertical and horizontal transmission. Infection due to vertical transmission tends to be more severe and earlier in onset.

Echovirus

Many neonatal echovirus infections are asymptomatic, but some antigenic types, for example 6, 7, 11, 12, 14 and 17, can cause serious disease. Most commonly the infant presents with fever, malaise and mild gastrointestinal upset lasting for 3 or 4 days, and a full recovery is made. Infants can also present with viral meningitis, usually mild, and usually with a good outcome. Severe viraemic illness is most often caused by serotypes 6, 7 and 11, and is often acquired vertically. It is a serious infection, usually associated with hepatitis and often with meningoencephalitis, pneumonitis, myocarditis, gastroenteritis and DIC (Tebruegge and Curtis 2009). There is often rapid deterioration, with acidaemia, jaundice, apnoea, internal and external haemorrhage, and profound hypotension resistant to volume expansion and inotropic drugs. Renal failure often develops and bone marrow failure has been reported. A large survey found an overall mortality rate of 31% (Abzug 2001). The autopsy findings are characteristic, with massive hepatic necrosis and haemorrhagic necrosis of adrenals, renal tubules and myocardium.

Coxsackievirus

Coxsackievirus infections can be acquired by both vertical and horizontal transmission. Most neonatal infections are due to type B. The spectrum ranges from a mild febrile illness, with or without diarrhoea, to meningoencephalitis, myocarditis and a severe viraemic illness similar to that seen with the echoviruses. Sometimes a biphasic illness is seen, with apparent recovery in between a mild illness and a fatal myocarditis. Coxsackievirus infections are often accompanied by a rash, which is sometimes petechial.

Coxsackievirus B myocarditis may present gradually with tachycardia, breathlessness and poor feeding, or acutely with circulatory collapse. There is invariably cardiomegaly, often a murmur, and the electrocardiogram shows ST-segment depression and sometimes a supraventricular tachycardia. Viral RNA can be demonstrated in the myocardium using PCR. This illness carries a high mortality rate and is often associated with signs of encephalitis or hepatitis.

Meningoencephalitis usually occurs in small epidemics, and outbreaks due to many group A and B serotypes have been reported. The CSF shows a typical picture of viral meningitis and the virus can be grown from a throat swab, stools or CSF. The infant is rarely severely ill and usually recovers completely within 7–10 days. Neurological sequelae are extremely unusual.

Poliomyelitis

Neonatal polio is rare outside the developing world, typically presenting with fever, listlessness, poor feeding, diarrhoea and flaccid paralysis of one or more limbs. There is often a CSF pleocytosis, and virus can usually be grown from the stools and CSF.

Treatment of enterovirus infections

The only antiviral agent that has been used with apparent success in severe neonatal enteroviral infection is pleconaril, given enterally at a dose of 5 mg/kg 8-hourly (Aradottir et al. 2001). Injections of pooled IVIG have had variable success (Abzug 2001). Fulminant liver failure may occasionally be managed by liver transplantation.

Measles

Measles in pregnancy is rare outside the devleoping world. There is a substantial complication rate among pregnant women with measles, with high hospitalisation rates and pneumonia in around a quarter of cases. Measles in pregnancy causes high rates of fetal loss and prematurity. Maternal infection around delivery may cause illness in the infant during the first 10 days; this is usually mild but sometimes may be severe with pneumonia (Narita et al. 1997).

Neonatal hepatitis

Neonatal hepatitis can be due to congenital, perinatal or postnatal infections. The main congenital causes are rubella, CMV, HSV, toxoplasmosis and syphilis. Perinatal infections include HSV, CMV, enteroviruses, varicella, adenovirus and specific hepatitis viruses. CMV is the only common postnatal cause of viral hepatitis.

Clinical presentation

Infants with congenital infective hepatitis are usually jaundiced within 24 hours of birth. Of the perinatally acquired causes of hepatitis, only HSV is likely to present within the first week. Hepatitis A, B and C usually present towards the end of the neonatal period. Acquired CMV usually comes from blood transfusion and often presents in the postneonatal period in transfused infants.

Babies with hepatitis are jaundiced and unwell. They usually have hepatosplenomegaly and often have dark urine and pale stools. A considerable proportion of the total bilirubin is conjugated and the liver enzymes are elevated. The commonest differential diagnosis is from conditions such as inspissated bile syndrome following haemolytic jaundice, TPN-related cholestasis and α_1-antitrypsin deficiency. The more complex metabolic possibilities and whether or not the infant has biliary atresia are outlined.

Hepatitis A

Transplacental and perinatal hepatitis A infection is rare. Epidemics of hepatitis A in neonatal units have been reported, some associated with transfusion and others with postnatal transmission from a mother. No treatment for hepatitis A is available, but prophylactic pooled immunoglobulin is usually given to exposed infants.

Hepatitis B

Epidemiology and vertical transmission

The majority of the 300 million asymptomatic carriers of hepatitis B virus (HBV) live in developing countries. Forty per cent of children with persistent infection eventually die as a result of chronic liver disease and carcinoma. The prevalence of hepatitis B surface antigen, (HBsAg) varies from 0.1% in parts of Europe and North America to around 20% in parts of Africa and East Asia. Transplacental passage of HBV is uncommon. Perinatal infection is caused by exposure to HBV-containing maternal blood or secretions. The risk of infection is high for babies born to carrier mothers in countries with high carrier rates, such as Taiwan, where the perinatal transmission rate is about 40%. Chinese HBsAg carrier mothers transmit infection more frequently to their infants than carriers among Africans, Asians or Caucasians in the UK. The presence of 'e' antigen, HBeAg, in the mother's blood greatly increases the risk of infection in the baby. More Chinese women carriers are HBeAg-positive than are African carrier mothers. Of children born to Chinese carrier mothers, between 40% and 70% become carriers; to African mothers, about 30%; to Indian mothers, 6–8%; and to European mothers, almost none.

Clinical picture

The majority of infected infants do not develop neonatal jaundice and remain asymptomatic. They seroconvert for HBsAg between 6 weeks and 4 months after birth, most becoming chronic carriers. A small number of infants develop fulminant hepatitis. The major long-term sequela is the devlopment of chronic liver disease and primary hepatic carcinoma in adulthood.

Management and prevention

Once the carrier state has developed, it cannot currently be terminated. Prevention is therefore extremely important, and regimens based on a combination of active and passive immunisation are most effective (Romano et al. 2011).

Current recommendations for preventing perinatal transmission of hepatitis B in the UK are shown in Table 39.9. The majority of hepatitis B-positive mothers are of low infectivity with hepatitis B e antigen-negative/e antibody-positive results. Babies born to those of high infectivity, i.e. with either positive hepatitis B e antigen or no hepatitis B eAg-antibody, should in addition receive hepatitis B immunoglcbulin as soon as possible after birth. If properly implemented, they are 85–95% effective in preventing perinatal transmission of the virus. The initial dose of vaccine should be given within 12 hours of birth. Immunisation with hepatitis B vaccine is very effective and serious adverse effects are extremely rare. Further doses of vaccine are given at 1, 2 and 12 months of age and a good deal of effort is required to ensure a complete and effective programme. Serological testing should be undertaken at 12–15 months of age, primarily to check that the baby has a negative hepatitis B surface antigen (HepBSAg) result, indicating success of vaccination at preventing viral transmission. If there is sufficient serum, it is also advisable to check the hepatitis B antibody status as a marker of immune response to vaccination. Babies in whom immunoglobulin as well as vaccine is indicated should receive 200 IU (one vial) of human hepatitis B immunoglobulin (HBIG) by intramuscular injection, within 12 hours of birth if possible.

Breastfeeding should not be discouraged, because transmission of the virus through breast milk or by ingestion of blood from excoriated nipples is negligible compared with the infant's exposure to contaminated maternal blood at delivery. Furthermore, the dangers of not breastfeeding in developing countries outweigh the very small chance of the baby becoming infected exclusively by the breast milk of the carrier mother.

Hepatitis C

Hepatitis C (HCV) can be transmitted vertically, especially when the mother is coinfected with HIV (Valladares et al. 2010). Breastfeeding, however, seems relatively safe (Lin et al. 1995). HCV RNA should be measured at 3–6 months and serology (and HCV RNA) at 12–18 months. This follow-up is recommended for all babies of all HCV mothers. Although maternal viral load in pregnancy determines the risk of transmission, negative results are reassuring and if the baby becomes infected with HCV, prompt referral to a children's liver unit is indicated.

Other hepatitis viruses

Vertical transmission of hepatitis E causing serious neonatal hepatitis is well documented in developing countries (Khuroo et al. 2009). Hepatitis E virus infection in those surviving the neonatal period appears to be self-limiting.

Parasitic infections

Pneumocystis carinii

Pneumocystis carinii infection in the developed world now occurs almost exclusively among babies with underlying

Table 39.9 Interpretation of hepatitis B serology markers

INTERPRETATION	HBsAg	HBeAg	ANTI-HBc	ANTI-HBc IgM	ANTI-HBs	ANTI-HBe
No previous infection with HBV or early incubation	−	NA	−		−	NA
Convalescent or past infection	−	NA	+	−	±	NA
Immunisation to HBsAg	−	NA	−	−	±	NA
Acute infection	+	−	−	±	−	−
Acute infection, high infectivity	+	+	±	+	−	−
Acute infection, low infectivity	+	−	±	+	−	+
Chronic infection, high infectivity	+	+	+			−
Chronic infection, low infectivity	+	−	+	−	−	+

HBV, hepatitis B virus; HBsAg, hepatitis B surface antigen, which is the envelope protein; anti-HBs, antibody to HBsAg; anti-HBc, antibody to hepatitis B core antigen; HBeAg, antigen associated with the nucleocapsid, also found as soluble protein in serum; anti-HBe, antibody to hepatitis Be antigen.
+ positive; − negative; ± positive or negative; NA, not applicable.

immunodeficiency, often in combination with CMV infection. The presentation is usually insidious, with progressive respiratory distress and a diffusely hazy CXR. The diagnosis requires a high level of clinical suspicion and may be confirmed by direct microscopy of bronchial lavage material, although lung biopsy is much more likely to be successful. Treatment is with high-dose co-trimoxazole or, if this is not successful, with pentamidine.

Malaria

Pregnancy is associated with an increased susceptibility to malaria and with more severe infection. Parasitaemia and parasite density are higher in primigravidae than in multigravidae, and both decline progressively with parity. Involvement of the placental tissue is common, but fetal infection is relatively uncommon in endemic areas where there are high rates of maternal immunity. The risk of fetal infection increases with both the density of maternal parasitaemia and the severity of involvement of the placenta. Simultaneous maternal HIV infection also increases the risk of fetal infection.

Congenital malaria

In endemic areas it is difficult to distinguish congenital malaria from malaria acquired soon after birth, because the life cycle of the protozoon means that symptoms from congenital malaria may be delayed for weeks or months. Infection may occur with *Plasmodium falciparum*, *P. vivax* and *P. malariae*, and there is no evidence that one of these organisms is more likely to cause a congenital infection than any of the others. Recent data from Indonesia suggest that *P. vivax* may cause particular clinical problems in young infants (Poespoprodjo et al. 2009). Congenital malaria is much more likely to occur when the mother has a clinical attack of malaria during pregnancy than when she has a chronic subclinical infection. This is mainly due to protection from maternally derived IgG antibody, which may protect the fetus even when there is major placental invasion.

Malarial parasites find it harder to thrive in erythrocytes containing fetal haemoglobin. This may explain the high gene frequencies of the thalassaemias and sickle-cell anaemias in malaria-endemic areas.

The prevalence of malaria in pregnancy in endemic countries has been reported to be in the range of 10–60%, depending on season and location. The incidence of parasitaemia in newborn infants may exceed 20%. Congenital malaria usually presents between 10 and 26 days of age, with the same symptoms as the acquired disease, i.e. fever, jaundice, severe anaemia and massive splenomegaly. Non-specific findings include poor feeding and failure to thrive, loose stools and diarrhoea. In the tropics, many infants with congenital malaria also suffer from other infections such as septicaemia and pneumonia. An exclusive breast milk diet may limit malarial infection in infants by depriving the parasite of *para*-aminobenzoic acid, which is required for its growth in the erythrocyte.

Treatment

Chloroquine is the drug of choice in the treatment of congenital malaria, particularly in regions of stable malaria. Quinine is preferred for treatment in regions of chloroquine-resistant *P. falciparum* malaria and in most regions of unstable (epidemic) malaria, but care is needed as cardiac arrhythmias (prolonged QT interval and T-wave flattening), hypotension and hypoglycaemia may follow rapid intravenous infusion.

Chloroquine will eliminate sensitive strains of *P. falciparum*, *P. vivax*, *P. malariae* and *P. ovale*, but it will not prevent relapses of

P. vivax and *P. ovale* infection. To ensure eradication of the exoerythrocytic forms of *P. vivax* and *P. ovale*, a 14-day course of primaquine is given following the chloroquine. Primaquine should not be administered to infants with G6PD deficiency, because of the danger of haemolysis.

Babies who require blood transfusions or exchange transfusion in areas in which malaria is endemic may be at risk of transfusion-acquired malaria. It is recommended that these infants receive a curative course of chloroquine following their transfusion. In areas now known to have chloroquine-resistant malaria, the treatment described above should be prescribed.

Trypanosomiasis

Trypanosomes are protozoa that cause two distinct diseases in humans. African sleeping sickness is caused by *Trypanosoma (brucei) gambiense* and *T. (brucei) rhodesiense* and is transmitted by *Glossina* (tsetse) flies. Chagas' disease, found in Latin America, is caused by *T. cruzi* and transmitted by large Triatomidae bugs.

African trypanosomiasis

Trypanosomiasis during pregnancy often leads to abortion, hydramnios and preterm delivery. Congenital African trypanosomiasis has been reported with both *T. gambiense* and *T. rhodesiense*, although most cases involve *T. gambiense*. Fever and anaemia, with trypanosomes in the blood and/or CSF of the infant in the first weeks of life, is the usual presentation of congenital infection. In congenital infection in endemic areas, trypanosomes are found in the CSF by the end of the first week even before they are detected in the blood. Increased rouleau formation in the blood should raise the suspicion of trypanosomiasis. IgM is usually high in the blood and low in the CSF during the neonatal period in infected infants. Lymphadenopathy is not a feature of the congenital disease, although it is characteristic of infection acquired after birth.

Management

Treatment is hazardous because highly toxic drugs such as suramin, an organic urea, and melarsoprol, an arsenical compound, have to be used.

Congenital Chagas' disease

Chagas' disease is a major public health problem in South and Central America. Studies in Chile, Argentina and Brazil have shown that 0.5–2% of low-birthweight infants have congenital Chagas' disease (Greene et al. 1990).

T. cruzi enters the fetal circulation through the placental trophoblast in acute, latent or chronic maternal disease. In most cases of transplacental infection the mother is asymptomatic. The diseased placenta is large and may be indistinguishable from the placentitis of syphilis or toxoplasmosis. Abortions occur when the placenta is massively diseased. Congenital Chagas' disease has been observed to recur in subsequent pregnancies.

Most newborn infants with Chagas' disease are of low birth-weight and may be either preterm or small for dates. Clinical manifestations of congenital infection may be obvious at birth or occur after a few months. Anaemia, jaundice, oedema, petechiae, hepatosplenomegaly, tremor and convulsions are common features. Dysphagia, with inflammatory infiltration of the oesophagus and absence of nerve cells of the myenteric plexus, interferes with feeding and has been described in a few cases. Prognosis of congenital infection depends upon the intensity of parasitaemia.

Several organs, including the heart, oesophagus, brain, skin and skeletal muscle, show pathological changes, with inflammation, giant cells (a distinctive feature) and granulomas. Parasites have been found either in the muscle fibres or in the reticuloendothelial system. Long-term follow-up has shown a high frequency of neurological sequelae, such as mental retardation or behavioural and learning disabilities.

Diagnosis

Diagnosis of congenital Chagas' disease in the newborn is made on the presence of *T. cruzi* amastigotes in the blood using a fresh thin blood smear or a thick drop preparation. An indirect immunofluorescence reaction detects IgM of fetal origin specific for *T. cruzi*. Direct agglutination testing and ELISA may also be used.

Management

No satisfactory treatment for Chagas' disease is currently available. Symptomatic treatment for heart failure may help, but the prognosis remains gloomy because *T. cruzi* invades many organs and there is no satisfactory drug to eradicate it. Nifurtimox, a nitrofuran derivative, has been used in the acute phase of the disease, with the elimination of parasitaemia and remission of clinical symptoms, but it is very toxic.

Amoebiasis

Entamoeba histolytica, a unicellular protozoal parasite, has a global distribution and frequently causes intestinal disease in warm climates in communities with poor sanitation. Pregnant women may transmit the parasite to their newborn infants through faecal contamination at birth. The infant will usually present with bloody diarrhoea within a few days of birth (Rennert and Ray 2000). Amoebic proctocolitis and liver abscess have been reported. Treatment is with metronidazole.

Non-bacterial congenital infections

Congenital rubella

The incidence of congenital rubella is now less than 2 cases per 100 000 births in countries with high rates of immunization, although the WHO (2005) estimates that there are currently 100 000 cases per year in the developing world. The effectiveness of the programme is monitored in the UK by the National Congenital Rubella Surveillance Programme (http://bpsu.inopsu.com/studies/congenital_rubella/protocol.pdf).

Pathogenesis

The embryo or fetus becomes infected with rubella virus transplacentally during maternal viraemia. The placenta often sustains cellular and tissue damage in the process, resulting in abortion, stillbirth or impaired fetal nutrition and oxygenation. In the embryo, the virus can cause widespread tissue injury and persists in the tissues until delivery and beyond. When infection occurs in the first 12–16 weeks of pregnancy there is virtually always embryonal or fetal infection. By the end of the second trimester, only a third of infected women transfer infection to their fetus. The risk of rubella-induced congenital abnormality also falls with advancing gestation. Malformations occur in 90% of infected infants whose mothers are infected in the first 2 months of pregnancy, but in only 50% of those infected in the third month and 20% of those infected

in the fourth and fifth months (Miller et al. 1982). Congenital rubella is rare after 20 weeks of gestation because of maturation of fetal immune mechanisms.

Clinical features

The extended rubella syndrome presents as a sick baby with jaundice, petechiae and hepatosplenomegaly. Eye and bone abnormalities may be found and a murmur heard. About one-third of affected babies are below the third centile for birthweight. A long-term follow-up of cases from the 1963–65 epidemic reported ocular disease in 78%, SNHL in 66%, psychomotor retardation in 62%, cardiac abnormalities in 58% and mental retardation in 42% (Givens et al. 1993).

Eye defects

Cataracts may be detected at birth and may affect the whole of the lens or be central. Glaucoma also occurs, and requires urgent treatment. Microphthalmia is common. A fine pigmentary retinopathy (pepper-and-salt retinopathy) may be seen.

Deafness

This is usually sensorineural and bilateral. It is caused by inflammatory changes within the cochlea or the organ of Corti and damage to these tissues is progressive. All babies suspected of congenital rubella should have auditory evoked responses checked as soon after delivery as possible.

Central nervous system

Microcephaly, delayed motor development, various types of cerebral palsy and mental retardation, often profound, are common in isolation or in combination.

Cardiovascular

Viral damage to the endothelium of large blood vessels results in a high incidence of patent ductus arteriosus and peripheral pulmonary artery stenosis.

Bone

In rubella osteitis there are irregular translucencies and an irregular trabecular pattern in the long bones. The radiological appearance is of a 'celery stick'.

Liver

Hepatitis causing prolonged jaundice is common in the extended rubella syndrome.

Thrombocytopenia

This is found in most neonatal cases of rubella, though rarely in cases presenting later.

Affected infants may present outside the neonatal period with neurological and eye defects, deafness and congenital heart disease. In infants presenting later with these conditions, it may not be possible to establish the diagnosis of congenital rubella by antibody studies, but culturing the virus from, for example, the lens at a cataract operation, strongly suggests prenatal infection. Infants presenting in the neonatal period, and those with a delayed presentation, may in later life develop a rubelliform rash, interstitial pneumonitis, hypogammaglobulinaemia, reduced cellular immunity, thyroid autoantibodies, thymic hypoplasia and diabetes mellitus.

Diagnosis

Congenital rubella is identified by culturing the virus from a throat swab or urine, and by demonstrating rubella-specific IgM in plasma. There is no value in screening otherwise normal small-for-dates babies for congenital rubella. Whenever the diagnosis is established in the UK, the baby must be notified to the Congenital Rubella Surveillance Programme.

Treatment

No specific treatment is available. Some babies with the extended rubella syndrome are quite ill and need intensive care. Platelet transfusion is often required, as is phototherapy or exchange transfusion. Cataracts and glaucoma must be treated early, and hearing aids fitted if there is any evidence of deafness.

The infants are highly infectious during the first few months of life and are a hazard to female members of the nursing and medical staff. Appropriate precautions should be taken, the most important of which is to ensure that these personnel are rubella-immune.

Prevention

In the UK in 1988, the immunisation policy was changed from one in which only schoolgirls were given monovalent rubella vaccine, to one of giving children of both sexes the rubella vaccine as part of the MMR vaccine (Tookey and Peckham 1999). The National Congenital Rubella Surveillance Programme survey in the UK has demonstrated the effectiveness of this change. The number of cases has dwindled to fewer than 10 cases annually since 1991, many in mothers born abroad who were not vaccinated. However, because of the risk to the fetus from secondary infection, pregnant women should avoid people with rubella.

Any woman who has a rubella contact or who develops a febrile, exanthematous illness in the first few months of pregnancy should have rubella serology checked as soon as possible, and again 2–3 weeks later. If both rubella IgM and IgG are present in the first sample, recent infection is very likely and termination of pregnancy should be offered. If there is a rising titre between the two samples, the same applies. If the IgG level shows no rise and the IgM level is low, the diagnosis of recent infection remains in doubt and decision-making should reflect this uncertainty. Rubella RNA may be detected by PCR on tissue obtained by chorionic villous sampling or amniocentesis early in the second trimester if confirmation of fetal infection is required.

Congenital cytomegalovirus

Epidemiology and incidence

CMV is the commonest cause of congenital infection in the developed world, affecting 1–2% of infants worldwide, and has recently been reviewed in full by Luck and Sharland (2009). Up to 20% of babies who acquire congenital CMV die. CMV is estimated to cause up to 12% of all SNHL (Peckham et al. 1987) and 10% of cerebral palsy. A high viral load is associated with a greater risk of SNHL, even if babies are clinically asymptomatic (Boppana et al. 2005). There are large international differences in incidence, and the estimated frequency in the UK is 0.3–0.4% (Griffiths et al. 1991). In the UK, just over half of all women presenting at antenatal clinics are seropositive for CMV (Tookey et al. 1992).

The European Congenital CMV Initiative is a network of professionals with a united interest in CMV infection aiming to promote awareness of CMV infection, support and encourage research initiatives and provide a platform for a UK National CMV registry (www.ecci.ac.uk and www.ecci.nhs.uk). It is anticipated that, in the absence of randomised controlled study results, a registry of all babies in the UK treated for CMV will provide information on the optimal drug levels to maintain viral suppression, reasons for commencing treatment and side-effects of treatment. An additional Viral load and Immunology in Congenital CMV study is prospectively analysing viral load in symptomatic versus asymptomatic and treated versus untreated babies (www.ecci.ac.uk and www.ecci.nhs.uk).

Transmission

Unlike rubella and toxoplasmosis, congenital acquisition of CMV occurs as a consequence of both recurrent and primary infection. Mothers are often asymptomatic with primary infection. Primary infection is more likely to cause symptomatic congenital CMV and long-term sequelae than reactivation of infection. Primary infection may also increase the risk of abortion, stillbirth and fetal hydrops. Primary infection in the first trimester is more likely to result in neurological complications and SNHL (Pass et al. 2006).

The risk of transplacental transmission during reactivated infection is around 1% (as opposed to as high as 40% during primary infection), but the high incidence of CMV seropositivity among pregnant women worldwide means that transplacental transmission during reactivated infection accounts for 30–50% of congenital infections, and there are well-documented cases of women having two affected infants.

Clinical signs

Over 90% of infants with congenital CMV (culture- and IgM-positive) are asymptomatic in the neonatal period, but SNHL may be delayed and progressive (Pass 2005). Jaundice and thrombocytopenia should alert clinicians, especially if the baby is small for gestation or has IUGR. In the minority who are symptomatic, severe multisystem disease may be present which is clinically similar to congenital rubella or toxoplasmosis. CMV hepatitis can lead to intrahepatic and extrahepatic bile duct destruction as well as haemochromatosis. CMV infection of the fetal brain causes microcephaly, with calcification in periventricular areas where the infection has caused brain necrosis. These lesions are clearly seen on ultrasound scanning. The pattern of CNS damage probably varies with the timing of injury, so that lissencephaly is a feature of early injury, and polymicrogyria of slightly later injury. When the gyral pattern is normal, the injury has probably occurred in the third trimester of pregnancy. Hydrocephalus has been reported. Eye involvement, with chorioretinitis, cataract and blindness, occurs in 10–20% of cases presenting in the neonatal period. Pneumonitis may develop in the first few months after birth, even in infants who were initially asymptomatic.

Diagnosis

Fetal infection can be confirmed by cordocentesis or amniocentesis (fetal urine) in the mid second trimester and neonatal infection by blood sampling. Viral load can be best estimated by PCR.

Treatment

The benefit of treatment for congenital CMV remains uncertain and there are ongoing studies assessing the potential benefits of ganciclovir and its prodrug valganciclovir (which can be given orally) in reducing SNHL and neurodevelopmental delay (Sharland et al. 2011). Intravenous ganciclovir does suppress viral load but has short-term risks of neutropenia and the need for prolonged intravenous access, and theoretical risks of teratogenicity.

A recent phase III study of intravenous ganciclovir given to symptomatic babies, involving the CNS, recruited in the neonatal period demonstrated a reduction in extent of delay (Oliver et al. 2009). Having previously demonstrated a reduction in SNHL with valganciclovir treatment for 6 weeks in symptomatic babies with CNS involvement, a phase II study is currently recruiting to a study comparing reduction in SNHL with 6 weeks versus 6 months' oral valganciclovir therapy in symptomatic infants (Collaborative Antiviral Study Group: http://medicine.uab.edu/peds/CASG/75308/).

Predicting long-term sequelae

The mortality from symptomatic neonatal CMV infection is between 10%[1] and 30%, although much higher if the baby is premature. Thrombocytopenia and IUGR are independent risk factors for SNHL (Rivera et al. 2002). An abnormal computed tomography, head ultrasound scan or abnormal brainstem auditory evoked response also predicts poor outcomes (Boppana et al. 1997; Luck and Sharland 2009).

Prevention

There is no successful CMV vaccine. If primary CMV infection is suspected in pregnancy, prenatal diagnosis may be attempted by examination of amniotic fluid, fetal blood or chorionic tissue for specific IgM and the presence of the virus, by PCR. CMV-infected infants excrete the virus for months or years, and should be segregated from potentially pregnant female members of staff.

Congenital toxoplasmosis

Toxoplasmosis is caused by the intracellular protozoan parasite *Toxoplasma gondii*. The definitive host is the cat, but all mammalian and bird species can be infected. *Toxoplasma* organisms exist in three forms: (1) the oocyst, excreted in cat faeces; (2) the tachyzoite, which is the active form and can migrate in tissues; and (3) cysts which are latent and may be located throughout the body, presenting no risk to health (Krick and Remington 1978). In immunocompetent individuals, *Toxoplasma* will result in no symptoms or a self-limiting flu-like illness. Although infection of the fetus is not an inevitable outcome of every maternal *Toxoplasma* infection, there is a significant risk of adverse fetal outcome if infection does occur. The risk of transmission from mother to fetus increases depending in which trimester maternal infection is acquired. Based on a range of reported studies, the mean risk of transmission in the first trimester is estimated to be 10–15%, rising to 70–80% in the third trimester (Dunn et al. 1999; Thulliez 2001). Transmission of *Toxoplasma* to the fetus typically occurs after the placenta has become infected and is influenced by the development of placental blood flow; this may well explain the increased rate of transmission later in pregnancy.

While the risk of transmission is low in the first trimester, the outcome is more severe than if infection is acquired later in pregnancy. Infection acquired in the 2–3 months prior to pregnancy rarely presents a risk of fetal damage. The incidence in England and Wales has been estimated as 3.4/100 000 births, with retinochoroiditis and intracranial abnormalities being the most common features amongst livebirths (Gilbert et al. 2006).

Pathogenesis

Humans become infected either by direct contamination from infected cats or their excreta, or as a result of *Toxoplasma* entering the human food chain. If meat is not adequately cooked, *Toxoplasma* cysts are not destroyed and the organism is liberated during digestion.

Clinical features

The classic tetrad of congenital toxoplasmosis is hydrocephalus, epilepsy, cerebral calcification and chorioretinitis. This is the result of CNS infection which causes extensive cortical and periventricular necrosis. Necrotic tissue becomes calcified, and can then be seen as diffuse intrahemispheric calcification on ultrasound. Periventricular damage around the aqueduct of the midbrain may obstruct CSF flow and lead to congenital hydrocephalus. Many babies are born with subtle signs or no signs. In the months or years following birth a child may present with hepatosplenomegaly, jaundice, rash, deafness, cataracts, developmental delay or seizures; patchy myelitis with ascending paralysis has been reported (Al Shawan et al. 1996).

About a third of congenitally infected infants, i.e. around 5–10% of all babies born to mothers infected during pregnancy, have neonatal symptoms and about 25% of these die as a result. These babies are often small for dates and can present with the classic tetrad. Hydrocephalus may obstruct delivery or be noted at birth. Eye abnormalities may occur, including microphthalmia and cataract. Congenital toxoplasmosis can also present with the typical congenital infection syndrome of jaundice, hepatosplenomegaly and petechiae.

Investigation

As the clinical features of acute *Toxoplasma* infection are non-specific, diagnosis relies primarily upon serological tests. It is always useful to compare results from serial maternal samples if available. IgM immunosorbent agglutination assay (IgM ISAGA) is more sensitive then standard IgM assay but may not help in distinguishing acute infection as it can detect IgM persisting for longer than 1 year after infection has been acquired. If the serum is found to be positive for IgM using an appropriate assay, further specialist investigation should be considered, including IgG avidity testing and comparison of both IgG and IgM levels in sequential samples (Roberts et al. 2001). In the UK, samples are sent to the Toxoplasma Reference Unit, where initial investigation is undertaken using the Sabin–Feldman dye test (DT) and IgM enzyme immunoassay. The DT is the international 'gold standard' reference test for *Toxoplasma*, detecting both IgG and IgM. The DT can confirm whether the pregnant woman has become infected at any time previously with *Toxoplasma* and the detection of IgM can identify infections probably (but not invariably) acquired within the past 6–9 months.

When IgG and IgM are confirmed as being positive, further laboratory testing is required in order to provide a more precise estimate of the duration of infection.

Neonatal

Direct detection of the parasite is attempted by culture and PCR of the amniotic fluid and cord blood. Investigation for placental infection is less helpful as detection of parasite in the placenta alone cannot be considered as unequivocal confirmation of fetal infection.

Detection of neonatal IgM and IgA by enzyme immunoassay and/or ISAGA is regarded as being diagnostic for neonatal infection. IgM and IgA may only be present in 50–60% of congenitally infected children in the first month of life but may appear subsequently. It is therefore essential to monitor the child serologically throughout the first year of life, by which time any passively acquired maternal IgG antibodies will decline and disappear. The disappearance of IgG within the first year of life excludes congenital infection. Persistence of positive DT after 12 months confirms infection.

Clinical and ophthalmological examinations of the neonate must be performed together with an ultrasound of the brain.

Treatment

Toxoplasmosis is a potentially treatable condition but precise choice of management option depends on a range of factors, including stage of pregnancy, clinical picture, results of serology tests and parental choice. Early treatment of congenital toxoplasmosis appears to decrease the frequency of chorioretinitis and be associated with the disappearance of cerebral opacities.

If clinical benefit can be achieved by appropriate treatment, then the diagnosis of neonatal infection becomes crucial. This can be straightforward in a child with characteristic clinical and serological findings that are confirmed by parasite detection. Unfortunately, in the majority of cases the diagnosis is less straightforward and should be discussed with a microbiologist and paediatric infectious diseases specialist.

Prognosis

For seropositive infants with no intracranial calcification and, at most, chorioretinitis in the neonatal period, the long-term prognosis is relatively good, although new areas of chorioretinitis may appear in untreated patients until early adult life. For those with neurological features or systemic disease, the outlook without treatment is bleak. About a quarter die and most of the survivors are handicapped.

Congenital varicella

Ninety-five per cent of women of childbearing age in the UK have had varicella in childhood and are immune. Varicella in pregnancy is therefore rare and prospective studies have shown it to be no more severe than at other times of life. The incidence of varicella in pregnancy is around 5 cases per 10 000, and among those who develop varicella in early pregnancy, the risk of fetal damage is around 2% (Pastuszak et al. 1994).

VZV is teratogenic and infection during early pregnancy can cause chromosomal aberrations as well as a host of congenital structural defects, affecting the brain, eye, skeleton, gastrointestinal tract and renal tract. A particular feature of congenital varicella is cutaneous scarring in a dermatomal distribution. Limb defects may be associated with severe cutaneous scarring.

Prevention

Pregnant women who are exposed to varicella but are uncertain of their immune status should have their antibody levels checked. Most will be found to be immune. Infection after 20 weeks of gestation seems not to cause congenital varicella (see above). With modern techniques of fetal imaging and blood sampling, it is now possible to assess the fetus for congenital infection in time to terminate the pregnancy if indicated.

Congenital Epstein–Barr virus infection

Maternal infection with the Epstein–Barr virus is uncommon, as most women of childbearing age are immune. Whether or not maternal Epstein–Barr virus infection can cause fetal malformations is still unclear, but rare cases have been described with low birthweight, abnormal facies, eye defects and congenital heart disease.

Congenital parvovirus B19 infection

Human parvovirus B19 is best known as the cause of erythema infectiosum (fifth disease) in children. The virus has a predilection for rapidly dividing cells, including erythrocyte precursors, and can cause haemolytic anaemia in the fetus (Ware 1989). The incidence of parvovirus infection in pregnancy is in the range 0.3–3.7%. In almost 50% of these cases there is serological evidence of fetal infection, and in 1–2% of these, the infection results in abortion, stillbirth or hydrops (Public Health Laboratory Service 1990; Koch et al. 1998). Between 10% and 25% of cases of non-immune hydrops are thought to be related to parvovirus. Maternal infection between 9 and 20 weeks gives the highest risk of fetal hydops, with later infections appearing safer to the infant (Enders et al. 2010). In a significant proportion of cases the hydrops resolves as the infection subsides, but in the remainder the prognosis seems to be very poor, with many infants dying. In some survivors the anaemia persists into childhood, but in others lasts only for a few weeks (Brown et al. 1994; Tugal et al. 1994). Parvovirus can cause myocarditis, cardiomyopathy and liver disease, and neonatal meningitis has been reported.

Congenital infections in the developing world

The intrauterine infections described in industrialised countries also occur in developing countries. Congenital rubella probably occurs more frequently in the absence of routine immunisation, but congenital CMV infection is relatively uncommon because most women of childbearing age in the developing world possess antibodies to CMV. *Toxoplasma gondii* infects the fetus in the pregnant mother who eats inadequately cooked infected meat. Syphilis and TB are rife in many cities in the developing world. Malaria is endemic throughout the tropics, HBV infection is a major public health problem in South-East Asia and trypanosomiasis is endemic in tropical Africa. Congenital infections caused by these agents are encountered, but in the cases of TB, malaria and trypanosomiasis, congenital infections occur much less frequently than might be anticipated from the prevalence of these diseases in the population at large.

The clinical manifestations of congenital rubella, CMV, herpes simplex and toxoplasmosis in the tropics show no essential differences from those described in industrial countries, and will not be further considered in this section.

Other congenital infections

Various other organisms have been shown to cause congenital infection by direct transplacental or intrapartum spread. For further information on these and a fuller overview of infections causing neonatal disease, please refer to the *Textbook of Pediatric Infectious Diseases* (Feigin et al. 2009).

Weblinks

British Association of Perinatal Medicine, 2001. Standard for Hospitals Providing Neonatal Intensive and High Dependency care. Available online at: http://www.bapm.org/media/documents/publications/hosp_standards.pdf. 1–17. 2001.

Children's HIV Association (CHIVA) standards of care for infants, children, and young people with HIV (including infants born to mothers with HIV). Available online at: www.chiva.org.uk/guidelines/2009/pdf/chiva-standards2009.pdf

Health Protection Agency, 2006. Investigation of toxoplasma in pregnancy. National Standard Method QSOP 59 Issue 1. Available online at: http://www. hpa-standardmethods.org.uk/pdf_sops.asp.

Mahon, C.R., Lehman, D.C., Manuselis, G. Textbook of Diagnositic Microbiology, third ed. Elsevier. http://evolve.com/mahon/microbiology/

References

Ablow, R.C., Driscoll, S.G., Effmann, E.L., et al., 1976. A comparison of early-onset group B steptococcal neonatal infection and the respiratory-distress syndrome of the newborn. N Engl J Med 294, 65–70.

Abzug, M.J., 2001. Prognosis for neonates with enterovirus hepatitis and coagulopathy. Pediatr Infect Dis J 20, 758–763.

Adams-Chapman, I., Stoll, B.J., 2006. Neonatal infection and long-term neurodevelopmental outcome in the preterm infant. Curr Opin Infect Dis 19, 290–297

Ahmed, A., Hickey, S.M., Ehrett, S., et al., 1996. Cerebrospinal fluid values in the term neonate. Pediatr Infect Dis J 15, 298–303.

Airede, A.I., 1993. Neonatal bacterial meningitis in the middle belt of Nigeria. Dev Med Child Neurol 35, 424–430.

Akinbi, H.T., Narendran, V., Pass, A.K., et al., 2004. Host defense proteins in vernix caseosa and amniotic fluid. Am J Obstet Gynecol 191, 2090–2096.

Alarcon, A., Pena, P., Salas, S., et al., 2004. Neonatal early onset Escherichia coli sepsis: trends in incidence and antimicrobial resistance in the era of intrapartum antimicrobial prophylaxis. Pediatr Infect Dis J 23, 295–299.

Al Shahwan, S., Rossi, M.L., al Thagafi, M.A., 1996. Ascending paralysis due to myelitis in a newborn with congenital toxoplasmosis. J Neurol Sci 139, 156–159.

Almuneef, M.A., Baltimore, R.S., Farrel, P.A., et al. 2001. Molecular typing demonstrating transmission of Gram-negative rods in a neonatal intensive care unit in the absence of a recognized epidemic. Clin Infect Dis 32, 220–227.

Anderson, M S., Abzug, M.J., 1999. Hydrops fetalis: an unusual presentation of intrauterine herpes simplex virus infection. Pediatr Infect Dis J 18, 837–839.

Austin, N.C., Darlow, B., 2009. Prophylactic oral/topical non-absorbed antifungal agents to prevent invasive fungal infection in very low birth weight infants. Cochrane Database Syst Rev 7, CD003478.

Babl, F.E., Ram, S., Barnett, E.D., et al., 2000. Neonatal gonococcal arthritis after negative prenatal screening and despite conjunctival prophylaxis. Pediatr Infect Dis J 19, 346–349.

Backhed, F., Ley, R.E., Sonnenburg, J.L., et al., 2005. Host–bacterial mutualism in the human intestine. Science 307, 1915–1920.

Badri, M.S., Zawaneh, S., Cruz, A.C., et al., 1977. Rectal colonization with group B streptococcus: relation to vaginal colonization of pregnant women. J Infect Dis 135, 308–312.

Bagci, S., Eis-Hübinger, A.M., Yassin, A.F., et al., 2010. Clinical characteristics of viral intestinal infection in preterm and term neonates. Eur J Clin Microbiol Infect Dis 29, 1079–1084.

Banerji, A., Noya, F.J., 1999. Brain abscess associated with neonatal listeriosis. Pediatr Infect Dis J 18, 305–307.

Barnhart, H.X., Caldwell, M.B., Thomas, P., et al., 1996. Natural history of human immunodeficiency virus disease in perinatally infected children: an analysis from the Pediatric Spectrum of Disease Project. Pediatrics 97, 710–716.

Bedford, H., de Louvois, J., Halket, S., et al., 2001. Meningitis in infancy in England and Wales: follow-up at 5 years of age. Br Med J 323, 533–536.

Bedford Russell, A.R., 2009. The role of granulocyte colony-stimulating factor in augmenting human neonatal neutrophil host defence. University of London, MD thesis, pp. 115–119.

Bedford Russell, A.R., Murch, S.H., 2006. Could peripartum antibiotics have delayed health consequences for the infant? Br J Obstet Gynaecol 113, 758–765.

Bedford Russell, A.R., Steer, P.J., 2008. Antibiotics in preterm labour – the ORACLE speaks. Lancet 372, 1276–1278.

Bedford Russell, A.R., Rivers, R.P.A., Davey, N., 1993. The development of anti-HLA antibodies in multiply transfused preterm infants. Arch Dis Child 68, 49–51.

Bedford Russell, A.R., Emmerson, A.J.B., Wilkinson, N., et al., 2000. A trial of recombinant human granulocyte colony stimulating factor for the treatment of very low birthweight infants with presumed sepsis and neutropenia. Arch Dis Child Fetal Neonatal Ed 84, 172–176.

Beiter, A., Lewis, K., Pineda, E.F., et al., 1993. Unrecognized maternal peripartum pertussis with subsequent fatal neonatal pertussis. Obstetr Gynecol 82, 691–693.

Beitzke, H., 1935. Uber die angeborne tuberculose infektion Ergebnisse der Gesamten. Tuberkulose-Forschung 7, 1–30.

Bell, C., Taxy, J., 2002. Pulmonary abscesses in congenital syphilis. Arch Pathol Lab Med 126, 484–486.

Bell, T.A., Stamm, W.E., Kuo, C.C., et al., 1994. Risk of perinatal transmission of Chlamydia trachomatis by mode of delivery. J Infect 29, 165–169.

Benjamin, D.K. Jr, Poole, C., Steinbach, W.J., et al., 2003. Neonatal candidemia and end-organ damage: a critical appraisal of the literature using meta-analytic techniques. Pediatrics 112, 634–640.

Benjamin, D.K. Jr, Stoll, B.J., Gantz, M.G., et al., 2010. Neonatal candidiasis: epidemiology, risk factors and clinical judgement. Pediatrics 126, e865–e873.

Benn, C.S., Thorsen, P., Jensen, J.S., et al., 2002. Maternal vaginal microflora during pregnancy and the risk of asthma hospitalization and use of anti-asthma medication in early childhood. J Allergy Clin Immunol 110, 72–77.

Bennett, M.L., Lynn, A.W., Klein, L.E., et al., 1997. Congenital syphilis: subtle presentation of fulminant disease. J Am Acad Dermatol 36, 351–354.

Berger, A., Salzer, H.R., Weninger, M., et al., 1998. Septicaemia in an Austrian neonatal intensive care unit: a 7-year analysis. Acta Paediatr 87, 1066–1069.

Bergström, A., Byaruhanga, R., Okong, P., 2005. The impact of newborn bathing on the prevalence of neonatal hypothermia in Uganda: a randomized, controlled trial. Acta Paediatr 94, 1462–1467.

Bernstein, H.M., Pollock, B.H., Calhoun, D.A., et al., 2001. Administration of recombinant G-CSF to neonates with septicaemia: a meta-analysis. Pediatrics 138, 917–920.

Bin-Nun, A., Bromiker, R., Wilshanki, M., et al., 2005. Oral probiotics prevent necrotizing enterocolitis in very low birthweight neonates. J Pediatr 147, 192–196.

Bitner-Glindzicz, M., Pembrey, M., Duncan, A., et al., 2009. Prevalence of mitochondrial 1555A–>G mutation in European children. N Engl J Med 360, 640–642.

Bjornvad, C.R., Schmidt, M., Petersen, Y.M., et al., 2005. Preterm birth makes the immature intestine sensitive to feeding-induced intestinal atrophy. Am J Physiol Regul Integr Comp Physiol 289, R1212–R1222.

Black, S., Kushner, I., Samols, D., 2004. C-reactive protein. J Biol Chem 279, 48487–48490.

Bloom, B.T., Craddock, A., Delmore, P.M., et al., 2003. Reducing acquired infections in the NICU: observing and implementing meaningful differences in process between high and low acquired infection rate centres. J Perinatol 23, 489–492.

Blume-Peytavi, U., Cork, M.J., Faergemann, J., et al., 2009. Bathing and cleansing in newborns from day 1 to first year of life: recommendations from a European round table meeting. J Eur Acad Dermatol Venereol 23, 751–759.

Bombell, S., McGuire, W., 2009. Early trophic feeding for very low birth weight infants. Cochrane Database Syst Rev Jul 8 (3), CD000504.

Boo, N.Y., Chor, C.Y., 1994. Six year trend of neonatal septicaemia in a large Malaysian maternity hospital. J Paediatr Child Health 30, 23–27.

Boppana, S.B., Fowler, K.B., Vaid, Y., et al., 1997. Neuroradiographic findings in the newborn period and long-term outcome in children with symptomatic congenital cytomegalovirus infection. Pediatrics 99, 409–414.

Boppana, S.B., Fowler, K.B., Pass, R.F., et al., 2005. Congenital cytomegalovirus infection: association between virus burden in infancy and hearing loss. J Pediatr 146, 817–823.

Borer, A., Livshiz-Riven, I., Golan, A., et al., 2010. Hospital-acquired conjunctivitis in a neonatal intensive care unit: bacterial etiology and susceptibility patterns. Am J Infect Control 38, 650–652.

Borkowsky, W., Paul, D., Bebenroth, D., 1987. Human immunodeficiency virus in infants negative for anti-HIV by enzyme-linked immunoassay. Lancet I, 1168–1171.

Bowdish, D.M., Davidson, D.J., Hancock, R.E., 2005. A re-evaluation of the role of host defence peptides in mammalian immunity. Curr Protein Pept Sci 6, 35–51.

Boyce, J.M., Cookson, B., Christiansen, K., et al., 2005. Meticillin-resistant Staphylococcus aureus. Lancet Infect Dis 5, 653–663.

Boyer, K.M., 1995. Neonatal group B streptococcal infections. Curr Opin Pediatr 7, 13–18.

Boyle, R.J., Chandler, B.D., Stonestreet, B.S., et al., 1978. Early identification of sepsis in infants with respiratory distress. Pediatrics 62, 744–750.

Boyle, E.M., Ainsworth, J.R., Levin, A.V., et al., 2001. Ophthalmic Pseudomonas infection in infancy. Arch Dis Child Fetal Neonat Ed 85, F139–F140.

Brazy, J.E., Grimm, J.K., Little, V.A., 1982. Neonatal manifestations of severe maternal hypertension occurring before the thirty-sixth week of pregnancy. J Pediatr 100, 25–271.

Brodie, S.B., Sands, K.E., Gray, J.E., et al., 2000. Occurrence of nosocomial bloodstream infections in six neonatal intensive care units. Pediatr Infect Dis J 19, 56–62.

Bromiker, R., Arad, I., Peleg, O., et al., 2001. Neonatal bacteremia: patterns of antibiotic resistance. Infect Control Hosp Epidemiol 22, 767–770.

Brown, Z.A., Vontver, L.A., Benedetti, J., 1987. Effects on infants of a first episode of genital herpes during pregnancy. N Engl J Med 317, 1246–1251.

Brown, Z.A., Benedetti, J., Ashley, R., et al., 1991. Neonatal herpes simplex virus infection in relation to asymptomatic maternal infection at the time of labor. N Engl J Med 324, 1247–1252.

Brown, K.E., Green, S.W., Antunez de Mayolo, J., et al., 1994. Congenital anaemia after transplacental B19 parvovirus infection. Lancet 343, 895–896.

Bryan, C.S., John, J.F., Jr., Pai, M.S., et al., 1985. Gentamicin vs cefotaxime for therapy of neonatal sepsis. Relationship to drug resistance. Am J Dis Child 139, 1086–1089.

Bryson, Y.J., Pang, S., Wei, M.S., 1995. Clearance of HIV infection in a perinatally infected infant. N Engl J Med 332, 833–838.

Buonocore, G., Gioia, D., De Filippo, M., et al., 1994. Superoxide anion release by polymorphonuclear leukocytes in whole blood of newborns and mothers during the peripartal period. Pediatr Res 36, 619–622.

Burgner, D., Levin, M., 2003. Genetic susceptibility to infectious diseases. Pediatr Infect Dis J 22, 1–9.

Buttery, J.P., 2002. Blood cultures in newborns and children: optimising an everyday test. Arch Dis Child Fetal Neonatal Ed 87, F25–F28.

Cadnapaphornchai, M., Faix, R.G., 1992. Increased nosocomial infection in neutropenic low birth weight (2000 grams or less) in infants of hypertensive mothers. J Pediatr 121, 956–961.

Cairo, M.S., Worcester, C.C., Rucker, R.W., et al., 1992. Randomized trial of granulocyte transfusions versus intravenous immune globulin therapy for neonatal neutropenia and sepsis. J Pediatr 120, 281–285.

Campbell, J.R., 1996. Neonatal pneumonia. Semin Respir Infect 11, 155–162.

Campbell, J.R., Diacovo, T., Baker, C.J., 1992. Serratia marcescens meningitis in neonates. Pediatr Infect Dis J 11, 881–886.

Carr, R., Modi, N., Doré, C.J., et al., 1999. A randomised controlled trial of prophylactic GM-CSF in human newborns less than 32 weeks gestation. Pediatrics 103, 796–802.

Carr, R., Modi, M., Dore, C., 2006. G-CSF and GM-CSF for treating or preventing neonatal infection. Cochrane Database of Systematic Reviews, Issue 3.

Carr, R., Brocklehurst, P., Doré, C.J., et al., 2009. Granulocyte–macrophage colony stimulating factor administered as prophylaxis for reduction of sepsis in extremely preterm, small for gestational age neonates (the PROGRAMS trial): a single-blind, multicentre, randomised controlled trial. Lancet 373, 226–233.

Cassell, G.H., Waites, K.B., Watson, H.L., et al., 1993. Ureaplasma urealyticum intrauterine infection: role in prematurity and disease in newborns. Clin Microbiol Rev 6, 69–87.

Cebon, J., Layton, J.E., Maher, D., et al., 1994. Endogenous haemopoietic growth factors in neutropenia and infection. Br J Haematol 86, 265.

Cederbaum, S.D., Kaitila, I., Rimoin, D.L., et al, 1976. The chondro-osseous dysplasia of adenosine deaminase deficiency with severe combined immunodeficiency. J Pediatr 89, 737–742.

Centers for Disease Control, 2002. Prevention of perinatal group B streptococcal disease – revised guidelines from CDC. MMWR Morb Mortal Wkly Rep 51 (RR11), 1–22.

Chequer, R.S., Tharp, B.R., Dreimane, D., et al., 1992. Prognostic value of EEG in neonatal meningitis: retrospective study of 29 infants. Pediatr Neurol 8, 417–422.

Chidekel, A.S., Rosen, C.L., Bazzy, A.R., 1997. Rhinovirus infection associated with serious lower respiratory illness in patients with bronchopulmonary dysplasia. Pediatr Infect Dis J 16, 43–47.

Chiou, C.C., Soong, W.J., Hwang, B., et al., 1994. Congenital adenoviral infection. Pediatr Infect Dis J 13, 664–665.

Chirico, G., Ciardelli, L., Cecchi, P., et al., 1997. Serum concentration of granulocyte colony stimulating factor in term and preterm infants. Eur J Pediatr 156, 269.

Christensen, R.D., Rothstein, G., 1980. Exhaustion of mature marrow neutrophils in neonates with sepsis. J Pediatr 96, 316–318.

Chun, C.S., Brady, L.J., Boyle, M.D., et al., 1991. Group B streptococcal C protein-associated antigens: association with neonatal sepsis. J Infect Dis 163, 786–791.

Cigni, A., Cossellu, S., Porcu, A., et al., 2004. Meningococcal osteomyelitis in a premature infant. Ann Ital Med Int 19, 280–282.

Cimolai, N., Roscoe, D.L., 1995. Contemporary context for early-onset group B streptococcal sepsis of the newborn. Am J Perinatol 12, 46–49.

Clerihew, L., Lamagni, T.L., Brocklehurst, P., et al., 2007. Prophylactic systemic antifungal agents to prevent mortality and morbidity in very low birth weight infants. Cochrane Database Syst Rev 17, CD003850.

Colbourn, T., Asseburg, C., Bojke, L., et al., 2007. Prenatal screening and treatment strategies to prevent group B streptococcal and other bacterial infections in early infancy: cost-effectiveness and expected value of information analyses. Health Technol Assess 11, 1–226.

Corey, L., Whitley, R.J., Stone, E.F., et al., 1988. Difference between herpes simplex type I and type II neonatal encephalitis in neurological outcome. Lancet i, 1–4.

Cotten, C.M., McDonald, S., Stoll, B., et al., 2006. The association of third-generation cephalosporin use and invasive candidiasis in extremely low birth-weight infants. Pediatrics 118, 717–722.

Cotten, C.M., Taylor, S., Stoll, B., et al., 2009. Prolonged duration of initial empirical antibiotic treatment is associated with increased rates of necrotizing enterocolitis and death in extremely low birth weight infants. Pediatrics 123, 58–66.

Coutsoudis, A., Pillay, K., Kuhn, L., et al., 2001. Method of feeding and transmission of HIV-1 from mothers to children by 15 months of age: prospective cohort study from Durban, South Africa. AIDS 15, 379–387.

Covert, R.F., Schreiber, M.D., 1993. Three different strains of heat-killed group B beta-hemolytic streptococcus cause different pulmonary and systemic hemodynamic responses in conscious neonatal lambs. Pediatr Res 33, 373–379.

Dale, D.C., Cottle, T.E., Fier, C.J., et al., 2003. Severe chronic neutropenia: treatment and follow-up of patients in the Severe Chronic Neutropenia International Registry. Am J Hematol 72, 82–93.

Dale, D.C., Rosenberg, P.S., Alter, B.P., 2006. Lineage-specific hematopoietic growth factors. N Engl J Med 355, 527–528.

Daley, A.J., Isaacs, D., 2004. Ten-year study on the effect of intrapartum antibiotic prophylaxis on early onset group B streptococcal and *Escherichia coli* neonatal sepsis in Australasia. Pediatr Infect Dis J 23, 630–634.

Dammann, O., Leviton, A., 1997. Maternal intrauterine infection, cytokines, and brain damage in the preterm newborn. Pediatr Res 42, 1–8.

Daoud, A.S., Batieha, A., Al-Sheyyab, M., et al., 1999. Lack of effectiveness of dexamethasone in neonatal bacterial meningitis. Eur J Pediatr 158, 230–233.

Darville, T., 2005. *Chlamydia trachomatis* infections in neonates and young children. Semin Pediatr Infect Dis 16, 235–244.

Da Silva, O., Gregson, D., Hammerberg, O., 1997. Role of *Ureaplasma urealyticum* and

Chlamydia trachomatis in development of bronchopulmonary dysplasia in very low birth weight infants. Pediatr Infect Dis J 16, 364–369.

de Haas, M., Kerst, J.M., van der Schoot, C.E., et al., 1994. Granulocyte colony-stimulating factor administration to healthy volunteers: analysis of the immediate activating effects on circulating neutrophils. Blood 84, 3885–3894.

De Jonge, M., Burchfield, D., Bloom, B., et al., 2007. Clinical trial of safety and efficacy of INH-A21 for the prevention of nosocomial staphylococcal bloodstream infection in premature infants. J Pediatr 51, 260–265, 265.e1.

De Louvois, J., Blackbourn, J., Hurley, R., et al., 1991. Infantile meningitis in England and Wales: a two-year study. Arch Dis Child 66, 603–607.

de Man, M.P., Verhoeven, B.A., Verbrugh, H.A., et al., 2000. An antibiotic policy to prevent emergence of resistant bacilli. Lancet 355, 973–978.

Dent, A., Toltzis, P., 2003. Descriptive and molecular epidemiology of Gram-negative bacilli infections in the neonatal intensive care unit. Curr Opin Infect Dis 16, 279–283.

de Ruiter, A., Mercey, D., Anderson, J., et al., 2008. British HIV Association and Children's HIV Association guidelines for the management of HIV infection in pregnant women 2008. HIV Med 9, 452–502.

Deshpande, G., Rao, S., Patole, S., 2007. Probiotics for prevention of necrotising enterocolitis in preterm neonates with very low birthweight: a systematic review of randomised controlled trials. Lancet 369, 1614–1620.

Dinger, J., Muller, D., Pargac, N., et al., 2002. 2002 Breast milk transmission of group B streptococcal infection. Pediatr Infect Dis J 21, 567–568.

Di Pentima, M.C., Chan, S., 2010. Impact of antimicrobial stewardship program on vancomycin use in a peadiatric teaching hospital. Pediatr Infect Dis J 29, 707–711.

Dobson, S.R., Isaacs, D., Wilkinson, A.R., et al., 1992. Reduced use of surface cultures for suspected neonatal sepsis and surveillance. Arch Dis Child 67, 44–47.

Doctor, B.A., Newman, N., Minich, N.M., et al., 2001. Clinical outcomes of neonatal meningitis in very-low birth-weight infants. Clin Pediatr (Phila) 40, 473–480.

Donnerstein, R.L., Berg, R.A., Shehab, Z., et al., 1994. Complex atrial tachycardias and respiratory syncytial virus infections in infants. J Pediatr 125, 23–28.

Dorschner, R.A., Lin, K.H., Murakami, M., et al., 2003. Neonatal skin in mice and humans expresses increased levels of antimicrobial peptides: innate immunity during development of the adaptive response. Pediatr Res 53, 566–572.

Duerkop, B.A., Vaishnava, S., Hooper, L.V., 2009. Immune responses to the microbiota at the intestinal mucosal surface. Immunity 31, 368–376.

Dunn, D., Wallon, M., Peyron, F., et al., 1999. Mother-to-child transmission of toxoplasmosis: risk estimates for clinical counselling. Lancet 353, 1829–1833.

Dworkin, L.D., Levine, G.M., Farber, N.J., et al., 1976. Small intestinal mass of the rat is partially determined by indirect effects of intraluminal nutrition. Gastroenterology 71, 626–630.

Dyke, M.P., Grauaug, A., Kohan, R., et al., 1993. *Ureaplasma urealyticum* in a neonatal intensive care population. J Paediatr Child Health 29, 295–297.

Early-onset and late-onset neonatal group B streptococcal disease – United States, 1996–2004. MMWR Morb Mortal Wkly Rep 54, 1205–1208. 2005.

Eastick, K., Leeming, J.P., Millar, M.R., 1996. Reservoirs of coagulase negative staphylococci in preterm infants. Arch Dis Child 74, F99–F104.

Edelman, C.M., Ogwo, J.E., Fine, B.P., 1973. The prevalence of bacteriuria in full-term and premature newborn infants. J Pediatr 82, 125–129.

Edelman, K., Nikkari, S., Ruuskanen, O., et al., 1996. Detection of *Bordetella pertussis* by polymerase chain reaction and culture in the nasopharynx of erythromycin-treated infants with pertussis. Pediatr Infect Dis J 15, 54–57.

Edelson, M.B., Bagwell, C.E., Rozycki, H.J., 1999. Circulating pro- and counterinflammatory cytokine levels and severity in necrotizing enterocolitis. Pediatrics 103, 766.

Edwards, M.S., Rench, M.A., Haffar, A.A., et al., 1985. Long-term sequelae of group B streptococcal meningitis in infants. J Pediatr 106, 717–722.

Edwards, W.H., Conner, J.M., Soll, R.F., 2004. The effect of prophylactic ointment therapy on nosocomial sepsis rates and skin integrity in infants with birth weights of 501 to 1000 g. Pediatrics 113, 1195–1203.

Eisenstein, E.M., Gesundheit, B., 1998. Neonatal hand abscess, osteomyelitis and meningitis caused by *Streptococcus pneumoniae*. Pediatr Infect Dis J 17, 760–761.

Elder, D.E., Zuccollo, J.M., Stanley, T.V., 2005. Neonatal death after hypoxic ischaemic encephalopathy: does a postmortem add to the final diagnoses? Br J Obstet Gynaecol 112, 935–940.

Embleton, N.D., 2001. Fetal and neonatal death from maternally acquired infection. Paediatr Perinat Epidemiol 15, 54–60.

Enders, M., Klingel, K., Weidner, A., et al., 2010. Risk of fetal hydrops and non-hydropic late intrauterine fetal death after gestational parvovirus B19 infection. J Clin Virol 49, 163–168.

Erdman, S.H., Christensen, R.D., Bradley, P.P., et al., 1982. Supply and release of storage neutrophils. Biol Neonate 41, 132–137.

Eriksson, M., Melen, B., Myrback, K.E., et al., 1982. Bacterial colonization of newborn infants in a neonatal intensive care unit. Acta Paediatr Scand 71, 779–783.

Eriksson, M., Bennett, R., Nord, C.E., et al., 1986. Fecal bacterial microflora of newborn infants during intensive care management and treatment with five antibiotic regimes. Pediatr Infect Dis J 5, 533–539.

Escobar, G.J., Li, D.K., Armstrong, M.A., et al., 2000. Neonatal sepsis work-ups in infants > 2000 grams at birth: a population based study. Pediatrics 106, 256–263.

European Collaborative Study, 1991. Children born to women with HIV-1 infection: natural history and risk of transmission. Lancet 337, 253–260.

Ewert, D.P., Lieb, L., Hayes, P.S., et al., 1995. Listeria monocytogenes infection and serotype distribution among HIV-infected persons in Los Angeles County, 1985–1992. J Acq Immun Defic Synd Hum Retrovirol 8, 461–465.

Fanaroff, A.A., Hack, M., 1999. Periventricular leukomalacia – prospects for prevention. N Engl J Med 341, 1229–1231.

Fanaroff, A.A., Korones, S.B., Wright, L.L., et al., 1994. A controlled trial of intravenous immune globulin to reduce nosocomial infections in very-low-birth-weight infants. N Engl J Med 330, 1107–1113.

Fanaroff, A.A., Korones, S.B., Wright, L.L., et al., 1998. Incidence, presenting features, risk factors and significance of late onset septicaemia in very low birth weight infants. Pediatr Infect Dis J 17, 593–598.

Fanaroff, A.A., Hack, M., Walsh, M.C., 2003. The NICHD neonatal research network: changes in practice and outcomes during the first 15 years. Semin Perinatol 281–287.

Farber, J.M., Peterkin, P.I., Carter, A.O., et al., 1991. Neonatal listeriosis due to cross-infection confirmed by isoenzyme typing and DNA fingerprinting. J Infect Dis 163, 927–928.

Feigin, R.D., Cherry, J.D., Demmler, G.J., et al., 2009. Textbook of Pediatric Infectious Diseases, sixth edn. Saunders, Philadelphia.

Feldman, W.E., 1979. Bacterial etiology and mortality of purulent pericarditis in paediatric patients. Review of 162 cases. Am J Dis Child 133, 641–647.

Feldman, E.J., Dowling, R.H., McNaughton, J., et al., 1976. Effects of oral versus intravenous nutrition on intestinal adaptation after small bowel resection in the dog. Gastroenterology 70, 712–719.

Fernandez, M., Rench, M.A., Baker, C.J., 1999. Neonatal sepsis caused simultaneously by two serotypes of group B Streptococcus. Pediatr Infect Dis J 18, 391–393.

Fernando, A.M., Heath, P.T., Menson, E.N., 2008. Antimicrobial policies in the neonatal units of the United Kingdom and Republic of Ireland. J Antimicrob Chemother 61, 743–745.

Ferretti, G., Papaldo, P., Cognetti, F., 2006. Lineage-specific hematopoietic growth factors. N Engl J Med 355, 527.

Field, C.J., 2005. The immunological components of human milk and their effect on immune development in infants. J Nutr 135, 1–4.

Figueroa-Damian, R., Arredondo-Garcia, J.L., 2001. Neonatal outcome of children born to women with tuberculosis. Arch Med Res 32, 66–69.

Fischer, E.G., McLennan, J.E., Suzuki, Y., 1981. Cerebral abscess in children. Am J Dis Child 135, 746–749.

Fischer, G.W., Cieslak, T.J., Wilson, S.R., et al., 1994b. Opsonic antibodies to Staphylococcus epidermidis: in vitro and in vivo studies using human intravenous immune globulin. J Infect Dis 169, 324–329.

Fitzgibbons, S.C., Ching, Y., Yu, D., et al., 2009. Mortality of necrotizing enterocolitis expressed by birth weight categories. J Pediatr Surg 44, 1072–1075.

Fleming, D.W., Cochi, S.L., MacDonald, K.L., 1985. Pasteurised milk as a vehicle of infection in an outbreak of listeriosis. N Engl J Med 312, 404–407.

Flidel-Rimon, O., Friedman, S., Lev, E., et al., 2004. Early enteral feeding and nosocomial sepsis in very low birthweight infants. Arch Dis Child Fetal Neonatal Ed 89, F289–F292.

Fraser, N., Davies, B.W., Cusack, J., 2006. Neonatal omphalitis: a review of its serious complications. Acta Paediatr 95, 519–522.

Frederiksen, B., Samuelsson, S., 1992. Feto-maternal listeriosis in Denmark 1981–1988. J Infect 24, 277–287.

Freeman, J., Platt, R., Sidebottom, D.G., et al., 1987. Coagulase-negative staphylococcal bacteremia in the changing neonatal intensive care unit population. Is there an epidemic? JAMA 258, 2548–2552.

Freund, M.W., Kleinveld, G., Krediet, T.G., et al., 2010. Prognosis for neonates with enterovirus myocarditis. Arch Dis Child Fetal Neonatal Ed 95, F206–F212.

Fridkin, S.K., Edwards, J.R., Courval, J.M., et al., 2001. Intensive Care Antimicrobial Resistance Epidemiology (ICARE) Project and the National Nosocomial Infections Surveillance (NNIS) System Hospitals. The effect of vancomycin and third-generation cephalosporins on prevalence of vancomycin-resistant enterococci in 126 U.S. adult intensive care units. Ann Intern Med 13, 175–183.

Fridkin, S.K., Lawton, R., Edwards, J.R., et al., 2002. Intensive Care Antimicrobial Resistance Epidemiology Project; National Nosocomial Infections Surveillance Systems Hospitals. Monitoring antimicrobial use and resistance: comparison with a national benchmark on reducing vancomycin use and vancomycin-resistant enterococci. Emerg Infect Dis 8, 702–707.

Fortnum, H., Davis, A., 1997. Epidemiology of permanent childhood hearing impairment in Trent Region, 1985–1993. Br J Audiol 31, 409–446. Erratum in Br J Audiol 1998, 32, 63.

Fowlie, P.W., Schmidt, B. 1998. Diagnostic tests for bacterial infection from birth to 90 days – a systematic review. Arch Dis Child Fetal Neonatal Ed, 78, F92–F98.

Gallo, R.L., Murakami, M., Ohtake, T., et al., 2002. Biology and clinical relevance of naturally occurring antimicrobial peptides. J Allergy Clin Immunol 110, 823–831.

Gastmeier, P., Geffers, C., Schwab, F., et al., 2004. Development of a surveillance system for nosocomial infections: the component for neonatal intensive care units in Germany. J Hosp Infect 57, 126–131.

Geffers, C., Baerwolff, S., Schwab, F., et al., 2008. Incidence of healthcare-associated infections in high-risk neonates: results from the German surveillance system for very-low-birthweight infants. J Hosp Infect 68, 214–221.

Gellin, B.G., Broome, C.V., 1989. Listeriosis. JAMA 261, 1313–1319.

Gendrel, D., Bohuon, C., 2000. Procalcitonin as a marker of bacterial infection. Pediatr Infect Dis J, 19, 679–687.

Gessler, P., Kirchmann, N., Kientsch-Engel, R., et al., 1993. Serum concentrations of granulocyte colony-stimulating factor in healthy term and preterm neonates and in those with various diseases including bacterial infections. Blood 82, 3177.

Gewolb, I.H., Schwalbe, R.S., Taciak, V.L., et al., 1999. Stool microflora in extremely low birthweight infants. Arch Dis Child Fetal Neonatal Ed 80, F167–F173.

Gfatter, R., Hackl, P., Braun, F., 1997. Effects of soap and detergents on skin surface pH, stratum corneum hydration and fat content in infants. Dermatology 195, 258–262.

Gibbs, R.S., McDuffie, R.S.J., McNabb, F., et al., 1994. Neonatal group B streptococcal sepsis during 2 years of a universal screening program. Obstetr Gynecol 84, 496–500.

Gibson, R.L., Soderland, C., Henderson, W.R.J., et al., 1995. Group B streptococci (GBS) injure lung endothelium in vitro: GBS invasion and GBS-induced eicosanoid production is greater with microvascular than with pulmonary artery cells. Infect Immun 63, 271–279.

Gilbert, R., 2004. Prenatal screening for group B streptococcal infection: gaps in the evidence. Int J Epidemiol 33, 2–8.

Gilbert, R., Tan, H.K., Cliffe, S., et al., 2006. Symptomatic toxoplasma infection due to congenital and postnatally acquired infection. Arch Dis Child 91, 495–498.

Gilbert, D.N., Moellering, R.C., Eliopoulos, G.M., et al., 2008. Comparison of antimicrobial spectra. In: The Sanford Guide to Antimicrobial Therapy 2008. Antimicrobial Therapy, Sperryville, pp. 65–70.

Gillan, E.R.,Christensen, R.D., Suen, Y., et al., 1994. A randomized, placebo-controlled trial of recombinant human granulocyte colony-stimulating factor administration in newborn infants with presumed sepsis: significant induction of peripheral and bone marrow neutrophilia. Blood 84, 1427–1433.

Ginsberg, I., 2002. Role of lipoteichoic acid in infection and inflammation. Lancet Infect Dis 2 171–179.

Girardin, E.P., Berner, M.E., Grau, G.E., et al., 1990. Serum tumour necrosis factor in newborns at risk for infections. Eur J Pediatr 149, 645–647.

Givens, K.T., Lee, D.A., Jones, T., et al., 1993. Congenital rubella syndrome: ophthalmic manifestations and associated systemic disorders. Br J Ophthalmol 77, 358–363

Gogus, S., Umer, H., Akcoren, Z., et al., 1993. Neonatal tuberculosis. Pediatr Pathol 13, 299–304.

Gomez, M., Alter, S., Kumar, M.L., et al., 1999. Neonatal Streptococcus pneumoniae infection: case reports and review of the literature. Pediatr Infect Dis J 18, 1014–1018.

Gorgen, I., Hartung, T., Leist, M., et al., 1999. Granulocyte colony-stimulating factor treatment protects rodents against lipopolysaccharide-induced toxicity via suppression of systemic tumor necrosis factor-alpha. Immunol 142, 918–923.

Gottbrath Flaherty, E.K., Agrawal, R., Thaker, V., et al., 1995. Urinary tract infections in cocaine-exposed infants. J Perinatol 15, 203–207.

Gray, M.L., 1960. Genital Listeriosis as a cause of repeated abortion. Lancet 2, 296–297.

Gray, J.W., 2007. Surveillance of infection in neonatal intensive care units. Early Hum Dev 83, 157–163.

Gray, J.E., Richardson, D.K., McCormick, M.C., et al., 1995. Coagulase-negative staphylococcal bacteremia among very low birth weight infants: relation to admission illness severity, resource use and outcome. Pediatrics 95, 225–230.

Green, M., Dashefsky, B., Wald, E.R., et al., 1993. Comparison of two antigen assays for rapid intrapartum detection of vaginal group B streptococcal colonization. J Clin Microbiol 31, 78–82.

Green, P.A., Singh, K.V., Murray, B.E., et al., 1994. Recurrent group B streptococcal infections in infants: clinical and microbiologic aspects. J Pediatr 125, 931–938.

Greene, K.A., Rhine, W.D., Starnes, V.A., et al., 1990. Fatal postoperative Legionella pneumonia in a newborn. J Perinatol 10, 183–184.

Greenough, A., 2009. Role of ventilation in RSV disease: CPAP, ventilation, HFO, ECMO. Paediatr Respir Rev 10 (Suppl 1), 26–28.

Gregory, J., Hey, E., 1972. Blood neutrophil response to bacterial infection in the first month of life. Arch Dis Child 47, 747–753.

Grether, J.K., Nelson, K., 1997. Maternal infection and cerebral palsy infants of normal birthweight. JAMA 278, 207–211.

Griffiths, P., Baboonian, C., Rutter, D., et al., 1991. Congenital maternal cytomegalovirus infections in a London population. Br J Obstet Gynaecol 98, 135–140.

Grigg, J.M., Barber, A., Silverman, M., 1992. Increased levels of bronchoalveolar lavage fluid interleukin-6 in preterm ventilated infants after prolonged rupture of membranes. Am Rev Respir Dis 145, 782–786.

Grio, R., Porpiglia, M., Vetro, E., et al., 1994. Asymptomatic bacteriuria in pregnancy: maternal and fetal complications. Panminerva Med 36, 198–200.

Gupta, S.D., Keyl, P.M., 1998. Effectiveness of prenatal tetanus toxoid immunization against neonatal tetanus in a rural area in India. Pediatr Infect Dis J 17, 316–321.

Hague, R.A., Rassam, S., Morgan, G., et al., 1994. Early diagnosis of severe combined immunodeficiency syndrome. Arch Dis Child 70, 260–263.

Halliday, H.L., 1989. When to do a lumbar puncture in a neonate. Arch Dis Child 64, 313–316.

Halliday, H.L., McClure, B.G., Reid, D., et al., 1984. Controlled trial of artificial surfactant to prevent respiratory distress syndrome. Lancet 1, 476–478.

Hampl, S.D., Olson, L.C., 1995. Pertussis in the young infant. Semin Respir Infect 10, 58–62.

Hanson, L.A., Korotkova, M., 2002. The role of breastfeeding in prevention of neonatal infection. Semin Neonatol 7, 275–281.

Hanson, L.A., Korotkova, M., Lundin, S., et al., 2003. The transfer of immunity from mother to child. Ann N Y Acad Sci 987, 199–206.

Haque, K.N., Khan, M.A., Kerry, S., et al., 2004. Pattern of culture-proven neonatal sepsis in a district general hospital in the United Kingdom 20. Infect Control Hosp Epidemiol 25, 759–764.

Harris, M.C., Costarino, A.T. Jr, Sullivan, J.S., et al., 1994. Cytokine elevations in critically ill infants with sepsis and necrotizing enterocolitis. J Pediatr 124, 105.

Hartung, T., Docke, W.D., Gantner, F., et al., 1995. Effect of granulocyte colony-stimulating factor treatment on ex vivo blood cytokine response in human volunteers. Blood 85, 2482.

Health Protection Agency, 2007. Pyogenic and non-pyogenic streptococcal bacteraemias. England, Wales and Northern Ireland 2, 1–16.

Heath, P.T., Feldman, R., 2005. Vaccination against group B streptococcus. Exp Rev Vaccines 4, 207–218.

Heath, P.T., Nik Yusoff, N.K., Baker, C.J., 2003. Neonatal meningitis. Arch Dis Child Fetal Neonatal Ed 88, F173–F178.

Heath, P.T., Balfour, G., Weisner, A.M., et al., 2004. Group B streptococcal disease in UK and Irish infants younger than 90 days. Lancet 363, 292–294.

Hedberg, C.L., Adcock, K., Martin, J., et al., 2004. Tumor necrosis factor α-308 polymorphism associated with increased sepsis mortality in ventilated very low birth weight infants. Pediatr Infect Dis J 23, 424–428.

Heininger, A., Binder, M., Schmidt, S., et al., 1999. PCR and blood culture for detection of Escherichia coli bacteremia in rats. J Clin Microbiol 37, 2479–2482.

Hemming, V.G., Overall, J.C. Jr, Britt, M.R., 1976. Nosocomial infections in a newborn intensive-care unit. Results of forty-one months of surveillance. N Engl J Med 294, 1310–13166.

Hendricks Munoz, K.D., Shapiro, D.L., 1990. The role of the lumbar puncture in the admission sepsis evaluation of the premature infant. J Perinatol 10, 60–64.

Hervas, J.A., Gonzalez, L., Gil, J., et al., 1993. Neonatal group B streptococcal infection in Mallorca, Spain. Clin Infect Dis 16, 714–718.

Hervas, J.A., Ballesteros, F., Alomar, A., et al., 2001. Increase of Enterobacter in neonatal sepsis: a twenty-two-year study. Pediatr Infect Dis J 20, 134–140.

Hintz, S.R., Kendrick, D.E., Stoll, B.J., et al., 2005. Neurodevelopmental and growth outcomes of extremely low-birthweight infants after necrotising enterocolitis. Pediatrics 115, 696–703.

Hirschl, R.B., Butler, M., Coburn, C.E., et al., 1994. Listeria monocytogenes and severe newborn respiratory failure supported with extracorporeal membrane oxygenation. Arch Pediatr Adolesc Med 148, 513–517.

Ho, N.K., Low, Y.P., See, H.F., 1989. Septic arthritis in the newborn – a 17 years' clinical experience. Singapore Med J 30, 356–358.

Holmberg, R.E.J., Pavia, A.T., Montgomery, D., et al., 1993. Nosocomial Legionella pneumonia in the neonate. Pediatrics 92, 450–453.

Holland, P., Isaacs, D., Moxon, E.R., 1986. Fatal neonatal varicella infection. Lancet ii, 1156.

Holt, D.E., Halket, S., de Louvois, J., et al., 2001. Neonatal meningitis in England and Wales: 10 years on. Arch Dis Child Fetal Neonatal Ed 84, F85–F89.

Honest, H., Sharma, S., Khan, K.S., 2006. Rapid tests for group B streptococcus colonization in laboring women: a systematic review. Pediatrics 117, 1055–1066.

Hooper, L.V., 2004. Bacterial contributions to mammalian gut development. Trends Microbiol 12, 129–134.

Hooper, L.V., Wong, M.H., Thelin, A., et al., 2001. Molecular analysis of commensal host–microbial relationships in the intestine. Science 291, 881–884.

Horbar, J.D., Rogowski, J., Plsek, P.E., et al., 2001. Collaborative quality improvement for neonatal intensive care. NIC/Q Project Investigators of the Vermont Oxford Network. Pediatrics 107, 14–22.

Howell, A., Isaacs, D., Halliday, R., 2009. Oral nystatin prophylaxis and neonatal fungal infections. Arch Dis Child Fetal Neonatal Ed 94, F429–F433.

Hristeva, L., Bowle, I., Booy, R., et al., 2003. Value of cerebrospinal fluid examination in the diagnosis of meningitis in the newborn. Arch Dis Child 69, 514–517.

Huang, S.Y., Tang, R.B., Chen, S.J., et al., 2003. Coagulase-negative staphylococcal bacteremia in critically ill children: risk factors and antimicrobial susceptibility. J Microbiol Immunol Infect 36, 51–55.

Hughes, C.A., Dowling, R.H., 1980. Speed of onset of adaptive mucosal hypoplasia and hypofunction in the intestine of parenterally fed rats. Clin Sci 59, 317–327.

Hughes, R., Brocklehurst, P., Heath, P., et al., Prevention of Neonatal Early Onset Group B Streptococcal Disease. RCOG Guideline No 36, 1–10. 2003. London: RCOG.

Hyde, T.B., Hilger, T.M., Reingold, A., et al., 2002. Trends in incidence and antimicrobial resistance of early-onset sepsis: population-based surveillance in San Francisco and Atlanta. Pediatrics 110, 690–695.

Inder, T.E., Volpe, J.J., 2000. Mechanisms of perinatal brain injury. Semin Neonatol 5, 3–15.

International Neonatal Immunotherapy Study (INIS) Collaborative Group, 2011. Treatment of neonatal sepsis with intravenous Immune Globulin. N Engl J Med 365, 1201–1211.

Isaacman, D.J., Karasic, R.B., Reynolds, E.A., Kost, S.I., 1996. Effect of number of blood cultures and volume of blood on detection of bacteremia in children. J Pediatr 128, 190–195.

Isaacs, D., 2000. Rationing antibiotic use in neonatal units. Arch Dis Child Fetal Neonatal Ed 82, F1–F2.

Isaacs, D., 2003. A ten year, multicentre study of coagulase negative staphylococcal infections in Australasian neonatal units. Arch Dis Child Fetal Neonatal Ed 88, F89–F93.

Isaacs, D., Moxon, E.R., 1991. Neonatal infections. Butterworth Heinemann, Oxford, pp. 149–166.

Isaacs, D., Royle, J.A., 1999. Intrapartum antibiotics and early onset neonatal sepsis caused by group B Streptococcus and by other organisms in Australia. Australasian Study Group for Neonatal Infections. Pediatr Infect Dis J 18, 524–528.

Isaacs, D., Barfield, C.P., Grimwood, K., et al., 1995. Systemic bacterial and fungal infections in infants in Australian neonatal units. Australian Study Group for Neonatal Infections. Med J Austral 162, 198–201.

Isaacs, D., Barfield, C., Clothier, T., et al., 1996. Late-onset infections of infants in neonatal units. J Paediatr Child Health 32, 158–161.

Isaacs, D., Fraser, S., Hogg, G., et al., 2004. Staphylococcus aureus infections in Australasian neonatal nurseries. Arch Dis Child Fetal Neonatal Ed 89, F331–F335.

Ish Horowicz, M.R., McIntyre, P., Nade, S., 1992. Bone and joint infections caused by multiply resistant Staphylococcus aureus in a neonatal intensive care unit. Pediatr Infect Dis J 11, 82–87.

Israels, J., Frakking, F.N., Kremer, L.C., et al., 2010. Mannose-binding lectin and infection risk in newborns: a systematic review. Arch Dis Child Fetal Neonatal Ed 95, F452–F461.

Jacob, J., Edwards, D., Gluck, L., 1980. Early-onset sepsis and pneumonia observed as respiratory distress syndrome: assessment of lung maturity. Am J Dis Child 134, 766–768.

Jacobs, J., Garmyn, K., Verhaegen, J., et al., 1990. Neonatal sepsis due to Streptococcus pneumoniae. Scand J Infect Dis 22, 493–497.

Jacobsson, B., Hagberg, G., 2004. Antenatal risk factors for cerebral palsy. Best Pract Res Clin Obstet Gynaecol 18, 425–436.

Jeffery, H.E., McIntosh, E.D., 1994. Antepartum screening and non-selective intrapartum chemoprophylaxis for group B streptococcus. Aust N Z J Obstet Gynaecol 34, 14–19.

Jeffery, H.E., Mitchison, R., Wigglesworth, J.S., et al., 1977. Early neonatal bacteraemia: comparison of group B streptococcal, other Gram-positive and Gram-negative infections. Arch Dis Child 52, 683–686.

Johnson, C.E., Whitwell, J.K., Pethe, K., et al., 1997. Term newborns who are at risk for sepsis: are lumbar punctures necessary? Pediatrics 99, e10.

Johnson, A.P., Sharland, M., Goodall, C.M., et al., 2010. Enhanced surveillance of methicillin-resistant Staphylococcus aureus (MRSA) bacteraemia in children in the UK and Ireland. Arch Dis Child 95, 781–785.

Jones, E.M., McCulloch, S.Y., Reeves, D.S., et al., 1994. A 10 year survey of the epidemiology and clinical aspects of listeriosis in a provincial English city. J Infect 29, 91–103.

Jones, C.E., Naidoo, S., De Beer, C., et al., 2011. Maternal HIV infection and antibody responses against vaccine-preventable diseases in uninfected infants. JAMA 305, 576–584.

Joynson, D.H., Guy, E., 1999. Investigation and management of Toxoplasma infection in pregnancy. CME Bull Med Microbiol 3, 8–11.

Kalliola, S., Vuopio-Varkila, J., Takala, A.K., et al., 1999. Neonatal group B streptococcal disease in Finland: a ten-year nationwide study. Pediatr Infect Dis J 18, 806–810.

Kang, C.I., Kim, S.H., Park, W.B., et al., 2005. Bloodstream infections caused by antibiotic-resistant Gram-negative bacilli: risk factors for mortality and impact of inappropriate initial antimicrobial therapy on outcome. Antimicrob Agents Chemother 49, 760–766.

Karlowicz, G., et al., 2000. Should central venous catheters be removed as soon as candidemia is detected in neonates? Pediatrics 106, 63.

Karlsson, H., Hessle, C., Rudin, A., 2002. Innate immune responses of human neonatal cells to bacteria from the normal gastrointestinal flora. Infect Immun 6688–6696.

Kartali, G., Tzelepi, E., Pournaras, S., et al., 2002. Outbreak of infections caused by Enterobacter cloacae producing the integron-associated beta-lactamase IBC-1 in a neonatal intensive care unit of a Greek hospital. Antimicrob Agents Chemother 46, 1577–1580.

Kaushansky, K., 2006. Lineage-specific hematopoietic growth factors. N Engl J Med 354, 2034–2045.

Kenyon, S.L., Taylor, D.J., Tarnow-Mordi, W., et al., 2001. Broad-spectrum antibiotics for preterm, prelabour rupture of fetal membranes: the ORACLE I randomised trial. ORACLE Collaborative Group. Lancet 357, 979–988.

Kenyon, S., Pike, K., Jones, D.R., et al., 2008. Childhood outcomes following prescription of antibiotics with spontaneous preterm labour: 7 year follow-up of the ORACLE II. Lancet 372, 1319–1327.

Keyworth, N., Millar, M.R., Holland, K.T., 1992. Development of cutaneous microflora in premature neonates. Arch Dis Child 67, 797–801.

Khan, E.A., Wafelman, L.S., Garcia-Prats, J.A., et al., 1997. Serratia marcescens pneumonia, empyema and pneumatocele in a preterm neonate. Pediatr Infect Dis J 16, 1003–1005.

Khuroo, M.S., Kamili, S., Khuroo, M.S., 2009. Clinical course and duration of viremia in vertically transmitted hepatitis E virus (HEV) infection in babies born to HEV-infected mothers. J Viral Hepat 16, 519–523.

Kinney, J.S., Johnson, K., Papasian, C., et al., 1993. Early onset *Haemophilus influenzae* sepsis in the newborn infant. Pediatr Infect Dis J 12, 739–743.

Klagsbrun, M., 1978. Human milk stimulates DNA synthesis and cellular proliferation in cultured fibroblasts. Proc Natl Acad Sci U S A 75, 5057–5061.

Klinger, G., Chin, C.N., Beyene, J., et al., 2000. Predicting the outcome of neonatal bacterial meningitis. Pediatrics 106, 477–482.

Koch, W.C., Harger, J.H., Barnstein, B., et al., 1998. Serologic and virologic evidence for frequent intrauterine transmission of human parvovirus B19 with a primary maternal infection during pregnancy. Pediatr Infect Dis J 17, 489–494.

Kocherlakota, P., La Gamma, E.F., 1997. Human granulocyte colony-stimulating factor may improve outcome attributable to neonatal sepsis complicated by neutropenia. Pediatrics 100, e1–e6.

Kocherlakota, P., La Gamma, E.F., 1998. Preliminary report: rhG-CSF may reduce the incidence of neonatal sepsis in prolonged pre-eclampsia associated neutropenia. Pediatrics 102, 1107–1111.

Koenig, J.M., Christensen, R.D., 1989. Incidence, neutrophil kinetics, and natural history of neonatal neutropenia associated with maternal hypertension. N Engl J Med 321, 557–562.

Koenig, J.M., Christensen, R.D., 1991. The mechanism responsible for diminished neutrophil production in neonates delivered of women with pregnancy-induced hypertension. Am J Obstet Gynecol 165, 467–473.

Kovacs, A., Schluchter, M., Easley, K., et al., 1999. Cytomegalovirus infection and HIV-1 disease progression in infants born to HIV-1-infected women. N Engl J Med 341, 77–84.

Krick, J.A., Remington, J.S., 1978. Toxoplasmosis in the adult – an overview. N Engl J Med 298, 550–553.

Krüger, C., Malleyeck, I., 2010. Congenital syphilis: still a serious, under-diagnosed threat for children in resource-poor countries. World J Pediatr 6, 125–131.

Kumar, Y., Qunibi, M., Neal, T.J., et al., 2001. Time to positivity of neonatal blood cultures. Arch Dis Child F182–F186.

Kurtoglu, S., Caksen, H., Ozturk, A., et al., 1998. A review of 207 newborn with tetanus. J Pakistan Med Assoc 48, 93–98.

Lachman, P., 2009. Using care bundles to prevent infection in neonatal and paediatric ICUs. Curr Opin Infect Dis 22, 224–228.

La Gamma, E.F., Ostertag, S.G., Birenbaum, H., 1985. Failure of delayed oral feedings to prevent necrotizing enterocolitis. Results of study in very-low-birth-weight neonates. Am J Dis Child 139, 385–389.

Larsen, B., Hwang, J., 2010. *Mycoplasma, Ureaplasma*, and adverse pregnancy outcomes: a fresh look. Infect Dis Obstet Gynecol pii, 521921.

Le, J., Nguyen, T., Okamoto, M., et al., 2008. Impact of empiric antibiotic use on development of infections caused by extended-spectrum beta-lactamase bacteria in a neonatal intensive care unit. Pediatr Infect Dis J 27, 314–318.

Leaf, A., Dorling, J., Kempley, S., et al., 2009. ADEPT – Abnormal Doppler Enteral Prescription Trial. BMC Pediatr 9, 63.

Lee, D.R., Moore, G.W., Hutchins, G.M., 1991. Lattice theory analysis of the relationship of hyaline membrane disease and fetal pneumonia in 96 perinatal autopsies. Pediatr Pathol 11, 223–233.

Lee, S.K., McMillan, D.D., Ohlsson, A., et al., 2000. Variations in practice and outcomes in the Canadian NICU network: 1996–1997. Pediatrics 106, 1070–1079.

Lee, L., Girish, S., van den Berg, E., et al., 2009. Random safety audits in the neonatal unit. Arch Dis Child Fetal Neonatal Ed, 94, F116–F119.

Lesprit, P., Brun-Buisson, C., 2008. Hospital antibiotic stewardship. Curr Opin Infect Dis 21, 344–349.

Levy, S.B., 1998. Multidrug resistance – a sign of the times. N Engl J Med 338, 1376–1378.

Levy, I., Comarsca, J., Davidovits, M., et al., 2009. Urinary tract infection in preterm infants: the protective role of breastfeeding. Pediatr Nephrol 24, 527–531.

Lin, F.Y., Troendle, J.F., 2006. Hypothesis: neonatal respiratory distress may be related to asymptomatic colonization with group B streptococci. Pediatr Infect Dis J 25, 884–888.

Lin, H.H., Kao, J.H., Hsu, H.Y., et al., 1995. Absence of infection in breast-fed infants born to hepatitis C virus-infected mothers. J Pediatr 126, 589–591.

Lin, H.C., Su, B.H., Chen, A.C., et al., 2005. Oral probiotics reduce the incidence and severity of necrotizing enterocolitis in very low birth weight infants. Pediatrics 115, 1–4.

Linder, N., Hernandez, A., Amit, L., et al., 2011. Persistent coagulase-negative staphylococci bacteremia in very-low-birth-weight infants. EurJ Pediatr Jan 8. [Epub ahead of print].

López Sastre, J.B., Coto Cotallo, G.D., Fernández Colomer, B., 2000. Neonatal sepsis of vertical transmission: an epidemiological study from the 'Grupo de Hospitales Castrillo'. J Perinat Med 28, 309–315.

López Sastre, J.B., Coto, C.D., Fernandez, C.B., 2002. Neonatal sepsis of nosocomial origin: an epidemiological study from the 'Grupo de Hospitales Castrillo'. J Perinatal Med 30, 149–157.

Lorenz, E., Hallman, M., Marttila, R., et al., 2002. Association between the Asp 299Gly polymorphisms in the Toll-like receptor 4 and premature births in the Finnish population. Pediatr Res 52, 373–376.

Lucas, A., Cole, T.J., 1990. Breast milk and neonatal necrotising enterocolitis. Lancet 336, 1519–1523.

Luck, S., Sharland, M., 2009. Congenital cytomegalovirus: new progress in an old disease. Paediatr Child Health 19, 178–184.

Luck, P.C., Dinger, E., Helbig, J.H., et al., 1994. Analysis of *Legionella pneumophila* strains associated with nosocomial pneumonia in a neonatal intensive care unit. Eur J Clin Microb Infect Dis 13, 565–571.

Luck, S., Torry, M., d'Agapeyeff, K., et al., 2003. Estimated early-onset group B streptococcal neonatal disease. Lancet 361, 1953–1954.

Lutsar, I., McCracken, G.H. Jr, Friedland, I.R., 1998. Antibiotic pharmacodynamics in cerebrospinal fluid. Clin Infect Dis 27, 1117–1129.

Madge, P., Paton, J.Y., McColl, J.H., et al., 1992. Prospective controlled study of four infection-control procedures to prevent nosocomial infection with respiratory syncytial virus. Lancet 340, 1079–1083.

Mahdavi, S., Malyuta, R., Semenenko, I., et al., 2010. Treatment and disease progression in a birth cohort of vertically HIV-1 infected children in Ukraine. BMC Pediatr 10, 85.

Makhoul, I.R., Sujov, P., Smolkin, T., et al., 2005. Pathogen-specific early mortality in very low birth weight infants with late-onset sepsis: a national survey. Clin Infect Dis 40, 218–224.

Malik, R.K., Montecalvo, M.A., Reale, M.R., et al., 1999. Epidemiology and control of vancomycin-resistant enterococci in a regional neonatal intensive care unit. Pediatr Infect Dis J 18, 352–356.

Manroe, B.L., Weinberg, A.G., Rosenfeld, C.R., et al., 1979. The neonatal blood count in health and disease. I. Reference values for neutrophilic cells. J Pediatr 95, 89–98.

Marchini, G., Lindow, S., Brismar, H., et al., 2002. The newborn infant is protected by an innate antimicrobial barrier: peptide antibiotics are present in the skin and vernix caseosa. Br J Dermatol 147, 1127–1134.

Marshall, D.D., Kotelchuck, M., Young, T.E., et al., 1999. Risk factors for chronic lung disease in the surfactant era: a North Carolina population-based study of very low birth weight infants. North Carolina Neonatologists Association. Pediatrics 104, 1345–1350.

Marwick, C., Davey, P., 2009. Care bundles: the Holy Grail of infectious risk management in hospital? Curr Opin Infect Dis 22, 364–369.

Maxwell, N.C., Nuttall, D., Kotecha, S., 2009. Does Ureaplasma spp. cause chronic lung disease of prematurity: ask the audience? Early Hum Dev 85, 291–296.

May, M., Daley, A.J., Donath, S., et al., 2005. Early onset neonatal meningitis in Australia and New Zealand, 1992–2002. Arch Dis Child Fetal Neonatal Ed 90, F324–F327.

Maymon, E., Chaim, W., Furman, B., et al., 1998. Meconium stained amniotic fluid in very low risk pregnancies at term gestation. Eur J Obst Gynaecol Reproduct Biol, 80, 169–173.

Mazade, M.A., Evans, E.M., Starke, J.R., et al., 2001. Congenital tuberculosis presenting as sepsis syndrome: case report and review of the literature. Pediatr Infect Dis J 20, 439–442.

Mazur, J.M., Ross, G., Cummings, J., et al., 1995. Usefulness of magnetic resonance imaging for the diagnosis of acute musculoskeletal infections in children. J Pediatr Orthoped 15, 144–147.

McCracken, G.H. Jr, Mize, S.G., Threlkeld, N., 1980. Intraventricular gentamicin therapy in Gram-negative bacillary meningitis of infancy. Report of the Second Neonatal Meningitis Cooperative Study Group. Lancet 1, 787–791.

McDuffie, R.S., Jr., McGregor, J.A., Gibbs, R.S., 1993. Adverse perinatal outcome and resistant Enterobacteriaceae after antibiotic usage for premature rupture of the membranes and group B streptococcus carriage. Obstet Gynecol 82, 487–489.

MacGowan, A.P., Cartlidge, P.H., MacLeod, F., et al., 1991. Maternal listeriosis in pregnancy without fetal or neonatal infection. J Infect 22, 53–57.

McGuire, W., Anthony, M., 2003. Donor human milk versus formula for preventing necrotisisng enterocolitis in preterm infants: systematic review. Arch Dis Child Fetal Neonatal Ed 88, F11–F14.

McGuire, W., Clerihew, L., Fowlie, P.W., 2004a. Infection in the preterm infant. Br Med J 329, 1277–1280.

McGuire, W., et al., 2004b. Prophylactic intravenous antifungal agents to prevent mortality and morbidity in very low birth weight infants. The Cochrane Database of Systematic Reviews (1), CD003850.

McIntosh, N., Kempson, C., Tyler, R.M., 1988. Blood counts in extremely low birth weight infants. Arch Dis Child 63, 74–76.

McKeever, T.M., Lewis, S.A., Smith, C., et al., 2002. The importance of prenatal exposures on the development of allergic disease: a birth cohort study with the West Midlands General Practice Research Database. Am J Crit Care Med 166, 827–832.

Mecrow, I.K., Ladusans, E.J., 1994. Infective endocarditis in newborn infants with structurally normal hearts. Acta Paediatr 83, 35–39.

Medves, J.M., O'Brien, B., 2001. Does bathing newborns remove potentially harmful pathogens from the skin? Birth 28, 161–165.

Mehr, S., Doyle, L.W., 2000. Cytokines as markers of bacterial sepsis in newborn infants: a review. Pediatr Infect Dis J 19, 879–887.

Meinzen-Derr, J.B., Poindexter, B., Wrage, L., et al., 2009. Role of human milk in extremely low birth weight infants' risk of necrotizing enterocolitis or death. J Perinatol 29, 57–62.

Mepham, S.O., Bland, R.M., Newell, M.L., 2011. Prevention of mother-to-child transmission of HIV in resource-rich and -poor settings. Br J Obstet Gynaecol 118, 202–218.

Metsvaht, T., Pisarev, H., Ilmoja, M.-L., et al., 2009. Clinical parameters predicting failure of empirical antibacterial therapy in early onset neonatal sepsis, identified by classification and regression tree analysis. BMC Pediatr 9, 72.

Millar, M., Philpott, A., Wilks, M., et al., 2008. Colonization and persistence of antibiotic-resistant Enterobacteriaceae strains in infants nursed in two neonatal intensive care units in East London, United Kingdom. J Clin Microbiol 6, 560–567.

Miller, E., Craddock-Watson, J.E. Pollock, T.M., 1982. Consequences of confirmed maternal rubella at successive stages of pregnancy. Lancet i, 781–784.

Miller, E., Craddock-Watson, J.E., Ridehalgh, M.K., 1989. Outcome in newborn babies given anti-varicella-zoster immunoglobulin after perinatal maternal infection with varicella-zoster virus. Lancet 2, 371–373.

Mnyani, C.N., McIntyre, J.A., 2011. Tuberculosis in pregnancy. Br J Obstet Gynaecol 118, 226–231.

Modi, N., Damjanovic, V., Cooke, R.W., 1987. Outbreak of cephalosporin resistant Enterobacter cloacae infection in a neonatal intensive care unit. Arch Dis Child 62, 148–151.

Modi, N., Dore, C.J., Saraswatula, A., et al., 2009. A case definition for national and international neonatal bloodstream infection surveillance. Arch Dis Child Fetal Neonatal Ed 94, F8–12.

Moore, M.R., Schrag, S.J., Schuchat, A., 2003. Effects of intrapartum antimicrobial prophylaxis for prevention of GBS disease on the ecology of early-onset neonatal sepsis. Lancet Infect Dis 3, 201–213.

Mouzinho, A., Rosenfeld, C.R., Sanchez, P.J., et al., 1992. Effect of maternal hypertension on neonatal neutropenia and risk of nosocomial infection. Pediatrics 90, 430–435.

Mouzinho, A., Rosenfeld, C.R., Sanchez, P.J., et al., 1994. Revised reference ranges for circulating neutrophils in very-low-birth-weight neonates. Pediatrics 94, 76–82.

Mulder, C.J.J., Zanen, H.C., 1984. A study of 280 cases of neonatal meningitis in the Netherlands. J Infect 9, 177–184.

Muller-Pebody, B., Johnson, A.P., Heath, P.T., et al., 2011. Empirical treatment of septic neonates, – are the current guidelines adequate? Arch Dis Child Fetal Neonatal Ed 96, F4–F8.

Murch, S., 2011. Gastrointestinal mucosal immunology and mechanisms of inflammation. In: Wyllie, R., Hyams, J.S., Kay, M. (Eds.), Pediatric gastrointestinal and liver disease, fourth ed. Elsevier, Philadelphia, pp. 50–63.

Murphy, D.J., Sellers, S., MacKenzie, I.Z., et al., 1995. Case-control study of antenatal and intrapartum risk factors for cerebral palsy in very preterm singleton babies. Lancet 346, 1449–1454.

Musoke, R.N., Revathi, G., 2000. Emergence of multidrug-resistant Gram-negative organisms in a neonatal unit and the therapeutic implications. J Trop Pediatr 46, 86–91.

Nambiar, S., Singh, N., 2002. Change in epidemiology of health care-associated infections in a neonatal intensive care unit. Pediatr Infect Dis J 21, 839–842.

Nambiar, S., Herwaldt, L.A., Singh, N., 2003. Outbreak of invasive disease caused by methicillin-resistant Staphylococcus aureus in neonates and prevalence in the neonatal intensive care unit. Pediatr Crit Care Med 4, 220–226.

Narita, M., Togashi, T., Kikuta, H., 1997. Neonatal measles in Hokkaido, Japan. Pediatr Infect Dis J 16, 908–909.

Natarajan, G., Johnson, Y.R., Zhang, F., et al., 2006. Real-time polymerase chain reaction for the detection of group B streptococcus colonization in neonates. Pediatrics 118, 14–22.

National Patient Safety Agency, 2010. Safer use of intravenous gentamicin for neonates. NPSA/2010/PSA001 Accessed 09 February.

Nduati, R.W., John, G.C., Richardson, B.A., et al., 1995. Human immunodeficiency virus type 1-infected cells in breast milk: association with immunosuppression and vitamin A deficiency. J Infect Dis 172, 1461–1468.

Neurath, M.F., Finotto, S., Glimcher, L.H., 2002. The role of Th1/Th2 polarization in mucosal immunity. Nat Med 8, 567–573.

Newell, M.L., Dunn, D.T., De Maria, A., 1996. Detection of virus in vertically exposed HIV antibody negative children. Lancet 347, 213–215.

Ng, P.C., Siu, Y.K., Lewindon, P.J., et al., 1994. Congenital Candida pneumonia in a preterm infant. J Paediatr Child Health 30, 552–554.

NICE clinical guideline 55. Intrapartum care: care of healthy women and their babies during childbirth. 2007. http://www.nice.org.uk/CG055

Nielubowicz, G.R., Mobley, H.L., 2010. Host–pathogen interactions in urinary tract infection. Nat Rev Urol 7, 430–441.

Nyambi, P.N., Ville, Y., Louwagie, J., et al., 1996. Mother-to-child transmission of human T-cell lymphotropic virus types I and II (HTLV-I/II) in Gabon: a prospective follow-up of 4 years. J Acq Immun Defic Syndr Hum Retrovirol 12, 187–192.

Ohlsson, A., Lacy, J.B., 2006. Intravenous immunoglobulins for treatment of suspected or subsequently proven infection in neonates. Cochrane Database of Systematic Reviews, Issue 3.

Oliver, S.E., Cloud, G.A., Sánchez, P.J., et al., 2009. Neurodevelopmental outcomes following ganciclovir therapy in symptomatic congenital cytomegalovirus infections involving the central nervous system. J Clin Virol 46 (Suppl 4), S22–S26

Ollikainen, J., Hiekkaniemi, H., Korppi, M., et al., 1993. Ureaplasma urealyticum infection associated with acute respiratory insufficiency and death in premature infants [see comments]. J Pediatr 122, 756–760.

Olver, W.J., Bond, D.W., Boswell, T.C., et al., 2000. Neonatal group B streptococcal disease associated with infected breast milk. Arch Dis Child Fetal Neonatal Ed 83, F48–F49.

Orsi, G.B., d'Ettorre, G., Panero, A., et al., 2009. Hospital-acquired infection surveillance in a neonatal intensive care unit. Am J Infect Control 37, 201–203.

Oste, M., Van Ginneken, C.J., Van Haver, E.R., et al., 2005. The intestinal trophic response to enteral food is reduced in parenterally fed preterm pigs and is associated with more nitrergic neurons. J Nutr 135, 2657–2663.

Oste, M., De Vos, M., Van Haver, E., et al. 2010a. Parenteral and enteral feeding in preterm piglets differently affects extracellular matrix proteins, enterocyte proliferation and apoptosis in the small intestine. Br J Nutr 104, 989–997.

Oste, M., Van Haver, E., Thymann, T., et al., 2010b. Formula induces intestinal apoptosis in preterm pigs within a few hours of feeding. JPEN J Parenter Enteral Nutr 34, 271–279.

Pang, Y., Rodts-Palenik, S.Z., et al., 2005. Suppression of glial activation is involved in the protection of IL-10 on maternal E. coli induced neonatal white matter injury. Brain Res Dev Brain Res 157, 141–149.

Pappas, P.G., Kauffman, C.A., Andes, D., et al., 2009. Clinical practice guidelines for the management of candidiasis: 2009 update by the Infectious Diseases Society of America. Clin Infect Dis 48, 503–535.

Paramore, L.C., Mahadevia, P.J., Piedra, P.A., 2010. Outpatient RSV lower respiratoryinfections among high-risk infants and other pediatric populations. Pediatr Pulmonol 45, 578–584.

Pass, R.F., 2005. Congenital cytomegalovirus infection and hearing loss. Herpes 12, 50–55. Review.

Pass, R.F., Fowler, K.B., Boppana, S.B., et al., 2006. Congenital cytomegalovirus infection following first trimester maternal infection: Symptoms at birth and outcome. J Clin Virol 35, 216–220.

Pastuszak, A.L., Levy, M., Schick, B., et al., 1994. Outcome after maternal varicella infection in the first 20 weeks of pregnancy. N Engl J Med 330, 901–905.

Peckham, C.S., Stark, O., Dudgein, J.A., et al., 1987. Congenital CMV infection: a cause of sensorineural hearing loss. Arch Dis Child 62, 1233–1237.

PENTA, 2009. Guidelines for the use of antiretroviral therapy in paediatric HIV-1 infection, PENTA Steering Committee. HIV Med 10, 591–613.

Peters, W., Irving, J., Letts, M., 1992. Long-term effects of neonatal bone and joint infection on adjacent growth plates. J Pediatr Orthoped 12, 806–810.

Petersen, Y.M., Hartmann, B., Holst, J.J., et al., 2003. Introduction of enteral food increases plasma GLP-2 and decreases GLP-2 receptor mRNA abundance during pig development. J Nutr 133, 1781–1786.

Petersen, E., Borobio, M.V., Guy, E., et al., 2005. European multicenter study of the LIAISON automated diagnostic system for determination of Toxoplasma gondii-specific immunoglobulin G (IgG) and IgM and the IgG avidity index. J Clin Microbiol 43, 1570–1574.

Philip, A.G.S., 1982. Detection of neonatal sepsis of late onset. JAMA 247, 489–492.

Philip, A.G., 1994. The changing face of neonatal infection: experience at a regional medical center. Pediatr Infect Dis J 13, 1098–1102.

Phillips, J.R., Karlowicz, M.G., 1997. Prevalence of Candida species in hospital-acquired urinary tract infections in a neonatal intensive care unit. Pediatr Infect Dis J 16, 190–194.

Piedra, P.A., Kasel, J.A., Norton, H.J., et al., 1992. Description of an adenovirus type 8 outbreak in hospitalized neonates born prematurely. Pediatr Infect Dis J 11, 460–465.

Pierro, A., van Saene, H.K.F., Donnell, S.C., et al., 1996. Microbial translocation in neonates and infants receiving long-term parenteral nutrition. Arch Surg 131, 176–179.

Pinna, G.S., Skevaki, C.L., Kafetzis, D.A., 2006. The significance of Ureaplasma urealyticum as a pathogenic agent in the paediatric population. Curr Opin Infect Dis 19, 283–289.

Plenge-Bönig, A., Soto-Ramírez, N., Karmaus, W., et al., 2010. Breastfeeding protects against acute gastroenteritis due to rotavirus in infants. Eur J Pediatr 169, 1471–1476.

Poespoprodjo, J.R., Fobia, W., Kenangalem, E., et al., 2009. Vivax malaria: a major cause of morbidity in early infancy. Clin Infect Dis 48, 1704–1712.

Public Health Laboratory Service Working Party on Fifth Disease, 1990. Prospective study of human parvovirus B19 infection in pregnancy. Br Med J 300, 1166–1170.

Puri, J., Revathi, G., Faridi, M.M., et al., 1995. Role of body surface cultures in prediction of sepsis in a neonatal intensive care unit. Ann Trop Paediatr 15, 307–311.

Quinn, D., Newton, N., Piecuch, R., 2005. Effect of less frequent bathing on premature infant skin. J Obstet Gynecol Neonatal Nurs 34, 741–746.

Raad, I.I., Sabbagh, M.F., 1992. Optimal duration of therapy for catheter-related Staphylococcus aureus bacteremia: a study of 55 cases and review. Clin Infect Dis 14, 75–82.

Ragnarsdóttir, B., Fischer, H., Godaly, G., et al., 2008. TLR- and CXCR1-dependent innate immunity: insights into the genetics of urinary tract infections. Eur J Clin Invest 38 (Suppl 2), 12–20.

Rao, S.C., Ahmed, M., Hagan, R., 2006. One dose per day compared to multiple doses per day of gentamicin for treatment of suspected or proven sepsis in neonates. Cochrane Database of Systematic Reviews Issue 1. Art. No.: CD005091.

Rastogi, A., Luken, J.A., Pildes, R.S., et al., 1993. Endocarditis in neonatal intensive care unit. Pediatr Cardiol 14, 183–186.

Rennert, W., Ray, C., 2000. Fulminant amebic colitis in a ten-day-old infant. Pediatr Infect Dis J 19, 1111–1112.

Report of working group of the British Association of Perinatal Medicine and Neonatal Nurses Association on categories of babies requiring neonatal care. 1992. Arch Dis Child 67, 868–869.

Rivera, L.B., Boppana, S.B., Fowler, K.B., et al., 2002. Predictors of hearing loss in children with symptomatic congenital cytomegalovirus infection. Pediatrics 110, 762–767.

Roberts, A.W., 2005. G-CSF: a key regulator of neutrophil production, but that's not all! Growth Factors 23, 33–41.

Roberts, A., Hedman, K., Luyasu, V., et al., 2001. Multicenter evaluation of strategies for serodiagnosis of primary infection with Toxoplasma gondii. Eur J Clin Microbiol Infect Dis 20, 467–474.

Robinson, J.L., Davies, H.D., Barton, M., et al., 2009. Characteristics and outcome of infants with candiduria in neonatal intensive care – a Paediatric Investigators Collaborative Network on Infections in Canada (PICNIC) study. BMC Infect Dis 9, 183.

Rodwell, R.L., Leslie, A.L., Tudehope, D.I., 1988. Early diagnosis of neonatal sepsis using a hematologic scoring system. J Pediatr 112, 761–767.

Rodwell, R.L., Faims, P.H.D., Taylor, K.M.C.D., et al., 1993. Hematologic scoring system in early diagnosis of sepsis in neutropenic newborns. Pediatr Infect Dis J 12, 372–376.

Rojas, J., Stahlman, M., 1984. The effects of group B streptococcus and other organisms on the pulmonary vasculature. Clin Perinatol 11, 591–599.

Roman, J., Fernandez, F., Velasco, F., et al., 1993. Serum TNF levels in neonatal sepsis and septic shock. Acta Paediatr 82, 352–354.

Romano, L., Paladini, S., Van Damme, P., et al., 2011. The worldwide impact of vaccination on the control and protection of viral hepatitis B. Dig Liver Dis 43 (Suppl 1), S2–S7.

Rombaldi, R.L., Serafini, E.P., Mandelli, J., et al., 2009. Perinatal transmission of human papillomavirus DNA. Virol J 6, 83.

Romero, R., Hanaoka, S., Mazor, M., et al., 1991. Meconium-stained amniotic fluid: a risk factor for microbial invasion of the amniotic cavity. Am J Obstet Gynecol 164, 859–862.

Rønnestad, A., Abrahamsen, T.G., Gaustad, P., et al., 1998. Blood culture isolates during 6 years in a tertiary neonatal intensive care unit. Scand J Infect Dis 30, 245–251.

Rønnestad, A., Abrahamsen, T.G., Medbø, S., et al., 2005. Late-onset septicemia in a norwegian national cohort of extremely premature infants receiving very early full human milk feeding. Pediatrics 115, e269–e276.

Rosenberg, P.S., Alter, B.P., Bolyard, A.A., et al., 2006. The incidence of leukaemia and mortality from sepsis in patients with severe congenital neutropenia receiving long-term G-CSF therapy. Blood 107, 4628–4635.

Royal College of Obstetricians and Gynaecologists (RCOG) Greentop guideline, Prevention of early onset group B streptococcal disease. 2003. No 36. Available online at: http://www.rcog.org.uk/guidelines

Rusin, P., Adam, R.D., Peterson, E.A., et al., 1991. *Haemophilus influenzae*: an important cause of maternal and neonatal infections. Obstet Gynecol 77, 92–96.

Saltigeral Simental, P., Macias Parra, M., Mejía Valdéz, J., et al., 1993. Neonatal tetanus experience at the National Institute of Pediatrics in Mexico City. Pediatr Infect Dis J 12, 722–725.

Samson, L., MacDonald, N.E., 1995. Management of infants born to mothers who have *Chlamydia* infection. Pediatr Infect Dis J 14, 407–408.

Sangild, P.T., Schmidt, M., Elnif, J., et al., 2002. Prenatal development of gastrointestinal function in the pig and the effects of fetal esophageal obstruction. Pediatr Res 52, 416–424.

Sawyer, M.H., 1999. Enterovirus infections: diagnosis and treatment. Pediatr Infect Dis J 18, 1033–1039.

Schanler, R.J., 2006. Probiotics and necrotizing enterocolitis in premature infants. Arch Dis Child Fetal Neonatal Ed 91, F395–F397.

Schelonka, R.L., Yoder, B.A., desJardins, S.E., et al., 1994. Peripheral leukocyte count and leukocyte indexes in healthy and newborn term infants. J Pediatr 125, 603–606.

Schwebke, K., Henry, K., Balfour, H.H.J., et al., 1995. Congenital cytomegalovirus infection as a result of nonprimary cytomegalovirus disease in a mother with acquired immunodeficiency syndrome. J Pediatr 126, 293–295.

Schwersenski, J., McIntyre, L., Bauer, C.R., 1991. Lumbar puncture frequency and cerebrospinal fluid analysis in the neonate. Am J Dis Child 145, 54–58.

Shalak, L.F., Perlman, J.M., 2002. Infection markers and early signs of neonatal encephalopathy in the term infant. Mental Retard Devel Disabil Res Rev 8, 14–19.

Shan, F., 2009. Sepsis in babies: should we stimulate the phagocytes? Lancet 373, 188–190.

Sharland, M., 2007. The use of antibacterials in children: a report of the Specialist Advisory Committee on Antimicrobial Resistance (SACAR) Paediatric Subgroup [supplement]. J Antimicrob Chemother 60 (Suppl 1), i15–i26.

Sharland, M., Bedford Russell, A.R., 2001. Preventing respiratory syncitial virus bronchiolitis. Br Med J 322, 62–63.

Sharland, M., Luck, S., Griffiths, P., et al., 2011. Antiviral therapy of CMV disease in children. Adv Exp Med Biol 697, 243–260.

Sharma, R., Hudak, M.L., Premachandra, B.R., et al., 2002. Clinical manifestations of rotavirus infection in the neonatal intensive care unit. Pediatr Infect Dis J 21, 1099–1105.

Sherer, C.R., Sprague, B.M., Campos, J.M., et al., 2005. Characterizing vancomycin-resistant enterococci in neonatal intensive care. Emerg Infect Dis 11, 1470–1472.

Silveira, R.C., Procianoy, R.S., 2003. Il-6 and TNF levels in plasma and cerebrospinal fluid of term newborn infants with HIE. J Pediatr 143, 625–629.

Simon, L., Gauvin, F., Amre, D.K., et al., 2004. Serum procalcitonin and C-reactive protein levels as markers of bacterial infection: a systematic review and meta-analysis. Clin Infect Dis 39, 206–217.

Singh, N., Patel, K.M., Leger, M.M., et al., 2002. Risk of resistant infections with Enterobacteriaceae in hospitalized neonates. Pediatr Infect Dis J 21, 1029–1033.

Sizun, J., Soupre, D., Legrand, M.C., et al., 1995. Neonatal nosocomial respiratory infection with coronavirus: a prospective study in a neonatal intensive care unit. Acta Paediatr 84, 617–620.

Smith, R., Malee, K., Charurat, M., et al., 2000. Timing of perinatal human immunodeficiency virus type 1 infection and rate of neurodevelopment. The Women and Infant Transmission Study Group. Pediatr Infect Dis J 19, 862–871.

So, A.D., Gupta, N., Cars, O., 2010. Tackling antibiotic resistance. Br Med J 340, 2071.

Sohn, A.H., Garrett, D.O., Sinkowitz-Cochran, R.L., et al., 2001. Prevalence of nosocomial infections in neonatal intensive care unit patients: results from the First National Point-Prevalence Survey. J Pediatr 139, 821–827.

Steele, A.D., Sears, J.F., 1996. Characterisation of rotaviruses recovered from neonates with symptomatic infection. South Afr Med J 86, 1546–1549.

Stenger, M.R., Reber, K.M., Giannone, P.J., et al., 2011. Probiotics and prebiotics for the prevention of necrotizing enterocolitis. Curr Infect Dis Rep 13, 13–20.

Stenson, B.J., Heath, P.T., Bedford Russell, A.R., 2007. Respiratory distress related to asymptomatic colonization with group B streptococci. Pediatr Infect Dis J 8, 765.

Stoll, B.J., Hansen, N., 2003. Infections in VLBW infants: studies from the NICHD Neonatal Research Network. Semin Perinatol 27, 293–301.

Stoll, B.J., Schuchat, A., 1998. Maternal carriage of group B streptococci in developing countries. Pediatr Infect Dis J 17, 499–503.

Stoll, B.J., Gordon, T., Korones, S.B., et al. 1996a. Early-onset sepsis in very low birth-weight neonates: a report from the National Institute of Child Health and Human Development Neonatal Research Network. J Pediatr 129, 72–80.

Stoll, B.J., Gordon, T., Korones, S.B., et al. 1996b. Late-onset sepsis in very low birth weight neonates: a report from the National Institute of Child Health and Human Development Neonatal Research Network. J Pediatr 129, 63–71.

Stoll, B.J., Hansen, N., Fanaroff, A.A., et al. 2002a. Late-onset sepsis in very low birth weight neonates: the experience of the NICHD Neonatal Research Network. Pediatrics 110, 285–291.

Stoll, B.J., Hansen, N., Fanaroff, A.A., et al. 2002b. Changes in pathogens causing early-onset sepsis in very-low-birth-weight infants. N Engl J Med 347, 240–247.

Stoll, B.J., Hansen, N., Adams-Chapman, I., et al., 2004. Neurodevelopmental and growth impairment amongst extremely low birth weight infants with neonatal infection. JAMA 292, 2357–2365.

Stoll, B.J., Hansen, N.I., Higgins, R.D., et al., 2005. Very low birth weight preterm infants with early onset neonatal sepsis: the predominance of Gram-negative infections continues in the National Institute of Child Health and Human Development Neonatal Research Network, 2002–2003. Pediatr Infect Dis J 24, 635–639.

Straka, M., Cruz, W.D., Blackmon, C., et al., 2004. Rapid detection of group B streptococcus and *Escherichia coli* in amniotic fluid using real-time fluorescent PCR. Infect Dis Obst Gynecol 12, 109–113.

Tan, N.W., Sriram, B., Tan-Kendrick, A.P., et al., 2005. Neonatal hepatic abscess in preterm infants: a rare entity? Ann Acad Med Singapore 34, 558–564.

Tarnow-Mordi, W., Isaacs, D., Dutta, S., 2010a. Adjunctive immunologic interventions in neonatal sepsis. Clin Perinatol 37, 481–499.

Tarnow-Mordi, W.O., Wilkinson, D., Trivedi, A., et al., 2010b. Probiotics reduce all-cause mortality and necrotizing enterocolitis: it is time to change practice? Pediatrics 125, 1068–1070.

Tebruegge, M., Curtis, N., 2009. Enterovirus infections in neonates. Semin Fetal Neonatal Med 14, 222–227.

Tenover, F.C., Mohammed, M.J., Stelling, J., et al., 2001. Ability of laboratories to detect emerging antimicrobial resistance: proficiency testing and quality control results from the World Health Organization's external quality assurance system for antimicrobial susceptibility testing. J Clin Microbiol, 39, 241–250.

The Paediatric Formulary Committee. BNF for children. British Medical Association, Royal Pharmaceutical Society of Great Britain, Royal College of Paediatrics and Child Health, Neonatal and Paediatric Pharmacists Group, 2008.

Thompson, C., Whitley, R., 2011. Neonatal herpes simplex virus infections: where are we now? Adv Exp Med Biol 697, 221–230.

Thompson, P.J., Greenough, A., Hird, M.F., et al., 1992. Nosocomial bacterial infections in very low birth weight infants. Eur J Pediatr 151, 451–454.

Thorp, J.M. Jr, Katz, V.L., Fowler, L.J., et al., 1989. Fetal death from chlamydial infection across intact amniotic membranes. Am J Obs Gynecol 161, 1245–1246.

Thulliez, P., 2001. Maternal and foetal infection. In: Joynson, D.H.M., Wreghitt, T.G. (Eds.), Toxoplasmosis: A Comprehensive Clinical Guide. Cambridge University Press, Cambridge, pp. 193–213.

TINN, 2010. Evaluation of antibiotics (ciprofloxacin and fluconazole) for the treatment of infections in preterm and term neonates (TINN). Funded under Seventh Framework Programme. Available online at: http://cordis.europa.eu/fp7/projects_en.html. Accessed 3/6/10

Toltzis, P., 2004. Antibiotic-resistant Gram-negative bacteria in hospitalized children. Clin Lab Med 24, 363–380.

Tookey, P., Peckham, C.S., 1996. Neonatal herpes simplex virus infection in the British Isles. Paediatr Perinat Epidemiol 10, 432–442.

Tookey, P.A., Peckham, C.S., 1999. Surveillance of congenital rubella in Great Britain, 1971-96. BMJ 318, 769–707.

Tookey, P.A., Ades, A.E., Peckham, C.S., 1992. Cytomegalovirus prevalence in pregnant women: the influence of parity. Arch Dis Child, 67, 779–783.

Trotter, S., 2006. Neonatal skincare: why change is vital. RCM Midwives 9, 134–138.

Tucker, J., UK Neonatal Staffing Study Group, 2002. Patient volume, staffing, and workload in relation to risk-adjusted outcomes in a random stratified sample of UK neonatal intensive care units: a prospective evaluation. Lancet 359, 99–107.

Tugal, O., Pallant, B., Shebarek, N., et al., 1994. Transient erythroblastopenia of the newborn caused by human parvovirus. Am J Pediatr Hematol Oncol 16, 352–355.

Umasankar, S., Mridha, E.U., Hannan, M.M., et al., 1996. An outbreak of *Salmonella enteritidis* in a maternity and neonatal intensive care unit. J Hosp Infect 34, 117–122.

Unahand, M., Mustafa, M.M., McCracken, G.H., et al., 1993. Gram-negative bacillary meningitis: a twenty-one year experience. J Pediatr 122, 15–21.

Valencia, G.B., Banzon, F., Cummings, M., et al., 1993. *Mycoplasma hominis* and *Ureaplasma urealyticum* in neonates with suspected infection. Pediatr Infect Dis J 12, 571–573.

Valladares, G., Chacaltana, A., Sjogren, M.H., 2010. The management of HCV-infected pregnant women. Ann Hepatol 9 (Suppl), 92–97.

Van Camp, J.M., Tomaselli, V., Coran, A.G., 1994. Bacterial translocation in the neonate. Curr Opin Pediatr 6, 327–333.

Vandebona, H., Mitchell, P., Manwaring, N., et al., 2009. Prevalence of mitochondrial 1555A–>G mutation in adults of European descent. N Engl J Med 60, 642–644.

Van Houten, M.A., Uiterwaal, C.S., Heesan, G., et al., 2001. Does the empiric use of vancomycin in pediatrics increase the risk of Gram-negative bacteraemia? Pediatr Infect Dis J 20, 171–177.

Vergnano, S., Embleton, N.D., Collinson, A., et al., 2009. Missed opportunities for preventing GBS infections. Arch Dis Child Fetal Neonatal Ed 95, F72–F73.

Vergnano, S., Menson, E., Kennea, N., et al., 2011. Neonatal infections in England: the NeonIN surveillance network, Arch Dis Child Fetal Neonatal Ed 96, F9–F14.

Verma, A., Dhawan, A., Zuckerman, M., et al., 2006. Neonatal herpes simplex virus infection presenting as acute liver failure: prevalent role of herpes simplex virus type I. J Pediatr Gastroenterol Nutr 42, 282–286.

Viscardi, R.M., 2010. *Ureaplasma* species: role in diseases of prematurity. Clin Perinatol 37, 393–409.

Viscardi, R.M., Hasday, J.D., 2009. Role of *Ureaplasma* species in neonatal chronic lung disease: epidemiologic and experimental evidence. Pediatr Res 65, 84R–90R.

Visser, V.E., Hall, R.T., 1980. Lumbar puncture in the evaluation of suspected neonatal sepsis. J Pediatr 96, 1063–1067.

Waites, K.B., Crouse, D.T., Cassell, G.H., 1993. Therapeutic considerations for Ureaplasma urealyticum infections in neonates. Clin Infect Dis 17, S208–S214.

Walker, V.P., Akinbi, H.T., Meinzen-Derr, J., et al., 2008. Host defense proteins on the surface of neonatal skin: implications for innate immunity. J Pediatr 152, 777–781.

Walsh, M.C., Kliegman, R.M., 1986. Necrotizing enterocolitis: treatment based on staging criteria. Pediatr Clin North Am 33, 179.

Walter, C., Noguera, A., Gene, A., et al., 2009. Group B streptococcal late-onset disease presenting with parotitis. J Paediatr Child Health 45, 764–766.

Ware, R., 1989. Human parvovirus infection. J Pediatr 114, 343–348.

Webber, S., Wilkinson, A.R., Lindsell, D., et al., 1990. Neonatal pneumonia. Arch Dis Child 65, 207–211.

Weisman, L.E., Cruess, D.F., 1994. Opsonic activity of commercially available standards intravenous immunglobulin preparations. Pediatr Infect Dis J 13, 1122–1125.

Weisman, L.E., Wilson, S.R., Fischer, G.W., 1996. Intravenous immunoglobulin (IV IGG) lots used in clinical trials to prevent late-onset infection in the high risk neonate contained variable *Staphylococcus epidermidis* antibody activity. Pediatr Res 39, 304A.

Weisman, L.E., Thackray, H.M., Garcia-Prats, J.A., et al., 2009. Phase 1/2 double-blind, placebo-controlled, dose escalation safety and pharmacokinetic study of pagibaximab (BSYX-A110), an anti-staphylococcal monoclonal antibody for the prevention of bloodstream infections in very low birth weoght neonates. Antimicrob Agents Chemother 53, 2879–2886.

Weisner, A.M., Johnson, A.P., Lamagni, T.L., et al., 2004. Characterisation of group B streptococcus recovered from infants with invasive disease in England and Wales. Clin Infect Dis 38, 1203–1208.

Weisse, M.E., Person, D.A., Berkenbaugh, J.T.J., 1993. Treatment of *Candida* arthritis with flucytosine and amphotericin. J Perinatol 13, 402–404.

Wershil, B.K., Furuta, G.T., 2008. 4. Gastrointestinal mucosal immunity. J Allergy Clin Immunol 121, S380–S383.

Wettergren, B., Jodal, U., Jonasson, G., 1985. Epidemiology of bacteriuria during the first year of life. Acta Paediatr Scand 74, 925–930.

Whitley, R.J., 1993. Neonatal herpes simplex virus infections. J Med Virol 1 (suppl), 13–21.

WHO, 2005. Progress towards elimination of measles and prevention of congenital rubella infection in the WHO European Region, 1990-2004. Weekly. Epidemiol Rec 80, 66–71.

WHO, 2011. Global HIV/AIDS response: epidemic update and health sector progress towards universal access: progress report 2011. http://www.who.int/publications/2011/9789241502986_eng.pdf.

Wiswell, T.E., Baumgart, S., Gannon, C.M., et al., 1995. No lumbar puncture in the evaluation for early neonatal sepsis: will meningitis be missed? Pediatrics 95, 803–806.

Woldensbet, M., Rosenfeld, C.R., Ramilo, O., et al., 2008. Severe neonatal hypoxic respiratory failure correlates with histopathological chorioamnionitis and raised concentrations of interleukin 6 (IL-6), IL-8 and C-reactive protein. Arch Dis Child Fetal Neonatal Ed 93, F413–F417.

Wong, S.N., Ng, T.L., 1991. *Haemophilus influenzae* septicaemia in the neonate: report of two cases and review of the English literature. J Paediatr Child Health 27, 113–115.

Woods, C.R., 2005. Gonococcal infections in neonates and young children. Semin Pediatr Infect Dis 16, 258–270.

World Health Organization, 2006. Antiretroviral drugs for treating pregnant women and preventing HIV infection in infants: towards universal access. Recommendations for a public health approach (2006 revision). Available online at: http://www.who.int/hiv/pub/mtct/antiretroviral/en/index.html

Yagupsky, P., Menegus, M.A., Powell, K.R., 1991. The changing spectrum of group B streptococcal disease in infants: an eleven-year experience in a tertiary care hospital. Pediatr Infect Dis J 10, 801–808.

Yuksel, B., Greenough, A., 1994. Viral infections acquired during neonatal intensive care and lung function of preterm infants at follow-up. Acta Paediatrica 83, 117–118.

Zaidi, A.K., Huskins, W.C., Thaver, D., et al., 2005. Hospital-acquired neonatal infections in developing countries. Lancet 365, 1175–1188.

Zar, H.J., 2005. Neonatal chlamydial infections: prevention and treatment. Paediatr Drugs 7, 103–110.

Zaoutis, T.E., Goyal, M., Chu, J.H., et al., 2005. Risk factors for and outcomes of bloodstream infection caused by extended-spectrum beta-lactamase-producing *Escherichia coli* and *Klebsiella* species in children. Pediatrics 115, 942–949.

Neurological problems in the newborn

Janet M Rennie   Angela Huertas-Ceballos   Geraldine B Boylan
Divyen K Shah   Nicola J Robertson   Floris Groenendaal
Leigh E Dyet   Peter G Barth   Adnan Y Manzur
Stephanie A Robb   Francesco Muntoni   Cornelia Hagmann

40

CHAPTER OUTLINE

© 2012 Elsevier Ltd

Part 1: **Examination of the nervous system**

Janet M Rennie   Angela Huertas-Ceballos

Introduction

Suspicion of neurological illness in the neonatal period is always important. As in any organ system disease, diagnosis and prognosis must be based on the findings of a full examination together with the results of appropriate investigation. Neonatal neurological assessment should include sequential careful examinations, which of necessity are dominated by examination of the baby's state of alertness and the motor system. Neurological examination of a baby receiving intensive care is difficult, but not impossible, and can be supplemented by a wide range of diagnostic tests. Cranial ultrasound scanning is now standard in neonatal units, and atlases have been published which can help clinicians interpret the findings

(Rennie et al. 2008; Govaert and de Vries 2010). Much valuable experience has been gained with magnetic resonance imaging scanning of the neonatal brain (Barkovich 1999; Rutherford 2002). Normal ranges exist for somatosensory, auditory and visual evoked potentials, and recording the electroencephalogram (EEG) can prove extremely helpful. The information in this short chapter can be supplemented by further reading from more detailed texts (Amiel-Tison 1994b, 2001, 2002; Dubowitz et al. 1999; Volpe 2001, 2008; Rennie et al. 2008). Much of the modern work on examination of the neonatal nervous system has built on that of the earlier teaching of Andre-Thomas Chesni and Saint-Anne Dargassies (1960), Illingworth (1960, 1980) and Prechtl (1977). For advice on general examination of the newborn, see Chapter 14.

Examination systems

The endless fascination which observing babies provides is reflected in the number of schemes which have been developed for assessment of the neonatal nervous system. Majnemer and Mazer (1998) reviewed nine different systems, many of which require special training and take up to an hour to carry out. This is not practical in clinical practice, or possible in sick babies. The recommendations vary from a detailed 'cut-down' version of an adult-style neurological examination (Mercuri et al. 2007) to a more general approach involving scoring of videos of general spontaneous movement (Prechtl and Nolte 1984; Cioni et al. 1997) or scoring of behavioural states (Lester et al. 2004). We agree with Amiel-Tison (2001) that the allocation of a numbered score implies a degree of standardisation and accuracy which does not exist.

Our own current system is illustrated in Figure 40.1, and can be carried out quickly and adapted for babies in intensive care. This scheme includes many of the items from the original Dubowitz system (Dubowitz et al. 1998, 1999) updated by Eugenio Mercuri et al. (2007), which has been developed after a great deal of careful research, and was designed to be taught to junior resident staff and to be reproducible and quick to carry out. The updated scheme takes into account the newer emphasis on the importance of hand posture and presence or absence of individual finger movements, and has reduced duplication. In addition to completing a suitable proforma, there is no substitute for a short and pithy narrative note. For example:

At the start of the examination, Tom was lying prone in his incubator in a flexed posture with his knees tucked up under his abdomen, eyes closed and breathing regularly. His head circumference was 35 cm and his fontanelle felt normal.

When stroked lightly on his back he awoke and began fussing, with normal facial and body movements and a normal cry, but he soon calmed when stroked again. He sucked vigorously on a finger with a stripping action of his tongue, made eye contact readily and followed a target horizontally through 90° in each direction with ease. When observed lying on his back he kicked with both legs, and his truncal and limb tone and reflexes were normal. His hands were relaxed and open and he made individual movements of his fingers. He could not be taken out of the incubator to test stepping or ventral suspension today but his Moro response appeared full and symmetrical, although it was not possible to test head lag. As far as I can assess, Tom's neurological state was normal today.

Alice's head circumference is small for a term baby at 32 cm, and her ears appear prominent – they are not low-set. Her skull is a normal shape and, although her fontanelle was small (little-fingertip size), the tension felt normal. When observed at the start, Alice was lying on her back, with outstretched arms and extended legs; she had a high-pitched scream and was arching her back at times, digging her heels into the cot mattress. Her hands were fisted with the thumbs in both palms all the time and I did not observe her to open them. She could be consoled by swaddling and rocking but this took patience, and when she was handled her tone was high in both the trunk and the limbs. After some persuasion Alice fixed on a red woolly ball but did not track it consistently or through a wide range of arc. Alice did not make eye contact with me; she chomped on my finger and I note that the nurses are tube-feeding her at the moment. Tendon reflexes were easy to obtain but I could not elicit a stepping or root reflex and

her Moro was incomplete with a brisk adduction phase. I am concerned about Alice, whose neurological assessment was not normal today, and in my view a re-examination should be carried out before she is discharged home.

Scheme of neonatal neurological examination

General observations

Head size and shape

The head circumference should be measured as part of routine examination of the newborn (Ch. 14), and the importance of documenting head size and head growth as part of neurological assessment cannot be overstressed. Fontanelle size and tension must be recorded.

The newborn skull is not fused, and it is possible to palpate the cranial sutures which should not be ridged or separated too far (Fig. 40.2). Observe any superficial swellings such as cephalhaematoma or subgaleal collections. Fused sutures (craniosynostosis) may need treatment, or may be a clue to an underlying disorder such as Apert's syndrome. Advice may need to be obtained from a neurosurgeon.

Orientation and behaviour

Behavioural states

The initial assessment of the baby's nervous system should involve evaluation of state of alertness, a sensitive indicator of neural integrity. Alertness or behavioural states can be described on the basis of four features (Table 40.1 and Fig. 40.1) (Prechtl 1974; Prechtl and O'Brien 1982; Brazelton and Nugent 1995).

Term babies spend about 50 minutes of each hour asleep and about 50% of the time in quiet sleep (state 1). Babies usually cycle between states, and failure to do so is abnormal; examples of conditions that cause this are drug withdrawal and hypoxic–ischaemic encephalopathy.

State 1: deep or quiet sleep

Quiet sleep begins when a baby who keeps his eyes closed begins to breathe regularly. Eye movements under the closed eyelids are not present. The baby is generally still and not moving. Rhythmical mouthing movements can appear, lasting a few seconds up to a maximum of a few minutes. Although gross motor movements are rare, startles do occur in this phase of sleep.

State 2: light or rapid eye movement sleep

In this phase of sleep respirations are irregular. The transition from state 1 into state 2 is frequently marked with a startle, gross movements or a sigh. Under the closed eyelids, slow eye movements can be observed. Small twitches are common in state 2 and are visible in the face, hands and feet. Grimaces, smiles and rhythmical mouthing are observable at times. The many movements result in frequently changing postures.

State 3: awake, drowsy, dozing

In state 3, the baby lies still and keeps his eyes open, although they may be heavy-lidded. Although there may be moments of staring, most of the time the baby seems to scan the environment with rapid eye movements. A stable posture and regular respiration are usual. Babies have a dazed look in this half-awake state. The longest such periods occur after a feed.

Neonatal CNS examination

Name: _____ Date of Exam: __/__/__

DOB: __/__/__ Examiner: _____

GA: _____ weeks

modified from Dubowitz 1981 and other sources ā JMR 2004

States:
0. Coma: no/little response to pain
1. Deep sleep, no movement, regular breathing
2. Light sleep, eyes shut, some movement
3. Dozing, eyes opening and closing
4. Awake, eyes open, minimal movement
5. Wide awake, vigorous movement
6. Crying

* Do not examine starred items * in ventilated or very ill babies

Orientation and behaviour; note any adverse circumstances e.g. excessive noise

State at start	0	1 or 2	3 or 4	5 or 6
and end of exam	0	1 or 2	3 or 4	5 or 6
Level of consciousness	Comatose	Lethargic	Hyperalert, stary-eyed	Normal, easily aroused
Consolability	High pitched cry, continuous	Cries, difficult to console	Cries, easy to console	Not crying, consoling not needed
Irritability	Cries when not handled	Cries often and easily	Cries sometimes when handled, not irritable	Quiet all the time – too quiet
Visual orientation	Doesn't fix or follow, or roving eye movements	Fixes and follows but loses interest	Fixes and follows up to 90° horizontally	Fixes and follows reliably horizontally
Social interaction	Cannot engage at all	Tries to engage but does not succeed	Brief interest in stimuli or face of examiner	Easy to engage and makes eye contact

Posture and movement (normal and abnormal)

Posture: draw here	Opistotonus, or flexed arms extended legs 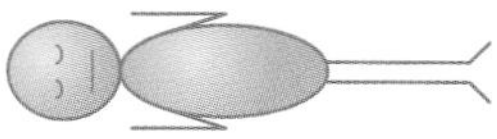	Arms + legs extended 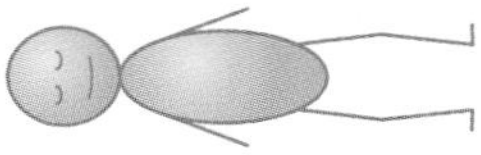	Legs flexed but not adducted 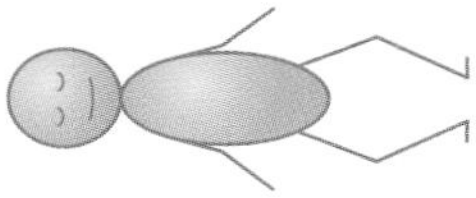	Normal, legs flexed. Legs well flexed near abdomen 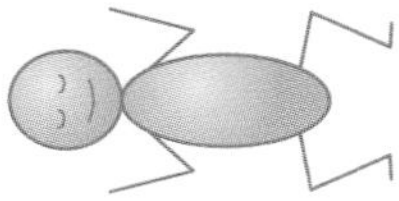
Spontaneous movements Observe quality and quantity	No spontaneous movement	Paucity of movement, occasional random jerky movement, only stretching	Stereotyped or monotonous	Rich variety, smooth, fluent, good variability and range
Hand movements	Thumb fixed in palm, hand fisted all the time	No finger movements, intermittent fisting	Some occasional finger movements	Fine elegant finger movements, hands open
Tremours/startles	None, no reaction to loud noise or stimuli	Continuous tremours and startles	Frequent spontaneous startles and tremours when awake	Tremour after Moro. occasional spontaneous startle
Clinical seizures – describe	More than 6/day	3–6/day	<3/day	None

(A)

Fig. 40.1 A system for neonatal neurological examination, adapted from several sources, including Dubowitz, Prechtl, Amiel-Tison and others. CNS, central nervous system; DOB, date of birth; GA, gestational age; OFC, occipitofrontal circumference; IPPV, intermittent positive-pressure ventilation.

Trunk and limb tone

Head control/head lag* draw here	No attempt to raise head, complete lag	Tries to lift head but effort better felt than seen, head drops back	Raises head very briefly, in line with body	Raises head – remains vertical and in front of body for brief time

Ventral suspension* draw here	Back curved head and limbs hang straight	Back curved limbs slightly flexed	Back straight head in line limbs flexed	Back straight head above body

Leg recoil	No flexion	Incomplete	Complete, but slow	Complete and fast
Take both ankles with one hand, flex hips and knees, quickly extend, let go. Repeat × 3				
Truncal tone	Flaccid	Hyotonic	Hypertonic	Normal
Limb tone	Flaccid	Hyotonic	Hypertonic	Normal

Reflexes

Tendon reflexes	Absent	Exaggerated	Clonus	Normal
Stepping*	No attempt to lift leg over the edge of the couch	Dorsiflexion of ankle	Flexes hip and knee and places sole on couch	Automatic walking easy to obtain
Moro*	Absent	Incomplete	Asymmetrical	Normal
Root*	Absent	Weak	Some head turning and mouth opening	Searches and localises
Asymmetric tonic neck	Absent			Present
Sucking	Absent	Bites, clenches	Weak irregular suck	Strong suck, strips

General observations

Fontanelle/OFC	OFC: cm	Tense	Full	Normal
Skull	Caput	Subgaleal haematoma	Sutures overriding	Cephalhaematoma
Respiration	IPPV for apnoea	Brief apnoeas	Hyperventilation	Normal
Stability during exam	Unstable	Abnormal state throughout, no change	Little transition of state, slow transition	Rapid transition of state, well tolerated

Comments:

(B)

Fig. 40.1, cont'd

Table 40.1 Features of neonatal behavioural states

STATE	EYES OPEN	RESPIRATION REGULAR	GROSS MOVEMENTS	VOCALISATION
1	−1	+1	−1	−1
2	−1	−1	0	−1
3	+1	+1	−1	−1
4	+1	−1	+1	−1
5	0	−1	+1	+1

Modified frcm Prechtl and O'Brien (1982).
+1, present; −1, absent; 0, present or absent.

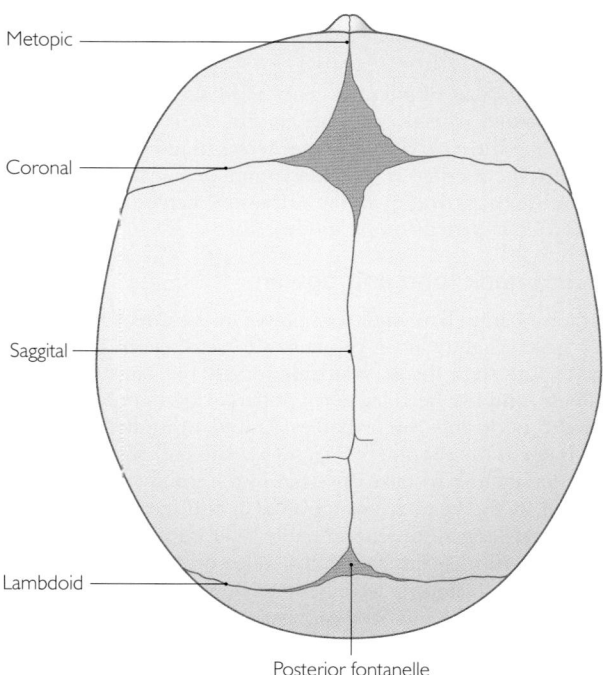

Fig. 40.2 Diagram to show the position of the cranial sutures and the fontanelles.

Metopic

Coronal

Saggital

Lambdoid

Posterior fontanelle

State 4: quiet alertness

In state 4, the baby is alert with eyes open and minimal motor activity; there can be a glazed look that is easily changed into a brighter look with appropriate visual or auditory stimulation.

State 5: alert

The baby is alert and content with bright open eyes. Posture changes frequently ard sequential, fluent movements of all four limbs (also known as writhing movements) are seen.

State 6: crying

Crying is a communication signal, and it is clear that parents and nurses can often discriminate between cries of discomfort, hunger and pain.

Behavioural state of the neonate less mature than 36 weeks' gestation

Babies born before 36 weeks' gestation spend a great deal of time asleep, but their sleep states cannot be classified so easily. Prechtl et al. (1979), on the basis of a longitudinal study of very low-risk preterm infants, came to the following conclusion: 'Cycles of rest and activity, regular and irregular breathing, and epochs with and without eye movements may alternate independently and may accidentally overlap, but often do not coincide at all before 35–37 weeks'.

Abnormal states, abnormal state cycling and coma

Nearly every disorder that affects the central nervous system disturbs the level of alertness at some time. Babies are usually arousable, that is, they will awaken to the sound of a bell or a bright light. Failure to arouse means that a baby is stuporose or comatose. Both in utero (Prechtl and Nolte 1984) and after birth stereotyped movements are an indicator of disease, and a rich variety of movement is an indicator of health.

In conclusion, in healthy newborns, both full-term and preterm, cycles of activity should be present. After 36 weeks these are recognised as distinct behavioural state cycles as described above; before 36 weeks these consist of more or less independently occurring cycles of activity and quiescence, of regular and irregular breathing, and of periods with and without rapid eye movements. Recognition of these cycles can be helped by looking at the electrocardiogram, respiratory pattern and TcPo$_2$. Attention to assessment of behavioural state and behavioural state cycling may be the single most sensitive way to assess the integrity of the neonatal central nervous system, and should be the starting point for examination of the nervous system.

Consolability/cuddliness

During an examination, or when they are cold or hungry, babies often cry but are usually consolable. Brazelton and Nugent (1995) stress that normal babies are 'cuddly' and will mould into the crook of an arm or nestle in the examiner's neck. Persistent, high-pitched crying is abnormal, as is the stiff 'uncuddly' behaviour of a baby with encephalopathy.

Posture, spontaneous movement and tone

Active tone and movements

Normal muscle offers a resistance to stretch which is felt by the examiner as tone. Active flexor tone appears between 28 and 34 weeks and matures from the feet and legs upwards (Amiel-Tison 1994b, 2001). This is clearly seen by watching the posture adopted by term babies, who lie with their limbs flexed and adducted, unlike preterm babies who adopt an extended posture. Asymmetrical tone does not always indicate asymmetrical pathology in the newborn period. A pattern of persistent mixed change in tone with hypertonia in the limbs and hypotonia in the trunk is abnormal, as is arching of the trunk at any age. When the whole body is arched, the term 'opisthotonos' is used. Tone can alter considerably in relation to medication, feeds and sleep state, and sequential examinations are required to confirm physical signs.

A term newborn makes smooth, varied, spontaneous and symmetrical limb movements which stop when the baby's attention is diverted (Prechtl 1990). Finger movements are elegant and varied, involving the thumb, which can be abducted away from the palm by term (Ferrari et al. 1990). A persistently adducted thumb (cortical thumb) in a tightly fisted hand is abnormal (Illingworth 1980; Dubowitz et al. 1999), and babies with brain injury often have this sign, with a paucity of fine finger movements.

Facial expression

Spontaneous facial movements are frequently seen in the normal newborn, although bilateral facial paralysis (as in Moebius syndrome) is much more difficult to diagnose than the more common unilateral facial palsy. Normal facial expression in an otherwise hypotonic and flaccid newborn baby suggests a spinal cord problem. Babies of just a few days old will often imitate facial gestures, for example putting out their tongues.

Limb movement, passive tone and power

Before passive movements are used to assess tone it may be possible to observe spontaneous movements of the limbs against gravity. Failure to move part or all of a limb may be due to pain or paralysis. Limb tone is influenced by the tonic neck reflex in newborns which means it is important to have the head in the midline before beginning to elicit passive movements. These involve gentle flexion of the upper and lower limbs, then rapid extension and observation of recoil. A summary is contained within the protocol suggested by Dubowitz et al. (1999). This examination system, like that of Amiel-Tison (1994b, 2001), involves assessing angles made by bending and manipulating the limbs and trunk. These include the popliteal angle (Fig. 40.3), the foot dorsiflexion angle and the scarf sign. A reduced popliteal angle and clusters of abnormal signs are sensitive indicators of later outcome (Dubowitz et al. 1984).

Jitteriness

The normal term newborn is in a state of relative hypertonicity, with brisk reflexes tending to clonus. This high tone can lead to the clinical sign of jittering. Jittering is a high-frequency, generalised, symmetrical tremor of the limbs which is stilled by flexion or by inducing the baby to suck on a finger. Jittering is common in the first 2 or 3 days in term babies and is generally benign (Shuper et al. 1991) but if it is excessive or persistent it deserves investigation (see seizures, p. 1080). Repetitive chewing movements or tongue

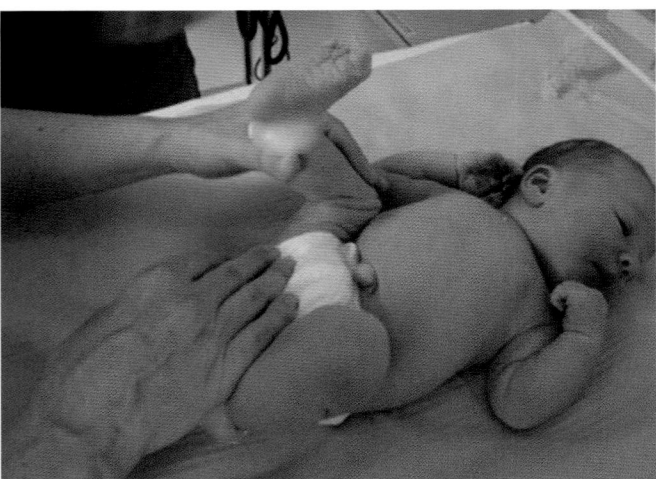

Fig. 40.3 Assessment of popliteal angle. Note that the ipsilateral hip joint should be fixed.

thrusting are not part of jitteriness and imply seizures. Jitteriness is stimulus-sensitive, whereas seizures are not. In seizure the movement has a fast and slow component whereas in jittering the tremor is symmetrical. Jittering is never accompanied by physiological changes due to the activation of the autonomic nervous system such as tachycardia, hypertension or apnoea.

Trunk and neck tone and power

Normal term babies have sufficient power in their neck muscles to lift their heads slightly when prone or supine. Preterm babies can manage to turn their heads from side to side but have much less power, with complete head lag when pulled to sit. In order to judge tone in the neck and trunk, babies should be pulled to sit by holding them at the shoulders (Fig. 40.4). The pull-to-sit manoeuvre elicits an attempt to raise the head in a normal term newborn (Fig. 40.4a). If the head is unsupported it will gradually fall forwards or backwards: normal term babies will be able to raise their heads to the vertical again from either direction (Fig. 40.4b), but it is normal for the head of a term baby to wobble. Truncal tone can be assessed by placing the baby on his side, with one hand on the back and the other manipulating the legs. It is normally easier to flex a baby's trunk than to extend it.

Reflexes

Tendon and Babinski reflexes

Eliciting tendon reflexes is of less value in the newborn period than later in childhood. Knee and biceps jerks can usually be obtained. Reflexes at term are very brisk due to the high tone, and a few beats of clonus at the ankle are usual. Very brisk reflexes and clonus are not reliable indicators of an upper motor neurone lesion until about 6 months of age (Amiel-Tison and Stewart 1994b). A crossed adductor response to the knee jerk (see below) is also usual in the first months of life whereas the sign is abnormal later on. The plantar reflex of Babinski is always extensor in babies, and this test is best omitted as the stimulus is painful and often results in a withdrawal response.

Primary neonatal reflexes

Whilst these responses are intriguing to doctors and parents alike it is necessary to have a working knowledge of only a few. Primitive

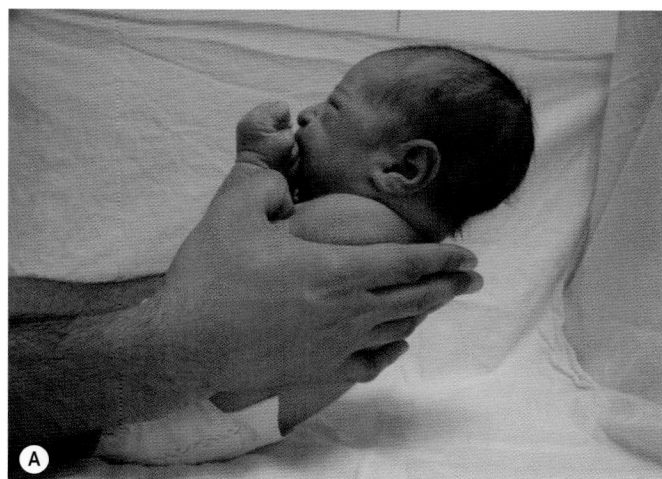

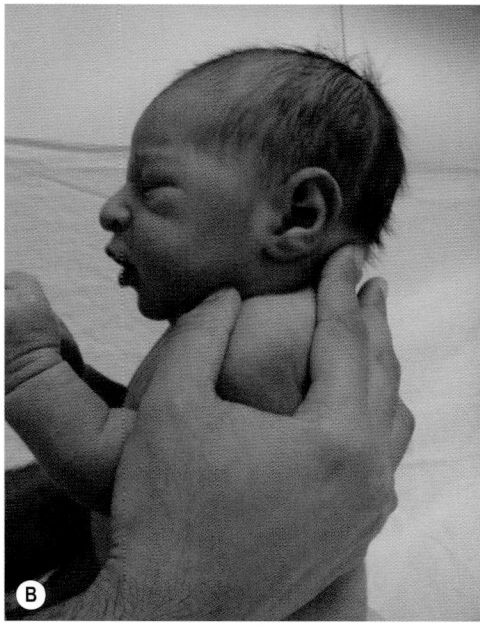

Fig. 40.4 (a) Pull-to-sit manoeuvre: this full-term baby is attempting to raise his head. (b) After being pulled to sit the baby has raised his head to the vertical position.

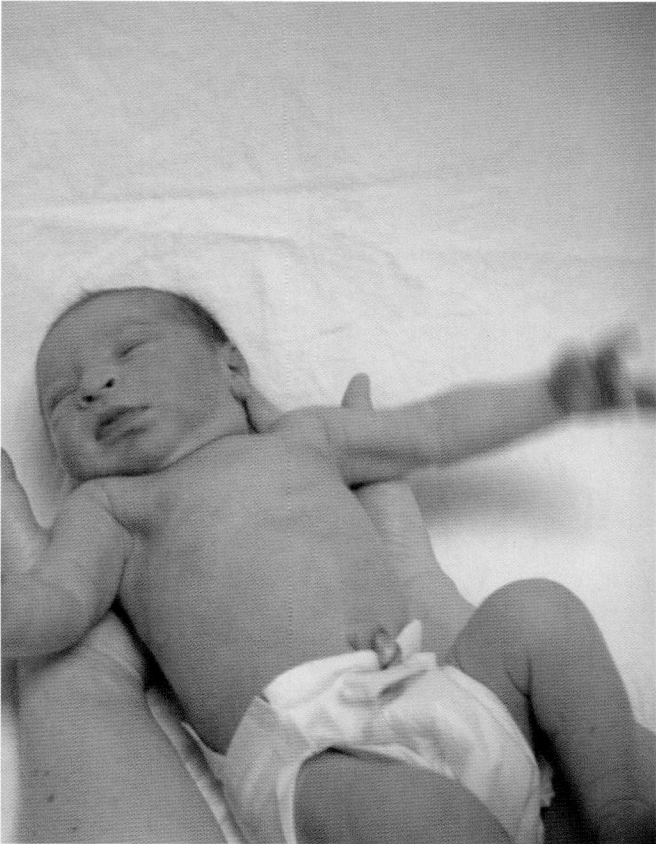

Fig. 40.5 The abduction phase of the Moro response: the baby's head has been allowed to fall back slightly but is then supported by the examiner's hand.

reflexes normally habituate after repeated performance. Persistence of primitive reflexes can inhibit normal movement in children with cerebral palsy.

Moro reflex

This reflex is usually elicited by allowing the previously supported head of a baby to fall backwards slightly, whereupon the baby extends and adducts both upper limbs, opening the hands (Fig. 40.5). Babies of greater than 33 weeks' gestation subsequently adduct their arms. The Moro response is present from 28 weeks of gestation and usually disappears by 4 months. Persistence beyond 6 months is always abnormal.

Asymmetric tonic neck reflex

Starting with the baby supine and the head in the midline the head is slowly turned to one side. This results in increased extensor tone in the arm on the side to which the head is turned and increased

flexor tone in the arm on the opposite side (fencing posture). The reflex appears by 35 weeks' gestation, is very prominent by about 1 month of age and disappears by about 7 months.

Crossed extension (adduction) reflex

One leg is held in extension and the sole of the foot is rubbed. The other leg first withdraws and then extends with fanning of the toes. The third and final component of the fully developed reflex brings the other foot towards the side which was stimulated. Eliciting the knee jerk often produces this reflex in the neonatal period, which should not persist after 8 months of age.

Placing and stepping

By stimulating the dorsum of the foot, usually by bringing it into contact with the edge of the couch, a mature baby can be induced to 'step' over the edge (Fig. 40.6). The baby's toes fan out and he lifts his foot up and then places it on the surface. Babies will extend their legs on to a flat surface and 'support' their weight when held under the arms. With the feet in contact with a solid surface and the body tilted forwards the baby will 'walk'.

Rooting, sucking and swallowing

Stroking the upper lip of a baby of 28 weeks' gestation and above results in the baby searching for the nipple and opening the mouth.

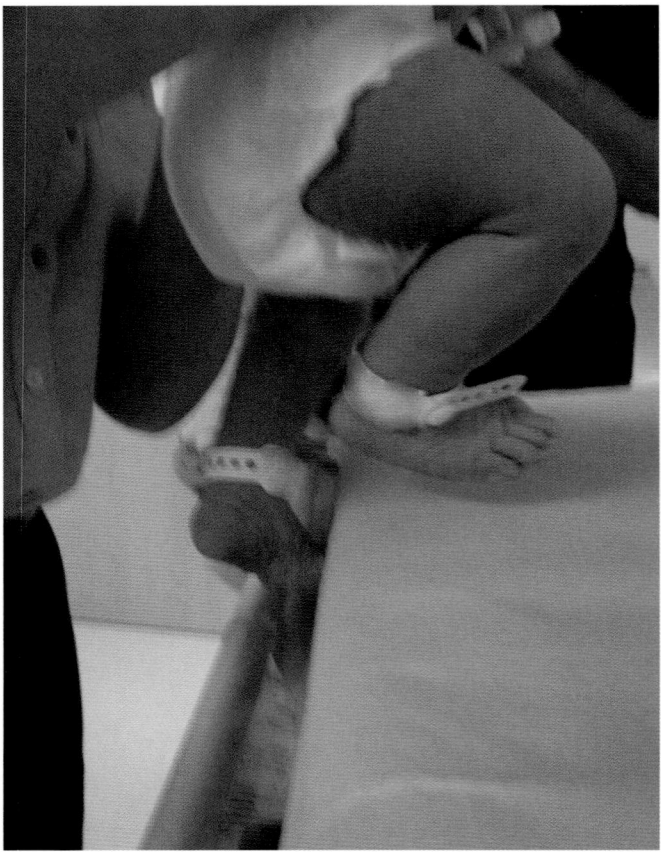

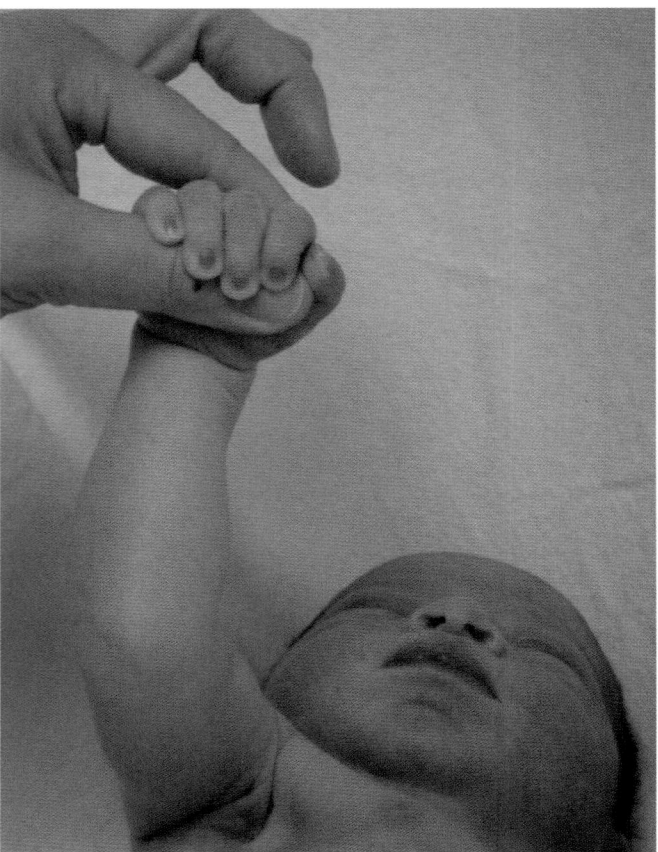

Fig. 40.6 The stepping reflex, elicited by bringing the dorsum of the baby's foot into contact with the couch.

Fig. 40.7 The palmar grasp reflex.

This reflex tests the sensation in the distribution of the fifth cranial nerve and the motor pathways of cranial nerves V, VII, XII. Swallowing also involves cranial nerves IX and X. The sensory input for the sucking reflex comes from the hard palate, not the tongue or cheek. Sucking begins during the 11th week of intrauterine life. Coordination between sucking and swallowing exists from 28 weeks' gestation but the strength to sustain it and to synchronise the process with breathing is only adequate after 32–34 weeks' gestation. Sucking gradually builds up from bursts of three sucks at a time to eight or more, with a reduction in the interburst interval. If sucking is absent, test the gag reflex by gently stroking the soft palate with a cotton bud.

Palmar and plantar

The palmar reflex results from stroking the palmar surface of the hand, eliciting a grasp that is often strong enough to lift the baby from the crib (Fig. 40.7). It is present from 26 weeks' gestation and persists up to 4 months. Stroking the plantar surface of the foot results in curling of the toes in a similar manner to the palmar response (Fig. 40.8).

Pupillary reflex

The pupils respond to light only after 30 weeks' gestation, and the response was present in all infants after 35 weeks (Robinson and Fielder 1990). Babies of less than 30 weeks' gestation do respond

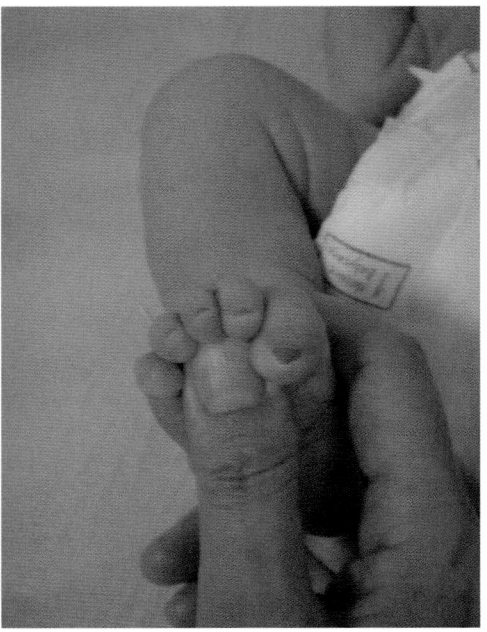

Fig. 40.8 The plantar grasp reflex.

to a bright light, by blinking or averting their eyes. The size of the pupil gradually decreases after the development of the light reflex. The amplitude of the response, that is, the difference in size of the pupil before and after the light exposure, increases up to term. A small pupil on the side of an Erb's palsy suggests Horner's sydrome due to involvement of C8 and T1 nerve roots. A large pupil can indicate a congenital or acquired third-nerve palsy.

Neonatal neurological alarm signals

Certain neonatal neurological signs are generally recognised as potential indicators of serious disease. These 'alarm signs', derived from the work of many authors (Joppich and Schulte 1968; Brown et al. 1974; Touwen 1976; Saint-Anne Dargassies 1977; Amiel-Tison and Grenier 1980; Dubowitz et al. 1999; Volpe 2001; Amiel-Tison 2002), are:

- persistent irritability
- difficulty in feeding
- persistent deviation of head and/or eyes
- persistent asymmetry in posture and movements
- persistently adducted thumbs in a fisted hand
- opisthotonos
- persistent posture of flexed arms and extended legs
- apathy and immobility
- floppiness, severe generalised hypotonia
- convulsions
- abnormal cry
- the combination of setting-sun sign, vomiting, wide sutures and/or abnormal increase in skull circumference.

Respiratory difficulties and apnoea can be signs of neurological dysfunction, although apnoea of prematurity is the commonest cause on a modern neonatal unit (Ch. 27, part 4). In one large study, recurrent apnoea (i.e. three or more episodes of apnoea of longer than 20 seconds' duration) occurred in 1% of 25 154 babies evaluated between 1974 and 1979 (Henderson-Smart 1981). Of the affected babies, apnoea commenced in the first 2 days of life in 77% and was unlikely to commence after 7 days (Henderson-Smart 1981). The gestational age at birth had a major impact with respect to the postnatal age when the last apnoea was detected.

Special senses

Examination of vision, visual evoked potentials

The assessment of visual function in newborn babies includes behavioural and electrophysiological techniques.

Behavioural techniques are based on the observation of spontaneous or elicited visual behaviours in the baby. The 26-week gestation preterm baby blinks in response to light; by 32 weeks there is eye closure; by 34 weeks a baby is able to fix and track a bright object briefly. By 37 weeks a baby will turn to soft light, and can track reliably (Fig. 40.9). Optokinetic horizontal nystagmus is present when a term baby looks at a striped rotating drum or a striped tape is moved in front of the baby's eyes. Changing the width of the stripes or forced-choice preferential looking at striped grids can be used to test visual acuity, which is equivalent to 20/150 vision at term. Vertical or asymmetrical nystagmus should always be investigated (Shawkat et al. 2000).

The interpretation of deficient neonatal visual responses, however, is much more difficult. Dubowitz stresses the importance of the loss

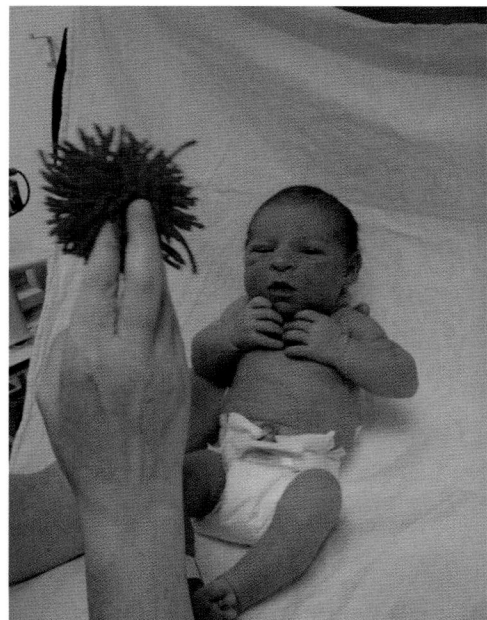

Fig. 40.9 Fixing and tracking a red pom-pom.

of previously good visual performance as a disturbing sign. Babies' eyes are usually in alignment, although a slight horizontal divergence is normal until 6 weeks of age, particularly in preterm babies. Vertical or skew deviation is always abnormal and has been seen in association with germinal matrix haemorrhage/intraventricular haemorrhage (Volpe 2001). For more information on abnormal and delayed visual development, and squint, see Chapter 33.

Electrophysiological techniques measure the visual evoked potentials which are produced within the occipital cortex as a result of repeatedly applying an appropriate visual stimulus so that the minute electrical response to it, which will be identical each time, can be extracted from the random background electrical noise (EEG) by computerised averaging. Strobosocopic or flashing red lights are used which can penetrate closed eyelids. The electrical response 'matures' with advancing gestation and can be detected from 25 weeks. Study of visual evoked potentials has been found to be of value in predicting outcome after birth asphyxia (Taylor et al. 1992), and is a sensitive test for the integrity of the visual pathway. Absent visual evoked potentials predicts cortical blindness in preterm infants with extensive cystic leukomalacia (de Vries et al. 1987), and visual impairment is the most important variable in determining the neurodevelopmental scores in these infants (Cioni 2000).

Auditory testing in the neonatal period

The fetus responds to sound from 19 weeks of gestation (Hepper and Shahidullah 1994). Babies from 28 weeks of gestation respond to noise by turning their heads, arousing from sleep or increasing their body movements. Bilateral sensorineural deafness occurs in about 1.5 per 1000 children. Successful universal neonatal screening programmes developed for use in the UK (Watkin 1996; Wessex Universal Neonatal Hearing Screening Trial Group 1998) have been rolled out gradually since 2000. Universal neonatal hearing screening is now established in the UK (www.hearing.screening.nhs.uk). Universal neonatal hearing screening is more cost-effective than the infant distraction test and children treated early have better speech and language skills, although debate continues about the strength of the evidence (Thompson et al. 2001).

Otoacoustic emissions

Otoacoustic emissions were discovered in 1978. Otoacoustic emissions are low-amplitude sound waves which are produced by the inner ear; they occur spontaneously as well as in response to a click stimulus. The automated method depends on the fact that a click stimulus, when presented to an intact hearing ear, evokes an otoacoustic emission which can be detected by a probe lying in the ear canal. Testing with otoacoustic emissions is quicker to administer than with an automated evoked brainstem response method but there are more false-positive results.

Brainstem auditory evoked potential

These indicate electrical events generated in the brainstem auditory pathway in response to sound (usually a click) presented at the ear. The electrical signals are recorded with EEG electrodes on the scalp. The results of many click stimulations are summed by a computer which uses coherent averaging to eliminate the background noise generated by the local EEG signal. The mature pattern consists of seven waves, but these are poorly developed with increased latency and require a larger stimulus in order to elicit them in babies, in whom the response is present from 24 weeks. Automated brainstem response equipment eliminates the need for extensive operator training and is a widely used method of hearing screening.

Imaging

For advice on the best imaging modality to choose when investigating the central nervous system, see Chapter 43.

Examination of cerebrospinal fluid and intracranial pressure

There should be a low threshold for performing lumbar puncture in babies because the signs of meningitis are subtle. For practical advice on how to perform the procedure, see Chapter 44. In the neonatal period cerebrospinal fluid may be xanthochromic because of jaundice or old germinal matrix haemorrhage/intraventricular haemorrhage. The mean and median white cell count is less than 10 cells per mm^3 and the upper limit of normal is around 21 (Appendix 1). Red cell counts of around 100 per mm^3 in the preterm baby are considered normal and counts more than 1000 per mm^3 make the interpretation of cerebrospinal fluid results very difficult: applying correction factors using the ratio of white cells to red cells has been shown to be inaccurate. The only course of action is to repeat the lumbar puncture after 24 hours.

Measured accurately with pressure transducers at lumbar puncture, the intracranial pressure was 0–5.5 mmHg (Kaiser and Whitelaw 1986) and 2 mmHg (Minns 1984).

Electroencephalography

Conventional multichannel EEG recordings are difficult to obtain in newborn babies, but the results can provide very valuable information (D'Allest and Andre 2002; Pressler et al. 2003). Short recordings are of less value than prolonged ones as the EEG shows wide variability and changes not only with sleep state but also with

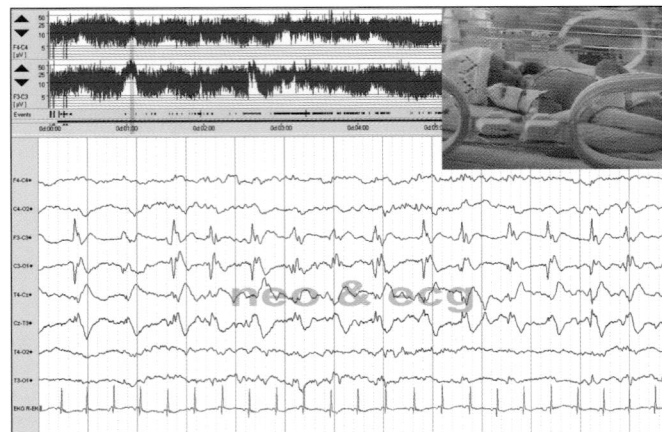

Fig. 40.10 Monitoring cerebral function with raw electroencephalogram (EEG), compressed and filtered EEG and digital video monitoring.

the length of the preceding sleep epoch and the degree of maturity of the baby (Roffwarg et al. 1966; Eyre et al. 1988; Pressler et al. 2003). Continuous monitoring is possible with a cerebral function monitor, which displays the amplitude of one or more channels of processed EEG, and modern equipment offers the opportunity to obtain multiple channels of raw EEG and a digital video signal in addition to a compressed and filtered amplitude-integrated EEG (Fig. 40.10). Cerebral function monitoring has drawbacks, but the advantages include continuous monitoring and relative ease of interpretation (Hellstrom-Westas 2002).

Maturation of EEG

The EEG of very preterm babies is markedly discontinuous with a pattern of high-voltage slow activity with suppressed EEG activity, termed 'tracé discontinu' (Boylan et al. 2008). Preterm babies also exhibit a pattern, called 'delta brush', of fast waves superimposed on delta waves, which can be misinterpreted as convulsive activity. Delta brush is most abundant at 32 weeks' gestation, and is very rarely seen after term. With increasing gestation the interburst intervals decrease and the record becomes more continuous (Fig. 40.11). Abnormal background EEG activity, such as severe amplitude depression or burst suppression, correlates well with later adverse outcome in both preterm and asphyxiated term babies (Watanabe et al. 1980; Holmes et al. 1982; Eken et al. 1995; Hellstrom-Westas et al. 1995; Murray et al. 2009). See part 2 and part 4 of this chapter for the role of the EEG in neonatal encephalopathy and page 1084 for its use in seizure detection.

Neurological examination before discharge, and follow-up

A complete neurological examination including assessment of movements is the best way of assessing the neurological status of a high-risk infant as long as is performed in a sequential way because it is the pattern of change that gives away the diagnosis and improves the accuracy of prediction. Therefore, good practice demands that high-risk babies should be closely monitored after discharge and during infancy. In high-risk preterm infants Touwen (1978) found a high correlation between the neonatal and follow-up examinations during infancy. Cramped synchronised movements on video assessments at term followed by absent or abnormal fidgety

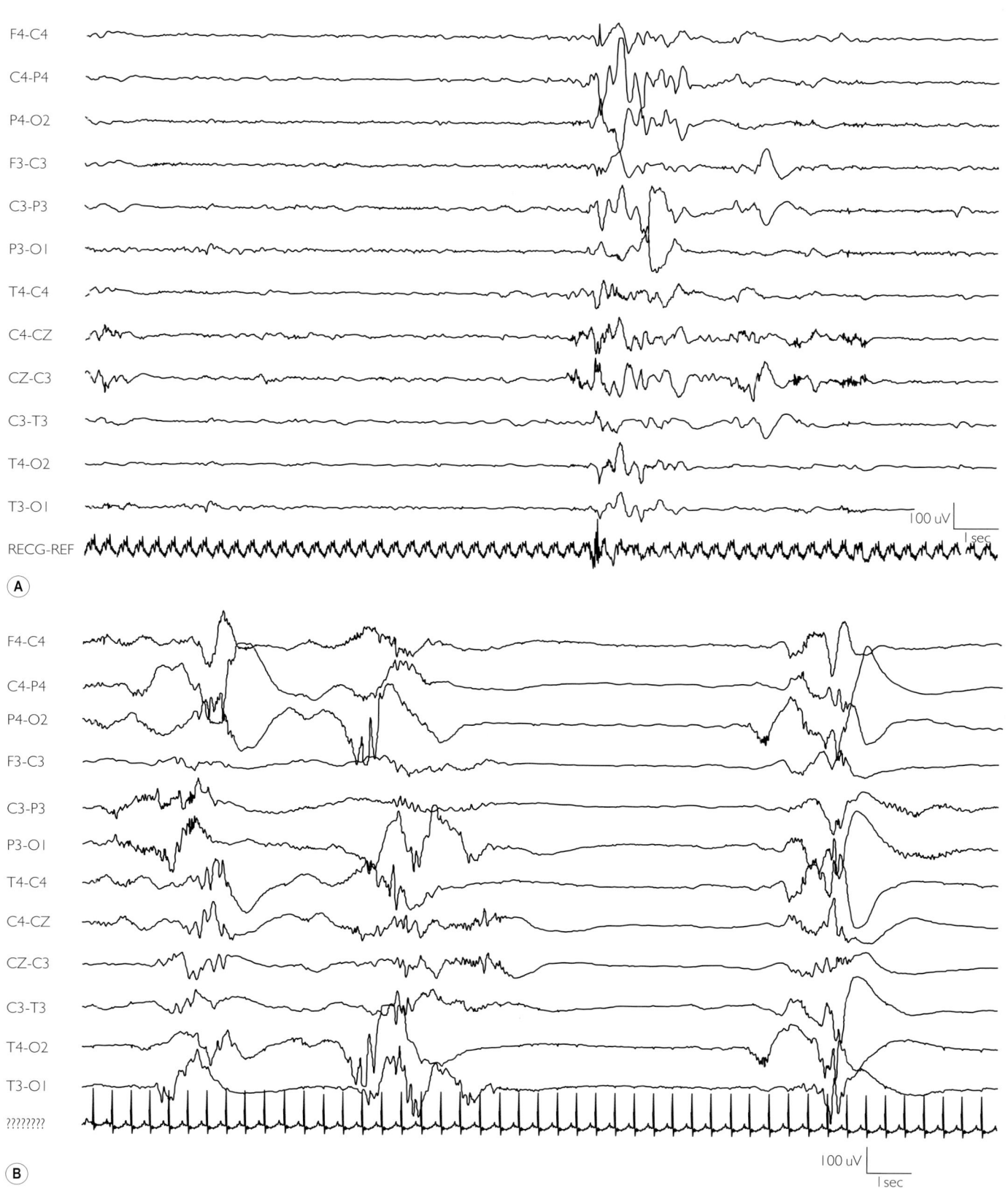

F4-C4

C4-P4

P4-O2

F3-C3

C3-P3

P3-O1

T4-C4

C4-CZ

CZ-C3

C3-T3

T4-O2

T3-O1

RECG-REF

100 uV

1 sec

(A)

F4-C4

C4-P4

P4-O2

F3-C3

C3-P3

P3-O1

T4-C4

C4-CZ

CZ-C3

C3-T3

T4-O2

T3-O1

????????

100 uV

1 sec

(B)

Fig. 40.11 Maturation of the electroencephalogram: (a) at 25 weeks; (b) at 29 weeks;

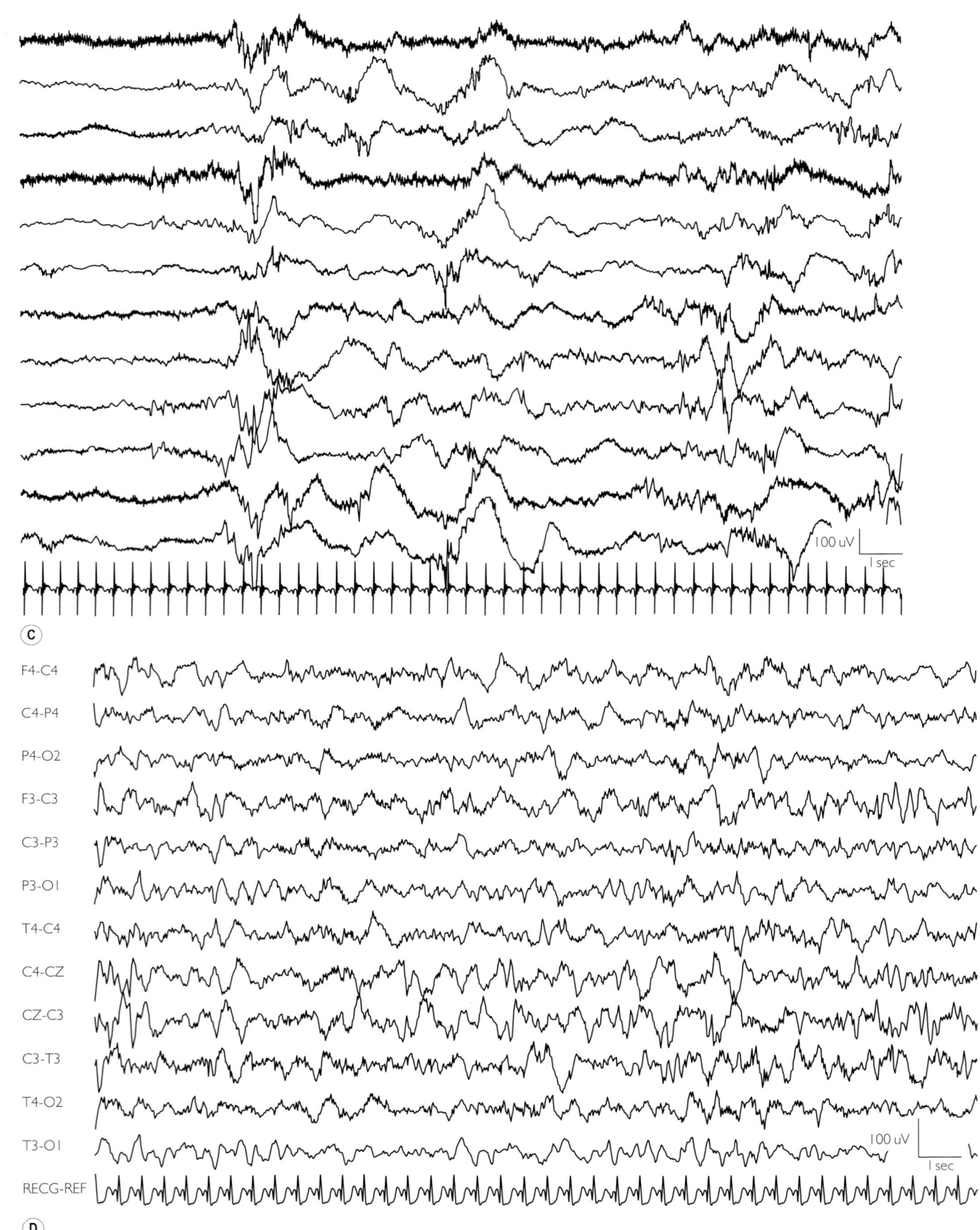

Fig. 40.11, cont'd (c) at 35 weeks; and (d) at 40 weeks.

movements at 3 months of age are known to be extremely sensitive and specific for early diagnosis of cerebral palsy (Einspeler and Prechtl 2005). The neonatal hemisyndrome and hypertonia syndrome have distinct prognostic value, whereas hypotonia does not. With asphyxia, however, hypotonia which evolves to hypertonia correlates significantly with subsequent neurological disorders (Brown et al. 1974). The neonatal hyperexcitability syndrome appears to correlate with subsequent developmental difficulties only when it persists for more than 6 weeks. If, upon discharge from the neonatal unit, it is concluded that the baby is definitely neurologically abnormal, on the basis of established abnormalities such as microcephaly or seizures, a nearly 100-fold increased risk of cerebral palsy does exist (Nelson and Ellenberg 1979).

Follow-up of high-risk infants is an important part of neonatal intensive care provision (Ch. 19). Monitoring of head growth and neurodevelopment over the first months can give early warning of neurodevelopmental problems. A failure to achieve a normal pattern of head growth is an ominous sign.

References

Amiel-Tison, C., 2001. Clinical Assessment of the infant nervous system. In: Levene, M.I., Chervenak, F.A., Whitte, M. (Eds.), Fetal and Neonatal Neurology and Neurosurgery, thrid ed. Churchill Livingstone, Edinburgh, pp. 99–120.

Amiel-Tison, C., 2002. Update of the Amiel-Tison neurologic assessment for the term neonate or at 40 weeks corrected age. Pediatr Neurol 27, 196–212.

Amiel-Tison, C., Grenier, A., 1980. Evaluation neurologique du nouveau-né et du nourisson. Masson, Paris.

Amiel-Tison. C., Stewart, A., 1994a. Apparently normal survivors: neuromotor and cognitive function as they grow older. In: Amiel-Tison, C., Stewart, A. (Eds.), The newborn infant: one brain for life. INSERM-Doin, Paris, pp. 227–237.

Amiel-Tison, C., Stewart, A., 1994b. The newborn infant: One brain for life. Les Editions INSERM, Publication office of the French National Institute of Health and Medical Research, Paris.

Andre-Thomas Chesni, Y., Saint-Anne Dargassies, S., 1960. The neurological examination of the infant. Clinics in Developmental Medicine, No 1. McKeith Press, Cambridge.

Barkovich, J.A., 1999. Pediatric Neuroimaging. Lippincott Williams Wilkins, Philadelphia.

Brazelton, T.B., Nugent, J.K., 1995. Neonatal behavioural assessment scale, third ed. Clinics in Developmental Medicine, No 137. MacKeith Press, London.

Brown, J.K., Purvis, R.J., Forfar, J.O., et al., 1974. Neurological aspects of perinatal asphyxia. Dev Med Child Neurol 16, 567–580.

Boylan, G., Murray, D., Rennie, J.M., 2008. In: Rennie, J., Hagmann, C.F., Robertson, N.J. (Eds.). The normal EEG. Cambridge University Press. pp. 83–91.

Cioni, G., Ferrari, F., Einspieler, C., et al., 1997. Comparison between observation of spontaneous movements and neurologic examination in preterm infants. J Pediatr 139, 704–711.

Cioni, G., Bertucelli, B., Boldrini, A., et al., 2000. Correlation between visual function, neurodevelopmental outcome, and magnetic resonance imaging findings in infants with periventricular leucomalacia. Arch Dis Child Fetal Neonatal Ed 82, F134–F140.

D'Allest, A.M., Andre, M., 2002. Electroencephalography. In: Lagercrantz, H., Hanson, M., Evrard, P., et al. (Eds.) The Newborn Brain: neuroscience and clinical applications. Cambridge University Press, Cambridge, pp. 339–367.

de Vries, L.S., Connell, J., Dubowitz, L.M.S., et al., 1987. Neurological, electrophysiological and MRI abnormalities in infants with extensive cystic leukomalacia. Neuropediatrics 18, 61–66.

Dubowitz, L.M.S., Dubowitz, V., Palmer P.G., et al., 1984. Correlation of neurological assessment in the preterm newborn infant with outcome at 1 year. J Pediatr 105, 452–456.

Dubowitz, L., Mercuri, E., Dubowitz, V., 1998. An optimality score for the neurological examination of the term newborn. J Pediatr 133, 406–416.

Dubowitz, L., Dubowitz, V., Mercuri, E., 1999. The neurological assessment of the preterm and full term newborn infant. second ed. Clinics in Developmental Medicine, No 148. MacKeith Press, Cambridge.

Dubowitz, L.M.S., Dubowitz, V., Mercuri, E., 1999. The Neurological Assessment of the Preterm and Full term newborn infant, second ed. Clinics in Developmental Medicine No 148 MacKeith Press, Cambridge.

Einspeler, C., Prechtl, H.F., 2005. Prechtl's assessment of general movements: a diagnostic tool for the functional assessment of the young nervous system. Ment Retard Dev Disabil Res Rev 11, 61–67.

Eken, P., Toet, M.C., Groenendaal, F., et al., 1995. Predictive value of early neuroimaging, pulsed Doppler and neurophysiology in full term infants with hypoxic-ischaemic encephalopathy. Arch Dis Child 73, F75–F80.

Eyre, J.A., Nanei, S., Wilkinson, A.R., 1988. Quantification of changes in normal neonatal EEGs with gestation from continuous 5 day recordings. Dev Med Child Neurol 30, 599–607.

Ferrari, F., Cioni, G., Prechtl, H.F.R., 1990. Qualitative changes of general movements in preterm infants with brain lesions. Early Hum Dev 23, 193–231.

Govaert, P., de Vries, L.S., 1997. An Atlas of Neonatal Brain Sonography. Clinics in Developmental Medicine, No 141–142. MacKeith Press, London.

Hellstrom-Westas, L., 2002. Cerebral Function Monitoring. In: Lagercrantz, H., Hanson, M., Evrard, P., et al. (Eds.), The Newborn Brain: neuroscience and clinical applications. Cambridge University Press, Cambridge, pp. 368–384.

Hellstrom-Westas, L., Rosen, I., Svenningsen, N.W., 1995. Predictive value of early continuous amplitude integrated EEG recordings on outcome after severe birth asphyxia in full term infants. Arch Dis Child 72, F34–F38.

Henderson-Smart, D.J., 1981. The effect of gestational age on the incidence and duration of recurrent apnoea in newborn babies. Aust Paediatr J 17, 273–276.

Hepper, P.G., Shahidullah, B.S., 1994. Development of fetal hearing. Arch Dis Child 71, F81–F87.

Holmes, G., Rowe, J., Hafford, J., et al., 1982. Prognostic value of the electroencephalogram in neonatal seizures. Electroencephalogr Clin Neurophysiol 53, 60–72.

Illingworth, R.S., 1960. The development of the infant and young child. Churchill Livingstone, Edinburgh.

Illingworth, R.S., 1980. The development of the infant and young child. seventh ed. Churchill Livingstone, Edinburgh.

Joppich, G., Schulte, F.J., 1968. Neurologie des Neugeborenen. Springer, Berlin.

Kaiser, A.M., Whitelaw, A.G.L., 1986. Normal cerebrospinal fluid pressure in the newborn. Neuropaediatrics 17, 100–102.

Lester, B.M., Tronik, E.Z., Brazelton, T.B., 2004. The Neonatal Intensive Care Unit Network Neurobehavioural Scale Procedures. Pediatrics 113, 641–667.

Majnemer, A., Mazer, B., 1998. Neurologic evaluation of the newborn infant: definition and psychometric properties. Dev Med Child Neurol 40, 708–715.

Mercuri, E., Haataja, L., Dubowitz, L., 2007. Neurological assessment in normal young infants. In Neurological Assessment in the First Two years of Life. Clinics in

Developmental Medicine, No 17, MacKeith Press, UK, pp. 24–37.

Minns, R.A., 1984. Intracranial pressure monitoring. Arch Dis Child 59, 486–488.

Murray, D.M., Boylan, G.B., Ryan, C.A., et al., 2009. Early EEG findings in hypoxic ischaemic encephalopathy predict outcomes at 2 years. Pediatrics 124, e459–e467.

Nelson, K.B., Ellenberg, J.H., 1979. Neonatal signs as predictors of cerebral palsy. Pediatrics 64, 225–232.

Prechtl, H.F.R., 1974. The behavioural states of the newborn infant. Brain Res 76, 185–212.

Prechtl, H.F.R., 1977. The neurological examination of the full term newborn infant, second ed. Clinics in Developmental Medicine, No 63. MacKeith Press, London.

Prechtl, H.F.R., 1990. Qualitative changes of spontaneous movements in fetus and preterm infant as a marker of neurological dysfunction. Early Hum Dev 23, 151–158.

Prechtl, H.F.R., O'Brien, M.J., 1982. Behavioural states of the full term newborn. The emergence of a concept. In: Stratton, P (ed.), Psychobiology of the human newborn. John Wiley, New York, pp. 53–73.

Prechtl, H.F.R., Nolte, R., 1984. Motor behaviour of preterm infants. In Prechtl, HFR (ed.), Continuity of neural functions from prenatal to postnatal life. Clinics in Developmental Medicine, No 84 MacKeith Press, London.

Prechtl, H.F.R., Fargel, V.W., Weinaman, H.M., et al., 1979. Postures, motility and respiration of low risk preterm infants. Dev Med Child Neurol 21, 3–7.

Pressler, R., Bady, B., Binnie, C.D., et al., 2003. Neurophysiology of the Neonatal Period. In: Binnie, C.D., Cooper, R., Mauguiere, F., et al. (Eds.), Clinical Neurophysiology, vol. 2. Elsevier, London.

Rennie, J.M., Hagmann, C.F., Robertson, N.J., 2008. Neonatal Cerebral Investigation. Cambridge University Press, New York.

Robinson, J., Fielder, A.R., 1990. Pupillary diameter and reaction to light in preterm neonates. Arch Dis Child 65, 35–38.

Roffwarg, H.P., Muzio, J.N., Dement, W.C., 1966. Ontogenetic development of human sleep dream cycles. Science 152, 604–619.

Rutherford, M.A., 2002. MRI of the neonatal brain. W B Saunders, London.

Saint-Anne Dargassies, S., 1977. Neurological development in the full term and premature neonate. Elsevier North Holland, Amsterdam.

Shawkat, F.S., Kriss, A., Thompson, D., et al., 2000. Vertical or asymmetric nystagmus need not imply neurological disease. Br J Ophthalmol 84, 175–180.

Shuper, A., Zalzberg, J., Weitz, R., et al., 1991. Jitteriness beyond the neonatal period: a benign pattern of movement in infancy. J Child Neurol 6, 243–245.

Taylor, M.J., Murphy, W.J., Whyte, H.E., 1992. Prognostic reliability of SEPs and VEPs in asphyxiated newborn infants. Dev Med Child Neurol 34, 507–515.

Thompson, D.C., McPhillips, H., Davis, R.L., et al., 2001. Universal newborn hearing screening: summary of evidence. JAMA 286, 2000–2010.

Touwen, B., 1976. Neurological development in infancy. Clinics in developmental medicine, No 58. Spastics International Medical Publications. Heinemann, London.

Touwen, B.C.L., 1978. Early detection of developmental neurological disorders. In: Jonxis, J.H.P. (ed.), Growth and development of the full term and premature infant. The Jonxis Lectures, Excerpta Medica, Amsterdam, pp. 244–261.

Volpe, 2001. The Neurological Examination: normal and abnormal features. In: Volpe, J.J. (ed.), Neonatal Neurology, fourth ed. WB Saunders, Philadelphia, pp. 103–133.

Volpe, J.J., 2008. Neurological evaluation. Unit II. In: Volpe, J.J. (ed.), Neonatal Neurology, fifth ed, WB Saunders, Philadelphia, pp. 121–203.

Watanabe, K., Miyazaki, S., Hara, K., et al., 1980. Behavioural state cycles, background EEGs and prognosis of newborns with perinatal hypoxia. Electroencephalogr Clin Neurophysiol 49, 618–625.

Watkin, P.M., 1996. Neonatal otoacoustic emission screening and the identification of deafness. Arch Dis Child 74, F16–F25.

Wessex Universal Neonatal Hearing Screening Trial Group, 1998. Controlled trial of universal neonatal screening for early identification of permanent childhood hearing impairment. Lancet 352, 1957–1964.

Part 2: **Neonatal seizures**

Geraldine Boylan   Janet M Rennie

Introduction

Seizures are the most common neurological emergency in the neonatal period and present a diagnostic and therapeutic challenge to clinicians worldwide. The neonatal brain is uniquely vulnerable to seizures and, as a result, seizures are more common in the neonatal period than at any other time of life. There is now convincing evidence that seizure can damage the brain and exacerbate pre-existing injury. Therefore it is imperative that seizures are identified and treated as soon as possible. However neonatal seizures differ in etiology, semiology, and electroencephalographic (EEG) characteristics to seizures in older children and adults and antiepileptic drugs (AEDs) do not work very well. There is also concern about the potential adverse effects of currently used AEDs on brain development.

All those who care for the newborn need a working knowledge of the likely causes and a management plan for this important emergency. Prompt diagnosis, investigation and treatment are vital as delayed recognition of a treatable cause can have a significant impact on the child's subsequent neurological outcome.

In neonates seizures are associated with conditions such as periventricular haemorrhage, cerebral infarction (stroke), hypoglycaemia, infection, cerebral malformations and hypoxic–ischaemic encephalopathy.

There is increasing evidence that neonatal seizures have an adverse effect on neurodevelopmental outcome and predispose to cognitive, behavioural or epileptic complications in later life (Levene 2002). Seizures cause synaptic reorganisation with aberrant growth (mossy fibres), and may interfere with the normal synaptic pruning which takes place during development (McCabe et al. 2001). If seizures are not controlled the electrical activity can continue to circulate, a phenomenon known as kindling. Prolonged seizures cause progressive cerebral hypoxia, changes in cerebral blood flow, cerebral oedema and lactic acidosis; changes have been shown in human babies with Doppler ultrasound and using magnetic resonance spectroscopy (Boylan et al. 1999a; Miller et al. 2002). Status epilepticus worsened the outcome for neonatal rats with hypoxic ischaemia (Wirrell et al. 2001). Some clinical studies have shown a correlation between the number of seizures and outcome, but others have not, although very few neonatal studies

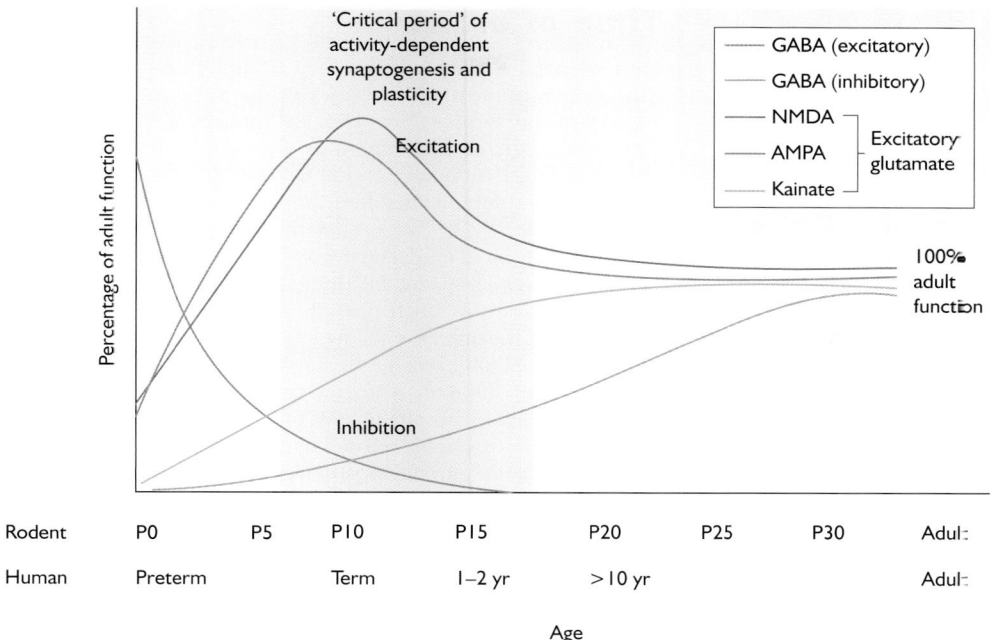

Fig. 40.12 Developmental profile of glutamate and gamma-aminobutyric acid (GABA) receptor expression and function. Equivalent developmental periods are displayed for rats and humans on the top and bottom x-axes. Activation of GABA receptors is depolarising in rats early in the first postnatal week and in humans up to and including the neonatal period. Neonatal seizures emerge within the critical period of synaptogenesis. NMDA, *N*-methyl-D-aspartate; AMPA, alpha-amino 3-hydroxy-5-methyl-4-isoxazole propionate. *(Modified from Rakhade and Jensen 2009 with permission.)*

have been done using EEG quantification of the seizure burden (McBride et al. 2000).

Pathophysiology

There have been substantial recent advances in our understanding of the pathophysiology of neonatal seizures and more specifically in the developmental age-specific factors that influence mechanisms of seizure generation, response to AEDs and neurodevelopmental outcome. The neonatal period is also a period of intense physiological synaptic excitability as the balance between excitatory versus inhibitory synapses is tipped in the favour of excitation to permit robust activity-dependent synaptic formation, plasticity and remodelling (Jensen 2009) (Fig. 40.12). Glutamate receptors are essential for plasticity and are transiently overexpressed in the neonatal period. In addition both *N*-methyl-D-aspartate (NMDA) and alpha-amino 3-hydroxy-5-methyl-4-isoxazole propionate (AMPA) receptors are developmentally regulated and are expressed at levels and with specific subunit composition that enhances excitability in neuronal networks in the neonatal brain (Jensen 2009). AMPA receptors are not calcium-permeable in the adult; in the newborn the receptors are deficient in the Glu-R2 subunit which renders them calcium-permeable and enhances excitation. Gamma-aminobutyric acid (GABA) is excitatory rather than inhibitory in perinatal neurons because of elevated neuronal chloride. This in turn is due to the presence of the chloride channel NKCCl which mediates chloride influx. The expression of the NKCCl cotransporter is high in the perinatal period and the high levels of neuronal chloride lead to an efflux of chloride when GABA-A receptors are activated (Dzhala et al. 2005). Hypoxic ischaemia leads to a further upregulation of the NKCCl transporter and hence the response to GABA agonist drugs such as phenobarbital and the benzodiazepines is particularly poor in hypoxic–ischaemic encephalopathy. Ion channels also

regulate neuronal excitability and mutations and low expression of certain channels such as K+ and HCN lead to enhanced excitability. Neuropeptide systems are also implicated in enhanced neuronal excitation; for example, corticotrophin-releasing hormone and its receptors are expressed at higher levels in the postnatal period and are increased during stress.

Basic science research has shown that, in animals, status epilepticus causes neuronal loss in the hippocampus. Cell death occurs from excessive excitatory neurotransmitter release, which allows calcium to enter the cell and trigger a cascade of biochemical changes, including activation of nitric oxide synthase, and enzyme activation. Seizures also activate genes that can lead to abnormal axon growth and synaptic reorganisation. This has been seen as 'mossy fibre sprouting' in the hippocampus, and sprouting and neosynapse formation have been seen in other areas of the brain (Holmes et al. 1999). Holmes' group has also shown alterations of neural pathways in animals subjected to repeated seizures, with early gene activation of *c-fos* (Liu et al. 1999), and suggested that seizures in early life may modify a wide range of essential processes such as neuronal migration, aborisation and synaptogenesis, leading to permanent effects on seizure susceptibility, learning and memory (Holmes and Ben-Ari 1998). This fundamental work has helped to explain why anticonvulsant drugs which are effective in older individuals do not work well in babies (Fig. 40.13).

Incidence

There is now clear evidence that there is both under- and overreporting of neonatal seizures in the neonatal intensive care unit (NICU) when EEG monitoring is not available for confirmation (Mizrahi and Kellaway 1987; Boylan et al. 1999b; Murray et al. 2008). All of the epidemiological studies to date report the incidence of clinical seizures: an epidemiological study is impossible without current

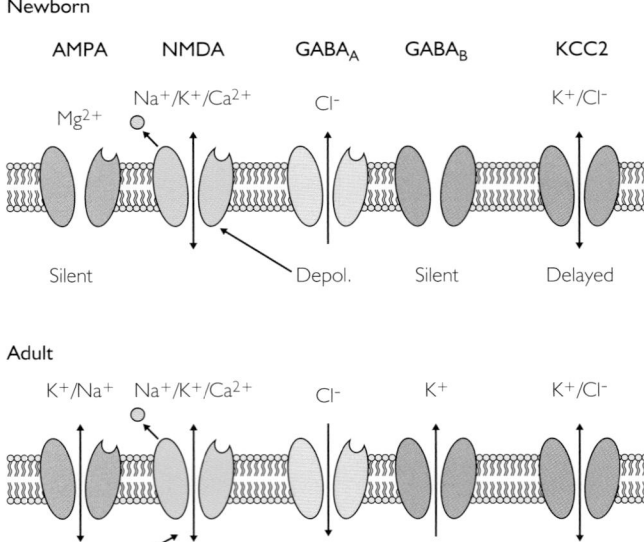

Newborn

AMPA   NMDA   GABA_A   GABA_B   KCC2

Silent   Depol.   Silent   Delayed

Adult

Depol.   Hyperpol.   Active

Fig. 40.13 Comparison of excitatory and inhibitory channels in neonate and adult. In the adult alpha-amino 3-hydroxy-5-methyl-4-isoxazole propionate (AMPA) responds to glutamate by opening and allowing Na^+ to enter cell. With depolarisation Mg^{2+} is displaced from the N-methyl-D-aspartate (NMDA) channel and Na^+ and Ca^{2+} enter the cell. $GABA_A$ and $GABA_B$, through Cl^- and K^+ ionic flow, serve to hyperpolarise the cell. In the neonate AMPA receptors, while present, are not functional (silent). NMDA channels, because of the block with Mg^{2+}, do not function at normal membrane resting potentials. Because of the higher Cl^- content of the immature brain, GABA activation results in an efflux of Cl^- which serves to depolarise the cell. With depolarisation, the NMDA and voltage-gated channels can open. $GABA_B$, like AMPA, develops later and provides little postsynaptic inhibition in the neonate. The K^+/Cl^- cotransporter (KCC2) which is responsible for controlling intracellular Cl^- is delayed in maturing, resulting in an increase in intracellular Cl^- in immature animals. Depol., depolarisation; Hyperpol., hyperpolarisation. *(Reproduced from Holmes et al. 2002 with permission.)*

EEG monitoring technology. Clinical neonatal seizures occur in 5–13% of very-low-birthweight infants, and in 1–3 per 1000 of infants born at term (Curtis et al. 1988; Watkins et al. 1988; Legido et al. 1991; Lanska et al. 1995; Lien et al. 1995; Lanska and Lanska 1996; Ronen et al. 1999; Saliba et al. 1999; Sheth et al. 1999; Kohelet et al. 2004). In a recent study of over 70 preterm babies monitored with amplitude-integrated EEG (aEEG) who had a formal EEG within 2–48 hours of birth, five were found to have definite seizures (West et al. 2010).

Many of the cases of clinical seizure reported in older studies were due to late-onset hypocalcaemia, which probably explains the higher incidence. The incidence of early (<48 hours) seizures in term infants has been proposed as an indicator of the quality of perinatal care because the most common cause in this group is hypoxic–ischaemic encephalopathy. The incidence of early seizures varies, being 0.87 per 1000 in Dublin between 1980 and 1984 (Curtis et al. 1988), 1.3 per 1000 in Cardiff during 1970–1979 (Minchom et al. 1987), 2.8 per 1000 in Fayette county, Kentucky in 1985–1989 (Lanska et al. 1995) and, in the most recent study, 1 per 1000 in California (Glass et al. 2008). There are many problems in the definition of neonatal seizures which will become apparent to the reader. When clinical signs of seizures are present they are commonly subtle in nature, particularly in premature infants, being present in 75% of the cases described by Scher et al. (1993a).

Time of onset

Most neonatal seizures start between 12 and 48 hours after birth; babies rarely present with seizures in the delivery room. In our experience, full-term babies who are thought to be seizing on admission to the neonatal unit after a difficult delivery often have abnormal jittery movements without electrographic seizures. This is particularly common after moderate or severe hypoxic–ischaemic injury.

With the advent of moderate hypothermia treatment for hypoxic–ischaemic encephalopathy, EEG monitoring generally commences earlier and it is now often possible to capture the true onset of electrographic seizure in neonates. In a study by Wusthoff et al. (2011), electrographic seizures began at a mean time of 9 hours and 30 minutes in full-term neonates treated with hypothermia for hypoxic–ischaemic encephalopathy. In a study by Nash et al. (2011) the onset of electrographic seizures in the majority of neonates with hypoxic–ischaemic encephalopathy, also treated with hypothermia, was within 18 hours of birth. Low and colleagues (2012) compared the seizure characteristics of two full-term cohorts of neonates with hypoxic–ischaemic encephalopathy: one group had received therapeutic hypothermia and the other group did not. The onset of electrographic seizures in both groups was not significantly different, with a mean of 18 hours in the non-cooled group and 13 hours in the cooled group. A study by Filan et al. (2005) in non-cooled term neonates with hypoxic–ischaemic encephalopathy showed electrographic seizure onset before 20 hours.

Animal work shows that seizures emerge 7–13 hours after a hypoxic–ischaemic insult (Williams et al. 1991), and this fits with what is known about glutamate release and damage during the secondary reperfusion phase in this situation. Late-onset seizures suggest meningitis, benign familial seizures or hypocalcaemia. Figure 40.14 shows the time of onset recorded in 277 neonatal cases (Holden et al. 1982). A study carried out 17 years later shows a very similar pattern (Saliba et al. 1999).

Diagnosis and classification

In 1870 J Hughlings Jackson described a seizure as 'an excessive discharge of nerve tissue on muscle'. Today this definition is expanded to include the effects on the sensory and autonomic nervous systems, including paroxysmal alterations in behavioural state. Four main seizure types are recognised (Table 40.2) and within each type the seizures can be unifocal, multifocal or generalised. Classic tonic-clonic seizures are very rare in babies, in whom there is the additional problem of electroclinical dissociation (Weiner et al. 1991).

Subtle

The clinical manifestations of seizures in infants can be extremely subtle. They can be divided into orofacial manifestations, including fixed eye opening, eye deviation, eyelid blinking, sucking, chewing and lip smacking, and limb movements (often described as swimming, boxing or cycling). In addition, apnoeic episodes can be due to seizure and this diagnosis should be considered if there is slow response to bag-and-mask ventilation, particularly in a preterm neonate with an intracranial lesion. Another clue may be associated movements such as eyelid or mouth opening and a bradycardia which starts soon after the collapse. Autonomic changes, such as a change in blood pressure or increased salivation, often accompany subtle seizures and these may provide a clue to the correct diagnosis in the absence of EEG confirmation.

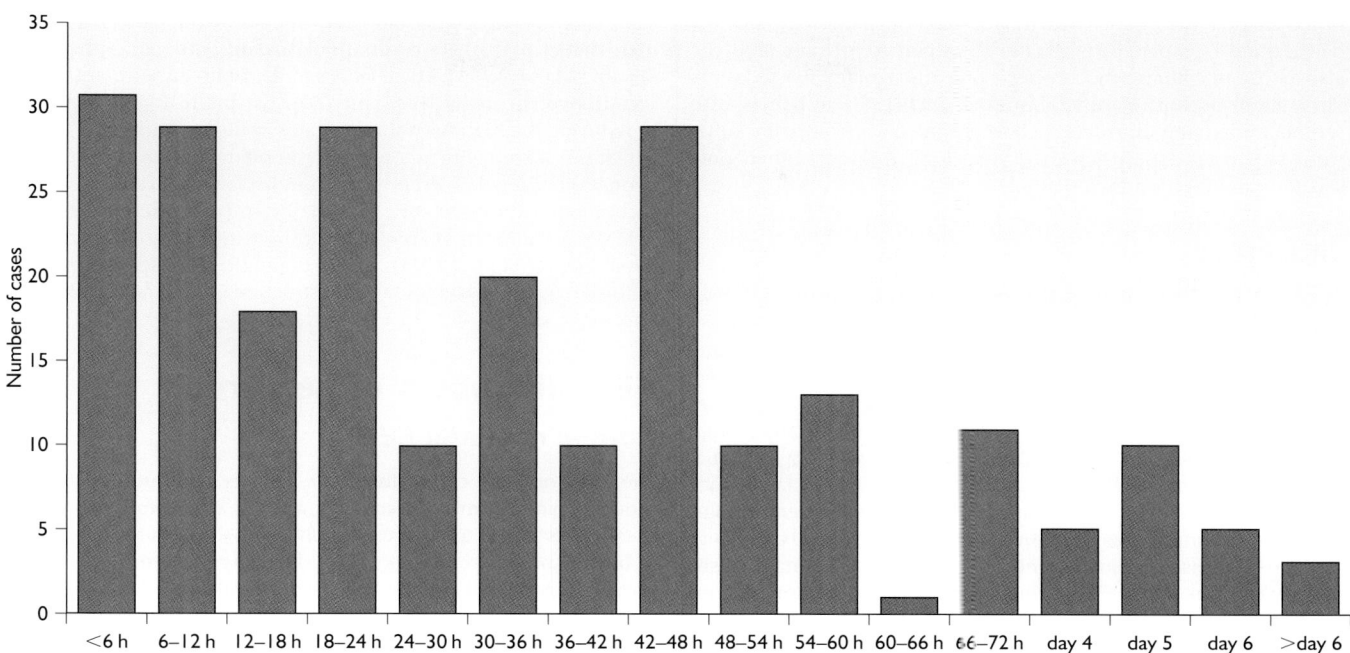

Fig. 40.14 Time of onset of seizures in 277 neonatal cases. Data from the National Collaborative Perinatal Project (Holden et al. 1982). Note the scale on the x-axis starts as 6-hourly periods, and is then grouped by days.

Table 40.2 Types of seizure in the newborn

TYPE	CLINICAL MANIFESTATION	FREQUENCY AND EEG CORRELATE
Subtle	Eye signs: eyelid fluttering, eye deviation, fixed open stare, blinking. Apnoea. Cycling, boxing, stepping, swimming movements of limbs. Mouthing, chewing, lip smacking, smiling	About 50% of neonatal seizures; EEG correlation variable. EEG changes most likely with ocular manifestations
Tonic	Stiffening. decerebrate posturing	About 5% of neonatal seizures. EEG correlation variable
Clonic	Repetitive jerking, distinct from jittering. Can be unifocal or multifocal	25–30% of neonatal seizures. EEG correlation highly likely, especially if focal
Myoclonic	Myoclonic jerks; sleep myoclonus can be benign	15–20% of neonatal seizures. EEG normal if focal, or sleep myoclonus

EEG, electroencephalogram.

Clonic

Clonic seizures usually involve one limb or one side of the face or body jerking rhythmically, usually at a frequency of 1–4 times per second. This type of seizure is associated with a characteristic EEG discharge consisting of runs of sharp slow-wave complexes which spread ipsilaterally from the hemisphere in which they originate. Clonic seizures in the neonate can have more than one focus or migrate in a non-jacksonian fashion; for example, jerking of one leg can be followed by similar movements in the opposite hand. Clonic seizures are often a clue to an underlying focal lesion such as a cortical infarction and are frequently associated with neonatal stroke (Selton et al. 2003). They may also occur in association with a metabolic cause and occasionally herpes encephalitis. Infants are not usually unconscious during clonic seizures.

Tonic

Tonic seizures are much less common than either subtle or clonic seizures in the newborn. Sustained posturing of the limbs or trunk or deviation of the head or eyes are the usual manifestations of tonic seizures in the newborn.

Myoclonic

Myoclonus is characterised by sudden brief and jerky movements which tend to occur in the flexor muscle groups. It can be localised to one muscle group or it may be generalised. It is irregular and arrhythmic and is of high amplitude. Generalised myoclonic seizures resemble salaam spasms and are the type most likely to be associated with EEG change. Myoclonic seizures are most frequently noted in preterm infants with major cerebral pathology and the background EEG pattern is usually abnormal. Myoclonic jerks can also occur in babies who are receiving midazolam for sedation, particularly during weaning (Lee et al. 1994). Some babies with serious underlying disorders such as glycine encephalopathy suffer from very troublesome repetitive myoclonic jerking as their only seizure manifestation (Scher 1985).

Jitteriness

Jitteriness is an extremely common phenomenon in normal newborns, being observed in 44% of a sample of 936 babies (Parker et al. 1990). It is defined as involuntary rhythmic oscillatory movement around a fixed axis that can be either fine (fast (>6 Hz) and of low amplitude) or coarse (slow and of high amplitude) (Huntsman et al. 2008). Fine jittery movements are usually benign or associated with a metabolic disturbance such as hypoglycaemia. Coarse jittery movements are more commonly associated with hypoxic–ischaemic encephalopathy or intracranial haemorrhage. Excessive jitteriness has also been reported in infants born to mothers who use marijuana, and can be a sign of neonatal abstinence syndrome (Ch. 26). Jittering is a symmetrical tremor, without the fast and slow component of a clonic or myoclonic seizure, and occurs at a faster rate of 5–6 times per second. Jittering does not involve the face (unlike subtle seizures), is markedly stimulus-sensitive, and ceases when the limb is held. The autonomic nervous system changes of a seizure, such as tachycardia or hypertension, are never seen in jittering. The EEG does not display electrographic seizure activity and fast-frequency movement artefact is common, synchronous with jittering movements.

Hyperekplexia

Hyperekplexia is a rare disorder caused by autosomal-dominant or recessive modes of inheritance and characterised by generalised muscle rigidity, nocturnal myoclonus and a very exaggerated startle response to auditory, visual and tactile stimuli (Tohier et al. 1991; Huntsman et al. 2008). The startles can look like myoclonic jerks, and the high tone, hyperreflexia and jitteriness can lead to an erroneous diagnosis of seizure (Gordon 1993). Hyperekplexia is probably the same condition previously known as hereditary stiff-baby syndrome (Lingham et al. 1981). Although the EEG is normal, the tonic spasms can be dangerous. Severe cases can lead to neonatal cardiac arrest and treatment is warranted. Treatment with clonazepam (0.05–0.2 mg/kg/day) or low-dose clobazam (0.25–0.3 mg/kg/day) usually results in marked improvement, and the episodes usually disappear by the age of 2 years (Stewart et al. 2002). The disorder is caused by mutations in the alpha subunit of the inhibitory glycine receptor (Shiang et al. 1995) and has been mapped to chromosome 5 (de Koning-Tijssen and Rees 2007); it can be inherited in an autosomal-dominant fashion, although some forms are autosomal-recessive (Lapunzina et al. 2003).

Physiological changes during seizures

Neonatal seizures cause an increase in metabolic rate, a decline in energy reserves, including brain glucose, and an increase in lactate (Wasterlain et al. 2010). This implies that brain transport mechanisms are unable to match the increased demand. The demand for oxygen is also increased, and cerebral blood flow rises to try to meet the need for oxygen and glucose. That metabolic demand outstrips supply in the newborn is supported by magnetic resonance spectroscopic data showing a shift in spectra from the high-energy phosphate compounds towards inorganic phosphate (Younkin et al. 1986). The changes in the brain are similar to those seen in hypoxic–ischaemic injury. Glucose pretreatment is effective in reducing the high mortality of status epilepticus in rats, a benefit which is not seen with ketone body supplementation, although the neonatal brain is known be able to utilise alternative fuels. Lactate accumulates during seizure, and the brain (and often the arterial) pH falls. Systemic blood pressure increases, and cerebral blood flow rises (Boylan et al. 1999a). These dramatic short-term effects are followed by the changes in cell structure and synaptic linkages referred to earlier.

EEG diagnosis of seizures

Normal neonatal EEG

The EEG of the normal full-term baby is continuous, contains moderate-voltage mixed-frequency activity, shows fully developed sleep cycles and is reactive to stimuli even within the first 12 hours of birth (Korotchikova et al. 2009). The type of continuous activity present depends on whether the baby is awake or in active or quiet sleep (this chapter, part 1). During quiet sleep the EEG may show a pattern called high-voltage slow-wave sleep that consists of continuous medium- to high-voltage delta waves. As quiet sleep continues this pattern may become somewhat discontinuous with periods of low-amplitude beta and theta activity, alternating with 3–5-second bursts of higher-voltage 1–3 Hz activity occurring at 3–10-second intervals. This pattern is called 'tracé alternant'. In active sleep, the EEG is continuous, of lower voltage and contains mixed-frequency activity. In wakefulness the EEG also shows a lower-voltage mixed-frequency pattern referred to as 'activité moyenne'. The EEG of a full-term baby is illustrated in Figure 40.15a. Specific normal maturational features that may be present in the full-term EEG are anterior slow dysrhythmia (first apparent from approximately 35 weeks) and frontal sharp transients.

The most striking feature of the very preterm EEG is long periods of quiescence interrupted only by bursts of high-voltage mixed-frequency waves (Fig. 40.15b). The length of quiescent periods (also referred to as interburst intervals) is directly proportional to the degree of prematurity and this normal background pattern is referred to as 'tracé discontinu' or discontinuous pattern. This pattern is different to the tracé alternant pattern seen in full-term babies because the periods of quiescence can be completely flat. True quiescence is always less than 15 µV. In tracé alternant the discontinuous pattern is characterised by periods of high-amplitude, mixed-frequency activity alternating with periods of lower-amplitude activity at 25–50 µV (it is never completely flat). The degree of discontinuity seen in the preterm EEG would be very abnormal at term (Connell et al. 1987). The maximum interburst interval falls from 60 seconds at 24–26 weeks, to 40 seconds at 27–29 weeks, and 20 seconds at 30–32 weeks (Anderson et al. 1985; Young and Da Silva 2000; Biagioni et al. 2001; Pressler et al. 2003). After 33–34 weeks and up to 37 weeks the EEG is discontinuous only in quiet sleep and the interburst interval should be no longer than 10 seconds (Pressler et al. 2003). After 37 weeks, the EEG is continuous in wakefulness and active sleep, and tracé alternant replaces tracé discontinu in quiet sleep. Specific normal maturational features of the preterm EEG include premature temporal theta activity, which is sharp activity with a characteristic 'saw-toothed' appearance seen from approximately 27 weeks, and delta brush activity, which is a combination of very slow delta activity with superimposed fast components, present from approximately 30 weeks.

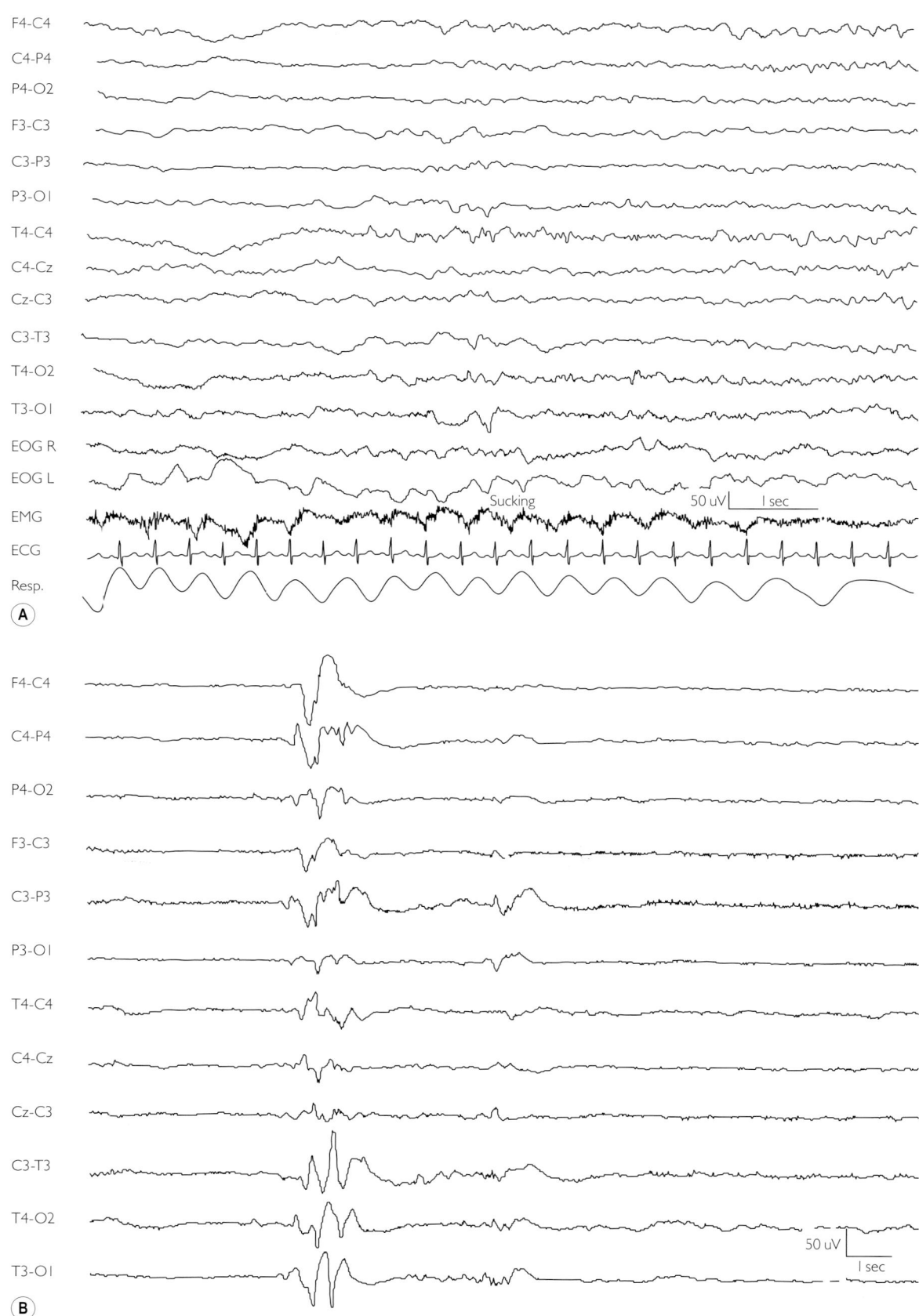

F4-C4
C4-P4
P4-O2
F3-C3
C3-P3
P3-O1
T4-C4
C4-Cz
Cz-C3
C3-T3
T4-O2
T3-O1
EOG R
EOG L
EMG
ECG
Resp.

Sucking
50 uV | sec

(A)

F4-C4
C4-P4
P4-O2
F3-C3
C3-P3
P3-O1
T4-C4
C4-Cz
Cz-C3
C3-T3
T4-O2
T3-O1

50 uV
| sec

(B)

Fig. 40.15 Electroencephalogram recordings showing: (a) normal term activity; (b) normal preterm activity;

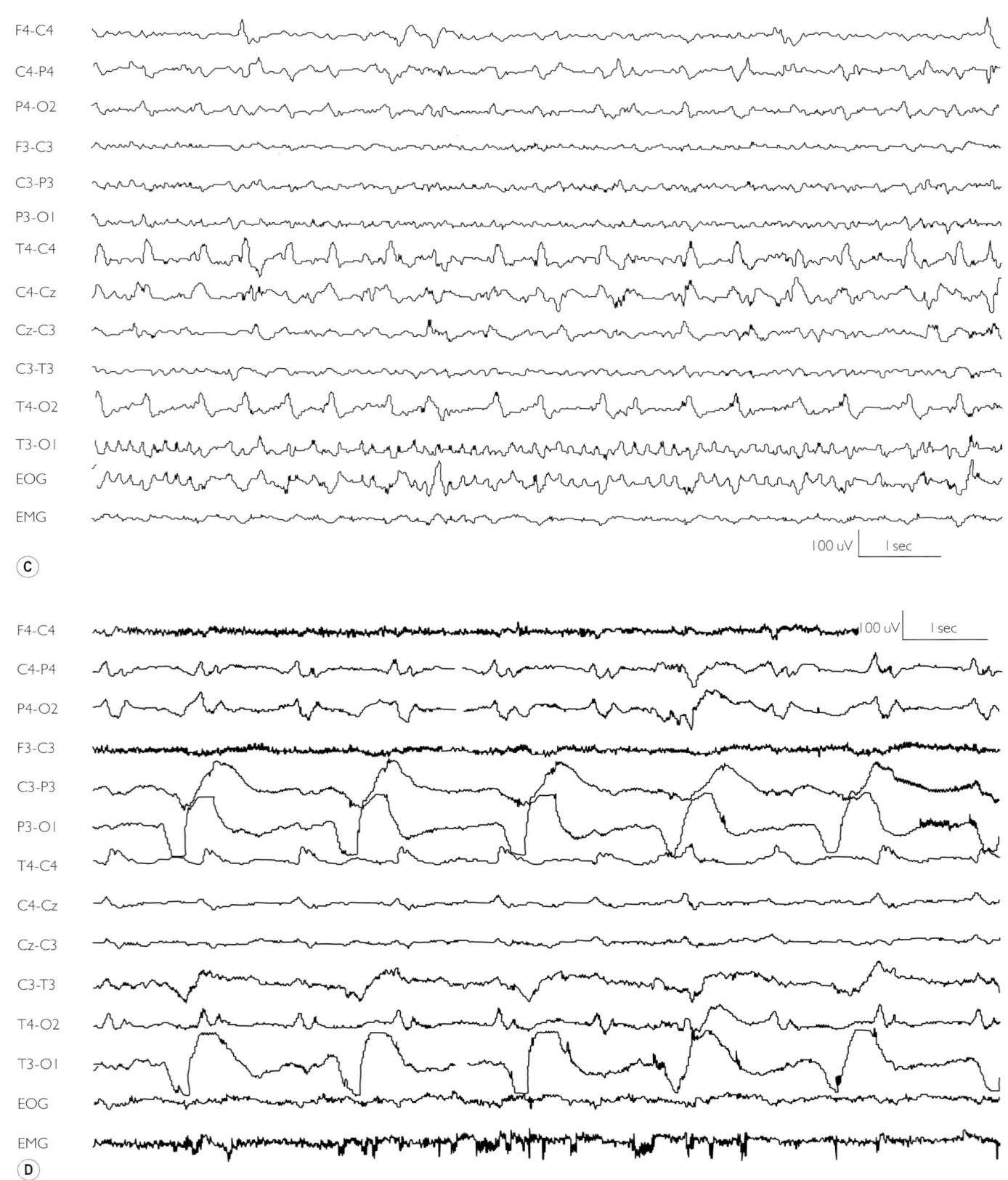

Fig. 40.15, cont'd and seizures in (c) a term baby and (d) a preterm baby.

The abnormal neonatal EEG

The neonatal EEG may be abnormal in a number of ways:

- disturbances of continuity, amplitude or frequency
- interhemispheric asymmetry or asynchrony
- abnormal waveforms may be present
- disturbances of sleep state
- seizure activity may be present.

Repetitive periods of true quiescence in the term newborn are abnormal. However anticonvulsants and sedation may induce some periods of quiescence in the term newborn and prolong periods in the preterm baby (Bell et al. 1993). Ellison et al. (1989) characterised the neonatal EEG mainly on the basis of the interburst interval, categorising the EEG of infants <30 weeks as abnormal if the interval was >60 seconds, using a figure of 30 seconds at term. Menache and colleagues (2002) confirmed that an interburst interval of more than 30 seconds was abnormal at term, and presaged a poor outcome.

Electrographic seizures

Electrographic seizures are typically defined as repetitive, rhythmic, stereotypic activity lasting at least 10 seconds that evolve in amplitude frequency and morphology (Patrizi et al. 2003). Both term and preterm infants have the ability to generate a multitude of ictal events but generally seizures originate in the central and temporal regions (Shellhaas et al. 2007; Bourez-Swart et al. 2009).

Few studies have quantified electrographic seizure duration in the newborn (Clancy and Ledigo 1987; Scher et al. 1993b; Bye and Flanagan 1995). Clancy and Ledigo (1987) used an arbitrary cut-off of 10 seconds as a minimum duration and this definition was also adopted by Scher et al. (1993b). Others have used 5 seconds (Schewman 1990). Very short bursts of abnormal rhythmic electrical activity have also been termed brief intermittent rhythmic discharges (BIRDS). Electrographic seizures characteristically consist of monophasic repetitive discharges or spike-and-wave activity (Fig. 40.15c and d) (Patrizi et al. 2003), but there is a rich variety in the onset, morphology and propagation patterns of neonatal seizures, which do not always correlate with the underlying pathology. An electrographic seizure should have a clear onset and conclusion, but these can be difficult to identify. Electrographic seizures may or may not be accompanied by steretoyped movements (see next section). Clancy and Ledigo (1987) found that the mean duration of electrographic seizures in the neonate was 2–3 minutes, with 97% of all seizures lasting 9 minutes or less and only 0.4% lasting 30 minutes or longer.

Electroclinical dissociation

There is asynchrony between the clinical and electrical representation of neonatal seizures: in only one-third of cases studied with video surveillance were the clinical and electrical manifestations simultaneous (Weiner et al. 1991; Mizrahi and Kellaway 1998). Murray et al. (2008) have shown that, on careful review of video EEG in neonates with electrographic seizures due to hypoxic–ischaemic encephalopathy, only 34% of seizures had concomitant clinical manifestations. When the medical charts of these neonates were reviewed, only 9% of seizures were actually documented during NICU stay, representing a significant gap between the electrographic, clinical and observed seizure burden.

Subtle stereotyped behaviour may or may not be associated with characteristic EEG changes, and continuous electrical monitoring detects many clinically silent seizures. One explanation is that the motor manifestations arise because of discharges from the brainstem and spinal cord which are 'released' because of lack of inhibition from higher centres (Mizrahi and Kellaway 1987). An alternative explanation is that scalp electrodes are incapable of recording from every part of the brain; depth electrodes reveal an otherwise unsuspected electrical focus in 10% of adult patients. The neurological effects of clinically silent (electrographic) seizures are not known, nor is it certain that treatment of clinically manifest seizures to electrical quiescence is required. This is an important question because phenobarbital treatment frequently abolishes the clinical manifestations whilst the electrical paroxysms continue (Painter et al. 1999; Boylan et al. 2002).

Current clinical practice is to commence anticonvulsant treatment without obtaining an EEG in the newborn. A study by Malone et al. (2009) has shown that there is both over- and underdiagnosis of neonatal seizures if EEG monitoring is not used, and we would advocate using EEG if at all possible to confirm the presence of true neonatal seizures. aEEG is now widely used in NICUs, especially since the introduction of therapeutic hypothermia for hypoxic–ischaemic encephalopathy. aEEG does have limitations, however, and short seizures, especially those less than 1 minute in duration, are missed, as are low-voltage seizures and seizures which remain localised (Rennie et al. 2004; Shellhaas and Clancy 2007). aEEG will usually detect seizures which are of high amplitude, generalised over a wide area and which are of long duration.

The lack of staff training and experience in aEEG interpretation is emerging as an important barrier to the effective adoption of aEEG monitoring in the NICU (Boylan et al. 2010). Nevertheless, the technique remains popular because it is easy to use and is useful for monitoring the response to antiepileptic treatment.

Many groups are now examining automated seizure detection algorithms for use in the NICU and promising results are emerging (Cherian et al. 2011; Temko et al. 2011a, b).

Evidence is scarce on the clinical benefits of treating electrographic seizures in neonates and, with the current state of knowledge, it is acceptable practice to aim to control clinically apparent seizures. In any case, it is virtually impossible to achieve electrical control in all cases with the anticonvulsants currently recommended for newborn use (Booth and Evans 2004).

Evidence is emerging from a small number of studies designed to measure the effect of treating electrographic seizures which does suggest a reduction in the severity of magnetic resonance imaging (MRI) injury when efforts are made to treat all such seizures (van Rooij et al. 2010). Evidence from large multicentre trials is essential before this practice can be recommended (Clancy 2006), and a number of such studies are currently under consideration.

Aetiology

Causes of neonatal seizures in current order of importance are shown in Table 40.3.

Hypoxic–ischaemic encephalopathy

This remains the most common cause of neonatal seizures at term, contributing over half the cases to most series. The characteristic time of onset is within 24 hours of birth, and seizures often begin in the first 12–18 hours. Seizures are rare in the first 6 hours unless there has been an antenatal insult (Filan et al. 2005). For more information on the management and prognosis of this condition, see pp. 1114–1150.

In moderate and severe hypoxic–ischaemic encephalopathy, the background EEG pattern can evolve over the first few days after

Table 40.3 Causes of neonatal seizure

	1	2	3	4	5*	6†	7	8
Number of cases			71	131	100	40	90	81
Hypoxic–ischaemic encephalopathy	53%	16%	49%	30%	49%	37%	40%	37%
Cerebral infarction (stroke)					12%	17%	1%	11%
Intracranial haemorrhage (includes intraventricular haemorrhage and subdural haematomas)	17%		14%		7%	12%	15%	9%
Meningitis	8%	3%	2%	7%	5%	5%	20% ~	9%
Maternal drug withdrawal				4%				
Hypoglycaemia	3%	2%	0.1%	5%	3%		3%	
Hypocalcaemia, hypomagnasaemia				22%			5%	
Rapidly changing serum sodium								
Congenitally abnormal brain		8%		4%	3%	17%	10%	6%
Fifth-day fits (benign non-familial)		52%						
Benign familial neonatal seizures							6%	1%
Pyridoxine-dependent seizures								
Hypertension				1.4%				
Kernicterus					1%			
Inborn errors of metabolism					3%			

Data in column 1 from Levene and Trounce (1986); column 2 from Goldberg (1983); column 3 from Andre et al. (1988); column 4 from Bergman et al. (1983); column 5 from Estan and Hope (1997); column 6 from Lien et al. (1995) column 7 from Ronen and Penney (1995); and column 8 from Ortibus et al. (1996).

birth. Very suppressed EEG activity is seen for a number of hours after birth and is often followed by a period of seizure activity that, depending on the severity of the insult, can be very difficult to control with anticonvulsants. The seizures also evolve in a characteristic manner in hypoxic–ischaemic encephalopathy over a number of days (Lynch et al. 2012). When seizures resolve, a burst suppression pattern can be seen for a number of days. Our group have reported delayed lactate clearance in neonates with hypoxic–ischaemic encephalopathy and a high EEG seizure burden (Murray et al. 2007b).

Intracranial haemorrhage

Intraventricular haemorrhage is the most important cause of seizures in preterm babies. A large parenchymal haemorrhage which causes seizures is associated with a poor outcome (Davis et al. 2010) (this chapter, part 5). Neonates of any gestation can have seizures because of bleeding into the subarachnoid space, the dural space, the cerebellum or cortex (Kohelet et al. 2004). A diagnosis of intracranial bleeding in a term baby should lead to a search for a coagulation disorder, including vitamin K deficiency, and testing for haemophilia in boys. MRI has shown that a small amount of subarachnoid or subdural bleeding is common in the newborn period, and these collections usually resolve without sequelae.

Focal cerebral infarction (stroke)

Seizures in term infants with normal Apgar scores who remain alert between spasms are likely to be due to focal lesions, most commonly middle cerebral artery infarction. Ten to 15% of seizures in full-term neonates are due to stroke (p. 1108). On EEG, the area of infarction is the focus of electrographic seizures that generally manifest as clonic seizures on the contralateral side. Seizures often require MRI for identification, and the prognosis is better than when the underlying cause is hypoxic–ischaemic encephalopathy.

The background EEG may be normal or show only mild focal abnormalities, though quiet sleep may enhance background abnormalities (Walsh et al. 2011). Diagnosis of arterial or venous occlusion in the newborn period should trigger investigations to rule out an underlying thrombotic tendency. EEG is useful for diagnosis and prognosis and should ideally be performed within 24 hours of signs; some neonates will have seizures early in the postnatal period (Estan and Hope 1997).

Seizures are also the most common presenting sign in cerebral venous sinus thrombosis (p. 1109). Associated lesions include thalamic haemorrhage, intraventricular haemorrhage and parenchymal haemorrhagic infarction (Berfelo et al. 2010). Ultrasound imaging is not reliable for the detection of stroke or sinus venous thrombosis, which often requires MRI for identification.

Meningitis

Intracranial infections, whether bacterial, non-bacterial or congenital, cause neonatal seizures usually after the first week of life. In a recent French study group B streptococci remained the most common cause of neonatal bacterial meningitis, causing 77% of early-onset and 50% of late-onset cases (Gaschignard et al. 2011). *Escherichia coli* was the most common cause of meningitis in preterm infants.

Aciclovir treatment should be started if the lumbar puncture reveals a high white-cell count in the cerebrospinal fluid (CSF), yet no organisms are seen on Gram stain in a baby who has not been treated with antibiotics, whilst awaiting the results of polymerase chain reaction for herpesvirus. The risks of starting treatment in this situation are minimal, whereas delay will worsen the prognosis. More information on the diagnosis and treatment of neonatal central nervous system infections can be found in Chapter 39, part 2.

Neonatal abstinence syndrome and other drug-related causes of neonatal seizure (Ch. 26)

Withdrawal seizures can occur for the first time at any age up to 3 weeks, with a median time of onset of 10 days. EEG abnormalities are present in 50% of cocaine-exposed neonates, persist up to 1 year, and are associated with an adverse neurodevelopmental outcome. Maternal methadone addiction is more likely to be associated with neonatal withdrawal seizures than heroin (Herzlinger et al. 1977). Tremors have been noted in children who received prolonged infusions of narcotics for analgesia (French and Nocera 1994), and there has been concern about the effects of midazolam for sedation in preterm babies (Montenegro et al. 2001). A high incidence of benign neonatal sleep myoclonus (BNSM) has been reported in the babies of opioid-dependent mothers (Held-Egli et al. 2009).

Metabolic causes

Hypoglycaemia

Hypoglycaemia can be the sole cause of neonatal seizures and other neurological signs such as apnoea, lethargy and jitteriness. Often hypoglycaemia complicates hypoxic–ischaemic encephalopathy or infection, and hypoglycaemia is common in infants who are small for gestational age (Ch. 10). The adverse outcome associated with the underlying cause makes it difficult to determine the prognosis of uncomplicated hypoglycaemia. However, animal evidence does show that if hypoglycaemia is present during seizures, the risk of brain injury is even higher (Wasterlain et al. 2010).There is no doubt that the finding of a low glucose level in a baby who is seizing is an indication for urgent intravenous treatment, and every effort should be made to normalise the glucose level as soon as possible.

Hypocalcaemia

Up until the late 1970s the high phosphate content in cow's milk-based formula for babies resulted in a high incidence of neonatal seizures due to hypocalaemia (Lynch and Rust 1994). Half the babies in the series of Brown et al. (1972) were hypocalcaemic (total serum calcium less than 1.75 mmol/L). Similarly high incidences of late hypocalcaemic seizures were reported prior to the introduction of modern low-phosphate milks; in the late 1960s infants were consuming doorstep cow's milk or a high-phosphate formula. A higher than usual level of hypocalcaemia has been found as the cause for neonatal seizures in an Indian population in more recent years (Sood et al. 2003).

A diagnosis of hypocalcaemia should lead to consideration of CATCH-22 (22q11.2 deletion syndrome), which can be diagnosed with fluorescent in situ hybridization genetic studies. Hypocalcaemic seizures occasionally occur secondary to maternal hypercalcaemia (prolonged intrauterine exposure to high levels) or maternal vitamin D deficiency and the neonatal diagnosis should prompt estimation of the maternal serum calcium. Low magnesium levels frequently accompany hypocalcaemia and require correction before the seizures will respond. Hypocalcaemia is common in ill very-low-birthweight babies and in babies with hypoxic–ischaemic encephalopathy and is probably not causally related to the seizures in these cases. Less often there is congenital hypoparathyroidism or calcium-sensing receptor defects.

Hypernatraemia and hyponatraemia

The most common cause of hypernatraemia is breast milk insufficiency and seizures can occur when the serum sodium level is very high or falls very rapidly. It is recommended that the level be reduced at a rate not exceeding 0.5 mmol/l/h when rehydrating hypernatraemic babies. Babies have also developed hyponatraemic seizures after being given excess solute-free water in intravenous solutions, or orally in the form of cheap alternatives to correctly balanced oral rehydration solutions. A very high, very low or rapidly changing serum sodium occurring in conditions such as the syndrome of inappropriate antidiuretic hormone secretion, Bartter's syndrome or severe dehydration can cause seizures.

Congenital malformations of the brain

Disorders of neuronal migration such as lissencephaly or schizencephaly can present with neonatal seizures. Diagnosis has been facilitated with the advent of MRI but is sometimes possible with ultrasound (pp. 1207–1212).

Inborn errors of metabolism

Pyridoxine-dependent seizures

The first case of an infant with intractable seizures controlled by pyridoxine was reported by Hunt et al. in 1954. It is a rare disorder and seizures can begin during intrauterine life (mothers describe 'hammering' movements lasting 15–20 minutes several times a day). Seizures are very resistant to conventional anticonvulsant treatments yet cease within minutes of parenteral pyridoxine (50–100 mg) and return within days of withdrawal. This therapeutic trial can cause hypotonia requiring ventilatory support and should be carried out in an intensive care unit (Kroll 1985). There is no other way to make the diagnosis, although characteristic EEG abnormalities have been recognised (Nabbout et al. 1999; Naasan et al. 2009). A more recent study has shown that some of the EEG changes seen after pyridoxine administration to neonates with pyridoxine-dependent seizures are also present in other treatment-resistant seizure disorders (Bok et al. 2010). Atypical cases that respond more slowly and that show late-onset seizures requiring unusually high doses of pyridoxine (up to 500 mg) have been described (Gospe 1998; Baxter 2001), and yet others respond to very small doses. Gospe suggests that a trial of pyridoxine should involve 100 mg intravenously every 10 minutes until the seizures stop or a total of 500 mg is reached.

The condition is caused by an inherited metabolic disorder of lysine degradation, resulting in increased urinary alpha-aminoadipic semialdehyde (α-AASA) excretion (Bok et al. 2007). In addition to increased urinary α-AASA concentrations, mutations in the ALDH7A1 (antiquitin) gene can also identify pyridoxine-resistant seizures (Mills et al. 2006; Been et al. 2008). The increased a-AASA concentrations in body fluids result in pyridoxal-5-phosphate deficiency. Pyridoxal-5-phosphate is responsible for converting glutamate into the inhibitory GABA. The condition is autosomal-recessive. Supplementation of the diet with pyridoxine (vitamin B_6) 20–100 mg bd is required for life, and the dose may need to be increased with age (Baxter 2001). Unfortunately, many of these children have severe cognitive disabilities despite early diagnosis and treatment. A better outcome has been achieved with higher doses of pyridoxine, leading to the suggestion that sufficient pyridoxine should be given to restore the CSF glutamate levels to normal.

Diagnostic tests such as measurements of urinary AASA and pipecolic acid, as well as gene testing for mutations in the antiquitin gene encoding for the AASA dehydrogenase enzyme, are now proving very useful for this disorder (Bok et al. 2007; Plecko et al. 2007).

Glycine encephalopathy

Non-ketotic hyperglycinaemia is an inborn error of glycine metabolism in which large quantities of glycine accumulate in all body tissues, including the brain. Neonates exhibit lethargy, hypotonia, apnoea, characteristic hiccups and intractable epileptic seizures that are not specific to this disease. Rapid progression can lead to intractable seizures, coma and respiratory failure. The outcome is invariably poor, and many die before the age of 1 year. Levels of glycine in blood, urine and CSF are very high. The EEG shows a generalised burst suppression pattern characterised by periodic high-amplitude bursts of activity on a near-silent background (Markand et al. 1982; Scher et al. 1986). Dextromethorphan monotherapy (35 mg/kg/day) was associated with cessation of seizures and normalisation of the EEG in a single case, but this regimen is not always successful (Schmitt et al. 1993). A recent report has shown an increase in seizure frequency following valproate treatment (Tsuyusaki et al. 2011).

Glucose transport across the blood–brain barrier is mediated by the facilitative glucose transporter isoform 1 (GLUT-1). A deficiency of this transporter results in impaired energy supply to the brain, and was recognised by De Vivo in 1991. This rare disorder is important because treatment has the potential to lead to a normal neurological outcome, and because the inheritance is autosomal-dominant (Fishman 1991). The interictal EEG is normal in this disorder, with spike-and-wave discharges generally only emerging during seizures (Leary et al. 2003). Babies have a low CSF glucose concentration, with low to normal CSF lactate levels despite normal blood glucose concentrations. Elevated lactate levels would suggest a mitochondrial disorder. The diagnosis should be suspected if the CSF glucose is less than a third of the blood glucose level, and GLUT-1 deficiency can be confirmed with an assay that measures the uptake of ^{14}C-O-methyl-D-glucose in erythrocytes. Treatment is with a ketogenic diet, which is usually successful in controlling the seizures but does not always prevent the microcephaly, developmental delay and ataxia. There may be a transient form of the disorder which does not require long-term treatment, but the three cases so far described may have had alternative explanations for the low CSF glucose levels, such as low-grade meningitis or subarachnoid haemorrhage (Klepper et al. 2003).

Biotinidase deficiency

This is one of the few treatable causes of resistant neonatal seizures, hence the importance of considering this rare autosomal-recessive condition. Biotinidase is responsible for biotin recycling and biotin is an essential cofactor for activation of the carboxylase enzymes. If biotinidase is absent, infantile or early-childhood encephalopathy, seizure disorder, dermatitis, alopecia, neural deafness and optic atrophy develop. In the neonatal period there is usually a skin rash, similar in appearance to seborrhoeic dermatitis. The disease can be diagnosed by simple fluorometric enzyme assay and treatment with biotin is cheap. The EEG shows a burst suppression pattern consistent with encephalopathy (Salbert et al. 1993).

Syndromic neonatal seizures

Benign familial neonatal seizures

This fascinating autosomal-dominant condition was first recognised in 1964 (Rett and Tuebel 1964). The onset is within the first week of life and seizures are dramatic, with 80% beginning on the second or third day of life. The seizures ceased after 6 weeks of age in 68% of the largest kindred reported, and rarely persist beyond 6 months (Ronen et al. 1993).

Seizures show an initial tonic phase with cyanosis followed by clonic movements of the whole body (Yamamoto et al. 2011). There is usually a family history of neonatal seizures but they are associated with normal psychomotor development, a normal interictal EEG and a favourable outcome. This rare condition has an autosomal-dominant inheritance with 85% penetrance, and mutations have been found in the genes situated on chromosomes 20q and 8q which code for a family of voltage-gated potassium channels (M (for muscarine) channels). Benign familial neonatal convulsions (BFNC) are thus an example of a 'channelopathy'. M channels can be kept open with a new AED, retigabine, and it has been suggested that this drug might hold promise for other types of neonatal seizure apart from those in BFNC.

In contrast to pyridoxine-dependent seizures, these fits can be controlled by conventional medication and the prognosis for development is excellent.

Benign non-familial neonatal seizures (fifth-day fits)

This benign self-limiting condition reached epidemic proportions in some Australian maternity units in the late 1970s (Pryor et al. 1981). Reports also came from France, but only two cases have been seen in Nancy since 1985 and the diagnosis has not been made in Camperdown since 1989 (North et al. 1989; Andre and Selton 1993). Seizures occur between day 1 and day 7 after birth and are usually partial clonic, rarely generalise and apnoea is common (North et al. 1989). Seizures last for 1–3 minutes but can become frequent, leading to status epilepticus. The neurological state is usually normal at the onset of seizures and there is no family history of seizures. The interictal EEG may be normal, show generalised or multifocal discharges or show characteristic bursts of sharp waves, sometimes called 'theta pointu alternant'.

The cause remains a mystery, although low CSF zinc was found in a few cases (Goldberg 1982). A few years ago we cared for a baby with this condition who had marked tonic-clonic seizures which are otherwise very unusual in the newborn period; she has thrived (Guerra et al. 2002).

Benign neonatal sleep myoclonus

Neurologically normal term neonates can present with BNSM, which is characterised by recurrent rhythmic jerks during sleep and a normal EEG. Jerks disappear during wakefulness and resolve within 3 months. A recent review of the literature which included 164 cases of BNSM found that repetitive jerks were located primarily in the distal part of the extremities, usually the arms but also the legs and very occasionally the face and abdomen (Maurer et al. 2010). Myoclonus was seen in quiet sleep predominantly but some reports did describe jerks during active sleep. There was also some evidence that an exacerbation of myoclonic jerks occurred when some infants were erroneously treated with AEDs. An interesting finding in this series was that the repetitive jerks did not always stop with gentle restraint and had not resolved by 3 months in one-third of cases. No treatment is required for BNSM and parents should be reassured that the jerks will cease eventually.

Epileptic encephalopathies

Ohtahara syndrome (early infantile epileptic encephalopathy)

This syndrome was first described by Ohtahara and colleagues in 1976 and is one of the age-dependent epileptic encephalopathies (the others being West's syndrome and Lennox–Gastaut syndrome). Seizures usually develop within the first 10 days of life and may occur as early as the first hour after delivery. The seizure types in Ohtahara syndrome are variable, with the most frequent type being spasms, which may be either generalised and symmetrical or lateralised. Spasms may occur singly or in clusters in both awake and asleep states. Generalised tonic-clonic seizures can develop later in the syndrome. Seizures are usually accompanied by a severe encephalopathy, and are resistant to treatment. Soon after the onset of seizures, the infants become inactive and hypotonic. The syndrome is now believed to be mainly attributable to a cerebral malformation (Yamamoto et al. 2011).

The EEG shows a characteristic burst suppression pattern and can be distinguished from the pattern seen in other encephalopathies (Ohtahara 1978). According to the Japanese group that has published most of the seminal works on this condition, the bursts must consist of high-amplitude non-synchronised paroxysms lasting 2–6 seconds and the suppression phase must show less than 10 μV or a flat tracing and continue for 3–5 seconds (Yamamoto et al. 2011). Suppression and burst phases must appear alternately and regularly every 5 seconds or more and should be seen in both sleep and wake states. During seizures, desynchronisation of the burst suppression pattern is seen. The prognosis is very poor: psychomotor development is arrested and severe neurological abnormalities such as spastic diplegia, hemiplegia, tetraplegia, ataxia, or dystonia develop (Yamamoto et al. 2011). Vigabatrin has been tried in a few cases (Baxter et al. 1995).

Early myoclonic epilepsy (EME)

This rare syndrome, originally described by Aicardi, presents with erratic, fragmentary myoclonus in the first month of life, evolving into focal seizures and infantile spasms. Seizure manifestations include partial or fragmented myoclonus, massive myoclonias, partial motor seizures and tonic spasms. Myoclonias may shift from one part of the body to another and usually persist in sleep. Normal background activity is absent. The background EEG shows a burst suppression pattern with complex bursts of spikes, sharp waves and slow waves lasting for 1–5 seconds in both waking and sleep. The burst suppression pattern seen in EME is similar to that in Ohtahara syndrome but the burst phase is shorter with longer periods of suppression than Ohtahara syndrome (Yamamoto et al. 2011). The

fragmented myoclonias usually have no EEG correlate, whereas massive myoclonias may be synchronous with the bursts. The clinical course of EME is severe and antiepileptic agents and corticosteroids or adrenocorticotrophic hormone have not been effective. Metabolic aetiologies are predominant in EME, whereas malformative aetiologies predominate in Ohtahara syndrome.

Investigation

Essential laboratory investigations include:

* blood glucose
* serum calcium, ionised calcium if possible
* serum magnesium
* arterial pH, blood gas
* lactate
* serum sodium
* serum urea and creatinine
* lumbar puncture
* blood culture
* cranial ultrasound scan.

If the cause is not revealed, second-line investigations are suggested in Table 40.4 and include specimens for virology and a congenital infection screen, MRI, samples such as hair or urine to look for maternal 'street' drugs, urinary and blood amino acid estimation, chromosomal analysis, blood ammonia and measurement of urinary organic acids. Consideration should be given to a trial of pyridoxine in resistant cases. The value of an EEG examination has already been discussed and an EEG should be obtained if at all possible, and certainly should be done in difficult cases. MRI is superior to computed tomography for most purposes, and should be considered in all cases, and certainly if the cause is not revealed by first-line investigations. Even if the cause is found, the information obtained from MRI can give valuable information about the prognosis.

Treatment

Indications for treatment

Most babies are still treated on the basis of a clinical diagnosis alone, and treatment is also monitored this way. Continuous EEG studies show that a considerable electrographic seizure burden often remains after anticonvulsant treatment begins, due to electroclinical dissociation (Boylan et al. 2002). Whether or not treating to electrical quiescence can improve the outcome is not known, and as yet there is no anticonvulsant regimen that will achieve this in all cases (Rennie and Boylan 2003). In the current state of knowledge most neonatologists would treat a baby who had more than three clinical seizures in an hour, or a single clinical seizure lasting more than 3 minutes; this remains reasonable practice, although every attempt should be made to obtain an EEG.

General guidelines

Treatment is best started intravenously as absorption is erratic from intramuscular or enteral administration, and the neonate has little muscle mass. Facilities to site and maintain intravenous lines and to institute artificial ventilation are necessary before treating seizures, as most of the available drugs depress respiration and ventilation can become inadequate due to frequent convulsions or the effects of treatment. The high total body water of the neonate means there is a large volume of distribution, hence the relatively large loading doses suggested in Table 40.4. Many of the drugs are

Table 40.4 Second-line investigations for seizures (not all are indicated in every case)

MRI brain
Ammonia
Urine organic acids and amino acids,
TORCH screen, viral cultures (herpes simplex virus)
Guthrie blood sample for acylcarnitine profile
Hair, urine, for drug screen
Urine: α-aminoadipic semialdehyde (AASA), reducing substances
Urine and blood creatine:creatinine ratio and guanidinoacetate compounds (GAMT), Urine NAG/RBP
Plasma biotinidase
Plasma urate/urine sulphite (fresh urine)
Transferrin isoforms/protein C
Very-long-chain fatty acids, cholesterol
White-cell ubiquinone
Immunoglobulins
Copper, caeruloplasmin
Lysosomal white-cell enzymes (neurodegenerative screen), vacuolated lymphocytes and chitotriosidase
Plasma (ethylene diaminetetraacetic acid) and urine purine/pyrimidine
Paired plasma (preferably fasting, take blood first) and CSF: glucose, lactate, amino acids
CSF viral studies, PCR for herpesvirus
CSF for neurotransmitters, including 5-methyltetrahydrofolate, pyridoxal phosphate, serum red cell folate and vitamin B₆
Consider karyotype, FISH for specific syndromes, CGH microarray
Careful examination of skin and consider Wood's light examination
Molecular: blood for DNA extraction and storage
Consider: i.e. SCN1A, CDKL4, PNPO (if low CSF PLP/PLP-responsive),
Antiquitin (if AASA-positive), mitochondrial DNA point mutations and rearrangements
POLG, RARS2 ± VRK1 and TSEN54, 2,34 if PCH on MRI
GLUT-1 if CSF:plasma ratio glucose <0.4

MRI, magnetic resonance imaging; TORCH, toxoplasmosis, rubella, cytomegalovirus, herpes; CSF, cerebrospinal fluid; PCR, polymerase chain reaction; PCH, pontocerebellar hypoplasia; PLP, proteolipid protein; FISH, fluorescence in situ hybridisation; GLUT-1, glucose transporter isoform 1.

protein-bound and can interact with other drugs and bilirubin. Therapeutic hypothermia does prolong the half-life of many drugs, including phenobarbital, and appropriate doses are still being worked out. In cooled babies we give a loading dose of 20 mg/kg phenobarbital with a maximum of two further doses of 10 mg/kg/dose and then check a level.

Initiating treatment

Phenobarbital remains the current first-line treatment of neonatal seizures worldwide, in spite of evidence that it is effective in only about a third of cases and there is concern about the effects of this drug on brain development, including apoptosis (Painter et al. 1999; Bittigau et al. 2002; Boylan et al. 2004; Kaindl et al. 2006; Ikonomidou and Turski 2010). Recently published surveys from Israel, Australia and the USA indicate that there are large variations in practice, both between neonatologists and neurologists and between countries (Bassan et al. 2008; Guillet et al. 2008). Off-label use of AEDs is not uncommon (Silverstein et al. 2008a, b). In a recent European survey, Vento and colleagues (2010) showed

almost unanimous use of phenobarbital as a first-line drug, followed by midazolam, phenytoin and lidocaine as second- and third-line drugs.

Phenobarbital enhances GABA actions. The qualitatively distinct action of GABA on the neuronal membrane in early development may explain why phenobarbital is often ineffective in newborns: it facilitates the passive outflow of chloride down its electrochemical gradient, depolarising and exciting neurons (as compared with its actions on mature neurons, which have low Cl⁻ concentrations).

Phenytoin is our current second-line choice, although this drug needs to be used with caution (and given slowly intravenously) in babies with hypoxic ischaemia who often have cardiac depression. About a third of babies fail to respond to a combination of phenobarbital and phenytoin: they are usually suffering from severe hypoxic–ischaemic encephalopathy and their prognosis is poor. The choice of third-line anticonvulsant varies, but one of the benzodiazepines is often chosen. Doses of commonly used anticonvulsant drugs are given in Table 40.5. Midazolam is effective for the control of status epilepticus in adults and children, but has shown varying results in babies (Boylan et al. 2004; Castro-Conde 2005; Sirsi et al. 2008). Recent evidence from a number of small studies does seem to indicate that midazolam may be a useful treatment for seizures in babies, but the exact dose and dosing regimen have not been established (Castro-Conde 2005; Sirsi et al. 2008). In addition, there are concerns about safety: midazolam can cause myoclonus in preterms (Montenegro et al. 2001).

Midazolam has been evaluated in an open comparison with lidocaine as a second-line treatment in babies whose seizures failed to respond to phenobarbital: seizures were monitored with continuous video-EEG (Boylan et al. 2004). Six babies received either clonazepam or midazolam, but none responded. Others have had better success with midazolam, one study using very high doses of 1000 µg/kg/h (Van Leuven et al. 2004; Castro Conde et al. 2005). An adequately powered randomised controlled trial of midazolam is clearly warranted.

Lorazepam is more popular in the USA (Maytal et al. 1991; Riviello 2004). Paraldehyde, formerly given rectally, can work well intravenously but is currently difficult to obtain in Europe and is not available in the USA. Those who have used intravenous paraldehyde as a third-line anticonvulsant report success in over 80% of cases with 200 mg/kg given intravenously as a single slow infusion repeated 12-hourly if required (Armstrong and Battin 2001). The problem with many of the studies which evaluate AED treatments in babies is that the outcome measure is clinical seizure control, which can be very misleading.

Lidocaine has a very narrow therapeutic range and accumulates in the blood, so that it can only be given as an infusion for 48 hours. There are reports of success with this agent, mainly from Scandinavia (Hellstrom-Westas et al. 1988; Kobayashi et al. 1999). Much more information is required before this drug can be recommended for routine use. A baby who has been given phenytoin already should not receive lidocaine because of the risk of cardiac toxicity: the drugs act on the same sodium channels (Table 40.5). Newer AEDs such as topiramate and levetiracetam have been anecdotally reported to improve acute neonatal seizures (Abend et al. 2011; Glass et al. 2011; Khan et al. 2011). It is also not known how long to continue treatment for neonatal seizures (see below), and how the length of treatment impacts outcome.

An age-dependent high expression of a chloride cotransporter is thought to be responsible for the high incidence of seizure in the newborn period and the lack of response to conventional drugs used in older children and adults (Dzhala et al 2005a). Bumetanide, a commonly used loop diuretic, blocks this specific age-dependent cotransporter and has been shown to reduce seizure

Table 40.5 Drug doses for seizure management in the newborn

DRUG	INITIAL DOSE	ROUTE	MAINTENANCE DOSE	ROUTE	HALF-LIFE	MODE OF EXCRETION	NOTES	THERAPEUTIC LEVEL
Phenobarbital	20–40 mg/kg	IV	4–5 mg/kg/24 h	O	100–200 h	Hepatic P$_{450}$ cytochrome oxidase	Slow oral absorption: liver enzyme inducer	20–40 mg/l 90–180 µmol/l
Phenytoin	20 mg/kg slowly (1 mg/kg/min)	IV	5 mg/kg/24 h in two doses	IV/O	20 h (75 prems)	Liver glucuronidation	Vitamin K antagonist; risk of extravasation, cardiac toxicity and purple-glove syndrome	10–20 mg/l 40–80 µmol/l
Paraldehyde	0.3 ml/kg (0.6 ml/kg mixture) PR	rectal	For rectal use dilute 1:1 with arachis oil, give no more than t.d.s.	Rectal	7–27 h	Mainly liver, some lungs	Protect from light and plastic	
Diazepam	0.3 mg/kg	IV	0.3 mg/kg	IV	20–60 h	Liver glucuronidation	Flumazenil is an antidote to diazepam and midazolam; rapid clearance from the brain limits value	
Clonazepam	100 µg/kg	IV	4 µg/kg/h	IV	30 h	Liver glucuronidation	Tends to increase salivation and bronchial secretions	30–100 mg/l
Midazolam	60 µg/kg	IV	150 µg/kg/h	IV	6–12 h	Liver glucuronidation	Reports of myoclonic jerks in preterm babies	
Valproate	20 mg/kg	IV	10 mg/kg/12-hourly	O	26–47 h	Hepatic	GABA modifier. Increased ammonia levels. Hepatotoxicity may be a problem but not yet described in babies	40–50 mg/l 275–350 µmol/l
Lidocaine	2–4 mg/kg	IV	2 mg/kg/h maximum 6 mg/kg/h and for no more than 48 hours	IV	200 min	Liver and kidney	Toxic metabolites accumulate in 24 hours	2.4–6 mg/l in adults; little known about therapeutic levels in babies
Pyridoxine	50–100 mg	IV	5–10 mg/kg/day	O			EEG monitoring in ICU for the initial dose	
Pyridoxal phosphate			30 mg/kg/day					
Folinic acid			4 mg/kg/day				Folinic acid-responsive Seizures are very rare	

GABA, gamma-aminobutyric acid; EEG, electroencephalogram; ICU, intensive care unit.

Table 40.6 Outcome of neonatal seizures by cause

	DEAD	HANDICAP	NORMAL	REFERENCE
HIE grade II, III	50%	25%	25%	
Preterm	58%	23%	18%	Scher et al. (1993a); Watkins et al. (1988); van Zeben-van der Aa et al. (1990)
Meningitis	20%	40%	40%	
Malformations	60%	40%		
Late-onset hypocalcaemia			100%	
Hypoglycaemia		50%	50%	Koivisto et al. (1972)
HIE, hypoxic–ischaemic encephalopathy.				

burden significantly in immature animals. More recently, animal experiments suggest that bumetanide in combination with phenobarbital may be even more effective in suppressing seizures in the immature brain (Dzhala et al 2008).

Bumetanide has been used as a diuretic in term and preterm babies for around 30 years and several studies have validated its efficacy and safety, including pharmacokinetics and dose-finding studies (Sullivan et al. 1996; Lopez-Samblas 1997). It is considered a safe drug in the neonatal period, even in critically ill infants (Ward & Lam 1977; Aranda et al. 1980; Turmen et al. 1982; Robertson et al. 1986; Walker et al. 1988; Walker et al. 1989; Wells et al. 1992; Shankaran et al. 1995; Sullivan et al. 1996 a and b; Lopez-Samblas et al. 1997; Clark et al. 2006). Studies in animals have suggested 0.1–0.2 mg/kg as the optimal dose to block the NKCC1 cotransporter, which is at the upper range of the dose used as a diuretic. Two randomised studies of bumetanide for neonatal seizure control are underway in the USA and Europe.

Duration of treatment

Concern about the effects of anticonvulsant treatment on the developing brain means that most British neonatologists would only discharge a baby on maintenance phenobarbital if the neurological examination was abnormal, although only 3% of US neonatologists discontinued treatment prior to discharge (Massingale and Boutross 1993). Only two of 55 Swedish infants discharged without medication relapsed (Hellstrom-Westas et al. 1995). Some perform an EEG at a month or prior to discharge, and discontinue anticonvulsants if this was normal. If babies are discharged on anticonvulsants, consider discontinuation of treatment if they remain seizure-free at 9 months. Babies can be allowed to 'grow out of' their dose, gradually reducing drug levels.

Maintenance anticonvulsants

Phenobarbital in a dose of 5 mg/kg/day is the usual maintenance anticonvulsant chosen for the newborn. There is very little experience with alternative maintenance therapy at the present time and combinations are best avoided. Phenytoin is not a good choice for long-term therapy. Resistant cases should be treated with a combination of phenobarbital and carbamazepine, although sodium valproate can be successful in some cases.

Prognosis

The prognosis depends largely on the cause of the seizures, being worse for those with hypoxic–ischaemic encephalopathy, meningitis and cerebral malformations than hypocalcaemia, benign familial neonatal seizures, subarachnoid haemorrhage or stroke (Tekgul et al. 2006) (Table 40.6). Mortality and morbidity are greater in preterm babies (Scher et al. 1993a; van Zeben et al. 1990). There is some evidence suggesting that seizures are independently associated with a poor outcome but recent evidence is conflicting (Glass et al. 2009; Kwon et al. 2011). The background EEG can be helpful, and a normal background EEG with well-organised sleep stages has consistently been shown to be associated with an 80% chance of normal development (Rose and Lombroso 1970; Holmes and Lombroso 1993; Tekgul et al. 2006). The background EEG features of encephalopathy evolve over time, and it is important not to prognosticate from a recording made too early; both we and others have shown that a low-voltage EEG seen in the first 6 hours of life can recover (Toet et al. 1999; Pressler et al. 2001; Murray et al. 2010).

This evolutionary pattern may have changed somewhat with the advent of therapeutic hypothermia and two studies using continuous aEEG monitoring have suggested that recovery of the EEG is delayed when babies with hypoxic–ischaemic encephalopathy are cooled (Hallberg et al. 2010; Thoresen et al. 2010). Rewarming seizures are occasionally seen (Battin et al. 2004). The number of electrographic seizures is not in general an indicator of prognosis, nor is the clinical seizure type. Some have suggested that the outcome is worse for babies with a large number of independent electrographic seizure foci, but this work requires confirmation (Bye et al. 1997). There is increasing consensus that seizures (including electrographic seizures which are clinically silent) which persist despite third-line AEDs carry a poor prognosis (McBride et al. 2000). Adverse outcomes include cerebral palsy and microcephaly with significant learning difficulties.

The risk of subsequent epilepsy after neonatal seizures also depends on the aetiology, and is more likely if spike and sharp-wave activity persists on the EEG at 3 months (Clancy and Legido 1991). The later seizure type includes infantile spasms, minor motor seizures, complex partial and tonic-clonic seizures, which often only emerge after a year or so. In a Dutch study, the incidence of postneonatal epilepsy after treatment of clinical and subclinical neonatal seizures detected with continuous aEEG was 9.4% (Toet et al 2005).

References

Abend, N.S., Gutierrez-Colina, A.M., Monk, H.M., et al., 2011. Levetiracetam for treatment of neonatal seizures. J Child Neurol 26, 465–470.

Anderson, C.M., Torres, F., Faoro, A., 1985. The EEG of the Early Premature. Electroencephalogr Clin Neurophysiol 60, 95–105.

Andre, M., Selton, D., 1993. Convulsions in the fifth day of life. A critical study. Arch Fr Pediatr 50, 197–200.

Andre, M., Matisse, M., Vert, P., et al., 1988. Neonatal seizures – recent aspects. Neuropediatrics 19, 201–207.

Aranda, J.V., Turmen, T., Sasyniuk, B.I., 1980 Jul. Pharmacokinetics of diuretics and methylxanthines in the baby. Eur J Clin Pharmacol 18 (1), 55–63.

Armstrong, D.L., Battin, M.R., 2001. Pervasive seizures caused by hypoxic-ischemic encephalopathy: treatment with intravenous paraldehyde. J Child Neurol 16, 915–917.

Bassan, Y., Bental, Y., Shany, E., 2008. Neonatal seizures: dilemmas in workup and management. Pediatric Neurology 38, 415–421.

Battin, M., Bennet, L., Gunn, A.J., 2004. Rebound seizures during rewarming. Pediatrics 114, 1369.

Baxter, P., 2001. Pyridoxine-dependent and pyridoxine-responsive seizures. Dev Med Child Neurol 43, 416–420.

Baxter, P.S., Gardner-Medwin, D., Barwick, D.D., et al., 1995. Vigabatrin monotherapy in resistant neonatal seizures. Seizure 4, 57–59.

Been, J.V., Bok, L.A., Willemsen, M.A.A.P., et al., 2008. Mutations in the aldh7a1 gene cause pyridoxine-dependent seizures. Arquivos neuro-psiquiatr 66, 288–289.

Bell, A.H., Greisen, G., Pryds, O., 1993. Comparison of the effects of phenobarbitone and morphine administration on EEG activity in preterm babies. Acta paediatr 82, 35–39.

Berfelo, F.J., Kersbergen, K.J., van Ommen, C.H., et al., 2010. Neonatal cerebral sinovenous thrombosis from symptom to outcome. Stroke 41, 1382–1388.

Bergman, I., Painter, M.J., Hirsch, R.P., et al., 1983. Outcome in neonates with convulsions treated in ICU. Ann Neurol 14, 642–647.

Biagioni, E., Mercuri, E., Rutherford, M., et al., 2001. Combined use of electroencephalogram and magnetic resonance imaging in full-term neonates with acute encephalopathy. Pediatrics 107, 461–468.

Bittigau, P., Sifringer, M., Genz, K., et al., 2002. Antiepileptic drugs and apoptotic neurodegeneration in the developing brain. Proceedings of the National Academy of Sciences of the United States of America 99 pp 15089–15094.

Bok, L.A., Struys, E., Willemsen, M.A., et al., 2007. Pyridoxine-dependent seizures in Dutch patients: diagnosis by elevated urinary alpha-aminoadipic semialdehyde levels. Arch Dis Child 92, 687–689.

Bok, L.A., Maurits, N.M., Willemsen, M.A., et al., 2010. The EEG response to pyridoxine-IV neither identifies nor excludes pyridoxine-dependent epilepsy. Epilepsia 51, 2406–2411.

Booth, D., Evans, D.J., 2004. Anticonvulsants for neonates with seizures. Cochrane Database Syst Rev (4), CD004218.

Bourez-Swart, M.D., van Rooij, L., Rizzo, C., et al., 2009. Detection of subclinical electroencephalographic seizure patterns with multichannel amplitude-integrated EEG in full-term neonates. Clin neurophysiol 120, 1916–1922.

Boylan, G.B., Panerai, R.B., Rennie, J.M., et al., 1999a. Cerebral blood flow velocity during neonatal seizures. Arch Dis Child 80, F105–F110.

Boylan, G.B., Pressler, R.M., Rennie, J.M., et al., 1999b, Outcome of electroclinical, electrographic, and clinical seizures in the newborn infant. Dev Med Child Neurol, 41, 819–825.

Boylan, G.B., Rennie, J.M., Pressler, R.M., et al., 2002. Phenobarbitone, neonatal seizures, and video-EEG. Arch Dis Child 86, 165–170.

Boylan, G., Rennie, J.M., Chorley, G., et al., 2004. Second line anticonvulsant treatment of neonatal seizures: a video-EEG monitoring study. Neurology 62, 486–488.

Boylan, G., Burgoyne, L., Moore, C., et al., 2010. An international survey of EEG use in the neonatal intensive care unit. Acta Paediatr 99, 1150–1155.

Brown, J.K., Cockburn, F., Forfar, J.O., 1972. Clinical and chemical correlates in convulsions of the newborn. Lancet 1, 135.

Bye, A.M.E., Cunningham, C.A., Chee, K.Y., Flanagan, D., 1997. Outcome of neonates with electrographically identified seizures, or at risk of seizures. Pediatr Neurol 16, 225–231.

Bye, A.M.E., Flanagan, D., 1995. Spatial and Temporal Characteristics of Neonatal Seizures. Epilepsia 36, 1009–1016.

Castro-Conde, J.R., Borges, A.A.H., Martinez, E.D., 2005. Midazolam in neonatal seizures with no response to phenobarbital. Neurology 64, 876–879.

Cherian, P.J., Deburchgraeve, W., Swarte, R.M., et al., 2011. Validation of a new automated neonatal seizure detection system: A clinician's perspective. Clin neurophysiol 122 (8), 1490–1499.

Clancy, R.R., 2006. Summary proceedings from the neurology group on neonatal seizures. Pediatrics 117 (3), S23–S27.

Clancy, R.R., Ledigo, A., 1987. The exact ictal and interictal duration of electroencephalographic neonatal seizures. Epilepsia 28, 537–541.

Clancy, R.R., Legido, A., 1991. Postnatal epilepsy after eeg-confirmed neonatal seizures. Epilepsia 21 (1) 69–76.

Clark, R.H., Bloom, B.T., Spitzer, A.R., Gerstmann, D.R., 2006 Jun. Reported medication use in the neonatal intensive care unit: data from a large national data set. Pediatrics 117 (6), 1979–1987.

Connell, J.A., Oozeer, R.C., Dubowitz, V., 1987. Continuous 4 channel EEG monitoring: a guide to interpretation, with normal values, in preterm infants. Neuropaediatrics 18, 138–145.

Curtis, P.D., Matthews, T.G., Clarke, T.A., et al., 1988. Neonatal seizures. Arch Dis Child 63, 1065–1067.

Davis, A.S., Hintz, S.R., Van Meurs, K.P., et al., 2010. Seizures in extremely low birth weight infants are associated with adverse outcome. J pediatr 157, 720–725.e1–2.

de Koning-Tijssen, M.A.J., Rees, M.I., 2007. Hyperekplexia. [Updated 2009 May 19]. In: Pagon, R.A., Bird, T.D., Dolan, C.R., et al., editors. GeneReviews™ [Internet]. University of Washington, Seattle, Seattle (WA), pp. 1993–2007.

De Vivo, D., Garcia-Alvarez, M., Ronen, G., et al., 1991. Defective glucose transport across the blood-brain barrier as a cause of persistent hypoglycorrhacia, seizures and developmental delay. N Engl J Med 325, 703–709.

Dzhala, V.I., Talos, D.M., Sdrulla, D.A., et al., 2005. NKCC1 transporter facilitates seizures in the developing brain. Nature Med 11, 1205–1213.

Dzhala, V.I., Talos, D.M., Sdrulla, D.A., Brumback, A.C., Mathews, G.C., Benke, T.A. et al., 2005a. NKCC1 transporter facilitates seizures in the developing brain. Nat Med 11 (11), 1205–1213.

Dzhala, V.I., Brumback, A.C., Staley, K.J., 2008. Bumetanide enhances phenobarbital efficacy in a neonatal seizure model. Ann Neurol 63 (2), 222–235.

Ellison, P., Franklin, S., Brown, P., et al., 1989. The evolution of a simplified method for interpretation of EEG in the preterm neonate. Acta Paediatr Scand 78, 210–216.

Estan, J., Hope, P.L., 1997. Unilateral neonatal cerebral infarction in full term infants. Arch Dis Child 76, F88–F93.

Filan, P., Boylan, G.B., Chorley, G., et al., 2005. The relationship between the onset of electrographic seizure activity after birth and the time of cerebral injury in utero. Br J Obstet Gynaecol 112, 504–507.

Fishman, R.A., 1992. The glucose transporter protein and gluconeogenic brain injury. N Engl J Med 325, 731–732.

French, J.P., Nocera, M., 1994. Drug withdrawal symptoms in children after continuous infusions of fentanyl. J Pediatr Nurs 9, 107–113.

Gaschignard, J., Levy, C., Romain, O., et al., 2011. Neonatal Bacterial Meningitis: 444 Cases in 7 Years. Pediatr infect dis j 30, 212–217.

Glass, H.C., Glidden, D., Jeremy, R.J., et al., 2009. Clinical Neonatal Seizures are Independently Associated with Outcome in Infants at Risk for Hypoxic-Ischemic Brain Injury. J Pediatr 155, 318–323.

Glass, H.C., Pham, T.N., Danielsen, B., et al., 2009b. Antenatal and intrapartum risk factors for seizures in term newborns: A population based study California 199802002. J Pediatr 154 (1), 24–28.

Glass, H.C., Poulin, C., Shevell, M.I., 2011. Topiramate for the treatment of neonatal seizures. Pediatr neurol 44, 439–442.

Goldberg, H.J., 1982. Fifth Day Fits – an acute zinc deficiency syndrome? Arch Dis Child 57, 633–635.

Goldberg, H.J., 1983. Neonatal convulsions – a ten year review. Arch Dis Child 57, 633–635.

Gordon, N., 1993. Startle disease or hyperexplexia. Dev Med Child Neurol 35, 1015–1024.

Gospe, S.M., 1998. Current perspectives on pyridoxine-dependent seizures. J Pediatr 132, 919–923.

Guerra, M.P., Wilson, G.A., Boylan, G.B., et al., 2002. An unusual presentation of fifth-day fits in the newborn. Pediatr neurol 26, 398–401.

Guillet, R., Kwon, J.M., 2008. Prophylactic phenobarbital administration after resolution of neonatal seizures: survey of current practice. Pediatrics 122 (4), 731–735.

Hallberg, B., Grossmann, K., Bartocci, M., et al., 2010. The prognostic value of early aEEG in asphyxiated infants undergoing systemic hypothermia treatment. Acta paediatr 99, 531–536.

Held-Egli, K., Rüegger, C., Das-Kundu, S., et al., 2009. Benign neonatal sleep myoclonus in newborn infants of opioid dependent mothers. Acta paediatr 98, 69–73.

Hellstrom-Westas, L., Blennow, G., Lindroth, M., et al., 1995. Low risk of seizure recurrence after early withdrawal of antiepileptic treatment in the neonatal period. Arch Dis Child 72, f97–f101.

Hellstrom-Westas, L., Westgren, U., Rosen, I., et al., 1988. Lidocaine for treatment of severe seizures in newborn infants. Acta Paediatr 77, 79–84.

Herzlinger, R.A., Kandall, S.R., Freeman, J.M., 1977. Neonatal seizures associated with drug withdrawal. J Pediatr 91, 638–641.

Holden, K.R., Mellits, E.D., Freeman, J.M., 1982. Neonatal seizures 1: correlation of prenatal and perinatal events with outcomes. Pediatrics 70, 165–176.

Holmes, G.L., Lombroso, C.T., 1993. Prognostic value of background patterns in the neonatal EEG Journal of Clinical Neurophysiology 10 (3), 323–352.

Holmes, G.L., Ben-Ari, Y., 1998. Seizures in the developing brain – perhaps not so benign after all? Neuron 21, 1231–1234.

Holmes, G.L., Sarkisian, M., Ben-Ari, Y., et al., 1999. Mossy fiber sprouting after recurrent seizures during early development in rats. J Comp Neurol 404, 537–553.

Hunt, A.D., Stokes, J., McCrory, W.W., et al., 1954. Pyridoxine dependency: report of a case of intractable convulsions in an infant controlled by pyridoxine. Pediatrics 13, 140–145.

Huntsman, R.J., Lowry, N.J., Sankaran, K., 2008. Nonepileptic motor phenomena in the neonate. Paediatr child health 13, 680–684.

Ikonomidou, C., Turski, L., 2010. Antiepileptic drugs and brain development. Epilepsy Research 88 (1), 11–22.

Jensen, F.E., 2009. Neonatal seizures: an update on mechanisms and management. Clin Perinatol 36, 881–900.

Kaindl, A.M., Asimiadou, S., Manthey, D., 2006. Antiepileptic drugs and the developing brain Cell and Molecular Life. Sciences 63, 399–413.

Khan, O., Chang, E., Cipriani, C., et al., 2011. Use of intravenous levetiracetam for management of acute seizures in neonates. Pediatr neurol 44, 265–269.

Klepper, J., De Vivi, D., Webb, D.W., et al., 2003. Reversible infantile hypoglycorrhachia: possible transient disturbance in glucose transport? Pediatr Neurol 29, 321–325.

Kobayashi, K., Ito, M., Miyajima, T., et al., 1999. Successful management of intractable epilepsy with intravenous lidocaine and lidocaine tapes. Pediatr Neurol 21, 476–480.

Kohelet, D., Shochat, R., Lusky, A., et al., 2004. Risk factors for neonatal seizures in very low birthweight infants: population-based survey. J Child Neurol 19, 1–9.

Korotchikova, I., Connolly, S., Ryan, C.A., et al., 2009. EEG in the healthy term newborn within 12 hours of birth. Clin neurophysiol 120, 1046–1053.

Kroll, J., 1985. Pyridoxine for neonatal seizures: an unexpected hazard. Dev Med Child Neurol 27, 369–382.

Kwon, J.M., Guillet, R., Shankaran, S., et al., 2011. Clinical seizures in neonatal hypoxic–ischemic encephalopathy have no independent impact on neurodevelopmental outcome: secondary analyses of data from the neonatal

research network hypothermia trial. J Child Neurol 26, 322–328.

Lanska, M.J., Lanska, D.J., 1996. Neonatal seizures in the United States: Results of the National Hospital Discharge Survey, 1980–1991. Neuroepidemiology 15, 117–125.

Lanska, M.J., Lanska, D.J., Baumann, R.J., et al., 1995. A population-based study of neonatal seizures in Fayette county, Kentucky. Neurology 45, 724–732.

Lapunzina, P., Sanchex, J.M., Cabrera, M., et al., 2003. Hyperekplexia (startle disease): a novel mutation (S270T) in the M2 domain of the GLRA1 gene and a molecular review of the disorder. Mol Diagn 7, 125–128.

Leary, L.D., Wang, D., Nordli, D.R., et al., 2003. Seizure characterization and electroencephalographic features in Glut-1 deficiency syndrome. Epilepsia 44, 701–707.

Lee, D.S., Wong, H.A., Knoppert, D.C., 1994. Myoclonus associated with lorazepam therapy in very-low-birth-weight infants. Biol neonate 66, 311–315.

Legido, A., Clancy, R.R., Berman, P.H., 1991. Neurological outcome after electroencephalographically proven neonatal seizures. Pediatrics 88, 583–595.

Levene, M., 2002. The clinical conundrum of neonatal seizures. Arch Dis Child 86, 75–77.

Levene, M.I., Trounce, J.Q., 1986. Cause of neonatal convulsions: towards more precise diagnosis. Arch Dis Child 61, 78–79.

Lien, J.M., Towers, C.V., Quilligan, E.J., et al., 1995. Term early-onset neonatal seizures: obstetric characteristics, etiologic classifications and perinatal care. Obstet Gynecol 85, 163–169.

Lingham, S., Wilson, J., Hart, E.W., 1981. Hereditary stiff baby syndrome. Am J Dis Child 135, 909–911.

Liu, Y., Yang, Y., Silveira, D.C., et al., 1999. Consequences of recurrent seizures during early brain development. Neuroscience 92 (4), 1443–1454.

Lopez-Samblas, A.M., Adams, J.A., Goldberg, R.N., Modi, M.W., 1997. The pharmacokinetics of bumetanide in the newborn infant. Biol Neonate 72 (5), 265–272.

Lopez-Samblas, A.M., Adams, J.A., Goldberg, R.N., Modi, M.W., 1997. The pharmacokinetics of bumetanide in the newborn infant. Biol Neonate 72 (5), 265–272.

Low, E., Boylan, G.B., Mathieson, S., et al., 2012. Cooling and seizure burden in term neonates: An observational study. Arch Dis Child Fetal Neonatal Ed, in press.

Lynch, B.J., Rust, R.S., 1994. Natural history and outcome of neonatal hypocalcemic and hypomagnesemic seizures. Pediatr neurol 11, 23–27.

Lynch, N.E., Stevenson, N.J., Livingstone, V., et al., 2012. The temporal evolution of electroencephalographic seizure burden in neonatal hypoxic ischaemic encephalopathy. Epilepsia 53 (3), 549–557.

Malone, A., Ryan, C.A., Fitzgerald, A., et al., 2009. Interobserver agreement in neonatal seizure identification. Epilepsia 50, 2097–2101.

Markand, O.N., Garg, B.P., Brandt, I.K., 1982. Nonketotic hyperglycinemia: electroencephalographic and evoked potential abnormalities. Neurology 32, 151–156

Massingale, T.W., Boutross, S., 1993. Survey of treatment practices for neonatal seizures. J Perinatol 13, 107–110.

Maurer, V.O., Rizzi, M., Bianchetti, M.G. et al., 2010. Benign neonatal sleep myoclonus: a review of the literature. Pediatrics 125, e919–24.

Maytal, J., Novak, G.P., King, K.C., 1991. Lorazepam in the treatment of refractory neonatal seizures. J Child Neurol 6, 319–323.

McBride, M.C., Laroia, N., Guillet, R., 2000. Electrographic seizures in neonates correlate with poor neurodevelopmental outcome. Neurology 55, 506–513.

McCabe, B.K., Silveira, D.C., Cilio, M.R., et al., 2001. Reduced neurogenesis after neonatal seizures. J neurosc 6, 2094–2103.

Menache, C.C., Bourgeois, B.F.D., Volpe, J.J., 2002. Prognostic value of the neonatal discontinuous EEG. Paediatr Neurol 27, 93–101.

Miller, S.P., Weiss, J., Barnwell, A., et al., 2002. Seizure-associated brain injury in term newborns with perinatal asphyxia. Neurology 58, 542–548.

Mills, P.B., Struys, E., Jakobs, C., et al., 2006. Mutations in antiquitin in individuals with pyridoxine-dependent seizures. Nature med 12, 307–309.

Minchom, P., Niswander, K., Chalmers, I., et al., 1987. Antecedents and outcome of very early neonatal seizures. Br J Obstet Gynaecol 94, 431–439.

Mizrahi, E.M., Kellaway, P., 1987. Characterization and classification of neonatal seizures. Neurology 37, 1837–1844.

Mizrahi, E.M., Kellaway, P., 1998. Diagnosis and management of neonatal seizures. Lippincott-Raven, Philadelphia.

Montenegro, M.A., Guerreiro, M.M., Cladas, J.P.S., et al., 2001. Epileptic manifestations induced by midazolam in the neonatal period. Arq Neuro-Psiquiat 59, 242–243.

Murray, D.M., Boylan, G.B., Ali, I., et al., 2008. Defining the gap between electro-graphic seizure burden, clinical expression and staff recognition of neonatal seizures. Arch Dis Child 93, F187–F191.

Murray, D.M., Boylan, G.B., Fitzgerald, A.P., et al., 2007. Persistent lactic acidosis in neonatal hypoxic ischaemic encephalopathy correlates with EEG grade and electrographic seizure burden. Arch Dis Child 93, F183–F185.

Murray, D.M., Bala, P., O'Connor, C.M., et al., 2010. The predictive value of early neurological examination in neonatal hypoxic-ischaemic encephalopathy and neurodevelopmental outcome at 24 months. Dev Med Child Neurol, 52, e55–9.

Naasan, G., Yabroudi, M., Rahi, A., et al., 2009. Electroencephalographic changes in pyridoxine-dependant epilepsy: new observations. Epileptic disorders 11, 293–300.

Nabbout, R., Soufflet, C., Plouin, P., et al., 1999. Pyridoxine dependent epilepsy: a suggestive electroclinical pattern. Arch Dis Child 81, F125–F129.

Nash, K.B., Bonifacio, S.L., Glass, H.C., et al., 2011. Video-EEG monitoring in newborns with hypoxic–ischemic encephalopathy treated with hypothermia. Neurology 76, 556–562.

North, K.N., Storey, G.N., Henderson-Smart, D.J., 1989. Fifth day fits in the newborn. Aust J Pediatr Child Health 25, 284–287.

Ohtahara, S., 1978. Clinico-electrical delineation of epileptic encephalopathies in childhood. Asian Medicine 21, 7–17.

Ortibus, E.L., Sum, J.M., Hahn, J.S., 1996. Predictive value of EEG for outcome and epilepsy following neonatal seizures. Electroencephalogr Clin Neurophysiol, 98, 175–185.

Painter, M.J., Scher, M.S., Stein, A.D., et al., 1999. Phenobarbital compared with phenytoin for the treatment of neonatal seizures. N Engl J Med 341, 485–489.

Parker, S., Zuckerman, B., Bauchner, H., et al., 1990. Jitteriness in full term neonates: prevalence and correlates. Pediatrics 85, 17–23.

Patrizi, S., Holmes, G.L., Orzalesi, M., et al., 2003. Neonatal seizures: characteristics of eeg ictal activity in preterm and fullterm infants. Brain dev 25, 427–437.

Plecko, B., Paul, K., Paschke, E., et al., 2007. Biochemical and molecular characterization of 18 patients with pyridoxine-dependent epilepsy and mutations of the antiquitin (ALDH7A1) gene. Hum mutat 28, 19–26.

Pressler, R., Bady, B., Binnie, C.D., et al., 2003. 'Neurophysiology of the neonatal period,' In Binnie C.B., Cooper R, Maguiere F, et al. (Eds.), Clinical Neurophysiology, Vol. 2: EEG, Paediatric neurophysiology, Special techniques and applications, second ed. London, Elsevier.

Pressler, R.M., Boylan, G.B., Morton, M., et al., 2001. Early serial EEG in hypoxic ischaemic encencephalopathy. Clin Neurophysiol 112, 31–37.

Pryor, D.S., Don, B., Macourt, D.C., 1981. Firth day fits: a syndrome of neonatal convulsions. Arch Dis Child 56, 753–758.

Rakhade, S.N., Jensen, F.E., 2009. Epilep-togenesis in the immature brain: emerging mechanisms. Nat Rev Neurol 5, 380–391.

Rennie, J.M., Boylan, G., 2003. Neonatal seizures and their treatment. Curr Opin Neurol 16, 177–181.

Rennie, J.M., Chorley, G., Boylan, G.B., et al., 2004. Non-expert use of the cerebral function nmonitor for neonatal seizure detection. Arch Dis Child 89, 37–40.

Rett, A., Tuebel, R., 1964. Neugeborenen Krampfe im Rohmen einer epiliptisch belasten familie. Wien Klin Wochenschr 76, 609–613.

Riviello, J.J., 2004. Drug therapy for neonatal seizures. Part 1. Neoreviews 5, e215–e220.

Robertson, A., Karp, W., 1986. Albumin binding of bumetanide. Dev Pharmacol Ther 9 (4), 241–248.

Ronen, G.M., Penney, S., 1995. The Epidemiology of Clinical Neonatal Seizures in Newfoundland, Canada: A Five-Year Cohort. Ann Neurol 38, 518–519.

Ronen, G.M., Penney, S., Andrews, W., 1999. The epidemiology of clinical neonatal seizures in Newfoundland: a population based study. J Pediatr 134, 71–75.

Ronen, G., Roslas, T.O., Connolly, M., et al., 1993. Seizure characteristics in chromosome 20 benign familial neonatal convulsions. Neurology 43, 1355–1360.

Rose, A., Lombroso, C.T., 1970. Neonatal seizure states: a study of clinical, pathological, and electroencephalographic features in 137 full-term babies with a long-term follow-up. Pediatrics 45, 404–425.

Salbert, B.A., Pellock, J.M., Wolf, B., 1993. Characterization of seizures associated with biotinidase deficiency. Neurology 43, 1351–1355.

Saliba, R.M., Annegers, J.F., Waller, D.K., et al., 1999. Incidence of neonatal seizures in Harris County, Texas, 1992–1994. Am J Epidemiol 150, 763–769.

Scher, M.S., 1985. Pathologic myoclonus of the newborn: electrographic and clinical correlations. Pediatr neurol 1, 342–348.

Scher, M.S., Bergman, I., Ahdab-Barmada, M. et al., 1986. Neurophysiological and anatomical correlations in neonatal nonketotic hyperglycinemia. Neuropediatrics. 17, 137–143.

Scher, M.S., Aso, K., Beggarly, M.E., et al., 1993a. Electrographic seizures in preterm and full-term neonates: clinical correlates, associated brain lesions, and risk for neurologic sequelae. Pediatrics. 91, 128–134.

Scher, M.S., Hamid, M.Y., Steppe, D.A., et al., 1993b. Ictal and interictal electrographic seizure durations in preterm and term neonates. Epilepsia. 34, 284–288.

Schewman, D.A., 1990. What is a neonatal seizure? Problems in definition and quantification for investigative and clinical purposes. J Clin Neurophysiol 7, 315–368.

Schmitt, B., Steinmann, B., Gitzelman, R., et al., 1993. Non-ketotic hyperglycinaemia: clinical and electrical effects of dextromethorphan, an antagonist of the NMDA receptor. Neurology 43, 421–424.

Selton, D., André, M., Hascoët, J.M., 2003. EEG et accident vasculaire cérébral ischémique du nouveau-né à terme: EEG and ischemic stroke in full-term newborns. Neurophysiol Clin/Clin Neurophysiol 33, 120–129.

Shankaran, S., Liang, K.C., Ilagan, N., Fleischmann, L., 1995. Mineral excretion following furosemide compared with bumetanide therapy in premature infants. Pediatr Nephrol 9 (2), 159–162.

Shellhaas, R.A., Clancy, R.R., 2007. Characterization of neonatal seizures by conventional EEG and single-channel EEG. Clin neurophysiol 118, 2156–2161.

Shellhaas, R.A., Soaita, A.I., Clancy, R.R., 2007. Sensitivity of amplitude-integrated electroencephalography for neonatal seizure detection. Pediatrics 120, 770–777.

Sheth, R.D., Hobbs, G.R., Mullett, M., 1999. Neonatal seizures: incidence, onset, and etiology by gestational age. J perinataol 19, 40–43.

Shiang, R., Ryan, S.G., Fielder, T.J., et al., 1995. Mutational analysis of familial and sporadic hyperekplexia. Ann Neurol 38, 85–91.

Silverstein, F.S., Ferriero, D.M., 2008. Off-label use of antiepileptic drugs for the treatment of neonatal seizures. Neurology 39, 77–79.

Silverstein, F.S., Jensen, F.E., Inder, T., 2008. Improving the treatment of neonatal seizures: national institute of neurological disorders and stroke workshop report. J Pediatr 153, 12–15.

Sood, A., Grover, N., Sharma, R., 2003. Biochemical abnormalities in neonatal seizures. Ind J Pediatr 70, 221–224.

Stewart, W.A., Wood, E.P., Gordon, K.E., et al., 2002. Successful treatment of severe infantile hyperekplexia with low dose clobazam. J Child Neurol 17, 154–156.

Sullivan, J.E., Witte, M.K., Yamashita, T.S., et al., 1996. Dose ranging evaluation of bumetanide pharmakokinetics in critically ill infants Clinical Pharmacology and. Therapeutics 60 (4), 424–434.

Sullivan, J.E., Witte, M.K., Yamashita, T.S., Myers, C.M., Blumer, J.L., 1996a Oct. Pharmacokinetics of bumetanide in critically ill infants. Clin Pharmacol Ther 60 (4), 405–413.

Sullivan, J.E., Witte, M.K., Yamashita, T.S., Myers, C.M., Blumer, J.L., 1996b Oct. Dose-ranging evaluation of bumetanide pharmacodynamics in critically ill infants. Clin Pharmacol Ther 60 (4), 424–434.

Tekgul, H., Gaubreau, K., Soul, L., et al., 2006. The current etiologic profile and neurodevelopmental outcome of seizures in term newborn infants. Pediatrics 117 (4), 1270–1280.

Temko, A., Thomas, E., Marnane, W., et al., 2011a. EEG-based neonatal seizure detection with Support Vector Machines. Clin neurophysiol 122, 464–473.

Temko, A., Thomas, E., Marnane, W., et al., 2011b. Performance assessment for EEG-based neonatal seizure detectors. Clin neurophysiol 122, 474–482.

Thoresen, M., Hellström-Westas, L., Liu, X., et al., 2010. Effect of hypothermia on amplitude-integrated electroencephalogram in infants with asphyxia. Pediatrics 126, e131–9.

Toet, M.C., Hellstrom-Westas, L., Groenendaal, F., De Vries, L.S., 1999. Amplitude integrated EEG 3 and 6 hours after birth in full term neonates with hypoxic-ischaemic encephalopathy. Arch Dis Child 81, F19–F23.

Toet, M.C., Groenendaal, F., Osredkar, D., van Huffelen, A.C., de Vries, L.S., 2005 Apr. Postneonatal epilepsy following amplitude-integrated EEG-detected neonatal seizures. Pediatr Neurol 32 (4), 241–247.

Tohier, C., Roze, J.C., David, A., et al., 1991. Hyperexplexia or stiff baby syndrome. Arch Dis Child 66, 460–461.

Tsuyusaki, Y., Shimbo, H., Wada, T., et al., 2011. Paradoxical increase in seizure frequency with valproate in nonketotic hyperglycinemia. Brain dev, 2012 34 (1), 75–76.

Turmen, T., Thom, P., Louridas, A.T., LeMorvan, P., Aranda, J.V., 1982. Protein binding and bilirubin displacing properties of bumetanide and furosemide. Clin Pharmacol 22 (11-12), 551–556.

Van Leuven, K., Toet, M.C., Schobben, A.F.A.M., et al., 2004. Midazolam and amplitude-integrated eeg in asphyxiated full-term neonates. Acta Paediatr 93, 1221–1227.

van Rooij, L.G., Toet, M.C., van Huffelen, A.C., et al., 2010. Effect of treatment of subclinical neonatal seizures detected with aEEG: randomized, controlled trial. Pediatrics 125, e358–e366.

van Zeben-van der Aa, D.M., Veerlove-Vanhorick, S.P., den Ouden, A.L., et al., 1990. Neonatal seizures in very preterm and low birthweight infants: mortality and handicaps at two years in a nationwide cohort. Neuropediatrics 21, 62–65.

Vento, M., De Vries, L.S., Alberola, A., 2010. Approach to seizures in the neonatal period: a european perspective. Acta Paediatr 99, 497–501.

Walker, P.C., Berry, N.S., Edwards, D.J., 1989. Protein binding characteristics of bumetanide. Dev Pharmacol Ther 12 (1), 13–18.

Walker, P.C., Shankaran, S., 1988. The bilirubin-displacing capacity of bumetanide in critically ill babys. Dev Pharmacol Ther 11 (5), 265–272.

Walsh, B.H., Low, E., Bogue, C.O., et al., 2011. Early continuous video electroencephalography in neonatal stroke. Dev Med Child Neurol 53, 89–92.

Ward, O.C., Lam, L.K., 1977. Bumetanide in heart failure in infancy. Arch Dis Child 52 (11), 877–882.

Wasterlain, C.G., Thompson, K.W., Suchomelova, L., et al., 2010. Brain energy metabolism during experimental neonatal seizures. Neurochem res 35, 2193–2198.

Watkins, A., Szymonowicz, W., Jin, X., et al., 1988. Significance of seizures in very low birthweight infants. Dev Med Child Neurol 30, 162–169.

Weiner, S.P., Painter, M.J., Geva, D., et al., 1991. Neonatal seizures electroclinical dissociation. Pediatr neurol 7, 363–368.

Wells, T.G., Fasules, J.W., Taylor, B.J., Kearns, G.L., 1992. Pharmacokinetics and pharmacodynamics of bumetanide in babys treated with extracorporeal membrane oxygenation. J Pediatr 121 (6), 974–980.

West, C.R., Harding, J.E., Williams, C.E., 2010. Cot-side electroencephalography for outcome prediction in preterm infants: observational study. Arch Dis Child Fetal Neonatal Ed 125, e358–e366.

Williams, C.E., Gunn, A., Gluckman, P.D., 1991. Time course of intracellular oedema and epileptiform activity following prenatal cerebral ischaemia in sheep. Stroke 22, 516–521.

Wirrell, E.C., Armstrong, E.A., Osman, L.D., et al., 2001. Prolonged seizures exacerbate perinatal hypoxic–ischemic brain damage. Pediatr Res 50, 445–454.

Wusthoff, C.J., Dlugos, D.J., Gutierrez-Colina, A., et al., 2011. Electrographic Seizures During Therapeutic Hypothermia for Neonatal Hypoxic–Ischemic Encephalopathy. J Child Neurol 26 (6), 724–728.

Yamamoto, H., Okumura, A., Fukuda, M., 2011. Epilepsies and epileptic syndromes starting in the neonatal period. Brain Dev 33, 213–220.

Young, G.B., Da Silva, O.P., 2000. Effects of morphine on the electroencephalograms of neonates: a prospective, observational study. Clin Neurophysiol 111, 1955–1960.

Younkin, D.P., Delivoria-Papadopoulos, M., Maris, J., et al., 1986. Cerebral metabolic effects of neonatal seizures measured with in vivo p 31 NMR spectroscopy. Ann Neurol 20, 513–519.

Part 3: **Intracranial haemorrhage and perinatal stroke (arterial and venous) at term**

Divyen K Shah   Janet M Rennie

Introduction

Intracranial haemorrhage (ICH) and stroke in term newborn represent an important and probably underrecognised group of conditions which require a high index of suspicion for diagnosis. The diagnosis should be considered in babies exhibiting neurological dysfunction such as seizures and encephalopathy. Symptomatic ICH can coexist with other pathologies such as hypoxic–ischaemic encephalopathy (HIE) or sepsis, and may be associated with serious consequences for the infant. Serious ICH following a difficult delivery is well recognised, and, although obstetric trauma is much less common than in the past, cases still occur, with disimpaction of the fetal head at caesarean section in the late second stage emerging as an increasing problem for the newborn, in our experience. With improved neuroimaging techniques, we now know that asymptomatic ICH is quite common and is generally associated with good outcome.

ICH may be classified according to the intracranial compartment in which the blood is found on imaging into extra-axial bleeds (outside the brain) which include subgaleal (subaponeurotic), extradural, subdural and subarachnoid, or intra-axial bleeds, including intraventricular and intraparenchymal bleeding (Fig. 40.16). Many babies will have haemorrhage in more than one location or compartment of the brain. ICH has also been categorised according to its position with respect to the tentorium cerebelli, an almost horizontal fold of dura, which separates the occipital cerebral lobes above from the cerebellum below into supratentorial and infratentorial compartments. Although subgaleal or subaponeurotic haemorrhage is extracranial, it will also be considered in this chapter because of its potentially serious nature.

Clinically, the subtype of ICH can be recognised by the site and pattern of distribution of the collection of blood on imaging. The subtypes of ICH will be considered together as a group initially because they may share similar aetiologies such as birth trauma and bleeding diatheses, they are often found to coexist and they all have the potential to cause permanent neurodisability.

Incidence and prevalence of intracranial haemorrhage

The true incidence of ICH is difficult to ascertain. Serious ICH related to traumatic birth is much less common with improved obstetric care (Govaert 1993). The prevalence of ICH revealed using magnetic resonance imaging (MRI) is much greater than ultrasound studies would suggest (Heibel et al. 1993). Recent MRI studies confirm the early pilot MRI results (Holden et al. 1999), showing that asymptomatic ICH is quite common. In an MRI study of 111 asymptomatic newborns in Sheffield, Whitby et al. (2004) used an 0.2 T magnet to detect subdural haemorrhage (SDH) in nine (8%) in the first 48 hours of life. In an American MRI study using a 1.5 T magnet in which 101 newborns were imaged in the first week of life, Rooks et al. (2008) found 46 (46%) had a supratentorial SDH; 20 infants also had an additional infratentorial SDH. In both studies, all haemorrhages had resolved by 1–3 months' age. At 2 years of age, no child followed up by Rooks and colleagues had a motor deficit, and the incidence of speech and language delay (6%) was no greater than expected. More recently, using a 3 T magnet, Looney et al. (2007) found 16 subdural, two subarachnoid and six parenchymal haemorrhages in 88 babies, giving a prevalence of 26%.

The incidence of symptomatic ICH is lower, and has been estimated at around 3 per 10 000 live births (Hanigan et al. 1995b). A large epidemiologic study of neonatal intracranial injury related to

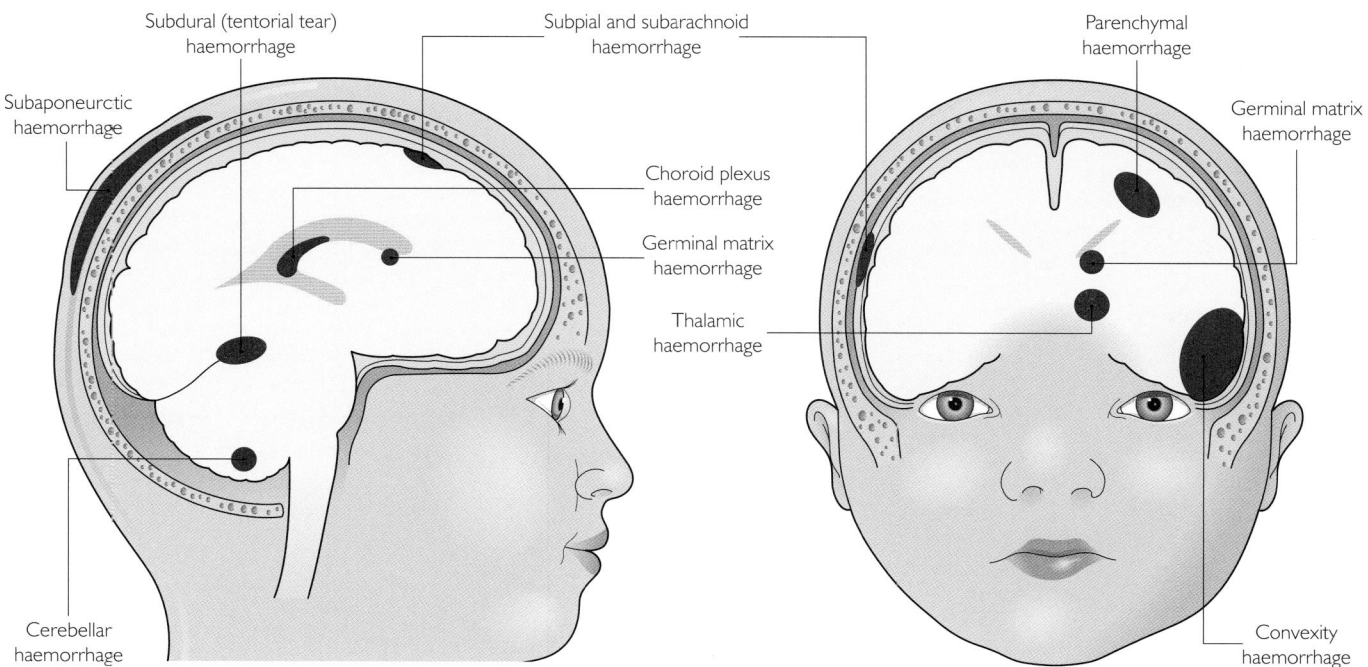

Fig. 40.16 Sites of intracranial haemorrhage.

the mode of delivery in almost 600 000 women from California suggested that the incidence of ICH varied from 1 in 664 infants delivered by forceps to 1 in 2750 delivered by caesarean section without labour (Towner et al. 1999). Subgaleal haemorrhage was not included in this study.

Risk factors for intracranial haemorrhage

Difficult delivery

The main risk factor for perinatal ICH is dystocia (difficult child birth: Table 40.7). Disimpaction of the fetal skull at caesarean section has become a more common cause of ICH due to trauma in our experience, and that of others, as more caesarean sections are performed in the second stage of labour when the head is deeply engaged (Tan 2007). There may be an associated skull fracture (Fig. 40.17). From an epidemiologic study from California, ICH occurred in 1 of 2750 infants delivered by caesarean section without labour, 1 in 1900 infants delivered by normal vaginal delivery, 1 in 907 infants delivered by caesarean section during labour, 1 in 860 infants delivered by vacuum extraction and 1 in 664 infants delivered by forceps, in nulliparous women (Towner et al. 1999). In a Sheffield study of asymptomatic infants (Whitby et al. 2004), five of nine infants with SDH were delivered by forceps after failed ventouse, one had had a traumatic ventouse delivery and the other three were born by normal vaginal delivery. Studies show that ICH is commoner after forceps delivery (Jhawar et al. 2003) when compared with vaginal delivery, and it is also commoner after a trial of forceps following a failed ventouse (Gardella et al. 2001) when compared with delivery by ventouse alone, forceps alone or a normal vaginal birth.

Maternal associations include primiparity, grand multiparity, pre-eclampsia and placental abruption. Neonatal factors include HIE, low Apgar scores and any bleeding disorder, including thrombocytopenia and haemophilia.

Neonatal bleeding disorders

ICH in babies with HIE or sepsis complicated by a coagulopathy is not uncommon. A study of 66 newborns with ICH showed that at least 12 (19%) had platelet counts of less than $50 \times 10^9/L$ within

Table 40.7 Risk factors for haemorrhage

Maternal
Primiparity
Grand mulitiparity
Mode of delivery
Difficult ventouse – multiple attempts, prolonged cup application time
Multiple application of instruments
Failed instrumentation followed by caesarean section
Infant
Hypoxic–ischaemic encephalopathy
Bleeding tendency
Tumour
Arteriovenous malformation
Venous thrombosis

the first 48 hours of life and were specifically associated with intraparenchymal haemorrhage and a more severe grade (Jhawar et al. 2003).

Neonatal alloimmune thrombocytopenia (Ch. 30) carries a substantial risk of ICH in the newborn, probably around 1 in 10, many of which occur during intrauterine life (Muller 1989; Williamson et al. 1999). These babies are prone to all types of extra-axial and intra-axial haemorrhage (Dale and Coleman 2002).

Primary inherited coagulation disorders are rare but may present with ICH in the newborn. Haemophilia A and B are the commonest of these (Kulkarni and Lusher 1999; Tarantino et al. 2007; Kulkarni et al. 2009). Recent studies suggest that 3.5–4% of all haemophilic boys develop ICH in the newborn period, a figure which represents a significantly increased risk compared to the normal population. Despite the poor outcome, the debate about prophylactic factor VIII still rages (Ch. 30) and of course many are first-born male babies, and the diagnosis is not suspected until the ICH is already very large. Very rarely, deficiency of factors X, VII, XIII and fibrinogen presents in the newborn period. These deficiencies are autosomal-recessive traits and as such are commoner in communities with consanguinity. Ineffective vitamin K prophylaxis, parental refusal of vitamin K and deficiency remain important causes of ICH. Babies with liver disease often present with vitamin K deficiency bleeding, usually intracranial (Danielsson et al. 2004; van Hasselt et al. 2009).

Structural anomalies

Arteriovenous malformations, aneurysms and tumours are rare causes of ICH at term.

Extracorporeal membrane oxygenation (ECMO)

The need for ECMO or cardiac surgery increases the risk that a term baby will develop symptomatic intraventricular haemorrhage (IVH) (Hanigan et al. 1995a; Wu et al. 2003).There are probably many reasons for this, including anticoagulation, sepsis and sinus thrombosis. Some forms of ECMO require ligation of one carotid artery.

Haemorrhage into an area of venous infarction

It is now appreciated that many parenchymal haemorrhages at term are due to bleeding into an area of venous infarction (Ramenghi et al. 2009). This is particularly likely in thalamic haemorrhage (see below) (Govaert et al. 2003). Hence, bleeding into the deep grey matter at term is often the first sign of a cerebral sinovenous thrombosis (CSVT: see below).

Clinical presentation of intracranial haemorrhage

When signs of ICH occur, the most commonly reported are seizures and apnoeas, but subtle clues such as poor temperature regulation or reluctance to feed can be present. Babies with focal lesions may be well at birth and present with focal seizures on the postnatal ward over the next 24–48 hours. All babies with neonatal encephalopathy should have a careful clinical neurologic examination; pupils and tone should be checked, paying particular attention to symmetry and focal signs.

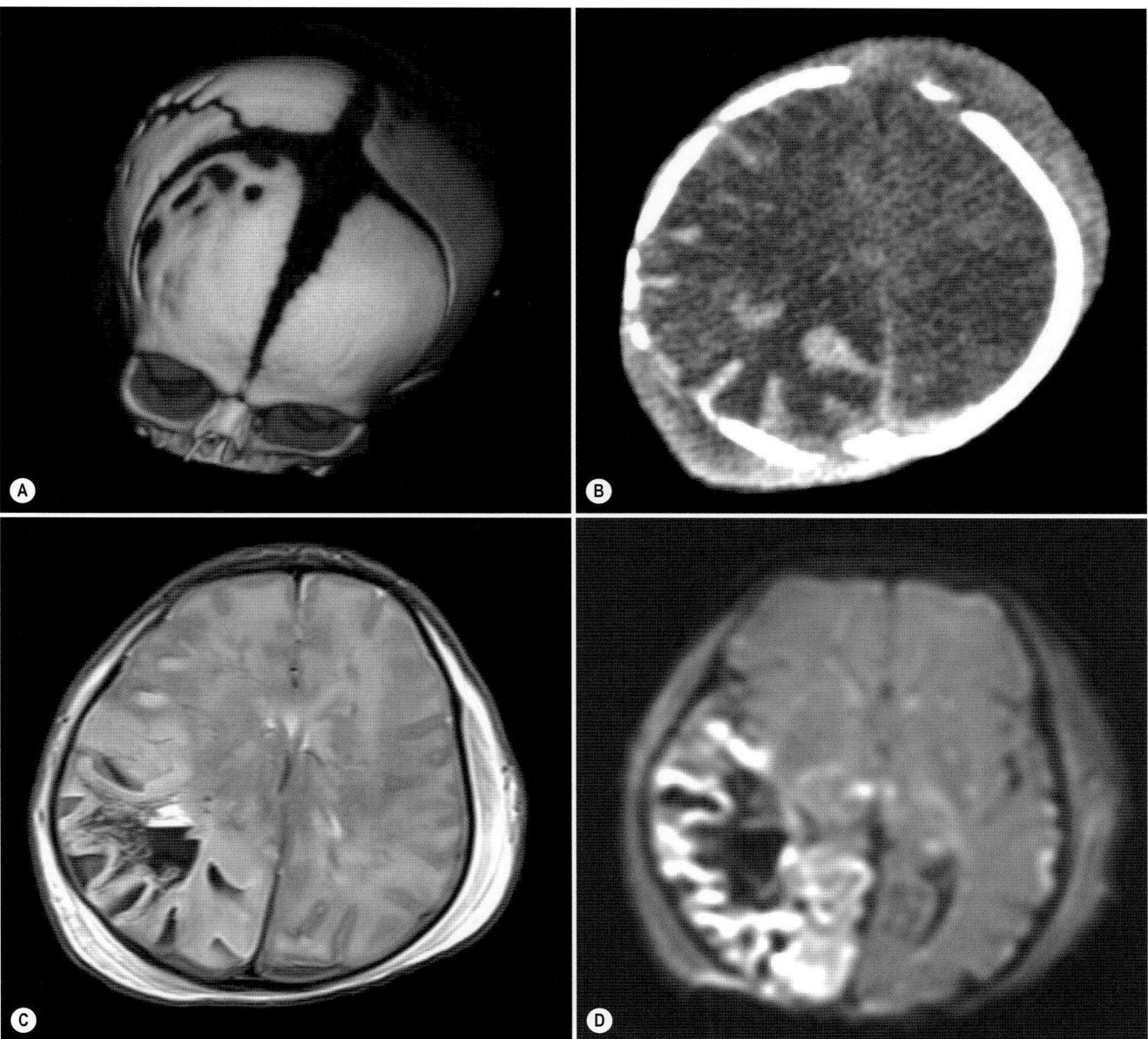

Fig. 40.17 Traumatic damage sustained at the time of disimpaction of the fetal head at caesarean section. (a) Computed tomography (CT) three-dimensional reconstruction of the skull showing a fracture of the right parietal bone. (b) CT scan at 16 hours of age showing subgaleal bleeding, the skull fracture and parenchymal bleeding. (c) T2-weighted axial image showing damage in the right parieto-occipital region with an area of deep haemorrhage. (d) Diffusion-weighted image confirming extensive cerebral trauma.

Investigations

A full blood count may reveal anaemia and thrombocytopenia; coagulation screen may be deranged.

Lumbar puncture

Lumbar puncture is not recommended to assist in the diagnosis of ICH. Clearly, in a sick infant with accompanying signs of neurological dysfunction such as encephalopathy and raised intracranial pressure, lumbar puncture is contraindicated.

If uniformly blood-stained cerebrospinal fluid (CSF) is obtained when a diagnostic lumbar puncture is undertaken it should raise a suspicion of ICH, particularly subarachnoid haemorrhage (SAH).

Electrophysiology

Digital bedside cerebral function monitoring carried out while a conventional multichannel electroencephalogram (EEG) is awaited may reveal electrographic seizures (p. 1084). Conventional multichannel EEG may show focal seizures localizing to the focus of the lesion.

Neuroimaging

Cranial ultrasound (CUS) remains the main modality of imaging of the newborn brain at the bedside and is generally a good technique for imaging intraventricular and parenchymal bleeds. In experienced hands, CUS allows visualisation of bleeds into the cerebellum as well as the basal ganglia and thalami. CUS is of limited value for the detection of subdural haemorrhage and SAH unless there is obvious midline shift.

Computed tomography (CT) scanning is easily available in most centres, where access to MRI may be more limited. CT entails a significant dose of X-ray irradiation, but provides images with a short acquisition time, albeit with low resolution. It is good for visualising skull fractures and will adequately detect modest-sized extra-axial bleeds, although MRI is likely to detect smaller bleeds. The radiation exposure of CT is justified when significant ICH is suspected, if MRI is not available.

MRI, where available, is the imaging modality of choice. A combination of MRI sequences such as T1, T2 and diffusion weighting will allow detection of most intra- and extra-axial bleeds at various stages of evolution. MR angiography, including the neck vessels, should be performed when stroke is suspected (see below).

Pathogenesis of subdural haemorrhage

Since SDH is a common finding after non-accidental injury, an understanding of SDH following birth trauma and its natural history is important (Table 40.8). SDH represents a collection of

Table 40.8 Risk factors for large subdural haemorrhage

When head is subjected to unusual deforming stresses such as face or brow presentation
When delivery requires multiple instrumentation, rotational manoeuvres or disimpaction of the fetal skull at caesarean section
Coagulation defect in the baby, e.g. haemophilia, so that a 'normal'-size subdural haemorrhage continues to enlarge because the blood does not clot

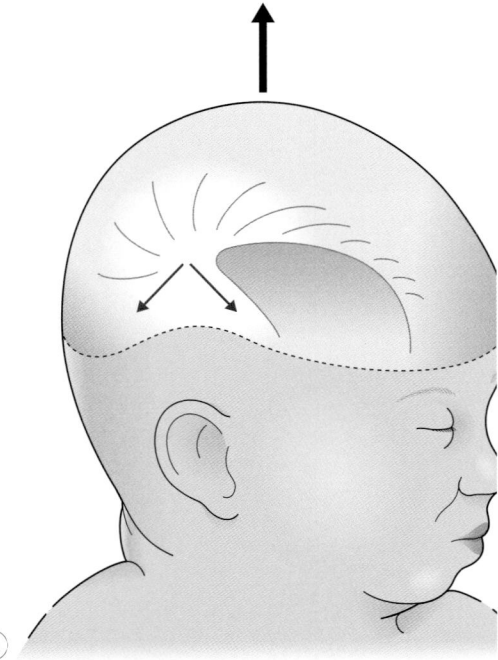

Fig. 40.18 (a) Forces on the tentorium (small arrows) as the result of traction on the vertex during delivery (large arrow).

blood in the dural border cell layer adjacent to the arachnoid membrane (Mack et al. 2009). Small veins from the dorsal convexity of the cerebral hemisphere drain into superficial cerebral veins, which in turn coalesce to form 10–18 bridging veins which cross the subarachnoid space through the arachnoid membrane into the dura and drain into the superior sagittal sinus. Traditionally, the mechanism ascribed to haemorrhagic collections on the surface of the brain such as subdural haemorrhage as well as SAH has been a tear in these bridging veins due to distorting forces.

Mechanism of subdural haemorrhage

Serious SDHs have been related to:
- tentorial and falx tears
- occipital diastasis
- convexity collections.

Tentorial and falx tears

Prolonged and difficult labour caused by cephalopelvic disproportion as the baby's head passes through the birth canal has been postulated to cause stretching of the dura and tears to the falx and tentorium (Fig. 40.18). The tentorium cerebelli has the transverse sinus running in the horizontal plane and the straight sinus running in the vertical plane (both posteriorly). The superior and inferior sagittal sinuses both meet the straight sinus within the tentorium. A severe tentorial tear can disrupt these large veins, causing haemorrhage into the posterior fossa. A tear to the falx is less common,

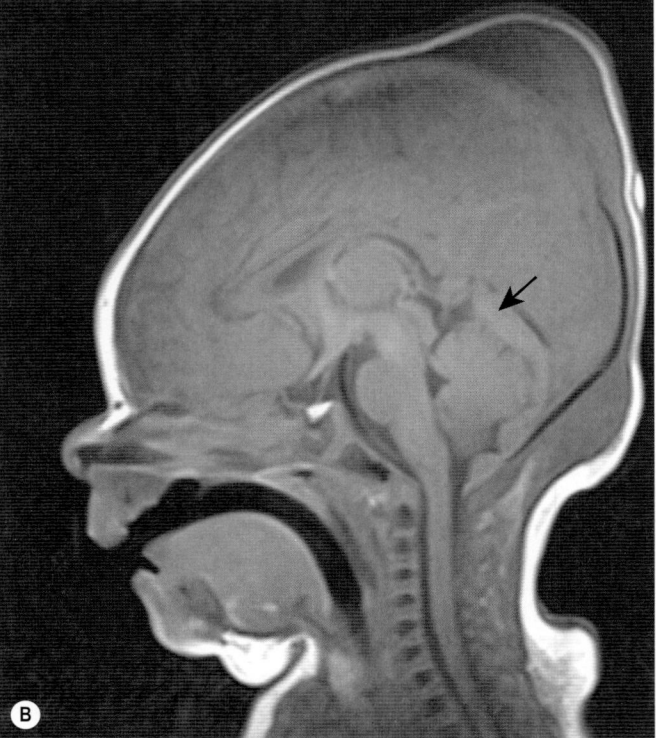

Fig. 40.18 (b) Sagittal magnetic resonance image showing a posterior fossa subdural collection (arrowed) in a baby delivered by forceps after failed ventouse.

causing damage to the inferior sagittal sinus, with blood seen above the corpus callosum on imaging. Most perinatal SDHs are peritentorial (Looney et al. 2007).

Occipital osteodiastasis

This is the result of serious trauma, and was often found in term infants who died after breech extraction, which is now rarely seen. The occipital bone has four parts which are not completely ossified at birth, and are separated by cartilage. Hyperextension of the head during breech extraction can exert enough pressure on the occipital bone to cause traumatic separation at the cartilaginous joint at the junction of the squamous and lateral or condylar parts, with injury to the occipital sinus causing haemorrhage into the posterior fossa (Wigglesworth and Husemeyer 1977). Volpe (2008) suggests that this lesion may be more common than has been recognised because it is easily missed at postmortem, in the absence of imaging.

Convexity haemorrhage

These are typically crescentic-shaped supratentorial collections lying on the convex surface of the brain which have traditionally been thought to be caused by ruptured bridging veins. Hence depending on the site of the rupture of the vessel, they may also be associated with SAH.

Asymptomatic subdural haemorrhage

In view of the fact that asymptomatic SDH is common, Mack et al. (2009) propose that the relatively large inner vascular plexus in the dura membrane of the newborn may be the origin of many SDHs, as opposed to the bridging veins.

Clinical features of subdural haemorrhage

Convexity haemorrhage

Most SDH is asymptomatic. Clinical signs may be non-specific and a high degree of vigilance and index of suspicion is important after a difficult delivery. The most common clinical features are seizures and apnoea. Seizures may be focal, particularly in cases of a supratentorial convexity haematoma overlying a cerebral contusion. Careful examination in such a baby may reveal neurological signs. A major convexity SDH may cause herniation of the temporal lobe through the tentorial notch and a distinct palsy of the third cranial nerve, with a dilated pupil that is poorly reactive to light.

Babies are often well in the first few hours of life but then go on to develop signs of raised intracranial pressure, including bulging fontanelle, poor feeding, irritability and seizures.

Infratentorial haemorrhage

Major infratentorial haemorrhage is now quite rare, although the MR studies mentioned above show that most subdural bleeding is peritentorial. Babies may be born with depressed Apgar scores or deteriorate later due to infratentorial clot swelling and compression of the brainstem. The clot may block free flow of CSF, causing hydrocephalus. These infants become obtunded, with opisthotonic posturing, bradycardia, loss of respiratory drive and dilated, poorly reactive pupils. Death may ensue over a matter of hours unless the pressure is relieved.

Clinical management and prognosis following subdural and intracranial haemorrhage

Medical management

Most ICHs can be managed conservatively. Seizures should be treated. Thrombocytopenia should be corrected with platelet transfusion and deranged coagulation should be treated with fresh frozen plasma, vitamin K and cryoprecipitate appropriately. Remember that a first-born male may be the first in his family with haemophilia, and if the diagnosis is missed and the baby dies, the family cannot benefit from antenatal diagnosis in future pregnancies. The baby may require respiratory and haemodynamic support.

Neurosurgical management

Neurosurgical input may be appropriate in cases of symptomatic ICH, particularly in the presence of an associated skull fracture, midline shift, signs of raised intracranial pressure and focal neurological signs. Sixteen of 53 infants with ICH in Holland (Brouwer et al. 2010) developed hydrocephalus due to obstruction of free flow of CSF. Imaging revealed midline shift in 21/53 infants, three of whom were treated with craniotomy.

The place of surgical intervention, particularly in infratentorial bleeds, is a subject for debate. The consensus view seems to be that, in the absence of brainstem compression or hydrocephalus, conservative management is appropriate. Indications for neurosurgery include the following (Perrin et al. 1997):

- signs of life-threatening brainstem compression such as apnoea, bradycardia and hypotension
- acute obstructive hydrocephalus with raised intracranial pressure
- a very large clot in the posterior fossa.

Neurosurgical procedures used in these circumstances include aspiration of clot using needle aspiration techniques or burrhole trephine, external ventricular drain for obstructive hydrocephalus and posterior fossa craniectomy. In a series of 15 infants with infratentorial SDH (Perrin et al. 1997) surgical evacuation was performed in eight. Outcomes were similar for both the conservatively managed and surgical intervention groups. Five of the 15 infants had moderate or profound delay.

Prognosis

Brouwer et al. (2010) reported cerebral palsy in four of 34 survivors of their series of 53 ICHs. Adverse outcome was associated with intraparenchymal bleeds and associated HIE. Other studies also show that coexisting HIE in infants with ICH puts them at increased risk of adverse outcome compared to infants with ICH alone (Hanigan et al. 1995a). Some children develop epilepsy.

Extradural haemorrhage

Extradural haemorrhage is rare in the newborn. It is typically a biconvex collection between the skull bone and the dura (Fig. 40.19). There may be a skull fracture immediately adjacent to the collection. On high-resolution imaging, the dura may be seen between the brain and such a collection. These collections do not cross suture lines, as dura attaches to the skull at these sites.

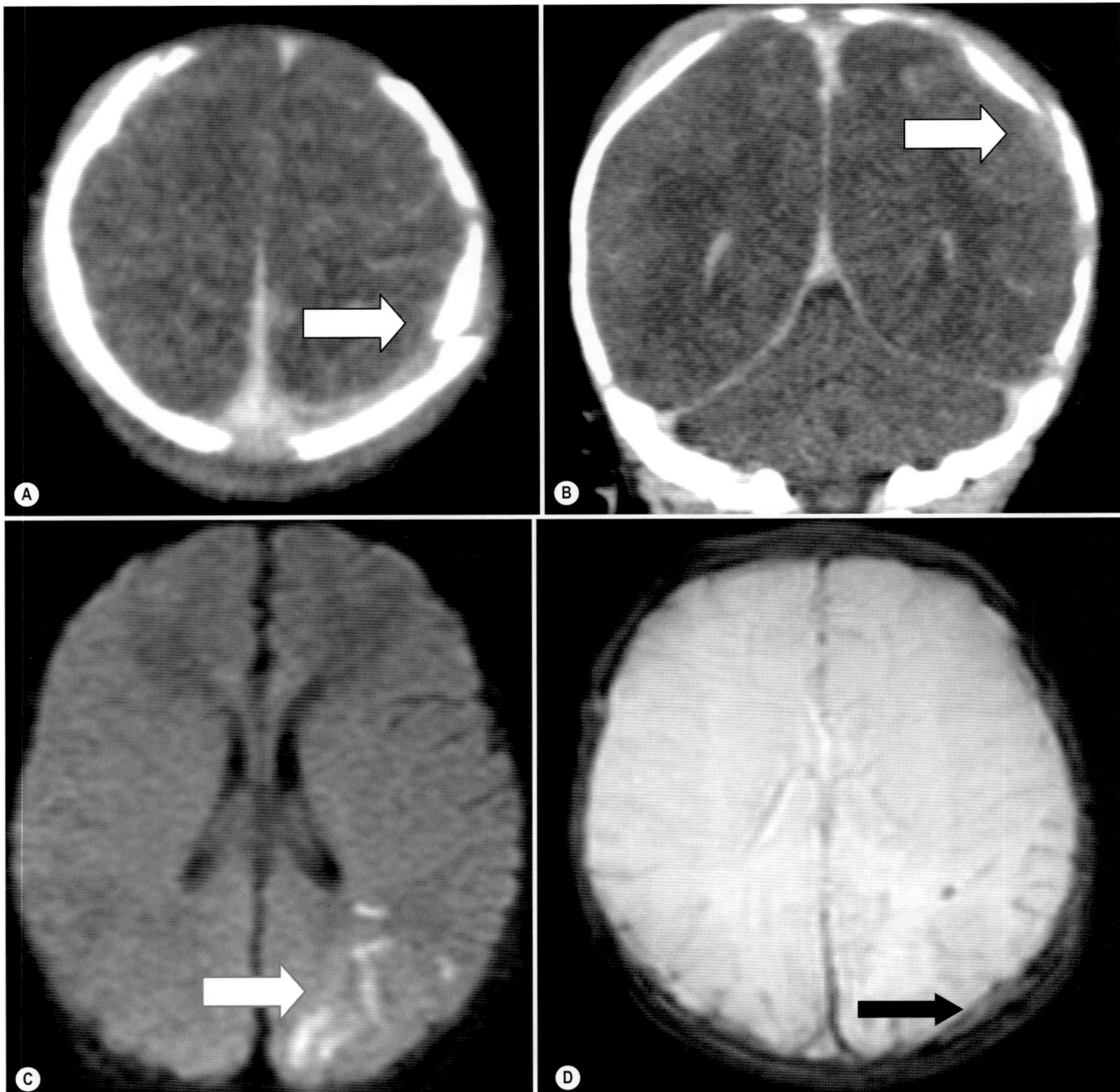

Fig. 40.19 (a and b) Computed tomography (CT) images at 18 hours of age, (c and d) magnetic resonance (MR) images at 3 days of age and (e) digital amplitude-integrated electroencephalogram (aEEG) recording of infant who was born at 41 weeks' gestation by caesarean section after failed ventouse delivery. The delivery was induced for postmaturity. Apgars were 9 and 10 at 1 and 5 minutes. The infant was admitted to the neonatal unit at 5 hours of age for respiratory distress and at 6 hours of age was noted to have focal seizures consisting of rhythmic jerking of right arm. The raw EEG trace on the digital aEEG (e) shows a seizure on the left hemisphere and the aEEG trace shows it lasted at least 15 minutes. CT scan shows a parietal skull fracture (a and b, arrows), with an underlying extradural haematoma on MRI (d, arrow).

Heyman et al. (2005) reported a series of 15 newborn infants with extradural haematoma. Eight had been delivered by instrumental delivery and five by caesarean section following a trial of vaginal delivery. Most presented within 24 hours with seizures (7/15) or hypotonia. Ten of the 15 had a skull fracture, most commonly of the parietal bone. All infants also had retinal haemorrhages. Seven infants were treated with craniotomy and two had ventriculoperitoneal shunts.

Subarachnoid haemorrhage

The pathogenesis of primary SAH is not well understood, but it probably represents bleeding into the subarachnoid space caused by ruptured blood vessels, including bridging veins, and may occur with convexity SDH. The incidence of SAH in the newborn is not known but is commonly noted at postmortem in babies who have died from unrelated causes.

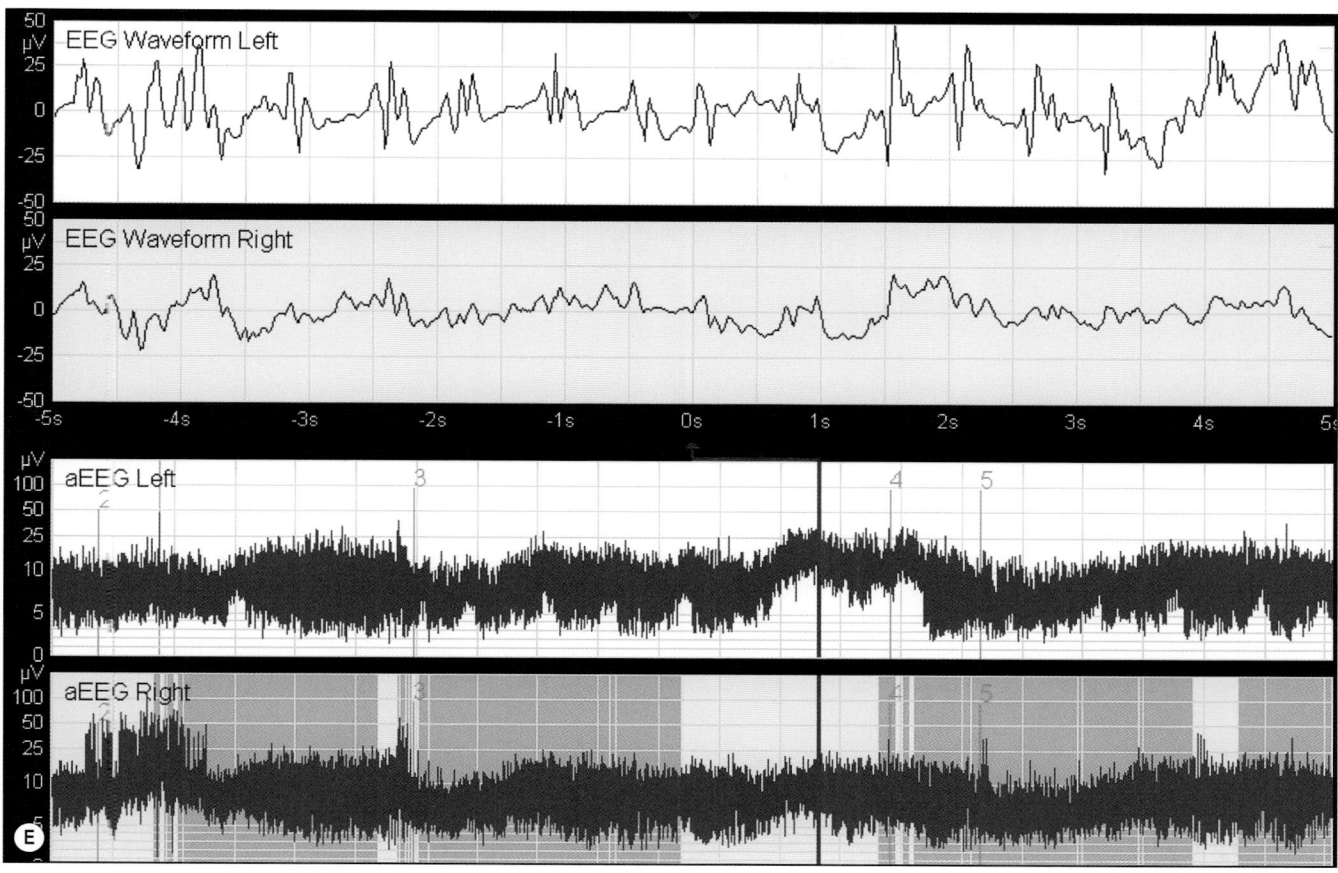

Fig. 40.19, cont'd

Babies may be asymptomatic. Seizures may be the main presenting feature and the infants may be well between seizures. Rarely, infants may die from a catastrophic SAH. SAH is recognised from CT and MR images as the blood fills CSF cavities, including sulci, cisterns and fissures. The diagnosis should be considered if blood-stained CSF is obtained from a lumbar puncture in an infant with cerebral dysfunction.

Intraventricular, intraparenchymal, thalamic and cerebellar haemorrhage

Intraventricular, intraparenchymal and cerebellar bleeds are commoner in preterm infants. In term infants the mechanism of the intraventricular and intraparenchymal bleeds is less well understood. IVH in term infants may occur in association with hypoxia–ischaemia, birth trauma, ECMO therapy, congenital heart disease, disseminated intravascular coagulation (DIC), sepsis and thrombophilic disorders. Intraventricular and parenchymal bleeds in term infants may occur with arterial and venous infarcts.

Thalamic haemorrhage at term typically presents with seizures, and unusual eye signs may be present (Trounce et al. 1985; Adams et al. 1988). Babies who were apparently well at birth can become lethargic, feed poorly and develop seizures (Rivkin et al. 1992). Figure 40.20 shows the characteristic imaging findings in a term baby with thalamic haemorrhage. From an early series of 19 term infants diagnosed with IVH on CT scan prior to 1 month of age, 12 were found to have thalamic haemorrhage, leading the authors to conclude that the thalamic haemorrhage was the source of the IVH (Roland et al. 1990). Bleeds into the choroid plexus are also thought to be a source of IVH in the term infant. A more recent case series of 29 term infants with IVH detected using CT and MRI associated the cause of IVH with sinus venous thrombosis in nine infants (Wu et al. 2003). Thalamic haemorrhage is probably due to sinovenous thrombosis in the majority of cases. As yet, there is little experience with anticoagulation in thalamic haemorrhage due to thrombosis of the deep venous system, or CSVT (see below) (Kersbergen et al. 2009).

IVH in term infants from sources such as the thalami, choroid plexus and sinus venous thrombosis lead us to conclude that IVH in term infants represents a different disease process to the common IVH in the preterm population, which is thought to arise mostly from the highly vascular germinal matrix near the subventricular zone.

In a series by Gardella et al. (2001), 14/29 (48%) had had perinatal complications such as fetal distress, low Apgar scores and HIE, 14/29 neonates had had major medical conditions such as congenital heart defects, the need for ECMO and DIC, and three neonates had thrombophilic disorders. In a third of the cases (9/29) there were no such associated perinatal or neonatal factors.

In the presence of HIE, term infants with IVH have a worse outcome than infants with IVH alone. Intraparenchymal haemorrhage is associated with a high risk of cerebral palsy (Brouwer et al. 2010). Our understanding of the role of the cerebellum for neurodevelopment has increased considerably over recent years, and explains why term infants with cerebellar bleeds have a guarded prognosis.

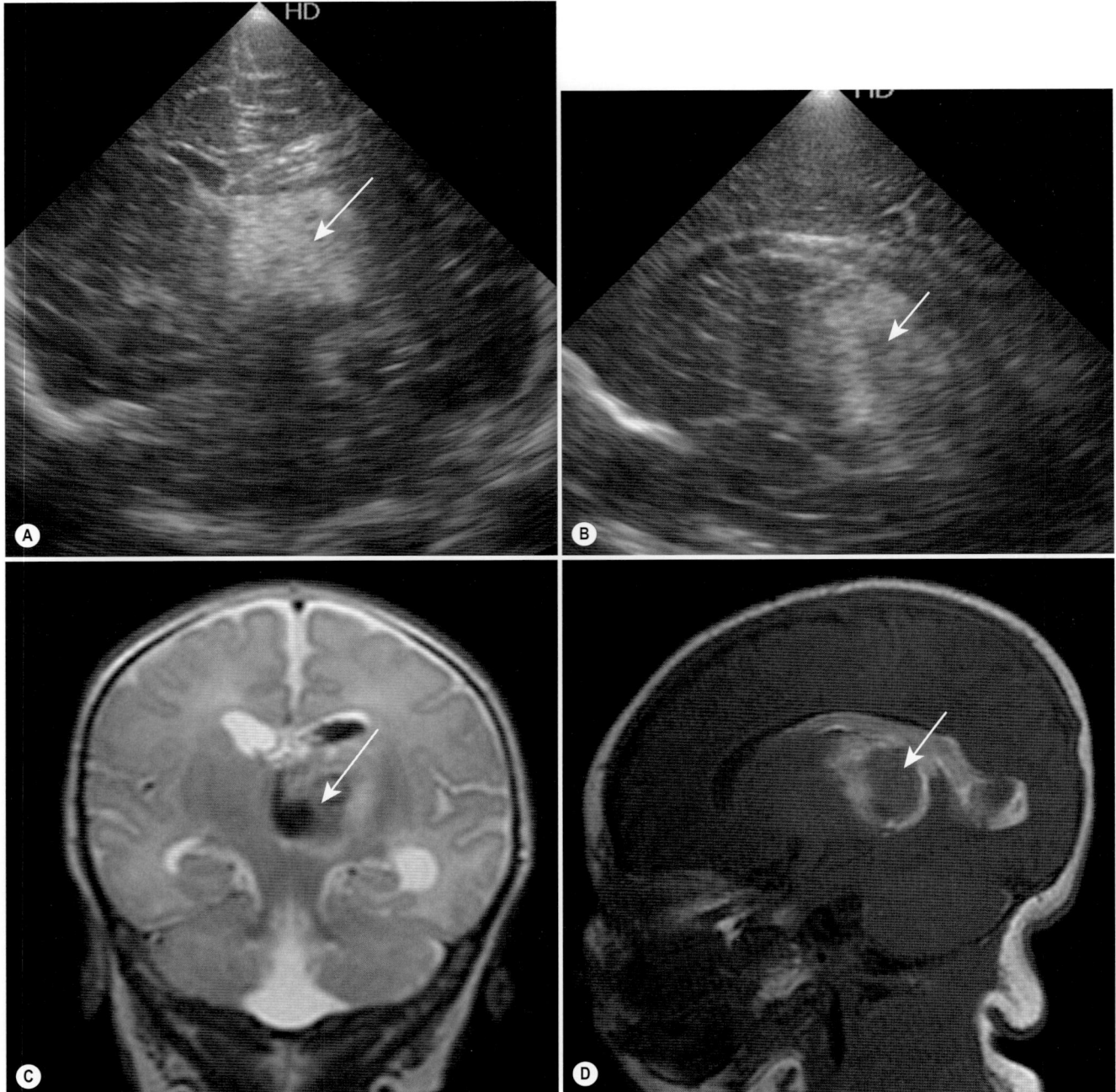

Fig. 40.20 Thalamic haemorrhage at term. (a) Coronal ultrasound image showing large globular echoreflectant area in the left thalamus (white arrow). (b) Corresponding parasagittal ultrasound image. (Courtesy of Silke Lee, King's College Hospital.) (c) Coronal and (d) parasagittal magnetic resonance image showing the lesion in the right thalamus (white arrow).

Subgaleal (subaponeurotic) haemorrhage

Subgaleal haemorrhage is rare, but a massive and expanding collection represents an emergency in the newborn, and can be fatal. It is thought to be caused by the rupture of emissary veins, which connect scalp veins to the dural sinuses, causing bleeding into the subaponeurotic space between the outer periosteum of the skull and the epicranial aponeurosis which extends from the orbital ridges anteriorly to the nuchal ridge posteriorly. This space can

hold up to 260 ml of blood (Davis 2001), which is almost as much as the total circulating volume of an average term newborn (Fig. 40.21).

Subgaleal haematomas are commoner in infants delivered by instrumental delivery, particularly ventouse (Govaert et al. 1992). In a case series of 34 infants from St Louis, Missouri, 31 had been delivered by instruments – 21 vacuum, eight vacuum followed by forceps and two forceps (Kilani and Wetmore 2006). Seventeen of the infants also had associated intracranial bleeds and six infants had skull fractures. The four (12%) infants who died had required large volumes of blood and blood products for treatment of

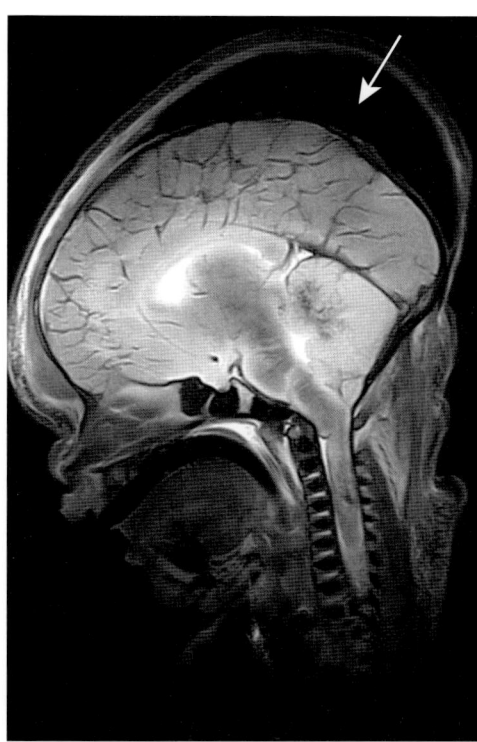

Fig. 40.21 T magnetic resonance image showing a massive subgaleal haematoma (white arrow). *(Reproduced with permission from Cheong et al. 2006.)*

coagulopathy and shock. In a prospective series from Malaysia, Boo et al. (2005) describe an incidence of 71/338 (21%) in babies born using the ventouse. These authors carefully examined all babies born by ventouse, checking head circumference and looking for fluctuant swellings several times over the first 24 hours of life. Two babies died, one from severe hypovolaemic shock and one from HIE. However, 58 (81%) developed some complication such as a coagulopathy, hyperbilirubinaemia or anaemia. The good outcome in this study was probably due to the active surveillance and increased awareness of the condition, which is often missed or appreciated too late.

Clinical presentation

A fluctuant swelling that crosses suture lines develops on the scalp after birth. Fluctuance, size and position help to distinguish subgaleal haemorrhage from cephalohaematoma, which does not cross the suture lines and does not become fluctuant until 48 hours of age. Some infants may deteriorate rapidly, sometimes when they are still in the labour ward. The head size may visibly increase and the infant becomes pale, sweaty and tachycardic. Some authors suggest that each centimetre increase in head circumference corresponds with a loss of 40 ml of blood into the subaponeurotic space (Plauche 1980). The baby may develop systemic shock with DIC and coagulopathy.

Investigations

The haematocrit may drop rapidly. The baby may develop a metabolic acidosis with a rising lactate. The infant may be anaemic and thrombocytopenic and have deranged coagulation. Measuring the head circumference at frequent intervals can help.

Management

The key to management of this condition is a high index of suspicion and prompt and early recognition (Smith et al. 1995; Gebremariam 1999). Delay in recognition of the condition may worsen outcome. Davis (2001) recommends at least 8 hours of observations for all babies following a difficult instrumental delivery regardless of the need for resuscitation or Apgar scores. Aggressive management of the blood loss with blood and blood products is essential to avoid death from hypovolaemic shock and DIC, and secondary hypoxic–ischaemic brain damage.

Prognosis

A study of 42 cases from Taiwan found that 13 (31%) had a poor outcome: five died, four had epilepsy, three had severe auditory impairment and two had cerebral palsy. Outcome is related to the size of the haemorrhage and hence the degree of supportive treatment required. Infants who need mechanical ventilation, pressor support and large volumes of blood products, all reflecting the severity of haemorrhage, are at risk of worse outcome, as are factors such as coagulopathy, metabolic acidosis and renal impairment (Chang et al. 2007). Good outcomes have been reported, as described above, following early recognition and aggressive replacement of blood and coagulation factors.

Perinatal stroke

Perinatal stroke can be defined as an area of damaged cerebral tissue resulting from focal disruption to cerebral blood flow secondary to arterial (perinatal arterial ischaemic stroke (PAIS): see below) or cerebral venous thrombosis (CSVT: see below) or embolisation, between 20 weeks of fetal life through the 28th postnatal day, confirmed by neuroimaging or neuropathological studies (Raju 2007). The growing importance of the topic was recognised by a recent National Institutes of Health workshop. Perinatal stroke is important because, apart from in later adult life, stroke is at no time more common than during this early period of development (Nelson 2007). Stroke is also thought to account for up to 30% of hemiplegic cerebral palsy in term-born infants (Kirton and deVeber 2009). Haemorrhagic transformation is common in CSVT and rare in PAIS.

In this chapter we discuss only PAIS and CSVT. Borderzone, or 'watershed', infarction is usually secondary to prolonged partial hypoxic ischaemia, is associated with HIE, and is covered in this chapter section 4. Central to both conditions is the thrombophilic state of the circulating blood of the infant. The most common site for neonatal stroke is in the territory of the left middle cerebral artery. Perhaps half the children with neonatal stroke present in the first 3 days with focal seizures. Others are diagnosed later (outside the neonatal period), presenting with asymmetric neurologic findings or early hand preference. This latter group is labelled as 'presumed perinatal stroke', presenting later in infancy with asymmetric neurologic examination and early hand preference, and a higher proportion of this group develop hemiplegic cerebral palsy compared to infants diagnosed in the neonatal period.

Depending on the age of presentation, neonatal stroke may be classified as follows (Raju 2007):

- fetal ischaemic stroke – diagnosed antenatally or at autopsy in a stillborn fetus
- neonatal ischaemic stroke – diagnosed after birth or during the first 28 days of postnatal life, including in preterm infants
- presumed perinatal ischaemic stroke – diagnosed after 28 days, in infants in whom the ischaemia is thought to

have occurred between 20 weeks' gestation and 28 days' postnatal age
- sinovenous thrombosis.

Thrombophilic state and the newborn

The newborn, like the pregnant woman, is in a thrombophilic state, as demonstrated in an elegant study that measured paired maternal and umbilical venous coagulation and anticoagulation factors (Lao et al. 1990). Protein C, protein S, antithrombin III, fibrinogen and plasminogen levels were all significantly lower in the cord specimens.

In the newborn, acquired thrombophilic risk factors include transplacental acquisition of maternal antiphospholipid antibodies and inherited thrombophilic tendencies. Prothrombotic coagulation factors are present in half of neonates with perinatal stroke (Cnossen et al. 2009). A meta-analysis of 22 cohort studies, with almost 2000 patients and 3000 controls, showed a statistically significant association between the thrombophilic traits of antithrombin deficiency, proteins C and S deficiency, factor V Leiden deficiency, factor II, methyltetrahydrofolate reductase (MTHFR) C677T mutation, antiphospholipid antibodies and elevated lipoprotein a with first stroke in childhood, with no difference found between PAIS and CSVT (Kenet et al. 2010). Children with combined thrombophilic disorders had the highest risk with an odds ratio of 11.86 (95% confidence interval 5.93–23.73).

Interestingly, in a study including 23 PAIS cases from the Israeli Paediatric Stroke registry in which the infants and parents had been screened for thrombophilic tendency, a risk factor was present in 18 mother–infant pairs but there was a mismatch in 15 cases so that the mother and the infant did not share one or more of the risk factors (Simchen et al. 2008). The most frequent risk factor in the study of Curry et al. (2007) was hetero- or homozygosity of the MTHFR C677T mutation, but this may only increase thrombogenesis when homocysteine levels are high. Inherited and acquired thrombophilic tendency is almost certainly important in neonatal stroke, but the whole story is, as yet, far from clear.

Perinatal arterial ischaemic stroke

PAIS is an increasingly recognised entity, largely due to increased use of MRI. PAIS is probably underrecognised, with incidences as high as 1 in 2300 live births quoted by centres with easy access to and frequent use of neonatal brain MRI, while other centres report lower incidences, of around 1 in 4000–5000 live births (Estan and Hope 1997; Lee et al. 2005a; Kirton and deVeber 2009). PAIS can affect both term and preterm babies (Benders et al. 2009).

Aetiology and pathogenesis

The cause of PAIS is not always clear. The most commonly cited hypothesis is that of a placental embolus travelling into the arterial tree as a paradoxical embolus, because of the frequency with which the left middle cerebral artery territory is involved and because of the presence of a patent foramen ovale in fetal and early neonatal life. There is an association with persistent pulmonary hypertension which tends to support this mechanism (Klesh et al. 1987). Other associations include meningitis (Fitzgerald and Golomb 2007), congenital heart disease, particularly if surgical repair is required (Chen et al. 2009), intravascular catheters and ECMO (Tables 40.9 and 40.10). Older studies report an association with perinatal hypoxic ischaemia, but these data are from the pre-MRI era and

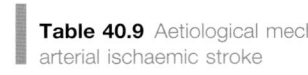

Table 40.9 Aetiological mechanisms of neonatal perinatal arterial ischaemic stroke

Embolism – a paradoxical venous embolism (from the placental bed) or from an extracorporeal membrane oxygenation circuit or central catheter, or during cardiac bypass surgery
Primary thrombosis – related to polycythaemia or prothrombotic tendency
Infection – endothelial injury and inflammation of arteries and veins associated with meningitis
Arterial dissection in the carotid artery
Arterial malformation – developmental abnormality
Arteriopathy – related to congenital infection with rubella, cytomegalovirus or *Toxoplasma*
Arterial spasm – induced by maternal cocaine or amphetamines

Table 40.10 Risk factors for perinatal arterial ischaemic stroke

Maternal risk factors
Primiparity
Infertility
Chorioamnionitis
Prolonged rupture of membranes
Pre-eclampsia
Intrauterine growth retardation
Drugs such as cocaine
Twin-to-twin transfusion
Gestational diabetes

Intrapartum factors
Long second stage of labour
Occiput posterior presentation

Neonatal factors
Prothrombotic states
Congenital heart disease
Diagnostic procedures and surgery for cardiac disease
Intravascular catheters, exchange transfusion
Persistent pulmonary hypertension
Extracorporeal membrane oxygenation
Meningitis
? Arterial dissection in the neck (few case reports)

there were no cases of PAIS in the TOBY trial, which had strict entry criteria for the definition of HIE (Rutherford et al. 2010). The previous association probably arose from the misclassification of babies with seizures; further, some babies with well-established infarction have developed acute neonatal signs. However, it remains the case that babies with stroke often have a complicated perinatal history (Chabrier et al. 2009; Cheong and Cowan 2009). Dissection of the internal carotid artery or its branches is very rare (Lequin et al. 2004): one of 215 German cases had arterial dissection demonstrated (Kurnik et al. 2003). There is a single case report of a 5-month-old child who presented with a left hemiplegia and a right Horner's syndrome. MRI revealed reduced blood flow in the internal carotid artery (Gupta et al. 2005). The cause was ascribed to a whiplash injury to the artery during fetal life, when the mother was involved in a road traffic accident. Congenital abnormalities of the neck vessels are also possible causes of PAIS.

Clinical presentation

Commoner in males, the commonest clinical feature of PAIS in the neonatal period is seizures, particularly focal seizures in the first 3 days of life. Babies with PAIS have usually been well before presentation, and often remain well between seizures. Infants diagnosed outside the neonatal period commonly present with abnormal hand preference or evolving hemiparesis.

Investigations

A full blood count and haematocrit may reveal polycythaemia. Conventional or amplitude-integrated EEG (aEEG) may identify focal or generalised seizures; the background activity is often normal, and can be a useful guide to prognosis (Mercuri et al. 1999). Echocardiography is indicated. An initial thrombophilia screen consisting of protein C, protein S, fibrinogen, antithrombin, lipoprotein a, anticardiolipin antibodies, lupus anticoagulant, partial thromboplastin time and international normalised ratio should be carried out, with a follow-up screen at 3–6 months (activated protein C resistance, factor V Leiden, prothrombin gene mutation, MTHFR, lipoprotein a, homocysteine, factors VIII/IX/X) (Nowak-Gottl et al. 2003).

Imaging

In experienced hands, CUS may reveal echogenic foci at sites of infarction (Cowan et al. 2005), but the gold-standard investigation for PAIS is MRI (Lequin et al. 2009) (Fig. 40.22). MR is preferable to CT, because of the radiation dosage associated with CT. CT is justified in an emergency, when it is important to determine whether or not there is a space-occupying subdural haematoma that might need neurosurgical intervention, or when there is thought to be significant ICH or trauma (bony windows can be obtained with CT). CT acquisition times are shorter and this can be a factor in critically ill babies.

Diffusion-weighted sequences may reveal restriction at affected territories of recent infarction (Fig. 40.22d) and sequences using MR angiography may reveal sites of arterial narrowing. Dudink et al. (2009) studied conventional T1 and T2 images and diffusion-weighted images (DWI) that were first imaged in the neonatal period, from 21 infants with unilateral PAIS. All DWI images showed high signal intensity in the affected region until day 4 (similar findings to Lequin's group in France). The cortex showed high signal intensity on T2 and low signal intensity on T1 until day 6, when the signal intensities reversed. Secondary changes in the thalamus and brainstem were seen in the first week of life and atrophic changes were seen after 4 weeks. These authors reported that the pattern of changes in signal intensities on conventional MRI and DWI were remarkably consistent in their patient group, leading them to conclude that PAIS in symptomatic term-born infants occurs within a very limited timeframe around birth. Govaert (2009) has provided helpful anatomical templates with which to identify the affected artery.

Management

During the acute phase of PAIS supportive measures such as adequate hydration, maintenance of normal glucose, pH and oxygen levels and anticonvulsants for seizures and antibiotics/antivirals for infection are important. Routine thrombolysis is not recommended as there are not sufficient data regarding its effectiveness or safety. In cases of PAIS with an ongoing documented cardioembolic source treatment with unfractionated heparin (UFH) or low-molecular-weight heparin (LMWH) may be appropriate (Cnossen et al. 2009), but specialist advice should be sought.

Outcome

PAIS in the middle cerebral artery territory may result in hemiplegia in up to 50% of children, the likelihood being predictable from neonatal MRI (Husson et al. 2009). Three-site involvement of the hemisphere, basal ganglia and posterior limb of the internal capsule is strongly associated with later contralateral hemiplegia irrespective of the size of the infarct (Mercuri et al. 1999; Boardman et al. 2005). The presence of pre-Wallerian degeneration in the cerebral peduncles also helps to predict the outcome (Fig. 40.22e) (Groenendaal 2006). Later cognitive impairments, epilepsy and behaviour problems remain relatively common adverse outcomes (Ricci et al. 2007), with language delay in 25% (Lee et al. 2005b). In one group of 63 term and preterm children with PAIS, 54% developed epilepsy in childhood (Chabrier et al. 2011), and cognitive difficulty is often present in those with epilepsy. Most children will walk, and recurrence is very rare in children without underlying cardiac disease.

Cerebral sinovenous thrombosis

Neonatal CSVT is rare, with a reported incidence of around 2.6 per 100 000 live births (Ramenghi et al. 2009). This is probably an underestimate, and the diagnosis is often missed due to the non-specific symptoms at presentation and the lack of sophisticated imaging in many centres (Sebire et al. 2005). CSVT can coexist with sepsis, meconium aspiration syndrome, meningitis and HIE. The commonest sinus to be involved is the superior sagittal sinus, but the transverse (lateral) or the straight sinus is also often thrombosed and many babies have more than one sinus involved (de Veber et al. 2001). CSVT propagation has been recognised with repeated MRI, and some would say that was an indication to consider anticoagulation (see below). Seizures are less commonly associated than with PAIS, and respiratory signs and hypotonia can be the clue to this diagnosis (Rivkin et al. 1992).

Aetiology and pathogenesis

Risk factors are similar to that for PAIS, with haemoconcentration and dehydration particularly important (Nwosu et al. 2008). Following CSVT venous pressure escalates in the occluded vessels and haemorrhagic infarction can develop in the region of brain drained by the sinus, because of venous congestion, vasogenic oedema, and increased capillary hydrostatic pressure (Diamini et al. 2010). The resulting brain injury may vary from venous congestion to the recognised ischaemic infarction involving the cortex, subcortical white matter and the deep nuclear grey matter. Haemorrhagic transformation of any infarcted cerebral tissue is the norm.

CSVT is frequently associated with secondary intraventricular, intraparenchymal and basal ganglia and thalami haemorrhage in term infants, and is thought to result from back pressure to distal draining veins. A 10-year review of patients from centres in the Netherlands (Berfelo et al. 2010) identified 52 neonates with CSVT, of whom half had associated thalamic haemorrhage, half had associated IVH and 79% had intraparenchymal haemorrhage. As discussed above, and as demonstrated in Figure 40.20, most term babies with thalamic haemorrhage have underlying CSVT.

Clinical features

In the Dutch study of 52 neonates with CSVT there was a male preponderance (75%) (Berfelo et al. 2010). The commonest symptoms were seizures (81%), focal in a fifth of patients, followed by apnoeas. Fifteen per cent of infants had suffered sepsis or

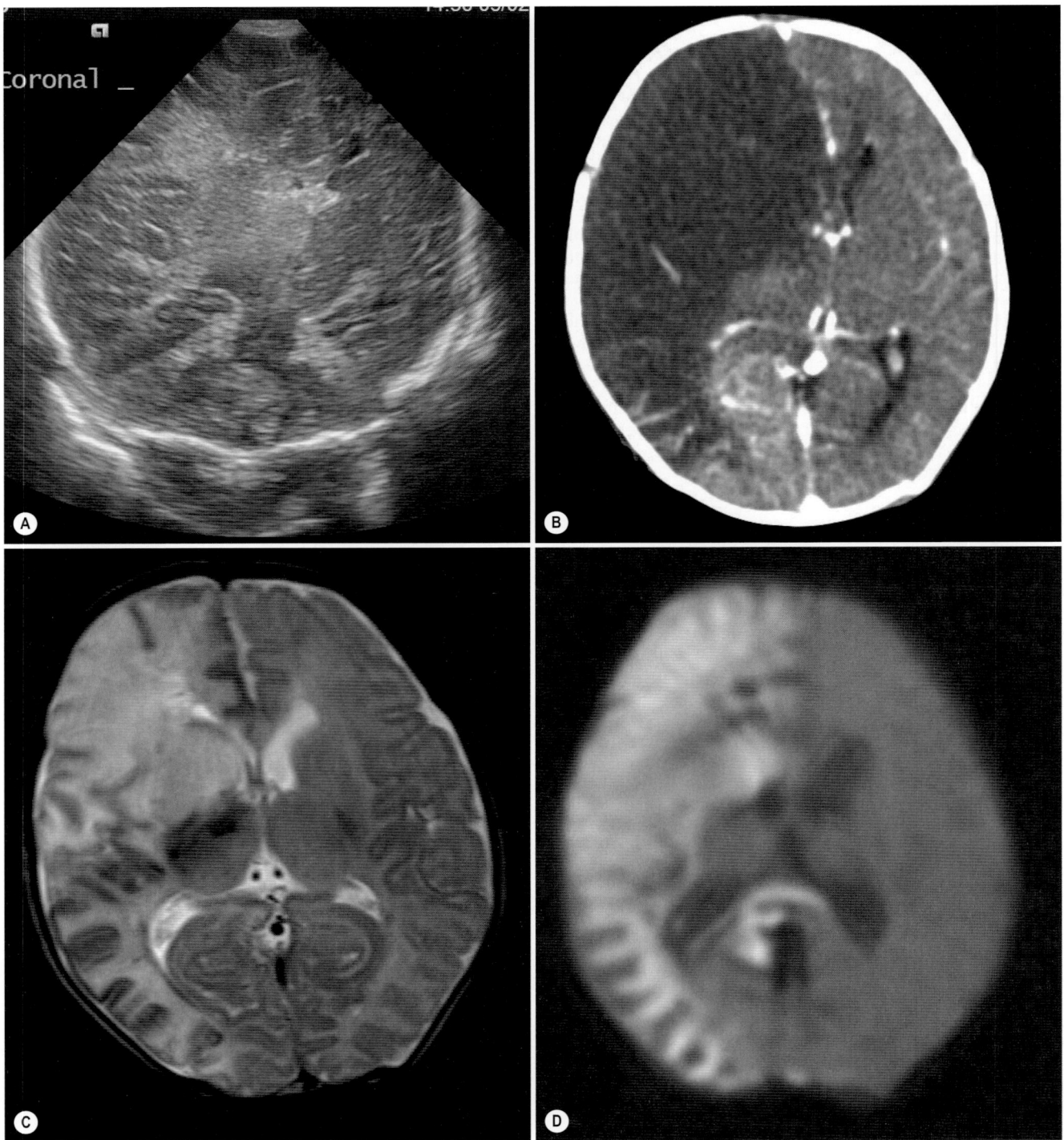

Fig. 40.22 Images from a baby with an extensive right middle cerebral artery stroke. (a) Ultrasound image showing midline shift, loss of normal anatomical detail and increased echodensity on the right. (b) Computed tomography scan the same day demonstrating an extensive region of loss of density. (c) Axial T2-weighted magnetic resonance image showing widespread area of abnormality involving the deep grey matter and posterior limb of the internal capsule. (d) Axial diffusion-weighted image (DWI) confirming the significant infarction.

meningitis and 13% were born to mothers with pregnancy-related hypertension.

Investigations

The key to diagnosis of CSVT (arguably even more so than with PAIS) is a high index of suspicion so that appropriate and specific investigation to demonstrate diminished blood flow through cerebral venous

sinuses can be carried out. Colour Doppler flow studies at the bedside may demonstrate reduced flow in affected venous sinuses. MR may show the clot, or venogram studies may identify regions of decreased flow-related enhancement in venous sinuses (Fig. 40.23). In the Dutch study (Berfelo et al. 2010), half of the infants had multiple sinus involvement, superior sagittal sinus was affected in 23% and straight sinus in 15%. In addition to the associated haemorrhage, infarcts may be seen in the parasagittal white matter and the basal ganglia. All other investigations are as for PAIS.

Management

Rehydration is necessary in a dehydrated newborn. In an infant with primary polycythaemia dilutional exchange transfusion may be needed. Seizures and infections will require treatment with anticonvulsants and antibiotics respectively.

At present there are few data on therapeutic efficacy and safety of antithrombotic treatment in newborns with CSVT (Moharir et al. 2010), and international practice is hugely variable (Jordan et al. 2010). In the absence of significant ICH, particularly if the thrombus is noted to propagate, anticoagulation with UFH or LMWH may be used with specialist haematology input and close monitoring of anti-Xa, heparin and activated partial thromboplastin time levels. The aim should be rapidly to achieve anti-Xa levels of 0.5–1.0 U/ml (Yang et al. 2010). Once commenced, treatment may need to be continued for several weeks until improved flow through the cerebral venous sinuses is established.

Outcome

Perinatal stroke is the leading known cause of hemiplegic cerebral palsy (Kirton and deVeber 2006). In all, 30–50% of infants with CSVT will go on to have a motor deficit (de Veber et al. 2001; Kersbergen et al. 2011). Other common deficits resulting from perinatal stroke include epilepsy, deficits in language, vision and cognitive outcomes.

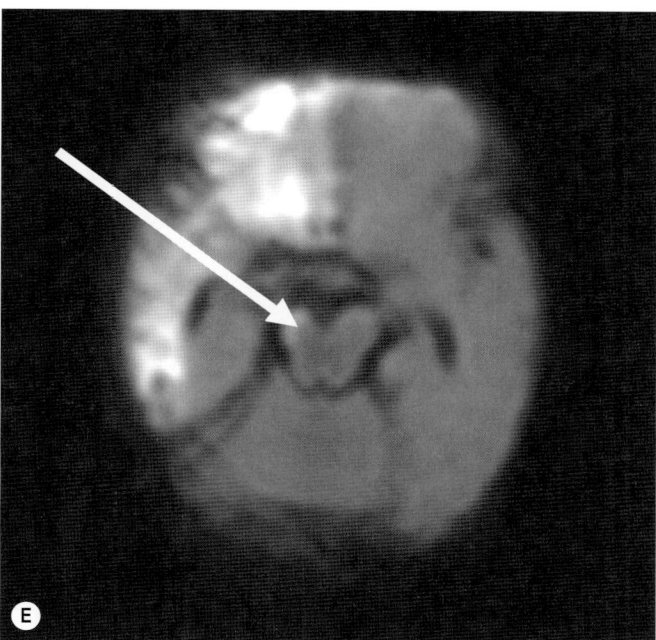

Fig. 40.22, cont'd (e) Axial DWI showing pre-Wallerian degeneration (arrowed).

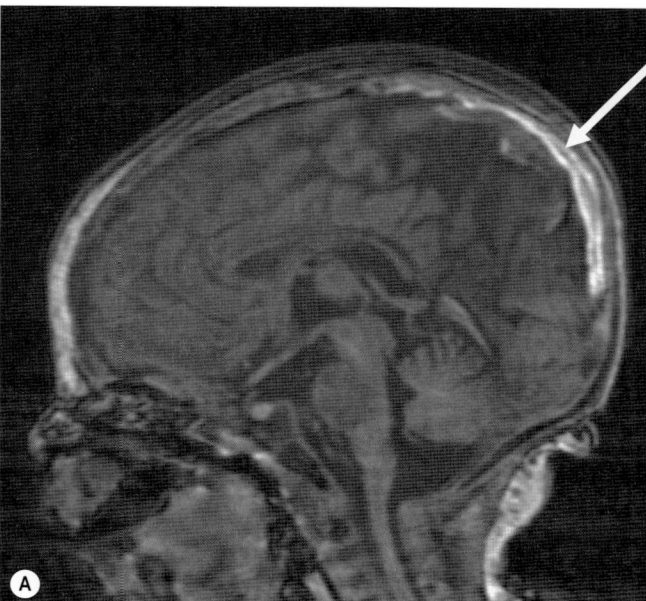
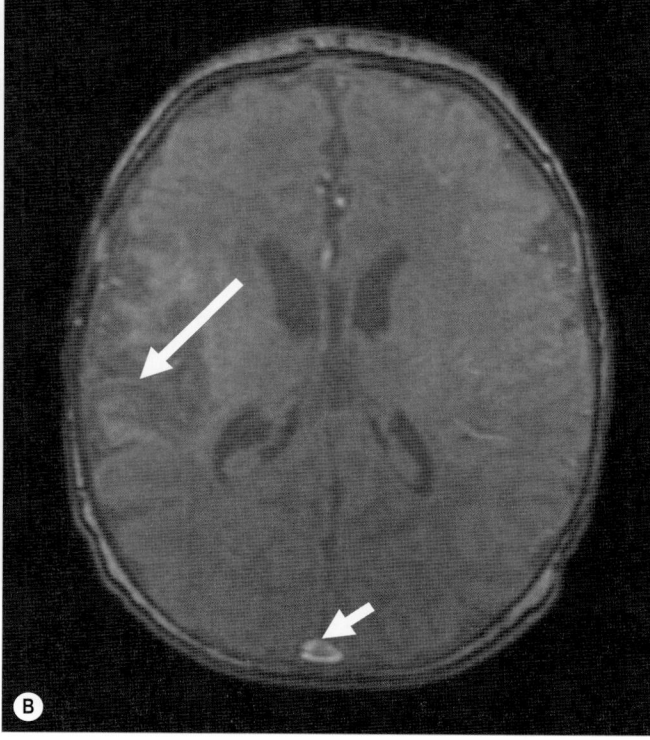

Fig. 40.23 (a) Midline sagittal T1-weighted magnetic resonance image (MRI) showing thrombus within the superior sagittal sinus (arrowed). (b) Axial T1-weighted MRI showing area of infarction in the right middle cerebral artery territory (white arrow) together with thrombus in the sagittal sinus (arrowhead).

References

Adams, C., Hochhauser, L., Logan, W.J., 1988. Primary thalamic and caudate hemorrhage in term neonates presenting with seizures. Pediatr Neurol 4, 175–177.

Benders, M.J.N.L., Groenendaal, F., de Vries, L.S., 2009. Preterm arterial ischemic stroke. Semin Fetal Neonat Med 14, 272–277.

Berfelo, F.J., Kersbergen, K.J., van Ommen, C.H., et al., 2010. Neonatal cerebral sinovenous thrombosis from symptom to outcome. Stroke 41, 1382–1388.

Boardman, J.P., Ganesan, V., Rutherford, M.A., et al., 2005. Magnetic resonance image correlates of hemiparesis after neonatal and childhood middle cerebral artery stroke. Pediatrics 115, 321–326.

Boo, N.Y., Foong, K.W., Mahdy, Z.A., et al., 2005. Risk factors associated with subaponeurotic haemorrhage in full-term infants exposed to vacuum extraction. British Journal of Obstetrics & Gynaecology 112, 1516–1521.

Brouwer, A.J., Groendaal, F., Koopman, C., et al., 2010. Intracranial hemorrhage in full-term newborns: a hospital-based cohort study. Neuroradiology 30 (5), 998–1004.

Chabrier, S., Saliba, E., Nguyen The Tich, S., et al., 2009. Obstetrical and neonatal characteristics vary with birthweight in a cohort of 100 term newborns with symptomatic arterial ischemic stroke. Eur J Paediatr Neurol 30, 1–8.

Chabrier, S., Husson, B., Dinomais, M., et al., 2011. New insights (and new interrogations) in perinatal arterial ischemic stroke. Thromb Res 127, 13–22.

Chang, H.Y., Peng, C.C., Kao, H.A., et al., 2007. Neonatal subgaleal hemorrhage: clinical presentation, treatment, and predictors of poor prognosis. Pediatr Int 49, 903–907.

Chen, J., Zimmerman, R.A., Jarvik, G.P., et al., 2009. Perioperative stroke in infants undergoing open heart operations for congenital heart disease. Ann Thorac Surg 88, 823–829.

Cheong, J.L.Y., Cowan, F.M., 2009. Neonatal arterial ischaemic stroke: obstetric issues. Semin Fetal Neonat Med 14, 267–271.

Cheong, J.L., Hagmann, C., Rennie, J.M., et al., 2006. Fatal newborn head enlargement: high resolution magnetic resonance imaging at 4.7 T. Arch Dis Child 91, F202–F203.

Cnossen, M.H., van Ommen, C.H., Appel, I.M., 2009. Etiology and treatment of perinatal stroke: a role for prothrombotic coagulation factors? Semin Fetal Neonat Med 14, 311–317.

Cowan, F., Mercuri, E., Groenendaal, F., et al., 2005. Does cranial ultrasound imaging identify arterial cerebral infarction in term neonates? Arch Dis Child 90, F252–F256.

Curry, C.J., Bhullar, S., Holmes, J., et al., 2007. Risk factors for perinatal arterial stroke: a study of 60 mother-child pairs. Paediatr Neurol 37, 99–107.

Dale, S.T., Coleman, L.T., 2002. Neonatal alloimmune thrombocytopenia: antenatal and postnatal imaging findings in the pediatric brain. Am J Neuroradiol 23, 1457–1465.

Danielsson, N., Hoa, D.P., Thang, N.V., et al., 2004. Intracranial haemorrhage due to late onset vitamin K deficiency bleeding in Hanoi province, Vietnam. Arch Dis Child 89 (6), 546–550.

Davis, D.J., 2001. Neonatal subgaleal hemorrhage: diagnosis and management. Can Med Assoc J 164, 1452–1454.

de Veber, G., Andrew, M., Adams, C., et al., 2001. Cerebral sinovenous thrombosis in children. N Engl J Med 345, 417–412.

Diamini, N., Billinghurst, L., Kirkham, F.J., 2010. Cerebral venous sinus (sinovenous) thrombosis in children. Neurosurg Clin North Am 21, 511–527.

Dudink, J., Mercuri, E., Al-Nakib, L., et al., 2009. Evolution of unilateral perinatal arterial ischemic stroke on conventional and diffusion-weighted mr imaging. Am J Neuroradiol 30 (5), 998–1004.

Estan, J., Hope, P.L., 1997. Unilateral neonatal cerebral infarction in full term infants. Arch Dis Child 76, F88–F93.

Fitzgerald, K.C., Golomb, M.R., 2007. Neonatal arterial ischemic stroke and sinovenous thrombosis associated with meningitis. J Child Neurol 22, 818–822.

Gardella, C., Taylor, M., Benedetti, T., et al., 2001. The effect of sequential l.use of vacuum and forceps for assited vaginal delivery on neonatal and maternal outcomes. Am J Obstet Gynecol 185, 896–902.

Gebremariam, A., 1999. Subgaleal haemorrhage: risk factors and neurological and developmental outcome in survivors. Ann Trop Paediatr 19, 45–50.

Govaert, P., 1993. Cranial haemorrhage in the term newborn infant. Mac Keith Press, London.

Govaert, P., 2009. Songraphic stroke templates. Semin Fetal Neonat Med 14, 284–298.

Govaert, P., Vanhaesebrouck, P., De Praeter, C., et al., 1992. Vacuum extraction, bone injury and neonatal subgaleal bleeding. Eur J Pediatr 151, 532–535.

Govaert, P., Swarte, R., Oostra, A., et al., 2003. Neonatal infarction within basal cerebral vein territory. Dev Med Child Neurol 43, 559–562.

Groenendaal, F., 2006. Pre-wallerian degeneration in the neonatal brain following perinatal cerebral hypoxia-ischemia demonstrated with MRI Groenendaal F Seminars in Perinatology 30 (3), 146–150.

Gupta, M., Dinakaran, S., Chan, T.K., 2005. Congenital Horner syndrome and hemiplegia secondary to carotid dissection. J Pediatr Ophthalmol Strabismus 42, 122–124.

Hanigan, W.C., Powell, F.C., Miller, T.C., et al., 1995a. Symptomatic intracranial hemorrhage in full-term infants. Child's Nerv System 11, 707.

Hanigan, W.C., Powell, F.C., Palagallo, G., et al., 1995b. Lobar hemorrhages in full term neonates. Child's Nerv System 11, 276–280.

Heibel, M., Heber, R., Bechinger, D., et al., 1993. Early diagnosis of perinatal cerebral lesions in apparently normal full term newborns by ultrasound of the brain. Neuroradiology 35, 85–91.

Heyman, R., Heckly, A., Magagi, J., et al., 2005. Intracranial epidural hematoma in newborn infants: clinical study of 15 cases. Neurosurgery 57, 924–929.

Holden, K.R., Titus, M.O., von Tassel, P., 1999. Cranial magnetic resonance imaging examination of normal term neonates: a pilot study. J Child Neurol 14, 708–710.

Husson, B., Hertz-Pannier, L., Renaud, C., et al., 2009. Motor outcomes after neonatal arterial ischemic stroke related to early MRI data in a prospective study. Pediatrics 126, e912–e918.

Jhawar, B.S., Ranger, A., Steven, D., et al., 2003. Risk factors for intracranial hemorrhage among full-term infants: a case-control study. Neurosurgery 52, 581–590.

Jordan, L.C., Rafay, M.F., Smith, S., et al., 2010. Antithrombotic treatment in neonatal cerebral sinovenous thrombosis: results of the international pediatric stroke study. J Pediatr 156, 704–710.

Kenet, G., Lutkoff, L.K., Albisetti, M., et al., 2010. Impact of thrombophilia on risk of arterial ischemic stroke or cerebral sinovenous thrombosis in neonates and children. Circulation 121, 1838–1847.

Kersbergen, K.J., de Vries, L.S., van Straaten, H.L.M., et al., 2009. Anticoagulation therapy and imaging in neonates with a unilaterael thalamic hemorrhage due to cerebral sinovenous thrombosis. Stroke 40, 2754–2760.

Kersbergen, K.J., Groenendaal, F., Benders, M.J.N.L., 2011. The spectrum of associated brain lesions in cerebral sinovenous thrombosis: relation to gestational age and outcome. Arch Dis Child Fetal Neonat Kersbergen 96 (6), F404–F409.

Kilani, R.A., Wetmore, J., 2006. Neonatal subgaleal hematoma: presentation and outcome – radiological findings and factors associated with mortality. Am J Perinatol 23, 41–47.

Kirton, A., deVeber, G., 2006. Cerebral palsy secondary to perinatal ischemic stroke. Clin Perinatol 33, 367–386.

Kirton, A., deVeber, G., 2009. Advances in perinatal ischemic stroke. Paediatr Neurol 40, 205–214.

Klesh, K.W., Murphy, T.F., Scher, M.S., et al., 1987. Cerebral infarction in persistent pulmonary hypertension of the newborn. Am J Dis Child 141, 852–857.

Kulkarni, R. Lusher, J.M., 1999. Intracranial and extracranial hemorrhages in newborns with hemophilia: a review of the literature. J Pediatr Hematol Oncol 21, 289–295.

Kulkarni, R., Soucie, J.M., Lusher, J., et al., 2009. Sites of initial bleeding episodes, mode of delivery and age of diagnosis in babies with haemophilia diagnosed before the age of 2 years: a report from the Centers for Disease Control and Prevention's (CDC) Universal Data Collection (UDC) project. Haemophilia 15, 1281–1290.

Kurnik, K., Kosch, A., Strater, R., et al., 2003. Recurrent thromboembolism in infants and children suffering from symptomatic neonatal arterial stroke. A prospective follow-up study. Stroke 34, 2887–2893.

Lao, T.T., Yin, J.A., Yuen, P.M., 1990. Coagulation and antiicoagulation systems in newborns – correlation with their mothers at delivery. Gynecol Obstet Invest 29, 181–184.

Lee, J., Croen, L.A., Backstrand, K.H., et al., 2005a. Maternal and infant characteristics associated with perinatal arterial stroke in the infant. Jama 293, 723–729.

Lee, J., Croen, L.A., Lindan, C., Nash, K.B., et al., 2005b. Predictors of outcome in perinatal arterial stroke: a population-based study. Ann Neurol 58, 303–308.

Lequin, M.H., Peeters, E.A.J., Holscher, H.C., et al., 2004. Arterial infarction caused by carotid artery dissection in the neonate. Eur J Paediatr Neurol 8, 155–160.

Lequin, M., Dudink, J., Tong, K.A., et al., 2009. Magnetic resonance imaging in neonatal stroke. Semin Fetal Neonat Med 14, 299–310.

Looney, C.B., Smith, J.K., Merck, L.H., et al., 2007. Intracranial hemorrhage in asymptomatic neonates: prevalence on MR images and relationship to obstetric and neonatal risk factors. Radiology 242, 535–541.

Mack, J., Squier, W., Eastman, J.T., 2009. Anatomy and development of the meninges: implictions for subdural collections and csf circulation. Pediatr Radiol 39, 200–210.

Mercuri, E., Rutherford, M., Cowan, F., et al., 1999. Early prognostic indicators of outcome in infants with neonatal cerebral infarction: a clinical, electroencephalogram, and magnetic resonance imaging study. Pediatrics 103, 39–46.

Moharir, M.D., Schroff, M., Stephens, D., et al., 2010. Anticoagulants in pediatric cerebral sinovenous thrombosis. A safety and outcome study. Ann Neurol 67, 590–599.

Muller, E., 1989. 348 cases of neonatal alloimmune thrombocytopaenia. Lancet i, 363–365.

Nelson, K., 2007. Perinatal ischemic stroke. Stroke 38, 742–745.

Nowak-Gottl, U., Gunther, G., Kurnik, K., et al., 2003. Arterial ischemic stroke in neonates, infants, and children: an overview of underlying conditions, imaging methods, and treatment modalities. Semin Thrombosis Hemost 29, 405–414.

Nwosu, M.E., Williams, L.S., Edwards-Brown, M., et al., 2008. Neonatal sinovenous thrombosis: presentation and association with imaging. Pediatr Neurol 39, 155–161.

Perrin, R.G., Rutka, J.T., Drake, J.M., et al., 1997. Management and outcomes of posterior fossa subdural hematomas in neonates. Neurosurgery 40, 1190–1200.

Plauche, W.C., 1980. Subgaleal haematoma: a complication of instrumental delivery. Jama 244, 1597–1598.

Raju, T.N.K., 2007. Ischemic perinatal stroke: summary of a workshop sponsored by the National Institute of Child Health and Human Development and the National Institute of Neurological Disorders and Stroke. Pediatrics 120, 609–616.

Ramenghi, L.A., Govaert, P., Fumagalli, M., et al., 2009. Neonatal cerebral sinovenous thrombosis. Semin Fetal Neonat Med 14, 278–283.

Ricci, D., Mercuri, E., Barnett, A., et al., 2008. Cognitive outcome at early school age in term-born children with perinatally acquired middle cerebral artery territory infarction. Stroke 39 (2), 403–410.

Rivkin, M.J., Anderson, M.L., Kaye, E.M., 1992. Neonatal idiopathic cerebral venous thrombosis: an unrecognised cause of transient seizures or lethargy. Ann Neurol 32, 51–56.

Roland, E.H., Flodmark, O., Hill, A., 1990. Thalamic haemorrhage with intraventricular haemorrhage in the full term newborn. Pediatrics 85, 737–742.

Rooks, V.J., Eaton, J.P., Ruess, L., et al., 2008. Prevalence and evolution of intracranial hemorrhage in asymptomatic term infants. Am J Neuroradiol 29, 1082–1089.

Rutherford, M., Ramenghi, L.A., Edwards, A.D., et al., 2010. Assesment of brain tissue injury after moderate hypothermia in neonates with hypoxic-ischaemic encephalopathy: a nested substudy of a randomised controlled trial. Lancet Neurol 9, 39–45.

Sebire, G., Tabarki, B., Saunders, D.E., et al., 2005. Cerebral venous sinus thrombosis in children: risk factors, presentation,

diagnosis and outcome. Brain 128, 477–489.

Simchen, M.J., Goldstein, G., Lubetsky, A., et al., 2009. Factor V Leiden and antiphospholipid antibodies in either mothers of infants increase the risk for perinatal arterial ischemic stroke. Stroke 40 (1), 65–70.

Smith, S.A., Jett, P.L., Jacobson, S.L., et al., 1995. Subgaleal haematoma – the need for increased awareness of risk. J Family Practice 41, 569–574.

Tan, E.K., 2007. Difficult caesarean delivery of an impacted head and neonatal skull fracture: can the morbidity be avoided? J Obstet Gynaecol 27, 427–428.

Tarantino, M.D., Gupta, S.L., Brusky, R.M., 2007. The incidence and outcome of intracranial haemorrhage in newborns with haemophilia: analysis of the nationwide inpatient sample database. Haemophilia 13, 380–382.

Towner, D., Castro, M.A., Evy-Wilkens, E., et al., 1999. Effect of mode of delivery in nulliparous women on neonatal intracranial injury. N Engl J Med 341, 1709–1714.

Trounce, J.Q., Fawer, C.L., Punt, J., et al., 1985. Primary thalamic haemorrhage in the newborn: a new clinical entity. Lancet 2, 190–192.

van Hasselt, P.M., Kok, K., Vorselaars, A., et al., 2009. Vitamin K deficiency bleeding in cholestatic infants with alpha-1-antitrypsin deficiency. Arch Dis Child Fetal Neonat 94, F456–F460.

Volpe, J.J., 2008. Intracranial hemorrhage: subdural, primary subarachnoid, cerebellar, intraventricular (term infant) and miscellaneous. In: Volpe J.J. (Ed.), Neurology of the Newborn, fifth ed. Saunders, Philadelphia, pp. 483–516.

Whitby, E.H., Griffiths, P.D., Rutter, S., et al., 2004. Frequency and natural history of subdural haemorrhages in babies and relation to obstetric factors. Lancet 363, 846–851.

Wigglesworth, J.S., Husemeyer, R.P., 1977. Intracranial birth trauma in vaginal breech delivery: the continued importance of injury to the occipital bone. Br J Obstet Gynaecol 84, 684–691.

Williamson, L.M., Lowe, S., Love, E.M., et al., 1999. Serious hazards of transfusion (SHOT) initiative: analysis of the first two annual reports. Br Med J 319, 16–19.

Wu, Y.W., Hamrick, S.E.G., Miller, S.P., et al., 2003. Intraventricular hemorrhage in term neonates caused by sinovenous thrombosis. Ann Neurol 54, 123–126.

Yang, J.Y.K., Chan, A.K.C., Callen, D.J.A., et al., 2010. Neonatal cerebral sinovenous thrombosis: sifting the evidence for a diagnostic plan and treatment strategy. Pediatrics 126, e693–e700.

Part 4: **Hypoxic–ischaemic brain injury**

Nicola J Robertson   Floris Groenendaal

Introduction

Definitions

Hypoxic–ischaemic brain injury of the term and near-term infant remains a significant problem throughout the world. Hypoxaemia is defined as the 'diminished amount of oxygen in the blood supply' and cerebral ischaemia as the 'diminished amount of blood perfusing the brain'; ischaemia is the more important of the two forms of oxygen deprivation since it also results in deprivation of glucose which is also crucial in the genesis of neuronal injury (Volpe 2001). Asphyxia is the result of an impairment of exchange of the respiratory gases oxygen and carbon dioxide. Thus, in addition to hypoxia, asphyxia has the important additional feature of producing elevated levels of carbon dioxide, which results in a number of additional metabolic and physiological features which include acidosis and increased cerebral blood flow (CBF) (Volpe 2001). Hypoxia–ischaemia may occur acutely or chronically and is most commonly associated with maternal factors (hypotension, severe hypoxia), cord factors (prolapse, occlusion), placental factors (insufficiency and abruption) and uterine factors (rupture). Neonatal postnatal events such as shock, respiratory or cardiac arrest can also lead to hypoxic–ischaemic injury.

Neonatal encephalopathy (NE) is the clinical manifestation of disordered neonatal brain function in the term infant in the early neonatal period, manifested by respiratory difficulties, depression of tone and reflexes, subnormal level of consciousness and often seizures (Nelson 1991). The aetiology of NE is varied, with many genetic, metabolic and infective conditions presenting with similar clinical signs (Hankins et al. 2003) (Tables 40.11 and 40.12). The disorder is termed hypoxic–ischaemic encephalopathy (HIE) if there is evidence that intrapartum asphyxia is the cause of the encephalopathy resulting in neurologic depression or seizures. An important concept that is recurrent in many studies is that the human injury of HIE does not follow a wholly reproducible pattern: the etiology, extent of hypoxia or ischaemia, maturational stage of the brain, regional CBF and general health of the infant prior to the injury can all impact on the extent of brain injury as well as the outcome following injury.

The term HIE is often incorrectly used synonymously with NE. The term NE is a clinical description of disordered neurological function that does not require assumptions about pathogenesis or aetiology. The diverse risk factors, causal pathways and aetiologies, which may lead to NE in a developed country such as Australia, are listed in Table 40.13. The case-control study of NE in Western Australia showed that many antecedents of NE are present before the onset of labour. Intrapartum risk factors included maternal pyrexia, persistent occipitoposterior position and acute intrapartum events; however in over 70% of cases of NE there was no evidence of intrapartum hypoxia (Badawi et al. 1998a, b). This is very different to the situation in many low-income countries where mothers are stunted, do not access antenatal care, have high stillbirth rates and receive poor obstetric care. Under these conditions intrapartum factors probably remain more important in the causation of NE (Ellis and Costello 1999). For example, in a case-controlled study in Kathmandu, there was evidence of intrapartum hypoxia–ischaemia in 60% of encephalopathic infants. Independent risk factors for NE included short maternal stature, high maternal age, lack of antenatal care and multiple birth (Ellis et al. 2000);

Table 40.11 Conditions causing neonatal depression and/or neonatal encephalopathy that mimic intrapartum asphyxia

CONDITION	EXAMPLE
Neonatal sepsis	Group B streptococcal septicaemia
Congenital infections	Viral, toxoplasmosis
Neuronal migration disorders	
Congenital myotonic disorders	Congenital and transient myasthenia gravis, nemaline myopathy, Prader–Willi syndrome, peroxisomal disorders
Lung or airway disorders	Pneumothorax sustained during birth or early resuscitation, congenital airway problem, congenital diaphragmatic hernia
Metabolic conditions	Non-ketotic hyperglycinaemia, mitochondrial myopathies, methylmalonic and propionic acidaemia, maple syrup urine disease
Extracranial trauma causing significant blood loss and/or pressure	Subgaleal, extradural and subdural haematomas
Genetic disorders associated with thrombotic or thrombophilic abnormalities	Protein C and protein S deficiencies, factor V Leiden deficiency, anticardiolipin antibodies

Table 40.12 Acute causes of brain injury – sentinel events

Prolapsed umbilical cord
   uterine rupture
Placental abruption
Amniotic fluid embolism
Acute maternal haemorrhage
Any condition causing a sudden decrease in maternal cardiac
   output and blood flow to the fetus (e.g. anaphylaxis)
Acute neonatal haemorrhage, e.g. vasa praevia, acute loss from
   cord, fetal–maternal haemorrhage

intrapartum risk factors included non-cephalic presentation, prolonged rupture of membranes, cord prolapse and uterine rupture.

Since 1996 there have been three consensus statements addressing the diagnosis of intrapartum asphyxia (Committee on Fetus and Newborn 1996; MacLennan 1999; American College of Obstetricians and Gynecologists Taskforce 2003). These consensus statements emphasise the use of multiple markers for the diagnosis – some signs are considered essential and others supportive. With advances in cerebral imaging technology, the two most recent

Staff Library
Singleton Hospital
Tel: 01792 205066 Ext. **5281**

Table 40.13 Risk factors for of neonatal encephalopathy

	ANTENATAL RISK FACTORS FOR NEONATAL ENCEPHALOPATHY	ADJUSTED ODDS RATIO (95% CONFIDENCE INTERVAL) ALL INCREASED RISK EXCEPT MARKED*
Maternal	History of seizures	2.6 (1.3–4.9)
	Older mother	6.0 (1.3–28.2)
	Decreased parity	1.8 (0.9–3.7)
	Infertility treatment	4.4 (1.1–17.6)
	Thyroid disease	9.7 (2–48)
	Bleeding	3.6 91.3–9.9)
	Viral illness during pregnancy	2.9 (1.5–5.8)
	Abnormal placenta at delivery	2.1 (1.2–3.7)
Infant	Weight < 3rd centile	38.2 (9.4–154.8)
Intrapartum risk factors		
	Maternal pyrexia	3.8 (1.4–10.1)
	Persistent occipitoposterior position	4.3 (1.7–10.5)
	Acute intrapartum event	4.4 (1.3–15.2)
	Instrumental vaginal delivery or emergency caesarean section	2.3 (1.2–4.7)
		2.2 (1.0–4.6)
	Elective caesarean section*	

*Reduced risk.
(Modified from population-based studies: Badawi et al. 1998a, b.)

Table 40.14 Three consensus statements on diagnosing intrapartum asphyxia

AMERICAN ACADEMY OF PEDIATRICS/AMERICAN COLLEGE OF OBSTETRICS AND GYNECOLOGY (1996)*	INTERNATIONAL CEREBRAL PALSY TASK FORCE (1999)†	AMERICAN COLLEGE OF OBSTETRICS AND GYNECOLOGY (2003)‡
Essential	Metabolic acidosis in early neonatal blood sample (pH <7.0 and base deficit >12 mmol/l)	Metabolic acidosis (pH <7.0 and base deficit >12 mmol/l
Profound metabolic acidosis (pH< 7.0)		
Apgar score <3 after 5 minutes	Moderate or severe encephalopathy	Moderate or severe encephalopathy
Neonatal encephalopathy	Cerebral palsy of spastic quadriplegia or dyskinetic type	Cerebral palsy of spastic quadriplegia or dyskinetic type
Multiorgan system dysfunction		
Criteria suggestive of intrapartum timing	Sentinel event	Exclusion of other pathologies of cerebral palsy
	Abrupt change in fetal heart rate	
	Apgar score <6 beyond 5 minutes	Sentinel event
	Multisystem involvement	Abrupt change in fetal heart rate
	Imaging evidence	Apgar score <3 beyond 5 minutes
		Multisystem failure within 72 hours of birth
		Imaging evidence

*Committee of Fetus and Newborn (1996).
†MacLennan (1999).
‡American College of Obstetricians and Gynecologists Taskforce (2003).

statements take the findings from cerebral imaging into consideration as supportive evidence of intrapartum asphyxia (MacLennan 1999; American College of Obstetricians and Gynecologists Taskforce 2003). This may cause problems, particularly in countries with poor access to this advanced technology. The diagnosis of intrapartum asphyxia has been restricted to certain types of cerebral palsy in these two most recent statements (Table 40.14). As cerebral palsy is an eventual outcome, which may take several years to be confirmed, it is difficult for this to be used as an essential diagnostic criterion for an acute condition such as intrapartum asphyxia.

Epidemiology

Industrialised countries

The lack of universal agreed definitions of NE and the subgroup with HIE make the estimation of the incidence and identification of risk factors problematic. Very few investigators use the same case definition for either NE or HIE. The reported incidence of NE ranges from 2 to 6/1000 live births (Badawi et al. 1998a; Evans et al. 2001) and that of HIE ranges from 1 to 8/1000 live births (Finer et al. 1981; Levene and Williams 1985; Thornberg et al. 1995; Badawi et al. 1998a). This wide range reflects a mix of population-based and hospital-based incidence figures (hospital-based figures tend to be higher as such studies tend to be conducted in referral centres and therefore referral bias is introduced) as well as different time periods when the data were collected. There is evidence of a reduction in the incidence from the late 1970s (7.6 per 1000 live births) (Hull 1992) through to the late 1980s (4.6) (Hull 1992) to the early 1990s (1.9) (Smith and Dodd 2000). Therefore the interpretation of older data in relation to the current situation is problematic. Not all investigators have access to population data by gestational age and the rates of HIE and NE may be quoted per 1000 births rather than 1000 term births, thus the denominator may differ between studies.

Based on population studies with similar inclusion and denominator criteria Kurinczuk et al. (2010) estimated the incidence of NE to be 3.0/1000 live births (95% confidence interval (CI) 2.7–3.3) (Badawi et al. 1998a) and HIE to be 1.5 per 1000 live births (95% CI 1.3–1.7) (Thornberg et al. 1995; Badawi et al. 1998a; Smith and Dodd 2000).

Role of hypoxia–ischaemia in the causation of NE in industrialised countries

Population-based studies have found intrapartum hypoxia–ischaemia to be present in a small percentage of term children with cerebral palsy, ranging from 8% in Australia (Blair 1988) to 28% in western Sweden (Hagberg et al. 2001). The most recent Swedish cohort suggests that an increasing number of term infants now fulfil the American College of Obstetricians and Gynecologists' criteria of intrapartum events severe enough to cause cerebral palsy (Himmelmann and Uvebrant 2010). However, a systematic review of the English-language literature on the association between intrapartum hypoxia–ischaemia and NE at term reported the proportion of cerebral palsy associated with intrapartum hypoxia–ischaemia was 14.5%, suggesting that most cases of cerebral palsy in term infants are not associated with intrapartum hypoxia–ischaemia (Graham et al. 2008). The incidence of an umbilical arterial pH <7.0 at birth was 3.7 per 1000 births, of which 17.2% survived with neonatal neurologic morbidity, 16.3% had seizures and 24 of 6% died during the neonatal period (Graham et al. 2008). In this meta-analysis the incidence of HIE was 2.5 of 1000 live births.

Conversely, although not population-based, a study of 351 term infants who presented within 72 hours of birth with NE or seizures or both at two tertiary referral intensive care units (Cowan et al. 2000) defined intrapartum asphyxia as the presence of at least three of the following: (1) late decelerations on fetal monitoring or meconium staining; (2) delayed onset of respiration; (3) arterial cord blood pH <7.1; (4) Apgar score <7 at 5 minutes; and (5) multiorgan damage (Cowan et al. 2000). On the basis of magnetic resonance imaging (MRI) within 2 weeks of birth or postmortem examination, 80% of the neonates with NE and asphyxia had lesions of the deep grey matter, cortex or white matter consistent with an evolving hypoxic–ischaemic insult and 69% of neonates with only seizures within 3 days of birth had acute ischaemic or haemorrhagic lesions. The authors concluded that events in the immediate perinatal period are most important in neonatal brain injury.

Mid- and low-resource settings

Infants born in the world's least developed countries have a high risk of intrapartum-related injury and of intrapartum stillbirth (Lawn et al. 2009). Almost one-quarter of the world's 4 million annual neonatal deaths are caused by perinatal asphyxia; 22% and 99% of these deaths occur in low- and mid-resource settings

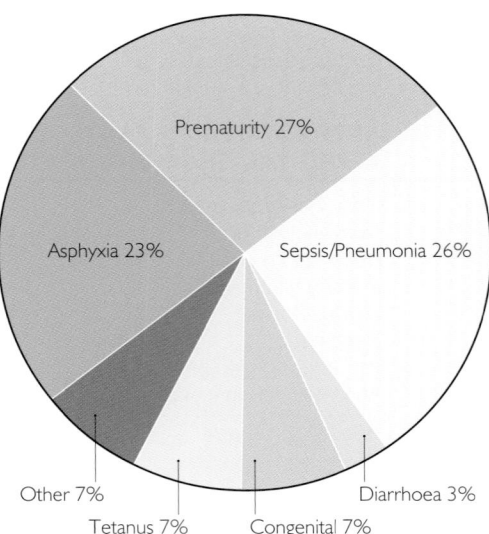

Fig. 40.24 Direct causes of neonatal death worldwide. Birth asphyxia is the direct cause of almost a quarter of the 4 million neonatal deaths worldwide. Infection is also a very significant problem. *(Adapted from Lawn et al. 2005.)*

respectively (Fig. 40.24). Severe infections are responsible for a further 26% of total estimated deaths (Lawn et al. 2005) and at times it is difficult to differentiate between the two conditions (Fig. 40.25). The World Health Organization *World Health Report* (2005) estimated that an annual 1 million survivors of 'birth asphyxia' may develop cerebral palsy, learning difficulties or other difficulties, although these numbers are difficult to estimate.

Precise estimates of NE and HIE incidence are uncertain as there is a lack of data from low- and mid-income countries and a complete absence of data from community-based settings where most of the burden of perinatal hypoxia–ischaemia falls. In 2006, an admission audit to the special care baby unit at Mulago Hospital, Kampala, Uganda revealed a moderate to severe NE incidence of 17.9/1000 term live births (M Nakakeeto, personal communication). In the Indian subcontinent, the Indian National Neonatal–Perinatal Database suggests an overall NE incidence of 14 per 1000 live births. As there is such a wide range in neonatal mortality rate (NMR) across countries throughout the world, a recent systematic review for the Global Burden of Disease Project estimated the incidence of NE by NMR category. In very-low-mortality settings (NMR< 5) (Fig. 40.25 and Table 40.15), the median incidence of NE is 1.9 per 1000 live births (range 0.7–6.0) compared with 26.5 per 1000 live births in the highest mortality settings (based on a single study) – a 14-fold disparity. Countries with NMR 6–15, 16–30 and 31–45 have an estimated median (range) incidence of NE of 6.7 (4.7–8.7), 9.8 (3.6–10.2) and 13.4 (5.5–22.2) (Lawn et al. 2009). South Asia and Africa, with large numbers of births and deaths, account for 73% of all intrapartum-related neonatal deaths worldwide.

Sensitising factors

Maternal pyrexia and maternal/fetal infection

Maternal intrapartum fever of >37.5°C has been shown to increase the risk of perinatal brain injury independently of infection (Badawi et al. 1998a) and increase the risk of early-onset neonatal seizures at term (Lieberman et al. 2000). There is also substantial experimental evidence that pre-existing intrauterine inflammation can

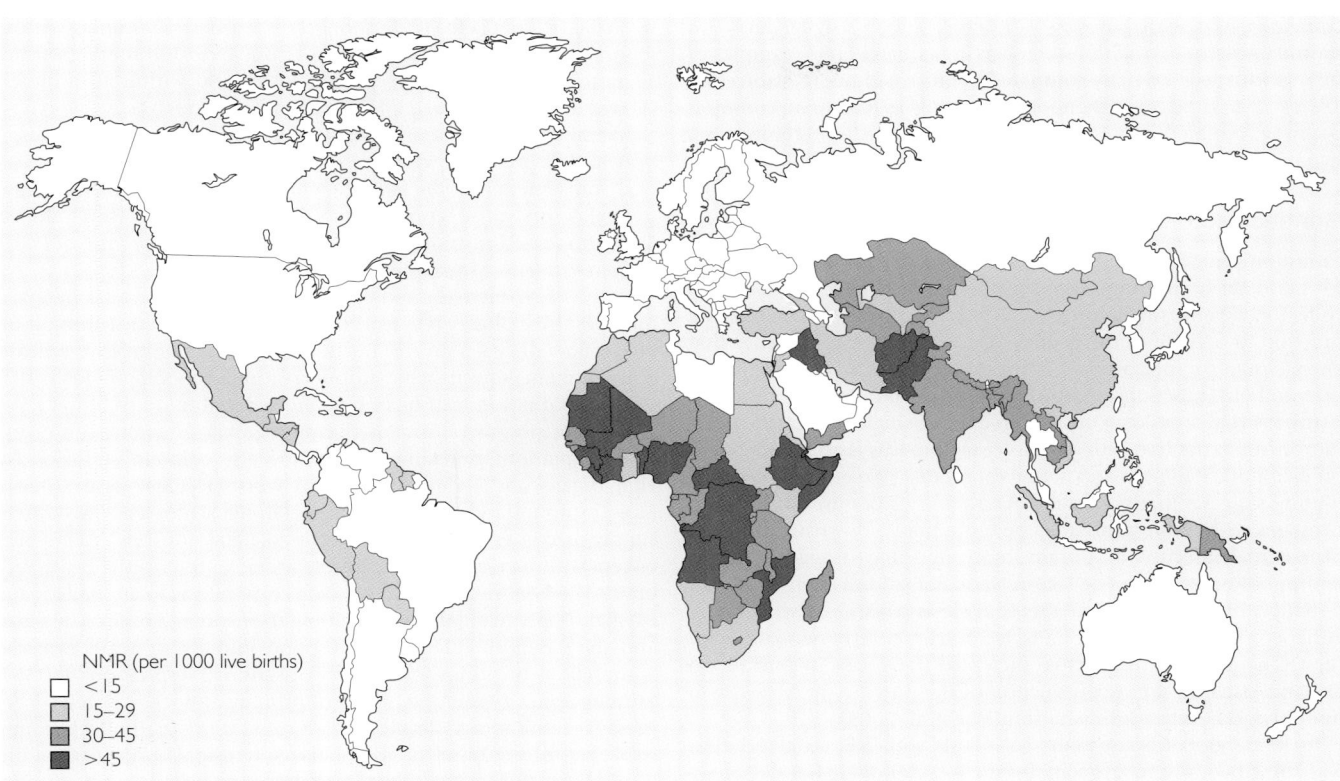

Fig. 40.25 Variation in neonatal mortality rate (NMR) between countries. *(Reproduced from Lawn et al. 2005, with permission.)*

NMR (per 1000 live births)
☐ <15
☐ 15–29
☐ 30–45
■ >45

Table 40.15 Variation in the incidence of neonatal encephalopathy (NE) and NE case-fatality for 193 countries organised according to five categories of neonatal mortality, as a marker of health system performance

	CATEGORY 1 VERY LOW MORTALITY NMR <5	CATEGORY 2 LOW MORTALITY NMR 6–15	CATEGORY 3 MODERATE MORTALITY	CATEGORY 4 HIGH MORTALITY NMR 31–45	CATEGORY 5 VERY HIGH MORTALITY NMR >45
Incidence of NE median (range)	1.9 (0.7–6.0)	6.7 (4.7–8.7)	9.8 (3.6–10.2)	13.4 (5.5–22.2)	26.5 (26.5)
NE case-fatality median (range)	21% (17–37)	12% (12%)	19% (10–28%)	31% (20–33%)	No data

Country groupings for neonatal mortality rates (NMRs) are adapted from the Lancet neonatal survival series (Lawn et al. 2005: Fig. 1). (Data adapted from Lawn et al. 2009.)

exacerbate hypoxic–ischaemic injury (Eklind et al. 2001; Lehnardt et al. 2003). A maternal intrapartum fever of > 38°C persisting >1 hour is usually considered a clinical indicator of chorioamnionitis; epidemiological studies suggest that chorioamnionitis is an independent risk factor for cerebral palsy among term and near-term infants (Wu et al. 2003). Indeed, term infants exposed to maternal infection are predisposed to delivery-room depression and NE (Nelson 2000). Convincing experimental (Eklind et al. 2001; Girard et al. 2009) and epidemiological evidence suggests that the 'dual hit' of combined infection and hypoxia–ischaemia results in more severe brain injury and increase in the risk of cerebral palsy (Longo and Hankins 2009). It is likely that this dual hit may be one of the

factors responsible for the worse neurological outcome even with mild or moderate NE reported from low and mid income countries (Ellis et al. 2000).

Cytokines are responsible for many normal cellular processes: the family of cytokines includes interleukins, interferons and the proinflammatory cytokines interleukin (IL)-1, 6, IL-8 and tumour necrosis factor-alpha (TNF-α). However, proinflammatory cyokines mediate a cascade of destructive cellular responses and higher levels of IL-6 and IL-8 were seen in the cerebrospinal fluid (CSF) of infants with HIE than control infants (Sävman et al. 1998). The levels of cytokines correlated with the NE stage and IL-6 correlated with outcome (Sävman et al. 1998). Other studies have shown that IL-1 correlated best with outcome (Aly et al. 2006). Higher levels of proinflammatory cytokines were seen in neonatal blood samples of infants with cerebral palsy compared to those without (Nelson et al. 1998). Cytokines may therefore be acting as the final common pathway initiated by a variety of insults, including infection, hypoxic–ischaemic injury and reperfusion injury.

Genetic factors

Common genetic variation has been implicated as a risk modulator for perinatal brain injury: specifically, minor changes in the DNA code for a gene single-nucleotide polymorphism that alters the function or activity of the gene product are reported in genes that encode putative mediators of brain injury. These include regulators of endothelial function, inflammation and thrombosis/thrombolysis pathways (Baier 2006). One example is the single-nucleotide polymorphism in the IL-6 gene promoter region: this is an independent predictor of CP in term and near-term infants (Wu et al. 2009). This finding suggests that the fetal inflammatory response observed in neonates with brain injury may be more than a downstream result of maternal infection and brain injury, and may instead represent an important pathogenetic factor. Neonatal studies of the IL-6-174 polymorphism suggest that the C allele is associated with either enhanced IL-6 production or adverse outcome. Term neonates with the CC genotype demonstrated increased IL-6 levels in cord blood and increased monocyte production of IL-6 in vitro, in response to lipopolysaccharide administration (Wu et al. 2009).

In severe global brain injury in infants with NE, an association was shown with homozygosity for the 677C>T allele (Dodelson de Kremer and Grosso 2005). The prevalence of the 677C>T allele was studied in 11 children with HIE, their mothers and 85 healthy individuals. Seven mothers were homozygous and four heterozygous for the 677C>T allele. Five of the children were homozygous and six heterozygous for this polymorphism. The variant allele frequency was higher in the group of mothers with affected children than in the controls and was associated with an increase in plasma homocysteine after methionine loading. The 677C>T mutation in mothers, either in a homozygous or heterozygous state, together with poor nutritional status (probable folate deficiency) may represent a risk factor for irreversible brain injury in the offspring (Dodelson de Kremer and Grosso 2005).

Impairment of fetal growth potential

Some epidemiological studies suggest that a significant proportion of neonates with NE demonstrate signs of antepartum injury, reflected in the impairment of their growth (Badawi et al. 1998b). In a case-controlled study to determine the frequency of growth impairment in NE, encephalopathic infants meeting criteria for an acute intrapartum hypoxic event (IHE, $n = 21$) and those who did not meet these criteria ($n = 20$) were compared with controls (Bukowski et al. 2003). More neonates with NE with and without IHE were below the 10th percentile of growth potential compared with controls. This association was similar in the presence or absence of IHE, which may suggest that antepartum injury has a causative rather than predisposing character in many cases of IHE.

Pathophysiology of hypoxia–ischaemia

Fetal responses to hypoxia–ischaemia

Animal models of acute, near-total hypoxia–ischaemia have demonstrated that fetal arterial P_{O_2} drops during acutely induced hypoxia–ischaemia from 25 mmHg to levels below 5 mmHg within 5 minutes, whereas arterial P_{CO_2} rises from 45 to 100 mmHg within 10 minutes, and pH drops from 7.30 to 6.80 within 10 minutes (Dawes 1969; Myers 1972). The fetus will respond to acute hypoxia–ischaemia in a number of ways, aiming to reduce energy consumption and to maintain cerebral oxygenation as much as possible. Body movements will be reduced, which is sometimes the first sign of fetal compromise reported by pregnant women. However, this is a very non-specific finding in term fetuses. With a lowering of Pa_{O_2}, oxygen extraction from the blood will increase.

In the experimental animal, the response to acute fetal hypoxia includes three phases (Peeters et al. 1979). First, a redistribution of blood flow directs a greater fraction of cardiac output to the heart and central nervous system without creating metabolic acidosis. The initial rapid fall in fetal heart rate and redistribution of blood flow away from peripheral organs during hypoxia or asphyxia are key fetal adaptations generally believed to help maintain perfusion of vital organs and reduce myocardial work (Fletcher et al. 2006). More profound hypoxia results in metabolic acidosis as the oxygen supply becomes inadequate to the skeletal muscles and some viscera with increasing diversion of cardiac output to the heart and brain. The final stage of fetal hypoxia corresponds to an inadequate oxygen supply to all organs, including the heart and brain. The fetus and the newborn infant both respond initially to acute hypoxia with shallow breathing followed by cessation of respirations, termed primary apnoea. After the period of primary apnoea, gasping (deep irregular respirations) develops, then respirations gradually become weaker until the onset of secondary or terminal apnoea when all respiratory effort ceases. Heart rate decreases from baseline during primary apnoea, decreases even lower during gasping and eventually ceases after several minutes of secondary apnoea. Blood pressure initially increases during primary apnoea and gasping, but then rapidly decreases during secondary apnoea (Fig. 40.26) (Wassink et al. 2007). Primary and secondary apnoea is not precisely distinguishable at birth – both present as a newborn who is not breathing and whose heart rate is slow. Tactile stimulation during primary apnoea can restore spontaneous respirations. Secondary apnoea requires assisted ventilation to restore spontaneous breathing (Dawes 1969).

Production of meconium can be induced by severe fetal hypoxia–ischaemia. In combination with gasping this may lead to meconium aspiration, and development of the meconium aspiration syndrome after birth (Ch. 27, part 2). In chronic fetal hypoxia, which may be the result of several maternal diseases such as severe anaemia, pregnancy-induced hypertension or pre-eclampsia, the fetus will produce erythropoietin to augment erythrocyte production through extramedullar haematopiesis. Increased numbers of erythroblasts have been reported to be a sign of chronic fetal hypoxia–ischaemia (Buonocore et al. 1999).

Mechanisms of brain injury

Initiating role of energy failure

Severe hypoxia–ischaemia rapidly results in cessation of cerebral oxidative metabolism, accumulation of cerebral lactate and rapid depletion of adenosine triphosphate (ATP). This initial decrease in ATP is capable of triggering a series of additional mechanisms that begin with failure of the ATP-dependent Na^+,K^+ pump (Fig. 40.27) (Volpe 2001). If the initial insult is very severe, the acute result is Na^+ influx followed by Cl^- and water influx, cell swelling, cell lysis and early death by necrosis. In the more usual less severe insult, membrane depolarisation occurs and is followed by extracellular accumulation of glutamate, increased cytosolic Ca^{2+} and a cascade

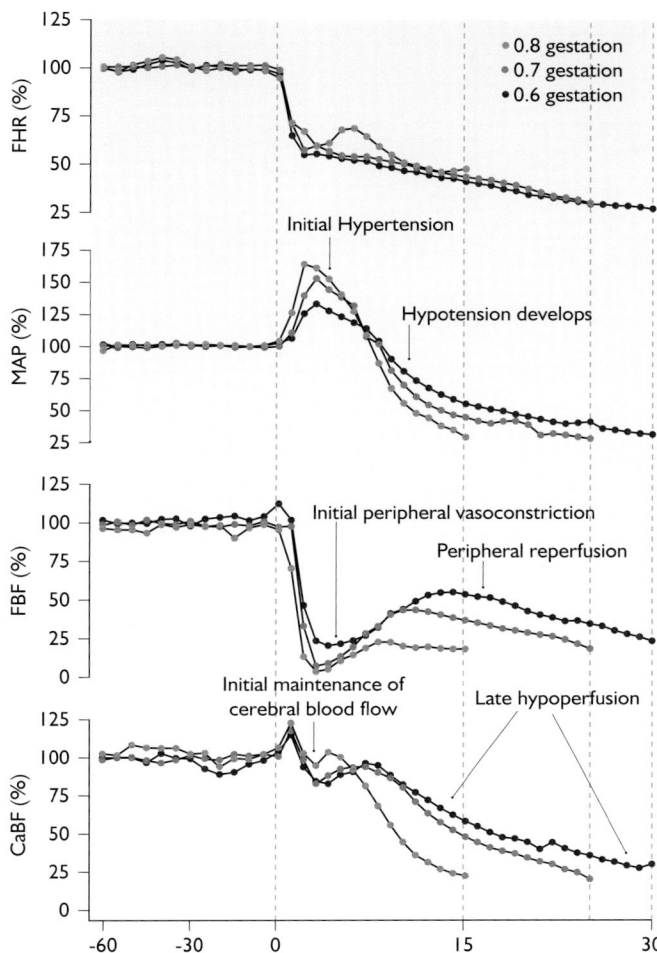

Fig. 40.26 Changes in fetal heart rate (FHR, bpm, top panel), mean arterial pressure (MAP, mmHg, second panel), femoral blood flow (FBF, ml/min, third panel) and carotid blood flow (CaBF, ml/min, bottom panel) in 0.6, 0.7 and 0.85 gestation fetuses during complete umbilical cord occlusion. FHR, MAP, FBF and CaBF data represent 1-minute averages and are expressed as a percentage of baseline. The period of umbilical cord occlusion for each group is indicated by the rectangles. Data are mean ± SE. *(Data from Wassink et al. 2007.)*

There is an initial period of compensation followed by progressive decompensation which ends by profound systemic hypotension and cerebral hypoperfusion. MAP initially rises with intense peripheral vasoconstriction; at this time CaBF is maintained at around baseline, but with suppression of electroencephalogram activity – although total brain flow does not change, within the brain, blood flow is diverted away from the cerebrum and increased in the brainstem. As umbilical cord occlusion was continued MAP eventually fell. The key mediators include impaired cardiac function secondary to hypoxia, acidosis, depletion of myocardial glycogen and cardiomyocyte injury and loss of the initial peripheral vasoconstriction. Once MAP falls below baseline, CaBF falls in parallel and there is loss of redistribution of flow within the brain.

of events leading to a more delayed cell death, principally apoptotic, although necrosis may also occur. Cell swelling can be demonstrated in vivo within 30 minutes using diffusion-weighted MRI techniques (Moseley et al. 1990). The details of the activated cascade of events are discussed below.

The accumulation of lactate and H^+ is initially beneficial as it leads to the generation of ATP from phosphocreatine (PCr) (due to the shift in creatine phosphokinase reaction) and an increase in CBF (due to the effect of acidosis on vascular smooth muscle). However, as severe tissue acidosis develops, detrimental effects of increased lactate and H^+ develop: autoregulation is lost, phosphofructokinase activity is inhibited, leading to reduced ATP production, and acidosis itself leads to neuronal injury and necrosis (Volpe 2001).

Release of excitatory amino acids

Excitotoxicity is an important mechanism of injury in the brain (Fatemi and Johnston 2009). Glutamate is the predominant excitatory amino acid neurotransmitter in the brain, and most neurons and many glia possess receptors for glutamate (Johnston 2005). Neuronal pathways mediating vision, hearing, somatosensory function, learning and memory use glutamate as their neurotransmitter (Johnston 2005). There are three major groups of glutamate receptors: (1) *N*-methyl-D-aspartate (NMDA); (2) α-amino-3-hydroxy-5-methylisoazole-4-propionic acid (AMPA); and (3) kainic acid. Normally, glutamate is contained within the presynaptic nerve terminal until release is stimulated by neuronal depolarisation (Santos and Voglmaier 2009); when release into the synaptic cleft does occur, the neurotransmitter is quickly taken up by high-capacity glutamate transporters in astroglia that surround synapses and nerve terminals (Santos et al. 2009).

Extracellular glutamate concentrations increase significantly with hypoxic–ischaemic insults (Hagberg et al. 1987; Silverstein et al. 1991) and CSF levels of glutamate of asphyxiated newborns are substantially higher than those of healthy newborn infants (Hagberg et al. 1991). Extracellular glutamate increases because of two reasons: firstly, impaired uptake of glutamate; and secondly, excessive release. Compared to the adult brain, the immature brain is especially vulnerable to activation of the NMDA receptor by glutamate (Calvert 2005). In addition the topography of glutamate receptors, particularly NMDA and APMA receptors, corresponds to the topography of the hypoxic–ischaemic neuronal injury (Johnston 1995). Further evidence of the central role that glutamate plays in hypoxic–ischaemic injury is the neuroprotection seen with the use of glutamate receptor blockers even when administered after termination of the insult (McDonald et al. 1990). Stimulation of the NMDA receptor leads to Ca^{2+} influx in to the cell and a large number of deleterious effects, described below (Fig. 40.28).

Calcium influx

There are many deleterious effects of increased cytosolic Ca^{2+} (Table 40.16) (Cheung et al. 1986). Different enzymes are activated, including proteases and lipases. Activation of lipases causes breakdown of cellular membranes and results in production of prostaglandins and leukotrienes. During this process oxygen free radicals are generated. Activation of proteases causes activation of the caspase cascade, leading to cellular apoptosis (see below). The utilisation of ATP by ATP-dependent Ca^{2+} transport systems, attempting to correct the Ca^{2+} accumulation, and the Ca^{2+}-mediated uncoupling of oxidative phosphorylation perpetuate the cycle. Another effect of calcium influx is activation of calcium-dependent isoforms of nitric oxide synthase (neuronal and endothelial forms).

Reactive oxygen and nitrogen species

Free radicals are highly reactive compounds with an uneven number of electrons in the outer orbital. During hypoxia–ischaemia, but even more so during reperfusion, reactive oxygen species (ROS) or oxygen free radicals and reactive nitrogen species (nitric oxide) are produced (Siesjö et al. 1989; Bågenholm et al. 1998). These highly

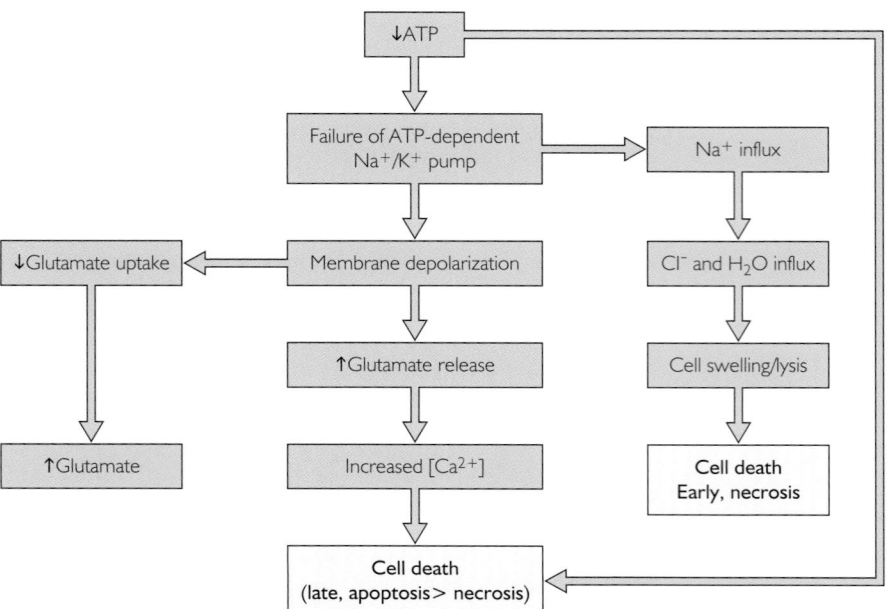

Fig. 40.27 Relation between energy depletion and cell death. Early cell death is mainly necrosis and the more important later cell death is mainly apoptosis. ATP, adenosine triphosphate.

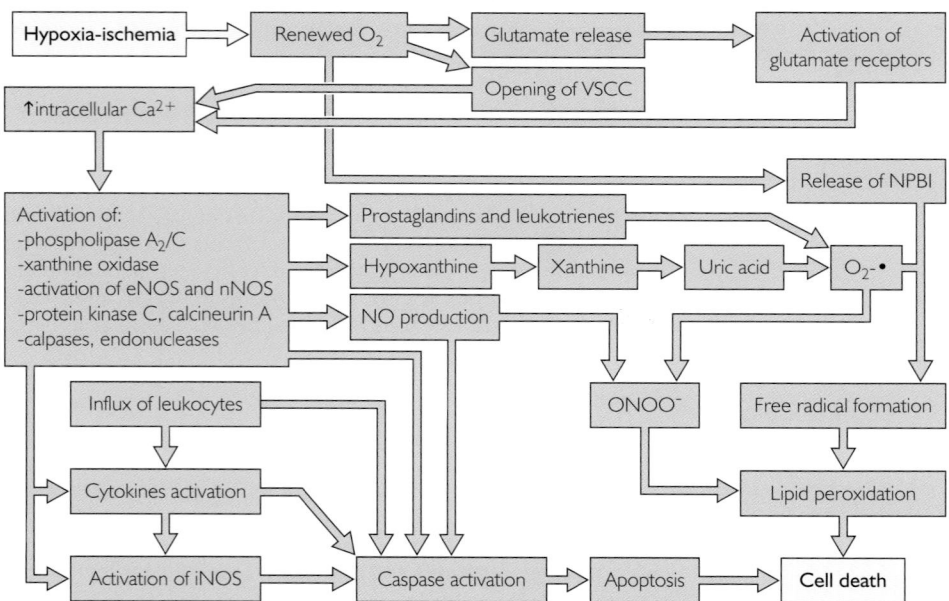

Fig. 40.28 A simplified diagram of the pathways leading to apoptotic cell death. VSCC, voltage-selective calcium channels; NPBI, non-protein-bound iron; eNOS, endothelial nitric oxide synthase; nNOS, neuronal nitric oxide synthase; O2⁻•, superoxide; ONOO⁻, peroxynitrite.

active chemical compounds react with cellular components and can generate new free radicals, thus producing a chain reaction, which results in irreversible injury (for example, peroxidation of fatty acids, membrane injury and cell necrosis). The body has enzyme systems, which defend the organism against injury by ROS, but these defence systems, including superoxide dismutase, may not be fully developed in the neonatal brain. Free radicals can lead to apoptotic cell death by activation of specific death genes (Blomgren 2006). The immature brain is also more vulnerable than adult brain to oxidative injury due to its pro-oxidant characteristics (high concentrations of polyunsaturated fatty acids and non-protein-bound iron) (McQuillen 2004). Production of ROS/oxygen free radicals is enhanced during resuscitation with 100% oxygen and may have long-term detrimental effects (Saugstad et al. 2008). For this reason current guidelines advise clinicians to resuscitate asphyxiated full-term neonates with room air.

Table 40.16 Damaging effects of increased [Ca^{2+}] due to hypoxia–ischaemia

CALCIUM ACTION	EFFECT
Activate phospholipases	Phospholipid hydrolysis and membrane injury Generation of free radicals by cyclooxygenase and lipoxygenase pathways
Activate proteases	Cellular skeleton disruption Proteolysis of other proteins
Activate nucleases	Nuclear injury
Activate calcium ATPase and other energy-dependent calcium extrusion mechanisms	Consumption of ATP at a time of deficient ATP
Uncouple mitochondrial oxidative phosphorylation	Decrease in ATP production
Increase glutamate and catecholamines	Activation of glutamate receptors
Activation of a protease that changes xanthine dehydrogenase to xanthine oxidase	Oxidation of hypoxanthine to xanthine and xanthine to uric acid with production of free radicals
Activate nitric oxide synthase	Generation of nitric oxide and peroxynitrite with toxicity to neurons

ATP, adenosine triphosphate.

Inflammation

Upon cerebral hypoxia–ischaemia and reperfusion many inflammatory pathways are activated, resulting in production of cytokines, infiltration of neutrophils into the brain and activation of microglia and macrophages (Hudome et al. 1997). Activated microglia begin to accumulate in the first 4 hours after reperfusion and continue to increase over the next 48 hours (Bona et al. 1999). Microglial cells release neurotoxic substances such as glutamate, cytokines, reactive oxygen and nitrogen species. Both IL-1β and TNF-α have been shown to increase in the brain 4–6 hours after the insult; an injection of IL-1β receptor antagonist ameliorates brain injury (Hagan et al. 1996). Antimicroglial agents such as minocycline are neuroprotective in several experimental paradigms of hypoxia–ischaemia, underlying the importance of microglia in the neurotoxic cascade (Arvin et al. 2002). As previously mentioned in the section on sensitising factors, activation of the immune response or coexisting infection (or exposure to molecular products of infection such as lipopolysaccharide) potentiates subthreshold hypoxic–ischaemic insults, leading to severe injury (Eklind et al. 2001; Lehnardt et al. 2003; Ikeda et al. 2004).

Pathways of cell death

Whilst necrotic cell death is prominent in the immediate and acute phases of severe cerebral insults, the predominant mode of cell death during the delayed phase of injury appears to be apoptosis (Northington et al. 2001a, b). This may be particularly true with less severe insults and apoptotic cell death seems to be more important in damage to the developing brain than after adult stroke (Northington et al. 2001a). In necrosis, death is triggered by an overwhelming insult, resulting in loss of membrane integrity and leaking cytoplasmic contents into the extracellular matrix. In contrast, cells dying by apoptosis carry out a highly conserved and regulated genetic programme (Fig. 40.29). They do not lose membrane integrity until late on and the organelles remain intact until the final stages when cell fragments are 'shrink-wrapped' in the contracting plasma membrane and bud off as apoptotic bodies, which are subsequently phagocytosed by healthy neighbouring cells. Apoptosis requires time and energy: although apoptosis and necrosis were considered distinct, there is a growing knowledge that dying cells may display a hybrid of apoptotic and necrotic features (Northington et al. 2007; 2011). The presence of a 'continuum' phenotype of cell death that varies on a cell-by-cell basis suggests that the phenotype of cell death is dependent on the energy available to drive the apoptotic pathways to completion (Northington et al. 2007).

Multiple apoptotic pathways have been shown to be involved in neonatal hypoxic–ischaemic cell death. As previously discussed, excitotoxicity, oxidative stress and other factors lead to injury of the mitochondrial membrane. An increase in the permeability of the mitochondrial membranes to molecules of less than 1500 Da in molecular weight (termed the mitochondrial permeability transition) plays an important role in multiple pathways to cell death (Blomgren 2006). Mitochondrial permeability transition leads to release of proapoptotic factors into the cytoplasm, including cytochrome c, apoptosis-inducing factor (AIF), caspase-9 and endonuclease G (Cao et al. 2007). Release of cytochrome c and procaspase-9 into the cytoplasm leads to activation of caspase-9 3–24 hours after the insult and is followed by conversion of procaspase-3 to active caspase-3 6–48 hours after injury (Gill et al. 2002). Caspase-3 activation results in proteolysis of essential cellular proteins, including cytoskeletal proteins and kinases, and can commit the cell to the morphological changes characteristic of apoptosis, including nuclear fragmentation (Wang et al. 2001). This cytochrome c-mediated pathway is also referred to as the intrinsic pathway. Activated caspase-3 has been shown in human postmortem brain tissue of full-term neonates with severe perinatal asphyxia.

Some cell surface receptors respond to cytokine (inflammatory) stimulation, resulting in activation of cell death signalling programmes. The TNF receptor superfamily (TNFRSF) belongs to this group of cytokine-responsive receptors. Fas death receptor is one of the most extensively studied TNFRSF members (Strasser and Nagata 2009). The apoptotic pathway that is regulated by Fas receptor involves caspase-8 and is referred to as the extrinsic pathway. Caspase-8 leads then to caspase-3 activation.

A caspase-independent apoptotic pathway has also been extensively studied. Poly(ADPribose) polymerase (PARP-1) is a nuclear enzyme that transfers adenosine diphosphate ribose groups from NAD+ to nuclear proteins and facilitates DNA repair. PARP activation consumes NAD+ needed for mitochondrial energy production, which in turn triggers release of cytochrome c and activation of caspases (Andrabi and Dawson 2008).

A knowledge of these pathways of cell death has led to a very important discovery about gender-specific cell death pathways: being male or female is likely to influence the efficacy of neuroprotective agents and the cells that are most at risk. Male neurons die mainly through activation of an AIF-dependent pathway while female neurons preferentially release cytochrome c from mitochondria and die as a result of subsequent activation of caspase 3 (Du

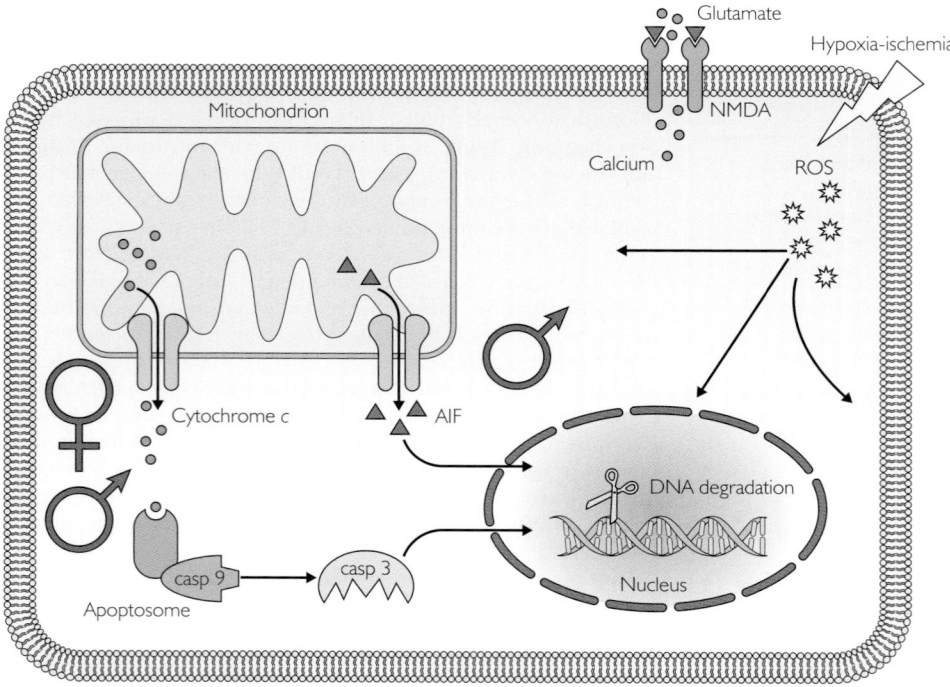

Fig. 40.29 Gender differences in neonatal apoptotic cell death after hypoxia–ischemia. Female neurons preferentially release cytochrome c from mitochondria and die as a result of subsequent activation of caspase 3. Male neurons are influenced more by the excitotoxic pathway and die mainly through the apoptosis-inducing factor (AIF)-dependent pathway. NMDA, *N*-methyl-D-aspartate; ROS, reactive oxygen species. *(Courtesy of Dr Cora Nijboer.)*

et al. 2009). Male neurons also have lower levels of glutathione following nitrosative stress than neurons from females. These sex-related differences in cell death pathways are present in neonatal mice and rats in vivo (Zhu et al. 2006). Gender influenced the neuroprotective efficacy of 2-iminobiotin treatment, which was neuroprotective and reduced cytochrome c release and caspase activation only in females (Nijboer et al. 2007). The glutamate antagonist dextromethorphan was protective against stroke in male but not female mice at 12 days of age – this supports the greater influence of the excitotoxic pathway in immature males (Comi et al. 2006).

This new information about gender differences in neuronal death pathways in experimental models is clinically relevant to perinatal asphyxia. The 2005 Surveillance of Cerebral Palsy in Europe study reported that male babies are at higher risk for cerebral palsy than females. In low-birthweight infants cognitive and motor outcome of brain injury is worse in males than in females (Johnston 2007). In future studies it will be important to determine the influence of gender in asphyxiated infants undergoing neuroprotective therapies and optimisation of therapy may require different agents for males and females.

Cerebral blood flow and autoregulation

In healthy neonates CBF is maintained within certain limits by autoregulation when arterial $P\text{CO}_2$ or blood pressure fluctuates. Studies using xenon clearance or Doppler ultrasound have demonstrated that autoregulation was impaired in full-term neonates with perinatal asphyxia, making cerebral perfusion pressure passive (Archer and Evans 1986; Pryds et al. 1990; Boylan et al. 2000). Infants with the poorest outcomes (isoelectric amplitude-integrated electroencephalogram (aEEG), death) had the highest values for

CBF and no autoregulation or CO_2 reactivity. Infants with burst suppression and moderate to severe brain injury had slightly elevated values for CBF and impaired autoregulation but sustained reactivity to CO_2. Infants without evidence of brain injury had normal values for CBF, intact autoregulation and reactivity to CO_2. This cerebral hyperaemia occurring in infants with perinatal asphyxia has been confirmed with Doppler studies and near-infrared spectroscopy studies. These studies showed an increase in CBF and decreased resistance between 6 and 130 hours. Other near-infrared spectroscopy studies have confirmed this loss of vascular reactivity, increase in cerebral blood volume and CBF (Wyatt 1993) as seen before in the fetal sheep (Marks et al. 1996). The postasphyxial newborn is in a state of vasoparesis and cerebral hyperaemia which correlates with the degree of brain injury. This state of maximal vasodilation may be related to the effects of elevated H^+, prostaglandins, adenosine, free radicals or nitric oxide. It is unknown, however, whether it is an adaptive mechanism to preserve brain injury or whether it causes additional injury.

Pathology

Animal models of term hypoxia–ischaemia

The use of animal models in the study of perinatal asphyxia has a long history. (LeGallois 1813) noted that, in newborn rabbits asphyxiated by submersion, respiration survived for 27 minutes, whereas in adult rabbits breathing ceased after 2 minutes. In 1870, Bert saw a similar resistance to asphyxia in the newborn rat submerged in water – respiratory movements lasted 30 minutes whereas in 20-day animals respirations ceased in 1.5 minutes (Bert 1870). Animal studies have shown that the premature animal is more tolerant of asphyxia than the term infant, which is in turn more resistant to asphyxia than the adult. These early studies have also shown that males appear to be less resistant than females and that high temperature, thyroxine, insulin or adrenalectomy reduces resistance to asphyxia.

The primate neonatal model shows very clearly that the pattern of brain injury is affected by the severity and type of hypoxia–ischaemia. Two distinct patterns of injury were described in the 1950s–1970s – acute total asphyxia (Ranck and Windle 1959) and chronic partial asphyxia (Brann and Myers 1975). Acute total asphyxia was induced in monkeys near term by detaching the placenta at hysterotomy under local anaesthesia, keeping the fetal membranes intact. Eleven to 16 minutes later the fetuses were delivered from their membranes and resuscitated. Two to 9 days later the monkeys were euthanised: there was a common pattern of symmetrical injury to the ventral posterior nuclei of the thalamus, putamen, globus pallidus, inferior colliculus, gracile and medial cuneate nuclei – a very similar topographical distribution to that seen in infants with basal ganglia and thalamus (BGT) injury following, for example, a sentinel event. The cerebral cortex was damaged in only one out of five monkeys and there was no relationship with cerebral vascular distribution. The injury began with primary nerve cells with secondary damage of myelin sheaths and astrocytic reaction.

In the mid-1970s, Brann and Myers (1975) established a different model of chronic partial asphyxia in the rhesus monkey to investigate the effect on the newborn monkey brain. Intrauterine asphyxia was produced in the pregnant term monkey by breathing halothane of a high enough concentration to cause a significant drop in mean blood pressure in the mother. Each fetus was exposed to asphyxia for 1–5 hours. At the end of the period of asphyxia, each fetus was delivered surgically, intubated and ventilated with 100% oxygen. Monkeys were given sodium bicarbonate and dextrose for correction of the acidosis and taken off the ventilator when able to breathe on their own. Five of the eight asphyxiated newborn monkeys exhibited low Apgar scores and delayed seizures starting from 14.5 hours after delivery. Following an average of 46 hours of survival the brains were perfusion-fixed and the pattern of brain injury assessed. A mainly symmetrical pattern of parasagittal injury was seen, involving the convexity of the hemispheres, particularly the paracentral and posterior parieto-occipital areas (Fig. 40.30a). In some newborn monkeys basal ganglia damage was present; however injury to brainstem structures was absent. In around half the animals there was an asymmetry and in these cases the left side was always more affected. A primate model of perinatal asphyxia is still used for neuroprotection studies (Juul et al. 2007). These findings are very similar to the pattern of injury in newborn infants who have experienced chronic partial asphyxia (Figs 40.30b and c and 40.31).

Patterns of injury

Using MRI, the patterns of hypoxic–ischaemic brain injury that have been described in pathology studies in the past can now be demonstrated with superb detail and resolution in vivo in human neonates (de Vries 2010a).

Basal ganglia/thalamus pattern

The BGT pattern of injury is the most common pattern seen in infants with HIE (Martinez-Biarge et al. 2010) when there has been a sentinel event such as a ruptured uterus or placental abruption during labour (Okereafor et al. 2008) involving 'acute near-total asphyxia'. This pattern is associated with more severe neonatal signs, more intensive resuscitation at birth, more severe encephalopathy

and more severe seizures (Miller et al. 2005). These deep nuclear structures are very susceptible to acute perinatal hypoxic–ischaemic injury because of their high metabolic rate and high concentration of NMDA receptors. BGT injury predominantly affects bilaterally the central grey nuclei (ventrolateral thalami and posterior putamina) and perirolandic cortex (especially around the central sulcus, interhemispheric fissure and insula) (Fig. 40.32). Brainstem injury often accompanies the BGT pattern of injury. Lesions are often seen in the midbrain (the inferior colliculus) and pons and the cerebellar vermis (Connolly and Griffiths 2007). This finding is in keeping with the studies of Ranck (1959) and (Faro and Windle, 1969) of asphyxiated monkeys with total asphyxia, and the primate studies of Juul et al. (2007) (see above).

BGT lesions vary in extent and severity (Fig. 40.33). Mild lesions are focal lesions in the ventrolateral nuclei of the thalamus and posterior putamen. Moderate lesions are defined as multifocal areas or more diffuse abnormalities on T2, involving several regions of the basal ganglia. In severe injury there is widespread abnormal signal intensity – this may involve the whole of the BGT area but often the caudate is spared. White-matter injury may occur with severe BGT injury as part of the original insult or occur secondarily to the BGT lesions and is seen later in infancy and associated with poor head growth (Mercuri et al. 2000).

The posterior limb of the internal capsule (PLIC) is actively myelinating at term-equivalent age and is also very susceptible to injury at this stage of development (Cowan 2005). Damage to the PLIC usually correlates with the severity of the BGT lesions. On MRI it can be described as normal, equivocal and abnormal. A normal PLIC is myelinating at term age and on MRI is seen as high signal on T1-weighted images and low signal but more ovoid shape on T2-weighted images (Fig. 40.33a). An abnormal PLIC has loss or reversed signal intensity on T1- and T2-weighted images (Fig. 40.33c,d); an equivocal PLIC is one with reduced or asymmetrical signal intensity (Fig. 40.33b).

Outcome

A total of 20–30% of infants with HIE die in the neonatal period and 15–20% of children may die in the first 2–3 years. Martinez-Biarge et al. (2010) have observed that the best predictor of death is the presence of brainstem lesions. They found that 50% of infants with brainstem lesions died in the neonatal or infant period.

Survivors face a range of functional impairments which include cerebral palsy, feeding problems, speech and language problems, visual and hearing impairment, later seizures and cognitive impairment. Cerebral palsy affects three-quarters of infants with HIE with BGT lesions and the severity of the BGT lesions is the best predictor of motor problems. The signal intensity of the PLIC is the best predictor of the ability to walk at 2 years (Martinez-Biarge et al. 2010). From their extensive experience in following infants with HIE, Martinez-Biarge et al. have produced very comprehensive flow charts for likely outcome for mild, moderate or severe BGT in surviving infants (Fig. 40.34a–c).

Watershed-predominant pattern

There are several terms for this pattern of injury – parasagittal cerebral injury or border zone injury. This injury pattern is thought to result from chronic partial hypoxia – in the primate model this injury was produced by several hours of maternal hypotension (see the section on animal models, above). The watershed pattern is also encountered after hypotension, infection and hypoglycaemia, all of which may be associated with a more chronic course and may be preceded by antenatal hypoxia. In one cohort representative of the spectrum of severity of term NE, the watershed-predominant injury pattern was the most common injury pattern, seen in 45% of the cohort (Miller et al. 2005); however a mixed pattern is often seen and watershed injury is often accompanied by less severe BGT injury.

The injury comprises cortical necrosis involving the immediately subjacent white matter with characteristic distribution, encompassing the parasagittal, superomedial areas of the convexities bilaterally, with posterior (parieto-occipital) more involved than anterior regions. The areas of necrosis in watershed injury are in the border zones between the major cerebral arteries. These border zones are the areas most susceptible to ischaemia from a fall in perfusion pressure (Fig. 40.30a–c). Another very vulnerable area for ischaemic cerebral injury is at the depth of the sulci.

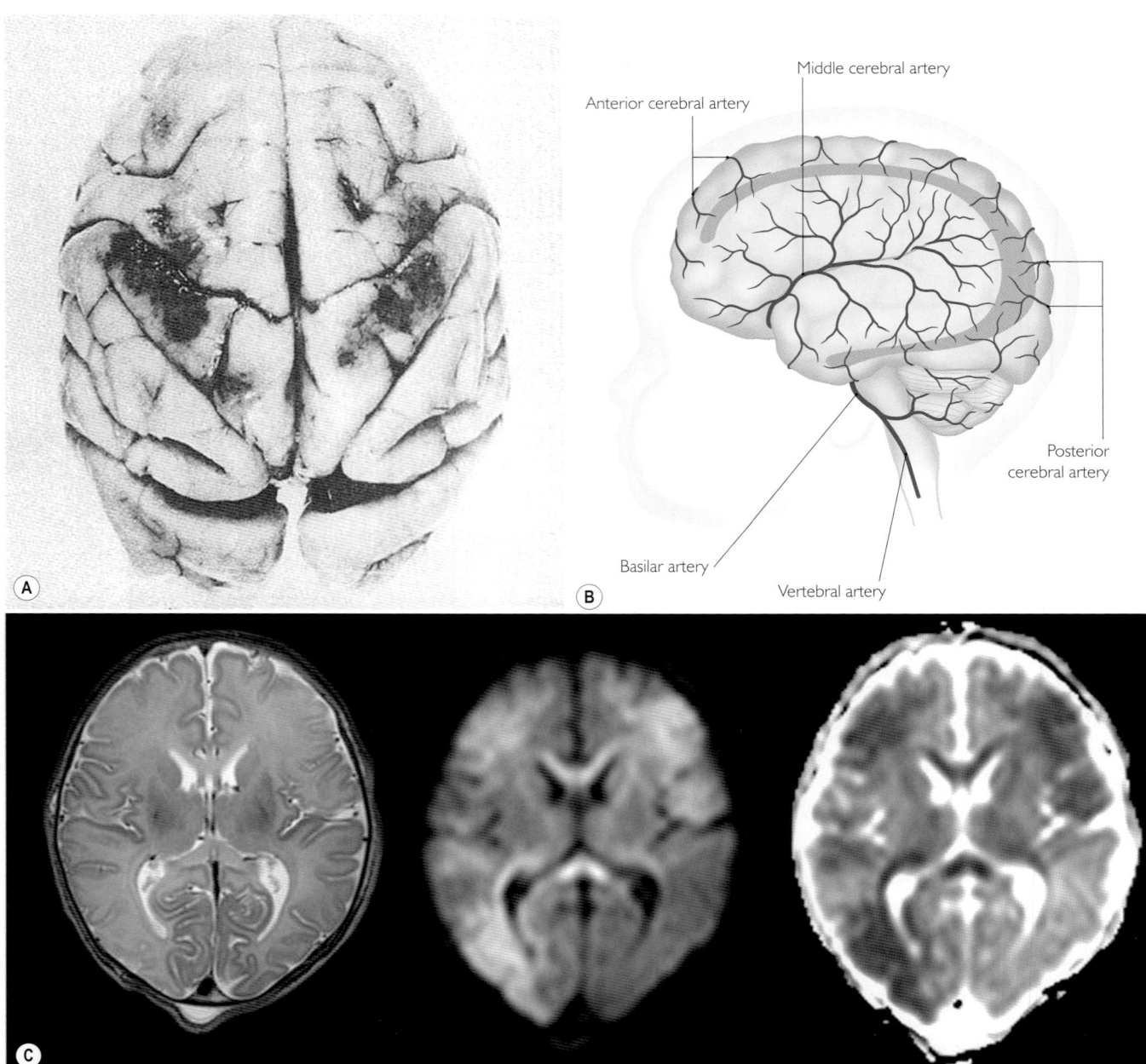

Fig. 40.30 (a) Symmetical foci of haemorrhagic injury of the newborn rhesus monkey following chronic partial hypoxia–ischaemia. Intrauterine asphyxia was produced in the pregnant term monkey by breathing halothane of a high enough concentration to cause a significant drop in mean blood pressure in the mother. Each fetus was exposed to asphyxia for 1–5 hours. A symmetrical pattern was seen involving the convexity of the hemispheres, particularly paracentral and posterior parieto-occipital. (Reproduced with permission from Brann and Myers 1975.) (b) Distribution of the major cerebral arteries. The distribution of injury as shown by the shaded area is in the border zones and end fields of these arteries. (c) Full-term neonate born after vacuum extraction for fetal bradycardia. Seizures occurred from 6 hours after birth. Magnetic resonance imaging at 3 T on day 4 showed watershed lesions on T2-weighted imaging (left), diffusion-weighted imaging (middle) and apparent diffusion coefficient map (right) in the area of the anterior and middle cerebral arteries, and middle and posterior cerebral arteries. Follow-up at 3 years showed a Griffiths developmental quotient of 97 and a preference for her left hand.

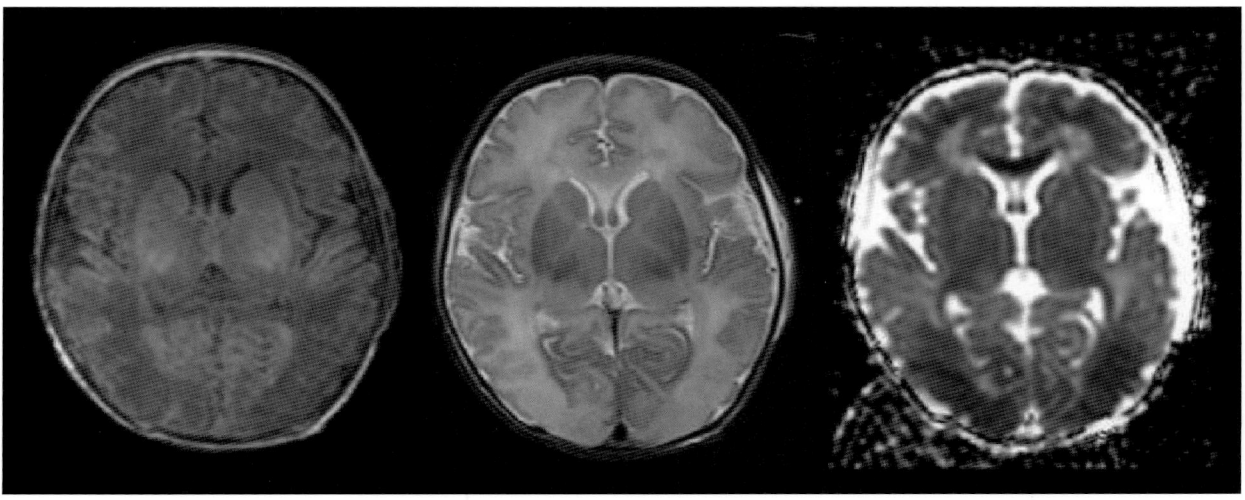

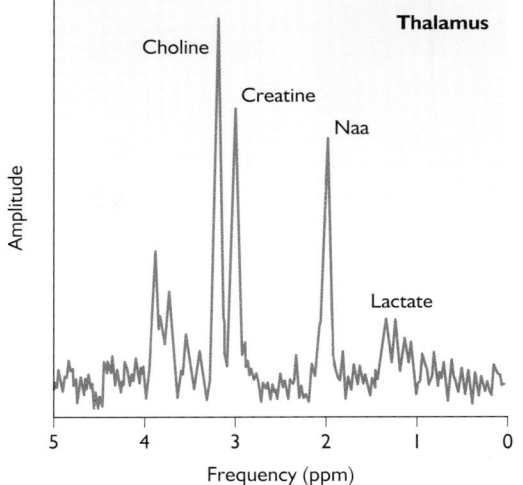

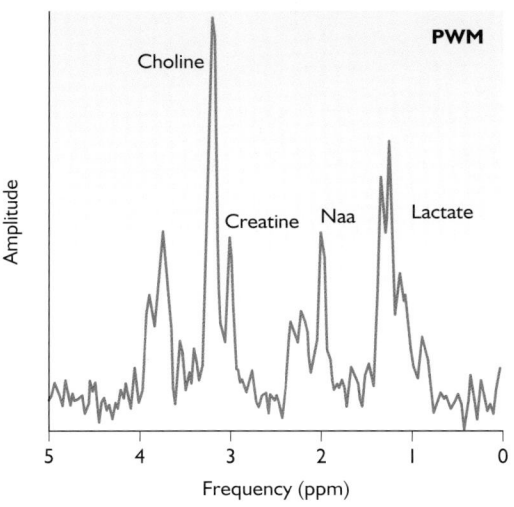

	Naa/Cho	Naa/Cr	Cho/Cr	Lac/Cho	Lac/Cr	Lac/Naa
Thalamus	0.71	1.18	1.65	0.28	0.46	0.39
PWM	0.46	1.36	2.97	0.95	2.83	2.08

Fig. 40.31 Magnetic resonance imaging at 1.5 T on day 3 of T1-weighted imaging (top left, movement artifacted), T2-weighted imaging (top middle) and apparent diffusion coefficient map (top right). There are bilateral parieto-occipital and frontal oedema with loss of the cortical ribbon and cortical restricted diffusion, in keeping with parasagittal watershed infarction. There is some oedema in the thalami and posterior limb of the internal capsule. Appearances are in keeping with a watershed-predominant pattern. Proton magnetic resonance spectroscopy (PRESS, TE 288 ms) of the left thalamus and basal ganglia (left) and left posterior white matter (PWM) (right) are shown below. The peak area ratios from the spectra are shown in the table. Although lactate/NAA peak area ratio is raised in both brain areas, the most significant changes are in the PWM voxel. Naa, *N*-acetyl aspartate; Cho, choline; Cr, creatine; Lac, lactate.

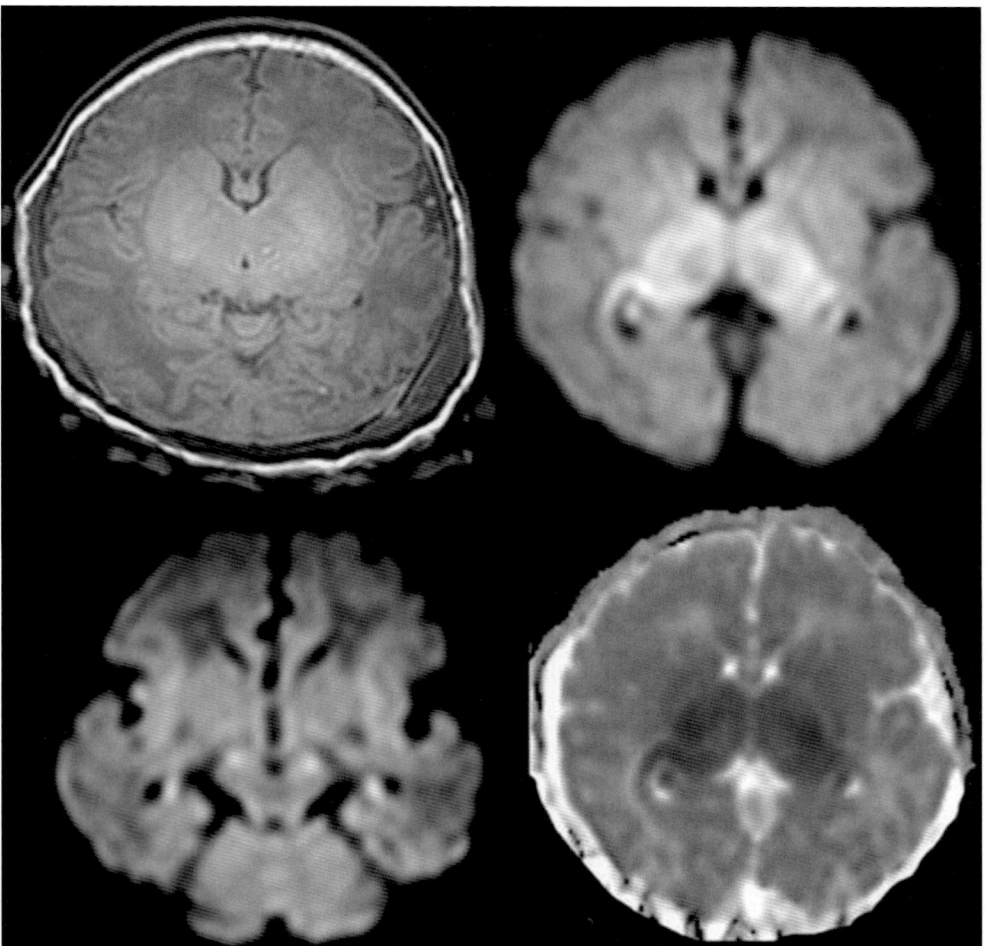

Fig. 40.32 Full-term neonate with severe perinatal asphyxia. Magnetic resonance imaging at 3 T on day 4 showing swelling of the basal ganglia on T1-weighted imaging (top left), signal changes in the basal ganglia and thalamus on diffusion-weighted imaging (top right), and apparent diffusion coefficient map (bottom right) and extension of the abnormalities into the cerebral peduncles (bottom left).

Takashima and Becker (1978) showed that, as sulci form and deepen near term in the human brain, the meningeal vessels are forced to bend acutely at the cortical–white-matter junction. This area represents 'a border zone within a border zone'. Therefore cerebral injury is more severe in the depths of the sulci; over time the cortex of the affected gyri shrinks and the term 'ulegyria' is used to define the type of cortical abnormality characterised by atrophy at the depth of the sulci and relative sparing of the crest of the gyri (Nikas et al. 2008). The term 'ulegyria' was introduced from the Greek word ουλη' (scar) and its presence suggests that the injury occurred around term age. With further development, additional vessels appear to supply this area.

Outcome

BGT and watershed injuries are associated with impairments in different developmental domains. Infants with a watershed pattern of injury have predominantly cognitive impairments, often without functional motor deficits. Cognitive deficits include memory impairments, visual–motor or visual–perceptive dysfunction, or increased hyperactivity, sometimes in the absence of functional motor problems (Gadian et al. 2000; Barnett et al. 2002; Marlow et al. 2005; Gonzalez 2006). These cognitive deficits often result in delayed school-readiness and a need for additional school-age

interventions (Armstrong-Wells et al. 2010). Cognitive deficits may not be detected at 12 months – therefore school-age assessment is needed, as are ongoing formal neuropsychological evaluation, as well as parental and teacher education, to help aid in the cognitive and behavioural rehabilitation resulting from perinatal hypoxic–ischaemic brain injury.

Global pattern

Involvement of the subcortical white matter and cortex can be seen, referred to as the 'white cerebrum', as diffusion-weighted imaging (DWI) shows an almost completely white cerebrum, in contrast with a normal-looking cerebellum. These patients show severe NE and the condition tends to be fatal. In the rare surviving neonate, multicystic encephalomalacia will develop (Fig. 40.35). Another important cause of multicystic encephalomalacia is central nervous system infection, especially with herpesvirus.

Cerebral energy metabolism associated with hypoxia–ischaemia

Magnetic resonance spectroscopy (MRS) has been used to study brain energy metabolism non-invasively; over the last 30 years

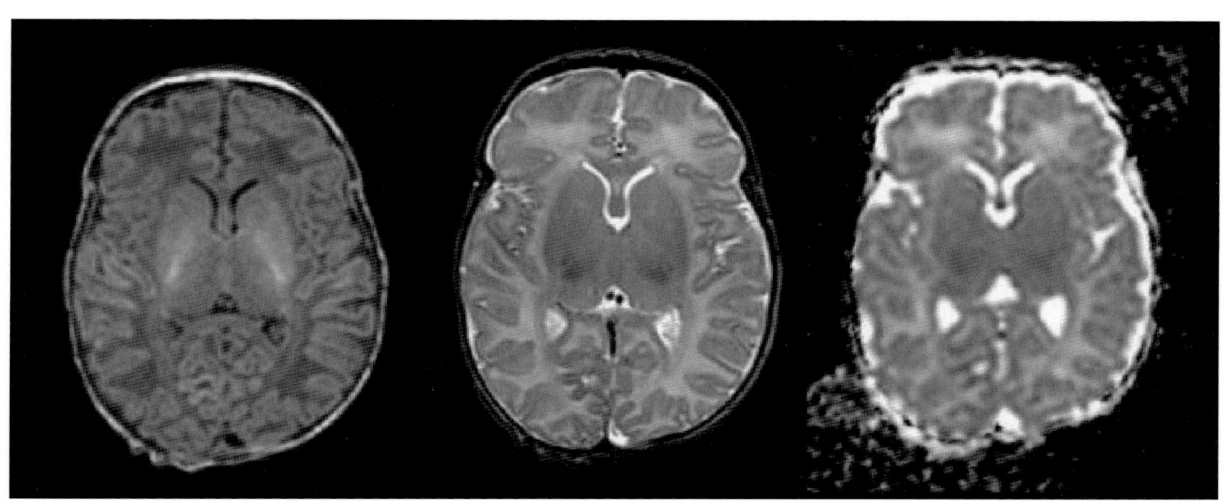

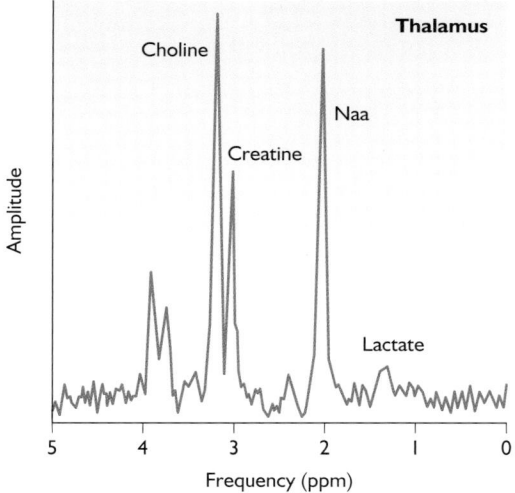

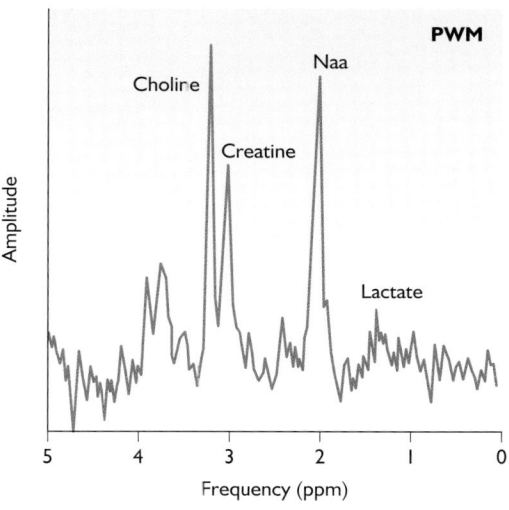

	Naa/Cho	Naa/Cr	Cho/Cr	Lac/Cho	Lac/Cr	Lac/Naa
Thalamus	1.04	1.72	1.65	0.15	0.24	0.14
PWM	1.19	2.12	1.78	0.16	0.28	0.13

(A)

Fig. 40.33 T1-weighted image (top left), T2-weighted image (top centre) apparent diffusion coefficient map (top right). Proton magnetic resonance spectroscopy (MRS) (PRESS, TE 288ms) spectra from basal ganglia and thalamus and posterior white matter (PWM). The ^{1}H MRS metabolite peak area ratios are shown in the table. (a) Normal full-term infant scanned at 1.5 T on day 4. The MRI and MRS findings are within the normal range. A normal PLIC is seen as high signal on T1-weighted images and low signal but a more cvoid shape on T2-weighted images.

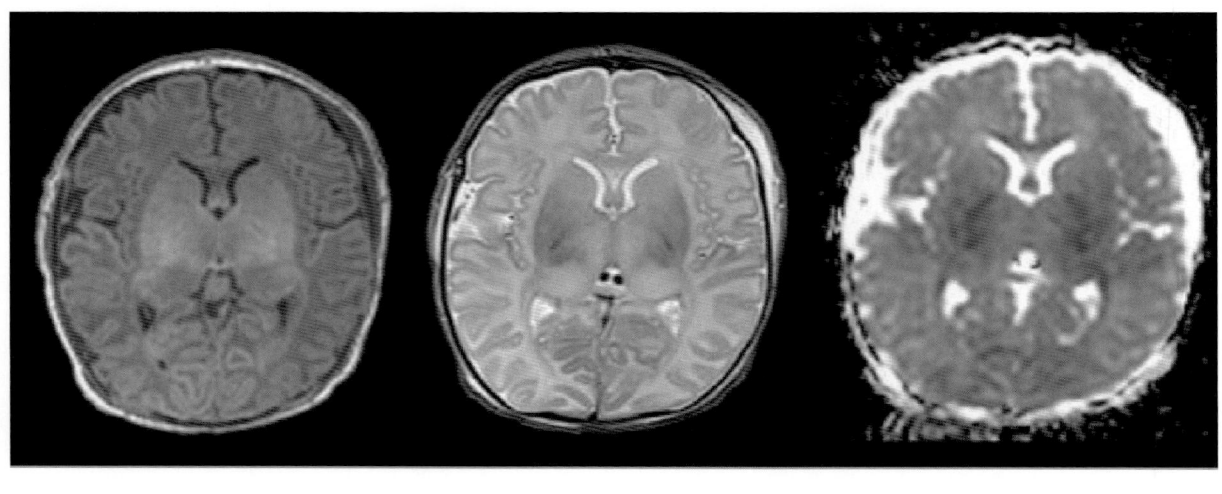

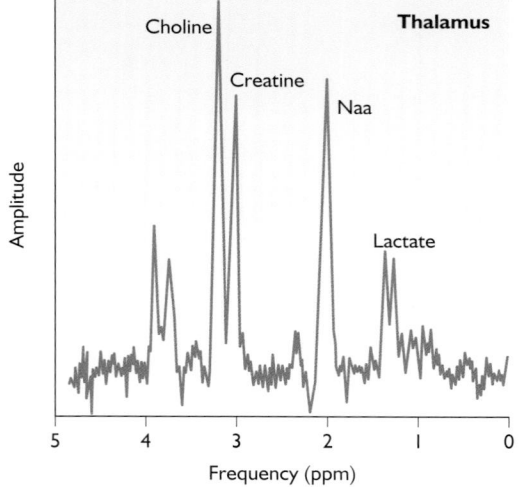

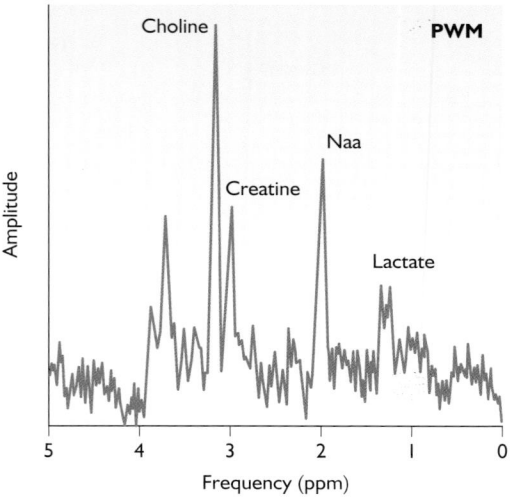

	Naa/Cho	Naa/Cr	Cho/Cr	Lac/Cho	Lac/Cr	Lac/Naa
Thalamus	0.83	1.40	1.69	0.53	0.90	0.64
PWM	0.77	1.63	2.13	0.47	1.00	0.62

(B)

Fig. 40.33, cont'd (b) Full-term infant with Sarnat Stage 2 neonatal encephalopathy scanned on day 4. Bilateral moderate basal ganglia swelling and oedema with restricted diffusion are seen on the apparent diffusion coefficient map. ^{1}H MRS peak area ratios demonstrate a raised lac/N-acetyl aspartate (NAA) peak area ratio in both the basal ganglia and thalamus (BGT) and PWM; the upright lactate doublet can be seen clearly at 1.3 ppm and the NAA peak height is reduced.

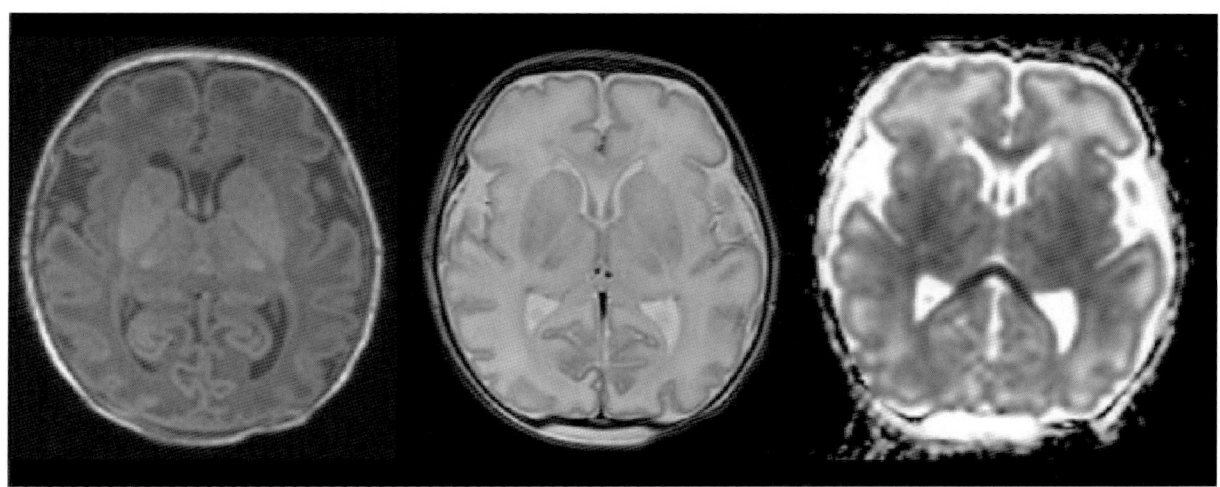

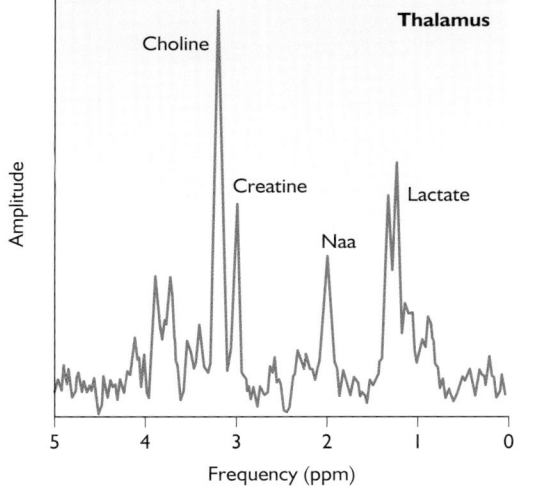

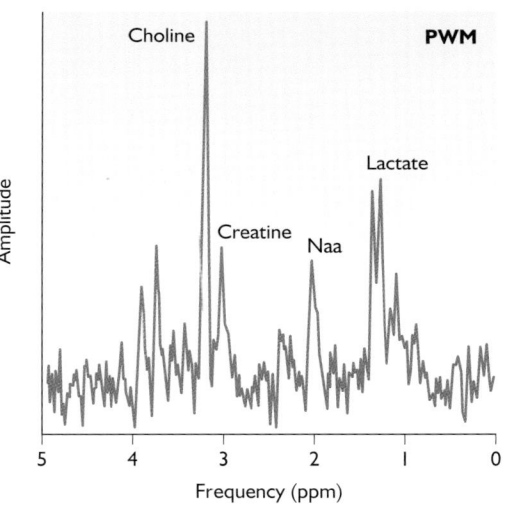

	Naa/Cho	Naa/Cr	Cho/Cr	Lac/Cho	Lac/Cr	Lac/Naa
Thalamus	0.43	1.14	2.66	0.79	2.11	1.85
PWM	0.37	1.35	3.63	0.84	3.04	2.26

(c)

Fig. 40.33, cont'd (c) Full-term infant with Sarnat Stage 3 neonatal encephalopathy scanned on day 6. There is marked swelling and oedema in the BGT, midbrain and pons, in keeping with profound hypoxic–ischaemic brain injury. There are also diffuse oedema and swelling in the cerebral hemisphere white matter. ^{1}H MRS peak area ratios show markedly raised lactate/NAA ratios due to a markedly raised lactate and reduced NAA. A peak is seen also at 1.1 ppm due to propan-1,2 diol, the carrier for phenobarbital.

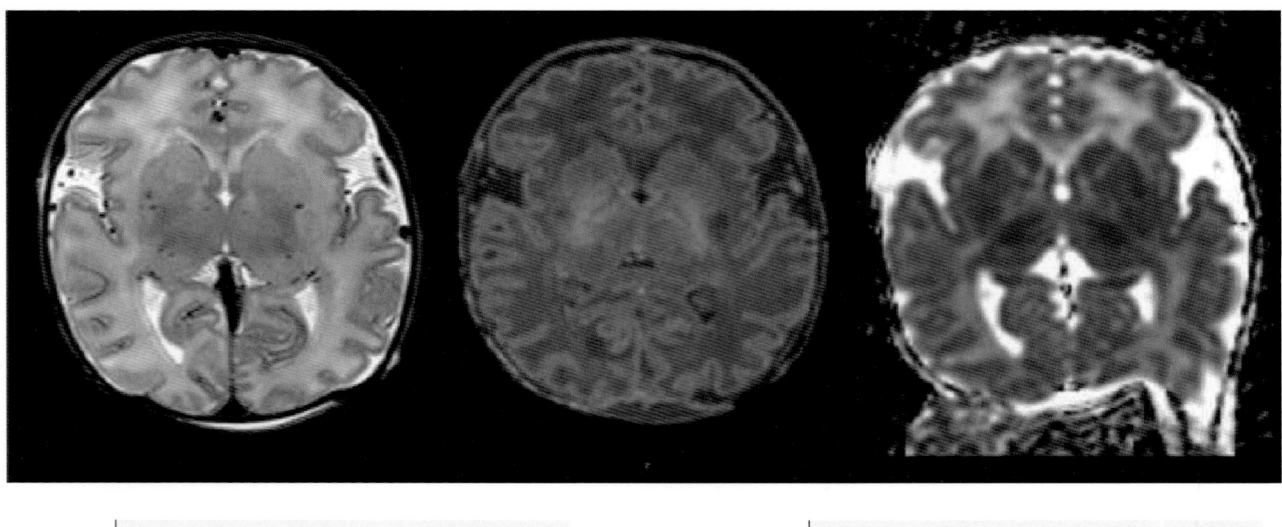

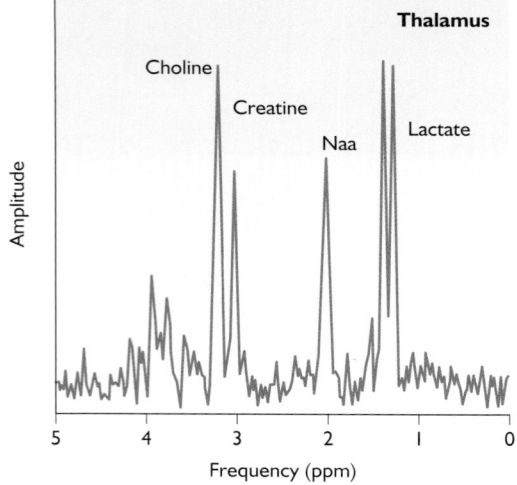

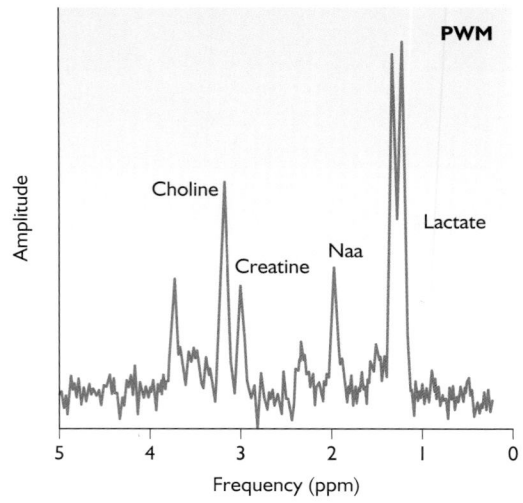

	Naa/Cho	Naa/Cr	Cho/Cr	Lac/Cho	Lac/Cr	Lac/Naa
Thalamus	0.68	1.10	1.63	1.71	2.78	2.52
PWM	0.65	2.07	3.20	2.65	8.48	4.10

(D)

Fig. 40.33, cont'd (d) Full-term infant with Sarnat Stage 3 neonatal encephalopathy scanned on day 1. There are bilateral BGT infarction (including lentiform and caudate nuclei), infarction of the perirolandic cortex and both hippocampi. There is involvement of both cerebral hemispheres, in keeping with very severe global hypoxic–ischaemic injury. The lactate doublet is significantly raised in both BGT and PWM.

phosphorus-31 (^{31}P) and proton (^{1}H) MRS have provided unique information on cerebral energy metabolism during the evolution of brain injury following hypoxia–ischaemia in the newborn infant (Azzopardi et al. 1989), neonatal rat (Blumberg et al. 1997) and newborn piglet (Lorek et al. 1994; Iwata et al. 2007). In human infants, shortly after intrapartum hypoxia–ischaemia ^{31}P MRS often reveals apparently normal cerebral energetics (Hope et al. 1984). However, in infants with adverse outcome, despite adequate oxygenation and circulation, PCr and nucleotide triphosphate (NTP, mainly ATP) decline, and Pi increases, in the first days of life (Hope et al. 1984; Azzopardi et al. 1989; Martin et al. 1996; Cady et al.

1997). These metabolic changes were termed 'secondary energy failure' (SEF) on the basis that they followed impaired intrapartum cerebral energy generation (resulting in transiently reduced PCr and NTP and increased Pi), which resolved following resuscitation (Lorek et al. 1994). It was assumed that SEF was consequential to a pathological mechanism initiated by intrapartum hypoxia–ischaemia and/or reperfusion/reoxygenation. ^{1}H MRS provides complementary information to ^{31}P MRS (in particular cerebral lactate, a marker of anaerobic metabolism and N-acetyl aspartate (NAA), an abundant amino acid found mostly in neurons in the central nervous system (Urenjak et al. 1992)) and because of the

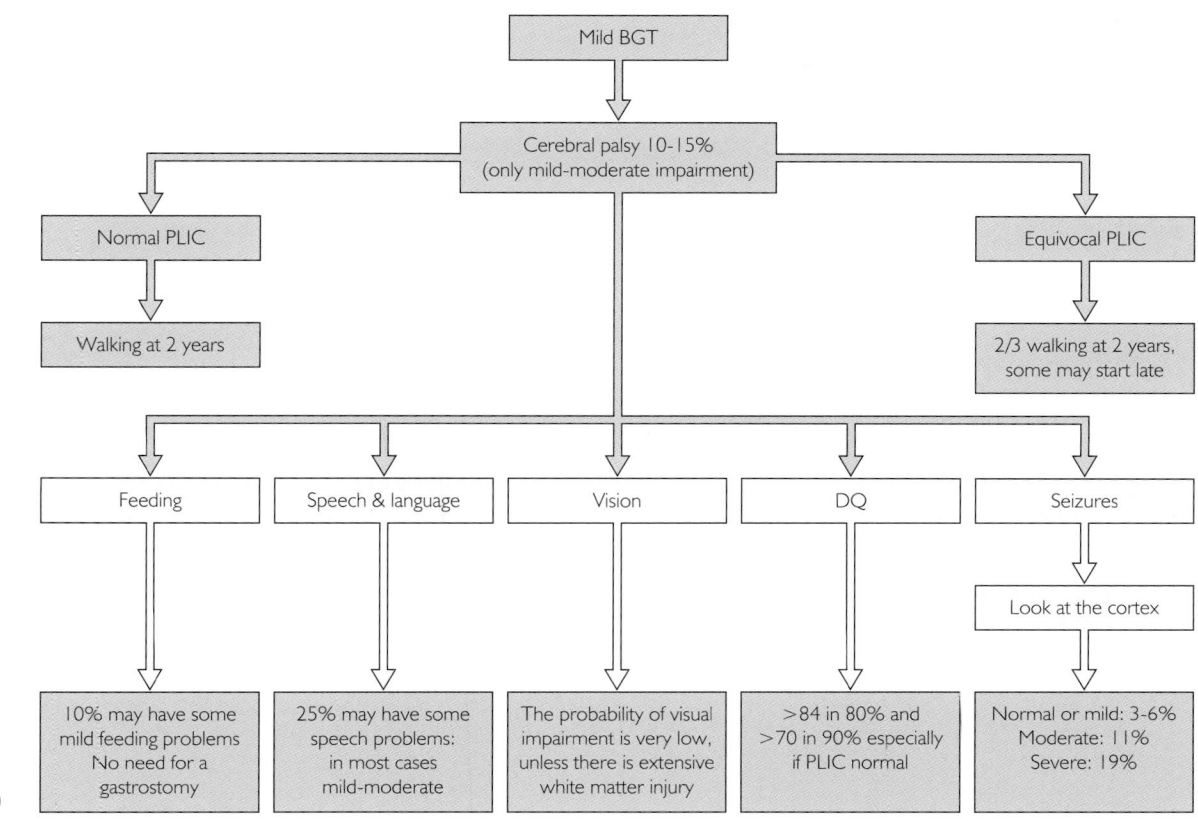

Fig. 40.34 (a) Flow chart showing patterns of outcome with mild basal ganglia and thalamus (BGT) injury.

greater sensitivity of the ¹H nucleus, data can be obtained from smaller regions of the brain. NAA appears as a singlet peak in the ¹H MR spectrum and is easier to quantify than lactate (Fig. 40.33a–d). The roles of NAA include action as: (1) an osmolyte (Baslow 2002); (2) a supplier of acetate for myelin sheath synthesis (Chakraborty et al. 2001); (3) a facilitator of mitochondrial energy generation (Madhavarao et al. 2003); and (4) a ligand for some metabotropic glutamate receptors (Yan et al. 2003). Cerebral lactate increases and NAA decreases during transient hypoxia–ischaemia; these metabolites return almost to baseline levels after successful resuscitation, only to be followed by a secondary increase in lactate and slower reduction in NAA in the hours that follow. These ¹H MRS changes occur in parallel with the energy disruption (reduction in PCr/exchangable phosphate pool (EPP) and NTP/EPP) seen on ³¹P MRS (Fig. 40.36).

We have used the composite biomarker consisting of the ratio of the cerebral lactate (Lac) and NAA peak areas at TE 288 ms (Lac/NAA) in our MRS studies of NE. The reciprocal changes in Lac and NAA concentrations increase the sensitivity to detect even minor neural injury, as well as enabling assessment of more severe injury. A recent meta-analysis of the prognostic accuracy of MR methods demonstrated that thalamic ¹H MRS Lac/NAA peak area ratio acquired between days 5 and 14 is a highly sensitive and specific biomarker of long-term neurodevelopmental outcome in infants with NE (Thayyil et al. 2010). Lac/NAA was more predictive than any other MRI technique including early and late conventional MRI, presence or absence of the normal signal from the PLIC and apparent diffusion coefficient (ADC) imaging.

Biphasic impairment of cerebral energy metabolism with transient hypoxia–ischaemia has been demonstrated in the newborn piglet (Lorek et al. 1994; Peeters-Scholte et al. 2003; Iwata et al. 2007); these studies provided a basis for the realisation that rescue treatment after hypoxia–ischaemia may reverse or ameliorate SEF. Experimental studies with moderate hypothermia (Thoresen et al. 1995) and other potential therapies soon followed (Peeters-Scholte et al. 2003). Recent work in the piglet model has shown that hypothermia extends the therapeutic window for other pharmacological therapies and the more severe the hypoxia–ischaemia, the shorter the therapeutic window (Iwata et al. 2007).

Biomarkers of brain injury

A biomarker is a characteristic that is objectively measured and evaluated as an indicator of normal biologic processes, pathogenic processes or pharmacologic responses to a therapeutic intervention. Biomarkers are needed in infants with HIE to predict which infants are most at risk of an abnormal outcome and who would benefit most from neuroprotective intervention (early biomarkers) and to predict long-term outcome following neuroprotective interventions (late biomarkers) (Azzopardi 2010a).

Markers of exposure to hypoxia–ischaemia

Markers of exposure to hypoxia–ischaemia are the obvious biomarkers to predict outcome; however many of these measures have low

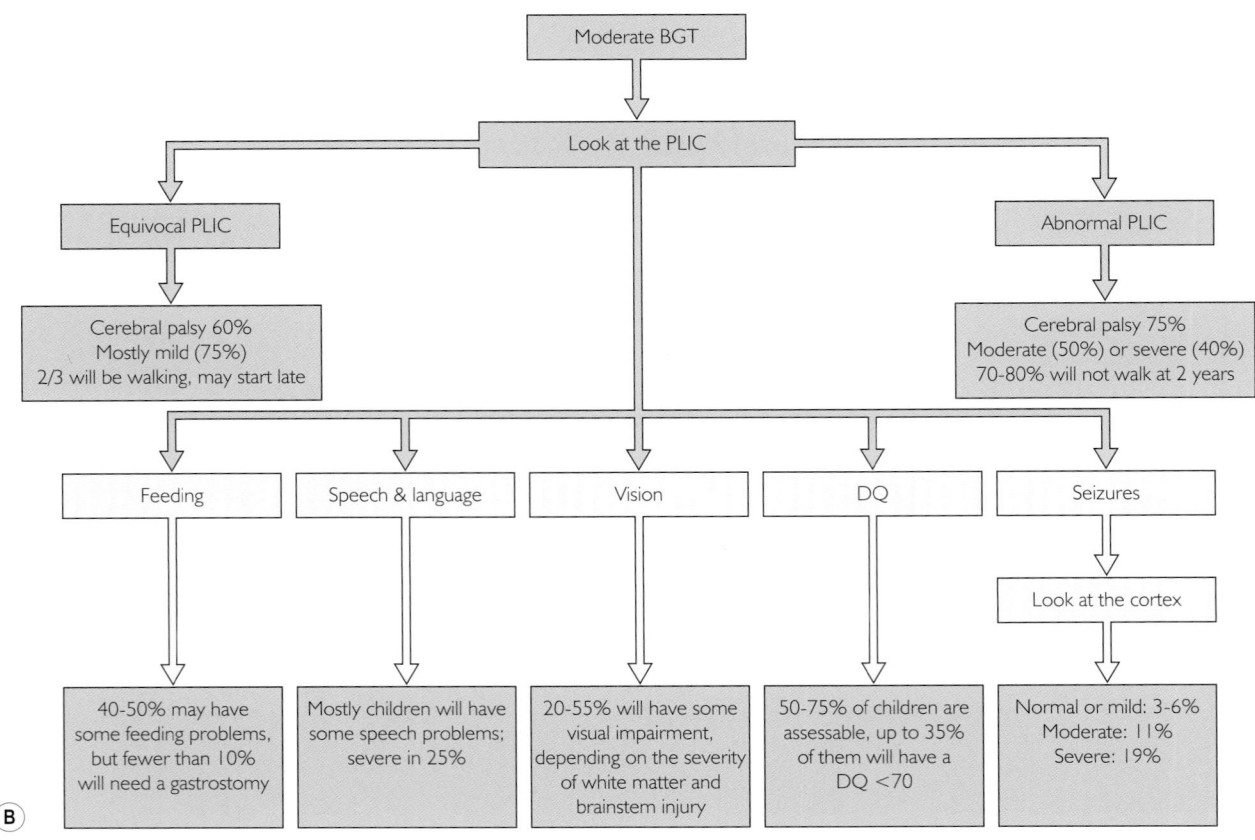

Fig. 40.34, cont'd (b) Flow chart showing patterns of outcome with moderate BGT injury.

predictive values for neural injury. For example, the presence of non-reassuring fetal heart changes, increased base deficit and blood lactate values on cord blood gases and need for resuscitation (i.e. Apgar score) infer exposure to hypoxia–ischaemia and are routinely recorded. However, non-reassuring heart rate changes are well known to have a very low positive predictive value for neural injury (Nelson et al. 1996). Base deficit (Low and Derrick 1997) and fetal lactate concentrations show an imprecise relationship with NE (Wiberg et al. 2010). Early neonatal lactate values in blood are predictive of encephalopathy stage (da Silva et al. 2000; Shah and Smyth 2004).

Biochemical biomarkers

Currently, many of the biochemical biomarkers can distinguish between mild and severe injury, but are not able to predict outcome accurately in infants with moderate or stage II encephalopathy. In a recent meta-analysis serum IL-1β and IL-6, and CSF IL-1β and NSE measured before 96 hours of age were predictive of long-term outcome (Ramaswamy et al. 2009). IL-6 (Chiesa et al. 2003), S100 beta (Qian and Wang 2009), Activin A (Florio et al. 2007), adrenomedullin and protein carbonyls are raised in the umbilical cord samples of hypoxic infants compared to controls. However so far only IL-6 and S100 beta have shown any ability to distinguish between grade of HIE (Qian and Wang 2009). Qian and Wang

(2009) showed that umbilical arterial S100 beta, at a cut-off of 2.02 µg/L, had a sensitivity of 86.7% and a specificity of 88.0% for predicting moderate or severe HIE, although an alternative grading system to the Sarnat system was used in this study. In another study a cut-off >1.0 µg/L urinary protein S100 beta had a sensitivity/ specificity of 100% for predicting neonatal death (Gazzolo et al. 2009). Nucleated red blood cells have been shown to be higher in encephalopathic infants with abnormal cerebral Doppler ultrasound, abnormal cranial ultrasound (cUS) and outcome at 2 and 3 years (Buonocore et al. 1999). A urinary lactate-to-creatinine ratio has been associated with adverse outcome in infants with HIE (Huang et al. 1999; Oh et al. 2008), but the significant overlap between normal/mild and moderate/severe disability groups limits the predictive value of this measure. Further research into the time course of changes in relation to the evolution of brain injury as well as into new methodologies such as bioinformatics and metabolomics (Chu et al. 2006) is needed before we can be sure that any of these measures can improve early outcome prediction.

Imaging biomarkers

In clinical practice, MRI is increasingly used after perinatal asphyxia as an effective tool for diagnosis and treatment efficacy assessment (Rutherford et al. 2010). To increase prognostic objectivity, quantitative cerebral biomarker modalities such as ^{1}H MRS have also been

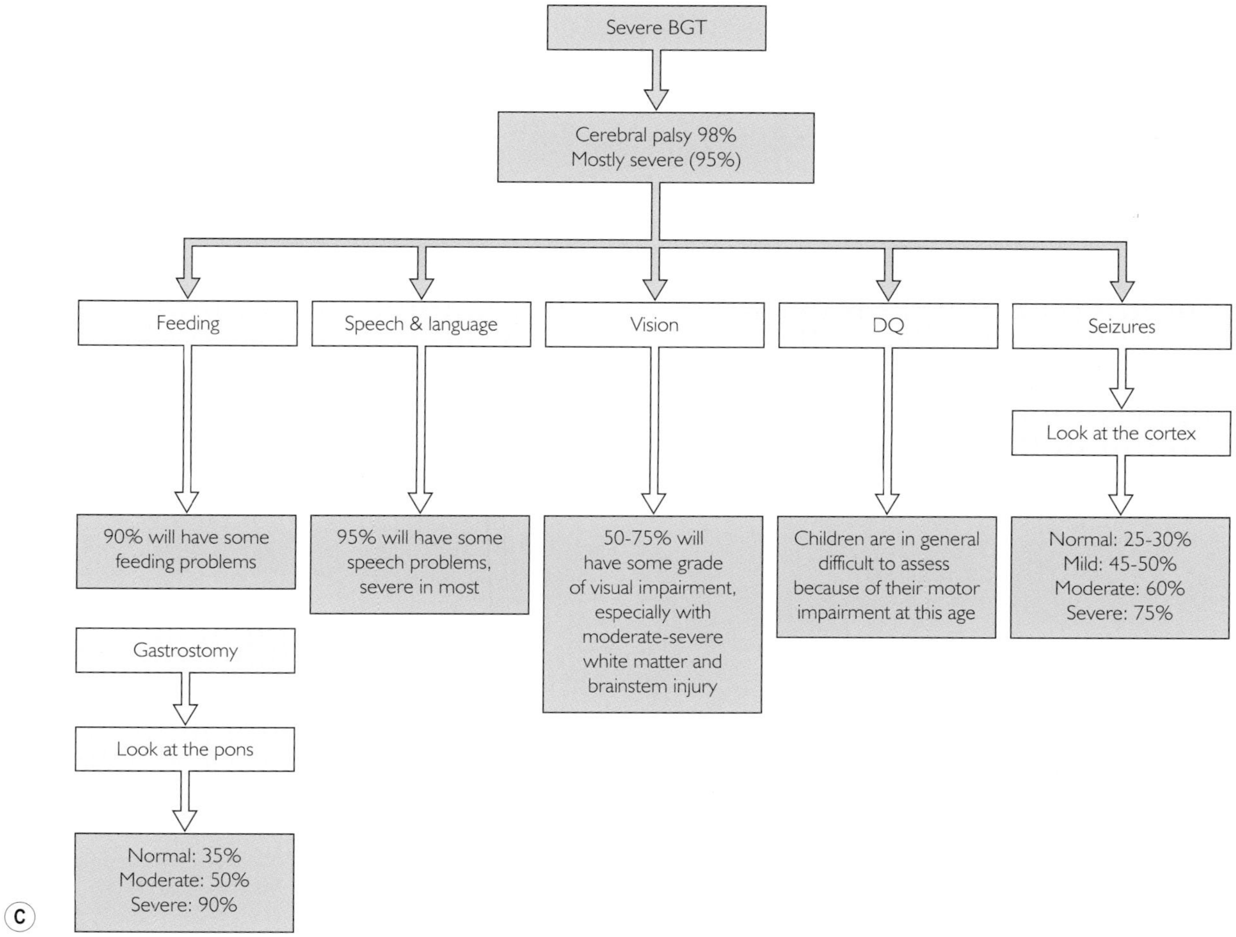

Severe BGT

↓

Cerebral palsy 98%
Mostly severe (95%)

```
Feeding          Speech & language     Vision              DQ                  Seizures
                                                                                 ↓
                                                                            Look at the cortex
```

90% will have some feeding problems	95% will have some speech problems, severe in most	50-75% will have some grade of visual impairment, especially with moderate-severe white matter and brainstem injury	Children are in general difficult to assess because of their motor impairment at this age	Normal: 25-30% Mild: 45-50% Moderate: 60% Severe: 75%

Gastrostomy

↓

Look at the pons

↓

Normal: 35%
Moderate: 50%
Severe: 90%

(C)

Fig. 40.34, cont'd (c) Flow chart showing patterns of outcome with severe BGT injury. DQ, developmental quotient; PLIC, posterior limb of internal capsule. *(Reproduced from Martinez-Biarge et al. 2010.)*

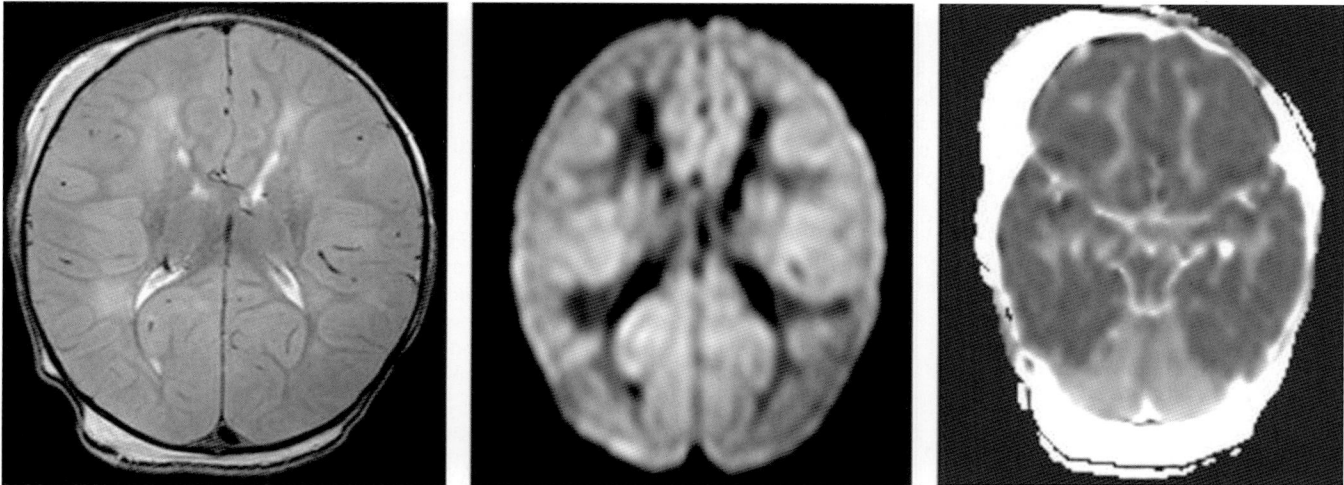

Fig. 40.35 Full-term neonate with severe perinatal asphyxia and 'white-brain' pattern of injury. Magnetic resonance imaging on day 3 shows diffuse swelling of the brain (T2-weighted image, left), elevated signal intensity in the whole cerebrum (diffusion-weighted imaging, middle) and a striking discrepancy between the severe abnormalities in the cerebrum and the spared cerebellum (apparent diffusion coefficient map, right).

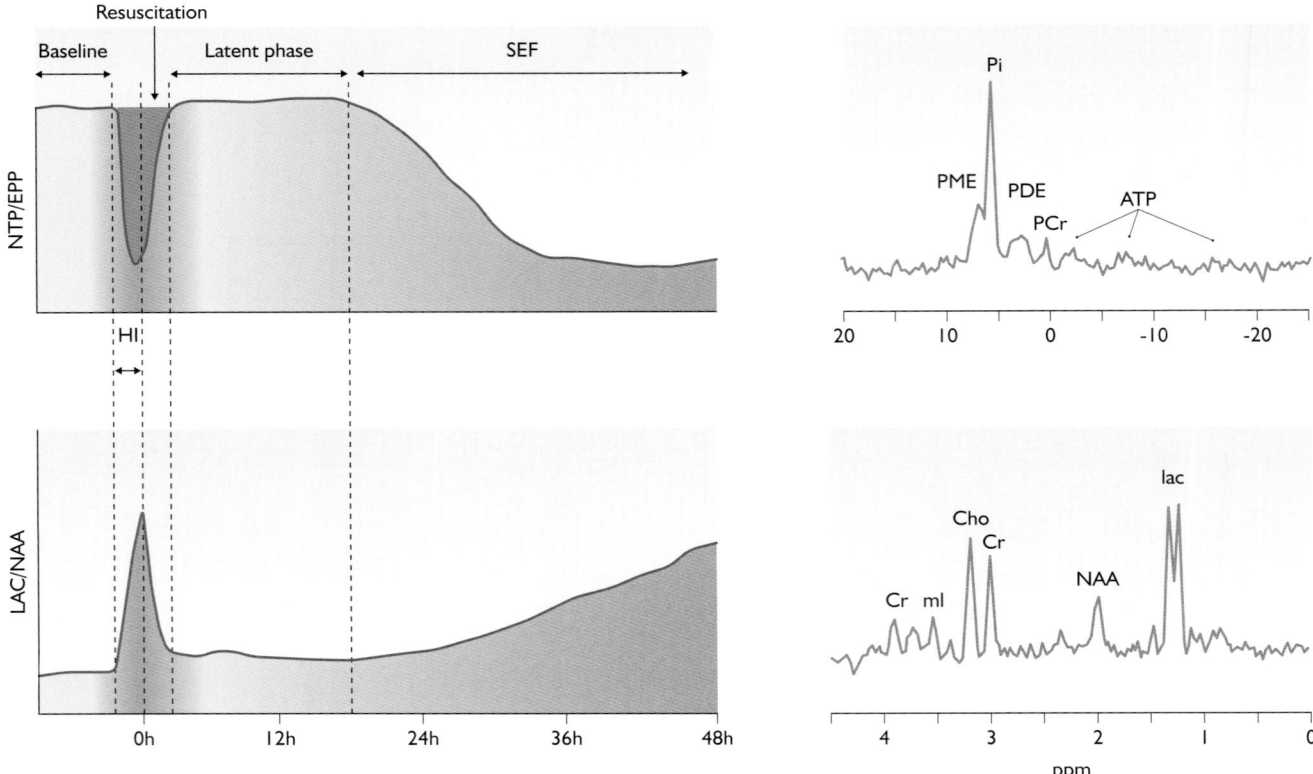

Fig. 40.36 The biphasic pattern of energy failure associated with a transient hypoxic–ischaemic insult visualised using ^{31}P MRS (top) and ^{1}H MRS (bottom) in the UCL piglet model. ^{31}P MRS: Nucleotide triphosphate (NTP)/exchangeable phosphate pool (EPP = Pi + PCr + NTP) is shown on the y-axis. The change in NTP/EPP during transient hypoxia–ischaemia (HI), resuscitation, the latent phase (period between the recovery from acute HI and the evolution of secondary energy failure (SEF)) and SEF itself are shown. A ^{31}P MR spectrum from a severely asphyxiated baby is shown on the top right. ^{1}H MRS: Lactate (Lac)/N-acetyl aspartate (NAA) is shown on the y-axis. The change in Lac/NAA during transient HI, resuscitation, latent phase and SEF are shown. A ^{1}H MR spectrum from a severely asphyxiated infant is shown on the bottom right.

During the acute energy depletion, some cells undergo primary cell death, the magnitude of which will depend on the severity and duration of HI. Following perfusion, the initial hypoxia-induced cytotoxic oedema and accumulation of excitatory amino acids typically resolve over 30–60 minutes with apparent recovery of cerebral oxidative metabolism (latent phase). It is thought that the neurotoxic cascade is largely inhibited during the latent phase and that this period provides a 'therapeutic window' for therapies such as hypothermia and other agents. Cerebral oxidative metabolism may then secondarily deteriorate 6–15 hours later (as SEF). This phase is marked by the onset of seizures, secondary cytotoxic oedema, accumulation of cytokines and mitochondrial failure. Mitochondrial failure is a key step leading to delayed cell death.

used (Robertson et al. 1999; Cheong et al. 2006; Azzopardi 2010a). As described above, a recent meta-analysis demonstrated that the cerebral ^{1}H-MRS Lac/NAA peak area ratio acquired 5–14 days after birth is the most sensitive and specific biomarker of long-term neurodevelopmental outcome in NE (Thayyil et al. 2010); this surrogate outcome measure is currently being used in a phase II clinical trial of hypothermia versus hypothermia plus inhaled xenon with the aim of speeding up clinical translation of effective therapies. The search for robust, sensitive and specific biomarkers is an important area for future research.

Clinical aspects

Fetal compromise

The intrapartum period is a time of risk for asphyxia; intrapartum care aims to identify those babies who are experiencing hypoxia–ischaemia. The fetus is generally well adapted to cope with the physiological stress normally imposed by labour, but on occasion the 'reserve capacity' is overwhelmed. The aim of intrapartum monitoring is to detect this.

Intrapartum fetal monitoring

When intermittent auscultation is used for low-risk pregnancies, twice as many babies will require admission to the neonatal intensive care unit (NICU) with NE than if electronic monitoring is used; however intermittent auscultation is supported by a Cochrane review (Alfirevic and Gyte 2006). Continuous cardiotocography during labour was associated with a reduction in neonatal seizures, but no significant differences in cerebral palsy, infant mortality or other standard measures of neonatal well-being (Alfirevic and Gyte 2006).

Some studies suggest electronic fetal monitoring correlates well with metabolic acidosis and neurological injury. The best intrapartum fetal heart rate parameter to predict development of acidaemia was minimal/absent variability for at least 1 hour (a single abnormal finding) or accompanied by late decelerations in the absence of accelerations (Williams 2003). However, although the sensitivity

Table 40.17 Clinical staging and typical outcome of hypoxic–ischaemic encephalopathy

	SEVERITY OF ENCEPHALOPATHY		
	Mild	**Moderate**	**Severe**
Level of consciousness	Alert or hyperalert	Lethargy	Stupor or coma
Spontaneous activity	May be normal	Decreased activity	No activity
Posture	May be normal	Distal flexion, complete extension	Decerebrate
Tone	Normal or hypertonia	Hypotonia (focal or generalised)	Flaccidity
Primitive reflexes			
Suck	Weak	Weak	Absent
Moro	Exaggerated	Incomplete	Absent
Autonomic function			
Pupils	Dilated	Constricted	Deviated, dilated or non-reactive to light
Heart rate	Tachycardia	Bradycardia	Variable
Respiration	Normal	Periodic breathing	Apnoea
Others	Irritability, jitteriness	Brainstem dysfunction	± elevated intracranial pressure
Seizures	Absent	±	Frequent, often refractory to anticonvulsants
EEG background	Normal	Low-voltage, periodic or paroxysmal	Periodic or isoelectric
Outcome	Normal	20–40% abnormal	Death or 100% abnormal

EEG, electroencephalogram.
Based on Sarnat and Sarnat (1976), Shankaran et al. (2005) and Hahn JS (2009).

of these electronic fetal monitoring abnormalities for identifying intrapartum asphyxia was 93%, the positive predictive value was only 3–18%. Neonates who developed seizures had a significantly longer duration of abnormal fetal heart rate patterns (72 ± 12 versus 48 ± 12 minutes, $P < 0.001$) (Williams 2004). In fetal monkeys, during the course of fetal hypoxia severe enough to cause death, fetal heart rate variability decreased, then disappeared; late decelerations preceded fetal acidaemia. Other studies have not found electronic fetal monitoring to be clinically helpful in the identification of fetal acidosis or neurological injury. Vigilance is a very important part of intrapartum fetal monitoring (Kumar 2010).

Caesarean section

Studies have shown an inverse relationship between elective caesarean section and NE (Badawi et al. 1998a). This is, however, a contentious issue – the risks of high rates of caesarean section to both mother and baby are considerable.

Staff training, guidelines and clinical governance

Several investigations suggest that intrapartum asphyxia is preventable (Draper et al. 2002). Suboptimal intrapartum care has been shown to occur in 40–50% of cases with metabolic acidosis at birth (Jonsson et al. 2009). It has been shown that intrapartum care protocols can decrease caesarean section rates and result in fewer adverse outcomes (Clark et al. 2008). In the UK, the Royal College of Obstetricians and Gynaecologists recommends that all obstetric services have robust and transparent clinical governance frameworks in place, with multidisciplinary care and good communication being key factors for good practice.

Clinical manifestations of hypoxic–ischaemic encephalopathy

Clinical features

Apgar scores

The original intent of the Apgar score was to provide a description of the newborn's physical condition and enable comparison of obstetric practice, maternal analgesia and resuscitation (Apgar 1953). A hypoxic–ischaemic insult may cause depression of the Apgar score, but this is not invariable and many other non-asphyxial factors can cause depression of the Apgar score, e.g. maternal analgesia, infection, prematurity. Nevertheless prolonged depression of the Apgar score is related to death or severe neurodevelopmental outcome (Nelson 1981).

Neurological syndrome and encephalopathy scores

NE is an evolving clinical illness typically with worsening of clinical signs (seizures and impaired conscious state) after the first 4–16 hours and a slow improvement after about 4–5 days. Sarnat and Sarnat (1976) introduced a grading system to describe the neurological abnormalities, which has been modified by Levene et al. (1986). An updated version has been used by the National Institute of Child Health and Human Development (NICHD) Neonatal Research Network to identify newborn infants who may be eligible for neuroprotection (Shankaran et al. 2005) (Table 40.17). Several other scoring systems now exist, all of which are based on that of Sarnat and Sarnat; recent modifications have been directed at developing quantifiable scores with good reproducibility

Table 40.18 The Thompson score, previously found to be of diagnostic and prognostic value in Africa, comprises nine clinical signs, giving a maximum score of 22

	SCORE			
Sign	0	1	2	3
Tone	Normal	Hypertonic	Hypotonic	Flaccid
conscious state	Normal	Hyperalert, stare	Lethargic	Comatose
Fits	Normal	Infrequent, <3/day	Frequent, >2/day	
Posture	Normal	Fisting, cycling	Strong distal flexion	Decerebrate
Moro	Normal	Partial	Absent	
Grasp	Normal	Poor	Absent	
Suck	Normal	Poor	Absent/bites	
Respiration	Normal	Hyperventilation	Brief apnoea	Apnoeic
Fontanelle	Normal	Full, not tense	Tense	

(Thompson et al. 1997; Dubowitz et al. 1998; Miller et al. 2004) (Table 40.18).

Stage 1 encephalopathy (mild)

Infants with the mildest degree of encephalopathy have transient irritability, hypertonia and poor feeding. Muscle tone is normal or increased and the deep tendon reflexes are hyperactive. The Moro reflex is often exaggerated. Pupillary dilatation and tachycardia are frequently seen. Mild encephalopathy usually lasts less than 24–48 hours and is associated with a good neurological outcome, although there are concerns about learning and memory difficulties in later childhood even in infants who appear to do well (Marlow and Budge 2005).

Stage 2 encephalopathy (moderate)

Newborn infants with moderate encephalopathy (stage 2) show lethargy, hypotonia, hyporeflexia and seizures. The EEG typically shows reduced background activity associated with a lowering of the lower baseline on the amplitude integrated EEG with seizures. Infants can typically be aroused with auditory stimuli or touch. Feeding is poor. Muscle tone is decreased with a prominent head lag. Exaggerated deep tendon reflexes are seen and clonus may be elicited. Cranial nerve examination reveals a weak suck and decreased gag reflex. Spontaneous movement is decreased. Pupils are often constricted and periodic breathing and bradycarida may occur. Seizures typically occur. Stage 2 encephalopathy is associated with a poor outcome in approximately 15–40% of the infants (Robertson 1993), especially if abnormal neurologic signs persist for over 1 week.

Stage 3 encephalopathy (severe)

The most severely affected infants have profound stupor or coma and the EEG is usually isoelectric, suppressed or shows burst suppression. Infants are flaccid and unresponsive to any stimuli. They also have episodic decerebrate (extensor) posturing and poor brainstem function. Deep tendon reflexes and sucking are absent. Seizures are common and may be difficult to treat. The infant often has bradycardia, hypotension, irregular respirations and apnoea. The mortality rate is high and nearly all survivors develop sequelae.

In many infants clinical features are intermediate between these stages or there is a transition from one stage to another over the first 1–3 days.

Multiorgan dysfunction

During hypoxia–ischaemia, the diving reflex is activated. This reflex shunts blood from the skin and splanchnic area to the heart, adrenals, and brain, ostensibly to protect these vital organs from hypoxic–ischaemic injury. It has been suggested that neonates with brain injury secondary to hypoxia–ischaemia would have activated the diving reflex for long enough to cause dysfunction of one or more nonessential organs, particularly kidney and liver. Multiorgan dysfunction has been considered a constant feature of the neonatal postasphyxial syndrome. However, in a retrospective cohort study of infants with HIE, there was no association between multiorgan dysfunction and outcome or between individual or combinations of organ involvements and outcome (Shah et al. 2004). In this study specific renal, cardiac, pulmonary and hepatic criteria for multiorgan dysfunction (Table 40.19) were used. All infants had evidence of multiorgan dysfunction (at least one organ dysfunction in addition to HIE). Renal, cardiovascular, pulmonary, and hepatic dysfunction was present in 58–88% of infants with good outcome and 64–86% of infants with adverse outcome.

Management of hypoxic–ischaemic encephalopathy

Resuscitation (Ch. 13.1)

In the UK, 10% of newborns (approximately 70 000 annually) require some form of resuscitaton after birth. Most infants respond quickly and make a full recovery, although it is concerning that infants who do not develop encephalopathy may have an increased risk of a low IQ score at 8 years if they required resuscitative efforts at birth, and infants with just brief depression of the Apgar score (<7 for 1 min after birth) may have poorer function in cognitive tests in later life (Odd et al. 2009).

A systematic review of the literature of surviving infants with Apgar zero at 10 minutes and who were resuscitated successfully, show that the outcomes for infants who do not respond to

Table 40.19 Criteria for organ/system dysfunction

SYSTEM/ORGAN	CRITERIA
Renal	Anuria or oliguria (< 1 ml/kg/h) for 24 hours or more, and a serum creatinine concentration >100 mmol/l; or anuria/oliguria for >36 hours; or any serum creatinine >125 mmol/l; or serial serum creatinine values that increased postnatally
Cardiovascular	Hypotension treated with an inotrope for more than 24 hours to maintain blood pressure within the normal range, or electrocardiographic evidence of transient myocardial ischaemia
Pulmonary	Need for ventilator support with oxygen requirement >40% for at least the first 4 hours after birth
Hepatic	Aspartate aminotransferase >100 IU/l or alanine aminotransferase >100 IU/l at any time during the first week after birth

(Modified from Shah et al. 2004.)

Ventilation and oxygenation

Inadequate ventilation and persistence of hypoxia can further aggravate cerebral injury and should be treated promptly. On the other hand, in many postasphyxial infants, cardiorespiratory function improves rapidly, outstripping weaning and resulting in unintentional hyperoxaemia and/or hypocapnia. Severe hyperoxaemia and severe hypocapnia have been associated with adverse outcome in infants with postasphyxial HIE, therefore during the first hours of life, oxygen supplementation and ventilation must be rigorously controlled (Klinger et al. 2005). In a study adjusting for the severity of birth asphyxia, peak Pa_{O_2} values exceeding 26.6 kPa (200 mmHg) and trough Pa_{CO_2} values of 2.6 kPa (20 mmHg) or lower during the first 20–120 minutes of life were associated with death or adverse neurodevelopmental outcome. The risk of adverse outcome was greatest in subjects who had both. Hypocapnia, by decreasing CBF, may increase the risk of injury in ischaemic cerebral disease states (Klinger et al. 2005); mechanisms of oxygen-induced brain damage are well established (Saugstad et al. 2008).

Cardiac dysfunction

Cardiovascular injury from hypoxia–ischaemia may be manifested as decreased ventricular function, abnormalities of rate and rhythm, tricuspid regurgitation and hypotension. Adequate perfusion of the brain is essential to prevent additional cerebral damage and inotropes and volume expanders may be necessary, especially if there is a transient hypoxia-induced myocardiopathy.

Metabolism

Normoglycaemia should be maintained, and adequate protein and caloric intake should be provided as soon as possible. Excessive early enteral feeding may facilitate the occurrence of necrotising enterocolitis, because the gut may be injured by hypoxic–ischaemic damage. Hypoglycaemia may aggravate the damage from hypoxic–ischaemic injury (Burns et al. 2008).

Coagulopathy and other organ damage

Birth asphyxia-related disseminated intravascular coagulation reduces levels of coagulation factors and thrombocytes, which can result in prolonged bleeding times. Renal dysfunction due to acute tubular necrosis is common, and is nearly always a temporary problem that resolves over the first week of life. Renal problems range from mild oliguria, proteinuria and haematuria to renal tubular acidosis and renal failure. However, permanent renal damage associated with HIE is very rare. Liver damage may exacerbate coagulation problems and may lead to elevated liver enzymes. Metabolic abnormalities are common and include hypoglycaemia, hypocalcaemia, hypomagnesaemia and sodium and potassium abnormalities.

Treatment of seizures

Seizures enhance the metabolic demand of the neonatal brain and independently exacerbate hypoxic–ischaemic injury (Glass et al. 2009). Therefore, early recognition of seizure activity is important. Phenobarbital is the most commonly used first-line anticonvulsant (Painter et al. 1999). In many units in Europe midazolam or lidocaine is used as add-on therapy. Elsewhere in the world phenytoin, lorazepam and primidone have been used. Future anticonvulsants for neonates may be topiramate, a blocker of the AMPA-type glutamate receptor, bumetanide, a blocker of NKCC1, a Cl⁻ cotransporter or levetiracetam. In most cases therapy can be limited to the first week after hypoxia–ischaemia. In neonates with severe brain injury maintenance of anticonvulsants may be indicated, but this is uncommon.

cardiopulmonary resuscitation by 10 minutes of age (Apgar scores of 0 at 10 minutes) are extremely poor, with a very low chance of surviving without severe disability (Harrington et al. 2007). These findings present strong evidence that adequate resuscitation beyond 10 minutes is not justified and form the basis for the ILCOR recommendation to discontinue resuscitation after 10 minutes of adequate resuscitation (International Liaison Committee on Resuscitation 2006). However, in a recent analysis of infants who qualified for the NICHD cooling trial, the outcome of survivors with an Apgar score of 0 at 10 minutes was more heterogeneous; 6 of the 13 survivors had either a mild or an absent disability at an 18–22-month assessment (Laptook et al. 2009).

Our practice is based on the 2006 International Liaison Committee on Resuscitation (ILCOR) guidelines, although it is important that experienced staff attend if the infant does not respond promptly to standard resuscitative measures. Complications such as a tension pneumothorax may be difficult to ascertain in the full-term infant in the delivery suite and some infants may have coexisting abnormalities that may be undetected by inexperienced personnel. Resuscitation in room air is advised – the use of 100% oxygen at birth is associated with worse outcomes than the use of room air, possibly because of free-radical injury and pulmonary atelectasis (Saugstad et al. 2008).

Clinical management in the NICU

Best-practice guidelines are available (Azzopardi 2010b). The initial management of infants with HIE following admission to the neonatal unit consists of standard neonatal intensive care measures, continuous core temperature monitoring using a rectal or oesophageal probe, initiation of therapeutic hypothermia if appropriate (see section on therapeutic hypothermia, below) and neurological monitoring by regular clinical examination, continuous EEG or aEEG and regular cUS examinations. Clinical management will depend on the severity of NE.

Table 40.20 Documentation and details needed in infants who present with neonatal encephalopathy

DOCUMENTATION	DETAILS
Maternal and family history	Maternal and paternal age and health, consanguinity, ethnic background, parity, details of previous pregnancies, health of other children, family history of thrombosis, thyroid disease, active herpes infection, neurological disease, cerebral palsy, seizures, neonatal or infant deaths, travel abroad before or during pregnancy
Details of current pregnancy	Last menstrual period and expected date of delivery and certainty, conception, whether natural or assisted, history of infertility, previous fetal losses and stillbirths, maternal medication/drugs, antenatal care, results of chorionic villous sampling/amniocentesis, results of antenatal scans, placental site, fetal position, fetal movements, including time of onset and any changes, chorionicity of twins, history of twin-to-twin transfusion syndrome, presence of oligo/polyhydramnios, growth pattern, infection, essential hypertension/pre-eclampsia, diabetes mellitus/gestational diabetes, accidental injury, rhesus incompatibility, results of any cardiotocogram in pregnancy
Details of resuscitation	Evidence for intrapartum fetal distress, cord blood gases and lactate from both arterial and venous samples, Apgar scores at 1, 5 and 10 minutes, need for intubation and duration, difficulties in intubation or ventilation, presence of meconium below the cord, onset of satisfactory heart rate, time to first gasp, onset of regular respirations, maximum ventilatory requirement, any drugs/fluids administered
Care in the NNU	Remember to inform registry, e.g. TOBY UK cooling register (www. npeu.ox.ac.uk/tobyregister)

NNU, neonatal unit.
(Adapted from Azzopardi et al. 2010.)

Table 40.21 Neurological monitoring required in the neonatal unit for infants with moderate to severe neonatal encephalopathy

NEUROLOGICAL MONITORING	ACTION
Daily neurological examinations	Document clinical encephalopathy score as HIE evolves over 1–4 days
Continuous aEEG or EEG	For a minimum of 48 hours
Monitor for clinical seizures	Correlate subtle signs such as lip smacking, head turning, eye turning, bradycardias and apnoeas with the aEEG. Subclinical seizures may be apparent on aEEG
Treat clinical (and subclinical) seizures	Phenobarbital 20 mg/kg first-line, repeated if necessary.
Daily cranial ultrasound	For first 4 days. Measure cerebral flow velocities and calculate pulsatility index during first 3 days
MRI/^{1}H MRS	If only one scan can be performed, the optimal timing is 5–14 days

HIE, hypoxic–ischaemic encephalopathy; aEEG, amplitude-integrated electroencephalogram; EEG, electroencephalogram; MRI, magnetic resonance imaging; MRS, magnetic resonance spectroscopy.
(Modified from Azzopardi et al. 2010.)

Documentation

It is important to obtain a detailed structured clinical history to identify risk factors for HIE, and evidence of alternative diagnoses and comorbidities. This information needs to be carefully documented so that it is readily available to multidisciplinary teams that are often involved in the long-term clinical management of affected children. The detail needed in the documentation is shown in Table 40.20 (Azzopardi 2010b).

Neurological monitoring

Regular neurological assessment is necessary to determine the severity of NE, detect deterioration and complications such as cerebral sinus thrombosis or haemorrhage, to assess the response to therapies such as anticonvulsant therapy and to assess likely neurological outcome to plan further clinical management. Details of neurological monitoring are given in Table 40.21 (Azzopardi 2010b).

Investigations

When encephalopathy has developed following resuscitative efforts at birth with evidence of perinatal asphyxia and following a sentinel event, a diagnosis of HIE is likely to be correct. Nevertheless, coexisting or predisposing conditions such as infection or trauma or metabolic disorder also need to be considered. A protocol will help ensure the most appropriate investigations are carried out and important ones not left out. Suggested first-, second- and third-line

Table 40.22 Suggested first-, second- and third-line investigatons for neonatal encephalopathy

INVESTIGATIONS	
First-line*	Cord blood gases and lactate Biochemistry, haematology and metabolic parameters Cardiac and hepatic enzymes Screen for infection (± lumbar puncture) Tests for congenital infection Cranial ultrasound EEG/aEEG MRI within 14 days
Second-line	Investigation for metabolic or genetic disorders if any dysmorphic features, parental consanguinity, abnormal intracranial anatomy, severe growth restriction, unusual pattern of injury on MRI scan, normal-looking MRI scan with ongoing neurological problems
Third-line	Consider further investigation for metabolic disorders (e.g. non-ketotic hyperglycinaemia, sulphite oxidase deficiency, biotidinase eficiency, mitochondrial disorders, peroxisomal disorders, carbohydrate glycosylation defects, carnitine or acyl carnitine disorders, disorders of lysosomal enzymes) Consider investigation for neuromuscular diseases (e.g. nerve conduction studies, electromyogram, muscle biopsy) Consider thrombophilia screen in cases with focal haemorrhage, infarction or thrombosis Store blood for future DNA analysis

*According to local protocols.
EEG, electroencephalogram; aEEG, amplitude-integrated electroencephalogram; MRI, magnetic resonance imaging.
(Modified from Azzopardi et al. 2010.)

investigations are described in recent reviews on NE and summarised in Table 40.22 (Azzopardi 2010b).

Cranial ultrasound

cUS has been used extensively in neonatal practice, since it is a convenient technique to visualise the neonatal brain through the anterior fontanelle serially without moving or disturbing the patient in a neonatal intensive care setting.

cUS scanning is helpful to exclude structural abnormality suggesting metabolic and other diagnoses, detect calcification and cysts suggestive of viral infection and detect atrophy suggestive of long-standing damage. It will also identify cerebral haemorrhage. Sequential observation of the evolution of injury following a recent hypoxic–ischaemic insult at birth is helpful both for defining the pattern of lesion and timing its onset. Brain swelling is a non-specific finding on cUS, which supports the diagnosis of hypoxia–ischaemia, but is not always present. The presence of 'slit-like' ventricles on the first day of life, however, is a very non-specific finding, since many healthy neonates have small ventricles. The ultrasound appearances of cerebral oedema include loss of the normal anatomical detail with obscuration of the sulcal markings and closure of the interhemispheric and sylvian fissures. The brain has a sparkly appearance with increased echoreflectance.

Following acute and severe hypoxia–ischaemia, echogenicity of the BGT may be seen to appear 24–48 hours after birth. The thalami appear egg-shaped and echoreflectant. In the coronal view the internal capsule remains of normal echogenicity and gives rise to a 'stripe' as it sits between the thalami and lentiform nuclei, both of which are abnormally echoreflectant (Rutherford et al. 1994). A clear and persistent abnormality of the thalami and basal ganglia on cUS correlates with MRI findings, which indicate a poor prognosis (Painter et al. 1999) (Fig. 40.37). Similarly, the appearance of a hyperechoic line running through the central grey matter is also a poor prognostic sign. Early detection may be facilitated by additional scanning with a low transducer frequency of 5 MHz – this

lower transducer frequency allows deeper penetration in larger infants or those with thick hair and enables visualisation of deeper structures (i.e. the BGT in large infants and the posterior fossa) (van Wezel-Meijler and Leijser 2010). MRI is necessary to determine the exact site and extent of injury and involvement of the PLIC.

Due to its localisation at the brain's convexity, the watershed or parasagittal injury pattern is not easily detectable with cUS. It often shows as a 'tramline' appearance of the cortex, that is, broadening of the hypoechogenic cortical rim combined with increased echogenicity of the subcortical white matter. Increasing the transducer frequency to 10 MHz will improve detection of this injury pattern with cUS; however, confirmation by MRI is indicated (van Wezel-Meijler and Leijser 2010). Doppler studies of CBF velocity showing a low resistance index are predictive of a poor outcome (Archer and Evans 1986).

Electrophysiology (EEG, aEEG, evoked responses)

Neurophysiology plays an important role in determining the severity of the insult in the newborn infant after hypoxia–ischaemia. In earlier studies the multichannel EEG was used to predict neurodevelopmental outcome (Monod and Guidasci 1972; Watanabe et al. 1980). In these studies, the EEG was usually performed after the first 12–24 hours. The electrical background activity was more predictive than the presence or absence of seizure activity. Since multichannel recordings have practical limitations, more compact systems, available within the intensive care unit, providing immediate access and storage of signals at the cot side over long period of time, are now increasingly being used. With this technique a single- or two-channel EEG is recorded from biparietal electrodes. The filtered signal is rectified, smoothed and amplitude-integrated before it is written out on a semilogarithmic scale at slow speed (6 cm/h). aEEG has a high concordance with the standard EEG (Hellström-Westas and Svenningsen 1995; Toet et al. 2002). The method is not always reliable for detection of seizures but works well in many babies and the neonatal staff can be taught to interpret the result.

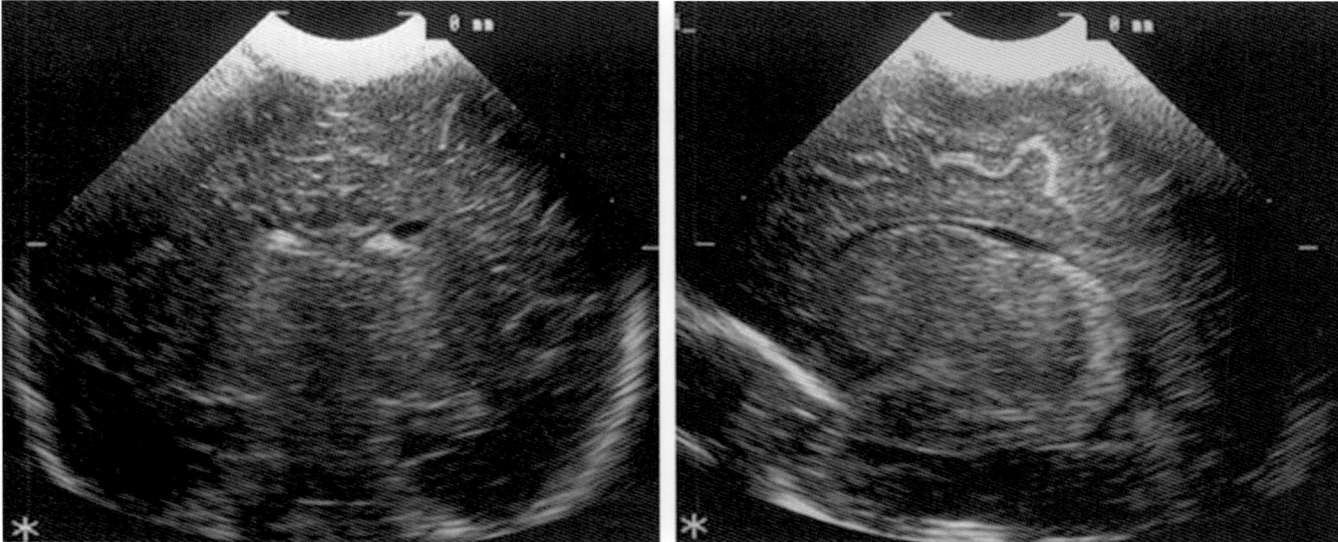

Fig. 40.37 Cranial ultrasound of a full-term neonate with severe perinatal asphyxia, day 3. Left: coronal image, right: parasagittal image. Both views show severe injury to the basal ganglia and thalamus.

The results obtained using aEEG to predict outcome are similar to those obtained using EEG: a very early trace showing burst suppression or no activity can normalise by 6 hours and the baby may do well, but persisting burst suppression or isoelectric activity carries a poor prognosis (Hellström-Westas and Svenningsen 1995; Toet et al. 1999; van Rooij et al. 2005).

Over the last 20 years several studies have confirmed that the aEEG pattern in the first 6 hours of life is strongly predictive of outcome in infants with NE (al Naqeeb et al. 1999; Toet et al. 1999). The speed of recovery, as well as the severity of the abnormality, in the aEEG trace is prognostically valuable (van Rooij et al. 2005). The predictive value of aEEG has been shown to extend to infants who were monitored after 24 hours of age and to infants with encephalopathy caused by conditions other than hypoxia–ischaemia, such as metabolic conditions (al Naqeeb et al. 1999), sepsis or meningitis (ter Horst et al. 2008).

Sleep–wake cycling (SWC) is present in healthy term newborns and is a sign of brain integrity. A good neurodevelopmental outcome was predicted by the onset of SWC before 36 hours in 82% of infants with NE in one study (Osredkar et al. 2005). Ideally, aEEG recording should be continued long enough for the onset of SWC to be determined.

The aEEG can be classified according to pattern or voltage criteria (de Vries and Hellström-Westas 2005; Shany et al. 2006). The voltage criteria are based on assessment of the lower and upper voltage margins of aEEG background (al Naqeeb et al. 1999) (Fig. 40.38). This method was used for selecting into the Cool-Cap and Whole Body Hypothermia for the Treatment of Perinatal Asphyxial Encephalopathy (TOBY) trials infants with encephalopathy (Gluckman et al. 2005; Azzopardi et al. 2009a). The voltage classification (Fig. 40.39a–d) is easier to use for clinicians with little experience in reading aEEG, but one should always try to assess the underlying pattern (Fig. 40.40a–e). It has been shown that a burst suppression pattern may be read as a normal voltage pattern when a 'drift of the baseline' brings the lower margin above 5 μV (Hagmann et al. 2006). The facility of inspecting the raw EEG in the new digital aEEG machines improves the accuracy of the interpretation of the aEEG. However, although some artifacts are easy to

recognise, in many cases the recognition of an artifact requires an ability to interpret the EEG.

Recent studies show that therapeutic hypothermia changes the predictive value of early aEEG (Hallberg et al. 2010; Thoresen et al. 2010). Normalisation of an infant's aEEG while being cooled occurs later: in an infant who develops normally and who is not cooled, the aEEG would be expected to return to normal by 24 hours, whereas in an infant who is cooled and develops normally, it may take as long as 48 hours for the aEEG to normalise. In one study the time to normal aEEG was a better predictor than time to SWC; however never achieving SWC always predicted poor outcome (Thoresen et al. 2010).

Computed tomography (CT)

CT scans have been used in the past in full-term neonates with hypoxia–ischaemia. MRI is superior to CT in all aspects and in most places CT has been replaced by MRI. Even the presence of calcifications, until recently only possible with ultrasound or CT scans, can be demonstrated with appropriate MRI sequences (susceptibility-weighted imaging). In a study comparing MRI with CT on day 3 in infants with NE, CT was able to detect the predominant pattern of injury with a 67% agreement with DWI MRI (Chau et al. 2009). The risk of exposure to ionising radiation with CT must be kept in mind and MRI used if at all possible.

MRI and MRS

MRI is the optimal imaging modality for the early evaluation of brain injury in full-term neonates with perinatal asphyxia. Hypoxic–ischaemic changes of the brain can be visualised with higher spatial resolution, sensitivity and specificity than with cUS and CT. The pattern of brain injury may not be fully apparent until after the first 4–7 days on conventional MRI, but may be seen with DWI. The main patterns of injury are: (1) basal ganglia-predominant; (2) watershed-predominant; or (3) severe global injury. The severity and duration of hypoxia–ischaemia (acute total or chronic partial) influence the pattern of injury; the patterns of injury and

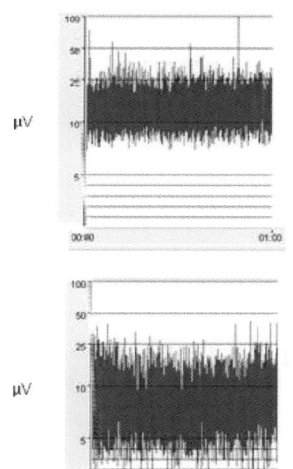

Normal voltage
Upper margin >10μV
Lower margin > 5 μV

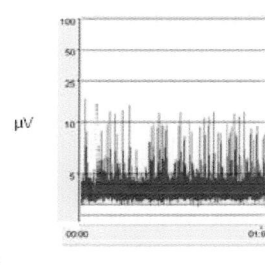

Moderately abnormal voltage
Upper margin > 10 μV
Lower margin ≤ 5 μV

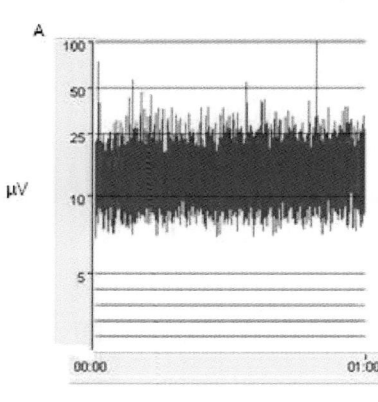

Severely abnormal voltage
Upper margin < 10 μV
Lower margin < 5 μV

μV

Time (hours)

(A)

Fig. 40.38 (a) Amplitude-integrated encephalogram (aEEG) classification based on voltage criteria. Based on assessment of the lower and upper voltage margins of aEEG background (al Naqeeb et al. 1999). (b) aEEG classification based on pattern. A, continuous normal voltage; B, discontinuous normal voltage; C, burst suppression; D, continuous low voltage; E, flat trace (de Vries and Hellström-Westas 2005).

A

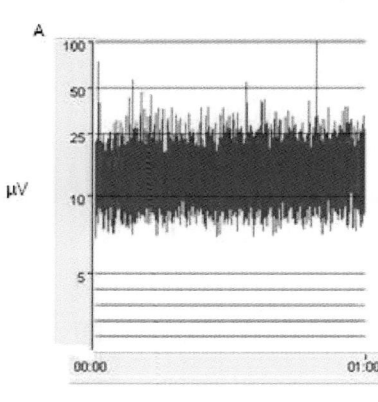

μV

Time (hours)

B

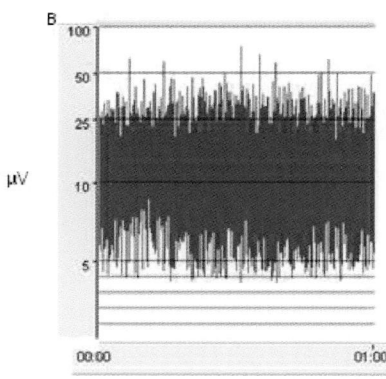

μV

Time (hours)

C

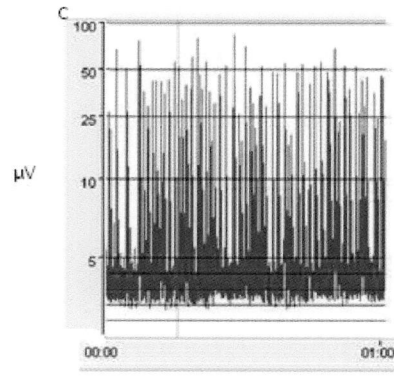

μV

Time (hours)

C

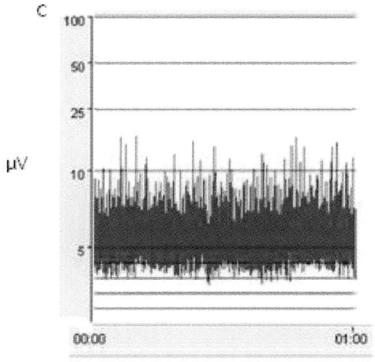

μV

Time (hours)

D

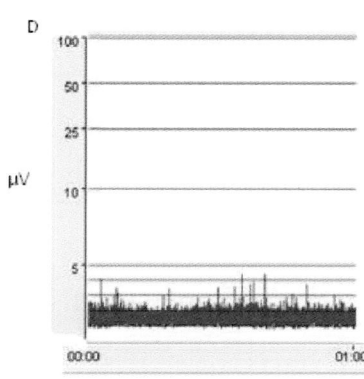

μV

Time (hours)

(B)

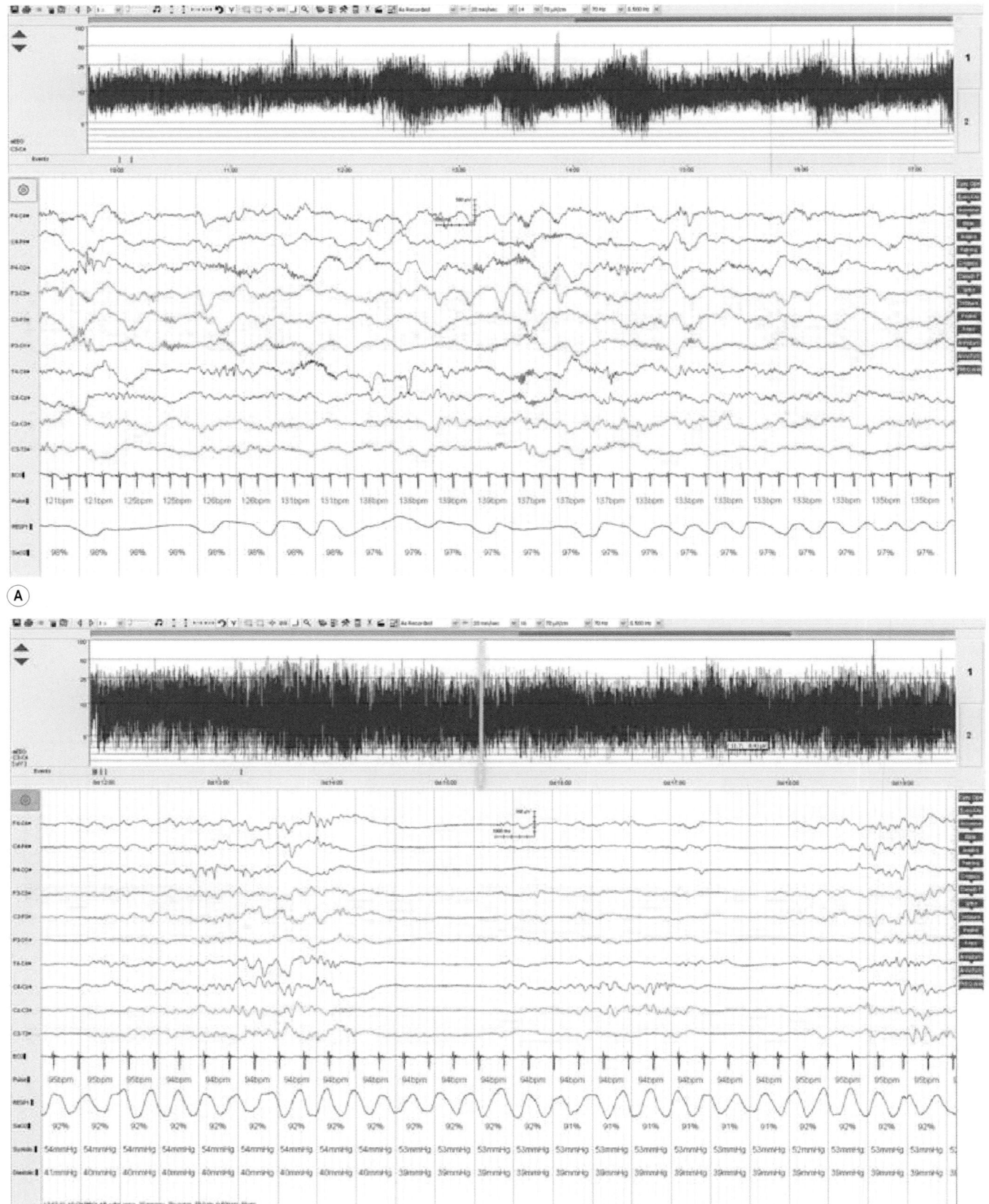

Fig. 40.39 (a) Normal voltage on amplitude-integrated encephalogram (aEEG: upper margin >10 μV, lower margin >5 μV) and sleep cycling. Continuous mixed-frequency activity on EEG. (b) Moderately abnormal voltage on aEEG (upper margin > 10 μV, lower margin <5 μV); EEG shows discontinuity.

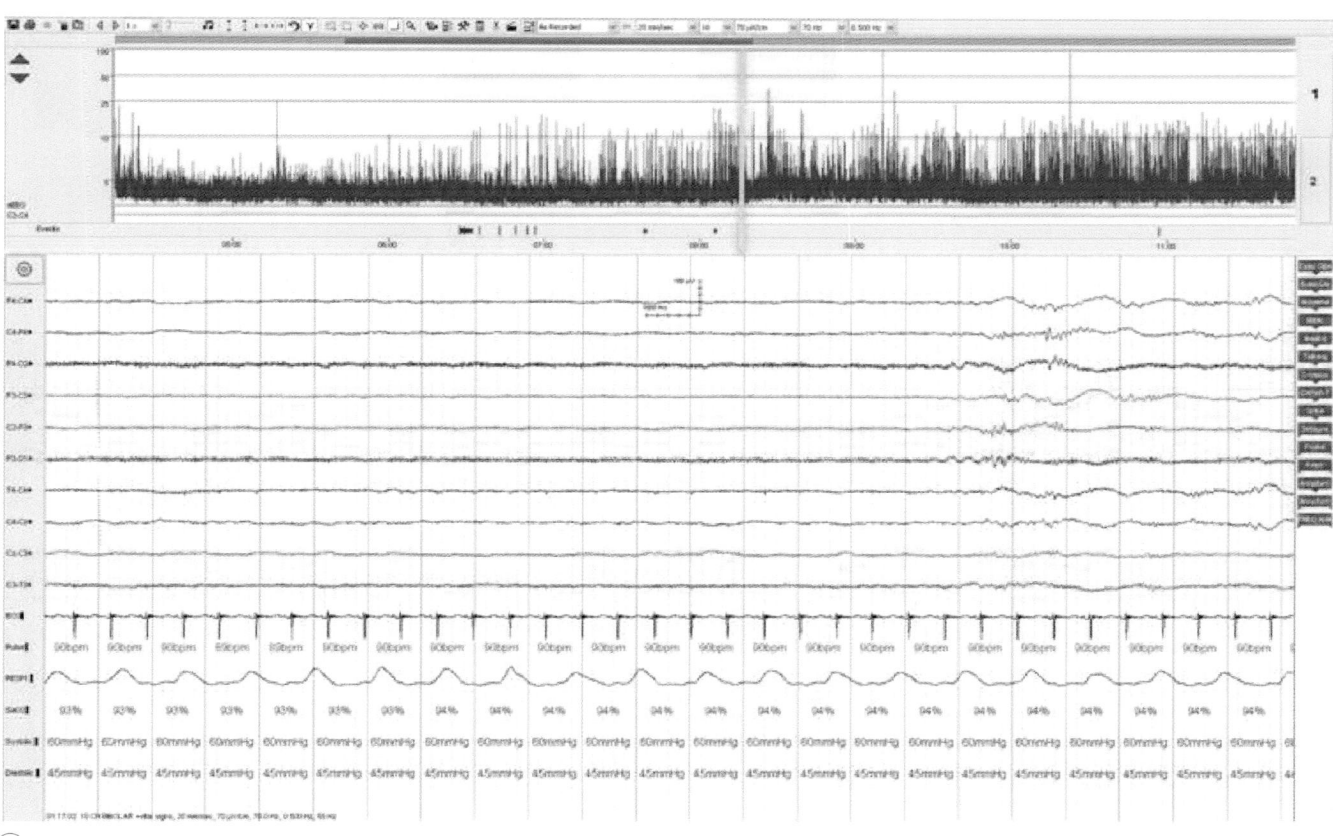

Fig. 40.39, cont'd (c) Severely abnormal voltage on aEEG (upper margin <10 μV, lower margin <5 μV), EEG shows infrequent bursts of low-amplitude activity. (d) Severely abnormal voltage plus seizures. Bilateral high-amplitude seizures on EEG cause transient upward deflection of upper and lower margin of aEEG.

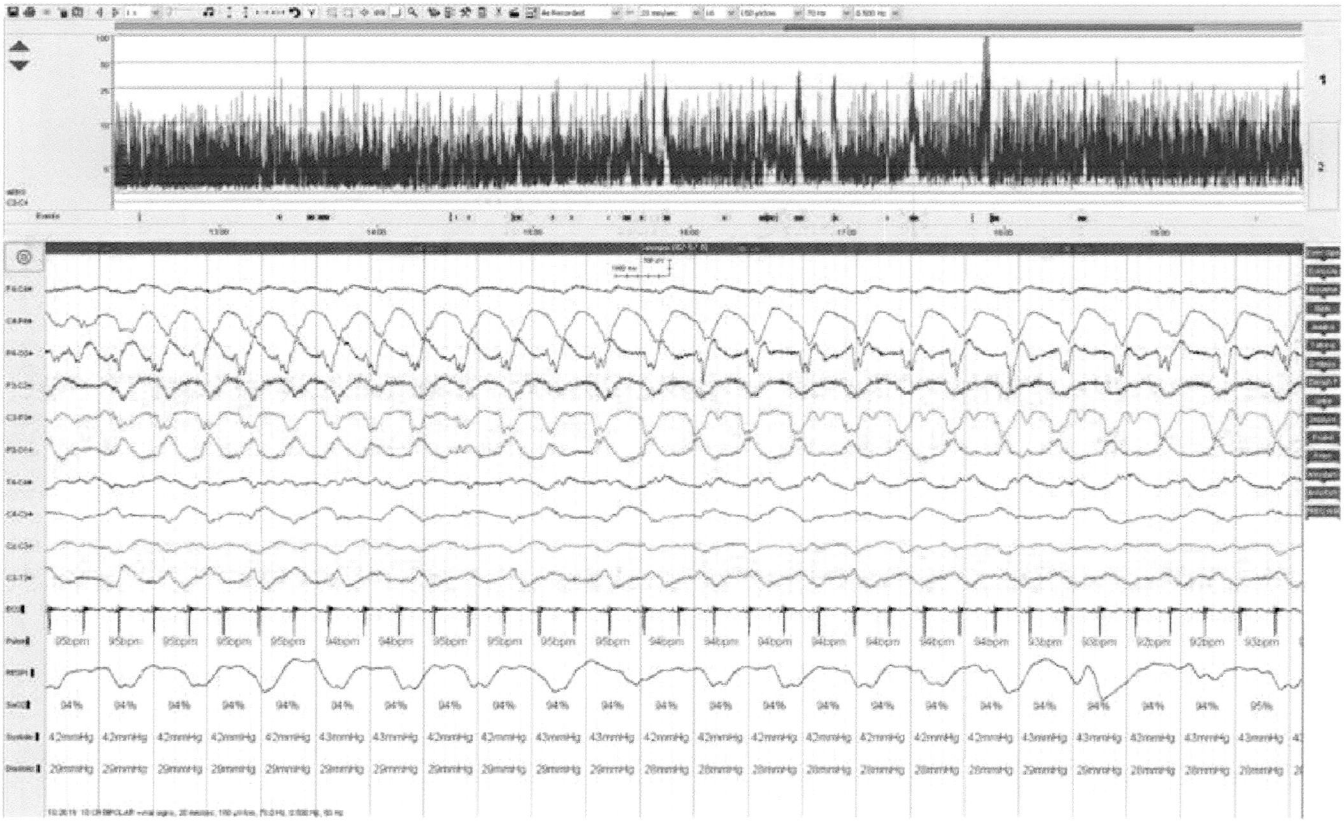

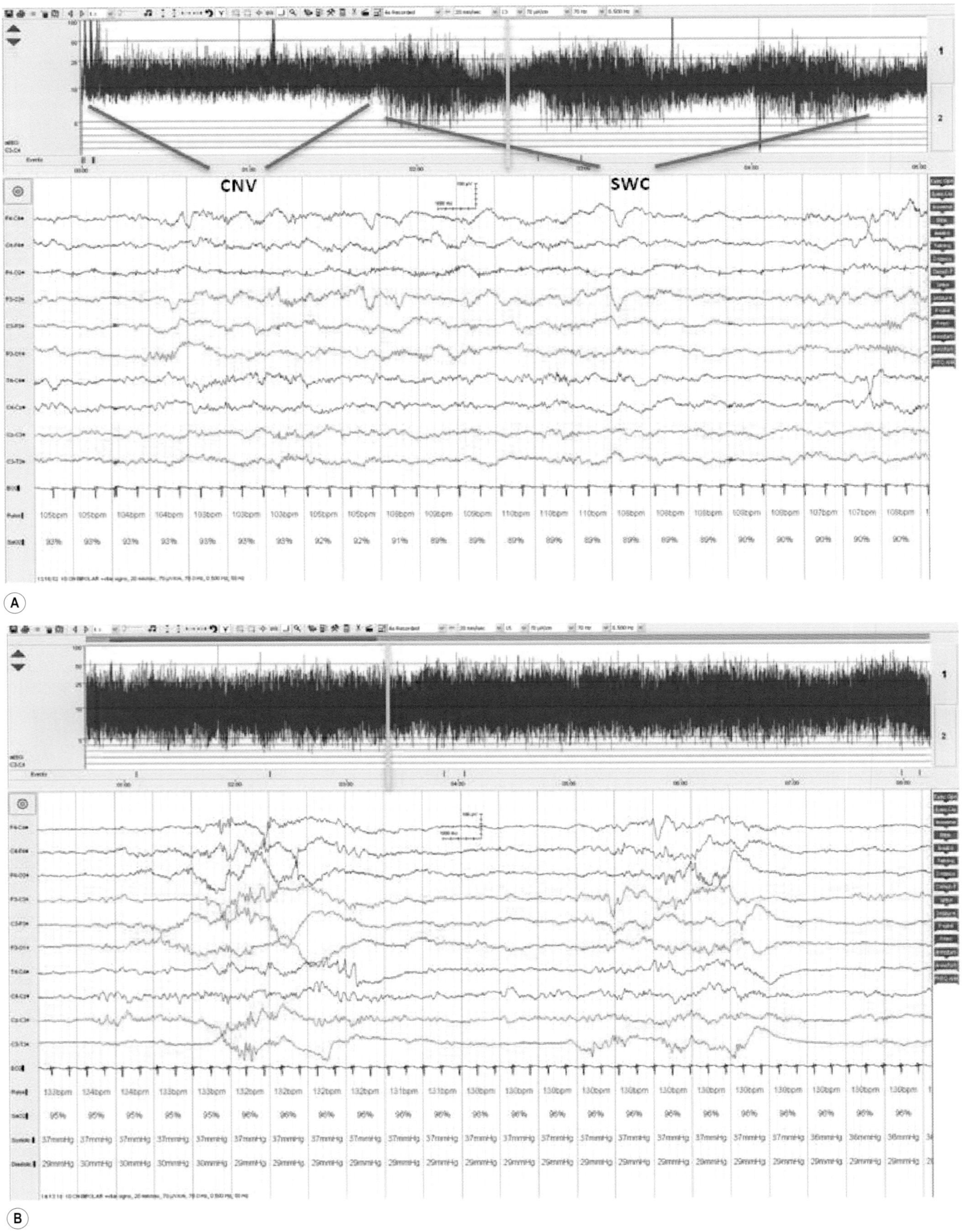

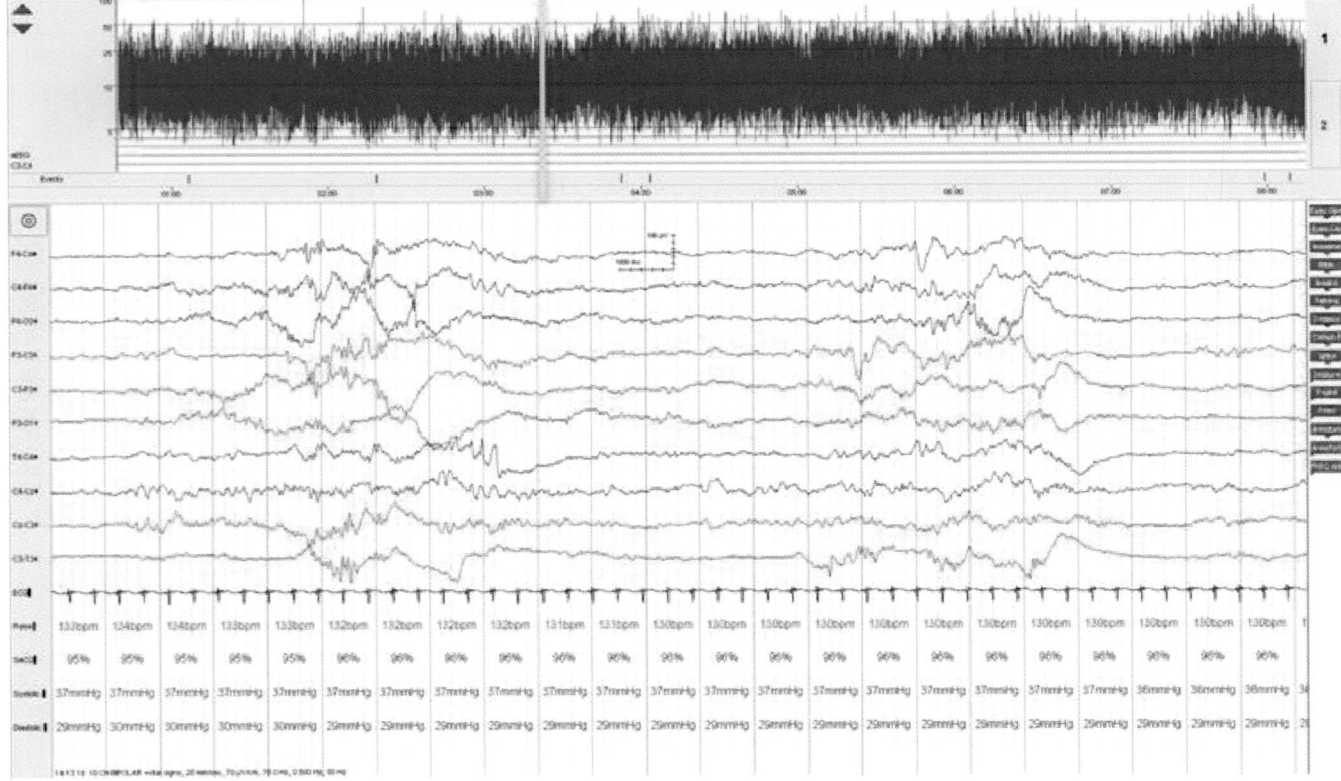

Fig. 40.40 (a) Continuous normal voltage (CNV) pattern on amplitude-integrated encephalogram (aEEG). Continuous activity with voltage 10–25 µV and sleep–wake cycling (SWC). EEG shows continuous mixed-frequency activity. (b) Discontinuous normal voltage pattern on aEEG (DNV, discontinuous trace, where the voltage is predominantly above 5 µV) with no sleep cycling. EEG shows low-amplitude activity alternating with higher-amplitude bursts.

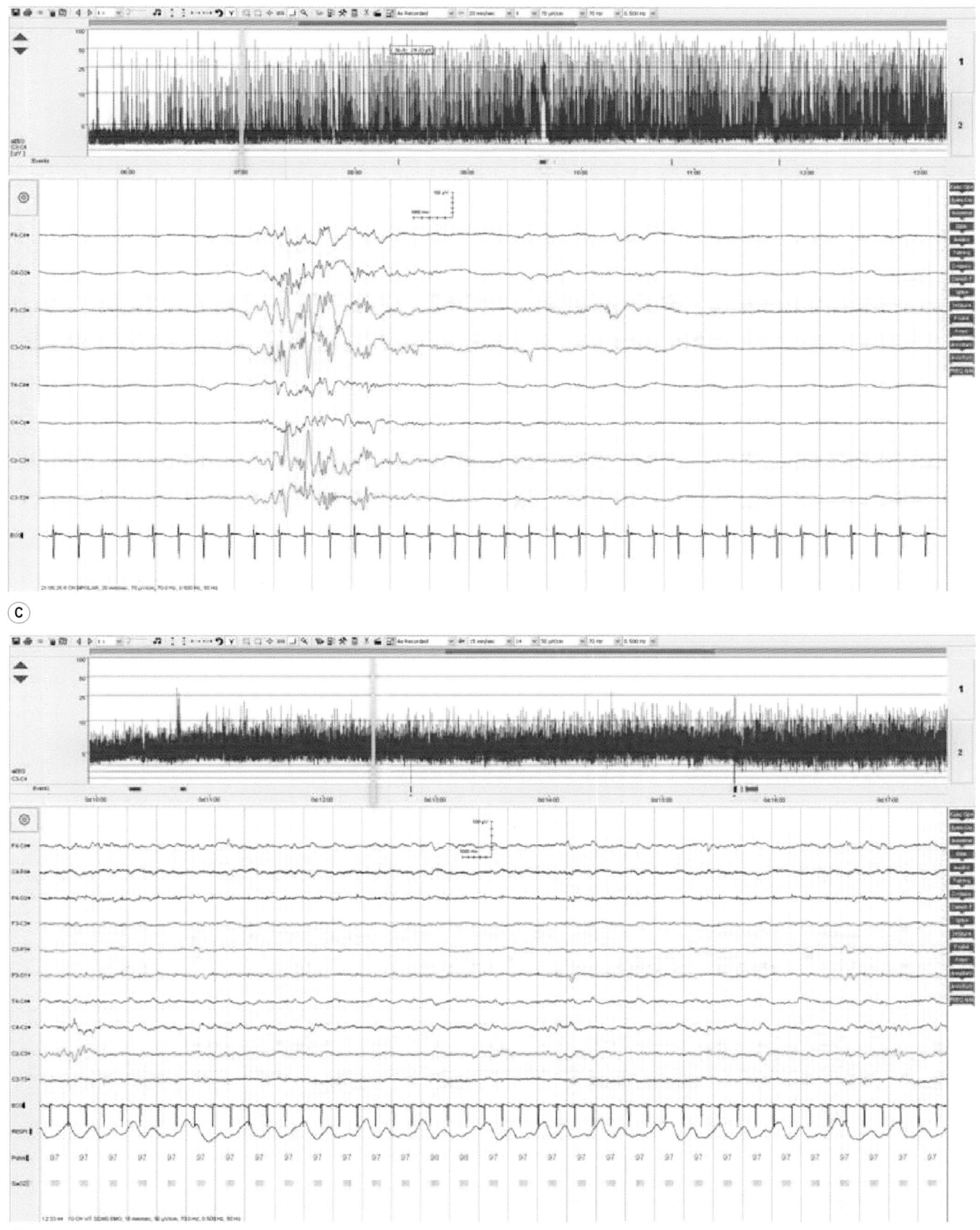

Fig. 40.40, cont'd (c) Burst suppression pattern on aEEG (BS, discontinuous background pattern; periods of very low voltage intermixed with bursts of higher amplitude). EEG shows transient isolated bursts of mixed-frequency activity with prolonged periods of inactivity. (d) Continuous low-voltage pattern on aEEG (CLV, continuous background pattern of very low voltage around 5 μV). EEG activities are continuous but low-amplitude.

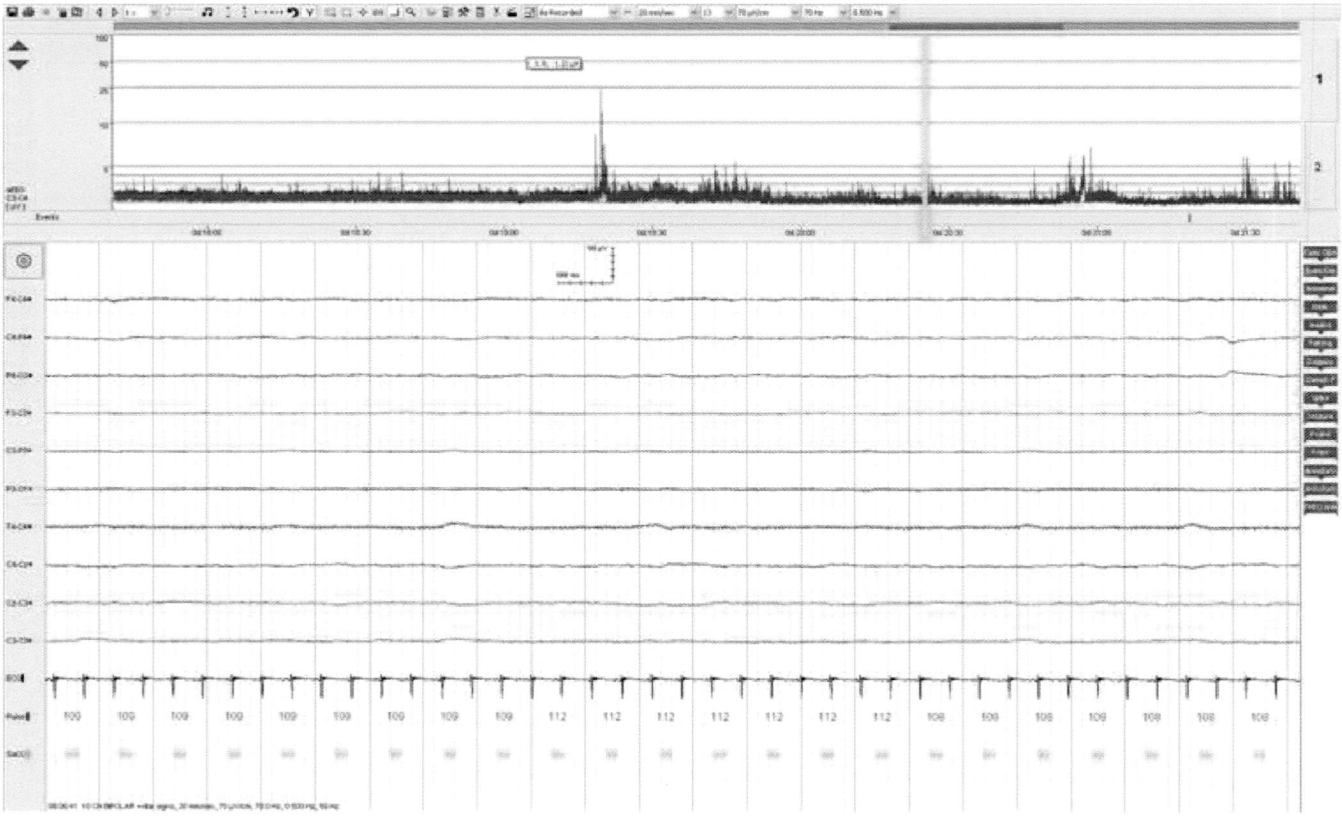

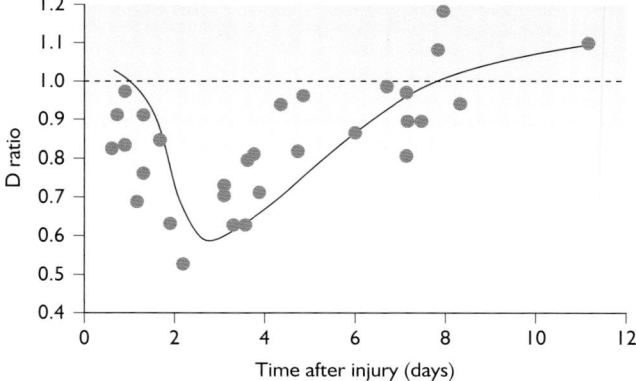

(E)

Fig. 40.40, cont'd (e) Flat trace pattern on aEEG (FT, inactive tracing with activity below 5 μV). EEG shows inactivity.

their likely outcome are discussed in the section on patterns of injury, above.

Proton MRS is increasingly available and provides important prognostic data during the first week (Cheong et al. 2006; Thayyil et al. 2010). A reduction in NAA and elevation of Lac in the thalamus/basal ganglia (an increased Lac/NAA peak area ratio) correlates with adverse outcome (Thayyil et al. 2010). Evolving abnormalities on MRS during the hours and days after birth and the use of MRS as a surrogate outcome measure are described in the section on cerebral energy metabolism associated with hypoxia–ischaemia, above.

DWI may help clinicians detect hypoxic–ischaemic lesions earlier than standard T1- or T2-weighted imaging. A reduced apparent diffusion coefficient can be calculated, showing reduced values (restricted diffusion) during the first few days after the insult, with pseudonormalisation by the end of the first week (McKinstry et al. 2002) (Fig. 40.41). Sequential imaging has shown that lesions in the basal ganglia may vary in size and site during the first week after birth (Barkovich et al. 2006). The appearance of new areas of reduced diffusion simultaneous with pseudonormalisation of areas that had reduced diffusion at earlier times results in entirely different patterns of injury on ADC maps acquired at different time points.

Counselling

The parents of a baby with HIE experience acute and terrible distress: after many months of waiting for their baby to be born they are faced with the possibility of their child either dying or surviving

Fig. 40.41 Time course of the diffusion abnormality following perinatal brain injury in newborn infants. D_{av} has been normalised to reference values for newborn infants (D_{av} ratio). The maximum reduction in D_{av} ratio of approximately 35% occurs between days 2 and 3. Pseudonormalisation is noted after the seventh day. (*Adapted from McKinstry et al. 2002.*)

with permanent disability. During the first few days after birth the senior attending physician, together with the nurse looking after the baby, should hold regular discussions with parents. A clear account of the baby's condition and prognosis and an explanation of the therapeutic options should be provided (see section on neurodevelopmental outcome, below, for neuroprotective therapies). Several meetings will be required, not least because it is not possible to give an accurate prognosis very early in the course of HIE. The parents' views are critical but the infant's best interests must be kept in mind; in our experience it is usual to reach a consensus decision.

Redirecting care

Around 30% of infants who meet the criteria used in the cooling trials die following moderate/severe HIE. Most of these babies die following a redirection of medical care and discontinuation of assisted ventilation. The longer the baby remains in a severe encephalopathic state (stage 3 encephalopathy) with a severely suppressed aEEG/EEG (EEG voltage extremely low or absent), the more likely it is that there will be a severely abnormal outcome. Persistence of this state beyond 48–72 hours indicates that further life-supporting treatment is futile. If possible we obtain an MRI to confirm the diagnosis and severity of brain injury. We would not rely on aEEG alone, in case of artifact, and would seek to confirm a low-voltage trace with formal multichannel EEG.

Some infants have a partial recovery but the level of encephalopathy persists at stage 2/3, with the aEEG/EEG remaining moderately or severely abnormal (e.g. burst suppression pattern or a severely discontinuous pattern). Clinical assessment of the prognosis is difficult; however the prognosis may be better than expected following therapeutic hypothermia (Gunn et al. 2008).

The preterm infant with hypoxic–ischaemic injury

Regional differences in the vulnerability of the preterm compared to the term brain exist. In two studies evaluating brain injury patterns in preterm infants with evidence of perinatal asphyxial encephalopathy (Barkovich 1995; Logitharajah et al. 2009), basal ganglia, thalamic and brainstem injury were seen with relative sparing of the perirolandic cortex. Cortical injury was commoner in older-gestation infants and less common in lower-gestation infants. Logitharajah et al. (2009) found that preterm infants with a presentation consistent with HIE have a high incidence of severe BGT and brainstem involvement associated with significant mortality and neurologic morbidity. White-matter lesions were common, though often mild, and cystic periventricular leukomalacia was not found. Placental abruption was a clear risk factor. As with term HIE, early MRI in preterm infants with HIE allows accurate prediction of neurological outcome and therefore may contribute significantly to the management and clinical decision-making in this preterm group.

Neuroprotective treatments

The seminal discovery about perinatal hypoxia–ischaemia in the last century was that, although some brain injury can occur during a sufficiently prolonged/severe episode of hypoxia–ischaemia, in many cases damage actually evolves for hours after resuscitation, during the recovery period (Lorek et al. 1994; Northington et al. 2001b, 2007). This evolution offers the prospect that there might be a 'window of opportunity' to provide treatment to reduce or prevent injury. This potential has been confirmed by the finding that therapeutic hypothermia can significantly reduce neurodevelopmental disability in infants with moderate to severe HIE at birth (Edwards et al. 2010).

Therapeutic hypothermia

A series of large randomised clinical trials has now shown that mild to moderate induced hypothermia (Gluckman et al. 2005; Shankaran et al. 2005; Azzopardi et al. 2009a; Simbruner et al. 2010) (also termed targeted temperature management): (1) decreases death and disability among infants with less severe aEEG abnormalities (Gluckman et al. 2005); (2) decreases death and moderate/severe disability; and (3) increases the number of survivors without disability (Shankaran et al. 2005; Azzopardi et al. 2009a; Simbruner et al. 2010). Therapeutic hypothermia under intensive care settings appears safe; although thrombocytopenia and arrhythmias are more frequent with therapeutic hypothermia, these can be corrected with appropriate clinical care (Shankaran et al. 2008; Shah 2010). Inotropic support was used more commonly in cooled infants but this may have been due to physician bias (Battin et al. 2009). Furthermore, there are suggestions that the favourable outcome of cooled infants at 18 months may be associated with favourable outcome at age 7–8 (Guillet et al. 2012).

Therapeutic hypothermia is now widely offered to infants with NE in high-income countries (Kapetanakis et al. 2009). In the UK, in May 2010, the National Institute for Health and Clinical Excellence recommended that therapeutic hypothermia with intracorporeal temperature monitoring for hypoxic perinatal brain injury should be offered to 'carefully selected infants … in units experienced in the care of severely asphyxiated infants [who] enter the details of infants undergoing cooling into the UK TOBY cooling register' (Azzopardi et al. 2009b; http://www.nice.org.uk/nicemedia/live/11315/48809/48809.pdf). No large trials have assessed the safety and efficacy of therapeutic hypothermia in neonatal encephalopathy in low resource settings and there is concern that risk factors and population differences may alter risks and benefits of this therapy in such settings (Robertson et al. 2008).

Meta-analysis of trials with 18 months of follow-up suggests a number needed to treat of approximately 9, with a relative risk for death or disability of 0.81 (95% CI 0.71–0.93; $P < 0.002$) (Edwards et al. 2010). This advance is the culmination of >40 years of basic and clinical research (Edwards 2009), and provides a strong platform from which to improve outcomes further. Eligibility criteria in the trials included a pH <7.0 or a base deficit of >16 mmol/L in umbilical cord blood or any blood during the first hour after birth. If blood gas was not available, additional criteria were required. These included an acute perinatal event and either a 10-minute Apgar score of 5 or less or assisted ventilation initiated at birth and continued for at least 10 minutes. A neurological exam with the presence of moderate to severe encephalopathy, and in some trials aEEG with specific findings, were required. Infants outside inclusion criteria for previously published clinical trials, including infants of 36 weeks' gestation, infants who present outside the previously studied 6-hour window and infants with encephalopathy not attributable to HIE, remain in the unstudied realm for cooling therapy. US studies are underway to determine whether cooling for longer and deeper (96 hours to 32°C) provides better neuroprotection or whether cooling initiated after 12 hours from birth is beneficial.

Experimental studies, however, indicate that the earlier cooling is commenced, the better the outcome (Gunn et al. 1998). This is particularly critical since the therapeutic window is substantially reduced with increasing severity of injury (Iwata et al. 2007). Guidelines are in place for cooling infants prior to and during transport to a cooling centre in the UK (Kendall et al. 2010). Once in a cooling centre, servo-controlled cooling devices are generally used (Tecotherm and Criticool) and whole-body cooling is practised more frequently than selective head cooling (Kapetanakis et al.

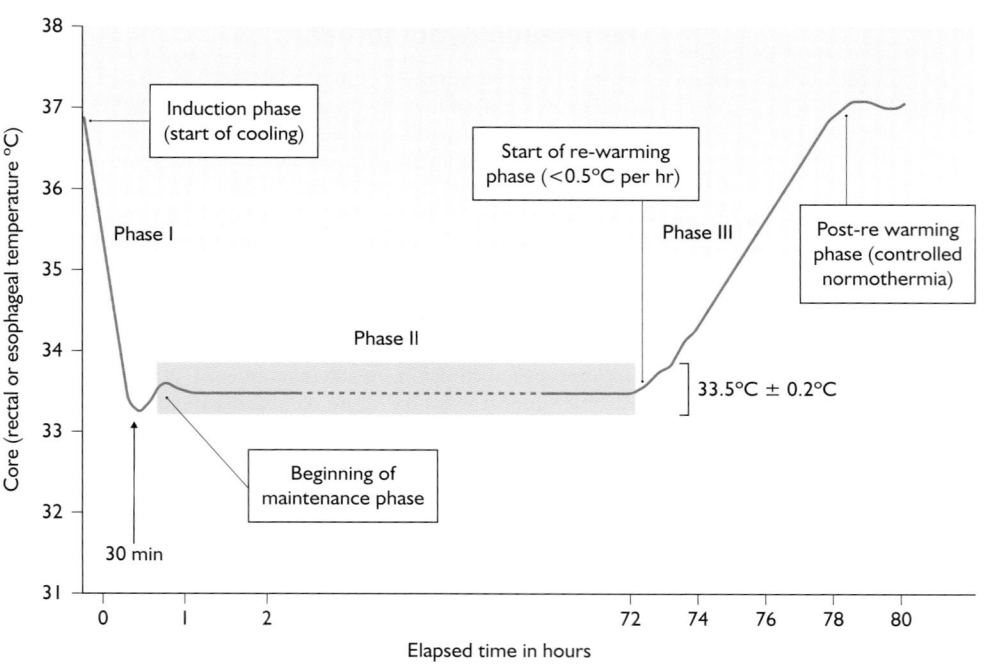

Fig. 40.42 The three phases of therapeutic hypothermia. The induction phase should be rapid and usually lasts between 30 and 120 minutes. Rapid cooling may lead to an overshoot which is acceptable if <1°C. The maintenance phase lasts for 72 hours and should have minimal fluctuations in temperature if possible (servo-controlled devices lead to most stable temperatures). The rewarming phase must be slow and controlled with rates of 0.2°C per hour. Temperature monitoring should continue to ensure that fever is prevented after rewarming. *(Reproduced from Robertson et al.)*

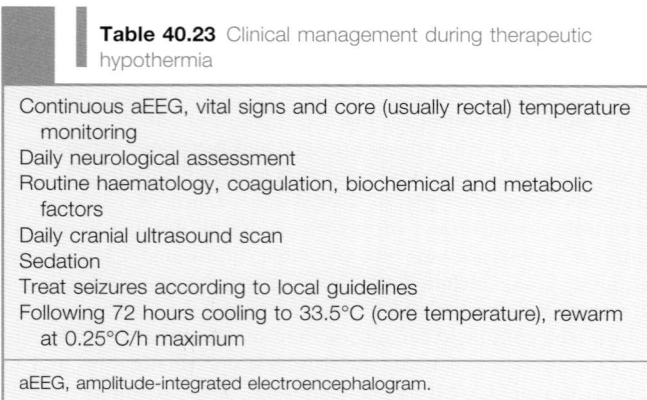

Table 40.23 Clinical management during therapeutic hypothermia

Continuous aEEG, vital signs and core (usually rectal) temperature monitoring
Daily neurological assessment
Routine haematology, coagulation, biochemical and metabolic factors
Daily cranial ultrasound scan
Sedation
Treat seizures according to local guidelines
Following 72 hours cooling to 33.5°C (core temperature), rewarm at 0.25°C/h maximum

aEEG, amplitude-integrated electroencephalogram.

2009; Robertson et al. 2010). Accumulating evidence from adult cooling studies emphasises the importance of rewarming as slowly as possible, by a maximum of 0.5°C over 2 hours. Key points in the clinical management during therapeutic hypothermia are shown in Table 40.23 and Figure 40.42. It is very important to avoid overcooling below 30°C, as this has been associated with adverse outcomes in experimental studies (Kerenyi et al. 2012). It is essential to monitor rectal temperature continuously, especially during transport. In the UK, continued surveillance via the national registry is needed to detect unusual complications and audit in therapeutic hypothermia. In particular, further experience needs to accumulate in understanding the safety of therapeutic hypothermia applied to infants with systemic complications associated with perinatal asphyxia, such as pulmonary hypertension or myocardial ischaemia; none of the trials were powered to study this.

Adjunct therapies

Despite therapeutic hypothermia, approximately half the infants who are cooled still have an abnormal outcome. Recent experimental data suggest that hypothermia extends the duration of the therapeutic window and that certain drugs given during this time may augment neuroprotection (Liu et al. 2004; O'Brien et al. 2006). Research is now being focused on preclinical studies of drugs (Kelen and Robertson 2010; Faulkner et al. 2011), which act synergistically or additively with hypothermia, with the hope that combination therapy might reduce the overall number of infants needed to treat to improve intact survival. Promising agents include erythropoietin, *N*-acetyl cysteine, melatonin, 2-immunobiotin and inhaled xenon.

Future research

It is important to make sure that the administration of individual drugs or combinations of drugs does not exacerbate neurodegeneration in the developing brain. Recent advances in regenerative medicine suggest that stem cell transplantation may improve repair of the damaged brain (van Velthoven et al. 2009). Novel interventions such as ischaemic postconditioning, which harness endogenous neuroprotective pathways, are very attractive. For all these studies, biomarkers will be needed to speed up clinical translation.

Neurodevelopmental outcome

Outcome following hypoxic–ischaemic brain injury in term or near-term infants has most frequently been studied in relation to clinical assessment of encephalopathy. Robertson and Finer (1989)

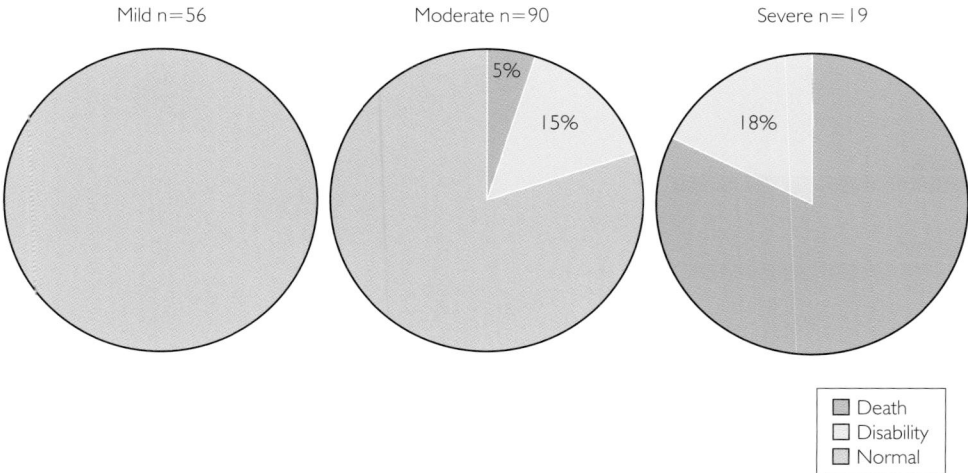

Mild n=56   Moderate n=90   Severe n=19

5%

15%

18%

☐ Death
☐ Disability
☐ Normal

Fig. 40.43 Proportion of non-disabled children in severe or moderate neonatal encephalopathy and comparison groups who failed to reach attainment level 2 (the expected level of achievement for age) for the national curriculum targets for English and mathematics. *$P < 0.05$; **$P < 0.01$; ***$P < 0.001$. *(Reproduced from Marlow et al 2005.)*

reported age-8 outcome data in a carefully staged group of children (Fig. 40.43). Their findings have been replicated in several subsequent studies. Pin and Galea (2009) have recently reviewed developmental outcomes following NE. No child had disability following mild NE and all children died or had severe disabilities following severe encephalopathy. The metaestimate of children with adverse outcomes following moderate NE (Sarnat stage 2) was 32%.

Adverse outcome is usually categorised in terms of severe cerebral palsy, which classically is a quadriplegic spastic palsy with dyskinetic features (American College of Obstetricians and Gynecologists Taskforce 2003). However NE arises from insults which are of different degrees of severity, with different time courses in relation to resuscitative efforts, and a much broader range of cerebral palsy is now evident (Cowan 2000).

Most studies of outcome following NE, including recent trials of neuroprotection, have concentrated on defining the prevalence of serious impairments such as cerebral palsy or severe cognitive deficit at 12–14 months of age. Survivors of NE without such deficits are often considered to be comparable to non-encephalopathic infants; this reflects the difficulty with assessing children in infancy. Few studies have reported outcomes into childhood and the definition of the populations studied varies widely. Indeed, an influential international taskforce on NE and cerebral palsy asserted that intrapartum hypoxia was not associated with isolated cognitive deficits (American College of Obstetricians and Gynecologists Taskforce 2003). However, it is becoming increasingly clear that significant deficits of cognitive and executive function, which lead to educational difficulties, are found more commonly amongst this group (Gonzalez 2006).

In a population tightly defined by Sarnat stage of encephalopathy, Robertson and Finer (1989) identified no deficits in association with mild encephalopathy and severe outcomes only among survivors with severe encephalopathy. In the moderate group, significantly reduced mean cognitive scores and a range of executive function deficits, with marked delays in reading, mathematics and spelling skills, were observed (Robertson and Finer 1989). More recently, a UK population-based study evaluated children following moderate encephalopathy defined as seizures with encephalopathic symptoms (Marlow et al. 2005). Within this

group, a 'severe' subgroup received more neonatal care but represented the more severe end of the 'moderate NE' spectrum. General cognitive scores were not significantly reduced compared to controls but encephalopathic infants had lower scores in language and sensorimotor function, and in narrative memory and sentence repetition. The 'severe' group had lower scores than the 'moderate' group, including everyday memory, memory for names and orientation, indicating a dose relationship with encephalopathy. These findings were reflected in the more functional measures of scholastic attainment (Fig. 40.44) (Marlow et al. 2005) and consistent with findings of greater frequency of grade repeats (Robertson and Finer 1989) and less kindergarten readiness (Robertson 1993).

The issue of specific memory deficits in association with hippocampal damage following anoxia is well described (Isaacs et al. 2003). Such injury is implicated in posthypoxic brain injury and others have identified memory impairment in children with moderate encephalopathy (Mañeru et al. 2001, 2003; van Handel et al. 2007, 2010). Behavioural problems overall and attentional problems were found more frequently among the Trent population with moderate encephalopathy (Marlow and Budge 2005) and in the Dutch cohort (van Handel et al. 2010), but no specific patterns of psychopathology are apparent.

Given the increased risk of cerebral palsy and poor outcome it is helpful to define outcome as precisely as possible for parents. MRI performed in the neonatal period has made a huge contribution to recognition of different patterns of injury. These different patterns of injury are related to the pattern and severity of later motor and cognitive disabilities (de Vries 2010b).

Basal ganglia-predominant injury

The detailed outcomes of mild, moderate and severe BGT injury are described in the section on patterns of injury, above (Martinez-Biarge et al. 2010). Dyskinetic tetraplegic cerebral palsy has the strongest causal link with intrapartum hypoxia. Intelligence may be preserved in some, particularly those with brief periods of anoxia (Rosenbloom 2003), and visual function is usually good. Many children can walk, although uncontrollable dystonic movements caused by damage to the deep grey matter can be disabling, speech

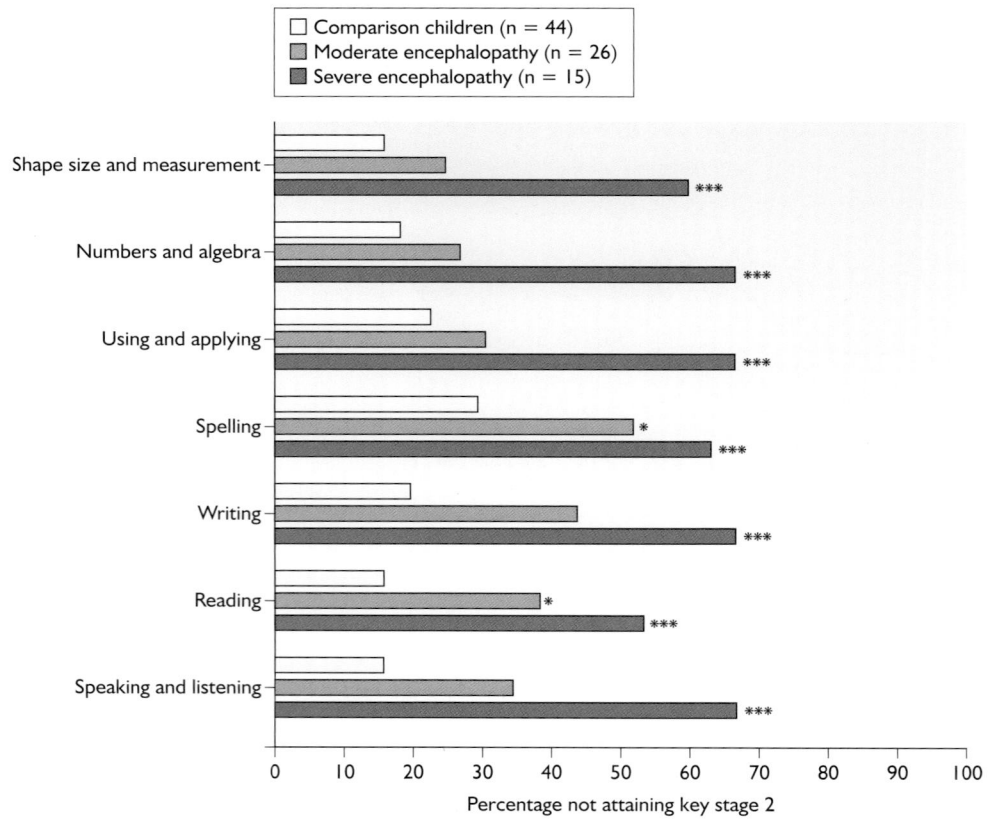

Legend:
- □ Comparison children (n = 44)
- ▨ Moderate encephalopathy (n = 26)
- ▦ Severe encephalopathy (n = 15)

Categories (top to bottom): Shape size and measurement, Numbers and algebra, Using and applying, Spelling, Writing, Reading, Speaking and listening

X-axis: Percentage not attaining key stage 2 (0 to 100)

Fig. 40.44 Eight-year overall outcome information on death and disability in cohort of infants with mild, moderate and severe neonatal encephalopathy (Marlow et al., 2005).

may be dysarthric and feeding a problem. In general, the degree of cognitive impairment reflects the severity of the motor impairment.

Parasagittal or watershed-predominant injury

Infants with a watershed pattern of injury have predominantly cognitive impairments, often without functional motor deficits (de Vries 2010b). Cognitive deficits include memory impairments, visual–motor or visual–perceptive dysfunction, difficulties in the reading, spelling and arithmetic/mathematics domains (Robertson 1993) and recognition of these deficits may be delayed beyond the first year of life (Miller et al. 2002). Some studies have reported increased hyperactivity or autism, but, as described above, there is no specific psychological behavioural pattern associated with hypoxia–ischaemia.

A recent MRI study described serial MRIs in a cohort of infants with NE (van Kooij et al. 2010): both neonatal and childhood MRIs were available in 33 children with NE. Comparable MRI patterns were seen in the scans done at different ages; as expected, BGT lesions were associated with more severe motor deficits compared to lesions in the watershed region. This study also confirmed the increased risk of cognitive deficits even without motor problems, as previously described (Marlow et al. 2005; Gonzalez 2006). Follow-up should be performed into school age for children with and without adverse neurological outcome following NE in early infancy, and include a detailed psychometric evaluation.

Intriguingly, a recent report has demonstrated an excess of low cognitive scores in association with low Apgar scores but without encephalopathy (Odd et al. 2008). This joins a large body of literature in which attempts have been made to correlate immediate neonatal outcomes (Apgar score, cord pH) or measures of fetal compromise with later outcomes (Low 1993, 2004). Although on an individual level the effect is likely to be difficult to show, and the effect size in population studies is small, this would seem to indicate a continuum of reproductive casualty as a result of perinatal hypoxia.

References

Alfirevic, Z., Devane, D., Gyte, G.M., 2006. 'Continuous cardiotocography (CTG) as a form of electronic fetal monitoring (EFM) for fetal assessment during labour.' Cochrane Database Syst Rev 19(3), CD006066.

al Naqeeb, N., Edwards, A., Cowan, F., et al., 1999. Assessment of neonatal encephalopathy by amplitude-integrated electroencephalography. Pediatrics 103, 1263–1271.

Aly, H., Khashaba, M., El-Ayouty, M., et al., 2006. IL-1beta, IL-6 and TNF-alpha and outcomes of neonatal hypoxic ischemic encephalopathy. Brain Dev 178–182.

American College of Obstetricians and Gynecologists Taskforce, 2003. Neonatal encephalopathy and cerebral palsy: defining the pathogenesis and pathophysiology. The American College of Obstetricians and Gynecologists, the American Academy of Pediatrics, Washington, DC, pp. 1–85.

Andrabi, S., Dawson, T., Dawson, V., 2008. Mitochondrial and nuclear cross talk in cell death: parthanatos. Ann N Y Acad Sci 1147, 233–241.

Apgar, V., 1953. A proposal for a new method of evaluation of the newborn infant. Curr Res Anesth Analg 32, 260–267.

Archer, L., Levene, M., Evans, D., 1986. Cerebral artery Doppler ultrasonography for prediction of outcome after perinatal asphyxia. Lancet 15, 1116–1118.

Armstrong-Wells, J., Bernard, T., Boada, R., et al., 2010. Neurocognitive outcomes following neonatal encephalopathy. Neurorehabilitation 26, 27–33.

Arvin, K., Han, B., Du, Y., et al., 2002. Minocycline markedly protects the neonatal brain against hypoxic-ischemic injury. Ann Neurol 52, 54–61.

Azzopardi, D., Edwards, A., 2010. Magnetic Resonance Biomarkers of Neuroprotective Effects in Infants with Hypoxic-ischaemic Encephalopathy. Semin Fetal Neonatal Med 15, 261–269.

Azzopardi, D., 2010. Clinical management of the baby with hypoxic ischaemic encephalopathy. Semin Fetal Neonatal Med 86, 345–350.

Azzopardi, D., Wyatt, J., Cady, E., et al., 1989. Prognosis of newborn infants with hypoxic–ischemic brain injury assessed by phosphorus magnetic resonance spectroscopy. Pediatr Res 25, 445–451.

Azzopardi, D., Strohm, B., Edwards, A., et al., 2009a. Moderate hypothermia to treat perinatal asphyxial encephalopathy. N Engl J Med 361, 1349–1358.

Azzopardi, D., Strohm, B., Edwards, A., et al., 2009b. Treatment of asphyxiated newborns with moderate hypothermia in routine clinical practice: how cooling is managed in the UK outside a clinical trial Arch Dis Child 94, F260–F264.

Badawi, N., Kurinczuk, J., Keogh, J., et al., 1998. Intrapartum risk factors for newborn encephalopathy: the Western Australian case-control study. BMJ 317, 1554–1558.

Badawi, N., Kurinczuk, J., Keogh, J., et al., 1998. Antepartum risk factors for newborn encephalopathy: the Western Australian case-control study. BMJ 317, 1549–1553.

Bågenholm, R., Nilsson, U., Götborg, C., et al., 1998. Free radicals are formed in the brain of fetal sheep during reperfusion after cerebral ischemia. Pediatr Res 43, 271–275.

Baier, R., 2006. Genetics of perinatal brain injury in the preterm infant. Front Biosci 1, 1371–1387.

Barkovich, A., Sargent, S., 1995. Profound asphyxia in the premature infant: imaging findings. AJNR Am J Neuroradiol 16, 1837–1846.

Barkovich, A., Miller, S., Bartha, A., et al., 2006. MR imaging, MR spectroscopy, and diffusion tensor imaging of sequential studies in neonates with encephalopathy. AJNR Am J Neuroradiol 27, 533–547.

Barnett, A., Mercuri, E., Rutherford, M., et al., 2002. Neurological and perceptual-motor outcome at 5-6 years of age in children with neonatal encephalopathy: relationship with neonatal brain MRI. Neuropediatrics 33, 242–248.

Baslow, M., 2002. Evidence supporting a role for N-acetyl-L-aspartate as a molecular water pump in myelinated neurons in the central nervous system. An analytical review. Neurochem Int 40, 295–300.

Battin, M., Thoresen, M., Robinson, E., et al., 2009. Does head cooling with mild systemic hypothermia affect requirement for blood pressure support? Pediatrics 123, 1031–1036.

Bert, P., 1870. Lecons sur La Physiologie Comparee de la Respiration. Kessinger Publishing, Paris.

Blair, E., Stanley, F., 1988. Intrapartum asphyxia: a rare cause of cerebral palsy. J Pediatr 112, 515–519.

Blomgren, K., Hagberg, H., 2006. Free radicals, mitochondria, and hypoxia-ischemia in the developing brain. Free Radic Biol Med 40, 388–397.

Blumberg, R.M., Cady, E.B., Wigglesworth, J.S., et al., 1997. Relation between delayed impairment of cerebral energy metabolism and infarction following transient focal hypoxia–ischaemia in the developing brain. Exp Brain Res 113, 130–137.

Bona, E., Andersson, A., Blomgren, K., et al., 1999. Chemokine and inflammatory cell response to hypoxia-ischemia in immature rats. Pediatr Res 45, 500–509.

Boylan, G., Young, K., Panerai, R., et al., 2000. Dynamic cerebral autoregulation in sick newborn infants. Pediatr Res 48, 12–17.

Brann, A., Myers, R., 1975. Central nervous system findings in the newborn monkey following severe in utero partial asphyxia. Neurology 25, 327–338.

Bukowski, R., Burgett, A., Gei, A., et al., 2003. Impairment of fetal growth potential and neonatal encephalopathy. Am J Obstet Gynaecol 188, 1011–1015.

Buonocore, G., Perrone, S., Gioia, D., et al., 1999. Nucleated red blood cell count at birth as an index of perinatal brain damage. Am J Obstet Gynecol 181, 1500–1505.

Burns, C., Rutherford, M., Boardman, J., et al., 2008. Patterns of cerebral injury and neurodevelopmental outcomes after symptomatic neonatal hypoglycemia. Pediatrics 12, 65–74.

Cady, E., Amess, P., Penrice, J., et al., 1997. Early cerebral-metabolite quantification in perinatal hypoxic–ischaemic encephalopathy by proton and phosphorus magnetic resonance spectroscopy. Magn Reson Imaging 15, 605–611.

Calvert, J., Zhang, J., 2005. Pathophysiology of an hypoxic-ischemic insult during the perinatal period. Neurol Res 27, 246–260.

Cao, G., Xing, J., Xiao, X., et al., 2007. Critical role of calpain I in mitochondrial release of apoptosis-inducing factor in ischemic neuronal injury. J Neurosci 27, 9278–9293.

Chakraborty, G., Mekala, P., Yahya, D., et al., 2001. Intraneuronal N-acetylaspartate supplies acetyl groups for myelin lipid synthesis: evidence for myelin-associated aspartoacylase. J Neurochem 78.

Chau, V., Poskitt, K., Sargent, M., et al., 2009. Comparison of computer tomography and magnetic resonance imaging scans on the third day of life in term newborns with neonatal encephalopathy. Pediatrics 123, 319–326.

Cheong, J., Cady, E., Penrice, J., et al., 2006. Proton MR spectroscopy in neonates with perinatal cerebral hypoxic–ischemic injury: metabolite peak-area ratios, relaxation times, and absolute concentrations. AJNR Am J Neuroradiol 27, 1546–1554.

Cheung, J., Bonventre, J., Malis, C., et al., 1986. Calcium and ischemic injury. N Engl J Med 314, 1670–1676.

Chiesa, C., Pellegrini, G., Panero, A., et al., 2003. Umbilical cord interleukin-6 levels are elevated in term neonates with perinatal asphyxia. Eur J Clin Invest 33, 352–358.

Chu, C., Xiao, X., Zhou, X., et al., 2006. Metabolomic and bioinformatic analyses in asphyxiated neonates. Clin Biochem 39, 203–209.

Clark, S., Belfort, M., Byrum, S., et al., 2008. Improved outcomes, fewer cesarean deliveries, and reduced litigation: results of a new paradigm in patient safety. Am J Obstet Gynecol 199, e1–e7.

Comi, A., Highet, B., Mehta, P., et al., 2006. Dextromethorphan protects male but not female mice with brain ischemia. Neuroreport 17, 1319–1322.

Committee on Fetus and Newborn American Academy of Pediatrics, 1996. Committee on Obstetric Practice American College of Obstetrics and Gynaecology. Use and abuse of the Apgar score. Pediatrics 98, 141–142.

Connolly, D., Widjaja, E., Griffiths, P., 2007. Involvement of the anterior lobe of the cerebellar vermis in perinatal profound hypoxia. Am J Neuroradiol 28, 16–19.

Cowan, F., 2000. Outcome after intrapartum asphyxia in term infants. Semin Neonatol 5, 127–140.

Cowan, F., de Vries, L., 2005. The internal capsule in neonatal imaging. Semin Fetal Neonatal Med 10, 461–474.

Cowan, F., Rutherford, M., Groenendaal, F., et al., 2000. Origin and timing of brain lesions in term infants with neonatal encephalopathy. Lancet 361, 736–742.

da Silva, S., Hennebert, N., Denis, R., et al., 2000. Clinical value of a single postnatal lactate measurement after intrapartum asphyxia. Acta Pediatr 89, 320–323.

Dawes, G., 1969. Birth Asphyxia, Resuscitation, and Brain Damage. In: Dawes, G. (Ed.), Foetal and Neonatal

Physiology. Year Book Medical Publishers, Chicago, pp. 141–159.

de Vries, L., Hellström-Westas, L., 2005. Role of cerebral function monitoring in the newborn. Arch Dis Child Fetal Neonatal Ed 90, F201–F207.

de Vries, L., Groenendaal, F., 2010. Patterns of neonatal hypoxic-ischaemic brain injury. Neuroradiology 52, 555–566.

de Vries, L., Jongmans, M., 2010. Long-term outcome after neonatal hypoxic-ischaemic encephalopathy. Archives Dis Child Fetal and Neonatal 95, F220–F224.

Dodelson de Kremer, R., Grosso, C., 2005. Maternal mutation 677C>T in the methylenetetrahydrofolate reductase gene associated with severe brain injury in offspring. Clin Genet 67, 69–80.

Draper, E., Kurinczuk, J., Lamming, C., et al., 2002. A confidential enquiry into cases of neonatal encephalopathy. Arch Dis Child Fetal Neonatal Ed 87, F176–F180.

Du, L., Hickey, R., Bayir, H., et al., 2009. Starving neurons show sex difference in autophagy. J Biol Chem 284, 2383–2396.

Dubowitz, L., Mercuri, E., Dubowitz, V., 1998. An optimality score for the neurologic examination of the term newborn. J Pediatr 133, 406–416.

Edwards, A., 2009. The discovery of hypothermic neural rescue therapy for perinatal hypoxic–ischemic encephalopathy. Semin Pediatr Neurol 16, 200–206.

Edwards, A., Brocklehurst, P., Gunn, A., et al., 2010. Neurological outcomes at 18 months of age after moderate hypothermia for perinatal hypoxic ischaemic encephalopathy: synthesis and meta-analysis of trial data. Br Med J 340, C363.

Eklind, S., Mallard, C., Leverin, A.L., et al., 2001. Bacterial endotoxin sensitizes the immature brain to hypoxic–ischaemic injury. Eur J Neurosci 13, 1101–1106.

Ellis, M., Costello, A., 1999. Antepartum risk factors for newborn encephalopathy. Intrapartum risk factors are important in developing world. Br Med J 318, 1414.

Ellis, M., Manandhar, N., Manandhar, D., et al., 2000. Risk factors for neonatal encephalopathy in Kathmandu, Nepal, a developing country: unmatched case-control study. Br Med J 320, 1229–1236.

Evans, K., Rigby, A., Hamilton, P., et al., 2001. The relationships between neonatal encephalopathy and cerebral palsy: a cohort study. J Obstet Gynaecol 21, 114–120.

Faro, M., Windle, W., 1969. Transneuronal degeneration in brains of monkeys asphyxiated at birth. Exp Neurol 24 (1), 38–53.

Fatemi, A., Wilson, M., Johnston, M., 2009. Hypoxic-ischemic encephalopathy in the term infant. Clin Perinatol 36, 835–858.

Faulkner, S., Bainbridge, A., Kato, T., et al., 2011. Xenon augmented hypothermia reduces early lactate/NAA and cell death

in Perinatal Asphyxia. Ann Neurol 70, 133–150.

Finer, N., Robertson, C., Richards, R., et al., 1981. Hypoxic-ischemic encephalopathy in term neonates: perinatal factors and outcome. J Pediatr 98, 112–117.

Fletcher, A., Gardner, D., Edwards, C., et al., 2006. Development of the ovine fetal cardiovascular defense to hypoxemia towards full term. Am J Physiol Heart Circ Physiol 291, H3023–H3034.

Florio, P., Luisi, S., Moataza, B., et al., 2007. High urinary concentrations of activin A in asphyxiated full-term newborns with moderate or severe hypoxic ischemic encephalopathy. Clin Chem 53, 520–522.

Gadian, D., Aicardi, J., Watkins, K., et al., 2000. Developmental amnesia associated with early hypoxic-ischaemic injury. Brain 123, 499–507.

Gazzolo, D., Abella, R., Marinoni, E., et al., 2009. New markers of neonatal neurology. J Matern Fetal Neonatal Med 22, 57–61.

Gill, R., Soriano, M., Blomgren, K., et al., 2002. Role of caspase-3 activation in cerebral ischemia-induced neurodegeneration in adult and neonatal brain. J Cereb Blood Flow Metab 22, 420–430.

Girard, S., Kadhim, H., Roy, M., et al., 2009. Role of perinatal inflammation in cerebral palsy. Pediatr Neurol 40, 168–174.

Glass, H.C., Glidden, D., Jeremy, R.J., et al., 2009. Clinical Neonatal Seizures are Independently Associated with Outcome in Infants at Risk for Hypoxic–ischemic Brain Injury. J Pediatr 155, 318–323.

Gluckman, P.D., Wyatt, J.S., Azzopardi, D., et al., 2005;Selective head cooling with mild systemic hypothermia after neonatal encephalopathy: multicentre randomised trial. Lancet 365, 663–670.

Gonzalez, F., Miller, S., 2006. Does Perinatal Asphyxia Impair Cognitive Function without Cerebral Palsy? Arch Dis Child Fetal Neonatal Ed 91, 454–459.

Graham, E., Ruis, K., Hartman, A., et al., 2008. A systematic review of the role of intrapartum hypoxia-ischemia in the causation of neonatal encephalopathy. Am J Obstet Gynaecol 199, 587–595.

Guillet, R., Edwards, A., Thoresen, M., et al., 2012. Seven- to eight-year follow-up of the CoolCap trial of head cooling for neonatal encephalopathy. Pediatr Res 71(2), 205–209.

Gunn, A., Gunn, T., Gunning, M., et al., 1998. Neuroprotection with prolonged head cooling started before postischemic seizures in fetal sheep. Pediatrics 102, 1098–1106.

Gunn, A., Wyatt, J., Whitelaw, A., et al., 2008. Therapeutic hypothermia changes the prognostic value of clinical evaluation of neonatal encephalopathy. J Pediatr 152, 55–58.

Hagan, P., Barks, J., Yabut, M., et al., 1996. Adenovirus-mediated over-expression of interleukin-1 receptor antagonist reduces

susceptibility to excitotoxic brain injury in perinatal rats. Neuroscience 75, 1033–1045.

Hagberg, H., Andersson, P., Kjellmer, I., et al., 1987. Extracellular overflow of glutamate, aspartate, GABA and taurine in the cortex and basal ganglia of fetal lambs during hypoxia-ischemia. Neurosci Lett 78, 311–317.

Hagberg, H., Thornberg, E., Blennow, M., et al., 1991. Excitatory amino acids in the cerebrospinal fluid of asphyxiated infants: relationship to hypoxic-ischemic encephalopathy. Acta Pediatr 82, 925–929.

Hagberg, B., Hagberg, G., Beckung, E., et al., 2001. Changing panorama of cerebral palsy in Sweden. VIII. Prevalence and origin in the birth year period 1991–1994. Acta Pediatr 90, 271–277.

Hagmann, C., Robertson, N., Azzopardi, D., 2006. Artifacts on electroencephalograms may influence the amplitude-integrated EEG classification: a qualitative analysis in neonatal encephalopathy. Pediatrics 118, 2552–2554.

Hahn, J., 2009. Clinical Manifestations of hypoxic-ischemic encephalopathy. In: Stevenson, B. Sunshine, Hintz, Druzin, editor. Fetal and Neonatal Brain Injury. Cambridge University Press, New York, 187–195.

Hallberg, B., Grossmann, K., Bartocci, M., et al., 2010. The prognostic value of early aEEG in asphyxiated infants undergoing systemic hypothermia treatment. Acta Pediatr 99, 531–536.

Hankins, G., 2003. The long journey: defining the true pathogenesis and pathophysiology of neonatal encephalopathy and cerebral palsy. Obstet Gynaecol Surv 58, 435–437.

Harrington, D., Redman, C., Moulden, M., et al., 2007. The long-term outcome in surviving infants with Apgar zero at 10 minutes: a systematic review of the literature and hospital-based cohort. Am J Obstet Gynaecol 196, 463. e461–465.

Hellström-Westas, L., Rosén, I., Svenningsen, N., 1995. Predictive value of early continuous amplitude integrated EEG recordings on outcome after severe birth asphyxia in full term infants. Arch Dis Child Fetal Neonatal Ed 72, F34–F38.

Himmelmann, K., Hagberg, G., Uvebrant, P., 2010. The changing panorama of cerebral palsy in Sweden. X. Prevalence and origin in the birth-year period 1999–2002. Acta Pediatr 99, 1337–1343.

Hope, P., Costello, A., Cady, E., et al., 1984. Cerebral energy metabolism studied with phosphorus NMR spectroscopy in normal and birth-asphyxiated infants. Lancet 18, 366–370.

Huang, C., Wang, S., Chang, Y., et al., 1999. Measurement of the urinary lactate:creatinine ratio for the early identification of newborn infants at risk for hypoxic-ischemic encephalopathy. N Engl J Med 341, 328–335.

Hudome, S., Palmer, C., Roberts, R., et al., 1997. The role of neutrophils in the production of hypoxic-ischemic brain injury in the neonatal rat. Pediatr Res 41, 607–616.

Hull, J., Dodd, K., 1992. Falling incidence of hypoxic-ischaemic encephalopathy in term infants. Br J Obstet Gynaecol 99, 386–391.

Ikeda, T., Mishima, K., Aoo, N., et al., 2004. Combination treatment of neonatal rats with hypoxia-ischemia and endotoxin induces long-lasting memory and learning impairment that is associated with extended cerebral damage. Am J Obstet Gynaecol 191, 2132–2141.

International Liaison Committee on Resuscitation, 2006. The International Liaison Committee on Resuscitation (ILCOR) consensus on science with treatment recommendations for pediatric and neonatal patients: pediatric basic and advanced life support. Pediatrics 117, e955–977.

Isaacs, E., Vargha-Khadem, F., Watkins, K., et al., 2003. Developmental amnesia and its relationship to degree of hippocampal atrophy. Proc Natl Acad Sci 100, 13060–13063.

Iwata, O., Iwata, S., Thornton, J., et al., 2007. "Therapeutic time window" duration decreases with increasing severity of cerebral hypoxia-ischaemia under normothermia and delayed hypothermia in newborn piglets. Brain Res 1154, 173–180.

Johnston, M., 1995. Neurotransmitters and vulnerability of the developing brain. Brain Dev 17, 301–306.

Johnston, M., 2005. Excitotoxicity in perinatal brain injury. Brain Pathol 15, 234–240.

Johnston, M., Hagberg, H., 2007. Sex and the pathogenesis of cerebral palsy. Dev Med Child Neurol 49, 74–78.

Jonsson, M., Nordén-Lindeberg, S., Ostlund, I., et al., 2009. Metabolic acidosis at birth and suboptimal care–illustration of the gap between knowledge and clinical practice. BJOG 116, 1453–1460.

Juul, S., Aylward, E., Richards, T., et al., 2007. Prenatal cord clamping in newborn Macaca nemestrina: a model of perinatal asphyxia. Dev Neurosci 29, 311–320.

Kapetanakis, A., Azzopardi, D., Wyatt, J., et al., 2009. Therapeutic hypothermia for neonatal encephalopathy: a UK survey of opinion, practice and neuro-investigation at the end of 2007. Acta Paediatr 98, 631–635.

Kelen, D., Robertson, N., 2010. Experimental treatments for hypoxic ischaemic encephalopathy. Early Hum Dev 86, 369–377.

Kendall, G., Kapetanakis, A., Ratnavel, N., et al., Cooling on Retrieval Group, 2010. Passive cooling for initiation of therapeutic hypothermia in neonatal encephalopathy. Arch Dis Child Fetal Neonatal Ed 95, F408–F412.

Kerenyi, A., Kelen, D., Faulkner, S., et al., 2012. Systemic effects of whole-body cooling to 35°C, 33.5°C, and 30°C in a piglet model of perinatal asphyxia: implications for therapeutic hypothermia. Pediatr Res 71, 573–582.

Klinger, G., Beyene, J., Shah, P., et al., 2005. Do hyperoxaemia and hypocapnia add to the risk of brain injury after intrapartum asphyxia? Arch Dis Child Fetal Neonatal Ed 90, F49–F52.

Kumar, S., Paterson-Brown, S., 2010. Obstetric aspects of hypoxic ischemic encephalopathy. Early Hum Dev 86, 339–344.

Kurinczuk, J., White-Koning, M., Badawi, N., 2010. Epidemiology of neonatal encephalopathy and hypoxic-ischaemic encephalopathy. Early Hum Dev 86, 329–338.

Laptook, A., Shankaran, S., Ambalavanan, N., et al., Network Hypothermia Subcommittee of the NICHD Neonatal Research Network, 2009. Outcome of term infants using apgar scores at 10 minutes following hypoxic-ischemic encephalopathy. Pediatrics 124, 1619–1626.

Lawn, J., Cousens, S., Zupan, J., Team for the Lancet Neonatal Survival Steering Team, 2005. 4 million neonatal deaths: When? Where? Why? Lancet 365, 891–900.

Lawn, J.E., Kinney, M., Lee, A.C., et al., 2009. Reducing intrapartum-related deaths and disability: can the health system deliver? Int J Gynaecol Obstet 107, S123–S142.

LeGallois, M., 1813. Experiments on the Principle of Life. Gryphon, Philadelphia.

Lehnardt, S., Massillon, L., Follett, P., et al., 2003. Activation of innate immunity in the CNS triggers neurodegeneration through a Toll-like receptor 4-dependent pathway. PNAS 100, 8514–8519.

Levene, M., Kornberg, J., Williams, T., 1985. The incidence and severity of post-asphyxial encephalopathy in full-term infants. Early Hum Dev 11, 21–26.

Levene, M., Sands, C., Grindulis, H., et al., 1986. Comparison of two methods of predicting outcome in perinatal asphyxia. Lancet 1, 67–69.

Lieberman, E., Eichenwald, E., Mathur, G., et al., 2000. Intrapartum fever and unexplained seizures in term infants. Pediatrics 106, 983–988.

Liu, Y., Barks, J., Xu, G., et al., 2004. Topiramate extends the therapeutic window for hypothermia-mediated neuroprotection after stroke in neonatal rats. Stroke 35, 1460–1465.

Logitharajah, P., Rutherford, M., Cowan, F., 2009. Hypoxic-ischemic encephalopathy in preterm infants: antecedent factors, brain imaging, and outcome. Pediatr Res 66, 222–229.

Longo, M., Hankins, G., 2009. Defining Cerebral Palsy: Pathogenesis, Pathophysiology and New Intervention. Minerva Ginecol 61, 421–429.

Lorek, A., Takei, Y., Cady, E., et al., 1994. Delayed ('secondary') cerebral energy failure after acute hypoxia–ischaemia in the newborn piglet: continuous 48-hour studies by phosphorus magnetic resonance spectroscopy. Pediatr Res 36, 699–706.

Low, J., 2004. Determining the contribution of asphyxia to brain damage in the neonate. J Obstet Gynaecol Res 30, 276–286.

Low, J., 1993. The relationship of asphyxia in the mature fetus to long-term neurologic function. Clin Obstet Gynaecol 36, 82–90.

Low, J., Lindsay, B., Derrick, E., 1997. Threshold of metabolic acidosis associated with newborn complications. Am J Obstet Gynaecol 177, 1391–1394.

MacLennan, A., 1999. A template for defining a causal relation between acute intrapartum events and cerebral palsy: international consensus statement. Br Med J 319, 1054–1059.

Madhavarao, C., Chinopoulos, C., Chandrasekaran, K., et al., 2003. Characterization of the N-acetylaspartate biosynthetic enzyme from rat brain. J Neurochem 86, 824–835.

Mañeru, C., Junqué, C., Botet, F., et al., 2001. Neuropsychological long-term sequelae of perinatal asphyxia. Brain Inj 15, 1029–1039.

Mañeru, C., Serra-Grabulosa, J., Junqué, C., et al., 2003. Residual hippocampal atrophy in asphyxiated term neonates. J Neuroimaging 13, 68–74.

Marks, K., Mallard, E., Roberts, I., et al., 1996. Delayed vasodilation and altered oxygenation after cerebral ischemia in fetal sheep. Pediatr Res 39, 48–54.

Marlow, N., Budge, H., 2005. Prevalence, causes, and outcome at 2 years of age of newborn encephalopathy. Arch Dis Child Fetal Neonatal Ed 90, F193–F194.

Marlow, N., Rose, A., Rands, C., et al., 2005. Neuropsychological and educational problems at school age associated with neonatal encephalopathy. Arch Dis Child Fetal Neonatal Ed 90, F380–F387.

Martin, E., Buchli, R., Ritter, S., et al., 1996. Diagnostic and prognostic value of cerebral ^{31}P magnetic resonance spectroscopy in neonates with perinatal asphyxia. Pediatr Res 40, 749–758.

Martinez-Biarge, M., Diez-Sebastian, J., Rutherford, M., et al., 2010. Outcomes after central grey matter injury in term perinatal hypoxic-ischaemic encephalopathy. Early Hum Dev 86, 675–682.

McDonald, J., Silverstein, F., Cardona, D., et al., 1990. Systemic administration of MK-801 protects against N-methyl-D-aspartate- and quisqualate-mediated neurotoxicity in perinatal rats. Neuroscience 36, 589–599.

McKinstry, R., Miller, J., Snyder, A., et al., 2002. A prospective, longitudinal diffusion tensor imaging study of brain injury in newborns. Neurology 59, 824–833.

McQuillen, P., Ferriero, D., 2004. Selective vulnerability in the developing central nervous system. Pediatr Neurol 15, 250–260.

Mercuri, E., Ricci, D., Cowan, F., et al., 2000. Head growth in infants with hypoxic–ischaemic encephalopathy: correlation with magnetic resonance imaging. Pediatrics 106, 235–243.

Miller, S., Newton, N., Ferriero, D., et al., 2002. Predictors of 30-month outcome after perinatal depression: role of proton MRS and socioeconomic factors. Pediatr Res 52, 71–77.

Miller, S., Latal, B., Clark, H., et al., 2004. Clinical signs predict 30-month neurodevelopmental outcome after neonatal encephalopathy. Am J Obstet Gynecol 190, 93–99.

Miller, S., Ramaswamy, V., Michelson, D., et al., 2005. Patterns of brain injury in term neonatal encephalopathy. J Pediatr 146, 453–460.

Monod, N., Pajot, N., Guidasci, S., 1972. The neonatal EEG: statistical studies and prognostic value in full-term and pre-term babies. Electroencephalogr Clin Neurophysiol 32, 529–544.

Moseley, M.E., Cohen, Y., Kucharczyk, J., et al., 1990. Diffusion-weighted MR imaging of anisotropic water diffusion in cat central nervous system. Radiology 176, 439–445.

Myers, R., 1972. Two patterns of perinatal brain damage and their conditions of occurrence. Am J Obstet Gynecol 112, 246–276.

Nelson, K., Ellenberg, J., 1981. Apgar scores as predictors of chronic neurologic disability. Pediatrics 68, 36–44.

Nelson, K., Leviton, A., 1991. How much of neonatal encephalopathy is due to birth asphyxia? Am J Dis Child 145, 1325–1331.

Nelson, K., Willoughby, R., 2000. Infection, inflammation and the risk of cerebral palsy. Curr Opin Neurol 13, 133–139.

Nelson, K., Dambrosia, J., Ting, T., et al., 1996. Uncertain value of electronic fetal monitoring in predicting cerebral palsy. N Engl J Med 334, 613–618.

Nelson, K., Dambrosia, J., Grether, J., et al., 1998. Neonatal cytokines and coagulation factors in children with cerebral palsy. Ann Neurol 44, 665–675.

Nijboer, C., Groenendaal, F., Kavelaars, A., et al., 2007. Gender-specific neuroprotection by 2-iminobiotin after hypoxia-ischemia in the neonatal rat via a nitric oxide independent pathway. J Cereb Blood Flow Metab 27, 282–292.

Nikas, I., Dermentzoglou, V., Theofanopoulou, M., et al., 2008. Parasagittal lesions and ulegyria in hypoxic-ischemic encephalopathy: neuroimaging findings and review of the pathogenesis. J Child Neurol 23, 51–58.

Northington, F., Chavez-Valdez, R., Martin, L., 2011. Neuronal cell death in neonatal hypoxia-ischemia. Ann Neurol 69, 743–758.

Northington, F., Ferriero, D., Graham, E., et al., 2001a. Early Neurodegeneration after Hypoxia–ischaemia in Neonatal Rat Is Necrosis while Delayed Neuronal Death Is Apoptosis. Neurobiol Dis 8, 207–219.

Northington, F., Ferriero, D., Flock, D., et al., 2001b. Delayed neurodegeneration in neonatal rat thalamus after hypoxia–ischaemia is apoptosis. J Neurosci 21, 1931–1938.

Northington, F., Zelaya, M., O'Riordan, D., et al., 2007. Failure to complete apoptosis following neonatal hypoxia-ischemia manifests as "continuum" phenotype of cell death and occurs with multiple manifestations of mitochondrial dysfunction in rodent forebrain. Neuroscience 149, 822–833.

O'Brien, F., Iwata, O., Thornton, J., et al., 2006. Delayed whole-body cooling to 33 or 35 degrees C and the development of impaired energy generation consequential to transient cerebral hypoxia–ischaemia in the newborn piglet. Pediatrics 117, 1549–1559.

Odd, D., Rasmussen, F., Gunnell, D., et al., 2008. A cohort study of low Apgar scores and cognitive outcomes. Arch Dis Child Fetal Neonatal Ed 93, F115–F120.

Odd, D., Lewis, G., Whitelaw, A., et al., 2009. Resuscitation at birth and cognition at 8 years of age: a cohort study. Lancet 373, 1615–1622.

Oh, W., Perritt, R., Shankaran, S., et al., 2008. Association between urinary lactate to creatinine ratio and neurodevelopmental outcome in term infants with hypoxic-ischemic encephalopathy. J Pediatr 153, 375–378.

Okereafor, A., Allsop, J., Counsell, S., et al., 2008. Patterns of brain injury in neonates exposed to perinatal sentinel events. Pediatrics 121, 906–914.

Osredkar, D., Toet, M., van Rooij, L., et al., 2005. Sleep-wake cycling on amplitude-integrated electroencephalography in term newborns with hypoxic-ischemic encephalopathy. Pediatrics 115, 327–332.

Painter, M.J., Scher, M.S., Stein, A.D., et al., 1999. Phenobarbital compared with phenytoin for the treatment of neonatal seizures. N Engl J Med 341, 485–489.

Peeters, L., Sheldon, R., Jones, M.J., et al., 1979. Blood flow to fetal organs as a function of arterial oxygen content. Obstet Gynaecol 135.

Peeters-Scholte, C., Braun, K., Koster, J., et al., 2003. Effects of allopurinol and deferoxamine on reperfusion injury of the brain in newborn piglets after neonatal hypoxia–ischaemia. Pediatr Res 54, 516–522.

Pin, T., Eldridge, B., Galea, M., 2009. A review of developmental outcomes of term infants with post-asphyxia neonatal encephalopathy. Eur J Pediatr Neurol 13, 224–234.

Pryds, O., Greisen, G., Lou, H., et al., 1990. Vasoparalysis associated with brain damage in asphyxiated term infants. J Pediatr 117, 119–125.

Qian, J., Zhou, D., Wang, Y., 2009. Umbilical artery blood S100beta protein: a tool for the early identification of neonatal hypoxic-ischemic encephalopathy. Eur J Pediatr 168, 71–77.

Ramaswamy, V., Horton, J., Vandermeer, B., et al., 2009. Systematic review of biomarkers of brain injury in term neonatal encephalopathy. Pediatr Neurol 40, 215–226.

Ranck, J.J., Windle, W., 1959. Brain damage in the monkey, macaca mulatta, by asphyxia neonatorum. Exp Neurol 1, 130–154.

Robertson, C., Finer, N., 1993. Long-term follow-up of term neonates with perinatal asphyxia. Clin Perinatol 20, 483–500.

Robertson, C.M., Finer, N.N., 1989. School performance of survivors of neonatal encephalopathy associated with birth asphyxia at term. J Pediatr 114, 753–760.

Robertson, N., Cox, I., Cowan, F., et al., 1999. Cerebral intracellular lactic alkalosis persisting months after neonatal encephalopathy measured by magnetic resonance spectroscopy. Pediatr Res 46, 287–296.

Robertson, N., Nakakeeto, M., Hagmann, C., et al., 2008. Therapeutic hypothermia for birth asphyxia in low-resource settings: a pilot randomised controlled trial. Lancet 372 (9641), 801–803.

Robertson, N., Kendall, G., Thayyil, S., 2010. Techniques for therapeutic hypothermia during transport and in hospital for perinatal asphyxial encephalopathy. Semin Fetal Neonatal Med 15, 276–286.

Rosenbloom, L., 2003. Dyskinetic cerebral palsy and birth asphyxia. Dev Med Child Neurol 36, 285–289.

Rutherford, M., Pennock, J., Dubowitz, L., 1994. Cranial ultrasound and magnetic resonance imaging in hypoxic-ischaemic encephalopathy: a comparison with outcome. Dev Med Child Neurol 36, 813–825.

Rutherford, M., Ramenghi, L., Edwards, A., et al., 2010. Assessment of brain tissue injury after moderate hypothermia in neonates with hypoxic–ischaemic encephalopathy: a nested substudy of a randomised controlled trial. Lancet Neurol 9, 39–45.

Santos, M., Li, H., Voglmaier, S., 2009. Synaptic vesicle protein trafficking at the glutamate synapse. Neuroscience 158, 189–203.

Sarnat, H., Sarnat, M., 1976. Neonatal encephalopathy following fetal distress. Arch Neurol 33.

Saugstad, O., Ramji, S., Soll, R., et al., 2008. Resuscitation of newborn infants with 21% or 100% oxygen: an updated systematic review and meta-analysis. Neonatology 94, 176–182.

Sävman, K., Blennow, M., Gustafson, K., et al., 1998. Cytokine response in cerebrospinal fluid after birth asphyxia. Pediatr Res 43, 746–751.

Shah, P., 2010. Hypothermia: a systematic review and meta-analysis of clinical trials. Semin Fetal Neonatal Med 15, 238–246.

Shah, S., Tracy, M., Smyth, J., 2004. Postnatal lactate as an early predictor of short-term outcome after intrapartum asphyxia. J Perinatol 24, 16–20.

Shah, P., Riphagen, S., Beyene, J., et al., 2004. Multiorgan dysfunction in infants with post-asphyxial hypoxic-ischaemic encephalopathy. Arch Dis Child Fetal Neonatal Ed 89, F152–F155.

Shankaran, S., Laptook, A., Ehrenkranz, R., et al., 2005. Whole-body hypothermia for neonates with hypoxic-ischemic encephalopathy. N Engl J Med; 353, 1574–1584.

Shankaran, S., Pappas, A., Laptook, A.R., et al., 2008. Outcomes of safety and effectiveness in a multicenter randomized, controlled trial of whole-body hypothermia for neonatal hypoxic-ischemic encephalopathy. Pediatrics 122, e79–798.

Shany, E., Goldstein, E., Khvatskin, S., et al., 2006. Predictive value of amplitude-integrated electroencephalography pattern and voltage in asphyxiated term infants. Pediatr Neurol 35, 335–342.

Siesjö, B., Agardh, C., Bengtsson, F., et al., 1989. Free radicals and brain damage. Cerebrovasc Brain Metab Rev 1, 165–211.

Silverstein, F., Naik, B., Simpson, J., 1991. Hypoxia-ischemia stimulates hippocampal glutamate efflux in perinatal rat brain: an in vivo microdialysis study. Pediatr Res 30, 587–590.

Simbruner, G., Mittal, R.A., Rohlmann, F., et al., 2010. Systemic hypothermia after neonatal encephalopathy: outcomes of neo.nEURO.network RC. Pediatrics 126, e771–778.

Smith, J., Wells, L., Dodd, K., 2000. The continuing fall in incidence of hypoxic-ischaemic encephalopathy in term infants. BJOG 107, 461–466.

Strasser, A., Jost, P., Nagata, S., 2009. The many roles of FAS receptor signaling in the immune system. Immunity 30, 180–192.

Takashima, S., Armstrong, D., Becker, L., 1978. Subcortical leukomalacia. Relationship to development of the cerebral sulcus and its vascular supply. Arch Neurol 35, 470–472.

ter Horst, H., van Olffen, M., Remmelts, H., et al., 2008. The prognostic value of amplitude integrated EEG in neonatal sepsis and/or meningitis. Acta Pediatr 99, 194–200.

Thayyil, S., Chandrasekaran, M., Taylor, A., et al., 2010. Cerebral magnetic resonance biomarkers in neonatal encephalopathy: a meta-analysis. Pediatrics 125, e382–395.

Thompson, C., Puterman, A., Linley, L., et al., 1997. The value of a scoring system for hypoxic-ischaemic encephalopathy in predicting neurodevelopmental outcome. Acta Pediatr 86, 757.

Thoresen, M., Hellström-Westas, L., Liu, X., et al., 2010. Effect of hypothermia on amplitude-integrated electroencephalogram in infants with asphyxia. Pediatrics 126, e131–139.

Thoresen, M., Penrice, J., Lorek, A., et al., 1995. Mild hypothermia after severe transient hypoxia–ischaemia ameliorates delayed cerebral energy failure in the newborn piglet. Pediatr Res 37, 667–670.

Thornberg, E., Thiringer, K., Odeback, A., et al., 1995. Birth asphyxia: incidence, clinical course and outcome in a Swedish population. Acta Pediatr 84, 927–932.

Toet, M., Hellström-Westas, L., Groenendaal, F., et al., 1999. Amplitude integrated EEG 3 and 6 hours after birth in full term neonates with hypoxic–ischaemic encephalopathy. Arch Dis Child Fetal Neonatal Ed 81, F19–F23.

Toet, M., van der Meij, W., de Vries, L., et al., 2002. Comparison between simultaneously recorded amplitude integrated electroencephalogram (cerebral function monitor) and standard electroencephalogram in neonates. Pediatrics 109, 772–779.

Urenjak, J., Williams, S., Gadian, D., et al., 1992. Specific expression of N-acetylaspartate in neurons, oligodendrocyte-type-2 astrocyte progenitors, and immature oligodendrocytes in vitro. J Neurochem 59, 55–61.

van Handel, M., Swaab, H., de Vries, L., et al., 2007. Long-term cognitive and behavioral consequences of neonatal encephalopathy following perinatal asphyxia: a review. Eur J Pediatr 166, 645–654.

van Handel, M., Swaab, H., de Vries, L., et al., 2010. Behavioral outcome in children with a history of neonatal encephalopathy following perinatal asphyxia. J Pediatr Psychol 35, 286–295.

van Kooij, B., van Handel, M., Nievelstein, R., et al., 2010. Serial MRI and neurodevelopmental outcome in 9- to 10-year-old children with neonatal encephalopathy. J Pediatr 157, 221–227.

van Rooij, L., Toet, M., Osredkar, D., et al., 2005. Recovery of amplitude integrated electroencephalographic background patterns within 24 hours of perinatal asphyxia. Arch Dis Child Fetal Neonatal Ed 90, F243–F251.

van Velthoven, C.T., Kavelaars, A., van Bel, F., et al., 2009. Regeneration of the ischemic brain by engineered stem cells: fuelling endogenous repair processes. Brain Res Rev 61, 1–13.

van Wezel-Meijler, G., Steggerda, S., Leijser, L., 2010. Cranial ultrasonography in neonates: role and limitations. Semin Perinatol 34, 28–38.

Volpe, J., 2001. Hypoxic–ischaemic encephalopathy: neuropathology and pathogenesis. In: Volpe, J. (Ed.), Neurology of the Newborn, fourth ed. Saunders, Philadelphia, pp. 497–520.

Wang, X., Karlsson, J., Zhu, C., et al., 2001. Caspase-3 activation after neonatal rat cerebral hypoxia-ischemia. Biol Neonate 79, 172–179.

Wassink, G., Bennet, L., Booth, L., et al., 2007. The ontogeny of hemodynamic responses to prolonged umbilical cord occlusion in fetal sheep. J Appl Physiol 103, 1311–1317.

Watanabe, K., Miyazaki, S., Hara, K., et al., 1980. Behavioral state cycles, background EEGs and prognosis of newborns with perinatal hypoxia. Electroencephalogr Clin Neurophysiol 49, 618–625.

Wiberg, N., Källén, K., Herbst, A., et al., 2010. Relation between umbilical cord blood pH, base deficit, lactate, 5-minute Apgar score and development of hypoxic ischemic encephalopathy. Acta Obstet Gynaecol Scand 89, 1263–1269.

Williams, K., Galerneau, F., 2003. Intrapartum fetal heart rate patterns in the prediction of neonatal acidemia. Am J Obstet Gynaecol 188, 820–823.

Williams, K., Galerneau, F., 2004. Comparison of intrapartum fetal heart rate tracings in patients with neonatal seizures vs. no seizures: what are the differences? J Perinat Med 32, 422–425.

World Health Organization, 2005. World Health Report: make every mother and child count. Geneva, Switzerland.

Wu, Y., Escobar, G., Grether, J., et al., 2003. Chorioamnionitis and cerebral palsy in term and near-term infants. JAMA 290, 2677–2684.

Wu, Y., Croen, L., Torres, A., et al., 2009. Interleukin-6 genotype and risk for cerebral palsy in term and near-term infants. Ann Neurol 66, 663–670.

Wyatt, J., 1993. Near-infrared spectroscopy in asphyxial brain injury. Clin Perinatol 20, 369–378.

Yan, H., Ishihara, K., Serikawa, T., et al., 2003. Activation by N-acetyl-L-aspartate of acutely dissociated hippocampal neurons in rats via metabotropic glutamate receptors. Epilepsia 44, 1153–1159.

Zhu, C., Xu, F., Wang, X., et al., 2006. Different apoptotic mechanisms are activated in male and female brains after neonatal hypoxia-ischaemia. J Neurochem 96, 1016–1027.

Leigh E Dyet   Janet M Rennie

Preterm cerebral haemorrhage

Introduction

The incidence of intracerebral haemorrhage has declined in the preterm population; however, it remains the most common type of neonatal intracranial lesion and is the main cause of cerebral palsy in preterm infants following the reduction in cystic periventricular leukomalacia (cPVL) (Hamrick et al. 2004). Cohort screening with ultrasound has provided information about the incidence, timing and evolution of neonatal cerebral lesions for over 30 years. Brain magnetic resonance imaging (MRI) is increasingly used, confirming the presence of germinal matrix–intraventricular haemorrhage (GMH-IVH) seen on ultrasound and providing some information on the prediction of outcome. However, MRI can pick up smaller GMH-IVHs not seen on ultrasound and in particular it identifies posterior fossa haemorrhage, including cerebellar haemorrhage, with greater accuracy.

Terminology

Classification of preterm cerebral haemorrhage has not changed significantly over the last decade. The Papile classification (Papile et al. 1978), which was based on computed tomography (CT) scan appearances, is outmoded, but to date none of the suggested alternatives has gained wide acceptance. The Papile classification was designed to grade a single CT 'snapshot' taken during the first week of life. In the Papile system grade I described a haemorrhage confined to the subependymal region, grade II was used for bleeding into the ventricular cavity but not distending it, grade III for an intraventricular bleed with ventricular enlargement due to blood clot and grade IV for any parenchymal lesion. There are several disadvantages to this system, including the fact that grade IV lumps all parenchymal lesions together, whereas modern neuroimaging can distinguish different types. The evolution of a parenchymal lesion often provides the best clue to which type of lesion it is.

All preterm infants should have early cranial ultrasound images obtained, but relatively few will have brain MRI and some will die before the evolving lesion can be studied. Hence, any system of classification must be applicable to the early ultrasound appearances. The term 'germinal matrix–intraventricular haemorrhage' remains the most appropriate generic term for the common form of intracranial haemorrhage seen in preterm infants that does not involve the brain parenchyma. The term 'intraparenchymal lesion' (IPL) is preferable to describe the early appearances of parenchymal lesions. Ultrasound cannot reliably distinguish between infarction and haemorrhage so we do not use the term 'haemorrhagic parenchymal infarction' (Kuban et al. 2001). This topic will be discussed in greater detail in the next section. A classification system based on the description of early and late ultrasound appearances, based on that suggested by Volpe (2008) and de Vries et al. (1992), is given in Table 40.24 and examples are provided in Table 40.25.

Cerebellar haemorrhage can be identified using cranial ultrasound, and the chance of detection is improved using alternative acoustic windows, such as the posterior fontanelle or mastoid window. It is only with brain MRI that the true incidence has become more apparent (Miall et al. 2003). Haemorrhage can be found within the cerebellum or within the posterior fossa and is frequently associated with GMH-IVH. There is no formal

Table 40.24 Description of preterm intracranial haemorrhagic lesions seen early in life with ultrasound

DESCRIPTION	GENERIC TERM
Germinal matrix haemorrhage	GMH
Intraventricular haemorrhage without ventricular dilatation	GMH-IVH
Intraventricular haemorrhage with acute ventricular dilatation (measure the ventricle)	GMH-IVH with ventricular dilatation

classification system to date, although a careful description of the site of the haemorrhage is helpful.

Germinal matrix–intraventricular haemorrhage

Incidence

In the late 1970s and early 1980s, initial studies using CT and ultrasound showed the incidence of all forms of intracranial haemorrhage (encompassing GMH-IVH and IPL) to be 40–50% in very-low-birthweight infants (VLBWI). In the 1990s many groups noted a decline in the incidence of GMH-IVH and IPL together, to about 20–30% of VLBWI (Philip et al. 1989; Batton et al. 1994; Lemons et al. 2001; Horbar et al. 2002). The incidence and severity of GMH-IVH remain tightly related to gestational age. It is more common in boys and the injury tends to be more severe (Mohamed and Aly 2010). About a quarter of cases are bilateral. The welcome reduction of GMH-IVH seen in the 1990s does not seem to have continued: the National Institute of Child Health and Human Development Neonatal Research Network reported a static incidence between 1990 and 2002 (Fanaroff et al. 2007) and similar findings were reported in Sweden between 1995 and 2004 (Lundqvist et al. 2009). The fact that studies use different descriptions makes comparisons difficult, but the incidence of grade III GMH-IVH and IPL together is currently approximately 10% in infants <1500 g (Sarkar et al. 2009).

Timing

Although GMH-IVH occasionally occurs antenatally, the vast majority of preterm infants develop the lesion after birth. Sequential ultrasound studies enabled accurate timing of the onset after birth (Funato et al. 1992). These studies showed that the majority of lesions occurred within 72 hours, with more than half occurring during the first 24 hours (Dolfin et al. 1983; McDonald et al. 1984; Ment et al. 1984; Paneth et al. 1993; Linder et al. 2003). In 10–20% of cases compression of the terminal vein occurs with development of an IPL due to haemorrhagic infarction over the next 24–48 hours (Levene and de Vries 1984). GMH-IVH often occurs very soon after birth in the least mature infants (Perlman and Volpe 1986; Leviton et al. 1991b) (Fig. 40.45). Only about 10% of GMH-IVH occurs beyond the end of the first week, in contrast to cPVL, where late onset is not uncommon (de Vries et al. 1986; Andre et al. 2001).

Table 40.2b Descriptions of preterm intracranial haemorrhagic lesions with equivalent terms and pictorial examples of early and late (term equivalent age) cranial ultrasounds and brain MRI where appropriate

DESCRIPTION OF ULTRASOUND APPEARANCES EQUIVALENT TERMS	NOMENCLATURE USED IN THIS CHAPTER	EXAMPLES OF IMAGING APPEARANCES
Germinal matrix haemorrhage that forms a subependymal cyst Subependymal haemorrhage Grade I IVH N.B. Not equivalent to a subependymal pseudocyst, which forms in a different place	GMH	
Intraventricular haemorrhage that resolves without ventricular enlargement Grade II IVH Intraventricular haemorrhage	Uncomplicated GMH-IVH	
Intraventricular haemorrhage that at some stage is associated with enlarged ventricles, which does not progress to hydrocephalus (<97th centile of Levene) Grade III IVH	Complicated GMH-IVH GMH-IVH with non-progressive ventricular dilatation	
Intraventricular haemorrhage with enlarged ventricles that progresses to hydrocephalus >97th centile of Levene) Posthaemorrhagic hydrocephalus	Complicated GMH-IVH GMH-IVH with progressive hydrocephalus Posthaemorrhagic hydrocephalus	

IVH, intraventricular haemorrhage.

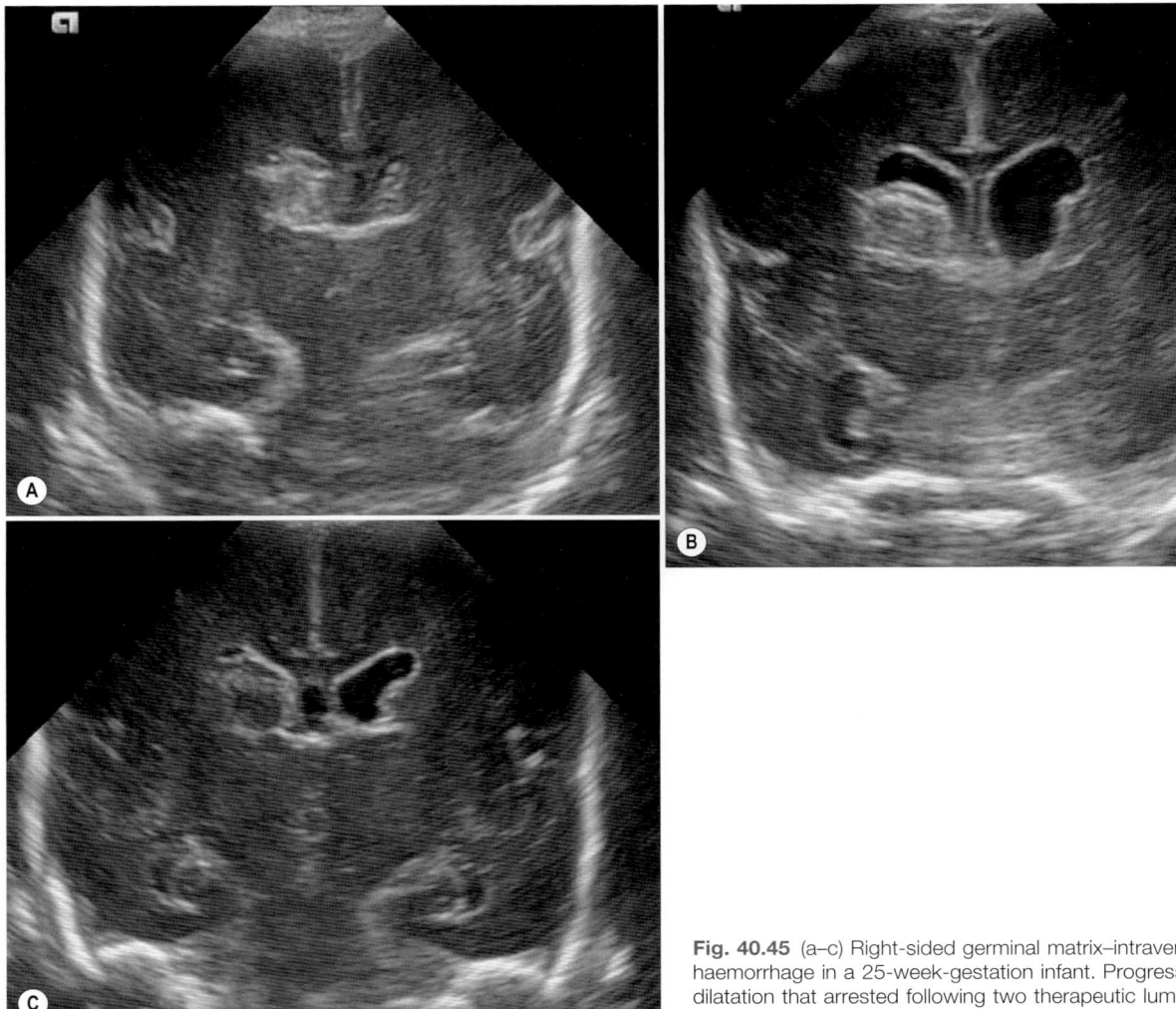

Fig. 40.45 (a–c) Right-sided germinal matrix–intraventricular haemorrhage in a 25-week-gestation infant. Progressive ventricular dilatation that arrested following two therapeutic lumbar punctures. No further treatment was required.

Pathogenesis

Anatomy and pathology of the preterm brain

Ruckensteiner and Zollner (1929) were the first to point out that GMH-IVH developed following haemorrhage in the subependymal germinal matrix, a structure that is most prominent between 24 and 34 weeks of gestation and has almost completely regressed by term. Germinal matrix tissue is abundant over the head of the caudate nucleus and can also be found in the periventricular zone. The germinal matrix contains neuroblasts and glioblasts, which undergo mitotic activity before the cells migrate to other parts of the cerebrum. Bleeding into the caudothalamic part of the germinal matrix was predominant in the large autopsy series from New Jersey but more than a third of cases also had bleeding into the temporal or occipital germinal matrix outer zones (Paneth et al. 1994). Choroid plexus bleeding was also common, particularly in more mature babies. Within the germinal matrix there is a rich capillary bed with large, irregular endothelial-lined vessels. The majority of haemorrhage is assumed to originate from this site, but there is evidence that it is actually at the capillary–venule junction (Nakamura et al. 1990).

The germinal matrix receives its blood supply from a branch of the anterior cerebral artery known as Heubner's artery. The rest of the blood supply is derived from the anterior choroidal artery and the terminal branches of the lateral striate arteries (Hambleton and Wigglesworth 1976). Venous drainage of the deep white matter occurs through a fan-shaped leash of short and long medullary veins which drain into the terminal vein which lies below the germinal matrix (Fig. 40.46) (Takashima et al. 1986). The blood can fill part of, or the entire ventricular system (Fig. 40.47), spreading through the foramen of Monro, the third ventricle, the aqueduct of Sylvius, the fourth ventricle and the foramina of Luschka and Magendie to collect around the brainstem in the posterior fossa.

Risk factors for GMH-IVH

Prematurity and the presence of respiratory distress syndrome are the main risk factors for GMH-IVH. The best unifying hypothesis (Fig. 40.48) is that GMH-IVH occurs as a result of a combination of vulnerable immature anatomy, haemodynamic instability and the propensity to bleeding which is intrinsic to the newborn (Pape and Wigglesworth 1979). Various prenatal and postnatal factors have been found to be associated with GMH-IVH in preterm infants (Table 40.26) (Hill et al. 1982a,b; Szymonowicz et al. 1984; Miall-Allen et al. 1987; Watkins et al. 1989; Wallin et al. 1990; Tsuji et al. 2000).

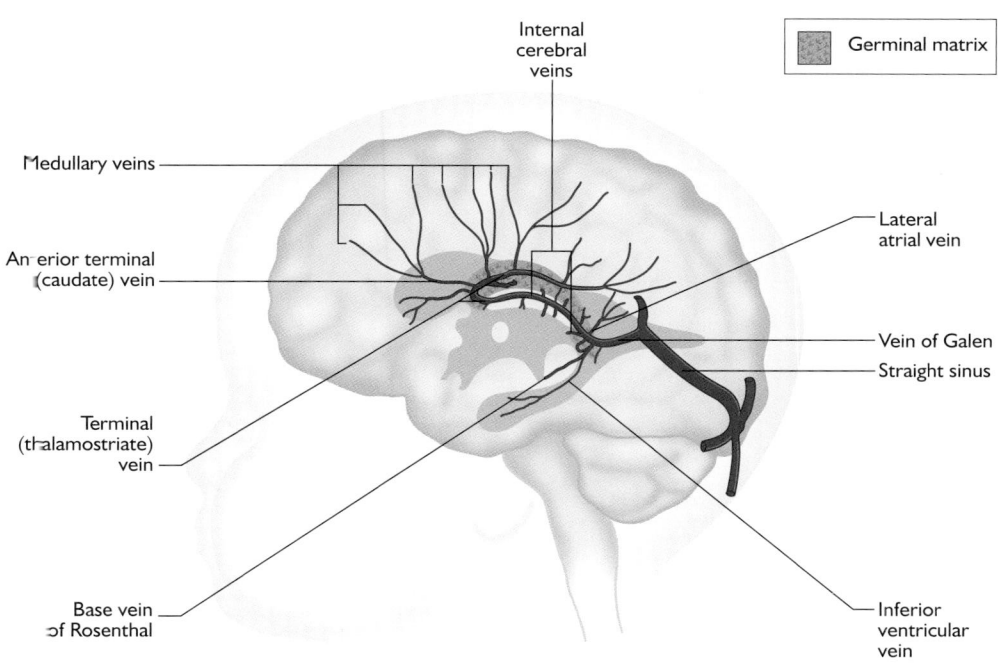

Fig. 40.46 Anatomy of the deep venous galenic system. Ant., anterior; Lat., lateral.

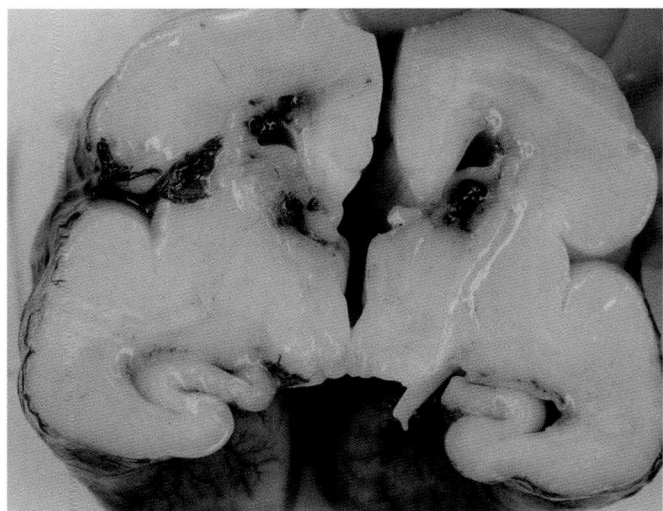

Fig. 40.47 Coronal section of the brain showing blood within the ventricular system.

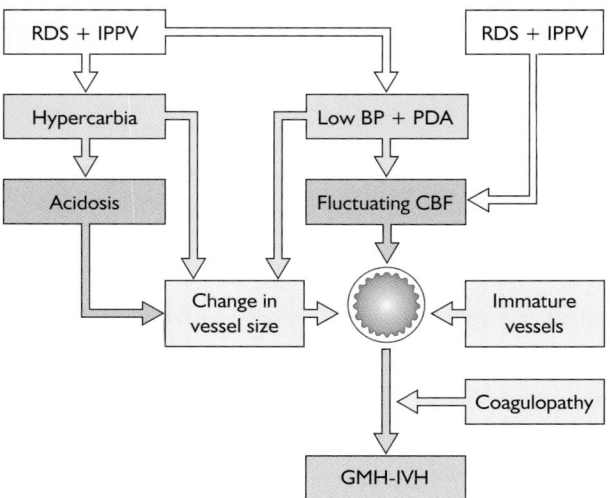

Fig. 40.48 Factors involved in the pathogenesis of germinal matrix–intraventricular haemorrhage (GMH-IVH). RDS, respiratory distress syndrome; IPPV, intermittent positive-pressure ventilation; BP, blood pressure; PDA, patent ductus arteriosus; CBF, cerebral blood flow.

Cerebral blood flow and autoregulation

Loss of autoregulation in sick preterm infants with a resultant 'pressure-passive' circulation is one of the hypotheses which have been generated to explain the development of GMH-IVH. Using radioactive xenon, Lou et al. (1979) showed a direct linear relationship between blood pressure and cerebral blood flow in a small number of babies. More recently, cerebral near-infrared spectroscopy, in conjunction with invasive arterial blood pressure monitoring, has shown the relationship between a pressure-passive circulation and GMH-IVH in infants <32 weeks' gestation (O'Leary et al. 2009). Loss of autoregulation leaves the brain unprotected against changes in blood pressure. The greater the change in cerebral blood flow in relation to a change in blood pressure, the

more likely GMH-IVH is to develop (Pryds et al. 1989). An increase in cerebral blood flow is also influenced by hypercarbia, hypoglycaemia (Pryds et al. 1990) and a reduced haematocrit, together with many of the day-to-day interventions carried out in these infants such as handling or tracheal suctioning (Perlman and Volpe 1983) plus complications such as pneumothoraces (Hill et al. 1982b).

Doppler ultrasound has been used to show cerebral blood flow fluctuations, mirroring changes in arterial blood pressure. This fluctuating pattern increased the risk of GMH-IVH (Perlman et al. 1983). The use of muscle paralysis stabilised cerebral blood flow

Table 40.26 Factors associated with an increased risk of germinal matrix–intraventricular haemorrhage in preterm infants

	REFERENCES
Prenatal	
Failure to give antenatal steroids	Synnes et al. 2001; Heuchan et al. 2002; Linder et al. 2003; Eriksson et al. 2009
Male sex	Heuchan et al. 2002; Lim et al. 2011; Mohamed and Aly 2010
Vaginal delivery	Dani et al. 2010; Lim et al. 2011
Very preterm delivery	Most studies
At delivery	
Birth depression, asphyxia	Synnes et al. 2001; Heuchan et al. 2002
Birth trauma, bruising	Arad et al. 2007
Postnatal	
Respiratory distress syndrome, particularly if complicated by pneumothorax	Hill et al. 1982; Perlman et al. 1983; Linder et al. 2003
Hypercarbia	Linder et al. 2003; Kaiser et al. 2006; Vela-Huerta et al. 2009
Acidosis	Synnes et al. 2001; Vela-Huerta et al. 2009; Lee et al. 2010
Hypotension, low superior cava flow	Klucklow and Evans 2000; Osborn et al. 2003; Miletin and Dempsey 2008; Vela-Huerta 2009
Fluctuating cerebral blood flow	Perlman et al. 1983; Van Bel et al. 1987
Low cerebral blood flow	Meek et al. 1999
Coagulation disturbance	Dani et al. 2009; Piotrowski et al. 2010
Patent ductus arteriosus	Evans and Kluckow 1996; Jim et al. 2005
Red blood cell transfusion	Baer et al. 2010
Hypernatraemia	Lim et al. 2011
Postnatal transfer	Synnes et al. 2001; Heuchan et al. 2002; Mohamed and Aly 2010

fluctuations and reduced the incidence of GMH-IVH (Perlman et al. 1985). The presence of hypercarbia, hypovolaemia, hypotension, a patent ductus arteriosus or a high inspired oxygen concentration all exacerbate cerebral blood flow fluctuations, the theory being that these fluctuations cause rupture of the vessels and subsequent bleeding. The initial studies showing these relationships were performed in the presurfactant era, although hypercarbia remains an important risk factor in the postsurfactant decades (Kaiser et al. 2006). Administration of surfactant has also been noted to cause a transient increase in cerebral blood flow by some (Van de Bor et al. 1991) but not by others (Cowan et al. 1991). Any increase is thought to be secondary to transient rising Pa_{CO_2}, rather than any effect of blood pressure (Kaiser et al. 2004). The benefits of surfactant therapy in ameliorating the severity of respiratory distress syndrome and hence reducing hypoxia, hypotension and hypercarbia clearly outweigh these theoretical risks, and surfactant therapy has been associated with fewer cases of GMH-IVH (Horbar et al. 1990; Long et al. 1991).

Hypotension and cerebral ischaemia

Hypotension is a common complication of severe respiratory distress syndrome, and in the presence of a pressure-passive cerebral circulation may lead to hypoxia–ischaemia of the germinal matrix and parenchyma. The brain may be damaged in the ischaemic phase or during subsequent reperfusion, and hypoxia–reperfusion probably underlies many of the early GMH-IVH lesions which occur in babies born in poor condition who require resuscitation. Several groups have shown that arterial hypotension precedes the development of both GMH-IVH and IPL (Miall-Allen et al. 1987; Watkins et al. 1989). It has been suggested that the protective effect of antenatal steroids is due to a reduction in the need for blood pressure support, or by direct stabilisation of the capillary endothelium (Moise et al. 1995). Early administration of gelofusin or fresh frozen plasma did not prevent either GMH-IVH or later handicap (Northern Neonatal Nursing Initiative 1996), perhaps because hypotension can be due to either cardiac dysfunction or hypovolaemia (Gill and Weindling 1993). Neither dopamine nor dobutamine reduced the incidence of GMH-IVH (Osborn et al. 2002). Nevertheless, a reduction in GMH-IVH has been seen during an era of closer attention to blood pressure, gentle handling, synchronous ventilation, less need for aggressive resuscitation at birth, better 'first-hour' care and less severe respiratory distress syndrome due to antenatal steroid and postnatal surfactant therapy, rather than to any specific drug used as prophylaxis (Philip et al. 1989; Wells and Ment 1995).

Cerebral venous pressure

Increases in cerebral venous pressure have been shown to be related to the development of GMH-IVH. Any external pressure on the neonatal skull can cause changes in venous pressure due to the malleability of the skull bones. Vaginal delivery potentially causes the greatest external forces on the neonatal brain and there is a significant relationship between the length of labour, subsequent vaginal delivery and the development of GMH-IVH (Leviton et al. 1991a). Cerebral venous pressure is also affected by mechanical ventilation, with a high peak inspiratory pressure having a much greater effect on flow than nasal continuous positive airway pressure (Cowan and Thoresen 1987), and this may also contribute to haemorrhage.

Coagulation and platelets

There is conflicting evidence concerning platelets and coagulation factors and their role in GMH-IVH. Platelet function rather than absolute number may be more important (Setzer et al. 1982). One study showed that the correction of abnormal coagulation results using fresh frozen plasma was associated with a lower incidence of GMH-IVH in babies less than 26 weeks' gestation, whereas there was no effect in more mature babies (Dani et al. 2009). This was a longitudinal study with historical controls and all babies with significant thrombocytopenia were treated. The results confirm one much older randomised controlled trial (Beverley et al. 1985), whereas a larger study of fresh frozen plasma showed no benefit (Northern Neonatal Nursing Initiative 1996). It has also recently been suggested that infants with GMH-IVH have a reduction in factor VII (Piotrowski et al. 2010) and there are currently ongoing studies investigating the use of factor VII in prevention. Whilst awaiting further studies, units should follow general guidelines regarding correction of thrombocytopenia and coagulopathy (Haematology chapter, 30).

Vascular and extravascular factors

Although the site of bleeding is probably the capillary–venule junction, the vessels within the germinal matrix are relatively fragile. They are temporary structures, as the germinal matrix will involute with time, and as such are poorly supported and immature. They are simple and endothelial-lined with little evidence of basement membrane protein, absent muscle and type IV collagen, and have a relatively large diameter (Grunnet 1989). These factors all contribute to an increased propensity to rupture due to many of the factors outlined above.

Diagnosis

Clinical diagnosis

Volpe (2008) describes three clinical syndromes, the first one being catastrophic deterioration. A sudden deterioration is noted in the baby's clinical state; examples include an increase in oxygen or ventilatory requirement, a fall in blood pressure and/or peripheral mottling, pallor, feed intolerance and acidosis. This change in condition is non-specific but, if accompanied by a drop in haematocrit, the occurrence of clinical seizures and a full fontanelle is very suggestive of GMH-IVH. The saltatory syndrome is more common and gradual in onset, presenting with a change in spontaneous general movements. The quality of the infant's movements may change from fluid and elegant to a paucity of cramped or stylised movements; there may be subtle seizures with eye deviation or lip smacking. The third and most frequent presentation is asymptomatic, with 25–50% of infants with GMH-IVH having no obvious clinical signs. Dubowitz et al. (1981) performed a careful neurological assessment on infants at different gestational ages with GMH-IVH. The most immature infants (31 weeks' gestation and below) had impaired visual tracking, an abnormal popliteal angle and subsequently developed roving eye movements and slightly more

Table 40.27 Cranial ultrasound screening protocol for preterm infants

	<30 WEEKS	31–35 WEEKS
As soon as possible after admission to intensive care	X	X
Day 1	X	
Day 2	X	
Day 3	X	
Day 7	X	X
Weekly to 32 weeks	X	
35 weeks	X	X
Term corrected	X	X
Discharge	X	

(Modified from Rennie et al. 2008.)

mature infants (32–35 weeks' gestation age) had decreased tone and poor motility. With the current ready availability of ultrasound in most neonatal units around the world, any abnormal central nervous system signs or a sudden unexplained deterioration in the general condition of a preterm neonate are indications for cranial imaging.

Ultrasound diagnosis

Cranial ultrasound is a reliable, portable and cheap non-invasive technique with which to diagnose GMH-IVH and IPL and to study their evolution over time. Good correlations with autopsy findings have been reported (Pape et al. 1983; Trounce et al. 1986; Carson et al. 1990). Most neonatal units routinely screen all VLBW admissions, partly as a form of audit and partly in order to provide an early warning of problems and to inform counselling about prognosis. The ideal protocol involves sequential scanning, with images taken at admission and serially throughout the neonatal period with a final scan at term or prior to discharge. An example of a cranial ultrasound protocol is given in Table 40.27.

Early imaging is particularly important in the extremely preterm baby, for whom continuation of intensive care may be inappropriate in the light of severe cranial ultrasound abnormalities. Frequent scans enable accurate timing of the onset of lesions and monitoring of their evolution to assist in the final classification. The records can be very helpful for audit and for medicolegal purposes, as lesions may have been evident before a given clinical event. If the available manpower or equipment allows for only a single scan then the optimal time is at the end of the first week, but repeated imaging is required to detect all lesions reliably. For more information on normal cranial ultrasound appearances, see Chapter 44. Several atlases exist (Rennie et al. 2008; Govaert and de Vries 2010).

A germinal matrix haemorrhage can most commonly be recognised as an echogenic area between the caudate nucleus and the ventricle, which evolves over a 2–4-week period into a cystic lesion that will eventually disappear. An intraventricular bleed is echogenic within the normally echolucent ventricle. When the amount of blood in the lateral ventricle is small, it is often difficult to make a distinction between a GMH and a GMH associated with a small IVH. A large IVH is easy to recognise and distends the ventricle in the acute stage. Babies with GMH-IVH that is sufficiently large to form a cast of the entire ventricle are almost certain to develop posthaemorrhagic ventricular dilatation (PHVD: see next section). A very large GMH-IVH that balloons the ventricle can be confused with an IPL.

Magnetic resonance imaging diagnosis

MRI is not infrequently used in the neonatal period; however, the majority of clinical scans are performed at term-equivalent age. There are a few groups that have performed imaging in the first few days of life and these scans have usually been for research purposes (Maalouf et al. 1999; Miller et al. 2005). The signal intensity of haemorrhage varies depending upon the timing of the scan, but initially blood will show as high signal intensity on T1-weighted imaging and low signal intensity on T2-weighted imaging (Rutherford 2002). Cranial ultrasound continues to be the mainstay of GMH-IVH diagnosis, although small amounts of blood in the posterior horn can sometimes be missed and can be easily identified as fluid levels using MRI (Maalouf et al. 1999). At term a previous GMH-IVH can often be identified due to the deposition of haemosiderin within the germinal matrix that is seen as low signal intensity on T2-weighted imaging (Fig. 40.49). There is a close correlation between cranial ultrasound and MRI for the detection of GMH-IVH (Maalouf et al. 2001) and MRI is rarely indicated to confirm the presence of haemorrhage. MRI has a greater role in assessing the complications of GMH-IVH and their prognostic significance.

Complications

Posthaemorrhagic ventricular dilatation

About 30% of infants with GMH-IVH go on to develop PHVD (Levene and Starte 1981; Lee et al. 2009); the more severe the GMH-IVH, the higher the risk of developing PHVD. This condition is considered to be due to an obliterative arachnoiditis in the majority of cases (Larroche 1972), although with large haemorrhages there can be acute PHVD due to obstruction with particulate matter. In obliterative arachnoiditis the arachnoid villi, situated over the vault of the brain, are damaged and cease to reabsorb cerebrospinal fluid (CSF), causing a communicating form of hydrocephalus. Some CSF is thought to be reabsorbed across the ependyma into small blood vessels, which become blocked with clot. Over time, transforming growth factor beta-1 may stimulate the production of extracellular matrix protein, which deposits and further blocks CSF pathways (Whitelaw et al. 2002).

Hydrocephalus usually develops between 10 and 20 days following the onset of the GMH-IVH (Fig. 40.50). Ventricular dilatation seen using cranial ultrasound precedes the development of clinical

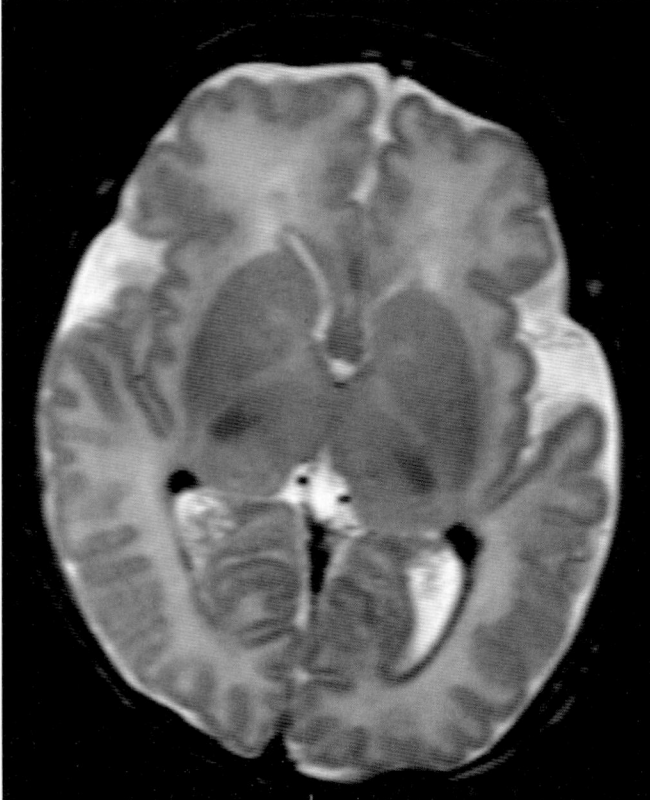

Fig. 40.49 T2-weighted brain magnetic resonance imaging in the axial plane showing residual haemosiderin at term-equivalent age following bilateral germinal matrix–intraventricular haemorrhage.

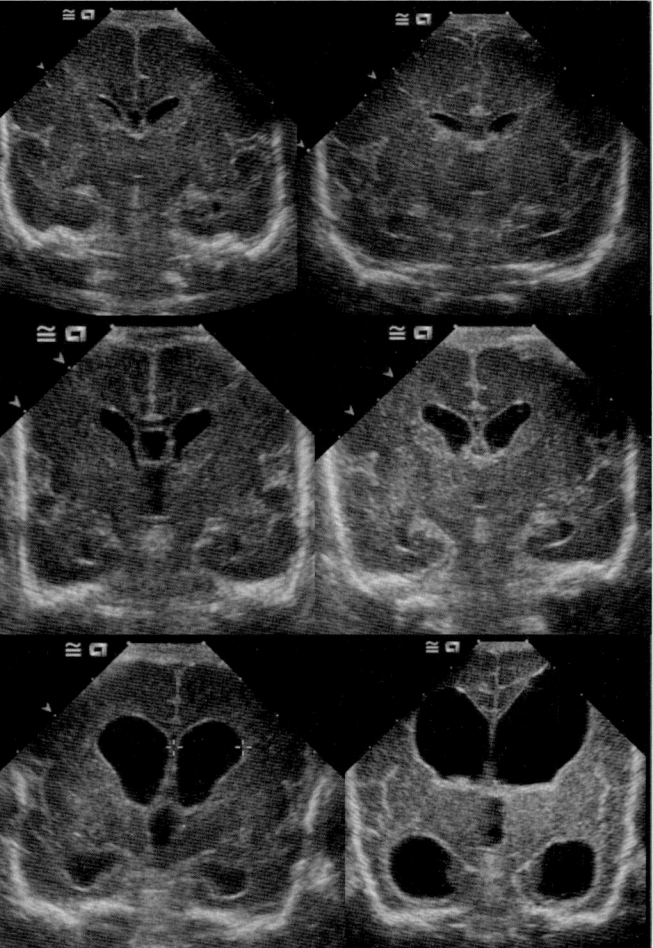

Fig. 40.50 Evolution of posthaemorrhagic ventricular dilatation in a single infant monitored over time using cranial ultrasound.

symptoms by days or even weeks. The clinical signs are a full fontanelle, diastasis of the sutures and an increase in head size. Sunsetting of the eyes is a late sign. Signs of raised intracranial pressure include seizures, feed intolerance and apnoea. The use of amplitude-integrated electroencephalogram (aEEG) monitoring has identified an increase in discontinuity without distinguishable sleep–wake cycling in association with increasing ventricular width (Olischar et al. 2004) and these abnormalities resolve following CSF drainage in the majority of infants (Olischar et al. 2009). In the long term, the associated destruction of neuronal tissue due to extravasation of CSF, free iron and pressure-induced neuronal necrosis can contribute to motor handicap and learning difficulties. Elasticity of the preterm skull limits the secondary damage and the main cause of disabilities is usually any associated parenchymal lesion or

cPVL. Short-term adverse effects on the nervous system have been confirmed using somatosensory and visual evoked potentials (de Vries et al. 1990), Doppler estimates of cerebral blood flow velocity (Saliba et al. 1985) and near-infrared spectroscopy (Casaer et al. 1992).

PHVD is transient in about half of the infants and is persistent or rapidly progressive in the remaining cases. Once it has been recognised that the ventricles are enlarged, the baseline size should be measured using ultrasound. The most widely adopted measurement system is that of Levene and Starte (1981). This 'ventricular index' is the distance between the midline and the lateral border of the ventricle measured in a coronal view in the plane of the foramina of Monro (Fig. 40.51). The measurement made from the scan image can then be compared to the chart of normal ranges

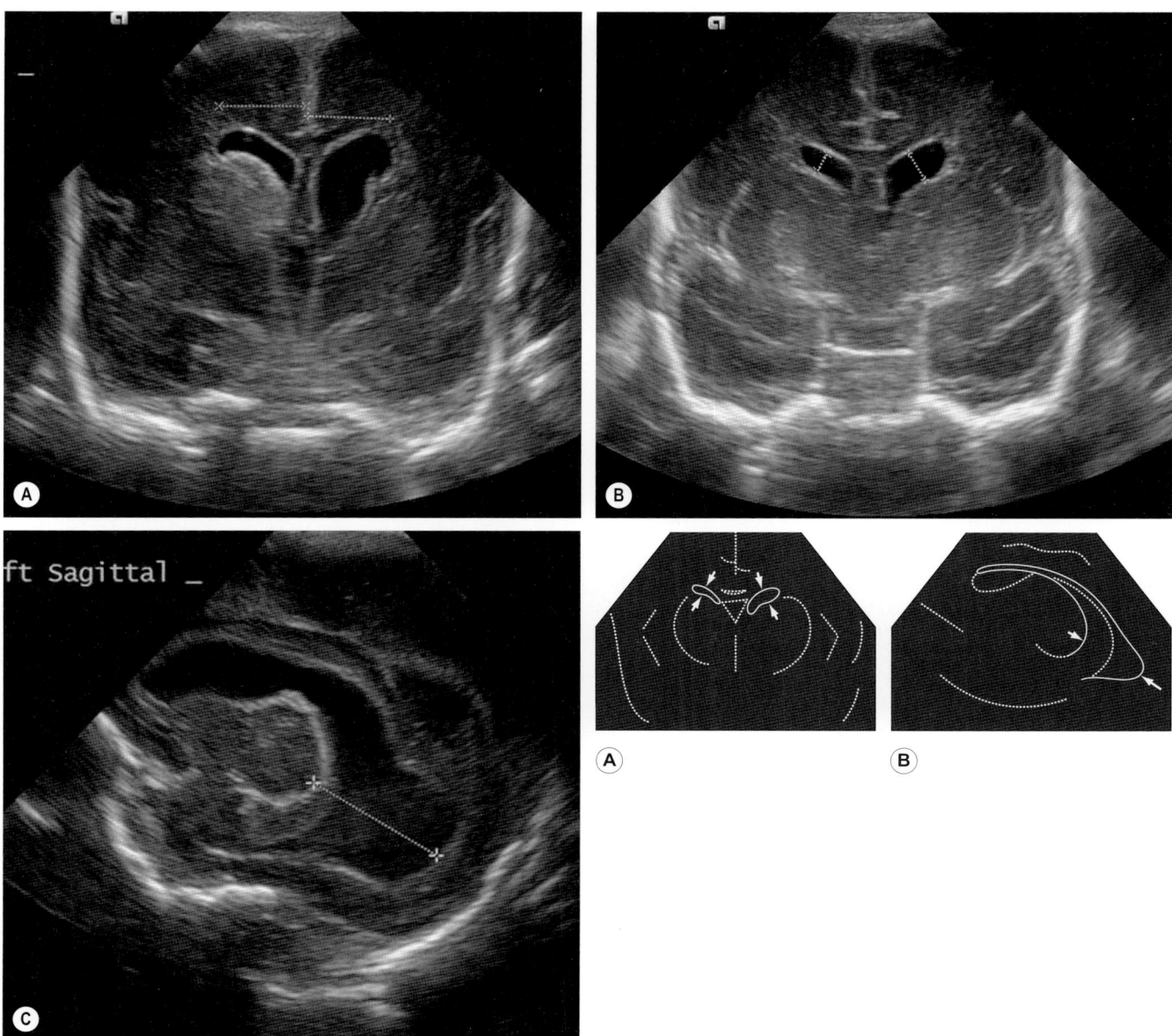

Fig. 40.51 Measurement of ventricular dilatation. (a) ventricular index of Levene, measured in the coronal plane at the level of the third ventricle as the distance from the midline to the lateral border of the lateral ventricle. (b) the height of the lateral ventricles. (c) the thalamo-occipital distance. Diagrams A and B show the ventricular width measured in the coronal plane at the level of the foramina of Monro and B the thalmo-occipital distance *(modified from Davies et al. 2000)*.

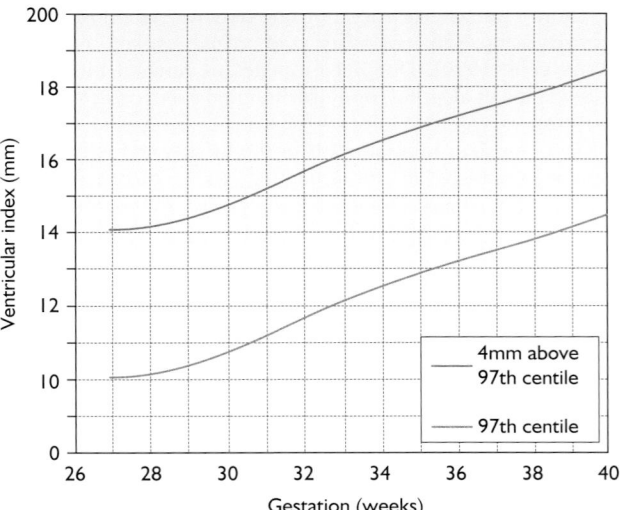

Fig. 40.52 Chart for normal ranges of the ventricular index. *(Modified from Levene and Starte 1981.)*

(Fig. 40.52). There are many other reported measurement systems, including area and volume estimation, but this simple linear index has proved repeatable and robust and has a well-established normal range. The ventricular index is a less sensitive measurement for identifying mild dilatation than other measurements such as the ventricular height and the diagonal width (Grasby et al. 2003), for which there are now published normal ranges (Davies et al. 2000; Sondhi et al. 2008), but as yet there is no published experience in using these measurements to identify infants requiring intervention for PHVD. The ventricular height is measured in the parasagittal plane just in front of the thalamic notch. A height of more than 3 mm is used to define ventriculomegaly and one of more than 8 mm suggests hydrocephalus; the ventricular width is taken in the coronal view in the same plane as the foramina of Monro and is the maximum width from the medial wall to the floor of the lateral ventricle (Fig. 40.51). As the ventricle can often dilate more significantly in the posterior regions a measurement of the thalamo-occipital distance can also be helpful, taken from the posterior aspect of the thalamus to the most posterior part of the posterior horn in the parasagittal view, and there are published normal ranges available (Davies et al. 2000) (Fig. 40.51).

In the early stages PHVD should be monitored with serial ultrasound scans and head circumference measurements at least thrice weekly. The key to management of PHVD is to distinguish between those cases who will require surgical treatment for progressive hydrocephalus (i.e. those with raised intracranial pressure) and those in whom the dilatation is due to cerebral atrophy (low pressure), who will not require surgery. Accurate measurement of pressure is a vital part of this assessment; the size of the ventricles cannot indicate the pressure, although their shape can sometimes provide a clue. Progressive hydrocephalus is very likely if the CSF pressure, measured via the lumbar route in communicating hydrocephalus or via the ventricle in non-communicating cases, is more than 1.6 kPa (12 mmHg or 15.6 cm CSF) (Ventriculomegaly Trial Group 1990, 1994) The upper limit of normal CSF pressure for newborns is 0.7 kPa (5.25 mmHg or 6.8 cm CSF) (Kaiser and Whitelaw 1986a, b). Performing a lumbar puncture also identifies whether there is communication between the lumbar and ventricular CSF and excludes low-grade meningitis as a cause for the ventriculomegaly.

If the pressure is low at lumbar puncture but the hydrocephalus is rapidly progressive, the cause is likely to be non-communicating hydrocephalus, and ventricular drainage through an external drain or via a surgically inserted subcutaneous reservoir should be considered. Repeated ventricular taps are not recommended as they can result in multiple needle tracks through the brain, and the need for a shunt will not be prevented by this treatment (Ventriculomegaly Trial Group 1990, 1994). In a large retrospective multicentre study from the Netherlands, 95 babies with large GMH-IVH and ventriculomegaly who received early or late treatment were compared (de Vries et al. 2002). The early-treated babies received treatment before their ventricular index reached 4 mm above the 97th centile of Levene and Starte; the late-treated babies were treated after their ventricles enlarged beyond this cut-off. There was a significantly reduced requirement for shunt insertion in the early-intervention group, who also did better at follow-up, although this finding was not statistically significant.

Acetazolamide cannot be recommended. Results of a European randomised trial of diuretic therapy with acetazolamide in PHVD have shown no benefit from this combination of treatment; in fact the treated group did worse, with 81% disabled at a year (International PHVD Drug Trial Group 1998; Kennedy et al. 2001). Fibrinolytic therapy in association with drainage and irrigation has been used in a randomised controlled trial setting. This strategy reduced the number of surviving infants with severe cognitive disability and reduced overall death and severe disability despite an increase in secondary intraventricular bleeding (Whitelaw et al. 2010). This is a relatively invasive therapy requiring close collaboration with neurosurgeons and at present is not available in the majority of centres. Endoscopic third ventriculostomy is unlikely to be an option for many babies in view of their small size and the communicating nature of the hydrocephalus, although in individual cases it has a role depending on the location of the obstruction (Peretta et al. 2007).

There remains no clear evidence that early drainage of CSF alters the natural history or outcome of PHVD, which is that about half of the infants will develop progressive hydrocephalus (Ventriculomegaly Trial Group 1990, 1994), although there is a general view that late treatment should be avoided. There is still no absolute consensus regarding the point at which drainage is indicated. Some would argue that the following indications, derived from the collaborative ventriculomegaly trials, let the situation deteriorate too far and that earlier treatment leads to better results. Others would say that waiting avoids the complications of surgery in some babies whose ventriculomegaly eventually stabilises. However there can be no doubt that absolute indications for CSF drainage include:

- symptoms such as apnoea, seizure, irritability or vomiting (visual deterioration in older infants) associated with an intracranial pressure of more than 10 cm CSF
- head circumference crossing two centile lines, or enlarging at twice the normal rate for more than 2 weeks.

Clues that the ventriculomegaly is likely to become progressive and that the child may need surgical drainage are a CSF pressure greater than 1.6 kPa at any stage (12 mmHg: 15.6 cm CSF) and a rapid progression of the ventricular index measurement. This knowledge may allow early transfer of an infant to a centre with a paediatric neurosurgeon before signs develop. Once it is established that treatment is required, the timing and nature of the intervention should be discussed with a neurosurgeon experienced in the management of small babies. Many neurosurgeons will insert ventricular drainage devices straight away, even in very small infants, but some advocate temporary external drainage or drainage via a surgically implanted subcutaneous reservoir in order to allow the baby to gain

Table 40.28 Neurodevelopmental impairment following germinal matrix–intraventricular haemorrhage (GMH-IVH), with and without shunt insertion

	N	NEURODEVELOPMENTAL IMPAIRMENT (%)
No GMH-IVH/no shunt	5163	35
GMH-IVH with ventricular dilatation/no shunt	459	55
GMH-IVH with ventricular dilatation/shunt	103	78

Neurodevelopmental impairment was defined as ≥1 of the following: MDI (Mental Development Index) <70, PDI (Psychomotor Development Index) <70, cerebral palsy, blind in both eyes or hearing aids in both ears.
(Derived from Adams-Chapman et al. 2008.)

weight (Hudgins et al. 1998; Shooman et al. 2009). Endoscopic ventriculostomy and choroid plexus ablation are now very rarely performed in this situation.

Temporary external drainage systems, with or without fibrinolytic agents, are prone to infection in this group, require on-site neurosurgical expertise and are probably less preferable to an indwelling device unless there is no alternative. Some neurosurgeons regard a high CSF protein level of more than 1.5 or 2 g/l as a contraindication for permanent shunt insertion and use repeated intermittent drainage until the protein level has reduced (Gaskill et al. 1988; Weninger et al. 1992). This can be achieved using a ventricular reservoir, which allows an infant to return to the referring hospital, but has an associated risk of infection, skin necrosis and tube migration. A subgaleal shunt can also be used, providing constant rather than intermittent drainage, but it will require replacement if the hydrocephalus does not arrest. The use of valveless shunts has made earlier surgery an option; however, they can still block and they require the infant to remain essentially flat and need replacing with a ventriculoperitoneal shunt prior to discharge (Vinchon et al. 2001).

It is important to note that late progression of PHVD has been described (Perlman 1990) and serial monitoring of head circumference is required for up to a year, with further ultrasound examinations if there is any concern about the pattern of head growth.

Prevention of GMH-IVH

A reduction in the incidence of GMH-IVH has been reported in many large neonatal units without any specific pharmacological prophylaxis, which is now largely historical. Details can be found in earlier editions of this book. The importance of good general care, with attention to careful control of blood pressure, coagulation defects, temperature and blood gases, gentle handling, gentle ventilation and the appropriate use of antenatal steroids and postnatal surfactant cannot be overemphasised (Volpe 1990). With the low incidence of parenchymal lesions seen in most neonatal units nowadays, the use of prophylaxis against GMH-IVH, which will benefit only a few infants whilst exposing many to potentially serious side-effects, is not recommended. The most promising specific prophylactic drug, excluding antenatal steroids, was indometacin (Ment et al. 1994; Fowlie 1996). Unfortunately a long-term outcome study (Ment et al. 1996) showed that no protection against neurodevelopmental handicap was gained, although there was a reduction in GMH-IVH in boys and an initial improvement in their language skills which did not persist (Ment et al. 2004; Luu et al. 2009), and this agent is generally not in widespread use for this purpose. There

has been some recent interest in the use of factor VII for the prevention of GMH-IVH as it has been shown to be reduced in infants with severe haemorrhage (Piotrowski et al. 2010); however, there have been few studies to date and the evidence is as yet limited for its role in prevention (Veldman et al. 2006).

Prognosis: neurodevelopmental outcome

Uncomplicated GMH-IVH has a good prognosis. The risk of handicap in VLBW survivors with uncomplicated GMH-IVH or normal cranial ultrasound scans at discharge is 4% (Stewart et al. 1983; Lowe and Papile 1990; Ment et al. 1998). Once ventricular dilatation develops, the risk of adverse neurodevelopmental outcome increases. It is speculated that this may be due to the presence of non-protein-bound iron as a generator of reactive oxygen species causing white-matter damage. Infants with GMH-IVH and moderate ventricular dilatation have impaired neurodevelopment compared to infants with GMH-IVH and no ventricular dilatation (Dyet et al. 2006; Vollmer et al. 2006). The risk of adverse outcome is approximately 50% and if ventricular dilatation progresses and shunting is required, this risk increases to 60–78% (Palmer et al. 1982; Shankaran et al. 1989; Fernell et al. 1993; Adams-Chapman et al. 2008) (Table 40.28). The outcome following shunting worsens if the baby suffers repeated episodes of shunt infection and revision.

Cerebellar haemorrhage

Cerebellar haemorrhages within the preterm population are being increasingly recognised following the more frequent use of brain MRI (Fig. 40.53). Cranial ultrasound using the anterior fontanelle as the acoustic window does not tend to provide adequate imaging of the posterior fossa (Miall et al. 2003; Sehgal et al. 2009). Imaging through the posterior fontanelle or mastoid improves detection (Merrill et al. 1998; Steggerda et al. 2009). Posterior fossa haemorrhages, including cerebellar haemorrhage, occur in 7–19% of preterm infants (Dyet et al. 2006; Steggerda et al. 2009). The haemorrhage has been described as occurring in six patterns: subarachnoid, lobar, folial, giant lobar, including the vermis, or contusional (Ecury-Goossen et al. 2010). These haemorrhages are often clinically silent, but there is some evidence that babies can develop unexplained motor agitation prior to a diagnosis being made (Ecury-Goossen et al. 2010). Cerebellar haemorrhage is often associated with supratentorial lesions and subsequent cerebellar atrophy is common. Generally infants with a cerebellar haemorrhage have a poorer prognosis, with an increased risk of mortality

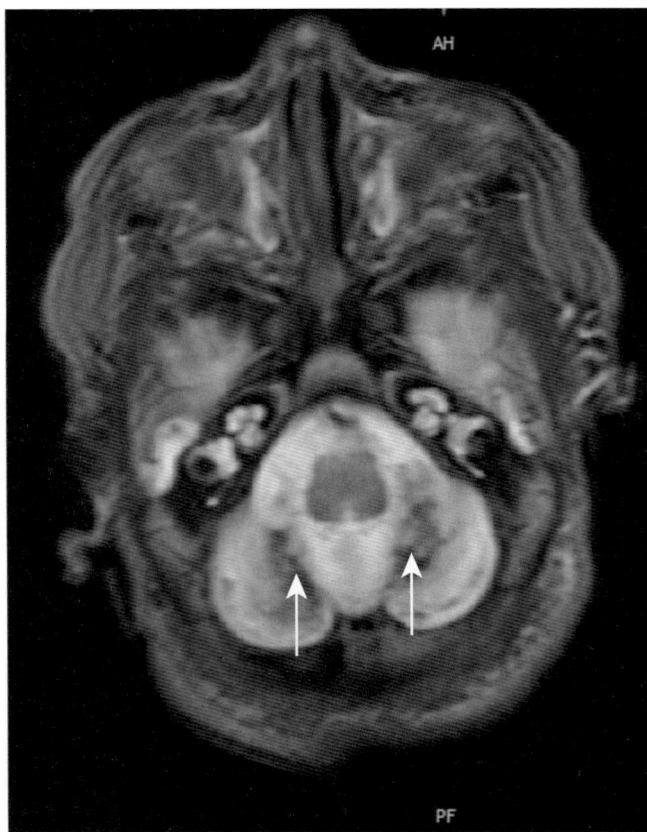

Fig. 40.53 T2-weighted magnetic resonance imaging in the axial plane showing bilateral cerebellar haemorrhage (arrowed).

and morbidity (Dyet et al. 2006). In particular, isolated cerebellar haemorrhage increases the risk of both motor and cognitive deficits in the preterm population and this is often more profound than in those with associated supratentorial injury (Limperopoulos et al. 2007). There is some evidence that involvement of the vermis in particular is associated with more severe deficits (Poretti et al. 2010). These infants do not tend to show the same cerebellar signs as more mature populations with cerebellar injury (Krageloh-Mann et al. 1999).

Preterm brain injury: white-matter disease of prematurity

Introduction

White-matter abnormalities are the most common finding within the preterm brain and our understanding of this disorder has changed significantly over the last 10 years. The focus on cPVL has shifted to the wider appreciation of the importance of diffuse white-matter abnormalities. The term 'white-matter disease of prematurity' encompasses IPLs identified on cranial ultrasound, in that their original aetiology is not always clear. As discussed, imaging (particularly early imaging) cannot always determine whether such lesions are haemorrhagic venous infarction or primary areas of ischaemic damage. This section discusses both focal and diffuse abnormalities of the white matter in the preterm infant.

History and terminology

White-matter damage in babies was observed by pathologists as early as 1867, when Virchow first described abnormal areas in the periventricular zone. The term 'periventricular leukomalacia' was coined in 1962 by Banker and Larroche, who described changes on histology in 51 infants. The name was chosen because white (*leukos*) spots and softening (*malacia*) were seen in the periventricular white matter.

Paneth et al. (1990) reported on autopsy findings in 22 very preterm infants who survived for at least 6 days. Although 15 of them had white-matter necrosis, only three had the classical changes of PVL. They subsequently published the autopsy findings from 25 infants with white-matter damage (Paneth et al. 1994). Only one had 'classic' PVL but the pathological changes of PVL were associated with GMH-IVH in 20 babies. Thirteen had been noted to have an increase in echogenicity in the periventricular white matter on ultrasound, and nine had ventriculomegaly apparently without GMH-IVH, both suggesting a more diffuse component to the white-matter injury.

PVL has been graded on cranial ultrasound images by de Vries et al. (1992) and this classification provides a guide to severity and can help with prognosis. In this system grade I PVL refers to periventricular echogenicities that last for 7 days or more, grade II PVL refers to transient periventricular echodensities evolving into small localised cysts, grade III PVL is defined as areas of periventricular echodensities evolving into extensive periventricular cystic lesions and grade IV PVL describes densities extending into the deep white matter evolving into extensive cystic lesions (Table 40.29).

Grading of the echogenicity within the white matter using ultrasound has also been carried out (van Wezel-Meijler et al. 1998). Grade 0 is normal echogenicity of the white matter (less than choroid plexus), grade 1 is moderately increased echogenicity (the affected region or smaller regions within the affected region are equal to the choroid plexus) and grade 2 is severely increased echogenicity (the affected region or smaller regions within the affected region are more echogenic than the choroid plexus). Grading of the severity of white-matter abnormalities using brain MRI has also been published in order to provide a score of severity for clinical and research purposes (Woodward et al. 2006).

Outlining appropriate terminology for the extremely common diffuse white-matter abnormalities seen on conventional MRI and diffusion-weighted imaging (DWI) as well as on pathological specimens remains an area of debate. Diffuse excessive high signal intensity (DEHSI) has been used to describe one common finding on brain MRI (Fig. 40.54), but this does not provide any explanation as to the pathological processes involved. One suggestion was to use the term 'cerebral leucoencephalopathy' to describe both the focal and diffuse white-matter abnormalities seen in the preterm brain. Volpe (2005) has coined the term 'encephalopathy of prematurity', which is an encompassing term intended to include PVL and the associated diffuse axonal/neuronal injury involving the cerebral white matter, thalamus, basal ganglia, cerebral cortex, brainstem and cerebellum sustained by these infants.

The other cause of focal white-matter damage is an IPL. As discussed earlier, most authorities now agree that a unilateral parenchymal lesion accompanying GMH-IVH is usually caused by the presence of haemorrhage compressing the terminal vein and leading to impaired venous drainage of the medullary veins and subsequent venous infarction (Fig. 40.46) (Gould et al. 1987). Ischaemic white-matter damage can be associated with secondary haemorrhage. IPLs seen early in life using ultrasound should be carefully described as to size, laterality, echogenicity and location. The evolution of the

Table 40.29 Descriptions of preterm white-matter lesions with equivalent terms and pictorial examples of early and late (term-equivalent age) cranial ultrasounds and brain magnetic resonance imaging

DESCRIPTION OF ULTRASOUND IMAGING APPEARANCES EQUIVALENT TERMS	NOMENCLATURE USED IN THIS CHAPTER	EXAMPLES OF IMAGING APPEARANCES
IPL (usually globular and unilateral, and usually associated with GMH-IVH) evolving to a single large porencephalic cyst	IPL with GMH-IVH evolving into porencephalic cyst	
Grade IV IVH		
Haemorrhagic parenchymal/periventricular infarction		
IPL (usually fan-shaped and unilateral, and usually associated with GMH-IVH, but partially separate from the ventricle) evolving into multiple cysts	IPL, separate from ventricle, evolving into multiple cysts – describe location	
IPL (usually bilateral) without cystic evolution usually lasting for at least 48 hours	IPL persisting for at least 48 hours	
Transient flare	Transient flare	
Periventricular flare		
IPL (usually bilateral) persisting for at least 7 days without cystic evolution	IPL persisting for 7 days	
Grade I PVL	Grade I PVL	
Persistent flare		

Continued

Table 40.29 Continued

DESCRIPTION OF ULTRASOUND IMAGING APPEARANCES EQUIVALENT TERMS	NOMENCLATURE USED IN THIS CHAPTER	EXAMPLES OF IMAGING APPEARANCES
IPL persisting for 7 days and evolving into localised small frontoparietal cysts; lesions not involving the occipital cortex	IPL persisting for 7 days and evolving into localised small frontoparietal cysts	
Cystic PVL	Frontoparietal cystic PVL	
Grade II PVL	Grade II PVL	
IPL persisting for days and evolving into multiple cysts in the parieto-occipital white matter	IPL evolving into multiple cysts in the parieto-occipital white matter	
Cystic PVL	Parieto-occipital PVL	
Grade III PVL	Grade III PVL	
IPL persisting for days and evolving into multiple subcortical cysts in the deep white matter	IPL persisting and evolving into multicystic leukoencephalomalacia	
Cystic PVL	Subcortical cystic PVL	
Grade IV PVL	Grade IV PVL	
Enlarged ventricles without preceding GMH-IVH	Enlarged ventricles without GMH-IVH	
Cerebral atrophy	Cerebral atrophy	
Ventriculomegaly		

IPL, intraparenchymal lesion; GMH-IVH, germinal matrix–intraventricular haemorrhage; PVL, periventricular leukomalacia.

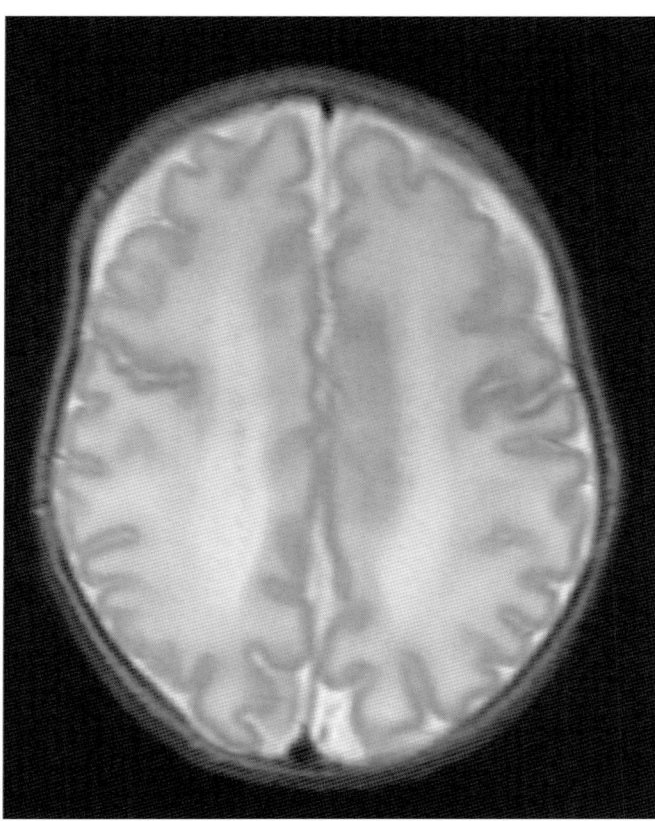

Fig. 40.54 T2-weighted magnetic resonance imaging in the axial plane showing bilateral diffuse increase in signal intensity within the white matter at term-equivalent. Previously described as diffuse excessive high signal intensity.

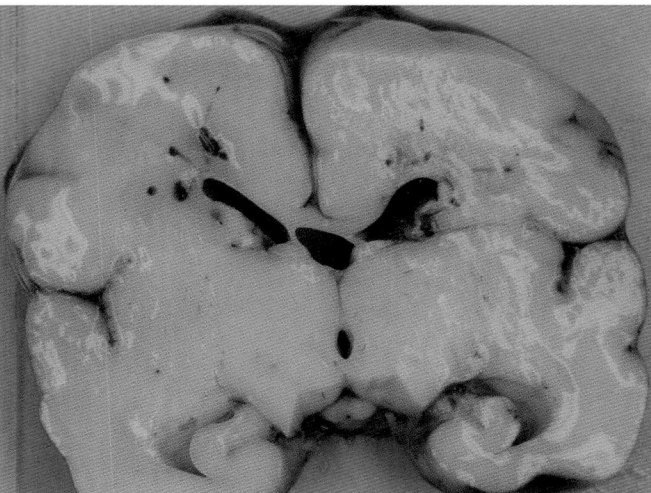

Fig. 40.55 Coronal section of the brain showing the cystic lesions of periventricular leukomalacia.

parenchymal lesion should then be followed. When first seen with ultrasound most parenchymal lesions are echoreflectant, or 'bright'. Over the next weeks some resolve, many evolve into multiple small cysts and others evolve into single large cysts (Table 40.29). Using ultrasound it is not possible to make a certain pathological diagnosis so the terms 'grade IV intraventricular haemorrhage' and 'haemorrhagic parenchymal infarction' should be abandoned and the more generic term of IPL should be used instead.

Periventricular leukomalacia: focal and diffuse white-matter injury

Incidence

The classic findings of cPVL have fortunately become less common over the last two decades, with a reduction from about 5% of infants born between 25 and 30 weeks' gestational age to less than 2% (Groenendaal et al. 2010). If infants at lower gestational ages are studied the incidence is slightly higher during the same time period; for example, 5.6% of infants born at <27 weeks' gestation in Sweden developed ultrasound evidence of cPVL (Fellman et al. 2009). The incidence of other grades of PVL are approximately 25% grade I, 1.4% grade II and 2.5% grade III in infants <32 weeks' gestational age (de Vries et al. 2004), revealed with cranial ultrasound.

Diffuse white-matter abnormalities identified on brain MRI are much more common: the incidence ranges from 50% to 75% of

preterm infants studied at term-equivalent age (Maalouf et al. 1999; Inder et al. 2003c; Skiold et al. 2010).

Timing

The timing of cPVL is much more variable than that of GMH-IVH. The onset can be antenatal, peripartum or postnatal. If the injury is of antenatal onset, depending upon the timing of the insult, fully developed cysts can be seen on the first image made shortly after birth. This can occur in situations such as twin-to-twin transfusion syndrome with or without the death of one twin, chorioamnionitis, prolonged rupture of membranes or antepartum haemorrhage (Murphy et al. 1995; Grether et al. 1996; Perlman et al. 1996; Denbow et al. 1998; Haverkamp et al. 2001; Bauer et al. 2009). Some of these factors may also be relevant in cPVL of peripartum onset. The time taken for an IPL of the 'flare' category (Table 40.29) to develop into cystic PVL is usually 2 weeks, although one Japanese study suggested that it might take longer: the median date of cyst formation was 18 days but the range was 10–39 days (Kubota et al. 2001). There is a clear relation between the severity of cPVL and the time it takes for the cysts to develop, i.e. the more localised the cysts, the longer it takes for the cysts to develop (Pierrat et al. 2001). Sometimes the initial IPL develops several weeks after birth following an acute clinical deterioration such as septicaemia or necrotising enterocolitis (de Vries et al. 1986; Andre et al. 2001; Kobayashi et al. 2008).

Pathology

Pathological changes include coagulation necrosis at 3–6 hours, followed by microglial activation at 6–8 hours. Several days later there is astrocytic degeneration and karyorrhexis with macrophage infiltration. Precisely when the earliest changes can be seen with ultrasound is not known; certainly a 'flare' can be seen 24–48 hours after a hypoxic–ischaemic insult in many cases. Less severe injury may not ever be detectable with ultrasound, although some babies develop late ventriculomegaly, and in others earlier imaging may show changes. Microcavities appear in the brain between 8 and 12 days with macroscopic cavities by 2 weeks (Fig. 40.55), and these can be imaged with ultrasound. The pathological hallmark of cPVL is coagulation necrosis. Liquefaction of the centre of the necrotic area can occur after 10–20 days and these small cavities are usually not in communication with the lateral ventricle when imaged with ultrasound. The abnormalities reflect a response to tissue injury that is specific to highly metabolically active white matter that is undergoing rapid myelination.

Diffuse white-matter abnormalities associated with PVL are characterised neuropathologically by diffuse activated microgliosis. Microglia are essential for axonal guidance and white-matter tract modelling and abnormal activation in the presence of injury may disrupt the normal developmental trajectory of the white matter. Assumptions have been made that DEHSI on MRI is equivalent to diffuse PVL; however, histological correlations are difficult to obtain as neonates with this milder abnormality are less likely to die and undergo postmortem. A rat model of gestational hypoxia has been used to produce milder white-matter injury and imaging of the brain showed an increase in apparent diffusion coefficient (ADC), a finding common to DEHSI and diffuse PVL, and at histology there were increased numbers of activated microglia (Baud et al. 2004).

Pathogenesis

The pathogenesis of PVL is multifactorial and is less well understood than for GMH-IVH. There seems to be a developmental window of vulnerability when white-matter damage is most likely. Pre-oligodendrocytes (OLs) are the predominant oligodendroglial cell present between 23 and 32 weeks' gestational age (Back et al. 2001) and these cells are much more sensitive to toxic effects than the earlier OL progenitors or the mature OLs (Back et al. 2002). Subplate neurons are another vulnerable population of cells that peak in density at 24–32 weeks' gestational age. They act as a 'waiting zone' for afferents from the thalamus and other cortical areas on their pathway to reach the cortex. They provide axonal guidance and also facilitate cortical organisation and synaptic development (Volpe 1996; Kostovic and Judas 2002). Subplate neurons are selectively sensitive to hypoxia–ischaemia (McQuillen et al. 2003) and there is increased apoptosis in the subplate of infants with PVL (Robinson et al. 2006). There are reductions in cortical (Inder et al. 1999b) and thalamic (Nagasunder et al. 2010) volumes in infants with PVL and subplate neuronal injury is a potential mechanism to account for these deficits. A simplistic way of considering the pathogenetic mechanisms involved is that there are two upstream initiating factors, ischaemia and inflammation, that activate two downstream mechanisms, excitotoxicity and free radical attack by reactive oxygen and nitrogen species (Khwaja and Volpe 2008) (Fig. 40.56). In turn this leads to pre-OL death and white-matter injury with cell death and subsequent abnormalities in myelination.

Ischaemia

The preterm brain is at risk from ischaemia due to impairment in the autoregulation of cerebral blood flow (as outlined in the previous section) and also the fact that there are arterial border and end zones within white matter. The periventricular region is probably vulnerable because the deep white matter is perfused by long penetrators forming distal arterial fields that are sensitive to falls in cerebral perfusion (Rorke 1992; Inage et al. 2000). Diffuse white-matter injury may in part be due to poor perfusion from shorter penetrators that anastomose with the long penetrators. The numbers of these short penetrators and their anastomoses increase within the third trimester, thereby decreasing white-matter vulnerability. Hypotension will tend to reduce the already low preterm cerebral blood flow and increase the potential for ischaemia if autoregulation is absent, although evidence that hypotension is actually linked to preterm white-matter injury is hard to find (Martens et al. 2003).

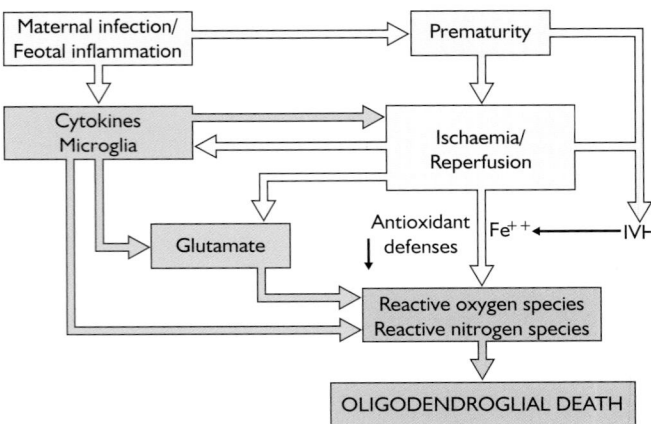

Fig. 40.56 Pathogenesis of periventricular leukomalacia. IVH, interventricular haemorrhage. *(Modified from Khwaja and Volpe 2008.)*

This may be because blood pressure is a poor index of circulating blood flow, and some have suggested that measurement of superior vena caval flow is a better marker of the state of the systemic circulation in preterm babies (Evans 2006). Hypocarbia has a similar end result, but as a consequence of vascular constriction, and is a very potent risk factor for PVL (Wiswell et al. 1996b; Okumura et al. 2001; Giannakopoulou et al. 2004; Murase and Ishida 2005; Shankaran et al. 2006). The cerebral 'steal' effect can occur when there is a large patent ductus arteriosus with an abnormal reversal of cerebral blood flow in diastole, rather than the normal situation of continuous forward flow. This particular flow pattern has been linked to PVL (Shortland et al. 1990).

Inflammation

Any infective or inflammatory process can lead to the systemic upregulation of proinflammatory cytokines and diffuse activation of microglia within the immature white matter. This includes maternal intrauterine infection and fetal or neonatal infection as well as ischaemia-induced inflammation (Folkerth 2005). There is significant evidence implicating ascending intrauterine infection with the subsequent production of proinflammatory cytokines and white-matter injury (Murphy et al. 1995; Perlman et al. 1996; Minagawa et al. 2002; Leviton et al. 2005). However, no direct relationship has been found between the levels of cytokines within neonatal blood or CSF and subsequent development of PVL (Ellison et al. 2005), so the associated microglial response and free radical generation may be more important. In particular interferon-γ and tumour necrosis factor, primarily expressed in microglia/macrophages, have been implicated in PVL lesions (Kadhim et al. 2001). The relationship between chorioamnionitis and cPVL is clear (Wu 2002), but it has not been shown to be a risk factor for more diffuse white-matter abnormalities (Inder et al. 2005; Dyet et al. 2006). There is also significant evidence for the effect of postnatal sepsis on white-matter injury (Wheater and Rennie 2000), with recurrent culture-positive infections increasing the risk of progressive white-matter abnormalities (Graham et al. 2004; Glass et al. 2008). This is one potential area for prevention.

Excitotoxicity

Excitotoxicity and free radical attack as mechanisms of cell injury are linked, with excitotoxicity probably leading to pre-OL injury due to calcium influx with resultant generation of reactive oxygen and nitrogen species, although free radical generation can also occur via microglial activation. In particular pre-OL excitotoxicity is thought to result from interferon-γ, tumour necrosis factor-α and glutamate. There is significant interferon-γ expression in astrocytes in the diffuse white-matter injury of PVL. Interferon-γ receptors have been identified in pre-OLs and toxicity is much greater than in more mature OLs. The toxicity also appears to be potentiated by tumour necrosis factor-α (Agresti et al. 1996; Andrews et al. 1998). Pre-OLs express glutamate transporters (Desilva et al. 2007) that are energy-dependent and fail in the face of hypoxia–ischaemia, resulting in increases in extracellular glutamate. Axons may also provide extracellular glutamate during hypoxia–ischaemia (Back et al. 2007). In a sheep hypoxia-ischaemia model of PVL, increased extracellular glutamate levels correlated directly with the extent of white-matter injury (Loeliger et al. 2003). This excitotoxicity and cell injury is mediated via the excessive activation of pre-OL glutamate receptors (Jensen 2005; Karadottir and Attwell 2007), with both receptors in the soma and in the oligodendroglial processes, activation of which leads to cell death (Matute 2006) or loss of cell processes (Karadottir et al. 2005; Salter and Fern 2005), respectively.

Free radical attack

In an immunocytochemical study by Haynes et al. (2003), staining for markers of oxidative and nitrative attack was found within pre-OLs and reactive astrocytes in the diffuse white-matter lesions associated with PVL. In vivo, infants who subsequently had MRI evidence of PVL had higher levels of oxidative products within their CSF early in the neonatal period compared to infants who did not develop PVL (Inder et al. 2002a). There is also a potential delay in the development of superoxide dismutase enzymes increasing the vulnerability of pre-OLs to free radical toxicity (Folkerth et al. 2004). There has been a significant focus on non-protein-bound iron and its role in white-matter injury. Pre-OLs accumulate iron for differentiation (Connor and Menzies 1996) and in the presence of excess hydrogen peroxide the iron is converted into the hydroxyl radical (Ozawa et al. 1994; Iida et al. 1995), again another potential agent of oxidative attack. Microglia also contain Toll-like receptors, activation of which releases free radicals.

Diagnosis and evolution

Clinical diagnosis

Compared with large GMH-IVH, the clinical signs occurring in infants who develop cystic PVL are less obvious and may easily go unnoticed, and often this devastating damage is clinically silent. In the acute phase, hypotonia and some degree of lethargy can be observed. Some 6–10 weeks later a characteristic clinical picture emerges. Infants become irritable and hard to pacify. They are hypertonic and show increased flexion of the arms and extension of the legs. Frequent tremors and startles can be noted and the Moro reaction is usually abnormal. General movement studies have reported these infants to have a 'cramped synchronised' movement pattern (Cioni and Prechtl 1990). In spite of the cortical visual impairment that is often noted in later infancy in this group, visual tracking still appears normal at this stage (Eken et al. 1994).

Electrographic diagnosis

Positive rolandic sharp waves on the EEG are an abnormal finding. These transient sharp waves are specifically associated with PVL in preterm infants and may assist in distinguishing those with a poor prognosis (Marret et al. 1992). According to one study, the sensitivity is higher in the more mature babies (Baud et al. 1998). Others were able to make a distinction between acute and non-acute EEG changes, which was helpful in timing the onset of PVL to the antenatal or perinatal period (Hayakawa et al. 1999). Prediction of the development of PVL in the first few days of life has been studied using both EEG and flash visual evoked potentials (fVEP). A total of 92% of infants with subsequent PVL had EEG and/or fVEP abnormalities (Kidokoro et al. 2008b). One group described a lower spectral edge frequency in the EEG of preterm babies who went on to develop white-matter injury (Inder et al. 2003b).

Ultrasound diagnosis

Since 1982 many groups have shown that cPVL can be diagnosed using cranial ultrasound scans (Hill et al. 1982a; Levene et al. 1983; Bozynski et al. 1985). The angle of insonation should be wide enough to visualise the periventricular white matter and the resolution of the transducer should be high (7.5–10 MHz) in order to detect small cystic lesions (de Vries et al. 1992). Serial ultrasound scans are essential for case ascertainment. These should initially be weekly, and can then be undertaken less frequently; however, an ultrasound at term is mandatory to prevent late-onset cystic pathology from being missed (Perlman and Rollins 2000; de Vries et al. 2004).

Correlation with both autopsy and MRI findings has shown that ultrasound is less sensitive for the detection of PVL than for GMH-IVH, and is particularly poor at detecting non-cavitating PVL (Hope et al. 1988; Paneth et al. 1990; Maalouf et al. 2001). Small areas of diffuse gliosis have often been seen at autopsy that were not identified using cranial ultrasound (Hope et al. 1988; Paneth et al. 1990). In the series described by Paneth et al., most of the cases with haemorrhagic PVL were correctly diagnosed with ultrasound but those with focal non-haemorrhagic PVL were frequently missed (Trounce et al. 1986; de Vries et al. 1988; Inder et al. 2003a). Similar findings have been shown comparing cranial ultrasound and MRI, with mild or moderate white-matter injury being identified with lower sensitivity on ultrasound than cystic disease.

The main difficulty with ultrasound diagnosis of early white-matter damage occurs with the requirement for a distinction between a genuinely echogenic patch and the normal peritrigonal 'blush' which is often seen in the brain of the very preterm infant. Ultrasound interpretation is prone to artefact due to poor transducer–skin contact and excessive gain settings and requires experience; even then, interpretation is still subjective.

A truly abnormal echogenic area is as bright as the choroid plexus, and the abnormality can be confirmed in more than one scan plane on more than one occasion. It can be graded as discussed earlier (van Wezel-Meijler et al. 1998). The genuinely abnormal area of confluent high-intensity echoes completely obliterates the normal pattern of finely interlaced echogenic and echopoor lines that fan out from the periventricular zone. These gracile lines, which can normally be seen in the periventricular region, are thought to represent interfaces between the neural and vascular bundles.

The presence of echogenicity within the white matter on sequential cranial ultrasound does not correlate well with white-matter abnormalities on MRI at term (Inder et al. 2003a) but this is hardly surprising as scans in this study were not acquired contemporaneously. The ability of cranial ultrasound to detect white-matter abnormalities on MR acquired at a similar time has proved variable, with a poor correlation in the study by Maalouf et al. in 2001 and better correlation in the study by Leijser et al. in 2008. Both of these studies looked at mild and severe white-matter abnormalities, although there were no cystic lesions in the former study. Interestingly the correlation of abnormalities in echogenicity with ultrasound and white-matter abnormalities on MRI improves when ultrasound abnormalities persist for more than 7 days (positive predictive value 0.72 with 95% confidence interval (CI) 0.58–0.87) (Maalouf et al. 2001), reinforcing the benign nature of transient white-matter echogenicity. A recent small study of MRI and cranial ultrasound at term-equivalent age has shown that a normal cranial ultrasound at term is relatively reassuring, as none of 28 infants with this finding had moderate or severe white-matter abnormalities on MRI (Horsch et al. 2010). Areas of increased echodensity persisting beyond day 7, but not becoming cystic, have been associated with subsequent mild ventricular dilatation and widening of the interhemispheric fissure, suggesting a degree of cerebral atrophy. Gliosis has indeed been found in a few cases who died after neonatal cranial ultrasound appearances of flare evolved into mild ventriculomegaly (Fawer et al. 1985; Trounce et al. 1986).

The sensitivity of ultrasound is very high in infants with cystic lesions (Nwaesei et al. 1984; Debillon et al. 2003). In some cases the echogenic area on ultrasound evolves into localised small cysts a few millimetres in diameter over 2–3 weeks (Pierrat et al. 2001). These are often located in the frontoparietal periventricular white matter. In a minority of the infants extensive cystic lesions develop. These are often especially prominent in the parieto-occipital periventricular white matter and do not communicate with the lateral ventricle. They collapse after several weeks and are no longer visible with cranial ultrasound once the child is 2–3 months old. At this stage, irregular ventricular dilatation can be noted due to atrophy of the periventricular white matter.

MRI performed in the second year of life or even much later confirms the triad of reduced white-matter volume, reduction in myelination and angular dilatation of the posterior lateral ventricles. There is often extensive gliosis in the areas where the cysts were initially seen (Flodmark et al. 1989). These findings are sometimes seen in infants who did not have cysts identified during the neonatal period; this may be because they were not imaged at the appropriate time or perhaps because the damage to the oligodendroglia was too subtle to be detected with ultrasound.

Magnetic resonance imaging diagnosis

As discussed above, ultrasonography has limitations in the diagnosis of non-cystic PVL. Even for babies with cystic PVL, MRI is able to identify the cysts earlier, often in larger numbers, plus more extensive cysts can be seen compared to ultrasonography (Sie et al. 2000; Roelants-van Rijn et al. 2001a). DWI enables identification of areas with cytotoxic oedema within hours of an insult. DWI has been performed in preterm infants who subsequently developed PVL (Inder et al. 1999a; Bozzao et al. 2003; Kidokoro et al. 2008a; Fu et al. 2009). Reductions in diffusion have been found throughout the periventricular white matter soon after birth (Fu et al. 2009) and the conventional MRI performed at the same time is often normal (Bozzao et al. 2003; Fu et al. 2009). More severe restrictions in diffusion are predominantly seen in the posterior white matter where cysts subsequently develop (Kidokoro et al. 2008a). There are also diffusion abnormalities within the posterior limb of the internal capsule (PLIC) and the corpus callosum (Kidokoro et al. 2008a) and the ADC in the PLIC is related to the subsequent severity of PVL (Bozzao et al. 2003; Kidokoro et al. 2008a). The early areas of abnormality identified by diffusion have been shown to develop into cystic areas on later conventional brain MRI, suggesting that DWI has a role in early identification of PVL (Kidokoro et al. 2008a; Fu et al. 2009). The abnormalities detected within the white matter on DWI have been confirmed with histopathlological studies (Roelants-van Rijn et al. 2001b).

Diffuse changes within the white matter, often referred to as DEHSI on MRI, are commonly seen at term-equivalent age in the preterm population (Maalouf et al. 2001; Counsell et al. 2003a, b; Dyet et al. 2006). This can be seen in association with focal white-matter injury, such as cystic PVL or with GMH-IVH, but also as an isolated abnormality. In particular, infants with diffuse white-matter abnormalities, characterised by abnormal apparent diffusion coefficients, have volume reduction within the thalamus, the globus pallidus, the periventricular white matter and the centrum semiovale (Boardman et al. 2006, 2010; Srinivasan et al. 2007). In particular thalamocortical connectivity is thought to be impaired, with a resultant decrease in thalamic volume. This is also found in infants with cPVL (Counsell et al. 2007; Srinivasan et al. 2007), but to a greater extent, as well as a reduction in cerebral cortical grey-matter volume (Inder et al. 1999c).

There is additional value of MRI in infants with non-cystic PVL. Other abnormalities are often noted, in particular focal areas of abnormal signal intensity, referred to as punctate white-matter lesions (see later section) (Childs et al. 2001; Maalouf et al. 2001; Roelants-van Rijn et al. 2001a), but also incidental findings of basal ganglia abnormalities and cerebellar haemorrhage have also been identified.

Prevention

In contrast to GMH-IVH, where many intervention studies have been performed both before and after delivery, hardly any studies are available with regard to the prevention of PVL. Prevention of systemic hypotension is considered to be important, in spite of the lack of convincing evidence that it is implicated.

Antenatal steroids are probably effective in helping to reduce the incidence of postnatal PVL, although one important study showed that it was only betamethasone that had a beneficial effect (Baud et al. 1999; Canterino et al. 2001; Agarwal et al. 2002). The lack of benefit for dexamethasone has been attributed to the presence of sulphite as a preservative (Baud et al. 2001). Given the wealth of evidence that maternal chorioamnionitis is important, it is perhaps surprising that there is no evidence (as yet) that antibiotics given antenatally are protective (Kenyon et al. 2001).

Adjusting ventilatory settings in order to avoid severe hypocarbia is essential, based on evidence both from animal studies and in human babies (Graziani et al. 1992; Wiswell et al. 1996a, b; Okumura et al. 2001). This may be especially important in infants ventilated with high-frequency oscillation (Wiswell et al. 1996a).

A retrospective case-control study showed that infants who were exposed to magnesium sulphate in utero were less likely to develop cPVL (Finesmith et al. 1997). Magnesium sulphate during preterm labour has been shown to reduce the rates of moderate to severe cerebral palsy (relative risk 0.55, 95% CI 0.32–0.95) (Crowther et al. 2003; Rouse et al. 2008; Costantine and Weiner 2009) and its routine use during preterm labour is gaining acceptance. However, the studies have not shown a specific reduction in cPVL or GMH-IVH (Crowther et al. 2003).

High hypoxanthine and protein carbonyl levels were present at birth in infants who went on to develop PVL, suggesting that free radical damage might be important (Russell et al. 1992; Inder et al. 2002b). One randomised double-blind study used allopurinol, an inhibitor of xanthine oxidase, but no protective effect could be shown (Russell and Cooke 1995). A prospective cohort study of infants <28 weeks' gestational age identified a prolonged indometacin course as a significant factor associated with a reduction in moderate to severe white-matter disease (Miller et al. 2006). There are a number of other potential neuroprotective agents that have been shown to be effective in animal studies, but the results of human studies are awaited. These include erythropoietin (Kumral et al. 2007; Mizuno et al. 2008), topiramate (Sfaello et al. 2005) and melatonin (Olivier et al. 2009; Kaur et al. 2010).

Prognosis: neurodevelopmental outcome

Bilateral occipitoparietal cPVL is a powerful predictor of cerebral palsy (usually spastic diplegia) (Han et al. 2002; de Vries et al. 2004; Bax et al. 2006). In many preterm cohort follow-up studies, almost all the cases of cerebral palsy had bilateral occipital cPVL in the neonatal period (Graham et al. 1987; Bennett et al. 1990; Fazzi et al. 1994; Rogers et al. 1994; Pinto-Martin et al. 1995). Earlier studies, reporting an association between ventricular dilatation and adverse outcome (Catto-Smith et al. 1985), probably included some undiagnosed cases of PVL due to poor resolution of the older ultrasound scanners. Single cysts and cysts confined to the frontal region appear to have a better outcome than multiple bilateral occipital cysts (Catto-Smith et al. 1985). Cystic PVL also has an impact on cognitive outcome, although this is probably related to the diffuse component of PVL. The cognitive profile of these children is quite uneven and language is less affected, with greater impairment of visuospatial skills (Jacobson et al. 2002).

Some prognostic information can be gathered from brain MRI at term-equivalent, where abnormal myelination of the PLIC is a poor prognostic sign (Roelants-van Rijn et al. 2001a; Woodward et al. 2006). Bilateral occipital cystic white-matter damage carries a significantly higher risk of developing a major handicap than a large unilateral parenchymal infarction (de Vries et al. 1985). As cPVL is almost always bilateral there is little scope for compensation by the contralateral hemisphere.

Cerebral visual impairment is another important sequel and attempts should be made to recognise this early in infancy (Eken et al. 1994; Cioni et al. 1997; Ricci et al. 2006). Abnormalities within the optic radiation on brain MRI predict visual impairment in this population, with more severe damage being related to more severe impairment of the optic radiation and also atrophy of the thalami (Ricci et al. 2006).

A number of studies have identified a relationship between diffuse white-matter abnormalities on MRI and cognitive deficits (Dyet et al. 2006; Krishnan et al. 2007; Boardman et al. 2010). Overall, infants with DEHSI alone on term imaging have been shown to have a statistical reduction in their developmental quotient using the Griffiths Mental Development Scales (Dyet et al. 2006; Krishnan et al. 2007), although approximately 50% of these infants' scores will still lie within the normal spectrum (Dyet et al. 2006). Diffuse white-matter abnormalities alone therefore cannot explain the large burden of neurodevelopmental impairments in this population; however, associated axonal/neuronal abnormalities, as described by 'encephalopathy of prematurity', may explain why some fare better than others. Longer-term follow-up studies are awaited.

Punctate white-matter lesions

Punctate lesions are small areas of increased signal intensity on T1-weighted MRI (Fig. 40.57) and can sometimes be identified as echogenic areas on cranial ultrasound. They were identified in 26% of 119 infants born at <30 weeks' gestational age and serially imaged between birth and term, but were not present on the first scan in the majority of cases (Dyet et al. 2006). They can still be seen at term and on later imaging in some. They are most frequently found along the corona radiata, in the posterior periventricular white matter and in the optic radiation. They are often assumed to

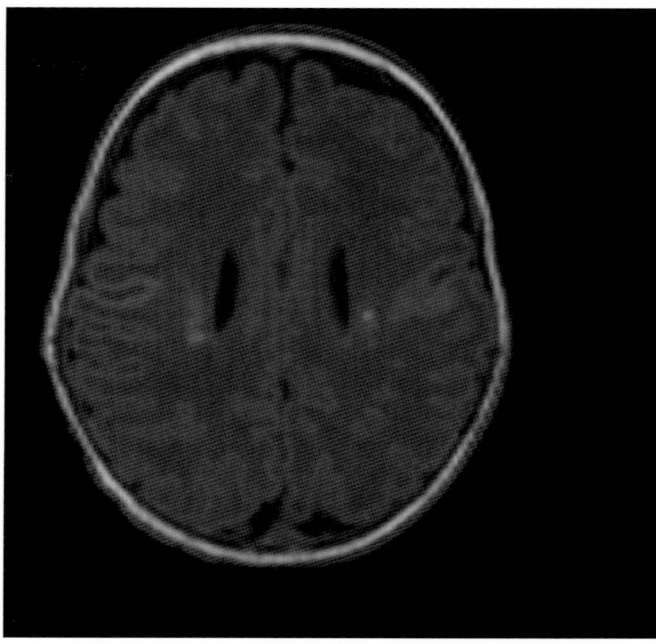

Fig. 40.57 T1-weighted axial magnetic resonance imaging scan showing small punctate white-matter lesions seen as small areas of high signal intensity.

represent haemorrhage, but their signal characteristics on MRI do not confirm this and abnormal DWI points more towards infarction (Rutherford et al. 2010). Studies have so far shown that the outcome for babies with punctate lesions is good (Cornette et al. 2002; Dyet et al. 2006) but these studies are small and the follow-up is short-term. Lesions in more critical positions, such as the PLIC or optic radiation, may have a more specific effect on neurodevelopment. One study has shown a reduction in myelination and cortical folding in infants with punctate white-matter lesions (Ramenghi et al. 2007), but this requires confirmation and the significance is not yet clear.

Haemorrhagic parenchymal infarction

Incidence

The incidence of IPLs secondary to haemorrhagic parenchymal infarction has fallen (Hamrick et al. 2004) in line with the reduction in GMH-IVH. There is an incidence of approximately 17% in infants <26 weeks' gestational age, which decreases to 1% at 30 weeks' gestational age (Larroque et al. 2003). IPLs are often included with grade III GMH-IVH in many studies so the incidence is not easy to identify (Ancel et al. 2006). The Australian and New Zealand neonatal network reported that their IPL rate had fallen to 24% (in babies of 24–30 weeks' gestation) by 1997 but that large interunit variation existed (Heuchan et al. 2002). Variation in incidence between centres has also been reported from the Vermont-Oxford and National Institutes of Health neonatal networks in the USA, in Canada (Synnes et al. 2001) and in the Pacific Rim (Martinez et al. 2002). In the Canadian study, 40% of the variance was explained by differences in illness severity measured with SNAP-II, but there are also concerns that significant variance is related to neonatal unit characteristics with lower rates in units with a high throughput of infants and high staffing ratios (Synnes et al. 2006).

Timing

Most IPLs secondary to venous infarction are present by 96 hours of age. They occur following significant GMH-IVH and many will develop 12–24 hours after this injury (Perlman et al. 1993). Some IPLs can be present at birth and this obviously indicates an antenatal insult, the timing of which can sometimes be estimated from the echogenicity of the white matter and any cystic components.

Pathogenesis

The most common cause of IPL is venous infarction following GMH-IVH, with or without a haemorrhagic component. The term grade IV IVH has now been superseded by the knowledge that it is not an extension of haemorrhage, but compression of the terminal vein within the germinal matrix by haemorrhage with subsequent obstruction of the medullary veins within the white matter (Gould et al. 1987) (Fig. 40.46). This has been shown histologically (Gould et al. 1987) and also using Doppler ultrasound (Taylor 1995). Histopathology of the regions of infarction shows that the white matter is oedematous and contains congested radial blood vessels which are cuffed by macrophages containing red blood cells. These changes form a well-defined wedge extending from the site of the haemorrhage in the germinal matrix out to the cortex. In the adjacent white matter there are oedema and axon retraction balls, consistent with infarction. Following this injury there is interruption of projection and association fibres and oligodendrocyte damage with resultant disruption in myelination.

Diagnosis

Clinical diagnosis

Infants with an IPL have bilateral abnormal general movements during the neonatal period irrespective of outcome (Cioni et al. 2000), although only those with an unfavourable outcome will have absent fidgety movements between 9 and 16 weeks postterm (Cioni et al. 2000). Standard neurological examination will identify abnormalities in many, but not all, infants with an IPL. In particular asymmetries can be noted.

Ultrasound diagnosis

Unilateral IPLs associated with GMH-IVH are due to venous infarction. This type of lesion is classically triangular or fan-shaped with the apex at the outer border of the lateral ventricle. In some cases the lesion is globular, with the apex of the triangle at the midline and a smooth outer border. This globular type of lesion (usually unilateral) evolves over 2–3 weeks into a porencephalic cyst, whereas those IPLs that are clearly separate from the ventricle at the start often form multiple small cysts (Rademaker et al. 1994). Porencephalic cysts do not disappear with time, unlike those of PVL. IPLs due to haemorrhage, such as following cerebral contusion, are seen as echogenic areas within the parenchyma that change over time, often with heterogeneous echogenicity, before developing cystic components.

MR diagnosis

The presence of large IPLs is clearly seen using brain MRI. In infants with a GMH-IVH, linear abnormalities can occasionally be seen within the white matter of the centrum semiovale, suggesting distended or obstructed veins (Counsell et al. 1999). Later imaging confirms the presence of porencephalic cysts and imaging at term-equivalent age is helpful prognostically, as outlined below.

Prognosis: neurodevelopmental outcome

The outcome following an IPL of any aetiology is dependent upon its site and extent. Large frontal lesions can have little clinical impact, whereas a small lesion at the site of the corticospinal tracts can be devastating. Single large porencephalic cysts are now less common and smaller IPLs that are only partly communicating with the lateral ventricle are more often seen, in our experience. In the study by Rademaker et al. (1994), using cranial ultrasound in the parasagittal plane, motor impairment was uncommon in infants with cysts anterior to the ventricular trigone, whereas all infants with cysts posterior to the trigone either died or developed a motor handicap. Involvement of more than two areas, bilateral lesions and midline shift in the early stages are adverse prognostic features (Bassan et al. 2006). Brain MRI at term-corrected age provides further prognostic information using assessment of myelination of the PLIC. Infants with asymmetrical myelination are likely to develop hemiplegia (de Vries et al. 1999). The impact on the PLIC is thought to be a secondary phenomenon related to wallerian degeneration rather than direct injury (de Vries et al. 1999). Diffusion tensor imaging has identified abnormal diffusion in the internal capsule in infants with cystic white-matter abnormalities, reinforcing this hypothesis (Huppi et al. 2001). Anterior cysts do not cause motor problems, but they may impact on more subtle function such as attention and concentration. Infants with bilateral extensive IPLs have the potential to develop spastic quadriplegia and this is generally regarded as an indication for withdrawal of intensive care at an early stage in many units following discussion with the parents. Fortunately this is not a common occurrence and is usually a complication in extremely preterm infants.

Infants with an IPL are unfortunately at risk of later epilepsy and those with haemorrhagic infarction and seizures have greater cognitive impairment than those with an IPL alone (Amess et al. 1998). The seizures can develop relatively late in childhood in some cases.

Conclusion

For over 30 years the use of cranial ultrasound imaging has allowed documentation of a changing pattern of brain injury in preterm infants and MRI has added to our understanding of this injury. The recognition that the majority of white-matter disease of prematurity is diffuse and that it is inextricably linked to the development of the cerebral cortex, cerebellum, thalamus, basal ganglia and brainstem is an important breakthrough and may explain the high levels of cognitive and behavioural difficulties that are seen in this population. The next challenge is to develop 'preterm neuroprotection' to try to alter the developmental trajectory of preterm white matter and initial studies are now underway.

References

Adams-Chapman, I., Hansen, N.I., Stoll, B.J., et al., 2008. Neurodevelopmental outcome of extremely low birth weight infants with posthemorrhagic hydrocephlus requiring shunt insertion. Pediatrics 121, e1167–e1177.

Agarwal, R., Chiswick, M.L., Rimmer, S., et al., 2002. Antenatal steroids are associated with a reduction in the incidence of cerebral white matter lesions in very low birthweight infants. Arch Dis Child Fetal Neonat Ed 86, F96–F101.

Agresti, C., D'Urso, D., Levi, G., 1996. Reversible inhibitory effects of interferon-gamma and tumour necrosis factor-alpha on oligodendroglial lineage cell proliferation and differentiation in vitro. Eur J Neurosci 8, 1106–1116.

Amess, P.N., Baudin, J., Townsend, J., et al., 1998. Epilepsy in very preterm infants: neonatal cranial ultrasound reveals a high-risk subcategory. Dev Med Child Neurol 40, 724–730.

Ancel, P.-Y., Livinec, L., Larroque, B., et al., 2006. Cerebral palsy among very preterm children in relation to gestational age and neonatal ultrasound abnormalities: the EPIPAGE cohort study. Pediatrics 117, 828–835.

Andre, P., Thebaud, B., Delavaucoupet, J., et al., 2001. Late-onset cystic periventricular leukomalacia in premature infants: a threat until term. Am J Perinatol 18, 79–86.

Andrews, T., Zhang, P., Bhat, N.R., 1998. TNFalpha potentiates IFNgamma-induced cell death in oligodendrocyte progenitors. J Neurosc Res 54, 574–583.

Arad, I., Braunstein, R., Ergaz, Z., et al., 2007. Bruising at birth: antenatal associations and neonatal outcome of extremely low birth weight infants. Neonatology 92, 258–263.

Back, S.A., Luo, N.L., Borenstein, N.S., et al., 2001. Late oligodendrocyte progenitors coincide with the developmental window of vulnerability for human perinatal white matter injury. J Neurosci 21, 1302–1312.

Back, S.A., Han, B.H., Luo, N.L., et al., 2002. Selective vulnerability of late oligodendrocyte progenitors to hypoxia-ischaemia. J Neurosci 22, 455–463.

Back, S.A., Craig, A., Kayton, R.J., et al., 2007. Hypoxic–ischaema preferentially triggers glutamate depletion from oligodendroglia and axons in perinatal cerebral white matter. J Cereb Blood Flow Metab 27, 334–347.

Baer, V.L., Lambert, D.K., Henry, E., et al., 2011. Among very low birth weight neonates is red blood cell transfusion an independent risk factor for subsequently developing a severe intraventricular haemorrhage? Transfusion 51, 1170–1178.

Banker, B.Q., Larroche, J.C., 1962. Periventricular leukomalacia of infancy. A form of neonatal anoxic encephalopathy. Arch Neurol 7, 386–410.

Bassan, H., Benson, C.B., Limperopoulos, C., et al., 2006. Ultrasonographic features and severity scoring of periventricular hemorrhagic infarction in relation to risk factors and outcome. Pediatrics 117, 2111–2117.

Batton, D.G., Holtrop, P., DeWitte, D., et al., 1994. Current gestational age-related incidence of major intraventricular hemorrhage. J Pediatr 125, 623–625.

Baud, O., d'Allest, A.-M., Lacaze-Masmonteio, T., et al., 1998. The early diagnosis of periventricular leukomalacia in premature infants with positive rolandic sharp waves on serial electroencephalography. J Pediatr 132, 813–817.

Baud, O., Foix-L'Helias, L., Kaminski, M., et al., 1999. Antenatal glucocorticoid treatment and cystic periventricular leukomalacia in very premature infants. N Engl J Med 341, 1190–1196.

Baud, O., Laudenbach, V., Evrard, P., et al., 2001. Neurotoxic effects of fluorinated glucocorticoid preparations on the developing mouse brain: role of preservatives. Pediatr Res 50, 706–711.

Baud, O., Daire, J.-L., Dalmaz, Y., et al., 2004. Gestational hypoxia induces white matter damage in neonatal rats: a new model of periventricular leukomalacia. Brain Pathol 14, 1–10.

Bauer, M., Fast, C., Haas, J., et al., 2009. Cystic periventricular leukomalacia in preterm infants: an analysis of obstetric risk factors. Early Hum Dev 85, 163–169.

Bax, M., Tydeman, C., Flodmark, O., 2006. Clinical and MRI correlates of cerebral palsy. JAMA 296, 1602–1608.

Bennett, F.C., Silver, G., Leung, E.J., et al., 1990. Periventricular echodensities detected by cranial ultrasound: usefulness in predicting neurodevelopmental outcome in low birthweight, preterm infants. Pediatrics 85, 400–404.

Beverley, D.W., Pitts-Tucker, T.J., Congdon, P.J., et al., 1985. Prevention of intraventricular haemorrhage by fresh frozen plasma. Arch. Dis Child 60, 710–713.

Boardman, J.P., Counsell, S.J., Rueckert, D., et al., 2006. Abnormal deep grey matter development following preterm birth detected using deformation based morphometry. NeuroImage 32, 70–78.

Boardman, J.P., Craven, C., Valappil, S., et al., 2010. A common neonatal image phenotype predicts adverse neurodevelopmental outcome in children born preterm. Neuroimage 52, 409–414.

Bozynski, M.E.A., Nelson, M.N., Matalon, T.A.S., et al., 1985. Cavitary periventricular leukomalacia: incidence and short-term outcome in infants weighing less than or greater than 1200 grams at birth. Dev Med Child Neurol 27, 572–577.

Bozzao, A., Di Paolo, A., Mazzoleni, C., et al., 2003. Diffusion-weighted MR imaging in the early diagnosis of periventricular leukomalacia. Eur Radiol 13, 1571–1576.

Canterino, J.C., Verma, U., Visintainer, P.F., et al., 2001. Antenatal steroids and neonatal periventricular leukomalacia. Obstet Gynecol 97, 135–139.

Carson, S.C., Hertzberg, B.S., Bowie, J.D., et al., 1990. Value of sonography in the diagnosis of intracranial hemorrhage and periventricular leukomalacia: a postmortem study of 35 cases. Am J Radiol 155, 595–601.

Casaer, P., von Siebenthal, K., van der Vlugt, A., et al., 1992. Cytochrome aa3 and intracranial pressure in newborn infants; a near infrared spectroscopy study. Neuropediatrics 23, 111.

Catto-Smith, A.G., Yu, V.Y.H., Bajuk, B., et al., 1985. Effect of neonatal periventricular haemorrhage on neurodevelopmental outcome. Arch Dis Child 60, 8–11.

Childs, A.-M., Cornette, L., Ramenghi, L.A., et al., 2001. Magnetic resonance and cranial ultrasound characteristics of periventricular white matter abnormalities in newborn infants. Clin Radiol 56, 647–655.

Cioni, G., Prechtl, H.F., 1990. Preterm and early postterm motor behaviour in low-risk premature infants. Early Hum Dev 23, 159–191.

Cioni, G., Fazzi, B., Coluccini, M., et al., 1997. Cerebral visual impairment in preterm infants with periventricular leukomalacia. Pediatr Neurol 17, 331–338.

Cioni, G., Bos, A.F., Einspieler, C., et al., 2000. Early neurological signs in preterm infants with unilateral intraparenchymal echodensities. Neuropediatrics 31, 240–251.

Connor, J.R., Menzies, S.L., 1996. Relationship of iron to oligodendrocytes and myelination. Glia 17, 83–93.

Cornette, L.G., Tanner, S.F., Ramenghi, L.A., et al., 2002. Magnetic resonance imaging of the infant brain: anatomical characteristics and clinical significance of punctate lesions. Arch Dis Child 86, 171–177.

Costantine, M.M., Weiner, S.J., 2009. Effects of antenatal exposure to magnesium sulfate on neuroprotection and mortality in preterm infants: a meta-analysis. Obstet Gynecol 114, 354–364.

Counsell, S., Maalouf, E.F., Rutherford, M.A., et al., 1999. Periventricular haemorrhagic infarct in a preterm neonate. Eur J Pediatr Neurol 3, 25–28.

Counsell, S.J., Allsop, J.M., Harrison, M.C., et al., 2003a. Diffusion-weighted imaging of the brain in preterm infants with focal and diffuse white matter abnormality. Pediatrics 112, 1–7.

Counsell, S.J., Rutherford, M.A., Cowan, F.M., et al., 2003b. Magnetic resonance imaging of preterm brain injury. Arch Dis Child Fetal Neonatal Ed 88, 269–274.

Counsell, S.J., Dyet, L.E., Larkman, D.J., et al., 2007. Thalamo-cortical connectivity in children born preterm mapped using probabilistic magnetic resonance tractography. NeuroImage 34, 896–904.

Cowan, F., Thoresen, M., 1987. The effects of intermittent positive pressure ventilation on cerebral arterial and venous blood velocities in the newborn infant. Acta Paediatr Scand 76, 239–247.

Cowan, F., Whitelaw, A., Wertheim, D., et al., 1991. Cerebral blood flow velocity changes after rapid administration of surfactant. Arch Dis Child 66, 1105–1109.

Crowther, C.A., Hiller, J.E., Doyle, L.W., et al., 2003. Effect of magnesium sulfate given for neuroprotection before preterm birth: a randomized controlled trial. JAMA 290, 2669–2676.

Dani, C., Poggi, C., Ceciarini, F., et al., 2009. Coagulopathy screening and early plasma treatment for the prevention of intraventricular hemorrhage in preterm infants. Transfusion 49, 2637–2644.

Dani, C., Poggi, C., Bertini, G., et al., 2010. Method of delivery and intraventircular haemorrhage in extremely preterm infants. J Matern Fetal Neonatal Med 23, 1419–1423.

Davies, M.W., Swaminathan, M., Chuang, S.L., et al., 2000. References ranges for the linear dimensions of the intracranial ventricles in preterm neonates. Arch Dis Child 82, F218–F223.

Debillon, T., N'Guyen, S., Quere, M.P., et al., 2003. Limitations of ultrasonography for diagnosing white matter damage in preterm infants. Arch Dis Child 88, 275–279.

de Vries, L.S., Dubowitz, L.M.S., Dubowitz, V., 1985. Predictive value of cranial ultrasound in the newborn baby: a reappraisal. Lancet 2, 137–140.

de Vries, L.S., Regev, R., Dubowitz, L.M.S., 1986. Late onset cystic leukomalacia. Arch Dis Child 61, 298–299.

de Vries, L.S., Wigglesworth, J.S., Regev, R., et al., 1988. Evolution of periventricular leukomalacia during the neonatal period and infancy: correlation of imaging and postmortem findings. Early Hum Dev 17, 205–219.

de Vries, L.S., Pierrat, V., Minami, T., et al., 1990. The role of short latency somatosensory evoked responses in infants with rapidly progressive ventricular dilatation. Neuropediatrics 21, 136–139.

de Vries, L.S., Eken, P., Dubowitz, L.M.S. 1992. The spectrum of leukomalacia using cranial ultrasound. Behav Brain Res 49, 1–6.

de Vries, L.S., Groenendaal, F., van Haastert, I.C., et al., 1999. Asymmetrical myelination of the posterior limb of the internal capsule in infants with periventricular haemorrhagic infarcction: an early predictor of hemiplegia. Neuropediatrics 30, 314–319.

de Vries, L.S., Liem, K.D., van Dijk, K., et al., 2002. Early versus late treatment of posthaemorrhagic ventricular dilatation: results of a retrospective study from five neonatal intensive care units in the Netherlands. Acta Paediatrica 91, 212–217.

de Vries, L.S., van Haastert, I.L., Rademaker, K.J., et al., 2004. Ultrasound abnormalities preceding cerebral palsy in high-risk preterm infants. J Pediatr 144, 815–820.

Denbow, M.L., Battin, M.R., Cowan, F., et al., 1998. Neonatal cranial ultrasonographic findings in preterm twins complicated by severe fetofetal transfusion syndrome. Am J Obstet Gynecol 178, 479–483.

Desilva, T.M., Kinney, H.C., Borenstein, N.S., et al., 2007. The glutamate transporter EAAT2 is transiently expressed in developing human cerebral white matter. J Comp Neurol 501, 879–890.

Dolfin, T., Skidmore, M.B., Fong, K.W., et al., 1983. Incidence, severity, and timing of subependymal and intraventricular hemorrhages in preterm infants born in a perinatal unit as detected by serial real-time ultrasound. Pediatrics 71, 541–546.

Dubowitz, L.M.S., Levene, M.I., Morante, A., et al., 1981. Neurological signs in neonatal intraventricular hemorrhage: correlation with real time ultrasound. J Pediatr 99, 127–133.

Dyet, L.E., Kennea, N., Counsell, S.J., et al., 2006. Natural history of brain lesions in extremely preterm infants studied with serial magnetic resonance imaging from birth and neurodevelopmental assessment. Pediatrics 118, 536–548.

Ecury-Goossen, G.M., Dudink, J., Lequin, M., et al., 2010. The clinical presentation of preterm cerebellar haemorrhage. Eur J Pediatr 169, 1249–1253.

Eken, P., van Nieuwenhuizen, O., van der Graag, Y., et al., 1994. Relation between neonatal cranial ultrasound abnormalities and cerebral visual impairment in infancy. Dev Med Child Neurol 36, 3–15.

Ellison, V.J., Mocatta, T.J., Winterbourn, C.C., et al., 2005. The relationship of CSF and plasma cytokine levels to cerebral white matter injury in the premature newborn. Pediatr Res 57, 282–286.

Eriksson, L., Haglund, B., Ewald, U., et al., 2009. Short and long-term effects of antenatal corticosteroids assessed in a cohort of 7,827 children born preterm. Acta Obstet Gynecol Scand 88, 933–938.

Evans, N., Kluckow, M., 1996. Early ductal shunting and intraventricular haemorrhage in ventilated preterm infants. Arch Dis Child Fetal Neonatal Ed 75, F183–F186.

Evans, N., 2006. Assessment and support of the preterm circulation. Early Hum Dev 82, 803–810.

Fanaroff, A.A., Stoll, B.J., Wright, L.L., et al., 2007. Trends in neonatal morbidity and mortality for very low birthweight infants. Am J Obstet Gynecol 196, 147.e1–e8.

Fawer, C.L., Calame, A., Perentes, E., et al., 1985. Periventricular leukomalacia: a correlation study between real time ultrasound and autopsy findings. Neuroradiology 27, 292–230.

Fazzi, E., Orcesi, S., Caffi, L., et al., 1994. Neurodevelopmental outcome at 5–7 years in preterm infants with periventricular leukomalacia. Neuropediatrics 25, 134–139.

Fellman, V., Hellström-Westas, L., Norman, M., et al., 2009. One-year survival of extremely preterm infants after active perinatal care in Sweden. JAMA 301, 2225–2233.

Fernell, E., Hagberg, G., Hagberg, B., 1993. Infantile hydrocephalus in preterm, low-birth-weight infants – a nationwide Swedish cohort study 1979–1988. Acta Pediatrica 82, 45–48.

Finesmith, R.B., Roche, K., Yellin, P.B., et al., 1997. Effect of magnesium sulfate on the development of cystic periventricular leukomalacia in preterm infants. Am J Perinatol 14, 303–307.

Flodmark, O., Lupton, B., Li, D., et al., 1989. MR imaging of periventricular leukomalacia in childhood. Am J Neuroradiol 10, 111–118.

Folkerth, R.D., 2005. Neuropathologic substrate of cerebral palsy. J Child Neurol 20, 940–949.

Folkerth, R.D., Haynes, R.L., Borenstein, N.S., et al., 2004. Developmental lag in superoxide dismutases relative to other antioxidant enzymes in premyelinated human telencephalic white matter. J Neuropathol Exp Neurol 63, 990–999.

Fowlie, P.W., 1996. Prophylactic indomethacin: systematic review and a meta-analysis. Arch Dis Child 74, F81–F86.

Fu, J., Xue, X., Chen, L., et al., 2009. Studies on the value of diffusion-weighted MR imaging in the early prediction of periventricular leukomalacia. J Neuroimaging 19, 13–18.

Funato, M., Tamai, H., Noma, K., et al., 1992. Clinical events in association with timing of intraventricular hemorrhage in preterm infants. J Pediatr 121, 614–619.

Gaskill, S.J., Marlin, A.E., Rivera, S., 1988. The subcutaneous ventricular reservoir: an effective treatment for posthemorrhagic hydrocephalus. Childs Nerv Syst 4, 291–295.

Giannakopoulou, C., Korakaki, E., Manoura, A., et al., 2004. Significance of hypocarbia in the development of periventricular leukomalacia in preterm infants. Pediatr Int 46, 268–273.

Gill, A.B., Weindling, A.M., 1993. Randomised controlled trial of plasma protein fraction versus dopamine in hypotensive very low birthweight infants. Arch Dis Child 69, 284–287.

Glass, H.C., Bonifacio, S.L., Chau, V., et al., 2008. Recurrent postnatal infections are associated with progressive white matter injury in premature infants. Paediatrics 122, 299–305.

Gould, S.J., Howard, S., Hope, P.L., et al., 1987. Periventricular intraparenchymal cerebral haemorrhage in preterm infants: the role of venous infarction. J Pathol 151, 197–202.

Govaert, P., de Vries, L.S., 2010. An Atlas of Neonatal Brain Sonography, second ed. MacKeith Press, London.

Graham, M., Levene, M.I., Trounce, J.Q., et al., 1987. Prediction of cerebral palsy in very low birthweight infants: prospective ultrasound study. Lancet ii, 593–594.

Graham, E.M., Holcroft, C.J., Rai, K.K., et al., 2004. Neonatal cerebral white matter injury in preterm infants is associated with culture positive infections and only rarely with metabolic acidosis. Am J Obstet Gynecol 191, 1305–1310.

Grasby, D.C., Esterman, A., Marshall, P., 2003. Ultrasound grading of cerebral ventricular dilatation in preterm neonates. J Paediatr Child Health 39, 186–190.

Graziani, L.J., Spitzer, A.R., Mitchell, D.G., et al., 1992. Mechanical ventilation in preterm infants: neurosonographic and developmental studies. Pediatrics 90, 515–522.

Grether, J.K., Nelson, K.B., Emery, E.S., et al., 1996. Prenatal and perinatal factors and cerebral palsy in very low birth weight infants. J Pediatr 128, 407–414.

Groenendaal, F., Termote, J.U., Heide-Jalving, M., et al., 2010. Complications affecting preterm neonates from 1991 to 2006: what have we gained? Acta Paediatr 99, 354–358.

Grunnet, M.L., 1989. Morphometry of blood vessels in the cortex and germinal plate of premature neonates. Pediatr Neurol 5, 12–16.

Hambleton, G., Wigglesworth, J.S., 1976. Origin of intraventricular haemorrhage in the preterm infant. Arch Dis Child 51, 651–659.

Hamrick, S.E.G., Miller, S.P., Leonard, C., et al., 2004. Trends in severe brain injury and neurodevelopmental outcome in premature newborn infants: the role of cystic periventricular leukomalacia. J Pediatrics 145, 593–599.

Han, T.R., Bang, M.S., Lim, J.Y., et al., 2002. Risk factors of cerebral palsy in preterm infants. Am J Phys Med Rehab 81, 297–303.

Haverkamp, F., Lex, C., Hanisch, C., et al., 2001. Neurodevelopmental risks in

twin-to-twin transfusion syndrome: preliminary findings. Eur J Paediatr Neurol 5, 221–227.

Hayakawa, F., Okumura, A., Kato, T., et al., 1999. Determination of timing of brain injury in preterm infants with periventricular leukomalacia with serial neonatal electroencephalography. Pediatrics 104, 1077–1088.

Haynes, R.L., Folkerth, R.D., Keeff, R.J., et al., 2003. Nitrosative and oxidative injury to premyelinating oligodendrocytes in periventricular leukomalacia. J Neuropathol Exp Neurol 62, 441–450.

Heuchan, A.M., Evans, N., Henderson-Smart, D.J., et al., 2002. Perinatal risk factors for major intraventricular haemorrhage in the Australian and New Zealand neonatal network, 1995–1997. Arch Dis Child 86, F86–F90.

Hill, A., Melson, G.L., Clark, H.B., et al., 1982a. Haemorrhagic periventricular leukomalacia: diagnosis by real time ultrasound and correlation with autopsy findings. Pediatrics 69, 282–284.

Hill, A., Perlman, J.M., Volpe, J.J., 1982b. Relationship of pneumothorax to occurence of intraventricular hemorrhage in the premature newborn. Pediatrics 69, 144–145.

Hope, P.L., Gould, S.J., Howard, S., et al., 1988. Precision of ultrasound diagnosis of pathologically verified lesions in the brains of very preterm infants. Dev Med Child Neurol 30, 457–471.

Horbar, J.D., Soll, R.F., Schaginger, H., 1990. A European multicentre randomized controlled trial of single dose surfactant therapy for idiopathic respiratory distress syndrome. Eur J Pediatr 149, 416–423.

Horbar, J.D., Badger, G.J., Carpenter, J.H., et al., 2002. Trends in mortality and morbidity for very low birth weight infants, 1991–1999. Pediatrics 110, 143–151.

Horsch, S., Skiold, B., Hallberg, B., et al., 2010. Cranial ultrasound and MRI at term age in extremely preterm infants. Arch Dis Child Fetal Neonatal Ed 95, F310–F314.

Hudgins, R.J., Boydston, W.R., Gilreath, C.L., 1998. Treatment of posthemorrhagic hydrocephalus in the preterm infant with a ventricular access device. Pediatr Neurosurg 29, 309–313.

Huppi, P.S., Murphy, B., Maier, S.E., et al., 2001. Microstructural brain development after perinatal cerebral white matter injury assessed by diffusion tensor magnetic resonance imaging. Pediatrics 107, 455–460.

Iida, K., Takashima, S., Ueda, K., 1995. Immunohistochemical study of myelination and oligodendrocyte in infants with periventricular leukomalacia. Pediatr Neurol 13, 296–304.

Inage, Y.W., Itoh, M., Takashima, S., 2000. Correlation between cerebrovascular maturity and periventricular leukomalacia. Pediatr Neurol 22, 204–208.

Inder, T., Huppi, P.S., Zientara, G.P., et al., 1999a. Early detection of periventricular leukomalacia by diffusion-weighted magnetic resonance imaging techniques. J Pediatr 134, 631–634.

Inder, T.E., Huppi, P.S., Warfield, S., et al., 1999b. Periventricular white matter injury in the premature infant is followed by reduced cerebral cortical gray matter volume at term. Ann Neurol 46, 755–760.

Inder, T.E., Huppi, P.S., Warfield, S., et al., 1999c. Periventricular white matter injury in the premature infant is followed by reduced cerebral cortical gray matter volume at term. Ann Neurol 46, 755–760.

Inder, T., Mocatta, T., Darlow, B., et al., 2002a. Elevated free radical products in the cerebrospinal fluid of VLBW infants with cerebral white matter injury. Pediatr Res 52, 213–218.

Inder, T., Mocatta, T., Darlow, B., et al., 2002b. Elevated free radical products in the cerebrospinal fluid of VLBW infants with cerebral white matter injury. Pediatr Res 52, 213–218.

Inder, T.E., Anderson, N.J., Spencer, C., et al., 2003a. White matter injury in the premature infant: a comparison between serial cranial sonographic and MR findings at term. AJNR Am J Neuroradiol 24, 805–809.

Inder, T.E., Buckland, L., Williams, C.E., et al., 2003b. Lowered electroencephalographic spectral edge frequency predicts the presence of cerebral white matter injury in premature infants. Pediatrics 111, 27–33.

Inder, T.E., Wells, S.J., Mogridge, N.B., et al., 2003c. Defining the nature of the cerebral abnormalities in the premature infant: a qualitative magnetic resonance imaging study. J Pediatr 143, 171–179.

Inder, T.E., Warfield, S.K., Wang, H., et al., 2005. Abnormal cerebral structure is present at term in premature infants. Pediatrics 115, 286–294.

International PHVD Drug Trial Group. 1998. International randomised controlled trial of acetazolamide and furosemide in posthaemorrhagic ventricular dilatation in infancy. Lancet 352, 433–440.

Jacobson, L., Ygge, J., Flodmark, O., et al., 2002. Visual and perceptual characteristics, ocular motility and strabismus in children with periventricular leukomalacia. Strabismus 10, 179–183.

Jensen, F.E., 2005. Role of glutamate receptors in periventricular leukomalacia. J Child Neurol 20, 950–959.

Jim, W.T., Chiu, N.C., Chen, M.R., et al., 2005. Cerebral hemodynamic change and intravnetricular haemorrhage in very low birth weight infants with patent ductus arteriosus. Ultrasound Med Biol 31, 197–202.

Kadhim, H., Tabarki, B., Verellen, G., et al., 2001. Inflammatory cytokines in the pathogenesis of periventricular leukomalacia. Neurology 56, 1278–1284.

Kaiser, A.M., Whitelaw, A., 1986a. Cerebrospinal fluid pressure during post haemorrhagic ventricular dilatation in newborn infants. Arch Dis Child 60, 920–924.

Kaiser, A.M., Whitelaw, A.G.L., 1986b. Normal cerebrospinal fluid pressure in the newborn. Neuropediatrics 17, 100–102.

Kaiser, J.R., Gauss, C.H., Williams, D.K., 2004. Surfactant administration acutely affects cerebral and systemic hemodynamics and gas exchange in very-low-birth-weight infants. J Paediatr 144, 809–814.

Kaiser, J.R., Gauss, C.H., Pont, M.M., et al., 2006. Hypercapnia during the first 3 days of life is associated with severe intraventricular hemorrhage in very low birth weight infants. J Perinatol 26, 279–285.

Karadottir, R., Attwell, D., 2007. Neurotransmitter receptors in the life and death of oligodendrocytes. Neuroscience 145, 1426–1438.

Karadottir, R., Cavelier, P., Bergersen, L.H., et al., 2005. NMDA receptors are expressed in oligodendrocytes and activated in ischaemia. Nature 438, 1162–1166.

Kaur, C., Sivakumar, V., Ling, E.A., 2010. Melatonin protects periventricular white matter from damage due to hypoxia. J Pineal Res 48, 185–193.

Kennedy, C.R., Ayers, S., Campbell, M.J., et al., 2001. Randomized, controlled trial of acetazolamide and furosemide in posthemorrhagic ventricular dilation in infancy: follow-up at 1 year. Pediatrics 108, 597–607.

Kenyon, S.L., Taylor, D.J., Tarnow-Mordi, W., 2001. Broad-spectrum antibiotics for preterm, prelabour rupture of fetal membranes: the ORACLE 1 randomised trial. Lancet 357, 979–988.

Khwaja, O., Volpe, J.J., 2008. Pathogenesis of cerebral white matter injury of prematurity. Arch Dis Child Fetal Neonatal Ed 93, F153–F161.

Kidokoro, H., Kubota, T., Ohe, H., et al., 2008a. Diffusion-weighted magnetic resonance imaging in infants with periventricular leukomalacia. Neuropediatrics 39, 233–238.

Kidokoro, H., Okumura, A., Kato, T., et al., 2008b. Electroencephalogram and flash visual evoked potentials for detecting periventricular leukomalacia. Neuropediatrics 39, 226–232.

Kluckow, M., Evans, N., 2000. Low superior vena cava flow and intraventricular haemorrhage in preterm infants. Arch Dis Child Fetal Neonatal Ed 82, F188–F194.

Kobayashi, S., Fujimoto, S., Koyama, N., et al., 2008. Late-onset circulatory dysfunction of premature infants and late-onset periventricular leukomalacia. Pediatr Int 50, 225–231.

Kostovic, I., Judas, M., 2002. Correlation between the sequential ingrowth of afferents and transient patterns of cortical lamination in preterm infants. Anatom Record 267, 1–6.

Krageloh-Mann, I., Toft, P., Lunding, L., et al., 1999. Brain lesions in preterms: origin, consequences and compensation. Acta Paediatr 88, 897–908.

Krishnan, M.L., Dyet, L.E., Boardman, J.P., et al., 2007. Relationship between white matter apparent diffusion coefficients in preterm infants at term-equivalent age and developmental outcome at 2 years. Pediatrics 120, e604–e609.

Kuban, K.C.K., Allred, E.N., Dammann, O., et al., 2001. Topography of cerebral white-matter disease of prematurity studied prospectively in 1607 very-low-birthweight infants. J Child Neurol 16, 401–408.

Kubota, T., Okumura, A., Hayakaa, F., et al., 2001. Relation between the date of cyst formation observable on ultrasonography and the timing of injury determined by serial electroencephalography in preterm infants with periventricular leukomalacia. Brain Dev 23, 390–394.

Kumral, A., Baskin, H., Yesilirmak, D.C., et al., 2007. Erythropoietin attenuates lipopolysaccharide-induced white matter injury in the neonatal rat brain. Neonatology 92, 269–278.

Larroche, J.-C., 1972. Post haemorrhagic hydrocephalus in infancy. Biol Neonate 20, 287–299.

Larroque, B., Marret, S., Ancel, P.Y., et al., 2003. White matter damage and intraventricular hemorrhage in very preterm infants: the EPIPAGE study. J Paediatr 143, 477–483.

Lee, I.C., Lee, H.S., Su, P.H., et al., 2009. Posthemorrhagic hydrocephalus in newborns: clinical characteristics and role of ventriculoperitoneal shunts. Pediatr Neonatol 50, 26–32.

Lee, J.Y., Kim, H.S., Jung, E., et al., 2010. Risk factors for periventricular-intraventricular haemorrhage in premature infants. J Korean Med Sci 25, 418–424.

Leijser, L.M., Liauw, L., Veen, S., et al., 2008. Comparing brain white matter on sequential cranial ultrasound and MRI in very preterm infants. Neuroradiology 50 (9), 799–811.

Lemons, J.A., Bauer, C.R., Oh, W., et al., 2001. Very low birth weight outcomes of the National Institute of Child Health and Human Development neonatal research network, January 1995 through December 1996. Pediatrics 107, e1–e8.

Levene, M.I., de Vries, L.S., 1984. Extension of neonatal intraventricular haemorrhage. Arch Dis Child 59, 631–636.

Levene, M.I., Starte, D.R., 1981. A longitudinal study of post haemorrhagic ventricular dilatation in the newborn. Arch Dis Child 56, 905–910.

Levene, M.I., Wigglesworth, J.S., Dubowitz, V., 1983. Haemorrhagic periventricular leukomalacia in the neonate: a real time ultrasound study. Pediatrics 71, 794–797.

Leviton, A., Fenton, T., Kuban, K.C., et al., 1991a. Labor and delivery characteristics and the risk of germinal matrix hemorrhage in low birth weight infants. J Child Neurol 6, 35–40.

Leviton, A., Pagano, M., Kuban, K.C.K., et al., 1991b. The epidemiology of germinal matrix haemorrhage during the first half day of life. Dev Med Child Neurol 33, 138–145.

Leviton, A., Dammann, O., Durum, S.K., 2005. The adaptive immune response in neonatal cerebral white matter damage. Ann Neurol 58, 821–828.

Lim, W.H., Lien, R., Chiang, M.C., et al., 2011. Hypernatraemia and grade III/IV intraventricular hemorrhage among extremely low birth weight infants. J Perinatol 31, 193–198.

Limperopoulos, C., Bassan, H., Gauvreau, K., et al., 2007. Does cerebellar injury in premature infants contribute to the high prevalence of long-term cognitive, learning, and behavioral disability in survivors? Pediatrics 120, 584–593.

Linder, N., Haskin, O., Levit, O., et al., 2003. Risk factors for intraventricular hemorrhage in very low birth weight premature infants: a retrospective case-control study. Pediatrics 111, e590–e595.

Loeliger, M., Watson, C.S., Reynolds, J.D., et al., 2003. Extracellular glutamate levels and neuropathology in cerebral white matter following repeated umbilical cord occlusion in the near term fetal sheep. Neuroscience 116, 705–714.

Long, W., Corbet, A., Cotton, R., 1991. A controlled trial of synthetic surfactant (Exosurf) in infants weighing 1250g or more with respiratory distress syndrome. N Engl J Med 325, 1696–1703.

Lou, H.C., Lassen, N.A., Friis-Hansen, B., 1979. Impaired ability of autoregulation of cerebral blood flow in the distressed newborn infant. J Pediatr 94, 118–121.

Lowe, J., Papile, J.A., 1990. Neurodevelopmental performance of very low birth weight infants with mild periventricular, intraventricular haemorrhage. Am J Dis Child 144, 1242–1245.

Lundqvist, P., Kallen, K., Hallstrom, I., et al., 2009. Trends in outcomes for very preterm infants in the southern region of Sweden over a 10-year period. Acta Paediat 98, 648–653.

Luu, T.M., Ment, L.R., Schneider, K.C., et al., 2009. Lasting effects of preterm birth and neonatal brain hemorhage at 12 years of age. Pediatrics 123, 1037–1044.

Maalouf, E.F., Duggan, P.J., Rutherford, M.A., et al., 1999. Magnetic resonance imaging of the brain in a cohort of extremely preterm infants. J Pediatr 135, 351–357.

Maalouf, E.F., Duggan, P.J., Counsell, S.J., et al., 2001. Comparison of findings on cranial ultrasound and magnetic resonance imaging in preterm infants. Pediatrics 107, 719–727.

Marret, S., Parain, D., Jeannot, E., et al., 1992. Positive rolandic sharp waves in the EEG of the premature newborn: a five year prospective study. Arch Dis Child 67, 948–951.

Martens, S.E., Rujken, M., Stoelhorst, G.M., et al., 2003. Is hypotension a major risk factor for neurological morbidity at term age in very preterm infants? Early Hum Dev 75, 79–89.

Martinez, A., Taeusch, H.W., Yu, V., et al., 2002. Variation in mortality and intraventricular haemorrhage in occupants of Pacific Rim nurseries. J Paediatr Child Health 38, 235–240.

Matute, C., 2006. Oligodendrocyte NMDA receptors: a novel therapeutic target. Trends Mol Med 12, 289–292.

McDonald, M.M., Koops, B.L., Johnson, M.L., et al., 1984. Timing and antecedents of intracranial hemorrhage in the newborn. Pediatrics 74, 32–36.

McQuillen, P.S., Sheldon, R.A., Shatz, C.J., et al., 2003. Selective vulnerability of subplate neurons after early neonatal hypoxia-ischemia. J Neurosci 23, 3308–3315.

Meek, J.H., Tyszczuk, L., Elwell, C.E., Wyatt, J.S., 1999. Low cerebral blood flow is a risk factor for severe intraventricular haemorrhage. Arch Dis Child Fetal Neonatal Ed 81, F15–F18.

Ment, L.R., Duncan, C.C., Ehrenkrantz, R.A., et al., 1984. Intraventricular haemorrhage in the neonate: timing and cerebral blood flow changes. J Pediatr 104, 419–425.

Ment, L.R., Oh, W., Ehrenkranz, R.A., et al., 1994. Low-dose indomethacin and prevention of intraventricular hemorrhage: a multicentre randomised trial. Pediatrics 93, 543–550.

Ment, L.R., Vohr, B., Oh, W., et al., 1996. Neurodevelopmental outcome at 36 months' corrected age of preterm infant in the multicenter indomethacin intraventricular hemorrhage prevention trial. Pediatrics 98, 714–718.

Ment, L.R., Westerveld, M., Makuch, R., et al., 1998. Cognitive outcome at 4 1/2 years of very low birth weight infants enrolled in the multicenter indomethacin intraventricular hemorrhage prevention trial. Pediatrics 102, 159–160.

Ment, L.R., Vohr, B.R., Makuch, R.W., et al., 2004. Prevention of intraventricular hemorrhage by indomethacin in male preterm infants. J Paediatr 145, 832–834.

Merrill, J.D., Piecuch, R.E., Fell, S.C., et al., 1998. A new pattern of cerebellar hemorrhages in preterm infants. Pediatrics 102, 1–5.

Miall, L.S., Cornette, L.G., Tanner, S.F., 2003. Posterior fossa abnormalities seen on magnetic resonance brain imaging in a cohort of newborn infants. J Perinatol 23, 396–403.

Miall-Allen, V.M., de Vries, L.S., Whitelaw, A.G., 1987. Mean arterial blood pressure and neonatal cerebral lesions. Arch Dis Child 62, 1068–1069.

Miletin, J., Dempsey, E.M., 2008. Low superior vena cava flow on day 1 and adverse outcome in the very low birthweight infant. Arch Dis Child Fetal Neonatal Ed 93, F368–F371.

Miller, S.P., Ferriero, D.M., Leonard, C., et al., 2005. Early brain injury in premature newborns detected with magnetic resonance imaging is associated with adverse early neurodevelopmental outcome. J Paediatr 147, 609–616.

Miller, S.P., Mayer, E.E., Clyman, R.I., et al., 2006. Prolonged indomethacin exposure is associated with decreased white matter injury detected with magnetic resonance imaging in premature newborns at 24 to 28 weeks' gestation at birth. Pediatrics 177, 1626–1631.

Minagawa, K., Tsuji, Y., Ueda, H., et al., 2002. Possible correlation between high levels of IL-18 in the cord blood of pre-term infants and neonatal development of periventricular leukomalacia and cerebral palsy. Cytokine 17, 164–170.

Mizuno, K., Hida, H., Masuda, T., et al., 2008. Pretreatment with low doses of erythropoietin ameliorates brain damage in periventricular leukomalacia by targeting late oligodendrocyte progenitors: a rat model. Neonatology 94, 255–266.

Mohamed, M.A., Aly, H., 2010. Male gender is associated with intraventricular hemorrhage. Pediatrics 125, e333–e339.

Moise, A.A., Wearden, M.E., Kozinetz, C.A., et al., 1995. Antenatal steroids are associated with less need for blood pressure support in extremely premature infants. Pediatrics 95, 845–850.

Murase, M., Ishida, A., 2005. Early hypocarbia of preterm infants: its relationship to periventricular leukomalacia and cerebral palsy, and its perinatal risk factors. Acta Paediat 94, 85–91.

Murphy, D.J., Sellers, S., MacKenzie, I.Z., et al., 1995. Case-control study of antenatal and intrapartum risk factors for cerebral palsy in very preterm singleton babies. Lancet 346, 1449–1454.

Nagasunder, A.C., Kinney, H.C., Bluml, S., et al., 2011. Abnormal microstructure of the atrophic thalamus in preterm survivors with periventricular leukomalacia. AJNR Am J Neuroradiol, 32, 185–191.

Nakamura, Y., Okudera, T., Fukunde, S., et al., 1990. Germinal matrix haemorrhage of venous origin in preterm neonates. Hum Pathol 21, 1059.

Northern Neonatal Nursing Initiative, 1996. Randomised trial of prophylactic early fresh-frozen plasma or gelatin or glucose in preterm babies outcome at 2 years. Lancet 348, 229–232.

Nwaesei, C.G., Pape, K.E., Martin, D.J., et al., 1984. Periventricular infarction diagnosed by ultrasound: a postmortem correlation. J Pediatr 105, 106–110.

Okumura, A., Hayakawa, F., Itomi, K., et al., 2001. Hypocarbia in preterm infants with periventricular leukomalacia: the relation between hypocarbia and mechanical ventilation. Pediatrics 107, 469–475.

O'Leary, H., Gregas, M.C., Limperopoulos, C., et al., 2009. Elevated cerebral pressure passivity is associated with prematurity-related intracranial hemorrhage. Pediatrics 124, 302–309.

Olischar, M., Klebermass, K., Kuhle, S., et al., 2004. Reference values for amplitude-integrated electroencephalographic activity in preterm infants younger than 30 weeks' gestational age. Pediatrics 113, e61–e66.

Olischar, M., Klebermass, K., Hengl, B., et al., 2009. Cerebrospinal fluid drainage in posthaemorrhagic ventricular dilatation leads to improvement in amplitude-integrated electroencephalographic activity. Acta Paediatr 98, 1002–1009.

Olivier, P., Fontaine, R.H., Loron, G., et al., 2009. Melatonin promotes oligodendroglial maturation of injured white matter in neonatal rats. PLoS One 4, e7128.

Osborn, D., Evans, N., Kluckow, M., 2002. Randomized trial of dobutamine versus dopamine in preterm infants with low systemic blood flow. J Pediatr 140, 183–191.

Osborn, D.A., Evans, N., Kluckow, M., 2003. Hemodynamic and antecedent risk factors of early and late periventricular / intraventricular haemorrhage in premature infants. Pediatrics 112, 33–39.

Ozawa, H., Nishida, A., Mito, T., et al., 1994. Development of ferritin-positive cells in cerebrum of human brain. Pediatr Neurol 10, 44–48.

Palmer, P., Dubowitz, L.M.S., Levene, M.I., et al., 1982. Developmental and neurological progress of preterm infants with intraventricular haemorrhage and ventricular dilatation. Arch Dis Child 57, 748–752.

Paneth, N., Rudelli, R., Monte, W., et al., 1990. White matter necrosis in very low birthweight infants: neuropathologic and ultrasonographic findings in infants surviving six days or longer. J Pediatr 116, 975–984.

Paneth, N., Pinto-Martin, J., Gardiner, J., et al., 1993. Incidence and timing of germinal matrix/intraventricular hemorrhage in low birth weight infants. Am J Epidemiol 137, 1167–1176.

Paneth, N., Kazam, E., Monte, W., 1994. Brain Damage in the Preterm Infant. MacKeith Press, London.

Pape, K.E., Wiglesworth, J.S., 1979. Haemorrhage, Ischaemia and the Perinatal Brain. MacKeith Press, London.

Pape, K.E., Bennett-Britton, S., Szymonowicz, W., et al., 1983. Diagnostic accuracy of neonatal brain imaging: a postmortem correlation of computed tomography and ultrasound scans. J Pediatr 102, 275–280.

Papile, L.-A., Burstein, J., Burstein, R., et al., 1978. Incidence and evolution of subependymal and intraventricular haemorhage: a study of infants with birthweights less than 1500g. J Pediatr 92, 529–534.

Peretta, P., Ragazzi, P., Carlino, C.F., et al., 2007. The role of Ommaya reservoir and endoscopic third ventriculostomy in the management of post-hemorrhagic hydrocephalus of prematurity. Childs Nerv Syst 23, 765–771.

Perlman, J.M., 1990. Late hydrocephalus after arrest and resolution of neonatal post haemorrhagic hydrocephalus. Dev Med Child Neurol 32, 725–742.

Perlman, J.M., Rollins, N., 2000. Surveillance protocol for the detection of intracranial abnormalities in premature neonates. Arch Pediatr Adolesc Med 154, 822–826.

Perlman, J.M., Volpe, J.J., 1983. Suctioning the preterm infant: effects on cerebral blood flow velocity, intracranial pressure and arterial blood pressure. Pediatrics 72, 329–334.

Perlman, J.M., Volpe, J.J., 1986. Intraventricular haemorrhage in extremely small preterm infants. Am J Dis Child 140, 1112–1114.

Perlman, J.M., McMenamin, J.B., Volpe, J.J., 1983. Fluctuating cerebral blood flow velocity in respiratory distress syndrome: relation to the development of intraventricular hemorrhage. N Engl J Med 309, 204–209.

Perlman, J.M., Goodman, S., Kreusser, K.L., et al., 1985. Reduction in intraventricular hemorrhage by elimination of fluctuating cerebral blood flow velocity in preterm infants with respiratory distress syndrome. N Engl J Med 312, 1353–1357.

Perlman, J.M., Rollins, N., Burns, D., et al., 1993. Relationship between periventricular intraparenchymal echodensities and germinal matrix-intraventricular hemorrhage in the very low birthweight neonate. Pediatrics 91, 474–480.

Perlman, J.M., Risser, R., Broyles, R.S., 1996. Bilateral cystic periventricular leukomalacia in the premature infant: associated risk factors. Pediatrics 97, 822–827.

Philip, A.G.S., Allan, W.C., Tito, A.M., et al., 1989. Intraventricular hemorrhage in preterm infants: declining incidence in the 1980s. Pediatrics 84, 797–801.

Pierrat, V., Duquennoy, C., van Haastertt, I.C., et al., 2001. Ultrasound diagnosis and neurodevelopmental outcome of localised and extensive cystic periventricular leucomalacia. Arch Dis Child 84, F151–F156.

Pinto-Martin, J.A., Riolo, S., Cnaan, A., et al., 1995. Cranial ultrasound prediction of disabling and nondisabling cerebral palsy at age two in a low birth weight population. Pediatrics 95, 249–254.

Piotrowski, A., Dabrowska-Wojciak, I., Mikinka, M., et al., 2010. Coagulation abnormalities and severe intraventricular hemorrhage in extremely low birth weight infants. J Matern Fetal Neonatal Med 23, 601–606.

Poretti, A., Limperopoulos, C., Roulet-Perez, E., et al., 2010. Outcome of severe unilateral cerebellar hypoplasia. Dev Med Child Neurol 52, 718–724.

Pryds, O., Greisen, G., Lou, H., et al., 1989. Heterogeneity of cerebral vasoreactivity in preterm infants supported by mechanical ventilation. J Pediatr 115, 638–645.

Pryds, O., Greisen, G., Lou, H., et al., 1990. Increased cerebral blood flow and plasma epinephrine in hypoglycaemic, preterm neonates. Pediatrics 85, 172–176.

Rademaker, K.J., Groenendaal, F., Jansen, G.H., et al., 1994. Unilateral haemorrhagic parenchymal lesions in the preterm infant: shape site and prognosis. Acta Paediatr Scand 83(6), 602–608.

Ramenghi, L.A., Fumagalli, M., Righini, A., et al., 2007. Magnetic resonance imaging assessment of brain maturation in preterm neonates with punctate white matter lesions. Neuroradiology 49, 161–167.

Rennie, J.M., Hagmann, C.F., Robertson, N.J., 2008. Neonatal Cerebral Investigation, 2nd ed., Cambridge University Press, Cambridge.

Ricci, D., Anker, S., Cowan, F., et al., 2006. Thalamic atrophy in infants with PVL and cerebral visual impairment. Early Hum Dev 82, 591–595.

Robinson, S., Li, Q., Dechant, A., et al., 2006. Neonatal loss of gamma-aminobutyric acid pathway expression after human perinatal brain injury. J Neurosurg 104 (Suppl), 396–408.

Roelants-van Rijn, A.M., Croenendaal, F., Beek, F.J.A., et al., 2001a. Parenchymal brain injury in the preterm infant: comparison of cranial ultrasound, MRI and neurodevelopmental outcome. Neuropediatrics 32, 80–89.

Roelants-van Rijn, A.M., Nikkels, P.G., Groenendaal, F., et al., 2001b. Neonatal diffusion-weighted MR imaging: relation with histopathology or follow-up MR examination. Neuropediatrics 32, 286–294.

Rogers, B., Msall, M., Owens, T., et al., 1994. Cystic periventricular leukomalacia and type of cerebral palsy in preterm infants. J Pediatr 125, S1–S8.

Rorke, L.B., 1992. Anatomical features of the developing brain implicated in pathogenesis of hypoxic–ischemic injury. Brain Pathology 2, 211–221.

Rouse, D.J., Hirtz, D.G., Thom, E., et al., 2008. A randomized, controlled trial of magnesium sulfate for the prevention of cerebral palsy. N Engl J Med 359, 895–905.

Ruckensteiner, E., Zollner, F., 1929. Uber die Blutngen im Gebiete der vena terminalis bei Neugeborenen. Frankfurt Z Pathol 37, 568–578.

Russell, G.A.B., Cooke, R.W.I., 1995. Randomised controlled trial of allpurinol prophylaxis in very preterm infants. Arch Dis Child 73, F27–F31.

Russell, G.A.B., Jeffers, G., Cooke, R.W.I., 1992. Plasma hypoxanthine: a marker for hypoxic ischaemic induced periventricular leukomalacia. Arch Dis Child 67, 388–392.

Rutherford, M.A., 2002. Hemorrhagic lesions of the newborn brain. In: Rutherford, M.A. (Ed.), MRI of the Neonatal Brain. W.B. Saunders, London, pp. 171–200.

Rutherford, M.A., Supramaniam, V., Ederies, A., et al., 2010. Magnetic resonance imaging of white matter diseases of prematurity. Neuroradiology 52, 505–521.

Saliba, E., Santini, J.J., Arbeille, Ph. 1985. Mesure non invasive du flux sanguin cérébral chez le nourisson hydrocéphale. Arch Fr Pediatr 42, 97–102.

Salter, M.G., Fern, R., 2005. NMDA receptors are expressed in developing oligodendrocyte processes and mediate injury. Nature 438, 1167–1171.

Sarkar, S., Bhagat, I., Dechert, R., et al., 2009. Severe intraventricular hemorrhage in preterm infants: comparison of risk factors and short-term neonatal morbidities between grade 3 and grade 4 intraventricular hemorrhage. Am J Perinatol 26, 419–424.

Sehgal, A., El Naggar, W., Glanc, P., et al., 2009. Risk factors and ultrasonographic profile of posterior fossa haemorrhages in preterm infants. J Paediatr Child Health 45, 215–218.

Setzer, E.S., Webb, I.B., Wassenaar, J.W., et al., 1982. Platelet dysfunction and coagulopathy in intraventricular hemorrhage in the premature infant. J Pediatr 100, 599–605.

Sfaello, I., Baud, O., Arzimanoglou, A., et al., 2005. Topiramate prevents excitotoxic damage in the newborn rodent brain. Neurobiol Dis 20, 837–848.

Shankaran, S., Koepke, T., Woldt, E., et al., 1989. Outcome after posthemorrhagic ventriculomegaly in comparison with mild hemorrhage without ventriculomegaly. J Pediatr 114, 109–114.

Shankaran, S., Langer, J.C., Kazzi, S.N., et al., 2006. Cumulative index of exposure to hypocarbia and hyperoxia as risk factors for periventricular leukomalacia in low birth weight infants. Pediatrics 118, 1654–1659.

Shooman, D., Portess, H., Sparrow, O., 2009. A review of the current treatment methods for posthaemorrhagic hydrocephalus of infants. Cerebrospinal Fluid Res 6, 1.

Shortland, D.B., Trounce, J.Q., Levene, M.I., et al., 1990. Patent ductus arteriosus and cerebral circulation in preterm circulation in preterm infants. Dev Med Child Neurol 32, 386–393.

Sie, L.T., van der Knaap, M.S., van Wezel-Meijler, G., et al., 2000. Early MR features of hypoxic-ischemic brain injury in neonates with periventricular densities on sonograms. Am J Neuroradiol 21, 852–861.

Skiold, B., Horsch, S., Hallberg, B., et al., 2010. White matter changes in extremely preterm infants, a population-based diffusion tensor imaging study. Acta Paediat 99, 842–849.

Sondhi, V., Gupta, G., Gupta, P.K., et al., 2008. Establishment of nomograms and reference ranges for intra-cranial ventricular dimensions and ventriculo-hemispheric ratio in newborns by ultrasonography. Acta Paediat 97, 738–744.

Srinivasan, L., Dutta, R., Counsell, S.J., et al., 2007. Quantification of deep gray matter in preterm infants at term-equivalent age using manual volumetry of 3-Tesla magnetic resonance images. Am Acad Pediatr 119, 759–765.

Steggerda, S.J., Leijser, L.M., Wiggers-de Bruine, F.T., et al., 2009. Cerebellar injury in preterm infants: incidence and findings on US and MR images. Radiology 252, 190–199.

Stewart, A.L., Thorburn, R.J., Hope, P.L., et al., 1983. Ultrasound appearance of the brain in very preterm infants and neurodevelopmental outcome at 18 months of age. Arch Dis Child 58, 598–604.

Synnes, A.R., Chien, L.-Y., Peliowski, A., et al., 2001. Variations in intraventricular hemorrhage incidence rates among Canadian neonatal intensive care units. J Pediatr 138, 525–531.

Synnes, A.R., Macnab, Y.C., Qiu, Z., et al., 2006. Neonatal intensive care unit characteristics affect the incidence of severe intraventricular hemorrhage. Medical Care 44, 754–759.

Szymonowicz, W., Yu, V.Y.H., Wilson, F.E., 1984. Antecedents of periventricular haemorrhage in infants weighing 1250 g or less at birth. Arch Dis Child 59, 13–17.

Takashima, S., Takashi, M., Ando, Y., 1986. Pathogenesis of periventricular white matter haemorrhage in preterm infants. Brain Dev 8, 25–30.

Taylor, G.A., 1995. Effect of germinal matrix hemorrhage on terminal vein position and patency. Pediatr Radiol 25 (Suppl 1), S37–S40.

Trounce, J.Q., Fagan, D., Levene, M.I., 1986. Intraventricular haemorrhage and periventricular leukomalacia in the preterm neonate: ultrasound and autopsy correlation. Arch Dis Child 61, 1203–1207.

Tsuji, M., Saul, P., du Plessis, A., et al., 2000. Cerebral intravascular oxygenation correlates with mean arterial pressure in critically ill premature infants. Pediatrics 108, 625–632.

Van Bel, F., Van de Bor, M., Stijnen, T., et al., 1987. Aetiological role of cerebral blood-flow alterations in development and extension of peri-intraventricular haemorrhage. Dev Med Child Neurol 29, 601–614.

Van de Bor, M., Ma, E.J., Walther, F.J., 1991. Cerebral blood flow velocity after surfactant instillation in preterm infants. J Pediatr 118, 285–287.

van Wezel-Meijler, F., van der Knaap, M.S., Sie, L.T., et al., 1998. Magnetic resonance imaging of the brain in premature infants during the neonatal period. Normal phenomena and reflection of mild ultrasound abnormalities. Neuropediatrics 29, 89–96.

Vela-Huerta, M.M., Amador-Licona, M., Medina-Ovando, N., et al., 2009. Factors associated with early severe intraventricular haemorrhage in very low birth weight infants. Neuropediatrics 40, 224–227.

Veldman, A., Josef, J., Fischer, D., et al., 2006. A prospective pilot study of prophylactic treatment of preterm neonates with recombinant activated factor VII during the first 72 hours of life. Pediatr Crit Care Med 7, 34–39.

Ventriculomegaly Trial Group, 1990. Randomised trial of early tapping in neonatal posthaemorrhagic ventricular dilatation. Arch Dis Child 65, 3–10.

Ventriculomegaly Trial Group, 1994. Randomised trial of early tapping in neonatal posthaemorrhagic periventricular dilatation: results at 30 months. Arch Dis Child 70, F129–F136.

Vinchon, M., Lapeyre, F., Duquennoy, C., et al., 2001. Early treatment of posthemorrhagic hydrocephalus in low-birth-weight infants with valveless ventriculoperitoneal shunts. Pediatr Neurosurg 35, 299–304.

Virchow, R., 1867. Zur pathologischen Anatomie des Gehirns I:congenitale encephalitis und myelitis. Virchows Arch 38, 129–142.

Vollmer, B., Roth, S., Riley, K., et al., 2006. Neurodevelopmental outcome of preterm infants with ventricular dilatation with and without associated haemorrhage. Dev Med Child Neurol 48, 348–352.

Volpe, J.J., 1990. Brain injury in the premature infant: is it preventable? Pediatr Res 27 (Suppl), S28–S33.

Volpe, J.J., 1996. Subplate neurons – missing link in brain injury of the premature infant? Pediatrics 97, 112–113.

Volpe, J.J., 2005. Encephalopathy of prematurity includes neuronal abnormalities. Pediatrics 116, 221–225.

Volpe, J.J., 2008. Intracranial haemorrhage: germinal matrix – intraventricular hemorrhage of the premature infant. In: Volpe, J.J. (Ed.), Neurology of the Newborn, fourth ed. W.B. Saunders, Philadelphia, pp. 517–588.

Wallin, L.A., Rosenfeld, C.R., Laptook, A.R., et al., 1990. Neonatal intracranial haemorrhage II: risk factor analysis in an inborn population. Early Hum Dev 23, 129–137.

Watkins, A.M.C., West, C.R., Cooke, R.W.I., 1989. Blood pressure and cerebral haemorrhage and ischaemia in very low birthweight infants. Early Hum Dev 19, 103–110.

Wells, J.T., Ment, L.R., 1995. Prevention of intraventricular hemorrhage in preterm infants. Early Hum Dev 42, 209–233.

Weninger, M., Salzer, H.R., Pollak, A., et al., 1992. External ventricular drainage for treatment of rapidly progressive posthemorrhagic hydrocephalus. Neurosurgery 31, 52–57.

Wheater, M., Rennie, J.M., 2000. Perinatal infection is an important risk factor for cerebral palsy in very-low-birthweight infants. Dev Med Child Neurol 42, 364–367.

Whitelaw, A., Thoresen, M., Pople, I., 2002. Posthaemorrhagic ventricular dilatation. Arch Dis Child 86, 72–74.

Whitelaw, A., Jary, S., Kmita, G., et al., 2010. Randomized trial of drainage, irrigation and fibrinolytic therapy for premature infants with posthemorrhagic ventricular dilatation: developmental outcome at 2 years. Pediatrics 125, e852–e858.

Wiswell, T.E., Graziani, L.J., Kornhauser, M.S., et al., 1996a. High-frequency jet ventilation in the early management of respiratory distress syndrome is associated with a greater risk for adverse outcomes. Pediatrics 98, 1035–1043.

Wiswell, T.E., Graziani, L.J., Kornhauser, M.S., et al., 1996b. Effects of hypocarbia on the development of cystic periventricular leukomalacia in premature infants treated with high-frequency jet ventilation. Pediatrics 98, 918–924.

Woodward, L.J., Anderson, P.J., Austin, N.C., et al., 2006. Neonatal MRI to predict neurodevelopmental outcomes in preterm infants. N Engl J Med 355, 685–694.

Wu, Y.W., 2002. Systematic review of chorioamnionitis and cerebral palsy. Ment Retard Dev Disabil Res Rev 8, 25–29.

Peter G Barth

Introduction

A number of inherited neurodegenerative diseases affect the central nervous system during the fetal period. Signs at the time of birth may include disturbed swallowing, stridor, abnormal posturing, nystagmus, seizures, hyperexcitation (clonus), polyhydramnios and arthrogryposis. External dysmorphic signs may be present. Results of routine neuroimaging by ultrasound or magnetic resonance imaging (MRI) of the brain may cause confusion with acquired disorders. For example, intracranial calcification may suggest congenital viral infection. The finding of an 'empty' space in the posterior fossa may invite a diagnosis of Dandy–Walker syndrome unless more thorough evaluation corrects this to pontocerebellar hypoplasia (PCH). Included in this chapter are some disorders that usually present during infancy, because they may start at birth.

Since these disorders are genetically determined, an accurate diagnosis allows appropriate genetic counselling. Genes have been identified for many of the disorders described here, allowing prenatal diagnosis in subsequent pregnancies.

Disorders of myelin and myelination

Myelination of the brain in the full-term newborn is largely limited to the brainstem and has hardly proceeded to the supratentorial structures at this stage of development. MRI at birth will show myelin in the cerebellar white matter, the dorsal (tegmental) part of the pons, the mesencephalon, the posterior limbs of the internal capsules and the postcentral parasagittal areas. The optic radiation is myelinated by the end of the first month.

Disorders of myelination are generally divided into three groups: delayed myelination, dysmyelination and demyelination. Delayed myelination (as observed by MRI) is a non-specific finding due to a variety of causes, including axonal loss in perinatal hypoxic–ischaemic encephalopathies, some defined metabolic disorders, including disorders of serine biosynthesis and cholesterol biosynthesis, and also chromosome disorders. Dysmyelination refers to the formation of a biochemically and ultrastructurally unstable kind of myelin, appearing on MRI or in neuropathological sections as delayed myelination. This is followed in later stages of the disease by active demyelination.

Pelizaeus–Merzbacher disease

Pelizaeus–Merzbacher disease is an X-linked dysmyelination. Mutations to the associated *PLP* gene are of two types: intragenic and gene duplications. The latter is the most common (Sistermans et al. 1998; Wolf et al. 2005).

Proteolipid protein is a transmembrane protein that spans the myelin lipid bilayer. It is assumed to provide stability to myelin by connecting the myelin layers and causing compaction as they become wrapped around the axon during the myelination process. Absence of proteolipid protein does not lead to absence of myelin but to impairment of the compaction process, causing instability, to be followed at a later stage by disintegration.

Symptoms may start at birth or in the first months of life, following a latent asymptomatic period. Typical nystagmoid eye movements may be present in the first weeks after birth and are often the presenting sign. Another early symptom, often encountered, is stridor. At this stage other findings are normal, including feeding behaviour and neonatal motor patterns (Renier et al. 1981; Scheffer et al. 1991). At a later stage, lack of proper head control and delayed motor milestones become prominent, followed by spastic paresis. Because of the physiological lack of myelin in the cerebral hemispheres at the time of birth MRI findings may not be helpful. A useful diagnostic instrument is the brainstem acoustic evoked response, by which decreased or absent responses past wave II may be found in Pelizaeus–Merzbacher disease, even in the newborn period (Garg et al. 1983).

A severe neonatal phenotype including neonatal nystagmus, hypotonia and stridor has been found in association with increased *PLP* copy number exceeding two (Wolf et al. 2005). Recently attention has become focused on phenocopies of Pelizaeus–Merzbacher disease, called PMD-like disease. An autosomal-recessive PMD-like disease is due to mutations of *GJA2* gene, and includes patients with severe neonatal-onset disease (Bugiani et al. 2006).

Vanishing white-matter disease

Demyelination accompanied by rarefaction and cavitation results from vanishing white-matter disease, a group of autosomal-recessive disorders associated with mutations in any of five genes encoding subunits of the translation initiation factor IF2B, which is necessary for protein synthesis and the regulation of this protein synthesis under different stress conditions. Though exceptional, signs may be present in the newborn such as contractures and hyperexcitation beside oligohydramnios, intrauterine growth retardation, cataracts, pancreatitis, hepatosplenomegaly, hypoplasia of the kidneys and ovarian dysgenesis (Boltshauser et al. 2002; Van der Knaap et al. 2003). MRI abnormalities may date from birth (Figs 40.58 and 40.59).

Krabbe's disease

Krabbe's disease is an autosomal-recessive deficiency of lysosomal galactosylceramidase. It typically presents in the first half-year, usually in the first months of life, with cerebral and peripheral nerve demyelination. The first signs are irritability and spasticity. While the usual onset is after the first months of life, some babies present as early as the first few days (Hagberg et al. 1963; Clarke et al. 1981; Rafi et al. 1995). The main signs are irritability and feeding difficulty. Early routine MRI findings in presymptomatic infants include mild signal abnormalities in the internal capsule and dentate nucleus (McGraw et al. 2005). Calcification was noted on computed tomographic (CT) scanning in the thalami and putamina with signal abnormalities in these regions on the MRI in a symptomatic neonatal case (Sahai et al. 2005). Diminished peripheral nerve conduction velocity, a sign of denervation, provides a useful clue to differential diagnosis. The ultimate diagnostic tool is either determination of lysosomal galactosylceramidase in leukocytes or cultured skin fibroblasts or identifying mutations/deletions in the *GALC* gene (Rafi et al. 1995).

Peroxisomal disorders

Neonatal adrenoleukodystrophy (NALD), Zellweger's syndrome and infantile Refsum disease together comprise the Zellweger

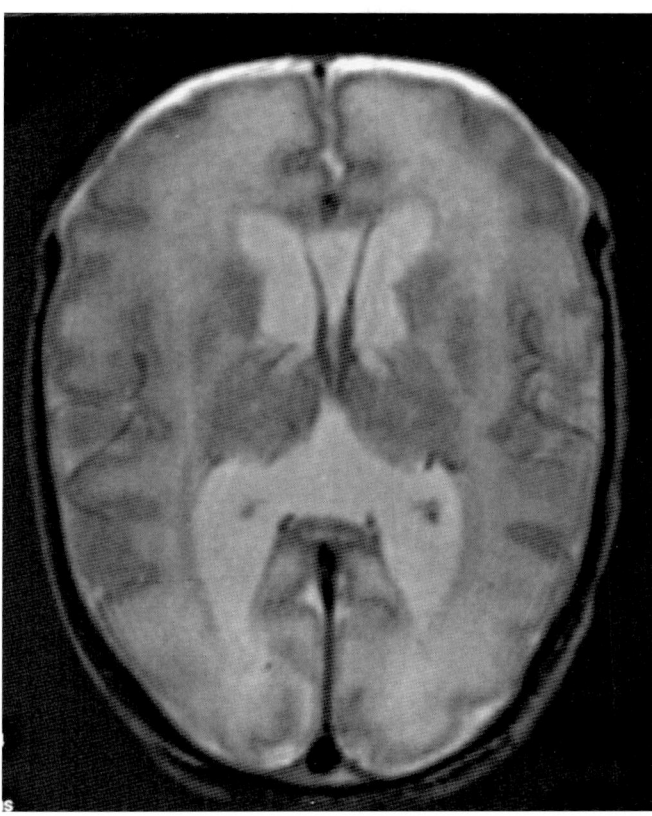

Fig. 40.58 Vanishing white-matter disease. Magnetic resonance imaging at 1 week. Mild ventricular dilatation. Abnormal (increased) signal of white matter. Axial T2w image. *(Adapted from Boltshauser et al. 2002, with permission from Thieme Verlag.)*

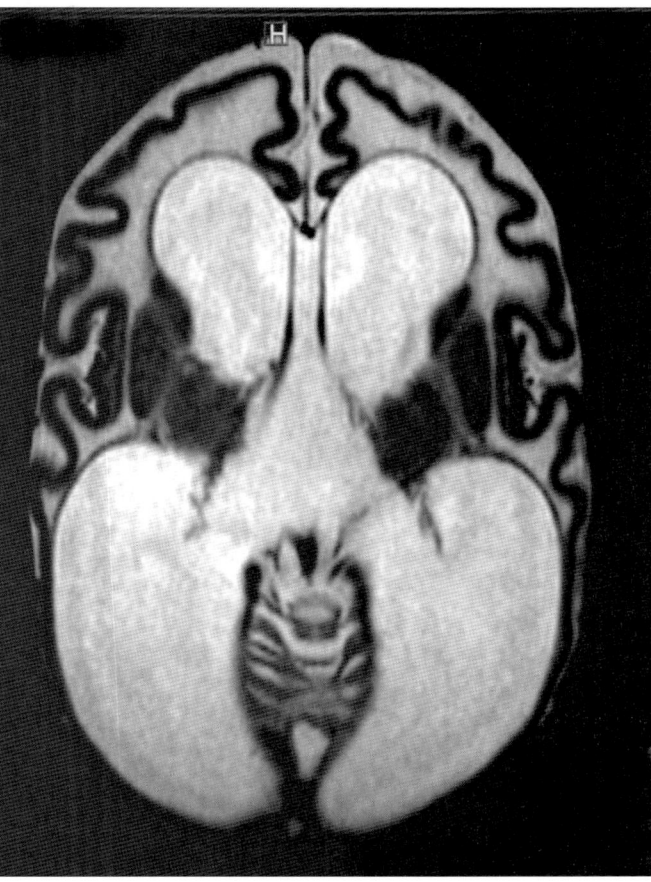

Fig. 40.59 Same patient as Figure 40.58 Magnetic resonance imaging at 6 months. Marked ventricular enlargement. Dilatation of extracerebral cerebrospinal fluid spaces. Bulk of white matter greatly reduced. No evidence of myelin. Axial T2w image. *(Adapted from Boltshauser et al. 2002, with permission from Thieme Verlag.)*

spectrum. The first two are symptomatic in the neonatal period. Biochemically they belong to the peroxisome biogenesis disorders (Shimozawa 2007) caused by impaired import of enzymes into the peroxisome or failure of its assembly. Normal peroxisomal assembly and carrier-mediated protein import require 13 *PEX* ('peroxin') genes (Shimozawa 2007). The difference between NALD and Zellweger's syndrome is phenotypical, with their underlying gene defects largely overlapping. Whereas in Zellweger's syndrome facial dysmorphic signs and neuronal migration disorder are prominent, these signs are less obvious or absent in NALD. Very large fontanelles and periarticular calcifications surrounding the large joints, especially the knees, are typical of Zellweger's syndrome but are not found in NALD. Liver enlargement and liver dysfunction are seen in both. Severe neonatal hypotonia is found in both disorders, and may necessitate gavage feeding. Examination of the eyes may reveal typical dot-like peripheral retinal pigmentary deposits in both disorders. Cataracts occur in a minority of both disorders. Neocortical polymicrogyria, a vertical upsweep of the sylvian fissure and subependymal germinolytic cysts (Barth et al. 1995) are typically found in Zellweger's syndrome (Figs 40.60 and 40.61). Zellweger's syndrome patients have delayed myelination (Barkovich and Peck 1997); NALD patients have early demyelination also involving the brainstem (Aubourg et al. 1986; Kelley et al. 1986). No neonatal MRI studies are available on NALD. On the basis of neuropathological studies and previous CT studies, signal changes of the white matter would be expected in NALD. Proton magnetic resonance spectroscopy may give additional clues leading to the

diagnosis of a progressive neurodegenerative disorder (Groenendaal et al. 2001).

Confirmation of the diagnosis of NALD or Zellweger's syndrome requires the finding in plasma of increased levels of very-long-chain fatty acids, the bile acid precursors trihydroxycholestanoic acid and dihydroxycholestanoic acid, pristanic acid, phytanic acid and pipecolic acid. Etherphospholipids (plasmalogens) are decreased in blood cells (Shimozawa 2007). Because 13 proteins are involved in peroxisomal assembly, the defective gene has to be identified first by complementation studies, to be followed by mutation analysis.

Life expectation in Zellweger's syndrome patients is limited. Most babies die before the age of 6 months and survival beyond a year is rare. NALD patients have a slightly better prognosis but usually die in infancy or early childhood.

A second group of peroxisomal disorders is caused by single-enzyme deficiencies. Deficient peroxisomal beta or peroxisomal alpha fatty acid oxidation defects largely overlap with the former group of peroxisome biogenesis disorders in symptomatology and clinical biochemical findings (Ferdinandusse et al. 2006; Wanders and Waterham 2006). Acyl-coenzyme A (CoA) oxidase-1 deficiency clinically mimics NALD with early signs of demyelination (Poll-Thé et al. 1988; Watkins et al. 1995; Wanders and

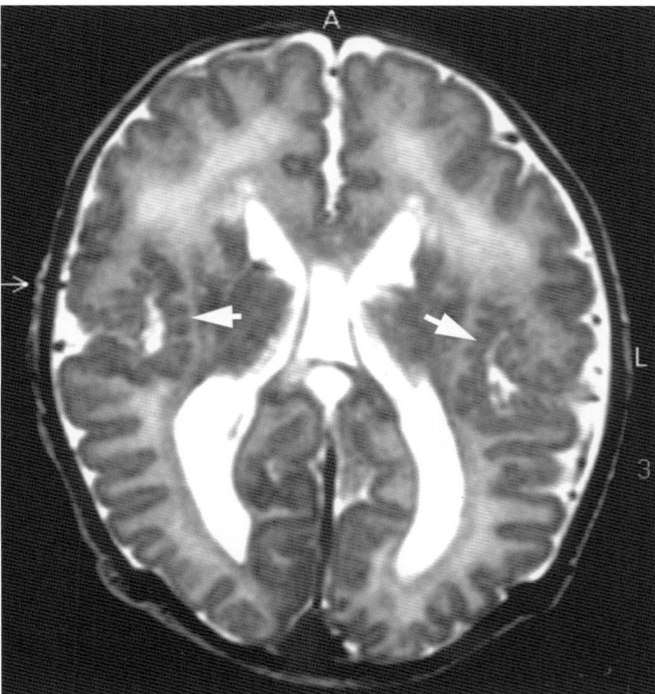

Fig. 40.60 Zellweger's syndrome. Transverse T2-weighted magnetic resonance image. The sylvian fissure extends to a higher level than normal and is bordered by an abnormally structured cortex composed of minuscule gyri with absence of intervening sulci: polymicrogyria (arrows). The ventricular system is moderately enlarged. *(Courtesy of Professor LS de Vries.)*

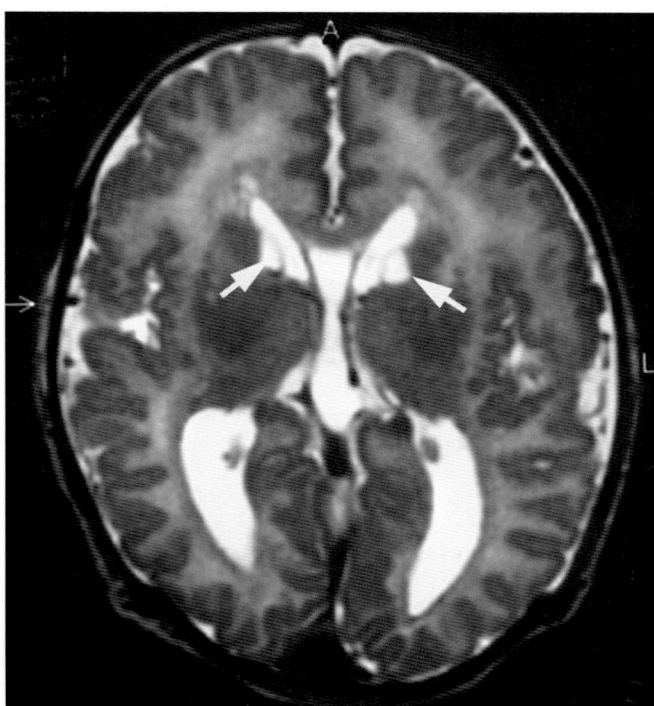

Fig. 40.61 Zellweger's syndrome. Transverse T2-weighted magnetic resonance image. Germinolytic cysts are present in the caudate–thalamic triangles (arrows). *(Courtesy of Professor LS de Vries.)*

Waterman 2006). Deficiency of d-bifunctional protein leads to a neuronal migration disorder similar to Zellweger's syndrome (Watkins et al. 1995). In acyl-CoA oxidase-1 deficiency, as well as in d-bifunctional protein deficiency, peroxisomal import is normal but these single-enzyme deficiencies retain many of the characteristics of NALD and Zellweger's syndrome. A detailed biochemical and molecular genetic work-up is necessary in each case presenting phenotypical features of either NALD or Zellweger's syndrome to differentiate peroxisome biogenesis disorders from the mentioned single-enzyme disorders. Their main difference in biochemical expression is the decrease of plasmalogens in the peroxisome biogenesis group and their normal presence in the single-enzyme group.

Alexander's disease

Alexander's disease, or leukodystrophy, is a disease of astrocytes and a de novo dominant mutation of the gene encoding glial fibrillary acidic protein (Brenner et al. 2001), resulting in abnormal thick glial filaments and proliferation of astrocytes. The disease has its clinical onset in the first months of life, sometimes at the time of birth. Hydrocephalus, probably due to aqueductal stenosis, megalencephaly and cystic disintegration of affected brain tissue, especially in the frontal lobes, are common findings. Seizures are common and their treatment is difficult. There is white-matter involvement on MRI with frontal-lobe predominance (Van der Knaap et al. 2001, 2005). MRI criteria for the diagnosis of Alexander's disease have been formulated and include white-matter involvement with frontal predominance, a periventricular rim of signal change, involvement of basal ganglia and thalami, brainstem lesions and contrast enhancement of affected regions. These criteria may not all be met in the neonate with Alexander's disease (Van der Knaap et al. 2001, 2005).

Neuroaxonal dystrophies

Axonal swellings ('spheroids') with stored tubular and filamentous structures are the morphological marker of a heterogeneous group of progressive inherited disorders of central and peripheral axons. Spheroids (Fig. 40.62) are found in the brain and spinal cord and

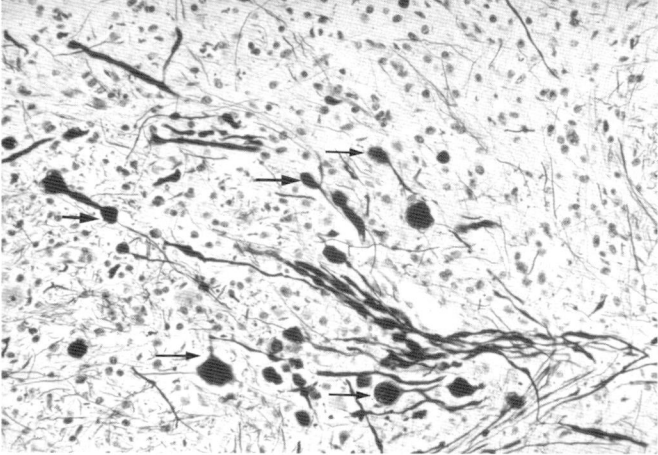

Fig. 40.62 Axonal spheroids present as solid round structures (arrows) on silver staining. Lumbar anterior horn. Autopsy of a newborn with atypical neuroaxonal dystrophy. Glees–Marsland stain. *(Adapted from Jennekens et al. 1984; copyright Springer Verlag.)*

may also be found in peripheral nerve endings, allowing a group diagnosis by biopsy (skin, conjunctiva).

The most common representative is infantile neuroaxonal dystrophy, with onset in the second half of the first year. Several axonopathies, probably unrelated to infantile neuroaxonal dystrophy, have their onset around or before birth as part of a multisystem disorder with extracerebral involvement. These include combinations with osteopetrosis (Steward 2003), cutis laxa (Shintaku et al. 2000) and cardiomyopathy and ophthalmic disease (Lyon et al. 1990). Some reported patients had mineralisation (calcification) of the thalamus and brainstem or basal ganglia combined with axonal neuropathy (Jennekens et al. 1984; Venkatesh et al. 1994). Diagnosis in this category may be difficult to establish by clinical means and eventually requires neuropathological confirmation. Mutations of the *PLA2G6* gene are associated with classic infantile neuroaxonal dystrophy (Kurian et al. 2008). So far no mutations have been found in congenital cases.

Neuronal degeneration

Progressive cortical atrophy with massive loss of cortical neurons, together with spongiform changes and involvement of the basal ganglia, is characteristic of Alpers' syndrome, an inherited disorder that usually starts in the first months of life and is rapidly progressive with acquired microcephaly and intractable epileptic seizures. This disease may start at birth. It was first described as a neuropathological entity. Accompanying liver cirrhosis is found in a significant proportion (Blackwood et al. 1963; Huttenlocher et al. 1976). Varous degrees of lactic acidosis occur as well as dysfunction

of the respiratory chain in muscle or liver biopsies (Tulinius et al. 1991). Insufficient maintenance of mitochondrial DNA by deficiency of the polymerase-gamma gene *POLG* is the most frequent cause of Alpers' syndrome (Hudson and Chinnery 2006). One reported family with progressive cortical degeneration starting before birth and presenting at birth with fetal akinesia sequence had a thorough biochemical study that did not reveal mitochondrial involvement (Frydman et al. 1993). Cortical degeneration during the period of cerebral growth spurt will lead to microcephaly at birth and sometimes to a 'walnut' brain with huge craniocerebral disproportion. When such loss precedes cortical folding the process can result in a smooth brain surface, superficially resembling lissencephaly but differing in histopathology because neuronal migration is not involved in its pathogenesis and the smooth cortical surface is the result of a disruptive process rather than malformation. This type of cortical pathology has been referred to as lissencephaly type III (Encha Razavi et al. 1996; Attia-Sobol et al. 2001) by different authors. The cause of this type of cortical degeneration is heterogeneous and no specific molecular causes have been defined yet.

Pontocerebellar hypoplasias

Pontocerebellar hypoplasia (PCH) describes a heterogeneous condition in which the cerebellum and pons are small. The cerebellar hemispheres are reduced in size and the ventral pons is reduced in size compared to the pontine tegmentum and flattened at its base (Figs 40.63 and 40.64). Importantly, the size of the posterior fossa is not enlarged, excluding Dandy–Walker syndrome.

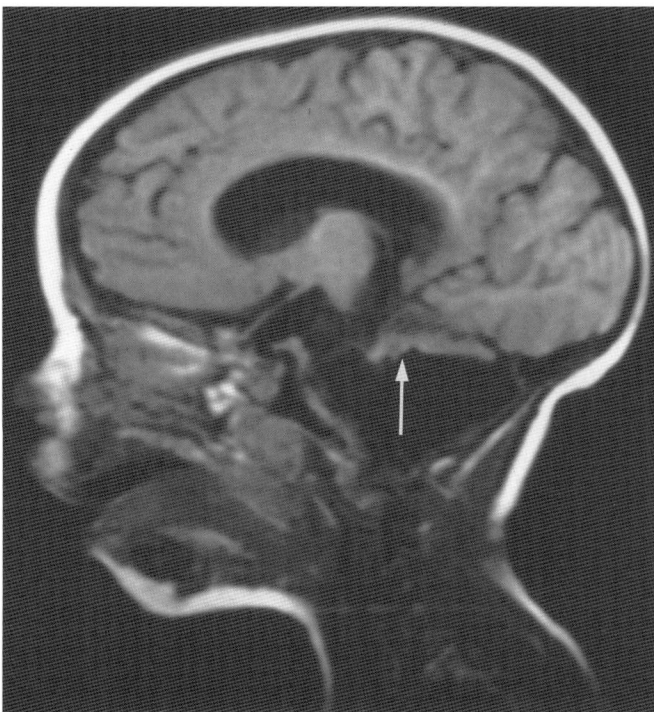

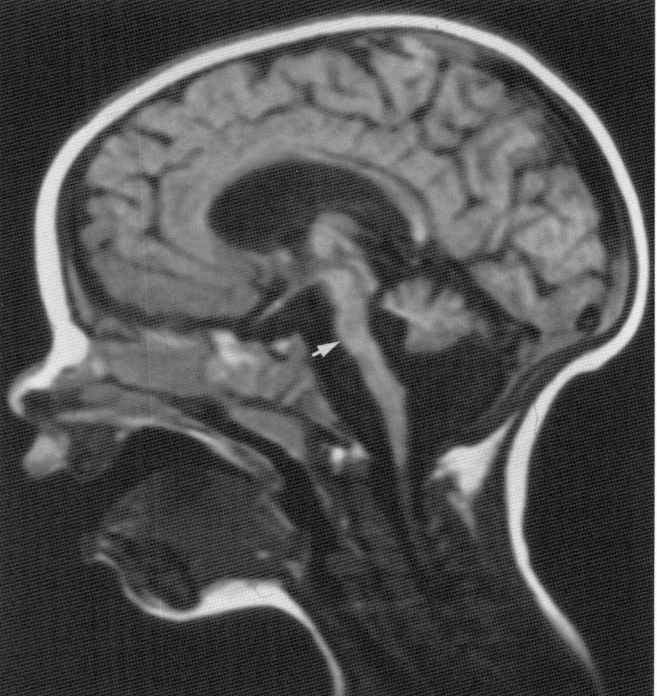

Fig. 40.63 Pontocerebellar hypoplasia. Sagittal T1-weighted magnetic resonance image showing the hypoplastic cerebellar hemisphere lying under the tentorium (arrow), and leaving an empty space in the posterior fossa. *(Adapted from Barth 1993; copyright Elsevier 1993.)*

Fig. 40.64 Pontocerebellar hypoplasia. Midsagittal T1-weighted magnetic resonance image showing the hypoplastic vermis and the flattening of the ventral pons (arrow). *(Adapted from Barth 1993; copyright Elsevier 1993.)*

These features are not specific for a particular diagnosis or subtype. They may be encountered in defined genetic disorders with neocortical dysplasia, which includes lissencephalies such as Walker–Warburg syndrome, lissencephaly with cerebellar hypoplasia (Ross et al. 2001) and, rarely, merosin-deficient congenital muscular dystrophy (Philpot et al. 1999). They have also been described in congenital disorders of glycosylation, especially type 1A (Horslen et al. 1991), but the usual MRI finding of CDG 1A is cerebellar hypoplasia rather than PCH. The designation PCH is made for a distinct group of autosomal recessive diseases. The initial classification (Barth 1993) with type 1 (PCH1) involving spinal anterior horn involvement and type 2 (PCH2) manifesting chorea/dyskinesia or spasticity has been extended to five (Patel et al. 2006), and lately to six subtypes (Edvardson et al. 2007).

The commonest are types 1, 2 and 4 (PCH4). Causative gene defects have been established in types 2, 4 and 6 (PCH6).

Pontocerebellar hypoplasia type 1

Affected babies often have polyhydramnios and/or contractures at birth, poor respiration and ventilator dependence as a result of generalised muscle weakness. When they survive the neonatal period mental and motor milestones are almost absent, and they usually die in infancy (Goutières et al. 1977; Barth 1993). Neuropathology shows PCH with degenerative changes mainly affecting the cerebellum, the ventral pons as well as spinal anterior horn involvement similar to spinal muscular atrophy type I. Gene studies have excluded PCH1 from the *SMA* gene on chromosome 5 (Muntoni et al. 1999).

There appears to be variability in the expression of this disease, with an overlapping spectrum from prenatal onset to onset within the first postnatal months (Rudnik-Schöneborn et al. 2003). Neuroimaging by ultrasound may show dilatation of the ventricular system but no other abnormalities above the tentorium. Images of the posterior fossa may reveal an enlarged fourth ventricle and disproportion between the size of the posterior fossa and its contents. No associated gene defects are known.

Pontocerebellar hypoplasia type 2

Progressive microcephaly from birth, severely impaired mental and motor development and chorea/dystonia together with MR or neuropathological features of PCH characterise PCH2 (Barth et al. 1995). The absence of neurogenic muscular atrophy distinguishes this disorder from PCH1. Survival in PCH2 is better than in PCH1 and patients may even reach young adulthood (Barth et al. 1995).

Newborns with PCH2 have a normal size at term birth and have no distinguishing external dysmorphic signs. Head circumference is below the 50th percentile and decreases progressively after birth. The presenting signs are restlessness, jitteriness and poor swallowing. MRI shows moderate ventricular widening, especially the anterior horns, and there may be some cortical atrophy. Typical findings are a flattened ventral pons and cerebellar hypoplasia with the vermis relatively spared and the cerebellar hemispheres hypotrophic with dorsoventral flattening (Figs 40.63 and 40.64). Sialotransferrin electrophoresis in plasma and lactate determination in the cerebrospinal fluid or by magnetic resonance spectroscopy may help to exclude CDG1A and mitochondrial PCHs. Final diagnosis rests with gene sequencing of tRNA endonuclease subunits. The most common mutation present in over 90% of PCH2 patients is a homozygous amino acid substitution in TSEN54: p.ala307ser (Budde et al. 2008).

Pontocerebellar hypoplasia type 4

Patients with PCH4, formerly also known as olivopontocerebellar cerebellar hypoplasia, present before birth with contractures and/or polyhydramnios, need prolonged artificial respiration and often cannot be weaned from the respirator (Albrecht et al. 1993; Chaves-Vischer et al. 2000). These signs are identical to what is often found in PCH1. Hypertonia (rather than hypotonia) and severe clonus are found, except when the disease leads to birth asphyxia, and distinguish this disease from PCH1. MRI findings are essentially similar to PCH1 and PCH2. Differential diagnostics is similar to type 2. Sequencing of tRNA endonuclease subunits may reveal double heterozygous mutations in TSEN54, usually with the classical TSEN54: p.ala307ser on one allelle and a more severe mutation, e.g. a stop codon, on the other (Budde et al. 2008).

Pontocerebellar hypoplasia type 6 and unclassified mitochondrial PCH

Autosomal-recessive PCH with lactic acidosis and multiple respiratory chain defects occurs as a defect in the arginyl-transfer RNA synthetase or *RARS2* gene in a single family (Edvardson et al. 2007). In an earlier described family with PCH, subependymal cysts and multiple respiratory chain defects, no associated gene defects were identified (De Koning et al. 1999).

Intracerebral calcification

Cerebral calcification in the neonate is usually associated with perinatal infections, especially cytomegalovirus or toxoplasmosis, or with hypoxic–ischaemic damage. Some cases are due to genetic disorders.

Aicardi–Goutières syndrome

Aicardi–Goutières syndrome is an autosomal-recessive disorder (Aicardi and Goutières 1984; Goutières et al. 1998) with the following main features:

- progressive microcephaly, but normal head circumference at birth
- developmental delay and regression, dystonia and mental handicap
- cerebral and brainstem atrophy, loss of white matter and progressive calcification affecting the cerebral white matter, basal ganglia, thalamus and dentate nuclei. Cerebrospinal fluid lymphocytosis and increase of alpha-interferon and pterins in cerebrospinal fluid may aid in diagnosis.

Clinical onset is in the first months of life. In a series of 27 patients (Goutières et al. 1998), four had onset at birth with irritability and feeding difficulties. In another case prenatal deceleration of head growth was documented. Early in the course of the disease calcifications may not be conspicuous. Cerebrospinal fluid findings (lymphocytosis), together with cerebral calcifications, may closely mimic an intrauterine infectious disease (Fig. 40.65). Most, but not all, patients with autosomal-recessive Aicardi–Goutières syndrome carry mutations in *TREX1* 3'→5' exonuclease gene or the three subunits of the RNASEH2 endonuclease complex. Patients with congenital onset mostly have *TREX1* mutations (Rice et al. 2007).

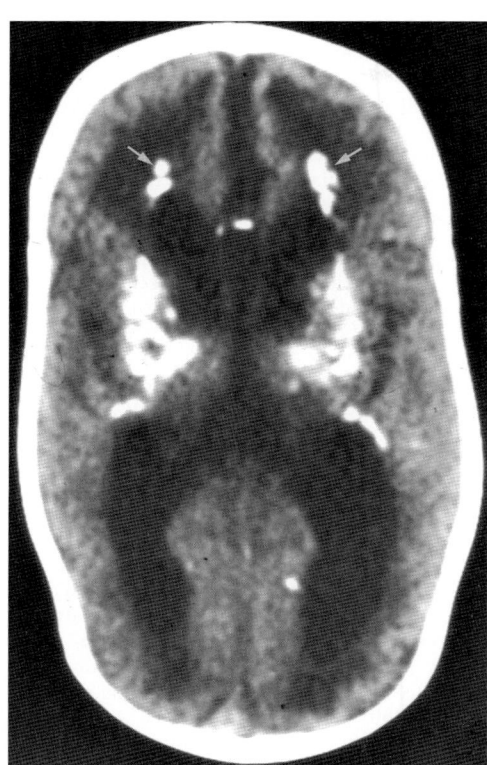

Fig. 40.65 Aicardi–Goutières syndrome. Computed tomographic scan at 3 months of age showing characteristic distribution of calcifications. Arrows point to calcifications in the frontal white matter. Decreased density in this area is close to the density of cerebrospinal fluid because of tissue damage.

Cerebro-oculo-facio-skeletal syndrome/ Cockayne's syndrome type B

Cerebro-oculo-facio-skeletal syndrome (Lowry et al. 1971) is an autosomal-recessive disorder with multiple dysmorphia that includes abnormalities of the brain (microcephaly) and eyes (microphthalmia, cataracts, blepharophimosis), facial dysmorphia (large ears, prominent root of the nose, micrognathia) and abnormalities of the skeletal system (flexion contractures at the elbows and knees) (Peña and Shokeir 1974). Other findings are generalised osteoporosis, failure to thrive and early death. A neuropathological study revealed the degenerative nature of this disease (Del Bigio et al. 1997). Findings besides microencephaly and widened ventricles are: dysmyelination, pericapillary and parenchymal mineralisation in the globus pallidus, putamen and cerebral cortex and degenerative changes in the cerebellum. Findings suggest a relation to Cockayne's syndrome (Lowry 1982). Cockayne's syndrome belongs to a group of nucleotide excision repair disorders together

with xeroderma pigmentosum and the photosensitive form of trichothiodystrophy. Nucleotide excision repair is the mechanism by which DNA is repaired following the formation of so-called adducts, compounds that bind adjacent pyrimidines under influence of ultraviolet light and carcinogens and distort the helical structure (Bootsma et al. 2001). Absence of a repair mechanism known as transcription-coupled repair leads to hypersensitivity to sunlight, a typical finding in Cockayne's syndrome. Cockayne's syndrome patients are defective in the preferential removal of oxidative damage from the transcribed strand of active genes by RA polymerase II. Two complementation groups exist in Cockayne's syndrome: CS A and CS B. Cerebro-oculo-facio-skeletal syndrome and CS B share mutations in the *ERCC6* gene (Meira et al. 2000), proving their aetiological identity.

Cerebral pathology to be found on MRI or CT in cerebro-oculo-facio-skeletal syndrome includes subcortical calcifications due to perivascular accumulation of calcium. Definite diagnosis requires mutation analysis of the *ERCC6* gene.

Differential diagnosis of cerebro-oculo-facio-skeletal syndrome/ CS B includes Raine's syndrome (Rickert et al. 2002), a rare autosomal-recessive syndrome with microcephaly from birth with supratentorial calcified brain lesions, osteosclerosis and external dysmorphic signs.

Cerebral cystic degeneration, calcifications and multicomplex mitochondrial disease

A severe and fatal neonatal-onset disease with lactic acidosis, neuronal migration disorder, multiple cerebral calcifications, cystic necroses of the cerebral hemispheres and overmigration of the cerebral cortex into the meningeal space has been reported twice. Typical findings include:

- severe lactic acidosis and combined deficiency of respiratory chain complexes I and IV and pyruvate dehydrogenase. Inheritance is autosomal-recessive (Samsom et al. 1994; Van Straaten et al. 2005)
- polymicrogyria and band-like cerebral calcifications. Polymicrogyria and band-like calcifications of the cortex and brainstem has recently been described in 5 patients, probably representing a new autosomal-recessive entity (Briggs et al. 2008).

Vasculopathies

Fowler's disease

Fowler's disease is an autosomal-recessive disorder presenting as fetal akinesia sequence and pterygia, possibly due to a severe prenatal brain degeneration resulting in hydrocephaly, hydranencephaly and cerebral calcifications. Microscopic tufts of abnormal blood vessels, called glomeruli, are an important marker of this disease, allowing neuropathological differentiation from acquired fetal disorders (Fowler et al. 1972; Harding et al. 1995).

References

Aicardi, J., Goutières, F., 1984. A progressive familial encephalopathy in infancy with calcifications of the basal ganglia and chronic cerebrospinal fluid lymphocytosis. Ann Neurol 15, 49–54.

Albrecht, S., Schneider, M.C., Belmont, J., 1993. Fatal infantile encephalopathy with

olivopontocerebellar hypoplasia and micrencephaly. Acta Neuropathol 85, 394–399.

Attia-Sobol, J., Encha-Razavi, F., Hermier, M., et al., 2001. Lissencephaly type III, stippled epiphyses and loose, thick skin: a new recessively inherited syndrome. Am J Med Genet 99, 14–20.

Aubourg, P., Scotto, J., Rocchiccioli, F., et al., 1986. Neonatal adrenoleukodystrophy. J Neurol Neurosurg Psychiatry 49, 77–86.

Barkovich, A.J., Peck, W.W., 1997. MR of Zellweger syndrome. Am J Neuroradiol 18, 1163–1170.

Barth, P.G., 1993. Pontocerebellar hypoplasias. An overview of a group of inherited neurodegenerative disorders with fetal onset. Brain Dev 15, 411–422.

Barth, P.G., Blennow, G., Lenard, H.-G., et al., 1995. The syndrome of autosomal recessive pontocerebellar hypoplasia, microcephaly and extrapyramidal dyskinesia (pontocerebellar hypoplasia type 2): compiled data from ten pedigrees. Neurology 45, 311–317.

Blackwood, W., Buxton, P.H., Cumings, J.N., et al., 1963. Diffuse cerebral degeneration in infancy (Alpers' disease). Arch Dis Child 38, 193–204.

Boltshauser, E., Barth, P.G., Troost, D., et al., 2002. 'Vanishing white matter' and ovarian dysgenesis in an infant with cerebro-oculo-facio-skeletal phenotype. Neuropediatrics 33, 57–62.

Bootsma, D., Kraemer, K.H., Cleaver, J.E., et al., 2001. Nucleotide excision repair syndromes: xeroderma pigmentosum, Cockayne syndrome, and trichothiodystrophy. In: Scriver, C.R., Beaudet, A.L., Sly, W.S., et al. (Eds.), The Metabolic and Molecular Bases of Inherited Disease, eighth ed. McGraw-Hill, New York, pp. 677–703.

Brenner, M., Johnson, A.B., Boespflug-Tanguy, O., et al., 2001. Mutations in GFAP, encoding glial fibrillary acidic protein, are associated with Alexander disease. Nat Genet 27, 117–120.

Briggs, T.A., Wolf, N.I., D'Arrigo, S., et al., 2008. Band-like intracranial calcification with simplified gyration and polymicrogyria: a distinct 'pseudo-TORCH' phenotype. Am J Med Genet A 146A, 3173–3180.

Budde, B.S., Namavar, Y., Barth, P.G., et al., 2008. tRNA splicing endonuclease mutations cause pontocerebellar hypoplasia. Nat Genet 40, 1113–1118.

Bugiani, M., Al Shahwan, S., Lamantea, E., et al., 2006. GJA12 mutations in children with recessive hypomyelinating leukoencephalopathy. Neurology 67, 273–279.

Chaves-Vischer, V., Pizzolato, G.P., Hanquinet, S., et al., 2000. Early fatal pontocerebellar hypoplasia in premature twin sisters. Eur J Paediatr Neurol 4, 171–176.

Clarke, J.T.R., Ozere, R.L., Krause, V.W., 1981. Early infantile variant of Krabbe globoid cell leucodystrophy with lung involvement. Arch Dis Child 56, 640–642.

De Koning, T.J., de Vries, L.S., Groenendaal, F., et al., 1999. Pontocerebellar hypoplasia associated with respiratory-chain defects. Neuropediatrics 30, 93–95.

Del Bigio, M.R., Greenberg, C.R., Rorke, L.B., et al., 1997. Neuropathological findings in eight children with cerebro-oculo-facio-skeletal (COFS) syndrome. J Neuropathol Exp Neurol 56, 1147–1157.

Edvardson, S., Shaag, A., Kolesnikova, O., et al., 2007. Deleterious mutation in the mitochondrial arginyl-transfer RNA synthetase gene is associated with pontocerebellar hypoplasia. Am J Hum Genet 81, 857–862.

Encha Razavi, F., Larroche, J.C., Roume, J., et al., 1996. Lethal familial fetal akinesia sequence (FAS) with distinct neuropathological pattern: type III lissencephaly syndrome. Am J Med Genet 62, 16.

Ferdinandusse, S., Denis, S., Mooyer, P.A.W., et al., 2006. Clinical and biochemical spectrum of D-bifunctional protein deficiency. Ann Neurol 59, 92–104.

Fowler, M., Dow, R., White, T.A., et al., 1972. Congenital hydrocephalus–hydrencephaly in five siblings, with autopsy studies: a new disease. Dev Med Child Neurol 14, 173–188.

Frydman, M., Jager-Roman, E., deVries, L., et al., 1993. Alpers progressive infantile neuronal poliodystrophy: an acute neonatal form with findings of the fetal akinesia syndrome. Am J Med Genet 47, 31–36.

Garg, B.P., Markand, O.N., DeMyer, W.E., 1983. Usefulness of BAER studies in the early diagnosis of Pelizaeus–Merzbacher disease. Neurology 33, 955–956.

Goutières, F., Aicardi, J., Farkas, E., 1977. Anterior horn cell disease associated with pontocerebellar hypoplasia in infants. J Neurol Neurosurg Psychiatry 40, 370–378.

Goutières, F., Aicardi, J., Barth, P.G., et al., 1998. Aicardi–Goutières syndrome: an update end results of interferon-α studies. Ann Neurol 44, 900–907.

Groenendaal, F., Bianchi, M.C., Battini, R., et al., 2001. Proton magnetic resonance spectroscopy (^{1}H-MRS) of the cerebrum in two young infants with Zellweger syndrome. Neuropediatrics 32, 23–27.

Hagberg, B., Sourander, P., Svennerholm, L., 1963. Diagnosis of Krabbe's infantile leucodystrophy. J Neurol Neurosurg Psychiatry 26, 195–198.

Harding, B.N., Ramani, P., Thurley, P., 1995. The familial syndrome of proliferative vasculopathy and hydranencephaly-hydrocephaly: immunocytochemical and ultrastructural evidence for endothelial proliferation. Neuropathol Appl Neurobiol 21, 61–67.

Horslen, S.P., Clayton, P.T., Harding, B.N., et al., 1991. Olivopontocerebellar atrophy of neonatal onset and disialotransferrin developmental deficiency syndrome. Arch Dis Child 66, 1027–1032.

Hudson, G., Chinnery, P.F., 2006. Mitochondrial DNA polymerase-γ and human disease. Hum Mol Genet 15, R244–R252.

Huttenlocher, P.R., Solitare, G.B., Adams, G., 1976. Infantile diffuse cerebral degeneration with hepatic cirrhosis. Arch Neurol 33, 186–192.

Jennekens, F.G.I., Barth, P.G., Fleury, P., et al., 1984. Axonal dystrophy in a case of connatal thalamic and brain stem degeneration. Acta Neuropathol 64, 68–71.

Kelley, R.I., Datta, N.S., Dobyns, W.B., et al., 1986. Neonatal adrenoleukodystrophy: new cases, biochemical studies, and differentiation from Zellweger and related peroxisomal polydystrophy syndromes. Am J Med Genet 23, 869–890.

Kurian, M.A., Morgan, N.V., MacPherson, L., et al., 2008. Phenotypic spectrum of neurodegeneration associated with mutations in the PLA2G6 gene (PLAN). Neurology 70, 1623–1629.

Lowry, R.B., 1982. Early onset of Cockayne syndrome. Am J Med Genet 13, 209–210.

Lowry, R.B., MacLean, R., McLean, D.M., et al., 1971. Cataracts, microcephaly, kyphosis, and limited joint movement in two siblings: a new syndrome. J Pediatr 79, 282–284.

Lyon, G., Arita, F., Le Galloudec, E., et al., 1990. A disorder of axonal development, necrotizing myopathy, cardiomyopathy and cataracts: a new familial disease. Ann Neurol 27, 193–199.

McGraw, P., Liang, L., Escolar, M., et al., 2005. Krabbe disease treated with hematopoietic stem cell transplantation: serial assessment of anisotropy measurements – initial experience. Radiology 236, 221–230.

Meira, L.B., Graham Jr., J.M., Greenberg, C.R., et al., 2000. Manitoba aboriginal kindred with original cerebro-oculo-facio-skeletal syndrome has a mutation in the Cockayne syndrome group B (CSB) gene. Am J Hum Genet 66, 1221–1228.

Muntoni, F., Goodwin, F., Sewry, C., et al., 1999. Clinical spectrum and diagnostic difficulties of infantile ponto-cerebellar hypoplasia type 1. Neuropediatrics 30, 243–248.

Patel, M.S., Becker, L.E., Toi, A., et al., 2006. Severe, fetal-onset form of olivopontocerebellar hypoplasia in three sibs: PCH type 5? Am J Med Genet A 140, 594–603.

Peña, S.D.J., Shokeir, M.H.K., 1974. Autosomal recessive cerebro-oculo-facio-skeletal syndrome. Clin Genet 5, 285–293.

Philpot, J., Cowan, F., Pennock, J., et al., 1999. Merosin-deficient congenital muscular dystrophy: the spectrum of brain involvement on magnetic resonance imaging. Neuromuscul Disord 9, 81–85.

Poll-Thé, B.T., Roels, F., Ogier, H., et al., 1988. A new peroxisomal disorder with enlarged peroxisomes and a specific deficiency of acyl-CoA oxidase (pseudo-neonatal adrenoleukodystrophy). Am J Hum Genet 42, 422–434.

Rafi, M.A., Luzi, P., Chen, Y.Q., et al., 1995. A large deletion together with a point mutation in the GALC gene is a common mutant allelel in patients with infantile

Krabbe disease. Hum Mol Genet 4, 1285–1289.

Renier, W.O., Gabreëls, F.J.M., Hustinx, T.W.J., et al., 1981. Connatal Pelizaeus–Merzbacher disease with congenital stridor in two maternal cousins. Acta Neuropathol (Berlin) 54, 11–17.

Rice, G., Patrick, T., Parmar, R., et al., 2007. Clinical and molecular phenotype of Aicardi–Goutière's syndrome. Am J Hum Genet 81, 713–725.

Rickert, C.H., Rieder, H., Rehder, H., et al., 2002. Neuropathology of Raine syndrome. Acta Neuropathol (Berlin) 103, 281–287.

Ross, M.E., Swanson, K., Dobyns, W.B., 2001. Lissencephaly with cerebellar hypoplasia (LCH): a heterogeneous group of cortical malformations. Neuropediatrics 32, 256–263.

Rudnik-Schöneborn, S., Sztriha, L., Aithala, G.R., et al., 2003. Extended phenotype of pontocerebellar hypoplasia with infantile spinal muscular atrophy. Am J Med Genet 117A, 10–17.

Sahai, I., Baris, H., Kimonis, V., et al., 2005. Krabbe disease: severe neonatal presentation with a family history of multiple sclerosis. J Child Neurol 20, 826–828.

Samsom, J.F., Barth, P.G., de Vries, J.I.P., et al., 1994. Familial mitochondrial encephalopathy with fetal

ultrasonographic ventriculomegaly and intracerebral calcifications. Eur J Paediatr 153, 510–516.

Scheffer, I.E., Baraitser, M., Wilson, J., et al., 1991. Pelizaeus–Merzbacher disease: classical or connatal? Neuropediatrics 22, 71–78.

Shimozawa, N., 2007. Molecular and clinical aspects of peroxisomal diseases. Journal of Inherited Metabolic Disease 30, 193–197.

Shintaku, M., Uemura, Y., Fujii, I., et al., 2000. Neuroaxonal leukodystrophy associated with congenital cutis laxa: report of an autopsy case. Acta Neuropathol 99, 420–424.

Sistermans, E.A., de Coo, R.F., De Wijs, I.J., et al., 1998. Duplication of the proteolipid protein gene is the major cause of Pelizaeus–Merzbacher disease. Neurology 50, 1749–1754.

Steward, C.G., 2003. Neurological aspects of osteopetrosis. Neuropathol Appl Neurobiol 29, 87–97.

Tulinius, M.H., Holme, E., Kristinasson, B., et al., 1991. Mitochondrial encephalomyelopathies in childhood. II. Clinical manifestations and syndromes. J Pediatr 119, 251–259.

Van der Knaap, M.S., Naidu, S., Breiter, S.N., et al., 2001. Alexander disease: diagnosis with MR imaging. Am J Neuroradiol 22, 541–552.

Van der Knaap, M.S., Van Berkel, C.G., Herms, J., et al., 2003. eIF2B-related disorders: antenatal onset and involvement of multiple organs. Am J Hum Genet 73, 1199–1207.

Van der Knaap, M.S., Salomons, G.S., Li, R., et al., 2005. Unusual variants of Alexander's disease. Ann Neurol 57, 327–338.

Van Straaten, H.L., van Tintelen, J.P., Trijbels, J.M., et al., 2005. Neonatal lactic acidosis, complex I/IV deficiency, and fetal cerebral disruption. Neuropediatrics 36, 193–199.

Venkatesh, S., Coulter, D., Kemper, T.D., 1994. Neuroaxonal dystrophy at birth with hypertonicity and basal ganglia mineralization. J Child Neurol 9, 74–76.

Wanders, R.J.A., Waterham, 2006. Peroxisomal disorders: the single peroxisomal enzyme deficiencies. Biochim Biophys Acta-Molecular Cell Research 1763, 1707–1720.

Watkins, P.A., McGuinness, M.C., Raymond, G.V., et al., 1995. Distinction between peroxisomal bifunctional enzyme and acyl-CoA oxidase deficiencies. Ann Neurol 38, 472–477.

Wolf, N.I., Sistermans, E.A., Cundall, M., et al., 2005. Three or more copies of the proteolipid gene PLP1 cause severe Pelizaeus–Merzbacher disease. Brain 128, 743–751.

Part 7: **Muscle disease in the newborn**

Adnan Y Manzur   Stephanie A Robb   Francesco Muntoni

Introduction

The field of neuromuscular disorders (conditions affecting the lower motor unit) is one of the fastest growing in medicine. This mainly reflects the impact of our improved understanding of the genetic basis of these conditions, with more than 200 responsible loci having been identified so far (see Weblinks section). This has allowed a much better definition of the clinical phenotypes associated with involvement of individual genes, and an improved diagnostic approach to these disorders. In this chapter we will review the current state of knowledge of the neuromuscular disorders with clinical onset in the neonatal period, focusing on their clinical presentation and giving an update on the rational approach to the diagnosis for each form.

Clinical presentation

Hypotonia is the most typical and common symptom of neuromuscular involvement in the newborn infant (Dubowitz 1969). There are, however, many non-neuromuscular disorders that can also present with profound hypotonia and, in some cases, the differential diagnosis can be quite difficult. A detailed clinical examination and a good clinical and obstetric history provide the foundation to distinguish infants with a peripheral neuromuscular involvement from those with central nervous system (CNS) involvement, and, in some cases, yield important clues to a more specific diagnosis. Common associated features of neuromuscular disorders include arthrogryposis, feeding difficulties, sudden episodes of 'collapse', and unexplained respiratory failure.

Obstetric history

Reduced fetal movements throughout the pregnancy, or normal movements initially followed by later reduction, are frequently observed in infants with neuromuscular disorders and suggest weakness with onset in utero. The presence of polyhydramnios is also common in some conditions and indicates antenatal involvement of the swallowing muscles. Breech presentation is a common feature.

Birth history

Profound osteopenia predisposing to 'spontaneous' fractures can occur in any condition which causes a severe paucity of movement in utero. It is seen particularly frequently in nemaline myopathy and centronuclear myopathy, and in patients at the severe end of

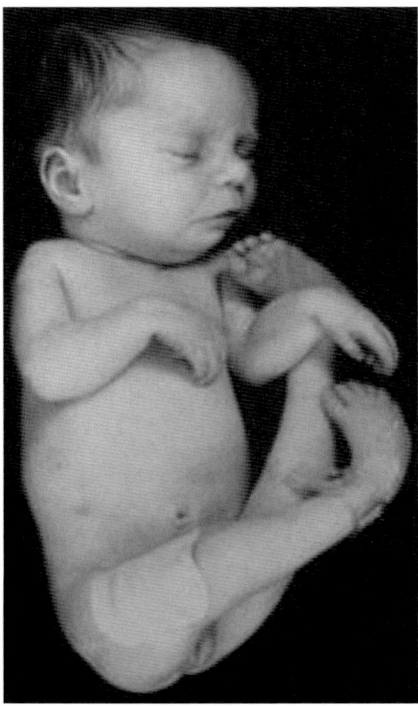

Fig. 40.66 Elbow, wrist and hip flexion contractures with extended knees in arthrogryposis.

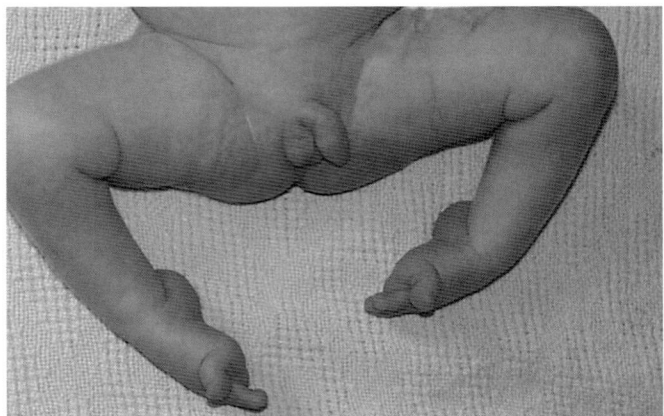

Fig. 40.67 Bilateral talipes equinovarus.

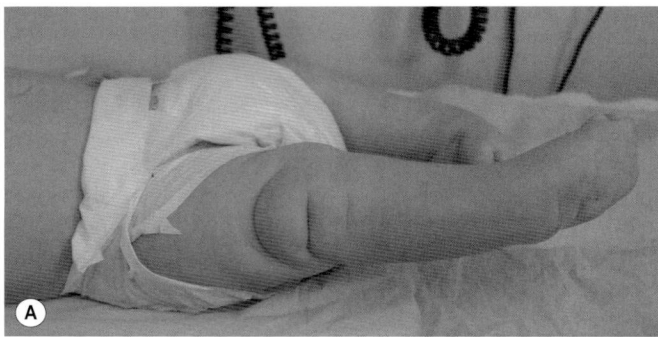

A

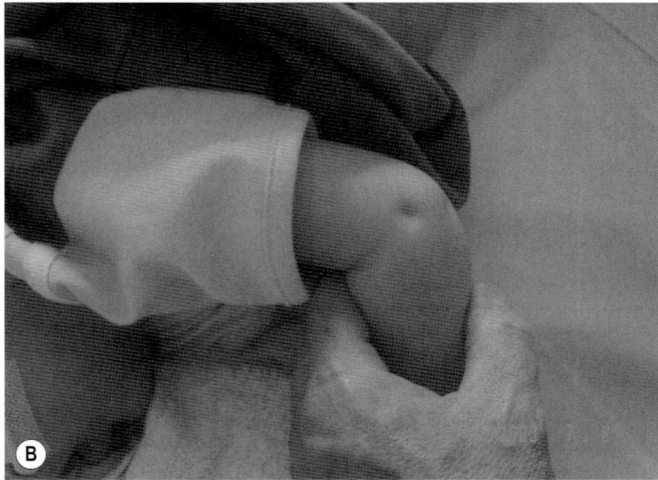

B

Fig. 40.68 Skin dimpling in arthrogryposis. (a) Knees. (b) Elbow.

the spinal muscular atrophy (SMA) spectrum. Poor respiration at birth requiring intubation and mechanical ventilation is also a feature of babies with severe congenital neuromuscular disorders; at times rigidity of the cervical spine, micrognathia and limited mandibulotemporal joint movement may complicate the intubation process.

Clinical examination

- Fixed joint contractures can be observed in patients with intrauterine immobility. Common patterns include flexion contractures at the elbows, knees, ankles and hips, or adducted thumbs, finger flexion contractures with poorly developed digits or extended talipes, extended-knee deformity with knee dislocation and hip dislocation (Fig. 40.66). Scoliosis and rigidity of the spine can also be present.
- Arthrogryposis, the term used for restricted movement at two or more joints at birth secondary to immobility in utero (Hageman and Willemse 1983), is not a diagnosis but a description of features which can result from several different types of pathological process. Electromyogram (EMG) and muscle biopsy are essential for the diagnosis, identifying neurogenic or myopathic patterns (Strehl and Vanasse 1985).
- Bilateral talipes equinovarus (Fig. 40.67) is classically described in infants with congenital myotonic dystrophy but can also be found in congenital myopathies, congenital muscular dystrophy (CMD) and congenital myasthenia; extended talipes is more rarely observed, and when present can suggest central core disease (CCD) and Ullrich CMD.
- Skin dimpling (Fig. 40.68) and poor dermatoglyphic pattern formation (Fig. 40.69) suggest immobility from the first trimester of pregnancy and are also indicators of reduced fetal movements.

- Thin osteopenic ribs on chest X-ray reflect poor respiratory muscle function in utero and are usually found in primary neuromuscular disorders (Fig. 40.70). Osteopenic ribs can rarely be found; insults of the CNS occur in the first trimester of pregnancy, or genetically determined neuronal migration disorders (pp. 1200–1218).
- The presence or absence of antigravity movements is one of the key elements in the detection of weakness (Vasta et al. 2005). It is important to observe the baby for a while

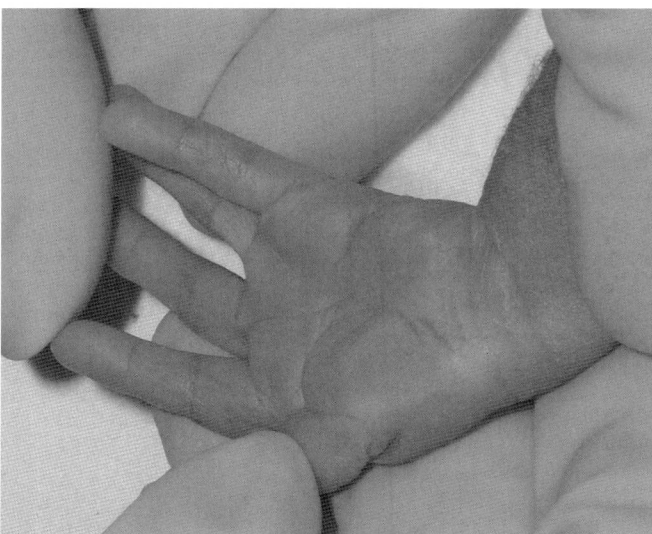

Fig. 40.69 Poor hand dermatoglyphic pattern secondary to immobility.

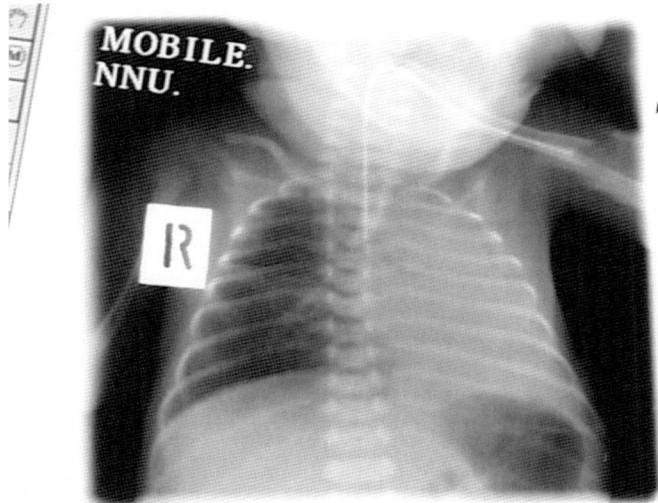

Fig. 40.70 Thin ribs and collapsed left lung in a ventilated infant with congenital myotonic dystrophy.

and judge movement at the peak of activity, such as when crying or stimulated. Weak children, such as those with neuromuscular involvement, will show little movement, even in response to stimulation. Children with CNS lesions or with syndromic conditions, who may be equally hypotonic, will show occasional antigravity movements or 'unexpectedly good' resistance and antigravity movement to painful stimuli or, for example, during a seizure. Fluctuations of weakness and the relationship with the sleep–wake cycle should be noted, as this may be significant in myasthenia.

- Facial weakness is often observed in infants with muscle diseases, such as myotonic dystrophy, congenital myopathies, congenital myasthenic syndromes (CMS) and CMD, while infants with the severe type of SMA, despite being very weak,

typically do not show significant facial weakness and, in contrast, appear to be alert and bright.

- Ophthalmoplegia is a feature of some of the congenital myopathies (typically centronuclear myopathy) and can be present in CMS and in mitochondrial diseases.
- Swallowing difficulties are often observed. Babies with severe weakness can be totally unable to swallow their own secretions and require regular suctioning; feeding difficulties are also common and generally in keeping with the swallowing difficulties observed. Infants with Prader–Willi syndrome show poor feeding and sucking, but are invariably able to manage their salivary secretions, as swallowing is not affected.
- Stridor can also be present in a few conditions, suggesting poor laryngeal muscle tone or vocal cord paralysis. Conditions in which bulbar function is more severely affected than other muscles include pontocerebellar hypoplasia type I (p. 1186), diaphragmatic SMA (or SMARD1) and some CMS.
- The assessment of the respiratory muscle movement is also important. In most muscle disorders there is diaphragmatic weakness with abdominal paradox (inward abdominal wall movement during inspiration). In some conditions, such as diaphragmatic SMA (SMARD1), the diaphragm is selectively affected. In typical chromosome 5-linked SMA, the weakness mainly affects intercostal muscles and the breathing pattern is abdominal, with the ribcage indrawing paradoxically during inspiration.
- Deep tendon reflexes are usually absent or reduced in neuromuscular disorders. Normal tendon reflexes in a floppy infant can almost exclude SMA or severe peripheral neuropathy but their absence does not necessarily suggest a muscle disorder. Brisk reflexes can be observed in CMS, in addition to conditions affecting the upper motor neuron.
- Visual and auditory attention and level of alertness are generally preserved in infants with neuromuscular disorders, although very sick infants with severe respiratory compromise will often have reduced level of consciousness. If encephalopathy is present in a weak infant, the possibility of the association of CNS involvement with a neuromuscular disorder (such as in mitochondrial disorders or muscle–eye brain disorders) should be considered, in addition to the possibility of a coincidental CNS involvement related to birth asphyxia.

Family history and examination

As most neonatal neuromuscular disorders are genetic, it is important to draw a pedigree going back three generations and to inquire about consanguinity and family history of neuromuscular diseases, stillbirth and neonatal death. When a dominant or an X-linked disorder is suspected, it is important to assess possible subclinical manifestations in the family. For example, myotonic dystrophy is inherited as an autosomal-dominant trait and is almost invariably inherited via an affected mother. In this condition the mother and other affected family members may be so mildly affected as to be unaware they have the disease. In these cases the examination of family members may detect abnormal physical signs, such as facial weakness (which may only consist of inability to bury the eyelashes), wasting of the facial muscles, percussion myotonia of the hands and relaxation myotonia of the hands. A history of cataracts and early diabetes may also be present. Other familial neuromuscular disorders that need to be considered are the myasthenias, including the acquired transient neonatal myasthenia or arthrogryposis due to passive transfer of maternal acetylcholine receptor (AChR) antibodies across the placenta (even in the absence of maternal symptoms) and the inherited CMS, where there may be parental consanguinity and/or a family history of unexplained infant deaths.

Clinical investigations

The determination of serum creatine kinase (CK) levels can be an important marker of possible muscle involvement. Serum CK levels are normally increased in cord blood up to five times the normal levels for adults as a reflection of muscle damage during labour and reach normal values by 5–10 days of age. Measurement of serum CK activity is likely to be of most value in some forms of muscular dystrophy, such as merosin-deficient CMD (MDC1A), or in the variants of CMD associated with brain malformation and defective glycosylation of α-dystroglycan, such as Walker–Warburg syndrome. However, in congenital myopathies or other forms of CMD and in motor neuron disorders, CK levels can be normal or mildly elevated.

EMG can be difficult to interpret in the neonatal period, and is not a reliable screen for congenital myopathies (Hellmann et al. 2005; Rabie et al. 2007). However, in experienced hands stimulation single-fibre EMG (stimSF-EMG) and/or repetitive nerve stimulation may help in the assessment of a child with suspected myasthenia (Tidswell and Pitt 2007). Peripheral motor nerve conduction studies are easier to perform and to interpret. A slow nerve conduction velocity may point to a hereditary motor neuropathy which may rarely present in early infancy, or to a neurometabolic disorder. Congenital but acquired variants of inflammatory demyelinating neuropathies have also been rarely observed.

Ultrasound imaging of muscle can help to demonstrate the presence of muscle involvement, and, in some cases, the selective involvement or sparing of muscles can be of considerable practical importance when taking a biopsy.

Muscle biopsy can be done using either an open technique or a needle. In our experience, a needle technique is well tolerated and we have an excellent success rate. However, an open technique is necessary when dealing with babies in whom metabolic myopathy is suspected, as for example in mitochondrial encephalomyopathies, and is the technique of choice in children with severe contractures and bone fractures. While a muscle biopsy is indicated whenever the clinical examination suggests a peripheral involvement, in a few conditions such as myotonic dystrophy and SMA the diagnosis can be reached rapidly and reliably using genetic analysis. When these conditions are suspected it is important to proceed quickly to obtain results from non-invasive genetic testing before considering a muscle biopsy, which may not be necessary if SMA is confirmed.

Brain imaging (cranial ultrasound and/or brain magnetic resonance imaging (MRI)) can help to identify structural brain lesions, such as cerebellar hypoplasia, cysts or cortical dysplasias, which are features of some conditions such as the α-dystroglycanopathies (including Walker–Warburg syndrome, muscle–eye–brain disease), mitochondrial disorders or pontocerebellar hypoplasia type I, with both central and peripheral involvement. Brain imaging can also help to identify brain haemorrhage and/or ischaemic lesions or ventricular dilatation, which commonly complicate the clinical picture of congenital myotonic dystrophy and other severe congenital myopathies such as centronuclear myopathy.

Congenital myotonic dystrophy

This is the commonest neuromuscular disorder occurring in the neonatal period.

Classically, infants with congenital myotonic dystrophy are born following a pregnancy complicated by reduced fetal movements and polyhydramnios. If the polyhydramnios is severe, premature delivery can further complicate the picture. Affected infants typically have hypotonia, bilateral talipes equinovarus and other contractures affecting mostly the legs (flexion deformity of the knees and hips) in association with marked difficulty in sucking and swallowing. Other features which are invariably present are facial weakness, characterised by a striking facial diplegia, with a triangular-shaped open mouth. The severity of the weakness is variable and, while children at the severe end of the spectrum can be totally paralysed, children at the milder end of the spectrum can show partial antigravity power in the limbs. Respiratory muscle weakness is frequent and ventilation is often required to sustain these infants in the first weeks of life. The severity of the respiratory involvement is the most important determinant of survival and previous studies have indicated that ventilation for more than 4 weeks in a term infant is a negative prognostic factor (Rutherford et al. 1989). Prematurity should also be taken into account and additional time allowed before assigning severity and considering discontinuation of care. The overall figures indicate a mortality of approximately 40% in the more severely affected patients (Mercuri et al. 2001).

Severe neonatal feeding difficulties are often present and nasogastric tube feeding is usually required for several months, even in those babies who breathe spontaneously. Feeding difficulties tend to improve over the first months of life in the survivors and gastrostomy feeding is rarely needed.

Learning difficulty is a frequent feature of children with congenital myotonic dystrophy. Recent studies suggest that the mean IQ of patients with this form varies between 50 and 65 and less than 10% of the survivors achieve normal education and employment (O'Brien and Harper 1984; Echenne et al. 2008).

It is important to realise that clinically evident myotonia is invariably absent in the neonatal period but can start to appear later on in childhood, when the progressive symptoms typical of the adult form of the disease become apparent. Children affected by the congenital variant of myotonic dystrophy who survive after the first months generally improve in the first 10 years of life. This is followed by a period of plateau and eventually by slow progression of weakness from the late teens onwards. Myotonia will usually appear in the first decade of life. Cardiac involvement, invariably present in older individuals with myotonic dystrophy, is rare in the neonatal period. A few cases of severe hypertrophic cardiomyopathy in infancy have, however, been reported (Igarashi et al. 1998).

Neuroimaging in the neonatal period often shows non-specific abnormalities such as ventricular dilatation, small haemorrhages or, in some cases, periventricular leukomalacia (Regev et al. 1987; Hashimoto et al. 1995).

A detailed pedigree, specifically seeking information about other children born with similar problems, is helpful for individuals with cognitive impairment, hand weakness and myotonia, cataracts and diabetes, but it is often the examination of the mother that suggests the diagnosis. There is no direct correlation between the severity of the condition in the mother and that in the baby, so that it is not unusual to find mothers who are unaware of being affected. Myotonia is best evaluated by asking the mother to clench her fists for a few seconds and observing the delay in fist releasing. Percussion myotonia can also be demonstrated in the thenar eminence or in the tongue. The EMG will invariably demonstrate myotonic discharge in the mother and the diagnosis is confirmed by molecular genetic testing, which reveals expansion (increase in the number of CTG trinucleotide repeats) in the *DMPK* gene on chromosome 19. The genetic diagnosis is essential for counselling as both prenatal and preimplantation diagnoses are available (Kakourou et al. 2008). A negative expansion study in the mother and the baby excludes the diagnosis of myotonic dystrophy. Muscle biopsy is not necessary in children with the congenital form of myotonic dystrophy; it is important to be aware that there is a significant pathological overlap between congenital myotonic dystrophy and centronuclear myopathy, and this has led to diagnostic confusion in several cases in the past (Dubowitz 1992).

Congenital muscular dystrophy

The term 'congenital muscular dystrophy' includes a heterogeneous group of muscle disorders characterised by weakness, usually from birth, and dystrophic changes on muscle biopsy. The classification of CMD has evolved to take into consideration the large number of genes and proteins identified, and the recognition that one CMD phenotype may be caused by many different genes, and that mutations in one gene can cause multiple phenotypes (Muntoni and Voit 2004; Godfrey et al. 2007).

The early classification of CMD was mainly based on the involvement of the CNS and on the presence or absence of merosin, an extracellular matrix protein found to be missing in approximately 35–45% of the cases with CMD. The current nomenclature is based on the protein product deficient in the patient, and the resulting clinical phenotype (Table 40.30). Despite the genetic heterogeneity, a restricted number of mechanisms responsible for CMD have been identified in the last decade. One important mechanism of disease is the reduction in glycosylated alpha-dystroglycan (αDG) expression, and its role in the pathogenesis of muscular dystrophy and the associated brain neuronal migration (Muntoni et al. 2002; Clement et al. 2008). A comprehensive panel of proteins studied using immunocytochemistry, including αDG (Dubowitz and Sewry 2007), on the muscle biopsy sample is now necessary for CMD classification and, together with brain imaging, directs diagnostic gene testing.

From a practical point of view, it is useful for the clinician to separate forms with CNS involvement from those in which CNS involvement is absent or rare, and to refer to the forms summarised in Table 40.30 for a first orientation. We will describe the most frequent forms of CMD observable in the neonatal period, separating the three forms associated with structural brain changes and eye abnormalities (Fukuyama CMD, muscle–eye–brain disease, Walker–Warburg syndrome) from other forms of CMD which can be observed in the neonatal period, providing clinical, pathological and imaging details to help their identification.

Forms of congenital muscular dystrophy with structural brain changes and eye involvement

Walker–Warburg syndrome

This is the most severe CMD with CNS involvement. Severe neonatal hypotonia, weakness, poor visual attention and decreased alertness are invariably present (Dobyns et al. 1989) and accompanied by ocular abnormalities, including retinal dysgenesis, microphthalmia, buphthalmos or anterior-chamber malformations.

Brain MRI shows a type II lissencephaly with the typical polymicrogyric cobblestone cortex and the white matter is also severely abnormal, showing dysmyelination or cystic changes (Dobyns et al. 1989). Cerebellar hypoplasia is also always present, associated with brainstem hypoplasia, Dandy–Walker syndrome or encephaloceles. Progressive hydrocephalus often develops. Cerebral ventricular dilatation is at times detected with antenatal ultrasonography. These infants are often considered only to have a CNS malformation until a markedly elevated serum CK indicates the coexistent skeletal muscle involvement. The presence of a muscular dystrophy is confirmed by muscle biopsy. In a few cases, normal CK in the neonatal period has been documented, followed by progressive and marked subsequent elevation with time.

The Walker–Warburg syndrome phenotype, originally associated with mutations in *POMT1* and *POMT2*, can be caused by recessive mutations in any of the genes encoding glycosyltransferase enzymes, as indicated in Table 40.30.

Muscle–eye–brain disease

This rare form of CMD was initially described in Finland. Hypotonia and weakness are usually present at birth or in the first months of life. Ocular abnormalities may become evident only after the first years of life. These children invariably develop severe mental retardation and, often, epilepsy (Santavuori et al. 1989); approximately a quarter of children eventually learn to walk.

Brain MRI shows extensive abnormalities of neuronal migration, such as pachygyria and polymicrogyria and often brainstem and cerebellar hypoplasia and periventricular white-matter changes. Recessive mutations in the *POMGTn1*, another glycosyltransferase, are responsible most cases of muscle–eye–brain disease (Hehr et al. 2007). Phenocopies can, however, be determined by mutations in any of the remaining putative glycosyltransferases.

Fukuyama congenital muscular dystrophy

This form is very frequent in Japan. The gene responsible for Fukuyama CMD is a glycosyltransferase, named fukutin (Osawa et al. 1997). The clinical features of Fukuyama CMD are almost identical those of muscle–eye–brain disease, with mild to moderate hypotonia at birth and a progressive course with increasing weakness, joint contractures, high CK levels, moderate to severe learning difficulties and frequent association with epilepsy. Ocular abnormalities occur in approximately 70% of these children but are rarely severe.

Brain MRI shows structural changes consisting of pachygyria and polymicrogyria and low-density white-matter areas. As in muscle–eye–brain disease, mutations in any of the putative glycosyltransferases can determine a Fukuyama CMD-like picture.

Congenital muscular dystrophy type 1C

This form was originally described associated with mutations in the putative glycosyltransferase fukutin-related protein gene. In its classical form, congenital muscular dystrophy type 1C (MDC1C) is associated with congenital onset of weakness, affecting the proximal limb muscles, muscle hypertrophy and markedly elevated serum CK. At variance with the conditions described above, there is no associated brain involvement in MDC1C.

Table 40.30 Genetically recognised forms of congenital muscular dystrophy (CMD) with presentation in the neonatal period

PROTEIN CATEGORY	DISEASE	ABBREVIATION	GENE SYMBOL*	GENE LOCATION	PROTEIN
Extracellular matrix and external membrane proteins	Merosin-deficient CMD	MDC1A	LAMA2	6q2	Laminin α2
	Ullrich CMD (Camacho-Vanegas et al. 2001; Mercuri et al. 2002)	UCMD	COL 6A1	21q2	Collagen VI
			COL 6A2	21q2	Collagen VI
			COL 6A3	2q3	Collagen VI
	Integrin α7-deficient CMD (Hayashi et al. 1998)		ITGA7	12q13	Integrin α7
	Integrin α9-deficient CMD		ITGA9	3p21	Integrin α9
Glycosyltransferases (variants with abnormal glycosylation of α-dystroglycan)	Fukuyama CMD	FCMD	FKTN	9q3	Fukutin
	Walker–Warburg syndrome*	WWS	POMT1	9q34	O-mannosyltransferase
			FKRP	19q	Fukutin-related protein
			POMT2	14q24.3	O-mannosyltransferase 2
			POMGnT1	1p3	Acetylglucosaminyltransferase
			LARGE	22q	Large
			FKTN	9q3	Fukutin
	Muscle-eye–brain disease	MEB	POMGnT1	1p3	O-linked mannose beta 1,2-N-acetylglucosaminyltransferase
	CMD + secondary merosin deficiency type C (Brockington et al. 2001)	MDC1C	FKRP	19q13.3	Fukutin-related protein
	CMD with mental retardation and pachygyria, type D (Longman et al. 2003)	MDC1D	LARGE	22q	Large
Endoplasmic reticulum proteins	Rigid-spine syndrome (Schara et al. 2008)	RSMD1	SEPN1	1p3	Selenoprotein N
Nuclear proteins	Lamin A/C-related CMD (Quijano-Roy et al. 2008)		LMNA	1q21.2	Lamin A/C
	CMD with adducted thumbs (Attali et al. 2009)		SYNE1	6q25	Nesprin 1

*Note that one disease phenotype may be caused by mutations in more than one gene, and, conversely, one gene may be causative for multiple phenotypes. The α dystroglycanopathies illustrate this concept well.

Other forms of congenital muscular dystrophies

Merosin-deficient congenital muscular dystrophy

This form, classified as MDC1A, is an autosomal-recessive form due to mutations in the *LAMA2* gene on chromosome 6, encoding laminin α₂, one of the components of the trieric protein merosin, an extracellular matrix protein (Tome et al. 1994).

Children with MDC1A are usually symptomatic at birth or in the first few weeks of life with hypotonia and muscle weakness, weak cry and, in 10–30% of cases, with contractures. These infants have associated feeding and respiratory problems, though these tend to recover in the first months. CK levels are grossly elevated (10 times the normal values). These children will show severe motor delay and never acquire independent ambulation (Philpot et al. 1995).

Brain MRI diffuse white-matter changes are a typical feature of MDC1A, and may be mistaken for a 'leukodystrophy'. These changes, however, become evident around 6 months and are not obvious on the conventional scans performed in the first months of life (Mercuri et al. 1996), though they can be suspected using more T2-weighted images (Mercuri et al. 2000a). Cerebellar hypoplasia and/or posterior cortical dysplasia (Sunada et al. 1995) can be observed in approximately 1 in 10 children with MDC1A.

CMD forms with normal merosin

Until recently the diagnosis of merosin-positive CMD was usually made after having excluded all the then known forms of CMD (Dubowitz 1993). It is now obvious that this group is heterogeneous and a number of forms have been mapped to specific genes. In addition, a number of syndromes have been described on the basis of clinical, imaging and pathological findings (Muntoni and Voit 2004). Table 47.30 lists the forms more often observed in the neonatal period, together with some relevant references for the rare forms not discussed in the text.

Ullrich CMD (UCMD) is the most common of these variants and it represents the most common CMD variant, followed by MDC1A. Presentation is with hypotonia, weakness and often contractures or dislocated hips, torticollis, kyphosis and extended talipes. The brain is not affected and serum CK is normal or moderately elevated. UCMD is the result of either recessive or de novo dominant mutations in one of the genes encoding collagen VI (Santavuori et al. 1989; Mercuri et al. 2006).

Muscle biopsy, followed by molecular genetic studies, leads to a form-specific CMD diagnosis which is important for genetic counselling and long-term prognosis. The short-term prognosis mainly depends on the severity of respiratory involvement, while the long-term prognosis is better discussed when the form of CMD has been identified.

Motor neuron disorders

Spinal muscular atrophy

SMA is the most common disease of the motor neuron in the newborn. The form affecting the newborn is the most severe of the subtypes of SMA and is classified as SMA type 1 or Werdnig–Hoffmann disease. Infants affected by this form are very weak, never acquire the ability to sit, have severe respiratory muscle weakness and usually die before the age of 1 year of an intercurrent respiratory infection.

The posture of the upper limbs in these infants is described as 'jug-handle' with a characteristic internal rotation of the shoulders and pronation of the forearms. There is a clear discordance between the weakness in the limbs, with little spontaneous activity, mainly limited to the feet and hands, and the sparing of the facial muscles, as infants with SMA generally show a bright expression and are very alert. Bulbar involvement can be present but is generally mild. Tongue fasciculations are frequent.

The intercostal muscles are always affected while the diaphragm is relatively spared. The combination of severe hypotonia with bright and alert face, tongue fasciculations and the respiratory pattern are generally strongly suggestive of the diagnosis. EMG showing fibrillation potentials further supports the diagnosis. The diagnosis is confirmed by *SMN1* (survival motor neuron 1) gene study, which shows homozygous deletion of exon 7 in 98% of cases and point mutations in the rest (Ogino and Wilson 2004).

SMA type 0

A few cases of prenatal-onset SMA with reduced fetal movements, severe weakness and asphyxia at birth have been reported (MacLeod et al. 1999). These infants also show signs of CNS involvement due to the birth asphyxia, which can be associated with non-specific signs of asphyxia on brain MRI. The survival time in these infants is short and because they appear to be more severely affected than the typical SMA type I, have been described as type 0. This form, confirmed by *SMN1* gene deletion studies, suggests that the phenotype of SMA is still expanding (Dubowitz 1999).

Other forms of motor neuron disease

Motor neuron involvement can also be present in other forms not linked to chromosome 5. Three of these forms have onset in early infancy: diaphragmatic SMA (Mercuri et al. 2000b; Grohmann et al. 2001), a form predominantly affecting the lower limbs (Van der Vleuten et al. 1998) and the form with pontocerebellar hypoplasia.

Pontocerebellar hypoplasia type 1 (p. 1186)

In this form, known as pontocerebellar hypoplasia type 1 (PCH1), SMA is associated with pontocerebellar hypoplasia (Barth 1993). These infants have most of the motor features of typical SMA 1, but in addition have reduced alertness and poor visual behaviour. The clinical course is progressive and respiratory and feeding difficulties, already present at birth or in early infancy, become more severe.

The diagnosis is mainly based on the association of clinical signs and MRI findings, of hypoplasia of cerebellar vermis, and often, hemispheres, and a thin brainstem and pons (Fig. 40.63). This form is not allelic to SMA (Dubowitz et al. 1995) and homozygous mutations in the vaccinia-related kinase 1 gene (*VKR1*) have recently been described in PCH1 (Renbaum et al. 2009).

Congenital myopathies

Four conditions, classified as structural congenital myopathies can present in the neonatal period (Dubowitz 1995). In order of frequency, these are nemaline myopathy; CCD; myotubular myopathy; minicore disease; their names derive from the typical muscle histopathological changes. Both minicore and CCD present more frequently in early infancy as opposed to the neonatal period, although earlier presentation is possible.

Nemaline myopathy

The clinical spectrum of nemaline myopathy is wide and, in the neonatal period, the two most common forms are the severe

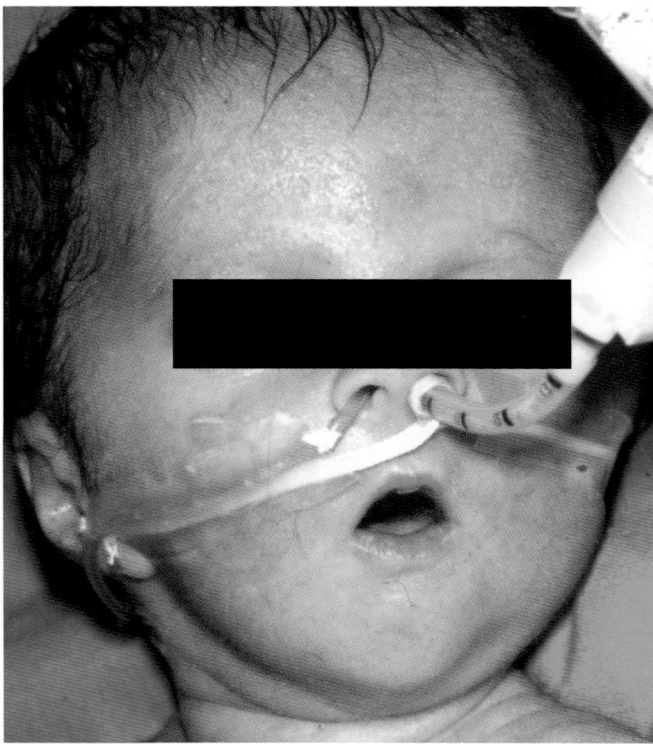

Fig. 40.71 Facies in a ventilated baby with congenital myotonic dystrophy showing the smooth forehead and triangular mouth.

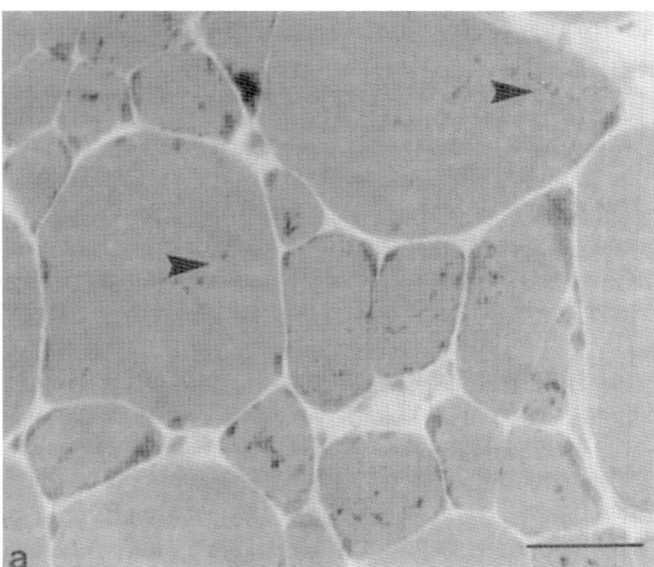

Fig. 40.72 Muscle biopsy showing nemaline rods (arrow).

congenital form, in which affected infants present with the classical fetal akinesia sequence (polyhydramnios/arthrogryposis/respiratory failure/complete immobility) to the so-called classical congenital form, characterised by hypotonia, general weakness predominantly affecting facial and axial muscles and disproportionately severe bulbar and feeding difficulties, requiring frequent suctioning, tube feeding and gastrostomy. In our clinical experience the frequency of these two conditions is quite similar; rare children might present with intermediate clinical features (for example, only mild contractures at birth, and significant weakness, with transient respiratory failure).

The serum CK levels are usually normal, the EMG myopathic and the nerve conduction studies normal. The muscle biopsy shows an abundance of rod-like structures in muscle and these stain red with the modified Gomori trichrome technique (Fig. 40.71) (Jungbluth et al. 2003).

The prognosis is invariably dismal for babies belonging to the severe congenital category, as these children do not appear to make any significant improvement of their limb, axial, bulbar and respiratory function even after several months. On the contrary, the prognosis for children with the classical form is much better, with most affected children acquiring independent ambulation. Frequent later complications are failure to thrive, scoliosis and nocturnal hypoventilation even in ambulant cases.

The condition is genetically heterogeneous with at least six genes implicated in its pathogenesis. However, with regard to the neonatal forms, de novo dominant mutations in the *ACTA1* gene account for a significant proportion of the severe form, while the rest are due to mutations in one or more, as yet unidentified, genes (Wallgren-Pettersson et al. 2004). Most of the classical milder congenital forms are due to recessive mutations in the *NEB* gene (Wallgren-Pettersson et al. 2004). Prenatal diagnosis is therefore available for the genetically defined variants.

Central core disease

CCD is characterised by a variable degree of hypotonia and axial and proximal muscle weakness predominantly affecting the hip girdle. Presentation with weakness is usually in infancy or early childhood, although contractures at birth (equinovarus foot deformity; hip dislocation) are frequently found. Some patients at the severe end of the spectrum may present with severe arthrogryposis and scoliosis. Severe facial and respiratory muscle weakness and bulbar dysfunction are not a common feature. Serum CK activity is usually normal or only moderately elevated. Most affected individuals achieve the ability to walk. The natural course is static or only slowly progressive. Malignant hyperthermia susceptibility is a common complication and all cases should be considered at risk.

The biopsy typically shows predominantly central, core-like areas on oxidative stains (Fig. 40.72); however, these striking abnormalities can be absent in the infantile period and only develop later on in life (Sewry et al. 2002). As the condition is often inherited in an autosomal-dominant way, careful examination of the parents might help to clarify the diagnosis in cases in which pathological changes are not clear. The gene responsible for CCD is the skeletal muscle ryanodine receptor (*RYR1*). Both dominant missense mutations (familial or de novo dominant mutations) and recessive mutations have been reported (Monnier et al. 2008).

Myotubular (centronuclear) myopathy

This term derives from the numerous centrally placed nuclei (Fig. 40.73) with a surrounding central zone devoid of oxidative enzyme activity seen on muscle biopsy. A similar histological picture can be found in patients with congenital myotonic dystrophy, and this may lead to diagnostic confusion if muscle biopsy is interpreted independently of the pedigree and clinical features in the affected infant and mother. The clinical phenotype of myotubular (centronuclear) myopathy is highly variable, depending on the mode of inheritance.

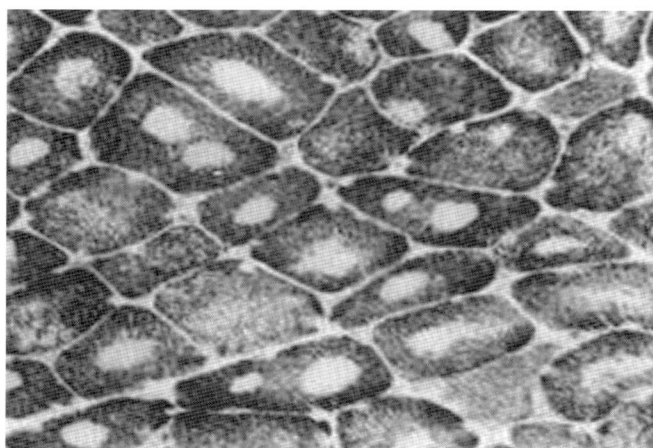

Fig. 40.73 Muscle biopsy showing central cores due to absent oxidative enzyme staining of the centre of the fibres (NADH).

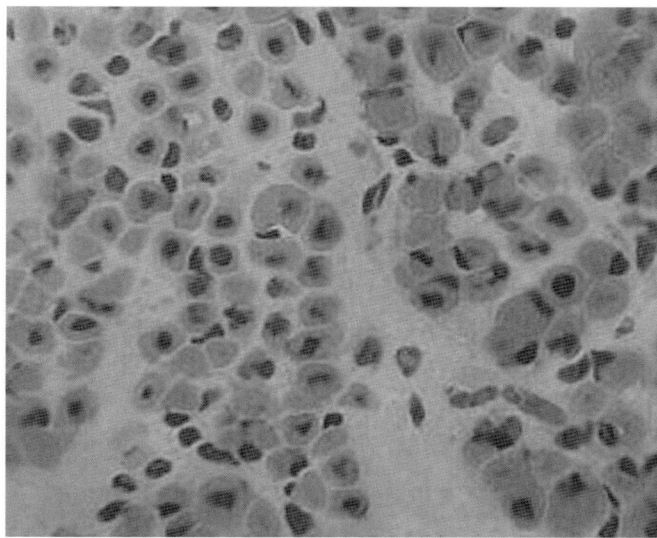

Fig. 40.74 Muscle biopsy showing multiple centrally placed nuclei in an infant with myotubular myopathy.

The more common X-linked form usually results in a severe phenotype in males presenting with polyhydramnios, reduced fetal movements, marked hypotonia, a variable degree of external ophthalmoplegia, respiratory failure at birth and an often fatal course. Severely affected infants who are ventilator-dependent in the neonatal period may survive if receiving continuous invasive ventilation, but show almost complete lack of motor developmental progress. The gene for the X-linked variant is the myotubularin gene (*MTM1*) on chromosome Xq28 (McEntagart et al. 2002) (Fig. 40.74).

The phenotype in the autosomal-recessive forms can range from early presentation with marked proximal weakness and inability to walk to milder variants characterised by generalised weakness and a variable degree of external ophthalmoplegia. Recently, dominant Dynamin 2 mutations or recessive Amphiphysin 2 (*BIN1*) gene mutations have been described as causative in some families (Nicot et al. 2007).

Minicore myopathy (multicore disease)

This is a rare condition, usually not presenting in the neonatal period. The most common phenotype features marked axial weakness with spinal rigidity, scoliosis and respiratory failure in late childhood. Another group of patients have associated partial or complete external ophthalmoplegia, and this is the variant that in our experience can present in the neonatal period. The name of the condition derives from the multifocal areas of myofibrillar disruption on oxidative enzyme staining. At least two genes are responsible for minicore disease: the *SEPN1* gene (which, when disrupted, can give rise to rigid spine CMD) and recessive *RYR1* gene mutations.

Myasthenia gravis

Transient neonatal myasthenia

This self-limiting but potentially life-threatening immune-mediated disorder occurs in approximately 20% of infants born to mothers with acquired myasthenia gravis, and is due to transplacental transfer of maternal antibodies directed against AChR. The diagnosis in mothers is often known, with the myasthenia active or in remission. Transient myasthenia rarely may occur in infants born to undiagnosed mothers with subclinical disease, but positive AChR antibodies (Papazian 1992). There is no direct relation between severity of maternal myasthenia and symptoms in the infant.

The onset occurs within a few hours of birth and always within the first 3 days. Typical features include poor sucking/swallowing, generalised hypotonia, facial weakness and weak cry. Fatigability, especially during feeds, may be present. Respiratory difficulties may require mechanical ventilation. Ptosis and ophthalmoparesis are less common, but diagnostically helpful, especially if variable. Recovery is anticipated by 2 months in 90% and by 4 months in all infants. Atypical presentation, in addition to the above symptoms, includes antenatal onset with polyhydramnios, decreased fetal movements and multiple joint contractures. Recurrent stillbirths with severe arthrogryposis secondary to maternal antibodies to the fetal γ AChR subunit have been described (Barnes et al. 1995).

Infants born to mothers with acquired myasthenia, either active or in remission, with or without measurable AChR antibodies, should be considered at risk for developing neonatal myasthenia. Prenatal care includes surveillance for polyhydramnios, decreased fetal movements and consideration of maternal plasma exchange to prevent fetal arthrogryposis. Infants should be observed for 3 days for development of symptoms. Once the first signs appear, diagnosis can be confirmed by anticholinesterase administration. Intramuscular neostigmine (single dose 0.15 mg/kg body weight) results in improvement in 15–30 minutes and lasts for 1–3 hours, allowing ample observation of infants feeding, crying, antigravity limb movements and respiration. This test should always be performed on the neonatal intensive care unit and a prior dose of atropine is useful in reducing muscarinic side-effects. Positive AChR antibodies in the infant or the mother are further evidence, but their absence does not rule out the diagnosis. In case of doubt, abnormal jitter on stimulation SF-EMG or an electrodecremental response on repetitive nerve stimulation at 3 Hz may be confirmatory.

Management aims at supporting feeding and maintaining adequate ventilation until spontaneous recovery occurs. In symptomatic infants, neostigmine (or pyridostigmine) is given orally or by nasogastric tube 30 minutes before 4-hourly feeds. Nasogastric feeding and mechanical ventilation may be required in more severely affected infants. Anticholinesterases are gradually weaned off when the infant is no longer symptomatic, between 1 and 4 months of age.

Congenital myasthenic syndromes

CMS are genetic disorders resulting in impaired neuromuscular transmission and fatigable weakness. Inheritance is autosomal-recessive, except for slow channel syndromes which are usually autosomal-dominant. CMS may be classified according to the site of the defect, into presynaptic, synaptic and postsynaptic categories. Mutations in at least 13 CMS genes have been identified, many with distinctive phenotypes and differing responses to medication, which may aid diagnosis (Burke et al. 2004; Palace and Beeson 2008).

Many CMS infants have symptoms from birth (Kinali et al. 2008), but diagnosis is often delayed. CMS should be considered in neonates with weakness affecting ocular (ptosis, ophthalmoplegia), bulbar (weak, fatigable suck and swallow), limb and respiratory muscles, with normal CK and negative AChR antibodies. Episodic apnoea, occurring in response to fever, intercurrent infection or stress, suggests *RAPSN* or *CHAT* mutations; arthrogryposis is common with *RAPSN* mutations, ophthalmoplegia occurs with AChR epsilon subunit mutations and also (together with a slow pupillary response to light) with acetylcholinesterase deficiency (*COLQ* mutations). Feeding difficulty with congenital stridor and vocal cord palsy may be an early diagnostic clue, notably in *DOK7* CMS, where limb girdle weakness may develop months or years later.

Confirmation of a CMS diagnosis requires neurophysiology by an experienced operator, demonstrating decrement on repetitive nerve stimulation or increased jitter on stimSF-EMG and/or genetic mutation analysis. If neonatal EMG facilities are not available, a trial of anticholinesterases may be considered whilst awaiting genetic confirmation. Importantly, subtypes such as acetylcholinesterase deficiency, slow-channel syndromes and *DOK7* CMS may be unresponsive or worsened by anticholinesterases. Medication trials must be given on a neonatal unit with the availability of full resuscitation facilities.

Neostigmine or pyridostigmine may significantly improve strength in AChR deficiency, fast-channel syndromes and *RAPSN* CMS. Increased secretions are helped by glycopyrrolate therapy. If *COLQ* or *DOK7* is suspected, anticholinesterases should be avoided; treatment with ephedrine or salbutamol may produce significant benefit, but experience in very young infants is limited. 3,4 diaminopyridine, which enhances acetylcholine release at the presynaptic nerve terminal, may be useful in addition to pyridostigmine in older children with *RAPSN*, AChR deficiency and fast-channel syndromes, but caution is advised with young infants. Electroencephalogram and electrocardiogram are recommended prior to 3,4 diaminopyridine therapy (Engel 2007). Supportive treatment with nasogastric feeding and ventilation may be necessary. Rarely, tracheostomy may be required if the airway is compromised by bilateral vocal cord paralysis, but the majority of CMS infants can be successfully extubated. All CMS infants are at risk of rapid respiratory decompensation, particularly *RAPSN* and *CHAT* genotypes and the fast-channel syndromes. Parents should be taught cardiopulmonary resuscitation before discharge and susceptible infants referred to specialist respiratory centres for provision of non-invasive ventilation for emergency use. Feeding gastrostomy may be needed for ongoing feeding difficulties and failure to thrive.

The prognosis for CMS is variable. Some subtypes improve (*RAPSN*), some remain stable and relatively mild (*CHRNE*), whereas those associated with progressive end-plate myopathy (*COLQ*, *DOK7* and severe slow-channel syndromes) may show gradual worsening with respiratory failure, necessitating nocturnal non-invasive ventilation in childhood.

Weblinks

http://www.elsevier.com/homepage/sah/nmd/menu.html: List of all neuromuscular disorders.

http://www.musclegenetable.org: From World Muscle Society. Neuromuscular focus on genes identified – very up to date.

http://www.ncbi.nlm.nih.gov/omim: OMIM from Johns Hopkins University. Industry standard, good for detail and also clinical synopsis of individual conditions.

http://neuromuscular.wustl.edu: Homepage from Neuromuscular Disease Center, Washington University, St Louis, MO, USA. Informative for overall neuromuscular conditions.

References

Barnes, P.R., Kanabar, D.J., Brueton, L., et al., 1995. Recurrent congenital arthrogryposis leading to a diagnosis of myasthenia gravis in an asymptomatic mother. Neuromuscul Disord 5, 59–65.

Barth, P.G., 1993. Pontocerebellar hypoplasia. An overview of a group of inherited neurodegenerative disorders with fetal onset. Brain Dev 15, 411–422.

Brockington, M., Blake, D.J., Prandini, P., et al., 2001. Mutations in the fukutin-related protein gene (FKRP) cause a form of congenital muscular dystrophy with secondary laminin α2 deficiency and abnormal glycosylation of α-dystroglycan. Am J Hum Genet 69, 1198–1209.

Burke, G., Cossins, J., Maxwell, S., et al., 2004. Distinct phenotypes of congenital acetylcholine receptor deficiency. Neuromuscul Disord 4, 356–364.

Camacho-Vanegas, O., Bertini, E., Zhang, R.Z., et al., 2001. Ullrich scleroatonic muscular dystrophy is caused by recessive mutations in collagen type VI. PNAS 98, 7516–7521.

Clement, E., Mercuri, E., Godfrey, et al., 2008. Brain involvement in muscular dystrophies with defective dystroglycan glycosylation. Ann Neurol 64, 573–582.

Dobyns, W.B., Pagon, R.A., Armstrong, D., et al., 1989. Diagnostic criteria for Walker–Warburg syndrome. Am J Med Genet 32, 195–210.

Dubowitz, V., 1969. The floppy infant. Clinics in Developmental Medicine, 31. Spastics International/Heinemann, London.

Dubowitz, V., 1992. Genetic counselling. Neuromuscul Disord 2, 85–86.

Dubowitz, V., 1994. Workshop report on 22nd ENMC-sponsored meeting on congenital muscular dystrophy held in Baarn, The Netherlands, May 14–16 1993. Neuromuscul Disord 4, 75–81.

Dubowitz, V., 1995. Muscle Disorders in Childhood, second ed. WB Saunders, London.

Dubowitz, V., 1999. Very severe spinal muscular atrophy (SMA type 0): an expanding clinical phenotype. Eur J Paediatr Neurol 3, 49–52.

Dubowitz, V., Sewry, C.A., 2007. Muscle biopsy – a practical approach. Saunders, Philadelphia.

Dubowitz, V., Daniels, R.J., Davies, K.E., 1995c. Olivopontocerebellar hypoplasia with anterior horn cell involvement (SMA) does not localize to chromosome 5q. Neuromusc Disord 5, 25–29.

Echenne, B., Rideau, A., Roubertie, A., et al., 2008. Myotonic dystrophy type I in childhood. Eur J Paediatr Neurol 12, 210–223.

Engel, A.G., 2007. The therapy of congenital myasthenic syndromes. Neurotherapeutics 4, 186–197.

Godfrey, C., Clement, E., Mein, R., et al., 2007. Refining genotype phenotype correlations in muscular dystrophies with defective glycosylation of dystroglycan. Brain 130, 2725–2735.

Grohmann, K., Schuelke, M., Diers, A., et al., 2001. Mutations in the gene encoding immunoglobulin mu-binding protein 2 cause spinal muscular atrophy with respiratory distress type 1. Nat Genet 29, 75–77.

Hageman, G., Willemse, J., 1983. Arthrogryposis multiplex congenita. Neuropediatrics 14, 6–11.

Hashimoto, T., Tayama, M., Myazaki, M., et al., 1995. Neuroimaging study of myotonic dystrophy I. Magnetic resonance imaging of the brain. Brain Dev 17, 24–27.

Hayashi, Y.K., Chou, F.L., Engvall, E., et al., 1998. Mutations in the integrin alpha7 gene cause congenital myopathy. Nat Genet 19, 94–97.

Hehr, U., Uyanik, G., Gross, C., et al., 2007. Novel POMGnT1 mutations define broader phenotypic spectrum of muscle–eye–brain disease. Neurogenetics 8, 279–288.

Hellmann, M., von Kleist-Retzow, J.C., Haupt, W.F., et al., 2005. Diagnostic value of electromyography in children and adolescents. J Clin Neurophysiol 22, 43–48.

Igarashi, H., Momoi, M.Y., Yamagata, T., et al., 1998. Hypertrophic cardiomyopathy in congenital myotonic dystrophy. Pediatr Neurol 18, 366–369.

Jungbluth, H., Sewry, C.A., Muntoni, F., 2003. What's new in neuromuscular disorders? The congenital myopathies. Eur J Paediatr Neurol 7, 23–30.

Kakourou, G., Dhanjal, S., Mamas, T., et al., 2008. Preimplantation genetic diagnosis for myotonic dystrophy type 1 in the UK. Neuromuscul Disord 18, 131–136.

Kinali, M., Beeson, D., Pitt, M.C., et al., 2008. Congenital myasthenic syndromes in childhood: diagnostic and management challenges. J Neuroimmunol 201–202, 6–12.

Longman, C., Brockington, M., Torelli, S., et al., 2003. Mutations in the human LARGE gene cause MDC1D, a novel form of congenital muscular dystrophy with severe mental retardation and abnormal glycosylation of alpha-dystroglycan. Hum Mol Genet 12, 2853–2861.

MacLeod, M.J., Taylor, J.E., Lunt, P.W., et al., 1999. Prenatal onset spinal muscular atrophy. Eur J Paediatr Neurol 3, 65–72.

McEntagart, M., Parsons, G., Buj-Bello, A., et al., 2002. Genotype–phenotype correlations in X-linked myotubular myopathy. Neuromuscul Disord 12, 939–946.

Mercuri, E., Pennock, J., Goodwin, F., et al., 1996. Sequential study of central and peripheral nervous system involvement in an infant with merosin-deficient CMD. Neuromuscul Disord 6, 425–429.

Mercuri, E., Rutherford, M., DeVile, C., et al., 2000a. Early white matter changes on brain magnetic resonance imaging in a newborn affected by merosin-deficient congenital muscular dystrophy. Neuromuscul Disord 11, 297–299.

Mercuri, E., Goodwin, F., Sewry, C., et al., 2000b. Diaphragmatic spinal muscular atrophy with bulbar weakness. Eur J Paediatr Neurol 4, 69–72.

Mercuri, E., Heckmatt, J., Dubowitz, V., 2001. The newborn with neuromuscular disorders. In: Levene, M.I., Chervenak, F.A., Whittle, M. (Eds.), Fetal and Neonatal Neurology and Neurosurgery, third ed. Churchill Livingstone, London.

Mercuri, E., Yuva, Y., Brown, S.C., et al., 2002. Collagen VI involvement in Ullrich syndrome: a clinical, genetic and immunohistochemical study. Neurology 58, 1354–1359.

Mercuri, E., Topaloglu, H., Brockington, M., et al., 2006. Spectrum of brain changes in patients with congenital muscular dystrophy and FKRP gene mutations. Arch Neurol 63, 251–257.

Monnier, N., Marty, I., Faure, J., et al., 2008. Null mutations causing depletion of the type 1 ryanodine receptor (RYR1) are commonly associated with recessive structural congenital myopathies with cores. Hum Mutat 29, 670–678.

Muntoni, F., Voit, T., 2004. The congenital muscular dystrophies in 2004: a century of exciting progress. Neuromuscul Disord 14, 635–649.

Muntoni, F., Brockington, M., Blake, D., et al., 2002. Defective glycosylation in muscular dystrophy. Lancet 360, 1419–1421.

Nicot, A.-S., Toussaint, A., Tosch, V., et al., 2007. Mutations in amphiphysin 2 (BIN1) disrupt interaction with dynamin 2 and cause autosomal recessive centronuclear myopathy. Nature Genet 39, 1134–1139.

O'Brien, J.A., Harper, P.S., 1984. Course prognosis and complications of childhood onset myotonic dystrophy. Dev Med Child Neurol 26, 62–67.

Ogino, S., Wilson, R.B., 2004. Spinal muscular atrophy: molecular genetics and diagnostics. Expert Rev Mol Diagn 4, 15–29.

Osawa, M., Sumida, S., Suzuki, N., et al., 1997. Fukuyama type congenital progressive muscular dystrophy. In: Fukuyama, Y., Osawa, M., Saito, K. (Eds.), Congenital Muscular Dystrophies. Elsevier Science, London.

Palace, J., Beeson, D., 2008. The congenital myasthenic syndromes. J Neuroimmunol 201–202, 2–5.

Papazian, O., 1992. Transient neonatal myasthenia gravis. J Child Neurol 7, 135–141.

Philpot, J., Sewry, C., Pennock, J., et al., 1995. Clinical phenotype in congenital muscular dystrophy: correlation with expression of merosin in skeletal muscle. Neuromusc Disord 5, 301–305.

Quijano-Roy, S., Mbieleu, B., Bönnemann, C.G., et al., 2008. De novo LMNA mutations cause a new form of congenital muscular dystrophy. Ann Neurol 64, 177–186.

Rabie, M., Jossiphov, J., Nevo, Y., 2007. Electromyography (EMG) accuracy compared to muscle biopsy in childhood. J Child Neurol 22, 803–808.

Regev, R., de Vries, L.S., Heckmatt, J.Z. et al., 1987. Cerebral ventricular dilation in congenital myotonic dystrophy. J Pediatr 111, 372–376.

Renbaum, P., Kellerman, E., Jaron, R., et al., 2009. Spinal muscular atrophy with pontocerebellar hypoplasia is caused by a mutation in the VRK1 gene. Am J Hum Genet 85, 281–289.

Rutherford, M.A., Heckmatt, J.Z., Dubowitz, V., 1989. Congenital myotonic dystrophy: respiratory function at birth determines survival. Arch Dis Child 64, 191–195.

Santavuori, P., Somer, H., Saino, K., et al., 1989. Muscle eye brain disease (MEB). Brain Dev 11, 147–153.

Schara, U., Kress, W., Bönnemann, C.G., et al., 2008. The phenotype and long-term follow-up in 11 patients with juvenile selenoprotein N1-related myopathy. Eur J Paediatr Neurol 12, 224–230.

Sewry, C.A., Muller, C., Davis, M., et al., 2002. The spectrum of pathology in central core disease. Neuromuscul Disord 12, 930–938.

Strehl, E., Vanasse, M., 1985. EMG and needle muscle biopsy studies in arthrogryposis multiplex congenita. Neuropediatrics 16, 225–227.

Sunada, Y., Edgar, T.S., Lotz, B.P., et al., 1995. Merosin-negative congenital muscular dystrophy associated with extensive brain abnormalities. Neurology 45, 2084–2089.

Tidswell, T., Pitt, M.C., 2007. A new analytical method to diagnose congenital myasthenia with stimulated single-fiber electromyography. Muscle Nerve 35, 107–110.

Tome, F.M., Evangelista, T., Leclerc, A., et al., 1994. Congenital muscular dystrophy with merosin deficiency. C R Acad Sci III 317, 351–357.

Van der Vleuten, A.J.W., van Ravenswaaij-Arts, C.M.A., Frijns, C.J.M., et al., 1998. Localisation of the gene for a dominant congenital spinal muscular atrophy predominantly affecting the lower limbs to chromosome 12q23-q24. Eur J Hum Genet 6, 376–382.

Vasta, I., Kinali, M., Messina, S., et al., 2005. Can clinical signs identify newborns with neuromuscular disorders? J Pediatr 146, 73–79.

Wallgren-Pettersson, C., Pelin, K., et al., 2004. ENMC International Consortium on Nemaline Myopathy. Genotype–

phenotype correlations in nemaline myopathy caused by mutations in the genes for nebulin and skeletal muscle alpha-actin. Neuromuscul Disord 14, 461–470.

Part 8: Central nervous system malformations

Cornelia Hagmann   Janet M Rennie

Introduction

The spectrum of central nervous system (CNS) malformations presenting in the neonatal period has changed dramatically since the first edition of this textbook. Antenatal diagnosis and termination of affected pregnancies have reduced the number of live-born babies with myelomeningocele, hydrocephalus, anencephaly and holoprosencephaly. The most challenging area of practice at the moment is counselling women (and their families) when an antenatal diagnosis of an abnormality such as ventriculomegaly, agenesis of the corpus callosum (ACC) or posterior fossa abnormality is made. Magnetic resonance imaging (MRI) has increased recognition of problems such as lissencephaly, previously thought to be very rare. Antenatal counselling is fraught with difficulty given the rapidly developing fetal CNS (grey-matter heterotopia and small areas of polymicrogyria cannot reliably be detected even with fetal MRI) and uncertainty about the natural history of conditions such as Dandy–Walker variant. The emphasis on detection of congenital abnormalities of the spine has shifted from spina bifida to occult spinal dysraphism.

Epidemiology of CNS malformations

In England and Wales, the National Congenital Anomaly system was set up in 1964. In 2007, a new classification was adopted, based on the Eurocat classification (see Weblinks).

In 1974, almost 5000 babies were conceived with CNS defects of all types. By 1993, this figure had reduced to just over 1000, and amongst live births CNS defects had reduced 10-fold. During the same period, other malformations increased from 159 to 191 per 10 000 deliveries (OPCS 1982–1987; see weblinks). Anencephalic births fell from 13.1 to 0.5 per 10 000 between 1974 and 1993, and the rate has remained stable since then; births of babies with any neural tube defects (NTDs) have fallen from 18.3 to around 2.0 per 10 000 and hydrocephalus from 4.8 to around 2.0 per 10 000. The rates of CNS abnormalities per 10 000 total births between 1988 and 2008 are shown in Table 40.31. No new data have been added to the Office for National Statistics website on CNS malformations since 2008. Eurocat produces annual tables, and reports about 3000 cases of CNS malformations per year for 2007 and 2008, a prevalence (excluding chromosomal malformations) of 17 per 10 000 births. About one-third of the cases were terminations of pregnancy.

There are large variations in the incidence of CNS defects in different parts of the world. NTDs are common in the USA and Europe, whereas encephalocele is more common in Asia. Periconceptional folate can reduce the incidence of NTDs, whereas drugs which are folate antagonists, such as phenobarbital or carbamazepine, increase the risk. Current recommendations are that women planning to become pregnant should take a vitamin supplement containing at least 400 µg folate daily, from before conception to the 12th week of pregnancy. Women with an affected child, who are taking antiepileptic drugs or are affected by a disorder such as an NTD, diabetes or coeliac disease are advised to take a larger dose of 5 mg.

Cephaloceles

Cranial encephalocele is rare in Europe, and more common in South-East Asia. In cranial encephalocele the skull is deficient and a cystic swelling protrudes through the defect, usually in the occipital region (Figs 40.75 and 40.76). Occasionally a frontal encephalocele protrudes into the upper nasal cavity, causing diagnostic

Table 40.31 Rates of central nervous system (CNS) abnormalities per 10 000 births in England and Wales 1988–2008

MALFORMATION	YEAR OF BIRTH									
	1988	1990	1992	1994	1996	1997	1998	1999	2002	2008
All CNS	7.3	5.1	4.6	4.0	3.9	3.5	4.5	4.8	11.5	6.9
Anencephalus	0.6	0.4	0.5	0.4	0.4	0.5	0.3	0.4	0.9	0.5
Spina bifida	2.3	1.7	1.2	0.7	0.9	0.8	1.0	1.0	1.9	1.3
Hydrocephalus	2.0	1.3	1.4	1.2	1.2	1.0	1.2	1.0	2.4	2.3

(Data from Office for National Statistics: http://www.statistics.gov.uk.)

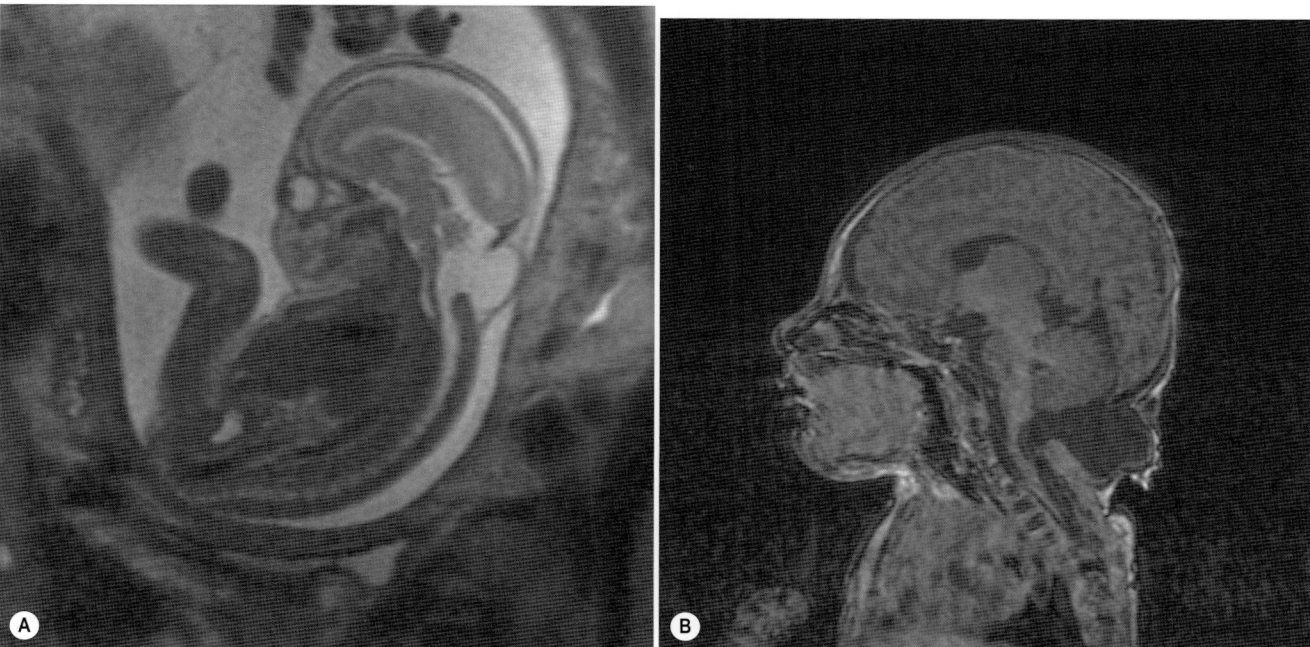

Fig. 40.75 (a) Fetal magnetic resonance imaging (MRI) sagittal section showing occipital cephalocele. (b) Postnatal MRI sagittal section, same case.

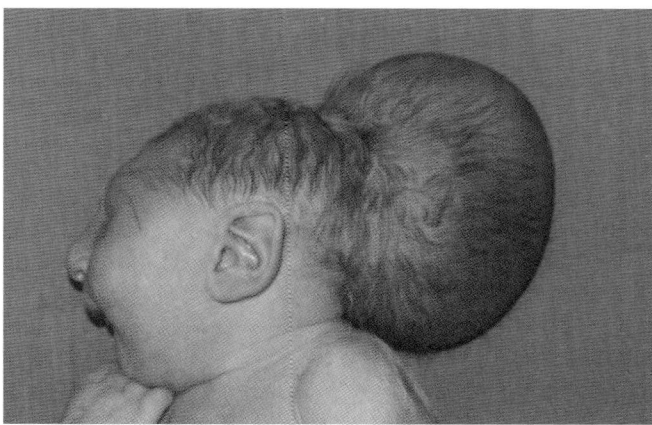

Fig. 40.76 Large occipital encephalocele.

difficulty. Some cephaloceles contain only cerebrospinal fluid (CSF), but most contain brain. The rest of the brain is often abnormal and associated microcephaly is common.

The Meckel–Gruber syndrome is an autosomal-recessive disorder in which there is an encephalocele with multicystic kidneys, and other malformations, including hepatic duct dysplasia and cysts. The genetic abnormality has been mapped in several populations. The prognosis of an encephalocele is generally poor: many succumb in early infancy and the overwhelming majority of the survivors are physically and mentally disabled. Walker–Warburg syndrome (p. 1193) is another disorder in which encephalocele is seen (see section on malformations due to abnormal neuronal migration, lissencephaly, below).

Neural tube defects

NTDs are believed to result from failure of fusion of the neural tube during embryogenesis. Based on the embryogenesis the most common spinal anomalies can be divided into five groups (Duczkowska et al. 2011), and others:

1. anomalies of notochord formation (diastematomyelia)
2. anomalies of premature dysjunction (lipomyelomeningocele, intradural lipomas, fibrolipomas of the filum terminale)
3. anomalies of nondysjunction (meningocele, myelomeningocele)
4. anomalies of the caudal cell mass (tight filum terminale, sacrococcygeal teratomas, dermoids, epidermoids and hamartomas)
5. anomalies of unknown origin (syringohydromyelia).

The most common NTDs are anencephaly and myelomeningocele (commonly called spina bifida). These two defects are often referred to as open defects whereas skin-covered or closed defects include encephalocele, meningocele, lipomeningocele, sacral agenesis and occult spinal dysraphism (Lemire 1988). The birth prevalence of NTDs is influenced by the availability of prenatal diagnosis and elective pregnancy termination (Palomaki et al. 1999; Rankin et al. 2000).

Anencephaly

Anencephaly results from failure of anterior neural tube closure. Anencephaly is a lethal condition, although some babies survive for weeks and one child who was ventilated survived for several years. Live birth with anencephaly is now very rare, due to prenatal detection and the acceptance of termination of pregnancy.

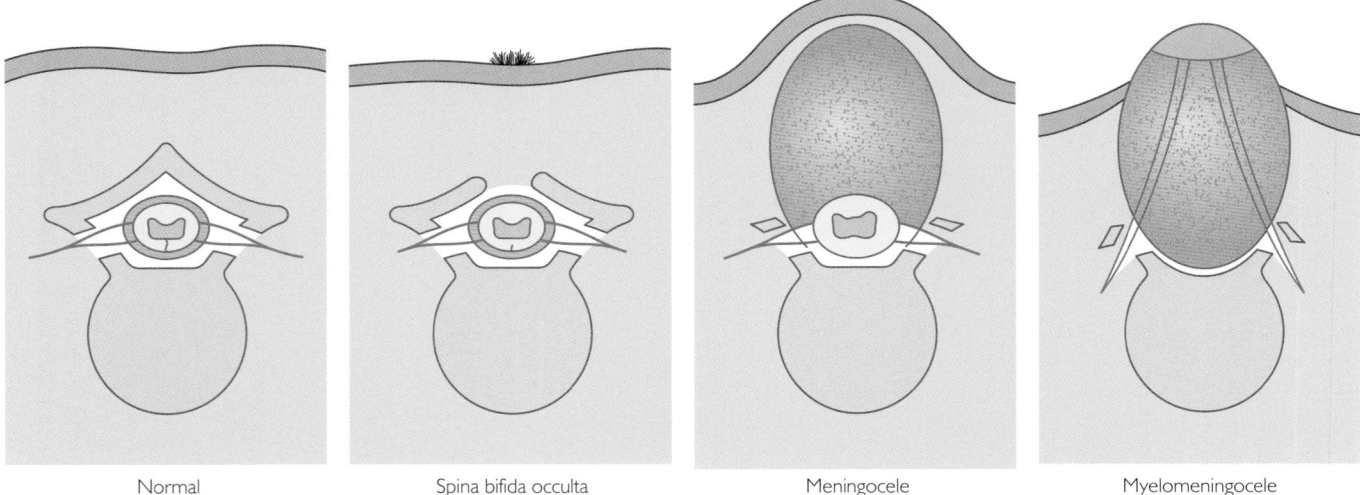

Normal   Spina bifida occulta   Meningocele   Myelomeningocele

Fig. 40.77 Classification of spina bifida. *(Redrawn from Forfar & Arneil's Textbook of Pediatrics, 4th edn).*

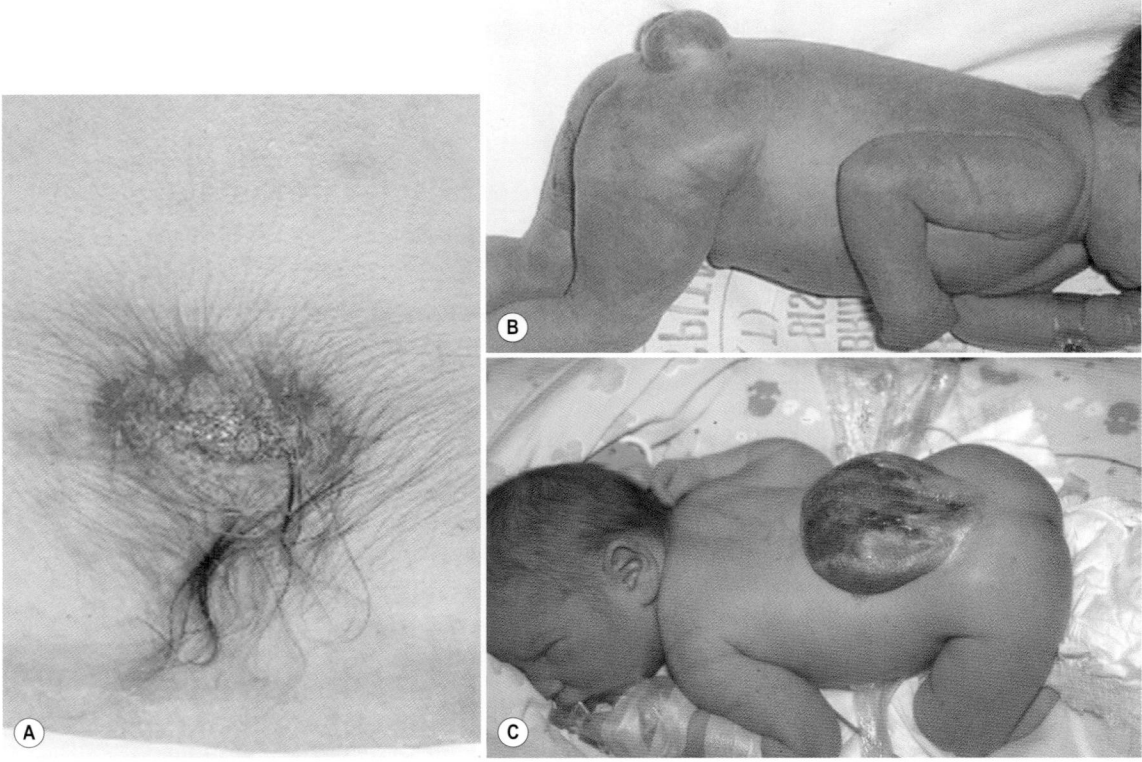

Fig. 40.78 Clinical appearances of the types of lesion shown in Figure 40.77. (a) Hairy patch with a skin defect over a spina bifida occulta; (b) small skin-covered sacral meningocele; (c) large thoracolumbar myelomeningocele.

Myelomeningocele

This disorder is due to failure of closure of the posterior neural tube. NTDs remain one of the most common congenital CNS defects, in spite of attempts to encourage women to take preconceptional folate. The general term 'spina bifida' encompasses both 'closed' spinal dysraphism (see below), meningocele, and 'open' spina bifida, or myelomeningoele (Fig 40.77). Figure 40.78 shows the clinical appearances of the three types of lesion shown in Figure 40.77. Figure 40.78a shows a hairy patch with a skin defect over a spina bifida occulta (an indication for spinal imaging, see below); Figure 40.78b shows a small skin-covered sacral meningocele and Figure 40.78c is a baby with a large thoracolumbar myelomeningocele.

About 80% of myelomeningoceles occur in the lumbar (thoraco-lumbar, lumbar, lumbosacral) area. The neurological function depends on the level of the lesion. Prenatal detection is possible in about 90% of cases. In a recent series from Bristol, UK, 72% of mothers whose fetus was diagnosed with myelomeningocele chose termination of pregnancy (Aguilera et al. 2009). The survival rate for the live-born group was 86%, in keeping with reports from other groups (87% at 1 year and 78% at 17 years) (Wong and Paulozzi 2001). All of the six cases of meningocele in the Bristol series walked independently, but half of them developed a neuropathic bladder. For most, postnatal repair remains the only option, although attempts at fetal repair continue. Adzick and colleagues (2011) have pioneered attempts at fetal surgery, and recently reported the results of a randomised trial of fetal repair of spina bifida before 26 weeks. Prenatal surgery was associated with a lower rate of shunt surgery (40% versus 82%) and improved ambulation at 30 months but the risk of precipitating a preterm birth, with all that entails, remains considerable. Of the 78 cases treated with fetal surgery, 10 delivered before 30 weeks and a further 26 before 34 weeks. The treatment was not without complications for the mothers either: those with a body mass index of over 35 were excluded from the trial but even so, 35% had a hysterotomy site that was either very thin or had actually dehisced at the time of delivery, and there were more cases of abruption of the placenta.

Individuals affected by myelomeningocele remain at high risk for physical and developmental disabilities such as motor deficits, skeletal deformities, bladder and bowel incontinence, sensory deficits below the level of the spinal lesion and sexual dysfunction (Table 40.32) (Bowman et al. 2001). Most patients with lesions below S1 are able to walk unaided, whereas those with lesions above L2 are usually wheelchair-dependent for a major portion of their daily activities (Coniglio et al. 1996; Williams et al. 1999). Muscle tests performed early in life can predict future use of wheelchair and ambulation to some extent (Seitzberg et al. 2008). However, a recent study showed that in children with levels between L3 and L5 adult ambulatory function could not be determined from muscle strength in early life (Seitzberg et al. 2008). When counselling antenatally it is important to remember that antenatal diagnosis is often wrong by at least one vertebral body, and the eventual functional spinal cord level may not correspond to the anatomical level of the defect. The postnatally determined sensory level was the best guide to prognosis in one carefully studied series (Hunt and Oakeshott 2003; Fig. 40.79).

Neurological deficit in infancy in 117 consecutive cases of open spina bifida and outcome in 54 people who survived to mean age 35 years

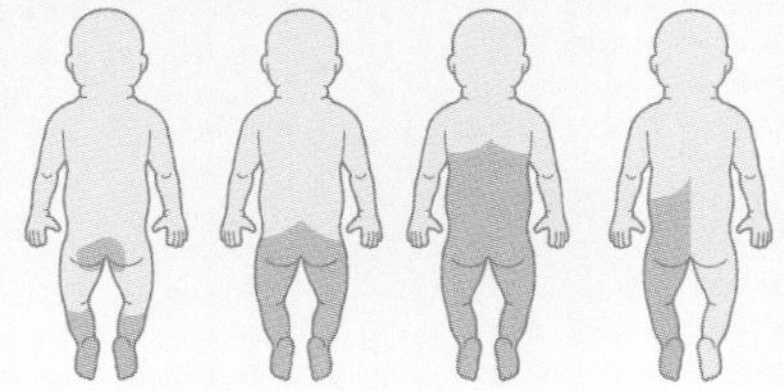

Sensory level in infancy

	Below L3	L3–T11	Above T11	Asymmetrical	P value for trend*
Whole cohort	38	32	42	5	
Those who died (n = 63)	14	17	30	2	<0.01

Disability and lifestyle in survivors (mean age 35):

	Below L3	L3–T11	Above T11	Asymmetrical	P value for trend*
Survivors	24	15	12	3	
No CSF shunt (n = 8)	7	0	1	0	<0.05
IQ ≥ 80 (n = 39)Á	21	11	6	1	0.05
Community walker (n = 16)#	16	0	0	0	<0.0001
Continent (n = 11)ξ	8	2	0	1	<0.05
Live independently (n = 22)λ	14	5	2	1	<0.05
Drive cars (n = 20)	14	4	2	0	<0.05
Open employment (n = 13)	9	2	2	0	0.18

* X^2 test. Asymmetrical sensory level excluded from analysis.
Á IQ recorded at age 5–15 years.
\# Able to walk ≥50 metres with aids if required.
ξ Continent without catheters or appliances.
λ Living in the community without help or supervision.

Fig. 40.79 Neurological deficit in infancy in 117 consecutive cases of open spina bifida and outcome in 54 people who survived to mean age 35 years. *(Reproduced from Hunt and Oakeshott 2003, with permission).*

Table 40.32 Evaluation of motor level according to muscle strength, based on Sharrard and Seitzberg

MOTOR LEVEL	MUSCLE FUNCTION	DESCRIPTION OF EXPECTED AMBULATION STATUS
At or above L2	No muscle activity in the lower limbs or hip flexors poor. No knee extension	Wheelchair use for mobility ambulation during therapy
L3	Good to normal hip flexion. Knee extension moderate	Household ambulation with leg callipers. Mainly wheelchair user
L4	Hip flexors normal. Knee extension good to normal. Dorsiflexion of foot good to normal	Community ambulation with need of ankle–foot orthoses and need for walking aid
L5	Hip flexors and knee extension normal. Normal dorsiflexors and good to normal evertors and invertors of the foot	Community ambulation with ankle–foot orthoses
S1	Good to normal plantar flexion	Community ambulation, no orthoses

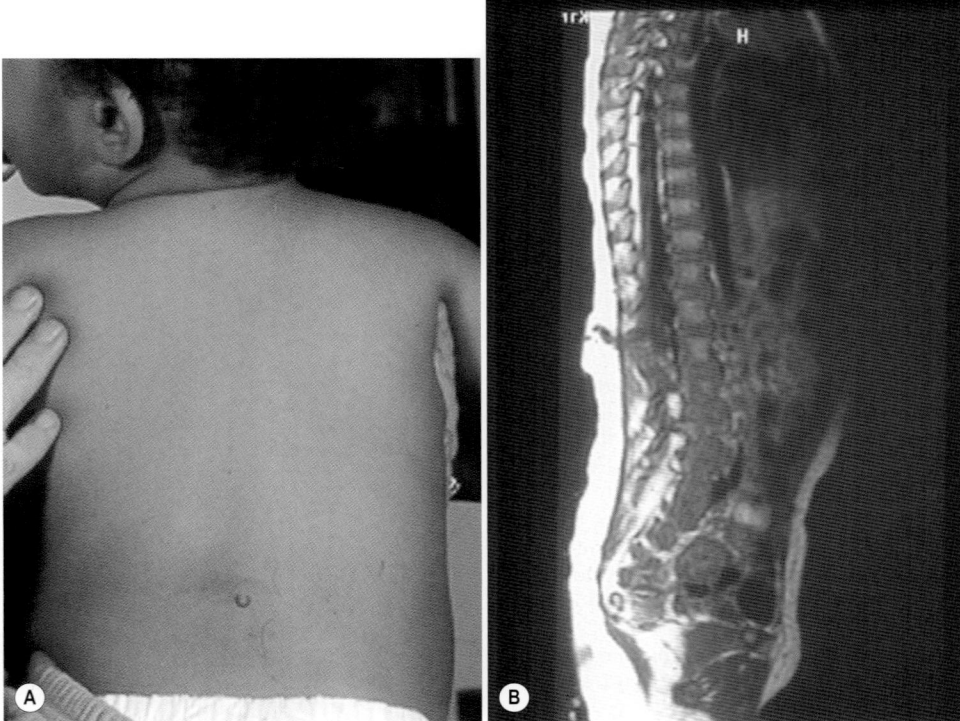

Fig. 40.80 (a) Midline skin lesion over the lumbar spine in an asymptomatic infant. (b) Magnetic resonance imaging scan of the same child revealed a tethered spinal cord and a dermal sinus, requiring surgery.

Arnold–Chiari malformation

In addition to the above-mentioned complications, some complications are caused by hydrocephalus. The incidence of hydrocephalus associated with spina bifida is site-dependent to some extent: with occipital, cervical, thoracic or sacral lesions, the incidence of hydrocephalus is about 60% whereas with thoracolumbar, lumbar or lumbosacral lesions, the incidence of hydrocephalus is about 85–90% (Stein and Schut 1979). Serial cranial ultrasound scans are important to evaluate the presence and progression of hydrocephalus. The most common time for symptomatic hydrocephalus with myelomeningocele is 2–3 weeks after birth (Stein and Schut 1979; Rintoul et al. 2002). The usual cause of hydrocephalus in babies with spina bifida is the Chiari type II malformation with obstruction of the fourth ventricular outflow or an associated aqueductal stenosis. Nearly every case of thoracolumbar, lumbar or lumbosacral myelomeningocele is accompanied by the Chiari type II malformation. This malformation includes inferior displacement of the medulla and fourth ventricle into cervical canal, elongation and thinning of the upper medulla and lower pons, inferior displacement of the lower cerebellum through the foramen magnum and bony defects of the foramen magnum and upper cervical vertebrae. The Arnold–Chiari malformation is associated with an aqueductal stenosis in up to 80% of cases (Stein and Schut 1979) and with aqueductal atresia in an additional 10%. The Arnold–Chiari malformation is usually diagnosed because of the association with an NTD. On occasion imaging performed for other signs – apnoea or swallowing problems – reveals the abnormality. In a carefully studied series of infants with Arnold–Chiari syndrome, one-third exhibited feeding disturbance (reflux, aspiration), laryngeal stridor, or apnoeic episode. The median age of onset of midbrain symptoms was 3.2 months (Worley et al. 1996).

Occult spinal dysraphism

Recognition of the importance of midline 'markers' of underlying spinal problems (Figs 40.78a, and 40.80) can make all the difference to a child's quality of life. Whilst 'simple dimples' just above the natal cleft are common (for definition, see Ch.14) any midline lesion more than 1 cm away from the natal cleft, and any lesion associated with a hairy patch, subcutaneous fatty tissue, skin tags or areas of atretic skin must be taken seriously and investigated. The same is true for babies with anorectal and urogenital anomalies such as VATER (Ch. 34). These anomalies have a high incidence of associated spinal cord tethering which justifies investigation.

Dermal sinuses course inward from the skin, ending in the spinal canal in 50–70% of cases and many are associated with dermoid or epidermoid tumours. If these are ignored they can become infected, worsening any spinal tethering and making subsequent surgery more difficult. When the condition is recognised, most paediatric neurosurgeons would recommend early surgery in order to preserve urologic sphincter function.

Ultrasound of the spine can be very useful in the newborn (Ch. 43), whereas X-ray is of no value and even MRI may need to be repeated. The conus is usually above L2 and rarely below L3, and most would consider that if the conus is at or below the level of the L2–3 disc space it should be considered abnormal, and a search should be made for a tethering mass. Most paediatric radiologists would say that a high-quality normal spinal ultrasound can exclude spinal dysraphism, and this is the first-line investigation (Ch. 43).

Diastomyelia refers to 'split cord', probably due to splitting of the notochord early in development. This condition is also associated with cutaneous stigmata and/or orthopaedic problems of the feet. About 50% of individuals with the Klippel–Feil abnormality have an associated diastomyelia.

Disorders of prosencephalic development

Prosencephalic development can be considered in terms of three sequential events:

1. prosencephalic formation (aprosencephaly, atelencephaly)
2. prosencephalic cleavage (holoprosencephaly, holotelencephaly)
3. midline prosencephalic development (ACC, agenesis of the septum pellucidum, septo-optic dysplasia).

Advances in genetics have revealed that homeobox genes, including sonic hedgehog (SHH) at the HPE3 locus causing an autosomal-dominant from of holoprosencephaly, are important in prosencephalic development (Roessler et al. 1996).

Holoprosencephaly

Holoprosencephaly is a complex brain malformation characterised by failure of the forebrain to bifurcate into two hemispheres. Three main variants are distinguished in holoprosencephaly: (1) alobar (the most severe form); (2) semilobar: (3) lobar holoprosencephaly; and (4) the middle interhemispheric variant of holoprosencephaly (Lewis et al. 2002; Simon et al. 2002). These subtypes are defined primarily by the degree and region of neocortical separation (Hahn and Barnes 2010).

Alobar holoprosencephaly is characterized by a single-sphered cerebral structure with a common ventricle, a membranous roof over the third ventricle that is often distended into a large cyst posteriorly, absence of olfactory bulbs and optic bulbs, usually accompanied by facial anomaly such as a single median eye ('cyclops'), or severe hypotelorism, a single-nostril nose (cebocephaly) with or without a proboscis and/or a cleft lip and palate. Abnormalities of other organs are frequent and include cardiac, skeletal, genitourinary and gastrointestinal malformations. Seizures occur in most cases; there is abnormal hypothalamic function and failure of normal neurological development (Hahn and Plawner 2004). Children with alobar holoprosencephaly make minimal developmental progress and generally have profound global impairment (Plawner et al. 2002).

Semilobar holoprosencephaly is a form in which there is a partial separation of the hemispheres posteriorly, and there are almost fully developed cerebral hemispheres, but with some continuity across the frontal cortex. Takahashi et al. (2003) have described a helpful classification of semilobar holoprosencephaly based on MRI morphology (Fig. 40.81a). Mortality is high for newborns with holoprosencephaly; however, some will survive beyond the neonatal period and maybe even for some years. The middle interhemispheric variant of holoprosencephaly involves failure of separation of the posterior frontal and parietal lobes and is the least severe form (Fig. 40.81b) (Hahn and Barnes 2010; Lewis et al. 2002; Simon et al. 2002). Prenatal diagnosis is possible (Fig. 40.81b).

Higher mortality correlates with the severity of the brain malformation, the presence of chromosomal abnormalities and the presence of a multiple congenital anomaly syndrome or other organ involvement (Whiteford and Tolmie 1996). Developmental disabilities are present in virtually all children with holoprosencephaly (Levey et al. 2010). The range of developmental outcome for children with semilobar holoprosencephaly is very wide.

Absence of the septum pellucidum

Absence of the septum pellucidum is rare, occurring in about 2–3/10 000 individuals (Fig. 40.82) (Barkovich and Norman 1989). More often it occurs with brain abnormalities such as schizencephaly, ACC, hydrocephalus, holoprosencephaly, Chiari II malformation, polymicrogyria and septo-optic dysplasia (Barkovich and Norman 1989; Kuhn et al. 1993; Belhocine et al. 2005). The full syndrome of septo-optic dysplasia includes absence of the septum pellucidum, optic nerve hypoplasia, absence or thinning of the corpus callosum and hypothalamic–pituitary dysfunction.

The corpus callosum is the largest interhemispheric commissure (containing around 800 million fibres) that connects neocortical areas, integrating their functions. Development of the corpus callosum is a late event in ontogenesis, taking place between 12 and 18 weeks (Volpe 2008). The corpus callosum may be completely absent (agenesis) or partially formed. If it is partially formed, the portions that form earlier (posterior genu, anterior body) will be formed but the portions formed later (posterior body, splenium, anterior/inferior genu and rostrum) will not be formed.

Agenesis of the corpus callosum

ACC is more correctly termed dysgenesis because the fibres that normally cross the midline are not absent, but remain forming the bundles of Probst on the internal aspect of the homolateral hemisphere (Fig. 40.83a–f). It is one of the most common brain abnormalities, with an incidence of 0.05–0.7% in the general population and in 2–5% in patients with mental retardation (Jeret et al. 1985). It is recognised that the diagnosis of isolated ACC is relatively unusual as it is frequently associated with a range of brain abnormalities such as ventriculomegaly, Dandy–Walker syndrome, Chiari II malformation, holoprosencephaly, encephalocele and cortical developmental abnormalities (with grey-matter heterotopia being the most common) (Parrish et al. 1979; Barkovich and Norman 1988; Goldstein et al. 1990; Barkovich and Kjos 1992a; d'Ercole et al. 1998; Fratelli et al. 2007; Tang et al. 2009). More recently, delayed sulcation was shown in fetuses with ACC, suggesting that there is more global white-matter dysgenesis (Warren et al. 2010; Tang et al. 2009).

One important disorder characterised by ACC in females is the Aicardi syndrome. Aicardi syndrome is defined as a triad of partial or complete ACC, infantile spasms and chorioretinal lacunae (Aicardi 2005).

While ACC is often associated with mental retardation, a significant proportion of individuals with ACC have intelligence quotients within normal range and no neurological impairment (Badaruddin et al. 2007; Paul et al. 2007). Indeed, if ACC is a genuinely isolated finding, then neurodevelopmental outcome is normal in 80–85% of patients (Goodyear et al. 2001; Francesco et al. 2006; Fratelli et al. 2007; Chadie et al. 2008). Gupta and Lilford (1995) reported a 56% risk of developmental delay for children with ACC when associated with other cerebral abnormalities, and an 85% chance of a normal outcome in isolated ACC. Despite normal intelligence, more subtle cognitive deficits have been reported in areas such as, for example, interhemispheric transfer complex sensory information and learning (Sauerwein and Lassonde 1983; Mueller et al. 2009) and bimanual motor coordination (Mueller et al. 2009). Symington et al. (2010) showed recently that there seems to be a combination of difficulty integrating information from multiple sources resulting in a less robust theory of mind. The difficulty

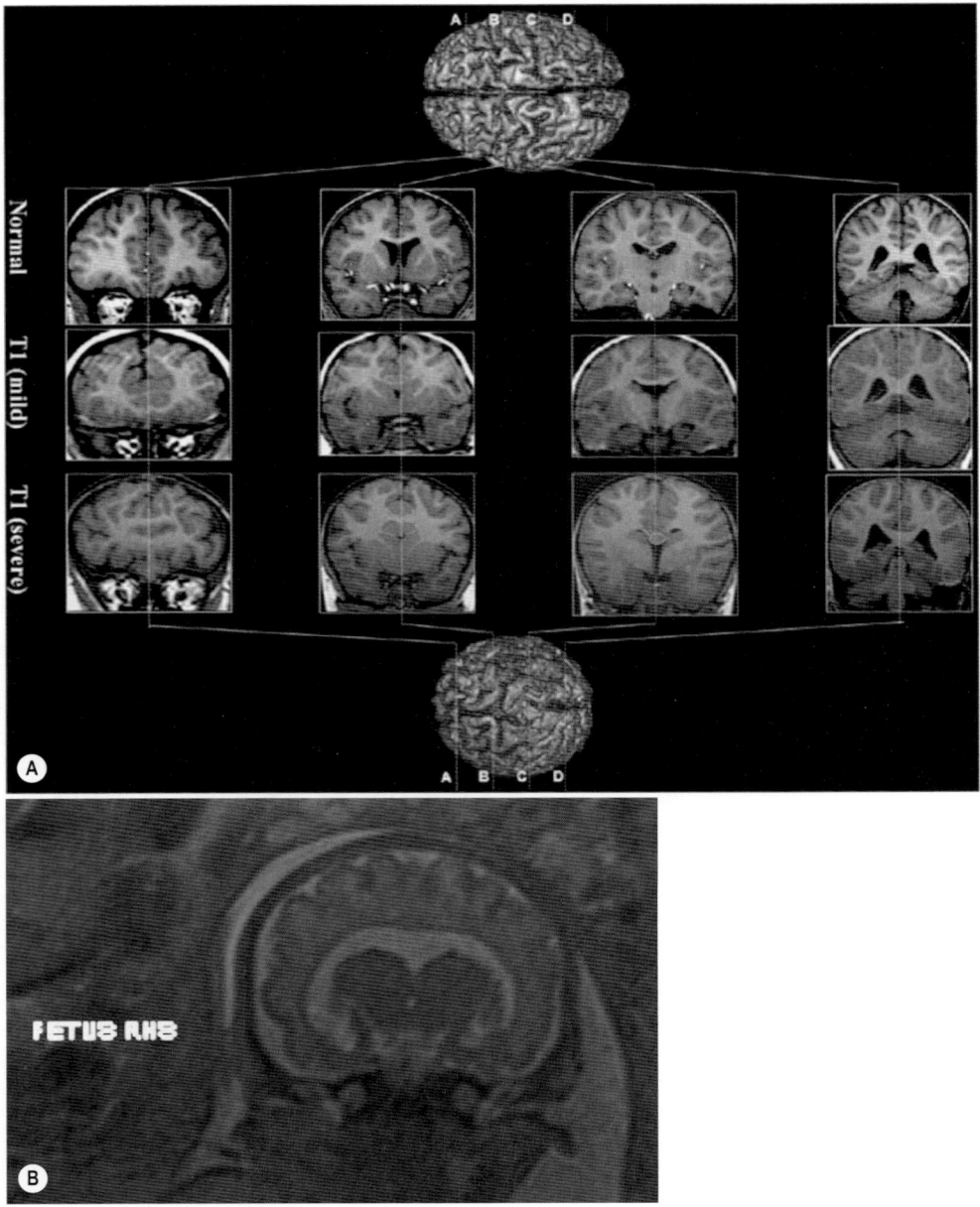

Fig. 40.81 (a) Coronal images of control and holoprosencephaly brain, referenced to cerebral exterior, with minimal and maximal degrees of malformation. The midforebrain images (B–D) of the control brain illustrate discontinuity of neocortical faces of interhemispheric fissure in superior relation to corpus callosum. The fornices are separated from thalamus by closed choroid fissure and choroid plexus (B–D). Rostrally in the two brains with holoprosencephaly, left and right cortex are continuous at the fundus of a partial-depth interhemispheric fissure (A, B). There are no evident septal nuclei, fornix or septal choroid plexus and the ventricular system is continuous through the open septal limbs of the choroid fissures (B, C). Caudally the interhemispheric fissure becomes full-depth and left and right cortical faces are bridged at the fundus by a seam of grey matter (C) (masks). The seam may be traced rostrally to where it becomes continuous with the conjoined heads of the caudate encapsulating the anterior tip of a probe-shaped tip of the forebrain ventricle. In caudal relation to the corpus callosum, left and right cortex are normally discontinuous in the fundus of the full-depth interhemispheric fissure. Occipital and temporal structures are topologically normal (D). In contrast to the abnormal structures of the septal limb, the temporal limb of choroid fissure and hippocampus extending from amygdala to hippocampal commissure (B–D) as well as the topology of internal capsules, thalamus (B), subthalamus, penduncles (C) and lower brainstem and cerebellum (D), are normal. *(Reproduced from Takahashi et al. 2003 with permission.)* (b) *Fetus with the middle interhemispheric variant of holoprosencephaly (sytelencephaly).* There is failure of separation of the cerebral hemispheres in the midzone.

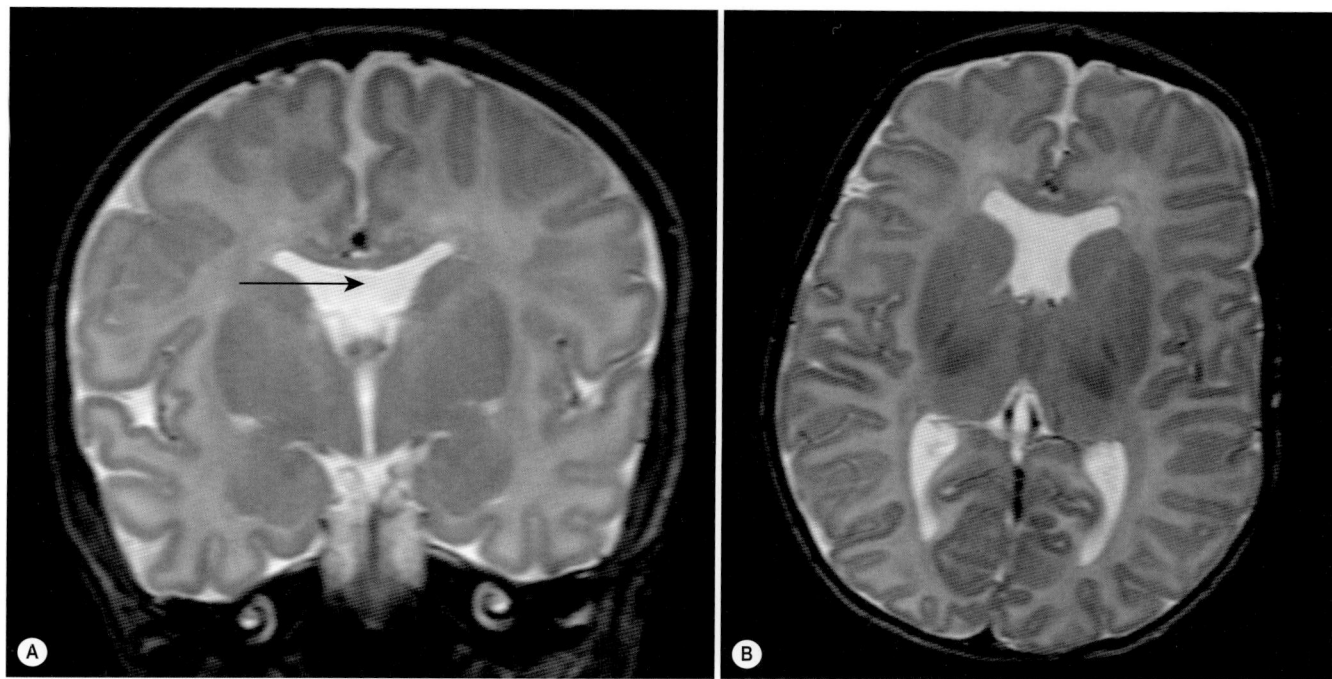

Fig. 40.82 (a) Coronal T2-weighted magnetic resonance imaging (MRI) showing absence of the septum pellucidum in the midline (arrow). (b) Axial T2-weighted MR image showing absence of the septum pellucidum.

in counselling antenatally is that it is not possible reliably to exclude grey-matter heterotopia or polymicrogyria. Figure 40.83g shows the MRI of a baby with an interhemispheric cyst, ACC and an area of polymicrogyria and grey-matter heterotopia in the right frontal lobe.

Malformation of cortical development

Cortical malformations are divided into three groups based upon the step that is likely first disturbed:

1. stem cell proliferation or apoptosis
2. neuronal migration
3. late migration and cortical organisation (Table 40.33) (Barkovich 2005; Volpe 2008).

Many causes that inhibit normal glial or neuronal proliferation, neuronal migration or organisation can result in a cortical malformation. The causes of cortical malformations can be chromosomal mutations, infections or ischaemia and/or exogenous toxins such as drugs or alcohol, endogenous toxins from metabolic disorders such as pyruvate dehydrogenase deficiency or non-ketotic hyperglycinaemia. In the next few paragraphs we discuss in more detail hemimegalencephaly, lissencephaly, heterotopia, polymicrogyria and schizencephaly.

Malformation due to abnormal proliferation

Hemimegalencephaly or unilateral megalencephaly is a rare hamartomatous malformation of the brain, involving excessive growth of one cerebral hemisphere with defects in neuronal proliferation,

migration and organisation. The brain can be affected in isolation (isolated hemimegalencephaly) or in association with cutaneous abnormalities, or sometimes there is also enlargement of the ipsilateral half of the body. In total hemimegalencephaly there is also enlargement of the ipsilateral cerebellar hemisphere and brainstem (Flores-Sarnat 2002).

Neurocutaneous syndromes associated with hemimegalencephaly include epidermal naevus syndrome, proteus syndrome, Klippel–Trenaunay–Weber syndrome (Fig. 40.84), hypomelanosis of Ito, neurofibromatosis and tuberous sclerosis (Dermatology chapter). Hemimegalencephaly can occur in either side of the brain and macrocephaly can be the first clinical sign, noted at birth or during fetal life. Some affected newborn infants present with intractable seizures that begin at a very early age, with hemiplegia and severe developmental delay (Barkovich and Chuang 1990). Epilepsy occurs in up to 93% of infants with hemimegalencephaly, and is the most frequent and severe neurological manifestation (Vigevano et al. 1989). The seizures are usually refractory to treatment and evolve into severe epilepsy in infancy (Vigevano et al. 1989). Hemimegalencephaly must be suspected early from the clinical picture. MRI can confirm hemimegalencephaly and rule out any other reason for macrocephaly. Electroencephalogram (EEG) is mandatory in every patient with megalencephaly because of the high incidence of epilepsy. Hemispherectomy within the first few months of life has been shown to improve outcome (Vigevano and Di Rocco 1990; Battaglia et al. 1999; Lettori et al. 2008).

Microcephaly is often defined as a head circumference of 3 SD or more below the mean. Microcephaly can be divided into primary and secondary, where primary is used to imply a static developmental anomaly whereas secondary microcephaly indicates a progressive neurodegenerative condition (Dobyns 2002). There are many genetic and non-genetic causes for microcephaly, such as congenital

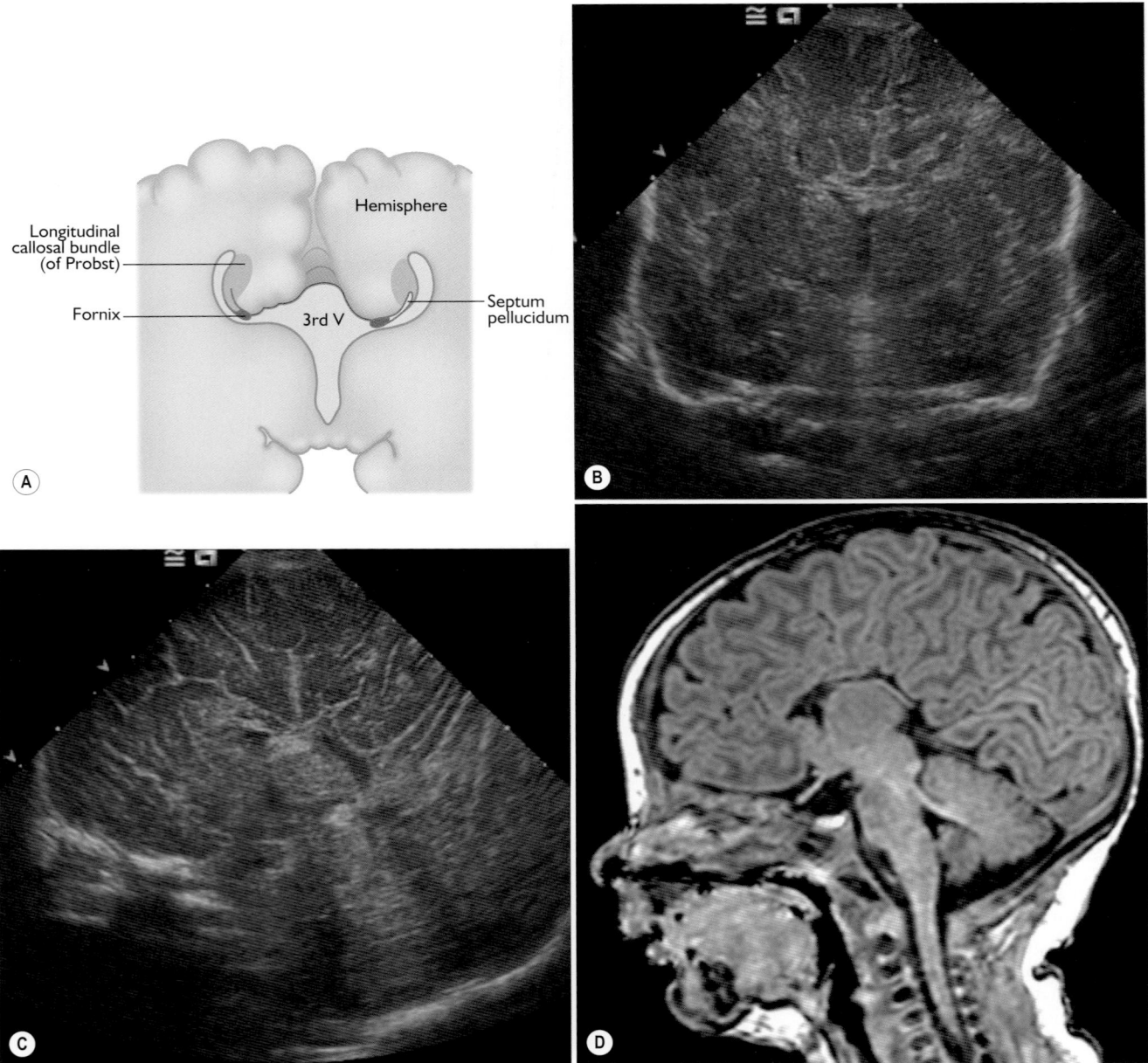

Fig. 40.83 (a) Schematic illustrating the findings in callosal agenesis. The lateral ventricles have a crescentic shape secondary to the medially located bundles of Probst. The third ventricle extends upward between the lateral ventricles into the interhemispheric fissure. The cingulated gyri remain everted and the cingulated sulci do not form. *(Reproduced from Barkovich 2005, with permission.)* (b) Coronal cranial ultrasound image showing characteristic features of agenesis of the corpus callosum (ACC) with the lateral ventricles appearing like butterfly wings. (c) Midline sagittal ultrasound image showing agenesis of the corpus callosum, with 'sunburst' gyri. (d) Midline sagittal T1-weighted image showing medial hemispheric sulci radiating into the third ventricle because of lack of cingulate gyrus.

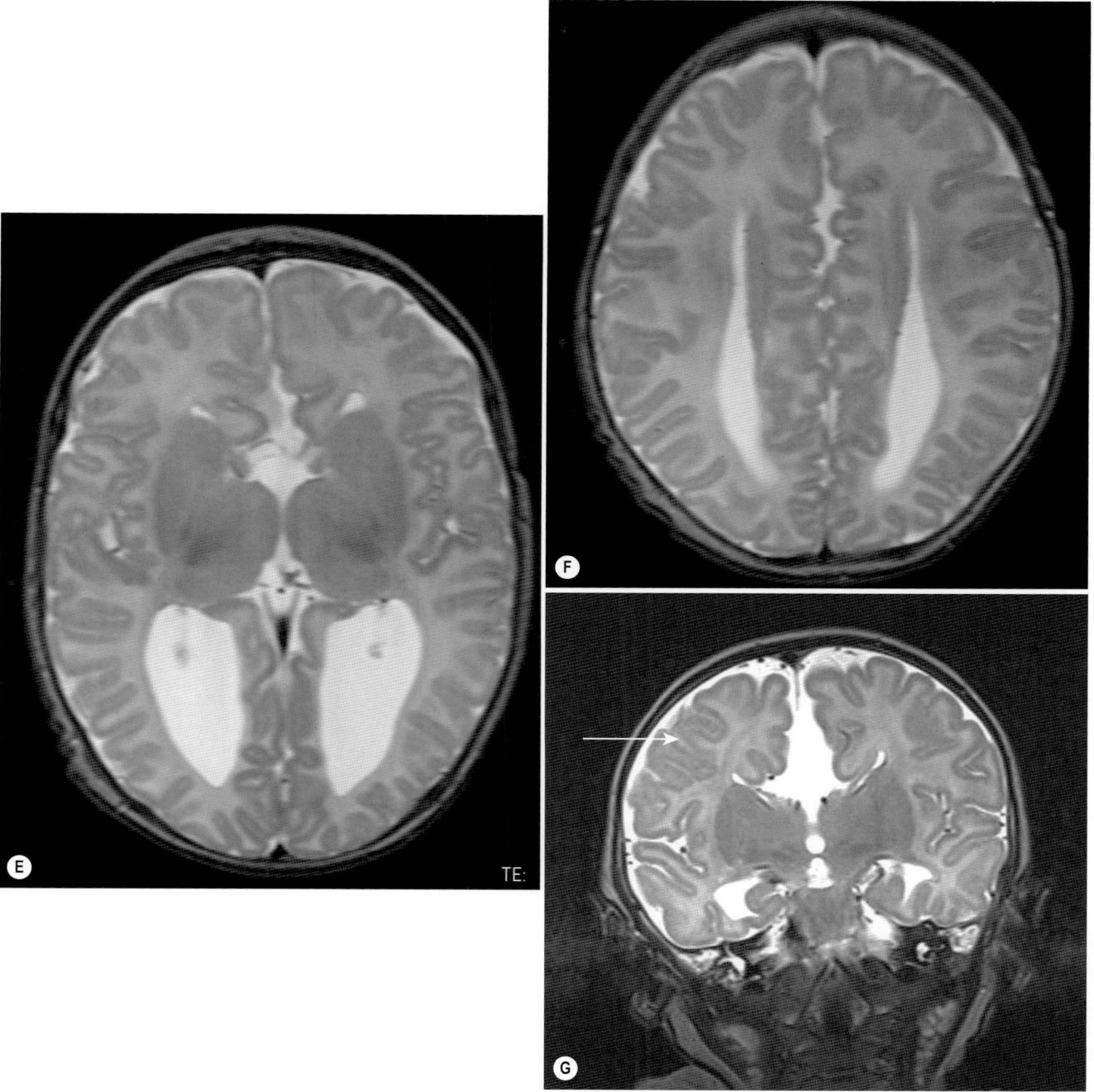

Fig. 40.83, cont'd (e and f) Axial T2-weighted images showing the colpocephaly secondary to large trigones and occipital horns in ACC (e) and that the bodies of the lateral ventricles are parallel (f). (g) Magnetic resonance imaging of a baby with an interhemispheric cyst, agenesis of the corpus callosum and an area of polymicrogyria and grey-matter heterotopia in the right frontal lobe (arrow).

Table 40.33 Classification of cortical malformations

1. Malformations due to abnormal neuronal and glial proliferation or apoptosis
   a. Decreased proliferation
      i. Microcephalies
   b. Increased proliferation
      i. Megalencephalies
   c. Abnormal proliferation
      i. Non-neoplastic
         1. Cortical hamartomas of tuberous sclerosis
         2. Cortical dysplasia with balloon cells
         3. Hemimegalencephaly
      ii. Neoplastic
         1. Dysembryoplastic neuroepithelial tumour
         2. Ganglioglioma
         3. Gangliocytoma
2. Malformation due to abnormal neuronal migration
   a. Lissencephaly/subcortical band heterotopia spectrum
   b. Cobblestone complex
      i. Congenital muscular dystrophy syndromes
      ii. Syndromes with no involvement of muscle
   c. Heterotopia
      i. Subependymal periventricular
      ii. Subcortical
      iii. Marginal glioneuronal
3. Malformations due to abnormal cortical organisation
   a. Polymicrogyria and schizencephaly
      i. Bilateral polymicrogyria syndromes
      ii. Schizencephaly
      iii. Polymicrogyria
   b. Cortical dysplasia without balloon cells
   c. Microdysgenesis
4. Malformations of cortical development, not otherwise classified
   a. Malformations secondary to inborn errors of metabolism
      i. Mitochondrial and pyruvate metabolic disorders
      ii. Peroxisomal disorders
   b. Other unclassified malformations
      i. Sublobar dysplasia
      ii. Others

(Modified from Barkovich et al. 2001.)

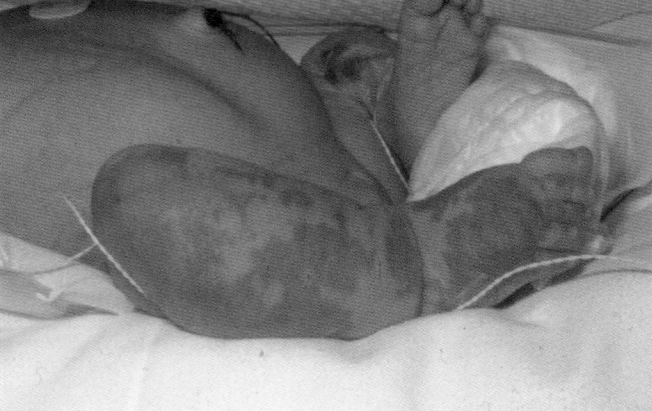

Fig. 40.84 Appearance of Klippel–Trenaunay syndrome, a neurocutaneous syndrome associated with hemimegalencephaly.

infections (toxoplasmosis, cytomegalovirus infection) and fetal alcohol syndrome.

In autosomal-recessive primary microcephaly (MCPH), the initial defining features are microcephaly at least 4 SD below the mean for age and sex, mental retardation, but no other neurological findings, such as spasticity or progressive cognitive decline. The diagnosis rests on the finding of a very small head in a baby of normal height, weight, appearance, karyotype and brain scan (Jackson et al. 2002; Roberts et al. 2002; Woods et al. 2005). Some MCPH1 children may show periventricular heterotopia, suggesting a migration disorder (Woods et al. 2005). MCPH genes have been identified which are available for prenatal or postnatal diagnosis and carrier testing. There are at least seven genes, of which four have been identified, suggesting that MCPH is probably a disorder of neurogenic mitosis (Woods et al. 2005). Microcephaly with simplified gyral pattern is diagnosed on imaging with too few gyri and abnormally shaped shallow sulci. Six different patient groups based on the neonatal course and neuroimaging have been described (Barkovich 2005).

Malformations due to abnormal neuronal migration

Lissencephaly means 'smooth brain' and refers to a paucity of gyral and sulcal development. It includes agyria and pachygyria and is the most severe form of neuronal migration malformation. Agyria is defined as an absence of gyri on the surface of the brain in association with thick cortex and is synonymous with 'complete lissencephaly'. Pachygyria is defined as the presence of few, flat gyri with thickened cortex and is synonymous with 'incomplete lissencephaly'. A finding of broad gyri and shallow sulci in the absence of thickened cortex should be considered as simplified gyral pattern.

Lissencephaly is believed to result from a complete interruption of normal neuronal migration. Type I lissencephaly is also known as classical lissencephaly. The cerebral structure in type I lissencephaly is similar to that of an approximately 12-week-old fetus. About 60% of cases with classical lissencephaly (agyria–pachygyria complex) have a defect of the lissencephaly1 (LIS1) gene at locus 17p13.3; a subset of the group with chromosome 17 mutations has characteristic facies and is classified as having the Miller–Dieker syndrome. About one-half of the remaining patients with classical lissencephaly have mutations of the doublecortin (DCX) gene at chromosome Xq22.3-q23; these patients are typically boys whose mothers have heterotopia (Gambello et al. 2003). Lissencephaly with cerebellar hypoplasia and X-linked lissencephaly are less common. X-linked lissencephaly is associated with absent corpus callosum and ambiguous genitalia, caused by mutations of the ARX gene on chromosome Xp22.13 (Kitamura et al. 2002).

Type II (also known as cobblestone lissencephaly), is characterised as HARD(E) syndrome (hydrocephaly, agyria and retinal dysplasia) with or without encephalocele (Pagon et al. 1978). The three syndromes associated with lissencephaly type II are Fukuyama congenital muscular dystrophy, Finnish muscle–eye–brain disorder and Walker–Warburg syndrome. The major clinical features of Walker–Warburg syndrome (Fig. 40.85a and b) are macrocephaly, congenital hydrocephalus, retinal malformations, congenital muscular dystrophy, cerebellar malformations and type II lissencephaly (Dobyns et al. 1985). Four genes have been associated with type II lissencephaly (POMT1 and POMT2 for Walker–Warburg, POMGnT1 for the Finnish muscle–eye–brain disease and fukutin for Fukuyama congenital muscular dystrophy).

Usually microcephaly is not present at birth, but characteristically develops during the first year of life; marked hypotonia and paucity

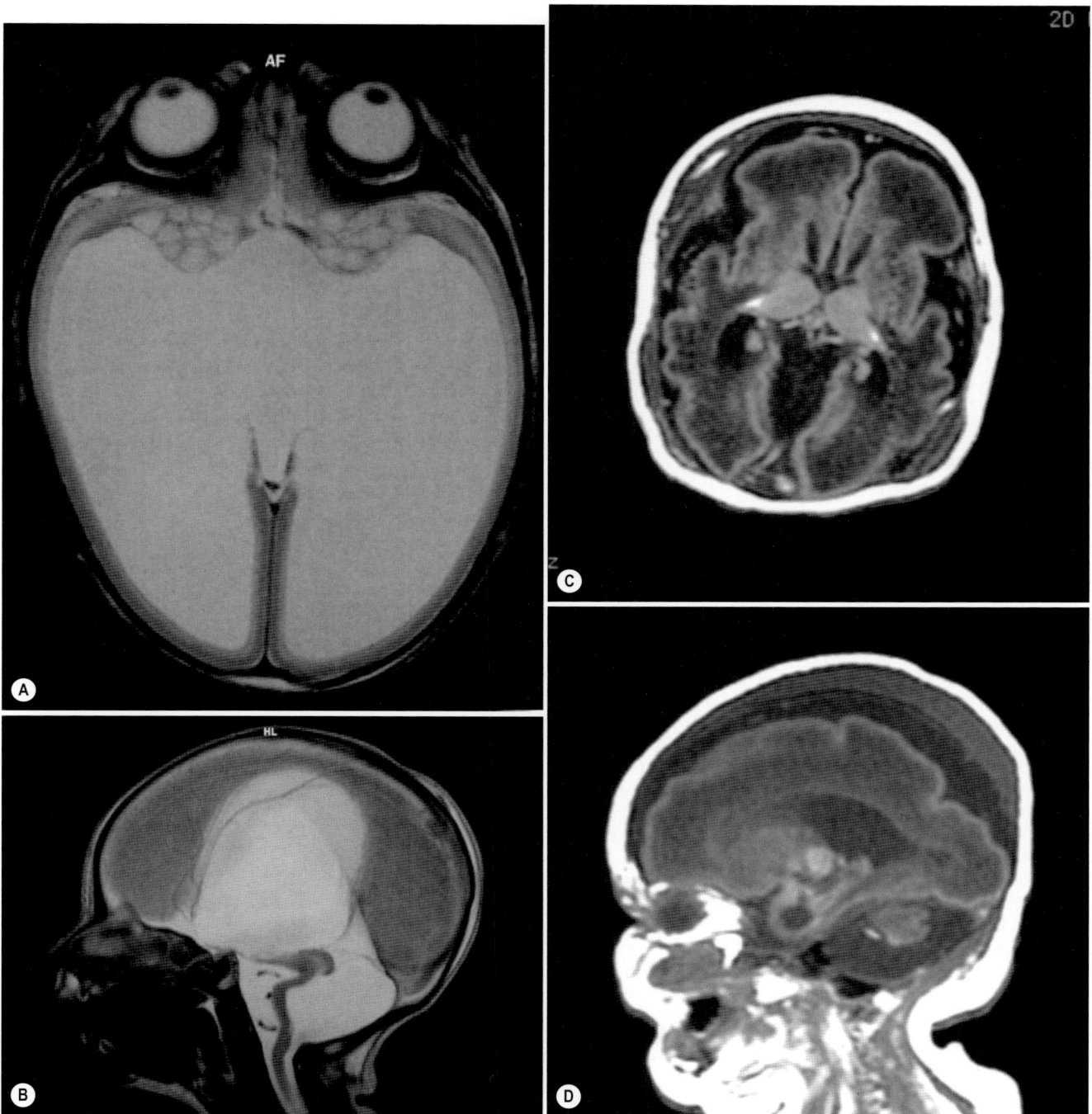

Fig. 40.85 Walker–Warburg syndrome. (a) T2-weighted axial magnetic resonance (MR) image showing massive hydrocephalus. (b) T1-weighted MR image showing very thin pons, dorsal 'kink' at the mesencephalic–pontine junction and absent vermis. *(Reproduced from www.neonet.ch, with permission.)* (c and d) Axial and parasagittal MR image showing lissencephaly.

of movements are typical. Infantile spasms are the rule and the EEG is always abnormal (Volpe 2008). There is always severe mental retardation, diplegia and seizure disorder in classical lissencephaly (Fig. 40.85 c and d).

Heterotopia refers to grey-matter collection (in nodular or laminar form) in an abnormal location (other than the cortex) due to arrest of radial migration of neurons. Heterotopia can be isolated or in association with other cerebral abnormalities.

Heterotopia is divided into three groups:

1. subependymal heterotopia
2. focal subcortical heterotopia
3. band heterotopia.

Subependymal heterotopia can be asymmetric and confined to the trigones and the temporal and occipital horns or can completely line the walls of the ventricles. They can be familial, with both

X-linked and autosomal-recessive pattern of inheritance (Sheen et al. 2003). Mutation of Filamin-1 at chromosome Xq28 has been identified (Dobyns et al. 1997). Children with isolated heterotopia usually manifest mild clinical symptoms with normal motor function and development and late seizure onset during the second decade of life (Barkovich and Kjos 1992a). Infants with focal subcortical heterotopia, however, have variable outcome depending on the size and location of the affected cortex. Those with large or thick unilateral lesions can have hemiplegia and less severe intellectual delay, whereas children with small or thin lesions may have normal motor function and normal development (Barkovich and Kjos 1992a). Almost all affected infants develop seizures, usually during the first or second decade of life (Barkovich and Kjos 1992a). Infants with band heterotopia (double cortex) may present with developmental delay and mixed seizure disorder. It mainly occurs in females and this is consistent with the report of a genetic locus on chromosome Xq22.3-q23 coding for DXC (doublecortin) gene (Ross et al. 1997).

Malformations due to abnormal cortical organisation

Polymicrogyria is characterised by a great number of small plications in the cortical surface (Figs 40.83g). The multitude of small gyri are arranged in complicated festoon-like formations (Volpe 2008). It is thought that polymicrogyria results from an insult to the brain that occurs toward the end of the neuronal migration period, during the early phase of cortical organisation (Ferrer and Catala 1991; Barkovich et al. 1995).

The two major histological variants are layered and unlayered polymicrogyria. The non-layered type represents a disorder of neuronal migration, thus appears no later than the fourth or fifth month of gestation. The layered type is a postmigrational disorder (Volpe 2008). The layered type has four distinct layers and often coexists with more severe ischaemic destructive lesions such as hydrancephaly, or in association with destructive infectious processes such as cytomegalovirus or toxoplasmosis infections (Marques Dias et al. 1984; de Vries et al. 2004).

Several syndromes have been associated with cerebral polymicrogyria, including bilateral opercular polymicrogyria (Guerreiro et al. 2000), the bilateral symmetrical frontoparietal polymicrogyria (Guerrini et al. 2000), syndrome of congenital hemiplegia and epilepsy (Pascual-Castroviejo et al. 2001) and the syndrome of megalencephaly with polymicrogyria and hydrocephalus (Barkovich et al. 2001). Epilepsy syndromes such as the Aicardi syndrome can be associated with polymicrogyria. A broad range of clinical features have been described, and the disability ranges from a severely neurologically abnormal infant with intractable epilepsy to a child with only mild neurological abnormalities. The outcome depends on the location and extent of the microgyri and the association with other brain abnormalities (corpus callosum abnormalities, cerebellar hypoplasia, periventricular nodular and sucortical heterotopia) (Barkovich 2010; Guerrini and Filippi 2005). Polymicrogyria may be focal, multifocal or diffuse; it may be unilateral, bilateral and asymmetrical; or bilateral and symmetrical. The most common location is around the sylvian fissure (Fig. 40.86) (Barkovich 2010).

Schizencephaly is the term used to describe grey-matter-lined clefts that extend through the entire hemisphere, from the ependymal lining of the lateral ventricles to the pial covering of the cortex (Yakolev and Wadsworth 1946a, b). They tend to occur in the regions of the rolandic and sylvian fissures, and involve predominantly frontal areas. Some cases are caused by an environmental insult in the second trimester; in other cases the disorder is familial

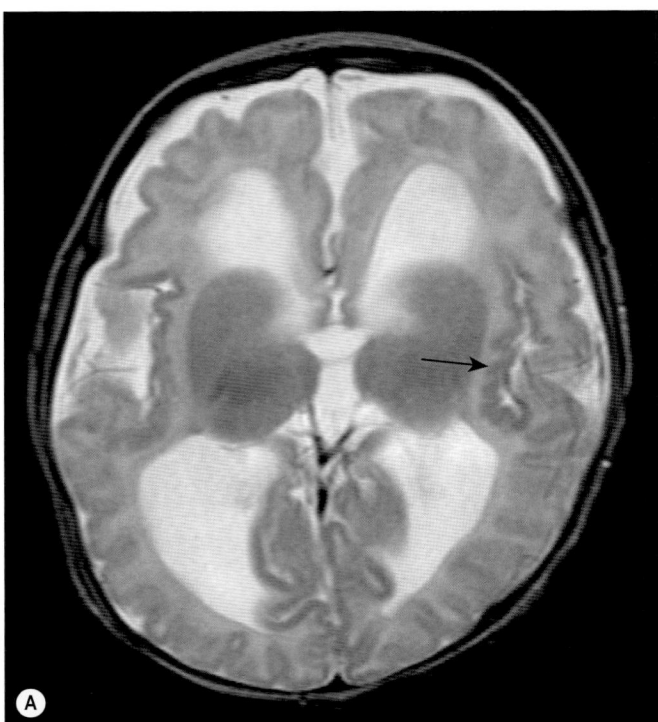

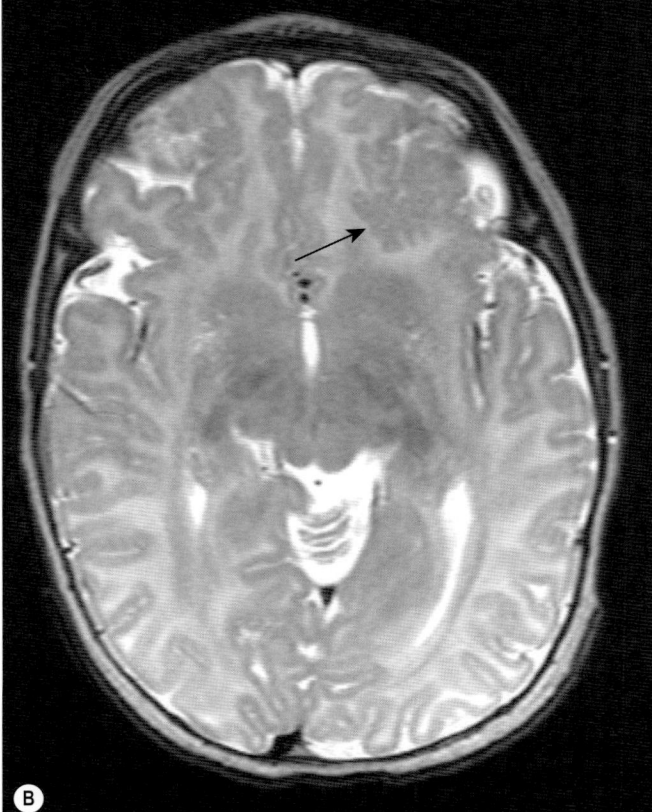

Fig. 40.86 Polymicrogyria. Axial T2-weighted magnetic resonance images showing (a) severe ventriculomegaly and bilateral perisylvian polymicrogyria (arrow) and (b) polymicrogyria in the frontal cortex (arrow).

and may be associated with mutations of the EMX2 homeobox gene, located on chromosome 10q26 (Brunelli et al. 1996; Granata et al. 1997). For prognostic purposes patients with schizencephaly are divided first into those with unilateral and bilateral clefts, then into fused or separated lips. The clinical (motor and cognitive outcome) features of schizencephaly are extremely variable and their severity is closely related to the size and bilaterality of the cleft. Children with unilateral schizencephaly often present with hemiparesis and mild mental delay. Children with bilateral cleft are usually tetraplegic with severe mental deficits and blindness (Barkovich and Kjos 1992b; Granata et al. 1997; Denis et al. 2000). Seizures can be the first neurological sign. Epilepsy is noted in 50–80% of cases of schizencephaly, with onset before the age of 3 years in 81% of cases (Granata et al. 1996, 2005). In most reports, seizures begin earlier and have worse outcome in patients with bilateral cleft, although seizures in unilateral ones are more frequent (Granata et al. 1996).

Ventriculomegaly

Fetal ventriculomegaly is the most common cerebral malformation found in fetal life, occurring in 1–2 per 1000 newborn infants (Achiron et al. 1993). Fetal ventriculomegaly is a sensitive marker for cerebral abnormalities (Filly et al. 1989). It is defined as the width of the atria of the lateral ventricles greater than 10 mm, which is 4 SD above the mean atrial width (Cardoza et al. 1988). The severity is said to be mild if the atrial width is 10–12 mm, moderate if 12–15 mm and severe if the atrial width is more than 15 mm. Male infants tend to have larger ventricles than female fetuses (Patel et al. 1994; Nadel and Benacerraf 1995) and male infants are more often found to have mild ventriculomegaly than female infants (Vergani et al. 1998; Gaglioti et al. 2005). Fetal ventriculomegaly can be due to many causes, such as an obstruction to CSF flow, loss of brain volume or secondary to cerebral malformations. Other causes of ventriculomegaly are intracerebral haemorrhage or periventricular leukomalacia.

In some cases, ventriculomegaly is the only abnormality (isolated ventriculomegaly). However, additional cerebral abnormalities can be found in about 41–78% of fetuses with ventriculomegaly (Cardoza et al. 1988; Kelly et al. 2001; Garel et al. 2003; Salomon et al. 2006, 2007). There seems to be a clear relationship between degree of ventriculomegaly and the risk of additional cerebral abnormalities. A recent study showed that fetuses with severe ventriculomegaly have a 10 times increased risk for an additional abnormality than fetuses with mild ventriculomegaly (Griffiths et al. 2010). Isolated ventriculomegaly is a diagnosis of exclusion, and certain exclusion of associated CNS or other problems remains difficult. Most studies have used fetal MRI to define isolated ventriculomegaly, as fetal MRI seems to detect more additional cerebral abnormalities than prenatal sonography (Levine et al. 1997; Simon et al. 2000; Launay et al. 2002; Garel et al. 2003; Whitby et al. 2004; Griffiths et al. 2005, 2010; Salomon et al. 2006; Hagmann et al. 2008). Excluding meningoceles, Garel et al. (2003) found additional brain abnormalities in 44% of fetuses with ventriculomegaly, including ACC in 9.5%, ischaemic injury in 7%, posterior fossa abnormality in 7% and many other causes. Vergani et al. (1998) found that an atrial width <12 mm was associated with other anomalies in only 6% of cases, compared with 56% when the atrial width was >12 mm. Other studies found that the incidence of associated anomalies was higher in fetuses having atria measuring 11–15 mm than those with atria measuring 10 mm (Tomlinson et al. 1997; Gaglioti et al. 2005; Morris et al. 2007). Data from several studies indicate that the associated anomalies account for

most of the increased mortality and morbidity in fetuses with ventriculomegaly (Chervenak et al. 1984; Nyberg et al. 1987; Mahony et al. 1988; Pilu et al. 1989; Goldstein et al. 1990; Bromley et al. 1991; Filly et al. 1991; Achiron et al. 1993; Patel et al. 1994; Vergani et al. 1998).

Comprehensive and detailed fetal ultrasound imaging is the primary investigation in a fetus found to have ventriculomegaly, in order to detect associated fetal abnormalities. The importance of separating the cases of isolated mild ventriculomegaly from those with associated abnormalities in order to counsel accordingly about the prognosis is essential. If mild fetal ventriculomegaly is found, investigation should include targeted ultrasound imaging aimed at the detection of associated CNS and other anomalies, karyotyping and screening for congenital infections and the presence of alloimmune thrombocytopenia (Hagmann and Rennie 2008).

Before beginning counselling parents whose fetus is found to have fetal ventriculomegaly it is important to establish the following facts as far as possible (Hagmann and Rennie 2008):

- the severity of the ventriculomegaly (10–12 mm; 12–15 mm; >15 mm)
- the gestation at which the diagnosis was first made and if there has been any progression
- the presence of any other abnormality (based on detailed ultrasound imaging of the fetus with MRI in appropriate cases)
- the karyotype and sex of the fetus
- whether there is any evidence of alloimmune thrombocytopenia
- whether there is any evidence of congenital infection.

If ventriculomegaly is isolated, then counselling is based on the severity of the ventriculomegaly. The prognosis for fetuses with severe ventriculomegaly (>15 mm) is poor, particularly when the ventriculomegaly is associated with other abnormalities (Chervenak et al. 1984; Twining et al. 1994; Graham et al. 2001; Gaglioti et al. 2005; Breeze et al. 2007; Joo et al. 2008; Nomura et al. 2010).

In a recent large study the neurodevelopmental outcome of 253 fetuses which were classified into four diagnostic groups – (1) normal; (2) isolated mild ventriculomegaly; (3) ventriculomegaly >12 mm; and (4) ventriculomegaly with other cerebral abnormalities – was examined at 6 months, 1 and/or 2 years (Beeghly et al. 2010). Fetuses with severe ventriculomegaly and those associated with additional cerebral abnormalities were less likely to proceed to a live birth with survival beyond the neonatal period. Among live-borns, neither ventriculomegaly group nor prenatal atrial width was related to postnatal developmental outcome. The mental developmental index was within the normal range in most infants in each group; however, the psychomotor scores were only within normal range in 47–60% of infants, suggesting that infants with ventriculomegaly are at increased risk for neuromotor delays regardless of the severity of the ventriculomegaly or the presence of additional cerebral abnormalities (Ouahba et al. 2006; Beeghly et al. 2010).

Mortality rate ranging between 20% and 40% is reported in infants with severe ventriculomegaly (Levitsky et al. 1995; Breeze et al. 2005; Kennelly et al. 2009); normal outcome occurs in 10–11% of infants with severe ventriculomegaly, and hence, abnormal neurodevelopmental outcome is from mild to severe in 90% (Levitsky et al. 1995; Graham et al. 2001; Breeze et al. 2005). Independent risk factors for perinatal loss and adverse outcome are early gestation at diagnosis, associated cerebral abnormalities, chromosomal abnormalities, malformation of cortical development and in utero progression of the ventriculomegaly (Kennelly et al. 2009; Nomura et al. 2010).

Table 40.34 Causes of neonatal hydrocephalus

Congenital malformations	Congenital aqueduct stenosis Chiari II malformation X-linked aqueduct stenosis Dandy–Walker malformation
Posthaemorrhagic	Intraventricular haemorrhage preterm Intraventricular haemorrhage at term Vitamin K deficiency bleeding
Postinfective	Neonatal meningitis Intrauterine viral infection
Neoplastic lesions	
Vascular malformations	Aneurysm of the vein of Galen Arteriovenous malformations
Choroid plexus papilloma	
Skull defects	Osteogenesis imperfecta Craniosynostosis

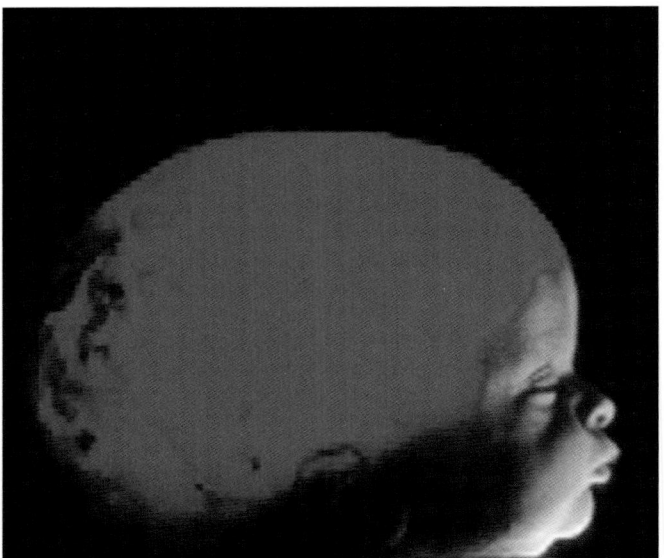

Fig. 40.87 Transillumination of the head in a case of hydrocephalus.

There is general agreement that the vast majority of children who had mild fetal ventriculomegaly function entirely normally, although as a population they are at an increased risk of developmental delay (Mahony et al. 1988; Bromley et al. 1991; Bloom et al. 1997; Goldstein et al. 2005; Laskin et al. 2005; Melchiorre et al. 2009).

Postnatal hydrocephalus is eventually always accompanied by progressive enlargement of the head size. Chiari II malformation, aqueductal stenosis and aqueductal gliosis account for about 80% of hydrocephalus in this group age (Barkovich 2005). Other causes of hydrocephalus in infancy are fetal/neonatal infections and fetal/neonatal haemorrhages (Table 40.34). Rare causes are choroid plexus papillomas (hydrocephalus resulting from excessive formation of CSF), midline tumours (hydrocephalus secondary to obstruction of CSF flow), other brain malformation such as arachnoid cysts, and vein of Galen malformation. X-linked hydrocephalus (X-linked aqueductal stenosis) is a rare hereditary disorder with mental retardation, hydrocephalus, spasticity of the lower extremities and clasped adducted thumbs (Bickers and Adams 1949). Mutation of the L1CAM genes has been localised to Xq28 (Willems et al. 1990). X-linked hydrocephalus is part of the CRASH syndrome (corpus callosum hypoplasia, retardation, adducted thumbs, spastic paraparesis and hydrocephalus), which seems to be the result of a mutation within the L1 protein (Fransen et al. 1995).

The most important clinical sign of hydrocephalus is excessive head growth. A large head size in itself might be not of any concern but serial occipitofrontal head circumference measurements that demonstrate an excessive rate of head growth require further investigation, such as cranial ultrasound and/or brain MRI. Diagnosis with transillumination of the head (Fig. 40.87) is now largely historical, and ultrasound is the method of choice for investigation of a baby with a large head. See this chapter section 5 for advice on monitoring and management of posthaemorrhagic ventricular dilatation in preterm babies.

Enlarged CSF spaces with normal or slightly normal ventricular sizes in infants without evidence of head trauma are common, and the affected infants are usually neurologically normal (Briner and Bodensteiner 1981; Ment et al. 1981; Nickel and Gallenstein 1987; Suara et al. 2001; Hellbusch 2007). The phenomenon of large CSF spaces in normal children with macrocephaly has been called benign extra-axial collections of infancy, benign external hydrocephalus and benign subdural effusions of infancy. We agree with Barkovich (2005) that the term 'benign enlargement of the subarachnoid spaces' is most appropriate and can be applied to children with large CSF with or without macrocephaly and normal neurology.

Posterior fossa abnormalities

The cerebellum begins development at approximately 5 weeks of gestation as two symmetrical thickenings on either side of the rhombencephalon (Fig. 40.88) (ten Donkelaar et al. 2003). At this time the fourth ventricle has a thin roof and laterally positioned dorsal plates, which then proliferate to form the rhombic lips. The neuroepithelial zones, in the roof of the fourth ventricle and the rhombic lips, are the location of part of the germinal matrix capillary bed. The glial and neuronal cells that compose the cerebellum migrate to their final destination in the cerebellar hemisphere by two general pathways. The neurons of the deep cerebellar nuclei and the Purkinje layer of the cerebellar cortex migrate radially outward from the germinal matrix in the wall of the fourth ventricle. The neurons of the granular layer of the cerebellar cortex migrate tangentially from the germinal zone over the cerebellar surface, forming the transitory external granular layer (Rakic and Sidman 1970). By approximately 7 weeks of gestation the cerebellar hemispheres are joined in the midline in only the rostral medullary vellum. At about 8 weeks of gestation the cerebellar hemispheres unite at the midline to form the vermis, which at this point is present rostrally but underdeveloped caudally. The vermis closes the vallecula between 14 and 17 weeks of gestation. Thereafter the vermis grows linearly with gestational age (Malinger et al. 2001).

The normal adult vermis has nine lobules. By week 8 choroid plexus can be seen with ultrasound in the fourth ventricular roof dividing the roof into area membranaceae rostralis and caudalis (Nelson et al. 2004). The area evaginates, creating the Blake's pouch, which is thin and normally disappears (Fig. 40.88) (Nelson et al. 2004).

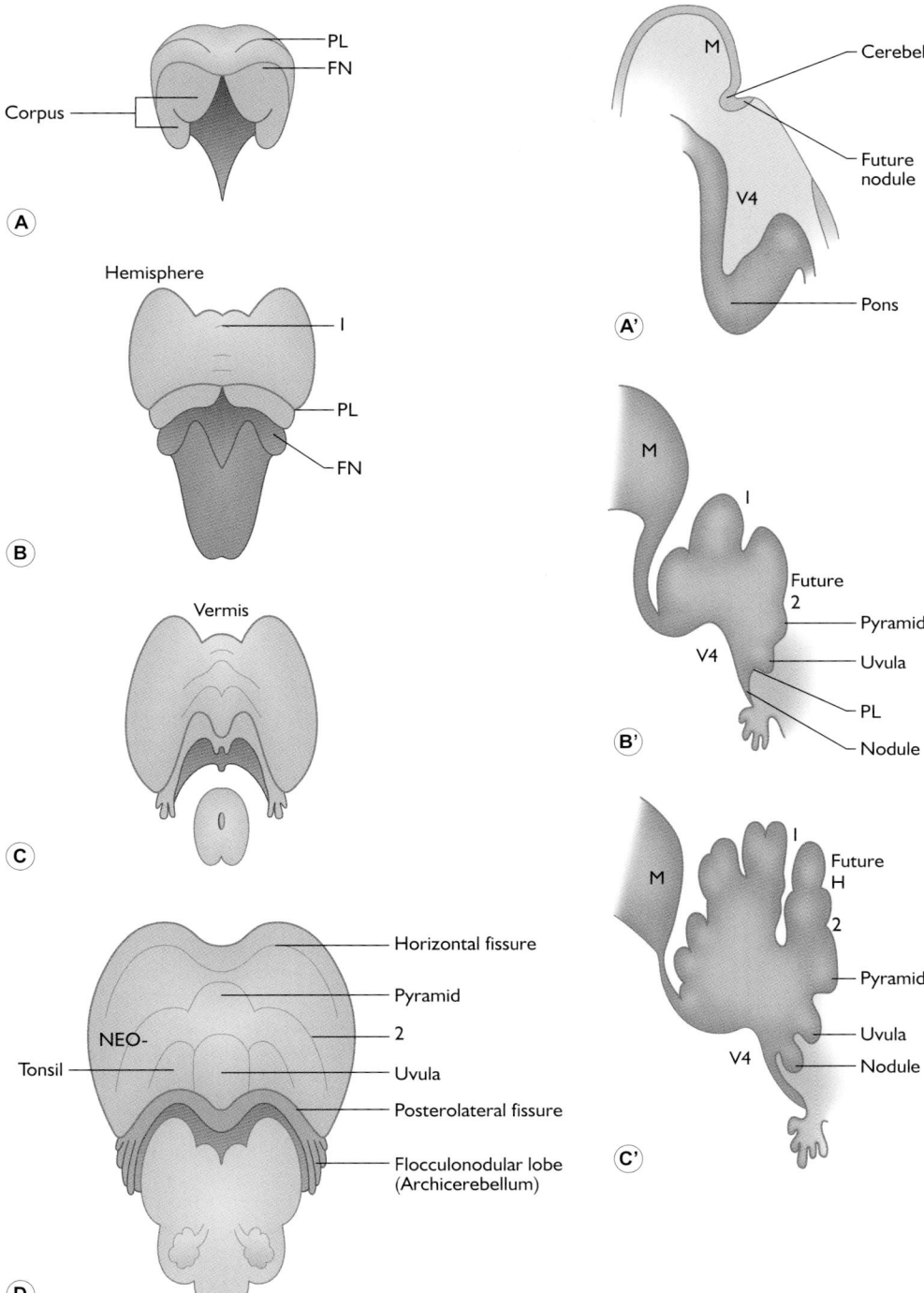

Fig. 40.88 Normal development of the cerebellum. (a) 8 weeks; (b) 13 weeks; (c) 14 weeks; (d) 19 weeks. Black-shaded areas represent the fourth ventricle. *(Reproduced from Nelson et al. 2004, with permission.)*

In 1969, Joubert et al. described five children with episodic hyperpnoea, abnormal eye movement, ataxia and mental retardation associated with agenesis of the cerebellar vermis and inherited in an autosomal-recessive manner. Since then, many children with Joubert syndrome have been described in the literature, confirming the original findings and establishing the 'molar tooth sign' as the cardinal diagnostic imaging feature (Kendall et al. 1990; Maria et al. 1999a, b). The Joubert syndrome ('molar tooth midbrain–hindbrain malformation') is associated with small dysplastic cerebellar vermis with midline clefting, dysplasia and heterotopia of cerebellar nuclei,

near-total absence of the pyramidal decussations and anomalies in the inferior olivary nuclei, descending trigeminal tract and dorsal column nuclei (Yachnis and Rorke 1999). Multiple syndromes have posterior fossa findings which are similar to those of Joubert syndrome, hence, all patients with molar tooth findings should be screened for any supratentorial anomalies and malformations in the liver, eyes and kidneys (Gleeson et al. 2004).

Complete absence of the cerebellar vermis with fusion of the cerebellar hemispheres is termed rhomboencephalosynapsis (Fig. 40.89). The prognosis for neurodevelopment is very poor.

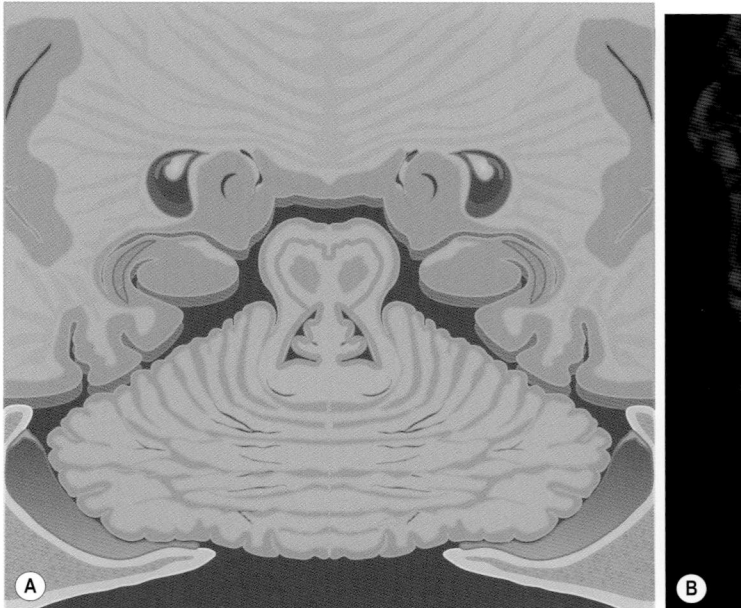
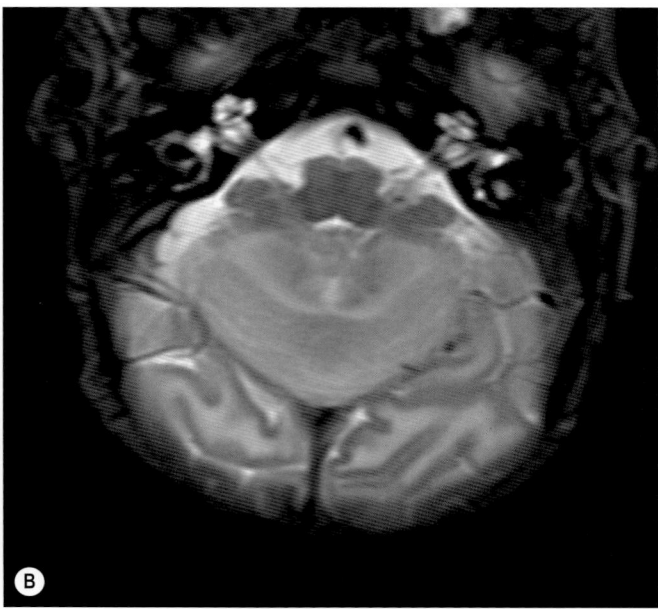

Fig. 40.89 (a) Rhomboencephalosynapsis showing absence of the cerebellar vermis. *(redrawn based on Barkovich 2007)* (b) Corresponding axial magnetic resonance imaging from a case of rhomboencephalosynapsis.

Table 40.35 Classification of cerebellar malformations

1. Cerebellar hypoplasia with cysts
   a. Focal hypoplasia
   b. Generalised hypoplasia
      i. With enlarged fourth ventricle: Dandy–Walker continuum
      ii. Normal fourth ventricle
         1. with normal pons
         2. with small pons
            a. Normal foliation
               i. Pontocerebellar hyoplasia of Barth
               ii. Cerebellar hypoplasia
2. Cerebellar dysplasia
   a. Focal dysplasia
      i. Isolated vermian dysplasia
         1. Molar tooth malformations
         2. Rhombencephalosynapsis
      ii. Isolated hemispheric dysplasia
         1. Focal cerebellar cortical dysplasias/heterotopia
         2. Lhermitte–Duclos–Cowden syndrome
   b. Generalised dysplasia
      i. Congenital muscular dystrophies
      ii. Congenital cytomegalovirus infection
      iii. Lissencephaly with rELN mutation
      iv. Lissencephaly with agenesis of the corpus callosum and cerebellar dysplasia
      v. Associated with diffuse cereberal polymicrogyria
      vi. Diffusely abnormal foliation

(Modified from Barkovich 2005.)

Classically, posterior fossa cystic abnormalities have been divided into the Dandy–Walker malformation, the Dandy–Walker variant, and the mega cisterna magna (Table 40.35). However, recent classifications are based on the morphology of the cerebellum (Barkovich 2005), as CSF collection can result from abnormal development of the cerebellum or fourth ventricle, from degeneration of the cerebellum or from formation of arachnoid cysts. The classification proposed by Barkovich (2005) is morphology-based and depends on the initial separation of cerebellar dysplasia from hypoplasia. On imaging studies, incompletely formed or small but otherwise normal-appearing cerebella are classified as hypoplastic whereas cerebella with abnormally formed folia and fissures are classified dysplastic. After the separation of incomplete formation (hypoplasia) from abnormal formation (dysplasia), the site of the abnormalities is evaluated into focal or generalised (Table 40.36) (Barkovich 2005).

Barkovich (2005) suggested using the term 'Dandy–Walker complex' to account for various imaging manifestations of this malformation. In the classification scheme of cerebellar malformation, Dandy–Walker complex falls within the classification of 'undergeneralised cerebellar hypoplasia with enlarged fourth ventricle'. The diagnosis of 'classic' Dandy–Walker malformation consists of three major abnormalities (Fig. 40.90):

1. enlarged posterior fossa with a high insertion of the tentorium cerebelli
2. complete or partial agenesis of the cerebellar vermis
3. cystic dilatation of the fourth ventricle that nearly fills the posterior fossa.

A tentorium in the correct anatomical position, not high, rules out a Dandy–Walker malformation. At the other end of the spectrum is a mildly hypoplastic vermis with a large fourth ventricle filling a normal-sized posterior fossa. The normal-sized posterior fossa Dandy–Walker cyst may simulate an arachnoid cyst or Blake's pouch cyst. However, the identification of a normal fourth ventricular choroid plexus rules out a Dandy–Walker malformation (Table 40.36) (Nelson et al. 2004).

Associated abnormalities in Dandy–Walker complex occur in up to 70% of cases and consist of ACC, aqueductal stenosis, cerebral neuronal heterotopias and abnormalities of inferior olivary or dentate nuclei (Volpe 2008). Hydrocephalus may not become apparent for months or years after birth; however, it is present in

Table 40.36 Imaging characteristics of posterior fossa cysts

TYPE	POSTERIOR FOSSA	FOURTH VENTRICULAR CHOROID PLEXUS	TORCULA	OCCIPITAL BONE	FALX CEREBELLI	CENTRAL NERVOUS SYSTEM MALFORMATION
Dandy–Walker	Normal to very large	Absent	Normal to elevated	Normal to thinned	Usually absent	Frequent
Blake's pouch	Usually normal to large	Normal to displaced	Usually normal to elevated	Normal to thinned	Usually present	Rare
Arachnoid cyst	Usually normal to large	Normal	Usually normal to elevated	Normal to thinned	Usually present	Rare

(Modified from Nelson et al. 2004.)

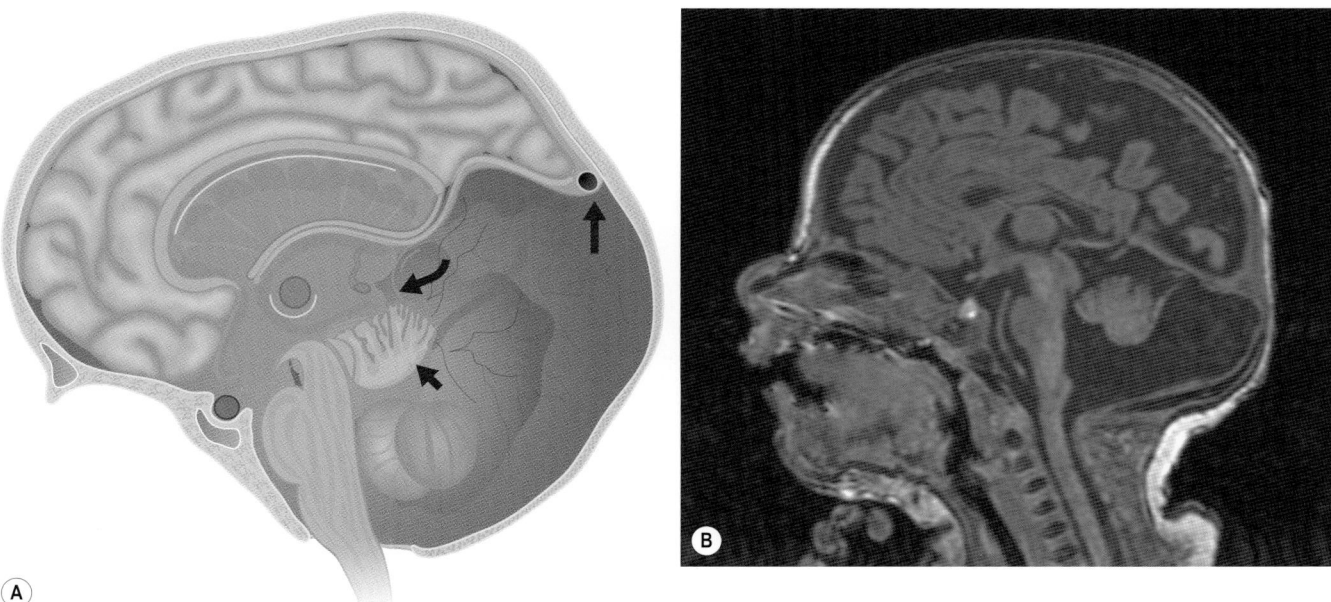

Fig. 40.90 (a) The components of the Dandy–Walker malformation. *(redrawn based on Barkovich, 2007)* The diagram shows an enlarged posterior fossa, elevated torcular heterophili, superior rotation of a hypoplastic cerebellar vermis and an overexpanded fourth ventricle with a thin wall. (b) Midline sagittal magnetic resonance imaging from a baby with Dandy–Walker variant. The cerebellar vermis is superiorly rotated but the torcular heterophili are not elevated; the fourth ventricle is expanded.

about 75% by 3 months of age (Volpe 2008). Hence, after birth the baby should be referred to a neurosurgeon and regular head circumference measurements should be performed. If undiagnosed antenatally, children under 1 year most often present with symptoms and signs of hydrocephalus and increased intracranial pressure whereas children beyond 1 year usually present with delayed achievement of milestones, particularly walking and coordination (Osenbach and Menezes 1992). Outcome is related to the severity of both the malformation and the associated anomalies, and the degree of hydrocephalus (Hirsch et al. 1984; Estroff et al. 1992; Ulm et al. 1997). Most large follow-up series of cases of Dandy–Walker complex report that most affected children have developmental delay, although the severity varies, and about a third of survivors are said to have an IQ of over 80 (Hirsch et al. 1984; Estroff et al. 1992). In other series, IQ was reported as normal in

54% of children with isolated Dandy–Walker complex (Bernard et al. 2001). Normal lobulation of the vermis, in the absence of any supratentorial anomaly, appears to be a good prognostic factor in Dandy–Walker malformation (Boddaert et al. 2003; Klein et al. 2003), whereas a dysgenetic vermis with only one or two recognisable lobes seems to be associated with not only poor neurodevelopmental outcome but also other brain malformations (Klein et al. 2003).

The term 'cisterna magna' refers to the portion of the wide subarachnoid space below the inferior cerebellar surface, behind the medulla (Robertson 1949). There is considerable variation in the size of the cisterna magna. The fetal cisterna magna is naturally wide (Haimovici et al. 1997) and widens throughout gestation before regressing postnatally. Generally in cases with mega cisterna magna the posterior fossa is wider than normal and in some cases the torcula is displaced cranially so that the posterior fossa is shaped approximately as in Dandy–Walker complex. The cerebellum, however, is not affected by any gross structural abnormalities, although in some cases hemispheric or vermian hypoplasia can be seen (Tortori-Donati et al. 1996). Mega cisterna magna is usually an incidental finding and it is not associated with hydrocephalus (Tortori-Donati et al. 1996). CSF collection in the posterior fossa should be termed mega cisterna magna only if there is no hydrocephalus or symptoms secondary to compression of the ventricular system (Tortori-Donati et al. 1996).

Persisting Blake's pouch is defined by failure of regression of Blake's pouch itself secondary to non-perforation of the foramen of Magendie (Strand et al. 1993; Tortori-Donati et al. 1996; Calabro et al. 2000). The cerebellar hemispheres and vermis can appear hypoplastic. This indicates a relaxation by the mass effect of the persisting Blake's pouch; however, some degree of cerebellar atrophy can be present due to pressure (Calabro et al. 2000). Shunting of either the lateral ventricles or the pouch restores the ventricle system to normal size and allows re-expansion of the compressed cerebellum (Tortori-Donati et al. 1996).

Arachnoid cysts

The differential diagnosis of persisting Blake's pouch includes arachnoid cyst. Arachnoid cysts are benign congenital collections of fluid that develop within the arachnoid membrane. Ultrastructural studies have shown that the cells lining true arachnoid cysts contain specialised membranes and enzymes for secretory activity (Go et al. 1984). If the arachnoid cysts expand, it seems to be an accumulation of CSF secreted by cells of the cyst wall rather than by osmotic filtration or ball-valve mechanism (Go et al. 1984; Barkovich 2005).

In many instances arachnoid cysts may be an incidental finding in children examined for head injury. But in recent years, the widespread use of antenatal ultrasound and the increasing use of fetal MRI have resulted in the frequent antenatal diagnosis of arachnoid cyst. They have a higher incidence in patients with autosomal-dominant polycystic kidney disease, in which they have been reported in as many as 8.1% of patients (Schievink et al. 1995). They are also very common in Aicardi syndrome.

The most common location is supratentorial (90%) within the middle cranial fossa (60%), with predominance of the left hemisphere and along the sylvian fissure (Wang et al. 1998; Gosalakkal 2002). Arachnoid cysts in the middle cranial fossa are usually of moderate size, and only 30% are reported to be large, occupying nearly the whole temporal fossa. Posterior fossa cysts are usually large and it is important to differentiate them from cysts of the Dandy–Walker malformation. Arachnoid cysts in the middle cranial fossa do not usually lead to dilatation of the fourth ventricle and postnatal evolving hydrocephalus is rare (Pierre-Kahn and Sonigo 2003). Suprasellar and posterior fossa cysts can lead to obstructive hydrocephalus. Interhemispheric cysts often reach a large size and are associated with dysgenesis or ACC (Griebel et al. 1995; Lena et al. 1995; Epelman et al. 2006). Spontaneous resolution of arachnoid cysts is rare; however, if the baby is asymptomatic, a wait-and-see policy may be adopted even for posterior fossa cysts (Russo et al. 2008). Although most arachnoid cysts remain static, some become enlarged, exerting a mass effect on adjacent neural structures and CSF circulation. After treatment of the cysts, the cognitive and motor outcome is generally excellent (Boltshauser et al. 2002).

Cerebrovascular malformations

There are a number of rare congenital cerebrovascular malformations, but few are recognisable in the newborn. These include the Sturge–Weber syndrome and arteriovenous aneurysms, including the aneurysm of the vein of Galen, which is characterised by heart failure and an intracranial murmur.

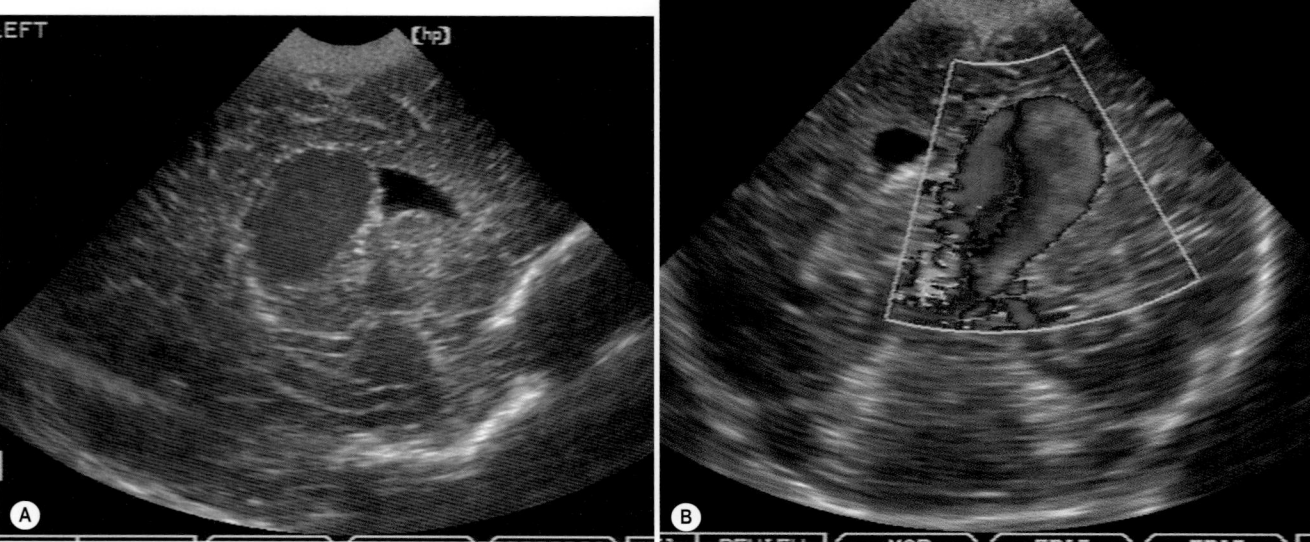

Fig. 40.91 Ultrasound appearance of vein of Galen malformation. (a) Black and white picture in the sagittal plane, with the malformation appearing as an ovoid shape filling the posterior part of the lateral ventricle. (b) Colour Doppler image in the coronal plane. The abnormal flow within the malformation is clearly seen.

Vein of Galen malformation

Aneurysms of the vein of Galen are dilatations of the vein, which range from a large single malformation to multiple smaller communications. Antenatal diagnosis is possible, giving forewarning and allowing counselling and delivery in a centre with interventional radiology. Fetuses with hydrops and babies requiring ventilation for heart failure in the neonatal period usually die, although some groups report success with very aggressive management (Frawley et al. 2002). In the neonatal period, ultrasound (Fig. 40.91) and MRI confirm the diagnosis and allow assessment of the feeder vessels. Therapeutic options now include the transarterial insertion of coils in the abnormal vessels. Lylyk et al. (1993) treated 28 children this way, 11 of whom were neonates; 17 had a good long-term outcome. Of 21 neonates (five diagnosed antenatally) treated in California between 1983 and 2002, four died in the neonatal period; seven had no abnormality at follow-up, two had minor sequelae and eight had significant neurodevelopmental problems, including epilepsy (Fullerton et al. 2003). The Great Ormond Street Hospital experience was similar, with most neonatal cases presenting in heart failure (McSweeney et al. 2010). This team treated 26 neonates between 2003 and 2008: seven died (five were not treated) and there was a high incidence of procedural-related complications, including hydrocephalus and intracranial haemorrhage. However, 14 had a good outcome. The Great Ormond Street Hospital team found that the Bicêtre score, devised in Paris by the group formerly led by Pierre Lasjaunias, did not reliably predict an adverse outcome.

Weblinks

European surveillance of congenital anomalies (Eurocat): www.eurocat-network.eu.

Office for National Statistics (UK): http://www.statistics.gov.uk. The repository of all UK national statistical data.

References

Achiron, R., Schimmel, M., et al., 1993. Fetal mild idiopathic lateral ventriculomegaly: is there a correlation with fetal trisomy? Ultrasound Obstet Gynecol 3, 89–92.

Adzick, N.S., Thom, E.A., Spong, C.Y., et al., 2011. A randomised trial of prenatal versus postnatal repair of myelomeningocele. N Engl J Med 364, 993–1004.

Aicardi, J., 2005. Aicardi syndrome. Brain Dev 27, 164–171.

Aguilera, S., Soothill, P., Denbow, M., et al., 2009. Prognosis of spina bifida in the era of prenatal diagnosis and termination of pregnancy. Fetal Diagn Ther 26, 68–74.

Badaruddin, D.H., Andrews, G.L., et al., 2007. Social and behavioral problems of children with agenesis of the corpus callosum. Child Psychiatry Hum Dev 38, 287–302.

Barkovich, A.J., 1992. Current concepts of polymicrogyria. Neuroradiology 52, 479–487.

Barkovich, A.J., 2005. Congenital malformations of the brain and skull. In: Barkovich, A.J. (Ed.), Pediatric Neuroimaging. Lippincott Williams & Wilkins, Philadelphia, pp. 291–439.

Barkovich, A.J., Chuang, S.H., 1990. Unilateral megalencephaly: correlation of MR imaging and pathologic characteristics. AJNR Am J Neuroradiol 11, 523–531.

Barkovich, A.J., Edwards, M.S., 1992. Applications of neuroimaging in hydrocephalus. Pediatr Neurosurg 18, 65–83.

Barkovich, A.J., Kjos, B.O., 1992a. Gray matter heterotopias: MR characteristics and correlation with developmental and neurologic manifestations. Radiology 182, 493–499.

Barkovich, A.J., Kjos, B.O., 1992b. Schizencephaly: correlation of clinical findings with MR characteristics. AJNR Am J Neuroradiol 13, 85–94.

Barkovich, A.J., Norman, D., 1988. Anomalies of the corpus callosum: correlation with further anomalies of the brain. AJR Am J Roentgenol 151, 171–179.

Barkovich, A.J., Norman, D., 1989. Absence of the septum pellucidum: a useful sign in the diagnosis of congenital brain malformations. AJR Am J Roentgenol 152, 353–360.

Barkovich, A.J., Rowley, H., et al., 1995. Correlation of prenatal events with the development of polymicrogyria. AJNR Am J Neuroradiol 16 (Suppl), 822–827.

Barkovich, A.J., Kuzniecky, R.I., et al., 2001. Classification system for malformations of cortical development: update 2001. Neurology 57, 2168–2178.

Battaglia, D., Di Rocco, C., et al., 1999. Neuro-cognitive development and epilepsy outcome in children with surgically treated hemimegalencephaly. Neuropediatrics 30, 307–313.

Beeghly, M., Ware, J., Soul, J., et al., 2010. Neurodevelopmental outcomes of fetuses referred for ventriculomegaly. Ultrasound Obstet Gynecol 35, 405–416.

Belhocine, O., Andre, C., et al., 2005. Does asymptomatic septal agenesis exist? A review of 34 cases. Pediatr Radiol 35, 410–418.

Bernard, J.P., Moscoso, G., et al., 2001. Cystic malformations of the posterior fossa. Prenat Diagn 21, 1064–1069.

Bickers, D.S., Adams, R.D., 1949. Hereditary stenosis of the aqueduct of Sylvius as a cause of congenital hydrocephalus. Brain 72, 246–262.

Bloom, S.L., Bloom, D.D., et al., 1997. The developmental outcome of children with antenatal mild isolated ventriculomegaly. Obstet Gynecol 90, 93–97.

Boddaert, N., Klein, O., et al., 2003. Intellectual prognosis of the Dandy–Walker malformation in children: the importance of vermian lobulation. Neuroradiology 45, 320–324.

Boltshauser, E., Martin, F., et al., 2002. Outcome in children with space-occupying posterior fossa arachnoid cysts. Neuropediatrics 33, 118–121.

Bowman, R.M., McLone, D.G., et al., 2001. Spina bifida outcome: a 25-year prospective. Pediatr Neurosurg 34, 114–120.

Breeze, A.C., Dey, P.K., et al., 2005. Obstetric and neonatal outcomes in apparently isolated mild fetal ventriculomegaly. J Perinat Med 33, 236–240.

Breeze, A.C., Alexander, P.M., Murdoch, E.M., et al., 2007. Obstetric and neonatal outcomes in severe fetal ventriculomegaly. Prenat Diagn 27, 124–129.

Briner, S., Bodensteiner, J., 1981. Benign subdural collections of infancy. Pediatrics 67, 802–804.

Bromley, B., Frigoletto Jr., F.D., et al., 1991. Mild fetal lateral cerebral ventriculomegaly: clinical course and outcome. Am J Obstet Gynecol 164, 863–867.

Brunelli, S., Faiella, A., et al., 1996. Germline mutations in the homeobox gene EMX2 in patients with severe schizencephaly. Nat Genet 12, 94–96.

Caemaert, J., Abdullah, J., et al., 1992. Endoscopic treatment of suprasellar arachnoid cysts. Acta Neurochir (Wien) 119, 68–73.

Calabro, F., Arcuri, T., et al., 2000. Blake's pouch cyst: an entity within the Dandy–Walker continuum. Neuroradiology 42, 290–295.

Cardoza, J.D., Goldstein, R.B., et al., 1988. Exclusion of fetal ventriculomegaly with a single measurement: the width of the lateral ventricular atrium. Radiology 169, 711–714.

Chadie, A., Radi, S., et al., 2008. Neurodevelopmental outcome in prenatally diagnosed isolated agenesis of the corpus callosum. Acta Paediatr 97, 420–424.

Chervenak, F.A., Duncan, C., et al., 1984. Outcome of fetal ventriculomegaly. Lancet 2, 179–181.

Coniglio, S.J., Anderson, S.M., et al., 1996. Functional motor outcome in children with myelomeningocele: correlation with anatomic level on prenatal ultrasound. Dev Med Child Neurol 38, 675–680.

d'Ercole, C., Girard, N., et al., 1998. Prenatal diagnosis of fetal corpus callosum agenesis by ultrasonography and magnetic resonance imaging. Prenat Diagn 18, 247–253.

Denis, D., Chateil, J.F., et al., 2000. Schizencephaly: clinical and imaging features in 30 infantile cases. Brain Dev 22, 475–483.

de Vries, L.S., Gunardi, H., et al., 2004. The spectrum of cranial ultrasound and magnetic resonance imaging abnormalities in congenital cytomegalovirus infection. Neuropediatrics 35, 113–119.

Dobyns, W.B., 2002. Primary microcephaly: new approaches for an old disorder. Am J Med Genet 112, 315–317.

Dobyns, W.B., Kirkpatrick, J.B., et al., 1985. Syndromes with lissencephaly. II: Walker–Warburg and cerebro-oculo-muscular syndromes and a new syndrome with type II lissencephaly. Am J Med Genet 22, 157–195.

Dobyns, W.B., Guerrini, R., et al., 1997. Bilateral periventricular nodular heterotopia with mental retardation and syndactyly in boys: a new X-linked mental retardation syndrome. Neurology 49, 1042–1047.

Duczkowska, A., Bekiesinska-Figatowska, M., Herman-Sucharska, I., et al., 2011. Magnetic resonance imaging in the evaluation of the fetal spinal canal contents. Brain Dev 33, 10–20.

Epelman, M., Daneman, A., et al., 2006. Differential diagnosis of intracranial cystic lesions at head US: correlation with CT and MR imaging. Radiographics 26, 173–196.

Estroff, J.A., Scott, M.R., et al., 1992. Dandy–Walker variant: prenatal sonographic features and clinical outcome. Radiology 185, 755–758.

Falip, C., Blanc, N., et al., 2007. Postnatal clinical and imaging follow-up of infants with prenatal isolated mild ventriculomegaly: a series of 101 cases. Pediatr Radiol 37, 981–989.

Ferrer, I., Catala I., 1991. Unlayered polymicrogyria: structural and developmental aspects. Anat Embryol (Berl) 184, 517–528.

Filly, R.A., Cardoza, J.D., et al., 1989. Detection of fetal central nervous system anomalies: a practical level of effort for a routine sonogram. Radiology 172, 403–408.

Filly, R.A., Goldstein, R.B., et al., 1991. Fetal ventricle: importance in routine obstetric sonography. Radiology 181, 1–7.

Flores-Sarnat, L., 2002. Hemimegalencephaly: part 1. Genetic, clinical, and imaging aspects. J Child Neurol 17, 373–384; discussion 384.

Francesco, P., Maria-Edgarda, B., et al., 2006. Prenatal diagnosis of agenesis of corpus callosum: what is the neurodevelopmental outcome? Pediatr Int 48, 298–304.

Fransen, E., Lemmon, V., et al., 1995. CRASH syndrome: clinical spectrum of corpus callosum hypoplasia, retardation, adducted thumbs, spastic paraparesis and hydrocephalus due to mutations in one single gene, L1. Eur J Hum Genet 3, 273–284.

Fratelli, N., Papageorghiou, A.T., et al., 2007. Outcome of prenatally diagnosed agenesis of the corpus callosum. Prenat Diagn 27, 512–517.

Frawley, G.P., Dargaville, P.A., Mitchell, P.J., et al., 2002. Clinical course and medical management of neonates with severe cardiac failure related to vein of Galen malformation. Arch Dis Child 87, F144–F149.

Fullerton, H.J., Aminoff, A.R., Ferriero, D.M., et al., 2003. Neurodevelopmental outcome after endovascular treatment of vein of Galen malformations. Neurology 61, 1386–1390.

Gaglioti, P., Danelon, D., et al., 2005. Fetal cerebral ventriculomegaly: outcome in 176 cases. Ultrasound Obstet Gynecol 25, 372–377.

Gambello, M.J., Darling, D.L., et al., 2003. Multiple dose-dependent effects of Lis1 on cerebral cortical development. J Neurosci 23, 1719–1729.

Garel, C., Luton, D., et al., 2003. Ventricular dilatations. Childs Nerv Syst 19, 517–523.

Germano, A., Caruso, G., et al., 2003. The treatment of large supratentorial arachnoid cysts in infants with cyst-peritoneal shunting and Hakim programmable valve. Childs Nerv Syst 19, 166–173.

Gleeson, J.G., Keeler, L.C., et al., 2004. Molar tooth sign of the midbrain–hindbrain junction: occurrence in multiple distinct syndromes. Am J Med Genet A 125A, 125–134; discussion 117.

Go, K.G., Houthoff, H.J., et al., 1984. Arachnoid cysts of the sylvian fissure. Evidence of fluid secretion. J Neurosurg 60, 803–813.

Goldstein, R.B., La Pidus, A.S., et al., 1990. Mild lateral cerebral ventricular dilatation in utero: clinical significance and prognosis. Radiology 176, 237–242.

Goldstein, I., Copel, J.A., et al., 2005. Mild cerebral ventriculomegaly in fetuses: characteristics and outcome. Fetal Diagn Ther 20, 281–284.

Goodyear, P.W., Bannister, C.M., et al., 2001. Outcome in prenatally diagnosed fetal agenesis of the corpus callosum. Fetal Diagn Ther 16, 139–145.

Gosalakkal, J.A., 2002. Intracranial arachnoid cysts in children: a review of pathogenesis, clinical features, and management. Pediatr Neurol 26, 93–98.

Graham, E., Duhl, A., et al., 2001. The degree of antenatal ventriculomegaly is related to pediatric neurological morbidity. J Matern Fetal Med 10, 258–263.

Granata, T., Battaglia, G., et al., 1996. Schizencephaly: neuroradiologic and epileptologic findings. Epilepsia 37, 1185–1193.

Granata, T., Farina, L., et al., 1997. Familial schizencephaly associated with EMX2 mutation. Neurology 48, 1403–1406.

Granata, T., Freri, E., et al., 2005. Schizencephaly: clinical spectrum, epilepsy, and pathogenesis. J Child Neurol 20, 313–318.

Griebel, M.L., Williams, J.P., et al., 1995. Clinical and developmental findings in children with giant interhemispheric cysts and dysgenesis of the corpus callosum. Pediatr Neurol 13, 119–124.

Griffiths, P.D., Paley, M.N., et al., 2005. In utero magnetic resonance imaging for brain and spinal abnormalities in fetuses. BMJ 331, 562–565.

Griffiths, P.D., Reeves, M.J., et al., 2010. A prospective study of fetuses with isolated ventriculomegaly investigated by antenatal sonography and in utero MR imaging. AJNR Am J Neuroradiol 31, 106–111.

Guerreiro, M.M., Andermann, E., et al., 2000. Familial perisylvian polymicrogyria: a new familial syndrome of cortical maldevelopment. Ann Neurol 48, 39–48.

Guerrini, R., Filippi, T., 2005. Neuronal migration disorders, genetics, and epileptogenesis. J Child Neurol 20, 287–299.

Guerrini, R., Barkovich, A.J., et al., 2000. Bilateral frontal polymicrogyria: a newly recognized brain malformation syndrome. Neurology 54, 909–913.

Gupta, J.K., Lilford, R.J., 1995. Assessment and management of fetal agenesis of the corpus callosum. Prenat Diagn 15, 301–312.

Hagmann, C.F., Rennie, J.M., 2008. The baby/fetus with large cerebral ventricles. In:

Rennie, J.M., Hagmann, C.F., Robertson, N.J. (Eds.), Neonatal Cerebral Investigation. Cambridge University Press, Cambridge, pp. 234–239.

Hagmann, C.F., Robertson, N.J., et al., 2008. Foetal brain imaging: ultrasound or MRI. A comparison between magnetic resonance imaging and a dedicated multidisciplinary neurosonographic opinion. Acta Paediatr 97, 414–419.

Hahn, J.S., Barnes, P.D., 2010. Neuroimaging advances in holoprosencephaly: refining the spectrum of the midline malformation. Am J Med Genet C Semin Med Genet 154C, 120–132.

Hahn, J.S., Plawner, L.L., 2004. Evaluation and management of children with holoprosencephaly. Pediatr Neurol 31, 79–88.

Haimovici, J.A., Doubilet, P.M., et al., 1997. Clinical significance of isolated enlargement of the cisterna magna (> 10 mm) on prenatal sonography. J Ultrasound Med 16, 731–734; quiz 735-6.

Heinz, E.R., Ward, A., et al., 1980. Distinction between obstructive and atrophic dilatation of ventricles in children. J Comput Assist Tomogr 4, 320–325.

Hellbusch, L.C., 2007. Benign extracerebral fluid collections in infancy: clinical presentation and long-term follow-up. J Neurosurg 107 (Suppl), 119–125.

Hirsch, J.F., Pierre-Kahn, A., et al., 1984. The Dandy–Walker malformation. A review of 40 cases. J Neurosurg 61, 515–522.

Hunt, G., Oakeshott, P., 2003. Outcome in people with open spina bifida at age 35: prospective community based study. BMJ 326, 1365–1366.

Jackson, A.P., Eastwood, H., et al., 2002. Identification of microcephalin, a protein implicated in determining the size of the human brain. Am J Hum Genet 71, 136–142.

Jeret, J.S., Serur, D., et al., 1985. Frequency of agenesis of the corpus callosum in the developmentally disabled population as determined by computerized tomography. Pediatr Neurosci 12, 101–103.

Joo, J.G., Toth, Z., et al., 2008. Etiology, prenatal diagnostics and outcome of ventriculomegaly in 230 cases. Fetal Diagn Ther 24, 254–263.

Joubert, M., Eisenring, J.J., et al., 1969. Familial agenesis of the cerebellar vermis. A syndrome of episodic hyperpnea, abnormal eye movements, ataxia, and retardation. Neurology 19, 813–825.

Kelly, E.N., Allen, V.M., et al., 2001. Mild ventriculomegaly in the fetus, natural history, associated findings and outcome of isolated mild ventriculomegaly: a literature review. Prenat Diagn 21, 697–700.

Kendall, B., Kingsley, D., et al., 1990. Joubert syndrome: a clinico-radiological study. Neuroradiology 31, 502–506.

Kennelly, M.M., Cooley, S.M., et al., 2009. Natural history of apparently isolated severe fetal ventriculomegaly: perinatal survival and neurodevelopmental outcome. Prenat Diagn 29, 1135–1140.

Kinzler, W.L., Smulian, J.C., et al., 2001. Outcome of prenatally diagnosed mild unilateral cerebral ventriculomegaly. J Ultrasound Med 20, 257–262.

Kitamura, K., Yanazawa, M., et al., 2002. Mutation of ARX causes abnormal development of forebrain and testes in mice and X-linked lissencephaly with abnormal genitalia in humans. Nat Genet 32, 359–369.

Klein, O., Pierre-Kahn, A., et al., 2003. Dandy–Walker malformation: prenatal diagnosis and prognosis. Childs Nerv Syst 19, 484–489.

Kuhn, M.J., Swenson, L.C., et al., 1993. Absence of the septum pellucidum and related disorders. Comput Med Imaging Graph 17, 137–147.

Laskin, M.D., Kingdom, J., et al., 2005. Perinatal and neurodevelopmental outcome with isolated fetal ventriculomegaly: a systematic review. J Matern Fetal Neonatal Med 18, 289–298.

Launay, S., Robert, Y., et al., 2002. [Cerebral fetal MRI and ventriculomegaly]. J Radiol 83, 723–730.

Leitner, Y., Stolar, O., et al., 2009. The neurocognitive outcome of mild isolated fetal ventriculomegaly verified by prenatal magnetic resonance imaging. Am J Obstet Gynecol 201, 215, e1–e6.

Lemire, R.J., 1988. Neural tube defects. JAMA 259, 558–562.

Lena, G., van Calenberg, F., et al., 1995. Supratentorial interhemispheric cysts associated with callosal agenesis: surgical treatment and outcome in 16 children. Childs Nerv Syst 11, 568–573.

Lettori, D., Battaglia, D., et al., 2008. Early hemispherectomy in catastrophic epilepsy: a neuro-cognitive and epileptic long-term follow-up. Seizure 17, 49–63.

Levey, E.B., Stashinko, E., Clegg, N.J., et al., 2010. Management of children with holoprosencephaly. Am J Med Genet C Semin Med Genet 154C, 183–190.

Levine, D., Barnes, P.D., et al., 1997. Fetal central nervous system anomalies: MR imaging augments sonographic diagnosis. Radiology 204, 635–642.

Levitsky, D.B., Mack, L.A., et al., 1995. Fetal aqueductal stenosis diagnosed sonographically: how grave is the prognosis? AJR Am J Roentgenol 164, 725–730.

Lewis, A.J., Simon, E.M., et al., 2002. Middle interhemispheric variant of holoprosencephaly: a distinct cliniconeuroradiologic subtype. Neurology 59, 1860–1865.

Lipitz, S., Yagel, S., et al., 1998. Outcome of fetuses with isolated borderline unilateral ventriculomegaly diagnosed at mid-gestation. Ultrasound Obstet Gynecol 12, 23–26.

Lylyk P., Vineula, F., Dion, J.E., et al., 1993. Therapeutic alternatives for vein of Galen vascular malformations. J Neurosurg 78, 438–445.

Mahony, B.S., Nyberg, D.A., et al., 1988. Mild idiopathic lateral cerebral ventricular dilatation in utero: sonographic evaluation. Radiology 169, 715–721.

Malinger, G., Ginath, S., et al., 2001. The fetal cerebellar vermis: normal development as shown by transvaginal ultrasound. Prenat Diagn 21, 687–692.

Maria, B.L., Boltshauser, E., et al., 1999a. Clinical features and revised diagnostic criteria in Joubert syndrome. J Child Neurol 14, 583–590; discussion 590-1.

Maria, B.L., Quisling, R.G., et al., 1999b. Molar tooth sign in Joubert syndrome: clinical, radiologic, and pathologic significance. J Child Neurol 14, 368–376.

Marques Dias, M.J., Harmant-van Rijckevorsel, G., et al., 1984. Prenatal cytomegalovirus disease and cerebral microgyria: evidence for perfusion failure, not disturbance of histogenesis, as the major cause of fetal cytomegalovirus encephalopathy. Neuropediatrics 15, 18–24.

Mazurkiewicz-Beldzinska, M., Dilling-Ostrowska, E., 2002. Presentation of intracranial arachnoid cysts in children: correlation between localization and clinical symptoms. Med Sci Monit 8, CR462–5.

McSweeney, N., Brew, S., Bhate, S., et al., 2010. Management and outcome of vein of Galen malformation. Arch Dis Child 95, 903–909.

Melchiorre, K., Liberati, M., et al., 2009. Neurological outcome following isolated 10–12 mm fetal ventriculomegaly. Arch Dis Child Fetal Neonatal Ed 94, F311-F312.

Ment, L.R., Duncan, C.C., et al., 1981. Benign enlargement of the subarachnoid spaces in the infant. J Neurosurg 54, 504–508.

Morris, J.E., Rickard, S., et al., 2007. The value of in-utero magnetic resonance imaging in ultrasound diagnosed foetal isolated cerebral ventriculomegaly. Clin Radiol 62, 140–144.

Mueller, K.L., Marion, S.D., et al., 2009. Bimanual motor coordination in agenesis of the corpus callosum. Behav Neurosci 123, 1000–1011.

Nadel, A.S., Benacerraf, B.R., 1995. Lateral ventricular atrium: larger in male than female fetuses. Int J Gynaecol Obstet 51, 123–126.

Nelson Jr., M.D., Maher, K., et al., 2004. A different approach to cysts of the posterior fossa. Pediatr Radiol 34, 720–732.

Nickel, R.E., Gallenstein, J.S., 1987. Developmental prognosis for infants with benign enlargement of the subarachnoid spaces. Dev Med Child Neurol 29, 181–186.

Nomura, M.L., Barini, R., De Andrade, K.C., et al., 2010. Congenital hydrocephalus: gestational and neonatal outcomes. Arch Gynecol Obstet 282, 607–611.

Nyberg, D.A., Mack, L.A., et al., 1987. Fetal hydrocephalus: sonographic detection and clinical significance of associated anomalies. Radiology 163, 187–191.

Osenbach, R.K., Menezes, A.H., 1992. Diagnosis and management of the Dandy–Walker malformation: 30 years of experience. Pediatr Neurosurg 18, 179–189.

Ouahba, J., Luton, D., et al., 2006. Prenatal isolated mild ventriculomegaly: outcome in 167 cases. B J Obstet Gynaecol 113, 1072–1079.

Pagon, R.A., Chandler, J.W., et al., 1978. Hydrocephalus, agyria, retinal dysplasia, encephalocele (HARD +/- E) syndrome: an autosomal recessive condition. Birth Defects Orig Artic Ser 14, 233–241.

Palomaki, G.E., Williams, J.R., et al., 1999. Prenatal screening for open neural-tube defects in Maine. N Engl J Med 340, 1049–1050.

Parrish, M.L., Roessmann, U., et al., 1979. Agenesis of the corpus callosum: a study of the frequency of associated malformations. Ann Neurol 6, 349–354.

Pascual-Castroviejo, I., Pascual-Pascual, S.I., et al., 2001. Unilateral polymicrogyria: a common cause of hemiplegia of prenatal origin. Brain Dev 23, 216–222.

Patel, M.D., Filly, A.L., et al., 1994. Isolated mild fetal cerebral ventriculomegaly: clinical course and outcome. Radiology 192, 759–764.

Paul, L.K., Brown, W.S., et al., 2007. Agenesis of the corpus callosum: genetic, developmental and functional aspects of connectivity. Nat Rev Neurosci 8, 287–299.

Pierre-Kahn, A., Sonigo, P., 2003. Malformative intracranial cysts: diagnosis and outcome. Childs Nerv Syst 19, 477–483.

Pilu, G., Reece, E.A., et al., 1989. Sonographic evaluation of the normal developmental anatomy of the fetal cerebral ventricles: II. The atria. Obstet Gynecol 73, 250–256.

Pilu, G., Falco, P., et al., 1999. The clinical significance of fetal isolated cerebral borderline ventriculomegaly: report of 31 cases and review of the literature. Ultrasound Obstet Gynecol 14, 320–326.

Plawner, L.L., Delgado, M.R., et al., 2002. Neuroanatomy of holoprosencephaly as predictor of function: beyond the face

predicting the brain. Neurology 59, 1058–1066.

Rakic, P., Sidman, R.L., 1970. Histogenesis of cortical layers in human cerebellum, particularly the lamina dissecans. J Comp Neurol 139, 473–500.

Rankin, J., Glinianaia, S., et al., 2000. The changing prevalence of neural tube defects: a population-based study in the north of England, 1984–96. Northern Congenital Abnormality Survey Steering Group. Paediatr Perinat Epidemiol 14, 104–110.

Rintoul, N.E., Sutton, L.N., et al., 2002. A new look at myelomeningoceles: functional level, vertebral level, shunting, and the implications for fetal intervention. Pediatrics 109, 409–413.

Roberts, E., Hampshire, D.J., et al., 2002. Autosomal recessive primary microcephaly: an analysis of locus heterogeneity and phenotypic variation. J Med Genet 39, 718–721.

Robertson, E.G., 1949. Developmental defects of the cisterna magna and dura mater. J Neurol Neurosurg Psychiatry 12, 39–51.

Roessler, E., Belloni, E., et al., 1996. Mutations in the human Sonic Hedgehog gene cause holoprosencephaly. Nat Genet 14, 357–360.

Ross, M.E., Allen, K.M., et al., 1997. Linkage and physical mapping of X-linked lissencephaly/SBH (XLIS): a gene causing neuronal migration defects in human brain. Hum Mol Genet 6, 555–562.

Russo, N., Domenicucci, M., et al., 2008. Spontaneous reduction of intracranial arachnoid cysts: a complete review. Br J Neurosurg 22, 626–629.

Salomon, L.J., Ouahba, J., et al., 2006. Third-trimester fetal MRI in isolated 10- to 12-mm ventriculomegaly: is it worth it? Br J Obstet Gynaecol 113, 942–947.

Salomon, L.J., Bernard, J.P., et al., 2007. Reference ranges for fetal ventricular width: a non-normal approach. Ultrasound Obstet Gynecol 30, 61–66.

Sauerwein, H., Lassonde, M.C., 1983. Intra- and interhemispheric processing of visual information in callosal agenesis. Neuropsychologia 21, 167–171.

Schievink, W.I., Huston 3rd, J., et al., 1995. Intracranial cysts in autosomal dominant polycystic kidney disease. J Neurosurg 83, 1004–1007.

Seitzberg, A., Lind, M., et al., 2008. Ambulation in adults with myelomeningocele. Is it possible to predict the level of ambulation in early life? Childs Nerv Syst 24, 231–237.

Senat, M.V., Bernard, J.P., et al., 1999. Prenatal diagnosis and follow-up of 14 cases of unilateral ventriculomegaly. Ultrasound Obstet Gynecol 14, 327–332.

Sheen, V.L., Topcu, M., et al., 2003. Autosomal recessive form of periventricular heterotopia. Neurology 60, 1108–1112.

Simon, E.M., Goldstein, R.B., et al., 2000. Fast MR imaging of fetal CNS anomalies in utero. AJNR Am J Neuroradiol 21, 1688–1698.

Simon, E.M., Hevner, R.F., et al., 2002. The middle interhemispheric variant of holoprosencephaly. AJNR Am J Neuroradiol 23, 151–156.

Sommer, I.E., 2010. The continuum hypothesis of psychosis: David's criticisms are timely. Psychol Med 40, 1959–1961.

Stein, S.C., Schut, L., 1979. Hydrocephalus in myelomeningocele. Childs Brain 5, 413–419.

Strand, R.D., Barnes, P.D., et al., 1993. Cystic retrocerebellar malformations: unification of the Dandy–Walker complex and the Blake's pouch cyst. Pediatr Radiol 23, 258–260.

Suara, R.O., Trouth, A.J., et al., 2001. Benign subarachnoid space enlargement of infancy. J Natl Med Assoc 93, 70–73.

Symington, S.H., Paul, L.K., Symington, M.F., et al., 2010. Social cognition in individuals with agenesis of the corpus callosum. Soc Neurosci 5, 296–308.

Takahashi, T., Kinsman, S., Makris, N., et al., 2003. Semilobar holoprosencephaly with midline 'seam'; a topologic and morphogenetic model based on MRI analysis. Cereb Cortex 13, 1299–1312.

Tamburrini, G., Caldarelli, M., et al., 2003. Subdural hygroma: an unwanted result of sylvian arachnoid cyst marsupialization. Childs Nerv Syst 19, 159–165.

Tang, P.H., Bartha, A.I., et al., 2009. Agenesis of the corpus callosum: an MR imaging analysis of associated abnormalities in the fetus. AJNR Am J Neuroradiol 30, 257–263.

ten Donkelaar, H.J., Lammens, M., et al., 2003. Development and developmental disorders of the human cerebellum. J Neurol 250, 1025–1036.

Tomlinson, M.W., Treadwell, M.C., et al., 1997. Isolated mild ventriculomegaly: associated karyotypic abnormalities and in utero observations. J Matern Fetal Med 6, 241–244.

Tortori-Donati, P., Fondelli, M.P., et al., 1996. Cystic malformations of the posterior cranial fossa originating from a defect of the posterior membranous area. Mega cisterna magna and persisting Blake's pouch: two separate entities. Childs Nerv Syst 12, 303–308.

Twining, P., Jaspan, T., et al., 1994. The outcome of fetal ventriculomegaly. Br J Radiol 67, 26–31.

Ulm, B., Ulm, M.R., et al., 1997. Dandy–Walker malformation diagnosed before 21 weeks of gestation: associated malformations and chromosomal abnormalities. Ultrasound Obstet Gynecol 10, 167–170.

Vergani, P., Locatelli, A., et al., 1998. Clinical outcome of mild fetal ventriculomegaly. Am J Obstet Gynecol 178, 218–222.

Vigevano, F., Di Rocco, C., 1990. Effectiveness of hemispherectomy in hemimegalencephaly with intractable seizures. Neuropediatrics 21, 222–223.

Vigevano, F., Bertini, E., et al., 1989. Hemimegalencephaly and intractable epilepsy: benefits of hemispherectomy. Epilepsia 30, 833–843.

Volpe, J., 2008. Neurology of the Newborn. Saunders, Philadelphia.

Wang, P.J., Lin, H.C., et al., 1998. Intracranial arachnoid cysts in children: related signs and associated anomalies. Pediatr Neurol 19, 100–104.

Warren, D.J., Connolly, D.J., Griffiths, P.D., 2010. Assessment of sulcation of the fetal brain in cases of isolated agenesis of the corpus callosum using in utero MR imaging. AJNR Am J Neuroradiol 31, 1085–1090.

Whitby, E.H., Paley, M.N., et al., 2004. Comparison of ultrasound and magnetic resonance imaging in 100 singleton pregnancies with suspected brain abnormalities. Br J Obstet Gynaecol 111, 784–792.

Whiteford, M.L., Tolmie, J.L., 1996. Holoprosencephaly in the west of Scotland 1975–1994. J Med Genet 33, 578–584.

Willems, P.J., Dijkstra, I., et al., 1990. Assignment of X-linked hydrocephalus to Xq28 by linkage analysis. Genomics 8, 367–370.

Williams, E.N., Broughton, N.S., et al., 1999. Age-related walking in children with spina bifida. Dev Med Child Neurol 41, 446–449.

Wong, L.Y., Paulozzi, L.J., 2001. Survival of infants with spina bifida: a population study, 1979–94. Paediatr Perinat Epidemiol 15, 374–378.

Woods, C.G., Bond, J., et al., 2005. Autosomal recessive primary microcephaly (MCPH): a review of clinical, molecular, and evolutionary findings. Am J Hum Genet 76, 717–728.

Worley, G., Schuster, J.M., et al., 1996. Survival at 5 years of a cohort of newborn infants with myelomeningocele. Dev Med Child Neurol 38, 816–822.

Yachnis, A.T., Rorke, L.B., 1999. Neuropathology of Joubert syndrome. J Child Neurol 14, 655–659; discussion 669–72.

Yakolev, P., Wadsworth, R., 1946a. Schizencephalies. A study of the congenital clefts in the cerebral mantle. 1. Clefts with fused lips. J Neuropathol Exp Neurol 5, 116–130.

Yakolev, P., Wadsworth, R., 1946b. Schizencephalies. A study of the congenital clefts in the cerebral mantle. 1. Clefts with hydrocephalus and lips separated. J Neuropathol Exp Neurol 5, 169–296.

section 6

Pathology, radiology and biochemistry

The perinatal postmortem examination

Martin A Weber   Sudhin Thayyil   Neil J Sebire

41

Introduction

Current guidelines in the UK (Royal College of Obstetricians and Gynaecologists, and Royal College of Pathologists 2001; Royal College of Paediatrics and Child Health 2002) recommend that an autopsy is offered to all parents who have experienced a perinatal death, ideally performed by specialist paediatric/perinatal pathologists. Following recent inquiries regarding organ retention, there has been a consistent decline in the number of consented perinatal autopsies performed in the UK (Confidential Enquiry into Maternal and Child Health 2005). Nevertheless, the perinatal autopsy remains an important component of perinatal and neonatal medicine, providing information for counselling, clinical governance, teaching and education, and recognition of iatrogenic complications.

This chapter will address the role of the perinatal autopsy, issues surrounding consent, the differences between consented (hospital) and coronial autopsies, the postmortem procedure itself, and recent developments such as postmortem magnetic resonance imaging (MRI) and the minimally invasive/endoscopic autopsy.

Role of the perinatal autopsy

Recent data from a systematic review of adult autopsies demonstrated that there remains substantial discrepancy between clinical diagnoses and autopsy findings. 'Major errors', defined as a previously unrecognised diagnosis, occur in almost one-quarter of cases, around 10% being 'class I errors', which may have directly affected patient management (Shojania et al. 2003). In a contemporary US institution, the estimated major error rate was 8–25%, with a class I error rate of around 4–7%. Despite rigorous investigations in life

© 2012 Elsevier Ltd

as part of current perinatal/neonatal care, similar data are available for perinatal autopsies (Table 41.1). In a review of 27 studies, autopsy resulted in a 'change in diagnosis' or 'additional findings' which might have influenced management or counselling in 22–76% (Gordijn et al. 2002); rates varied from 28% to 75% for stillbirths, from 22% to 49% for terminations of pregnancy and from 22% to 81% for neonatal deaths.

Contribution of autopsy findings

Determination of cause of death

In many cases a postmortem examination will establish the cause of death. However, it is noteworthy that the majority of clinically unexpected stillbirths remain unexplained even after postmortem examination, highlighting the need for further research in this area (Confidential Enquiry into Maternal and Child Health 2009). Similarly, up to half of all sudden unexpected early neonatal deaths will remain unexplained following detailed postmortem examination, a situation analogous to sudden infant death syndrome in older infants (Weber et al. 2009). Whilst the currently available evidence suggests that additional information will be revealed in a significant proportion of perinatal and neonatal autopsies (see Table 41.1), it is important to recognise that even negative findings may prove reassuring to parents and clinicians.

Future pregnancies and siblings

As outlined in Table 41.1, in around 20% of cases, additional information will become available following autopsy which may directly affect siblings or the recurrence risk and counselling of future pregnancies. Placental examination may reveal potentially recurrent disorders, including massive perivillous fibrin deposition and chronic histiocytic intervillositis, both of which are associated with an adverse pregnancy outcome and carry a high risk of recurrence (Weber et al. 2006).

Research and clinical practice development

Postmortem studies have led to a better understanding of a variety of neonatal diseases, including pulmonary hypoplasia, bronchopulmonary dysplasia and patterns of hypoxic–ischaemic brain injury. Moreover, autopsy-based research contributes to the assessment of new diagnostic procedures and the effects of new treatment modalities and therapeutic interventions, including complications and side-effects (Nikkels 2004), as well as providing important epidemiological information regarding the pathological spectrum of rare or emerging new infectious diseases, such as viral epidemics (Johnson et al. 2009; Gill et al. 2010).

Audit, quality control and teaching

Autopsy plays an important role in audit: comparisons between postmortem findings and imaging during life, including antenatal ultrasonography, are imperative in order to improve diagnostic accuracy (Boyd et al. 2004; Amini et al. 2006; Antonsson et al. 2008), and regular discussion and feedback at multidisciplinary meetings will improve patient care and service provision. Furthermore, the postmortem examination remains an invaluable resource for teaching medical staff, including surgeons, pathologists and undergraduates (Burton and Underwood 2007).

Medicolegal issues/malpractice litigation

Increasingly, the perinatal pathologist is requested to perform a coronial autopsy if there is risk of litigation relating to an intrapartum or neonatal death. In such instances, questions usually relate to the timing of events, such as hypoxic–ischaemic brain injury or iatrogenic injury, such as that related to placement of long lines or other therapeutic interventions. If litigation is thought likely, the case should be referred to HM Coroner (see below).

Factors influencing the value of the perinatal autopsy

Sophisticated antemortem imaging and clinical expertise may decrease the likelihood of identifying additional findings at postmortem, although tertiary care centres are likely to be referred more complex cases, which tend to yield more additional information (Gordijn et al. 2002). Similarly, the results of the postmortem examination are affected by the expertise of the pathologist, with autopsies performed by specialist perinatal/paediatric pathologists being more likely to reveal significantly useful information (Gordijn et al. 2002).

Unsurprisingly, technical factors (such as the extent of maceration) may limit the pathologist's ability to identify subtle abnormalities. In one study, almost 8% of antenatally detected brain abnormalities could not be confirmed at autopsy owing to maceration and/or postmortem autolysis (Piercecchi-Marti et al. 2004). Significant findings may also remain undetected if the autopsy is limited to a specific body region, or ancillary investigations are not performed; for example, microbiological investigations or tandem mass spectrometric analysis of postmortem blood and bile in sudden unexpected early neonatal deaths (Weber et al. 2009).

Changes in perinatal autopsy rates

Despite the potential benefits of the autopsy outlined above, postmortem rates have decreased over recent years. According to data released by the Confidential Enquiry into Maternal and Child Health (2005), perinatal autopsy rates fell from 48% in 2000 to 39% in 2003. Current data reveal a plateau in the proportion of neonatal deaths referred for consented postmortem examination: 28% in 2000, 22% in 2003 and 21% in 2007 (Confidential Enquiry into Maternal and Child Health 2009). However, the proportion of neonatal autopsies not offered by clinicians, and that declined by parents, has changed dramatically: from 29% in 2002 to 18% in 2007 (option of autopsy not offered to parents), and from 40% in 2002 to 52% in 2007 (autopsy declined by parents). Whilst it is reassuring that the proportion of postmortem examinations not offered to parents has fallen, it remains unclear why the proportion of parents declining an autopsy has increased to over 50%; possible reasons are discussed below.

Attitudes to the perinatal postmortem examination

Bereaved parents

Parents' opinions are undoubtedly influenced by the organ retention issues that surrounded Bristol and Alder Hey hospitals: parents are concerned about the unauthorised and/or undisclosed retention and use of tissues and organs (Snowdon et al. 2004; Gordijn et al.

Table 41.1 Contribution of the perinatal autopsy: selected recent postmortem series

STUDY	SAMPLE SIZE	SAMPLE GROUP	CONTRIBUTION OF AUTOPSY
Antonsson et al. 2008	112	TOPs (second trimester)	40% additional findings 'of clinical importance' 11% partial discrepancy, and 4% complete discrepancy, between antenatal ultrasound and postmortem findings
Amini et al. 2006	328	TOPs	47% 'further diagnostic findings' In 10% this allowed syndromic diagnosis 9% discrepancy with antenatal ultrasound findings
Elder and Zuccollo 2005	29	Neonatal deaths <28 weeks' gestation	79% new findings 28% change of diagnosis 41% iatrogenic lesions
Elder et al. 2005	16	Neonatal deaths (≥37 weeks' gestation) with HIE	63% significant new information
Boyd et al. 2004	132	TOPs for structural malformations with no abnormal karyotype	72% confirmed suspected antenatal ultrasound findings 27% changed recurrence risk (in 8% recurrence risk was increased to one in four)
Newton et al. 2004	61	Perinatal and paediatric deaths	20% major new finding 28% additional minor findings 34% information regarding treatment effects
Killeen et al. 2004	213	Perinatal deaths	18% additional relevant findings 11% changed recurrence risk
Johns et al. 2004	47	TOPs	28% significant additional findings 23% minor additional findings 2% complete discrepancy with antenatal ultrasound findings
Piercecchi-Marti et al. 2004	352	TOPs	51% autopsy findings considered 'decisive for genetic counselling' 9% additional major malformations
Feria-Kaiser et al. 2002	75	Neonatal deaths	40% additional findings 28% additional findings that may have contributed to death
Brodlie et al. 2002	209	Neonatal deaths	26% new information 3% new information 'crucial for future counselling'
Kabra and Udani 2001	197	Neonatal deaths	12% class I errors, likely to have affected patient outcome 27% additional major findings (class II errors, unlikely to have altered patient management)

TOPs, terminations of pregnancy; HIE, hypoxic–ischaemic encephalopathy.

2007). In addition, McHaffie (2001) identified two main reasons for parents declining the autopsy: first, the 'dread of the child being mutilated', often coupled with the notion that, in deaths where the child was in the intensive care unit, the infant had been 'through enough' already; and second, the feeling by parents that there were 'no unanswered questions', an attitude that may be more likely to reflect the opinion of the consenting clinician (see later).

Parents' decision not to consent to a postmortem examination may also be influenced by cultural and religious considerations, although most major religions do not explicitly prohibit the autopsy (Gordijn et al. 2007). Recent data from the UK show that the proportion of parents declining an autopsy following a neonatal death is similar among most ethnic groups – 52% of white parents, 55% of Asian parents and 56% of Chinese and black parents (Confidential Enquiry into Maternal and Child Health 2009). It is also noteworthy that 30% of women who refused an autopsy subsequently regretted this choice (Rahman and Khong 1995).

Clinicians' attitudes

There is little doubt that neonatologists may find discussing the option of a postmortem examination with bereaved parents difficult, 'distasteful and distressing' (McDermott 2004). Clinicians' attitudes may be further exacerbated by the lengthy consent forms now required in the UK, which are very detailed, time-consuming and possibly confusing. It has been reported that younger clinicians regard the autopsy as less useful compared with their senior colleagues (Snowdon et al. 2004). Clinicians' perceptions are probably also influenced by pathologists' attitudes, with delays in issuing a final postmortem report, lack of clinicopathological correlation and paucity of appropriate multidisciplinary team meetings undoubtedly contributing to the notion that the autopsy is of limited value in the immediate and subsequent management of the patient and/or parents (McDermott 2004).

Consented versus coronial autopsies

The majority of neonatal postmortem examinations will require consent by one or both parents since the likely cause of death will be known. Occasionally, intrapartum and neonatal deaths may be referred to HM Coroner, who may decide to instruct a perinatal/paediatric pathologist to perform a (coroner's) autopsy on his/her behalf; in these circumstances, parental consent is not required and the coroner's decision overrides that of the parents. Neonatal deaths that should be referred to the coroner include cases in which (The Registration of Births and Deaths Regulations 1987):

- cause of death is unknown, or sudden and unexpected
- death occurred during an operation or before recovery from the effects of an anaesthetic
- deceased infant was not seen by the certifying medical practitioner, either after death or within 14 days of death
- death may have been caused by violence or neglect
- death may have been due to an accident
- death may have been in any other way unnatural or there are suspicious circumstances.

Once the coroner has completed the investigation, samples taken as part of the autopsy fall under the Human Tissue Act (see below) and should be handled according to parents' wishes. If there is a potential issue of litigation owing to neglect by hospital staff, the case should always be discussed with HM Coroner.

Consent

The Human Tissue Act 2004 came into force on 1 September 2006; its implementation was overseen by the Human Tissue Authority (HTA). In addition, the HTA oversees the licensing of organisations and establishments that deal with human tissue (http://www.hta.gov.uk). The Act requires consent for the removal, storage and use of human tissue for any 'scheduled purpose', including determination of the cause of death and tissue for research, clinical audit, education and quality assurance. This applies to all tissue removed at postmortem, including small samples such as blocks and slides (see below), and samples that might be kept as part of the infant's medical record. The Act applies to all stillbirths and neonatal deaths.

The Act (HTA Code of Practice 1 2009) defines the giving of consent as a positive action; the absence of refusal is not evidence of adequate consent. In order for consent to be valid, it must be given voluntarily by an appropriately informed person with the capacity to agree. The Act defines who may give consent, which for perinatal postmortem examinations will usually be parents. For stillbirths and neonatal deaths, it is recommended that, if possible, consent is obtained from the mother, and that, where appropriate, both parents are involved. It is usually the treating clinician's responsibility to seek consent; the clinician should be sufficiently senior and with knowledge of the postmortem procedure. It is recommended that he or she be trained in the management of bereavement and should have witnessed a postmortem examination.

As valid consent can only be given if appropriate communication has taken place, information leaflets and consent forms should be available in the main local community languages for patients whose first language is not English, and interpreters should be used. Written consent is not required by law, although it is usually required by the local hospital policy.

The postmortem examination

External and macroscopic examination

Once the clinical details have been reviewed by the pathologist, and, ideally, the case discussed with the requesting clinician, the consent status verified and the body correctly identified, a careful external examination is performed. The infant is weighed and basic measurements taken, which are compared with standard reference tables. Assessment of fetal biometry allows identification of intrauterine growth restriction/small-for-gestational-age infants and macrosomic/large-for-gestational-age infants.

The degree of postmortem change is assessed, which includes documenting the extent of skin discoloration, blistering and skin slippage, allowing the pathologist to make an approximate estimate of the duration of time since death, although it must be emphasised that such estimates are not precise and may be affected by various factors, including duration of the interval between delivery and postmortem examination, the size of the fetus, storage of the body and the presence of (ascending amniotic fluid) infection or maternal pyrexia (Genest and Singer 1992; Wigglesworth and Singer 1998).

Particular emphasis is placed on identifying possible dysmorphic features, although the external appearances should be interpreted in the context of the gestational age and subtle syndromic abnormalities may not be readily discernible in mid-trimester fetuses.

The fetus or infant is assessed for other general features such as pallor, oedema and traumatic or iatrogenic lesions. Routine photographs are usually taken and stored as part of the infant's medical record, with more detailed photographs to document specific abnormalities; these may prove invaluable, not only for multidisciplinary team meetings and as teaching aids but also for review by clinical geneticists to enable direct assessment of possible dysmorphic features.

External examination is followed by a detailed macroscopic investigation of the body. Access to the thoracic and abdominal viscera is traditionally gained via a midline incision through the anterior thorax and abdomen. Careful inspection and dissection of the internal organs are performed, and the organs are then removed, weighed and further dissected. If the brain is to be examined, the scalp is incised posteriorly, and the skull opened by following the nonfused cranial suture lines, although in older infants cranial bones may have to be cut. The brain can either be examined immediately ('fresh') or following a period of formalin fixation, which may require several weeks for complex brain anomalies.

Abnormalities are described and documented, after which small samples are routinely taken for histological examination. The organs are then returned to the body, which is reconstructed prior to release. All organs are routinely weighed, and the weights compared with reference tables against the gestational age; more helpful are weight ratios, such as the brain:liver weight ratio and combined lung : body weight ratio (De Paepe et al. 2005; Cox and Marton 2009).

Microscopic examination

The standard postmortem examination involves taking small tissue samples of organs for microscopic examination to confirm or exclude the presence of disease. It is well recognised that many conditions will only be apparent on histological examination, and that in a significant proportion of cases an organ may be normal on macroscopic examination despite significant pathology on histological examination, for example the heart in myocarditis (Weber et al. 2008).

The tissue samples taken for microscopic examination are processed into small paraffin wax blocks and glass microscope slides (Fig. 41.1). The average size of these tissue samples is that of a standard postage stamp and measures around 3–5 mm in thickness; in small fetuses, the samples are considerably smaller. The tissue section on the glass slide, which measures around 3–5 μm in thickness, is stained with haematoxylin and eosin (Fig. 41.2), as well as a range of histochemical and immunohistochemical stains in selected cases to allow for detailed characterisation of the underlying disease process; other options include in situ hybridisation techniques and occasionally electron microscopy.

Ancillary investigations

Radiology

Most perinatal autopsies are usually preceded by whole-body X-ray examination, usually by using a Faxitron radiographic unit. If there are suspected skeletal abnormalities, particularly of suspected skeletal dysplasias, detailed whole-body radiography is mandatory. Other imaging modalities include postmortem computed tomography (CT) and MRI. The latter has been shown to be useful in examining the brain of babies with suspected brain abnormalities and intracranial haemorrhage.

Other

Other important ancillary investigations include microbiological and virological analyses, as well as metabolic studies (blood and bile spots for acylcarnitine profiling by tandem mass spectrometry, or enzyme assays using cultured fibroblasts harvested from a postmortem skin biopsy), and cytogenetic and DNA analysis.

Retention of organs

Occasionally it may be beneficial to retain an organ temporarily for further examination. This usually involves fixing the organ in formalin prior to examination; this process hardens the tissues by cross-linking intracellular enzymes and other proteins, thus facilitating a more detailed macroscopic examination and allowing better quality histological sections to be obtained. Temporary retention of an organ for formalin fixation prior to examination is especially useful for the brain, which is very friable and soft and prone to disintegrate on handling, thus limiting the extent of the examination. Formalin fixation is also recommended for detailed examination of the heart in cases with suspected structural cardiac malformations, especially if the tissues are macerated and/ or examination is required with the aid of a dissecting microscope (Fig. 41.3).

It is, however, worth emphasising that the retention of an organ for formalin fixation and further examination does not mean that the organ has be retained indefinitely; in the majority of cases in

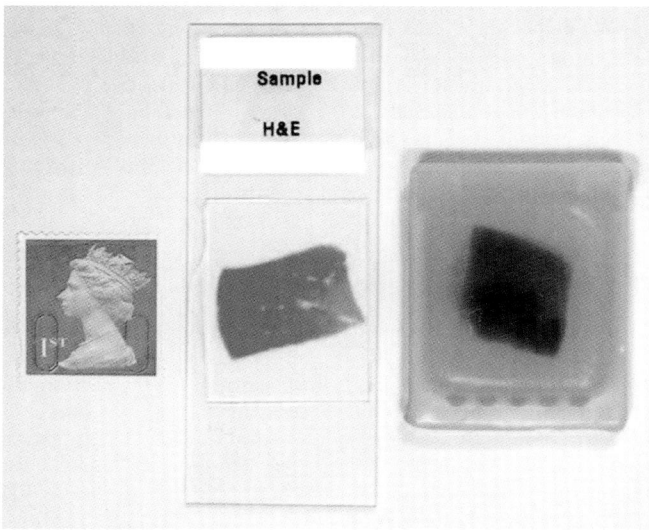

Fig. 41.1 Paraffin wax block and glass microscope slide.

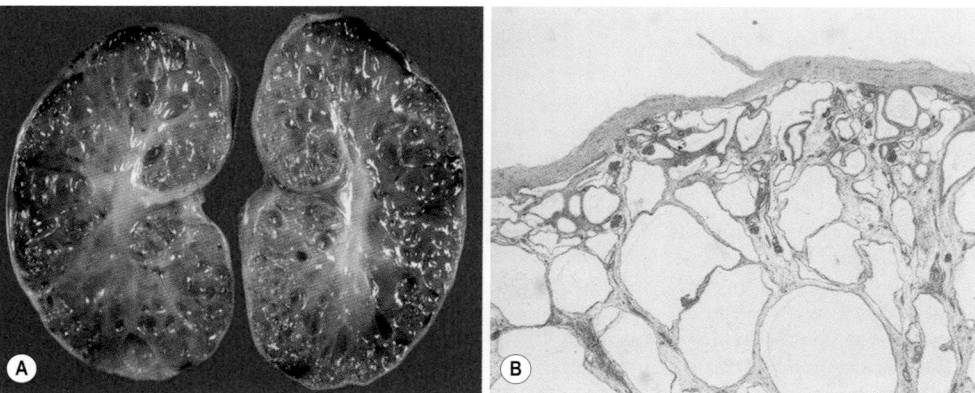

Fig. 41.2 Autosomal dominant polycystic kidney disease. (A) Macroscopic appearances. (B) Histological appearances (haematoxylin and eosin stain). Histological examination is required to confirm the diagnosis.

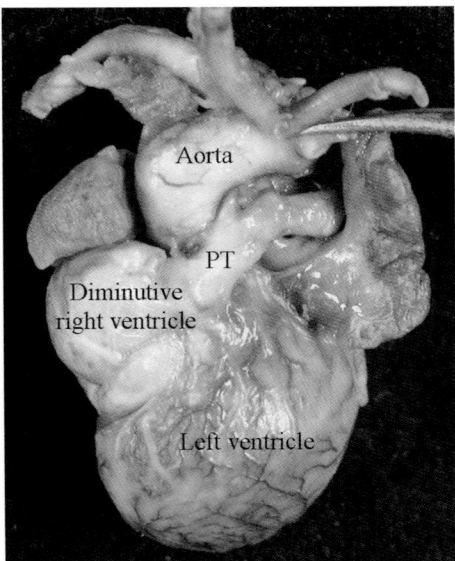

Fig. 41.3 Structural congenital heart disease: pulmonary atresia with intact ventricular septum (post-formalin fixation). Note that the diameter of the pulmonary trunk (PT) is approximately half that of the aorta. *(Courtesy of Dr Michael Ashworth.)*

our centre (Great Ormond Street Hospital, London, UK), the organ is reunited with the body after fixation and examination, prior to release of the body, although this may delay the funeral to allow for adequate fixation. Organs other than the brain can usually be examined after 24 hours of formalin fixation. If parents do not wish to delay the funeral, the retained organs can be returned to them at a later stage, usually via their undertakers, for subsequent burial or cremation. Alternatively, parents have the option of requesting the hospital to dispose of the organ on their behalf or to donate the organ to the hospital for research, audit and training purposes. Temporary retention of organs requires specific additional consent, but parents should be informed that in certain cases, such as terminations of pregnancy or neonatal deaths with a suspected brain abnormality, the value of the autopsy is likely to be significantly reduced if the brain is not fixed prior to examination.

Disposal of retained tissue samples, including blocks and slides

It is recommended that the blocks and slides containing tissue taken as part of the postmortem examination be kept indefinitely by the hospital as part of the baby's permanent medical record in order that they can be reviewed in the future. Parents have the option to consent to the use of tissue for research and all research must be approved by a research ethics committee. Consenting to the use of tissue for research may help other families in the future, and surveys of bereaved parents have shown that the majority of parents are keen to participate in research (Cohen et al. 2009).

All tissue samples taken during a coroner's autopsy are done so under the authority of HM Coroner. According to The Coroners (Amendment) Rules (2005), only samples that have a bearing on the cause of death, or help to establish the identity of the deceased, may be taken during a coronial autopsy; these samples remain under the coroner's jurisdiction until he/she has concluded the investigation, after which the tissue samples are subject to the Human Tissue Act and require parental consent for further handling. Parents then have the same options as for consented

postmortem examinations (i.e. retention and use for research or other purposes, disposal by the hospital or return to the family), but it is noteworthy that, if no communication has been received by the family within 3 months of the coroner's function having ceased, the tissue samples, including all blocks and slides, must be disposed of by the hospital according to current legislation in the UK (HTA Code of Practice 5 2009).

The limited/partial postmortem examination

Parents have the option to choose a limited or partial postmortem examination, which can take several forms. The postmortem examination may be limited to an external examination only, postmortem radiology only, or restricted to a particular body region (such as the chest, abdomen or head) or specific organ (for example, heart only). The information obtained by a limited postmortem examination may in some instances, if appropriately directed, yield sufficient information to allow for a definitive diagnosis or appropriate genetic counselling for future pregnancies.

Limitations of the postmortem examination

Despite the potential benefits of the postmortem examination, as outlined above, it is important to manage parents' expectations. The postmortem examination may not always answer all their questions, and in a significant number of cases may not establish a cause of death, especially for stillbirths and sudden unexpected early neonatal deaths (Weber et al. 2009). As outlined above, the postmortem examination may find no additional unsuspected abnormalities, but this, too, may be clinically helpful, providing reassurance to both clinicians and parents that nothing important had been overlooked during life.

The postmortem report

Current guidelines recommend that a preliminary report is submitted to the clinician within 24–48 hours of the postmortem examination, followed by a final report which incorporates the histological findings and results of further investigations (Royal College of Obstetricians and Gynaecologists, and Royal College of Pathologists 2001), usually within 4–6 weeks. The postmortem report must document macroscopic and microscopic findings, as well as the results of ancillary investigations. Importantly, the salient (positive and negative) findings should be summarised, followed by an appropriate clinicopathological correlation. If possible, photographs of macroscopic or histological abnormalities, as well as copies of X-rays or MRI images, should be incorporated into the postmortem report. Parents are entitled to a copy of the report, but it is recommended that the contents of the report be discussed with them by their clinician prior to receipt, preferably in person, as some parents may find the technical language (and photographs) insensitive and distressing.

The minimally invasive autopsy

As previously noted, two issues that appear to be significant contributors to parents not agreeing to autopsy are the dislike of large incisions (the fear of 'disfigurement') and concerns regarding organ retention. In view of this, there has been recent interest in developing alternative methods of determining or confirming diagnoses at postmortem. Several small studies have anecdotally suggested that postmortem MRI may be a useful investigation, either as an adjunct to traditional autopsy or as an alternative for those cases in which

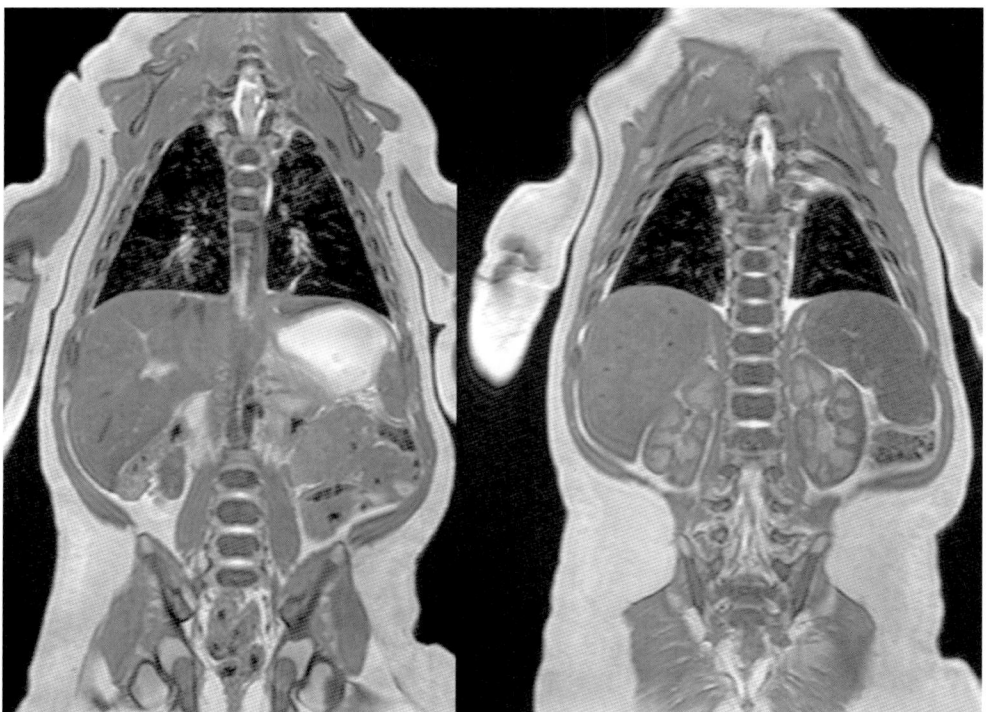

Fig. 41.4 Postmortem magnetic resonance imaging demonstrating excellent soft-tissue resolution and clear visualisation of the structure of internal organs.

parents do not consent to a standard postmortem examination (Cohen et al. 2008). The UK Department of Health has funded two large studies to investigate the possible role of postmortem MRI compared with traditional postmortem examination, and the paediatric/perinatal component of this study is nearing completion (Thayyil et al. 2009a).

Postmortem MRI, particularly when combined with postmortem CT scanning, can provide very high-quality images of both bony and soft-tissue elements, and, with acquisition protocols optimised for the specific postmortem setting, excellent tissue resolution is achievable (Fig. 41.4). With the development of high-field 9.4 T magnetic resonance scanners, even higher spatial resolutions will be possible (Thayyil et al. 2009b).

At present, there are no high-quality published data on the accuracy of postmortem MRI versus traditional autopsy for the detection of abnormalities in a blinded setting, but current experience suggests that postmortem MRI will provide reliable detection of the vast majority of structural abnormalities, being particularly good for central nervous system defects (Thayyil et al. 2009c). However, since a significant proportion of causes of death and other significant pathologies at autopsy can only be detected following direct inspection of organs and the use of ancillary investigations, such as histological sampling or microbiological investigations, postmortem imaging alone cannot replace traditional autopsies.

Nevertheless, there are several settings in which the development of postmortem MRI is likely to change future autopsy practice significantly. First, since anatomical detail is excellent with MRI, with the added advantage that an original dataset is captured that can be reviewed at a later date, postmortem MRI is likely to provide significant adjunctive information. This is particularly important in cases of fetal neuroimaging, where the brain may be autolysed and conventional histopathology uninformative, but in which postmortem MRI may still be useful in identifying the abnormality;

furthermore, abnormalities on antenatal ultrasound imaging, particularly relating to posterior fossa pathology, may not be adequately demonstrated at autopsy, but postmortem MRI may allow visualisation of this area. Second, for those parents who would find a traditional autopsy unacceptable, a non-invasive postmortem examination that may detect additional information may prove superior to doing nothing at all. Third, accurate three-dimensional reconstruction of internal organs and skeletal injuries can be done by rapid prototyping of three-dimensional MR and CT datasets, and these may be extremely useful for both teaching and explaining findings to parents.

Finally, it is likely that the use of postmortem imaging modalities in conjunction with modified tissue-sampling techniques, such as endoscopic examination, could revolutionise the way many autopsies are performed. The combination of these two modalities would allow the acquisition of datasets for review, reconstructions and determination of accurate anatomical information, whilst maintaining the ability to examine organs and tissues directly, and taking appropriate samples for histological examination or other ancillary investigations. Great Ormond Street Hospital, London, UK, is currently developing the infant minimally invasive autopsy (postmortem MRI with subsequent endoscopic-assisted internal examination and tissue sampling), with the aim of potentially replacing the conventional autopsy in selected cases.

Placental examination

Placental examination forms an integral part of the perinatal postmortem examination, and it is important that the placenta be transferred with the body to the pathologist (Table 41.2). In a significant proportion of cases, the cause of intrauterine fetal demise is only revealed by examination of the placenta (Korteweg et al. 2009).

Placental examination may also reveal potentially recurrent disorders, such as massive perivillous fibrin deposition, chronic intervillositis or villitis of unknown aetiology, and may confirm the presence of chorioamnionitis and funisitis, viral pathogens or fetal thrombotic vasculopathy, some of which may have implications for future siblings or pregnancies (Fox and Sebire 2007). Moreover, targeted specialist investigations can be performed, such as vascular injection studies in complicated monochorionic twin placentas.

Specific neonatal autopsy scenarios and common associated autopsy findings

Selected neonatal disorders and their major associated morphological findings at postmortem examination are summarised in Table 41.3.

Table 41.2 Indications for placental examination

FETAL INDICATIONS	NEONATAL INDICATIONS	MATERNAL INDICATIONS
IUGR/low birthweight (<2.5 kg/ <3rd centile)	Requiring admission to neonatal intensive care unit	Maternal pyrexia/maternal carriage of GBS
Prematurity (<37 weeks' gestation)	Infection	Pre-eclampsia/hypertension
Abruption	Neurological abnormalities	Severe diabetes mellitus
Fetal hydrops		Maternal thrombophilia
Fetal abnormality/chromosome abnormality		Maternal autoimmune disease
Stillbirth		Tumour
Severe fetal distress requiring admission to neonatal intensive care unit		Maternal metabolic disorder
Rhesus and other isoimmunisation		
Multiple pregnancy		
Placenta accreta		
Abnormal placental shape or other macroscopic placental abnormality (infarction, haematoma, two-vessel cord)		
Prolonged rupture of membranes (>36 hours)		

IUGR, intrauterine growth restriction; GBS, group B beta-haemolytic *Streptococcus*.
Adapted from Hargitai et al. (2004).

Table 41.3 Common autopsy findings and associated clinicopathological issues in selected neonatal disorders

CLINICAL PRESENTATION	PATHOLOGICAL FINDINGS	SPECIALIST INVESTIGATIONS	CLINICOPATHOLOGICAL CORRELATION/ POTENTIAL CONTRIBUTION OF AUTOPSY
Birth asphyxia/ neonatal hypoxic–ischaemic encephalopathy	Morphological evidence of hypoxic–ischaemic brain injury Associated findings: • Intracranial haemorrhage • Meconium aspiration • Pulmonary haemorrhage • Persistent pulmonary hypertension of the newborn • Myocardial necrosis • Acute tubular damage/cortical necrosis of the kidneys • Adrenal gland haemorrhage/ necrosis • Iatrogenic lesions (see below)	Fixation of the brain is highly recommended Referral of the brain to a paediatric neuropathologist should be considered in selected cases If there is a risk of litigation, the case should be discussed with HM Coroner Placental examination, if available	Approximate timing of insult (days versus weeks) Extent and distribution of injury Exclusion of differential diagnoses: • Metabolic disorders • Infection • Neuromuscular disorders • Congenital brain tumour

Table 41.3 Continued

CLINICAL PRESENTATION	PATHOLOGICAL FINDINGS	SPECIALIST INVESTIGATIONS	CLINICOPATHOLOGICAL CORRELATION/ POTENTIAL CONTRIBUTION OF AUTOPSY
Respiratory insufficiency	Pulmonary hypoplasia Malformations: • Laryngeal atresia • Tracheo-oesophageal fistula • CPAM • Pulmonary sequestration • Structural congenital heart disease Congenital lobar overinflation Congenital surfactant deficiency Persistent pulmonary hypertension of the newborn Meconium aspiration Pneumonia Hyaline membrane disease	Fixation of the lungs and/or heart is recommended for suspected malformations For suspected cardiac malformations, referral to a paediatric cardiac pathologist should be considered	Causes and severity of pulmonary hypoplasia (lung weights; combined lung:body weight ratio; histology, including radial alveolar counts) Characterisation of malformations and other associated structural abnormalities Referral of parents to a clinical geneticist should be considered in selected cases
Congenital renal diseases	Urogenital malformations Renal cystic disease: • Renal dysplasia • Autosomal recessive polycystic kidney disease • Autosomal dominant polycystic kidney disease • Glomerulocystic kidney disease • Nephronophthisis Congenital nephrotic syndrome: • Finnish type • Diffuse mesangial sclerosis Renal tubular dysgenesis	DNA mutation analysis available for selected disorders	Differential diagnosis of renal cystic disease and congenital nephrotic syndrome Characterisation of malformations and other associated structural abnormalities Referral of parents to a clinical geneticist should be considered in selected cases
Skeletal dysplasias	Wide range of lethal skeletal dysplasias with specific features	Radiology is mandatory and will establish the diagnosis in the majority of cases Histological sampling of cartilage and bone highly recommended as may be diagnostic in selected cases; usually requires head of humerus and/or femur, including metaphysis and part of diaphysis; parents should thus be counselled appropriately when taking consent for postmortem examination	Interpretation of radiological appearances usually requires paediatric radiologist with specialist interest in skeletal dysplasias Characterisation of other associated structural abnormalities Referral of parents to a clinical geneticist
Congenital tumours	Teratoma (majority are sacrococcygeal; other sites include orbit; and head and neck, including brain and pharynx; may contain yolk sac tumour or other malignant germ cell tumour elements) Congenital neuroblastoma Congenital mesoblastic nephroma Langerhans cell histiocytosis Juvenile xanthogranuloma Rhabdoid tumour Rhabdomyosarcoma Infantile haemangioendothelioma	Require histological examination, with molecular studies in selected cases	Some tumours are inherited and others may have syndromic associations; referral of parents to a clinical geneticist should be considered in selected cases

Table 41.3 Continued

CLINICAL PRESENTATION	PATHOLOGICAL FINDINGS	SPECIALIST INVESTIGATIONS	CLINICOPATHOLOGICAL CORRELATION/ POTENTIAL CONTRIBUTION OF AUTOPSY
Prematurity-related deaths	Hyaline membrane disease Intraventricular haemorrhage Periventricular leukomalacia Necrotising enterocolitis Infection Iatrogenic lesions (see below): • TPN-associated liver disease • Chronic lung disease/ bronchopulmonary dysplasia • Metabolic bone disease	Usually multiple pathologies present Fixation of the brain is recommended in selected cases, and referral of the brain to a paediatric neuropathologist should be considered If there is a risk of litigation, the case should be discussed with HM Coroner	Characterisation of extent and distribution of pathologies present
Iatrogenic lesions	Vascular access-related (thrombosis, embolism, infarction, infection) TPN-associated liver disease Injuries secondary to intubation Pneumothorax Effects of drugs Fractures following instrumental delivery Subaponeurotic haemorrhage secondary to ventouse delivery	If there is a risk of litigation, the case should be discussed with HM Coroner	Extent and distribution of injuries/lesions, and assessment of relative contribution to cause of death
Suspected metabolic disorder	Evidence of abnormal storage material on histological examination Brain malformations Syndromic associations	Biochemical investigations in life (blood, urine, CSF – these can also be collected at postmortem but interpretation is difficult) Specific postmortem investigations usually limited to: • Histology and electron microscopy for abnormal storage material, e.g. glycogen and lysosomal storage disorders, fatty acid oxidation defects • Blood and bile spot collection (Guthrie cards) for acylcarnitine profiling (fatty acid oxidation defects) • Postmortem skin, muscle and liver biopsy for enzyme assays, histochemistry and (nuclear and/or mitochondrial) DNA mutation analysis (must be taken as soon as possible after death, if not taken during life) Fixation of the brain is highly recommended, including referral to a paediatric neuropathologist	Correlation with antemortem investigations mandatory Referral of parents to a clinical geneticist If metabolic disease is suspected, samples should be taken in life or immediately postmortem as many metabolic studies are uninterpretable after a period of death
SUEND/SUDI	Unsuspected structural congenital heart disease Infection Metabolic disorder (usually fatty acid oxidation defect) Persistent pulmonary hypertension of the newborn	These deaths must be referred to HM Coroner	In around 40% of SUEND, the postmortem examination will not reveal a cause of death, analogous to SUDI/SIDS in older infants

CPAM, congenital pulmonary airway malformation; CSF, cerebrospinal fluid; SIDS, sudden infant death syndrome; SUDI, sudden unexpected death in infancy (7–365 days); SUEND, sudden unexpected early neonatal death (i.e. in the first week of life); TPN, total parenteral nutrition.

Conclusion

The perinatal postmortem examination continues to play an important role in the 21st century. However, the value of the perinatal autopsy may be further improved by better communication between clinicians and pathologists, the issuing of standardised, high-quality postmortem reports with appropriate clinicopathological correlation, shorter turnaround times, regular multidisciplinary team meetings and the further development of novel postmortem techniques, such as the minimally invasive autopsy, which give parents additional choices. Furthermore, a commitment to ongoing research is vital to further our understanding of possible underlying pathogeneses of otherwise unexplained deaths such as late still-births and sudden unexpected neonatal deaths.

References

Amini, H., Antonsson, P., Papadogiannakis, N., et al., 2006. Comparison of ultrasound and autopsy findings in pregnancies terminated due to fetal anomalies. Acta Obstet Gynecol Scand 85, 1208–1216.

Antonsson, P., Sundberg, A., Kublickas, M., et al., 2008. Correlation between ultrasound and autopsy findings after 2nd trimester terminations of pregnancy. J Perinat Med 36, 59–69.

Boyd, P.A., Tondi, F., Hicks, N.R., et al., 2004. Autopsy after termination of pregnancy for fetal anomaly: retrospective cohort study. BMJ 328, 137.

Brodlie, M., Laing, I.A., Keeling, J.W., et al., 2002. Ten years of neonatal autopsies in tertiary referral centre, retrospective study. BMJ 324, 761–763.

Burton, J.L., Underwood, J. 2007. Clinical, educational, and epidemiological value of autopsy. Lancet 369, 1471–1480.

Cohen, M.C., Paley, M.N., Griffiths, P.D., et al., 2008. Less invasive autopsy: benefits and limitations of the use of magnetic resonance imaging in the perinatal postmortem. Pediatr Dev Pathol 11, 1–9.

Cohen, M.C., Blakey, S., Donn, T., et al., 2009. An audit of parents'/guardians' wishes recorded after coronial autopsies in cases of sudden unexpected death in infancy, issues raised and future directions. Med Sci Law 49, 179–184.

Confidential Enquiry into Maternal and Child Health (CEMACH), 2005. Stillbirth, Neonatal and Post-Neonatal Mortality 2000–2003: England, Wales and Northern Ireland. RCOG Press, London.

Confidential Enquiry into Maternal and Child Health (CEMACH), 2009. Perinatal Mortality 2007: United Kingdom. Dorset Press, Dorchester.

Cox, P., Marton, T., 2009. Pathological assessment of intrauterine growth restriction. Best Pract Res Clin Obstet Gynaecol 23, 751–764.

De Paepe, M.E., Friedman, R.M., Gundogan, F., et al., 2005. Postmortem lung weight/body weight standards for term and preterm infants. Pediatr Pulmonol 40, 445–448.

Elder, D.E., Zuccollo, J.M., 2005. Autopsy after death due to extreme prematurity. Arch Dis Child Fetal Neonatal Ed 90, F270–F272.

Elder, D.E., Zuccollo, J.M., Stanley, T.V., 2005. Neonatal death after hypoxic ischaemic encephalopathy: does a postmortem add to the final diagnoses? Br J Obstet Gynaecol 112, 935–940.

Feria-Kaiser, C., Furuya, M.E., Vargas, M.H., et al., 2002. Main diagnosis and cause of death in a neonatal intensive care unit, do clinicians and pathologists agree? Acta Paediatr 91, 453–458.

Fox, H., Sebire, N.J., 2007. Pathology of the Placenta, third ed. Saunders Elsevier, Philadelphia.

Genest, D.R., Singer, D.B., 1992. Estimating the time of death in stillborn fetuses. III. External fetal examination; a study of 86 stillborns. Obstet Gynecol 80, 593–600.

Gill, J.R., Sheng, Z.M., Ely, S.F., et al., 2010. Pulmonary pathologic findings of fatal 2009 pandemic influenza A/H1N1 viral infections. Arch Pathol Lab Med 134, 235–243.

Gordijn, S.J., Erwich, J.J.H.M., Khong, T.Y., 2002. Value of the perinatal autopsy, critique. Pediatr Dev Pathol 5, 480–488.

Gordijn, S.J., Erwich, J.J., Khong, T.Y., 2007. The perinatal autopsy: pertinent issues in multicultural Western Europe. Eur J Obstet Gynecol Reprod Biol 132, 3–7.

Hargitai, B., Marton, T., Cox, P.M., 2004. Best Practice No 178. Examination of the human placenta. J Clin Pathol 57, 785–792.

HTA Code of Practice 1: Consent. 2009. Available online at: http://www.hta.gov.uk/legislationpoliciesandcodesofpractice/codesofpractice/code1consent.cfm.

HTA Code of Practice 5: Disposal of Human Tissue. 2009. Available online at: http://www.hta.gov.uk/legislationpoliciesandcodesofpractice/codesofpractice/code5disposal.cfm.

Human Tissue Act 2004. Available online at: http://www.opsi.gov.uk/acts/acts2004/pdf/ukpga_20040030_en.pdf.

Johns, N., Al-Salti, W., Cox, P., et al., 2004. A comparative study of prenatal ultrasound findings and post-mortem examination in a tertiary referral centre. Prenat Diagn 24, 339–346.

Johnson, B.F., Wilson, L.E., Ellis, J., et al., 2009. Fatal cases of influenza A in childhood. PLoS One 4, e7671.

Kabra, N.S., Udani, R.H., 2001. Correlation between clinical diagnoses at the time of death and autopsy findings in critically sick neonates at a regional neonatal intensive care unit in India. J Trop Pediatr 47, 295–300.

Killeen, O.G., Burke, C., Devaney, D., et al., 2004. The value of the perinatal and neonatal autopsy. Ir Med J 97, 241–244.

Korteweg, F.J., Erwich, J.J., Holm, J.P., et al., 2009. Diverse placental pathologies as the main causes of fetal death. Obstet Gynecol 114, 809–817.

McDermott, M., 2004. The continuing decline of autopsies in clinical trials, is there any way back? Arch Dis Child Fetal Neonatal Ed 89, F198–F199.

McHaffie, H.E., 2001. Crucial Decisions at the Beginning of Life. Parents' Experiences of Treatment Withdrawals from Infants. Radcliffe Medical Press, Abingdon.

Newton, D., Coffin, C.M., Clark, E.B., et al., 2004. How the pediatric autopsy yields valuable information in a vertically integrated health care system. Arch Pathol Lab Med 128, 1239–1246.

Nikkels, P.G., 2004. Iatrogenic damage in the neonatal period. Semin Neonatol 9, 303–310.

Piercecchi-Marti, M.D., Liprandi, A., Sigaudy, S., et al., 2004. Value of fetal autopsy after medical termination of pregnancy. Forensic Sci Int 144, 7–10.

Rahman, H.A., Khong, T.Y., 1995. Survey of women's reactions to perinatal necropsy. BMJ 310, 870–871.

Royal College of Obstetricians and Gynaecologists, Royal College of Pathologists. 2001. Fetal and Perinatal Pathology. RCPCH, London.

Royal College of Paediatrics and Child Health. 2002. The Future of Paediatric Pathology Services. RCPCH, London. Available online at: www.rcpch.ac.uk/doc.aspx?id_Resource=1742.

Shojania, K.G., Burton, E.C., McDonald, K.M., et al., 2003. Changes in rates of autopsy-detected diagnostic errors over time: a systematic review. JAMA 289, 2849–2856.

Snowdon, C., Elbourne, D.R., Garcia, J., 2004. Perinatal pathology in the context of a clinical trial, a review of the literature. Arch Dis Child Fetal Neonatal Ed 89, F200–F203.

Thayyil, S., Robertson, N.J., Chitty, L.S., et al., 2009a. Protocol 08PRT/5409: Postmortem magnetic resonance imaging in the fetus, infant, and child: a comparative study with conventional autopsy (UKCRN: 6794). Available online at: http://

www.lancet.com/protocol-reviews/08PRT-5409.

Thayyil, S., Cleary, J.O., Sebire, N.J., et al., 2009b. Post-mortem examination of human fetuses: a comparison of whole-body high-field MRI at 9.4T with conventional MRI and invasive autopsy. Lancet 374, 467–475.

Thayyil, S., Chandrasekaran, M., Chitty, L.S., et al., 2009c. Diagnostic accuracy of post-mortem magnetic resonance imaging in fetuses, children and adults: A systematic review. Eur J Radiol 75: 142–148.

The Coroners (Amendment) Rules, 2005. Statutory Instrument 2005, No. 420. Available online at: http://www.opsi. gov.uk/SI/si2005/20050420.htm.

The Registration of Births and Deaths Regulations, 1987. Statutory Instrument 1987, No. 2088. Available online at: http://www.opsi.gov.uk/SI/si1987/Uksi_19872088_en_1.htm.

Weber, M.A., Nikkels, P.G., Hamoen, K., et al., 2006. Co-occurrence of massive perivillous fibrin deposition and chronic intervillositis: case report. Pediatr Dev Pathol 9, 234–238.

Weber, M.A., Ashworth, M.T., Risdon, R.A., et al., 2008. Clinicopathological features of paediatric deaths due to myocarditis: an autopsy series. Arch Dis Child 93, 594–598.

Weber, M.A., Ashworth, M.T., Risdon, R.A., et al., 2009. Sudden unexpected neonatal death in the first week of life: autopsy findings from a specialist centre. J Matern Fetal Neonatal Med 22, 398–404.

Wigglesworth, J.S., Singer, D.B., 1998. Textbook of Fetal and Perinatal Pathology, second ed. Blackwell Science, Malden.

The clinical biochemistry laboratory

Ruth M Ayling

42

Introduction

In neonatology, biochemical tests are used for screening, diagnosis and monitoring the effect of treatment, and the laboratory may already have been involved in antenatal testing of maternal and fetal samples.

Successful working relationships between neonatologists and the staff of clinical biochemistry departments require a mutual understanding of clinical and laboratory problems, which is often best achieved by the nomination of a designated clinical biochemist with a responsibility for the neonatal unit. Some laboratory tests considered 'routine' in hospitals with specialist neonatal units may be unusual, challenging or unavailable in other settings.

Centralisation of laboratory services features on some management agendas. Any changes should be planned with involvement of users taking into account all aspects of the laboratory service, not just the analytical component, so that there is no detrimental effect on service delivery.

Specimen collection

Before requesting a biochemical investigation, the neonatologist should define the question to which the analysis will help provide an answer. Various specimens can be used for biochemical tests (Box 42.1), although the majority of requests are for analysis of blood. The laboratory must be provided with the correct specimen and sufficient clinical information to ensure that the correct tests can be performed and that results will be interpreted appropriately and returned correctly.

Blood

It is essential to ensure that the correct sample is taken for the test required; this may be plasma, serum or whole blood. Plasma refers to the aqueous phase of the blood in vivo and to the supernatant obtained after centrifugation of a blood sample collected into a tube containing an anticoagulant, most commonly lithium heparin. Blood collected into a plain tube clots, and, after centrifugation, serum is obtained. Certain tests require plasma samples (e.g. ammonia), but the majority can be performed on either plasma or serum. There may be differences between the results obtained from plasma and serum samples; for example, the potassium concentration is higher in serum owing to release from platelets during clotting. If results are required with particular urgency, it is preferable to send a plasma sample, as it can be centrifuged and analysed immediately, without having to wait for the blood to clot in order to obtain the serum. Some analyses require whole blood, that is, blood collected into anticoagulant but not centrifuged, for example genetic studies and investigations of white or red cell enzymes.

Blood samples from neonates are often obtained by heel puncture ('capillary samples'), venepuncture or from indwelling catheters, usually sited in arteries. Capillary samples contain blood from arterioles, venules and capillaries together with interstitial and intracellular fluids and are not appropriate for all tests – for example, contamination from sweat can cause spurious elevation of ammonia concentration and they should not be used to provide meaningful

© 2012 Elsevier Ltd

Table 42.1 Examples of sampling errors which may cause spurious results

ERROR	MECHANISM	RESULT
Blood sampling site	Dilution of sample by intravenous fluid	Variable depending on intravenous fluid
Blood sampling technique	Difficulty in obtaining sample leads to haemolysis, resulting in release of red cells Components	↑ Potassium ↑ Phosphate and AST
Stasis during venepuncture	Diffusion of plasma water from intravascular compartment and concentration of plasma	↑ Protein, albumin and protein-bound components, e.g. calcium
Incorrect specimen container	Glycolysis will not be inhibited unless a fluoride/oxalate preservative is used Effect of even a slight amount of potassium EDTA (the anticoagulant in a 'full blood count bottle')	↓ Glucose ↑ Potassium ↓ Calcium, ↓ ALP ↓ Magnesium
Delay in transit to laboratory	Metabolism of glucose Leakage of cellular components	↓ Glucose ↑ Potassium, ↑ Phosphate

ALP, alkaline phosphatase; AST, aspartate transaminase; EDTA, ethylene diaminetetraacetic acid.

Box 42.1 Specimens used for biochemical analysis

Blood
  Capillary
  Venous
  Arterial
Urine
Faeces
Cerebrospinal fluid
Saliva

Other fluid
  Synovial
  Pleural
  Ascitic
Calculi
Biopsy specimens
  Skin
  Liver
  Muscle

---

estimates of arterial P_{AO_2}. Venepuncture has been assessed to be less painful than skin puncture sampling (Shah and Ohlsson 2007). To prevent contamination from infusate prior to taking blood from an indwelling catheter, ideally three to five times the dead-space volume should be withdrawn prior to sampling. This may not be practical in the very tiny baby. This volume should be reinfused afterwards, preferably into a peripheral intravenous line.

Sampling errors

A number of preanalytical variables can have an effect on the integrity of the sample and affect the quality of testing. These include the way in which phlebotomy is performed, the nature of the specimen tube and the way in which the sample is transported to the laboratory. Errors in standard procedure may prevent the laboratory from producing meaningful results; examples of those arising most often are shown in Table 42.1.

Sample volume

A disadvantage of frequent biochemical investigation in the neonate is that the volume of blood withdrawn may necessitate subsequent blood transfusion. It may be helpful for the laboratory to provide an indication of sample volume requirements and for clinicians and clinical biochemists to work together to provide guidelines for the frequency of biochemical monitoring.

Non-invasive techniques are obviously an attractive alternative to blood sampling and pulse oximetry and transcutaneous P_{O_2} monitors are important management tools. Transcutaneous glucose monitoring and bilirubinometry are under development but are not yet sufficiently reliable to be incorporated into routine practice.

Urine

Urine can be collected from babies by using plastic urine bags secured to the perineal area, but the adhesive used can cause irritation. Proprietary urine pads placed inside a nappy can be used to facilitate collection, the urine being aspirated from the pad and placed in a suitable container. Collection directly from a nappy is not generally recommended as contamination from constituents within the nappy may affect test results, but can be of use when the method has been suitably adapted (Heckmann et al. 2005). Timed urine collections should be performed accurately in neonates as, owing to the small volumes passed, any losses are highly significant.

If a small sample of urine or other fluid is obtained, it may be preferable to send it to the laboratory in a bottle intended for serum collection, as all the available sample can be amalgamated by centrifugation. The same amount of fluid arriving in small drops on the sides of a universal (urine) container that is too large to centrifuge may be deemed insufficient for analysis.

Cerebrospinal fluid

Cerebrospinal fluid for glucose analysis should be sent in a bottle containing fluoride/oxalate to prevent a result that is spuriously low. Samples for protein analysis should be sent in a plain container.

Faeces

Samples of faeces can generally be obtained from a nappy.

Reference ranges

Biochemical tests are interpreted in the light of a quoted reference range or, more correctly, reference interval. The reference range is usually determined as the interval into which the central 95% of apparently healthy individuals fall. If the distribution is gaussian, this is the range two standard deviations above and below the mean. With non-gaussian distributions, this range is obtained by deleting the 2.5% at the upper and lower ends of ranked values. One in 20 (i.e. 5%) of apparently healthy babies will therefore have a value outside this range. The finding of a value outside the quoted reference range does not necessarily indicate the presence of a pathological cause, and the more tests performed which are independent variables, the greater the probability of finding a result outside the reference range. Similarly, the presence of abnormality is not excluded by a result within the reference range. When monitoring trends, it should be remembered that a difference in results could be due to a genuine change in biochemical status, itself the result of biological variation or pathological change, or to laboratory imprecision. A significant change is likely to have occurred when two results differ by more than 2.8 times the analytical standard deviation. Reference ranges may vary between laboratories, and reference ranges from other institutions and the literature should not be used to interpret a result without prior consultation with the clinical biochemist from the laboratory that performed the analysis.

Historically, laboratory testing for the newborn was performed in specialised laboratories using procedures and instruments suitable for the small volume of available samples. Different reference ranges were often necessitated by the differences in methodology. Technological advances have led to more widespread ability to use small sample volumes, and different reference intervals for neonates now tend to reflect their physiological differences from adult populations. These differences must be interpreted in the context of a patient's growth and development. Particularly in the neonatal population physiology and development may not be synchronous with age.

Outside children's hospitals, the reference ranges appended to laboratory reports tend to refer to adult populations. Neonatal reference ranges are required for optimal diagnosis and monitoring, yet obtaining them is difficult. Collecting suitable samples is fraught with ethical problems in children and additional issues are raised by blood collection from healthy newborns or stable premature infants. Even if such ranges were available laboratory information systems do not generally have the functionality to enable the automatic calculation of gestational age and addition of the appropriate reference range.

Although there are problems associated with obtaining valid reference ranges, not providing them has potential for inappropriate interpretation of results with either delayed diagnosis or misclassification with incorrect treatment and unnecessary further investigation. Alternative methods for developing reference ranges based on mathematical modelling using large databases may prove useful in the future (Schnabl et al. 2008).

Alert limits

Most laboratories have a clear system in place to enable clinicians to be alerted to grossly abnormal results, usually by a telephone call to the requestor or ward triggered by the finding of a result outside predetermined limits. For optimum effectiveness these limits should be specifically relevant to a neonatal population, for example a lower action limit for creatinine and a higher one for potassium would be appropriate in a neonatal population compared with adults.

Quality control, accreditation and clinical governance

Hospital laboratories should be accredited by a relevant professional organisation. For clinical biochemistry in the UK this is usually Clinical Pathology Accreditation (CPA (UK)). To ensure the quality of the work they produce, accredited laboratories run regular internal quality controls, i.e. standards with known values, at regular intervals each day. They also participate in regular, often monthly, external quality assessment schemes in which samples containing unknown amounts of a substance must be measured and the concentration reported back to an external assessor. Laboratories that fail to reach satisfactory standards have their practice reviewed. In addition to these quality standards laboratories should also have a programme of departmental audit and be proactive in involving clinical colleagues.

Point-of-care testing

Point-of-care testing (POCT) is defined as any analytical test undertaken by a member of the healthcare team or by a non-medical individual in a setting distinct from a hospital laboratory (Royal College of Pathologists 2004). Such testing encompasses disposable systems such as urinalysis reagent strips, small hand-held devices such as blood glucose meters and desktop analysers, for example, for measurement of blood gases or electrolytes.

The use of POCT is well established in many neonatal units, particularly with respect to blood gas and glucose measurement. The small sample size required by such systems may offer a particular benefit in neonatology, in addition to the immediacy of results.

However, before establishing any new POCT activity a business case must be produced and the cost of POCT, which is likely to exceed that performed in the laboratory, must be justified by real clinical need. Once need has been established the relevant equipment must be selected. The contribution of laboratory personnel familiar with the evaluation of such equipment is often invaluable at this stage. Implementation of POCT should be part of a clinical total quality assurance package overseen by the laboratory and managerially accountable to a POCT committee to ensure clinical governance needs are fulfilled. A standard operating procedure should be in place for any test performed, covering all aspects of its use (Box 42.2).

Inherited metabolic disease

The clinical biochemistry laboratory has a pivotal role in the investigation of suspected inherited metabolic disease, and neonatologists and clinical biochemists should work together to agree protocols for investigation. Laboratories require an adequate number of samples to ensure technical and interpretative performance. Thus even large specialised children's hospitals are likely to outsource some rarely performed tests to other hospital laboratories. Complex sample-handling procedures may be required prior to dispatch and it is essential for both neonatologists and all laboratory personnel to ensure that robust mechanisms are in place, for example on call and when the designated liaison individual is on leave, to ensure that these valuable specimens are dealt with correctly.

Box 42.2 Aspects to be covered in a standard operating procedure for a point-of-care testing device

Clinical background
Analytical principle
Health and safety, including:
   Information on Control of Substances Hazardous to Health
   Safe disposal of waste
   Control of infection
Adverse incident reporting
Preanalytical considerations
Equipment
Reagents, standards, controls and quality assurance
Test procedure
Sample analysis
Calculation of results
Assay performance
Maintenance
Record-keeping

To enable full interpretation of the results it is important to provide with the specimens accurate details regarding the date and time of sampling, and of feeding and treatment regimens. If a dying infant is suspected of having a metabolic disorder, it may be helpful to obtain tissue specimens to facilitate diagnosis and therefore provide the opportunity for genetic counselling during future pregnancies. It is preferable to take such samples before death, although skin biopsies for fibroblast culture can be obtained up to 24 hours and liver and muscle samples up to 2 hours after death. Skin samples should be placed in a sterile container in transport medium and stored at 4°C. Culture medium should be available from virology or cytogenetics departments; if not, isotonic (N/Saline) can be used. Liver and muscle biopsies should be placed in a plastic tube, snap-frozen in liquid nitrogen and stored as cold as possible. Care should be taken that erroneous diagnoses are not made on samples of blood showing postmortem changes, as results may reveal hypoglycaemia as well as spurious increases in serum potassium, phosphate, aspartate transaminase, lactate, ammonia and amino acids, owing to protein autolysis and cellular breakdown.

Neonatal screening

Clinical biochemists are involved in testing all babies in the UK via the national neonatal screening programme. Screening is carried out in the first week of life using a sample of capillary blood placed on to a blood spot (Guthrie) card. This is usually performed by a community midwife in the child's home and it is important for hospital staff to remember to perform the test on babies who remain inpatients. In the UK, screening for phenylketonuria was introduced in the early 1960s and that for congenital hypothyroidism was added in the mid-1970s. An increase in thyroid-stimulating hormone concentration is used as the screening test for congenital hypothyroidism: this will fail to detect hypothyroidism secondary to hypothalamopituitary disease. More recent additions to the neonatal screening programme include sickle-cell disease, cystic fibrosis using immunoreactive trypsin and medium-chain acyl-coenzyme A dehydrogenase deficiency using acyl carnitines. Clinical biochemists now have the capability to use tandem mass spectrometry and molecular genetics to screen for a number of other inherited metabolic disorders (Tarini 2007).

The neonatal screening programme is carried out at regional centres and the blood spot cards are retained there for some time, so can be obtained for later use, after appropriate discussion with parents, for example for metabolic or genetic studies in cases of sudden infant death when no other appropriate samples are available.

Conclusion

The neonatal unit provides unique challenges for the clinical biochemistry laboratory, and mutual understanding of each other's resources and limitations should lead to the best possible diagnostic service. As changes occur in neonatal practice and advances are made in diagnostic technology, close contact with the clinical biochemistry laboratory will ensure that appropriate arrangements are made for service provision to take account of developments in neonatal screening, diagnosis and monitoring.

References

Heckmann, M., Hartmann, M.F., Kampschutte, B., et al., 2005. Assessing cortisol production in preterm infants: do not dispose of the nappies. Pediatr Res 57, 412–418.

Royal College of Pathologists, 2004. Guidelines on Point of Care Testing. Available online at: www.rcpath.org/resources/pdf/Point-of-CareTestingOct04.pdf.

Schnabl, K., Chan, M.K., Gong, Y., et al., 2008. Closing the gaps in paediatric reference intervals: the CALIPER initiative. Clin Biochem Rev 29, 89–96.

Shah, V., Ohlsson, A., 2007. Venepuncture versus heel lance for blood sampling in term neonates. Cochrane Database Syst Rev (2), CD001452.

Tarini, B.A., 2007. The current revolution in newborn screening: new technology old controversies. Arch Pediatr Adolesc Med 161, 767–772.

Neonatal imaging

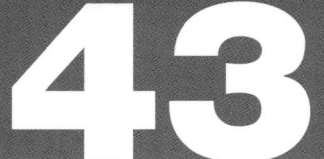

Paul Humphries

Introduction

Imaging in the neonate includes the whole range of imaging investigations available in the older child and adult. The cornerstone of imaging is still conventional radiography but ultrasound plays an important part. Most neonatal imaging is undertaken on very sick and usually very small neonates in the intensive care unit. This requires portable X-ray equipment of a very high specification that is capable of using very short exposure times. In the main computerised radiography has now largely replaced conventional film radiographs, maintaining high-quality imaging and providing several advantages, with postprocessing being one example. The advent of picture archiving and communication systems has allowed images to be available for viewing on monitors within the intensive care unit or transmitted electronically if a further opinion is required. Interpretation of intensive care radiology is often done on the spot by clinicians, who must receive appropriate training. Regular multidisciplinary meetings between clinical and radiology staff are essential for audit, training and maintenance of skills.

Radiation safety

All involved in the management of neonates should sign up to the ALARA (as low as reasonably achievable) principle with regard to radiation dose. In the European Union legislation has been enacted which, in the UK, has led to the IR(ME)R 2000 regulations (HMSO 2000) governing both the justification, i.e. clinical needs, for an examination and optimisation (obtaining the best images with the lowest possible radiation dose).

© 2012 Elsevier Ltd

Chest imaging

Almost every baby admitted to a neonatal intensive care unit will have one or more chest radiographs. It is most important that these answer the clinical question posed by the requesting doctor and that all those requesting such radiographs are able to interpret them. The film must be technically satisfactory with the appropriate radiation exposure so that the lungs, soft tissues and bones can be adequately visualised on the radiograph produced.

A systematic approach to reviewing the chest radiograph enables consistent interpretation, which should lead to accurate diagnosis. Routine review of any available older films is mandatory to place current radiological findings in context. A suggested routine for chest radiograph evaluation is as follows:

1. Check the patient's name, date of birth and the date of the radiograph.
2. Assess the technical quality of the radiograph – degree of rotation, degree of penetration and degree of inspiration – all of which may influence the interpretation of the film.
3. Check the position of lines and tubes to ensure that they are in the expected place and have not become displaced since the last radiograph.
4. Check heart size and position, site of aortic knuckle and tracheal position.
5. Is there normal, increased or decreased vascularity? This can be quite subjective if not grossly abnormal.
6. Is there lung transradiancy? Is it equal or asymmetrical? If asymmetrical, evaluate for increased lucency versus increased density and try to determine which side you feel is abnormal. If there is increased transradiancy, the side with fewer visible vessels is abnormal.
7. Review the upper abdomen – check beneath both hemidiaphragms for free air and the liver shadow for evidence of portal venous gas.
8. Review the bones – the bone density, signs of metabolic bone disease, fractures and congenital malformations.

Technical considerations

The chest should be straight so that the hemithoraces in the normal situation would appear isodense. In the neonate evaluating the relative positions of the anterior ribs on both sides most easily assesses this. It is also important that the film is taken in full inspiration (Fig. 43.1). Films that are grossly rotated, expiratory or under-penetrated can be very difficult to interpret and caution is advised when reviewing such radiographs.

Lines and tubes

Whilst most chest radiographs are taken to assess lung or intrapleural pathology or cardiac shape and size, a significant number are taken either solely for or additionally to demonstrate the positions of various lines and tubes inserted in the treatment of the baby. It is most important that all those managing such neonates are aware of the appearances of these.

Endotracheal tube

The endotracheal tube (ETT) is usually clearly visible on a plain X-ray. The tip of the tube should lie between the level of the seventh cervical vertebra (C7) (just below the larynx) and the level of the carina, which is usually around about the level of the fourth thoracic vertebra (T4). The vertebrae should be used as landmarks

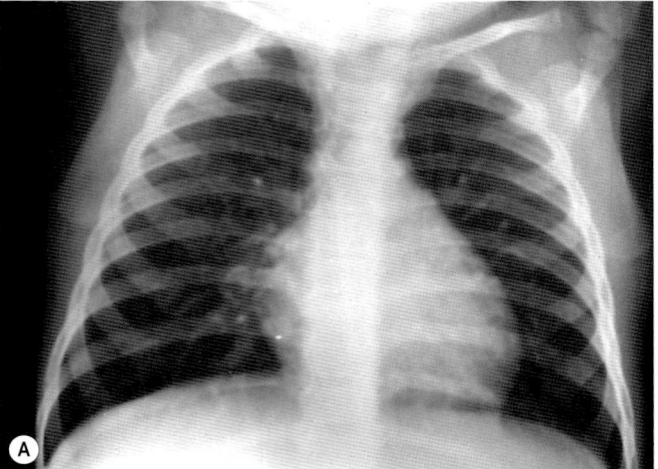
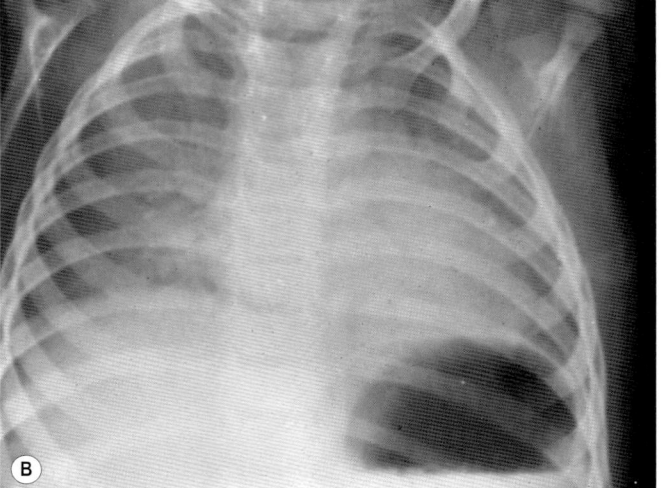

Fig. 43.1 Same-day films of the same patient with a normal chest. (A) Inspiration. (B) Expiration.

when assessing tube position rather than the clavicles, and the tip of the ETT is best placed opposite the body of the first thoracic vertebra (Blayney and Logan 1994). Head flexion will effectively advance the ETT and head extension will withdraw the tube, hence an acceptable ETT tube position can be rendered apparently unacceptable by either of these manoeuvres.

Umbilical venous and arterial catheters

Umbilical venous catheters (UVCs) pass from the umbilical vein to the left portal vein and thence through the ductus venosus (up to 2 cm in length in term babies), middle or left hepatic vein, inferior vena cava (IVC) and into the right atrium. The ideal tip position is at the junction of the IVC and the right atrium. Advancement past the ductus venosus is not possible in 11% and the line terminates in the liver or below in 24% (Khilani et al. 1991). Based on radiographic correlation, optimum tip position is considered to be opposite T8–9 on an anteroposterior film, but the right atrium–IVC junction is not always consistent with these bony landmarks (Raval et al. 1995). A line at the T6 or higher level is within the heart and if the tip lies below T11 the catheter is proximal to the ductus venosus (Greenberg et al. 1995).

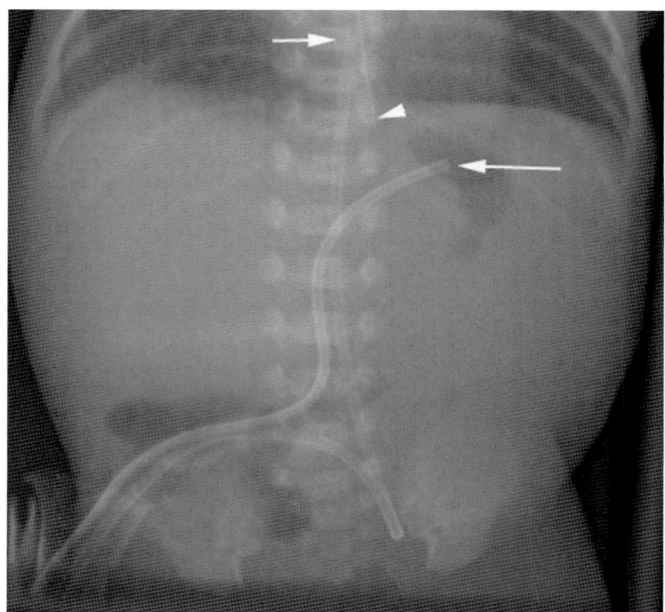

Fig. 43.2 Anteroposterior abdominal radiograph demonstrating a malpositioned umbilical venous catheter, with the tip lying projected over the left lobe of the liver, probably within the left portal vein (arrow). Note also the umbilical venous catheter in a 'high' position, with its tip at T9 (short arrow) and the nasogastric tube lying short, within the distal oesophagus (arrowhead).

If the UVC is placed too far in, the tip may enter the superior vena cava, pass through the foramen ovale (and potentially into the pulmonary outflow tract) or through the tricuspid valve into the right ventricle. Low abnormal catheter positions can be seen with the UVC positioned within the portal venous system, the hepatic veins, ductus venosus or within the umbilical vein (Schlesinger et al. 2003) (Fig. 43.2). For more information on complications of UVCs and umbilical arterial catheters (UACs), see Chapter 44.

Either umbilical artery can be utilised for umbilical arterial line placement, with the catheter passing into the internal iliac artery, the common iliac artery and thence into the aorta (Fig. 43.2). Owing to the course of the catheter, there is an apparent loop in the catheter on radiographs, passing into the pelvis before ascending. This 'loop' is the hallmark of a UAC and is important to establish its presence when checking UAC placement, which hence requires a chest and abdominal film. Optimal placement is away from the visceral aortic branch vessels (which usually lie opposite T12) and this can be achieved through either a 'low' or 'high' placement. With 'low' placement the line tip should lie between L3 and L5; 'high' placement should (ideally) leave the tip between T7 and T9 (Scanlon et al. 1982) (Fig. 43.2). A Cochrane Review concluded that the evidence is strongly in favour of a high catheter position (Barrington 1999).

Long lines

Small peripheral venous catheters are frequently used for venous access and these may be inserted in any of the four limbs or sometimes via a scalp vein (see Ch. 44). The tip of such catheters should be in a large central vein but outside the heart. The tip of one of these catheters should not lie more centrally than the inferior limit of the superior vena cava or the superior limit of the IVC. As with a UVC, if the tip of the line lies opposite T6 it is within the heart

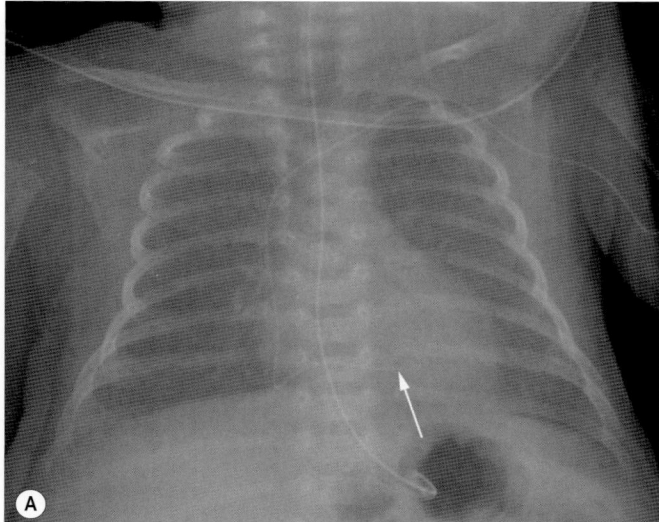

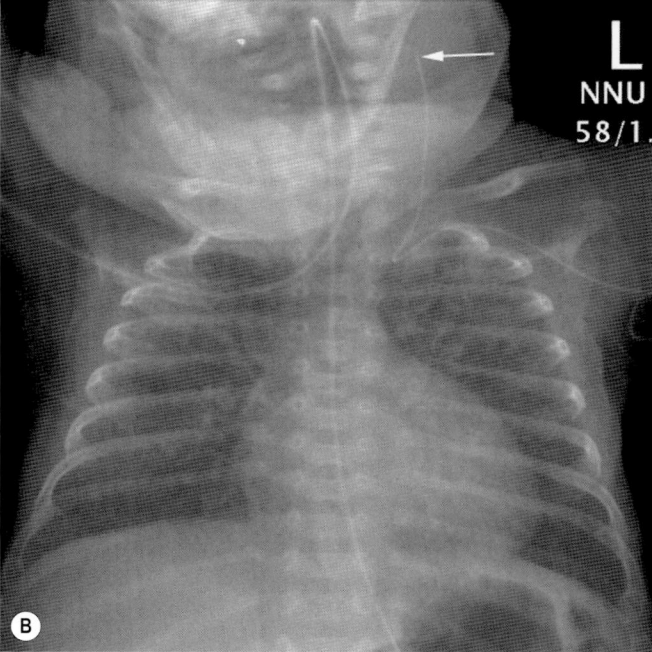

Fig. 43.3 Malpositioned long lines. These thin catheters are very difficult to see without contrast administration. Undesired placements include (A) intracardiac position, with the tip projected over the right atrium, and (B) jugular position. Lines may also be seen coiled within the arm/leg used for access or within the subclavian vein.

and should be withdrawn. These catheters are very fine and are not usually radiopaque. Their position must be confirmed by radiography after insertion by injecting 0.5 ml of intravenous contrast medium (such as Omnipaque or Niopam) to confirm the position of the tip of the catheter (Fig. 43.3). The question of how often the position of a catheter position should be checked after insertion is a difficult one, about which there is no consensus, but all clinicians must be aware that catheter migration both distally and proximally can occur. The tip of the catheter can be extremely difficult to identify without contrast medium, particularly over the chest or abdomen when overlying mediastinal structures or bowel can be extremely confusing. The positions of lines within the abdomen can

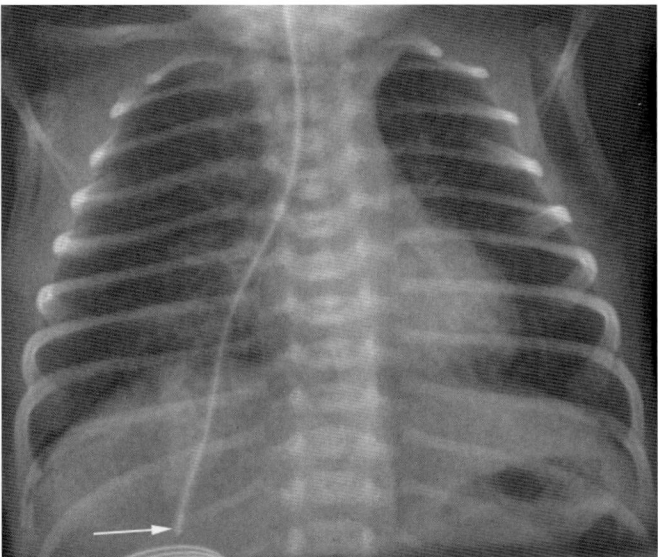

Fig. 43.4 Chest X-ray showing a malpositioned nasogastric tube, with the tip (arrow) lying within a right lower lobe bronchus in the costodiaphragmatic recess. Note how inferior the posterior costodiaphragmatic recess extends.

also be determined by ultrasound and, whilst this is potentially an attractive option, it has not found favour owing to difficulties with overlying bowel gas.

Enteral feeding tube(s)

Frequently a nasogastric tube has been placed to assist feeding on the neonatal unit and the position of such tubes should be reviewed on each chest or abdominal film. The optimal position is within the stomach bubble. If the tube is not projected there consider the following:

- Is the tube simply short, within the distal oesophagus, or long, lying within the proximal small bowel?
- Is the tube projected away from the expected course of the oesophagus? Possibilities would then include intubation of the tracheobronchial tree (most likely: Fig. 43.4) or oesophageal perforation.
- Is the tube tip projected higher and more laterally than expected despite following an appropriate oesophageal course? If so, a congenital diaphragmatic hernia needs to be considered.
- Is the tube coiled up, projected over the cervical/upper thoracic region? If so, oesophageal atresia needs to be considered.

Heart size, position, aortic arch and pulmonary vasculature

Many congenital cardiac lesions are diagnosed prior to birth (Ch. 28). However there are frequent occasions when a lesion is detected antenatally and the chest radiograph may provide some important clues to the presence of congenital heart disease.

Assessment of cardiac size may be challenging, given the widely variable appearances of the thymus in neonates. The thymus can fill the whole of the upper mediastinum or be prominent on the right or the left. Typical normal thymic features include an

undulating margin or the 'sail sign'. In preterm neonates the thymic shadow may be very difficult to identify or be apparently absent. A cardiothoracic ratio of 60% is the accepted upper limit of normal on a frontal radiograph. Apparent cardiomegaly caused by a prominent thymic shadow can be evaluated further using either a lateral chest radiograph or an ultrasound to look for prominent thymic tissue. When there is true cardiomegaly the heart shadow extends posterior to a line drawn from the trachea to the diaphragm on the lateral radiograph.

A right-sided aortic arch is associated with underlying congenital heart disease, including tetralogy of Fallot (25%), truncus arteriosus (35%) and pulmonary atresia with ventricular septal defect. Identification of the aortic arch position can be difficult. It may be possible to visualise the arch or the descending aorta or alternatively use leftward displacement of the tracheal position (which should normally be slightly to the right of the midline) or right-sided tracheal indentation to determine if a right-sided arch is present.

Assessment of pulmonary vasculature is challenging and can be quite subjective, with different observers having differing opinions! Essentially the aim here is to decide if there is increased, normal or reduced vascularity. For the differential diagnosis of congenital heart disease, see Chapter 28.

Lung appearances

The lung parenchymal appearances should be evaluated not only by comparing each hemithorax with the other but also by comparing the overall appearances with a mental picture of what the normal appearances should be. This clearly requires a degree of experience, but with practice a mental 'reference image' will become easier to define. This is particularly important when assessing neonatal chest radiographs as many of the disease processes seen in this population lead to bilateral radiographic abnormalities. With improved perinatal care 'classical' appearances are less frequently encountered; however, the following is a rough rule of thumb.

Increased opacity

- Technical – an underpenetrated radiograph will lead to globally increased lung density.
- Respiratory distress syndrome (RDS) – classically small-volume lungs with a bilateral ground-glass infiltrate (Fig. 43.5), often with a nodular pattern. Can have air bronchograms. May be asymmetric following administration of surfactant, with the right lower zone typically being better aerated than the remainder of the lung parenchyma.
- Transient tachypnoea of the newborn – classically normal-volume lungs with increased vascular and interstitial markings. May have small effusions and mild cardiomegaly. Usually resolves within 72 hours.
- Meconium aspiration syndrome – coarse 'rope-like' opacities emanating from the hila. Overinflation and areas of atelectasis (Fig. 43.6). There may be a pneumothorax present also.
- Congenital pneumonia – segmental or lobar consolidation, sometimes with effusions, which may be large.
- Pulmonary haemorrhage – varied appearance. Can mimic meconium aspiration or RDS.
- Pleural effusion – homogeneous increased density on a supine film. Without any distinguishing features (for example, air bronchograms) it may be impossible to differentiate fluid from air-space processes. When an effusion tracks laterally along the chest wall the lung edge may be displaced, allowing positive identification (Fig. 43.7). Clearly both consolidation

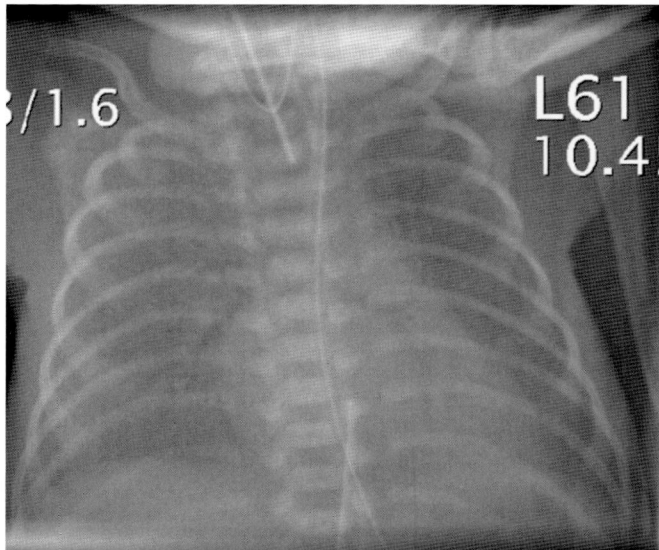

Fig. 43.5 Chest X-ray showing classical respiratory distress syndrome pattern with bilateral, relatively symmetrical, nodular ground-glass infiltrates, with air bronchograms.

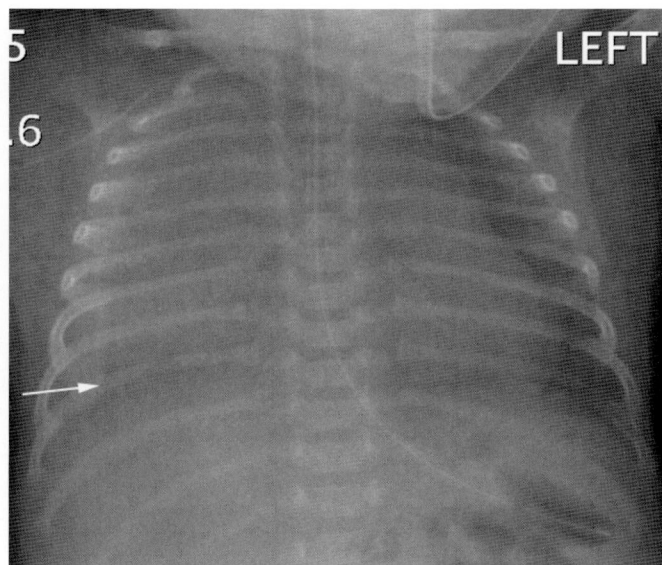

Fig. 43.7 Chest X-ray showing generalised increased density within the right hemithorax, with a definite fluid–lung interface (arrow), consistent with a pleural effusion.

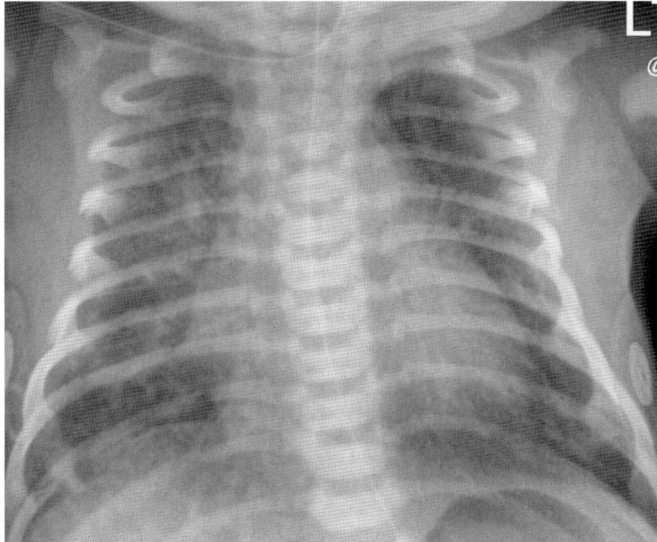

Fig. 43.6 Chest X-ray showing typical features of meconium aspiration syndrome, with hyperinflation and coarse linear opacities.

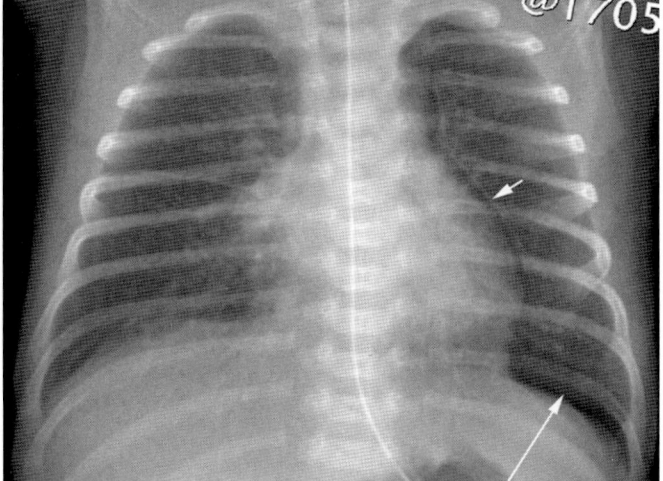

Fig. 43.8 Chest X-ray showing increased transradiancy and sharp lower left heart border and hemidiaphragm (arrow), consistent with a pneumothorax. Additionally there is an etched appearance to the upper left heart border and superior mediastinum (short arrow). Differentiating pneumothorax and pneumomediastinum can be difficult in this situation.

and effusion may coexist, further confusing the radiological appearances.

- Lung aplasia/agenesis – increased density on the abnormal side, with volume loss, manifesting as mediastinal shift, elevation of the hemidiaphragm or both. May be difficult to differentiate from collapse – previous films are helpful to assess if the lungs previously appeared normal or not.

Increased transradiancy

- Technical – a rotated radiograph will lead to discrepancy between the transradiancy of the two hemithoraces. An overpenetrated film will cause both lungs to appear hyperlucent.
- Pneumothorax – as films are taken with the neonate in a supine position, free pleural air rises anteriorly, hence a lung edge may not be visible. Signs that suggest a pneumothorax are:
  - sharp ipsilateral heart border or diaphragm (Fig. 43.8)
  - depression of the ipsilateral hemidiaphragm, if under tension
  - deviation of the ipsilateral thymic lobe
  - mediastinal shift away from the affected side.

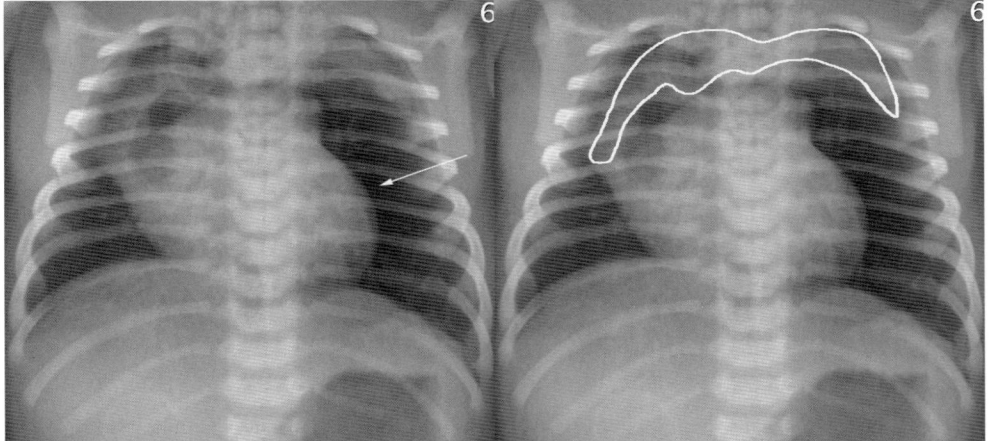

Fig. 43.9 Chest X-ray showing increased transradiancy and sharp left heart border (arrow), consistent with a pneumothorax. Additionally air outlines and elevates the thymus, creating an 'angel wing' appearance (outlined).

- Pneumomediastinum – air may outline the thymus, the so-called angel wing sign (Fig. 43.9) or etch around the heart with pneumopericardium, which can be challenging to differentiate from pneumothorax (Fig. 43.8).
- Congenital lobar overinflation – increased lucency, reduced vessels and a variable degree of mass effect. Involves left upper, right upper and right middle lobes in decreasing order of frequency. May initially appear as a density, becoming aerated (and therefore lucent) over time.
- Congenital pulmonary airway malformation (CPAM) – see below and Chapter 27.

Mixed lucency and opacity

- Pulmonary interstitial emphysema – branching irregular lucencies, with atelectatic areas interposed. The radiographic appearances are easy to misinterpret as multiple increased densities – beware! Often associated increased volume of the segment of the lung or hemithorax (Fig. 43.10). May be complicated by pneumothorax.
- Congenital diaphragmatic hernia – if air is contained within the bowel loops it will appear as a cystic area, with associated mass effect. The more non-aerated loops present, the denser the appearance.
- Chronic lung disease – increased reticular (linear) markings, which appear thickened and irregular. Areas of air trapping and overinflation.
- CPAM – previously known as congenital cystic adenomatoid malformations, CPAMs may radiologically appear as one or more large air- or air/fluid-filled cysts, measuring up to 10 cm in size, with associated mass effect (type 1 and type 4); one or more smaller cysts, measuring up to 2 cm in size (type 2); or a solid lesion (type 3) (Stocker 2009) (Fig. 43.11).
- There is recognition that there may be overlap between lesions traditionally thought to represent separate entities, such as congenital lobar overinflation, pulmonary sequestrations and CPAM lesions; so-called hybrid lesions (Zeidan et al. 2009).

Computed tomography (CT) is used to define the anatomy of any feeding arterial vessels, draining veins and the lung parenchymal appearances to characterise congenital lung lesions and aid treatment planning (Frush 2005) (Fig. 43.12). There are few other

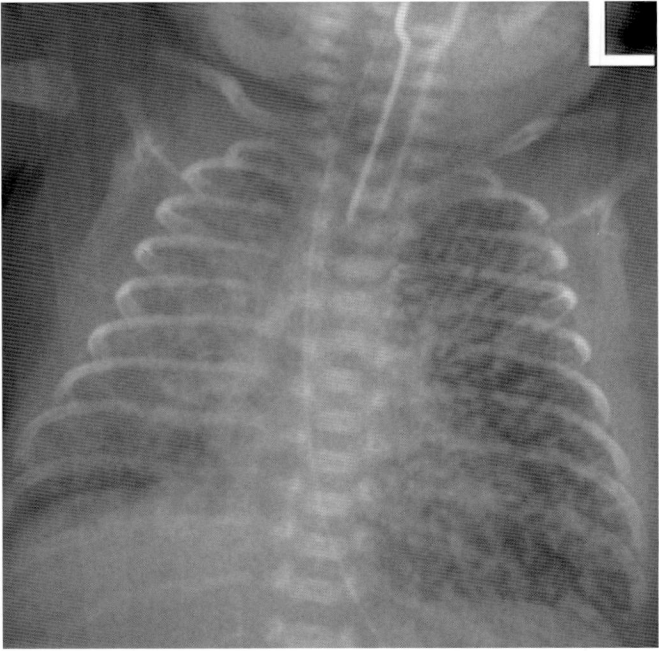

Fig. 43.10 Chest X-ray demonstrating multiple branching linear lucencies within the left lung, with associated hyperinflation, consistent with pulmonary interstitial emphysema.

indications for CT examination of the thorax in the neonatal period, as transfer from the neonatal unit and the radiation dose imparted necessarily limit its use.

Chest ultrasonography

The lack of ionising radiation makes ultrasound an ideal modality for use in neonates; however, it is operator-dependent and prolonged examinations may not be well tolerated by a sick ventilated baby. Ultrasound can be employed to help differentiate between pleural fluid and lung consolidation, thymus and an anterior mediastinal mass and to look for feeding vessels related to lung masses.

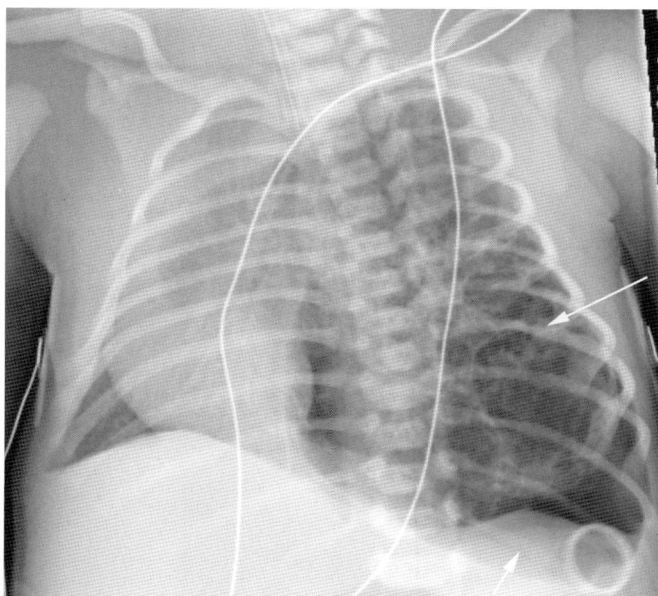

Fig. 43.11 Chest X-ray demonstrating a large multicystic lesion within the left hemithorax (arrow), pathologically proven to be a type 1 congenital pulmonary airway malformation. Note also a loculated left basal pneumothorax, with flattening of the left hemidiaphragm (short arrow).

Magnetic resonance imaging of the chest

Magnetic resonance imaging (MRI) of the lungs is not currently the modality of choice but MRI of the mediastinum and particularly of the heart and vascular structures is often very helpful in assessing the cardiovascular anatomy. Echocardiography however should always be the first choice for examination of the cardiovascular system, supplemented by MRI where there are particular questions, such as evaluating the presence of a vascular ring.

Abdominal imaging

Plain abdominal radiography is often obtained to evaluate the position of long lines, umbilical catheters or in the setting of a possible surgical abdominal condition presenting with distension, bile-stained aspirates or passage of blood per rectum. Once again, having a checklist aids interpretation:

1. Check the patient's name, date of birth and the date of the radiograph.
2. Assess the technical quality of the radiograph – degree of rotation and degree of penetration.
3. Check lines and tubes to ensure that they are in the expected positions and have not become displaced since the last radiograph.
4. Are there aerated bowel loops and is the pattern appropriate for the age of the neonate? In a term neonate one would expect gas through to the rectum by the end of day 1 of life; in a preterm neonate it can take several days for this to occur.
5. Are the bowel loops dilated? Bowel loops are considered dilated if they are greater in size than the width of a vertebral body.

6. Is there any free air (Fig. 43.13)? This can be difficult to evaluate but the key review areas are:
   - Is there a diffuse radiolucency overlying the upper abdomen, particularly overlying the liver?
   - Is the falciform ligament visible?
   - Does the diaphragm appear as a continuous line?
   - Are both sides of bowel wall visible (Rigler's sign)? This can be difficult to determine when there are dilated loops abutting each other (Rigler 1941).
   - Are there any triangular lucencies interposed between bowel loops? (Triangular lucency does not conform to any normal structure and must be free.)
7. Are there any features to suggest necrotising enterocolitis?
   - This is often a very difficult question in the small premature neonate. The classical appearance of necrotising enterocolitis with gas in the bowel wall appearing as linear streaks or 'bubbles' is not often seen in the premature neonate (Fig. 43.14). The condition is suggested on plain radiographs by some dilated loops of bowel (paralytic ileus). If these appear fixed from one radiograph to another, this is very suggestive of necrotising enterocolitis (Fig. 43.15). Sometimes the bowel loops have an unusual contour to them, suggesting oedema, which can be a sign of necrotising enterocolitis. This diagnosis is however usually a clinical one and radiology is of limited value, often only confirming the diagnosis on those uncommon occasions when there is a pneumoperitoneum due to perforation. Some authors have advocated the use of ultrasound to identify pneumatosis and fluid collections that are otherwise not evident on plain X-ray (Epelman et al. 2007; Silva et al. 2007); however this has yet to gain widespread clinical use.
8. Is there any calcification present? Spotty or linear calcification suggests meconium peritonitis. Calcification conforming to the colonic lumen suggests bowel/urinary tract communication. Calcification overlying the renal outlines suggests nephrocalcinosis.
9. Review the lung bases – check for basal lung changes and pneumothorax.
10. Review the hernial orifices – is there any sign of a hernia?
11. Review the bones – the bone density, signs of metabolic bone disease, fractures and congenital malformations.

Radiological differential diagnosis for abdominal appearances

Dilated bowel loops

In neonates it is usually impossible to differentiate large from small bowel on radiographic grounds. Topography can sometimes be of use, with large bowel tending to be located within the periphery of the abdomen; however very dilated small bowel can mimic these appearances.

Radiologically dilated loops can be due to:

- Continuous positive airway pressure administration – thin-walled, with no secondary features
- Ileus – uniform appearance. Seen in sepsis, necrotising enterocolitis and electrolyte disturbance
- Gastrointestinal (GI) obstruction – see below.

In the setting of GI obstruction, the key decision is to determine if there are relatively few dilated loops, or many dilated loops:

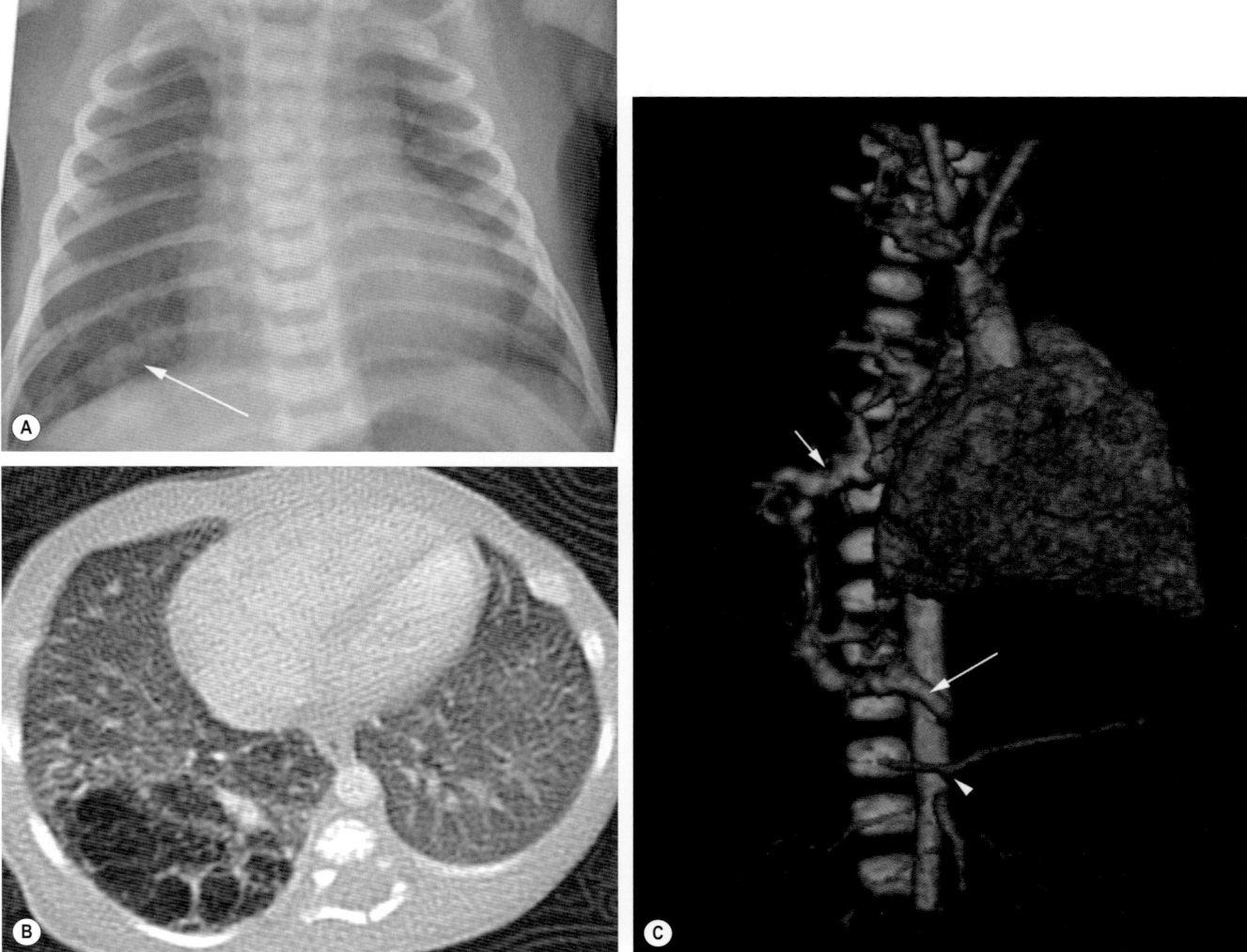

Fig. 43.12 Hybrid lesion. Chest X-ray (A) demonstrating a cystic abnormality within the right lower lobe (arrow). Computed tomography (lung window settings) (B) reveals the extent of the cystic components of the lesion. Surface-shaded display of post-intravenous contrast dataset (C) elegantly demonstrates that there is a large arterial feeding vessel (arrow) and venous drainage from the lesion (short arrow) into the right inferior pulmonary vein – features consistent with an intrapulmonary sequestration. Note the relative size of the feeding vessel to the coeliac axis (arrowhead).

- Relatively few dilated loops = 'upper GI obstruction' (presents with vomiting, often bilious)
  - pyloric or prepyloric membrane/antral web
  - duodenal atresia/stenosis/web – 'double-bubble sign' with no distal gas if complete atresia and variable amount of distal gas if a stenosis
  - malrotation and volvulus – sudden onset of bilious vomiting. No reliable plain film signs to make this diagnosis
  - jejunal atresia – 'triple-bubble' sign of dilated bowel. May show signs of antenatal perforation, with calcified meconium peritonitis.

As stated above, it is not possible to confirm clinical suspicion of malrotation and volvulus on plain X-ray, hence in the appropriate clinical setting an upper GI contrast study is needed. In this circumstance it is usual to use water-soluble contrast media. The examination should usually be undertaken using fluoroscopy so that the dynamic aspects of the examination can be followed as far as the duodenum. The stomach is examined and gastric emptying into the duodenum noted. It is important to obtain an anteroposterior view of the duodenojejunal flexure, which should be to the left of the midline and at the level of the pylorus to exclude malrotation (Fig. 43.16). Volvulus with incomplete obstruction appears as a corkscrew configuration of the duodenum (Fig. 43.17). Complete obstruction secondary to volvulus produces a beaking appearance of the duodenum. Aside from evaluating potential upper GI obstruction, the upper GI contrast series may also be used to assess gastro-oesophageal reflux, which can usually be demonstrated when the baby stops swallowing and either cries or is tilted gently head-down, but often occurs spontaneously. It is important to exclude the presence of hiatus hernia at this stage.

- Relatively many dilated loops = 'low GI obstruction' (typically presents with failure to pass meconium)
  - meconium ileus – may have a bubbly appearance. Peritoneal calcification seen in 30%
  - ileal atresia (Fig. 43.18)
  - incarcerated inguinal hernia
  - functional immaturity of the left hemicolon

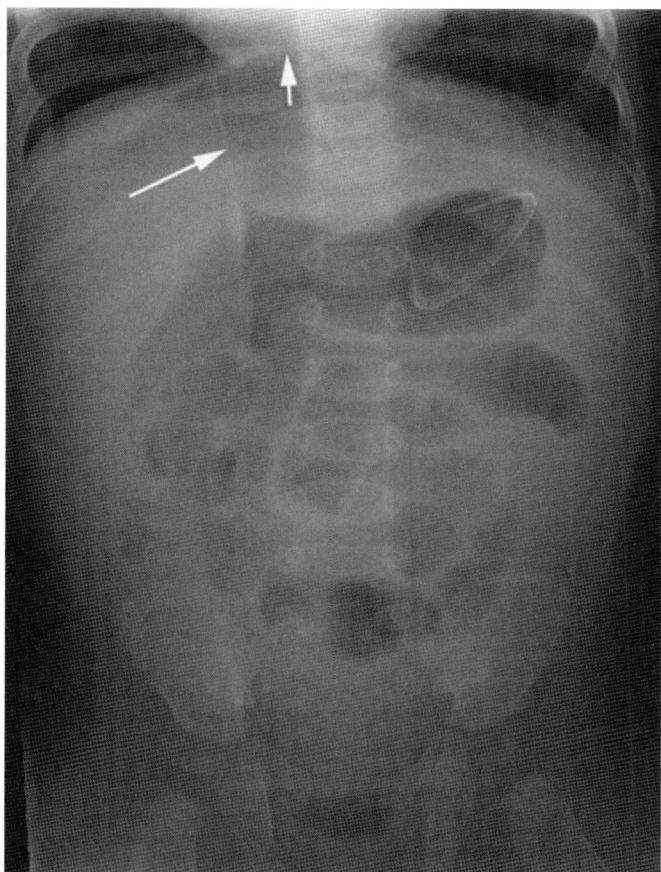

Fig. 43.13 Perforation. Note increased lucency projected over the liver, with the falciform ligament outlined by air (arrow). Additionally the diaphragm is visibly outlined by air (short arrow).

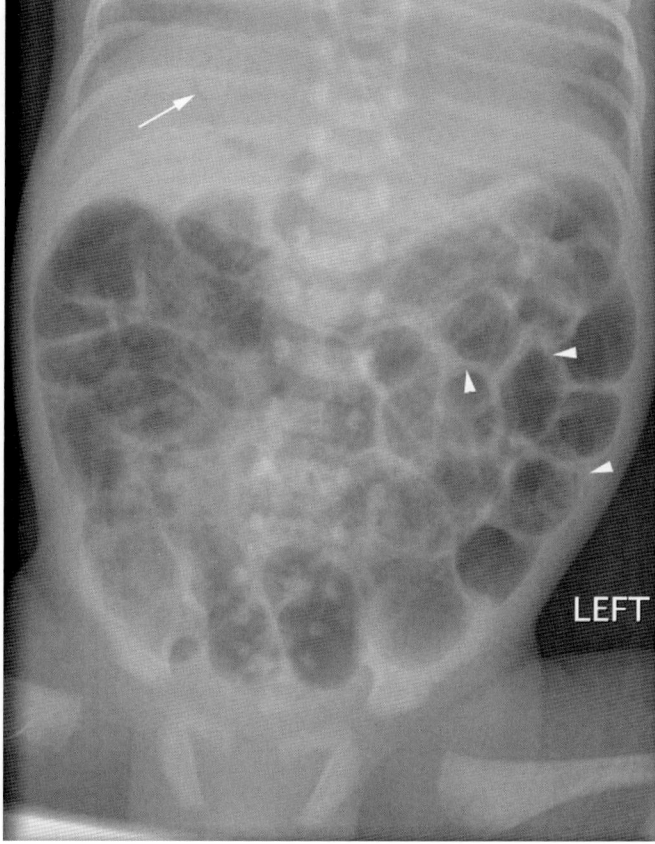

Fig. 43.14 Abdominal X-ray showing extensive intramural gas in a neonate with necrotising enterocolitis (arrowheads). Note also portal venous gas (arrow).

- Hirschsprung disease
- meconium plug syndrome
- inspissated milk
- colonic atresia
- anorectal malformation.

With the exception of anorectal malformations (see below), the neonate with potential low GI obstruction will usually be further evaluated with a contrast enema in an attempt to ascertain the cause. A small catheter (about 8 French) can be inserted into the rectum and contrast instilled using a syringe until the large bowel has been demonstrated with reflux into the terminal ileum. The level of obstruction can usually easily be identified and appropriate films obtained (Fig. 43.19). This technique can also be used to instil dilute Gastrografin as a means of treating meconium ileus.

Neonates with anorectal malformation will usually be defunctioned via a loop colostomy on day 1 of life. Prior to definitive surgery a loopogram will be performed to examine the distal limb of the stoma for its position relative to the expected normal anal position and to look for an associated fistula with the genitourinary tract. There is no place for inverted X-rays to evaluate anorectal malformations as this will not define any associated fistula and imparts an additional radiation burden. Loopograms are also used to assess distal bowel for stricture(s) following resection for necrotising enterocolitis.

Gasless abdomen/paucity of bowel gas

- Fluid-filled bowel loops – for example, with an ileus (see above).
- Ascites – any aerated loops will tend to sit centrally when significant ascites is present (Fig. 43.20).

Ultrasound is useful in this situation, enabling differentation between the two possibilities.

Portal venous gas (Fig. 43.21)

- Necrotising enterocolitis.
- Following umbilical vein catheterisation – no intestinal pneumatosis present when this is the cause.
- Erythroblastosis fetalis.

Imaging in the neonate with abnormal liver function tests

There is a wide differential diagnosis for neonatal jaundice (Ch. 29, part 1), with causes such as neonatal hepatitis, sepsis and total parenteral nutrition administration showing minimal changes on imaging investigations, such as biliary sludge or gallbladder wall thickening. The role of imaging in the setting of neonatal jaundice

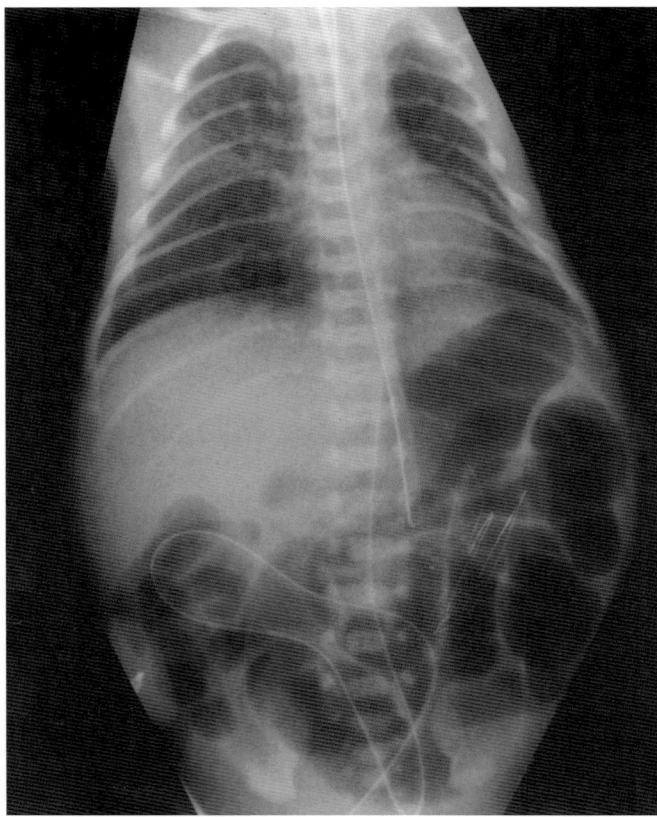

Fig. 43.15 Dilated loops of small and large bowel due to paralytic ileus. These loops did not change configuration over a period of several days. The clinical diagnosis was necrotising enterocolitis.

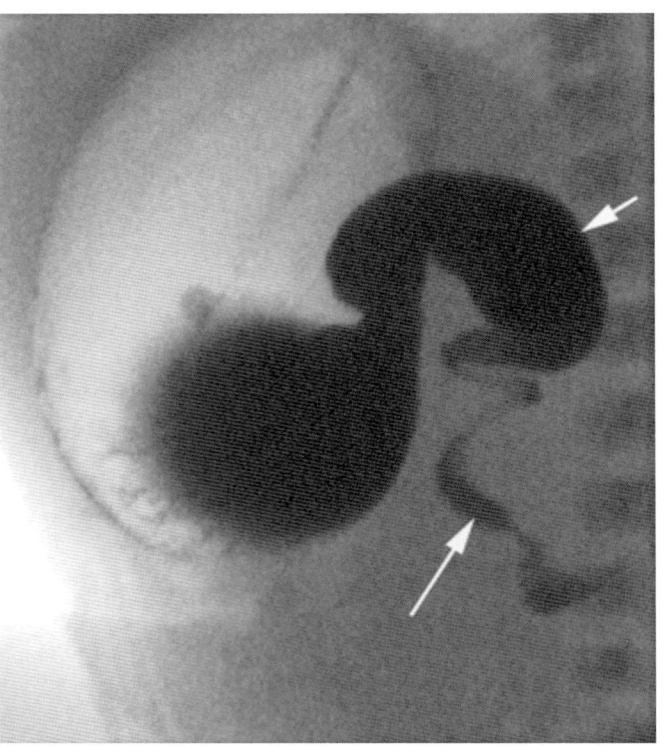

Fig. 43.17 Fluoroscopic capture from an upper gastrointestinal series (lateral view) demonstrating proximal duodenal dilatation (short arrow) and a corkscrew appearance (arrow), consistent with malrotation and volvulus.

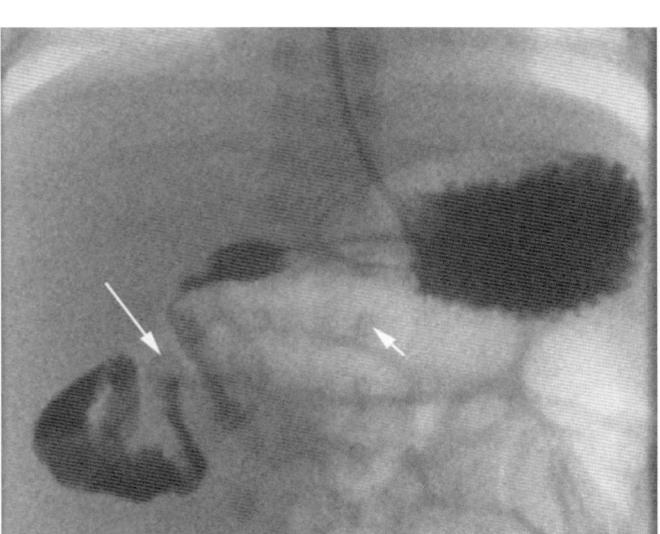

Fig. 43.16 Fluoroscopic capture from an upper gastrointestinal series. The duodenojejunal flexure (arrow) lies to the right of the spine, opposite and inferior to its expected position at or to the left of the left pedicle of L1 (short arrow). There is no dilatation or hold-up of contrast, consistent with malrotation without volvulus present.

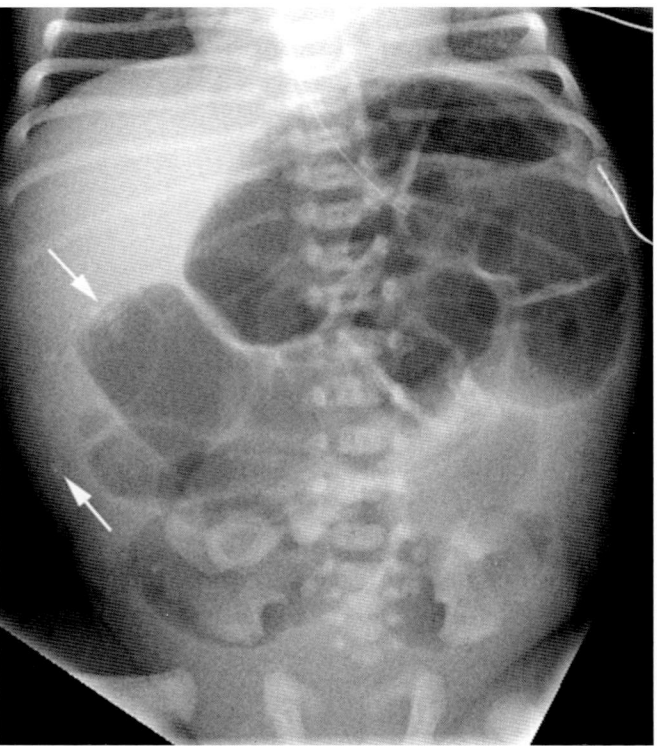

Fig. 43.18 Ileal atresia. Abdominal X-ray showing multiple dilated loops of bowel, with punctate peritoneal calcification (arrows) in keeping with in utero perforation and meconium peritonitis.

Staff Library
Singleton Hospital
Tel: 01792 205666 Ext. 5281

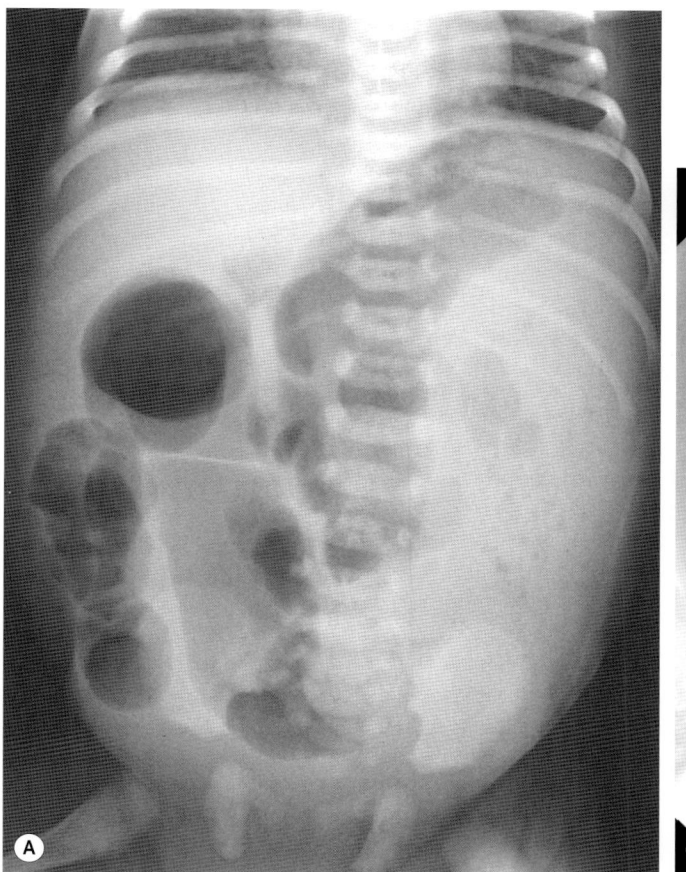

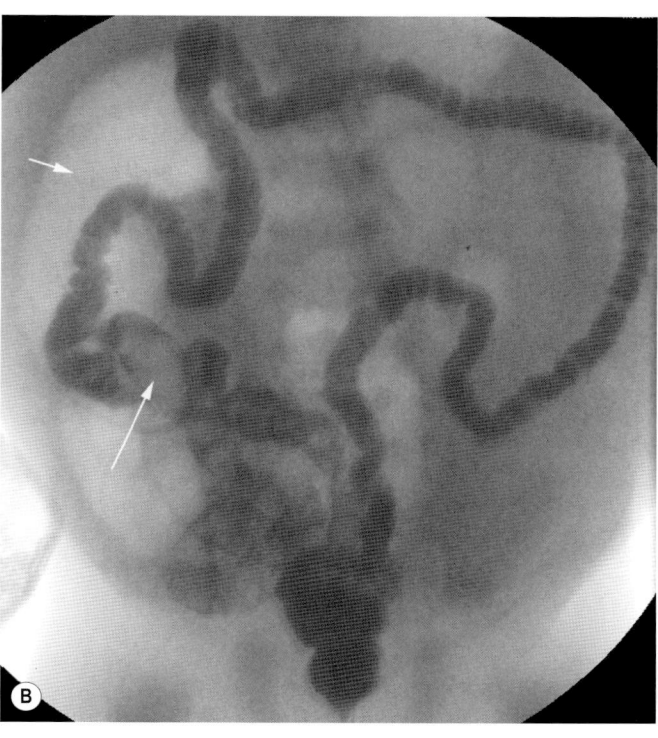

Fig. 43.19 Meconium ileus. Abdominal X-ray (A) showing markedly dilated bowel loops within the central and right hemiabdomen. Fluoroscopic capture (B) from subsequent contrast enema showing a microcolon and filling defects within the terminal ileum (arrow). Note that the peripherally located dilated viscus (short arrow) is small bowel.

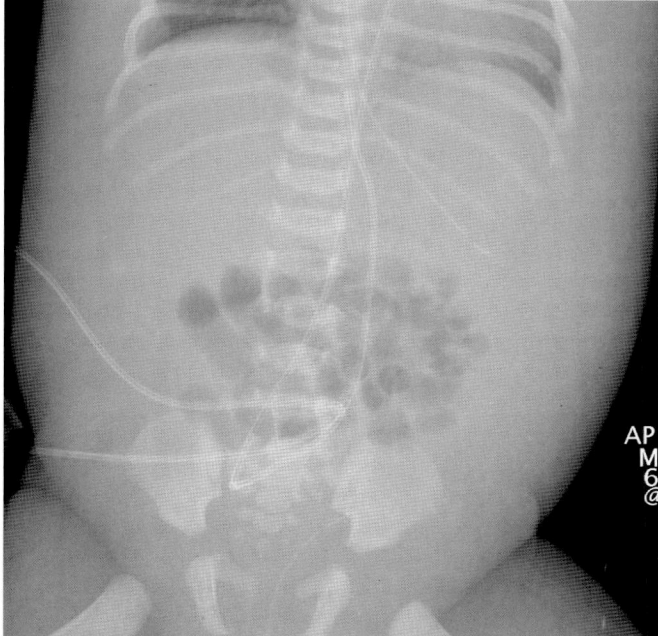

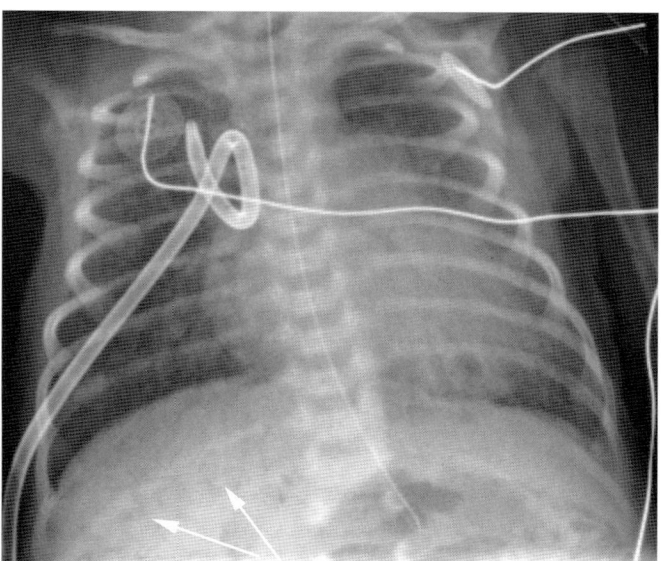

Fig. 43.21 Portal venous gas. Chest X-ray performed for assessment of intercostal drain position. Note branching linear lucencies within the liver that extend to the liver periphery (arrows). This was the first indication of necrotising enterocolitis in this case, highlighting the importance of reviewing the upper abdomen on chest radiographs.

Fig. 43.20 Abdominal X-ray demonstrating centrally positioned bowel loops with ground-glass appearance at the periphery of the abdomen, consistent with ascites. Note also the marked subcutaneous oedema.

is to look for surgically correctable causes such as biliary atresia and choledochal cysts. Ultrasound provides a quick and safe means of evaluating the liver parenchyma and biliary tree. The most reliable ultrasound signs of biliary atresia are said to be the 'triangular cord sign', abnormal gallbladder wall and shape, and absence of the common bile duct (Kim et al. 2000; Humphrey and Stringer 2007). It must be remembered that ultrasound is both operator- and experience-dependent and combination with ^{99m}Tc-labelled trimethyl-bromo-hepatobiliary iminodiacetic acid scanning further refines the differential diagnosis between neonatal hepatitis and biliary atresia, although biopsy is the ultimate arbiter. It is important to exclude the diagnosis of biliary atresia before 6 weeks of life.

Imaging in the neonate with an abdominal mass

Abdominal masses may be either diagnosed antenatally or present in the postnatal period. The majority of such masses will be benign in nature, although malignant lesions can also occur. The majority of neonatal masses arise from the kidney (55%). The differential diagnoses to be considered are listed in Table 43.1.

Once again, ultrasound is the front-line imaging investigation, and can usually identify the organ of origin, and either provide a firm diagnosis or narrow the differential diagnosis considerably. Where there remains diagnostic uncertainty and cross-sectional imaging is felt necessary, MRI is the modality of choice thanks to its excellent soft-tissue characterisation, non-ionising nature and multiplanar capabilities (Donoghue et al. 2008).

Genitourinary imaging

Imaging investigation of the genitourinary tract may be driven either by findings identified on antenatal ultrasound or by the baby's postnatal clinical condition (Ch. 35, part 2).

Ultrasound remains the most commonly utilised imaging modality for genitourinary evaluation in the neonate, with excellent resolution and real-time evaluation. The haste with which investigations are performed depends on the clinical scenario, with bilateral antenatal anomalies, possible posterior urethral valves and complex duplex systems requiring early imaging assessment. Neonates with suspected renal vein thrombosis are also a priority. Owing to relative dehydration in the first 24–48 hours, it is possible to underestimate the degree of dilatation present. Similarly, when a baby is virtually anuric, dilatation may not be evident.

There is a trend towards reduced use of micturating cystourethrograms (MCUGs). MCUGs require bladder catheterisation, either per urethram or via a suprapubic catheter, and require antibiotic cover. Water-soluble contrast material is then introduced and the bladder outline, bladder emptying and urethral appearances evaluated. The presence or absence of reflux is documented. If there is any suspicion of posterior urethral valves or bladder pathology an MCUG should be performed.

Musculoskeletal imaging

Most of the indications for skeletal radiographs in neonates are related to birth trauma.

Metabolic bone disease of prematurity has become less frequent in recent years (Ch. 34, part 4) but isolated rib fractures are still quite often seen in extremely preterm babies who spend many months in neonatal intensive care. Osteomyelitis is an infrequent complication of neonatal intensive care. It is often clinically

Table 43.1 Differential diagnosis of an abdominal mass based on imaging studies

Renal (55%)
Hydronephrosis
Multicystic dysplastic kidney
Polycystic kidney
Mesoblastic nephroma
Wilms' tumour
Renal vein thrombosis
Crossed fused renal ectopia

Genital (15%)
Hydrometrocolpos
Ovarian cyst

Gastrointestinal (15%)
Duplication cyst
Omental/mesenteric cyst
Splenic cyst

Adrenal (5%)
Adrenal haemorrhage
Congenital neuroblastoma (NBL)

Liver/biliary (5%)
Hepatic cyst
Hepatic tumour
■ Benign infantile haemangioendothelioma
■ Mesenchymal hamartoma
■ Malignant hepatoblastoma
Choledochal cyst
NBL metastases

Retroperitoneal masses (5%)
Lymphangioma
Extra-adrenal NBL
Anterior meningomyelocele
Teratoma
Rhabdomyosarcoma

asymptomatic and may only be recognised when the plain X-ray findings are fairly advanced. Isotope bone scans using ^{99m}Tc-methylene diphosphonate may be positive but a normal or negative isotope bone scan does not exclude the diagnosis. The late changes will be seen on plain X-ray usually undertaken for unexplained limb swelling.

Hip ultrasound

Following upon the work of Graf and others, the technique of ultrasound of the neonatal hip has been developed. The aim is to detect developmental dysplasia of the hip and to guide management. Normal measurements of the angles of the acetabulum, both bony and the cartilaginous labrum, are well documented. The technique requires considerable attention to detail. Applying ultrasound as a screening test to a whole population has been tried in continental Europe and in Coventry, UK, with some success. Selective use of the technique in a high-risk population is the usual current UK strategy.

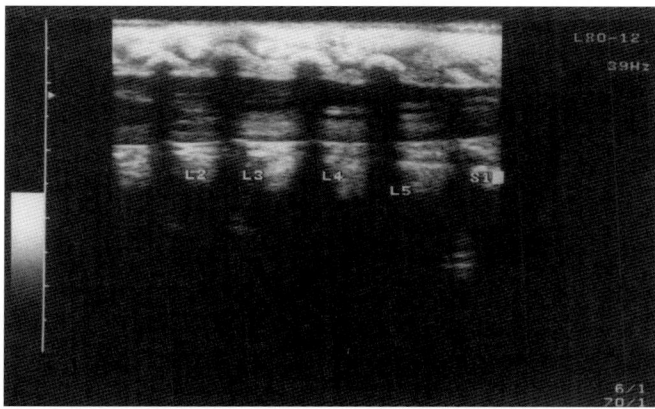

Fig. 43.22 Longitudinal section of the spinal canal showing the cord finishing at the L2 level. The nerve roots are seen lying against the anterior wall of the spinal canal. These are normal appearances.

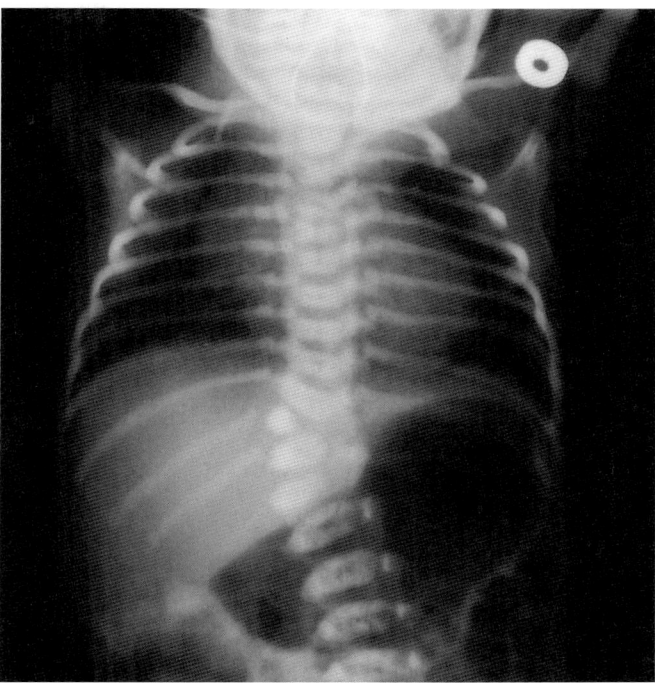

Fig. 43.23 VATER (vertebral defects, anal atresia, tracheo-oesophageal fistula, oesophageal atresia, and renal/radial defects) anomaly. Note the thoracic and lumbar vertebral anomalies. The stomach is filled with gas owing to an associated tracheo-oesophageal fistula.

Spinal imaging

In the neonate ultrasound of the spine is a very effective way of demonstrating the cord and spinal canal contents. It is efficient because the vertebral arches are not ossified at this age and good access of ultrasound to the spine is therefore possible (Fig. 43.22). This can be used to demonstrate the cord, nerve roots and spinal contents very effectively and is indicated in babies whose spinal dimples are not 'simple'. MRI, which is considered the gold standard, often does not give images that are as detailed as ultrasound at this age and is a second-line investigation. Plain X-rays of the spine are unhelpful except for documenting segmentation defects (Fig. 43.23).

Central nervous system imaging

Ultrasound

Neonatal cranial ultrasound has developed dramatically in the last 30 years. A standard examination is undertaken with a small footprint probe of 5 or 7.5 MHz. The anterior fontanelle is used almost exclusively as the portal of entry of ultrasound. The standard views are coronal, midline, sagittal and parasagittal (Figs 43.24 and 43.25). Most views are coronal oblique, angled from the anterior fontanelle anteriorly or posteriorly and not true coronal. Whilst the concept of standard views is often used for the purpose of documentation the examination is a dynamic one, with the probe sweeping from anterior to posterior and from side to side to obtain as full a view of the head as possible. Obviously the areas under the parietal convexities are not as well demonstrated as other areas using this approach and it must be appreciated that small subdural collections in this site will not be excluded by ultrasound.

Computed tomography

With modern helical and multislice CT scanners the quality of resolution of the neonatal brain is exceptional. Obviously the

examination has the disadvantage of the requirements to move the baby from its more controlled environment to the CT scanner and this is therefore somewhat restricted. The length of time of the examination has been reduced to a few seconds so that movement is considerably reduced and sedation is not usually needed. It is usual just to obtain axial sections of the brain as these give most of the relevant information with the lowest radiation dose. CT is the only diagnostic modality that confidently diagnoses calcification. However changes relating to bleeding and particularly extra-axial bleeds are best assessed by CT, much better than ultrasound and at least equal to MRI.

Magnetic resonance imaging

The length of time taken for MR examinations and poor availability of scanning time restrict the use of MRI to a very small number of neonates. The lack of radiation, multiplanar capabilities and exquisite demonstration of differences in tissue density make this the gold standard for brain imaging. As well as being very efficient at assessing haemorrhage, hypoxia–ischaemia and maturation of the neonatal brain can be most accurately assessed using MRI and this will continue to evolve with more sophisticated software. The fact that the neonatal brain has a high water content means that specific sequences have been devised to maximise the information from MRI scans, especially using long T2 relaxation times.

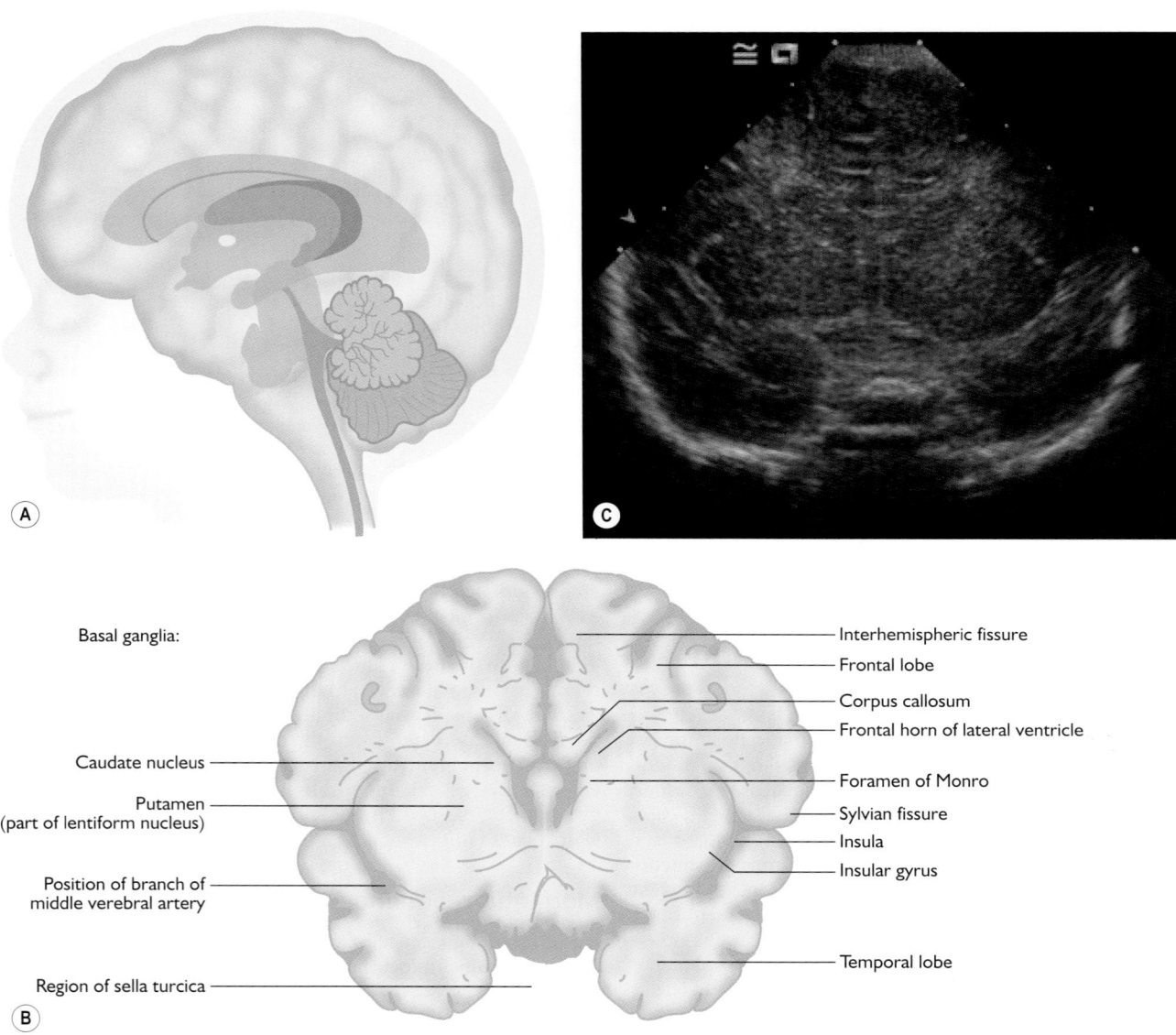

Basal ganglia:

Caudate nucleus

Putamen
(part of lentiform nucleus)

Position of branch of
middle verebral artery

Region of sella turcica

Interhemispheric fissure

Frontal lobe

Corpus callosum

Frontal horn of lateral ventricle

Foramen of Monro

Sylvian fissure

Insula

Insular gyrus

Temporal lobe

Fig. 43.24 Standard coronal section of the neonatal head imaged with ultrasound: (A) plane of scanning; (B) labelled diagram; and (C) corresponding scan picture. *(Reproduced with permission from (Rennie et al. 2008).)*

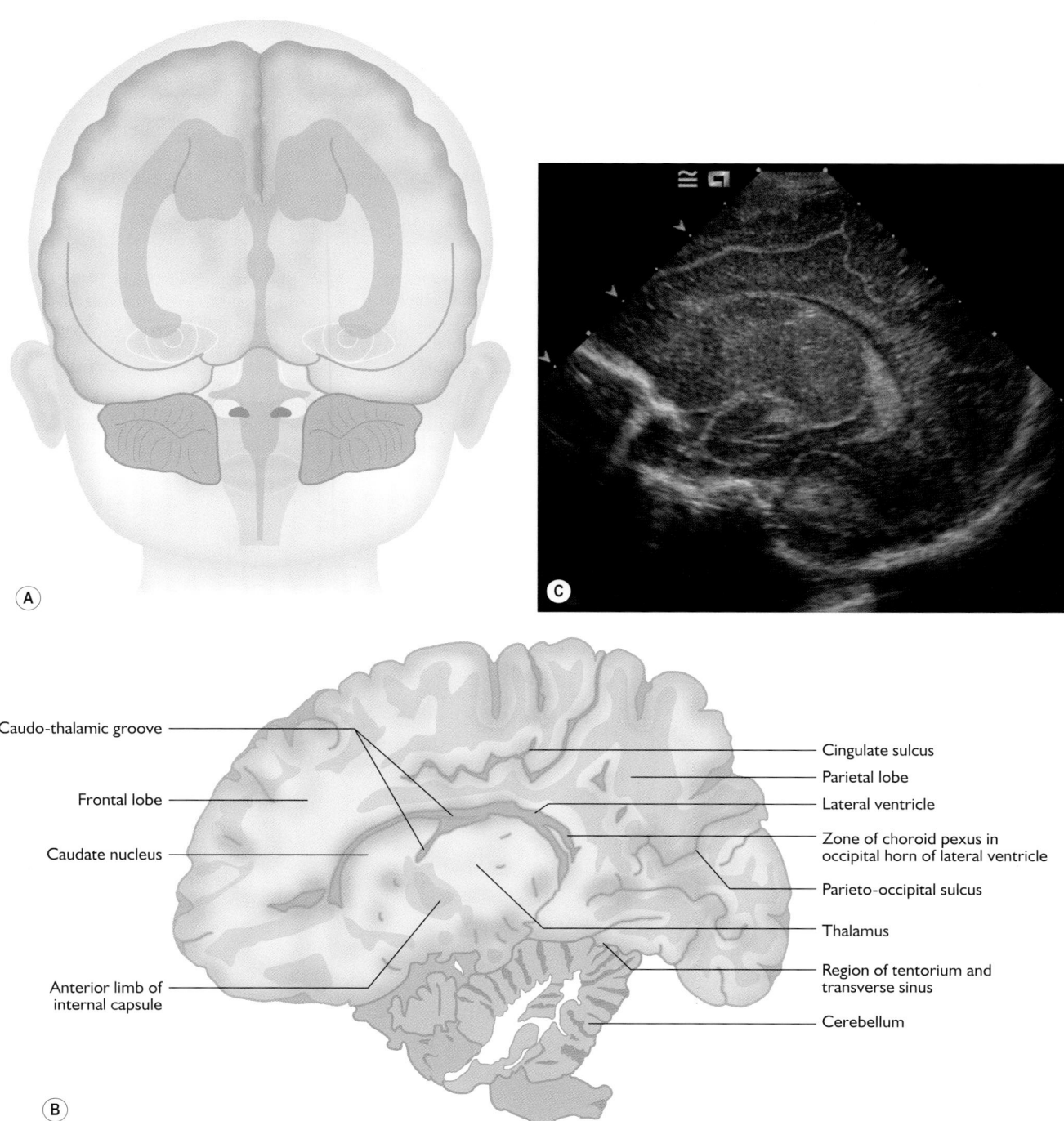

Caudo-thalamic groove

Frontal lobe

Caudate nucleus

Anterior limb of
internal capsule

Cingulate sulcus

Parietal lobe

Lateral ventricle

Zone of choroid pexus in
occipital horn of lateral ventricle

Parieto-occipital sulcus

Thalamus

Region of tentorium and
transverse sinus

Cerebellum

Fig. 43.25 Standard parasagittal section of the neonatal head imaged with ultrasound: (A) plane of scanning; (B) labelled diagram; and (C) corresponding scan picture. *(Reproduced with permission from (Rennie 1997).)*

References

Barrington, K.J., 1999. Umbilical artery catheters in the newborn; effects of position of the catheter tip. Cochrane Database Syst Rev (1), CD000505.

Blayney, M.P., Logan, D.R., 1994. First thoracic body as reference for endotracheal tube placement. Arch Dis Child Fetal Neonatal Ed 71, F32–F35.

Donoghue, V., Ryan, S., Twomey, E., 2008. Perinatal tumours: the contribution of radiology to management. Pediatr Radiol 38 (Suppl. 3), S477–S483.

Epelman, M., Daneman, A., Navarro, O.M., et al., 2007. Necrotizing enterocolitis: review of state-of-the-art imaging findings with pathologic correlation. Radiographics 27, 285–305.

Frush, D.P., 2005. Technique of pediatric thoracic CT angiography. Radiol Clin North Am 43, 419–433.

Greenberg, M., Movahed, H., Peterson, B., et al., 1995. Placement of umbilical venous catheters with use of bedside real-time ultrasonography. J Pediatr 126, 633.

HMSO, 2000. Ionising Radiation (Medical Examinations) Regulations. HMSO, London.

Humphrey, T.M., Stringer, M.D., 2007. Biliary atresia: US diagnosis. Radiology 244, 845–851.

Khilani, P., Goldstein, B., Todres, I.D., 1991. Double lumen umbilical venous catheters in critically ill neonates: A randomized prospective study. Crit Care Med 19, 1348.

Kim, M.J., Park, Y.N., Han, S.J., et al., 2000. Biliary atresia in neonates and infants: triangular area of high signal intensity in the portahepatis on T2 weighted magnetic resonance cholangiography with US and histopathologic correlation. Radiology 215, 395–401.

Raval, N.C., Gonzalez, E., Bhat, A.M., et al., 1995. Umbilical venous catheters: Evaluation of radiographs to determine position and associated complications of malpositioned umbilical venous catheters. Am J Perinatol 12, 201.

Rennie, J.M., 1997. Neonatal Cerebral Ultrasound. Cambridge University Press, Cambridge.

Rennie, J.M., Hagmann, C.F., Robertson, N.J., 2008. Neonatal Cerebral Investigation. Cambridge University Press, Cambridge.

Rigler, L.G., 1941. Spontaneous pneumoperitoneum. Rontgenologic sign found in the supine position. Radiology 37, 604–607.

Scanlon, K.B., Grylack, L.J., Borten, M., 1982. Placement of umbilical artery catheters: High vs. low. JOGN Nursing 11, 355.

Schlesinger, A.E., Braverman, R.M., DiPietro, M.A., 2003. Pictorial essay. Neonates and umbilical venous catheters: normal appearance, anomalous positions, complications, and potential aid to diagnosis. AJR Am J Roentgenol 180, 1147–1153.

Silva, C.T., Daneman, A., Navarro, O.M., et al., 2007. Correlation of sonographic findings and outcome in necrotizing enterocolitis. Pediatr Radiol 37, 274–282.

Stocker, J.T., 2009. Cystic lung disease in infants and children. Fetal Pediatr Pathol 28, 155–184.

Zeidan, S., Hery, G., Lacroix, F., et al., 2009. Intralobar sequestration associated with cystic adenomatoid malformation: diagnostic and thoracoscopic pitfalls. Surg Endosc 23, 1750–1753.

Further reading

Carty, H., Brunelle, F., Stringer, D.A., et al., 2004. Imaging Children. Churchill Livingstone, Edinburgh.

Graf, R., Scott, S., Lercher, K., et al., 2006. Hip Sonography: Diagnosis and Management of Infant Hip Dysplasia, second edn. Springer, Berlin.

Rennie, J.M., Hagmann, C.F., Robertson, N.J., 2008. Neonatal Cerebral Investigation. Cambridge University Press, Cambridge.

section 7

Practical procedures

Procedures and iatrogenic disorders

Sian Harding

44

Introduction

The word 'iatrogenic' is derived from the Greek 'iatros', meaning physician, and 'genic', meaning produced by. An iatrogenic disorder is any adverse condition that occurs as a result of a diagnostic procedure or therapeutic intervention that is not the natural consequence of the underlying disease. 'Pathos' is Greek for suffering, hence the term 'iatropathic', meaning suffering caused by medical examination or treatment.

Many iatrogenic events in neonatology are avoidable. The most commonly reported iatrogenic events in neonates include

© 2012 Elsevier Ltd

nosocomial infections, catheter-related complications, medication errors and respiratory events, including intubation injury and unplanned extubations. Low birthweight and gestational age, length of stay, presence of a central venous line, mechanical ventilation and support with continuous positive airway pressure have been identified as major risk factors for iatrogenic events (Ligi et al. 2008).

Good infection control and safe drug-prescribing and administration practices must be established to ensure that vulnerable infants are exposed to a minimum of hazards during their admission to neonatal intensive care. Considerable progress is being made in reducing nosocomial infection rates in intensive care units across the world. In 2009, The UK National Patient Safety Agency began a quality improvement project, Matching Michigan, in adult and paediatric intensive care units with the aim of reducing catheter-associated bloodstream infections (Pronovost et al. 2006; Matching Michigan 2009). This quality improvement project has now been rolled out to neonatal units across the UK. The Matching Michigan model incorporates electronic reporting of infections with a number of technical and non-technical interventions that are aimed at promoting a safety culture within the critical care environment.

Medication errors occur all too frequently in busy neonatal units. A neonatal clinical pharmacist is a valuable addition to a multidisciplinary team caring for sick neonates. Medication errors will be minimised if the pharmacist attends daily rounds, checks drug and total parenteral nutrition (TPN) prescription charts and is available to give advice about therapeutic drug monitoring and pharmacokinetics. Errors can also be reduced by using electronic prescribing and smart infusion pumps (Sekar 2010). Individualised, computer-generated emergency medication sheets decrease the risk of errors in emergency situations and using standardised drug infusion concentrations should eliminate the risk of 10-fold dosing errors. There should also be clear procedures in every neonatal unit to ensure that the right patient receives the right drug, in the right dose, by the right route, at the right time (Chief Pharmaceutical Officer 2004).

The remainder of this chapter deals with how and when to perform many of the practical procedures that are undertaken during neonatal intensive care and describes the most important complications that are associated with each procedure. Every procedure performed on a baby carries risks. Knowledge of anatomy and standardised operating procedures, meticulous hand hygiene (Pessoa-Silva et al. 2007) and careful observation will help to reduce many of the procedure-related iatrogenic events in neonatal intensive care units. It is imperative that doctors and nurses performing practical procedures receive training and supervision until they are competent at performing the necessary tasks.

Consent for procedures

Implicit consent is considered acceptable for many of the routine, low-risk procedures performed in neonatology (Consent for Common Neonatal Investigations, Interventions and Treatments 2004). However, explicit verbal or written consent should be taken for complex procedures, procedures involving significant risks and procedures that require general or regional anaesthesia or sedation.

In an emergency, when informed consent cannot be, or has not been, obtained, procedures considered to be in the best interests of the baby should be performed without delay, but clinical staff should always notify the parents as soon as possible after an emergency procedure has been performed.

Pain management (Ch. 25)

The American Academy of Pediatrics (2006) recommends that neonatal units should develop strategies to minimise the number of minor painful or stressful procedures and to provide effective non-pharmacological and/or pharmacological pain relief for all procedures. The continuous infusion of morphine in ventilated neonates may not effectively prevent acute pain from minor painful procedures.

'Kangaroo care' (skin-to-skin contact), swaddling and developmental care have been shown to reduce the response to pain from minor procedures. If available, breastfeeding or breast milk should be administered to neonates undergoing single painful procedures. Sucrose (0.05–0.50 ml of 24% sucrose), given approximately 2 minutes before and 1–2 minutes after a single heelprick or venepuncture, also modifies the response to pain in neonates (Slater et al. 2010).

Topical anaesthetics, such as 4% tetracaine gel (Ametop), reduce pain from procedures such as venepuncture (Jain and Rutter 2000), lumbar puncture and intravenous catheter insertion. The gel must be applied for 30–45 minutes before the procedure and appears to be ineffective for heelpricks (Jain et al. 2001). In practice, topical anaesthesia is not much used in the newborn because of the time taken for it to work, and because it is not always possible to achieve cannulation in a single attempt.

Aseptic technique and skin preparation

Gloves should be used for all procedures. Consider using restraints (e.g. swaddling or immobilisation of one or more of the limbs) in order to maintain asepsis.

Preparation for minor procedures

- Blood taking.
- Insertion of peripheral venous or arterial catheters.
- Suprapubic aspiration.

Wash hands with an antibacterial soap and apply alcohol gel. Put on disposable non-sterile gloves. Clean the baby's skin with antiseptic or alcohol and allow to dry. Use a no-touch technique during the procedure.

Preparation for a major procedure

- Central line placement.
- Insertion of umbilical lines.
- Insertion of chest drains.
- Lumbar puncture or ventricular tap.

Wear a cap and mask. Scrub up for 4–5 minutes using antiseptic solution. Hands should be dried thoroughly with sterile towels. Put on sterile gown and sterile gloves.

Apply antiseptic to the skin, cleaning from the centre of a circle and working out to a diameter of ~5 cm. 10% Povidone-iodine and 0.5% chlorhexidine/70% isopropyl alcohol solution (Hydrex) are the most widely used antiseptic solutions. 2% Chlorhexidine/70% isopropyl alcohol solution has been shown to enhance skin antisepsis; however, the manufacturer does not recommended its use in infants <2 months of age. In extremely preterm babies, 0.5% chlorhexidine in aqueous solution (Sterexidine 200) may reduce

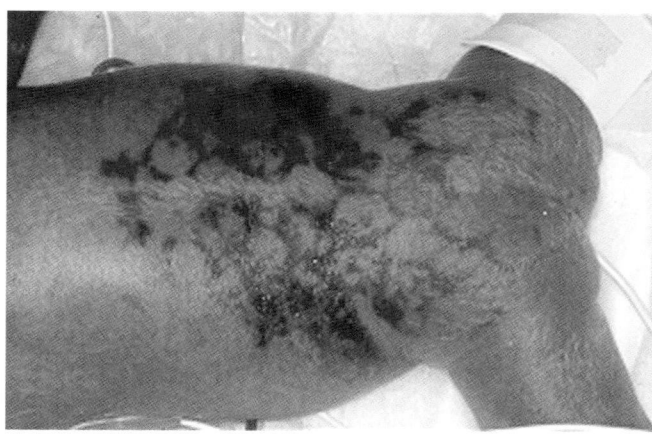

Fig. 44.1 Chemical burn from pooling of antiseptic solution under a premature baby who was lying on bubble wrap. Fortunately the burn healed without scarring.

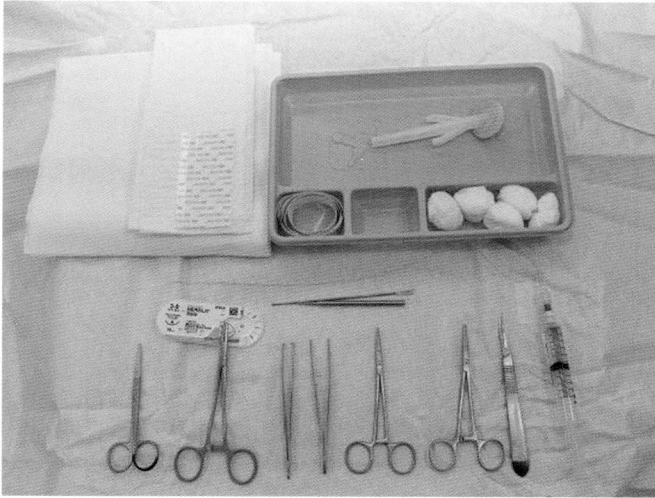

Fig. 44.2 Arrange instruments/equipment in the order of use and avoid contaminating the sterile equipment with dirty swabs.

the risk of chemical burns, but limited data exist to indicate the best preparation for this group of babies.

- Always allow antiseptics to dry for at least 30 seconds before starting any procedure.
- Avoid chemical burns (Fig. 44.1) by ensuring that there is no pooling of the antiseptic solution under the baby.

Equipment

Where possible, use disposable sterile instruments. Many manufacturers provide procedure-specific trays, which contain all of the required instruments and accessories. Always lay out the equipment trolley so that the sterile instruments and accessories are near to hand (Fig. 44.2). Assemble equipment and flush lines with saline before commencing the procedure.

Dressings

Transparent, semipermeable adhesive dressings have become a popular means of dressing catheter insertion sites. Ensure good

haemostasis and minimise the amount of dressing that adheres to the baby's skin. Never allow tapes or dressings to extend around an extremity as they will act as a tourniquet if there is venous congestion. Change dressings if they become damp, soiled or non-adherent.

Procedures and their complications

Airway

Endotracheal intubation

This is one of the most commonly performed life-saving procedures.

It is generally accepted that premedication drugs should be used for all elective or semielective intubations where intravenous access is established or can easily be obtained. Drugs that are commonly used include:

- fentanyl 4 µg/kg (give slowly over 30 seconds)
- suxamethonium 2 mg/kg or Atracurium 300 µg/kg
- atropine 20 µg/kg.

Fentanyl has a nearly immediate onset of action, with duration of 1–2 hours. Adverse effects include chest wall rigidity and laryngospasm. Suxamethonium must be drawn up and ready for immediate administration, in case chest wall rigidity occurs. Do not give Suxamethonium if there is significant hyperkalaemia.

Indications

- Stabilisation of the airway to allow tracheal suctioning and removal of meconium or other secretions.
- The administration of surfactant.
- When mechanical ventilation is required for babies with respiratory failure, circulatory problems or neurological dysfunction, or during intra- or interhospital transfers.

Equipment

A complete set of equipment for endotracheal intubation must be kept together in an intubation tray or resuscitation trolley and should be available for immediate use in every delivery room, neonatal nursery and emergency room.

- Neopuff circuit or resuscitation bag and mask.
- 2 × straight-blade laryngoscopes, Miller size 0 for a preterm baby and 1 for a term baby (International Guidelines for Neonatal Resuscitation 2000). Disposable blades are recommended.
- Suction equipment with 8–10 F suction catheters.
- Endotracheal tubes (ETTs), straight or shouldered tubes, with internal diameters of 2.0–4.0 mm.
- An introducer (optional – if used the introducer must not extend beyond the tip of the ETT).
- Magill forceps and lubricating jelly (for nasal intubation)
- Fixation devices, hydrocolloid dressing, adhesive tapes or bonnet and ties.

Procedure

Prepare all equipment and select an appropriate-size ETT (Table 44.1). If gestation/weight is unknown the distance from the base of the nasal septum to the tragus +1 cm is a reasonable guide for the length of an oral ETT (Whyte et al. 2007).

Table 44.1 Oral endotracheal tube (ETT) size and approximate length by gestational age and weight

GESTATIONAL AGE (weeks)	WEIGHT (grams)	ETT SIZE (INTERNAL DIAMETER: mm)	APPROX. LENGTH FOR OROTRACHEAL ROUTE (cm)
23–24	500–600	2.0–2.5	5.5
25–26	700–800	2.5	6.0
27–29	900–1000	2.5	6.5
30–34	1000–2000	3.0	7.0–7.5
34–38	2000–3500	3.0–3.5	7.5–8.0
>38	>3500	3.5–4.0	8.5–9.0

(Adapted from Kempley et al. (2008).)

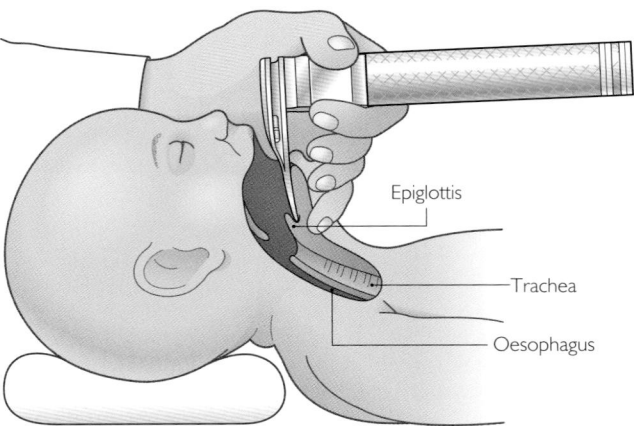

Fig. 44.3 The tip of the laryngoscope should be placed in the vallecula.

Orotracheal intubation

The orotracheal route is best for emergency intubations. To minimise hypoxia, each intubation attempt should last no more than 20–30 seconds.

1. Position the baby's head in the midline in a neutral position. Do not hyperextend the neck as this makes visualisation of the cords more difficult.
2. Use gentle suctioning to clear the oropharynx.
3. Hold the laryngoscope in the left hand and introduce the blade into the right-hand side of the mouth, sweeping the tongue to the left as the blade is advanced.
4. The tip of the blade should be introduced into the vallecula (Fig. 44.3).
5. In extremely preterm infants, the vallecula may be too small, in which case gently elevate the epiglottis with the laryngoscope blade.
6. Apply gentle anterior traction to the laryngoscope (in the direction of the handle). Do not use the upper gum as a fulcrum, as this will not produce a clear view of the glottis and will traumatise the gum. Applying cricoid pressure will help to bring the vocal cords into view (Fig. 44.4).
7. Under direct vision, the ETT tip should be inserted about 1 cm below the cords. Do not try to pass the ETT down the

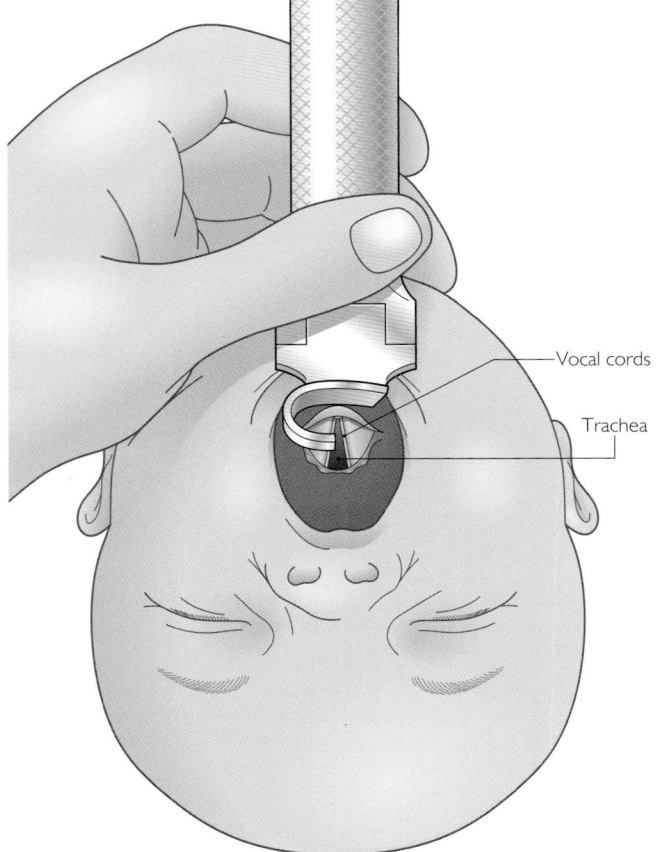

Fig. 44.4 Visualisation of the vocal cords.

laryngoscope blade as this will obstruct your line of sight. Do not force the ETT through closed cords. Wait for the cords to open. If necessary, stop, mask ventilate the baby and try again.

8. Confirm the position of the tube by looking for symmetrical chest wall movement and listening for equal breath sounds over both lung fields. Colorimetric end-tidal CO_2 detectors can be used to confirm that the tube is lying within the trachea.

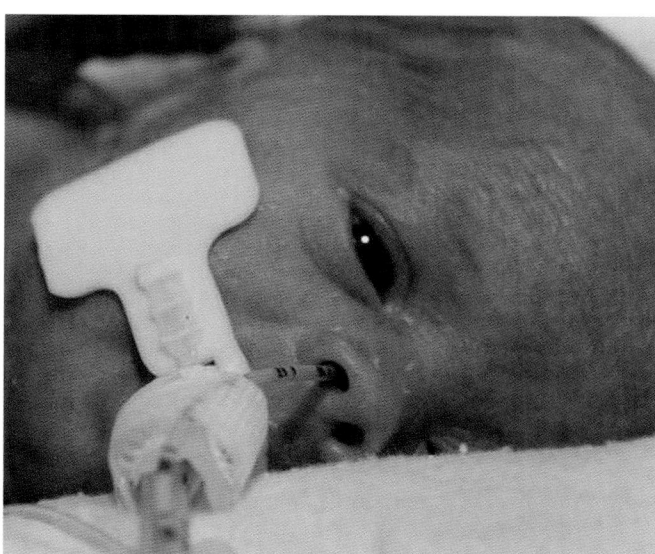

Fig. 44.5 Fixation device for oral endotracheal tube.

9. Secure the ETT using adhesive tape or a purpose-made fixation device (Fig. 44.5).
10. After fixation, listen to the breath sounds again and observe chest wall movement. Shorten the ETT to reduce dead space.
11. The ETT position must be confirmed with a chest X-ray. The tip of the ETT is best placed opposite the body of the first thoracic vertebra (T1) (Blayney and Logan 1994). Note that the carina lies variably between T3 and T5.
12. Note the final length of the tube at the lips.

Nasotracheal intubation

Nasotracheal tubes may be preferred in infants who are very active on the ventilator. Foot length has been reported as an accurate predictor of nasotracheal tube length in neonates (Embleton et al. 2001).

Do not use an introducer.

1. Insert the laryngoscope to visualise the oropharynx. Avoid hyperextending the neck.
2. Insert a lubricated straight ETT through the nostril, following the curve of the nasopharynx, until the tip is in line with the glottis.
3. Apply gentle cricoid pressure and advance the tube through the cords under direct vision. Magill forceps can be used in larger babies to thread the tip of the ETT through the cords.
4. Nasal ETTs are commonly secured with two half split tapes. One-half of each split tape is used to encircle the tube, while the remainder of the tape adheres to a hydrocolloid dressing on the upper lip and cheek.

Complications of intubation

Minor degrees of stridor secondary to laryngeal oedema are common in the first 24 hours following extubation. At present there is no evidence to support the routine use of corticosteroids prior to elective extubation. However, a trend towards reduced rates of reintubation or postextubation stridor following administration of steroids has been demonstrated in high-risk neonates (Khemani et al. 2009).

The risk of iatrogenic injury increases with decreasing gestational age and birthweight. Damage to the pharynx or oesophagus has been reported to occur in 0.44% of babies born at 1000–1500 g

and 0.47% of babies born at <1000 g (Schuman et al. 2010). This complication can usually be treated conservatively with intravenous antibiotics and withholding of oral feeds; however, many of the complications of intubation will require referral to a paediatric ENT, plastic or dental surgeon for more definitive management (Table 44.2).

Breathing

Needle thoracocentesis

Indications

- Emergency drainage of a simple or tension pneumothorax.
- Diagnostic tap of a pleural effusion.

Equipment

- Cold light, with sterile glove to cover the tip of the fibreoptic lead.
- 21–25 G butterfly needle, three-way tap, universal container, sterile water.
- If draining an effusion: 21–25 G venous cannula (Venflon), extension set, three-way tap and syringe.

Procedure

Simple or tension pneumothorax

1. Confirm the diagnosis:
   (a) Clinical examination: look for signs of mediastinal shift, abdominal distension and increasing oxygen requirement.
   (b) Transilluminate the chest.
   (c) Perform a chest X-ray if unsure of the diagnosis, but do not delay treatment of clinically obvious tension pneumothorax.
2. Prepare equipment. Attach the three-way tap, open to air, to the tubing of the butterfly needle and place under water. The weight of the three-way tap will keep the end of the tubing submerged.
3. Clean the skin.
4. Using a no-touch technique, insert the needle into the second intercostal space in the midclavicular line.
5. Air will bubble out, confirming the diagnosis of a pneumothorax. If the pneumothorax was under tension, leave the needle in situ, while preparing to insert a formal chest drain.
6. In the case of a simple pneumothorax, a syringe can be attached to the three-way tap to remove any residual air. When all the air has been aspirated, remove the needle and repeat a chest X-ray.

Diagnostic pleural tap

1. Confirm the diagnosis:
   (a) Examination: reduced/absent breath sounds.
   (b) Chest X-ray to assess the size of the effusion.
2. Prepare the equipment. Clean and drape the skin.
3. Using a no-touch technique, insert the catheter needle into the fourth to fifth intercostal space in the midaxillary line, keeping the catheter needle at right angles to the skin until the pleural space is penetrated. Advance the catheter over the needle and withdraw the needle. Attach a short extension to the catheter and aspirate the pleural fluid slowly with a syringe.
4. When enough fluid has been aspirated, remove the catheter and apply a sterile gauze dressing.

Table 44.2 Complications of intubation

INJURY	PRESENTING SIGNS	MANAGEMENT
Nasal damage	Erosion of nasal septum. Nasal cartilage necrosis	Nasal damage more likely in infants <1000 g. Avoid upward traction on the nostril. Damage more likely from nasal ETT than CPAP tubes. Refer to plastic surgeon
Pharyngeal tear (Meyers et al. 1978)	Respiratory distress, difficulty passing a nasogastric tube. Ectopic nasogastric tube. Pneumomediastinum, pneumothorax, surgical emphysema and pleural effusion	The site most commonly perforated is the pharynx, posterior to the cricopharyngeal muscle; the second most common site is the piriform sinus. Remove ectopic NG tube. Seek expert ENT advice. May require early surgical exploration. Treat with antibiotics
Laryngeal injury including trauma to vocal cords and arytenoids (Fan et al. 1983; Roberts et al. 1988)	Weak cry, aphonia, respiratory distress, stridor, poor feeding. Risk of injury increased if intubation for more than 7 days and 3 or more intubations	Refer to ENT for diagnostic laryngoscopy
SGS (Walner et al. 2001)	Biphasic stridor and airway obstruction. Acquired SGS occurs in ~1–2% of intubated neonates	Once SGS is mature, medical therapy (oral or inhaled steroids) is almost always unsuccessful. Treat suspected gastro-oesophageal reflux preoperatively and postoperatively for optimal surgical results
Subglottic granuloma or cysts (Lim et al. 2003)	Upper airway obstruction	May require tracheostomy and laser therapy
Tracheal tear (Serlin and Daily 1975; Ammari et al. 2002)	Surgical emphysema, pneumomediastinum, pneumothorax, respiratory distress	Secure airway: tip of the ETT must lie distal to the tear. Tracheotomy may be required. Manage small tears conservatively with antibiotic cover. Large tears usually require primary closure. Seek expert ENT advice
Palatal grooves (Erenberg and Nowak 1984; Hohoff et al. 2005)	Narrow channel of variable depth near midline of the palate	Role of palatal protection plates remains unclear. Nasal intubation protects against palatal grooving. Palatal appearance usually normalises within 2 years
Defective dentition (Mason et al. 1994; Harila-Kaera et al. 2002)	Altered dental arch dimensions in premature infants. Malocclusion, delayed eruption of maxillary central incisors. Enamel hypoplasia	Minimise trauma during intubation. Referral to paediatric dentist once teeth have started to erupt
Acquired oral commissure defect (Kahn and Spinazzola 2005)	Lateral placement of the ETT holder against the oral commissure	Prevent by maintaining the ETT in the desired position. Refer to plastic surgeon

ETT, endotracheal tube; CPAP, continuous positive airway pressure; NG, nasogastric; ENT, ear, nose and throat; SGS, subglottic stenosis.

Complications

See complications of chest drains, below.

Chest drain insertion

This procedure is often performed as an emergency. The majority of infants requiring a chest drain for treatment of a pneumothorax will need ventilation. Remember that positive-pressure ventilation may convert a simple pneumothorax into a tension pneumothorax.

Insertion of a chest drain for pneumothorax or pleural fluid drainage is painful. The American Academy of Pediatrics (2006) recommends infiltration of the skin site with a local anaesthetic before incision and the use of opioids before or after chest drain insertion.

Indications

- Drainage of a pneumothorax that is causing significant respiratory or haemodynamic compromise.
- Drainage of a large pleural effusion or chylothorax.

Note that rapid and complete drainage of a large pleural effusion may cause haemodynamic compromise: if possible drain enough fluid to improve respiratory status and then consider clamping the tube and draining the effusion intermittently over the next few hours.

Equipment

- Chest drain insertion pack containing drapes, intercostal drains, scalpel, forceps if using blunt dissection technique, silk suture, Steri-Strips, gauze, adhesive dressings.

- Chest drains – select according to the preferred technique:
  - Classic method: 8 or 10 Fr chest tubes.
  - Seldinger method: Fuhrman straight or pigtail chest tubes (5, 6 or 8.5 Fr gauge).
- Underwater sealed drainage system or a Heimlich valve.

Procedure

Classic (blunt dissection) method

1. Position the infant with a towel under the back so the affected side is raised ~30° above the horizontal. Ask an assistant to hold, or secure, the arm above the infant's head.
2. Clean the skin with antiseptic solution, taking care not to allow the solution to pool under the baby's back.
3. Identify the fourth or fifth intercostal space, midaxillary line. Infiltrate 1% lidocaine into the skin and subcutaneous tissues.
4. Assemble the equipment and remove the trochar from the chest drain tube.
5. Using a no. 11 scalpel blade, make a 1-cm-long incision in the skin, parallel to and just above the rib. Insert a pair of artery forceps into the incision, and, keeping the forceps perpendicular to the chest wall, use blunt dissection to penetrate the muscle layer.
6. The pleura can be incised with the scalpel or opened by applying pressure with the closed tip of the forceps. A definite give will be felt as the tip of the forceps pierces the pleura. Use your index finger as a guard to prevent the forceps from penetrating too deeply.
7. Keep the forceps in place and thread the chest drain tube between the opened tips of the forceps and advance it 2–3 cm into the pleural space. Alternatively, withdraw the artery forceps and clip the chest tube via the side hole and advance the chest drain into the pleural space. The disadvantage of this second technique is that it is not always easy to relocate the tract through the intercostal muscles.
8. Direct the chest drain anteriorly and apically to drain a pneumothorax and posteriorly to drain a pleural effusion. Ensure that all of the side holes in the chest drain tube are contained within the pleural cavity.
9. Connect the tube to the drainage system with an underwater seal and look for bubbling and/or a swinging meniscus.
10. Secure the chest drain to the skin with a simple suture: the ends of the suture should be tied around the chest drain tube four or five times and knotted securely. An additional suture may be required to close the incision. Do not use a pursestring suture as this leaves an unsightly scar.
11. Apply a small square of gauze to the insertion site and secure the chest drain tube at right angles to the skin with two transparent adhesive dressings, applied to the tube and chest wall in an inverted T.
12. X-ray to confirm the position of the chest drain and that the pneumothorax has resolved.
13. A low-pressure vacuum (−5–10 cmH₂O) can be applied to the drainage system to assist with drainage of a pneumothorax.
14. If a large pleural effusion is present, control the rate of drainage by intermittent clamping of the drain.

Seldinger technique

If appropriate equipment is available, this is a less traumatic procedure. Straight or pigtail chest drain tubes are available for use in neonates.

1. Position the baby and clean and drape the skin as before.
2. Infiltrate the skin and subcutaneous tissues with local anaesthetic and make a 0.5-cm incision in the skin.

Remember to aspirate on the needle before infiltrating the local anaesthetic.
3. Attach a saline-filled syringe on to the introducer needle and insert the introducer needle into the pleural space, keeping the needle at right angles to the skin. Fluid or bubbles of air should be aspirated into the syringe to confirm that the needle lies in the pleural space.
4. Remove the syringe and pass the guidewire into the pleural space and remove the introducer needle.
5. Thread a dilator over the guidewire and gently dilate the tract, using a twisting motion.
6. Remove the dilator and thread the chest drain tube over the guidewire, angling the tube anteriorly for a pneumothorax and posteriorly for a pleural effusion.
7. Withdraw the guidewire, secure the chest drain in place, connect to the underwater drain and apply an adhesive dressing as described above.
8. Confirm the position of the tube with an X-ray.

Complications of chest drains

See Table 44.3 and Figure 44.6.

Chest drain removal

Once the pneumothorax or pleural effusion has resolved, clamp the tube for several hours. Removal of the chest drain is known to be very painful and a short-acting, rapid-onset systemic analgesic should be given before proceeding.

Equipment

- Dressing pack, stitch cutter, suture or Steri-Strips, sterile dressing.

Procedure

1. Remove dressings and clean the skin in the area of the chest drain with antiseptic solution.
2. Remove any sutures.
3. Pull the chest drain out, keeping the edges of the wound approximated. Apply Steri-Strips to close the wound. Use a simple suture if the wound is gaping or if the Steri-Strips do not stick. Dress with sterile gauze and cover with a transparent dressing.
4. Perform a chest X-ray to exclude reaccumulation of the pneumothorax.

Drainage of pneumomediastinum

Pneumomediastinum may occur in association with birth injury, pneumonia, meconium aspiration syndrome and following tracheal injury. X-ray appearances include the spinnaker-sail sign (upwards and outwards deviation of the thymic lobes) and continuous-diaphragm sign (due to the interposition of air between the pericardium and diaphragm) (Hauri-Hohla et al. 2008). The presence of free air in the mediastinum can usually be managed conservatively, with resolution of the pneumomediastinum within 72 hours. Tension pneumomediastinum associated with mechanical ventilation may compress the heart and large blood vessels, leading to cardiorespiratory compromise. High-frequency oscillatory ventilation may help to reduce tension within the mediastinum (Miyahara et al. 1999).

Indications for drainage

- Tension pneumomediastinum with major cardiorespiratory compromise.

Table 44.3 Complications of chest drains

COMPLICATION	COMMENTS	PRECAUTIONS AND MANAGEMENT
Haemorrhage	The intercostal artery and vein lie in the intercostal groove below the rib The internal thoracic artery runs down the inside of the chest wall, ~1 cm from the sternum	During insertion try to roll the dissecting forceps or introducer needle over the top of the rib Use the midclavicular line as the anatomical landmark for needle thoracocentesis
Trauma	Lung perforation or laceration (Moessinger et al. 1978) Pericardial damage (Quak et al. 1993), including haemorrhagic pericardial effusion and tamponade Thoracic duct damage with resultant chylothorax (Kumar and Belik 1984) Phrenic nerve injury (Ayra et al. 1991) Permanent damage to breast tissue (Rainer et al. 2003)	The risk of lung perforation is reduced by removing the trochar from a conventional chest drain prior to insertion. Be careful not to push the introducer needle too far into the chest when using the Seldinger technique Confirm diagnosis urgently with ultrasound if baby develops signs of reduced cardiac output. Proceed to pericardiocentesis if tamponade is confirmed Avoid inserting the chest drain in too far. The chylothorax usually resolves with conservative management Avoid inserting the chest drain in too far Phrenic nerve injury may lead to diaphragmatic paralysis or eventration of the diaphragm. Nerve injury may recover following removal of the chest drain In term infants, breast tissue extends from the second to sixth rib and almost to the anterior axillary line. Use the midaxillary line, and avoid the anterior approach for formal chest drains
Infection	Inoculation of pleura with skin organisms/local cellulitis	Meticulous skin care. Change dressings if soiled
Failure to drain/ reaccumulation of the pneumothorax		Check all connections are tight and open to the water trap. Look to see if the drain has fallen out, or if the side holes are outside the chest – if so, it will bubble continuously if under suction. There may be surgical emphysema on chest X-ray. If the chest drain is misplaced or blocked with blood or protein, it will require replacement. Consider intubation of the main bronchus and unilateral lung ventilation for 48 hours for recalcitrant pneumothorax (Joseph et al. 2011)

Equipment

- 21–25 G venous cannula (Venflon), extension set, three-way tap and syringe.

Procedure

1. Clean the skin.
2. Assemble equipment. Depending on how the mediastinal air is distributed, either insert the cannula via the second intercostal space, midclavicular line, or use the subxiphoid approach: insert the cannula just below the xiphoid cartilage, 0.5 cm to the left of the midline, and advance the cannula towards the left shoulder whilst aspirating gently on the syringe.
3. Once the needle is within the collection of air, slide the catheter forward and remove the needle. Reconnect the syringe and aspirate as much air as possible.
4. Withdraw the catheter and X-ray.

Complications

1. Cardiac puncture.
2. Pneumopericardium.
3. Pneumothorax.
4. Arrhythmias.

Access to the circulation

Capillary heelpricks

Capillary blood samples are easy to obtain, conserve the veins in critically ill infants and can be used for most haematological and biochemical tests. However, capillary samples cannot be used for blood cultures and the capillary Po_2 value bears little relationship to the arterial Pao_2.

Indications

- Capillary blood gas sampling.
- Routine haematology and biochemistry analyses requiring a limited amount of blood (i.e. less than 1.5 ml).
- Bilirubin and glucose measurements.
- Newborn screening tests (Guthrie card).

Equipment

- Automated heel-lancing device (Tenderfoot, Minilet or Glucolet lancets).
- Heparinised capillary blood gas tubes, sample bottles.

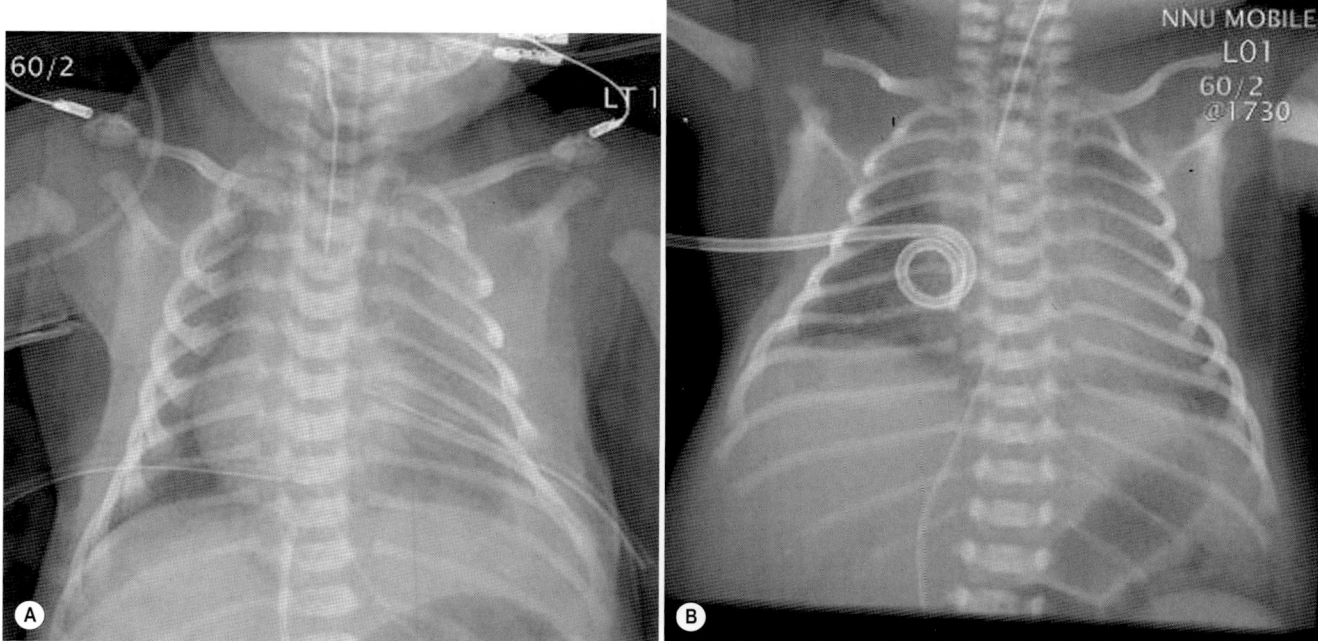

Fig. 44.6 (A) Bilateral chest drains. The drains have been inserted in the seventh intercostal space and are too long, risking injuries to the liver, diaphragm and mediastinal structures, including phrenic nerves and thoracic duct. The drains should have been inserted in the fourth or fifth intercostal space. Note the endotracheal tube is at T3 and should be shortened. The nasogastric tube is in the stomach. The umbilical venous line is in a satisfactory position at T9. (B) Right pigtail chest drain has been inserted via the fourth intercostal space and is in a satisfactory position. Endotracheal tube at T2. The umbilical venous line is at T6, and is lying within the right atrium.

Procedure

1. The foot must be warm and well perfused.
2. Clean the heel with an antibacterial swab.
3. The preferred areas for capillary sampling are the outer aspects of the heel (Fig. 44.7). Do not sample from the end of the heel because the perichondrium of the calcaneum lies superficially and the risk of osteomyelitis is increased.
4. Dorsiflex the foot, hold the automated device against the skin and activate. Apply gentle pressure and allow a drop of blood to form.
5. When samples have been collected, apply pressure with sterile cotton wool or gauze and dress with a plaster.

Complications

1. Pain.
2. Scarring.
3. Infection, including osteomyelitis of the calcaneum (Lilien et al. 1976).

Venepuncture blood samples

Use veins in the dorsum of the hand or feet. Try to conserve the long saphenous veins and veins in the antecubital fossa in babies who are likely to need a long line.

Indications

- Larger volumes of blood for laboratory analyses.
- Samples for coagulation.
- Blood cultures.

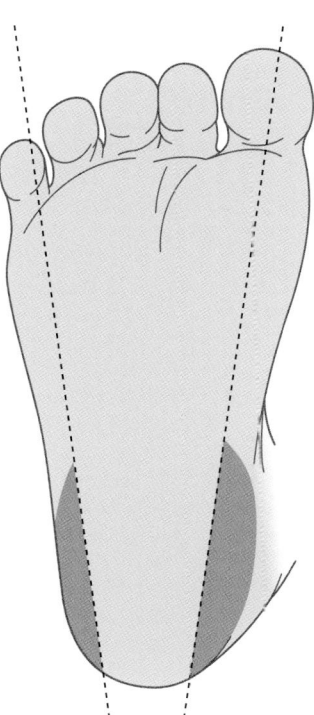

Fig. 44.7 The shaded areas indicate the lateral and medial aspects of the heel, which are suitable for heelpricks.

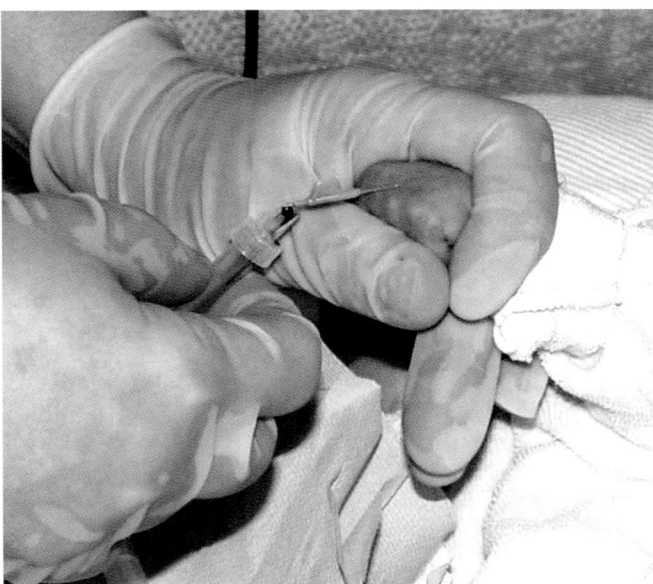

Fig. 44.8 Venous blood sampling from a flanged needle.

Equipment

- 23 G flanged collection needle.
- Specimen bottles.

Procedure

1. Clean skin with antiseptic or with an alcohol swab and allow to dry.
2. Occlude the vein proximally, using gentle pressure
3. Insert the needle or butterfly at an angle of 30–45° to the skin. Inserting the needle where the vein bifurcates prevents the vein rolling away from the point of the needle.
4. Allow blood to drip into the specimen bottles from the needle (Fig. 44.8).
5. After needle removal, apply gentle pressure with sterile gauze to prevent bruising/haematoma formation.

Complications

1. Pain.
2. Scarring.
3. Infection.

Arterial puncture

The radial artery is most commonly used, providing the ulnar collateral circulation is intact. The posterior tibial and dorsalis pedis arteries can also be used. Avoid using the brachial or femoral arteries, as they are end-arteries.

Indications

- Arterial blood gas sampling.
- Large volumes of blood for laboratory analyses when venous and capillary samples are unsuitable or unobtainable.

Equipment

- 24 G needle or cannula.
- Heparinised blood gas syringes, capillary tubes, sample bottles.

> **Box 44.1** Management of digital ischaemia
>
> 1. Remove the needle or cannula.
> 2. Application of 1/4 of a cutaneous glyceryl trinitrate patch over the ipsilateral brachial or popliteal artery may improve the distal circulation.

Procedure

Radial artery puncture

1. Before proceeding, perform the modified Allen's test:
    - Elevate the arm.
    - Occlude both the radial and ulnar arteries at the wrist.
    - Release pressure from over the ulnar artery: colour should be restored to the hand in less than 10 seconds.
2. Identify the artery, using palpation and/or transillumination with a cold light.
3. Extend the wrist in a supine position, but do not overextend the wrist.
4. Clean skin with antiseptic and allow to dry.
5. Insert the needle at an angle of ~30°; blood should flow freely into the needle.
6. Blood can be collected with a syringe or by the drip method.
7. Remove the needle and apply compression with a sterile gauze swab for 5 minutes, or until haemostasis is achieved.

Complications

See complications of peripheral arterial cannulation (Box 44.1).

Peripheral venous cannulation

Veins in the back of the hand, forearm and foot should be used first. Confirm that the vessel empties following proximal occlusion and fills distally. Limit the number of attempts at cannulation to two or three per person.

Indications

- Administration of intravenous medications, fluids, blood products and short-term parenteral nutrition.

Equipment

- 24 G cannula.
- Extension tube with Luer-Lok and valved connector.
- 0.9% saline in 5-ml syringe.
- Steri-Strips, transparent dressing.

Procedure

1. Flush the extension tubing with saline.
2. Clean skin with antiseptic and allow to dry.
3. Occlude the vessel proximally and apply gentle traction to the skin.
4. Insert the cannula at an angle of 30–45° to the skin. As the needle pierces the vein, blood will appear in the hub of the cannula. Push the cannula in a further 1–2 mm, partially withdraw the needle and advance the cannula forward into the vessel. Remove the needle. Collect blood samples by the drip method or by aspirating blood from the hub of the cannula with a needle and syringe.
5. Connect the extension tubing to the cannula and flush gently with saline.

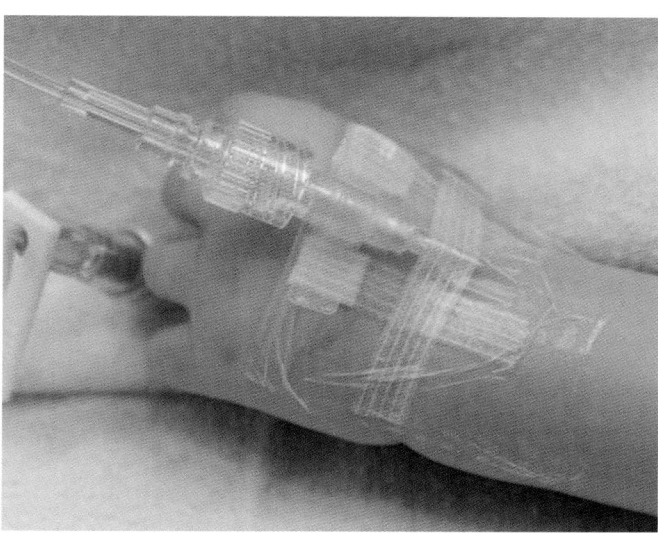

Fig. 44.9 Fixation of a peripheral venous catheter.

Table 44.4 Staging of extravasation injuries

STAGE	CHARACTERISTIC
I	Painful intravenous site, no erythema or swelling
II	Painful intravenous site, slight swelling, no blanching. Good pulse and brisk capillary refill below extravasation site
III	Painful intravenous site. Marked swelling. Blanching. Skin cool to touch. Good pulse and brisk capillary refill below extravasation site
IV	Painful intravenous site. Very marked swelling. Blanching. Cool to touch. Decreased or absent pulse. Capillary refill >4 seconds. Skin breakdown or necrosis

(Adapted from Ramesthu (2004).)

6. Secure the cannula using Steri-Strips and a transparent adhesive dressing to allow inspection of the cannula site (Fig. 44.9). Do not apply the dressing around the whole circumference of the limb.
7. Use a size-appropriate splint if the cannula is inserted over the elbow or ankle joint. Do not fix the limb too tightly to the splint.
8. Intravenous infusions should be infused via pressure-sensitive pumps and cannula sites must be checked hourly.
9. Cannulae should be removed promptly if the insertion site or vein becomes erythematous or if the limb becomes swollen.

Complications

1. Haematoma formation: apply gentle pressure to secure haemostasis before applying the dressing.
2. Thrombophlebitis occurs in ~13% of babies with a peripheral intravenous infusion (Cronin et al. 1990). Redness and tenderness over the course of the vein usually resolve with removal of the cannula.
3. Infection: *Staphylococcus epidermidis* may be grown from the site and the cannula. Septicaemia from peripheral intravenous sites is uncommon in paediatric populations (Garland et al. 1992); however, any breach in the integrity of the skin can predispose to infection in the newborn.
4. Extravasation injury is a common complication, presenting with pain and swelling that progress to superficial blistering, ischaemia and tissue necrosis.

Management of extravasation injury

Extravasation injuries must be treated promptly in order to mini- mise tissue damage and subsequent scarring. Seek specialist advice for stage III and IV extravasations (Table 44.4).

1. Stop the intravenous infusion immediately, but do not remove the cannula.
2. Remove the dressing and elevate the limb.
3. Try to aspirate fluid from the extravasated area via the cannula, using a 1-ml syringe.
4. In more severe extravasation injuries, where there is blistering or discoloration of the skin or if the infusion contained calcium, potassium, sodium bicarbonate, antibiotics or inotropes, inform the plastic surgeons and seek their advice regarding the following treatments:
   (a) Multiple puncture technique (Chandavasu et al. 1986): applying a strict aseptic technique, use a blood-drawing stylet or scalpel to make multiple punctures over the most oedematous area. Gently express the extravasated fluid. Dress the area with room-temperature saline soaks to aid drainage.
   (b) Hyaluronidase + saline flush-out (Davies et al. 1994): hyaluronidase is a dispersing agent that is effective in extravasations involving calcium, TPN, antibiotics and sodium bicarbonate. It is most effective if administered within 1 hour of the injury but may be used up to 12 hours:
   - After cleaning and infiltrating the area with 1% lidocaine, inject 500–1000 units of hyaluronidase subcutaneously. Make 2–4 small stab incisions at the periphery of the injury.
   - Inject up to 500 ml of saline through a blunt cannula inserted through one of the puncture sites and flush the saline towards the other incisions to wash out the extravasated material (Fig. 44.10).
   (c) Topical nitroglycerine 2% ointment 4 mm/kg body weight applied 8-hourly to the affected area has been shown to be effective in extravasation injuries involving dopamine (Denkler and Cohen 1989).
5. Elevate the limb to reduce oedema.
6. Dress with Jelonet and sterile gauze.
7. Review daily: complete healing may take up to 3 months.

Percutaneous central venous catheters

The veins most commonly used for peripheral inserted central venous catheters (CVCs) are shown in Table 44.5.

Indications

- Long-term administration of TPN.
- Drug infusions such as inotropes.

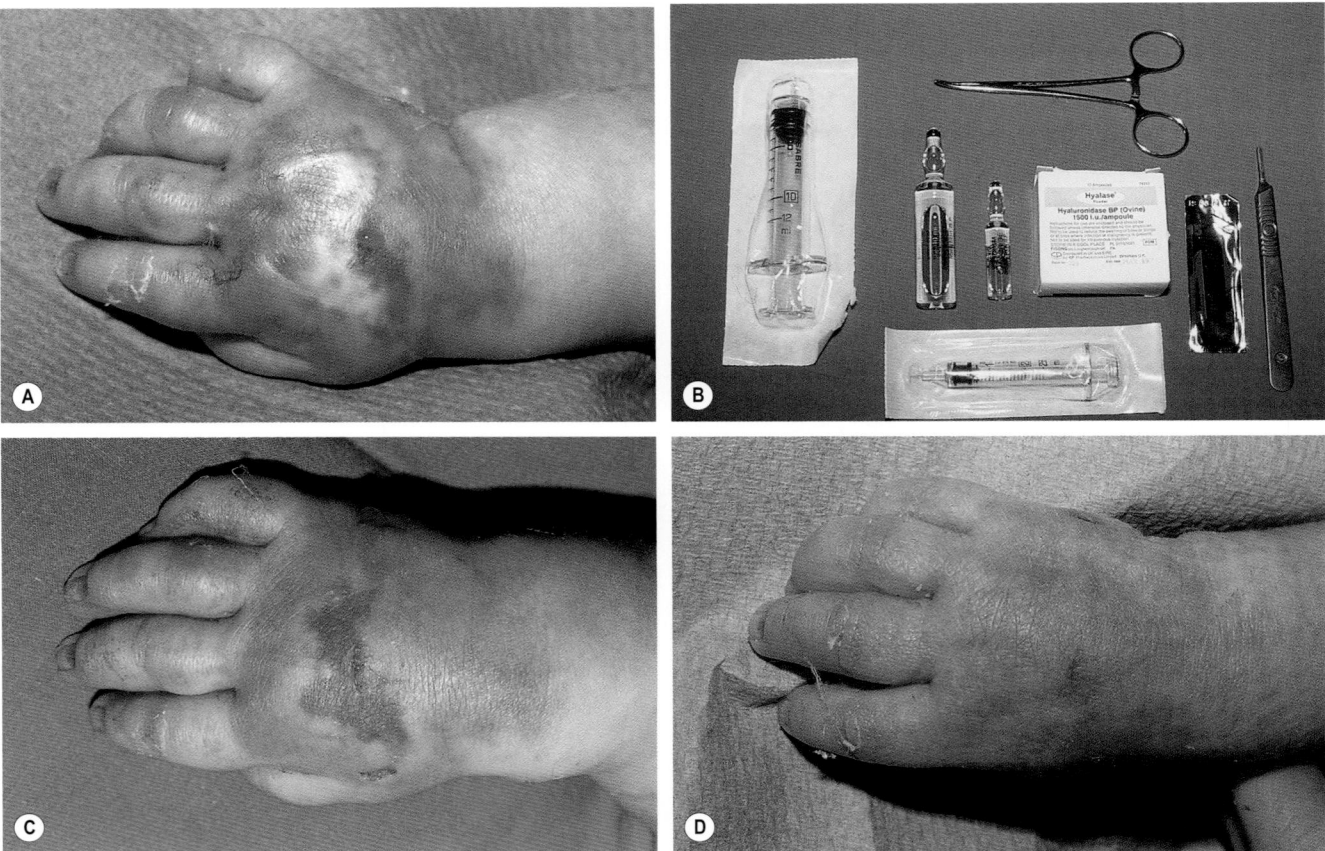

Fig. 44.10 (A) An acute extravasation injury to the dorsum of the hand. (B) Kit required for hyaluronidase + saline flush-out. There is marked improvement (C) immediately following irrigation and (D) at 24 hours.

Table 44.5 Veins commonly used for peripherally inserted central venous catheters

SITE	VEIN	COMMENTS
Upper limb	Median cubital and basilic veins	These veins lie medially in the antecubital fossa and drain directly into the axillary vein. They are the best veins to use in the upper limb
	Cephalic vein	Lies laterally in the antecubital fossa. It often divides into a number of branches before joining the axillary vein just below the clavicle. If this vein is used, lines tend to get caught around the shoulder or below the clavicle
	Axillary vein	If the arm is raised and abducted, the axillary vein lies anteriorly and inferiorly to the axillary artery and nerves of the brachial plexus
Lower limb	Long saphenous vein	Lies anterior to the medial malleolus and runs up the medial aspect of the leg to join the femoral vein. Vein of choice in the lower limb
	Short saphenous vein	Lies inferior and posterior to the lateral malleolus and runs up the posterior aspect of the leg passing between the heads of the gastrocnemius muscle and drains into the popliteal vein, around the level of the knee joint
Scalp	Preauricular veins or superficial temporal vein	These drain via the deep facial vein into the internal jugular. Avoid using the posterior auricular vein, as lines tends to get stuck in the external jugular vein at the root of the neck

Equipment

- Instrument pack containing drapes, fine non-toothed forceps and artery forceps.
- Long line with insertion butterfly, splitting needle or cannula.
- Gauze, Steri-Strips, transparent adhesive dressing.
- Luer-Lok connectors and extension sets.
- Injectable X-ray contrast.

Procedure

1. Identify the vein. If an upper limb or scalp vein is being catheterised, measure the distance to the third intercostal space to the right of the sternum. If a lower limb vein is used, measure from the insertion site to the inguinal ligament, across to the umbilicus and up to the xiphoid cartilage.
2. Restrain the limb if necessary.

3. If the CVC is inserted via a vein in the upper limb, turn the baby's head towards that arm to reduce the likelihood of the line entering the external jugular vein.
4. Clean and drape the skin. Apply a sterile tourniquet (a piece of sterile gauze can be wrapped around the limb and secured tightly with the artery forceps).
5. Flush the CVC with saline.
6. Insert the introducer needle into the vein. Release the tourniquet and thread the catheter into position with non-toothed fine forceps. Attach the extension set to the catheter. If the CVC is correctly sited, it should be easy to aspirate blood back down the line.
7. Remove the introducer needle. Secure the line with Steri-Strips and apply pressure over the insertion site to secure haemostasis.
8. Neatly coil the external length catheter and fix to the skin with Steri-Strips. Place a small square of gauze under the hub to protect the skin and apply a temporary sterile dressing to the insertion site.
9. Flush the line with 0.5 ml of contrast material and X-ray to confirm the position of the catheter tip. If the line has been inserted via an arm or scalp vein, the tip of the CVC should lie in the superior vena cava, ideally above T2 on X-ray, outside the cardiac silhouette. If the line has been inserted via the leg, the tip of the catheter should lie just below the diaphragm (T9–10).
10. Maintain a sterile field whilst the X-ray is taken.
11. Shorten the CVC if it is too long. If the line has coiled back on itself or is kinked or misplaced (Fig. 44.11), replace the line or pull it back to midhumerus or midfemur and use as a short line for a few days. The only exception to this rule is that CVCs that inadvertently enter the jugular vein from the upper limb often 'flip' into the correct position if they are left overnight. Run an infusion of heparinised saline at 0.5 ml/h through the line and repeat X-ray with contrast the following morning (Fig. 44.12).
12. Finally apply a transparent adhesive dressing to cover the insertion site, catheter and hub of the extension set (Fig. 44.13).

Complications

See Table 44.6.

Peripheral arterial cannulation

Indications

- Continuous monitoring of arterial blood pressure.
- Frequent monitoring of blood gases or other blood parameters.

Equipment

- 24 G cannula.
- Steri-Strips, transparent dressing, splint.
- Extension set with valved connector.
- Heparinised 0.45% or 0.9% saline (0.5 IU heparin/ml).

Procedure

Identify a suitable peripheral artery, usually the radial or posterior tibial arteries. Do not use the ulnar artery if the radial artery in that arm has been punctured or cannulated previously.

Avoid using the brachial or femoral arteries, as they are end-arteries with limited collateral circulation (Fig. 44.14).

Always perform the modified Allen's test before cannulating the radial artery:

- elevate the arm.
- occlude both the radial and ulnar arteries at the wrist
- release pressure from over the ulnar artery: colour should be restored to the hand in less than 10 seconds.

Failure to perform this simple test may result in ischaemia with loss of fingers or part of the hand (Fig. 44.15).

1. Clean the skin with antiseptic solution or alcohol. Using a no-touch technique, insert the cannula into the artery at an angle of 30–45°; as blood flushes into the chamber, advance the needle 1–2 mm and then slide the catheter forward into the artery.
2. Apply pressure proximal to the cannula and remove the needle. Attach a preflushed Luer-Lok extension set.
3. The cannula should sample easily. Flush slowly with 0.5 ml of heparinised saline. There is usually an area of transient blanching of the skin close to the injection site.
4. Secure the cannula with Steri-Strips or tape and dress with Tegaderm or similar transparent dressing.
5. Apply a splint to the limb and ensure that the tips of fingers or toes are easily visible.
6. A heparinised saline infusion should be commenced.
7. Remove the cannula without delay if it stops sampling or if there is loss of the arterial pressure waveform. Do not flush the cannula to remove clots.

Complications

Major complications of peripheral arterial lines are reported to occur in less than 2% of babies (Randel et al. 1987).

Complications include:

1. haemorrhage/haematoma formation
2. trauma:
   (a) to the vessel wall with aneurysm formation (Rey et al. 1987)
   (b) to adjacent nerves, e.g. to median, ulnar and posterior tibial nerves (Pape et al. 1987)
3. thromboembolism/vasospasm and distal ischaemia (Cartwright and Schreiner 1980)
4. infection.

Remove the arterial line immediately if distal perfusion is compromised or if the line stops sampling or fails to give a reliable blood pressure trace (Box 44.1).

Umbilical artery catheterisation

The umbilical artery is the terminal branch of the anterior division of the internal iliac artery. The internal iliac artery gives rise to a number of arteries that supply the viscera and walls of the pelvis and the buttocks.

If correctly inserted, an umbilical artery catheter (UAC) will always appear to form a loop in the pelvis as it passes down the umbilical artery and then turns upwards into the internal iliac and common iliac arteries before entering the aorta.

An UAC provides relatively long-term access to the circulation, but usually should not remain in place for longer than 10–14 days.

Catheters must be inserted using full aseptic precautions.

Before you scrub up for the procedure, estimate how far to insert the line by:

- measuring the distance from the tip of the left shoulder to the base of the umbilicus + stump length (cm) (Dunn 1966), or

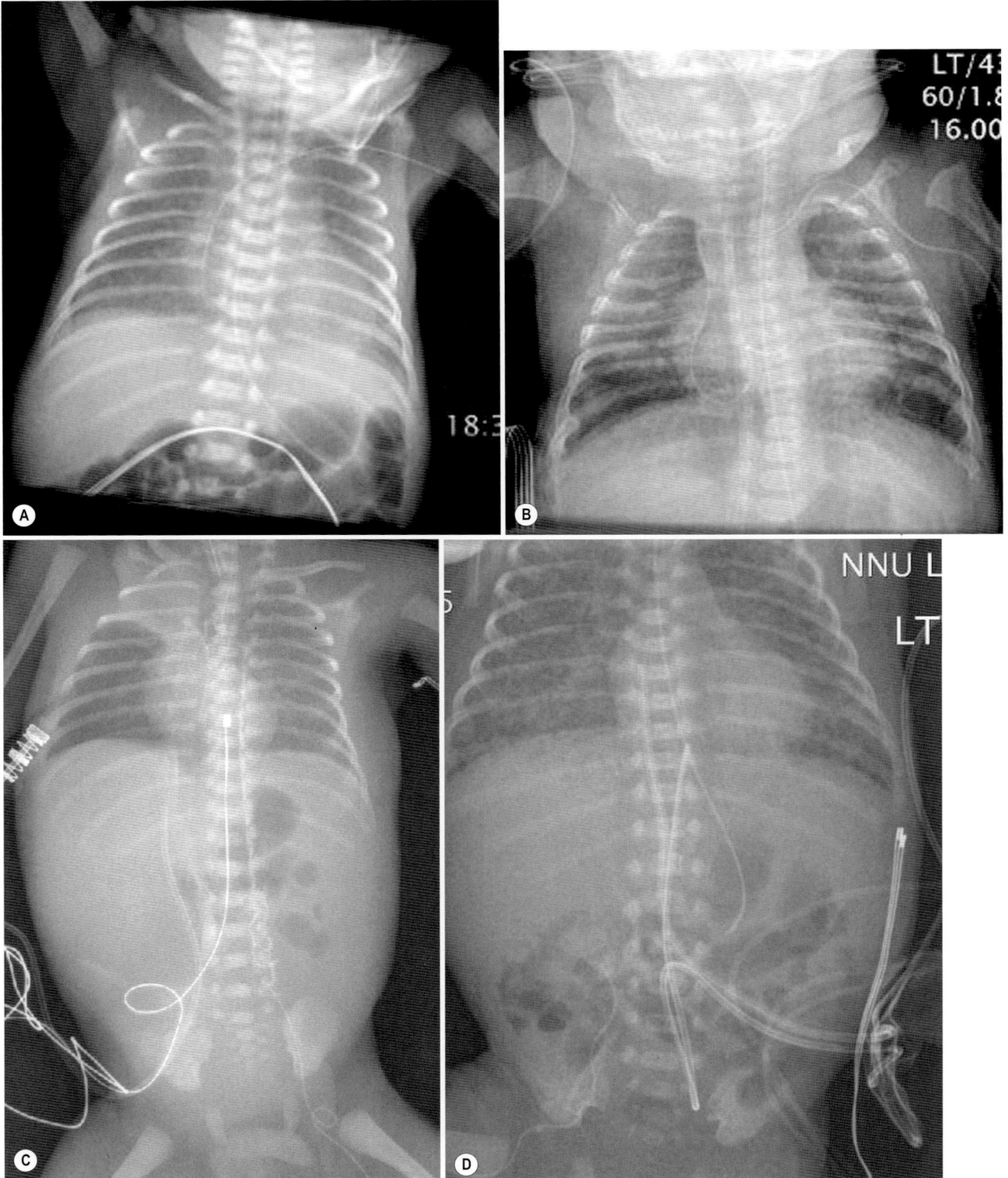

Fig. 44.11 Misplaced central venous catheters (CVCs). (A) The tip of the long line is in the right atrium and should be pulled back to T2/just outside the cardiac silhouette. (B) The tip of the CVC has traversed the foramen ovale and is lying in the left atrium. (C) The CVC tip is lying in the iliolumbar vein, which is a branch of the external iliac vein. Contrast outlines the lumbar plexus. Note how the CVC line curls in the groin (the 'hump' sign). Lines that curl or kink are almost always wrongly sited. Note the tip of the ETT is correctly placed at T1; the umbilical arterial catheter is T8. The umbilical venous catheter is short and the tip should lie just below the diaphragm (T9). (D) The peripherally inserted long line is in the inferior epigastric vein and must be removed. The umbilical arterial catheter position is satisfactory. The umbilical venous catheter is long and is best positioned at T9.

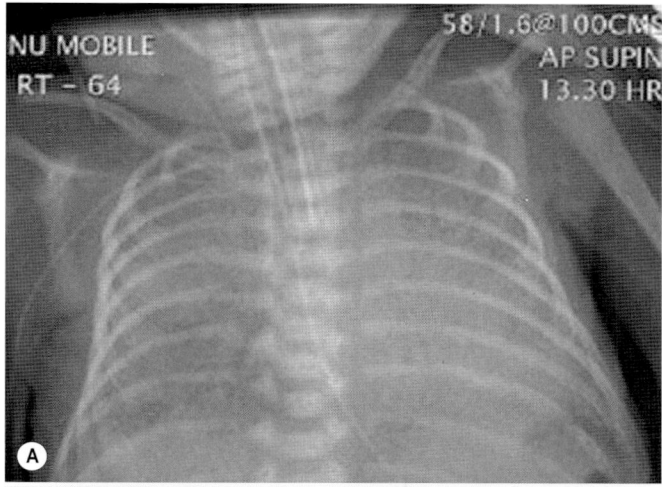

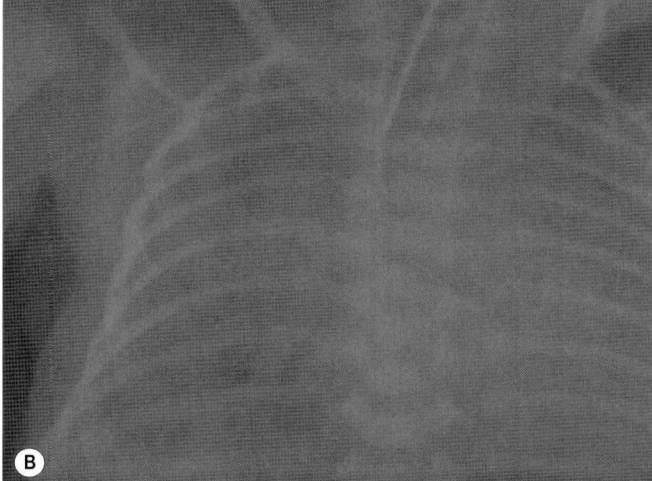

Fig. 44.12 (A) The central venous catheter is lying in the right external jugular vein. Heparinised saline is infused overnight. (B) The following morning, a repeat X-ray shows the line has flipped into the superior vena cava. Note that the endotracheal tube in the first film lies just above the carina and has been shortened.

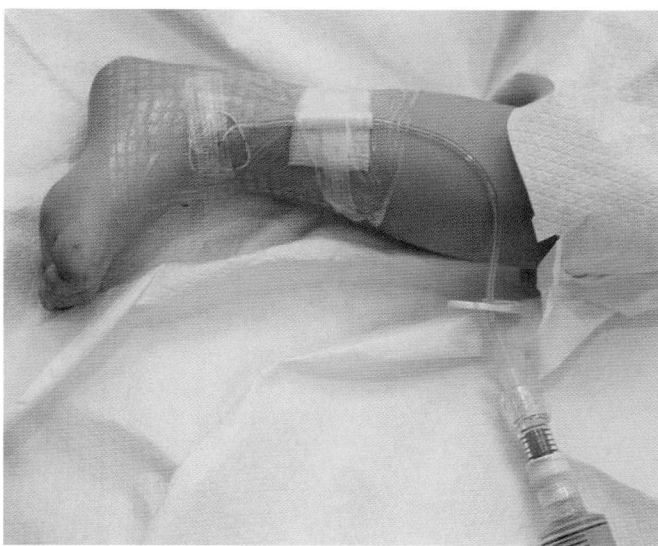

Fig. 44.13 Central venous catheter dressing.

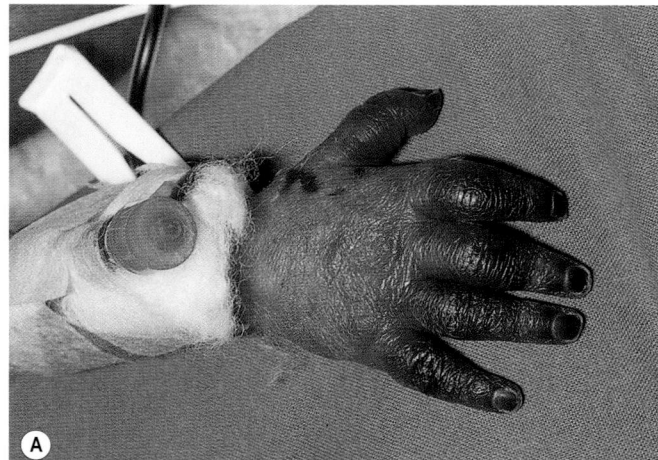

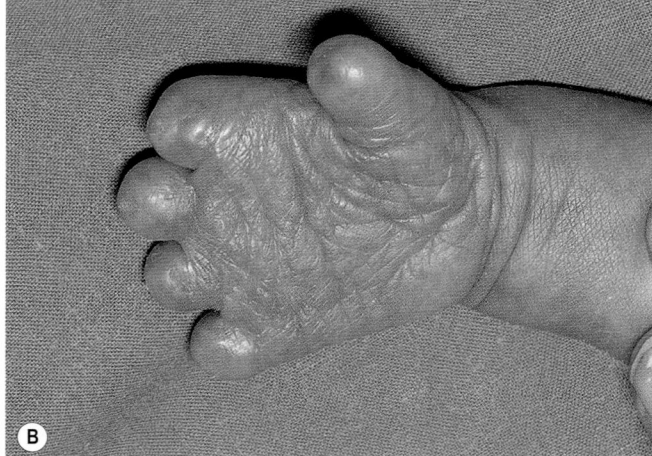

Fig. 44.15 (A, B) Irreversible digital ischaemia following radial artery catheterisation.

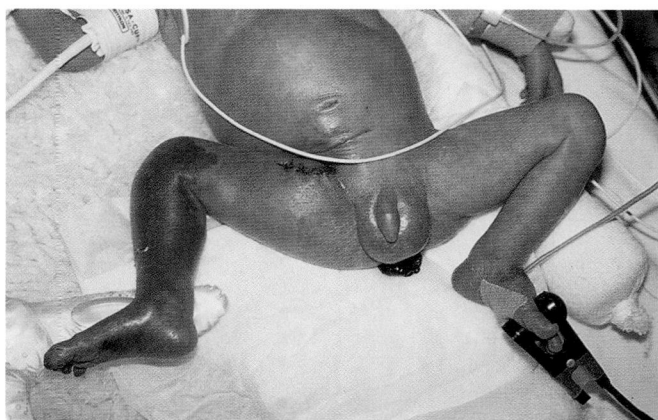

Fig. 44.14 Ischaemic injury to the right leg following insertion of a femoral arterial line.

Table 44.6 Complications of central venous catheter (CVC) lines

COMPLICATION	COMMENTS	PRECAUTIONS AND MANAGEMENT
Trauma during insertion	Includes damage to vessels, nerves and other organs during placement	Before insertion, occlude the vein and ensure that it fills from a distal direction to avoid inadvertent cannulation of an artery. Remember that the sural nerve lies in close proximity to the short saphenous vein, the median nerve and brachial artery lie deep to the median cubital nerve and the nerves of the brachial plexus can be traumatised if the axillary vein is used
Catheter-related sepsis	Recent studies have reported the incidence of CVC-related bloodstream infection as 4–14 per 1000 catheter-days (Hsu et al. 2010; Chien et al. 2002). The incidence is highest in babies with a birthweight of <1000 g	Higher incidence of infection with CVC inserted via the femoral vein. Aim to complete placement of the line within 30 minutes. Strict protocols for CVC care. If the line is infected, remove CVC if possible. The line can sometimes be preserved by locking it with antibiotics, but if cultures remain positive the line must be removed
Bacterial or fungal endocarditis	In association with CVC and *Staphylococcus aureus* septicaemia (Armstron et al. 2002)	Remove the catheter. Treat staphylococcal endocarditis with intravenous antibiotics for up to 6 weeks. Give fluconazole prophylaxis to highest risk infants (<1500 g) (Clerihew et al. 2007)
Thrombosis	Relatively rare with peripherally inserted CVC. SVC obstruction reported with Broviac lines (Mulvihill and Fonkalsrud 1984), cardiac thrombus, renal vein thrombosis, deep-vein thrombosis	SVC obstruction presents with mild to moderate oedema and venous suffusion of the head and upper extremities. Renal vein thrombosis is only infrequently associated with the presence of a catheter (Kuhle et al. 2004). Remove the CVC. Screen for prothrombotic condition
Misplacement or line migration	Tissue extravasation, pleural effusion, pericardial effusion (Cartwright 2004) and tamponade, cardiac arrhythmias (Daniels et al. 1984)	At the end of the procedure, ensure that the tip of the CVC is correctly placed. Check that you can withdraw blood from the CVC. Use just enough injectable contrast to fill the catheter. Do not use lines that are kinked or looped as they are usually misplaced. Fix the line securely to reduce the risk of migration. Check the position of the line on any subsequent X-rays. Confirm pericardial effusion with ultrasound and perform emergency pericardiocentesis if tamponade is present. If the tip of the line is abnormally sited in the heart it may provoke arrhythmias. Be aware that a CVC in the inferior epigastric vein can appear well positioned on an anteroposterior X-ray (Baker and Imong 2002) – if in doubt, obtain a lateral view
Catheter dysfunction	Increased pump pressure, inability to infuse fluids	Select correct-size catheter. Do not use 27 G line in babies >1500 g, as the high flow rates will generate high pump pressures. If the line has clotted, consider using alteplase 1 mg/ml or 5000–10 000 units of urokinase in normal saline to fill catheter dead space. Aspirate the lysate after 2–4 hours, then flush with normal saline
Catheter breakage	The intravascular remnant of the CVC may embolise to the heart	Avoid using toothed forceps to handle the line. If the CVC is too long, do not pull the line back through a needle, as this may sever the line. If the catheter breaks and is not visible, apply pressure over the distal vein to prevent embolisation. Confirm where the catheter is on X-ray and refer to a paediatric or cardiothoracic surgeon for urgent removal of the catheter remnant
Arachnoiditis and paraplegia from lines in the lumbar venous plexus (Chen et al. 2001)	May present with paraplegia, urinary retention and milky CSF	This has been reported following insertion of long lines via the left long saphenous vein. Beware of lines that fail to insert beyond or appear to kink around L2/3. Use contrast to check the position of the line and take a lateral abdominal X-ray if there is any doubt about the position of the line

SVC, superior vena cava; CSF, cerebrospinal fluid.

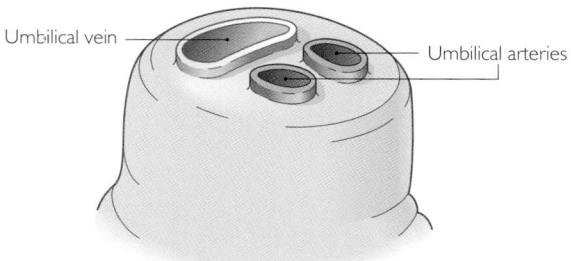

Fig. 44.16 Cut surface of the umbilical cord.

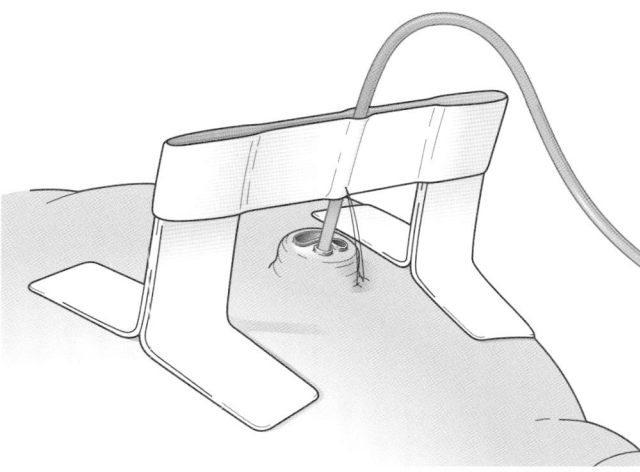

Fig. 44.17 Using an H-tape bridge to secure an umbilical catheter.

- using the following calculations to estimate insertion length:
  Infants >1500 g = (birthweight in kg × 3) + 9 cm + stump length (cm) (Shukla and Ferrara 1986)
  Infants <1500 g = (birthweight in kg × 4) + 7 cm + stump length (cm) (Wright et al. 2008).

Indications
- Repeated intermittent sampling for blood gases and laboratory assays.
- Continuous monitoring of blood gas parameters via indwelling electrodes.
- Continuous monitoring of blood pressure.
- Exchange transfusion.

Equipment
- Sterile gown and gloves.
- Sterile instrument pack containing drapes, scalpel, needle holder, artery clamps, fine forceps, dilating probes, scissors.
- Umbilical catheters:
  (a) Single-lumen, end-hole (Barrington 1999a), radiopaque, with Luer-Lok connector.
  (b) 2.5 Fr for babies <1000 g, 3.5 Fr for babies <1500 g and 5.0 Fr for those >1500 g.
- Sterile cord tie, three-way tap, Luer-Lok extension set, syringes, sutures.
- Heparinised saline (0.25–1.0 units/ml).

Procedure
1. Flush the catheter and three-way tap with saline.
2. Clean the umbilical cord and skin of the anterior abdominal wall with antiseptic solution and allow to dry.
3. Drape the skin.
4. Place the sterile cord tie loosely around the base of the stump. This can be tightened to control blood loss.
5. Use a scalpel to cut the umbilical cord horizontally 1–2 cm above the skin margin.
6. Apply two artery forceps to, and evert the edge of, the cord. Identify the two thick-walled arteries and a single thin-walled gaping umbilical vein (Fig. 44.16).
7. The artery should be gently dilated with a probe or an iris dilator. Try to avoid using the non-toothed forceps, as they are not designed for this purpose and you are more likely to make a false passage. Once the artery is dilated, use the non-toothed forceps to introduce the catheter into the artery. Gently insert the catheter to the calculated length. It should be easy to aspirate blood when the catheter is in the correct position.

8. The catheter should be secured using a suture that is carefully inserted into the umbilical stump. H-tape bridges or commercial devices can be attached to the abdominal wall to secure the line (Fig. 44.17).
9. A chest and abdominal X-ray must be taken to confirm the position of the line. The tip of the UAC can be safely positioned above the diaphragm at a level between the sixth and ninth thoracic vertebrae, which is below the level of the ductus arteriosus (T4–T5) and above the origin of the coeliac axis (T12) (Fig. 44.18). UACs can also be positioned between the third and fifth lumbar vertebrae (just above the aortic bifurcation). The higher position is associated with a lower incidence of clinical vascular complications, and should be used in preference to the low position (Barrington 1999b).
10. If the line is too long or misplaced, reposition or insert a new line.
11. Beware of kinked catheters or catheters that appear to take a convoluted route: the catheter is not likely to be lying in the aorta.
12. Heparinised saline is the infusion of choice.
13. Monitor perfusion to the lower limbs and skin of the buttocks whilst the UAC is in situ.
14. The UAC must be removed if perfusion problems persist or if it is no longer clinically required. Heparinised fluids are stopped 30 minutes before removal; the line is withdrawn with gentle traction, the last 5 cm removed over several minutes, to minimise bleeding. Pressure on the stump and suture insertion will control bleeding. Keep the umbilicus for a few hours after line removal.

Complications
See Tables 44.7 and 44.8.

Umbilical venous catheterisation

The umbilical vein is 2–3 cm long. It passes from the umbilicus within the layers of the falciform ligament and joins the left branch of the portal vein. It continues for another 2–3 cm as the ductus venosus, which drains into the subdiaphragmatic venous confluence along with the inferior vena cava and hepatic veins (Fig. 44.18).

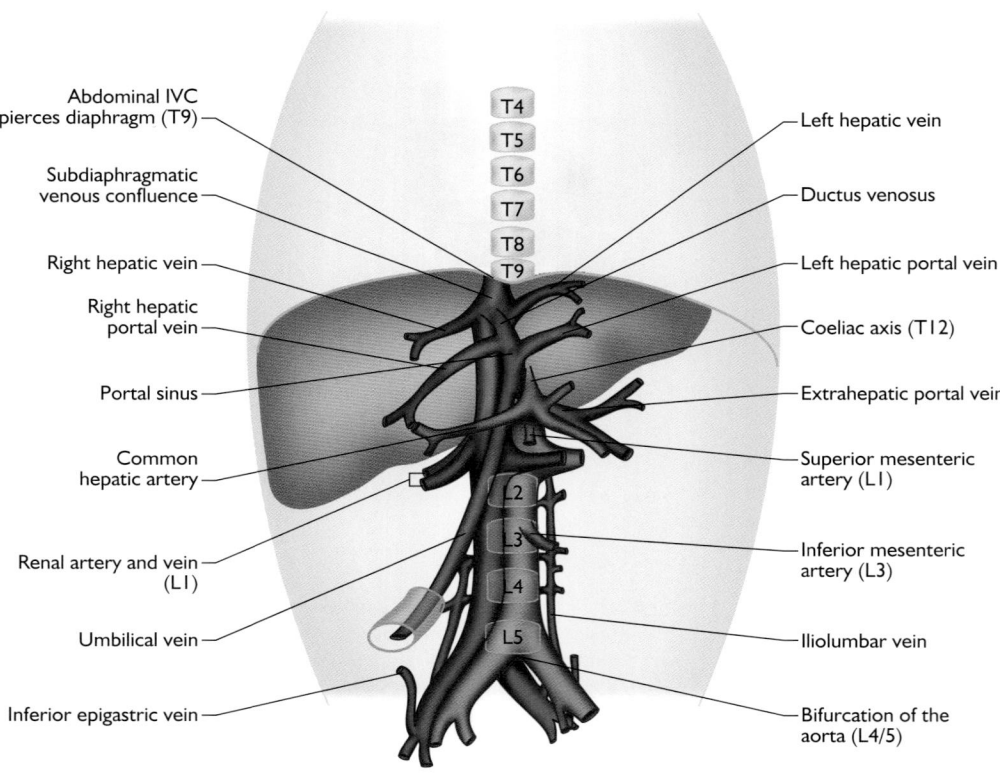

Fig. 44.18 Anatomy of the abdominal aorta, inferior vena cava and ductus venosus.

Table 44.7 Vertebral levels of the major branches of the aorta and potential complications if the umbilical artery catheter (UAC) is not correctly sited

BRANCHES OF THE AORTA	VERTEBRAL LEVEL	COMPLICATIONS ASSOCIATED WITH MISPLACED UAC
Coeliac axis	T12	Infusion of glucose at the level of the coeliac axis may cause hypoglycaemia
Superior mesenteric artery	T12–L1	? Risk of NEC
Renal artery	L1–2	Microemboli to kidney
Inferior mesenteric artery	L3	
Artery of Adamkiewitz (aka anterior radiculomedullary artery)	At or between T10–L2	This artery most commonly arises at T10. It supplies the anterior spinal artery. Vasospasm or thromboembolism of this artery may cause infarction of the spinal cord and paralysis (Brown and Phipps 1988)
Aortic bifurcation	L4–5	
Inferior gluteal artery	<L5	Thrombosis causes gluteoperineal necrosis and ischaemic injury to the sciatic nerve

NEC, necrotising enterocolitis.

1. The catheter must be inserted using full aseptic precautions.
2. Before you scrub up for the procedure, estimate how far to insert the line by:
   (a) measuring the distance from the base of the umbilicus to the xiphisternum (remember to add the remaining length of the umbilical stump), or
   (b) using the following calculation:

$$\text{Estimated insertion length} = (\text{birthweight in kg} \times 2) + 5\,\text{cm} + \text{stump length (cm)}$$

There is insufficient evidence from randomised trials to support the use of prophylactic antibiotics when umbilical vein catheters (UVCs) are inserted in newborn infants. There is no evidence to support continuing antibiotics once initial cultures rule out infection in newborn infants.

Indications

- Emergency vascular access during resuscitation.
- Long-term central venous access for administration of parenteral nutrition, inotropic drugs, hyperosmolar solutions and blood products.
- Exchange transfusion.

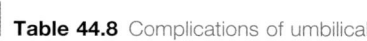

Table 44.8 Complications of umbilical lines

COMPLICATION	COMMENTS	PRECAUTIONS AND MANAGEMENT
Trauma during insertion	Creation of false passage, haematoma, peritoneal perforation, vessel perforation. Damage to or transection of the urachus (Hepworth and Milstein 1984), bladder injury, vesicoumbilical fistula	Use the correct instruments to dilate vessels. There is often a feeling of resistance as the umbilical ring is penetrated; apply gentle steady pressure. Minimise risks of damage to the urachus and bladder by the avoiding subumbilical cut-down method
Vasospasm	This is the most frequent complication seen with UACs, presenting with blanching or duskiness of the lower limbs or toes	Remove the UAC if perfusion has not improved within 10–15 minutes
Air embolism	Take particular care when instrumenting the umbilical vein	Ensure all lines are properly flushed before commencing the procedure. Transient portal venous gas can be seen following insertion of a UVC and should not be mistaken for NEC
Arterial thromboembolism	May involve the aorta (Vailas et al. 1986), iliac, renal (Marsh et al. 1975) and mesenteric or other vessels. Symptoms include pallor or coldness of the lower limbs, gluteal skin necrosis (Mann 1980), absent pulses, haematuria, systemic hypertension and renal failure	Low-dose heparin (0.25–1.0 unit/ml/h) should be infused via the UAC to reduce the risk of catheter occlusion. It may reduce the risk of thromboembolism but has not been shown to lower the rates of aortic thrombosis (Barrington 1999a). Use of fibrinolytic treatment is controversial and depends on the risk to organs and limbs. For intravascular thrombosis consider intravenous infusion of alteplase (rt-PA) 100–500 µg/kg/h for 3–6 hours. Side-effects include intracerebral haemorrhage and bleeding from other sites
Misplacement of UVC and venous thromboembolism	UVCs placed in the right atrium can provoke arrhythmias and perforate the myocardium, resulting in tamponade. UVCs that are malpositioned in the liver can cause portal vein thrombosis or hepatic vein thrombosis and hepatic necrosis RVT	The IVC pierces the diaphragm at T8. Remove lines that are kinked or are sited in the right atrium or liver RVT presents with flank mass, haematuria, hypertension or renal failure Predisposing factors include dehydration, sepsis, polycythaemia and indwelling umbilical venous catheter. Diagnose with ultrasound. Seek expert advice. Rapid collateralisation of RVT in neonates has been described. If bilateral, RVT may require peritoneal dialysis or haemodialysis/filtration and consider thrombolysis (Jaako Dardashti et al. 2009) if the thrombosis has originated in the IVC
Catheter breakage	The line may be cut or snap during removal leading to embolisation of the catheter remnant into the arterial tree	The catheter remnant must be removed by an interventional radiologist or cardiologist whenever possible (Simon-Fayard et al. 1997)

UAC, umbilical artery catheter; UVC, umbilical vein catheter; NEC, necrotising enterocolitis; IVC, inferior vena cava; RVT, renal vein thrombosis.

Equipment

As for UAC insertion, but use a larger catheter, e.g. 4.5–5.0 G. Double-lumen catheters are available and can be useful in babies likely to require multiple infusions.

Procedure

1. Clean the umbilical cord and skin of the anterior abdominal wall with antiseptic solution. Avoid any pooling of the solution under the baby. Allow the solution to dry. Drape the skin.
2. Flush the catheter and three-way tap with saline.
3. Place the sterile cord tie loosely around the base of the stump. This can be tightened to control blood loss.
4. Use a scalpel to cut the umbilical cord horizontally 1–2 cm above the skin margin.
5. Apply artery forceps to the edge of the cord and evert the rim of the cord. Identify the single thin-walled gaping umbilical vein.
6. Gently dilate the vein and insert the catheter the appropriate distance. Using a syringe, gently aspirate: blood will usually flow smoothly down the line if it is correctly sited.
7. Secure the UVC with a suture and confirm the position of the UVC with a chest/abdominal X-ray.
8. When correctly positioned, the tip of the UVC should lie at the level of the ninth to 10th thoracic vertebra.
9. Remove the UVC if it is in the liver.

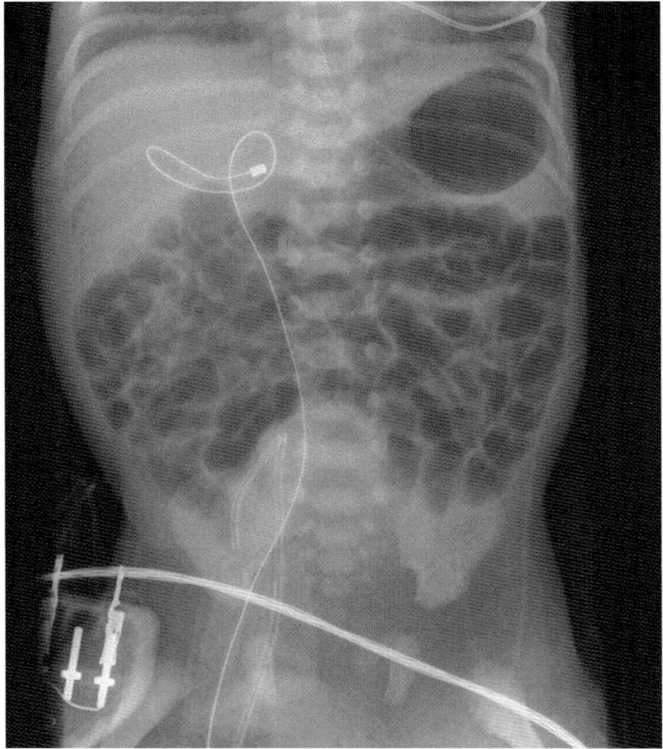

Fig. 44.19 The larger catheter has been inadvertently positioned in the umbilical artery (below L5) and should be removed. The smaller calibre line has been inserted via the umbilical vein line and is coiled in the right portal vein. Select the right-size line for the baby. Lines that are too small are more likely to coil within the vessels.

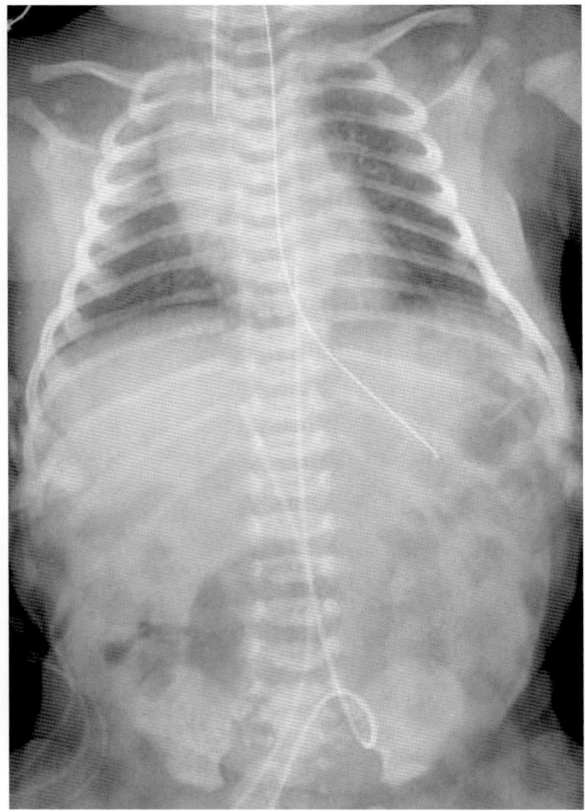

Fig. 44.20 Baby receiving therapeutic hypothermia (hence the cool wrap artefact). The umbilical arterial catheter is positioned correctly at T7. The umbilical venous catheter is short, sitting near the origin of the right portal vein.

Complications

See Table 44.8 and Figures 44.19–44.26.

Exchange transfusion

Indications

- Infants with severe unconjugated hyperbilirubinaemia:
  - refer to the bilirubin threshold graphs in the National Institute for Health and Clinical Excellence neonatal jaundice guideline (http://guidance.nice.org.uk/CG98) and Chapter 29.1.
- Infants with haemolysis, where the rate of rise of bilirubin exceeds 8.5 μmol/l/h despite double phototherapy.
- Hydropic infants with severe anaemia at birth.
- Severe sepsis or disseminated intravascular coagulation.

Equipment

- Oxygen saturation and cardiorespiratory monitors.
- Equipment for umbilical arterial and venous lines.
- Blood administration sets, warming coils.
- Sterile exchange transfusion set with two three-way taps (or one four-way tap) and waste bag.
- Cross-matched, cytomegalovirus-negative, irradiated plasma-reduced red cells (use within 24 hours of irradiation). The blood should be as fresh as possible (<5 days old).
- Volume of exchange = 160 ml/kg + an extra 30 ml for dead space in the tubing.

Procedure

1. Empty the infant's stomach and give maintenance intravenous fluids via a peripheral line.
2. Scrub up and put on sterile gown, mask and gloves.
3. Use drapes to ensure that all equipment is kept within a sterile field.
4. Insert umbilical catheters and take bloods from the baby for any serological, metabolic or genetic tests and check:
   (a) full blood count (FBC), packed cell volume (PCV), clotting studies
   (b) urea and electrolytes (U&E), Ca^{2+}
   (c) bilirubin
   (d) blood gas
   (e) blood glucose.
5. Start the exchange transfusion.
   (a) Isovolumetric technique: administer blood as a continuous infusion via the umbilical venous line, whilst blood is withdrawn slowly from the umbilical arterial line at a rate of 5 ml/kg every 5 minutes.
   (b) Pull–push technique: withdraw 5 ml/kg of blood from the umbilical venous line over 1 minute and discard, then inject 5 ml/kg of blood over 4 minutes.
6. Every 5 minutes, the nurse responsible for the baby must record the vital signs and document the total volume of blood that has been removed and replaced.

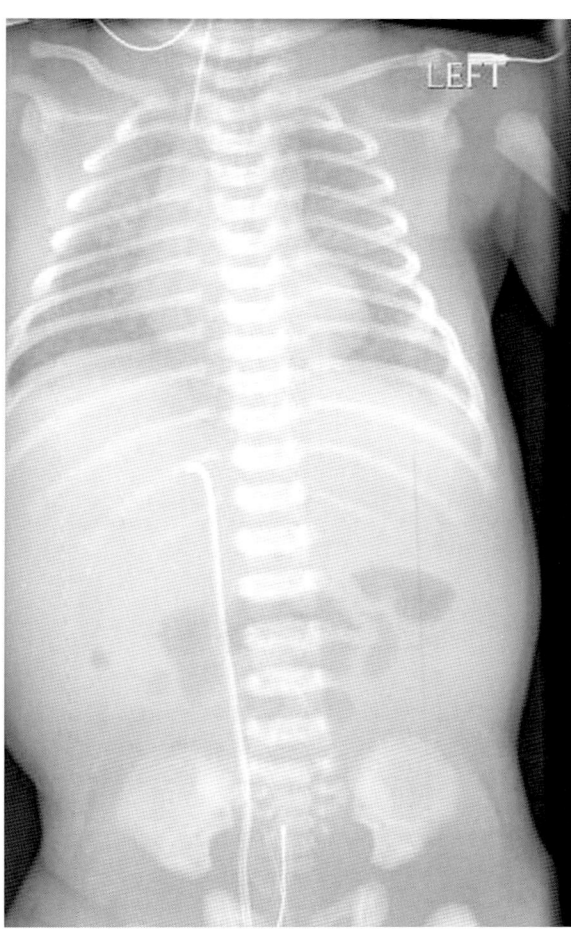

Fig. 44.21 This umbilical venous catheter is kinked and the tip is just entering the right portal vein. The tip of the line should lie at T9, immediately below the diaphragm. The line should be removed as there is a risk of portal vein thrombosis and liver injury.

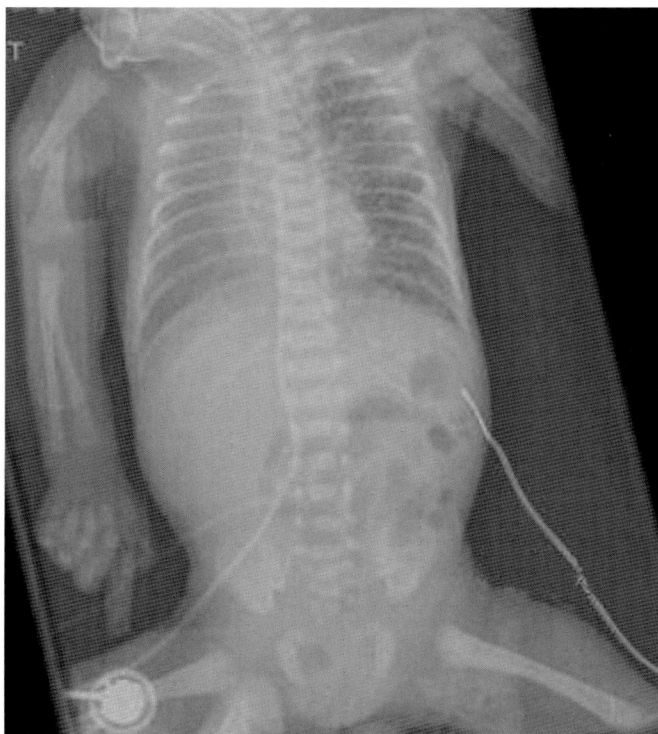

Fig. 44.22 The umbilical venous catheter is lying in the right atrium and must be withdrawn to T9. The tip of the endotracheal tube is lying at T4/5, abutting the carina, and there is evidence of pulmonary interstitial emphysema in the left lung. Note the right humerus is fractured.

7. Halfway through the procedure, check:
   (a) PCV
   (b) U&E, Ca²⁺
   (c) blood gas
   (d) blood glucose.
8. The procedure should be completed in ~2 hours.
9. If the baby shows any signs of cardiorespiratory decompensation during the procedure, consider slowing down the rate of exchange and using smaller aliquots. If the baby develops any serious complication stop the procedure immediately.
10. At the end of the procedure, recheck:
    (a) FBC, PCV, clotting studies
    (b) U&E, Ca²⁺
    (c) blood gas
    (d) blood glucose
    (e) bilirubin.
11. Leave the catheters in situ. Check the rate of rise of the bilirubin 2 hours after the procedure.

Complications

1. Hypoglycaemia, acid–base and electrolyte abnormalities.
2. Abnormal coagulation and thrombocytopenia.
3. Transfusion reaction.
4. Complications from the intravascular lines, including infection and thromboembolism.

Partial dilutional exchange transfusion

This procedure is probably not necessary in entirely well polycythaemic babies or those with mild transient problems, but most recommend treatment for babies with complications such as hypoglycaemia. Partial dilutional exchange transfusion usually improves the acute symptoms of hyperviscosity, but there is no evidence that it improves long-term outcome in asymptomatic polycythaemic infants (Dempsey and Barrington 2006).

Indications

Whilst the serious complications of polycythaemia, including renal vein thrombosis or cerebral venous sinus thrombosis, are rare, most clinicians will proceed with dilutional exchange if:

• the PCV is >70–75% in asymptomatic infants or >65% in symptomatic infants; symptoms include lethargy, hypotonia, irritability, hypoglycaemia, respiratory distress and poor feeding.

Equipment

• As for peripheral arterial and venous lines.
• 0.9% saline is cheap, widely available and as effective as using plasma, albumin or crystalloid (De Waal et al. 2006).

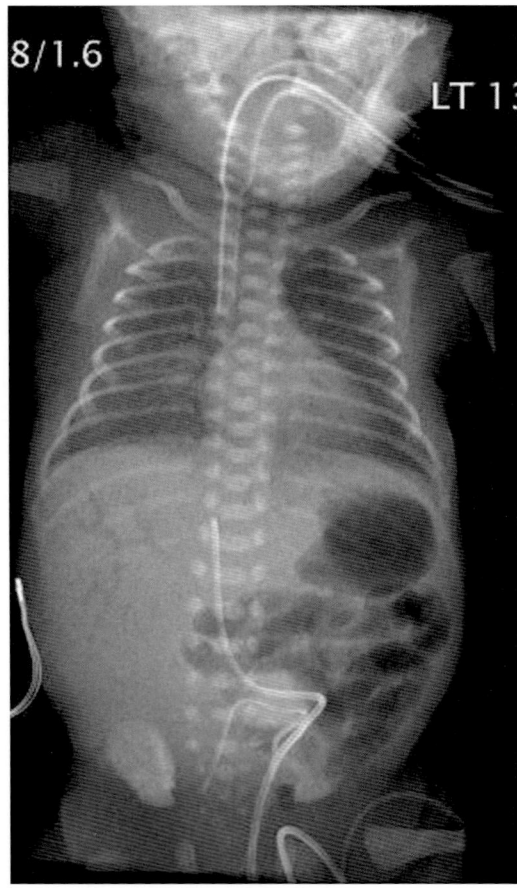

Fig. 44.23 The endotracheal tube should be shortened. Transient portal venous gas following insertion of umbilical venous catheter. The tip of the umbilical vein catheter should lie at T9 but is at T11–12. The umbilical artery catheter is very short (<L5) and should be removed.

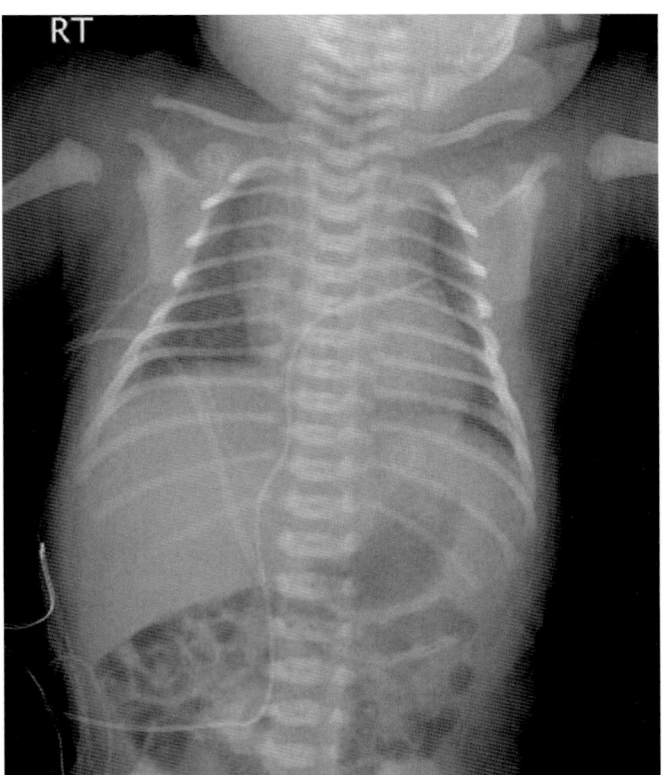

Fig. 44.24 The umbilical vein catheter has traversed the foramen ovale and is in the left atrium. It must be pulled back to T9 or replaced.

Intraosseous lines

Indications

* Emergency access to the circulation when other routes have failed.
* Administration of resuscitation fluids, blood products and drugs.

Equipment

* 18 G intraosseous needle or 20 G, 3.75 cm spinal needle.
* Luer-Lok extension sets.

Procedure

1. Clean and drape the skin.
2. Using full aseptic precautions, insert the intraosseous needle into the anterior medial aspect of the tibia, 1–2 cm below the tuberosity, at an angle of 10–15° towards the foot. Using a twisting motion, insert the needle to a depth of ~1 cm. You should feel a sudden give as the needle enters the marrow cavity.
3. Remove the trochar; the needle should stay in place without support.
4. Aspirate a sample of marrow for cross-match and culture.
5. Attach a syringe and inject 2–3 ml of saline to ensure the needle has penetrated the bone correctly.
6. Start infusing drugs and fluids to restore circulation. Observe for signs of extravasation.
7. Secure venous access as soon as possible.

Procedure

Calculate volume of blood to be removed and replaced using the formula:

$$\text{Volume (ml)} = \text{Total blood volume} \times \frac{(\text{Observed PCV} - \text{Desired PCV})}{\text{Observed PCV}}$$

This usually equates to around 20 ml/kg of saline.

1. Insert peripheral arterial and venous lines.
2. Start the saline infusion via the venous line.
3. Withdraw 5 ml/kg aliquots of blood slowly from the arterial line every 5 minutes.
4. During the procedure, keep a record of the volume of saline infused and the volume of blood removed.
5. Aim to complete the dilutional exchange over 20–30 minutes.
6. Check the PCV at the end of the procedure.

Complications

* See complications of peripheral arterial and venous lines.
* Transfusion-related risks are avoided if saline is used.

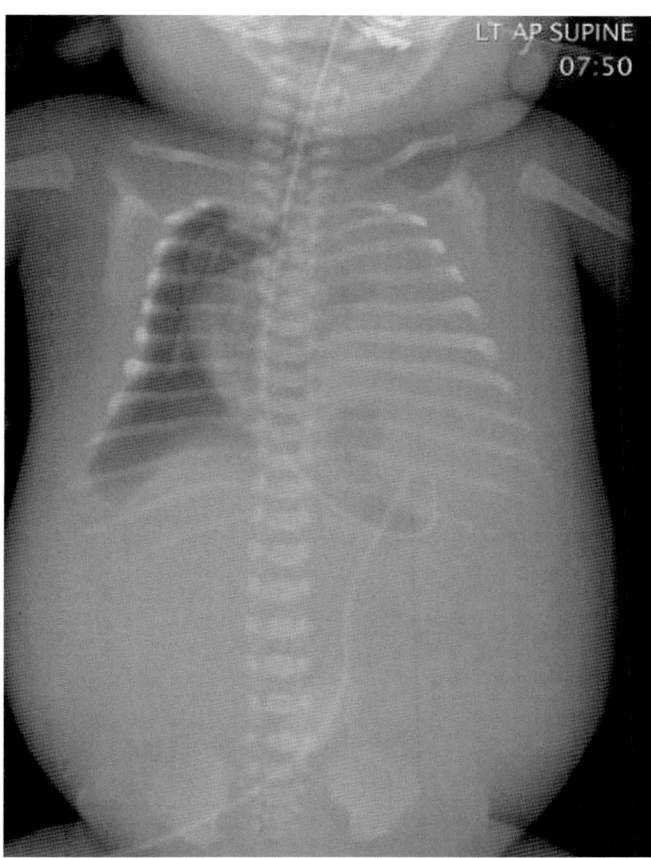

LT AP SUPINE
07:50

Fig. 44.25 Hydropic baby with left congenital diaphragmatic hernia. The endotracheal tube is at T1. There is a right pneumothorax. Note how the distorted anatomy is reflected in the position of the umbilical venous catheter.

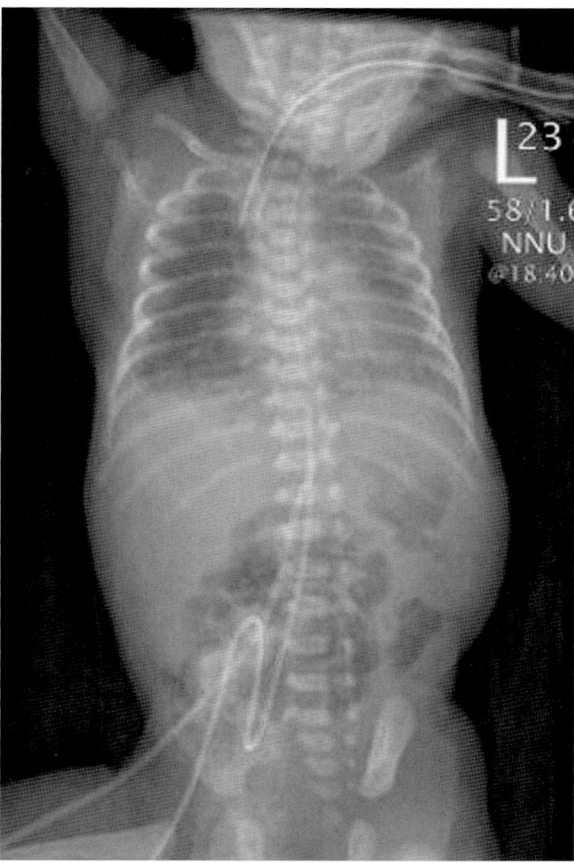

L 23
58/1.6
NNU
@18:40

Fig. 44.26 The umbilical artery catheter is at T10 (ideal position T6–9). The film is rotated and the UVC, which is little short, appears to cross the midline. The endotracheal tube is slightly long at T3.

Complications

1. Fracture – should be excluded once the baby is stable.
2. Damage to the growth plate of the tibia: minimise risk by angling the needle towards the foot.
3. Infection, including osteomyelitis, cellulitis and abscess.
4. Extravasation.
5. Compartment syndrome.

Bone marrow aspiration

Indications

- Investigation of marrow dysfunction.
- Diagnosis of marrow involvement in malignancies.

Equipment

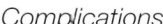

- Dressing pack.
- 22 G, 3.75 cm spinal needle, bone marrow aspiration needle.
- Appropriate slides and assay bottles.

Procedure

1. Using full aseptic technique, infiltrate local anaesthetic into the skin and subcutaneous tissues overlying the tibial tuberosity, anterior iliac spine or posterior iliac crests.
2. The needle is held perpendicular to the bone, and carefully screwed into the bone marrow cavity.

3. Marrow should be aspirated and prepared as directed by the haematologist.

Complications

See intraosseous line insertion.

Needle pericardiocentesis

Consider a diagnosis of tamponade in any baby with a central venous or arterial access who presents with severe cardiorespiratory compromise. Confirm the diagnosis with ultrasound, but do not delay the procedure if the baby is in extremis.

Indications

- Emergency treatment of pericardial tamponade due to fluid or air.

Equipment

- 21–25 G venous cannula (Venflon), extension set, three-way tap and syringe.

Procedure

1. Clean the skin.
2. Using a no-touch technique, insert the venous cannula just below the xiphoid cartilage and 0.5 cm to the left of the

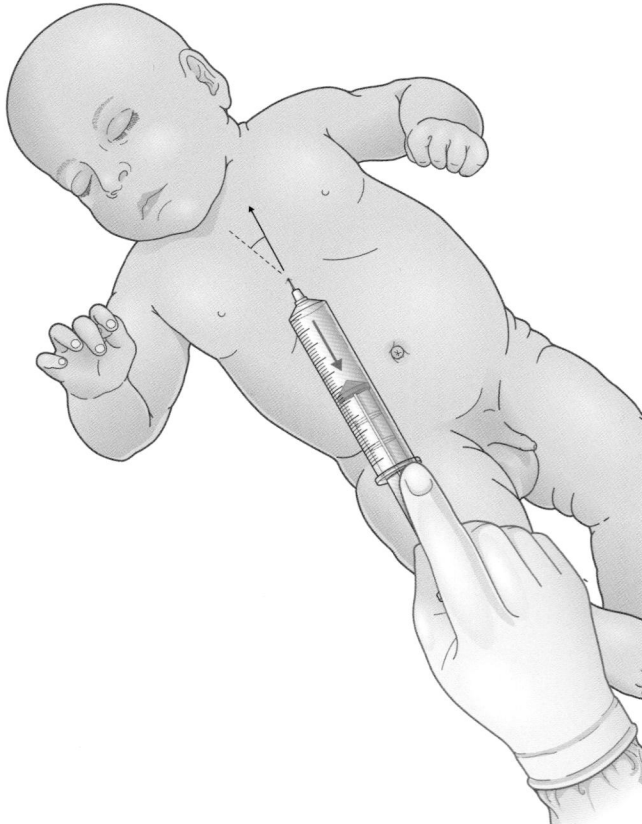

Fig. 44.27 Needle pericardiocentesis. Subxiphoid approach.

midline, directing the needle towards the left shoulder whilst aspirating gently on the syringe (Fig. 44.27).
3. Continue advancing the needle until air or fluid is obtained, usually at a depth of 1–2 cm. Slide the catheter over the needle and remove the needle to avoid traumatising the heart as the fluid or air is removed.
4. Evacuate as much air or fluid as possible from the pericardial sac. Removal of 5–10 ml of fluid will effect a significant improvement in cardiac output within seconds.

Complications

1. Cardiac puncture.
2. Pneumopericardium.
3. Pneumothorax.
4. Arrhythmias.

Feeding tubes

Nasogastric/orogastric feeding tubes

Colour-coded feeding tubes and syringes should be used to minimise the risk of 'wrong route' enteral nutrition and medication errors.

Indications

- Enteral nutrition in infants who are unable to feed normally.
- Decompression of the stomach.

Equipment

1. Colour-coded feeding tubes (4 Fr for babies <1000 g, 6 Fr for babies >1000 g, 8–10 Fr for decompression of stomach).
2. pH paper.
3. Hydrocolloid dressing and tape.

Procedure

1. Wash hands and put on gloves. Place the baby in a supine position.
2. Measure the distance from the nose to ear to halfway between the xiphisternum and umbilicus.
3. Lubricate the gastric tube and insert through the nostril, or over the tongue and into the oropharynx. Advance the tube to the predetermined length. Do not push against resistance. Monitor the baby's heart rate and breathing during the procedure.
4. Confirm that the tube is in the stomach by aspirating fluid and checking that the pH is less than 6. If there is no aspirate or the pH is above 6, take an X-ray to confirm the position of the tube.
5. Tape the tube to a hydrocolloid dressing on the baby's cheek or chin.
6. If the baby is on continuous positive airway pressure, leave on free drainage to decompress the stomach.
7. Tubes should be changed every 7 days to prevent bacterial contamination.

Nasojejunal feeding tubes

Indications

- Intolerance to nasogastric feeds.
- Severe gastro-oesophageal reflux with risk of aspiration (Misra et al. 2007).

Equipment

- Nasojejunal feeding tube.
- As for nasogastric/orogastric tubes.

Procedure

1. Measure the length for insertion: orogastric length + 8 cm, or nares to ankle, and mark the length on the nasojejunal tube with tape.
2. Insert an orogastric tube. Turn the baby on to the right side and advance the nasojejunal tube into the stomach. Allow time for peristalsis to carry the weighted tip through the pylorus.
3. When the nasojejunal marker reaches the nares, X-ray to confirm that the tip of the tube is lying just beyond the second part of the duodenum.
4. Secure the tube as described for nasogastric tubes and commence continuous milk feeds. Milk aspirates from the stomach indicate that the tube has slipped back.

Complications from nasogastric and nasojejunal tubes

See Table 44.9 and Figures 44.28–44.31.

Table 44.9 Complications of feeding tubes

COMPLICATION	PRESENTING SIGNS	MANAGEMENT
Misplacement on insertion	Apnoea, bradycardia or desaturation during insertion or subsequent feeding. Coiling in the oropharynx or oesophagus on X-ray. Pneumonia	Replace the tube X-ray to check position if any concern
Perforation of pharynx or oesophagus (Shah et al. 2003; Schuman et al. 2010)	Consider the diagnosis in any infant who presents with sudden/acute respiratory deterioration following intubation or passage of gastric/jejunal tube. Signs include surgical emphysema, pneumothorax, pneumomediastinum, pleural effusion and respiratory distress. Incidence of injury increases with decreasing gestational age and weight	Risk of perforation reduced if Silastic rather than PVC tubes are used (Filippi et al. 2005). Treat air leak/drain effusion. Refer to surgeon. May respond to conservative management: 7–10 days nil by mouth and antibiotics followed by contrast study to confirm healing
Perforation of stomach or duodenum (Abadir et al. 2005)	Pneumoperitoneum and signs of perionitis	Risk of duodenal perforation increased with PVC tubes. Refer to paediatric surgeon for laparotomy and primary repair
Sepsis and necrotising enterocolitis (Dallagrammaticas et al. 1983)	Nasojejunal feeding is associated with a predominance of Gram-negative organisms in upper GI flora	Apnoeas and bradycardias, abdominal distension, bilious aspirates, GI bleeding

PVC, polyvinyl chloride; GI, gastrointestinal.

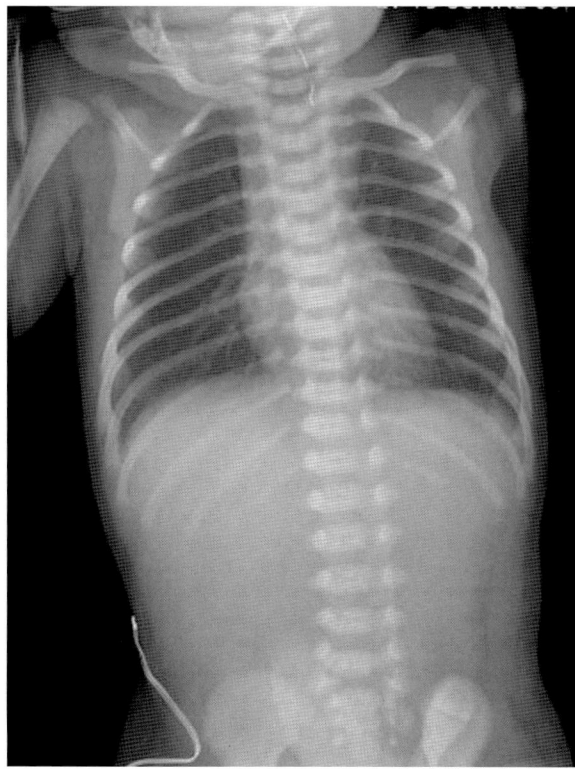

Fig. 44.28 High oesophageal atresia. Note that the tip of the large-bore nasogastric tube is level with the clavicles and the absence of gas in the stomach and bowel.

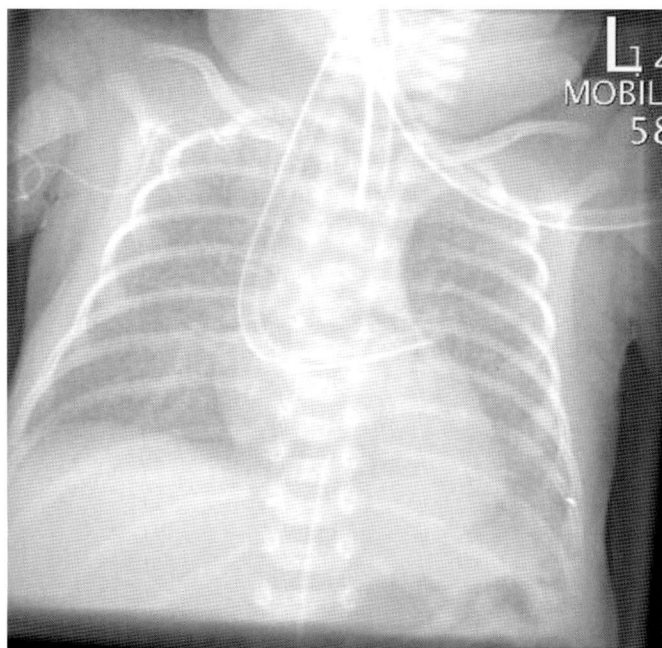

Fig. 44.29 Misplaced nasogastric tube secondary to pharyngo-oesophageal tear. The endotracheal tube and umbilical lines are in satisfactory positions. The central venous catheter is kinked in the right subclavian vein and should be pulled back to midhumerus or replaced.

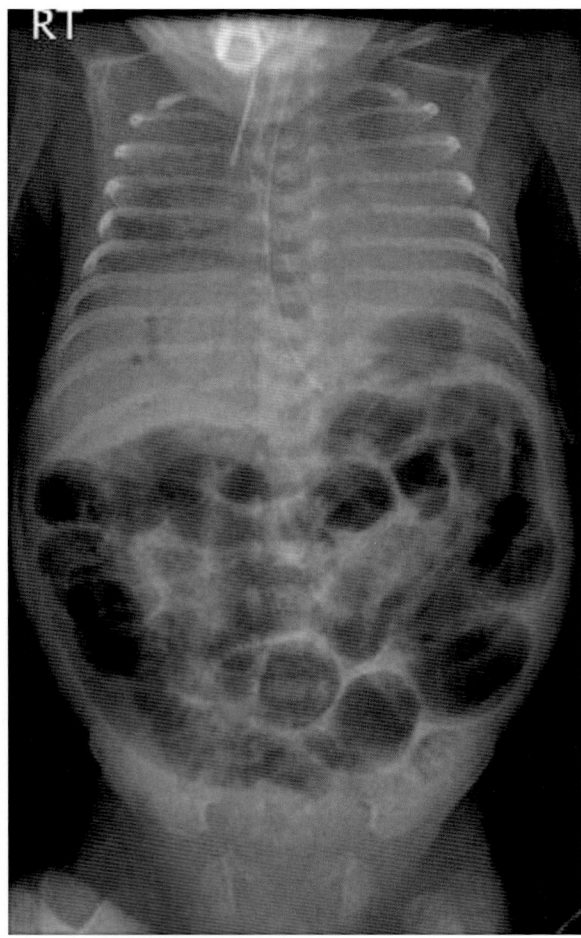

Fig. 44.30 Coiled nasogastric tube in a baby with extensive necrotising enterocolitis. The nasogastric tube should be resited in order to decompress the bowel. The endotracheal tube is just above the carina and should be shortened. Note the extensive pneumatosis intestinalis and portal venous gas.

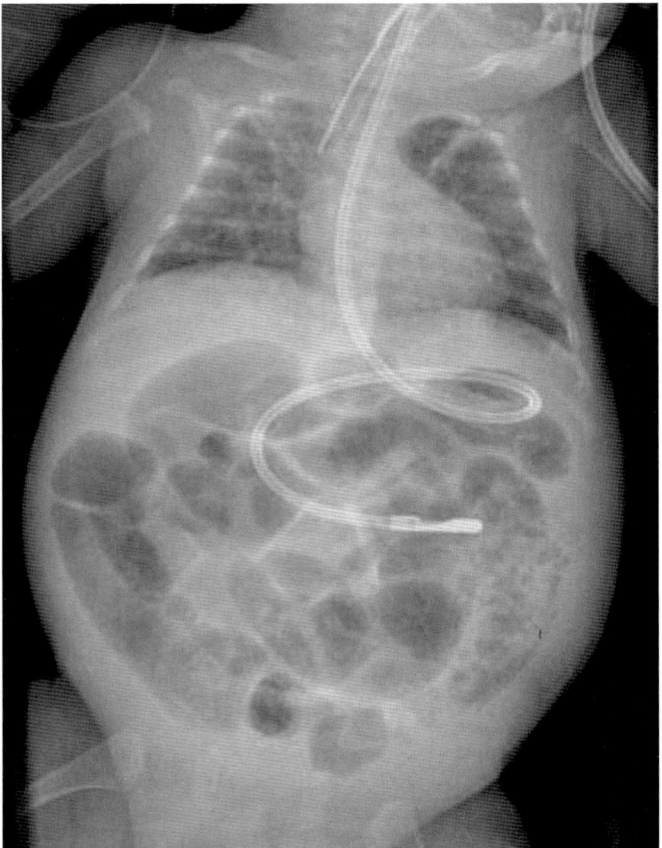

Fig. 44.31 Necrotising enterocolitis in a baby who was fed via a nasojejunal tube.

Urine collection

Suprapubic aspiration

Indications

* To obtain uncontaminated urine for culture.

Equipment

* Sterile dressing pack.
* Syringes (5 ml), 25 G needle.

Procedure

1. An assistant should hold the baby in a supine, frog-leg position. If the baby passes urine unexpectedly, the assistant should be prepared to catch a clean sample in a sterile container.
2. Using ultrasound, confirm that the bladder is full.
3. Clean the skin between the umbilicus and symphysis pubis with antiseptic solution.
4. Insert the needle through the anterior abdominal wall in the midline, 1 cm above the pubic symphysis. Apply

gentle suction with the syringe and advance the needle at a perpendicular angle to a depth of 1–2 cm until urine is obtained (Fig. 44.32). Withdraw the needle and apply pressure over the puncture site with sterile gauze.

Complications

1. Haemorrhage: transient microscopic haematuria occurs in 0.6–10% of cases. Gross haematuria, abdominal and bladder wall haematomas are rare.
2. Perforation of the bowel. If a 25 G needle is used, this should heal without complication.
3. Infection.

Suprapubic catheterisation

This procedure should only be performed after consultation with a paediatric urologist.

Indications

* Posterior urethral valves.
* Urethral trauma or surgery.

Equipment

* Sterile dressing pack, local anaesthetic.
* Suprapubic catheterisation pack and collection system.

3. Injury to an abdominal viscus.
4. Extravasation of urine.

Transurethral catheterisation

Indications
- In/out catheterisation to obtain urine for culture.
- Monitoring of urine output in a critically ill neonate.

Equipment
- Sterile dressing pack, Steri-Strips.
- Urinary catheter or fine feeding tube and collection system.

Procedure
1. Clean the external genitalia with antiseptic solution and allow to dry.
2. Lubricate the outside of the catheter with sterile K-Y jelly.
3. Using a no-touch technique, insert the catheter through the urethral meatus into the bladder.
4. Urine should drain freely.
5. Fix the catheter to the thigh with adhesive tape and attach to the collecting system.
6. Remove the catheters as soon as possible to minimise the risk of infection.

Complications
1. Trauma to the urethra with risk of subsequent stricture formation.
2. Haemorrhage.
3. Infection.

Abdominal paracentesis

Indications
- Emergency drainage of massive ascites.
- Diagnostic tap.

Equipment
- Sterile gloves and gown.
- Sterile dressing pack containing drapes.
- 1% lidocaine.
- 24 G venous catheter.
- 10-ml syringe.

Procedure
1. Position the baby with the right flank slightly elevated to encourage fluid to drain to the left lower quadrant of the abdomen. Empty the bladder.
2. Clean the skin and drape.
3. Identify the point at the junction of the middle and outer third of the distance along a line between the umbilicus and left anterior superior iliac spine. If this is an elective procedure, infiltrate the skin with local anaesthetic.
4. Push the catheter gently into the peritoneal cavity while applying gentle suction on the syringe. When peritoneal fluid is aspirated, advance the catheter over the needle and withdraw the needle.
5. Reconnect the syringe to the catheter and aspirate slowly.
6. Remove the catheter when the fluid stops flowing and apply a dressing.

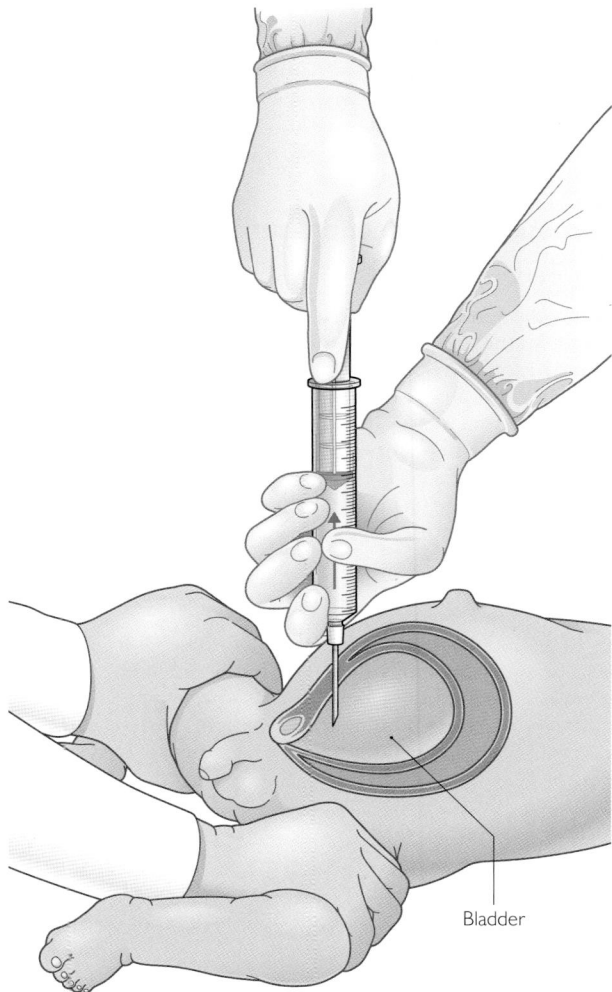

Fig. 44.32 Suprapubic aspiration.

Bladder

Procedure
1. Confirm that the bladder is full using ultrasound.
2. An assistant should hold the baby in a supine, frog-leg position.
3. Scrub up and put on sterile gloves and gown.
4. Clean the skin between the umbilicus and symphysis pubis with antiseptic solution and allow to dry.
5. Infiltrate the skin and subcutaneous tissue with local anaesthetic and make a small incision 1 cm above the symphysis in the midline.
6. Using a Seldinger technique, insert the introducer needle at right angles to the skin and aspirate gently as the needle is advanced. When urine is obtained, remove the needle from the introducer and insert a guidewire into the bladder.
7. Remove the introducer, and thread the suprapubic catheter over the guidewire and into the bladder.
8. Secure the catheter to the abdominal wall and attach the collecting system.

Complications
1. Haematuria.
2. Infection.

Complications

- Perforation of the bladder or bowel: this can usually be managed conservatively as a small-gauge needle is used.
- Haemorrhage (ensure clotting is normal if this is an elective procedure).
- Injury to the liver – avoid using the right lower quadrant to drain ascites if there is significant hepatomegaly.

Peritoneal dialysis

The management of renal failure should be discussed with a paediatric nephrologist.

Peritoneal dialysis (PD) is a relatively safe and easy method of renal replacement therapy in neonates. It is contraindicated in babies with acute abdominal pathology and should be avoided in babies with abdominal adhesions or significant respiratory compromise.

Surgical insertion of a permanent Tenchkoff PD catheter is the preferred option if dialysis is indicated for more than 3–5 days. Tunnelling of the catheter from the skin to the peritoneum reduces the risk of leak and infection.

If surgical insertion is not possible a temporary PD catheter can be inserted using the Seldinger technique.

Indications

- Renal failure secondary to acute tubular necrosis, renal cortical necrosis, obstructive uropathy or bilateral renal dysplasia.
- Metabolic disorders, although haemofiltration is considered to be more effective.

Equipment

- Sterile gloves and gown.
- Sterile instrument pack containing drapes, scalpel, needle holder, artery clamps, fine scissors.
- 1% lidocaine.
- 8.5 Fr acute PD catheter.
- Dialysis solution.

Procedure

1. Weigh the baby and measure the abdominal girth.
2. Empty the stomach and catheterise the bladder.
3. Clean the abdominal skin and drape with sterile towels.
4. Identify the insertion site: level with the umbilicus and just lateral to the rectus sheath, or in the midline below the umbilicus.
5. Infiltrate the skin with 0.5 ml of 1% lidocaine.
6. Make a 4-mm incision with the scalpel. Carefully advance the introducer needle into the peritoneum. Insert the flexible guidewire through the hub of the needle into the peritoneal cavity. Remove the needle, leaving the guidewire in place. Use the dilator to enlarge the tract and then introduce the catheter into the peritoneal cavity. Remove the guidewire.
7. Attach the connecting tubing and secure the catheter to the abdominal wall with a suture and adhesive dressing.
8. The volumes and duration of dialysate cycles should be discussed with a nephrologist. Starting volume is usually 20 ml/kg and cycle length 60 minutes: fill by gravity, dwell time of 40 minutes and then drain by gravity.

Complications

- Perforation of the bladder or bowel (3–7%).
- Leakage.
- Outflow obstruction (usually from omentum), leading to retention of >10% of solution in each of several consecutive cycles.
- Peritonitis.
- Wound infection.
- Electrolyte disturbance and hyperglycaemia.

Cerebrospinal fluid collection

Lumbar puncture

In fetal life, the vertebral column elongates more rapidly than the spinal cord, so the level of the conus medullaris (lower end of the spinal cord) ascends relative to the lumbar vertebrae. The conus medullaris lies above L2/3 in 98% of term infants and in ~90% of preterm infants from 31 to 37 weeks' gestation (Sahin et al. 1997). It is considered safer to perform the lumbar puncture at L4/5 or L5/S1 in very preterm infants.

Ensure that the baby has normal clotting studies and a normal platelet count before proceeding.

Indications

- Suspected central nervous system infection.
- For the investigation of seizures and neurometabolic disease.
- Removal of cerebrospinal fluid (CSF) in babies with symptoms of raised intracranial pressure secondary to posthaemorrhagic hydrocephalus. Symptoms include full or tense anterior fonatanelle, separation of sutures, apnoea and bradycardia, vomiting and poor feeding.

Equipment

- Dressing pack, universal sterile containers.
- 22 or 25 G, 3.75 cm spinal needle with short bevel.

Procedure

1. An experienced assistant should restrain the baby on a firm surface, in a left-side-down or sitting position.
2. Scrub up and put on gown and sterile gloves.
3. Using a full aseptic technique, clean the skin and drape.
4. Ask the assistant to flex the spine to open the intervertebral spaces. Identify the L4 spinous process, which lies on an imaginary line joining the top of the right and left iliac crests.
5. In a term infant, insert the needle through the midline of the intervertebral space at L3/4 or L4/5, aiming towards the umbilicus. A change in resistance can be felt as the ligamentum flavum and dura are penetrated.
6. Remove the stylet and attach a three-way tap and manometer to the hub of the spinal needle to measure the opening pressure.
7. Allow CSF to drip into the universal containers. If there is no flow, carefully rotate the needle. A traumatic tap (with blood-stained CSF that clears as the samples are collected) occurs when the needle damages the epidural venous plexus on the posterior surface of the vertebral bodies. Uniformly blood-stained CSF is seen with intraventricular and, more rarely, subarachnoid haemorrhages.
8. At the end of the procedure, replace the stylet before removing the needle. Apply a sterile dressing.

Ventricular tap

There is no evidence that early tapping of CSF by lumbar puncture or ventricular tap reduces the risk of shunt dependence, disability or death (Whitelaw 2001). The use of repeated taps is associated with an increased risk of central nervous system infection, so it is essential that full aseptic precautions are taken during this procedure.

Equipment

- As for lumbar puncture.

Procedure

1. Confirm that there is progressive ventriculomegaly on cranial ultrasound examination and estimate the depth for needle insertion.
2. Use scissors to trim any hair that overlies the lateral angle of the fontanelle. Do not shave the scalp.
3. An assistant should hold the baby's head in the neutral position. Clean the skin with antiseptic solution and drape with sterile towels. Insert the spinal needle at the lateral angle of the fontanelle and advance to the required depth, aiming towards the inner canthus of the eye.
4. Remove the stylet from the needle and attach a three-way tap and manometer to measure the opening pressure.
5. Allow the CSF to drain, or aspirate slowly at a rate of 1–2 ml/min. Remove a maximum of 10–15 ml/kg of CSF.
6. Remove the needle and apply pressure for 2–3 minutes until CSF stops leaking from the puncture site. Dress with sterile gauze.

Complications of cerebrospinal fluid drainage

1. Infection – there is a risk of introducing microorganisms during CSF sampling.
2. Haemorrhage – usually local and settles spontaneously.
3. Trauma to brain tissue with repeated venticular taps – parenchymal cysts frequently develop along the needle track.

Tapping ventricular reservoirs

Ventricular reservoirs are used to drain CSF in preterm infants with posthaemorrhagic hydrocephalus who are too small for formal ventriculoperitoneal shunting.

Maintain strict asepsis during this procedure.

Procedure

1. Clean the skin and drape with sterile towels.
2. Insert a 25 G butterfly at an angle of 45° through the skin and into the dome of the reservoir. Use a different insertion site each time the procedure is performed to reduce the risk of tearing the dome of the reservoir.
3. Aspirate CSF at a rate of 1–2 ml/min. Remove a maximum of 10–15 ml/kg of fluid.
4. Remove the butterfly and apply pressure for 2–3 minutes. Dress with sterile gauze.

Complications

1. Hyponatraemia and hypoproteinaemia if regular drainage is performed.
2. Infection.
3. Skin breakdown over the reservoir.

Punch skin biopsy

Indications

- Diagnosis of skin lesions.
- Fibroblast culture for suspected genetic or metabolic disorders.
- Consult a trained dermatologist before taking a biopsy of any skin lesion. Try to biopsy early or fully established lesions, but not excoriated, crusted or traumatised lesions. The biopsy may need to include some normal skin.
- If the skin biopsy is performed in a neonate with a suspected underlying genetic or metabolic disorder, seek expert advice regarding transport medium and handling of the specimen.
- Excision of larger lesions should be performed by a dermatologist or surgeon.

Equipment

- Sterile gloves and gown.
- Sterile instrument pack containing drapes, scalpel, needle holder, artery clamps, fine scissors.
- 1% lidocaine.
- 3–4-mm disposable cylindrical punch (Steifel).
- 5-0 Prolene suture on a curved needle.
- Sterile container with appropriate transport medium.

Procedure

1. Choose the biopsy site and clean and drape the skin.
2. Infiltrate the skin with 0.25–0.5 ml of 1% lidocaine and wait 2–3 minutes.
3. Stretch the skin and cut through the skin with the punch, using a twisting motion.
4. Remove the punch and lift the biopsy up gently, using non-toothed forceps. The biopsy should include some subcutaneous fat. Use scissors to cut the specimen at its base and place in transport medium.
5. Apply gentle pressure to control the bleeding.
6. Use a single suture to approximate the wound edges.

Complications

1. Infection.
2. Bleeding (rare, unless there is a coagulation defect).
3. Keloid scarring.

References

Abadir, J., Emil, S., Nguyen, N., 2005. Abdominal foregut perforations in children: a 10-year experience. J Pediatr Surg 40, 1903–1907.

American Academy of Pediatrics and Canadian pediatric society, 2006. Prevention and management of pain in the neonate. Pediatrics 118, 2231–2241.

Ammari, A.N., Jen, A., Towers, H., et al., 2002. Subcutaneous emphysema and pneumomediastinum as presenting manifestations of neonatal tracheal injury. J Perinatol 22, 499–501.

Armstron, D., Battin, M.R., Knight, D., et al., 2002. Staphylococcus aureus endocarditis in preterm neonates. Am J Perinatol 19, 247–251.

Ayra, H., Williams, J., Ponsford, S.N., et al., 1991. Neonatal diaphragmatic paralysis caused by chest drains. Arch Dis Child 66, 441–442.

Baker, J., Imong, S., 2002. A rare complication of neonatal central venous access. Arch Dis Child Fetal Neonatal Ed 86, F61–F62.

Barrington, K.J., 1999a. Umbilical artery catheters in the newborn: effects of catheter design (end vs. side hole). Cochrane Database Syst Rev (1), CD000508.

Barrington, K.J., 1999b. Umbilical artery catheters in the newborn: effects of position of the catheter tip. Cochrane Database Syst Rev (1), CD000505.

Blayney, M.P., Logan, D.R., 1994. First thoracic body as reference for endotracheal tube placement. Arch Dis Child Fetal Neonatal Ed 71, F32–F35.

Brown, M.S., Phipps, R.H., 1988. Spinal cord injury in newborns from use of umbilical artery catheters: a report of 2 cases and a review of the literature. J Perinatol 8, 105–110.

Cartwright, D.W., 2004. Central venous lines in neonates: a study of 2186 catheters. Arch Dis Child Fetal Neonatal Ed 89, F504–F508.

Cartwright, G.W., Schreiner, R.L., 1980. Major complications secondary to percutaneous radial artery catheterization in the neonate. Pediatrics 65, 139–141.

Chandavasu, O., Garrow, E., Valda, V., et al., 1986. A new method for the prevention of skin sloughs and necrosis secondary to intravenous infiltration. Am J Perinatol 3, 4–5.

Chen, C.C., Tsao, P.N., Yau, K.I., 2001. Paraplegia: complication of percutaneous central venous line malposition. Pediatr Neurol 23, 65–68.

Chief Pharmaceutical Officer, 2004. Building a safer NHS for patients: Improving Medication Safety. Department for Health, London.

Chien, L.Y., Ying, M., Aziz, K., et al., 2002 Jun. Variations in central venous catheter-related infection risks among Canadian neonatal intensive care units. Pediatr Infect Dis J 21(6), 505–511.

Clerihew, L., Austin, N., McGuire, W., 2007. Prophylactic systemic antifungal agents to prevent mortality and morbidity in very low birth weight infants. Cochrane Database Syst Rev (4), CD003850.

Consent for Common Neonatal Investigations, Interventions and Treatments. s.l.: BAPM Working Party. Publications, BAPM.org/publications. 2004.

Cronin, W.A., Germanson, T.P., Donowitz, L.G., 1990. Intravascular catheter colonization and related bloodstream infection in critically ill neonates. Infect Control Hosp Epidemiol 11, 301.

Daniels, S.R., Hannon, D., Meyer, R.A., et al., 1984. Paroxysmal supraventricular tachycardia: a complication of jugular central venous catheters in neonates. Am J Dis Child 138, 474–475.

Davies, J., Gault, D., Buchdahl, R., 1994. Preventing the scars of neonatal intensive care. Arch Dis Child 70, F50–F51.

Dellagrammaticas, H.D., Duerden, B.I., Milner, R.D., 1983. Upper intestinal bacterial flora during transpyloric feeding. Arch Dis Child 58, 115–119.

De Waal, K.A., Baerts, W., Offringa, M., 2006. Systematic review of the optimal fluid for dilutional exchange transfusion in neonatal polycythaemia. Arch Dis Child Fetal Neonatal Ed 91, F7–F10.

Dempsey, E.M., Barrington, K., 2006. Short and long term outcomes following partial exchange transfusion in the polycythaemic newborn. Arch Dis Child Fetal Neonatal Ed 91, F2–F6.

Denkler, K.A., Cohen, B.E., 1989. Reversal of dopamine extravasation injury with topical nitroglycerin ointment. Plast Reconstruct Surg 84, 811–813.

Department of Health, 2001. Good Practice in Consent Implementation Guide: Consent to Examination or Treatment. s.l.: Department for Health Publications, London.

Dunn, P., 1966. Localization of the umbilical catheter by post-mortem measurement. Arch Dis Child 41, 69–75.

Embleton, N.D., Deshpande, S.A., Scott, D., et al., 2001. Foot length, an accurate predictor of nasotracheal tube length in neonates. Arch Dis Child Fetal Neonatal Ed 85, F60–F64.

Erenberg, A., Nowak, A.J., 1984. Palatal groove formation in neonates with orotracheal tubes. Am J Dis Child 138, 974–975.

Fan, L., Flynn, J.W., Pathak, D.R., 1983. Risk factors predicting laryngeal injury in intubated neonates. Crit Care Med 11, 431–433.

Filippi, L., Pezzati, M., Poggi, C., 2005. Use of polyvinyl feeding tubes and iatrogenic pharyngo-oesophageal perforation in very-low-birthweight infants. Acta Paediatr 94, 1825–1828.

Garland, J.S., Havens, P., Dunne, W.M., et al., 1992. Peripheral intravenous catheter complications in critically ill children: a prospective study. Pediatrics 89, 1145–1150.

Harila-Kaera, V., Gron, M., Heikkinen, T., et al., 2002. Saggittal occlusal relationships and asymmetry in prematurely born children. Eur J Orthodont 24, 615–625.

Hauri-Hohla, A., Baenziger, O., Frey, B., 2008. Pneumomediastinum in the neonatal and paediatric intensive care unit. Eur J Pediatr 167, 415–418.

Hepworth, R., Milstein, J.M., 1984. The transected urachus: an unusual cause of neonatal ascites. Pediatrics 73, 397–400.

Hohoff, A., Rabe, H., Ehmer, U., et al., 2005. Palatal development of preterm and low birthweight infants compared to term infants – What do we know? Part 2: The palate of the preterm/low birthweight infant. Head Face Med 1, 9.

Hsu, J.F., Tsai, M.H., Huang, H.R., et al., 2010. Risk factors for catheter-related bloodstream infections in very low birthweight infants: a center's experience in Taiwan. Pediatr Neonataol 51, 336–342.

International Guidelines for Neonatal Resuscitation, 2000. An Excerpt from the Guidelines 2000 for CPR and emergency cardiovascular care: international consensus on science. Pediatrics 106.

Jaako Dardashti, V., Bekassy, Z.D., Ljung, R., et al., 2009. Successful thrombolysis of neonatal bilateral renal vein thrombosis originating in the IVC. Pediatr Nephrol 24, 2069–2071.

Jain, A., Rutter, N., 2000. Does topical amethocaine gel reduce the pain of venepuncture in newborn infants? A randomised double blind controlled trial. Arch Dis Child Fetal Neonatal Ed 83, F207–F210.

Jain, A., Rutter, N., Ratnayaka, M., 2001. Topical amethocaine gel for pain relief of heel prick blood sampling: a randomised double blind controlled trial. Arch Dis Child Fetal Neonatal Ed 84, F56–F59.

Joseph, L.J., Bromiker, R., Toker, O., et al., 2011. Unilateral lung intubation for pulmonary air leak syndrome in neonates: a case series and a review of the literature. Am J Perinatol 28, 151–156.

Kahn, D.J., Spinazzola, R., 2005. Acquired oral commissure defect: a complication of prolonged endotracheal intubation. J Perinatol 25, 612–614.

Kempley, S.T., Moreiras, J.W., Petrone, F.L., 2008. Endotracheal tube length for neonatal intubation. Resuscitation 77, 369–373.

Khemani, R.G., Randolph, A., Markovitz, B., 2009. Corticosteroids for the prevention and treatment of postextubation stridor in neonates, children and adults. Cochrane Database Syst Rev (3), CD001000.

Kuhle, S., Massicotte, P., Chan, A., et al., 2004. Antithrombotic therapy in Neonates and Children. Thromb haemostas 92, 729–733.

Kumar, S.P., Belik, J., 1984. Chylothorax – a complication of tube placement in the neonate. Crit Care Med 12, 411–412.

Ligi, I., Arnaud, F., Jouve, E., et al., 2008. Iatrogenic events in admitted neonates: a prospective cohort study. Lancet 371, 404–410.

Lilien, L.D., Harris, V.J., Ramamurthy, R.S., et al., 1976. Neonatal osteomyelitis of the calcaneus: complication of heel puncture. J Pediatr 88, 478–480.

Lim, J., Hellier, W., Harcourt, J., et al., 2003. Subglottic cysts: the Great Ormond Street experience. Int J Pediatr Otorhinolaryngol 67, 461–465.

Mann, N.P., 1980. Gluteal skin necrosis after umbilical arterial catheterisation. Arch Dis Child 55, 815–817.

Marsh, J.L., King, W., Barrett, C., et al., 1975. Serious complications after umbilical artery catheterization for neonatal monitoring. Arch Surg 110, 1203–1205.

Mason, C., Odell, E.W., Longhurst, P., 1994. Dental complications associated with repeated orotracheal intubation in infancy: a case report. Int J Pediatr Dent 4, 257–264.

Matching Michigan, 2009. Patient Safety First Campaign. Available online at: www.patientsafetyfirst.nhs.uk.

Meyers, A., Lillydahl, P., Brown, G., 1978. Hypopharyngeal perforations in neonates. Arch Otolaryngol 104, 51–54.

Misra, S., Macwan, K., Albert, V., 2007. Transpyloric feeding in gastroesophageal-reflux-associated apnea in premature infants. Acta Paediatr 96, 1426–1429.

Miyahara, K., Ichihara, T., Watanabe, T., 1999. Successful use of high frequency oscillatory ventilation for pneumomediastinum. Ann Thorac Cardiovasc Surg 5, 49–51.

Moessinger, A.C., Driscoll, J.M., Wigger, H.J., 1978. High incidence of lung perforation by chest tube in neonatal pneumothorax. J Pediatr 92, 635–637.

Mulvihill, S.J., Fonkalsrud, E.W., 1984. Complications of superior versus inferior vena cava occlusion in infants receiving central total parenteral nutrition. J Pediatr Surg 19, 752–757.

Pape, K.E., Armstrong, D.L., Fitzhardinge, P.M., 1987. Peripheral median nerve damage secondary to brachial artery blood gas sampling. J Pediatr 93, 852–856.

Pessoa-Silva, C., Hugonnet, S., Pfister, R., et al., 2007. Reduction of health care-associated infection risk in neonates by successful hand hygiene promotion. Pediatrics 120, e382–e390.

Pronovost, P., Needham, D., Berenholtz, S., et al., 2006. An intervention to decrease catheter-related bloodstream infections in the ICU. N Engl J Med 355, 2725–2732.

Quak, J.M., Szatmari, A., van den Anker, J.N., 1993. Cardiac tamponade in a preterm neonate secondary to a chest tube. Acta Paediatr 82, 490–491.

Rainer, C., Gardetto, A., Fruhwirth, M., et al., 2003. Breast deformity in adolescence as a result of pneumothorax drainage during neonatal intensive care. Pediatrics 111, 80–86.

Ramasethu, J., 2004. Prevention and management of extravasation injuries in neonates. Neoreviews 5, 491–497.

Randel, S.N., Tang, B.H., Wung, J.T., et al., 1987. Experience with percutaneous indwelling peripheral arterial catheterization in neonates. Am J Dis Child 141, 848–851.

Rey, C., Marache, P., Watel, A., et al., 1987. Iatrogenic false aneurysm of the brachial artery in an infant. Eur J Pediatr 146, 438–439.

Roberts, D., McQuinn, T., Beckerman, R.C., 1988. Neonatal arytenoid dislocation. Pediatrics 81, 580–582.

Sahin, F., Selçuki, M., Ecin, N., et al., 1997. Level of conus medullaris in term and preterm neonates. Arch Dis Child 77, F67–F69.

Schuman, T.A., Jacobs, B., Walsh, W., et al., 2010. Iatrogenic perinatal pharyngoesophageal injury: a disease of prematurity. Int J Pediatr Otorhinolaryngol 74, 393–397.

Sekar, K.C., 2010. Iatrogenic complications in the neonatal intensive care unit. J Perinatol 30, S51–S56.

Serlin, S.P., Daily, W.J.R., 1975. Tracheal perforation in a neonate: a complication of tracheal intubation. J Pediatr 86, 596–597.

Shah, P.S., Dunn, M.S., Shah, V.S., 2003. Oesophageal perforation in preterm neonates: not an innocent bystander. J Paediatr Child Health 39, 697–699.

Shukla, H., Ferrara, A., 1986. Rapid estimation of intentional length of umbilical catheters in newborns. Am J Dis Child 140, 786–788.

Sirnon-Fayard, E.E., Kroncke, R.S., Solarte, D., et al., 1997. Non-surgical retrieval of embolised umbilical catheters in premature infants. J Perinatol 17, 143–147.

Slater, R., Cornelissen, L., Fabrizi, L., et al., 2010. Oral sucrose as an analgesic drug for procedural pain in newborn infants: a randomised controlled trial. Lancet 376, 1225–1232.

Vailas, G.N., Brouilette, R.T., Scott, J.P., et al., 1986. Neonatal aortic thrombosis: recent experience. J Pediatr 109, 101–108.

Walner, D.L., Loewen, M.S., Kimura, R.E., 2001. Neonatal subglottic stenosis: incidence and trends. Laryngoscope 111, 48–51.

Whitelaw, A., 2001. Repeated lumbar or ventricular punctures in newborns with intraventricular hemorrhage. Cochrane Database Syst Rev (1), CD000216.

Whyte, K., Levin, R., Powls, A., 2007. Clinical audit: optimal positioning of endotracheal tubes in neonates. Scot Med J 52, 25–27.

Wright, M.R., Owers, M., Wagner, M., 2008. The umbilical arterial catheter: a formula for improved positioning in the very low birth weight infant. Pediatr Crit Care Med 9, 498–501.

Irene A G Roberts
Neil A Murray

Appendix 1

Haematological values in the newborn

Table A1.1 Red cell parameters in the fetus

AGE (weeks)	Hb (g/dl)	PCV	RBC (×10¹²/l)	MCV (fl)	MCH (pg)	MCHC (g/dl)	NUCLEATED RBC (% OF WBC)	RETICULOCYTES (%)
12	8.0–10.0	0.33	1.5	180	60	34	5.0–8.0	40
16	10.0	0.35	2.0	140	45	33	2.0–4.0	10–25
20	11.0	0.37	2.5	135	44	33	1.0	10–20
24	14.0	0.40	3.5	123	38	31	1.0	5–10
28	14.5	0.45	4.0	120	40	31	0.5	5–20
34	15.0	0.47	4.4	118	38	32	0.2	3–10
Term 40 cord	16.8	0.53	5.25	107	34	31.7	0.01	3–7

Hb, haemoglobin; MCH, mean corpuscular haemoglobin; MCHC, mean corpuscular haemoglobin concentration; MCV, mean cell volume; PCV, packed cell volume; RBC, red blood cells; WBC, white blood cells.
Adapted from Oski, F.A., Naiman, J.L., 1982. Hematologic Problems in the Newborn, third ed. WB Saunders, New York.

Table A1.2 Normal leukocyte counts (×10⁹/l) in the first month of life

AGE	TOTAL LEUKOCYTES, MEAN (RANGE)	NEUTROPHILS, MEAN (RANGE)	%	LYMPHOCYTES, MEAN (RANGE)	%	MONOCYTES, MEAN	%	EOSINOPHILS, (MEAN)	%
Birth	18.1 (9.0–30.0)	11.1 (6.0–26.0)	61	5.5 (2.0–11.0)	31	1.1	6	0.4	2
12 h	22.8 (13.0–38.0)	15.5 (6.0–28.0)	68	5.5 (2.0–11.0)	24	1.2	5	0.5	2
24 h	18.9 (9.4–34.0)	11.5 (5.0–21.0)	61	5.8 (2.0–11.5)	31	1.1	6	0.5	2
1 week	12.2 (5.0–21.0)	5.5 (1.5–10.0)	45	5.0 (2.0–17.0)	41	1.1	9	0.5	4
2 weeks	11.4 (5.0–20.0)	4.5 (1.0–9.5)	40	5.5 (2.0–17.0)	48	1.0	9	0.4	3
1 month	10.8 (5.0–19.5)	3.8 (1.0–9.0)	35	6.0 (2.5–16.5)	56	0.7	7	0.3	3

Neutrophils include band forms and a small number of metamyelocytes and myelocytes in the first few days of life.
With permission from Dallman, P.R., 1977. Reference ranges for leukocyte counts in children. In: Rudolph, A.M. (Ed.), Pediatrics, sixteenth ed. Appleton-Century-Crofts, New York, p. 1178.

© 2012 Elsevier Ltd

Appendix 2

Coagulation values in term and preterm infants

Table A2.1 Reference values for coagulation tests in healthy term infants and in the adult (means and standard deviations)

TEST	DAY 1	DAY 5	DAY 30	ADULT
PT (s)	13 ± 1.43	12.4 ± 1.46	11.8 ± 1.25	12.4 ± 0.78
APPT (s)	42.9 ± 5.8	42.6 ± 8.62	40.4 ± 7.42	33.5 ± 3.44
TCT (s)	23.5 ± 2.38	23.1 ± 3.07	24.3 ± 2.44	25 ± 2.66
Fibrinogen (g/l)	2.83 ± 0.58	3.12 ± 0.75	2.7 ± 0.54	2.78 ± 0.61
II (U/ml)	0.48 ± 0.11	0.63 ± 0.15	0.68 ± 0.17	1.08 ± 0.19
V (U/ml)	0.72 ± 0.18	0.95 ± 0.25	0.98 ± 0.18	1.06 ± 0.22
VII (U/ml)	0.66 ± 0.19	0.89 ± 0.27	0.9 ± 0.24	1.05 ± 0.19
VIII (U/ml)	1.00 ± 0.39	0.88 ± 0.33	0.91 ± 0.33	0.99 ± 0.25
vWF (U/ml)	1.53 ± 0.67	1.40 ± 0.57	1.28 ± 0.59	0.92 ± 0.33
IX (U/ml)	0.53 ± 0.19	0.53 ± 0.19	0.51 ± 0.15	1.09 ± 0.27
X (U/ml)	0.40 ± 0.14	0.49 ± 0.15	0.59 ± 0.14	1.06 ± 0.23
XI (U/ml)	0.38 ± 0.14	0.55 ± 0.16	0.53 ± 0.13	0.97 ± 0.15
XII (U/ml)	0.53 ± 0.20	0.47 ± 0.18	0.49 ± 0.16	1.08 ± 0.28
Plasminogen (U/ml)	1.95 ± 0.35	2.17 ± 0.38	1.98 ± 0.36	3.36 ± 0.44

All factors except fibrinogen and plasminogen are expressed as units per millilitre where pooled plasma contains 1.0 U/ml. Plasminogen units are those recommended by the Committee on Thrombolytic Agents.
APPT, activated partial thromboplastin time; PT, prothrombin time; TCT, thrombin clotting time; vWF, von Willebrand factor.
From Andrew, M., Paes, B., Milner, R., et al., 1987. Development of the human coagulation system in the full term infant. Blood 70, 165–172.

© 2012 Elsevier Ltd

Table A2.2 Reference values for coagulation tests in preterm infants (means and boundaries given, where the boundaries encompass 95% of the observations)

TEST	DAY 1	DAY 5	DAY 30	ADULT
PT (s)	13 (10.6–16.2)	12.5 (10.0–15.3)	11.8 (10.0–13.6)	12.4 (10.8–13.9)
APPT (s)	53.6 (27.5–79.4)	50.5 (26.9–74.1)	44.7 (26.9–62.5)	33.5 (26.6–40.3)
TCT (s)	24.8 (19.2–30.4)	24.1 (18.8–29.4)	24.4 (18.8–29.9)	25.0 (19.7–30.3)
Fibrinogen (g/l)	2.43 (1.5–3.73)	2.8 (1.6–4.2)	2.54 (1.5–4.14)	2.78 (1.56–4.0)
II (U/ml)	0.45 (0.41–1.44)	0.57 (0.29–0.85)	0.57 (0.36–0.95)	1.08 (0.71–1.46)
V (U/ml)	0.88 (0.41–1.44)	1.0 (0.46–1.54)	1.02 (0.48–1.56)	1.06 (0.62–1.50)
VII (U/ml)	0.67 (0.21–1.13)	0.84 (0.3–1.38)	0.83 (0.21–1.45)	1.05 (0.67–1.43)
VIII (U/ml)	1.11 (0.50–2.13)	1.15 (0.53–2.05)	1.11 (0.5–1.99)	0.99 (0.5–1.49)
vWF (U/ml)	1.36 (0.78–2.1)	1.33 (0.72–2.19)	1.36 (0.66–2.16)	0.92 (0.5–1.58)
IX (U/ml)	0.35 (0.19–0.65)	0.42 (0.14–0.74)	0.44 (0.13–0.8)	1.09 (0.55–1.63)
X (U/ml)	0.41 (0.11–0.71)	0.51 (0.19–0.83)	0.56 (0.20–0.92)	1.06 (0.7–1.52)
XI (U/ml)	0.30 (0.08–0.52)	0.41 (0.13–0.69)	0.43 (0.15–0.71)	0.97 (0.67–1.27)
XII (U/ml)	0.38 (0.10–0.66)	0.39 (0.09–0.69)	0.43 (0.11–0.75)	1.08 (0.52–1.64)
Plasminogen (U/ml)	1.70 (1.12–2.48)	1.91 (1.21–2.61)	1.81 (1.09–2.53)	3.36 (2.48–4.24)

APPT, activated partial thromboplastin time; PT, prothrombin time; TCT, thrombin clotting time; vWF, von Willebrand factor.
From Andrew, M., Paes, B., Milner, R., et al., 1988. Development of the coagulation system in the healthy premature infant. Blood 72, 1651–1657.

Table A2.3 Reference values for the inhibitors of coagulation in healthy full-term infants (means and standard deviations)

COAGULATION INHIBITOR (U/ml)	DAY 1	DAY 5	DAY 30	ADULT
AT III	0.63 ± 0.12	0.67 ± 0.13	0.78 ± 0.15	1.05 ± 0.13
α_2 M	1.39 ± 0.22	1.48 ± 0.25	1.50 ± 0.22	0.86 ± 0.17
α_2 AP	0.85 ± 0.15	1.0 ± 0.15	1.0 ± 0.12	1.02 ± 0.17
C_1-INH	0.72 ± 0.18	0.9 ± 0.15	0.89 ± 0.21	1.01 ± 0.15
α_1 AT	0.83 ± 0.22	0.89 ± 0.20	0.62 ± 0.13	0.93 ± 0.19
Protein C	0.35 ± 0.09	0.42 ± 0.11	0.43 ± 0.11	0.96 ± 0.16
Protein S	0.36 ± 0.12	0.50 ± 0.14	0.63 ± 0.15	0.92 ± 0.16

α_1 AT, α_1 antitrypsin; α_2 AP, α_2 antiplasmin; α_2 M, α_2 macroglobulin; AT III, antithrombin III; C_1-INH, C_1 esterase inhibitor.
From Andrew, M., Paes, B., Milner, R., et al., 1987. Development of the human coagulation system in the full term infant. Blood 70, 165–172.

Table A2.4 Reference values for the inhibitors of coagulation in preterm infants (means and boundaries given, where the boundaries encompass 95% of the observations)

COAGULATION INHIBITOR (U/ml)	DAY 1	DAY 5	DAY 30	ADULT
AT II	0.38 (0.14–0.62)	0.56 (0.30–0.82)	0.59 (0.37–0.81)	1.05 (0.79–1.31)
α_2 M	1.10 (0.56–1.82)	1.25 (0.71–0.77)	1.38 (0.72–2.04)	0.86 (0.52–1.2)
α_2 AP	0.78 (0.40–1.16)	0.81 (0.49–1.13)	0.89 (0.55–1.23)	1.02 (0.68–1.36)
C_1–INH	0.65 (0.31–0.99)	0.83 (0.45–1.21)	0.74 (0.40–1.24)	1.01 (0.71–1.31)
α_1 AT	0.90 (0.36–1.44)	0.94 (0.42–1.46)	0.76 (0.38–1.12)	0.93 (0.55–1.31)
Protein C	0.28 (0.12–0.44)	0.31 (0.11–0.51)	0.37 (0.15–0.59)	0.96 (0.64–1.28)
Protein S	0.26 (0.14–0.38)	0.37 (0.13–0.61)	0.56 (0.22–0.90)	0.92 (0.60–1.24)

α_1 AT, α_1 antitrypsin; α_2 AP, α_2 antiplasmin; α_2 M, α_2 macroglobulin; AT III, antithrombin III; C_1-INH, C_1 esterase inhibitor.
From Andrew, M., Paes, B., Milner, R., et al., 1988. Development of the coagulation system in the healthy premature infant. Blood 72, 1651–1657.

Rob Yates
Nick Archer

Appendix 3

Normal ranges for commonly assessed ECG values in the newborn

Table A3.1 Normal ranges for commonly assessed ECG values in the newborn

	<1 DAY	1–3 DAYS	4–7 DAYS	8–10 DAYS
Heart rate (beats/min)	94–155	92–158	90–166	106–182
PR lead II (ms)	80–100	81–139	74–136	72–138
QRS duration V5 (ms)	21–75	22–67	21–68	22–79
Frontal QRS axis (degrees)	+60 to +190	+62 to +196	+75 to +190	+65 to +160
QRS size (mV)				
V1				
Q	0	0	0	0
R	0.5–2.6	0.5–2.6	0.3–2.4	0.3–2.1
S	0–2.3	0–2.1	0–1.7	0–1.1
T	−0.3 to 4	−0.4 to 4	−0.45 to 2.5	−5 to −1
V6				
Q	0–0.17	0–0.21	0–0.28	0–0.28
R	0–1.1	0–1.2	0–1.2	0.25–1.6
S	0–1.0	0–0.9	0–1.0	0–1.0
R/S V1	0.2–9.8	0.2–6	0.2–9.8	1–7
R/S V6	0.2–10	0.2–1	0.2–10	0.2–12

Ranges given are approximately 2nd and 98th centiles, derived from Davignon et al. (1979/80). Qtc = QT/√RR, using lead II and where the RR interval is the one preceding the QRS complex in which the QT interval is measured. Qtc 98th centile figure from Davigncn and colleagues is <0.48, except in the first few days of life, when higher values may transiently be found. Other authors consider persistent values above 0.46 to be abnormal (Garson 1990).

References

Davignon, A., Rautaharju, P., Boisselle, E., et al., 1979/80. Normal ECG standards for infants and children. Pediatr Cardiol 1, 123–131.

Garson, A., 1990. Ventricular arrhythmias. In: Gillette, P.C., Garson, A. (Eds.), Pediatric Arrhythmias: Electrophysiology and Pacing. WB Saunders, Philadelphia, pp. 427–500.

© 2012 Elsevier Ltd

Rob Yates
Janet M Rennie

Appendix 4

Normal values for neonatal blood pressure

Good normative data on blood pressure in healthy newborns are surprisingly hard to find. A recent study (2003–2005) of 406 healthy Australian newborns using an oscillometric method, averaging three readings for each baby, confirmed previous work showing that there is a relationship with postnatal age, particularly between day 1 and 2 of life, but failed to demonstrate a significant relationship with weight (Kent et al. 2007a). The values are shown in Table A4.1 and Figure A4.1.

While an indwelling arterial catheter is undoubtedly the 'gold standard' method for measurement of blood pressure, the data produced from studies using this method inevitably reflect the sick nature of the population. Over 12 552 blood pressure measurements were made with oscillometry in 373 stable infants (292 preterm) born in Belgrade over a period of 27 months (Pejovic et al. 2007). These data confirmed other studies, again showing a relationship with postnatal age, gestational age, and weight (Fig. A4.2). The mean blood pressure at each gestation was slightly lower than the gestational age in weeks between 24 and 32 weeks (Pejovic et al. 2007, Table 6), but this remains a useful aide-memoire in an emergency, particularly as others have found the 10th centile for the mean BP to be a little higher than this (Fig. A4.3) (Kent et al. 2009). In other words, the mean BP of a 28-weeks' gestation baby is generally above 28 mmHg in the first few days of life. It is important to appreciate that this is not the case after a week or two (see below). The data of Zubrow et al. (1995) are also valuable for preterms, but do not give a value for the mean BP (Fig. A4.4).

Several studies, including that of Zubrow et al. (1995), have shown that the blood pressure of preterm babies rises quite rapidly over the first few days (and first 2 weeks) of life, with the systolic blood pressure increasing by about 2.5 mmHg/day for the first 5 days and then at about 0.25 mmHg/day. This has led Dionne et al. (2012) to devise a helpful table of values of normal blood pressure after the first 2 weeks of life (Table A4.2). For older infants, the data of the Second Task Force of the National High Blood Pressure Education Programme, published in 1987, remain the most widely available reference data, but were based on a single Doppler measurement in awake infants, and a revision is awaited. In the meanwhile, helpful data for monitoring infants with chronic lung disease (who can develop hypertension) are provided by Kent et al. (2007b) (Fig. A4.5).

Blood pressure in term babies

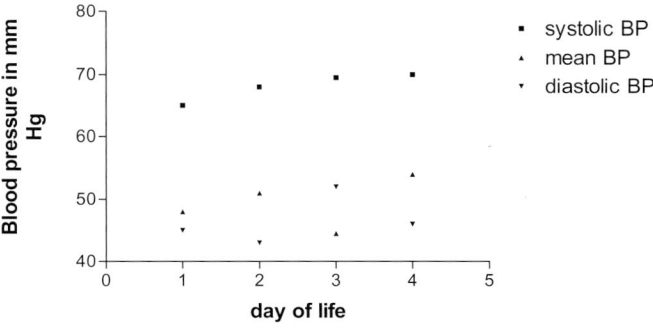

- systolic BP
- mean BP
- diastolic BP

Fig. A4.1 Blood pressure in healthy term newborns; graph of data derived from Table A4.1.

Table A4.1 Normal blood pressure by day of life in 406 healthy term newborns (Kent et al 2007a)

BP IN mmHg	DAY 1 (RANGE)	DAY 2 (RANGE)	DAY 3 (RANGE)	DAY 4 (RANGE)
Systolic	65 (46–94)	68 (46–91)	69.5 (51–93)	70 (60–88)
Mean	48 (31–63)	51 (37–68)	44.5 (26–61)	54 (41–65)
Diastolic	45 (24–57)	43 (27–58)	52 (36–70)	46 (34–57)

© 2012 Elsevier Ltd

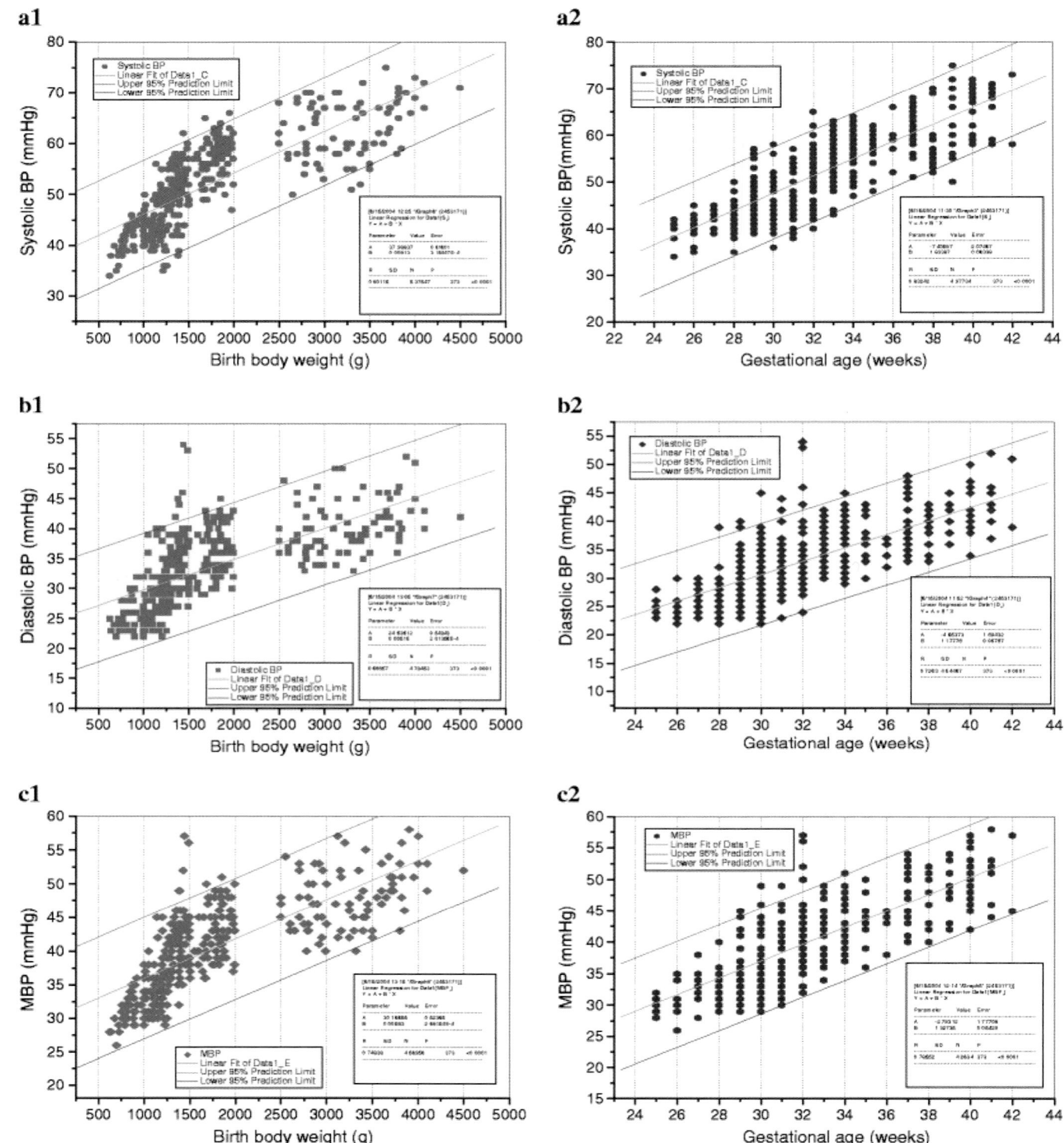

Fig. A4.2 Linear regression of a systolic b diastolic and c mean blood pressure according to birthweight and gestational age on day 1 of life with 95% confidence limits *(from Pejovic et al. 2007, with permission)*.

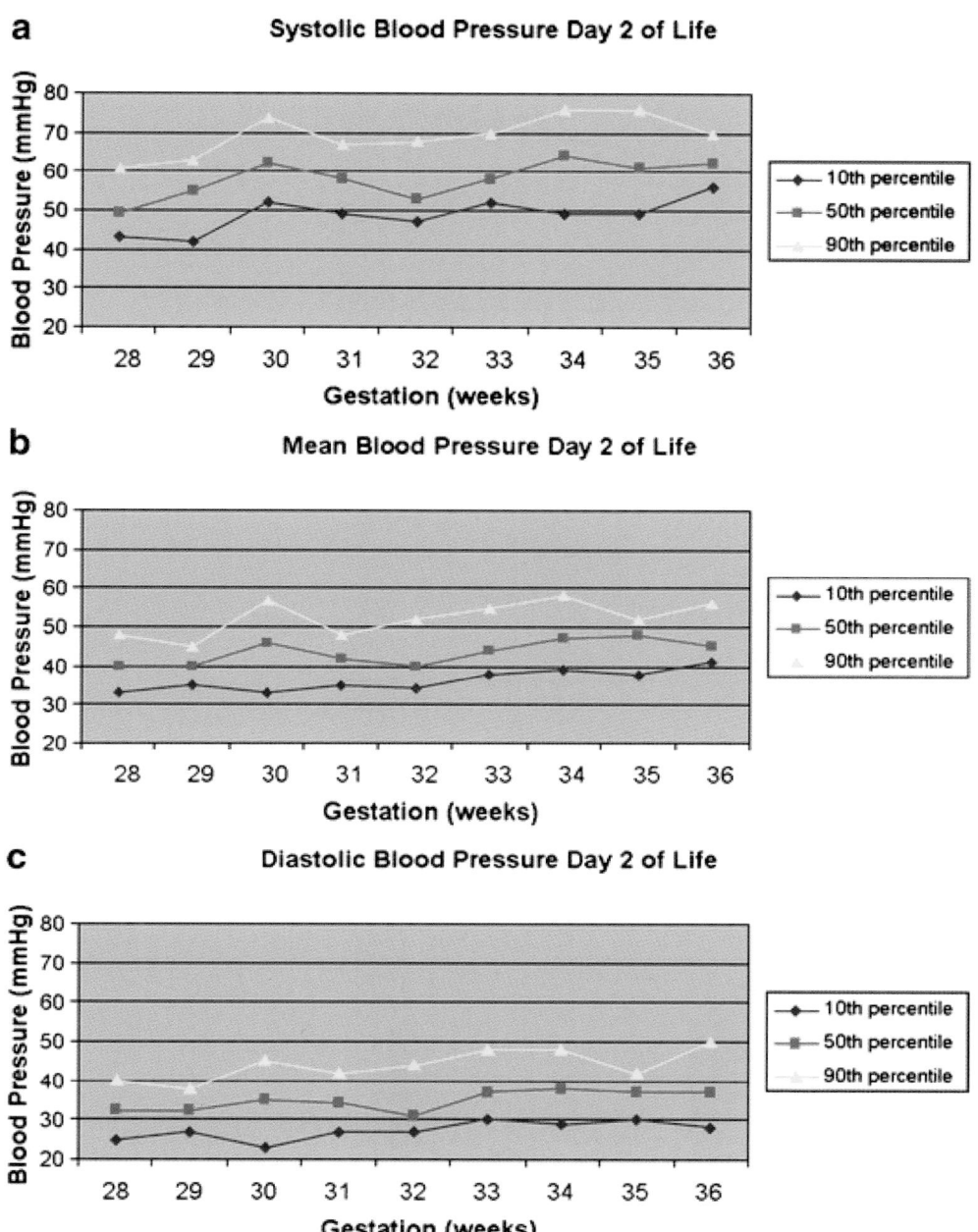

a

Systolic Blood Pressure Day 2 of Life

b

Mean Blood Pressure Day 2 of Life

c

Diastolic Blood Pressure Day 2 of Life

Fig. A4.3 Tenth, 50th and 90th percentiles of systolic, mean, and diastolic blood pressure plotted for each week of gestation on day 2 of life *(from Kent et al. 2009, with permission).*

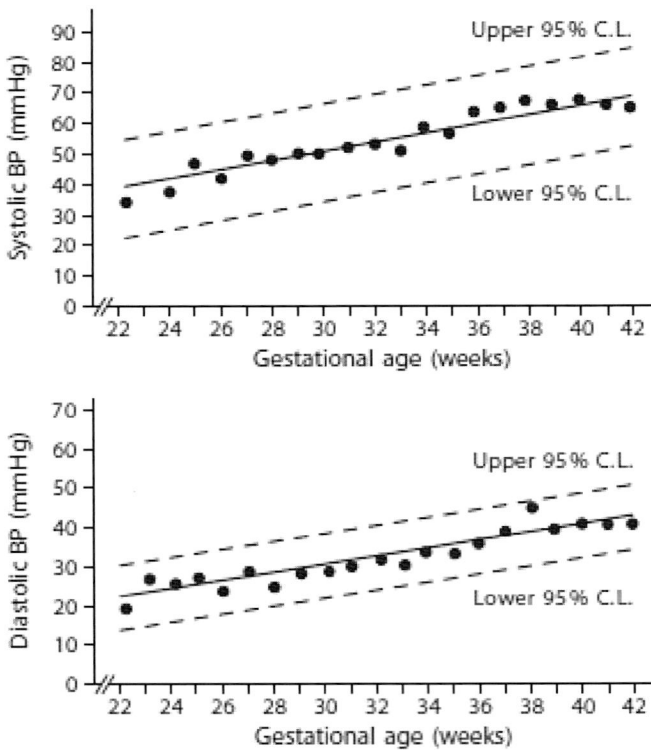

Fig. A4.4 Linear regression of mean systolic and diastolic blood pressure by gestational age on day 1 of life, with 95% confidence limits (upper and lower dashed lines). *(Reproduced from Zubrow et al. 1995 with permission.)*

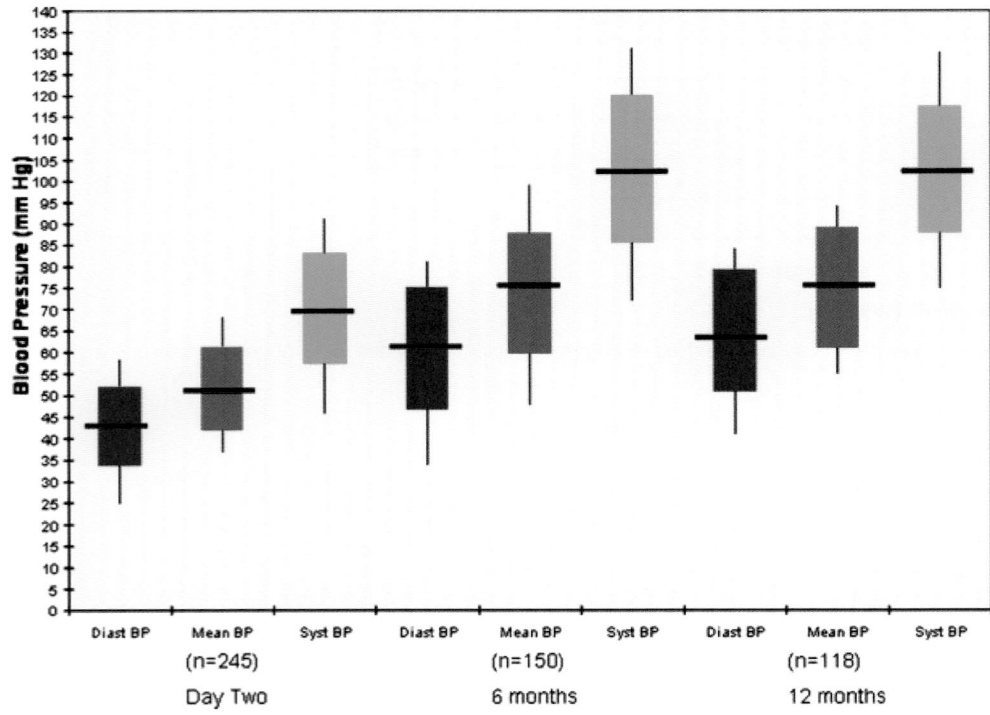

Fig. A4.5 Diastolic, mean and systolic measurements at 2 days, 6 months and 12 months of age. The boxes show 5th and 95th percentiles, the horizontal bar indicates the median, and the longitudinal lines represent the range of values; blue diastolic BP, red mean BP, green systolic BP. *(Data from Kent et al. 2007b, with permission.)*

Table A4.2 Estimated BP values after 2 weeks of age in infants from 26 to 44 weeks postconceptional age (from Dionne et al 2011, with permission)

POSTCONCEPTIONAL AGE	50TH PERCENTILE	95TH PERCENTILE	99TH PERCENTILE
44 weeks			
SBP	88	105	110
DBP	50	68	73
MAP	**63**	**80**	**85**
42 weeks			
SBP	85	98	102
DBP	50	65	70
MAP	**62**	**76**	**81**
40 weeks			
SBP	80	95	100
DBP	50	65	70
MAP	**60**	**75**	**80**
38 weeks			
SBP	77	92	97
DBP	50	65	70
MAP	**59**	**74**	**79**
36 weeks			
SBP	72	87	92
DBP	50	65	70
MAP	**57**	**72**	**71**
34 weeks			
SBP	70	85	90
DBP	40	55	60
MAP	**50**	**65**	**70**
32 weeks			
SBP	68	83	88
DBP	40	55	60
MAP	**48**	**62**	**69**
30 weeks			
SBP	65	80	85
DBP	40	55	60
MAP	**48**	**65**	**68**
28 weeks			
SBP	60	75	80
DBP	38	50	54
MAP	**48**	**58**	**63**
26 weeks			
SBP	55	72	77
DBP	30	50	56
MAP	**38**	**57**	**63**

References

Dionne, J.M., Abitbol, C.L., Flynn, J.T., 2012. Hypertension in infancy: diagnosis, management and outcome. Pediatr Nephrol 27, 17–32.

Kent, A.L., Kecskes, Z., Shadbolt, B., et al., 2007a. Normative blood pressure data in the early neonatal period. Pediatr Nephrol 22, 1335–1341.

Kent, A.L., Kecskes, Z., Shadbolt, B., et al., 2007b. Blood pressure in the first year of life in healthy infants born at term. Pediatr Nephrol 22, 1743–1749.

Kent, A.L., Meskell, S., Falk, M.C., et al., 2009. Normative blood pressure data in non-ventilated premature neonates from 28–36 weeks gestation. Pediatr Nephrol 24, 141–146.

Pejovic, B., Peco-Antic, A., Marinkovic-Eric, J., 2007. Blood pressure in non-critically ill preterm and full term neonates. Pediatr Nephrol 22, 249–257.

Zubrow, A.B., Hulman, S., Kushner, H., et al., 1995. Determinants of blood pressure in infants admitted to neonatal intensive care units: a prospective multicentre study. J Perinatol 15, 470–479.

Appendix 5

Tim Cole

UK-WHO chart source data

Introduction

The UK–World Health Organization (UK-WHO) 0–4-year-old charts were officially launched on 11 May 2009. Any child born after that date should be plotted on a UK-WHO growth chart. Children born before 11 May 2009 are already plotted on British 1990 (UK90) charts, and subsequent measurements will continue to be plotted using those charts. There will be no switchover of existing children to the new UK-WHO charts. After age 4 we will revert to using UK90 charts.

The source data for these charts are included in two spreadsheets as LMS tables. Together they define the UK-WHO growth charts, containing LMS values by age. If the data are needed in centile or SDS look-up format they can be accessed via the LMSgrowth Excel add in (see below). We have also included data not yet incorporated into a paper chart – for example, body mass index (BMI) and head circumference beyond 2 years.

These data and the LMSgrowth software can be freely used without charge as long as their source is acknowledged in any publications or products using them. Users may not claim any IP rights over them, derive financial gain from supplying the data to others, seek to restrict use of the data by others or use them for the purposes of advertising or promoting other products. Notwithstanding this limited grant of rights, the original copyright notices must continue to be reproduced in any copies of these materials.

Data files

There are two data files, each made up of three sections: a birth section, based on UK90 reference data, a postnatal section from 2 weeks to 4 years copied from the WHO standard, and for completeness the 4–20 years section from the UK90 reference.

UK_WHO_term.xls

Average values at birth for weight, length and head circumference (not BMI) for all term births (gestations 37–42 weeks) computed from the UK90 reference data base (Cole et al. 1998).

Acknowledgement statements using these data should specify the data source as: British 1990 reference data, reanalysed 2009.

This is combined with the WHO standard for weight, BMI and head circumference from 2 weeks to 4 years, for length from 2 weeks to 2 years and height from 2 to 4 years. It is shown by week to 13 weeks and then by calendar month. They are exactly the same data as the LMS tables accessed from the WHO website (http://www.who.int/childgrowth/standards/) except that the data from birth to 2 weeks are omitted.

Acknowledgement statements using these data should specify the data source as: WHO Child Growth Standards (WHO 2006, 2007).

The British 1990 section runs from 4 to 20 years by month, and includes height, weight, BMI and head circumference (to 18/17 years in boys/girls).

Acknowledgement statements using these data should specify the data source as: British 1990 reference data (Cole et al. 1998).

UK_WHO_preterm.xls

Weight and head circumference at birth by gestation from 23 to 42 weeks and length at birth from 25 to 42 weeks, computed from the UK90 reference database and shown by week (Cole et al. 2011).

Acknowledgement statements using these data should specify the data source as: British 1990 reference data, reanalysed 2009.

This is combined with the WHO standard from 2 weeks post-term, and the British 1990 reference from 4 years, as described above.

Use of data files

These files should be used as follows:

Term infants

These are infants born at or beyond 37 completed weeks' gestation. UK_WHO_term.xls should be used for all term infants, with no adjustment for gestation. Centiles should not be computed between birth and 2 weeks.

Preterm infants

These are infants born before 37 completed weeks' gestation. UK_WHO_preterm.xls should be used for all preterm infants

© 2012 Elsevier Ltd

for birth and subsequent measurements, using gestationally corrected age.

Gestationally corrected age

This is actual age – (40 – gestation at birth).

Note this age will be negative until the expected date of delivery is reached.

Use of LMSgrowth software

This software can be used to access the above files and manipulate growth data as required.

Files required for this are downloadable from:

http://www.healthforallchildren.com/index.php/shop/category-list/Software

Instructions on installation of Excel add-in LMSgrowth

1. Copy the data files above to the Excel start-up folder c:\Program Files\Microsoft Office\Office\XLStart for Windows 2000/XP or earlier versions of Office c:\Program Files\Microsoft Office\Office 10\XLStart for Office XP or /Applications/Microsoft Office/Office/Startup/Excel for Mac OS X
2. Copy growth.xla, growth.hlp and growth.cnt to another directory, e.g. c:\growth in Windows
3. Start Excel, click File|New, then click Tools|Add-ins|Browse to locate growth.xla and click OK to confirm.

The Growth add-in program is then installed. You will see the LMSgrowth menu appear on the menu bar. Acknowledgement

statements for this add-in should read: LMSgrowth programme version x.xx, authors Huiqi Pan and Tim Cole, copyright MRC 2002–10.

What LMSgrowth does

For those wanting to reproduce the workings of LMSgrowth in software, its algorithm to convert measurements to z-scores is as follows:

1. Look up in the LMS table for the relevant measurement (height or weight, etc.) the age/sex-specific values of L, M and S for the child, using either linear or cubic interpolation to get the exact age.
2. To obtain the z-score, plug the LMS values with the child's measurement into the formula

$$z = \frac{\left[\left(\frac{\text{Measurement}}{M}\right)^L - 1\right]}{L \times S}$$

3. If required, convert the z-score to a centile using normal distribution tables.

The algorithm for the reverse process, from z-score or centile back to measurement, is as follows:

4. Repeat step 1 to obtain the LMS values for the child's measurement, age and sex.
5. The z-score is then converted back to a measurement with the formula

$$\text{Measurement} = M\left(1 + L \times S \times z\right)^{1/L}$$

6. This conversion is useful, for example, to obtain centiles to plot growth charts, where each centile is defined by its corresponding z-score.

References

Cole, T.J., Freeman, J.V., Preece, M.A., 1998. British 1990 growth reference centiles for weight, height, body mass index and head circumference fitted by maximum penalized likelihood. Stat Med 17, 407–429.

Cole, T.J., Williams, A.E., Wright, C.M., RCPCH Growth Chart Expert Group, 2011. Revised birth centiles for weight, length and head circumference in the UK-WHO growth charts. Ann Hum Biol 38, 7–11.

WHO Multicentre Growth Reference Study Group, 2006. WHO Child Growth Standards: Length/Height-for-age, Weight-for-age, Weight-for-length, Weight-for-height and Body Mass Index-for age. Methods and Development. World Health Organization, Geneva. ISBN 92 4 154693 X.

WHO Multicentre Growth Reference Study Group, 2007. WHO Child Growth Standards: Head Circumference-for-age, Arm Circumference-for-age, Triceps Skinfold-for-age and Subscapular Skinfold-for age. Methods and Development. World Health Organization, Geneva. ISBN 978 92 4 1547185.

Ruth M Ayling
Ann Bowron

Appendix 6

Neonatal biochemical reference ranges

Table A6.1 Plasma/serum

ANALYTE	UNIT	REFERENCE RANGE						COMMENT
		Preterm			**Term**			
		Gestational age (weeks)	Age	Reference range	Age	Reference range		
Alanine aminotransferase (ALT) (Soldin et al. 1997c)	IU/l				1–7 d	M 6–40	F 7–40	Range dependent on methodology
					8–30 d	10–40	8–32	
Albumin (Zlotkin and Casselman 1987; Ghoshal and Soldin 2003)	g/l	27		21–33		M	F	
		29		23–34	1–7 d	24–39	19–40	
		31		22–35	8–30 d	21–45	19–44	
		33		22–35				
		35		22–36				
Alkaline phosphatase (ALP) (Ghoshal and Soldin 2003)	IU/l				1–7 d	M 107–357	F	Range dependent on methodology
					8–30 d	107–474		
α₁-antitrypsin (Davis et al. 1996)	g/l				0–30 d	0.79–2.23		'Adult' concentrations at birth, falling after 2 weeks. To assess possible deficiency, phenotype should be determined

© 2012 Elsevier Ltd

Table A6.1 Continued

ANALYTE	UNIT	REFERENCE RANGE					COMMENT
		Preterm			**Term**		
		Gestational age (weeks)	Age	Reference range	Age	Reference range	
α-fetoprotein (AFP) (Blohm et al. 1998)	U/ml				Birth 1 d 2 d 3 d 4 d 5 d 6 d 7 d 8–14 d 15–21 d 22–28 d	7533–157390 6561–137082 5741–119393 4977–103988 4375–90569 3819–79796 3335–69660 2911–60811 1222–48640 475–18924 261–5212	Range dependent on methodology Higher in premature babies Half-life 5.1 days
Aldosterone (Soldin et al. 1999a)	ng/dL	26–28 31–35	4 d 4 d	5–635 19–141	3 d 1 w 1 m	7–184 5–175 5–90	
Aluminium (NHS Supraregional Assay Service Handbook 1998)	µmol/l					0.07–0.80	
Ammonia (Diaz et al. 1995)	µmol/l				0–30 d	21–95	Preterm and/or sick babies may have concentrations up to 200 µmol/l
Amylase (Soldin et al. 1995a)	IU/l				0–30 d	<30	Range dependent on methodology
Androstenedione (Garagorri et al. 2008)	nmol/l				0 d 15 d 30 d	M 1.47–13 1.0–8.7 0.6–5.9 F 0.8–12 0.7–7.9 0.5–5.3	
Aspartate transaminase (AST) (Ghoshal and Soldin 2003)	IU/l				1–7 d 8–30 d	M 26–98 16–67 F 20–93 20–69	Range dependent on methodology
Bilirubin (Soldin et al. 1999a) Total Conjugated	µmol/l				Birth–1 d 1–2 d 3–5 d 0–30 d	<100 <140 <200 <10	Refer to neonatal treatment charts for further details
Caeruloplasmin (Soldin et al. 1997a)	mg/l				1–30 d	M 77–253 F 33–275	Increases from birth throughout first year
Calcium Total (Thalme 1962; Ghoshal and Soldin 2003)	mmol/l	21–28		2.14–2.65	0–7 d 8–30 d	M 1.83–2.85 2.15–2.93 1.05–1.37 1.10–1.44 1.20–1.48 F 1.88–2.83 2.10–2.98	Results should be interpreted in conjunction with serum albumin concentration
Ionised (Wandrup et al. 1988; Nelson et al. 1989)	mmol/l	25–36	1 d 2 d 3 d	0.81–1.41 0.72–1.44 1.04–1.52	1 d 3 d 5 d		

Staff Library
Singleton Hospital
Tel: 01792 205666 Ext. 5281

Table A6.1 Continued

ANALYTE	UNIT	Gestational age (weeks)	Age	Reference range	Age	Reference range		COMMENT
		Preterm			**Term**			
Chloride (Ghoshal and Soldin 2003)	mmol/l				0–30 d	97–108		
Cholesterol (Hicks et al. 1996)	mmol/l				1–30 d	M 1.4–3.9	F 1.6–4.0	Gradual increase from birth
Copper (Lockitch et al. 1988)	µmol/l	28–34		3.0–8.3	0–5 d 5–28 d	1.4–7.2 4.0–11.0		Rapid increase during first week
Cortisol (Heckmann et al. 1991; Garagorri et al. 2008)	mmol/l	24	0–14 d	73–562	0 d 3 d 15 d 30 d	54–839 54–814 54–728 55–645		If there is doubt about the integrity of the hypothalamo-pituitary adrenal axis, a short Synacthen test should be performed
C-reactive protein (CRP) (Soldin et al. 2004)	mg/l					<16		
Creatine kinase (CK) (Jedeikin et al. 1982)	IU/l				Cord blood 5–8 h 24–33 h 72–100 h	70–380 214–1175 130–1200 87–725		Range dependent on methodology
Creatinine (Rudd et al. 1983; Sonntag et al. 1996; Finney et al. 2000)	µmol/l	24–28 29–36 26–34	1 d 1 d 1 w 2 w 3–4 w 5–6 w 7–9 w	35–136 27–175 69–141 45–99 39–71 42–62 39–48	2 d 7 d 14 d 21 d 28 d	37–113 14–86 18–58 15–55 12–48		Creatinine rises in the first 48 h, especially in infants <30 weeks' gestation (Miall et al., 1999)
Cystatin C (Finney et al. 2000)	mg/l	24–28 29–36		0.65–3.37 0.62–4.42	0–28 d	0.81–2.32		
Dehydroepiandrosterone sulphate (DHEAS) (Garagorri et al. 2008)	µmol/l				0 d 3 d 15 d 30 d	M 0.7–8.9 0.7–8.4 0.6–6.6 0.5–4.8	F 0.8–10 0.9–9.6 0.7–8.1 0.6–6.3	
Ferritin (Murthy et al. 1995)	µg/l				1–30 d	M 36–381	F 36–483	
Glucose (Ghoshal and Soldin 2003)	mmol/l				1–7 d 8–30 d	2.71–6.11 3.00–6.49		
γ-Glutamyltransferase (GGT) (Ghoshal and Soldin 2003)	IU/l				1–7 d 8–30 d	18–148 16–140		Results depend on methodology
17α-Hydroxyprogesterone (17-OHP) (Garagorri et al. 2008)	nmol/l				0 d 3 d 15 d 30 d	17.2–252 9.9–33.1 8.8–29.2 7.4–24.5		Premature and/or sick infants may have concentrations 2–3-fold higher

Table A6.1 Continued

ANALYTE	UNIT	REFERENCE RANGE						COMMENT
		Preterm			Term			
		Gestational age (weeks)	Age	Reference range	Age	Reference range		
Immunoglobulins (Soldin et al. 1995b, 1999a)						M	F	Lower in premature infants
IgG	g/l				1–30 d	2.21–8.38	1.88–8.76	
IgA	g/l					0.01–0.17	0.01–0.16	
IgM	g/l					0.08–0.78	0.13–0.70	
IgD	mg/l					none detected		
IgE	kIU/l				0–12 m	2–24	0–20	
Immunoreactive trypsin (Heeley and Bangert 1992)	µg/l					<60		Blood spot
Insulin								Should be measured during documented hypoglycaemia. There may be cross-reactivity with proinsulins and values may be higher in premature infants, hence results should always be interpreted in light of clinical features and intravenous glucose requirements
Insulin-like growth factor-1 (IGF-1) (Soldin et al. 1997b)	ng/ml				0 d / 1–30 d	22.8–100.9 / 7–92		
Insulin-like growth factor binding protein-3 (IGFBP-3) (Blum et al. 1990)	mg/l				0–1 w / 1–4 w	0.42–1.39 / 0.77–2.09		
Iron (Soldin et al. 1999b)	µmol/l				0–30 d	M 5.7–20.0	F 5.2–22.7	
Lactate (Ghoshal and Soldin 2003)	mmol/l				0–90 d	1.0–3.5		
Lactate dehydrogenase (LDH) (Ghoshal and Soldin 2003)	U/l				1–30 d / 1–3 m	M 178–629 / 158–373	F 187–600 / 152–353	Results depend on methodology

Table A6.1 Continued

		REFERENCE RANGE					
		Preterm			**Term**		
ANALYTE	**UNIT**	**Gestational age (weeks)**	**Age**	**Reference range**	**Age**	**Reference range**	**COMMENT**
Magnesium (Meites 1989; Nelson et al. 1989)	mmol/l	25–36	1 d 3 d 5 d 7–28 d	0.62–1.02 0.66–1.10 0.68–1.24 0.75–1.00	1 d 3 d 5 d 7–28 d	0.72–1.00 0.81–1.05 0.78–1.02 0.65–1.00	
Manganese (NHS Supraregional Assay Service Handbook 1998)	nmol/l					>360	Risk of toxicity
Non-esterified fatty acids (Hawdon et al. 1992)	mmol/l	26–36	3 d	0.01–1.04	3 d	0.04–1.34	
Osmolality (Davies 1973)	mosmol/kg		Birth 7 d 28 d	275–300 276–305 274–305		275–295	
Phenylalanine (Hommes 1991)	µmol/l			98–213		38–137	
Phosphate (Thalme 1962)	mmol/l				2–3 d 3–4 d 4–6 d 6–12 d 21 d	1.81–3.00 1.74–2.76 1.64–2.70 1.39–3.03 1.74–2.66	Tends to be higher in babies fed formula milk
Potassium (Greeley et al. 1993; Ghoshal and Soldin 2003)	mmol/l		7 d	4.6–6.7	0–1 w 1 w–1 m	3.2–5.7 3.4–6.2	Results from capillary blood tend to be higher. Serum potassium concentrations are higher than those of plasma due to potassium released from platelets during clotting
Prolactin (Cook et al. 1992)	mU/l				0–30 d	9–2850	May be considerably higher in the first 2 weeks
Protein (Zlotkin and Casselman 1987; Hicks et al. 1995) (total)	g/l	22–36		36–63	1–30 d	41–63	
Pyruvate (Soldin et al. 1999a)	µmol/l				1–30 d	80–150	
Selenium (Muntau et al. 2002)	µmol/l				0–4 w	0.19–1.35	
Sodium (Ghoshal and Soldin 2003)	mmol/l				0–7 d 7–31 d	131–144 132–142	

Table A6.1 Continued

ANALYTE	UNIT	REFERENCE RANGE Preterm Gestational age (weeks)	Age	Reference range	Term Age	Reference range	COMMENT
Testosterone (Soldin et al. 1999a)	nmol/l	26–28 31–35	4 d 4 d	M 2.1–4.4 F 0.18–0.6 1.3–6.9 0.18–0.8		M 2.6–14 F 0.7–2.2	
Thyroid-stimulating hormone (TSH) (Cuestas 1978; Clark et al. 2001; Dugaw et al. 2001)	mU/l	28–40	>7 d	0.8–12.0	1 d 2 d 3–30 d	3.0–120 3.0–30 0.5–6.0	Rapid increase during the first 24 h
Thyroxine (Adams et al. 1995; Dugaw et al. 2001) free (FT$_4$)	pmol/l	25–30 31–36	0–7 0–7	6.4–42.5 16.7–60.6	1–3 d 1–4 w	25.7–68.2	
Triiodothyronine (Cuestas 1978; John and Bamforth, 1987; Adams et al. 1995) free (FT$_3$)	pmol/l	29–36	1–3 d 4–10 d	1.2–7.3 1.2–4.9	1–3 d 4–10 d	2.5–9.3 2.8–5.7	Lower in small sick infants
Triglyceride (Soldin and Morse 1998)	mmol/l				0–7 d 8–30 d	M 0.24–2.06 F 0.32–1.88 0.34–2.08 0.34–1.86	
Urate (Soldin et al. 1997d)	µmol/l				0–1 d 1–2 d 2–3 d 3–7 d	300–505 200–490 190–395 150–290	
Urea (Soldin et al. 1997e)	mmol/l				1–7 d 8–30 d	0.7–4.6 0.7–5.7	May be higher in infants fed formula milk
Zinc (Rükgauer et al. 1997; Lockitch et al. 1998)	µmol/l	28–34		10–24	0–5 d	9.9–21.4	Higher in preterms. Concentration decreases during first week

h = hour(s), d = day(s), w= week(s), m = month(s).

Table A6.2 Urine

ANALYTE	UNIT	Preterm			Term		COMMENT
		Gestational age	Age	Reference range	Age	Reference range	
Calcium (Karlen et al. 1985)	mmol/l		0–7 d	0.2–1.6	0–1 w	<0.6	
Calcium:creatinine ratio (Sargent et al. 1993)	mmol/mmol				1–4 w	<2.4	
Creatinine clearance (Sonntag et al. 1996)	ml/mim/1.73 m²		1 w 2 w 2–4 w	7–22 10–28 11–34			
Fractional sodium excretion (Rossi et al. 1994)	%				0–3 d	<0.72	$\dfrac{\text{Urinary[Sodium]} \times \text{Serum[Creatinine]}}{\text{Serum[Sodium]} \times \text{Urinary[Creatinine]}}$
Phosphate (Rossi et al. 1994)	mmol/24 h		1–2 w 3–4 w	<0.5–9.9 0.5–12	0–7 d	<18	
Potassium (Wilkins 1992)	mmol/l mmol/kg/24 h		0–30 d	2–28 0.2–1.2		<5	Dependent upon intake
Sodium (Wilkins 1992)	mmol/l		0–30 d	1–15		<1	Dependent upon intake
Transport maximum of phosphate in relation to GFR (TmP/GFR) (Bistarakis et al. 1986; Rossi et al. 1994)	µmol/ml				0–30 d	1.89–2.37	Tubular phosphate reabsorption/ml GFR: $P[\text{Phos}] - \left(U[\text{Phos}] \times \dfrac{P[\text{Creat}]}{\text{Ur}[\text{Creat}]}\right)$
Urate:creatinine ratio (Kaufman et al. 1968)	mmol/mmol					0.1–2.0	The ratio is generally elevated in Lesch-Nyhan syndrome and <0.03 mmol/mmol in sulphite oxidase deficiency

References

Adams, L.M., Emery, J.R., Clark, S.J., et al., 1995. Reference ranges for newer thyroid function tests in premature infants. J Pediatr 126, 122–127.

Bistarakis, L., Voskaki, I., Lambadaridis, J., et al., 1986. Renal handling of phosphate in the first six months of life. Arch Dis Child 61, 677–681.

Blohm, M.E., Vesterling-Horner, D., Calaminus, G., et al., 1998. Alpha 1-fetoprotein (AFP) reference range values in infants up to 2 years of age. Pediatr Hematol Oncol 15, 135–142.

Blum, W.F., Ranke, M.B., Kietzmann, K., et al., 1990. A specific radio-immunoassay for the growth hormone (GH)-dependent somatomedin-binding protein: its use for diagnosis of GH deficiency. J Clin Endocrinol Metab 70, 1292–1298.

Clark, S.J., Deming, D.D., Emery, J.R., et al., 2001. Reference ranges for thyroid function tests in premature infants beyond the first week of life. J Perinatol 21, 531–536.

Cook, J.F., Hicks, J.M., Godwin, I.D., et al., 1992. Pediatric reference ranges for prolactin. Clin Chem 38, 959.

Cuestas, R.A., 1978. Thyroid function in preterm infants. J Pediatr 92, 963–967.

Davies, D.P., 1973. Plasma osmolality and protein intake in preterm infants. Arch Dis Child 48, 575–579.

Davis, M.L., Austin, C., Messmer, B.L., et al., 1996. IFCC-standardized pediatric reference intervals for 10 serum proteins using Beckman Array 360 system. Clin Biochem 29, 489–492.

Diaz, J., Tornel, P.L., Martinez, P., 1995. Reference intervals for blood ammonia in healthy subjects, determined by microdiffusion. Clin Chem 41, 1048.

Dugaw, K.A., Jack, R.M., Rutledge, J., 2001. Pediatric reference ranges for TSH, free T4, total T4, total T3 and T3 uptake on the Vitros ECi analyzer. Clin Chem 47, A108.

Finney, H., Newman, D.J., Thakkar, H., et al., 2000. Reference ranges for plasma cystatin C and creatinine measurements in premature infants, neonates and older children. Arch Dis Child 82, 71–75.

Garagorri, J., Rodriguez, G., Lario-Elboj, A.J., et al., 2008. Reference levels for 17-hydroxyprogesterone, 11-desoxycortisol, cortisol, testosterone, dehydroepiandrosterone sulphate and androsterone in infants from birth to six months of age. Eur J Paediatr 167, 647–653.

Ghoshal, A.K., Soldin, S.J., 2003. Evaluation of the Dade Behring Dimension RxL:integrated chemistry system – pediatric reference ranges. Clin Chim Acta 331, 135–146.

Greeley, C., Snell, J., Colaco, A., et al., 1993. Pediatric reference ranges for electrolytes and creatinine. Clin Chem 39, 1172.

Hawdon, J.M., Ward Platt, M.P., Aynsley-Green, A., 1992. Patterns of metabolic adaptation for preterm and term infants in the first week of life. Arch Dis Child 68, 274–279.

Heckmann, M., Wudy, S.A., Haack, D., Pohlandt, F., 1991. Reference range for serum cortisol in well preterm infants. Arch Dis Child Fetal Neonatal Ed 81, F171–F174.

Heeley, A.F., Bangert, S.K., 1992. The neonatal detection of cystic fibrosis by measurement of immunoreactive trypsin in blood. Ann Clin Biochem 29, 464–467.

Hicks, J.M., Bjorn, S., Beatey, J., 1995. Pediatric reference ranges for albumin, globulin and total protein on the Hitachi 747. Clin Chem 41, S93.

Hicks, J.M., Bailey, J., Beatey, J., 1996. Pediatric reference ranges for cholesterol. Clin Chem 42, S307.

Hommes, F.A. (Ed.), 1991. Techniques in Diagnostic Human Biochemical Genetics – A Laboratory Manual. Wiley Liss, New York.

Jedeikin, R., Makela, S.K., Shennan, A.T., et al., 1982. Creatine kinase isoenzymes in serum from cord blood and the blood of healthy full-term infants during the first three postnatal days. Clin Chem 28, 317–322.

John, R., Bamforth, F.J., 1987. Serum free thyroxine and free triiodothyronine concentrations in healthy full term, pre-term and sick pre-term neonates. Ann Clin Biochem 24, 461–465.

Karlen, J., Aperia, A., Zetterstrom, R., 1985. Renal excretion of calcium and phosphate in preterm and term infants. J Pediatr 106, 814–819.

Kaufman, J.M., Greene, M.L., Seegmiller, J.E., 1968. Urine uric acid:creatinine ratio – a screening test for inherited disorders of purine metabolism. J Pediatr 73, 583–592.

Lockitch, G., Halstead, A.C., Wadsworth, L., et al., 1988. Age and sex specific pediatric reference intervals and correlations for zinc, copper, selenium, iron, vitamins A and E and related proteins. Clin Chem 34, 1625–1628.

Meites, S. (Ed.), 1989. Pediatric Clinical Chemistry, third ed. AACCPress, Washington DC, p. 191.

Miall, L.S., Henderson, M.J., Turner, A.J., et al., 1999. Plasma creatinine rises dramatically in the first 48 hours of life in preterm infants. Pediatrics 104, e76.

Muntau, A.C., Streiter, M., Kappler, M., et al., 2002. Age-related reference ranges for serum selenium concentrations in infants and children. Clin Chem 48, 555–560.

Murthy, J.N., Hicks, J.N., Soldin, S.J., 1995. Evaluation of the Technicon Immuno I random access immunoassay analyser and calculation of pediatric reference ranges for endocrine tests, T-uptake and ferritin. Clin Biochem 28, 181–185.

Nelson, N., Finnstrom, O., Larsson, L., 1989. Plasma ionised calcium, phosphate and magnesium in pre-term and small for gestational age infants. Acta Paediatr Scand 78, 351–357.

NHS, 1998. Supraregional Assay Service Handbook, third ed.

Rossi, R., Danzebrink, S., Linnenburger, K., et al., 1994. Assessment of tubular reabsorption on sodium, glucose, phosphate and amino acids based on spot urine samples. Acta Paediatr 83, 1282–1286.

Rudd, P.T., Hughes, E.A., Placzek, M.M., et al., 1983. Reference ranges for plasma creatinine during the first month of life. Arch Dis Child 58, 212–215.

Rükgauer, M., Klein, J., Kruse-Jarres, J.D., 1997. Reference values for the trace elements copper, manganese, selenium and zinc in the serum/plasma of children, adolescents and adults. J Trace Elem Med Biol 11, 92–98.

Sargent, J.D., Strukel, T.A., Kresel, J., et al., 1993. Normal values for random urinary calcium to creatinine ratios in infancy. J Paediatr 123, 393–397.

Soldin, S.J., Morse, A.S., 1998. Pediatric reference ranges for calcium and triglycerides in children < 1 year old using the Vitros 500 analyser. Clin Chem 44, A16.

Soldin, S.J., Hickson, J.M., Bailey, J., et al., 1995a. Pediatric reference ranges for amylase. Clin Chem 41, S94.

Soldin, S.J., Morales, A., Albalos, F., et al., 1995b. Pediatric reference ranges on the Abbott Imx for FSH, LH, prolactin, TSH, T4, T3, free T4, free T3, T-uptake, IgE and ferritin. Clin Biochem 28, 603–606.

Soldin, S.J., Hicks, J.M., Bailey, J., 1997a. Pediatric reference ranges for β2-microglobulin and ceruloplasmin. Clin Chem 43, S199.

Soldin, S.J., Hicks, J.M., Bailey, J., 1997b. Pediatric reference ranges for creatinine kinase and insulin-like growth factor I. Clin Chem 43, S199.

Soldin, S.J., Savwoir, T.V., Guo, Y., 1997c. Pediatric reference ranges for alkaline phosphatase, aspartate aminotransferase, and alanine aminotransferase in children less than 1 year old on the Vitros 500. Clin Chem 43, S199.

Soldin, S.J., Savwoir, T.V., Guo, Y., 1997d. Pediatric reference ranges for lactate dehydrogenase and uric acid during the first year of life on the Vitros 500 analyzer. Clin Chem 43, S199.

Soldin, S.J., Savwoir, T.V., Guo, Y., 1997e. Pediatric reference ranges for gamma-glutamyltransferase and urea nitrogen during the first year of life on the Vitros 500 analyser. Clin Chem 43, S199.

Soldin, S.J., Brugnara, C., Hichs, J.M. (Eds.), 1999a. Pediatric reference ranges, third ed. AACC Press, Washington DC.

Soldin, S.J., Bailey, J., Bjorn, J., 1999b. Pediatric reference ranges for iron on the Hitachi 747 with Boehringer Mannheim reagents. Clin Chem 45, A22.

Soldin, O.P., Bierbower, L.H., Choi, J.J., et al., 2004. Serum iron, ferritin, transferrin, total iron binding capacity, hs-CRP, LDL cholesterol and magnesium in children; new reference intervals using the Dade Dimension Clinical Chemistry System. Clin Chim Acta 342, 211–217.

Sonntag, J., Prankel, B., Waltz, S., 1996. Serum creatinine concentration, urinary creatinine excretion and creatinine clearance during the first 9 weeks in preterm infants with a birth weight below 1500g. Eur J Paediatr 155, 815–819.

Thalme, B., 1962. Calcium, chloride, cholesterol, inorganic phosphorus and total protein in blood plasma during the early neonatal period studied with ultramicrochemical methods. Acta Paediatr Scand 51, 649–660.

Wandrup, J., Kroner, J., Pryds, O., et al., 1988. Age related reference values for ionized calcium in the first week of life in premature and full term neonates. Scand J Clin Lab Invest 48, 255–260.

Wilkins, B.H., 1992. Renal function in sick, very low birthweight infants: 3. Sodium, potassium and water excretion. Arch Dis Child 67, 1154–1161.

Zlotkin, S.H., Casselman, C.W., 1987. Percentile estimates of reference values for total protein and albumin in sera of premature infants (<37 weeks of gestation). Clin Chem 33, 411–413.

N R C Roberton
Janet M Rennie

Appendix 7

Normal blood gas values

Table A7.1 Normal blood gas values

	PaO$_2$				PaCO$_2$				H$^+$			
	kPa	mmHg	kPa	mmHg	kPa	mmHg	kPa	mmHg	nmol/l	pH	nmol/l	pH
15 min	11.6	87			3.7	28			48	7.32		
30 min	11.4	86			4.3	32			43	7.37		
60 min	10.8	81			4.1	31			40	7.40		
1–6 h	8.0–10.6	60–80	*8.0–9.3*	*60–70*	4.7–6.0	35–45	*4.7–6.0*	*35–45*	46–49	7.31–7.34	*42–48*	*7.32–7.38*
6–24 h	9.3–10	70–75	*8.0–9.3*	*60–70*	4.4–4.8	33–36	*3.6–5.3*	*27–40*	37–43	7.37–7.43	*35–45*	*7.36–7.45*
48 h–1 week	9.3–11.3	70–85	*10.0–10.6*	*75–80*	4.4–4.8	33–36	*4.3–4.5*	*32–36*	42–44	7.36–7.38	*40–48*	*7.32–7.40*
2 weeks					4.8–5.2	36–39	*5.1*	*38*	43	7.37	*48*	*7.32*
3 weeks					5.3	40	*5.1*	*38*	42	7.38	*49*	*7.31*
1 month					5.2	39	*4.9*	*37*	41	7.39	*49*	*7.31*

The values at 15, 30 and 60 minutes are from our own unpublished observations on full-term infants. Data from 1 hour to 1 week are drawn from the literature on arterial samples. Data beyond 1 week are on capillary samples. Values in the table which are in *italics* are those for premature infants; those not in italics are for full-term infants.

Reproduced from Rennie, J.M., Roberton, N.R.C., 2002. Manual of Neonatal Intensive Care, fourth ed. Edward Arnold, London.

© 2012 Elsevier Ltd

Appendix 8

Normal cerebrospinal fluid values

TYPE OF INFANT	WHITE CELL COUNT (COUNT/mm³)	PROTEIN (g/l)	GLUCOSE (mmol/l)
Preterm <28 days	9 (0–30)	1 (0.5–2.5)*	3 (1.5–5.5)
Term <28 days	6 (0–21)	0.6 (0.3–2.0)*	3 (1.5–5.5)

All values are given as mean and range.
Table combined from a review of the literature (see reference list).
*Protein values are higher in the first week of life and depend on the red cell count. A white cell count of more than 21/mm³ with a protein value of more than 1 g/l with less than 1000 red cells is suspicious of meningitis.

No value is given for a normal red cell count, because the definition of a 'traumatic tap' varies from 500 to 1000 red blood cells (RBC)/mm³. Byington used a definition of <1000/mm³, and found that the mean red cell count was 95 RBC/mm³, the median value was 5 with a range of 0–236 (Byington et al. 2011).

More recent studies tend to give lower white cell counts (WCCs) than older studies, and as a result the upper limit of normal for the WCC in neonatal cerebrospinal fluid (CSF) has gradually been revised down in successive editions of this textbook. Gyllensward and Malmstrom (1962) give values of up to 112 white blood cells (WBC)/mm³ in preterm and 90 in term babies, but the study included babies with over 1000 RBC/mm³ and was done before routine ultrasound was available. The results are so much higher than other more recent studies that they now appear historical. Recent studies have used polymerase chain reaction to exclude viral infection, which was not available in the past.

In 278 babies less than a month old who did not have meningitis the mean WCC was 6.1 with a median of only 5 WBC/mm³ (Byington et al. 2011). Babies less than a month old have higher cell counts than older babies. Similar low values were reported by Kestenbaum et al. (2010). The 95th percentile value for CSF WCCs in the newborn babies in this study was 19/mm³. The results were not different in the preterm group, but only 22 preterm babies less than a month old were included. Garges et al. (2006) found that using 21 WBC/mm³ as the upper limit of the threshold led to a sensitivity of 79% and a specificity of 81% for the diagnosis of meningitis; in this study there were 95 babies with meningitis, of whom 12 had a WCC ≤21 cells/mm³. Chadwick et al. (2011) found that the 90th percentile value for CSF WCC was 26 cells/mm³ in the first week of life, and 9 cells/mm³ thereafter. Occasionally babies with meningitis have falsely reassuring CSF WCCs (Garges et al. 2006; Greenberg et al. 2008). Sometimes CSF obtained very early after meningeal invasion may not reflect the inflammatory response, and brain abscess or other parenchymal foci may not trigger a CSF pleocytosis. Viral encephalitis can also be present even when there is no CSF pleocytosis.

Protein values also fall after the first week of life (Chadwick et al. 2011). These authors found that the mean CSF protein in the first week was 1.06 g/l, with the 90th percentile 1.53 g/l. The value fell to around 0.6 g/l thereafter, with the 90th percentile less than 1 g/l. The protein value does depend on the red cell count, and in older children it has been said that every additional 1000 RBC/mm³ adds 1 mg/dl (0.1 g/l) to the protein concentration.

CSF glucose is usually 70–80% of plasma glucose, and at least 50%. Take the plasma glucose sample *before* doing the lumbar puncture to avoid the effect of stress. The concentration of glucose does not seem to be affected in the short term by the presence of red cells, but low CSF glucose levels can develop and persist for weeks after intraventricular haemorrhage (Deonna et al. 1977).

Traumatic lumbar puncture

Traumatic lumbar puncture is common in the newborn. The incidence varies depending on the definition. Greenberg et al. (2008) defined a traumatic tap as one with more than 500 RBC/mm³ and reported an incidence of 40%; Byington et al. (2011) chose a threshold of 1000 RBC/mm³ and reported an incidence of 10%.

Osborne and Pizer (1981) and Byington et al. (2011) considered that contamination with less than 10 000 RBC/mm³ did not influence the WCC, and at these levels of red cell contamination blood in the CSF is not sufficient to explain CSF pleocytosis.

It has been suggested that it is possible to apply a formula to compare observed with predicted WCCs in CSF samples with high

© 2012 Elsevier Ltd

red cell counts thought to be due to a 'traumatic tap'. None of the formulas can be used with confidence, and most recent reports doubt their value (Greenberg et al. 2008). They cannot be recommended. Several authors have pointed out that the use of ratios 'overcorrects' the CSF WCC in newborn infants (Osborne and Pizer 1981; Novak 1984; Rubenstein and Yogev 1985). In suspicious clinical cases the only course is to repeat the lumbar puncture after 24–48 hours and to treat for meningitis in the meanwhile. A normal CSF result obtained on the repeat specimen probably excludes meningitis.

References and further reading

Ahmed, A., Hickey, S.M., Ehrett, S., et al., 1996. Cerebrospinal fluid values in the term neonate. Pediatr Infect Dis J 15, 298–303.

Bonadio, W.A., Smith, D.S., Goddard, S., et al., 1990. Distinguishing cerebrospinal fluid abnormalities in children with bacterial meningitis and traumatic lumbar puncture. J Infect Dis 162, 251–254.

Bonadio, W.A., Stanco, L., Bruce, R., et al., 1992. Reference values of normal cerebrospinal fluid composition in infants ages 0 to 8 weeks. Pediatr Infect Dis J 11, 589–591.

Byington, C., Kendwick, J., Sheng, X., 2011. Normative cerebrospinal fluid profiles in febrile infants. J Pediatr 158, 130–134.

Chadwick, S.L., Wilson, J.W., Levin, J.E., et al., 2011. Cerebrospinal fluid characteristics of infants who present to the emergency department with fever. Pediatr Infect Dis J 30, e63–e67.

Deonna, T., Calame, A., van Melle, G., et al., 1977. Hypoglycorrhachia in neonatal intracranial haemorrage. Relationship to posthaemorrhagic hydrocephalus. Helvet Paediatr Acta 32, 351–361.

Escobedo, M., Barton, L.L., Volpe, J.J., 1975. Cerebrospinal fluid studies in an intensive care nursery. J Perinat Med 3, 204–210.

Garges, H.P., Moody, A., Cotton, C.M., et al., 2006. Neonatal meningitis: what is the correlation among cerebrospinal fluid cultures, blood cultures, and the cerebrospinal fluid parameters? Pediatrics 117, 1094–1100.

Greenberg, R.G., Smith, P.B., Cotton, C.M., et al., 2008. Adjustment of cerebrospinal fluid cell counts for a traumatic lumbar puncture does not aid diagnosis of meningitis in neonates. Pediatr Infect Dis J 27, 1047–1051.

Gyllensward, A., Malmstrom, S., 1962. The cerebrospinal fluid in immature infants. Acta Paediatr Scand 51 (Suppl. 135), 54–62.

Kestenbaum, L.A., Ebberson, J., Zorc, J.J., et al., 2010. Defining cerebrospinal fluid white blood cell count reference values in neonates and young infants. Pediatrics 125, 257–264.

Martin-Ancel, M., Garcia-Alix, A., Salas, S., et al., 2006. Cerebrospinal fluid leucocyte counts in healthy neonates. Arch Dis Child 91, F357–F358.

Naidoo, B.T., 1968. The cerebrospinal fluid in the healthy newborn infant. S Afr Med J 42, 933–935.

Novak, R.W., 1984. Lack of validity of standard corrections for white blood cell counts of blood-contaminated cerebrospinal fluid in infants. Am J Clin Pathol 82, 95–97.

Osborne, J.P., Pizer, B., 1981. Effect on the white cell count of contaminating cerebrospinal fluid with blood. Arch Dis Child 56, 400–401.

Otila, E., 1948. Studies on the cerebrospinal fluid in premature infants. Acta Paediatr Scand 35 (Suppl. 9), 7–97.

Portnoy, J.M., Olson, L.C., 1985. Normal cerebrospinal fluid values in children: another look. Pediatrics 75, 484–487.

Rodriguez, A.F., Kaplan, S.L., Mason, E.O., 1990. Cerebrospinal fluid values in the very low birthweight infant. J Pediatr 116, 971–974.

Rubenstein, J.S., Yogev, R., 1985. What represents pleocytosis in blood contaminated ('traumatic tap') cerebrospinal fluid in children? J Pediatr 107, 249–252.

Sarff, L.D., Platt, L.H., McCracken Jr., G.H., 1976. Cerebrospinal fluid evaluation in neonates: comparison of high risk infants with and without meningitis. J Pediatr 88, 473–477.

Widell, S., 1958. On the cerebrospinal fluid in normal children and in patients with acute abacterial meningoencephalitis. Acta Paediatr Scand 47 (Suppl. 115), 1–102.

Wolf, H., Hoepffner, L., 1961. The cerebrospinal fluid in the newborn and premature infant. World Neurol 2, 871–877.

Janet M Rennie

Appendix 9

Oxyhaemoglobin dissociation curve

Oxyhaemoglobin dissociation curves for adult blood and neonatal blood. The dotted lines dropping from 50% saturation give the p50 values for neonatal blood (19 mmHg) and of adult blood (28 mmHg).

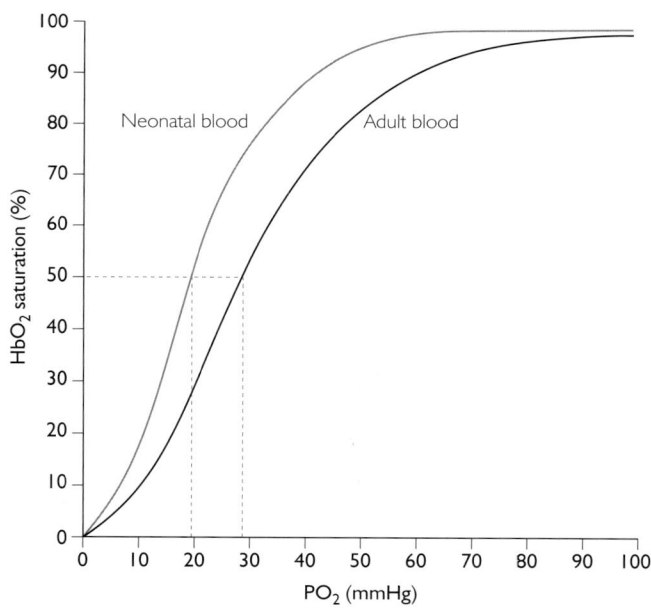

© 2012 Elsevier Ltd

Janet M Rennie

Appendix 10

The Siggaard-Andersen nomogram

By knowing any two values of an acid–base measurement, the other values can be derived by connecting the two known points on this nomogram. For newborn babies, the haemoglobin can be assumed to be 15 g/100 ml. Reproduced from Siggaard-Andersen, O., 1963. Blood acid-base alignment nomogram. Scandinavian Journal of Clinical and Laboratory Investigation 15, 211–217.

© 2012 Elsevier Ltd

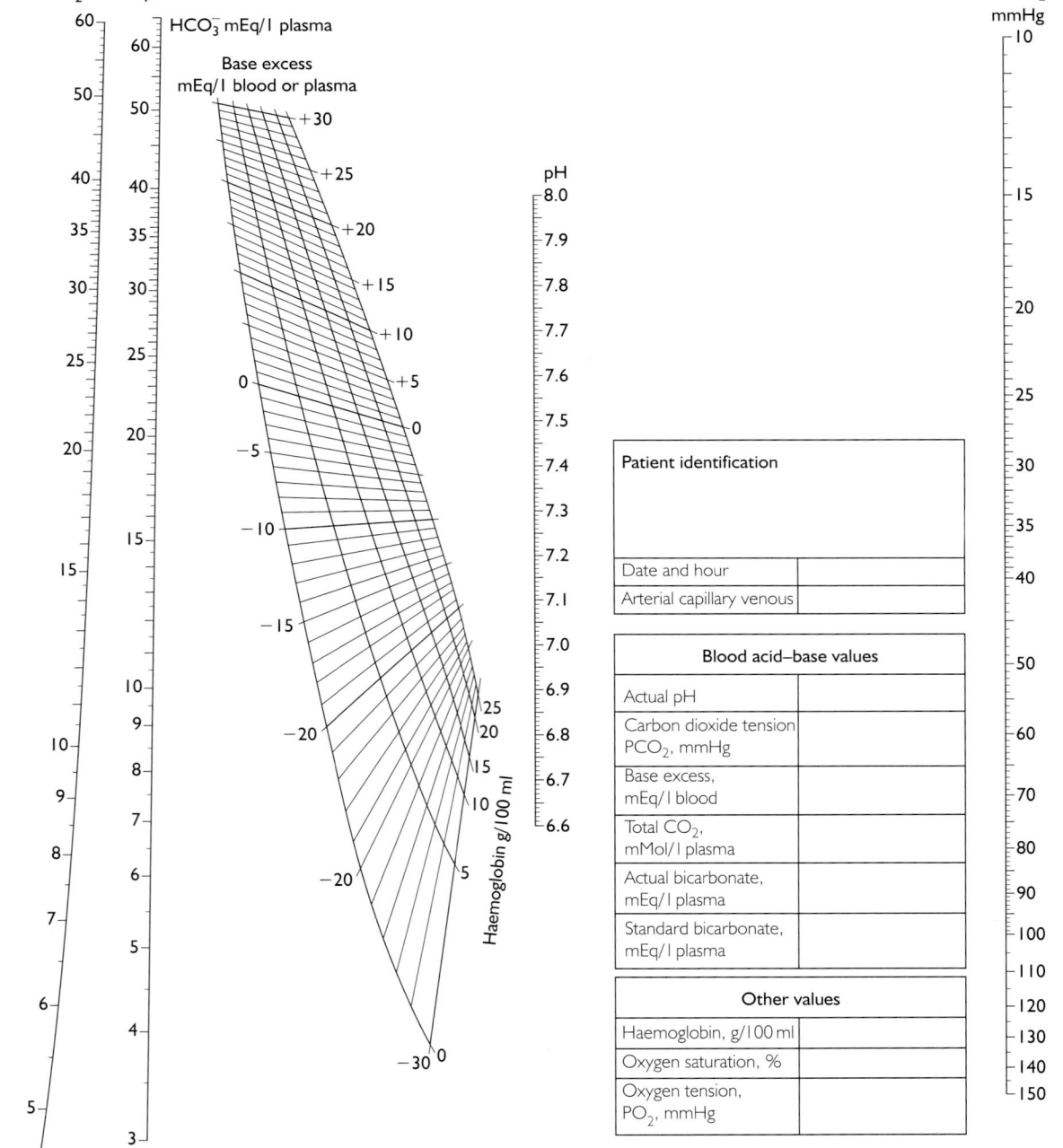

Total-CO₂ mMol/l plasma

T-37°C

PCO₂ mmHg

Patient identification	
Date and hour	
Arterial capillary venous	

Blood acid–base values	
Actual pH	
Carbon dioxide tension PCO₂, mmHg	
Base excess, mEq/l blood	
Total CO₂, mMol/l plasma	
Actual bicarbonate, mEq/l plasma	
Standard bicarbonate, mEq/l plasma	

Other values	
Haemoglobin, g/100 ml	
Oxygen saturation, %	
Oxygen tension, PO₂, mmHg	

Index

Staff Library
Singleton Hospital
Tel: 01792 206666 Ext. 5281

Thumb, persistently adducted, 1072

Thyroid disease

abnormalities of function in neonatal period, 876–877

abnormal thyroid hormone transport into cell, 877

binding proteins, abnormalities, 877

congenital hypothyroidism, 368, 873–876

delayed TSH rise, 876

low T₃ syndrome, 877

neonatal screening and preterm infant, 876

peripheral abnormalities of thyroid hormone binding, transport or action, 877

in pregnancy, 195–196, 878

thyroid dysgenesis, 873

thyroid hormone resistance, 877

see also Endocrine disorders; Hyperthyroidism; Hypothyroidism

Thyroid gland

function in neonatal period, 873

function in utero, 872–873

iodine in, 291

normal function, 872–873

Thyroid hormones, surfactant maturation, 462

Thyroid-stimulating hormone (TSH), 195, 368

Thyrotoxicosis, in pregnancy, 196

Thyrotrophin-releasing hormone (TRH), 474

Thyroxine, 203, 462, 477

Thyroxine-binding globulin deficiency, 877

Tibiae, bowed, 257

Tibial hemimelia, 976–977

Tibial kyphosis (posteromedial bowing of tibia), 978–979

Tidal volume, saturation monitoring, 352

Tissue factor pathway inhibitor (TFPI), 772

Tissue factor (TF), 771

Tissue plasminogen activator, 192

Tissue samples, 1232

T lymphocytes, 304, 998

Tocolysis, 217

Tolazoline, 499

Tolerance, 423

Tongue tie (ankyloglossia), 371

Tonic neck reflex, 1072

Tonic seizures, 1083

Tooley, M., 103

Topical administration of drugs, 406, 412

Total anomalous pulmonary venous connection (TAPVC), 620–621, 649

Total fertility rate, 5, 7f, 8t

Total parenteral nutrition (TPN), 285, 322t

Toxic erythema of newborn, 821

Toxicity

bilirubin, 676, 679

in breastfed infants, 414–415

cardiovascular, 438

drug

antibiotic therapy, 406

cocaine, 438

metabolic acidosis, 407

mortality, 406

multiorgan failure, 407

retinopathy of prematurity, 407

seizures, 407

history in neonates, 406–407

important examples, neonates, 406t

local anaesthesia, 425

oxygen, 553

oxygen therapy, 516

percutaneous, 406

see also Drugs; Drugs of abuse; Substance abuse

Toxoplasmosis, 156, 842, 1051–1052

T-piece ventilation devices, 233

Trace alternant/discontinuous EEG patterns, 1084

Trace metals

in breast milk, 301

parenteral nutrition, 324

requirements, 289t, 290–291

Trachea

development, 604

postnatal function, 452

Tracheal secretions, sepsis investigations, 1022

Tracheobronchomalacia, 613

Tracheomalacia, 612–613

Tracheo-oesophageal fistula, 507, 730

Tracheoscopy, 731f

Tracheostomy

complications, 614

decannulation from, 614–615

home care, 614

indications for, 613–615

mortality, 614

post-tracheostomy ward care, 614

Tracheotomy, changes in, 604

Training

hypoxia–ischaemia, 1135

resuscitation of the newborn, 224, 237, 382

transport, neonatal, 241

Transcription, gene, 139

Transcutaneous CO₂ monitoring, 350, 351f

Transcutaneous monitoring, 348

Transcutaneous PO₂ (TCO₂), 348

Transepidermal water loss (TEWL)

non-renal influences, 332–334, 333f, 333t

water evaporation, 266

Transfer RNAs (tRNAs), 131

Transfers, organisation of care, 56–57

Transfusion-associated graft-versus-host disease (TA-GVHD), 763

Transient abnormal myelopoiesis (TAM), 770

Transient myeloproliferative disorder, and Down syndrome, 960–961

Transient neonatal myasthenia, 1197–1198

Transient neonatal pustular dermatosis/melanosis, 821–822

Transient tachypnoea of the newborn (TTN), 485–486, 485f

Transitional care areas, 108

Transitional care units (TCUs)

categories of babies suitable for transitional care, 376t

decline of availability, 376

feeding on, 378–379

infection control, 379

observation and monitoring on, 376–378, 377f

and special baby care units, 376

Translation, in genetics, 131, 139

Transplacental infection

herpesviruses, 1044

Listeria monocytogenes, 1018

Transport, neonatal

air transport, 242

care at receiving hospital, 241

clinical and physiological stresses, 240

clinical care, 240–241

communication, 241

equipment and vehicles, 242

governance, 242

importance of, 239

organisation of services, 241–242

and parents, 242

pretransport stabilisation, 240

process, 240f

remit, 240

staffing, 241

thermal environment, 272

training, 241

see also Resuscitation of the newborn

Transposition, heart disease, 649

Transpyloric feeding, 315

Transurethral catheterisation, 1287

Transvaginal ultrasound, 147, 161f

Traumatic cyanosis, 250

Treatment

consent to see Consent to treatment

discontinuation where futile, 112–113

refusal of, 111–112

unrealistic expectations regarding, 112–113

withholding and withdrawing, 104, 112–113

Trend monitoring, continuous, 356–357

Triacylglycerols, 460

Triclofos sodium, 424

Tricuspid atresia, 648–649

Tricyclic antidepressants, 432, 440

Trigger thumb, 979

Tri-iodothyronine (T₃), 477, 563

Triplet and higher-order births, 18–21, 22f, 23t

multifetal pregnancy reduction, 160

see also Multiple births

Triploidy (69 chromosomes), 133, 139

Trishydroxymethylaminomethane (THAM), 481

Trisomies

haematological abnormalities in, 770

trisomy 13 (Patau syndrome) see Patau syndrome

trisomy 18 (Edward syndrome) see Edward syndrome

trisomy 21 (Down syndrome) see Down syndrome

Trophic feeding, 279, 711

Trouble, anticipating/averting, 98

Truncus arteriosus, 650

Trunk

hypotonia, 1072

tone and power, 1072, 1073f

Trypanosomiasis, 1048

Tube feeding

on transitional care units, 378

see also Feeding tubes

1372

Staff Library
Singleton Hospital
Tel: 01792 ___666 Ext. 5281

Vomiting
  aspiration pneumonia, 509
  congenital defects/surgical problems, 725
  drug toxicity, 406
  fetal, 209
  milk protein intolerance, 719
  necrotising enterocolitis, 707–708
  in pregnancy, 202
  as sign of disorder, 707–708
  see also Nausea and vomiting
von Willebrand disease, 773–775
Vulva
  examination, 255
  problems, 990

W

Waardenburg syndrome type IV, 803f, 810
Walker–Warburg syndrome, 807–809, 1186,
    1193, 1200–1201, 1211f
Warfarin, 192
Warm environment, response to, 264
Warming tub, 116
Water, requirements, 288
Water evaporation, heat loss, 266–267
Watering eyes, 844
Water-soluble drugs, 409
Waveforms, saturation monitoring, 352–353
Weaning
  from PPHN therapy, 500
  recurrent failure to wean from ventilation,
    530
  solid foods, introduction, 317–318
  from ventilation, 528–530, 557
Webbed neck, 253
Webs, airway, 609
Weight gain
  composition, 287f
  poor, 372, 381
  small baby, normal, 380–381
  third-trimester intrauterine, 322
  twins, 400
Weight loss
  early postnatal, 331, 365, 379
  macrosomia, 389
  small baby, normal, 379

Weight of newborn
  gain *see* Weight gain
  loss *see* Weight loss
  small baby, normal, 379
Well-baby care, 367
White blood cells
  CSF examination, 1076, 1089
  disorders
    Down syndrome, congenital leukaemias
      and haematological abnormalities
      associated with, 770
    neutropenia, 769–770
    sepsis, 1023
  normal values, 768–769
  production in fetus and newborn, 757–758
  total count, in sepsis, 1023
  see also Red blood cells (RBCs)
White-matter disease of prematurity
  focal and diffuse *see* Periventricular
    leukomalacia (PVL)
  haemorrhagic parenchymal infarction,
    1156, 1173–1174
  history and terminology, 1159f, 1166–1169,
    1167t–1168t
  periventricular leukomalacia *see*
    Periventricular leukomalacia (PVL)
  punctuate white-matter lesions, 1173
White-matter injury
  hypoxia–ischaemia, 1123, 1133f
  see also White-matter disease of prematurity
WHO *see* World Health Organization (WHO)
Wilhelmy balance, 117–118
Williams syndrome, 622, 884
Wilms' tumours, 961
Wilson–Mikity syndrome, 564–565
Wind, 371–372
Wiskott–Aldrich syndrome, 1003, 1007
Withdrawal, neonatal
  assessment, 436, 437f
  clinical analgesia, 423
  general outline of drugs associated with,
    434t
  neonatal abstinence syndrome, 1089
  opioids/opiates, 432–438, 434t
  sleep–wake cycles, abnormal, 1068
  treatment agents, 432–435, 435t

Wolff–Parkinson–White syndrome, 662–663
Wolf–Hirschorn syndrome, 803f, 805–806
Wolman disease, 890–891
World Health Organization (WHO)
  on breastfeeding, 303
  impairments, classification, 66t
  on iron intake, 302
  morbidity definitions, 66
  on prematurity, 83
  on preterm births and low birthweight, 12
  SGA assessment, 175
  UK-WHO reference chart, 1307–1308
Writhing movements, 1071
WT-1 gene, bipotential urogenital ridge
    formation, 894

X

X-linked hyper-IgM syndrome, 1007
X-linked ichthyosis, 829
X-linked recessive inheritance, 135–136, 136f,
    136t, 139
X-rays
  chest *see* Chest X-ray
  clinical and laboratory monitoring, 356
  high-resolution (phase contrast), 234f
  see also Ultrasound assessment
XX karyotype, patients exposed to excess
    androgen, 896–897
XY karyotype, incomplete virilisation in baby
    with, 895–896

Z

Zafirlukast, 199
Zellweger syndrome, 1182–1183
Zero heat flux temperature, 354
Zinc, 290–291
Zinc-deficiency dermatosis, 826–827
Zoster immune globulin (ZIG), 1045
Zygosity, 396
  flow chart for determining, 398f
  paternal, 154
  postnatal determination of, 397,
    398f
  see also Twins

Staff Library
Singleton Hospital
Tel: 01792 205666 Ext. 5281